ICD·10·CM

International Classification of Diseases
10th Revision

Clinical Modification

Color Coded

2022

Office, Hospital and Payer Edition

ISBN 978-1-946868-32-9 (Perfect Bound)
ISBN 978-1-57066-086-3 (Spiral Bound)
ISBN 978-1-57066-024-5 (e-Book)

Practice Management Information Corporation (PMIC)
4727 Wilshire Boulevard
Los Angeles, California 90010
http://www.pmiconline.com

Preface

On October 1, 2015, a key element of the data foundation of the United States' health care system underwent a major transformation…the transition from the decades-old Ninth Edition of the International Classification of Diseases (ICD-9) set of diagnosis and inpatient procedure codes to the far more contemporary, vastly larger, and much more detailed Tenth Edition of those code sets—or ICD-10—used by most developed countries throughout the world. The transition had a major impact on any person or entity recording health care information containing a diagnosis and/or inpatient procedure code.

All "covered entities"—as defined by the Health Insurance Portability and Accountability Act of 1996 (HIPAA)—were required to adopt ICD-10 codes for use in all HIPAA transactions with dates of service on or after the October 1, 2015 compliance date. for HIPAA inpatient claims, ICD-10 diagnosis and procedure codes are required for all inpatient stays with discharge dates on or after October 1, 2015.

This Fiscal Year (FY) update of the International Statistical Classification of Diseases and Related Health Problems, 10th revision, Clinical Modification (ICD-10-CM) is being published by PMIC to promulgate this classification throughout the United States for morbidity coding. The International Statistical Classification of Diseases and Related Health Problems, 10th Revision (ICD-10), published by the World Health Organization (WHO), is the foundation of ICD-10-CM. ICD-10 continues to be the classification used in cause-of-death coding in the United States. The ICD-10-CM is comparable with the ICD-10.

The WHO Collaborating Center for the Family of International Classifications in North America, housed at the Centers for Disease Control and Prevention's National Center for Health Statistics (NCHS), has responsibility for the implementation of ICD and other WHO-FIC classifications and serves as a liaison with the WHO, fulfilling international obligations for comparable classifications and the national health data needs of the United States.

This edition of ICD-10-CM includes all official codes, descriptions, guidelines, tables and indexes. A new edition is available approximately mid-September of each year. New editions may be purchased from:

Practice Management Information Corporation
4727 Wilshire Boulevard, Suite 300
Los Angeles, CA 90010
1-800-MED-SHOP
http://pmiconline.com

Disclaimer

This publication includes all official ICD-10-CM codes, descriptions, annotations and guidelines. This publication is revised annually so that we may present the most current information possible. Though all of the information is carefully researched and checked for accuracy and completeness, the publisher accepts no responsibility with regard to errors, omissions, misuse or misinterpretation.

Table of Contents

TABLE OF CONTENTS

Introduction to ICD-10-CM

On October 1, 2015, a key element of the data foundation of the United States' health care system underwent a major transformation, the transition from the decades-old Ninth Edition of the International Classification of Diseases (ICD-9) set of diagnosis and inpatient procedure codes to the far more contemporary, vastly larger, and much more detailed Tenth Edition of those code sets—or ICD-10—used by most developed countries throughout the world. The transition had a major impact on any person or entity recording health care information containing a diagnosis and/or inpatient procedure code.

HISTORY OF THE INTERNATIONAL CLASSIFICATION OF DISEASES

For students of medical nomenclature and coding systems, the following history of the International Classification of Diseases excerpted from Wikipedia may be interesting.

HISTORICAL SYNOPSIS

In 1893, a French physician, Jacques Bertillon, introduced the *Bertillon Classification of Causes of Death* at a congress of the International Statistical Institute in Chicago. a number of countries and cities adopted Dr. Bertillon's system, which was based on the principle of distinguishing between general diseases and those localized to a particular organ or anatomical site, as used by the City of Paris for classifying deaths. Subsequent revisions represented a synthesis of English, German and Swiss classifications, expanding from the original 44 titles to 161 titles. in 1898, the American Public Health Association (APHA) recommended that the registrars of Canada, Mexico, and the United States also adopt it. The APHA also recommended revising the system every ten years to ensure the system remained current with medical practice advances. As a result, the first international conference to revise the International Classification of Causes of Death convened in 1900; with revisions occurring every ten years thereafter. At that time the classification system was contained in one book, which included an Alphabetic Index as well as a Tabular List. The book was small compared with current coding texts.

The revisions that followed contained minor changes, until the sixth revision of the classification system. with the sixth revision, the classification system expanded to two volumes. The sixth revision included morbidity and mortality conditions, and its title was modified to reflect the changes: *International Statistical Classification of Diseases, Injuries and Causes of Death (ICD)*. Prior to the sixth revision, responsibility for ICD revisions fell to the Mixed Commission, a group composed of representatives from the International Statistical Institute and the Health Organization of the League of Nations. in 1948, the World Health Organization (WHO) assumed responsibility for preparing and publishing the revisions to the ICD every ten years. WHO sponsored the seventh and eighth revisions in 1957 and 1968, respectively. It later become clear that the established ten-year interval between revisions was too short.

The ICD is currently the most widely used statistical classification system for diseases in the world. International health statistics using this system are available at the WHO Statistical Information System (WHOSIS). in addition, some countries—including Australia, Canada and the United States—have developed their own adaptations of ICD, with more procedure for classification of operative or diagnostic procedures.

HISTORY AND USAGE IN THE UNITED STATES

In the United States, the U.S. Public Health Service published the *International Classification of Diseases, Adapted for Indexing of Hospital Records and Operation Classification (ICDA),* completed in 1962 and expanding the ICD-7 in a number of areas to more completely meet the indexing needs of hospitals. The U.S. Public Health Service later published the *Eighth Revision, International Classification of Diseases, Adapted for Use in the United States,* commonly referred to as ICDA-8, for official national morbidity and mortality statistics. This was followed by the *ICD, 9th Revision, Clinical Modification,* known as ICD-9-CM, published by the U.S. Department of Health and Human Services and used by hospitals and other healthcare facilities to better describe the clinical picture of the patient. The diagnosis component of ICD-9-CM is completely consistent with ICD-9 codes and remained the data standard for reporting morbidity until 2015. National adaptations of the ICD-10 progressed to incorporate both clinical code (ICD-10-CM) and procedure code (ICD-10-PCS) with the revisions completed in 2003. in 2009, the U.S. Centers for Medicare and Medicaid Services announced that it would begin using ICD-10 on April 1, 2010, with full compliance by all involved parties by 2013. Implementation of ICD-10 was ultimately delayed until 2015.

BRIEF HISTORY OF ICD-10

ICD-10 was first published by the World Health Organization (WHO) in 1992. The National Center for Health Statistics (NCHS), the Federal agency responsible for use of the International Statistical Classification of Diseases and Related Health

Problems, 10th revision (ICD-10) in the United States, has developed a clinical modification of the classification for morbidity purposes. The ICD-10 is used to code and classify mortality data from death certificates, having replaced ICD-9 for this purpose as of January 1, 1999. ICD-10-CM is planned as the replacement for ICD-9-CM, volumes 1 and 2. ICD-10-PCS is the replacement for ICD-9-CM volume 3, Procedures.

ICD-10-CM was developed following a thorough evaluation by a Technical Advisory Panel and extensive additional consultation with physician groups, clinical coders, and others to assure clinical accuracy and utility. Notable improvements in the content and format include: the addition of information relevant to ambulatory and managed care encounters; expanded injury codes; the creation of combination diagnosis/symptom codes to reduce the number of codes needed to fully describe a condition; the addition of a sixth character; incorporation of common 4th and 5th digit subclassifications; laterality; and greater specificity in code assignment. After several delays, ICD-10 was officially implemented on October 1, 2015.

TERMINOLOGY

ACI	Advancing Care Information. Replaces Meaningful Use. It features more reasonable reporting features, including base and performance scoring, fewer measures and 90-day reporting periods.
acute conditions	The medical conditions characterized by sudden onset, severe change, and/or short duration.
additional diagnosis	The secondary diagnosis code used, if available, to provide a more complete picture of the primary diagnosis.
alteration	Modifying the anatomic structure of a body part without affecting the function of the body part
APMs	Alternative payment models. APMs typically have shared savings, flexible payment bundles and other desirable features. There are two APM participation classifications— Advanced APMs, which have their own reporting requirements and are exempt from MIPS reporting, and MIPS APMs.
applied mapping	Distillation of a reference mapping to conform to the needs of a particular application (e.g., data quality, research).
approach (5th character)	Defines the technique used to reach the site of the procedure.
backward mapping	Mapping that proceeds from a newer code set to an older code set, for example from ICD-10-CM to ICD-9-CM.
bilateral	For bilateral sites, the final character of the codes in the ICD-10-CM indicates laterality. an unspecified side code is also provided should the side not be identified in the medical record. If no bilateral code is provided and the condition is bilateral, assign separate codes for both the left and right side.
body part or region (4th character)	Defines the specific anatomical site where the procedure is performed.
body system (2nd character)	Defines the general physiological system on which the procedure is performed or anatomical region where the procedure is performed.
bypass	Altering the route of passage of the contents of a tubular body part.
category	The three-digit diagnosis code classifications that broadly define each condition (e.g., 250 for diabetes mellitus).
Centers for Disease Control and Prevention (CDC)	A federal health data organization that helps maintain several code sets included in the HIPAA standards, including the ICD-9-CM codes. a division of the Department of Health and Human Services responsible for monitoring, researching and developing public health policies for the prevention of disease, injury and disability and the promotion of healthy behaviors. The National Center for Health Statistics is the part of the CDC that maintains health related statistics including the coordination with World Health Organization (WHO) on use of International Classification of Diseases (ICD) in North America.
Centers for Medicare & Medicaid Services (CMS)	The federal agency that runs the Medicare program. in addition, CMS works with the States to run the Medicaid program. CMS works to make sure that the beneficiaries in these programs are able to get high quality healthcare.

change	Taking out or off a device from a body part and putting back an identical or similar device in or on the same body part without cutting or puncturing the skin or a mucous membrane
character	One of the seven components that comprise an ICD-10-PCS procedure code.
chronic conditions	Medical conditions characterized by long duration, frequent recurrence over a long period of time, and/or slow progression over time.
cluster	In a combination entry, one instance where a code is chosen from each of the choice lists in the target system entry, that when combined satisfies the equivalent meaning of the corresponding code in the source system
combination codes	A single code used to classify any of the following: two diagnoses; a diagnosis with an associated secondary process (manifestation); or a diagnosis with an associated complication.
control	Stopping, or attempting to stop, postprocedural bleeding.
Conventions of ICD-10	The general rules for use of the classification independent of guidelines. These conventions are incorporated within the Index and Tabular of the ICD-10-CM as instructional notes.
creation	Making a new genital structure that does not take over the function of a body part.
crosswalk/mapping	A new test is determined to be similar to an existing test, multiple existing test codes, or a portion of an existing test code. The new test code is then assigned to the related existing local fee schedule amounts and resulting national limitation amount. in some instances, a test may only equate to a portion of a test, and, in those instances, payment at an appropriate percentage of the payment for the existing test is assigned.
Current Procedural Terminology (CPT) Codes	This is the procedural coding system that is currently used in America primarily to report physician professional services. Frequently called "CPT", the Current Procedural Terminology, is a code set, developed in 1966 and maintained by the American Medical Association (AMA), used to describe what healthcare professional services were provided or utilized by healthcare professionals. CPT codes are also known as "Level I" codes. Additional codes to describe use of healthcare facilities and services provided by healthcare professionals are known as "Level II" or "Healthcare Common Procedure Coding System" (HCPCS). Level II codes were developed are maintained by CMS.
destruction	Physical eradication of all or a portion of a body part by the direct use of energy, force or a destructive agent.
detachment	Cutting off all or a portion of the upper or lower extremities.
dilation	Expanding an orifice or the lumen of a tubular body part.
division	Cutting into a body part without draining fluids and/or gases from the body part in order to separate or transect a body part.
drainage	Taking or letting out fluids and/or gases from a body part.
excision	Cutting out or off, without replacement, a portion of a body part.
external (approach)	Procedures performed directly on the skin or mucous membrane and procedures performed indirectly by the application of external force through the skin or mucous membrane.
extirpation	Taking or cutting out solid matter from a body part.
extraction	Pulling or stripping out or off all or a portion of a body part by the use of force.
Federal Register	The "Federal Register" is the official daily publication for rules, proposed rules and notices of federal agencies and organizations, as well as Executive Orders and other Presidential documents.
forward mapping	Mapping that proceeds from an older code set to a newer code set, for example from ICD-9-CM Volume 3 to ICD-10-PCS.
fragmentation	Breaking solid matter in a body part into pieces.
GEMs	This reference mapping attempts to include all valid relationships between the codes in the ICD-9-CM diagnosis classification and the ICD-10-CM diagnosis classification.

General Equivalence Map (GEM)	Reference mapping that attempts to include all valid relationships between the codes in the ICD-9- CM diagnosis classification and the ICD-10-CM diagnosis classification
Health Insurance Portability & Accountability Act (HIPAA)	A law passed in 1996 which is also sometimes called the "Kassebaum-Kennedy" law. This law expands healthcare coverage for patients who have lost or changed jobs or have pre-existing conditions. HIPAA does not replace the states' roles as primary regulators of insurance. The HIPAA legislation has the following broad goals, to provide: 1) a way to uniquely identify providers, employers and health plans, 2) a uniform level of protection of health information, known as the "Security Rule," 3) a uniform level of protection of the privacy of health data associated with patients, known as the "Privacy Rule" and 4) a simpler healthcare electronic transaction process by describing standards by which all healthcare administrative entities would use, which is known as the "Transactions and Code Sets Rule".
Healthcare Common Procedure Coding System (HCPCS)	A medical code set that identifies healthcare procedures, equipment, and supplies for claim submission purposes. It has been selected for use in the HIPAA transactions. HCPCS Level I contains numeric CPT codes which are maintained by the AMA. HCPCS Level II contains alphanumeric codes used to identify various items and services that are not included in the CPT medical code set. These are maintained by Health Care Financing Administration (HCFA), Blue Cross and Blue Shield Association (BCBSA), and the Health Insurance Association of America (HIAA). HCPCS Level III contains alphanumeric codes that are assigned by Medicaid state agencies to identify additional items and services not included in levels I or II. These are usually called "local codes", and must have "W", "X", "Y", or "Z" in the first position. HCPCS Procedure Modifier Codes can be used with all three levels, with the WA - ZY range used for locally assigned procedure modifiers.
Hierarchical condition category (HCC)	Hierarchical condition category (HCC) coding is a risk-adjustment model originally designed to estimate future health care costs for patients. Approximately 9,000 ICD-10-CM codes are designated as HCC category codes.
HIPAA 4010	The original healthcare transactions version of HIPAA (officially known as Version 004010 of the ASC X12 transaction implementation guides) named as part of HIPAA's Electronic Transaction Standards regulation. Version 4010 was required to be used by HIPAA covered healthcare entities by Oct. 16, 2003.
HIPAA 5010	Required by Jan. 1, 2012 to be the new version of the HIPAA healthcare transactions. Officially known as Version 005010 of the ASC X12 transaction Technical Report Type 3. This new version was required as a result of Department of Health and Human Services (HHS) final rules published on Jan. 6, 2009.
ICD-10	The mortality and morbidity classification coding system implemented by WHO in 1993 to replace ICD-9.
ICD-10-CM	The updated version of the clinical modification coding set defined by the National Center for Health Statistics that will replace ICD-9-CM on Oct. 1, 2013.
ICD-10-PCS	The updated procedural coding system defined by CMS that will replace Volume 3 of ICD-9-CM for hospital inpatient services.
ICD-9	The mortality and morbidity classification coding system used prior to ICD-10. Replaced by ICD-10 in October 2015.
ICD-9-CM	The "clinical modification" to the ICD-9 code used prior to ICD-10-CM in America to report medical diagnoses. Replaced by ICD-10 in October 2015.
index (to diseases)	The ICD-10-CM is divided into the Alphabetic Index, an alphabetical list of terms and their corresponding code, and the Tabular List, a chronological list of codes divided into chapters based on body system or condition. The Alphabetic Index consists of the following parts: the Index of Diseases and Injury, the Index of External Causes of Injury, the Table of Neoplasms and the Table of Drugs and Chemicals.
insertion	Putting in a nonbiological device that monitors, assists, performs or prevents a physiological function but does not physically take the place of a body part.
inspection	Visually and/or manually exploring a body part.

International Classification of Diseases (ICD)	A medical code set maintained by the World Health Organization (WHO). The primary purpose of this code set is to classify both causes of death or mortality and diseases or morbidity. A U.S. version, known as ICD-CM, "Clinical Modification," is maintained by the NCHS within the CDC to more precisely define ICD use in the U.S.
Low-volume threshold	Physicians with less than $30,000 in annual Medicare revenue or fewer than 100 Part B-enrolled Medicare beneficiaries will be exempt from all MIPS reporting.
MACRA	Acronym for the Medicare Access and CHIP Reauthorization Act of 2015. This is the law passed to reform the Medicare payment system. It repealed the sustainable growth rate formula, which calculated payment cuts for physicians. It also created a new framework for rewarding physicians who provide higher-value care.
manifestation codes	Certain conditions have both an underlying etiology and multiple body system manifestations due to the underlying etiology. for such conditions, the ICD-10-CM has a coding convention that requires the underlying condition be sequenced first followed by the manifestation. Wherever such a combination exists, there is a "use additional code" note at the etiology code, and a "code first" note at the manifestation code. These instructional notes indicate the proper sequencing order of the codes, etiology followed by manifestation.
map	Locating the route of passage of electrical impulses and/or locating functional areas in a body part.
medical necessity	Services or supplies that: are proper and needed for the diagnosis or treatment of a medical condition; are provided for the diagnosis, direct care, and treatment of a medical condition; meet the standards of good medical practice in the local area; and are not mainly for the convenience of the patient or doctor.
MIPS	Acronym for Merit-based Incentive Payment System. MIPS aims to align three currently independent programs—quality reporting (what physicians know now as PQRS), Advancing Care Information (now known as EHR Meaningful Use), and cost (now known as the value-based modifier)—and adds a fourth component, Improvement Activities, designed to promote practice improvement and innovation.
morbidity	Term refers to the disease rate or number of cases of a particular disease in a given age range, gender, occupation, or other relevant population based grouping.
mortality	Term refers to the death rate reflected by the population in a given region, age range, or other relevant statistical grouping
National Center for Health Statistics (NCHS)	A federal organization within the CDC that collects, analyzes, and distributes healthcare statistics. The NCHS helps maintain the ICD-CM codes.
No Map Flag	attribute in a GEM that when turned on indicates that a code in the source system is not linked to any code in the target system .
occlusion	Completely closing an orifice or the lumen of a tubular body part.
open (approach)	Cutting through the skin or mucous membrane and any other body layers necessary to expose the site of the procedure.
percutaneous (approach)	Entry, by puncture or minor incision, of instrumentation through the skin or mucous membrane and any other body layers necessary to reach the site of the procedure.
percutaneous endoscopic (approach)	Entry, by puncture or minor incision, of instrumentation through the skin or mucous membrane and any other body layers necessary to reach and visualize the site of the procedure.
principle diagnosis	First-listed/primary diagnosis code. The code sequenced first on a medical record defines the primary reason for the encounter as determined at the end of the encounter.
procedure	The complete specification of the ICD-10-PCS seven characters.
reattachment	Putting back in or on all or a portion of a separated body part to its normal location or other suitable location.
release	Freeing a body part from an abnormal physical constraint by cutting or by use of force.
removal	Taking out or off a device from a body part.

repair	Restoring, to the extent possible, a body part to its normal anatomic structure and function.
replacement	Putting in or on biological or synthetic material that physically takes the place and/or function of all or a portion of a body part.
Reporting option	Requirement for physicians to decide whether to report as an individual or as part of a group. A group is defined as two or more eligible clinicians. A physician in a group may choose to participate as an individual under MIPS.
reposition	Moving to its normal location, or other suitable location, all or a portion of a body part.
resection	Cutting out or off, without replacement, all of a body part.
restriction	Partially closing an orifice or the lumen of a tubular body part.
reverse lookup	Using a GEM by looking up a target system code to see all the codes in the source system that translate to it.
revision	Correcting, to the extent possible, a portion of a malfunctioning device or the position of a displaced device.
root operation/type (3rd character)	Defines the objective of the procedure.
section (1st character)	Defines the general type of procedure.
sequelae	A late effect is the residual effect (condition produced) after the acute phase of an illness or injury has terminated. There is no time limit on when a late effect code can be used. The residual may be apparent early, such as in cerebral infarction, or it may occur months or years later, such as that due to a previous injury.
signs/symptoms	Codes that describe symptoms and signs, as opposed to diagnoses, are acceptable for reporting purposes when a related definitive diagnosis has not been established (confirmed) by the provider.
source system	Code set of origin in the mapping; the set being mapped 'from'
supplement	Putting in or on biological or synthetic material that physically reinforces and/or augments the function of a portion of a body part
Tabular List	It is essential to use both the Alphabetic Index and Tabular List when locating and assigning a code. The Alphabetic Index does not always provide the full code. Selection of the full code, including laterality and any applicable 7th character can only be done in the Tabular List. a dash (-) at the end of an Alphabetic Index entry indicates that additional characters are required. Even if a dash is not included at the Alphabetic Index entry, it is necessary to refer to the Tabular List to verify that no 7th character is required.
target system	Destination code set in the mapping; the set being mapped 'to'.
transfer	Moving, without taking out, all or a portion of a body part to another location to take over the function of all or a portion of a body part.
transplantation	Putting in or on all or a portion of a living body part taken from another individual or animal to physically take the place and/or function of all or a portion of a similar body part.
Uniform Hospital Discharge Data Set (UHDDS)	The UHDDS definitions are used by hospitals to report inpatient data elements in a standardized manner. These data elements and their definitions can be found in the July 31, 1985, Federal Register (Vol. 50, No, 147), pp. 31038-40.
value	Individual units defined for each character of ICD-10-PCS and represented by a number or letter.
via natural or artificial opening (approach)	Entry of instrumentation through a natural or artificial external opening to reach the site of the procedure.
via natural or artificial opening endoscopic (approach)	Entry of instrumentation through a natural or artificial external opening to reach and visualize the site of the procedure.
via natural or artificial opening with percutaneous endoscopic assistance (approach)	Entry of instrumentation through a natural or artificial external opening and entry, by puncture or minor incision, of instrumentation through the skin or mucous membrane and any other body layers necessary to aid in the performance of the procedure.

Volume I	The detailed, tabular list of diagnosis codes in the ICD-9-CM manual.
Volume II	The alphabetical index to diseases in the ICD-9-CM diagnosis coding manual.
Volume III	The ICD-9/ICD-10 list of procedure codes, used in inpatient settings.
World Health Organization (WHO)	An organization that maintains the International Classification of Diseases (ICD) medical code set.

ICD-10-CM OVERVIEW

WHAT IS ICD-10-CM?

ICD-10-CM is an acronym for *International Classification of Diseases, 10th Revision, Clinical Modification*, published under different names since 1900. ICD-10-CM is a statistical classification system that arranges diseases and injuries into groups according to established criteria. Most ICD-9-CM codes are numeric and consist of three seven digits and a description. The codes are revised approximately every 10 years by the World Health Organization and annual updates are published by Center for Medicare and Medicaid Services (CMS).

ICD-10-CM is the United States' clinical modification of the World Health Organization's ICD-10. The term "clinical" is used to emphasize the modification's intent: to serve as a useful tool in the area of classification of morbidity data for indexing of health records, medical care review, and ambulatory and other health care programs, as well as for basic health statistics. To describe the clinical picture of the patient the codes must be more precise than those needed only for statistical groupings and trend analysis.

ICD-10-CM far exceeds its predecessors in the number of concepts and codes provided. The disease classification has been expanded to include health-related conditions and to provide greater specificity at the sixth and seventh character level. The sixth and seventh characters are not optional and are intended for use in recording the information documented in the clinical record.

KEY POINTS REGARDING ICD-10-CM

1. ICD-10-CM codes are three (3) to seven (7) digit alphanumeric codes.

2. ICD-10-CM codes describe illnesses, injuries, signs and symptoms, and procedures.

3. ICD-10-CM codes must be used on all health insurance claims as of October 1, 2014 (subject to extension by CMS).

4. Most ICD-10-CM codes have a specific definition; however, some ICD-10-CM codes have more than one definition.

5. Correct ICD-10-CM coding can make a significant difference in your reimbursement.

6. Accurate ICD-10-CM coding puts you in control of the reimbursement process.

STRUCTURE OF AN ICD-10-CM CODE

S32.010A   Wedge compression fracture of first lumbar vertebra, initial encounter for closed fracture

Letter	Number or Letter					
1ST Digit	2nd Digit	3rd Digit	4th Digit	5th Digit	6th Digit	7th Digit
S	**3**	**2**	**.0**	**1**	**0**	**A**
Category			Etiology, anatomic site, severity			Added code extensions for obstetrics, injuries and external causes of injury

ITEM	DESCRIPTION
Length:	ICD-10-CM codes are from 3-7 digits
First character:	The first character of all ICD-10-CM codes is a Letter only (all letters except U are used)
Character 2:	The second character of all ICD-10-CM codes is a Number only
Characters 3-7:	The 3rd through 7th characters of an ICD-10-CM codes may be Numbers or letter
Decimal:	The decimal for all ICD-10-CM codes occurs after the 3rd character
Placeholder:	In cases where a 7th digit is required on an ICD-10-CM codes of less than 6 digits, the character "X" is used as a dummy placeholder
Letter format:	Letters are case-sensitive

FORMAT OF ICD-10-CM

The Tabular List (Volume 1)

The ICD-10-CM Tabular List contains categories, subcategories and codes. Characters for categories, subcategories and codes may be either a letter or a number. All categories are 3 characters. a three-character category that has no further subdivision is equivalent to a code. Subcategories are either 4 or 5 characters. Codes may be 3, 4, 5, 6 or 7 characters. That is, each level of subdivision after a category is a subcategory. The final level of subdivision is a code. Codes that have applicable 7th characters are still referred to as codes, not subcategories. a code that has an applicable 7th character is considered invalid without the 7th character.

The Alphabetic Index (Volume 2)

The Alphabetic Index consists of the following parts: the Index of Diseases and Injury, the Index of External Causes of Injury, the Table of Neoplasms and the Table of Drugs and Chemicals.

CONVENTIONS USED IN THE TABULAR LIST

The ICD-10-CM Tabular List (Volume 1) makes use of certain abbreviations, punctuation, symbols, and other conventions that must be clearly understood. The purpose of these conventions is to provide special coding instructions and conserve space. Most of the conventions are defined in the ICD-10-CM Official Guidelines to Coding and Reporting following this chapter.

COLOR CODING AND SYMBOLS

All PMIC versions of ICD-10-CM include color-coding to alert the user to special coding situations or conditions that require additional attention. The use of color-coding is found in the Tabular List (Volume 1). The color is applied as solid rectangular bars over the codes only so that the descriptions remain clear and legible. The color codes and definitions are printed at the bottom of all right-sided pages of the Tabular List (Volume 1)

Color Coding

Three digit code that requires the addition of 4th – 7th digits. Coding to higher level of specificity is required.

Unspecified code. Descriptions include the term "unspecified." Use only if a more specific diagnosis is not known or available.

Nonspecific code. Descriptions include the term "nonspecific, unspecified, other specified or other." A report *may* be required by insurance carriers.

Manifestation codes. Used only to code the manifestation of an underlying disease. Code the underlying disease first.

Symbols

●   A filled BLACK CIRCLE preceding a code indicates that the code is new to this revision of ICD-9-CM. A symbol key appears on all left-hand pages of the Tabular List, Volume 1.

▲   A filled BLACK TRIANGLE preceding a code indicates that there is a revision to the text of an existing code. A symbol key appears on all left-hand pages of the Tabular List, Volume 1.

⑦   A red circle containing the number 7 preceding a code indicates that a seventh digit is required for coding to the highest level of specificity. The appropriate 7th character is to be added to each code from category. Definitions of valid seventh digits are found under the major category. If a code that requires a 7th character is not 6 characters, a placeholder X must be used to fill in the empty characters.

⊗   A red circle containing the letter P preceding a code indicates that a placeholder character "X" is required for the code to be complete. An example of this is at the poisoning, adverse effect and underdosing codes, categories T36-T50. Where a place holder exists, the X must be used in order for the code to be considered a valid code.

[HCC]   Hierarchal Condition Category code indicator. These indicators appear at the end of the diagnosis description for approximately 9,000 ICD-10-CM codes defined as HCC codes by CMS.

Sex Specific Diagnosis Codes

Some ICD-10-CM codes apply only to female or male patients. Some ICD-10-CM codes include the word "male" or "female" in the diagnosis description, while others are known to apply to female or male because of sex specific terms such as ovary, vagina, prostate, testes, etc. For chapters or sections where all of the diagnosis codes are sex specific, the following alerts appear at the beginning of the section:

> NOTE: ALL DIAGNOSIS CODES IN THIS SECTION APPLY TO FEMALE PATIENTS ONLY

> NOTE: ALL DIAGNOSIS CODES IN THIS SECTION APPLY TO MALE PATIENTS ONLY

Age Specific Diagnosis Codes

Some ICD-10-CM codes apply to patients of general age ranges. These codes are identified by the inclusion of the following terms within the diagnosis description: "adult", "child", "infant", "juvenile", or "newborn".

ALPHABETIC INDEX INDENTATION

The alphabetic index of ICD-10-CM lists main terms and subterms. The main terms are in **Bold**. A main term may have as many as six levels of subterms and each subterm may have its own levels of subterms. The PMIC ICD-10-CM includes a unique pipe delimitation character "|" to clearly indicate the indentation levels of the index terms. Lines without the pipe character are wrapped text from the previous line. Following is an example of an index entry illustrating the pipe delimited format

```
Abscess (connective tissue) (embolic) (fistulous)
    (infective) (metastatic) (multiple) (pernicious)
    (pyogenic) (septic) L02.91
|with
  |diverticular disease (intestine) K57.80
    |with bleeding K57.81
    |large intestine K57.20
      |with
        |bleeding K57.21
        |small intestine K57.40
          |with bleeding K57.41
```

HIERARCHICAL CONDITION CATEGORIES AND RISK ADJUSTMENT FACTORS

On November 30, 2017, the Centers for Medicare & Medicaid Services (CMS) announced a revised hierarchical condition category (HCC) risk adjustment model. There were no clinical changes to the HCCs as part of the model revision, but updates were made to reflect new, revised, and deleted ICD-10-CM codes implemented on October 1, 2019

There are over 9,500 ICD-10-CM codes that map to one or more of the 79 HCC codes included in the CMS-HCC Risk Adjustment Model (Version 22). A code can map to more than one HCC as ICD-10-CM contains combination codes (i.e., one code can represent two diagnoses or a diagnosis with a complication).

What Does HCC Mean?

- HCC (Hierarchical Condition Categories) is a model implemented by Medicare in 2004 to adjust capitation payments to private healthcare plans for the health expenditure risk of their enrollees

- The CMS risk adjustment model measures the disease burden that includes 70 HCC categories, which are correlated to diagnosis codes

What Is An HCC Code?

The HCC model is made up of about 9,000 ICD-10-CM codes that typically represent costly, chronic diseases such as:

- Diabetes
- Chronic kidney disease
- Congestive heart failure
- Chronic obstructive pulmonary disease
- Malignant neoplasms
- Some acute conditions (MI, CVA, hip fx)

How Are HCC Codes Identified In The PMIC ICD-10-CM?

All ICD-10-CM codes cross-referenced to a Heirarchal Condition Category code include the symbol [HCC] at the end of the diagnosis description. These indicators appear at the end of the diagnosis description for approximately 9,500 ICD-10-CM codes defined as HCC codes by CMS.

How Is The Risk Score Developed?

The Risk Adjustment Factor (RAF score) is set for each patient and includes:

- Baseline demographic elements (age/sex, dual eligibility status)

- Incremental increases based on HCC diagnoses submitted on claims from face to face encounters with qualified practitioners during the calendar year

- HCC coding is prospective in nature - the work you do in this year sets the RAF and subsequent funding for next year

- All models include chronic conditions that do not change from year to year, i.e., diabetes, COPD, CHF, Atrial-Fib, MS, Parkinson's, Chronic Hepatitis

ICD-10-CM Official Guidelines for Coding and Reporting

The Centers for Medicare and Medicaid Services (CMS) and the National Center for Health Statistics (NCHS), two departments within the U.S. Federal Government's Department of Health and Human Services (DHHS) provide the following guidelines for coding and reporting using the International Classification of Diseases, 10th Revision, Clinical Modification (ICD-10-CM). These guidelines should be used as a companion document to the official version of the ICD-10-CM as published on the NCHS website. The ICD-10-CM is a morbidity classification published by the United States for classifying diagnoses and reason for visits in all health care settings. The ICD-10-CM is based on the ICD-10, the statistical classification of disease published by the World Health Organization (WHO).

These guidelines have been approved by the four organizations that make up the Cooperating Parties for the ICD-10-CM: the American Hospital Association (AHA), the American Health Information Management Association (AHIMA), CMS, and NCHS.

These guidelines are a set of rules that have been developed to accompany and complement the official conventions and instructions provided within the ICD-10-CM itself. The instructions and conventions of the classification take precedence over guidelines. These guidelines are based on the coding and sequencing instructions in the Tabular List and Alphabetic Index of ICD-10-CM but provide additional instruction. Adherence to these guidelines when assigning ICD-10-CM diagnosis codes is required under the Health Insurance Portability and Accountability Act (HIPAA). The diagnosis codes (Tabular List and Alphabetic Index) have been adopted under HIPAA for all healthcare settings. A joint effort between the healthcare provider and the coder is essential to achieve complete and accurate documentation, code assignment, and reporting of diagnoses and procedures. These guidelines have been developed to assist both the healthcare provider and the coder in identifying those diagnoses that are to be reported. The importance of consistent, complete documentation in the medical record cannot be overemphasized. Without such documentation accurate coding cannot be achieved. The entire record should be reviewed to determine the specific reason for the encounter and the conditions treated.

The term encounter is used for all settings, including hospital admissions. In the context of these guidelines, the term provider is used throughout the guidelines to mean physician or any qualified health care practitioner who is legally accountable for establishing the patient's diagnosis. Only this set of guidelines, approved by the Cooperating Parties, is official.

The guidelines are organized into sections. Section I includes the structure and conventions of the classification and general guidelines that apply to the entire classification, and chapter-specific guidelines that correspond to the chapters as they are arranged in the classification. Section II includes guidelines for selection of principal diagnosis for non-outpatient settings. Section III includes guidelines for reporting additional diagnoses in non-outpatient settings. Section IV is for outpatient coding and reporting. It is necessary to review all sections of the guidelines to fully understand all of the rules and instructions needed to code properly.

Section I. Conventions, General Coding Guidelines and Chapter Specific Guidelines

The conventions, general guidelines and chapter-specific guidelines are applicable to all health care settings unless otherwise indicated. The conventions and instructions of the classification take precedence over guidelines.

A. Conventions for the ICD-10-CM

The conventions for the ICD-10-CM are the general rules for use of the classification independent of the guidelines. These conventions are incorporated within the Alphabetic Index and Tabular List of the ICD-10-CM as instructional notes.

1. The Alphabetic Index and Tabular List

The ICD-10-CM is divided into the Alphabetic Index, an alphabetical list of terms and their corresponding code, and the Tabular List, a structured list of codes divided into chapters based on body system or condition. The Alphabetic Index consists of the following parts: the Index of Diseases and Injury, the Index of External Causes of Injury, the Table of Neoplasms and the Table of Drugs and Chemicals.

See Section I.C2. General guidelines
See Section I.C.19. Adverse effects, poisoning, underdosing and toxic effects

2. **Format and Structure:**

The ICD-10-CM Tabular List contains categories, subcategories and codes. Characters for categories, subcategories and codes may be either a letter or a number. All categories are 3 characters. A three-character category that has no further subdivision is equivalent to a code. Subcategories are either 4 or 5 characters. Codes may be 3, 4, 5, 6 or 7 characters. That is, each level of subdivision after a category is a subcategory. The final level of subdivision is a code. Codes that have applicable 7th characters are still referred to as codes, not subcategories. A code that has an applicable 7th character is considered invalid without the 7th character.

The ICD-10-CM uses an indented format for ease in reference.

3. **Use of codes for reporting purposes**

For reporting purposes only codes are permissible, not categories or subcategories, and any applicable 7th character is required.

4. **Placeholder character**

The ICD-10-CM utilizes a placeholder character "X". The "X" is used as a placeholder at certain codes to allow for future expansion. An example of this is at the poisoning, adverse effect and underdosing codes, categories T36-T50.

Where a placeholder exists, the X must be used in order for the code to be considered a valid code.

5. **7th Characters**

Certain ICD-10-CM categories have applicable 7th characters. The applicable 7th character is required for all codes within the category, or as the notes in the Tabular List instruct. The 7th character must always be the 7th character in the data field. If a code that requires a 7th character is not 6 characters, a placeholder X must be used to fill in the empty characters.

6. **Abbreviations**

   a. **Alphabetic Index abbreviations**

   NEC "Not elsewhere classifiable"

   This abbreviation in the Alphabetic Index represents "other specified." When a specific code is not available for a condition, the Alphabetic Index directs the coder to the "other specified" code in the Tabular List.

   NOS "Not otherwise specified"

   This abbreviation is the equivalent of unspecified.

   b. **Tabular List abbreviations**

   NEC "Not elsewhere classifiable"

   This abbreviation in the Tabular List represents "other specified". When a specific code is not available for a condition, the Tabular List includes an NEC entry under a code to identify the code as the "other specified" code.

   NOS "Not otherwise specified"

   This abbreviation is the equivalent of unspecified.

7. **Punctuation**

   [ ] Brackets are used in the Tabular List to enclose synonyms, alternative wording or explanatory phrases. Brackets are used in the Alphabetic Index to identify manifestation codes.

   ( ) Parentheses are used in both the Alphabetic Index and Tabular List to enclose supplementary words that may be present or absent in the statement of a disease or procedure without affecting the code number to which it is assigned. The terms within the parentheses are referred to as nonessential modifiers. The nonessential modifiers in the Alphabetic Index to Diseases apply to subterms following a main term except when a nonessential modifier and a subentry are mutually exclusive, the subentry takes precedence. For example, in the ICD-10-CM Alphabetic Index under the main term Enteritis, "acute" is a nonessential modifier and "chronic" is a subentry. In this case, the nonessential modifier "acute" does not apply to the subentry "chronic".

   : Colons are used in the Tabular List after an incomplete term which needs one or more of the modifiers following the colon to make it assignable to a given category.

8. **Use of "and".**

   See Section I.A.14. Use of the term "And"

9. **Other and Unspecified codes**

   a. **"Other" codes**

      Codes titled "other" or "other specified" are for use when the information in the medical record provides detail for which a specific code does not exist. Alphabetic Index entries with NEC in the line designate "other" codes in the Tabular List. These Alphabetic Index entries represent specific disease entities for which no specific code exists, so the term is included within an "other" code.

   b. **"Unspecified" codes**

      Codes titled "unspecified" are for use when the information in the medical record is insufficient to assign a more specific code. For those categories for which an unspecified code is not provided, the "other specified" code may represent both other and unspecified.

      See Section I.B.18 Use of Signs/Symptom/Unspecified Codes

10. **Includes Notes**

    This note appears immediately under a three-character code title to further define, or give examples of, the content of the category.

11. **Inclusion terms**

    List of terms is included under some codes. These terms are the conditions for which that code is to be used. The terms may be synonyms of the code title, or, in the case of "other specified" codes, the terms are a list of the various conditions assigned to that code. The inclusion terms are not necessarily exhaustive. Additional terms found only in the Alphabetic Index may also be assigned to a code.

12. **Excludes Notes**

    The ICD-10-CM has two types of excludes notes. Each type of note has a different definition for use, but they are all similar in that they indicate that codes excluded from each other are independent of each other.

    a. **Excludes1:**
       A type 1 Excludes note is a pure excludes note. It means "NOT CODED HERE!" An Excludes1 note indicates that the code excluded should never be used at the same time as the code above the Excludes1 note. An Excludes1 is used when two conditions cannot occur together, such as a congenital form versus an acquired form of the same condition.

An exception to the Excludes1 definition is the circumstance when the two conditions are unrelated to each other. If it is not clear whether the two conditions involving an Excludes1 note are related or not, query the provider. For example, code F45.8, Other somatoform disorders, has an Excludes1 note for "sleep related teeth grinding (G47.63)," because "teeth grinding" is an inclusion term under F45.8. Only one of these two codes should be assigned for teeth grinding. However psychogenic dysmenorrhea is also an inclusion term under F45.8, and a patient could have both this condition and sleep related teeth grinding. In this case, the two conditions are clearly unrelated to each other, and so it would be appropriate to report F45.8 and G47.63 together.

b. **Excludes2:**

A type 2 Excludes note represents "Not included here." An Excludes2 note indicates that the condition excluded is not part of the condition represented by the code, but a patient may have both conditions at the same time. When an Excludes2 note appears under a code, it is acceptable to use both the code and the excluded code together, when appropriate.

13. **Etiology/manifestation convention ("code first", "use additional code" and "in diseases classified elsewhere" notes)**

Certain conditions have both an underlying etiology and multiple body system manifestations due to the underlying etiology. For such conditions, the ICD-10-CM has a coding convention that requires the underlying condition be sequenced first, if applicable, followed by the manifestation. Wherever such a combination exists, there is a "use additional code" note at the etiology code, and a "code first" note at the manifestation code. These instructional notes indicate the proper sequencing order of the codes, etiology followed by manifestation.

In most cases the manifestation codes will have in the code title, "in diseases classified elsewhere." Codes with this title are a component of the etiology/ manifestation convention. The code title indicates that it is a manifestation code. "In diseases classified elsewhere" codes are never permitted to be used as first listed or principal diagnosis codes. They must be used in conjunction with an underlying condition code, and they must be listed following the underlying condition. See category F02, Dementia in other diseases classified elsewhere, for an example of this convention.

There are manifestation codes that do not have "in diseases classified elsewhere" in the title. For such codes, there is a "use additional code" note at the etiology code and a "code first" note at the manifestation code, and the rules for sequencing apply.

In addition to the notes in the Tabular List, these conditions also have a specific Alphabetic Index entry structure. In the Alphabetic Index both conditions are listed together with the etiology code first followed by the manifestation codes in brackets. The code in brackets is always to be sequenced second.

An example of the etiology/manifestation convention is dementia in Parkinson's disease. In the Alphabetic Index, code G20 is listed first, followed by code F02.80 or F02.81 in brackets. Code G20 represents the underlying etiology, Parkinson's disease, and must be sequenced first, whereas code F02.80 and F02.81 represent the manifestation of dementia in diseases classified elsewhere, with or without behavioral disturbance.

"Code first" and "Use additional code" notes are also used as sequencing rules in the classification for certain codes that are not part of an etiology/ manifestation combination.

See Section I.B.7. Multiple coding for a single condition.

14. **"And"**

The word "and" should be interpreted to mean either "and" or "or" when it appears in a title.

For example, cases of "tuberculosis of bones", "tuberculosis of joints" and "tuberculosis of bones and joints" are classified to subcategory A18.0, Tuberculosis of bones and joints.

15. **"With"**

The word "with" or "in" should be interpreted to mean "associated with" or "due to" when it appears in a code title, the Alphabetic Index (either under a main term or subterm), or an instructional note in the Tabular List. The classification presumes a causal relationship between the two conditions linked by these terms in the Alphabetic Index or Tabular List. These conditions should be coded as related even in the absence of provider documentation explicitly linking them, unless the documentation clearly states the conditions are unrelated or when another guideline exists that specifically requires a documented linkage between two conditions (e.g., sepsis guideline for "acute organ dysfunction that is not clearly associated with the sepsis").

For conditions not specifically linked by these relational terms in the classification or when a guideline requires that a linkage between two conditions be explicitly documented, provider documentation must link the conditions in order to code them as related.

The word "with" in the Alphabetic Index is sequenced immediately following the main term or subterm, not in alphabetical order.

16. "See" and "See Also"

The "see" instruction following a main term in the Alphabetic Index indicates that another term should be referenced. It is necessary to go to the main term referenced with the "see" note to locate the correct code.

A "see also" instruction following a main term in the Alphabetic Index instructs that there is another main term that may also be referenced that may provide additional Alphabetic Index entries that may be useful. It is not necessary to follow the "see also" note when the original main term provides the necessary code.

17. "Code also" note

A "code also" note instructs that two codes may be required to fully describe a condition, but this note does not provide sequencing direction. The sequencing depends on the circumstances of the encounter.

18. Default codes

A code listed next to a main term in the ICD-10-CM Alphabetic Index is referred to as a default code. The default code represents that condition that is most commonly associated with the main term or is the unspecified code for the condition. If a condition is documented in a medical record (for example, appendicitis) without any additional information, such as acute or chronic, the default code should be assigned.

19. Code assignment and Clinical Criteria

The assignment of a diagnosis code is based on the provider's diagnostic statement that the condition exists. The provider's statement that the patient has a particular condition is sufficient. Code assignment is not based on clinical criteria used by the provider to establish the diagnosis.

B. General Coding Guidelines

1. Locating a code in the ICD-10-CM

To select a code in the classification that corresponds to a diagnosis or reason for visit documented in a medical record, first locate the term in the Alphabetic Index, and then verify the code in the Tabular List. Read and be guided by instructional notations that appear in both the Alphabetic Index and the Tabular List.

It is essential to use both the Alphabetic Index and Tabular List when locating and assigning a code. The Alphabetic Index does not always provide the full code. Selection of the full code, including laterality and any applicable 7th character can only be done in the Tabular List. A dash (-) at the end of an Alphabetic Index entry indicates that additional characters are required. Even if a dash is not included at the Alphabetic Index entry, it is necessary to refer to the Tabular List to verify that no 7th character is required.

2. Level of Detail in Coding

Diagnosis codes are to be used and reported at their highest number of characters available and to the highest level of specificity documented in the medical record.

ICD-10-CM diagnosis codes are composed of codes with 3, 4, 5, 6 or 7 characters. Codes with three characters are included in ICD-10-CM as the heading of a category of codes that may be further subdivided by the use of fourth and/or fifth characters and/or sixth characters, which provide greater detail.

A three-character code is to be used only if it is not further subdivided. A code is invalid if it has not been coded to the full number of characters required for that code, including the 7th character, if applicable.

3. **Code or codes from A00.0 through T88.9, Z00-Z99.8, U00-U85**

The appropriate code or codes from A00.0 through T88.9, Z00-Z99.8, and U00-U85 must be used to identify diagnoses, symptoms, conditions, problems, complaints or other reason(s) for the encounter/visit.

4. **Signs and symptoms**

Codes that describe symptoms and signs, as opposed to diagnoses, are acceptable for reporting purposes when a related definitive diagnosis has not been established (confirmed) by the provider. Chapter 18 of ICD-10-CM, Symptoms, Signs, and Abnormal Clinical and Laboratory Findings, Not Elsewhere Classified (codes R00.0 - R99) contains many, but not all, codes for symptoms.

See Section I.B.18 Use of Signs/Symptom/Unspecified Codes

5. **Conditions that are an integral part of a disease process**

Signs and symptoms that are associated routinely with a disease process should not be assigned as additional codes, unless otherwise instructed by the classification.

6. **Conditions that are not an integral part of a disease process**

Additional signs and symptoms that may not be associated routinely with a disease process should be coded when present.

7. **Multiple coding for a single condition**

In addition to the etiology/manifestation convention that requires two codes to fully describe a single condition that affects multiple body systems, there are other single conditions that also require more than one code. "Use additional code" notes are found in the Tabular List at codes that are not part of an etiology/manifestation pair where a secondary code is useful to fully describe a condition. The sequencing rule is the same as the etiology/manifestation pair, "use additional code" indicates that a secondary code should be added, if known.

For example, for bacterial infections that are not included in chapter 1, a secondary code from category B95, Streptococcus, Staphylococcus, and Enterococcus, as the cause of diseases classified elsewhere, or B96, Other bacterial agents as the cause of diseases classified elsewhere, may be required to identify the bacterial organism causing the infection. A "use additional code" note will normally be found at the infectious disease code, indicating a need for the organism code to be added as a secondary code.

"Code first" notes are also under certain codes that are not specifically manifestation codes but may be due to an underlying cause. When there is a "code first" note and an underlying condition is present, the underlying condition should be sequenced first, if known.

"Code, if applicable, any causal condition first" notes indicate that this code may be assigned as a principal diagnosis when the causal condition is unknown or not applicable. If a causal condition is known, then the code for that condition should be sequenced as the principal or first-listed diagnosis.

Multiple codes may be needed for sequela, complication codes and obstetric codes to more fully describe a condition. See the specific guidelines for these conditions for further instruction.

8. **Acute and Chronic Conditions**

If the same condition is described as both acute (subacute) and chronic, and separate subentries exist in the Alphabetic Index at the same indentation level, code both and sequence the acute (subacute) code first.

9. **Combination Code**

A combination code is a single code used to classify:

- Two diagnoses, or
- A diagnosis with an associated secondary process (manifestation)
- A diagnosis with an associated complication

Combination codes are identified by referring to subterm entries in the Alphabetic Index and by reading the inclusion and exclusion notes in the Tabular List.

Assign only the combination code when that code fully identifies the diagnostic conditions involved or when the Alphabetic Index so directs. Multiple coding should not be used when the classification provides a combination code that clearly identifies all of the elements documented in the diagnosis. When the combination code lacks necessary specificity in describing the manifestation or complication, an additional code should be used as a secondary code.

10. **Sequela (Late Effects)**

A sequela is the residual effect (condition produced) after the acute phase of an illness or injury has terminated. There is no time limit on when a sequela code can be used. The residual may be apparent early, such as in cerebral infarction, or it may occur months or years later, such as that due to a previous injury. Examples of sequela include scar formation resulting from a burn, deviated septum due to a nasal fracture, and infertility due to tubal occlusion from old tuberculosis. Coding of sequela generally requires two codes sequenced in the following order: the condition or nature of the sequela is sequenced first. The sequela code is sequenced second.

An exception to the above guidelines are those instances where the code for the sequela is followed by a manifestation code identified in the Tabular List and title, or the sequela code has been expanded (at the fourth, fifth or sixth character levels) to include the manifestation(s). The code for the acute phase of an illness or injury that led to the sequela is never used with a code for the late effect.

See Section I.C.9. Sequelae of cerebrovascular disease
See Section I.C.15. Sequelae of complication of pregnancy, childbirth and the puerperium
See Section I.C.19. Application of 7th characters for Chapter 19

11. **Impending or Threatened Condition**

Code any condition described at the time of discharge as "impending" or "threatened" as follows:

If it did occur, code as confirmed diagnosis.

If it did not occur, reference the Alphabetic Index to determine if the condition has a subentry term for "impending" or "threatened" and also reference main term entries for "Impending" and for "Threatened."
If the subterms are listed, assign the given code.

If the subterms are not listed, code the existing underlying condition(s) and not the condition described as impending or threatened.

12. **Reporting Same Diagnosis Code More than Once**

Each unique ICD-10-CM diagnosis code may be reported only once for an encounter. This applies to bilateral conditions when there are no distinct codes identifying laterality or two different conditions classified to the same ICD-10-CM diagnosis code.

13. **Laterality**

Some ICD-10-CM codes indicate laterality, specifying whether the condition occurs on the left, right or is bilateral. If no bilateral code is provided and the condition is bilateral, assign separate codes for both the left and right side. If the side is not identified in the medical record, assign the code for the unspecified side.

When a patient has a bilateral condition and each side is treated during separate encounters, assign the "bilateral" code (as the condition still exists on both sides), including for the encounter to treat the first side. For the second encounter for treatment after one side has previously been treated and the condition no longer exists on that side, assign the appropriate unilateral code for the side where the condition still exists (e.g., cataract surgery performed on each eye in separate encounters). The bilateral code would not be assigned for the subsequent encounter, as the patient no longer has the condition in the previously-treated site. If the treatment on the first side did not completely resolve the condition, then the bilateral code would still be appropriate.

14. **Documentation by Clinicians Other than the Patient's Provider**

Code assignment is based on the documentation by the patient's provider (i.e., physician or other qualified healthcare practitioner legally accountable for establishing the patient's diagnosis). There are a few exceptions when code assignment may be based on medical record documentation from clinicians who are not the patient's provider (i.e., physician or other qualified healthcare practitioner legally accountable for establishing the patient's diagnosis). In this context, "clinicians" other than the patient's provider refer to healthcare professionals permitted, based on regulatory or accreditation requirements or internal hospital policies, to document in a patient's official medical record.

These exceptions include codes for:
- **Body Mass Index (BMI)**
- **Depth of non-pressure chronic ulcers**
- **Pressure ulcer stage**
- **Coma scale**
- **NIH stroke scale (NIHSS)**
- **Social determinants of health (SDOH)**
- **Laterality**
- **Blood alcohol level**

This information is typically, or may be, documented by other clinicians involved in the care of the patient (e.g., a dietitian often documents the BMI, a nurse often documents the pressure ulcer stages, and an emergency medical technician often documents the coma scale). However, the associated diagnosis (such as overweight, obesity, acute stroke, pressure ulcer, or a condition classifiable to category F10, Alcohol related disorders) must be documented by the patient's provider. If there is conflicting medical record documentation, either from the same clinician or different clinicians, the patient's attending provider should be queried for clarification.

The BMI, coma scale, NIHSS, blood alcohol level codes and codes for social determinants of health should only be reported as secondary diagnoses.

See Section I.C.21.c.17 for additional information regarding coding social determinants of health.

15. **Syndromes**

Follow the Alphabetic Index guidance when coding syndromes. In the absence of Alphabetic Index guidance, assign codes for the documented manifestations of the syndrome. Additional codes for manifestations that are not an integral part of the disease process may also be assigned when the condition does not have a unique code.

16. **Documentation of Complications of Care**

Code assignment is based on the provider's documentation of the relationship between the condition and the care or procedure, unless otherwise instructed by the classification. The guideline extends to any complications of care, regardless of the chapter the code is located in. It is important to note that not all conditions that occur during or following medical care or surgery are classified as complications. There must be a cause-and-effect relationship between the care provided and the condition, and an indication in the documentation that it is a complication. Query the provider for clarification, if the complication is not clearly documented.

17. **Borderline Diagnosis**

If the provider documents a "borderline" diagnosis at the time of discharge, the diagnosis is coded as confirmed, unless the classification provides a specific entry (e.g., borderline diabetes). If a borderline condition has a specific index entry in ICD-10-CM, it should be coded as such. Since borderline conditions are not uncertain diagnoses, no distinction is made between the care setting (inpatient versus outpatient). Whenever the documentation is unclear regarding a borderline condition, coders are encouraged to query for clarification.

18. **Use of Sign/Symptom/Unspecified Codes**

Sign/symptom and "unspecified" codes have acceptable, even necessary, uses. While specific diagnosis codes should be reported when they are supported by the available medical record documentation and clinical knowledge of the patient's health condition, there are instances when signs/symptoms or unspecified codes are the best choices for accurately reflecting the healthcare encounter. Each healthcare encounter should be coded to the level of certainty known for that encounter.

As stated in the introductory section of these official coding guidelines, a joint effort between the healthcare provider and the coder is essential to achieve complete and accurate documentation, code assignment, and reporting of diagnoses and procedures. The importance of consistent, complete documentationin the medical record cannot be overemphasized. Without such documentation accurate coding cannot be achieved. The entire record should be reviewed to determine the specific reason for the encounter and the conditions treated.

If a definitive diagnosis has not been established by the end of the encounter, it is appropriate to report codes for sign(s) and/or symptom(s) in lieu of a definitive diagnosis. When sufficient clinical information isn't known or available about a particular health condition to assign a more specific code, it is acceptable to report the appropriate "unspecified" code (e.g., a diagnosis of pneumonia has been determined, but not the specific type). Unspecified codes should be reported when they are the codes that most accurately reflect what is known about the patient's condition at the time of that particular encounter. It would be inappropriate to select a specific code that is not supported by the medical record documentation or conduct medically unnecessary diagnostic testing in order to determine a more specific code.

19. **Coding for Healthcare Encounters in Hurricane Aftermath**

    a. **Use of External Cause of Morbidity Codes**

    An external cause of morbidity code should be assigned to identify the cause of the injury(ies) incurred as a result of the hurricane. The use of external cause of morbidity codes is supplemental to the application of ICD-10-CM codes. External cause of morbidity codes are never to be recorded as a principal diagnosis (first-listed in non-inpatient settings). The appropriate injury code should be sequenced before any external cause codes. The external cause of morbidity codes capture how the injury or health condition happened (cause), the intent (unintentional or accidental; or intentional, such as suicide or assault), the place where the event occurred, the activity of the patient at the time of the event, and the person's status (e.g., civilian, military). They should not be assigned for encounters to treat hurricane victims' medical conditions when no injury, adverse effect or poisoning is involved. External cause of morbidity codes should be assigned for each encounter for care and treatment of the injury. External cause of morbidity codes may be assigned in all health care settings. For the purpose of capturing complete and accurate ICD-10-CM data in the aftermath of the hurricane, a healthcare setting should be considered as any location where medical care is provided by licensed healthcare professionals.

    b. **Sequencing of External Causes of Morbidity Codes**

    Codes for cataclysmic events, such as a hurricane, take priority over all other external cause codes except child and adult abuse and terrorism and should be sequenced before other external cause of injury codes. Assign as many external cause of morbidity codes as necessary to fully explain each cause. For example, if an injury occurs as a result of a building collapse during the hurricane, external cause codes for both the hurricane and the building collapse should be assigned, with the external causes code for hurricane being sequenced as the first external cause code. For injuries incurred as a direct result of the hurricane, assign the appropriate code(s) for the injuries, followed by the code X37.0-, Hurricane (with the appropriate 7th character), and any other applicable external cause of injury codes. Code X37.0- also should be assigned when an injury is incurred as a result of flooding caused by a levee breaking related to the hurricane. Code X38.-, Flood (with the appropriate 7th character), should be assigned when an injury is from flooding resulting directly from the storm. Code X36.0-, Collapse of dam or man-made structure, should not be assigned when the cause of the collapse is due to the hurricane. Use of code X36.0- is limited to collapses of man-made structures due to earth surface movements, not due to storm surges directly from a hurricane.

c. **Other External Causes of Morbidity Code Issues**

For injuries that are not a direct result of the hurricane, such as an evacuee that has incurred an injury as a result of a motor vehicle accident, assign the appropriate external cause of morbidity code(s) to describe the cause of the injury, but do not assign code X37.0-, Hurricane. If it is not clear whether the injury was a direct result of the hurricane, assume the injury is due to the hurricane and assign code X37.0-, Hurricane, as well as any other applicable external cause of morbidity codes. In addition to code X37.0-, Hurricane, other possible applicable external cause of morbidity codes include:

W54.0- Bitten by dog
X30- Exposure to excessive natural heat
X31- Exposure to excessive natural cold
X38- Flood

d. **Use of Z codes**

Z codes (other reasons for healthcare encounters) may be assigned as appropriate to further explain the reasons for presenting for healthcare services, including transfers between healthcare facilities, or provide additional information relevant to a patient encounter. The identify which codes maybe assigned as principal or first-listed diagnosis only, secondary diagnosis only, or principal/first-listed or secondary (depending on the circumstances). Possible applicable Z codes include:

Z59.0 Homelessness
Z59.1 Inadequate housing
Z59.5 Extreme poverty
Z75.1 Person awaiting admission to adequate facility elsewhere
Z75.3 Unavailability and inaccessibility of health-care facilities
Z75.4 Unavailability and inaccessibility of other helping agencies
Z76.2 Encounter for health supervision and care of other healthy infant and child
Z99.12 Encounter for respirator [ventilator] dependence during power failure

The external cause of morbidity codes and the Z codes listed above are not an all-inclusive list. Other codes may be applicable to the encounter based upon the documentation. Assign as many codes as necessary to fully explain each healthcare encounter. Since patient history information may be very limited, use any available documentation to assign the appropriate external cause of morbidity and Z codes.

C. Chapter-Specific Coding Guidelines

In addition to general coding guidelines, there are guidelines for specific diagnoses and/or conditions in the classification. Unless otherwise indicated, these guidelines apply to all health care settings. Please refer to Section II for guidelines on the selection of principal diagnosis.

1. Chapter 1: Certain Infectious and Parasitic Diseases (A00-B99), U07.1

a. **Human Immunodeficiency Virus (HIV) Infections**

1) Code only confirmed cases

Code only confirmed cases of HIV infection/illness. This is an exception to the hospital inpatient guideline Section II, H.

In this context, "confirmation" does not require documentation of positive serology or culture for HIV; the provider's diagnostic statement that the patient is HIV positive or has an HIV-related illness is sufficient.

2) Selection and sequencing of HIV codes

(a) Patient admitted for HIV-related condition

If a patient is admitted for an HIV-related condition, the principal diagnosis should be B20, Human immunodeficiency virus [HIV] disease followed by additional diagnosis codes for all reported HIV-related conditions.

(b) Patient with HIV disease admitted for unrelated condition

If a patient with HIV disease is admitted for an unrelated condition (such as a traumatic injury), the code for the unrelated condition (e.g., the nature of injury code) should be the principal diagnosis. Other diagnoses would be B20 followed by additional diagnosis codes for all reported HIV-related conditions.

(c) Whether the patient is newly diagnosed

Whether the patient is newly diagnosed or has had previous admissions/encounters for HIV conditions is irrelevant to the sequencing decision.

(d) Asymptomatic human immunodeficiency virus

Z21, Asymptomatic human immunodeficiency virus [HIV] infection status, is to be applied when the patient without any documentation of symptoms is listed as being "HIV positive," "known HIV," "HIV test positive," or similar terminology. Do not use this code if the term "AIDS" or "HIV disease" is used or if the patient is treated for any HIV-related illness or is described as having any condition(s) resulting from his/her HIV positive status; use B20 in these cases.

(e) Patients with inconclusive HIV serology, but no definitive diagnosis or manifestations of the illness, may be assigned code R75, Inconclusive laboratory evidence of human immunodeficiency virus [HIV].

(f) Previously diagnosed HIV-related illness

Patients with any known prior diagnosis of an HIV-related illness should be coded to B20. Once a patient has developed an HIV-related illness, the patient should always be assigned code B20 on every subsequent admission/encounter. Patients previously diagnosed with any HIV illness (B20) should never be assigned to R75 or Z21, Asymptomatic human immunodeficiency virus [HIV] infection status.

(g) HIV Infection in Pregnancy, Childbirth and the Puerperium

During pregnancy, childbirth or the puerperium, a patient admitted (or presenting for a health care encounter) because of an HIV-related illness should receive a principal diagnosis code of O98.7-, Human immunodeficiency [HIV] disease complicating pregnancy, childbirth and the puerperium, followed by B20 and the code(s) for the HIV-related illness(es). Codes from Chapter 15 always take sequencing priority.

Patients with asymptomatic HIV infection status admitted (or presenting for a health care encounter) during pregnancy, childbirth, or the puerperium should receive codes of O98.7- and Z21.

(h) **Encounters for testing for HIV**

If a patient is being seen to determine his/her HIV status, use code Z11.4, Encounter for screening for human immunodeficiency virus [HIV]. Use additional codes for any associated high-risk behavior, if applicable.

If a patient with signs or symptoms is being seen for HIV testing, code the signs and symptoms. An additional counseling code Z71.7, Human immunodeficiency virus [HIV] counseling, may be used if counseling is provided during the encounter for the test.

When a patient returns to be informed of his/her HIV test results and the test result is negative, use code Z71.7, Human immunodeficiency virus [HIV] counseling.

If the results are positive, see previous guidelines and assign codes as appropriate.

(i) **History of HIV managed by medication**

If a patient with documented history of HIV disease is currently managed on antiretroviral medications, assign codeB20, Human immunodeficiency virus [HIV] disease. Code Z79.899, Other long term (current) drug therapy, may be assigned as an additional code to identify the long-term (current) use of antiretroviral medications.

b. **Infectious agents as the cause of diseases classified to other chapters**

Certain infections are classified in chapters other than Chapter 1 and no organism is identified as part of the infection code. In these instances, it is necessary to use an additional code from Chapter 1 to identify the organism. A code from category B95, Streptococcus, Staphylococcus, and Enterococcus as the cause of diseases classified to other chapters, B96, Other bacterial agents as the cause of diseases classified to other chapters, or B97, Viral agents as the cause of diseases classified to other chapters, is to be used as an additional code to identify the organism. An instructional note will be found at the infection code advising that an additional organism code is required.

c. **Infections resistant to antibiotics**

Many bacterial infections are resistant to current antibiotics. It is necessary to identify all infections documented as antibiotic resistant. Assign a code from category Z16, Resistance to antimicrobial drugs, following the infection code only if the infection code does not identify drug resistance.

d. **Sepsis, Severe Sepsis, and Septic Shock**

1) **Coding of Sepsis and Severe Sepsis**

(a) **Sepsis**
For a diagnosis of sepsis, assign the appropriate code for the underlying systemic infection. If the type of infection or causal organism is not further specified, assign code A41.9, Sepsis, unspecified organism.

A code from subcategory R65.2, Severe sepsis, should not be assigned unless severe sepsis or an associated acute organ dysfunction is documented.

(i) Negative or inconclusive blood cultures and sepsis

Negative or inconclusive blood cultures do not preclude a diagnosis of sepsis in patients with clinical evidence of the condition; however, the provider should be queried.

(ii) Urosepsis

The term urosepsis is a nonspecific term. It is not to be considered synonymous with sepsis. It has no default code in the Alphabetic Index. Should a provider use this term, he/she must be queried for clarification.

(iii) Sepsis with organ dysfunction

If a patient has sepsis and associated acute organ dysfunction or multiple organ dysfunction (MOD), follow the instructions for coding severe sepsis.

(iv) Acute organ dysfunction that is not clearly associated with the sepsis

If a patient has sepsis and an acute organ dysfunction, but the medical record documentation indicates that the acute organ dysfunction is related to a medical condition other than the sepsis, do not assign a code from subcategory R65.2, Severe sepsis. An acute organ dysfunction must be associated with the sepsis in order to assign the severe sepsis code.

If the documentation is not clear as to whether an acute organ dysfunction is related to the sepsis or another medical condition, query the provider.

(b) **Severe sepsis**

The coding of severe sepsis requires a minimum of 2 codes: first a code for the underlying systemic infection, followed by a code from subcategory R65.2, Severe sepsis. If the causal organism is not documented, assign code A41.9, Sepsis, unspecified organism, for the infection. Additional code(s) for the associated acute organ dysfunction are also required.

Due to the complex nature of severe sepsis, some cases may require querying the provider prior to assignment of the codes.

2) **Septic shock**

(a) Septic shock generally refers to circulatory failure associated with severe sepsis, and therefore, it represents a type of acute organ dysfunction.

For cases of septic shock, the code for the systemic infection should be sequenced first, followed by code R65.21, Severe sepsis with septic shock or code T81.12, Postprocedural septic shock. Any additional codes for the other acute organ dysfunctions should also be assigned. As noted in the sequencing instructions in the Tabular List, the code for septic shock cannot be assigned as a principal diagnosis.

3) **Sequencing of severe sepsis**

If severe sepsis is present on admission, and meets the definition of principal diagnosis, the underlying systemic infection should be assigned as principal diagnosis followed by the appropriate code from subcategory R65.2 as required by the sequencing rules in the Tabular List. A code from subcategory R65.2 can never be assigned as a principal diagnosis.

When severe sepsis develops during an encounter (it was not present on admission), the underlying systemic infection and the appropriate code from subcategory R65.2 should be assigned as secondary diagnoses.

Severe sepsis may be present on admission, but the diagnosis may not be confirmed until sometime after admission. If the documentation is not clear whether severe sepsis was present on admission, the provider should be queried.

4) **Sepsis or severe sepsis with a localized infection**

If the reason for admission is sepsis or severe sepsis and a localized infection, such as pneumonia or cellulitis, a code(s) for the underlying systemic infection should be assigned first and the code for the localized infection should be assigned as a secondary diagnosis. If the patient has severe sepsis, a code from subcategory R65.2 should also be assigned as a secondary diagnosis. If the patient is admitted with a localized infection, such as pneumonia, and sepsis/severe sepsis doesn't develop until after admission, the localized infection should be assigned first, followed by the appropriate sepsis/severe sepsis codes.

5) **Sepsis due to a postprocedural infection**

(a) **Documentation of causal relationship**

As with all postprocedural complications, code assignment is based on the provider's documentation of the relationship between the infection and the procedure.

(b) **Sepsis due to a postprocedural infection**

For infections following a procedure, a code from T81.40, to T81.43 Infection following a procedure, or a code from O86.00 to O86.03, Infection of obstetric surgical wound, that identifies the site of the infection should be coded first, if known. Assign an additional code for sepsis following a procedure (T81.44) or sepsis following an obstetrical procedure (O86.04). Use an additional code to identify the infectious agent. If the patient has severe sepsis, the appropriate code from subcategory R65.2 should also be assigned with the additional code(s) for any acute organ dysfunction.

For infections following infusion, transfusion, therapeutic injection, or immunization, a code from subcategory T80.2, Infections following infusion, transfusion, and therapeutic injection, or code T88.0-, Infection following immunization, should be coded first, followed by the code for the specific infection. If the patient has severe sepsis, the appropriate code from subcategory R65.2 should also be assigned, with the additional codes(s) for any acute organ dysfunction.

(c) **Postprocedural infection and postprocedural septic shock**

If a postprocedural infection has resulted in postprocedural septic shock, assign the codes indicated above for sepsis due to a postprocedural infection, followed by code T81.12-, Postprocedural septic shock. Do not assign code R65.21, Severe sepsis with septic shock. Additional code(s) should be assigned for any acute organ dysfunction.

6) **Sepsis and severe sepsis associated with a noninfectious process (condition)**

In some cases, a noninfectious process (condition) such as trauma, may lead to an infection which can result in sepsis or severe sepsis. If sepsis or severe sepsis is documented as associated with a noninfectious condition, such as a burn or serious injury, and this condition meets the definition for principal diagnosis, the code for the noninfectious condition should be sequenced first, followed by the code for the resulting infection. If severe sepsis is present, a code from subcategory R65.2 should also be assigned with any associated organ dysfunction(s) codes. It is not necessary to assign a code from subcategory R65.1, Systemic inflammatory response syndrome (SIRS) of non-infectious origin, for these cases.

If the infection meets the definition of principal diagnosis, it should be sequenced before the non-infectious condition. When both the associated non-infectious condition and the infection meet the definition of principal diagnosis, either may be assigned as principal diagnosis.

Only one code from category R65, Symptoms and signs specifically associated with systemic inflammation and infection, should be assigned. Therefore, when a non-infectious condition leads to an infection resulting in severe sepsis, assign the appropriate code from subcategory R65.2, Severe sepsis. Do not additionally assign a code from subcategory R65.1, Systemic inflammatory response syndrome (SIRS) of non-infectious origin.

See Section I.C.18. SIRS due to non-infectious process

7) **Sepsis and septic shock complicating abortion, pregnancy, childbirth, and the puerperium**

See Section I.C.15. Sepsis and septic shock complicating abortion, pregnancy, childbirth and the puerperium

8) Newborn sepsis

See Section I.C.16. f. Bacterial sepsis of Newborn

e. Methicillin Resistant Staphylococcus aureus (MRSA) Conditions

1) Selection and sequencing of MRSA codes

(a) Combination codes for MRSA infection

When a patient is diagnosed with an infection that is due to methicillin resistant *Staphylococcus aureus* (MRSA), and that infection has a combination code that includes the causal organism (e.g., sepsis, pneumonia) assign the appropriate combination code for the condition (e.g., code A41.02, Sepsis due to Methicillin resistant Staphylococcus aureus or code J15.212, Pneumonia due to Methicillin resistant Staphylococcus aureus). Do not assign code B95.62, Methicillin resistant Staphylococcus aureus infection as the cause of diseases classified elsewhere, as an additional code, because the combination code includes the type of infection and the MRSA organism. Do not assign a code from subcategory Z16.11, Resistance to penicillins, as an additional diagnosis.

See Section C.1. for instructions on coding and sequencing of sepsis and severe sepsis.

(b) Other codes for MRSA infection

When there is documentation of a current infection (e.g., wound infection, stitch abscess, urinary tract infection) due to MRSA, and that infection does not have a combination code that includes the causal organism, assign the appropriate code to identify the condition along with code B95.62, Methicillin resistant

Staphylococcus aureus infection as the cause of diseases classified elsewhere for the MRSA infection. Do not assign a code from subcategory Z16.11, Resistance to penicillins.

(c) Methicillin susceptible Staphylococcus aureus (MSSA) and MRSA colonization

The condition or state of being colonized or carrying MSSA or MRSA is called colonization or carriage, while an individual person is described as being colonized or being a carrier. Colonization means that MSSA or MSRA is present on or in the body without necessarily causing illness. A positive MRSA colonization test might be documented by the provider as "MRSA screen positive" or "MRSA nasal swab positive".

Assign code Z22.322, Carrier or suspected carrier of Methicillin resistant Staphylococcus aureus, for patients documented as having MRSA colonization. Assign code Z22.321, Carrier or suspected carrier of Methicillin susceptible Staphylococcus aureus, for patients documented as having MSSA colonization. Colonization is not necessarily indicative of a disease process or as the cause of a specific condition the patient may have unless documented as such by the provider.

(d MRSA colonization and infection

If a patient is documented as having both MRSA colonization and infection during a hospital admission, code Z22.322, Carrier or suspected carrier of Methicillin resistant Staphylococcus aureus, and a code for the MRSA infection may both be assigned.

f. Zika virus infections

1) Code only confirmed cases

Code only a confirmed diagnosis of Zika virus (A92.5, Zika virus disease) as documented by the provider. This is an exception to the hospital inpatient guideline Section II, H. In this context, "confirmation" does not require documentation of the type of test performed; the provider's diagnostic statement that the condition is confirmed is sufficient. This code should be assigned regardless of the stated mode of transmission.

If the provider documents "suspected", "possible" or "probable" Zika, do not assign code A92.5. Assign a code(s) explaining the reason for encounter (such as fever, rash, or joint pain) or Z20.821, Contact with and (suspected) exposure to Zika virus.

g. **Coronavirus infections**

1) COVID-19 infection (infection due to SARS-CoV-2)

    (a) Code only confirmed cases

Code only a confirmed diagnosis of the 2019 novel coronavirus disease (COVID-19) as documented by the provider or documentation of a positive COVID-19 test result. For a confirmed diagnosis, assign code U07.1, COVID-19. This is an exception to the hospital inpatient guideline Section II, H. In this context, "confirmation" does not require documentation of a positive test result for COVID-19; the provider's documentation that the individual has COVID-19 is sufficient.

If the provider documents "suspected," "possible," "probable," or "inconclusive" COVID-19, do not assign code U07.1. Instead, code the signs and symptoms reported. See guideline I.C.1.g.1.g.

    (b) Sequencing of codes

When COVID-19 meets the definition of principal diagnosis, code U07.1, COVID-19, should be sequenced first, followed by the appropriate codes for associated manifestations, except when another guideline requires that certain codes be sequenced first, such as obstetrics, sepsis, or transplant complications.

For a COVID-19 infection that progresses to sepsis, see Section I.C.1.d. Sepsis, Severe Sepsis, and Septic Shock

See Section I.C.15.s. for COVID-19 infection in pregnancy,childbirth, and the puerperium

See Section I.C.16.h. for COVID-19 infection in newborn

For a COVID-19 infection in a lung transplant patient, see Section I.C.19.g.3.a. Transplant complications other than kidney.

    (c) Acute respiratory manifestations of COVID-19

When the reason for the encounter/admission is a respiratory manifestation of COVID-19, assign code U07.1, COVID-19, as the principal/first-listed diagnosis and assign code(s) for the respiratory manifestation(s) as additional diagnoses.

The following conditions are examples of common respiratory manifestations of COVID-19.

    (i) Pneumonia

For a patient with pneumonia confirmed as due to COVID-19, assign codes U07.1, COVID-19, and J12.89, Other viral pneumonia.

    (ii) Acute bronchitis

For a patient with acute bronchitis confirmed as due to COVID-19, assign codes U07.1, and J20.8, Acute bronchitis due to other specified organisms.

Bronchitis not otherwise specified (NOS) due to COVID-19 should be coded using code U07.1 and J40, Bronchitis, not specified as acute or chronic.

(iii) Lower respiratory infection

If the COVID-19 is documented as being associated with a lower respiratory infection, not otherwise specified (NOS), or an acute respiratory infection, NOS, codes U07.1 and J22, Unspecified acute lower respiratory infection, should be assigned.

If the COVID-19 is documented as being associated with a respiratory infection, NOS, codes U07.1 and J98.8, Other specified respiratory disorders, should be assigned.

(iv) Acute respiratory distress syndrome

For acute respiratory distress syndrome (ARDS) due to COVID-19, assign codes U07.1, and J80, Acute respiratory distress syndrome.

(v) Acute respiratory failure

For acute respiratory failure due to COVID-19, assign code U07.1, and code J96.0-, Acute respiratory failure.

(d) Non-respiratory manifestations of COVID-19

When the reason for the encounter/admission is a non-respiratory manifestation (e.g., viral enteritis) of COVID-19, assign code U07.1, COVID-19, as the principal/first-listed diagnosis and assign code(s) for the manifestation(s) as additional diagnoses.

(e) Exposure to COVID-19

For asymptomatic individuals with actual or suspected exposure to COVID-19, assign code Z20.828, Contact with and (suspected) exposure to other viral communicable diseases.

For symptomatic individuals with actual or suspected exposure to COVID-19 and the infection has been ruled out, or test results are inconclusive or unknown, assign code Z20.828, Contact with and (suspected) exposure to other viral communicable diseases. See guideline I.C.21.c.1, Contact/Exposure, for additional guidance regarding the use of category Z20 codes. If COVID-19 is confirmed, see guideline I.C.1.g.1.a.

(f) Screening for COVID-19

During the COVID-19 pandemic, a screening code is generally not appropriate. For encounters for COVID-19 testing, including preoperative testing, code as exposure to COVID-19 (guideline I.C.1.g.1.e).

Coding guidance will be updated as new information concerning any changes in the pandemic status becomes available.

(g) Signs and symptoms without definitive diagnosis of COVID-19

For patients presenting with any signs/symptoms associated with COVID-19 (such as fever, etc.) but a definitive diagnosis has not been established, assign the appropriate code(s) for each of the presenting signs and symptoms such as:

- R05.1, Acute cough, or R05.9, Cough, unspecified
- R06.02 Shortness of breath
- R50.9 Fever, unspecified

If a patient with signs/symptoms associated with COVID-19 also has an actual or suspected contact with or exposure to COVID-19, assign Z20.828, Contact with and (suspected) exposure to other viral communicable diseases, as an additional code.

(h) Asymptomatic individuals who test positive for COVID-19

For asymptomatic individuals who test positive for COVID-19, see guideline I.C.1.g.1.a. Although the individual is asymptomatic, the individual has tested positive and is considered to have the COVID-19 infection.

(i) Personal history of COVID-19

For patients with a history of COVID-19, assign code Z86.19, Personal history of other infectious and parasitic diseases.

(j) Follow-up visits after COVID-19 infection has resolved

For individuals who previously had COVID-19, **without residual symptom(s) or condition(s)**, and are being seen for follow-up evaluation, and COVID-19 test results are negative, assign codes Z09, Encounter for follow-up examination after completed treatment for conditions other than malignant neoplasm, and Z86.19, Personal history of other infectious and parasitic diseases.

For follow-up visits for individuals with symptom(s) or condition(s) related to a previous COVID-19 infection, see guideline I.C.1.g.1.m.

See Section I.C.21.c.8, Factors influencing health states and contact with health services, Follow-up

(k) Encounter for antibody testing

For an encounter for antibody testing that is not being performed to confirm a current COVID-19 infection, nor is a follow-up test after resolution of COVID-19, assign Z01.84, Encounter for antibody response examination.

Follow the applicable guidelines above if the individual is being tested to confirm a current COVID-19 infection.

For follow-up testing after a COVID-19 infection, see guideline I.C.1.g.1.j.

(l) Multisystem Inflammatory Syndrome

For individuals with multisystem inflammatory syndrome (MIS) and COVID-19, assign code U07.1, COVID-19, as the principal/first-listed diagnosis and assign code M35.81, Multisystem inflammatory syndrome, as an additional diagnosis.

If an individual with a history of COVID-19 develops MIS, assign codes M35.81, Multisystem inflammatory syndrome, and U09.9, Post COVID-19 condition, unspecified.

If an individual with a known or suspected exposure to COVID- 19, and no current COVID-19 infection or history of COVID-19, develops MIS, assign codes M35.81, Multisystem inflammatory syndrome, and Z20.822, Contact with and (suspected) exposure to COVID-19.

Additional codes should be assigned for any associated complications of MIS.

(m) **Post COVID-19 Condition**

For sequela of COVID-19, or associated symptoms or conditions that develop following a previous COVID-19 infection, assign a code(s) for the specific symptom(s) or condition(s) related to the previous COVID-19 infection, if known, and code U09.9, Post COVID-19 condition, unspecified.

Code U09.9 should not be assigned for manifestations of anactive (current) COVID-19 infection.

If a patient has a condition(s) associated with a previous COVID-19 infection and develops a new active (current) COVID-19 infection, code U09.9 may be assigned in conjunction with code U07.1, COVID-19, to identify that the patient also has a condition(s) associated with a previous COVID-19 infection. Code(s) for the specific condition(s) associated with the previous COVID-19 infection and code(s)for manifestation(s) of the new active (current) COVID-19 infection should also be assigned.

2. Chapter 2: Neoplasms (C00-D49)

General guidelines

Chapter 2 of the ICD-10-CM contains the codes for most benign and all malignant neoplasms. Certain benign neoplasms, such as prostatic adenomas, may be found in the specific body system chapters. To properly code a neoplasm, it is necessary to determine from the record if the neoplasm is benign, in-situ, malignant, or of uncertain histologic behavior. If malignant, any secondary (metastatic) sites should also be determined.

Primary malignant neoplasms overlapping site boundaries

A primary malignant neoplasm that overlaps two or more contiguous (next to each other) sites should be classified to the subcategory/code .8 ('overlapping lesion'), unless the combination is specifically indexed elsewhere. For multiple neoplasms of the same site that are not contiguous such as tumors in different quadrants of the same breast, codes for each site should be assigned.

Malignant neoplasm of ectopic tissue

Malignant neoplasms of ectopic tissue are to be coded to the site of origin mentioned, e.g., ectopic pancreatic malignant neoplasms involving the stomach are coded to malignant neoplasm of pancreas, unspecified (C25.9).

The neoplasm table in the Alphabetic Index should be referenced first. However, if the histological term is documented, that term should be referenced first, rather than going immediately to the Neoplasm Table, in order to determine which column in the Neoplasm Table is appropriate. For example, if the documentation indicates "adenoma," refer to the term in the Alphabetic Index to review the entries under this term and the instructional note to "see also neoplasm, by site, benign." The table provides the proper code based on the type of neoplasm and the site. It is important to select the proper column in the table that corresponds to the type of neoplasm. The Tabular List should then be referenced to verify that the correct code has been selected from the table and that a more specific site code does not exist.

See Section I.C.21. Factors influencing health status and contact with health services, Status, for information regarding Z15.0, codes for genetic susceptibility to cancer.

a. Treatment directed at the malignancy

If the treatment is directed at the malignancy, designate the malignancy as the principal diagnosis.

The only exception to this guideline is if a patient admission/encounter is solely for the administration of chemotherapy, immunotherapy or external beam radiation therapy, assign the appropriate Z51.-- code as the first-listed or principal diagnosis, and the diagnosis or problem for which the service is being performed as a secondary diagnosis.

b. Treatment of secondary site

When a patient is admitted because of a primary neoplasm with metastasis and treatment is directed toward the secondary site only, the secondary neoplasm is designated as the principal diagnosis even though the primary malignancy is still present.

c. Coding and sequencing of complications

Coding and sequencing of complications associated with the malignancies or with the therapy thereof are subject to the following guidelines:

1) **Anemia associated with malignancy**

When admission/encounter is for management of an anemia associated with the malignancy, and the treatment is only for anemia, the appropriate code for the malignancy is sequenced as the principal or first-listed diagnosis followed by the appropriate code for the anemia (such as code D63.0, Anemia in neoplastic disease).

2) **Anemia associated with chemotherapy, immunotherapy and radiation therapy**

When the admission/encounter is for management of an anemia associated with an adverse effect of the administration of chemotherapy or immunotherapy and the only treatment is for the anemia, the anemia code is sequenced first followed by the appropriate codes for the neoplasm and the adverse effect (T45.1X5-, Adverse effect of antineoplastic and immunosuppressive drugs).

When the admission/encounter is for management of an anemia associated with an adverse effect of radiotherapy, the anemia code should be sequenced first, followed by the appropriate neoplasm code and code Y84.2, Radiological procedure and radiotherapy as the cause of abnormal reaction of the patient, or of later complication, without mention of misadventure at the time of the procedure.

3) **Management of dehydration due to the malignancy**

When the admission/encounter is for management of dehydration due to the malignancy and only the dehydration is being treated (intravenous rehydration), the dehydration is sequenced first, followed by the code(s) for the malignancy.

4) **Treatment of a complication resulting from a surgical procedure**

When the admission/encounter is for treatment of a complication resulting from a surgical procedure, designate the complication as the principal or first-listed diagnosis if treatment is directed at resolving the complication.

d. **Primary malignancy previously excised**

When a primary malignancy has been previously excised or eradicated from its site and there is no further treatment directed to that site and there is no evidence of any existing primary malignancy at that site, a code from category Z85, Personal history of malignant neoplasm, should be used to indicate the former site of the malignancy. Any mention of extension, invasion, or metastasis to another site is coded as a secondary malignant neoplasm to that site. The secondary site may be the principal or first-listed diagnosis with the Z85 code used as a secondary code.

e. **Admissions/Encounters involving chemotherapy, immunotherapy and radiation therapy**

1) **Episode of care involves surgical removal of neoplasm**

When an episode of care involves the surgical removal of a neoplasm, primary or secondary site, followed by adjunct chemotherapy or radiation treatment during the same episode of care, the code for the neoplasm should be assigned as principal or first-listed diagnosis.

2) **Patient admission/encounter solely for administration of chemotherapy, immunotherapy and radiation therapy**

If a patient admission/encounter is solely for the administration of chemotherapy, immunotherapy or external beam radiation therapy assign code Z51.0, Encounter for antineoplastic radiation therapy, or Z51.11, Encounter for antineoplastic chemotherapy, or Z51.12, Encounter for antineoplastic immunotherapy as the first-listed or principal diagnosis. If a patient receives more than one of these therapies during the same admission more than one of these codes may be assigned, in any sequence.

The malignancy for which the therapy is being administered should be assigned as a secondary diagnosis.

If a patient admission/encounter is for the insertion or implantation of radioactive elements (e.g., brachytherapy) the appropriate code for the malignancy is sequenced as the principal or first-listed diagnosis. Code Z51.0 should not be assigned.

3) Patient admitted for radiation therapy, chemotherapy or immunotherapy and develops complications

When a patient is admitted for the purpose of external beam radiotherapy, immunotherapy or chemotherapy and develops complications such as uncontrolled nausea and vomiting or dehydration, the principal or first-listed diagnosis is Z51.0, Encounter for antineoplastic radiation therapy, or Z51.11, Encounter for antineoplastic chemotherapy, or Z51.12, Encounter for antineoplastic immunotherapy followed by any codes for the complications.

When a patient is admitted for the purpose of insertion or implantation of radioactive elements (e.g., brachytherapy) and develops complications such as uncontrolled nausea and vomiting or dehydration, the principal or first-listed diagnosis is the appropriate code for the malignancy followed by any codes for the complications.

f. Admission/encounter to determine extent of malignancy

When the reason for admission/encounter is to determine the extent of the malignancy, or for a procedure such as paracentesis or thoracentesis, the primary malignancy or appropriate metastatic site is designated as the principal or first-listed diagnosis, even though chemotherapy or radiotherapy is administered.

g. Symptoms, signs, and abnormal findings listed in Chapter 18 associated with neoplasms

Symptoms, signs, and ill-defined conditions listed in Chapter 18 characteristic of, or associated with, an existing primary or secondary site malignancy cannot be used to replace the malignancy as principal or first-listed diagnosis, regardless of the number of admissions or encounters for treatment and care of the neoplasm.

See section I.C.21. Factors influencing health status and contact with health services, Encounter for prophylactic organ removal.

h. Admission/encounter for pain control/management

See Section I.C.6. for information on coding admission/encounter for pain control/management.

i. Malignancy in two or more noncontiguous sites

A patient may have more than one malignant tumor in the same organ. These tumors may represent different primaries or metastatic disease, depending on the site. Should the documentation be unclear, the provider should be queried as to the status of each tumor so that the correct codes can be assigned.

j. Disseminated malignant neoplasm, unspecified

Code C80.0, Disseminated malignant neoplasm, unspecified, is for use only in those cases where the patient has advanced metastatic disease, and no known primary or secondary sites are specified. It should not be used in place of assigning codes for the primary site and all known secondary sites.

k. Malignant neoplasm without specification of site

Code C80.1, Malignant (primary) neoplasm, unspecified, equates to Cancer, unspecified. This code should only be used when no determination can be made as to the primary site of a malignancy. This code should rarely be used in the inpatient setting.

l. Sequencing of neoplasm codes

1) Encounter for treatment of primary malignancy

If the reason for the encounter is for treatment of a primary malignancy, assign the malignancy as the principal/first-listed diagnosis. The primary site is to be sequenced first, followed by any metastatic sites.

2) **Encounter for treatment of secondary malignancy**

When an encounter is for a primary malignancy with metastasis and treatment is directed toward the metastatic (secondary) site(s) only, the metastatic site(s) is designated as the principal/first-listed diagnosis. The primary malignancy is coded as an additional code.

3) **Malignant neoplasm in a pregnant patient**

When a pregnant patient has a malignant neoplasm, a code from subcategory O9A.1-, Malignant neoplasm complicating pregnancy, childbirth, and the puerperium, should be sequenced first, followed by the appropriate code from Chapter 2 to indicate the type of neoplasm.

4) **Encounter for complication associated with a neoplasm**

When an encounter is for management of a complication associated with a neoplasm, such as dehydration, and the treatment is only for the complication, the complication is coded first, followed by the appropriate code(s) for the neoplasm.

The exception to this guideline is anemia. When the admission/encounter is for management of an anemia associated with the malignancy, and the treatment is only for anemia, the appropriate code for the malignancy is sequenced as the principal or first-listed diagnosis followed by code D63.0, Anemia in neoplastic disease.

5) **Complication from surgical procedure for treatment of a neoplasm**

When an encounter is for treatment of a complication resulting from a surgical procedure performed for the treatment of the neoplasm, designate the complication as the principal/first-listed diagnosis. See the guideline regarding the coding of a current malignancy versus personal history to determine if the code for the neoplasm should also be assigned.

6) **Pathologic fracture due to a neoplasm**

When an encounter is for a pathological fracture due to a neoplasm, and the focus of treatment is the fracture, a code from subcategory M84.5, Pathological fracture in neoplastic disease, should be sequenced first, followed by the code for the neoplasm.

If the focus of treatment is the neoplasm with an associated pathological fracture, the neoplasm code should be sequenced first, followed by a code from M84.5 for the pathological fracture.

m. **Current malignancy versus personal history of malignancy**

When a primary malignancy has been excised but further treatment, such as an additional surgery for the malignancy, radiation therapy or chemotherapy is directed to that site, the primary malignancy code should be used until treatment is completed.

When a primary malignancy has been previously excised or eradicated from its site, there is no further treatment (of the malignancy) directed to that site, and there is no evidence of any existing primary malignancy at that site, a code from category Z85, Personal history of malignant neoplasm, should be used to indicate the former site of the malignancy.

Codes from subcategories Z85.0 – Z85.85 should only be assigned for the former site of a primary malignancy, not the site of a secondary malignancy. Code Z85.89 may be assigned for the former site(s) of either a primary or secondary malignancy .

See Section I.C.21. Factors influencing health status and contact with health services, History (of)

n. **Leukemia, Multiple Myeloma, and Malignant Plasma Cell Neoplasms in remission versus personal history**

The categories for leukemia, and category C90, Multiple myeloma and malignant plasma cell neoplasms, have codes indicating whether or not the leukemia has achieved remission. There are also codes Z85.6, Personal history of leukemia, and Z85.79, Personal history of other malignant neoplasms of lymphoid, hematopoietic and related tissues. If the documentation is unclear as to whether the leukemia has achieved remission, the provider should be queried.

See Section I.C.21. Factors influencing health status and contact with health services, History (of)

o. **Aftercare following surgery for neoplasm**

See Section I.C.21. Factors influencing health status and contact with health services, Aftercare

p. **Follow-up care for completed treatment of a malignancy**

See Section I.C.21. Factors influencing health status and contact with health services, Follow-up

q. **Prophylactic organ removal for prevention of malignancy**

See Section I.C. 21, Factors influencing health status and contact with health services, Prophylactic organ removal

r. **Malignant neoplasm associated with transplanted organ**

A malignant neoplasm of a transplanted organ should be coded as a transplant complication. Assign first the appropriate code from category T86.-, Complications of transplanted organs and tissue, followed by code C80.2, Malignant neoplasm associated with transplanted organ. Use an additional code for the specific malignancy.

s. **Breast Implant Associated Anaplastic Large Cell Lymphoma**

Breast implant associated anaplastic large cell lymphoma (BIA-ALCL) is a type of lymphoma that can develop around breast implants. Assign code C84.7A, Anaplastic large cell lymphoma, ALK-negative, breast, for BIA-ALCL. Do not assign a complication code from chapter 19.

3. Chapter 3: Disease of the blood and blood-forming organs and certain disorders involving the immune mechanism (D50-D89)

Reserved for future guideline expansion

4. Chapter 4: Endocrine, Nutritional, and Metabolic Diseases (E00-E89)

a. **Diabetes mellitus**

The diabetes mellitus codes are combination codes that include the type of diabetes mellitus, the body system affected, and the complications affecting that body system. As many codes within a particular category as are necessary to describe all of the complications of the disease may be used. They should be sequenced based on the reason for a particular encounter. Assign as many codes from categories E08 – E13 as needed to identify all of the associated conditions that the patient has.

1) **Type of diabetes**

The age of a patient is not the sole determining factor, though most type 1 diabetics develop the condition before reaching puberty. For this reason, type 1 diabetes mellitus is also referred to as juvenile diabetes.

2) **Type of diabetes mellitus not documented**

If the type of diabetes mellitus is not documented in the medical record the default is E11.-, Type 2 diabetes mellitus.

3) **Diabetes mellitus and the use of insulin, oral hypoglycemics, and injectable non-insulin drugs**

If the documentation in a medical record does not indicate the type of diabetes but does indicate that the patient uses insulin, code E11-, Type 2diabetes mellitus, should be assigned. Additional code(s) should be assigned from category Z79 to identify the long-term (current) use of insulin, oral hypoglycemic drugs, or injectable non-insulin antidiabetic, as follows:

If the patient is treated with both oral medications and insulin, both codeZ79.4, Long term (current) use of insulin, and code Z79.84, Long term (current) use of oral hypoglycemic drugs, should be assigned.

If the patient is treated with both insulin and an injectable non-insulin antidiabetic drug, assign codes Z79.4, Long term (current) use of insulin,and Z79.899, Other long term (current) drug therapy.

If the patient is treated with both oral hypoglycemic drugs and an injectable non-insulin antidiabetic drug, assign codes Z79.84, Long term(current) use of oral hypoglycemic drugs, and Z79.899, Other long term (current) drug therapy.

Code Z79.4 should not be assigned if insulin is given temporarily to bring a type 2 patient's blood sugar under control during an encounter.

4) **Diabetes mellitus in pregnancy and gestational diabetes**

   See Section I.C.15. Diabetes mellitus in pregnancy.
   See Section I.C.15. Gestational (pregnancy induced) diabetes

5) **Complications due to insulin pump malfunction**

   (a) **Underdose of insulin due to insulin pump failure**

   An underdose of insulin due to an insulin pump failure should be assigned to a code from subcategory T85.6, Mechanical complication of other specified internal and external prosthetic devices, implants and grafts, that specifies the type of pump malfunction, as the principal or first-listed code, followed by code T38.3X6-, Underdosing of insulin and oral hypoglycemic [antidiabetic] drugs. Additional codes for the type of diabetes mellitus and any associated complications due to the underdosing should also be assigned.

   (b) **Overdose of insulin due to insulin pump failure**

   The principal or first-listed code for an encounter due to an insulin pump malfunction resulting in an overdose of insulin, should also be T85.6-, Mechanical complication of other specified internal and external prosthetic devices, implants and grafts, followed by code T38.3X1-, Poisoning by insulin and oral hypoglycemic [antidiabetic] drugs, accidental (unintentional).

6) **Secondary diabetes mellitus**

   Codes under categories E08, Diabetes mellitus due to underlying condition, E09, Drug or chemical induced diabetes mellitus, and E13, Other specified diabetes mellitus, identify complications/manifestations associated with secondary diabetes mellitus. Secondary diabetes is always caused by another condition or event (e.g., cystic fibrosis, malignant neoplasm of pancreas, pancreatectomy, adverse effect of drug, or poisoning).

   (a) **Secondary diabetes mellitus and the use of insulin or oral hypoglycemic drugs**

   For patients with secondary diabetes mellitus who routinely useinsulin, oral hypoglycemic drugs, or injectable non-insulin drugs, additional code(s) from category Z79 should be assignedto identify the long-term (current) use of insulin, oral hypoglycemic drugs, or non-injectable non-insulin drugs as follows:

   If the patient is treated with both oral medications and insulin,both code Z79.4, Long term (current) use of insulin, and code Z79.84, Long term (current) use of oral hypoglycemic drugs, should be assigned.

   If the patient is treated with both insulin and an injectable non- insulin antidiabetic drug, assign codes Z79.4, Long- term (current) use of insulin, and Z79.899, Other long term(current) drug therapy.

If the patient is treated with both oral hypoglycemic drugs and an injectable non-insulin antidiabetic drug, assign codes Z79.84, Long-term (current) use of oral hypoglycemic drugs,and Z79.899, Other long-term (current) drug therapy.

Code Z79.4 should not be assigned if insulin is given temporarily to bring a secondary diabetic patient's bloodsugar under control during an encounter.

(b) **Assigning and sequencing secondary diabetes codes and its causes**

The sequencing of the secondary diabetes codes in relationship to codes for the cause of the diabetes is based on the Tabular List instructions for categories E08, E09 and E13.

(i) **Secondary diabetes mellitus due to pancreatectomy**

For postpancreatectomy diabetes mellitus (lack of insulin due to the surgical removal of all or part of the pancreas), assign code E89.1, Postprocedural hypoinsulinemia. Assign a code from category E13 and a code from subcategory Z90.41, Acquired absence of pancreas, as additional codes.

(ii) **Secondary diabetes due to drugs**

Secondary diabetes may be caused by an adverse effect of correctly administered medications, poisoning or sequela of poisoning.

See section I.C.19.e for coding of adverse effects and poisoning, and section I.C.20 for external cause code reporting.

5. Chapter 5: Mental, Behavioral and Neurodevelopmental disorders (F01 – F99)

a. **Pain disorders related to psychological factors**

Assign code F45.41, for pain that is exclusively related to psychological disorders. As indicated by the Excludes 1 note under category G89, a code from category G89 should not be assigned with code F45.41.

Code F45.42, Pain disorders with related psychological factors, should be used with a code from category G89, Pain, not elsewhere classified, if there is documentation of a psychological component for a patient with acute or chronic pain.

See Section I.C.6. Pain

b. **Mental and behavioral disorders due to psychoactive substance use**

1) **In Remission**

Selection of codes for "in remission" for categories F10-F19, Mental and behavioral disorders due to psychoactive substance use (categories F10-F19 with -.11, -.21) requires the provider's clinical judgment. The appropriate codes for "in remission" are assigned only on the basis of provider documentation (as defined in the Official Guidelines for Coding and Reporting), unless otherwise instructed by the classification.

Mild substance use disorders in early or sustained remission are classified to the appropriate codes for substance abuse in remission, and moderate or severe substance use disorders in early or sustained remission are classified to the appropriate codes for substance dependence in remission.

2) **Psychoactive Substance Use, Abuse and Dependence**

When the provider documentation refers to use, abuse and dependence of the same substance (e.g., alcohol, opioid, cannabis, etc.), only one code should be assigned to identify the pattern of use based on the following hierarchy:

- If both use and abuse are documented, assign only the code for abuse

- If both abuse and dependence are documented, assign only the code for dependence
- If use, abuse and dependence are all documented, assign only the code for dependence
- If both use and dependence are documented, assign only the code for dependence.

3) **Psychoactive Substance Use, Unspecified**

As with all other unspecified diagnoses, the codes for unspecified psychoactive substance use (F10.9-, F11.9-, F12.9-, F13.9-, F14.9-, F15.9-, F16.9-, F18.9-, F19.9-) should only be assigned based on provider documentation and when they meet the definition of a reportable diagnosis (see Section III, Reporting Additional Diagnoses).

These codes are to be used only when the psychoactive substance use is associated with a substance related disorder (chapter 5 disorders such as sexual dysfunction, sleep disorder, or a mental or behavioral disorder)or medical condition, and such a relationship is documented by the provider.

4) **Medical Conditions Due to Psychoactive Substance Use, Abuseand Dependence**

Medical conditions due to substance use, abuse, and dependence arenot classified as substance-induced disorders. Assign the diagnosis code for the medical condition as directed by the Alphabetical Index along with the appropriate psychoactive substance use, abuse or dependence code. For example, for alcoholic pancreatitis due to alcohol dependence, assign the appropriate code from subcategory K85.2, Alcohol induced acute pancreatitis, and the appropriate codefrom subcategory F10.2, such as code F10.20, Alcohol dependence, uncomplicated. It would not be appropriate to assign code F10.288, Alcohol dependence with other alcohol-induced disorder.

5) **Blood Alcohol Level**

A code from category Y90, Evidence of alcohol involvement determined by blood alcohol level, may be assigned when this information is documented and the patient's provider has documented a condition classifiable to category F10, Alcohol relateddisorders. The blood alcohol level does not need to be documented by the patient's provider in order for it to be coded.

c. **Factitious Disorder**

Factitious disorder imposed on self or Munchausen's syndrome is a disorder in which a person falsely reports or causes his or her own physical or psychological signs or symptoms. For patients with documented factitious disorder on self or Munchausen's syndrome, assign the appropriate code from subcategory F68.1-, Factitious disorder imposed on self.

Munchausen's syndrome by proxy (MSBP) is a disorder in which a caregiver (perpetrator) falsely reports or causes an illness or injury in another person (victim) under his or her care, such as a child, an elderly adult, or a person who has a disability. The condition is also referred to as "factitious disorder imposed on another" or "factitious disorder by proxy." The perpetrator, not the victim, receives this diagnosis. Assign code F68.A, Factitious disorder imposed on another, to the perpetrator's record. For the victim of a patient suffering from MSBP, assign the appropriate code from categories T74, Adult and child abuse, neglect and other maltreatment, confirmed, or T76, Adult and child abuse, neglect and other maltreatment, suspected.

See Section I.C.19.f. Adult and child abuse, neglect and other maltreatment

6. Chapter 6: Diseases of the Nervous System (G00-G99)

a. **Dominant/nondominant side**

Codes from category G81, Hemiplegia and hemiparesis, and subcategories G83.1, Monoplegia of lower limb, G83.2, Monoplegia of upper limb, and G83.3, Monoplegia, unspecified, identify whether the dominant or nondominant side is affected. Should the affected side be documented, but not specified as dominant or nondominant, and the classification system does not indicate a default, code selection is as follows:

- For ambidextrous patients, the default should be dominant.
- If the left side is affected, the default is non-dominant.
- If the right side is affected, the default is dominant.

b. **Pain - Category G89**

1) **General coding information**

Codes in category G89, Pain, not elsewhere classified, may be used in conjunction with codes from other categories and chapters to provide more detail about acute or chronic pain and neoplasm-related pain, unless otherwise indicated below.

If the pain is not specified as acute or chronic, post-thoracotomy, postprocedural, or neoplasm-related, do not assign codes from category G89.

A code from category G89 should not be assigned if the underlying (definitive) diagnosis is known, unless the reason for the encounter is pain control/ management and not management of the underlying condition.

When an admission or encounter is for a procedure aimed at treating the underlying condition (e.g., spinal fusion, kyphoplasty), a code for the underlying condition (e.g., vertebral fracture, spinal stenosis) should be assigned as the principal diagnosis. No code from category G89 should be assigned.

(a) **Category G89 Codes as Principal or First-Listed Diagnosis**

Category G89 codes are acceptable as principal diagnosis or the first-listed code:

- When pain control or pain management is the reason for the admission/encounter (e.g., a patient with displaced intervertebral disc, nerve impingement and severe back pain presents for injection of steroid into the spinal canal). The underlying cause of the pain should be reported as an additional diagnosis, if known.

- When a patient is admitted for the insertion of a neurostimulator for pain control, assign the appropriate pain code as the principal or first-listed diagnosis. When an admission or encounter is for a procedure aimed at treating the underlying condition and a neurostimulator is inserted for pain control during the same admission/encounter, a code for the underlying condition should be assigned as the principal diagnosis and the appropriate pain code should be assigned as a secondary diagnosis.

(b) **Use of Category G89 Codes in Conjunction with Site Specific Pain Codes**

(i) **Assigning Category G89 and Site-Specific Pain Codes**

Codes from category G89 may be used in conjunction with codes that identify the site of pain (including codes from chapter 18) if the category G89 code provides additional information. For example, if the code describes the site of the pain, but does not fully describe whether the pain is acute or chronic, then both codes should be assigned.

(ii) **Sequencing of Category G89 Codes with Site-Specific Pain Codes**

The sequencing of category G89 codes with site-specific pain codes (including chapter 18 codes), is dependent on the circumstances of the encounter/admission as follows:

- If the encounter is for pain control or pain management, assign the code from category G89 followed by the code identifying the specific site of pain (e.g., encounter for pain management for acute neck pain from trauma is assigned code G89.11, Acute pain due to trauma, followed by code M54.2, Cervicalgia, to identify the site of pain).

- If the encounter is for any other reason except pain control or pain management, and a related definitive diagnosis has not been established (confirmed) by the provider, assign the code for the specific site of pain first, followed by the appropriate code from category G89.

2) Pain due to devices, implants and grafts

See Section I.C.19. Pain due to medical devices

3) Postoperative Pain

The provider's documentation should be used to guide the coding of postoperative pain, as well as *Section III. Reporting Additional Diagnoses* and *Section IV. Diagnostic Coding and Reporting in the Outpatient Setting.*

The default for post-thoracotomy and other postoperative pain not specified as acute or chronic is the code for the acute form.

Routine or expected postoperative pain immediately after surgery should not be coded.

(a) **Postoperative pain not associated with specific postoperative complication**

Postoperative pain not associated with a specific postoperative complication is assigned to the appropriate postoperative pain code in category G89.

(b) **Postoperative pain associated with specific postoperative complication**

Postoperative pain associated with a specific postoperative complication (such as painful wire sutures) is assigned to the appropriate code(s) found in Chapter 19, Injury, poisoning, and certain other consequences of external causes. If appropriate, use additional code(s) from category G89 to identify acute or chronic pain (G89.18 or G89.28).

4) Chronic pain

Chronic pain is classified to subcategory G89.2. There is no time frame defining when pain becomes chronic pain. The provider's documentation should be used to guide use of these codes.

5) Neoplasm Related Pain

Code G89.3 is assigned to pain documented as being related, associated or due to cancer, primary or secondary malignancy, or tumor. This code is assigned regardless of whether the pain is acute or chronic.

This code may be assigned as the principal or first-listed code when the stated reason for the admission/encounter is documented as pain control/pain management. The underlying neoplasm should be reported as an additional diagnosis.

When the reason for the admission/encounter is management of the neoplasm and the pain associated with the neoplasm is also documented, code G89.3 may be assigned as an additional diagnosis. It is not necessary to assign an additional code for the site of the pain.

See Section I.C.2 for instructions on the sequencing of neoplasms for all other stated reasons for the admission/encounter (except for pain control/pain management).

6) Chronic pain syndrome

Central pain syndrome (G89.0) and chronic pain syndrome (G89.4) are different than the term "chronic pain," and therefore codes should only be used when the provider has specifically documented this condition.

See Section I.C.5. Pain disorders related to psychological factors

7. Chapter 7: Diseases of the Eye and Adnexa (H00-H59)

a. Glaucoma

1) Assigning Glaucoma Codes

Assign as many codes from category H40, Glaucoma, as needed to identify the type of glaucoma, the affected eye, and the glaucoma stage.

2) **Bilateral glaucoma with same type and stage**

When a patient has bilateral glaucoma and both eyes are documented as being the same type and stage, and there is a code for bilateral glaucoma, report only the code for the type of glaucoma, bilateral, with the seventh character for the stage.

When a patient has bilateral glaucoma and both eyes are documented as being the same type and stage, and the classification does not provide a code for bilateral glaucoma (i.e., subcategories H40.10, and H40.20) report only one code for the type of glaucoma with the appropriate seventh character for the stage.

3) **Bilateral glaucoma stage with different types or stages**

When a patient has bilateral glaucoma and each eye is documented as having a different type or stage, and the classification distinguishes laterality, assign the appropriate code for each eye rather than the code for bilateral glaucoma.

When a patient has bilateral glaucoma and each eye is documented as having a different type, and the classification does not distinguish laterality (i.e., subcategories H40.10, and H40.20), assign one code for each type of glaucoma with the appropriate seventh character for the stage.

When a patient has bilateral glaucoma and each eye is documented as having the same type, but different stage, and the classification does not distinguish laterality (i.e., subcategories H40.10 and H40.20), assign a code for the type of glaucoma for each eye with the seventh character for the specific glaucoma stage documented for each eye.

4) **Patient admitted with glaucoma and stage evolves during the admission**

If a patient is admitted with glaucoma and the stage progresses during the admission, assign the code for highest stage documented.

5) **Indeterminate stage glaucoma**

Assignment of the seventh character "4" for "indeterminate stage" should be based on the clinical documentation. The seventh character "4" is used for glaucomas whose stage cannot be clinically determined. This seventh character should not be confused with the seventh character "0", unspecified, which should be assigned when there is no documentation regarding the stage of the glaucoma.

b. **Blindness**

If "blindness" or "low vision" of both eyes is documented but the visual impairment category is not documented, assign code H54.3, Unqualified visual loss, both eyes. If "blindness" or "low vision" in one eye is documented but the visual impairment category is not documented, assign a code from H54.6-, Unqualified visual loss, one eye. If "blindness" or "visual loss" is documented without any information about whether one or both eyes are affected, assign code H54.7, Unspecified visual loss.

8. Chapter 8: Diseases of the Ear and Mastoid Process (H60-H95)

Reserved for future guideline expansion

9. Chapter 9: Diseases of the Circulatory System (I00-I99)

a. **Hypertension**

The classification presumes a causal relationship between hypertension and heart involvement and between hypertension and kidney involvement, as the two conditions are linked by the term "with" in the Alphabetic

Index. These conditions should be coded as related even in the absence of provider documentation explicitly linking them, unless the documentation clearly states the conditions are unrelated.

For hypertension and conditions not specifically linked by relational terms such as "with," "associated with" or "due to" in the classification, provider documentation must link the conditions in order to code them as related.

1) **Hypertension with Heart Disease**

Hypertension with heart conditions classified to I50.- or I51.4-I51.7, I51.89, I51.9, are assigned to a code from category I11, Hypertensive heart disease. Use additional code(s) from category I50, Heart failure, to identify the type(s) of heart failure in those patients with heart failure.

The same heart conditions (I50.-, I51.4-I51.7, I51.89, I51.9) with hypertension are coded separately if the provider has documented they are unrelated to the hypertension. Sequence according to the circumstances of the admission/encounter.

2) **Hypertensive Chronic Kidney Disease**

Assign codes from category I12, Hypertensive chronic kidney disease, when both hypertension and a condition classifiable to category N18, Chronic kidney disease (CKD), are present. CKD should not be coded as hypertensive if the provider indicates the CKD is not related to the hypertension.

The appropriate code from category N18 should be used as a secondary code with a code from category I12 to identify the stage of chronic kidney disease.

See Section I.C.14. Chronic kidney disease.

If a patient has hypertensive chronic kidney disease and acute renal failure, the acute renal failure should also be coded.

Sequence according to the circumstances of the admission/encounter.

3) **Hypertensive Heart and Chronic Kidney Disease**

Assign codes from combination category I13, Hypertensive heart and chronic kidney disease, when there is hypertension with both heart and kidney involvement. If heart failure is present, assign an additional code from category I50 to identify the type of heart failure.

The appropriate code from category N18, Chronic kidney disease, should be used as a secondary code with a code from category I13 to identify the stage of chronic kidney disease.

See Section I.C.14. Chronic kidney disease.

The codes in category I13, Hypertensive heart and chronic kidney disease, are combination codes that include hypertension, heart disease and chronic kidney disease. The Includes note at I13 specifies that the conditions included at I11 and I12 are included together in I13. If a patient has hypertension, heart disease and chronic kidney disease, then a code from I13 should be used, not individual codes for hypertension, heart disease and chronic kidney disease, or codes from I11 or I12.

For patients with both acute renal failure and chronic kidney disease, the acute renal failure should also be coded. Sequence according to the circumstances of the admission/encounter.

4) **Hypertensive Cerebrovascular Disease**

For hypertensive cerebrovascular disease, first assign the appropriate code from categories I60-I69, followed by the appropriate hypertension code.

5) **Hypertensive Retinopathy**

Subcategory H35.0, Background retinopathy and retinal vascular changes, should be used with a code from category I10 – I15, Hypertensive disease to include the systemic hypertension. The sequencing is based on the reason for the encounter.

6) Hypertension, Secondary

Secondary hypertension is due to an underlying condition. Two codes are required: one to identify the underlying etiology and one from category I15 to identify the hypertension. Sequencing of codes is determined by the reason for admission/encounter.

7) Hypertension, Transient

Assign code R03.0, Elevated blood pressure reading without diagnosis of hypertension, unless patient has an established diagnosis of hypertension. Assign code O13.-, Gestational [pregnancy-induced] hypertension without significant proteinuria, or O14.-, Pre-eclampsia, for transient hypertension of pregnancy.

8) Hypertension, Controlled

This diagnostic statement usually refers to an existing state of hypertension under control by therapy. Assign the appropriate code from categories I10-I15, Hypertensive diseases.

9) Hypertension, Uncontrolled

Uncontrolled hypertension may refer to untreated hypertension or hypertension not responding to current therapeutic regimen. In either case, assign the appropriate code from categories I10-I15, Hypertensive diseases.

10) Hypertensive Crisis

Assign a code from category I16, Hypertensive crisis, for documented hypertensive urgency, hypertensive emergency or unspecified hypertensive crisis. Code also any identified hypertensive disease (I10-I15). The sequencing is based on the reason for the encounter.

11) Pulmonary Hypertension

Pulmonary hypertension is classified to category I27, Other pulmonary heart diseases. For secondary pulmonary hypertension (I27.1, I27.2-), code also any associated conditions or adverse effects of drugs or toxins. The sequencing is based on the reason for the encounter, except for adverse effects of drugs (See Section I.C.19.e.).

b. Atherosclerotic Coronary Artery Disease and Angina

ICD-10-CM has combination codes for atherosclerotic heart disease with angina pectoris. The subcategories for these codes are I25.11, Atherosclerotic heart disease of native coronary artery with angina pectoris and I25.7, Atherosclerosis of coronary artery bypass graft(s) and coronary artery of transplanted heart with angina pectoris.

When using one of these combination codes it is not necessary to use an additional code for angina pectoris. A causal relationship can be assumed in a patient with both atherosclerosis and angina pectoris, unless the documentation indicates the angina is due to something other than the atherosclerosis.

If a patient with coronary artery disease is admitted due to an acute myocardial infarction (AMI), the AMI should be sequenced before the coronary artery disease.

See Section I.C.9. Acute myocardial infarction (AMI)

c. Intraoperative and Postprocedural Cerebrovascular Accident

Medical record documentation should clearly specify the cause- and-effect relationship between the medical intervention and the cerebrovascular accident in order to assign a code for intraoperative or postprocedural cerebrovascular accident.

Proper code assignment depends on whether it was an infarction or hemorrhage and whether it occurred intraoperatively or postoperatively. If it was a cerebral hemorrhage, code assignment depends on the type of procedure performed.

d. Sequelae of Cerebrovascular Disease

1) Category I69, Sequelae of Cerebrovascular disease

Category I69 is used to indicate conditions classifiable to categories I60-I67 as the causes of sequela (neurologic deficits), themselves classified elsewhere. These "late effects" include neurologic deficits that persist after initial onset of conditions classifiable to categories I60-I67. The neurologic deficits caused by cerebrovascular disease may be present from the onset or may arise at any time after the onset of the condition classifiable to categories I60-I67.

Codes from category I69, Sequelae of cerebrovascular disease, that specify hemiplegia, hemiparesis and monoplegia identify whether the dominant or nondominant side is affected. Should the affected side be documented, but not specified as dominant or nondominant, and the classification system does not indicate a default, code selection is as follows:

- For ambidextrous patients, the default should be dominant.
- If the left side is affected, the default is non-dominant.
- If the right side is affected, the default is dominant.

2) Codes from category I69 with codes from I60-I67

Codes from category I69 may be assigned on a health care record with codes from I60-I67, if the patient has a current cerebrovascular disease and deficits from an old cerebrovascular disease.

3) Codes from category I69 and Personal history of transient ischemic attack (TIA) and cerebral infarction (Z86.73)

Codes from category I69 should not be assigned if the patient does not have neurologic deficits.

See Section I.C.21. 4. History (of) for use of personal history codes

e. Acute myocardial infarction (AMI)

1) Type 1 ST elevation myocardial infarction (STEMI) and non-ST elevation myocardial infarction (NSTEMI)

The ICD-10-CM codes for type 1 acute myocardial infarction (AMI) identify the site, such as anterolateral wall or true posterior wall. Subcategories I21.0-I21.2 and code I21.3 are used for type 1 ST elevation myocardial infarction (STEMI). Code I21.4, Non-ST elevation (NSTEMI) myocardial infarction, is used for type 1 non-ST elevation myocardial infarction (NSTEMI) and nontransmural MIs.

If a type 1 NSTEMI evolves to STEMI, assign the STEMI code. If a type 1 STEMI converts to NSTEMI due to thrombolytic therapy, it is still coded as STEMI.

For encounters occurring while the myocardial infarction is equal to, or less than, four weeks old, including transfers to another acute setting or a postacute setting, and the myocardial infarction meets the definition for "other diagnoses" (see Section III, Reporting Additional Diagnoses), codes from category I21 may continue to be reported. For encounters after the 4 week time frame and the patient is still receiving care related to the myocardial infarction, the appropriate aftercare code should be assigned, rather than a code from category I21. For old or healed myocardial infarctions not requiring further care, code I25.2, Old myocardial infarction, may be assigned.

2) **Acute myocardial infarction, unspecified**

Code I21.9, Acute myocardial infarction, unspecified, is the default for unspecified acute myocardial infarction or unspecified type. If only type 1 STEMI or transmural MI without the site is documented, assign code I21.3, ST elevation (STEMI) myocardial infarction of unspecified site.

3) **AMI documented as nontransmural or subendocardial, but site provided**

If an AMI is documented as nontransmural or subendocardial, but the site is provided, it is still coded as a subendocardial AMI.

See Section I.C.21.3 for information on coding status post administration of tPA in a different facility within the last 24 hours.

4) **Subsequent acute myocardial infarction**

A code from category I22, Subsequent ST elevation (STEMI) and non-ST elevation (NSTEMI) myocardial infarction, is to be used when a patient who has suffered a type 1 or unspecified AMI has a new AMI within the 4 week time frame of the initial AMI. A code from category I22 must be used in conjunction with a code from category I21. The sequencing of the I22 and I21 codes depends on the circumstances of the encounter.

Do not assign code I22 for subsequent myocardial infarctions other than type 1 or unspecified. For subsequent type 2 AMI assign only code I21.A1. For subsequent type 4 or type 5 AMI, assign only code I21.A9.

If a subsequent myocardial infarction of one type occurs within 4 weeks of a myocardial infarction of a different type, assign the appropriate codes from category I21 to identify each type. Do not assign a code from I22. Codes from category I22 should only be assigned if both the initial and subsequent myocardial infarctions are type 1 or unspecified.

5) **Other Types of Myocardial Infarction**

The ICD-10-CM provides codes for different types of myocardial infarction. Type 1 myocardial infarctions are assigned to codes I21.0-I21.4.

Type 2 myocardial infarction (myocardial infarction due to demand ischemia or secondary to ischemic imbalance) is assigned to code I21.A1, Myocardial infarction type 2 with the underlying cause coded first. Do not assign code I24.8, Other forms of acute ischemic heart disease, for the demand ischemia.

If a type 2 AMI is described as NSTEMI or STEMI, only assign code I21.A1. Codes I21.01-I21.4 should only be assigned for type 1 AMIs.

Acute myocardial infarctions type 3, 4a, 4b, 4c and 5 are assigned to code I21.A9, Other myocardial infarction type.

The "Code also" and "Code first" notes should be followed related to complications, and for coding of postprocedural myocardial infarctions during or following cardiac surgery.

10. Chapter 10: Diseases of the Respiratory System (J00-J99), U07.0

a. **Chronic Obstructive Pulmonary Disease [COPD] and Asthma**

1) **Acute exacerbation of chronic obstructive bronchitis and asthma**

The codes in categories J44 and J45 distinguish between uncomplicated cases and those in acute exacerbation. An acute exacerbation is a worsening or a decompensation of a chronic condition. An acute exacerbation is not equivalent to an infection superimposed on a chronic condition, though an exacerbation may be triggered by an infection.

b. **Acute Respiratory Failure**

1) **Acute respiratory failure as principal diagnosis**

A code from subcategory J96.0, Acute respiratory failure, or subcategory J96.2, Acute and chronic respiratory failure, may be assigned as a principal diagnosis when it is the condition established after study to be chiefly responsible for occasioning the admission to the hospital, and the selection is supported by the Alphabetic Index and Tabular List. However, chapter-specific coding guidelines (such as obstetrics, poisoning, HIV, newborn) that provide sequencing direction take precedence.

2) **Acute respiratory failure as secondary diagnosis**

Respiratory failure may be listed as a secondary diagnosis if it occurs after admission, or if it is present on admission, but does not meet the definition of principal diagnosis.

3) **Sequencing of acute respiratory failure and another acute condition**

When a patient is admitted with respiratory failure and another acute condition, (e.g., myocardial infarction, cerebrovascular accident, aspiration pneumonia), the principal diagnosis will not be the same in every situation. This applies whether the other acute condition is a respiratory or nonrespiratory condition. Selection of the principal diagnosis will be dependent on the circumstances of admission. If both the respiratory failure and the other acute condition are equally responsible for occasioning the admission to the hospital, and there are no chapter-specific sequencing rules, the guideline regarding two or more diagnoses that equally meet the definition for principal diagnosis (Section II, C.) may be applied in these situations.

If the documentation is not clear as to whether acute respiratory failure and another condition are equally responsible for occasioning the admission, query the provider for clarification.

c. **Influenza due to certain identified influenza viruses**

Code only confirmed cases of influenza due to certain identified influenza viruses (category J09), and due to other identified influenza virus (category J10). This is an exception to the hospital inpatient guideline Section II, H. (Uncertain Diagnosis).

In this context, "confirmation" does not require documentation of positive laboratory testing specific for avian or other novel influenza A or other identified influenza virus. However, coding should be based on the provider's diagnostic statement that the patient has avian influenza, or other novel influenza A, for category J09, or has another particular identified strain of influenza, such as H1N1 or H3N2, but not identified as novel or variant, for category J10.

If the provider records "suspected" or "possible" or "probable" avian influenza, or novel influenza, or other identified influenza, then the appropriate influenza code from category J11, Influenza due to unidentified influenza virus, should be assigned. A code from category J09, Influenza due to certain identified influenza viruses, should not be assigned nor should a code from category J10, Influenza due to other identified influenza virus.

d. **Ventilator associated Pneumonia**

1) **Documentation of Ventilator associated Pneumonia**

As with all procedural or postprocedural complications, code assignment is based on the provider's documentation of the relationship between the condition and the procedure.

Code J95.851, Ventilator associated pneumonia, should be assigned only when the provider has documented ventilator associated pneumonia (VAP). An additional code to identify the organism (e.g., Pseudomonas aeruginosa, code B96.5) should also be assigned. Do not assign an additional code from categories J12-J18 to identify the type of pneumonia.

Code J95.851 should not be assigned for cases where the patient has pneumonia and is on a mechanical ventilator and the provider has not specifically stated that the pneumonia is ventilator-associated pneumonia. If the documentation is unclear as to whether the patient has a pneumonia that is a complication attributable to the mechanical ventilator, query the provider.

2) Ventilator associated Pneumonia Develops after Admission

A patient may be admitted with one type of pneumonia (e.g., code J13, Pneumonia due to Streptococcus pneumonia) and subsequently develop VAP. In this instance, the principal diagnosis would be the appropriate code from categories J12-J18 for the pneumonia diagnosed at the time of admission. Code J95.851, Ventilator associated pneumonia, would be assigned as an additional diagnosis when the provider has also documented the presence of ventilator associated pneumonia.

e. Vaping-related disorders
For patients presenting with condition(s) related to vaping, assign code U07.0, Vaping-related disorder, as the principal diagnosis. For lung injury due to vaping, assign only code U07.0. Assign additional codes for other manifestations, such as acute respiratory failure (subcategory J96.0-) or pneumonitis (code J68.0).

Associated respiratory signs and symptoms due to vaping, such as cough, shortness of breath, etc., are not coded separately, when a definitive diagnosis has been established. However, it would be appropriate to code separately any gastrointestinal symptoms, such as diarrhea and abdominal pain.

11. Chapter 11: Diseases of the Digestive System (K00-K95)

Reserved for future guideline expansion

12. Chapter 12: Diseases of the Skin and Subcutaneous Tissue (L00-L99)

a. **Pressure ulcer stage codes**

1) **Pressure ulcer stages**

Codes in category L89, Pressure ulcer, identify the site and stage of the pressure ulcer.

The ICD-10-CM classifies pressure ulcer stages based on severity, which is designated by stages 1-4, deep tissue pressure injury, unspecified stage, and unstageable.

Assign as many codes from category L89 as needed to identify all the pressure ulcers the patient has, if applicable.
See Section I.B.14 for pressure ulcer stage documentation by clinicians other than patient's provider.

2) **Unstageable pressure ulcers**

Assignment of the code for unstageable pressure ulcer (L89.--0) should be based on the clinical documentation. These codes are used for pressure ulcers whose stage cannot be clinically determined (e.g., the ulcer is covered by eschar or has been treated with a skin or muscle graft). This code should not be confused with the codes for unspecified stage (L89.--9). When there is no documentation regarding the stage of the pressure ulcer, assign the appropriate code for unspecified stage (L89.--9)**.**

3) **Documented pressure ulcer stage**

Assignment of the pressure ulcer stage code should be guided by clinical documentation of the stage or documentation of the terms found in the Alphabetic Index. For clinical terms describing the stage that are not found in the Alphabetic Index, and there is no documentation of the stage, the provider should be queried.

4) **Patients admitted with pressure ulcers documented as healed**

No code is assigned if the documentation states that the pressure ulcer is completely healed at the time of admission.

5) **Pressure ulcers documented as healing**

Pressure ulcers described as healing should be assigned the appropriate pressure ulcer stage code based on the documentation in the medical record. If the documentation does not provide information about the stage of the healing pressure ulcer, assign the appropriate code for unspecified stage.

If the documentation is unclear as to whether the patient has a current (new) pressure ulcer or if the patient is being treated for a healing pressure ulcer, query the provider.

For ulcers that were present on admission but healed at the time of discharge, assign the code for the site and stage of the pressure ulcer at the time of admission.

6) **Patient admitted with pressure ulcer evolving into another stage during the admission**

If a patient is admitted to an inpatient hospital with a pressure ulcer at one stage and it progresses to a higher stage, two separate codes should be assigned: one code for the site and stage of the ulcer on admission and a second code for the same ulcer site and the highest stage reported during the stay.

7) **Pressure-induced deep tissue damage**

For pressure-induced deep tissue damage or deep tissue pressure injury, assign only the appropriate code for pressure-induced deep tissue damage (L89.--6).

b. **Non-Pressure Chronic Ulcers**

1) **Patients admitted with non-pressure ulcers documented as healed**

No code is assigned if the documentation states that the non-pressure ulcer is completely healed at the time of admission.

2) **Non-pressure ulcers documented as healing**

Non-pressure ulcers described as healing should be assigned the appropriate non-pressure ulcer code based on the documentation in the medical record. If the documentation does not provide information about the severity of the healing non-pressure ulcer, assign the appropriate code for unspecified severity.

If the documentation is unclear as to whether the patient has a current (new) non-pressure ulcer or if the patient is being treated for a healing non-pressure ulcer, query the provider.
For ulcers that were present on admission but healed at the time of discharge, assign the code for the site and severity of the non-pressure ulcer at the time of admission.

3) **Patient admitted with non-pressure ulcer that progresses to another severity level during the admission**

If a patient is admitted to an inpatient hospital with a non-pressure ulcer at one severity level and it progresses to a higher severity level, two separate codes should be assigned: one code for the site and severity level of the ulcer on admission and a second code for the same ulcer site and the highest severity level reported during the stay.

See Section I.B.14 for pressure ulcer stage documentation by clinicians other than patient's provider

13. Chapter 13: Diseases of the Musculoskeletal System and Connective Tissue (M00-M99)

a. **Site and laterality**

Most of the codes within Chapter 13 have site and laterality designations. The site represents the bone, joint or the muscle involved. For some conditions where more than one bone, joint or muscle is usually involved, such as osteoarthritis, there is a "multiple sites" code available. For categories where no multiple site code is provided and more than one bone, joint or muscle is involved, multiple codes should be used to indicate the different sites involved.

1) Bone versus joint

For certain conditions, the bone may be affected at the upper or lower end, (e.g., avascular necrosis of bone, M87, Osteoporosis, M80, M81). Though the portion of the bone affected may be at the joint, the site designation will be the bone, not the joint.

b. Acute traumatic versus chronic or recurrent musculoskeletal conditions

Many musculoskeletal conditions are a result of previous injury or trauma to a site or are recurrent conditions. Bone, joint or muscle conditions that are the result of a healed injury are usually found in chapter 13. Recurrent bone, joint or muscle conditions are also usually found in chapter 13. Any current, acute injury should be coded to the appropriate injury code from chapter 19. Chronic or recurrent conditions should generally be coded with a code from chapter 13. If it is difficult to determine from the documentation in the record which code is best to describe a condition, query the provider.

c. Coding of Pathologic Fractures

7th character A is for use as long as the patient is receiving active treatment for the fracture. While the patient may be seen by a new or different provider over the course of treatment for a pathological fracture, assignment of the 7th character is based on whether the patient is undergoing active treatment and not whether the provider is seeing the patient for the first time.

7th character D is to be used for encounters after the patient has completed active treatment for the fracture and is receiving routine care for the fracture during the healing or recovery phase. The other 7th characters, listed under each subcategory in the Tabular List, are to be used for subsequent encounters for treatment of problems associated with the healing, such as malunions, nonunions, and sequelae.

Care for complications of surgical treatment for fracture repairs during the healing or recovery phase should be coded with the appropriate complication codes.

See Section I.C.19. Coding of traumatic fractures.

d. Osteoporosis

Osteoporosis is a systemic condition, meaning that all bones of the musculoskeletal system are affected. Therefore, site is not a component of the codes under category M81, Osteoporosis without current pathological fracture. The site codes under category M80, Osteoporosis with current pathological fracture, identify the site of the fracture, not the osteoporosis.

1) Osteoporosis without pathological fracture

Category M81, Osteoporosis without current pathological fracture, is for use for patients with osteoporosis who do not currently have a pathologic fracture due to the osteoporosis, even if they have had a fracture in the past. For patients with a history of osteoporosis fractures, status code Z87.310, Personal history of (healed) osteoporosis fracture, should follow the code from M81.

2) Osteoporosis with current pathological fracture

Category M80, Osteoporosis with current pathological fracture, is for patients who have a current pathologic fracture at the time of an encounter. The codes under M80 identify the site of the fracture. A code from category M80, not a traumatic fracture code, should be used for any patient with known osteoporosis who suffers a fracture, even if the patient had a minor fall or trauma, if that fall or trauma would not usually break a normal, healthy bone.

14. Chapter 14: Diseases of Genitourinary System (N00-N99)

a. Chronic kidney disease

1) Stages of chronic kidney disease (CKD)

The ICD-10-CM classifies CKD based on severity. The severity of CKD is designated by stages 1-5. Stage 2, code N18.2, equates to mild CKD; stage 3, codes N18.30-N18.32, equate to moderate CKD; and stage 4, code N18.4, equates to severe CKD. Code N18.6, End stage renal disease (ESRD), is assigned when the provider has documented end-stage renal disease (ESRD).

If both a stage of CKD and ESRD are documented, assign code N18.6 only.

2) Chronic kidney disease and kidney transplant status

Patients who have undergone kidney transplant may still have some form of chronic kidney disease (CKD) because the kidney transplant may not fully restore kidney function. Therefore, the presence of CKD alone does not constitute a transplant complication. Assign the appropriate N18 code for the patient's stage of CKD and code Z94.0, Kidney transplant status. If a transplant complication such as failure or rejection or other transplant complication is documented, see section I.C.19.g for information on coding complications of a kidney transplant. If the documentation is unclear as to whether the patient has a complication of the transplant, query the provider.

3) Chronic kidney disease with other conditions

Patients with CKD may also suffer from other serious conditions, most commonly diabetes mellitus and hypertension. The sequencing of the CKD code in relationship to codes for other contributing conditions is based on the conventions in the Tabular List.

See I.C.9. Hypertensive chronic kidney disease.
See I.C.19. Chronic kidney disease and kidney transplant complications.

15. Chapter 15: Pregnancy, Childbirth, and the Puerperium (O00-O9A)

a. General Rules for Obstetric Cases

1) Codes from chapter 15 and sequencing priority

Obstetric cases require codes from chapter 15, codes in the range O00-O9A, Pregnancy, Childbirth, and the Puerperium. Chapter 15 codes have sequencing priority over codes from other chapters. Additional codes from other chapters may be used in conjunction with chapter 15 codes to further specify conditions. Should the provider document that the pregnancy is incidental to the encounter, then code Z33.1, Pregnant state, incidental, should be used in place of any chapter 15 codes. It is the provider's responsibility to state that the condition being treated is not affecting the pregnancy.

2) Chapter 15 codes used only on the maternal record

Chapter 15 codes are to be used only on the maternal record, never on the record of the newborn.

3) Final character for trimester

The majority of codes in Chapter 15 have a final character indicating the trimester of pregnancy. The timeframes for the trimesters are indicated at the beginning of the chapter. If trimester is not a component of a code, it is because the condition always occurs in a specific trimester, or the concept of trimester of pregnancy is not applicable. Certain codes have characters for only certain trimesters because the condition does not occur in all trimesters, but it may occur in more than just one.

Assignment of the final character for trimester should be based on the provider's documentation of the trimester (or number of weeks) for the current admission/encounter. This applies to the assignment of trimester for pre-existing conditions as well as those that develop during or are due to the pregnancy. The provider's documentation of the number of weeks may be used to assign the appropriate code identifying the trimester.

Whenever delivery occurs during the current admission, and there is an "in childbirth" option for the obstetric complication being coded, the "in childbirth" code should be assigned. When the classification does not provide an obstetric code with an "in childbirth" option, it is appropriate to assign a code describing the current trimester.

4) **Selection of trimester for inpatient admissions that encompass more than one trimester**

In instances when a patient is admitted to a hospital for complications of pregnancy during one trimester and remains in the hospital into a subsequent trimester, the trimester character for the antepartum complication code should be assigned on the basis of the trimester when the complication developed, not the trimester of the discharge. If the condition developed prior to the current admission/encounter or represents a pre-existing condition, the trimester character for the trimester at the time of the admission/encounter should be assigned.

5) **Unspecified trimester**

Each category that includes codes for trimester has a code for "unspecified trimester." The "unspecified trimester" code should rarely be used, such as when the documentation in the record is insufficient to determine the trimester and it is not possible to obtain clarification.

6) **7th character for Fetus Identification**

Where applicable, a 7th character is to be assigned for certain categories (O31, O32, O33.3 - O33.6, O35, O36, O40, O41, O60.1, O60.2, O64, and O69) to identify the fetus for which the complication code applies.

Assign 7th character "0":

- For single gestations
- When the documentation in the record is insufficient to determine the fetus affected and it is not possible to obtain clarification.
- When it is not possible to clinically determine which fetus is affected.

b. **Selection of OB Principal or First-listed Diagnosis**

1) **Routine outpatient prenatal visits**

For routine outpatient prenatal visits when no complications are present, a code from category Z34, Encounter for supervision of normal pregnancy, should be used as the first-listed diagnosis. These codes should not be used in conjunction with chapter 15 codes.

2) **Supervision of High-Risk Pregnancy**

Codes from category O09, Supervision of high-risk pregnancy, are intended for use only during the prenatal period. For complications during the labor or delivery episode as a result of a high-risk pregnancy, assign the applicable complication codes from Chapter 15. If there are no complications during the labor or delivery episode, assign code O80, Encounter for full-term uncomplicated delivery.

For routine prenatal outpatient visits for patients with high-risk pregnancies, a code from category O09, Supervision of high-risk pregnancy, should be used as the first-listed diagnosis. Secondary chapter 15 codes may be used in conjunction with these codes if appropriate.

3) **Episodes when no delivery occurs**

In episodes when no delivery occurs, the principal diagnosis should correspond to the principal complication of the pregnancy which necessitated the encounter. Should more than one complication exist, all of which are treated or monitored, any of the complication codes may be sequenced first.

4) When a delivery occurs

When an obstetric patient is admitted and delivers during that admission, the condition that prompted the admission should be sequenced as the principal diagnosis. If multiple conditions prompted the admission, sequence the one most related to the delivery as the principal diagnosis. A code for any complication of the delivery should be assigned as an additional diagnosis. In cases of cesarean delivery, if the patient was admitted with a condition that resulted in the performance of a cesarean procedure, that condition should be selected as the principal diagnosis. If the reason for the admission was unrelated to the condition resulting in the cesarean delivery, the condition related to the reason for the admission should be selected as the principal diagnosis.

5) Outcome of delivery

A code from category Z37, Outcome of delivery, should be included on every maternal record when a delivery has occurred. These codes are not to be used on subsequent records or on the newborn record.

c. Pre-existing conditions versus conditions due to the pregnancy

Certain categories in Chapter 15 distinguish between conditions of the mother that existed prior to pregnancy (pre-existing) and those that are a direct result of pregnancy. When assigning codes from Chapter 15, it is important to assess if a condition was pre-existing prior to pregnancy or developed during or due to the pregnancy in order to assign the correct code.

Categories that do not distinguish between pre-existing and pregnancy-related conditions may be used for either. It is acceptable to use codes specifically for the puerperium with codes complicating pregnancy and childbirth if a condition arises postpartum during the delivery encounter.

d. Pre-existing hypertension in pregnancy

Category O10, Pre-existing hypertension complicating pregnancy, childbirth and the puerperium, includes codes for hypertensive heart and hypertensive chronic kidney disease. When assigning one of the O10 codes that includes hypertensive heart disease or hypertensive chronic kidney disease, it is necessary to add a secondary code from the appropriate hypertension category to specify the type of heart failure or chronic kidney disease.

See Section I.C.9. Hypertension.

e. Fetal Conditions Affecting the Management of the Mother

1) Codes from categories O35 and O36

Codes from categories O35, Maternal care for known or suspected fetal abnormality and damage, and O36, Maternal care for other fetal problems, are assigned only when the fetal condition is actually responsible for modifying the management of the mother, i.e., by requiring diagnostic studies, additional observation, special care, or termination of pregnancy. The fact that the fetal condition exists does not justify assigning a code from this series to the mother's record.

2) In utero surgery

In cases when surgery is performed on the fetus, a diagnosis code from category O35, Maternal care for known or suspected fetal abnormality and damage, should be assigned identifying the fetal condition. Assign the appropriate procedure code for the procedure performed.

No code from Chapter 16, the perinatal codes, should be used on the mother's record to identify fetal conditions. Surgery performed in utero on a fetus is still to be coded as an obstetric encounter.

f. HIV Infection in Pregnancy, Childbirth and the Puerperium

During pregnancy, childbirth or the puerperium, a patient admitted because of an HIV-related illness should receive a principal diagnosis from subcategory O98.7-, Human immunodeficiency [HIV] disease complicating pregnancy, childbirth and the puerperium, followed by the code(s) for the HIV-related illness(es).

Patients with asymptomatic HIV infection status admitted during pregnancy, childbirth, or the puerperium should receive codes of O98.7- and Z21, Asymptomatic human immunodeficiency virus [HIV] infection status.

g. Diabetes mellitus in pregnancy

Diabetes mellitus is a significant complicating factor in pregnancy. Pregnant women who are diabetic should be assigned a code from category O24, Diabetes mellitus in pregnancy, childbirth, and the puerperium, first, followed by the appropriate diabetes code(s) (E08-E13) from Chapter 4.

h. Long term use of insulin and oral hypoglycemics

See section I.C.4.a.3 for information on the long-term use of insulin and oral hypoglycemics.

i. Gestational (pregnancy induced) diabetes

Gestational (pregnancy induced) diabetes can occur during the second and thirdtrimester of pregnancy in patients who were not diabetic prior to pregnancy. Gestational diabetes can cause complications in the pregnancy similar to thoseof pre-existing diabetes mellitus. It also puts the patient at greater risk of developing diabetes after the pregnancy.

Codes for gestational diabetes are in subcategory O24.4, Gestational diabetes mellitus. No other code from category O24, Diabetes mellitus in pregnancy, childbirth, and the puerperium, should be used with a code from O24.4.

The codes under subcategory O24.4 include diet controlled, insulin controlled, and controlled by oral hypoglycemic drugs. If a patient with gestational diabetes is treated with both diet and insulin, only the code for insulin-controlled is required. If a patient with gestational diabetes is treated with both diet and oral hypoglycemic medications, only the code for "controlled by oral hypoglycemic drugs" is required. Code Z79.4, Long-term (current) use of insulin or code Z79.84, Long-term (current) use of oral hypoglycemic drugs, should not be assigned with codes from subcategory O24.4.

An abnormal glucose tolerance in pregnancy is assigned a code from subcategory O99.81, Abnormal glucose complicating pregnancy, childbirth, and the puerperium.

j. Sepsis and septic shock complicating abortion, pregnancy, childbirth and the puerperium

When assigning a chapter 15 code for sepsis complicating abortion, pregnancy, childbirth, and the puerperium, a code for the specific type of infection should be assigned as an additional diagnosis. If severe sepsis is present, a code from subcategory R65.2, Severe sepsis, and code(s) for associated organ dysfunction(s) should also be assigned as additional diagnoses.

k. Puerperal sepsis

Code O85, Puerperal sepsis, should be assigned with a secondary code to identify the causal organism (e.g., for a bacterial infection, assign a code from category B95-B96, Bacterial infections in conditions classified elsewhere). A code from category A40, Streptococcal sepsis, or A41, Other sepsis, should not be used for puerperal sepsis. If applicable, use additional codes to identify severe sepsis (R65.2-) and any associated acute organ dysfunction.

Code O85 should not be assigned for sepsis following an obstetrical procedure (See Section I.C.1.d.5.b., Sepsis due to a postprocedural infection).

l. Alcohol, tobacco and drug use during pregnancy, childbirth and the puerperium

1) Alcohol use during pregnancy, childbirth and the puerperium

Codes under subcategory O99.31, Alcohol use complicating pregnancy, childbirth, and the puerperium, should be assigned for any pregnancy case when a patient uses alcohol during the pregnancy or postpartum. A secondary code from category F10, Alcohol related disorders, should also be assigned to identify manifestations of the alcohol use.

2) Tobacco use during pregnancy, childbirth and the puerperium

Codes under subcategory O99.33, Smoking (tobacco) complicating pregnancy, childbirth, and the puerperium, should be assigned for any pregnancy case when a mother uses any type of tobacco product during the pregnancy or postpartum.

A secondary code from category F17, Nicotine dependence, should also be assigned to identify the type of nicotine dependence.

3) Drug use during pregnancy, childbirth and the puerperium

Codes under subcategory O99.32, Drug use complicating pregnancy, childbirth, and the puerperium, should be assigned for any pregnancy case when a patient uses drugs during the pregnancy or postpartum. This can involve illegal drugs, or inappropriate use or abuse of prescription drugs. Secondary code(s) from categories F11-F16 and F18-F19 should also be assigned to identify manifestations of the drug use.

m. Poisoning, toxic effects, adverse effects and underdosing in a pregnant patient

A code from subcategory O9A.2, Injury, poisoning and certain other consequences of external causes complicating pregnancy, childbirth, and the puerperium, should be sequenced first, followed by the appropriate injury, poisoning, toxic effect, adverse effect or underdosing code, and then the additional code(s) that specifies the condition caused by the poisoning, toxic effect, adverse effect or underdosing.

See Section I.C.19. Adverse effects, poisoning, underdosing and toxic effects.

n. Normal Delivery, Code O80

1) Encounter for full term uncomplicated delivery

Code O80 should be assigned when a patient is admitted for a full-term normal delivery and delivers a single, healthy infant without any complications antepartum, during the delivery, or postpartum during the delivery episode. Code O80 is always a principal diagnosis. It is not to be used if any other code from chapter 15 is needed to describe a current complication of the antenatal, delivery, or postnatal period. Additional codes from other chapters may be used with code O80 if they are not related to or are in any way complicating the pregnancy.

2) Uncomplicated delivery with resolved antepartum complication

Code O80 may be used if the patient had a complication at some point during the pregnancy, but the complication is not present at the time of the admission for delivery.

3) Outcome of delivery for O80

Z37.0, Single live birth, is the only outcome of delivery code appropriate for use with O80.

o. The Peripartum and Postpartum Periods

1) Peripartum and Postpartum periods

The postpartum period begins immediately after delivery and continues for six weeks following delivery. The peripartum period is defined as the last month of pregnancy to five months postpartum.

2) Peripartum and postpartum complication

A postpartum complication is any complication occurring within the six-week period.

3) Pregnancy-related complications after 6-week period

Chapter 15 codes may also be used to describe pregnancy-related complications after the peripartum or postpartum period if the provider documents that a condition is pregnancy related.

4) Admission for routine postpartum care following delivery outside hospital

When the mother delivers outside the hospital prior to admission and is admitted for routine postpartum care and no complications are noted, code Z39.0, Encounter for care and examination of mother immediately after delivery, should be assigned as the principal diagnosis.

5) Pregnancy associated cardiomyopathy

Pregnancy associated cardiomyopathy, code O90.3, is unique in that it may be diagnosed in the third trimester of pregnancy but may continue to progress months after delivery. For this reason, it is referred to as peripartum cardiomyopathy. Code O90.3 is only for use when the cardiomyopathy develops as a result of pregnancy in a woman who did not have pre-existing heart disease.

p. Code O94, Sequelae of complication of pregnancy, childbirth, and the puerperium

1) Code O94

Code O94, Sequelae of complication of pregnancy, childbirth, and the puerperium, is for use in those cases when an initial complication of a pregnancy develops a sequela or sequelae requiring care or treatment at a future date.

2) After the initial postpartum period

This code may be used at any time after the initial postpartum period.

3) Sequencing of Code O94

This code, like all sequela codes, is to be sequenced following the code describing the sequelae of the complication.

q. Termination of Pregnancy and Spontaneous abortions

1) Abortion with Liveborn Fetus

When an attempted termination of pregnancy results in a liveborn fetus, assign code Z33.2, Encounter for elective termination of pregnancy and a code from category Z37, Outcome of Delivery.

2) Retained Products of Conception following an abortion

Subsequent encounters for retained products of conception following a spontaneous abortion or elective termination of pregnancy, without complications are assigned O03.4, Incomplete spontaneous abortion without complication, or code O07.4, Failed attempted termination of pregnancy without complication. This advice is appropriate even when the patient was discharged previously with a discharge diagnosis of complete abortion. If the patient has a specific complication associated with the spontaneous abortion or elective termination of pregnancy in addition to retained products of conception, assign the appropriate complication code (e.g., O03.-, O04.-, O07.-) instead of code O03.4 or O07.4.

3) Complications leading to abortion

Codes from Chapter 15 may be used as additional codes to identify any documented complications of the pregnancy in conjunction with codes in categories in O04, O07 and O08.

r. Abuse in a pregnant patient

For suspected or confirmed cases of abuse of a pregnant patient, a code(s) from subcategories O9A.3, Physical abuse complicating pregnancy, childbirth, and the puerperium, O9A.4, Sexual abuse complicating pregnancy, childbirth, and the puerperium, and O9A.5, Psychological abuse complicating pregnancy, childbirth, and the puerperium, should be sequenced first, followed by the appropriate codes (if applicable) to identify any associated current injury due to physical abuse, sexual abuse, and the perpetrator of abuse.

See Section I.C.19. Adult and child abuse, neglect and other maltreatment.

s. COVID-19 infection in pregnancy, childbirth, and the puerperium

During pregnancy, childbirth or the puerperium, when COVID-19 is the reason for admission/encounter, code O98.5-, Other viral diseases complicating pregnancy, childbirth and the puerperium, should be sequenced as the principal/first-listed diagnosis, and code U07.1, COVID-19, and the appropriate codes for associated manifestation(s) should be assigned as additional diagnoses. Codes from Chapter 15 always take sequencing priority.

If the reason for admission/encounter is unrelated to COVID-19 but the patient tests positive for COVID-19 during the admission/encounter, the appropriate code for the reason for admission/encounter should be sequenced as the principal/first-listed diagnosis, and codes O98.5- and U07.1, as well as the appropriate codes for associated COVID-19 manifestations, should be assigned as additional diagnoses.

16. Chapter 16: Certain Conditions Originating in the Perinatal Period (P00-P96)

For coding and reporting purposes the perinatal period is defined as before birth through the 28th day following birth. The following guidelines are provided for reporting purposes.

a. **General Perinatal Rules**

1) **Use of Chapter 16 Codes**

Codes in this chapter are never for use on the maternal record. Codes from Chapter 15, the obstetric chapter, are never permitted on the newborn record. Chapter 16 codes may be used throughout the life of the patient if the condition is still present.

2) **Principal Diagnosis for Birth Record**

When coding the birth episode in a newborn record, assign a code from category Z38, Liveborn infants according to place of birth and type of delivery, as the principal diagnosis. A code from category Z38 is assigned only once, to a newborn at the time of birth. If a newborn is transferred to another institution, a code from category Z38 should not be used at the receiving hospital.

A code from category Z38 is used only on the newborn record, not on the mother's record.

3) **Use of Codes from other Chapters with Codes from Chapter 16**

Codes from other chapters may be used with codes from chapter 16 if the codes from the other chapters provide more specific detail. Codes for signs and symptoms may be assigned when a definitive diagnosis has not been established. If the reason for the encounter is a perinatal condition, the code from chapter 16 should be sequenced first.

4) **Use of Chapter 16 Codes after the Perinatal Period**

Should a condition originate in the perinatal period, and continue throughout the life of the patient, the perinatal code should continue to be used regardless of the patient's age.

5) **Birth process or community acquired conditions**

If a newborn has a condition that may be either due to the birth process or community acquired and the documentation does not indicate which it is, the default is due to the birth process and the code from

Chapter 16 should be used. If the condition is community-acquired, a code from Chapter 16 should not be assigned.

For COVID-19 infection in a newborn, see guideline I.C.16.h.

6) Code all clinically significant conditions

All clinically significant conditions noted on routine newborn examination should be coded. A condition is clinically significant if it requires:

- clinical evaluation; or
- therapeutic treatment; or
- diagnostic procedures; or
- extended length of hospital stay; or
- increased nursing care and/or monitoring; or
- has implications for future health care needs

Note: The perinatal guidelines listed above are the same as the general coding guidelines for "additional diagnoses," except for the final point regarding implications for future health care needs. Codes should be assigned for conditions that have been specified by the provider as having implications for future health care needs.

b. Observation and Evaluation of Newborns for Suspected Conditions not Found

1) Use of Z05 codes

Assign a code from category Z05, Observation and evaluation of newborns and infants for suspected conditions ruled out, to identify those instances when a healthy newborn is evaluated for a suspected condition that is determined after study not to be present. Do not use a code from category Z05 when the patient has identified signs or symptoms of a suspected problem; in such cases code the sign or symptom.

2) Z05 on other than the birth record

A code from category Z05 may also be assigned as a principal or first-listed code for readmissions or encounters when the code from category Z38 code no longer applies. Codes from category Z05 are for use only for healthy newborns and infants for which no condition after study is found to be present.

3) Z05 on a birth record

A code from category Z05 is to be used as a secondary code after the code from category Z38, Liveborn infants according to place of birth and type of delivery.

c. Coding Additional Perinatal Diagnoses

1) Assigning codes for conditions that require treatment

Assign codes for conditions that require treatment or further investigation, prolong the length of stay, or require resource utilization.

2) Codes for conditions specified as having implications for future health care needs

Assign codes for conditions that have been specified by the provider as having implications for future health care needs.

Note: This guideline should not be used for adult patients.

d. Prematurity and Fetal Growth Retardation

Providers utilize different criteria in determining prematurity. A code for prematurity should not be assigned unless it is documented. Assignment of codes in categories P05, Disorders of newborn related to slow fetal growth and fetal malnutrition, and P07, Disorders of newborn related to short gestation and low birth weight, not elsewhere classified, should be based on the recorded birth weight and estimated gestational age.

When both birth weight and gestational age are available, two codes from category P07 should be assigned, with the code for birth weight sequenced before the code for gestational age.

e. Low birth weight and immaturity status

Codes from category P07, Disorders of newborn related to short gestation and low birth weight, not elsewhere classified, are for use for a child or adult who was premature or had a low birth weight as a newborn and this is affecting the patient's current health status.

See Section I.C.21. Factors influencing health status and contact with health services, Status.

f. Bacterial Sepsis of Newborn

Category P36, Bacterial sepsis of newborn, includes congenital sepsis. If a perinate is documented as having sepsis without documentation of congenital or community acquired, the default is congenital and a code from category P36 should be assigned. If the P36 code includes the causal organism, an additional code from category B95, Streptococcus, Staphylococcus, and Enterococcus as the cause of diseases classified elsewhere, or B96, Other bacterial agents as the cause of diseases classified elsewhere, should not be assigned. If the P36 code does not include the causal organism, assign an additional code from category B96. If applicable, use additional codes to identify severe sepsis (R65.2-) and any associated acute organ dysfunction.

g. Stillbirth

Code P95, Stillbirth, is only for use in institutions that maintain separate records for stillbirths. No other code should be used with P95. Code P95 should not be used on the mother's record.

h. COVID-19 Infection in Newborn

For a newborn that tests positive for COVID-19, assign code U07.1, COVID-19, and the appropriate codes for associated manifestation(s) in neonates/newborns in the absence of documentation indicating a specific type of transmission. For a newborn that tests positive for COVID-19 and the provider documents the condition was contracted in utero or during the birth process, assign codes P35.8, Other congenital viral diseases, and U07.1, COVID-19. When coding the birth episode in a newborn record, the appropriate code from category Z38, Liveborn infants according to place of birth and type of delivery, should be assigned as the principal diagnosis.

17. Chapter 17: Congenital malformations, deformations, and chromosomal abnormalities (Q00-Q99)

Assign an appropriate code(s) from categories Q00-Q99, Congenital malformations, deformations, and chromosomal abnormalities when a malformation/deformation or chromosomal abnormality is documented. A malformation/deformation/or chromosomal abnormality may be the principal/first-listed diagnosis on a record or a secondary diagnosis.

When a malformation/deformation or chromosomal abnormality does not have a unique code assignment, assign additional code(s) for any manifestations that may be present.

When the code assignment specifically identifies the malformation/deformation or chromosomal abnormality, manifestations that are an inherent component of the anomaly should not be coded separately. Additional codes should be assigned for manifestations that are not an inherent component.

Codes from Chapter 17 may be used throughout the life of the patient. If a congenital malformation or deformity has been corrected, a personal history code should be used to identify the history of the malformation or deformity. Although present at birth, a malformation/deformation/or chromosomal abnormality may not be identified until later in life. Whenever the condition is diagnosed by the provider, it is appropriate to assign a code from codes Q00-Q99.

For the birth admission, the appropriate code from category Z38, Liveborn infants, according to place of birth and type of delivery, should be sequenced as the principal diagnosis, followed by any congenital anomaly codes, Q00-Q99.

18. Chapter 18: Symptoms, signs, and abnormal clinical and laboratory findings, not elsewhere classified (R00-R99)

Chapter 18 includes symptoms, signs, abnormal results of clinical or other investigative procedures, and ill-defined conditions regarding which no diagnosis classifiable elsewhere is recorded. Signs and symptoms that point to a specific diagnosis have been assigned to a category in other chapters of the classification.

a. Use of symptom codes

Codes that describe symptoms and signs are acceptable for reporting purposes when a related definitive diagnosis has not been established (confirmed) by the provider.

b. Use of a symptom code with a definitive diagnosis code

Codes for signs and symptoms may be reported in addition to a related definitive diagnosis when the sign or symptom is not routinely associated with that diagnosis, such as the various signs and symptoms associated with complex syndromes. The definitive diagnosis code should be sequenced before the symptom code.

Signs or symptoms that are associated routinely with a disease process should not be assigned as additional codes, unless otherwise instructed by the classification.

c. Combination codes that include symptoms

ICD-10-CM contains a number of combination codes that identify both the definitive diagnosis and common symptoms of that diagnosis. When using one of these combination codes, an additional code should not be assigned for the symptom.

d. Repeated falls

Code R29.6, Repeated falls, is for use for encounters when a patient has recently fallen and the reason for the fall is being investigated.

Code Z91.81, History of falling, is for use when a patient has fallen in the past and is at risk for future falls. When appropriate, both codes R29.6 and Z91.81 may be assigned together.

e. Coma scale

Code R40.20, Unspecified coma, may be assigned in conjunction with codesfor any medical condition.

Do not report codes for unspecified coma, individual or total Glasgow comascale scores for a patient with a medically induced coma or a sedated patient.

The coma scale codes (R40.21- to R40.24-) can be used in conjunction with traumatic brain injury codes. These codes are primarily for use by trauma registries, but they may be used in any setting where this information is collected. The coma scale codes should be sequenced afterthe diagnosis code(s).

These codes, one from each subcategory, are needed to complete the scale. The 7th character indicates when the scale was recorded. The 7thcharacter should match for all three codes.

At a minimum, report the initial score documented on presentation at your facility. This may be a score from the emergency medicine technician (EMT) or in the emergency department. If desired, a facility may choose to capture multiple coma scale scores.

Assign code R40.24-, Glasgow coma scale, total score, when only the total score is documented in the medical record and not the individual score(s).
If multiple coma scores are captured within the first 24 hours after hospital admission, assign only the code for the score at the time of admission. ICD-10-CM does not classify coma scores that are reported after admission but less than 24 hours later.

See Section I.B.14 for coma scale documentation by clinicians other than patient's provider

f. **Functional quadriplegia**

GUIDELINE DELETED EFFECTIVE OCTOBER 1, 2017

g. **SIRS due to Non-Infectious Process**

The systemic inflammatory response syndrome (SIRS) can develop as a result of certain non-infectious disease processes, such as trauma, malignant neoplasm, or pancreatitis. When SIRS is documented with a noninfectious condition, and no subsequent infection is documented, the code for the underlying condition, such as an injury, should be assigned, followed by code R65.10, Systemic inflammatory response syndrome (SIRS) of non-infectious origin without acute organ dysfunction, or code R65.11, Systemic inflammatory response syndrome (SIRS) of non-infectious origin with acute organ dysfunction. If an associated acute organ dysfunction is documented, the appropriate code(s) for the specific type of organ dysfunction(s) should be assigned in addition to code R65.11. If acute organ dysfunction is documented, but it cannot be determined if the acute organ dysfunction is associated with SIRS or due to another condition (e.g., directly due to the trauma), the provider should be queried.

h. **Death NOS**

Code R99, Ill-defined and unknown cause of mortality, is only for use in the very limited circumstance when a patient who has already died is brought into an emergency department or other healthcare facility and is pronounced dead upon arrival. It does not represent the discharge disposition of death.

i. **NIHSS Stroke Scale**

The NIH stroke scale (NIHSS) codes (R29.7- -) can be used in conjunction with acute stroke codes (I63) to identify the patient's neurological status and the severity of the stroke. The stroke scale codes should be sequenced after the acute stroke diagnosis code(s).

At a minimum, report the initial score documented. If desired, a facility may choose to capture multiple stroke scale scores.

See Section I.B.14 for NIHSS stroke scale documentation by clinicians other than patient's provider

19. Chapter 19: Injury, poisoning, and certain other consequences of external causes (S00-T88)

a. **Application of 7th Characters in Chapter 19**

Most categories in chapter 19 have a 7th character requirement for each applicable code. Most categories in this chapter have three 7th character values (with the exception of fractures): A, initial encounter, D, subsequent encounter and S, sequela. Categories for traumatic fractures have additional 7th character values. While the patient may be seen by a new or different provider over the course of treatment for an injury, assignment of the 7th character is based on whether the patient is undergoing active treatment and not whether the provider is seeing the patient for the first time.

For complication codes, active treatment refers to treatment for the condition described by the code, even though it may be related to an earlier precipitating problem. For example, code T84.50XA, Infection and inflammatory reaction due to unspecified internal joint prosthesis, initial encounter, is used when active treatment is provided for the infection, even though the condition relates to the prosthetic device, implant or graft that was placed at a previous encounter.

7th character "A", initial encounter is used for each encounter where the patient is receiving active treatment for the condition.

7th character "D" subsequent encounter is used for encounters after the patient has completed active treatment of the condition and is receiving routine care for the condition during the healing or recovery phase.

The aftercare Z codes should not be used for aftercare for conditions such as injuries or poisonings, where 7th characters are provided to identify subsequent care. For example, for aftercare of an injury, assign the acute injury code with the 7th character "D" (subsequent encounter).

7th character "S", sequela, is for use for complications or conditions that arise as a direct result of a condition, such as scar formation after a burn. The scars are sequelae of the burn. When using 7th character "S", it is necessary to use both the injury code that precipitated the sequela and the code for the sequela itself. The "S" is added only to the injury code, not the sequela code. The 7th character "S" identifies the injury responsible for the sequela. The specific type of sequela (e.g., scar) is sequenced first, followed by the injury code.

See Section I.B.10 Sequelae, (Late Effects)

b. Coding of Injuries

When coding injuries, assign separate codes for each injury unless a combination code is provided, in which case the combination code is assigned. Codes from category T07, Unspecified multiple injuries should not be assigned in the inpatient setting unless information for a more specific code is not available. Traumatic injury codes (S00-T14.9) are not to be used for normal, healing surgical wounds or to identify complications of surgical wounds.

The code for the most serious injury, as determined by the provider and the focus of treatment, is sequenced first.

1) Superficial injuries

Superficial injuries such as abrasions or contusions are not coded when associated with more severe injuries of the same site.

2) Primary injury with damage to nerves/blood vessels

When a primary injury results in minor damage to peripheral nerves or blood vessels, the primary injury is sequenced first with additional code(s) for injuries to nerves and spinal cord (such as category S04), and/or injury to blood vessels (such as category S15). When the primary injury is to the blood vessels or nerves, that injury should be sequenced first.

3) Iatrogenic injuries

Injury codes from Chapter 19 should not be assigned for injuries that occur during, or as a result of, a medical intervention. Assign the appropriate complication code(s).

c. Coding of Traumatic Fractures

The principles of multiple coding of injuries should be followed in coding fractures. Fractures of specified sites are coded individually by site in accordance with both the provisions within categories S02, S12, S22, S32, S42, S49, S52, S59, S62, S72, S79, S82, S89, S92 and the level of detail furnished by medical record content.

A fracture not indicated as open or closed should be coded to closed. A fracture not indicated whether displaced or not displaced should be coded to displaced.

More specific guidelines are as follows:

1) Initial vs. subsequent encounter for fractures

Traumatic fractures are coded using the appropriate 7th character for initial encounter (A, B, C) for each encounter where the patient is receiving active treatment for the fracture. The appropriate 7th character for initial encounter should also be assigned for a patient who delayed seeking treatment for the fracture or nonunion.

Fractures are coded using the appropriate 7th character for subsequent care for encounters after the patient has completed active treatment of the fracture and is receiving routine care for the fracture during the healing or recovery phase.

Care for complications of surgical treatment for fracture repairs during the healing or recovery phase should be coded with the appropriate complication codes.

Care of complications of fractures, such as malunion and nonunion, should be reported with the appropriate 7th character for subsequent care with nonunion (K, M, N,) or subsequent care with malunion (P, Q, R).

Malunion/nonunion: The appropriate 7th character for initial encounter should also be assigned for a patient who delayed seeking treatment for the fracture or nonunion.

The open fracture designations in the assignment of the 7th character for fractures of the forearm, femur and lower leg, including ankle are based on the Gustilo open fracture classification. When the Gustilo classification type is not specified for an open fracture, the 7th character for open fracture type I or II should be assigned (B, E, H, M, Q).

A code from category M80, not a traumatic fracture code, should be used for any patient with known osteoporosis who suffers a fracture, even if the patient had a minor fall or trauma, if that fall or trauma would not usually break a normal, healthy bone.

See Section I.C.13. Osteoporosis.

The aftercare Z codes should not be used for aftercare for traumatic fractures. For aftercare of a traumatic fracture, assign the acute fracture code with the appropriate 7th character.

2) Multiple fractures sequencing

Multiple fractures are sequenced in accordance with the severity of the fracture.

3) Physeal fractures

For physeal fractures, assign only the code identifying the type of physeal fracture. Do not assign a separate code to identify the specific bone that is fractured.

d. Coding of Burns and Corrosions

The ICD-10-CM makes a distinction between burns and corrosions. The burn codes are for thermal burns, except sunburns, that come from a heat source, such as a fire or hot appliance. The burn codes are also for burns resulting from electricity and radiation. Corrosions are burns due to chemicals. The guidelines are the same for burns and corrosions.

Current burns (T20-T25) are classified by depth, extent and by agent (X code). Burns are classified by depth as first degree (erythema), second degree (blistering), and third degree (full-thickness involvement). Burns of the eye and internal organs (T26-T28) are classified by site, but not by degree.

1) Sequencing of burn and related condition codes

Sequence first the code that reflects the highest degree of burn when more than one burn is present.

a. When the reason for the admission or encounter is for treatment of external multiple burns, sequence first the code that reflects the burn of the highest degree.

b. When a patient has both internal and external burns, the circumstances of admission govern the selection of the principal diagnosis or first-listed diagnosis.

c. When a patient is admitted for burn injuries and other related conditions such as smoke inhalation and/or respiratory failure, the circumstances of admission govern the selection of the principal or first-listed diagnosis.

2) Burns of the same anatomic site

Classify burns of the same anatomic site and on the same side but of different degrees to the subcategory identifying the highest degree recorded in the diagnosis (e.g., for second and third degree burns of right thigh, assign only code T24.311-).

3) Non-healing burns

Non-healing burns are coded as acute burns.

Necrosis of burned skin should be coded as a non-healed burn.

4) Infected burn

For any documented infected burn site, use an additional code for the infection.

5) Assign separate codes for each burn site

When coding burns, assign separate codes for each burn site. Category T30, Burn and corrosion, body region unspecified is extremely vague and should rarely be used.

Codes for burns of "multiple sites" should only be assigned when the medical record documentation does not specify the individual sites.

6) Burns and corrosions classified according to extent of body surface involved

Assign codes from category T31, Burns classified according to extent of body surface involved, or T32, Corrosions classified according to extent of body surface involved, for acute burns or corrosions when the site of the burn or corrosion is not specified or when there is a need for additional data. It is advisable to use category T31 as additional coding when needed to provide data for evaluating burn mortality, such as that needed by burn units. It is also advisable to use category T31 as an additional code for reporting purposes when there is mention of a third-degree burn involving 20 percent or more of the body surface. Codes from categories T31 and T32 should not be used for sequelae of burns or corrosions.

Categories T31 and T32 are based on the classic "rule of nines" in estimating body surface involved: head and neck are assigned nine percent, each arm nine percent, each leg 18 percent, the anterior trunk 18 percent, posterior trunk 18 percent, and genitalia one percent. Providers may change these percentage assignments where necessary to accommodate infants and children who have proportionately larger heads than adults, and patients who have large buttocks, thighs, or abdomen that involve burns.

7) Encounters for treatment of sequela of burns

Encounters for the treatment of the late effects of burns or corrosions (i.e., scars or joint contractures) should be coded with a burn or corrosion code with the 7th character "S" for sequela.

8) Sequelae with a late effect code and current burn

When appropriate, both a code for a current burn or corrosion with 7th character "A" or "D" and a burn or corrosion code with 7th character "S" may be assigned on the same record (when both a current burn and

sequelae of an old burn exist). Burns and corrosions do not heal at the same rate and a current healing wound may still exist with sequela of a healed burn or corrosion.
See Section I.B.10 Sequela (Late Effects)

9) Use of an external cause code with burns and corrosions

An external cause code should be used with burns and corrosions to identify the source and intent of the burn, as well as the place where it occurred.

e. Adverse Effects, Poisoning, Underdosing and Toxic Effects

Codes in categories T36-T65 are combination codes that include the substance that was taken as well as the intent. No additional external cause code is required for poisonings, toxic effects, adverse effects and underdosing codes.

1) Do not code directly from the Table of Drugs

Do not code directly from the Table of Drugs and Chemicals. Always refer back to the Tabular List.

2) Use as many codes as necessary to describe

Use as many codes as necessary to describe completely all drugs, medicinal or biological substances.

3) If the same code would describe the causative agent

If the same code would describe the causative agent for more than one adverse reaction, poisoning, toxic effect or underdosing, assign the code only once.

4) If two or more drugs, medicinal or biological substances

If two or more drugs, medicinal or biological substances are taken, code each individually unless a combination code is listed in the Table of Drugs and Chemicals.

If multiple unspecified drugs, medicinal or biological substances were taken, assign the appropriate code from subcategory T50.91, Poisoning by, adverse effect of and underdosing of multiple unspecified drugs, medicaments and biological substances.

5) The occurrence of drug toxicity is classified in ICD-10-CM as follows:

(a) Adverse Effect

When coding an adverse effect of a drug that has been correctly prescribed and properly administered, assign the appropriate code for the nature of the adverse effect followed by the appropriate code for the adverse effect of the drug (T36-T50). The code for the drug should have a 5th or 6th character "5" (for example T36.0X5-) Examples of the nature of an adverse effect are tachycardia, delirium, gastrointestinal hemorrhaging, vomiting, hypokalemia, hepatitis, renal failure, or respiratory failure.

(b) Poisoning

When coding a poisoning or reaction to the improper use of a medication (e.g., overdose, wrong substance given or taken in error, wrong route of administration), first assign the appropriate code from categories T36-T50. The poisoning codes have an associated intent as their 5th or 6th character (accidental, intentional self-harm, assault and undetermined. If the intent of the poisoning is unknown or unspecified, code the intent as accidental intent. The undetermined intent is only for use if the documentation in the record specifies that the intent cannot be determined. Use additional code(s) for all manifestations of poisonings.

If there is also a diagnosis of abuse or dependence of the substance, the abuse or dependence is assigned as an additional code.

Examples of poisoning include:

(i) Error was made in drug prescription

Errors made in drug prescription or in the administration of the drug by provider, nurse, patient, or other person.

(ii) Overdose of a drug intentionally taken

If an overdose of a drug was intentionally taken or administered and resulted in drug toxicity, it would be coded as a poisoning.

(iii) Nonprescribed drug taken with correctly prescribed and properly administered drug

If a nonprescribed drug or medicinal agent was taken in combination with a correctly prescribed and properly administered drug, any drug toxicity or other reaction resulting from the interaction of the two drugs would be classified as a poisoning.

(iv) Interaction of drug(s) and alcohol

When a reaction results from the interaction of a drug(s) and alcohol, this would be classified as poisoning.

See Section I.C.4. if poisoning is the result of insulin pump malfunctions.

(c) **Underdosing**

Underdosing refers to taking less of a medication than is prescribed by a provider or a manufacturer's instruction. Discontinuing the use of a prescribed medication on the patient's own initiative (not directed by the patient's provider) is also classified as an underdosing. For underdosing, assign the code from categories T36-T50 (fifth or sixth character "6").

Codes for underdosing should never be assigned as principal or first-listed codes. If a patient has a relapse or exacerbation of the medical condition for which the drug is prescribed because of the reduction in dose, then the medical condition itself should be coded.

Noncompliance (Z91.12-, Z91.13- and Z91.14-) or complication of care (Y63.6-Y63.9) codes are to be used with an underdosing code to indicate intent, if known.

(d) **Toxic Effects**

When a harmful substance is ingested or comes in contact with a person, this is classified as a toxic effect. The toxic effect codes are in categories T51-T65.

Toxic effect codes have an associated intent: accidental, intentional self-harm, assault and undetermined.

f. **Adult and child abuse, neglect and other maltreatment**

Sequence first the appropriate code from categories T74, Adult and child abuse, neglect and other maltreatment, confirmed) or T76, Adult and child abuse, neglect and other maltreatment, suspected) for abuse, neglect and other maltreatment, followed by any accompanying mental health or injury code(s).

If the documentation in the medical record states abuse or neglect it is coded as confirmed (T74.-). It is coded as suspected if it is documented as suspected (T76.-).

For cases of confirmed abuse or neglect an external cause code from the assault section (X92-Y09) should be added to identify the cause of any physical injuries. A perpetrator code (Y07) should be added when the perpetrator of the abuse is known. For suspected cases of abuse or neglect, do not report external cause or perpetrator code.

If a suspected case of abuse, neglect or mistreatment is ruled out during an encounter code Z04.71, Encounter for examination and observation following alleged physical adult abuse, ruled out, or code Z04.72, Encounter for examination and observation following alleged child physical abuse, ruled out, should be used, not a code from T76.

If a suspected case of alleged rape or sexual abuse is ruled out during an encounter code Z04.41, Encounter for examination and observation following alleged adult rape or code Z04.42, Encounter for examination and observation following alleged child rape, should be used, not a code from T76.

If a suspected case of forced sexual exploitation or forced labor exploitation is ruled out during an encounter, code Z04.81, Encounter for examination and observation of victim following forced sexual exploitation, or code Z04.82, Encounter for examination and observation of victim following forced labor exploitation, should be used, not a code from T76.

See Section I.C.15. Abuse in a pregnant patient.

g. **Complications of care**

1) **General guidelines for complications of care**

(a) **Documentation of complications of care**

See Section I.B.16. for information on documentation of complications of care.

2) **Pain due to medical devices**

Pain associated with devices, implants or grafts left in a surgical site (for example painful hip prosthesis) is assigned to the appropriate code(s) found in Chapter 19, Injury, poisoning, and certain other consequences of external causes. Specific codes for pain due to medical devices are found in the T code section of the ICD-10-CM. Use additional code(s) from category G89 to identify acute or chronic pain due to presence of the device, implant or graft (G89.18 or G89.28).

3) **Transplant complications**

(a) **Transplant complications other than kidney**

Codes under category T86, Complications of transplanted organs and tissues, are for use for both complications and rejection of transplanted organs. A transplant complication code is only assigned if the complication affects the function of the transplanted organ. Two codes are required to fully describe a transplant complication: the appropriate code from category T86 and a secondary code that identifies the complication.

Pre-existing conditions or conditions that develop after the transplant are not coded as complications unless they affect the function of the transplanted organs.

See I.C.21. for transplant organ removal status See I.C.2. for malignant neoplasm associated with transplanted organ.

(b) **Kidney transplant complications**

Patients who have undergone kidney transplant may still have some form of chronic kidney disease (CKD) because the kidney transplant may not fully restore kidney function. Code T86.1- should be assigned for documented complications of a kidney transplant, such as transplant failure or rejection or other transplant complication. Code T86.1- should not be assigned for post kidney transplant patients who have chronic kidney (CKD) unless a transplant complication such as transplant failure or rejection is documented. If the documentation is unclear as to whether the patient has a complication of the transplant, query the provider.

Conditions that affect the function of the transplanted kidney, other than CKD, should be assigned a code from subcategory T86.1, Complications of transplanted organ, Kidney, and a secondary code that identifies the complication.

For patients with CKD following a kidney transplant, but who do not have a complication such as failure or rejection, *see section I.C.14. Chronic kidney disease and kidney transplant status*.

4) Complication codes that include the external cause

As with certain other T codes, some of the complications of care codes have the external cause included in the code. The code includes the nature of the complication as well as the type of procedure that caused the complication. No external cause code indicating the type of procedure is necessary for these codes.

5) Complications of care codes within the body system chapters

Intraoperative and postprocedural complication codes are found within the body system chapters with codes specific to the organs and structures of that body system. These codes should be sequenced first, followed by a code(s) for the specific complication, if applicable.

Complication codes from the body system chapters should be assigned for intraoperative and post-procedural complications (e.g., the appropriate complication code from chapter 9 would be assigned for a vascular intraoperative or postprocedural complication) unless the complication is specifically indexed to a T code in chapter 19.

20. Chapter 20: External Causes of Morbidity (V00-Y99)

The external causes of morbidity codes should never be sequenced as the first-listed or principal diagnosis.

External cause codes are intended to provide data for injury research and evaluation of injury prevention strategies. These codes capture how the injury or health condition happened (cause), the intent (unintentional or accidental; or intentional, such as suicide or assault), the place where the event occurred the activity of the patient at the time of the event, and the person's status (e.g., civilian, military).

There is no national requirement for mandatory ICD-10-CM external cause code reporting. Unless a provider is subject to a state-based external cause code reporting mandate or these codes are required by a particular payer, reporting of ICD-10-CM codes in Chapter 20, External Causes of Morbidity, is not required. In the absence of a mandatory reporting requirement, providers are encouraged to voluntarily report external cause codes, as they provide valuable data for injury research and evaluation of injury prevention strategies.

a. General External Cause Coding Guidelines

1) Used with any code in the range of A00.0-T88.9, Z00-Z99

An external cause code may be used with any code in the range of A00.0-T88.9, Z00-Z99, classification that represents a health condition due to an external cause. Though they are most applicable to injuries, they are also valid for use with such things as infections or diseases due to an external source, and other health conditions, such as a heart attack that occurs during strenuous physical activity.

2) External cause code used for length of treatment

Assign the external cause code, with the appropriate 7th character (initial encounter, subsequent encounter or sequela) for each encounter for which the injury or condition is being treated.

Most categories in chapter 20 have a 7th character requirement for each applicable code. Most categories in this chapter have three 7th character values: A, initial encounter, D, subsequent encounter and S, sequela. While the patient may be seen by a new or different provider over the course of treatment for an injury or condition, assignment of the 7th character for external cause should match the 7th character of the code assigned for the associated injury or condition for the encounter.

3) Use the full range of external cause codes

Use the full range of external cause codes to completely describe the cause, the intent, the place of occurrence, and if applicable, the activity of the patient at the time of the event, and the patient's status, for all injuries, and other health conditions due to an external cause.

4) Assign as many external cause codes as necessary

Assign as many external cause codes as necessary to fully explain each cause. If only one external code can be recorded, assign the code most related to the principal diagnosis.

5) The selection of the appropriate external cause code

The selection of the appropriate external cause code is guided by the Alphabetic Index of External Causes and by Inclusion and Exclusion notes in the Tabular List.

6) External cause code can never be a principal diagnosis

An external cause code can never be a principal (first-listed) diagnosis.

7) Combination external cause codes

Certain of the external cause codes are combination codes that identify sequential events that result in an injury, such as a fall which results in striking against an object. The injury may be due to either event or both. The combination external cause code used should correspond to the sequence of events regardless of which caused the most serious injury.

8) No external cause code needed in certain circumstances

No external cause code from Chapter 20 is needed if the external cause and intent are included in a code from another chapter (e.g., T36.0X1- Poisoning by penicillins, accidental (unintentional)).

b. Place of Occurrence Guideline

Codes from category Y92, Place of occurrence of the external cause, are secondary codes for use after other external cause codes to identify the location of the patient at the time of injury or other condition.

Generally, a place of occurrence code is assigned only once, at the initial encounter for treatment. However, in the rare instance that a new injury occurs during hospitalization, an additional place of occurrence code may be assigned. No 7th characters are used for Y92.

Do not use place of occurrence code Y92.9 if the place is not stated or is not applicable.

c. Activity Code

Assign a code from category Y93, Activity code, to describe the activity of the patient at the time the injury or other health condition occurred.

An activity code is used only once, at the initial encounter for treatment. Only one code from Y93 should be recorded on a medical record.

The activity codes are not applicable to poisonings, adverse effects, misadventures or sequela.

Do not assign Y93.9, Unspecified activity, if the activity is not stated.

A code from category Y93 is appropriate for use with external cause and intent codes if identifying the activity provides additional information about the event.

d. **Place of Occurrence, Activity, and Status Codes Used with other External Cause Code**
When applicable, place of occurrence, activity, and external cause status codes are sequenced after the main external cause code(s). Regardless of the number of external cause codes assigned, generally there should be only one place of occurrence code, one activity code, and one external cause status code assigned to an encounter. However, in the rare instance that a new injury occurs during hospitalization, an additional place of occurrence code may be assigned.

e. **If the Reporting Format Limits the Number of External Cause Codes**

If the reporting format limits the number of external cause codes that can be used in reporting clinical data, report the code for the cause/intent most related to the principal diagnosis. If the format permits capture of additional external cause codes, the cause/intent, including medical misadventures, of the additional events should be reported rather than the codes for place, activity, or external status.

f. **Multiple External Cause Coding Guidelines**

More than one external cause code is required to fully describe the external cause of an illness or injury. The assignment of external cause codes should be sequenced in the following priority:

If two or more events cause separate injuries, an external cause code should be assigned for each cause. The first-listed external cause code will be selected in the following order:

External codes for child and adult abuse take priority over all other external cause codes.

See Section I.C.19., Child and Adult abuse guidelines.

External cause codes for terrorism events take priority over all other external cause codes except child and adult abuse.

External cause codes for cataclysmic events take priority over all other external cause codes except child and adult abuse and terrorism.

External cause codes for transport accidents take priority over all other external cause codes except cataclysmic events, child and adult abuse and terrorism.

Activity and external cause status codes are assigned following all causal (intent) external cause codes.

The first-listed external cause code should correspond to the cause of the most serious diagnosis due to an assault, accident, or self-harm, following the order of hierarchy listed above.

g. **Child and Adult Abuse Guideline**

Adult and child abuse, neglect and maltreatment are classified as assault. Any of the assault codes may be used to indicate the external cause of any injury resulting from the confirmed abuse.
For confirmed cases of abuse, neglect and maltreatment, when the perpetrator is known, a code from Y07, Perpetrator of maltreatment and neglect, should accompany any other assault codes.

See Section I.C.19. Adult and child abuse, neglect and other maltreatment

h. **Unknown or Undetermined Intent Guideline**

If the intent (accident, self-harm, assault) of the cause of an injury or other condition is unknown or unspecified, code the intent as accidental intent. All transport accident categories assume accidental intent.

1) **Use of undetermined intent**

External cause codes for events of undetermined intent are only for use if the documentation in the record specifies that the intent cannot be determined.

i. Sequelae (Late Effects) of External Cause Guidelines

1) Sequelae external cause codes

Sequela are reported using the external cause code with the 7th character "S" for sequela. These codes should be used with any report of a late effect or sequela resulting from a previous injury.

See Section I.B.10 Sequela (Late Effects)

2) Sequela external cause code with a related current injury

A sequela external cause code should never be used with a related current nature of injury code.

3) Use of sequela external cause codes for subsequent visits

Use a late effect external cause code for subsequent visits when a late effect of the initial injury is being treated. Do not use a late effect external cause code for subsequent visits for follow-up care (e.g., to assess healing, to receive rehabilitative therapy) of the injury when no late effect of the injury has been documented.

j. Terrorism Guidelines

1) Cause of injury identified by the Federal Government (FBI) as terrorism

When the cause of an injury is identified by the Federal Government (FBI) as terrorism, the first-listed external cause code should be a code from category Y38, Terrorism. The definition of terrorism employed by the FBI is found at the

inclusion note at the beginning of category Y38. Use additional code for place of occurrence (Y92.-). More than one Y38 code may be assigned if the injury is the result of more than one mechanism of terrorism.

2) Cause of an injury is suspected to be the result of terrorism

When the cause of an injury is suspected to be the result of terrorism a code from category Y38 should not be assigned. Suspected cases should be classified as assault.

3) Code Y38.9, Terrorism, secondary effects

Assign code Y38.9, Terrorism, secondary effects, for conditions occurring subsequent to the terrorist event. This code should not be assigned for conditions that are due to the initial terrorist act.

It is acceptable to assign code Y38.9 with another code from Y38 if there is an injury due to the initial terrorist event and an injury that is a subsequent result of the terrorist event.

k. External Cause Status

A code from category Y99, External cause status, should be assigned whenever any other external cause code is assigned for an encounter, including an Activity code, except for the events noted below. Assign a code from category Y99, External cause status, to indicate the work status of the person at the time the event occurred. The status code indicates whether the event occurred during military activity, whether a non-military person was at work, whether an individual including a student or volunteer was involved in a non-work activity at the time of the causal event.

A code from Y99, External cause status, should be assigned, when applicable, with other external cause codes, such as transport accidents and falls. The external cause status codes are not applicable to poisonings, adverse effects, misadventures or late effects.

Do not assign a code from category Y99 if no other external cause codes (cause, activity) are applicable for the encounter.

An external cause status code is used only once, at the initial encounter for treatment. Only one code from Y99 should be recorded on a medical record.

Do not assign code Y99.9, Unspecified external cause status, if the status is not stated.

21. Chapter 21: Factors influencing health status and contact with health services (Z00-Z99)

Note: The chapter specific guidelines provide additional information about the use of Z codes for specified encounters.

a. Use of Z Codes in Any Healthcare Setting

Z codes are for use in any healthcare setting. Z codes may be used as either a first-listed (principal diagnosis code in the inpatient setting) or secondary code, depending on the circumstances of the encounter. Certain Z codes may only be used as first-listed or principal diagnosis.

b. Z Codes Indicate a Reason for an Encounter

Z codes are not procedure codes. A corresponding procedure code must accompany a Z code to describe any procedure performed.

c. Categories of Z Codes

1) Contact/Exposure

Category Z20 indicates contact with, and suspected exposure to, communicable diseases. These codes are for patients who are suspected to have been exposed to a disease by close personal contact with an infected individual or are in an area where a disease is epidemic.

Category Z77, Other contact with and (suspected) exposures hazardous to health, indicates contact with and suspected exposures hazardous to health.

Contact/exposure codes may be used as a first-listed code to explain an encounter for testing, or, more commonly, as a secondary code to identify a potential risk.

2) Inoculations and vaccinations

Code Z23 is for encounters for inoculations and vaccinations. It indicates that a patient is being seen to receive a prophylactic inoculation against a disease. Procedure codes are required to identify the actual administration of the injection and the type(s) of immunizations given. Code Z23 may be used as a secondary code if the inoculation is given as a routine part of preventive health care, such as a well-baby visit.

3) Status

Status codes indicate that a patient is either a carrier of a disease or has the sequelae or residual of a past disease or condition.

This includes such things as the presence of prosthetic or mechanical devices resulting from past treatment. A status code is informative, because the status may affect the course of treatment and its outcome. A status code is distinct from a history code. The history code indicates that the patient no longer has the condition.

A status code should not be used with a diagnosis code from one of the body system chapters, if the diagnosis code includes the information provided by the status code. For example, code Z94.1, Heart transplant status, should not be used with a code from subcategory T86.2, Complications of heart transplant. The status code does not provide additional information. The complication code indicates that the patient is a heart transplant patient.

For encounters for weaning from a mechanical ventilator, assign a code from subcategory J96.1, Chronic respiratory failure, followed by code Z99.11, Dependence on respirator [ventilator] status.
The status Z codes/categories are: Z14 Genetic carrier

Genetic carrier status indicates that a person carries a gene, associated with a particular disease, which may be passed to offspring who may develop that disease. The person does not have the disease and is not at risk of developing the disease.

Z15 Genetic susceptibility to disease

Genetic susceptibility indicates that a person has a gene that increases the risk of that person developing the disease.

Codes from category Z15 should not be used as principal or first-listed codes. If the patient has the condition to which he/she is susceptible, and that condition is the reason for the encounter, the code for the current condition should be sequenced first. If the patient is being seen for follow-up after completed treatment for this condition, and the condition no longer exists, a follow-up code should be sequenced first, followed by the appropriate personal history and genetic susceptibility codes. If the purpose of the encounter is genetic counseling associated with procreative management, code Z31.5, Encounter for genetic counseling, should be

assigned as the first-listed code, followed by a code from category Z15. Additional codes should be assigned for any applicable family or personal history.

Z16   Resistance to antimicrobial drugs

        This code indicates that a patient has a condition that is resistant to antimicrobial drug treatment. Sequence the infection code first.

Z17   Estrogen receptor status

Z18   Retained foreign body fragments

Z19   Hormone sensitivity malignancy status Z21 Asymptomatic HIV infection status

        This code indicates that a patient has tested positive for HIV but has manifested no signs or symptoms of the disease.

Z22   Carrier of infectious disease

        Carrier status indicates that a person harbors the specific organisms of a disease without manifest symptoms and is capable of transmitting the infection.

Z28.3   Underimmunization status

Z33.1   Pregnant state, incidental

        This code is a secondary code only for use when the pregnancy is in no way complicating the reason for visit. Otherwise, a code from the obstetric chapter is required.

Z66   Do not resuscitate

        This code may be used when it is documented by the provider that a patient is on do not resuscitate status at any time during the stay.

Z67   Blood type

Z68   Body mass index (BMI)

BMI codes should only be assigned when there is an associated, reportable diagnosis (such as obesity). Do not assign BMI codes during pregnancy.
See Section I.B.14 for BMI documentation by clinicians other than the patient's provider.

Z74.01   Bed confinement status

Z76.82   Awaiting organ transplant status

Z78   Other specified health status

Code Z78.1, Physical restraint status, may be used when it is documented by the provider that a patient has been put in restraints during the current encounter. Please note that this code should not be reported when it is documented by the provider that a patient is temporarily restrained during a procedure.

Z79   Long-term (current) drug therapy

Codes from this category indicate a patient's continuous use of a prescribed drug (including such things as aspirin therapy) for the long-term treatment of a condition or for prophylactic use. It is not for use for patients who have addictions to drugs. This subcategory is not for use of medications for detoxification or maintenance programs to prevent withdrawal symptoms (e.g., methadone maintenance for opiate dependence). Assign the appropriate code for the drug use, abuse, or dependence instead.

Assign a code from Z79 if the patient is receiving a medication for an extended period as a prophylactic measure (such as for the prevention of deep vein thrombosis) or as treatment of a chronic condition (such as arthritis) or a disease requiring a lengthy course of treatment (such as cancer). Do not assign a code from category Z79 for medication being administered for a brief period of time to treat an acute illness or injury (such as a course of antibiotics to treat acute bronchitis).

Z88   Allergy status to drugs, medicaments and biological substances

Except: Z88.9, Allergy status to unspecified drugs, medicaments and biological substances status

Z89   Acquired absence of limb

Z90   Acquired absence of organs, not elsewhere classified

Z91.0-   Allergy status, other than to drugs and biological substances

Z92.82   Status post administration of tPA (rtPA) in a different facility within the last 24 hours prior to admission to a current facility

Assign code Z92.82, Status post administration of tPA (rtPA) in a different facility within the last 24 hours prior to admission to current facility, as a secondary diagnosis when a patient is received by transfer into a facility and documentation indicates they were administered tissue plasminogen activator (tPA) within the last 24 hours prior to admission to the current facility.

This guideline applies even if the patient is still receiving the tPA at the time they are received into the current facility.

The appropriate code for the condition for which the tPA was administered (such as cerebro-vascular disease or myocardial infarction) should be assigned first.

Code Z92.82 is only applicable to the receiving facility record and not to the transferring facility record.

Z93   Artificial opening status

Z94   Transplanted organ and tissue status

Z95   Presence of cardiac and vascular implants and grafts Z96 Presence of other functional implants

Z97   Presence of other devices

Z98   Other postprocedural states

Assign code Z98.85, Transplanted organ removal status, to indicate that a transplanted organ has been previously removed. This code should not be assigned for the encounter in which the transplanted organ is removed. The complication necessitating removal of the transplant organ should be assigned for that encounter.

See section I.C19. for information on the coding of organ transplant complications.

Z99   Dependence on enabling machines and devices, not elsewhere classified

Note: Categories Z89-Z90 and Z93-Z99 are for use only if there are no complications or malfunctions of the organ or tissue replaced, the amputation site or the equipment on which the patient is dependent.

4) **History (of)**

There are two types of history Z codes, personal and family. Personal history codes explain a patient's past medical condition that no longer exists and is not receiving any treatment, but that has the potential for recurrence, and therefore may require continued monitoring.

Family history codes are for use when a patient has a family member(s) who has had a particular disease that causes the patient to be at higher risk of also contracting the disease.

Personal history codes may be used in conjunction with follow-up codes and family history codes may be used in conjunction with screening codes to explain the need for a test or procedure. History codes are also acceptable on any medical record regardless of the reason for visit. A history of an illness, even if no longer present, is important information that may alter the type of treatment ordered.

The reason for the encounter (for example, screening or counseling)should be sequenced first and the appropriate personal and/or family history code(s) should be assigned as additional diagnos(es).

The history Z code categories are:

Z80   Family history of primary malignant neoplasm

Z81   Family history of mental and behavioral disorders

Z82   Family history of certain disabilities and chronic diseases (leading to disablement)

Z83   Family history of other specific disorders

Z84   Family history of other conditions

Z85   Personal history of malignant neoplasm

Z86   Personal history of certain other diseases

Z87   Personal history of other diseases and conditions

Z91.4- Personal history of psychological trauma, not elsewhere classified

Z91.5	Personal history of self-harm
Z91.81	History of falling
Z91.82	Personal history of military deployment
Z92	Personal history of medical treatment
	Except: Z92.0, Personal history of contraception
	Except: Z92.82, Status post administration of tPA (rtPA) in a different facility within the last 24 hours prior to admission to a current facility

5) **Screening**

Screening is the testing for disease or disease precursors in seemingly well individuals so that early detection and treatment can be provided for those who test positive for the disease (e.g., screening mammogram).

The testing of a person to rule out or confirm a suspected diagnosis because the patient has some sign or symptom is a diagnostic examination, not a screening. In these cases, the sign or symptom is used to explain the reason for the test.

A screening code may be a first-listed code if the reason for the visit is specifically the screening exam. It may also be used as an additional code if the screening is done during an office visit for other health problems. A screening code is not necessary if the screening is inherent to a routine examination, such as a pap smear done during a routine pelvic examination.

Should a condition be discovered during the screening then the code for the condition may be assigned as an additional diagnosis.

The Z code indicates that a screening exam is planned. A procedure code is required to confirm that the screening was performed.

The screening Z codes/categories:

Z11	Encounter for screening for infectious and parasitic diseases
Z12	Encounter for screening for malignant neoplasms
Z13	Encounter for screening for other diseases and disorders
	Except: Z13.9, Encounter for screening, unspecified
Z36	Encounter for antenatal screening for mother

6) **Observation**

There are three observation Z code categories. They are for use in very limited circumstances when a person is being observed for a suspected condition that is ruled out. The observation codes are not for use if an injury or illness or any signs or symptoms related to the suspected condition are present. In such cases the diagnosis/symptom code is used with the corresponding external cause code.

The observation codes are primarily to be used as a principal/first-listed diagnosis. An observation code may be assigned as a secondary diagnosis code when the patient is being observed for a condition that is ruled out and is unrelated to the principal/first-listed diagnosis (e.g., patient presents for treatment following injuries sustained in a motor vehicle accident and is also observed for suspected COVID-19 infection that is subsequently ruled out). Also, when the principal diagnosis is required to be a code from category Z38, Liveborn infants according to place of birth and type of delivery, then a code from category Z05, Encounter for observation and evaluation of newborn for suspected diseases and conditions ruled out, is sequenced after the Z38 code. Additional codes may be used in addition to the observation code, but only if they are unrelated to the suspected condition being observed.

Codes from subcategory Z03.7, Encounter for suspected maternal and fetal conditions ruled out, may either be used as a first-listed or as an additional code assignment depending on the case. They are for use in very limited circumstances on a maternal record when an encounter is for a suspected maternal or fetal condition that is ruled out during that encounter (for example, a maternal or fetal condition may be suspected due to an abnormal test result). These codes should not be used when the condition is confirmed. In those cases, the confirmed condition should be coded. In addition, these codes are not for use if an illness or any signs or symptoms related to the suspected condition or problem are present. In such cases the diagnosis/symptom code is used.

Additional codes may be used in addition to the code from subcategory Z03.7, but only if they are unrelated to the suspected condition being evaluated.

Codes from subcategory Z03.7 may not be used for encounters for antenatal screening of mother.

See Section I.C.21. Screening.

For encounters for suspected fetal condition that are inconclusive following testing and evaluation, assign the appropriate code from category O35, O36, O40 or O41.

The observation Z code categories:

Z03 Encounter for medical observation for suspected diseases and conditions ruled out

Z04 Encounter for examination and observation for other reasons

   Except: Z04.9, Encounter for examination and observation for unspecified reason

Z05 Encounter for observation and evaluation of newborn for suspected diseases and conditions ruled out

7) Aftercare

Aftercare visit codes cover situations when the initial treatment of a disease has been performed and the patient requires continued care during the healing or recovery phase, or for the long-term consequences of the disease. The aftercare Z code should not be used if treatment is directed at a current, acute disease. The diagnosis code is to be used in these cases. Exceptions to this rule are codes Z51.0, Encounter for antineoplastic radiation therapy, and codes from subcategory Z51.1, Encounter for antineoplastic chemotherapy and immunotherapy. These codes are to be first listed, followed by the diagnosis code when a patient's encounter is solely to receive radiation therapy, chemotherapy, or immunotherapy for the treatment of a neoplasm. If the reason for the encounter is more than one type of antineoplastic therapy, code Z51.0 and a code from subcategory Z51.1 may be assigned together, in which case one of these codes would be reported as a secondary diagnosis.

The aftercare Z codes should also not be used for aftercare for injuries. For aftercare of an injury, assign the acute injury code with the appropriate 7th character (for subsequent encounter).

The aftercare codes are generally first listed to explain the specific reason for the encounter. An aftercare code may be used as an additional code when some type of aftercare is provided in addition to the reason for admission and no diagnosis code is applicable. An example of this would be the closure of a colostomy during an encounter for treatment of another condition.

Aftercare codes should be used in conjunction with other aftercare codes or diagnosis codes to provide better detail on the specifics of an aftercare encounter visit, unless otherwise directed by the classification. The sequencing of multiple aftercare codes depends on the circumstances of the encounter.

Certain aftercare Z code categories need a secondary diagnosis code to describe the resolving condition or sequelae. For others, the condition is included in the code title.

Additional Z code aftercare category terms include fitting and adjustment, and attention to artificial openings.

Status Z codes may be used with aftercare Z codes to indicate the nature of the aftercare. For example, code Z95.1, Presence of aortocoronary bypass graft, may be used with code Z48.812, Encounter for surgical aftercare following surgery on the circulatory system, to indicate the surgery for which the aftercare is being performed. A status code should not be used when the aftercare code indicates the type of status, such as using Z43.0, Encounter for attention to tracheostomy, with Z93.0, Tracheostomy status.

The aftercare Z category/codes:

Z42   Encounter for plastic and reconstructive surgery following medical procedure or healed injury

Z43   Encounter for attention to artificial openings

Z44   Encounter for fitting and adjustment of external prosthetic device

Z45   Encounter for adjustment and management of implanted device

Z46   Encounter for fitting and adjustment of other devices

Z47   Orthopedic aftercare

Z48   Encounter for other postprocedural aftercare

Z49   Encounter for care involving renal dialysis

Z51   Encounter for other aftercare and medical care

8) Follow-up

The follow-up codes are used to explain continuing surveillance following completed treatment of a disease, condition, or injury. They imply that the condition has been fully treated and no longer exists. They should not be confused with aftercare codes, or injury codes with a 7th character for subsequent encounter, that explain ongoing care of a healing condition or its sequelae. Follow-up codes may be used in conjunction with history codes to provide the full picture of the healed condition and its treatment. The follow-up code is sequenced first, followed by the history code.

A follow-up code may be used to explain multiple visits. Should a condition be found to have recurred on the follow-up visit, then the diagnosis code for the condition should be assigned in place of the follow-up code.

The follow-up Z code categories:

Z08   Encounter for follow-up examination after completed treatment for malignant neoplasm

Z09   Encounter for follow-up examination after completed treatment for conditions other than malignant neoplasm

Z39   Encounter for maternal postpartum care and examination

9) Donor

Codes in category Z52, Donors of organs and tissues, are used for living individuals who are donating blood or other body tissue. These codes are for individuals donating for others, as well as for self-donations. They are not used to identify cadaveric donations.

10) Counseling

Counseling Z codes are used when a patient or family member receives assistance in the aftermath of an illness or injury, or when support is required in coping with family or social problems.

The counseling Z codes/categories:

Z30.0-   Encounter for general counseling and advice on contraception

Z31.5   Encounter for procreative genetic counseling

Z31.6-   Encounter for general counseling and advice on procreation

Z32.2   Encounter for childbirth instruction

Z32.3   Encounter for childcare instruction

Z69   Encounter for mental health services for victim and perpetrator of abuse

Z70   Counseling related to sexual attitude, behavior and orientation

Z71   Persons encountering health services for other counseling and medical advice, not elsewhere classified

Note: Code Z71.84, Encounter for health counseling related to travel, is to be used for health risk and safety counseling for future travel purposes.

Code Z71.85, Encounter for immunization safety counseling, is to be used for counseling of the patient or caregiver regarding the safety of a vaccine. This code should not be used for the provision of general information regarding risks and potential side effects during routine encounters for the administration of vaccines.

Z76.81   Expectant mother prebirth pediatrician visit

11) Encounters for Obstetrical and Reproductive Services

See Section I.C.15. Pregnancy, Childbirth, and the Puerperium, for further instruction on the use of these codes.

Z codes for pregnancy are for use in those circumstances when none of the problems or complications included in the codes from the Obstetrics chapter exist (a routine prenatal visit or postpartum care). Codes in category Z34, Encounter for supervision of normal pregnancy, are always first listed and are not to be used with any other code from the OB chapter.

Codes in category Z3A, Weeks of gestation, may be assigned to provide additional information about the pregnancy. Category Z3A codes should not be assigned for pregnancies with abortive outcomes (categories O00-O08), elective termination of pregnancy (code Z33.2), nor for postpartum conditions, as category Z3A is not applicable to these conditions. The date of the admission should be used to determine weeks of gestation for inpatient admissions that encompass more than one gestational week.

The outcome of delivery, category Z37, should be included on all maternal delivery records. It is always a secondary code.

Codes in category Z37 should not be used on the newborn record.

Z codes for family planning (contraceptive) or procreative management and counseling should be included on an obstetric record either during the pregnancy or the postpartum stage, if applicable.

Z codes/categories for obstetrical and reproductive services:

Z30   Encounter for contraceptive management

Z31   Encounter for procreative management

Z32.2   Encounter for childbirth instruction

Z32.3   Encounter for childcare instruction

Z33   Pregnant state

Z34   Encounter for supervision of normal pregnancy

Z36   Encounter for antenatal screening of mother

Z3A   Weeks of gestation

Z37   Outcome of delivery

Z39   Encounter for maternal postpartum care and examination

Z76.81 Expectant mother prebirth pediatrician visit

12) Newborns and Infants

See Section I.C.16. Newborn (Perinatal) Guidelines, for further instruction on the use of these codes.

Newborn Z codes/categories:

Z76.1   Encounter for health supervision and care of foundling

Z00.1- Encounter for routine child health examination

Z38   Liveborn infants according to place of birth and type of delivery

13) Routine and Administrative Examinations

The Z codes allow for the description of encounters for routine examinations, such as, a general check-up, or examinations for administrative purposes, such as, a pre-employment physical. The codes are not to be used if the examination is for diagnosis of a suspected condition or for treatment purposes. In such cases the diagnosis code is used. During a routine exam, should a diagnosis or condition be discovered, it should be coded as an additional code. Pre-existing and chronic conditions and history codes may also be included as additional codes as long as the examination is for administrative purposes and not focused on any particular condition.

Some of the codes for routine health examinations distinguish between "with" and "without" abnormal findings. Code assignment depends on the information that is known at the time the encounter is being coded. For example, if no abnormal findings were found during the examination, but the encounter is being coded before test results are back, it is acceptable to assign the code for "without abnormal findings." When assigning a code for "with abnormal findings," additional code(s) should be assigned to identify the specific abnormal finding(s).

Pre-operative examination and pre-procedural laboratory examination Z codes are for use only in those situations when a patient is being cleared for a procedure or surgery and no treatment is given.

The Z codes/categories for routine and administrative examinations:

Z00   Encounter for general examination without complaint, suspected or reported diagnosis

Z01   Encounter for other special examination without complaint, suspected or reported diagnosis

Z02   Encounter for administrative examination

          Except: Z02.9, Encounter for administrative examinations, unspecified

Z32.0- Encounter for pregnancy test

14) Miscellaneous Z Codes

The miscellaneous Z codes capture a number of other health care encounters that do not fall into one of the other categories. Certain of these codes identify the reason for the encounter; others are for use as additional codes that provide useful information on circumstances that may affect a patient's care and treatment.

Prophylactic Organ Removal

For encounters specifically for prophylactic removal of an organ (such as prophylactic removal of breasts due to a genetic susceptibility to cancer or a family history of cancer), the principal or first-listed code should be a code from category Z40, Encounter for prophylactic surgery, followed by the appropriate codes to identify the associated risk factor (such as genetic susceptibility or family history).

If the patient has a malignancy of one site and is having prophylactic removal at another site to prevent either a new primary malignancy or metastatic disease, a code for the malignancy should also be assigned in addition to a code from subcategory Z40.0, Encounter for prophylactic surgery for risk factors related to malignant neoplasms. A Z40.0 code should not be assigned if the patient is having organ removal for treatment of a malignancy, such as the removal of the testes for the treatment of prostate cancer.

Miscellaneous Z codes/categories:

Z28   Immunization not carried out

          Except: Z28.3, Underimmunization status

Z29   Encounter for other prophylactic measures

Z40   Encounter for prophylactic surgery

Z41   Encounter for procedures for purposes other than remedying health state
          Except: Z41.9, Encounter for procedure for purposes other than remedying health state, unspecified

Z53   Persons encountering health services for specific procedures and treatment, not carried out

Z55   Problems related to education and literacy

Z56   Problems related to employment and unemployment

Z57   Occupational exposure to risk factors

Z58   Problems related to physical environment

Z59   Problems related to housing and economic circumstances

Z60   Problems related to social environment

Z62   Problems related to upbringing

Z63   Other problems related to primary support group, including family circumstances

Z64   Problems related to certain psychosocial circumstances
Z65   Problems related to other psychosocial circumstances

Z72   Problems related to lifestyle

        Note: These codes should be assigned only when the documentation specifies that the patient has an associated problem

Z73   Problems related to life management difficulty

Z74   Problems related to care provider dependency

        Except: Z74.01, Bed confinement status

Z75   Problems related to medical facilities and other health care

Z76.0   Encounter for issue of repeat prescription

Z76.3   Healthy person accompanying sick person

Z76.4   Other boarder to healthcare facility

Z76.5   Malingerer [conscious simulation]

Z91.1- Patient's noncompliance with medical treatment and regimen

Z91.83 Wandering in diseases classified elsewhere

Z91.84 - Oral health risk factors

Z91.89 Other specified personal risk factors, not elsewhere classified

See Section I.B.14 for Z55-Z65 Persons with potential health hazards related to socioeconomic and psychosocial circumstances, documentation by clinicians other than the patient's provider

15) Nonspecific Z Codes

Certain Z codes are so non-specific, or potentially redundant with other codes in the classification, that there can be little justification for their use in the inpatient setting. Their use in the outpatient setting should be limited to those instances when there is no further documentation to permit more precise coding. Otherwise, any sign or symptom or any other reason for visit that is captured in another code should be used.

Nonspecific Z codes/categories:

Z02.9   Encounter for administrative examinations, unspecified

Z04.9   Encounter for examination and observation for unspecified reason

Z13.9   Encounter for screening, unspecified

Z41.9   Encounter for procedure for purposes other than remedying health state, unspecified

Z52.9   Donor of unspecified organ or tissue

Z86.59 Personal history of other mental and behavioral disorders

Z88.9   Allergy status to unspecified drugs, medicaments and biological substances status

Z92.0   Personal history of contraception

16) Z Codes That May Only be Principal/First-Listed Diagnosis

The following Z codes/categories may only be reported as the principal/first-listed diagnosis, except when there are multiple encounters on the same day and the medical records for the encounters are combined:

Z00   Encounter for general examination without complaint, suspected or reported diagnosis

       Except: Z00.6

Z01   Encounter for other special examination without complaint, suspected or reported diagnosis

Z02   Encounter for administrative examination

Z04   Encounter for examination and observation for other reasons

Z33.2   Encounter for elective termination of pregnancy

Z31.81   Encounter for male factor infertility in female patient

Z31.83   Encounter for assisted reproductive fertility procedure cycle

Z31.84   Encounter for fertility preservation procedure

Z34   Encounter for supervision of normal pregnancy

Z39   Encounter for maternal postpartum care and examination

Z38   Liveborn infants according to place of birth and type of delivery

Z40   Encounter for prophylactic surgery

Z42   Encounter for plastic and reconstructive surgery following medical procedure or healed injury

Z51.0   Encounter for antineoplastic radiation therapy

Z51.1-   Encounter for antineoplastic chemotherapy and immunotherapy

Z52   Donors of organs and tissues

       Except: Z52.9, Donor of unspecified organ or tissue

Z76.1   Encounter for health supervision and care of foundling

Z76.2   Encounter for health supervision and care of other healthy infant and child

Z99.12   Encounter for respirator [ventilator] dependence during power failure

17) Social Determinants of Health

Codes describing social determinants of health (SDOH) should be assigned when this information is documented.

For social determinants of health, such as information found in categories Z55-Z65, Persons with potential health hazards related to socioeconomic and psychosocial circumstances, code assignment may be based on medical record documentation from clinicians involved in the care of the patient who are not the patient's provider since this information represents social information, rather than medical diagnoses. For example, coding professionals may utilize documentation of social information from social workers, community health workers, case managers, or nurses, if their documentation is included in the official medical record.

Patient self-reported documentation may be used to assign codes for social determinants of health, as long as the patient self-reported information is signed-off by and incorporated into the medical record by either a clinician or provider.

Social determinants of health codes are located primarily in these Z code categories:

Z55	Problems related to education and literacy
Z56	Problems related to employment and unemployment
Z57	Occupational exposure to risk factors
Z58	Problems related to physical environment
Z59	Problems related to housing and economic circumstances
Z60	Problems related to social environment
Z62	Problems related to upbringing
Z63	Other problems related to primary support group, including family circumstances
Z64	Problems related to certain psychosocial circumstances
Z65	Problems related to other psychosocial circumstances

See Section I.B.14. Documentation by Clinicians Other than thePatient's Provider.

22. Chapter 22: Codes for Special Purposes (U00-U85)

U07.0   Vaping-related disorder (see Section I.C.10.e., Vaping-related disorders)

U07.1   COVID-19 (see Section I.C.1.g.1., COVID-19 infection)

U09.9   Post COVID-19 condition, unspecified (see Section I.C.1.g.1.m)

Section II. Selection of Principal Diagnosis

The circumstances of inpatient admission always govern the selection of principal diagnosis. The principal diagnosis is defined in the Uniform Hospital Discharge Data Set (UHDDS) as "that condition established after study to be chiefly responsible for occasioning the admission of the patient to the hospital for care."

The UHDDS definitions are used by hospitals to report inpatient data elements in a standardized manner. These data elements and their definitions can be found in the July 31, 1985, Federal Register (Vol. 50, No, 147), pp. 31038-40.

Since that time, the application of the UHDDS definitions has been expanded to include all non-outpatient settings (acute care, short term, long term care and psychiatric hospitals; home health agencies; rehab facilities; nursing homes, etc.). The UHDDS definitions also apply to hospice services (all levels of care).

In determining principal diagnosis, coding conventions in the ICD-10-CM, the Tabular List and Alphabetic Index take precedence over these official coding guidelines.

(See Section I.A., Conventions for the ICD-10-CM)

The importance of consistent, complete documentation in the medical record cannot be overemphasized. Without such documentation the application of all coding guidelines is a difficult, if not impossible, task.

A. **Codes for symptoms, signs, and ill-defined conditions**

Codes for symptoms, signs, and ill-defined conditions from Chapter 18 are not to be used as principal diagnosis when a related definitive diagnosis has been established.

B. **Two or more interrelated conditions, each potentially meeting the definition for principal diagnosis.**

When there are two or more interrelated conditions (such as diseases in the same ICD-10-CM chapter or manifestations characteristically associated with a certain disease) potentially meeting the definition of principal diagnosis, either condition may be sequenced first, unless the circumstances of the admission, the therapy provided, the Tabular List, or the Alphabetic Index indicate otherwise.

C. Two or more diagnoses that equally meet the definition for principal diagnosis

In the unusual instance when two or more diagnoses equally meet the criteria for principal diagnosis as determined by the circumstances of admission, diagnostic workup and/or therapy provided, and the Alphabetic Index, Tabular List, or another coding guidelines does not provide sequencing direction, any one of the diagnoses may be sequenced first.

D. Two or more comparative or contrasting conditions

In those rare instances when two or more contrasting or comparative diagnoses are documented as "either/or" (or similar terminology), they are coded as if the diagnoses were confirmed, and the diagnoses are sequenced according to the circumstances of the admission. If no further determination can be made as to which diagnosis should be principal, either diagnosis may be sequenced first.

E. A symptom(s) followed by contrasting/comparative diagnoses

GUIDELINE DELETED EFFECTIVE OCTOBER 1, 2014

F. Original treatment plan not carried out

Sequence as the principal diagnosis the condition, which after study occasioned the admission to the hospital, even though treatment may not have been carried out due to unforeseen circumstances.

G. Complications of surgery and other medical care

When the admission is for treatment of a complication resulting from surgery or other medical care, the complication code is sequenced as the principal diagnosis. If the complication is classified to the T80-T88 series and the code lacks the necessary specificity in describing the complication, an additional code for the specific complication should be assigned.

H. Uncertain Diagnosis

If the diagnosis documented at the time of discharge is qualified as "probable," "suspected," "likely," "questionable," "possible," or "still to be ruled out," "compatible with," "consistent with," or other similar terms indicating uncertainty, code the condition as if it existed or was established. The bases for these guidelines are the diagnostic workup, arrangements for further workup or observation, and initial therapeutic approach that correspond most closely with the established diagnosis.

Note: This guideline is applicable only to inpatient admissions to short-term, acute, long-term care and psychiatric hospitals.

I. Admission from Observation Unit

1. Admission Following Medical Observation

When a patient is admitted to an observation unit for a medical condition, which either worsens or does not improve, and is subsequently admitted as an inpatient of the same hospital for this same medical condition, the principal diagnosis would be the medical condition which led to the hospital admission.

2. Admission Following Post-Operative Observation

When a patient is admitted to an observation unit to monitor a condition (or complication) that develops following outpatient surgery, and then is subsequently admitted as an inpatient of the same hospital, hospitals should apply the Uniform Hospital Discharge Data Set (UHDDS) definition of principal diagnosis as "that condition established after study to be chiefly responsible for occasioning the admission of the patient to the hospital for care."

J. Admission from Outpatient Surgery

When a patient receives surgery in the hospital's outpatient surgery department and is subsequently admitted for continuing inpatient care at the same hospital, the following guidelines should be followed in selecting the principal diagnosis for the inpatient admission:

- If the reason for the inpatient admission is a complication, assign the complication as the principal diagnosis.
- If no complication, or other condition, is documented as the reason for the inpatient admission, assign the reason for the outpatient surgery as the principal diagnosis.
- If the reason for the inpatient admission is another condition unrelated to the surgery, assign the unrelated condition as the principal diagnosis.

K. Admissions/Encounters for Rehabilitation

When the purpose for the admission/encounter is rehabilitation, sequence first the code for the condition for which the service is being performed. For example, for an admission/encounter for rehabilitation for right-sided dominant hemiplegia following a cerebrovascular infarction, report code I69.351, Hemiplegia and hemiparesis following cerebral infarction affecting right dominant side, as the first-listed or principal diagnosis.

If the condition for which the rehabilitation service is being provided is no longer present, report the appropriate aftercare code as the first-listed or principal diagnosis, unless the rehabilitation service is being provided following an injury. For rehabilitation services following active treatment of an injury, assign the injury code with the appropriate seventh character for subsequent encounter as the first-listed or principal diagnosis. For example, if a patient with severe degenerative osteoarthritis of the hip, underwent hip replacement and the current encounter/admission is for rehabilitation, report code Z47.1, Aftercare following joint replacement surgery, as the first-listed or principal diagnosis. If the patient requires rehabilitation post hip replacement for right intertrochanteric femur fracture, report code S72.141D, Displaced intertrochanteric fracture of right femur, subsequent encounter for closed fracture with routine healing, as the first-listed or principal diagnosis.

See Section I.C.21.c.7, Factors influencing health states and contact with health services, Aftercare.
See Section I.C.19.a, for additional information about the use of 7th characters for injury codes.

Section III. Reporting Additional Diagnoses

GENERAL RULES FOR OTHER (ADDITIONAL) DIAGNOSES

For reporting purposes, the definition for "other diagnoses" is interpreted as additional conditions that affect patient care in terms of requiring:

- clinical evaluation; or therapeutic treatment;
- or diagnostic procedures; or
- extended length of hospital stay; or
- increased nursing care and/or monitoring.

The UHDDS item #11-b defines Other Diagnoses as "all conditions that coexist at the time of admission, that develop subsequently, or that affect the treatment received and/or the length of stay. Diagnoses that relate to an earlier episode which have no bearing on the current hospital stay are to be excluded." UHDDS definitions apply to inpatients in acute care, short-term, long term care and psychiatric hospital setting. The UHDDS definitions are used by acute care short-term hospitals to report inpatient data elements in a standardized manner. These data elements and their definitions can be found in the July 31, 1985, Federal Register (Vol. 50, No, 147), pp. 31038-40.

Since that time, the application of the UHDDS definitions has been expanded to include all non-outpatient settings (acute care, short term, long term care and psychiatric hospitals; home health agencies; rehab facilities; nursing homes, etc.). The UHDDS definitions also apply to hospice services (all levels of care).

The following guidelines are to be applied in designating "other diagnoses" when neither the Alphabetic Index nor the Tabular List in ICD-10-CM provide direction. The listing of the diagnoses in the patient record is the responsibility of the attending provider.

A. Previous conditions

If the provider has included a diagnosis in the final diagnostic statement, such as the discharge summary or the face sheet, it should ordinarily be coded. Some providers include in the diagnostic statement resolved conditions or diagnoses and status-post procedures from previous admissions that have no bearing on the current stay. Such conditions are not to be reported and are coded only if required by hospital policy.

However, history codes (categories Z80-Z87) may be used as secondary codes if the historical condition or family history has an impact on current care or influences treatment.

B. Abnormal findings

Abnormal findings (laboratory, x-ray, pathologic, and other diagnostic results) are not coded and reported unless the provider indicates their clinical significance. If the findings are outside the normal range and the attending provider has ordered other tests to evaluate the condition or prescribed treatment, it is appropriate to ask the provider whether the abnormal finding should be added.

Please note: This differs from the coding practices in the outpatient setting for coding encounters for diagnostic tests that have been interpreted by a provider.

C. Uncertain Diagnosis

If the diagnosis documented at the time of discharge is qualified as "probable," "suspected," "likely," "questionable," "possible," or "still to be ruled out," "compatible with," "consistent with," or other similar terms indicating uncertainty, code the condition as if it existed or was established. The bases for these guidelines are the diagnostic workup, arrangements for further workup or observation, and initial therapeutic approach that correspond most closely with the established diagnosis.

Note: This guideline is applicable only to inpatient admissions to short-term, acute, long-term care and psychiatric hospitals.

Section IV. Diagnostic Coding and Reporting Guidelines for Outpatient Services

These coding guidelines for outpatient diagnoses have been approved for use by hospitals/ providers in coding and reporting hospital-based outpatient services and provider-based office visits. Guidelines in Section I, Conventions, general coding guidelines and chapter-specific guidelines, should also be applied for outpatient services and office visits.

Information about the use of certain abbreviations, punctuation, symbols, and other conventions used in the ICD-10-CM Tabular List (code numbers and titles), can be found in Section IA of these guidelines, under "Conventions Used in the Tabular List." Section I.B. contains general guidelines that apply to the entire classification. Section I.C. contains chapter-specific guidelines that correspond to the chapters as they are arranged in the classification. Information about the correct sequence to use in finding a code is also described in Section I.

The terms encounter and visit are often used interchangeably in describing outpatient service contacts and, therefore, appear together in these guidelines without distinguishing one from the other.

Though the conventions and general guidelines apply to all settings, coding guidelines for outpatient and provider reporting of diagnoses will vary in a number of instances from those for inpatient diagnoses, recognizing that:

The Uniform Hospital Discharge Data Set (UHDDS) definition of principal diagnosis does not apply to hospital-based outpatient services and provider-based office visits.

Coding guidelines for inconclusive diagnoses (probable, suspected, rule out, etc.) were developed for inpatient reporting and do not apply to outpatients.

A. Selection of first-listed condition

In the outpatient setting, the term first-listed diagnosis is used in lieu of principal diagnosis.

In determining the first-listed diagnosis the coding conventions of ICD-10-CM, as well as the general and disease specific guidelines take precedence over the outpatient guidelines.
Diagnoses often are not established at the time of the initial encounter/visit. It may take two or more visits before the diagnosis is confirmed.

The most critical rule involves beginning the search for the correct code assignment through the Alphabetic Index. Never begin searching initially in the Tabular List as this will lead to coding errors.

1. Outpatient Surgery

When a patient presents for outpatient surgery (same day surgery), code the reason for the surgery as the first-listed diagnosis (reason for the encounter), even if the surgery is not performed due to a contraindication.

2. Observation Stay

When a patient is admitted for observation for a medical condition, assign a code for the medical condition as the first-listed diagnosis.

When a patient presents for outpatient surgery and develops complications requiring admission to observation, code the reason for the surgery as the first reported diagnosis (reason for the encounter), followed by codes for the complications as secondary diagnoses.

B. Codes from A00.0 through T88.9, Z00-Z99, U00-U85

The appropriate code(s) from A00.0 through T88.9, Z00-Z99 and U00-U85 must be used to identify diagnoses, symptoms, conditions, problems, complaints, or other reason(s) for the encounter/visit.

C. Accurate reporting of ICD-10-CM diagnosis codes

For accurate reporting of ICD-10-CM diagnosis codes, the documentation should describe the patient's condition, using terminology which includes specific diagnoses as well as symptoms, problems, or reasons for the encounter. There are ICD-10-CM codes to describe all of these.

D. Codes that describe symptoms and signs

Codes that describe symptoms and signs, as opposed to diagnoses, are acceptable for reporting purposes when a diagnosis has not been established (confirmed) by the provider. Chapter 18 of ICD-10-CM, Symptoms, Signs, and Abnormal Clinical and Laboratory Findings Not Elsewhere Classified (codes R00-R99) contain many, but not all codes for symptoms.

E. Encounters for circumstances other than a disease or injury

ICD-10-CM provides codes to deal with encounters for circumstances other than a disease or injury. The Factors Influencing Health Status and Contact with Health Services codes (Z00-Z99) are provided to deal with occasions when circumstances other than a disease or injury are recorded as diagnosis or problems.

See Section I.C.21. Factors influencing health status and contact with health services.

F. Level of Detail in Coding

1. ICD-10-CM codes with 3, 4, 5, 6 or 7 characters

ICD-10-CM is composed of codes with 3, 4, 5, 6 or 7 characters. Codes with three characters are included in ICD-10-CM as the heading of a category of codes that may be further subdivided by the use of fourth, fifth, sixth or seventh characters to provide greater specificity.

2. **Use of full number of characters required for a code**

A three-character code is to be used only if it is not further subdivided. A code is invalid if it has not been coded to the full number of characters required for that code, including the 7th character, if applicable.

3. **Highest level of specificity**

Code to the highest level of specificity when supported by the medical recorddocumentation.

G. **ICD-10-CM code for the diagnosis, condition, problem, or other reason for encounter/visit**

List first the ICD-10-CM code for the diagnosis, condition, problem, or other reason for encounter/visit shown in the medical record to be chiefly responsible for the services provided. List additional codes that describe any coexisting conditions. In some cases, the first-listed diagnosis may be a symptom when a diagnosis has not been established (confirmed) by the provider.

H. **Uncertain diagnosis**

Do not code diagnoses documented as "probable", "suspected," "questionable," "rule out," "compatible with," "consistent with," or "working diagnosis" or other similar terms indicating uncertainty. Rather, code the condition(s) to the highest degree of certainty for that encounter/visit, such as symptoms, signs, abnormal test results, or other reason for the visit.

Please note: This differs from the coding practices used by short-term, acute care, long-term care and psychiatric hospitals.

I. **Chronic diseases**

Chronic diseases treated on an ongoing basis may be coded and reported as many times as the patient receives treatment and care for the condition(s)

J. **Code all documented conditions that coexist**

Code all documented conditions that coexist at the time of the encounter/visit and require or affect patient care treatment or management. Do not code conditions that were previously treated and no longer exist. However, history codes (categories Z80-Z87) may be used as secondary codes if the historical condition or family history has an impact on current care or influences treatment.

K. **Patients receiving diagnostic services only**

For patients receiving diagnostic services only during an encounter/visit, sequence first the diagnosis, condition, problem, or other reason for encounter/visit shown in the medical record to be chiefly responsible for the outpatient services provided during the encounter/visit. Codes for other diagnoses (e.g., chronic conditions) may be sequenced as additional diagnoses.

For encounters for routine laboratory/radiology testing in the absence of any signs, symptoms, or associated diagnosis, assign Z01.89, Encounter for other specified special examinations. If routine testing is performed during the same encounter as a test to evaluate a sign, symptom, or diagnosis, it is appropriate to assign both the Z code and the code describing the reason for the non-routine test.

For outpatient encounters for diagnostic tests that have been interpreted by a physician, and the final report is available at the time of coding, code any confirmed or definitive diagnosis(es) documented in the interpretation. Do not code related signs and symptoms as additional diagnoses.

Please note: This differs from the coding practice in the hospital inpatient setting regarding abnormal findings on test results.

L. **Patients receiving therapeutic services only**

For patients receiving therapeutic services only during an encounter/visit, sequence first the diagnosis, condition, problem, or other reason for encounter/visit shown in the medical record to be chiefly responsible for the outpatient services provided during the encounter/visit. Codes for other diagnoses (e.g., chronic conditions) may be sequenced as additional diagnoses.

The only exception to this rule is that when the primary reason for the admission/encounter is chemotherapy or radiation therapy, the appropriate Z code for the service is listed first, and the diagnosis or problem for which the service is being performed listed second.

M. Patients receiving preoperative evaluations only

For patients receiving preoperative evaluations only, sequence first a code from subcategory Z01.81, Encounter for pre-procedural examinations, to describe the pre-op consultations. Assign a code for the condition to describe the reason for the surgery as an additional diagnosis. Code also any findings related to the pre-op evaluation.

N. Ambulatory surgery

For ambulatory surgery, code the diagnosis for which the surgery was performed. If the postoperative diagnosis is known to be different from the preoperative diagnosis at the time the diagnosis is confirmed, select the postoperative diagnosis for coding, since it is the most definitive.

O. Routine outpatient prenatal visits

See Section I.C.15. Routine outpatient prenatal visits.

P. Encounters for general medical examinations with abnormal findings

The subcategories for encounters for general medical examinations, Z00.0- and encounter for routine child health examination, Z00.12-, provide codes for with and without abnormal findings. Should a general medical examination result in an abnormal finding, the code for general medical examination with abnormal finding should be assigned as the first-listed diagnosis. An examination with abnormal findings refers to a condition/diagnosis that is newly identified or a change in severity of a chronic condition (such as uncontrolled hypertension, or an acute exacerbation of chronic obstructive pulmonary disease) during a routine physical examination. A secondary code for the abnormal finding should also be coded.

Q. Encounters for routine health screenings

See Section I.C.21. Factors influencing health status and contact with health services, Screening

Appendix I

Present on Admission Reporting Guidelines

Introduction

These guidelines are to be used as a supplement to the to facilitate the assignment of the Present on Admission (POA) indicator for each diagnosis and external cause of injury code reported on claim forms (UB-04 and 837 Institutional).

These guidelines are not intended to replace any guidelines in the main body of the . The POA guidelines are not intended to provide guidance on when a condition should be coded, but rather, how to apply the POA indicator to the final set of diagnosis codes that have been assigned in accordance with Sections I, II, and III of the official coding guidelines. Subsequent to the assignment of the ICD-10-CM codes, the POA indicator should then be assigned to those conditions that have been coded.

As stated in the Introduction to the , a joint effort between the healthcare provider and the coder is essential to achieve complete and accurate documentation, code assignment, and reporting of diagnoses and procedures. The importance of consistent, complete documentation in the medical record cannot be overemphasized. Medical record documentation from any provider involved in the care and treatment of the patient may be used to support the determination of whether a condition was present on admission or not. In the context of the official coding guidelines, the term "provider" means a physician or any qualified healthcare practitioner who is legally accountable for establishing the patient's diagnosis.

These guidelines are not a substitute for the provider's clinical judgment as to the determination of whether a condition was/was not present on admission. The provider should be queried regarding issues related to the linking of signs/symptoms, timing of test results, and the timing of findings.

Please see the CDC website for the detailed list of ICD-10-CM codes that do not require the use of a POA indicator (https://www.cdc.gov/nchs/icd/icd10cm.htm). The codes and categories on this exempt list are for circumstances regarding the healthcare encounter or factors influencing health status that do not represent a current disease or injury or that describe conditions that are always present on admission.

General Reporting Requirements

All claims involving inpatient admissions to general acute care hospitals or other facilities that are subject to a law or regulation mandating collection of present on admission information.

Present on admission is defined as present at the time the order for inpatient admission occurs -- conditions that develop during an outpatient encounter, including emergency department, observation, or outpatient surgery, are considered as present on admission.

POA indicator is assigned to principal and secondary diagnoses (as defined in Section II of the Official Guidelines for Coding and Reporting) and the external cause of injury codes.

Issues related to inconsistent, missing, conflicting or unclear documentation must still be resolved by the provider.

If a condition would not be coded and reported based on UHDDS definitions and current official coding guidelines, then the POA indicator would not be reported.

Reporting Options

Y - Yes
N - No
U - Unknown
W – Clinically undetermined

Unreported/Not used – (Exempt from POA reporting)

Reporting Definitions

Y = present at the time of inpatient admission
N = not present at the time of inpatient admission
U = documentation is insufficient to determine if condition is present on admission
W = provider is unable to clinically determine whether condition was present on admission or not

Timeframe for POA Identification and Documentation

There is no required timeframe as to when a provider (per the definition of "provider" used in these guidelines) must identify or document a condition to be present on admission. In some clinical situations, it may not be possible for a provider to make a definitive diagnosis (or a condition may not be recognized or reported by the patient) for a period of time after admission. In some cases, it may be several days before the provider arrives at a definitive diagnosis. This does not mean that the condition was not present on admission. Determination of whether the condition was present on admission or not will be based on the applicable POA guideline as identified in this document, or on the provider's best clinical judgment.

If at the time of code assignment, the documentation is unclear as to whether a condition was present on admission or not, it is appropriate to query the provider for clarification.

Assigning the POA Indicator

Condition is on the "Exempt from Reporting" list

Leave the "present on admission" field blank if the condition is on the list of ICD-10-CM codes for which this field is not applicable. This is the only circumstance in which the field may be left blank.

POA Explicitly Documented

Assign Y for any condition the provider explicitly documents as being present on admission.

Assign N for any condition the provider explicitly documents as not present at the time of admission.

Conditions diagnosed prior to inpatient admission

Assign "Y" for conditions that were diagnosed prior to admission (example: hypertension, diabetes mellitus, asthma)

Conditions diagnosed during the admission but clearly present before admission

Assign "Y" for conditions diagnosed during the admission that were clearly present but not diagnosed until after admission occurred.

Diagnoses subsequently confirmed after admission are considered present on admission if at the time of admission, they are documented as suspected, possible, rule out, differential diagnosis, or constitute an underlying cause of a symptom that is present at the time of admission.

Condition develops during outpatient encounter prior to inpatient admission

Assign Y for any condition that develops during an outpatient encounter prior to a written order for inpatient admission.

Documentation does not indicate whether condition was present on admission

Assign "U" when the medical record documentation is unclear as to whether the condition was present on admission. "U" should not be routinely assigned and used only in very limited circumstances. Coders are encouraged to query the providers when the documentation is unclear.

Documentation states that it cannot be determined whether the condition was or was not present on admission

Assign "W" when the medical record documentation indicates that it cannot be clinically determined whether or not the condition was present on admission.

Chronic condition with acute exacerbation during the admission

If a single code identifies both the chronic condition and the acute exacerbation, see POA guidelines pertaining to codes that contain multiple clinical concepts.

If a single code only identifies the chronic condition and not the acute exacerbation (e.g., acute exacerbation of chronic leukemia), assign "Y."

Conditions documented as possible, probable, suspected, or rule out at the time of discharge

If the final diagnosis contains a possible, probable, suspected, or rule out diagnosis, and this diagnosis was based on signs, symptoms or clinical findings suspected at the time of inpatient admission, assign "Y."

If the final diagnosis contains a possible, probable, suspected, or rule out diagnosis, and this diagnosis was based on signs, symptoms or clinical findings that were not present on admission, assign "N".

Conditions documented as impending or threatened at the time of discharge

If the final diagnosis contains an impending or threatened diagnosis, and this diagnosis is based on symptoms or clinical findings that were present on admission, assign "Y".

If the final diagnosis contains an impending or threatened diagnosis, and this diagnosis is based on symptoms or clinical findings that were not present on admission, assign "N".

Acute and Chronic Conditions

Assign "Y" for acute conditions that are present at time of admission and N for acute conditions that are not present at time of admission.

Assign "Y" for chronic conditions, even though the condition may not be diagnosed until after admission.

If a single code identifies both an acute and chronic condition, see the POA guidelines for codes that contain multiple clinical concepts.

Codes That Contain Multiple Clinical Concepts

Assign "N" if at least one of the clinical concepts included in the code was not present on admission (e.g., COPD with acute exacerbation and the exacerbation was not present on admission; gastric ulcer that does not start bleeding until after admission; asthma patient develops status asthmaticus after admission).

Assign "Y" if all of the clinical concepts included in the code were present on admission (e.g., duodenal ulcer that perforates prior to admission).

For infection codes that include the causal organism, assign "Y" if the infection (or signs of the infection) were present on admission, even though the culture results may not be known until after admission (e.g., patient is admitted with pneumonia and the provider documents Pseudomonas as the causal organism a few days later).

Same Diagnosis Code for Two or More Conditions

When the same ICD-10-CM diagnosis code applies to two or more conditions during the same encounter (e.g., two separate conditions classified to the same ICD-10-CM diagnosis code):

Assign "Y" if all conditions represented by the single ICD-10-CM code were present on admission (e.g., bilateral unspecified age-related cataracts).

Assign "N" if any of the conditions represented by the single ICD-10-CM code was not present on admission (e.g., traumatic secondary and recurrent hemorrhage and seroma is assigned to a single code T79.2, but only one of the conditions was present on admission).

Obstetrical conditions

Whether or not the patient delivers during the current hospitalization does not affect assignment of the POA indicator. The determining factor for POA assignment is whether the pregnancy complication or obstetrical condition described by the code was present at the time of admission or not.

If the pregnancy complication or obstetrical condition was present on admission (e.g., patient admitted in preterm labor), assign "Y".

If the pregnancy complication or obstetrical condition was not present on admission (e.g., 2nd degree laceration during delivery, postpartum hemorrhage that occurred during current hospitalization, fetal distress develops after admission), assign "N".

If the obstetrical code includes more than one diagnosis and any of the diagnoses identified by the code were not present on admission assign "N". (e.g., Category O11, Pre-existing hypertension with pre-eclampsia)

Perinatal conditions

Newborns are not considered to be admitted until after birth. Therefore, any condition present at birth or that developed in utero is considered present at admission and should be assigned "Y". This includes conditions that occur during delivery (e.g., injury during delivery, meconium aspiration, exposure to streptococcus B in the vaginal canal).

Congenital conditions and anomalies

Assign "Y" for congenital conditions and anomalies except for categories Q00-Q99, Congenital anomalies, which are on the exempt list. Congenital conditions are always considered present on admission.

External cause of injury codes

Assign "Y" for any external cause code representing an external cause of morbidity that occurred prior to inpatient admission (e.g., patient fell out of bed at home, patient fell out of bed in emergency room prior to admission)

Assign "N" for any external cause code representing an external cause of morbidity that occurred during inpatient hospitalization (e.g., patient fell out of hospital bed during hospital stay, patient experienced an adverse reaction to a medication administered after inpatient admission).

Anatomical Illustrations

A fundamental knowledge and understanding of basic human anatomy and physiology is a prerequisite for accurate diagnosis coding. While a comprehensive treatment of anatomy and physiology is beyond the scope of this text, the large scale, full color anatomical illustrations on the following pages are designed to facilitate the procedure coding process for both beginning and experienced coders.

The illustrations provide an anatomical perspective of procedure coding by providing a side-by-side view of the major systems of the human body and a corresponding list of the most common ICD-10-CM categories used to report medical, surgical and diagnostic services performed on the illustrated system.

The ICD-10-CM categories listed on the left facing page of each anatomical illustration are code ranges only and should not be used for coding. These categories are provided as "pointers" to the appropriate section of ICD-10-CM, where the definitive code may be found.

PLATE 1. SKIN AND SUBCUTANEOUS TISSUE – MALE

Viral infections characterized by skin and mucous membrane lesions	**B00-B09**
Bacterial and viral infectious agents	**B95-B97**
Melanoma and other malignant neoplasms of skin	**C43-C44**
Malignant neoplasms of mesothelial and soft tissue	**C45-C49**
Malignant neoplasms of ill-defined, other secondary and unspecified sites	**C76-C80**
In situ neoplasms	**D00-D09**
Benign neoplasms, except benign neuroendocrine tumors	**D10-D36**
Neoplasms of uncertain behavior, polycythemia vera and myelodysplastic syndromes	**D37-D48**
Neoplasms of unspecified behavior	**D49**
Infections of the skin and subcutaneous tissue	**L00-L08**
Bullous disorders	**L10-L14**
Dermatitis and eczema	**L20-L30**
Papulosquamous disorders	**L40-L45**
Urticaria and erythema	**L49-L54**
Radiation-related disorders of the skin and subcutaneous tissue	**L55-L59**
Disorders of skin appendages	**L60-L75**
Intraoperative and postprocedural complications of skin and subcutaneous tissue	**L76**
Other disorders of the skin and subcutaneous tissue	**L80-L99**
Symptoms and signs involving the skin and subcutaneous tissue	**R20-R23**
General symptoms and signs	**R50-R69**
Abnormal findings on diagnostic imaging and in function studies, without diagnosis	**R90-R94**
Burns and corrosions of external body surface, specified by site	**T20-T25**
Burns and corrosions	**T20-T32**
Burns and corrosions of multiple and unspecified body regions	**T30-T32**
Persons encountering health services for examinations	**Z00-Z13**
Encounters for other specific health care	**Z40-Z53**

Male Figure
(Anterior View)

Partietal region

Frontal region

Temporal region

Orbital region

Nasal region

Oral region

Mental region

Anterior neck region

Lateral neck region

Infraclavicular region

Deltoid region

Sternal region

Pectoral region

Axillary region

Brachial region

Hypochondriac region

Epigastric region

Cubital region

Umbilical region

Antebrachial region

Lateral abdominal region

Inguinal region

Pubic region

Femoral region

Knee region

Crural region

©Practice Management Information Corp., Los Angeles, CA

PLATE 2. SKIN AND SUBCUTANEOUS TISSUE - FEMALE

Viral infections characterized by skin and mucous membrane lesions	**B00-B09**
Bacterial and viral infectious agents	**B95-B97**
Melanoma and other malignant neoplasms of skin	**C43-C44**
Malignant neoplasms of mesothelial and soft tissue	**C45-C49**
Malignant neoplasms of ill-defined, other secondary and unspecified sites	**C76-C80**
In situ neoplasms	**D00-D09**
Benign neoplasms, except benign neuroendocrine tumors	**D10-D36**
Neoplasms of uncertain behavior, polycythemia vera and myelodysplastic syndromes	**D37-D48**
Neoplasms of unspecified behavior	**D49**
Infections of the skin and subcutaneous tissue	**L00-L08**
Bullous disorders	**L10-L14**
Dermatitis and eczema	**L20-L30**
Papulosquamous disorders	**L40-L45**
Urticaria and erythema	**L49-L54**
Radiation-related disorders of the skin and subcutaneous tissue	**L55-L59**
Disorders of skin appendages	**L60-L75**
Intraoperative and postprocedural complications of skin and subcutaneous tissue	**L76**
Other disorders of the skin and subcutaneous tissue	**L80-L99**
Symptoms and signs involving the skin and subcutaneous tissue	**R20-R23**
General symptoms and signs	**R50-R69**
Abnormal findings on diagnostic imaging and in function studies, without diagnosis	**R90-R94**
Burns and corrosions of external body surface, specified by site	**T20-T25**
Burns and corrosions	**T20-T32**
Burns and corrosions of multiple and unspecified body regions	**T30-T32**
Persons encountering health services for examinations	**Z00-Z13**
Encounters for other specific health care	**Z40-Z53**

Female Figure
(Anterior View)

Partietal region

Temporal region

Frontal region

Orbital region

Nasal region

Oral region

Mental region

Anterior neck region

Lateral neck region

Infraclavicular region

Deltoid region

Sternal region

Pectoral region

Axillary region

Brachial region

Hypochondriac region

Epigastric region

Cubital region

Antebrachial region

Umbilical region

Lateral abdominal region

Inguinal region

Pubic region

Femoral region

Knee region

Crural region

PLATE 3. FEMALE BREAST

Bacterial and viral infectious agents	**B95-B97**
Malignant neoplasms of breast	**C50**
Malignant neoplasms of ill-defined, other secondary and unspecified sites	**C76-C80**
In situ neoplasms	**D00-D09**
Benign neoplasms, except benign neuroendocrine tumors	**D10-D36**
Neoplasms of uncertain behavior, polycythemia vera and myelodysplastic syndromes	**D37-D48**
Neoplasms of unspecified behavior	**D49**
Disorders of breast	**N60-N65**
General symptoms and signs	**R50-R69**
Abnormal findings on diagnostic imaging and in function studies, without diagnosis	**R90-R94**
Persons encountering health services for examinations	**Z00-Z13**
Encounters for other specific health care	**Z40-Z53**

Female Breast

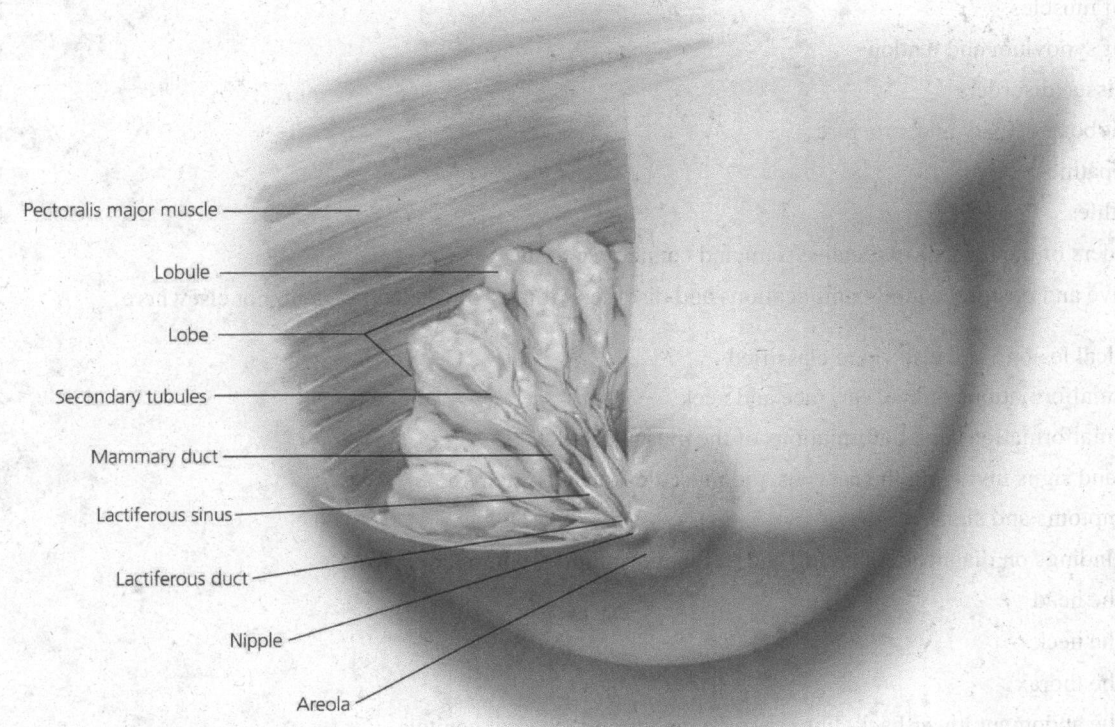

Pectoralis major muscle

Lobule

Lobe

Secondary tubules

Mammary duct

Lactiferous sinus

Lactiferous duct

Nipple

Areola

PLATE 4. MUSCULAR SYSTEM AND CONNECTIVE TISSUE – ANTERIOR VIEW

Malignant neoplasms of bone and articular cartilage	**C40-C41**
Infectious arthropathies	**M00-M02**
Inflammatory polyarthropathies	**M05-M14**
Osteoarthritis	**M15-M19**
Other joint disorders	**M20-M25**
Dentofacial anomalies [including malocclusion] and other disorders of jaw	**M26-M27**
Systemic connective tissue disorders	**M30-M36**
Deforming dorsopathies	**M40-M43**
Spondylopathies	**M45-M49**
Other dorsopathies	**M50-M54**
Disorders of muscles	**M60-M63**
Disorders of synovium and tendon	**M65-M67**
Other soft tissue disorders	**M70-M79**
Disorders of bone density and structure	**M80-M85**
Other osteopathies	**M86-M90**
Chondropathies	**M91-M94**
Other disorders of the musculoskeletal system and connective tissue	**M95**
Intraoperative and postprocedural complications and disorders of musculoskeletal system, not elsewhere classified	**M96**
Biomechanical lesions, not elsewhere classified	**M99**
Congenital malformations of eye, ear, face and neck	**Q10-Q18**
Congenital malformations and deformations of the musculoskeletal system	**Q65-Q79**
Symptoms and signs involving the nervous and musculoskeletal systems	**R25-R29**
General symptoms and signs	**R50-R69**
Abnormal findings on diagnostic imaging and in function studies, without diagnosis	**R90-R94**
Injuries to the head	**S00-S09**
Injuries to the neck	**S10-S19**
Injuries to the thorax	**S20-S29**
Injuries to the abdomen, lower back, lumbar spine, pelvis and external genitals	**S30-S39**
Injuries to the shoulder and upper arm	**S40-S49**
Injuries to the elbow and forearm	**S50-S59**
Injuries to the wrist, hand and fingers	**S60-S69**
Injuries to the hip and thigh	**S70-S79**
Injuries to the knee and lower leg	**S80-S89**
Injuries to the ankle and foot	**S90-S99**
Injuries involving multiple body regions	**T07**
Certain early complications of trauma	**T79**
Accidents	**V00-X58**
Persons encountering health services for examinations	**Z00-Z13**
Encounters for other specific health care	**Z40-Z53**

Muscular System
(Anterior View)

Temporalis m.
Orbicularis oculi m.
Masseter m.
Sternocleidomastoid m.
Trapezius m.
Levator scapulae m.
Deltoid m.
Pectoralis major m.
Serratus anterior m.
Biceps m.
External abdominal oblique m.
Brachialis m.
Brachioradialis m.
Extensor carpi radialis longus m.
Palmaris longus m.
Flexor carpi radialis m.
Superficial inguinal ring
Tensor fasciae latae m.
Sartorius m.
Rectus femoris m.
Adductor longus m.
Vastus lateralis m.
Iliotibial tract
Vastus medialis m.
Lateral patellar retinaculum
Tibialis anterior m.
Gastrocnemius m.
Extensor digitorum longus m.
Peroneus longus m.
Soleus m.
Peroneus brevis m.
Extensor hallucis longus m.
Extensor hallucis brevis m.
Extensor digitorum brevis m.

Frontalis m.
Buccinator
Orbicularis oris m.
Depressor anguli oris m.
Pectoralis minor m.
Internal intercostal m.
Coracobrachialis m.
Brachialis m.
Rectus sheath
Rectus abdominis m.
Linea alba
Internal abdominal oblique m.
Transversus abdominis m.
Flexor digitorum superficialis m.
Flexor pollicis longus m.
Abductor digiti minimi m.
Abductor pollicis brevis m.
Flexor pollicis brevis m.
Iliopsoas m.
Pectineus m.
Adductor brevis m.
Gracilis m.
Adductor magnus m.
Vastus medialis m.
Vastus lateralis m.
Sartorius m.
Patella
Patellar ligament
Medial patellar retinaculum
Gastrocnemius m.
Soleus m.
Tibia
Flexor digitorum longus m.
Extensor hallucis brevis m.
Abductor hallucis m.

PLATE 5. MUSCULAR SYSTEM AND CONNECTIVE TISSUE – POSTERIOR VIEW

Malignant neoplasms of bone and articular cartilage	**C40-C41**
Infectious arthropathies	**M00-M02**
Inflammatory polyarthropathies	**M05-M14**
Osteoarthritis	**M15-M19**
Other joint disorders	**M20-M25**
Dentofacial anomalies [including malocclusion] and other disorders of jaw	**M26-M27**
Systemic connective tissue disorders	**M30-M36**
Deforming dorsopathies	**M40-M43**
Spondylopathies	**M45-M49**
Other dorsopathies	**M50-M54**
Disorders of muscles	**M60-M63**
Disorders of synovium and tendon	**M65-M67**
Other soft tissue disorders	**M70-M79**
Disorders of bone density and structure	**M80-M85**
Other osteopathies	**M86-M90**
Chondropathies	**M91-M94**
Other disorders of the musculoskeletal system and connective tissue	**M95**
Intraoperative and postprocedural complications and disorders of musculoskeletal system, not elsewhere classified	**M96**
Biomechanical lesions, not elsewhere classified	**M99**
Congenital malformations of eye, ear, face and neck	**Q10-Q18**
Congenital malformations and deformations of the musculoskeletal system	**Q65-Q79**
Symptoms and signs involving the nervous and musculoskeletal systems	**R25-R29**
General symptoms and signs	**R50-R69**
Abnormal findings on diagnostic imaging and in function studies, without diagnosis	**R90-R94**
Injuries to the head	**S00-S09**
Injuries to the neck	**S10-S19**
Injuries to the thorax	**S20-S29**
Injuries to the abdomen, lower back, lumbar spine, pelvis and external genitals	**S30-S39**
Injuries to the shoulder and upper arm	**S40-S49**
Injuries to the elbow and forearm	**S50-S59**
Injuries to the wrist, hand and fingers	**S60-S69**
Injuries to the hip and thigh	**S70-S79**
Injuries to the knee and lower leg	**S80-S89**
Injuries to the ankle and foot	**S90-S99**
Injuries involving multiple body regions	**T07**
Certain early complications of trauma	**T79**
Accidents	**V00-X58**
Persons encountering health services for examinations	**Z00-Z13**
Encounters for other specific health care	**Z40-Z53**

Muscular System
(Posterior View)

Frontalis m.
Temporoparietalis m.
Zygomaticus major m.
Masseter m.
Risorius m.
Trapezius m.
Deltoid m.
Infraspinatus m.
Teres minor m.
Teres major m.
Triceps m.
Latissimus dorsi m.
Brachialis m.
Brachioradialis m.
Extensor carpi radialis longus m.
Flexor carpi ulnaris m.
Extensor digitorum m.
Extensor carpi radialis brevis m.
Extensor carpi ulnaris m.
Abductor pollicis longus m.
Extensor pollicis brevis m.
Gluteus medius m.
Gluteus maximus m.

Biceps femoris m.
Adductor magnus m.
Iliotibial tract
Vastus lateralis m.
Semimembranosus m.
Semitendinosus m.

Gastrocnemius m.
Peroneus longus m.

Soleus m.
Calcaneal t. (Achilles)

Galea aponeurotica
Occipitalis m.
Sternocleidomastoid m.
Splenius capitis m.
Splenius cervicis m.
Levator scapulae m.
Supraspinatus m.
Rhomboid minor m.
Rhomboid major m.
Spinalis thoracis m.
Iliocostalis thoracis m.
Longissimus thoracis m.
Serratus posterior inferior m.
Brachioradialis m.
Extensor carpi radialis longus m.
External abdominal oblique m.
Supinator m.
Gluteus medius m.
Extensor pollicis longus m.
Gluteus minimus m.
Piriformis m.
Superior gemellus m.
Obturator internus m.
Inferior gemellus m.
Quadratus femoris m.
Adductor magnus m.

Gracilis m.
Biceps femoris m.
Semimembranosus m.

Plantaris m.
Popliteus m.
Soleus m.

Flexor digitorum longus m.
Peroneus longus m.
Flexor hallucis longus m.
Peroneus brevis m.

PLATE 6. MUSCULAR SYSTEM - SHOULDER AND ELBOW

Malignant neoplasms of bone and articular cartilage	**C40-C41**
Infectious arthropathies	**M00-M02**
Inflammatory polyarthropathies	**M05-M14**
Osteoarthritis	**M15-M19**
Other joint disorders	**M20-M25**
Dentofacial anomalies [including malocclusion] and other disorders of jaw	**M26-M27**
Systemic connective tissue disorders	**M30-M36**
Deforming dorsopathies	**M40-M43**
Spondylopathies	**M45-M49**
Other dorsopathies	**M50-M54**
Disorders of muscles	**M60-M63**
Disorders of synovium and tendon	**M65-M67**
Other soft tissue disorders	**M70-M79**
Disorders of bone density and structure	**M80-M85**
Other osteopathies	**M86-M90**
Chondropathies	**M91-M94**
Other disorders of the musculoskeletal system and connective tissue	**M95**
Intraoperative and postprocedural complications and disorders of musculoskeletal system, not elsewhere classified	**M96**
Biomechanical lesions, not elsewhere classified	**M99**
Congenital malformations and deformations of the musculoskeletal system	**Q65-Q79**
Symptoms and signs involving the nervous and musculoskeletal systems	**R25-R29**
General symptoms and signs	**R50-R69**
Abnormal findings on diagnostic imaging and in function studies, without diagnosis	**R90-R94**
Injuries to the shoulder and upper arm	**S40-S49**
Injuries to the elbow and forearm	**S50-S59**
Injuries involving multiple body regions	**T07**
Certain early complications of trauma	**T79**
Accidents	**V00-X58**
Persons encountering health services for examinations	**Z00-Z13**
Encounters for other specific health care	**Z40-Z53**

Shoulder and Elbow
(Anterior View)

Coracoclavicular ligament
Acromioclavicular ligament
Coracoacromial ligament
Supraspinatus tendon
Coracohumeral ligament
Transverse humeral ligament
Tendon of long head of biceps muscle
Subscapularis tendon
Articular capsule

Acromion
Clavicle

Coracoid process
Scapular notch
Subscapular fossa
Head of humerus
Lesser tubercle
Greater tubercle
Scapula
Nutrient foramen
Humerus
Deltoid tuberosity

Articular capsule
Radial collateral ligament
Annular ligament
Ulnar collateral ligament

Interosseous membrane
Radius
Ulna

Lateral epicondyle
Capitulum
Coronoid fossa
Medal epicondyle
Trochlea
Coronoid process
Head of radius
Ulnar tuberosity
Radial tuberosity

PLATE 7. MUSCULAR SYSTEM - HAND AND WRIST

Malignant neoplasms of bone and articular cartilage	**C40-C41**
Infectious arthropathies	**M00-M02**
Inflammatory polyarthropathies	**M05-M14**
Osteoarthritis	**M15-M19**
Other joint disorders	**M20-M25**
Dentofacial anomalies [including malocclusion] and other disorders of jaw	**M26-M27**
Systemic connective tissue disorders	**M30-M36**
Deforming dorsopathies	**M40-M43**
Spondylopathies	**M45-M49**
Other dorsopathies	**M50-M54**
Disorders of muscles	**M60-M63**
Disorders of synovium and tendon	**M65-M67**
Other soft tissue disorders	**M70-M79**
Disorders of bone density and structure	**M80-M85**
Other osteopathies	**M86-M90**
Chondropathies	**M91-M94**
Other disorders of the musculoskeletal system and connective tissue	**M95**
Intraoperative and postprocedural complications and disorders of musculoskeletal system, not elsewhere classified	**M96**
Biomechanical lesions, not elsewhere classified	**M99**
Congenital malformations and deformations of the musculoskeletal system	**Q65-Q79**
Symptoms and signs involving the nervous and musculoskeletal systems	**R25-R29**
General symptoms and signs	**R50-R69**
Abnormal findings on diagnostic imaging and in function studies, without diagnosis	**R90-R94**
Injuries to the wrist, hand and fingers	**S60-S69**
Injuries involving multiple body regions	**T07**
Certain early complications of trauma	**T79**
Accidents	**V00-X58**
Persons encountering health services for examinations	**Z00-Z13**
Encounters for other specific health care	**Z40-Z53**

Hand and Wrist

Abductor pollicis longus muscle

Extensor pollicis brevis muscle

Extensor digitorum tendons

Extensor pollicis brevis tendon

Extensor pollicis longus tendon

Extensor carpi radialis brevis tendon

Extensor carpi radialis longus tendon

1st dorsal interosseous muscle

Extensor digiti minimi muscle

Extensor carpi ulnaris muscle

Extensor retinaculum

Extensor digiti minimi tendons

Extensor digitorum tendons

2nd, 3rd, 4th dorsal interosseous muscles

Brachioradialis tendon

Flexor carpi radialis tendon

Flexor pollicis longus muscle

Abductor pollicis longus tendon

Opponens pollicis muscle

Abductor pollicis brevis muscle

Flexor pollicis brevis muscle

Flexor digitorum superficialis muscle & tendons

Flexor carpi ulnaris tendon

Palmaris longus tendon

Opponens digiti minimi muscle

Flexor digiti minimi brevis muscle

Abductor digiti minimi muscle

Flexor digitorum superficialis tendons

Palmar interosseous muscles

Fibrous digital sheath:
anular part
cruciform part

Adductor pollicis muscle

Lumbrical muscles

Flexor digitorum profundus tendon

PLATE 8. MUSCULOSKELETAL SYSTEM - HIP AND KNEE

Malignant neoplasms of bone and articular cartilage	**C40-C41**
Infectious arthropathies	**M00-M02**
Inflammatory polyarthropathies	**M05-M14**
Osteoarthritis	**M15-M19**
Other joint disorders	**M20-M25**
Dentofacial anomalies [including malocclusion] and other disorders of jaw	**M26-M27**
Systemic connective tissue disorders	**M30-M36**
Deforming dorsopathies	**M40-M43**
Spondylopathies	**M45-M49**
Other dorsopathies	**M50-M54**
Disorders of muscles	**M60-M63**
Disorders of synovium and tendon	**M65-M67**
Other soft tissue disorders	**M70-M79**
Disorders of bone density and structure	**M80-M85**
Other osteopathies	**M86-M90**
Chondropathies	**M91-M94**
Other disorders of the musculoskeletal system and connective tissue	**M95**
Intraoperative and postprocedural complications and disorders of musculoskeletal system, not elsewhere classified	**M96**
Biomechanical lesions, not elsewhere classified	**M99**
Congenital malformations and deformations of the musculoskeletal system	**Q65-Q79**
Symptoms and signs involving the nervous and musculoskeletal systems	**R25-R29**
General symptoms and signs	**R50-R69**
Abnormal findings on diagnostic imaging and in function studies, without diagnosis	**R90-R94**
Injuries to the hip and thigh	**S70-S79**
Injuries to the knee and lower leg	**S80-S89**
Injuries involving multiple body regions	**T07**
Certain early complications of trauma	**T79**
Accidents	**V00-X58**
Persons encountering health services for examinations	**Z00-Z13**
Encounters for other specific health care	**Z40-Z53**

Hip and Knee
(Anterior View)

Sacral promontory
Sacrum
Iliac crest
Ilium
Anterior superior iliac spine
Spine of ischium
Anterior inferior iliac spine
Head of femur
Greater trochanter
Obturator foramen
Pubis
Lesser trochanter

Anterior longitudinal ligament
Iliolumbar ligament
Anterior sacroiliac ligament
Coccyx
Sacrotuberous ligament
Sacrospinous ligament
Inguinal ligament
Iliofemoral ligament
Pubofemoral ligament
Obturator membrane
Pubic symphysis
Femur

Medial epicondyle
Lateral epicondyle
Patella
Lateral condyles
Head of fibula
Tibial tuberosity
Medial condyles
Tibia
Fibula

Quadriceps femoris tendon
Medial patellar retinaculum
Fibular collateral ligament
Tibial collateral ligament
Lateral patellar retinaculum
Patellar ligament
Interosseous membrane

PLATE 9. MUSCULOSKELETAL SYSTEM – FOOT AND ANKLE

Malignant neoplasms of bone and articular cartilage	**C40-C41**
Infectious arthropathies	**M00-M02**
Inflammatory polyarthropathies	**M05-M14**
Osteoarthritis	**M15-M19**
Other joint disorders	**M20-M25**
Dentofacial anomalies [including malocclusion] and other disorders of jaw	**M26-M27**
Systemic connective tissue disorders	**M30-M36**
Deforming dorsopathies	**M40-M43**
Spondylopathies	**M45-M49**
Other dorsopathies	**M50-M54**
Disorders of muscles	**M60-M63**
Disorders of synovium and tendon	**M65-M67**
Other soft tissue disorders	**M70-M79**
Disorders of bone density and structure	**M80-M85**
Other osteopathies	**M86-M90**
Chondropathies	**M91-M94**
Other disorders of the musculoskeletal system and connective tissue	**M95**
Intraoperative and postprocedural complications and disorders of musculoskeletal system, not elsewhere classified	**M96**
Biomechanical lesions, not elsewhere classified	**M99**
Congenital malformations of eye, ear, face and neck	**Q10-Q18**
Congenital malformations and deformations of the musculoskeletal system	**Q65-Q79**
Symptoms and signs involving the nervous and musculoskeletal systems	**R25-R29**
General symptoms and signs	**R50-R69**
Abnormal findings on diagnostic imaging and in function studies, without diagnosis	**R90-R94**
Injuries to the ankle and foot	**S90-S99**
Injuries involving multiple body regions	**T07**
Certain early complications of trauma	**T79**
Accidents	**V00-X58**
Persons encountering health services for examinations	**Z00-Z13**
Encounters for other specific health care	**Z40-Z53**

Foot and Ankle

Soleus muscle

Tibia

Flexor digitorum
longus muscle

Flexor hallucis tendon

Achilles tendon

Medial malleolus

Tibialis posterior tendon

Retinaculum

Tibialis posterior tendon

Tibialis anterior tendon

Extensor hallucis
brevis muscle

Abductor hallucis
muscle

Tibialis anterior
muscle

Peroneus brevis muscle

Peroneus longus tendon

Extensor digitorum
longus muscle

Tibia

Fibula

Extensor hallucis
longus muscle

Lateral malleous

Retinaculum

Peroneus
longus tendon

Extensor digitorum
brevis muscle

Calcaneus

Peroneus
brevis tendon

Peroneus
tertius tendon

Opponens digiti
minimi muscle

Dorsal interosseous muscles

Extensor hallucis
longus tendon

Extensor hallucis
brevis muscle

Extensor digitorum
longus tendons

PLATE 10. SKELETAL SYSTEM - ANTERIOR VIEW

Malignant neoplasms of bone and articular cartilage	**C40-C41**
Infectious arthropathies	**M00-M02**
Inflammatory polyarthropathies	**M05-M14**
Osteoarthritis	**M15-M19**
Other joint disorders	**M20-M25**
Dentofacial anomalies [including malocclusion] and other disorders of jaw	**M26-M27**
Systemic connective tissue disorders	**M30-M36**
Deforming dorsopathies	**M40-M43**
Spondylopathies	**M45-M49**
Other dorsopathies	**M50-M54**
Disorders of muscles	**M60-M63**
Disorders of synovium and tendon	**M65-M67**
Other soft tissue disorders	**M70-M79**
Disorders of bone density and structure	**M80-M85**
Other osteopathies	**M86-M90**
Chondropathies	**M91-M94**
Other disorders of the musculoskeletal system and connective tissue	**M95**
Intraoperative and postprocedural complications and disorders of musculoskeletal system, not elsewhere classified	**M96**
Biomechanical lesions, not elsewhere classified	**M99**
Congenital malformations of eye, ear, face and neck	**Q10-Q18**
Congenital malformations and deformations of the musculoskeletal system	**Q65-Q79**
Symptoms and signs involving the nervous and musculoskeletal systems	**R25-R29**
General symptoms and signs	**R50-R69**
Abnormal findings on diagnostic imaging and in function studies, without diagnosis	**R90-R94**
Injuries to the head	**S00-S09**
Injuries to the neck	**S10-S19**
Injuries to the thorax	**S20-S29**
Injuries to the abdomen, lower back, lumbar spine, pelvis and external genitals	**S30-S39**
Injuries to the shoulder and upper arm	**S40-S49**
Injuries to the elbow and forearm	**S50-S59**
Injuries to the wrist, hand and fingers	**S60-S69**
Injuries to the hip and thigh	**S70-S79**
Injuries to the knee and lower leg	**S80-S89**
Injuries to the ankle and foot	**S90-S99**
Injuries involving multiple body regions	**T07**
Certain early complications of trauma	**T79**
Accidents	**V00-X58**
Persons encountering health services for examinations	**Z00-Z13**
Encounters for other specific health care	**Z40-Z53**

Skeletal System
(Anterior View)

Frontal bone
Parietal bone
Temporal bone
Orbit
Nasal conchae
Zygomatic bone
Maxilla
Nasal septum
Manubrium of sternum
Mandible
Coracoid process
Hyoid bone
Acromion
Clavicle
Greater tubercle
Coracoclavicular ligament
Head of humerus
Supraspinatus tendon
Scapula
Subscapularis tendon
Humerus
Body of sternum
Xiphoid process
True ribs (1–7)
Costal cartilages
False ribs (8–12)
Anterior longitudinal ligament
Medial epicondyle
Ulnar collateral ligament
Lateral epicondyle
Radial collateral ligament
Radius
Annular ligament
Ulna
L3
Iliac crest
Sacrum
Anterior sacroiliac ligament
Anterior superior iliac spine
Interosseous membrane
Head of femur
Inguinal ligament
Greater trochanter
Coccyx
Iliofemoral ligament
Pubic symphysis
Metacarpals
Proximal phalanges
Middle phalanges
Femur
Distal phalanges

Key to Carpal Bones
A Scaphoid
B Trapezium
C Trapezoid
D Capitate
E Lunate
F Pisiform
G Triquetral
H Hamate

Medial epicondyle
Quadriceps femoris tendon
Lateral epicondyle
Tibial collateral ligament
Patella
Fibular collateral ligament
Head of fibula
Patellar ligament
Tibial tuberosity
Tibia
Fibula
Interosseous membrane

Key to Tarsal Bones
J Intermediate cuneiform
K Lateral cuneiform
L Cuboid
M Talus
N Navicular
O Calcaneus
P Medial cuneiform

Medial malleolus
Lateral malleolus

PLATE 11. SKELETAL SYSTEM - POSTERIOR VIEW

Malignant neoplasms of bone and articular cartilage	**C40-C41**
Infectious arthropathies	**M00-M02**
Inflammatory polyarthropathies	**M05-M14**
Osteoarthritis	**M15-M19**
Other joint disorders	**M20-M25**
Dentofacial anomalies [including malocclusion] and other disorders of jaw	**M26-M27**
Systemic connective tissue disorders	**M30-M36**
Deforming dorsopathies	**M40-M43**
Spondylopathies	**M45-M49**
Other dorsopathies	**M50-M54**
Disorders of muscles	**M60-M63**
Disorders of synovium and tendon	**M65-M67**
Other soft tissue disorders	**M70-M79**
Disorders of bone density and structure	**M80-M85**
Other osteopathies	**M86-M90**
Chondropathies	**M91-M94**
Other disorders of the musculoskeletal system and connective tissue	**M95**
Intraoperative and postprocedural complications and disorders of musculoskeletal system, not elsewhere classified	**M96**
Biomechanical lesions, not elsewhere classified	**M99**
Congenital malformations of eye, ear, face and neck	**Q10-Q18**
Congenital malformations and deformations of the musculoskeletal system	**Q65-Q79**
Symptoms and signs involving the nervous and musculoskeletal systems	**R25-R29**
General symptoms and signs	**R50-R69**
Abnormal findings on diagnostic imaging and in function studies, without diagnosis	**R90-R94**
Injuries to the head	**S00-S09**
Injuries to the neck	**S10-S19**
Injuries to the thorax	**S20-S29**
Injuries to the abdomen, lower back, lumbar spine, pelvis and external genitals	**S30-S39**
Injuries to the shoulder and upper arm	**S40-S49**
Injuries to the elbow and forearm	**S50-S59**
Injuries to the wrist, hand and fingers	**S60-S69**
Injuries to the hip and thigh	**S70-S79**
Injuries to the knee and lower leg	**S80-S89**
Injuries to the ankle and foot	**S90-S99**
Injuries involving multiple body regions	**T07**
Certain early complications of trauma	**T79**
Accidents	**V00-X58**
Persons encountering health services for examinations	**Z00-Z13**
Encounters for other specific health care	**Z40-Z53**

Skeletal System
(Posterior View)

PLATE 12. SKELETAL SYSTEM - VERTEBRAL COLUMN

Malignant neoplasms of bone and articular cartilage	**C40-C41**
Infectious arthropathies	**M00-M02**
Inflammatory polyarthropathies	**M05-M14**
Osteoarthritis	**M15-M19**
Other joint disorders	**M20-M25**
Dentofacial anomalies [including malocclusion] and other disorders of jaw	**M26-M27**
Systemic connective tissue disorders	**M30-M36**
Deforming dorsopathies	**M40-M43**
Spondylopathies	**M45-M49**
Other dorsopathies	**M50-M54**
Disorders of muscles	**M60-M63**
Disorders of synovium and tendon	**M65-M67**
Other soft tissue disorders	**M70-M79**
Disorders of bone density and structure	**M80-M85**
Other osteopathies	**M86-M90**
Chondropathies	**M91-M94**
Other disorders of the musculoskeletal system and connective tissue	**M95**
Intraoperative and postprocedural complications and disorders of musculoskeletal system, not elsewhere classified	**M96**
Biomechanical lesions, not elsewhere classified	**M99**
Congenital malformations of eye, ear, face and neck	**Q10-Q18**
Congenital malformations and deformations of the musculoskeletal system	**Q65-Q79**
Symptoms and signs involving the nervous and musculoskeletal systems	**R25-R29**
General symptoms and signs	**R50-R69**
Abnormal findings on diagnostic imaging and in function studies, without diagnosis	**R90-R94**
Injuries to the head	**S00-S09**
Injuries to the neck	**S10-S19**
Injuries to the thorax	**S20-S29**
Injuries to the abdomen, lower back, lumbar spine, pelvis and external genitals	**S30-S39**
Injuries involving multiple body regions	**T07**
Certain early complications of trauma	**T79**
Accidents	**V00-X58**
Persons encountering health services for examinations	**Z00-Z13**
Encounters for other specific health care	**Z40-Z53**

Vertebral Column
(Lateral View)

Atlas (C1)

Axis (C2)

Cervical
vertebrae
(C1–C7)

Cervical
curve

C7

T1

Intervertebral
discs

Thoracic
vertebrae
(T1–T12)

Thoracic
curve

Foveae for
ribs

T12

L1

Lumbar
curve

Lumbar
vertebrae
(L1–L5)

Intervertebral
foramina

L5

Sacrum

Pelvic
curve

Coccyx

©Scientific Publishing Ltd., Rolling Meadows, IL

PLATE 13. RESPIRATORY SYSTEM

Respiratory System

Frontal sinus
Superior nasal concha
Middle nasal concha
Inferior nasal concha
Sphenoid sinus
Nasopharynx
Soft palate
Oropharynx
Epiglottis
Esophagus
Thyroid cartilage
Cricoid cartilage
Trachea
Right lung
Superior lobe
Left lung
Superior lobe
Aortic arch
Left pulmonary artery
Superior lobar bronchus
Superior lobar bronchus
Superior vena cava
Left superior pulmonary vein
Middle lobar bronchus
Inferior lobar bronchus
Right atrium
Left inferior pulmonary vein
Left ventricle
Right ventricle
Oblique fissure
Middle lobe
Inferior lobe
Pericardium
Inferior lobe
Diaphragmatic pleura
Diaphragm

PLATE 14. HEART AND PERICARDIUM

Heart
(External View)

Left common
carotid artery
Left subclavian artery
Brachiocephalic
artery
Aortic arch
Ligamentum arteriosum
Superior vena cava
Left pulmonary artery
Ascending aorta
Pulmonary trunk
Left auricle
Right coronary artery
Circumflex artery
Right atrium
Great cardiac vein
Right ventricle
Anterior descending
(interventricular) artery
Anterior cardiac vein
Left ventricle
Right marginal artery
Small cardiac vein
Apex

Heart
(Internal View)

Superior vena cava
Left pulmonary artery
Right pulmonary
artery branches
Aorta
Left pulmonary veins
Pulmonary trunk
Right pulmonary
veins
Left atrium
Pulmonary
semilunar valve
Aortic semilunar
valve
Right atrium
Bicuspid
(left AV) valve
Tricuspid
(right AV) valve
Left ventricle
Papillary muscle
Chordae tendineae
Interventricular septum
Inferior vena cava
Myocardium
Right ventricle
Trabeculae carneae

PLATE 15. VASCULAR SYSTEM

Bacterial and viral infectious agents	**B95-B97**
Malignant neoplasms of ill-defined, other secondary and unspecified sites	**C76-C80**
In situ neoplasms	**D00-D09**
Benign neoplasms, except benign neuroendocrine tumors	**D10-D36**
Neoplasms of uncertain behavior, polycythemia vera and myelodysplastic syndromes	**D37-D48**
Neoplasms of unspecified behavior	**D49**
Cerebrovascular diseases	**I60-I69**
Diseases of arteries, arterioles and capillaries	**I70-I79**
Diseases of veins, lymphatic vessels and lymph nodes, not elsewhere classified	**I80-I89**
Other and unspecified disorders of the circulatory system	**I95-I99**
General symptoms and signs	**R50-R69**
Abnormal findings on diagnostic imaging and in function studies, without diagnosis	**R90-R94**
Persons encountering health services for examinations	**Z00-Z13**
Encounters for other specific health care	**Z40-Z53**

Vascular System

©Practice Management Information Corp., Los Angeles, CA

PLATE 16. DIGESTIVE SYSTEM

Intestinal infectious diseases	**A00-A09**
Bacterial and viral infectious agents	**B95-B97**
Malignant neoplasms of lip, oral cavity and pharynx	**C00-C14**
Malignant neoplasms of digestive organs	**C15-C26**
Malignant neoplasms of ill-defined, other secondary and unspecified sites	**C76-C80**
In situ neoplasms	**D00-D09**
Benign neoplasms, except benign neuroendocrine tumors	**D10-D36**
Neoplasms of uncertain behavior, polycythemia vera and myelodysplastic syndromes	**D37-D48**
Neoplasms of unspecified behavior	**D49**
Diseases of oral cavity and salivary glands	**K00-K14**
Diseases of esophagus, stomach and duodenum	**K20-K31**
Diseases of appendix	**K35-K38**
Hernia	**K40-K46**
Noninfective enteritis and colitis	**K50-K52**
Other diseases of intestines	**K55-K64**
Diseases of peritoneum and retroperitoneum	**K65-K68**
Diseases of liver	**K70-K77**
Disorders of gallbladder, biliary tract and pancreas	**K80-K87**
Other diseases of the digestive system	**K90-K95**
Cleft lip and cleft palate	**Q35-Q37**
Other congenital malformations of the digestive system	**Q38-Q45**
Symptoms and signs involving the digestive system and abdomen	**R10-R19**
General symptoms and signs	**R50-R69**
Abnormal findings on diagnostic imaging and in function studies, without diagnosis	**R90-R94**
Persons encountering health services for examinations	**Z00-Z13**
Encounters for other specific health care	**Z40-Z53**

Digestive System

Teeth

Tongue

Epiglottis

Pharynx

Larynx

Esophagus

Liver, left lobe

Liver, right lobe

Stomach

Common hepatic duct

Rugae

Aorta

Cystic duct

Portal vein

Common bile duct

Celiac trunk

Muscularis:
Oblique
Circular
Longitudinal

Pancreas

Superior mesenteric
vein & artery

Free tenia

Circular folds

Iliocecal valve

Semilunar fold

Cecum

Opening of appendix

Appendix

Levator ani muscle

External anal
sphincter muscles

©Practice Management Information Corp., Los Angeles, CA

PLATE 17. GENITOURINARY SYSTEM

Bacterial and viral infectious agents	**B95-B97**
Malignant neoplasms of urinary tract	**C64-C68**
Malignant neoplasms of ill-defined, other secondary and unspecified sites	**C76-C80**
In situ neoplasms	**D00-D09**
Benign neoplasms, except benign neuroendocrine tumors	**D10-D36**
Neoplasms of uncertain behavior, polycythemia vera and myelodysplastic syndromes	**D37-D48**
Neoplasms of unspecified behavior	**D49**
Glomerular diseases	**N00-N08**
Renal tubulointerstitial diseases	**N10-N16**
Acute kidney failure and chronic kidney disease	**N17-N19**
Urolithiasis	**N20-N23**
Other disorders of kidney and ureter	**N25-N29**
Other diseases of the urinary system	**N30-N39**
Congenital malformations of the urinary system	**Q60-Q64**
Symptoms and signs involving the genitourinary system	**R30-R39**
General symptoms and signs	**R50-R69**
Abnormal findings on examination of urine, without diagnosis	**R80-R82**
Abnormal findings on diagnostic imaging and in function studies, without diagnosis	**R90-R94**
Persons encountering health services for examinations	**Z00-Z13**
Encounters for other specific health care	**Z40-Z53**

Urinary System

Inferior vena cava

Adrenal gland

Cortex

Medulla

Kidney

Fibrous capsule

Major calyx

Minor calyx

Renal artery

Cortex

Renal vein

Renal pyramid

Renal pelvis

Renal column

Ureter

Abdominal aorta

Right common iliac vein

Left common iliac artery

Right common iliac artery

Left common iliac vein

Urinary bladder

Opening of ureter

Trigone

Urethra

PLATE 18. MALE REPRODUCTIVE SYSTEM

Male Reproductive System

Bladder
Trigone
Prostatic utricle
Prostatic urethra
Prostate
Bulbourethral gland
Membranous urethra
Bulb of penis
Crus of penis
Opening of bulbourethral gland
Corpus cavernosum
Deep artery of penis
Corpus spongiosum
Penile urethra
Corona
Glans penis
Prepuce
Urethral opening

Sigmoid colon

Peritoneum
Ampulla of ductus deferens
Urinary bladder
Seminal vesicle
Pubic symphysis
Ejaculatory duct
Prostate gland
Urogenital diaphragm
Corpus cavernosum
Corpus spongiosum
Urethra
Ductus deferens
Glans of penis
Rectum
Anus
Testis
Epididymis

PLATE 19. FEMALE REPRODUCTIVE SYSTEM

Infections with a predominantly sexual mode of transmission	**A50-A64**
Other diseases caused by chlamydiae	**A70-A74**
Bacterial and viral infectious agents	**B95-B97**
Malignant neoplasms of female genital organs	**C51-C58**
Malignant neoplasms of ill-defined, other secondary and unspecified sites	**C76-C80**
In situ neoplasms	**D00-D09**
Benign neoplasms, except benign neuroendocrine tumors	**D10-D36**
Neoplasms of uncertain behavior, polycythemia vera and myelodysplastic syndromes	**D37-D48**
Neoplasms of unspecified behavior	**D49**
Inflammatory diseases of female pelvic organs	**N70-N77**
Noninflammatory disorders of female genital tract	**N80-N98**
Intraoperative and postprocedural complications and disorders of genitourinary system, not elsewhere classified	**N99**
Congenital malformations of genital organs	**Q50-Q56**
General symptoms and signs	**R50-R69**
Abnormal findings on diagnostic imaging and in function studies, without diagnosis	**R90-R94**
Persons encountering health services for examinations	**Z00-Z13**
Estrogen receptor status	**Z17**
Persons encountering health services in circumstances related to reproduction	**Z30-Z39**
Encounters for other specific health care	**Z40-Z53**

Female Reproductive System

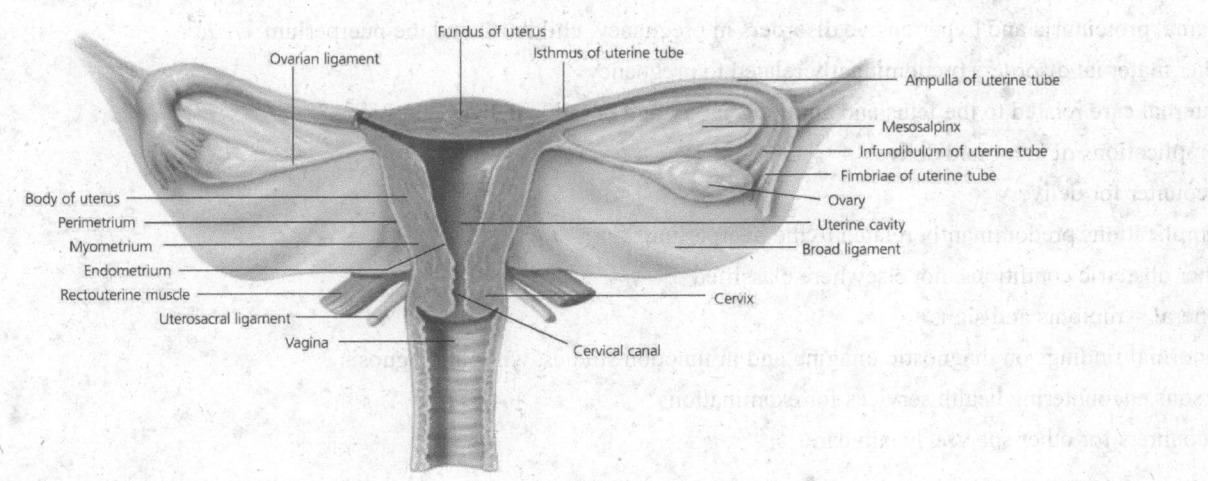

Ovarian ligament
Fundus of uterus
Isthmus of uterine tube
Ampulla of uterine tube
Mesosalpinx
Infundibulum of uterine tube
Fimbriae of uterine tube
Ovary
Body of uterus
Perimetrium
Myometrium
Uterine cavity
Endometrium
Broad ligament
Rectouterine muscle
Uterosacral ligament
Cervix
Vagina
Cervical canal

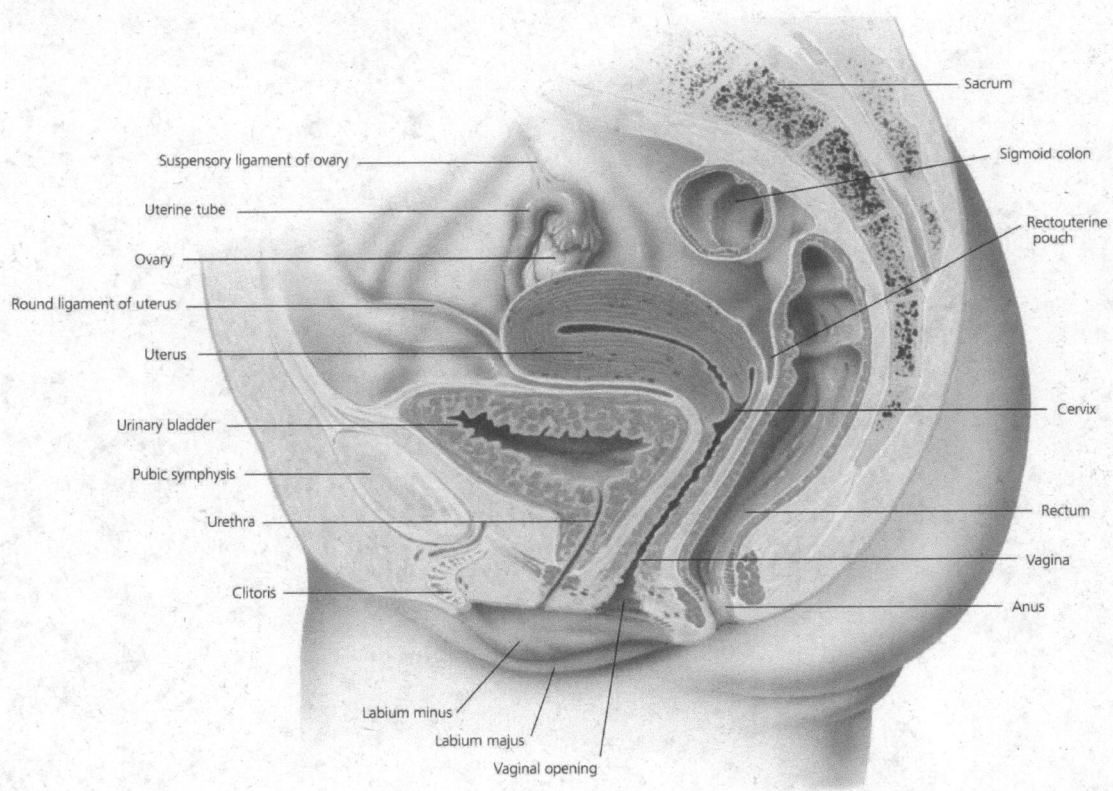

Sacrum
Sigmoid colon
Suspensory ligament of ovary
Uterine tube
Rectouterine pouch
Ovary
Round ligament of uterus
Uterus
Urinary bladder
Cervix
Pubic symphysis
Urethra
Rectum
Clitoris
Vagina
Anus
Labium minus
Labium majus
Vaginal opening

PLATE 20. PREGNANCY, CHILDBIRTH AND THE PUERPERIUM

Female Reproductive System: Pregnancy
(Lateral View)

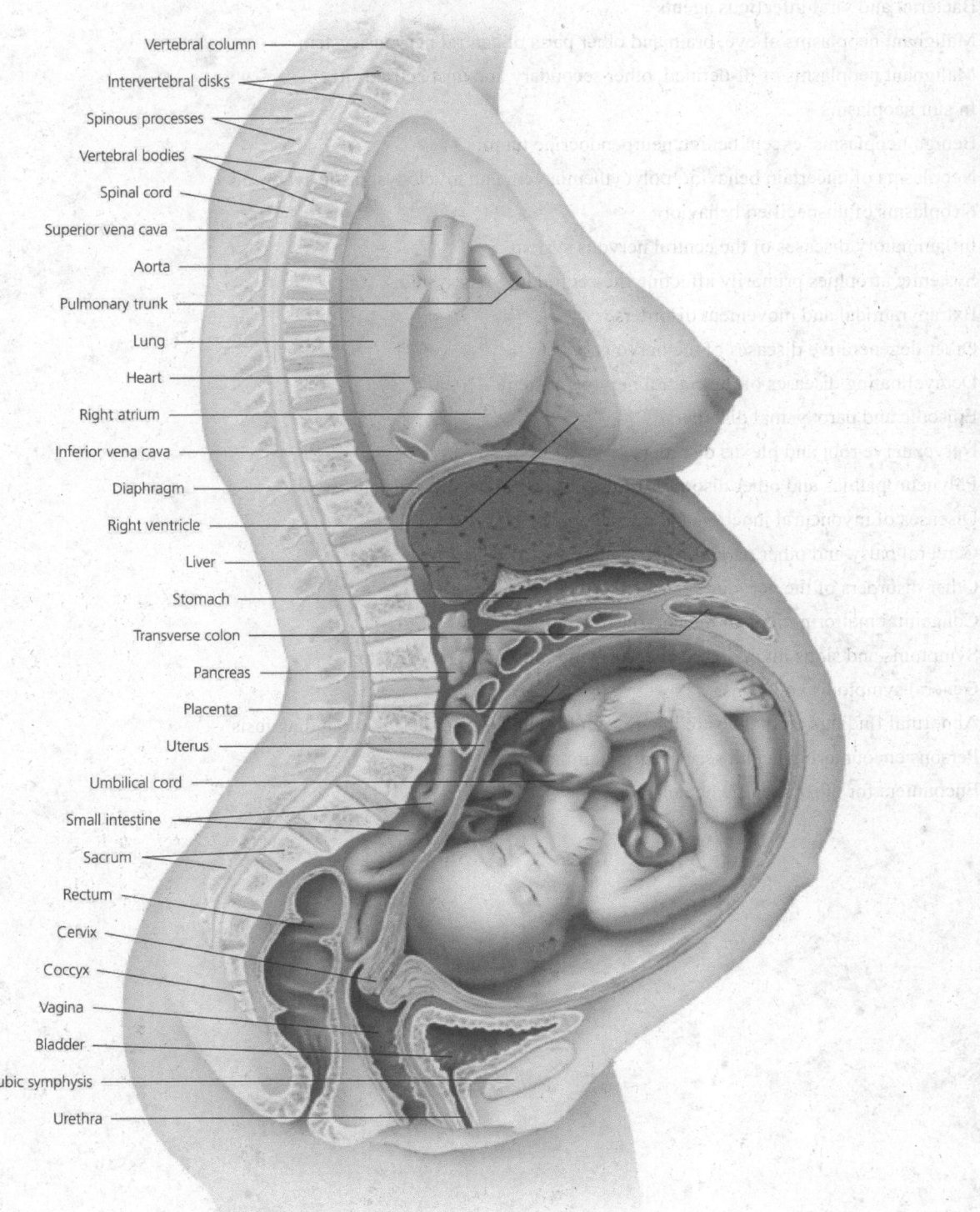

Vertebral column
Intervertebral disks
Spinous processes
Vertebral bodies
Spinal cord
Superior vena cava
Aorta
Pulmonary trunk
Lung
Heart
Right atrium
Inferior vena cava
Diaphragm
Right ventricle
Liver
Stomach
Transverse colon
Pancreas
Placenta
Uterus
Umbilical cord
Small intestine
Sacrum
Rectum
Cervix
Coccyx
Vagina
Bladder
Pubic symphysis
Urethra

PLATE 21. NERVOUS SYSTEM – BRAIN

Viral and prion infections of the central nervous system	**A80-A89**
Bacterial and viral infectious agents	**B95-B97**
Malignant neoplasms of eye, brain and other parts of central nervous system	**C69-C72**
Malignant neoplasms of ill-defined, other secondary and unspecified sites	**C76-C80**
In situ neoplasms	**D00-D09**
Benign neoplasms, except benign neuroendocrine tumors	**D10-D36**
Neoplasms of uncertain behavior, polycythemia vera and myelodysplastic syndromes	**D37-D48**
Neoplasms of unspecified behavior	**D49**
Inflammatory diseases of the central nervous system	**G00-G09**
Systemic atrophies primarily affecting the central nervous system	**G10-G14**
Extrapyramidal and movement disorders	**G20-G26**
Other degenerative diseases of the nervous system	**G30-G32**
Demyelinating diseases of the central nervous system	**G35-G37**
Episodic and paroxysmal disorders	**G40-G47**
Nerve, nerve root and plexus disorders	**G50-G59**
Polyneuropathies and other disorders of the peripheral nervous system	**G60-G65**
Diseases of myoneural junction and muscle	**G70-G73**
Cerebral palsy and other paralytic syndromes	**G80-G83**
Other disorders of the nervous system	**G89-G99**
Congenital malformations of the nervous system	**Q00-Q07**
Symptoms and signs involving the nervous and musculoskeletal systems	**R25-R29**
General symptoms and signs	**R50-R69**
Abnormal findings on diagnostic imaging and in function studies, without diagnosis	**R90-R94**
Persons encountering health services for examinations	**Z00-Z13**
Encounters for other specific health care	**Z40-Z53**

Brain
(Base View)

Cerebrum

Anterior communicating artery

Anterior cerebral artery

Middle cerebral artery

Posterior communicating artery

Posterior cerebral artery

Superior cerebellar artery

Basilar artery

Abducens nerve

Hypoglossal nerve (XII)

Accessory nerve (XI)

Vertebral artery

Anterior spinal artery

Spinal cord

Olfactory bulb

Olfactory tract (I)

Optic nerve (II)

Optic chiasm

Internal carotid artery

Pituitary gland

Oculomotor nerve (III)

Troclear nerve (IV)

Trigeminal nerve (V)

Pons

Abducens nerve (VI)

Facial nerve (VII)

Vestibulocochlear nerve (VIII)

Glossopharyngeal nerve (IX)

Vagus nerve (X)

Anterior inferior cerebellar artery

Medulla oblongata

Cerebellum

Posterior inferior cerebellar artery

PLATE 22. NERVOUS SYSTEM

Viral and prion infections of the central nervous system	**A80-A89**
Bacterial and viral infectious agents	**B95-B97**
Malignant neoplasms of eye, brain and other parts of central nervous system	**C69-C72**
Malignant neoplasms of ill-defined, other secondary and unspecified sites	**C76-C80**
In situ neoplasms	**D00-D09**
Benign neoplasms, except benign neuroendocrine tumors	**D10-D36**
Neoplasms of uncertain behavior, polycythemia vera and myelodysplastic syndromes	**D37-D48**
Neoplasms of unspecified behavior	**D49**
Inflammatory diseases of the central nervous system	**G00-G09**
Systemic atrophies primarily affecting the central nervous system	**G10-G14**
Extrapyramidal and movement disorders	**G20-G26**
Other degenerative diseases of the nervous system	**G30-G32**
Demyelinating diseases of the central nervous system	**G35-G37**
Episodic and paroxysmal disorders	**G40-G47**
Nerve, nerve root and plexus disorders	**G50-G59**
Polyneuropathies and other disorders of the peripheral nervous system	**G60-G65**
Diseases of myoneural junction and muscle	**G70-G73**
Cerebral palsy and other paralytic syndromes	**G80-G83**
Other disorders of the nervous system	**G89-G99**
Congenital malformations of the nervous system	**Q00-Q07**
Symptoms and signs involving the nervous and musculoskeletal systems	**R25-R29**
General symptoms and signs	**R50-R69**
Abnormal findings on diagnostic imaging and in function studies, without diagnosis	**R90-R94**
Persons encountering health services for examinations	**Z00-Z13**
Encounters for other specific health care	**Z40-Z53**

Nervous System

- Brain
- Cerebrum
- Cerebellum
- Brain stem
- Cervical plexus
- Lateral cord
- Medial cord
- Spinal cord
- Posterior cord
- Brachial plexus
- Musculocutaneous nerve
- Phrenic nerve
- Intercostal nerves
- Ulnar nerve
- Median nerve
- Subcostal nerve
- Radial nerve
- Iliohypogastric nerve
- Lumbar plexus
- Ilioinguinal nerve
- Genitofemoral nerve
- Deep branch of radial nerve
- Sacral plexus
- Lateral femoral cutaneous nerve
- Coccygeal plexus
- Superficial branch of radial nerve
- Femoral nerve
- Obturator nerve
- Pudendal nerve
- Sciatic nerve
- Muscular branches of femoral nerve
- Saphenous nerve
- Common peroneal nerve
- Deep peroneal nerve
- Superficial peroneal nerve
- Tibial nerve

©Practice Management Information Corp., Los Angeles, CA

PLATE 23. EYE AND OCULAR ADNEXA

Bacterial and viral infectious agents	**B95-B97**
Malignant neoplasms of eye, brain and other parts of central nervous system	**C69-C72**
Malignant neoplasms of ill-defined, other secondary and unspecified sites	**C76-C80**
In situ neoplasms	**D00-D09**
Benign neoplasms, except benign neuroendocrine tumors	**D10-D36**
Neoplasms of uncertain behavior, polycythemia vera and myelodysplastic syndromes	**D37-D48**
Neoplasms of unspecified behavior	**D49**
Disorders of eyelid, lacrimal system and orbit	**H00-H05**
Disorders of conjunctiva	**H10-H11**
Disorders of sclera, cornea, iris and ciliary body	**H15-H22**
Disorders of lens	**H25-H28**
Disorders of choroid and retina	**H30-H36**
Glaucoma	**H40-H42**
Disorders of vitreous body and globe	**H43-H44**
Disorders of optic nerve and visual pathways	**H46-H47**
Disorders of ocular muscles, binocular movement, accommodation and refraction	**H49-H52**
Visual disturbances and blindness	**H53-H54**
Other disorders of eye and adnexa	**H55-H57**
Intraoperative and postprocedural complications and disorders of eye and adnexa, not elsewhere classified	**H59**
Congenital malformations of eye, ear, face and neck	**Q10-Q18**
General symptoms and signs	**R50-R69**
Abnormal findings on diagnostic imaging and in function studies, without diagnosis	**R90-R94**
Burns and corrosions confined to eye and internal organs	**T26-T28**
Persons encountering health services for examinations	**Z00-Z13**
Encounters for other specific health care	**Z40-Z53**

Right Eye
(Horizontal Section)

Lateral rectus muscle

Conjunctiva

Canal of Schlemm

Zonular fibers

Iris

Lens

Cornea

Pupil

Aqueous humor

Anterior chamber

Posterior chamber

Ciliary body

Sclera

Ora serrata

Choroid

Medial rectus muscle

Vitreous body

Hyaloid canal

Macula lutea

Optic disc

Retinal vessels

Optic nerve

Nerve sheath

Retina

PLATE 24. AUDITORY SYSTEM

Bacterial and viral infectious agents **B95-B97**

Malignant neoplasms of ill-defined, other secondary and unspecified sites **C76-C80**

In situ neoplasms **D00-D09**

Benign neoplasms, except benign neuroendocrine tumors **D10-D36**

Neoplasms of uncertain behavior, polycythemia vera and myelodysplastic syndromes **D37-D48**

Neoplasms of unspecified behavior **D49**

Diseases of external ear **H60-H62**

Diseases of middle ear and mastoid **H65-H75**

Diseases of inner ear **H80-H83**

Other disorders of ear **H90-H94**

Intraoperative and postprocedural complications and disorders of ear and mastoid process, not elsewhere classified **H95**

Congenital malformations of eye, ear, face and neck **Q10-Q18**

General symptoms and signs **R50-R69**

Abnormal findings on diagnostic imaging and in function studies, without diagnosis **R90-R94**

Persons encountering health services for examinations **Z00-Z13**

Encounters for other specific health care **Z40-Z53**

The Ear

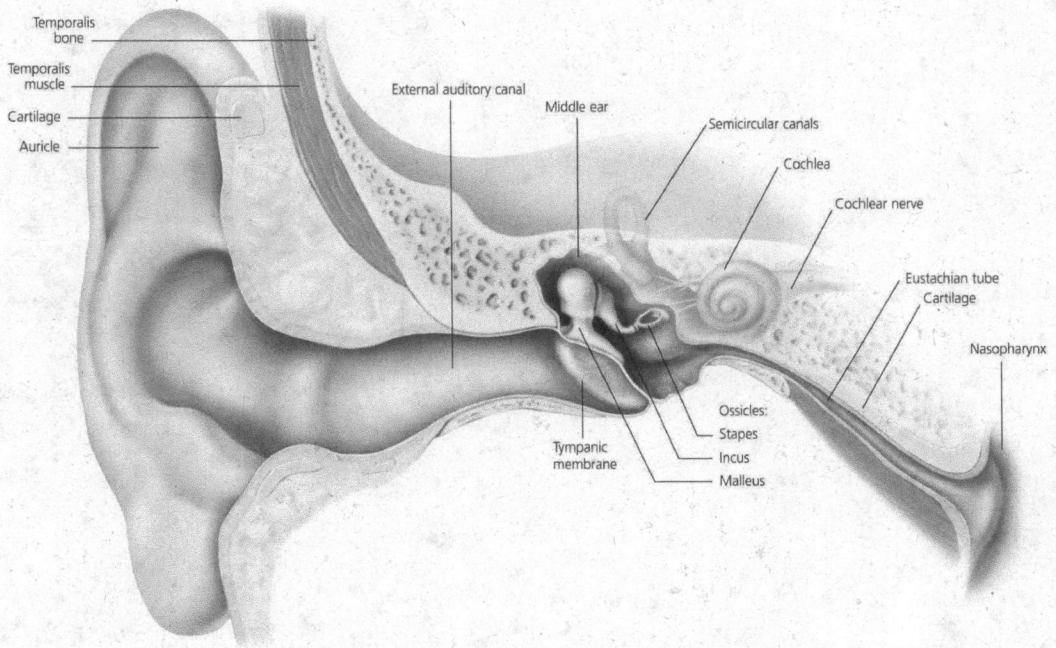

1: Certain Infectious and Parasitic Diseases (A00-B99)

DEFINITIONS

This chapter includes definitions of selected key words, terms and phrases and coding alerts for adding points to the clinical domain, and references to coding late effects where appropriate. An example from this chapter is as follows:

A01   Typhoid and paratyphoid fevers
    Definition: Typhoid fever, aka enteric fever, salmonella typhi is an illness caused by the bacterium salmonella enterica serovar typhi.

MULTIPLE CODING FOR A SINGLE CONDITION

In addition to the etiology/manifestation convention that requires two codes to fully describe a single condition that affects multiple body systems, there are other single conditions that also require more than one code. "**Use Additional Code**" notes are found in the Tabular List at codes that are not part of an etiology/manifestation pair where a secondary code is useful to fully describe a condition. The sequencing rule is the same as the etiology/manifestation pair, "**Use Additional Code**" indicates that a secondary code should be added.

For example, for bacterial infections that are not included in chapter 1, a secondary code from category B95, Streptococcus, Staphylococcus, and Enterococcus, as the cause of diseases classified elsewhere, or B96, Other bacterial agents as the cause of diseases classified elsewhere, may be required to identify the bacterial organism causing the infection. A "**Use Additional Code**" note will normally be found at the infectious disease code, indicating a need for the organism code to be added as a secondary code.

"Code first" notes are also under certain codes that are not specifically manifestation codes but may be due to an underlying cause. When there is a "Code first" note and an underlying condition is present, the underlying condition should be sequenced first.

"Code, if applicable, any causal condition first", notes indicate that this code may be assigned as a principal diagnosis when the causal condition is unknown or not applicable. If a causal condition is known, then the code for that condition should be sequenced as the principal or first-listed diagnosis.

Multiple codes may be needed for sequela, complication codes and obstetric codes to more fully describe a condition. See the specific guidelines for these conditions for further instruction.

COMBINATION CODE

A combination code is a single code used to classify: Two diagnoses, or a diagnosis with an associated secondary process (manifestation) A diagnosis with an associated complication

Combination codes are identified by referring to subterm entries in the Alphabetic Index and by reading the inclusion and exclusion notes in the Tabular List.

Assign only the combination code when that code fully identifies the diagnostic conditions involved or when the Alphabetic Index so directs. Multiple coding should not be used when the classification provides a combination code that clearly identifies all of the elements documented in the diagnosis. When the combination code lacks necessary specificity in describing the manifestation or complication, an additional code should be used as a secondary code.

SEQUELA (LATE EFFECTS)

A sequela is the residual effect (condition produced) after the acute phase of an illness or injury has terminated. There is no time limit on when a sequela code can be used. The residual may be apparent early, such as in cerebral infarction, or it may occur months or years later, such as that due to a previous injury. Coding of sequela generally requires two codes sequenced in the following order: The condition or nature of the sequela is sequenced first.

The sequela code is sequenced second.

An exception to the above guidelines are those instances where the code for the sequela is followed by a manifestation code identified in the Tabular List and title, or the sequela code has been expanded (at the fourth, fifth or sixth character levels) to

include the manifestation(s). The code for the acute phase of an illness or injury that led to the sequela is never used with a code for the late effect.

In addition to general coding guidelines, there are guidelines for specific diagnoses and/or conditions in the classification. Unless otherwise indicated, these guidelines apply to all health care settings. Please refer to Section II for guidelines on the selection of principal diagnosis.

HUMAN IMMUNODEFICIENCY VIRUS (HIV) INFECTIONS

1) **Code only confirmed cases**

   Code only confirmed cases of HIV infection/illness. This is an exception to the hospital inpatient guideline Section II, H.

   In this context, "confirmation" does not require documentation of positive serology or culture for HIV; the provider's diagnostic statement that the patient is HIV positive or has an HIV-related illness is sufficient.

2) **Selection and sequencing of HIV codes**

   (a) Patient admitted for HIV-related condition

      If a patient is admitted for an HIV-related condition, the principal diagnosis should be B20, Human immunodeficiency virus [HIV] disease followed by additional diagnosis codes for all reported HIV-related conditions.

   (b) Patient with HIV disease admitted for unrelated condition

      If a patient with HIV disease is admitted for an unrelated condition (such as a traumatic injury), the code for the unrelated condition (e.g., the nature of injury code) should be the principal diagnosis. Other diagnoses would be B20 followed by additional diagnosis codes for all reported HIV-related conditions.

   (c) Whether the patient is newly diagnosed

      Whether the patient is newly diagnosed or has had previous admissions/encounters for HIV conditions is irrelevant to the sequencing decision.

   (d) Asymptomatic human immunodeficiency virus

      Z21, Asymptomatic human immunodeficiency virus [HIV] infection status, is to be applied when the patient without any documentation of symptoms is listed as being "HIV positive," "known HIV," "HIV test positive," or similar terminology. Do not use this code if the term "AIDS" is used or if the patient is treated for any HIV-related illness or is described as having any condition(s) resulting from his/her HIV positive status; use B20 in these cases.

   (e) Patients with inconclusive HIV serology

      Patients with inconclusive HIV serology, but no definitive diagnosis or manifestations of the illness, may be assigned code R75, Inconclusive laboratory evidence of human immunodeficiency virus [HIV].

   (f) Previously diagnosed HIV-related illness

      Patients with any known prior diagnosis of an HIV-related illness should be coded to B20. Once a patient has developed an HIV-related illness, the patient should always be assigned code B20 on every subsequent admission/encounter. Patients previously diagnosed with any HIV illness (B20) should never be assigned to R75 or Z21, Asymptomatic human immunodeficiency virus [HIV] infection status.

   (g) HIV Infection in Pregnancy, Childbirth and the Puerperium

      During pregnancy, childbirth or the puerperium, a patient admitted (or presenting for a health care encounter) because of an HIV-related illness should receive a principal diagnosis code of O98.7-, Human immunodeficiency [HIV] disease complicating pregnancy, childbirth and the puerperium, followed by B20 and the code(s) for the HIV-related illness(es). Codes from Chapter 15 always take sequencing priority.

Patients with asymptomatic HIV infection status admitted (or presenting for a health care encounter) during pregnancy, childbirth, or the puerperium should receive codes of O98.7- and Z21.

(h) **Encounters for testing for HIV**

If a patient is being seen to determine his/her HIV status, use code Z11.4, Encounter for screening for human immunodeficiency virus [HIV]. Use additional codes for any associated high-risk behavior, **if applicable.**

If a patient with signs or symptoms is being seen for HIV testing, code the signs and symptoms. An additional counseling code Z71.7, Human immunodeficiency virus [HIV] counseling, may be used if counseling is provided during the encounter for the test.

When a patient returns to be informed of his/her HIV test results and the test result is negative, use code Z71.7, Human immunodeficiency virus [HIV] counseling.

If the results are positive, see previous guidelines and assign codes as appropriate.

(i) **History of HIV managed by medication**

If a patient with documented history of HIV disease is currently managed on antiretroviral medications, assign codeB20, Human immunodeficiency virus [HIV] disease. Code Z79.899, Other long term (current) drug therapy, may be assigned as an additional code to identify the long-term (current) use of antiretroviral medications.

INFECTIOUS AGENTS AS THE CAUSE OF DISEASES CLASSIFIED TO OTHER CHAPTERS

Certain infections are classified in chapters other than Chapter 1 and no organism is identified as part of the infection code. In these instances, it is necessary to use an additional code from Chapter 1 to identify the organism. A code from category B95, Streptococcus, Staphylococcus, and Enterococcus as the cause of diseases classified to other chapters, B96, Other bacterial agents as the cause of diseases classified to other chapters, or B97, Viral agents as the cause of diseases classified to other chapters, is to be used as an additional code to identify the organism. An instructional note will be found at the infection code advising that an additional organism code is required.

INFECTIONS RESISTANT TO ANTIBIOTICS

Many bacterial infections are resistant to current antibiotics. It is necessary to identify all infections documented as antibiotic resistant. Assign a code from category Z16, Resistance to antimicrobial drugs, following the infection code only if the infection code does not identify drug resistance.

SEPSIS, SEVERE SEPSIS, AND SEPTIC SHOCK

1) **Coding of Sepsis and Severe Sepsis**

(a) Sepsis

For a diagnosis of sepsis, assign the appropriate code for the underlying systemic infection. If the type of infection or causal organism is not further specified, assign code A41.9, Sepsis, unspecified organism.

A code from subcategory R65.2, Severe sepsis, should not be assigned unless severe sepsis or an associated acute organ dysfunction is documented.

(i) Negative or inconclusive blood cultures and sepsis

Negative or inconclusive blood cultures do not preclude a diagnosis of sepsis in patients with clinical evidence of the condition; however, the provider should be queried.

(ii) Urosepsis

The term urosepsis is a nonspecific term. It is not to be considered synonymous with sepsis. It has no default code in the Alphabetic Index. Should a provider use this term, he/she must be queried for clarification.

(iii) Sepsis with organ dysfunction

If a patient has sepsis and associated acute organ dysfunction or multiple organ dysfunction (MOD), follow the instructions for coding severe sepsis.

(iv) Acute organ dysfunction that is not clearly associated with the sepsis

If a patient has sepsis and an acute organ dysfunction, but the medical record documentation indicates that the acute organ dysfunction is related to a medical condition other than the sepsis, do not assign a code from subcategory R65.2, Severe sepsis. An acute organ dysfunction must be associated with the sepsis in order to assign the severe sepsis code.

If the documentation is not clear as to whether an acute organ dysfunction is related to the sepsis or another medical condition, query the provider.

(b) Severe sepsis

The coding of severe sepsis requires a minimum of 2 codes: first a code for the underlying systemic infection, followed by a code from subcategory R65.2, Severe sepsis. If the causal organism is not documented, assign code A41.9, Sepsis, unspecified organism, for the infection. Additional code(s) for the associated acute organ dysfunction are also required.

Due to the complex nature of severe sepsis, some cases may require querying the provider prior to assignment of the codes.

2) **Septic shock**

(a) Septic shock generally refers to circulatory failure associated with severe sepsis, and therefore, it represents a type of acute organ dysfunction.

For cases of septic shock, the code for the systemic infection should be sequenced first, followed by code R65.21, Severe sepsis with septic shock or code T81.12, Postprocedural septic shock. Any additional codes for the other acute organ dysfunctions should also be assigned. As noted in the sequencing instructions in the Tabular List, the code for septic shock cannot be assigned as a principal diagnosis.

3) **Sequencing of severe sepsis**

If severe sepsis is present on admission, and meets the definition of principal diagnosis, the underlying systemic infection should be assigned as principal diagnosis followed by the appropriate code from subcategory R65.2 as required by the sequencing rules in the Tabular List. A code from subcategory R65.2 can never be assigned as a principal diagnosis.

When severe sepsis develops during an encounter (it was not present on admission), the underlying systemic infection and the appropriate code from subcategory R65.2 should be assigned as secondary diagnoses.

Severe sepsis may be present on admission, but the diagnosis may not be confirmed until sometime after admission. If the documentation is not clear whether severe sepsis was present on admission, the provider should be queried.

4) **Sepsis and severe sepsis with a localized infection**

If the reason for admission is both sepsis or severe sepsis and a localized infection, such as pneumonia or cellulitis, a code(s) for the underlying systemic infection should be assigned first and the code for the localized infection should be assigned as a secondary diagnosis. If the patient has severe sepsis, a code from subcategory R65.2 should also be assigned as a secondary diagnosis. If the patient is admitted with a localized infection, such as pneumonia, and sepsis/severe sepsis does not develop until after admission, the localized infection should be assigned first, followed by the appropriate sepsis/severe sepsis codes.

5) **Sepsis due to a postprocedural infection**

   (a) Documentation of causal relationship

   As with all postprocedural complications, code assignment is based on the provider's documentation of the relationship between the infection and the procedure.

   (b) Sepsis due to a postprocedural infection

   For infections following a procedure, a code from T81.40, to T81.43 Infection following a procedure, or a code from O86.00 to O86.03, Infection of obstetric surgical wound, that identifies the site of the infection should be coded first, if known. Assign an additional code for sepsis following a procedure (T81.44) or sepsis following an obstetrical procedure (O86.04). Use an additional code to identify the infectious agent. If the patient has severe sepsis, the appropriate code from subcategory R65.2 should also be assigned with the additional code(s) for any acute organ dysfunction.

   For infections following infusion, transfusion, therapeutic injection, or immunization, a code from subcategory T80.2, Infections following infusion, transfusion, and therapeutic injection, or code T88.0-, Infection following immunization, should be coded first, followed by the code for the specific infection. If the patient has severe sepsis, the appropriate code from subcategory R65.2 should also be assigned, with the additional codes(s) for any acute organ dysfunction.

   (c) Postprocedural infection and postprocedural septic shock

   If a postprocedural infection has resulted in postprocedural septic shock, assign the codes indicated above for sepsis due to a postprocedural infection, followed by code T81.12-, Postprocedural septic shock. Do not assign code R65.21, Severe sepsis with septic shock. Additional code(s)should be assigned for any acute organ dysfunction.

6) **Sepsis and severe sepsis associated with a noninfectious process (condition)**

   In some cases, a noninfectious process (condition), such as trauma, may lead to an infection which can result in sepsis or severe sepsis. If sepsis or severe sepsis is documented as associated with a noninfectious condition, such as a burn or serious injury, and this condition meets the definition for principal diagnosis, the code for the noninfectious condition should be sequenced first, followed by the code for the resulting infection. If severe sepsis is present, a code from subcategory R65.2 should also be assigned with any associated organ dysfunction(s) codes. It is not necessary to assign a code from subcategory R65.1, Systemic inflammatory response syndrome (SIRS) of non-infectious origin, for these cases.

   If the infection meets the definition of principal diagnosis, it should be sequenced before the non-infectious condition. When both the associated non-infectious condition and the infection meet the definition of principal diagnosis, either may be assigned as principal diagnosis.

   Only one code from category R65, Symptoms and signs specifically associated with systemic inflammation and infection, should be assigned. Therefore, when a non-infectious condition leads to an infection resulting in severe sepsis, assign the appropriate code from subcategory R65.2, Severe sepsis. Do not additionally assign a code from subcategory R65.1, Systemic inflammatory response syndrome (SIRS) of non-infectious origin.

   See Section I.C.18. SIRS due to non-infectious process

7) **Sepsis and septic shock complicating abortion, pregnancy, childbirth, and the puerperium**

   See Section I.C.15. Sepsis and septic shock complicating abortion, pregnancy, childbirth and the puerperium

8) **Newborn sepsis**

   See Section I.C.16. f. Bacterial sepsis of Newborn

METHICILLIN RESISTANT STAPHYLOCOCCUS AUREUS (MRSA) CONDITIONS

1) **Selection and sequencing of MRSA codes**

(a) Combination codes for MRSA infection

When a patient is diagnosed with an infection that is due to methicillin resistant *Staphylococcus aureus* (MRSA), and that infection has a combination code that includes the causal organism (e.g., sepsis, pneumonia) assign the appropriate combination code for the condition (e.g., code A41.02, Sepsis due to Methicillin resistant Staphylococcus aureus or code J15.212, Pneumonia due to Methicillin resistant Staphylococcus aureus). Do not assign code B95.62, Methicillin resistant Staphylococcus aureus infection as the cause of diseases classified elsewhere, as an additional code, because the combination code includes the type of infection and the MRSA organism. Do not assign a code from subcategory Z16.11, Resistance to penicillins, as an additional diagnosis.

See Section C.1. for instructions on coding and sequencing of sepsis and severe sepsis.

(b) Other codes for MRSA infection

When there is documentation of a current infection (e.g., wound infection, stitch abscess, urinary tract infection) due to MRSA, and that infection does not have a combination code that includes the causal organism, assign the appropriate code to identify the condition along with code B95.62, Methicillin resistant Staphylococcus aureus infection as the cause of diseases classified elsewhere for the MRSA infection. Do not assign a code from subcategory Z16.11, Resistance to penicillins.

(c) Methicillin susceptible Staphylococcus aureus (MSSA) and MRSA colonization

The condition or state of being colonized or carrying MSSA or MRSA is called colonization or carriage, while an individual person is described as being colonized or being a carrier. Colonization means that MSSA or MSRA is present on or in the body without necessarily causing illness. A positive MRSA colonization test might be documented by the provider as "MRSA screen positive" or "MRSA nasal swab positive".

Assign code Z22.322, Carrier or suspected carrier of Methicillin resistant Staphylococcus aureus, for patients documented as having MRSA colonization. Assign code Z22.321, Carrier or suspected carrier of Methicillin susceptible Staphylococcus aureus, for patient documented as having MSSA colonization. Colonization is not necessarily indicative of a disease process or as the cause of a specific condition the patient may have unless documented as such by the provider.

(d) MRSA colonization and infection

If a patient is documented as having both MRSA colonization and infection during a hospital admission, code Z22.322, Carrier or suspected carrier of Methicillin resistant Staphylococcus aureus, and a code for the MRSA infection may both be assigned.

ZIKA VIRUS INFECTIONS

1) Code only confirmed cases

Code only a confirmed diagnosis of Zika virus (A92.5, Zika virus disease) as documented by the provider. This is an exception to the hospital inpatient guideline Section II, H. In this context, "confirmation" does not require documentation of the type of test performed; the provider's diagnostic statement that the condition is confirmed is sufficient. This code should be assigned regardless of the stated mode of transmission.

If the provider documents "suspected", "possible" or "probable" Zika, do not assign code A92.5. Assign a code(s) explaining the reason for encounter (such as fever, rash, or joint pain) or Z20.821, Contact with and (suspected) exposure to Zika virus.

CORONAVIRUS INFECTIONS

1) COVID-19 infection (infection due to SARS-CoV-2)

(a) Code only confirmed cases

Code only a confirmed diagnosis of the 2019 novel coronavirus disease (COVID-19) as documented by the provider or documentation of a positive COVID-19 test result. For a confirmed diagnosis, assign code U07.1, COVID-19. This

● New code ▲ Revised code **Excludes1:** Not coded here **Excludes2:** Not included here ⊗ Placeholder required ⑦7th digit required

is an exception to the hospital inpatient guideline Section II, H. In this context, "confirmation" does not require documentation of a positive test result for COVID-19; the provider's documentation that the individual has COVID-19 is sufficient.

If the provider documents "suspected," "possible," "probable," or "inconclusive" COVID-19, do not assign code U07.1. Instead, code the signs and symptoms reported. See guideline I.C.1.g.1.g.

(b) **Sequencing of codes**

When COVID-19 meets the definition of principal diagnosis, code U07.1, COVID-19, should be sequenced first, followed by the appropriate codes for associated manifestations, except when another guideline requires that certain codes be sequenced first, such as obstetrics, sepsis, or transplant complications.

For a COVID-19 infection that progresses to sepsis, see Section I.C.1.d. Sepsis, Severe Sepsis, and Septic Shock
See Section I.C.15.s. for COVID-19 infection in pregnancy, childbirth, and the puerperium
See Section I.C.16.h. for COVID-19 infection in newborn
For a COVID-19 infection in a lung transplant patient, see Section I.C.19.g.3.a. Transplant complications other than kidney.

(c) **Acute respiratory manifestations of COVID-19**

When the reason for the encounter/admission is a respiratory manifestation of COVID-19, assign code U07.1, COVID-19, as the principal/first-listed diagnosis and assign code(s) for the respiratory manifestation(s) as additional diagnoses.
The following conditions are examples of common respiratory manifestations of COVID-19.

(i) Pneumonia

For a patient with pneumonia confirmed as due to COVID-19, assign codes U07.1, COVID-19, and J12.89, Other viral pneumonia.

(ii) Acute bronchitis

For a patient with acute bronchitis confirmed as due to COVID-19, assign codes U07.1, and J20.8, Acute bronchitis due to other specified organisms.

Bronchitis not otherwise specified (NOS) due to COVID-19 should be coded using code U07.1 and J40, Bronchitis, not specified as acute or chronic.

(iii) Lower respiratory infection

If the COVID-19 is documented as being associated with a lower respiratory infection, not otherwise specified (NOS), or an acute respiratory infection, NOS, codes U07.1 and J22, Unspecified acute lower respiratory infection, should be assigned.

If the COVID-19 is documented as being associated with a respiratory infection, NOS, codes U07.1 and J98.8, Other specified respiratory disorders, should be assigned.

(iv) Acute respiratory distress syndrome

For acute respiratory distress syndrome (ARDS) due to COVID-19, assign codes U07.1, and J80, Acute respiratory distress syndrome.

(v) Acute respiratory failure

For acute respiratory failure due to COVID-19, assign code U07.1, and code J96.0-, Acute respiratory failure.

(d) Non-respiratory manifestations of COVID-19

When the reason for the encounter/admission is a non-respiratory manifestation (e.g., viral enteritis) of COVID-19, assign code U07.1, COVID-19, as the principal/first-listed diagnosis and assign code(s) for the manifestation(s) as additional diagnoses.

(e) Exposure to COVID-19

For asymptomatic individuals with actual or suspected exposure to COVID-19, assign code Z20.828, Contact with and (suspected) exposure to other viral communicable diseases.

For symptomatic individuals with actual or suspected exposure to COVID-19 and the infection has been ruled out, or test results are inconclusive or unknown, assign code Z20.828, Contact with and (suspected) exposure to other viral communicable diseases. See guideline I.C.21.c.1, Contact/Exposure, for additional guidance regarding the use of category Z20 codes.

If COVID-19 is confirmed, see guideline I.C.1.g.1.a.

(f) Screening for COVID-19

During the COVID-19 pandemic, a screening code is generally not appropriate. For encounters for COVID-19 testing, including preoperative testing, code as exposure to COVID-19 (guideline I.C.1.g.1.e).

Coding guidance will be updated as new information concerning any changes in the pandemic status becomes available.

(g) Signs and symptoms without definitive diagnosis of COVID-19

For patients presenting with any signs/symptoms associated with COVID-19 (such as fever, etc.) but a definitive diagnosis has not been established, assign the appropriate code(s) for each of the presenting signs and symptoms such as:

- R05.1, Acute cough, or R05.9, Cough, unspecified
- R06.02   Shortness of breath
- R50.9   Fever, unspecified

If a patient with signs/symptoms associated with COVID-19 also has an actual or suspected contact with or exposure to COVID-19, assign Z20.828, Contact with and (suspected) exposure to other viral communicable diseases, as an additional code.

(h) Asymptomatic individuals who test positive for COVID-19

For asymptomatic individuals who test positive for COVID-19, see guideline I.C.1.g.1.a. Although the individual is asymptomatic, the individual has tested positive and is considered to have the COVID-19 infection.

(i) Personal history of COVID-19

For patients with a history of COVID-19, assign code Z86.19, Personal history of other infectious and parasitic diseases.

(j) Follow-up visits after COVID-19 infection has resolved

For individuals who previously had COVID-19, without residual symptom(s) or condition(s), and are being seen for follow-up evaluation, and COVID-19 test results are negative, assign codes Z09, Encounter for follow-up examination after completed treatment for conditions other than malignant neoplasm, and Z86.19, Personal history of other infectious and parasitic diseases.

For follow-up visits for individuals with symptom(s) or condition(s) related to a previous COVID-19 infection, seeguideline I.C.1.g.1.m.

See Section I.C.21.c.8, Factors influencing health states andcontact with health services, Follow-up

(k) Encounter for antibody testing

For an encounter for antibody testing that is not being performed to confirm a current COVID-19 infection, nor is a follow-up test after resolution of COVID-19, assign Z01.84, Encounter for antibody response examination.

Follow the applicable guidelines above if the individual is being tested to confirm a current COVID-19 infection.

For follow-up testing after a COVID-19 infection, see guideline I.C.1.g.1.j.

(l) Multisystem Inflammatory Syndrome

For individuals with multisystem inflammatory syndrome (MIS)and COVID-19, assign code U07.1, COVID-19, as the principal/first-listed diagnosis and assign code M35.81, Multisystem inflammatory syndrome, as an additional diagnosis.

If an individual with a history of COVID-19 develops MIS, assign codes M35.81, Multisystem inflammatory syndrome, andU09.9, Post COVID-19 condition, unspecified.

If an individual with a known or suspected exposure to COVID- 19, and no current COVID-19 infection or history of COVID-19,develops MIS, assign codes M35.81, Multisystem inflammatory syndrome, and Z20.822, Contact with and (suspected) exposure to COVID-19.

Additional codes should be assigned for any associatedcomplications of MIS.

(m) Post COVID-19 Condition

For sequela of COVID-19, or associated symptoms or conditions that develop following a previous COVID-19 infection, assign a code(s) for the specific symptom(s) or condition(s) related to the previous COVID-19 infection, ifknown, and code U09.9, Post COVID-19 condition, unspecified.

Code U09.9 should not be assigned for manifestations of anactive (current) COVID-19 infection.

If a patient has a condition(s) associated with a previous COVID-19 infection and develops a new active (current) COVID-19 infection, code U09.9 may be assigned in conjunction with code U07.1, COVID-19, to identify that the patient also has a condition(s) associated with a previous COVID-19 infection. Code(s) for the specific condition(s) associated with the previous COVID-19 infection and code(s)for manifestation(s) of the new active (current) COVID-19 infection should also be assigned.

Chapter 1

Certain Infectious and Parasitic Diseases (A00-B99)

Includes: diseases generally recognized as communicable or transmissible

Use Additional Code to identify resistance to antimicrobial drugs (Z16.-)

Excludes1: certain localized infections - see body system-related chapters

Excludes2: carrier or suspected carrier of infectious disease (Z22.-)

infectious and parasitic diseases complicating pregnancy, childbirth and the puerperium (O98.-)

infectious and parasitic diseases specific to the perinatal period (P35-P39)

influenza and other acute respiratory infections (J00-J22)

This chapter contains the following blocks:

A00-A09	Intestinal infectious diseases
A15-A19	Tuberculosis
A20-A28	Certain zoonotic bacterial diseases
A30-A49	Other bacterial diseases
A50-A64	Infections with a predominantly sexual mode of transmission
A65-A69	Other spirochetal diseases
A70-A74	Other diseases caused by chlamydiae
A75-A79	Rickettsioses
A80-A89	Viral and prion infections of the central nervous system
A90-A99	Arthropod-borne viral fevers and viral hemorrhagic fevers
B00-B09	Viral infections characterized by skin and mucous membrane lesions
B10	Other human herpesviruses
B15-B19	Viral hepatitis
B20	Human immunodeficiency virus [HIV] disease
B25-B34	Other viral diseases
B35-B49	Mycoses
B50-B64	Protozoal diseases
B65-B83	Helminthiases
B85-B89	Pediculosis, acariasis and other infestations
B90-B94	Sequelae of infectious and parasitic diseases
B95-B97	Bacterial and viral infectious agents
B99	Other infectious diseases

INTESTINAL INFECTIOUS DISEASES (A00-A09)

A00 Cholera

Definition: Cholera, aka Asiatic or epidemic cholera, is an infectious gastroenteritis caused by enterotoxin-producing strains of the bacterium vibrio cholerae.

A00.0 Cholera due to Vibrio cholerae 01, biovar cholerae

Classical cholera

A00.1 Cholera due to Vibrio cholerae 01, biovar eltor

Cholera eltor

A00.9 Cholera, unspecified

A01 Typhoid and paratyphoid fevers

A01.0 Typhoid fever

Definition: Typhoid fever, aka enteric fever, salmonella typhi is an illness caused by the bacterium salmonella enterica serovar typhi.

Infection due to Salmonella typhi

A01.00 Typhoid fever, unspecified

A01.01 Typhoid meningitis

A01.02 Typhoid fever with heart involvement

Typhoid endocarditis

Typhoid myocarditis

A01.03 Typhoid pneumonia [HCC]

A01.04 Typhoid arthritis [HCC]

A01.05 Typhoid osteomyelitis [HCC]

A01.09 Typhoid fever with other complications

A01.1 Paratyphoid fever A

A01.2 Paratyphoid fever B

A01.3 Paratyphoid fever C

A01.4 Paratyphoid fever, unspecified

Infection due to Salmonella paratyphi NOS

A02 Other salmonella infections

Definition: Salmonellosis is an infection with salmonella bacteria. Most persons infected with salmonella develop diarrhea, fever, vomiting, and abdominal cramps.

Includes: infection or foodborne intoxication due to any Salmonella species other than S. typhi and S. paratyphi

A02.0 Salmonella enteritis

Salmonellosis

A02.1 Salmonella sepsis [HCC]

A02.2 Localized salmonella infections

A02.20 Localized salmonella infection, unspecified

A02.21 Salmonella meningitis

A02.22 Salmonella pneumonia [HCC]

A02.23 Salmonella arthritis [HCC]

A02.24 Salmonella osteomyelitis [HCC]

A02.25 Salmonella pyelonephritis

Salmonella tubulo-interstitial nephropathy

A02.29 Salmonella with other localized infection

A02.8 Other specified salmonella infections

A02.9 Salmonella infection, unspecified

A03 Shigellosis

Definition: Shigellosis, aka bacillary dysentery, is a food borne illness caused by infection by bacteria of the genus shigella.

A03.0 Shigellosis due to Shigella dysenteriae

Group A shigellosis [Shiga-Kruse dysentery]

A03.1 Shigellosis due to Shigella flexneri

Group B shigellosis

A03.2 Shigellosis due to Shigella boydii

Group C shigellosis

A03.3 Shigellosis due to Shigella sonnei

Group D shigellosis

A03.8 Other shigellosis

A03.9 Shigellosis, unspecified

Bacillary dysentery NOS

A04 Other bacterial intestinal infections

Excludes1: bacterial foodborne intoxications, NEC (A05.-)

tuberculous enteritis (A18.32)

A04.0 Enteropathogenic Escherichia coli infection

A04.1 Enterotoxigenic Escherichia coli infection

A04.2 Enteroinvasive Escherichia coli infection

A04.3 Enterohemorrhagic Escherichia coli infection

A04.4 Other intestinal Escherichia coli infections

Escherichia coli enteritis NOS

A04.5 **Campylobacter enteritis**

A04.6 **Enteritis due to Yersinia enterocolitica**

Excludes1: extraintestinal yersiniosis (A28.2)

A04.7 **Enterocolitis due to Clostridium difficile**

Foodborne intoxication by Clostridium difficile

Pseudomembranous colitis

A04.71 **Enterocolitis due to Clostridium difficile, recurrent**

A04.72 **Enterocolitis due to Clostridium difficile, not specified as recurrent**

A04.8 Other specified bacterial intestinal infections

A04.9 Bacterial intestinal infection, unspecified

Bacterial enteritis NOS

A05 **Other bacterial foodborne intoxications, not elsewhere classified**

Excludes1: Clostridium difficile foodborne intoxication and infection (A04.7-)

Escherichia coli infection (A04.0-A04.4)

listeriosis (A32.-)

salmonella foodborne intoxication and infection (A02.-)

toxic effect of noxious foodstuffs (T61-T62)

A05.0 **Foodborne staphylococcal intoxication**

A05.1 **Botulism food poisoning**

Botulism NOS

Classical foodborne intoxication due to Clostridium botulinum

Excludes1: infant botulism (A48.51)

wound botulism (A48.52)

A05.2 **Foodborne Clostridium perfringens [Clostridium welchii] intoxication**

Enteritis necroticans

Pig-bel

A05.3 **Foodborne Vibrio parahaemolyticus intoxication**

A05.4 **Foodborne Bacillus cereus intoxication**

A05.5 **Foodborne Vibrio vulnificus intoxication**

A05.8 **Other specified bacterial foodborne intoxications**

A05.9 **Bacterial foodborne intoxication, unspecified**

A06 **Amebiasis**

Definition: Amebiasis is an inflammation of the intestines caused by infection with entamoeba histolytica characterized by frequent, loose stools flecked with blood and mucus.

Includes: infection due to Entamoeba histolytica

Excludes1: Other protozoal intestinal diseases (A07.-)

Excludes2: acanthamebiasis (B60.1-)

Naegleriasis (B60.2)

A06.0 **Acute amebic dysentery**

Acute amebiasis

Intestinal amebiasis NOS

A06.1 **Chronic intestinal amebiasis**

A06.2 **Amebic nondysenteric colitis**

A06.3 **Ameboma of intestine**

Ameboma NOS

A06.4 **Amebic liver abscess**

Hepatic amebiasis

A06.5 **Amebic lung abscess** [HCC]

Amebic abscess of lung (and liver)

A06.6 **Amebic brain abscess**

Amebic abscess of brain (and liver) (and lung)

A06.7 **Cutaneous amebiasis**

A06.8 **Amebic infection of other sites**

A06.81 **Amebic cystitis**

A06.82 **Other amebic genitourinary infections**

Amebic balanitis

Amebic vesiculitis

Amebic vulvovaginitis

A06.89 **Other amebic infections**

Amebic appendicitis

Amebic splenic abscess

A06.9 **Amebiasis, unspecified**

A07 **Other protozoal intestinal diseases**

Definition: Protozoal intestinal diseases refers to diseases of the intestinal system caused by protozoa, which are single-cell organisms that can only divide within a host organism. Malaria , Giardia and toxoplasmosis are examples of diseases caused by protozoa.

A07.0 **Balantidiasis**

Balantidial dysentery

A07.1 **Giardiasis [lambliasis]**

A07.2 **Cryptosporidiosis** [HCC]

A07.3 **Isosporiasis**

Infection due to Isospora belli and Isospora hominis

Intestinal coccidiosis

Isosporosis

A07.4 **Cyclosporiasis**

A07.8 **Other specified protozoal intestinal diseases**

Intestinal microsporidiosis

Intestinal trichomoniasis

Sarcocystosis

Sarcosporidiosis

A07.9 **Protozoal intestinal disease, unspecified**

Flagellate diarrhea

Protozoal colitis

Protozoal diarrhea

Protozoal dysentery

A08 **Viral and other specified intestinal infections**

Excludes1: influenza with involvement of gastrointestinal tract (J09.X3, J10.2, J11.2)

A08.0 **Rotaviral enteritis**

A08.1 **Acute gastroenteropathy due to Norwalk agent and other small round viruses**

A08.11 **Acute gastroenteropathy due to Norwalk agent**

Acute gastroenteropathy due to Norovirus

Acute gastroenteropathy due to Norwalk-like agent

A08.19 **Acute gastroenteropathy due to other small round viruses**

Acute gastroenteropathy due to small round virus [SRV] NOS

A08.2 **Adenoviral enteritis**

A08.3 **Other viral enteritis**

A08.31 **Calicivirus enteritis**

A08.32 **Astrovirus enteritis**

A08.39 **Other viral enteritis**

Coxsackie virus enteritis

● New code ▲ Revised code Excludes1: Not coded here Excludes2: Not included here ⊗ Placeholder required ⑦7th digit required

Echovirus enteritis

Enterovirus enteritis NEC

Torovirus enteritis

A08.4 **Viral intestinal infection, unspecified**

Viral enteritis NOS

Viral gastroenteritis NOS

Viral gastroenteropathy NOS

A08.8 **Other specified intestinal infections**

A09 **Infectious gastroenteritis and colitis, unspecified**

Infectious colitis NOS

Infectious enteritis NOS

Infectious gastroenteritis NOS

Excludes1: colitis NOS (K52.9)

diarrhea NOS (R19.7)

enteritis NOS (K52.9)

gastroenteritis NOS (K52.9)

noninfective gastroenteritis and colitis, unspecified (K52.9)

TUBERCULOSIS (A15-A19)

Definition: Tuberculosis is a common and often deadly infectious disease caused by mycobacteria, in humans mainly mycobacterium tuberculosis. Tuberculosis usually attacks the lungs but can also affect the central nervous system, the lymphatic system, the circulatory system, the genitourinary system, the gastrointestinal system, bones, joints, and even the skin.

Includes: infections due to Mycobacterium tuberculosis and Mycobacterium bovis

Excludes1: congenital tuberculosis (P37.0)

nonspecific reaction to test for tuberculosis without active tuberculosis (R76.1-)

pneumoconiosis associated with tuberculosis, any type in A15 (J65)

positive PPD (R76.11)

positive tuberculin skin test without active tuberculosis (R76.11)

sequelae of tuberculosis (B90.-)

silicotuberculosis (J65)

A15 **Respiratory tuberculosis**

A15.0 **Tuberculosis of lung**

Tuberculous bronchiectasis

Tuberculous fibrosis of lung

Tuberculous pneumonia

Tuberculous pneumothorax

A15.4 **Tuberculosis of intrathoracic lymph nodes**

Tuberculosis of hilar lymph nodes

Tuberculosis of mediastinal lymph nodes

Tuberculosis of tracheobronchial lymph nodes

Excludes1: tuberculosis specified as primary (A15.7)

A15.5 **Tuberculosis of larynx, trachea and bronchus**

Tuberculosis of bronchus

Tuberculosis of glottis

Tuberculosis of larynx

Tuberculosis of trachea

A15.6 **Tuberculous pleurisy**

Tuberculosis of pleura

Tuberculous empyema

Excludes1: primary respiratory tuberculosis (A15.7)

A15.7 **Primary respiratory tuberculosis**

A15.8 **Other respiratory tuberculosis**

Mediastinal tuberculosis

Nasopharyngeal tuberculosis

Tuberculosis of nose

Tuberculosis of sinus [any nasal]

A15.9 **Respiratory tuberculosis unspecified**

A17 **Tuberculosis of nervous system**

A17.0 **Tuberculous meningitis**

Tuberculosis of meninges (cerebral)(spinal)

Tuberculous leptomeningitis

Excludes1: tuberculous meningoencephalitis (A17.82)

A17.1 **Meningeal tuberculoma**

Tuberculoma of meninges (cerebral) (spinal)

Excludes2: tuberculoma of brain and spinal cord (A17.81)

A17.8 **Other tuberculosis of nervous system**

A17.81 **Tuberculoma of brain and spinal cord**

Tuberculous abscess of brain and spinal cord

A17.82 **Tuberculous meningoencephalitis**

Tuberculous myelitis

A17.83 **Tuberculous neuritis**

Tuberculous mononeuropathy

A17.89 **Other tuberculosis of nervous system**

Tuberculous polyneuropathy

A17.9 **Tuberculosis of nervous system, unspecified**

A18 **Tuberculosis of other organs**

A18.0 **Tuberculosis of bones and joints**

A18.01 **Tuberculosis of spine**

Pott's disease or curvature of spine

Tuberculous arthritis

Tuberculous osteomyelitis of spine

Tuberculous spondylitis

A18.02 **Tuberculous arthritis of other joints**

Tuberculosis of hip (joint)

Tuberculosis of knee (joint)

A18.03 **Tuberculosis of other bones**

Tuberculous mastoiditis

Tuberculous osteomyelitis

A18.09 **Other musculoskeletal tuberculosis**

Tuberculous myositis

Tuberculous synovitis

Tuberculous tenosynovitis

A18.1 **Tuberculosis of genitourinary system**

A18.10 **Tuberculosis of genitourinary system, unspecified**

A18.11 **Tuberculosis of kidney and ureter**

A18.12 **Tuberculosis of bladder**

A18.13 **Tuberculosis of other urinary organs**

Tuberculous urethritis

A18.14 **Tuberculosis of prostate**

A18.15 **Tuberculosis of other male genital organs**

A18.16 **Tuberculosis of cervix**

A18.17 **Tuberculous female pelvic inflammatory disease**

Tuberculous endometritis

Tuberculous oophoritis and salpingitis

A18.18 **Tuberculosis of other female genital organs**

Tuberculous ulceration of vulva

A18.2 **Tuberculous peripheral lymphadenopathy**

Tuberculous adenitis

Excludes2: tuberculosis of bronchial and mediastinal lymph nodes (A15.4)

tuberculosis of mesenteric and retroperitoneal lymph nodes (A18.39)

tuberculous tracheobronchial adenopathy (A15.4)

A18.3 **Tuberculosis of intestines, peritoneum and mesenteric glands**

A18.31 **Tuberculous peritonitis**

Tuberculous ascites

A18.32 **Tuberculous enteritis**

Tuberculosis of anus and rectum

Tuberculosis of intestine (large) (small)

A18.39 **Retroperitoneal tuberculosis**

Tuberculosis of mesenteric glands

Tuberculosis of retroperitoneal (lymph glands)

A18.4 **Tuberculosis of skin and subcutaneous tissue**

Erythema induratum, tuberculous

Lupus exedens

Lupus vulgaris NOS

Lupus vulgaris of eyelid

Scrofuloderma

Tuberculosis of external ear

Excludes2: lupus erythematosus (L93.-)

Systemic lupus erythematosus (M32.-)

A18.5 **Tuberculosis of eye**

Excludes2: lupus vulgaris of eyelid (A18.4)

A18.50 **Tuberculosis of eye, unspecified**

A18.51 **Tuberculous episcleritis**

A18.52 **Tuberculous keratitis**

Tuberculous interstitial keratitis

Tuberculous keratoconjunctivitis (interstitial) (phlyctenular)

A18.53 **Tuberculous chorioretinitis**

A18.54 **Tuberculous iridocyclitis**

A18.59 **Other tuberculosis of eye**

Tuberculous conjunctivitis

A18.6 **Tuberculosis of (inner) (middle) ear**

Tuberculous otitis media

Excludes2: tuberculosis of external ear (A18.4)

tuberculous mastoiditis (A18.03)

A18.7 **Tuberculosis of adrenal glands**

Tuberculous Addison's disease

A18.8 **Tuberculosis of other specified organs**

A18.81 **Tuberculosis of thyroid gland**

A18.82 **Tuberculosis of other endocrine glands**

Tuberculosis of pituitary gland

Tuberculosis of thymus gland

A18.83 **Tuberculosis of digestive tract organs, not elsewhere classified**

Excludes1: tuberculosis of intestine (A18.32)

A18.84 **Tuberculosis of heart**

Tuberculous cardiomyopathy

Tuberculous endocarditis

Tuberculous myocarditis

Tuberculous pericarditis

A18.85 **Tuberculosis of spleen**

A18.89 **Tuberculosis of other sites**

Tuberculosis of muscle

Tuberculous cerebral arteritis

A19 **Miliary tuberculosis**

Definition: Miliary tuberculosis acute tuberculosis characterized by the appearance of tiny tubercles on one or more organs of the body.

Includes: disseminated tuberculosis

generalized tuberculosis tuberculous polyserositis

A19.0 **Acute miliary tuberculosis of a single specified site**

A19.1 **Acute miliary tuberculosis of multiple sites**

A19.2 **Acute miliary tuberculosis, unspecified**

A19.8 **Other miliary tuberculosis**

A19.9 **Miliary tuberculosis, unspecified**

CERTAIN ZOONOTIC BACTERIAL DISEASES (A20-A28)

A20 **Plague**

Definition: Plague is a deadly infectious disease caused by the enterobacteria yersinia pestis (pasteurella pestis).

Includes: infection due to Yersinia pestis

A20.0 **Bubonic plague**

A20.1 **Cellulocutaneous plague**

A20.2 **Pneumonic plague** [HCC]

A20.3 **Plague meningitis**

A20.7 **Septicemic plague** [HCC]

A20.8 **Other forms of plague**

Abortive plague

Asymptomatic plague

Pestis minor

A20.9 **Plague, unspecified**

A21 **Tularemia**

Definition: Tularemia, aka rabbit fever, deer fly fever, O'Hara's fever is a serious infectious disease caused by the bacterium Francisella tularensis.

Includes: deer-fly fever

infection due to Francisella tularensis rabbit fever

A21.0 **Ulceroglandular tularemia**

A21.1 **Oculoglandular tularemia**

Ophthalmic tularemia

A21.2 **Pulmonary tularemia** [HCC]

A21.3 **Gastrointestinal tularemia**

Abdominal tularemia

A21.7 **Generalized tularemia**

A21.8 **Other forms of tularemia**

A21.9 **Tularemia, unspecified**

A22 **Anthrax**

Definition: Anthrax is an acute disease in humans and animals caused by the bacterium bacillus anthracis which is highly lethal in some forms.

Includes: infection due to Bacillus anthracis

A22.0 **Cutaneous anthrax**

Malignant carbuncle

Malignant pustule

A22.1 **Pulmonary anthrax** [HCC]

Inhalation anthrax

Ragpicker's disease

Woolsorter's disease

A22.2   **Gastrointestinal anthrax**

A22.7   **Anthrax sepsis** [HCC]

A22.8   **Other forms of anthrax**

Anthrax meningitis

A22.9   **Anthrax, unspecified**

A23   **Brucellosis**

Definition: Brucellosis, aka undulant fever, or Malta fever is a highly contagious zoonosis caused by ingestion of unsterilized milk or meat from infected animals, or close contact with their secretions.

Includes: Malta fever

Mediterranean fever undulant fever

A23.0   **Brucellosis due to Brucella melitensis**

A23.1   **Brucellosis due to Brucella abortus**

A23.2   **Brucellosis due to Brucella suis**

A23.3   **Brucellosis due to Brucella canis**

A23.8   **Other brucellosis**

A23.9   **Brucellosis, unspecified**

A24   **Glanders and melioidosis**

Definition: Glanders is an infectious disease that occurs primarily in horses, mules, and donkeys and other animals such as dogs, cats and goats that can be transmitted to humans. It is caused by infection with the bacterium Burkholderia mallei.

A24.0   **Glanders**

Infection due to Pseudomonas mallei

Malleus

A24.1   **Acute and fulminating melioidosis**

Melioidosis pneumonia

Melioidosis sepsis

A24.2   **Subacute and chronic melioidosis**

A24.3   **Other melioidosis**

A24.9   **Melioidosis, unspecified**

Infection due to Pseudomonas pseudomallei NOS
Whitmore's disease

A25   **Rat-bite fevers**

A25.0   **Spirillosis**

Sodoku

A25.1   **Streptobacillosis**

Epidemic arthritic erythema

Haverhill fever

Streptobacillary rat-bite fever

A25.9   **Rat-bite fever, unspecified**

A26   **Erysipeloid**

A26.0   **Cutaneous erysipeloid**

Erythema migrans

A26.7   **Erysipelothrix sepsis** [HCC]

A26.8   **Other forms of erysipeloid**

A26.9   **Erysipeloid, unspecified**

A27   **Leptospirosis**

A27.0   **Leptospirosis icterohemorrhagica**

Leptospiral or spirochetal jaundice (hemorrhagic) Weil's disease

A27.8   **Other forms of leptospirosis**

A27.81   **Aseptic meningitis in leptospirosis**

A27.89   **Other forms of leptospirosis**

A27.9   **Leptospirosis, unspecified**

A28   **Other zoonotic bacterial diseases, not elsewhere classified**

Definition: Zoonotic refers to other diseases that can be passed from animals, whether wild or domesticated, to humans.

A28.0   **Pasteurellosis**

A28.1   **Cat-scratch disease**

Cat-scratch fever

A28.2   **Extraintestinal yersiniosis**

Excludes1: enteritis due to Yersinia
enterocolitica (A04.6)
plague (A20.-)

A28.8   **Other specified zoonotic bacterial diseases, not elsewhere classified**

A28.9   **Zoonotic bacterial disease, unspecified**

OTHER BACTERIAL DISEASES (A30-A49)

A30   **Leprosy [Hansen's disease]**

Definition: Leprosy is an infectious disease characterized by disfiguring skin sores, nerve damage, and progressive debilitation. Leprosy is caused by the organism mycobacterium leprae.

Includes: infection due to Mycobacterium leprae

Excludes1: sequelae of leprosy (B92)

A30.0   **Indeterminate leprosy**

I leprosy

A30.1   **Tuberculoid leprosy**

TT leprosy

A30.2   **Borderline tuberculoid leprosy**

BT leprosy

A30.3   **Borderline leprosy**

BB leprosy

A30.4   **Borderline lepromatous leprosy**

BL leprosy

A30.5   **Lepromatous leprosy**

LL leprosy

A30.8   **Other forms of leprosy**

A30.9   **Leprosy, unspecified**

A31   **Infection due to other mycobacteria**

Excludes2: leprosy (A30.-)
tuberculosis (A15-A19)

A31.0   **Pulmonary mycobacterial infection** [HCC]

Infection due to Mycobacterium avium

Infection due to Mycobacterium intracellulare [Battey bacillus]

Infection due to Mycobacterium kansasii

A31.1   **Cutaneous mycobacterial infection**

Buruli ulcer

Infection due to Mycobacterium marinum

Infection due to Mycobacterium ulcerans

A31.2   **Disseminated mycobacterium avium-intracellulare complex (DMAC)** [HCC]

MAC sepsis

A31.8   **Other mycobacterial infections**

A31.9   **Mycobacterial infection, unspecified**

Atypical mycobacterial infection NOS

Mycobacteriosis NOS

A32   **Listeriosis**

Includes: listerial foodborne infection

Excludes1: neonatal (disseminated) listeriosis (P37.2)

A32.0   **Cutaneous listeriosis**

A32.1   **Listerial meningitis and meningoencephalitis**

A32.11   **Listerial meningitis**

A32.12   **Listerial meningoencephalitis**

A32.7   **Listerial sepsis** [HCC]

A32.8   **Other forms of listeriosis**

    A32.81   **Oculoglandular listeriosis**

    A32.82   **Listerial endocarditis**

    A32.89   **Other forms of listeriosis**

        Listerial cerebral arteritis

A32.9   **Listeriosis, unspecified**

A33   **Tetanus neonatorum**

A34   **Obstetrical tetanus**

A35   **Other tetanus**

   Tetanus NOS

   Excludes1: obstetrical tetanus (A34)

        tetanus neonatorum (A33)

A36   **Diphtheria**

   Definition: Diphtheria is a highly infectious disease of the upper respiratory tract characterized by a sore throat, fever and causing difficulty in breathing.

A36.0   **Pharyngeal diphtheria**

   Diphtheritic membranous angina

   Tonsillar diphtheria

A36.1   **Nasopharyngeal diphtheria**

A36.2   **Laryngeal diphtheria**

   Diphtheritic laryngotracheitis

A36.3   **Cutaneous diphtheria**

   Excludes2: erythrasma (L08.1)

A36.8   **Other diphtheria**

    A36.81   **Diphtheritic cardiomyopathy** [HCC]

        Diphtheritic myocarditis

    A36.82   **Diphtheritic radiculomyelitis**

    A36.83   **Diphtheritic polyneuritis**

    A36.84   **Diphtheritic tubulo-interstitial nephropathy**

    A36.85   **Diphtheritic cystitis**

    A36.86   **Diphtheritic conjunctivitis**

    A36.89   **Other diphtheritic complications**

        Diphtheritic peritonitis

A36.9   **Diphtheria, unspecified**

A37   **Whooping cough**

   Definition: Whooping cough, aka pertussis, is a highly contagious disease caused by bacteria. The most prominent symptom of whooping cough is a distinctive, uncontrollable cough, followed by a sharp, high-pitched intake of air.

A37.0   **Whooping cough due to Bordetella pertussis**

    A37.00   **Whooping cough due to Bordetella pertussis without pneumonia**

        Paroxysmal cough due to Bordetella pertussis without pneumonia

    A37.01   **Whooping cough due to Bordetella pertussis with pneumonia**

        Paroxysmal cough due to Bordetella pertussis with pneumonia

A37.1   **Whooping cough due to Bordetella parapertussis**

    A37.10   **Whooping cough due to Bordetella parapertussis without pneumonia**

    A37.11   **Whooping cough due to Bordetella parapertussis with pneumonia**

A37.8   **Whooping cough due to other Bordetella species**

    A37.80   **Whooping cough due to other Bordetella species without pneumonia**

    A37.81   **Whooping cough due to other Bordetella species with pneumonia**

A37.9   **Whooping cough, unspecified species**

    A37.90   **Whooping cough, unspecified species without pneumonia**

    A37.91   **Whooping cough, unspecified species with pneumonia**

A38   **Scarlet fever**

   Includes: scarlatina

   Excludes2: streptococcal sore throat (J02.0)

A38.0   **Scarlet fever with otitis media**

A38.1   **Scarlet fever with myocarditis**

A38.8   **Scarlet fever with other complications**

A38.9   **Scarlet fever, uncomplicated**

   Scarlet fever, NOS

A39   **Meningococcal infection**

A39.0   **Meningococcal meningitis**

A39.1   **Waterhouse-Friderichsen syndrome** [HCC]

   Meningococcal hemorrhagic adrenalitis

   Meningococcic adrenal syndrome

A39.2   **Acute meningococcemia** [HCC]

A39.3   **Chronic meningococcemia** [HCC]

A39.4   **Meningococcemia, unspecified** [HCC]

A39.5   **Meningococcal heart disease**

    A39.50   **Meningococcal carditis, unspecified**

    A39.51   **Meningococcal endocarditis**

    A39.52   **Meningococcal myocarditis**

    A39.53   **Meningococcal pericarditis**

A39.8   **Other meningococcal infections**

    A39.81   **Meningococcal encephalitis**

    A39.82   **Meningococcal retrobulbar neuritis**

    A39.83   **Meningococcal arthritis** [HCC]

    A39.84   **Postmeningococcal arthritis** [HCC]

    A39.89   **Other meningococcal infections**

        Meningococcal conjunctivitis

A39.9   **Meningococcal infection, unspecified**

   Meningococcal disease NOS

A40   **Streptococcal sepsis**

   Code first postprocedural streptococcal sepsis (T81.4-)

   streptococcal sepsis during labor (O75.3)

   streptococcal sepsis following abortion or ectopic or molar pregnancy (O03-O07, O08.0)

   streptococcal sepsis following immunization (T88.0)

   streptococcal sepsis following infusion, transfusion or therapeutic injection (T80.2-)

   Excludes1: neonatal (P36.0-P36.1)

        puerperal sepsis (O85)

        sepsis due to Streptococcus, group D (A41.81)

A40.0   **Sepsis due to streptococcus, group A** [HCC]

A40.1   **Sepsis due to streptococcus, group B** [HCC]

A40.3   **Sepsis due to Streptococcus pneumoniae** [HCC]

   Pneumococcal sepsis

A40.8   **Other streptococcal sepsis** [HCC]

A40.9   **Streptococcal sepsis, unspecified** [HCC]

A41   **Other sepsis**

   Code first postprocedural sepsis (T81.4-)

   sepsis during labor (O75.3)

sepsis following abortion, ectopic or molar pregnancy (O03-O07, O08.0)

sepsis following immunization (T88.0)

sepsis following infusion, transfusion or therapeutic injection (T80.2-)

Excludes1: bacteremia NOS (R78.81)

neonatal (P36.-) puerperal sepsis (O85)

streptococcal sepsis (A40.-)

Excludes2: sepsis (due to) (in) actinomycotic (A42.7)

sepsis (due to) (in) anthrax (A22.7)

sepsis (due to) (in) candidal (B37.7)

sepsis (due to) (in) Erysipelothrix (A26.7)

sepsis (due to) (in) extraintestinal yersiniosis (A28.2)

sepsis (due to) (in) gonococcal (A54.86)

sepsis (due to) (in) herpesviral (B00.7)

sepsis (due to) (in) listerial (A32.7)

sepsis (due to) (in) melioidosis (A24.1)

sepsis (due to) (in) meningococcal (A39.2-A39.4)

sepsis (due to) (in) plague (A20.7)

sepsis (due to) (in) tularemia (A21.7)

toxic shock syndrome (A48.3)

A41.0   Sepsis due to Staphylococcus aureus

    A41.01   Sepsis due to Methicillin susceptible Staphylococcus aureus [HCC]

        MSSA sepsis

        Staphylococcus aureus sepsis NOS

    A41.02   Sepsis due to Methicillin resistant Staphylococcus aureus [HCC]

A41.1   Sepsis due to other specified staphylococcus [HCC]

    Coagulase negative staphylococcus sepsis

A41.2   Sepsis due to unspecified staphylococcus [HCC]

A41.3   Sepsis due to Hemophilus influenzae [HCC]

A41.4   Sepsis due to anaerobes [HCC]

    Excludes1: gas gangrene (A48.0)

A41.5   Sepsis due to other Gram-negative organisms

    A41.50   Gram-negative sepsis, unspecified [HCC]

        Gram-negative sepsis NOS

    A41.51   Sepsis due to Escherichia coli [E. coli] [HCC]

    A41.52   Sepsis due to Pseudomonas [HCC]

        Pseudomonas aeruginosa

    A41.53   Sepsis due to Serratia [HCC]

    A41.59   Other Gram-negative sepsis [HCC]

A41.8   Other specified sepsis

    A41.81   Sepsis due to Enterococcus [HCC]

    A41.89   Other specified sepsis [HCC]

A41.9   Sepsis, unspecified organism

    Septicemia NOS

A42   Actinomycosis

Definition: Actinomycosis is an infection primarily caused by the bacterium actinomyces israelii. Infection most often occurs in the face and neck region and is characterized by the presence of a slowly enlarging, hard, red lump.

Excludes1: actinomycetoma (B47.1)

A42.0   Pulmonary actinomycosis [HCC]

A42.1   Abdominal actinomycosis

A42.2   Cervicofacial actinomycosis

A42.7   Actinomycotic sepsis [HCC]

A42.8   Other forms of actinomycosis

    A42.81   Actinomycotic meningitis

    A42.82   Actinomycotic encephalitis

    A42.89   Other forms of actinomycosis

A42.9   Actinomycosis, unspecified

A43   Nocardiosis

A43.0   Pulmonary nocardiosis [HCC]

A43.1   Cutaneous nocardiosis

A43.8   Other forms of nocardiosis

A43.9   Nocardiosis, unspecified

A44   Bartonellosis

A44.0   Systemic bartonellosis

    Oroya fever

A44.1   Cutaneous and mucocutaneous bartonellosis

    Verruga peruana

A44.8   Other forms of bartonellosis

A44.9   Bartonellosis, unspecified

A46   Erysipelas

Definition: Erysipelas is an acute febrile disease that is associated with intense often vesicular and edematous local inflammation of the skin and subcutaneous tissues and that is caused by a hemolytic streptococcus.

Excludes1: postpartum or puerperal erysipelas (O86.89)

A48   Other bacterial diseases, not elsewhere classified

Excludes1: actinomycetoma (B47.1)

A48.0   Gas gangrene [HCC]

    Clostridial cellulitis

    Clostridial myonecrosis

A48.1   Legionnaires' disease [HCC]

A48.2   Nonpneumonic Legionnaires' disease [Pontiac fever]

A48.3   Toxic shock syndrome [HCC]

    Use Additional Code to identify the organism (B95, B96)

    Excludes1: endotoxic shock NOS (R57.8)

        sepsis NOS (A41.9)

A48.4   Brazilian purpuric fever

    Systemic Hemophilus aegyptius infection

A48.5   Other specified botulism

    Non-foodborne intoxication due to toxins of Clostridium botulinum [C. botulinum]

    Excludes1: food poisoning due to toxins of Clostridium botulinum (A05.1)

    A48.51   Infant botulism

    A48.52   Wound botulism

        Non-foodborne botulism NOS

        Use Additional Code for associated wound

A48.8   Other specified bacterial diseases

A49   Bacterial infection of unspecified site

Excludes1: bacterial agents as the cause of diseases classified elsewhere (B95-B96)

chlamydial infection NOS (A74.9)

meningococcal infection NOS (A39.9)

rickettsial infection NOS (A79.9)

spirochetal infection NOS (A69.9)

A49.0   Staphylococcal infection, unspecified site

    A49.01   Methicillin susceptible Staphylococcus aureus infection, unspecified site

        Methicillin susceptible Staphylococcus aureus (MSSA) infection

Staphylococcus aureus infection NOS

A49.02 **Methicillin resistant Staphylococcus aureus infection, unspecified site**

Methicillin resistant Staphylococcus aureus (MRSA) infection

A49.1 **Streptococcal infection, unspecified site**

A49.2 **Hemophilus influenzae infection, unspecified site**

A49.3 **Mycoplasma infection, unspecified site**

A49.8 **Other bacterial infections of unspecified site**

A49.9 **Bacterial infection, unspecified**

Excludes1: bacteremia NOS (R78.81)

INFECTIONS WITH A PREDOMINANTLY SEXUAL MODE OF TRANSMISSION (A50-A64)

Excludes1: human immunodeficiency virus [HIV] disease (B20)

nonspecific and nongonococcal urethritis (N34.1)

Reiter's disease (M02.3-)

A50 **Congenital syphilis**

Definition: Congenital syphilis is syphilis present in utero and at birth, and occurs when a child is born to a mother with secondary or tertiary syphilis.

A50.0 **Early congenital syphilis, symptomatic**

Any congenital syphilitic condition specified as early or manifest less than two years after birth.

A50.01 **Early congenital syphilitic oculopathy**

A50.02 **Early congenital syphilitic osteochondropathy**

A50.03 **Early congenital syphilitic pharyngitis**

Early congenital syphilitic laryngitis

A50.04 **Early congenital syphilitic pneumonia**

A50.05 **Early congenital syphilitic rhinitis**

A50.06 **Early cutaneous congenital syphilis**

A50.07 **Early mucocutaneous congenital syphilis**

A50.08 **Early visceral congenital syphilis**

A50.09 **Other early congenital syphilis, symptomatic**

A50.1 **Early congenital syphilis, latent**

Congenital syphilis without clinical manifestations, with positive serological reaction and negative

spinal fluid test, less than two years after birth.

A50.2 **Early congenital syphilis, unspecified**

Congenital syphilis NOS less than two years after birth.

A50.3 **Late congenital syphilitic oculopathy**

Excludes1: Hutchinson's triad (A50.53)

A50.30 **Late congenital syphilitic oculopathy, unspecified**

A50.31 **Late congenital syphilitic interstitial keratitis**

A50.32 **Late congenital syphilitic chorioretinitis**

A50.39 **Other late congenital syphilitic oculopathy**

A50.4 **Late congenital neurosyphilis [juvenile neurosyphilis]**

Use Additional Code to identify any associated mental disorder

Excludes1: Hutchinson's triad (A50.53)

A50.40 **Late congenital neurosyphilis, unspecified**

Juvenile neurosyphilis NOS

A50.41 **Late congenital syphilitic meningitis**

A50.42 **Late congenital syphilitic encephalitis**

A50.43 **Late congenital syphilitic polyneuropathy**

A50.44 **Late congenital syphilitic optic nerve atrophy**

A50.45 **Juvenile general paresis**

Dementia paralytica juvenilis

Juvenile tabetoparetic neurosyphilis

A50.49 **Other late congenital neurosyphilis**

Juvenile tabes dorsalis

A50.5 **Other late congenital syphilis, symptomatic**

Any congenital syphilitic condition specified as late or manifest two years or more after birth.

A50.51 **Clutton's joints**

A50.52 **Hutchinson's teeth**

A50.53 **Hutchinson's triad**

A50.54 **Late congenital cardiovascular syphilis**

A50.55 **Late congenital syphilitic arthropathy** [HCC]

A50.56 **Late congenital syphilitic osteochondropathy**

A50.57 **Syphilitic saddle nose**

A50.59 **Other late congenital syphilis, symptomatic**

A50.6 **Late congenital syphilis, latent**

Congenital syphilis without clinical manifestations, with positive serological reaction and negative spinal fluid test, two years or more after birth.

A50.7 **Late congenital syphilis, unspecified**

Congenital syphilis NOS two years or more after birth.

A50.9 **Congenital syphilis, unspecified**

A51 **Early syphilis**

Definition: Early syphilis is defined as the stages of syphilis (primary, secondary, and early latent syphilis) that typically occur within the first year after acquisition of the infection.

A51.0 **Primary genital syphilis**

Syphilitic chancre NOS

A51.1 **Primary anal syphilis**

A51.2 **Primary syphilis of other sites**

A51.3 **Secondary syphilis of skin and mucous membranes**

A51.31 **Condyloma latum**

A51.32 **Syphilitic alopecia**

A51.39 **Other secondary syphilis of skin**

Syphilitic leukoderma

Syphilitic mucous patch

Excludes1: late syphilitic leukoderma (A52.79)

A51.4 **Other secondary syphilis**

A51.41 **Secondary syphilitic meningitis**

A51.42 **Secondary syphilitic female pelvic disease**

A51.43 **Secondary syphilitic oculopathy**

Secondary syphilitic chorioretinitis

Secondary syphilitic iridocyclitis, iritis

Secondary syphilitic uveitis

A51.44 **Secondary syphilitic nephritis**

A51.45 **Secondary syphilitic hepatitis**

A51.46 **Secondary syphilitic osteopathy**

A51.49 **Other secondary syphilitic conditions**

Secondary syphilitic lymphadenopathy

Secondary syphilitic myositis

A51.5 **Early syphilis, latent**

Syphilis (acquired) without clinical manifestations, with positive serological reaction and negative spinal fluid test, less than two years after infection.

A51.9 **Early syphilis, unspecified**

A52 **Late syphilis**

A52.0 **Cardiovascular and cerebrovascular syphilis**

Definition: Cardiovascular syphilis refers to the involvement of the cardiovascular system in late syphilis usually resulting in aortitis aneurysm formation, and aortic valvular insufficiency.

A52.00 **Cardiovascular syphilis, unspecified**

A52.01 **Syphilitic aneurysm of aorta**

A52.02 **Syphilitic aortitis**

A52.03 **Syphilitic endocarditis**

Syphilitic aortic valve incompetence or stenosis

Syphilitic mitral valve stenosis

Syphilitic pulmonary valve regurgitation

A52.04 **Syphilitic cerebral arteritis**

A52.05 **Other cerebrovascular syphilis**

Syphilitic cerebral aneurysm (ruptured) (non-ruptured)

Syphilitic cerebral thrombosis

A52.06 **Other syphilitic heart involvement**

Syphilitic coronary artery disease

Syphilitic myocarditis

Syphilitic pericarditis

A52.09 **Other cardiovascular syphilis**

A52.1 **Symptomatic neurosyphilis**

Definition: Neurosyphilis, aka tabes dorsalis, is the slowly progressive degeneration of the spinal cord that occurs in the late (tertiary) phase of syphilis a decade or more after contracting the infection.

A52.10 **Symptomatic neurosyphilis, unspecified**

A52.11 **Tabes dorsalis**

Locomotor ataxia (progressive)

Tabetic neurosyphilis

A52.12 **Other cerebrospinal syphilis**

A52.13 **Late syphilitic meningitis**

A52.14 **Late syphilitic encephalitis**

A52.15 **Late syphilitic neuropathy**

Late syphilitic acoustic neuritis

Late syphilitic optic (nerve) atrophy

Late syphilitic polyneuropathy

Late syphilitic retrobulbar neuritis

A52.16 **Charcôt's arthropathy (tabetic)**

A52.17 **General paresis**

Dementia paralytica

A52.19 **Other symptomatic neurosyphilis**

Syphilitic parkinsonism

A52.2 **Asymptomatic neurosyphilis**

A52.3 **Neurosyphilis, unspecified**

Gumma (syphilitic)

Syphilis (late)

Syphiloma

A52.7 **Other symptomatic late syphilis**

Definition: Late syphilis is defined as involvement of the cardiovascular or central nervous system, or the development of a gumma in any organ, due to infection with treponema pallidum; usually several years to 2-3 decades after the initial infection. Also known as tertiary syphilis.

A52.71 **Late syphilitic oculopathy**

Late syphilitic chorioretinitis

Late syphilitic episcleritis

A52.72 **Syphilis of lung and bronchus**

A52.73 **Symptomatic late syphilis of other respiratory organs**

A52.74 **Syphilis of liver and other viscera**

Late syphilitic peritonitis

A52.75 **Syphilis of kidney and ureter**

Syphilitic glomerular disease

A52.76 **Other genitourinary symptomatic late syphilis**

Late syphilitic female pelvic inflammatory disease

A52.77 **Syphilis of bone and joint**

A52.78 **Syphilis of other musculoskeletal tissue**

Late syphilitic bursitis

Syphilis [stage unspecified] of bursa

Syphilis [stage unspecified] of muscle

Syphilis [stage unspecified] of synovium

Syphilis [stage unspecified] of tendon

A52.79 **Other symptomatic late syphilis**

Late syphilitic leukoderma

Syphilis of adrenal gland

Syphilis of pituitary gland

Syphilis of thyroid gland

Syphilitic splenomegaly

Excludes1: syphilitic leukoderma (secondary) (A51.39)

A52.8 **Late syphilis, latent**

Syphilis (acquired) without clinical manifestations, with positive serological reaction and negative spinal fluid test, two years or more after infection

A52.9 **Late syphilis, unspecified**

A53 **Other and unspecified syphilis**

A53.0 **Latent syphilis, unspecified as early or late**

Latent syphilis NOS

Positive serological reaction for syphilis

A53.9 **Syphilis, unspecified**

Infection due to Treponema pallidum NOS

Syphilis (acquired) NOS

Excludes1: syphilis NOS under two years of age (A50.2)

A54 **Gonococcal infection**

Definition: Gonococcal infection is a sexually transmitted disease caused by gonococcal bacteria that affects the mucous membrane chiefly of the genital and urinary tracts and is characterized by an acute purulent discharge and painful or difficult urination, though women often have no symptoms.

A54.0 **Gonococcal infection of lower genitourinary tract without periurethral or accessory gland abscess**

Excludes1: gonococcal infection with genitourinary gland abscess (A54.1)

gonococcal infection with periurethral abscess (A54.1)

A54.00 **Gonococcal infection of lower genitourinary tract, unspecified**

A54.01 **Gonococcal cystitis and urethritis, unspecified**

A54.02 **Gonococcal vulvovaginitis, unspecified**

A54.03 **Gonococcal cervicitis, unspecified**

A54.09 **Other gonococcal infection of lower genitourinary tract**

A54.1 **Gonococcal infection of lower genitourinary tract with periurethral and accessory gland abscess**

Gonococcal Bartholin's gland abscess

A54.2 **Gonococcal pelviperitonitis and other gonococcal genitourinary infection**

A54.21 **Gonococcal infection of kidney and ureter**

A54.22 **Gonococcal prostatitis**

A54.23 **Gonococcal infection of other male genital organs**

Gonococcal epididymitis

Gonococcal orchitis

A54.24 **Gonococcal female pelvic inflammatory disease**

Gonococcal pelviperitonitis

Excludes1: gonococcal peritonitis (A54.85)

A54.29 **Other gonococcal genitourinary infections**

A54.3 **Gonococcal infection of eye**

A54.30 **Gonococcal infection of eye, unspecified**

A54.31 **Gonococcal conjunctivitis**

Ophthalmia neonatorum due to gonococcus

A54.32 **Gonococcal iridocyclitis**

A54.33 **Gonococcal keratitis**

A54.39 **Other gonococcal eye infection**

Gonococcal endophthalmia

A54.4 **Gonococcal infection of musculoskeletal system**

A54.40 **Gonococcal infection of musculoskeletal system, unspecified** [HCC]

A54.41 **Gonococcal spondylopathy** [HCC]

A54.42 **Gonococcal arthritis** [HCC]

Excludes2: gonococcal infection of spine (A54.41)

A54.43 **Gonococcal osteomyelitis** [HCC]

Excludes2: gonococcal infection of spine (A54.41)

A54.49 **Gonococcal infection of other musculoskeletal tissue** [HCC]

Gonococcal bursitis

Gonococcal myositis

Gonococcal synovitis

Gonococcal tenosynovitis

A54.5 **Gonococcal pharyngitis**

A54.6 **Gonococcal infection of anus and rectum**

A54.8 **Other gonococcal infections**

A54.81 **Gonococcal meningitis**

A54.82 **Gonococcal brain abscess**

A54.83 **Gonococcal heart infection**

Gonococcal endocarditis

Gonococcal myocarditis

Gonococcal pericarditis

A54.84 **Gonococcal pneumonia** [HCC]

A54.85 **Gonococcal peritonitis** [HCC]

Excludes1: gonococcal pelviperitonitis (A54.24)

A54.86 **Gonococcal sepsis** [HCC]

A54.89 **Other gonococcal infections**

Gonococcal keratoderma

Gonococcal lymphadenitis

A54.9 **Gonococcal infection, unspecified**

A55 **Chlamydial lymphogranuloma (venereum)**

Climatic or tropical bubo

Durand-Nicolas-Favre disease

Esthiomene

Lymphogranuloma inguinale

A56 **Other sexually transmitted chlamydial diseases**

Includes: sexually transmitted diseases due to Chlamydia trachomatis

Excludes1: neonatal chlamydial conjunctivitis (P39.1)

neonatal chlamydial pneumonia (P23.1)

Excludes2: chlamydial lymphogranuloma (A55)

conditions classified to A74.-

A56.0 **Chlamydial infection of lower genitourinary tract**

A56.00 **Chlamydial infection of lower genitourinary tract, unspecified**

A56.01 **Chlamydial cystitis and urethritis**

A56.02 **Chlamydial vulvovaginitis**

A56.09 **Other chlamydial infection of lower genitourinary tract**

Chlamydial cervicitis

A56.1 **Chlamydial infection of pelviperitoneum and other genitourinary organs**

A56.11 **Chlamydial female pelvic inflammatory disease**

A56.19 **Other chlamydial genitourinary infection**

Chlamydial epididymitis

Chlamydial orchitis

A56.2 **Chlamydial infection of genitourinary tract, unspecified**

A56.3 **Chlamydial infection of anus and rectum**

A56.4 **Chlamydial infection of pharynx**

A56.8 **Sexually transmitted chlamydial infection of other sites**

A57 **Chancroid**

Ulcus molle

A58 **Granuloma inguinale**

Donovanosis

A59 **Trichomoniasis**

Definition: Trichomoniasis is a common sexually transmitted disease caused by the parasite trichomonas vaginalis and infecting the urinary tract or vagina.

Excludes2: intestinal trichomoniasis (A07.8)

A59.0 **Urogenital trichomoniasis**

A59.00 **Urogenital trichomoniasis, unspecified**

Fluor (vaginalis) due to Trichomonas

Leukorrhea (vaginalis) due to Trichomonas

A59.01 **Trichomonal vulvovaginitis**

A59.02 **Trichomonal prostatitis**

A59.03 **Trichomonal cystitis and urethritis**

A59.09 **Other urogenital trichomoniasis**

Trichomonas cervicitis

A59.8 **Trichomoniasis of other sites**

A59.9 **Trichomoniasis, unspecified**

A60 **Anogenital herpesviral [herpes simplex] infections**

A60.0 **Herpesviral infection of genitalia and urogenital tract**

A60.00 **Herpesviral infection of urogenital system, unspecified**

A60.01 **Herpesviral infection of penis**

A60.02 **Herpesviral infection of other male genital organs**

A60.03 **Herpesviral cervicitis**

A60.04 **Herpesviral vulvovaginitis**

Herpesviral [herpes simplex] ulceration

Herpesviral [herpes simplex] vaginitis

Herpesviral [herpes simplex] vulvitis

A60.09 **Herpesviral infection of other urogenital tract**

A60.1 **Herpesviral infection of perianal skin and rectum**

A60.9   **Anogenital herpesviral infection, unspecified**

A63   **Other predominantly sexually transmitted diseases, not elsewhere classified**

Excludes2: molluscum contagiosum (B08.1)

papilloma of cervix (D26.0)

A63.0   **Anogenital (venereal) warts**

Anogenital warts due to (human) papillomavirus [HPV]

Condyloma acuminatum

A63.8   **Other specified predominantly sexually transmitted diseases**

A64   **Unspecified sexually transmitted disease**

OTHER SPIROCHETAL DISEASES (A65-A69)

Excludes2: leptospirosis (A27.-)

syphilis (A50-A53)

A65   **Nonvenereal syphilis**

Bejel

Endemic syphilis

Njovera

A66   **Yaws**

Definition: Yaws is a contagious tropical disease caused by the spirochete treponema pertenue, characterized by yellowish or reddish tumors, which often resemble currants, strawberries, or raspberries.

Includes: bouba

frambesia (tropica) pian

A66.0   **Initial lesions of yaws**

Chancre of yaws

Frambesia, initial or primary

Initial frambesial ulcer

Mother yaw

A66.1   **Multiple papillomata and wet crab yaws**

Frambesioma

Pianoma

Plantar or palmar papilloma of yaws

A66.2   **Other early skin lesions of yaws**

Cutaneous yaws, less than five years after infection

Early yaws (cutaneous)(macular)(maculopapular)(micropapular)(papular)

Frambeside of early yaws

A66.3   **Hyperkeratosis of yaws**

Ghoul hand

Hyperkeratosis, palmar or plantar (early) (late) due to yaws

Worm-eaten soles

A66.4   **Gummata and ulcers of yaws**

Gummatous frambeside

Nodular late yaws (ulcerated)

A66.5   **Gangosa**

Rhinopharyngitis mutilans

A66.6   **Bone and joint lesions of yaws** [HCC]

Yaws ganglion

Yaws goundou

Yaws gumma, bone

Yaws gummatous osteitis or periostitis

Yaws hydrarthrosis

Yaws osteitis

Yaws periostitis (hypertrophic)

A66.7   **Other manifestations of yaws**

Juxta-articular nodules of yaws

Mucosal yaws

A66.8   **Latent yaws**

Yaws without clinical manifestations, with positive serology

A66.9   **Yaws, unspecified**

A67   **Pinta [carate]**

A67.0   **Primary lesions of pinta**

Chancre (primary) of pinta

Papule (primary) of pinta

A67.1   **Intermediate lesions of pinta**

Erythematous plaques of pinta

Hyperchromic lesions of pinta

Hyperkeratosis of pinta

Pintids

A67.2   **Late lesions of pinta**

Achromic skin lesions of pinta

Cicatricial skin lesions of pinta

Dyschromic skin lesions of pinta

A67.3   **Mixed lesions of pinta**

Achromic with hyperchromic skin lesions of pinta [carate]

A67.9   **Pinta, unspecified**

A68   **Relapsing fevers**

Definition: Relapsing fever is an infection caused by certain bacteria in the genus Borrelia. It is a vector-borne disease that is transmitted through louse or soft-bodied tick bites.

Includes: recurrent fever

Excludes2: Lyme disease (A69.2-)

A68.0   **Louse-borne relapsing fever**

Relapsing fever due to Borrelia recurrentis

A68.1   **Tick-borne relapsing fever**

Relapsing fever due to any Borrelia species other than Borrelia recurrentis

A68.9   **Relapsing fever, unspecified**

A69   **Other spirochetal infections**

A69.0   **Necrotizing ulcerative stomatitis**

Cancrum oris

Fusospirochetal gangrene Noma

Stomatitis gangrenosa

A69.1   **Other Vincent's infections**

Fusospirochetal pharyngitis

Necrotizing ulcerative (acute) gingivitis

Necrotizing ulcerative (acute) gingivostomatitis

Spirochetal stomatitis

Trench mouth

Vincent's angina

Vincent's gingivitis

A69.2   **Lyme disease**

Erythema chronicum migrans due to Borrelia burgdorferi

A69.20   **Lyme disease, unspecified**

A69.21   **Meningitis due to Lyme disease**

A69.22   **Other neurologic disorders in Lyme disease**

Cranial neuritis

Meningoencephalitis

Polyneuropathy

A69.23   **Arthritis due to Lyme disease** [HCC]

A69.29   **Other conditions associated with Lyme disease**

Myopericarditis due to Lyme disease

A69.8 Other specified spirochetal infections

A69.9 Spirochetal infection, unspecified

OTHER DISEASES CAUSED BY CHLAMYDIAE (A70-A74)

Excludes1: sexually transmitted chlamydial diseases (A55-A56)

A70 Chlamydia psittaci infections

Ornithosis

Parrot fever

Psittacosis

A71 Trachoma

Excludes1: sequelae of trachoma (B94.0)

A71.0 Initial stage of trachoma

Trachoma dubium

A71.1 Active stage of trachoma

Granular conjunctivitis (trachomatous)

Trachomatous follicular conjunctivitis

Trachomatous pannus

A71.9 Trachoma, unspecified

A74 Other diseases caused by chlamydiae

Excludes1: neonatal chlamydial conjunctivitis (P39.1)

neonatal chlamydial pneumonia (P23.1)

Reiter's disease (M02.3-)

sexually transmitted chlamydial diseases (A55-A56)

Excludes2: chlamydial pneumonia (J16.0)

A74.0 Chlamydial conjunctivitis

Paratrachoma

A74.8 Other chlamydial diseases

A74.81 Chlamydial peritonitis

A74.89 Other chlamydial diseases

A74.9 Chlamydial infection, unspecified

Chlamydiosis NOS

RICKETTSIOSES (A75-A79)

Definition: Rickettsioses is a disease caused by intracellular bacteria. Examples of rickettsioses include typhus, Rocky Mountain spotted fever, and Rickettsialpox.

A75 Typhus fever

Excludes1: rickettsiosis due to Ehrlichia sennetsu (A79.81)

A75.0 Epidemic louse-borne typhus fever due to Rickettsia prowazekii

Classical typhus (fever)

Epidemic (louse-borne) typhus

A75.1 Recrudescent typhus [Brill's disease]

Brill-Zinsser disease

A75.2 Typhus fever due to Rickettsia typhi

Murine (flea-borne) typhus

A75.3 Typhus fever due to Rickettsia tsutsugamushi

Scrub (mite-borne) typhus

Tsutsugamushi fever

Typhus fever due to Orientia Tsutsugamushi (scrub typhus)

A75.9 Typhus fever, unspecified

Typhus (fever) NOS

A77 Spotted fever [tick-borne rickettsioses]

A77.0 Spotted fever due to Rickettsia rickettsii

Rocky Mountain spotted fever

Sao Paulo fever

A77.1 Spotted fever due to Rickettsia conorii

African tick typhus

Boutonneuse fever

India tick typhus

Kenya tick typhus

Marseilles fever

Mediterranean tick fever

A77.2 Spotted fever due to Rickettsia siberica

North Asian tick fever

Siberian tick typhus

A77.3 Spotted fever due to Rickettsia australis

Queensland tick typhus

A77.4 Ehrlichiosis

Excludes1: anaplasmosis [A. phagocytophilum] (A79.82)

rickettsiosis due to Ehrlichia sennetsu (A79.81

A77.40 Ehrlichiosis, unspecified

A77.41 Ehrlichiosis chafeensis [E. chafeensis]

A77.49 Other ehrlichiosis

Ehrlichiosis due to E. ewingii

Ehrlichiosis due to E. muris euclairensis

A77.8 Other spotted fevers

Rickettsia 364D/R. philipii (Pacific Coast tick fever)

Spotted fever due to Rickettsia africae (African tick bite fever)

Spotted fever due to Rickettsia parkeri

A77.9 Spotted fever, unspecified

Tick-borne typhus NOS

A78 Q fever

Infection due to Coxiella burnetii

Nine Mile fever

Quadrilateral fever

A79 Other rickettsioses

A79.0 Trench fever

Quintan fever

Wolhynian fever

A79.1 Rickettsialpox due to Rickettsia akari

Kew Garden fever

Vesicular rickettsiosis

A79.8 Other specified rickettsioses

A79.81 Rickettsiosis due to Ehrlichia sennetsu

Rickettsiosis due to Neorickettsia sennetsu

●**A79.82 Anaplasmosis [A. phagocytophilum]**

Transfusion transmitted A. phagocytophilum

A79.89 Other specified rickettsioses

A79.9 Rickettsiosis, unspecified

Rickettsial infection NOS

VIRAL AND PRION INFECTIONS OF THE CENTRAL NERVOUS SYSTEM (A80-A89)

Excludes1: postpolio syndrome (G14)

sequelae of poliomyelitis (B91)

sequelae of viral encephalitis (B94.1)

A80   Acute poliomyelitis

Excludes1: acute flaccid myelitis (G04.82)

A80.0   Acute paralytic poliomyelitis, vaccine-associated

A80.1   Acute paralytic poliomyelitis, wild virus, imported

A80.2   Acute paralytic poliomyelitis, wild virus, indigenous

A80.3   Acute paralytic poliomyelitis, other and unspecified

    A80.30   Acute paralytic poliomyelitis, unspecified

    A80.39   Other acute paralytic poliomyelitis

A80.4   Acute nonparalytic poliomyelitis

A80.9   Acute poliomyelitis, unspecified

A81   Atypical virus infections of central nervous system

Includes: diseases of the central nervous system caused by prions

Use Additional Code to identify:

dementia with behavioral disturbance (F02.81)

dementia without behavioral disturbance (F02.80)

A81.0   Creutzfeldt-Jakob disease

    A81.00   Creutzfeldt-Jakob disease, unspecified

        Jakob-Creutzfeldt disease, unspecified

    A81.01   Variant Creutzfeldt-Jakob disease

        vCJD

    A81.09   Other Creutzfeldt-Jakob disease

        CJD

        Familial Creutzfeldt-Jakob disease

        Iatrogenic Creutzfeldt-Jakob disease

        Sporadic Creutzfeldt-Jakob disease

        Subacute spongiform encephalopathy (with dementia)

A81.1   Subacute sclerosing panencephalitis

    Dawson's inclusion body encephalitis

    Van Bogaert's sclerosing leukoencephalopathy

A81.2   Progressive multifocal leukoencephalopathy

    Multifocal leukoencephalopathy NOS

A81.8   Other atypical virus infections of central nervous system

    A81.81   Kuru

    A81.82   Gerstmann-Sträussler-Scheinker syndrome

        GSS syndrome

    A81.83   Fatal familial insomnia

        FFI

    A81.89   Other atypical virus infections of central nervous system

A81.9   Atypical virus infection of central nervous system, unspecified

    Prion diseases of the central nervous system NOS

A82   Rabies

Definition: Rabies is a viral disease that causes acute encephalitis in warm-blooded animals and people, characterized by abnormal behavior such as excitement, aggressiveness, and dementia, followed by paralysis and death.

A82.0   Sylvatic rabies

A82.1   Urban rabies

A82.9   Rabies, unspecified

A83   Mosquito-borne viral encephalitis

Includes: mosquito-borne viral meningoencephalitis

Excludes2: Venezuelan equine encephalitis (A92.2)

West Nile fever (A92.3-) West Nile virus (A92.3-)

A83.0   Japanese encephalitis

A83.1   Western equine encephalitis

A83.2   Eastern equine encephalitis

A83.3   St Louis encephalitis

A83.4   Australian encephalitis

    Kunjin virus disease

A83.5   California encephalitis

    California meningoencephalitis

    La Crosse encephalitis

A83.6   Rocio virus disease

A83.8   Other mosquito-borne viral encephalitis

A83.9   Mosquito-borne viral encephalitis, unspecified

A84   Tick-borne viral encephalitis

Includes: tick-borne viral meningoencephalitis

A84.0   Far Eastern tick-borne encephalitis [Russian spring-summer encephalitis]

A84.1   Central European tick-borne encephalitis

A84.8   Other tick-borne viral encephalitis

    A84.81   Powassan virus disease

    A84.89   Other tick-borne viral encephalitis

        Louping ill

        Code first, if applicable, transfusion related infection (T80.22-)

A84.9   Tick-borne viral encephalitis, unspecified

A85   Other viral encephalitis, not elsewhere classified

Includes: specified viral encephalomyelitis NEC

specified viral meningoencephalitis NEC

Excludes1: benign myalgic encephalomyelitis (G93.3)

    encephalitis due to cytomegalovirus (B25.8)

    encephalitis due to herpesvirus NEC (B10.0-)

    encephalitis due to herpesvirus [herpes simplex] (B00.4)

    encephalitis due to measles virus (B05.0)

    encephalitis due to mumps virus (B26.2)

    encephalitis due to poliomyelitis virus (A80.-)

    encephalitis due to zoster (B02.0)

    lymphocytic choriomeningitis (A87.2)

A85.0   Enteroviral encephalitis

    Enteroviral encephalomyelitis

A85.1   Adenoviral encephalitis

    Adenoviral meningoencephalitis

A85.2   Arthropod-borne viral encephalitis, unspecified

    Excludes1: West Nile virus with encephalitis (A92.31)

A85.8   Other specified viral encephalitis

    Encephalitis lethargica

    Von Economo-Cruchet disease

A86   Unspecified viral encephalitis

Viral encephalomyelitis NOS

Viral meningoencephalitis NOS

A87   Viral meningitis

Definition: Meningitis due to enterovirus refers to any of a subgroup of picornaviruses, including polioviruses, coxsackie viruses, and echoviruses, that infect the gastrointestinal tract and often spread to other areas of the body, especially the nervous system

Excludes1: meningitis due to herpesvirus [herpes simplex] (B00.3)

    meningitis due to herpesvirus [herpes simplex] (B00.3)

meningitis due to measles virus (B05.1)

meningitis due to mumps virus (B26.1)

meningitis due to poliomyelitis virus (A80.-)

meningitis due to zoster (B02.1)

A87.0 **Enteroviral meningitis**

Coxsackievirus meningitis

Echovirus meningitis

A87.1 **Adenoviral meningitis**

A87.2 **Lymphocytic choriomeningitis**

Lymphocytic meningoencephalitis

A87.8 **Other viral meningitis**

A87.9 **Viral meningitis, unspecified**

A88 **Other viral infections of central nervous system, not elsewhere classified**

Excludes1: viral encephalitis NOS (A86)

viral meningitis NOS (A87.9)

A88.0 **Enteroviral exanthematous fever [Boston exanthem]**

A88.1 **Epidemic vertigo**

A88.8 **Other specified viral infections of central nervous system**

A89 **Unspecified viral infection of central nervous system**

ARTHROPOD-BORNE VIRAL FEVERS AND VIRAL HEMORRHAGIC FEVERS (A90-A99)

Definition: Hemorrhagic fever is a group of viral infections characterized by fever, chills, headache, malaise, and respiratory or gastrointestinal symptoms, followed by capillary hemorrhages and, in severe infection, by oliguria, kidney failure, hypotension, and possibly death.

A90 **Dengue fever [classical dengue]**

Excludes1: dengue hemorrhagic fever (A91)

A91 **Dengue hemorrhagic fever**

A92 **Other mosquito-borne viral fevers**

Excludes1: Ross River disease (B33.1)

A92.0 **Chikungunya virus disease**

Chikungunya (hemorrhagic) fever

A92.1 **O'nyong-nyong fever**

A92.2 **Venezuelan equine fever**

Venezuelan equine encephalitis

Venezuelan equine encephalomyelitis virus disease

A92.3 **West Nile virus infection**

West Nile fever

A92.30 **West Nile virus infection, unspecified**

West Nile fever NOS

West Nile fever without complications

West Nile virus NOS

A92.31 **West Nile virus infection with encephalitis**

West Nile encephalitis

West Nile encephalomyelitis

A92.32 **West Nile virus infection with other neurologic manifestation**

Use Additional Code to specify the neurologic manifestation

A92.39 **West Nile virus infection with other complications**

Use Additional Code to specify the other conditions

A92.4 **Rift Valley fever**

A92.5 **Zika virus disease**

Excludes1: congenital Zika virus disease (P35.4)

Zika virus fever

Zika virus infection

Zika NOS

A92.8 **Other specified mosquito-borne viral fevers**

A92.9 **Mosquito-borne viral fever, unspecified**

A93 **Other arthropod-borne viral fevers, not elsewhere classified**

A93.0 **Oropouche virus disease**

Oropouche fever

A93.1 **Sandfly fever**

Pappataci fever

Phlebotomus fever

A93.2 **Colorado tick fever**

A93.8 **Other specified arthropod-borne viral fevers**

Piry virus disease

Vesicular stomatitis virus disease [Indiana fever]

A94 **Unspecified arthropod-borne viral fever**

Arboviral fever NOS

Arbovirus infection NOS

A95 **Yellow fever**

Definition: Yellow fever is an acute systemic (body wide) illness caused by a virus called a flavivirus. In severe cases, the viral infection causes a high fever, bleeding into the skin, and necrosis (death) of cells in the kidney and liver.

A95.0 **Sylvatic yellow fever**

Jungle yellow fever

A95.1 **Urban yellow fever**

A95.9 **Yellow fever, unspecified**

A96 **Arenaviral hemorrhagic fever**

A96.0 **Junin hemorrhagic fever**

Argentinian hemorrhagic fever

A96.1 **Machupo hemorrhagic fever**

Bolivian hemorrhagic fever

A96.2 **Lassa fever**

A96.8 **Other arenaviral hemorrhagic fevers**

A96.9 **Arenaviral hemorrhagic fever, unspecified**

A98 **Other viral hemorrhagic fevers, not elsewhere classified**

Excludes1: chikungunya hemorrhagic fever (A92.0)

dengue hemorrhagic fever (A91)

A98.0 **Crimean-Congo hemorrhagic fever**

Central Asian hemorrhagic fever

A98.1 **Omsk hemorrhagic fever**

A98.2 **Kyasanur Forest disease**

A98.3 **Marburg virus disease**

A98.4 **Ebola virus disease**

A98.5 **Hemorrhagic fever with renal syndrome**

Epidemic hemorrhagic fever

Korean hemorrhagic fever

Russian hemorrhagic fever

Hantaan virus disease

Hantavirus disease with renal manifestations

Nephropathia epidemica

Songo fever

Excludes1: hantavirus (cardio)-pulmonary syndrome (B33.4)

A98.8 **Other specified viral hemorrhagic fevers**

● New code   ▲ Revised code   **Excludes1:** Not coded here   **Excludes2:** Not included here   ⊗ Placeholder required   ⑦7th digit required

A99   Unspecified viral hemorrhagic fever

VIRAL INFECTIONS CHARACTERIZED BY SKIN AND MUCOUS MEMBRANE LESIONS (B00-B09)

B00   Herpesviral [herpes simplex] infections

Definition: Herpes simplex is an infection caused by the herpes simplex virus; affects the skin and nervous system; produces small temporary blisters on the skin and mucous membranes.

Excludes1: congenital herpesviral infections (P35.2)

Excludes2: anogenital herpesviral infection (A60.-)

gammaherpesviral mononucleosis (B27.0-)

herpangina (B08.5)

B00.0   Eczema herpeticum

Kaposi's varicelliform eruption

B00.1   Herpesviral vesicular dermatitis

Herpes simplex facialis

Herpes simplex labialis

Herpes simplex otitis externa

Vesicular dermatitis of ear

Vesicular dermatitis of lip

B00.2   Herpesviral gingivostomatitis and pharyngotonsillitis

Herpesviral pharyngitis

B00.3   Herpesviral meningitis

B00.4   Herpesviral encephalitis

Herpesviral meningoencephalitis

Simian B disease

Excludes1: herpesviral encephalitis due to herpesvirus 6 and 7 (B10.01, B10.09)

non-simplex herpesviral encephalitis (B10.0-)

B00.5   Herpesviral ocular disease

B00.50   Herpesviral ocular disease, unspecified

B00.51   Herpesviral iridocyclitis

Herpesviral iritis

Herpesviral uveitis, anterior

B00.52   Herpesviral keratitis

Herpesviral keratoconjunctivitis

B00.53   Herpesviral conjunctivitis

B00.59   Other herpesviral disease of eye

Herpesviral dermatitis of eyelid

B00.7   Disseminated herpesviral disease [HCC]

Herpesviral sepsis

B00.8   Other forms of herpesviral infections

B00.81   Herpesviral hepatitis

B00.82   Herpes simplex myelitis [HCC]

B00.89   Other herpesviral infection

Herpesviral whitlow

B00.9   Herpesviral infection, unspecified

Herpes simplex infection NOS

B01   Varicella [chickenpox]

Definition: Chickenpox is an acute contagious disease caused by herpes varicella zoster virus; causes a rash of vesicles on the face and body.

B01.0   Varicella meningitis

B01.1   Varicella encephalitis, myelitis and encephalomyelitis

Post chickenpox encephalitis, myelitis and encephalomyelitis

B01.11   Varicella encephalitis and encephalomyelitis

Post chickenpox encephalitis and encephalomyelitis

B01.12   Varicella myelitis [HCC]

Post chickenpox myelitis

B01.2   Varicella pneumonia

B01.8   Varicella with other complications

B01.81   Varicella keratitis

B01.89   Other varicella complications

B01.9   Varicella without complication

Varicella NOS

B02   Zoster [herpes zoster]

Definition: Herpes zoster is a viral disease characterized by a painful skin rash with blisters in a limited area on one side of the body, often in a stripe.

Includes: shingles

zona

B02.0   Zoster encephalitis

Zoster meningoencephalitis

B02.1   Zoster meningitis

B02.2   Zoster with other nervous system involvement

B02.21   Postherpetic geniculate ganglionitis

B02.22   Postherpetic trigeminal neuralgia

B02.23   Postherpetic polyneuropathy

B02.24   Postherpetic myelitis [HCC]

Herpes zoster myelitis

B02.29   Other postherpetic nervous system involvement

Postherpetic radiculopathy

B02.3   Zoster ocular disease

B02.30   Zoster ocular disease, unspecified

B02.31   Zoster conjunctivitis

B02.32   Zoster iridocyclitis

B02.33   Zoster keratitis

Herpes zoster keratoconjunctivitis

B02.34   Zoster scleritis

B02.39   Other herpes zoster eye disease

Zoster blepharitis

B02.7   Disseminated zoster

B02.8   Zoster with other complications

Herpes zoster otitis externa

B02.9   Zoster without complications

Zoster NOS

B03   Smallpox

Note: In 1980 the 33rd World Health Assembly declared that smallpox had been eradicated.

The classification is maintained for surveillance purposes.

B04   Monkeypox

B05   Measles

Definition: Measles is a viral infection which causes an illness displaying a characteristic skin rash. Measles is also sometimes called rubeola, 5-day measles, or hard measles.

Includes: morbilli

Excludes1: subacute sclerosing panencephalitis (A81.1)

B05.0   Measles complicated by encephalitis

Post measles encephalitis

B05.1   Measles complicated by meningitis

Post measles meningitis

B05.2   Measles complicated by pneumonia

Post measles pneumonia

B05.3 Measles complicated by otitis media

Post measles otitis media

B05.4 Measles with intestinal complications

B05.8 Measles with other complications

B05.81 Measles keratitis and keratoconjunctivitis

B05.89 Other measles complications

B05.9 Measles without complication

Measles NOS

B06 Rubella [German measles]

Definition: Rubella is a highly contagious viral disease, aka German measles. The symptoms include swollen glands, joint pain, low fever, and a fine red rash.

Excludes1: congenital rubella (P35.0)

B06.0 Rubella with neurological complications

B06.00 Rubella with neurological complication, unspecified

B06.01 Rubella encephalitis

Rubella meningoencephalitis

B06.02 Rubella meningitis

B06.09 Other neurological complications of rubella

B06.8 Rubella with other complications

B06.81 Rubella pneumonia

B06.82 Rubella arthritis [HCC]

B06.89 Other rubella complications

B06.9 Rubella without complication

Rubella NOS

B07 Viral warts

Includes: verruca simplex

verruca vulgaris

viral warts due to human papillomavirus

Excludes2: anogenital (venereal) warts (A63.0)

papilloma of bladder (D41.4)

papilloma of cervix (D26.0)

papilloma larynx (D14.1)

B07.0 Plantar wart

Verruca plantaris

B07.8 Other viral warts

Common wart

Flat wart

Verruca plana

B07.9 Viral wart, unspecified

B08 Other viral infections characterized by skin and mucous membrane lesions, not elsewhere classified

Excludes1: vesicular stomatitis virus disease (A93.8)

B08.0 Other orthopoxvirus infections

Excludes2: monkeypox (B04)

B08.01 Cowpox and vaccinia not from vaccine

B08.010 Cowpox

B08.011 Vaccinia not from vaccine

Excludes1: vaccinia (from vaccination) (generalized) (T88.1)

B08.02 ORF virus disease

Contagious pustular dermatitis

Ecthyma contagiosum

B08.03 Pseudocowpox [milker's node]

B08.04 Paravaccinia, unspecified

B08.09 Other orthopoxvirus infections

Orthopoxvirus infection NOS

B08.1 Molluscum contagiosum

B08.2 Exanthema subitum [sixth disease]

Roseola infantum

B08.20 Exanthema subitum [sixth disease], unspecified

Roseola infantum, unspecified

B08.21 Exanthema subitum [sixth disease] due to human herpesvirus 6

Roseola infantum due to human herpesvirus 6

B08.22 Exanthema subitum [sixth disease] due to human herpesvirus 7

Roseola infantum due to human herpesvirus 7

B08.3 Erythema infectiosum [fifth disease]

B08.4 Enteroviral vesicular stomatitis with exanthem

Hand, foot and mouth disease

B08.5 Enteroviral vesicular pharyngitis

Herpangina

B08.6 Parapoxvirus infections

B08.60 Parapoxvirus infection, unspecified

B08.61 Bovine stomatitis

B08.62 Sealpox

B08.69 Other parapoxvirus infections

B08.7 Yatapoxvirus infections

B08.70 Yatapoxvirus infection, unspecified

B08.71 Tanapox virus disease

B08.72 Yaba pox virus disease

Yaba monkey tumor disease

B08.79 Other yatapoxvirus infections

B08.8 Other specified viral infections characterized by skin and mucous membrane lesions

Enteroviral lymphonodular pharyngitis

Foot-and-mouth disease

Poxvirus NEC

B09 Unspecified viral infection characterized by skin and mucous membrane lesions

Viral enanthema NOS

Viral exanthema NOS

OTHER HUMAN HERPESVIRUSES (B10)

Definition: Human herpes viruses, refers to a family of viruses including herpes simplex, varicella zoster, and Epstein-Barr.

B10 Other human herpesviruses

Excludes2: cytomegalovirus (B25.9)

Epstein-Barr virus (B27.0-)

herpes NOS (B00.9)

herpes simplex (B00.-)

herpes zoster (B02.-)

human herpesvirus NOS (B00.-)

human herpesvirus 1 and 2 (B00.-)

human herpesvirus 3 (B01.-, B02.-)

human herpesvirus 4 (B27.0-)

human herpesvirus 5 (B25.-)

varicella (B01.-)

zoster (B02.-)

B10.0 Other human herpesvirus encephalitis

● New code ▲ Revised code **Excludes1:** Not coded here **Excludes2:** Not included here ⊗ Placeholder required ⑦ 7th digit required

Excludes2: herpes encephalitis NOS (B00.4)

herpes simplex encephalitis (B00.4)

human herpesvirus encephalitis (B00.4)

simian B herpes virus encephalitis (B00.4)

B10.01   Human herpesvirus 6 encephalitis

B10.09   Other human herpesvirus encephalitis

Human herpesvirus 7 encephalitis

B10.8   Other human herpesvirus infection

B10.81   Human herpesvirus 6 infection

B10.82   Human herpesvirus 7 infection

B10.89   Other human herpesvirus infection

Human herpesvirus 8 infection

Kaposi's sarcoma-associated herpesvirus infection

VIRAL HEPATITIS (B15-B19)

Definition: Viral hepatitis is a liver inflammation due to a viral infection. It may present in acute or chronic forms. The most common causes of viral hepatitis are the five unrelated hepatotropic viruses hepatitis A, hepatitis B, hepatitis C, hepatitis D, and hepatitis E.

Excludes1: sequelae of viral hepatitis (B94.2)

Excludes2: cytomegaloviral hepatitis (B25.1)

herpesviral [herpes simplex] hepatitis (B00.81)

B15   Acute hepatitis A

B15.0   Hepatitis A with hepatic coma

B15.9   Hepatitis A without hepatic coma

Hepatitis A (acute)(viral) NOS

B16   Acute hepatitis B

B16.0   Acute hepatitis B with delta-agent with hepatic coma

B16.1   Acute hepatitis B with delta-agent without hepatic coma

B16.2   Acute hepatitis B without delta-agent with hepatic coma

B16.9   Acute hepatitis B without delta-agent and without hepatic coma

Hepatitis B (acute) (viral) NOS

B17   Other acute viral hepatitis

B17.0   Acute delta-(super) infection of hepatitis B carrier

B17.1   Acute hepatitis C

B17.10   Acute hepatitis C without hepatic coma

Acute hepatitis C NOS

B17.11   Acute hepatitis C with hepatic coma

B17.2   Acute hepatitis E

B17.8   Other specified acute viral hepatitis

Hepatitis non-A non-B (acute) (viral) NEC

B17.9   Acute viral hepatitis, unspecified

Acute hepatitis NOS

Acute infectious hepatitis NOS

B18   Chronic viral hepatitis

Includes: Carrier of viral hepatitis

B18.0   Chronic viral hepatitis B with delta-agent [HCC]

B18.1   Chronic viral hepatitis B without delta-agent [HCC]

Carrier of viral hepatitis B

Chronic (viral) hepatitis B

B18.2   Chronic viral hepatitis C [HCC]

Carrier of viral hepatitis C

B18.8   Other chronic viral hepatitis

Carrier of other viral hepatitis

B18.9   Chronic viral hepatitis, unspecified [HCC]

Carrier of unspecified viral hepatitis

B19   Unspecified viral hepatitis

B19.0   Unspecified viral hepatitis with hepatic coma

B19.1   Unspecified viral hepatitis B

B19.10   Unspecified viral hepatitis B without hepatic coma

Unspecified viral hepatitis B NOS

B19.11   Unspecified viral hepatitis B with hepatic coma

B19.2   Unspecified viral hepatitis C

B19.20   Unspecified viral hepatitis C without hepatic coma

Viral hepatitis C NOS

B19.21   Unspecified viral hepatitis C with hepatic coma

B19.9   Unspecified viral hepatitis without hepatic coma

Viral hepatitis NOS

HUMAN IMMUNODEFICIENCY VIRUS [HIV] DISEASE (B20)

Definition: Human immunodeficiency virus (HIV) disease is a virus that can lead to acquired immunodeficiency syndrome (AIDS), a condition in humans in which the immune system begins to fail, leading to life-threatening opportunistic infections.

B20   Human immunodeficiency virus [HIV] disease [HCC]

Includes: acquired immune deficiency syndrome [AIDS]

AIDS-related complex [ARC]

HIV infection, symptomatic

Code first Human immunodeficiency virus [HIV] disease complicating pregnancy, childbirth and the puerperium, if applicable (O98.7-)

Use Additional Code(s) to identify all manifestations of HIV infection

Excludes1: asymptomatic human immunodeficiency virus [HIV] infection status (Z21)

exposure to HIV virus (Z20.6)

inconclusive serologic evidence of HIV (R75)

OTHER VIRAL DISEASES (B25-B34)

B25   Cytomegaloviral disease

Excludes1: congenital cytomegalovirus infection (P35.1)

cytomegaloviral mononucleosis (B27.1-)

B25.0   Cytomegaloviral pneumonitis [HCC]

B25.1   Cytomegaloviral hepatitis [HCC]

B25.2   Cytomegaloviral pancreatitis [HCC]

B25.8   Other cytomegaloviral diseases [HCC]

Cytomegaloviral encephalitis

B25.9   Cytomegaloviral disease, unspecified [HCC]

B26   Mumps

Includes: epidemic parotitis

infectious parotitis

B26.0   Mumps orchitis

B26.1   Mumps meningitis

B26.2   Mumps encephalitis

B26.3   Mumps pancreatitis

B26.8   Mumps with other complications

B26.81   Mumps hepatitis

B26.82   Mumps myocarditis

B26.83   Mumps nephritis

B26.84   Mumps polyneuropathy

B26.85   Mumps arthritis [HCC]

B26.89   Other mumps complications

B26.9   **Mumps without complication**

Mumps NOS

Mumps parotitis NOS

B27   **Infectious mononucleosis**

Definition: Infectious mononucleosis, aka mono, glandular fever, kissing disease is an acute disease characterized by fever and swollen lymph nodes and an abnormal increase of mononuclear leucocytes or monocytes in the bloodstream.

Includes: glandular fever

monocytic angina

Pfeiffer's disease

B27.0   **Gammaherpesviral mononucleosis**

Mononucleosis due to Epstein-Barr virus

B27.00   **Gammaherpesviral mononucleosis without complication**

B27.01   **Gammaherpesviral mononucleosis with polyneuropathy**

B27.02   **Gammaherpesviral mononucleosis with meningitis**

B27.09   **Gammaherpesviral mononucleosis with other complications**

Hepatomegaly in gammaherpesviral mononucleosis

B27.1   **Cytomegaloviral mononucleosis**

B27.10   **Cytomegaloviral mononucleosis without complications**

B27.11   **Cytomegaloviral mononucleosis with polyneuropathy**

B27.12   **Cytomegaloviral mononucleosis with meningitis**

B27.19   **Cytomegaloviral mononucleosis with other complication**

Hepatomegaly in cytomegaloviral mononucleosis

B27.8   **Other infectious mononucleosis**

B27.80   **Other infectious mononucleosis without complication**

B27.81   **Other infectious mononucleosis with polyneuropathy**

B27.82   **Other infectious mononucleosis with meningitis**

B27.89   **Other infectious mononucleosis with other complication**

Hepatomegaly in other infectious mononucleosis

B27.9   **Infectious mononucleosis, unspecified**

B27.90   **Infectious mononucleosis, unspecified without complication**

B27.91   **Infectious mononucleosis, unspecified with polyneuropathy**

B27.92   **Infectious mononucleosis, unspecified with meningitis**

B27.99   **Infectious mononucleosis, unspecified with other complication**

Hepatomegaly in unspecified infectious mononucleosis

B30   **Viral conjunctivitis**

Excludes1: herpesviral [herpes simplex] ocular disease (B00.5)

ocular zoster (B02.3)

B30.0   **Keratoconjunctivitis due to adenovirus**

Epidemic keratoconjunctivitis

Shipyard eye

B30.1   **Conjunctivitis due to adenovirus**

Acute adenoviral follicular conjunctivitis

Swimming-pool conjunctivitis

B30.2   **Viral pharyngoconjunctivitis**

B30.3   **Acute epidemic hemorrhagic conjunctivitis (enteroviral)**

Conjunctivitis due to coxsackievirus 24

Conjunctivitis due to enterovirus 70

Hemorrhagic conjunctivitis (acute)(epidemic)

B30.8   **Other viral conjunctivitis**

Newcastle conjunctivitis

B30.9   **Viral conjunctivitis, unspecified**

B33   **Other viral diseases, not elsewhere classified**

B33.0   **Epidemic myalgia**

Bornholm disease

B33.1   **Ross River disease**

Epidemic polyarthritis and exanthema

Ross River fever

B33.2   **Viral carditis**

Coxsackie (virus) carditis

B33.20   **Viral carditis, unspecified**

B33.21   **Viral endocarditis**

B33.22   **Viral myocarditis**

B33.23   **Viral pericarditis**

B33.24   **Viral cardiomyopathy** [HCC]

B33.3   **Retrovirus infections, not elsewhere classified**

Retrovirus infection NOS

B33.4   **Hantavirus (cardio)-pulmonary syndrome [HPS] [HCPS]**

Hantavirus disease with pulmonary manifestations

Sin nombre virus disease

Use Additional Code to identify any associated acute kidney failure (N17.9)

Excludes1: hantavirus disease with renal manifestations (A98.5)

hemorrhagic fever with renal manifestations (A98.5)

B33.8   **Other specified viral diseases**

Excludes1: anogenital human papillomavirus infection (A63.0)

viral warts due to human papillomavirus infection (B07)

B34   **Viral infection of unspecified site**

Excludes1: anogenital human papillomavirus infection (A63.0)

cytomegaloviral disease NOS (B25.9)

herpesvirus [herpes simplex] infection NOS (B00.9)

retrovirus infection NOS (B33.3)

viral agents as the cause of diseases classified elsewhere (B97.-)

viral warts due to human papillomavirus infection (B07)

B34.0   **Adenovirus infection, unspecified**

B34.1   **Enterovirus infection, unspecified**

Coxsackievirus infection NOS

Echovirus infection NOS

B34.2   **Coronavirus infection, unspecified**

Excludes1:

COVID-19 (U07.1)

pneumonia due to SARS-associated coronavirus (J12.81)

B34.3   **Parvovirus infection, unspecified**

B34.4   **Papovavirus infection, unspecified**

B34.8   **Other viral infections of unspecified site**

B34.9   **Viral infection, unspecified**

Viremia NOS

MYCOSES (B35-B49)

Excludes2: hypersensitivity pneumonitis due to organic dust (J67.-)

mycosis fungoides (C84.0-)

B35 Dermatophytosis

Definition: Dermatophytosis, aka tinea or ringworm, is a disease that can affect the scalp (tinea capitis), body (tinea corporis), nails (tinea unguium), feet (tinea pedis), groin (tinea cruris), and bearded skin (tinea hebrae).

Includes: favus infections due to species of Epidermophyton, Micro-sporum and Trichophyton tinea, any type except those in B36.-

B35.0 Tinea barbae and tinea capitis

Beard ringworm

Kerion

Scalp ringworm

Sycosis, mycotic

B35.1 Tinea unguium

Dermatophytic onychia

Dermatophytosis of nail

Onychomycosis

Ringworm of nails

B35.2 Tinea manuum

Dermatophytosis of hand ringworm

B35.3 Tinea pedis

Athlete's foot

Dermatophytosis of foot ringworm

B35.4 Tinea corporis

Ringworm of the body

B35.5 Tinea imbricata

Tokelau

B35.6 Tinea cruris

Dhobi itch Groin ringworm Jock itch

B35.8 Other dermatophytoses

Disseminated dermatophytosis

Granulomatous dermatophytosis

B35.9 Dermatophytosis, unspecified

Ringworm NOS

B36 Other superficial mycoses

B36.0 Pityriasis versicolor

Tinea flava

Tinea versicolor

B36.1 Tinea nigra

Keratomycosis nigricans palmaris

Microsporosis nigra

Pityriasis nigra

B36.2 White piedra

Tinea blanca

B36.3 Black piedra

B36.8 Other specified superficial mycoses

B36.9 Superficial mycosis, unspecified

B37 Candidiasis

Definition: Candidiasis is an infection caused by a species of the yeast candida, usually candida albicans. Candidiasis is a common cause of vaginal infections in women.

Includes: candidosis

moniliasis

Excludes1: neonatal candidiasis (P37.5)

B37.0 Candidal stomatitis

Oral thrush

B37.1 Pulmonary candidiasis [HCC]

Candidal bronchitis

Candidal pneumonia

B37.2 Candidiasis of skin and nail

Candidal onychia

Candidal paronychia

Excludes2: diaper dermatitis (L22)

B37.3 Candidiasis of vulva and vagina

Candidal vulvovaginitis

Monilial vulvovaginitis

Vaginal thrush

B37.4 Candidiasis of other urogenital sites

B37.41 Candidal cystitis and urethritis

B37.42 Candidal balanitis

B37.49 Other urogenital candidiasis

Candidal pyelonephritis

B37.5 Candidal meningitis

B37.6 Candidal endocarditis

B37.7 Candidal sepsis [HCC]

Disseminated candidiasis

Systemic candidiasis

B37.8 Candidiasis of other sites

B37.81 Candidal esophagitis [HCC]

B37.82 Candidal enteritis

Candidal proctitis

B37.83 Candidal cheilitis

B37.84 Candidal otitis externa

B37.89 Other sites of candidiasis

Candidal osteomyelitis

B37.9 Candidiasis, unspecified

Thrush NOS

B38 Coccidioidomycosis

B38.0 Acute pulmonary coccidioidomycosis [HCC]

B38.1 Chronic pulmonary coccidioidomycosis [HCC]

B38.2 Pulmonary coccidioidomycosis, unspecified [HCC]

B38.3 Cutaneous coccidioidomycosis

B38.4 Coccidioidomycosis meningitis

B38.7 Disseminated coccidioidomycosis

Generalized coccidioidomycosis

B38.8 Other forms of coccidioidomycosis

B38.81 Prostatic coccidioidomycosis

B38.89 Other forms of coccidioidomycosis

B38.9 Coccidioidomycosis, unspecified

B39 Histoplasmosis

Definition: Histoplasmosis, aka Darling's disease, is a disease caused by the fungus histoplasma capsulatum. Symptoms vary greatly, but the disease primarily affects the lungs. Histoplasmosis is common among aids patients because of their lowered immune system.

Code first associated AIDS (B20)

Use Additional Code for any associated manifestations, such as:

endocarditis (I39)

meningitis (G02)

pericarditis (I32)

retinitis (H32)

B39.0 Acute pulmonary histoplasmosis capsulati [HCC]

B39.1 **Chronic pulmonary histoplasmosis capsulati** [HCC]

B39.2 **Pulmonary histoplasmosis capsulati, unspecified** [HCC]

B39.3 **Disseminated histoplasmosis capsulati**

Generalized histoplasmosis capsulati

B39.4 **Histoplasmosis capsulati, unspecified**

American histoplasmosis

B39.5 **Histoplasmosis duboisii**

African histoplasmosis

B39.9 **Histoplasmosis, unspecified**

B40 **Blastomycosis**

Definition: Blastomycotic infection, aka North American blastomycosis, blastomycetic dermatitis, and Gilchrist's disease, is a fungal infection caused by the organism Blastomyces dermatitidis. Endemic to portions of north America, blastomycosis causes clinical symptoms similar to histoplasmosis.

Excludes1: Brazilian blastomycosis (B41.-)

keloidal blastomycosis (B48.0)

B40.0 **Acute pulmonary blastomycosis** [HCC]

B40.1 **Chronic pulmonary blastomycosis** [HCC]

B40.2 **Pulmonary blastomycosis, unspecified** [HCC]

B40.3 **Cutaneous blastomycosis**

B40.7 **Disseminated blastomycosis**

Generalized blastomycosis

B40.8 **Other forms of blastomycosis**

B40.81 **Blastomycotic meningoencephalitis**

Meningomyelitis due to blastomycosis

B40.89 **Other forms of blastomycosis**

B40.9 **Blastomycosis, unspecified**

B41 **Paracoccidioidomycosis**

Includes: Brazilian blastomycosis

Lutz' disease

B41.0 **Pulmonary paracoccidioidomycosis** [HCC]

B41.7 **Disseminated paracoccidioidomycosis**

Generalized paracoccidioidomycosis

B41.8 **Other forms of paracoccidioidomycosis**

B41.9 **Paracoccidioidomycosis, unspecified**

B42 **Sporotrichosis**

B42.0 **Pulmonary sporotrichosis**

B42.1 **Lymphocutaneous sporotrichosis**

B42.7 **Disseminated sporotrichosis**

Generalized sporotrichosis

B42.8 **Other forms of sporotrichosis**

B42.81 **Cerebral sporotrichosis**

Meningitis due to sporotrichosis

B42.82 **Sporotrichosis arthritis** [HCC]

B42.89 **Other forms of sporotrichosis**

B42.9 **Sporotrichosis, unspecified**

B43 **Chromomycosis and pheomycotic abscess**

B43.0 **Cutaneous chromomycosis**

Dermatitis verrucosa

B43.1 **Pheomycotic brain abscess**

Cerebral chromomycosis

B43.2 **Subcutaneous pheomycotic abscess and cyst**

B43.8 **Other forms of chromomycosis**

B43.9 **Chromomycosis, unspecified**

B44 **Aspergillosis**

Includes: aspergilloma

B44.0 **Invasive pulmonary aspergillosis** [HCC]

B44.1 **Other pulmonary aspergillosis** [HCC]

B44.2 **Tonsillar aspergillosis** [HCC]

B44.7 **Disseminated aspergillosis** [HCC]

Generalized aspergillosis

B44.8 **Other forms of aspergillosis**

B44.81 **Allergic bronchopulmonary aspergillosis** [HCC]

B44.89 **Other forms of aspergillosis** [HCC]

B44.9 **Aspergillosis, unspecified** [HCC]

B45 **Cryptococcosis**

B45.0 **Pulmonary cryptococcosis** [HCC]

B45.1 **Cerebral cryptococcosis** [HCC]

Cryptococcal meningitis

Cryptococcosis meningocerebralis

B45.2 **Cutaneous cryptococcosis** [HCC]

B45.3 **Osseous cryptococcosis** [HCC]

B45.7 **Disseminated cryptococcosis** [HCC]

Generalized cryptococcosis

B45.8 **Other forms of cryptococcosis** [HCC]

B45.9 **Cryptococcosis, unspecified** [HCC]

B46 **Zygomycosis**

B46.0 **Pulmonary mucormycosis** [HCC]

B46.1 **Rhinocerebral mucormycosis** [HCC]

B46.2 **Gastrointestinal mucormycosis** [HCC]

B46.3 **Cutaneous mucormycosis** [HCC]

Subcutaneous mucormycosis

B46.4 **Disseminated mucormycosis** [HCC]

Generalized mucormycosis

B46.5 **Mucormycosis, unspecified** [HCC]

B46.8 **Other zygomycoses** [HCC]

Entomophthoromycosis

B46.9 **Zygomycosis, unspecified** [HCC]

Phycomycosis NOS

B47 **Mycetoma**

B47.0 **Eumycetoma**

Madura foot, mycotic

Maduromycosis

B47.1 **Actinomycetoma**

B47.9 **Mycetoma, unspecified**

Madura foot NOS

B48 **Other mycoses, not elsewhere classified**

B48.0 **Lobomycosis**

Keloidal blastomycosis Lobo's disease

B48.1 **Rhinosporidiosis**

B48.2 **Allescheriasis**

Infection due to Pseudallescheria boydii

Excludes1: eumycetoma (B47.0)

B48.3 **Geotrichosis**

Geotrichum stomatitis

B48.4 **Penicillosis** [HCC]

Talaromycosis

B48.8 **Other specified mycoses** [HCC]

Adiaspiromycosis

Infection of tissue and organs by Alternaria

Infection of tissue and organs by Drechslera

Infection of tissue and organs by Fusarium

Infection of tissue and organs by saprophytic fungi NEC

B49 **Unspecified mycosis**

Fungemia NOS

PROTOZOAL DISEASES (B50-B64)

Excludes1: amebiasis (A06.-)

Other protozoal intestinal diseases (A07.-)

B50 **Plasmodium falciparum malaria**

Includes: mixed infections of Plasmodium falciparum with any other Plasmodium species

B50.0 **Plasmodium falciparum malaria with cerebral complications**

Cerebral malaria NOS

B50.8 **Other severe and complicated Plasmodium falciparum malaria**

Severe or complicated Plasmodium falciparum malaria NOS

B50.9 **Plasmodium falciparum malaria, unspecified**

B51 **Plasmodium vivax malaria**

Includes: mixed infections of Plasmodium vivax with other Plasmodium species, except Plasmodium falciparum

Excludes1: plasmodium vivax with Plasmodium falciparum (B50.-)

B51.0 **Plasmodium vivax malaria with rupture of spleen**

B51.8 **Plasmodium vivax malaria with other complications**

B51.9 **Plasmodium vivax malaria without complication**

Plasmodium vivax malaria NOS

B52 **Plasmodium malariae malaria**

Includes: mixed infections of Plasmodium malariae with other Plasmodium species, except Plasmodium falciparum and Plasmodium vivax

Excludes1: Plasmodium falciparum (B50.-)

Plasmodium vivax (B51.-)

B52.0 **Plasmodium malariae malaria with nephropathy**

B52.8 **Plasmodium malariae malaria with other complications**

B52.9 **Plasmodium malariae malaria without complication**

Plasmodium malariae malaria NOS

B53 **Other specified malaria**

B53.0 **Plasmodium ovale malaria**

Excludes1: Plasmodium ovale with Plasmodium falciparum (B50.-)

Plasmodium ovale with Plasmodium malariae (B52.-)

Plasmodium ovale with Plasmodium vivax (B51.-)

B53.1 **Malaria due to simian plasmodia**

Excludes1: Malaria due to simian plasmodia with Plasmodium falciparum (B50.-)

Malaria due to simian plasmodia with Plasmodium malariae (B52.-)

Malaria due to simian plasmodia with Plasmodium ovale (B53.0)

Malaria due to simian plasmodia with Plasmodium vivax (B51.-)

B53.8 **Other malaria, not elsewhere classified**

B54 **Unspecified malaria**

B55 **Leishmaniasis**

B55.0 **Visceral leishmaniasis**

Kala-azar

Post-kala-azar dermal leishmaniasis

B55.1 **Cutaneous leishmaniasis**

B55.2 **Mucocutaneous leishmaniasis**

B55.9 **Leishmaniasis, unspecified**

B56 **African trypanosomiasis**

B56.0 **Gambiense trypanosomiasis**

Infection due to Trypanosoma brucei gambiense

West African sleeping sickness

B56.1 **Rhodesiense trypanosomiasis**

East African sleeping sickness

Infection due to Trypanosoma brucei rhodesiense

B56.9 **African trypanosomiasis, unspecified**

Sleeping sickness NOS

B57 **Chagas' disease**

Includes: American trypanosomiasis

infection due to Trypanosoma cruzi

B57.0 **Acute Chagas' disease with heart involvement**

Acute Chagas' disease with myocarditis

B57.1 **Acute Chagas' disease without heart involvement**

Acute Chagas' disease NOS

B57.2 **Chagas' disease (chronic) with heart involvement**

American trypanosomiasis NOS

Chagas' disease (chronic) NOS

Chagas' disease (chronic) with myocarditis

Trypanosomiasis NOS

B57.3 **Chagas' disease (chronic) with digestive system involvement**

B57.30 **Chagas' disease with digestive system involvement, unspecified**

B57.31 **Megaesophagus in Chagas' disease**

B57.32 **Megacolon in Chagas' disease**

B57.39 **Other digestive system involvement in Chagas' disease**

B57.4 **Chagas' disease (chronic) with nervous system involvement**

B57.40 **Chagas' disease with nervous system involvement, unspecified**

B57.41 **Meningitis in Chagas' disease**

B57.42 **Meningoencephalitis in Chagas' disease**

B57.49 **Other nervous system involvement in Chagas' disease**

B57.5 **Chagas' disease (chronic) with other organ involvement**

B58 **Toxoplasmosis**

Definition: Toxoplasmosis is an infection caused by the parasite named toxoplasma gondii that can invade tissues and damage the brain, especially in a fetus and in a newborn baby. Symptoms include fever, fatigue, headache, swollen lymph glands, and muscle aches and pains.

Includes: infection due to Toxoplasma gondii

Excludes1: congenital toxoplasmosis (P37.1)

B58.0 **Toxoplasma oculopathy**

B58.00 **Toxoplasma oculopathy, unspecified**

B58.01 **Toxoplasma chorioretinitis**

B58.09 **Other toxoplasma oculopathy**

Toxoplasma uveitis

B58.1 **Toxoplasma hepatitis**

B58.2 **Toxoplasma meningoencephalitis** [HCC]

B58.3 **Pulmonary toxoplasmosis** [HCC]

B58.8 **Toxoplasmosis with other organ involvement**

B58.81 **Toxoplasma myocarditis**

B58.82   **Toxoplasma myositis**

B58.83   **Toxoplasma tubulo-interstitial nephropathy**

       Toxoplasma pyelonephritis

B58.89   **Toxoplasmosis with other organ involvement**

B58.9   **Toxoplasmosis, unspecified**

B59   **Pneumocystosis** [HCC]

Pneumonia due to Pneumocystis carinii

Pneumonia due to Pneumocystis jiroveci

B60   **Other protozoal diseases, not elsewhere classified**

Excludes1: cryptosporidiosis (A07.2)

       intestinal microsporidiosis (A07.8)

       isosporiasis (A07.3)

B60.0   **Babesiosis**

B60.00   **Babesiosis, unspecified**

       Babesiosis due to unspecified Babesia species

       Piroplasmosis, unspecified

B60.01   **Babesiosis due to Babesia microti**

       Infection due to B. microti

B60.02   **Babesiosis due to Babesia duncani**

       Infection due to B. duncani and B. duncani-type species

B60.03   **Babesiosis due to Babesia divergens**

       Babesiosis due to Babesia MO-1

       Infection due to B. divergens and B. divergens-like strains

B60.09   **Other babesiosis**

       Babesiosis due to Babesia KO-1

       Babesiosis due to Babesia venatorum

       Infection due to other Babesia species

       Infection due to other protozoa of the order Piroplasmida

       Other piroplasmosis

B60.1   **Acanthamebiasis**

B60.10   **Acanthamebiasis, unspecified**

B60.11   **Meningoencephalitis due to Acanthamoeba (culbertsoni)**

B60.12   **Conjunctivitis due to Acanthamoeba**

B60.13   **Keratoconjunctivitis due to Acanthamoeba**

B60.19   **Other acanthamebic disease**

B60.2   **Naegleriasis**

       Primary amebic meningoencephalitis

B60.8   **Other specified protozoal diseases**

       Microsporidiosis

B64   **Unspecified protozoal disease**

HELMINTHIASES (B65-B83)

B65   **Schistosomiasis [bilharziasis]**

Definition: Schistosomiasis [bilharziasis], aka bilharzia, bilharziosis or snail fever, is a parasitic disease caused by several species of fluke of the genus Schistosoma. Schistosomiasis often is a chronic illness that can damage internal organs and, in children, impair growth and cognitive development.

Includes: snail fever

B65.0   **Schistosomiasis due to Schistosoma haematobium [urinary schistosomiasis]**

B65.1   **Schistosomiasis due to Schistosoma mansoni [intestinal schistosomiasis]**

B65.2   **Schistosomiasis due to Schistosoma japonicum**

       Asiatic schistosomiasis

B65.3   **Cercarial dermatitis**

       Swimmer's itch

B65.8   **Other schistosomiasis**

       Infection due to Schistosoma intercalatum

       Infection due to Schistosoma mattheei

       Infection due to Schistosoma mekongi

B65.9   **Schistosomiasis, unspecified**

B66   **Other fluke infections**

B66.0   **Opisthorchiasis**

       Infection due to cat liver fluke

       Infection due to Opisthorchis (felineus)(viverrini)

B66.1   **Clonorchiasis**

       Chinese liver fluke disease

       Infection due to Clonorchis sinensis

       Oriental liver fluke disease

B66.2   **Dicroceliasis**

       Infection due to Dicrocoelium dendriticum

       Lancet fluke infection

B66.3   **Fascioliasis**

       Infection due to Fasciola gigantica

       Infection due to Fasciola hepatica

       Infection due to Fasciola indica

       Sheep liver fluke disease

B66.4   **Paragonimiasis** [HCC]

       Infection due to Paragonimus species

       Lung fluke disease

       Pulmonary distomiasis

B66.5   **Fasciolopsiasis**

       Infection due to Fasciolopsis buski

       Intestinal distomiasis

B66.8   **Other specified fluke infections**

       Echinostomiasis

       Heterophyiasis

       Metagonimiasis Nanophyetiasis Watsoniasis

B66.9   **Fluke infection, unspecified**

B67   **Echinococcosis**

Includes: hydatidosis

B67.0   **Echinococcus granulosus infection of liver**

B67.1   **Echinococcus granulosus infection of lung** [HCC]

B67.2   **Echinococcus granulosus infection of bone**

B67.3   **Echinococcus granulosus infection, other and multiple sites**

B67.31   **Echinococcus granulosus infection, thyroid gland**

B67.32   **Echinococcus granulosus infection, multiple sites**

B67.39   **Echinococcus granulosus infection, other sites**

B67.4   **Echinococcus granulosus infection, unspecified**

       Dog tapeworm (infection)

B67.5   **Echinococcus multilocularis infection of liver**

B67.6   **Echinococcus multilocularis infection, other and multiple sites**

B67.61   **Echinococcus multilocularis infection, multiple sites**

B67.69   **Echinococcus multilocularis infection, other sites**

B67.7   **Echinococcus multilocularis infection, unspecified**

B67.8   **Echinococcosis, unspecified, of liver**

B67.9 **Echinococcosis, other and unspecified**

    B67.90 **Echinococcosis, unspecified**

        Echinococcosis NOS

    B67.99 **Other echinococcosis**

B68 **Taeniasis**

    Excludes1: cysticercosis (B69.-)

B68.0 **Taenia solium taeniasis**

    Pork tapeworm (infection)

B68.1 **Taenia saginata taeniasis**

    Beef tapeworm (infection)

    Infection due to adult tapeworm

    Taenia saginata

B68.9 **Taeniasis, unspecified**

B69 **Cysticercosis**

    Includes: cysticerciasis infection due to larval form of Taenia solium

B69.0 **Cysticercosis of central nervous system**

B69.1 **Cysticercosis of eye**

B69.8 **Cysticercosis of other sites**

    B69.81 **Myositis in cysticercosis**

    B69.89 **Cysticercosis of other sites**

B69.9 **Cysticercosis, unspecified**

B70 **Diphyllobothriasis and sparganosis**

B70.0 **Diphyllobothriasis**

    Diphyllobothrium (adult) (latum) (pacificum) infection

    Fish tapeworm (infection)

    Excludes2: larval diphyllobothriasis (B70.1)

B70.1 **Sparganosis**

    Infection due to Sparganum (mansoni) (proliferum)

    Infection due to Spirometra larva

    Larval diphyllobothriasis

    Spirometrosis

B71 **Other cestode infections**

B71.0 **Hymenolepiasis**

    Dwarf tapeworm infection

    Rat tapeworm (infection)

B71.1 **Dipylidiasis**

B71.8 **Other specified cestode infections**

    Coenurosis

B71.9 **Cestode infection, unspecified**

    Tapeworm (infection) NOS

B72 **Dracunculiasis**

    Includes: guinea worm infection

  infection due to Dracunculus medinensis

B73 **Onchocerciasis**

    Includes: onchocerca volvulus infection

  onchocercosis river blindness

B73.0 **Onchocerciasis with eye disease**

    B73.00 **Onchocerciasis with eye involvement, unspecified**

    B73.01 **Onchocerciasis with endophthalmitis**

    B73.02 **Onchocerciasis with glaucoma**

    B73.09 **Onchocerciasis with other eye involvement**

        Infestation of eyelid due to onchocerciasis

B73.1 **Onchocerciasis without eye disease**

B74 **Filariasis**

    Excludes2: onchocerciasis (B73)

    tropical (pulmonary) eosinophilia NOS (J82.89)

B74.0 **Filariasis due to Wuchereria bancrofti**

    Bancroftian elephantiasis

    Bancroftian filariasis

B74.1 **Filariasis due to Brugia malayi**

B74.2 **Filariasis due to Brugia timori**

B74.3 **Loiasis**

    Calabar swelling

    Eyeworm disease of Africa

    Loa Loa infection

B74.4 **Mansonelliasis**

    Infection due to Mansonella ozzardi

    Infection due to Mansonella perstans

    Infection due to Mansonella streptocerca

B74.8 **Other filariases**

    Dirofilariasis

B74.9 **Filariasis, unspecified**

B75 **Trichinellosis**

    Includes: infection due to Trichinella species

    trichiniasis

B76 **Hookworm diseases**

    Includes: uncinariasis

B76.0 **Ancylostomiasis**

    Infection due to Ancylostoma species

B76.1 **Necatoriasis**

    Infection due to Necator americanus

B76.8 **Other hookworm diseases**

B76.9 **Hookworm disease, unspecified**

    Cutaneous larva migrans NOS

B77 **Ascariasis**

    Includes: ascaridiasis

    roundworm infection

B77.0 **Ascariasis with intestinal complications**

B77.8 **Ascariasis with other complications**

    B77.81 **Ascariasis pneumonia**

    B77.89 **Ascariasis with other complications**

B77.9 **Ascariasis, unspecified**

B78 **Strongyloidiasis**

    Excludes1: trichostrongyliasis (B81.2)

B78.0 **Intestinal strongyloidiasis**

B78.1 **Cutaneous strongyloidiasis**

B78.7 **Disseminated strongyloidiasis**

B78.9 **Strongyloidiasis, unspecified**

B79 **Trichuriasis**

    Includes: trichocephaliasis

  whipworm (disease)(infection)

B80 **Enterobiasis**

    Includes: oxyuriasis

    pinworm infection threadworm infection

B81 **Other intestinal helminthiases, not elsewhere classified**

    Definition: Helminthiases is a disease in which a part of the body is infested with worms such as pinworm, roundworm or tapeworm.

    Excludes1: angiostrongyliasis due to:

      Angiostrongylus cantonensis (B83.2)

      Parastrongylus cantonensis (B83.2)

B81.0 **Anisakiasis**

Infection due to Anisakis larva

B81.1 **Intestinal capillariasis**

Capillariasis NOS

Infection due to Capillaria philippinensis

Excludes2: hepatic capillariasis (B83.8)

B81.2 **Trichostrongyliasis**

B81.3 **Intestinal angiostrongyliasis**

Angiostrongyliasis due to:

Angiostrongylus costaricensis

Parastrongylus costaricensis

B81.4 **Mixed intestinal helminthiases**

Infection due to intestinal helminths classified to more than one of the categories B65.0-B81.3 and B81.8

Mixed helminthiasis NOS

B81.8 **Other specified intestinal helminthiases**

Infection due to Oesophagostomum species [esophagostomiasis]

Infection due to Ternidens diminutus [Ternidensiasis]

B82 **Unspecified intestinal parasitism**

B82.0 **Intestinal helminthiasis, unspecified**

B82.9 **Intestinal parasitism, unspecified**

B83 **Other helminthiases**

Excludes1: capillariasis NOS (B81.1)

Excludes2: intestinal capillariasis (B81.1)

B83.0 **Visceral larva migrans**

Toxocariasis

B83.1 **Gnathostomiasis**

Wandering swelling

B83.2 **Angiostrongyliasis due to Parastrongylus cantonensis**

Eosinophilic meningoencephalitis due to Parastrongylus cantonensis

Excludes2: intestinal angiostrongyliasis (B81.3)

B83.3 **Syngamiasis**

Syngamosis

B83.4 **Internal hirudiniasis**

Excludes2: external hirudiniasis (B88.3)

B83.8 **Other specified helminthiases**

Acanthocephaliasis

Gongylonemiasis

Hepatic capillariasis

Metastrongyliasis

Thelaziasis

B83.9 **Helminthiasis, unspecified**

Worms NOS

Excludes1: intestinal helminthiasis NOS (B82.0)

PEDICULOSIS, ACARIASIS AND OTHER INFESTATIONS (B85-B89)

Definition: Pediculosis and Phthirus infestation is an infestation with lice (pediculus humanus) or true lice or crab lice (Phthirus) resulting in severe itching.

Definition: Acariasis is an infestation with arthropod parasites of the order Acarina including the ticks and mites.

B85 **Pediculosis and phthiriasis**

B85.0 **Pediculosis due to Pediculus humanus capitis**

Head-louse infestation

B85.1 **Pediculosis due to Pediculus humanus corporis**

Body-louse infestation

B85.2 **Pediculosis, unspecified**

B85.3 **Phthiriasis**

Infestation by crab-louse

Infestation by Phthirus pubis

B85.4 **Mixed pediculosis and phthiriasis**

Infestation classifiable to more than one of the categories B85.0-B85.3

B86 **Scabies**

Sarcoptic itch

B87 **Myiasis**

Includes: infestation by larva of flies

B87.0 **Cutaneous myiasis**

Creeping myiasis

B87.1 **Wound myiasis**

Traumatic myiasis

B87.2 **Ocular myiasis**

B87.3 **Nasopharyngeal myiasis**

Laryngeal myiasis

B87.4 **Aural myiasis**

B87.8 **Myiasis of other sites**

B87.81 **Genitourinary myiasis**

B87.82 **Intestinal myiasis**

B87.89 **Myiasis of other sites**

B87.9 **Myiasis, unspecified**

B88 **Other infestations**

B88.0 **Other acariasis**

Acarine dermatitis

Dermatitis due to Demodex species

Dermatitis due to Dermanyssus gallinae

Dermatitis due to Liponyssoides sanguineus

Trombiculosis

Excludes2: scabies (B86)

B88.1 **Tungiasis [sandflea infestation]**

B88.2 **Other arthropod infestations**

Scarabiasis

B88.3 **External hirudiniasis**

Leech infestation NOS

Excludes2: internal hirudiniasis (B83.4)

B88.8 **Other specified infestations**

Ichthyoparasitism due to Vandellia cirrhosa

Linguatulosis

Porocephaliasis

B88.9 **Infestation, unspecified**

Infestation (skin) NOS

Infestation by mites NOS

Skin parasites NOS

B89 **Unspecified parasitic disease**

SEQUELAE OF INFECTIOUS AND PARASITIC DISEASES (B90-B94)

Note: Categories B90-B94 are to be used to indicate conditions in categories A00-B89 as the cause of sequelae, which are themselves classified elsewhere. The 'sequelae' include conditions specified as such; they also include residuals of diseases classifiable to the above categories if there is evidence that the disease itself is no longer present. Codes from these categories are not to be used for chronic infections. Code chronic current infections to active infectious disease as appropriate.

Code first condition resulting from (sequela) the infectious or parasitic disease

B90 **Sequelae of tuberculosis**

B90.0 Sequelae of central nervous system tuberculosis

B90.1 Sequelae of genitourinary tuberculosis

B90.2 Sequelae of tuberculosis of bones and joints

B90.8 Sequelae of tuberculosis of other organs

Excludes2: sequelae of respiratory tuberculosis (B90.9)

B90.9 Sequelae of respiratory and unspecified tuberculosis

Sequelae of tuberculosis NOS

B91 Sequelae of poliomyelitis

Excludes1: postpolio syndrome (G14)

B92 Sequelae of leprosy

B94 **Sequelae of other and unspecified infectious and parasitic diseases**

B94.0 Sequelae of trachoma

B94.1 Sequelae of viral encephalitis

B94.2 Sequelae of viral hepatitis

B94.8 Sequelae of other specified infectious and parasitic diseases

B94.9 Sequelae of unspecified infectious and parasitic disease

Excludes2: post COVID-19 condition (U09.9)

BACTERIAL AND VIRAL INFECTIOUS AGENTS (B95-B97)

Note: These categories are provided for use as supplementary or additional codes to identify the infectious agent(s) in diseases classified elsewhere.

B95 **Streptococcus, Staphylococcus, and Enterococcus as the cause of diseases classified elsewhere**

B95.0 Streptococcus, group A, as the cause of diseases classified elsewhere

B95.1 Streptococcus, group B, as the cause of diseases classified elsewhere

B95.2 Enterococcus as the cause of diseases classified elsewhere

B95.3 Streptococcus pneumoniae as the cause of diseases classified elsewhere

B95.4 Other streptococcus as the cause of diseases classified elsewhere

B95.5 Unspecified streptococcus as the cause of diseases classified elsewhere

B95.6 Staphylococcus aureus as the cause of diseases classified elsewhere

B95.61 Methicillin susceptible Staphylococcus aureus infection as the cause of diseases classified elsewhere

Methicillin susceptible Staphylococcus aureus (MSSA) infection as the cause of diseases classified elsewhere

Staphylococcus aureus infection NOS as the cause of diseases classified elsewhere

B95.62 Methicillin resistant Staphylococcus aureus infection as the cause of diseases classified elsewhere

Methicillin resistant staphylococcus aureus (MRSA) infection as the cause of diseases classified elsewhere

B95.7 Other staphylococcus as the cause of diseases classified elsewhere

B95.8 Unspecified staphylococcus as the cause of diseases classified elsewhere

B96 **Other bacterial agents as the cause of diseases classified elsewhere**

B96.0 Mycoplasma pneumoniae [M. pneumoniae] as the cause of diseases classified elsewhere

Pleuro-pneumonia-like-organism [PPLO]

B96.1 Klebsiella pneumoniae [K. pneumoniae] as the cause of diseases classified elsewhere

B96.2 Escherichia coli [E. coli] as the cause of diseases classified elsewhere

B96.20 Unspecified Escherichia coli [E. coli] as the cause of diseases classified elsewhere

Escherichia coli [E. coli] NOS

B96.21 Shiga toxin-producing Escherichia coli [E. coli] (STEC) O157 as the cause of diseases classified elsewhere

E. coli O157:H- (nonmotile) with confirmation of Shiga toxin

E. coli O157 with confirmation of Shiga toxin when H antigen is unknown, or is not H7 O157:H7

Escherichia coli [E. coli] with or without confirmation of Shiga toxin-production

Shiga toxin-producing Escherichia coli [E. coli] O157:H7 with or without confirmation of Shiga toxin-production

STEC O157:H7 with or without confirmation of Shiga toxin-production

B96.22 Other specified Shiga toxin-producing Escherichia coli [E. coli] (STEC) as the cause of diseases classified elsewhere

Non-O157 Shiga toxin-producing Escherichia coli [E. coli]

Non-O157 Shiga toxin-producing Escherichia coli [E. coli] with known O group

B96.23 Unspecified Shiga toxin-producing Escherichia coli [E. coli] (STEC) as the cause of diseases classified elsewhere

Shiga toxin-producing Escherichia coli [E. coli] with unspecified O group STEC NOS

B96.29 Other Escherichia coli [E. coli] as the cause of diseases classified elsewhere

Non-Shiga toxin-producing E. coli

B96.3 Hemophilus influenzae [H. influenzae] as the cause of diseases classified elsewhere

B96.4 Proteus (mirabilis) (morganii) as the cause of diseases classified elsewhere

B96.5 Pseudomonas (aeruginosa) (mallei) (pseudomallei) as the cause of diseases classified elsewhere

B96.6 Bacteroides fragilis [B. fragilis] as the cause of diseases classified elsewhere

B96.7 Clostridium perfringens [C. perfringens] as the cause of diseases classified elsewhere

B96.8 Other specified bacterial agents as the cause of diseases classified elsewhere

B96.81 Helicobacter pylori [H. pylori] as the cause of diseases classified elsewhere

B96.82 Vibrio vulnificus as the cause of diseases classified elsewhere

B96.89 Other specified bacterial agents as the cause of diseases classified elsewhere

B97 **Viral agents as the cause of diseases classified elsewhere**

B97.0 Adenovirus as the cause of diseases classified elsewhere

B97.1 Enterovirus as the cause of diseases classified elsewhere

B97.10 Unspecified enterovirus as the cause of diseases classified elsewhere

B97.11 Coxsackievirus as the cause of diseases classified elsewhere

B97.12   Echovirus as the cause of diseases classified
elsewhere

B97.19   Other enterovirus as the cause of diseases
classified elsewhere

B97.2   Coronavirus as the cause of diseases classified elsewhere

B97.21   SARS-associated coronavirus as the cause of
diseases classified elsewhere

Excludes1: pneumonia due to SARS-associated
coronavirus (J12.81)

B97.29   Other coronavirus as the cause of diseases
classified elsewhere

B97.3   Retrovirus as the cause of diseases classified elsewhere

Excludes1: Human immunodeficiency virus [HIV] disease
(B20)

B97.30   Unspecified retrovirus as the cause of diseases
classified elsewhere

B97.31   Lentivirus as the cause of diseases classified
elsewhere

B97.32   Oncovirus as the cause of diseases classified
elsewhere

B97.33   Human T-cell lymphotrophic virus, type I
[HTLV-I] as the cause of diseases classified
elsewhere

B97.34   Human T-cell lymphotrophic virus, type II
[HTLV-II] as the cause of diseases classified
elsewhere

B97.35   Human immunodeficiency virus, type 2 [HIV 2]
as the cause of diseases classified elsewhere
[HCC]

B97.39   Other retrovirus as the cause of diseases
classified elsewhere

B97.4   Respiratory syncytial virus as the cause of diseases
classified elsewhere

RSV as the cause of diseases classified elsewhere
Code first related disorders, such as:
otitis media (H65.-)
upper respiratory infection (J06.9)

Excludes1: acute bronchiolitis due to respiratory syncytial
virus (RSV) (J21.0)
acute bronchitis due to respiratory syncytial virus
(RSV) (J20.5)
respiratory syncytial virus (RSV) pneumonia
(J12.1)

B97.5   Reovirus as the cause of diseases classified elsewhere

B97.6   Parvovirus as the cause of diseases classified elsewhere

B97.7   Papillomavirus as the cause of diseases classified
elsewhere

B97.8   Other viral agents as the cause of diseases classified
elsewhere

B97.81   Human metapneumovirus as the cause of
diseases classified elsewhere

B97.89   Other viral agents as the cause of diseases
classified elsewhere

OTHER INFECTIOUS DISEASES (B99)

B99   Other and unspecified infectious diseases

B99.8   Other infectious disease

B99.9   Unspecified infectious disease

Chapter 2: Neoplasms (C00-D49)

DEFINITIONS

This chapter includes definitions of selected key words, terms and phrases and coding alerts for adding points to the clinical domain, and references to coding late effects where appropriate. An example from this chapter is as follows:

C46   Kaposi's sarcoma
> **Definition:** Kaposi's sarcoma is a form of skin cancer that can involve internal organs. It is most often found in patients with acquired immunodeficiency syndrome (AIDS) and can be fatal.

MULTIPLE CODING FOR A SINGLE CONDITION

In addition to the etiology/manifestation convention that requires two codes to fully describe a single condition that affects multiple body systems, there are other single conditions that also require more than one code. "**Use Additional Code**" notes are found in the Tabular List at codes that are not part of an etiology/manifestation pair where a secondary code is useful to fully describe a condition. The sequencing rule is the same as the etiology/manifestation pair, "**Use Additional Code**" indicates that a secondary code should be added.

For example, for bacterial infections that are not included in chapter 1, a secondary code from category B95, Streptococcus, Staphylococcus, and Enterococcus, as the cause of diseases classified elsewhere, or B96, Other bacterial agents as the cause of diseases classified elsewhere, may be required to identify the bacterial organism causing the infection. A "**Use Additional Code**" note will normally be found at the infectious disease code, indicating a need for the organism code to be added as a secondary code.

"Code first" notes are also under certain codes that are not specifically manifestation codes but may be due to an underlying cause. When there is a "Code first" note and an underlying condition is present, the underlying condition should be sequenced first.

"Code, if applicable, any causal condition first", notes indicate that this code may be assigned as a principal diagnosis when the causal condition is unknown or not applicable. If a causal condition is known, then the code for that condition should be sequenced as the principal or first-listed diagnosis.

Multiple codes may be needed for sequela, complication codes and obstetric codes to more fully describe a condition. See the specific guidelines for these conditions for further instruction.

COMBINATION CODE

A combination code is a single code used to classify: Two diagnoses, or a diagnosis with an associated secondary process (manifestation) A diagnosis with an associated complication

Combination codes are identified by referring to subterm entries in the Alphabetic Index and by reading the inclusion and exclusion notes in the Tabular List.

Assign only the combination code when that code fully identifies the diagnostic conditions involved or when the Alphabetic Index so directs. Multiple coding should not be used when the classification provides a combination code that clearly identifies all of the elements documented in the diagnosis. When the combination code lacks necessary specificity in describing the manifestation or complication, an additional code should be used as a secondary code.

SEQUELA (LATE EFFECTS)

A sequela is the residual effect (condition produced) after the acute phase of an illness or injury has terminated. There is no time limit on when a sequela code can be used. The residual may be apparent early, such as in cerebral infarction, or it may occur months or years later, such as that due to a previous injury. Coding of sequela generally requires two codes sequenced in the following order: The condition or nature of the sequela is sequenced first.

The sequela code is sequenced second.

An exception to the above guidelines are those instances where the code for the sequela is followed by a manifestation code identified in the Tabular List and title, or the sequela code has been expanded (at the fourth, fifth or sixth character levels) to

---

include the manifestation(s). The code for the acute phase of an illness or injury that led to the sequela is never used with a code for the late effect.

GENERAL GUIDELINES

Chapter 2 of the ICD-10-CM contains the codes for most benign and all malignant neoplasms. Certain benign neoplasms, such as prostatic adenomas, may be found in the specific body system chapters. To properly code a neoplasm, it is necessary to determine from the record if the neoplasm is benign, in-situ, malignant, or of uncertain histologic behavior. If malignant, any secondary (metastatic) sites should also be determined.

PRIMARY MALIGNANT NEOPLASMS OVERLAPPING SITE BOUNDARIES

A primary malignant neoplasm that overlaps two or more contiguous (next to each other) sites should be classified to the subcategory/code .8 ('overlapping lesion'), unless the combination is specifically indexed elsewhere. For multiple neoplasms of the same site that are not contiguous such as tumors in different quadrants of the same breast, codes for each site should be assigned.

MALIGNANT NEOPLASM OF ECTOPIC TISSUE

Malignant neoplasms of ectopic tissue are to be coded to the site of origin mentioned, e.g., ectopic pancreatic malignant neoplasms involving the stomach are coded to malignant neoplasm of pancreas, unspecified (C25.9).

The neoplasm table in the Alphabetic Index should be referenced first. However, if the histological term is documented, that term should be referenced first, rather than going immediately to the Neoplasm Table, in order to determine which column in the Neoplasm Table is appropriate. For example, if the documentation indicates "adenoma," refer to the term in the Alphabetic Index to review the entries under this term and the instructional note to "see also neoplasm, by site, benign." The table provides the proper code based on the type of neoplasm and the site. It is important to select the proper column in the table that corresponds to the type of neoplasm. The Tabular List should then be referenced to verify that the correct code has been selected from the table and that a more specific site code does not exist.

See Section I.C.21. Factors influencing health status and contact with health services, Status, for information regarding Z15.0, codes for genetic susceptibility to cancer.

a. **Treatment directed at the malignancy**

If the treatment is directed at the malignancy, designate the malignancy as the principal diagnosis.

The only exception to this guideline is if a patient admission/encounter is solely for the administration of chemotherapy, immunotherapy or external beam radiation therapy, assign the appropriate Z51.-- code as the first-listed or principal diagnosis, and the diagnosis or problem for which the service is being performed as a secondary diagnosis.

b. **Treatment of secondary site**

When a patient is admitted because of a primary neoplasm with metastasis and treatment is directed toward the secondary site only, the secondary neoplasm is designated as the principal diagnosis even though the primary malignancy is still present.

c. **Coding and sequencing of complications**

Coding and sequencing of complications associated with the malignancies or with the therapy thereof are subject to the following guidelines:

1) **Anemia associated with malignancy**

When admission/encounter is for management of an anemia associated with the malignancy, and the treatment is only for anemia, the appropriate code for the malignancy is sequenced as the principal or first-listed diagnosis followed by the appropriate code for the anemia (such as code D63.0, Anemia in neoplastic disease).

2) **Anemia associated with chemotherapy, immunotherapy and radiation therapy**

● New code   ▲ Revised code   **Excludes1:** Not coded here   **Excludes2:** Not included here   ⊗ Placeholder required   ⑦ 7th digit required

When the admission/encounter is for management of an anemia associated with an adverse effect of the administration of chemotherapy or immunotherapy and the only treatment is for the anemia, the anemia code is sequenced first followed by the appropriate codes for the neoplasm and the adverse effect (T45.1X5-, Adverse effect of antineoplastic and immunosuppressive drugs).

When the admission/encounter is for management of an anemia associated with an adverse effect of radiotherapy, the anemia code should be sequenced first, followed by the appropriate neoplasm code and code Y84.2, Radiological procedure and radiotherapy as the cause of abnormal reaction of the patient, or of later complication, without mention of misadventure at the time of the procedure.

3)   Management of dehydration due to the malignancy

When the admission/encounter is for management of dehydration due to the malignancy and only the dehydration is being treated (intravenous rehydration), the dehydration is sequenced first, followed by the code(s) for the malignancy.

4)   Treatment of a complication resulting from a surgical procedure

When the admission/encounter is for treatment of a complication resulting from a surgical procedure, designate the complication as the principal or first-listed diagnosis if treatment is directed at resolving the complication.

d.   Primary malignancy previously excised

When a primary malignancy has been previously excised or eradicated from its site and there is no further treatment directed to that site and there is no evidence of any existing primary malignancy at that site, a code from category Z85, Personal history of malignant neoplasm, should be used to indicate the former site of the malignancy. Any mention of extension, invasion, or metastasis to another site is coded as a secondary malignant neoplasm to that site. The secondary site may be the principal or first-listed diagnosis with the Z85 code used as a secondary code.

e.   Admissions/Encounters involving chemotherapy, immunotherapy and radiation therapy

1)   Episode of care involves surgical removal of neoplasm

When an episode of care involves the surgical removal of a neoplasm, primary or secondary site, followed by adjunct chemotherapy or radiation treatment during the same episode of care, the code for the neoplasm should be assigned as principal or first-listed diagnosis.

2)   Patient admission/encounter solely for administration of chemotherapy, immunotherapy and radiation therapy

If a patient admission/encounter is solely for the administration of chemotherapy, immunotherapy or external beam radiation therapy assign code Z51.0, Encounter for antineoplastic radiation therapy, or Z51.11, Encounter for antineoplastic chemotherapy, or Z51.12, Encounter for antineoplastic immunotherapy as the first-listed or principal diagnosis. If a patient receives more than one of these therapies during the same admission more than one of these codes may be assigned, in any sequence.

The malignancy for which the therapy is being administered should be assigned as a secondary diagnosis.

If a patient admission/encounter is for the insertion or implantation of radioactive elements (e.g., brachytherapy) the appropriate code for the malignancy is sequenced as the principal or first-listed diagnosis. Code Z51.0 should not be assigned.

3)   Patient admitted for radiation therapy, chemotherapy or immunotherapy and develops complications

When a patient is admitted for the purpose of external beam radiotherapy, immunotherapy or chemotherapy and develops complications such as uncontrolled nausea and vomiting or dehydration, the principal or first-listed diagnosis is Z51.0, Encounter for antineoplastic radiation therapy, or Z51.11, Encounter for antineoplastic chemotherapy, or Z51.12,

Encounter for antineoplastic immunotherapy followed by any codes for the complications.

When a patient is admitted for the purpose of insertion or implantation of radioactive elements (e.g., brachytherapy) and develops complications such as uncontrolled nausea and vomiting or dehydration, the principal or first-listed diagnosis is the appropriate code for the malignancy followed by any codes for the complications.

f.   Admission/encounter to determine extent of malignancy

When the reason for admission/encounter is to determine the extent of the malignancy, or for a procedure such as paracentesis or thoracentesis, the primary malignancy or appropriate metastatic site is designated as the principal or first-listed diagnosis, even though chemotherapy or radiotherapy is administered.

g.   Symptoms, signs, and abnormal findings listed in Chapter 18 associated with neoplasms

Symptoms, signs, and ill-defined conditions listed in Chapter 18 characteristic of, or associated with, an existing primary or secondary site malignancy cannot be used to replace the malignancy as principal or first-listed diagnosis, regardless of the number of admissions or encounters for treatment and care of the neoplasm.

See section I.C.21. Factors influencing health status and contact with health services, Encounter for prophylactic organ removal.

h.   Admission/encounter for pain control/management

See Section I.C.6. for information on coding admission/encounter for pain control/management.

i.   Malignancy in two or more noncontiguous sites

A patient may have more than one malignant tumor in the same organ. These tumors may represent different primaries or metastatic disease, depending on the site. Should the documentation be unclear, the provider should be queried as to the status of each tumor so that the correct codes can be assigned.

j.   Disseminated malignant neoplasm, unspecified

Code C80.0, Disseminated malignant neoplasm, unspecified, is for use only in those cases where the patient has advanced metastatic disease, and no known primary or secondary sites are specified. It should not be used in place of assigning codes for the primary site and all known secondary sites.

k.   Malignant neoplasm without specification of site

Code C80.1, Malignant (primary) neoplasm, unspecified, equates to Cancer, unspecified. This code should only be used when no determination can be made as to the primary site of a malignancy. This code should rarely be used in the inpatient setting.

l.   Sequencing of neoplasm codes

1)   Encounter for treatment of primary malignancy

If the reason for the encounter is for treatment of a primary malignancy, assign the malignancy as the principal/first-listed diagnosis. The primary site is to be sequenced first, followed by any metastatic sites.

2)   Encounter for treatment of secondary malignancy

When an encounter is for a primary malignancy with metastasis and treatment is directed toward the metastatic (secondary) site(s) only, the metastatic site(s) is designated as the principal/first-listed diagnosis. The primary malignancy is coded as an additional code.

3)   Malignant neoplasm in a pregnant patient

When a pregnant patient has a malignant neoplasm, a code from subcategory O9A.1-, Malignant neoplasm complicating pregnancy, childbirth, and the puerperium, should be sequenced first, followed by the appropriate code from Chapter 2 to indicate the type of neoplasm.

4) Encounter for complication associated with a neoplasm

When an encounter is for management of a complication associated with a neoplasm, such as dehydration, and the treatment is only for the complication, the complication is coded first, followed by the appropriate code(s) for the neoplasm.

The exception to this guideline is anemia. When the admission/encounter is for management of an anemia associated with the malignancy, and the treatment is only for anemia, the appropriate code for the malignancy is sequenced as the principal or first-listed diagnosis followed by code D63.0, Anemia in neoplastic disease.

5) Complication from surgical procedure for treatment of a neoplasm

When an encounter is for treatment of a complication resulting from a surgical procedure performed for the treatment of the neoplasm, designate the complication as the principal/first-listed diagnosis. See the guideline regarding the coding of a current malignancy versus personal history to determine if the code for the neoplasm should also be assigned.

6) Pathologic fracture due to a neoplasm

When an encounter is for a pathological fracture due to a neoplasm, and the focus of treatment is the fracture, a code from subcategory M84.5, Pathological fracture in neoplastic disease, should be sequenced first, followed by the code for the neoplasm.

If the focus of treatment is the neoplasm with an associated pathological fracture, the neoplasm code should be sequenced first, followed by a code from M84.5 for the pathological fracture.

m. Current malignancy versus personal history of malignancy

When a primary malignancy has been excised but further treatment, such as an additional surgery for the malignancy, radiation therapy or chemotherapy is directed to that site, the primary malignancy code should be used until treatment is completed.

When a primary malignancy has been previously excised or eradicated from its site, there is no further treatment (of the malignancy) directed to that site, and there is no evidence of any existing primary malignancy at that site, a code from category Z85, Personal history of malignant neoplasm, should be used to indicate the former site of the malignancy.

Subcategories Z85.0 – Z85.7 should only be assigned for the former site of a primary malignancy, not the site of a secondary malignancy. Codes from subcategory Z85.8-, may be assigned for the former site(s) of either a primary or secondary malignancy included in this subcategory.

See Section I.C.21. Factors influencing health status and contact with health services, History (of)

n. Leukemia, Multiple Myeloma, and Malignant Plasma Cell Neoplasms in remission versus personal history

The categories for leukemia, and category C90, Multiple myeloma and malignant plasma cell neoplasms, have codes indicating whether or not the leukemia has achieved remission. There are also codes Z85.6, Personal history of leukemia, and Z85.79, Personal history of other malignant neoplasms of lymphoid, hematopoietic and related tissues. If the documentation is unclear as to whether the leukemia has achieved remission, the provider should be queried.

See Section I.C.21. Factors influencing health status and contact with health services, History (of)

o. Aftercare following surgery for neoplasm

See Section I.C.21. Factors influencing health status and contact with health services, Aftercare

p. Follow-up care for completed treatment of a malignancy

See Section I.C.21. Factors influencing health status and contact with health services, Follow-up

q. **Prophylactic organ removal for prevention of malignancy**

See Section I.C. 21, Factors influencing health status and contact with health services, Prophylactic organ removal

r. **Malignant neoplasm associated with transplanted organ**

A malignant neoplasm of a transplanted organ should be coded as a transplant complication. Assign first the appropriate code from category T86.-, Complications of transplanted organs and tissue, followed by code C80.2, Malignant neoplasm associated with transplanted organ. Use an additional code for the specific malignancy.

s. **Breast Implant Associated Anaplastic Large Cell Lymphoma**

Breast implant associated anaplastic large cell lymphoma (BIA-ALCL) is a type of lymphoma that can develop around breast implants. Assign code C84.7A, Anaplastic large cell lymphoma, ALK-negative, breast, for BIA-ALCL. Do not assign a complication code from chapter 19.

Chapter 2
Neoplasms (C00-D49)

This chapter contains the following blocks:

C00-C14	Malignant neoplasms of lip, oral cavity and pharynx
C15-C26	Malignant neoplasms of digestive organs
C30-C39	Malignant neoplasms of respiratory and intrathoracic organs
C40-C41	Malignant neoplasms of bone and articular cartilage
C43-C44	Melanoma and other Malignant neoplasms of skin
C45-C49	Malignant neoplasms of Mesothelial and soft tissue
C50	Malignant neoplasms of breast
C51-C58	Malignant neoplasms of female genital organs
C60-C63	Malignant neoplasms of Male genital organs
C64-C68	Malignant neoplasms of urinary tract
C69-C72	Malignant neoplasms of eye, brain and other parts of central nervous system
C73-C75	Malignant neoplasms of thyroid and other endocrine glands
C7A	Malignant neuroendocrine tumors
C7B	Secondary neuroendocrine tumors
C76-C80	Malignant neoplasms of ill-defined, other secondary and unspecified sites
C81-C96	Malignant neoplasms of lymphoid, hematopoietic and related tissue
D00-D09	In situ neoplasms
D10-D36	Benign neoplasms, except benign neuroendocrine tumors
D3A	Benign neuroendocrine tumors
D37-D48	Neoplasms of uncertain behavior, polycythemia vera and Myelodysplastic syndromes
D49	Neoplasms of unspecified behavior

Note: Functional activity

All neoplasms are classified in this chapter, whether they are functionally active or not. An additional code from Chapter 4 may be used, to identify functional activity associated with any neoplasm. Morphology [Histology]

Chapter 2 classifies neoplasms primarily by site (topography), with broad groupings for behavior, malignant, in situ, benign, etc. The Table of Neoplasms should be used to identify the correct topography code. In a few cases, such as for malignant melanoma and certain neuroendocrine tumors, the morphology (histologic type) is included in the category and codes.

Primary malignant neoplasms overlapping site boundaries

A primary malignant neoplasm that overlaps two or more contiguous (next to each Other) sites should be classified to the subcategory/code .8 ('overlapping lesion'), unless the combination is specifically indexed elsewhere. For multiple neoplasms of the same site that are not contiguous, such as tumors in different quadrants of the same breast, codes for each site should be assigned.

Malignant neoplasm of ectopic tissue

Malignant neoplasms of ectopic tissue are to be coded to the site mentioned, e.g., ectopic pancreatic malignant neoplasms are coded to pancreas, unspecified (C25.9).

MALIGNANT NEOPLASMS (C00-C96)

Definition: Malignant neoplasm refers to a tumor that tends to grow, invade, and metastasize. The tumor usually has an irregular shape and is composed of poorly differentiated cells. If untreated, it may result in death.

MALIGNANT NEOPLASMS, STATED OR PRESUMED TO BE PRIMARY (OF SPECIFIED SITES), AND CERTAIN SPECIFIED HISTOLOGIES, EXCEPT NEUROENDOCRINE, AND OF LYMPHOID, HEMATOPOIETIC AND RELATED TISSUE (C00-C75)

MALIGNANT NEOPLASMS OF LIP, ORAL CAVITY AND PHARYNX (C00-C14)

C00 **Malignant neoplasm of lip**

Use Additional Code to identify:

alcohol abuse and dependence (F10.-)

history of tobacco dependence (Z87.891)

tobacco dependence (F17.-)

tobacco use (Z72.0)

Excludes1: malignant melanoma of lip (C43.0)

Merkel cell carcinoma of lip (C4A.0)

Other and unspecified malignant neoplasm of skin of lip (C44.0-)

C00.0 **Malignant neoplasm of external upper lip**

Malignant neoplasm of lipstick area of upper lip

Malignant neoplasm of upper lip NOS

Malignant neoplasm of vermilion border of upper lip

C00.1 **Malignant neoplasm of external lower lip**

Malignant neoplasm of lower lip NOS

Malignant neoplasm of lipstick area of lower lip

Malignant neoplasm of vermilion border of lower lip

C00.2 **Malignant neoplasm of external lip, unspecified**

Malignant neoplasm of vermilion border of lip NOS

C00.3 **Malignant neoplasm of upper lip, inner aspect**

Malignant neoplasm of buccal aspect of upper lip

Malignant neoplasm of frenulum of upper lip

Malignant neoplasm of mucosa of upper lip

Malignant neoplasm of oral aspect of upper lip

C00.4 **Malignant neoplasm of lower lip, inner aspect**

Malignant neoplasm of buccal aspect of lower lip

Malignant neoplasm of frenulum of lower lip

Malignant neoplasm of mucosa of lower lip

Malignant neoplasm of oral aspect of lower lip

C00.5 **Malignant neoplasm of lip, unspecified, inner aspect**

Malignant neoplasm of buccal aspect of lip, unspecified

Malignant neoplasm of frenulum of lip, unspecified

Malignant neoplasm of mucosa of lip, unspecified

Malignant neoplasm of oral aspect of lip, unspecified

C00.6 **Malignant neoplasm of commissure of lip, unspecified**

C00.8 **Malignant neoplasm of overlapping sites of lip**

C00.9 **Malignant neoplasm of lip, unspecified**

C01 **Malignant neoplasm of base of tongue** [HCC]

Malignant neoplasm of dorsal surface of base of tongue

Malignant neoplasm of fixed part of tongue NOS

Malignant neoplasm of posterior third of tongue

Use Additional Code to identify:

alcohol abuse and dependence (F10.-)

history of tobacco dependence (Z87.891)

tobacco dependence (F17.-)

tobacco use (Z72.0)

C02 **Malignant neoplasm of other and unspecified parts of tongue**

Use Additional Code to identify:

alcohol abuse and dependence (F10.-)

history of tobacco dependence (Z87.891)

tobacco dependence (F17.-)

tobacco use (Z72.0)

C02.0 **Malignant neoplasm of dorsal surface of tongue** [HCC]

Malignant neoplasm of anterior two-thirds of tongue, dorsal surface

Excludes2: malignant neoplasm of dorsal surface of base of tongue (C01)

C02.1 **Malignant neoplasm of border of tongue** [HCC]

Malignant neoplasm of tip of tongue

C02.2 **Malignant neoplasm of ventral surface of tongue** [HCC]

Malignant neoplasm of anterior two-thirds of tongue, ventral surface

Malignant neoplasm of frenulum linguae

C02.3 **Malignant neoplasm of anterior two-thirds of tongue, part unspecified** [HCC]

Malignant neoplasm of middle third of tongue NOS

Malignant neoplasm of mobile part of tongue NOS

C02.4 **Malignant neoplasm of lingual tonsil** [HCC]

Excludes2: malignant neoplasm of tonsil NOS (C09.9)

C02.8 **Malignant neoplasm of overlapping sites of tongue** [HCC]

Malignant neoplasm of two or more contiguous sites of tongue

C02.9 **Malignant neoplasm of tongue, unspecified** [HCC]

C03 **Malignant neoplasm of gum**

Includes: malignant neoplasm of alveolar (ridge) mucosa

malignant neoplasm of gingiva

Use Additional Code to identify:

alcohol abuse and dependence (F10.-)

history of tobacco dependence (Z87.891)

tobacco dependence (F17.-)

tobacco use (Z72.0)

Excludes2: malignant odontogenic neoplasms (C41.0-C41.1)

C03.0 **Malignant neoplasm of upper gum** [HCC]

C03.1 **Malignant neoplasm of lower gum** [HCC]

C03.9 **Malignant neoplasm of gum, unspecified** [HCC]

C04 **Malignant neoplasm of floor of mouth**

Use Additional Code to identify:

alcohol abuse and dependence (F10.-)

history of tobacco dependence (Z87.891)

tobacco dependence (F17.-)

tobacco use (Z72.0)

C04.0 **Malignant neoplasm of anterior floor of mouth** [HCC]

Malignant neoplasm of anterior to the premolar-canine junction

C04.1 **Malignant neoplasm of lateral floor of mouth** [HCC]

C04.8 **Malignant neoplasm of overlapping sites of floor of mouth** [HCC]

C04.9 **Malignant neoplasm of floor of mouth, unspecified** [HCC]

C05 **Malignant neoplasm of palate**

Use Additional Code to identify:

alcohol abuse and dependence (F10.-)

history of tobacco dependence (Z87.891)

tobacco dependence (F17.-)

tobacco use (Z72.0)

Excludes1: Kaposi's sarcoma of palate (C46.2)

C05.0 **Malignant neoplasm of hard palate** [HCC]

C05.1 **Malignant neoplasm of soft palate** [HCC]

Excludes2: malignant neoplasm of nasopharyngeal surface of soft palate (C11.3)

C05.2 **Malignant neoplasm of uvula** [HCC]

C05.8 **Malignant neoplasm of overlapping sites of palate** [HCC]

C05.9 **Malignant neoplasm of palate, unspecified**

Malignant neoplasm of roof of mouth

C06 **Malignant neoplasm of other and unspecified parts of mouth**

Use Additional Code to identify:

alcohol abuse and dependence (F10.-)

history of tobacco dependence (Z87.891)

tobacco dependence (F17.-)

tobacco use (Z72.0)

C06.0 **Malignant neoplasm of cheek mucosa** [HCC]

Malignant neoplasm of buccal mucosa NOS

Malignant neoplasm of internal cheek

C06.1 **Malignant neoplasm of vestibule of mouth** [HCC]

Malignant neoplasm of buccal sulcus (upper) (lower)

Malignant neoplasm of labial sulcus (upper) (lower)

C06.2 **Malignant neoplasm of retromolar area** [HCC]

C06.8 **Malignant neoplasm of overlapping sites of other and unspecified parts of mouth**

C06.80 **Malignant neoplasm of overlapping sites of unspecified parts of mouth** [HCC]

C06.89 **Malignant neoplasm of overlapping sites of other parts of mouth** [HCC]

'book leaf' neoplasm [ventral surface of tongue and floor of mouth]

C06.9 **Malignant neoplasm of mouth, unspecified** [HCC]

Malignant neoplasm of minor salivary gland, unspecified site

Malignant neoplasm of oral cavity NOS

C07 **Malignant neoplasm of parotid gland** [HCC]

Use Additional Code to identify:

alcohol abuse and dependence (F10.-)

exposure to environmental tobacco smoke (Z77.22)

exposure to tobacco smoke in the perinatal period (P96.81)

history of tobacco dependence (Z87.891)

occupational exposure to environmental tobacco smoke (Z57.31)

tobacco dependence (F17.-)

tobacco use (Z72.0)

C08 **Malignant neoplasm of other and unspecified major salivary glands**

Includes: malignant neoplasm of salivary ducts

Use Additional Code to identify:

alcohol abuse and dependence (F10.-)

exposure to environmental tobacco smoke (Z77.22)

exposure to tobacco smoke in the perinatal period (P96.81)

history of tobacco dependence (Z87.891)

occupational exposure to environmental tobacco smoke (Z57.31)

tobacco dependence (F17.-)

tobacco use (Z72.0)

Excludes1: malignant neoplasms of specified minor salivary glands which are classified according to their anatomical location

Excludes2: malignant neoplasms of minor salivary glands NOS (C06.9)

malignant neoplasm of parotid gland (C07)

C08.0 **Malignant neoplasm of submandibular gland** [HCC]

Malignant neoplasm of submaxillary gland

C08.1 **Malignant neoplasm of sublingual gland** [HCC]

C08.9 **Malignant neoplasm of major salivary gland, unspecified** [HCC]

Malignant neoplasm of salivary gland (major) NOS

● New code ▲ Revised code **Excludes1:** Not coded here **Excludes2:** Not included here ⊗ Placeholder required ⑦ᵗʰ digit required

C09 **Malignant neoplasm of tonsil** [HCC]

Use Additional Code to identify:

alcohol abuse and dependence (F10.-)

exposure to environmental tobacco smoke (Z77.22)

exposure to tobacco smoke in the perinatal period (P96.81)

history of tobacco dependence (Z87.891)

occupational exposure to environmental tobacco smoke (Z57.31)

tobacco dependence (F17.-)

tobacco use (Z72.0)

Excludes2: malignant neoplasm of lingual tonsil (C02.4)

malignant neoplasm of pharyngeal tonsil (C11.1)

C09.0 **Malignant neoplasm of tonsillar fossa** [HCC]

C09.1 **Malignant neoplasm of tonsillar pillar (anterior) (posterior)** [HCC]

C09.8 **Malignant neoplasm of overlapping sites of tonsil** [HCC]

C09.9 **Malignant neoplasm of tonsil, unspecified** [HCC]

Malignant neoplasm of tonsil NOS

Malignant neoplasm of faucial tonsils

Malignant neoplasm of palatine tonsils

C10 **Malignant neoplasm of oropharynx** [HCC]

Use Additional Code to identify:

alcohol abuse and dependence (F10.-)

exposure to environmental tobacco smoke (Z77.22)

exposure to tobacco smoke in the perinatal period (P96.81)

history of tobacco dependence (Z87.891)

occupational exposure to environmental tobacco smoke (Z57.31)

tobacco dependence (F17.-)

tobacco use (Z72.0)

Excludes2: malignant neoplasm of tonsil (C09.-)

C10.0 **Malignant neoplasm of vallecula**

C10.1 **Malignant neoplasm of anterior surface of epiglottis** [HCC]

Malignant neoplasm of epiglottis, free border [margin]

Malignant neoplasm of glossoepiglottic fold(s)

Excludes2: malignant neoplasm of epiglottis (suprahyoid portion) NOS (C32.1)

C10.2 **Malignant neoplasm of lateral wall of oropharynx** [HCC]

C10.3 **Malignant neoplasm of posterior wall of oropharynx** [HCC]

C10.4 **Malignant neoplasm of branchial cleft** Malignant neoplasm of branchial cyst [site of neoplasm]

C10.8 **Malignant neoplasm of overlapping sites of oropharynx** [HCC]

Malignant neoplasm of junctional region of oropharynx

C10.9 **Malignant neoplasm of oropharynx, unspecified** [HCC]

C11 **Malignant neoplasm of nasopharynx**

Use Additional Code to identify:

exposure to environmental tobacco smoke (Z77.22)

exposure to tobacco smoke in the perinatal period (P96.81)

history of tobacco dependence (Z87.891)

occupational exposure to environmental tobacco smoke (Z57.31)

tobacco dependence (F17.-)

tobacco use (Z72.0)

C11.0 **Malignant neoplasm of superior wall of nasopharynx** [HCC]

Malignant neoplasm of roof of nasopharynx

C11.1 **Malignant neoplasm of posterior wall of nasopharynx** [HCC]

Malignant neoplasm of adenoid

Malignant neoplasm of pharyngeal tonsil

C11.2 **Malignant neoplasm of lateral wall of nasopharynx** [HCC]

Malignant neoplasm of fossa of Rosenmüller

Malignant neoplasm of opening of auditory tube

Malignant neoplasm of pharyngeal recess

C11.3 **Malignant neoplasm of anterior wall of nasopharynx** [HCC]

Malignant neoplasm of floor of nasopharynx

Malignant neoplasm of nasopharyngeal (anterior) (posterior) surface of soft palate

Malignant neoplasm of posterior margin of nasal choana

Malignant neoplasm of posterior margin of nasal septum

C11.8 **Malignant neoplasm of overlapping sites of nasopharynx** [HCC]

C11.9 **Malignant neoplasm of nasopharynx, unspecified** [HCC]

Malignant neoplasm of nasopharyngeal wall NOS

C12 **Malignant neoplasm of pyriform sinus** [HCC]

Malignant neoplasm of pyriform fossa

Use Additional Code to identify:

exposure to environmental tobacco smoke (Z77.22)

exposure to tobacco smoke in the perinatal period (P96.81)

history of tobacco dependence (Z87.891)

occupational exposure to environmental tobacco smoke (Z57.31)

tobacco dependence (F17.-)

tobacco use (Z72.0)

C13 **Malignant neoplasm of hypopharynx**

Use Additional Code to identify:

exposure to environmental tobacco smoke (Z77.22)

exposure to tobacco smoke in the perinatal period (P96.81)

history of tobacco dependence (Z87.891)

occupational exposure to environmental tobacco smoke (Z57.31)

tobacco dependence (F17.-)

tobacco use (Z72.0)

Excludes2: malignant neoplasm of pyriform sinus (C12)

C13.0 **Malignant neoplasm of postcricoid region** [HCC]

C13.1 **Malignant neoplasm of aryepiglottic fold, hypopharyngeal aspect** [HCC]

Malignant neoplasm of aryepiglottic fold, marginal zone

Malignant neoplasm of aryepiglottic fold NOS

Malignant neoplasm of interarytenoid fold, marginal zone

Malignant neoplasm of interarytenoid fold NOS

Excludes2: malignant neoplasm of aryepiglottic fold or interarytenoid fold, laryngeal aspect (C32.1)

C13.2 **Malignant neoplasm of posterior wall of hypopharynx** [HCC]

C13.8 **Malignant neoplasm of overlapping sites of hypopharynx** [HCC]

C13.9 **Malignant neoplasm of hypopharynx, unspecified** [HCC]

Malignant neoplasm of hypopharyngeal wall NOS

C14 **Malignant neoplasm of other and ill-defined sites in the lip, oral cavity and pharynx**

Use Additional Code to identify:

alcohol abuse and dependence (F10.-)

exposure to environmental tobacco smoke (Z77.22)

exposure to tobacco smoke in the perinatal period (P96.81)

history of tobacco dependence (Z87.891)

occupational exposure to environmental tobacco smoke (Z57.31) tobacco dependence (F17.-)

tobacco use (Z72.0)

Excludes1: malignant neoplasm of oral cavity NOS (C06.9)

C14.0   **Malignant neoplasm of pharynx, unspecified** [HCC]

C14.2   **Malignant neoplasm of Waldeyer's ring** [HCC]

C14.8   **Malignant neoplasm of overlapping sites of lip, oral cavity and pharynx** [HCC]

Primary malignant neoplasm of two or more contiguous sites of lip, oral cavity and pharynx

Excludes1: 'book leaf' neoplasm [ventral surface of tongue and floor of mouth] (C06.89)

MALIGNANT NEOPLASMS OF DIGESTIVE ORGANS (C15-C26)

Excludes1: Kaposi's sarcoma of gastrointestinal sites (C46.4)

Excludes2: gastrointestinal stromal tumors (C49.A-)

C15   **Malignant neoplasm of esophagus**

Use Additional Code to identify:

alcohol abuse and dependence (F10.-)

C15.3   **Malignant neoplasm of upper third of esophagus**

C15.4   **Malignant neoplasm of middle third of esophagus** [HCC]

C15.5   **Malignant neoplasm of lower third of esophagus** [HCC]

Excludes1: malignant neoplasm of cardio-esophageal junction (C16.0)

C15.8   **Malignant neoplasm of overlapping sites of esophagus** [HCC]

C15.9   **Malignant neoplasm of esophagus, unspecified** [HCC]

C16   **Malignant neoplasm of stomach**

Use Additional Code to identify:

alcohol abuse and dependence (F10.-)

Excludes2: malignant carcinoid tumor of the stomach (C7A.092)

C16.0   **Malignant neoplasm of cardia** [HCC]

Malignant neoplasm of cardiac orifice

Malignant neoplasm of cardio-esophageal junction

Malignant neoplasm of esophagus and stomach

Malignant neoplasm of gastro-esophageal junction

C16.1   **Malignant neoplasm of fundus of stomach** [HCC]

C16.2   **Malignant neoplasm of body of stomach** [HCC]

C16.3   **Malignant neoplasm of pyloric antrum** [HCC]

Malignant neoplasm of gastric antrum

C16.4   **Malignant neoplasm of pylorus** [HCC]

Malignant neoplasm of prepylorus

Malignant neoplasm of pyloric canal

C16.5   **Malignant neoplasm of lesser curvature of stomach, unspecified** [HCC]

Malignant neoplasm of lesser curvature of stomach, not classifiable to C16.1-C16.4

C16.6   **Malignant neoplasm of greater curvature of stomach, unspecified** [HCC]

Malignant neoplasm of greater curvature of stomach, not classifiable to C16.0-C16.4

C16.8   **Malignant neoplasm of overlapping sites of stomach** [HCC]

C16.9   **Malignant neoplasm of stomach, unspecified** [HCC]

Gastric cancer NOS

C17   **Malignant neoplasm of small intestine**

Excludes1: malignant carcinoid tumors of the small intestine (C7A.01)

C17.0   **Malignant neoplasm of duodenum** [HCC]

C17.1   **Malignant neoplasm of jejunum** [HCC]

C17.2   **Malignant neoplasm of ileum** [HCC]

Excludes1: malignant neoplasm of ileocecal valve (C18.0)

C17.3   **Meckel's diverticulum, malignant** [HCC]

Excludes1: Meckel's diverticulum, congenital (Q43.0)

C17.8   **Malignant neoplasm of overlapping sites of small intestine** [HCC]

C17.9   **Malignant neoplasm of small intestine, unspecified**

C18   **Malignant neoplasm of colon**

Excludes1: malignant carcinoid tumors of the colon (C7A.02-)

C18.0   **Malignant neoplasm of cecum** [HCC]

Malignant neoplasm of ileocecal valve

C18.1   **Malignant neoplasm of appendix** [HCC]

C18.2   **Malignant neoplasm of ascending colon** [HCC]

C18.3   **Malignant neoplasm of hepatic flexure** [HCC]

C18.4   **Malignant neoplasm of transverse colon** [HCC]

C18.5   **Malignant neoplasm of splenic flexure** [HCC]

C18.6   **Malignant neoplasm of descending colon** [HCC]

C18.7   **Malignant neoplasm of sigmoid colon** [HCC]

Malignant neoplasm of sigmoid (flexure)

Excludes1: malignant neoplasm of rectosigmoid junction (C19)

C18.8   **Malignant neoplasm of overlapping sites of colon** [HCC]

C18.9   **Malignant neoplasm of colon, unspecified** [HCC]

Malignant neoplasm of large intestine NOS

C19   **Malignant neoplasm of rectosigmoid junction** [HCC]

Malignant neoplasm of colon with rectum

Malignant neoplasm of rectosigmoid (colon)

Excludes1: malignant carcinoid tumors of the colon (C7A.02-)

C20   **Malignant neoplasm of rectum** [HCC]

Malignant neoplasm of rectal ampulla

Excludes1: malignant carcinoid tumor of the rectum (C7A.026)

C21   **Malignant neoplasm of anus and anal canal**

Excludes2: malignant carcinoid tumors of the colon (C7A.02-)

malignant melanoma of anal margin (C43.51)

malignant melanoma of anal skin (C43.51)

malignant melanoma of perianal skin (C43.51)

Other and unspecified malignant neoplasm of anal margin (C44.500, C44.510, C44.520, C44.590)

Other and unspecified malignant neoplasm of anal skin (C44.500, C44.510, C44.520, C44.590)

Other and unspecified malignant neoplasm of perianal skin (C44.500, C44.510, C44.520, C44.590)

C21.0   **Malignant neoplasm of anus, unspecified** [HCC]

C21.1   **Malignant neoplasm of anal canal** [HCC]

Malignant neoplasm of anal sphincter

C21.2   **Malignant neoplasm of cloacogenic zone** [HCC]

C21.8   **Malignant neoplasm of overlapping sites of rectum, anus and anal canal** [HCC]

Malignant neoplasm of anorectal junction

Malignant neoplasm of anorectum

Primary malignant neoplasm of two or more contiguous sites of rectum, anus and anal canal

C22   **Malignant neoplasm of liver and intrahepatic bile ducts**

Excludes1: malignant neoplasm of biliary tract NOS (C24.9)

secondary malignant neoplasm of liver and intrahepatic bile duct (C78.7)

Use Additional Code to identify:

alcohol abuse and dependence (F10.-)

hepatitis B (B16.-, B18.0-B18.1)

hepatitis C (B17.1-, B18.2)

C22.0 Liver cell carcinoma [HCC]

Hepatocellular carcinoma

Hepatoma

C22.1 Intrahepatic bile duct carcinoma [HCC]

Cholangiocarcinoma

Excludes1: malignant neoplasm of hepatic duct (C24.0)

C22.2 Hepatoblastoma [HCC]

C22.3 Angiosarcoma of liver [HCC]

Kupffer cell sarcoma

C22.4 Other sarcomas of liver [HCC]

C22.7 Other specified carcinomas of liver [HCC]

C22.8 Malignant neoplasm of liver, primary, unspecified as to type [HCC]

C22.9 Malignant neoplasm of liver, not specified as primary or secondary [HCC]

C23 Malignant neoplasm of gallbladder [HCC]

C24 Malignant neoplasm of other and unspecified parts of biliary tract

Excludes1: malignant neoplasm of intrahepatic bile duct (C22.1)

C24.0 Malignant neoplasm of extrahepatic bile duct [HCC]

Malignant neoplasm of biliary duct or passage NOS

Malignant neoplasm of common bile duct

Malignant neoplasm of cystic duct

Malignant neoplasm of hepatic duct

C24.1 Malignant neoplasm of ampulla of Vater [HCC]

C24.8 Malignant neoplasm of overlapping sites of biliary tract [HCC]

Malignant neoplasm involving both intrahepatic and extrahepatic bile ducts

Primary malignant neoplasm of two or more contiguous sites of biliary tract

C24.9 Malignant neoplasm of biliary tract, unspecified [HCC]

C25 Malignant neoplasm of pancreas

Code also if applicable exocrine pancreatic insufficiency (K86.81)

Use Additional Code to identify:

alcohol abuse and dependence (F10.-)

C25.0 Malignant neoplasm of head of pancreas [HCC]

C25.1 Malignant neoplasm of body of pancreas [HCC]

C25.2 Malignant neoplasm of tail of pancreas [HCC]

C25.3 Malignant neoplasm of pancreatic duct

C25.4 Malignant neoplasm of endocrine pancreas [HCC]

Malignant neoplasm of islets of Langerhans

Use Additional Code to identify any functional activity.

C25.7 Malignant neoplasm of other parts of pancreas [HCC]

Malignant neoplasm of neck of pancreas

C25.8 Malignant neoplasm of overlapping sites of pancreas [HCC]

C25.9 Malignant neoplasm of pancreas, unspecified [HCC]

C26 Malignant neoplasm of other and ill-defined digestive organs

Excludes1: malignant neoplasm of peritoneum and retroperitoneum (C48.-)

C26.0 Malignant neoplasm of intestinal tract, part unspecified [HCC]

Malignant neoplasm of intestine NOS

C26.1 Malignant neoplasm of spleen [HCC]

Excludes1: Hodgkin lymphoma (C81.-)

non-Hodgkin lymphoma (C82-C85)

C26.9 Malignant neoplasm of ill-defined sites within the digestive system [HCC]

Malignant neoplasm of alimentary canal or tract NOS

Malignant neoplasm of gastrointestinal tract NOS

Excludes1: malignant neoplasm of abdominal NOS (C76.2)

malignant neoplasm of intra-abdominal NOS (C76.2)

MALIGNANT NEOPLASMS OF RESPIRATORY AND INTRATHORACIC ORGANS (C30-C39)

Includes: malignant neoplasm of middle ear

Excludes1: mesothelioma (C45.-)

C30 Malignant neoplasm of nasal cavity and middle ear [HCC]

C30.0 Malignant neoplasm of nasal cavity [HCC]

Malignant neoplasm of cartilage of nose

Malignant neoplasm of nasal concha

Malignant neoplasm of internal nose

Malignant neoplasm of septum of nose

Malignant neoplasm of vestibule of nose

Excludes1: malignant neoplasm of nasal bone (C41.0)

malignant neoplasm of nose NOS (C76.0)

malignant neoplasm of olfactory bulb (C72.2-)

malignant neoplasm of posterior margin of nasal septum and choana (C11.3)

malignant melanoma of skin of nose (C43.31)

malignant neoplasm of turbinates (C41.0)

other and unspecified malignant neoplasm of skin of nose (C44.301, C44.311, C44.321, C44.391)

C30.1 Malignant neoplasm of middle ear [HCC]

Malignant neoplasm of antrum tympanicum

Malignant neoplasm of auditory tube

Malignant neoplasm of eustachian tube

Malignant neoplasm of inner ear

Malignant neoplasm of mastoid air cells

Malignant neoplasm of tympanic cavity

Excludes1: malignant neoplasm of auricular canal (external) (C43.2-,C44.2-)

malignant neoplasm of bone of ear (meatus) (C41.0)

malignant neoplasm of cartilage of ear (C49.0)

malignant melanoma of skin of (external) ear (C43.2-)

Other and unspecified malignant neoplasm of skin of (external) ear (C44.2-)

C31 Malignant neoplasm of accessory sinuses

C31.0 Malignant neoplasm of maxillary sinus [HCC]

Malignant neoplasm of antrum (Highmore) (maxillary)

C31.1 Malignant neoplasm of ethmoidal sinus [HCC]

C31.2 Malignant neoplasm of frontal sinus [HCC]

C31.3 Malignant neoplasm of sphenoid sinus [HCC]

C31.8 Malignant neoplasm of overlapping sites of accessory sinuses [HCC]

C31.9 Malignant neoplasm of accessory sinus, unspecified [HCC]

C32 Malignant neoplasm of larynx

Use Additional Code to identify:

alcohol abuse and dependence (F10.-)

exposure to environmental tobacco smoke (Z77.22)

exposure to tobacco smoke in the perinatal period (P96.81)

history of tobacco dependence (Z87.891)

■ Add 4th-7th digits ■ Nonspecific code ■ Unspecified code ■ Manifestation code [HCC] Hierarchical Condition Code occupational exposure to environmental tobacco smoke (Z57.31)

tobacco dependence (F17.-)

tobacco use (Z72.0)

C32.0 **Malignant neoplasm of glottis** [HCC]

Malignant neoplasm of intrinsic larynx

Malignant neoplasm of laryngeal commissure (anterior)(posterior)

Malignant neoplasm of vocal cord (true) NOS

C32.1 **Malignant neoplasm of supraglottis** [HCC]

Malignant neoplasm of aryepiglottic fold or interarytenoid fold, laryngeal aspect

Malignant neoplasm of epiglottis (suprahyoid portion) NOS

Malignant neoplasm of extrinsic larynx

Malignant neoplasm of false vocal cord

Malignant neoplasm of posterior (laryngeal) surface of epiglottis

Malignant neoplasm of ventricular bands

Excludes2: malignant neoplasm of anterior surface of epiglottis (C10.1)

malignant neoplasm of aryepiglottic fold or interarytenoid fold, hypopharyngeal aspect (C13.1)

malignant neoplasm of aryepiglottic fold or interarytenoid fold, marginal zone (C13.1)

malignant neoplasm of aryepiglottic fold or interarytenoid fold NOS (C13.1)

C32.2 **Malignant neoplasm of subglottis** [HCC]

C32.3 **Malignant neoplasm of laryngeal cartilage** [HCC]

C32.8 **Malignant neoplasm of overlapping sites of larynx** [HCC]

C32.9 **Malignant neoplasm of larynx, unspecified** [HCC]

C33 **Malignant neoplasm of trachea** [HCC]

Use Additional Code to identify:

exposure to environmental tobacco smoke (Z77.22)

exposure to tobacco smoke in the perinatal period (P96.81)

history of tobacco dependence (Z87.891)

occupational exposure to environmental tobacco smoke (Z57.31)

tobacco dependence (F17.-)

tobacco use (Z72.0)

C34 **Malignant neoplasm of bronchus and lung**

Use Additional Code to identify:

exposure to environmental tobacco smoke (Z77.22)

exposure to tobacco smoke in the perinatal period (P96.81)

history of tobacco dependence (Z87.891)

occupational exposure to environmental tobacco smoke (Z57.31)

tobacco dependence (F17.-)

tobacco use (Z72.0)

Excludes1: Kaposi's sarcoma of lung (C46.5-)

malignant carcinoid tumor of the bronchus and lung (C7A.090)

C34.0 **Malignant neoplasm of main bronchus**

Malignant neoplasm of carina

Malignant neoplasm of hilus (of lung)

C34.00 **Malignant neoplasm of unspecified main bronchus** [HCC]

C34.01 **Malignant neoplasm of right main bronchus** [HCC]

C34.02 **Malignant neoplasm of left main bronchus** [HCC]

C34.1 **Malignant neoplasm of upper lobe, bronchus or lung**

C34.10 **Malignant neoplasm of upper lobe, unspecified bronchus or lung** [HCC]

C34.11 **Malignant neoplasm of upper lobe, right bronchus or lung** [HCC]

C34.12 **Malignant neoplasm of upper lobe, left bronchus or lung** [HCC]

C34.2 **Malignant neoplasm of middle lobe, bronchus or lung**

C34.3 **Malignant neoplasm of lower lobe, bronchus or lung**

C34.30 **Malignant neoplasm of lower lobe, unspecified bronchus or lung** [HCC]

C34.31 **Malignant neoplasm of lower lobe, right bronchus or lung** [HCC]

C34.32 **Malignant neoplasm of lower lobe, left bronchus or lung** [HCC]

C34.8 **Malignant neoplasm of overlapping sites of bronchus and lung**

C34.80 **Malignant neoplasm of overlapping sites of unspecified bronchus and lung** [HCC]

C34.81 **Malignant neoplasm of overlapping sites of right bronchus and lung** [HCC]

C34.82 **Malignant neoplasm of overlapping sites of left bronchus and lung** [HCC]

C34.9 **Malignant neoplasm of unspecified part of bronchus or lung**

C34.90 **Malignant neoplasm of unspecified part of unspecified bronchus or lung** [HCC]

Lung cancer NOS

C34.91 **Malignant neoplasm of unspecified part of right bronchus or lung** [HCC]

C34.92 **Malignant neoplasm of unspecified part of left bronchus or lung** [HCC]

C37 **Malignant neoplasm of thymus**

Excludes1: malignant carcinoid tumor of the thymus (C7A.091)

C38 **Malignant neoplasm of heart, mediastinum and pleura**

Excludes1: mesothelioma (C45.-)

C38.0 **Malignant neoplasm of heart** [HCC]

Malignant neoplasm of pericardium

Excludes1: malignant neoplasm of great vessels (C49.3)

C38.1 **Malignant neoplasm of anterior mediastinum** [HCC]

C38.2 **Malignant neoplasm of posterior mediastinum** [HCC]

C38.3 **Malignant neoplasm of mediastinum, part unspecified** [HCC]

C38.4 **Malignant neoplasm of pleura** [HCC]

C38.8 **Malignant neoplasm of overlapping sites of heart, mediastinum and pleura** [HCC]

C39 **Malignant neoplasm of other and ill-defined sites in the respiratory system and intrathoracic organs** [HCC]

Use Additional Code to identify:

exposure to environmental tobacco smoke (Z77.22)

exposure to tobacco smoke in the perinatal period (P96.81)

history of tobacco dependence (Z87.891)

occupational exposure to environmental tobacco smoke (Z57.31)

tobacco dependence (F17.-)

tobacco use (Z72.0)

Excludes1: intrathoracic malignant neoplasm NOS (C76.1)

thoracic malignant neoplasm NOS (C76.1)

C39.0 **Malignant neoplasm of upper respiratory tract, part unspecified** [HCC]

C39.9 **Malignant neoplasm of lower respiratory tract, part unspecified** [HCC]

Malignant neoplasm of respiratory tract NOS

MALIGNANT NEOPLASMS OF BONE AND ARTICULAR CARTILAGE (C40-C41)

Includes: malignant neoplasm of cartilage (articular) (joint)

malignant neoplasm of periosteum

Excludes1: malignant neoplasm of bone marrow NOS (C96.9)

malignant neoplasm of synovia (C49.-)

C40 **Malignant neoplasm of bone and articular cartilage of limbs**

<u>Use Additional Code</u> to identify major osseous defect, if applicable (M89.7-)

C40.0 **Malignant neoplasm of scapula and long bones of upper limb**

C40.00 **Malignant neoplasm of scapula and long bones of unspecified upper limb** [HCC]

C40.01 **Malignant neoplasm of scapula and long bones of right upper limb** [HCC]

C40.02 **Malignant neoplasm of scapula and long bones of left upper limb** [HCC]

C40.1 **Malignant neoplasm of short bones of upper limb**

C40.10 **Malignant neoplasm of short bones of unspecified upper limb** [HCC]

C40.11 **Malignant neoplasm of short bones of right upper limb**

C40.12 **Malignant neoplasm of short bones of left upper limb** [HCC]

C40.2 **Malignant neoplasm of long bones of lower limb**

C40.20 **Malignant neoplasm of long bones of unspecified lower limb** [HCC]

C40.21 **Malignant neoplasm of long bones of right lower limb** [HCC]

C40.22 **Malignant neoplasm of long bones of left lower limb** [HCC]

C40.3 **Malignant neoplasm of short bones of lower limb**

C40.30 **Malignant neoplasm of short bones of unspecified lower limb** [HCC]

C40.31 **Malignant neoplasm of short bones of right lower limb** [HCC]

C40.32 **Malignant neoplasm of short bones of left lower limb** [HCC]

C40.8 **Malignant neoplasm of overlapping sites of bone and articular cartilage of limb**

C40.80 **Malignant neoplasm of overlapping sites of bone and articular cartilage of unspecified limb** [HCC]

C40.81 **Malignant neoplasm of overlapping sites of bone and articular cartilage of right limb** [HCC]

C40.82 **Malignant neoplasm of overlapping sites of bone and articular cartilage of left limb** [HCC]

C40.9 **Malignant neoplasm of unspecified bones and articular cartilage of limb**

C40.90 **Malignant neoplasm of unspecified bones and articular cartilage of unspecified limb** [HCC]

C40.91 **Malignant neoplasm of unspecified bones and articular cartilage of right limb** [HCC]

C40.92 **Malignant neoplasm of unspecified bones and articular cartilage of left limb** [HCC]

C41 **Malignant neoplasm of bone and articular cartilage of other and unspecified sites**

Excludes1: malignant neoplasm of bones of limbs (C40.-)

malignant neoplasm of cartilage of ear (C49.0)

malignant neoplasm of cartilage of eyelid (C49.0)

malignant neoplasm of cartilage of larynx (C32.3)

malignant neoplasm of cartilage of limbs (C40.-)

malignant neoplasm of cartilage of nose (C30.0)

C41.0 **Malignant neoplasm of bones of skull and face** [HCC]

Malignant neoplasm of maxilla (superior)

Malignant neoplasm of orbital bone

Excludes2: carcinoma, any type except intraosseous or odontogenic of:

maxillary sinus (C31.0)

upper jaw (C03.0)

malignant neoplasm of jaw bone (lower) (C41.1)

C41.1 **Malignant neoplasm of mandible** [HCC]

Malignant neoplasm of inferior maxilla

Malignant neoplasm of lower jaw bone

Excludes2: carcinoma, any type except intraosseous or odontogenic of:

jaw NOS (C03.9)

lower (C03.1)

malignant neoplasm of upper jaw bone (C41.0)

C41.2 **Malignant neoplasm of vertebral column** [HCC]

Excludes1: malignant neoplasm of sacrum and coccyx (C41.4)

C41.3 **Malignant neoplasm of ribs, sternum and clavicle** [HCC]

C41.4 **Malignant neoplasm of pelvic bones, sacrum and coccyx** [HCC]

C41.9 **Malignant neoplasm of bone and articular cartilage, unspecified** [HCC]

MELANOMA AND OTHER MALIGNANT NEOPLASMS OF SKIN (C43-C44)

C43 **Malignant melanoma of skin**

Excludes1: melanoma in situ (D03.-)

Excludes2: malignant melanoma of skin of genital organs (C51-C52, C60.-, C63.-)

Merkel cell carcinoma (C4A.-)

sites other than skin-code to malignant neoplasm of the site

C43.0 **Malignant melanoma of lip** [HCC]

Excludes1: malignant neoplasm of vermilion border of lip (C00.0-C00.2)

C43.1 **Malignant melanoma of eyelid, including canthus**

C43.10 **Malignant melanoma of unspecified eyelid, including canthus** [HCC]

C43.11 **Malignant melanoma of right eyelid, including canthus** [HCC]

C43.111 **Malignant melanoma of right upper eyelid, including canthus** [HCC]

C43.112 **Malignant melanoma of right lower eyelid, including canthus** [HCC]

C43.12 **Malignant melanoma of left eyelid, including canthus**

C43.121 **Malignant melanoma of left upper eyelid, including canthus** [HCC]

C43.122 **Malignant melanoma of left lower eyelid, including canthus** [HCC]

C43.2 **Malignant melanoma of ear and external auricular canal**

C43.20 **Malignant melanoma of unspecified ear and external auricular canal** [HCC]

C43.21 **Malignant melanoma of right ear and external auricular canal** [HCC]

C43.22 **Malignant melanoma of left ear and external auricular canal** [HCC]

C43.3 **Malignant melanoma of other and unspecified parts of face**

C43.30 Malignant melanoma of unspecified part of face [HCC]

C43.31 Malignant melanoma of nose [HCC]

C43.39 Malignant melanoma of other parts of face [HCC]

C43.4 Malignant melanoma of scalp and neck [HCC]

C43.5 Malignant melanoma of trunk [HCC]

Excludes2: malignant neoplasm of anus NOS (C21.0)

malignant neoplasm of scrotum (C63.2)

C43.51 Malignant melanoma of anal skin [HCC]

Malignant melanoma of anal margin

Malignant melanoma of perianal skin

C43.52 Malignant melanoma of skin of breast [HCC]

C43.59 Malignant melanoma of other part of trunk [HCC]

C43.6 Malignant melanoma of upper limb, including shoulder

C43.60 Malignant melanoma of unspecified upper limb, including shoulder [HCC]

C43.61 Malignant melanoma of right upper limb, including shoulder

C43.62 Malignant melanoma of left upper limb, including shoulder [HCC]

C43.7 Malignant melanoma of lower limb, including hip

C43.70 Malignant melanoma of unspecified lower limb, including hip [HCC]

C43.71 Malignant melanoma of right lower limb, including hip [HCC]

C43.72 Malignant melanoma of left lower limb, including hip [HCC]

C43.8 Malignant melanoma of overlapping sites of skin [HCC]

C43.9 Malignant melanoma of skin, unspecified [HCC]

Malignant melanoma of unspecified site of skin

Melanoma (malignant) NOS

C4A Merkel cell carcinoma

C4A.0 Merkel cell carcinoma of lip [HCC]

Excludes1: malignant neoplasm of vermilion border of lip (C00.0-C00.2)

C4A.1 Merkel cell carcinoma of eyelid, including canthus

C4A.10 Merkel cell carcinoma of unspecified eyelid, including canthus [HCC]

C4A.11 Merkel cell carcinoma of right eyelid, including canthus

C4A.111 Merkel cell carcinoma of right upper eyelid, including canthus [HCC]

C4A.112 Merkel cell carcinoma of right lower eyelid, including canthus [HCC]

C4A.12 Merkel cell carcinoma of left eyelid, including canthus

C4A.121 Merkel cell carcinoma of left upper eyelid, including canthus [HCC]

C4A.122 Merkel cell carcinoma of left lower eyelid, including canthus [HCC]

C4A.2 Merkel cell carcinoma of ear and external auricular canal

C4A.20 Merkel cell carcinoma of unspecified ear and external auricular canal [HCC]

C4A.21 Merkel cell carcinoma of right ear and external auricular canal [HCC]

C4A.22 Merkel cell carcinoma of left ear and external auricular canal [HCC]

C4A.3 Merkel cell carcinoma of other and unspecified parts of face

C4A.30 Merkel cell carcinoma of unspecified part of face [HCC]

C4A.31 Merkel cell carcinoma of nose [HCC]

C4A.39 Merkel cell carcinoma of other parts of face [HCC]

C4A.4 Merkel cell carcinoma of scalp and neck [HCC]

C4A.5 Merkel cell carcinoma of trunk [HCC]

Excludes2: malignant neoplasm of anus NOS (C21.0)

malignant neoplasm of scrotum (C63.2)

C4A.51 Merkel cell carcinoma of anal skin [HCC]

Merkel cell carcinoma of anal margin

Merkel cell carcinoma of perianal skin

C4A.52 Merkel cell carcinoma of skin of breast [HCC]

C4A.59 Merkel cell carcinoma of other part of trunk [HCC]

C4A.6 Merkel cell carcinoma of upper limb, including shoulder

C4A.60 Merkel cell carcinoma of unspecified upper limb, including shoulder

C4A.61 Merkel cell carcinoma of right upper limb, including shoulder [HCC]

C4A.62 Merkel cell carcinoma of left upper limb, including shoulder [HCC]

C4A.7 Merkel cell carcinoma of lower limb, including hip

C4A.70 Merkel cell carcinoma of unspecified lower limb, including hip [HCC]

C4A.71 Merkel cell carcinoma of right lower limb, including hip [HCC]

C4A.72 Merkel cell carcinoma of left lower limb, including hip [HCC]

C4A.8 Merkel cell carcinoma of overlapping sites [HCC]

C4A.9 Merkel cell carcinoma, unspecified [HCC]

Merkel cell carcinoma of unspecified site

Merkel cell carcinoma NOS

C44 Other and unspecified malignant neoplasm of skin

Includes: malignant neoplasm of sebaceous glands

malignant neoplasm of sweat glands

Excludes1: Kaposi's sarcoma of skin (C46.0)

malignant melanoma of skin (C43.-)

malignant neoplasm of skin of genital organs (C51-C52, C60.-, C63.2)

Merkel cell carcinoma (C4A.-)

C44.0 Other and unspecified malignant neoplasm of skin of lip

Excludes1: malignant neoplasm of lip (C00.-)

C44.00 Unspecified malignant neoplasm of skin of lip [HCC]

C44.01 Basal cell carcinoma of skin of lip [HCC]

C44.02 Squamous cell carcinoma of skin of lip [HCC]

C44.09 Other specified malignant neoplasm of skin of lip [HCC]

C44.1 Other and unspecified malignant neoplasm of skin of eyelid, including canthus

Excludes1: connective tissue of eyelid (C49.0)

C44.10 Unspecified malignant neoplasm of skin of eyelid, including canthus

C44.101 Unspecified malignant neoplasm of skin of unspecified eyelid, including canthus [HCC]

C44.102 Unspecified malignant neoplasm of skin of right eyelid, including canthus [HCC]

● New code   ▲ Revised code   **Excludes1:** Not coded here   **Excludes2:** Not included here   ⊗ Placeholder required   ⑦ 7th digit required

C44.1021   Unspecified malignant neoplasm of skin of right upper eyelid, including canthus [HCC]

C44.1022   Unspecified malignant neoplasm of skin of right lower eyelid, including canthus [HCC]

C44.109   Unspecified malignant neoplasm of skin of left eyelid, including canthus

C44.1091   Unspecified malignant neoplasm of skin of left upper eyelid, including canthus [HCC]

C44.1092   Unspecified malignant neoplasm of skin of left lower eyelid, including canthus [HCC]

C44.11   Basal cell carcinoma of skin of eyelid, including canthus

C44.111   Basal cell carcinoma of skin of unspecified eyelid, including canthus [HCC]

C44.112   Basal cell carcinoma of skin of right eyelid, including canthus

C44.1121   Basal cell carcinoma of skin of right upper eyelid, including canthus [HCC]

C44.1122   Basal cell carcinoma of skin of right lower eyelid, including canthus [HCC]

C44.119   Basal cell carcinoma of skin of left eyelid, including canthus

C44.1191   Basal cell carcinoma of skin of left upper eyelid, including canthus [HCC]

C44.1192   Basal cell carcinoma of skin of left lower eyelid, including canthus [HCC]

C44.12   Squamous cell carcinoma of skin of eyelid, including canthus

C44.121   Squamous cell carcinoma of skin of unspecified eyelid, including canthus

C44.122   Squamous cell carcinoma of skin of right eyelid, including canthus

C44.1221   Squamous cell carcinoma of skin of right upper eyelid, including canthus [HCC]

C44.1222   Squamous cell carcinoma of skin of right lower eyelid, including canthus [HCC]

C44.129   Squamous cell carcinoma of skin of left eyelid, including canthus [HCC]

C44.1291   Squamous cell carcinoma of skin of left upper eyelid, including canthus [HCC]

C44.1292   Squamous cell carcinoma of skin of left lower eyelid, including canthus [HCC]

C44.13   Sebaceous cell carcinoma of skin of eyelid, including canthus

C44.131   Sebaceous cell carcinoma of skin of unspecified eyelid, including canthus [HCC]

C44.132   Sebaceous cell carcinoma of skin of right eyelid, including canthus [HCC]

C44.1321   Sebaceous cell carcinoma of skin of right upper eyelid, including canthus [HCC]

C44.1322   Sebaceous cell carcinoma of skin of right lower eyelid, including canthus [HCC]

C44.139   Sebaceous cell carcinoma of skin of left eyelid, including canthus

C44.1391   Sebaceous cell carcinoma of skin of left upper eyelid, including canthus [HCC]

C44.1392   Sebaceous cell carcinoma of skin of left lower eyelid, including canthus [HCC]

C44.19   Other specified malignant neoplasm of skin of eyelid, including canthus

C44.191   Other specified malignant neoplasm of skin of unspecified eyelid, including canthus [HCC]

C44.192   Other specified malignant neoplasm of skin of right eyelid, including canthus

C44.1921   Other specified malignant neoplasm of skin of right upper eyelid, including canthus [HCC]

C44.1922   Other specified malignant neoplasm of skin of right lower eyelid, including canthus [HCC]

C44.199   Other specified malignant neoplasm of skin of left eyelid, including canthus

C44.1991   Other specified malignant neoplasm of skin of left upper eyelid, including canthus [HCC]

C44.1992   Other specified malignant neoplasm of skin of left lower eyelid, including canthus [HCC]

C44.2   Other and unspecified malignant neoplasm of skin of ear and external auricular canal

Excludes1: connective tissue of ear (C49.0)

C44.20   Unspecified malignant neoplasm of skin of ear and external auricular canal

C44.201   Unspecified malignant neoplasm of skin of unspecified ear and external auricular canal [HCC]

C44.202   Unspecified malignant neoplasm of skin of right ear and external auricular canal [HCC]

C44.209   Unspecified malignant neoplasm of skin of left ear and external auricular canal [HCC]

C44.21   Basal cell carcinoma of skin of ear and external auricular canal

C44.211   Basal cell carcinoma of skin of unspecified ear and external auricular canal [HCC]

C44.212 **Basal cell carcinoma of skin of right ear and external auricular canal** [HCC]

C44.219 **Basal cell carcinoma of skin of left ear and external auricular canal** [HCC]

C44.22 **Squamous cell carcinoma of skin of ear and external auricular canal**

C44.221 **Squamous cell carcinoma of skin of unspecified ear and external auricular canal** [HCC]

C44.222 **Squamous cell carcinoma of skin of right ear and external auricular canal** [HCC]

C44.229 **Squamous cell carcinoma of skin of left ear and external auricular canal** [HCC]

C44.29 **Other specified malignant neoplasm of skin of ear and external auricular canal**

C44.291 **Other specified malignant neoplasm of skin of unspecified ear and external auricular canal** [HCC]

C44.292 **Other specified malignant neoplasm of skin of right ear and external auricular canal** [HCC]

C44.299 **Other specified malignant neoplasm of skin of left ear and external auricular canal** [HCC]

C44.3 **Other and unspecified malignant neoplasm of skin of other and unspecified parts of face**

C44.30 **Unspecified malignant neoplasm of skin of other and unspecified parts of face**

C44.300 **Unspecified malignant neoplasm of skin of unspecified part of face** [HCC]

C44.301 **Unspecified malignant neoplasm of skin of nose** [HCC]

C44.309 **Unspecified malignant neoplasm of skin of other parts of face** [HCC]

C44.31 **Basal cell carcinoma of skin of other and unspecified parts of face**

C44.310 **Basal cell carcinoma of skin of unspecified parts of face** [HCC]

C44.311 **Basal cell carcinoma of skin of nose**

C44.319 **Basal cell carcinoma of skin of other parts of face** [HCC]

C44.32 **Squamous cell carcinoma of skin of other and unspecified parts of face**

C44.320 **Squamous cell carcinoma of skin of unspecified parts of face** [HCC]

C44.321 **Squamous cell carcinoma of skin of nose** [HCC]

C44.329 **Squamous cell carcinoma of skin of other parts of face** [HCC]

C44.39 **Other specified malignant neoplasm of skin of other and unspecified parts of face**

C44.390 **Other specified malignant neoplasm of skin of unspecified parts of face** [HCC]

C44.391 **Other specified malignant neoplasm of skin of nose** [HCC]

C44.399 **Other specified malignant neoplasm of skin of other parts of face** [HCC]

C44.4 **Other and unspecified malignant neoplasm of skin of scalp and neck**

C44.40 **Unspecified malignant neoplasm of skin of scalp and neck** [HCC]

C44.41 **Basal cell carcinoma of skin of scalp and neck** [HCC]

C44.42 **Squamous cell carcinoma of skin of scalp and neck** [HCC]

C44.49 **Other specified malignant neoplasm of skin of scalp and neck** [HCC]

C44.5 **Other and unspecified malignant neoplasm of skin of trunk**

Excludes1: anus NOS (C21.0)

scrotum (C63.2)

C44.50 **Unspecified malignant neoplasm of skin of trunk**

C44.500 **Unspecified malignant neoplasm of anal skin** [HCC]

Unspecified malignant neoplasm of anal margin

Unspecified malignant neoplasm of perianal skin

C44.501 **Unspecified malignant neoplasm of skin of breast** [HCC]

C44.509 **Unspecified malignant neoplasm of skin of other part of trunk** [HCC]

C44.51 **Basal cell carcinoma of skin of trunk**

C44.510 **Basal cell carcinoma of anal skin** [HCC]

Basal cell carcinoma of anal margin

Basal cell carcinoma of perianal skin

C44.511 **Basal cell carcinoma of skin of breast** [HCC]

C44.519 **Basal cell carcinoma of skin of other part of trunk** [HCC]

C44.52 **Squamous cell carcinoma of skin of trunk**

C44.520 **Squamous cell carcinoma of anal skin** [HCC]

Squamous cell carcinoma of anal margin

Squamous cell carcinoma of perianal skin

C44.521 **Squamous cell carcinoma of skin of breast** [HCC]

C44.529 **Squamous cell carcinoma of skin of other part of trunk** [HCC]

C44.59 **Other specified malignant neoplasm of skin of trunk**

C44.590 **Other specified malignant neoplasm of anal skin** [HCC]

Other specified malignant neoplasm of anal margin

Other specified malignant neoplasm of perianal skin

C44.591 **Other specified malignant neoplasm of skin of breast** [HCC]

C44.599 **Other specified malignant neoplasm of skin of other part of trunk** [HCC]

C44.6 **Other and unspecified malignant neoplasm of skin of upper limb, including shoulder**

C44.60 **Unspecified malignant neoplasm of skin of upper limb, including shoulder**

C44.601 **Unspecified malignant neoplasm of skin of unspecified upper limb, including shoulder** [HCC]

C44.602 **Unspecified malignant neoplasm of skin of right upper limb, including shoulder** [HCC]

C44.609 Unspecified malignant neoplasm of skin of left upper limb, including shoulder [HCC]

C44.61 Basal cell carcinoma of skin of upper limb, including shoulder

  C44.611 Basal cell carcinoma of skin of unspecified upper limb, including shoulder [HCC]

  C44.612 Basal cell carcinoma of skin of right upper limb, including shoulder [HCC]

  C44.619 Basal cell carcinoma of skin of left upper limb, including shoulder [HCC]

C44.62 Squamous cell carcinoma of skin of upper limb, including shoulder

  C44.621 Squamous cell carcinoma of skin of unspecified upper limb, including shoulder [HCC]

  C44.622 Squamous cell carcinoma of skin of right upper limb, including shoulder [HCC]

  C44.629 Squamous cell carcinoma of skin of left upper limb, including shoulder [HCC]

C44.69 Other specified malignant neoplasm of skin of upper limb, including shoulder

  C44.691 Other specified malignant neoplasm of skin of unspecified upper limb, including shoulder [HCC]

  C44.692 Other specified malignant neoplasm of skin of right upper limb, including shoulder [HCC]

  C44.699 Other specified malignant neoplasm of skin of left upper limb, including shoulder [HCC]

C44.7 Other and unspecified malignant neoplasm of skin of lower limb, including hip

  C44.70 Unspecified malignant neoplasm of skin of lower limb, including hip

    C44.701 Unspecified malignant neoplasm of skin of unspecified lower limb, including hip [HCC]

    C44.702 Unspecified malignant neoplasm of skin of right lower limb, including hip [HCC]

    C44.709 Unspecified malignant neoplasm of skin of left lower limb, including hip [HCC]

  C44.71 Basal cell carcinoma of skin of lower limb, including hip

    C44.711 Basal cell carcinoma of skin of unspecified lower limb, including hip [HCC]

    C44.712 Basal cell carcinoma of skin of right lower limb, including hip [HCC]

    C44.719 Basal cell carcinoma of skin of left lower limb, including hip [HCC]

  C44.72 Squamous cell carcinoma of skin of lower limb, including hip

    C44.721 Squamous cell carcinoma of skin of unspecified lower limb, including hip

    C44.722 Squamous cell carcinoma of skin of right lower limb, including hi [HCC]

    C44.729 Squamous cell carcinoma of skin of left lower limb, including hip [HCC]

  C44.79 Other specified malignant neoplasm of skin of lower limb, including hip

    C44.791 Other specified malignant neoplasm of skin of unspecified lower limb, including hip [HCC]

    C44.792 Other specified malignant neoplasm of skin of right lower limb, including hip [HCC]

    C44.799 Other specified malignant neoplasm of skin of left lower limb, including hip [HCC]

C44.8 Other and unspecified malignant neoplasm of overlapping sites of skin

  C44.80 Unspecified malignant neoplasm of overlapping sites of skin [HCC]

  C44.81 Basal cell carcinoma of overlapping sites of skin [HCC]

  C44.82 Squamous cell carcinoma of overlapping sites of skin [HCC]

  C44.89 Other specified malignant neoplasm of overlapping sites of skin [HCC]

C44.9 Other and unspecified malignant neoplasm of skin, unspecified

  C44.90 Unspecified malignant neoplasm of skin, unspecified [HCC]

  Malignant neoplasm of unspecified site of skin

  C44.91 Basal cell carcinoma of skin, unspecified [HCC]

  C44.92 Squamous cell carcinoma of skin, unspecified [HCC]

  C44.99 Other specified malignant neoplasm of skin, unspecified [HCC]

MALIGNANT NEOPLASMS OF MESOTHELIAL AND SOFT TISSUE (C45-C49)

C45 Mesothelioma

  C45.0 Mesothelioma of pleura [HCC]

  Excludes1: Other malignant neoplasm of pleura (C38.4)

  C45.1 Mesothelioma of peritoneum [HCC]

  Mesothelioma of cul-de-sac

  Mesothelioma of mesentery

  Mesothelioma of mesocolon

  Mesothelioma of omentum

  Mesothelioma of peritoneum (parietal) (pelvic)

  Excludes1: Other malignant neoplasm of soft tissue of peritoneum (C48.-)

  C45.2 Mesothelioma of pericardium [HCC]

  Excludes1: Other malignant neoplasm of pericardium (C38.0)

  C45.7 Mesothelioma of other sites [HCC]

  C45.9 Mesothelioma, unspecified [HCC]

C46 Kaposi's sarcoma [HCC]

  Definition: Kaposi's sarcoma is a form of skin cancer that can involve internal organs. It is most often found in patients with acquired immunodeficiency syndrome (AIDS) and can be fatal.

  Code first any human immunodeficiency virus [HIV] disease (B20)

  C46.0 Kaposi's sarcoma of skin

  C46.1 Kaposi's sarcoma of soft tissue [HCC]

  Kaposi's sarcoma of blood vessel

  Kaposi's sarcoma of connective tissue

  Kaposi's sarcoma of fascia

  Kaposi's sarcoma of ligament

  Kaposi's sarcoma of lymphatic(s) NEC

  Kaposi's sarcoma of muscle

Excludes2: Kaposi's sarcoma of lymph glands and nodes (C46.3)

C46.2 Kaposi's sarcoma of palate [HCC]

C46.3 Kaposi's sarcoma of lymph nodes [HCC]

C46.4 Kaposi's sarcoma of gastrointestinal sites [HCC]

C46.5 Kaposi's sarcoma of lung

    C46.50 Kaposi's sarcoma of unspecified lung [HCC]

    C46.51 Kaposi's sarcoma of right lung [HCC]

    C46.52 Kaposi's sarcoma of left lung [HCC]

C46.7 Kaposi's sarcoma of other sites [HCC]

C46.9 Kaposi's sarcoma, unspecified [HCC]

    Kaposi's sarcoma of unspecified site

C47 Malignant neoplasm of peripheral nerves and autonomic nervous system

Includes: malignant neoplasm of sympathetic and parasympathetic nerves and ganglia

Excludes1: Kaposi's sarcoma of soft tissue (C46.1)

C47.0 Malignant neoplasm of peripheral nerves of head, face and neck [HCC]

    Excludes1: malignant neoplasm of peripheral nerves of orbit (C69.6-)

C47.1 Malignant neoplasm of peripheral nerves of upper limb, including shoulder

    C47.10 Malignant neoplasm of peripheral nerves of unspecified upper limb, including shoulder [HCC]

    C47.11 Malignant neoplasm of peripheral nerves of right upper limb, including shoulder [HCC]

    C47.12 Malignant neoplasm of peripheral nerves of left upper limb, including shoulder [HCC]

C47.2 Malignant neoplasm of peripheral nerves of lower limb, including hip

    C47.20 Malignant neoplasm of peripheral nerves of unspecified lower limb, including hip [HCC]

    C47.21 Malignant neoplasm of peripheral nerves of right lower limb, including hip [HCC]

    C47.22 Malignant neoplasm of peripheral nerves of left lower limb, including hip [HCC]

C47.3 Malignant neoplasm of peripheral nerves of thorax [HCC]

C47.4 Malignant neoplasm of peripheral nerves of abdomen [HCC]

C47.5 Malignant neoplasm of peripheral nerves of pelvis [HCC]

C47.6 Malignant neoplasm of peripheral nerves of trunk, unspecified [HCC]

    Malignant neoplasm of peripheral nerves of unspecified part of trunk

C47.8 Malignant neoplasm of overlapping sites of peripheral nerves and autonomic nervous system [HCC]

C47.9 Malignant neoplasm of peripheral nerves and autonomic nervous system, unspecified [HCC]

    Malignant neoplasm of unspecified site of peripheral nerves and autonomic nervous system

C48 Malignant neoplasm of retroperitoneum and peritoneum

Excludes1: Kaposi's sarcoma of connective tissue (C46.1)

    mesothelioma (C45.-)

C48.0 Malignant neoplasm of retroperitoneum [HCC]

C48.1 Malignant neoplasm of specified parts of peritoneum [HCC]

    Malignant neoplasm of cul-de-sac

    Malignant neoplasm of mesentery

    Malignant neoplasm of mesocolon

    Malignant neoplasm of omentum

    Malignant neoplasm of parietal peritoneum

    Malignant neoplasm of pelvic peritoneum

C48.2 Malignant neoplasm of peritoneum, unspecified [HCC]

C48.8 Malignant neoplasm of overlapping sites of retroperitoneum and peritoneum [HCC]

C49 Malignant neoplasm of other connective and soft tissue

Includes: malignant neoplasm of blood vessel

malignant neoplasm of bursa

malignant neoplasm of cartilage

malignant neoplasm of fascia

malignant neoplasm of fat

malignant neoplasm of ligament, except uterine

malignant neoplasm of lymphatic vessel

malignant neoplasm of muscle

malignant neoplasm of synovia

malignant neoplasm of tendon (sheath)

Excludes1: malignant neoplasm of cartilage (of):

    articular (C40-C41)

    larynx (C32.3)

    nose (C30.0)

    malignant neoplasm of connective tissue of breast (C50.-)

Excludes2: Kaposi's sarcoma of soft tissue (C46.1)

    malignant neoplasm of heart (C38.0)

    malignant neoplasm of peripheral nerves and autonomic nervous system (C47.-)

    malignant neoplasm of peritoneum (C48.2)

    malignant neoplasm of retroperitoneum (C48.0)

    malignant neoplasm of uterine ligament (C57.3)

    mesothelioma (C45.-)

C49.0 Malignant neoplasm of connective and soft tissue of head, face and neck [HCC]

    Malignant neoplasm of connective tissue of ear

    Malignant neoplasm of connective tissue of eyelid

    Excludes1: connective tissue of orbit (C69.6-)

C49.1 Malignant neoplasm of connective and soft tissue of upper limb, including shoulder

    C49.10 Malignant neoplasm of connective and soft tissue of unspecified upper limb, including shoulder [HCC]

    C49.11 Malignant neoplasm of connective and soft tissue of right upper limb, including shoulder [HCC]

    C49.12 Malignant neoplasm of connective and soft tissue of left upper limb, including shoulder [HCC]

C49.2 Malignant neoplasm of connective and soft tissue of lower limb, including hip

    C49.20 Malignant neoplasm of connective and soft tissue of unspecified lower limb, including hip [HCC]

    C49.21 Malignant neoplasm of connective and soft tissue of right lower limb, including hip [HCC]

    C49.22 Malignant neoplasm of connective and soft tissue of left lower limb, including hip [HCC]

C49.3 Malignant neoplasm of connective and soft tissue of thorax [HCC]

    Malignant neoplasm of axilla

    Malignant neoplasm of diaphragm

    Malignant neoplasm of great vessels

    Excludes1: malignant neoplasm of breast (C50.-)

malignant neoplasm of heart (C38.0)

malignant neoplasm of mediastinum (C38.1-C38.3)

malignant neoplasm of thymus (C37)

C49.4 **Malignant neoplasm of connective and soft tissue of abdomen** [HCC]

Malignant neoplasm of abdominal wall

Malignant neoplasm of hypochondrium

C49.5 **Malignant neoplasm of connective and soft tissue of pelvis** [HCC]

Malignant neoplasm of buttock

Malignant neoplasm of groin

Malignant neoplasm of perineum

C49.6 **Malignant neoplasm of connective and soft tissue of trunk, unspecified** [HCC]

Malignant neoplasm of back NOS

C49.8 **Malignant neoplasm of overlapping sites of connective and soft tissue** [HCC]

Primary malignant neoplasm of two or more contiguous sites of connective and soft tissue

C49.9 **Malignant neoplasm of connective and soft tissue, unspecified** [HCC]

C49.A **Gastrointestinal stromal tumor**

　C49.A0 **Gastrointestinal stromal tumor, unspecified site** [HCC]

　C49.A1 **Gastrointestinal stromal tumor of esophagus** [HCC]

　C49.A2 **Gastrointestinal stromal tumor of stomach** [HCC]

　C49.A3 **Gastrointestinal stromal tumor of small intestine** [HCC]

　C49.A4 **Gastrointestinal stromal tumor of large intestine** [HCC]

　C49.A5 **Gastrointestinal stromal tumor of rectum** [HCC]

　C49.A9 **Gastrointestinal stromal tumor of other sites** [HCC]

MALIGNANT NEOPLASMS OF BREAST (C50) [HCC]

C50 **Malignant neoplasm of breast** [HCC]

Includes: connective tissue of breast

Paget's disease of breast

Paget's disease of nipple

Use Additional Code to identify estrogen receptor status (Z17.0, Z17.1)

Excludes1: skin of breast (C44.501, C44.511, C44.521, C44.591)

C50.0 **Malignant neoplasm of nipple and areola**

　C50.01 **Malignant neoplasm of nipple and areola, female**

　　C50.011 **Malignant neoplasm of nipple and areola, right female breast** [HCC]

　　C50.012 **Malignant neoplasm of nipple and areola, left female breast** [HCC]

　　C50.019 **Malignant neoplasm of nipple and areola, unspecified female breast** [HCC]

　C50.02 **Malignant neoplasm of nipple and areola, male**

　　C50.021 **Malignant neoplasm of nipple and areola, right male breast** [HCC]

　　C50.022 **Malignant neoplasm of nipple and areola, left male breast** [HCC]

　　C50.029 **Malignant neoplasm of nipple and areola, unspecified male breast** [HCC]

C50.1 **Malignant neoplasm of central portion of breast**

　C50.11 **Malignant neoplasm of central portion of breast, female**

　　C50.111 **Malignant neoplasm of central portion of right female breast** [HCC]

　　C50.112 **Malignant neoplasm of central portion of left female breast** [HCC]

　　C50.119 **Malignant neoplasm of central portion of unspecified female breast** [HCC]

　C50.12 **Malignant neoplasm of central portion of breast, male**

　　C50.121 **Malignant neoplasm of central portion of right male breast** [HCC]

　　C50.122 **Malignant neoplasm of central portion of left male breast** [HCC]

　　C50.129 **Malignant neoplasm of central portion of unspecified male breast** [HCC]

C50.2 **Malignant neoplasm of upper-inner quadrant of breast**

　C50.21 **Malignant neoplasm of upper-inner quadrant of breast, female**

　　C50.211 **Malignant neoplasm of upper-inner quadrant of right female breast** [HCC]

　　C50.212 **Malignant neoplasm of upper-inner quadrant of left female breast** [HCC]

　　C50.219 **Malignant neoplasm of upper-inner quadrant of unspecified female breast** [HCC]

　C50.22 **Malignant neoplasm of upper-inner quadrant of breast, male**

　　C50.221 **Malignant neoplasm of upper-inner quadrant of right male breast** [HCC]

　　C50.222 **Malignant neoplasm of upper-inner quadrant of left male breast** [HCC]

　　C50.229 **Malignant neoplasm of upper-inner quadrant of unspecified male breast** [HCC]

C50.3 **Malignant neoplasm of lower-inner quadrant of breast**

　C50.31 **Malignant neoplasm of lower-inner quadrant of breast, female**

　　C50.311 **Malignant neoplasm of lower-inner quadrant of right female breast** [HCC]

　　C50.312 **Malignant neoplasm of lower-inner quadrant of left female breast**

　　C50.319 **Malignant neoplasm of lower-inner quadrant of unspecified female breast** [HCC]

　C50.32 **Malignant neoplasm of lower-inner quadrant of breast, male**

　　C50.321 **Malignant neoplasm of lower-inner quadrant of right male breast** [HCC]

　　C50.322 **Malignant neoplasm of lower-inner quadrant of left male breast** [HCC]

　　C50.329 **Malignant neoplasm of lower-inner quadrant of unspecified male breast** [HCC]

C50.4 **Malignant neoplasm of upper-outer quadrant of breast**

　C50.41 **Malignant neoplasm of upper-outer quadrant of breast, female**

　　C50.411 **Malignant neoplasm of upper-outer quadrant of right female breast** [HCC]

　　C50.412 **Malignant neoplasm of upper-outer quadrant of left female breast** [HCC]

　　C50.419 **Malignant neoplasm of upper-outer quadrant of unspecified female breast** [HCC]

C50.42 **Malignant neoplasm of upper-outer quadrant of breast, male**

   C50.421 **Malignant neoplasm of upper-outer quadrant of right male breast** [HCC]

   C50.422 **Malignant neoplasm of upper-outer quadrant of left male breast** [HCC]

   C50.429 **Malignant neoplasm of upper-outer quadrant of unspecified male breast** [HCC]

C50.5 **Malignant neoplasm of lower-outer quadrant of breast**

  C50.51 **Malignant neoplasm of lower-outer quadrant of breast, female**

   C50.511 **Malignant neoplasm of lower-outer quadrant of right female breast** [HCC]

   C50.512 **Malignant neoplasm of lower-outer quadrant of left female breast** [HCC]

   C50.519 **Malignant neoplasm of lower-outer quadrant of unspecified female breast** [HCC]

  C50.52 **Malignant neoplasm of lower-outer quadrant of breast, male**

   C50.521 **Malignant neoplasm of lower-outer quadrant of right male breast** [HCC]

   C50.522 **Malignant neoplasm of lower-outer quadrant of left male breast** [HCC]

   C50.529 **Malignant neoplasm of lower-outer quadrant of unspecified male breast** [HCC]

C50.6 **Malignant neoplasm of axillary tail of breast** [HCC]

  C50.61 **Malignant neoplasm of axillary tail of breast, female**

   C50.611 **Malignant neoplasm of axillary tail of right female breast** [HCC]

   C50.612 **Malignant neoplasm of axillary tail of left female breast** [HCC]

   C50.619 **Malignant neoplasm of axillary tail of unspecified female breast** [HCC]

  C50.62 **Malignant neoplasm of axillary tail of breast, male**

   C50.621 **Malignant neoplasm of axillary tail of right male breast** [HCC]

   C50.622 **Malignant neoplasm of axillary tail of left male breast** [HCC]

   C50.629 **Malignant neoplasm of axillary tail of unspecified male breast** [HCC]

C50.8 **Malignant neoplasm of overlapping sites of breast**

  C50.81 **Malignant neoplasm of overlapping sites of breast, female**

   C50.811 **Malignant neoplasm of overlapping sites of right female breast** [HCC]

   C50.812 **Malignant neoplasm of overlapping sites of left female breast** [HCC]

   C50.819 **Malignant neoplasm of overlapping sites of unspecified female breast** [HCC]

  C50.82 **Malignant neoplasm of overlapping sites of breast, male**

   C50.821 **Malignant neoplasm of overlapping sites of right male breast** [HCC]

   C50.822 **Malignant neoplasm of overlapping sites of left male breast** [HCC]

   C50.829 **Malignant neoplasm of overlapping sites of unspecified male breast** [HCC]

C50.9 **Malignant neoplasm of breast of unspecified site** [HCC]

  C50.91 **Malignant neoplasm of breast of unspecified site, female**

   C50.911 **Malignant neoplasm of unspecified site of right female breast** [HCC]

   C50.912 **Malignant neoplasm of unspecified site of left female breast** [HCC]

   C50.919 **Malignant neoplasm of unspecified site of unspecified female breast** [HCC]

  C50.92 **Malignant neoplasm of breast of unspecified site, male**

   C50.921 **Malignant neoplasm of unspecified site of right male breast** [HCC]

   C50.922 **Malignant neoplasm of unspecified site of left male breast** [HCC]

   C50.929 **Malignant neoplasm of unspecified site of unspecified male breast** [HCC]

MALIGNANT NEOPLASMS OF FEMALE GENITAL ORGANS (C51-C58)

NOTE: ALL DIAGNOSIS CODES IN THIS SECTION APPLY TO FEMALE PATIENTS ONLY

Includes: malignant neoplasm of skin of female genital organs

C51 **Malignant neoplasm of vulva**

Excludes1: carcinoma in situ of vulva (D07.1)

  C51.0 **Malignant neoplasm of labium majus** [HCC]

    Malignant neoplasm of Bartholin's [greater vestibular] gland

  C51.1 **Malignant neoplasm of labium minus** [HCC]

  C51.2 **Malignant neoplasm of clitoris** [HCC]

  C51.8 **Malignant neoplasm of overlapping sites of vulva** [HCC]

  C51.9 **Malignant neoplasm of vulva, unspecified** [HCC]

    Malignant neoplasm of external female genitalia NOS

    Malignant neoplasm of pudendum

C52 **Malignant neoplasm of vagina** [HCC]

Excludes1: carcinoma in situ of vagina (D07.2)

C53 **Malignant neoplasm of cervix uteri**

Excludes1: carcinoma in situ of cervix uteri (D06.-)

  C53.0 **Malignant neoplasm of endocervix**

  C53.1 **Malignant neoplasm of exocervix** [HCC]

  C53.8 **Malignant neoplasm of overlapping sites of cervix uteri** [HCC]

  C53.9 **Malignant neoplasm of cervix uteri, unspecified** [HCC]

C54 **Malignant neoplasm of corpus uteri**

  C54.0 **Malignant neoplasm of isthmus uteri** [HCC]

    Malignant neoplasm of lower uterine segment

  C54.1 **Malignant neoplasm of endometrium** [HCC]

  C54.2 **Malignant neoplasm of myometrium** [HCC]

  C54.3 **Malignant neoplasm of fundus uteri** [HCC]

  C54.8 **Malignant neoplasm of overlapping sites of corpus uteri** [HCC]

  C54.9 **Malignant neoplasm of corpus uteri, unspecified** [HCC]

C55 **Malignant neoplasm of uterus, part unspecified** [HCC]

C56 **Malignant neoplasm of ovary**

Use Additional Code to identify any functional activity

  C56.1 **Malignant neoplasm of right ovary** [HCC]

  C56.2 **Malignant neoplasm of left ovary** [HCC]

  ●C56.3 **Malignant neoplasm of bilateral ovaries** [HCC]

  C56.9 **Malignant neoplasm of unspecified ovary** [HCC]

C57 **Malignant neoplasm of other and unspecified female genital organs**

  C57.0 **Malignant neoplasm of fallopian tube**

● New code ▲ Revised code Excludes1: Not coded here Excludes2: Not included here ⊗ Placeholder required ⑦7th digit required

Malignant neoplasm of oviduct

Malignant neoplasm of uterine tube

- **C57.00** **Malignant neoplasm of unspecified fallopian tube** [HCC]
- **C57.01** **Malignant neoplasm of right fallopian tube** [HCC]
- **C57.02** **Malignant neoplasm of left fallopian tube** [HCC]

C57.1 **Malignant neoplasm of broad ligament**

- **C57.10** **Malignant neoplasm of unspecified broad ligament** [HCC]
- **C57.11** **Malignant neoplasm of right broad ligament** [HCC]
- **C57.12** **Malignant neoplasm of left broad ligament** [HCC]

C57.2 **Malignant neoplasm of round ligament**

- **C57.20** **Malignant neoplasm of unspecified round ligament** [HCC]
- **C57.21** **Malignant neoplasm of right round ligament** [HCC]
- **C57.22** **Malignant neoplasm of left round ligament** [HCC]

C57.3 **Malignant neoplasm of parametrium** [HCC]

Malignant neoplasm of uterine ligament NOS

C57.4 **Malignant neoplasm of uterine adnexa, unspecified**

C57.7 **Malignant neoplasm of other specified female genital organs** [HCC]

Malignant neoplasm of wolffian body or duct

C57.8 **Malignant neoplasm of overlapping sites of female genital organs** [HCC]

Primary malignant neoplasm of two or more contiguous sites of the female genital organs whose point of origin cannot be determined

Primary tubo-ovarian malignant neoplasm whose point of origin cannot be determined Primary utero-ovarian malignant neoplasm whose point of origin cannot be determined

C57.9 **Malignant neoplasm of female genital organ, unspecified** [HCC]

Malignant neoplasm of female genitourinary tract NOS

C58 **Malignant neoplasm of placenta** [HCC]

Includes: choriocarcinoma NOS

chorionepithelioma NOS

Excludes1: chorioadenoma (destruens) (D39.2)

hydatidiform mole NOS (O01.9)

invasive hydatidiform mole (D39.2)

male choriocarcinoma NOS (C62.9-)

malignant hydatidiform mole (D39.2)

MALIGNANT NEOPLASMS OF MALE GENITAL ORGANS (C60-C63)

> NOTE: ALL DIAGNOSIS CODES IN THIS SECTION APPLY TO MALE PATIENTS ONLY

Includes: malignant neoplasm of skin of male genital organs

C60 **Malignant neoplasm of penis**

C60.0 **Malignant neoplasm of prepuce** [HCC]

Malignant neoplasm of foreskin

C60.1 **Malignant neoplasm of glans penis** [HCC]

C60.2 **Malignant neoplasm of body of penis** [HCC]

Malignant neoplasm of corpus cavernosum

C60.8 **Malignant neoplasm of overlapping sites of penis** [HCC]

C60.9 **Malignant neoplasm of penis, unspecified** [HCC]

Malignant neoplasm of skin of penis NOS

C61 **Malignant neoplasm of prostate** [HCC]

Use Additional Code to identify:

hormone sensitivity status (Z19.1-Z19.2)

rising PSA following treatment for malignant neoplasm of prostate (R97.21)

Excludes1: malignant neoplasm of seminal vesicle (C63.7)

C62 **Malignant neoplasm of testis**

Use Additional Code to identify any functional activity

C62.0 **Malignant neoplasm of undescended testis** [HCC]

Malignant neoplasm of ectopic testis

Malignant neoplasm of retained testis

- **C62.00** **Malignant neoplasm of unspecified undescended testis** [HCC]
- **C62.01** **Malignant neoplasm of undescended right testis** [HCC]
- **C62.02** **Malignant neoplasm of undescended left testis**

C62.1 **Malignant neoplasm of descended testis**

Malignant neoplasm of scrotal testis

- **C62.10** **Malignant neoplasm of unspecified descended testis** [HCC]
- **C62.11** **Malignant neoplasm of descended right testis** [HCC]
- **C62.12** **Malignant neoplasm of descended left testis** [HCC]

C62.9 **Malignant neoplasm of testis, unspecified whether descended or undescended**

- **C62.90** **Malignant neoplasm of unspecified testis, unspecified whether descended or undescended** [HCC]

  Malignant neoplasm of testis NOS

- **C62.91** **Malignant neoplasm of right testis, unspecified whether descended or undescended** [HCC]
- **C62.92** **Malignant neoplasm of left testis, unspecified whether descended or undescended** [HCC]

C63 **Malignant neoplasm of other and unspecified male genital organs**

C63.0 **Malignant neoplasm of epididymis**

- **C63.00** **Malignant neoplasm of unspecified epididymis** [HCC]
- **C63.01** **Malignant neoplasm of right epididymis** [HCC]
- **C63.02** **Malignant neoplasm of left epididymis** [HCC]

C63.1 **Malignant neoplasm of spermatic cord**

- **C63.10** **Malignant neoplasm of unspecified spermatic cord** [HCC]
- **C63.11** **Malignant neoplasm of right spermatic cord** [HCC]
- **C63.12** **Malignant neoplasm of left spermatic cord** [HCC]

C63.2 **Malignant neoplasm of scrotum** [HCC]

Malignant neoplasm of skin of scrotum

C63.7 **Malignant neoplasm of other specified male genital organs** [HCC]

Malignant neoplasm of seminal vesicle

Malignant neoplasm of tunica vaginalis

C63.8 **Malignant neoplasm of overlapping sites of male genital organs** [HCC]

Primary malignant neoplasm of two or more contiguous sites of male genital organs whose point of origin cannot be determined

C63.9 **Malignant neoplasm of male genital organ, unspecified** [HCC]

Malignant neoplasm of male genitourinary tract NOS

MALIGNANT NEOPLASMS OF URINARY TRACT (C64-C68)

C64 **Malignant neoplasm of kidney, except renal pelvis** [HCC]

Excludes1: malignant carcinoid tumor of the kidney (C7A.093)

malignant neoplasm of renal calyces (C65.-)

malignant neoplasm of renal pelvis (C65.-)

C64.1 **Malignant neoplasm of right kidney, except renal pelvis** [HCC]

C64.2 **Malignant neoplasm of left kidney, except renal pelvis** [HCC]

C64.9 **Malignant neoplasm of unspecified kidney, except renal pelvis**

C65 **Malignant neoplasm of renal pelvis**

Includes: malignant neoplasm of pelviureteric junction

malignant neoplasm of renal calyces

C65.1 **Malignant neoplasm of right renal pelvis** [HCC]

C65.2 **Malignant neoplasm of left renal pelvis** [HCC]

C65.9 **Malignant neoplasm of unspecified renal pelvis** [HCC]

C66 **Malignant neoplasm of ureter**

Excludes1: malignant neoplasm of ureteric orifice of bladder (C67.6)

C66.1 **Malignant neoplasm of right ureter** [HCC]

C66.2 **Malignant neoplasm of left ureter** [HCC]

C66.9 **Malignant neoplasm of unspecified ureter** [HCC]

C67 **Malignant neoplasm of bladder**

C67.0 **Malignant neoplasm of trigone of bladder** [HCC]

C67.1 **Malignant neoplasm of dome of bladder** [HCC]

C67.2 **Malignant neoplasm of lateral wall of bladder** [HCC]

C67.3 **Malignant neoplasm of anterior wall of bladder** [HCC]

C67.4 **Malignant neoplasm of posterior wall of bladder** [HCC]

C67.5 **Malignant neoplasm of bladder neck** [HCC]

Malignant neoplasm of internal urethral orifice

C67.6 **Malignant neoplasm of ureteric orifice** [HCC]

C67.7 **Malignant neoplasm of urachus** [HCC]

C67.8 **Malignant neoplasm of overlapping sites of bladder** [HCC]

C67.9 **Malignant neoplasm of bladder, unspecified** [HCC]

C68 **Malignant neoplasm of other and unspecified urinary organs**

Excludes1: malignant neoplasm of female genitourinary tract NOS (C57.9)

malignant neoplasm of male genitourinary tract NOS (C63.9)

C68.0 **Malignant neoplasm of urethra** [HCC]

Excludes1: malignant neoplasm of urethral orifice of bladder (C67.5)

C68.1 **Malignant neoplasm of paraurethral glands** [HCC]

C68.8 **Malignant neoplasm of overlapping sites of urinary organs** [HCC]

Primary malignant neoplasm of two or more contiguous sites of urinary organs whose point of origin cannot be determined

C68.9 **Malignant neoplasm of urinary organ, unspecified** [HCC]

Malignant neoplasm of urinary system NOS

MALIGNANT NEOPLASMS OF EYE, BRAIN AND OTHER PARTS OF CENTRAL NERVOUS SYSTEM (C69-C72)

C69 **Malignant neoplasm of eye and adnexa**

Excludes1: malignant neoplasm of connective tissue of eyelid (C49.0)

malignant neoplasm of eyelid (skin) (C43.1-, C44.1-)

malignant neoplasm of optic nerve (C72.3-)

C69.0 **Malignant neoplasm of conjunctiva**

C69.00 **Malignant neoplasm of unspecified conjunctiva** [HCC]

C69.01 **Malignant neoplasm of right conjunctiva** [HCC]

C69.02 **Malignant neoplasm of left conjunctiva** [HCC]

C69.1 **Malignant neoplasm of cornea**

C69.10 **Malignant neoplasm of unspecified cornea** [HCC]

C69.11 **Malignant neoplasm of right cornea** [HCC]

C69.12 **Malignant neoplasm of left cornea** [HCC]

C69.2 **Malignant neoplasm of retina**

Excludes1: dark area on retina (D49.81)

neoplasm of unspecified behavior of retina and choroid (D49.81)

retinal freckle (D49.81)

C69.20 **Malignant neoplasm of unspecified retina** [HCC]

C69.21 **Malignant neoplasm of right retina** [HCC]

C69.22 **Malignant neoplasm of left retina** [HCC]

C69.3 **Malignant neoplasm of choroid**

C69.30 **Malignant neoplasm of unspecified choroid** [HCC]

C69.31 **Malignant neoplasm of right choroid** [HCC]

C69.32 **Malignant neoplasm of left choroid** [HCC]

C69.4 **Malignant neoplasm of ciliary body** [HCC]

C69.40 **Malignant neoplasm of unspecified ciliary body** [HCC]

C69.41 **Malignant neoplasm of right ciliary body** [HCC]

C69.42 **Malignant neoplasm of left ciliary body** [HCC]

C69.5 **Malignant neoplasm of lacrimal gland and duct** [HCC]

Malignant neoplasm of lacrimal sac

Malignant neoplasm of nasolacrimal duct

C69.50 **Malignant neoplasm of unspecified lacrimal gland and duct** [HCC]

C69.51 **Malignant neoplasm of right lacrimal gland and duct** [HCC]

C69.52 **Malignant neoplasm of left lacrimal gland and duct** [HCC]

C69.6 **Malignant neoplasm of orbit**

Malignant neoplasm of connective tissue of orbit

Malignant neoplasm of extraocular muscle

Malignant neoplasm of peripheral nerves of orbit

Malignant neoplasm of retrobulbar tissue

Malignant neoplasm of retro-ocular tissue

Excludes1: malignant neoplasm of orbital bone (C41.0)

C69.60 **Malignant neoplasm of unspecified orbit** [HCC]

C69.61 **Malignant neoplasm of right orbit** [HCC]

C69.62 **Malignant neoplasm of left orbit** [HCC]

C69.8 **Malignant neoplasm of overlapping sites of eye and adnexa**

C69.80 **Malignant neoplasm of overlapping sites of unspecified eye and adnexa** [HCC]

C69.81 **Malignant neoplasm of overlapping sites of right eye and adnexa** [HCC]

C69.82 **Malignant neoplasm of overlapping sites of left eye and adnexa** [HCC]

C69.9 **Malignant neoplasm of unspecified site of eye**

Malignant neoplasm of eyeball

C69.90 **Malignant neoplasm of unspecified site of unspecified eye** [HCC]

C69.91 **Malignant neoplasm of unspecified site of right eye** [HCC]

● New code   ▲ Revised code   **Excludes1:** Not coded here   **Excludes2:** Not included here   ⊗ Placeholder required   ⑦7th digit required

C69.92 **Malignant neoplasm of unspecified site of left eye** [HCC]

C70 **Malignant neoplasm of meninges** [HCC]

C70.0 **Malignant neoplasm of cerebral meninges** [HCC]

C70.1 **Malignant neoplasm of spinal meninges** [HCC]

C70.9 **Malignant neoplasm of meninges, unspecified** [HCC]

C71 **Malignant neoplasm of brain**

Excludes1: malignant neoplasm of cranial nerves (C72.2-C72.5)

retrobulbar malignant neoplasm (C69.6-)

C71.0 **Malignant neoplasm of cerebrum, except lobes and ventricles** [HCC]

Malignant neoplasm of supratentorial NOS

C71.1 **Malignant neoplasm of frontal lobe** [HCC]

C71.2 **Malignant neoplasm of temporal lobe** [HCC]

C71.3 **Malignant neoplasm of parietal lobe** [HCC]

C71.4 **Malignant neoplasm of occipital lobe** [HCC]

C71.5 **Malignant neoplasm of cerebral ventricle** [HCC]

Excludes1: malignant neoplasm of fourth cerebral ventricle (C71.7)

C71.6 **Malignant neoplasm of cerebellum** [HCC]

C71.7 **Malignant neoplasm of brain stem** [HCC]

Malignant neoplasm of fourth cerebral ventricle

Infratentorial malignant neoplasm NOS

C71.8 **Malignant neoplasm of overlapping sites of brain**

C71.9 **Malignant neoplasm of brain, unspecified** [HCC]

C72 **Malignant neoplasm of spinal cord, cranial nerves and other parts of central nervous system**

Excludes1: malignant neoplasm of meninges (C70.-)

malignant neoplasm of peripheral nerves and autonomic nervous system (C47.-)

C72.0 **Malignant neoplasm of spinal cord** [HCC]

C72.1 **Malignant neoplasm of cauda equina** [HCC]

C72.2 **Malignant neoplasm of olfactory nerve**

Malignant neoplasm of olfactory bulb

C72.20 **Malignant neoplasm of unspecified olfactory nerve** [HCC]

C72.21 **Malignant neoplasm of right olfactory nerve** [HCC]

C72.22 **Malignant neoplasm of left olfactory nerve** [HCC]

C72.3 **Malignant neoplasm of optic nerve**

C72.30 **Malignant neoplasm of unspecified optic nerve** [HCC]

C72.31 **Malignant neoplasm of right optic nerve** [HCC]

C72.32 **Malignant neoplasm of left optic nerve** [HCC]

C72.4 **Malignant neoplasm of acoustic nerve**

C72.40 **Malignant neoplasm of unspecified acoustic nerve** [HCC]

C72.41 **Malignant neoplasm of right acoustic nerve** [HCC]

C72.42 **Malignant neoplasm of left acoustic nerve** [HCC]

C72.5 **Malignant neoplasm of other and unspecified cranial nerves**

C72.50 **Malignant neoplasm of unspecified cranial nerve** [HCC]

Malignant neoplasm of cranial nerve NOS

C72.59 **Malignant neoplasm of other cranial nerves** [HCC]

C72.9 **Malignant neoplasm of central nervous system, unspecified** [HCC]

Malignant neoplasm of unspecified site of central nervous system

Malignant neoplasm of nervous system NOS

MALIGNANT NEOPLASMS OF THYROID AND OTHER ENDOCRINE GLANDS (C73-C75)

C73 **Malignant neoplasm of thyroid gland** [HCC]

Use Additional Code to identify any functional activity

C74 **Malignant neoplasm of adrenal gland**

C74.0 **Malignant neoplasm of cortex of adrenal gland**

C74.00 **Malignant neoplasm of cortex of unspecified adrenal gland** [HCC]

C74.01 **Malignant neoplasm of cortex of right adrenal gland** [HCC]

C74.02 **Malignant neoplasm of cortex of left adrenal gland** [HCC]

C74.1 **Malignant neoplasm of medulla of adrenal gland**

C74.10 **Malignant neoplasm of medulla of unspecified adrenal gland** [HCC]

C74.11 **Malignant neoplasm of medulla of right adrenal gland** [HCC]

C74.12 **Malignant neoplasm of medulla of left adrenal gland** [HCC]

C74.9 **Malignant neoplasm of unspecified part of adrenal gland**

C74.90 **Malignant neoplasm of unspecified part of unspecified adrenal gland** [HCC]

C74.91 **Malignant neoplasm of unspecified part of right adrenal gland** [HCC]

C74.92 **Malignant neoplasm of unspecified part of left adrenal gland** [HCC]

C75 **Malignant neoplasm of other endocrine glands and related structures**

Excludes1: malignant carcinoid tumors (C7A.0-)

malignant neoplasm of adrenal gland (C74.-)

malignant neoplasm of endocrine pancreas (C25.4)

malignant neoplasm of islets of Langerhans (C25.4)

malignant neoplasm of ovary (C56.-)

malignant neoplasm of testis (C62.-)

malignant neoplasm of thymus (C37)

malignant neoplasm of thyroid gland (C73)

malignant neuroendocrine tumors (C7A.-)

C75.0 **Malignant neoplasm of parathyroid gland** [HCC]

C75.1 **Malignant neoplasm of pituitary gland** [HCC]

C75.2 **Malignant neoplasm of craniopharyngeal duct** [HCC]

C75.3 **Malignant neoplasm of pineal gland** [HCC]

C75.4 **Malignant neoplasm of carotid body** [HCC]

C75.5 **Malignant neoplasm of aortic body and other paraganglia** [HCC]

C75.8 **Malignant neoplasm with pluriglandular involvement, unspecified** [HCC]

C75.9 **Malignant neoplasm of endocrine gland, unspecified** [HCC]

MALIGNANT NEUROENDOCRINE TUMORS (C7A) [HCC]

C7A **Malignant neuroendocrine tumors**

Code also any associated multiple endocrine neoplasia [MEN] syndromes (E31.2-)

Use Additional Code to identify any associated endocrine syndrome, such as:

carcinoid syndrome (E34.0)

Excludes2: malignant pancreatic islet cell tumors (C25.4)

Merkel cell carcinoma (C4A.-)

C7A.0 **Malignant carcinoid tumors**

C7A.00 **Malignant carcinoid tumor of unspecified site** [HCC]

C7A.01 **Malignant carcinoid tumors of the small intestine**

C7A.010 **Malignant carcinoid tumor of the duodenum** [HCC]

C7A.011 **Malignant carcinoid tumor of the jejunum**

C7A.012 **Malignant carcinoid tumor of the ileum** [HCC]

C7A.019 **Malignant carcinoid tumor of the small intestine, unspecified portion** [HCC]

C7A.02 **Malignant carcinoid tumors of the appendix, large intestine, and rectum**

C7A.020 **Malignant carcinoid tumor of the appendix** [HCC]

C7A.021 **Malignant carcinoid tumor of the cecum** [HCC]

C7A.022 **Malignant carcinoid tumor of the ascending colon** [HCC]

C7A.023 **Malignant carcinoid tumor of the transverse colon** [HCC]

C7A.024 **Malignant carcinoid tumor of the descending colon** [HCC]

C7A.025 **Malignant carcinoid tumor of the sigmoid colon** [HCC]

C7A.026 **Malignant carcinoid tumor of the rectum** [HCC]

C7A.029 **Malignant carcinoid tumor of the large intestine, unspecified portion** [HCC]

Malignant carcinoid tumor of the colon NOS

C7A.09 **Malignant carcinoid tumors of other sites**

C7A.090 **Malignant carcinoid tumor of the bronchus and lung** [HCC]

C7A.091 **Malignant carcinoid tumor of the thymus** [HCC]

C7A.092 **Malignant carcinoid tumor of the stomach** [HCC]

C7A.093 **Malignant carcinoid tumor of the kidney** [HCC]

C7A.094 **Malignant carcinoid tumor of the foregut, unspecified** [HCC]

C7A.095 **Malignant carcinoid tumor of the midgut, unspecified** [HCC]

C7A.096 **Malignant carcinoid tumor of the hindgut, unspecified** [HCC]

C7A.098 **Malignant carcinoid tumors of other sites** [HCC]

C7A.1 **Malignant poorly differentiated neuroendocrine tumors** [HCC]

Malignant poorly differentiated neuroendocrine tumor NOS

Malignant poorly differentiated neuroendocrine carcinoma, any site

High grade neuroendocrine carcinoma, any site

C7A.8 **Other malignant neuroendocrine tumors** [HCC]

SECONDARY NEUROENDOCRINE TUMORS (C7B)

C7B **Secondary neuroendocrine tumors**

Use Additional Code to identify any functional activity

C7B.0 **Secondary carcinoid tumors**

C7B.00 **Secondary carcinoid tumors, unspecified site** [HCC]

C7B.01 **Secondary carcinoid tumors of distant lymph nodes** [HCC]

C7B.02 **Secondary carcinoid tumors of liver** [HCC]

C7B.03 **Secondary carcinoid tumors of bone**

C7B.04 **Secondary carcinoid tumors of peritoneum** [HCC]

Mesentery metastasis of carcinoid tumor

C7B.09 **Secondary carcinoid tumors of other sites** [HCC]

C7B.1 **Secondary Merkel cell carcinoma** [HCC]

Merkel cell carcinoma nodal presentation

Merkel cell carcinoma visceral metastatic presentation

C7B.8 **Other secondary neuroendocrine tumors** [HCC]

MALIGNANT NEOPLASMS OF ILL-DEFINED, OTHER SECONDARY AND UNSPECIFIED SITES (C76-C80)

C76 **Malignant neoplasm of other and ill-defined sites**

Excludes1: malignant neoplasm of female genitourinary tract NOS (C57.9)

malignant neoplasm of male genitourinary tract NOS (C63.9)

malignant neoplasm of lymphoid, hematopoietic and related tissue (C81-C96)

malignant neoplasm of skin (C44.-)

malignant neoplasm of unspecified site NOS (C80.1)

C76.0 **Malignant neoplasm of head, face and neck** [HCC]

Malignant neoplasm of cheek NOS

Malignant neoplasm of nose NOS

C76.1 **Malignant neoplasm of thorax** [HCC]

Intrathoracic malignant neoplasm NOS

Malignant neoplasm of axilla NOS

Thoracic malignant neoplasm NOS

C76.2 **Malignant neoplasm of abdomen** [HCC]

C76.3 **Malignant neoplasm of pelvis** [HCC]

Malignant neoplasm of groin NOS

Malignant neoplasm of sites overlapping systems within the pelvis

Rectovaginal (septum) malignant neoplasm

Rectovesical (septum) malignant neoplasm

C76.4 **Malignant neoplasm of upper limb**

C76.40 **Malignant neoplasm of unspecified upper limb** [HCC]

C76.41 **Malignant neoplasm of right upper limb** [HCC]

C76.42 **Malignant neoplasm of left upper limb** [HCC]

C76.5 **Malignant neoplasm of lower limb**

C76.50 **Malignant neoplasm of unspecified lower limb** [HCC]

C76.51 **Malignant neoplasm of right lower limb** [HCC]

C76.52 **Malignant neoplasm of left lower limb** [HCC]

C76.8 **Malignant neoplasm of other specified ill-defined sites** [HCC]

Malignant neoplasm of overlapping ill-defined sites

C77 **Secondary and unspecified malignant neoplasm of lymph nodes**

Excludes1: malignant neoplasm of lymph nodes, specified as primary (C81-C86, C88, C96.-)

mesentery metastasis of carcinoid tumor (C7B.04)

secondary carcinoid tumors of distant lymph nodes (C7B.01)

C77.0 **Secondary and unspecified malignant neoplasm of lymph nodes of head, face and neck** [HCC]

● New code   ▲ Revised code   **Excludes1:** Not coded here   **Excludes2:** Not included here   ⊗ Placeholder required   ⑦7th digit required

Secondary and unspecified malignant neoplasm of supraclavicular lymph nodes

C77.1 **Secondary and unspecified malignant neoplasm of intrathoracic lymph nodes** [HCC]

C77.2 **Secondary and unspecified malignant neoplasm of intra-abdominal lymph nodes** [HCC]

C77.3 **Secondary and unspecified malignant neoplasm of axilla and upper limb lymph nodes** [HCC]

Secondary and unspecified malignant neoplasm of pectoral lymph nodes

C77.4 **Secondary and unspecified malignant neoplasm of inguinal and lower limb lymph nodes** [HCC]

C77.5 **Secondary and unspecified malignant neoplasm of intrapelvic lymph nodes** [HCC]

C77.8 **Secondary and unspecified malignant neoplasm of lymph nodes of multiple regions** [HCC]

C77.9 **Secondary and unspecified malignant neoplasm of lymph node, unspecified** [HCC]

C78 **Secondary malignant neoplasm of respiratory and digestive organs**

Excludes1: secondary carcinoid tumors of liver (C7B.02)

secondary carcinoid tumors of peritoneum (C7B.04)

Excludes2: lymph node metastases (C77.0)

C78.0 **Secondary malignant neoplasm of lung**

C78.00 **Secondary malignant neoplasm of unspecified lung** [HCC]

C78.01 **Secondary malignant neoplasm of right lung** [HCC]

C78.02 **Secondary malignant neoplasm of left lung** [HCC]

C78.1 **Secondary malignant neoplasm of mediastinum** [HCC]

C78.2 **Secondary malignant neoplasm of pleura** [HCC]

C78.3 **Secondary malignant neoplasm of other and unspecified respiratory organs**

C78.30 **Secondary malignant neoplasm of unspecified respiratory organ** [HCC]

C78.39 **Secondary malignant neoplasm of other respiratory organs** [HCC]

C78.4 **Secondary malignant neoplasm of small intestine** [HCC]

C78.5 **Secondary malignant neoplasm of large intestine and rectum** [HCC]

C78.6 **Secondary malignant neoplasm of retroperitoneum and peritoneum** [HCC]

C78.7 **Secondary malignant neoplasm of liver and intrahepatic bile duct** [HCC]

C78.8 **Secondary malignant neoplasm of other and unspecified digestive organs**

C78.80 **Secondary malignant neoplasm of unspecified digestive organ** [HCC]

C78.89 **Secondary malignant neoplasm of other digestive organs** [HCC]

Code also exocrine pancreatic insufficiency (K86.81)

C79 **Secondary malignant neoplasm of other and unspecified sites**

Excludes1: secondary carcinoid tumors (C7B.-)

secondary neuroendocrine tumors (C7B.-)

C79.0 **Secondary malignant neoplasm of kidney and renal pelvis**

C79.00 **Secondary malignant neoplasm of unspecified kidney and renal pelvis** [HCC]

C79.01 **Secondary malignant neoplasm of right kidney and renal pelvis** [HCC]

C79.02 **Secondary malignant neoplasm of left kidney and renal pelvis** [HCC]

C79.1 **Secondary malignant neoplasm of bladder and other and unspecified urinary organs** [HCC]

C79.10 **Secondary malignant neoplasm of unspecified urinary organs** [HCC]

C79.11 **Secondary malignant neoplasm of bladder** [HCC]

Excludes2: lymph node metastases (C77.0)

C79.19 **Secondary malignant neoplasm of other urinary organs** [HCC]

C79.2 **Secondary malignant neoplasm of skin** [HCC]

Excludes1: secondary Merkel cell carcinoma (C7B.1)

C79.3 **Secondary malignant neoplasm of brain and cerebral meninges**

C79.31 **Secondary malignant neoplasm of brain** [HCC]

C79.32 **Secondary malignant neoplasm of cerebral meninges** [HCC]

C79.4 **Secondary malignant neoplasm of other and unspecified parts of nervous system**

C79.40 **Secondary malignant neoplasm of unspecified part of nervous system** [HCC]

C79.49 **Secondary malignant neoplasm of other parts of nervous system** [HCC]

C79.5 **Secondary malignant neoplasm of bone and bone marrow**

Excludes1: secondary carcinoid tumors of bone (C7B.03)

C79.51 **Secondary malignant neoplasm of bone** [HCC]

C79.52 **Secondary malignant neoplasm of bone marrow** [HCC]

C79.6 **Secondary malignant neoplasm of ovary**

C79.60 **Secondary malignant neoplasm of unspecified ovary** [HCC]

C79.61 **Secondary malignant neoplasm of right ovary** [HCC]

C79.62 **Secondary malignant neoplasm of left ovary** [HCC]

●**C79.63** **Secondary malignant neoplasm of bilateral ovaries** [HCC]

C79.7 **Secondary malignant neoplasm of adrenal gland**

C79.70 **Secondary malignant neoplasm of unspecified adrenal gland** [HCC]

C79.71 **Secondary malignant neoplasm of right adrenal gland** [HCC]

C79.72 **Secondary malignant neoplasm of left adrenal gland** [HCC]

C79.8 **Secondary malignant neoplasm of other specified sites**

C79.81 **Secondary malignant neoplasm of breast** [HCC]

C79.82 **Secondary malignant neoplasm of genital organs** [HCC]

C79.89 **Secondary malignant neoplasm of other specified sites** [HCC]

C79.9 **Secondary malignant neoplasm of unspecified site**

Metastatic cancer NOS

Metastatic disease NOS

Excludes1: carcinomatosis NOS (C80.0)

generalized cancer NOS (C80.0)

malignant (primary) neoplasm of unspecified site (C80.1)

C80 **Malignant neoplasm without specification of site**

Excludes1: malignant carcinoid tumor of unspecified site (C7A.00)

malignant neoplasm of specified multiple sites- code to each site

C80.0 **Disseminated malignant neoplasm, unspecified** [HCC]

Carcinomatosis NOS

Generalized cancer, unspecified site (primary) (secondary)

Generalized malignancy, unspecified site (primary) (secondary)

C80.1 **Malignant (primary) neoplasm, unspecified** [HCC]

Cancer NOS

Cancer unspecified site (primary)

Carcinoma unspecified site (primary)

Malignancy unspecified site (primary)

Excludes1: secondary malignant neoplasm of unspecified site (C79.9)

C80.2 **Malignant neoplasm associated with transplanted organ** [HCC]

Code first complication of transplanted organ (T86.-)

Use Additional Code to identify the specific malignancy

MALIGNANT NEOPLASMS OF LYMPHOID, HEMATOPOIETIC AND RELATED TISSUE (C81-C96)

Excludes2: Kaposi's sarcoma of lymph nodes (C46.3)

secondary and unspecified neoplasm of lymph nodes (C77.-)

secondary neoplasm of bone marrow (C79.52)

secondary neoplasm of spleen (C78.89)

C81 **Hodgkin lymphoma**

Definition: Hodgkin's disease is a malignant disease of the lymphatic system is characterized by painless enlargement of lymph nodes, the spleen, or other lymphatic tissue. It is sometimes accompanied by symptoms such as fever, weight loss, fatigue and night sweats.

Excludes1: personal history of Hodgkin lymphoma (Z85.71)

C81.0 **Nodular lymphocyte predominant Hodgkin lymphoma**

C81.00 **Nodular lymphocyte predominant Hodgkin lymphoma, unspecified site** [HCC]

C81.01 **Nodular lymphocyte predominant Hodgkin lymphoma, lymph nodes of head, face, and neck** [HCC]

C81.02 **Nodular lymphocyte predominant Hodgkin lymphoma, intrathoracic lymph nodes** [HCC]

C81.03 **Nodular lymphocyte predominant Hodgkin lymphoma, intra-abdominal lymph nodes** [HCC]

C81.04 **Nodular lymphocyte predominant Hodgkin lymphoma, lymph nodes of axilla and upper limb** [HCC]

C81.05 **Nodular lymphocyte predominant Hodgkin lymphoma, lymph nodes of inguinal region and lower limb** [HCC]

C81.06 **Nodular lymphocyte predominant Hodgkin lymphoma, intrapelvic lymph nodes** [HCC]

C81.07 **Nodular lymphocyte predominant Hodgkin lymphoma, spleen** [HCC]

C81.08 **Nodular lymphocyte predominant Hodgkin lymphoma, lymph nodes of multiple sites** [HCC]

C81.09 **Nodular lymphocyte predominant Hodgkin lymphoma, extranodal and solid organ sites** [HCC]

C81.1 **Nodular sclerosis Hodgkin lymphoma**

Nodular sclerosis classical Hodgkin lymphoma

C81.10 **Nodular sclerosis Hodgkin lymphoma, unspecified site** [HCC]

C81.11 **Nodular sclerosis Hodgkin lymphoma, lymph nodes of head, face, and neck** [HCC]

C81.12 **Nodular sclerosis Hodgkin lymphoma, intrathoracic lymph nodes** [HCC]

C81.13 **Nodular sclerosis Hodgkin lymphoma, intra-abdominal lymph nodes** [HCC]

C81.14 **Nodular sclerosis Hodgkin lymphoma, lymph nodes of axilla and upper limb** [HCC]

C81.15 **Nodular sclerosis Hodgkin lymphoma, lymph nodes of inguinal region and lower limb** [HCC]

C81.16 **Nodular sclerosis Hodgkin lymphoma, intrapelvic lymph nodes** [HCC]

C81.17 **Nodular sclerosis Hodgkin lymphoma, spleen** [HCC]

C81.18 **Nodular sclerosis Hodgkin lymphoma, lymph nodes of multiple sites** [HCC]

C81.19 **Nodular sclerosis Hodgkin lymphoma, extranodal and solid organ sites** [HCC]

C81.2 **Mixed cellularity Hodgkin lymphoma**

Mixed cellularity classical Hodgkin lymphoma

C81.20 **Mixed cellularity Hodgkin lymphoma, unspecified site** [HCC]

C81.21 **Mixed cellularity Hodgkin lymphoma, lymph nodes of head, face, and neck** [HCC]

C81.22 **Mixed cellularity Hodgkin lymphoma, intrathoracic lymph nodes** [HCC]

C81.23 **Mixed cellularity Hodgkin lymphoma, intra-abdominal lymph nodes** [HCC]

C81.24 **Mixed cellularity Hodgkin lymphoma, lymph nodes of axilla and upper limb** [HCC]

C81.25 **Mixed cellularity Hodgkin lymphoma, lymph nodes of inguinal region and lower limb** [HCC]

C81.26 **Mixed cellularity Hodgkin lymphoma, intrapelvic lymph nodes** [HCC]

C81.27 **Mixed cellularity Hodgkin lymphoma, spleen** [HCC]

C81.28 **Mixed cellularity Hodgkin lymphoma, lymph nodes of multiple sites** [HCC]

C81.29 **Mixed cellularity Hodgkin lymphoma, extranodal and solid organ sites** [HCC]

C81.3 **Lymphocyte depleted Hodgkin lymphoma**

Lymphocyte depleted classical Hodgkin lymphoma

C81.30 **Lymphocyte depleted Hodgkin lymphoma, unspecified site** [HCC]

C81.31 **Lymphocyte depleted Hodgkin lymphoma, lymph nodes of head, face, and neck** [HCC]

C81.32 **Lymphocyte depleted Hodgkin lymphoma, intrathoracic lymph nodes** [HCC]

C81.33 **Lymphocyte depleted Hodgkin lymphoma, intra-abdominal lymph nodes** [HCC]

C81.34 **Lymphocyte depleted Hodgkin lymphoma, lymph nodes of axilla and upper limb** [HCC]

C81.35 **Lymphocyte depleted Hodgkin lymphoma, lymph nodes of inguinal region and lower limb** [HCC]

C81.36 **Lymphocyte depleted Hodgkin lymphoma, intrapelvic lymph nodes**

C81.37 **Lymphocyte depleted Hodgkin lymphoma, spleen** [HCC]

C81.38 **Lymphocyte depleted Hodgkin lymphoma, lymph nodes of multiple sites** [HCC]

C81.39 **Lymphocyte depleted Hodgkin lymphoma, extranodal and solid organ sites** [HCC]

C81.4 **Lymphocyte-rich Hodgkin lymphoma**

Lymphocyte-rich classical Hodgkin lymphoma

Excludes1: nodular lymphocyte predominant Hodgkin lymphoma (C81.0-)

C81.40 **Lymphocyte-rich Hodgkin lymphoma, unspecified site** [HCC]

C81.41 **Lymphocyte-rich Hodgkin lymphoma, lymph nodes of head, face, and neck** [HCC]

C81.42 **Lymphocyte-rich Hodgkin lymphoma, intrathoracic lymph nodes** [HCC]

C81.43 **Lymphocyte-rich Hodgkin lymphoma, intra-abdominal lymph nodes** [HCC]

C81.44 **Lymphocyte-rich Hodgkin lymphoma, lymph nodes of axilla and upper limb** [HCC]

C81.45 **Lymphocyte-rich Hodgkin lymphoma, lymph nodes of inguinal region and lower limb** [HCC]

C81.46 **Lymphocyte-rich Hodgkin lymphoma, intrapelvic lymph nodes** [HCC]

C81.47 **Lymphocyte-rich Hodgkin lymphoma, spleen** [HCC]

C81.48 **Lymphocyte-rich Hodgkin lymphoma, lymph nodes of multiple sites** [HCC]

C81.49 **Lymphocyte-rich Hodgkin lymphoma, extranodal and solid organ sites** [HCC]

C81.7 **Other Hodgkin lymphoma**

Classical Hodgkin lymphoma NOS

Other classical Hodgkin lymphoma

C81.70 **Other Hodgkin lymphoma, unspecified site** [HCC]

C81.71 **Other Hodgkin lymphoma, lymph nodes of head, face, and neck** [HCC]

C81.72 **Other Hodgkin lymphoma, intrathoracic lymph nodes** [HCC]

C81.73 **Other Hodgkin lymphoma, intra-abdominal lymph nodes** [HCC]

C81.74 **Other Hodgkin lymphoma, lymph nodes of axilla and upper limb** [HCC]

C81.75 **Other Hodgkin lymphoma, lymph nodes of inguinal region and lower limb** [HCC]

C81.76 **Other Hodgkin lymphoma, intrapelvic lymph nodes** [HCC]

C81.77 **Other Hodgkin lymphoma, spleen** [HCC]

C81.78 **Other Hodgkin lymphoma, lymph nodes of multiple sites** [HCC]

C81.79 **Other Hodgkin lymphoma, extranodal and solid organ sites** [HCC]

C81.9 **Hodgkin lymphoma, unspecified**

C81.90 **Hodgkin lymphoma, unspecified, unspecified site** [HCC]

C81.91 **Hodgkin lymphoma, unspecified, lymph nodes of head, face, and neck** [HCC]

C81.92 **Hodgkin lymphoma, unspecified, intrathoracic lymph nodes** [HCC]

C81.93 **Hodgkin lymphoma, unspecified, intra-abdominal lymph nodes**

C81.94 **Hodgkin lymphoma, unspecified, lymph nodes of axilla and upper limb** [HCC]

C81.95 **Hodgkin lymphoma, unspecified, lymph nodes of inguinal region and lower limb** [HCC]

C81.96 **Hodgkin lymphoma, unspecified, intrapelvic lymph nodes** [HCC]

C81.97 **Hodgkin lymphoma, unspecified, spleen** [HCC]

C81.98 **Hodgkin lymphoma, unspecified, lymph nodes of multiple sites** [HCC]

C81.99 **Hodgkin lymphoma, unspecified, extranodal and solid organ sites** [HCC]

C82 **Follicular lymphoma**

Includes: follicular lymphoma with or without diffuse areas

Excludes1: mature T/NK-cell lymphomas (C84.-)

personal history of non-Hodgkin lymphoma (Z85.72)

C82.0 **Follicular lymphoma grade I**

C82.00 **Follicular lymphoma grade I, unspecified site** [HCC]

C82.01 **Follicular lymphoma grade I, lymph nodes of head, face, and neck** [HCC]

C82.02 **Follicular lymphoma grade I, intrathoracic lymph nodes** [HCC]

C82.03 **Follicular lymphoma grade I, intra-abdominal lymph nodes** [HCC]

C82.04 **Follicular lymphoma grade I, lymph nodes of axilla and upper limb** [HCC]

C82.05 **Follicular lymphoma grade I, lymph nodes of inguinal region and lower limb** [HCC]

C82.06 **Follicular lymphoma grade I, intrapelvic lymph nodes** [HCC]

C82.07 **Follicular lymphoma grade I, spleen** [HCC]

C82.08 **Follicular lymphoma grade I, lymph nodes of multiple sites** [HCC]

C82.09 **Follicular lymphoma grade I, extranodal and solid organ sites** [HCC]

C82.1 **Follicular lymphoma grade II**

C82.10 **Follicular lymphoma grade II, unspecified site** [HCC]

C82.11 **Follicular lymphoma grade II, lymph nodes of head, face, and neck** [HCC]

C82.12 **Follicular lymphoma grade II, intrathoracic lymph nodes** [HCC]

C82.13 **Follicular lymphoma grade II, intra-abdominal lymph nodes** [HCC]

C82.14 **Follicular lymphoma grade II, lymph nodes of axilla and upper limb** [HCC]

C82.15 **Follicular lymphoma grade II, lymph nodes of inguinal region and lower limb** [HCC]

C82.16 **Follicular lymphoma grade II, intrapelvic lymph nodes** [HCC]

C82.17 **Follicular lymphoma grade II, spleen** [HCC]

C82.18 **Follicular lymphoma grade II, lymph nodes of multiple sites** [HCC]

C82.19 **Follicular lymphoma grade II, extranodal and solid organ sites** [HCC]

C82.2 **Follicular lymphoma grade III, unspecified**

C82.20 **Follicular lymphoma grade III, unspecified, unspecified site** [HCC]

C82.21 **Follicular lymphoma grade III, unspecified, lymph nodes of head, face, and neck** [HCC]

C82.22 **Follicular lymphoma grade III, unspecified, intrathoracic lymph nodes** [HCC]

C82.23 **Follicular lymphoma grade III, unspecified, intra-abdominal lymph nodes** [HCC]

C82.24 **Follicular lymphoma grade III, unspecified, lymph nodes of axilla and upper limb** [HCC]

C82.25 **Follicular lymphoma grade III, unspecified, lymph nodes of inguinal region and lower limb** [HCC]

C82.26 **Follicular lymphoma grade III, unspecified, intrapelvic lymph nodes** [HCC]

C82.27 **Follicular lymphoma grade III, unspecified, spleen** [HCC]

C82.28 **Follicular lymphoma grade III, unspecified, lymph nodes of multiple sites** [HCC]

C82.29 **Follicular lymphoma grade III, unspecified, extranodal and solid organ sites** [HCC]

C82.3 **Follicular lymphoma grade IIIa**

 C82.30 **Follicular lymphoma grade IIIa, unspecified site** [HCC]

 C82.31 **Follicular lymphoma grade IIIa, lymph nodes of head, face, and neck** [HCC]

 C82.32 **Follicular lymphoma grade IIIa, intrathoracic lymph nodes** [HCC]

 C82.33 **Follicular lymphoma grade IIIa, intra-abdominal lymph nodes** [HCC]

 C82.34 **Follicular lymphoma grade IIIa, lymph nodes of axilla and upper limb** [HCC]

 C82.35 **Follicular lymphoma grade IIIa, lymph nodes of inguinal region and lower limb** [HCC]

 C82.36 **Follicular lymphoma grade IIIa, intrapelvic lymph nodes** [HCC]

 C82.37 **Follicular lymphoma grade IIIa, spleen** [HCC]

 C82.38 **Follicular lymphoma grade IIIa, lymph nodes of multiple sites** [HCC]

 C82.39 **Follicular lymphoma grade IIIa, extranodal and solid organ sites** [HCC]

C82.4 **Follicular lymphoma grade IIIb**

 C82.40 **Follicular lymphoma grade IIIb, unspecified site** [HCC]

 C82.41 **Follicular lymphoma grade IIIb, lymph nodes of head, face, and neck** [HCC]

 C82.42 **Follicular lymphoma grade IIIb, intrathoracic lymph nodes** [HCC]

 C82.43 **Follicular lymphoma grade IIIb, intra-abdominal lymph nodes** [HCC]

 C82.44 **Follicular lymphoma grade IIIb, lymph nodes of axilla and upper limb** [HCC]

 C82.45 **Follicular lymphoma grade IIIb, lymph nodes of inguinal region and lower limb** [HCC]

 C82.46 **Follicular lymphoma grade IIIb, intrapelvic lymph nodes** [HCC]

 C82.47 **Follicular lymphoma grade IIIb, spleen** [HCC]

 C82.48 **Follicular lymphoma grade IIIb, lymph nodes of multiple sites** [HCC]

 C82.49 **Follicular lymphoma grade IIIb, extranodal and solid organ sites** [HCC]

C82.5 **Diffuse follicle center lymphoma**

 C82.50 **Diffuse follicle center lymphoma, unspecified site** [HCC]

 C82.51 **Diffuse follicle center lymphoma, lymph nodes of head, face, and neck** [HCC]

 C82.52 **Diffuse follicle center lymphoma, intrathoracic lymph nodes** [HCC]

 C82.53 **Diffuse follicle center lymphoma, intra-abdominal lymph nodes** [HCC]

 C82.54 **Diffuse follicle center lymphoma, lymph nodes of axilla and upper limb** [HCC]

 C82.55 **Diffuse follicle center lymphoma, lymph nodes of inguinal region and lower limb** [HCC]

 C82.56 **Diffuse follicle center lymphoma, intrapelvic lymph nodes** [HCC]

 C82.57 **Diffuse follicle center lymphoma, spleen** [HCC]

 C82.58 **Diffuse follicle center lymphoma, lymph nodes of multiple sites** [HCC]

 C82.59 **Diffuse follicle center lymphoma, extranodal and solid organ sites** [HCC]

C82.6 **Cutaneous follicle center lymphoma**

 C82.60 **Cutaneous follicle center lymphoma, unspecified site** [HCC]

 C82.61 **Cutaneous follicle center lymphoma, lymph nodes of head, face, and neck** [HCC]

 C82.62 **Cutaneous follicle center lymphoma, intrathoracic lymph nodes** [HCC]

 C82.63 **Cutaneous follicle center lymphoma, intra-abdominal lymph nodes** [HCC]

 C82.64 **Cutaneous follicle center lymphoma, lymph nodes of axilla and upper limb** [HCC]

 C82.65 **Cutaneous follicle center lymphoma, lymph nodes of inguinal region and lower limb** [HCC]

 C82.66 **Cutaneous follicle center lymphoma, intrapelvic lymph nodes** [HCC]

 C82.67 **Cutaneous follicle center lymphoma, spleen** [HCC]

 C82.68 **Cutaneous follicle center lymphoma, lymph nodes of multiple sites** [HCC]

 C82.69 **Cutaneous follicle center lymphoma, extranodal and solid organ sites** [HCC]

C82.8 **Other types of follicular lymphoma**

 C82.80 **Other types of follicular lymphoma, unspecified site** [HCC]

 C82.81 **Other types of follicular lymphoma, lymph nodes of head, face, and neck** [HCC]

 C82.82 **Other types of follicular lymphoma, intrathoracic lymph nodes** [HCC]

 C82.83 **Other types of follicular lymphoma, intra-abdominal lymph nodes** [HCC]

 C82.84 **Other types of follicular lymphoma, lymph nodes of axilla and upper limb** [HCC]

 C82.85 **Other types of follicular lymphoma, lymph nodes of inguinal region and lower limb** [HCC]

 C82.86 **Other types of follicular lymphoma, intrapelvic lymph nodes** [HCC]

 C82.87 **Other types of follicular lymphoma, spleen** [HCC]

 C82.88 **Other types of follicular lymphoma, lymph nodes of multiple sites** [HCC]

 C82.89 **Other types of follicular lymphoma, extranodal and solid organ sites** [HCC]

C82.9 **Follicular lymphoma, unspecified**

 C82.90 **Follicular lymphoma, unspecified, unspecified site** [HCC]

 C82.91 **Follicular lymphoma, unspecified, lymph nodes of head, face, and neck** [HCC]

 C82.92 **Follicular lymphoma, unspecified, intrathoracic lymph nodes** [HCC]

 C82.93 **Follicular lymphoma, unspecified, intra-abdominal lymph nodes** [HCC]

 C82.94 **Follicular lymphoma, unspecified, lymph nodes of axilla and upper limb** [HCC]

 C82.95 **Follicular lymphoma, unspecified, lymph nodes of inguinal region and lower limb** [HCC]

 C82.96 **Follicular lymphoma, unspecified, intrapelvic lymph nodes** [HCC]

 C82.97 **Follicular lymphoma, unspecified, spleen** [HCC]

 C82.98 **Follicular lymphoma, unspecified, lymph nodes of multiple sites** [HCC]

 C82.99 **Follicular lymphoma, unspecified, extranodal and solid organ sites** [HCC]

C83 **Non-follicular lymphoma**

 Excludes1: personal history of non-Hodgkin lymphoma (Z85.72)

C83.0 **Small cell B-cell lymphoma**

 Lymphoplasmacytic lymphoma

 Nodal marginal zone lymphoma

 ● New code ▲ Revised code Excludes1: Not coded here Excludes2: Not included here ⊗ Placeholder required ⑦ 7th digit required

Non-leukemic variant of B-CLL

Splenic marginal zone lymphoma

Excludes1: chronic lymphocytic leukemia (C91.1)

mature T/NK-cell lymphomas (C84.-)

Waldenström macroglobulinemia (C88.0)

C83.00 **Small cell B-cell lymphoma, unspecified site** [HCC]

C83.01 **Small cell B-cell lymphoma, lymph nodes of head, face, and neck** [HCC]

C83.02 **Small cell B-cell lymphoma, intrathoracic lymph nodes** [HCC]

C83.03 **Small cell B-cell lymphoma, intra-abdominal lymph nodes** [HCC]

C83.04 **Small cell B-cell lymphoma, lymph nodes of axilla and upper limb** [HCC]

C83.05 **Small cell B-cell lymphoma, lymph nodes of inguinal region and lower limb** [HCC]

C83.06 **Small cell B-cell lymphoma, intrapelvic lymph nodes** [HCC]

C83.07 **Small cell B-cell lymphoma, spleen** [HCC]

C83.08 **Small cell B-cell lymphoma, lymph nodes of multiple sites** [HCC]

C83.09 **Small cell B-cell lymphoma, extranodal and solid organ sites** [HCC]

C83.1 **Mantle cell lymphoma**

Centrocytic lymphoma

Malignant lymphomatous polyposis

C83.10 **Mantle cell lymphoma, unspecified site** [HCC]

C83.11 **Mantle cell lymphoma, lymph nodes of head, face, and neck** [HCC]

C83.12 **Mantle cell lymphoma, intrathoracic lymph nodes**

C83.13 **Mantle cell lymphoma, intra-abdominal lymph nodes** [HCC]

C83.14 **Mantle cell lymphoma, lymph nodes of axilla and upper limb** [HCC]

C83.15 **Mantle cell lymphoma, lymph nodes of inguinal region and lower limb** [HCC]

C83.16 **Mantle cell lymphoma, intrapelvic lymph nodes** [HCC]

C83.17 **Mantle cell lymphoma, spleen** [HCC]

C83.18 **Mantle cell lymphoma, lymph nodes of multiple sites** [HCC]

C83.19 **Mantle cell lymphoma, extranodal and solid organ sites** [HCC]

C83.3 **Diffuse large B-cell lymphoma**

Anaplastic diffuse large B-cell lymphoma

CD30-positive diffuse large B-cell lymphoma

Centroblastic diffuse large B-cell lymphoma

Diffuse large B-cell lymphoma, subtype not specified

Immunoblastic diffuse large B-cell lymphoma

Plasmablastic diffuse large B-cell lymphoma

Diffuse large B-cell lymphoma, subtype not specified

T-cell rich diffuse large B-cell lymphoma

Excludes1: mediastinal (thymic) large B-cell lymphoma (C85.2-)

mature T/NK-cell lymphomas (C84.-)

C83.30 **Diffuse large B-cell lymphoma, unspecified site** [HCC]

C83.31 **Diffuse large B-cell lymphoma, lymph nodes of head, face, and neck** [HCC]

C83.32 **Diffuse large B-cell lymphoma, intrathoracic lymph nodes** [HCC]

C83.33 **Diffuse large B-cell lymphoma, intra-abdominal lymph nodes** [HCC]

C83.34 **Diffuse large B-cell lymphoma, lymph nodes of axilla and upper limb** [HCC]

C83.35 **Diffuse large B-cell lymphoma, lymph nodes of inguinal region and lower limb** [HCC]

C83.36 **Diffuse large B-cell lymphoma, intrapelvic lymph nodes** [HCC]

C83.37 **Diffuse large B-cell lymphoma, spleen** [HCC]

C83.38 **Diffuse large B-cell lymphoma, lymph nodes of multiple sites** [HCC]

C83.39 **Diffuse large B-cell lymphoma, extranodal and solid organ sites** [HCC]

C83.5 **Lymphoblastic (diffuse) lymphoma**

B-precursor lymphoma

Lymphoblastic B-cell lymphoma

Lymphoblastic lymphoma NOS

Lymphoblastic T-cell lymphoma

T-precursor lymphoma

C83.50 **Lymphoblastic (diffuse) lymphoma, unspecified site** [HCC]

C83.51 **Lymphoblastic (diffuse) lymphoma, lymph nodes of head, face, and neck** [HCC]

C83.52 **Lymphoblastic (diffuse) lymphoma, intrathoracic lymph nodes** [HCC]

C83.53 **Lymphoblastic (diffuse) lymphoma, intra-abdominal lymph nodes** [HCC]

C83.54 **Lymphoblastic (diffuse) lymphoma, lymph nodes of axilla and upper limb**

C83.55 **Lymphoblastic (diffuse) lymphoma, lymph nodes of inguinal region and lower limb** [HCC]

C83.56 **Lymphoblastic (diffuse) lymphoma, intrapelvic lymph nodes** [HCC]

C83.57 **Lymphoblastic (diffuse) lymphoma, spleen** [HCC]

C83.58 **Lymphoblastic (diffuse) lymphoma, lymph nodes of multiple sites** [HCC]

C83.59 **Lymphoblastic (diffuse) lymphoma, extranodal and solid organ sites** [HCC]

C83.7 **Burkitt lymphoma**

Atypical Burkitt lymphoma Burkitt-like lymphoma

Excludes1: mature B-cell leukemia Burkitt type (C91.A-)

C83.70 **Burkitt lymphoma, unspecified site** [HCC]

C83.71 **Burkitt lymphoma, lymph nodes of head, face, and neck** [HCC]

C83.72 **Burkitt lymphoma, intrathoracic lymph nodes** [HCC]

C83.73 **Burkitt lymphoma, intra-abdominal lymph nodes** [HCC]

C83.74 **Burkitt lymphoma, lymph nodes of axilla and upper limb** [HCC]

C83.75 **Burkitt lymphoma, lymph nodes of inguinal region and lower limb** [HCC]

C83.76 **Burkitt lymphoma, intrapelvic lymph nodes** [HCC]

C83.77 **Burkitt lymphoma, spleen** [HCC]

C83.78 **Burkitt lymphoma, lymph nodes of multiple sites** [HCC]

C83.79 **Burkitt lymphoma, extranodal and solid organ sites** [HCC]

C83.8 **Other non-follicular lymphoma**

Intravascular large B-cell lymphoma Lymphoid granulomatosis

Primary effusion B-cell lymphoma

Excludes1: mediastinal (thymic) large B-cell lymphoma (C85.2-)

T-cell rich B-cell lymphoma (C83.3-)

C83.80 Other non-follicular lymphoma, unspecified site [HCC]

C83.81 Other non-follicular lymphoma, lymph nodes of head, face, and neck [HCC]

C83.82 Other non-follicular lymphoma, intrathoracic lymph nodes [HCC]

C83.83 Other non-follicular lymphoma, intra-abdominal lymph nodes [HCC]

C83.84 Other non-follicular lymphoma, lymph nodes of axilla and upper limb [HCC]

C83.85 Other non-follicular lymphoma, lymph nodes of inguinal region and lower limb [HCC]

C83.86 Other non-follicular lymphoma, intrapelvic lymph nodes [HCC]

C83.87 Other non-follicular lymphoma, spleen [HCC]

C83.88 Other non-follicular lymphoma, lymph nodes of multiple sites [HCC]

C83.89 Other non-follicular lymphoma, extranodal and solid organ sites

C83.9 Non-follicular (diffuse) lymphoma, unspecified

C83.90 Non-follicular (diffuse) lymphoma, unspecified, unspecified site [HCC]

C83.91 Non-follicular (diffuse) lymphoma, unspecified, lymph nodes of head, face, and neck [HCC]

C83.92 Non-follicular (diffuse) lymphoma, unspecified, intrathoracic lymph nodes [HCC]

C83.93 Non-follicular (diffuse) lymphoma, unspecified, intra-abdominal lymph nodes [HCC]

C83.94 Non-follicular (diffuse) lymphoma, unspecified, lymph nodes of axilla and upper limb [HCC]

C83.95 Non-follicular (diffuse) lymphoma, unspecified, lymph nodes of inguinal region and lower limb [HCC]

C83.96 Non-follicular (diffuse) lymphoma, unspecified, intrapelvic lymph nodes [HCC]

C83.97 Non-follicular (diffuse) lymphoma, unspecified, spleen [HCC]

C83.98 Non-follicular (diffuse) lymphoma, unspecified, lymph nodes of multiple sites [HCC]

C83.99 Non-follicular (diffuse) lymphoma, unspecified, extranodal and solid organ sites [HCC]

C84 Mature T/NK-cell lymphomas

Excludes1: personal history of non-Hodgkin lymphoma (Z85.72)

C84.0 Mycosis fungoides

Excludes1: peripheral T-cell lymphoma, not classified (C84.4-)

C84.00 Mycosis fungoides, unspecified site [HCC]

C84.01 Mycosis fungoides, lymph nodes of head, face, and neck [HCC]

C84.02 Mycosis fungoides, intrathoracic lymph nodes [HCC]

C84.03 Mycosis fungoides, intra-abdominal lymph nodes [HCC]

C84.04 Mycosis fungoides, lymph nodes of axilla and upper limb [HCC]

C84.05 Mycosis fungoides, lymph nodes of inguinal region and lower limb [HCC]

C84.06 Mycosis fungoides, intrapelvic lymph nodes [HCC]

C84.07 Mycosis fungoides, spleen [HCC]

C84.08 Mycosis fungoides, lymph nodes of multiple sites [HCC]

C84.09 Mycosis fungoides, extranodal and solid organ sites [HCC]

C84.1 Sézary disease

C84.10 Sézary disease, unspecified site [HCC]

C84.11 Sézary disease, lymph nodes of head, face, and neck [HCC]

C84.12 Sézary disease, intrathoracic lymph nodes [HCC] ♦

C84.13 Sézary disease, intra-abdominal lymph nodes [HCC]

C84.14 Sézary disease, lymph nodes of axilla and upper limb [HCC]

C84.15 Sézary disease, lymph nodes of inguinal region and lower limb [HCC]

C84.16 Sézary disease, intrapelvic lymph nodes

C84.17 Sézary disease, spleen [HCC]

C84.18 Sézary disease, lymph nodes of multiple sites [HCC]

C84.19 Sézary disease, extranodal and solid organ sites [HCC]

C84.4 Peripheral T-cell lymphoma, not classified

Lennert's lymphoma

Lymphoepithelioid lymphoma

Mature T-cell lymphoma, not elsewhere classified

C84.40 Peripheral T-cell lymphoma, not classified, unspecified site [HCC]

C84.41 Peripheral T-cell lymphoma, not classified, lymph nodes of head, face, and neck [HCC]

C84.42 Peripheral T-cell lymphoma, not classified, intrathoracic lymph nodes [HCC]

C84.43 Peripheral T-cell lymphoma, not classified, intra-abdominal lymph nodes [HCC]

C84.44 Peripheral T-cell lymphoma, not classified, lymph nodes of axilla and upper limb [HCC]

C84.45 Peripheral T-cell lymphoma, not classified, lymph nodes of inguinal region and lower limb [HCC]

C84.46 Peripheral T-cell lymphoma, not classified, intrapelvic lymph nodes [HCC]

C84.47 Peripheral T-cell lymphoma, not classified, spleen [HCC]

C84.48 Peripheral T-cell lymphoma, not classified, lymph nodes of multiple sites [HCC]

C84.49 Peripheral T-cell lymphoma, not classified, extranodal and solid organ sites [HCC]

C84.6 Anaplastic large cell lymphoma, ALK-positive

Anaplastic large cell lymphoma, CD30-positive

C84.60 Anaplastic large cell lymphoma, ALK-positive, unspecified site [HCC]

C84.61 Anaplastic large cell lymphoma, ALK-positive, lymph nodes of head, face, and neck [HCC]

C84.62 Anaplastic large cell lymphoma, ALK-positive, intrathoracic lymph nodes [HCC]

C84.63 Anaplastic large cell lymphoma, ALK-positive, intra-abdominal lymph nodes [HCC]

C84.64 Anaplastic large cell lymphoma, ALK-positive, lymph nodes of axilla and upper limb [HCC]

C84.65 Anaplastic large cell lymphoma, ALK-positive, lymph nodes of inguinal region and lower limb [HCC]

● New code   ▲ Revised code   Excludes1: Not coded here   Excludes2: Not included here   ⊗ Placeholder required   ⑦7th digit required

C84.66 **Anaplastic large cell lymphoma, ALK-positive, intrapelvic lymph nodes** [HCC]

C84.67 **Anaplastic large cell lymphoma, ALK-positive, spleen** [HCC]

C84.68 **Anaplastic large cell lymphoma, ALK-positive, lymph nodes of multiple sites** [HCC]

C84.69 **Anaplastic large cell lymphoma, ALK-positive, extranodal and solid organ sites** [HCC]

C84.7 **Anaplastic large cell lymphoma, ALK-negative**

Excludes1: primary cutaneous CD30-positive T-cell proliferations (C86.6-)

●C84.7A **Anaplastic large cell lymphoma, ALK-negative, breast**
Breast implant associated anaplastic large cell lymphoma (BIA-ALCL)
Use Additional Code to identify:
breast implant status (Z98.82)
personal history of breast implant removal (Z98.86)

C84.70 **Anaplastic large cell lymphoma, ALK-negative, unspecified site** [HCC]

C84.71 **Anaplastic large cell lymphoma, ALK-negative, lymph nodes of head, face, and neck** [HCC]

C84.72 **Anaplastic large cell lymphoma, ALK-negative, intrathoracic lymph nodes** [HCC]

C84.73 **Anaplastic large cell lymphoma, ALK-negative, intra-abdominal lymph nodes**

C84.74 **Anaplastic large cell lymphoma, ALK-negative, lymph nodes of axilla and upper limb** [HCC]

C84.75 **Anaplastic large cell lymphoma, ALK-negative, lymph nodes of inguinal region and lower limb** [HCC]

C84.76 **Anaplastic large cell lymphoma, ALK-negative, intrapelvic lymph nodes** [HCC]

C84.77 **Anaplastic large cell lymphoma, ALK-negative, spleen** [HCC]

C84.78 **Anaplastic large cell lymphoma, ALK-negative, lymph nodes of multiple sites** [HCC]

C84.79 **Anaplastic large cell lymphoma, ALK-negative, extranodal and solid organ sites** [HCC]

C84.A **Cutaneous T-cell lymphoma, unspecified**

C84.A0 **Cutaneous T-cell lymphoma, unspecified, unspecified site** [HCC]

C84.A1 **Cutaneous T-cell lymphoma, unspecified lymph nodes of head, face, and neck** [HCC]

C84.A2 **Cutaneous T-cell lymphoma, unspecified, intrathoracic lymph nodes** [HCC]

C84.A3 **Cutaneous T-cell lymphoma, unspecified, intra-abdominal lymph nodes** [HCC]

C84.A4 **Cutaneous T-cell lymphoma, unspecified, lymph nodes of axilla and upper limb** [HCC]

C84.A5 **Cutaneous T-cell lymphoma, unspecified, lymph nodes of inguinal region and lower limb** [HCC]

C84.A6 **Cutaneous T-cell lymphoma, unspecified, intrapelvic lymph nodes** [HCC]

C84.A7 **Cutaneous T-cell lymphoma, unspecified, spleen** [HCC]

C84.A8 **Cutaneous T-cell lymphoma, unspecified, lymph nodes of multiple sites** [HCC]

C84.A9 **Cutaneous T-cell lymphoma, unspecified, extranodal and solid organ sites** [HCC]

C84.Z **Other mature T/NK-cell lymphomas** [HCC]

Note: If T-cell lineage or involvement is mentioned in conjunction with a specific lymphoma, code to the more specific description.

Excludes1: angioimmunoblastic T-cell lymphoma (C86.5)
blastic NK-cell lymphoma (C86.4)
enteropathy-type T-cell lymphoma (C86.2)
extranodal NK-cell lymphoma, nasal type (C86.0)
hepatosplenic T-cell lymphoma (C86.1)
primary cutaneous CD30-positive T-cell proliferations (C86.6)
subcutaneous panniculitis-like T-cell lymphoma (C86.3)
T-cell leukemia (C91.1-)

C84.Z0 **Other mature T/NK-cell lymphomas, unspecified site** [HCC]

C84.Z1 **Other mature T/NK-cell lymphomas, lymph nodes of head, face, and neck** [HCC]

C84.Z2 **Other mature T/NK-cell lymphomas, intrathoracic lymph nodes** [HCC]

C84.Z3 **Other mature T/NK-cell lymphomas, intra-abdominal lymph nodes** [HCC]

C84.Z4 **Other mature T/NK-cell lymphomas, lymph nodes of axilla and upper limb** [HCC]

C84.Z5 **Other mature T/NK-cell lymphomas, lymph nodes of inguinal region and lower limb** [HCC]

C84.Z6 **Other mature T/NK-cell lymphomas, intrapelvic lymph nodes** [HCC]

C84.Z7 **Other mature T/NK-cell lymphomas, spleen**

C84.Z8 **Other mature T/NK-cell lymphomas, lymph nodes of multiple sites** [HCC]

C84.Z9 **Other mature T/NK-cell lymphomas, extranodal and solid organ sites** [HCC]

C84.9 **Mature T/NK-cell lymphomas, unspecified**

NK/T cell lymphoma NOS

Excludes1: mature T-cell lymphoma, not elsewhere classified (C84.4-)

C84.90 **Mature T/NK-cell lymphomas, unspecified, unspecified site** [HCC]

C84.91 **Mature T/NK-cell lymphomas, unspecified, lymph nodes of head, face, and neck** [HCC]

C84.92 **Mature T/NK-cell lymphomas, unspecified, intrathoracic lymph nodes** [HCC]

C84.93 **Mature T/NK-cell lymphomas, unspecified, intra-abdominal lymph nodes** [HCC]

C84.94 **Mature T/NK-cell lymphomas, unspecified, lymph nodes of axilla and upper limb** [HCC]

C84.95 **Mature T/NK-cell lymphomas, unspecified, lymph nodes of inguinal region and lower limb** [HCC]

C84.96 **Mature T/NK-cell lymphomas, unspecified, intrapelvic lymph nodes** [HCC]

C84.97 **Mature T/NK-cell lymphomas, unspecified, spleen** [HCC]

C84.98 **Mature T/NK-cell lymphomas, unspecified, lymph nodes of multiple sites** [HCC]

C84.99 **Mature T/NK-cell lymphomas, unspecified, extranodal and solid organ sites** [HCC]

C85 **Other specified and unspecified types of non-Hodgkin lymphoma**

Excludes1: Other specified types of T/NK-cell lymphoma (C86.-)
personal history of non-Hodgkin lymphoma (Z85.72)

C85.1 **Unspecified B-cell lymphoma**

Note: If B-cell lineage or involvement is mentioned in conjunction with a specific lymphoma, code to the more specific description.

C85.10 **Unspecified B-cell lymphoma, unspecified site** [HCC]

C85.11 **Unspecified B-cell lymphoma, lymph nodes of head, face, and neck** [HCC]

C85.12 **Unspecified B-cell lymphoma, intrathoracic lymph nodes** [HCC]

C85.13 **Unspecified B-cell lymphoma, intra-abdominal lymph nodes** [HCC]

C85.14 **Unspecified B-cell lymphoma, lymph nodes of axilla and upper limb** [HCC]

C85.15 **Unspecified B-cell lymphoma, lymph nodes of inguinal region and lower limb** [HCC]

C85.16 **Unspecified B-cell lymphoma, intrapelvic lymph nodes** [HCC]

C85.17 **Unspecified B-cell lymphoma, spleen** [HCC]

C85.18 **Unspecified B-cell lymphoma, lymph nodes of multiple sites** [HCC]

C85.19 **Unspecified B-cell lymphoma, extranodal and solid organ sites** [HCC]

C85.2 **Mediastinal (thymic) large B-cell lymphoma**

C85.20 **Mediastinal (thymic) large B-cell lymphoma, unspecified site** [HCC]

C85.21 **Mediastinal (thymic) large B-cell lymphoma, lymph nodes of head, face, and neck**

C85.22 **Mediastinal (thymic) large B-cell lymphoma, intrathoracic lymph nodes** [HCC]

C85.23 **Mediastinal (thymic) large B-cell lymphoma, intra-abdominal lymph nodes** [HCC]

C85.24 **Mediastinal (thymic) large B-cell lymphoma, lymph nodes of axilla and upper limb** [HCC]

C85.25 **Mediastinal (thymic) large B-cell lymphoma, lymph nodes of inguinal region and lower limb** [HCC]

C85.26 **Mediastinal (thymic) large B-cell lymphoma, intrapelvic lymph nodes** [HCC]

C85.27 **Mediastinal (thymic) large B-cell lymphoma, spleen** [HCC]

C85.28 **Mediastinal (thymic) large B-cell lymphoma, lymph nodes of multiple sites** [HCC]

C85.29 **Mediastinal (thymic) large B-cell lymphoma, extranodal and solid organ sites** [HCC]

C85.8 **Other specified types of non-Hodgkin lymphoma**

C85.80 **Other specified types of non-Hodgkin lymphoma, unspecified site** [HCC]

C85.81 **Other specified types of non-Hodgkin lymphoma, lymph nodes of head, face, and neck** [HCC]

C85.82 **Other specified types of non-Hodgkin lymphoma, intrathoracic lymph nodes** [HCC]

C85.83 **Other specified types of non-Hodgkin lymphoma, intra-abdominal lymph nodes** [HCC]

C85.84 **Other specified types of non-Hodgkin lymphoma, lymph nodes of axilla and upper limb** [HCC]

C85.85 **Other specified types of non-Hodgkin lymphoma, lymph nodes of inguinal region and lower limb** [HCC]

C85.86 **Other specified types of non-Hodgkin lymphoma, intrapelvic lymph nodes** [HCC]

C85.87 **Other specified types of non-Hodgkin lymphoma, spleen** [HCC]

C85.88 **Other specified types of non-Hodgkin lymphoma, lymph nodes of multiple sites** [HCC]

C85.89 **Other specified types of non-Hodgkin lymphoma, extranodal and solid organ sites** [HCC]

C85.9 **Non-Hodgkin lymphoma, unspecified**

Lymphoma NOS

Malignant lymphoma NOS

Non-Hodgkin lymphoma NOS

C85.90 **Non-Hodgkin lymphoma, unspecified, unspecified site** [HCC]

C85.91 **Non-Hodgkin lymphoma, unspecified, lymph nodes of head, face, and neck** [HCC]

C85.92 **Non-Hodgkin lymphoma, unspecified, intrathoracic lymph nodes** [HCC]

C85.93 **Non-Hodgkin lymphoma, unspecified, intra-abdominal lymph nodes** [HCC]

C85.94 **Non-Hodgkin lymphoma, unspecified, lymph nodes of axilla and upper limb** [HCC]

C85.95 **Non-Hodgkin lymphoma, unspecified, lymph nodes of inguinal region and lower limb** [HCC]

C85.96 **Non-Hodgkin lymphoma, unspecified, intrapelvic lymph nodes** [HCC]

C85.97 **Non-Hodgkin lymphoma, unspecified, spleen** [HCC]

C85.98 **Non-Hodgkin lymphoma, unspecified, lymph nodes of multiple sites** [HCC]

C85.99 **Non-Hodgkin lymphoma, unspecified, extranodal and solid organ sites** [HCC]

C86 **Other specified types of T/NK-cell lymphoma**

Excludes1: anaplastic large cell lymphoma, ALK negative (C84.7-)

anaplastic large cell lymphoma, ALK positive (C84.6-)

mature T/NK-cell lymphomas (C84.-)

Other specified types of non-Hodgkin lymphoma (C85.8-)

C86.0 **Extranodal NK/T-cell lymphoma, nasal type** [HCC]

C86.1 **Hepatosplenic T-cell lymphoma** [HCC]

Alpha-beta and gamma delta types

C86.2 **Enteropathy-type (intestinal) T-cell lymphoma** [HCC]

Enteropathy associated T-cell lymphoma

C86.3 **Subcutaneous panniculitis-like T-cell lymphoma** [HCC]

C86.4 **Blastic NK-cell lymphoma** [HCC]

Blastic plasmacytoid dendritic cell neoplasm (BPDCN)

C86.5 **Angioimmunoblastic T-cell lymphoma** [HCC]

Angioimmunoblastic lymphadenopathy with dysproteinemia (AILD)

C86.6 **Primary cutaneous CD30-positive T-cell proliferations** [HCC]

Lymphomatoid papulosis

Primary cutaneous anaplastic large cell lymphoma

Primary cutaneous CD30-positive large T-cell lymphoma

C88 **Malignant immunoproliferative diseases and certain other B-cell lymphomas** [HCC]

Excludes1: B-cell lymphoma, unspecified (C85.1-)

personal history of other malignant neoplasms of lymphoid, hematopoietic and related tissues (Z85.79)

C88.0 **Waldenström macroglobulinemia** [HCC]

Lymphoplasmacytic lymphoma with IgM-production

Macroglobulinemia (idiopathic) (primary)

Excludes1: small cell B-cell lymphoma (C83.0)

C88.2 **Heavy chain disease** [HCC]

Franklin disease

Gamma heavy chain disease

Mu heavy chain disease

C88.3 **Immunoproliferative small intestinal disease** [HCC]

Alpha heavy chain disease

Mediterranean lymphoma

C88.4 **Extranodal marginal zone B-cell lymphoma of mucosa-associated lymphoid tissue [MALT-lymphoma]** [HCC]

Lymphoma of skin-associated lymphoid tissue [SALT-lymphoma]

Lymphoma of bronchial-associated lymphoid tissue [BALT-lymphoma]

Excludes1: high malignant (diffuse large B-cell) lymphoma (C83.3-)

C88.8 **Other malignant immunoproliferative diseases** [HCC]

C88.9 **Malignant immunoproliferative disease, unspecified** [HCC]

Immunoproliferative disease NOS

C90 **Multiple myeloma and malignant plasma cell neoplasms**

Definition: Multiple myeloma and immunoproliferative neoplasms is a cancer in which there is a uncontrolled proliferation and disordered function of cells called plasma cells in the bone marrow., aka a plasma cell neoplasm.

Excludes1: personal history of other malignant neoplasms of lymphoid, hematopoietic and related tissues (Z85.79)

C90.0 **Multiple myeloma**

Kahler's disease

Medullary plasmacytoma

Myelomatosis

Plasma cell myeloma

Excludes1: solitary myeloma (C90.3-)

solitary plasmacytoma (C90.3-)

C90.00 **Multiple myeloma not having achieved remission** [HCC]

Multiple myeloma with failed remission

Multiple myeloma NOS

C90.01 **Multiple myeloma in remission** [HCC]

C90.02 **Multiple myeloma in relapse** [HCC]

C90.1 **Plasma cell leukemia**

Plasmacytic leukemia

C90.10 **Plasma cell leukemia not having achieved remission** [HCC]

Plasma cell leukemia with failed remission

Plasma cell leukemia NOS

C90.11 **Plasma cell leukemia in remission** [HCC]

C90.12 **Plasma cell leukemia in relapse** [HCC]

C90.2 **Extramedullary plasmacytoma**

C90.20 **Extramedullary plasmacytoma not having achieved remission** [HCC]

Extramedullary plasmacytoma with failed remission

Extramedullary plasmacytoma NOS

C90.21 **Extramedullary plasmacytoma in remission** [HCC]

C90.22 **Extramedullary plasmacytoma in relapse** [HCC]

C90.3 **Solitary plasmacytoma**

Localized malignant plasma cell tumor NOS

Plasmacytoma NOS

Solitary myeloma

C90.30 **Solitary plasmacytoma not having achieved remission** [HCC]

Solitary plasmacytoma with failed remission

Solitary plasmacytoma NOS

C90.31 **Solitary plasmacytoma in remission** [HCC]

C90.32 **Solitary plasmacytoma in relapse** [HCC]

C91 **Lymphoid leukemia**

Excludes1: personal history of leukemia (Z85.6)

C91.0 **Acute lymphoblastic leukemia [ALL]**

Note: Codes in subcategory C91.0- should only be used for T-cell and B-cell precursor leukemia

C91.00 **Acute lymphoblastic leukemia not having achieved remission** [HCC]

Acute lymphoblastic leukemia with failed remission

Acute lymphoblastic leukemia NOS

C91.01 **Acute lymphoblastic leukemia, in remission** [HCC]

C91.02 **Acute lymphoblastic leukemia, in relapse**

C91.1 **Chronic lymphocytic leukemia of B-cell type**

Lymphoplasmacytic leukemia

Richter syndrome

Excludes1: lymphoplasmacytic lymphoma (C83.0-)

C91.10 **Chronic lymphocytic leukemia of B-cell type not having achieved remission** [HCC]

Chronic lymphocytic leukemia of B-cell type with failed remission

Chronic lymphocytic leukemia of B-cell type NOS

C91.11 **Chronic lymphocytic leukemia of B-cell type in remission** [HCC]

C91.12 **Chronic lymphocytic leukemia of B-cell type in relapse** [HCC]

C91.3 **Prolymphocytic leukemia of B-cell type**

C91.30 **Prolymphocytic leukemia of B-cell type not having achieved remission** [HCC]

Prolymphocytic leukemia of B-cell type with failed remission

Prolymphocytic leukemia of B-cell type NOS

C91.31 **Prolymphocytic leukemia of B-cell type, in remission** [HCC]

C91.32 **Prolymphocytic leukemia of B-cell type, in relapse** [HCC]

C91.4 **Hairy cell leukemia**

Leukemic reticuloendotheliosis

C91.40 **Hairy cell leukemia not having achieved remission** [HCC]

Hairy cell leukemia with failed remission

Hairy cell leukemia NOS

C91.41 **Hairy cell leukemia, in remission** [HCC]

C91.42 **Hairy cell leukemia, in relapse** [HCC]

C91.5 **Adult T-cell lymphoma/leukemia (HTLV-1-associated)**

Acute variant of adult T-cell lymphoma/leukemia (HTLV-1-associated)

Chronic variant of adult T-cell lymphoma/leukemia (HTLV-1-associated)

Lymphomatoid variant of adult T-cell lymphoma/leukemia (HTLV-1-associated)

Smouldering variant of adult T-cell lymphoma/leukemia (HTLV-1-associated)

C91.50 **Adult T-cell lymphoma/leukemia (HTLV-1-associated) not having achieved remission** [HCC]

Adult T-cell lymphoma/leukemia (HTLV-1-associated) with failed remission

Adult T-cell lymphoma/leukemia (HTLV-1-associated) NOS

C91.51 **Adult T-cell lymphoma/leukemia (HTLV-1-associated), in remission** [HCC]

C91.52 **Adult T-cell lymphoma/leukemia (HTLV-1-associated), in relapse** [HCC]

C91.6 **Prolymphocytic leukemia of T-cell type**

C91.60 **Prolymphocytic leukemia of T-cell type not having achieved remission** [HCC]

Prolymphocytic leukemia of T-cell type with failed remission

Prolymphocytic leukemia of T-cell type NOS

C91.61 **Prolymphocytic leukemia of T-cell type, in remission** [HCC]

C91.62 **Prolymphocytic leukemia of T-cell type, in relapse** [HCC]

C91.A **Mature B-cell leukemia Burkitt-type**

Excludes1: Burkitt lymphoma (C83.7-)

C91.A0 **Mature B-cell leukemia Burkitt-type not having achieved remission** [HCC]

Mature B-cell leukemia Burkitt-type with failed remission

Mature B-cell leukemia Burkitt-type NOS

C91.A1 **Mature B-cell leukemia Burkitt-type, in remission** [HCC]

C91.A2 **Mature B-cell leukemia Burkitt-type, in relapse** [HCC]

C91.Z **Other lymphoid leukemia**

T-cell large granular lymphocytic leukemia (associated with rheumatoid arthritis)

C91.Z0 **Other lymphoid leukemia not having achieved remission** [HCC]

Other lymphoid leukemia with failed remission

Other lymphoid leukemia NOS

C91.Z1 **Other lymphoid leukemia, in remission** [HCC]

C91.Z2 **Other lymphoid leukemia, in relapse** [HCC]

C91.9 **Lymphoid leukemia, unspecified**

C91.90 **Lymphoid leukemia, unspecified not having achieved remission** [HCC]

Lymphoid leukemia with failed remission

Lymphoid leukemia NOS

C91.91 **Lymphoid leukemia, unspecified, in remission** [HCC]

C91.92 **Lymphoid leukemia, unspecified, in relapse** [HCC]

C92 **Myeloid leukemia**

Includes: granulocytic leukemia

myelogenous leukemia

Excludes1: personal history of leukemia (Z85.6)

C92.0 **Acute myeloblastic leukemia**

Acute myeloblastic leukemia, minimal differentiation

Acute myeloblastic leukemia (with maturation)

Acute myeloblastic leukemia 1/ETO

Acute myeloblastic leukemia M0

Acute myeloblastic leukemia M1

Acute myeloblastic leukemia M2

Acute myeloblastic leukemia with t(8;21)

Acute myeloblastic leukemia (without a FAB classification) NOS

Refractory anemia with excess blasts in transformation [RAEB T]

Excludes1: acute exacerbation of chronic myeloid leukemia (C92.10)

refractory anemia with excess of blasts not in transformation (D46.2-)

C92.00 **Acute myeloblastic leukemia, not having achieved remission** [HCC]

Acute myeloblastic leukemia with failed remission

Acute myeloblastic leukemia NOS

C92.01 **Acute myeloblastic leukemia, in remission** [HCC]

C92.02 **Acute myeloblastic leukemia, in relapse** [HCC]

C92.1 **Chronic myeloid leukemia, BCR/ABL-positive** [HCC]

Chronic myelogenous leukemia, Philadelphia chromosome (Ph1) positive

Chronic myelogenous leukemia, t(9;22) (q34;q11)

Chronic myelogenous leukemia with crisis of blast cells

Excludes1: atypical chronic myeloid leukemia BCR/ABL-negative (C92.2-)

chronic myelomonocytic leukemia (C93.1-)

chronic myeloproliferative disease (D47.1)

C92.10 **Chronic myeloid leukemia, BCR/ABL-positive, not having achieved remission** [HCC]

Chronic myeloid leukemia, BCR/ABL-positive with failed remission

Chronic myeloid leukemia, BCR/ABL-positive NOS

C92.11 **Chronic myeloid leukemia, BCR/ABL-positive, in remission** [HCC]

C92.12 **Chronic myeloid leukemia, BCR/ABL-positive, in relapse** [HCC]

C92.2 **Atypical chronic myeloid leukemia, BCR/ABL-negative**

C92.20 **Atypical chronic myeloid leukemia, BCR/ABL-negative, not having achieved remission** [HCC]

Atypical chronic myeloid leukemia, BCR/ABL-negative with failed remission

Atypical chronic myeloid leukemia, BCR/ABL-negative NOS

C92.21 **Atypical chronic myeloid leukemia, BCR/ABL-negative, in remission** [HCC]

C92.22 **Atypical chronic myeloid leukemia, BCR/ABL-negative, in relapse** [HCC]

C92.3 **Myeloid sarcoma**

A malignant tumor of immature myeloid cells

Chloroma

Granulocytic sarcoma

C92.30 **Myeloid sarcoma, not having achieved remission** [HCC]

Myeloid sarcoma with failed remission

Myeloid sarcoma NOS

C92.31 **Myeloid sarcoma, in remission** [HCC]

C92.32 **Myeloid sarcoma, in relapse** [HCC]

C92.4 **Acute promyelocytic leukemia**

AML M3

AML Me with t(15;17) and variants

C92.40 **Acute promyelocytic leukemia, not having achieved remission** [HCC]

Acute promyelocytic leukemia with failed remission

Acute promyelocytic leukemia NOS

C92.41 **Acute promyelocytic leukemia, in remission** [HCC]

C92.42 **Acute promyelocytic leukemia, in relapse** [HCC]

C92.5 **Acute myelomonocytic leukemia**

AML M4

AML M4 EO with inv(16) or t(16;16)

C92.50 **Acute myelomonocytic leukemia, not having achieved remission** [HCC]

Acute myelomonocytic leukemia with failed remission

Acute myelomonocytic leukemia NOS

C92.51 **Acute myelomonocytic leukemia, in remission** [HCC]

C92.52 **Acute myelomonocytic leukemia, in relapse** [HCC]

C92.6 **Acute myeloid leukemia with 11q23-abnormality** [HCC]

Acute myeloid leukemia with variation of MLL-gene

C92.60 **Acute myeloid leukemia with 11q23-abnormality not having achieved remission**

Acute myeloid leukemia with 11q23-abnormality with failed remission

Acute myeloid leukemia with 11q23-abnormality NOS

C92.61 **Acute myeloid leukemia with 11q23-abnormality in remission** [HCC]

C92.62 **Acute myeloid leukemia with 11q23-abnormality in relapse** [HCC]

C92.A **Acute myeloid leukemia with multilineage dysplasia**

Acute myeloid leukemia with dysplasia of remaining hematopoesis and/or myelodysplastic disease in its history

C92.A0 **Acute myeloid leukemia with multilineage dysplasia, not having achieved remission** [HCC]

Acute myeloid leukemia with multilineage dysplasia with failed remission

Acute myeloid leukemia with multilineage dysplasia NOS

C92.A1 **Acute myeloid leukemia with multilineage dysplasia, in remission** [HCC]

C92.A2 **Acute myeloid leukemia with multilineage dysplasia, in relapse** [HCC]

C92.Z **Other myeloid leukemia**

C92.Z0 **Other myeloid leukemia not having achieved remission** [HCC]

Myeloid leukemia NEC with failed remission

Myeloid leukemia NEC

C92.Z1 **Other myeloid leukemia, in remission** [HCC]

C92.Z2 **Other myeloid leukemia, in relapse** [HCC]

C92.9 **Myeloid leukemia, unspecified**

C92.90 **Myeloid leukemia, unspecified, not having achieved remission** [HCC]

Myeloid leukemia, unspecified with failed remission

Myeloid leukemia, unspecified NOS

C92.91 **Myeloid leukemia, unspecified in remission** [HCC]

C92.92 **Myeloid leukemia, unspecified in relapse** [HCC]

C93 **Monocytic leukemia**

Includes: monocytoid leukemia

Excludes1: personal history of leukemia (Z85.6)

C93.0 **Acute monoblastic/monocytic leukemia**

AML M5 AML M5a AML M5b

C93.00 **Acute monoblastic/monocytic leukemia, not having achieved remission** [HCC]

Acute monoblastic/monocytic leukemia with failed remission

Acute monoblastic/monocytic leukemia NOS

C93.01 **Acute monoblastic/monocytic leukemia, in remission** [HCC]

C93.02 **Acute monoblastic/monocytic leukemia, in relapse** [HCC]

C93.1 **Chronic myelomonocytic leukemia**

Code also, if applicable, eosinophilia (D72.18)

Chronic monocytic leukemia CMML-1

CMML-2

CMML with eosinophilia

C93.10 **Chronic myelomonocytic leukemia not having achieved remission** [HCC]

Chronic myelomonocytic leukemia with failed remission

Chronic myelomonocytic leukemia NOS

C93.11 **Chronic myelomonocytic leukemia, in remission** [HCC]

C93.12 **Chronic myelomonocytic leukemia, in relapse** [HCC]

C93.3 **Juvenile myelomonocytic leukemia**

C93.30 **Juvenile myelomonocytic leukemia, not having achieved remission** [HCC]

Juvenile myelomonocytic leukemia with failed remission Juvenile myelomonocytic leukemia NOS

C93.31 **Juvenile myelomonocytic leukemia, in remission** [HCC]

C93.32 **Juvenile myelomonocytic leukemia, in relapse** [HCC]

C93.Z **Other monocytic leukemia]**

C93.Z0 **Other monocytic leukemia, not having achieved remission** [HCC]

Other monocytic leukemia NOS

C93.Z1 **Other monocytic leukemia, in remission** [HCC]

C93.Z2 **Other monocytic leukemia, in relapse** [HCC]

C93.9 **Monocytic leukemia, unspecified**

C93.90 **Monocytic leukemia, unspecified, not having achieved remission** [HCC]

Monocytic leukemia, unspecified with failed remission

Monocytic leukemia, unspecified NOS

C93.91 **Monocytic leukemia, unspecified in remission** [HCC]

C93.92 **Monocytic leukemia, unspecified in relapse** [HCC]

C94 **Other leukemias of specified cell type**

Excludes1: leukemic reticuloendotheliosis (C91.4-)

myelodysplastic syndromes (D46.-)

personal history of leukemia (Z85.6)

plasma cell leukemia (C90.1-)

C94.0 **Acute erythroid leukemia**

Acute myeloid leukemia M6(a)(b)

Erythroleukemia

C94.00 **Acute erythroid leukemia, not having achieved remission** [HCC]

Acute erythroid leukemia with failed remission

Acute erythroid leukemia NOS

C94.01 **Acute erythroid leukemia, in remission** [HCC]

C94.02 **Acute erythroid leukemia, in relapse** [HCC]

C94.2 **Acute megakaryoblastic leukemia**

Acute myeloid leukemia M7

Acute megakaryocytic leukemia

C94.20 **Acute megakaryoblastic leukemia not having achieved remission** [HCC]

Acute megakaryoblastic leukemia with failed remission

Acute megakaryoblastic leukemia NOS

C94.21 **Acute megakaryoblastic leukemia, in remission** [HCC]

C94.22 **Acute megakaryoblastic leukemia, in relapse** [HCC]

C94.3 **Mast cell leukemia**

C94.30 **Mast cell leukemia not having achieved remission** [HCC]

Mast cell leukemia with failed remission

Mast cell leukemia NOS

C94.31 **Mast cell leukemia, in remission** [HCC]

C94.32 **Mast cell leukemia, in relapse** [HCC]

C94.4 **Acute panmyelosis with myelofibrosis**

Acute myelofibrosis

Excludes1: myelofibrosis NOS (D75.81)

secondary myelofibrosis NOS (D75.81)

C94.40 **Acute panmyelosis with myelofibrosis not having achieved remission** [HCC]

Acute myelofibrosis NOS

Acute panmyelosis with myelofibrosis with failed remission

Acute panmyelosis NOS

C94.41 **Acute panmyelosis with myelofibrosis, in remission** [HCC]

C94.42 **Acute panmyelosis with myelofibrosis, in relapse** [HCC]

C94.6 **Myelodysplastic disease, not classified** [HCC]

Myeloproliferative disease, not classified

C94.8 **Other specified leukemias** [HCC]

Aggressive NK-cell leukemia

Acute basophilic leukemia

C94.80 **Other specified leukemias not having achieved remission** [HCC]

Other specified leukemia with failed remission

Other specified leukemias NOS

C94.81 **Other specified leukemias, in remission** [HCC]

C94.82 **Other specified leukemias, in relapse** [HCC]

C95 **Leukemia of unspecified cell type**

Excludes1: personal history of leukemia (Z85.6)

C95.0 **Acute leukemia of unspecified cell type**

Acute bilineal leukemia

Acute mixed lineage leukemia

Biphenotypic acute leukemia

Stem cell leukemia of unclear lineage

Excludes1: acute exacerbation of unspecified chronic leukemia (C95.10)

C95.00 **Acute leukemia of unspecified cell type not having achieved remission** [HCC]

Acute leukemia of unspecified cell type with failed remission

Acute leukemia NOS

C95.01 **Acute leukemia of unspecified cell type, in remission** [HCC]

C95.02 **Acute leukemia of unspecified cell type, in relapse**

C95.1 **Chronic leukemia of unspecified cell type**

C95.10 **Chronic leukemia of unspecified cell type not having achieved remission** [HCC]

Chronic leukemia of unspecified cell type with failed remission

Chronic leukemia NOS

C95.11 **Chronic leukemia of unspecified cell type, in remission** [HCC]

C95.12 **Chronic leukemia of unspecified cell type, in relapse** [HCC]

C95.9 **Leukemia, unspecified**

C95.90 **Leukemia, unspecified not having achieved remission** [HCC]

Leukemia, unspecified with failed remission

Leukemia NOS

C95.91 **Leukemia, unspecified, in remission** [HCC]

C95.92 **Leukemia, unspecified, in relapse** [HCC]

C96 **Other and unspecified malignant neoplasms of lymphoid, hematopoietic and related tissue**

Excludes1: personal history of other malignant neoplasms of lymphoid, hematopoietic and related tissues (Z85.79)

C96.0 **Multifocal and multisystemic (disseminated) Langerhans-cell histiocytosis** [HCC]

Histiocytosis X, multisystemic Letterer-Siwe disease

Excludes1: adult pulmonary Langerhans cell histiocytosis J84.82)

multifocal and unisystemic Langerhans-cell histiocytosis (C96.5)

unifocal Langerhans-cell histiocytosis (C96.6)

C96.2 **Malignant mast cell neoplasm**

Excludes1: indolent mastocytosis (D47.02)

mast cell leukemia (C94.30)

mastocytosis (congenital) (cutaneous) (Q82.2)

C96.20 **Malignant mast cell neoplasm, unspecified** [HCC]

C96.21 **Aggressive systemic mastocytosis** [HCC]

C96.22 **Mast cell sarcoma** [HCC]

C96.29 **Other malignant mast cell neoplasm** [HCC]

C96.4 **Sarcoma of dendritic cells (accessory cells)** [HCC]

Follicular dendritic cell sarcoma

Interdigitating dendritic cell sarcoma Langerhans cell sarcoma

C96.5 **Multifocal and unisystemic Langerhans-cell histiocytosis** [HCC]

Hand-Schüller-Christian disease

Histiocytosis X, multifocal

Excludes1: multifocal and multisystemic (disseminated) Langerhans-cell histiocytosis (C96.0)

unifocal Langerhans-cell histiocytosis (C96.6)

C96.6 **Unifocal Langerhans-cell histiocytosis** [HCC]

Eosinophilic granuloma

Histiocytosis X, unifocal

Histiocytosis X NOS

Langerhans-cell histiocytosis NOS

Excludes1: multifocal and multisystemic (disseminated) Langerhans-cell histiocytosis (C96.0)

multifocal and unisystemic Langerhans-cell histiocytosis (C96.5)

C96.A **Histiocytic sarcoma** [HCC]

Malignant histiocytosis

C96.Z **Other specified malignant neoplasms of lymphoid, hematopoietic and related tissue** [HCC]

C96.9 **Malignant neoplasm of lymphoid, hematopoietic and related tissue, unspecified** [HCC]

IN SITU NEOPLASMS (D00-D09)

Definition: Carcinoma in situ is a cluster of malignant cells that has not yet invaded the deeper epithelial tissue or spread to other parts of the body.

Includes: Bowen's disease

erythroplasia

grade III intraepithelial neoplasia

Queyrat's erythroplasia

D00 Carcinoma in situ of oral cavity, esophagus and stomach

Excludes1: melanoma in situ (D03.-)

D00.0 Carcinoma in situ of lip, oral cavity and pharynx

Use Additional Code to identify:

exposure to environmental tobacco smoke (Z77.22)

exposure to tobacco smoke in the perinatal period (P96.81)

history of tobacco dependence (Z87.891)

occupational exposure to environmental tobacco smoke (Z57.31)

tobacco dependence (F17.-)

tobacco use (Z72.0)

Excludes1: carcinoma in situ of aryepiglottic fold or interarytenoid fold, laryngeal aspect (D02.0)

carcinoma in situ of epiglottis NOS (D02.0)

carcinoma in situ of epiglottis suprahyoid portion (D02.0)

carcinoma in situ of skin of lip (D03.0, D04.0)

D00.00 Carcinoma in situ of oral cavity, unspecified site

D00.01 Carcinoma in situ of labial mucosa and vermilion border

D00.02 Carcinoma in situ of buccal mucosa

D00.03 Carcinoma in situ of gingiva and edentulous alveolar ridge

D00.04 Carcinoma in situ of soft palate

D00.05 Carcinoma in situ of hard palate

D00.06 Carcinoma in situ of floor of mouth

D00.07 Carcinoma in situ of tongue

D00.08 Carcinoma in situ of pharynx

Carcinoma in situ of aryepiglottic fold NOS

Carcinoma in situ of hypopharyngeal aspect of aryepiglottic fold

Carcinoma in situ of marginal zone of aryepiglottic fold

D00.1 Carcinoma in situ of esophagus

D00.2 Carcinoma in situ of stomach

D01 Carcinoma in situ of other and unspecified digestive organs

Excludes1: melanoma in situ (D03.-)

D01.0 Carcinoma in situ of colon

Excludes1: carcinoma in situ of rectosigmoid junction (D01.1)

D01.1 Carcinoma in situ of rectosigmoid junction

D01.2 Carcinoma in situ of rectum

D01.3 Carcinoma in situ of anus and anal canal

Anal intraepithelial neoplasia III [AIN III]

Severe dysplasia of anus

Excludes1: anal intraepithelial neoplasia I and II [AIN I and AIN II] (K62.82)

carcinoma in situ of anal margin (D04.5)

carcinoma in situ of anal skin (D04.5)

carcinoma in situ of perianal skin (D04.5)

D01.4 Carcinoma in situ of other and unspecified parts of intestine

Excludes1: carcinoma in situ of ampulla of Vater (D01.5)

D01.40 Carcinoma in situ of unspecified part of intestine

D01.49 Carcinoma in situ of other parts of intestine

D01.5 Carcinoma in situ of liver, gallbladder and bile ducts

Carcinoma in situ of ampulla of Vater

D01.7 Carcinoma in situ of other specified digestive organs

Carcinoma in situ of pancreas

D01.9 Carcinoma in situ of digestive organ, unspecified

D02 Carcinoma in situ of middle ear and respiratory system

Use Additional Code to identify:

exposure to environmental tobacco smoke (Z77.22)

exposure to tobacco smoke in the perinatal period (P96.81)

history of tobacco dependence (Z87.891)

occupational exposure to environmental tobacco smoke (Z57.31)

tobacco dependence (F17.-)

tobacco use (Z72.0)

Excludes1: melanoma in situ (D03.-)

D02.0 Carcinoma in situ of larynx

Carcinoma in situ of aryepiglottic fold or interarytenoid fold, laryngeal aspect

Carcinoma in situ of epiglottis (suprahyoid portion)

Excludes1: carcinoma in situ of aryepiglottic fold or interarytenoid fold NOS (D00.08)

carcinoma in situ of hypopharyngeal aspect (D00.08)

carcinoma in situ of marginal zone (D00.08)

D02.1 Carcinoma in situ of trachea

D02.2 Carcinoma in situ of bronchus and lung

D02.20 Carcinoma in situ of unspecified bronchus and lung

D02.21 Carcinoma in situ of right bronchus and lung

D02.22 Carcinoma in situ of left bronchus and lung

D02.3 Carcinoma in situ of other parts of respiratory system

Carcinoma in situ of accessory sinuses

Carcinoma in situ of middle ear

Carcinoma in situ of nasal cavities

Excludes1: carcinoma in situ of ear (external) (skin) (D04.2-)

carcinoma in situ of nose NOS (D09.8)

carcinoma in situ of skin of nose (D04.3)

D02.4 Carcinoma in situ of respiratory system, unspecified

D03 Melanoma in situ

D03.0 Melanoma in situ of lip [HCC]

D03.1 Melanoma in situ of eyelid, including canthus

D03.10 Melanoma in situ of unspecified eyelid, including canthus

D03.11 Melanoma in situ of right eyelid, including canthus

D03.111 Melanoma in situ of right upper eyelid, including canthus [HCC]

D03.112 Melanoma in situ of right lower eyelid, including canthus [HCC]

D03.12 Melanoma in situ of left eyelid, including canthus

D03.121 Melanoma in situ of left upper eyelid, including canthus [HCC]

D03.122   Melanoma in situ of left lower eyelid, including canthus [HCC]

D03.2   **Melanoma in situ of ear and external auricular canal**

D03.20   Melanoma in situ of unspecified ear and external auricular canal [HCC]

D03.21   Melanoma in situ of right ear and external auricular canal [HCC]

D03.22   Melanoma in situ of left ear and external auricular canal [HCC]

D03.3   **Melanoma in situ of other and unspecified parts of face**

D03.30   Melanoma in situ of unspecified part of face [HCC]

D03.39   Melanoma in situ of other parts of face [HCC]

D03.4   **Melanoma in situ of scalp and neck** [HCC]

D03.5   **Melanoma in situ of trunk**

D03.51   Melanoma in situ of anal skin [HCC]

Melanoma in situ of anal margin

Melanoma in situ of perianal skin

D03.52   Melanoma in situ of breast (skin) (soft tissue) [HCC]

D03.59   Melanoma in situ of other part of trunk [HCC]

D03.6   **Melanoma in situ of upper limb, including shoulder**

D03.60   Melanoma in situ of unspecified upper limb, including shoulder [HCC]

D03.61   Melanoma in situ of right upper limb, including shoulder [HCC]

D03.62   Melanoma in situ of left upper limb, including shoulder [HCC]

D03.7   **Melanoma in situ of lower limb, including hip**

D03.70   Melanoma in situ of unspecified lower limb, including hip [HCC]

D03.71   Melanoma in situ of right lower limb, including hip [HCC]

D03.72   Melanoma in situ of left lower limb, including hip [HCC]

D03.8   **Melanoma in situ of other sites** [HCC]

Melanoma in situ of scrotum

Excludes1: carcinoma in situ of scrotum (D07.61)

D03.9   **Melanoma in situ, unspecified** [HCC]

D04   **Carcinoma in situ of skin**

Excludes1: erythroplasia of Queyrat (penis) NOS (D07.4)

melanoma in situ (D03.-)

D04.0   **Carcinoma in situ of skin of lip**

Excludes 2: carcinoma in situ of vermilion border of lip (D00.01)

D04.1   **Carcinoma in situ of skin of eyelid, including canthus**

D04.10   Carcinoma in situ of skin of unspecified eyelid, including canthus

D04.11   Carcinoma in situ of skin of right eyelid, including canthus

D04.111   Carcinoma in situ of skin of right upper eyelid, including canthus

D04.112   Carcinoma in situ of skin of right lower eyelid, including canthus

D04.12   Carcinoma in situ of skin of left eyelid, including canthus

D04.121   Carcinoma in situ of skin of left upper eyelid, including canthus

D04.122   Carcinoma in situ of skin of left lower eyelid, including canthus

D04.2   **Carcinoma in situ of skin of ear and external auricular canal**

D04.20   Carcinoma in situ of skin of unspecified ear and external auricular canal

D04.21   Carcinoma in situ of skin of right ear and external auricular canal

D04.22   Carcinoma in situ of skin of left ear and external auricular canal

D04.3   **Carcinoma in situ of skin of other and unspecified parts of face**

D04.30   Carcinoma in situ of skin of unspecified part of face

D04.39   Carcinoma in situ of skin of other parts of face

D04.4   **Carcinoma in situ of skin of scalp and neck**

D04.5   **Carcinoma in situ of skin of trunk**

Carcinoma in situ of anal margin

Carcinoma in situ of anal skin

Carcinoma in situ of perianal skin

Carcinoma in situ of skin of breast

Excludes1: carcinoma in situ of anus NOS (D01.3)

carcinoma in situ of scrotum (D07.61)

carcinoma in situ of skin of genital organs (D07.-)

D04.6   **Carcinoma in situ of skin of upper limb, including shoulder**

D04.60   Carcinoma in situ of skin of unspecified upper limb, including shoulder

D04.61   Carcinoma in situ of skin of right upper limb, including shoulder

D04.62   Carcinoma in situ of skin of left upper limb, including shoulder

D04.7   **Carcinoma in situ of skin of lower limb, including hip**

D04.70   Carcinoma in situ of skin of unspecified lower limb, including hip

D04.71   Carcinoma in situ of skin of right lower limb, including hip

D04.72   Carcinoma in situ of skin of left lower limb, including hip

D04.8   **Carcinoma in situ of skin of other sites**

D04.9   **Carcinoma in situ of skin, unspecified**

D05   **Carcinoma in situ of breast**

Excludes1: carcinoma in situ of skin of breast (D04.5)

melanoma in situ of breast (skin) (D03.5)

Paget's disease of breast or nipple (C50.-)

D05.0   **Lobular carcinoma in situ of breast**

D05.00   Lobular carcinoma in situ of unspecified breast

D05.01   Lobular carcinoma in situ of right breast

D05.02   Lobular carcinoma in situ of left breast

D05.1   **Intraductal carcinoma in situ of breast**

D05.10   Intraductal carcinoma in situ of unspecified breast

D05.11   Intraductal carcinoma in situ of right breast

D05.12   Intraductal carcinoma in situ of left breast

D05.8   **Other specified type of carcinoma in situ of breast**

D05.80   Other specified type of carcinoma in situ of unspecified breast

D05.81   Other specified type of carcinoma in situ of right breast

D05.82   Other specified type of carcinoma in situ of left breast

D05.9   **Unspecified type of carcinoma in situ of breast**

D05.90   Unspecified type of carcinoma in situ of unspecified breast

D05.91   Unspecified type of carcinoma in situ of right breast

D05.92   Unspecified type of carcinoma in situ of left breast

D06   Carcinoma in situ of cervix uteri

Includes: cervical adenocarcinoma in situ

cervical intraepithelial glandular neoplasia

cervical intraepithelial neoplasia III [CIN III]

severe dysplasia of cervix uteri

Excludes1: cervical intraepithelial neoplasia II [CIN II] (N87.1)

cytologic evidence of malignancy of cervix without histologic confirmation (R87.614)

high grade squamous intraepithelial lesion (HGSIL) of cervix (R87.613)

melanoma in situ of cervix (D03.5)

moderate cervical dysplasia (N87.1)

D06.0   Carcinoma in situ of endocervix

D06.1   Carcinoma in situ of exocervix

D06.7   Carcinoma in situ of other parts of cervix

D06.9   Carcinoma in situ of cervix, unspecified

D07   Carcinoma in situ of other and unspecified genital organs

Excludes1: melanoma in situ of trunk (D03.5)

D07.0   Carcinoma in situ of endometrium

D07.1   Carcinoma in situ of vulva

Severe dysplasia of vulva

Vulvar intraepithelial neoplasia III [VIN III]

Excludes1: moderate dysplasia of vulva (N90.1)

vulvar intraepithelial neoplasia II [VIN II] (N90.1)

D07.2   Carcinoma in situ of vagina

Severe dysplasia of vagina

Vaginal intraepithelial neoplasia III [VAIN III]

Excludes1: moderate dysplasia of vagina (N89.1)

vaginal intraepithelial neoplasia II [VIN II] (N89.1)

D07.3   Carcinoma in situ of other and unspecified female genital organs

D07.30   Carcinoma in situ of unspecified female genital organs

D07.39   Carcinoma in situ of other female genital organs

D07.4   Carcinoma in situ of penis

Erythroplasia of Queyrat NOS

D07.5   Carcinoma in situ of prostate

Prostatic intraepithelial neoplasia III (PIN III)

Severe dysplasia of prostate

Excludes1: dysplasia (mild) (moderate) of prostate (N42.3-)

prostatic intraepithelial neoplasia II [PIN II] (N42.3-)

D07.6   Carcinoma in situ of other and unspecified male genital organs

D07.60   Carcinoma in situ of unspecified male genital organs

D07.61   Carcinoma in situ of scrotum

D07.69   Carcinoma in situ of other male genital organs

D09   Carcinoma in situ of other and unspecified sites

Excludes1: melanoma in situ (D03.-)

D09.0   Carcinoma in situ of bladder

D09.1   Carcinoma in situ of other and unspecified urinary organs

D09.10   Carcinoma in situ of unspecified urinary organ

D09.19   Carcinoma in situ of other urinary organs

D09.2   Carcinoma in situ of eye

Excludes1: carcinoma in situ of skin of eyelid (D04.1-)

D09.20   Carcinoma in situ of unspecified eye

D09.21   Carcinoma in situ of right eye

D09.22   Carcinoma in situ of left eye

D09.3   Carcinoma in situ of thyroid and other endocrine glands

Excludes1: carcinoma in situ of endocrine pancreas (D01.7)

carcinoma in situ of ovary (D07.39)

carcinoma in situ of testis (D07.69)

D09.8   Carcinoma in situ of other specified sites

D09.9   Carcinoma in situ, unspecified

BENIGN NEOPLASMS, EXCEPT BENIGN NEUROENDOCRINE TUMORS (D10-D36)

Definition: A benign neoplasm is a localized tumor that has a fibrous capsule, limited potential for growth, a regular shape, and cells that are well differentiated. A benign neoplasm does not invade surrounding tissue or metastasize to distant sites. Some kinds of benign neoplasms are adenoma, fibroma, hemangioma, and lipoma.

D10 Benign neoplasm of mouth and pharynx

D10   Benign neoplasm of mouth and pharynx

D10.0   Benign neoplasm of lip

Benign neoplasm of lip (frenulum) (inner aspect) (mucosa) (vermilion border)

Excludes1: benign neoplasm of skin of lip (D22.0, D23.0)

D10.1   Benign neoplasm of tongue

Benign neoplasm of lingual tonsil

D10.2   Benign neoplasm of floor of mouth

D10.3   Benign neoplasm of other and unspecified parts of mouth

D10.30   Benign neoplasm of unspecified part of mouth

D10.39   Benign neoplasm of other parts of mouth

Benign neoplasm of minor salivary gland NOS

Excludes1: benign odontogenic neoplasms (D16.4-D16.5)

benign neoplasm of mucosa of lip (D10.0)

benign neoplasm of nasopharyngeal surface of soft palate (D10.6)

D10.4   Benign neoplasm of tonsil

Benign neoplasm of tonsil (faucial) (palatine)

Excludes1: benign neoplasm of lingual tonsil (D10.1)

benign neoplasm of pharyngeal tonsil (D10.6)

benign neoplasm of tonsillar fossa (D10.5)

benign neoplasm of tonsillar pillars (D10.5)

D10.5   Benign neoplasm of other parts of oropharynx

Benign neoplasm of epiglottis, anterior aspect

Benign neoplasm of tonsillar fossa

Benign neoplasm of tonsillar pillars

Benign neoplasm of vallecula

Excludes1: benign neoplasm of epiglottis NOS (D14.1)

benign neoplasm of epiglottis, suprahyoid portion (D14.1)

D10.6   Benign neoplasm of nasopharynx

Benign neoplasm of pharyngeal tonsil

Benign neoplasm of posterior margin of septum and choanae

D10.7   **Benign neoplasm of hypopharynx**

D10.9   **Benign neoplasm of pharynx, unspecified**

D11   **Benign neoplasm of major salivary glands**

Excludes1: benign neoplasms of specified minor salivary glands which are classified according to their anatomical location

benign neoplasms of minor salivary glands NOS (D10.39)

D11.0   **Benign neoplasm of parotid gland**

D11.7   **Benign neoplasm of other major salivary glands**

Benign neoplasm of sublingual salivary gland

Benign neoplasm of submandibular salivary gland

D11.9   **Benign neoplasm of major salivary gland, unspecified**

D12   **Benign neoplasm of colon, rectum, anus and anal canal**

Excludes1: benign carcinoid tumors of the large intestine, and rectum (D3A.02-)

D12.0   **Benign neoplasm of cecum**

Benign neoplasm of ileocecal valve

D12.1   **Benign neoplasm of appendix**

Excludes1: benign carcinoid tumor of the appendix (D3A.020)

D12.2   **Benign neoplasm of ascending colon**

D12.3   **Benign neoplasm of transverse colon**

Benign neoplasm of hepatic flexure

Benign neoplasm of splenic flexure

D12.4   **Benign neoplasm of descending colon**

D12.5   **Benign neoplasm of sigmoid colon**

D12.6   **Benign neoplasm of colon, unspecified**

Adenomatosis of colon

Benign neoplasm of large intestine NOS

Polyposis (hereditary) of colon

Excludes1: inflammatory polyp of colon (K51.4-)

D12.7   **Benign neoplasm of rectosigmoid junction**

D12.8   **Benign neoplasm of rectum**

Excludes1: benign carcinoid tumor of the rectum (D3A.026)

D12.9   **Benign neoplasm of anus and anal canal**

Benign neoplasm of anus NOS

Excludes1: benign neoplasm of anal margin (D22.5, D23.5)

benign neoplasm of anal skin (D22.5, D23.5)

benign neoplasm of perianal skin (D22.5, D23.5)

D13   **Benign neoplasm of other and ill-defined parts of digestive system**

Excludes1: benign stromal tumors of digestive system (D21.4)

D13.0   **Benign neoplasm of esophagus**

D13.1   **Benign neoplasm of stomach**

Excludes1: benign carcinoid tumor of the stomach (D3A.092)

D13.2   **Benign neoplasm of duodenum**

Excludes1: benign carcinoid tumor of the duodenum (D3A.010)

D13.3   **Benign neoplasm of other and unspecified parts of small intestine**

Excludes1: benign carcinoid tumors of the small intestine (D3A.01-)

benign neoplasm of ileocecal valve (D12.0)

D13.30   **Benign neoplasm of unspecified part of small intestine**

D13.39   **Benign neoplasm of other parts of small intestine**

D13.4   **Benign neoplasm of liver**

Benign neoplasm of intrahepatic bile ducts

D13.5   **Benign neoplasm of extrahepatic bile ducts**

D13.6   **Benign neoplasm of pancreas**

Excludes1: benign neoplasm of endocrine pancreas (D13.7)

D13.7   **Benign neoplasm of endocrine pancreas**

Islet cell tumor Benign neoplasm of islets of Langerhans

Use Additional Code to identify any functional activity.

D13.9   **Benign neoplasm of ill-defined sites within the digestive system**

Benign neoplasm of digestive system NOS

Benign neoplasm of intestine NOS

Benign neoplasm of spleen

D14   **Benign neoplasm of middle ear and respiratory system**

D14.0   **Benign neoplasm of middle ear, nasal cavity and accessory sinuses**

Benign neoplasm of cartilage of nose

Excludes1: benign neoplasm of auricular canal (external) (D22.2-, D23.2-)

benign neoplasm of bone of ear (D16.4)

benign neoplasm of bone of nose (D16.4)

benign neoplasm of cartilage of ear (D21.0)

benign neoplasm of ear (external)(skin) (D22.2-, D23.2-)

benign neoplasm of nose NOS (D36.7)

benign neoplasm of skin of nose (D22.39, D23.39)

benign neoplasm of olfactory bulb (D33.3)

benign neoplasm of posterior margin of septum and choanae (D10.6)

polyp of accessory sinus (J33.8)

polyp of ear (middle) (H74.4)

polyp of nasal (cavity) (J33.-)

D14.1   **Benign neoplasm of larynx**

Adenomatous polyp of larynx

Benign neoplasm of epiglottis (suprahyoid portion)

Excludes1: benign neoplasm of epiglottis, anterior aspect (D10.5)

polyp (nonadenomatous) of vocal cord or larynx (J38.1)

D14.2   **Benign neoplasm of trachea**

D14.3   **Benign neoplasm of bronchus and lung**

Excludes1: benign carcinoid tumor of the bronchus and lung (D3A.090)

D14.30   **Benign neoplasm of unspecified bronchus and lung**

D14.31   **Benign neoplasm of right bronchus and lung**

D14.32   **Benign neoplasm of left bronchus and lung**

D14.4   **Benign neoplasm of respiratory system, unspecified**

D15   **Benign neoplasm of other and unspecified intrathoracic organs**

Excludes1: benign neoplasm of mesothelial tissue (D19.-)

D15.0   **Benign neoplasm of thymus**

Excludes1: benign carcinoid tumor of the thymus (D3A.091)

D15.1   **Benign neoplasm of heart**

Excludes1: benign neoplasm of great vessels (D21.3)

D15.2   Benign neoplasm of mediastinum

D15.7   Benign neoplasm of other specified intrathoracic organs

D15.9   Benign neoplasm of intrathoracic organ, unspecified

D16   Benign neoplasm of bone and articular cartilage

Excludes1: benign neoplasm of connective tissue of ear (D21.0)

benign neoplasm of connective tissue of eyelid (D21.0)

benign neoplasm of connective tissue of larynx (D14.1)

benign neoplasm of connective tissue of nose (D14.0)

benign neoplasm of synovia (D21.-)

D16.0   Benign neoplasm of scapula and long bones of upper limb

     D16.00   Benign neoplasm of scapula and long bones of unspecified upper limb

     D16.01   Benign neoplasm of scapula and long bones of right upper limb

     D16.02   Benign neoplasm of scapula and long bones of left upper limb

D16.1   Benign neoplasm of short bones of upper limb

     D16.10   Benign neoplasm of short bones of unspecified upper limb

     D16.11   Benign neoplasm of short bones of right upper limb

     D16.12   Benign neoplasm of short bones of left upper limb

D16.2   Benign neoplasm of long bones of lower limb

     D16.20   Benign neoplasm of long bones of unspecified lower limb

     D16.21   Benign neoplasm of long bones of right lower limb

     D16.22   Benign neoplasm of long bones of left lower limb

D16.3   Benign neoplasm of short bones of lower limb

     D16.30   Benign neoplasm of short bones of unspecified lower limb

     D16.31   Benign neoplasm of short bones of right lower limb

     D16.32   Benign neoplasm of short bones of left lower limb

D16.4   Benign neoplasm of bones of skull and face

Benign neoplasm of maxilla (superior)

Benign neoplasm of orbital bone

Keratocyst of maxilla

Keratocystic odontogenic tumor of maxilla

Excludes2: benign neoplasm of lower jaw bone (D16.5)

D16.5   Benign neoplasm of lower jaw bone

Keratocyst of mandible

Keratocystic odontogenic tumor of mandible

D16.6   Benign neoplasm of vertebral column

Excludes1: benign neoplasm of sacrum and coccyx (D16.8)

D16.7   Benign neoplasm of ribs, sternum and clavicle

D16.8   Benign neoplasm of pelvic bones, sacrum and coccyx

D16.9   Benign neoplasm of bone and articular cartilage, unspecified

D17   Benign lipomatous neoplasm

D17.0   Benign lipomatous neoplasm of skin and subcutaneous tissue of head, face and neck

D17.1   Benign lipomatous neoplasm of skin and subcutaneous tissue of trunk

D17.2   Benign lipomatous neoplasm of skin and subcutaneous tissue of limb

     D17.20   Benign lipomatous neoplasm of skin and subcutaneous tissue of unspecified limb

     D17.21   Benign lipomatous neoplasm of skin and subcutaneous tissue of right arm

     D17.22   Benign lipomatous neoplasm of skin and subcutaneous tissue of left arm

     D17.23   Benign lipomatous neoplasm of skin and subcutaneous tissue of right leg

     D17.24   Benign lipomatous neoplasm of skin and subcutaneous tissue of left leg

D17.3   Benign lipomatous neoplasm of skin and subcutaneous tissue of other and unspecified sites

     D17.30   Benign lipomatous neoplasm of skin and subcutaneous tissue of unspecified sites

     D17.39   Benign lipomatous neoplasm of skin and subcutaneous tissue of other sites

D17.4   Benign lipomatous neoplasm of intrathoracic organs

D17.5   Benign lipomatous neoplasm of intra-abdominal organs

Excludes1: benign lipomatous neoplasm of peritoneum and retroperitoneum (D17.79)

D17.6   Benign lipomatous neoplasm of spermatic cord

D17.7   Benign lipomatous neoplasm of other sites

     D17.71   Benign lipomatous neoplasm of kidney

     D17.72   Benign lipomatous neoplasm of other genitourinary organ

     D17.79   Benign lipomatous neoplasm of other sites

       Benign lipomatous neoplasm of peritoneum

       Benign lipomatous neoplasm of retroperitoneum

D17.9   Benign lipomatous neoplasm, unspecified

Lipoma NOS

D18   Hemangioma and lymphangioma, any site

Definition: Hemangioma is a benign skin lesion consisting of dense, usually elevated masses of dilated blood vessels. Lymphangioma is a benign neoplasm characterized by lymph vessel proliferation.

Excludes1: benign neoplasm of glomus jugulare (D35.6)

blue or pigmented nevus (D22.-) nevus NOS (D22.-)

vascular nevus (Q82.5)

D18.0   Hemangioma

Angioma NOS

Cavernous nevus

     D18.00   Hemangioma unspecified site

     D18.01   Hemangioma of skin and subcutaneous tissue

     D18.02   Hemangioma of intracranial structures [HCC]

     D18.03   Hemangioma of intra-abdominal structures

     D18.09   Hemangioma of other sites

D18.1   Lymphangioma, any site

D19   Benign neoplasm of mesothelial tissue

D19.0   Benign neoplasm of mesothelial tissue of pleura

D19.1   Benign neoplasm of mesothelial tissue of peritoneum

D19.7   Benign neoplasm of mesothelial tissue of other sites

D19.9   Benign neoplasm of mesothelial tissue, unspecified

Benign mesothelioma NOS

D20   Benign neoplasm of soft tissue of retroperitoneum and peritoneum

Excludes1: benign lipomatous neoplasm of peritoneum and retroperitoneum (D17.79)

benign neoplasm of mesothelial tissue (D19.-)

D20.0   Benign neoplasm of soft tissue of retroperitoneum

D20.1   Benign neoplasm of soft tissue of peritoneum

D21 **Other benign neoplasms of connective and other soft tissue**

Includes: benign neoplasm of blood vessel

benign neoplasm of bursa

benign neoplasm of cartilage

benign neoplasm of fascia

benign neoplasm of fat

benign neoplasm of ligament, except uterine

benign neoplasm of lymphatic channel

benign neoplasm of muscle

benign neoplasm of synovia

benign neoplasm of tendon (sheath)

benign stromal tumors

Excludes1: benign neoplasm of articular cartilage (D16.-)

benign neoplasm of cartilage of larynx (D14.1)

benign neoplasm of cartilage of nose (D14.0)

benign neoplasm of connective tissue of breast (D24.-)

benign neoplasm of peripheral nerves and autonomic nervous system (D36.1-)

benign neoplasm of peritoneum (D20.1)

benign neoplasm of retroperitoneum (D20.0)

benign neoplasm of uterine ligament, any (D28.2)

benign neoplasm of vascular tissue (D18.-)

hemangioma (D18.0-)

lipomatous neoplasm (D17.-)

lymphangioma (D18.1)

D22.2 **Mela**

uterine leiomyoma (D25.-)

D21.0 **Benign neoplasm of connective and other soft tissue of head, face and neck**

Benign neoplasm of connective tissue of ear

Benign neoplasm of connective tissue of eyelid

Excludes1: benign neoplasm of connective tissue of orbit (D31.6-)

D21.1 **Benign neoplasm of connective and other soft tissue of upper limb, including shoulder**

   D21.10 Benign neoplasm of connective and other soft tissue of unspecified upper limb, including shoulder

   D21.11 Benign neoplasm of connective and other soft tissue of right upper limb, including shoulder

   D21.12 Benign neoplasm of connective and other soft tissue of left upper limb, including shoulder

D21.2 **Benign neoplasm of connective and other soft tissue of lower limb, including hip**

   D21.20 Benign neoplasm of connective and other soft tissue of unspecified lower limb, including hip

   D21.21 Benign neoplasm of connective and other soft tissue of right lower limb, including hip

   D21.22 Benign neoplasm of connective and other soft tissue of left lower limb, including hip

D21.3 **Benign neoplasm of connective and other soft tissue of thorax**

Benign neoplasm of axilla

Benign neoplasm of diaphragm

Benign neoplasm of great vessels

Excludes1: benign neoplasm of heart (D15.1)

benign neoplasm of mediastinum (D15.2)

benign neoplasm of thymus (D15.0)

D21.4 **Benign neoplasm of connective and other soft tissue of abdomen**

Benign stromal tumors of abdomen

D21.5 **Benign neoplasm of connective and other soft tissue of pelvis**

Excludes1: benign neoplasm of any uterine ligament (D28.2)

uterine leiomyoma (D25.-)

D21.6 **Benign neoplasm of connective and other soft tissue of trunk, unspecified**

Benign neoplasm of connective and other soft tissue of back NOS

D21.9 **Benign neoplasm of connective and other soft tissue, unspecified**

D22 **Melanocytic nevi**

Includes: atypical nevus

blue hairy pigmented nevus NOS

D22.0 **Melanocytic nevi of lip**

D22.1 **Melanocytic nevi of eyelid, including canthus**

   D22.10 Melanocytic nevi of unspecified eyelid, including canthus

   D22.11 Melanocytic nevi of right eyelid, including canthus

      D22.111 Melanocytic nevi of right upper eyelid, including canthus

      D22.112 Melanocytic nevi of right lower eyelid, including canthus

   D22.12 Melanocytic nevi of left eyelid, including canthus

      D22.121 Melanocytic nevi of left upper eyelid, including canthus

      D22.122 Melanocytic nevi of left lower eyelid, including canthus

   D22.20 Melanocytic nevi of unspecified ear and external auricular canal

   D22.21 Melanocytic nevi of right ear and external auricular canal

   D22.22 Melanocytic nevi of left ear and external auricular canal

D22.3 **Melanocytic nevi of other and unspecified parts of face**

   D22.30 Melanocytic nevi of unspecified part of face

   D22.39 Melanocytic nevi of other parts of face

D22.4 **Melanocytic nevi of scalp and neck**

D22.5 **Melanocytic nevi of trunk**

Melanocytic nevi of anal margin

Melanocytic nevi of anal skin

Melanocytic nevi of perianal skin

Melanocytic nevi of skin of breast

D22.6 **Melanocytic nevi of upper limb, including shoulder**

   D22.60 Melanocytic nevi of unspecified upper limb, including shoulder

   D22.61 Melanocytic nevi of right upper limb, including shoulder

   D22.62 Melanocytic nevi of left upper limb, including shoulder

D22.7 **Melanocytic nevi of lower limb, including hip**

   D22.70 Melanocytic nevi of unspecified lower limb, including hip

   D22.71 Melanocytic nevi of right lower limb, including hip

   D22.72 Melanocytic nevi of left lower limb, including hip

D22.9 Melanocytic nevi, unspecified

D23 Other benign neoplasms of skin

Includes: benign neoplasm of hair follicles

benign neoplasm of sebaceous glands

benign neoplasm of sweat glands

Excludes2: benign lipomatous neoplasms of skin (D17.0-D17.3)

melanocytic nevi (D22.-)

D23.0 Other benign neoplasm of skin of lip

Excludes1: benign neoplasm of vermilion border of lip (D10.0)

D23.1 Other benign neoplasm of skin of eyelid, including canthus

D23.10 Other benign neoplasm of skin of unspecified eyelid, including canthus

D23.11 Other benign neoplasm of skin of right eyelid, including canthus

D23.111 Other benign neoplasm of skin of right upper eyelid, including canthus

D23.112 Other benign neoplasm of skin of right lower eyelid, including canthus

D23.12 Other benign neoplasm of skin of left eyelid, including canthus

D23.121 Other benign neoplasm of skin of left upper eyelid, including canthus

D23.122 Other benign neoplasm of skin of left lower eyelid, including canthus

D23.2 Other benign neoplasm of skin of ear and external auricular canal

D23.20 Other benign neoplasm of skin of unspecified ear and external auricular canal

D23.21 Other benign neoplasm of skin of right ear and external auricular canal

D23.22 Other benign neoplasm of skin of left ear and external auricular canal

D23.3 Other benign neoplasm of skin of other and unspecified parts of face

D23.30 Other benign neoplasm of skin of unspecified part of face

D23.39 Other benign neoplasm of skin of other parts of face

D23.4 Other benign neoplasm of skin of scalp and neck

D23.5 Other benign neoplasm of skin of trunk

Other benign neoplasm of anal margin

Other benign neoplasm of anal skin

Other benign neoplasm of perianal skin

Other benign neoplasm of skin of breast

Excludes1: benign neoplasm of anus NOS (D12.9)

D23.6 Other benign neoplasm of skin of upper limb, including shoulder

D23.60 Other benign neoplasm of skin of unspecified upper limb, including shoulder

D23.61 Other benign neoplasm of skin of right upper limb, including shoulder

D23.62 Other benign neoplasm of skin of left upper limb, including shoulder

D23.7 Other benign neoplasm of skin of lower limb, including hip

D23.70 Other benign neoplasm of skin of unspecified lower limb, including hip

D23.71 Other benign neoplasm of skin of right lower limb, including hip

D23.72 Other benign neoplasm of skin of left lower limb, including hip

D23.9 Other benign neoplasm of skin, unspecified

D24 Benign neoplasm of breast

Includes: benign neoplasm of connective tissue of breast

benign neoplasm of soft parts of breast

fibroadenoma of breast

Excludes2: adenofibrosis of breast (N60.2)

benign cyst of breast (N60.-)

benign mammary dysplasia (N60.-)

benign neoplasm of skin of breast (D22.5, D23.5)

fibrocystic disease of breast (N60.-)

D24.1 Benign neoplasm of right breast

D24.2 Benign neoplasm of left breast

D24.9 Benign neoplasm of unspecified breast

D25 Leiomyoma of uterus

Includes: uterine fibroid

uterine fibromyoma

uterine myoma

D25.0 Submucous leiomyoma of uterus

D25.1 Intramural leiomyoma of uterus

Interstitial leiomyoma of uterus

D25.2 Subserosal leiomyoma of uterus

Subperitoneal leiomyoma of uterus

D25.9 Leiomyoma of uterus, unspecified

D26 Other benign neoplasms of uterus

D26.0 Other benign neoplasm of cervix uteri

D26.1 Other benign neoplasm of corpus uteri

D26.7 Other benign neoplasm of other parts of uterus

D26.9 Other benign neoplasm of uterus, unspecified

D27 Benign neoplasm of ovary

Use Additional Code to identify any functional activity.

Excludes2: corpus albicans cyst (N83.2-)

corpus luteum cyst (N83.1-)

endometrial cyst (N80.1)

follicular (atretic) cyst (N83.0-)

graafian follicle cyst (N83.0-)

ovarian cyst NEC (N83.2-)

ovarian retention cyst (N83.2-)

D27.0 Benign neoplasm of right ovary

D27.1 Benign neoplasm of left ovary

D27.9 Benign neoplasm of unspecified ovary

D28 Benign neoplasm of other and unspecified female genital organs

Includes: adenomatous polyp

benign neoplasm of skin of female genital organs

benign teratoma

Excludes1: epoophoron cyst (Q50.5)

fimbrial cyst (Q50.4)

Gartner's duct cyst (Q52.4)

parovarian cyst (Q50.5)

D28.0 Benign neoplasm of vulva

D28.1 Benign neoplasm of vagina

D28.2 Benign neoplasm of uterine tubes and ligaments

Benign neoplasm of fallopian tube

Benign neoplasm of uterine ligament (broad) (round)

D28.7 Benign neoplasm of other specified female genital organs

D28.9   Benign neoplasm of female genital organ, unspecified

D29   Benign neoplasm of male genital organs

    Includes: benign neoplasm of skin of male genital organs

    D29.0   Benign neoplasm of penis

    D29.1   Benign neoplasm of prostate

      Excludes1: enlarged prostate (N40.-)

    D29.2   Benign neoplasm of testis

      Use Additional Code to identify any functional activity.

      D29.20   Benign neoplasm of unspecified testis

      D29.21   Benign neoplasm of right testis

      D29.22   Benign neoplasm of left testis

    D29.3   Benign neoplasm of epididymis

      D29.30   Benign neoplasm of unspecified epididymis

      D29.31   Benign neoplasm of right epididymis

      D29.32   Benign neoplasm of left epididymis

    D29.4   Benign neoplasm of scrotum

      Benign neoplasm of skin of scrotum

    D29.8   Benign neoplasm of other specified male genital organs

      Benign neoplasm of seminal vesicle

      Benign neoplasm of spermatic cord

      Benign neoplasm of tunica vaginalis

    D29.9   Benign neoplasm of male genital organ, unspecified

D30   Benign neoplasm of urinary organs

    D30.0   Benign neoplasm of kidney

      Excludes1: benign carcinoid tumor of the kidney (D3A.093)

        benign neoplasm of renal calyces (D30.1-)

        benign neoplasm of renal pelvis (D30.1-)

      D30.00   Benign neoplasm of unspecified kidney

      D30.01   Benign neoplasm of right kidney

      D30.02   Benign neoplasm of left kidney

    D30.1   Benign neoplasm of renal pelvis

      D30.10   Benign neoplasm of unspecified renal pelvis

      D30.11   Benign neoplasm of right renal pelvis

      D30.12   Benign neoplasm of left renal pelvis

    D30.2   Benign neoplasm of ureter

      Excludes1: benign neoplasm of ureteric orifice of bladder (D30.3)

      D30.20   Benign neoplasm of unspecified ureter

      D30.21   Benign neoplasm of right ureter

      D30.22   Benign neoplasm of left ureter

    D30.3   Benign neoplasm of bladder

      Benign neoplasm of ureteric orifice of bladder

      Benign neoplasm of urethral orifice of bladder

    D30.4   Benign neoplasm of urethra

      Excludes1: benign neoplasm of urethral orifice of bladder (D30.3)

    D30.8   Benign neoplasm of other specified urinary organs

      Benign neoplasm of paraurethral glands

    D30.9   Benign neoplasm of urinary organ, unspecified

      Benign neoplasm of urinary system NOS

D31   Benign neoplasm of eye and adnexa

    Excludes1: benign neoplasm of connective tissue of eyelid (D21.0)

      benign neoplasm of optic nerve (D33.3)

      benign neoplasm of skin of eyelid (D22.1-, D23.1-)

    D31.0   Benign neoplasm of conjunctiva

      D31.00   Benign neoplasm of unspecified conjunctiva

      D31.01   Benign neoplasm of right conjunctiva

      D31.02   Benign neoplasm of left conjunctiva

    D31.1   Benign neoplasm of cornea

      D31.10   Benign neoplasm of unspecified cornea

      D31.11   Benign neoplasm of right cornea

      D31.12   Benign neoplasm of left cornea

    D31.2   Benign neoplasm of retina

      Excludes1: dark area on retina (D49.81)

        hemangioma of retina (D49.81)

        neoplasm of unspecified behavior of retina and choroid (D49.81)

        retinal freckle (D49.81)

      D31.20   Benign neoplasm of unspecified retina

      D31.21   Benign neoplasm of right retina

      D31.22   Benign neoplasm of left retina

    D31.3   Benign neoplasm of choroid

      D31.30   Benign neoplasm of unspecified choroid

      D31.31   Benign neoplasm of right choroid

      D31.32   Benign neoplasm of left choroid

    D31.4   Benign neoplasm of ciliary body

      D31.40   Benign neoplasm of unspecified ciliary body

      D31.41   Benign neoplasm of right ciliary body

      D31.42   Benign neoplasm of left ciliary body

    D31.5   Benign neoplasm of lacrimal gland and duct

      Benign neoplasm of lacrimal sac

      Benign neoplasm of nasolacrimal duct

      D31.50   Benign neoplasm of unspecified lacrimal gland and duct

      D31.51   Benign neoplasm of right lacrimal gland and duct

      D31.52   Benign neoplasm of left lacrimal gland and duct

    D31.6   Benign neoplasm of unspecified site of orbit

      Benign neoplasm of connective tissue of orbit

      Benign neoplasm of extraocular muscle

      Benign neoplasm of peripheral nerves of orbit

      Benign neoplasm of retrobulbar tissue

      Benign neoplasm of retro-ocular tissue

      Excludes1: benign neoplasm of orbital bone (D16.4)

      D31.60   Benign neoplasm of unspecified site of unspecified orbit

      D31.61   Benign neoplasm of unspecified site of right orbit

      D31.62   Benign neoplasm of unspecified site of left orbit

    D31.9   Benign neoplasm of unspecified part of eye

      Benign neoplasm of eyeball

      D31.90   Benign neoplasm of unspecified part of unspecified eye

      D31.91   Benign neoplasm of unspecified part of right eye

      D31.92   Benign neoplasm of unspecified part of left eye

D32   Benign neoplasm of meninges

    D32.0   Benign neoplasm of cerebral meninges [HCC]

    D32.1   Benign neoplasm of spinal meninges [HCC]

    D32.9   Benign neoplasm of meninges, unspecified [HCC]

      Meningioma NOS

D33   Benign neoplasm of brain and other parts of central nervous system

    Excludes1: angioma (D18.0-)

● New code   ▲ Revised code   **Excludes1:** Not coded here   **Excludes2:** Not included here   ⊗ Placeholder required   ⑦ 7th digit required

benign neoplasm of meninges (D32.-)

benign neoplasm of peripheral nerves and autonomic nervous system (D36.1-)

hemangioma (D18.0-)

neurofibromatosis (Q85.0-)

retro-ocular benign neoplasm (D31.6-)

D33.0 **Benign neoplasm of brain, supratentorial** [HCC]

Benign neoplasm of cerebral ventricle

Benign neoplasm of cerebrum

Benign neoplasm of frontal lobe

Benign neoplasm of occipital lobe

Benign neoplasm of parietal lobe

Benign neoplasm of temporal lobe

Excludes1: benign neoplasm of fourth ventricle (D33.1)

D33.1 **Benign neoplasm of brain, infratentorial** [HCC]

Benign neoplasm of brain stem

Benign neoplasm of cerebellum

Benign neoplasm of fourth ventricle

D33.2 **Benign neoplasm of brain, unspecified** [HCC]

D33.3 **Benign neoplasm of cranial nerves** [HCC]

Benign neoplasm of olfactory bulb

D33.4 **Benign neoplasm of spinal cord** [HCC]

D33.7 **Benign neoplasm of other specified parts of central nervous system** [HCC]

D33.9 **Benign neoplasm of central nervous system, unspecified** [HCC]

Benign neoplasm of nervous system (central) NOS

D34 **Benign neoplasm of thyroid gland**

Use Additional Code to identify any functional activity

D35 **Benign neoplasm of other and unspecified endocrine glands**

Use Additional Code to identify any functional activity

Excludes1: benign neoplasm of endocrine pancreas (D13.7)

benign neoplasm of ovary (D27.-)

benign neoplasm of testis (D29.2.-)

benign neoplasm of thymus (D15.0)

D35.0 **Benign neoplasm of adrenal gland**

D35.00 **Benign neoplasm of unspecified adrenal gland**

D35.01 **Benign neoplasm of right adrenal gland**

D35.02 **Benign neoplasm of left adrenal gland**

D35.1 **Benign neoplasm of parathyroid gland**

D35.2 **Benign neoplasm of pituitary gland** [HCC]

D35.3 **Benign neoplasm of craniopharyngeal duct** [HCC]

D35.4 **Benign neoplasm of pineal gland** [HCC]

D35.5 **Benign neoplasm of carotid body**

D35.6 **Benign neoplasm of aortic body and other paraganglia**

Benign tumor of glomus jugulare

D35.7 **Benign neoplasm of other specified endocrine glands**

D35.9 **Benign neoplasm of endocrine gland, unspecified**

Benign neoplasm of unspecified endocrine gland

D36 **Benign neoplasm of other and unspecified sites**

D36.0 **Benign neoplasm of lymph nodes**

Excludes1: lymphangioma (D18.1)

D36.1 **Benign neoplasm of peripheral nerves and autonomic nervous system**

Excludes1: benign neoplasm of peripheral nerves of orbit (D31.6-)

neurofibromatosis (Q85.0-)

D36.10 **Benign neoplasm of peripheral nerves and autonomic nervous system, unspecified**

D36.11 **Benign neoplasm of peripheral nerves and autonomic nervous system of face, head, and neck**

D36.12 **Benign neoplasm of peripheral nerves and autonomic nervous system, upper limb, including shoulder**

D36.13 **Benign neoplasm of peripheral nerves and autonomic nervous system of lower limb, including hip**

D36.14 **Benign neoplasm of peripheral nerves and autonomic nervous system of thorax**

D36.15 **Benign neoplasm of peripheral nerves and autonomic nervous system of abdomen**

D36.16 **Benign neoplasm of peripheral nerves and autonomic nervous system of pelvis**

D36.17 **Benign neoplasm of peripheral nerves and autonomic nervous system of trunk, unspecified**

D36.7 **Benign neoplasm of other specified sites**

Benign neoplasm of back NOS

Benign neoplasm of nose NOS

D36.9 **Benign neoplasm, unspecified site**

BENIGN NEUROENDOCRINE TUMORS (D3A)

Definition: Neuroendocrine tumor is a tumor derived from cells that release a hormone in response to a signal from the nervous system. Examples of neuroendocrine tumors include carcinoid tumors islet cell tumors, medullary thyroid carcinoma, and pheochromocytoma.

D3A **Benign neuroendocrine tumors**

Code also any associated multiple endocrine neoplasia [MEN] syndromes (E31.2-)

Use Additional Code to identify any associated endocrine syndrome, such as:

carcinoid syndrome (E34.0)

Excludes2: benign pancreatic islet cell tumors (D13.7)

D3A.0 **Benign carcinoid tumors**

D3A.00 **Benign carcinoid tumor of unspecified site**

Carcinoid tumor NOS

D3A.01 **Benign carcinoid tumors of the small intestine**

D3A.010 **Benign carcinoid tumor of the duodenum**

D3A.011 **Benign carcinoid tumor of the jejunum**

D3A.012 **Benign carcinoid tumor of the ileum**

D3A.019 **Benign carcinoid tumor of the small intestine, unspecified portion**

D3A.020 **Benign carcinoid tumor of the appendix**

D3A.021 **Benign carcinoid tumor of the cecum**

D3A.022 **Benign carcinoid tumor of the ascending colon**

D3A.023 **Benign carcinoid tumor of the transverse colon**

D3A.024 **Benign carcinoid tumor of the descending colon**

D3A.025 **Benign carcinoid tumor of the sigmoid colon**

D3A.026 **Benign carcinoid tumor of the rectum**

D3A.029 **Benign carcinoid tumor of the large intestine, unspecified portion**

Benign carcinoid tumor of the colon NOS

D3A.09   Benign carcinoid tumors of other sites

D3A.090   Benign carcinoid tumor of the bronchus and lung

D3A.091   Benign carcinoid tumor of the thymus

D3A.092   Benign carcinoid tumor of the stomach

D3A.093   Benign carcinoid tumor of the kidney

D3A.094   Benign carcinoid tumor of the foregut, unspecified

D3A.095   Benign carcinoid tumor of the midgut, unspecified

D3A.096   Benign carcinoid tumor of the hindgut, unspecified

D3A.098   Benign carcinoid tumors of other sites

D3A.8   Other benign neuroendocrine tumors

Neuroendocrine tumor NOS

NEOPLASMS OF UNCERTAIN BEHAVIOR, POLYCYTHEMIA VERA AND MYELODYSPLASTIC SYNDROMES (D37-D48)

Note: Categories D37-D44, and D48 classify by site neoplasms of uncertain behavior, i.e., histologic confirmation whether the neoplasm is malignant or benign cannot be made.

Excludes1: neoplasms of unspecified behavior (D49.-)

D37   Neoplasm of uncertain behavior of oral cavity and digestive organs

Excludes1: stromal tumors of uncertain behavior of digestive system (D48.1)

D37.0   Neoplasm of uncertain behavior of lip, oral cavity and pharynx

Excludes1: neoplasm of uncertain behavior of aryepiglottic fold or interarytenoid fold, laryngeal aspect (D38.0)

neoplasm of uncertain behavior of epiglottis NOS (D38.0)

neoplasm of uncertain behavior of skin of lip (D48.5)

neoplasm of uncertain behavior of suprahyoid portion of epiglottis (D38.0)

D37.01   Neoplasm of uncertain behavior of lip

Neoplasm of uncertain behavior of vermilion border of lip

D37.02   Neoplasm of uncertain behavior of tongue

D37.03   Neoplasm of uncertain behavior of the major salivary glands

D37.030   Neoplasm of uncertain behavior of the parotid salivary glands

D37.031   Neoplasm of uncertain behavior of the sublingual salivary glands

D37.032   Neoplasm of uncertain behavior of the submandibular salivary glands

D37.039   Neoplasm of uncertain behavior of the major salivary glands, unspecified

D37.04   Neoplasm of uncertain behavior of the minor salivary glands

Neoplasm of uncertain behavior of submucosal salivary glands of lip

Neoplasm of uncertain behavior of submucosal salivary glands of cheek

Neoplasm of uncertain behavior of submucosal salivary glands of hard palate

Neoplasm of uncertain behavior of submucosal salivary glands of soft palate

D37.05   Neoplasm of uncertain behavior of pharynx

Neoplasm of uncertain behavior of aryepiglottic fold of pharynx NOS

Neoplasm of uncertain behavior of hypopharyngeal aspect of aryepiglottic fold of pharynx

Neoplasm of uncertain behavior of marginal zone of aryepiglottic fold of pharynx

D37.09   Neoplasm of uncertain behavior of other specified sites of the oral cavity

D37.1   Neoplasm of uncertain behavior of stomach

D37.2   Neoplasm of uncertain behavior of small intestine

D37.3   Neoplasm of uncertain behavior of appendix

D37.4   Neoplasm of uncertain behavior of colon

D37.5   Neoplasm of uncertain behavior of rectum

Neoplasm of uncertain behavior of rectosigmoid junction

D37.6   Neoplasm of uncertain behavior of liver, gallbladder and bile ducts

Neoplasm of uncertain behavior of ampulla of Vater

D37.8   Neoplasm of uncertain behavior of other specified digestive organs

Neoplasm of uncertain behavior of anal canal

Neoplasm of uncertain behavior of anal sphincter

Neoplasm of uncertain behavior of anus NOS

Neoplasm of uncertain behavior of esophagus

Neoplasm of uncertain behavior of intestine NOS

Neoplasm of uncertain behavior of pancreas

Excludes1: neoplasm of uncertain behavior of anal margin (D48.5)

neoplasm of uncertain behavior of anal skin (D48.5)

neoplasm of uncertain behavior of perianal skin (D48.5)

D37.9   Neoplasm of uncertain behavior of digestive organ, unspecified

D38   Neoplasm of uncertain behavior of middle ear and respiratory and intrathoracic organs

Excludes1: neoplasm of uncertain behavior of heart (D48.7)

D38.0   Neoplasm of uncertain behavior of larynx

Neoplasm of uncertain behavior of aryepiglottic fold or interarytenoid fold, laryngeal aspect

Neoplasm of uncertain behavior of epiglottis (suprahyoid portion)

Excludes1: neoplasm of uncertain behavior of aryepiglottic fold or interarytenoid fold NOS (D37.05)

neoplasm of uncertain behavior of hypopharyngeal aspect of aryepiglottic fold (D37.05)

neoplasm of uncertain behavior of marginal zone of aryepiglottic fold (D37.05)

D38.1   Neoplasm of uncertain behavior of trachea, bronchus and lung

D38.2   Neoplasm of uncertain behavior of pleura

D38.3   Neoplasm of uncertain behavior of mediastinum

D38.4   Neoplasm of uncertain behavior of thymus

D38.5   Neoplasm of uncertain behavior of other respiratory organs

Neoplasm of uncertain behavior of accessory sinuses

Neoplasm of uncertain behavior of cartilage of nose

● New code   ▲ Revised code   **Excludes1:** Not coded here   **Excludes2:** Not included here   ⊗ Placeholder required   ⑦ 7th digit required

Neoplasm of uncertain behavior of middle ear

Neoplasm of uncertain behavior of nasal cavities

Excludes1: neoplasm of uncertain behavior of ear (external) (skin) (D48.5)

neoplasm of uncertain behavior of nose NOS (D48.7)

neoplasm of uncertain behavior of skin of nose (D48.5)

D38.6 **Neoplasm of uncertain behavior of respiratory organ, unspecified**

D39 **Neoplasm of uncertain behavior of female genital organs**

D39.0 **Neoplasm of uncertain behavior of uterus**

D39.1 **Neoplasm of uncertain behavior of ovary**

Use Additional Code to identify any functional activity.

D39.10 **Neoplasm of uncertain behavior of unspecified ovary**

D39.11 **Neoplasm of uncertain behavior of right ovary**

D39.12 **Neoplasm of uncertain behavior of left ovary**

D39.2 **Neoplasm of uncertain behavior of placenta**

Chorioadenoma destruens

Invasive hydatidiform mole

Malignant hydatidiform mole

Excludes1: hydatidiform mole NOS (O01.9)

D39.8 **Neoplasm of uncertain behavior of other specified female genital organs**

Neoplasm of uncertain behavior of skin of female genital organs

D39.9 **Neoplasm of uncertain behavior of female genital organ, unspecified**

D40 **Neoplasm of uncertain behavior of male genital organs**

D40.0 **Neoplasm of uncertain behavior of prostate**

D40.1 **Neoplasm of uncertain behavior of testis**

D40.10 **Neoplasm of uncertain behavior of unspecified testis**

D40.11 **Neoplasm of uncertain behavior of right testis**

D40.12 **Neoplasm of uncertain behavior of left testis**

D40.8 **Neoplasm of uncertain behavior of other specified male genital organs**

Neoplasm of uncertain behavior of skin of male genital organs

D40.9 **Neoplasm of uncertain behavior of male genital organ, unspecified**

D41 **Neoplasm of uncertain behavior of urinary organs**

D41.0 **Neoplasm of uncertain behavior of kidney**

Excludes1: neoplasm of uncertain behavior of renal pelvis (D41.1-)

D41.00 **Neoplasm of uncertain behavior of unspecified kidney**

D41.01 **Neoplasm of uncertain behavior of right kidney**

D41.02 **Neoplasm of uncertain behavior of left kidney**

D41.1 **Neoplasm of uncertain behavior of renal pelvis**

D41.10 **Neoplasm of uncertain behavior of unspecified renal pelvis**

D41.11 **Neoplasm of uncertain behavior of right renal pelvis**

D41.12 **Neoplasm of uncertain behavior of left renal pelvis**

D41.2 **Neoplasm of uncertain behavior of ureter**

D41.20 **Neoplasm of uncertain behavior of unspecified ureter**

D41.21 **Neoplasm of uncertain behavior of right ureter**

D41.22 **Neoplasm of uncertain behavior of left ureter**

D41.3 **Neoplasm of uncertain behavior of urethra**

D41.4 **Neoplasm of uncertain behavior of bladder**

D41.8 **Neoplasm of uncertain behavior of other specified urinary organs**

D41.9 **Neoplasm of uncertain behavior of unspecified urinary organ**

D42 **Neoplasm of uncertain behavior of meninges**

D42.0 **Neoplasm of uncertain behavior of cerebral meninges** [HCC]

D42.1 **Neoplasm of uncertain behavior of spinal meninges** [HCC]

D42.9 **Neoplasm of uncertain behavior of meninges, unspecified** [HCC]

D43 **Neoplasm of uncertain behavior of brain and central nervous system**

Excludes1: neoplasm of uncertain behavior of peripheral nerves and autonomic nervous system (D48.2)

D43.0 **Neoplasm of uncertain behavior of brain, supratentorial** [HCC]

Neoplasm of uncertain behavior of cerebral ventricle

Neoplasm of uncertain behavior of cerebrum

Neoplasm of uncertain behavior of frontal lobe

Neoplasm of uncertain behavior of occipital lobe

Neoplasm of uncertain behavior of parietal lobe

Neoplasm of uncertain behavior of temporal lobe

Excludes1: neoplasm of uncertain behavior of fourth ventricle (D43.1)

D43.1 **Neoplasm of uncertain behavior of brain, infratentorial** [HCC]

Neoplasm of uncertain behavior of brain stem Neoplasm of uncertain behavior of cerebellum Neoplasm of uncertain behavior of fourth ventricle

D43.2 **Neoplasm of uncertain behavior of brain, unspecified** [HCC]

D43.3 **Neoplasm of uncertain behavior of cranial nerves** [HCC]

D43.4 **Neoplasm of uncertain behavior of spinal cord** [HCC]

D43.8 **Neoplasm of uncertain behavior of other specified parts of central nervous system** [HCC]

D43.9 **Neoplasm of uncertain behavior of central nervous system, unspecified** [HCC]

Neoplasm of uncertain behavior of nervous system (central) NOS

D44 **Neoplasm of uncertain behavior of endocrine glands**

Excludes1: multiple endocrine adenomatosis (E31.2-)

multiple endocrine neoplasia (E31.2-)

neoplasm of uncertain behavior of endocrine pancreas (D37.8)

neoplasm of uncertain behavior of ovary (D39.1-)

neoplasm of uncertain behavior of testis (D40.1-)

neoplasm of uncertain behavior of thymus (D38.4)

D44.0 **Neoplasm of uncertain behavior of thyroid gland**

D44.1 **Neoplasm of uncertain behavior of adrenal gland**

Use Additional Code to identify any functional activity.

D44.10 **Neoplasm of uncertain behavior of unspecified adrenal gland**

D44.11 **Neoplasm of uncertain behavior of right adrenal gland**

D44.12 **Neoplasm of uncertain behavior of left adrenal gland**

D44.2 **Neoplasm of uncertain behavior of parathyroid gland**

D44.3 **Neoplasm of uncertain behavior of pituitary gland** [HCC]

Use Additional Code to identify any functional activity.

D44.4 **Neoplasm of uncertain behavior of craniopharyngeal duct** [HCC]

D44.5 **Neoplasm of uncertain behavior of pineal gland** [HCC]

D44.6 **Neoplasm of uncertain behavior of carotid body** [HCC]

D44.7 **Neoplasm of uncertain behavior of aortic body and other paraganglia** [HCC]

D44.9 **Neoplasm of uncertain behavior of unspecified endocrine gland**

D45 **Polycythemia vera**

Excludes1: familial polycythemia (D75.0)

secondary polycythemia (D75.1)

D46 **Myelodysplastic syndromes**

Use Additional Code for adverse effect, if applicable, to identify drug (T36-T50 with fifth or sixth character 5)

Excludes2: drug-induced aplastic anemia (D61.1)

D46.0 **Refractory anemia without ring sideroblasts, so stated** [HCC]

Refractory anemia without sideroblasts, without excess of blasts

D46.1 **Refractory anemia with ring sideroblasts** [HCC]

RARS

D46.2 **Refractory anemia with excess of blasts [RAEB]**

D46.20 **Refractory anemia with excess of blasts, unspecified** [HCC]

RAEB NOS

D46.21 **Refractory anemia with excess of blasts 1** [HCC]

RAEB 1

D46.22 **Refractory anemia with excess of blasts 2** [HCC]

RAEB 2

D46.4 **Refractory anemia, unspecified** [HCC]

D46.9 **Myelodysplastic syndrome, unspecified** [HCC]

Myelodysplasia NOS

D46.A **Refractory cytopenia with multilineage dysplasia** [HCC]

D46.B **Refractory cytopenia with multilineage dysplasia and ring sideroblasts** [HCC]

RCMD RS

D46.C **Myelodysplastic syndrome with isolated del(5q) chromosomal abnormality** [HCC]

Myelodysplastic syndrome with 5q deletion 5q minus syndrome NOS

D46.Z **Other myelodysplastic syndromes** [HCC]

Excludes1: chronic myelomonocytic leukemia (C93.1-)

D47 **Other neoplasms of uncertain behavior of lymphoid, hematopoietic and related tissue**

D47.0 **Mast cell neoplasms of uncertain behavior**

Excludes1: congenital cutaneous mastocytosis (Q82.2)

histiocytic neoplasms of uncertain behavior (D47.Z9)

malignant mast cell neoplasm (C96.2-)

D47.01 **Cutaneous mastocytosis**

Diffuse cutaneous mastocytosis

Maculopapular cutaneous mastocytosis

Solitary mastocytoma

Telangiectasia macularis eruptiva perstans

Urticaria pigmentosa

Excludes1: congenital (diffuse) (maculopapular) cutaneous mastocytosis (Q82.2)

congenital urticaria pigmentosa (Q82.2)

extracutaneous mastocytoma (D47.09)

D47.02 **Systemic mastocytosis**

Indolent systemic mastocytosis

Isolated bone marrow mastocytosis

Smoldering systemic mastocytosis

Systemic mastocytosis, with an associated hematological non-mast cell lineage disease (SM-AHNMD)

Code also, if applicable, any associated hematological non-mast cell lineage disease, such as:

acute myeloid leukemia (C92.6-, C92.A-)

chronic myelomonocytic leukemia (C93.1-)

essential thrombocytosis (D47.3)

hypereosinophilic syndrome (D72.1)

myelodysplastic syndrome (D46.9)

myeloproliferative syndrome (D47.1)

non-Hodgkin lymphoma (C82-C85)

plasma cell myeloma (C90.0-)

polycythemia vera (D45)

Excludes1: aggressive systemic mastocytosis (C96.21)

mast cell leukemia (C94.3-)

D47.09 **Other mast cell neoplasms of uncertain behavior**

Extracutaneous mastocytoma

Mast cell tumor NOS

Mastocytoma NOS

Mastocytosis NOS Monoclonal gammopathy of undetermined significance [MGUS]

D47.3 **Essential (hemorrhagic) thrombocythemia**

Essential thrombocytosis

Idiopathic hemorrhagic thrombocythemia

D47.4 **Osteomyelofibrosis**

Chronic idiopathic myelofibrosis

Myelofibrosis (idiopathic) (with myeloid metaplasia)

Myelosclerosis (megakaryocytic) with myeloid metaplasia

Secondary myelofibrosis in myeloproliferative disease

Excludes1: acute myelofibrosis (C94.4-)

D47.1 **Chronic myeloproliferative disease** [HCC]

Chronic neutrophilic leukemia

Myeloproliferative disease, unspecified

Excludes1: atypical chronic myeloid leukemia BCR/ABL-negative (C92.2-)

chronic myeloid leukemia BCR/ABL-positive (C92.1-)

myelofibrosis NOS (D75.81)

myelophthisic anemia (D61.82)

myelophthisis (D61.82)

secondary myelofibrosis NOS (D75.81)

D47.2 **Monoclonal gammopathy**

D47.3 **Essential (hemorrhagic) thrombocythemia** [HCC]

Essential thrombocytosis

Idiopathic hemorrhagic thrombocythemia

Primary thrombocytosis

Excludes2: reactive thrombocytosis (D75.838)

secondary thrombocytosis (D75.838)

thrombocythemia NOS (D75.839)

thrombocytosis NOS (D75.839)

● New code ▲ Revised code Excludes1: Not coded here Excludes2: Not included here ⊗ Placeholder required ⑦7th digit required

D47.4 **Osteomyelofibrosis** [HCC]

Chronic idiopathic myelofibrosis

Myelofibrosis (idiopathic) (with myeloid metaplasia)

Myelosclerosis (megakaryocytic) with myeloid metaplasia

Secondary myelofibrosis in myeloproliferative disease

Excludes1: acute myelofibrosis (C94.4-)

D47.9 **Neoplasm of uncertain behavior of lymphoid, hematopoietic and related tissue, unspecified** [HCC]

Lymphoproliferative disease NOS

D47.Z **Other specified neoplasms of uncertain behavior of lymphoid, hematopoietic and related tissue**

D47.Z1 **Post-transplant lymphoproliferative disorder (PTLD)** [HCC]

Code first complications of transplanted organs and tissue (T86.-)

D47.Z2 **Castleman disease** [HCC]

Code also, if applicable, human herpesvirus 8 infection (B10.89)

Excludes2: Kaposi's sarcoma (C46.-)

D47.Z9 **Other specified neoplasms of uncertain behavior of lymphoid, hematopoietic and related tissue** [HCC]

Histiocytic tumors of uncertain behavior

D48 **Neoplasm of uncertain behavior of other and unspecified sites**

Excludes1: neurofibromatosis (nonmalignant) (Q85.0-)

D48.0 **Neoplasm of uncertain behavior of bone and articular cartilage**

Excludes1: neoplasm of uncertain behavior of cartilage of ear (D48.1)

neoplasm of uncertain behavior of cartilage of larynx (D38.0)

neoplasm of uncertain behavior of cartilage of nose (D38.5)

neoplasm of uncertain behavior of connective tissue of eyelid (D48.1)

neoplasm of uncertain behavior of synovia (D48.1)

D48.1 **Neoplasm of uncertain behavior of connective and other soft tissue**

Neoplasm of uncertain behavior of connective tissue of ear

Neoplasm of uncertain behavior of connective tissue of eyelid

Stromal tumors of uncertain behavior of digestive system

Excludes1: neoplasm of uncertain behavior of articular cartilage (D48.0)

neoplasm of uncertain behavior of cartilage of larynx (D38.0)

neoplasm of uncertain behavior of cartilage of nose (D38.5)

neoplasm of uncertain behavior of connective tissue of breast (D48.6-)

D48.2 **Neoplasm of uncertain behavior of peripheral nerves and autonomic nervous system**

Excludes1: neoplasm of uncertain behavior of peripheral nerves of orbit (D48.7)

D48.3 **Neoplasm of uncertain behavior of retroperitoneum**

D48.4 **Neoplasm of uncertain behavior of peritoneum**

D48.5 **Neoplasm of uncertain behavior of skin**

Neoplasm of uncertain behavior of anal margin

Neoplasm of uncertain behavior of anal skin

Neoplasm of uncertain behavior of perianal skin

Neoplasm of uncertain behavior of skin of breast

Excludes1: neoplasm of uncertain behavior of anus NOS (D37.8)

neoplasm of uncertain behavior of skin of genital organs (D39.8, D40.8)

neoplasm of uncertain behavior of vermilion border of lip (D37.0)

D48.6 **Neoplasm of uncertain behavior of breast**

Neoplasm of uncertain behavior of connective tissue of breast

Cystosarcoma phyllodes

Excludes1: neoplasm of uncertain behavior of skin of breast (D48.5)

D48.60 **Neoplasm of uncertain behavior of unspecified breast**

D48.61 **Neoplasm of uncertain behavior of right breast**

D48.62 **Neoplasm of uncertain behavior of left breast**

D48.7 **Neoplasm of uncertain behavior of other specified sites**

Neoplasm of uncertain behavior of eye Neoplasm of uncertain behavior of heart

Neoplasm of uncertain behavior of peripheral nerves of orbit

Excludes1: neoplasm of uncertain behavior of connective tissue (D48.1)

neoplasm of uncertain behavior of skin of eyelid (D48.5)

D48.9 **Neoplasm of uncertain behavior, unspecified**

NEOPLASMS OF UNSPECIFIED BEHAVIOR (D49)

D49 **Neoplasms of unspecified behavior Note:**

Category D49 classifies by site neoplasms of unspecified morphology and behavior. The term 'mass', unless otherwise stated, is not to be regarded as a neoplastic growth.

Includes: 'growth' NOS

neoplasm NOS

new growth NOS

tumor NOS

Excludes1: neoplasms of uncertain behavior (D37-D44, D48)

D49.0 **Neoplasm of unspecified behavior of digestive system**

Excludes1: neoplasm of unspecified behavior of margin of anus (D49.2)

neoplasm of unspecified behavior of perianal skin (D49.2)

neoplasm of unspecified behavior of skin of anus (D49.2)

D49.1 **Neoplasm of unspecified behavior of respiratory system**

D49.2 **Neoplasm of unspecified behavior of bone, soft tissue, and skin**

Excludes1: neoplasm of unspecified behavior of anal canal (D49.0)

neoplasm of unspecified behavior of anus NOS (D49.0)

neoplasm of unspecified behavior of bone marrow (D49.89)

neoplasm of unspecified behavior of cartilage of larynx (D49.1)

neoplasm of unspecified behavior of cartilage of nose (D49.1)

neoplasm of unspecified behavior of connective tissue of breast (D49.3)

neoplasm of unspecified behavior of skin of genital organs (D49.59)

neoplasm of unspecified behavior of vermilion border of lip (D49.0)

D49.3 **Neoplasm of unspecified behavior of breast**

Excludes1: neoplasm of unspecified behavior of skin of breast (D49.2)

D49.4 **Neoplasm of unspecified behavior of bladder**

D49.5 **Neoplasm of unspecified behavior of other genitourinary organs**

D49.51 **Neoplasm of unspecified behavior of kidney**

D49.511 Neoplasm of unspecified behavior of right kidney

D49.512 Neoplasm of unspecified behavior of left kidney

D49.519 Neoplasm of unspecified behavior of unspecified kidney

D49.59 **Neoplasm of unspecified behavior of other genitourinary organ**

D49.6 **Neoplasm of unspecified behavior of brain** [HCC]

Excludes1: neoplasm of unspecified behavior of cerebral meninges (D49.7)

neoplasm of unspecified behavior of cranial nerves (D49.7)

D49.7 **Neoplasm of unspecified behavior of endocrine glands and other parts of nervous system**

Excludes1: neoplasm of unspecified behavior of peripheral, sympathetic, and parasympathetic nerves and ganglia (D49.2)

D49.8 **Neoplasm of unspecified behavior of other specified sites**

Excludes1: neoplasm of unspecified behavior of eyelid (skin) (D49.2)

neoplasm of unspecified behavior of eyelid cartilage (D49.2)

neoplasm of unspecified behavior of great vessels (D49.2)

neoplasm of unspecified behavior of optic nerve (D49.7)

D49.81 **Neoplasm of unspecified behavior of retina and choroid**

Dark area on retina

Retinal freckle

D49.89 **Neoplasm of unspecified behavior of other specified sites**

D49.9 **Neoplasm of unspecified behavior of unspecified site**

Chapter 3: Diseases of the Blood and Blood-Forming Organs and Certain Disorders Involving the Immune Mechanism (D50-D89)

DEFINITIONS AND CODING ALERTS

This chapter includes definitions of selected key words, terms and phrases and coding alerts for adding points to the clinical domain, and references to coding late effects where appropriate. An example from this chapter is as follows:

D50   Iron deficiency anemia
   Definition: Iron deficiency anemia is a form of anemia due to lack of iron in the diet or to iron loss as a result of chronic bleeding.

MULTIPLE CODING FOR A SINGLE CONDITION

In addition to the etiology/manifestation convention that requires two codes to fully describe a single condition that affects multiple body systems, there are other single conditions that also require more than one code. "**Use Additional Code**" notes are found in the Tabular List at codes that are not part of an etiology/manifestation pair where a secondary code is useful to fully describe a condition. The sequencing rule is the same as the etiology/manifestation pair, "**Use Additional Code**" indicates that a secondary code should be added.

For example, for bacterial infections that are not included in chapter 1, a secondary code from category B95, Streptococcus, Staphylococcus, and Enterococcus, as the cause of diseases classified elsewhere, or B96, Other bacterial agents as the cause of diseases classified elsewhere, may be required to identify the bacterial organism causing the infection. A "**Use Additional Code**" note will normally be found at the infectious disease code, indicating a need for the organism code to be added as a secondary code.

"Code first" notes are also under certain codes that are not specifically manifestation codes but may be due to an underlying cause. When there is a "Code first" note and an underlying condition is present, the underlying condition should be sequenced first.

"Code, if applicable, any causal condition first", notes indicate that this code may be assigned as a principal diagnosis when the causal condition is unknown or not applicable. If a causal condition is known, then the code for that condition should be sequenced as the principal or first-listed diagnosis.

Multiple codes may be needed for sequela, complication codes and obstetric codes to more fully describe a condition. See the specific guidelines for these conditions for further instruction.

COMBINATION CODE

A combination code is a single code used to classify: Two diagnoses, or a diagnosis with an associated secondary process (manifestation) A diagnosis with an associated complication

Combination codes are identified by referring to subterm entries in the Alphabetic Index and by reading the inclusion and exclusion notes in the Tabular List.

Assign only the combination code when that code fully identifies the diagnostic conditions involved or when the Alphabetic Index so directs. Multiple coding should not be used when the classification provides a combination code that clearly identifies all of the elements documented in the diagnosis. When the combination code lacks necessary specificity in describing the manifestation or complication, an additional code should be used as a secondary code.

SEQUELA (LATE EFFECTS)

A sequela is the residual effect (condition produced) after the acute phase of an illness or injury has terminated. There is no time limit on when a sequela code can be used. The residual may be apparent early, such as in cerebral infarction, or it may occur months or years later, such as that due to a previous injury. Coding of sequela generally requires two codes sequenced in the following order: The condition or nature of the sequela is sequenced first.

The sequela code is sequenced second.

An exception to the above guidelines are those instances where the code for the sequela is followed by a manifestation code identified in the Tabular List and title, or the sequela code has been expanded (at the fourth, fifth or sixth character levels) to include the manifestation(s). The code for the acute phase of an illness or injury that led to the sequela is never used with a code for the late effect.

● New code   ▲ Revised code   **Excludes1:** Not coded here   **Excludes2:** Not included here   ⊗ Placeholder required   ⑦7ᵗʰ digit required

Chapter 3

Diseases of the Blood and Blood-Forming Organs and Certain Disorders Involving the Immune Mechanism (D50-D89)

Excludes2: autoimmune disease (systemic) NOS (M35.9)

certain conditions originating in the perinatal period (P00-P96)

complications of pregnancy, childbirth and the puerperium (O00-O9A)

congenital malformations, deformations and chromosomal abnormalities (Q00-Q99)

endocrine, nutritional and metabolic diseases (E00-E88)

human immunodeficiency virus [HIV] disease (B20)

injury, poisoning and certain other consequences of external causes (S00-T88)

neoplasms (C00-D49)

symptoms, signs and abnormal clinical and laboratory findings, not elsewhere classified (R00-R94)

This chapter contains the following blocks:

D50-D53	Nutritional anemias
D55-D59	Hemolytic anemias
D60-D64	Aplastic and other anemias and other bone marrow failure syndromes
D65-D69	Coagulation defects, purpura and other hemorrhagic conditions
D70-D77	Other disorders of blood and blood-forming organs
D78	Intraoperative and postprocedural complications of the spleen
D80-D89	Certain disorders involving the immune mechanism

NUTRITIONAL ANEMIAS (D50-D53)

D50 Iron deficiency anemia

Includes: asiderotic anemia

hypochromic anemia

D50.0 Iron deficiency anemia secondary to blood loss (chronic)

Posthemorrhagic anemia (chronic)

Excludes1: acute posthemorrhagic anemia (D62)

congenital anemia from fetal blood loss (P61.3)

D50.1 Sideropenic dysphagia

Kelly-Paterson syndrome

Plummer-Vinson syndrome

D50.8 Other iron deficiency anemias

Iron deficiency anemia due to inadequate dietary iron intake

D50.9 Iron deficiency anemia, unspecified

D51 Vitamin B12 deficiency anemia

Excludes1: vitamin B12 deficiency (E53.8)

D51.0 Vitamin B12 deficiency anemia due to intrinsic factor deficiency

Addison anemia

Biermer anemia

Pernicious (congenital) anemia

Congenital intrinsic factor deficiency

D51.1 Vitamin B12 deficiency anemia due to selective vitamin B12 malabsorption with proteinuria

Imerslund (Gräsbeck) syndrome

Megaloblastic hereditary anemia

D51.2 Transcobalamin II deficiency

D51.3 Other dietary vitamin B12 deficiency anemia

Vegan anemia

D51.8 Other vitamin B12 deficiency anemias

D51.9 Vitamin B12 deficiency anemia, unspecified

D52 Folate deficiency anemia

Excludes1: folate deficiency without anemia (E53.8)

D52.0 Dietary folate deficiency anemia

Nutritional megaloblastic anemia

D52.1 Drug-induced folate deficiency anemia

Use Additional Code for adverse effect, if applicable, to identify drug (T36-T50 with fifth or sixth character 5)

D52.8 Other folate deficiency anemias

D52.9 Folate deficiency anemia, unspecified

Folic acid deficiency anemia NOS

D53 Other nutritional anemias

Includes: megaloblastic anemia unresponsive to vitamin B12 o folate therapy

D53.0 Protein deficiency anemia

Amino-acid deficiency anemia

Orotaciduric anemia

Excludes1: Lesch-Nyhan syndrome (E79.1)

D53.1 Other megaloblastic anemias, not elsewhere classified

Megaloblastic anemia NOS

Excludes1: Di Guglielmo's disease (C94.0)

D53.2 Scorbutic anemia

Excludes1: scurvy (E54)

D53.8 Other specified nutritional anemias

Anemia associated with deficiency of copper

Anemia associated with deficiency of molybdenum

Anemia associated with deficiency of zinc

Excludes1: nutritional deficiencies without anemia, such as:

copper deficiency NOS (E61.0)

molybdenum deficiency NOS (E61.5)

zinc deficiency NOS (E60)

D53.9 Nutritional anemia, unspecified

Simple chronic anemia

Excludes1: anemia NOS (D64.9)

HEMOLYTIC ANEMIAS (D55-D59)

D55 Anemia due to enzyme disorders

Excludes1: drug-induced enzyme deficiency anemia (D59.2)

D55.0 Anemia due to glucose-6-phosphate dehydrogenase [G6PD] deficiency [HCC]

Favism

G6PD deficiency anemia

Excludes1: glucose-6-phosphate dehydrogenase (G6PD) deficiency without anemia (D75.A)

D55.1 Anemia due to other disorders of glutathione metabolism [HCC]

Anemia (due to) enzyme deficiencies, except G6PD, related to the hexose monophosphate [HMP] shunt pathway

Anemia (due to) hemolytic nonspherocytic (hereditary), type I

D55.2 Anemia due to disorders of glycolytic enzymes [HCC]

Excludes1: disorders of glycolysis not associated with
●anemia (E74.81-)

● **D55.21 Anemia due to pyruvate kinase deficiency**

PK deficiency anemia

Pyruvate kinase deficiency anemia

● **D55.29   Anemia due to other disorders of glycolytic enzymes**

Hexokinase deficiency anemia

Triose-phosphate isomerase deficiency anemia

D55.3   Anemia due to disorders of nucleotide metabolism [HCC]

D55.8   Other anemias due to enzyme disorders [HCC]

D55.9   Anemia due to enzyme disorder, unspecified [HCC]

D56   Thalassemia

Excludes1: sickle-cell thalassemia (D57.4-)

D56.0   Alpha thalassemia [HCC]

Alpha thalassemia major

Hemoglobin H Constant Spring

Hemoglobin H disease

Hydrops fetalis due to alpha thalassemia

Severe alpha thalassemia

Triple gene defect alpha thalassemia

Use Additional Code, if applicable, for hydrops fetalis due to alpha thalassemia (P56.99)

Excludes1: alpha thalassemia trait or minor (D56.3)

asymptomatic alpha thalassemia (D56.3)

hydrops fetalis due to isoimmunization (P56.0)

hydrops fetalis not due to immune hemolysis (P83.2)

D56.1   Beta thalassemia [HCC]

Beta thalassemia major Cooley's anemia

Homozygous beta thalassemia

Severe beta thalassemia

Thalassemia intermedia

Thalassemia major

Excludes1: beta thalassemia minor (D56.3)

beta thalassemia trait (D56.3)

delta-beta thalassemia (D56.2)

hemoglobin E-beta thalassemia (D56.5)

sickle-cell beta thalassemia (D57.4-)

D56.2   Delta-beta thalassemia [HCC]

Homozygous delta-beta thalassemia

Excludes1: delta-beta thalassemia minor (D56.3)

delta-beta thalassemia trait (D56.3)

D56.3   Thalassemia minor Alpha thalassemia minor Alpha thalassemia silent carrier

Alpha thalassemia trait

Beta thalassemia minor Beta thalassemia trait

Delta-beta thalassemia minor

Delta-beta thalassemia trait

Thalassemia trait NOS

Excludes1: alpha thalassemia (D56.0)

beta thalassemia (D56.1)

delta-beta thalassemia (D56.2)

hemoglobin E-beta thalassemia (D56.5)

sickle-cell trait (D57.3)

D56.4   Hereditary persistence of fetal hemoglobin [HPFH] [HCC]

D56.5   Hemoglobin E-beta thalassemia [HCC]

Excludes1: beta thalassemia (D56.1)

beta thalassemia minor (D56.3)

beta thalassemia trait (D56.3)

delta-beta thalassemia (D56.2)

delta-beta thalassemia trait (D56.3)

hemoglobin E disease (D58.2)

Other hemoglobinopathies (D58.2)

sickle-cell beta thalassemia (D57.4-)

D56.8   Other thalassemias [HCC]

Dominant thalassemia

Hemoglobin C thalassemia

Mixed thalassemia

Thalassemia with other hemoglobinopathy

Excludes1: hemoglobin C disease (D58.2)

hemoglobin E disease (D58.2)

Other hemoglobinopathies (D58.2)

sickle-cell anemia (D57.-)

sickle-cell thalassemia (D57.4)

D56.9   Thalassemia, unspecified

Mediterranean anemia (with other hemoglobinopathy)

D57   Sickle-cell disorders

Use Additional Code for any associated fever (R50.81)

Excludes1: Other hemoglobinopathies (D58.-)

D57.0   Hb-SS disease with crisis

Sickle-cell disease with crisis

Hb-SS disease with vasoocclusive pain

D57.00   Hb-SS disease with crisis, unspecified [HCC]

Hb-SS disease with (painful) crisis NOS

Hb-SS disease with vasoocclusive pain NOS

D57.01   Hb-SS disease with acute chest syndrome [HCC]

D57.02   Hb-SS disease with splenic sequestration [HCC]

D57.03   Hb-SS disease with cerebral vascular involvement

Code also, if applicable, cerebral infarction (I63.-)

D57.09   Hb-SS disease with crisis with other specified complication

Use Additional Code to identify complications, such as:

cholelithiasis (K80.-)

priapism (N48.32)

D57.1   Sickle-cell disease without crisis [HCC]

Hb-SS disease without crisis

Sickle-cell anemia NOS

Sickle-cell disease NOS

Sickle-cell disorder NOS

D57.2   Sickle-cell/Hb-C disease

Hb-SC disease

Hb-S/Hb-C disease

D57.20   Sickle-cell/Hb-C disease without crisis

D57.21   Sickle-cell/Hb-C disease with crisis

D57.211   Sickle-cell/Hb-C disease with acute chest syndrome [HCC]

D57.212   Sickle-cell/Hb-C disease with splenic sequestration [HCC]

D57.213   Sickle-cell/Hb-C disease with cerebral vascular involvement

Code also, if applicable, cerebral infarction (I63.-)

D57.218   Sickle-cell/Hb-C disease with crisis with other specified complication

Use Additional Code to identify complications, such as:

cholelithiasis (K80.-)

priapism (N48.32)

D57.219 **Sickle-cell/Hb-C disease with crisis, unspecified** [HCC]

Sickle-cell/Hb-C disease with crisis NOS

Sickle-cell/Hb-C disease with vasoocclusive pain NOS

D57.3 **Sickle-cell trait** [HCC]

Hb-S trait

Heterozygous hemoglobin S

D57.4 **Sickle-cell thalassemia**

Sickle-cell beta thalassemia

Thalassemia Hb-S disease

D57.40 **Sickle-cell thalassemia without crisis** [HCC]

Microdrepanocytosis

Sickle-cell thalassemia NOS

D57.41 **Sickle-cell thalassemia, unspecified, with crisis**

Sickle-cell thalassemia with (painful) crisis NOS

Sickle-cell thalassemia with vasoocclusive pain NOS

D57.411 **Sickle-cell thalassemia, unspecified, with acute chest syndrome** [HCC]

D57.412 **Sickle-cell thalassemia, unspecified, with splenic sequestration** [HCC]

D57.419 **Sickle-cell thalassemia, unspecified, with crisis** [HCC]

Sickle-cell thalassemia with (painful) crisis NOS

Sickle-cell thalassemia with vasoocclusive pain NOS

D57.42 **Sickle-cell thalassemia beta zero without crisis**

HbS-beta zero without crisis

Sickle-cell beta zero without crisis

D57.43 **Sickle-cell thalassemia beta zero with crisis**

HbS-beta zero with crisis

Sickle-cell beta zero with crisis

D57.431 **Sickle-cell thalassemia beta zero with acute chest syndrome**

HbS-beta zero with acute chest syndrome

Sickle-cell beta zero with acute chest syndrome

D57.432 **Sickle-cell thalassemia beta zero with splenic sequestration**

HbS-beta zero with splenic sequestration

Sickle-cell beta zero with splenic sequestration

D57.433 **Sickle-cell thalassemia beta zero with cerebral vascular involvement**

HbS-beta zero with cerebral vascular involvement

Sickle-cell beta zero with cerebral vascular involvement

Code also, if applicable cerebral infarction (I63.-)

D57.438 **Sickle-cell thalassemia beta zero with crisis with other specified complication**

HbS-beta zero with other specified complication

Sickle-cell beta zero with other specified complication

Use Additional Code to identify complications, such as:

cholelithiasis (K80.-)

priapism (N48.32)

D57.439 **Sickle-cell thalassemia beta zero with crisis, unspecified**

HbS-beta zero with other specified complication

Sickle-cell beta zero with crisis unspecified

Sickle-cell thalassemia beta zero with (painful) crisis NOS

Sickle-cell thalassemia beta zero with vasoocclusive pain NOS

D57.44 **Sickle-cell thalassemia beta plus without crisis**

HbS-beta plus without crisis

Sickle-cell beta plus without crisis

D57.45 **Sickle-cell thalassemia beta plus with crisis**

HbS-beta plus with crisis

Sickle-cell beta plus with crisis

D57.451 **Sickle-cell thalassemia beta plus with acute chest syndrome**

HbS-beta plus with acute chest syndrome

Sickle-cell beta plus with acute chest syndrome

D57.452 **Sickle-cell thalassemia beta plus with splenic sequestration**

HbS-beta plus with splenic sequestration

Sickle-cell beta plus with splenic sequestration

D57.453 **Sickle-cell thalassemia beta plus with cerebral vascular involvement**

HbS-beta plus with cerebral vascular involvement

Sickle-cell beta plus with cerebral vascular involvement

Code also, if applicable cerebral infarction (I63.-)

D57.458 **Sickle-cell thalassemia beta plus with crisis with other specified complication**

HbS-beta plus with crisis with other specified complication

Sickle-cell beta plus with crisis with other specified complication

Use Additional Code to identify complications, such as:

cholelithiasis (K80.-)

priapism (N48.32)

D57.459 **Sickle-cell thalassemia beta plus with crisis, unspecified**

HbS-beta plus with crisis with unspecified complication

Sickle-cell beta plus with crisis with unspecified complication

Sickle-cell thalassemia beta plus with (painful) crisis NOS

Sickle-cell thalassemia beta plus with vasoocclusive pain NOS

D57.8 **Other sickle-cell disorders**

Hb-SD disease Hb-SE disease

> **D57.80** **Other sickle-cell disorders without crisis** [HCC]
>
> **D57.81** **Other sickle-cell disorders with crisis**
>
> > **D57.811** **Other sickle-cell disorders with acute chest syndrome** [HCC]
> >
> > **D57.812** **Other sickle-cell disorders with splenic sequestration** [HCC]
> >
> > **D57.813** **Other sickle-cell disorders with cerebral vascular involvement**
> >
> > **Code also**, if applicable: cerebral infarction (I63.-)
> >
> > **D57.818** **Other sickle-cell disorders with crisis with other specified complication**
> >
> > **Use Additional Code** to identify complications, such as:
> >
> > cholelithiasis (K80.-)
> >
> > priapism (N48.32)
> >
> > **D57.819** **Other sickle-cell disorders with crisis, unspecified** [HCC]
> >
> > Other sickle-cell disorders with crisis NOS
> >
> > Other sickle-cell disorders with vasoocclusive pain NOS

D58 **Other hereditary hemolytic anemias**

Excludes1: hemolytic anemia of the newborn (P55.-)

> **D58.0** **Hereditary spherocytosis** [HCC]
>
> Acholuric (familial) jaundice
>
> Congenital (spherocytic) hemolytic icterus
>
> Minkowski-Chauffard syndrome
>
> **D58.1** **Hereditary elliptocytosis** [HCC]
>
> Elliptocytosis (congenital)
>
> Ovalocytosis (congenital) (hereditary)
>
> **D58.2** **Other hemoglobinopathies** [HCC]
>
> Abnormal hemoglobin NOS
>
> Congenital Heinz body anemia
>
> Hb-C disease
>
> Hb-D disease
>
> Hb-E disease
>
> Hemoglobinopathy NOS
>
> Unstable hemoglobin hemolytic disease
>
> **Excludes1:** familial polycythemia (D75.0)
>
> Hb-M disease (D74.0)
>
> hemoglobin E-beta thalassemia (D56.5)
>
> hereditary persistence of fetal hemoglobin [HPFH] (D56.4)
>
> high-altitude polycythemia (D75.1)
>
> methemoglobinemia (D74.-)
>
> Other hemoglobinopathies with thalassemia (D56.8)
>
> **D58.8** **Other specified hereditary hemolytic anemias** [HCC]
>
> Stomatocytosis
>
> **D58.9** **Hereditary hemolytic anemia, unspecified** [HCC]

D59 **Acquired hemolytic anemia**

> **D59.0** **Drug-induced autoimmune hemolytic anemia** [HCC]
>
> **Use Additional Code** for adverse effect, if applicable, to identify drug (T36-T50 with fifth or sixth character 5)
>
> **D59.1** **Other autoimmune hemolytic anemias** [HCC]
>
> **Excludes2:** Evans syndrome (D69.41)

hemolytic disease of newborn (P55.-)

paroxysmal cold hemoglobinuria (D59.6)

> **D59.10** **Autoimmune hemolytic anemia, unspecified**
>
> **D59.11** **Warm autoimmune hemolytic anemia**
>
> Warm type (primary) (secondary) (symptomatic) autoimmune hemolytic anemia
>
> Warm type autoimmune hemolytic disease
>
> **D59.12** **Cold autoimmune hemolytic anemia**
>
> Chronic cold hemagglutinin disease
>
> Cold agglutinin disease
>
> Cold agglutinin hemoglobinuria
>
> Cold type (primary) (secondary) (symptomatic) autoimmune hemolytic anemia
>
> Cold type autoimmune hemolytic disease
>
> **D59.13** **Mixed type autoimmune hemolytic anemia**
>
> Mixed type autoimmune hemolytic disease
>
> Mixed type, cold and warm, (primary) (secondary) (symptomatic) autoimmune hemolyticanemia
>
> **D59.19** **Other autoimmune hemolytic anemia**

D59.2 **Drug-induced nonautoimmune hemolytic anemia** [HCC]

Drug-induced enzyme deficiency anemia

Use Additional Code for adverse effect, if applicable, to identify drug (T36-T50 with fifth or sixth character 5)

D59.3 **Hemolytic-uremic syndrome** [HCC]

Use Additional Code to identify associated:

E. coli infection (B96.2-)

Pneumococcal pneumonia (J13)

Shigella dysenteriae (A03.9)

D59.4 **Other nonautoimmune hemolytic anemias** [HCC]

Mechanical hemolytic anemia

Microangiopathic hemolytic anemia

Toxic hemolytic anemia

D59.5 **Paroxysmal nocturnal hemoglobinuria [Marchiafava-Micheli]** [HCC]

Excludes1: hemoglobinuria NOS (R82.3)

D59.6 **Hemoglobinuria due to hemolysis from other external causes** [HCC]

Hemoglobinuria from exertion

March hemoglobinuria

Paroxysmal cold hemoglobinuria

Use Additional Code (Chapter 20) to identify external cause

Excludes1: hemoglobinuria NOS (R82.3)

D59.8 **Other acquired hemolytic anemias** [HCC]

D59.9 **Acquired hemolytic anemia, unspecified** [HCC]

Idiopathic hemolytic anemia, chronic

APLASTIC AND OTHER ANEMIAS AND OTHER BONE MARROW FAILURE SYNDROMES (D60-D64)

D60 **Acquired pure red cell aplasia [erythroblastopenia]**

Includes: red cell aplasia (acquired) (adult) (with thymoma)

Excludes1: congenital red cell aplasia (D61.01)

> **D60.0** **Chronic acquired pure red cell aplasia** [HCC]
>
> **D60.1** **Transient acquired pure red cell aplasia** [HCC]
>
> **D60.8** **Other acquired pure red cell aplasias** [HCC]
>
> **D60.9** **Acquired pure red cell aplasia, unspecified** [HCC]

D61 **Other aplastic anemias and other bone marrow failure syndromes**

Excludes2: neutropenia (D70.-)

D61.0 **Constitutional aplastic anemia**

    D61.01 **Constitutional (pure) red blood cell aplasia** [HCC]

      Blackfan-Diamond syndrome

      Congenital (pure) red cell aplasia

      Familial hypoplastic anemia

      Primary (pure) red cell aplasia

      Red cell (pure) aplasia of infants

      Excludes1: acquired red cell aplasia (D60.9)

    D61.09 **Other constitutional aplastic anemia** [HCC]

      Fanconi's anemia

      Pancytopenia with malformations

D61.1 **Drug-induced aplastic anemia** [HCC]

    Use Additional Code for adverse effect, if applicable, to identify drug (T36-T50 with fifth or sixth character 5)

D61.2 **Aplastic anemia due to other external agents** [HCC]

    Code first, if applicable, toxic effects of substances chiefly nonmedicinal as to source (T51-T65)

D61.3 **Idiopathic aplastic anemia** [HCC]

D61.8 **Other specified aplastic anemias and other bone marrow failure syndromes**

    D61.81 **Pancytopenia**

      Excludes1: pancytopenia (due to) (with) aplastic anemia (D61.9)

      pancytopenia (due to) (with) bone marrow infiltration (D61.82)

      pancytopenia (due to) (with) congenital (pure) red cell aplasia (D61.01)

      pancytopenia (due to) (with) hairy cell leukemia (C91.4-)

      pancytopenia (due to) (with) human immunodeficiency virus disease (B20.-)

      pancytopenia (due to) (with) leukoerythroblastic anemia (D61.82)

      pancytopenia (due to) (with) myeloproliferative disease (D47.1)

      Excludes2: pancytopenia (due to) (with) myelodysplastic syndromes (D46.-)

      D61.810 **Antineoplastic chemotherapy induced pancytopenia** [HCC]

        Excludes2: aplastic anemia due to antineoplastic chemotherapy (D61.1)

      D61.811 **Other drug-induced pancytopenia** [HCC]

        Excludes2: aplastic anemia due to drugs (D61.1)

      D61.818 **Other pancytopenia** [HCC]

    D61.82 **Myelophthisis** [HCC]

      Leukoerythroblastic anemia

      Myelophthisic anemia

      Panmyelophthisis

      Code also the underlying disorder, such as:

      malignant neoplasm of breast (C50.-)

      tuberculosis (A15.-)

      Excludes1: idiopathic myelofibrosis (D47.1)

      myelofibrosis NOS (D75.81)

      myelofibrosis with myeloid metaplasia (D47.4)

      primary myelofibrosis (D47.1)

secondary myelofibrosis (D75.81)

    D61.89 **Other specified aplastic anemias and other bone marrow failure syndromes** [HCC]

D61.9 **Aplastic anemia, unspecified** [HCC]

    Hypoplastic anemia NOS

    Medullary hypoplasia

D62 **Acute posthemorrhagic anemia**

Excludes1: anemia due to chronic blood loss (D50.0)

    blood loss anemia NOS (D50.0)

    congenital anemia from fetal blood loss (P61.3)

D63 **Anemia in chronic diseases classified elsewhere**

D63.0 **Anemia in neoplastic disease**

    Code first neoplasm (C00-D49)

    Excludes2: anemia due to antineoplastic chemotherapy (D64.81)

    aplastic anemia due to antineoplastic chemotherapy (D61.1)

D63.1 **Anemia in chronic kidney disease**

    Erythropoietin resistant anemia (EPO resistant anemia)

    Code first underlying chronic kidney disease (CKD) (N18.-)

D63.8 **Anemia in other chronic diseases classified elsewhere**

    Code first underlying disease, such as:

    diphyllobothriasis (B70.0)

    hookworm disease (B76.0-B76.9)

    hypothyroidism (E00.0-E03.9)

    malaria (B50.0-B54)

    symptomatic late syphilis (A52.79)

    tuberculosis (A18.89)

D64 **Other anemias**

Excludes1: refractory anemia (D46.-)

    refractory anemia with excess blasts in transformation [RAEB T] (C92.0-)

D64.0 **Hereditary sideroblastic anemia** [HCC]

    Sex-linked hypochromic sideroblastic anemia

D64.1 **Secondary sideroblastic anemia due to disease** [HCC]

    Code first underlying disease

D64.2 **Secondary sideroblastic anemia due to drugs and toxins** [HCC]

    Code first poisoning due to drug or toxin, if applicable (T36-T65 with fifth or sixth character 1-4 or 6)

    Use Additional Code for adverse effect, if applicable, to identify drug (T36-T50 with fifth or sixth character 5)

D64.3 **Other sideroblastic anemias** [HCC]

    Sideroblastic anemia NOS

    Pyridoxine-responsive sideroblastic anemia NEC

D64.4 **Congenital dyserythropoietic anemia**

    Dyshematopoietic anemia (congenital)

    Excludes1: Blackfan-Diamond syndrome (D61.01)

      Di Guglielmo's disease (C94.0)

D64.8 **Other specified anemias**

    D64.81 **Anemia due to antineoplastic chemotherapy**

      Antineoplastic chemotherapy induced anemia

      Excludes2: aplastic anemia due to antineoplastic chemotherapy (D61.1)

      Excludes2: anemia in neoplastic disease (D63.0)

    D64.89 **Other specified anemias**

      Infantile pseudoleukemia

D64.9 **Anemia, unspecified**

COAGULATION DEFECTS, PURPURA AND OTHER HEMORRHAGIC CONDITIONS (D65-D69)

D65 **Disseminated intravascular coagulation [defibrination syndrome]** [HCC]

Afibrinogenemia, acquired

Consumption coagulopathy

Diffuse or disseminated intravascular coagulation [DIC]

Fibrinolytic hemorrhage, acquired

Fibrinolytic purpura

Purpura fulminans

Excludes1: disseminated intravascular coagulation (complicating):

abortion or ectopic or molar pregnancy (O00-O07, O08.1)

in newborn (P60)

pregnancy, childbirth and the puerperium (O45.0, O46.0, O67.0, O72.3)

D66 **Hereditary factor VIII deficiency** [HCC]

Classical hemophilia

Deficiency factor VIII (with functional defect)

Hemophilia NOS

Hemophilia A

Excludes1: factor VIII deficiency with vascular defect (D68.0)

D67 **Hereditary factor IX deficiency** [HCC]

Christmas disease

Factor IX deficiency (with functional defect)

Hemophilia B

Plasma thromboplastin component [PTC] deficiency

D68 **Other coagulation defects**

Excludes1: abnormal coagulation profile (R79.1)

coagulation defects complicating abortion or ectopic or molar pregnancy (O00-O07, O08.1)

coagulation defects complicating pregnancy, childbirth and the puerperium (O45.0, O46.0, O67.0, O72.3)

D68.0 **Von Willebrand's disease** [HCC]

Angiohemophilia

Factor VIII deficiency with vascular defect

Vascular hemophilia

Excludes1: capillary fragility (hereditary) (D69.8)

factor VIII deficiency NOS (D66)

factor VIII deficiency with functional defect (D66)

D68.1 **Hereditary factor XI deficiency** [HCC]

Hemophilia C

Plasma thromboplastin antecedent [PTA] deficiency

Rosenthal's disease

D68.2 **Hereditary deficiency of other clotting factors** [HCC]

AC globulin deficiency

Congenital afibrinogenemia

Deficiency of factor I [fibrinogen]

Deficiency of factor II [prothrombin]

Deficiency of factor V [labile]

Deficiency of factor VII [stable]

Deficiency of factor X [Stuart-Prower]

Deficiency of factor XII [Hageman]

Deficiency of factor XIII [fibrin stabilizing]

Dysfibrinogenemia (congenital)

Hypoproconvertinemia

Owren's disease

Proaccelerin deficiency

D68.3 **Hemorrhagic disorder due to circulating anticoagulants**

D68.31 **Hemorrhagic disorder due to intrinsic circulating anticoagulants, antibodies, or inhibitors**

D68.311 **Acquired hemophilia** [HCC]

Autoimmune hemophilia

Autoimmune inhibitors to clotting factors

Secondary hemophilia

D68.312 **Antiphospholipid antibody with hemorrhagic disorder** [HCC]

Lupus anticoagulant (LAC) with hemorrhagic disorder

Systemic lupus erythematosus [SLE] inhibitor with hemorrhagic disorder

Excludes1: antiphospholipid antibody, finding without diagnosis (R76.0)

antiphospholipid antibody syndrome (D68.61)

antiphospholipid antibody with hypercoagulable state (D68.61)

lupus anticoagulant (LAC) finding without diagnosis (R76.0)

lupus anticoagulant (LAC) with hypercoagulable state (D68.62)

systemic lupus erythematosus [SLE] inhibitor finding without diagnosis (R76.0)

systemic lupus erythematosus [SLE] inhibitor with hypercoagulable state (D68.62)

D68.318 **Other hemorrhagic disorder due to intrinsic circulating anticoagulants, antibodies, or inhibitors** [HCC]

Antithromboplastinemia

Antithromboplastinogenemia

Hemorrhagic disorder due to intrinsic increase in antithrombin

Hemorrhagic disorder due to intrinsic increase in anti-VIIIa

Hemorrhagic disorder due to intrinsic increase in anti-IXa

Hemorrhagic disorder due to intrinsic increase in anti-XIa

D68.32 **Hemorrhagic disorder due to extrinsic circulating anticoagulants** [HCC]

Drug-induced hemorrhagic disorder

Hemorrhagic disorder due to increase in anti-IIa

Hemorrhagic disorder due to increase in anti-Xa

Hyperheparinemia

Use Additional Code for adverse effect, if applicable, to identify drug (T45.515, T45.525)

D68.4 **Acquired coagulation factor deficiency** [HCC]

Deficiency of coagulation factor due to liver disease

Deficiency of coagulation factor due to vitamin K deficiency

Excludes1: vitamin K deficiency of newborn (P53)

D68.5 **Primary thrombophilia**

Primary hypercoagulable states

Excludes1: antiphospholipid syndrome (D68.61)

● New code ▲ Revised code **Excludes1:** Not coded here **Excludes2:** Not included here ⊗ Placeholder required ⑦7th digit required

lupus anticoagulant (D68.62)

secondary activated protein C resistance (D68.69)

secondary antiphospholipid antibody syndrome (D68.69)

secondary lupus anticoagulant with hypercoagulable state (D68.69)

secondary systemic lupus erythematosus [SLE] inhibitor with hypercoagulable state (D68.69)

systemic lupus erythematosus [SLE] inhibitor finding without diagnosis (R76.0)

systemic lupus erythematosus [SLE] inhibitor with hemorrhagic disorder (D68.312)

thrombotic thrombocytopenic purpura (M31.19)

D68.51 Activated protein C resistance [HCC]

Factor V Leiden mutation

D68.52 Prothrombin gene mutation [HCC]

D68.59 Other primary thrombophilia [HCC]

Antithrombin III deficiency

Hypercoagulable state NOS

Primary hypercoagulable state NEC

Primary thrombophilia NEC

Protein C deficiency

Protein S deficiency

Thrombophilia NOS

D68.6 Other thrombophilia

Other hypercoagulable states

Excludes1: diffuse or disseminated intravascular coagulation [DIC] (D65)

heparin induced thrombocytopenia (HIT) (D75.82)

hyperhomocysteinemia (E72.11)

D68.61 Antiphospholipid syndrome [HCC]

Anticardiolipin syndrome

Antiphospholipid antibody syndrome

Excludes1: anti-phospholipid antibody, finding without diagnosis (R76.0)

anti-phospholipid antibody with hemorrhagic disorder (D68.312)

lupus anticoagulant syndrome (D68.62)

D68.62 Lupus anticoagulant syndrome [HCC]

Lupus anticoagulant

Presence of systemic lupus erythematosus [SLE] inhibitor

Excludes1: anticardiolipin syndrome (D68.61)

antiphospholipid syndrome (D68.61)

lupus anticoagulant (LAC) finding without diagnosis (R76.0)

lupus anticoagulant (LAC) with hemorrhagic disorder (D68.312)

D68.69 Other thrombophilia [HCC]

Hypercoagulable states NEC

Secondary hypercoagulable state NOS

D68.8 Other specified coagulation defects [HCC]

Excludes1: hemorrhagic disease of newborn (P53)

D68.9 Coagulation defect, unspecified [HCC]

D69 Purpura and other hemorrhagic conditions

Excludes1: benign hypergammaglobulinemic purpura (D89.0)

cryoglobulinemic purpura (D89.1)

essential (hemorrhagic) thrombocythemia (D47.3)

hemorrhagic thrombocythemia (D47.3)

purpura fulminans (D65)

thrombotic thrombocytopenic purpura (M31.1)

Waldenström hypergammaglobulinemic purpura (D89.0)

D69.0 Allergic purpura [HCC]

Allergic vasculitis

Nonthrombocytopenic hemorrhagic purpura

Nonthrombocytopenic idiopathic purpura

Purpura anaphylactoid

Purpura Henoch(-Schönlein)

Purpura rheumatica

Vascular purpura

Excludes1: thrombocytopenic hemorrhagic purpura (D69.3)

D69.1 Qualitative platelet defects [HCC]

Bernard-Soulier [giant platelet] syndrome Glanzmann's disease

Grey platelet syndrome

Thromboasthenia (hemorrhagic) (hereditary)

Thrombocytopathy

Excludes1: von Willebrand's disease (D68.0)

D69.2 Other nonthrombocytopenic purpura [HCC]

Purpura NOS

Purpura simplex

Senile purpura

D69.3 Immune thrombocytopenic purpura [HCC]

Hemorrhagic (thrombocytopenic) purpura

Idiopathic thrombocytopenic purpura

Tidal platelet dysgenesis

D69.4 Other primary thrombocytopenia

Excludes1: transient neonatal thrombocytopenia (P61.0)

Wiskott-Aldrich syndrome (D82.0)

D69.41 Evans syndrome [HCC]

D69.42 Congenital and hereditary thrombocytopenia purpura [HCC]

Congenital thrombocytopenia

Hereditary thrombocytopenia

Code first congenital or hereditary disorder, such as:

thrombocytopenia with absent radius (TAR syndrome) (Q87.2)

D69.49 Other primary thrombocytopenia [HCC]

Megakaryocytic hypoplasia

Primary thrombocytopenia NOS

D69.5 Secondary thrombocytopenia

Excludes1: heparin induced thrombocytopenia (HIT) (D75.82)

transient thrombocytopenia of newborn (P61.0)

D69.51 Posttransfusion purpura

Posttransfusion purpura from whole blood (fresh) or blood products PTP

D69.59 Other secondary thrombocytopenia

D69.6 Thrombocytopenia, unspecified [HCC]

D69.8 Other specified hemorrhagic conditions [HCC]

Capillary fragility (hereditary)

Vascular pseudohemophilia

D69.9 Hemorrhagic condition, unspecified [HCC]

OTHER DISORDERS OF BLOOD AND BLOOD-FORMING ORGANS (D70-D77)

D70 **Neutropenia**

Includes: agranulocytosis

decreased absolute neutrophile count (ANC)

Use Additional Code for any associated:

fever (R50.81)

mucositis (J34.81, K12.3-, K92.81, N76.81)

Excludes1: neutropenic splenomegaly (D73.81)

transient neonatal neutropenia (P61.5)

D70.0 **Congenital agranulocytosis** [HCC]

Congenital neutropenia

Infantile genetic agranulocytosis

Kostmann's disease

D70.1 **Agranulocytosis secondary to cancer chemotherapy** [HCC]

Code also underlying neoplasm

Use Additional Code for adverse effect, if applicable, to identify drug (T45.1X5)

D70.2 **Other drug-induced agranulocytosis** [HCC]

Use Additional Code for adverse effect, if applicable, to identify drug (T36-T50 with fifth or sixth character 5)

D70.3 **Neutropenia due to infection** [HCC]

D70.4 **Cyclic neutropenia** [HCC]

Cyclic hematopoiesis

Periodic neutropenia

D70.8 **Other neutropenia** [HCC]

D70.9 **Neutropenia, unspecified** [HCC]

D71 **Functional disorders of polymorphonuclear neutrophils** [HCC]

Cell membrane receptor complex [CR3] defect

Chronic (childhood) granulomatous disease

Congenital dysphagocytosis

Progressive septic granulomatosis

D72 **Other disorders of white blood cells**

Definition: White blood cells, aka leukocyte, refers to any of various blood cells that help protect the body from infection and disease. White blood cells include neutrophils, eosinophils, basophils, lymphocytes, and monocytes

Excludes1: basophilia (D72.824)

immunity disorders (D80-D89)

neutropenia (D70)

preleukemia (syndrome) (D46.9)

D72.0 **Genetic anomalies of leukocytes** [HCC]

Alder (granulation) (granulocyte) anomaly

Alder syndrome

Hereditary leukocytic hypersegmentation

Hereditary leukocytic hyposegmentation

Hereditary Leukomelanopathy

May-Hegglin (granulation) (granulocyte) anomaly

May-Hegglin syndrome

Pelger-Huët (granulation) (granulocyte anomaly

Pelger-Huët syndrome

Excludes1: Chédiak (-Steinbrinck)-Higashi syndrome(E70.330)

D72.1 **Eosinophilia**

Excludes2: Löffler's syndrome (J82.89)

pulmonary eosinophilia (J82.-)

D72.10 **Eosinophilia, unspecified**

D72.11 **Hypereosinophilic syndrome [HES]**

D72.110 **Idiopathic hypereosinophilic syndrome [IHES]**

D72.111 **Lymphocytic Variant Hypereosinophilic Syndrome [LHES]**

Lymphocyte variant hypereosinophilia

Code also, if applicable, any associated lymphocytic neoplastic disorder

D72.118 **Other hypereosinophilic syndrome**

Episodic angioedema with eosinophilia

Gleich's syndrome

D72.119 **Hypereosinophilic syndrome [HES], unspecified**

D72.12 **Drug rash with eosinophilia and systemic symptoms syndrome**

DRESS syndrome

Use Additional Code for adverse effect, if applicable, to identify drug (T36-T50 with fifth or sixth character 5)

D72.18 **Eosinophilia in diseases classified elsewhere**

Code first underlying disease, such as:

chronic myelomonocytic leukemia (C93.1-)

D72.19 **Other eosinophilia**

Familial eosinophilia

Hereditary eosinophilia

D72.8 **Other specified disorders of white blood cells**

Excludes1: leukemia (C91-C95)

D72.81 **Decreased white blood cell count**

Excludes1: neutropenia (D70.-)

D72.810 **Lymphocytopenia**

Decreased lymphocytes

D72.818 **Other decreased white blood cell count**

Basophilic leukopenia Eosinophilic leukopenia

Monocytopenia

Other decreased leukocytes

Plasma cytopenia

D72.819 **Decreased white blood cell count, unspecified**

Decreased leukocytes, unspecified

Leukocytopenia, unspecified

Leukopenia

Excludes1: malignant leukopenia (D70.9)

D72.82 **Elevated white blood cell count**

Excludes1: eosinophilia (D72.1)

D72.820 **Lymphocytosis (symptomatic)**

Elevated lymphocytes

D72.821 **Monocytosis (symptomatic)**

Excludes1: infectious mononucleosis (B27.-)

D72.822 **Plasmacytosis**

D72.823 **Leukemoid reaction**

Basophilic leukemoid reaction

Leukemoid reaction NOS

Lymphocytic leukemoid reaction

Monocytic leukemoid reaction

Myelocytic leukemoid reaction

Neutrophilic leukemoid reaction

D72.824 **Basophilia**

D72.825 **Bandemia**

Bandemia without diagnosis of specific infection

Excludes1: confirmed infection - code to infection

leukemia (C91.-, C92.-, C93.-, C94.-, C95.-)

D72.828 **Other elevated white blood cell count**

D72.829 **Elevated white blood cell count, unspecified**

Elevated leukocytes, unspecified

Leukocytosis, unspecified

D72.89 **Other specified disorders of white blood cells**

Abnormality of white blood cells NEC

D72.9 **Disorder of white blood cells, unspecified**

Abnormal leukocyte differential NOS

D73 **Diseases of spleen**

D73.0 **Hyposplenism**

Atrophy of spleen

Excludes1: asplenia (congenital) (Q89.01)

postsurgical absence of spleen (Z90.81)

D73.1 **Hypersplenism**

Excludes1: neutropenic splenomegaly (D73.81)

primary splenic neutropenia (D73.81)

splenitis, splenomegaly in late syphilis (A52.79)

splenitis, splenomegaly in tuberculosis (A18.85)

splenomegaly NOS (R16.1)

splenomegaly congenital (Q89.0)

D73.2 **Chronic congestive splenomegaly**

D73.3 **Abscess of spleen**

D73.4 **Cyst of spleen**

D73.5 **Infarction of spleen**

Splenic rupture, nontraumatic

Torsion of spleen

Excludes1: rupture of spleen due to Plasmodium vivax malaria (B51.0)

traumatic rupture of spleen (S36.03-)

D73.8 **Other diseases of spleen**

D73.81 **Neutropenic splenomegaly**

Werner-Schultz disease

D73.89 **Other diseases of spleen**

Fibrosis of spleen NOS

Perisplenitis

Splenitis NOS

D73.9 **Disease of spleen, unspecified**

D74 **Methemoglobinemia**

D74.0 **Congenital methemoglobinemia**

Congenital NADH-methemoglobin reductase deficiency

Hemoglobin-M [Hb-M] disease

Methemoglobinemia, hereditary

D74.8 **Other methemoglobinemias**

Acquired methemoglobinemia (with sulfhemoglobinemia)

Toxic methemoglobinemia

D74.9 **Methemoglobinemia, unspecified**

D75 **Other and unspecified diseases of blood and blood-forming organs**

Excludes2: acute lymphadenitis (L04.-)

chronic lymphadenitis (I88.1)

enlarged lymph nodes (R59.-)

hypergammaglobulinemia NOS (D89.2)

lymphadenitis NOS (I88.9)

mesenteric lymphadenitis (acute) (chronic) (I88.0)

D75.0 **Familial erythrocytosis**

Benign polycythemia

Familial polycythemia

Excludes1: hereditary ovalocytosis (D58.1)

D75.1 **Secondary polycythemia**

Acquired polycythemia

Emotional polycythemia

Erythrocytosis NOS

Hypoxemic polycythemia

Nephrogenous polycythemia

Polycythemia due to erythropoietin

Polycythemia due to fall in plasma volume

Polycythemia due to high altitude

Polycythemia due to stress

Polycythemia NOS

Relative polycythemia

Excludes1: polycythemia neonatorum (P61.1)

polycythemia vera (D45)

D75.8 **Other specified diseases of blood and blood-forming organs**

D75.81 **Myelofibrosis** [HCC]

Myelofibrosis NOS

Secondary myelofibrosis NOS

Code first the underlying disorder, such as:

malignant neoplasm of breast (C50.-)

Use Additional Code, if applicable, for associated therapy-related myelodysplastic syndrome (D46.-)

Use Additional Code for adverse effect, if applicable, to identify drug (T45.1X5)

Excludes1: acute myelofibrosis (C94.4-)

idiopathic myelofibrosis (D47.1)

leukoerythroblastic anemia (D61.82)

myelofibrosis with myeloid metaplasia (D47.4)

myelophthisic anemia (D61.82)

myelophthisis (D61.82)

primary myelofibrosis (D47.1)

D75.82 **Heparin induced thrombocytopenia (HIT)** [HCC]

● **D75.83** **Thrombocytosis**

Excludes2 essential thrombocythemia (D47.3)

● **D75.838** **Other thrombocytosis**

Reactive thrombocytosis

Secondary thrombocytosis

Code also underlying condition, if known and applicable

● **D75.839** **Thrombocytosis, unspecified**

Thrombocythemia NOS

Thrombocytosis NOS

D75.89 **Other specified diseases of blood and blood-forming organs**

D75.9 **Disease of blood and blood-forming organs, unspecified**

D75.A **Glucose-6-phosphate dehydrogenase (G6PD) deficiency without anemia**

glucose-6-phosphate dehydrogenase (G6PD) deficiency with anemia (D55.0)

D76 **Other specified diseases with participation of lymphoreticular and reticulohistiocytic tissue**

Excludes1: (Abt-) Letterer-Siwe disease (C96.0)

eosinophilic granuloma (C96.6)

Hand-Schüller-Christian disease (C96.5)

histiocytic medullary reticulosis (C96.9)

histiocytic sarcoma (C96.A)

histiocytosis X, multifocal (C96.5)

histiocytosis X, unifocal (C96.6)

Langerhans-cell histiocytosis, multifocal (C96.5)

Langerhans-cell histiocytosis NOS (C96.6)

Langerhans-cell histiocytosis, unifocal (C96.6)

leukemic reticuloendotheliosis (C91.4-)

lipomelanotic reticulosis (I89.8)

malignant histiocytosis (C96.A)

malignant reticulosis (C86.0)

nonlipid reticuloendotheliosis (C96.0)

D76.1 **Hemophagocytic lymphohistiocytosis** [HCC]

Familial hemophagocytic reticulosis

Histiocytoses of mononuclear phagocytes

D76.2 **Hemophagocytic syndrome, infection-associated** [HCC]

Use Additional Code to identify infectious agent or disease.

D76.3 **Other histiocytosis syndromes** [HCC]

Reticulohistiocytoma (giant-cell)

Sinus histiocytosis with massive lymphadenopathy Xanthogranuloma

D77 **Other disorders of blood and blood-forming organs in diseases classified elsewhere**

Code first underlying disease, such as:

amyloidosis (E85.-)

congenital early syphilis (A50.0)

echinococcosis (B67.0-B67.9)

malaria (B50.0-B54)

schistosomiasis [bilharziasis] (B65.0-B65.9)

vitamin C deficiency (E54)

Excludes1: rupture of spleen due to Plasmodium vivax malaria (B51.0)

splenitis, splenomegaly in late syphilis (A52.79)

splenitis, splenomegaly in tuberculosis (A18.85)

INTRAOPERATIVE AND POSTPROCEDURAL COMPLICATIONS OF THE SPLEEN (D78)

D78 **Intraoperative and postprocedural complications of the spleen**

D78.0 **Intraoperative hemorrhage and hematoma of the spleen complicating a procedure**

Excludes1: intraoperative hemorrhage and hematoma of the spleen due to accidental puncture or laceration during a procedure (D78.1-)

D78.01 **Intraoperative hemorrhage and hematoma of the spleen complicating a procedure on the spleen**

D78.02 **Intraoperative hemorrhage and hematoma of the spleen complicating other procedure**

D78.1 **Accidental puncture and laceration of the spleen during a procedure**

D78.11 **Accidental puncture and laceration of the spleen during a procedure on the spleen**

D78.12 **Accidental puncture and laceration of the spleen during other procedure**

D78.2 **Postprocedural hemorrhage of the spleen following a procedure**

D78.21 **Postprocedural hemorrhage of the spleen following a procedure on the spleen**

D78.22 **Postprocedural hemorrhage of the spleen following other procedure**

D78.3 **Postprocedural hematoma and seroma of the spleen following a procedure**

D78.31 **Postprocedural hematoma of the spleen following a procedure on the spleen**

D78.32 **Postprocedural hematoma of the spleen following other procedure**

D78.33 **Postprocedural seroma of the spleen following a procedure on the spleen**

D78.34 **Postprocedural seroma of the spleen following other procedure**

D78.8 **Other intraoperative and postprocedural complications of the spleen**

Use Additional Code, if applicable, to further specify disorder

D78.81 **Other intraoperative complications of the spleen**

D78.89 **Other postprocedural complications of the spleen**

CERTAIN DISORDERS INVOLVING THE IMMUNE MECHANISM (D80-D89)

Includes: defects in the complement system

immunodeficiency disorders, except human immunodeficiency virus [HIV] disease sarcoidosis

Excludes1: autoimmune disease (systemic) NOS (M35.9)

functional disorders of polymorphonuclear neutrophils (D71)

human immunodeficiency virus [HIV] disease (B20)

D80 **Immunodeficiency with predominantly antibody defects**

D80.0 **Hereditary hypogammaglobulinemia** [HCC]

Autosomal recessive agammaglobulinemia (Swiss type)

X-linked agammaglobulinemia [Bruton] (with growth hormone deficiency)

D80.1 **Nonfamilial hypogammaglobulinemia** [HCC]

Agammaglobulinemia with immunoglobulin-bearing B-lymphocytes

Common variable agammaglobulinemia [CVA gamma]

Hypogammaglobulinemia NOS

D80.2 **Selective deficiency of immunoglobulin A [IgA]** [HCC]

D80.3 **Selective deficiency of immunoglobulin G [IgG] subclasses** [HCC]

D80.4 **Selective deficiency of immunoglobulin M [IgM]** [HCC]

D80.5 **Immunodeficiency with increased immunoglobulin M [IgM]** [HCC]

D80.6 **Antibody deficiency with near-normal immunoglobulins or with hyperimmunoglobulinemia** [HCC]

D80.7 **Transient hypogammaglobulinemia of infancy** [HCC]

D80.8 **Other immunodeficiencies with predominantly antibody defects** [HCC]

Kappa light chain deficiency

D80.9 **Immunodeficiency with predominantly antibody defects, unspecified** [HCC]

D81 **Combined immunodeficiencies**

Excludes1: autosomal recessive agammaglobulinemia (Swiss type) (D80.0)

D81.0 **Severe combined immunodeficiency [SCID] with reticular dysgenesis** [HCC]

D81.1 **Severe combined immunodeficiency [SCID] with low T- and B-cell numbers** [HCC]

D81.2 **Severe combined immunodeficiency [SCID] with low or normal B-cell numbers** [HCC]

D81.3 **Adenosine deaminase [ADA] deficiency** [HCC]

D81.30 **Adenosine deaminase deficiency, unspecified** [HCC]

ADA deficiency NOS

D81.31 **Severe combined immunodeficiency due to adenosine deaminase deficiency** [HCC]

ADA deficiency with SCID

Adenosine deaminase [ADA] deficiency with severe combined immunodeficiency

D81.32 **Adenosine deaminase 2 deficiency** [HCC]

ADA2 deficiency

Adenosine deaminase deficiency type 2

Code also, if applicable, any associated manifestations, such as:

polyarteritis nodosa (M30.0)

stroke (I63.-)

D81.39 **Other adenosine deaminase deficiency** [HCC]

Adenosine deaminase [ADA] deficiency type 1, NOS

Adenosine deaminase [ADA] deficiency type 1, without SCID

Adenosine deaminase [ADA] deficiency type 1, without severe combined immunodeficiency

Partial ADA deficiency (type 1)

Partial adenosine deaminase deficiency (type 1)

D81.4 **Nezelof's syndrome**

D81.5 **Purine nucleoside phosphorylase [PNP] deficiency** [HCC]

D81.6 **Major histocompatibility complex class I deficiency** [HCC]

Bare lymphocyte syndrome

D81.7 **Major histocompatibility complex class II deficiency** [HCC]

D81.8 **Other combined immunodeficiencies**

D81.81 **Biotin-dependent carboxylase deficiency**

Multiple carboxylase deficiency

Excludes1: biotin-dependent carboxylase deficiency due to dietary deficiency of biotin (E53.8)

D81.810 **Biotinidase deficiency**

D81.818 **Other biotin-dependent carboxylase deficiency**

Holocarboxylase synthetase deficiency

Other multiple carboxylase deficiency

D81.819 **Biotin-dependent carboxylase deficiency, unspecified**

Multiple carboxylase deficiency, unspecified

D81.89 **Other combined immunodeficiencies** [HCC]

D81.9 **Combined immunodeficiency, unspecified** [HCC]

Severe combined immunodeficiency disorder [SCID] NOS

D82 **Immunodeficiency associated with other major defects**

Excludes1: ataxia telangiectasia [Louis-Bar] (G11.3)

D82.0 **Wiskott-Aldrich syndrome** [HCC]

Immunodeficiency with thrombocytopenia and eczema

D82.1 **Di George's syndrome** [HCC]

Pharyngeal pouch syndrome

Thymic alymphoplasia

Thymic aplasia or hypoplasia with immunodeficiency

D82.2 **Immunodeficiency with short-limbed stature** [HCC]

D82.3 **Immunodeficiency following hereditary defective response to Epstein-Barr virus** [HCC]

X-linked lymphoproliferative disease

D82.4 **Hyperimmunoglobulin E [IgE] syndrome** [HCC]

D82.8 **Immunodeficiency associated with other specified major defects** [HCC]

D82.9 **Immunodeficiency associated with major defect, unspecified** [HCC]

D83 **Common variable immunodeficiency**

D83.0 **Common variable immunodeficiency with predominant abnormalities of B-cell numbers and function** [HCC]

D83.1 **Common variable immunodeficiency with predominant immunoregulatory T-cell disorders** [HCC]

D83.2 **Common variable immunodeficiency with autoantibodies to B- or T-cells** [HCC]

D83.8 **Other common variable immunodeficiencies** [HCC]

D83.9 **Common variable immunodeficiency, unspecified** [HCC]

D84 **Other immunodeficiencies**

D84.0 **Lymphocyte function antigen-1[LFA-1] defect** [HCC]

D84.1 **Defects in the complement system** [HCC]

C1 esterase inhibitor [C1-INH] deficiency

D84.8 **Other specified immunodeficiencies** [HCC]

Code first underlying condition, such as:

chromosomal abnormalities (Q90-Q99)

diabetes mellitus (E08-E13)

malignant neoplasms (C00-C96)

Excludes1: certain disorders involving the immune mechanism (D80-D83, D84.0, D84.1,D84.9)

human immunodeficiency virus [HIV] disease (B20)

D84.82 **Immunodeficiency due to drugs and external causes**

D84.821 **Immunodeficiency due to drugs**

Immunodeficiency due to (current or past) medication

Use Additional Code for adverse effect if applicable, to identify adverse effect of drug (T36-T50 with fifth or six character 5)

Use Additional Code, if applicable, for associated long term (current) drug therapy drug or medication such as:

long term (current) drug therapy systemic steroids (Z79.52)

other long term (current) drug therapy (Z79.899)

D84.822 **Immunodeficiency due to external causes**

Code also, if applicable, radiological procedure and radiotherapy (Y84.2)

Use Additional Code for external cause such as:

exposure to ionizing radiation (W88)

D84.89 **Other immunodeficiencies** [HCC]

D84.9 **Immunodeficiency, unspecified** [HCC]

Immunocompromised NOS

Immunodeficient NOS

Immunosuppressed NOS

D86   **Sarcoidosis**

D86.0   **Sarcoidosis of lung** [HCC]

D86.1   **Sarcoidosis of lymph nodes**

D86.2   **Sarcoidosis of lung with sarcoidosis of lymph nodes** [HCC]

D86.3   **Sarcoidosis of skin**

D86.8   **Sarcoidosis of other sites**

D86.81   **Sarcoid meningitis**

D86.82   **Multiple cranial nerve palsies in sarcoidosis** [HCC]

D86.83   **Sarcoid iridocyclitis**

D86.84   **Sarcoid pyelonephritis**

Tubulo-interstitial nephropathy in sarcoidosis

D86.85   **Sarcoid myocarditis**

D86.86   **Sarcoid arthropathy**

Polyarthritis in sarcoidosis

D86.87   **Sarcoid myositis**

D86.89   **Sarcoidosis of other sites**

Hepatic granuloma

Uveoparotid fever [Heerfordt]

D86.9   **Sarcoidosis, unspecified**

D89   **Other disorders involving the immune mechanism, not elsewhere classified**

Excludes1: hyperglobulinemia NOS (R77.1)

monoclonal gammopathy (of undetermined significance) (D47.2)

Excludes2: transplant failure and rejection (T86.-)

D89.0   **Polyclonal hypergammaglobulinemia**

Benign hypergammaglobulinemic purpura

Polyclonal gammopathy NOS

D89.1   **Cryoglobulinemia** [HCC]

Cryoglobulinemic purpura

Cryoglobulinemic vasculitis

Essential cryoglobulinemia

Idiopathic cryoglobulinemia

Mixed cryoglobulinemia

Primary cryoglobulinemia

Secondary cryoglobulinemia

D89.2   **Hypergammaglobulinemia, unspecified**

D89.3   **Immune reconstitution syndrome** [HCC]

Immune reconstitution inflammatory syndrome [IRIS]

Use Additional Code for adverse effect, if applicable, to identify drug (T36-T50 with fifth or sixth character 5)

D89.4   **Mast cell activation syndrome and related disorders**

Excludes1: aggressive systemic mastocytosis (C96.21)

congenital cutaneous mastocytosis (Q82.2)

(non-congenital) cutaneous mastocytosis (D47.01)

(indolent) systemic mastocytosis (D47.02)

malignant mast cell neoplasm (C96.2-)

malignant mastocytoma (C96.29)

mast cell leukemia (C94.3-)

mast cell sarcoma (C96.22)

mastocytoma NOS (D47.09)

other mast cell neoplasms of uncertain behavior (D47.09)systemic mastocytosis associated with a clonal hematologic non-mast cell lineage disease (SM-AHNMD) (D47.02)

D89.40   **Mast cell activation, unspecified** [HCC]

Mast cell activation disorder, unspecified

Mast cell activation syndrome, NOS

D89.41   **Monoclonal mast cell activation syndrome** [HCC]

D89.42   **Idiopathic mast cell activation syndrome** [HCC]

D89.43   **Secondary mast cell activation** [HCC]

Secondary mast cell activation syndrome

Code also underlying etiology, if known

• **D89.44**   **Hereditary alpha tryptasemia**

Use Additional Code, if applicable, for:

allergy status, other than to drugs and biological substances (Z91.0-)

personal history of anaphylaxis (Z87.892)

D89.49   **Other mast cell activation disorder** [HCC]

Other mast cell activation syndrome

D89.8   **Other specified disorders involving the immune mechanism, not elsewhere classified**

D89.81   **Graft-versus-host disease**

Code first underlying cause, such as:

complications of transplanted organs and tissue (T86.-)

complications of blood transfusion (T80.89)

Use Additional Code to identify associated manifestations, such as:

desquamative dermatitis (L30.8)

diarrhea (R19.7)

elevated bilirubin (R17)

hair loss (L65.9)

D89.810   **Acute graft-versus-host disease** [HCC]

D89.811   **Chronic graft-versus-host disease** [HCC]

D89.812   **Acute on chronic graft-versus-host disease** [HCC]

D89.813   **Graft-versus-host disease, unspecified** [HCC]

D89.82   **Autoimmune lymphoproliferative syndrome [ALPS]** [HCC]

D89.89   **Other specified disorders involving the immune mechanism, not elsewhere classified** [HCC]

Excludes1: human immunodeficiency virus disease (B20)

D89.83   **Cytokine release syndrome**

Code first underlying cause, such as:

complications following infusion, transfusion and therapeutic injection (T80.89-)

complications of transplanted organs and tissue (T86.-)

Use Additional Code to identify associated manifestations

D89.831   **Cytokine release syndrome, grade 1**

D89.832   **Cytokine release syndrome, grade 2**

D89.833   **Cytokine release syndrome, grade 3**

D89.834   **Cytokine release syndrome, grade 4**

D89.835   **Cytokine release syndrome, grade 5**

D89.839   **Cytokine release syndrome, grade unspecified**

D89.9   **Disorder involving the immune mechanism, unspecified** [HCC]

Immune disease NOS

● New code   ▲ Revised code   **Excludes1:** Not coded here   **Excludes2:** Not included here   ⊗ Placeholder required   ⑦7th digit required

Chapter 4: Endocrine, Nutritional and Metabolic Diseases (E00-E89)

DEFINITIONS

This chapter includes definitions of selected key words, terms and phrases and coding alerts for adding points to the clinical domain, and references to coding late effects where appropriate. An example from this chapter is as follows:

 E20 Hypoparathyroidism

Definition: Parathyroid glands are small endocrine glands in the neck that produce parathyroid hormone. Humans have four parathyroid glands, which are usually located behind the thyroid gland.

MULTIPLE CODING FOR A SINGLE CONDITION

In addition to the etiology/manifestation convention that requires two codes to fully describe a single condition that affects multiple body systems, there are other single conditions that also require more than one code. "**Use Additional Code**" notes are found in the Tabular List at codes that are not part of an etiology/manifestation pair where a secondary code is useful to fully describe a condition. The sequencing rule is the same as the etiology/manifestation pair, "**Use Additional Code**" indicates that a secondary code should be added.

For example, for bacterial infections that are not included in chapter 1, a secondary code from category B95, Streptococcus, Staphylococcus, and Enterococcus, as the cause of diseases classified elsewhere, or B96, Other bacterial agents as the cause of diseases classified elsewhere, may be required to identify the bacterial organism causing the infection. A "**Use Additional Code**" note will normally be found at the infectious disease code, indicating a need for the organism code to be added as a secondary code.

 "Code first" notes are also under certain codes that are not specifically manifestation codes but may be due to an underlying cause. When there is a "Code first" note and an underlying condition is present, the underlying condition should be sequenced first.

"Code, if applicable, any causal condition first", notes indicate that this code may be assigned as a principal diagnosis when the causal condition is unknown or not applicable. If a causal condition is known, then the code for that condition should be sequenced as the principal or first-listed diagnosis.

Multiple codes may be needed for sequela, complication codes and obstetric codes to more fully describe a condition. See the specific guidelines for these conditions for further instruction.

COMBINATION CODE

A combination code is a single code used to classify: Two diagnoses, or a diagnosis with an associated secondary process (manifestation) A diagnosis with an associated complication

Combination codes are identified by referring to subterm entries in the Alphabetic Index and by reading the inclusion and exclusion notes in the Tabular List.

Assign only the combination code when that code fully identifies the diagnostic conditions involved or when the Alphabetic Index so directs. Multiple coding should not be used when the classification provides a combination code that clearly identifies all of the elements documented in the diagnosis. When the combination code lacks necessary specificity in describing the manifestation or complication, an additional code should be used as a secondary code.

SEQUELA (LATE EFFECTS)

A sequela is the residual effect (condition produced) after the acute phase of an illness or injury has terminated. There is no time limit on when a sequela code can be used. The residual may be apparent early, such as in cerebral infarction, or it may occur months or years later, such as that due to a previous injury. Coding of sequela generally requires two codes sequenced in the following order: The condition or nature of the sequela is sequenced first.

The sequela code is sequenced second.

An exception to the above guidelines are those instances where the code for the sequela is followed by a manifestation code identified in the Tabular List and title, or the sequela code has been expanded (at the fourth, fifth or sixth character levels) to include the manifestation(s). The code for the acute phase of an illness or injury that led to the sequela is never used with a code for the late effect.

DIABETES MELLITUS

The diabetes mellitus codes are combination codes that include the type of diabetes mellitus, the body system affected, and the complications affecting that body system. As many codes within a particular category as are necessary to describe all of the complications of the disease may be used. They should be sequenced based on the reason for a particular encounter. Assign as many codes from categories E08 – E13 as needed to identify all of the associated conditions that the patient has.

1) **Type of diabetes**

   The age of a patient is not the sole determining factor, though most type 1 diabetics develop the condition before reaching puberty. For this reason, type 1 diabetes mellitus is also referred to as juvenile diabetes.

2) **Type of diabetes mellitus not documented**

   If the type of diabetes mellitus is not documented in the medical record the default is E11.-, Type 2 diabetes mellitus.

3) **Diabetes mellitus and the use of insulin, oral hypoglycemics, and injectable non-insulin drugs**

   If the documentation in a medical record does not indicate the type of diabetes but does indicate that the patient uses insulin, code E11-, Type 2diabetes mellitus, should be assigned. Additional code(s) should be assigned from category Z79 to identify the long-term (current) use of insulin, oral hypoglycemic drugs, or injectable non-insulin antidiabetic, as follows:

   If the patient is treated with both oral medications and insulin, both codeZ79.4, Long term (current) use of insulin, and code Z79.84, Long term (current) use of oral hypoglycemic drugs, should be assigned.

   If the patient is treated with both insulin and an injectable non-insulin antidiabetic drug, assign codes Z79.4, Long term (current) use of insulin,and Z79.899, Other long term (current) drug therapy.

   If the patient is treated with both oral hypoglycemic drugs and an injectable non-insulin antidiabetic drug, assign codes Z79.84, Long term(current) use of oral hypoglycemic drugs, and Z79.899, Other long term(current) drug therapy.

   Code Z79.4 should not be assigned if insulin is given temporarily to bring a type 2 patient's blood sugar under control during an encounter.

4) **Diabetes mellitus in pregnancy and gestational diabetes**

   See Section I.C.15. Diabetes mellitus in pregnancy.

   See Section I.C.15. Gestational (pregnancy induced) diabetes

5) **Complications due to insulin pump malfunction**

   (a) Underdose of insulin due to insulin pump failure

   An underdose of insulin due to an insulin pump failure should be assigned to a code from subcategory T85.6, Mechanical complication of other specified internal and external prosthetic devices, implants and grafts, that specifies the type of pump malfunction, as the principal or first-listed code, followed by code T38.3X6-, Underdosing of insulin and oral hypoglycemic [antidiabetic] drugs. Additional codes for the type of diabetes mellitus and any associated complications due to the underdosing should also be assigned.

   (b) Overdose of insulin due to insulin pump failure

● New code   ▲ Revised code   **Excludes1:** Not coded here   **Excludes2:** Not included here   ⊗ Placeholder required   ⑦7ᵗʰ digit required

The principal or first-listed code for an encounter due to an insulin pump malfunction resulting in an overdose of insulin, should also be T85.6-, Mechanical complication of other specified internal and external prosthetic devices, implants and grafts, followed by code T38.3X1-, Poisoning by insulin and oral hypoglycemic [antidiabetic] drugs, accidental (unintentional).

6) **Secondary diabetes mellitus**

Codes under categories E08, Diabetes mellitus due to underlying condition, E09, Drug or chemical induced diabetes mellitus, and E13, Other specified diabetes mellitus, identify complications/manifestations associated with secondary diabetes mellitus. Secondary diabetes is always caused by another condition or event (e.g., cystic fibrosis, malignant neoplasm of pancreas, pancreatectomy, adverse effect of drug, or poisoning).

(a) **Secondary diabetes mellitus and the use of insulin or oral hypoglycemic drugs**

For patients with secondary diabetes mellitus who routinely useinsulin, oral hypoglycemic drugs, or injectable non-insulin drugs, additional code(s) from category Z79 should be assignedto identify the long-term (current) use of insulin, oral hypoglycemic drugs, or non-injectable non-insulin drugs as follows:

If the patient is treated with both oral medications and insulin,both code Z79.4, Long term (current) use of insulin, and code Z79.84, Long term (current) use of oral hypoglycemic drugs, should be assigned.

If the patient is treated with both insulin and an injectable non- insulin antidiabetic drug, assign codes Z79.4, Long- term (current) use of insulin, and Z79.899, Other long term(current) drug therapy.

If the patient is treated with both oral hypoglycemic drugs and an injectable non-insulin antidiabetic drug, assign codes Z79.84, Long-term (current) use of oral hypoglycemic drugs,and Z79.899, Other long-term (current) drug therapy.

Code Z79.4 should not be assigned if insulin is given temporarily to bring a secondary diabetic patient's blood sugar under control during an encounter.

(b) Assigning and sequencing secondary diabetes codes and its causes

The sequencing of the secondary diabetes codes in relationship to codes for the cause of the diabetes is based on the Tabular List instructions for categories E08, E09 and E13.

(i) Secondary diabetes mellitus due to pancreatectomy

For postpancreatectomy diabetes mellitus (lack of insulin due to the surgical removal of all or part of the pancreas), assign code E89.1, Postprocedural hypoinsulinemia. Assign a code from category E13 and a code from subcategory Z90.41, Acquired absence of pancreas, as additional codes.

(ii) Secondary diabetes due to drugs

Secondary diabetes may be caused by an adverse effect of correctly administered medications, poisoning or sequela of poisoning.

See section I.C.19.e for coding of adverse effects and poisoning, and section I.C.20 for external cause code reporting.

● New code   ▲ Revised code   Excludes1: Not coded here   Excludes2: Not included here   ⊗ Placeholder required   ⑦7th digit required

Chapter 4

Endocrine, Nutritional and Metabolic Diseases (E00-E89)

Note: All neoplasms, whether functionally active or not, are classified in Chapter 2. Appropriate codes in this chapter (i.e., E05.8, E07.0, E16-E31, E34.-) may be used as additional codes to indicate either functional activity by neoplasms and ectopic endocrine tissue or hyperfunction and hypofunction of endocrine glands associated with neoplasms and other conditions classified elsewhere.

Excludes1: transitory endocrine and metabolic disorders specific to newborn (P70-P74)

This chapter contains the following blocks:

E00-E07	Disorders of thyroid gland
E08-E13	Diabetes mellitus
E15-E16	Other disorders of glucose regulation and pancreatic internal secretion
E20-E35	Disorders of other endocrine glands
E36	Intraoperative complications of endocrine system
E40-E46	Malnutrition
E50-E64	Other nutritional deficiencies
E65-E68	Overweight, obesity and other hyperalimentation
E70-E88	Metabolic disorders
E89	Postprocedural endocrine and metabolic complications and disorders, not elsewhere classified

DISORDERS OF THYROID GLAND (E00-E07)

E00 **Congenital iodine-deficiency syndrome**

Use Additional Code (F70-F79) to identify associated intellectual disabilities.

Excludes1: subclinical iodine-deficiency hypothyroidism (E02)

E00.0 **Congenital iodine-deficiency syndrome, neurological type**

Endemic cretinism, neurological type

E00.1 **Congenital iodine-deficiency syndrome, myxedematous type**

Endemic hypothyroid cretinism

Endemic cretinism, myxedematous type

E00.2 **Congenital iodine-deficiency syndrome, mixed type**

Endemic cretinism, mixed type

E00.9 **Congenital iodine-deficiency syndrome, unspecified**

Congenital iodine-deficiency hypothyroidism NOS

Endemic cretinism NOS

E01 **Iodine-deficiency related thyroid disorders and allied conditions**

Excludes1: congenital iodine-deficiency syndrome (E00.-)

subclinical iodine-deficiency hypothyroidism (E02)

E01.0 **Iodine-deficiency related diffuse (endemic) goiter**

E01.1 **Iodine-deficiency related multinodular (endemic) goiter**

Iodine-deficiency related nodular goiter

E01.2 **Iodine-deficiency related (endemic) goiter, unspecified**

Endemic goiter NOS

E01.8 **Other iodine-deficiency related thyroid disorders and allied conditions**

Acquired iodine-deficiency hypothyroidism NOS

E02 **Subclinical iodine-deficiency hypothyroidism**

E03 **Other hypothyroidism**

Excludes1: iodine-deficiency related hypothyroidism (E00-E02)

postprocedural hypothyroidism (E89.0)

E03.0 **Congenital hypothyroidism with diffuse goiter**

Congenital parenchymatous goiter (nontoxic)

Congenital goiter (nontoxic) NOS

Excludes1: transitory congenital goiter with normal function (P72.0)

E03.1 **Congenital hypothyroidism without goiter**

Aplasia of thyroid (with myxedema)

Congenital atrophy of thyroid

Congenital hypothyroidism NOS

E03.2 **Hypothyroidism due to medicaments and other exogenous substances**

Code first poisoning due to drug or toxin, if applicable (T36-T65 with fifth or sixth character 1-4 or 6)

Use Additional Code for adverse effect, if applicable, to identify drug (T36-T50 with fifth or sixth character 5)

E03.3 **Postinfectious hypothyroidism**

E03.4 **Atrophy of thyroid (acquired)**

Excludes1: congenital atrophy of thyroid (E03.1)

E03.5 **Myxedema coma** [HCC]

E03.8 **Other specified hypothyroidism**

E03.9 **Hypothyroidism, unspecified**

Myxedema NOS

E04 **Other nontoxic goiter**

Definition: Nontoxic nodular goiter is a type of simple goiter with enlargement caused by nodules, or lumps, on the thyroid.

Excludes1: congenital goiter (NOS) (diffuse) (parenchymatous) (E03.0)

iodine-deficiency related goiter (E00-E02)

E04.0 **Nontoxic diffuse goiter**

Diffuse (colloid) nontoxic goiter

Simple nontoxic goiter

E04.1 **Nontoxic single thyroid nodule**

Colloid nodule (cystic) (thyroid)

Nontoxic uninodular goiter

Thyroid (cystic) nodule NOS

E04.2 **Nontoxic multinodular goiter**

Cystic goiter NOS

Multinodular (cystic) goiter NOS

E04.8 **Other specified nontoxic goiter**

E04.9 **Nontoxic goiter, unspecified**

Goiter NOS

Nodular goiter (nontoxic) NOS

E05 **Thyrotoxicosis [hyperthyroidism]**

Definition: Thyrotoxicosis with or without goiter is a condition resulting from excessive concentrations of thyroid hormones in the body, as in hyperthyroidism.

Excludes1: chronic thyroiditis with transient thyrotoxicosis (E06.2)

neonatal thyrotoxicosis (P72.1)

E05.0 **Thyrotoxicosis with diffuse goiter**

Exophthalmic or toxic goiter NOS Graves' disease

Toxic diffuse goiter

E05.00 **Thyrotoxicosis with diffuse goiter without thyrotoxic crisis or storm**

E05.01 **Thyrotoxicosis with diffuse goiter with thyrotoxic crisis or storm**

E05.1 **Thyrotoxicosis with toxic single thyroid nodule**

Thyrotoxicosis with toxic uninodular goiter

E05.10 **Thyrotoxicosis with toxic single thyroid nodule without thyrotoxic crisis or storm**

E05.11 **Thyrotoxicosis with toxic single thyroid nodule with thyrotoxic crisis or storm**

E05.2 **Thyrotoxicosis with toxic multinodular goiter**

Toxic nodular goiter NOS

    E05.20 **Thyrotoxicosis with toxic multinodular goiter without thyrotoxic crisis or storm**

    E05.21 **Thyrotoxicosis with toxic multinodular goiter with thyrotoxic crisis or storm**

E05.3 **Thyrotoxicosis from ectopic thyroid tissue**

    E05.30 **Thyrotoxicosis from ectopic thyroid tissue without thyrotoxic crisis or storm**

    E05.31 **Thyrotoxicosis from ectopic thyroid tissue with thyrotoxic crisis or storm**

E05.4 **Thyrotoxicosis factitia**

    E05.40 **Thyrotoxicosis factitia without thyrotoxic crisis or storm**

    E05.41 **Thyrotoxicosis factitia with thyrotoxic crisis or storm**

E05.8 **Other thyrotoxicosis**

Overproduction of thyroid-stimulating hormone

    E05.80 **Other thyrotoxicosis without thyrotoxic crisis or storm**

    E05.81 **Other thyrotoxicosis with thyrotoxic crisis or storm**

E05.9 **Thyrotoxicosis, unspecified**

Hyperthyroidism NOS

    E05.90 **Thyrotoxicosis, unspecified without thyrotoxic crisis or storm**

    E05.91 **Thyrotoxicosis, unspecified with thyrotoxic crisis or storm**

E06 **Thyroiditis**

Excludes1: postpartum thyroiditis (O90.5)

E06.0 **Acute thyroiditis**

Abscess of thyroid

Pyogenic thyroiditis

Suppurative thyroiditis

Use Additional Code (B95-B97) to identify infectious agent.

E06.1 **Subacute thyroiditis**

de Quervain thyroiditis

Giant-cell thyroiditis

Granulomatous thyroiditis

Nonsuppurative thyroiditis

Viral thyroiditis

Excludes1: autoimmune thyroiditis (E06.3)

E06.2 **Chronic thyroiditis with transient thyrotoxicosis**

Excludes1: autoimmune thyroiditis (E06.3)

E06.3 **Autoimmune thyroiditis**

Hashimoto's thyroiditis

Hashitoxicosis (transient)

Lymphadenoid goiter

Lymphocytic thyroiditis

Struma lymphomatosa

E06.4 **Drug-induced thyroiditis**

Use Additional Code for adverse effect, if applicable, to identify drug (T36-T50 with fifth or sixth character 5)

E06.5 **Other chronic thyroiditis**

Chronic fibrous thyroiditis

Chronic thyroiditis NOS

Ligneous thyroiditis

Riedel thyroiditis

E06.9 **Thyroiditis, unspecified**

E07 **Other disorders of thyroid**

E07.0 **Hypersecretion of calcitonin**

C-cell hyperplasia of thyroid

Hypersecretion of thyrocalcitonin

E07.1 **Dyshormogenetic goiter**

Familial Dyshormogenetic goiter

Pendred's syndrome

Excludes1: transitory congenital goiter with normal function (P72.0)

E07.8 **Other specified disorders of thyroid**

    E07.81 **Sick-euthyroid syndrome**

Euthyroid sick-syndrome

    E07.89 **Other specified disorders of thyroid**

Abnormality of thyroid-binding globulin

Hemorrhage of thyroid

Infarction of thyroid

E07.9 **Disorder of thyroid, unspecified**

DIABETES MELLITUS (E08-E13)

Definition: Diabetes mellitus is a condition in which the pancreas no longer produces enough insulin or cells stop responding to the insulin that is produced, so that glucose in the blood cannot be absorbed into the cells of the body. Symptoms include frequent urination, lethargy, excessive thirst, and hunger.

E08 **Diabetes mellitus due to underlying condition**

Code first the underlying condition, such as:

congenital rubella (P35.0)

Cushing's syndrome (E24.-)

cystic fibrosis (E84.-)

malignant neoplasm (C00-C96)

malnutrition (E40-E46)

pancreatitis **and other** diseases of the pancreas (K85-K86.-)

Use Additional Code to identify control using:

insulin (Z79.4)

oral antidiabetic drugs (Z79.84)

oral hypoglycemic drugs (Z79.84)

Excludes1: drug or chemical induced diabetes mellitus (E09.-)

gestational diabetes (O24.4-)

neonatal diabetes mellitus (P70.2)

postpancreatectomy diabetes mellitus (E13.-)

postprocedural diabetes mellitus (E13.-)

secondary diabetes mellitus NEC (E13.-)

type 1 diabetes mellitus (E10.-)

type 2 diabetes mellitus (E11.-)

E08.0 **Diabetes mellitus due to underlying condition with hyperosmolarity**

    E08.00 **Diabetes mellitus due to underlying condition with hyperosmolarity without nonketotic** [HCC] hyperglycemic-hyperosmolar coma (NKHHC)

    E08.01 **Diabetes mellitus due to underlying condition with hyperosmolarity with coma** [HCC]

E08.1 **Diabetes mellitus due to underlying condition with ketoacidosis**

    E08.10 **Diabetes mellitus due to underlying condition with ketoacidosis without coma** [HCC]

   ● New code   ▲ Revised code   Excludes1: Not coded here   Excludes2: Not included here   ⊗ Placeholder required   ⑦ 7th digit required

E08.11   Diabetes mellitus due to underlying condition with ketoacidosis with coma [HCC]

E08.2   **Diabetes mellitus due to underlying condition with kidney complications**

E08.21   Diabetes mellitus due to underlying condition with diabetic nephropathy [HCC]

Diabetes mellitus due to underlying condition with intercapillary glomerulosclerosis

Diabetes mellitus due to underlying condition with intracapillary glomerulonephrosis

Diabetes mellitus due to underlying condition with Kimmelstiel-Wilson disease

E08.22   Diabetes mellitus due to underlying condition with diabetic chronic kidney disease [HCC]

Use Additional Code to identify stage of chronic kidney disease (N18.1-N18.6)

E08.29   Diabetes mellitus due to underlying condition with other diabetic kidney complication [HCC]

Renal tubular degeneration in diabetes mellitus due to underlying condition

E08.3   **Diabetes mellitus due to underlying condition with ophthalmic complications**

E08.31   Diabetes mellitus due to underlying condition with unspecified diabetic retinopathy

E08.311   Diabetes mellitus due to underlying condition with unspecified diabetic retinopathy with macular edema [HCC]

E08.319   Diabetes mellitus due to underlying condition with unspecified diabetic retinopathy without macular edema [HCC]

E08.32   Diabetes mellitus due to underlying condition with mild nonproliferative diabetic retinopathy

Diabetes mellitus due to underlying condition with nonproliferative diabetic retinopathy NOS

One of the following 7th characters is to be assigned to codes in subcategory E08.32 to designate laterality of the disease:

1 - right eye

2 - left eye

3 – bilateral

9 - unspecified eye

⑦E08.321   Diabetes mellitus due to underlying condition with mild nonproliferative diabetic retinopathy with macular edema [HCC]

⑦E08.329   Diabetes mellitus due to underlying condition with mild nonproliferative diabetic retinopathy without macular edema [HCC]

E08.33   Diabetes mellitus due to underlying condition with moderate nonproliferative diabetic retinopathy

One of the following 7th characters is to be assigned to codes in subcategory E08.33 to designate laterality of the disease:

1 - right eye

2 - left eye

3 - bilateral

9 - unspecified eye

⑦E08.331   Diabetes mellitus due to underlying condition with moderate nonproliferative diabetic retinopathy with macular edema [HCC]

⑦E08.339   Diabetes mellitus due to underlying condition with moderate nonproliferative diabetic retinopathy without macular edema [HCC]

E08.34   Diabetes mellitus due to underlying condition with severe nonproliferative diabetic retinopathy

One of the following 7th characters is to be assigned to codes in subcategory E08.34 to designate laterality of the disease:

1 - right eye

2 - left eye

3 - bilateral

9 - unspecified eye

⑦E08.341   Diabetes mellitus due to underlying condition with severe nonproliferative diabetic retinopathy with macular edema [HCC]

⑦E08.349   Diabetes mellitus due to underlying condition with severe nonproliferative diabetic retinopathy without macular edema [HCC]

E08.35   Diabetes mellitus due to underlying condition with proliferative diabetic retinopathy

One of the following 7th characters is to be assigned to codes in subcategory E08.35 to designate laterality of the disease:

1 - right eye

2 - left eye

3 - bilateral

9 - unspecified eye

⑦E08.351   Diabetes mellitus due to underlying condition with proliferative diabetic retinopathy with macular edema [HCC]

⑦E08.352   Diabetes mellitus due to underlying condition with proliferative diabetic retinopathy with traction retinal detachment involving the macula [HCC]

⑦E08.353   Diabetes mellitus due to underlying condition with proliferative diabetic retinopathy with traction retinal detachment not involving the macula [HCC]

⑦E08.354   Diabetes mellitus due to underlying condition with proliferative diabetic retinopathy with combined traction retinal detachment and rhegmatogenous retinal detachment [HCC]

⑦E08.355   Diabetes mellitus due to underlying condition with stable proliferative diabetic retinopathy [HCC]

⑦E08.359   Diabetes mellitus due to underlying condition with proliferative diabetic retinopathy without macular edema [HCC]

E08.36   Diabetes mellitus due to underlying condition with diabetic cataract [HCC]

⊗⑦E08.37   Diabetes mellitus due to underlying condition with diabetic macular edema, resolved following treatment [HCC]

One of the following 7th characters is to be assigned to code E08.37 to designate laterality of the disease:

1 - right eye

2 - left eye

---

3 - bilateral

9 - unspecified eye

E08.39 **Diabetes mellitus due to underlying condition with other diabetic ophthalmic complication** [HCC]

Use Additional Code to identify manifestation, such as:

diabetic glaucoma (H40-H42)

E08.4 **Diabetes mellitus due to underlying condition with neurological complications**

E08.40 **Diabetes mellitus due to underlying condition with diabetic neuropathy, unspecified** [HCC]

E08.41 **Diabetes mellitus due to underlying condition with diabetic mononeuropathy** [HCC]

E08.42 **Diabetes mellitus due to underlying condition with diabetic polyneuropathy** [HCC]

Diabetes mellitus due to underlying condition with diabetic neuralgia

E08.43 **Diabetes mellitus due to underlying condition with diabetic autonomic (poly)neuropathy** [HCC]

Diabetes mellitus due to underlying condition with diabetic gastroparesis

E08.44 **Diabetes mellitus due to underlying condition with diabetic amyotrophy** [HCC]

E08.49 **Diabetes mellitus due to underlying condition with other diabetic neurological complication** [HCC]

E08.5 **Diabetes mellitus due to underlying condition with circulatory complications**

E08.51 **Diabetes mellitus due to underlying condition with diabetic peripheral angiopathy without gangrene** [HCC]

E08.52 **Diabetes mellitus due to underlying condition with diabetic peripheral angiopathy with gangrene** [HCC]

Diabetes mellitus due to underlying condition with diabetic gangrene

E08.59 **Diabetes mellitus due to underlying condition with other circulatory complications** [HCC]

E08.6 **Diabetes mellitus due to underlying condition with other specified complications**

E08.61 **Diabetes mellitus due to underlying condition with diabetic arthropathy**

E08.610 **Diabetes mellitus due to underlying condition with diabetic neuropathic arthropathy** [HCC]

Diabetes mellitus due to underlying condition with Charcôt's joints

E08.618 **Diabetes mellitus due to underlying condition with other diabetic arthropathy** [HCC]

E08.62 **Diabetes mellitus due to underlying condition with skin complications**

E08.620 **Diabetes mellitus due to underlying condition with diabetic dermatitis** [HCC]

Diabetes mellitus due to underlying condition with diabetic necrobiosis lipoidica

E08.621 **Diabetes mellitus due to underlying condition with foot ulcer** [HCC]

Use Additional Code to identify site of ulcer (L97.4-, L97.5-)

E08.622 **Diabetes mellitus due to underlying condition with other skin ulcer** [HCC]

Use Additional Code to identify site of ulcer (L97.1-L97.9, L98.41-L98.49)

E08.628 **Diabetes mellitus due to underlying condition with other skin complications** [HCC]

E08.63 **Diabetes mellitus due to underlying condition with oral complications**

E08.630 **Diabetes mellitus due to underlying condition with periodontal disease** [HCC]

E08.638 **Diabetes mellitus due to underlying condition with other oral complications** [HCC]

E08.64 **Diabetes mellitus due to underlying condition with hypoglycemia**

E08.641 **Diabetes mellitus due to underlying condition with hypoglycemia with coma** [HCC]

E08.649 **Diabetes mellitus due to underlying condition with hypoglycemia without coma** [HCC]

E08.65 **Diabetes mellitus due to underlying condition with hyperglycemia** [HCC]

E08.69 **Diabetes mellitus due to underlying condition with other specified complication** [HCC]

Use Additional Code to identify complication

E08.8 **Diabetes mellitus due to underlying condition with unspecified complications** [HCC]

E08.9 **Diabetes mellitus due to underlying condition without complications** [HCC]

E09 **Drug or chemical induced diabetes mellitus**

Code first poisoning due to drug or toxin, if applicable (T36-T65 with fifth or sixth character 1-4 or 6)

Use Additional Code for adverse effect, if applicable, to identify drug (T36-T50 with fifth or sixth character 5)

Use Additional Code to identify control using:

insulin (Z79.4)

oral antidiabetic drugs (Z79.84)

oral hypoglycemic drugs (Z79.84)

Excludes1: diabetes mellitus due to underlying condition (E08.-)

gestational diabetes (O24.4-)

neonatal diabetes mellitus (P70.2)

postpancreatectomy diabetes mellitus (E13.-)

postprocedural diabetes mellitus (E13.-)

secondary diabetes mellitus NEC (E13.-)

type 1 diabetes mellitus (E10.-)

type 2 diabetes mellitus (E11.-)

E09.0 **Drug or chemical induced diabetes mellitus with hyperosmolarity**

E09.00 **Drug or chemical induced diabetes mellitus with hyperosmolarity without nonketotic hyperglycemic-hyperosmolar coma (NKHHC)** [HCC]

E09.01 **Drug or chemical induced diabetes mellitus with hyperosmolarity with coma** [HCC]

E09.1 **Drug or chemical induced diabetes mellitus with ketoacidosis**

E09.10 **Drug or chemical induced diabetes mellitus with ketoacidosis without coma** [HCC]

E09.11 **Drug or chemical induced diabetes mellitus with ketoacidosis with coma** [HCC]

E09.2 **Drug or chemical induced diabetes mellitus with kidney complications**

● New code   ▲ Revised code   **Excludes1:** Not coded here   **Excludes2:** Not included here   ⊗ Placeholder required   ⑦ 7th digit required

E09.21 **Drug or chemical induced diabetes mellitus with diabetic nephropathy** [HCC]

Drug or chemical induced diabetes mellitus with intercapillary glomerulosclerosis

Drug or chemical induced diabetes mellitus with intracapillary glomerulonephrosis

Drug or chemical induced diabetes mellitus with Kimmelstiel-Wilson disease

E09.22 **Drug or chemical induced diabetes mellitus with diabetic chronic kidney disease** [HCC]

Use Additional Code to identify stage of chronic kidney disease (N18.1-N18.6)

E09.29 **Drug or chemical induced diabetes mellitus with other diabetic kidney complication** [HCC]

Drug or chemical induced diabetes mellitus with renal tubular degeneration

E09.3 **Drug or chemical induced diabetes mellitus with ophthalmic complications**

E09.31 **Drug or chemical induced diabetes mellitus with unspecified diabetic retinopathy**

E09.311 **Drug or chemical induced diabetes mellitus with unspecified diabetic retinopathy with macular edema** [HCC]

E09.319 **Drug or chemical induced diabetes mellitus with unspecified diabetic retinopathy without macular edema** [HCC]

E09.32 **Drug or chemical induced diabetes mellitus with mild nonproliferative diabetic retinopathy**

Drug or chemical induced diabetes mellitus with nonproliferative diabetic retinopathy NOS

One of the following 7th characters is to be assigned to codes in subcategory E09.32 to designate laterality of the disease:

1 - right eye 2 - left eye

3 - bilateral

9 - unspecified eye

⑦E09.321 **Drug or chemical induced diabetes mellitus with mild nonproliferative diabetic retinopathy with macular edema** [HCC]

⑦E09.329 **Drug or chemical induced diabetes mellitus with mild nonproliferative diabetic retinopathy without macular edema** [HCC]

E09.33 **Drug or chemical induced diabetes mellitus with moderate nonproliferative diabetic retinopathy**

One of the following 7th characters is to be assigned to codes in subcategory E09.33 to designate laterality of the disease:

1 - right eye

2 - left eye

3 - bilateral

9 - unspecified eye

⑦E09.331 **Drug or chemical induced diabetes mellitus with moderate nonproliferative diabetic retinopathy with macular edema** [HCC]

⑦E09.339 **Drug or chemical induced diabetes mellitus with moderate nonproliferative diabetic retinopathy without macular edema** [HCC]

E09.34 **Drug or chemical induced diabetes mellitus with severe nonproliferative diabetic retinopathy**

One of the following 7th characters is to be assigned to codes in subcategory E09.34 to designate laterality of the disease:

1 - right eye

2 - left eye

3 - bilateral

9 - unspecified eye

⑦E09.341 **Drug or chemical induced diabetes mellitus with severe nonproliferative diabetic retinopathy with macular edema** [HCC]

⑦E09.349 **Drug or chemical induced diabetes mellitus with severe nonproliferative diabetic retinopathy without macular edema** [HCC]

E09.35 **Drug or chemical induced diabetes mellitus with proliferative diabetic retinopathy**

One of the following 7th characters is to be assigned to codes in subcategory E09.35 to designate laterality of the disease:

1 - right eye

2 - left eye

3 - bilateral

9 - unspecified eye

⑦E09.351 **Drug or chemical induced diabetes mellitus with proliferative diabetic retinopathy with macular edema** [HCC]

⑦E09.352 **Drug or chemical induced diabetes mellitus with proliferative diabetic retinopathy with traction retinal detachment involving the macula** [HCC]

⑦E09.353 **Drug or chemical induced diabetes mellitus with proliferative diabetic retinopathy with traction retinal detachment not involving the macula** [HCC]

⑦E09.354 **Drug or chemical induced diabetes mellitus with proliferative diabetic retinopathy with combined traction retinal detachment and rhegmatogenous retinal detachment** [HCC]

⑦E09.355 **Drug or chemical induced diabetes mellitus with stable proliferative diabetic retinopathy** [HCC]

⑦E09.359 **Drug or chemical induced diabetes mellitus with proliferative diabetic retinopathy without macular edema** [HCC]

E09.36 **Drug or chemical induced diabetes mellitus with diabetic cataract** [HCC]

⊗⑦E09.37 **Drug or chemical induced diabetes mellitus with diabetic macular edema, resolved following treatment** [HCC]

One of the following 7th characters is to be assigned to code E09.37 to designate laterality of the disease:

1 - right eye

2 - left eye

3 - bilateral

9 - unspecified eye

ENDOCRINE, NUTRITIONAL AND METABOLIC DISEASES

E09.39   **Drug or chemical induced diabetes mellitus with other diabetic ophthalmic complication** [HCC]

> **Use Additional Code** to identify manifestation, such as: diabetic glaucoma (H40-H42)

E09.4   **Drug or chemical induced diabetes mellitus with neurological complications**

E09.40   **Drug or chemical induced diabetes mellitus with neurological complications with diabetic neuropathy, unspecified** [HCC]

E09.41   **Drug or chemical induced diabetes mellitus with neurological complications with diabetic mononeuropathy** [HCC]

E09.42   **Drug or chemical induced diabetes mellitus with neurological complications with diabetic polyneuropathy** [HCC]

> Drug or chemical induced diabetes mellitus with diabetic neuralgia

E09.43   **Drug or chemical induced diabetes mellitus with neurological complications with diabetic autonomic (poly)neuropathy**

> Drug or chemical induced diabetes mellitus with diabetic gastroparesis

E09.44   **Drug or chemical induced diabetes mellitus with neurological complications with diabetic amyotrophy** [HCC]

E09.49   **Drug or chemical induced diabetes mellitus with neurological complications with other diabetic neurological complication** [HCC]

E09.5   **Drug or chemical induced diabetes mellitus with circulatory complications**

E09.51   **Drug or chemical induced diabetes mellitus with diabetic peripheral angiopathy without gangrene** [HCC]

E09.52   **Drug or chemical induced diabetes mellitus with diabetic peripheral angiopathy with gangrene** [HCC]

> Drug or chemical induced diabetes mellitus with diabetic gangrene

E09.59   **Drug or chemical induced diabetes mellitus with other circulatory complications** [HCC]

E09.6   **Drug or chemical induced diabetes mellitus with other specified complications**

E09.61   **Drug or chemical induced diabetes mellitus with diabetic arthropathy**

E09.610   **Drug or chemical induced diabetes mellitus with diabetic neuropathic arthropathy** [HCC]

> Drug or chemical induced diabetes mellitus with Charcôt's joints

E09.618   **Drug or chemical induced diabetes mellitus with other diabetic arthropathy** [HCC]

E09.62   **Drug or chemical induced diabetes mellitus with skin complications**

E09.620   **Drug or chemical induced diabetes mellitus with diabetic dermatitis** [HCC]

> Drug or chemical induced diabetes mellitus with diabetic necrobiosis lipoidica

E09.621   **Drug or chemical induced diabetes mellitus with foot ulcer** [HCC]

> **Use Additional Code** to identify site of ulcer (L97.4-, L97.5-)

E09.622   **Drug or chemical induced diabetes mellitus with other skin ulcer** [HCC]

> **Use Additional Code** to identify site of ulcer (L97.1-L97.9, L98.41-L98.49)

E09.628   **Drug or chemical induced diabetes mellitus with other skin complications** [HCC]

E09.63   **Drug or chemical induced diabetes mellitus with oral complications**

E09.630   **Drug or chemical induced diabetes mellitus with periodontal disease** [HCC]

E09.638   **Drug or chemical induced diabetes mellitus with other oral complications** [HCC]

E09.64   **Drug or chemical induced diabetes mellitus with hypoglycemia**

E09.641   **Drug or chemical induced diabetes mellitus with hypoglycemia with coma** [HCC]

E09.649   **Drug or chemical induced diabetes mellitus with hypoglycemia without coma** [HCC]

E09.65   **Drug or chemical induced diabetes mellitus with hyperglycemia** [HCC]

E09.69   **Drug or chemical induced diabetes mellitus with other specified complication** [HCC]

> **Use Additional Code** to identify complication

E09.8   **Drug or chemical induced diabetes mellitus with unspecified complications** [HCC]

E09.9   **Drug or chemical induced diabetes mellitus without complications** [HCC]

E10   **Type 1 diabetes mellitus**

> **Includes:** brittle diabetes (mellitus)
>
> diabetes (mellitus) due to autoimmune process
>
> diabetes (mellitus) due to immune mediated pancreatic islet beta-cell destruction idiopathic diabetes (mellitus)
>
> juvenile onset diabetes (mellitus)
>
> ketosis-prone diabetes (mellitus)
>
> **Excludes1:** diabetes mellitus due to underlying condition (E08.-)
>
> drug or chemical induced diabetes mellitus (E09.-)
>
> gestational diabetes (O24.4-)
>
> hyperglycemia NOS (R73.9)
>
> neonatal diabetes mellitus (P70.2)
>
> postpancreatectomy diabetes mellitus (E13.-)
>
> postprocedural diabetes mellitus (E13.-)
>
> secondary diabetes mellitus NEC (E13.-)
>
> type 2 diabetes mellitus (E11.-)

E10.1   **Type 1 diabetes mellitus with ketoacidosis**

E10.10   **Type 1 diabetes mellitus with ketoacidosis without coma** [HCC]

E10.11   **Type 1 diabetes mellitus with ketoacidosis with coma** [HCC]

E10.2   **Type 1 diabetes mellitus with kidney complications**

E10.21   **Type 1 diabetes mellitus with diabetic nephropathy** [HCC]

> Type 1 diabetes mellitus with intercapillary glomerulosclerosis
>
> Type 1 diabetes mellitus with intracapillary glomerulonephrosis
>
> Type 1 diabetes mellitus with Kimmelstiel-Wilson disease

E10.22   **Type 1 diabetes mellitus with diabetic chronic kidney disease** [HCC]

   ● New code   ▲ Revised code   **Excludes1:** Not coded here   **Excludes2:** Not included here   ⊗ Placeholder required   ⑦7th digit required

Use Additional Code to identify stage of chronic kidney disease (N18.1-N18.6)

E10.29   Type 1diabetes mellitus with other diabetic kidney complication [HCC]

Type 1 diabetes mellitus with renal tubular degeneration

E10.3   Type 1 Diabetes mellitus with ophthalmic complications

E10.31   Type 1diabetes mellitus with unspecified diabetic retinopathy

E10.311   Type 1 diabetes mellitus with unspecified diabetic retinopathy with macular edema [HCC]

E10.319   Type 1 diabetes mellitus with unspecified diabetic retinopathy without macular edema [HCC]

E10.32   Type 1 diabetes mellitus with mild nonproliferative diabetic retinopathy

Type 1 diabetes mellitus with nonproliferative diabetic retinopathy NOS

One of the following 7th characters is to be assigned to codes in subcategory E10.32 to designate laterality of the disease:

1 - right eye

2 - left eye

3 - bilateral

9 - unspecified eye

⑦E10.321   Type 1 diabetes mellitus with mild nonproliferative diabetic retinopathy with macular edema [HCC]

⑦E10.329   Type 1 diabetes mellitus with mild nonproliferative diabetic retinopathy without macular edema [HCC]

E10.33   Type 1 diabetes mellitus with moderate nonproliferative diabetic retinopathy

One of the following 7th characters is to be assigned to codes in subcategory E10.33 to designate laterality of the disease:

1 - right eye

2 - left eye

3 - bilateral

9 - unspecified eye

⑦E10.331   Type 1 diabetes mellitus with moderate nonproliferative diabetic retinopathy with macular edema [HCC]

⑦E10.339   Type 1 diabetes mellitus with moderate nonproliferative diabetic retinopathy without macular edema [HCC]

E10.34   Type 1 diabetes mellitus with severe nonproliferative diabetic retinopathy

One of the following 7th characters is to be assigned to codes in subcategory E10.34 to designate laterality of the disease:

1 - right eye

2 - left eye

3 - bilateral

9 - unspecified eye

⑦E10.341   Type 1 diabetes mellitus with severe nonproliferative diabetic retinopathy with macular edema [HCC]

⑦E10.349   Type 1 diabetes mellitus with severe nonproliferative diabetic retinopathy without macular edema [HCC]

E10.35   Type 1 diabetes mellitus with proliferative diabetic retinopathy

One of the following 7th characters is to be assigned to codes in subcategory E10.35 to designate laterality of the disease:

1 - right eye

2 - left eye

3 - bilateral

9 - unspecified eye

⑦E10.351   Type 1 diabetes mellitus with proliferative diabetic retinopathy with macular edema [HCC]

⑦E10.352   Type 1 diabetes mellitus with proliferative diabetic retinopathy with traction retinal detachment involving the macula [HCC]

⑦E10.353   Type 1 diabetes mellitus with proliferative diabetic retinopathy with traction retinal detachment not involving the macula [HCC]

⑦E10.354   Type 1 diabetes mellitus with proliferative diabetic retinopathy with combined traction retinal detachment and rhegmatogenous retinal detachment [HCC]

⑦E10.355   Type 1 diabetes mellitus with stable proliferative diabetic retinopathy [HCC]

⑦E10.359   Type 1 diabetes mellitus with proliferative diabetic retinopathy without macular edema [HCC]

⊗⑦E10.36   Type 1 diabetes mellitus with diabetic cataract [HCC]

⊗⑦E10.37   Type 1 diabetes mellitus with diabetic macular edema, resolved following treatment [HCC]

One of the following 7th characters is to be assigned to code E10.37 to designate laterality of the disease:

1 - right eye

2 - left eye

3 - bilateral

9 - unspecified eye

E10.39   Type 1 diabetes mellitus with other diabetic ophthalmic complication [HCC]

Use Additional Code to identify manifestation, such as:

diabetic glaucoma (H40-H42)

E10.4   Type 1 diabetes mellitus with neurological complications

E10.40   Type 1 diabetes mellitus with diabetic neuropathy, unspecified [HCC]

E10.41   Type 1 diabetes mellitus with diabetic mononeuropathy [HCC]

E10.42   Type 1 diabetes mellitus with diabetic polyneuropathy [HCC]

Type 1 diabetes mellitus with diabetic neuralgia

E10.43   Type 1 diabetes mellitus with diabetic autonomic (poly)neuropathy [HCC]

Type 1 diabetes mellitus with diabetic gastroparesis

E10.44   Type 1 diabetes mellitus with diabetic amyotrophy [HCC]

E10.49   Type 1 diabetes mellitus with other diabetic neurological complication

E10.5   Type 1 diabetes mellitus with circulatory complications

E10.51 **Type 1 diabetes mellitus with diabetic peripheral angiopathy without gangrene** [HCC]

E10.52 **Type 1 diabetes mellitus with diabetic peripheral angiopathy with gangrene** [HCC]

Type 1 diabetes mellitus with diabetic gangrene

E10.59 **Type 1 diabetes mellitus with other circulatory complications** [HCC]

E10.6 **Type 1 diabetes mellitus with other specified complications**

E10.61 **Type 1 diabetes mellitus with diabetic arthropathy**

E10.610 **Type 1 diabetes mellitus with diabetic neuropathic arthropathy** [HCC]

Type 1 diabetes mellitus with Charcôt's joints

E10.618 **Type 1 diabetes mellitus with other diabetic arthropathy** [HCC]

E10.62 **Type 1 diabetes mellitus with skin complications**

E10.620 **Type 1 diabetes mellitus with diabetic dermatitis** [HCC]

Type 1 diabetes mellitus with diabetic necrobiosis lipoidica

E10.621 **Type 1 diabetes mellitus with foot ulcer** [HCC]

Use Additional Code to identify site of ulcer (L97.4-, L97.5-)

E10.622 **Type 1 diabetes mellitus with other skin ulcer** [HCC]

Use Additional Code to identify site of ulcer (L97.1-L97.9, L98.41-L98.49)

E10.628 **Type 1 diabetes mellitus with other skin complications** [HCC]

E10.63 **Type 1 diabetes mellitus with oral complications**

E10.630 **Type 1 diabetes mellitus with periodontal disease** [HCC]

E10.638 **Type 1 diabetes mellitus with other oral complications** [HCC]

E10.64 **Type 1 diabetes mellitus with hypoglycemia**

E10.641 **Type 1 diabetes mellitus with hypoglycemia with coma** [HCC]

E10.649 **Type 1 diabetes mellitus with hypoglycemia without coma** [HCC]

E10.65 **Type 1 diabetes mellitus with hyperglycemia** [HCC]

E10.69 **Type 1 diabetes mellitus with other specified complication** [HCC]

Use Additional Code to identify complication

E10.8 **Type 1 diabetes mellitus with unspecified complications** [HCC]

E10.9 **Type 1 diabetes mellitus without complications** [HCC]

E11 **Type 2 diabetes mellitus**

Includes: diabetes (mellitus) due to insulin secretory defect

diabetes NOS

insulin resistant diabetes (mellitus)

Use Additional Code to identify control using:

insulin (Z79.4)

oral antidiabetic drugs (Z79.84)

oral hypoglycemic drugs (Z79.84)

Excludes1: diabetes mellitus due to underlying condition (E08.-)

drug or chemical induced diabetes mellitus (E09.-)

gestational diabetes (O24.4-)

neonatal diabetes mellitus (P70.2)

postpancreatectomy diabetes mellitus (E13.-)

postprocedural diabetes mellitus (E13.-)

secondary diabetes mellitus NEC (E13.-)

type 1 diabetes mellitus (E10.-)

E11.0 **Type 2 diabetes mellitus with hyperosmolarity**

E11.00 **Type 2 diabetes mellitus with hyperosmolarity without nonketotic hyperglycemic-hyperosmolar coma (NKHHC)** [HCC]

E11.01 **Type 2 diabetes mellitus with hyperosmolarity with coma** [HCC]

E11.1 **Type 2 diabetes mellitus with ketoacidosis**

E11.10 **Type 2 diabetes mellitus with ketoacidosis without coma** [HCC]

E11.11 **Type 2 diabetes mellitus with ketoacidosis with coma** [HCC]

E11.2 **Type 2 diabetes mellitus with kidney complications**

E11.21 **Type 2 diabetes mellitus with diabetic nephropathy** [HCC]

Type 2 diabetes mellitus with intercapillary glomerulosclerosis

Type 2 diabetes mellitus with intracapillary glomerulonephrosis

Type 2 diabetes mellitus with Kimmelstiel-Wilson disease

E11.22 **Type 2 diabetes mellitus with diabetic chronic kidney disease** [HCC]

Use Additional Code to identify stage of chronic kidney disease (N18.1-N18.6)

E11.29 **Type 2 diabetes mellitus with other diabetic kidney complication** [HCC]

Type 2 diabetes mellitus with renal tubular degeneration

E11.3 **Type 2 diabetes mellitus with ophthalmic complications**

E11.31 **Type 2 diabetes mellitus with unspecified diabetic retinopathy**

E11.311 **Type 2 diabetes mellitus with unspecified diabetic retinopathy with macular edema** [HCC]

E11.319 **Type 2 diabetes mellitus with unspecified diabetic retinopathy without macular edema** [HCC]

E11.32 **Type 2 diabetes mellitus with mild nonproliferative diabetic retinopathy**

Type 2 diabetes mellitus with nonproliferative diabetic retinopathy NOS

One of the following 7th characters is to be assigned to codes in subcategory E11.32 to designate laterality of the disease:

1 - right eye

2 - left eye

3 – bilateral

9 - unspecified eye

⑦E11.321 **Type 2 diabetes mellitus with mild nonproliferative diabetic retinopathy with macular edema** [HCC]

⑦E11.329 **Type 2 diabetes mellitus with mild nonproliferative diabetic retinopathy without macular edema** [HCC]

E11.33 **Type 2 diabetes mellitus with moderate nonproliferative diabetic retinopathy**

● New code ▲ Revised code **Excludes1:** Not coded here **Excludes2:** Not included here ⊗ Placeholder required ⑦7ᵗʰ digit required

One of the following 7th characters is to be assigned to codes in subcategory E11.33 to designate laterality of the disease:

1 - right eye

2 - left eye

3 - bilateral

9 - unspecified eye

⑦**E11.331** **Type 2 diabetes mellitus with moderate nonproliferative diabetic retinopathy with macular edema** [HCC]

⑦**E11.339** **Type 2 diabetes mellitus with moderate nonproliferative diabetic retinopathy without macular edema** [HCC]

E11.34 **Type 2 diabetes mellitus with severe nonproliferative diabetic retinopathy**

One of the following 7th characters is to be assigned to codes in subcategory E11.34 to designate laterality of the disease:

1 - right eye

2 - left eye

3 - bilateral

9 - unspecified eye

⑦**E11.341** **Type 2 diabetes mellitus with severe nonproliferative diabetic retinopathy with macular edema** [HCC]

⑦**E11.349** **Type 2 diabetes mellitus with severe nonproliferative diabetic retinopathy without macular edema** [HCC]

E11.35 **Type 2 diabetes mellitus with proliferative diabetic retinopathy**

One of the following 7th characters is to be assigned to codes in subcategory E11.35 to designate laterality of the disease:

1 - right eye

2 - left eye

3 - bilateral

9 - unspecified eye

⑦**E11.351** **Type 2 diabetes mellitus with proliferative diabetic retinopathy with macular edema** [HCC]

⑦**E11.352** **Type 2 diabetes mellitus with proliferative diabetic retinopathy with traction retinal detachment involving the macula** [HCC]

⑦**E11.353** **Type 2 diabetes mellitus with proliferative diabetic retinopathy with traction retinal detachment not involving the macula**

⑦**E11.354** **Type 2 diabetes mellitus with proliferative diabetic retinopathy with combined traction retinal detachment and rhegmatogenous retinal detachment** [HCC]

⑦**E11.355** **Type 2 diabetes mellitus with stable proliferative diabetic retinopathy** [HCC]

⑦**E11.359** **Type 2 diabetes mellitus with proliferative diabetic retinopathy without macular edema** [HCC]

E11.36 **Type 2 diabetes mellitus with diabetic cataract** [HCC]

⊗⑦**E11.37** **Type 2 diabetes mellitus with diabetic macular edema, resolved following treatment** [HCC]

One of the following 7th characters is to be assigned to code E11.37 to designate laterality of the disease:

1 - right eye

2 - left eye

3 - bilateral

9 - unspecified eye

E11.39 **Type 2 diabetes mellitus with other diabetic ophthalmic complication** [HCC]

Use Additional Code to identify manifestation, such as: diabetic glaucoma (H40-H42)

E11.4 **Type 2 diabetes mellitus with neurological complications**

E11.40 **Type 2 diabetes mellitus with diabetic neuropathy, unspecified** [HCC]

E11.41 **Type 2 diabetes mellitus with diabetic mononeuropathy** [HCC]

E11.42 **Type 2 diabetes mellitus with diabetic polyneuropathy** [HCC]

Type 2 diabetes mellitus with diabetic neuralgia

E11.43 **Type 2 diabetes mellitus with diabetic autonomic (poly)neuropathy** [HCC]

Type 2 diabetes mellitus with diabetic gastroparesis

E11.44 **Type 2 diabetes mellitus with diabetic amyotrophy** [HCC]

E11.49 **Type 2 diabetes mellitus with other diabetic neurological complication** [HCC]

E11.5 **Type 2 diabetes mellitus with circulatory complications**

E11.51 **Type 2 diabetes mellitus with diabetic peripheral angiopathy without gangrene** [HCC]

E11.52 **Type 2 diabetes mellitus with diabetic peripheral angiopathy with gangrene** [HCC]

Type 2 diabetes mellitus with diabetic gangrene

E11.59 **Type 2 diabetes mellitus with other circulatory complications** [HCC]

E11.6 **Type 2 diabetes mellitus with other specified complications**

E11.61 **Type 2 diabetes mellitus with diabetic arthropathy** [HCC]

E11.610 **Type 2 diabetes mellitus with diabetic neuropathic arthropathy** [HCC]

Type 2 diabetes mellitus with Charcôt's joints

E11.618 **Type 2 diabetes mellitus with other diabetic arthropathy** [HCC]

E11.62 **Type 2 diabetes mellitus with skin complications**

E11.620 **Type 2 diabetes mellitus with diabetic dermatitis** [HCC]

Type 2 diabetes mellitus with diabetic necrobiosis lipoidica

E11.621 **Type 2 diabetes mellitus with foot ulcer**

Use Additional Code to identify site of ulcer (L97.4-, L97.5-)

E11.622 **Type 2 diabetes mellitus with other skin ulcer** [HCC]

Use Additional Code to identify site of ulcer (L97.1-L97.9, L98.41-L98.49)

E11.628 **Type 2 diabetes mellitus with other skin complications** [HCC]

E11.63 **Type 2 diabetes mellitus with oral complications**

E11.630   **Type 2 diabetes mellitus with periodontal disease** [HCC]

E11.638   **Type 2 diabetes mellitus with other oral complications** [HCC]

E11.64   **Type 2 diabetes mellitus with hypoglycemia**

E11.641   **Type 2 diabetes mellitus with hypoglycemia with coma** [HCC]

E11.649   **Type 2 diabetes mellitus with hypoglycemia without coma** [HCC]

E11.65   **Type 2 diabetes mellitus with hyperglycemia**

E11.69   **Type 2 diabetes mellitus with other specified complication** [HCC]

   Use Additional Code to identify complication

E11.8   **Type 2 diabetes mellitus with unspecified complications** [HCC]

E11.9   **Type 2 diabetes mellitus without complications** [HCC]

E13   **Other specified diabetes mellitus**

Includes: diabetes mellitus due to genetic defects of beta-cell function

diabetes mellitus due to genetic defects in insulin action

postpancreatectomy diabetes mellitus

postprocedural diabetes mellitus secondary diabetes mellitus NEC

Use Additional Code to identify control using:

insulin (Z79.4)

oral antidiabetic drugs (Z79.84)

oral hypoglycemic drugs (Z79.84)

Excludes1: diabetes (mellitus) due to autoimmune process (E10.-)

diabetes (mellitus) due to immune mediated pancreatic islet beta-cell destruction (E10.-)

diabetes mellitus due to underlying condition (E08.-)

drug or chemical induced diabetes mellitus (E09.-)

gestational diabetes (O24.4-)

neonatal diabetes mellitus (P70.2)

type 1 diabetes mellitus (E10.-)

E13.0   **Other specified diabetes mellitus with hyperosmolarity**

E13.00   **Other specified diabetes mellitus with hyperosmolarity without nonketotic hyperglycemic-hyperosmolar coma (NKHHC)** [HCC]

Excludes2: type 2 diabetes mellitus (E11.-)

E13.01   **Other specified diabetes mellitus with hyperosmolarity with coma** [HCC]

E13.1   **Other specified diabetes mellitus with ketoacidosis**

E13.10   **Other specified diabetes mellitus with ketoacidosis without coma** [HCC]

E13.11   **Other specified diabetes mellitus with ketoacidosis with coma**

E13.2   **Other specified diabetes mellitus with kidney complications**

E13.21   **Other specified diabetes mellitus with diabetic nephropathy** [HCC]

Other specified diabetes mellitus with intercapillary glomerulosclerosis

Other specified diabetes mellitus with intracapillary glomerulonephrosis

Other specified diabetes mellitus with Kimmelstiel-Wilson disease

E13.22   **Other specified diabetes mellitus with diabetic chronic kidney disease** [HCC]

Use Additional Code to identify stage of chronic kidney disease (N18.1-N18.6)

E13.29   **Other specified diabetes mellitus with other diabetic kidney complication** [HCC]

Other specified diabetes mellitus with renal tubular degeneration

E13.3   **Other specified diabetes mellitus with ophthalmic complications**

E13.31   **Other specified diabetes mellitus with unspecified diabetic retinopathy** [HCC]

E13.311   **Other specified diabetes mellitus with unspecified diabetic retinopathy with macular edema** [HCC]

E13.319   **Other specified diabetes mellitus with unspecified diabetic retinopathy without macular edema** [HCC]

E13.32   **Other specified diabetes mellitus with mild nonproliferative diabetic retinopathy**

Other specified diabetes mellitus with nonproliferative diabetic retinopathy NOS

One of the following 7th characters is to be assigned to codes in subcategory E13.32 to designate laterality of the disease:

1 - right eye

2 - left eye

3 - bilateral

9 - unspecified eye

⑦**E13.321**   **Other specified diabetes mellitus with mild nonproliferative diabetic retinopathy with macular edema** [HCC]

⑦**E13.329**   **Other specified diabetes mellitus with mild nonproliferative diabetic retinopathy without macular edema** [HCC]

E13.33   **Other specified diabetes mellitus with moderate nonproliferative diabetic retinopathy**

One of the following 7th characters is to be assigned to codes in subcategory E13.33 to designate laterality of the disease:

1 - right eye

2 - left eye

3 - bilateral

9 - unspecified eye

⑦**E13.331**   **Other specified diabetes mellitus with moderate nonproliferative diabetic retinopathy with macular edema** [HCC]

⑦**E13.339**   **Other specified diabetes mellitus with moderate nonproliferative diabetic retinopathy without macular edema** [HCC]

E13.34   **Other specified diabetes mellitus with severe nonproliferative diabetic retinopathy**

One of the following 7th characters is to be assigned to codes in subcategory E13.34 to designate laterality of the disease:

1 - right eye

2 - left eye

3 - bilateral

9 - unspecified eye

⑦**E13.341**   **Other specified diabetes mellitus with severe nonproliferative diabetic retinopathy with macular edema** [HCC]

   ● New code   ▲ Revised code   **Excludes1:** Not coded here   **Excludes2:** Not included here   ⊗ Placeholder required   ⑦7th digit required

⑦ **E13.349** **Other specified diabetes mellitus with severe nonproliferative diabetic retinopathy without macular edema** [HCC]

E13.35 **Other specified diabetes mellitus with proliferative diabetic retinopathy**

One of the following 7th characters is to be assigned to codes in subcategory E13.35 to designate laterality of the disease:

1 - right eye

2 - left eye

3 - bilateral

9 - unspecified eye

⑦ **E13.351** **Other specified diabetes mellitus with proliferative diabetic retinopathy with macular edema** [HCC]

⑦ **E13.352** **Other specified diabetes mellitus with proliferative diabetic retinopathy with traction retinal detachment involving the macula** [HCC]

⑦ **E13.353** **Other specified diabetes mellitus with proliferative diabetic retinopathy with traction retinal detachment not involving the macula** [HCC]

⑦ **E13.354** **Other specified diabetes mellitus with proliferative diabetic retinopathy with combined traction retinal detachment and rhegmatogenous retinal detachment** [HCC]

⑦ **E13.355** **Other specified diabetes mellitus with stable proliferative diabetic retinopathy** [HCC]

⑦ **E13.359** **Other specified diabetes mellitus with proliferative diabetic retinopathy without macular edema** [HCC]

E13.36 **Other specified diabetes mellitus with diabetic cataract** [HCC]

⊗⑦ **E13.37** **Other specified diabetes mellitus with diabetic macular edema, resolved following treatment** [HCC]

One of the following 7th characters is to be assigned to code E13.37 to designate laterality of the disease:

1 - right eye

2 - left eye

3 - bilateral

9 - unspecified eye

E13.39 **Other specified diabetes mellitus with other diabetic ophthalmic complication** [HCC]

Use Additional Code to identify manifestation, such as:

diabetic glaucoma (H40-H42)

E13.4 **Other specified diabetes mellitus with neurological complications**

E13.40 **Other specified diabetes mellitus with diabetic neuropathy, unspecified** [HCC]

E13.41 **Other specified diabetes mellitus with diabetic mononeuropathy** [HCC]

E13.42 **Other specified diabetes mellitus with diabetic polyneuropathy** [HCC]

Other specified diabetes mellitus with diabetic neuralgia

E13.43 **Other specified diabetes mellitus with diabetic autonomic (poly)neuropathy** [HCC]

Other specified diabetes mellitus with diabetic gastroparesis

E13.44 **Other specified diabetes mellitus with diabetic amyotrophy** [HCC]

E13.49 **Other specified diabetes mellitus with other diabetic neurological complication**

E13.5 **Other specified diabetes mellitus with circulatory complications**

E13.51 **Other specified diabetes mellitus with diabetic peripheral angiopathy without gangrene** [HCC]

E13.52 **Other specified diabetes mellitus with diabetic peripheral angiopathy with gangrene** [HCC]

Other specified diabetes mellitus with diabetic gangrene

E13.59 **Other specified diabetes mellitus with other circulatory complications** [HCC]

E13.6 **Other specified diabetes mellitus with other specified complications**

E13.61 **Other specified diabetes mellitus with diabetic arthropathy**

E13.610 **Other specified diabetes mellitus with diabetic neuropathic arthropathy** [HCC]

Other specified diabetes mellitus with Charcôt's joints

E13.618 **Other specified diabetes mellitus with other diabetic arthropathy** [HCC]

E13.62 **Other specified diabetes mellitus with skin complications**

E13.620 **Other specified diabetes mellitus with diabetic dermatitis** [HCC]

Other specified diabetes mellitus with diabetic necrobiosis lipoidica

E13.621 **Other specified diabetes mellitus with foot ulcer** [HCC]

Use Additional Code to identify site of ulcer (L97.4-, L97.5-)

E13.622 **Other specified diabetes mellitus with other skin ulcer** [HCC]

Use Additional Code to identify site of ulcer (L97.1-L97.9, L98.41-L98.49)

E13.628 **Other specified diabetes mellitus with other skin complications** [HCC]

E13.63 **Other specified diabetes mellitus with oral complications**

E13.630 **Other specified diabetes mellitus with periodontal disease** [HCC]

E13.638 **Other specified diabetes mellitus with other oral complications** [HCC]

E13.64 **Other specified diabetes mellitus with hypoglycemia**

E13.641 **Other specified diabetes mellitus with hypoglycemia with coma** [HCC]

E13.649 **Other specified diabetes mellitus with hypoglycemia without coma** [HCC]

E13.65 **Other specified diabetes mellitus with hyperglycemia** [HCC]

E13.69 **Other specified diabetes mellitus with other specified complication** [HCC]

Use Additional Code to identify complication

E13.8 **Other specified diabetes mellitus with unspecified complications** [HCC]

E13.9 Other specified diabetes mellitus without complications [HCC]

OTHER DISORDERS OF GLUCOSE REGULATION AND PANCREATIC INTERNAL SECRETION (E15-E16)

E15 Nondiabetic hypoglycemic coma [HCC]

Includes: drug-induced insulin coma in nondiabetic

hyperinsulinism with hypoglycemic coma hypoglycemic coma NOS

E16 Other disorders of pancreatic internal secretion

E16.0 Drug-induced hypoglycemia without coma

Excludes1: diabetes with hypoglycemia without coma (E09.649)

Use Additional Code for adverse effect, if applicable, to identify drug (T36-T50 with fifth or sixth character 5)

E16.1 Other hypoglycemia

Functional hyperinsulinism

Functional nonhyperinsulinemic hypoglycemia

Hyperinsulinism NOS

Hyperplasia of pancreatic islet beta cells NOS

Excludes1: diabetes with hypoglycemia (E08.649, E10.649, E11.649, E13.649)

hypoglycemia in infant of diabetic mother (P70.1)

neonatal hypoglycemia (P70.4)

E16.2 Hypoglycemia, unspecified

Definition: Hypoglycemia is the medical term for abnormally low blood sugar usually resulting from excessive insulin or a poor diet.

Excludes1: diabetes with hypoglycemia (E08.649, E10.649, E11.649, E13.649)

E16.3 Increased secretion of glucagon

Hyperplasia of pancreatic endocrine cells with glucagon excess

E16.4 Increased secretion of gastrin

Hypergastrinemia

Hyperplasia of pancreatic endocrine cells with gastrin excess Zollinger-Ellison syndrome

E16.8 Other specified disorders of pancreatic internal secretion

Increased secretion from endocrine pancreas of growth hormone-releasing hormone

Increased secretion from endocrine pancreas of pancreatic polypeptide

Increased secretion from endocrine pancreas of somatostatin

Increased secretion from endocrine pancreas of vasoactive-intestinal polypeptide

E16.9 Disorder of pancreatic internal secretion, unspecified

Islet-cell hyperplasia NOS

Pancreatic endocrine cell hyperplasia NOS

DISORDERS OF OTHER ENDOCRINE GLANDS (E20-E35)

Excludes1: galactorrhea (N64.3)

gynecomastia (N62)

E20 Hypoparathyroidism

Excludes1: Di George's syndrome (D82.1)

postprocedural hypoparathyroidism (E89.2)

tetany NOS (R29.0)

transitory neonatal hypoparathyroidism (P71.4)

E20.0 Idiopathic hypoparathyroidism [HCC]

E20.1 Pseudohypoparathyroidism

E20.8 Other hypoparathyroidism [HCC]

E20.9 Hypoparathyroidism, unspecified [HCC]

Parathyroid tetany

E21 Hyperparathyroidism and other disorders of parathyroid gland

Excludes1: adult osteomalacia (M83.-)

ectopic hyperparathyroidism (E34.2)

hungry bone syndrome (E83.81)

infantile and juvenile osteomalacia (E55.0)

Excludes2: familial hypocalciuric hypercalcemia (E83.52)

E21.0 Primary hyperparathyroidism [HCC]

Hyperplasia of parathyroid

Osteitis fibrosa cystica generalisata [von Recklinghausen's disease of bone]

E21.1 Secondary hyperparathyroidism, not elsewhere classified [HCC]

Excludes1: secondary hyperparathyroidism of renal origin (N25.81)

E21.2 Other hyperparathyroidism [HCC]

Tertiary hyperparathyroidism

Excludes1: familial hypocalciuric hypercalcemia (E83.52)

E21.3 Hyperparathyroidism, unspecified [HCC]

E21.4 Other specified disorders of parathyroid gland [HCC]

E21.5 Disorder of parathyroid gland, unspecified [HCC]

E22 Hyperfunction of pituitary gland

Excludes1: Cushing's syndrome (E24.-)

Nelson's syndrome (E24.1)

overproduction of ACTH not associated with Cushing's disease (E27.0)

overproduction of pituitary ACTH (E24.0)

overproduction of thyroid-stimulating hormone (E05.8-)

E22.0 Acromegaly and pituitary gigantism

Overproduction of growth hormone

Excludes1: constitutional gigantism (E34.4)

constitutional tall stature (E34.4)

increased secretion from endocrine pancreas of growth hormone-releasing hormone (E16.8)

E22.1 Hyperprolactinemia [HCC]

Use Additional Code for adverse effect, if applicable, to identify drug (T36-T50 with fifth or sixth character 5)

E22.2 Syndrome of inappropriate secretion of antidiuretic hormone [HCC]

E22.8 Other hyperfunction of pituitary gland [HCC]

Central precocious puberty

E22.9 Hyperfunction of pituitary gland, unspecified [HCC]

E23 Hypofunction and other disorders of the pituitary gland

Includes: the listed conditions whether the disorder is in the pituitary or the hypothalamus

Excludes1: postprocedural hypopituitarism (E89.3)

E23.0 Hypopituitarism [HCC]

Fertile eunuch syndrome

Hypogonadotropic hypogonadism

Idiopathic growth hormone deficiency

Isolated deficiency of gonadotropin

Isolated deficiency of growth hormone

Isolated deficiency of pituitary hormone

Kallmann's syndrome

Lorain-Levi short stature

Necrosis of pituitary gland (postpartum)

Panhypopituitarism

Pituitary cachexia

Pituitary insufficiency NOS

Pituitary short stature

Sheehan's syndrome

Simmonds' disease

E23.1 **Drug-induced hypopituitarism** [HCC]

Use Additional Code for adverse effect, if applicable, to identify drug (T36-T50 with fifth or sixth character 5)

E23.2 **Diabetes insipidus** [HCC]

Excludes1: nephrogenic diabetes insipidus (N25.1)

E23.3 **Hypothalamic dysfunction, not elsewhere classified** [HCC]

Excludes1: Prader-Willi syndrome (Q87.11)

Russell-Silver syndrome (Q87.11)

E23.6 **Other disorders of pituitary gland** [HCC]

Abscess of pituitary

Adiposogenital dystrophy

E23.7 **Disorder of pituitary gland, unspecified**

E24 **Cushing's syndrome**

Definition: Cushing's syndrome is a condition due to tumors of the adrenal cortex or the anterior lobe of the pituitary gland.

Excludes1: congenital adrenal hyperplasia (E25.0)

E24.0 **Pituitary-dependent Cushing's disease** [HCC]

Overproduction of pituitary ACTH

Pituitary-dependent hypercorticalism

E24.1 **Nelson's syndrome** [HCC]

E24.2 **Drug-induced Cushing's syndrome** [HCC]

Use Additional Code for adverse effect, if applicable, to identify drug (T36-T50 with fifth or sixth character 5)

E24.3 **Ectopic ACTH syndrome** [HCC]

E24.4 **Alcohol-induced pseudo-Cushing's syndrome** [HCC]

E24.8 **Other Cushing's syndrome** [HCC]

E24.9 **Cushing's syndrome, unspecified** [HCC]

E25 **Adrenogenital disorders**

Includes: adrenogenital syndromes, virilizing or feminizing, whether acquired or due to adrenal hyperplasia consequent on inborn enzyme defects in hormone synthesis

Female adrenal pseudohermaphroditism

Female heterosexual precocious pseudopuberty

Male isosexual precocious pseudopuberty

Male macrogenitosomia praecox

Male sexual precocity with adrenal hyperplasia

Male virilization (female)

Excludes1: indeterminate sex and pseudohermaphroditism (Q56)

chromosomal abnormalities (Q90-Q99)

E25.0 **Congenital adrenogenital disorders associated with enzyme deficiency** [HCC]

Congenital adrenal hyperplasia 21-Hydroxylase deficiency

Salt-losing congenital adrenal hyperplasia

E25.8 **Other adrenogenital disorders** [HCC]

Idiopathic adrenogenital disorder

Use Additional Code for adverse effect, if applicable, to identify drug (T36-T50 with fifth or sixth character 5)

E25.9 **Adrenogenital disorder, unspecified**

Adrenogenital syndrome NOS

E26 **Hyperaldosteronism**

E26.0 **Primary hyperaldosteronism**

E26.01 **Conn's syndrome** [HCC]

Code also adrenal adenoma (D35.0-)

E26.02 **Glucocorticoid-remediable aldosteronism** [HCC]

Familial aldosteronism type I

E26.09 **Other primary hyperaldosteronism** [HCC]

Primary aldosteronism due to adrenal hyperplasia (bilateral)

E26.1 **Secondary hyperaldosteronism** [HCC]

E26.8 **Other hyperaldosteronism**

E26.81 **Bartter's syndrome** [HCC]

E26.89 **Other hyperaldosteronism** [HCC]

E26.9 **Hyperaldosteronism, unspecified** [HCC]

Aldosteronism NOS

Hyperaldosteronism NOS

E27 **Other disorders of adrenal gland**

E27.0 **Other adrenocortical overactivity** [HCC]

Overproduction of ACTH, not associated with Cushing's disease

Premature adrenarche

Excludes1: Cushing's syndrome (E24.-)

E27.1 **Primary adrenocortical insufficiency** [HCC]

Addison's disease

Autoimmune adrenalitis

Excludes1: Addison only phenotype adrenoleukodystrophy (E71.528)

amyloidosis (E85.-)

tuberculous Addison's disease (A18.7)

Waterhouse-Friderichsen syndrome (A39.1)

E27.2 **Addisonian crisis** [HCC]

Adrenal crisis

Adrenocortical crisis

E27.3 **Drug-induced adrenocortical insufficiency** [HCC]

Use Additional Code for adverse effect, if applicable, to identify drug (T36-T50 with fifth or sixth character 5)

E27.4 **Other and unspecified adrenocortical insufficiency**

Excludes1: adrenoleukodystrophy [Addison-Schilder] (E71.528)

Waterhouse-Friderichsen syndrome (A39.1)

E27.40 **Unspecified adrenocortical insufficiency** [HCC]

Adrenocortical insufficiency NOS

Hypoaldosteronism

E27.49 **Other adrenocortical insufficiency** [HCC]

Adrenal hemorrhage

Adrenal infarction

E27.5 **Adrenomedullary hyperfunction** [HCC]

Adrenomedullary hyperplasia

Catecholamine hypersecretion

E27.8 **Other specified disorders of adrenal gland** [HCC]

Abnormality of cortisol-binding globulin

E27.9 **Disorder of adrenal gland, unspecified** [HCC]

E28 **Ovarian dysfunction**

Excludes1: isolated gonadotropin deficiency (E23.0)

postprocedural ovarian failure (E89.4-)

E28.0 **Estrogen excess**

Use Additional Code for adverse effect, if applicable, to identify drug (T36-T50 with fifth or sixth character 5)

E28.1 **Androgen excess**

Hypersecretion of ovarian androgens

Use Additional Code for adverse effect, if applicable, to identify drug (T36-T50 with fifth or sixth character 5)

E28.2   **Polycystic ovarian syndrome**

Sclerocystic ovary syndrome

Stein-Leventhal syndrome

E28.3   **Primary ovarian failure**

Excludes1: pure gonadal dysgenesis (Q99.1)

Turner's syndrome (Q96.-)

E28.31   **Premature menopause**

E28.310   **Symptomatic premature menopause**

Symptoms such as flushing, sleeplessness, headache, lack of concentration, associated with premature menopause

E28.319   **Asymptomatic premature menopause**

Premature menopause NOS

E28.39   **Other primary ovarian failure**

Decreased estrogen

Resistant ovary syndrome

E28.8   **Other ovarian dysfunction**

Ovarian hyperfunction NOS

Excludes1: postprocedural ovarian failure (E89.4-)

E28.9   **Ovarian dysfunction, unspecified**

E29   **Testicular dysfunction**

Excludes1: androgen insensitivity syndrome (E34.5-)

azoospermia or oligospermia NOS (N46.0-N46.1)

isolated gonadotropin deficiency (E23.0)

Klinefelter's syndrome (Q98.0-Q98.1, Q98.4)

E29.0   **Testicular hyperfunction**

Hypersecretion of testicular hormones

E29.1   **Testicular hypofunction**

Defective biosynthesis of testicular androgen NOS

5-delta-Reductase deficiency (with male pseudohermaphroditism)

Testicular hypogonadism NOS

Use Additional Code for adverse effect, if applicable, to identify drug (T36-T50 with fifth or sixth character 5)

Excludes1: postprocedural testicular hypofunction (E89.5)

E29.8   **Other testicular dysfunction**

E29.9   **Testicular dysfunction, unspecified**

E30   **Disorders of puberty, not elsewhere classified**

E30.0   **Delayed puberty**

Constitutional delay of puberty

Delayed sexual development

E30.1   **Precocious puberty**

Precocious menstruation

Excludes1: Albright (-McCune) (-Sternberg) syndrome (Q78.1)

central precocious puberty (E22.8)

congenital adrenal hyperplasia (E25.0)

female heterosexual precocious pseudopuberty (E25.-)

male isosexual precocious pseudopuberty (E25.-)

E30.8   **Other disorders of puberty**

Premature thelarche

E30.9   **Disorder of puberty, unspecified**

E31   **Polyglandular dysfunction**

Excludes1: ataxia telangiectasia [Louis-Bar] (G11.3)

dystrophia myotonica [Steinert] (G71.11)

pseudohypoparathyroidism (E20.1)

E31.0   **Autoimmune polyglandular failure** [HCC]

Schmidt's syndrome

E31.1   **Polyglandular hyperfunction** [HCC]

Excludes1: multiple endocrine adenomatosis (E31.2-)

multiple endocrine neoplasia (E31.2-)

E31.2   **Multiple endocrine neoplasia [MEN] syndromes**

Multiple endocrine adenomatosis

Code also any associated malignancies **and other** conditions associated with the syndromes

E31.20   **Multiple endocrine neoplasia [MEN] syndrome, unspecified** [HCC]

Multiple endocrine adenomatosis NOS

Multiple endocrine neoplasia [MEN] syndrome NOS

E31.21   **Multiple endocrine neoplasia [MEN] type I** [HCC]

Wermer's syndrome

E31.22   **Multiple endocrine neoplasia [MEN] type IIA** [HCC]

Sipple's syndrome

E31.23   **Multiple endocrine neoplasia [MEN] type IIB** [HCC]

E31.8   **Other polyglandular dysfunction** [HCC]

E31.9   **Polyglandular dysfunction, unspecified** [HCC]

E32   **Diseases of thymus**

Definition: The thymus is a gland located behind the breastbone that functions in the development of the immune system. The thymus is large in infancy and early childhood but begins to atrophy between ages eight and ten.

Excludes1: aplasia or hypoplasia of thymus with immunodeficiency (D82.1)

myasthenia gravis (G70.0)

E32.0   **Persistent hyperplasia of thymus** [HCC]

Hypertrophy of thymus

E32.1   **Abscess of thymus** [HCC]

E32.8   **Other diseases of thymus** [HCC]

Excludes1: aplasia or hypoplasia with immunodeficiency (D82.1)

thymoma (D15.0)

E32.9   **Disease of thymus, unspecified** [HCC]

E34   **Other endocrine disorders**

Definition: Endocrine disorders refers to disorders which involve the over-production or under-production of hormone substances from an endocrine gland. Examples include diabetes, hypothyroidism, hyperthyroidism, hyperparathyroidism, Cushing's disease, Cushing's syndrome and acromegaly.

Excludes1: pseudohypoparathyroidism (E20.1)

E34.0   **Carcinoid syndrome** [HCC]

Note: May be used as an additional code to identify functional activity associated with a carcinoid tumor.

E34.1   **Other hypersecretion of intestinal hormones**

E34.2   **Ectopic hormone secretion, not elsewhere classified**

Excludes1: ectopic ACTH syndrome (E24.3)

E34.3   **Short stature due to endocrine disorder**

Constitutional short stature

Laron-type short stature

Excludes1: achondroplastic short stature (Q77.4)

hypochondroplastic short stature (Q77.4)

nutritional short stature (E45)

pituitary short stature (E23.0)

progeria (E34.8)

renal short stature (N25.0)

Russell-Silver syndrome (Q87.11)

short-limbed stature with immunodeficiency (D82.2)

short stature in specific dysmorphic syndromes - code to syndrome - see Alphabetical

Index short stature NOS (R62.52)

E34.4 **Constitutional tall stature** [HCC]

Constitutional gigantism

E34.5 **Androgen insensitivity syndrome**

E34.50 **Androgen insensitivity syndrome, unspecified**

Androgen insensitivity NOS

E34.51 **Complete androgen insensitivity syndrome**

Complete androgen insensitivity de Quervain syndrome

Goldberg-Maxwell syndrome

E34.52 **Partial androgen insensitivity syndrome**

Partial androgen insensitivity

Reifenstein syndrome

E34.8 **Other specified endocrine disorders**

Pineal gland dysfunction

Progeria

Excludes2: pseudohypoparathyroidism (E20.1)

E34.9 **Endocrine disorder, unspecified**

Endocrine disturbance NOS

Hormone disturbance NOS

E35 **Disorders of endocrine glands in diseases classified elsewhere**

Code first underlying disease, such as:

late congenital syphilis of thymus gland [Dubois disease] (A50.5)

Use Additional Code, if applicable, to identify:

sequelae of tuberculosis of other organs (B90.8)

Excludes1: Echinococcus granulosus infection of thyroid gland (B67.3)

meningococcal hemorrhagic adrenalitis (A39.1)

syphilis of endocrine gland (A52.79)

tuberculosis of adrenal gland, except calcification (A18.7)

tuberculosis of endocrine gland NEC (A18.82)

tuberculosis of thyroid gland (A18.81)

Waterhouse-Friderichsen syndrome (A39.1)

INTRAOPERATIVE COMPLICATIONS OF ENDOCRINE SYSTEM (E36)

E36 **Intraoperative complications of endocrine system**

Excludes2: postprocedural endocrine and metabolic complications and disorders, not elsewhere classified (E89.-)

E36.0 **Intraoperative hemorrhage and hematoma of an endocrine system organ or structure complicating a procedure**

Excludes1: intraoperative hemorrhage and hematoma of an endocrine system organ or structure due to accidental puncture or laceration during a procedure (E36.1-)

E36.01 **Intraoperative hemorrhage and hematoma of an endocrine system organ or structure complicating an endocrine system procedure**

E36.02 **Intraoperative hemorrhage and hematoma of an endocrine system organ or structure complicating other procedure**

E36.1 **Accidental puncture and laceration of an endocrine system organ or structure during a procedure**

E36.11 **Accidental puncture and laceration of an endocrine system organ or structure during an endocrine system procedure**

E36.12 **Accidental puncture and laceration of an endocrine system organ or structure during other procedure**

E36.8 **Other intraoperative complications of endocrine system**

Use Additional Code, if applicable, to further specify disorder

MALNUTRITION (E40-E46)

Excludes1: intestinal malabsorption (K90.-)

sequelae of protein-calorie malnutrition (E64.0)

Excludes2: nutritional anemias (D50-D53)

starvation (T73.0)

E40 **Kwashiorkor** [HCC]

Severe malnutrition with nutritional edema with dyspigmentation of skin and hair

Excludes1: marasmic kwashiorkor (E42)

E41 **Nutritional marasmus** [HCC]

Severe malnutrition with marasmus

Excludes1: marasmic kwashiorkor (E42)

E42 **Marasmic kwashiorkor** [HCC]

Intermediate form severe protein-calorie malnutrition

Severe protein-calorie malnutrition with signs of both kwashiorkor and marasmus

E43 **Unspecified severe protein-calorie malnutrition** [HCC]

Starvation edema

E44 **Protein-calorie malnutrition of moderate and mild degree**

E44.0 **Moderate protein-calorie malnutrition** [HCC]

E44.1 **Mild protein-calorie malnutrition** [HCC]

E45 **Retarded development following protein-calorie malnutrition** [HCC]

Nutritional short stature

Nutritional stunting

Physical retardation due to malnutrition

E46 **Unspecified protein-calorie malnutrition** [HCC]

Malnutrition NOS

Protein-calorie imbalance NOS

Excludes1: nutritional deficiency NOS (E63.9)

OTHER NUTRITIONAL DEFICIENCIES (E50-E64)

Excludes2: nutritional anemias (D50-D53)

E50 **Vitamin A deficiency**

Definition: Vitamin A deficiency (VAD) occurs where diets contain insufficient vitamin A for meeting the needs associated with growth and development, physiological functions, and periods of added stress due to illness.

Excludes1: sequelae of vitamin A deficiency (E64.1)

E50.0 **Vitamin A deficiency with conjunctival xerosis**

E50.1 **Vitamin A deficiency with Bitot's spot and conjunctival xerosis**

Bitot's spot in the young child

E50.2 **Vitamin A deficiency with corneal xerosis**

E50.3 **Vitamin A deficiency with corneal ulceration and xerosis**

E50.4 **Vitamin A deficiency with keratomalacia**

E50.5 **Vitamin A deficiency with night blindness**

E50.6 Vitamin A deficiency with xerophthalmic scars of cornea

E50.7 Other ocular manifestations of vitamin A deficiency

Xerophthalmia NOS

E50.8 Other manifestations of vitamin A deficiency

Follicular keratosis Xeroderma

E50.9 Vitamin A deficiency, unspecified

Hypovitaminosis A NOS

E51 Thiamine deficiency

Excludes1: sequelae of thiamine deficiency (E64.8)

E51.1 Beriberi

E51.11 Dry beriberi

Beriberi NOS

Beriberi with polyneuropathy

E51.12 Wet beriberi

Beriberi with cardiovascular manifestations

Cardiovascular beriberi

Shoshin disease

E51.2 Wernicke's encephalopathy

E51.8 Other manifestations of thiamine deficiency

E51.9 Thiamine deficiency, unspecified

E52 Niacin deficiency [pellagra]

Niacin (-tryptophan) deficiency

Nicotinamide deficiency

Pellagra (alcoholic)

Excludes1: sequelae of niacin deficiency (E64.8)

E53 Deficiency of other B group vitamins

Excludes1: sequelae of vitamin B deficiency (E64.8)

E53.0 Riboflavin deficiency

Ariboflavinosis

Vitamin B2 deficiency

E53.1 Pyridoxine deficiency

Vitamin B6 deficiency

Excludes1: pyridoxine-responsive sideroblastic anemia (D64.3)

E53.8 Deficiency of other specified B group vitamins

Biotin deficiency

Cyanocobalamin deficiency

Folate deficiency

Folic acid deficiency

Pantothenic acid deficiency

Vitamin B12 deficiency

Excludes1: folate deficiency anemia (D52.-)

vitamin B12 deficiency anemia (D51.-)

E53.9 Vitamin B deficiency, unspecified

E54 Ascorbic acid deficiency

Deficiency of vitamin C

Scurvy

Excludes1: scorbutic anemia (D53.2)

sequelae of vitamin C deficiency (E64.2)

E55 Vitamin D deficiency

Excludes1: adult osteomalacia (M83.-)

osteoporosis (M80.-)

sequelae of rickets (E64.3)

E55.0 Rickets, active

Infantile osteomalacia Juvenile osteomalacia

Excludes1: celiac rickets (K90.0)

Crohn's rickets (K50.-)

hereditary vitamin D-dependent rickets (E83.32)

inactive rickets (E64.3)

renal rickets (N25.0)

sequelae of rickets (E64.3)

vitamin D-resistant rickets (E83.31)

E55.9 Vitamin D deficiency, unspecified

Avitaminosis D

E56 Other vitamin deficiencies

Excludes1: sequelae of other vitamin deficiencies (E64.8)

E56.0 Deficiency of vitamin E

E56.1 Deficiency of vitamin K

Excludes1: deficiency of coagulation factor due to vitamin K deficiency (D68.4)

vitamin K deficiency of newborn (P53)

E56.8 Deficiency of other vitamins

E56.9 Vitamin deficiency, unspecified

E58 Dietary calcium deficiency

Excludes1: disorders of calcium metabolism (E83.5-)

sequelae of calcium deficiency (E64.8)

E59 Dietary selenium deficiency

Keshan disease

Excludes1: sequelae of selenium deficiency (E64.8)

E60 Dietary zinc deficiency

E61 Deficiency of other nutrient elements

Use Additional Code for adverse effect, if applicable, to identify drug (T36-T50 with fifth or sixth character 5)

Excludes1: disorders of mineral metabolism (E83.-)

iodine deficiency related thyroid disorders (E00-E02)

sequelae of malnutrition and other nutritional deficiencies (E64.-)

E61.0 Copper deficiency

E61.1 Iron deficiency

Excludes1: iron deficiency anemia (D50.-)

E61.2 Magnesium deficiency

E61.3 Manganese deficiency

E61.4 Chromium deficiency

E61.5 Molybdenum deficiency

E61.6 Vanadium deficiency

E61.7 Deficiency of multiple nutrient elements

E61.8 Deficiency of other specified nutrient elements

E61.9 Deficiency of nutrient element, unspecified

E63 Other nutritional deficiencies

Excludes2: dehydration (E86.0)

failure to thrive, adult (R62.7)

failure to thrive, child (R62.51)

feeding problems in newborn (P92.-)

sequelae of malnutrition and other nutritional deficiencies (E64.-)

E63.0 Essential fatty acid [EFA] deficiency

E63.1 Imbalance of constituents of food intake

E63.8 Other specified nutritional deficiencies

E63.9 Nutritional deficiency, unspecified

E64 Sequelae of malnutrition and other nutritional deficiencies

Note: This category is to be used to indicate conditions in categories E43, E44, E46, E50-E63 as the cause of sequelae, which are themselves classified elsewhere. The 'sequelae' include conditions

● New code   ▲ Revised code   **Excludes1:** Not coded here   **Excludes2:** Not included here   ⊗ Placeholder required   ⑦7th digit required

specified as such; they also include the late effects of diseases classifiable to the above categories if the disease itself is no longer present

Code first condition resulting from (sequela) of malnutrition **and other** nutritional deficiencies

E64.0 **Sequelae of protein-calorie malnutrition** [HCC]

> **Excludes2:** retarded development following protein-calorie malnutrition (E45)

E64.1 **Sequelae of vitamin A deficiency**

E64.2 **Sequelae of vitamin C deficiency**

E64.3 **Sequelae of rickets**

E64.8 **Sequelae of other nutritional deficiencies**

E64.9 **Sequelae of unspecified nutritional deficiency**

OVERWEIGHT, OBESITY AND OTHER HYPERALIMENTATION (E65-E68)

E65 **Localized adiposity**

Fat pad

E66 **Overweight and obesity**

Code first obesity complicating pregnancy, childbirth and the puerperium, if applicable (O99.21-)

Use Additional Code to identify body mass index (BMI), if known (Z68.-)

Excludes1: adiposogenital dystrophy (E23.6)

> lipomatosis NOS (E88.2)

> lipomatosis dolorosa [Dercum] (E88.2)

> Prader-Willi syndrome (Q87.11)

E66.0 **Obesity due to excess calories**

E66.01 **Morbid (severe) obesity due to excess calories** [HCC]

> **Excludes1:** morbid (severe) obesity with alveolar hypoventilation (E66.2)

E66.09 **Other obesity due to excess calories**

E66.1 **Drug-induced obesity**

Use Additional Code for adverse effect, if applicable, to identify drug (T36-T50 with fifth or sixth character 5)

E66.2 **Morbid (severe) obesity with alveolar hypoventilation** [HCC]

Obesity hypoventilation syndrome (OHS)

Pickwickian syndrome

E66.3 **Overweight**

E66.8 **Other obesity**

E66.9 **Obesity, unspecified**

Obesity NOS

E67 **Other hyperalimentation**

Excludes1: hyperalimentation NOS (R63.2)

> sequelae of hyperalimentation (E68)

E67.0 **Hypervitaminosis A**

E67.1 **Hypercarotenemia**

E67.2 **Megavitamin-B6 syndrome**

E67.3 **Hypervitaminosis D**

E67.8 **Other specified hyperalimentation**

E68 **Sequelae of hyperalimentation**

Code first condition resulting from (sequela) of hyperalimentation

METABOLIC DISORDERS (E70-E88)

Excludes1: androgen insensitivity syndrome (E34.5-)

> congenital adrenal hyperplasia (E25.0)

> hemolytic anemias attributable to enzyme disorders (D55.-)

Marfan's syndrome (Q87.4)

5-alpha-reductase deficiency (E29.1)

Excludes2: Ehlers-Danlos syndromes (Q79.6-)

E70 **Disorders of aromatic amino-acid metabolism**

E70.0 **Classical phenylketonuria** [HCC]

E70.1 **Other hyperphenylalaninemias** [HCC]

E70.2 **Disorders of tyrosine metabolism**

> **Excludes1:** transitory tyrosinemia of newborn (P74.5)

E70.20 **Disorder of tyrosine metabolism, unspecified** [HCC]

E70.21 **Tyrosinemia** [HCC]

Hypertyrosinemia

E70.29 **Other disorders of tyrosine metabolism** [HCC]

Alkaptonuria

Ochronosis

E70.3 **Albinism**

E70.30 **Albinism, unspecified** [HCC]

E70.31 **Ocular albinism**

E70.310 **X-linked ocular albinism** [HCC]

E70.311 **Autosomal recessive ocular albinism** [HCC]

E70.318 **Other ocular albinism** [HCC]

E70.319 **Ocular albinism, unspecified** [HCC]

E70.32 **Oculocutaneous albinism**

> **Excludes1:** Chediak-Higashi syndrome (E70.330)

> Hermansky-Pudlak syndrome (E70.331)

E70.320 **Tyrosinase negative oculocutaneous albinism** [HCC]

Albinism I

Oculocutaneous albinism ty-neg

E70.321 **Tyrosinase positive oculocutaneous albinism** [HCC]

Albinism II

Oculocutaneous albinism ty-pos

E70.328 **Other oculocutaneous albinism** [HCC]

Cross syndrome

E70.329 **Oculocutaneous albinism, unspecified** [HCC]

E70.33 **Albinism with hematologic abnormality**

E70.330 **Chediak-Higashi syndrome** [HCC]

E70.331 **Hermansky-Pudlak syndrome** [HCC]

E70.338 **Other albinism with hematologic abnormality** [HCC]

E70.339 **Albinism with hematologic abnormality, unspecified** [HCC]

E70.39 **Other specified albinism** [HCC]

Piebaldism

E70.4 **Disorders of histidine metabolism**

E70.40 **Disorders of histidine metabolism, unspecified** [HCC]

E70.41 **Histidinemia** [HCC]

E70.49 **Other disorders of histidine metabolism** [HCC]

E70.5 **Disorders of tryptophan metabolism** [HCC]

E70.8 **Other disorders of aromatic amino-acid metabolism** [HCC]

E70.81 **Aromatic L-amino acid decarboxylase deficiency**

AADC deficiency

E70.89   Other disorders of aromatic amino-acid metabolism

E70.9   Disorder of aromatic amino-acid metabolism, unspecified [HCC]

E71   Disorders of branched-chain amino-acid metabolism and fatty-acid metabolism

E71.0   Maple-syrup-urine disease

E71.1   Other disorders of branched-chain amino-acid metabolism

E71.11   Branched-chain organic acidurias

E71.110   Isovaleric acidemia [HCC]

E71.111   3-methylglutaconic aciduria [HCC]

E71.118   Other branched-chain organic acidurias

E71.12   Disorders of propionate metabolism

E71.120   Methylmalonic acidemia [HCC]

E71.121   Propionic acidemia [HCC]

E71.128   Other disorders of propionate metabolism [HCC]

E71.19   Other disorders of branched-chain amino-acid metabolism [HCC]

Hyperleucine-isoleucinemia

Hypervalinemia

E71.2   Disorder of branched-chain amino-acid metabolism, unspecified [HCC]

E71.3   Disorders of fatty-acid metabolism

Excludes1: peroxisomal disorders (E71.5)

Refsum's disease (G60.1)

Schilder's disease (G37.0)

Excludes2: carnitine deficiency due to inborn error of metabolism (E71.42)

E71.30   Disorder of fatty-acid metabolism, unspecified

E71.31   Disorders of fatty-acid oxidation

E71.310   Long chain/very long chain acyl CoA dehydrogenase deficiency

LCAD

VLCAD

E71.311   Medium chain acyl CoA dehydrogenase deficiency [HCC]

MCAD

E71.312   Short chain acyl CoA dehydrogenase deficiency [HCC]

SCAD

E71.313   Glutaric aciduria type II [HCC]

Glutaric aciduria type II A

Glutaric aciduria type II B

Glutaric aciduria type II C

Excludes1: glutaric aciduria (type 1) NOS (E72.3)

E71.314   Muscle carnitine palmitoyltransferase deficiency [HCC]

E71.318   Other disorders of fatty-acid oxidation [HCC]

E71.32   Disorders of ketone metabolism [HCC]

E71.39   Other disorders of fatty-acid metabolism [HCC]

E71.4   Disorders of carnitine metabolism

Excludes1: Muscle carnitine palmitoyltransferase deficiency (E71.314)

E71.40   Disorder of carnitine metabolism, unspecified [HCC]

E71.41   Primary carnitine deficiency [HCC]

E71.42   Carnitine deficiency due to inborn errors of metabolism [HCC]

<u>Code also</u> associated inborn error or metabolism

E71.43   Iatrogenic carnitine deficiency [HCC]

Carnitine deficiency due to hemodialysis

Carnitine deficiency due to Valproic acid therapy

E71.44   Other secondary carnitine deficiency

E71.440   Ruvalcaba-Myhre-Smith syndrome [HCC]

E71.448   Other secondary carnitine deficiency [HCC]

E71.5   Peroxisomal disorders

Excludes1: Schilder's disease (G37.0)

E71.50   Peroxisomal disorder, unspecified [HCC]

E71.51   Disorders of peroxisome biogenesis

Group 1 peroxisomal disorders

Excludes1: Refsum's disease (G60.1)

E71.510   Zellweger syndrome [HCC]

E71.511   Neonatal adrenoleukodystrophy [HCC]

Excludes1: X-linked adrenoleukodystrophy (E71.42-)

E71.518   Other disorders of peroxisome biogenesis [HCC]

E71.52   X-linked adrenoleukodystrophy

E71.520   Childhood cerebral X-linked adrenoleukodystrophy [HCC]

E71.521   Adolescent X-linked adrenoleukodystrophy [HCC]

E71.522   Adrenomyeloneuropathy [HCC]

E71.528   Other X-linked adrenoleukodystrophy [HCC]

Addison only phenotype adrenoleukodystrophy

Addison-Schilder adrenoleukodystrophy

E71.529   X-linked adrenoleukodystrophy, unspecified type [HCC]

E71.53   Other group 2 peroxisomal disorders [HCC]

E71.54   Other peroxisomal disorders

E71.540   Rhizomelic chondrodysplasia punctata [HCC]

Excludes1: chondrodysplasia punctata NOS (Q77.3)

E71.541   Zellweger-like syndrome [HCC]

E71.542   Other group 3 peroxisomal disorders [HCC]

E71.548   Other peroxisomal disorders [HCC]

E72   Other disorders of amino-acid metabolism

Excludes1: disorders of:

aromatic amino-acid metabolism (E70.-)

branched-chain amino-acid metabolism (E71.0-E71.2)

fatty-acid metabolism (E71.3)

purine and pyrimidine metabolism (E79.-)

gout (M1A.-, M10.-)

E72.0   Disorders of amino-acid transport

Excludes1: disorders of tryptophan metabolism (E70.5)

E72.00   Disorders of amino-acid transport, unspecified [HCC]

E72.01   **Cystinuria** [HCC]

E72.02   **Hartnup's disease** [HCC]

E72.03   **Lowe's syndrome** [HCC]

Use Additional Code for associated glaucoma (H42)

E72.04   **Cystinosis** [HCC]

Fanconi (-de Toni) (-Debré) syndrome with cystinosis

Excludes1: Fanconi (-de Toni) (-Debré) syndrome without cystinosis (E72.09)

E72.09   **Other disorders of amino-acid transport** [HCC]

Fanconi (-de Toni) (-Debré) syndrome, unspecified

E72.1   **Disorders of sulfur-bearing amino-acid metabolism**

Excludes1: cystinosis (E72.04)

cystinuria (E72.01)

transcobalamin II deficiency (D51.2)

E72.10   **Disorders of sulfur-bearing amino-acid metabolism, unspecified** [HCC]

E72.11   **Homocystinuria** [HCC]

Cystathionine synthase deficiency

E72.12   **Methylenetetrahydrofolate reductase deficiency** [HCC]

E72.19   **Other disorders of sulfur-bearing amino-acid metabolism** [HCC]

Cystathioninuria

Methioninemia

Sulfite oxidase deficiency

E72.2   **Disorders of urea cycle metabolism**

Excludes1: disorders of ornithine metabolism (E72.4)

E72.20   **Disorder of urea cycle metabolism, unspecified** [HCC]

Hyperammonemia

Excludes1: hyperammonemia-hyperornithinemia-homocitrullinemia syndrome E72.4

transient hyperammonemia of newborn (P74.6)

E72.21   **Argininemia** [HCC]

E72.22   **Arginosuccinic aciduria** [HCC]

E72.23   **Citrullinemia** [HCC]

E72.29   **Other disorders of urea cycle metabolism** [HCC]

E72.3   **Disorders of lysine and hydroxylysine metabolism** [HCC]

Glutaric aciduria NOS Glutaric aciduria (type I)

Hydroxylysinemia

Hyperlysinemia

Excludes1: glutaric aciduria type II (E71.313)

Refsum's disease (G60.1)

Zellweger syndrome (E71.510)

E72.4   **Disorders of ornithine metabolism** [HCC]

Hyperammonemia-Hyperornithinemia-Homocitrullinemia syndrome

Ornithinemia (types I, II)

Ornithine transcarbamylase deficiency

Excludes1: hereditary choroidal dystrophy (H31.2-)

E72.5   **Disorders of glycine metabolism**

E72.50   **Disorder of glycine metabolism, unspecified** [HCC]

E72.51   **Non-ketotic hyperglycinemia** [HCC]

E72.52   **Trimethylaminuria** [HCC]

E72.53   **Primary hyperoxaluria** [HCC]

Oxalosis

Oxaluria

E72.59   **Other disorders of glycine metabolism** [HCC]

D-glyceric acidemia

Hyperhydroxyprolinemia

Hyperprolinemia (types I, II)

Sarcosinemia

E72.8   **Other specified disorders of amino-acid metabolism**

E72.81   **Disorders of gamma aminobutyric acid metabolism** [HCC]

4-hydroxybutyric aciduria

Disorders of GABA metabolism

GABA metabolic defect

GABA transaminase deficiency

GABA-T deficiency

Gamma-hydroxybutyric aciduria

SSADHD

Succinic semialdehyde dehydrogenase deficiency

E72.89   **Other specified disorders of amino-acid metabolism** [HCC]

Disorders of beta-amino-acid metabolism

Disorders of gamma-glutamyl cycle

E72.9   **Disorder of amino-acid metabolism, unspecified** [HCC]

E73   **Lactose intolerance**

E73.0   **Congenital lactase deficiency**

E73.1   **Secondary lactase deficiency**

E73.8   **Other lactose intolerance**

E73.9   **Lactose intolerance, unspecified**

E74   **Other disorders of carbohydrate metabolism**

Excludes1: diabetes mellitus (E08-E13)

hypoglycemia NOS (E16.2)

increased secretion of glucagon (E16.3)

mucopolysaccharidosis (E76.0-E76.3)

E74.0   **Glycogen storage disease**

E74.00   **Glycogen storage disease, unspecified** [HCC]

E74.01   **von Gierke disease** [HCC]

Type I glycogen storage disease

E74.02   **Pompe disease** [HCC]

Cardiac glycogenosis

Type II glycogen storage disease

E74.03   **Cori disease** [HCC]

Forbes disease

Type III glycogen storage disease

E74.04   **McArdle disease** [HCC]

Type V glycogen storage disease

E74.09   **Other glycogen storage disease** [HCC]

Andersen disease

Hers disease

Tarui disease

Glycogen storage disease, types 0, IV, VI-XI

Liver phosphorylase deficiency

Muscle phosphofructokinase deficiency

E74.1   **Disorders of fructose metabolism**

Excludes1: muscle phosphofructokinase deficiency (E74.09)

E74.10   **Disorder of fructose metabolism, unspecified**

E74.11 **Essential fructosuria**

Fructokinase deficiency

E74.12 **Hereditary fructose intolerance**

Fructosemia

E74.19 **Other disorders of fructose metabolism**

Fructose-1, 6-diphosphatase deficiency

E74.2 **Disorders of galactose metabolism**

E74.20 **Disorders of galactose metabolism, unspecified**
[HCC]

E74.21 **Galactosemia** [HCC]

E74.29 **Other disorders of galactose metabolism**

Galactokinase deficiency

E74.3 **Other disorders of intestinal carbohydrate absorption**

Excludes2: lactose intolerance (E73.-)

E74.31 **Sucrase-isomaltase deficiency**

E74.39 **Other disorders of intestinal carbohydrate absorption**

Disorder of intestinal carbohydrate absorption NOS

Glucose-galactose malabsorption

Sucrase deficiency

E74.4 **Disorders of pyruvate metabolism and gluconeogenesis**

Deficiency of phosphoenolpyruvate carboxykinase

Deficiency of pyruvate carboxylase

Deficiency of pyruvate dehydrogenase

Excludes1: disorders of pyruvate metabolism and gluconeogenesis with anemia (D55.-)

Leigh's syndrome (G31.82)

E74.8 **Other specified disorders of carbohydrate metabolism**

E74.81 **Disorders of glucose transport, not elsewhere classified**

E74.810 **Glucose transporter protein type 1 deficiency**

De Vivo syndrome

Glucose transport defect, blood-brain barrier

Glut1 deficiency

GLUT1 deficiency syndrome 1, infantile onset

GLUT1 deficiency syndrome 2, childhood onset

E74.818 **Other disorders of glucose transport**

(Familial) renal glycosuria

E74.819 **Disorders of glucose transport, unspecified**

E74.89 **Other specified disorders of carbohydrate metabolism**

Essential pentosuria

E74.9 **Disorder of carbohydrate metabolism, unspecified**

E75 **Disorders of sphingolipid metabolism and other lipid storage disorders**

Excludes1: mucolipidosis, types I-III (E77.0-E77.1)

Refsum's disease (G60.1)

E75.0 **GM2 gangliosidosis**

E75.00 **GM2 gangliosidosis, unspecified**

E75.01 **Sandhoff disease**

E75.02 **Tay-Sachs disease**

E75.09 **Other GM2 gangliosidosis**

Adult GM2 gangliosidosis

Juvenile GM2 gangliosidosis

E75.1 **Other and unspecified gangliosidosis**

E75.10 **Unspecified gangliosidosis**

Gangliosidosis NOS

E75.11 **Mucolipidosis IV**

E75.19 **Other gangliosidosis**

GM1 gangliosidosis

GM3 gangliosidosis

E75.2 **Other sphingolipidosis**

Excludes1: adrenoleukodystrophy [Addison-Schilder] (E71.528)

E75.21 **Fabry (-Anderson) disease** [HCC]

E75.22 **Gaucher disease** [HCC]

E75.23 **Krabbe disease**

E75.24 **Niemann-Pick disease**

Acid sphingomyelinase deficiency (ASMD)

E75.240 **Niemann-Pick disease type A** [HCC]

Acid sphingomyelinase deficiency type A (ASMD type A)

Infantile neurovisceral acid sphingomyelinase deficiency

E75.241 **Niemann-Pick disease type B** [HCC]

Acid sphingomyelinase deficiency type B (ASMD type B)

Chronic visceral acid sphingomyelinase deficiency

E75.242 **Niemann-Pick disease type C** [HCC]

E75.243 **Niemann-Pick disease type D** [HCC]

● E75.244 **Niemann-Pick disease type A/B** [HCC]

Acid sphingomyelinase deficiency type A/B (ASMD type A/B)

Chronic neurovisceral acid sphingomyelinase deficiency

E75.248 **Other Niemann-Pick disease** [HCC]

E75.249 **Niemann-Pick disease, unspecified** [HCC]

Acid sphingomyelinase deficiency (ASMD) NOS

E75.25 **Metachromatic leukodystrophy**

E75.26 **Sulfatase deficiency**

E75.29 **Other sphingolipidosis**

Farber's syndrome

Sulfatide lipidosis

E75.3 **Sphingolipidosis, unspecified** [HCC]

E75.4 **Neuronal ceroid lipofuscinosis**

Batten disease

Bielschowsky-Jansky disease

Kufs disease

Spielmeyer-Vogt disease

E75.5 **Other lipid storage disorders**

Cerebrotendinous cholesterosis [van Bogaert-Scherer-Epstein]

Wolman's disease

E75.6 **Lipid storage disorder, unspecified**

E76 **Disorders of glycosaminoglycan metabolism**

E76.0 **Mucopolysaccharidosis, type I**

E76.01 **Hurler's syndrome** [HCC]

● New code ▲ Revised code **Excludes1:** Not coded here **Excludes2:** Not included here ⊗ Placeholder required ⑦7th digit required

E76.02 **Hurler-Scheie syndrome** [HCC]

E76.03 **Scheie's syndrome** [HCC]

E76.1 **Mucopolysaccharidosis, type II** [HCC]

Hunter's syndrome

E76.2 **Other mucopolysaccharidoses**

E76.21 **Morquio mucopolysaccharidoses**

E76.210 **Morquio A mucopolysaccharidoses** [HCC]

Classic Morquio syndrome

Morquio syndrome A

Mucopolysaccharidosis, type IVA

E76.211 **Morquio B mucopolysaccharidoses** [HCC]

Morquio-like mucopolysaccharidoses

Morquio-like syndrome

Morquio syndrome B

Mucopolysaccharidosis, type IVB

E76.219 **Morquio mucopolysaccharidoses, unspecified** [HCC]

Morquio syndrome

Mucopolysaccharidosis, type IV

E76.22 **Sanfilippo mucopolysaccharidoses** [HCC]

Mucopolysaccharidosis, type III (A) (B) (C) (D)

Sanfilippo A syndrome

Sanfilippo B syndrome

Sanfilippo C syndrome

Sanfilippo D syndrome

E76.29 **Other mucopolysaccharidoses** [HCC]

beta-Glucuronidase deficiency

Maroteaux-Lamy (mild) (severe) syndrome

Mucopolysaccharidosis, types VI, VII

E76.3 **Mucopolysaccharidosis, unspecified** [HCC]

E76.8 **Other disorders of glucosaminoglycan metabolism** [HCC]

E76.9 **Glucosaminoglycan metabolism disorder, unspecified** [HCC]

E77 **Disorders of glycoprotein metabolism**

E77.0 **Defects in post-translational modification of lysosomal enzymes** [HCC]

Mucolipidosis II [I-cell disease]

Mucolipidosis III [pseudo-Hurler polydystrophy]

E77.1 **Defects in glycoprotein degradation** [HCC]

Aspartylglucosaminuria

Fucosidosis

Mannosidosis

Sialidosis [mucolipidosis I]

E77.8 **Other disorders of glycoprotein metabolism** [HCC]

E77.9 **Disorder of glycoprotein metabolism, unspecified** [HCC]

E78 **Disorders of lipoprotein metabolism and other lipidemias**

Excludes1: sphingolipidosis (E75.0-E75.3)

E78.0 **Pure hypercholesterolemia**

E78.00 **Pure hypercholesterolemia, unspecified**

(Pure) hypercholesterolemia NOS

Fredrickson's hyperlipoproteinemia, type IIa

Hyperbetalipoproteinemia

Low-density-lipoprotein-type [LDL] hyperlipoproteinemia

E78.01 **Familial hypercholesterolemia**

E78.1 **Pure hyperglyceridemia**

Elevated fasting triglycerides

Endogenous hyperglyceridemia

Fredrickson's hyperlipoproteinemia, type IV

Hyperlipidemia, group B

Hyperprebetalipoproteinemia

Very-low-density-lipoprotein-type [VLDL] hyperlipoproteinemia

E78.2 **Mixed hyperlipidemia**

Broad- or floating-betalipoproteinemia

Combined hyperlipidemia NOS

Elevated cholesterol with elevated triglycerides NEC

Fredrickson's hyperlipoproteinemia, type IIb or III

Hyperbetalipoproteinemia with prebetalipoproteinemia

Hypercholesteremia with endogenous hyperglyceridemia

Hyperlipidemia, group C

Tubo-eruptive xanthoma

Xanthoma tuberosum

Excludes1: cerebrotendinous cholesterosis [van Bogaert-Scherer- Epstein] (E75.5)

familial combined hyperlipidemia (E78.4)

E78.3 **Hyperchylomicronemia**

Chylomicron retention disease

Fredrickson's hyperlipoproteinemia, type I or V

Hyperlipidemia, group D

Mixed hyperglyceridemia

E78.4 **Other hyperlipidemia**

E78.41 **Elevated Lipoprotein(a)**

Elevated Lp(a)

E78.49 **Other hyperlipidemia**

Familial combined hyperlipidemia

E78.5 **Hyperlipidemia, unspecified**

E78.6 **Lipoprotein deficiency**

Abetalipoproteinemia

Depressed HDL cholesterol

High-density lipoprotein deficiency

Hypoalphalipoproteinemia

Hypobetalipoproteinemia (familial)

Lecithin cholesterol acyltransferase deficiency

Tangier disease

E78.7 **Disorders of bile acid and cholesterol metabolism**

Excludes1: Niemann-Pick disease type C (E75.242)

E78.70 **Disorder of bile acid and cholesterol metabolism, unspecified**

E78.71 **Barth syndrome**

E78.72 **Smith-Lemli-Opitz syndrome**

E78.79 **Other disorders of bile acid and cholesterol metabolism**

E78.8 **Other disorders of lipoprotein metabolism**

E78.81 **Lipoid dermatoarthritis**

E78.89 **Other lipoprotein metabolism disorders**

E78.9 **Disorder of lipoprotein metabolism, unspecified**

E79 **Disorders of purine and pyrimidine metabolism**

Excludes1: Ataxia-telangiectasia (Q87.19)

Bloom's syndrome (Q82.8)

Cockayne's syndrome (Q87.19)

calculus of kidney (N20.0)

combined immunodeficiency disorders (D81.-)

Fanconi's anemia (D61.09)

gout (M1A.-, M10.-)

orotaciduric anemia (D53.0)

progeria (E34.8)

Werner's syndrome (E34.8)

xeroderma pigmentosum (Q82.1)

E79.0 **Hyperuricemia without signs of inflammatory arthritis and tophaceous disease**

Asymptomatic hyperuricemia

E79.1 **Lesch-Nyhan syndrome** [HCC]

HGPRT deficiency

E79.2 **Myoadenylate deaminase deficiency** [HCC]

E79.8 **Other disorders of purine and pyrimidine metabolism** [HCC]

Hereditary xanthinuria

E79.9 **Disorder of purine and pyrimidine metabolism, unspecified** [HCC]

E80 **Disorders of porphyrin and bilirubin metabolism**

Includes: defects of catalase and peroxidase

E80.0 **Hereditary erythropoietic porphyria** [HCC]

Congenital erythropoietic porphyria

Erythropoietic protoporphyria

E80.1 **Porphyria cutanea tarda** [HCC]

E80.2 **Other and unspecified porphyria**

E80.20 **Unspecified porphyria** [HCC]

Porphyria NOS

E80.21 **Acute intermittent (hepatic) porphyria** [HCC]

E80.29 **Other porphyria** [HCC]

Hereditary coproporphyria

E80.3 **Defects of catalase and peroxidase** [HCC]

Acatalasia [Takahara]

E80.4 **Gilbert syndrome**

E80.5 **Crigler-Najjar syndrome**

E80.6 **Other disorders of bilirubin metabolism**

Dubin-Johnson syndrome

Rotor's syndrome

E80.7 **Disorder of bilirubin metabolism, unspecified**

E83 **Disorders of mineral metabolism**

Excludes1: dietary mineral deficiency (E58-E61)

parathyroid disorders (E20-E21)

vitamin D deficiency (E55.-)

E83.0 **Disorders of copper metabolism**

E83.00 **Disorder of copper metabolism, unspecified**

E83.01 **Wilson's disease**

Code also associated Kayser Fleischer ring (H18.04-)

E83.09 **Other disorders of copper metabolism**

Menkes' (kinky hair) (steely hair) disease

E83.1 **Disorders of iron metabolism**

Excludes1: iron deficiency anemia (D50.-)

sideroblastic anemia (D64.0-D64.3)

E83.10 **Disorder of iron metabolism, unspecified**

E83.11 **Hemochromatosis**

Excludes1: GALD (P78.84)

Gestational alloimmune liver disease (P78.84)

Neonatal hemochromatosis (P78.84)

E83.110 **Hereditary hemochromatosis** [HCC]

Bronzed diabetes

Pigmentary cirrhosis (of liver)

Primary (hereditary) hemochromatosis

E83.111 **Hemochromatosis due to repeated red blood cell transfusions**

Iron overload due to repeated red blood cell transfusions

Transfusion (red blood cell) associated hemochromatosis

E83.118 **Other hemochromatosis**

E83.119 **Hemochromatosis, unspecified**

E83.19 **Other disorders of iron metabolism**

Use Additional Code, if applicable, for idiopathic pulmonary hemosiderosis (J84.03)

E83.2 **Disorders of zinc metabolism**

Acrodermatitis enteropathica

E83.3 **Disorders of phosphorus metabolism and phosphatases**

Excludes1: adult osteomalacia (M83.-)

osteoporosis (M80.-)

E83.30 **Disorder of phosphorus metabolism, unspecified**

E83.31 **Familial hypophosphatemia**

Vitamin D-resistant osteomalacia

Vitamin D-resistant rickets

Excludes1: vitamin D-deficiency rickets (E55.0)

E83.32 **Hereditary vitamin D-dependent rickets (type 1) (type 2)**

25-hydroxyvitamin D 1-alpha-hydroxylase deficiency

Pseudovitamin D deficiency

Vitamin D receptor defect

E83.39 **Other disorders of phosphorus metabolism**

Acid phosphatase deficiency

Hypophosphatasia

E83.4 **Disorders of magnesium metabolism**

E83.40 **Disorders of magnesium metabolism, unspecified**

E83.41 **Hypermagnesemia**

E83.42 **Hypomagnesemia**

E83.49 **Other disorders of magnesium metabolism**

E83.5 **Disorders of calcium metabolism**

Excludes1: chondrocalcinosis (M11.1-M11.2)

hungry bone syndrome (E83.81)

hyperparathyroidism (E21.0-E21.3)

E83.50 **Unspecified disorder of calcium metabolism**

E83.51 **Hypocalcemia**

E83.52 **Hypercalcemia**

Familial hypocalciuric hypercalcemia

E83.59 **Other disorders of calcium metabolism**

E83.8 **Other disorders of mineral metabolism**

E83.81 **Hungry bone syndrome**

E83.89 **Other disorders of mineral metabolism**

E83.9 **Disorder of mineral metabolism, unspecified**

E84 **Cystic fibrosis**

Includes: mucoviscidosis

Code also exocrine pancreatic insufficiency (K86.81)

E84.0 Cystic fibrosis with pulmonary manifestations [HCC]

    Use Additional Code to identify any infectious organism present, such as:

    Pseudomonas (B96.5)

E84.1 Cystic fibrosis with intestinal manifestations

    E84.11 Meconium ileus in cystic fibrosis [HCC]

        Excludes1: meconium ileus not due to cystic fibrosis (P76.0)

    E84.19 Cystic fibrosis with other intestinal manifestations [HCC]

        Distal intestinal obstruction syndrome

E84.8 Cystic fibrosis with other manifestations [HCC]

E84.9 Cystic fibrosis, unspecified [HCC]

E85 Amyloidosis

    Excludes2: Alzheimer's disease (G30.0-)

E85.0 Non-neuropathic heredofamilial amyloidosis [HCC]

    Hereditary amyloid nephropathy

    Code also associated disorders, such as:

    Autoinflammatory syndromes (M04.-)

    Transthyretin-related (ATTR) familial amyloid cardiomyopathy (E85.4)

E85.1 Neuropathic heredofamilial amyloidosis

    Amyloid polyneuropathy (Portuguese)

    Transthyretin-related (ATTR) familial amyloid polyneuropathy

E85.2 Heredofamilial amyloidosis, unspecified [HCC]

E85.3 Secondary systemic amyloidosis [HCC]

    Hemodialysis-associated amyloidosis

E85.4 Organ-limited amyloidosis [HCC]

    Localized amyloidosis

    Transthyretin-related (ATTR) familial amyloid cardiomyopathy

E85.8 Other amyloidosis

    E85.81 Light chain (AL) amyloidosis [HCC]

    E85.82 Wild-type transthyretin-related (ATTR) amyloidosis [HCC]

        Senile systemic amyloidosis (SSA)

    E85.89 Other amyloidosis [HCC]

E85.9 Amyloidosis, unspecified [HCC]

E86 Volume depletion

    Use Additional Code(s) for any associated disorders of electrolyte and acid-base balance (E87.-)

    Excludes1: dehydration of newborn (P74.1)

        postprocedural hypovolemic shock (T81.19)

        traumatic hypovolemic shock (T79.4)

    Excludes2: hypovolemic shock NOS (R57.1)

E86.0 Dehydration

E86.1 Hypovolemia

    Depletion of volume of plasma

E86.9 Volume depletion, unspecified

E87 Other disorders of fluid, electrolyte and acid-base balance

    Excludes1: diabetes insipidus (E23.2)

        electrolyte imbalance associated with hyperemesis gravidarum (O21.1)

        electrolyte imbalance following ectopic or molar pregnancy (O08.5)

        familial periodic paralysis (G72.3)

E87.0 Hyperosmolality and hypernatremia

    Sodium [Na] excess

    Sodium [Na] overload

E87.1 Hypo-osmolality and hyponatremia

    Sodium [Na] deficiency

    Excludes1: syndrome of inappropriate secretion of antidiuretic hormone (E22.2)

E87.2 Acidosis

    Acidosis NOS

    Lactic acidosis

    Metabolic acidosis

    Respiratory acidosis

    Excludes1: diabetic acidosis - see categories E08-E10, E11, E13 with ketoacidosis

E87.3 Alkalosis

    Alkalosis NOS

    Metabolic alkalosis

    Respiratory alkalosis

E87.4 Mixed disorder of acid-base balance

E87.5 Hyperkalemia

    Potassium [K] excess

    Potassium [K] overload

E87.6 Hypokalemia

    Potassium [K] deficiency

E87.7 Fluid overload

    Excludes1: edema NOS (R60.9)

        fluid retention (R60.9)

    E87.70 Fluid overload, unspecified

    E87.71 Transfusion associated circulatory overload

        Fluid overload due to transfusion (blood) (blood components) TACO

    E87.79 Other fluid overload

E87.8 Other disorders of electrolyte and fluid balance, not elsewhere classified

    Electrolyte imbalance NOS

    Hyperchloremia

    Hypochloremia

E88 Other and unspecified metabolic disorders

    Use Additional Codes for associated conditions

    Excludes1: histiocytosis X (chronic) (C96.6)

E88.0 Disorders of plasma-protein metabolism, not elsewhere classified

    Excludes1: monoclonal gammopathy (of undetermined significance) (D47.2)

        polyclonal hypergammaglobulinemia (D89.0)

        Waldenström macroglobulinemia (C88.0)

    Excludes2: disorder of lipoprotein metabolism (E78.-)

    E88.01 Alpha-1-antitrypsin deficiency [HCC]

        AAT deficiency

    E88.02 Plasminogen deficiency

        Dysplasminogenemia

        Hypoplasminogenemia

        Type 1 plasminogen deficiency

        Type 2 plasminogen deficiency

        Code also, if applicable, ligneous conjunctivitis (H10.51)

        Use Additional Code for associated findings, such as:

hydrocephalus (G91.4)

ligneous conjunctivitis (H10.51)

otitis media (H67.-)

respiratory disorder related to plasminogen deficiency (J99)

E88.09 **Other disorders of plasma-protein metabolism, not elsewhere classified**

Bisalbuminemia

E88.1 **Lipodystrophy, not elsewhere classified**

Lipodystrophy NOS

Excludes1: Whipple's disease (K90.81)

E88.2 **Lipomatosis, not elsewhere classified**

Lipomatosis NOS

Lipomatosis (Check) dolorosa [Dercum]

E88.3 **Tumor lysis syndrome**

Tumor lysis syndrome (spontaneous)

Tumor lysis syndrome following antineoplastic drug chemotherapy

Use Additional Code for adverse effect, if applicable, to identify drug (T45.1X5)

E88.4 **Mitochondrial metabolism disorders**

Excludes1: disorders of pyruvate metabolism (E74.4)

Kearns-Sayre syndrome (H49.81)

Leber's disease (H47.22)

Leigh's encephalopathy (G31.82)

Mitochondrial myopathy, NEC (G71.3)

Reye's syndrome (G93.7)

E88.40 **Mitochondrial metabolism disorder, unspecified** [HCC]

E88.41 **MELAS syndrome** [HCC]

Mitochondrial myopathy, encephalopathy, lactic acidosis and stroke-like episodes

E88.42 **MERRF syndrome** [HCC]

Myoclonic epilepsy associated with ragged-red fibers

Code also progressive myoclonic epilepsy (G40.3-)

E88.49 **Other mitochondrial metabolism disorders** [HCC]

E88.8 **Other specified metabolic disorders**

E88.81 **Metabolic syndrome**

Dysmetabolic syndrome X

Use Additional Codes for associated manifestations, such as:

obesity (E66.-)

E88.89 **Other specified metabolic disorders**

Launois-Bensaude adenolipomatosis

Excludes1: adult pulmonary Langerhans cell histiocytosis (J84.82)

E88.9 **Metabolic disorder, unspecified**

POSTPROCEDURAL ENDOCRINE AND METABOLIC COMPLICATIONS AND DISORDERS, NOT ELSEWHERE CLASSIFIED (E89)

E89 **Postprocedural endocrine and metabolic complications and disorders, not elsewhere classified**

Excludes2: intraoperative complications of endocrine system organ or structure (E36.0-, E36.1-, E36.8)

E89.0 **Postprocedural hypothyroidism**

Postirradiation hypothyroidism

Postsurgical hypothyroidism

E89.1 **Postprocedural hypoinsulinemia**

Postpancreatectomy hyperglycemia

Postsurgical hypoinsulinemia

Use Additional Code, if applicable, to identify:

acquired absence of pancreas (Z90.41-)

diabetes mellitus (postpancreatectomy) (postprocedural) (E13.-)

insulin use (Z79.4)

Excludes1: transient postprocedural hyperglycemia (R73.9)

transient postprocedural hypoglycemia (E16.2)

E89.2 **Postprocedural hypoparathyroidism** [HCC]

Parathyroprival tetany

E89.3 **Postprocedural hypopituitarism** [HCC]

Postirradiation hypopituitarism

E89.4 **Postprocedural ovarian failure**

E89.40 **Asymptomatic postprocedural ovarian failure**

Postprocedural ovarian failure NOS

E89.41 **Symptomatic postprocedural ovarian failure**

Symptoms such as flushing, sleeplessness, headache, lack of concentration, associated with postprocedural menopause

E89.5 **Postprocedural testicular hypofunction**

E89.6 **Postprocedural adrenocortical (-medullary) hypofunction** [HCC]

E89.8 **Other postprocedural endocrine and metabolic complications and disorders**

E89.81 **Postprocedural hemorrhage of an endocrine system organ or structure following a procedure**

E89.810 **Postprocedural hemorrhage of an endocrine system organ or structure following an endocrine system procedure**

E89.811 **Postprocedural hemorrhage of an endocrine system organ or structure following other procedure**

E89.82 **Postprocedural hematoma and seroma of an endocrine system organ or structure**

E89.820 **Postprocedural hematoma of an endocrine system organ or structure following an endocrine system procedure**

E89.821 **Postprocedural hematoma of an endocrine system organ or structure following other procedure**

E89.822 **Postprocedural seroma of an endocrine system organ or structure following an endocrine system procedure**

E89.823 **Postprocedural seroma of an endocrine system organ or structure following other procedure**

E89.89 **Other postprocedural endocrine and metabolic complications and disorders**

Use Additional Code, if applicable, to further specify disorder

● New code ▲ Revised code Excludes1: Not coded here Excludes2: Not included here ⊗ Placeholder required ⑦7th digit required

Chapter 5: Mental, Behavioral and Neurodevelopmental Disorders (F01-F99)

DEFINITIONS

This chapter includes definitions of selected key words, terms and phrases and coding alerts for adding points to the clinical domain, and references to coding late effects where appropriate. An example from this chapter is as follows:

F02   Dementia in other diseases classified elsewhere

Definition: Dementia refers to a group of symptoms caused by disorders that affect the brain. It is not a specific disease.

MULTIPLE CODING FOR A SINGLE CONDITION

In addition to the etiology/manifestation convention that requires two codes to fully describe a single condition that affects multiple body systems, there are other single conditions that also require more than one code. "**Use Additional Code**" notes are found in the Tabular List at codes that are not part of an etiology/manifestation pair where a secondary code is useful to fully describe a condition. The sequencing rule is the same as the etiology/manifestation pair, "**Use Additional Code**" indicates that a secondary code should be added.

For example, for bacterial infections that are not included in chapter 1, a secondary code from category B95, Streptococcus, Staphylococcus, and Enterococcus, as the cause of diseases classified elsewhere, or B96, Other bacterial agents as the cause of diseases classified elsewhere, may be required to identify the bacterial organism causing the infection. A "**Use Additional Code**" note will normally be found at the infectious disease code, indicating a need for the organism code to be added as a secondary code.

"Code first" notes are also under certain codes that are not specifically manifestation codes but may be due to an underlying cause. When there is a "Code first" note and an underlying condition is present, the underlying condition should be sequenced first.

"Code, if applicable, any causal condition first", notes indicate that this code may be assigned as a principal diagnosis when the causal condition is unknown or not applicable. If a causal condition is known, then the code for that condition should be sequenced as the principal or first-listed diagnosis.

Multiple codes may be needed for sequela, complication codes and obstetric codes to more fully describe a condition. See the specific guidelines for these conditions for further instruction.

COMBINATION CODE

A combination code is a single code used to classify: Two diagnoses, or a diagnosis with an associated secondary process (manifestation) A diagnosis with an associated complication

Combination codes are identified by referring to subterm entries in the Alphabetic Index and by reading the inclusion and exclusion notes in the Tabular List.

Assign only the combination code when that code fully identifies the diagnostic conditions involved or when the Alphabetic Index so directs. Multiple coding should not be used when the classification provides a combination code that clearly identifies all of the elements documented in the diagnosis. When the combination code lacks necessary specificity in describing the manifestation or complication, an additional code should be used as a secondary code.

SEQUELA (LATE EFFECTS)

A sequela is the residual effect (condition produced) after the acute phase of an illness or injury has terminated. There is no time limit on when a sequela code can be used. The residual may be apparent early, such as in cerebral infarction, or it may occur months or years later, such as that due to a previous injury. Coding of sequela generally requires two codes sequenced in the following order: The condition or nature of the sequela is sequenced first.

The sequela code is sequenced second.

An exception to the above guidelines are those instances where the code for the sequela is followed by a manifestation code identified in the Tabular List and title, or the sequela code has been expanded (at the fourth, fifth or sixth character levels) to

F01-F99

include the manifestation(s). The code for the acute phase of an illness or injury that led to the sequela is never used with a code for the late effect.

Pain disorders related to psychological factors

Assign code F45.41, for pain that is exclusively related to psychological disorders. As indicated by the Excludes 1 note under category G89, a code from category G89 should not be assigned with code F45.41.

Code F45.42, Pain disorders with related psychological factors, should be used with a code from category G89, Pain, not elsewhere classified, if there is documentation of a psychological component for a patient with acute or chronic pain.

See Section I.C.6. Pain

Mental and behavioral disorders due to psychoactive substance use

1) In Remission

Selection of codes for "in remission" for categories F10-F19, Mental and behavioral disorders due to psychoactive substance use (categories F10-F19 with -.11, -.21) requires the provider's clinical judgment. The appropriate codes for "in remission" are assigned only on the basis of provider documentation (as defined in the Official Guidelines for Coding and Reporting), unless otherwise instructed by the classification.

Mild substance use disorders in early or sustained remission are classified to the appropriate codes for substance abuse in remission, and moderate or severe substance use disorders in early or sustained remission are classified to the appropriate codes for substance dependence in remission.

2) Psychoactive Substance Use, Abuse and Dependence

When the provider documentation refers to use, abuse and dependence of the same substance (e.g., alcohol, opioid, cannabis, etc.), only one code should be assigned to identify the pattern of use based on the following hierarchy:

- If both use and abuse are documented, assign only the code for abuse

- If both abuse and dependence are documented, assign only the code for dependence

- If use, abuse and dependence are all documented, assign only the code for dependence

- If both use and dependence are documented, assign only the code for dependence.

3) Psychoactive Substance Use, Unspecified

As with all other unspecified diagnoses, the codes for unspecified psychoactive substance use (F10.9-, F11.9-, F12.9-, F13.9-, F14.9-, F15.9-, F16.9-, F18.9-, F19.9-) should only be assigned based on provider documentation and when they meet the definition of a reportable diagnosis (see Section III, Reporting Additional Diagnoses).

These codes are to be used only when the psychoactive substance use is associated with a substance related disorder (chapter 5 disorders such as sexual dysfunction, sleep disorder, or a mental or behavioral disorder)or medical condition, and such a relationship is documented by the provider.

4) Medical Conditions Due to Psychoactive Substance Use, Abuseand Dependence

Medical conditions due to substance use, abuse, and dependence arenot classified as substance-induced disorders. Assign the diagnosis code for the medical condition as directed by the Alphabetical Indexalong with the appropriate psychoactive substance use, abuse or dependence code. For example, for alcoholic pancreatitis due to alcohol dependence, assign the appropriate code from subcategory K85.2, Alcohol induced acute pancreatitis, and the appropriate codefrom subcategory F10.2, such as code F10.20, Alcohol dependence, uncomplicated. It would not be appropriate to assign code F10.288, Alcohol dependence with other alcohol-induced disorder.

5) Blood Alcohol Level

A code from category Y90, Evidence of alcohol involvement determined by blood alcohol level, may be assigned when this information is documented and the patient's provider has documented a condition classifiable to category F10, Alcohol relateddisorders. The blood alcohol level does not need to be documented by the patient's provider in order for it to be coded.

FACTITIOUS DISORDER

Factitious disorder imposed on self or Munchausen's syndrome is a disorder in which a person falsely reports or causes his or her own physical or psychological signs or symptoms. For patients with documented factitious disorder on self or Munchausen's syndrome, assign the appropriate code from subcategory F68.1-, Factitious disorder imposed on self.

Munchausen's syndrome by proxy (MSBP) is a disorder in which a caregiver (perpetrator) falsely reports or causes an illness or injury in another person (victim) under his or her care, such as a child, an elderly adult, or a person who has a disability. The condition is also referred to as "factitious disorder imposed on another" or "factitious disorder by proxy." The perpetrator, not the victim, receives this diagnosis. Assign code F68.A, Factitious disorder imposed on another, to the perpetrator's record. For the victim of a patient suffering from MSBP, assign the appropriate code from categories T74, Adult and child abuse, neglect and other maltreatment, confirmed, or T76, Adult and child abuse, neglect and other maltreatment, suspected.

See Section I.C.19.f. Adult and child abuse, neglect and other maltreatment

Chapter 5

Mental, Behavioral and Neurodevelopmental Disorders (F01-F99)

Includes: disorders of psychological development

Excludes2: symptoms, signs and abnormal clinical laboratory findings, not elsewhere classified (R00-R99)

This chapter contains the following blocks:

F01-F09	Mental disorders due to known physiological conditions
F10-F19	Mental and behavioral disorders due to psychoactive substance use
F20-F29	Schizophrenia, schizotypal, delusional, and other non-mood psychotic disorders
F30-F39	Mood [affective] disorders
F40-F48	Anxiety, dissociative, stress-related, somatoform and other nonpsychotic mental disorders
F50-F59	Behavioral syndromes associated with physiological disturbances and physical factors
F60-F69	Disorders of adult personality and behavior
F70-F79	Intellectual disabilities
F80-F89	Pervasive and specific developmental disorders
F90-F98	Behavioral and emotional disorders with onset usually occurring in childhood and adolescence
F99	Unspecified mental disorder

MENTAL DISORDERS DUE TO KNOWN PHYSIOLOGICAL CONDITIONS (F01-F09)

Note: This block comprises a range of mental disorders grouped together on the basis of their having in common a demonstrable etiology in cerebral disease, brain injury, or other insult leading to cerebral dysfunction. The dysfunction may be primary, as in diseases, injuries, and insults that affect the brain directly and selectively; or secondary, as in systemic diseases and disorders that attack the brain only as one of the multiple organs or systems of the body that are involved.

F01   Vascular dementia

Vascular dementia as a result of infarction of the brain due to vascular disease, including hypertensive cerebrovascular disease.

Includes: arteriosclerotic dementia

Code first the underlying physiological condition or sequelae of cerebrovascular disease.

F01.5   Vascular dementia

F01.50   Vascular dementia without behavioral disturbance

Major neurocognitive disorder without behavioral disturbance

F01.51   Vascular dementia with behavioral disturbance

Major neurocognitive disorder due to vascular disease, with behavioral disturbance

Major neurocognitive disorder with aggressive behavior

Major neurocognitive disorder with combative behavior

Major neurocognitive disorder with violent behavior

Vascular dementia with aggressive behavior

Vascular dementia with combative behavior

Vascular dementia with violent behavior

Use Additional Code, if applicable, to identify wandering in vascular dementia (Z91.83)

F02   Dementia in other diseases classified elsewhere

Definition: Dementia refers to a group of symptoms caused by disorders that affect the brain. It is not a specific disease.

Includes: Major neurocognitive disorder **in other** diseases classified elsewhere

Code first the underlying physiological condition, such as:

Alzheimer's (G30.-)

cerebral lipidosis (E75.4)

Creutzfeldt-Jakob disease (A81.0-)

dementia with Lewy bodies (G31.83)

dementia with Parkinsonism (G31.83)

epilepsy and recurrent seizures (G40.-)

frontotemporal dementia (G31.09)

hepatolenticular degeneration (E83.0)

human immunodeficiency virus [HIV] disease (B20)

Huntington's disease (G10)

hypercalcemia (E83.52)

hypothyroidism, acquired (E00-E03.-)

intoxications (T36-T65)

Jakob-Creutzfeldt disease (A81.0-)

multiple sclerosis (G35)

neurosyphilis (A52.17)

niacin deficiency [pellagra] (E52)

Parkinson's disease (G20)

Pick's disease (G31.01)

polyarteritis nodosa (M30.0)

prion disease (A81.9)

systemic lupus erythematosus (M32.-)

traumatic brain injury (S06.-)

trypanosomiasis (B56.-, B57.-)

vitamin B deficiency (E53.8)

Excludes2: dementia in alcohol and psychoactive substance disorders (F10-F19, with .17, .27, .97)

vascular dementia (F01.5-)

F02.8   Dementia in other diseases classified elsewhere

F02.80   Dementia in other diseases classified elsewhere without behavioral disturbance

Dementia in other diseases classified elsewhere NOS

Major neurocognitive disorder **in other** diseases classified elsewhere

F02.81   Dementia in other diseases classified elsewhere with behavioral disturbance

Dementia in other diseases classified elsewhere with aggressive behavior

Dementia in other diseases classified elsewhere with combative behavior

Dementia in other diseases classified elsewhere with violent behavior

Major neurocognitive disorder in other diseases classified elsewhere with aggressive behavior

Major neurocognitive disorder in other diseases classified elsewhere with combative behavior

Major neurocognitive disorder in other diseases classified elsewhere with violent behavior

Use Additional Code, if applicable, to identify wandering in dementia in conditions classified elsewhere (Z91.83)

F03   Unspecified dementia

Presenile dementia NOS

Add 4th-7th digits	Nonspecific code	Unspecified code	Manifestation code	[HCC] Hierarchical Condition Code

Presenile psychosis NOS

Primary degenerative dementia NOS

Senile dementia NOS

Senile dementia depressed or paranoid type

Senile psychosis NOS

Excludes1: senility NOS (R41.81)

Excludes2: mild memory disturbance due to known physiological condition (F06.8)

senile dementia with delirium or acute confusional state (F05)

F03.9   Unspecified dementia

F03.90   Unspecified dementia without behavioral disturbance

Dementia NOS

F03.91   Unspecified dementia with behavioral disturbance

Unspecified dementia with aggressive behavior

Unspecified dementia with combative behavior

Unspecified dementia with violent behavior

Use Additional Code, if applicable, to identify wandering in unspecified dementia (Z91.83)

F04   Amnestic disorder due to known physiological condition

Korsakov's psychosis or syndrome, nonalcoholic

Code first the underlying physiological condition

Excludes1: amnesia NOS (R41.3)

anterograde amnesia (R41.1)

dissociative amnesia (F44.0)

retrograde amnesia (R41.2)

Excludes2: alcohol-induced or unspecified Korsakov's syndrome (F10.26, F10.96)

Korsakov's syndrome induced by other psychoactive substances (F13.26, F13.96, F19.16, F19.26, F19.96)

F05   Delirium due to known physiological condition

Acute or subacute brain syndrome

Acute or subacute confusional state (nonalcoholic)

Acute or subacute infective psychosis

Acute or subacute organic reaction

Acute or subacute psycho-organic syndrome

Delirium of mixed etiology

Delirium superimposed on dementia

Sundowning

Code first the underlying physiological condition

Excludes1: delirium NOS (R41.0)

Excludes2: delirium tremens alcohol-induced or unspecified (F10.231, F10.921)

F06   Other mental disorders due to known physiological condition

Includes: mental disorders due to endocrine disorder

mental disorders due to exogenous hormone

mental disorders due to exogenous toxic substance

mental disorders due to primary cerebral disease

mental disorders due to somatic illness

mental disorders due to systemic disease affecting the brain

Code first the underlying physiological condition

Excludes1: unspecified dementia (F03)

Excludes2: delirium due to known physiological condition (F05)

dementia as classified in F01-F02

Other mental disorders associated with alcohol and other psychoactive substances (F10-F19)

F06.0   Psychotic disorder with hallucinations due to known physiological condition

Organic hallucinatory state (nonalcoholic)

Excludes2: hallucinations and perceptual disturbance induced by alcohol and other psychoactive substances (F10-F19 with .151, .251, .951)

schizophrenia (F20.-)

F06.1   Catatonic disorder due to known physiological condition

Catatonia associated with another mental disorder

Catatonia NOS

Excludes1: catatonic stupor (R40.1)

stupor NOS (R40.1)

Excludes2: catatonic schizophrenia (F20.2)

dissociative stupor (F44.2)

F06.2   Psychotic disorder with delusions due to known physiological condition

Paranoid and paranoid-hallucinatory organic states

Schizophrenia-like psychosis in epilepsy

Excludes2: alcohol and drug-induced psychotic disorder (F10-F19 with .150, .250, .950)

brief psychotic disorder (F23)

delusional disorder (F22)

schizophrenia (F20.-)

F06.3   Mood disorder due to known physiological condition

Excludes2: mood disorders due to alcohol and other psychoactive substances (F10-F19 with .14, .24, .94)

mood disorders, not due to known physiological condition or unspecified (F30-F39)

F06.30   Mood disorder due to known physiological condition, unspecified

F06.31   Mood disorder due to known physiological condition with depressive features

Depressive disorder due to known physiological condition, with depressive features

F06.32   Mood disorder due to known physiological condition with major depressive-like episode

Depressive disorder due to known physiological condition, with major depressive-like episode

F06.33   Mood disorder due to known physiological condition with manic features

Bipolar and related disorder due to a known physiological condition, with manic features

Bipolar and related disorder due to known physiological condition, with manic- or hypomanic-like episodes

F06.34   Mood disorder due to known physiological condition with mixed features

Bipolar and related disorder due to known physiological condition, with mixed features

Depressive disorder due to known physiological condition, with mixed features

F06.4   Anxiety disorder due to known physiological condition

Excludes2: anxiety disorders due to alcohol and other psychoactive substances (F10-F19 with .180, .280, .980)

anxiety disorders, not due to known physiological condition or unspecified (F40.-, F41.-)

F06.8   Other specified mental disorders due to known physiological condition

Epileptic psychosis NOS

Obsessive-compulsive and related disorder due to a known physiological condition

Organic dissociative disorder

Organic emotionally labile [asthenic] disorder

F07 Personality and behavioral disorders due to known physiological condition

Code first the underlying physiological condition

F07.0 Personality change due to known physiological condition

Frontal lobe syndrome

Limbic epilepsy personality syndrome

Lobotomy syndrome

Organic personality disorder

Organic pseudopsychopathic personality

Organic pseudoretarded personality

Postleucotomy syndrome

Code first underlying physiological condition

Excludes1: mild cognitive impairment (G31.84)

postconcussional syndrome (F07.81)

postencephalitic syndrome (F07.89)

signs and symptoms involving emotional state (R45.-)

Excludes2: specific personality disorder (F60.-)

F07.8 Other personality and behavioral disorders due to known physiological condition

F07.81 Postconcussional syndrome

Postcontusional syndrome (encephalopathy)

Post-traumatic brain syndrome, nonpsychotic

Use Additional Code to identify associated post-traumatic headache, if applicable (G44.3-)

Excludes1: current concussion (brain) (S06.0-)

postencephalitic syndrome (F07.89)

F07.89 Other personality and behavioral disorders due to known physiological condition

Postencephalitic syndrome

Right hemispheric organic affective disorder

F07.9 Unspecified personality and behavioral disorder due to known physiological condition

Organic psychosyndrome

F09 Unspecified mental disorder due to known physiological condition

Mental disorder NOS due to known physiological condition

Organic brain syndrome NOS

Organic mental disorder NOS

Organic psychosis NOS

Symptomatic psychosis NOS

Code first the underlying physiological condition

Excludes1: psychosis NOS (F29)

MENTAL AND BEHAVIORAL DISORDERS DUE TO PSYCHOACTIVE SUBSTANCE USE (F10-F19)

F10 Alcohol related disorders

Definition: Alcohol-induced mental disorders is an alcohol-induced psychological or behavioral pattern that occurs in an individual and is thought to cause distress or disability that is not expected as part of normal development or culture.

Use Additional Code for blood alcohol level, if applicable (Y90.-)

F10.1 Alcohol abuse

Excludes1: alcohol dependence (F10.2-)

alcohol use, unspecified (F10.9-)

F10.10 Alcohol abuse, uncomplicated

Alcohol use disorder, mild

F10.11 Alcohol abuse, in remission

Alcohol use disorder, mild, in early remission

Alcohol use disorder, mild, in sustained remission

F10.12 Alcohol abuse with intoxication

F10.120 Alcohol abuse with intoxication, uncomplicated [HCC]

F10.121 Alcohol abuse with intoxication delirium [HCC]

F10.129 Alcohol abuse with intoxication, unspecified [HCC]

F10.13 Alcohol abuse, with withdrawal

F10.130 Alcohol abuse with withdrawal, uncomplicated [HCC]

F10.131 Alcohol abuse with withdrawal delirium [HCC]

F10.132 Alcohol abuse with withdrawal with perceptual disturbance [HCC]

F10.139 Alcohol abuse with withdrawal, unspecified

F10.14 Alcohol abuse with alcohol-induced mood disorder [HCC]

Alcohol use disorder, mild, with alcohol-induced bipolar or related disorder

Alcohol use disorder, mild, with alcohol-induced depressive disorder

F10.15 Alcohol abuse with alcohol-induced psychotic disorder

F10.150 Alcohol abuse with alcohol-induced psychotic disorder with delusions [HCC]

F10.151 Alcohol abuse with alcohol-induced psychotic disorder with hallucinations [HCC]

F10.159 Alcohol abuse with alcohol-induced psychotic disorder, unspecified [HCC]

F10.18 Alcohol abuse with other alcohol-induced disorders

F10.180 Alcohol abuse with alcohol-induced anxiety disorder [HCC]

F10.181 Alcohol abuse with alcohol-induced sexual dysfunction [HCC]

F10.182 Alcohol abuse with alcohol-induced sleep disorder [HCC]

F10.188 Alcohol abuse with other alcohol-induced disorder [HCC]

F10.19 Alcohol abuse with unspecified alcohol-induced disorder [HCC]

F10.2 Alcohol dependence

Excludes1: alcohol abuse (F10.1-)

alcohol use, unspecified (F10.9-)

Excludes2: toxic effect of alcohol (T51.0-)

F10.20 Alcohol dependence, uncomplicated [HCC]

Alcohol use disorder, moderate

Alcohol use disorder, severe

F10.21 Alcohol dependence, in remission [HCC]

Alcohol use disorder, moderate, in early remission

Alcohol use disorder, moderate, in sustained remission

Alcohol use disorder, severe, in early remission

Alcohol use disorder, severe, in sustained remission

F10.22　**Alcohol dependence with intoxication**

Acute drunkenness (in alcoholism)

Excludes2: alcohol dependence with withdrawal (F10.23-)

　　F10.220　**Alcohol dependence with intoxication, uncomplicated** [HCC]

　　F10.221　**Alcohol dependence with intoxication delirium** [HCC]

　　F10.229　**Alcohol dependence with intoxication, unspecified** [HCC]

F10.23　**Alcohol dependence with withdrawal**

Excludes2: Alcohol dependence with intoxication (F10.22-)

　　F10.230　**Alcohol dependence with withdrawal, uncomplicated** [HCC]

　　F10.231　**Alcohol dependence with withdrawal delirium** [HCC]

　　F10.232　**Alcohol dependence with withdrawal with perceptual disturbance** [HCC]

　　F10.239　**Alcohol dependence with withdrawal, unspecified** [HCC]

F10.24　**Alcohol dependence with alcohol-induced mood disorder** [HCC]

Alcohol use disorder, moderate, with alcohol-induced bipolar or related disorder

Alcohol use disorder, moderate, with alcohol-induced depressive disorder

Alcohol use disorder, severe, with alcohol-induced bipolar or related disorder

Alcohol use disorder, severe, with alcohol-induced depressive disorder

F10.25　**Alcohol dependence with alcohol-induced psychotic disorder**

　　F10.250　**Alcohol dependence with alcohol-induced psychotic disorder with delusions** [HCC]

　　F10.251　**Alcohol dependence with alcohol-induced psychotic disorder with hallucinations** [HCC]

　　F10.259　**Alcohol dependence with alcohol-induced psychotic disorder, unspecified** [HCC]

F10.26　**Alcohol dependence with alcohol-induced persisting amnestic disorder** [HCC]

Alcohol use disorder, moderate, with alcohol-induced major neurocognitive disorder, amnestic-confabulatory type

Alcohol use disorder, severe, with alcohol-induced major neurocognitive disorder, amnestic-confabulatory type

F10.27　**Alcohol dependence with alcohol-induced persisting dementia** [HCC]

Alcohol use disorder, moderate, with alcohol-induced major neurocognitive disorder, non amnestic-confabulatory type

Alcohol use disorder, severe, with alcohol-induced major neurocognitive disorder, non amnestic-confabulatory type

F10.28　**Alcohol dependence with other alcohol-induced disorders**

　　F10.280　**Alcohol dependence with alcohol-induced anxiety disorder** [HCC]

　　F10.281　**Alcohol dependence with alcohol-induced sexual dysfunction** [HCC]

　　F10.282　**Alcohol dependence with alcohol-induced sleep disorder** [HCC]

　　F10.288　**Alcohol dependence with other alcohol-induced disorder** [HCC]

Alcohol use disorder, moderate, with alcohol-induced mild neurocognitive disorder

Alcohol use disorder, severe, with alcohol-induced mild neurocognitive disorder

F10.29　**Alcohol dependence with unspecified alcohol-induced disorder** [HCC]

F10.9　**Alcohol use, unspecified**

Excludes1: alcohol abuse (F10.1-)

alcohol dependence (F10.2-)

F10.92　**Alcohol use, unspecified with intoxication**

　　F10.920　**Alcohol use, unspecified with intoxication, uncomplicated** [HCC]

　　F10.921　**Alcohol use, unspecified with intoxication delirium** [HCC]

　　F10.929　**Alcohol use, unspecified with intoxication, unspecified** [HCC]

F10.93　**Alcohol use, unspecified with withdrawal**

　　F10.930　**Alcohol use, unspecified with withdrawal, uncomplicated**

　　F10.931　**Alcohol use, unspecified with withdrawal delirium**

　　F10.932　**Alcohol use, unspecified with withdrawal with perceptual disturbance**

　　F10.939　**Alcohol use, unspecified with withdrawal, unspecified**

F10.94　**Alcohol use, unspecified with alcohol-induced mood disorder** [HCC]

Alcohol induced bipolar or related disorder, without use disorder

Alcohol induced depressive disorder, without use disorder

F10.95　**Alcohol use, unspecified with alcohol-induced psychotic disorder**

　　F10.950　**Alcohol use, unspecified with alcohol-induced psychotic disorder with delusions** [HCC]

　　F10.951　**Alcohol use, unspecified with alcohol-induced psychotic disorder with hallucinations** [HCC]

　　F10.959　**Alcohol use, unspecified with alcohol-induced psychotic disorder, unspecified** [HCC]

Alcohol-induced psychotic disorder without use disorder

F10.96　**Alcohol use, unspecified with alcohol-induced persisting amnestic disorder** [HCC]

Alcohol-induced major neurocognitive disorder, amnestic-confabulatory type, without use disorder

F10.97　**Alcohol use, unspecified with alcohol-induced persisting dementia** [HCC]

Alcohol-induced major neurocognitive disorder, non amnestic-confabulatory type, without use disorder

F10.98　**Alcohol use, unspecified with other alcohol-induced disorders**

　　F10.980　**Alcohol use, unspecified with alcohol-induced anxiety disorder** [HCC]

● New code　▲ Revised code　Excludes1: Not coded here　Excludes2: Not included here　⊗ Placeholder required　⑦7th digit required

Alcohol induced anxiety disorder, without use disorder

F10.981 **Alcohol use, unspecified with alcohol-induced sexual dysfunction** [HCC]

Alcohol induced sexual dysfunction, without use disorder

F10.982 **Alcohol use, unspecified with alcohol-induced sleep disorder** [HCC]

Alcohol induced sleep disorder, without use disorder

F10.988 **Alcohol use, unspecified with other alcohol-induced disorder** [HCC]

Alcohol induced mild neurocognitive disorder, without use disorder

F10.99 **Alcohol use, unspecified with unspecified alcohol-induced disorder** [HCC]

F11 **Opioid related disorders**

Definition: Opioids are medications that relieve pain. They reduce the intensity of pain signals reaching the brain and affect those brain areas controlling emotion, which diminishes the effects of a painful stimulus. Medications that fall within this class include hydrocodone (e.g., Vicodin), oxycodone (e.g., OxyContin, Percocet), morphine (e.g., Kadian, Avinza), codeine, and related drugs.

F11.1 **Opioid abuse**

Excludes1: opioid dependence (F11.2-)

opioid use, unspecified (F11.9-)

F11.10 **Opioid abuse, uncomplicated** [HCC]

Opioid use disorder, mild

F11.11 **Opioid abuse, in remission** [HCC]

Opioid use disorder, mild, in early remission

Opioid use disorder, mild, in sustained remission

F11.12 **Opioid abuse with intoxication**

F11.120 **Opioid abuse with intoxication, uncomplicated** [HCC]

F11.121 **Opioid abuse with intoxication delirium** [HCC]

F11.122 **Opioid abuse with intoxication with perceptual disturbance** [HCC]

F11.129 **Opioid abuse with intoxication, unspecified** [HCC]

F11.13 **Opioid abuse with withdrawal**

F11.14 **Opioid abuse with opioid-induced mood disorder** [HCC]

Opioid use disorder, mild, with opioid-induced depressive disorder

F11.15 **Opioid abuse with opioid-induced psychotic disorder**

F11.150 **Opioid abuse with opioid-induced psychotic disorder with delusions** [HCC]

F11.151 **Opioid abuse with opioid-induced psychotic disorder with hallucinations** [HCC]

F11.159 **Opioid abuse with opioid-induced psychotic disorder, unspecified** [HCC]

F11.18 **Opioid abuse with other opioid-induced disorder**

F11.181 **Opioid abuse with opioid-induced sexual dysfunction** [HCC]

F11.182 **Opioid abuse with opioid-induced sleep disorder** [HCC]

F11.188 **Opioid abuse with other opioid-induced disorder** [HCC]

F11.19 **Opioid abuse with unspecified opioid-induced disorder** [HCC]

F11.2 **Opioid dependence**

Excludes1: opioid abuse (F11.1-)

opioid use, unspecified (F11.9-)

Excludes2: opioid poisoning (T40.0-T40.2-)

F11.20 **Opioid dependence, uncomplicated** [HCC]

Opioid use disorder, moderate

Opioid use disorder, severe

F11.21 **Opioid dependence, in remission** [HCC]

Opioid use disorder, moderate, in early remission

Opioid use disorder, moderate, in sustained remission

Opioid use disorder, severe, in early remission

Opioid use disorder, severe, in sustained remission

F11.22 **Opioid dependence with intoxication**

Excludes1: opioid dependence with withdrawal (F11.23)

F11.220 **Opioid dependence with intoxication, uncomplicated** [HCC]

F11.221 **Opioid dependence with intoxication delirium** [HCC]

F11.222 **Opioid dependence with intoxication with perceptual disturbance** [HCC]

F11.229 **Opioid dependence with intoxication, unspecified** [HCC]

F11.23 **Opioid dependence with withdrawal** [HCC]

Excludes1: opioid dependence with intoxication (F11.22-)

F11.24 **Opioid dependence with opioid-induced mood disorder** [HCC]

Opioid use disorder, moderate, with opioid induced depressive disorder

F11.25 **Opioid dependence with opioid-induced psychotic disorder**

F11.250 **Opioid dependence with opioid-induced psychotic disorder with delusions** [HCC]

F11.251 **Opioid dependence with opioid-induced psychotic disorder with hallucinations** [HCC]

F11.259 **Opioid dependence with opioid-induced psychotic disorder, unspecified** [HCC]

F11.28 **Opioid dependence with other opioid-induced disorder**

F11.281 **Opioid dependence with opioid-induced sexual dysfunction** [HCC]

F11.282 **Opioid dependence with opioid-induced sleep disorder** [HCC]

F11.288 **Opioid dependence with other opioid-induced disorder** [HCC]

F11.29 **Opioid dependence with unspecified opioid-induced disorder** [HCC]

F11.9 **Opioid use, unspecified**

Excludes1: opioid abuse (F11.1-)

opioid dependence (F11.2-)

F11.90 **Opioid use, unspecified, uncomplicated**

F11.92 **Opioid use, unspecified with intoxication**

Excludes1: opioid use, unspecified with withdrawal (F11.93)

F11.920 **Opioid use, unspecified with intoxication, uncomplicated** [HCC]

F11.921 **Opioid use, unspecified with intoxication delirium** [HCC]

Opioid-induced delirium

F11.922 **Opioid use, unspecified with intoxication with perceptual disturbance** [HCC]

F11.929 **Opioid use, unspecified with intoxication, unspecified** [HCC] [HCC]

F11.93 **Opioid use, unspecified with withdrawal** [HCC]

Excludes1: opioid use, unspecified with intoxication (F11.92-)

F11.94 **Opioid use, unspecified with opioid-induced mood disorder** [HCC]

Opioid induced depressive disorder, without use disorder

F11.95 **Opioid use, unspecified with opioid-induced psychotic disorder**

F11.950 **Opioid use, unspecified with opioid-induced psychotic disorder with delusions** [HCC]

F11.951 **Opioid use, unspecified with opioid-induced psychotic disorder with hallucinations** [HCC]

F11.959 **Opioid use, unspecified with opioid-induced psychotic disorder, unspecified** [HCC]

F11.98 **Opioid use, unspecified with other specified opioid-induced disorder**

F11.981 **Opioid use, unspecified with opioid-induced sexual dysfunction** [HCC]

Opioid induced sexual dysfunction, without use disorder

F11.982 **Opioid use, unspecified with opioid-induced sleep disorder** [HCC]

Opioid induced sleep disorder, without use disorder

F11.988 **Opioid use, unspecified with other opioid-induced disorder** [HCC]

Opioid induced anxiety disorder, without use disorder

F11.99 **Opioid use, unspecified with unspecified opioid-induced disorder** [HCC]

F12 **Cannabis related disorders**

Includes: marijuana

F12.1 **Cannabis abuse**

Excludes1: cannabis dependence (F12.2-)

cannabis use, unspecified (F12.9-)

F12.10 **Cannabis abuse, uncomplicated**

Cannabis use disorder, mild

F12.11 **Cannabis abuse, in remission**

Cannabis use disorder, mild, in early remission

Cannabis use disorder, mild, in sustained remission

F12.12 **Cannabis abuse with intoxication**

F12.120 **Cannabis abuse with intoxication, uncomplicated** [HCC]

F12.121 **Cannabis abuse with intoxication delirium** [HCC]

F12.122 **Cannabis abuse with intoxication with perceptual disturbance** [HCC]

F12.129 **Cannabis abuse with intoxication, unspecified** [HCC]

F12.13 **Cannabis abuse with withdrawal unspecified** [HCC]

F12.15 **Cannabis abuse with psychotic disorder**

F12.150 **Cannabis abuse with psychotic disorder with delusions** [HCC]

F12.151 **Cannabis abuse with psychotic disorder with hallucinations** [HCC]

F12.159 **Cannabis abuse with psychotic disorder, unspecified** [HCC]

F12.18 **Cannabis abuse with other cannabis-induced disorder**

F12.180 **Cannabis abuse with cannabis-induced anxiety disorder** [HCC]

F12.188 **Cannabis abuse with other cannabis-induced disorder** [HCC]

Cannabis use disorder, mild, with cannabis-induced sleep disorder

F12.19 **Cannabis abuse with unspecified cannabis-induced disorder** [HCC]

F12.2 **Cannabis dependence**

Excludes1: cannabis abuse (F12.1-)

cannabis use, unspecified (F12.9-)

Excludes2: cannabis poisoning (T40.7-)

F12.20 **Cannabis dependence, uncomplicated** [HCC]

Cannabis use disorder, moderate

Cannabis use disorder, severe

F12.21 **Cannabis dependence, in remission** [HCC]

Cannabis use disorder, moderate, in early remission

Cannabis use disorder, moderate, in sustained remission

Cannabis use disorder, severe, in early remission

Cannabis use disorder, severe, in sustained remission

F12.22 **Cannabis dependence with intoxication**

F12.220 **Cannabis dependence with intoxication, uncomplicated** [HCC]

F12.221 **Cannabis dependence with intoxication delirium** [HCC]

F12.222 **Cannabis dependence with intoxication with perceptual disturbance** [HCC]

F12.229 **Cannabis dependence with intoxication, unspecified** [HCC]

F12.23 **Cannabis dependence with withdrawal** [HCC]

F12.25 **Cannabis dependence with psychotic disorder**

F12.250 **Cannabis dependence with psychotic disorder with delusions** [HCC]

F12.251 **Cannabis dependence with psychotic disorder with hallucinations** [HCC]

F12.259 **Cannabis dependence with psychotic disorder, unspecified** [HCC]

F12.28 **Cannabis dependence with other cannabis-induced disorder**

F12.280 **Cannabis dependence with cannabis-induced anxiety disorder** [HCC]

F12.288 **Cannabis dependence with other cannabis-induced disorder** [HCC]

Cannabis use disorder, moderate, with cannabis-induced sleep disorder

● New code   ▲ Revised code   Excludes1: Not coded here   Excludes2: Not included here   ⊗ Placeholder required   ⑦7th digit required

Cannabis use disorder, severe, with cannabis-induced sleep disorder

Cannabis withdrawal

F12.29 **Cannabis dependence with unspecified cannabis-induced disorder** [HCC]

F12.9 **Cannabis use, unspecified**

Excludes1: cannabis abuse (F12.1-)

cannabis dependence (F12.2-)

F12.90 **Cannabis use, unspecified, uncomplicated** [HCC]

F12.92 **Cannabis use, unspecified with intoxication**

F12.920 **Cannabis use, unspecified with intoxication, uncomplicated** [HCC]

F12.921 **Cannabis use, unspecified with intoxication delirium** [HCC]

F12.922 **Cannabis use, unspecified with intoxication with perceptual disturbance** [HCC]

F12.929 **Cannabis use, unspecified with intoxication, unspecified** [HCC]

F12.93 **Cannabis use, unspecified with withdrawal**

F12.95 **Cannabis use, unspecified with psychotic disorder**

F12.950 **Cannabis use, unspecified with psychotic disorder with delusions** [HCC]

F12.951 **Cannabis use, unspecified with psychotic disorder with hallucinations** [HCC]

F12.959 **Cannabis use, unspecified with psychotic disorder, unspecified** [HCC]

Cannabis induced psychotic disorder, without use disorder

F12.98 **Cannabis use, unspecified with other cannabis-induced disorder**

F12.980 **Cannabis use, unspecified with anxiety disorder** [HCC]

Cannabis induced anxiety disorder, without use disorder

F12.988 **Cannabis use, unspecified with other cannabis-induced disorder** [HCC]

Cannabis induced sleep disorder, without use disorder

F12.99 **Cannabis use, unspecified with unspecified cannabis-induced disorder** [HCC]

F13 **Sedative, hypnotic, or anxiolytic related disorders**

F13.1 **Sedative, hypnotic or anxiolytic-related abuse**

Excludes1: sedative, hypnotic or anxiolytic-related dependence (F13.2-)

sedative, hypnotic, or anxiolytic use, unspecified (F13.9-)

F13.10 **Sedative, hypnotic or anxiolytic abuse, uncomplicated** [HCC]

Sedative, hypnotic, or anxiolytic use disorder, mild

F13.11 **Sedative, hypnotic or anxiolytic abuse, in remission** [HCC]

Sedative, hypnotic or anxiolytic use disorder, mild, in early remission

Sedative, hypnotic or anxiolytic use disorder, mild, in sustained remission

F13.12 **Sedative, hypnotic or anxiolytic abuse with intoxication** [HCC]

F13.120 **Sedative, hypnotic or anxiolytic abuse with intoxication, uncomplicated** [HCC]

F13.121 **Sedative, hypnotic or anxiolytic abuse with intoxication delirium** [HCC]

F13.129 **Sedative, hypnotic or anxiolytic abuse with intoxication, unspecified** [HCC]

F13.14 **Sedative, hypnotic or anxiolytic abuse with sedative, hypnotic or anxiolytic-induced mood disorder** [HCC]

Sedative, hypnotic, or anxiolytic use disorder, mild, with sedative, hypnotic, or anxiolytic-induced bipolar or related disorder

Sedative, hypnotic, or anxiolytic use disorder, mild, with sedative, hypnotic, or anxiolytic-induced depressive disorder

F13.15 **Sedative, hypnotic or anxiolytic abuse with sedative, hypnotic or anxiolytic-induced psychotic disorder**

F13.150 **Sedative, hypnotic or anxiolytic abuse with sedative, hypnotic or anxiolytic-induced psychotic disorder with delusions** [HCC]

F13.151 **Sedative, hypnotic or anxiolytic abuse with sedative, hypnotic or anxiolytic-induced psychotic disorder with hallucinations** [HCC]

F13.159 **Sedative, hypnotic or anxiolytic abuse with sedative, hypnotic or anxiolytic-induced psychotic disorder, unspecified** [HCC]

F13.18 **Sedative, hypnotic or anxiolytic abuse with other sedative, hypnotic or anxiolytic-induced disorders**

F13.180 **Sedative, hypnotic or anxiolytic abuse with sedative, hypnotic or anxiolytic-induced anxiety disorder** [HCC]

F13.181 **Sedative, hypnotic or anxiolytic abuse with sedative, hypnotic or anxiolytic-induced sexual dysfunction** [HCC]

F13.182 **Sedative, hypnotic or anxiolytic abuse with sedative, hypnotic or anxiolytic-induced sleep disorder** [HCC]

F13.188 **Sedative, hypnotic or anxiolytic abuse with other sedative, hypnotic or anxiolytic-induced disorder** [HCC]

F13.19 **Sedative, hypnotic or anxiolytic abuse with unspecified sedative, hypnotic or anxiolytic-induced disorder** [HCC]

F13.2 **Sedative, hypnotic or anxiolytic-related dependence**

Excludes1: sedative, hypnotic or anxiolytic-related abuse (F13.1-)

sedative, hypnotic, or anxiolytic use, unspecified (F13.9-)

Excludes2: sedative, hypnotic, or anxiolytic poisoning (T42.-)

F13.20 **Sedative, hypnotic or anxiolytic dependence, uncomplicated** [HCC]

F13.21 **Sedative, hypnotic or anxiolytic dependence, in remission** [HCC]

Sedative, hypnotic or anxiolytic use disorder, moderate, in early remission

Sedative, hypnotic or anxiolytic use disorder, moderate, in sustained remission

Sedative, hypnotic or anxiolytic use disorder, severe, in early remission

Sedative, hypnotic or anxiolytic use disorder, severe, in sustained remission

F13.22 **Sedative, hypnotic or anxiolytic dependence with intoxication**

> **Excludes1:** sedative, hypnotic or anxiolytic dependence with withdrawal (F13.23-)

F13.220 **Sedative, hypnotic or anxiolytic dependence with intoxication, uncomplicated** [HCC]

F13.221 **Sedative, hypnotic or anxiolytic dependence with intoxication delirium** [HCC]

F13.229 **Sedative, hypnotic or anxiolytic dependence with intoxication, unspecified** [HCC]

F13.23 **Sedative, hypnotic or anxiolytic dependence with withdrawal**

Sedative, hypnotic, or anxiolytic use disorder, moderate

Sedative, hypnotic, or anxiolytic use disorder, severe

> **Excludes1:** sedative, hypnotic or anxiolytic dependence with intoxication (F13.22-)

F13.230 **Sedative, hypnotic or anxiolytic dependence with withdrawal, uncomplicated** [HCC]

F13.231 **Sedative, hypnotic or anxiolytic dependence with withdrawal delirium** [HCC]

F13.232 **Sedative, hypnotic or anxiolytic dependence with withdrawal with perceptual disturbance** [HCC]

Sedative, hypnotic, or anxiolytic withdrawal with perceptual disturbances

F13.239 **Sedative, hypnotic or anxiolytic dependence with withdrawal, unspecified** [HCC]

Sedative, hypnotic, or anxiolytic withdrawal without perceptual disturbances

F13.24 **Sedative, hypnotic or anxiolytic dependence with sedative, hypnotic or anxiolytic-induced mood disorder** [HCC]

Sedative, hypnotic, or anxiolytic use disorder, moderate, with sedative, hypnotic, or anxiolytic-induced bipolar or related disorder

Sedative, hypnotic, or anxiolytic use disorder, moderate, with sedative, hypnotic, or anxiolytic-induced depressive disorder

Sedative, hypnotic, or anxiolytic use disorder, severe, with sedative, hypnotic, or anxiolytic-induced depressive disorder

F13.25 **Sedative, hypnotic or anxiolytic dependence with sedative, hypnotic or anxiolytic-induced psychotic disorder**

F13.250 **Sedative, hypnotic or anxiolytic dependence with sedative, hypnotic or anxiolytic-induced psychotic disorder with delusions** [HCC]

F13.251 **Sedative, hypnotic or anxiolytic dependence with sedative, hypnotic or anxiolytic-induced psychotic disorder with hallucinations** [HCC]

F13.259 **Sedative, hypnotic or anxiolytic dependence with sedative, hypnotic**

or anxiolytic-induced psychotic disorder, unspecified [HCC]

F13.26 **Sedative, hypnotic or anxiolytic dependence with sedative, hypnotic or anxiolytic-induced persisting amnestic disorder** [HCC]

F13.27 **Sedative, hypnotic or anxiolytic dependence with sedative, hypnotic or anxiolytic-induced persisting dementia** [HCC]

Sedative, hypnotic, or anxiolytic use disorder, moderate, with sedative, hypnotic, or anxiolytic-induced major neurocognitive disorder

Sedative, hypnotic, or anxiolytic use disorder, severe, with sedative, hypnotic, or anxiolytic-induced major neurocognitive disorder

F13.28 **Sedative, hypnotic or anxiolytic dependence with other sedative, hypnotic or anxiolytic-induced disorders**

F13.280 **Sedative, hypnotic or anxiolytic dependence with sedative, hypnotic or anxiolytic-induced anxiety disorder** [HCC]

F13.281 **Sedative, hypnotic or anxiolytic dependence with sedative, hypnotic or anxiolytic-induced sexual dysfunction** [HCC]

F13.282 **Sedative, hypnotic or anxiolytic dependence with sedative, hypnotic or anxiolytic-induced sleep disorder** [HCC]

F13.288 **Sedative, hypnotic or anxiolytic dependence with other sedative, hypnotic or anxiolytic-induced disorder** [HCC]

Sedative, hypnotic, or anxiolytic use disorder, moderate, with sedative, hypnotic, or anxiolytic-induced mild neurocognitive disorder

Sedative, hypnotic, or anxiolytic use disorder, severe, with sedative, hypnotic, or anxiolytic-induced mild neurocognitive disorder

F13.29 **Sedative, hypnotic or anxiolytic dependence with unspecified sedative, hypnotic or anxiolytic-induced disorder** [HCC]

F13.9 **Sedative, hypnotic or anxiolytic-related use, unspecified**

> **Excludes1:** sedative, hypnotic or anxiolytic-related abuse (F13.1-)
>
> sedative, hypnotic or anxiolytic-related dependence (F13.2-)

F13.90 **Sedative, hypnotic, or anxiolytic use, unspecified, uncomplicated**

F13.92 **Sedative, hypnotic or anxiolytic use, unspecified with intoxication**

> **Excludes1:** sedative, hypnotic or anxiolytic use, unspecified with withdrawal (F13.93-)

F13.920 **Sedative, hypnotic or anxiolytic use, unspecified with intoxication, uncomplicated** [HCC]

F13.921 **Sedative, hypnotic or anxiolytic use, unspecified with intoxication delirium** [HCC]

Sedative, hypnotic, or anxiolytic-induced delirium

F13.929 **Sedative, hypnotic or anxiolytic use, unspecified with intoxication, unspecified** [HCC]

● New code ▲ Revised code **Excludes1:** Not coded here **Excludes2:** Not included here ⊗ Placeholder required ⑦ 7th digit required

F13.93　Sedative, hypnotic or anxiolytic use, unspecified with withdrawal

Excludes1: sedative, hypnotic or anxiolytic use, unspecified with intoxication (F13.92-)

F13.930　Sedative, hypnotic or anxiolytic use, unspecified with withdrawal, uncomplicated [HCC]

F13.931　Sedative, hypnotic or anxiolytic use, unspecified with withdrawal delirium [HCC]

F13.932　Sedative, hypnotic or anxiolytic use, unspecified with withdrawal with perceptual disturbances [HCC]

F13.939　Sedative, hypnotic or anxiolytic use, unspecified with withdrawal, unspecified [HCC]

F13.94　Sedative, hypnotic or anxiolytic use, unspecified with sedative, hypnotic or anxiolytic-induced mood disorder [HCC]

Sedative, hypnotic, or anxiolytic-induced bipolar or related disorder, without use disorder

Sedative, hypnotic, or anxiolytic-induced depressive disorder, without use disorder

F13.95　Sedative, hypnotic or anxiolytic use, unspecified with sedative, hypnotic or anxiolytic-induced psychotic disorder

F13.950　Sedative, hypnotic or anxiolytic use, unspecified with sedative, hypnotic or anxiolytic-induced psychotic disorder with delusions [HCC]

F13.951　Sedative, hypnotic or anxiolytic use, unspecified with sedative, hypnotic or anxiolytic-induced psychotic disorder with hallucinations [HCC]

F13.959　Sedative, hypnotic or anxiolytic use, unspecified with sedative, hypnotic or anxiolytic-induced psychotic disorder, unspecified [HCC]

Sedative, hypnotic, or anxiolytic-induced psychotic disorder, without use disorder

F13.96　Sedative, hypnotic or anxiolytic use, unspecified with sedative, hypnotic or anxiolytic-induced persisting amnestic disorder [HCC]

F13.97　Sedative, hypnotic or anxiolytic use, unspecified with sedative, hypnotic or anxiolytic-induced persisting dementia [HCC]

Sedative, hypnotic, or anxiolytic-induced major neurocognitive disorder, without use disorder

F13.98　Sedative, hypnotic or anxiolytic use, unspecified with other sedative, hypnotic or anxiolytic-induced disorders

F13.980　Sedative, hypnotic or anxiolytic use, unspecified with sedative, hypnotic or anxiolytic-induced anxiety disorder [HCC]

Sedative, hypnotic, or anxiolytic-induced anxiety disorder, without use disorder

F13.981　Sedative, hypnotic or anxiolytic use, unspecified with sedative, hypnotic or anxiolytic-induced sexual dysfunction [HCC]

Sedative, hypnotic, or anxiolytic-induced sexual dysfunction disorder, without use disorder

F13.982　Sedative, hypnotic or anxiolytic use, unspecified with sedative, hypnotic or anxiolytic-induced sleep disorder [HCC]

Sedative, hypnotic, or anxiolytic-induced sleep disorder, without use disorder

F13.988　Sedative, hypnotic or anxiolytic use, unspecified with other sedative, hypnotic or anxiolytic-induced disorder [HCC]

Sedative, hypnotic, or anxiolytic-induced mild neurocognitive disorder

F13.99　Sedative, hypnotic or anxiolytic use, unspecified with unspecified sedative, hypnotic or anxiolytic-induced disorder [HCC]

F14　Cocaine related disorders

Excludes2: Other stimulant-related disorders (F15.-)

F14.1　Cocaine abuse

Excludes1: cocaine dependence (F14.2-)

cocaine use, unspecified (F14.9-)

F14.10　Cocaine abuse, uncomplicated [HCC]

Cocaine use disorder, mild

F14.11　Cocaine abuse, in remission [HCC]

Cocaine use disorder, mild, in early remission

Cocaine use disorder, mild, in sustained remission

F14.12　Cocaine abuse with intoxication

F14.120　Cocaine abuse with intoxication, uncomplicated [HCC]

F14.121　Cocaine abuse with intoxication with delirium [HCC]

F14.122　Cocaine abuse with intoxication with perceptual disturbance [HCC]

F14.129　Cocaine abuse with intoxication, unspecified [HCC]

F14.13　Cocaine abuse, unspecified with withdrawal

F14.14　Cocaine abuse with cocaine-induced mood disorder [HCC]

Cocaine use disorder, mild, with cocaine-induced bipolar or related disorder

Cocaine use disorder, mild, with cocaine-induced depressive disorder

F14.15　Cocaine abuse with cocaine-induced psychotic disorder

F14.150　Cocaine abuse with cocaine-induced psychotic disorder with delusions [HCC]

F14.151　Cocaine abuse with cocaine-induced psychotic disorder with hallucinations [HCC]

F14.159　Cocaine abuse with cocaine-induced psychotic disorder, unspecified [HCC]

F14.18　Cocaine abuse with other cocaine-induced disorder

F14.180　Cocaine abuse with cocaine-induced anxiety disorder [HCC]

F14.181　Cocaine abuse with cocaine-induced sexual dysfunction [HCC]

F14.182　Cocaine abuse with cocaine-induced sleep disorder [HCC]

F14.188　Cocaine abuse with other cocaine-induced disorder [HCC]

Cocaine use disorder, mild, with cocaine-induced obsessive compulsive or related disorder

F14.19   Cocaine abuse with unspecified cocaine-induced disorder [HCC]

F14.2   Cocaine dependence

> Excludes1: cocaine abuse (F14.1-)
>
> cocaine use, unspecified (F14.9-)
>
> Excludes2: cocaine poisoning (T40.5-)

F14.20   Cocaine dependence, uncomplicated [HCC]

Cocaine use disorder, moderate

Cocaine use disorder, severe

F14.21   Cocaine dependence, in remission [HCC]

Cocaine use disorder, moderate, in early remission

Cocaine use disorder, moderate, in sustained remission

Cocaine use disorder, severe, in early remission

Cocaine use disorder, severe, in sustained remission

F14.22   Cocaine dependence with intoxication

> Excludes1: cocaine dependence with withdrawal (F14.23)

F14.220   Cocaine dependence with intoxication, uncomplicated [HCC]

F14.221   Cocaine dependence with intoxication delirium [HCC]

F14.222   Cocaine dependence with intoxication with perceptual disturbance [HCC]

F14.229   Cocaine dependence with intoxication, unspecified [HCC]

F14.23   Cocaine dependence with withdrawal [HCC]

> Excludes1: cocaine dependence with intoxication (F14.22-)

F14.24   Cocaine dependence with cocaine-induced mood disorder [HCC]

Cocaine use disorder, moderate, with cocaine-induced bipolar or related disorder

Cocaine use disorder, moderate, with cocaine-induced depressive disorder

Cocaine use disorder, severe, with cocaine-induced bipolar or related disorder

Cocaine use disorder, severe, with cocaine-induced depressive disorder

F14.25   Cocaine dependence with cocaine-induced psychotic disorder

F14.250   Cocaine dependence with cocaine-induced psychotic disorder with delusions [HCC]

F14.251   Cocaine dependence with cocaine-induced psychotic disorder with hallucinations [HCC]

F14.259   Cocaine dependence with cocaine-induced psychotic disorder, unspecified [HCC]

F14.28   Cocaine dependence with other cocaine-induced disorder

F14.280   Cocaine dependence with cocaine-induced anxiety disorder [HCC]

F14.281   Cocaine dependence with cocaine-induced sexual dysfunction [HCC]

F14.282   Cocaine dependence with cocaine-induced sleep disorder [HCC]

F14.288   Cocaine dependence with other cocaine-induced disorder [HCC]

Cocaine use disorder, moderate, with cocaine-induced obsessive compulsive or related disorder

Cocaine use disorder, severe, with cocaine-induced obsessive compulsive or related disorder

F14.29   Cocaine dependence with unspecified cocaine-induced disorder [HCC]

F14.9   Cocaine use, unspecified

> Excludes1: cocaine abuse (F14.1-)
>
> cocaine dependence (F14.2-)

F14.90   Cocaine use, unspecified, uncomplicated [HCC]

F14.92   Cocaine use, unspecified with intoxication

F14.920   Cocaine use, unspecified with intoxication, uncomplicated [HCC]

F14.921   Cocaine use, unspecified with intoxication delirium [HCC]

F14.922   Cocaine use, unspecified with intoxication with perceptual disturbance [HCC]

F14.929   Cocaine use, unspecified with intoxication, unspecified [HCC]

F14.93   Cocaine use, unspecified with withdrawal

F14.94   Cocaine use, unspecified with cocaine-induced mood disorder [HCC]

Cocaine induced bipolar or related disorder, without use disorder

Cocaine induced depressive disorder, without use disorder

F14.95   Cocaine use, unspecified with cocaine-induced psychotic disorder

F14.950   Cocaine use, unspecified with cocaine-induced psychotic disorder with delusions [HCC]

F14.951   Cocaine use, unspecified with cocaine-induced psychotic disorder with hallucinations [HCC]

F14.959   Cocaine use, unspecified with cocaine-induced psychotic disorder, unspecified [HCC]

Cocaine induced psychotic disorder, without use disorder

F14.98   Cocaine use, unspecified with other specified cocaine-induced disorder

F14.980   Cocaine use, unspecified with cocaine-induced anxiety disorder [HCC]

Cocaine induced anxiety disorder, without use disorder

F14.981   Cocaine use, unspecified with cocaine-induced sexual dysfunction [HCC]

Cocaine induced sexual dysfunction, without use disorder

F14.982   Cocaine use, unspecified with cocaine-induced sleep disorder [HCC]

Cocaine induced sleep disorder, without use disorder

F14.988   Cocaine use, unspecified with other cocaine-induced disorder [HCC]

Cocaine induced obsessive compulsive or related disorder

● New code   ▲ Revised code   Excludes1: Not coded here   Excludes2: Not included here   ⊗ Placeholder required   ⑦ 7th digit required

F14.99 **Cocaine use, unspecified with unspecified cocaine-induced disorder**

F15 **Other stimulant related disorders**

Includes: amphetamine-related disorders

caffeine

Excludes2: cocaine-related disorders (F14.-)

F15.1 **Other stimulant abuse**

Excludes1: Other stimulant dependence (F15.2-)

Other stimulant use, unspecified (F15.9-)

F15.10 **Other stimulant abuse, uncomplicated** [HCC]

Amphetamine type substance use disorder, mild

Other or unspecified stimulant use disorder, mild

F15.11 **Other stimulant abuse, in remission** [HCC]

Amphetamine type substance use disorder, mild, in early remission

Amphetamine type substance use disorder, mild, in sustained remission

Other or unspecified stimulant use disorder, mild, in early remission

Other or unspecified stimulant use disorder, mild, in sustained remission

F15.12 **Other stimulant abuse with intoxication**

F15.120 **Other stimulant abuse with intoxication, uncomplicated** [HCC]

F15.121 **Other stimulant abuse with intoxication delirium** [HCC]

F15.122 **Other stimulant abuse with intoxication with perceptual disturbance** [HCC]

Amphetamine or other stimulant use disorder, mild, with amphetamine or other stimulant intoxication, with perceptual disturbances

F15.129 **Other stimulant abuse with intoxication, unspecified** [HCC]

Amphetamine or other stimulant use disorder, mild, with amphetamine or other stimulant intoxication, without perceptual disturbances

F15.13 **Other stimulant abuse with withdrawal**

F15.14 **Other stimulant abuse with stimulant-induced mood disorder** [HCC]

Amphetamine or other stimulant use disorder, mild, with amphetamine or other stimulant induced bipolar or related disorder

Amphetamine or other stimulant use disorder, mild, with amphetamine or other stimulant induced depressive disorder

F15.15 **Other stimulant abuse with stimulant-induced psychotic disorder**

F15.150 **Other stimulant abuse with stimulant-induced psychotic disorder with delusions** [HCC]

F15.151 **Other stimulant abuse with stimulant-induced psychotic disorder with hallucinations** [HCC]

F15.159 **Other stimulant abuse with stimulant-induced psychotic disorder, unspecified** [HCC]

F15.18 **Other stimulant abuse with other stimulant-induced disorder**

F15.180 **Other stimulant abuse with stimulant-induced anxiety disorder** [HCC]

F15.181 **Other stimulant abuse with stimulant-induced sexual dysfunction** [HCC]

F15.182 **Other stimulant abuse with stimulant-induced sleep disorder** [HCC]

F15.188 **Other stimulant abuse with other stimulant-induced disorder** [HCC]

Amphetamine or other stimulant use disorder, mild, with amphetamine or other stimulant induced obsessive-compulsive or related disorder

F15.19 **Other stimulant abuse with unspecified stimulant-induced disorder** [HCC]

F15.2 **Other stimulant dependence**

Excludes1: Other stimulant abuse (F15.1-)

Other stimulant use, unspecified (F15.9-)

F15.20 **Other stimulant dependence, uncomplicated** [HCC]

Amphetamine type substance use disorder, moderate

Amphetamine type substance use disorder, severe

Other or unspecified stimulant use disorder, moderate

Other or unspecified stimulant use disorder, severe

F15.21 **Other stimulant dependence, in remission** [HCC]

Amphetamine type substance use disorder, moderate, in early remission

Amphetamine type substance use disorder, moderate, in sustained remission

Amphetamine type substance use disorder, severe, in early remission

Amphetamine type substance use disorder, severe, in sustained remission

Other or unspecified stimulant use disorder, moderate, in early remission

Other or unspecified stimulant use disorder, moderate, in sustained remission

Other or unspecified stimulant use disorder, severe, in early remission

Other or unspecified stimulant use disorder, severe, in sustained remission

F15.22 **Other stimulant dependence with intoxication**

Excludes1: Other stimulant dependence with withdrawal (F15.23)

F15.220 **Other stimulant dependence with intoxication, uncomplicated** [HCC]

F15.221 **Other stimulant dependence with intoxication delirium** [HCC]

F15.222 **Other stimulant dependence with intoxication with perceptual disturbance** [HCC]

Amphetamine or other stimulant use disorder, moderate, with amphetamine or other stimulant intoxication, with perceptual disturbances

Amphetamine or other stimulant use disorder, severe, with amphetamine or other stimulant intoxication, with perceptual disturbances

F15.229 **Other stimulant dependence with intoxication, unspecified** [HCC]

Amphetamine or other stimulant use disorder, moderate, with amphetamine or other stimulant intoxication, without perceptual disturbances

Amphetamine **or other** stimulant use disorder, severe, with amphetamine **or other** stimulant intoxication, without perceptual disturbances

F15.23 **Other stimulant dependence with withdrawal** [HCC]

Amphetamine **or other** stimulant withdrawal

Excludes1: Other stimulant dependence with intoxication (F15.22-)

F15.24 **Other stimulant dependence with stimulant-induced mood disorder** [HCC]

Amphetamine or other stimulant use disorder, moderate, with amphetamine or other stimulant-induced bipolar or related disorder

Amphetamine or other stimulant use disorder, moderate, with amphetamine or other stimulant induced depressive disorder

Amphetamine or other stimulant use disorder, severe, with amphetamine or other stimulant-induced bipolar or related disorder

Amphetamine or other stimulant use disorder, severe, with amphetamine or other stimulant-induced depressive disorder

F15.25 **Other stimulant dependence with stimulant-induced psychotic disorder**

F15.250 **Other stimulant dependence with stimulant-induced psychotic disorder with delusions** [HCC]

F15.251 **Other stimulant dependence with stimulant-induced psychotic disorder with hallucinations** [HCC]

F15.259 **Other stimulant dependence with stimulant-induced psychotic disorder, unspecified** [HCC]

F15.28 **Other stimulant dependence with other stimulant-induced disorder**

F15.280 **Other stimulant dependence with stimulant-induced anxiety disorder** [HCC]

F15.281 **Other stimulant dependence with stimulant-induced sexual dysfunction** [HCC]

F15.282 **Other stimulant dependence with stimulant-induced sleep disorder** [HCC]

F15.288 **Other stimulant dependence with other stimulant-induced disorder** [HCC]

Amphetamine or other stimulant use disorder, moderate, with amphetamine or other stimulant induced obsessive compulsive or related disorder

Amphetamine or other stimulant use disorder, severe, with amphetamine or other stimulant induced obsessive compulsive or related disorder

F15.29 **Other stimulant dependence with unspecified stimulant-induced disorder** [HCC]

F15.9 **Other stimulant use, unspecified**

Excludes1: Other stimulant abuse (F15.1-)

Other stimulant dependence (F15.2-)

F15.90 **Other stimulant use, unspecified, uncomplicated** [HCC]

F15.92 **Other stimulant use, unspecified with intoxication**

Excludes1: Other stimulant use, unspecified with withdrawal (F15.93)

F15.920 **Other stimulant use, unspecified with intoxication, uncomplicated** [HCC]

F15.921 **Other stimulant use, unspecified with intoxication delirium** [HCC]

Amphetamine or other stimulant-induced delirium

F15.922 **Other stimulant use, unspecified with intoxication with perceptual disturbance** [HCC]

F15.929 **Other stimulant use, unspecified with intoxication, unspecified** [HCC]

Caffeine intoxication

F15.93 **Other stimulant use, unspecified with withdrawal** [HCC]

Caffeine withdrawal

Excludes1: Other stimulant use, unspecified with intoxication (F15.92-)

F15.94 **Other stimulant use, unspecified with stimulant-induced mood disorder** [HCC]

Amphetamine or other stimulant-induced bipolar or related disorder, without use disorder

Amphetamine or other stimulant-induced depressive disorder, without use disorder

F15.95 **Other stimulant use, unspecified with stimulant-induced psychotic disorder** [HCC]

F15.950 **Other stimulant use, unspecified with stimulant-induced psychotic disorder with delusions** [HCC]

F15.951 **Other stimulant use, unspecified with stimulant-induced psychotic disorder with hallucinations** [HCC]

F15.959 **Other stimulant use, unspecified with stimulant-induced psychotic disorder, unspecified** [HCC]

Amphetamine or other stimulant-induced psychotic disorder, without use disorder

F15.98 **Other stimulant use, unspecified with other stimulant-induced disorder**

F15.980 **Other stimulant use, unspecified with stimulant-induced anxiety disorder** [HCC]

Amphetamine or other stimulant-induced anxiety disorder, without use disorder

Caffeine induced anxiety disorder, without use disorder

F15.981 **Other stimulant use, unspecified with stimulant-induced sexual dysfunction** [HCC]

Amphetamine or other stimulant-induced sexual dysfunction, without use disorder

F15.982 **Other stimulant use, unspecified with stimulant-induced sleep disorder** [HCC]

Amphetamine or other stimulant-induced sleep disorder, without use disorder

Caffeine induced sleep disorder, without use disorder

F15.988 **Other stimulant use, unspecified with other stimulant-induced disorder** [HCC]

● New code   ▲ Revised code   **Excludes1:** Not coded here   **Excludes2:** Not included here   ⊗ Placeholder required   ⑦7th digit required

Amphetamine or other stimulant-induced obsessive compulsive or related disorder, without use disorder

F15.99   Other stimulant use, unspecified with unspecified stimulant-induced disorder

F16   Hallucinogen related disorders

Includes: ecstasy

PCP phencyclidine

F16.1   Hallucinogen abuse

Excludes1: hallucinogen dependence (F16.2-)

hallucinogen use, unspecified (F16.9-)

F16.10   Hallucinogen abuse, uncomplicated [HCC]

Other hallucinogen use disorder, mild

Phencyclidine use disorder, mild

F16.11   Hallucinogen abuse, in remission [HCC]

Other hallucinogen use disorder, mild, in early remission

Other hallucinogen use disorder, mild, in sustained remission

Phencyclidine use disorder, mild, in early remission

Phencyclidine use disorder, mild, in sustained remission

F16.12   Hallucinogen abuse with intoxication

F16.120   Hallucinogen abuse with intoxication, uncomplicated [HCC]

F16.121   Hallucinogen abuse with intoxication with delirium [HCC]

F16.122   Hallucinogen abuse with intoxication with perceptual disturbance [HCC]

F16.129   Hallucinogen abuse with intoxication, unspecified [HCC]

F16.14   Hallucinogen abuse with hallucinogen-induced mood disorder [HCC]

Other hallucinogen use disorder, mild, with other hallucinogen induced bipolar or related disorder

Other hallucinogen use disorder, mild, with other hallucinogen induced depressive disorder

Phencyclidine use disorder, mild, with phencyclidine induced bipolar or related disorder

Phencyclidine use disorder, mild, with phencyclidine induced depressive disorder

F16.15   Hallucinogen abuse with hallucinogen-induced psychotic disorder

F16.150   Hallucinogen abuse with hallucinogen-induced psychotic disorder with delusions [HCC]

F16.151   Hallucinogen abuse with hallucinogen-induced psychotic disorder with hallucinations [HCC]

F16.159   Hallucinogen abuse with hallucinogen-induced psychotic disorder, unspecified [HCC]

F16.18   Hallucinogen abuse with other hallucinogen-induced disorder

F16.180   Hallucinogen abuse with hallucinogen-induced anxiety disorder [HCC]

F16.183   Hallucinogen abuse with hallucinogen persisting perception disorder (flashbacks) [HCC]

F16.188   Hallucinogen abuse with other hallucinogen-induced disorder [HCC]

F16.19   Hallucinogen abuse with unspecified hallucinogen-induced disorder [HCC]

F16.2   Hallucinogen dependence

Excludes1: hallucinogen abuse (F16.1-)

hallucinogen use, unspecified (F16.9-)

F16.20   Hallucinogen dependence, uncomplicated [HCC]

Other hallucinogen use disorder, moderate

Other hallucinogen use disorder, severe

Phencyclidine use disorder, moderate

Phencyclidine use disorder, severe

F16.21   Hallucinogen dependence, in remission [HCC]

Other hallucinogen use disorder, moderate, in early remission

Other hallucinogen use disorder, moderate, in sustained remission

Other hallucinogen use disorder, severe, in early remission

Other hallucinogen use disorder, severe, in sustained remission

Phencyclidine use disorder, moderate, in early remission

Phencyclidine use disorder, moderate, in sustained remission

Phencyclidine use disorder, severe, in early remission

Phencyclidine use disorder, severe, in sustained remission

F16.22   Hallucinogen dependence with intoxication

F16.220   Hallucinogen dependence with intoxication, uncomplicated [HCC]

F16.221   Hallucinogen dependence with intoxication with delirium [HCC]

F16.229   Hallucinogen dependence with intoxication, unspecified [HCC]

F16.24   Hallucinogen dependence with hallucinogen-induced mood disorder [HCC]

Other hallucinogen use disorder, moderate, with other hallucinogen induced bipolar or related disorder

Other hallucinogen use disorder, moderate, with other hallucinogen induced depressive disorder

Other hallucinogen use disorder, severe, with other hallucinogen-induced bipolar or related disorder

Other hallucinogen use disorder, severe, with other hallucinogen-induced depressive disorder

Phencyclidine use disorder, moderate, with phencyclidine induced bipolar or related disorder

Phencyclidine use disorder, moderate, with phencyclidine induced depressive disorder

Phencyclidine use disorder, severe, with phencyclidine induced bipolar or related disorder

Phencyclidine use disorder, severe, with phencyclidine-induced depressive disorder

F16.25   Hallucinogen dependence with hallucinogen-induced psychotic disorder

F16.250   Hallucinogen dependence with hallucinogen-induced psychotic disorder with delusions [HCC]

F16.251   Hallucinogen dependence with hallucinogen-induced psychotic disorder with hallucinations [HCC]

F16.259 Hallucinogen dependence with hallucinogen-induced psychotic disorder, unspecified [HCC]

F16.28 Hallucinogen dependence with other hallucinogen-induced disorder

F16.280 Hallucinogen dependence with hallucinogen-induced anxiety disorder [HCC]

F16.283 Hallucinogen dependence with hallucinogen persisting perception disorder (flashbacks) [HCC]

F16.288 Hallucinogen dependence with other hallucinogen-induced disorder [HCC]

F16.29 Hallucinogen dependence with unspecified hallucinogen-induced disorder [HCC]

F16.9 Hallucinogen use, unspecified

Excludes1: hallucinogen abuse (F16.1-)

hallucinogen dependence (F16.2-)

F16.90 Hallucinogen use, unspecified, uncomplicated [HCC]

F16.92 Hallucinogen use, unspecified with intoxication

F16.920 Hallucinogen use, unspecified with intoxication, uncomplicated [HCC]

F16.921 Hallucinogen use, unspecified with intoxication with delirium [HCC]

Other hallucinogen intoxication delirium

F16.929 Hallucinogen use, unspecified with intoxication, unspecified [HCC]

F16.94 Hallucinogen use, unspecified with hallucinogen-induced mood disorder [HCC]

Other hallucinogen induced bipolar or related disorder, without use disorder

Other hallucinogen induced depressive disorder, without use disorder

Phencyclidine induced bipolar or related disorder, without use disorder

Phencyclidine induced depressive disorder, without use disorder

F16.95 Hallucinogen use, unspecified with hallucinogen-induced psychotic disorder

F16.950 Hallucinogen use, unspecified with hallucinogen-induced psychotic disorder with delusions [HCC]

F16.951 Hallucinogen use, unspecified with hallucinogen-induced psychotic disorder with hallucinations [HCC]

F16.959 Hallucinogen use, unspecified with hallucinogen-induced psychotic disorder, unspecified [HCC]

Other hallucinogen induced psychotic disorder, without use disorder

Phencyclidine induced psychotic disorder, without use disorder

F16.98 Hallucinogen use, unspecified with other specified hallucinogen-induced disorder [HCC]

F16.980 Hallucinogen use, unspecified with hallucinogen-induced anxiety disorder [HCC]

Other hallucinogen-induced anxiety disorder, without use disorder

Phencyclidine induced anxiety disorder, without use disorder

F16.983 Hallucinogen use, unspecified with hallucinogen persisting perception disorder (flashbacks) [HCC]

F16.988 Hallucinogen use, unspecified with other hallucinogen-induced disorder [HCC]

F16.99 Hallucinogen use, unspecified with unspecified hallucinogen-induced disorder [HCC]

F17 Nicotine dependence

Excludes1: history of tobacco dependence (Z87.891)

tobacco use NOS (Z72.0)

Excludes2: tobacco use (smoking) during pregnancy, childbirth and the puerperium (O99.33-)

toxic effect of nicotine (T65.2-)

F17.2 Nicotine dependence

F17.20 Nicotine dependence, unspecified [HCC]

F17.200 Nicotine dependence, unspecified, uncomplicated [HCC]

Tobacco use disorder, mild

Tobacco use disorder, moderate

Tobacco use disorder, severe

F17.201 Nicotine dependence, unspecified, in remission [HCC]

Tobacco use disorder, mild, in early remission

Tobacco use disorder, mild, in sustained remission

Tobacco use disorder, moderate, in early remission

Tobacco use disorder, moderate, in sustained remission

Tobacco use disorder, severe, in early remission

Tobacco use disorder, severe, in sustained remission

F17.203 Nicotine dependence unspecified, with withdrawal [HCC]

Tobacco withdrawal

F17.208 Nicotine dependence, unspecified, with other nicotine-induced disorders [HCC]

F17.209 Nicotine dependence, unspecified, with unspecified nicotine-induced disorders [HCC]

F17.21 Nicotine dependence, cigarettes

F17.210 Nicotine dependence, cigarettes, uncomplicated [HCC]

F17.211 Nicotine dependence, cigarettes, in remission [HCC]

Tobacco use disorder, cigarettes, mild, in early remission

Tobacco use disorder, cigarettes, mild, in sustained remission

Tobacco use disorder, cigarettes, moderate, in early remission

Tobacco use disorder, cigarettes, moderate, in sustained remission

Tobacco use disorder, cigarettes, severe, in early remission

Tobacco use disorder, cigarettes, severe, in sustained remission

F17.213 Nicotine dependence, cigarettes, with withdrawal [HCC]

● New code   ▲ Revised code   **Excludes1:** Not coded here   **Excludes2:** Not included here   ⊗ Placeholder required   ⑦7th digit required

F17.218   **Nicotine dependence, cigarettes, with other nicotine-induced disorders** [HCC]

F17.219   **Nicotine dependence, cigarettes, with unspecified nicotine-induced disorders** [HCC]

F17.22   **Nicotine dependence, chewing tobacco**

F17.220   **Nicotine dependence, chewing tobacco, uncomplicated** [HCC]

F17.221   **Nicotine dependence, chewing tobacco, in remission** [HCC]

Tobacco use disorder, chewing tobacco, mild, in early remission

Tobacco use disorder, chewing tobacco, mild, in sustained remission

Tobacco use disorder, chewing tobacco, moderate, in early remission

Tobacco use disorder, chewing tobacco, moderate, in sustained remission

Tobacco use disorder, chewing tobacco, severe, in early remission

Tobacco use disorder, chewing tobacco, severe, in sustained remission

F17.223   **Nicotine dependence, chewing tobacco, with withdrawal** [HCC]

F17.228   **Nicotine dependence, chewing tobacco, with other nicotine-induced disorders** [HCC]

F17.229   **Nicotine dependence, chewing tobacco, with unspecified nicotine-induced disorders** [HCC]

F17.29   **Nicotine dependence, other tobacco product** [HCC]

F17.290   **Nicotine dependence, other tobacco product, uncomplicated** [HCC]

F17.291   **Nicotine dependence, other tobacco product, in remission** [HCC]

Tobacco use disorder, other tobacco product, mild, in early remission

Tobacco use disorder, other tobacco product, mild, in sustained remission

Tobacco use disorder, other tobacco product, moderate, in early remission

Tobacco use disorder, other tobacco product, moderate, in sustained remission

Tobacco use disorder, other tobacco product, severe, in early remission

Tobacco use disorder, other tobacco product, severe, in sustained remission

F17.293   **Nicotine dependence, other tobacco product, with withdrawal** [HCC]

F17.298   **Nicotine dependence, other tobacco product, with other nicotine-induced disorders** [HCC]

F17.299   **Nicotine dependence, other tobacco product, with unspecified nicotine-induced disorders** [HCC]

F18   **Inhalant related disorders**

Includes: volatile solvents

F18.1   **Inhalant abuse**

Excludes1: inhalant dependence (F18.2-)

inhalant use, unspecified (F18.9-)

F18.10   **Inhalant abuse, uncomplicated** [HCC]

Inhalant use disorder, mild

F18.11   **Inhalant abuse, in remission** [HCC]

Inhalant use disorder, mild, in early remission

Inhalant use disorder, mild, in sustained remission

F18.12   **Inhalant abuse with intoxication**

F18.120   **Inhalant abuse with intoxication, uncomplicated** [HCC]

F18.121   **Inhalant abuse with intoxication delirium** [HCC]

F18.129   **Inhalant abuse with intoxication, unspecified** [HCC]

F18.14   **Inhalant abuse with inhalant-induced mood disorder** [HCC]

Inhalant use disorder, mild, with inhalant induced depressive disorder

F18.15   **Inhalant abuse with inhalant-induced psychotic disorder**

F18.150   **Inhalant abuse with inhalant-induced psychotic disorder with delusions** [HCC]

F18.151   **Inhalant abuse with inhalant-induced psychotic disorder with hallucinations** [HCC]

F18.159   **Inhalant abuse with inhalant-induced psychotic disorder, unspecified** [HCC]

F18.17   **Inhalant abuse with inhalant-induced dementia** [HCC]

Inhalant use disorder, mild, with inhalant induced major neurocognitive disorder

F18.18   **Inhalant abuse with other inhalant-induced disorders**

F18.180   **Inhalant abuse with inhalant-induced anxiety disorder** [HCC]

F18.188   **Inhalant abuse with other inhalant-induced disorder** [HCC]

Inhalant use disorder, mild, with inhalant induced mild neurocognitive disorder

F18.19   **Inhalant abuse with unspecified inhalant-induced disorder** [HCC]

F18.2   **Inhalant dependence**

Excludes1: inhalant abuse (F18.1-)

inhalant use, unspecified (F18.9-)

F18.20   **Inhalant dependence, uncomplicated** [HCC]

Inhalant use disorder, moderate

Inhalant use disorder, severe

F18.21   **Inhalant dependence, in remission** [HCC]

Inhalant use disorder, moderate, in early remission

Inhalant use disorder, moderate, in sustained remission

Inhalant use disorder, severe, in early remission

Inhalant use disorder, severe, in sustained remission

F18.22   **Inhalant dependence with intoxication**

F18.220   **Inhalant dependence with intoxication, uncomplicated** [HCC]

F18.221   **Inhalant dependence with intoxication delirium** [HCC]

F18.229   **Inhalant dependence with intoxication, unspecified** [HCC]

F18.24   **Inhalant dependence with inhalant-induced mood disorder** [HCC]

Inhalant use disorder, moderate, with inhalant induced depressive disorder

Inhalant use disorder, severe, with inhalant induced depressive disorder

F18.25 **Inhalant dependence with inhalant-induced psychotic disorder**

F18.250 **Inhalant dependence with inhalant-induced psychotic disorder with delusions** [HCC]

F18.251 **Inhalant dependence with inhalant-induced psychotic disorder with hallucinations** [HCC]

F18.259 **Inhalant dependence with inhalant-induced psychotic disorder, unspecified** [HCC]

F18.27 **Inhalant dependence with inhalant-induced dementia** [HCC]

Inhalant use disorder, moderate, with inhalant induced major neurocognitive disorder

Inhalant use disorder, severe, with inhalant induced major neurocognitive disorder

F18.28 **Inhalant dependence with other inhalant-induced disorders**

F18.280 **Inhalant dependence with inhalant-induced anxiety disorder** [HCC]

F18.288 **Inhalant dependence with other inhalant-induced disorder** [HCC]

Inhalant use disorder, moderate, with inhalant-induced mild neurocognitive disorder

Inhalant use disorder, severe, with inhalant-induced mild neurocognitive disorder

F18.29 **Inhalant dependence with unspecified inhalant-induced disorder** [HCC]

F18.9 **Inhalant use, unspecified**

Excludes1: inhalant abuse (F18.1-)

inhalant dependence (F18.2-)

F18.90 **Inhalant use, unspecified, uncomplicated** [HCC]

F18.92 **Inhalant use, unspecified with intoxication**

F18.920 **Inhalant use, unspecified with intoxication, uncomplicated** [HCC]

F18.921 **Inhalant use, unspecified with intoxication with delirium** [HCC]

F18.929 **Inhalant use, unspecified with intoxication, unspecified** [HCC]

F18.94 **Inhalant use, unspecified with inhalant-induced mood disorder** [HCC]

Inhalant induced depressive disorder

F18.95 **Inhalant use, unspecified with inhalant-induced psychotic disorder**

F18.950 **Inhalant use, unspecified with inhalant-induced psychotic disorder with delusions**

F18.951 **Inhalant use, unspecified with inhalant-induced psychotic disorder with hallucinations** [HCC]

F18.959 **Inhalant use, unspecified with inhalant-induced psychotic disorder, unspecified** [HCC]

F18.97 **Inhalant use, unspecified with inhalant-induced persisting dementia** [HCC]

Inhalant-induced major neurocognitive disorder

F18.98 **Inhalant use, unspecified with other inhalant-induced disorders**

F18.980 **Inhalant use, unspecified with inhalant-induced anxiety disorder** [HCC]

F18.988 **Inhalant use, unspecified with other inhalant-induced disorder** [HCC]

Inhalant-induced mild neurocognitive disorder

F18.99 **Inhalant use, unspecified with unspecified inhalant-induced disorder** [HCC]

F19 **Other psychoactive substance related disorders**

Includes: polysubstance drug use (indiscriminate drug use)

F19.1 **Other psychoactive substance abuse**

Excludes1: Other psychoactive substance dependence (F19.2-)

Other psychoactive substance use, unspecified (F19.9-)

F19.10 **Other psychoactive substance abuse, uncomplicated** [HCC]

Other (or unknown) substance use disorder, mild

F19.11 **Other psychoactive substance abuse, in remission** [HCC]

Other (or unknown) substance use disorder, mild, in early remission

Other (or unknown) substance use disorder, mild, in sustained remission

F19.12 **Other psychoactive substance abuse with intoxication** [HCC]

F19.120 **Other psychoactive substance abuse with intoxication, uncomplicated** [HCC]

F19.121 **Other psychoactive substance abuse with intoxication delirium** [HCC]

F19.122 **Other psychoactive substance abuse with intoxication with perceptual disturbances** [HCC]

F19.129 **Other psychoactive substance abuse with intoxication, unspecified** [HCC]

F19.13 **Other psychoactive substance abuse with withdrawal**

F19.130 **Other psychoactive substance abuse with withdrawal, uncomplicated**

F19.131 **Other psychoactive substance abuse with withdrawal delirium**

F19.132 **Other psychoactive substance abuse with withdrawal with perceptual disturbance**

F19.139 **Other psychoactive substance abuse with withdrawal, unspecified**

F19.14 **Other psychoactive substance abuse with psychoactive substance-induced mood disorder** [HCC]

Other (or unknown) substance use disorder, mild, with other (or unknown) substance-induced bipolar or related disorder

Other (or unknown) substance use disorder, mild, with other (or unknown) substance-induced depressive disorder

F19.15 **Other psychoactive substance abuse with psychoactive substance-induced psychotic disorder**

F19.150 **Other psychoactive substance abuse with psychoactive substance-induced psychotic disorder with delusions** [HCC]

F19.151 **Other psychoactive substance abuse with psychoactive substance-induced psychotic disorder with hallucinations** [HCC]

F19.159 **Other psychoactive substance abuse with psychoactive substance-induced psychotic disorder, unspecified** [HCC]

F19.16 **Other psychoactive substance abuse with psychoactive substance-induced persisting amnestic disorder** [HCC]

F19.17 **Other psychoactive substance abuse with psychoactive substance-induced persisting dementia** [HCC]

Other (or unknown) substance use disorder, mild, with other (or unknown) substance-induced major neurocognitive disorder

F19.18 **Other psychoactive substance abuse with other psychoactive substance-induced disorders**

F19.180 **Other psychoactive substance abuse with psychoactive substance-induced anxiety disorder** [HCC]

F19.181 **Other psychoactive substance abuse with psychoactive substance-induced sexual dysfunction** [HCC]

F19.182 **Other psychoactive substance abuse with psychoactive substance-induced sleep disorder** [HCC]

F19.188 **Other psychoactive substance abuse with other psychoactive substance-induced disorder** [HCC]

Other (or unknown) substance use disorder, mild, with other (or unknown) substance induced mild neurocognitive disorder

Other (or unknown) substance use disorder, mild, with other (or unknown) substance induced obsessive-compulsive or elated disorder

F19.19 **Other psychoactive substance abuse with unspecified psychoactive substance-induced disorder** [HCC]

F19.2 **Other psychoactive substance dependence**

Excludes1: Other psychoactive substance abuse (F19.1-)
Other psychoactive substance use, unspecified (F19.9-)

F19.20 **Other psychoactive substance dependence, uncomplicated** [HCC]

Other (or unknown) substance use disorder, moderate **Other** (or unknown) substance use disorder, severe

F19.21 **Other psychoactive substance dependence, in remission** [HCC]

Other (or unknown) substance use disorder, moderate, in early remission

Other (or unknown) substance use disorder, moderate, in sustained remission

Other (or unknown) substance use disorder, severe, in early remission

Other (or unknown) substance use disorder, severe, in sustained remission

F19.22 **Other psychoactive substance dependence with intoxication**

Excludes1: Other psychoactive substance dependence with withdrawal (F19.23-)

F19.220 **Other psychoactive substance dependence with intoxication, uncomplicated** [HCC]

F19.221 **Other psychoactive substance dependence with intoxication delirium** [HCC]

F9.2122 **Other psychoactive substance dependence with intoxication with perceptual disturbance** [HCC]

F19.229 **Other psychoactive substance dependence with intoxication, unspecified** [HCC]

F19.23 **Other psychoactive substance dependence with withdrawal**

Excludes1: Other psychoactive substance dependence with intoxication (F19.22-)

F19.230 **Other psychoactive substance dependence with withdrawal, uncomplicated** [HCC]

F19.231 **Other psychoactive substance dependence with withdrawal delirium** [HCC]

F19.232 **Other psychoactive substance dependence with withdrawal with perceptual disturbance** [HCC]

F19.239 **Other psychoactive substance dependence with withdrawal, unspecified** [HCC]

F19.24 **Other psychoactive substance dependence with psychoactive substance-induced mood disorder** [HCC]

Other (or unknown) substance use disorder, moderate, with other (or unknown) substance induced bipolar or related disorder

Other (or unknown) substance use disorder, moderate, with other (or unknown) substance induced depressive disorder

Other (or unknown) substance use disorder, severe, with other (or unknown) substance induced bipolar or related disorder

Other (or unknown) substance use disorder, severe, with other (or unknown) substance induced depressive disorder

F19.25 **Other psychoactive substance dependence with psychoactive substance-induced psychotic disorder**

F19.250 **Other psychoactive substance dependence with psychoactive substance-induced psychotic disorder with delusions** [HCC]

F19.251 **Other psychoactive substance dependence with psychoactive substance-induced psychotic disorder with hallucinations** [HCC]

F19.259 **Other psychoactive substance dependence with psychoactive substance-induced psychotic disorder, unspecified** [HCC]

F19.26 **Other psychoactive substance dependence with psychoactive substance-induced persisting amnestic disorder** [HCC]

F19.27 **Other psychoactive substance dependence with psychoactive substance-induced persisting dementia** [HCC]

Other (or unknown) substance use disorder, moderate, with other (or unknown) substance induced major neurocognitive disorder

Other (or unknown) substance use disorder, severe, with other (or unknown) substance induced major neurocognitive disorder

F19.28 Other psychoactive substance dependence with other psychoactive substance-induced disorders

F19.280 Other psychoactive substance dependence with psychoactive substance-induced anxiety disorder [HCC]

F19.281 Other psychoactive substance dependence with psychoactive substance-induced sexual dysfunction [HCC]

F19.282 Other psychoactive substance dependence with psychoactive substance-induced sleep disorder [HCC]

F19.288 Other psychoactive substance dependence with other psychoactive substance-induced disorder [HCC]

Other (or unknown) substance use disorder, moderate, with other (or unknown) substance induced mild neurocognitive disorder

Other (or unknown) substance use disorder, severe, with other (or unknown) substance induced mild neurocognitive disorder

Other (or unknown) substance use disorder, moderate, with other (or unknown) substance induced obsessive compulsive or related disorder

Other (or unknown) substance use disorder, severe, with other (or unknown) substance induced obsessive-compulsive or related disorder

F19.29 Other psychoactive substance dependence with unspecified psychoactive substance-induced disorder [HCC]

F19.9 Other psychoactive substance use, unspecified

Excludes1: Other psychoactive substance abuse (F19.1-)

Other psychoactive substance dependence (F19.2-)

F19.90 Other psychoactive substance use, unspecified, uncomplicated [HCC]

F19.92 Other psychoactive substance use, unspecified with intoxication

Excludes1: Other psychoactive substance use, unspecified with withdrawal (F19.93)

F19.920 Other psychoactive substance use, unspecified with intoxication, uncomplicated

F19.921 Other psychoactive substance use, unspecified with intoxication with delirium [HCC]

Other (or unknown) substance-induced delirium

F19.922 Other psychoactive substance use, unspecified with intoxication with perceptual disturbance [HCC]

F19.929 Other psychoactive substance use, unspecified with intoxication, unspecified [HCC]

F19.93 Other psychoactive substance use, unspecified with withdrawal

Excludes1: Other psychoactive substance use, unspecified with intoxication (F19.92-)

F19.930 Other psychoactive substance use, unspecified with withdrawal, uncomplicated [HCC]

F19.931 Other psychoactive substance use, unspecified with withdrawal delirium [HCC]

F19.932 Other psychoactive substance use, unspecified with withdrawal with perceptual disturbance [HCC]

F19.939 Other psychoactive substance use, unspecified with withdrawal, unspecified [HCC]

F19.94 Other psychoactive substance use, unspecified with psychoactive substance-induced mood disorder

Other (or unknown) substance-induced bipolar or related disorder, without use disorder

Other (or unknown) substance-induced depressive disorder, without use disorder

F19.95 Other psychoactive substance use, unspecified with psychoactive substance-induced psychotic disorder

F19.950 Other psychoactive substance use, unspecified with psychoactive substance-induced psychotic disorder with delusions [HCC]

F19.951 Other psychoactive substance use, unspecified with psychoactive substance-induced psychotic disorder with hallucinations [HCC]

F19.959 Other psychoactive substance use, unspecified with psychoactive substance-induced psychotic disorder, unspecified [HCC]

Other or unknown substance-induced psychotic disorder, without use disorder

F19.96 Other psychoactive substance use, unspecified with psychoactive substance-induced persisting amnestic disorder [HCC]

F19.97 Other psychoactive substance use, unspecified with psychoactive substance-induced persisting dementia [HCC]

Other (or unknown) substance-induced major neurocognitive disorder, without use disorder

F19.98 Other psychoactive substance use, unspecified with other psychoactive substance-induced disorders

F19.980 Other psychoactive substance use, unspecified with psychoactive substance-induced anxiety disorder [HCC]

Other (or unknown) substance-induced anxiety disorder, without use disorder

F19.981 Other psychoactive substance use, unspecified with psychoactive substance-induced sexual dysfunction [HCC]

Other (or unknown) substance-induced sexual dysfunction, without use disorder

F19.982 Other psychoactive substance use, unspecified with psychoactive substance-induced sleep disorder [HCC]

Other (or unknown) substance-induced sleep disorder, without use disorder

F19.988 Other psychoactive substance use, unspecified with other psychoactive substance-induced disorder

Other (or unknown) substance-induced obsessive-compulsive or related disorder, without use disorder

F19.99 **Other psychoactive substance use, unspecified with unspecified psychoactive substance-induced disorder** [HCC]

SCHIZOPHRENIA, SCHIZOTYPAL, DELUSIONAL, AND OTHER NON-MOOD PSYCHOTIC DISORDERS (F20-F29)

F20 **Schizophrenia**

Definition: Schizophrenia is a psychotic disorder marked by severely impaired thinking, emotions, and behaviors. Schizophrenic patients are typically unable to filter sensory stimuli and may have enhanced perceptions of sounds, colors, and other features of their environment.

Excludes1: brief psychotic disorder (F23)

cyclic schizophrenia (F25.0)

mood [affective] disorders with psychotic symptoms (F30.2, F31.2, F31.5, F31.64, F32.3, F33.3)

schizoaffective disorder (F25.-)

schizophrenic reaction NOS (F23)

Excludes2: schizophrenic reaction in:

alcoholism (F10.15-, F10.25-, F10.95-)

brain disease (F06.2)

epilepsy (F06.2)

psychoactive drug use (F11-F19 with .15, .25, .95)

schizotypal disorder (F21)

F20.0 **Paranoid schizophrenia** [HCC]

Paraphrenic schizophrenia

Excludes1: involutional paranoid state (F22)

paranoia (F22)

F20.1 **Disorganized schizophrenia** [HCC]

Hebephrenic schizophrenia

Hebephrenia

F20.2 **Catatonic schizophrenia** [HCC]

Schizophrenic catalepsy

Schizophrenic catatonia

Schizophrenic flexibilitas cerea

Excludes1: catatonic stupor (R40.1)

F20.3 **Undifferentiated schizophrenia** [HCC]

Atypical schizophrenia

Excludes1: acute schizophrenia-like psychotic disorder (F23)

Excludes2: post-schizophrenic depression (F32.89)

F20.5 **Residual schizophrenia** [HCC]

Restzustand (schizophrenic)

Schizophrenic residual state

F20.8 **Other schizophrenia**

F20.81 **Schizophreniform disorder** [HCC]

Schizophreniform psychosis NOS

F20.89 **Other schizophrenia** [HCC]

Cenesthopathic schizophrenia

Simple schizophrenia

F20.9 **Schizophrenia, unspecified** [HCC]

F21 **Schizotypal disorder** [HCC]

Borderline schizophrenia

Latent schizophrenia

Latent schizophrenic reaction

Prepsychotic schizophrenia

Prodromal schizophrenia

Pseudoneurotic schizophrenia

Pseudopsychopathic schizophrenia

Schizotypal personality disorder

Excludes2: Asperger's syndrome (F84.5)

schizoid personality disorder (F60.1)

F22 **Delusional disorders** [HCC]

Delusional dysmorphophobia

Involutional paranoid state

Paranoia

Paranoia querulans

Paranoid psychosis

Paranoid state

Paraphrenia (late)

Sensitiver Beziehungswahn

Excludes1: mood [affective] disorders with psychotic symptoms (F30.2, F31.2, F31.5, F31.64, F32.3, F33.3)

paranoid schizophrenia (F20.0)

Excludes2: paranoid personality disorder (F60.0)

paranoid psychosis, psychogenic (F23)

paranoid reaction (F23)

F23 **Brief psychotic disorder** [HCC]

Paranoid reaction

Psychogenic paranoid psychosis

Excludes2: mood [affective] disorders with psychotic symptoms (F30.2, F31.2, F31.5, F31.64, F32.3, F33.3)

F24 **Shared psychotic disorder** [HCC]

Folie à deux

Induced paranoid disorder

Induced psychotic disorder

F25 **Schizoaffective disorders**

Excludes1: mood [affective] disorders with psychotic symptoms (F30.2, F31.2, F31.5, F31.64, F32.3, F33.3)

schizophrenia (F20.-)

F25.0 **Schizoaffective disorder, bipolar type** [HCC]
Cyclic schizophrenia

Schizoaffective disorder, mixed type

Schizoaffective psychosis, bipolar type

Schizophreniform psychosis, manic type

F25.1 **Schizoaffective disorder, depressive type** [HCC]

Schizophreniform psychosis, depressive type

F25.8 **Other schizoaffective disorders** [HCC]

F25.9 **Schizoaffective disorder, unspecified** [HCC]

Schizoaffective psychosis NOS

F28 **Other psychotic disorder not due to a substance or known physiological condition** [HCC]

Chronic hallucinatory psychosis

F29 **Unspecified psychosis not due to a substance or known physiological condition** [HCC]

Psychosis NOS

Excludes1: mental disorder NOS (F99)

unspecified mental disorder due to known physiological condition (F09)

MOOD [AFFECTIVE] DISORDERS (F30-F39)

Definition: A mood disorder, also referred to as an affective disorder, is a condition impacting mood and related functions. In a mood disorder, moods range from extremely low (depressed) to extremely high or irritable (manic).

F30 Manic episode

Includes: bipolar disorder, single manic episode

mixed affective episode

Excludes1: bipolar disorder (F31.-)

> major depressive disorder, single episode (F32.-)

> major depressive disorder, recurrent (F33.-)

F30.1 Manic episode without psychotic symptoms

> **F30.10 Manic episode without psychotic symptoms, unspecified** [HCC]

> **F30.11 Manic episode without psychotic symptoms, mild** [HCC]

> **F30.12 Manic episode without psychotic symptoms, moderate** [HCC]

> **F30.13 Manic episode, severe, without psychotic symptoms** [HCC]

F30.2 Manic episode, severe with psychotic symptoms

> Manic stupor

> Mania with mood-congruent psychotic symptoms

> Mania with mood-incongruent psychotic symptoms

F30.3 Manic episode in partial remission

F30.4 Manic episode in full remission

F30.8 Other manic episodes

> Hypomania

F30.9 Manic episode, unspecified

> Mania NOS

F31 Bipolar disorder

Definition: Bipolar disorder, formerly called manic depression, is a mental illness that brings severe high and low moods and changes in sleep, energy, thinking, and behavior.

Includes: bipolar I disorder

bipolar type I disorder

manic-depressive illness

manic-depressive psychosis manic-depressive reaction

Excludes1: bipolar disorder, single manic episode (F30.-)

> major depressive disorder, single episode (F32.-)

> major depressive disorder, recurrent (F33.-)

Excludes2: cyclothymia (F34.0)

F31.0 Bipolar disorder, current episode hypomanic [HCC]

F31.1 Bipolar disorder, current episode manic without psychotic features

> **F31.10 Bipolar disorder, current episode manic without psychotic features, unspecified**

> **F31.11 Bipolar disorder, current episode manic without psychotic features, mild** [HCC]

> **F31.12 Bipolar disorder, current episode manic without psychotic features, moderate** [HCC]

> **F31.13 Bipolar disorder, current episode manic without psychotic features, severe** [HCC]

F31.2 Bipolar disorder, current episode manic severe with psychotic features [HCC]

> Bipolar disorder, current episode manic with mood-congruent psychotic symptoms

> Bipolar disorder, current episode manic with mood-incongruent psychotic symptoms

F31.3 Bipolar disorder, current episode depressed, mild or moderate severity

> **F31.30 Bipolar disorder, current episode depressed, mild or moderate severity, unspecified** [HCC]

> **F31.31 Bipolar disorder, current episode depressed, mild** [HCC]

> **F31.32 Bipolar disorder, current episode depressed, moderate** [HCC]

F31.4 Bipolar disorder, current episode depressed, severe, without psychotic features [HCC]

F31.5 Bipolar disorder, current episode depressed, severe, with psychotic features [HCC]

> Bipolar disorder, current episode depressed with mood-incongruent psychotic symptoms

> Bipolar disorder, current episode depressed with mood-congruent psychotic symptoms

> Bipolar I disorder, current or most recent episode depressed, with psychotic features

F31.6 Bipolar disorder, current episode mixed

> **F31.60 Bipolar disorder, current episode mixed, unspecified** [HCC]

> **F31.61 Bipolar disorder, current episode mixed, mild** [HCC]

> **F31.62 Bipolar disorder, current episode mixed, moderate** [HCC]

> **F31.63 Bipolar disorder, current episode mixed, severe, without psychotic features** [HCC]

> **F31.64 Bipolar disorder, current episode mixed, severe, with psychotic features** [HCC]

> > Bipolar disorder, current episode mixed with mood-congruent psychotic symptoms

> > Bipolar disorder, current episode mixed with mood-incongruent psychotic symptoms

F31.7 Bipolar disorder, currently in remission

> **F31.70 Bipolar disorder, currently in remission, most recent episode unspecified** [HCC]

> **F31.71 Bipolar disorder, in partial remission, most recent episode hypomanic** [HCC]

> **F31.72 Bipolar disorder, in full remission, most recent episode hypomanic** [HCC]

> **F31.73 Bipolar disorder, in partial remission, most recent episode manic** [HCC]

> **F31.74 Bipolar disorder, in full remission, most recent episode manic** [HCC]

> **F31.75 Bipolar disorder, in partial remission, most recent episode depressed** [HCC]

> **F31.76 Bipolar disorder, in full remission, most recent episode depressed** [HCC]

> **F31.77 Bipolar disorder, in partial remission, most recent episode mixed** [HCC]

> **F31.78 Bipolar disorder, in full remission, most recent episode mixed** [HCC]

F31.8 Other bipolar disorders

> **F31.81 Bipolar II disorder** [HCC]

> > Bipolar disorder, type 2

> **F31.89 Other bipolar disorder** [HCC]

> > Recurrent manic episodes NOS

F31.9 Bipolar disorder, unspecified [HCC]

> Manic depression

F32 Depressive episode

Includes: single episode of agitated depression

single episode of depressive reaction single episode of major depression

single episode of psychogenic depression single episode of reactive depression single episode of vital depression

Excludes1: bipolar disorder (F31.-)

> manic episode (F30.-)

> recurrent depressive disorder (F33.-)

● New code ▲ Revised code **Excludes1:** Not coded here **Excludes2:** Not included here ⊗ Placeholder required ⑦7th digit required

Excludes2: adjustment disorder (F43.2)

F32.0 Major depressive disorder, single episode, mild [HCC]

F32.1 Major depressive disorder, single episode, moderate [HCC]

F32.2 Major depressive disorder, single episode, severe without psychotic features [HCC]

F32.3 Major depressive disorder, single episode, severe with psychotic features [HCC]

Single episode of major depression with mood-congruent psychotic symptoms

Single episode of major depression with mood-incongruent psychotic symptoms

Single episode of major depression with psychotic symptoms

Single episode of psychogenic depressive psychosis

Single episode of psychotic depression

Single episode of reactive depressive psychosis

F32.4 Major depressive disorder, single episode, in partial remission [HCC]

F32.5 Major depressive disorder, single episode, in full remission [HCC]

F32.8 Other depressive episodes

F32.81 Premenstrual dysphoric disorder

Excludes1: premenstrual tension syndrome (N94.3)

F32.89 Other specified depressive episodes

Atypical depression

Post-schizophrenic depression

Single episode of 'masked' depression NOS

F32.9 Major depressive disorder, single episode, unspecified

Major depression NOS

• **F32.A Depression, unspecified**

Depression NOS

Depressive disorder NOS

F33 Major depressive disorder, recurrent

Includes: recurrent episodes of depressive reaction

recurrent episodes of endogenous depression recurrent episodes of major depression

recurrent episodes of psychogenic depression recurrent episodes of reactive depression

recurrent episodes of seasonal depressive disorder recurrent episodes of vital depression

Excludes1: bipolar disorder (F31.-)

manic episode (F30.-)

F33.0 Major depressive disorder, recurrent, mild [HCC]

F33.1 Major depressive disorder, recurrent, moderate [HCC]

F33.2 Major depressive disorder, recurrent severe without psychotic features [HCC]

F33.3 Major depressive disorder, recurrent, severe with psychotic symptoms [HCC]

Endogenous depression with psychotic symptoms

Major depressive disorder, recurrent, with psychotic features

Recurrent severe episodes of major depression with mood-congruent psychotic symptoms

Recurrent severe episodes of major depression with mood-incongruent psychotic symptoms

Recurrent severe episodes of major depression with psychotic symptoms

Recurrent severe episodes of psychogenic depressive psychosis

Recurrent severe episodes of psychotic depression

Recurrent severe episodes of reactive depressive psychosis

F33.4 Major depressive disorder, recurrent, in remission

F33.40 Major depressive disorder, recurrent, in remission, unspecified [HCC]

F33.41 Major depressive disorder, recurrent, in partial remission [HCC]

F33.42 Major depressive disorder, recurrent, in full remission [HCC]

F33.8 Other recurrent depressive disorders [HCC]

Recurrent brief depressive episodes

F33.9 Major depressive disorder, recurrent, unspecified [HCC]

Monopolar depression NOS

F34 Persistent mood [affective] disorders

F34.0 Cyclothymic disorder

Affective personality disorder

Cycloid personality

Cyclothymia

Cyclothymic personality

F34.1 Dysthymic disorder

Depressive neurosis

Depressive personality disorder

Dysthymia

Neurotic depression

Persistent anxiety depression

Persistent depressive disorder

Excludes2: anxiety depression (mild or not persistent) (F41.8)

F34.8 Other persistent mood [affective] disorders

F34.81 Disruptive mood dysregulation disorder [HCC]

F34.89 Other specified persistent mood disorders [HCC]

F34.9 Persistent mood [affective] disorder, unspecified [HCC]

F39 Unspecified mood [affective] disorder [HCC]

Affective psychosis NOS

ANXIETY, DISSOCIATIVE, STRESS-RELATED, SOMATOFORM AND OTHER NONPSYCHOTIC MENTAL DISORDERS (F40-F48)

Definition: Anxiety disorders are a group of mental disorders characterized by feelings of anxiety and fear, where anxiety is a worry about future events and fear is a reaction to current events.

F40 Phobic anxiety disorders

F40.0 Agoraphobia

F40.00 Agoraphobia, unspecified

F40.01 Agoraphobia with panic disorder

Panic disorder with agoraphobia

Excludes1: panic disorder without agoraphobia (F41.0)

F40.02 Agoraphobia without panic disorder

F40.1 Social phobias

Anthropophobia

Social anxiety disorder

Social anxiety disorder of childhood

Social neurosis

F40.10 Social phobia, unspecified

F40.11 Social phobia, generalized

F40.2 Specific (isolated) phobias

Excludes2: dysmorphophobia (nondelusional) (F45.22)

nosophobia (F45.22)

F40.21 Animal type phobia

	F40.210	**Arachnophobia**
		Fear of spiders
	F40.218	**Other animal type phobia**
F40.22		**Natural environment type phobia**
	F40.220	**Fear of thunderstorms**
	F40.228	**Other natural environment type phobia**
F40.23		**Blood, injection, injury type phobia**
	F40.230	**Fear of blood**
	F40.231	**Fear of injections and transfusions**
	F40.232	**Fear of other medical care**
	F40.233	**Fear of injury**
F40.24		**Situational type phobia**
	F40.240	**Claustrophobia**
	F40.241	**Acrophobia**
	F40.242	**Fear of bridges**
	F40.243	**Fear of flying**
	F40.248	**Other situational type phobia**
F40.29		**Other specified phobia**
	F40.290	**Androphobia**
		Fear of men
	F40.291	**Gynephobia**
		Fear of women
	F40.298	**Other specified phobia**

F40.8 **Other phobic anxiety disorders**

Phobic anxiety disorder of childhood

F40.9 **Phobic anxiety disorder, unspecified**

Phobia NOS

Phobic state NOS

F41 **Other anxiety disorders**

Excludes2: anxiety in:

acute stress reaction (F43.0)

transient adjustment reaction (F43.2)

neurasthenia (F48.8)

psychophysiologic disorders (F45.-)

separation anxiety (F93.0)

F41.0 **Panic disorder [episodic paroxysmal anxiety]**

Panic attack

Panic state

Excludes1: panic disorder with agoraphobia (F40.01)

F41.1 **Generalized anxiety disorder**

Anxiety neurosis

Anxiety reaction

Anxiety state

Overanxious disorder

Excludes2: neurasthenia (F48.8)

F41.3 **Other mixed anxiety disorders**

F41.8 **Other specified anxiety disorders**

Anxiety depression (mild or not persistent)

Anxiety hysteria

Mixed anxiety and depressive disorder

F41.9 **Anxiety disorder, unspecified**

Anxiety NOS

F42 **Obsessive-compulsive disorder**

Excludes2: obsessive-compulsive personality (disorder) (F60.5)

obsessive-compulsive symptoms occurring in depression (F32-F33)

obsessive-compulsive symptoms occurring in schizophrenia (F20.-)

F42.2 **Mixed obsessional thoughts and acts**

F42.3 **Hoarding disorder**

F42.4 **Excoriation (skin-picking) disorder**

Excludes1: factitial dermatitis (L98.1)

Other specified behavioral and emotional disorders with onset usually occurring in early childhood and adolescence (F98.8)

F42.8 **Other obsessive-compulsive disorder**

Anancastic neurosis

Obsessive-compulsive neurosis

F42.9 **Obsessive-compulsive disorder, unspecified**

F43 **Reaction to severe stress, and adjustment disorders**

F43.0 **Acute stress reaction**

Acute crisis reaction

Acute reaction to stress

Combat and operational stress reaction

Combat fatigue

Crisis state

Psychic shock

F43.1 **Post-traumatic stress disorder (PTSD)**

Traumatic neurosis

F43.10 **Post-traumatic stress disorder, unspecified**

F43.11 **Post-traumatic stress disorder, acute**

F43.12 **Post-traumatic stress disorder, chronic**

F43.2 **Adjustment disorders**

Culture shock Grief reaction

Hospitalism in children

Excludes2: separation anxiety disorder of childhood (F93.0)

F43.20 **Adjustment disorder, unspecified**

F43.21 **Adjustment disorder with depressed mood**

F43.22 **Adjustment disorder with anxiety**

F43.23 **Adjustment disorder with mixed anxiety and depressed mood**

F43.24 **Adjustment disorder with disturbance of conduct**

F43.25 **Adjustment disorder with mixed disturbance of emotions and conduct**

F43.29 **Adjustment disorder with other symptoms**

F43.8 **Other reactions to severe stress**

Other specified trauma and stressor-related disorder

F43.9 **Reaction to severe stress, unspecified**

Trauma and stressor-related disorder, NOS

F44 **Dissociative and conversion disorders**

Includes: conversion hysteria

conversion reaction hysteria

hysterical psychosis

Excludes2: malingering [conscious simulation] (Z76.5)

F44.0 **Dissociative amnesia** [HCC]

Excludes1: amnesia NOS (R41.3)

anterograde amnesia (R41.1)

dissociative amnesia with dissociative fugue (F44.1)

retrograde amnesia (R41.2)

● New code ▲ Revised code **Excludes1:** Not coded here **Excludes2:** Not included here ⊗ Placeholder required ⑦7th digit required

Excludes2: alcohol-**or other** psychoactive substance-induced amnestic disorder (F10, F13, F19 with .26, .96)

amnestic disorder due to known physiological condition (F04)

postictal amnesia in epilepsy (G40.-)

F44.1 Dissociative fugue [HCC]

Dissociative amnesia with dissociative fugue

Excludes2: postictal fugue in epilepsy (G40.-)

F44.2 Dissociative stupor

Excludes1: catatonic stupor (R40.1)

stupor NOS (R40.1)

Excludes2: catatonic disorder due to known physiological condition (F06.1)

depressive stupor (F32, F33)

manic stupor (F30, F31)

F44.4 Conversion disorder with motor symptom or deficit

Conversion disorder with abnormal movement

Conversion disorder with speech symptoms

Conversion disorder with swallowing symptoms

Conversion disorder with weakness/paralysis

Dissociative motor disorders

Psychogenic aphonia

Psychogenic dysphonia

F44.5 Conversion disorder with seizures or convulsions

Conversion disorder with attacks or seizures

Dissociative convulsions

F44.6 Conversion disorder with sensory symptom or deficit

Conversion disorder with anesthesia or sensory loss

Conversion disorder with special sensory symptoms

Dissociative anesthesia and sensory loss

Psychogenic deafness

F44.7 Conversion disorder with mixed symptom presentation

F44.8 Other dissociative and conversion disorders

F44.81 Dissociative identity disorder [HCC]

Multiple personality disorder

F44.89 Other dissociative and conversion disorders

Ganser's syndrome

Psychogenic confusion

Psychogenic twilight state

Trance and possession disorders

F44.9 Dissociative and conversion disorder, unspecified

Dissociative disorder NOS

F45 Somatoform disorders

Definition: Somatoform disorder is the name for a group of conditions in which the physical pain and symptoms a person feels are related to psychological factors. These symptoms cannot be traced
to a specific physical cause.

Excludes2: dissociative and conversion disorders (F44.-)

factitious disorders (F68.1-, F68.A)

hair-plucking (F63.3)

lalling (F80.0)

lisping (F80.0)

malingering [conscious simulation] (Z76.5)

nail-biting (F98.8)

psychological or behavioral factors associated with disorders or diseases classified elsewhere (F54)

sexual dysfunction, not due to a substance or known physiological condition (F52.-)

thumb-sucking (F98.8)

tic disorders (in childhood and adolescence) (F95.-)

Tourette's syndrome (F95.2)

trichotillomania (F63.3)

F45.0 Somatization disorder

Briquet's disorder

Multiple psychosomatic disorder

F45.1 Undifferentiated somatoform disorder

Somatic symptom disorder

Undifferentiated psychosomatic disorder

F45.2 Hypochondriacal disorders

Excludes2: delusional dysmorphophobia (F22)

fixed delusions about bodily functions or shape (F22)

F45.20 Hypochondriacal disorder, unspecified

F45.21 Hypochondriasis

Hypochondriacal neurosis

Illness anxiety disorder

F45.22 Body dysmorphic disorder

Dysmorphophobia (nondelusional)

Nosophobia

F45.29 Other hypochondriacal disorders

F45.4 Pain disorders related to psychological factors

Excludes1: pain NOS (R52)

F45.41 Pain disorder exclusively related to psychological factors

Somatoform pain disorder (persistent)

F45.42 Pain disorder with related psychological factors

Code also associated acute or chronic pain (G89.-)

F45.8 Other somatoform disorders

Psychogenic dysmenorrhea

Psychogenic dysphagia, including 'globus hystericus'

Psychogenic pruritus

Psychogenic torticollis

Somatoform autonomic dysfunction

Teeth grinding

Excludes1: sleep related teeth grinding (G47.63)

F45.9 Somatoform disorder, unspecified

Psychosomatic disorder NOS

F48 Other nonpsychotic mental disorders

F48.1 Depersonalization-derealization syndrome [HCC]

F48.2 Pseudobulbar affect

Involuntary emotional expression disorder

Code first underlying cause, if known, such as:

amyotrophic lateral sclerosis (G12.21)

multiple sclerosis (G35)

sequelae of cerebrovascular disease (I69.-)

sequelae of traumatic intracranial injury (S06.-)

F48.8 Other specified nonpsychotic mental disorders

Dhat syndrome Neurasthenia

Occupational neurosis, including writer's cramp

Psychasthenia

Psychasthenic neurosis

Psychogenic syncope

F48.9 Nonpsychotic mental disorder, unspecified

Neurosis NOS

BEHAVIORAL SYNDROMES ASSOCIATED WITH PHYSIOLOGICAL DISTURBANCES AND PHYSICAL FACTORS (F50-F59)

F50   Eating disorders

Excludes1: anorexia NOS (R63.0)

feeding problems of newborn (P92.-)

polyphagia (R63.2)

Excludes2: feeding difficulties (R63.3)

feeding disorder in infancy or childhood (F98.2-)

F50.0   Anorexia nervosa

Excludes1: loss of appetite (R63.0)

psychogenic loss of appetite (F50.89)

F50.00   Anorexia nervosa, unspecified

F50.01   Anorexia nervosa, restricting type

F50.02   Anorexia nervosa, binge eating/purging type

Excludes1: bulimia nervosa (F50.2)

F50.2   Bulimia nervosa

Bulimia NOS

Hyperorexia nervosa

Excludes1: anorexia nervosa, binge eating/purging type (F50.02)

F50.8   Other eating disorders

Excludes2: pica of infancy and childhood (F98.3)

F50.81   Binge eating disorder

F50.82   Avoidant/restrictive food intake disorder

F50.89   Other specified eating disorder

Pica in adults

Psychogenic loss of appetite

F50.9   Eating disorder, unspecified

Atypical anorexia nervosa

Atypical bulimia nervosa

Feeding or eating disorder, unspecified

Other specified feeding disorder

F51   Sleep disorders not due to a substance or known physiological condition

Excludes2: organic sleep disorders (G47.-)

F51.0   Insomnia not due to a substance or known physiological condition

Excludes2: alcohol related insomnia (F10.182, F10.282, F10.982)

drug-related insomnia (F11.182, F11.282, F11.982, F13.182, F13.282, F13.982, F14.182, F14.282, F14.982, F15.182, F15.282, F15.982, F19.182, F19.282, F19.982)

insomnia NOS (G47.0-)

insomnia due to known physiological condition (G47.0-)

organic insomnia (G47.0-)

sleep deprivation (Z72.820)

F51.01   Primary insomnia

Idiopathic insomnia

F51.02   Adjustment insomnia

F51.03   Paradoxical insomnia

F51.04   Psychophysiologic insomnia

F51.05   Insomnia due to other mental disorder

Code also associated mental disorder

F51.09   Other insomnia not due to a substance or known physiological condition

F51.1   Hypersomnia not due to a substance or known physiological condition

Excludes2: alcohol related hypersomnia (F10.182, F10.282, F10.982)

drug-related hypersomnia (F11.182, F11.282, F11.982, F13.182, F13.282, F13.982, F14.182, F14.282, F14.982, F15.182, F15.282, F15.982, F19.182, F19.282, F19.982)

hypersomnia NOS (G47.10)

hypersomnia due to known physiological condition (G47.10)

idiopathic hypersomnia (G47.11, G47.12)

narcolepsy (G47.4-)

F51.11   Primary hypersomnia

F51.12   Insufficient sleep syndrome

Excludes1: sleep deprivation (Z72.820)

F51.13   Hypersomnia due to other mental disorder

Code also associated mental disorder

F51.19   Other hypersomnia not due to a substance or known physiological condition

F51.3   Sleepwalking [somnambulism]

Non-rapid eye movement sleep arousal disorders, sleepwalking type

Non-rapid eye movement sleep arousal disorders, sleep terror type

F51.4   Sleep terrors [night terrors]

Non-rapid eye movement sleep arousal disorders, sleep terror type

F51.5   Nightmare disorder

Dream anxiety disorder

F51.8   Other sleep disorders not due to a substance or known physiological condition

F51.9   Sleep disorder not due to a substance or known physiological condition, unspecified

Emotional sleep disorder NOS

F52   Sexual dysfunction not due to a substance or known physiological condition

Excludes2: Dhat syndrome (F48.8)

F52.0   Hypoactive sexual desire disorder

Lack or loss of sexual desire

Male hypoactive sexual desire disorder

Sexual anhedonia

Excludes1: decreased libido (R68.82)

F52.1   Sexual aversion disorder

Sexual aversion and lack of sexual enjoyment

F52.2   Sexual arousal disorders

Failure of genital response

F52.21   Male erectile disorder

Erectile disorder

Psychogenic impotence

Excludes1: impotence of organic origin (N52.-)

impotence NOS (N52.-)

F52.22   Female sexual arousal disorder

Female sexual interest/arousal disorder

F52.3   Orgasmic disorder

Inhibited orgasm

Psychogenic anorgasmy

F52.31   Female orgasmic disorder

F52.32   Male orgasmic disorder

Delayed ejaculation

F52.4 **Premature ejaculation**

F52.5 **Vaginismus not due to a substance or known physiological condition**

Psychogenic vaginismus

Excludes2: vaginismus (due to a known physiological condition) (N94.2)

F52.6 **Dyspareunia not due to a substance or known physiological condition**

Genito-pelvic pain penetration disorder

Psychogenic dyspareunia

Excludes2: dyspareunia (due to a known physiological condition) (N94.1-)

F52.8 **Other sexual dysfunction not due to a substance or known physiological condition**

Excessive sexual drive

Nymphomania

Satyriasis

F52.9 **Unspecified sexual dysfunction not due to a substance or known physiological condition**

Sexual dysfunction NOS

F53 **Mental and behavioral disorders associated with the puerperium, not elsewhere classified**

Postpartum depression

Excludes1: mood disorders with psychotic features (F30.2, F31.5, F31.64, F32.3, F33.3)

psychosis in schizophrenia, schizotypal, delusional, and other psychotic disorders (F20-F29)

F53.0 **Postpartum depression**

Postnatal depression, NOS

Postpartum depression, NOS

F53.1 **Puerperal psychosis**

Postpartum psychosis

Puerperal psychosis, NOS

F54 **Psychological and behavioral factors associated with disorders or diseases classified elsewhere**

Psychological factors affecting physical conditions

Code first the associated physical disorder, such as:

asthma (J45.-)

dermatitis (L23-L25)

gastric ulcer (K25.-)

mucous colitis (K58.-)

ulcerative colitis (K51.-)

urticaria (L50.-)

Excludes2: tension-type headache (G44.2)

F55 **Abuse of non-psychoactive substances**

Excludes2: abuse of psychoactive substances (F10-F19)

F55.0 **Abuse of antacids**

F55.1 **Abuse of herbal or folk remedies**

F55.2 **Abuse of laxatives**

F55.3 **Abuse of steroids or hormones**

F55.4 **Abuse of vitamins**

F55.8 **Abuse of other non-psychoactive substances**

F59 **Unspecified behavioral syndromes associated with physiological disturbances and physical factors**

Psychogenic physiological dysfunction NOS

DISORDERS OF ADULT PERSONALITY AND BEHAVIOR
(F60-F69)

F60 **Specific personality disorders**

F60.0 **Paranoid personality disorder** [HCC]

Expansive paranoid personality (disorder)

Fanatic personality (disorder)

Querulant personality (disorder)

Paranoid personality (disorder)

Sensitive paranoid personality (disorder)

Excludes2: paranoia (F22)

paranoia querulans (F22)

paranoid psychosis (F22)

paranoid schizophrenia (F20.0)

paranoid state (F22)

F60.1 **Schizoid personality disorder** [HCC]

Excludes2: Asperger's syndrome (F84.5)

delusional disorder (F22)

schizoid disorder of childhood (F84.5)

schizophrenia (F20.-)

schizotypal disorder (F21)

F60.2 **Antisocial personality disorder** [HCC]

Amoral personality (disorder)

Asocial personality (disorder)

Dissocial personality disorder

Psychopathic personality (disorder)

Sociopathic personality (disorder)

Excludes1: conduct disorders (F91.-)

Excludes2: borderline personality disorder (F60.3)

F60.3 **Borderline personality disorder** [HCC]

Aggressive personality (disorder)

Emotionally unstable personality disorder

Explosive personality (disorder)

Excludes2: antisocial personality disorder (F60.2)

F60.4 **Histrionic personality disorder**

Hysterical personality (disorder)

Psychoinfantile personality (disorder)

F60.5 **Obsessive-compulsive personality disorder** [HCC]

Anankastic personality (disorder)

Compulsive personality (disorder)

Obsessional personality (disorder)

Excludes2: obsessive-compulsive disorder (F42.-)

F60.6 **Avoidant personality disorder** [HCC]

Anxious personality disorder

F60.7 **Dependent personality disorder** [HCC]

Asthenic personality (disorder)

Inadequate personality (disorder)

Passive personality (disorder)

F60.8 **Other specific personality disorders**

F60.81 **Narcissistic personality disorder** [HCC]

F60.89 **Other specific personality disorders** [HCC]

Eccentric personality disorder

'Haltlose' type personality disorder

Immature personality disorder

Passive-aggressive personality disorder

Psychoneurotic personality disorder

Self-defeating personality disorder

F60.9 **Personality disorder, unspecified** [HCC]

Character disorder NOS

Character neurosis NOS

Pathological personality NOS

F63   Impulse disorders

Excludes2: habitual excessive use of alcohol or psychoactive substances (F10-F19)

impulse disorders involving sexual behavior (F65.-)

F63.0   Pathological gambling

Compulsive gambling

Gambling disorder

Excludes1: gambling and betting NOS (Z72.6)

Excludes2: excessive gambling by manic patients (F30, F31)

gambling in antisocial personality disorder (F60.2)

F63.1   Pyromania

Pathological fire-setting

Excludes2: fire-setting (by) (in):

adult with antisocial personality disorder (F60.2)

alcohol or psychoactive substance intoxication (F10-F19)

conduct disorders (F91.-)

mental disorders due to known physiological condition (F01-F09)

schizophrenia (F20.-)

F63.2   Kleptomania

Pathological stealing

Excludes1: shoplifting as the reason for observation for suspected mental disorder (Z03.8)

Excludes2: depressive disorder with stealing (F31-F33)

stealing due to underlying mental condition-code to mental condition stealing in mental disorders due to known physiological condition (F01-F09)

F63.3   Trichotillomania

Hair plucking

Excludes2: Other stereotyped movement disorder (F98.4)

F63.8   Other impulse disorders

F63.81   Intermittent explosive disorder

F63.89   Other impulse disorders

F63.9   Impulse disorder, unspecified

Impulse control disorder NOS

F64   Gender identity disorders

F64.0   Transsexualism

Gender identity disorder in adolescence and adulthood

Gender dysphoria in adolescents and adults

F64.1   Dual role transvestism

Use Additional Code to identify sex reassignment status (Z87.890)

Excludes1: gender identity disorder in childhood (F64.2)

Excludes2: fetishistic transvestism (F65.1)

F64.2   Gender identity disorder of childhood

Gender dysphoria in children

Excludes1: gender identity disorder in adolescence and adulthood (F64.0)

Excludes2: sexual maturation disorder (F66)

F64.8   Other gender identity disorders

Other specified gender dysphoria

F64.9   Gender identity disorder, unspecified

Gender dysphoria, unspecified

Gender-role disorder NOS

F65   Paraphilias

F65.0   Fetishism

Fetishistic disorder

F65.1   Transvestic Fetishism

Transvestic disorder

Fetishistic transvestism

F65.2   Exhibitionism

Exhibitionistic disorder

F65.3   Voyeurism

Voyeuristic disorder

F65.4   Pedophilia

Pedophilic disorder

F65.5   Sadomasochism

F65.50   Sadomasochism, unspecified

F65.51   Sexual masochism

Sexual masochism disorder

F65.52   Sexual sadism

Sexual sadism disorder

F65.8   Other paraphilias

F65.81   Frotteurism

Frotteuristic disorder

F65.89   Other paraphilias

Necrophilia

Other specified paraphilic disorder

F65.9   Paraphilia, unspecified

Paraphilic disorder, unspecified

Sexual deviation NOS

F66   Other sexual disorders

Sexual maturation disorder

Sexual relationship disorder

F68   Other disorders of adult personality and behavior

F68.1   Factitious disorder imposed on self

Compensation neurosis

Elaboration of physical symptoms for psychological reasons

Hospital hopper syndrome

Munchausen's syndrome

Peregrinating patient

Excludes2: factitial dermatitis (L98.1)

person feigning illness (with obvious motivation) (Z76.5)

F68.10   Factitious disorder imposed on self, unspecified

F68.11   Factitious disorder imposed on self, with predominantly psychological signs and symptoms

F68.12   Factitious disorder imposed on self, with predominantly physical signs and symptoms

F68.13   Factitious disorder imposed on self, with combined psychological and physical signs and symptoms

F68.8   Other specified disorders of adult personality and behavior

F68.A   Factitious disorder imposed on another

Factitious disorder by proxy

Munchausen's by proxy

F69   Unspecified disorder of adult personality and behavior

● New code   ▲ Revised code   **Excludes1:** Not coded here   **Excludes2:** Not included here   ⊗ Placeholder required   ⑦7th digit required

INTELLECTUAL DISABILITIES (F70-F79)

Code first any associated physical or developmental disorders

Excludes1: borderline intellectual functioning, IQ above 70 to 84 (R41.83)

F70 Mild intellectual disabilities
IQ level 50-55 to approximately 70
Mild mental subnormality

F71 Moderate intellectual disabilities
IQ level 35-40 to 50-55
Moderate mental subnormality

F72 Severe intellectual disabilities
IQ 20-25 to 35-40
Severe mental subnormality

F73 Profound intellectual disabilities
IQ level below 20-25 Profound mental subnormality

F78 Other intellectual disabilities

- **F78.A Other genetic related intellectual disabilities**

  - **F78.A1 SYNGAP1-related intellectual disability**

    Code also, if applicable, any associated:

    autism spectrum disorder (F84.0)

    autistic disorder (F84.0)

    encephalopathy (G93.4-)

    epilepsy and recurrent seizures (G40.-)

    other pervasive developmental disorders (F84.8)

    pervasive developmental disorder, NOS (F84.9)

  - **F78.A9 Other genetic related intellectual disability**

    Code also, if applicable, any associated disorders

F79 Unspecified intellectual disabilities
Mental deficiency NOS
Mental subnormality NOS

PERVASIVE AND SPECIFIC DEVELOPMENTAL DISORDERS (F80-F89)

F80 Specific developmental disorders of speech and language

F80.0 Phonological disorder
Dyslalia
Functional speech articulation disorder
Lalling
Lisping
Phonological developmental disorder
Speech articulation developmental disorder
Speech-sound disorder

Excludes1: speech articulation impairment due to aphasia NOS (R47.01)

speech articulation impairment due to apraxia (R48.2)

Excludes2: speech articulation impairment due to hearing loss (F80.4)

speech articulation impairment due to intellectual disabilities (F70-F79)

speech articulation impairment with expressive language developmental disorder (F80.1)

speech articulation impairment with mixed receptive expressive language developmental disorder (F80.2)

F80.1 Expressive language disorder
Developmental dysphasia or aphasia, expressive type

Excludes1: mixed receptive-expressive language disorder (F80.2)

dysphasia and aphasia NOS (R47.-)

Excludes2: acquired aphasia with epilepsy [Landau-Kleffner] (G40.80-)

selective mutism (F94.0)

intellectual disabilities (F70-F79)

pervasive developmental disorders (F84.-)

F80.2 Mixed receptive-expressive language disorder
Developmental dysphasia or aphasia, receptive type
Developmental Wernicke's aphasia

Excludes1: central auditory processing disorder (H93.25)

dysphasia or aphasia NOS (R47.-)

expressive language disorder (F80.1)

expressive type dysphasia or aphasia (F80.1)

word deafness (H93.25)

Excludes2: acquired aphasia with epilepsy [Landau-Kleffner] (G40.80-)

pervasive developmental disorders (F84.-)

selective mutism (F94.0)

intellectual disabilities (F70-F79)

F80.4 Speech and language development delay due to hearing loss
Code also type of hearing loss (H90.-, H91.-)

F80.8 Other developmental disorders of speech and language

F80.81 Childhood onset fluency disorder
Cluttering NOS
Stuttering NOS

Excludes1: adult onset fluency disorder (F98.5)

fluency disorder in conditions classified elsewhere (R47.82)

fluency disorder (stuttering) following cerebrovascular disease (I69. with final characters - 23)

F80.82 Social pragmatic communication disorder

Excludes1: Asperger's syndrome (F84.5)

autistic disorder (F84.0)

F80.89 Other developmental disorders of speech and language

F80.9 Developmental disorder of speech and language, unspecified
Communication disorder NOS
Language disorder NOS

F81 Specific developmental disorders of scholastic skills

F81.0 Specific reading disorder
Backward reading'
Developmental dyslexia
Specific learning disorder, with impairment in reading
Specific reading retardation

Excludes1: alexia NOS (R48.0)

dyslexia NOS (R48.0)

F81.2 Mathematics disorder
Developmental acalculia
Developmental arithmetical disorder
Developmental Gerstmann's syndrome
Specific learning disorder, with impairment in mathematics

Excludes1: acalculia NOS (R48.8)

Excludes2: arithmetic difficulties associated with a reading disorder (F81.0) arithmetical difficulties associated with a spelling disorder (F81.81)

arithmetical difficulties due to inadequate teaching (Z55.8)

F81.8 Other developmental disorders of scholastic skills

> **F81.81 Disorder of written expression**
>
> Specific learning disorder, with impairment in written expression
>
> Specific spelling disorder
>
> **F81.89 Other developmental disorders of scholastic skills**

F81.9 Developmental disorder of scholastic skills, unspecified

Knowledge acquisition disability NOS

Learning disability NOS

Learning disorder NOS

F82 Specific developmental disorder of motor function

Clumsy child syndrome

Developmental coordination disorder

Developmental dyspraxia

> **Excludes1:** abnormalities of gait and mobility (R26.-)
>
> lack of coordination (R27.-)
>
> **Excludes2:** lack of coordination secondary to intellectual disabilities (F70-F79)

F84 Pervasive developmental disorders

Code also any associated medical condition and intellectual disabilities.

F84.0 Autistic disorder

Autism spectrum disorder

Infantile autism

Infantile psychosis

Kanner's syndrome

> **Excludes1:** Asperger's syndrome (F84.5)

F84.2 Rett's syndrome

> **Excludes1:** Asperger's syndrome (F84.5)
>
> Autistic disorder (F84.0)
>
> Other childhood disintegrative disorder (F84.3)

F84.3 Other childhood disintegrative disorder

Dementia infantilis

Disintegrative psychosis

Heller's syndrome

Symbiotic psychosis

Use Additional Code to identify any associated neurological condition.

> **Excludes1:** Asperger's syndrome (F84.5)
>
> Autistic disorder (F84.0)
>
> Rett's syndrome (F84.2)

F84.5 Asperger's syndrome

Asperger's disorder

Autistic psychopathy

Schizoid disorder of childhood

F84.8 Other pervasive developmental disorders

Overactive disorder associated with intellectual disabilities and stereotyped movements

F84.9 Pervasive developmental disorder, unspecified

Atypical autism

F88 Other disorders of psychological development

Developmental agnosia Global developmental delay

Other specified neurodevelopmental disorder

F89 Unspecified disorder of psychological development

Developmental disorder NOS

Neurodevelopmental disorder NOS

BEHAVIORAL AND EMOTIONAL DISORDERS WITH ONSET USUALLY OCCURRING IN CHILDHOOD AND ADOLESCENCE (F90-F98)

Note: Codes within categories F90-F98 may be used regardless of the age of a patient. These disorders generally have onset within the childhood or adolescent years, but may continue throughout life or not be diagnosed until adulthood

F90 Attention-deficit hyperactivity disorders

Definition: Attention deficit hyperactivity disorder refers to any of a range of behavioral disorders occurring primarily in children, including such symptoms as poor concentration, hyperactivity, and impulsivity.

Includes: attention deficit disorder with hyperactivity

attention deficit syndrome with hyperactivity

> **Excludes2:** anxiety disorders (F40.-, F41.-)
>
> mood [affective] disorders (F30-F39)
>
> pervasive developmental disorders (F84.-)
>
> schizophrenia (F20.-)

F90.0 Attention-deficit hyperactivity disorder, predominantly inattentive type

F90.1 Attention-deficit hyperactivity disorder, predominantly hyperactive type

Attention-deficit/hyperactivity disorder, predominantly hyperactive impulsive presentation

F90.2 Attention-deficit hyperactivity disorder, combined type

Attention-deficit/hyperactivity disorder, combined presentation

F90.8 Attention-deficit hyperactivity disorder, other type

F90.9 Attention-deficit hyperactivity disorder, unspecified type

Attention-deficit hyperactivity disorder of childhood or adolescence NOS

Attention-deficit hyperactivity disorder NOS

F91 Conduct disorders

> **Excludes1:** antisocial behavior (Z72.81-)
>
> antisocial personality disorder (F60.2)
>
> **Excludes2:** conduct problems associated with attention-deficit hyperactivity disorder (F90.-)
>
> mood [affective] disorders (F30-F39)
>
> pervasive developmental disorders (F84.-)
>
> schizophrenia (F20.-)

F91.0 Conduct disorder confined to family context

F91.1 Conduct disorder, childhood-onset type

Unsocialized conduct disorder

Conduct disorder, solitary aggressive type

Unsocialized aggressive disorder

F91.2 Conduct disorder, adolescent-onset type

Socialized conduct disorder

Conduct disorder, group type

F91.3 Oppositional defiant disorder

F91.8 Other conduct disorders

Other specified conduct disorder

Other specified disruptive disorder

F91.9 Conduct disorder, unspecified

Behavioral disorder NOS

Conduct disorder NOS

Disruptive behavior disorder NOS

Disruptive disorder NOS

F93 **Emotional disorders with onset specific to childhood**

F93.0 **Separation anxiety disorder of childhood**

Excludes2: mood [affective] disorders (F30-F39)

nonpsychotic mental disorders (F40-F48)

phobic anxiety disorder of childhood (F40.8)

social phobia (F40.1)

F93.8 **Other childhood emotional disorders**

Identity disorder

Excludes2: gender identity disorder of childhood (F64.2)

F93.9 **Childhood emotional disorder, unspecified**

F94 **Disorders of social functioning with onset specific to childhood and adolescence**

F94.0 **Selective mutism**

Elective mutism

Excludes2: pervasive developmental disorders (F84.-)

schizophrenia (F20.-)

specific developmental disorders of speech and language (F80.-)

transient mutism as part of separation anxiety in young children (F93.0)

F94.1 **Reactive attachment disorder of childhood**

Use Additional Code to identify any associated failure to thrive or growth retardation

Excludes1: disinhibited attachment disorder of childhood (F94.2)

normal variation in pattern of selective attachment

Excludes2: Asperger's syndrome (F84.5)

maltreatment syndromes (T74.-)

sexual or physical abuse in childhood, resulting in psychosocial problems (Z62.81-)

F94.2 **Disinhibited attachment disorder of childhood**

Affectionless psychopathy

Institutional syndrome

Excludes1: reactive attachment disorder of childhood (F94.1)

Excludes2: Asperger's syndrome (F84.5)

attention-deficit hyperactivity disorders (F90.-)

hospitalism in children (F43.2-)

F94.8 **Other childhood disorders of social functioning**

F94.9 **Childhood disorder of social functioning, unspecified**

F95 **Tic disorder**

F95.0 **Transient tic disorder**

Provisional tic disorder

F95.1 **Chronic motor or vocal tic disorder**

F95.2 **Tourette's disorder**

Combined vocal and multiple motor tic disorder [de la Tourette]

Tourette's syndrome

F95.8 **Other tic disorders**

F95.9 **Tic disorder, unspecified**

Tic NOS

F98 **Other behavioral and emotional disorders with onset usually occurring in childhood and adolescence**

Excludes2: breath-holding spells (R06.89)

gender identity disorder of childhood (F64.2)

Kleine-Levin syndrome (G47.13)

obsessive-compulsive disorder (F42.-)

sleep disorders not due to a substance or known physiological condition (F51.-)

F98.0 **Enuresis not due to a substance or known physiological condition**

Enuresis (primary) (secondary) of nonorganic origin Functional enuresis

Psychogenic enuresis

Urinary incontinence of nonorganic origin

Excludes1: enuresis NOS (R32)

F98.1 **Encopresis not due to a substance or known physiological condition**

Functional encopresis

Incontinence of feces of nonorganic origin

Psychogenic encopresis

Use Additional Code to identify the cause of any coexisting constipation.

Excludes1: encopresis NOS (R15.-)

F98.2 **Other feeding disorders of infancy and childhood**

Excludes2: anorexia nervosa and other eating disorders (F50.-)

feeding difficulties (R63.3)

feeding problems of newborn (P92.-)

pica of infancy or childhood (F98.3)

F98.21 **Rumination disorder of infancy**

F98.29 **Other feeding disorders of infancy and early childhood**

F98.3 **Pica of infancy and childhood**

F98.4 **Stereotyped movement disorders**

Stereotype/habit disorder

Excludes1: abnormal involuntary movements (R25.-)

Excludes2: compulsions in obsessive-compulsive disorder (F42.-)

hair plucking (F63.3)

movement disorders of organic origin (G20-G25)

nail-biting (F98.8)

nose-picking (F98.8)

stereotypies that are part of a broader psychiatric condition (F01-F95)

thumb-sucking (F98.8)

tic disorders (F95.-)

trichotillomania (F63.3)

F98.5 **Adult onset fluency disorder**

Excludes1: childhood onset fluency disorder (F80.81)

dysphasia (R47.02)

fluency disorder in conditions classified elsewhere (R47.82)

fluency disorder (stuttering)

following cerebrovascular disease (I69. with final characters -23)

tic disorders (F95.-)

F98.8 **Other specified behavioral and emotional disorders with onset usually occurring in childhood and adolescence**

Excessive masturbation Nail-biting

Nose-picking

Thumb-sucking

F98.9 **Unspecified behavioral and emotional disorders with onset usually occurring in childhood and adolescence**

UNSPECIFIED MENTAL DISORDER (F99)

F99   **Mental disorder, not otherwise specified**

Mental illness NOS

Excludes1: unspecified mental disorder due to known physiological
condition (F09)

Chapter 6: Diseases of the Nervous System (G00-G99)

DEFINITIONS

This chapter includes definitions of selected key words, terms and phrases and coding alerts for adding points to the clinical domain, and references to coding late effects where appropriate. An example from this chapter is as follows:

G00   Bacterial meningitis, not elsewhere classified

> **Definition:** Meningitis is an infectious disease characterized by inflammation of the meninges (the tissues that surround the brain or spinal cord) usually caused by a bacterial infection; symptoms include headache and stiff neck and fever and nausea.

MULTIPLE CODING FOR A SINGLE CONDITION

In addition to the etiology/manifestation convention that requires two codes to fully describe a single condition that affects multiple body systems, there are other single conditions that also require more than one code. "**Use Additional Code**" notes are found in the Tabular List at codes that are not part of an etiology/manifestation pair where a secondary code is useful to fully describe a condition. The sequencing rule is the same as the etiology/manifestation pair, "**Use Additional Code**" indicates that a secondary code should be added.

For example, for bacterial infections that are not included in chapter 1, a secondary code from category B95, Streptococcus, Staphylococcus, and Enterococcus, as the cause of diseases classified elsewhere, or B96, Other bacterial agents as the cause of diseases classified elsewhere, may be required to identify the bacterial organism causing the infection. A "**Use Additional Code**" note will normally be found at the infectious disease code, indicating a need for the organism code to be added as a secondary code.

"Code first" notes are also under certain codes that are not specifically manifestation codes but may be due to an underlying cause. When there is a "Code first" note and an underlying condition is present, the underlying condition should be sequenced first.

"Code, if applicable, any causal condition first", notes indicate that this code may be assigned as a principal diagnosis when the causal condition is unknown or not applicable. If a causal condition is known, then the code for that condition should be sequenced as the principal or first-listed diagnosis.

Multiple codes may be needed for sequela, complication codes and obstetric codes to more fully describe a condition. See the specific guidelines for these conditions for further instruction.

COMBINATION CODE

A combination code is a single code used to classify: Two diagnoses, or a diagnosis with an associated secondary process (manifestation) A diagnosis with an associated complication

Combination codes are identified by referring to subterm entries in the Alphabetic Index and by reading the inclusion and exclusion notes in the Tabular List.

Assign only the combination code when that code fully identifies the diagnostic conditions involved or when the Alphabetic Index so directs. Multiple coding should not be used when the classification provides a combination code that clearly identifies all of the elements documented in the diagnosis. When the combination code lacks necessary specificity in describing the manifestation or complication, an additional code should be used as a secondary code.

SEQUELA (LATE EFFECTS)

A sequela is the residual effect (condition produced) after the acute phase of an illness or injury has terminated. There is no time limit on when a sequela code can be used. The residual may be apparent early, such as in cerebral infarction, or it may occur months or years later, such as that due to a previous injury. Coding of sequela generally requires two codes sequenced in the following order: The condition or nature of the sequela is sequenced first.

The sequela code is sequenced second.

An exception to the above guidelines are those instances where the code for the sequela is followed by a manifestation code identified in the Tabular List and title, or the sequela code has been expanded (at the fourth, fifth or sixth character levels) to

include the manifestation(s). The code for the acute phase of an illness or injury that led to the sequela is never used with a code for the late effect.

DOMINANT/NONDOMINANT SIDE

]Codes from category G81, Hemiplegia and hemiparesis, and subcategories G83.1, Monoplegia of lower limb, G83.2, Monoplegia of upper limb, and G83.3, Monoplegia, unspecified, identify whether the dominant or nondominant side is affected. Should the affected side be documented, but not specified as dominant or nondominant, and the classification system does not indicate a default, code selection is as follows:

- For ambidextrous patients, the default should be dominant.

- If the left side is affected, the default is non-dominant.

- If the right side is affected, the default is dominant.

PAIN - CATEGORY G89

1) General coding information

Codes in category G89, Pain, not elsewhere classified, may be used in conjunction with codes from other categories and chapters to provide more detail about acute or chronic pain and neoplasm-related pain, unless otherwise indicated below.

If the pain is not specified as acute or chronic, post-thoracotomy, postprocedural, or neoplasm-related, do not assign codes from category G89.

A code from category G89 should not be assigned if the underlying (definitive) diagnosis is known, unless the reason for the encounter is pain control/ management and not management of the underlying condition.

When an admission or encounter is for a procedure aimed at treating the underlying condition (e.g., spinal fusion, kyphoplasty), a code for the underlying condition (e.g., vertebral fracture, spinal stenosis) should be assigned as the principal diagnosis. No code from category G89 should be assigned.

(a) Category G89 Codes as Principal or First-Listed Diagnosis

Category G89 codes are acceptable as principal diagnosis or the first-listed code:

When pain control or pain management is the reason for the admission/encounter (e.g., a patient with displaced intervertebral disc, nerve impingement and severe back pain presents for injection of steroid into the spinal canal). The underlying cause of the pain should be reported as an additional diagnosis, if known.

When a patient is admitted for the insertion of a neurostimulator for pain control, assign the appropriate pain code as the principal or first-listed diagnosis. When an admission or encounter is for a procedure aimed at treating the underlying condition and a neurostimulator is inserted for pain control during the same admission/encounter, a code for the underlying condition should be assigned as the principal diagnosis and the appropriate pain code should be assigned as a secondary diagnosis.

(b) Use of Category G89 Codes in Conjunction with Site Specific Pain Codes

(i) Assigning Category G89 and Site-Specific Pain Codes

Codes from category G89 may be used in conjunction with codes that identify the site of pain (including codes from chapter 18) if the category G89 code provides additional information. For example, if the code describes the site of the pain, but does not fully describe whether the pain is acute or chronic, then both codes should be assigned.

(ii) Sequencing of Category G89 Codes with Site-Specific Pain Codes

The sequencing of category G89 codes with site-specific pain codes (including chapter 18 codes), is dependent on the circumstances of the encounter/admission as follows:

- If the encounter is for pain control or pain management, assign the code from category G89 followed by the code identifying the specific site of pain (e.g., encounter for pain management for acute neck pain from trauma is assigned code G89.11, Acute pain due to trauma, followed by code M54.2, Cervicalgia, to identify the site of pain).

- If the encounter is for any other reason except pain control or pain management, and a related definitive diagnosis has not been established (confirmed) by the provider, assign the code for the specific site of pain first, followed by the appropriate code from category G89.

2) Pain due to devices, implants and grafts

See Section I.C.19. Pain due to medical devices

3) Postoperative Pain

The provider's documentation should be used to guide the coding of postoperative pain, as well as *Section III. Reporting Additional Diagnoses* and *Section IV. Diagnostic Coding and Reporting in the Outpatient Setting*.

The default for post-thoracotomy and other postoperative pain not specified as acute or chronic is the code for the acute form.

Routine or expected postoperative pain immediately after surgery should not be coded.

(a) Postoperative pain not associated with specific postoperative complication

Postoperative pain not associated with a specific postoperative complication is assigned to the appropriate postoperative pain code in category G89.

(b) Postoperative pain associated with specific postoperative complication

Postoperative pain associated with a specific postoperative complication (such as painful wire sutures) is assigned to the appropriate code(s) found in Chapter 19, Injury, poisoning, and certain other consequences of external causes. If appropriate, **Use Additional Code**(s) from category G89 to identify acute or chronic pain (G89.18 or G89.28).

4) Chronic pain

Chronic pain is classified to subcategory G89.2. There is no time frame defining when pain becomes chronic pain. The provider's documentation should be used to guide use of these codes.

5) Neoplasm Related Pain

Code G89.3 is assigned to pain documented as being related, associated or due to cancer, primary or secondary malignancy, or tumor. This code is assigned regardless of whether the pain is acute or chronic.

This code may be assigned as the principal or first-listed code when the stated reason for the admission/encounter is documented as pain control/pain management. The underlying neoplasm should be reported as an additional diagnosis.

When the reason for the admission/encounter is management of the neoplasm and the pain associated with the neoplasm is also documented, code G89.3 may be assigned as an additional diagnosis. It is not necessary to assign an additional code for the site of the pain.

See Section I.C.2 for instructions on the sequencing of neoplasms for all other stated reasons for the admission/encounter (except for pain control/pain management).

6) Chronic pain syndrome

Central pain syndrome (G89.0) and chronic pain syndrome (G89.4) are different than the term "chronic pain," and therefore codes should only be used when the provider has specifically documented this condition.

See Section I.C.5. Pain disorders related to psychological factors

● New code ▲ Revised code **Excludes1:** Not coded here **Excludes2:** Not included here ⊗ Placeholder required ⑦7ᵗʰ digit required

Chapter 6
Diseases of the Nervous System (G00-G99)

Excludes2: certain conditions originating in the perinatal period (P04-P96)

certain infectious and parasitic diseases (A00-B99)

complications of pregnancy, childbirth and the puerperium (O00-O9A)

congenital malformations, deformations, and chromosomal abnormalities (Q00-Q99)

endocrine, nutritional and metabolic diseases (E00-E88)

injury, poisoning and certain other consequences of external causes (S00-T88)

neoplasms (C00-D49)

symptoms, signs and abnormal clinical and laboratory findings, not elsewhere classified (R00-R94)

This chapter contains the following blocks:

G00-G09	Inflammatory diseases of the central nervous system
G10-G14	Systemic atrophies primarily affecting the central nervous system
G20-G26	Extrapyramidal and movement disorders
G30-G32	Other degenerative diseases of the nervous system
G35-G37	Demyelinating diseases of the central nervous system
G40-G47	Episodic and paroxysmal disorders
G50-G59	Nerve, nerve root and plexus disorders
G60-G65	Polyneuropathies and other disorders of the peripheral nervous system
G70-G73	Diseases of myoneural junction and muscle
G80-G83	Cerebral palsy and other paralytic syndromes
G89-G99	Other disorders of the nervous system

INFLAMMATORY DISEASES OF THE CENTRAL NERVOUS SYSTEM (G00-G09)

G00 **Bacterial meningitis, not elsewhere classified**

Definition: Meningitis is an infectious disease characterized by inflammation of the meninges (the tissues that surround the brain or spinal cord) usually caused by a bacterial infection, symptoms include headache and stiff neck and fever and nausea.

Includes: bacterial arachnoiditis

bacterial leptomeningitis

bacterial meningitis

bacterial pachymeningitis

Excludes1: bacterial meningoencephalitis (G04.2)

bacterial meningomyelitis (G04.2)

G00.0 **Hemophilus meningitis**

Meningitis due to Hemophilus influenzae

G00.1 **Pneumococcal meningitis**

Meningitis due to

Streptococcal pneumoniae

G00.2 **Streptococcal meningitis**

Use Additional Code to further identify organism (B95.0-B95.5)

G00.3 **Staphylococcal meningitis**

Use Additional Code to further identify organism (B95.61-B95.8)

G00.8 **Other bacterial meningitis**

Meningitis due to Escherichia coli

Meningitis due to Friedländer's bacillus

Meningitis due to Klebsiella

Use Additional Code to further identify organism (B96.-)

G00.9 **Bacterial meningitis, unspecified**

Meningitis due to gram-negative bacteria, unspecified

Purulent meningitis NOS

Pyogenic meningitis NOS

Suppurative meningitis NOS

G01 **Meningitis in bacterial diseases classified elsewhere**

Code first underlying disease

Excludes1: meningitis (in):

gonococcal (A54.81)

leptospirosis (A27.81)

listeriosis (A32.11)

Lyme disease (A69.21)

meningococcal (A39.0)

neurosyphilis (A52.13)

tuberculosis (A17.0)

meningoencephalitis and meningomyelitis in bacterial diseases classified elsewhere (G05)

G02 **Meningitis in other infectious and parasitic diseases classified elsewhere**

Code first underlying disease, such as:

African trypanosomiasis (B56.-)

poliovirus infection (A80.-)

Excludes1: candidal meningitis (B37.5)

coccidioidomycosis meningitis (B38.4)

cryptococcal meningitis (B45.1)

herpesviral [herpes simplex] meningitis (B00.3)

infectious mononucleosis complicated by meningitis (B27.- with fifth character 2)

measles complicated by meningitis (B05.1)

meningoencephalitis and meningomyelitis in other infectious and parasitic diseases classified elsewhere (G05)

mumps meningitis (B26.1)

rubella meningitis (B06.02)

varicella [chickenpox] meningitis (B01.0)

zoster meningitis (B02.1)

G03 **Meningitis due to other and unspecified causes**

Includes: arachnoiditis NOS

leptomeningitis NOS

meningitis NOS

pachymeningitis NOS

Excludes1: meningoencephalitis (G04.-)

meningomyelitis (G04.-)

G03.0 **Nonpyogenic meningitis**

Aseptic meningitis Nonbacterial meningitis

G03.1 **Chronic meningitis**

G03.2 **Benign recurrent meningitis [Mollaret]**

G03.8 **Meningitis due to other specified causes**

G03.9 **Meningitis, unspecified**

Arachnoiditis (spinal) NOS

G04 **Encephalitis, myelitis and encephalomyelitis**

Definition: Encephalitis is an inflammation of the brain, usually caused by a direct viral infection or a hypersensitivity reaction to a virus or foreign protein. Myelitis is an inflammation of the spinal column. Encephalomyelitis is an inflammation of the brain and spinal cord.

Includes: acute ascending myelitis

meningoencephalitis meningomyelitis

Excludes1: encephalopathy NOS (G93.40)

Excludes2: acute transverse myelitis (G37.3-)

    alcoholic encephalopathy (G31.2)

    benign myalgic encephalomyelitis (G93.3)

    multiple sclerosis (G35)

    subacute necrotizing myelitis (G37.4)

    toxic encephalitis (G92.8)

    toxic encephalopathy (G92.8)

G04.0 **Acute disseminated encephalitis and encephalomyelitis (ADEM)**

    Excludes1: acute necrotizing hemorrhagic encephalopathy (G04.3-)

      Other noninfectious acute disseminated encephalomyelitis (noninfectious ADEM) (G04.81)

  G04.00 **Acute disseminated encephalitis and encephalomyelitis, unspecified**

  G04.01 **Postinfectious acute disseminated encephalitis and encephalomyelitis (postinfectious ADEM)**

    Excludes1: post chickenpox encephalitis (B01.1)

      post measles encephalitis (B05.0)

      post measles myelitis (B05.1)

  G04.02 **Postimmunization acute disseminated encephalitis, myelitis and encephalomyelitis**

    Encephalitis, post immunization

    Encephalomyelitis, post immunization

    Use Additional Code to identify the vaccine (T50.A-, T50.B-, T50.Z-)

G04.1 **Tropical spastic paraplegia** [HCC]

G04.2 **Bacterial meningoencephalitis and meningomyelitis, not elsewhere classified**

G04.3 **Acute necrotizing hemorrhagic encephalopathy**

  Excludes1: acute disseminated encephalitis and encephalomyelitis (G04.0-)

  G04.30 **Acute necrotizing hemorrhagic encephalopathy, unspecified**

  G04.31 **Postinfectious acute necrotizing hemorrhagic encephalopathy**

  G04.32 **Postimmunization acute necrotizing hemorrhagic encephalopathy**

    Use Additional Code to identify the vaccine (T50.A-, T50.B-, T50.Z-)

  G04.39 **Other acute necrotizing hemorrhagic encephalopathy**

    Code also underlying etiology, if applicable

G04.8 **Other encephalitis, myelitis and encephalomyelitis**

  Code also any associated seizure (G40.-, R56.9)

  G04.81 **Other encephalitis and encephalomyelitis**

    Noninfectious acute disseminated encephalomyelitis (noninfectious ADEM)

  • **G04.82** **Acute flaccid myelitis**

    Excludes1: transverse myelitis (G37.3)

  G04.89 **Other myelitis** [HCC]

G04.9 **Encephalitis, myelitis and encephalomyelitis, unspecified**

  G04.90 **Encephalitis and encephalomyelitis, unspecified**

    Ventriculitis (cerebral) NOS

  G04.91 **Myelitis, unspecified** [HCC]

G05 **Encephalitis, myelitis and encephalomyelitis in diseases classified elsewhere**

Code first underlying disease, such as:

  congenital toxoplasmosis encephalitis, myelitis and encephalomyelitis (P37.1)

  cytomegaloviral encephalitis, myelitis and encephalomyelitis (B25.8)

  encephalitis, myelitis and encephalomyelitis (in) systemic lupus erythematosus (M32.19)

  eosinophilic meningoencephalitis (B83.2)

  human immunodeficiency virus [HIV] disease (B20)

  poliovirus (A80.-)

  suppurative otitis media (H66.01-H66.4)

  trichinellosis (B75)

Excludes1: adenoviral encephalitis, myelitis and encephalomyelitis (A85.1)

  enteroviral encephalitis, myelitis and encephalomyelitis (A85.0)

  herpesviral [herpes simplex] encephalitis, myelitis and encephalomyelitis (B00.4)

  listerial encephalitis, myelitis and encephalomyelitis (A32.12)

  meningococcal encephalitis, myelitis and encephalomyelitis (A39.81)

  mumps encephalitis, myelitis and encephalomyelitis (B26.2)

  post chickenpox encephalitis, myelitis and encephalomyelitis (B01.1-)

  rubella encephalitis, myelitis and encephalomyelitis (B06.01)

  toxoplasmosis encephalitis, myelitis and encephalomyelitis (B58.2)

  zoster encephalitis, myelitis and encephalomyelitis (B02.0)

G05.3 **Encephalitis and encephalomyelitis in diseases classified elsewhere**

  Meningoencephalitis in diseases classified elsewhere

G05.4 **Myelitis in diseases classified elsewhere** [HCC]

  Meningomyelitis in diseases classified elsewhere

G06 **Intracranial and intraspinal abscess and granuloma**

Use Additional Code (B95-B97) to identify infectious agent.

G06.0 **Intracranial abscess and granuloma**

  Brain [any part] abscess (embolic)

  Cerebellar abscess (embolic)

  Cerebral abscess (embolic)

  Intracranial epidural abscess or granuloma

  Intracranial extradural abscess or granuloma

  Intracranial subdural abscess or granuloma

  Otogenic abscess (embolic)

  Excludes1: tuberculous intracranial abscess and granuloma (A17.81)

G06.1 **Intraspinal abscess and granuloma**

  Abscess (embolic) of spinal cord [any part]

  Intraspinal epidural abscess or granuloma

  Intraspinal extradural abscess or granuloma

  Intraspinal subdural abscess or granuloma

  Excludes1: tuberculous intraspinal abscess and granuloma (A17.81)

G06.2 **Extradural and subdural abscess, unspecified**

G07 **Intracranial and intraspinal abscess and granuloma in diseases classified elsewhere**

Code first underlying disease, such as:

  schistosomiasis granuloma of brain (B65.-)

Excludes1: abscess of brain:

● New code   ▲ Revised code   **Excludes1:** Not coded here   **Excludes2:** Not included here   ⊗ Placeholder required   ⑦ 7th digit required

amebic (A06.6)

chromomycotic (B43.1)

gonococcal (A54.82)

tuberculous (A17.81)

tuberculoma of meninges (A17.1)

G08   Intracranial and intraspinal phlebitis and thrombophlebitis

Septic embolism of intracranial or intraspinal venous sinuses and veins

Septic endophlebitis of intracranial or intraspinal venous sinuses and veins

Septic phlebitis of intracranial or intraspinal venous sinuses and veins

Septic thrombophlebitis of intracranial or intraspinal venous sinuses and veins

Septic thrombosis of intracranial or intraspinal venous sinuses and veins

Excludes1: intracranial phlebitis and thrombophlebitis complicating:

abortion, ectopic or molar pregnancy (O00-O07, O08.7)

pregnancy, childbirth and the puerperium (O22.5, O87.3)

nonpyogenic intracranial phlebitis and thrombophlebitis (I67.6)

Excludes2: intracranial phlebitis and thrombophlebitis complicating nonpyogenic intraspinal phlebitis and thrombophlebitis (G95.1)

G09   Sequelae of inflammatory diseases of central nervous system

Note: Category G09 is to be used to indicate conditions whose primary classification is to G00-G08 as the cause of sequelae, themselves classifiable elsewhere. The 'sequelae' include conditions specified as residuals.

Code first condition resulting from (sequela) of inflammatory diseases of central nervous system

SYSTEMIC ATROPHIES PRIMARILY AFFECTING THE CENTRAL NERVOUS SYSTEM (G10-G14)

G10   Huntington's disease [HCC]

Huntington's chorea

Huntington's dementia

Code also dementia in other diseases classified elsewhere without behavioral disturbance (F02.80)

G11   Hereditary ataxia

Excludes2: cerebral palsy (G80.-)

hereditary and idiopathic neuropathy (G60.-)

metabolic disorders (E70-E88)

G11.0   Congenital nonprogressive ataxia [HCC]

G11.1   Early-onset cerebellar ataxia [HCC]

G11.10   Early-onset cerebellar ataxia, unspecified [HCC]

G11.11   Friedreich ataxia [HCC]

Autosomal recessive Friedreich ataxia

Friedreich ataxia with retained reflexes

G11.19   Other early-onset cerebellar ataxia [HCC]

Early-onset cerebellar ataxia with essential tremor

Early-onset cerebellar ataxia with myoclonus [Hunt's ataxia]

Early-onset cerebellar ataxia with retained tendon reflexes

X-linked recessive spinocerebellar ataxia

G11.2   Late-onset cerebellar ataxia [HCC]

G11.3   Cerebellar ataxia with defective DNA repair [HCC]

Ataxia telangiectasia [Louis-Bar]

Excludes2: Cockayne's syndrome (Q87.19)

Other disorders of purine and pyrimidine metabolism (E79.-)

xeroderma pigmentosum (Q82.1)

G11.4   Hereditary spastic paraplegia [HCC]

G11.8   Other hereditary ataxias [HCC]

G11.9   Hereditary ataxia, unspecified [HCC]

Hereditary cerebellar ataxia NOS

Hereditary cerebellar degeneration

Hereditary cerebellar disease

Hereditary cerebellar syndrome

G12   Spinal muscular atrophy and related syndromes

G12.0   Infantile spinal muscular atrophy, type I [Werdnig-Hoffman] [HCC]

G12.1   Other inherited spinal muscular atrophy [HCC]

Adult form spinal muscular atrophy

Childhood form, type II spinal muscular atrophy

Distal spinal muscular atrophy

Juvenile form, type III spinal muscular atrophy [Kugelberg-Welander]

Progressive bulbar palsy of childhood [Fazio-Londe]

Scapuloperoneal form spinal muscular atrophy

G12.2   Motor neuron disease

G12.20   Motor neuron disease, unspecified [HCC]

G12.21   Amyotrophic lateral sclerosis [HCC]

G12.22   Progressive bulbar palsy [HCC]

G12.23   Primary lateral sclerosis [HCC]

G12.24   Familial motor neuron disease [HCC]

G12.25   Progressive spinal muscle atrophy [HCC]

G12.29   Other motor neuron disease [HCC]

G12.8   Other spinal muscular atrophies and related syndromes [HCC]

G12.9   Spinal muscular atrophy, unspecified [HCC]

G13   Systemic atrophies primarily affecting central nervous system in diseases classified elsewhere

G13.0   Paraneoplastic neuromyopathy and neuropathy [HCC]

Carcinomatous neuromyopathy

Sensorial paraneoplastic neuropathy [Denny Brown]

Code first underlying neoplasm (C00-D49)

G13.1   Other systemic atrophy primarily affecting central nervous system in neoplastic disease [HCC]

Paraneoplastic limbic encephalopathy

Code first underlying neoplasm (C00-D49)

G13.2   Systemic atrophy primarily affecting the central nervous system in myxedema

Code first underlying disease, such as:

hypothyroidism (E03.-)

myxedematous congenital iodine deficiency (E00.1)

G13.8   Systemic atrophy primarily affecting central nervous system in other diseases classified elsewhere

Code first underlying disease

G14   Postpolio syndrome

Includes: postpolio myelitic syndrome

Excludes1: sequelae of poliomyelitis (B91)

EXTRAPYRAMIDAL AND MOVEMENT DISORDERS (G20-G26)

Definition: Extrapyramidal symptoms (EPS) are various movement disorders such as acute dystonic reactions, pseudoparkinsonism, Tardive dyskinesia or akathisia suffered as a result of taking dopamine antagonists, usually antipsychotic (neuroleptic) drugs, which are often used to control psychosis.

G20 **Parkinson's disease** [HCC]

Use Additional Code to identify:

dementia with behavioral disturbance (F02.81)

dementia without behavioral disturbance (F02.80)

Hemiparkinsonism

Idiopathic Parkinsonism or Parkinson's disease

Paralysis agitans

Parkinsonism or Parkinson's disease NOS

Primary Parkinsonism or Parkinson's disease

Excludes1: dementia with Parkinsonism (G31.83)

G21 **Secondary parkinsonism**

Excludes1: dementia with Parkinsonism (G31.83)

Huntington's disease (G10)

Shy-Drager syndrome (G90.3)

syphilitic Parkinsonism (A52.19)

G21.0 **Malignant neuroleptic syndrome**

Use Additional Code for adverse effect, if applicable, to identify drug (T43.3X5, T43.4X5, T43.505, T43.595)

Excludes1: neuroleptic induced parkinsonism (G21.11)

G21.1 **Other drug-induced secondary parkinsonism**

G21.11 **Neuroleptic induced parkinsonism** [HCC]

Use Additional Code for adverse effect, if applicable, to identify drug (T43.3X5, T43.4X5, T43.505, T43.595)

Excludes1: malignant neuroleptic syndrome (G21.0)

G21.19 **Other drug induced secondary parkinsonism** [HCC]

Other medication-induced parkinsonism

Use Additional Code for adverse effect, if applicable, to identify drug (T36-T50 with fifth or sixth character 5)

G21.2 **Secondary parkinsonism due to other external agents** [HCC]

Code first (T51-T65) to identify external agent

G21.3 **Postencephalitic parkinsonism** [HCC]

G21.4 **Vascular parkinsonism** [HCC]

G21.8 **Other secondary parkinsonism** [HCC]

G21.9 **Secondary parkinsonism, unspecified** [HCC]

G23 **Other degenerative diseases of basal ganglia**

Excludes2: multi-system degeneration of the autonomic nervous system (G90.3)

G23.0 **Hallervorden-Spatz disease** [HCC]

Pigmentary pallidal degeneration

G23.1 **Progressive supranuclear ophthalmoplegia [Steele-Richardson-Olszewski]** [HCC]

Progressive supranuclear palsy

G23.2 **Striatonigral degeneration** [HCC]

G23.8 **Other specified degenerative diseases of basal ganglia** [HCC]

Calcification of basal ganglia

G23.9 **Degenerative disease of basal ganglia, unspecified** [HCC]

G24 **Dystonia**

Includes: dyskinesia

Excludes2: athetoid cerebral palsy (G80.3)

G24.0 **Drug induced dystonia**

Use Additional Code for adverse effect, if applicable, to identify drug (T36-T50 with fifth or sixth character 5)

G24.01 **Drug induced subacute dyskinesia**

Drug induced blepharospasm

Drug induced orofacial dyskinesia

Neuroleptic induced tardive dyskinesia

Tardive dyskinesia

G24.02 **Drug induced acute dystonia**

Acute dystonic reaction to drugs

Neuroleptic induced acute dystonia

G24.09 **Other drug induced dystonia**

G24.1 **Genetic torsion dystonia**

Dystonia deformans progressiva

Dystonia musculorum deformans

Familial torsion dystonia

Idiopathic familial dystonia

Idiopathic (torsion) dystonia NOS (Schwalbe-) Ziehen-Oppenheim disease

G24.2 **Idiopathic nonfamilial dystonia**

G24.3 **Spasmodic torticollis**

Excludes1: congenital torticollis (Q68.0)

hysterical torticollis (F44.4)

ocular torticollis (R29.891)

psychogenic torticollis (F45.8)

torticollis NOS (M43.6)

traumatic recurrent torticollis (S13.4)

G24.4 **Idiopathic orofacial dystonia**

Orofacial dyskinesia

Excludes1: drug induced orofacial dyskinesia (G24.01)

G24.5 **Blepharospasm**

Excludes1: drug induced blepharospasm (G24.01)

G24.8 **Other dystonia**

Acquired torsion dystonia NOS

G24.9 **Dystonia, unspecified**

Dyskinesia NOS

G25 **Other extrapyramidal and movement disorders**

Definition: Extrapyramidal disease is a general term for a number of disorders caused by abnormalities of the basal ganglia or certain brain stem or thalamic nuclei; characterized by motor deficits, loss of postural reflexes, bradykinesia, tremor, rigidity, and various involuntary movements.

Excludes2: sleep related movement disorders (G47.6-)

G25.0 **Essential tremor** Familial tremor

Excludes1: tremor NOS (R25.1)

G25.1 **Drug-induced tremor**

Use Additional Code for adverse effect, if applicable, to identify drug (T36-T50 with fifth or sixth character 5)

G25.2 **Other specified forms of tremor**

Intention tremor

G25.3 **Myoclonus**

Drug-induced myoclonus

Palatal myoclonus

Use Additional Code for adverse effect, if applicable, to identify drug (T36-T50 with fifth or sixth character 5)

Excludes1: facial myokymia (G51.4)

myoclonic epilepsy (G40.-)

G25.4 **Drug-induced chorea**

● New code ▲ Revised code **Excludes1:** Not coded here **Excludes2:** Not included here ⊗ Placeholder required ⑦7th digit required

Use Additional Code for adverse effect, if applicable, to identify drug (T36-T50 with fifth or sixth character 5)

G25.5 **Other chorea**

Chorea NOS

Excludes1: chorea NOS with heart involvement (I02.0)

Huntington's chorea (G10)

rheumatic chorea (I02.-)

Sydenham's chorea (I02.-)

G25.6 **Drug induced tics and other tics of organic origin**

G25.61 **Drug induced tics**

Use Additional Code for adverse effect, if applicable, to identify drug (T36-T50 with fifth or sixth character 5)

G25.69 **Other tics of organic origin**

Excludes1: habit spasm (F95.9)

tic NOS (F95.9)

Tourette's syndrome (F95.2)

G25.7 **Other and unspecified drug induced movement disorders**

Use Additional Code for adverse effect, if applicable, to identify drug (T36-T50 with fifth or sixth character 5)

G25.70 **Drug induced movement disorder, unspecified**

G25.71 **Drug induced akathisia**

Drug induced acathisia

Neuroleptic induced acute akathisia

Tardive akathisia

G25.79 **Other drug induced movement disorders**

G25.8 **Other specified extrapyramidal and movement disorders**

G25.81 **Restless legs syndrome**

G25.82 **Stiff-man syndrome**

G25.83 **Benign shuddering attacks**

G25.89 **Other specified extrapyramidal and movement disorders**

G25.9 **Extrapyramidal and movement disorder, unspecified**

G26 **Extrapyramidal and movement disorders in diseases classified elsewhere**

Code first underlying disease

OTHER DEGENERATIVE DISEASES OF THE NERVOUS SYSTEM (G30-G32)

G30 **Alzheimer's disease**

Includes: Alzheimer's dementia senile and presenile forms

Use Additional Code to identify:

delirium, if applicable (F05)

dementia with behavioral disturbance (F02.81)

dementia without behavioral disturbance (F02.80)

Excludes1: senile degeneration of brain NEC (G31.1)

senile dementia NOS (F03)

senility NOS (R41.81)

G30.0 **Alzheimer's disease with early onset**

G30.1 **Alzheimer's disease with late onset**

G30.8 **Other Alzheimer's disease**

G30.9 **Alzheimer's disease, unspecified**

G31 **Other degenerative diseases of nervous system, not elsewhere classified**

Use Additional For codes G31.0-G31.83, G31.85-G31.9, **Use Additional Code** to identify:

dementia with behavioral disturbance (F02.81)

dementia without behavioral disturbance (F02.80)

Excludes2: Reye's syndrome (G93.7)

G31.0 **Frontotemporal dementia**

G31.01 **Pick's disease**

Primary progressive aphasia

Progressive isolated aphasia

G31.09 **Other frontotemporal dementia**

Frontal dementia

G31.1 **Senile degeneration of brain, not elsewhere classified**

Excludes1: Alzheimer's disease (G30.-)

senility NOS (R41.81)

G31.2 **Degeneration of nervous system due to alcohol**

Alcoholic cerebellar ataxia

Alcoholic cerebellar degeneration

Alcoholic cerebral degeneration

Alcoholic encephalopathy

Dysfunction of the autonomic nervous system due to alcohol

Code also associated alcoholism (F10.-)

G31.8 **Other specified degenerative diseases of nervous system**

G31.81 **Alpers disease**

Grey-matter degeneration

G31.82 **Leigh's disease**

Subacute necrotizing encephalopathy

G31.83 **Dementia with Lewy bodies**

Dementia with Parkinsonism

Lewy body dementia

Lewy body disease

G31.84 **Mild cognitive impairment, so stated**

Mild neurocognitive disorder

Excludes1: age related cognitive decline (R41.81)

altered mental status (R41.82)

cerebral degeneration (G31.9)

change in mental status (R41.82)

cognitive deficits following (sequelae of) cerebral hemorrhage or infarction (I69.01-, I69.11-, I69.21-, I69.31-, I69.81-, I69.91-)

cognitive impairment due to intracranial or head injury (S06.-)

dementia (F01.-, F02.-, F03)

mild memory disturbance (F06.8)

neurologic neglect syndrome (R41.4)

personality change, nonpsychotic (F68.8)

G31.85 **Corticobasal degeneration**

G31.89 **Other specified degenerative diseases of nervous system**

G31.9 **Degenerative disease of nervous system, unspecified**

G32 **Other degenerative disorders of nervous system in diseases classified elsewhere**

G32.0 **Subacute combined degeneration of spinal cord in diseases classified elsewhere** [HCC]

Dana-Putnam syndrome

Sclerosis of spinal cord (combined) (dorsolateral) (posterolateral)

Code first underlying disease, such as:

anemia (D51.9)

dietary (D51.3)

pernicious (D51.0)

vitamin B12 deficiency (E53.8)

Excludes1: syphilitic combined degeneration of spinal cord (A52.11)

G32.8 **Other specified degenerative disorders of nervous system in diseases classified elsewhere**

Code first underlying disease, such as:

amyloidosis cerebral degeneration (E85.-)

cerebral degeneration (due to) hypothyroidism (E00.0-E03.9)

cerebral degeneration (due to) neoplasm (C00-D49)

cerebral degeneration (due to) vitamin B deficiency, except thiamine (E52-E53.-)

Excludes1: superior hemorrhagic polioencephalitis [Wernicke's encephalopathy] (E51.2)

G32.81 **Cerebellar ataxia in diseases classified elsewhere** [HCC]

Code first underlying disease, such as:

celiac disease (with gluten ataxia) (K90.0)

cerebellar ataxia (in) neoplastic disease (paraneoplastic cerebellar degeneration) (C00-D49)

non-celiac gluten ataxia (M35.9)

Excludes1: systemic atrophy primarily affecting the central nervous system in alcoholic cerebellar ataxia (G31.2)

systemic atrophy primarily affecting the central nervous system in myxedema (G13.2)

G32.89 **Other specified degenerative disorders of nervous system in diseases classified elsewhere**

Degenerative encephalopathy in diseases classified elsewhere

DEMYELINATING DISEASES OF THE CENTRAL NERVOUS SYSTEM (G35-G37)

Definition: A demyelinating disease is any condition that results in damage to the protective covering (myelin sheath) that surrounds nerve fibers in your brain and spinal cord. When the myelin sheath is damaged, nerve impulses slow or even stop, causing neurological problems.

G35 **Multiple sclerosis** [HCC]

Definition: Multiple sclerosis is a chronic autoimmune disorder affecting movement, sensation, and bodily functions. It is caused by destruction of the myelin insulation covering nerve fibers in the central nervous system.

Disseminated multiple sclerosis

Generalized multiple sclerosis

Multiple sclerosis NOS

Multiple sclerosis of brain stem

Multiple sclerosis of cord

G36 **Other acute disseminated demyelination**

Excludes1: postinfectious encephalitis and encephalomyelitis NOS (G04.01)

G36.0 **Neuromyelitis optica [Devic]** [HCC]

Demyelination in optic neuritis

Excludes1: optic neuritis NOS (H46)

G36.1 **Acute and subacute hemorrhagic leukoencephalitis [Hurst]** [HCC]

G36.8 **Other specified acute disseminated demyelination** [HCC]

G36.9 **Acute disseminated demyelination, unspecified** [HCC]

G37 **Other demyelinating diseases of central nervous system**

Definition: Demyelinating diseases of the central nervous system is any disease of the nervous system in which the myelin sheath of

neurons is damaged.

G37.0 **Diffuse sclerosis of central nervous system** [HCC]

Periaxial encephalitis

Schilder's disease

Excludes1: X linked adrenoleukodystrophy (E71.52-)

G37.1 **Central demyelination of corpus callosum** [HCC]

G37.2 **Central pontine myelinolysis** [HCC]

G37.3 **Acute transverse myelitis in demyelinating disease of central nervous system** [HCC]

Acute transverse myelitis NOS

Acute transverse myelopathy

Excludes1: acute flaccid myelitis (G04.82)

multiple sclerosis (G35)

neuromyelitis optica [Devic] (G36.0)

G37.4 **Subacute necrotizing myelitis of central nervous system** [HCC]

G37.5 **Concentric sclerosis [Balo] of central nervous system** [HCC]

G37.8 **Other specified demyelinating diseases of central nervous system** [HCC]

G37.9 **Demyelinating disease of central nervous system, unspecified** [HCC]

EPISODIC AND PAROXYSMAL DISORDERS (G40-G47)

G40 **Epilepsy and recurrent seizures**

Definition: Epilepsy and recurrent seizures is a common chronic neurological disorder characterized by recurrent unprovoked seizures. These seizures are transient signs and/or symptoms of abnormal, excessive or synchronous neuronal activity in the brain.

Note: the following terms are to be considered equivalent to intractable: pharmacoresistent (pharmacologically resistant), treatment resistant, refractory (medically) and poorly controlled

Excludes1: conversion disorder with seizures (F44.5)

convulsions NOS (R56.9)

post traumatic seizures (R56.1)

seizure (convulsive) NOS (R56.9)

seizure of newborn (P90)

Excludes2: hippocampal sclerosis (G93.81)

mesial temporal sclerosis (G93.81)

temporal sclerosis (G93.81)

Todd's paralysis (G83.84)

G40.0 **Localization-related (focal) (partial) idiopathic epilepsy and epileptic syndromes with seizures of localized onset**

Benign childhood epilepsy with centrotemporal EEG spikes

Childhood epilepsy with occipital EEG paroxysms

Excludes1: adult onset localization-related epilepsy (G40.1-, G40.2-)

G40.00 **Localization-related (focal) (partial) idiopathic epilepsy and epileptic syndromes with seizures of localized onset, not intractable**

Localization-related (focal) (partial) idiopathic epilepsy and epileptic syndromes with seizures of localized onset without intractability

G40.001 **Localization-related (focal) (partial) idiopathic epilepsy and epileptic syndromes with seizures of localized onset, not intractable, with status epilepticus** [HCC]

G40.009 **Localization-related (focal) (partial) idiopathic epilepsy and epileptic syndromes with seizures of localized**

onset, not intractable, without status epilepticus [HCC]

Localization-related (focal) (partial) idiopathic epilepsy and epileptic syndromes with seizures of localized onset NOS

G40.01 Localization-related (focal) (partial) idiopathic epilepsy and epileptic syndromes with seizures of localized onset, intractable

G40.011 Localization-related (focal) (partial) idiopathic epilepsy and epileptic syndromes with seizures of localized onset, intractable, with status epilepticus [HCC]

G40.019 Localization-related (focal) (partial) idiopathic epilepsy and epileptic syndromes with seizures of localized onset, intractable, without status epilepticus [HCC]

G40.1 Localization-related (focal) (partial) symptomatic epilepsy and epileptic syndromes with simple partial seizures

Attacks without alteration of consciousness

Epilepsia partialis continua [Koshevnikoff]

Simple partial seizures developing into secondarily generalized seizures

G40.10 Localization-related (focal) (partial) symptomatic epilepsy and epileptic syndromes with simple partial seizures, not intractable

Localization-related (focal) (partial) symptomatic epilepsy and epileptic syndromes with simple partial seizures without intractability

G40.101 Localization-related (focal) (partial) symptomatic epilepsy and epileptic syndromes with simple partial seizures, not intractable, with status epilepticus [HCC]

G40.109 Localization-related (focal) (partial) symptomatic epilepsy and epileptic syndromes with simple partial seizures, not intractable, without status epilepticus [HCC]

Localization-related (focal) (partial) symptomatic epilepsy and epileptic syndromes with simple partial seizures NOS

G40.11 Localization-related (focal) (partial) symptomatic epilepsy and epileptic syndromes with simple partial seizures, intractable

G40.111 Localization-related (focal) (partial) symptomatic epilepsy and epileptic syndromes with simple partial seizures, intractable, with status epilepticus [HCC]

G40.119 Localization-related (focal) (partial) symptomatic epilepsy and epileptic syndromes with simple partial seizures, intractable, without status epilepticus [HCC]

G40.2 Localization-related (focal) (partial) symptomatic epilepsy and epileptic syndromes with complex partial seizures

Attacks with alteration of consciousness, often with automatisms

Complex partial seizures developing into secondarily generalized seizures

G40.20 Localization-related (focal) (partial) symptomatic epilepsy and epileptic syndromes with complex partial seizures, not intractable

Localization-related (focal) (partial) symptomatic epilepsy and epileptic syndromes with complex partial seizures without intractability

G40.201 Localization-related (focal) (partial) symptomatic epilepsy and epileptic syndromes with complex partial seizures, not intractable, with status epilepticus [HCC]

G40.209 Localization-related (focal) (partial) symptomatic epilepsy and epileptic syndromes with complex partial seizures, not intractable, without status epilepticus [HCC]

Localization-related (focal) (partial) symptomatic epilepsy and epileptic syndromes with complex partial seizures NOS

G40.21 Localization-related (focal) (partial) symptomatic epilepsy and epileptic syndromes with complex partial seizures, intractable

G40.211 Localization-related (focal) (partial) symptomatic epilepsy and epileptic syndromes with complex partial seizures, intractable, with status epilepticus [HCC]

G40.219 Localization-related (focal) (partial) symptomatic epilepsy and epileptic syndromes with complex partial seizures, intractable, without status epilepticus [HCC]

G40.3 Generalized idiopathic epilepsy and epileptic syndromes

Code also MERRF syndrome, if applicable (E88.42)

G40.30 Generalized idiopathic epilepsy and epileptic syndromes, not intractable

Generalized idiopathic epilepsy and epileptic syndromes without intractability

G40.301 Generalized idiopathic epilepsy and epileptic syndromes, not intractable, with status epilepticus [HCC]

G40.309 Generalized idiopathic epilepsy and epileptic syndromes, not intractable, without status epilepticus [HCC]

Generalized idiopathic epilepsy and epileptic syndromes NOS

G40.31 Generalized idiopathic epilepsy and epileptic syndromes, intractable

G40.311 Generalized idiopathic epilepsy and epileptic syndromes, intractable, with status epilepticus [HCC]

G40.319 Generalized idiopathic epilepsy and epileptic syndromes, intractable, without status epilepticus [HCC]

G40.A Absence epileptic syndrome

Childhood absence epilepsy [pyknolepsy]

Juvenile absence epilepsy

Absence epileptic syndrome, NOS

G40.A0 Absence epileptic syndrome, not intractable

G40.A01 Absence epileptic syndrome, not intractable, with status epilepticus [HCC]

G40.A09 Absence epileptic syndrome, not intractable, without status epilepticus [HCC]

G40.A1 Absence epileptic syndrome, intractable

G40.A11   **Absence epileptic syndrome, intractable, with status epilepticus** [HCC]

G40.A19   **Absence epileptic syndrome, intractable, without status epilepticus** [HCC]

G40.B   **Juvenile myoclonic epilepsy [impulsive petit mal]**

   G40.B0   **Juvenile myoclonic epilepsy, not intractable**

     G40.B01   **Juvenile myoclonic epilepsy, not intractable, with status epilepticus** [HCC]

     G40.B09   **Juvenile myoclonic epilepsy, not intractable, without status epilepticus** [HCC]

   G40.B1   **Juvenile myoclonic epilepsy, intractable**

     G40.B11   **Juvenile myoclonic epilepsy, intractable, with status epilepticus** [HCC]

     G40.B19   **Juvenile myoclonic epilepsy, intractable, without status epilepticus** [HCC]

G40.4   **Other generalized epilepsy and epileptic syndromes**

   Epilepsy with grand mal seizures on awakening

   Epilepsy with myoclonic absences

   Epilepsy with myoclonic-astatic seizures

   Grand mal seizure NOS

   Nonspecific atonic epileptic seizures

   Nonspecific clonic epileptic seizures

   Nonspecific myoclonic epileptic seizures

   Nonspecific tonic epileptic seizures

   Nonspecific tonic-clonic epileptic seizures

   Symptomatic early myoclonic encephalopathy

   G40.40   **Other generalized epilepsy and epileptic syndromes, not intractable**

     Other generalized epilepsy and epileptic syndromes without intractability

     Other generalized epilepsy and epileptic syndromes NOS

     G40.401   **Other generalized epilepsy and epileptic syndromes, not intractable, with status epilepticus** [HCC]

     G40.409   **Other generalized epilepsy and epileptic syndromes, not intractable, without status epilepticus** [HCC]

   G40.41   **Other generalized epilepsy and epileptic syndromes, intractable**

     G40.411   **Other generalized epilepsy and epileptic syndromes, intractable, with status epilepticus** [HCC]

     G40.419   **Other generalized epilepsy and epileptic syndromes, intractable, without status epilepticus** [HCC]

   G40.42   **Cyclin-Dependent Kinase-Like 5 Deficiency Disorder**

     CDKL5

     <u>Use Additional Code</u>, if known, to identify associated manifestations, such as:

     cortical blindness (H47.61-)

     global developmental delay (F88)

G40.5   **Epileptic seizures related to external causes**

   Epileptic seizures related to alcohol

   Epileptic seizures related to drugs

   Epileptic seizures related to hormonal changes

Epileptic seizures related to sleep deprivation

Epileptic seizures related to stress

<u>Code also</u>, if applicable, associated epilepsy and recurrent seizures (G40.-)

<u>Use Additional Code</u> for adverse effect, if applicable, to identify drug (T36-T50 with fifth or sixth character 5)

   G40.50   **Epileptic seizures related to external causes, not intractable**

     G40.501   **Epileptic seizures related to external causes, not intractable, with status epilepticus** [HCC]

     G40.509   **Epileptic seizures related to external causes, not intractable, without status epilepticus** [HCC]

     Epileptic seizures related to external causes, NOS

G40.8   **Other epilepsy and recurrent seizures**

   Epilepsies and epileptic syndromes undetermined as to whether they are focal or generalized Landau-Kleffner syndrome

   G40.80   **Other epilepsy**

     G40.801   **Other epilepsy, not intractable, with status epilepticus** [HCC]

     Other epilepsy without intractability with status epilepticus

     G40.802   **Other epilepsy, not intractable, without status epilepticus** [HCC]

     Other epilepsy NOS

     Other epilepsy without intractability without status epilepticus

     G40.803   **Other epilepsy, intractable, with status epilepticus** [HCC]

     G40.804   **Other epilepsy, intractable, without status epilepticus** [HCC]

   G40.81   **Lennox-Gastaut syndrome**

     G40.811   **Lennox-Gastaut syndrome, not intractable, with status epilepticus** [HCC]

     G40.812   **Lennox-Gastaut syndrome, not intractable, without status epilepticus** [HCC]

     G40.813   **Lennox-Gastaut syndrome, intractable, with status epilepticus** [HCC]

     G40.814   **Lennox-Gastaut syndrome, intractable, without status epilepticus** [HCC]

   G40.82   **Epileptic spasms**

     Infantile spasms

     Salaam attacks West's syndrome

     G40.821   **Epileptic spasms, not intractable, with status epilepticus** [HCC]

     G40.822   **Epileptic spasms, not intractable, without status epilepticus** [HCC]

     G40.823   **Epileptic spasms, intractable, with status epilepticus** [HCC]

     G40.824   **Epileptic spasms, intractable, without status epilepticus** [HCC]

   G40.83   **Dravet syndrome**

     Polymorphic epilepsy in infancy (PMEI)

     Severe myoclonic epilepsy in infancy (SMEI)

     G40.833   **Dravet syndrome, intractable, with status epilepticus**

   ● New code   ▲ Revised code   **Excludes1:** Not coded here   **Excludes2:** Not included here   ⊗ Placeholder required   ⑦7th digit required

G40.834 **Dravet syndrome, intractable, without status epilepticus**

Dravet syndrome NOS

G40.89 **Other seizures** [HCC]

Excludes1: post traumatic seizures (R56.1)

recurrent seizures NOS (G40.909)

seizure NOS (R56.9)

G40.9 **Epilepsy, unspecified**

G40.90 **Epilepsy, unspecified, not intractable**

Epilepsy, unspecified, without intractability

G40.901 **Epilepsy, unspecified, not intractable, with status epilepticus** [HCC]

G40.909 **Epilepsy, unspecified, not intractable, without status epilepticus** [HCC]

Epilepsy NOS

Epileptic convulsions NOS

Epileptic fits NOS

Epileptic seizures NOS

Recurrent seizures NOS

Seizure disorder NOS

G40.91 **Epilepsy, unspecified, intractable**

Intractable seizure disorder NOS

G40.911 **Epilepsy, unspecified, intractable, with status epilepticus** [HCC]

G40.919 **Epilepsy, unspecified, intractable, without status epilepticus** [HCC]

G43 **Migraine**

Definition: Migraine is a severe, disabling headache, usually affecting only one side of the head, and often accompanied by nausea, vomiting, photophobia and visual disturbances.

Note: the following terms are to be considered equivalent to intractable: pharmacoresistent (pharmacologically resistant), treatment resistant, refractory (medically) and poorly controlled

Use Additional Code for adverse effect, if applicable, to identify drug (T36-T50 with fifth or sixth character 5)

Excludes1: headache NOS (R51.9)

lower half migraine (G44.00)

Excludes2: headache syndromes (G44.-)

G43.0 **Migraine without aura**

Common migraine

Excludes1: chronic migraine without aura (G43.7-)

G43.00 **Migraine without aura, not intractable**

Migraine without aura without mention of refractory migraine

G43.001 **Migraine without aura, not intractable, with status migrainosus**

G43.009 **Migraine without aura, not intractable, without status migrainosus**

Migraine without aura NOS

G43.01 **Migraine without aura, intractable**

Migraine without aura with refractory migraine

G43.011 **Migraine without aura, intractable, with status migrainosus**

G43.019 **Migraine without aura, intractable, without status migrainosus**

G43.1 **Migraine with aura**

Basilar migraine

Classical migraine

Migraine equivalents

Migraine preceded or accompanied by transient focal neurological phenomena

Migraine triggered seizures

Migraine with acute-onset aura

Migraine with aura without headache (migraine equivalents)

Migraine with prolonged aura

Migraine with typical aura

Retinal migraine

Code also any associated seizure (G40.-, R56.9)

Excludes1: persistent migraine aura (G43.5-, G43.6-)

G43.10 **Migraine with aura, not intractable**

Migraine with aura without mention of refractory migraine

G43.101 **Migraine with aura, not intractable, with status migrainosus**

G43.109 **Migraine with aura, not intractable, without status migrainosus**

Migraine with aura NOS

G43.11 **Migraine with aura, intractable**

Migraine with aura with refractory migraine

G43.111 **Migraine with aura, intractable, with status migrainosus**

G43.119 **Migraine with aura, intractable, without status migrainosus**

G43.4 **Hemiplegic migraine**

Familial migraine

Sporadic migraine

G43.40 **Hemiplegic migraine, not intractable**

Hemiplegic migraine without refractory migraine

G43.401 **Hemiplegic migraine, not intractable, with status migrainosus**

G43.409 **Hemiplegic migraine, not intractable, without status migrainosus**

Hemiplegic migraine NOS

G43.41 **Hemiplegic migraine, intractable**

Hemiplegic migraine with refractory migraine

G43.411 **Hemiplegic migraine, intractable, with status migrainosus**

G43.419 **Hemiplegic migraine, intractable, without status migrainosus**

G43.5 **Persistent migraine aura without cerebral infarction**

G43.50 **Persistent migraine aura without cerebral infarction, not intractable**

Persistent migraine aura without cerebral infarction, without refractory migraine

G43.501 **Persistent migraine aura without cerebral infarction, not intractable, with status migrainosus**

G43.509 **Persistent migraine aura without cerebral infarction, not intractable, without status migrainosus**

Persistent migraine aura NOS

G43.51 **Persistent migraine aura without cerebral infarction, intractable**

Persistent migraine aura without cerebral infarction, with refractory migraine

G43.511 **Persistent migraine aura without cerebral infarction, intractable, with status migrainosus**

G43.519 Persistent migraine aura without cerebral infarction, intractable, without status migrainosus

G43.6 Persistent migraine aura with cerebral infarction

Code also the type of cerebral infarction (I63.-)

G43.60 Persistent migraine aura with cerebral infarction, not intractable

Persistent migraine aura with cerebral infarction, without refractory migraine

G43.601 Persistent migraine aura with cerebral infarction, not intractable, with status migrainosus

G43.609 Persistent migraine aura with cerebral infarction, not intractable, without status migrainosus

G43.61 Persistent migraine aura with cerebral infarction, intractable

Persistent migraine aura with cerebral infarction, with refractory migraine

G43.611 Persistent migraine aura with cerebral infarction, intractable, with status migrainosus

G43.619 Persistent migraine aura with cerebral infarction, intractable, without status migrainosus

G43.7 Chronic migraine without aura

Transformed migraine

Excludes1: migraine without aura (G43.0-)

G43.70 Chronic migraine without aura, not intractable

Chronic migraine without aura, without refractory migraine

G43.701 Chronic migraine without aura, not intractable, with status migrainosus

G43.709 Chronic migraine without aura, not intractable, without status migrainosus

Chronic migraine without aura NOS

G43.71 Chronic migraine without aura, intractable

Chronic migraine without aura, with refractory migraine

G43.711 Chronic migraine without aura, intractable, with status migrainosus

G43.719 Chronic migraine without aura, intractable, without status migrainosus

G43.A Cyclical vomiting

Excludes1: cyclical vomiting syndrome unrelated to migraine (R11.15)

G43.A0 Cyclical vomiting, in migraine, not intractable

Cyclical vomiting, without refractory migraine

G43.A1 Cyclical vomiting, in migraine, intractable

Cyclical vomiting, with refractory migraine

G43.B Ophthalmoplegic migraine

G43.B0 Ophthalmoplegic migraine, not intractable

Ophthalmoplegic migraine, without refractory migraine

G43.B1 Ophthalmoplegic migraine, intractable

Ophthalmoplegic migraine, with refractory migraine

G43.C Periodic headache syndromes in child or adult

G43.C0 Periodic headache syndromes in child or adult, not intractable

Periodic headache syndromes in child or adult, without refractory migraine

G43.C1 Periodic headache syndromes in child or adult, intractable

Periodic headache syndromes in child or adult, with refractory migraine

G43.D Abdominal migraine

G43.D0 Abdominal migraine, not intractable

Abdominal migraine, without refractory migraine

G43.D1 Abdominal migraine, intractable

Abdominal migraine, with refractory migraine

G43.8 Other migraine

G43.80 Other migraine, not intractable

Other migraine, without refractory migraine

G43.801 Other migraine, not intractable, with status migrainosus

G43.809 Other migraine, not intractable, without status migrainosus

G43.81 Other migraine, intractable

Other migraine, with refractory migraine

G43.811 Other migraine, intractable, with status migrainosus

G43.819 Other migraine, intractable, without status migrainosus

G43.82 Menstrual migraine, not intractable

Menstrual headache, not intractable

Menstrual migraine, without refractory migraine

Menstrually related migraine, not intractable

Pre-menstrual headache, not intractable

Pre-menstrual migraine, not intractable

Pure menstrual migraine, not intractable

Code also associated premenstrual tension syndrome (N94.3)

G43.821 Menstrual migraine, not intractable, with status migrainosus

G43.829 Menstrual migraine, not intractable, without status migrainosus

Menstrual migraine NOS

G43.83 Menstrual migraine, intractable

Menstrual headache, intractable

Menstrual migraine, with refractory migraine

Menstrually related migraine, intractable

Pre-menstrual headache, intractable

Pre-menstrual migraine, intractable

Pure menstrual migraine, intractable

Code also associated premenstrual tension syndrome (N94.3)

G43.831 Menstrual migraine, intractable, with status migrainosus

G43.839 Menstrual migraine, intractable, without status migrainosus

G43.9 Migraine, unspecified

G43.90 Migraine, unspecified, not intractable

Migraine, unspecified, without refractory migraine

G43.901 Migraine, unspecified, not intractable, with status migrainosus

Status migrainosus NOS

G43.909 Migraine, unspecified, not intractable, without status migrainosus

Migraine NOS

G43.91   Migraine, unspecified, intractable

Migraine, unspecified, with refractory migraine

    G43.911   Migraine, unspecified, intractable, with status migrainosus

    G43.919   Migraine, unspecified, intractable, without status migrainosus

G44   Other headache syndromes

Excludes1: headache NOS (R51.9)

Excludes2: atypical facial pain (G50.1)

headache due to lumbar puncture (G97.1)

migraines (G43.-)

trigeminal neuralgia (G50.0)

G44.0   Cluster headaches and other trigeminal autonomic cephalgias (TAC)

  G44.00   Cluster headache syndrome, unspecified

Ciliary neuralgia

Cluster headache NOS

Histamine cephalgia

Lower half migraine

Migrainous neuralgia

    G44.001   Cluster headache syndrome, unspecified, intractable

    G44.009   Cluster headache syndrome, unspecified, not intractable

Cluster headache syndrome NOS

  G44.01   Episodic cluster headache

    G44.011   Episodic cluster headache, intractable

    G44.019   Episodic cluster headache, not intractable

Episodic cluster headache NOS

  G44.02   Chronic cluster headache

    G44.021   Chronic cluster headache, intractable

    G44.029   Chronic cluster headache, not intractable

Chronic cluster headache NOS

  G44.03   Episodic paroxysmal hemicrania

Paroxysmal hemicrania NOS

    G44.031   Episodic paroxysmal hemicrania, intractable

    G44.039   Episodic paroxysmal hemicrania, not intractable

Episodic paroxysmal hemicrania NOS

  G44.04   Chronic paroxysmal hemicrania

    G44.041   Chronic paroxysmal hemicrania, intractable

    G44.049   Chronic paroxysmal hemicrania, not intractable

Chronic paroxysmal hemicrania NOS

  G44.05   Short lasting unilateral neuralgiform headache with conjunctival injection and tearing (SUNCT)

    G44.051   Short lasting unilateral neuralgiform headache with conjunctival injection and tearing (SUNCT), intractable

    G44.059   Short lasting unilateral neuralgiform headache with conjunctival injection and tearing (SUNCT), not intractable

Short lasting unilateral neuralgiform headache with conjunctival injection and tearing (SUNCT) NOS

  G44.09   Other trigeminal autonomic cephalgias (TAC)

    G44.091   Other trigeminal autonomic cephalgias (TAC), intractable

    G44.099   Other trigeminal autonomic cephalgias (TAC), not intractable

G44.1   Vascular headache, not elsewhere classified

Excludes2: cluster headache (G44.0)

complicated headache syndromes (G44.5-)

drug-induced headache (G44.4-)

migraine (G43.-)

Other specified headache syndromes (G44.8-)

post-traumatic headache (G44.3-)

tension-type headache (G44.2-)

G44.2   Tension-type headache

  G44.20   Tension-type headache, unspecified

    G44.201   Tension-type headache, unspecified, intractable

    G44.209   Tension-type headache, unspecified, not intractable

Tension headache NOS

  G44.21   Episodic tension-type headache

    G44.211   Episodic tension-type headache, intractable

    G44.219   Episodic tension-type headache, not intractable

Episodic tension-type headache NOS

  G44.22   Chronic tension-type headache

    G44.221   Chronic tension-type headache, intractable

    G44.229   Chronic tension-type headache, not intractable

Chronic tension-type headache NOS

G44.3   Post-traumatic headache

  G44.30   Post-traumatic headache, unspecified

    G44.301   Post-traumatic headache, unspecified, intractable

    G44.309   Post-traumatic headache, unspecified, not intractable

Post-traumatic headache NOS

  G44.31   Acute post-traumatic headache

    G44.311   Acute post-traumatic headache, intractable

    G44.319   Acute post-traumatic headache, not intractable

Acute post-traumatic headache NOS

  G44.32   Chronic post-traumatic headache

    G44.321   Chronic post-traumatic headache, intractable

    G44.329   Chronic post-traumatic headache, not intractable

Chronic post-traumatic headache NOS

G44.4   Drug-induced headache, not elsewhere classified

Medication overuse headache

Use Additional Code for adverse effect, if applicable, to identify drug (T36-T50 with fifth or sixth character 5)

  G44.40   Drug-induced headache, not elsewhere classified, not intractable

G44.41 Drug-induced headache, not elsewhere classified, intractable

G44.5 Complicated headache syndromes

G44.51 Hemicrania continua

G44.52 New daily persistent headache (NDPH)

G44.53 Primary thunderclap headache

G44.59 Other complicated headache syndrome

G44.8 Other specified headache syndromes

Excludes2: headache with orthostatic or positional component, not elsewhere classified

G44.81 Hypnic headache

G44.82 Headache associated with sexual activity

Orgasmic headache

Preorgasmic headache

G44.83 Primary cough headache

G44.84 Primary exertional headache

G44.85 Primary stabbing headache

● **G44.86** Cervicogenic headache

Code also associated cervical spinal condition, if known

G44.89 Other headache syndrome

G45 Transient cerebral ischemic attacks and related syndromes

Definition: Transient cerebral ischemic attack is a brief episode of neurological dysfunction resulting from an interruption in the blood supply to the brain or the eye, sometimes as a precursor to a stroke.

Excludes1: neonatal cerebral ischemia (P91.0)

transient retinal artery occlusion (H34.0-)

G45.0 Vertebro-basilar artery syndrome

G45.1 Carotid artery syndrome (hemispheric)

G45.2 Multiple and bilateral precerebral artery syndromes

G45.3 Amaurosis fugax

G45.4 Transient global amnesia

Excludes1: amnesia NOS (R41.3)

G45.8 Other transient cerebral ischemic attacks and related syndromes

G45.9 Transient cerebral ischemic attack, unspecified

Spasm of cerebral artery TIA

Transient cerebral ischemia NOS

G46 Vascular syndromes of brain in cerebrovascular diseases

Code first underlying cerebrovascular disease (I60-I69)

G46.0 Middle cerebral artery syndrome

G46.1 Anterior cerebral artery syndrome

G46.2 Posterior cerebral artery syndrome

G46.3 Brain stem stroke syndrome

Benedikt syndrome

Claude syndrome

Foville syndrome

Millard-Gubler syndrome

Wallenberg syndrome

Weber syndrome

G46.4 Cerebellar stroke syndrome

G46.5 Pure motor lacunar syndrome

G46.6 Pure sensory lacunar syndrome

G46.7 Other lacunar syndromes

G46.8 Other vascular syndromes of brain in cerebrovascular diseases

G47 Sleep disorders

Excludes2: nightmares (F51.5)

nonorganic sleep disorders (F51.-)

sleep terrors (F51.4)

sleepwalking (F51.3)

G47.0 Insomnia

Excludes2: alcohol related insomnia (F10.182, F10.282, F10.982)

drug-related insomnia (F11.182, F11.282, F11.982, F13.182, F13.282, F13.982, F14.182, F14.282, F14.982, F15.182, F15.282, F15.982, F19.182, F19.282, F19.982)

idiopathic insomnia (F51.01)

insomnia due to a mental disorder (F51.05)

insomnia not due to a substance or known physiological condition (F51.0-)

nonorganic insomnia (F51.0-)

primary insomnia (F51.01)

sleep apnea (G47.3-)

G47.00 Insomnia, unspecified

Insomnia NOS

G47.01 Insomnia due to medical condition

Code also associated medical condition

G47.09 Other insomnia

G47.1 Hypersomnia

Excludes2: alcohol-related hypersomnia (F10.182, F10.282, F10.982)

drug-related hypersomnia (F11.182, F11.282, F11.982, F13.182, F13.282, F13.982, F14.182, F14.282, F14.982, F15.182, F15.282, F15.982, F19.182, F19.282, F19.982)

hypersomnia due to a mental disorder (F51.13)

hypersomnia not due to a substance or known physiological condition (F51.1-)

primary hypersomnia (F51.11)

sleep apnea (G47.3-)

G47.10 Hypersomnia, unspecified

Hypersomnia NOS

G47.11 Idiopathic hypersomnia with long sleep time

Idiopathic hypersomnia NOS

G47.12 Idiopathic hypersomnia without long sleep time

G47.13 Recurrent hypersomnia

Kleine-Levin syndrome

Menstrual related hypersomnia

G47.14 Hypersomnia due to medical condition

Code also associated medical condition

G47.19 Other hypersomnia

G47.2 Circadian rhythm sleep disorders

Disorders of the sleep wake schedule

Inversion of nyctohemeral rhythm

Inversion of sleep rhythm

G47.20 Circadian rhythm sleep disorder, unspecified type

Sleep wake schedule disorder NOS

G47.21 Circadian rhythm sleep disorder, delayed sleep phase type

Delayed sleep phase syndrome

G47.22 Circadian rhythm sleep disorder, advanced sleep phase type

G47.23 Circadian rhythm sleep disorder, irregular sleep wake type

Irregular sleep-wake pattern

● New code ▲ Revised code Excludes1: Not coded here Excludes2: Not included here ⊗ Placeholder required ⑦7th digit required

G47.24 **Circadian rhythm sleep disorder, free running type**

Circadian rhythm sleep disorder, non-24-hour sleep-wake type

G47.25 **Circadian rhythm sleep disorder, jet lag type**

G47.26 **Circadian rhythm sleep disorder, shift work type**

G47.27 **Circadian rhythm sleep disorder in conditions classified elsewhere**

Code first underlying condition

G47.29 **Other circadian rhythm sleep disorder**

G47.3 **Sleep apnea**

Definition: Sleep apnea is a potentially serious sleep disorder in which breathing repeatedly stops and starts. **Code also** any associated underlying condition

Excludes1: apnea NOS (R06.81)

Cheyne-Stokes breathing (R06.3)

pickwickian syndrome (E66.2)

sleep apnea of newborn (P28.3)

G47.30 **Sleep apnea, unspecified**

Sleep apnea NOS

G47.31 **Primary central sleep apnea**

Idiopathic central sleep apnea

G47.32 **High altitude periodic breathing**

G47.33 **Obstructive sleep apnea (adult) (pediatric)**

Obstructive sleep apnea hypopnea

Excludes1: obstructive sleep apnea of newborn (P28.3)

G47.34 **Idiopathic sleep related nonobstructive alveolar hypoventilation**

Sleep related hypoxia

G47.35 **Congenital central alveolar hypoventilation syndrome**

G47.36 **Sleep related hypoventilation in conditions classified elsewhere**

Sleep related hypoxemia in conditions classified elsewhere

Code first underlying condition

G47.37 **Central sleep apnea in conditions classified elsewhere**

Code first underlying condition

G47.39 **Other sleep apnea**

G47.4 **Narcolepsy and cataplexy**

G47.41 **Narcolepsy**

G47.411 **Narcolepsy with cataplexy**

G47.419 **Narcolepsy without cataplexy**

Narcolepsy NOS

G47.42 **Narcolepsy in conditions classified elsewhere**

Code first underlying condition

G47.421 **Narcolepsy in conditions classified elsewhere with cataplexy**

G47.429 **Narcolepsy in conditions classified elsewhere without cataplexy**

G47.5 **Parasomnia**

Excludes1: alcohol induced parasomnia (F10.182, F10.282, F10.982)

drug induced parasomnia (F11.182, F11.282, F11.982, F13.182, F13.282, F13.982, F14.182, F14.282, F14.982, F15.182, F15.282, F15.982, F19.182, F19.282, F19.982)

parasomnia not due to a substance or known physiological condition (F51.8)

G47.50 **Parasomnia, unspecified**

Parasomnia NOS

G47.51 **Confusional arousals**

G47.52 **REM sleep behavior disorder**

G47.53 **Recurrent isolated sleep paralysis**

G47.54 **Parasomnia in conditions classified elsewhere**

Code first underlying condition

G47.59 **Other parasomnia**

G47.6 **Sleep related movement disorders**

Excludes2: restless legs syndrome (G25.81)

G47.61 **Periodic limb movement disorder**

G47.62 **Sleep related leg cramps**

G47.63 **Sleep related bruxism**

Excludes1: psychogenic bruxism (F45.8)

G47.69 **Other sleep related movement disorders**

G47.8 **Other sleep disorders**

Other specified sleep-wake disorder

G47.9 **Sleep disorder, unspecified**

Sleep disorder NOS

Unspecified sleep-wake disorder

NERVE, NERVE ROOT AND PLEXUS DISORDERS (G50-G59)

Excludes1: current traumatic nerve, nerve root and plexus disorders - see Injury, nerve by body region

neuralgia NOS (M79.2)

neuritis NOS (M79.2)

peripheral neuritis in pregnancy (O26.82-)

radiculitis NOS (M54.1-)

G50 **Disorders of trigeminal nerve**

Includes: disorders of 5th cranial nerve

G50.0 **Trigeminal neuralgia**

Syndrome of paroxysmal facial pain

Tic douloureux

G50.1 **Atypical facial pain**

G50.8 **Other disorders of trigeminal nerve**

G50.9 **Disorder of trigeminal nerve, unspecified**

G51 **Facial nerve disorders**

Definition: Facial nerve disorders refers to a disorder resulting from a weakness of the facial nerve. Bell's palsy is an example of a facial nerve disorder.

Includes: disorders of 7th cranial nerve

G51.0 **Bell's palsy**

Facial palsy

G51.1 **Geniculate ganglionitis**

Excludes1: postherpetic geniculate ganglionitis (B02.21)

G51.2 **Melkersson's syndrome**

Melkersson-Rosenthal syndrome

G51.3 **Clonic hemifacial spasm**

G51.31 **Clonic hemifacial spasm, right**

G51.32 **Clonic hemifacial spasm, left**

G51.33 **Clonic hemifacial spasm, bilateral**

G51.39 **Clonic hemifacial spasm, unspecified**

G51.4 **Facial myokymia**

G51.8 **Other disorders of facial nerve**

G51.9 **Disorder of facial nerve, unspecified**

G52 **Disorders of other cranial nerves**
Excludes2: disorders of acoustic [8th] nerve (H93.3)
disorders of optic [2nd] nerve (H46, H47.0)
paralytic strabismus due to nerve palsy (H49.0-H49.2)

G52.0 **Disorders of olfactory nerve**
Disorders of 1st cranial nerve

G52.1 **Disorders of glossopharyngeal nerve**
Disorder of 9th cranial nerve
Glossopharyngeal neuralgia

G52.2 **Disorders of vagus nerve**
Disorders of pneumogastric [10th] nerve

G52.3 **Disorders of hypoglossal nerve**
Disorders of 12th cranial nerve

G52.7 **Disorders of multiple cranial nerves**
Polyneuritis cranialis

G52.8 **Disorders of other specified cranial nerves**

G52.9 **Cranial nerve disorder, unspecified**

G53 **Cranial nerve disorders in diseases classified elsewhere**
Code first underlying disease, such as:
neoplasm (C00-D49)
Excludes1: multiple cranial nerve palsy in sarcoidosis (D86.82)
multiple cranial nerve palsy in syphilis (A52.15)
postherpetic geniculate ganglionitis (B02.21)
postherpetic trigeminal neuralgia (B02.22)

G54 **Nerve root and plexus disorders**
Definition: A nerve root is the initial segment of a nerve leaving the central nervous system. Plexus refers to a network of intersecting nerves and blood vessels or of lymphatic vessels. The body contains many plexuses, such as the brachial plexus, the cardiac plexus, the cervical plexus, and the lumbar plexus.
Excludes1: current traumatic nerve root and plexus disorders - see nerve injury by body region
intervertebral disc disorders (M50-M51)
neuralgia or neuritis NOS (M79.2)
neuritis or radiculitis brachial NOS (M54.13)
neuritis or radiculitis lumbar NOS (M54.16)
neuritis or radiculitis lumbosacral NOS (M54.17)
neuritis or radiculitis thoracic NOS (M54.14)
radiculitis NOS (M54.10)
radiculopathy NOS (M54.10)
spondylosis (M47.-)

G54.0 **Brachial plexus disorders**
Thoracic outlet syndrome

G54.1 **Lumbosacral plexus disorders**

G54.2 **Cervical root disorders, not elsewhere classified**

G54.3 **Thoracic root disorders, not elsewhere classified**

G54.4 **Lumbosacral root disorders, not elsewhere classified**

G54.5 **Neuralgic amyotrophy**
Parsonage-Aldren-Turner syndrome
Shoulder-girdle neuritis
Excludes1: neuralgic amyotrophy in diabetes mellitus (E08-E13 with .44)

G54.6 **Phantom limb syndrome with pain** [HCC]

G54.7 **Phantom limb syndrome without pain** [HCC]
Phantom limb syndrome NOS

G54.8 **Other nerve root and plexus disorders**

G54.9 **Nerve root and plexus disorder, unspecified**

G55 **Nerve root and plexus compressions in diseases classified elsewhere**
Code first underlying disease, such as:
neoplasm (C00-D49)
Excludes1: nerve root compression (due to) (in) ankylosing spondylitis (M45.-)
nerve root compression (due to) (in) dorsopathies (M53.-, M54.-)
nerve root compression (due to) (in) intervertebral disc disorders (M50.1.-, M51.1.-)
nerve root compression (due to) (in) spondylopathies (M46.-, M48.-)
nerve root compression (due to) (in) spondylosis (M47.0-, M47.2.-)

G56 **Mononeuropathies of upper limb**
Definition: Mononeuropathy: A disorder of a single nerve or nerve trunk. Mononeuropathies may be due to entrapment, compression, stretch injury, ischemia, infection, or inflammation of a nerve.
Excludes1: current traumatic nerve disorder - see nerve injury by body region

G56.0 **Carpal tunnel syndrome**
G56.00 **Carpal tunnel syndrome, unspecified upper limb**
G56.01 **Carpal tunnel syndrome, right upper limb**
G56.02 **Carpal tunnel syndrome, left upper limb**
G56.03 **Carpal tunnel syndrome, bilateral upper limbs**

G56.1 **Other lesions of median nerve**
G56.10 **Other lesions of median nerve, unspecified upper limb**
G56.11 **Other lesions of median nerve, right upper limb**
G56.12 **Other lesions of median nerve, left upper limb**
G56.13 **Other lesions of median nerve, bilateral upper limbs**

G56.2 **Lesion of ulnar nerve**
Tardy ulnar nerve palsy
G56.20 **Lesion of ulnar nerve, unspecified upper limb**
G56.21 **Lesion of ulnar nerve, right upper limb**
G56.22 **Lesion of ulnar nerve, left upper limb**
G56.23 **Lesion of ulnar nerve, bilateral upper limbs**

G56.3 **Lesion of radial nerve**
G56.30 **Lesion of radial nerve, unspecified upper limb**
G56.31 **Lesion of radial nerve, right upper limb**
G56.32 **Lesion of radial nerve, left upper limb**
G56.33 **Lesion of radial nerve, bilateral upper limbs**

G56.4 **Causalgia of upper limb**
Complex regional pain syndrome II of upper limb
Excludes1: complex regional pain syndrome I of lower limb (G90.52-)
complex regional pain syndrome I of upper limb (G90.51-)
complex regional pain syndrome II of lower limb (G57.7-)
reflex sympathetic dystrophy of lower limb (G90.52-)
reflex sympathetic dystrophy of upper limb (G90.51-)
G56.40 **Causalgia of unspecified upper limb**
G56.41 **Causalgia of right upper limb**
G56.42 **Causalgia of left upper limb**

G56.43   Causalgia of bilateral upper limbs

G56.8   Other specified mononeuropathies of upper limb

Interdigital neuroma of upper limb

G56.80   Other specified mononeuropathies of unspecified upper limb

G56.81   Other specified mononeuropathies of right upper limb

G56.82   Other specified mononeuropathies of left upper limb

G56.83   Other specified mononeuropathies of bilateral upper limbs

G56.9   Unspecified mononeuropathy of upper limb

G56.90   Unspecified mononeuropathy of unspecified upper limb

G56.91   Unspecified mononeuropathy of right upper limb

G56.92   Unspecified mononeuropathy of left upper limb

G56.93   Unspecified mononeuropathy of bilateral upper limbs

G57   Mononeuropathies of lower limb

Excludes1: current traumatic nerve disorder - see nerve injury by body region

G57.0   Lesion of sciatic nerve

Excludes1: sciatica NOS (M54.3-)

Excludes2: sciatica attributed to intervertebral disc disorder (M51.1.-)

G57.00   Lesion of sciatic nerve, unspecified lower limb

G57.01   Lesion of sciatic nerve, right lower limb

G57.02   Lesion of sciatic nerve, left lower limb

G57.03   Lesion of sciatic nerve, bilateral lower limbs

G57.1   Meralgia paresthetica

Lateral cutaneous nerve of thigh syndrome

G57.10   Meralgia paresthetica, unspecified lower limb

G57.11   Meralgia paresthetica, right lower limb

G57.12   Meralgia paresthetica, left lower limb

G57.13   Meralgia paresthetica, bilateral lower limbs

G57.2   Lesion of femoral nerve

G57.20   Lesion of femoral nerve, unspecified lower limb

G57.21   Lesion of femoral nerve, right lower limb

G57.22   Lesion of femoral nerve, left lower limb

G57.23   Lesion of femoral nerve, bilateral lower limbs

G57.3   Lesion of lateral popliteal nerve

Peroneal nerve palsy

G57.30   Lesion of lateral popliteal nerve, unspecified lower limb

G57.31   Lesion of lateral popliteal nerve, right lower limb

G57.32   Lesion of lateral popliteal nerve, left lower limb

G57.33   Lesion of lateral popliteal nerve, bilateral lower limbs

G57.4   Lesion of medial popliteal nerve

G57.40   Lesion of medial popliteal nerve, unspecified lower limb

G57.41   Lesion of medial popliteal nerve, right lower limb

G57.42   Lesion of medial popliteal nerve, left lower limb

G57.43   Lesion of medial popliteal nerve, bilateral lower limbs

G57.5   Tarsal tunnel syndrome

G57.50   Tarsal tunnel syndrome, unspecified lower limb

G57.51   Tarsal tunnel syndrome, right lower limb

G57.52   Tarsal tunnel syndrome, left lower limb

G57.53   Tarsal tunnel syndrome, bilateral lower limbs

G57.6   Lesion of plantar nerve

Morton's metatarsalgia

G57.60   Lesion of plantar nerve, unspecified lower limb

G57.61   Lesion of plantar nerve, right lower limb

G57.62   Lesion of plantar nerve, left lower limb

G57.63   Lesion of plantar nerve, bilateral lower limbs

G57.7   Causalgia of lower limb

Complex regional pain syndrome II of lower limb

Excludes1: complex regional pain syndrome I of lower limb (G90.52-)

complex regional pain syndrome I of upper limb (G90.51-)

complex regional pain syndrome II of upper limb (G56.4-)

reflex sympathetic dystrophy of lower limb (G90.52-)

reflex sympathetic dystrophy of upper limb (G90.51-)

G57.70   Causalgia of unspecified lower limb

G57.71   Causalgia of right lower limb

G57.72   Causalgia of left lower limb

G57.73   Causalgia of bilateral lower limbs

G57.8   Other specified mononeuropathies of lower limb

Interdigital neuroma of lower limb

G57.80   Other specified mononeuropathies of unspecified lower limb

G57.81   Other specified mononeuropathies of right lower limb

G57.82   Other specified mononeuropathies of left lower limb

G57.83   Other specified mononeuropathies of bilateral lower limbs

G57.9   Unspecified mononeuropathy of lower limb

G57.90   Unspecified mononeuropathy of unspecified lower limb

G57.91   Unspecified mononeuropathy of right lower limb

G57.92   Unspecified mononeuropathy of left lower limb

G57.93   Unspecified mononeuropathy of bilateral lower limbs

G58   Other mononeuropathies

G58.0   Intercostal neuropathy

G58.7   Mononeuritis multiplex

G58.8   Other specified mononeuropathies

G58.9   Mononeuropathy, unspecified

G59   Mononeuropathy in diseases classified elsewhere

Code first underlying disease

Excludes1: diabetic mononeuropathy (E08-E13 with .41)

syphilitic nerve paralysis (A52.19)

syphilitic neuritis (A52.15)

tuberculous mononeuropathy (A17.83)

POLYNEUROPATHIES AND OTHER DISORDERS OF THE PERIPHERAL NERVOUS SYSTEM (G60-G65)

Definition: Polyneuropathy is damage or disease affecting peripheral nerves (peripheral neuropathy) in roughly the same areas on both sides of the body, featuring weakness, numbness, pins-and-needles and burning pain.

Excludes1: neuralgia NOS (M79.2)

neuritis NOS (M79.2)

peripheral neuritis in pregnancy (O26.82-)

radiculitis NOS (M54.10)

G60   Hereditary and idiopathic neuropathy

    G60.0   Hereditary motor and sensory neuropathy

        Charcot-Marie-Tooth disease

        Déjérine-Sottas disease

        Hereditary motor and sensory neuropathy, types I-IV

        Hypertrophic neuropathy of infancy

        Peroneal muscular atrophy (axonal type) (hypertrophic type)

        Roussy-Levy syndrome

    G60.1   Refsum's disease

        Infantile Refsum disease

    G60.2   Neuropathy in association with hereditary ataxia

    G60.3   Idiopathic progressive neuropathy

    G60.8   Other hereditary and idiopathic neuropathies

        Dominantly inherited sensory neuropathy

        Morvan's disease

        Nélaton's syndrome

        Recessively inherited sensory neuropathy

    G60.9   Hereditary and idiopathic neuropathy, unspecified

G61   Inflammatory polyneuropathy

    G61.0   Guillain-Barre syndrome [HCC]

        Acute (post-)infective polyneuritis

        Miller Fisher Syndrome

    G61.1   Serum neuropathy [HCC]

        Use Additional Code for adverse effect, if applicable, to identify serum (T50.-)

    G61.8   Other inflammatory polyneuropathies

        G61.81   Chronic inflammatory demyelinating polyneuritis [HCC]

        G61.82   Multifocal motor neuropathy [HCC]

            MMN

        G61.89   Other inflammatory polyneuropathies [HCC]

    G61.9   Inflammatory polyneuropathy, unspecified [HCC]

G62   Other and unspecified polyneuropathies

    G62.0   Drug-induced polyneuropathy [HCC]

        Use Additional Code for adverse effect, if applicable, to identify drug (T36-T50 with fifth or sixth character 5)

    G62.1   Alcoholic polyneuropathy [HCC]

    G62.2   Polyneuropathy due to other toxic agents [HCC]

        Code first (T51-T65) to identify toxic agent

    G62.8   Other specified polyneuropathies

        G62.81   Critical illness polyneuropathy [HCC]

            Acute motor neuropathy

        G62.82   Radiation-induced polyneuropathy [HCC]

            Use additional external cause code (W88-W90, X39.0-) to identify cause

        G62.89   Other specified polyneuropathies

    G62.9   Polyneuropathy, unspecified

        Neuropathy NOS

G63   Polyneuropathy in diseases classified elsewhere [HCC]

    Code first underlying disease, such as:

    amyloidosis (E85.-)

    endocrine disease, except diabetes (E00-E07, E15-E16, E20-E34)

    metabolic diseases (E70-E88)

neoplasm (C00-D49)

nutritional deficiency (E40-E64)

Excludes1: polyneuropathy (in):

    diabetes mellitus (E08-E13 with .42)

    diphtheria (A36.83)

    infectious mononucleosis complicated by polyneuropathy (B27.0-B27.9 with fifth character 1)

    Lyme disease (A69.22)

    mumps (B26.84)

    postherpetic (B02.23)

    rheumatoid arthritis (M05.5-)

    scleroderma (M34.83)

    systemic lupus erythematosus (M32.19)

G64   Other disorders of peripheral nervous system

Disorder of peripheral nervous system NOS

G65   Sequelae of inflammatory and toxic polyneuropathies

Code first condition resulting from (sequela) of inflammatory and toxic polyneuropathies

    G65.0   Sequelae of Guillain-Barré syndrome [HCC]

    G65.1   Sequelae of other inflammatory polyneuropathy [HCC]

    G65.2   Sequelae of toxic polyneuropathy [HCC]

DISEASES OF MYONEURAL JUNCTION AND MUSCLE (G70-G73)

G70   Myasthenia gravis and other myoneural disorders

Excludes1: botulism (A05.1, A48.51-A48.52)

    transient neonatal myasthenia gravis (P94.0)

    G70.0   Myasthenia gravis

        G70.00   Myasthenia gravis without (acute) exacerbation [HCC]

            Myasthenia gravis NOS

        G70.01   Myasthenia gravis with (acute) exacerbation [HCC]

            Myasthenia gravis in crisis

    G70.1   Toxic myoneural disorders [HCC]

        Code first (T51-T65) to identify toxic agent

    G70.2   Congenital and developmental myasthenia [HCC]

    G70.8   Other specified myoneural disorders

        G70.80   Lambert-Eaton syndrome, unspecified [HCC]

            Lambert-Eaton syndrome NOS

        G70.81   Lambert-Eaton syndrome in disease classified elsewhere [HCC]

            Code first underlying disease

            Excludes1: Lambert-Eaton syndrome in neoplastic disease (G73.1)

        G70.89   Other specified myoneural disorders [HCC]

    G70.9   Myoneural disorder, unspecified

G71   Primary disorders of muscles

Excludes2: arthrogryposis multiplex congenita (Q74.3)

    metabolic disorders (E70-E88)

    myositis (M60.-)

    G71.0   Muscular dystrophy

        Definition: Muscular dystrophy refers to a group of genetic, hereditary muscle diseases that weaken the muscles that move the human body. Muscular dystrophies are characterized by progressive skeletal muscle weakness, defects in muscle proteins, and the death of muscle cells and tissue.

        G71.00   Muscular dystrophy, unspecified [HCC]

G71.01 **Duchenne or Becker muscular dystrophy** [HCC]

Autosomal recessive, childhood type, muscular dystrophy resembling Duchenne or Becker muscular dystrophy

Benign [Becker] muscular dystrophy

Severe [Duchenne] muscular dystrophy

G71.02 **Facioscapulohumeral muscular dystrophy** [HCC]

Scapulohumeral muscular dystrophy

G71.09 **Other specified muscular dystrophies** [HCC]

Benign scapuloperoneal muscular dystrophy with early contractures [Emery-Dreifuss]

Congenital muscular dystrophy NOS

Congenital muscular dystrophy with specific morphological abnormalities of the muscle fiber

Distal muscular dystrophy

Limb-girdle muscular dystrophy

Ocular muscular dystrophy

Oculopharyngeal muscular dystrophy

Scapuloperoneal muscular dystrophy

G71.1 **Myotonic disorders**

G71.11 **Myotonic muscular dystrophy** [HCC]

Dystrophia myotonica [Steinert]

Myotonia atrophica

Myotonic dystrophy

Proximal myotonic myopathy (PROMM)

Steinert disease

G71.12 **Myotonia congenita**

Acetazolamide responsive myotonia congenita

Dominant myotonia congenita [Thomsen disease]

Myotonia levior

Recessive myotonia congenita [Becker disease]

G71.13 **Myotonic chondrodystrophy**

Chondrodystrophic myotonia

Congenital myotonic chondrodystrophy

Schwartz-Jampel disease

G71.14 **Drug induced myotonia**

Use Additional Code for adverse effect, if applicable, to identify drug (T36-T50 with fifth or sixth

character 5)

G71.19 **Other specified myotonic disorders**

Myotonia fluctuans

Myotonia permanens Neuromyotonia [Isaacs]

Paramyotonia congenita (of von Eulenburg)

Pseudomyotonia

Symptomatic myotonia

G71.2 **Congenital myopathies** [HCC]

Excludes2: arthrogryposis multiplex congenita (Q74.3)

▲ **G71.20** **Congenital myopathy, unspecified**

G71.21 **Nemaline myopathy**

G71.22 **Centronuclear myopathy**

G71.220 **X-linked myotubular myopathy**

Myotubular (centronuclear) myopathy

G71.228 **Other centronuclear myopathy**

Autosomal centronuclear myopathy

Autosomal dominant centronuclear myopathy

Autosomal recessive centronuclear myopathy

Centronuclear myopathy, NOS

G71.29 **Other congenital myopathy**

Central core disease

Minicore disease

Multicore disease

Multiminicore disease

G71.3 **Mitochondrial myopathy, not elsewhere classified** [HCC]

Excludes1: Kearns-Sayre syndrome (H49.81)

Leber's disease (H47.21)

Leigh's encephalopathy (G31.82)

mitochondrial metabolism disorders (E88.4.-)

Reye's syndrome (G93.7)

G71.8 **Other primary disorders of muscles**

G71.9 **Primary disorder of muscle, unspecified**

Hereditary myopathy NOS

G72 **Other and unspecified myopathies**

Excludes1: arthrogryposis multiplex congenita (Q74.3)

dermatopolymyositis (M33.-)

ischemic infarction of muscle (M62.2-)

myositis (M60.-)

polymyositis (M33.2.-)

G72.0 **Drug-induced myopathy**

Use Additional Code for adverse effect, if applicable, to identify drug (T36-T50 with fifth or sixth character 5)

G72.1 **Alcoholic myopathy**

Use Additional Code to identify alcoholism (F10.-)

G72.2 **Myopathy due to other toxic agents**

Code first (T51-T65) to identify toxic agent

G72.3 **Periodic paralysis**

Familial periodic paralysis

Hyperkalemic periodic paralysis (familial)

Hypokalemic periodic paralysis (familial)

Myotonic periodic paralysis (familial)

Normokalemic paralysis (familial)

Potassium sensitive periodic paralysis

Excludes1: paramyotonia congenita (of von Eulenburg) (G71.19)

G72.4 **Inflammatory and immune myopathies, not elsewhere classified**

G72.41 **Inclusion body myositis [IBM]**

G72.49 **Other inflammatory and immune myopathies, not elsewhere classified**

Inflammatory myopathy NOS

G72.8 **Other specified myopathies**

G72.81 **Critical illness myopathy**

Acute necrotizing myopathy

Acute quadriplegic myopathy

Intensive care (ICU) myopathy

Myopathy of critical illness

G72.89 **Other specified myopathies**

G72.9 **Myopathy, unspecified**

G73 **Disorders of myoneural junction and muscle in diseases classified elsewhere**

G73.1 **Lambert-Eaton syndrome in neoplastic disease** [HCC]

Code first underlying neoplasm (C00-D49)

Add 4th-7th digits   Nonspecific code   Unspecified code   Manifestation code   [HCC] Hierarchical Condition Code

Excludes1: Lambert-Eaton syndrome not associated with neoplasm (G70.80-G70.81)

G73.3 Myasthenic syndromes in other diseases classified elsewhere [HCC]

Code first underlying disease, such as:

neoplasm (C00-D49)

thyrotoxicosis (E05.-)

G73.7 Myopathy in diseases classified elsewhere

Code first underlying disease, such as:

hyperparathyroidism (E21.0, E21.3)

hypoparathyroidism (E20.-)

glycogen storage disease (E74.0)

lipid storage disorders (E75.-)

Excludes1: myopathy in:

rheumatoid arthritis (M05.32)

sarcoidosis (D86.87)

scleroderma (M34.82)

Sjögren syndrome (M35.03)

systemic lupus erythematosus (M32.19)

CEREBRAL PALSY AND OTHER PARALYTIC SYNDROMES (G80-G83)

Definition: Cerebral palsy is a condition marked by impaired muscle coordination (spastic paralysis) and/or other disabilities, typically caused by damage to the brain before or at birth.

G80 Cerebral palsy

Excludes1: hereditary spastic paraplegia (G11.4)

G80.0 Spastic quadriplegic cerebral palsy [HCC]

Congenital spastic paralysis (cerebral)

G80.1 Spastic diplegic cerebral palsy [HCC]

Spastic cerebral palsy NOS

G80.2 Spastic hemiplegic cerebral palsy [HCC]

G80.3 Athetoid cerebral palsy [HCC]

Double athetosis (syndrome)

Dyskinetic cerebral palsy

Dystonic cerebral palsy

Vogt disease

G80.4 Ataxic cerebral palsy [HCC]

G80.8 Other cerebral palsy [HCC]

Mixed cerebral palsy syndromes

G80.9 Cerebral palsy, unspecified [HCC]

Cerebral palsy NOS

G81 Hemiplegia and hemiparesis

Definition: Hemiplegia is defined as paralysis or loss of voluntary motion, on one side of the body; may include head and neck, trunk and/or limbs. Hemiparesis is weakness on one side of the body.

Note: This category is to be used only when hemiplegia (complete) (incomplete) is reported without further specification or is stated to be old or longstanding but of unspecified cause. The category is also for use in multiple coding to identify these types of hemiplegia resulting from any cause.

Excludes1: congenital cerebral palsy (G80.-)

hemiplegia and hemiparesis due to sequela of cerebrovascular disease (I69.05-, I69.15-, I69.25-I69.35-, I69.85-, I69.95-)

G81.0 Flaccid hemiplegia

G81.00 Flaccid hemiplegia affecting unspecified side [HCC]

G81.01 Flaccid hemiplegia affecting right dominant side [HCC]

G81.02 Flaccid hemiplegia affecting left dominant side [HCC]

G81.03 Flaccid hemiplegia affecting right nondominant side [HCC]

G81.04 Flaccid hemiplegia affecting left nondominant side [HCC]

G81.1 Spastic hemiplegia

G81.10 Spastic hemiplegia affecting unspecified side [HCC]

G81.11 Spastic hemiplegia affecting right dominant side [HCC]

G81.12 Spastic hemiplegia affecting left dominant side [HCC]

G81.13 Spastic hemiplegia affecting right nondominant side [HCC]

G81.14 Spastic hemiplegia affecting left nondominant side [HCC]

G81.9 Hemiplegia, unspecified

G81.90 Hemiplegia, unspecified affecting unspecified side [HCC]

G81.91 Hemiplegia, unspecified affecting right dominant side [HCC]

G81.92 Hemiplegia, unspecified affecting left dominant side [HCC]

G81.93 Hemiplegia, unspecified affecting right nondominant side [HCC]

G81.94 Hemiplegia, unspecified affecting left nondominant side [HCC]

G82 Paraplegia (paraparesis) and quadriplegia (quadriparesis)

Note: This category is to be used only when the listed conditions are reported without further specification or are stated to be old or longstanding but of unspecified cause. The category is also for use in multiple coding to identify these conditions resulting from any cause

Excludes1: congenital cerebral palsy (G80.-)

functional quadriplegia (R53.2)

hysterical paralysis (F44.4)

G82.2 Paraplegia

Paralysis of both lower limbs NOS

Paraparesis (lower) NOS

Paraplegia (lower) NOS

G82.20 Paraplegia, unspecified [HCC]

G82.21 Paraplegia, complete [HCC]

G82.22 Paraplegia, incomplete [HCC]

G82.5 Quadriplegia

G82.50 Quadriplegia, unspecified [HCC]

G82.51 Quadriplegia, C1-C4 complete [HCC]

G82.52 Quadriplegia, C1-C4 incomplete [HCC]

G82.53 Quadriplegia, C5-C7 complete [HCC]

G82.54 Quadriplegia, C5-C7 incomplete [HCC]

G83 Other paralytic syndromes [HCC]

Note: This category is to be used only when the listed conditions are reported without further specification or are stated to be old or longstanding but of unspecified cause. The category is also for use in multiple coding to identify these conditions resulting from any cause.

Includes: paralysis (complete) (incomplete), except as in G80-G82

G83.0 Diplegia of upper limbs

Diplegia (upper)

Paralysis of both upper limbs

G83.1 Monoplegia of lower limb

Paralysis of lower limb

Excludes1: monoplegia of lower limbs due to sequela of cerebrovascular disease (I69.04-, I69.14-, I69.24-, I69.34-, I69.84-, I69.94-)

G83.10 **Monoplegia of lower limb affecting unspecified side** [HCC]

G83.11 **Monoplegia of lower limb affecting right dominant side** [HCC]

G83.12 **Monoplegia of lower limb affecting left dominant side** [HCC]

G83.13 **Monoplegia of lower limb affecting right nondominant side** [HCC]

G83.14 **Monoplegia of lower limb affecting left nondominant side** [HCC]

G83.2 **Monoplegia of upper limb** [HCC]

Paralysis of upper limb

Excludes1: monoplegia of upper limbs due to sequela of cerebrovascular disease (I69.03-, I69.13-, I69.23-, I69.33-, I69.83-, I69.93-)

G83.20 **Monoplegia of upper limb affecting unspecified side** [HCC]

G83.21 **Monoplegia of upper limb affecting right dominant side** [HCC]

G83.22 **Monoplegia of upper limb affecting left dominant side** [HCC]

G83.23 **Monoplegia of upper limb affecting right nondominant side** [HCC]

G83.24 **Monoplegia of upper limb affecting left nondominant side** [HCC]

G83.3 **Monoplegia, unspecified**

G83.30 **Monoplegia, unspecified affecting unspecified side** [HCC]

G83.31 **Monoplegia, unspecified affecting right dominant side** [HCC]

G83.32 **Monoplegia, unspecified affecting left dominant side** [HCC]

G83.33 **Monoplegia, unspecified affecting right nondominant side** [HCC]

G83.34 **Monoplegia, unspecified affecting left nondominant side** [HCC]

G83.4 **Cauda equina syndrome** [HCC]

Neurogenic bladder due to cauda equina syndrome

Excludes1: cord bladder NOS (G95.89)

neurogenic bladder NOS (N31.9)

G83.5 **Locked-in state** [HCC]

G83.8 **Other specified paralytic syndromes**

Excludes1: paralytic syndromes due to current spinal cord injury-code to spinal cord injury (S14, S24, S34)

G83.81 **Brown-Séquard syndrome** [HCC]

G83.82 **Anterior cord syndrome** [HCC]

G83.83 **Posterior cord syndrome** [HCC]

G83.84 **Todd's paralysis (postepileptic)** [HCC]

G83.89 **Other specified paralytic syndromes** [HCC]

G83.9 **Paralytic syndrome, unspecified** [HCC]

OTHER DISORDERS OF THE NERVOUS SYSTEM (G89-G99)

G89 **Pain, not elsewhere classified**

Code also related psychological factors associated with pain (F45.42)

Excludes1: generalized pain NOS (R52)

pain disorders exclusively related to psychological factors (F45.41)

pain NOS (R52)

Excludes2: atypical face pain (G50.1)

headache syndromes (G44.-)

localized pain, unspecified type - code to pain by site, such as: abdomen pain (R10.-)

back pain (M54.9)

breast pain (N64.4)

chest pain (R07.1-R07.9)

ear pain (H92.0-)

eye pain (H57.1)

headache (R51.9)

joint pain (M25.5-)

limb pain (M79.6-)

lumbar region pain (M54.5-)

painful urination (R30.9)

pelvic and perineal pain (R10.2)

shoulder pain (M25.51-)

spine pain (M54.-)

throat pain (R07.0)

tongue pain (K14.6)

tooth pain (K08.8)

renal colic (N23)

migraines (G43.-)

myalgia (M79.1)

pain from prosthetic devices, implants, and grafts (T82.84, T83.84, T84.84, T85.84-)

phantom limb syndrome with pain (G54.6)

vulvar vestibulitis (N94.810)

vulvodynia (N94.81-)

G89.0 **Central pain syndrome**

Déjérine-Roussy syndrome

Myelopathic pain syndrome

Thalamic pain syndrome (hyperesthetic)

G89.1 **Acute pain, not elsewhere classified**

G89.11 **Acute pain due to trauma**

G89.12 **Acute post-thoracotomy pain**

Post-thoracotomy pain NOS

G89.18 **Other acute postprocedural pain**

Postoperative pain NOS

Postprocedural pain NOS

G89.2 **Chronic pain, not elsewhere classified**

Excludes1: causalgia, lower limb (G57.7-)

causalgia, upper limb (G56.4-)

central pain syndrome (G89.0)

chronic pain syndrome (G89.4)

complex regional pain syndrome II, lower limb (G57.7-)

complex regional pain syndrome II, upper limb (G56.4-)

neoplasm related chronic pain (G89.3)

reflex sympathetic dystrophy (G90.5-)

G89.21 **Chronic pain due to trauma**

G89.22 **Chronic post-thoracotomy pain**

G89.28 **Other chronic postprocedural pain**

Other chronic postoperative pain

G89.29 **Other chronic pain**

G89.3 **Neoplasm related pain (acute) (chronic)**

Cancer associated pain

Pain due to malignancy (primary) (secondary)

Tumor associated pain

G89.4 Chronic pain syndrome

Chronic pain associated with significant psychosocial dysfunction

G90 Disorders of autonomic nervous system

Excludes1: dysfunction of the autonomic nervous system due to alcohol (G31.2)

G90.0 Idiopathic peripheral autonomic neuropathy

G90.01 Carotid sinus syncope

Carotid sinus syndrome

G90.09 Other idiopathic peripheral autonomic neuropathy

Idiopathic peripheral autonomic neuropathy NOS

G90.1 Familial dysautonomia [Riley-Day] [HCC]

G90.2 Horner's syndrome

Bernard(-Horner) syndrome

Cervical sympathetic dystrophy or paralysis

G90.3 Multi-system degeneration of the autonomic nervous system [HCC]

Neurogenic orthostatic hypotension [Shy-Drager]

Excludes1: orthostatic hypotension NOS (I95.1)

G90.4 Autonomic dysreflexia

Use Additional Code to identify the cause, such as:

fecal impaction (K56.41)

pressure ulcer (pressure area) (L89.-)

urinary tract infection (N39.0)

G90.5 Complex regional pain syndrome I (CRPS I)

Reflex sympathetic dystrophy

Excludes1: causalgia of lower limb (G57.7-)

causalgia of upper limb (G56.4-)

complex regional pain syndrome II of lower limb (G57.7-)

complex regional pain syndrome II of upper limb (G56.4-)

G90.50 Complex regional pain syndrome I, unspecified

G90.51 Complex regional pain syndrome I of upper limb

G90.511 Complex regional pain syndrome I of right upper limb

G90.512 Complex regional pain syndrome I of left upper limb

G90.513 Complex regional pain syndrome I of upper limb, bilateral

G90.519 Complex regional pain syndrome I of unspecified upper limb

G90.52 Complex regional pain syndrome I of lower limb

G90.521 Complex regional pain syndrome I of right lower limb

G90.522 Complex regional pain syndrome I of left lower limb

G90.523 Complex regional pain syndrome I of lower limb, bilateral

G90.529 Complex regional pain syndrome I of unspecified lower limb

G90.59 Complex regional pain syndrome I of other specified site

G90.8 Other disorders of autonomic nervous system

G90.9 Disorder of the autonomic nervous system, unspecified

G91 Hydrocephalus

Includes: acquired hydrocephalus

Excludes1: Arnold-Chiari syndrome with hydrocephalus (Q07.-)

congenital hydrocephalus (Q03.-)

spina bifida with hydrocephalus (Q05.-)

G91.0 Communicating hydrocephalus

Secondary normal pressure hydrocephalus

G91.1 Obstructive hydrocephalus

G91.2 (Idiopathic) normal pressure hydrocephalus

Normal pressure hydrocephalus NOS

G91.3 Post-traumatic hydrocephalus, unspecified

G91.4 Hydrocephalus in diseases classified elsewhere

Code first underlying condition, such as:

congenital syphilis (A50.4-)

neoplasm (C00-D49)

plasminogen deficiency (E88.02)

Excludes1: hydrocephalus due to congenital toxoplasmosis (P37.1)

G91.8 Other hydrocephalus

G91.9 Hydrocephalus, unspecified

G92 Toxic encephalopathy

● **G92.0 Immune effector cell-associated neurotoxicity syndrome**

Code first underlying cause such as:

complications of immune effector cellular therapy (T80.82)

Code also associated signs and symptoms, such as seizures and cerebral edema

Code also, if applicable:

cerebral edema (G93.6)

unspecified convulsions (R56.9)

● **G92.00 Immune effector cell-associated neurotoxicity syndrome, grade unspecified**

ICANS, grade unspecified

● **G92.01 Immune effector cell-associated neurotoxicity syndrome, grade 1**

ICANS, grade 1

● **G92.02 Immune effector cell-associated neurotoxicity syndrome, grade 2**

ICANS, grade 2

● **G92.03 Immune effector cell-associated neurotoxicity syndrome, grade 3**

ICANS, grade 3

● **G92.04 Immune effector cell-associated neurotoxicity syndrome, grade 4**

ICANS, grade 4

● **G92.05 Immune effector cell-associated neurotoxicity syndrome, grade 5**

ICANS, grade 5

● **G92.8 Other toxic encephalopathy**

Toxic encephalitis

Toxic metabolic encephalopathy

Code first poisoning due to drug or toxin, if applicable, (T36-T65 with fifth or sixth character 1-4 or 6)

Use Additional Code for adverse effect, if applicable, to identify drug (T36-T50 with fifth or sixth character 5)

● **G92.9 Unspecified toxic encephalopathy**

Code first poisoning due to drug or toxin, if applicable, (T36-T65 with fifth or sixth character 1-4 or 6)

Use Additional Code for adverse effect, if applicable, to identify drug (T36-T50 with fifth or sixth character 5)

G93 **Other disorders of brain**

  G93.0 **Cerebral cysts**

    Arachnoid cyst

    Porencephalic cyst, acquired

    Excludes1: acquired periventricular cysts of newborn (P91.1)

      congenital cerebral cysts (Q04.6)

  G93.1 **Anoxic brain damage, not elsewhere classified** [HCC]

    Excludes1: cerebral anoxia due to anesthesia during labor and delivery (O74.3)

      cerebral anoxia due to anesthesia during the puerperium (O89.2)

      neonatal anoxia (P84)

  G93.2 **Benign intracranial hypertension**

    Pseudotumor

    Excludes1: hypertensive encephalopathy (I67.4)

      obstructive hydrocephalus (G91.1)

  G93.3 **Postviral fatigue syndrome**

    Benign myalgic encephalomyelitis

    Excludes1: chronic fatigue syndrome NOS (R53.82)

  G93.4 **Other and unspecified encephalopathy**

    Excludes1: alcoholic encephalopathy (G31.2)

      encephalopathy in diseases classified elsewhere (G94)

      hypertensive encephalopathy (I67.4)

    Excludes2: toxic (metabolic) encephalopathy (G92.8)

    G93.40 **Encephalopathy, unspecified**

    G93.41 **Metabolic encephalopathy**

      Septic encephalopathy

    G93.49 **Other encephalopathy**

      Encephalopathy NEC

  G93.5 **Compression of brain** [HCC]

    Arnold-Chiari type 1 compression of brain

    Compression of brain (stem)

    Herniation of brain (stem)

    Excludes1: traumatic compression of brain (S06.A-)

  G93.6 **Cerebral edema** [HCC]

    Excludes1: cerebral edema due to birth injury (P11.0)

      traumatic cerebral edema (S06.1-)

  G93.7 **Reye's syndrome**

    Code first poisoning due to salicylates, if applicable (T39.0-, with sixth character 1-4)

    Use Additional Code for adverse effect due to salicylates, if applicable (T39.0-, with sixth character 5)

  G93.8 **Other specified disorders of brain**

    G93.81 **Temporal sclerosis**

      Hippocampal sclerosis

      Mesial temporal sclerosis

    G93.82 **Brain death**

    G93.89 **Other specified disorders of brain**

      Postradiation encephalopathy

  G93.9 **Disorder of brain, unspecified**

G94 **Other disorders of brain in diseases classified elsewhere**

  Code first underlying disease

  Excludes1: encephalopathy in congenital syphilis (A50.49)

    encephalopathy in influenza (J09.X9, J10.81, J11.81)

    encephalopathy in syphilis (A52.19)

    hydrocephalus in diseases classified elsewhere (G91.4)

G95 **Other and unspecified diseases of spinal cord**

  Excludes2: myelitis (G04.-)

  G95.0 **Syringomyelia and syringobulbia** [HCC]

  G95.1 **Vascular myelopathies**

    Excludes2: intraspinal phlebitis and thrombophlebitis, except non-pyogenic (G08)

    G95.11 **Acute infarction of spinal cord (embolic) (nonembolic)** [HCC]

      Anoxia of spinal cord

      Arterial thrombosis of spinal cord

    G95.19 **Other vascular myelopathies** [HCC]

      Edema of spinal cord

      Hematomyelia

      Nonpyogenic intraspinal phlebitis and thrombophlebitis

      Subacute necrotic myelopathy

  G95.2 **Other and unspecified cord compression**

    G95.20 **Unspecified cord compression** [HCC]

    G95.29 **Other cord compression** [HCC]

  G95.8 **Other specified diseases of spinal cord**

    Excludes1: neurogenic bladder NOS (N31.9)

      neurogenic bladder due to cauda equina syndrome (G83.4)

      neuromuscular dysfunction of bladder without spinal cord lesion (N31.-)

    G95.81 **Conus medullaris syndrome** [HCC]

    G95.89 **Other specified diseases of spinal cord** [HCC]

      Cord bladder NOS

      Drug-induced myelopathy

      Radiation-induced myelopathy

      Excludes1: myelopathy NOS (G95.9)

  G95.9 **Disease of spinal cord, unspecified** [HCC]

    Myelopathy NOS

G96 **Other disorders of central nervous system**

  G96.0 **Cerebrospinal fluid leak**

    Code also if applicable:

    intracranial hypotension (G96.81-)

    Excludes1: cerebrospinal fluid leak from spinal puncture (G97.0)

    G96.00 **Cerebrospinal fluid leak, unspecified**

    Code also if applicable:

    head injury (S00.- to S09.-)

    G96.01 **Cranial cerebrospinal fluid leak, spontaneous**

      Otorrhea due to spontaneous cerebrospinal fluid CSF leak

      Rhinorrhea due to spontaneous cerebrospinal fluid CSF leak

      Spontaneous cerebrospinal fluid leak from skull base

    G96.02 **Spinal cerebrospinal fluid leak, spontaneous**

      Spontaneous cerebrospinal fluid leak from spine

    G96.08 **Other cranial cerebrospinal fluid leak**

      Postoperative cranial cerebrospinal fluid leak

      Traumatic cranial cerebrospinal fluid leak

      Code also if applicable:

      head injury (S00.- to S09.-)

    G96.09 **Other spinal cerebrospinal fluid leak**

Other spinal CSF leak

Postoperative spinal cerebrospinal fluid leak

Traumatic spinal cerebrospinal fluid leak

Code also if applicable:

head injury (S00.- to S09.-)

G96.1 **Disorders of meninges, not elsewhere classified**

G96.11 **Dural tear**

Code also intracranial hypotension, if applicable (G96.81-)

Excludes1: accidental puncture or laceration of dura during a procedure (G97.41)

G96.12 **Meningeal adhesions (cerebral) (spinal)**

G96.19 **Other disorders of meninges, not elsewhere classified**

G96.191 **Perineural cyst**

Cervical nerve root cyst

Lumbar nerve root cyst

Sacral nerve root cyst

Tarlov cyst

Thoracic nerve root cyst

G96.198 **Other disorders of meninges, not elsewhere classified**

G96.8 **Other specified disorders of central nervous system**

G96.81 **Intracranial hypotension**

Code also any associated diagnoses, such as:

Brachial amyotrophy (G54.5)

Cerebrospinal fluid leak from spine (G96.02)

Cranial nerve disorders in diseases classified elsewhere (G53)

Nerve root and compressions in diseases classified elsewhere (G55)

Nonpyogenic thrombosis of intracranial venous system (I67.6)

Nontraumatic intracerebral hemorrhage (I61.-)

Nontraumatic subdural hemorrhage (I62.0-)

Other and unspecified cord compression (G95.2-)

Other secondary parkinsonism (G21.8)

Reversible cerebrovascular vasoconstriction syndrome (I67.841)

Spinal cord herniation (G95.89)

Stroke (I63.-)

Syringomyelia (G95.0)

G96.810 **Intracranial hypotension, unspecified**

G96.811 **Intracranial hypotension, spontaneous**

G96.819 **Other intracranial hypotension**

G96.89 **Other specified disorders of central nervous system**

G96.9 **Disorder of central nervous system, unspecified**

G97 **Intraoperative and postprocedural complications and disorders of nervous system, not elsewhere classified**

Excludes2: intraoperative and postprocedural cerebrovascular infarction (I97.81-, I97.82-)

G97.0 **Cerebrospinal fluid leak from spinal puncture**

Code also any associated diagnoses or complications, such as:

intracranial hypotension following a procedure (G97.83-G97.84)

G97.1 **Other reaction to spinal and lumbar puncture**

Headache due to lumbar puncture

G97.2 **Intracranial hypotension following ventricular shunting**

Code also any associated diagnoses or complications

G97.3 **Intraoperative hemorrhage and hematoma of a nervous system organ or structure complicating a procedure**

Excludes1: intraoperative hemorrhage and hematoma of a nervous system organ or structure due to accidental puncture and laceration during a procedure (G97.4-)

G97.31 **Intraoperative hemorrhage and hematoma of a nervous system organ or structure complicating a nervous system procedure**

G97.32 **Intraoperative hemorrhage and hematoma of a nervous system organ or structure complicating other procedure**

G97.4 **Accidental puncture and laceration of a nervous system organ or structure during a procedure**

G97.41 **Accidental puncture or laceration of dura during a procedure**

Code also any associated diagnoses or complications

Incidental (inadvertent) durotomy

G97.48 **Accidental puncture and laceration of other nervous system organ or structure during a nervous system procedure**

G97.49 **Accidental puncture and laceration of other nervous system organ or structure during other procedure**

G97.5 **Postprocedural hemorrhage of a nervous system organ or structure following a procedure**

G97.51 **Postprocedural hemorrhage of a nervous system organ or structure following a nervous system procedure**

G97.52 **Postprocedural hemorrhage of a nervous system organ or structure following other procedure**

G97.6 **Postprocedural hematoma and seroma of a nervous system organ or structure following a procedure**

G97.61 **Postprocedural hematoma of a nervous system organ or structure following a nervous system procedure**

G97.62 **Postprocedural hematoma of a nervous system organ or structure following other procedure**

G97.63 **Postprocedural seroma of a nervous system organ or structure following a nervous system procedure**

G97.64 **Postprocedural seroma of a nervous system organ or structure following other procedure**

G97.8 **Other intraoperative and postprocedural complications and disorders of nervous system**

Use Additional Code to further specify disorder

G97.81 **Other intraoperative complications of nervous system**

G97.82 **Other postprocedural complications and disorders of nervous system**

G97.83 **Intracranial hypotension following lumbar cerebrospinal fluid shunting**

Code also any associated diagnoses or complications

G97.84 **Intracranial hypotension following other procedure**

Code also, if applicable:

accidental puncture or laceration of dura during a procedure (G97.41)

cerebrospinal fluid leak from spinal puncture (G97.0)

G98 **Other disorders of nervous system not elsewhere classified**

Includes: nervous system disorder NOS

    G98.0 **Neurogenic arthritis, not elsewhere classified**

        Nonsyphilitic neurogenic arthropathy NEC

        Nonsyphilitic neurogenic spondylopathy NEC

        Excludes1: spondylopathy (in):

            syringomyelia and syringobulbia (G95.0)

            tabes dorsalis (A52.11)

    G98.8 **Other disorders of nervous system**

        Nervous system disorder NOS

G99 **Other disorders of nervous system in diseases classified elsewhere**

    G99.0 **Autonomic neuropathy in diseases classified elsewhere**

        Code first underlying disease, such as:

        amyloidosis (E85.-)

        gout (M1A.-, M10.-)

        hyperthyroidism (E05.-)

        Excludes1: diabetic autonomic neuropathy (E08-E13 with .43)

    G99.2 **Myelopathy in diseases classified elsewhere** [HCC]

        Code first underlying disease, such as:

        neoplasm (C00-D49)

        Excludes1: myelopathy in:

        intervertebral disease (M50.0-, M51.0-)

        spondylosis (M47.0-, M47.1-)

    G99.8 **Other specified disorders of nervous system in diseases classified elsewhere**

        Code first underlying disorder, such as:

        amyloidosis (E85.-)

        avitaminosis (E56.9)

        Excludes1: nervous system involvement in:

            cysticercosis (B69.0)

            rubella (B06.0-)

            syphilis (A52.1-)

● New code ▲ Revised code **Excludes1:** Not coded here **Excludes2:** Not included here ⊗ Placeholder required ⑦7th digit required

Chapter 7: Diseases of the Eye and Adnexa (H00-H59)

DEFINITIONS

This chapter includes definitions of selected key words, terms and phrases and coding alerts for adding points to the clinical domain, and references to coding late effects where appropriate. An example from this chapter is as follows:

H16   **Keratitis**

Definition: Keratitis is an infection or inflammation of the cornea which can be caused by a variety of conditions, including infections, dry eyes, foreign objects, contact lenses, intense light, vitamin a deficiency or allergies.

MULTIPLE CODING FOR A SINGLE CONDITION

In addition to the etiology/manifestation convention that requires two codes to fully describe a single condition that affects multiple body systems, there are other single conditions that also require more than one code. "**Use Additional Code**" notes are found in the Tabular List at codes that are not part of an etiology/manifestation pair where a secondary code is useful to fully describe a condition. The sequencing rule is the same as the etiology/manifestation pair, "**Use Additional Code**" indicates that a secondary code should be added.

For example, for bacterial infections that are not included in chapter 1, a secondary code from category B95, Streptococcus, Staphylococcus, and Enterococcus, as the cause of diseases classified elsewhere, or B96, Other bacterial agents as the cause of diseases classified elsewhere, may be required to identify the bacterial organism causing the infection. A "**Use Additional Code**" note will normally be found at the infectious disease code, indicating a need for the organism code to be added as a secondary code.

"Code first" notes are also under certain codes that are not specifically manifestation codes but may be due to an underlying cause. When there is a "Code first" note and an underlying condition is present, the underlying condition should be sequenced first.

"Code, if applicable, any causal condition first", notes indicate that this code may be assigned as a principal diagnosis when the causal condition is unknown or not applicable. If a causal condition is known, then the code for that condition should be sequenced as the principal or first-listed diagnosis.

Multiple codes may be needed for sequela, complication codes and obstetric codes to more fully describe a condition. See the specific guidelines for these conditions for further instruction.

COMBINATION CODE

A combination code is a single code used to classify: Two diagnoses, or a diagnosis with an associated secondary process (manifestation) A diagnosis with an associated complication

Combination codes are identified by referring to subterm entries in the Alphabetic Index and by reading the inclusion and exclusion notes in the Tabular List.

Assign only the combination code when that code fully identifies the diagnostic conditions involved or when the Alphabetic Index so directs. Multiple coding should not be used when the classification provides a combination code that clearly identifies all of the elements documented in the diagnosis. When the combination code lacks necessary specificity in describing the manifestation or complication, an additional code should be used as a secondary code.

SEQUELA (LATE EFFECTS)

A sequela is the residual effect (condition produced) after the acute phase of an illness or injury has terminated. There is no time limit on when a sequela code can be used. The residual may be apparent early, such as in cerebral infarction, or it may occur months or years later, such as that due to a previous injury. Coding of sequela generally requires two codes sequenced in the following order: The condition or nature of the sequela is sequenced first.

The sequela code is sequenced second.

H00-H95

An exception to the above guidelines are those instances where the code for the sequela is followed by a manifestation code identified in the Tabular List and title, or the sequela code has been expanded (at the fourth, fifth or sixth character levels) to include the manifestation(s). The code for the acute phase of an illness or injury that led to the sequela is never used with a code for the late effect.

GLAUCOMA

1) Assigning Glaucoma Codes

Assign as many codes from category H40, Glaucoma, as needed to identify the type of glaucoma, the affected eye, and the glaucoma stage.

2) Bilateral glaucoma with same type and stage

When a patient has bilateral glaucoma and both eyes are documented as being the same type and stage, and there is a code for bilateral glaucoma, report only the code for the type of glaucoma, bilateral, with the seventh character for the stage.

When a patient has bilateral glaucoma and both eyes are documented as being the same type and stage, and the classification does not provide a code for bilateral glaucoma (i.e., subcategories H40.10, and H40.20) report only one code for the type of glaucoma with the appropriate seventh character for the stage.

3) Bilateral glaucoma stage with different types or stages

When a patient has bilateral glaucoma and each eye is documented as having a different type or stage, and the classification distinguishes laterality, assign the appropriate code for each eye rather than the code for bilateral glaucoma.

When a patient has bilateral glaucoma and each eye is documented as having a different type, and the classification does not distinguish laterality (i.e., subcategories H40.10, and H40.20), assign one code for each type of glaucoma with the appropriate seventh character for the stage.

When a patient has bilateral glaucoma and each eye is documented as having the same type, but different stage, and the classification does not distinguish laterality (i.e., subcategories H40.10 and H40.20), assign a code for the type of glaucoma for each eye with the seventh character for the specific glaucoma stage documented for each eye.

4) Patient admitted with glaucoma and stage evolves during the admission

If a patient is admitted with glaucoma and the stage progresses during the admission, assign the code for highest stage documented.

5) Indeterminate stage glaucoma

Assignment of the seventh character "4" for "indeterminate stage" should be based on the clinical documentation. The seventh character "4" is used for glaucomas whose stage cannot be clinically determined. This seventh character should not be confused with the seventh character "0", unspecified, which should be assigned when there is no documentation regarding the stage of the glaucoma.

BLINDNESS

If "blindness" or "low vision" of both eyes is documented but the visual impairment category is not documented, assign code H54.3, Unqualified visual loss, both eyes. If "blindness" or "low vision" in one eye is documented but the visual impairment category is not documented, assign a code from H54.6-, Unqualified visual loss, one eye. If "blindness" or "visual loss" is documented without any information about whether one or both eyes are affected, assign code H54.7, Unspecified visual loss.

Chapter 7

Diseases of The Eye and Adnexa (H00-H59)

Note: Use an external cause code following the code for the eye condition, if applicable, to identify the cause of the eye condition

Excludes2: certain conditions originating in the perinatal period (P04-P96)

certain infectious and parasitic diseases (A00-B99)

complications of pregnancy, childbirth and the puerperium (O00-O9A)

congenital malformations, deformations, and chromosomal abnormalities (Q00-Q99)

diabetes mellitus related eye conditions (E09.3-, E10.3-, E11.3-, E13.3-)

endocrine, nutritional and metabolic diseases (E00-E88)

injury (trauma) of eye and orbit (S05.-)

injury, poisoning and certain other consequences of external causes (S00-T88)

neoplasms (C00-D49)

symptoms, signs and abnormal clinical and laboratory findings, not elsewhere classified (R00-R94)

syphilis related eye disorders (A50.01, A50.3-, A51.43, A52.71)

This chapter contains the following blocks:

H00-H05	Disorders of eyelid, lacrimal system and orbit
H10-H11	Disorders of conjunctiva
H15-H22	Disorders of sclera, cornea, iris and ciliary body
H25-H28	Disorders of lens
H30-H36	Disorders of choroid and retina
H40-H42	Glaucoma
H43-H44	Disorders of vitreous body and globe
H46-H47	Disorders of optic nerve and visual pathways
H49-H52	Disorders of ocular muscles, binocular movement, accommodation and refraction
H53-H54	Visual disturbances and blindness
H55-H57	Other disorders of eye and adnexa
H59	Intraoperative and postprocedural complications and disorders of eye and adnexa, not elsewhere classified

DISORDERS OF EYELID, LACRIMAL SYSTEM AND ORBIT (H00-H05)

Excludes2: open wound of eyelid (S01.1-)

superficial injury of eyelid (S00.1-, S00.2-)

H00 Hordeolum and chalazion

H00.0 Hordeolum (externum) (internum) of eyelid

H00.01 Hordeolum externum

Hordeolum NOS

Stye

H00.011 Hordeolum externum right upper eyelid

H00.012 Hordeolum externum right lower eyelid

H00.013 Hordeolum externum right eye, unspecified eyelid

H00.014 Hordeolum externum left upper eyelid

H00.015 Hordeolum externum left lower eyelid

H00.016 Hordeolum externum left eye, unspecified eyelid

H00.019 Hordeolum externum unspecified eye, unspecified eyelid

H00.02 Hordeolum internum

Infection of meibomian gland

H00.021 Hordeolum internum right upper eyelid

H00.022 Hordeolum internum right lower eyelid

H00.023 Hordeolum internum right eye, unspecified eyelid

H00.024 Hordeolum internum left upper eyelid

H00.025 Hordeolum internum left lower eyelid

H00.026 Hordeolum internum left eye, unspecified eyelid

H00.029 Hordeolum internum unspecified eye, unspecified eyelid

H00.03 Abscess of eyelid

Furuncle of eyelid

H00.031 Abscess of right upper eyelid

H00.032 Abscess of right lower eyelid

H00.033 Abscess of eyelid right eye, unspecified eyelid

H00.034 Abscess of left upper eyelid

H00.035 Abscess of left lower eyelid

H00.036 Abscess of eyelid left eye, unspecified eyelid

H00.039 Abscess of eyelid unspecified eye, unspecified eyelid

H00.1 Chalazion

Meibomian (gland) cyst

Excludes2: infected meibomian gland (H00.02-)

H00.11 Chalazion right upper eyelid

H00.12 Chalazion right lower eyelid

H00.13 Chalazion right eye, unspecified eyelid

H00.14 Chalazion left upper eyelid

H00.15 Chalazion left lower eyelid

H00.16 Chalazion left eye, unspecified eyelid

H00.19 Chalazion unspecified eye, unspecified eyelid

H01 Other inflammation of eyelid

H01.0 Blepharitis

Excludes1: blepharoconjunctivitis (H10.5-)

H01.00 Unspecified blepharitis

H01.001 Unspecified blepharitis right upper eyelid

H01.002 Unspecified blepharitis right lower eyelid

H01.003 Unspecified blepharitis right eye, unspecified eyelid

H01.004 Unspecified blepharitis left upper eyelid

H01.005 Unspecified blepharitis left lower eyelid

H01.006 Unspecified blepharitis left eye, unspecified eyelid

H01.009 Unspecified blepharitis unspecified eye, unspecified eyelid

H01.00A Unspecified blepharitis right eye, upper and lower eyelids

H01.00B Unspecified blepharitis left eye, upper and lower eyelids

---

Add 4th-7th digits   Nonspecific code   Unspecified code   Manifestation code   [HCC] Hierarchical Condition Code

H01.01 Ulcerative blepharitis

- H01.011 Ulcerative blepharitis right upper eyelid
- H01.012 Ulcerative blepharitis right lower eyelid
- H01.013 Ulcerative blepharitis right eye, unspecified eyelid
- H01.014 Ulcerative blepharitis left upper eyelid
- H01.015 Ulcerative blepharitis left lower eyelid
- H01.016 Ulcerative blepharitis left eye, unspecified eyelid
- H01.019 Ulcerative blepharitis unspecified eye, unspecified eyelid
- H01.01A Ulcerative blepharitis right eye, upper and lower eyelids
- H01.01B Ulcerative blepharitis left eye, upper and lower eyelids

H01.02 Squamous blepharitis

- H01.021 Squamous blepharitis right upper eyelid
- H01.022 Squamous blepharitis right lower eyelid
- H01.023 Squamous blepharitis right eye, unspecified eyelid
- H01.024 Squamous blepharitis left upper eyelid
- H01.025 Squamous blepharitis left lower eyelid
- H01.026 Squamous blepharitis left eye, unspecified eyelid
- H01.029 Squamous blepharitis unspecified eye, unspecified eyelid
- H01.02A Squamous blepharitis right eye, upper and lower eyelids
- H01.02B Squamous blepharitis left eye, upper and lower eyelids

H01.1 Noninfectious dermatoses of eyelid

H01.11 Allergic dermatitis of eyelid

Contact dermatitis of eyelid

- H01.111 Allergic dermatitis of right upper eyelid
- H01.112 Allergic dermatitis of right lower eyelid
- H01.113 Allergic dermatitis of right eye, unspecified eyelid
- H01.114 Allergic dermatitis of left upper eyelid
- H01.115 Allergic dermatitis of left lower eyelid
- H01.116 Allergic dermatitis of left eye, unspecified eyelid
- H01.119 Allergic dermatitis of unspecified eye, unspecified eyelid

H01.12 Discoid lupus erythematosus of eyelid

- H01.121 Discoid lupus erythematosus of right upper eyelid
- H01.122 Discoid lupus erythematosus of right lower eyelid
- H01.123 Discoid lupus erythematosus of right eye, unspecified eyelid
- H01.124 Discoid lupus erythematosus of left upper eyelid
- H01.125 Discoid lupus erythematosus of left lower eyelid
- H01.126 Discoid lupus erythematosus of left eye, unspecified eyelid
- H01.129 Discoid lupus erythematosus of unspecified eye, unspecified eyelid

H01.13 Eczematous dermatitis of eyelid

- H01.131 Eczematous dermatitis of right upper eyelid
- H01.132 Eczematous dermatitis of right lower eyelid
- H01.133 Eczematous dermatitis of right eye, unspecified eyelid
- H01.134 Eczematous dermatitis of left upper eyelid
- H01.135 Eczematous dermatitis of left lower eyelid
- H01.136 Eczematous dermatitis of left eye, unspecified eyelid
- H01.139 Eczematous dermatitis of unspecified eye, unspecified eyelid

H01.14 Xeroderma of eyelid

- H01.141 Xeroderma of right upper eyelid
- H01.142 Xeroderma of right lower eyelid
- H01.143 Xeroderma of right eye, unspecified eyelid
- H01.144 Xeroderma of left upper eyelid
- H01.145 Xeroderma of left lower eyelid
- H01.146 Xeroderma of left eye, unspecified eyelid
- H01.149 Xeroderma of unspecified eye, unspecified eyelid

H01.8 Other specified inflammations of eyelid

H01.9 Unspecified inflammation of eyelid

Inflammation of eyelid NOS

H02 Other disorders of eyelid

Excludes1: congenital malformations of eyelid (Q10.0-Q10.3)

H02.0 Entropion and trichiasis of eyelid

H02.00 Unspecified entropion of eyelid

- H02.001 Unspecified entropion of right upper eyelid
- H02.002 Unspecified entropion of right lower eyelid
- H02.003 Unspecified entropion of right eye, unspecified eyelid
- H02.004 Unspecified entropion of left upper eyelid
- H02.005 Unspecified entropion of left lower eyelid
- H02.006 Unspecified entropion of left eye, unspecified eyelid
- H02.009 Unspecified entropion of unspecified eye, unspecified eyelid

H02.01 Cicatricial entropion of eyelid

- H02.011 Cicatricial entropion of right upper eyelid
- H02.012 Cicatricial entropion of right lower eyelid
- H02.013 Cicatricial entropion of right eye, unspecified eyelid
- H02.014 Cicatricial entropion of left upper eyelid

H02.015   Cicatricial entropion of left lower eyelid

H02.016   Cicatricial entropion of left eye, unspecified eyelid

H02.019   Cicatricial entropion of unspecified eye, unspecified eyelid

H02.02   Mechanical entropion of eyelid

H02.021   Mechanical entropion of right upper eyelid

H02.022   Mechanical entropion of right lower eyelid

H02.023   Mechanical entropion of right eye, unspecified eyelid

H02.024   Mechanical entropion of left upper eyelid

H02.025   Mechanical entropion of left lower eyelid

H02.026   Mechanical entropion of left eye, unspecified eyelid

H02.029   Mechanical entropion of unspecified eye, unspecified eyelid

H02.03   Senile entropion of eyelid

H02.031   Senile entropion of right upper eyelid

H02.032   Senile entropion of right lower eyelid

H02.033   Senile entropion of right eye, unspecified eyelid

H02.034   Senile entropion of left upper eyelid

H02.035   Senile entropion of left lower eyelid

H02.036   Senile entropion of left eye, unspecified eyelid

H02.039   Senile entropion of unspecified eye, unspecified eyelid

H02.04   Spastic entropion of eyelid

H02.041   Spastic entropion of right upper eyelid

H02.042   Spastic entropion of right lower eyelid

H02.043   Spastic entropion of right eye, unspecified eyelid

H02.044   Spastic entropion of left upper eyelid

H02.045   Spastic entropion of left lower eyelid

H02.046   Spastic entropion of left eye, unspecified eyelid

H02.049   Spastic entropion of unspecified eye, unspecified eyelid

H02.05   Trichiasis without entropion

H02.051   Trichiasis without entropion right upper eyelid

H02.052   Trichiasis without entropion right lower eyelid

H02.053   Trichiasis without entropion right eye, unspecified eyelid

H02.054   Trichiasis without entropion left upper eyelid

H02.055   Trichiasis without entropion left lower eyelid

H02.056   Trichiasis without entropion left eye, unspecified eyelid

H02.059   Trichiasis without entropion unspecified eye, unspecified eyelid

H02.1   Ectropion of eyelid

H02.10   Unspecified ectropion of eyelid

H02.101   Unspecified ectropion of right upper eyelid

H02.102   Unspecified ectropion of right lower eyelid

H02.103   Unspecified ectropion of right eye, unspecified eyelid

H02.104   Unspecified ectropion of left upper eyelid

H02.105   Unspecified ectropion of left lower eyelid

H02.106   Unspecified ectropion of left eye, unspecified eyelid

H02.109   Unspecified ectropion of unspecified eye, unspecified eyelid

H02.11   Cicatricial ectropion of eyelid

H02.111   Cicatricial ectropion of right upper eyelid

H02.112   Cicatricial ectropion of right lower eyelid

H02.113   Cicatricial ectropion of right eye, unspecified eyelid

H02.114   Cicatricial ectropion of left upper eyelid

H02.115   Cicatricial ectropion of left lower eyelid

H02.116   Cicatricial ectropion of left eye, unspecified eyelid

H02.119   Cicatricial ectropion of unspecified eye, unspecified eyelid

H02.12   Mechanical ectropion of eyelid

H02.121   Mechanical ectropion of right upper eyelid

H02.122   Mechanical ectropion of right lower eyelid

H02.123   Mechanical ectropion of right eye, unspecified eyelid

H02.124   Mechanical ectropion of left upper eyelid

H02.125   Mechanical ectropion of left lower eyelid

H02.126   Mechanical ectropion of left eye, unspecified eyelid

H02.129   Mechanical ectropion of unspecified eye, unspecified eyelid

H02.13   Senile ectropion of eyelid

H02.131   Senile ectropion of right upper eyelid

H02.132   Senile ectropion of right lower eyelid

H02.133   Senile ectropion of right eye, unspecified eyelid

H02.134   Senile ectropion of left upper eyelid

H02.135   Senile ectropion of left lower eyelid

H02.136   Senile ectropion of left eye, unspecified eyelid

H02.139   Senile ectropion of unspecified eye, unspecified eyelid

H02.14   Spastic ectropion of eyelid

H02.141   Spastic ectropion of right upper eyelid

H02.142   Spastic ectropion of right lower eyelid

H02.143   Spastic ectropion of right eye, unspecified eyelid

H02.144   Spastic ectropion of left upper eyelid

H02.145   Spastic ectropion of left lower eyelid

H02.146   Spastic ectropion of left eye, unspecified eyelid

H02.149   Spastic ectropion of unspecified eye, unspecified eyelid

H02.15   Paralytic ectropion of eyelid

H02.151   Paralytic ectropion of right upper eyelid

H02.152   Paralytic ectropion of right lower eyelid

H02.153   Paralytic ectropion of right eye, unspecified eyelid

H02.154   Paralytic ectropion of left upper eyelid

H02.155   Paralytic ectropion of left lower eyelid

H02.156   Paralytic ectropion of left eye, unspecified eyelid

H02.159   Paralytic ectropion of unspecified eye, unspecified eyelid

H02.2   Lagophthalmos

H02.20   Unspecified lagophthalmos

H02.201   Unspecified lagophthalmos right upper eyelid

H02.202   Unspecified lagophthalmos right lower eyelid

H02.203   Unspecified lagophthalmos right eye, unspecified eyelid

H02.204   Unspecified lagophthalmos left upper eyelid

H02.205   Unspecified lagophthalmos left lower eyelid

H02.206   Unspecified lagophthalmos left eye, unspecified eyelid

H02.209   Unspecified lagophthalmos unspecified eye, unspecified eyelid

H02.20A   Unspecified lagophthalmos right eye, upper and lower eyelids

H02.20B   Unspecified lagophthalmos left eye, upper and lower eyelids

H02.20C   Unspecified lagophthalmos, bilateral, upper and lower eyelids

H02.21   Cicatricial lagophthalmos

H02.211   Cicatricial lagophthalmos right upper eyelid

H02.212   Cicatricial lagophthalmos right lower eyelid

H02.213   Cicatricial lagophthalmos right eye, unspecified eyelid

H02.214   Cicatricial lagophthalmos left upper eyelid

H02.215   Cicatricial lagophthalmos left lower eyelid

H02.216   Cicatricial lagophthalmos left eye, unspecified eyelid

H02.219   Cicatricial lagophthalmos unspecified eye, unspecified eyelid

H02.21A   Cicatricial lagophthalmos right eye, upper and lower eyelids

H02.21B   Cicatricial lagophthalmos left eye, upper and lower eyelids

H02.21C   Cicatricial lagophthalmos, bilateral, upper and lower eyelids

H02.22   Mechanical lagophthalmos

H02.221   Mechanical lagophthalmos right upper eyelid

H02.222   Mechanical lagophthalmos right lower eyelid

H02.223   Mechanical lagophthalmos right eye, unspecified eyelid

H02.224   Mechanical lagophthalmos left upper eyelid

H02.225   Mechanical lagophthalmos left lower eyelid

H02.226   Mechanical lagophthalmos left eye, unspecified eyelid

H02.229   Mechanical lagophthalmos unspecified eye, unspecified eyelid

H02.22A   Mechanical lagophthalmos right eye, upper and lower eyelids

H02.22B   Mechanical lagophthalmos left eye, upper and lower eyelids

H02.22C   Mechanical lagophthalmos, bilateral, upper and lower eyelids

H02.23   Paralytic lagophthalmos

H02.231   Paralytic lagophthalmos right upper eyelid

H02.232   Paralytic lagophthalmos right lower eyelid

H02.233   Paralytic lagophthalmos right eye, unspecified eyelid

H02.234   Paralytic lagophthalmos left upper eyelid

H02.235   Paralytic lagophthalmos left lower eyelid

H02.236   Paralytic lagophthalmos left eye, unspecified eyelid

H02.239   Paralytic lagophthalmos unspecified eye, unspecified eyelid

H02.23A   Paralytic lagophthalmos right eye, upper and lower eyelids

H02.23B   Paralytic lagophthalmos left eye, upper and lower eyelids

H02.23C   Paralytic lagophthalmos, bilateral, upper and lower eyelids

H02.3   Blepharochalasis

Pseudoptosis

H02.30   Blepharochalasis unspecified eye, unspecified eyelid

H02.31   Blepharochalasis right upper eyelid

H02.32   Blepharochalasis right lower eyelid

H02.33   Blepharochalasis right eye, unspecified eyelid

H02.34   Blepharochalasis left upper eyelid

H02.35   Blepharochalasis left lower eyelid

H02.36   Blepharochalasis left eye, unspecified eyelid

H02.4   Ptosis of eyelid

H02.40   Unspecified ptosis of eyelid

H02.401   Unspecified ptosis of right eyelid

H02.402   Unspecified ptosis of left eyelid

H02.403   Unspecified ptosis of bilateral eyelids

H02.409   Unspecified ptosis of unspecified eyelid

H02.41   Mechanical ptosis of eyelid

H02.411   Mechanical ptosis of right eyelid

H02.412   Mechanical ptosis of left eyelid

H02.413   Mechanical ptosis of bilateral eyelids

● New code   ▲ Revised code   **Excludes1:** Not coded here   **Excludes2:** Not included here   ⊗ Placeholder required   ⑦7ᵗʰ digit required

H02.419   Mechanical ptosis of unspecified eyelid

H02.42   Myogenic ptosis of eyelid

     H02.421   Myogenic ptosis of right eyelid

     H02.422   Myogenic ptosis of left eyelid

     H02.423   Myogenic ptosis of bilateral eyelids

     H02.429   Myogenic ptosis of unspecified eyelid

H02.43   Paralytic ptosis of eyelid

     Neurogenic ptosis of eyelid

     H02.431   Paralytic ptosis of right eyelid

     H02.432   Paralytic ptosis of left eyelid

     H02.433   Paralytic ptosis of bilateral eyelids

     H02.439   Paralytic ptosis unspecified eyelid

H02.5   **Other disorders affecting eyelid function**

     Excludes2:   blepharospasm (G24.5)

       organic tic (G25.69)

       psychogenic tic (F95.-)

H02.51   Abnormal innervation syndrome

     H02.511   Abnormal innervation syndrome right upper eyelid

     H02.512   Abnormal innervation syndrome right lower eyelid

     H02.513   Abnormal innervation syndrome right eye, unspecified eyelid

     H02.514   Abnormal innervation syndrome left upper eyelid

     H02.515   Abnormal innervation syndrome left lower eyelid

     H02.516   Abnormal innervation syndrome left eye, unspecified eyelid

     H02.519   Abnormal innervation syndrome unspecified eye, unspecified eyelid

H02.52   Blepharophimosis

     Ankyloblepharon

     H02.521   Blepharophimosis right upper eyelid

     H02.522   Blepharophimosis right lower eyelid

     H02.523   Blepharophimosis right eye, unspecified eyelid

     H02.524   Blepharophimosis left upper eyelid

     H02.525   Blepharophimosis left lower eyelid

     H02.526   Blepharophimosis left eye, unspecified eyelid

     H02.529   Blepharophimosis unspecified eye, unspecified lid

H02.53   Eyelid retraction

     Eyelid lag

     H02.531   Eyelid retraction right upper eyelid

     H02.532   Eyelid retraction right lower eyelid

     H02.533   Eyelid retraction right eye, unspecified eyelid

     H02.534   Eyelid retraction left upper eyelid

     H02.535   Eyelid retraction left lower eyelid

     H02.536   Eyelid retraction left eye, unspecified eyelid

     H02.539   Eyelid retraction unspecified eye, unspecified lid

H02.59   Other disorders affecting eyelid function

     Deficient blink reflex

     Sensory disorders

H02.6   **Xanthelasma of eyelid**

H02.60   Xanthelasma of unspecified eye, unspecified eyelid

H02.61   Xanthelasma of right upper eyelid

H02.62   Xanthelasma of right lower eyelid

H02.63   Xanthelasma of right eye, unspecified eyelid

H02.64   Xanthelasma of left upper eyelid

H02.65   Xanthelasma of left lower eyelid

H02.66   Xanthelasma of left eye, unspecified eyelid

H02.7   **Other and unspecified degenerative disorders of eyelid and periocular area**

H02.70   Unspecified degenerative disorders of eyelid and periocular area

H02.71   Chloasma of eyelid and periocular area

     Dyspigmentation of eyelid

     Hyperpigmentation of eyelid

     H02.711   Chloasma of right upper eyelid and periocular area

     H02.712   Chloasma of right lower eyelid and periocular area

     H02.713   Chloasma of right eye, unspecified eyelid and periocular area

     H02.714   Chloasma of left upper eyelid and periocular area

     H02.715   Chloasma of left lower eyelid and periocular area

     H02.716   Chloasma of left eye, unspecified eyelid and periocular area

     H02.719   Chloasma of unspecified eye, unspecified eyelid and periocular area

H02.72   Madarosis of eyelid and periocular area

     Hypotrichosis of eyelid

     H02.721   Madarosis of right upper eyelid and periocular area

     H02.722   Madarosis of right lower eyelid and periocular area

     H02.723   Madarosis of right eye, unspecified eyelid and periocular area

     H02.724   Madarosis of left upper eyelid and periocular area

     H02.725   Madarosis of left lower eyelid and periocular area

     H02.726   Madarosis of left eye, unspecified eyelid and periocular area

     H02.729   Madarosis of unspecified eye, unspecified eyelid and periocular area

H02.73   Vitiligo of eyelid and periocular area

     Hypopigmentation of eyelid

     H02.731   Vitiligo of right upper eyelid and periocular area

     H02.732   Vitiligo of right lower eyelid and periocular area

     H02.733   Vitiligo of right eye, unspecified eyelid and periocular area

     H02.734   Vitiligo of left upper eyelid and periocular area

     H02.735   Vitiligo of left lower eyelid and periocular area

     H02.736   Vitiligo of left eye, unspecified eyelid and periocular area

H02.739 Vitiligo of unspecified eye, unspecified eyelid and periocular area

H02.79 **Other degenerative disorders of eyelid and periocular area**

H02.8 **Other specified disorders of eyelid**

H02.81 **Retained foreign body in eyelid**

Use Additional Code to identify the type of retained foreign body (Z18.-)

Excludes1: laceration of eyelid with foreign body (S01.12-)

retained intraocular foreign body (H44.6-, H44.7-)

superficial foreign body of eyelid and periocular area (S00.25-)

H02.811 **Retained foreign body in right upper eyelid**

H02.812 **Retained foreign body in right lower eyelid**

H02.813 **Retained foreign body in right eye, unspecified eyelid**

H02.814 **Retained foreign body in left upper eyelid**

H02.815 **Retained foreign body in left lower eyelid**

H02.816 **Retained foreign body in left eye, unspecified eyelid**

H02.819 **Retained foreign body in unspecified eye, unspecified eyelid**

H02.82 **Cysts of eyelid**

Sebaceous cyst of eyelid

H02.821 **Cysts of right upper eyelid**

H02.822 **Cysts of right lower eyelid**

H02.823 **Cysts of right eye, unspecified eyelid**

H02.824 **Cysts of left upper eyelid**

H02.825 **Cysts of left lower eyelid**

H02.826 **Cysts of left eye, unspecified eyelid**

H02.829 **Cysts of unspecified eye, unspecified eyelid**

H02.83 **Dermatochalasis of eyelid**

H02.831 **Dermatochalasis of right upper eyelid**

H02.832 **Dermatochalasis of right lower eyelid**

H02.833 **Dermatochalasis of right eye, unspecified eyelid**

H02.834 **Dermatochalasis of left upper eyelid**

H02.835 **Dermatochalasis of left lower eyelid**

H02.836 **Dermatochalasis of left eye, unspecified eyelid**

H02.839 **Dermatochalasis of unspecified eye, unspecified eyelid**

H02.84 **Edema of eyelid**

Hyperemia of eyelid

H02.841 **Edema of right upper eyelid**

H02.842 **Edema of right lower eyelid**

H02.843 **Edema of right eye, unspecified eyelid**

H02.844 **Edema of left upper eyelid**

H02.845 **Edema of left lower eyelid**

H02.846 **Edema of left eye, unspecified eyelid**

H02.849 **Edema of unspecified eye, unspecified eyelid**

H02.85 **Elephantiasis of eyelid**

H02.851 **Elephantiasis of right upper eyelid**

H02.852 **Elephantiasis of right lower eyelid**

H02.853 **Elephantiasis of right eye, unspecified eyelid**

H02.854 **Elephantiasis of left upper eyelid**

H02.855 **Elephantiasis of left lower eyelid**

H02.856 **Elephantiasis of left eye, unspecified eyelid**

H02.859 **Elephantiasis of unspecified eye, unspecified eyelid**

H02.86 **Hypertrichosis of eyelid**

H02.861 **Hypertrichosis of right upper eyelid**

H02.862 **Hypertrichosis of right lower eyelid**

H02.863 **Hypertrichosis of right eye, unspecified eyelid**

H02.864 **Hypertrichosis of left upper eyelid**

H02.865 **Hypertrichosis of left lower eyelid**

H02.866 **Hypertrichosis of left eye, unspecified eyelid**

H02.869 **Hypertrichosis of unspecified eye, unspecified eyelid**

H02.87 **Vascular anomalies of eyelid**

H02.871 **Vascular anomalies of right upper eyelid**

H02.872 **Vascular anomalies of right lower eyelid**

H02.873 **Vascular anomalies of right eye, unspecified eyelid**

H02.874 **Vascular anomalies of left upper eyelid**

H02.875 **Vascular anomalies of left lower eyelid**

H02.876 **Vascular anomalies of left eye, unspecified eyelid**

H02.879 **Vascular anomalies of unspecified eye, unspecified eyelid**

H02.88 **Meibomian gland dysfunction of eyelid**

H02.881 **Meibomian gland dysfunction right upper eyelid**

H02.882 **Meibomian gland dysfunction right lower eyelid**

H02.883 **Meibomian gland dysfunction of right eye, unspecified eyelid**

H02.884 **Meibomian gland dysfunction left upper eyelid**

H02.885 **Meibomian gland dysfunction left lower eyelid**

H02.886 **Meibomian gland dysfunction of left eye, unspecified eyelid**

H02.889 **Meibomian gland dysfunction of unspecified eye, unspecified eyelid**

H02.88A **Meibomian gland dysfunction right eye, upper and lower eyelids**

H02.88B **Meibomian gland dysfunction left eye, upper and lower eyelids**

H02.89 **Other specified disorders of eyelid**

Hemorrhage of eyelid

H02.9 **Unspecified disorder of eyelid**

Disorder of eyelid NOS

H04 **Disorders of lacrimal system**

Excludes1: congenital malformations of lacrimal system (Q10.4-Q10.6)

H04.0 **Dacryoadenitis**

H04.00 **Unspecified dacryoadenitis**

H04.001 Unspecified dacryoadenitis, right lacrimal gland

H04.002 Unspecified dacryoadenitis, left lacrimal gland

H04.003 Unspecified dacryoadenitis, bilateral lacrimal glands

H04.009 Unspecified dacryoadenitis, unspecified lacrimal gland

H04.01 **Acute dacryoadenitis**

H04.011 Acute dacryoadenitis, right lacrimal gland

H04.012 Acute dacryoadenitis, left lacrimal gland

H04.013 Acute dacryoadenitis, bilateral lacrimal glands

H04.019 Acute dacryoadenitis, unspecified lacrimal gland

H04.02 **Chronic dacryoadenitis**

H04.021 Chronic dacryoadenitis, right lacrimal gland

H04.022 Chronic dacryoadenitis, left lacrimal gland

H04.023 Chronic dacryoadenitis, bilateral lacrimal gland

H04.029 Chronic dacryoadenitis, unspecified lacrimal gland

H04.03 **Chronic enlargement of lacrimal gland**

H04.031 Chronic enlargement of right lacrimal gland

H04.032 Chronic enlargement of left lacrimal gland

H04.033 Chronic enlargement of bilateral lacrimal glands

H04.039 Chronic enlargement of unspecified lacrimal gland

H04.1 **Other disorders of lacrimal gland**

H04.11 **Dacryops**

H04.111 Dacryops of right lacrimal gland

H04.112 Dacryops of left lacrimal gland

H04.113 Dacryops of bilateral lacrimal glands

H04.119 Dacryops of unspecified lacrimal gland

H04.12 **Dry eye syndrome**

Tear film insufficiency, NOS

H04.121 Dry eye syndrome of right lacrimal gland

H04.122 Dry eye syndrome of left lacrimal gland

H04.123 Dry eye syndrome of bilateral lacrimal glands

H04.129 Dry eye syndrome of unspecified lacrimal gland

H04.13 **Lacrimal cyst**

Lacrimal cystic degeneration

H04.131 Lacrimal cyst, right lacrimal gland

H04.132 Lacrimal cyst, left lacrimal gland

H04.133 Lacrimal cyst, bilateral lacrimal glands

H04.139 Lacrimal cyst, unspecified lacrimal gland

H04.14 **Primary lacrimal gland atrophy**

H04.141 Primary lacrimal gland atrophy, right lacrimal gland

H04.142 Primary lacrimal gland atrophy, left lacrimal gland

H04.143 Primary lacrimal gland atrophy, bilateral lacrimal glands

H04.149 Primary lacrimal gland atrophy, unspecified lacrimal gland

H04.15 **Secondary lacrimal gland atrophy**

H04.151 Secondary lacrimal gland atrophy, right lacrimal gland

H04.152 Secondary lacrimal gland atrophy, left lacrimal gland

H04.153 Secondary lacrimal gland atrophy, bilateral lacrimal glands

H04.159 Secondary lacrimal gland atrophy, unspecified lacrimal gland

H04.16 **Lacrimal gland dislocation**

H04.161 Lacrimal gland dislocation, right lacrimal gland

H04.162 Lacrimal gland dislocation, left lacrimal gland

H04.163 Lacrimal gland dislocation, bilateral lacrimal glands

H04.169 Lacrimal gland dislocation, unspecified lacrimal gland

H04.19 **Other specified disorders of lacrimal gland**

H04.2 **Epiphora**

H04.20 **Unspecified epiphora**

H04.201 Unspecified epiphora, right side

H04.202 Unspecified epiphora, left side

H04.203 Unspecified epiphora, bilateral

H04.209 Unspecified epiphora, unspecified side

H04.21 **Epiphora due to excess lacrimation**

H04.211 Epiphora due to excess lacrimation, right lacrimal gland

H04.212 Epiphora due to excess lacrimation, left lacrimal gland

H04.213 Epiphora due to excess lacrimation, bilateral lacrimal glands

H04.219 Epiphora due to excess lacrimation unspecified lacrimal gland

H04.22 **Epiphora due to insufficient drainage**

H04.221 Epiphora due to insufficient drainage, right side

H04.222 Epiphora due to insufficient drainage, left side

H04.223 Epiphora due to insufficient drainage, bilateral

H04.229 Epiphora due to insufficient drainage, unspecified side

H04.3 **Acute and unspecified inflammation of lacrimal passages**

Excludes1: neonatal dacryocystitis (P39.1)

H04.30 **Unspecified dacryocystitis**

H04.301 Unspecified dacryocystitis of right lacrimal passage

H04.302 Unspecified dacryocystitis of left lacrimal passage

H04.303 Unspecified dacryocystitis of bilateral lacrimal passages

H04.309 Unspecified dacryocystitis of unspecified lacrimal passage

H04.31 Phlegmonous dacryocystitis

H04.311 Phlegmonous dacryocystitis of right lacrimal passage

H04.312 Phlegmonous dacryocystitis of left lacrimal passage

H04.313 Phlegmonous dacryocystitis of bilateral lacrimal passages

H04.319 Phlegmonous dacryocystitis of unspecified lacrimal passage

H04.32 Acute dacryocystitis

Acute dacryopericystitis

H04.321 Acute dacryocystitis of right lacrimal passage

H04.322 Acute dacryocystitis of left lacrimal passage

H04.323 Acute dacryocystitis of bilateral lacrimal passages

H04.329 Acute dacryocystitis of unspecified lacrimal passage

H04.33 Acute lacrimal canaliculitis

H04.331 Acute lacrimal canaliculitis of right lacrimal passage

H04.332 Acute lacrimal canaliculitis of left lacrimal passage

H04.333 Acute lacrimal canaliculitis of bilateral lacrimal passages

H04.339 Acute lacrimal canaliculitis of unspecified lacrimal passage

H04.4 Chronic inflammation of lacrimal passages

H04.41 Chronic dacryocystitis

H04.411 Chronic dacryocystitis of right lacrimal passage

H04.412 Chronic dacryocystitis of left lacrimal passage

H04.413 Chronic dacryocystitis of bilateral lacrimal passages

H04.419 Chronic dacryocystitis of unspecified lacrimal passage

H04.42 Chronic lacrimal canaliculitis

H04.421 Chronic lacrimal canaliculitis of right lacrimal passage

H04.422 Chronic lacrimal canaliculitis of left lacrimal passage

H04.423 Chronic lacrimal canaliculitis of bilateral lacrimal passages

H04.429 Chronic lacrimal canaliculitis of unspecified lacrimal passage

H04.43 Chronic lacrimal mucocele

H04.431 Chronic lacrimal mucocele of right lacrimal passage

H04.432 Chronic lacrimal mucocele of left lacrimal passage

H04.433 Chronic lacrimal mucocele of bilateral lacrimal passages

H04.439 Chronic lacrimal mucocele of unspecified lacrimal passage

H04.5 Stenosis and insufficiency of lacrimal passages

H04.51 Dacryolith

H04.511 Dacryolith of right lacrimal passage

H04.512 Dacryolith of left lacrimal passage

H04.513 Dacryolith of bilateral lacrimal passages

H04.519 Dacryolith of unspecified lacrimal passage

H04.52 Eversion of lacrimal punctum

H04.521 Eversion of right lacrimal punctum

H04.522 Eversion of left lacrimal punctum

H04.523 Eversion of bilateral lacrimal punctum

H04.529 Eversion of unspecified lacrimal punctum

H04.53 Neonatal obstruction of nasolacrimal duct

Excludes1: congenital stenosis and stricture of lacrimal duct (Q10.5)

H04.531 Neonatal obstruction of right nasolacrimal duct

H04.532 Neonatal obstruction of left nasolacrimal duct

H04.533 Neonatal obstruction of bilateral nasolacrimal duct

H04.539 Neonatal obstruction of unspecified nasolacrimal duct

H04.54 Stenosis of lacrimal canaliculi

H04.541 Stenosis of right lacrimal canaliculi

H04.542 Stenosis of left lacrimal canaliculi

H04.543 Stenosis of bilateral lacrimal canaliculi

H04.549 Stenosis of unspecified lacrimal canaliculi

H04.55 Acquired stenosis of nasolacrimal duct

H04.551 Acquired stenosis of right nasolacrimal duct

H04.552 Acquired stenosis of left nasolacrimal duct

H04.553 Acquired stenosis of bilateral nasolacrimal duct

H04.559 Acquired stenosis of unspecified nasolacrimal duct

H04.56 Stenosis of lacrimal punctum

H04.561 Stenosis of right lacrimal punctum

H04.562 Stenosis of left lacrimal punctum

H04.563 Stenosis of bilateral lacrimal punctum

H04.569 Stenosis of unspecified lacrimal punctum

H04.57 Stenosis of lacrimal sac

H04.571 Stenosis of right lacrimal sac

H04.572 Stenosis of left lacrimal sac

H04.573 Stenosis of bilateral lacrimal sac

H04.579 Stenosis of unspecified lacrimal sac

H04.6 Other changes of lacrimal passages

H04.61 Lacrimal fistula

H04.611 Lacrimal fistula right lacrimal passage

H04.612 Lacrimal fistula left lacrimal passage

H04.613   Lacrimal fistula bilateral lacrimal passages

H04.619   Lacrimal fistula unspecified lacrimal passage

H04.69   Other changes of lacrimal passages

H04.8   Other disorders of lacrimal system

H04.81   Granuloma of lacrimal passages

H04.811   Granuloma of right lacrimal passage

H04.812   Granuloma of left lacrimal passage

H04.813   Granuloma of bilateral lacrimal passages

H04.819   Granuloma of unspecified lacrimal passage

H04.89   Other disorders of lacrimal system

H04.9   Disorder of lacrimal system, unspecified

H05   Disorders of orbit

Excludes1: congenital malformation of orbit (Q10.7)

H05.0   Acute inflammation of orbit

H05.00   Unspecified acute inflammation of orbit

H05.01   Cellulitis of orbit

Abscess of orbit

H05.011   Cellulitis of right orbit

H05.012   Cellulitis of left orbit

H05.013   Cellulitis of bilateral orbits

H05.019   Cellulitis of unspecified orbit

H05.02   Osteomyelitis of orbit

H05.021   Osteomyelitis of right orbit

H05.022   Osteomyelitis of left orbit

H05.023   Osteomyelitis of bilateral orbits

H05.029   Osteomyelitis of unspecified orbit

H05.03   Periostitis of orbit

H05.031   Periostitis of right orbit

H05.032   Periostitis of left orbit

H05.033   Periostitis of bilateral orbits

H05.039   Periostitis of unspecified orbit

H05.04   Tenonitis of orbit

H05.041   Tenonitis of right orbit

H05.042   Tenonitis of left orbit

H05.043   Tenonitis of bilateral orbits

H05.049   Tenonitis of unspecified orbit

H05.1   Chronic inflammatory disorders of orbit

H05.10   Unspecified chronic inflammatory disorders of orbit

H05.11   Granuloma of orbit

Pseudotumor (inflammatory) of orbit

H05.111   Granuloma of right orbit

H05.112   Granuloma of left orbit

H05.113   Granuloma of bilateral orbits

H05.119   Granuloma of unspecified orbit

H05.12   Orbital myositis

H05.121   Orbital myositis, right orbit

H05.122   Orbital myositis, left orbit

H05.123   Orbital myositis, bilateral

H05.129   Orbital myositis, unspecified orbit

H05.2   Exophthalmic conditions

H05.20   Unspecified exophthalmos

H05.21   Displacement (lateral) of globe

H05.211   Displacement (lateral) of globe, right eye

H05.212   Displacement (lateral) of globe, left eye

H05.213   Displacement (lateral) of globe, bilateral

H05.219   Displacement (lateral) of globe, unspecified eye

H05.22   Edema of orbit

Orbital congestion

H05.221   Edema of right orbit

H05.222   Edema of left orbit

H05.223   Edema of bilateral orbit

H05.229   Edema of unspecified orbit

H05.23   Hemorrhage of orbit

H05.231   Hemorrhage of right orbit

H05.232   Hemorrhage of left orbit

H05.233   Hemorrhage of bilateral orbit

H05.239   Hemorrhage of unspecified orbit

H05.24   Constant exophthalmos

H05.241   Constant exophthalmos, right eye

H05.242   Constant exophthalmos, left eye

H05.243   Constant exophthalmos, bilateral

H05.249   Constant exophthalmos, unspecified eye

H05.25   Intermittent exophthalmos

H05.251   Intermittent exophthalmos, right eye

H05.252   Intermittent exophthalmos, left eye

H05.253   Intermittent exophthalmos, bilateral

H05.259   Intermittent exophthalmos, unspecified eye

H05.26   Pulsating exophthalmos

H05.261   Pulsating exophthalmos, right eye

H05.262   Pulsating exophthalmos, left eye

H05.263   Pulsating exophthalmos, bilateral

H05.269   Pulsating exophthalmos, unspecified eye

H05.3   Deformity of orbit

Excludes1: congenital deformity of orbit (Q10.7)

hypertelorism (Q75.2)

H05.30   Unspecified deformity of orbit

H05.31   Atrophy of orbit

H05.311   Atrophy of right orbit

H05.312   Atrophy of left orbit

H05.313   Atrophy of bilateral orbit

H05.319   Atrophy of unspecified orbit

H05.32   Deformity of orbit due to bone disease

Code also associated bone disease

H05.321   Deformity of right orbit due to bone disease

H05.322   Deformity of left orbit due to bone disease

H05.323   Deformity of bilateral orbits due to bone disease

H05.329   Deformity of unspecified orbit due to bone disease

H05.33   Deformity of orbit due to trauma or surgery

H05.331   Deformity of right orbit due to trauma or surgery

H05.332　Deformity of left orbit due to trauma or surgery

H05.333　Deformity of bilateral orbits due to trauma or surgery

H05.339　Deformity of unspecified orbit due to trauma or surgery

H05.34　Enlargement of orbit

H05.341　Enlargement of right orbit

H05.342　Enlargement of left orbit

H05.343　Enlargement of bilateral orbits

H05.349　Enlargement of unspecified orbit

H05.35　Exostosis of orbit

H05.351　Exostosis of right orbit

H05.352　Exostosis of left orbit

H05.353　Exostosis of bilateral orbits

H05.359　Exostosis of unspecified orbit

H05.4　Enophthalmos

H05.40　Unspecified enophthalmos

H05.401　Unspecified enophthalmos, right eye

H05.402　Unspecified enophthalmos, left eye

H05.403　Unspecified enophthalmos, bilateral

H05.409　Unspecified enophthalmos, unspecified eye

H05.41　Enophthalmos due to atrophy of orbital tissue

H05.411　Enophthalmos due to atrophy of orbital tissue, right eye

H05.412　Enophthalmos due to atrophy of orbital tissue, left eye

H05.413　Enophthalmos due to atrophy of orbital tissue, bilateral

H05.419　Enophthalmos due to atrophy of orbital tissue, unspecified eye

H05.42　Enophthalmos due to trauma or surgery

H05.421　Enophthalmos due to trauma or surgery, right eye

H05.422　Enophthalmos due to trauma or surgery, left eye

H05.423　Enophthalmos due to trauma or surgery, bilateral

H05.429　Enophthalmos due to trauma or surgery, unspecified eye

H05.5　Retained (old) foreign body following penetrating wound of orbit

Retrobulbar foreign body

Use Additional Code to identify the type of retained foreign body (Z18.-)

Excludes1: current penetrating wound of orbit (S05.4-)

Excludes2: retained foreign body of eyelid (H02.81-)

retained intraocular foreign body (H44.6-, H44.7-)

H05.50　Retained (old) foreign body following penetrating wound of unspecified orbit

H05.51　Retained (old) foreign body following penetrating wound of right orbit

H05.52　Retained (old) foreign body following penetrating wound of left orbit

H05.53　Retained (old) foreign body following penetrating wound of bilateral orbits

H05.8　Other disorders of orbit

H05.81　Cyst of orbit

Encephalocele of orbit

H05.811　Cyst of right orbit

H05.812　Cyst of left orbit

H05.813　Cyst of bilateral orbits

H05.819　Cyst of unspecified orbit

H05.82　Myopathy of extraocular muscles

H05.821　Myopathy of extraocular muscles, right orbit

H05.822　Myopathy of extraocular muscles, left orbit

H05.823　Myopathy of extraocular muscles, bilateral

H05.829　Myopathy of extraocular muscles, unspecified orbit

H05.89　Other disorders of orbit

H05.9　Unspecified disorder of orbit

DISORDERS OF CONJUNCTIVA (H10-H11)

Definition: Disorders of conjunctiva are disorders of the mucous membrane that lines the inner surface of the eyelid and the exposed surface of the eyeball.

H10　Conjunctivitis

Excludes1: keratoconjunctivitis (H16.2-)

H10.0　Mucopurulent conjunctivitis

H10.01　Acute follicular conjunctivitis

H10.011　Acute follicular conjunctivitis, right eye

H10.012　Acute follicular conjunctivitis, left eye

H10.013　Acute follicular conjunctivitis, bilateral

H10.019　Acute follicular conjunctivitis, unspecified eye

H10.02　Other mucopurulent conjunctivitis

H10.021　Other mucopurulent conjunctivitis, right eye

H10.022　Other mucopurulent conjunctivitis, left eye

H10.023　Other mucopurulent conjunctivitis, bilateral

H10.029　Other mucopurulent conjunctivitis, unspecified eye

H10.1　Acute atopic conjunctivitis

Acute papillary conjunctivitis

H10.10　Acute atopic conjunctivitis, unspecified eye

H10.11　Acute atopic conjunctivitis, right eye

H10.12　Acute atopic conjunctivitis, left eye

H10.13　Acute atopic conjunctivitis, bilateral

H10.2　Other acute conjunctivitis

H10.21　Acute toxic conjunctivitis

Acute chemical conjunctivitis

Code first (T51-T65) to identify chemical and intent

Excludes1: burn and corrosion of eye and adnexa (T26.-)

H10.211　Acute toxic conjunctivitis, right eye

H10.212　Acute toxic conjunctivitis, left eye

H10.213　Acute toxic conjunctivitis, bilateral

H10.219　Acute toxic conjunctivitis, unspecified eye

H10.22　Pseudomembranous conjunctivitis

H10.221　Pseudomembranous conjunctivitis, right eye

H10.222   Pseudomembranous conjunctivitis, left eye

H10.223   Pseudomembranous conjunctivitis, bilateral

H10.229   Pseudomembranous conjunctivitis, unspecified eye

H10.23   Serous conjunctivitis, except viral

Excludes1: viral conjunctivitis (B30.-)

H10.231   Serous conjunctivitis, except viral, right eye

H10.232   Serous conjunctivitis, except viral, left eye

H10.233   Serous conjunctivitis, except viral, bilateral

H10.239   Serous conjunctivitis, except viral, unspecified eye

H10.3   Unspecified acute conjunctivitis

Excludes1: ophthalmia neonatorum NOS (P39.1)

H10.30   Unspecified acute conjunctivitis, unspecified eye

H10.31   Unspecified acute conjunctivitis, right eye

H10.32   Unspecified acute conjunctivitis, left eye

H10.33   Unspecified acute conjunctivitis, bilateral

H10.4   Chronic conjunctivitis

H10.40   Unspecified chronic conjunctivitis

H10.401   Unspecified chronic conjunctivitis, right eye

H10.402   Unspecified chronic conjunctivitis, left eye

H10.403   Unspecified chronic conjunctivitis, bilateral

H10.409   Unspecified chronic conjunctivitis, unspecified eye

H10.41   Chronic giant papillary conjunctivitis

H10.411   Chronic giant papillary conjunctivitis, right eye

H10.412   Chronic giant papillary conjunctivitis, left eye

H10.413   Chronic giant papillary conjunctivitis, bilateral

H10.419   Chronic giant papillary conjunctivitis, unspecified eye

H10.42   Simple chronic conjunctivitis

H10.421   Simple chronic conjunctivitis, right eye

H10.422   Simple chronic conjunctivitis, left eye

H10.423   Simple chronic conjunctivitis, bilateral

H10.429   Simple chronic conjunctivitis, unspecified eye

H10.43   Chronic follicular conjunctivitis

H10.431   Chronic follicular conjunctivitis, right eye

H10.432   Chronic follicular conjunctivitis, left eye

H10.433   Chronic follicular conjunctivitis, bilateral

H10.439   Chronic follicular conjunctivitis, unspecified eye

H10.44   Vernal conjunctivitis

Excludes1: vernal keratoconjunctivitis with limbar and corneal involvement (H16.26-)

H10.45   Other chronic allergic conjunctivitis

H10.5   Blepharoconjunctivitis

H10.50   Unspecified blepharoconjunctivitis

H10.501   Unspecified blepharoconjunctivitis, right eye

H10.502   Unspecified blepharoconjunctivitis, left eye

H10.503   Unspecified blepharoconjunctivitis, bilateral

H10.509   Unspecified blepharoconjunctivitis, unspecified eye

H10.51   Ligneous conjunctivitis

Code also underlying condition if known, such as: plasminogen deficiency (E88.02)

H10.511   Ligneous conjunctivitis, right eye

H10.512   Ligneous conjunctivitis, left eye

H10.513   Ligneous conjunctivitis, bilateral

H10.519   Ligneous conjunctivitis, unspecified eye

H10.52   Angular blepharoconjunctivitis

H10.521   Angular blepharoconjunctivitis, right eye

H10.522   Angular blepharoconjunctivitis, left eye

H10.523   Angular blepharoconjunctivitis, bilateral

H10.529   Angular blepharoconjunctivitis, unspecified eye

H10.53   Contact blepharoconjunctivitis

H10.531   Contact blepharoconjunctivitis, right eye

H10.532   Contact blepharoconjunctivitis, left eye

H10.533   Contact blepharoconjunctivitis, bilateral

H10.539   Contact blepharoconjunctivitis, unspecified eye

H10.8   Other conjunctivitis

H10.81   Pingueculitis

Excludes1: pinguecula (H11.15-)

H10.811   Pingueculitis, right eye

H10.812   Pingueculitis, left eye

H10.813   Pingueculitis, bilateral

H10.819   Pingueculitis, unspecified eye

H10.82   Rosacea conjunctivitis

Code first underlying rosacea dermatitis (L71.-)

H10.821   Rosacea conjunctivitis, right eye

H10.822   Rosacea conjunctivitis, left eye

H10.823   Rosacea conjunctivitis, bilateral

H10.829   Rosacea conjunctivitis, unspecified eye

H10.89   Other conjunctivitis

H10.9   Unspecified conjunctivitis

H11   Other disorders of conjunctiva

Excludes1: keratoconjunctivitis (H16.2-)

H11.0   Pterygium of eye

Excludes1: pseudopterygium (H11.81-)

H11.00 Unspecified pterygium of eye
    H11.001 Unspecified pterygium of right eye
    H11.002 Unspecified pterygium of left eye
    H11.003 Unspecified pterygium of eye, bilateral
    H11.009 Unspecified pterygium of unspecified eye

H11.01 Amyloid pterygium
    H11.011 Amyloid pterygium of right eye
    H11.012 Amyloid pterygium of left eye
    H11.013 Amyloid pterygium of eye, bilateral
    H11.019 Amyloid pterygium of unspecified eye

H11.02 Central pterygium of eye
    H11.021 Central pterygium of right eye
    H11.022 Central pterygium of left eye
    H11.023 Central pterygium of eye, bilateral
    H11.029 Central pterygium of unspecified eye

H11.03 Double pterygium of eye
    H11.031 Double pterygium of right eye
    H11.032 Double pterygium of left eye
    H11.033 Double pterygium of eye, bilateral
    H11.039 Double pterygium of unspecified eye

H11.04 Peripheral pterygium of eye, stationary
    H11.041 Peripheral pterygium, stationary, right eye
    H11.042 Peripheral pterygium, stationary, left eye
    H11.043 Peripheral pterygium, stationary, bilateral
    H11.049 Peripheral pterygium, stationary, unspecified eye

H11.05 Peripheral pterygium of eye, progressive
    H11.051 Peripheral pterygium, progressive, right eye
    H11.052 Peripheral pterygium, progressive, left eye
    H11.053 Peripheral pterygium, progressive, bilateral
    H11.059 Peripheral pterygium, progressive, unspecified eye

H11.06 Recurrent pterygium of eye
    H11.061 Recurrent pterygium of right eye
    H11.062 Recurrent pterygium of left eye
    H11.063 Recurrent pterygium of eye, bilateral
    H11.069 Recurrent pterygium of unspecified eye

H11.1 Conjunctival degenerations and deposits
    Excludes2: pseudopterygium (H11.81)

H11.10 Unspecified conjunctival degenerations

H11.11 Conjunctival deposits
    H11.111 Conjunctival deposits, right eye
    H11.112 Conjunctival deposits, left eye .
    H11.113 Conjunctival deposits, bilateral
    H11.119 Conjunctival deposits, unspecified eye

H11.12 Conjunctival concretions
    H11.121 Conjunctival concretions, right eye
    H11.122 Conjunctival concretions, left eye

H11.123 Conjunctival concretions, bilateral
H11.129 Conjunctival concretions, unspecified eye

H11.13 Conjunctival pigmentations
    Conjunctival argyrosis [argyria]
    H11.131 Conjunctival pigmentations, right eye
    H11.132 Conjunctival pigmentations, left eye
    H11.133 Conjunctival pigmentations, bilateral
    H11.139 Conjunctival pigmentations, unspecified eye

H11.14 Conjunctival xerosis, unspecified
    Excludes1: xerosis of conjunctiva due to vitamin A deficiency (E50.0, E50.1)
    H11.141 Conjunctival xerosis, unspecified, right eye
    H11.142 Conjunctival xerosis, unspecified, left eye
    H11.143 Conjunctival xerosis, unspecified, bilateral
    H11.149 Conjunctival xerosis, unspecified, unspecified eye

H11.15 Pinguecula
    Excludes1: pingueculitis (H10.81-)
    H11.151 Pinguecula, right eye
    H11.152 Pinguecula, left eye
    H11.153 Pinguecula, bilateral
    H11.159 Pinguecula, unspecified eye

H11.2 Conjunctival scars
    H11.21 Conjunctival adhesions and strands (localized)
        H11.211 Conjunctival adhesions and strands (localized), right eye
        H11.212 Conjunctival adhesions and strands (localized), left eye
        H11.213 Conjunctival adhesions and strands (localized), bilateral
        H11.219 Conjunctival adhesions and strands (localized), unspecified eye

    H11.22 Conjunctival granuloma
        H11.221 Conjunctival granuloma, right eye
        H11.222 Conjunctival granuloma, left eye
        H11.223 Conjunctival granuloma, bilateral
        H11.229 Conjunctival granuloma, unspecified

    H11.23 Symblepharon
        H11.231 Symblepharon, right eye
        H11.232 Symblepharon, left eye
        H11.233 Symblepharon, bilateral
        H11.239 Symblepharon, unspecified eye

    H11.24 Scarring of conjunctiva
        H11.241 Scarring of conjunctiva, right eye
        H11.242 Scarring of conjunctiva, left eye
        H11.243 Scarring of conjunctiva, bilateral
        H11.249 Scarring of conjunctiva, unspecified eye

H11.3 Conjunctival hemorrhage
    Subconjunctival hemorrhage
    H11.30 Conjunctival hemorrhage, unspecified eye
    H11.31 Conjunctival hemorrhage, right eye
    H11.32 Conjunctival hemorrhage, left eye

● New code ▲ Revised code Excludes1: Not coded here Excludes2: Not included here ⊗ Placeholder required ⑦7th digit required

H11.33   Conjunctival hemorrhage, bilateral
H11.4   Other conjunctival vascular disorders and cysts
H11.41   Vascular abnormalities of conjunctiva
Conjunctival aneurysm
H11.411   Vascular abnormalities of conjunctiva, right eye
H11.412   Vascular abnormalities of conjunctiva, left eye
H11.413   Vascular abnormalities of conjunctiva, bilateral
H11.419   Vascular abnormalities of conjunctiva, unspecified eye
H11.42   Conjunctival edema
H11.421   Conjunctival edema, right eye
H11.422   Conjunctival edema, left eye
H11.423   Conjunctival edema, bilateral
H11.429   Conjunctival edema, unspecified eye
H11.43   Conjunctival hyperemia
H11.431   Conjunctival hyperemia, right eye
H11.432   Conjunctival hyperemia, left eye
H11.433   Conjunctival hyperemia, bilateral
H11.439   Conjunctival hyperemia, unspecified eye
H11.44   Conjunctival cysts
H11.441   Conjunctival cysts, right eye
H11.442   Conjunctival cysts, left eye
H11.443   Conjunctival cysts, bilateral
H11.449   Conjunctival cysts, unspecified eye
H11.8   Other specified disorders of conjunctiva
H11.81   Pseudopterygium of conjunctiva
H11.811   Pseudopterygium of conjunctiva, right eye
H11.812   Pseudopterygium of conjunctiva, left eye
H11.813   Pseudopterygium of conjunctiva, bilateral
H11.819   Pseudopterygium of conjunctiva, unspecified eye
H11.82   Conjunctivochalasis
H11.821   Conjunctivochalasis, right eye
H11.822   Conjunctivochalasis, left eye
H11.823   Conjunctivochalasis, bilateral
H11.829   Conjunctivochalasis, unspecified eye
H11.89   Other specified disorders of conjunctiva
H11.9   Unspecified disorder of conjunctiva

DISORDERS OF SCLERA, CORNEA, IRIS AND CILIARY BODY (H15-H22)

H15   Disorders of sclera
H15.0   Scleritis
H15.00   Unspecified scleritis
H15.001   Unspecified scleritis, right eye
H15.002   Unspecified scleritis, left eye
H15.003   Unspecified scleritis, bilateral
H15.009   Unspecified scleritis, unspecified eye
H15.01   Anterior scleritis
H15.011   Anterior scleritis, right eye
H15.012   Anterior scleritis, left eye
H15.013   Anterior scleritis, bilateral

H15.019   Anterior scleritis, unspecified eye
H15.02   Brawny scleritis
H15.021   Brawny scleritis, right eye
H15.022   Brawny scleritis, left eye
H15.023   Brawny scleritis, bilateral
H15.029   Brawny scleritis, unspecified eye
H15.03   Posterior scleritis
Sclerotenonitis
H15.031   Posterior scleritis, right eye
H15.032   Posterior scleritis, left eye
H15.033   Posterior scleritis, bilateral
H15.039   Posterior scleritis, unspecified eye
H15.04   Scleritis with corneal involvement
H15.041   Scleritis with corneal involvement, right eye
H15.042   Scleritis with corneal involvement, left eye
H15.043   Scleritis with corneal involvement, bilateral
H15.049   Scleritis with corneal involvement, unspecified eye
H15.05   Scleromalacia perforans
H15.051   Scleromalacia perforans, right eye
H15.052   Scleromalacia perforans, left eye
H15.053   Scleromalacia perforans, bilateral
H15.059   Scleromalacia perforans, unspecified eye
H15.09   Other scleritis
Scleral abscess
H15.091   Other scleritis, right eye
H15.092   Other scleritis, left eye
H15.093   Other scleritis, bilateral
H15.099   Other scleritis, unspecified eye
H15.1   Episcleritis
H15.10   Unspecified episcleritis
H15.101   Unspecified episcleritis, right eye
H15.102   Unspecified episcleritis, left eye
H15.103   Unspecified episcleritis, bilateral
H15.109   Unspecified episcleritis, unspecified eye
H15.11   Episcleritis periodica fugax
H15.111   Episcleritis periodica fugax, right eye
H15.112   Episcleritis periodica fugax, left eye
H15.113   Episcleritis periodica fugax, bilateral
H15.119   Episcleritis periodica fugax, unspecified eye
H15.12   Nodular episcleritis
H15.121   Nodular episcleritis, right eye
H15.122   Nodular episcleritis, left eye
H15.123   Nodular episcleritis, bilateral
H15.129   Nodular episcleritis, unspecified eye
H15.8   Other disorders of sclera
Excludes2: blue sclera (Q13.5)
degenerative myopia (H44.2-)
H15.81   Equatorial staphyloma
H15.811   Equatorial staphyloma, right eye
H15.812   Equatorial staphyloma, left eye
H15.813   Equatorial staphyloma, bilateral

H15.819   Equatorial staphyloma, unspecified eye

H15.82   Localized anterior staphyloma

H15.821   Localized anterior staphyloma, right eye

H15.822   Localized anterior staphyloma, left eye

H15.823   Localized anterior staphyloma, bilateral

H15.829   Localized anterior staphyloma, unspecified eye

H15.83   Staphyloma posticum

H15.831   Staphyloma posticum, right eye

H15.832   Staphyloma posticum, left eye

H15.833   Staphyloma posticum, bilateral

H15.839   Staphyloma posticum, unspecified eye

H15.84   Scleral ectasia

H15.841   Scleral ectasia, right eye

H15.842   Scleral ectasia, left eye

H15.843   Scleral ectasia, bilateral

H15.849   Scleral ectasia, unspecified eye

H15.85   Ring staphyloma

H15.851   Ring staphyloma, right eye

H15.852   Ring staphyloma, left eye

H15.853   Ring staphyloma, bilateral

H15.859   Ring staphyloma, unspecified eye

H15.89   Other disorders of sclera

H15.9   Unspecified disorder of sclera

H16   Keratitis

Definition: Keratitis is an infection or inflammation of the cornea which can be caused by a variety of conditions, including infections, dry eyes, foreign objects, contact lenses, intense light, vitamin a deficiency or allergies.

H16.0   Corneal ulcer

H16.00   Unspecified corneal ulcer

H16.001   Unspecified corneal ulcer, right eye

H16.002   Unspecified corneal ulcer, left eye

H16.003   Unspecified corneal ulcer, bilateral

H16.009   Unspecified corneal ulcer, unspecified eye

H16.01   Central corneal ulcer

H16.011   Central corneal ulcer, right eye

H16.012   Central corneal ulcer, left eye

H16.013   Central corneal ulcer, bilateral

H16.019   Central corneal ulcer, unspecified eye

H16.02   Ring corneal ulcer

H16.021   Ring corneal ulcer, right eye

H16.022   Ring corneal ulcer, left eye

H16.023   Ring corneal ulcer, bilateral

H16.029   Ring corneal ulcer, unspecified eye

H16.03   Corneal ulcer with hypopyon

H16.031   Corneal ulcer with hypopyon, right eye

H16.032   Corneal ulcer with hypopyon, left eye

H16.033   Corneal ulcer with hypopyon, bilateral

H16.039   Corneal ulcer with hypopyon, unspecified eye

H16.04   Marginal corneal ulcer

H16.041   Marginal corneal ulcer, right eye

H16.042   Marginal corneal ulcer, left eye

H16.043   Marginal corneal ulcer, bilateral

H16.049   Marginal corneal ulcer, unspecified eye

H16.05   Mooren's corneal ulcer

H16.051   Mooren's corneal ulcer, right eye

H16.052   Mooren's corneal ulcer, left eye

H16.053   Mooren's corneal ulcer, bilateral

H16.059   Mooren's corneal ulcer, unspecified eye

H16.06   Mycotic corneal ulcer

H16.061   Mycotic corneal ulcer, right eye

H16.062   Mycotic corneal ulcer, left eye

H16.063   Mycotic corneal ulcer, bilateral

H16.069   Mycotic corneal ulcer, unspecified eye

H16.07   Perforated corneal ulcer

H16.071   Perforated corneal ulcer, right eye

H16.072   Perforated corneal ulcer, left eye

H16.073   Perforated corneal ulcer, bilateral

H16.079   Perforated corneal ulcer, unspecified eye

H16.1   Other and unspecified superficial keratitis without conjunctivitis

H16.10   Unspecified superficial keratitis

H16.101   Unspecified superficial keratitis, right eye

H16.102   Unspecified superficial keratitis, left eye

H16.103   Unspecified superficial keratitis, bilateral

H16.109   Unspecified superficial keratitis, unspecified eye

H16.11   Macular keratitis

Areolar keratitis

Nummular keratitis \

Stellate keratitis \

Striate keratitis

H16.111   Macular keratitis, right eye

H16.112   Macular keratitis, left eye

H16.113   Macular keratitis, bilateral

H16.119   Macular keratitis, unspecified eye

H16.12   Filamentary keratitis

H16.121   Filamentary keratitis, right eye

H16.122   Filamentary keratitis, left eye

H16.123   Filamentary keratitis, bilateral

H16.129   Filamentary keratitis, unspecified eye

H16.13   Photokeratitis

Snow blindness Welders keratitis

H16.131   Photokeratitis, right eye

H16.132   Photokeratitis, left eye

H16.133   Photokeratitis, bilateral

H16.139   Photokeratitis, unspecified eye

H16.14   Punctate keratitis

H16.141   **Punctate keratitis, right eye**

H16.142   **Punctate keratitis, left eye**

H16.143   **Punctate keratitis, bilateral**

H16.149   **Punctate keratitis, unspecified eye**

H16.2   **Keratoconjunctivitis**

   H16.20   **Unspecified keratoconjunctivitis**

     Superficial keratitis with conjunctivitis NOS

     H16.201   **Unspecified keratoconjunctivitis, right eye**

     H16.202   **Unspecified keratoconjunctivitis, left eye**

     H16.203   **Unspecified keratoconjunctivitis, bilateral**

     H16.209   **Unspecified keratoconjunctivitis, unspecified eye**

   H16.21   **Exposure keratoconjunctivitis**

     H16.211   **Exposure keratoconjunctivitis, right eye**

     H16.212   **Exposure keratoconjunctivitis, left eye**

     H16.213   **Exposure keratoconjunctivitis, bilateral**

     H16.219   **Exposure keratoconjunctivitis, unspecified eye**

   H16.22   **Keratoconjunctivitis sicca, not specified as Sjögren's**

     Excludes1: Sjögren's syndrome (M35.01)

     H16.221   **Keratoconjunctivitis sicca, not specified as Sjögren's, right eye**

     H16.222   **Keratoconjunctivitis sicca, not specified as Sjögren's, left eye**

     H16.223   **Keratoconjunctivitis sicca, not specified as Sjögren's, bilateral**

     H16.229   **Keratoconjunctivitis sicca, not specified as Sjögren's, unspecified eye**

   H16.23   **Neurotrophic keratoconjunctivitis**

     H16.231   **Neurotrophic keratoconjunctivitis, right eye**

     H16.232   **Neurotrophic keratoconjunctivitis, left eye**

     H16.233   **Neurotrophic keratoconjunctivitis, bilateral**

     H16.239   **Neurotrophic keratoconjunctivitis, unspecified eye**

   H16.24   **Ophthalmia nodosa**

     H16.241   **Ophthalmia nodosa, right eye**

     H16.242   **Ophthalmia nodosa, left eye**

     H16.243   **Ophthalmia nodosa, bilateral**

     H16.249   **Ophthalmia nodosa, unspecified eye**

   H16.25   **Phlyctenular keratoconjunctivitis**

     H16.251   **Phlyctenular keratoconjunctivitis, right eye**

     H16.252   **Phlyctenular keratoconjunctivitis, left eye**

     H16.253   **Phlyctenular keratoconjunctivitis, bilateral**

     H16.259   **Phlyctenular keratoconjunctivitis, unspecified eye**

   H16.26   **Vernal keratoconjunctivitis, with limbar and corneal involvement**

     Excludes1: vernal conjunctivitis without limbar and corneal involvement (H10.44)

     H16.261   **Vernal keratoconjunctivitis, with limbar and corneal involvement, right eye**

     H16.262   **Vernal keratoconjunctivitis, with limbar and corneal involvement, left eye**

     H16.263   **Vernal keratoconjunctivitis, with limbar and corneal involvement, bilateral**

     H16.269   **Vernal keratoconjunctivitis, with limbar and corneal involvement, unspecified eye**

   H16.29   **Other keratoconjunctivitis**

     H16.291   **Other keratoconjunctivitis, right eye**

     H16.292   **Other keratoconjunctivitis, left eye**

     H16.293   **Other keratoconjunctivitis, bilateral**

     H16.299   **Other keratoconjunctivitis, unspecified eye**

H16.3   **Interstitial and deep keratitis**

   H16.30   **Unspecified interstitial keratitis**

     H16.301   **Unspecified interstitial keratitis, right eye**

     H16.302   **Unspecified interstitial keratitis, left eye**

     H16.303   **Unspecified interstitial keratitis, bilateral**

     H16.309   **Unspecified interstitial keratitis, unspecified eye**

   H16.31   **Corneal abscess**

     H16.311   **Corneal abscess, right eye**

     H16.312   **Corneal abscess, left eye**

     H16.313   **Corneal abscess, bilateral**

     H16.319   **Corneal abscess, unspecified eye**

   H16.32   **Diffuse interstitial keratitis**

     Cogan's syndrome

     H16.321   **Diffuse interstitial keratitis, right eye**

     H16.322   **Diffuse interstitial keratitis, left eye**

     H16.323   **Diffuse interstitial keratitis, bilateral**

     H16.329   **Diffuse interstitial keratitis, unspecified eye**

   H16.33   **Sclerosing keratitis**

     H16.331   **Sclerosing keratitis, right eye**

     H16.332   **Sclerosing keratitis, left eye**

     H16.333   **Sclerosing keratitis, bilateral**

     H16.339   **Sclerosing keratitis, unspecified eye**

   H16.39   **Other interstitial and deep keratitis**

     H16.391   **Other interstitial and deep keratitis, right eye**

     H16.392   **Other interstitial and deep keratitis, left eye**

     H16.393   **Other interstitial and deep keratitis, bilateral**

     H16.399   **Other interstitial and deep keratitis, unspecified eye**

H16.4   **Corneal neovascularization**

   H16.40   **Unspecified corneal neovascularization**

     H16.401   **Unspecified corneal neovascularization, right eye**

H16.402 Unspecified corneal neovascularization, left eye

H16.403 Unspecified corneal neovascularization, bilateral

H16.409 Unspecified corneal neovascularization, unspecified eye

H16.41 Ghost vessels (corneal)

H16.411 Ghost vessels (corneal), right eye

H16.412 Ghost vessels (corneal), left eye

H16.413 Ghost vessels (corneal), bilateral

H16.419 Ghost vessels (corneal), unspecified eye

H16.42 Pannus (corneal)

H16.421 Pannus (corneal), right eye

H16.422 Pannus (corneal), left eye

H16.423 Pannus (corneal), bilateral

H16.429 Pannus (corneal), unspecified eye

H16.43 Localized vascularization of cornea

H16.431 Localized vascularization of cornea, right eye

H16.432 Localized vascularization of cornea, left eye

H16.433 Localized vascularization of cornea, bilateral

H16.439 Localized vascularization of cornea, unspecified eye

H16.44 Deep vascularization of cornea

H16.441 Deep vascularization of cornea, right eye

H16.442 Deep vascularization of cornea, left eye

H16.443 Deep vascularization of cornea, bilateral

H16.449 Deep vascularization of cornea, unspecified eye

H16.8 Other keratitis

H16.9 Unspecified keratitis

H17 Corneal scars and opacities

H17.0 Adherent leukoma

H17.00 Adherent leukoma, unspecified eye

H17.01 Adherent leukoma, right eye

H17.02 Adherent leukoma, left eye

H17.03 Adherent leukoma, bilateral

H17.1 Central corneal opacity

Definition: Corneal opacity is a cloudy spot in the cornea, which is normally transparent. Causes include corneal scar tissue and infection.

H17.10 Central corneal opacity, unspecified eye

H17.11 Central corneal opacity, right eye

H17.12 Central corneal opacity, left eye

H17.13 Central corneal opacity, bilateral

H17.8 Other corneal scars and opacities

H17.81 Minor opacity of cornea

Corneal nebula

H17.811 Minor opacity of cornea, right eye

H17.812 Minor opacity of cornea, left eye

H17.813 Minor opacity of cornea, bilateral

H17.819 Minor opacity of cornea, unspecified eye

H17.82 Peripheral opacity of cornea

H17.821 Peripheral opacity of cornea, right eye

H17.822 Peripheral opacity of cornea, left eye

H17.823 Peripheral opacity of cornea, bilateral

H17.829 Peripheral opacity of cornea, unspecified eye

H17.89 Other corneal scars and opacities

H17.9 Unspecified corneal scar and opacity

H18 Other disorders of cornea

H18.0 Corneal pigmentations and deposits

H18.00 Unspecified corneal deposit

H18.001 Unspecified corneal deposit, right eye

H18.002 Unspecified corneal deposit, left eye

H18.003 Unspecified corneal deposit, bilateral

H18.009 Unspecified corneal deposit, unspecified eye

H18.01 Anterior corneal pigmentations

Staehlin's line

H18.011 Anterior corneal pigmentations, right eye

H18.012 Anterior corneal pigmentations, left eye

H18.013 Anterior corneal pigmentations, bilateral

H18.019 Anterior corneal pigmentations, unspecified eye

H18.02 Argentous corneal deposits

H18.021 Argentous corneal deposits, right eye

H18.022 Argentous corneal deposits, left eye

H18.023 Argentous corneal deposits, bilateral

H18.029 Argentous corneal deposits, unspecified eye

H18.03 Corneal deposits in metabolic disorders

Code also associated metabolic disorder

H18.031 Corneal deposits in metabolic disorders, right eye

H18.032 Corneal deposits in metabolic disorders, left eye

H18.033 Corneal deposits in metabolic disorders, bilateral

H18.039 Corneal deposits in metabolic disorders, unspecified eye

H18.04 Kayser-Fleischer ring

Code also associated Wilson's disease (E83.01)

H18.041 Kayser-Fleischer ring, right eye

H18.042 Kayser-Fleischer ring, left eye

H18.043 Kayser-Fleischer ring, bilateral

H18.049 Kayser-Fleischer ring, unspecified eye

H18.05 Posterior corneal pigmentations

Krukenberg's spindle

H18.051 Posterior corneal pigmentations, right eye

H18.052 Posterior corneal pigmentations, left eye

H18.053 Posterior corneal pigmentations, bilateral

H18.059 Posterior corneal pigmentations, unspecified eye

H18.06 Stromal corneal pigmentations

Hematocornea

H18.061   **Stromal corneal pigmentations, right eye**

H18.062   **Stromal corneal pigmentations, left eye**

H18.063   **Stromal corneal pigmentations, bilateral**

H18.069   **Stromal corneal pigmentations, unspecified eye**

H18.1   **Bullous keratopathy**

   H18.10   **Bullous keratopathy, unspecified eye**

   H18.11   **Bullous keratopathy, right eye**

   H18.12   **Bullous keratopathy, left eye**

   H18.13   **Bullous keratopathy, bilateral**

H18.2   **Other and unspecified corneal edema**

   H18.20   **Unspecified corneal edema**

   H18.21   **Corneal edema secondary to contact lens**

     Excludes2: Other corneal disorders due to contact lens (H18.82-)

     H18.211   **Corneal edema secondary to contact lens, right eye**

     H18.212   **Corneal edema secondary to contact lens, left eye**

     H18.213   **Corneal edema secondary to contact lens, bilateral**

     H18.219   **Corneal edema secondary to contact lens, unspecified eye**

   H18.22   **Idiopathic corneal edema**

     H18.221   **Idiopathic corneal edema, right eye**

     H18.222   **Idiopathic corneal edema, left eye**

     H18.223   **Idiopathic corneal edema, bilateral**

     H18.229   **Idiopathic corneal edema, unspecified eye**

   H18.23   **Secondary corneal edema**

     H18.231   **Secondary corneal edema, right eye**

     H18.232   **Secondary corneal edema, left eye**

     H18.233   **Secondary corneal edema, bilateral**

     H18.239   **Secondary corneal edema, unspecified eye**

H18.3   **Changes of corneal membranes**

   H18.30   **Unspecified corneal membrane change**

   H18.31   **Folds and rupture in Bowman's membrane**

     H18.311   **Folds and rupture in Bowman's membrane, right eye**

     H18.312   **Folds and rupture in Bowman's membrane, left eye**

     H18.313   **Folds and rupture in Bowman's membrane, bilateral**

     H18.319   **Folds and rupture in Bowman's membrane, unspecified eye**

   H18.32   **Folds in Descemet's membrane**

     H18.321   **Folds in Descemet's membrane, right eye**

     H18.322   **Folds in Descemet's membrane, left eye**

     H18.323   **Folds in Descemet's membrane, bilateral**

     H18.329   **Folds in Descemet's membrane, unspecified eye**

   H18.33   **Rupture in Descemet's membrane**

H18.331   **Rupture in Descemet's membrane, right eye**

H18.332   **Rupture in Descemet's membrane, left eye**

H18.333   **Rupture in Descemet's membrane, bilateral**

H18.339   **Rupture in Descemet's membrane, unspecified eye**

H18.4   **Corneal degeneration**

   Excludes1: Mooren's ulcer (H16.0-)

   recurrent erosion of cornea (H18.83-)

   H18.40   **Unspecified corneal degeneration**

   H18.41   **Arcus senilis**

   Senile corneal changes

     H18.411   **Arcus senilis, right eye**

     H18.412   **Arcus senilis, left eye**

     H18.413   **Arcus senilis, bilateral**

     H18.419   **Arcus senilis, unspecified eye**

   H18.42   **Band keratopathy**

     H18.421   **Band keratopathy, right eye**

     H18.422   **Band keratopathy, left eye**

     H18.423   **Band keratopathy, bilateral**

     H18.429   **Band keratopathy, unspecified eye**

   H18.43   **Other calcereous corneal degeneration**

   H18.44   **Keratomalacia**

     Excludes1: keratomalacia due to vitamin A deficiency (E50.4)

     H18.441   **Keratomalacia, right eye**

     H18.442   **Keratomalacia, left eye**

     H18.443   **Keratomalacia, bilateral**

     H18.449   **Keratomalacia, unspecified eye**

   H18.45   **Nodular corneal degeneration**

     H18.451   **Nodular corneal degeneration, right eye**

     H18.452   **Nodular corneal degeneration, left eye**

     H18.453   **Nodular corneal degeneration, bilateral**

     H18.459   **Nodular corneal degeneration, unspecified eye**

   H18.46   **Peripheral corneal degeneration**

     H18.461   **Peripheral corneal degeneration, right eye**

     H18.462   **Peripheral corneal degeneration, left eye**

     H18.463   **Peripheral corneal degeneration, bilateral**

     H18.469   **Peripheral corneal degeneration, unspecified eye**

   H18.49   **Other corneal degeneration**

H18.5   **Hereditary corneal dystrophies**

   H18.50   **Unspecified hereditary corneal dystrophies**

     H18.501   **Unspecified hereditary corneal dystrophies, right eye**

     H18.502   **Unspecified hereditary corneal dystrophies, left eye**

     H18.503   **Unspecified hereditary corneal dystrophies, bilateral**

     H18.509   **Unspecified hereditary corneal dystrophies, unspecified eye**

H18.51 **Endothelial corneal dystrophy**
Fuchs' dystrophy
    H18.511 **Endothelial corneal dystrophy, right eye**
    H18.512 **Endothelial corneal dystrophy, left eye**
    H18.513 **Endothelial corneal dystrophy, bilateral**
    H18.519 **Endothelial corneal dystrophy, unspecified eye**

H18.52 **Epithelial (juvenile) corneal dystrophy**
    H18.521 **Epithelial (juvenile) corneal dystrophy, right eye**
    H18.522 **Epithelial (juvenile) corneal dystrophy, left eye**
    H18.523 **Epithelial (juvenile) corneal dystrophy, bilateral**
    H18.529 **Epithelial (juvenile) corneal dystrophy, unspecified eye**

H18.53 **Granular corneal dystrophy**
    H18.531 **Granular corneal dystrophy, right eye**
    H18.532 **Granular corneal dystrophy, left eye**
    H18.533 **Granular corneal dystrophy, bilateral**
    H18.539 **Granular corneal dystrophy, unspecified eye**

H18.54 **Lattice corneal dystrophy**
    H18.541 **Lattice corneal dystrophy, right eye**
    H18.542 **Lattice corneal dystrophy, left eye**
    H18.543 **Lattice corneal dystrophy, bilateral**
    H18.549 **Lattice corneal dystrophy, unspecified eye**

H18.55 **Macular corneal dystrophy**
    H18.551 **Macular corneal dystrophy, right eye**
    H18.552 **Macular corneal dystrophy, left eye**
    H18.553 **Macular corneal dystrophy, bilateral**
    H18.559 **Macular corneal dystrophy, unspecified eye**

H18.59 **Other hereditary corneal dystrophies**
    H18.591 **Other hereditary corneal dystrophies, right eye**
    H18.592 **Other hereditary corneal dystrophies, left eye**
    H18.593 **Other hereditary corneal dystrophies, bilateral**
    H18.599 **Other hereditary corneal dystrophies, unspecified eye**

H18.6 **Keratoconus**
H18.60 **Keratoconus, unspecified**
    H18.601 **Keratoconus, unspecified, right eye**
    H18.602 **Keratoconus, unspecified, left eye**
    H18.603 **Keratoconus, unspecified, bilateral**
    H18.609 **Keratoconus, unspecified, unspecified eye**

H18.61 **Keratoconus, stable**
    H18.611 **Keratoconus, stable, right eye**
    H18.612 **Keratoconus, stable, left eye**
    H18.613 **Keratoconus, stable, bilateral**
    H18.619 **Keratoconus, stable, unspecified eye**

H18.62 **Keratoconus, unstable**

Acute hydrops
    H18.621 **Keratoconus, unstable, right eye**
    H18.622 **Keratoconus, unstable, left eye**
    H18.623 **Keratoconus, unstable, bilateral**
    H18.629 **Keratoconus, unstable, unspecified eye**

H18.7 **Other and unspecified corneal deformities**
Excludes1: congenital malformations of cornea (Q13.3-Q13.4)

H18.70 **Unspecified corneal deformity**
H18.71 **Corneal ectasia**
    H18.711 **Corneal ectasia, right eye**
    H18.712 **Corneal ectasia, left eye**
    H18.713 **Corneal ectasia, bilateral**
    H18.719 **Corneal ectasia, unspecified eye**

H18.72 **Corneal staphyloma**
    H18.721 **Corneal staphyloma, right eye**
    H18.722 **Corneal staphyloma, left eye**
    H18.723 **Corneal staphyloma, bilateral**
    H18.729 **Corneal staphyloma, unspecified eye**

H18.73 **Descemetocele**
    H18.731 **Descemetocele, right eye**
    H18.732 **Descemetocele, left eye**
    H18.733 **Descemetocele, bilateral**
    H18.739 **Descemetocele, unspecified eye**

H18.79 **Other corneal deformities**
    H18.791 **Other corneal deformities, right eye**
    H18.792 **Other corneal deformities, left eye**
    H18.793 **Other corneal deformities, bilateral**
    H18.799 **Other corneal deformities, unspecified eye**

H18.8 **Other specified disorders of cornea**
H18.81 **Anesthesia and hypoesthesia of cornea**
    H18.811 **Anesthesia and hypoesthesia of cornea, right eye**
    H18.812 **Anesthesia and hypoesthesia of cornea, left eye**
    H18.813 **Anesthesia and hypoesthesia of cornea, bilateral**
    H18.819 **Anesthesia and hypoesthesia of cornea, unspecified eye**

H18.82 **Corneal disorder due to contact lens**
Excludes2: corneal edema due to contact lens (H18.21-)
    H18.821 **Corneal disorder due to contact lens, right eye**
    H18.822 **Corneal disorder due to contact lens, left eye**
    H18.823 **Corneal disorder due to contact lens, bilateral**
    H18.829 **Corneal disorder due to contact lens, unspecified eye**

H18.83 **Recurrent erosion of cornea**
    H18.831 **Recurrent erosion of cornea, right eye**
    H18.832 **Recurrent erosion of cornea, left eye**
    H18.833 **Recurrent erosion of cornea, bilateral**
    H18.839 **Recurrent erosion of cornea, unspecified eye**

● New code   ▲ Revised code   **Excludes1:** Not coded here   **Excludes2:** Not included here   ⊗ Placeholder required   ⑦ 7th digit required

H18.89 Other specified disorders of cornea

    H18.891 Other specified disorders of cornea, right eye

    H18.892 Other specified disorders of cornea, left eye

    H18.893 Other specified disorders of cornea, bilateral

    H18.899 Other specified disorders of cornea, unspecified eye

H18.9 Unspecified disorder of cornea

H20 Iridocyclitis

  H20.0 Acute and subacute iridocyclitis

    Acute anterior uveitis

    Acute cyclitis

    Acute iritis

    Subacute anterior uveitis

    Subacute cyclitis

    Subacute iritis

    Excludes1: iridocyclitis, iritis, uveitis (due to) (in) diabetes mellitus (E08-E13 with .39)

    iridocyclitis, iritis, uveitis (due to) (in) diphtheria (A36.89)

    iridocyclitis, iritis, uveitis (due to) (in) gonococcal (A54.32)

    iridocyclitis, iritis, uveitis (due to) (in) herpes (simplex) (B00.51)

    iridocyclitis, iritis, uveitis (due to) (in) herpes zoster (B02.32)

    iridocyclitis, iritis, uveitis (due to) (in) late congenital syphilis (A50.39)

    iridocyclitis, iritis, uveitis (due to) (in) late syphilis (A52.71)

    iridocyclitis, iritis, uveitis (due to) (in) sarcoidosis (D86.83)

    iridocyclitis, iritis, uveitis (due to) (in) syphilis (A51.43)

    iridocyclitis, iritis, uveitis (due to) (in) toxoplasmosis (B58.09)

    iridocyclitis, iritis, uveitis (due to) (in) tuberculosis (A18.54)

    H20.00 Unspecified acute and subacute iridocyclitis

    H20.01 Primary iridocyclitis

      H20.011 Primary iridocyclitis, right eye

      H20.012 Primary iridocyclitis, left eye

      H20.013 Primary iridocyclitis, bilateral

      H20.019 Primary iridocyclitis, unspecified eye

    H20.02 Recurrent acute iridocyclitis

      H20.021 Recurrent acute iridocyclitis, right eye

      H20.022 Recurrent acute iridocyclitis, left eye

      H20.023 Recurrent acute iridocyclitis, bilateral

      H20.029 Recurrent acute iridocyclitis, unspecified eye

    H20.03 Secondary infectious iridocyclitis

      H20.031 Secondary infectious iridocyclitis, right eye

      H20.032 Secondary infectious iridocyclitis, left eye

      H20.033 Secondary infectious iridocyclitis, bilateral

      H20.039 Secondary infectious iridocyclitis, unspecified eye

    H20.04 Secondary noninfectious iridocyclitis

      H20.041 Secondary noninfectious iridocyclitis, right eye

      H20.042 Secondary noninfectious iridocyclitis, left eye

      H20.043 Secondary noninfectious iridocyclitis, bilateral

      H20.049 Secondary noninfectious iridocyclitis, unspecified eye

    H20.05 Hypopyon

      H20.051 Hypopyon, right eye

      H20.052 Hypopyon, left eye

      H20.053 Hypopyon, bilateral

      H20.059 Hypopyon, unspecified eye

  H20.1 Chronic iridocyclitis

    <u>Use Additional Code</u> for any associated cataract (H26.21-)

    Excludes2: posterior cyclitis (H30.2-)

    H20.10 Chronic iridocyclitis, unspecified eye

    H20.11 Chronic iridocyclitis, right eye

    H20.12 Chronic iridocyclitis, left eye

    H20.13 Chronic iridocyclitis, bilateral

  H20.2 Lens-induced iridocyclitis

    H20.20 Lens-induced iridocyclitis, unspecified eye

    H20.21 Lens-induced iridocyclitis, right eye

    H20.22 Lens-induced iridocyclitis, left eye

    H20.23 Lens-induced iridocyclitis, bilateral

  H20.8 Other iridocyclitis

    Excludes2: glaucomatocyclitic crises (H40.4-)

    posterior cyclitis (H30.2-) sympathetic uveitis (H44.13-)

    H20.81 Fuchs' heterochromic cyclitis

      H20.811 Fuchs' heterochromic cyclitis, right eye

      H20.812 Fuchs' heterochromic cyclitis, left eye

      H20.813 Fuchs' heterochromic cyclitis, bilateral

      H20.819 Fuchs' heterochromic cyclitis, unspecified eye

    H20.82 Vogt-Koyanagi syndrome

      H20.821 Vogt-Koyanagi syndrome, right eye

      H20.822 Vogt-Koyanagi syndrome, left eye

      H20.823 Vogt-Koyanagi syndrome, bilateral

      H20.829 Vogt-Koyanagi syndrome, unspecified eye

  H20.9 Unspecified iridocyclitis

    Uveitis NOS

H21 Other disorders of iris and ciliary body

  Excludes2: sympathetic uveitis (H44.1-)

  H21.0 Hyphema

    Excludes1: traumatic hyphema (S05.1-)

    H21.00 Hyphema, unspecified eye

    H21.01 Hyphema, right eye

    H21.02 Hyphema, left eye

    H21.03 Hyphema, bilateral

  H21.1 Other vascular disorders of iris and ciliary body

    Neovascularization of iris or ciliary body

Rubeosis iridis

Rubeosis of iris

H21.1X Other vascular disorders of iris and ciliary body

    H21.1X1 Other vascular disorders of iris and ciliary body, right eye

    H21.1X2 Other vascular disorders of iris and ciliary body, left eye

    H21.1X3 Other vascular disorders of iris and ciliary body, bilateral

    H21.1X9 Other vascular disorders of iris and ciliary body, unspecified eye

H21.2 Degeneration of iris and ciliary body

  H21.21 Degeneration of chamber angle

    H21.211 Degeneration of chamber angle, right eye

    H21.212 Degeneration of chamber angle, left eye

    H21.213 Degeneration of chamber angle, bilateral

    H21.219 Degeneration of chamber angle, unspecified eye

  H21.22 Degeneration of ciliary body

    H21.221 Degeneration of ciliary body, right eye

    H21.222 Degeneration of ciliary body, left eye

    H21.223 Degeneration of ciliary body, bilateral

    H21.229 Degeneration of ciliary body, unspecified eye

  H21.23 Degeneration of iris (pigmentary)

Translucency of iris

    H21.231 Degeneration of iris (pigmentary), right eye

    H21.232 Degeneration of iris (pigmentary), left eye

    H21.233 Degeneration of iris (pigmentary), bilateral

    H21.239 Degeneration of iris (pigmentary), unspecified eye

  H21.24 Degeneration of pupillary margin

    H21.241 Degeneration of pupillary margin, right eye

    H21.242 Degeneration of pupillary margin, left eye

    H21.243 Degeneration of pupillary margin, bilateral

    H21.249 Degeneration of pupillary margin, unspecified eye

  H21.25 Iridoschisis

    H21.251 Iridoschisis, right eye

    H21.252 Iridoschisis, left eye

    H21.253 Iridoschisis, bilateral

    H21.259 Iridoschisis, unspecified eye

  H21.26 Iris atrophy (essential) (progressive)

    H21.261 Iris atrophy (essential) (progressive), right eye

    H21.262 Iris atrophy (essential) (progressive), left eye

    H21.263 Iris atrophy (essential) (progressive), bilateral

    H21.269 Iris atrophy (essential) (progressive), unspecified eye

  H21.27 Miotic pupillary cyst

    H21.271 Miotic pupillary cyst, right eye

    H21.272 Miotic pupillary cyst, left eye

    H21.273 Miotic pupillary cyst, bilateral

    H21.279 Miotic pupillary cyst, unspecified eye

  H21.29 Other iris atrophy

H21.3 Cyst of iris, ciliary body and anterior chamber

Excludes2: miotic pupillary cyst (H21.27-)

  H21.30 Idiopathic cysts of iris, ciliary body or anterior chamber

Cyst of iris, ciliary body or anterior chamber NOS

    H21.301 Idiopathic cysts of iris, ciliary body or anterior chamber, right eye

    H21.302 Idiopathic cysts of iris, ciliary body or anterior chamber, left eye

    H21.303 Idiopathic cysts of iris, ciliary body or anterior chamber, bilateral

    H21.309 Idiopathic cysts of iris, ciliary body or anterior chamber, unspecified eye

  H21.31 Exudative cysts of iris or anterior chamber

    H21.311 Exudative cysts of iris or anterior chamber, right eye

    H21.312 Exudative cysts of iris or anterior chamber, left eye

    H21.313 Exudative cysts of iris or anterior chamber, bilateral

    H21.319 Exudative cysts of iris or anterior chamber, unspecified eye

  H21.32 Implantation cysts of iris, ciliary body or anterior chamber

    H21.321 Implantation cysts of iris, ciliary body or anterior chamber, right eye

    H21.322 Implantation cysts of iris, ciliary body or anterior chamber, left eye

    H21.323 Implantation cysts of iris, ciliary body or anterior chamber, bilateral

    H21.329 Implantation cysts of iris, ciliary body or anterior chamber, unspecified eye

  H21.33 Parasitic cyst of iris, ciliary body or anterior chamber

    H21.331 Parasitic cyst of iris, ciliary body or anterior chamber, right eye

    H21.332 Parasitic cyst of iris, ciliary body or anterior chamber, left eye

    H21.333 Parasitic cyst of iris, ciliary body or anterior chamber, bilateral

    H21.339 Parasitic cyst of iris, ciliary body or anterior chamber, unspecified eye

  H21.34 Primary cyst of pars plana

    H21.341 Primary cyst of pars plana, right eye

    H21.342 Primary cyst of pars plana, left eye

    H21.343 Primary cyst of pars plana, bilateral

    H21.349 Primary cyst of pars plana, unspecified eye

  H21.35 Exudative cyst of pars plana

    H21.351 Exudative cyst of pars plana, right eye

    H21.352 Exudative cyst of pars plana, left eye

H21.353 **Exudative cyst of pars plana, bilateral**

H21.359 **Exudative cyst of pars plana, unspecified eye**

H21.4 **Pupillary membranes**

Iris bombé

Pupillary occlusion

Pupillary seclusion

Excludes1: congenital pupillary membranes (Q13.8)

H21.40 **Pupillary membranes, unspecified eye**

H21.41 **Pupillary membranes, right eye**

H21.42 **Pupillary membranes, left eye**

H21.43 **Pupillary membranes, bilateral**

H21.5 **Other and unspecified adhesions and disruptions of iris and ciliary body**

Excludes1: corectopia (Q13.2)

H21.50 **Unspecified adhesions of iris**

Synechia (iris) NOS

H21.501 **Unspecified adhesions of iris, right eye**

H21.502 **Unspecified adhesions of iris, left eye**

H21.503 **Unspecified adhesions of iris, bilateral**

H21.509 **Unspecified adhesions of iris and ciliary body, unspecified eye**

H21.51 **Anterior synechiae (iris)**

H21.511 **Anterior synechiae (iris), right eye**

H21.512 **Anterior synechiae (iris), left eye**

H21.513 **Anterior synechiae (iris), bilateral**

H21.519 **Anterior synechiae (iris), unspecified eye**

H21.52 **Goniosynechiae**

H21.521 **Goniosynechiae, right eye**

H21.522 **Goniosynechiae, left eye**

H21.523 **Goniosynechiae, bilateral**

H21.529 **Goniosynechiae, unspecified eye**

H21.53 **Iridodialysis**

H21.531 **Iridodialysis, right eye**

H21.532 **Iridodialysis, left eye**

H21.533 **Iridodialysis, bilateral**

H21.539 **Iridodialysis, unspecified eye**

H21.54 **Posterior synechiae (iris)**

H21.541 **Posterior synechiae (iris), right eye**

H21.542 **Posterior synechiae (iris), left eye**

H21.543 **Posterior synechiae (iris), bilateral**

H21.549 **Posterior synechiae (iris), unspecified eye**

H21.55 **Recession of chamber angle**

H21.551 **Recession of chamber angle, right eye**

H21.552 **Recession of chamber angle, left eye**

H21.553 **Recession of chamber angle, bilateral**

H21.559 **Recession of chamber angle, unspecified eye**

H21.56 **Pupillary abnormalities**

Deformed pupil

Ectopic pupil

Rupture of sphincter, pupil

Excludes1: congenital deformity of pupil (Q13.2-)

H21.561 **Pupillary abnormality, right eye**

H21.562 **Pupillary abnormality, left eye**

H21.563 **Pupillary abnormality, bilateral**

H21.569 **Pupillary abnormality, unspecified eye**

H21.8 **Other specified disorders of iris and ciliary body**

H21.81 **Floppy iris syndrome**

Intraoperative floppy iris syndrome (IFIS)

Use Additional Code for adverse effect, if applicable, to identify drug (T36-T50 with fifth or sixth character 5)

H21.82 **Plateau iris syndrome (post-iridectomy) (postprocedural)**

H21.89 **Other specified disorders of iris and ciliary body**

H21.9 **Unspecified disorder of iris and ciliary body**

H22 **Disorders of iris and ciliary body in diseases classified elsewhere**

Code first underlying disease, such as:

gout (M1A.-, M10.-)

leprosy (A30.-)

parasitic disease (B89)

DISORDERS OF LENS (H25-H28)

H25 **Age-related cataract**

Definition: A cataract is a clouding that develops in the crystalline lens of the eye or in its envelope, varying in degree from slight to complete opacity and obstructing the passage of light. Senile cataract

Excludes2: capsular glaucoma with pseudoexfoliation of lens (H40.1-)

H25.0 **Age-related incipient cataract**

H25.01 **Cortical age-related cataract**

H25.011 **Cortical age-related cataract, right eye**

H25.012 **Cortical age-related cataract, left eye**

H25.013 **Cortical age-related cataract, bilateral**

H25.019 **Cortical age-related cataract, unspecified eye**

H25.03 **Anterior subcapsular polar age-related cataract**

H25.031 **Anterior subcapsular polar age-related cataract, right eye**

H25.032 **Anterior subcapsular polar age-related cataract, left eye**

H25.033 **Anterior subcapsular polar age-related cataract, bilateral**

H25.039 **Anterior subcapsular polar age-related cataract, unspecified eye**

H25.04 **Posterior subcapsular polar age-related cataract**

H25.041 **Posterior subcapsular polar age-related cataract, right eye**

H25.042 **Posterior subcapsular polar age-related cataract, left eye**

H25.043 **Posterior subcapsular polar age-related cataract, bilateral**

H25.049 **Posterior subcapsular polar age-related cataract, unspecified eye**

H25.09 **Other age-related incipient cataract**

Coronary age-related cataract

Punctate age-related cataract

Water clefts

H25.091	Other age-related incipient cataract, right eye
H25.092	Other age-related incipient cataract, left eye
H25.093	Other age-related incipient cataract, bilateral
H25.099	Other age-related incipient cataract, unspecified eye

H25.1   **Age-related nuclear cataract**

Cataracta brunescens Nuclear sclerosis cataract

H25.10	Age-related nuclear cataract, unspecified eye
H25.11	Age-related nuclear cataract, right eye
H25.12	Age-related nuclear cataract, left eye
H25.13	Age-related nuclear cataract, bilateral

H25.2   **Age-related cataract, morgagnian type**

Age-related hypermature cataract

H25.20	Age-related cataract, morgagnian type, unspecified eye
H25.21	Age-related cataract, morgagnian type, right eye
H25.22	Age-related cataract, morgagnian type, left eye
H25.23	Age-related cataract, morgagnian type, bilateral

H25.8   **Other age-related cataract**

| H25.81 | Combined forms of age-related cataract |

H25.811	Combined forms of age-related cataract, right eye
H25.812	Combined forms of age-related cataract, left eye
H25.813	Combined forms of age-related cataract, bilateral
H25.819	Combined forms of age-related cataract, unspecified eye

| H25.89 | Other age-related cataract |

H25.9   **Unspecified age-related cataract**

H26   **Other cataract**

Excludes1: congenital cataract (Q12.0)

H26.0   **Infantile and juvenile cataract**

| H26.00 | Unspecified infantile and juvenile cataract |

H26.001	Unspecified infantile and juvenile cataract, right eye
H26.002	Unspecified infantile and juvenile cataract, left eye
H26.003	Unspecified infantile and juvenile cataract, bilateral
H26.009	Unspecified infantile and juvenile cataract, unspecified eye

| H26.01 | Infantile and juvenile cortical, lamellar, or zonular cataract |

H26.011	Infantile and juvenile cortical, lamellar, or zonular cataract, right eye
H26.012	Infantile and juvenile cortical, lamellar, or zonular cataract, left eye
H26.013	Infantile and juvenile cortical, lamellar, or zonular cataract, bilateral
H26.019	Infantile and juvenile cortical, lamellar, or zonular cataract, unspecified eye

| H26.03 | Infantile and juvenile nuclear cataract |

H26.031	Infantile and juvenile nuclear cataract, right eye
H26.032	Infantile and juvenile nuclear cataract, left eye
H26.033	Infantile and juvenile nuclear cataract, bilateral
H26.039	Infantile and juvenile nuclear cataract, unspecified eye

| H26.04 | Anterior subcapsular polar infantile and juvenile cataract |

H26.041	Anterior subcapsular polar infantile and juvenile cataract, right eye
H26.042	Anterior subcapsular polar infantile and juvenile cataract, left eye
H26.043	Anterior subcapsular polar infantile and juvenile cataract, bilateral
H26.049	Anterior subcapsular polar infantile and juvenile cataract, unspecified eye

| H26.05 | Posterior subcapsular polar infantile and juvenile cataract |

H26.051	Posterior subcapsular polar infantile and juvenile cataract, right eye
H26.052	Posterior subcapsular polar infantile and juvenile cataract, left eye
H26.053	Posterior subcapsular polar infantile and juvenile cataract, bilateral
H26.059	Posterior subcapsular polar infantile and juvenile cataract, unspecified eye

| H26.06 | Combined forms of infantile and juvenile cataract |

H26.061	Combined forms of infantile and juvenile cataract, right eye
H26.062	Combined forms of infantile and juvenile cataract, left eye
H26.063	Combined forms of infantile and juvenile cataract, bilateral
H26.069	Combined forms of infantile and juvenile cataract, unspecified eye

| H26.09 | Other infantile and juvenile cataract |

H26.1   **Traumatic cataract**

Use Additional Code (Chapter 20) to identify external cause

| H26.10 | Unspecified traumatic cataract |

H26.101	Unspecified traumatic cataract, right eye
H26.102	Unspecified traumatic cataract, left eye
H26.103	Unspecified traumatic cataract, bilateral
H26.109	Unspecified traumatic cataract, unspecified eye

| H26.11 | Localized traumatic opacities |

H26.111	Localized traumatic opacities, right eye
H26.112	Localized traumatic opacities, left eye
H26.113	Localized traumatic opacities, bilateral
H26.119	Localized traumatic opacities, unspecified eye

| H26.12 | Partially resolved traumatic cataract |

| H26.121 | Partially resolved traumatic cataract, right eye |

   ● New code   ▲ Revised code   **Excludes1:** Not coded here   **Excludes2:** Not included here · ⊗ Placeholder required   ⑦7ᵗʰ digit required

H26.122 **Partially resolved traumatic cataract, left eye**

H26.123 **Partially resolved traumatic cataract, bilateral**

H26.129 **Partially resolved traumatic cataract, unspecified eye**

H26.13 **Total traumatic cataract**

H26.131 **Total traumatic cataract, right eye**

H26.132 **Total traumatic cataract, left eye**

H26.133 **Total traumatic cataract, bilateral**

H26.139 **Total traumatic cataract, unspecified eye**

H26.2 **Complicated cataract**

H26.20 **Unspecified complicated cataract**

Cataracta complicata NOS

H26.21 **Cataract with neovascularization**

Code also associated condition, such as:

chronic iridocyclitis (H20.1-)

H26.211 **Cataract with neovascularization, right eye**

H26.212 **Cataract with neovascularization, left eye**

H26.213 **Cataract with neovascularization, bilateral**

H26.219 **Cataract with neovascularization, unspecified eye**

H26.22 **Cataract secondary to ocular disorders (degenerative) (inflammatory)**

Code also associated ocular disorder

H26.221 **Cataract secondary to ocular disorders (degenerative) (inflammatory), right eye**

H26.222 **Cataract secondary to ocular disorders (degenerative) (inflammatory), left eye**

H26.223 **Cataract secondary to ocular disorders (degenerative) (inflammatory), bilateral**

H26.229 **Cataract secondary to ocular disorders (degenerative) (inflammatory), unspecified eye**

H26.23 **Glaucomatous flecks (subcapsular)**

Code first underlying glaucoma (H40-H42)

H26.231 **Glaucomatous flecks (subcapsular), right eye**

H26.232 **Glaucomatous flecks (subcapsular), left eye**

H26.233 **Glaucomatous flecks (subcapsular), bilateral**

H26.239 **Glaucomatous flecks (subcapsular), unspecified eye**

H26.3 **Drug-induced cataract**

Toxic cataract

Use Additional Code for adverse effect, if applicable, to identify drug (T36-T50 with fifth or sixth character 5)

H26.30 **Drug-induced cataract, unspecified eye**

H26.31 **Drug-induced cataract, right eye**

H26.32 **Drug-induced cataract, left eye**

H26.33 **Drug-induced cataract, bilateral**

H26.4 **Secondary cataract**

H26.40 **Unspecified secondary cataract**

H26.41 **Soemmering's ring**

H26.411 **Soemmering's ring, right eye**

H26.412 **Soemmering's ring, left eye**

H26.413 **Soemmering's ring, bilateral**

H26.419 **Soemmering's ring, unspecified eye**

H26.49 **Other secondary cataract**

H26.491 **Other secondary cataract, right eye**

H26.492 **Other secondary cataract, left eye**

H26.493 **Other secondary cataract, bilateral**

H26.499 **Other secondary cataract, unspecified eye**

H26.8 **Other specified cataract**

H26.9 **Unspecified cataract**

H27 **Other disorders of lens**

Excludes1: congenital lens malformations (Q12.-)

mechanical complications of intraocular lens implant (T85.2)

pseudophakia (Z96.1)

H27.0 **Aphakia**

Acquired absence of lens

Acquired aphakia

Aphakia due to trauma

Excludes1: cataract extraction status (Z98.4-)

congenital absence of lens (Q12.3)

congenital aphakia (Q12.3)

H27.00 **Aphakia, unspecified eye**

H27.01 **Aphakia, right eye**

H27.02 **Aphakia, left eye**

H27.03 **Aphakia, bilateral**

H27.1 **Dislocation of lens**

H27.10 **Unspecified dislocation of lens**

H27.11 **Subluxation of lens**

H27.111 **Subluxation of lens, right eye**

H27.112 **Subluxation of lens, left eye**

H27.113 **Subluxation of lens, bilateral**

H27.119 **Subluxation of lens, unspecified eye**

H27.12 **Anterior dislocation of lens**

H27.121 **Anterior dislocation of lens, right eye**

H27.122 **Anterior dislocation of lens, left eye**

H27.123 **Anterior dislocation of lens, bilateral**

H27.129 **Anterior dislocation of lens, unspecified eye**

H27.13 **Posterior dislocation of lens**

H27.131 **Posterior dislocation of lens, right eye**

H27.132 **Posterior dislocation of lens, left eye**

H27.133 **Posterior dislocation of lens, bilateral**

H27.139 **Posterior dislocation of lens, unspecified eye**

H27.8 **Other specified disorders of lens**

H27.9 **Unspecified disorder of lens**

H28 **Cataract in diseases classified elsewhere**

Code first underlying disease, such as:

hypoparathyroidism (E20.-)

myotonia (G71.1-)

myxedema (E03.-)

protein-calorie malnutrition (E40-E46)

Excludes1: cataract in diabetes mellitus (E08.36, E09.36, E10.36, E11.36, E13.36)

DISORDERS OF CHOROID AND RETINA (H30-H36)

H30 Chorioretinal inflammation

H30.0 Focal chorioretinal inflammation

Focal chorioretinitis

Focal choroiditis

Focal retinitis

Focal retinochoroiditis

H30.00 Unspecified focal chorioretinal inflammation

Focal chorioretinitis NOS

Focal choroiditis NOS

Focal retinitis NOS

Focal retinochoroiditis NOS

H30.001 Unspecified focal chorioretinal inflammation, right eye

H30.002 Unspecified focal chorioretinal inflammation, left eye

H30.003 Unspecified focal chorioretinal inflammation, bilateral

H30.009 Unspecified focal chorioretinal inflammation, unspecified eye

H30.01 Focal chorioretinal inflammation, juxtapapillary

H30.011 Focal chorioretinal inflammation, juxtapapillary, right eye

H30.012 Focal chorioretinal inflammation, juxtapapillary, left eye

H30.013 Focal chorioretinal inflammation, juxtapapillary, bilateral

H30.019 Focal chorioretinal inflammation, juxtapapillary, unspecified eye

H30.02 Focal chorioretinal inflammation of posterior pole

H30.021 Focal chorioretinal inflammation of posterior pole, right eye

H30.022 Focal chorioretinal inflammation of posterior pole, left eye

H30.023 Focal chorioretinal inflammation of posterior pole, bilateral

H30.029 Focal chorioretinal inflammation of posterior pole, unspecified eye

H30.03 Focal chorioretinal inflammation, peripheral

H30.031 Focal chorioretinal inflammation, peripheral, right eye

H30.032 Focal chorioretinal inflammation, peripheral, left eye

H30.033 Focal chorioretinal inflammation, peripheral, bilateral

H30.039 Focal chorioretinal inflammation, peripheral, unspecified eye

H30.04 Focal chorioretinal inflammation, macular or paramacular

H30.041 Focal chorioretinal inflammation, macular or paramacular, right eye

H30.042 Focal chorioretinal inflammation, macular or paramacular, left eye

H30.043 Focal chorioretinal inflammation, macular or paramacular, bilateral

H30.049 Focal chorioretinal inflammation, macular or paramacular, unspecified eye

H30.1 Disseminated chorioretinal inflammation

Disseminated chorioretinitis

Disseminated choroiditis

Disseminated retinitis

Disseminated retinochoroiditis

Excludes2: exudative retinopathy (H35.02-)

H30.10 Unspecified disseminated chorioretinal inflammation

Disseminated chorioretinitis NOS

Disseminated choroiditis NOS

Disseminated retinitis NOS

Disseminated retinochoroiditis NOS

H30.101 Unspecified disseminated chorioretinal inflammation, right eye

H30.102 Unspecified disseminated chorioretinal inflammation, left eye

H30.103 Unspecified disseminated chorioretinal inflammation, bilateral

H30.109 Unspecified disseminated chorioretinal inflammation, unspecified eye

H30.11 Disseminated chorioretinal inflammation of posterior pole

H30.111 Disseminated chorioretinal inflammation of posterior pole, right eye

H30.112 Disseminated chorioretinal inflammation of posterior pole, left eye

H30.113 Disseminated chorioretinal inflammation of posterior pole, bilateral

H30.119 Disseminated chorioretinal inflammation of posterior pole, unspecified eye

H30.12 Disseminated chorioretinal inflammation, peripheral

H30.121 Disseminated chorioretinal inflammation, peripheral right eye

H30.122 Disseminated chorioretinal inflammation, peripheral, left eye

H30.123 Disseminated chorioretinal inflammation, peripheral, bilateral

H30.129 Disseminated chorioretinal inflammation, peripheral, unspecified eye

H30.13 Disseminated chorioretinal inflammation, generalized

H30.131 Disseminated chorioretinal inflammation, generalized, right eye

H30.132 Disseminated chorioretinal inflammation, generalized, left eye

H30.133 Disseminated chorioretinal inflammation, generalized, bilateral

H30.139 Disseminated chorioretinal inflammation, generalized, unspecified eye

H30.14 Acute posterior multifocal placoid pigment epitheliopathy

H30.141 Acute posterior multifocal placoid pigment epitheliopathy, right eye

H30.142 Acute posterior multifocal placoid pigment epitheliopathy, left eye

H30.143   Acute posterior multifocal placoid pigment epitheliopathy, bilateral

H30.149   Acute posterior multifocal placoid pigment epitheliopathy, unspecified eye

H30.2   **Posterior cyclitis**

Pars planitis

H30.20   Posterior cyclitis, unspecified eye

H30.21   Posterior cyclitis, right eye

H30.22   Posterior cyclitis, left eye

H30.23   Posterior cyclitis, bilateral

H30.8   **Other chorioretinal inflammations**

H30.81   Harada's disease

H30.811   Harada's disease, right eye

H30.812   Harada's disease, left eye

H30.813   Harada's disease, bilateral

H30.819   Harada's disease, unspecified eye

H30.89   Other chorioretinal inflammations

H30.891   Other chorioretinal inflammations, right eye

H30.892   Other chorioretinal inflammations, left eye

H30.893   Other chorioretinal inflammations, bilateral

H30.899   Other chorioretinal inflammations, unspecified eye

H30.9   **Unspecified chorioretinal inflammation**

Chorioretinitis NOS

Choroiditis NOS Neuroretinitis NOS

Retinitis NOS

Retinochoroiditis NOS

H30.90   Unspecified chorioretinal inflammation, unspecified eye

H30.91   Unspecified chorioretinal inflammation, right eye

H30.92   Unspecified chorioretinal inflammation, left eye

H30.93   Unspecified chorioretinal inflammation, bilateral

H31   **Other disorders of choroid**

H31.0   **Chorioretinal scars**

Excludes2: postsurgical chorioretinal scars (H59.81-)

H31.00   Unspecified chorioretinal scars

H31.001   Unspecified chorioretinal scars, right eye

H31.002   Unspecified chorioretinal scars, left eye

H31.003   Unspecified chorioretinal scars, bilateral

H31.009   Unspecified chorioretinal scars, unspecified eye

H31.01   Macula scars of posterior pole (postinflammatory) (post-traumatic)

Excludes1: postprocedural chorioretinal scar (H59.81-)

H31.011   Macula scars of posterior pole (postinflammatory) (post-traumatic), right eye

H31.012   Macula scars of posterior pole (postinflammatory) (post-traumatic), left eye

H31.013   Macula scars of posterior pole (postinflammatory) (post-traumatic), bilateral

H31.019   Macula scars of posterior pole (postinflammatory) (post-traumatic), unspecified eye

H31.02   Solar retinopathy

H31.021   Solar retinopathy, right eye

H31.022   Solar retinopathy, left eye

H31.023   Solar retinopathy, bilateral

H31.029   Solar retinopathy, unspecified eye

H31.09   Other chorioretinal scars

H31.091   Other chorioretinal scars, right eye

H31.092   Other chorioretinal scars, left eye

H31.093   Other chorioretinal scars, bilateral

H31.099   Other chorioretinal scars, unspecified eye

H31.1   **Choroidal degeneration**

Excludes2: angioid streaks of macula (H35.33)

H31.10   Unspecified choroidal degeneration

Choroidal sclerosis NOS

H31.101   Choroidal degeneration, unspecified, right eye

H31.102   Choroidal degeneration, unspecified, left eye

H31.103   Choroidal degeneration, unspecified, bilateral

H31.109   Choroidal degeneration, unspecified, unspecified eye

H31.11   Age-related choroidal atrophy

H31.111   Age-related choroidal atrophy, right eye

H31.112   Age-related choroidal atrophy, left eye

H31.113   Age-related choroidal atrophy, bilateral

H31.119   Age-related choroidal atrophy, unspecified eye

H31.12   Diffuse secondary atrophy of choroid

H31.121   Diffuse secondary atrophy of choroid, right eye

H31.122   Diffuse secondary atrophy of choroid, left eye

H31.123   Diffuse secondary atrophy of choroid, bilateral

H31.129   Diffuse secondary atrophy of choroid, unspecified eye

H31.2   **Hereditary choroidal dystrophy**

Excludes2: hyperornithinemia (E72.4)

ornithinemia (E72.4)

H31.20   Hereditary choroidal dystrophy, unspecified

H31.21   Choroideremia

H31.22   Choroidal dystrophy (central areolar) (generalized) (peripapillary)

H31.23   Gyrate atrophy, choroid

H31.29   Other hereditary choroidal dystrophy

H31.3   **Choroidal hemorrhage and rupture**

H31.30   Unspecified choroidal hemorrhage

H31.301   Unspecified choroidal hemorrhage, right eye

H31.302 Unspecified choroidal hemorrhage, left eye

H31.303 Unspecified choroidal hemorrhage, bilateral

H31.309 Unspecified choroidal hemorrhage, unspecified eye

H31.31 Expulsive choroidal hemorrhage

H31.311 Expulsive choroidal hemorrhage, right eye

H31.312 Expulsive choroidal hemorrhage, left eye

H31.313 Expulsive choroidal hemorrhage, bilateral

H31.319 Expulsive choroidal hemorrhage, unspecified eye

H31.32 Choroidal rupture

H31.321 Choroidal rupture, right eye

H31.322 Choroidal rupture, left eye

H31.323 Choroidal rupture, bilateral

H31.329 Choroidal rupture, unspecified eye

H31.4 Choroidal detachment

H31.40 Unspecified choroidal detachment

H31.401 Unspecified choroidal detachment, right eye

H31.402 Unspecified choroidal detachment, left eye

H31.403 Unspecified choroidal detachment, bilateral

H31.409 Unspecified choroidal detachment, unspecified eye

H31.41 Hemorrhagic choroidal detachment

H31.411 Hemorrhagic choroidal detachment, right eye

H31.412 Hemorrhagic choroidal detachment, left eye

H31.413 Hemorrhagic choroidal detachment, bilateral

H31.419 Hemorrhagic choroidal detachment, unspecified eye

H31.42 Serous choroidal detachment

H31.421 Serous choroidal detachment, right eye

H31.422 Serous choroidal detachment, left eye

H31.423 Serous choroidal detachment, bilateral

H31.429 Serous choroidal detachment, unspecified eye

H31.8 Other specified disorders of choroid

H31.9 Unspecified disorder of choroid

H32 Chorioretinal disorders in diseases classified elsewhere

Code first underlying disease, such as:

congenital toxoplasmosis (P37.1)

histoplasmosis (B39.-)

leprosy (A30.-)

Excludes1: chorioretinitis (in):

toxoplasmosis (acquired) (B58.01)

tuberculosis (A18.53)

H33 Retinal detachments and breaks

Definition: Retinal detachment is a disorder of the eye in which the retina peels away from its underlying layer of support tissue.

Excludes1: detachment of retinal pigment epithelium (H35.72-, H35.73-)

H33.0 Retinal detachment with retinal break

Rhegmatogenous retinal detachment

Excludes1: serous retinal detachment (without retinal break) (H33.2-)

H33.00 Unspecified retinal detachment with retinal break

H33.001 Unspecified retinal detachment with retinal break, right eye

H33.002 Unspecified retinal detachment with retinal break, left eye

H33.003 Unspecified retinal detachment with retinal break, bilateral

H33.009 Unspecified retinal detachment with retinal break, unspecified eye

H33.01 Retinal detachment with single break

H33.011 Retinal detachment with single break, right eye

H33.012 Retinal detachment with single break, left eye

H33.013 Retinal detachment with single break, bilateral

H33.019 Retinal detachment with single break, unspecified eye

H33.02 Retinal detachment with multiple breaks

H33.021 Retinal detachment with multiple breaks, right eye

H33.022 Retinal detachment with multiple breaks, left eye

H33.023 Retinal detachment with multiple breaks, bilateral

H33.029 Retinal detachment with multiple breaks, unspecified eye

H33.03 Retinal detachment with giant retinal tear

H33.031 Retinal detachment with giant retinal tear, right eye

H33.032 Retinal detachment with giant retinal tear, left eye

H33.033 Retinal detachment with giant retinal tear, bilateral

H33.039 Retinal detachment with giant retinal tear, unspecified eye

H33.04 Retinal detachment with retinal dialysis

H33.041 Retinal detachment with retinal dialysis, right eye

H33.042 Retinal detachment with retinal dialysis, left eye

H33.043 Retinal detachment with retinal dialysis, bilateral

H33.049 Retinal detachment with retinal dialysis, unspecified eye

H33.05 Total retinal detachment

H33.051 Total retinal detachment, right eye

H33.052 Total retinal detachment, left eye

H33.053 Total retinal detachment, bilateral

H33.059 Total retinal detachment, unspecified eye

H33.1 Retinoschisis and retinal cysts

Excludes1: congenital retinoschisis (Q14.1)

microcystoid degeneration of retina (H35.42-)

H33.10 Unspecified retinoschisis

H33.101   Unspecified retinoschisis, right eye

H33.102   Unspecified retinoschisis, left eye

H33.103   Unspecified retinoschisis, bilateral

H33.109   Unspecified retinoschisis, unspecified eye

H33.11   **Cyst of ora serrata**

H33.111   Cyst of ora serrata, right eye

H33.112   Cyst of ora serrata, left eye

H33.113   Cyst of ora serrata, bilateral

H33.119   Cyst of ora serrata, unspecified eye

H33.12   **Parasitic cyst of retina**

H33.121   Parasitic cyst of retina, right eye

H33.122   Parasitic cyst of retina, left eye

H33.123   Parasitic cyst of retina, bilateral

H33.129   Parasitic cyst of retina, unspecified eye

H33.19   **Other retinoschisis and retinal cysts**

Pseudocyst of retina

H33.191   Other retinoschisis and retinal cysts, right eye

H33.192   Other retinoschisis and retinal cysts, left eye

H33.193   Other retinoschisis and retinal cysts, bilateral

H33.199   Other retinoschisis and retinal cysts, unspecified eye

H33.2   **Serous retinal detachment**

Retinal detachment NOS

Retinal detachment without retinal break

Excludes1: central serous chorioretinopathy (H35.71-)

H33.20   Serous retinal detachment, unspecified eye

H33.21   Serous retinal detachment, right eye

H33.22   Serous retinal detachment, left eye

H33.23   Serous retinal detachment, bilateral

H33.3   **Retinal breaks without detachment**

Excludes1: chorioretinal scars after surgery for detachment (H59.81-)

peripheral retinal degeneration without break (H35.4-)

H33.30   **Unspecified retinal break**

H33.301   Unspecified retinal break, right eye

H33.302   Unspecified retinal break, left eye

H33.303   Unspecified retinal break, bilateral

H33.309   Unspecified retinal break, unspecified eye

H33.31   **Horseshoe tear of retina without detachment**

Operculum of retina without detachment

H33.311   Horseshoe tear of retina without detachment, right eye

H33.312   Horseshoe tear of retina without detachment, left eye

H33.313   Horseshoe tear of retina without detachment, bilateral

H33.319   Horseshoe tear of retina without detachment, unspecified eye

H33.32   **Round hole of retina without detachment**

H33.321   Round hole, right eye

H33.322   Round hole, left eye

H33.323   Round hole, bilateral

H33.329   Round hole, unspecified eye

H33.33   **Multiple defects of retina without detachment**

H33.331   Multiple defects of retina without detachment, right eye

H33.332   Multiple defects of retina without detachment, left eye

H33.333   Multiple defects of retina without detachment, bilateral

H33.339   Multiple defects of retina without detachment, unspecified eye

H33.4   **Traction detachment of retina**

Proliferative vitreo-retinopathy with retinal detachment

H33.40   Traction detachment of retina, unspecified eye

H33.41   Traction detachment of retina, right eye

H33.42   Traction detachment of retina, left eye

H33.43   Traction detachment of retina, bilateral

H33.8   **Other retinal detachments**

H34   **Retinal vascular occlusions**

Excludes1: amaurosis fugax (G45.3)

H34.0   **Transient retinal artery occlusion**

H34.00   Transient retinal artery occlusion, unspecified eye

H34.01   Transient retinal artery occlusion, right eye

H34.02   Transient retinal artery occlusion, left eye

H34.03   Transient retinal artery occlusion, bilateral

H34.1   **Central retinal artery occlusion**

H34.10   Central retinal artery occlusion, unspecified eye

H34.11   Central retinal artery occlusion, right eye

H34.12   Central retinal artery occlusion, left eye

H34.13   Central retinal artery occlusion, bilateral

H34.2   **Other retinal artery occlusions**

H34.21   **Partial retinal artery occlusion**

Hollenhorst's plaque

Retinal microembolism

H34.211   Partial retinal artery occlusion, right eye

H34.212   Partial retinal artery occlusion, left eye

H34.213   Partial retinal artery occlusion, bilateral

H34.219   Partial retinal artery occlusion, unspecified eye

H34.23   **Retinal artery branch occlusion**

H34.231   Retinal artery branch occlusion, right eye

H34.232   Retinal artery branch occlusion, left eye

H34.233   Retinal artery branch occlusion, bilateral

H34.239   Retinal artery branch occlusion, unspecified eye

H34.8   **Other retinal vascular occlusions**

H34.81   **Central retinal vein occlusion**

One of the following 7th characters is to be assigned to codes in subcategory H34.81 to designate the severity of the occlusion:

0 - with macular edema

1 - with retinal neovascularization

2 – stable Old central retinal vein occlusion

---

⑦H34.811   **Central retinal vein occlusion, right eye**

⑦H34.812   **Central retinal vein occlusion, left eye**

⑦H34.813   **Central retinal vein occlusion, bilateral**

⑦H34.819   **Central retinal vein occlusion, unspecified eye**

H34.82   **Venous engorgement**

    Incipient retinal vein occlusion

    Partial retinal vein occlusion

    H34.821   **Venous engorgement, right eye**

    H34.822   **Venous engorgement, left eye**

    H34.823   **Venous engorgement, bilateral**

    H34.829   **Venous engorgement, unspecified eye**

H34.83   **Tributary (branch) retinal vein occlusion**

    One of the following 7th characters is to be assigned to codes in subcategory H34.83 to designate the severity of the occlusion:

    0 - with macular edema

    1 - with retinal neovascularization

    2 – stable Old tributary (branch) retinal vein occlusion

    ⑦H34.831   **Tributary (branch) retinal vein occlusion, right eye**

    ⑦H34.832   **Tributary (branch) retinal vein occlusion, left eye**

    ⑦H34.833   **Tributary (branch) retinal vein occlusion, bilateral**

    ⑦H34.839   **Tributary (branch) retinal vein occlusion, unspecified eye**

H34.9   **Unspecified retinal vascular occlusion**

H35   **Other retinal disorders**

    Excludes2: diabetic retinal disorders (E08.311-E08.359, E09.311-E09.359, E10.311-E10.359, E11.311-E11.359, E13.311-E13.359)

H35.0   **Background retinopathy and retinal vascular changes**

    Code also any associated hypertension (I10)

    H35.00   **Unspecified background retinopathy**

    H35.01   **Changes in retinal vascular appearance**

      Retinal vascular sheathing

      H35.011   **Changes in retinal vascular appearance, right eye**

      H35.012   **Changes in retinal vascular appearance, left eye**

      H35.013   **Changes in retinal vascular appearance, bilateral**

      H35.019   **Changes in retinal vascular appearance, unspecified eye**

    H35.02   **Exudative retinopathy**

      Coats retinopathy

      H35.021   **Exudative retinopathy, right eye**

      H35.022   **Exudative retinopathy, left eye**

      H35.023   **Exudative retinopathy, bilateral**

      H35.029   **Exudative retinopathy, unspecified eye**

    H35.03   **Hypertensive retinopathy**

      H35.031   **Hypertensive retinopathy, right eye**

      H35.032   **Hypertensive retinopathy, left eye**

      H35.033   **Hypertensive retinopathy, bilateral**

H35.039   **Hypertensive retinopathy, unspecified eye**

H35.04   **Retinal micro-aneurysms, unspecified**

    H35.041   **Retinal micro-aneurysms, unspecified, right eye**

    H35.042   **Retinal micro-aneurysms, unspecified, left eye**

    H35.043   **Retinal micro-aneurysms, unspecified, bilateral**

    H35.049   **Retinal micro-aneurysms, unspecified, unspecified eye**

H35.05   **Retinal neovascularization, unspecified**

    H35.051   **Retinal neovascularization, unspecified, right eye**

    H35.052   **Retinal neovascularization, unspecified, left eye**

    H35.053   **Retinal neovascularization, unspecified, bilateral**

    H35.059   **Retinal neovascularization, unspecified, unspecified eye**

H35.06   **Retinal vasculitis**

    Eales disease

    Retinal perivasculitis

    H35.061   **Retinal vasculitis, right eye**

    H35.062   **Retinal vasculitis, left eye**

    H35.063   **Retinal vasculitis, bilateral**

    H35.069   **Retinal vasculitis, unspecified eye**

H35.07   **Retinal telangiectasis**

    H35.071   **Retinal telangiectasis, right eye**

    H35.072   **Retinal telangiectasis, left eye**

    H35.073   **Retinal telangiectasis, bilateral**

    H35.079   **Retinal telangiectasis, unspecified eye**

H35.09   **Other intraretinal microvascular abnormalities**

    Retinal varices

H35.1   **Retinopathy of prematurity**

    H35.10   **Retinopathy of prematurity, unspecified**

      Retinopathy of prematurity NOS

      H35.101   **Retinopathy of prematurity, unspecified, right eye**

      H35.102   **Retinopathy of prematurity, unspecified, left eye**

      H35.103   **Retinopathy of prematurity, unspecified, bilateral**

      H35.109   **Retinopathy of prematurity, unspecified, unspecified eye**

    H35.11   **Retinopathy of prematurity, stage 0**

      H35.111   **Retinopathy of prematurity, stage 0, right eye**

      H35.112   **Retinopathy of prematurity, stage 0, left eye**

      H35.113   **Retinopathy of prematurity, stage 0, bilateral**

      H35.119   **Retinopathy of prematurity, stage 0, unspecified eye**

    H35.12   **Retinopathy of prematurity, stage 1**

      H35.121   **Retinopathy of prematurity, stage 1, right eye**

      H35.122   **Retinopathy of prematurity, stage 1, left eye**

      H35.123   **Retinopathy of prematurity, stage 1, bilateral**

H35.129 Retinopathy of prematurity, stage 1, unspecified eye

H35.13 **Retinopathy of prematurity, stage 2**

H35.131 Retinopathy of prematurity, stage 2, right eye

H35.132 Retinopathy of prematurity, stage 2, left eye

H35.133 Retinopathy of prematurity, stage 2, bilateral

H35.139 Retinopathy of prematurity, stage 2, unspecified eye

H35.14 **Retinopathy of prematurity, stage 3**

H35.141 Retinopathy of prematurity, stage 3, right eye

H35.142 Retinopathy of prematurity, stage 3, left eye

H35.143 Retinopathy of prematurity, stage 3, bilateral

H35.149 Retinopathy of prematurity, stage 3, unspecified eye

H35.15 **Retinopathy of prematurity, stage 4**

H35.151 Retinopathy of prematurity, stage 4, right eye

H35.152 Retinopathy of prematurity, stage 4, left eye

H35.153 Retinopathy of prematurity, stage 4, bilateral

H35.159 Retinopathy of prematurity, stage 4, unspecified eye

H35.16 **Retinopathy of prematurity, stage 5**

H35.161 Retinopathy of prematurity, stage 5, right eye

H35.162 Retinopathy of prematurity, stage 5, left eye

H35.163 Retinopathy of prematurity, stage 5, bilateral

H35.169 Retinopathy of prematurity, stage 5, unspecified eye

H35.17 **Retrolental fibroplasia**

H35.171 Retrolental fibroplasia, right eye

H35.172 Retrolental fibroplasia, left eye

H35.173 Retrolental fibroplasia, bilateral

H35.179 Retrolental fibroplasia, unspecified eye

H35.2 **Other non-diabetic proliferative retinopathy**

Proliferative vitreo-retinopathy

Excludes1: proliferative vitreo-retinopathy with retinal detachment (H33.4-)

H35.20 **Other non-diabetic proliferative retinopathy, unspecified eye**

H35.21 **Other non-diabetic proliferative retinopathy, right eye**

H35.22 **Other non-diabetic proliferative retinopathy, left eye**

H35.23 **Other non-diabetic proliferative retinopathy, bilateral**

H35.3 **Degeneration of macula and posterior pole**

H35.30 **Unspecified macular degeneration**

Age-related macular degeneration

H35.31 **Nonexudative age-related macular degeneration**

Atrophic age-related macular degeneration

Dry age-related macular degeneration

One of the following 7th characters is to be assigned to codes in subcategory H35.31 to designate the stage of the disease:

0 - stage unspecified

1 - early dry stage

2 - intermediate dry stage

3 - advanced atrophic without subfoveal involvement advanced dry stage

4 - advanced atrophic with subfoveal involvement

⑦**H35.311** Nonexudative age-related macular degeneration, right eye

⑦**H35.312** Nonexudative age-related macular degeneration, left eye

⑦**H35.313** Nonexudative age-related macular degeneration, bilateral

⑦**H35.319** Nonexudative age-related macular degeneration, unspecified eye

H35.32 **Exudative age-related macular degeneration**

Wet age-related macular degeneration

One of the following 7th characters is to be assigned to codes in subcategory H35.32 to designate the stage of the disease:

0 - stage unspecified

1 - with active choroidal neovascularization

2 - with inactive choroidal neovascularization with involuted or regressed neovascularization

3 - with inactive scar

⑦**H35.321** Exudative age-related macular degeneration, right eye [HCC]

⑦**H35.322** Exudative age-related macular degeneration, left eye [HCC]

⑦**H35.323** Exudative age-related macular degeneration, bilateral [HCC]

⑦**H35.329** Exudative age-related macular degeneration, unspecified eye [HCC]

H35.33 **Angioid streaks of macula**

H35.34 **Macular cyst, hole, or pseudohole**

H35.341 Macular cyst, hole, or pseudohole, right eye

H35.342 Macular cyst, hole, or pseudohole, left eye

H35.343 Macular cyst, hole, or pseudohole, bilateral

H35.349 Macular cyst, hole, or pseudohole, unspecified eye

H35.35 **Cystoid macular degeneration**

Excludes1: cystoid macular edema following cataract surgery (H59.03-)

H35.351 Cystoid macular degeneration, right eye

H35.352 Cystoid macular degeneration, left eye

H35.353 Cystoid macular degeneration, bilateral

H35.359 Cystoid macular degeneration, unspecified eye

H35.36 **Drusen (degenerative) of macula**

H35.361 Drusen (degenerative) of macula, right eye

H35.362 Drusen (degenerative) of macula, left eye

H35.363   Drusen (degenerative) of macula, bilateral

H35.369   Drusen (degenerative) of macula, unspecified eye

H35.37   Puckering of macula

H35.371   Puckering of macula, right eye

H35.372   Puckering of macula, left eye

H35.373   Puckering of macula, bilateral

H35.379   Puckering of macula, unspecified eye

H35.38   Toxic maculopathy

<u>Code first</u> poisoning due to drug or toxin, if applicable (T36-T65 with fifth or sixth character 1-4 or 6)

<u>Use Additional Code</u> for adverse effect, if applicable, to identify drug (T36-T50 with fifth or sixth character 5)

H35.381   Toxic maculopathy, right eye

H35.382   Toxic maculopathy, left eye

H35.383   Toxic maculopathy, bilateral

H35.389   Toxic maculopathy, unspecified eye

H35.4   Peripheral retinal degeneration

`Excludes1:` hereditary retinal degeneration (dystrophy) (H35.5-)

peripheral retinal degeneration with retinal break (H33.3-)

H35.40   Unspecified peripheral retinal degeneration

H35.41   Lattice degeneration of retina

Palisade degeneration of retina

H35.411   Lattice degeneration of retina, right eye

H35.412   Lattice degeneration of retina, left eye

H35.413   Lattice degeneration of retina, bilateral

H35.419   Lattice degeneration of retina, unspecified eye

H35.42   Microcystoid degeneration of retina

H35.421   Microcystoid degeneration of retina, right eye

H35.422   Microcystoid degeneration of retina, left eye

H35.423   Microcystoid degeneration of retina, bilateral

H35.429   Microcystoid degeneration of retina, unspecified eye

H35.43   Paving stone degeneration of retina

H35.431   Paving stone degeneration of retina, right eye

H35.432   Paving stone degeneration of retina, left eye

H35.433   Paving stone degeneration of retina, bilateral

H35.439   Paving stone degeneration of retina, unspecified eye

H35.44   Age-related reticular degeneration of retina

H35.441   Age-related reticular degeneration of retina, right eye

H35.442   Age-related reticular degeneration of retina, left eye

H35.443   Age-related reticular degeneration of retina, bilateral

H35.449   Age-related reticular degeneration of retina, unspecified eye

H35.45   Secondary pigmentary degeneration

H35.451   Secondary pigmentary degeneration, right eye

H35.452   Secondary pigmentary degeneration, left eye

H35.453   Secondary pigmentary degeneration, bilateral

H35.459   Secondary pigmentary degeneration, unspecified eye

H35.46   Secondary vitreoretinal degeneration

H35.461   Secondary vitreoretinal degeneration, right eye

H35.462   Secondary vitreoretinal degeneration, left eye

H35.463   Secondary vitreoretinal degeneration, bilateral

H35.469   Secondary vitreoretinal degeneration, unspecified eye

H35.5   Hereditary retinal dystrophy

`Excludes1:` dystrophies primarily involving Bruch's membrane (H31.1-)

H35.50   Unspecified hereditary retinal dystrophy

H35.51   Vitreoretinal dystrophy

H35.52   Pigmentary retinal dystrophy

Albipunctate retinal dystrophy

Retinitis pigmentosa

Tapetoretinal dystrophy

H35.53   Other dystrophies primarily involving the sensory retina

Stargardt's disease

H35.54   Dystrophies primarily involving the retinal pigment epithelium

Vitelliform retinal dystrophy

H35.6   Retinal hemorrhage

H35.60   Retinal hemorrhage, unspecified eye

H35.61   Retinal hemorrhage, right eye

H35.62   Retinal hemorrhage, left eye

H35.63   Retinal hemorrhage, bilateral

H35.7   Separation of retinal layers

`Excludes1:` retinal detachment (serous) (H33.2-)

rhegmatogenous retinal detachment (H33.0-)

H35.70   Unspecified separation of retinal layers

H35.71   Central serous chorioretinopathy

H35.711   Central serous chorioretinopathy, right eye

H35.712   Central serous chorioretinopathy, left eye

H35.713   Central serous chorioretinopathy, bilateral

H35.719   Central serous chorioretinopathy, unspecified eye

H35.72   Serous detachment of retinal pigment epithelium

H35.721   Serous detachment of retinal pigment epithelium, right eye

H35.722   Serous detachment of retinal pigment epithelium, left eye

H35.723   Serous detachment of retinal pigment epithelium, bilateral

  ● New code   ▲ Revised code   `Excludes1:` Not coded here   `Excludes2:` Not included here   ⊗ Placeholder required   ⑦7ᵗʰ digit required

H35.729 Serous detachment of retinal pigment epithelium, unspecified eye

H35.73 Hemorrhagic detachment of retinal pigment epithelium

> **H35.731** Hemorrhagic detachment of retinal pigment epithelium, right eye
>
> **H35.732** Hemorrhagic detachment of retinal pigment epithelium, left eye
>
> **H35.733** Hemorrhagic detachment of retinal pigment epithelium, bilateral
>
> **H35.739** Hemorrhagic detachment of retinal pigment epithelium, unspecified eye

H35.8 Other specified retinal disorders

> Excludes2: retinal hemorrhage (H35.6-)

H35.81 Retinal edema

> Retinal cotton wool spots

H35.82 Retinal ischemia

H35.89 Other specified retinal disorders

H35.9 Unspecified retinal disorder

H36 Retinal disorders in diseases classified elsewhere

Code first underlying disease, such as:

lipid storage disorders (E75.-)

sickle-cell disorders (D57.-)

Excludes1: arteriosclerotic retinopathy (H35.0-)

> diabetic retinopathy (E08.3-, E09.3-, E10.3-, E11.3-, E13.3-)

GLAUCOMA (H40-H42)

Definition: Glaucoma is a group of eye diseases characterized by damage to the optic nerve usually due to excessively high intraocular pressure.

H40 Glaucoma

> Excludes1: absolute glaucoma (H44.51-)
>
> congenital glaucoma (Q15.0)
>
> traumatic glaucoma due to birth injury (P15.3)

H40.0 Glaucoma suspect

H40.00 Preglaucoma, unspecified

> **H40.001** Preglaucoma, unspecified, right eye
>
> **H40.002** Preglaucoma, unspecified, left eye
>
> **H40.003** Preglaucoma, unspecified, bilateral
>
> **H40.009** Preglaucoma, unspecified, unspecified eye

H40.01 Open angle with borderline findings, low risk

> Open angle, low risk
>
> **H40.011** Open angle with borderline findings, low risk, right eye
>
> **H40.012** Open angle with borderline findings, low risk, left eye
>
> **H40.013** Open angle with borderline findings, low risk, bilateral
>
> **H40.019** Open angle with borderline findings, low risk, unspecified eye

H40.02 Open angle with borderline findings, high risk

> Open angle, high risk
>
> **H40.021** Open angle with borderline findings, high risk, right eye
>
> **H40.022** Open angle with borderline findings, high risk, left eye
>
> **H40.023** Open angle with borderline findings, high risk, bilateral
>
> **H40.029** Open angle with borderline findings, high risk, unspecified eye

H40.03 Anatomical narrow angle

> Primary angle closure suspect
>
> **H40.031** Anatomical narrow angle, right eye
>
> **H40.032** Anatomical narrow angle, left eye
>
> **H40.033** Anatomical narrow angle, bilateral
>
> **H40.039** Anatomical narrow angle, unspecified eye

H40.04 Steroid responder

> **H40.041** Steroid responder, right eye
>
> **H40.042** Steroid responder, left eye
>
> **H40.043** Steroid responder, bilateral
>
> **H40.049** Steroid responder, unspecified eye

H40.05 Ocular hypertension

> **H40.051** Ocular hypertension, right eye
>
> **H40.052** Ocular hypertension, left eye
>
> **H40.053** Ocular hypertension, bilateral
>
> **H40.059** Ocular hypertension, unspecified eye

H40.06 Primary angle closure without glaucoma damage

> **H40.061** Primary angle closure without glaucoma damage, right eye
>
> **H40.062** Primary angle closure without glaucoma damage, left eye
>
> **H40.063** Primary angle closure without glaucoma damage, bilateral
>
> **H40.069** Primary angle closure without glaucoma damage, unspecified eye

H40.1 Open-angle glaucoma

⊗⑦**H40.10** Unspecified open-angle glaucoma

> One of the following 7th characters is to be assigned to code H40.10 to designate the stage of glaucoma
>
> 0 - stage unspecified
>
> 1 - mild stage
>
> 2 - moderate stage
>
> 3 - severe stage
>
> 4 - indeterminate stage

H40.11 Primary open-angle glaucoma

> Chronic simple glaucoma
>
> One of the following 7th characters is to be assigned to each code in subcategory H40.11 to designate the stage of glaucoma
>
> 0 - stage unspecified
>
> 1 - mild stage
>
> 2 - moderate stage
>
> 3 - severe stage
>
> 4 - indeterminate stage
>
> ⑦**H40.111** Primary open-angle glaucoma, right eye
>
> ⑦**H40.112** Primary open-angle glaucoma, left eye
>
> ⑦**H40.113** Primary open-angle glaucoma, bilateral
>
> ⑦**H40.119** Primary open-angle glaucoma, unspecified eye

H40.12 Low-tension glaucoma

> One of the following 7th characters is to be assigned to each code in subcategory H40.12 to designate the stage of glaucoma
>
> 0 - stage unspecified

1 - mild stage

2 - moderate stage

3 - severe stage

4 - indeterminate stage

⑦H40.121　Low-tension glaucoma, right eye

⑦H40.122　Low-tension glaucoma, left eye

⑦H40.123　Low-tension glaucoma, bilateral

⑦H40.129　Low-tension glaucoma, unspecified eye

H40.13　Pigmentary glaucoma

One of the following 7th characters is to be assigned to each code in subcategory H40.13 to designate the stage of glaucoma

0 - stage unspecified

1 - mild stage

2 - moderate stage

3 - severe stage

4 - indeterminate stage

⑦H40.131　Pigmentary glaucoma, right eye

⑦H40.132　Pigmentary glaucoma, left eye

⑦H40.133　Pigmentary glaucoma, bilateral

⑦H40.139　Pigmentary glaucoma, unspecified eye

H40.14　Capsular glaucoma with pseudoexfoliation of lens

One of the following 7th characters is to be assigned to each code in subcategory H40.14 to designate the stage of glaucoma

0 - stage unspecified

1 - mild stage

2 - moderate stage

3 - severe stage

4 - indeterminate stage

⑦H40.141　Capsular glaucoma with pseudoexfoliation of lens, right eye

⑦H40.142　Capsular glaucoma with pseudoexfoliation of lens, left eye

⑦H40.143　Capsular glaucoma with pseudoexfoliation of lens, bilateral

⑦H40.149　Capsular glaucoma with pseudoexfoliation of lens, unspecified eye

H40.15　Residual stage of open-angle glaucoma

H40.151　Residual stage of open-angle glaucoma, right eye

H40.152　Residual stage of open-angle glaucoma, left eye

H40.153　Residual stage of open-angle glaucoma, bilateral

H40.159　Residual stage of open-angle glaucoma, unspecified eye

H40.2　Primary angle-closure glaucoma

Excludes1: aqueous misdirection (H40.83-)

malignant glaucoma (H40.83-)

⊗⑦H40.20　Unspecified primary angle-closure glaucoma

One of the following 7th characters is to be assigned to code H40.20 to designate the stage of glaucoma

0 - stage unspecified

1 - mild stage

2 - moderate stage

3 - severe stage

4 - indeterminate stage

H40.21　Acute angle-closure glaucoma

Acute angle-closure glaucoma attack

Acute angle-closure glaucoma crisis

H40.211　Acute angle-closure glaucoma, right eye

H40.212　Acute angle-closure glaucoma, left eye

H40.213　Acute angle-closure glaucoma, bilateral

H40.219　Acute angle-closure glaucoma, unspecified eye

H40.22　Chronic angle-closure glaucoma

Chronic primary angle closure glaucoma

One of the following 7th characters is to be assigned to each code in subcategory H40.22 to designate the stage of glaucoma

0 - stage unspecified

1 - mild stage

2 - moderate stage

3 - severe stage

4 - indeterminate stage

⑦H40.221　Chronic angle-closure glaucoma, right eye

⑦H40.222　Chronic angle-closure glaucoma, left eye

⑦H40.223　Chronic angle-closure glaucoma, bilateral

⑦H40.229　Chronic angle-closure glaucoma, unspecified eye

H40.23　Intermittent angle-closure glaucoma

H40.231　Intermittent angle-closure glaucoma, right eye

H40.232　Intermittent angle-closure glaucoma, left eye

H40.233　Intermittent angle-closure glaucoma, bilateral

H40.239　Intermittent angle-closure glaucoma, unspecified eye

H40.24　Residual stage of angle-closure glaucoma

H40.241　Residual stage of angle-closure glaucoma, right eye

H40.242　Residual stage of angle-closure glaucoma, left eye

H40.243　Residual stage of angle-closure glaucoma, bilateral

H40.249　Residual stage of angle-closure glaucoma, unspecified eye

H40.3　Glaucoma secondary to eye trauma

Code also underlying condition

One of the following 7th characters is to be assigned to each code in subcategory H40.3 to designate the stage of glaucoma

0 - stage unspecified

1 - mild stage

2 - moderate stage

3 - severe stage

4 - indeterminate stage

⊗⑦H40.30　Glaucoma secondary to eye trauma, unspecified eye

　● New code　▲ Revised code　Excludes1: Not coded here　Excludes2: Not included here　⊗ Placeholder required　⑦7th digit required

⊗⑦H40.31   Glaucoma secondary to eye trauma, right eye

⊗⑦H40.32   Glaucoma secondary to eye trauma, left eye

⊗⑦H40.33   Glaucoma secondary to eye trauma, bilateral

H40.4   Glaucoma secondary to eye inflammation

<u>Code also</u> underlying condition

One of the following 7th characters is to be assigned to each code in subcategory H40.4 to designate the stage of glaucoma

0 - stage unspecified

1 - mild stage

2 - moderate stage

3 - severe stage

4 - indeterminate stage

⊗⑦H40.40   Glaucoma secondary to eye inflammation, unspecified eye

⊗⑦H40.41   Glaucoma secondary to eye inflammation, right eye

⊗⑦H40.42   Glaucoma secondary to eye inflammation, left eye

⊗⑦H40.43   Glaucoma secondary to eye inflammation, bilateral

H40.5   Glaucoma secondary to other eye disorders

<u>Code also</u> underlying eye disorder

One of the following 7th characters is to be assigned to each code in subcategory H40.5 to designate the stage of glaucoma

0 - stage unspecified

1 - mild stage

2 - moderate stage

3 - severe stage

4 - indeterminate stage

⊗⑦H40.50   Glaucoma secondary to other eye disorders, unspecified eye

⊗⑦H40.51   Glaucoma secondary to other eye disorders, right eye

⊗⑦H40.52   Glaucoma secondary to other eye disorders, left eye

⊗⑦H40.53   Glaucoma secondary to other eye disorders, bilateral

H40.6   Glaucoma secondary to drugs

<u>Use Additional Code</u> for adverse effect, if applicable, to identify drug (T36-T50 with fifth or sixth character 5)

One of the following 7th characters is to be assigned to each code in subcategory H40.6 to designate the stage of glaucoma

0 - stage unspecified

1 - mild stage

2 - moderate stage

3 - severe stage

4 - indeterminate stage

⊗⑦H40.60   Glaucoma secondary to drugs, unspecified eye

⊗⑦H40.61   Glaucoma secondary to drugs, right eye

⊗⑦H40.62   Glaucoma secondary to drugs, left eye

⊗⑦H40.63   Glaucoma secondary to drugs, bilateral

H40.8   Other glaucoma

H40.81   Glaucoma with increased episcleral venous pressure

H40.811   Glaucoma with increased episcleral venous pressure, right eye

H40.812   Glaucoma with increased episcleral venous pressure, left eye

H40.813   Glaucoma with increased episcleral venous pressure, bilateral

H40.819   Glaucoma with increased episcleral venous pressure, unspecified eye

H40.82   Hypersecretion glaucoma

H40.821   Hypersecretion glaucoma, right eye

H40.822   Hypersecretion glaucoma, left eye

H40.823   Hypersecretion glaucoma, bilateral

H40.829   Hypersecretion glaucoma, unspecified eye

H40.83   Aqueous misdirection

Malignant glaucoma

H40.831   Aqueous misdirection, right eye

H40.832   Aqueous misdirection, left eye

H40.833   Aqueous misdirection, bilateral

H40.839   Aqueous misdirection, unspecified eye

H40.89   Other specified glaucoma

H40.9   Unspecified glaucoma

H42   Glaucoma in diseases classified elsewhere

<u>Code first</u> underlying condition, such as:

amyloidosis (E85.-)

aniridia (Q13.1)

Lowe's syndrome (E72.03)

Rieger's anomaly (Q13.81)

specified metabolic disorder (E70-E88)

Excludes1: glaucoma (in) onchocerciasis (B73.02)

glaucoma (in) syphilis (A52.71)

glaucoma (in) tuberculous (A18.59)

DISORDERS OF VITREOUS BODY AND GLOBE (H43-H44)

H43   Disorders of vitreous body

H43.0   Vitreous prolapse

Excludes1: vitreous syndrome following cataract surgery (H59.0-)

traumatic vitreous prolapse (S05.2-)

H43.00   Vitreous prolapse, unspecified eye

H43.01   Vitreous prolapse, right eye

H43.02   Vitreous prolapse, left eye

H43.03   Vitreous prolapse, bilateral

H43.1   Vitreous hemorrhage

H43.10   Vitreous hemorrhage, unspecified eye [HCC]

H43.11   Vitreous hemorrhage, right eye [HCC]

H43.12   Vitreous hemorrhage, left eye [HCC]

H43.13   Vitreous hemorrhage, bilateral [HCC]

H43.2   Crystalline deposits in vitreous body

H43.20   Crystalline deposits in vitreous body, unspecified eye

H43.21   Crystalline deposits in vitreous body, right eye

H43.22   Crystalline deposits in vitreous body, left eye

H43.23   Crystalline deposits in vitreous body, bilateral

H43.3   Other vitreous opacities

H43.31   Vitreous membranes and strands

H43.311   Vitreous membranes and strands, right eye

H43.312   Vitreous membranes and strands, left eye

H43.313 Vitreous membranes and strands, bilateral

H43.319 Vitreous membranes and strands, unspecified eye

H43.39 Other vitreous opacities

Vitreous floaters

H43.391 Other vitreous opacities, right eye

H43.392 Other vitreous opacities, left eye

H43.393 Other vitreous opacities, bilateral

H43.399 Other vitreous opacities, unspecified eye

H43.8 Other disorders of vitreous body

Excludes1: proliferative vitreo-retinopathy with retinal detachment (H33.4-)

Excludes2: vitreous abscess (H44.02-)

H43.81 Vitreous degeneration

Vitreous detachment

H43.811 Vitreous degeneration, right eye

H43.812 Vitreous degeneration, left eye

H43.813 Vitreous degeneration, bilateral

H43.819 Vitreous degeneration, unspecified eye

H43.82 Vitreomacular adhesion

Vitreomacular traction

H43.821 Vitreomacular adhesion, right eye

H43.822 Vitreomacular adhesion, left eye

H43.823 Vitreomacular adhesion, bilateral

H43.829 Vitreomacular adhesion, unspecified eye

H43.89 Other disorders of vitreous body

H43.9 Unspecified disorder of vitreous body

H44 Disorders of globe

Includes: disorders affecting multiple structures of eye

H44.0 Purulent endophthalmitis

Use Additional Code to identify organism

Excludes1: bleb associated endophthalmitis (H59.4-)

H44.00 Unspecified purulent endophthalmitis

H44.001 Unspecified purulent endophthalmitis, right eye

H44.002 Unspecified purulent endophthalmitis, left eye

H44.003 Unspecified purulent endophthalmitis, bilateral

H44.009 Unspecified purulent endophthalmitis, unspecified eye

H44.01 Panophthalmitis (acute)

H44.011 Panophthalmitis (acute), right eye

H44.012 Panophthalmitis (acute), left eye

H44.013 Panophthalmitis (acute), bilateral

H44.019 Panophthalmitis (acute), unspecified eye

H44.02 Vitreous abscess (chronic)

H44.021 Vitreous abscess (chronic), right eye

H44.022 Vitreous abscess (chronic), left eye

H44.023 Vitreous abscess (chronic), bilateral

H44.029 Vitreous abscess (chronic), unspecified eye

H44.1 Other endophthalmitis

Excludes1: bleb associated endophthalmitis (H59.4-)

Excludes2: ophthalmia nodosa (H16.2-)

H44.11 Panuveitis

H44.111 Panuveitis, right eye

H44.112 Panuveitis, left eye

H44.113 Panuveitis, bilateral

H44.119 Panuveitis, unspecified eye

H44.12 Parasitic endophthalmitis, unspecified

H44.121 Parasitic endophthalmitis, unspecified, right eye

H44.122 Parasitic endophthalmitis, unspecified, left eye

H44.123 Parasitic endophthalmitis, unspecified, bilateral

H44.129 Parasitic endophthalmitis, unspecified, unspecified eye

H44.13 Sympathetic uveitis

H44.131 Sympathetic uveitis, right eye

H44.132 Sympathetic uveitis, left eye

H44.133 Sympathetic uveitis, bilateral

H44.139 Sympathetic uveitis, unspecified eye

H44.19 Other endophthalmitis

H44.2 Degenerative myopia

Malignant myopia

H44.20 Degenerative myopia, unspecified eye

H44.21 Degenerative myopia, right eye

H44.22 Degenerative myopia, left eye

H44.23 Degenerative myopia, bilateral

H44.2A Degenerative myopia with choroidal neovascularization

Use Additional Code for any associated choroid disorders (H31.-)

H44.2A1 Degenerative myopia with choroidal neovascularization, right eye

H44.2A2 Degenerative myopia with choroidal neovascularization, left eye

H44.2A3 Degenerative myopia with choroidal neovascularization, bilateral eye

H44.2A9 Degenerative myopia with choroidal neovascularization, unspecified eye

H44.2B Degenerative myopia with macular hole

H44.2B1 Degenerative myopia with macular hole, right eye

H44.2B2 Degenerative myopia with macular hole, left eye

H44.2B3 Degenerative myopia with macular hole, bilateral eye

H44.2B9 Degenerative myopia with macular hole, unspecified eye

H44.2C Degenerative myopia with retinal detachment

Use Additional Code to identify the retinal detachment (H33.-)

H44.2C1 Degenerative myopia with retinal detachment, right eye

H44.2C2 Degenerative myopia with retinal detachment, left eye

H44.2C3 Degenerative myopia with retinal detachment, bilateral eye

H44.2C9   Degenerative myopia with retinal detachment, unspecified eye

H44.2D   Degenerative myopia with foveoschisis

     H44.2D1   Degenerative myopia with foveoschisis, right eye

     H44.2D2   Degenerative myopia with foveoschisis, left eye

     H44.2D3   Degenerative myopia with foveoschisis, bilateral eye

     H44.2D9   Degenerative myopia with foveoschisis, unspecified eye

H44.2E   Degenerative myopia with other maculopathy

     H44.2E1   Degenerative myopia with other maculopathy, right eye

     H44.2E2   Degenerative myopia with other maculopathy, left eye

     H44.2E3   Degenerative myopia with other maculopathy, bilateral eye

     H44.2E9   Degenerative myopia with other maculopathy, unspecified eye

H44.3   Other and unspecified degenerative disorders of globe

   H44.30   Unspecified degenerative disorder of globe

   H44.31   Chalcosis

     H44.311   Chalcosis, right eye

     H44.312   Chalcosis, left eye

     H44.313   Chalcosis, bilateral

     H44.319   Chalcosis, unspecified eye

   H44.32   Siderosis of eye

     H44.321   Siderosis of eye, right eye

     H44.322   Siderosis of eye, left eye

     H44.323   Siderosis of eye, bilateral

     H44.329   Siderosis of eye, unspecified eye

   H44.39   Other degenerative disorders of globe

     H44.391   Other degenerative disorders of globe, right eye

     H44.392   Other degenerative disorders of globe, left eye

     H44.393   Other degenerative disorders of globe, bilateral

     H44.399   Other degenerative disorders of globe, unspecified eye

H44.4   Hypotony of eye

   H44.40   Unspecified hypotony of eye

   H44.41   Flat anterior chamber hypotony of eye

     H44.411   Flat anterior chamber hypotony of right eye

     H44.412   Flat anterior chamber hypotony of left eye

     H44.413   Flat anterior chamber hypotony of eye, bilateral

     H44.419   Flat anterior chamber hypotony of unspecified eye

   H44.42   Hypotony of eye due to ocular fistula

     H44.421   Hypotony of right eye due to ocular fistula

     H44.422   Hypotony of left eye due to ocular fistula

     H44.423   Hypotony of eye due to ocular fistula, bilateral

     H44.429   Hypotony of unspecified eye due to ocular fistula

   H44.43   Hypotony of eye due to other ocular disorders

     H44.431   Hypotony of eye due to other ocular disorders, right eye

     H44.432   Hypotony of eye due to other ocular disorders, left eye

     H44.433   Hypotony of eye due to other ocular disorders, bilateral

     H44.439   Hypotony of eye due to other ocular disorders, unspecified eye

   H44.44   Primary hypotony of eye

     H44.441   Primary hypotony of right eye

     H44.442   Primary hypotony of left eye

     H44.443   Primary hypotony of eye, bilateral

     H44.449   Primary hypotony of unspecified eye

H44.5   Degenerated conditions of globe

   H44.50   Unspecified degenerated conditions of globe

   H44.51   Absolute glaucoma

     H44.511   Absolute glaucoma, right eye

     H44.512   Absolute glaucoma, left eye

     H44.513   Absolute glaucoma, bilateral

     H44.519   Absolute glaucoma, unspecified eye

   H44.52   Atrophy of globe

     Phthisis bulbi

     H44.521   Atrophy of globe, right eye

     H44.522   Atrophy of globe, left eye

     H44.523   Atrophy of globe, bilateral

     H44.529   Atrophy of globe, unspecified eye

   H44.53   Leucocoria

     H44.531   Leucocoria, right eye

     H44.532   Leucocoria, left eye

     H44.533   Leucocoria, bilateral

     H44.539   Leucocoria, unspecified eye

H44.6   Retained (old) intraocular foreign body, magnetic

   Use Additional Code to identify magnetic foreign body (Z18.11)

   Excludes1: current intraocular foreign body (S05.-)

   Excludes2: retained foreign body in eyelid (H02.81-)

     retained (old) foreign body following penetrating wound of orbit (H05.5-)

     retained (old) intraocular foreign body, nonmagnetic (H44.7-)

   H44.60   Unspecified retained (old) intraocular foreign body, magnetic

     H44.601   Unspecified retained (old) intraocular foreign body, magnetic, right eye

     H44.602   Unspecified retained (old) intraocular foreign body, magnetic, left eye

     H44.603   Unspecified retained (old) intraocular foreign body, magnetic, bilateral

     H44.609   Unspecified retained (old) intraocular foreign body, magnetic, unspecified eye

   H44.61   Retained (old) magnetic foreign body in anterior chamber

     H44.611   Retained (old) magnetic foreign body in anterior chamber, right eye

     H44.612   Retained (old) magnetic foreign body in anterior chamber, left eye

H44.613 Retained (old) magnetic foreign body in anterior chamber, bilateral

H44.619 Retained (old) magnetic foreign body in anterior chamber, unspecified eye

H44.62 Retained (old) magnetic foreign body in iris or ciliary body

H44.621 Retained (old) magnetic foreign body in iris or ciliary body, right eye

H44.622 Retained (old) magnetic foreign body in iris or ciliary body, left eye

H44.623 Retained (old) magnetic foreign body in iris or ciliary body, bilateral

H44.629 Retained (old) magnetic foreign body in iris or ciliary body, unspecified eye

H44.63 Retained (old) magnetic foreign body in lens

H44.631 Retained (old) magnetic foreign body in lens, right eye

H44.632 Retained (old) magnetic foreign body in lens, left eye

H44.633 Retained (old) magnetic foreign body in lens, bilateral

H44.639 Retained (old) magnetic foreign body in lens, unspecified eye

H44.64 Retained (old) magnetic foreign body in posterior wall of globe

H44.641 Retained (old) magnetic foreign body in posterior wall of globe, right eye

H44.642 Retained (old) magnetic foreign body in posterior wall of globe, left eye

H44.643 Retained (old) magnetic foreign body in posterior wall of globe, bilateral

H44.649 Retained (old) magnetic foreign body in posterior wall of globe, unspecified eye

H44.65 Retained (old) magnetic foreign body in vitreous body

H44.651 Retained (old) magnetic foreign body in vitreous body, right eye

H44.652 Retained (old) magnetic foreign body in vitreous body, left eye

H44.653 Retained (old) magnetic foreign body in vitreous body, bilateral

H44.659 Retained (old) magnetic foreign body in vitreous body, unspecified eye

H44.69 Retained (old) intraocular foreign body, magnetic, in other or multiple sites

H44.691 Retained (old) intraocular foreign body, magnetic, in other or multiple sites, right eye

H44.692 Retained (old) intraocular foreign body, magnetic, in other or multiple sites, left eye

H44.693 Retained (old) intraocular foreign body, magnetic, in other or multiple sites, bilateral

H44.699 Retained (old) intraocular foreign body, magnetic, in other or multiple sites, unspecified eye

H44.7 Retained (old) intraocular foreign body, nonmagnetic

Use Additional Code to identify nonmagnetic foreign body (Z18.01-Z18.10, Z18.12, Z18.2-Z18.9)

Excludes1: current intraocular foreign body (S05.-)

Excludes2: retained foreign body in eyelid (H02.81-)

retained (old) foreign body following penetrating wound of orbit (H05.5-)

retained (old) intraocular foreign body, magnetic (H44.6-)

H44.70 Unspecified retained (old) intraocular foreign body, nonmagnetic

H44.701 Unspecified retained (old) intraocular foreign body, nonmagnetic, right eye

H44.702 Unspecified retained (old) intraocular foreign body, nonmagnetic, left eye

H44.703 Unspecified retained (old) intraocular foreign body, nonmagnetic, bilateral

H44.709 Unspecified retained (old) intraocular foreign body, nonmagnetic, unspecified eye

Retained (old) intraocular foreign body NOS

H44.71 Retained (nonmagnetic) (old) foreign body in anterior chamber

H44.711 Retained (nonmagnetic) (old) foreign body in anterior chamber, right eye

H44.712 Retained (nonmagnetic) (old) foreign body in anterior chamber, left eye

H44.713 Retained (nonmagnetic) (old) foreign body in anterior chamber, bilateral

H44.719 Retained (nonmagnetic) (old) foreign body in anterior chamber, unspecified eye

H44.72 Retained (nonmagnetic) (old) foreign body in iris or ciliary body

H44.721 Retained (nonmagnetic) (old) foreign body in iris or ciliary body, right eye

H44.722 Retained (nonmagnetic) (old) foreign body in iris or ciliary body, left eye

H44.723 Retained (nonmagnetic) (old) foreign body in iris or ciliary body, bilateral

H44.729 Retained (nonmagnetic) (old) foreign body in iris or ciliary body, unspecified eye

H44.73 Retained (nonmagnetic) (old) foreign body in lens

H44.731 Retained (nonmagnetic) (old) foreign body in lens, right eye

H44.732 Retained (nonmagnetic) (old) foreign body in lens, left eye

H44.733 Retained (nonmagnetic) (old) foreign body in lens, bilateral

H44.739 Retained (nonmagnetic) (old) foreign body in lens, unspecified eye

H44.74 Retained (nonmagnetic) (old) foreign body in posterior wall of globe

H44.741 Retained (nonmagnetic) (old) foreign body in posterior wall of globe, right eye

H44.742 Retained (nonmagnetic) (old) foreign body in posterior wall of globe, left eye

H44.743 Retained (nonmagnetic) (old) foreign body in posterior wall of globe, bilateral

H44.749 Retained (nonmagnetic) (old) foreign body in posterior wall of globe, unspecified eye

H44.75   Retained (nonmagnetic) (old) foreign body in vitreous body

    H44.751   Retained (nonmagnetic) (old) foreign body in vitreous body, right eye

    H44.752   Retained (nonmagnetic) (old) foreign body in vitreous body, left eye

    H44.753   Retained (nonmagnetic) (old) foreign body in vitreous body, bilateral

    H44.759   Retained (nonmagnetic) (old) foreign body in vitreous body, unspecified eye

H44.79   Retained (old) intraocular foreign body, nonmagnetic, in other or multiple sites

    H44.791   Retained (old) intraocular foreign body, nonmagnetic, in other or multiple sites, right eye

    H44.792   Retained (old) intraocular foreign body, nonmagnetic, in other or multiple sites, left eye

    H44.793   Retained (old) intraocular foreign body, nonmagnetic, in other or multiple sites, bilateral

    H44.799   Retained (old) intraocular foreign body, nonmagnetic, in other or multiple sites, unspecified eye

H44.8   Other disorders of globe

  H44.81   Hemophthalmos

    H44.811   Hemophthalmos, right eye

    H44.812   Hemophthalmos, left eye

    H44.813   Hemophthalmos, bilateral

    H44.819   Hemophthalmos, unspecified eye

  H44.82   Luxation of globe

    H44.821   Luxation of globe, right eye

    H44.822   Luxation of globe, left eye

    H44.823   Luxation of globe, bilateral

    H44.829   Luxation of globe, unspecified eye

  H44.89   Other disorders of globe

H44.9   Unspecified disorder of globe

DISORDERS OF OPTIC NERVE AND VISUAL PATHWAYS (H46-H47)

H46   Optic neuritis

  Excludes2: ischemic optic neuropathy (H47.01-)

  neuromyelitis optica [Devic] (G36.0)

H46.0   Optic papillitis

  H46.00   Optic papillitis, unspecified eye

  H46.01   Optic papillitis, right eye

  H46.02   Optic papillitis, left eye

  H46.03   Optic papillitis, bilateral

H46.1   Retrobulbar neuritis

  Retrobulbar neuritis NOS

  Excludes1: syphilitic retrobulbar neuritis (A52.15)

  H46.10   Retrobulbar neuritis, unspecified eye

  H46.11   Retrobulbar neuritis, right eye

  H46.12   Retrobulbar neuritis, left eye

  H46.13   Retrobulbar neuritis, bilateral

H46.2   Nutritional optic neuropathy

H46.3   Toxic optic neuropathy

  Code first (T51-T65) to identify cause

H46.8   Other optic neuritis

H46.9   Unspecified optic neuritis

H47   Other disorders of optic [2nd] nerve and visual pathways

H47.0   Disorders of optic nerve, not elsewhere classified

  H47.01   Ischemic optic neuropathy

    H47.011   Ischemic optic neuropathy, right eye

    H47.012   Ischemic optic neuropathy, left eye

    H47.013   Ischemic optic neuropathy, bilateral

    H47.019   Ischemic optic neuropathy, unspecified eye

  H47.02   Hemorrhage in optic nerve sheath

    H47.021   Hemorrhage in optic nerve sheath, right eye

    H47.022   Hemorrhage in optic nerve sheath, left eye

    H47.023   Hemorrhage in optic nerve sheath, bilateral

    H47.029   Hemorrhage in optic nerve sheath, unspecified eye

  H47.03   Optic nerve hypoplasia

    H47.031   Optic nerve hypoplasia, right eye

    H47.032   Optic nerve hypoplasia, left eye

    H47.033   Optic nerve hypoplasia, bilateral

    H47.039   Optic nerve hypoplasia, unspecified eye

  H47.09   Other disorders of optic nerve, not elsewhere classified

    Compression of optic nerve

    H47.091   Other disorders of optic nerve, not elsewhere classified, right eye

    H47.092   Other disorders of optic nerve, not elsewhere classified, left eye

    H47.093   Other disorders of optic nerve, not elsewhere classified, bilateral

    H47.099   Other disorders of optic nerve, not elsewhere classified, unspecified eye

H47.1   Papilledema

  H47.10   Unspecified papilledema

  H47.11   Papilledema associated with increased intracranial pressure

  H47.12   Papilledema associated with decreased ocular pressure

  H47.13   Papilledema associated with retinal disorder

  H47.14   Foster-Kennedy syndrome

    H47.141   Foster-Kennedy syndrome, right eye

    H47.142   Foster-Kennedy syndrome, left eye

    H47.143   Foster-Kennedy syndrome, bilateral

    H47.149   Foster-Kennedy syndrome, unspecified eye

H47.2   Optic atrophy

  H47.20   Unspecified optic atrophy

  H47.21   Primary optic atrophy

    H47.211   Primary optic atrophy, right eye

    H47.212   Primary optic atrophy, left eye

    H47.213   Primary optic atrophy, bilateral

    H47.219   Primary optic atrophy, unspecified eye

  H47.22   Hereditary optic atrophy

    Leber's optic atrophy

  H47.23   Glaucomatous optic atrophy

H47.231 Glaucomatous optic atrophy, right eye

H47.232 Glaucomatous optic atrophy, left eye

H47.233 Glaucomatous optic atrophy, bilateral

H47.239 Glaucomatous optic atrophy, unspecified eye

H47.29 **Other optic atrophy**

Temporal pallor of optic disc

H47.291 Other optic atrophy, right eye

H47.292 Other optic atrophy, left eye

H47.293 Other optic atrophy, bilateral

H47.299 Other optic atrophy, unspecified eye

H47.3 **Other disorders of optic disc**

H47.31 **Coloboma of optic disc**

H47.311 Coloboma of optic disc, right eye

H47.312 Coloboma of optic disc, left eye

H47.313 Coloboma of optic disc, bilateral

H47.319 Coloboma of optic disc, unspecified eye

H47.32 **Drusen of optic disc**

H47.321 Drusen of optic disc, right eye

H47.322 Drusen of optic disc, left eye

H47.323 Drusen of optic disc, bilateral

H47.329 Drusen of optic disc, unspecified eye

H47.33 **Pseudopapilledema of optic disc**

H47.331 Pseudopapilledema of optic disc, right eye

H47.332 Pseudopapilledema of optic disc, left eye

H47.333 Pseudopapilledema of optic disc, bilateral

H47.339 Pseudopapilledema of optic disc, unspecified eye

H47.39 **Other disorders of optic disc**

H47.391 Other disorders of optic disc, right eye

H47.392 Other disorders of optic disc, left eye

H47.393 Other disorders of optic disc, bilateral

H47.399 Other disorders of optic disc, unspecified eye

H47.4 **Disorders of optic chiasm**

Code also underlying condition

H47.41 **Disorders of optic chiasm in (due to) inflammatory disorders**

H47.42 **Disorders of optic chiasm in (due to) neoplasm**

H47.43 **Disorders of optic chiasm in (due to) vascular disorders**

H47.49 **Disorders of optic chiasm in (due to) other disorders**

H47.5 **Disorders of other visual pathways**

Disorders of optic tracts, geniculate nuclei and optic radiations

Code also underlying condition

H47.51 **Disorders of visual pathways in (due to) inflammatory disorders**

H47.511 Disorders of visual pathways in (due to) inflammatory disorders, right side

H47.512 Disorders of visual pathways in (due to) inflammatory disorders, left side

H47.519 Disorders of visual pathways in (due to) inflammatory disorders, unspecified side

H47.52 **Disorders of visual pathways in (due to) neoplasm**

H47.521 Disorders of visual pathways in (due to) neoplasm, right side

H47.522 Disorders of visual pathways in (due to) neoplasm, left side

H47.529 Disorders of visual pathways in (due to) neoplasm, unspecified side

H47.53 **Disorders of visual pathways in (due to) vascular disorders**

H47.531 Disorders of visual pathways in (due to) vascular disorders, right side

H47.532 Disorders of visual pathways in (due to) vascular disorders, left side

H47.539 Disorders of visual pathways in (due to) vascular disorders, unspecified side

H47.6 **Disorders of visual cortex**

Code also underlying condition

Excludes1: injury to visual cortex S04.04-i82.819

H47.61 **Cortical blindness**

H47.611 Cortical blindness, right side of brain

H47.612 Cortical blindness, left side of brain

H47.619 Cortical blindness, unspecified side of brain

H47.62 **Disorders of visual cortex in (due to) inflammatory disorders**

H47.621 Disorders of visual cortex in (due to) inflammatory disorders, right side of brain

H47.622 Disorders of visual cortex in (due to) inflammatory disorders, left side of brain

H47.629 Disorders of visual cortex in (due to) inflammatory disorders, unspecified side of brain

H47.63 **Disorders of visual cortex in (due to) neoplasm**

H47.631 Disorders of visual cortex in (due to) neoplasm, right side of brain

H47.632 Disorders of visual cortex in (due to) neoplasm, left side of brain

H47.639 Disorders of visual cortex in (due to) neoplasm, unspecified side of brain

H47.64 **Disorders of visual cortex in (due to) vascular disorders**

H47.641 Disorders of visual cortex in (due to) vascular disorders, right side of brain

H47.642 Disorders of visual cortex in (due to) vascular disorders, left side of brain

H47.649 Disorders of visual cortex in (due to) vascular disorders, unspecified side of brain

H47.9 **Unspecified disorder of visual pathways**

DISORDERS OF OCULAR MUSCLES, BINOCULAR MOVEMENT, ACCOMMODATION AND REFRACTION (H49-H52)

Definition: Refraction is the ability of the eye to bend light so that an

● New code   ▲ Revised code   Excludes1: Not coded here   Excludes2: Not included here   ⊗ Placeholder required   ⑦7th digit required

image is focused on the retina. Accommodation is the automatic adjustment in focal length of the natural lens of the eye.

Excludes2: nystagmus and other irregular eye movements (H55)

H49   Paralytic strabismus

Definition: Strabismus, aka crossed eyes, is a visual defect in which the eyes are misaligned and point in different directions. Strabismus usually occurs in childhood but can occur later in life.

Excludes2: internal ophthalmoplegia (H52.51-)

internuclear ophthalmoplegia (H51.2-)

progressive supranuclear ophthalmoplegia (G23.1)

H49.0   Third [oculomotor] nerve palsy

H49.00   Third [oculomotor] nerve palsy, unspecified eye

H49.01   Third [oculomotor] nerve palsy, right eye

H49.02   Third [oculomotor] nerve palsy, left eye

H49.03   Third [oculomotor] nerve palsy, bilateral

H49.1   Fourth [trochlear] nerve palsy

H49.10   Fourth [trochlear] nerve palsy, unspecified eye

H49.11   Fourth [trochlear] nerve palsy, right eye

H49.12   Fourth [trochlear] nerve palsy, left eye

H49.13   Fourth [trochlear] nerve palsy, bilateral

H49.2   Sixth [abducent] nerve palsy

H49.20   Sixth [abducent] nerve palsy, unspecified eye

H49.21   Sixth [abducent] nerve palsy, right eye

H49.22   Sixth [abducent] nerve palsy, left eye

H49.23   Sixth [abducent] nerve palsy, bilateral

H49.3   Total (external) ophthalmoplegia

H49.30   Total (external) ophthalmoplegia, unspecified eye

H49.31   Total (external) ophthalmoplegia, right eye

H49.32   Total (external) ophthalmoplegia, left eye

H49.33   Total (external) ophthalmoplegia, bilateral

H49.4   Progressive external ophthalmoplegia

Excludes1: Kearns-Sayre syndrome (H49.81-)

H49.40   Progressive external ophthalmoplegia, unspecified eye

H49.41   Progressive external ophthalmoplegia, right eye

H49.42   Progressive external ophthalmoplegia, left eye

H49.43   Progressive external ophthalmoplegia, bilateral

H49.8   Other paralytic strabismus

H49.81   Kearns-Sayre syndrome

Progressive external ophthalmoplegia with pigmentary retinopathy

Use Additional Code for other manifestation, such as: heart block (I45.9)

H49.811   Kearns-Sayre syndrome, right eye [HCC]

H49.812   Kearns-Sayre syndrome, left eye [HCC]

H49.813   Kearns-Sayre syndrome, bilateral [HCC]

H49.819   Kearns-Sayre syndrome, unspecified eye [HCC]

H49.88   Other paralytic strabismus

External ophthalmoplegia NOS

H49.881   Other paralytic strabismus, right eye

H49.882   Other paralytic strabismus, left eye

H49.883   Other paralytic strabismus, bilateral

H49.889   Other paralytic strabismus, unspecified eye

H49.9   Unspecified paralytic strabismus

H50   Other strabismus

H50.0   Esotropia

Convergent concomitant strabismus

Excludes1: intermittent esotropia (H50.31-, H50.32)

H50.00   Unspecified esotropia

H50.01   Monocular esotropia

H50.011   Monocular esotropia, right eye

H50.012   Monocular esotropia, left eye

H50.02   Monocular esotropia with A pattern

H50.021   Monocular esotropia with A pattern, right eye

H50.022   Monocular esotropia with A pattern, left eye

H50.03   Monocular esotropia with V pattern

H50.031   Monocular esotropia with V pattern, right eye

H50.032   Monocular esotropia with V pattern, left eye

H50.04   Monocular esotropia with other noncomitancies

H50.041   Monocular esotropia with other noncomitancies, right eye

H50.042   Monocular esotropia with other noncomitancies, left eye

H50.05   Alternating esotropia

H50.06   Alternating esotropia with A pattern

H50.07   Alternating esotropia with V pattern

H50.08   Alternating esotropia with other noncomitancies

H50.1   Exotropia

Divergent concomitant strabismus

Excludes1: intermittent exotropia (H50.33-, H50.34)

H50.10   Unspecified exotropia

H50.11   Monocular exotropia

H50.111   Monocular exotropia, right eye

H50.112   Monocular exotropia, left eye

H50.12   Monocular exotropia with A pattern

H50.121   Monocular exotropia with A pattern, right eye

H50.122   Monocular exotropia with A pattern, left eye

H50.13   Monocular exotropia with V pattern

H50.131   Monocular exotropia with V pattern, right eye

H50.132   Monocular exotropia with V pattern, left eye

H50.14   Monocular exotropia with other noncomitancies

H50.141   Monocular exotropia with other noncomitancies, right eye

H50.142   Monocular exotropia with other noncomitancies, left eye

H50.15   Alternating exotropia

H50.16   Alternating exotropia with A pattern

H50.17   Alternating exotropia with V pattern

H50.18   Alternating exotropia with other noncomitancies

H50.2   Vertical strabismus

Hypertropia

H50.21   Vertical strabismus, right eye

H50.22   Vertical strabismus, left eye

H50.3   Intermittent heterotropia

    H50.30   Unspecified intermittent heterotropia

    H50.31   Intermittent monocular esotropia

        H50.311   Intermittent monocular esotropia, right eye

        H50.312   Intermittent monocular esotropia, left eye

    H50.32   Intermittent alternating esotropia

    H50.33   Intermittent monocular exotropia

        H50.331   Intermittent monocular exotropia, right eye

        H50.332   Intermittent monocular exotropia, left eye

    H50.34   Intermittent alternating exotropia

H50.4   Other and unspecified heterotropia

    H50.40   Unspecified heterotropia

    H50.41   Cyclotropia

        H50.411   Cyclotropia, right eye

        H50.412   Cyclotropia, left eye

    H50.42   Monofixation syndrome

    H50.43   Accommodative component in esotropia

H50.5   Heterophoria

    H50.50   Unspecified heterophoria

    H50.51   Esophoria

    H50.52   Exophoria

    H50.53   Vertical heterophoria

    H50.54   Cyclophoria

    H50.55   Alternating heterophoria

H50.6   Mechanical strabismus

    H50.60   Mechanical strabismus, unspecified

    H50.61   Brown's sheath syndrome

        H50.611   Brown's sheath syndrome, right eye

        H50.612   Brown's sheath syndrome, left eye

    H50.69   Other mechanical strabismus

        Strabismus due to adhesions

        Traumatic limitation of duction of eye muscle

H50.8   Other specified strabismus

    H50.81   Duane's syndrome

        H50.811   Duane's syndrome, right eye

        H50.812   Duane's syndrome, left eye

    H50.89   Other specified strabismus

H50.9   Unspecified strabismus

H51   Other disorders of binocular movement

H51.0   Palsy (spasm) of conjugate gaze

H51.1   Convergence insufficiency and excess

    H51.11   Convergence insufficiency

    H51.12   Convergence excess

H51.2   Internuclear ophthalmoplegia

    H51.20   Internuclear ophthalmoplegia, unspecified eye

    H51.21   Internuclear ophthalmoplegia, right eye

    H51.22   Internuclear ophthalmoplegia, left eye

    H51.23   Internuclear ophthalmoplegia, bilateral

H51.8   Other specified disorders of binocular movement

H51.9   Unspecified disorder of binocular movement

H52   Disorders of refraction and accommodation

H52.0   Hypermetropia

    H52.00   Hypermetropia, unspecified eye

    H52.01   Hypermetropia, right eye

    H52.02   Hypermetropia, left eye

    H52.03   Hypermetropia, bilateral

H52.1   Myopia

    Excludes1: degenerative myopia (H44.2-)

    H52.10   Myopia, unspecified eye

    H52.11   Myopia, right eye

    H52.12   Myopia, left eye

    H52.13   Myopia, bilateral

H52.2   Astigmatism

    H52.20   Unspecified astigmatism

        H52.201   Unspecified astigmatism, right eye

        H52.202   Unspecified astigmatism, left eye

        H52.203   Unspecified astigmatism, bilateral

        H52.209   Unspecified astigmatism, unspecified eye

    H52.21   Irregular astigmatism

        H52.211   Irregular astigmatism, right eye

        H52.212   Irregular astigmatism, left eye

        H52.213   Irregular astigmatism, bilateral

        H52.219   Irregular astigmatism, unspecified eye

    H52.22   Regular astigmatism

        H52.221   Regular astigmatism, right eye

        H52.222   Regular astigmatism, left eye

        H52.223   Regular astigmatism, bilateral

        H52.229   Regular astigmatism, unspecified eye

H52.3   Anisometropia and aniseikonia

    H52.31   Anisometropia

    H52.32   Aniseikonia

H52.4   Presbyopia

H52.5   Disorders of accommodation

    H52.51   Internal ophthalmoplegia (complete) (total)

        H52.511   Internal ophthalmoplegia (complete) (total), right eye

        H52.512   Internal ophthalmoplegia (complete) (total), left eye

        H52.513   Internal ophthalmoplegia (complete) (total), bilateral

        H52.519   Internal ophthalmoplegia (complete) (total), unspecified eye

    H52.52   Paresis of accommodation

        H52.521   Paresis of accommodation, right eye

        H52.522   Paresis of accommodation, left eye

        H52.523   Paresis of accommodation, bilateral

        H52.529   Paresis of accommodation, unspecified eye

    H52.53   Spasm of accommodation

        H52.531   Spasm of accommodation, right eye

        H52.532   Spasm of accommodation, left eye

        H52.533   Spasm of accommodation, bilateral

        H52.539   Spasm of accommodation, unspecified eye

H52.6   Other disorders of refraction

H52.7   Unspecified disorder of refraction

VISUAL DISTURBANCES AND BLINDNESS (H53-H54)

H53   Visual disturbances

H53.0 Amblyopia ex anopsia

Excludes1: amblyopia due to vitamin A deficiency (E50.5)

H53.00 Unspecified amblyopia

- **H53.001 Unspecified amblyopia, right eye**
- **H53.002 Unspecified amblyopia, left eye**
- **H53.003 Unspecified amblyopia, bilateral**
- **H53.009 Unspecified amblyopia, unspecified eye**

H53.01 Deprivation amblyopia

- **H53.011 Deprivation amblyopia, right eye**
- **H53.012 Deprivation amblyopia, left eye**
- **H53.013 Deprivation amblyopia, bilateral**
- **H53.019 Deprivation amblyopia, unspecified eye**

H53.02 Refractive amblyopia

- **H53.021 Refractive amblyopia, right eye**
- **H53.022 Refractive amblyopia, left eye**
- **H53.023 Refractive amblyopia, bilateral**
- **H53.029 Refractive amblyopia, unspecified eye**

H53.03 Strabismic amblyopia

Excludes1: strabismus (H50.-)

- **H53.031 Strabismic amblyopia, right eye**
- **H53.032 Strabismic amblyopia, left eye**
- **H53.033 Strabismic amblyopia, bilateral**
- **H53.039 Strabismic amblyopia, unspecified eye**

H53.04 Amblyopia suspect

- **H53.041 Amblyopia suspect, right eye**
- **H53.042 Amblyopia suspect, left eye**
- **H53.043 Amblyopia suspect, bilateral**
- **H53.049 Amblyopia suspect, unspecified eye**

H53.1 Subjective visual disturbances

subjective visual disturbances due to vitamin A deficiency (E50.5)

visual hallucinations (R44.1)

H53.10 Unspecified subjective visual disturbances

H53.11 Day blindness

Hemeralopia

H53.12 Transient visual loss

Scintillating scotoma amaurosis fugax (G45.3-)

transient retinal artery occlusion (H34.0-)

- **H53.121 Transient visual loss, right eye**
- **H53.122 Transient visual loss, left eye**
- **H53.123 Transient visual loss, bilateral**
- **H53.129 Transient visual loss, unspecified eye**

H53.13 Sudden visual loss

- **H53.131 Sudden visual loss, right eye**
- **H53.132 Sudden visual loss, left eye**
- **H53.133 Sudden visual loss, bilateral**
- **H53.139 Sudden visual loss, unspecified eye**

H53.14 Visual discomfort

Asthenopia

Photophobia

- **H53.141 Visual discomfort, right eye**
- **H53.142 Visual discomfort, left eye**
- **H53.143 Visual discomfort, bilateral**

- **H53.149 Visual discomfort, unspecified**

H53.15 Visual distortions of shape and size

Metamorphopsia

H53.16 Psychophysical visual disturbances

H53.19 Other subjective visual disturbances

Visual halos

H53.2 Diplopia

Double vision

H53.3 Other and unspecified disorders of binocular vision

H53.30 Unspecified disorder of binocular vision

H53.31 Abnormal retinal correspondence

H53.32 Fusion with defective stereopsis

H53.33 Simultaneous visual perception without fusion

H53.34 Suppression of binocular vision

H53.4 Visual field defects

H53.40 Unspecified visual field defects

H53.41 Scotoma involving central area

Central scotoma

- **H53.411 Scotoma involving central area, right eye**
- **H53.412 Scotoma involving central area, left eye**
- **H53.413 Scotoma involving central area, bilateral**
- **H53.419 Scotoma involving central area, unspecified eye**

H53.42 Scotoma of blind spot area

Enlarged blind spot

- **H53.421 Scotoma of blind spot area, right eye**
- **H53.422 Scotoma of blind spot area, left eye**
- **H53.423 Scotoma of blind spot area, bilateral**
- **H53.429 Scotoma of blind spot area, unspecified eye**

H53.43 Sector or arcuate defects

Arcuate scotoma

Bjerrum scotoma

- **H53.431 Sector or arcuate defects, right eye**
- **H53.432 Sector or arcuate defects, left eye**
- **H53.433 Sector or arcuate defects, bilateral**
- **H53.439 Sector or arcuate defects, unspecified eye**

H53.45 Other localized visual field defect

Peripheral visual field defect

Ring scotoma NOS

Scotoma NOS

- **H53.451 Other localized visual field defect, right eye**
- **H53.452 Other localized visual field defect, left eye**
- **H53.453 Other localized visual field defect, bilateral**
- **H53.459 Other localized visual field defect, unspecified eye**

H53.46 Homonymous bilateral field defects

Homonymous hemianopia

Homonymous hemianopsia

Quadrant anopia

Quadrant anopsia

H53.461 Homonymous bilateral field defects, right side

H53.462 Homonymous bilateral field defects, left side

H53.469 Homonymous bilateral field defects, unspecified side

Homonymous bilateral field defects NOS

H53.47 Heteronymous bilateral field defects

Heteronymous hemianop(s)ia

H53.48 Generalized contraction of visual field

H53.481 Generalized contraction of visual field, right eye

H53.482 Generalized contraction of visual field, left eye

H53.483 Generalized contraction of visual field, bilateral

H53.489 Generalized contraction of visual field, unspecified eye

H53.5 Color vision deficiencies

Color blindness

Excludes2: day blindness (H53.11)

H53.50 Unspecified color vision deficiencies

Color blindness NOS

H53.51 Achromatopsia

H53.52 Acquired color vision deficiency

H53.53 Deuteranomaly

Deuteranopia

H53.54 Protanomaly

Protanopia

H53.55 Tritanomaly

Tritanopia

H53.59 Other color vision deficiencies

H53.6 Night blindness

Excludes1: night blindness due to vitamin A deficiency (E50.5)

H53.60 Unspecified night blindness

H53.61 Abnormal dark adaptation curve

H53.62 Acquired night blindness

H53.63 Congenital night blindness

H53.69 Other night blindness

H53.7 Vision sensitivity deficiencies

H53.71 Glare sensitivity

H53.72 Impaired contrast sensitivity

H53.8 Other visual disturbances

H53.9 Unspecified visual disturbance

H54 **Blindness and low vision**

Note: For definition of visual impairment categories see table below

Code first any associated underlying cause of the blindness

Excludes1: amaurosis fugax (G45.3)

H54.0 Blindness, both eyes

Visual impairment categories 3, 4, 5 in both eyes.

H54.0X Blindness, both eyes, different category levels

H54.0X3 Blindness right eye, category 3

H54.0X33 Blindness right eye category 3, blindness left eye category 3

H54.0X34 Blindness right eye category 3, blindness left eye category 4

H54.0X35 Blindness right eye category 3, blindness left eye category 5

H54.0X4 Blindness right eye, category 4

H54.0X43 Blindness right eye category 4, blindness left eye category 3

H54.0X44 Blindness right eye category 4, blindness left eye category 4

H54.0X45 Blindness right eye category 4, blindness left eye category 5

H54.0X5 Blindness right eye, category 5

H54.0X53 Blindness right eye category 5, blindness left eye category 3

H54.0X54 Blindness right eye category 5, blindness left eye category 4

H54.0X55 Blindness right eye category 5, blindness left eye category 5

H54.1 Blindness, one eye, low vision other eye

Visual impairment categories 3, 4, 5 in one eye, with categories 1 or 2 in the other eye.

H54.10 Blindness, one eye, low vision other eye, unspecified eyes

H54.11 Blindness, right eye, low vision left eye

H54.113 Blindness right eye category 3, low vision left eye

H54.1131 Blindness right eye category 3, low vision left eye category 1

H54.1132 Blindness right eye category 3, low vision left eye category 2

H54.114 Blindness right eye category 4, low vision left eye

H54.1141 Blindness right eye category 4, low vision left eye category 1

H54.1142 Blindness right eye category 4, low vision left eye category 2

H54.115 Blindness right eye category 5, low vision left eye

H54.1151 Blindness right eye category 5, low vision left eye category 1

H54.1152 Blindness right eye category 5, low vision left eye category 2

H54.12 Blindness, left eye, low vision right eye

H54.121 Low vision right eye category 1, blindness left eye

H54.1213 Low vision right eye category 1, blindness left eye category 3

H54.1214 Low vision right eye category 1, blindness left eye category 4

● New code   ▲ Revised code   **Excludes1:** Not coded here   **Excludes2:** Not included here   ⊗ Placeholder required   ⑦7th digit required

H54.1215   **Low vision right eye category 1, blindness left eye category 5**

H54.122   **Low vision right eye category 2, blindness left eye**

H54.1223   **Low vision right eye category 2, blindness left eye category 3**

H54.1224   **Low vision right eye category 2, blindness left eye category 4**

H54.1225   **Low vision right eye category 2, blindness left eye category 5**

H54.2   Low vision, both eyes

Visual impairment categories 1 or 2 in both eyes.

H54.2X   Low vision, both eyes, different category levels

H54.2X1   **Low vision, right eye, category 1**

H54.2X11   **Low vision right eye category 1, low vision left eye category 1**

H54.2X12   **Low vision right eye category 1, low vision left eye category 2**

H54.2X2   **Low vision, right eye, category 2**

H54.2X21   **Low vision right eye category 2, low vision left eye category 1**

H54.2X22   **Low vision right eye category 2, low vision left eye category 2**

H54.3   Unqualified visual loss, both eyes

Visual impairment category 9 in both eyes.

H54.4   Blindness, one eye

Visual impairment categories 3, 4, 5 in one eye [normal vision in other eye]

H54.40   Blindness, one eye, unspecified eye

H54.41   Blindness, right eye, normal vision left eye

H54.413   **Blindness, right eye, category 3**

H54.413A   **Blindness right eye category 3, normal vision left eye**

H54.414   **Blindness, right eye, category 4**

H54.414A   **Blindness right eye category 4, normal vision left eye**

H54.415   **Blindness, right eye, category 5**

H54.415A   **Blindness right eye category 5, normal vision left eye**

H54.42   Blindness, left eye, normal vision right eye

H54.42A   **Blindness, left eye, category 3-5**

H54.42A3   **Blindness left eye category 3, normal vision right eye**

H54.42A4   **Blindness left eye category 4, normal vision right eye**

H54.42A5   **Blindness left eye category 5, normal vision right eye**

H54.5   Low vision, one eye

Visual impairment categories 1 or 2 in one eye [normal vision in other eye].

H54.50   Low vision, one eye, unspecified eye

H54.51   Low vision, right eye, normal vision left eye

H54.511   **Low vision, right eye, category 1-2**

H54.511A   **Low vision right eye category 1, normal vision left eye**

H54.512A   **Low vision right eye category 2, normal vision left eye**

H54.52   Low vision, left eye, normal vision right eye

H54.52A   **Low vision, left eye, category 1-2**

H54.52A1   **Low vision left eye category 1, normal vision right eye**

H54.52A2   **Low vision left eye category 2, normal vision right eye**

H54.414   **Blindness, right eye, category 4**

H54.414A   **Blindness right eye category 4, normal vision left eye**

H54.415   **Blindness, right eye, category 5**

H54.415A   **Blindness right eye category 5, normal vision left eye**

H54.6   Unqualified visual loss, one eye

Visual impairment category 9 in one eye [normal vision in other eye].

H54.60   Unqualified visual loss, one eye, unspecified

H54.61   Unqualified visual loss, right eye, normal vision left eye

H54.62   Unqualified visual loss, left eye, normal vision right eye

H54.7   Unspecified visual loss

Visual impairment category 9 NOS

H54.8   Legal blindness, as defined in USA

Blindness NOS according to USA definition legal blindness with specification of impairment level (H54.0-H54.7)

Note: The table below gives a classification of severity of visual impairment recommended by a WHO Study Group on the Prevention of Blindness, Geneva, 6-10 November 1972.

The term 'low vision' in category H54 comprises categories 1 and 2 of the table, the term 'blindness' categories 3, 4 and 5, and the term 'unqualified visual loss' category 9.

If the extent of the visual field is taken into account, patients with a field no greater than 10 but greater than 5 around central fixation should be placed in category 3 and patients with a field no greater than 5 around central fixation should be placed in category 4, even if the central acuity is not impaired. (Document 508 compliance requires all cells in the following table to be filled.)

Category of visual impairment	Visual acuity with best possible correction	
	Maximum less than:	**Minimum equal to or better than:**
-	6/18	6/60
3/10(0.3)	1/10(0.1)	-
20/70	20/200	-
-	6/60	3/60
1/10(0.1)	1/20(0.05)	-
20/200	20/400	-
-	3/60	1/60(finger counting at one meter)
1/200(0.05)	1/50(0.02)	-
20/400	5/300(20/1200)	-
-	1/60(finger counting at one	Light perception

	meter)	
1/50(0.02)	-	-
5/300	-	-
-	No light perception	-
-	Undetermined or unspecified	-

OTHER DISORDERS OF EYE AND ADNEXA (H55-H57)

H55   **Nystagmus and other irregular eye movements**

    H55.0   **Nystagmus**

        H55.00   **Unspecified nystagmus**

        H55.01   **Congenital nystagmus**

        H55.02   **Latent nystagmus**

        H55.03   **Visual deprivation nystagmus**

        H55.04   **Dissociated nystagmus**

        H55.09   **Other forms of nystagmus**

    H55.8   **Other irregular eye movements**

        ▲**H55.81**   **Deficient saccadic eye movements**

        H55.82   **Deficient smooth pursuit eye movements**

        H55.89   **Other irregular eye movements**

H57   **Other disorders of eye and adnexa**

    H57.0   **Anomalies of pupillary function**

        H57.00   **Unspecified anomaly of pupillary function**

        H57.01   **Argyll Robertson pupil, atypical**

           Excludes1: syphilitic Argyll Robertson pupil (A52.19)

        H57.02   **Anisocoria**

        H57.03   **Miosis**

        H57.04   **Mydriasis**

        H57.05   **Tonic pupil**

           H57.051   **Tonic pupil, right eye**

           H57.052   **Tonic pupil, left eye**

           H57.053   **Tonic pupil, bilateral**

           H57.059   **Tonic pupil, unspecified eye**

        H57.09   **Other anomalies of pupillary function**

    H57.1   **Ocular pain**

        H57.10   **Ocular pain, unspecified eye**

        H57.11   **Ocular pain, right eye**

        H57.12   **Ocular pain, left eye**

        H57.13   **Ocular pain, bilateral**

    H57.8   **Other specified disorders of eye and adnexa**

        H57.81   **Brow ptosis**

           H57.811   **Brow ptosis, right**

           H57.812   **Brow ptosis, left**

           H57.813   **Brow ptosis, bilateral**

           H57.819   **Brow ptosis, unspecified**

        H57.89   **Other specified disorders of eye and adnexa**

    H57.9   **Unspecified disorder of eye and adnexa**

INTRAOPERATIVE AND POSTPROCEDURAL COMPLICATIONS AND DISORDERS OF EYE AND ADNEXA, NOT ELSEWHERE CLASSIFIED (H59)

H59   **Intraoperative and postprocedural complications and disorders of eye and adnexa, not elsewhere classified**

    Excludes1: mechanical complication of intraocular lens (T85.2)

        mechanical complication of **other** ocular prosthetic devices, implants and grafts (T85.3)

        pseudophakia (Z96.1)

        secondary cataracts (H26.4-)

H59.0   **Disorders of the eye following cataract surgery**

    H59.01   **Keratopathy (bullous aphakic) following cataract surgery**

        Vitreal corneal syndrome

        Vitreous (touch) syndrome

        H59.011   **Keratopathy (bullous aphakic) following cataract surgery, right eye**

        H59.012   **Keratopathy (bullous aphakic) following cataract surgery, left eye**

        H59.013   **Keratopathy (bullous aphakic) following cataract surgery, bilateral**

        H59.019   **Keratopathy (bullous aphakic) following cataract surgery, unspecified eye**

    H59.02   **Cataract (lens) fragments in eye following cataract surgery**

        H59.021   **Cataract (lens) fragments in eye following cataract surgery, right eye**

        H59.022   **Cataract (lens) fragments in eye following cataract surgery, left eye**

        H59.023   **Cataract (lens) fragments in eye following cataract surgery, bilateral**

        H59.029   **Cataract (lens) fragments in eye following cataract surgery, unspecified eye**

    H59.03   **Cystoid macular edema following cataract surgery**

        H59.031   **Cystoid macular edema following cataract surgery, right eye**

        H59.032   **Cystoid macular edema following cataract surgery, left eye**

        H59.033   **Cystoid macular edema following cataract surgery, bilateral**

        H59.039   **Cystoid macular edema following cataract surgery, unspecified eye**

    H59.09   **Other disorders of the eye following cataract surgery**

        H59.091   **Other disorders of the right eye following cataract surgery**

        H59.092   **Other disorders of the left eye following cataract surgery**

        H59.093   **Other disorders of the eye following cataract surgery, bilateral**

        H59.099   **Other disorders of unspecified eye following cataract surgery**

H59.1   **Intraoperative hemorrhage and hematoma of eye and adnexa complicating a procedure**

    Excludes1: intraoperative hemorrhage and hematoma of eye and adnexa due to accidental puncture or laceration during a procedure (H59.2-)

    H59.11   **Intraoperative hemorrhage and hematoma of eye and adnexa complicating an ophthalmic procedure**

        H59.111   **Intraoperative hemorrhage and hematoma of right eye and adnexa complicating an ophthalmic procedure**

        H59.112   **Intraoperative hemorrhage and hematoma of left eye and adnexa complicating an ophthalmic procedure**

        H59.113   **Intraoperative hemorrhage and hematoma of eye and adnexa complicating an ophthalmic procedure, bilateral**

● New code   ▲ Revised code   **Excludes1:** Not coded here   **Excludes2:** Not included here   ⊗ Placeholder required   ⑦7th digit required

H59.119 Intraoperative hemorrhage and hematoma of unspecified eye and adnexa complicating an ophthalmic procedure

H59.12 Intraoperative hemorrhage and hematoma of eye and adnexa complicating other procedure

H59.121 Intraoperative hemorrhage and hematoma of right eye and adnexa complicating other procedure

H59.122 Intraoperative hemorrhage and hematoma of left eye and adnexa complicating other procedure

H59.123 Intraoperative hemorrhage and hematoma of eye and adnexa complicating other procedure, bilateral

H59.129 Intraoperative hemorrhage and hematoma of unspecified eye and adnexa complicating other procedure

H59.2 Accidental puncture and laceration of eye and adnexa during a procedure

H59.21 Accidental puncture and laceration of eye and adnexa during an ophthalmic procedure

H59.211 Accidental puncture and laceration of right eye and adnexa during an ophthalmic procedure

H59.212 Accidental puncture and laceration of left eye and adnexa during an ophthalmic procedure

H59.213 Accidental puncture and laceration of eye and adnexa during an ophthalmic procedure, bilateral

H59.219 Accidental puncture and laceration of unspecified eye and adnexa during an ophthalmic procedure

H59.22 Accidental puncture and laceration of eye and adnexa during other procedure

H59.221 Accidental puncture and laceration of right eye and adnexa during other procedure

H59.222 Accidental puncture and laceration of left eye and adnexa during other procedure

H59.223 Accidental puncture and laceration of eye and adnexa during other procedure, bilateral

H59.229 Accidental puncture and laceration of unspecified eye and adnexa during other procedure

H59.3 Postprocedural hemorrhage, hematoma, and seroma of eye and adnexa following a procedure

H59.31 Postprocedural hemorrhage of eye and adnexa following an ophthalmic procedure

H59.311 Postprocedural hemorrhage of right eye and adnexa following an ophthalmic procedure

H59.312 Postprocedural hemorrhage of left eye and adnexa following an ophthalmic procedure

H59.313 Postprocedural hemorrhage of eye and adnexa following an ophthalmic procedure, bilateral

H59.319 Postprocedural hemorrhage of unspecified eye and adnexa following an ophthalmic procedure

H59.32 Postprocedural hemorrhage of eye and adnexa following other procedure

H59.321 Postprocedural hemorrhage of right eye and adnexa following other procedure

H59.322 Postprocedural hemorrhage of left eye and adnexa following other procedure

H59.323 Postprocedural hemorrhage of eye and adnexa following other procedure, bilateral

H59.329 Postprocedural hemorrhage of unspecified eye and adnexa following other procedure

H59.33 Postprocedural hematoma of eye and adnexa following an ophthalmic procedure

H59.331 Postprocedural hematoma of right eye and adnexa following an ophthalmic procedure

H59.332 Postprocedural hematoma of left eye and adnexa following an ophthalmic procedure

H59.333 Postprocedural hematoma of eye and adnexa following an ophthalmic procedure, bilateral

H59.339 Postprocedural hematoma of unspecified eye and adnexa following an ophthalmic procedure

H59.34 Postprocedural hematoma of eye and adnexa following other procedure

H59.341 Postprocedural hematoma of right eye and adnexa following other procedure

H59.342 Postprocedural hematoma of left eye and adnexa following other procedure

H59.343 Postprocedural hematoma of eye and adnexa following other procedure, bilateral

H59.349 Postprocedural hematoma of unspecified eye and adnexa following other procedure

H59.35 Postprocedural seroma of eye and adnexa following an ophthalmic procedure

H59.351 Postprocedural seroma of right eye and adnexa following an ophthalmic procedure

H59.352 Postprocedural seroma of left eye and adnexa following an ophthalmic procedure

H59.353 Postprocedural seroma of eye and adnexa following an ophthalmic procedure, bilateral

H59.359 Postprocedural seroma of unspecified eye and adnexa following an ophthalmic procedure

H59.36 Postprocedural seroma of eye and adnexa following other procedure

H59.361 Postprocedural seroma of right eye and adnexa following other procedure

H59.362 Postprocedural seroma of left eye and adnexa following other procedure

H59.363 Postprocedural seroma of eye and adnexa following other procedure, bilateral

H59.369 Postprocedural seroma of unspecified eye and adnexa following other procedure

H59.4 **Inflammation (infection) of postprocedural bleb**

Postprocedural blebitis

Excludes1: filtering (vitreous) bleb after glaucoma surgery status (Z98.83)

H59.40 **Inflammation (infection) of postprocedural bleb, unspecified**

H59.41 **Inflammation (infection) of postprocedural bleb, stage 1**

H59.42 **Inflammation (infection) of postprocedural bleb, stage 2**

H59.43 **Inflammation (infection) of postprocedural bleb, stage 3**

Bleb endophthalmitis

H59.8 **Other intraoperative and postprocedural complications and disorders of eye and adnexa, not elsewhere classified**

H59.81 **Chorioretinal scars after surgery for detachment**

H59.811 Chorioretinal scars after surgery for detachment, right eye

H59.812 Chorioretinal scars after surgery for detachment, left eye

H59.813 Chorioretinal scars after surgery for detachment, bilateral

H59.819 Chorioretinal scars after surgery for detachment, unspecified eye

H59.88 **Other intraoperative complications of eye and adnexa, not elsewhere classified**

H59.89 **Other postprocedural complications and disorders of eye and adnexa, not elsewhere classified**

● New code   ▲ Revised code   Excludes1: Not coded here   Excludes2: Not included here   ⊗ Placeholder required   ⑦7th digit required

Chapter 8: Diseases of the Ear and Mastoid Process (H60-H95)

DEFINITIONS

This chapter includes definitions of selected key words, terms and phrases and coding alerts for adding points to the clinical domain, and references to coding late effects where appropriate. An example from this chapter is as follows:

H65 Nonsuppurative otitis media
Definition: Nonsuppurative otitis media and eustachian tube disorders, otitis media is an inflammation of the middle ear without the formation or discharge of pus.

MULTIPLE CODING FOR A SINGLE CONDITION

In addition to the etiology/manifestation convention that requires two codes to fully describe a single condition that affects multiple body systems, there are other single conditions that also require more than one code. "**Use Additional Code**" notes are found in the Tabular List at codes that are not part of an etiology/manifestation pair where a secondary code is useful to fully describe a condition. The sequencing rule is the same as the etiology/manifestation pair, "**Use Additional Code**" indicates that a secondary code should be added.

For example, for bacterial infections that are not included in chapter 1, a secondary code from category B95, Streptococcus, Staphylococcus, and Enterococcus, as the cause of diseases classified elsewhere, or B96, Other bacterial agents as the cause of diseases classified elsewhere, may be required to identify the bacterial organism causing the infection. A "**Use Additional Code**" note will normally be found at the infectious disease code, indicating a need for the organism code to be added as a secondary code.

 "Code first" notes are also under certain codes that are not specifically manifestation codes but may be due to an underlying cause. When there is a "Code first" note and an underlying condition is present, the underlying condition should be sequenced first.

"Code, if applicable, any causal condition first", notes indicate that this code may be assigned as a principal diagnosis when the causal condition is unknown or not applicable. If a causal condition is known, then the code for that condition should be sequenced as the principal or first-listed diagnosis.

Multiple codes may be needed for sequela, complication codes and obstetric codes to more fully describe a condition. See the specific guidelines for these conditions for further instruction.

COMBINATION CODE

A combination code is a single code used to classify: Two diagnoses, or a diagnosis with an associated secondary process (manifestation) A diagnosis with an associated complication

Combination codes are identified by referring to subterm entries in the Alphabetic Index and by reading the inclusion and exclusion notes in the Tabular List.

Assign only the combination code when that code fully identifies the diagnostic conditions involved or when the Alphabetic Index so directs. Multiple coding should not be used when the classification provides a combination code that clearly identifies all of the elements documented in the diagnosis. When the combination code lacks necessary specificity in describing the manifestation or complication, an additional code should be used as a secondary code.

SEQUELA (LATE EFFECTS)

A sequela is the residual effect (condition produced) after the acute phase of an illness or injury has terminated. There is no time limit on when a sequela code can be used. The residual may be apparent early, such as in cerebral infarction, or it may occur months or years later, such as that due to a previous injury. Coding of sequela generally requires two codes sequenced in the following order: The condition or nature of the sequela is sequenced first.

The sequela code is sequenced second.

An exception to the above guidelines are those instances where the code for the sequela is followed by a manifestation code identified in the Tabular List and title, or the sequela code has been expanded (at the fourth, fifth or sixth character levels) to include the manifestation(s). The code for the acute phase of an illness or injury that led to the sequela is never used with a code for the late effect.

● New code   ▲ Revised code   **Excludes1:** Not coded here   **Excludes2:** Not included here   ⊗ Placeholder required   ⑦7th digit required

Chapter 8

Diseases of The Ear and Mastoid Process (H60-H95)

Note: Use an external cause code following the code for the ear condition, if applicable, to identify the cause of the ear condition

Excludes2: certain conditions originating in the perinatal period (P04-P96)

certain infectious and parasitic diseases (A00-B99)

complications of pregnancy, childbirth and the puerperium (O00-O9A)

congenital malformations, deformations and chromosomal abnormalities (Q00-Q99)

endocrine, nutritional and metabolic diseases (E00-E88)

injury, poisoning and certain other consequences of external causes (S00-T88)

neoplasms (C00-D49)

symptoms, signs and abnormal clinical and laboratory findings, not elsewhere classified (R00-R94)

This chapter contains the following blocks:

H60-H62	Diseases of external ear
H65-H75	Diseases of middle ear and mastoid
H80-H83	Diseases of inner ear
H90-H94	Other disorders of ear
H95	Intraoperative and postprocedural complications and disorders of ear and mastoid process, not elsewhere classified

DISEASES OF EXTERNAL EAR (H60-H62)

H60 Otitis externa

H60.0 Abscess of external ear

Boil of external ear

Carbuncle of auricle or external auditory canal

Furuncle of external ear

H60.00 Abscess of external ear, unspecified ear

H60.01 Abscess of right external ear

H60.02 Abscess of left external ear

H60.03 Abscess of external ear, bilateral

H60.1 Cellulitis of external ear

Cellulitis of auricle

Cellulitis of external auditory canal

H60.10 Cellulitis of external ear, unspecified ear

H60.11 Cellulitis of right external ear

H60.12 Cellulitis of left external ear

H60.13 Cellulitis of external ear, bilateral

H60.2 Malignant otitis externa

H60.20 Malignant otitis externa, unspecified ear

H60.21 Malignant otitis externa, right ear

H60.22 Malignant otitis externa, left ear

H60.23 Malignant otitis externa, bilateral

H60.3 Other infective otitis externa

H60.31 Diffuse otitis externa

H60.311 Diffuse otitis externa, right ear

H60.312 Diffuse otitis externa, left ear

H60.313 Diffuse otitis externa, bilateral

H60.319 Diffuse otitis externa, unspecified ear

H60.32 Hemorrhagic otitis externa

H60.321 Hemorrhagic otitis externa, right ear

H60.322 Hemorrhagic otitis externa, left ear

H60.323 Hemorrhagic otitis externa, bilateral

H60.329 Hemorrhagic otitis externa, unspecified ear

H60.33 Swimmer's ear

H60.331 Swimmer's ear, right ear

H60.332 Swimmer's ear, left ear

H60.333 Swimmer's ear, bilateral

H60.339 Swimmer's ear, unspecified ear

H60.39 Other infective otitis externa

H60.391 Other infective otitis externa, right ear

H60.392 Other infective otitis externa, left ear

H60.393 Other infective otitis externa, bilateral

H60.399 Other infective otitis externa, unspecified ear

H60.4 Cholesteatoma of external ear

Keratosis obturans of external ear (canal)

Excludes2: cholesteatoma of middle ear (H71.-)

recurrent cholesteatoma of postmastoidectomy cavity (H95.0-)

H60.40 Cholesteatoma of external ear, unspecified ear

H60.41 Cholesteatoma of right external ear

H60.42 Cholesteatoma of left external ear

H60.43 Cholesteatoma of external ear, bilateral

H60.5 Acute noninfective otitis externa

H60.50 Unspecified acute noninfective otitis externa

Acute otitis externa NOS

H60.501 Unspecified acute noninfective otitis externa, right ear

H60.502 Unspecified acute noninfective otitis externa, left ear

H60.503 Unspecified acute noninfective otitis externa, bilateral

H60.509 Unspecified acute noninfective otitis externa, unspecified ear

H60.51 Acute actinic otitis externa

H60.511 Acute actinic otitis externa, right ear

H60.512 Acute actinic otitis externa, left ear

H60.513 Acute actinic otitis externa, bilateral

H60.519 Acute actinic otitis externa, unspecified ear

H60.52 Acute chemical otitis externa

H60.521 Acute chemical otitis externa, right ear

H60.522 Acute chemical otitis externa, left ear

H60.523 Acute chemical otitis externa, bilateral

H60.529 Acute chemical otitis externa, unspecified ear

H60.53 Acute contact otitis externa

H60.531 Acute contact otitis externa, right ear

H60.532 Acute contact otitis externa, left ear

H60.533 Acute contact otitis externa, bilateral

H60.539 Acute contact otitis externa, unspecified ear

H60.54 Acute eczematoid otitis externa

H60.541 Acute eczematoid otitis externa, right ear

H60.542 Acute eczematoid otitis externa, left ear

H60.543	Acute eczematoid otitis externa, bilateral	
H60.549	Acute eczematoid otitis externa, unspecified ear	

H60.55 Acute reactive otitis externa

H60.551 Acute reactive otitis externa, right ear

H60.552 Acute reactive otitis externa, left ear

H60.553 Acute reactive otitis externa, bilateral

H60.559 Acute reactive otitis externa, unspecified ear

H60.59 Other noninfective acute otitis externa

H60.591 Other noninfective acute otitis externa, right ear

H60.592 Other noninfective acute otitis externa, left ear

H60.593 Other noninfective acute otitis externa, bilateral

H60.599 Other noninfective acute otitis externa, unspecified ear

H60.6 Unspecified chronic otitis externa

H60.60 Unspecified chronic otitis externa, unspecified ear

H60.61 Unspecified chronic otitis externa, right ear

H60.62 Unspecified chronic otitis externa, left ear

H60.63 Unspecified chronic otitis externa, bilateral

H60.8 Other otitis externa

H60.8X Other otitis externa

H60.8X1 Other otitis externa, right ear

H60.8X2 Other otitis externa, left ear

H60.8X3 Other otitis externa, bilateral

H60.8X9 Other otitis externa, unspecified ear

H60.9 Unspecified otitis externa

H60.90 Unspecified otitis externa, unspecified ear

H60.91 Unspecified otitis externa, right ear

H60.92 Unspecified otitis externa, left ear

H60.93 Unspecified otitis externa, bilateral

H61 Other disorders of external ear

H61.0 Chondritis and perichondritis of external ear

Chondrodermatitis nodularis chronica helicis

Perichondritis of auricle

Perichondritis of pinna

H61.00 Unspecified perichondritis of external ear

H61.001 Unspecified perichondritis of right external ear

H61.002 Unspecified perichondritis of left external ear

H61.003 Unspecified perichondritis of external ear, bilateral

H61.009 Unspecified perichondritis of external ear, unspecified ear

H61.01 Acute perichondritis of external ear

H61.011 Acute perichondritis of right external ear

H61.012 Acute perichondritis of left external ear

H61.013 Acute perichondritis of external ear, bilateral

H61.019 Acute perichondritis of external ear, unspecified ear

H61.02 Chronic perichondritis of external ear

H61.021 Chronic perichondritis of right external ear

H61.022 Chronic perichondritis of left external ear

H61.023 Chronic perichondritis of external ear, bilateral

H61.029 Chronic perichondritis of external ear, unspecified ear

H61.03 Chondritis of external ear

Chondritis of auricle

Chondritis of pinna

H61.031 Chondritis of right external ear

H61.032 Chondritis of left external ear

H61.033 Chondritis of external ear, bilateral

H61.039 Chondritis of external ear, unspecified ear

H61.1 Noninfective disorders of pinna

Excludes2: cauliflower ear (M95.1-)

gouty tophi of ear (M1A.-)

H61.10 Unspecified noninfective disorders of pinna

Disorder of pinna NOS

H61.101 Unspecified noninfective disorders of pinna, right ear

H61.102 Unspecified noninfective disorders of pinna, left ear

H61.103 Unspecified noninfective disorders of pinna, bilateral

H61.109 Unspecified noninfective disorders of pinna, unspecified ear

H61.11 Acquired deformity of pinna

Acquired deformity of auricle

Excludes2: cauliflower ear (M95.1-)

H61.111 Acquired deformity of pinna, right ear

H61.112 Acquired deformity of pinna, left ear

H61.113 Acquired deformity of pinna, bilateral

H61.119 Acquired deformity of pinna, unspecified ear

H61.12 Hematoma of pinna

Hematoma of auricle

H61.121 Hematoma of pinna, right ear

H61.122 Hematoma of pinna, left ear

H61.123 Hematoma of pinna, bilateral

H61.129 Hematoma of pinna, unspecified ear

H61.19 Other noninfective disorders of pinna

H61.191 Noninfective disorders of pinna, right ear

H61.192 Noninfective disorders of pinna, left ear

H61.193 Noninfective disorders of pinna, bilateral

H61.199 Noninfective disorders of pinna, unspecified ear

H61.2 Impacted cerumen

Wax in ear

H61.20 Impacted cerumen, unspecified ear

H61.21 Impacted cerumen, right ear

H61.22 Impacted cerumen, left ear

H61.23   Impacted cerumen, bilateral

H61.3   **Acquired stenosis of external ear canal**

  Collapse of external ear canal

  Excludes1: postprocedural stenosis of external ear canal (H95.81-)

  H61.30   **Acquired stenosis of external ear canal, unspecified**

    H61.301   **Acquired stenosis of right external ear canal, unspecified**

    H61.302   **Acquired stenosis of left external ear canal, unspecified**

    H61.303   **Acquired stenosis of external ear canal, unspecified, bilateral**

    H61.309   **Acquired stenosis of external ear canal, unspecified, unspecified ear**

  H61.31   **Acquired stenosis of external ear canal secondary to trauma**

    H61.311   **Acquired stenosis of right external ear canal secondary to trauma**

    H61.312   **Acquired stenosis of left external ear canal secondary to trauma**

    H61.313   **Acquired stenosis of external ear canal secondary to trauma, bilateral**

    H61.319   **Acquired stenosis of external ear canal secondary to trauma, unspecified ear**

  H61.32   **Acquired stenosis of external ear canal secondary to inflammation and infection**

    H61.321   **Acquired stenosis of right external ear canal secondary to inflammation and infection**

    H61.322   **Acquired stenosis of left external ear canal secondary to inflammation and infection**

    H61.323   **Acquired stenosis of external ear canal secondary to inflammation and infection, bilateral**

    H61.329   **Acquired stenosis of external ear canal secondary to inflammation and infection, unspecified ear**

  H61.39   **Other acquired stenosis of external ear canal**

    H61.391   **Other acquired stenosis of right external ear canal**

    H61.392   **Other acquired stenosis of left external ear canal**

    H61.393   **Other acquired stenosis of external ear canal, bilateral**

    H61.399   **Other acquired stenosis of external ear canal, unspecified ear**

H61.8   **Other specified disorders of external ear**

  H61.81   **Exostosis of external canal**

    H61.811   **Exostosis of right external canal**

    H61.812   **Exostosis of left external canal**

    H61.813   **Exostosis of external canal, bilateral**

    H61.819   **Exostosis of external canal, unspecified ear**

  H61.89   **Other specified disorders of external ear**

    H61.891   **Other specified disorders of right external ear**

    H61.892   **Other specified disorders of left external ear**

    H61.893   **Other specified disorders of external ear, bilateral**

    H61.899   **Other specified disorders of external ear, unspecified ear**

H61.9   **Disorder of external ear, unspecified**

  H61.90   **Disorder of external ear, unspecified, unspecified ear**

  H61.91   **Disorder of right external ear, unspecified**

  H61.92   **Disorder of left external ear, unspecified**

  H61.93   **Disorder of external ear, unspecified, bilateral**

H62   **Disorders of external ear in diseases classified elsewhere**

H62.4   **Otitis externa in other diseases classified elsewhere**

  Code first underlying disease, such as:

  erysipelas (A46)

  impetigo (L01.0)

  Excludes1: otitis externa (in):

    candidiasis (B37.84)

    herpes viral [herpes simplex] (B00.1)

    herpes zoster (B02.8)

  H62.40   **Otitis externa in other diseases classified elsewhere, unspecified ear**

  H62.41   **Otitis externa in other diseases classified elsewhere, right ear**

  H62.42   **Otitis externa in other diseases classified elsewhere, left ear**

  H62.43   **Otitis externa in other diseases classified elsewhere, bilateral**

H62.8   **Other disorders of external ear in diseases classified elsewhere**

  Code first underlying disease, such as:

  gout (M1A.-, M10.-)

  H62.8X   **Other disorders of external ear in diseases classified elsewhere**

    H62.8X1   **Other disorders of right external ear in diseases classified elsewhere**

    H62.8X2   **Other disorders of left external ear in diseases classified elsewhere**

    H62.8X3   **Other disorders of external ear in diseases classified elsewhere, bilateral**

    H62.8X9   **Other disorders of external ear in diseases classified elsewhere, unspecified ear**

DISEASES OF MIDDLE EAR AND MASTOID (H65-H75)

H65   **Nonsuppurative otitis media**

  Definition: Nonsuppurative otitis media and eustachian tube disorders, otitis media is an inflammation of the middle ear without the formation or discharge of pus.

  Includes: nonsuppurative otitis media with myringitis

  Use Additional Code for any associated perforated tympanic membrane (H72.-)

  Use Additional Code, if applicable, to identify:

  exposure to environmental tobacco smoke (Z77.22)

  exposure to tobacco smoke in the perinatal period (P96.81)

  history of tobacco dependence (Z87.891)

  infectious agent (B95-B97)

  occupational exposure to environmental tobacco smoke (Z57.31)

  tobacco dependence (F17.-)

  tobacco use (Z72.0)

  H65.0   **Acute serous otitis media**

    Acute and subacute secretory otitis

H65.00 Acute serous otitis media, unspecified ear

H65.01 Acute serous otitis media, right ear

H65.02 Acute serous otitis media, left ear

H65.03 Acute serous otitis media, bilateral

H65.04 Acute serous otitis media, recurrent, right ear

H65.05 Acute serous otitis media, recurrent, left ear

H65.06 Acute serous otitis media, recurrent, bilateral

H65.07 Acute serous otitis media, recurrent, unspecified ear

H65.1 Other acute nonsuppurative otitis media

Excludes1: otitic barotrauma (T70.0)

otitis media (acute) NOS (H66.9)

H65.11 Acute and subacute allergic otitis media (mucoid) (sanguinous) (serous)

H65.111 Acute and subacute allergic otitis media (mucoid) (sanguinous) (serous), right ear

H65.112 Acute and subacute allergic otitis media (mucoid) (sanguinous) (serous), left ear

H65.113 Acute and subacute allergic otitis media (mucoid) (sanguinous) (serous), bilateral

H65.114 Acute and subacute allergic otitis media (mucoid) (sanguinous) (serous), recurrent, right ear

H65.115 Acute and subacute allergic otitis media (mucoid) (sanguinous) (serous), recurrent, left ear

H65.116 Acute and subacute allergic otitis media (mucoid) (sanguinous) (serous), recurrent, bilateral

H65.117 Acute and subacute allergic otitis media (mucoid) (sanguinous) (serous), recurrent, unspecified ear

H65.119 Acute and subacute allergic otitis media (mucoid) (sanguinous) (serous), unspecified ear

H65.19 Other acute nonsuppurative otitis media

Acute and subacute mucoid otitis media

Acute and subacute nonsuppurative otitis media NOS

Acute and subacute sanguinous otitis media

Acute and subacute seromucinous otitis media

H65.191 Other acute nonsuppurative otitis media, right ear

H65.192 Other acute nonsuppurative otitis media, left ear

H65.193 Other acute nonsuppurative otitis media, bilateral

H65.194 Other acute nonsuppurative otitis media, recurrent, right ear

H65.195 Other acute nonsuppurative otitis media, recurrent, left ear

H65.196 Other acute nonsuppurative otitis media, recurrent, bilateral

H65.197 Other acute nonsuppurative otitis media recurrent, unspecified ear

H65.199 Other acute nonsuppurative otitis media, unspecified ear

H65.2 Chronic serous otitis media

Chronic tubotympanal catarrh

H65.20 Chronic serous otitis media, unspecified ear

H65.21 Chronic serous otitis media, right ear

H65.22 Chronic serous otitis media, left ear

H65.23 Chronic serous otitis media, bilateral

H65.3 Chronic mucoid otitis media

Chronic mucinous otitis media

Chronic secretory otitis media

Chronic transudative otitis media Glue ear

Excludes1: adhesive middle ear disease (H74.1)

H65.30 Chronic mucoid otitis media, unspecified ear

H65.31 Chronic mucoid otitis media, right ear

H65.32 Chronic mucoid otitis media, left ear

H65.33 Chronic mucoid otitis media, bilateral

H65.4 Other chronic nonsuppurative otitis media

H65.41 Chronic allergic otitis media

H65.411 Chronic allergic otitis media, right ear

H65.412 Chronic allergic otitis media, left ear

H65.413 Chronic allergic otitis media, bilateral

H65.419 Chronic allergic otitis media, unspecified ear

H65.49 Other chronic nonsuppurative otitis media

Chronic exudative otitis media

Chronic nonsuppurative otitis media NOS

Chronic otitis media with effusion (nonpurulent)

Chronic seromucinous otitis media

H65.491 Other chronic nonsuppurative otitis media, right ear

H65.492 Other chronic nonsuppurative otitis media, left ear

H65.493 Other chronic nonsuppurative otitis media, bilateral

H65.499 Other chronic nonsuppurative otitis media, unspecified ear

H65.9 Unspecified nonsuppurative otitis media

Allergic otitis media NOS

Catarrhal otitis media NOS

Exudative otitis media NOS

Mucoid otitis media NOS

Otitis media with effusion (nonpurulent) NOS

Secretory otitis media NOS

Seromucinous otitis media NOS

Serous otitis media NOS

Transudative otitis media NOS

H65.90 Unspecified nonsuppurative otitis media, unspecified ear

H65.91 Unspecified nonsuppurative otitis media, right ear

H65.92 Unspecified nonsuppurative otitis media, left ear

H65.93 Unspecified nonsuppurative otitis media, bilateral

H66 **Suppurative and unspecified otitis media**

Definition: Suppurative and unspecified otitis media is an inflammation of the middle ear including the formation or discharge of pus.

Includes: suppurative and unspecified otitis media with myringitis

Use Additional Code to identify:

exposure to environmental tobacco smoke (Z77.22)

exposure to tobacco smoke in the perinatal period (P96.81)

history of tobacco dependence (Z87.891)

occupational exposure to environmental tobacco smoke (Z57.31)

tobacco dependence (F17.-)

tobacco use (Z72.0)

H66.0 **Acute suppurative otitis media**

H66.00 **Acute suppurative otitis media without spontaneous rupture of ear drum**

H66.001 Acute suppurative otitis media without spontaneous rupture of ear drum, right ear

H66.002 Acute suppurative otitis media without spontaneous rupture of ear drum, left ear

H66.003 Acute suppurative otitis media without spontaneous rupture of ear drum, bilateral

H66.004 Acute suppurative otitis media without spontaneous rupture of ear drum, recurrent, right ear

H66.005 Acute suppurative otitis media without spontaneous rupture of ear drum, recurrent, left ear

H66.006 Acute suppurative otitis media without spontaneous rupture of ear drum, recurrent, bilateral

H66.007 Acute suppurative otitis media without spontaneous rupture of ear drum, recurrent, unspecified ear

H66.009 Acute suppurative otitis media without spontaneous rupture of ear drum, unspecified ear

H66.01 **Acute suppurative otitis media with spontaneous rupture of ear drum**

H66.011 Acute suppurative otitis media with spontaneous rupture of ear drum, right ear

H66.012 Acute suppurative otitis media with spontaneous rupture of ear drum, left ear

H66.013 Acute suppurative otitis media with spontaneous rupture of ear drum, bilateral

H66.014 Acute suppurative otitis media with spontaneous rupture of ear drum, recurrent, right ear

H66.015 Acute suppurative otitis media with spontaneous rupture of ear drum, recurrent, left ear

H66.016 Acute suppurative otitis media with spontaneous rupture of ear drum, recurrent, bilateral

H66.017 Acute suppurative otitis media with spontaneous rupture of ear drum, recurrent, unspecified ear

H66.019 Acute suppurative otitis media with spontaneous rupture of ear drum, unspecified ear

H66.1 **Chronic tubotympanic suppurative otitis media**

Benign chronic suppurative otitis media

Chronic tubotympanic disease

Use Additional Code for any associated perforated tympanic membrane (H72.-)

H66.10 **Chronic tubotympanic suppurative otitis media, unspecified**

H66.11 **Chronic tubotympanic suppurative otitis media, right ear**

H66.12 **Chronic tubotympanic suppurative otitis media, left ear**

H66.13 **Chronic tubotympanic suppurative otitis media, bilateral**

H66.2 **Chronic atticoantral suppurative otitis media**

Chronic atticoantral disease

Use Additional Code for any associated perforated tympanic membrane (H72.-)

H66.20 **Chronic atticoantral suppurative otitis media, unspecified ear**

H66.21 **Chronic atticoantral suppurative otitis media, right ear**

H66.22 **Chronic atticoantral suppurative otitis media, left ear**

H66.23 **Chronic atticoantral suppurative otitis media, bilateral**

H66.3 **Other chronic suppurative otitis media**

Chronic suppurative otitis media NOS

Use Additional Code for any associated perforated tympanic membrane (H72.-)

Excludes1: tuberculous otitis media (A18.6)

H66.3X **Other chronic suppurative otitis media**

H66.3X1 Other chronic suppurative otitis media, right ear

H66.3X2 Other chronic suppurative otitis media, left ear

H66.3X3 Other chronic suppurative otitis media, bilateral

H66.3X9 Other chronic suppurative otitis media, unspecified ear

H66.4 **Suppurative otitis media, unspecified**

Purulent otitis media NOS

Use Additional Code for any associated perforated tympanic membrane (H72.-)

H66.40 **Suppurative otitis media, unspecified, unspecified ear**

H66.41 **Suppurative otitis media, unspecified, right ear**

H66.42 **Suppurative otitis media, unspecified, left ear**

H66.43 **Suppurative otitis media, unspecified, bilateral**

H66.9 **Otitis media, unspecified**

Otitis media NOS

Acute otitis media NOS

Chronic otitis media NOS

Use Additional Code for any associated perforated tympanic membrane (H72.-)

H66.90 **Otitis media, unspecified, unspecified ear**

H66.91 **Otitis media, unspecified, right ear**

H66.92 **Otitis media, unspecified, left ear**

H66.93 **Otitis media, unspecified, bilateral**

H67 **Otitis media in diseases classified elsewhere**

Code first underlying disease, such as:

plasminogen deficiency (E88.02)

viral disease NEC (B00-B34)

Use Additional Code for any associated perforated tympanic membrane (H72.-)

Excludes1: otitis media in:

influenza (J09.X9, J10.83, J11.83)

measles (B05.3)

scarlet fever (A38.0)

tuberculosis (A18.6)

H67.1 Otitis media in diseases classified elsewhere, right ear

H67.2 Otitis media in diseases classified elsewhere, left ear

H67.3 Otitis media in diseases classified elsewhere, bilateral

H67.9 Otitis media in diseases classified elsewhere, unspecified ear

H68 Eustachian salpingitis and obstruction

H68.0 Eustachian salpingitis

H68.00 Unspecified Eustachian salpingitis

H68.001 Unspecified Eustachian salpingitis, right ear

H68.002 Unspecified Eustachian salpingitis, left ear

H68.003 Unspecified Eustachian salpingitis, bilateral

H68.009 Unspecified Eustachian salpingitis, unspecified ear

H68.01 Acute Eustachian salpingitis

H68.011 Acute Eustachian salpingitis, right ear

H68.012 Acute Eustachian salpingitis, left ear

H68.013 Acute Eustachian salpingitis, bilateral

H68.019 Acute Eustachian salpingitis, unspecified ear

H68.02 Chronic Eustachian salpingitis

H68.021 Chronic Eustachian salpingitis, right ear

H68.022 Chronic Eustachian salpingitis, left ear

H68.023 Chronic Eustachian salpingitis, bilateral

H68.029 Chronic Eustachian salpingitis, unspecified ear

H68.1 Obstruction of Eustachian tube

Stenosis of Eustachian tube

Stricture of Eustachian tube

H68.10 Unspecified obstruction of Eustachian tube

H68.101 Unspecified obstruction of Eustachian tube, right ear

H68.102 Unspecified obstruction of Eustachian tube, left ear

H68.103 Unspecified obstruction of Eustachian tube, bilateral

H68.109 Unspecified obstruction of Eustachian tube, unspecified ear

H68.11 Osseous obstruction of Eustachian tube

H68.111 Osseous obstruction of Eustachian tube, right ear

H68.112 Osseous obstruction of Eustachian tube, left ear

H68.113 Osseous obstruction of Eustachian tube, bilateral

H68.119 Osseous obstruction of Eustachian tube, unspecified ear

H68.12 Intrinsic cartilaginous obstruction of Eustachian tube

H68.121 Intrinsic cartilaginous obstruction of Eustachian tube, right ear

H68.122 Intrinsic cartilaginous obstruction of Eustachian tube, left ear

H68.123 Intrinsic cartilaginous obstruction of Eustachian tube, bilateral

H68.129 Intrinsic cartilaginous obstruction of Eustachian tube, unspecified ear

H68.13 Extrinsic cartilaginous obstruction of Eustachian tube

Compression of Eustachian tube

H68.131 Extrinsic cartilaginous obstruction of Eustachian tube, right ear

H68.132 Extrinsic cartilaginous obstruction of Eustachian tube, left ear

H68.133 Extrinsic cartilaginous obstruction of Eustachian tube, bilateral

H68.139 Extrinsic cartilaginous obstruction of Eustachian tube, unspecified ear

H69 Other and unspecified disorders of Eustachian tube

H69.0 Patulous Eustachian tube

H69.00 Patulous Eustachian tube, unspecified ear

H69.01 Patulous Eustachian tube, right ear

H69.02 Patulous Eustachian tube, left ear

H69.03 Patulous Eustachian tube, bilateral

H69.8 Other specified disorders of Eustachian tube

H69.80 Other specified disorders of Eustachian tube, unspecified ear

H69.81 Other specified disorders of Eustachian tube, right ear

H69.82 Other specified disorders of Eustachian tube, left ear

H69.83 Other specified disorders of Eustachian tube, bilateral

H69.9 Unspecified Eustachian tube disorder

H69.90 Unspecified Eustachian tube disorder, unspecified ear

H69.91 Unspecified Eustachian tube disorder, right ear

H69.92 Unspecified Eustachian tube disorder, left ear

H69.93 Unspecified Eustachian tube disorder, bilateral

H70 Mastoiditis and related conditions

Definition: Mastoiditis is an infection of the spaces within the mastoid bone. It is almost always associated with otitis media, an infection of the middle ear. In the most serious cases, the bone itself becomes infected.

H70.0 Acute mastoiditis

Abscess of mastoid Empyema of mastoid

H70.00 Acute mastoiditis without complications

H70.001 Acute mastoiditis without complications, right ear

H70.002 Acute mastoiditis without complications, left ear

H70.003 Acute mastoiditis without complications, bilateral

H70.009 Acute mastoiditis without complications, unspecified ear

H70.01 Subperiosteal abscess of mastoid

H70.011 Subperiosteal abscess of mastoid, right ear

H70.012 Subperiosteal abscess of mastoid, left ear

H70.013 Subperiosteal abscess of mastoid, bilateral

H70.019 Subperiosteal abscess of mastoid, unspecified ear

H70.09 Acute mastoiditis with other complications

H70.091   Acute mastoiditis with other complications, right ear

H70.092   Acute mastoiditis with other complications, left ear

H70.093   Acute mastoiditis with other complications, bilateral

H70.099   Acute mastoiditis with other complications, unspecified ear

H70.1   **Chronic mastoiditis**

Caries of mastoid

Fistula of mastoid

Excludes1: tuberculous mastoiditis (A18.03)

H70.10   Chronic mastoiditis, unspecified ear

H70.11   Chronic mastoiditis, right ear

H70.12   Chronic mastoiditis, left ear

H70.13   Chronic mastoiditis, bilateral

H70.2   **Petrositis**

Inflammation of petrous bone

H70.20   Unspecified petrositis

    H70.201   Unspecified petrositis, right ear

    H70.202   Unspecified petrositis, left ear

    H70.203   Unspecified petrositis, bilateral

    H70.209   Unspecified petrositis, unspecified ear

H70.21   Acute petrositis

    H70.211   Acute petrositis, right ear

    H70.212   Acute petrositis, left ear

    H70.213   Acute petrositis, bilateral

    H70.219   Acute petrositis, unspecified ear

H70.22   Chronic petrositis

    H70.221   Chronic petrositis, right ear

    H70.222   Chronic petrositis, left ear

    H70.223   Chronic petrositis, bilateral

    H70.229   Chronic petrositis, unspecified ear

H70.8   **Other mastoiditis and related conditions**

Excludes1: preauricular sinus and cyst (Q18.1)

    sinus, fistula, and cyst of branchial cleft (Q18.0)

H70.81   Postauricular fistula

    H70.811   Postauricular fistula, right ear

    H70.812   Postauricular fistula, left ear

    H70.813   Postauricular fistula, bilateral

    H70.819   Postauricular fistula, unspecified ear

H70.89   Other mastoiditis and related conditions

    H70.891   Other mastoiditis and related conditions, right ear

    H70.892   Other mastoiditis and related conditions, left ear

    H70.893   Other mastoiditis and related conditions, bilateral

    H70.899   Other mastoiditis and related conditions, unspecified ear

H70.9   **Unspecified mastoiditis**

H70.90   Unspecified mastoiditis, unspecified ear

H70.91   Unspecified mastoiditis, right ear

H70.92   Unspecified mastoiditis, left ear

H70.93   Unspecified mastoiditis, bilateral

H71   **Cholesteatoma of middle ear**

Excludes2: cholesteatoma of external ear (H60.4-)

recurrent cholesteatoma of postmastoidectomy cavity (H95.0-)

H71.0   **Cholesteatoma of attic**

H71.00   Cholesteatoma of attic, unspecified ear

H71.01   Cholesteatoma of attic, right ear

H71.02   Cholesteatoma of attic, left ear

H71.03   Cholesteatoma of attic, bilateral

H71.1   **Cholesteatoma of tympanum**

H71.10   Cholesteatoma of tympanum, unspecified ear

H71.11   Cholesteatoma of tympanum, right ear

H71.12   Cholesteatoma of tympanum, left ear

H71.13   Cholesteatoma of tympanum, bilateral

H71.2   **Cholesteatoma of mastoid**

H71.20   Cholesteatoma of mastoid, unspecified ear

H71.21   Cholesteatoma of mastoid, right ear

H71.22   Cholesteatoma of mastoid, left ear

H71.23   Cholesteatoma of mastoid, bilateral

H71.3   **Diffuse cholesteatosis**

H71.30   Diffuse cholesteatosis, unspecified ear

H71.31   Diffuse cholesteatosis, right ear

H71.32   Diffuse cholesteatosis, left ear

H71.33   Diffuse cholesteatosis, bilateral

H71.9   **Unspecified cholesteatoma**

H71.90   Unspecified cholesteatoma, unspecified ear

H71.91   Unspecified cholesteatoma, right ear

H71.92   Unspecified cholesteatoma, left ear

H71.93   Unspecified cholesteatoma, bilateral

H72   **Perforation of tympanic membrane**

Includes: persistent post-traumatic perforation of ear drum

postinflammatory perforation of ear drum

Code first any associated otitis media (H65.-, H66.1-, H66.2-, H66.3-, H66.4-, H66.9-, H67.-)

Excludes1: acute suppurative otitis media with rupture of the tympanic membrane (H66.01-)

traumatic rupture of ear drum (S09.2-)

H72.0   **Central perforation of tympanic membrane**

H72.00   Central perforation of tympanic membrane, unspecified ear

H72.01   Central perforation of tympanic membrane, right ear

H72.02   Central perforation of tympanic membrane, left ear

H72.03   Central perforation of tympanic membrane, bilateral

H72.1   **Attic perforation of tympanic membrane**

Perforation of pars flaccida

H72.10   Attic perforation of tympanic membrane, unspecified ear

H72.11   Attic perforation of tympanic membrane, right ear

H72.12   Attic perforation of tympanic membrane, left ear

H72.13   Attic perforation of tympanic membrane, bilateral

H72.2   **Other marginal perforations of tympanic membrane**

H72.2X   Other marginal perforations of tympanic membrane

    H72.2X1   Other marginal perforations of tympanic membrane, right ear

---

Add 4th-7th digits   Nonspecific code   Unspecified code   Manifestation code   [HCC] Hierarchical Condition Code

H72.2X2   **Other marginal perforations of tympanic membrane, left ear**

H72.2X3   **Other marginal perforations of tympanic membrane, bilateral**

H72.2X9   **Other marginal perforations of tympanic membrane, unspecified ear**

H72.8   **Other perforations of tympanic membrane**

    H72.81   **Multiple perforations of tympanic membrane**

        H72.811   **Multiple perforations of tympanic membrane, right ear**

        H72.812   **Multiple perforations of tympanic membrane, left ear**

        H72.813   **Multiple perforations of tympanic membrane, bilateral**

        H72.819   **Multiple perforations of tympanic membrane, unspecified ear**

    H72.82   **Total perforations of tympanic membrane**

        H72.821   **Total perforations of tympanic membrane, right ear**

        H72.822   **Total perforations of tympanic membrane, left ear**

        H72.823   **Total perforations of tympanic membrane, bilateral**

        H72.829   **Total perforations of tympanic membrane, unspecified ear**

H72.9   **Unspecified perforation of tympanic membrane**

    H72.90   **Unspecified perforation of tympanic membrane, unspecified ear**

    H72.91   **Unspecified perforation of tympanic membrane, right ear**

    H72.92   **Unspecified perforation of tympanic membrane, left ear**

    H72.93   **Unspecified perforation of tympanic membrane, bilateral**

H73   **Other disorders of tympanic membrane**

H73.0   **Acute myringitis**

    Excludes1: acute myringitis with otitis media (H65, H66)

    H73.00   **Unspecified acute myringitis**

        Acute tympanitis NOS

        H73.001   **Acute myringitis, right ear**

        H73.002   **Acute myringitis, left ear**

        H73.003   **Acute myringitis, bilateral**

        H73.009   **Acute myringitis, unspecified ear**

    H73.01   **Bullous myringitis**

        H73.011   **Bullous myringitis, right ear**

        H73.012   **Bullous myringitis, left ear**

        H73.013   **Bullous myringitis, bilateral**

        H73.019   **Bullous myringitis, unspecified ear**

    H73.09 **Other acute myringitis**

        H73.091   **Other acute myringitis, right ear**

        H73.092   **Other acute myringitis, left ear**

        H73.093   **Other acute myringitis, bilateral**

        H73.099   **Other acute myringitis, unspecified ear**

H73.1   **Chronic myringitis**

    Chronic tympanitis

    Excludes1: chronic myringitis with otitis media (H65, H66)

    H73.10   **Chronic myringitis, unspecified ear**

    H73.11   **Chronic myringitis, right ear**

    H73.12   **Chronic myringitis, left ear**

    H73.13   **Chronic myringitis, bilateral**

H73.2   **Unspecified myringitis**

    H73.20   **Unspecified myringitis, unspecified ear**

    H73.21   **Unspecified myringitis, right ear**

    H73.22   **Unspecified myringitis, left ear**

    H73.23   **Unspecified myringitis, bilateral**

H73.8   **Other specified disorders of tympanic membrane**

    H73.81   **Atrophic flaccid tympanic membrane**

        H73.811   **Atrophic flaccid tympanic membrane, right ear**

        H73.812   **Atrophic flaccid tympanic membrane, left ear**

        H73.813   **Atrophic flaccid tympanic membrane, bilateral**

        H73.819   **Atrophic flaccid tympanic membrane, unspecified ear**

    H73.82   **Atrophic nonflaccid tympanic membrane**

        H73.821   **Atrophic nonflaccid tympanic membrane, right ear**

        H73.822   **Atrophic nonflaccid tympanic membrane, left ear**

        H73.823   **Atrophic nonflaccid tympanic membrane, bilateral**

        H73.829   **Atrophic nonflaccid tympanic membrane, unspecified ear**

    H73.89   **Other specified disorders of tympanic membrane**

        H73.891   **Other specified disorders of tympanic membrane, right ear**

        H73.892   **Other specified disorders of tympanic membrane, left ear**

        H73.893   **Other specified disorders of tympanic membrane, bilateral**

        H73.899   **Other specified disorders of tympanic membrane, unspecified ear**

H73.9   **Unspecified disorder of tympanic membrane**

    H73.90   **Unspecified disorder of tympanic membrane, unspecified ear**

    H73.91   **Unspecified disorder of tympanic membrane, right ear**

    H73.92   **Unspecified disorder of tympanic membrane, left ear**

    H73.93   **Unspecified disorder of tympanic membrane, bilateral**

H74   **OTHER DISORDERS OF MIDDLE EAR MASTOID**

    Definition: The middle ear is the space between the eardrum and the inner ear that contains the three auditory ossicles, which convey vibrations through the oval window to the cochlea. The mastoid is the bone located directly behind the external ear.

    Excludes2: mastoiditis (H70.-)

H74.0   **Tympanosclerosis**

    H74.01   **Tympanosclerosis, right ear**

    H74.02   **Tympanosclerosis, left ear**

    H74.03   **Tympanosclerosis, bilateral**

    H74.09   **Tympanosclerosis, unspecified ear**

H74.1   **Adhesive middle ear disease**

    Adhesive otitis

    Excludes1: glue ear (H65.3-)

    H74.11   **Adhesive right middle ear disease**

    H74.12   **Adhesive left middle ear disease**

    H74.13   **Adhesive middle ear disease, bilateral**

  ● New code   ▲ Revised code   **Excludes1:** Not coded here   **Excludes2:** Not included here   ⊗ Placeholder required   ⑦ 7th digit required

H74.19   Adhesive middle ear disease, unspecified ear

H74.2   Discontinuity and dislocation of ear ossicles

H74.20   Discontinuity and dislocation of ear ossicles, unspecified ear

H74.21   Discontinuity and dislocation of right ear ossicles

H74.22   Discontinuity and dislocation of left ear ossicles

H74.23   Discontinuity and dislocation of ear ossicles, bilateral

H74.3   Other acquired abnormalities of ear ossicles

H74.31   Ankylosis of ear ossicles

H74.311   Ankylosis of ear ossicles, right ear

H74.312   Ankylosis of ear ossicles, left ear

H74.313   Ankylosis of ear ossicles, bilateral

H74.319   Ankylosis of ear ossicles, unspecified ear

H74.32   Partial loss of ear ossicles

H74.321   Partial loss of ear ossicles, right ear

H74.322   Partial loss of ear ossicles, left ear

H74.323   Partial loss of ear ossicles, bilateral

H74.329   Partial loss of ear ossicles, unspecified ear

H74.39   Other acquired abnormalities of ear ossicles

H74.391   Other acquired abnormalities of right ear ossicles

H74.392   Other acquired abnormalities of left ear ossicles

H74.393   Other acquired abnormalities of ear ossicles, bilateral

H74.399   Other acquired abnormalities of ear ossicles, unspecified ear

H74.4   Polyp of middle ear

H74.40   Polyp of middle ear, unspecified ear

H74.41   Polyp of right middle ear

H74.42   Polyp of left middle ear

H74.43   Polyp of middle ear, bilateral

H74.8   Other specified disorders of middle ear and mastoid

H74.8X   Other specified disorders of middle ear and mastoid

H74.8X1   Other specified disorders of right middle ear and mastoid

H74.8X2   Other specified disorders of left middle ear and mastoid

H74.8X3   Other specified disorders of middle ear and mastoid, bilateral

H74.8X9   Other specified disorders of middle ear and mastoid, unspecified ear

H74.9   Unspecified disorder of middle ear and mastoid

H74.90   Unspecified disorder of middle ear and mastoid, unspecified ear

H74.91   Unspecified disorder of right middle ear and mastoid

H74.92   Unspecified disorder of left middle ear and mastoid

H74.93   Unspecified disorder of middle ear and mastoid, bilateral

H75   OTHER DISORDERS OF MIDDLE EAR AND MASTOID IN DISEASES CLASSIFIED ELSEWHERE

Code first underlying disease

H75.0   Mastoiditis in infectious and parasitic diseases classified elsewhere

Excludes1: mastoiditis (in):

syphilis (A52.77)

tuberculosis (A18.03)

H75.00   Mastoiditis in infectious and parasitic diseases classified elsewhere, unspecified ear

H75.01   Mastoiditis in infectious and parasitic diseases classified elsewhere, right ear

H75.02   Mastoiditis in infectious and parasitic diseases classified elsewhere, left ear

H75.03   Mastoiditis in infectious and parasitic diseases classified elsewhere, bilateral

H75.8   Other specified disorders of middle ear and mastoid in diseases classified elsewhere

H75.80   Other specified disorders of middle ear and mastoid in diseases classified elsewhere, unspecified ear

H75.81   Other specified disorders of right middle ear and mastoid in diseases classified elsewhere

H75.82   Other specified disorders of left middle ear and mastoid in diseases classified elsewhere

H75.83   Other specified disorders of middle ear and mastoid in diseases classified elsewhere, bilateral

DISEASES OF INNER EAR (H80-H83)

H80   Otosclerosis

Includes: Otospongiosis

H80.0   Otosclerosis involving oval window, nonobliterative

H80.00   Otosclerosis involving oval window, nonobliterative, unspecified ear

H80.01   Otosclerosis involving oval window, nonobliterative, right ear

H80.02   Otosclerosis involving oval window, nonobliterative, left ear

H80.03   Otosclerosis involving oval window, nonobliterative, bilateral

H80.1   Otosclerosis involving oval window, obliterative

H80.10   Otosclerosis involving oval window, obliterative, unspecified ear

H80.11   Otosclerosis involving oval window, obliterative, right ear

H80.12   Otosclerosis involving oval window, obliterative, left ear

H80.13   Otosclerosis involving oval window, obliterative, bilateral

H80.2   Cochlear otosclerosis

Otosclerosis involving otic capsule

Otosclerosis involving round window

H80.20   Cochlear otosclerosis, unspecified ear

H80.21   Cochlear otosclerosis, right ear

H80.22   Cochlear otosclerosis, left ear

H80.23   Cochlear otosclerosis, bilateral

H80.8   Other otosclerosis

H80.80   Other otosclerosis, unspecified ear

H80.81   Other otosclerosis, right ear

H80.82   Other otosclerosis, left ear

H80.83   Other otosclerosis, bilateral

H80.9   Unspecified otosclerosis

H80.90   Unspecified otosclerosis, unspecified ear

H80.91   Unspecified otosclerosis, right ear
H80.92   Unspecified otosclerosis, left ear
H80.93   Unspecified otosclerosis, bilateral

H81   Disorders of vestibular function

Excludes1: epidemic vertigo (A88.1)

vertigo NOS (R42)

H81.0   **Ménière's disease**

Labyrinthine hydrops

Ménière's syndrome or vertigo

H81.01   Ménière's disease, right ear
H81.02   Ménière's disease, left ear
H81.03   Ménière's disease, bilateral
H81.09   Ménière's disease, unspecified ear

H81.1   **Benign paroxysmal vertigo**

H81.10   Benign paroxysmal vertigo, unspecified ear
H81.11   Benign paroxysmal vertigo, right ear
H81.12   Benign paroxysmal vertigo, left ear
H81.13   Benign paroxysmal vertigo, bilateral

H81.2   **Vestibular neuronitis**

H81.20   Vestibular neuronitis, unspecified ear
H81.21   Vestibular neuronitis, right ear
H81.22   Vestibular neuronitis, left ear
H81.23   Vestibular neuronitis, bilateral

H81.3   **Other peripheral vertigo**

H81.31   **Aural vertigo**

H81.311   Aural vertigo, right ear
H81.312   Aural vertigo, left ear
H81.313   Aural vertigo, bilateral
H81.319   Aural vertigo, unspecified ear

H81.39   **Other peripheral vertigo**

Lermoyez' syndrome

Otogenic vertigo

Peripheral vertigo NOS

H81.391   Other peripheral vertigo, right ear
H81.392   Other peripheral vertigo, left ear
H81.393   Other peripheral vertigo, bilateral
H81.399   Other peripheral vertigo, unspecified ear

H81.4   **Vertigo of central origin**

Central positional nystagmus

H81.8   **Other disorders of vestibular function**

H81.8X   **Other disorders of vestibular function**

H81.8X1   Other disorders of vestibular function, right ear
H81.8X2   Other disorders of vestibular function, left ear
H81.8X3   Other disorders of vestibular function, bilateral
H81.8X9   Other disorders of vestibular function, unspecified ear

H81.9   **Unspecified disorder of vestibular function**

Vertiginous syndrome NOS

H81.90   Unspecified disorder of vestibular function, unspecified ear
H81.91   Unspecified disorder of vestibular function, right ear
H81.92   Unspecified disorder of vestibular function, left ear

H81.93   Unspecified disorder of vestibular function, bilateral

H82   Vertiginous syndromes in diseases classified elsewhere

Code first underlying disease

Excludes1: epidemic vertigo (A88.1)

H82.1   **Vertiginous syndromes in diseases classified elsewhere, right ear**

H82.2   **Vertiginous syndromes in diseases classified elsewhere, left ear**

H82.3   **Vertiginous syndromes in diseases classified elsewhere, bilateral**

H82.9   **Vertiginous syndromes in diseases classified elsewhere, unspecified ear**

H83   Other diseases of inner ear

H83.0   **Labyrinthitis**

H83.01   Labyrinthitis, right ear
H83.02   Labyrinthitis, left ear
H83.03   Labyrinthitis, bilateral
H83.09   Labyrinthitis, unspecified ear

H83.1   **Labyrinthine fistula**

H83.11   Labyrinthine fistula, right ear
H83.12   Labyrinthine fistula, left ear
H83.13   Labyrinthine fistula, bilateral
H83.19   Labyrinthine fistula, unspecified ear

H83.2   **Labyrinthine dysfunction**

Labyrinthine hypersensitivity

Labyrinthine hypofunction

Labyrinthine loss of function

H83.2X   **Labyrinthine dysfunction**

H83.2X1   Labyrinthine dysfunction, right ear
H83.2X2   Labyrinthine dysfunction, left ear
H83.2X3   Labyrinthine dysfunction, bilateral
H83.2X9   Labyrinthine dysfunction, unspecified ear

H83.3   **Noise effects on inner ear**

Acoustic trauma of inner ear

Noise-induced hearing loss of inner ear

H83.3X   **Noise effects on inner ear**

H83.3X1   Noise effects on right inner ear
H83.3X2   Noise effects on left inner ear
H83.3X3   Noise effects on inner ear, bilateral
H83.3X9   Noise effects on inner ear, unspecified ear

H83.8   **Other specified diseases of inner ear**

H83.8X   **Other specified diseases of inner ear**

H83.8X1   Other specified diseases of right inner ear
H83.8X2   Other specified diseases of left inner ear
H83.8X3   Other specified diseases of inner ear, bilateral
H83.8X9   Other specified diseases of inner ear, unspecified ear

H83.9   **Unspecified disease of inner ear**

H83.90   Unspecified disease of inner ear, unspecified ear
H83.91   Unspecified disease of right inner ear
H83.92   Unspecified disease of left inner ear
H83.93   Unspecified disease of inner ear, bilateral

   ● New code   ▲ Revised code   Excludes1: Not coded here   Excludes2: Not included here   ⊗ Placeholder required   ⑦ 7th digit required

OTHER DISORDERS OF EAR (H90-H94)

H90 **Conductive and sensorineural hearing loss**

Excludes1: deaf nonspeaking NEC (H91.3)

deafness NOS (H91.9-)

hearing loss NOS (H91.9-)

noise-induced hearing loss (H83.3-)

ototoxic hearing loss (H91.0-)

sudden (idiopathic) hearing loss (H91.2-)

H90.0 **Conductive hearing loss, bilateral**

H90.1 **Conductive hearing loss, unilateral with unrestricted hearing on the contralateral side**

H90.11 **Conductive hearing loss, unilateral, right ear, with unrestricted hearing on the contralateral side**

H90.12 **Conductive hearing loss, unilateral, left ear, with unrestricted hearing on the contralateral side**

H90.2 **Conductive hearing loss, unspecified**

Conductive deafness NOS

H90.3 **Sensorineural hearing loss, bilateral**

H90.4 **Sensorineural hearing loss, unilateral with unrestricted hearing on the contralateral side**

H90.41 **Sensorineural hearing loss, unilateral, right ear, with unrestricted hearing on the contralateral side**

H90.42 **Sensorineural hearing loss, unilateral, left ear, with unrestricted hearing on the contralateral side**

H90.5 **Unspecified sensorineural hearing loss**

Central hearing loss NOS

Congenital deafness NOS

Neural hearing loss NOS

Perceptive hearing loss NOS

Sensorineural deafness NOS

Sensory hearing loss NOS

Excludes1: abnormal auditory perception (H93.2-)

psychogenic deafness (F44.6)

H90.6 **Mixed conductive and sensorineural hearing loss, bilateral**

H90.7 **Mixed conductive and sensorineural hearing loss, unilateral with unrestricted hearing on the contralateral side**

H90.71 **Mixed conductive and sensorineural hearing loss, unilateral, right ear, with unrestricted hearing on the contralateral side**

H90.72 **Mixed conductive and sensorineural hearing loss, unilateral, left ear, with unrestricted hearing on the contralateral side**

H90.8 **Mixed conductive and sensorineural hearing loss, unspecified**

H90.A **Conductive and sensorineural hearing loss with restricted hearing on the contralateral side**

H90.A1 **Conductive hearing loss, unilateral, with restricted hearing on the contralateral side**

H90.A11 **Conductive hearing loss, unilateral, right ear with restricted hearing on the contralateral side**

H90.A12 **Conductive hearing loss, unilateral, left ear with restricted hearing on the contralateral side**

H90.A2 **Sensorineural hearing loss, unilateral, with restricted hearing on the contralateral side**

H90.A21 **Sensorineural hearing loss, unilateral, right ear, with restricted hearing on the contralateral side**

H90.A22 **Sensorineural hearing loss, unilateral, left ear, with restricted hearing on the contralateral side**

H90.A3 **Mixed conductive and sensorineural hearing loss, unilateral with restricted hearing on the contralateral side**

H90.A31 **Mixed conductive and sensorineural hearing loss, unilateral, right ear with restricted hearing on the contralateral side**

H90.A32 **Mixed conductive and sensorineural hearing loss, unilateral, left ear with restricted hearing on the contralateral side**

H91 **Other and unspecified hearing loss**

Excludes1: abnormal auditory perception (H93.2-)

hearing loss as classified in H90.-

impacted cerumen (H61.2-)

noise-induced hearing loss (H83.3-)

psychogenic deafness (F44.6)

transient ischemic deafness (H93.01-)

H91.0 **Ototoxic hearing loss**

Code first poisoning due to drug or toxin, if applicable (T36-T65 with fifth or sixth character 1-4 or 6)

Use Additional Code for adverse effect, if applicable, to identify drug (T36-T50 with fifth or sixth character 5)

H91.01 **Ototoxic hearing loss, right ear**

H91.02 **Ototoxic hearing loss, left ear**

H91.03 **Ototoxic hearing loss, bilateral**

H91.09 **Ototoxic hearing loss, unspecified ear**

H91.1 **Presbycusis**

Presbyacusia

H91.10 **Presbycusis, unspecified ear**

H91.11 **Presbycusis, right ear**

H91.12 **Presbycusis, left ear**

H91.13 **Presbycusis, bilateral**

H91.2 **Sudden idiopathic hearing loss**

Sudden hearing loss NOS

H91.20 **Sudden idiopathic hearing loss, unspecified ear**

H91.21 **Sudden idiopathic hearing loss, right ear**

H91.22 **Sudden idiopathic hearing loss, left ear**

H91.23 **Sudden idiopathic hearing loss, bilateral**

H91.3 **Deaf nonspeaking, not elsewhere classified**

H91.8 **Other specified hearing loss**

H91.8X **Other specified hearing loss**

H91.8X1 **Other specified hearing loss, right ear**

H91.8X2 **Other specified hearing loss, left ear**

H91.8X3 **Other specified hearing loss, bilateral**

H91.8X9 **Other specified hearing loss, unspecified ear**

H91.9 **Unspecified hearing loss**

Deafness NOS

High frequency deafness

Low frequency deafness

H91.90 **Unspecified hearing loss, unspecified ear**

H91.91 **Unspecified hearing loss, right ear**

H91.92 Unspecified hearing loss, left ear

H91.93 Unspecified hearing loss, bilateral

H92   Otalgia and effusion of ear

H92.0   Otalgia

H92.01 Otalgia, right ear

H92.02 Otalgia, left ear

H92.03 Otalgia, bilateral

H92.09 Otalgia, unspecified ear

H92.1   Otorrhea

Excludes1: leakage of cerebrospinal fluid through ear (G96.0)

H92.10 Otorrhea, unspecified ear

H92.11 Otorrhea, right ear

H92.12 Otorrhea, left ear

H92.13 Otorrhea, bilateral

H92.2   Otorrhagia

Excludes1: traumatic otorrhagia - code to injury

H92.20 Otorrhagia, unspecified ear

H92.21 Otorrhagia, right ear

H92.22 Otorrhagia, left ear

H92.23 Otorrhagia, bilateral

H93   Other disorders of ear, not elsewhere classified

H93.0   Degenerative and vascular disorders of ear

Excludes1: presbycusis (H91.1)

H93.01 Transient ischemic deafness

H93.011 Transient ischemic deafness, right ear

H93.012 Transient ischemic deafness, left ear

H93.013 Transient ischemic deafness, bilateral

H93.019 Transient ischemic deafness, unspecified ear

H93.09 Unspecified degenerative and vascular disorders of ear

H93.091 Unspecified degenerative and vascular disorders of right ear

H93.092 Unspecified degenerative and vascular disorders of left ear

H93.093 Unspecified degenerative and vascular disorders of ear, bilateral

H93.099 Unspecified degenerative and vascular disorders of unspecified ear

H93.1   Tinnitus

H93.11 Tinnitus, right ear

H93.12 Tinnitus, left ear

H93.13 Tinnitus, bilateral

H93.19 Tinnitus, unspecified ear

H93.A   Pulsatile tinnitus

H93.A1 Pulsatile tinnitus, right ear

H93.A2 Pulsatile tinnitus, left ear

H93.A3 Pulsatile tinnitus, bilateral

H93.A9 Pulsatile tinnitus, unspecified ear

H93.2   Other abnormal auditory perceptions

Excludes2: auditory hallucinations (R44.0)

H93.21 Auditory recruitment

H93.211 Auditory recruitment, right ear

H93.212 Auditory recruitment, left ear

H93.213 Auditory recruitment, bilateral

H93.219 Auditory recruitment, unspecified ear

H93.22 Diplacusis

H93.221 Diplacusis, right ear

H93.222 Diplacusis, left ear

H93.223 Diplacusis, bilateral

H93.229 Diplacusis, unspecified ear

H93.23 Hyperacusis

H93.231 Hyperacusis, right ear

H93.232 Hyperacusis, left ear

H93.233 Hyperacusis, bilateral

H93.239 Hyperacusis, unspecified ear

H93.24 Temporary auditory threshold shift

H93.241 Temporary auditory threshold shift, right ear

H93.242 Temporary auditory threshold shift, left ear

H93.243 Temporary auditory threshold shift, bilateral

H93.249 Temporary auditory threshold shift, unspecified ear

H93.25 Central auditory processing disorder

Congenital auditory imperception Word deafness

Excludes1: mixed receptive-expressive language disorder (F80.2)

H93.29 Other abnormal auditory perceptions

H93.291 Other abnormal auditory perceptions, right ear

H93.292 Other abnormal auditory perceptions, left ear

H93.293 Other abnormal auditory perceptions, bilateral

H93.299 Other abnormal auditory perceptions, unspecified ear

H93.3   Disorders of acoustic nerve

Disorder of 8th cranial nerve

Excludes1: acoustic neuroma (D33.3)

syphilitic acoustic neuritis (A52.15)

H93.3X Disorders of acoustic nerve

H93.3X1 Disorders of right acoustic nerve

H93.3X2 Disorders of left acoustic nerve

H93.3X3 Disorders of bilateral acoustic nerves

H93.3X9 Disorders of unspecified acoustic nerve

H93.8   Other specified disorders of ear

H93.8X Other specified disorders of ear

H93.8X1 Other specified disorders of right ear

H93.8X2 Other specified disorders of left ear

H93.8X3 Other specified disorders of ear, bilateral

H93.8X9 Other specified disorders of ear, unspecified ear

H93.9   Unspecified disorder of ear

H93.90 Unspecified disorder of ear, unspecified ear

H93.91 Unspecified disorder of right ear

H93.92 Unspecified disorder of left ear

H93.93 Unspecified disorder of ear, bilateral

H94   Other disorders of ear in diseases classified elsewhere

H94.0   Acoustic neuritis in infectious and parasitic diseases classified elsewhere

● New code   ▲ Revised code   **Excludes1:** Not coded here   **Excludes2:** Not included here   ⊗ Placeholder required   ⑦ 7th digit required

Code first underlying disease, such as:

parasitic disease (B65-B89)

Excludes1: acoustic neuritis (in):

herpes zoster (B02.29)

syphilis (A52.15)

H94.00 **Acoustic neuritis in infectious and parasitic diseases classified elsewhere, unspecified ear**

H94.01 **Acoustic neuritis in infectious and parasitic diseases classified elsewhere, right ear**

H94.02 **Acoustic neuritis in infectious and parasitic diseases classified elsewhere, left ear**

H94.03 **Acoustic neuritis in infectious and parasitic diseases classified elsewhere, bilateral**

H94.8 **Other specified disorders of ear in diseases classified elsewhere**

Code first underlying disease, such as:

congenital syphilis (A50.0)

Excludes1: aural myiasis (B87.4)

syphilitic labyrinthitis (A52.79)

H94.80 **Other specified disorders of ear in diseases classified elsewhere, unspecified ear**

H94.81 **Other specified disorders of right ear in diseases classified elsewhere**

H94.82 **Other specified disorders of left ear in diseases classified elsewhere**

H94.83 **Other specified disorders of ear in diseases classified elsewhere, bilateral**

INTRAOPERATIVE AND POSTPROCEDURAL COMPLICATIONS AND DISORDERS OF EAR AND MASTOID PROCESS, NOT ELSEWHERE CLASSIFIED (H95)

H95 **Intraoperative and postprocedural complications and disorders of ear and mastoid process, not elsewhere classified**

H95.0 **Recurrent cholesteatoma of postmastoidectomy cavity**

H95.00 **Recurrent cholesteatoma of postmastoidectomy cavity, unspecified ear**

H95.01 **Recurrent cholesteatoma of postmastoidectomy cavity, right ear**

H95.02 **Recurrent cholesteatoma of postmastoidectomy cavity, left ear**

H95.03 **Recurrent cholesteatoma of postmastoidectomy cavity, bilateral ears**

H95.1 **Other disorders of ear and mastoid process following mastoidectomy**

H95.11 **Chronic inflammation of postmastoidectomy cavity**

H95.111 **Chronic inflammation of postmastoidectomy cavity, right ear**

H95.112 **Chronic inflammation of postmastoidectomy cavity, left ear**

H95.113 **Chronic inflammation of postmastoidectomy cavity, bilateral ears**

H95.119 **Chronic inflammation of postmastoidectomy cavity, unspecified ear**

H95.12 **Granulation of postmastoidectomy cavity**

H95.121 **Granulation of postmastoidectomy cavity, right ear**

H95.122 **Granulation of postmastoidectomy cavity, left ear**

H95.123 **Granulation of postmastoidectomy cavity, bilateral ears**

H95.129 **Granulation of postmastoidectomy cavity, unspecified ear**

H95.13 **Mucosal cyst of postmastoidectomy cavity**

H95.131 **Mucosal cyst of postmastoidectomy cavity, right ear**

H95.132 **Mucosal cyst of postmastoidectomy cavity, left ear**

H95.133 **Mucosal cyst of postmastoidectomy cavity, bilateral ears**

H95.139 **Mucosal cyst of postmastoidectomy cavity, unspecified ear**

H95.19 **Other disorders following mastoidectomy**

H95.191 **Other disorders following mastoidectomy, right ear**

H95.192 **Other disorders following mastoidectomy, left ear**

H95.193 **Other disorders following mastoidectomy, bilateral ears**

H95.199 **Other disorders following mastoidectomy, unspecified ear**

H95.2 **Intraoperative hemorrhage and hematoma of ear and mastoid process complicating a procedure**

Excludes1: intraoperative hemorrhage and hematoma of ear and mastoid process due to accidental puncture or laceration during a procedure (H95.3-)

H95.21 **Intraoperative hemorrhage and hematoma of ear and mastoid process complicating a procedure on the ear and mastoid process**

H95.22 **Intraoperative hemorrhage and hematoma of ear and mastoid process complicating other procedure**

H95.3 **Accidental puncture and laceration of ear and mastoid process during a procedure**

H95.31 **Accidental puncture and laceration of the ear and mastoid process during a procedure on the ear and mastoid process**

H95.32 **Accidental puncture and laceration of the ear and mastoid process during other procedure**

H95.4 **Postprocedural hemorrhage of ear and mastoid process following a procedure**

H95.41 **Postprocedural hemorrhage of ear and mastoid process following a procedure on the ear and mastoid process**

H95.42 **Postprocedural hemorrhage of ear and mastoid process following other procedure**

H95.5 **Postprocedural hematoma and seroma of ear and mastoid process following a procedure**

H95.51 **Postprocedural hematoma of ear and mastoid process following a procedure on the ear and mastoid process**

H95.52 **Postprocedural hematoma of ear and mastoid process following other procedure**

H95.53 **Postprocedural seroma of ear and mastoid process following a procedure on the ear and mastoid process**

H95.54 **Postprocedural seroma of ear and mastoid process following other procedure**

H95.8 **Other intraoperative and postprocedural complications and disorders of the ear and mastoid process, not elsewhere classified**

Excludes2: postprocedural complications and disorders following mastoidectomy (H95.0-, H95.1-)

H95.81 **Postprocedural stenosis of external ear canal**

H95.811 **Postprocedural stenosis of right external ear canal**

H95.812 **Postprocedural stenosis of left external ear canal**

H95.813 **Postprocedural stenosis of external ear canal, bilateral**

H95.819 **Postprocedural stenosis of unspecified external ear canal**

H95.88 **Other intraoperative complications and disorders of the ear and mastoid process, not elsewhere classified**

Use Additional Code, if applicable, to further specify disorder

H95.89 **Other postprocedural complications and disorders of the ear and mastoid process, not elsewhere classified**

Use Additional Code, if applicable, to further specify disorder

Chapter 9: Diseases of the Circulatory System (I00-I99)

DEFINITIONS

This chapter includes definitions of selected key words, terms and phrases and coding alerts for adding points to the clinical domain, and references to coding late effects where appropriate. An example from this chapter is as follows:

I12   Hypertensive chronic kidney disease
    Definition: Hypertensive chronic kidney disease, refers to diseases of the kidney caused by high blood pressure.

MULTIPLE CODING FOR A SINGLE CONDITION

In addition to the etiology/manifestation convention that requires two codes to fully describe a single condition that affects multiple body systems, there are other single conditions that also require more than one code. "**Use Additional Code**" notes are found in the Tabular List at codes that are not part of an etiology/manifestation pair where a secondary code is useful to fully describe a condition. The sequencing rule is the same as the etiology/manifestation pair, "**Use Additional Code**" indicates that a secondary code should be added.

For example, for bacterial infections that are not included in chapter 1, a secondary code from category B95, Streptococcus, Staphylococcus, and Enterococcus, as the cause of diseases classified elsewhere, or B96, Other bacterial agents as the cause of diseases classified elsewhere, may be required to identify the bacterial organism causing the infection. A "**Use Additional Code**" note will normally be found at the infectious disease code, indicating a need for the organism code to be added as a secondary code.

"Code first" notes are also under certain codes that are not specifically manifestation codes but may be due to an underlying cause. When there is a "Code first" note and an underlying condition is present, the underlying condition should be sequenced first.

"Code, if applicable, any causal condition first", notes indicate that this code may be assigned as a principal diagnosis when the causal condition is unknown or not applicable. If a causal condition is known, then the code for that condition should be sequenced as the principal or first-listed diagnosis.

Multiple codes may be needed for sequela, complication codes and obstetric codes to more fully describe a condition. See the specific guidelines for these conditions for further instruction.

COMBINATION CODE

A combination code is a single code used to classify: Two diagnoses, or a diagnosis with an associated secondary process (manifestation) A diagnosis with an associated complication

Combination codes are identified by referring to subterm entries in the Alphabetic Index and by reading the inclusion and exclusion notes in the Tabular List.

Assign only the combination code when that code fully identifies the diagnostic conditions involved or when the Alphabetic Index so directs. Multiple coding should not be used when the classification provides a combination code that clearly identifies all of the elements documented in the diagnosis. When the combination code lacks necessary specificity in describing the manifestation or complication, an additional code should be used as a secondary code.

SEQUELA (LATE EFFECTS)

A sequela is the residual effect (condition produced) after the acute phase of an illness or injury has terminated. There is no time limit on when a sequela code can be used. The residual may be apparent early, such as in cerebral infarction, or it may occur months or years later, such as that due to a previous injury. Coding of sequela generally requires two codes sequenced in the following order: The condition or nature of the sequela is sequenced first.

The sequela code is sequenced second.

An exception to the above guidelines are those instances where the code for the sequela is followed by a manifestation code identified in the Tabular List and title, or the sequela code has been expanded (at the fourth, fifth or sixth character levels) to

include the manifestation(s). The code for the acute phase of an illness or injury that led to the sequela is never used with a code for the late effect.

HYPERTENSION

The classification presumes a causal relationship between hypertension and heart involvement and between hypertension and kidney involvement, as the two conditions are linked by the term "with" in the Alphabetic Index. These conditions should be coded as related even in the absence of provider documentation explicitly linking them, unless the documentation clearly states the conditions are unrelated.

For hypertension and conditions not specifically linked by relational terms such as "with," "associated with" or "due to" in the classification, provider documentation must link the conditions in order to code them as related.

1) **Hypertension with Heart Disease**

   Hypertension with heart conditions classified to I50.- or I51.4-I51.7, I51.89, I51.9, are assigned to a code from category I11, Hypertensive heart disease. <u>**Use Additional Code**</u>(s) from category I50, Heart failure, to identify the type(s) of heart failure in those patients with heart failure.

   The same heart conditions (I50.-, I51.4-I51.7, I51.89, I51.9) with hypertension are coded separately if the provider has documented they are unrelated to the hypertension. Sequence according to the circumstances of the admission/encounter.

2) **Hypertensive Chronic Kidney Disease**

   Assign codes from category I12, Hypertensive chronic kidney disease, when both hypertension and a condition classifiable to category N18, Chronic kidney disease (CKD), are present. CKD should not be coded as hypertensive if the **provider indicates the CKD is not related to the hypertension**.

   The appropriate code from category N18 should be used as a secondary code with a code from category I12 to identify the stage of chronic kidney disease.

   See Section I.C.14. Chronic kidney disease.

   If a patient has hypertensive chronic kidney disease and acute renal failure, an additional code for the acute renal failure is required.

3) **Hypertensive Heart and Chronic Kidney Disease**

   Assign codes from combination category I13, Hypertensive heart and chronic kidney disease, when there is hypertension with both heart and kidney involvement. If heart failure is present, assign an additional code from category I50 to identify the type of heart failure.

   The appropriate code from category N18, Chronic kidney disease, should be used as a secondary code with a code from category I13 to identify the stage of chronic kidney disease.

   See Section I.C.14. Chronic kidney disease.

   The codes in category I13, Hypertensive heart and chronic kidney disease, are combination codes that include hypertension, heart disease and chronic kidney disease. The Includes note at I13 specifies that the conditions included at I11 and I12 are included together in I13. If a patient has hypertension, heart disease and chronic kidney disease, then a code from I13 should be used, not individual codes for hypertension, heart disease and chronic kidney disease, or codes from I11 or I12.

   For patients with both acute renal failure and chronic kidney disease, **the** acute renal failure **should also be coded. Sequence according to the circumstances of the admission/encounter.**

4) **Hypertensive Cerebrovascular Disease**

   For hypertensive cerebrovascular disease, first assign the appropriate code from categories I60-I69, followed by the appropriate hypertension code.

---

5) Hypertensive Retinopathy

Subcategory H35.0, Background retinopathy and retinal vascular changes, should be used with a code from category I10 – I15, Hypertensive disease to include the systemic hypertension. The sequencing is based on the reason for the encounter.

6) Hypertension, Secondary

Secondary hypertension is due to an underlying condition. Two codes are required: one to identify the underlying etiology and one from category I15 to identify the hypertension. Sequencing of codes is determined by the reason for admission/encounter.

7) Hypertension, Transient

Assign code R03.0, Elevated blood pressure reading without diagnosis of hypertension, unless patient has an established diagnosis of hypertension. Assign code O13.-, Gestational [pregnancy-induced] hypertension without significant proteinuria, or O14.-, Pre-eclampsia, for transient hypertension of pregnancy.

8) Hypertension, Controlled

This diagnostic statement usually refers to an existing state of hypertension under control by therapy. Assign the appropriate code from categories I10-I15, Hypertensive diseases.

9) Hypertension, Uncontrolled

Uncontrolled hypertension may refer to untreated hypertension or hypertension not responding to current therapeutic regimen. In either case, assign the appropriate code from categories I10-I15, Hypertensive diseases.

10) Hypertensive Crisis

Assign a code from category I16, Hypertensive crisis, for documented hypertensive urgency, hypertensive emergency or unspecified hypertensive crisis. Code also any identified hypertensive disease (I10-I15). The sequencing is based on the reason for the encounter.

11) Pulmonary Hypertension

Pulmonary hypertension is classified to category I27, Other pulmonary heart diseases. For secondary pulmonary hypertension (I27.1, I27.2-), code also any associated conditions or adverse effects of drugs or toxins. The sequencing is based on the reason for the encounter, except for adverse effects of drugs (See Section I.C.19.e.).

ATHEROSCLEROTIC CORONARY ARTERY DISEASE AND ANGINA

ICD-10-CM has combination codes for atherosclerotic heart disease with angina pectoris. The subcategories for these codes are I25.11, Atherosclerotic heart disease of native coronary artery with angina pectoris and I25.7, Atherosclerosis of coronary artery bypass graft(s) and coronary artery of transplanted heart with angina pectoris.

When using one of these combination codes it is not necessary to use an additional code for angina pectoris. A causal relationship can be assumed in a patient with both atherosclerosis and angina pectoris, unless the documentation indicates the angina is due to something other than the atherosclerosis.

If a patient with coronary artery disease is admitted due to an acute myocardial infarction (AMI), the AMI should be sequenced before the coronary artery disease.

See Section I.C.9. Acute myocardial infarction (AMI)

INTRAOPERATIVE AND POSTPROCEDURAL CEREBROVASCULAR ACCIDENT

Medical record documentation should clearly specify the cause- and-effect relationship between the medical intervention and the cerebrovascular accident in order to assign a code for intraoperative or postprocedural cerebrovascular accident.

Proper code assignment depends on whether it was an infarction or hemorrhage and whether it occurred intraoperatively or postoperatively. If it was a cerebral hemorrhage, code assignment depends on the type of procedure performed.

SEQUELAE OF CEREBROVASCULAR DISEASE

1) Category I69, Sequelae of Cerebrovascular disease

Category I69 is used to indicate conditions classifiable to categories I60-I67 as the causes of sequela (neurologic deficits), themselves classified elsewhere. These "late effects" include neurologic deficits that persist after initial onset of conditions classifiable to categories I60-I67. The neurologic deficits caused by cerebrovascular disease may be present from the onset or may arise at any time after the onset of the condition classifiable to categories I60-I67.

Codes from category I69, Sequelae of cerebrovascular disease, that specify hemiplegia, hemiparesis and monoplegia identify whether the dominant or nondominant side is affected. Should the affected side be documented, but not specified as dominant or nondominant, and the classification system does not indicate a default, code selection is as follows:

- For ambidextrous patients, the default should be dominant.

- If the left side is affected, the default is non-dominant.

- If the right side is affected, the default is dominant.

2) Codes from category I69 with codes from I60-I67

Codes from category I69 may be assigned on a health care record with codes from I60-I67, if the patient has a current cerebrovascular disease and deficits from an old cerebrovascular disease.

3) Codes from category I69 and Personal history of transient ischemic attack (TIA) and cerebral infarction (Z86.73)

Codes from category I69 should not be assigned if the patient does not have neurologic deficits.

See Section I.C.21. 4. History (of) for use of personal history codes

ACUTE MYOCARDIAL INFARCTION (AMI)

1) Type 1 ST elevation myocardial infarction (STEMI) and non-ST elevation myocardial infarction (NSTEMI)

The ICD-10-CM codes for type 1 acute myocardial infarction (AMI) identify the site, such as anterolateral wall or true posterior wall. Subcategories I21.0-I21.2 and code I21.3 are used for type 1 ST elevation myocardial infarction (STEMI). Code I21.4, Non-ST elevation (NSTEMI) myocardial infarction, is used for type 1 non-ST elevation myocardial infarction (NSTEMI) and nontransmural MIs.

If a type 1 NSTEMI evolves to STEMI, assign the STEMI code. If a type 1 STEMI converts to NSTEMI due to thrombolytic therapy, it is still coded as STEMI.

For encounters occurring while the myocardial infarction is equal to, or less than, four weeks old, including transfers to another acute setting or a postacute setting, and the myocardial infarction meets the definition for "other diagnoses" (see Section III, Reporting Additional Diagnoses), codes from category I21 may continue to be reported. For encounters after the 4-week time frame and the patient is still receiving care related to the myocardial infarction, the appropriate aftercare code should be assigned, rather than a code from category I21. For old or healed myocardial infarctions not requiring further care, code I25.2, Old myocardial infarction, may be assigned.

2) Acute myocardial infarction, unspecified

Code I21.9, Acute myocardial infarction, unspecified, is the default for unspecified acute myocardial infarction or unspecified type. If only type 1 STEMI or transmural MI without the site is documented, assign code I21.3, ST elevation (STEMI) myocardial infarction of unspecified site.

3) AMI documented as nontransmural or subendocardial, but site provided

---

● New code   ▲ Revised code   **Excludes1:** Not coded here   **Excludes2:** Not included here   ⊗ Placeholder required   ⑦7th digit required

If an AMI is documented as nontransmural or subendocardial, but the site is provided, it is still coded as a subendocardial AMI.

See Section I.C.21.3 for information on coding status post administration of tPA in a different facility within the last 24 hours.

4) Subsequent acute myocardial infarction

A code from category I22, Subsequent ST elevation (STEMI) and non-ST elevation (NSTEMI) myocardial infarction, is to be used when a patient who has suffered a type 1 or unspecified AMI has a new AMI within the 4-week time frame of the initial AMI. A code from category I22 must be used in conjunction with a code from category I21. The sequencing of the I22 and I21 codes depends on the circumstances of the encounter.

Do not assign code I22 for subsequent myocardial infarctions other than type 1 or unspecified. For subsequent type 2 AMI assign only code I21.A1. For subsequent type 4 or type 5 AMI, assign only code I21.A9.

If a subsequent myocardial infarction of one type occurs within 4 weeks of a myocardial infarction of a different type, assign the appropriate codes from category I21 to identify each type. Do not assign a code from I22. Codes from category I22 should only be assigned if both the initial and subsequent myocardial infarctions are type 1 or unspecified.

5) Other Types of Myocardial Infarction

The ICD-10-CM provides codes for different types of myocardial infarction. Type 1 myocardial infarctions are assigned to codes I21.0-I21.4 and I21.9.

Type 2 myocardial infarction (myocardial infarction due to demand ischemia or secondary to ischemic imbalance) is assigned to code I21.A1, Myocardial infarction type 2 with a code for the underlying cause . coded first. Do not assign code I24.8, Other forms of acute ischemic heart disease, for the demand ischemia. Sequencing of type 2 AMI or the underlying cause is dependent on the circumstances of admission. If a type 2 AMI code is described as NSTEMI or STEMI, only assign code I21.A1. Codes I21.01-I21.4 should only be assigned for type 1 AMIs.

Acute myocardial infarctions type 3, 4a, 4b, 4c and 5 are assigned to code I21.A9, Other myocardial infarction type.

The "Code also" and "Code first" notes should be followed related to complications, and for coding of postprocedural myocardial infarctions during or following cardiac surgery.

Chapter 9

Diseases of The Circulatory System (I00-I99)

Excludes2: certain conditions originating in the perinatal period (P04-P96)

certain infectious and parasitic diseases (A00-B99)

complications of pregnancy, childbirth and the puerperium (O00-O9A)

congenital malformations, deformations, and chromosomal abnormalities (Q00-Q99)

endocrine, nutritional and metabolic diseases (E00-E88)

injury, poisoning and certain other consequences of external causes (S00-T88)

neoplasms (C00-D49)

symptoms, signs and abnormal clinical and laboratory findings, not elsewhere classified (R00-R94)

systemic connective tissue disorders (M30-M36)

transient cerebral ischemic attacks and related syndromes (G45.-)

This chapter contains the following blocks:

I00-I02	Acute rheumatic fever
I05-I09	Chronic rheumatic heart diseases
I10-I16	Hypertensive diseases
I20-I25	Ischemic heart diseases
I26-I28	Pulmonary heart disease and diseases of pulmonary circulation
I30-I5A	Other forms of heart disease
I60-I69	Cerebrovascular diseases
I70-I79	Diseases of arteries, arterioles and capillaries
I80-I89	Diseases of veins, lymphatic vessels and lymph nodes, not elsewhere classified
I95-I99	Other and unspecified disorders of the circulatory system

ACUTE RHEUMATIC FEVER (I00-I02)

I00   **Rheumatic fever without heart involvement**

Includes: arthritis, rheumatic, acute or subacute

Excludes1: rheumatic fever with heart involvement (I01.0 -I01.9)

I01   **Rheumatic fever with heart involvement**

Excludes1: chronic diseases of rheumatic origin (I05-I09) unless rheumatic fever is also present or there is evidence of reactivation or activity of the rheumatic process.

   I01.0   **Acute rheumatic pericarditis**

Any condition in I00 with pericarditis

Rheumatic pericarditis (acute)

Excludes1: acute pericarditis not specified as rheumatic (I30.-)

   I01.1   **Acute rheumatic endocarditis**

Any condition in I00 with endocarditis or valvulitis

Acute rheumatic valvulitis

   I01.2   **Acute rheumatic myocarditis**

Any condition in I00 with myocarditis

   I01.8   **Other acute rheumatic heart disease**

Any condition in I00 with other or multiple types of heart involvement

Acute rheumatic pancarditis

   I01.9   **Acute rheumatic heart disease, unspecified**

Any condition in I00 with unspecified type of heart involvement

Rheumatic carditis, acute

Rheumatic heart disease, active or acute

I02   **Rheumatic chorea**

Includes: Sydenham's chorea

Excludes1: chorea NOS (G25.5)

Huntington's chorea (G10)

   I02.0   **Rheumatic chorea with heart involvement**

Chorea NOS with heart involvement

Rheumatic chorea with heart involvement of any type classifiable under I01.-

   I02.9   **Rheumatic chorea without heart involvement**

Rheumatic chorea NOS

CHRONIC RHEUMATIC HEART DISEASES (I05-I09)

Definition: Rheumatic heart disease refers to a thickening and stenosis of one or more of the heart valves and often requires surgery to repair or replace the involved valve(s).

I05   **Rheumatic mitral valve diseases**

Includes: conditions classifiable to both I05.0 and I05.2-I05.9, whether specified as rheumatic or not

Excludes1: mitral valve disease specified as nonrheumatic (I34.-)

mitral valve disease with aortic and/or tricuspid valve involvement (I08.-)

   I05.0   **Rheumatic mitral stenosis**

Mitral (valve) obstruction (rheumatic)

   I05.1   **Rheumatic mitral insufficiency**

Rheumatic mitral incompetence

Rheumatic mitral regurgitation

Excludes1: mitral insufficiency not specified as rheumatic (I34.0)

   I05.2   **Rheumatic mitral stenosis with insufficiency**

Rheumatic mitral stenosis with incompetence or regurgitation

   I05.8   **Other rheumatic mitral valve diseases**

Rheumatic mitral (valve) failure

   I05.9   **Rheumatic mitral valve disease, unspecified**

Rheumatic mitral (valve) disorder (chronic) NOS

I06   **Rheumatic aortic valve diseases**

Excludes1: aortic valve disease not specified as rheumatic (I35.-)

aortic valve disease with mitral and/or tricuspid valve involvement (I08.-)

   I06.0   **Rheumatic aortic stenosis**

Rheumatic aortic (valve) obstruction

   I06.1   **Rheumatic aortic insufficiency**

Rheumatic aortic incompetence

Rheumatic aortic regurgitation

   I06.2   **Rheumatic aortic stenosis with insufficiency**

Rheumatic aortic stenosis with incompetence or regurgitation

   I06.8   **Other rheumatic aortic valve diseases**

   I06.9   **Rheumatic aortic valve disease, unspecified**

Rheumatic aortic (valve) disease NOS

I07   **Rheumatic tricuspid valve diseases**

Includes: rheumatic tricuspid valve diseases specified as rheumatic or unspecified

Excludes1: tricuspid valve disease specified as nonrheumatic (I36.-)

tricuspid valve disease with aortic and/or mitral valve involvement (I08.-)

   I07.0   **Rheumatic tricuspid stenosis**

Tricuspid (valve) stenosis (rheumatic)

I07.1   **Rheumatic tricuspid insufficiency**

Tricuspid (valve) insufficiency (rheumatic)

I07.2   **Rheumatic tricuspid stenosis and insufficiency**

I07.8   **Other rheumatic tricuspid valve diseases**

I07.9   **Rheumatic tricuspid valve disease, unspecified**

Rheumatic tricuspid valve disorder NOS

I08   **Multiple valve diseases**

Includes: multiple valve diseases specified as rheumatic or unspecified

Excludes1: endocarditis, valve unspecified (I38)

multiple valve disease specified a nonrheumatic (I34.-, I35.-, I36.-, I37.-, I38.-, Q22.-, Q23.-, Q24.8-)

rheumatic valve disease NOS (I09.1)

I08.0   **Rheumatic disorders of both mitral and aortic valves**

Involvement of both mitral and aortic valves specified as rheumatic or unspecified

I08.1   **Rheumatic disorders of both mitral and tricuspid valves**

I08.2   **Rheumatic disorders of both aortic and tricuspid valves**

I08.3   **Combined rheumatic disorders of mitral, aortic and tricuspid valves**

I08.8   **Other rheumatic multiple valve diseases**

I08.9   **Rheumatic multiple valve disease, unspecified**

I09   **Other rheumatic heart diseases**

I09.0   **Rheumatic myocarditis**

Excludes1: myocarditis not specified as rheumatic (I51.4)

I09.1   **Rheumatic diseases of endocardium, valve unspecified**

Rheumatic endocarditis (chronic)

Rheumatic valvulitis (chronic)

Excludes1: endocarditis, valve unspecified (I38)

I09.2   **Chronic rheumatic pericarditis**

Adherent pericardium, rheumatic

Chronic rheumatic mediastinopericarditis

Chronic rheumatic myopericarditis

Excludes1: chronic pericarditis not specified as rheumatic (I31.-)

I09.8   **Other specified rheumatic heart diseases**

I09.81   **Rheumatic heart failure** [HCC]

Use Additional Code to identify type of heart failure (I50.-)

I09.89   **Other specified rheumatic heart diseases**

Rheumatic disease of pulmonary valve

I09.9   **Rheumatic heart disease, unspecified**

Rheumatic carditis

Excludes1: rheumatoid carditis (M05.31)

HYPERTENSIVE DISEASES (I10-I16)

Definition: Hypertensive heart disease refers to heart disease caused by high blood pressure, especially localized high blood pressure.

Use Additional Code to identify:

exposure to environmental tobacco smoke (Z77.22)

history of tobacco dependence (Z87.891)

occupational exposure to environmental tobacco smoke (Z57.31)

tobacco dependence (F17.-)

tobacco use (Z72.0)

Excludes1: neonatal hypertension (P29.2)

primary pulmonary hypertension (I27.0)

Excludes2: hypertensive disease complicating pregnancy, childbirth and the puerperium (O10-O11, O13-O16)

I10   **Essential (primary) hypertension**

Includes: high blood pressure

hypertension (arterial) (benign) (essential) (malignant) (primary) (systemic)

Excludes1: hypertensive disease complicating pregnancy, childbirth and the puerperium (O10-O11, O13-O16)

Excludes2: essential (primary) hypertension involving vessels of brain (I60-I69)

essential (primary) hypertension involving vessels of eye (H35.0-)

I11   **Hypertensive heart disease**

Includes: any condition in I50.- or I51.4-I51.7, I51.89, I51.9 due to hypertension

I11.0   **Hypertensive heart disease with heart failure** [HCC]

Hypertensive heart failure

Use Additional Code to identify type of heart failure (I50.-)

I11.9   **Hypertensive heart disease without heart failure**

Hypertensive heart disease NOS

I12   **Hypertensive chronic kidney disease**

Includes: any condition in N18 and N26 - due to hypertension

arteriosclerosis of kidney

arteriosclerotic nephritis (chronic) (interstitial) hypertensive nephropathy

nephrosclerosis

Excludes1: hypertension due to kidney disease (I15.0, I15.1)

renovascular hypertension (I15.0) secondary hypertension (I15.-)

Excludes2: acute kidney failure (N17.-)

I12.0   **Hypertensive chronic kidney disease with stage 5 chronic kidney disease or end stage renal disease** [HCC]

Use Additional Code to identify the stage of chronic kidney disease (N18.5, N18.6)

I12.9   **Hypertensive chronic kidney disease with stage 1 through stage 4   chronic kidney disease, or unspecified chronic kidney disease**

Hypertensive chronic kidney disease NOS Hypertensive renal disease NOS

Use Additional Code to identify the stage of chronic kidney disease (N18.1-N18.4, N18.9)

I13   **Hypertensive heart and chronic kidney disease**

Includes: any condition in I11.- with any condition in I12.-

cardiorenal disease cardiovascular renal disease

I13.0   **Hypertensive heart and chronic kidney disease with heart failure and stage 1 through stage 4 chronic kidney disease, or unspecified chronic kidney disease** [HCC]

Use Additional Code to identify type of heart failure (I50.-)

Use Additional Code to identify stage of chronic kidney disease (N18.1-N18.4, N18.9)

I13.1   **Hypertensive heart and chronic kidney disease without heart failure**

I13.10   **Hypertensive heart and chronic kidney disease without heart failure, with stage 1 through stage 4 chronic kidney disease, or unspecified chronic kidney disease**

Hypertensive heart disease and hypertensive chronic kidney disease NOS

Use Additional Code to identify the stage of chronic kidney disease (N18.1-N18.4, N18.9)

I13.11   **Hypertensive heart and chronic kidney disease without heart failure, with stage 5 chronic kidney disease, or end stage renal disease** [HCC]

<u>Use Additional Code</u> to identify the stage of chronic kidney disease (N18.5, N18.6)

I13.2 **Hypertensive heart and chronic kidney disease with heart failure and with stage 5 chronic kidney disease, or end stage renal disease** [HCC]

<u>Use Additional Code</u> to identify type of heart failure (I50.-)

<u>Use Additional Code</u> to identify the stage of chronic kidney disease (N18.5, N18.6)

I15 **Secondary hypertension**

Definition: Secondary hypertension is a type of hypertension caused by an identifiable underlying secondary cause.

<u>Code also</u> underlying condition

Excludes1: postprocedural hypertension (I97.3)

Excludes2: secondary hypertension involving vessels of brain (I60-I69)

secondary hypertension involving vessels of eye (H35.0-)

I15.0 **Renovascular hypertension**

I15.1 **Hypertension secondary to other renal disorders**

I15.2 **Hypertension secondary to endocrine disorders**

I15.8 **Other secondary hypertension**

I15.9 **Secondary hypertension, unspecified**

I16 **Hypertensive crisis**

<u>Code also</u> any identified hypertensive disease (I10-I15)

I16.0 **Hypertensive urgency**

I16.1 **Hypertensive emergency**

I16.9 **Hypertensive crisis, unspecified**

ISCHEMIC HEART DISEASES (I20-I25)

Definition: Ischemic heart disease is a condition caused by a reduced amount of blood supplying the heart muscle. It can be caused by cholesterol and other lipids building up on the inner walls of arteries that supply the heart, forming a thick plaque that can reduce the amount of blood carrying nutrients and oxygen to heart tissue.

<u>Code also</u> the presence of hypertension (I10-I16)

I20 **Angina pectoris**

<u>Use Additional Code</u> to identify:

exposure to environmental tobacco smoke (Z77.22)

history of tobacco dependence (Z87.891)

occupational exposure to environmental tobacco smoke (Z57.31)

tobacco dependence (F17.-)

tobacco use (Z72.0)

Excludes1: angina pectoris with atherosclerotic heart disease of native coronary arteries (I25.1-)

atherosclerosis of coronary artery bypass graft(s) and coronary artery of transplanted heart with angina pectoris (I25.7-)

postinfarction angina (I23.7)

I20.0 **Unstable angina** [HCC]

Accelerated angina

Crescendo angina

De novo effort angina

Intermediate coronary syndrome

Preinfarction syndrome

Worsening effort angina

I20.1 **Angina pectoris with documented spasm** [HCC]

Angiospastic angina

Prinzmetal angina

Spasm-induced angina

Variant angina

I20.8 **Other forms of angina pectoris** [HCC]

Angina equivalent

Angina of effort

Coronary slow flow syndrome

Stenocardia

Stable angina

<u>Use Additional Code</u>(s) for symptoms associated with angina equivalent

I20.9 **Angina pectoris, unspecified** [HCC]

Angina NOS

Anginal syndrome

Cardiac angina

Ischemic chest pain

I21 **Acute myocardial infarction**

Definition: Myocardial infarction, commonly known as a heart attack, occurs when the blood supply to part of the heart is interrupted causing some heart cells to die.

Includes: cardiac infarction

coronary (artery) embolism

coronary (artery) occlusion

coronary (artery) rupture

coronary (artery) thrombosis

infarction of heart, myocardium, or ventricle

myocardial infarction specified as acute or with a stated duration of 4 weeks (28 days) or less from onset

<u>Use Additional Code</u>, if applicable, to identify:

exposure to environmental tobacco smoke (Z77.22)

history of tobacco dependence (Z87.891)

occupational exposure to environmental tobacco smoke (Z57.31)

status post administration of tPA (rtPA) in a different facility within the last 24 hours prior to admission to current facility (Z92.82)

tobacco dependence (F17.-)

tobacco use (Z72.0)

Excludes2: old myocardial infarction (I25.2)

postmyocardial infarction syndrome (I24.1)

subsequent type 1 myocardial infarction (I22.-)

I21.0 **ST elevation (STEMI) myocardial infarction of anterior wall**

Type 1 ST elevation myocardial infarction of anterior wall

I21.01 **ST elevation (STEMI) myocardial infarction involving left main coronary artery** [HCC]

I21.02 **ST elevation (STEMI) myocardial infarction involving left anterior descending coronary artery** [HCC]

ST elevation (STEMI) myocardial infarction involving diagonal coronary artery

I21.09 **ST elevation (STEMI) myocardial infarction involving other coronary artery of anterior wall** [HCC]

Acute transmural myocardial infarction of anterior wall

Anteroapical transmural (Q wave) infarction (acute)

Anterolateral transmural (Q wave) infarction (acute)

Anteroseptal transmural (Q wave) infarction (acute)

Transmural (Q wave) infarction (acute) (of) anterior (wall) NOS

I21.1 **ST elevation (STEMI) myocardial infarction of inferior wall**

Type 1 ST elevation myocardial infarction of inferior wall

I21.11 **ST elevation (STEMI) myocardial infarction involving right coronary artery** [HCC]

Inferoposterior transmural (Q wave) infarction (acute)

I21.19 **ST elevation (STEMI) myocardial infarction involving other coronary artery of inferior wall** [HCC]

Acute transmural myocardial infarction of inferior wall

Inferolateral transmural (Q wave) infarction (acute)

Transmural (Q wave) infarction (acute) (of) diaphragmatic wall

Transmural (Q wave) infarction (acute) (of) inferior (wall) NOS

Excludes2: ST elevation (STEMI) myocardial infarction involving left circumflex coronary artery (I21.21)

I21.2 **ST elevation (STEMI) myocardial infarction of other sites**

Type 1 ST elevation myocardial infarction of other sites

I21.21 **ST elevation (STEMI) myocardial infarction involving left circumflex coronary artery** [HCC]

ST elevation (STEMI) myocardial infarction involving oblique marginal coronary artery

I21.29 **ST elevation (STEMI) myocardial infarction involving other sites** [HCC]

Acute transmural myocardial infarction of other sites

Apical-lateral transmural (Q wave) infarction (acute)

Basal-lateral transmural (Q wave) infarction (acute)

High lateral transmural (Q wave) infarction (acute)

Lateral (wall) NOS transmural (Q wave) infarction (acute)

Posterior (true) transmural (Q wave) infarction (acute)

Posterobasal transmural (Q wave) infarction (acute)

Posterolateral transmural (Q wave) infarction (acute)

Posteroseptal transmural (Q wave) infarction (acute)

Septal transmural (Q wave) infarction (acute) NOS

I21.3 **ST elevation (STEMI) myocardial infarction of unspecified site** [HCC]

Acute transmural myocardial infarction of unspecified site

Type 1 ST elevation myocardial infarction of unspecified site

Transmural (Q wave) myocardial infarction NOS

I21.4 **Non-ST elevation (NSTEMI) myocardial infarction**

Acute subendocardial myocardial infarction

Non-Q wave myocardial infarction NOS

Nontransmural myocardial infarction NOS

Type 1 non-ST elevation myocardial infarction

I21.9 **Acute myocardial infarction, unspecified** [HCC]

Myocardial infarction (acute) NOS

I21.A **Other type of myocardial infarction**

I21.A1 **Myocardial infarction type 2** [HCC]

Myocardial infarction due to demand ischemia

Myocardial infarction secondary to ischemic imbalance

Code first the underlying cause, such as:

anemia (D50.0-D64.9)

chronic obstructive pulmonary disease (J44.-)

paroxysmal tachycardia (I47.0-I47.9)

shock (R57.0-R57.9)

I21.A9 **Other myocardial infarction type** [HCC]

Myocardial infarction associated with revascularization procedure

Myocardial infarction type 3

Myocardial infarction type 4a

Myocardial infarction type 4b

Myocardial infarction type 4c

Myocardial infarction type 5

Code first, if applicable, postprocedural myocardial infarction following cardiac surgery (I97.190), or postprocedural myocardial infarction during cardiac surgery (I97.790)

Code also complication, if known and applicable, such as:

(acute) stent occlusion (T82.897-)

(acute) stent stenosis (T82.855-)

(acute) stent thrombosis (T82.867-)

cardiac arrest due to underlying cardiac condition (I46.2)

complication of percutaneous coronary intervention (PCI) (I97.89)

occlusion of coronary artery bypass graft (T82.218-)

I22 **Subsequent ST elevation (STEMI) and non-ST elevation (NSTEMI) myocardial infarction**

Includes: acute myocardial infarction occurring within four weeks (28 days) of a previous acute myocardial infarction, regardless of site

cardiac infarction

coronary (artery) embolism coronary (artery) occlusion

coronary (artery) rupture coronary (artery) thrombosis

infarction of heart, myocardium, or ventricle recurrent myocardial infarction

reinfarction of myocardium

rupture of heart, myocardium, or ventricle

subsequent type 1 myocardial infarction

Excludes1: subsequent myocardial infarction, type 2 (I21.A1)

subsequent myocardial infarction of other type (type 3) (type 4) (type 5) (I21.A9)

Use Additional Code, if applicable, to identify:

exposure to environmental tobacco smoke (Z77.22)

history of tobacco dependence (Z87.891)

occupational exposure to environmental tobacco smoke (Z57.31)

status post administration of tPA (rtPA) in a different facility within the last 24 hours prior to admission to current facility (Z92.82)

tobacco dependence (F17.-)

tobacco use (Z72.0)

I22.0 **Subsequent ST elevation (STEMI) myocardial infarction of anterior wall** [HCC]

Subsequent acute transmural myocardial infarction of anterior wall

Subsequent transmural (Q wave) infarction (acute) (of) anterior (wall) NOS

Subsequent anteroapical transmural (Q wave) infarction (acute)

Subsequent anterolateral transmural (Q wave) infarction (acute)

Subsequent anteroseptal transmural (Q wave) infarction (acute)

I22.1 Subsequent ST elevation (STEMI) myocardial infarction of inferior wall [HCC]

Subsequent acute transmural myocardial infarction of inferior wall

Subsequent transmural (Q wave) infarction (acute)(of) diaphragmatic wall

Subsequent transmural (Q wave) infarction (acute)(of) inferior (wall) NOS

Subsequent inferolateral transmural (Q wave) infarction (acute)

Subsequent inferoposterior transmural (Q wave) infarction (acute)

I22.2 Subsequent non-ST elevation (NSTEMI) myocardial infarction [HCC]

Subsequent acute subendocardial myocardial infarction

Subsequent non-Q wave myocardial infarction NOS

Subsequent nontransmural myocardial infarction NOS

I22.8 Subsequent ST elevation (STEMI) myocardial infarction of other sites [HCC]

Subsequent acute transmural myocardial infarction of other sites

Subsequent apical-lateral transmural (Q wave) myocardial infarction (acute)

Subsequent basal-lateral transmural (Q wave) myocardial infarction (acute)

Subsequent high lateral transmural (Q wave) myocardial infarction (acute)

Subsequent transmural (Q wave) myocardial infarction (acute)(of) lateral (wall) NOS

Subsequent posterior (true) transmural (Q wave) myocardial infarction (acute)

Subsequent posterobasal transmural (Q wave) myocardial infarction (acute)

Subsequent posterolateral transmural (Q wave) myocardial infarction (acute)

Subsequent posteroseptal transmural (Q wave) myocardial infarction (acute)

Subsequent septal NOS transmural (Q wave) myocardial infarction (acute)

I22.9 Subsequent ST elevation (STEMI) myocardial infarction of unspecified site [HCC]

Subsequent acute myocardial infarction of unspecified site

Subsequent myocardial infarction (acute) NOS

I23 Certain current complications following ST elevation (STEMI) and non-ST elevation (NSTEMI) myocardial infarction (within the 28-day period)

I23.0 Hemopericardium as current complication following acute myocardial infarction [HCC]

Excludes1: hemopericardium not specified as current complication following acute myocardial infarction (I31.2)

I23.1 Atrial septal defect as current complication following acute myocardial infarction [HCC]

Excludes1: acquired atrial septal defect not specified as current complication following acute myocardial infarction (I51.0)

I23.2 Ventricular septal defect as current complication following acute myocardial infarction [HCC]

Excludes1: acquired ventricular septal defect not specified as current complication following acute myocardial infarction (I51.0)

I23.3 Rupture of cardiac wall without hemopericardium as current complication following acute myocardial infarction [HCC]

I23.4 Rupture of chordae tendineae as current complication following acute myocardial infarction [HCC]

Excludes1: rupture of chordae tendineae not specified as current complication following acute myocardial infarction (I51.1)

I23.5 Rupture of papillary muscle as current complication following acute myocardial infarction [HCC]

Excludes1: rupture of papillary muscle not specified as current complication following acute myocardial infarction (I51.2) [HCC]

I23.6 Thrombosis of atrium, auricular appendage, and ventricle as current complications following acute myocardial infarction [HCC]

Excludes1: thrombosis of atrium, auricular appendage, and ventricle not specified as current complication following acute myocardial infarction (I51.3)

I23.7 Postinfarction angina [HCC]

I23.8 Other current complications following acute myocardial infarction [HCC]

I24 Other acute ischemic heart diseases

Excludes1: angina pectoris (I20.-)

transient myocardial ischemia in newborn (P29.4)

Excludes2: non-ischemic myocardial injury (I5A)

I24.0 Acute coronary thrombosis not resulting in myocardial infarction [HCC]

Acute coronary (artery) (vein) embolism not resulting in myocardial infarction

Acute coronary (artery) (vein) occlusion not resulting in myocardial infarction

Acute coronary (artery) (vein) thromboembolism not resulting in myocardial infarction

Excludes1: atherosclerotic heart disease (I25.1-)

I24.1 Dressler's syndrome [HCC]

Postmyocardial infarction syndrome

Excludes1: postinfarction angina (I23.7)

I24.8 Other forms of acute ischemic heart disease [HCC]

Excludes1: myocardial infarction due to demand ischemia (I21.A1)

I24.9 Acute ischemic heart disease, unspecified [HCC]

Excludes1: ischemic heart disease (chronic) NOS (I25.9)

I25 Chronic ischemic heart disease

Use Additional Code to identify:

chronic total occlusion of coronary artery (I25.82)

exposure to environmental tobacco smoke (Z77.22)

history of tobacco dependence (Z87.891)

occupational exposure to environmental tobacco smoke (Z57.31)

tobacco dependence (F17.-)

tobacco use (Z72.0)

Excludes2: non-ischemic myocardial injury (I5A)

I25.1 Atherosclerotic heart disease of native coronary artery

Atherosclerotic cardiovascular disease

Coronary (artery) atheroma

Coronary (artery) atherosclerosis

Coronary (artery) disease

Coronary (artery) sclerosis

Use Additional Code, if applicable, to identify:

coronary atherosclerosis due to calcified coronary lesion (I25.84)

coronary atherosclerosis due to lipid rich plaque (I25.83)

Excludes2: atheroembolism (I75.-)

atherosclerosis of coronary artery bypass graft(s) and transplanted heart (I25.7-)

I25.10   Atherosclerotic heart disease of native coronary artery without angina pectoris

Atherosclerotic heart disease NOS

I25.11   Atherosclerotic heart disease of native coronary artery with angina pectoris

I25.110   Atherosclerotic heart disease of native coronary artery with unstable angina pectoris [HCC]

Excludes1: unstable angina without atherosclerotic heart disease (I20.0)

I25.111   Atherosclerotic heart disease of native coronary artery with angina pectoris with documented spasm [HCC]

Excludes1: angina pectoris with documented spasm without atherosclerotic heart disease (I20.1)

I25.118   Atherosclerotic heart disease of native coronary artery with other forms of angina pectoris [HCC]

Excludes1: Other forms of angina pectoris without atherosclerotic heart disease (I20.8)

I25.119   Atherosclerotic heart disease of native coronary artery with unspecified angina pectoris [HCC]

Atherosclerotic heart disease with angina NOS

Atherosclerotic heart disease with ischemic chest pain

Excludes1: unspecified angina pectoris without atherosclerotic heart disease (I20.9)

I25.2   Old myocardial infarction

Definition: Old myocardial infarction refers to an old occlusion or blockage of arteries supplying the muscles of the heart, resulting in injury or necrosis of the heart muscle. Healed myocardial infarction Past myocardial infarction diagnosed by ECG **or other** investigation, but currently presenting no symptoms

I25.3   Aneurysm of heart

Mural aneurysm

Ventricular aneurysm

I25.4   Coronary artery aneurysm and dissection

I25.41   Coronary artery aneurysm

Coronary arteriovenous fistula, acquired

Excludes1: congenital coronary (artery) aneurysm (Q24.5)

I25.42   Coronary artery dissection

I25.5   Ischemic cardiomyopathy

Excludes2: coronary atherosclerosis (I25.1-, I25.7-)

I25.6   Silent myocardial ischemia

I25.7   Atherosclerosis of coronary artery bypass graft(s) and coronary artery of transplanted heart with angina pectoris

Use Additional Code, if applicable, to identify:

coronary atherosclerosis due to calcified coronary lesion (I25.84)

coronary atherosclerosis due to lipid rich plaque (I25.83)

Excludes1: atherosclerosis of bypass graft(s) of transplanted heart without angina pectoris (I25.812)

atherosclerosis of coronary artery bypass graft(s) without angina pectoris (I25.810)

atherosclerosis of native coronary artery of transplanted heart without angina pectoris (I25.811)

I25.70   Atherosclerosis of coronary artery bypass graft(s), unspecified, with angina pectoris

I25.700   Atherosclerosis of coronary artery bypass graft(s), unspecified, with unstable angina pectoris [HCC]

Excludes1: unstable angina pectoris without atherosclerosis of coronary artery bypass graft (I20.0)

I25.701   Atherosclerosis of coronary artery bypass graft(s), unspecified, with angina pectoris with documented spasm [HCC]

Excludes1: angina pectoris with documented spasm without atherosclerosis of coronary artery bypass graft (I20.1)

I25.708   Atherosclerosis of coronary artery bypass graft(s), unspecified, with other forms of angina pectoris [HCC]

Excludes1: Other forms of angina pectoris without atherosclerosis of coronary artery bypass graft (I20.8)

I25.709   Atherosclerosis of coronary artery bypass graft(s), unspecified, with unspecified angina pectoris [HCC]

Excludes1: unspecified angina pectoris without atherosclerosis of coronary artery bypass graft (I20.9)

I25.71   Atherosclerosis of autologous vein coronary artery bypass graft(s) with angina pectoris

I25.710   Atherosclerosis of autologous vein coronary artery bypass graft(s) with unstable angina pectoris [HCC]

Excludes1: unstable angina without atherosclerosis of autologous vein coronary artery bypass graft(s) (I20.0)

embolism or thrombus of coronary artery bypass graft(s) (T82.8-)

I25.711   Atherosclerosis of autologous vein coronary artery bypass graft(s) with angina pectoris with documented spasm [HCC]

Excludes1: angina pectoris with documented spasm without atherosclerosis of autologous vein coronary artery bypass graft(s) (I20.1)

I25.718 **Atherosclerosis of autologous vein coronary artery bypass graft(s) with other forms of angina pectoris** [HCC]

Excludes1: Other forms of angina pectoris without athero-sclerosis of autologous vein coronary artery bypass graft(s) (I20.8)

I25.719 **Atherosclerosis of autologous vein coronary artery bypass graft(s) with unspecified angina pectoris** [HCC]

Excludes1: unspecified angina pectoris without athero-sclerosis of autologous vein coronary artery bypass graft(s) (I20.9)

I25.72 **Atherosclerosis of autologous artery coronary artery bypass graft(s) with angina pectoris**

Atherosclerosis of internal mammary artery graft with angina pectoris

I25.720 **Atherosclerosis of autologous artery coronary artery bypass graft(s) with unstable angina pectoris** [HCC]

Excludes1: unstable angina without atherosclerosis of autologous artery coronary artery bypass graft(s) (I20.0)

I25.721 **Atherosclerosis of autologous artery coronary artery bypass graft(s) with angina pectoris with documented spasm** [HCC]

Excludes1: angina pectoris with documented spasm without atherosclerosis of autologous artery coronary artery bypass graft(s) (I20.1)

I25.728 **Atherosclerosis of autologous artery coronary artery bypass graft(s) with other forms of angina pectoris** [HCC]

Excludes1: Other forms of angina pectoris without athero-sclerosis of autologous artery coronary artery bypass graft(s) (I20.8)

I25.729 **Atherosclerosis of autologous artery coronary artery bypass graft(s) with unspecified angina pectoris** [HCC]

Excludes1: unspecified angina pectoris without athero-sclerosis of autologous artery coronary artery bypass graft(s) (I20.9)

I25.73 **Atherosclerosis of nonautologous biological coronary artery bypass graft(s) with angina pectoris**

I25.730 **Atherosclerosis of nonautologous biological coronary artery bypass graft(s) with unstable angina pectoris** [HCC]

Excludes1: unstable angina without atherosclerosis of nonauto-logous biological coronary artery bypass graft(s) (I20.0)

I25.731 **Atherosclerosis of nonautologous biological coronary artery bypass**

graft(s) with angina pectoris with documented spasm [HCC]

Excludes1: angina pectoris with documented spasm without atherosclerosis of nonautologous biological coronary artery bypass graft(s) (I20.1)

I25.738 **Atherosclerosis of nonautologous biological coronary artery bypass graft(s) with other forms of angina pectoris** [HCC]

Excludes1: Other forms of angina pectoris without atherosclerosis of nonautologous biological coronary artery bypass graft(s) (I20.8)

I25.739 **Atherosclerosis of nonautologous biological coronary artery bypass graft(s) with unspecified angina pectoris** [HCC]

Excludes1: unspecified angina pectoris without atherosclerosis of nonautologous biological coronary artery bypass graft(s) (I20.9)

I25.75 **Atherosclerosis of native coronary artery of transplanted heart with angina pectoris**

Excludes1: atherosclerosis of native coronary artery of transplanted heart without angina pectoris (I25.811)

I25.750 **Atherosclerosis of native coronary artery of transplanted heart with unstable angina** [HCC]

I25.751 **Atherosclerosis of native coronary artery of transplanted heart with angina pectoris with documented spasm** [HCC]

I25.758 **Atherosclerosis of native coronary artery of transplanted heart with other forms of angina pectoris** [HCC]

I25.759 **Atherosclerosis of native coronary artery of transplanted heart with unspecified angina pectoris** [HCC]

I25.76 **Atherosclerosis of bypass graft of coronary artery of transplanted heart with angina pectoris**

Excludes1: atherosclerosis of bypass graft of coronary artery of transplanted heart without angina pectoris (I25.812)

I25.760 **Atherosclerosis of bypass graft of coronary artery of transplanted heart with unstable angina** [HCC]

I25.761 **Atherosclerosis of bypass graft of coronary artery of transplanted heart with angina pectoris with documented spasm** [HCC]

I25.768 **Atherosclerosis of bypass graft of coronary artery of transplanted heart with other forms of angina pectoris** [HCC]

I25.769 **Atherosclerosis of bypass graft of coronary artery of transplanted heart with unspecified angina pectoris** [HCC]

I25.79 **Atherosclerosis of other coronary artery bypass graft(s) with angina pectoris**

> **I25.790** **Atherosclerosis of other coronary artery bypass graft(s) with unstable angina pectoris** [HCC]
>
> > **Excludes1:** unstable angina without atherosclerosis of other coronary artery bypass graft(s) (I20.0)
>
> **I25.791** **Atherosclerosis of other coronary artery bypass graft(s) with angina pectoris with documented spasm** [HCC]
>
> > **Excludes1:** angina pectoris with documented spasm without atherosclerosis of other coronary artery bypass graft(s) (I20.1)
>
> **I25.798** **Atherosclerosis of other coronary artery bypass graft(s) with other forms of angina pectoris** [HCC]
>
> > **Excludes1:** Other forms of angina pectoris without atherosclerosis of other coronary artery bypass graft(s) (I20.8)
>
> **I25.799** **Atherosclerosis of other coronary artery bypass graft(s) with unspecified angina pectoris** [HCC]
>
> > **Excludes1:** unspecified angina pectoris without atherosclerosis of other coronary artery bypass graft(s) (I20.9)

I25.8 **Other forms of chronic ischemic heart disease**

> **I25.81** **Atherosclerosis of other coronary vessels without angina pectoris**
>
> > **Use Additional Code**, if applicable, to identify:
> >
> > coronary atherosclerosis due to calcified coronary lesion (I25.84)
> >
> > coronary atherosclerosis due to lipid rich plaque (I25.83)
> >
> > atherosclerotic heart disease of native coronary artery without angina pectoris (I25.10)
>
> **I25.810** **Atherosclerosis of coronary artery bypass graft(s) without angina pectoris**
>
> > Atherosclerosis of coronary artery bypass graft NOS
> >
> > **Excludes1:** atherosclerosis of coronary bypass graft(s) with angina pectoris (I25.70-I25.73-,I25.79-)
>
> **I25.811** **Atherosclerosis of native coronary artery of transplanted heart without angina pectoris**
>
> > Atherosclerosis of native coronary artery of transplanted heart NOS
> >
> > **Excludes1:** atherosclerosis of native coronary artery of transplanted heart with angina pectoris (I25.75-)
>
> **I25.812** **Atherosclerosis of bypass graft of coronary artery of transplanted heart without angina pectoris**

Atherosclerosis of bypass graft of transplanted heart NOS

> **Excludes1:** atherosclerosis of bypass graft of transplanted heart with angina pectoris (I25.76)

I25.82 **Chronic total occlusion of coronary artery**

Complete occlusion of coronary artery

Total occlusion of coronary artery

> **Code first** coronary atherosclerosis (I25.1-, I25.7-, I25.81-)
>
> **Excludes1:** acute coronary occlusion with myocardial infarction (I21.0-I21.9, I22.-) acute coronary occlusion without myocardial infarction (I24.0)

I25.83 **Coronary atherosclerosis due to lipid rich plaque**

> **Code first** coronary atherosclerosis (I25.1-, I25.7-, I25.81-)

I25.84 **Coronary atherosclerosis due to calcified coronary lesion**

Coronary atherosclerosis due to severely calcified coronary lesion

> **Code first** coronary atherosclerosis (I25.1-, I25.7-, I25.81-)

I25.89 **Other forms of chronic ischemic heart disease**

I25.9 **Chronic ischemic heart disease, unspecified**

Ischemic heart disease (chronic) NOS

PULMONARY HEART DISEASE AND DISEASES OF PULMONARY CIRCULATION (I26-I28)

Definition: Pulmonary heart disease is the enlargement and eventual failure of the right ventricle of the heart due to disorders of the lungs or their blood vessels or chest wall abnormalities.

Definition: Pulmonary circulation is the circulation of blood through the lungs for the purpose of oxygenation and the release of carbon dioxide. Also known as lesser circulation.

I26 **Pulmonary embolism**

> **Includes:** pulmonary (acute) (artery)(vein) infarction
>
> pulmonary (acute) (artery)(vein) thromboembolism pulmonary (acute) (artery)(vein) thrombosis
>
> **Excludes2:** chronic pulmonary embolism (I27.82)
>
> personal history of pulmonary embolism (Z86.711)
>
> pulmonary embolism complicating abortion, ectopic or molar pregnancy (O00-O07, O08.2)
>
> pulmonary embolism complicating pregnancy, childbirth and the puerperium (O88.-)
>
> pulmonary embolism due to trauma (T79.0, T79.1)
>
> pulmonary embolism due to complications of surgical and medical care (T80.0, T81.7-, T82.8-)
>
> septic (non-pulmonary) arterial embolism (I76)

I26.0 **Pulmonary embolism with acute cor pulmonale**

> **I26.01** **Septic pulmonary embolism with acute cor pulmonale** [HCC]
>
> > **Code first** underlying infection
>
> **I26.02** **Saddle embolus of pulmonary artery with acute cor pulmonale** [HCC]
>
> **I26.09** **Other pulmonary embolism with acute cor pulmonale** [HCC]
>
> > Acute cor pulmonale NOS

I26.9 **Pulmonary embolism without acute cor pulmonale**

> **I26.90** **Septic pulmonary embolism without acute cor pulmonale** [HCC]

● New code ▲ Revised code **Excludes1:** Not coded here **Excludes2:** Not included here ⊗ Placeholder required ⑦7th digit required

Code first underlying infection

I26.92   **Saddle embolus of pulmonary artery without acute cor pulmonale** [HCC]

I26.93   **Single subsegmental pulmonary embolism without acute cor pulmonale**

Subsegmental pulmonary embolism NOS

I26.94   **Multiple subsegmental pulmonary emboli without acute cor pulmonale**

I26.99   **Other pulmonary embolism without acute cor pulmonale** [HCC]

Acute pulmonary embolism NOS

Pulmonary embolism NOS

I27   **Other pulmonary heart diseases**

I27.0   **Primary pulmonary hypertension** [HCC]

Heritable pulmonary arterial hypertension

Idiopathic pulmonary arterial hypertension

Primary group 1 pulmonary hypertension

Primary pulmonary arterial hypertension

Excludes1: persistent pulmonary hypertension of newborn (P29.30)

pulmonary hypertension NOS (I27.20)

secondary pulmonary arterial hypertension (I27.21)

secondary pulmonary hypertension (I27.29)

I27.1   **Kyphoscoliotic heart disease** [HCC]

I27.2   **Other secondary pulmonary hypertension**

Code also associated underlying condition

Excludes1: Eisenmenger's syndrome (I27.83)

I27.20   **Pulmonary hypertension, unspecified** [HCC]

Pulmonary hypertension NOS

I27.21   **Secondary pulmonary arterial hypertension** [HCC]

(Associated) (drug-induced) (toxin-induced) pulmonary arterial hypertension NOS

(Associated) (drug-induced) (toxin-induced) (secondary) group 1 pulmonary hypertension

Code also associated conditions if applicable, or adverse effects of drugs or toxins, such as:

adverse effect of appetite depressants (T50.5X5)

congenital heart disease (Q20-Q28)

human immunodeficiency virus [HIV] disease (B20)

polymyositis (M33.2-)

portal hypertension (K76.6)

rheumatoid arthritis (M05.-)

schistosomiasis (B65.-)

Sjögren syndrome (M35.0-)

systemic sclerosis (M34.-)

I27.22   **Pulmonary hypertension due to left heart disease** [HCC]

Group 2 pulmonary hypertension

Code also associated left heart disease, if known, such as:

multiple valve disease (I08.-)

rheumatic mitral valve diseases (I05.-)

rheumatic aortic valve diseases (I06.-)

I27.23   **Pulmonary hypertension due to lung diseases and hypoxia** [HCC]

Group 3 pulmonary hypertension

Code also associated lung disease, if known, such as:

bronchiectasis (J47.-)

cystic fibrosis with pulmonary manifestations (E84.0)

interstitial lung disease (J84.-)

pleural effusion (J90)

sleep apnea (G47.3-)

I27.24   **Chronic thromboembolic pulmonary hypertension** [HCC]

Group 4 pulmonary hypertension

Code also associated pulmonary embolism, if applicable (I26.-, I27.82)

I27.29   **Other secondary pulmonary hypertension** [HCC]

Group 5 pulmonary hypertension

Pulmonary hypertension with unclear multifactorial mechanisms

Pulmonary hypertension due to hematologic disorders

Pulmonary hypertension due to metabolic disorders

Pulmonary hypertension due to other systemic disorders

Code also other associated disorders, if known, such as:

chronic myeloid leukemia (C92.10-C92.22)

essential thrombocythemia (D47.3)

Gaucher disease (E75.22)

hypertensive chronic kidney disease with end stage renal disease (I12.0, I13.11, I13.2)

hyperthyroidism (E05.-)

hypothyroidism (E00-E03)

polycythemia vera (D45)

sarcoidosis (D86.-)

I27.8   **Other specified pulmonary heart diseases**

I27.81   **Cor pulmonale (chronic)** [HCC]

Cor pulmonale NOS

Excludes1: acute cor pulmonale (I26.0-)

I27.82   **Chronic pulmonary embolism** [HCC]

Use Additional Code, if applicable, for associated long-term (current) use of anticoagulants (Z79.01)

Excludes1: personal history of pulmonary embolism (Z86.711)

I27.83   **Eisenmenger's syndrome** [HCC]

Eisenmenger's complex

(Irreversible) Eisenmenger's disease

Pulmonary hypertension with right to left shunt related to congenital heart disease

Code also underlying heart defect, if known, such as:

atrial septal defect (Q21.1)

Eisenmenger's defect (Q21.8)

patent ductus arteriosus (Q25.0)

ventricular septal defect (Q21.0)

I27.89   **Other specified pulmonary heart diseases** [HCC]

I27.9   **Pulmonary heart disease, unspecified** [HCC]

Chronic cardiopulmonary disease

I28   **Other diseases of pulmonary vessels**

I28.0   **Arteriovenous fistula of pulmonary vessels** [HCC]

Excludes1: congenital arteriovenous fistula (Q25.72)

I28.1   **Aneurysm of pulmonary artery** [HCC]

Excludes1: congenital aneurysm (Q25.79)

     congenital arteriovenous aneurysm (Q25.72)

I28.8   **Other diseases of pulmonary vessels** [HCC]

Pulmonary arteritis

Pulmonary endarteritis

Rupture of pulmonary vessels

Stenosis of pulmonary vessels

Stricture of pulmonary vessels

I28.9   **Disease of pulmonary vessels, unspecified** [HCC]

OTHER FORMS OF HEART DISEASE (I30-I52)

I30   **Acute pericarditis**

Definition: Pericarditis is an inflammation of the two layers of the thin, sac-like membrane that surrounds the heart.

Includes: acute mediastinopericarditis

acute myopericarditis

acute pericardial effusion

acute pleuropericarditis

acute pneumopericarditis

Excludes1: Dressler's syndrome (I24.1)

    rheumatic pericarditis (acute) (I01.0)

    viral pericarditis due to Coxsackie virus (B33.23)

I30.0   **Acute nonspecific idiopathic pericarditis**

I30.1   **Infective pericarditis**

Pneumococcal pericarditis

Pneumopyopericardium

Purulent pericarditis

Pyopericarditis

Pyopericardium

Pyopneumopericardium

Staphylococcal pericarditis

Streptococcal pericarditis

Suppurative pericarditis

Viral pericarditis

Use Additional Code (B95-B97) to identify infectious agent

I30.8   **Other forms of acute pericarditis**

I30.9   **Acute pericarditis, unspecified**

I31   **Other diseases of pericardium**

Excludes1: diseases of pericardium specified as rheumatic (I09.2)

    postcardiotomy syndrome (I97.0)

    traumatic injury to pericardium (S26.-)

I31.0   **Chronic adhesive pericarditis**

Accretio cordis

Adherent pericardium

Adhesive mediastinopericarditis

I31.1   **Chronic constrictive pericarditis**

Concretio cordis

Pericardial calcification

I31.2   **Hemopericardium, not elsewhere classified**

Excludes1: hemopericardium as current complication following acute myocardial infarction (I23.0)

I31.3   **Pericardial effusion (noninflammatory)**

Chylopericardium

Excludes1: acute pericardial effusion (I30.9)

I31.4   **Cardiac tamponade**

Code first underlying cause

I31.8   **Other specified diseases of pericardium**

Epicardial plaques

Focal pericardial adhesions

I31.9   **Disease of pericardium, unspecified**

Pericarditis (chronic) NOS

I32   **Pericarditis in diseases classified elsewhere**

Code first underlying disease

Excludes1: pericarditis (in):

    coxsackie (virus) (B33.23)

    gonococcal (A54.83)

    meningococcal (A39.53)

    rheumatoid (arthritis) (M05.31)

    syphilitic (A52.06)

    systemic lupus erythematosus (M32.12)

    tuberculosis (A18.84)

I33   **Acute and subacute endocarditis**

Definition: Endocarditis is an infection of the lining of the heart chambers and heart valves that is caused by bacteria, fungi, or other infectious substances.

Excludes1: acute rheumatic endocarditis (I01.1)

    endocarditis NOS (I38)

I33.0   **Acute and subacute infective endocarditis**

Bacterial endocarditis (acute) (subacute)

Infective endocarditis (acute) (subacute) NOS

Endocarditis lenta (acute) (subacute)

Malignant endocarditis (acute) (subacute)

Purulent endocarditis (acute) (subacute)

Septic endocarditis (acute) (subacute)

Ulcerative endocarditis (acute) (subacute)

Vegetative endocarditis (acute) (subacute)

Use Additional Code (B95-B97) to identify infectious agent

I33.9   **Acute and subacute endocarditis, unspecified**

Acute endocarditis NOS

Acute myoendocarditis NOS

Acute Periendocarditis NOS

Subacute endocarditis NOS

Subacute myoendocarditis NOS

Subacute Periendocarditis NOS

I34   **Nonrheumatic mitral valve disorders**

Excludes1: mitral valve disease (I05.9)

    mitral valve failure (I05.8)

    mitral valve stenosis (I05.0)

    mitral valve disorder of unspecified cause with diseases of aortic and/or tricuspid valve(s) (I08.-)

    mitral valve disorder of unspecified cause with mitral stenosis or obstruction (I05.0)

    mitral valve disorder specified as congenital (Q23.2, Q23.9)

    mitral valve disorder specified as rheumatic (I05.-)

I34.0   **Nonrheumatic mitral (valve) insufficiency**

Nonrheumatic mitral (valve) incompetence NOS

Nonrheumatic mitral (valve) regurgitation NOS

I34.1   **Nonrheumatic mitral (valve) prolapse**

Floppy nonrheumatic mitral valve syndrome

Excludes1: Marfan's syndrome (Q87.4-)

I34.2   **Nonrheumatic mitral (valve) stenosis**

● New code   ▲ Revised code   **Excludes1:** Not coded here   **Excludes2:** Not included here   ⊗ Placeholder required   ⑦7th digit required

I34.8   **Other nonrheumatic mitral valve disorders**

I34.9   **Nonrheumatic mitral valve disorder, unspecified**

I35   **Nonrheumatic aortic valve disorders**

Excludes1: aortic valve disorder of unspecified cause but with diseases of mitral and/or tricuspid valve(s) (I08.-)

aortic valve disorder specified as congenital (Q23.0, Q23.1)

aortic valve disorder specified as rheumatic (I06.-)

hypertrophic subaortic stenosis (I42.1)

I35.0   **Nonrheumatic aortic (valve) stenosis**

I35.1   **Nonrheumatic aortic (valve) insufficiency**

Nonrheumatic aortic (valve) incompetence NOS

Nonrheumatic aortic (valve) regurgitation NOS

I35.2   **Nonrheumatic aortic (valve) stenosis with insufficiency**

I35.8   **Other nonrheumatic aortic valve disorders**

I35.9   **Nonrheumatic aortic valve disorder, unspecified**

I36   **Nonrheumatic tricuspid valve disorders**

Excludes1: tricuspid valve disorders of unspecified cause (I07.-)

tricuspid valve disorders specified as congenital (Q22.4, Q22.8, Q22.9)

tricuspid valve disorders specified as rheumatic (I07.-)

tricuspid valve disorders with aortic and/or mitral valve involvement (I08.-)

I36.0   **Nonrheumatic tricuspid (valve) stenosis**

I36.1   **Nonrheumatic tricuspid (valve) insufficiency**

Nonrheumatic tricuspid (valve) incompetence

Nonrheumatic tricuspid (valve) regurgitation

I36.2   **Nonrheumatic tricuspid (valve) stenosis with insufficiency**

I36.8   **Other nonrheumatic tricuspid valve disorders**

I36.9   **Nonrheumatic tricuspid valve disorder, unspecified**

I37   **Nonrheumatic pulmonary valve disorders**

Excludes1: pulmonary valve disorder specified as congenital (Q22.1, Q22.2, Q22.3)

pulmonary valve disorder specified as rheumatic (I09.89)

I37.0   **Nonrheumatic pulmonary valve stenosis**

I37.1   **Nonrheumatic pulmonary valve insufficiency**

Nonrheumatic pulmonary valve incompetence

Nonrheumatic pulmonary valve regurgitation

I37.2   **Nonrheumatic pulmonary valve stenosis with insufficiency**

I37.8   **Other nonrheumatic pulmonary valve disorders**

I37.9   **Nonrheumatic pulmonary valve disorder, unspecified**

I38   **Endocarditis, valve unspecified**

Includes: endocarditis (chronic) NOS

valvular incompetence NOS

valvular insufficiency NOS

valvular regurgitation NOS

valvular stenosis NOS

valvulitis (chronic) NOS

Excludes1: congenital insufficiency of cardiac valve NOS (Q24.8)

congenital stenosis of cardiac valve NOS (Q24.8)

endocardial fibroelastosis (I42.4)

endocarditis specified as rheumatic (I09.1)

I39   **Endocarditis and heart valve disorders in diseases classified elsewhere**

Code first underlying disease, such as:

Q fever (A78)

Excludes1: endocardial involvement in:

candidiasis (B37.6) gonococcal infection (A54.83)

Libman-Sacks disease (M32.11)

listerosis (A32.82)

meningococcal infection (A39.51)

rheumatoid arthritis (M05.31)

syphilis (A52.03)

tuberculosis (A18.84)

typhoid fever (A01.02)

I40   **Acute myocarditis**

Includes: subacute myocarditis

Excludes1: acute rheumatic myocarditis (I01.2)

I40.0   **Infective myocarditis**

Septic myocarditis

Use Additional Code (B95-B97) to identify infectious agent

I40.1   **Isolated myocarditis**

Fiedler's myocarditis

Giant cell myocarditis

Idiopathic myocarditis

I40.8   **Other acute myocarditis**

I40.9   **Acute myocarditis, unspecified**

I41   **Myocarditis in diseases classified elsewhere**

Code first underlying disease, such as:

typhus (A75.0-A75.9)

Excludes1: myocarditis (in):

Chagas' disease (chronic) (B57.2)

acute (B57.0)

coxsackie (virus) infection (B33.22)

diphtheritic (A36.81)

gonococcal (A54.83)

influenzal (J09.X9, J10.82, J11.82)

meningococcal (A39.52)

mumps (B26.82)

rheumatoid arthritis (M05.31)

sarcoid (D86.85)

syphilis (A52.06)

toxoplasmosis (B58.81)

tuberculous (A18.84)

I42   **Cardiomyopathy**

Definition: Cardiomyopathy is a weakening of the heart muscle or a change in heart muscle structure. It is often associated with inadequate heart pumping or other heart function problems.

Includes: myocardiopathy

Code first pre-existing cardiomyopathy complicating pregnancy and puerperium (O99.4)

Excludes2: ischemic cardiomyopathy (I25.5)

peripartum cardiomyopathy (O90.3)

ventricular hypertrophy (I51.7)

I42.0   **Dilated cardiomyopathy** [HCC]

Congestive cardiomyopathy

I42.1   **Obstructive hypertrophic cardiomyopathy** [HCC]

Hypertrophic subaortic stenosis (idiopathic)

I42.2   **Other hypertrophic cardiomyopathy** [HCC]

Nonobstructive hypertrophic cardiomyopathy

I42.3   **Endomyocardial (eosinophilic) disease** [HCC]

Endomyocardial (tropical) fibrosis

Löffler's endocarditis

I42.4 **Endocardial fibroelastosis** [HCC]

Congenital cardiomyopathy

Elastomyofibrosis

I42.5 **Other restrictive cardiomyopathy** [HCC]

Constrictive cardiomyopathy NOS

I42.6 **Alcoholic cardiomyopathy** [HCC]

Code also presence of alcoholism (F10.-)

I42.7 **Cardiomyopathy due to drug and external agent** [HCC]

Code first poisoning due to drug or toxin, if applicable (T36-T65 with fifth or sixth character 1-4 or 6)

Use Additional Code for adverse effect, if applicable, to identify drug (T36-T50 with fifth or sixth character 5)

I42.8 **Other cardiomyopathies** [HCC]

I42.9 **Cardiomyopathy, unspecified** [HCC]

Cardiomyopathy (primary) (secondary) NOS

I43 **Cardiomyopathy in diseases classified elsewhere** [HCC]

Code first underlying disease, such as:

amyloidosis (E85.-)

glycogen storage disease (E74.0) gout (M10.0-)

thyrotoxicosis (E05.0-E05.9-)

Excludes1: cardiomyopathy (in):

coxsackie (virus) (B33.24)

diphtheria (A36.81)

sarcoidosis (D86.85)

tuberculosis (A18.84)

I44 **Atrioventricular and left bundle-branch block**

I44.0 **Atrioventricular block, first degree**

I44.1 **Atrioventricular block, second degree**

Atrioventricular block, type I and II

Mobitz block, type I and II

Second degree block, type I and II

Wenckebach's block

I44.2 **Atrioventricular block, complete** [HCC]

Complete heart block NOS

Third degree block

I44.3 **Other and unspecified atrioventricular block**

Atrioventricular block NOS

I44.30 **Unspecified atrioventricular block**

I44.39 **Other atrioventricular block**

I44.4 **Left anterior fascicular block**

I44.5 **Left posterior fascicular block**

I44.6 **Other and unspecified fascicular block**

I44.60 **Unspecified fascicular block**

Left bundle-branch hemiblock NOS

I44.69 **Other fascicular block**

I44.7 **Left bundle-branch block, unspecified**

I45 **Other conduction disorders**

I45.0 **Right fascicular block**

I45.1 **Other and unspecified right bundle-branch block**

I45.10 **Unspecified right bundle-branch block**

Right bundle-branch block NOS

I45.19 **Other right bundle-branch block**

I45.2 **Bifascicular block**

I45.3 **Trifascicular block**

I45.4 **Nonspecific intraventricular block**

Bundle-branch block NOS

I45.5 **Other specified heart block**

Sinoatrial block

Sinoauricular block

Excludes1: heart block NOS (I45.9)

I45.6 **Pre-excitation syndrome**

Accelerated atrioventricular conduction

Accessory atrioventricular conduction

Anomalous atrioventricular excitation

Lown-Ganong-Levine syndrome

Pre-excitation atrioventricular conduction

Wolff-Parkinson-White syndrome

I45.8 **Other specified conduction disorders**

I45.81 **Long QT syndrome**

I45.89 **Other specified conduction disorders**

Atrioventricular [AV] dissociation

Interference dissociation

Isorhythmic dissociation

Nonparoxysmal AV nodal tachycardia

I45.9 **Conduction disorder, unspecified**

Heart block NOS

Stokes-Adams syndrome

I46 **Cardiac arrest**

Excludes2: cardiogenic shock (R57.0)

I46.2 **Cardiac arrest due to underlying cardiac condition** [HCC]

Code first underlying cardiac condition

I46.8 **Cardiac arrest due to other underlying condition** [HCC]

Code first underlying condition

I46.9 **Cardiac arrest, cause unspecified** [HCC]

I47 **Paroxysmal tachycardia**

Code first tachycardia complicating:

abortion or ectopic or molar pregnancy (O00-O07, O08.8)

obstetric surgery and procedures (O75.4)

Excludes1: tachycardia NOS (R00.0)

sinoauricular tachycardia NOS (R00.0)

sinus [sinusal] tachycardia NOS (R00.0)

I47.0 **Re-entry ventricular arrhythmia** [HCC]

I47.1 **Supraventricular tachycardia** [HCC]

Atrial (paroxysmal) tachycardia

Atrioventricular [AV] (paroxysmal) tachycardia

Atrioventricular re-entrant (nodal) tachycardia [AVNRT] [AVRT]

Junctional (paroxysmal) tachycardia

Nodal (paroxysmal) tachycardia

I47.2 **Ventricular tachycardia** [HCC]

I47.9 **Paroxysmal tachycardia, unspecified** [HCC]

Bouveret (-Hoffman) syndrome

I48 **Atrial fibrillation and flutter**

I48.0 **Paroxysmal atrial fibrillation**

I48.1 **Persistent atrial fibrillation**

Excludes1: Permanent atrial fibrillation (I48.21)

I48.11 **Longstanding persistent atrial fibrillation** [HCC]

I48.19 **Other persistent atrial fibrillation** [HCC]

Chronic persistent atrial fibrillation

Persistent atrial fibrillation, NOS

I48.2 **Chronic atrial fibrillation**

I48.20 **Chronic atrial fibrillation, unspecified** [HCC]

Excludes1: Chronic persistent atrial fibrillation (I48.19)

 I48.21 **Permanent atrial fibrillation** [HCC]

I48.3 **Typical atrial flutter** [HCC]

 Type I atrial flutter

I48.4 **Atypical atrial flutter** [HCC]

 Type II atrial flutter

I48.9 **Unspecified atrial fibrillation and atrial flutter**

 I48.91 **Unspecified atrial fibrillation** [HCC]

 I48.92 **Unspecified atrial flutter** [HCC]

I49 **Other cardiac arrhythmias**

Code first cardiac arrhythmia complicating:

abortion or ectopic or molar pregnancy (O00-O07, O08.8)

obstetric surgery and procedures (O75.4)

Excludes1: neonatal dysrhythmia (P29.1-)

 sinoatrial bradycardia (R00.1)

 sinus bradycardia (R00.1)

 vagal bradycardia (R00.1)

Excludes2: bradycardia NOS (R00.1)

I49.0 **Ventricular fibrillation and flutter**

 I49.01 **Ventricular fibrillation** [HCC]

 I49.02 **Ventricular flutter** [HCC]

I49.1 **Atrial premature depolarization**

 Atrial premature beats

I49.2 **Junctional premature depolarization** [HCC]

I49.3 **Ventricular premature depolarization**

I49.4 **Other and unspecified premature depolarization**

 I49.40 **Unspecified premature depolarization**

  Premature beats NOS

 I49.49 **Other premature depolarization**

  Ectopic beats

  Extrasystoles

  Extrasystolic arrhythmias

  Premature contractions

I49.5 **Sick sinus syndrome** [HCC]

 Tachycardia-bradycardia syndrome

I49.8 **Other specified cardiac arrhythmias**

 Brugada syndrome

 Coronary sinus rhythm disorder

 Ectopic rhythm disorder

 Nodal rhythm disorder

I49.9 **Cardiac arrhythmia, unspecified**

 Arrhythmia (cardiac) NOS

I50 **Heart failure**

Definition: Heart failure is a condition where there is ineffective pumping of the heart leading to an accumulation of fluid in the lungs. Typical symptoms include shortness of breath with exertion, difficulty breathing when lying flat and leg or ankle swelling.

Code first heart failure complicating abortion or ectopic or molar pregnancy (O00-O07, O08.8)

heart failure due to hypertension (I11.0)

heart failure due to hypertension with chronic kidney disease (I13.-)

heart failure following surgery (I97.13-)

obstetric surgery and procedures (O75.4)

rheumatic heart failure (I09.81)

Excludes1: neonatal cardiac failure (P29.0)

Excludes2: cardiac arrest (I46.-)

I50.1 **Left ventricular failure, unspecified** [HCC]

Cardiac asthma

Edema of lung with heart disease NOS

Edema of lung with heart failure

Left heart failure

Pulmonary edema with heart disease NOS

Pulmonary edema with heart failure

Excludes1: edema of lung without heart disease or heart failure (J81.-)

 pulmonary edema without heart disease or failure (J81.-)

I50.2 **Systolic (congestive) heart failure**

Heart failure with reduced ejection fraction [HFrEF]

Systolic left ventricular heart failure

Code also end stage heart failure, if applicable (I50.84)

Excludes1: combined systolic (congestive) and diastolic (congestive) heart failure (I50.4-)

 I50.20 **Unspecified systolic (congestive) heart failure** [HCC]

 I50.21 **Acute systolic (congestive) heart failure** [HCC]

 I50.22 **Chronic systolic (congestive) heart failure** [HCC]

 I50.23 **Acute on chronic systolic (congestive) heart failure** [HCC]

I50.3 **Diastolic (congestive) heart failure**

Diastolic left ventricular heart failure

Heart failure with normal ejection fraction

Heart failure with preserved ejection fraction [HFpEF]

Code also end stage heart failure, if applicable (I50.84)

Excludes1: combined systolic (congestive) and diastolic (congestive) heart failure (I50.4-)

 I50.30 **Unspecified diastolic (congestive) heart failure** [HCC]

 I50.31 **Acute diastolic (congestive) heart failure** [HCC]

 I50.32 **Chronic diastolic (congestive) heart failure** [HCC]

 I50.33 **Acute on chronic diastolic (congestive) heart failure** [HCC]

I50.4 **Combined systolic (congestive) and diastolic (congestive) heart failure**

Combined systolic and diastolic left ventricular heart failure

Heart failure with reduced ejection fraction and diastolic dysfunction

Code also end stage heart failure, if applicable (I50.84)

 I50.40 **Unspecified combined systolic (congestive) and diastolic (congestive) heart failure** [HCC]

 I50.41 **Acute combined systolic (congestive) and diastolic (congestive) heart failure** [HCC]

 I50.42 **Chronic combined systolic (congestive) and diastolic (congestive) heart failure** [HCC]

 I50.43 **Acute on chronic combined systolic (congestive) and diastolic (congestive) heart failure** [HCC]

I50.8 **Other heart failure**

 I50.81 **Right heart failure**

 Right ventricular failure

  I50.810 **Right heart failure, unspecified** [HCC]

  Right heart failure without mention of left heart failure

  Right ventricular failure NOS

  I50.811 **Acute right heart failure** [HCC]

  Acute isolated right heart failure

Acute (isolated) right ventricular failure

I50.812 Chronic right heart failure [HCC]

Chronic isolated right heart failure

Chronic (isolated) right ventricular failure

I50.813 Acute on chronic right heart failure [HCC]

Acute on chronic isolated right heart failure

Acute on chronic (isolated) right ventricular failure

Acute decompensation of chronic (isolated) right ventricular failure

Acute exacerbation of chronic (isolated) right ventricular failure

I50.814 Right heart failure due to left heart failure [HCC]

Right ventricular failure secondary to left ventricular failure

Code also the type of left ventricular failure, if known (I50.2-I50.43)

Excludes1: Right heart failure with but not due to left heart failure (I50.82)

I50.82 Biventricular heart failure [HCC]

Code also the type of left ventricular failure as systolic, diastolic, or combined, if known (I50.2-I50.43)

I50.83 High output heart failure [HCC]

I50.84 End stage heart failure [HCC]

Stage D heart failure

Code also the type of heart failure as systolic, diastolic, or combined, if known (I50.2-I50.43)

I50.89 Other heart failure [HCC]

I50.9 Heart failure, unspecified [HCC]

Cardiac, heart or myocardial failure NOS

Congestive heart disease

Congestive heart failure NOS

Excludes2: fluid overload unrelated to congestive heart failure (E87.70)

I51 Complications and ill-defined descriptions of heart disease

Excludes1: any condition in I51.4-I51.9 due to hypertension (I11.-)

any condition in I51.4-I51.9 due to hypertension and chronic kidney disease (I13.-)

heart disease specified as rheumatic (I00-I09)

I51.0 Cardiac septal defect, acquired

Acquired septal atrial defect (old)

Acquired septal auricular defect (old)

Acquired septal ventricular defect (old)

Excludes1: cardiac septal defect as current complication following acute myocardial infarction (I23.1, I23.2)

I51.1 Rupture of chordae tendineae, not elsewhere classified [HCC]

Excludes1: rupture of chordae tendineae as current complication following acute myocardial infarction (I23.4)

I51.2 Rupture of papillary muscle, not elsewhere classified [HCC]

Excludes1: rupture of papillary muscle as current complication following acute myocardial infarction (I23.5)

I51.3 Intracardiac thrombosis, not elsewhere classified

Apical thrombosis (old)

Atrial thrombosis (old)

Auricular thrombosis (old)

Mural thrombosis (old)

Ventricular thrombosis (old)

Excludes1: intracardiac thrombosis as current complication following acute myocardial infarction (I23.6)

I51.4 Myocarditis, unspecified [HCC]

Chronic (interstitial) myocarditis

Myocardial fibrosis

Myocarditis NOS

Excludes1: acute or subacute myocarditis (I40.-)

I51.5 Myocardial degeneration [HCC]

Fatty degeneration of heart or myocardium

Myocardial disease

Senile degeneration of heart or myocardium

I51.7 Cardiomegaly

Cardiac dilatation

Cardiac hypertrophy

Ventricular dilatation

I51.8 Other ill-defined heart diseases

I51.81 Takotsubo syndrome

Reversible left ventricular dysfunction following sudden emotional stress

Stress induced cardiomyopathy

Takotsubo cardiomyopathy

Transient left ventricular apical ballooning syndrome

I51.89 Other ill-defined heart diseases

Carditis (acute)(chronic)

Pancarditis (acute)(chronic)

I51.9 Heart disease, unspecified

I52 Other heart disorders in diseases classified elsewhere

Code first underlying disease, such as:

congenital syphilis (A50.5)

mucopolysaccharidosis (E76.3)

schistosomiasis (B65.0-B65.9)

Excludes1: heart disease (in):

gonococcal infection (A54.83)

meningococcal infection (A39.50)

rheumatoid arthritis (M05.31)

syphilis (A52.06)

CEREBROVASCULAR DISEASES (I60-I69)

Use Additional Code to identify presence of:

alcohol abuse and dependence (F10.-)

exposure to environmental tobacco smoke (Z77.22)

history of tobacco dependence (Z87.891)

hypertension (I10-I16)

occupational exposure to environmental tobacco smoke (Z57.31)

tobacco dependence (F17.-)

tobacco use (Z72.0)

Excludes1: traumatic intracranial hemorrhage (S06.-)

I60 Nontraumatic subarachnoid hemorrhage

Definition: Subarachnoid hemorrhage refers to bleeding within the head into the space between two membranes that surround the brain.

Excludes1: syphilitic ruptured cerebral aneurysm (A52.05)

Excludes2: sequelae of subarachnoid hemorrhage (I69.0-)

I60.0 **Nontraumatic subarachnoid hemorrhage from carotid siphon and bifurcation**

I60.00 **Nontraumatic subarachnoid hemorrhage from unspecified carotid siphon and bifurcation** [HCC]

I60.01 **Nontraumatic subarachnoid hemorrhage from right carotid siphon and bifurcation** [HCC]

I60.02 **Nontraumatic subarachnoid hemorrhage from left carotid siphon and bifurcation** [HCC]

I60.1 **Nontraumatic subarachnoid hemorrhage from middle cerebral artery**

I60.10 **Nontraumatic subarachnoid hemorrhage from unspecified middle cerebral artery** [HCC]

I60.11 **Nontraumatic subarachnoid hemorrhage from right middle cerebral artery** [HCC]

I60.12 **Nontraumatic subarachnoid hemorrhage from left middle cerebral artery** [HCC]

I60.2 **Nontraumatic subarachnoid hemorrhage from anterior communicating artery** [HCC]

I60.3 **Nontraumatic subarachnoid hemorrhage from posterior communicating artery**

I60.30 **Nontraumatic subarachnoid hemorrhage from unspecified posterior communicating artery** [HCC]

I60.31 **Nontraumatic subarachnoid hemorrhage from right posterior communicating artery** [HCC]

I60.32 **Nontraumatic subarachnoid hemorrhage from left posterior communicating artery** [HCC]

I60.4 **Nontraumatic subarachnoid hemorrhage from basilar artery** [HCC]

I60.5 **Nontraumatic subarachnoid hemorrhage from vertebral artery**

I60.50 **Nontraumatic subarachnoid hemorrhage from unspecified vertebral artery** [HCC]

I60.51 **Nontraumatic subarachnoid hemorrhage from right vertebral artery** [HCC]

I60.52 **Nontraumatic subarachnoid hemorrhage from left vertebral artery** [HCC]

I60.6 **Nontraumatic subarachnoid hemorrhage from other intracranial arteries** [HCC]

I60.7 **Nontraumatic subarachnoid hemorrhage from unspecified intracranial artery** [HCC]

Ruptured (congenital) berry aneurysm

Ruptured (congenital) cerebral aneurysm

Subarachnoid hemorrhage (nontraumatic) from cerebral artery NOS

Subarachnoid hemorrhage (nontraumatic) from communicating artery NOS

Excludes1: berry aneurysm, nonruptured (I67.1)

I60.8 **Other nontraumatic subarachnoid hemorrhage** [HCC]

Meningeal hemorrhage

Rupture of cerebral arteriovenous malformation

I60.9 **Nontraumatic subarachnoid hemorrhage, unspecified** [HCC]

I61 **Nontraumatic intracerebral hemorrhage**

Definition: Intracerebral hemorrhage is a medical condition indicated by the rupturing of a blood vessel in the brain and the subsequent bleeding into the tissues of the brain.

Excludes2: sequelae of intracerebral hemorrhage (I69.1-)

I61.0 **Nontraumatic intracerebral hemorrhage in hemisphere, subcortical** [HCC]

Deep intracerebral hemorrhage (nontraumatic)

I61.1 **Nontraumatic intracerebral hemorrhage in hemisphere, cortical** [HCC]

Cerebral lobe hemorrhage (nontraumatic)

Superficial intracerebral hemorrhage (nontraumatic)

I61.2 **Nontraumatic intracerebral hemorrhage in hemisphere, unspecified** [HCC]

I61.3 **Nontraumatic intracerebral hemorrhage in brain stem** [HCC]

I61.4 **Nontraumatic intracerebral hemorrhage in cerebellum** [HCC]

I61.5 **Nontraumatic intracerebral hemorrhage, intraventricular** [HCC]

I61.6 **Nontraumatic intracerebral hemorrhage, multiple localized** [HCC]

I61.8 **Other nontraumatic intracerebral hemorrhage** [HCC]

I61.9 **Nontraumatic intracerebral hemorrhage, unspecified** [HCC]

I62 **Other and unspecified nontraumatic intracranial hemorrhage**

Definition: Intracranial hemorrhage is bleeding in the brain caused by the breaking (rupture) of a blood vessel in the head.

Excludes2: sequelae of intracranial hemorrhage (I69.2)

I62.0 **Nontraumatic subdural hemorrhage**

I62.00 **Nontraumatic subdural hemorrhage, unspecified** [HCC]

I62.01 **Nontraumatic acute subdural hemorrhage** [HCC]

I62.02 **Nontraumatic subacute subdural hemorrhage** [HCC]

I62.03 **Nontraumatic chronic subdural hemorrhage**

I62.1 **Nontraumatic extradural hemorrhage** [HCC]

Nontraumatic epidural hemorrhage

I62.9 **Nontraumatic intracranial hemorrhage, unspecified** [HCC]

I63 **Cerebral infarction**

Includes: occlusion and stenosis of cerebral and precerebral arteries, resulting in cerebral infarction

Use Additional Code, if applicable, to identify status post administration of tPA (rtPA) in a different facility within the last 24 hours prior to admission to current facility (Z92.82)

Use Additional Code, if known, to indicate National Institutes of Health Stroke Scale (NIHSS) score (R29.7-)

Excludes1: neonatal cerebral infarction (P91.82-)

Excludes2: sequelae of cerebral infarction (I69.3-)

I63.0 **Cerebral infarction due to thrombosis of precerebral arteries**

I63.00 **Cerebral infarction due to thrombosis of unspecified precerebral artery** [HCC]

I63.01 **Cerebral infarction due to thrombosis of vertebral artery**

I63.011 **Cerebral infarction due to thrombosis of right vertebral artery** [HCC]

I63.012 **Cerebral infarction due to thrombosis of left vertebral artery** [HCC]

I63.013 **Cerebral infarction due to thrombosis of bilateral vertebral arteries** [HCC]

I63.019 **Cerebral infarction due to thrombosis of unspecified vertebral artery** [HCC]

I63.02 **Cerebral infarction due to thrombosis of basilar artery** [HCC]

I63.03 Cerebral infarction due to thrombosis of carotid artery

I63.031 Cerebral infarction due to thrombosis of right carotid artery [HCC]

I63.032 Cerebral infarction due to thrombosis of left carotid artery [HCC]

I63.033 Cerebral infarction due to thrombosis of bilateral carotid arteries [HCC]

I63.039 Cerebral infarction due to thrombosis of unspecified carotid artery [HCC]

I63.09 Cerebral infarction due to thrombosis of other precerebral artery [HCC]

I63.1 Cerebral infarction due to embolism of precerebral arteries

I63.10 Cerebral infarction due to embolism of unspecified precerebral artery

I63.11 Cerebral infarction due to embolism of vertebral artery

I63.111 Cerebral infarction due to embolism of right vertebral artery [HCC]

I63.112 Cerebral infarction due to embolism of left vertebral artery [HCC]

I63.113 Cerebral infarction due to embolism of bilateral vertebral arteries [HCC]

I63.119 Cerebral infarction due to embolism of unspecified vertebral artery [HCC]

I63.12 Cerebral infarction due to embolism of basilar artery [HCC]

I63.13 Cerebral infarction due to embolism of carotid artery

I63.131 Cerebral infarction due to embolism of right carotid artery [HCC]

I63.132 Cerebral infarction due to embolism of left carotid artery

I63.133 Cerebral infarction due to embolism of bilateral carotid arteries [HCC]

I63.139 Cerebral infarction due to embolism of unspecified carotid artery [HCC]

I63.19 Cerebral infarction due to embolism of other precerebral artery [HCC]

I63.2 Cerebral infarction due to unspecified occlusion or stenosis of precerebral arteries

I63.20 Cerebral infarction due to unspecified occlusion or stenosis of unspecified precerebral artery [HCC]

I63.21 Cerebral infarction due to unspecified occlusion or stenosis of vertebral arteries

I63.211 Cerebral infarction due to unspecified occlusion or stenosis of right vertebral artery [HCC]

I63.212 Cerebral infarction due to unspecified occlusion or stenosis of left vertebral arteries [HCC]

I63.213 Cerebral infarction due to unspecified occlusion or stenosis of bilateral vertebral arteries [HCC]

I63.219 Cerebral infarction due to unspecified occlusion or stenosis of unspecified vertebral artery [HCC]

I63.22 Cerebral infarction due to unspecified occlusion or stenosis of basilar artery [HCC]

I63.23 Cerebral infarction due to unspecified occlusion or stenosis of carotid arteries

I63.231 Cerebral infarction due to unspecified occlusion or stenosis of right carotid arteries [HCC]

I63.232 Cerebral infarction due to unspecified occlusion or stenosis of left carotid arteries [HCC]

I63.233 Cerebral infarction due to unspecified occlusion or stenosis of bilateral carotid arteries [HCC]

I63.239 Cerebral infarction due to unspecified occlusion or stenosis of unspecified carotid arteries [HCC]

I63.29 Cerebral infarction due to unspecified occlusion or stenosis of other precerebral arteries [HCC]

I63.3 Cerebral infarction due to thrombosis of cerebral arteries

I63.30 Cerebral infarction due to thrombosis of unspecified cerebral artery [HCC]

I63.31 Cerebral infarction due to thrombosis of middle cerebral artery

I63.311 Cerebral infarction due to thrombosis of right middle cerebral artery [HCC]

I63.312 Cerebral infarction due to thrombosis of left middle cerebral artery [HCC]

I63.313 Cerebral infarction due to thrombosis of bilateral middle cerebral arteries [HCC]

I63.319 Cerebral infarction due to thrombosis of unspecified middle cerebral artery [HCC]

I63.32 Cerebral infarction due to thrombosis of anterior cerebral artery

I63.321 Cerebral infarction due to thrombosis of right anterior cerebral artery [HCC]

I63.322 Cerebral infarction due to thrombosis of left anterior cerebral artery [HCC]

I63.323 Cerebral infarction due to thrombosis of bilateral anterior cerebral arteries [HCC]

I63.329 Cerebral infarction due to thrombosis of unspecified anterior cerebral artery [HCC]

I63.33 Cerebral infarction due to thrombosis of posterior cerebral artery

I63.331 Cerebral infarction due to thrombosis of right posterior cerebral artery [HCC]

I63.332 Cerebral infarction due to thrombosis of left posterior cerebral artery

I63.333 Cerebral infarction due to thrombosis of bilateral posterior cerebral arteries [HCC]

I63.339 Cerebral infarction due to thrombosis of unspecified posterior cerebral artery

I63.34 Cerebral infarction due to thrombosis of cerebellar artery

I63.341 Cerebral infarction due to thrombosis of right cerebellar artery [HCC]

● New code ▲ Revised code **Excludes1:** Not coded here **Excludes2:** Not included here ⊗ Placeholder required ⑦ 7th digit required

I63.342   Cerebral infarction due to thrombosis of left cerebellar artery [HCC]

I63.343   Cerebral infarction due to thrombosis of bilateral cerebellar arteries [HCC]

I63.349   Cerebral infarction due to thrombosis of unspecified cerebellar artery [HCC]

I63.39   Cerebral infarction due to thrombosis of other cerebral artery [HCC]

I63.4   **Cerebral infarction due to embolism of cerebral arteries**

I63.40   Cerebral infarction due to embolism of unspecified cerebral artery [HCC]

I63.41   Cerebral infarction due to embolism of middle cerebral artery

     I63.411   Cerebral infarction due to embolism of right middle cerebral artery [HCC]

     I63.412   Cerebral infarction due to embolism of left middle cerebral artery [HCC]

     I63.413   Cerebral infarction due to embolism of bilateral middle cerebral arteries [HCC]

     I63.419   Cerebral infarction due to embolism of unspecified middle cerebral artery [HCC]

I63.42   Cerebral infarction due to embolism of anterior cerebral artery

     I63.421   Cerebral infarction due to embolism of right anterior cerebral artery [HCC]

     I63.422   Cerebral infarction due to embolism of left anterior cerebral artery [HCC]

     I63.423   Cerebral infarction due to embolism of bilateral anterior cerebral arteries [HCC]

     I63.429   Cerebral infarction due to embolism of unspecified anterior cerebral artery [HCC]

I63.43   Cerebral infarction due to embolism of posterior cerebral artery

     I63.431   Cerebral infarction due to embolism of right posterior cerebral artery [HCC]

     I63.432   Cerebral infarction due to embolism of left posterior cerebral artery [HCC]

     I63.433   Cerebral infarction due to embolism of bilateral posterior cerebral arteries [HCC]

     I63.439   Cerebral infarction due to embolism of unspecified posterior cerebral artery [HCC]

I63.44   Cerebral infarction due to embolism of cerebellar artery

     I63.441   Cerebral infarction due to embolism of right cerebellar artery [HCC]

     I63.442   Cerebral infarction due to embolism of left cerebellar artery [HCC]

     I63.443   Cerebral infarction due to embolism of bilateral cerebellar arteries [HCC]

     I63.449   Cerebral infarction due to embolism of unspecified cerebellar artery [HCC]

I63.49   Cerebral infarction due to embolism of other cerebral artery [HCC]

I63.5   **Cerebral infarction due to unspecified occlusion or stenosis of cerebral arteries** [HCC]

I63.50   Cerebral infarction due to unspecified occlusion or stenosis of unspecified cerebral artery

I63.51   Cerebral infarction due to unspecified occlusion or stenosis of middle cerebral artery

     I63.511   Cerebral infarction due to unspecified occlusion or stenosis of right middle cerebral artery [HCC]

     I63.512   Cerebral infarction due to unspecified occlusion or stenosis of left middle cerebral artery [HCC]

     I63.513   Cerebral infarction due to unspecified occlusion or stenosis of bilateral middle cerebral arteries [HCC]

     I63.519   Cerebral infarction due to unspecified occlusion or stenosis of unspecified middle cerebral artery [HCC]

I63.52   Cerebral infarction due to unspecified occlusion or stenosis of anterior cerebral artery

     I63.521   Cerebral infarction due to unspecified occlusion or stenosis of right anterior cerebral artery [HCC]

     I63.522   Cerebral infarction due to unspecified occlusion or stenosis of left anterior cerebral artery [HCC]

     I63.523   Cerebral infarction due to unspecified occlusion or stenosis of bilateral anterior cerebral arteries [HCC]

     I63.529   Cerebral infarction due to unspecified occlusion or stenosis of unspecified anterior cerebral artery [HCC]

I63.53   Cerebral infarction due to unspecified occlusion or stenosis of posterior cerebral artery

     I63.531   Cerebral infarction due to unspecified occlusion or stenosis of right posterior cerebral artery [HCC]

     I63.532   Cerebral infarction due to unspecified occlusion or stenosis of left posterior cerebral artery [HCC]

     I63.533   Cerebral infarction due to unspecified occlusion or stenosis of bilateral posterior cerebral arteries [HCC]

     I63.539   Cerebral infarction due to unspecified occlusion or stenosis of unspecified posterior cerebral artery [HCC]

I63.54   Cerebral infarction due to unspecified occlusion or stenosis of cerebellar artery

     I63.541   Cerebral infarction due to unspecified occlusion or stenosis of right cerebellar artery [HCC]

     I63.542   Cerebral infarction due to unspecified occlusion or stenosis of left cerebellar artery [HCC]

     I63.543   Cerebral infarction due to unspecified occlusion or stenosis of bilateral cerebellar arteries [HCC]

     I63.549   Cerebral infarction due to unspecified occlusion or stenosis of unspecified cerebellar artery [HCC]

I63.59   Cerebral infarction due to unspecified occlusion or stenosis of other cerebral artery [HCC]

I63.6   **Cerebral infarction due to cerebral venous thrombosis, nonpyogenic** [HCC]

I63.8   **Other cerebral infarction**

I63.81 **Other cerebral infarction due to occlusion or stenosis of small artery** [HCC]

Lacunar infarction

I63.89 **Other cerebral infarction** [HCC]

I63.9 **Cerebral infarction, unspecified** [HCC]

Stroke NOS

Excludes2: transient cerebral ischemic attacks and related syndromes (G45.-)

I65 **Occlusion and stenosis of precerebral arteries, not resulting in cerebral infarction**

Includes: embolism of precerebral artery

narrowing of precerebral artery

obstruction (complete) (partial) of precerebral artery

thrombosis of precerebral artery

Excludes1: insufficiency, NOS, of precerebral artery (G45.-)

insufficiency of precerebral arteries causing cerebral infarction (I63.0-I63.2)

I65.0 **Occlusion and stenosis of vertebral artery**

I65.01 **Occlusion and stenosis of right vertebral artery**

I65.02 **Occlusion and stenosis of left vertebral artery**

I65.03 **Occlusion and stenosis of bilateral vertebral arteries**

I65.09 **Occlusion and stenosis of unspecified vertebral artery**

I65.1 **Occlusion and stenosis of basilar artery**

I65.2 **Occlusion and stenosis of carotid artery**

I65.21 **Occlusion and stenosis of right carotid artery**

I65.22 **Occlusion and stenosis of left carotid artery**

I65.23 **Occlusion and stenosis of bilateral carotid arteries**

I65.29 **Occlusion and stenosis of unspecified carotid artery**

I65.8 **Occlusion and stenosis of other precerebral arteries**

I65.9 **Occlusion and stenosis of unspecified precerebral artery**

Occlusion and stenosis of precerebral artery NOS

I66 **Occlusion and stenosis of cerebral arteries, not resulting in cerebral infarction**

Includes: embolism of cerebral artery

narrowing of cerebral artery

obstruction (complete) (partial) of cerebral artery

thrombosis of cerebral artery

Excludes1: Occlusion and stenosis of cerebral artery causing cerebral infarction (I63.3-I63.5)

I66.0 **Occlusion and stenosis of middle cerebral artery**

I66.01 **Occlusion and stenosis of right middle cerebral artery**

I66.02 **Occlusion and stenosis of left middle cerebral artery**

I66.03 **Occlusion and stenosis of bilateral middle cerebral arteries**

I66.09 **Occlusion and stenosis of unspecified middle cerebral artery**

I66.1 **Occlusion and stenosis of anterior cerebral artery**

I66.11 **Occlusion and stenosis of right anterior cerebral artery**

I66.12 **Occlusion and stenosis of left anterior cerebral artery**

I66.13 **Occlusion and stenosis of bilateral anterior cerebral arteries**

I66.19 **Occlusion and stenosis of unspecified anterior cerebral artery**

I66.2 **Occlusion and stenosis of posterior cerebral artery**

I66.21 **Occlusion and stenosis of right posterior cerebral artery**

I66.22 **Occlusion and stenosis of left posterior cerebral artery**

I66.23 **Occlusion and stenosis of bilateral posterior cerebral arteries**

I66.29 **Occlusion and stenosis of unspecified posterior cerebral artery**

I66.3 **Occlusion and stenosis of cerebellar arteries**

I66.8 **Occlusion and stenosis of other cerebral arteries**

Occlusion and stenosis of perforating arteries

I66.9 **Occlusion and stenosis of unspecified cerebral artery**

I67 **Other cerebrovascular diseases**

Excludes2: sequelae of the listed conditions (I69.8)

I67.0 **Dissection of cerebral arteries, nonruptured** [HCC]

Excludes1: ruptured cerebral arteries (I60.7)

I67.1 **Cerebral aneurysm, nonruptured**

Cerebral aneurysm NOS

Cerebral arteriovenous fistula, acquired

Internal carotid artery aneurysm, intracranial portion

Internal carotid artery aneurysm, NOS

Excludes1: congenital cerebral aneurysm, nonruptured (Q28.-)

ruptured cerebral aneurysm (I60.7)

I67.2 **Cerebral atherosclerosis**

Atheroma of cerebral and precerebral arteries

I67.3 **Progressive vascular leukoencephalopathy**

Binswanger's disease

I67.4 **Hypertensive encephalopathy**

Excludes2: insufficiency, NOS, of precerebral arteries (G45.2)

I67.5 **Moyamoya disease**

I67.6 **Nonpyogenic thrombosis of intracranial venous system**

Nonpyogenic thrombosis of cerebral vein

Nonpyogenic thrombosis of intracranial venous sinus

Excludes1: nonpyogenic thrombosis of intracranial venous system causing infarction (I63.6)

I67.7 **Cerebral arteritis, not elsewhere classified**

Granulomatous angiitis of the nervous system

Excludes1: allergic granulomatous angiitis (M30.1)

I67.8 **Other specified cerebrovascular diseases**

I67.81 **Acute cerebrovascular insufficiency**

Acute cerebrovascular insufficiency unspecified as to location or reversibility

I67.82 **Cerebral ischemia**

Chronic cerebral ischemia

I67.83 **Posterior reversible encephalopathy syndrome**

PRES

I67.84 **Cerebral vasospasm and vasoconstriction**

I67.841 **Reversible cerebrovascular vasoconstriction syndrome**

Call-Fleming syndrome

Code first underlying condition, if applicable, such as eclampsia (O15.00-O15.9)

I67.848   **Other cerebrovascular vasospasm and vasoconstriction**

I67.85   **Hereditary cerebrovascular diseases**

I67.850   **Cerebral autosomal dominant arteriopathy with subcortical infarcts and leukoencephalopathy**

CADASIL

<u>Code also</u> any associated diagnoses, such as:

epilepsy (G40.-)

stroke (I63.-)

vascular dementia (F01.-)

I67.858   **Other hereditary cerebrovascular disease**

I67.89   **Other cerebrovascular disease**

I67.9   **Cerebrovascular disease, unspecified**

I68   **Cerebrovascular disorders in diseases classified elsewhere**

I68.0   **Cerebral amyloid angiopathy**

<u>Code first</u> underlying amyloidosis (E85.-)

I68.2   **Cerebral arteritis in other diseases classified elsewhere**

<u>Code first</u> underlying disease

Excludes1: cerebral arteritis (in):

listerosis (A32.89)

systemic lupus erythematosus (M32.19)

syphilis (A52.04)

tuberculosis (A18.89)

I68.8   **Other cerebrovascular disorders in diseases classified elsewhere**

<u>Code first</u> underlying disease

Excludes1: syphilitic cerebral aneurysm (A52.05)

I69   **Sequelae of cerebrovascular disease**

Note: Category I69 is to be used to indicate conditions in I60-I67 as the cause of sequelae. The 'sequelae' include conditions specified as such or as residuals which may occur at any time after the onset of the causal condition

Excludes1: personal history of cerebral infarction without residual deficit (Z86.73)

personal history of prolonged reversible ischemic neurologic deficit (PRIND) (Z86.73)

personal history of reversible ischemic neurological deficit (RIND) (Z86.73)

sequelae of traumatic intracranial injury (S06.-)

I69.0   **Sequelae of nontraumatic subarachnoid hemorrhage**

I69.00   **Unspecified sequelae of nontraumatic subarachnoid hemorrhage**

I69.01   **Cognitive deficits following nontraumatic subarachnoid hemorrhage**

I69.010   **Attention and concentration deficit following nontraumatic subarachnoid hemorrhage**

I69.011   **Memory deficit following nontraumatic subarachnoid hemorrhage**

I69.012   **Visuospatial deficit and spatial neglect following nontraumatic subarachnoid hemorrhage**

I69.013   **Psychomotor deficit following nontraumatic subarachnoid hemorrhage**

I69.014   **Frontal lobe and executive function deficit following nontraumatic subarachnoid hemorrhage**

I69.015   **Cognitive social or emotional deficit following nontraumatic subarachnoid hemorrhage**

I69.018   **Other symptoms and signs involving cognitive functions following nontraumatic subarachnoid hemorrhage**

I69.019   **Unspecified symptoms and signs involving cognitive functions following nontraumatic subarachnoid hemorrhage**

I69.02   **Speech and language deficits following nontraumatic subarachnoid hemorrhage**

I69.020   **Aphasia following nontraumatic subarachnoid hemorrhage**

I69.021   **Dysphasia following nontraumatic subarachnoid hemorrhage**

I69.022   **Dysarthria following nontraumatic subarachnoid hemorrhage**

I69.023   **Fluency disorder following nontraumatic subarachnoid hemorrhage**

Stuttering following nontraumatic subarachnoid hemorrhage

I69.028   **Other speech and language deficits following nontraumatic subarachnoid hemorrhage**

I69.03   **Monoplegia of upper limb following nontraumatic subarachnoid hemorrhage**

I69.031   **Monoplegia of upper limb following nontraumatic subarachnoid hemorrhage affecting right dominant side** [HCC]

I69.032   **Monoplegia of upper limb following nontraumatic subarachnoid hemorrhage affecting left dominant side** [HCC]

I69.033   **Monoplegia of upper limb following nontraumatic subarachnoid hemorrhage affecting right non-dominant side** [HCC]

I69.034   **Monoplegia of upper limb following nontraumatic subarachnoid hemorrhage affecting left non-dominant side** [HCC]

I69.039   **Monoplegia of upper limb following nontraumatic subarachnoid hemorrhage affecting unspecified side** [HCC]

I69.04   **Monoplegia of lower limb following nontraumatic subarachnoid hemorrhage** [HCC]

I69.041   **Monoplegia of lower limb following nontraumatic subarachnoid hemorrhage affecting right dominant side** [HCC]

I69.042   **Monoplegia of lower limb following nontraumatic subarachnoid hemorrhage affecting left dominant side** [HCC]

I69.043   **Monoplegia of lower limb following nontraumatic subarachnoid hemorrhage affecting right non-dominant side** [HCC]

I69.044   **Monoplegia of lower limb following nontraumatic subarachnoid hemorrhage affecting left non-dominant side** [HCC]

I69.049 Monoplegia of lower limb following nontraumatic subarachnoid hemorrhage affecting unspecified side [HCC]

I69.05 Hemiplegia and hemiparesis following nontraumatic subarachnoid hemorrhage [HCC]

I69.051 Hemiplegia and hemiparesis following nontraumatic subarachnoid hemorrhage affecting right dominant side [HCC]

I69.052 Hemiplegia and hemiparesis following nontraumatic subarachnoid hemorrhage affecting left dominant side [HCC]

I69.053 Hemiplegia and hemiparesis following nontraumatic subarachnoid hemorrhage affecting right non-dominant side [HCC]

I69.054 Hemiplegia and hemiparesis following nontraumatic subarachnoid hemorrhage affecting left non-dominant side [HCC]

I69.059 Hemiplegia and hemiparesis following nontraumatic subarachnoid hemorrhage affecting unspecified side [HCC]

I69.06 Other paralytic syndrome following nontraumatic subarachnoid hemorrhage [HCC]

Use Additional Code to identify type of paralytic syndrome, such as:

locked-in state (G83.5)

quadriplegia (G82.5-)

Excludes1: hemiplegia/hemiparesis following nontraumatic subarachnoid hemorrhage (I69.05-)

monoplegia of lower limb following nontraumatic subarachnoid hemorrhage (I69.04-)

monoplegia of upper limb following nontraumatic subarachnoid hemorrhage (I69.03-)

I69.061 Other paralytic syndrome following nontraumatic subarachnoid hemorrhage affecting right dominant side

I69.062 Other paralytic syndrome following nontraumatic subarachnoid hemorrhage affecting left dominant side

I69.063 Other paralytic syndrome following nontraumatic subarachnoid hemorrhage affecting right non-dominant side

I69.064 Other paralytic syndrome following nontraumatic subarachnoid hemorrhage affecting left non-dominant side

I69.065 Other paralytic syndrome following nontraumatic subarachnoid hemorrhage, bilateral

I69.069 Other paralytic syndrome following nontraumatic subarachnoid hemorrhage affecting unspecified side

I69.09 Other sequelae of nontraumatic subarachnoid hemorrhage

I69.090 Apraxia following nontraumatic subarachnoid hemorrhage

I69.091 Dysphagia following nontraumatic subarachnoid hemorrhage

Use Additional Code to identify the type of dysphagia, if known (R13.1-)

I69.092 Facial weakness following nontraumatic subarachnoid hemorrhage

Facial droop following nontraumatic subarachnoid hemorrhage

I69.093 Ataxia following nontraumatic subarachnoid hemorrhage

I69.098 Other sequelae following nontraumatic subarachnoid hemorrhage

Alterations of sensation following nontraumatic subarachnoid hemorrhage

Disturbance of vision following nontraumatic subarachnoid hemorrhage

Use Additional Code to identify the sequelae

I69.1 Sequelae of nontraumatic intracerebral hemorrhage

I69.10 Unspecified sequelae of nontraumatic intracerebral hemorrhage

I69.11 Cognitive deficits following nontraumatic intracerebral hemorrhage

I69.110 Attention and concentration deficit following nontraumatic intracerebral hemorrhage

I69.111 Memory deficit following nontraumatic intracerebral hemorrhage

I69.112 Visuospatial deficit and spatial neglect following nontraumatic intracerebral hemorrhage

I69.113 Psychomotor deficit following nontraumatic intracerebral hemorrhage

I69.114 Frontal lobe and executive function deficit following nontraumatic intracerebral hemorrhage

I69.115 Cognitive social or emotional deficit following nontraumatic intracerebral hemorrhage

I69.118 Other symptoms and signs involving cognitive functions following nontraumatic intracerebral hemorrhage

I69.119 Unspecified symptoms and signs involving cognitive functions following nontraumatic intracerebral hemorrhage

I69.12 Speech and language deficits following nontraumatic intracerebral hemorrhage

I69.120 Aphasia following nontraumatic intracerebral hemorrhage

I69.121 Dysphasia following nontraumatic intracerebral hemorrhage

I69.122 Dysarthria following nontraumatic intracerebral hemorrhage

I69.123 Fluency disorder following nontraumatic intracerebral hemorrhage

Stuttering following nontraumatic intracerebral hemorrhage

I69.128   **Other speech and language deficits following nontraumatic intracerebral hemorrhage**

I69.13   **Monoplegia of upper limb following nontraumatic intracerebral hemorrhage**

I69.131   **Monoplegia of upper limb following nontraumatic intracerebral hemorrhage affecting right dominant side** [HCC]

I69.132   **Monoplegia of upper limb following nontraumatic intracerebral hemorrhage affecting left dominant side** [HCC]

I69.133   **Monoplegia of upper limb following nontraumatic intracerebral hemorrhage affecting right non-dominant side** [HCC]

I69.134   **Monoplegia of upper limb following nontraumatic intracerebral hemorrhage affecting left non-dominant side** [HCC]

I69.139   **Monoplegia of upper limb following nontraumatic intracerebral hemorrhage affecting unspecified side** [HCC]

I69.14   **Monoplegia of lower limb following nontraumatic intracerebral hemorrhage**

I69.141   **Monoplegia of lower limb following nontraumatic intracerebral hemorrhage affecting right dominant side** [HCC]

I69.142   **Monoplegia of lower limb following nontraumatic intracerebral hemorrhage affecting left dominant side** [HCC]

I69.143   **Monoplegia of lower limb following nontraumatic intracerebral hemorrhage affecting right non-dominant side** [HCC]

I69.144   **Monoplegia of lower limb following nontraumatic intracerebral hemorrhage affecting left non-dominant side** [HCC]

I69.149   **Monoplegia of lower limb following nontraumatic intracerebral hemorrhage affecting unspecified side** [HCC]

I69.15   **Hemiplegia and hemiparesis following nontraumatic intracerebral hemorrhage**

I69.151   **Hemiplegia and hemiparesis following nontraumatic intracerebral hemorrhage affecting right dominant side** [HCC]

I69.152   **Hemiplegia and hemiparesis following nontraumatic intracerebral hemorrhage affecting left dominant side** [HCC]

I69.153   **Hemiplegia and hemiparesis following nontraumatic intracerebral hemorrhage affecting right non-dominant side** [HCC]

I69.154   **Hemiplegia and hemiparesis following nontraumatic intracerebral hemorrhage affecting left non-dominant side** [HCC]

I69.159   **Hemiplegia and hemiparesis following nontraumatic intracerebral hemorrhage affecting unspecified side** [HCC]

I69.16   **Other paralytic syndrome following nontraumatic intracerebral hemorrhage**

Use Additional Code to identify type of paralytic syndrome, such as:

locked-in state (G83.5)

quadriplegia (G82.5-)

Excludes1: hemiplegia/hemiparesis following nontraumatic intracerebral hemorrhage (I69.15-)

monoplegia of lower limb following nontraumatic intracerebral hemorrhage (I69.14-)

monoplegia of upper limb following nontraumatic intracerebral hemorrhage (I69.13-)

I69.161   **Other paralytic syndrome following nontraumatic intracerebral hemorrhage affecting right dominant side** [HCC]

I69.162   **Other paralytic syndrome following nontraumatic intracerebral hemorrhage affecting left dominant side** [HCC]

I69.163   **Other paralytic syndrome following nontraumatic intracerebral hemorrhage affecting right non-dominant side** [HCC]

I69.164   **Other paralytic syndrome following nontraumatic intracerebral hemorrhage affecting left non-dominant side** [HCC]

I69.165   **Other paralytic syndrome following nontraumatic intracerebral hemorrhage, bilateral** [HCC]

I69.169   **Other paralytic syndrome following nontraumatic intracerebral hemorrhage affecting unspecified side** [HCC]

I69.19   **Other sequelae of nontraumatic intracerebral hemorrhage**

I69.190   **Apraxia following nontraumatic intracerebral hemorrhage**

I69.191   **Dysphagia following nontraumatic intracerebral hemorrhage**

Use Additional Code to identify the type of dysphagia, if known (R13.1-)

I69.192   **Facial weakness following nontraumatic intracerebral hemorrhage**

Facial droop following nontraumatic intracerebral hemorrhage

I69.193   **Ataxia following nontraumatic intracerebral hemorrhage**

I69.198   **Other sequelae of nontraumatic intracerebral hemorrhage**

Alteration of sensations following nontraumatic intracerebral hemorrhage

Disturbance of vision following nontraumatic intracerebral hemorrhage

Use Additional Code to identify the sequelae

I69.2   **Sequelae of other nontraumatic intracranial hemorrhage**

I69.20   **Unspecified sequelae of other nontraumatic intracranial hemorrhage**

■ Add 4th-7th digits   ■ Nonspecific code   ■ Unspecified code   Manifestation code   [HCC] Hierarchical Condition Code

I69.21 Cognitive deficits following other nontraumatic intracranial hemorrhage

    I69.210 Attention and concentration deficit following other nontraumatic intracranial hemorrhage

    I69.211 Memory deficit following other nontraumatic intracranial hemorrhage

    I69.212 Visuospatial deficit and spatial neglect following other nontraumatic intracranial hemorrhage

    I69.213 Psychomotor deficit following other nontraumatic intracranial hemorrhage

    I69.214 Frontal lobe and executive function deficit following other nontraumatic intracranial hemorrhage

    I69.215 Cognitive social or emotional deficit following other nontraumatic intracranial hemorrhage

    I69.218 Other symptoms and signs involving cognitive functions following other nontraumatic intracranial hemorrhage

    I69.219 Unspecified symptoms and signs involving cognitive functions following other nontraumatic intracranial hemorrhage

I69.22 Speech and language deficits following other nontraumatic intracranial hemorrhage

    I69.220 Aphasia following other nontraumatic intracranial hemorrhage

    I69.221 Dysphasia following other nontraumatic intracranial hemorrhage

    I69.222 Dysarthria following other nontraumatic intracranial hemorrhage

    I69.223 Fluency disorder following other nontraumatic intracranial hemorrhage

        Stuttering following other nontraumatic intracranial hemorrhage

    I69.228 Other speech and language deficits following other nontraumatic intracranial hemorrhage

I69.23 Monoplegia of upper limb following other nontraumatic intracranial hemorrhage

    I69.231 Monoplegia of upper limb following other nontraumatic intracranial hemorrhage affecting right dominant side [HCC]

    I69.232 Monoplegia of upper limb following other nontraumatic intracranial hemorrhage affecting left dominant side [HCC]

    I69.233 Monoplegia of upper limb following other nontraumatic intracranial hemorrhage affecting right non-dominant side [HCC]

    I69.234 Monoplegia of upper limb following other nontraumatic intracranial hemorrhage affecting left non-dominant side [HCC]

    I69.239 Monoplegia of upper limb following other nontraumatic intracranial

hemorrhage affecting unspecified side [HCC]

I69.24 Monoplegia of lower limb following other nontraumatic intracranial hemorrhage [HCC]

    I69.241 Monoplegia of lower limb following other nontraumatic intracranial hemorrhage affecting right dominant side [HCC]

    I69.242 Monoplegia of lower limb following other nontraumatic intracranial hemorrhage affecting left dominant side [HCC]

    I69.243 Monoplegia of lower limb following other nontraumatic intracranial hemorrhage affecting right non-dominant side [HCC]

    I69.244 Monoplegia of lower limb following other nontraumatic intracranial hemorrhage affecting left non-dominant side [HCC]

    I69.249 Monoplegia of lower limb following other nontraumatic intracranial hemorrhage affecting unspecified side [HCC]

I69.25 Hemiplegia and hemiparesis following other nontraumatic intracranial hemorrhage

    I69.251 Hemiplegia and hemiparesis following other nontraumatic intracranial hemorrhage affecting right dominant side

    I69.252 Hemiplegia and hemiparesis following other nontraumatic intracranial hemorrhage affecting left dominant side [HCC]

    I69.253 Hemiplegia and hemiparesis following other nontraumatic intracranial hemorrhage affecting right non-dominant side [HCC]

    I69.254 Hemiplegia and hemiparesis following other nontraumatic intracranial hemorrhage affecting left non-dominant side [HCC]

    I69.259 Hemiplegia and hemiparesis following other nontraumatic intracranial hemorrhage affecting unspecified side [HCC]

I69.26 Other paralytic syndrome following other nontraumatic intracranial hemorrhage

    <u>Use Additional Code</u> to identify type of paralytic syndrome, such as:

    locked-in state (G83.5)

    quadriplegia (G82.5-)

    Excludes1: hemiplegia/hemiparesis following other nontraumatic intracranial hemorrhage (I69.25-)

        monoplegia of lower limb following other nontraumatic intracranial hemorrhage (I69.24-)

        monoplegia of upper limb following other nontraumatic intracranial hemorrhage (I69.23-)

    I69.261 Other paralytic syndrome following other nontraumatic intracranial hemorrhage affecting right dominant side [HCC]

    I69.262 Other paralytic syndrome following other nontraumatic intracranial hemorrhage affecting left dominant side [HCC]

I69.263 Other paralytic syndrome following other nontraumatic intracranial hemorrhage affecting right non-dominant side [HCC]

I69.264 Other paralytic syndrome following other nontraumatic intracranial hemorrhage affecting left non-dominant side [HCC]

I69.265 Other paralytic syndrome following other nontraumatic intracranial hemorrhage, bilateral [HCC]

I69.269 Other paralytic syndrome following other nontraumatic intracranial hemorrhage affecting unspecified side [HCC]

I69.29 Other sequelae of other nontraumatic intracranial hemorrhage

I69.290 Apraxia following other nontraumatic intracranial hemorrhage

I69.291 Dysphagia following other nontraumatic intracranial hemorrhage

Use Additional Code to identify the type of dysphagia, if known (R13.1-)

I69.292 Facial weakness following other nontraumatic intracranial hemorrhage

Facial droop following other nontraumatic intracranial hemorrhage

I69.293 Ataxia following other nontraumatic intracranial hemorrhage

I69.298 Other sequelae of other nontraumatic intracranial hemorrhage

Alteration of sensation following other nontraumatic intracranial hemorrhage

Disturbance of vision following other nontraumatic intracranial hemorrhage

Use Additional Code to identify the sequelae

I69.3 Sequelae of cerebral infarction

Sequelae of stroke NOS

I69.30 Unspecified sequelae of cerebral infarction

I69.31 Cognitive deficits following cerebral infarction

I69.310 Attention and concentration deficit following cerebral infarction

I69.311 Memory deficit following cerebral infarction

I69.312 Visuospatial deficit and spatial neglect following cerebral infarction

I69.313 Psychomotor deficit following cerebral infarction

I69.314 Frontal lobe and executive function deficit following cerebral infarction

I69.315 Cognitive social or emotional deficit following cerebral infarction

I69.318 Other symptoms and signs involving cognitive functions following cerebral infarction

I69.319 Unspecified symptoms and signs involving cognitive functions following cerebral infarction

I69.32 Speech and language deficits following cerebral infarction

I69.320 Aphasia following cerebral infarction

I69.321 Dysphasia following cerebral infarction

I69.322 Dysarthria following cerebral infarction

Excludes2: transient ischemic attack (TIA) (G45.9)

I69.323 Fluency disorder following cerebral infarction

Stuttering following cerebral infarction

I69.328 Other speech and language deficits following cerebral infarction

I69.33 Monoplegia of upper limb following cerebral infarction

I69.331 Monoplegia of upper limb following cerebral infarction affecting right dominant side [HCC]

I69.332 Monoplegia of upper limb following cerebral infarction affecting left dominant side [HCC]

I69.333 Monoplegia of upper limb following cerebral infarction affecting right non-dominant side [HCC]

I69.334 Monoplegia of upper limb following cerebral infarction affecting left non-dominant side [HCC]

I69.339 Monoplegia of upper limb following cerebral infarction affecting unspecified side [HCC]

I69.34 Monoplegia of lower limb following cerebral infarction [HCC]

I69.341 Monoplegia of lower limb following cerebral infarction affecting right dominant side [HCC]

I69.342 Monoplegia of lower limb following cerebral infarction affecting left dominant side [HCC]

I69.343 Monoplegia of lower limb following cerebral infarction affecting right non-dominant side [HCC]

I69.344 Monoplegia of lower limb following cerebral infarction affecting left non-dominant side [HCC]

I69.349 Monoplegia of lower limb following cerebral infarction affecting unspecified side [HCC]

I69.35 Hemiplegia and hemiparesis following cerebral infarction

I69.351 Hemiplegia and hemiparesis following cerebral infarction affecting right dominant side [HCC]

Excludes2: precerebral artery, congenital (nonruptured) (Q28.1)

I69.352 Hemiplegia and hemiparesis following cerebral infarction affecting left dominant side [HCC]

I69.353 Hemiplegia and hemiparesis following cerebral infarction affecting right non-dominant side [HCC]

I69.354 Hemiplegia and hemiparesis following cerebral infarction affecting left non-dominant side

I69.359 Hemiplegia and hemiparesis following cerebral infarction affecting unspecified side [HCC]

I69.36 Other paralytic syndrome following cerebral infarction

Use Additional Code to identify type of paralytic syndrome, such as:

locked-in state (G83.5)

quadriplegia (G82.5-)

Excludes1: hemiplegia/hemiparesis following cerebral infarction (I69.35-)

monoplegia of lower limb following cerebral infarction (I69.34-)

monoplegia of upper limb following cerebral infarction (I69.33-)

I69.361 Other paralytic syndrome following cerebral infarction affecting right dominant side [HCC]

I69.362 Other paralytic syndrome following cerebral infarction affecting left dominant side [HCC]

I69.363 Other paralytic syndrome following cerebral infarction affecting right non-dominant side [HCC]

I69.364 Other paralytic syndrome following cerebral infarction affecting left non-dominant side [HCC]

I69.365 Other paralytic syndrome following cerebral infarction, bilateral [HCC]

I69.369 Other paralytic syndrome following cerebral infarction affecting unspecified side [HCC]

I69.39 Other sequelae of cerebral infarction

I69.390 Apraxia following cerebral infarction

I69.391 Dysphagia following cerebral infarction

Use Additional Code to identify the type of dysphagia, if known (R13.1-)

I69.392 Facial weakness following cerebral infarction

Facial droop following cerebral infarction

I69.393 Ataxia following cerebral infarction

I69.398 Other sequelae of cerebral infarction

Alteration of sensation following cerebral infarction

Disturbance of vision following cerebral infarction

Use Additional Code to identify the sequelae

I69.8 Sequelae of other cerebrovascular diseases

Excludes1: sequelae of traumatic intracranial injury (S06.-)

I69.80 Unspecified sequelae of other cerebrovascular disease

I69.81 Cognitive deficits following other cerebrovascular disease

I69.810 Attention and concentration deficit following other cerebrovascular disease

I69.811 Memory deficit following other cerebrovascular disease

I69.812 Visuospatial deficit and spatial neglect following other cerebrovascular disease

I69.813 Psychomotor deficit following other cerebrovascular disease

I69.814 Frontal lobe and executive function deficit following other cerebrovascular disease

I69.815 Cognitive social or emotional deficit following other cerebrovascular disease

I69.818 Other symptoms and signs involving cognitive functions following other cerebrovascular disease

I69.819 Unspecified symptoms and signs involving cognitive functions following other cerebrovascular disease

I69.82 Speech and language deficits following other cerebrovascular disease

I69.820 Aphasia following other cerebrovascular disease

I69.821 Dysphasia following other cerebrovascular disease

I69.822 Dysarthria following other cerebrovascular disease

I69.823 Fluency disorder following other cerebrovascular disease

Stuttering following other cerebrovascular disease

I69.828 Other speech and language deficits following other cerebrovascular disease

I69.83 Monoplegia of upper limb following other cerebrovascular disease

I69.831 Monoplegia of upper limb following other cerebrovascular disease affecting right dominant side [HCC]

I69.832 Monoplegia of upper limb following other cerebrovascular disease affecting left dominant side [HCC]

I69.833 Monoplegia of upper limb following other cerebrovascular disease affecting right non-dominant side [HCC]

I69.834 Monoplegia of upper limb following other cerebrovascular disease affecting left non-dominant side [HCC]

I69.839 Monoplegia of upper limb following other cerebrovascular disease affecting unspecified side [HCC]

I69.84 Monoplegia of lower limb following other cerebrovascular disease

I69.841 Monoplegia of lower limb following other cerebrovascular disease affecting right dominant side [HCC]

I69.842 Monoplegia of lower limb following other cerebrovascular disease affecting left dominant side [HCC]

I69.843 Monoplegia of lower limb following other cerebrovascular disease affecting right non-dominant side [HCC]

● New code   ▲ Revised code   Excludes1: Not coded here   Excludes2: Not included here   ⊗ Placeholder required   ⑦7th digit required

I69.844   **Monoplegia of lower limb following other cerebrovascular disease affecting left non-dominant side** [HCC]

I69.849   **Monoplegia of lower limb following other cerebrovascular disease affecting unspecified side** [HCC]

I69.85   **Hemiplegia and hemiparesis following other cerebrovascular disease** [HCC]

I69.851   **Hemiplegia and hemiparesis following other cerebrovascular disease affecting right dominant side** [HCC]

I69.852   **Hemiplegia and hemiparesis following other cerebrovascular disease affecting left dominant side** [HCC]

I69.853   **Hemiplegia and hemiparesis following other cerebrovascular disease affecting right non-dominant side** [HCC]

I69.854   **Hemiplegia and hemiparesis following other cerebrovascular disease affecting left non-dominant side** [HCC]

I69.859   **Hemiplegia and hemiparesis following other cerebrovascular disease affecting unspecified side** [HCC]

I69.86   **Other paralytic syndrome following other cerebrovascular disease**

Use Additional Code to identify type of paralytic syndrome, such as:

locked-in state (G83.5)

quadriplegia (G82.5-)

Excludes1: hemiplegia/hemiparesis following other cerebrovascular disease (I69.85-)

monoplegia of lower limb following other cerebrovascular disease (I69.84-)

monoplegia of upper limb following other cerebrovascular disease (I69.83-)

I69.861   **Other paralytic syndrome following other cerebrovascular disease affecting right dominant side** [HCC]

I69.862   **Other paralytic syndrome following other cerebrovascular disease affecting left dominant side** [HCC]

I69.863   **Other paralytic syndrome following other cerebrovascular disease affecting right non-dominant side** [HCC]

I69.864   **Other paralytic syndrome following other cerebrovascular disease affecting left non-dominant side** [HCC]

I69.865   **Other paralytic syndrome following other cerebrovascular disease, bilateral** [HCC]

I69.869   **Other paralytic syndrome following other cerebrovascular disease affecting unspecified side** [HCC]

I69.89   **Other sequelae of other cerebrovascular disease**

I69.890   **Apraxia following other cerebrovascular disease**

I69.891   **Dysphagia following other cerebrovascular disease**

Use Additional Code to identify the type of dysphagia, if known (R13.1-)

I69.892   **Facial weakness following other cerebrovascular disease**

Facial droop following other cerebrovascular disease

I69.893   **Ataxia following other cerebrovascular disease**

I69.898   **Other sequelae of other cerebrovascular disease**

Alteration of sensation following other cerebrovascular disease

Disturbance of vision following other cerebrovascular disease

Use Additional Code to identify the sequelae

I69.9   **Sequelae of unspecified cerebrovascular diseases**

Excludes1: sequelae of stroke (I69.3)

sequelae of traumatic intracranial injury (S06.-)

I69.90   **Unspecified sequelae of unspecified cerebrovascular disease**

I69.91   **Cognitive deficits following unspecified cerebrovascular disease**

I69.910   **Attention and concentration deficit following unspecified cerebrovascular disease**

I69.911   **Memory deficit following unspecified cerebrovascular disease**

I69.912   **Visuospatial deficit and spatial neglect following unspecified cerebrovascular disease**

I69.913   **Psychomotor deficit following unspecified cerebrovascular disease**

I69.914   **Frontal lobe and executive function deficit following unspecified cerebrovascular disease**

I69.915   **Cognitive social or emotional deficit following unspecified cerebrovascular disease**

I69.918   **Other symptoms and signs involving cognitive functions following unspecified cerebrovascular disease**

I69.919   **Unspecified symptoms and signs involving cognitive functions following unspecified cerebrovascular disease**

I69.92   **Speech and language deficits following unspecified cerebrovascular disease**

I69.920   **Aphasia following unspecified cerebrovascular disease**

I69.921   **Dysphasia following unspecified cerebrovascular disease**

I69.922   **Dysarthria following unspecified cerebrovascular disease**

I69.923   **Fluency disorder following unspecified cerebrovascular disease**

Stuttering following unspecified cerebrovascular disease

I69.928   **Other speech and language deficits following unspecified cerebrovascular disease**

I69.93   **Monoplegia of upper limb following unspecified cerebrovascular disease**

I69.931 **Monoplegia of upper limb following unspecified cerebrovascular disease affecting right dominant side** [HCC]

I69.932 **Monoplegia of upper limb following unspecified cerebrovascular disease affecting left dominant side** [HCC]

I69.933 **Monoplegia of upper limb following unspecified cerebrovascular disease affecting right non-dominant side** [HCC]

I69.934 **Monoplegia of upper limb following unspecified cerebrovascular disease affecting left non-dominant side** [HCC]

I69.939 **Monoplegia of upper limb following unspecified cerebrovascular disease affecting unspecified side** [HCC]

I69.94 **Monoplegia of lower limb following unspecified cerebrovascular disease**

I69.941 **Monoplegia of lower limb following unspecified cerebrovascular disease affecting right dominant side** [HCC]

I69.942 **Monoplegia of lower limb following unspecified cerebrovascular disease affecting left dominant side** [HCC]

I69.943 **Monoplegia of lower limb following unspecified cerebrovascular disease affecting right non-dominant side** [HCC]

I69.944 **Monoplegia of lower limb following unspecified cerebrovascular disease affecting left non-dominant side** [HCC]

I69.949 **Monoplegia of lower limb following unspecified cerebrovascular disease affecting unspecified side** [HCC]

I69.95 **Hemiplegia and hemiparesis following unspecified cerebrovascular disease**

I69.951 **Hemiplegia and hemiparesis following unspecified cerebrovascular disease affecting right dominant side** [HCC]

I69.952 **Hemiplegia and hemiparesis following unspecified cerebrovascular disease affecting left dominant side** [HCC]

I69.953 **Hemiplegia and hemiparesis following unspecified cerebrovascular disease affecting right non-dominant side** [HCC]

I69.954 **Hemiplegia and hemiparesis following unspecified cerebrovascular disease affecting left non-dominant side** [HCC]

I69.959 **Hemiplegia and hemiparesis following unspecified cerebrovascular disease affecting unspecified side** [HCC]

I69.96 **Other paralytic syndrome following unspecified cerebrovascular disease**

Use Additional Code to identify type of paralytic syndrome, such as:

locked-in state (G83.5)

quadriplegia (G82.5-)

Excludes1: hemiplegia/hemiparesis following unspecified cerebrovascular disease (I69.95-)

monoplegia of lower limb following unspecified

cerebrovascular disease (I69.94-)

monoplegia of upper limb following unspecified cerebrovascular disease (I69.93-)

I69.961 **Other paralytic syndrome following unspecified cerebrovascular disease affecting right dominant side** [HCC]

I69.962 **Other paralytic syndrome following unspecified cerebrovascular disease affecting left dominant side** [HCC]

I69.963 **Other paralytic syndrome following unspecified cerebrovascular disease affecting right non-dominant side** [HCC]

I69.964 **Other paralytic syndrome following unspecified cerebrovascular disease affecting left non-dominant side** [HCC]

I69.965 **Other paralytic syndrome following unspecified cerebrovascular disease, bilateral** [HCC]

I69.969 **Other paralytic syndrome following unspecified cerebrovascular disease affecting unspecified side** [HCC]

I69.99 **Other sequelae of unspecified cerebrovascular disease**

I69.990 **Apraxia following unspecified cerebrovascular disease**

I69.991 **Dysphagia following unspecified cerebrovascular disease**

Use Additional Code to identify the type of dysphagia, if known (R13.1-)

I69.992 **Facial weakness following unspecified cerebrovascular disease**

Facial droop following unspecified cerebrovascular disease

I69.993 **Ataxia following unspecified cerebrovascular disease**

I69.998 **Other sequelae following unspecified cerebrovascular disease**

Alteration in sensation following unspecified cerebrovascular disease

Disturbance of vision following unspecified cerebrovascular disease

Use Additional Code to identify the sequelae

DISEASES OF ARTERIES, ARTERIOLES AND CAPILLARIES (I70-I79)

I70 **Atherosclerosis**

Definition: Atherosclerosis is a condition in which an artery wall thickens as the result of a buildup of fatty materials such as cholesterol. It is a syndrome affecting arterial blood vessels.

Includes: arteriolosclerosis

arterial degeneration arteriosclerosis

arteriosclerotic vascular disease

arteriovascular degeneration atheroma

endarteritis deformans or obliterans

senile arteritis

senile endarteritis vascular degeneration

Use Additional Code to identify:

exposure to environmental tobacco smoke (Z77.22)

history of tobacco dependence (Z87.891)

occupational exposure to environmental tobacco smoke (Z57.31) tobacco dependence (F17.-)

tobacco use (Z72.0)

Excludes2: arteriosclerotic cardiovascular disease (I25.1-)

arteriosclerotic heart disease (I25.1-)

atheroembolism (I75.-)

cerebral atherosclerosis (I67.2)

coronary atherosclerosis (I25.1-)

mesenteric atherosclerosis (K55.1)

precerebral atherosclerosis (I67.2)

primary pulmonary atherosclerosis (I27.0)

I70.0 **Atherosclerosis of aorta** [HCC]

I70.1 **Atherosclerosis of renal artery** [HCC]

Goldblatt's kidney

Excludes2: atherosclerosis of renal arterioles (I12.-)

I70.2 **Atherosclerosis of native arteries of the extremities**

Mönckeberg's (medial) sclerosis

Use Additional Code, if applicable, to identify chronic total occlusion of artery of extremity (I70.92)

Excludes2: atherosclerosis of bypass graft of extremities (I70.30-I70.79)

I70.20 **Unspecified atherosclerosis of native arteries of extremities**

I70.201 **Unspecified atherosclerosis of native arteries of extremities, right leg** [HCC]

I70.202 **Unspecified atherosclerosis of native arteries of extremities, left leg** [HCC]

I70.203 **Unspecified atherosclerosis of native arteries of extremities, bilateral legs** [HCC]

I70.208 **Unspecified atherosclerosis of native arteries of extremities, other extremity** [HCC]

I70.209 **Unspecified atherosclerosis of native arteries of extremities, unspecified extremity** [HCC]

I70.21 **Atherosclerosis of native arteries of extremities with intermittent claudication** [HCC]

I70.211 **Atherosclerosis of native arteries of extremities with intermittent claudication, right leg** [HCC]

I70.212 **Atherosclerosis of native arteries of extremities with intermittent claudication, left leg** [HCC]

I70.213 **Atherosclerosis of native arteries of extremities with intermittent claudication, bilateral legs** [HCC]

I70.218 **Atherosclerosis of native arteries of extremities with intermittent claudication, other extremity** [HCC]

I70.219 **Atherosclerosis of native arteries of extremities with intermittent claudication, unspecified extremity** [HCC]

I70.22 **Atherosclerosis of native arteries of extremities with rest pain**

Includes: any condition classifiable to I70.21-

chronic limb-threatening ischemia NOS of native arteries of extremities

chronic limb-threatening ischemia of native arteries of extremities with rest pain

critical limb ischemia NOS of native arteries of extremities

critical limb ischemia of native arteries of extremities with rest pain

I70.221 **Atherosclerosis of native arteries of extremities with rest pain, right leg** [HCC]

I70.222 **Atherosclerosis of native arteries of extremities with rest pain, left leg** [HCC]

I70.223 **Atherosclerosis of native arteries of extremities with rest pain, bilateral legs** [HCC]

I70.228 **Atherosclerosis of native arteries of extremities with rest pain, other extremity** [HCC]

I70.229 **Atherosclerosis of native arteries of extremities with rest pain, unspecified extremity** [HCC]

I70.23 **Atherosclerosis of native arteries of right leg with ulceration**

Includes: any condition classifiable to I70.211 and I70.221

chronic limb-threatening ischemia of native arteries of right leg with ulceration

critical limb ischemia of native arteries of right leg with ulceration

Use Additional Code to identify severity of ulcer (L97.-)

I70.231 **Atherosclerosis of native arteries of right leg with ulceration of thigh** [HCC]

I70.232 **Atherosclerosis of native arteries of right leg with ulceration of calf** [HCC]

I70.233 **Atherosclerosis of native arteries of right leg with ulceration of ankle** [HCC]

I70.234 **Atherosclerosis of native arteries of right leg with ulceration of heel and midfoot** [HCC]

Atherosclerosis of native arteries of right leg with ulceration of plantar surface of midfoot

I70.235 **Atherosclerosis of native arteries of right leg with ulceration of other part of foot** [HCC]

Atherosclerosis of native arteries of right leg extremities with ulceration of toe

I70.238 **Atherosclerosis of native arteries of right leg with ulceration of other part of lower leg** [HCC]

I70.239 **Atherosclerosis of native arteries of right leg with ulceration of unspecified site** [HCC]

I70.24 **Atherosclerosis of native arteries of left leg with ulceration**

Includes: any condition classifiable to I70.212 and I70.222

chronic limb-threatening ischemia of native arteries of left leg with ulceration

critical limb ischemia of native arteries of left leg with ulceration`

Use Additional Code to identify severity of ulcer (L97.-)

I70.241 **Atherosclerosis of native arteries of left leg with ulceration of thigh** [HCC]

I70.242 Atherosclerosis of native arteries of left leg with ulceration of calf [HCC]

I70.243 Atherosclerosis of native arteries of left leg with ulceration of ankle [HCC]

I70.244 Atherosclerosis of native arteries of left leg with ulceration of heel and midfoot [HCC]

Atherosclerosis of native arteries of left leg with ulceration of plantar surface of midfoot

I70.245 Atherosclerosis of native arteries of left leg with ulceration of other part of foot [HCC]

Atherosclerosis of native arteries of left leg extremities with ulceration of toe

I70.248 Atherosclerosis of native arteries of left leg with ulceration of other part of lower leg [HCC]

I70.249 Atherosclerosis of native arteries of left leg with ulceration of unspecified site [HCC]

I70.25 Atherosclerosis of native arteries of other extremities with ulceration

Includes: any condition classifiable to I70.218 and I70.228

Use Additional Code to identify the severity of the ulcer (L98.49-)

I70.26 Atherosclerosis of native arteries of extremities with gangrene [HCC]

Includes: any condition classifiable to I70.21-, I70.22-, I70.23-, I70.24-, and I70.25-

chronic limb-threatening ischemia of native arteries of extremities with gangrene

critical limb ischemia of native arteries of extremities with gangrene

Use Additional Code to identify the severity of any ulcer (L97.-, L98.49-), if applicable

I70.261 Atherosclerosis of native arteries of extremities with gangrene, right leg [HCC]

I70.262 Atherosclerosis of native arteries of extremities with gangrene, left leg [HCC]

I70.263 Atherosclerosis of native arteries of extremities with gangrene, bilateral legs [HCC]

I70.268 Atherosclerosis of native arteries of extremities with gangrene, other extremity [HCC]

I70.269 Atherosclerosis of native arteries of extremities with gangrene, unspecified extremity [HCC]

I70.29 Other atherosclerosis of native arteries of extremities

I70.291 Other atherosclerosis of native arteries of extremities, right leg [HCC]

I70.292 Other atherosclerosis of native arteries of extremities, left leg [HCC]

I70.293 Other atherosclerosis of native arteries of extremities, bilateral legs [HCC]

I70.298 Other atherosclerosis of native arteries of extremities, other extremity [HCC]

I70.299 Other atherosclerosis of native arteries of extremities, unspecified extremity [HCC]

I70.3 Atherosclerosis of unspecified type of bypass graft(s) of the extremities

Use Additional Code, if applicable, to identify chronic total occlusion of artery of extremity (I70.92)

Excludes1: embolism or thrombus of bypass graft(s) of extremities (T82.8-)

I70.30 Unspecified atherosclerosis of unspecified type of bypass graft(s) of the extremities [HCC]

I70.301 Unspecified atherosclerosis of unspecified type of bypass graft(s) of the extremities, right leg [HCC]

I70.302 Unspecified atherosclerosis of unspecified type of bypass graft(s) of the extremities, left leg [HCC]

I70.303 Unspecified atherosclerosis of unspecified type of bypass graft(s) of the extremities, bilateral legs [HCC]

I70.308 Unspecified atherosclerosis of unspecified type of bypass graft(s) of the extremities, other extremity [HCC]

I70.309 Unspecified atherosclerosis of unspecified type of bypass graft(s) of the extremities, unspecified extremity [HCC]

I70.31 Atherosclerosis of unspecified type of bypass graft(s) of the extremities with intermittent claudication

I70.311 Atherosclerosis of unspecified type of bypass graft(s) of the extremities with intermittent claudication, right leg [HCC]

I70.312 Atherosclerosis of unspecified type of bypass graft(s) of the extremities with intermittent claudication, left leg

I70.313 Atherosclerosis of unspecified type of bypass graft(s) of the extremities with intermittent claudication, bilateral legs [HCC]

I70.318 Atherosclerosis of unspecified type of bypass graft(s) of the extremities with intermittent claudication, other extremity [HCC]

I70.319 Atherosclerosis of unspecified type of bypass graft(s) of the extremities with intermittent claudication, unspecified extremity [HCC]

I70.32 Atherosclerosis of unspecified type of bypass graft(s) of the extremities with rest pain

Includes: any condition classifiable to I70.31-

chronic limb-threatening ischemia NOS of unspecified type of bypass graft(s) of the extremities

chronic limb-threatening ischemia of unspecified type of bypass graft(s) of the extremities with rest pain, right leg

critical limb ischemia NOS of unspecified type of bypass graft(s) of the extremities

critical limb ischemia of unspecified type of bypass graft(s) of the extremities with rest pain

I70.321 Atherosclerosis of unspecified type of bypass graft(s) of the extremities with rest pain, right leg [HCC]

● New code   ▲ Revised code   Excludes1: Not coded here   Excludes2: Not included here   ⊗ Placeholder required   ⑦7th digit required

I70.322   **Atherosclerosis of unspecified type of bypass graft(s) of the extremities with rest pain, left leg** [HCC]

I70.323   **Atherosclerosis of unspecified type of bypass graft(s) of the extremities with rest pain, bilateral legs** [HCC]

I70.328   **Atherosclerosis of unspecified type of bypass graft(s) of the extremities with rest pain, other extremity** [HCC]

I70.329   **Atherosclerosis of unspecified type of bypass graft(s) of the extremities with rest pain, unspecified extremity** [HCC]

I70.33   **Atherosclerosis of unspecified type of bypass graft(s) of the right leg with ulceration**

> **Includes:** any condition classifiable to I70.311 and I70.321
>
> chronic limb-threatening ischemia of unspecified type of bypass graft(s) of the right leg with ulceration
>
> critical limb ischemia of unspecified type of bypass graft(s) of the right leg with ulceration
>
> **Use Additional Code** to identify severity of ulcer (L97.-)

I70.331   **Atherosclerosis of unspecified type of bypass graft(s) of the right leg with ulceration of thigh** [HCC]

I70.332   **Atherosclerosis of unspecified type of bypass graft(s) of the right leg with ulceration of calf** [HCC]

I70.333   **Atherosclerosis of unspecified type of bypass graft(s) of the right leg with ulceration of ankle** [HCC]

I70.334   **Atherosclerosis of unspecified type of bypass graft(s) of the right leg with ulceration of heel and midfoot** [HCC]

> Atherosclerosis of unspecified type of bypass graft(s) of right leg with ulceration of plantar surface of midfoot

I70.335   **Atherosclerosis of unspecified type of bypass graft(s) of the right leg with ulceration of other part of foot** [HCC]

> Atherosclerosis of unspecified type of bypass graft(s) of the right leg with ulceration of toe

I70.338   **Atherosclerosis of unspecified type of bypass graft(s) of the right leg with ulceration of other part of lower leg** [HCC]

I70.339   **Atherosclerosis of unspecified type of bypass graft(s) of the right leg with ulceration of unspecified site** [HCC]

I70.34   **Atherosclerosis of unspecified type of bypass graft(s) of the left leg with ulceration**

> **Includes:** any condition classifiable to I70.312 and I70.322
>
> **Includes:** chronic limb-threatening ischemia of unspecified type of bypass graft(s) of the left leg with ulceration
>
> critical limb ischemia of unspecified type of bypass graft(s) of the left leg with ulceration
>
> **Use Additional Code** to identify severity of ulcer (L97.-)

I70.341   **Atherosclerosis of unspecified type of bypass graft(s) of the left leg with ulceration of thigh** [HCC]

I70.342   **Atherosclerosis of unspecified type of bypass graft(s) of the left leg with ulceration of calf** [HCC]

I70.343   **Atherosclerosis of unspecified type of bypass graft(s) of the left leg with ulceration of ankle** [HCC]

I70.344   **Atherosclerosis of unspecified type of bypass graft(s) of the left leg with ulceration of heel and midfoot** [HCC]

> Atherosclerosis of unspecified type of bypass graft(s) of left leg with ulceration of plantar surface of midfoot

I70.345   **Atherosclerosis of unspecified type of bypass graft(s) of the left leg with ulceration of other part of foot** [HCC]

> Atherosclerosis of unspecified type of bypass graft(s) of the left leg with ulceration of toe

I70.348   **Atherosclerosis of unspecified type of bypass graft(s) of the left leg with ulceration of other part of lower leg** [HCC]

I70.349   **Atherosclerosis of unspecified type of bypass graft(s) of the left leg with ulceration of unspecified site** [HCC]

I70.35   **Atherosclerosis of unspecified type of bypass graft(s) of other extremity with ulceration** [HCC]

> **Includes:** any condition classifiable to I70.318 and I70.328
>
> **Use Additional Code** to identify severity of ulcer (L98.49-)

I70.36   **Atherosclerosis of unspecified type of bypass graft(s) of the extremities with gangrene**

> **Includes:** any condition classifiable to I70.31-, I70.32-, I70.33-, I70.34-, I70.35
>
> chronic limb-threatening ischemia of unspecified type of bypass graft(s) of the extremities with gangrene
>
> critical limb ischemia of unspecified type of bypass graft(s) of the extremities with gangrene
>
> **Use Additional Code** to identify the severity of any ulcer (L97.-, L98.49-), if applicable

I70.361   **Atherosclerosis of unspecified type of bypass graft(s) of the extremities with gangrene, right leg** [HCC]

I70.362   **Atherosclerosis of unspecified type of bypass graft(s) of the extremities with gangrene, left leg** [HCC]

I70.363   **Atherosclerosis of unspecified type of bypass graft(s) of the extremities with gangrene, bilateral legs** [HCC]

I70.368   **Atherosclerosis of unspecified type of bypass graft(s) of the extremities with gangrene, other extremity** [HCC]

I70.369   **Atherosclerosis of unspecified type of bypass graft(s) of the extremities with gangrene, unspecified extremity** [HCC]

I70.39   **Other atherosclerosis of unspecified type of bypass graft(s) of the extremities**

I70.391   **Other atherosclerosis of unspecified type of bypass graft(s) of the extremities, right leg** [HCC]

I70.392   **Other atherosclerosis of unspecified type of bypass graft(s) of the extremities, left leg** [HCC]

I70.393 **Other atherosclerosis of unspecified type of bypass graft(s) of the extremities, bilateral legs** [HCC]

I70.398 **Other atherosclerosis of unspecified type of bypass graft(s) of the extremities, other extremity** [HCC]

I70.399 **Other atherosclerosis of unspecified type of bypass graft(s) of the extremities, unspecified extremity**

I70.4 **Atherosclerosis of autologous vein bypass graft(s) of the extremities**

Use Additional Code, if applicable, to identify chronic total occlusion of artery of extremity (I70.92)

I70.40 **Unspecified atherosclerosis of autologous vein bypass graft(s) of the extremities** [HCC]

I70.401 **Unspecified atherosclerosis of autologous vein bypass graft(s) of the extremities, right leg** [HCC]

I70.402 **Unspecified atherosclerosis of autologous vein bypass graft(s) of the extremities, left leg** [HCC]

I70.403 **Unspecified atherosclerosis of autologous vein bypass graft(s) of the extremities, bilateral legs** [HCC]

I70.408 **Unspecified atherosclerosis of autologous vein bypass graft(s) of the extremities, other extremity** [HCC]

I70.409 **Unspecified atherosclerosis of autologous vein bypass graft(s) of the extremities, unspecified extremity** [HCC]

I70.41 **Atherosclerosis of autologous vein bypass graft(s) of the extremities with intermittent claudication**

I70.411 **Atherosclerosis of autologous vein bypass graft(s) of the extremities with intermittent claudication, right leg** [HCC]

I70.412 **Atherosclerosis of autologous vein bypass graft(s) of the extremities with intermittent claudication, left leg** [HCC]

I70.413 **Atherosclerosis of autologous vein bypass graft(s) of the extremities with intermittent claudication, bilateral legs** [HCC]

I70.418 **Atherosclerosis of autologous vein bypass graft(s) of the extremities with intermittent claudication, other extremity** [HCC]

I70.419 **Atherosclerosis of autologous vein bypass graft(s) of the extremities with intermittent claudication, unspecified extremity** [HCC]

I70.42 **Atherosclerosis of autologous vein bypass graft(s) of the extremities with rest pain**

Includes: any condition classifiable to I70.41-

chronic limb-threatening ischemia NOS of autologous vein bypass graft(s) of the extremities

chronic limb-threatening ischemia of autologous vein bypass graft(s) of the extremities with rest pain

critical limb ischemia NOS of autologous vein bypass graft(s) of the extremities

critical limb ischemia of autologous vein bypass graft(s) of the extremities with rest pain

I70.421 **Atherosclerosis of autologous vein bypass graft(s) of the extremities with rest pain, right leg** [HCC]

I70.422 **Atherosclerosis of autologous vein bypass graft(s) of the extremities with rest pain, left leg** [HCC]

I70.423 **Atherosclerosis of autologous vein bypass graft(s) of the extremities with rest pain, bilateral legs** [HCC]

I70.428 **Atherosclerosis of autologous vein bypass graft(s) of the extremities with rest pain, other extremity** [HCC]

I70.429 **Atherosclerosis of autologous vein bypass graft(s) of the extremities with rest pain, unspecified extremity** [HCC]

I70.43 **Atherosclerosis of autologous vein bypass graft(s) of the right leg with ulceration**

Includes: any condition classifiable to I70.411 and I70.421

Use Additional Code to identify severity of ulcer (L97.-)

Includes: chronic limb-threatening ischemia of autologous vein bypass graft(s) of the right leg with ulceration

critical limb ischemia of autologous vein bypass graft(s) of the right leg with ulceration

I70.431 **Atherosclerosis of autologous vein bypass graft(s) of the right leg with ulceration of thigh** [HCC]

I70.432 **Atherosclerosis of autologous vein bypass graft(s) of the right leg with ulceration of calf**

I70.433 **Atherosclerosis of autologous vein bypass graft(s) of the right leg with ulceration of ankle** [HCC]

I70.434 **Atherosclerosis of autologous vein bypass graft(s) of the right leg with ulceration of heel and midfoot** [HCC]

Atherosclerosis of autologous vein bypass graft(s) of right leg with ulceration of plantar surface of midfoot

I70.435 **Atherosclerosis of autologous vein bypass graft(s) of the right leg with ulceration of other part of foot** [HCC]

Atherosclerosis of autologous vein bypass graft(s) of right leg with ulceration of toe

I70.438 **Atherosclerosis of autologous vein bypass graft(s) of the right leg with ulceration of other part of lower leg** [HCC]

I70.439 **Atherosclerosis of autologous vein bypass graft(s) of the right leg with ulceration of unspecified site** [HCC]

I70.44 **Atherosclerosis of autologous vein bypass graft(s) of the left leg with ulceration**

Includes: any condition classifiable to I70.412 and I70.422

chronic limb-threatening ischemia of autologous vein bypass graft(s) of the left leg with ulceration

● New code ▲ Revised code **Excludes1:** Not coded here **Excludes2:** Not included here ⊗ Placeholder required ⑦ 7th digit required

critical limb ischemia of autologous vein bypass graft(s) of the left leg with ulceration

Use Additional Code to identify severity of ulcer (L97.-)

I70.441 **Atherosclerosis of autologous vein bypass graft(s) of the left leg with ulceration of thigh** [HCC]

I70.442 **Atherosclerosis of autologous vein bypass graft(s) of the left leg with ulceration of calf** [HCC]

I70.443 **Atherosclerosis of autologous vein bypass graft(s) of the left leg with ulceration of ankle** [HCC]

I70.444 **Atherosclerosis of autologous vein bypass graft(s) of the left leg with ulceration of heel and midfoot** [HCC]

Atherosclerosis of autologous vein bypass graft(s) of left leg with ulceration of plantar surface of midfoot

I70.445 **Atherosclerosis of autologous vein bypass graft(s) of the left leg with ulceration of other part of foot** [HCC]

Atherosclerosis of autologous vein bypass graft(s) of left leg with ulceration of toe

I70.448 **Atherosclerosis of autologous vein bypass graft(s) of the left leg with ulceration of other part of lower leg** [HCC]

I70.449 **Atherosclerosis of autologous vein bypass graft(s) of the left leg with ulceration of unspecified site** [HCC]

I70.45 **Atherosclerosis of autologous vein bypass graft(s) of other extremity with ulceration** [HCC]

Includes: any condition classifiable to I70.418, I70.428, and I70.438

Use Additional Code to identify severity of ulcer (L98.49)

I70.46 **Atherosclerosis of autologous vein bypass graft(s) of the extremities with gangrene**

Includes: any condition classifiable to I70.41-, I70.42-, and I70.43-, I70.44-, I70.45

chronic limb-threatening ischemia of autologous vein bypass graft(s) of the extremities with gangrene

critical limb ischemia of autologous vein bypass graft(s) of the extremities with gangrene

Use Additional Code to identify the severity of any ulcer (L97.-, L98.49-), if applicable

I70.461 **Atherosclerosis of autologous vein bypass graft(s) of the extremities with gangrene, right leg** [HCC]

I70.462 **Atherosclerosis of autologous vein bypass graft(s) of the extremities with gangrene, left leg** [HCC]

I70.463 **Atherosclerosis of autologous vein bypass graft(s) of the extremities with gangrene, bilateral legs** [HCC]

I70.468 **Atherosclerosis of autologous vein bypass graft(s) of the extremities with gangrene, other extremity** [HCC]

I70.469 **Atherosclerosis of autologous vein bypass graft(s) of the extremities**

with gangrene, unspecified extremity [HCC]

I70.49 **Other atherosclerosis of autologous vein bypass graft(s) of the extremities**

I70.491 **Other atherosclerosis of autologous vein bypass graft(s) of the extremities, right leg** [HCC]

I70.492 **Other atherosclerosis of autologous vein bypass graft(s) of the extremities, left leg** [HCC]

I70.493 **Other atherosclerosis of autologous vein bypass graft(s) of the extremities, bilateral legs** [HCC]

I70.498 **Other atherosclerosis of autologous vein bypass graft(s) of the extremities, other extremity** [HCC]

I70.499 **Other atherosclerosis of autologous vein bypass graft(s) of the extremities, unspecified extremity** [HCC]

I70.5 **Atherosclerosis of nonautologous biological bypass graft(s) of the extremities**

Use Additional Code, if applicable, to identify chronic total occlusion of artery of extremity (I70.92)

I70.50 **Unspecified atherosclerosis of nonautologous biological bypass graft(s) of the extremities** [HCC]

I70.501 **Unspecified atherosclerosis of nonautologous biological bypass graft(s) of the extremities, right leg** [HCC]

I70.502 **Unspecified atherosclerosis of nonautologous biological bypass graft(s) of the extremities, left leg** [HCC]

I70.503 **Unspecified atherosclerosis of nonautologous biological bypass graft(s) of the extremities, bilateral legs** [HCC]

I70.508 **Unspecified atherosclerosis of nonautologous biological bypass graft(s) of the extremities, other extremity** [HCC]

I70.509 **Unspecified atherosclerosis of nonautologous biological bypass graft(s) of the extremities, unspecified extremity** [HCC]

I70.51 **Atherosclerosis of nonautologous biological bypass graft(s) of the extremities intermittent claudication**

I70.511 **Atherosclerosis of nonautologous biological bypass graft(s) of the extremities with intermittent claudication, right leg** [HCC]

I70.512 **Atherosclerosis of nonautologous biological bypass graft(s) of the extremities with intermittent claudication, left leg** [HCC]

I70.513 **Atherosclerosis of nonautologous biological bypass graft(s) of the extremities with intermittent claudication, bilateral legs** [HCC]

I70.518 **Atherosclerosis of nonautologous biological bypass graft(s) of the extremities with intermittent claudication, other extremity** [HCC]

I70.519 **Atherosclerosis of nonautologous biological bypass graft(s) of the extremities with intermittent**

claudication, unspecified extremity [HCC]

I70.52 **Atherosclerosis of nonautologous biological bypass graft(s) of the extremities with rest pain**

Includes: any condition classifiable to I70.51-

Includes: chronic limb-threatening ischemia NOS of nonautologous biological bypass graft(s) of the extremities

chronic limb-threatening ischemia of nonautologous biological bypass graft(s) of the extremities with rest pain

critical limb ischemia NOS of nonautologous biological bypass graft(s) of the extremities

critical limb ischemia of nonautologous biological bypass graft(s) of the extremities with rest pain

I70.521 **Atherosclerosis of nonautologous biological bypass graft(s) of the extremities with rest pain, right leg** [HCC]

I70.522 **Atherosclerosis of nonautologous biological bypass graft(s) of the extremities with rest pain, left leg** [HCC]

I70.523 **Atherosclerosis of nonautologous biological bypass graft(s) of the extremities with rest pain, bilateral legs** [HCC]

I70.528 **Atherosclerosis of nonautologous biological bypass graft(s) of the extremities with rest pain, other extremity** [HCC]

I70.529 **Atherosclerosis of nonautologous biological bypass graft(s) of the extremities with rest pain, unspecified extremity** [HCC]

I70.53 **Atherosclerosis of nonautologous biological bypass graft(s) of the right leg with ulceration**

Includes: any condition classifiable to I70.511 and I70.521

chronic limb-threatening ischemia of nonautologous biological bypass graft(s) of the right leg with ulceration

critical limb ischemia of nonautologous biological bypass graft(s) of the right leg with ulceration

Use Additional Code to identify severity of ulcer (L97.-)

I70.531 **Atherosclerosis of nonautologous biological bypass graft(s) of the right leg with ulceration of thigh** [HCC]

I70.532 **Atherosclerosis of nonautologous biological bypass graft(s) of the right leg with ulceration of calf** [HCC]

I70.533 **Atherosclerosis of nonautologous biological bypass graft(s) of the right leg with ulceration of ankle** [HCC]

I70.534 **Atherosclerosis of nonautologous biological bypass graft(s) of the right leg with ulceration of heel and midfoot** [HCC]

Atherosclerosis of nonautologous biological bypass graft(s) of right leg with ulceration of plantar surface of midfoot

I70.535 **Atherosclerosis of nonautologous biological bypass graft(s) of the right leg with ulceration of other part of foot** [HCC]

Atherosclerosis of nonautologous biological bypass graft(s) of the right leg with ulceration of toe

I70.538 **Atherosclerosis of nonautologous biological bypass graft(s) of the right leg with ulceration of other part of lower leg** [HCC]

I70.539 **Atherosclerosis of nonautologous biological bypass graft(s) of the right leg with ulceration of unspecified site** [HCC]

I70.54 **Atherosclerosis of nonautologous biological bypass graft(s) of the left leg with ulceration**

Includes: any condition classifiable to I70.512 and I70.522

chronic limb-threatening ischemia of nonautologous biological bypass graft(s) of the left leg with ulceration

critical limb ischemia of nonautologous biological bypass graft(s) of the left leg with ulceration

Use Additional Code to identify severity of ulcer (L97.-)

I70.541 **Atherosclerosis of nonautologous biological bypass graft(s) of the left leg with ulceration of thigh** [HCC]

I70.542 **Atherosclerosis of nonautologous biological bypass graft(s) of the left leg with ulceration of calf** [HCC]

I70.543 **Atherosclerosis of nonautologous biological bypass graft(s) of the left leg with ulceration of ankle** [HCC]

I70.544 **Atherosclerosis of nonautologous biological bypass graft(s) of the left leg with ulceration of heel and midfoot** [HCC]

Atherosclerosis of nonautologous biological bypass graft(s) of left leg with ulceration of plantar surface of midfoot

I70.545 **Atherosclerosis of nonautologous biological bypass graft(s) of the left leg with ulceration of other part of foot** [HCC]

Atherosclerosis of nonautologous biological bypass graft(s) of the left leg with ulceration of toe

I70.548 **Atherosclerosis of nonautologous biological bypass graft(s) of the left leg with ulceration of other part of lower leg** [HCC]

I70.549 **Atherosclerosis of nonautologous biological bypass graft(s) of the left leg with ulceration of unspecified site** [HCC]

I70.55 **Atherosclerosis of nonautologous biological bypass graft(s) of other extremity with ulceration** [HCC]

Includes: any condition classifiable to I70.518, I70.528, and I70.538

Use Additional Code to identify severity of ulcer (L98.49)

I70.56 **Atherosclerosis of nonautologous biological bypass graft(s) of the extremities with gangrene**

● New code ▲ Revised code Excludes1: Not coded here Excludes2: Not included here ⊗ Placeholder required ⑦7th digit required

Includes: any condition classifiable to I70.51-, I70.52-, and I70.53-, I70.54-, I70.55

chronic limb-threatening ischemia of nonautologous biological bypass graft(s) of the extremities with gangrene

critical limb ischemia of nonautologous biological bypass graft(s) of the extremities with gangrene

Use Additional Code to identify the severity of any ulcer (L97.-, L98.49-), if applicable

I70.561 **Atherosclerosis of nonautologous biological bypass graft(s) of the extremities with gangrene, right leg** [HCC]

I70.562 **Atherosclerosis of nonautologous biological bypass graft(s) of the extremities with gangrene, left leg** [HCC]

I70.563 **Atherosclerosis of nonautologous biological bypass graft(s) of the extremities with gangrene, bilateral legs** [HCC]

I70.568 **Atherosclerosis of nonautologous biological bypass graft(s) of the extremities with gangrene, other extremity** [HCC]

I70.569 **Atherosclerosis of nonautologous biological bypass graft(s) of the extremities with gangrene, unspecified extremity** [HCC]

I70.59 **Other atherosclerosis of nonautologous biological bypass graft(s) of the extremities**

I70.591 **Other atherosclerosis of nonautologous biological bypass graft(s) of the extremities, right leg** [HCC]

I70.592 **Other atherosclerosis of nonautologous biological bypass graft(s) of the extremities, left leg** [HCC]

I70.593 **Other atherosclerosis of nonautologous biological bypass graft(s) of the extremities, bilateral legs** [HCC]

I70.598 **Other atherosclerosis of nonautologous biological bypass graft(s) of the extremities, other extremity** [HCC]

I70.599 **Other atherosclerosis of nonautologous biological bypass graft(s) of the extremities, unspecified extremity** [HCC]

I70.6 **Atherosclerosis of nonbiological bypass graft(s) of the extremities**

Use Additional Code, if applicable, to identify chronic total occlusion of artery of extremity (I70.92)

I70.60 **Unspecified atherosclerosis of nonbiological bypass graft(s) of the extremities** [HCC]

I70.601 **Unspecified atherosclerosis of nonbiological bypass graft(s) of the extremities, right leg**

I70.602 **Unspecified atherosclerosis of nonbiological bypass graft(s) of the extremities, left leg** [HCC]

I70.603 **Unspecified atherosclerosis of nonbiological bypass graft(s) of the extremities, bilateral legs** [HCC]

I70.608 **Unspecified atherosclerosis of nonbiological bypass graft(s) of the extremities, other extremity** [HCC]

I70.609 **Unspecified atherosclerosis of nonbiological bypass graft(s) of the extremities, unspecified extremity** [HCC]

I70.61 **Atherosclerosis of nonbiological bypass graft(s) of the extremities with intermittent claudication**

I70.611 **Atherosclerosis of nonbiological bypass graft(s) of the extremities with intermittent claudication, right leg** [HCC]

I70.612 **Atherosclerosis of nonbiological bypass graft(s) of the extremities with intermittent claudication, left leg** [HCC]

I70.613 **Atherosclerosis of nonbiological bypass graft(s) of the extremities with intermittent claudication, bilateral legs** [HCC]

I70.618 **Atherosclerosis of nonbiological bypass graft(s) of the extremities with intermittent claudication, other extremity** [HCC]

I70.619 **Atherosclerosis of nonbiological bypass graft(s) of the extremities with intermittent claudication, unspecified extremity** [HCC]

I70.62 **Atherosclerosis of nonbiological bypass graft(s) of the extremities with rest pain**

Includes: any condition classifiable to I70.61-

chronic limb-threatening ischemia NOS of nonbiological bypass graft(s) of the extremities

chronic limb-threatening ischemia of nonbiological bypass graft(s) of the extremities with rest pain

critical limb ischemia NOS of nonbiological bypass graft(s) of the extremities

critical limb ischemia of nonbiological bypass graft(s) of the extremities with rest pain

I70.621 **Atherosclerosis of nonbiological bypass graft(s) of the extremities with rest pain, right leg** [HCC]

I70.622 **Atherosclerosis of nonbiological bypass graft(s) of the extremities with rest pain, left leg** [HCC]

I70.623 **Atherosclerosis of nonbiological bypass graft(s) of the extremities with rest pain, bilateral legs** [HCC]

I70.628 **Atherosclerosis of nonbiological bypass graft(s) of the extremities with rest pain, other extremity** [HCC]

I70.629 **Atherosclerosis of nonbiological bypass graft(s) of the extremities with rest pain, unspecified extremity** [HCC]

I70.63 **Atherosclerosis of nonbiological bypass graft(s) of the right leg with ulceration**

Includes: any condition classifiable to I70.611 and I70.621

chronic limb-threatening ischemia of nonbiological bypass graft(s) of the right leg with ulceration critical limb ischemia of nonbiological bypass graft(s) of the right leg with ulceration

Use Additional Code to identify severity of ulcer (L97.-)

I70.631 **Atherosclerosis of nonbiological bypass graft(s) of the right leg with ulceration of thigh** [HCC]

I70.632 **Atherosclerosis of nonbiological bypass graft(s) of the right leg with ulceration of calf** [HCC]

I70.633 **Atherosclerosis of nonbiological bypass graft(s) of the right leg with ulceration of ankle** [HCC]

I70.634 **Atherosclerosis of nonbiological bypass graft(s) of the right leg with ulceration of heel and midfoot** [HCC]

Atherosclerosis of nonbiological bypass graft(s) of right leg with ulceration of plantar surface of midfoot

I70.635 **Atherosclerosis of nonbiological bypass graft(s) of the right leg with ulceration of other part of foot** [HCC]

Atherosclerosis of nonbiological bypass graft(s) of the right leg with ulceration of toe

I70.638 **Atherosclerosis of nonbiological bypass graft(s) of the right leg with ulceration of other part of lower leg** [HCC]

I70.639 **Atherosclerosis of nonbiological bypass graft(s) of the right leg with ulceration of unspecified site** [HCC]

I70.64 **Atherosclerosis of nonbiological bypass graft(s) of the left leg with ulceration**

Includes: any condition classifiable to I70.612 and I70.622

chronic limb-threatening ischemia of nonbiological bypass graft(s) of the left leg with ulceration

critical limb ischemia of nonbiological bypass graft(s) of the left leg with ulceration

Use Additional Code to identify severity of ulcer (L97.-)

I70.641 **Atherosclerosis of nonbiological bypass graft(s) of the left leg with ulceration of thigh** [HCC]

I70.642 **Atherosclerosis of nonbiological bypass graft(s) of the left leg with ulceration of calf** [HCC]

I70.643 **Atherosclerosis of nonbiological bypass graft(s) of the left leg with ulceration of ankle** [HCC]

I70.644 **Atherosclerosis of nonbiological bypass graft(s) of the left leg with ulceration of heel and midfoot** [HCC]

Atherosclerosis of nonbiological bypass graft(s) of left leg with ulceration of plantar surface of midfoot

I70.645 **Atherosclerosis of nonbiological bypass graft(s) of the left leg with ulceration of other part of foot** [HCC]

Atherosclerosis of nonbiological bypass graft(s) of the left leg with ulceration of toe

I70.648 **Atherosclerosis of nonbiological bypass graft(s) of the left leg with ulceration of other part of lower leg** [HCC]

I70.649 **Atherosclerosis of nonbiological bypass graft(s) of the left leg with ulceration of unspecified site** [HCC]

I70.65 **Atherosclerosis of nonbiological bypass graft(s) of other extremity with ulceration** [HCC]

Includes: any condition classifiable to I70.618 and I70.628

Use Additional Code to identify severity of ulcer (L98.49)

I70.66 **Atherosclerosis of nonbiological bypass graft(s) of the extremities with gangrene**

Includes: any condition classifiable to I70.61-, I70.62-, I70.63-, I70.64-, I70.65

chronic limb-threatening ischemia of nonbiological bypass graft(s) of the extremities with gangrene

critical limb ischemia of nonbiological bypass graft(s) of the extremities with gangrene

Use Additional Code to identify the severity of any ulcer (L97.-, L98.49-), if applicable

I70.661 **Atherosclerosis of nonbiological bypass graft(s) of the extremities with gangrene, right leg** [HCC]

I70.662 **Atherosclerosis of nonbiological bypass graft(s) of the extremities with gangrene, left leg** [HCC]

I70.663 **Atherosclerosis of nonbiological bypass graft(s) of the extremities with gangrene, bilateral legs** [HCC]

I70.668 **Atherosclerosis of nonbiological bypass graft(s) of the extremities with gangrene, other extremity** [HCC]

I70.669 **Atherosclerosis of nonbiological bypass graft(s) of the extremities with gangrene, unspecified extremity** [HCC]

I70.69 **Other atherosclerosis of nonbiological bypass graft(s) of the extremities**

I70.691 **Other atherosclerosis of nonbiological bypass graft(s) of the extremities, right leg**

I70.692 **Other atherosclerosis of nonbiological bypass graft(s) of the extremities, left leg** [HCC]

I70.693 **Other atherosclerosis of nonbiological bypass graft(s) of the extremities, bilateral legs** [HCC]

I70.698 **Other atherosclerosis of nonbiological bypass graft(s) of the extremities, other extremity** [HCC]

I70.699 **Other atherosclerosis of nonbiological bypass graft(s) of the extremities, unspecified extremity** [HCC]

I70.7 **Atherosclerosis of other type of bypass graft(s) of the extremities**

Use Additional Code, if applicable, to identify chronic total occlusion of artery of extremity (I70.92)

I70.70 **Unspecified atherosclerosis of other type of bypass graft(s) of the extremities** [HCC]

I70.701   Unspecified atherosclerosis of other type of bypass graft(s) of the extremities, right leg [HCC]

I70.702   Unspecified atherosclerosis of other type of bypass graft(s) of the extremities, left leg [HCC]

I70.703   Unspecified atherosclerosis of other type of bypass graft(s) of the extremities, bilateral legs [HCC]

I70.708   Unspecified atherosclerosis of other type of bypass graft(s) of the extremities, other extremity [HCC]

I70.709   Unspecified atherosclerosis of other type of bypass graft(s) of the extremities, unspecified extremity [HCC]

I70.71   Atherosclerosis of other type of bypass graft(s) of the extremities with intermittent claudication

I70.711   Atherosclerosis of other type of bypass graft(s) of the extremities with intermittent claudication, right leg [HCC]

I70.712   Atherosclerosis of other type of bypass graft(s) of the extremities with intermittent claudication, left leg [HCC]

I70.713   Atherosclerosis of other type of bypass graft(s) of the extremities with intermittent claudication, bilateral legs [HCC]

I70.718   Atherosclerosis of other type of bypass graft(s) of the extremities with intermittent claudication, other extremity [HCC]

I70.719   Atherosclerosis of other type of bypass graft(s) of the extremities with intermittent claudication, unspecified extremity [HCC]

I70.72   Atherosclerosis of other type of bypass graft(s) of the extremities with rest pain

Includes: any condition classifiable to I70.71-

chronic limb-threatening ischemia NOS of other type of bypass graft(s) of the extremities

chronic limb-threatening ischemia of other type of bypass graft(s) of the extremities with rest pain

critical limb ischemia NOS of other type of bypass graft(s) of the extremities

critical limb ischemia of other type of bypass graft(s) of the extremities with rest pain

I70.721   Atherosclerosis of other type of bypass graft(s) of the extremities with rest pain, right leg [HCC]

I70.722   Atherosclerosis of other type of bypass graft(s) of the extremities with rest pain, left leg [HCC]

I70.723   Atherosclerosis of other type of bypass graft(s) of the extremities with rest pain, bilateral legs [HCC]

I70.728   Atherosclerosis of other type of bypass graft(s) of the extremities with rest pain, other extremity [HCC]

I70.729   Atherosclerosis of other type of bypass graft(s) of the extremities with rest pain, unspecified extremity [HCC]

I70.73   Atherosclerosis of other type of bypass graft(s) of the right leg with ulceration

Includes: any condition classifiable to I70.711 and I70.721

Includes: chronic limb-threatening ischemia of other type of bypass graft(s) of the right leg with ulceration

critical limb ischemia of other type of bypass graft(s) of the right leg with ulceration

Use Additional Code to identify severity of ulcer (L97.-)

I70.731   Atherosclerosis of other type of bypass graft(s) of the right leg with ulceration of thigh [HCC]

I70.732   Atherosclerosis of other type of bypass graft(s) of the right leg with ulceration of calf [HCC]

I70.733   Atherosclerosis of other type of bypass graft(s) of the right leg with ulceration of ankle [HCC]

I70.734   Atherosclerosis of other type of bypass graft(s) of the right leg with ulceration of heel and midfoot [HCC]

Atherosclerosis of other type of bypass graft(s) of right leg with ulceration of plantar surface of midfoot

I70.735   Atherosclerosis of other type of bypass graft(s) of the right leg with ulceration of other part of foot [HCC]

Atherosclerosis of other type of bypass graft(s) of right leg with ulceration of toe

I70.738   Atherosclerosis of other type of bypass graft(s) of the right leg with ulceration of other part of lower leg [HCC]

I70.739   Atherosclerosis of other type of bypass graft(s) of the right leg with ulceration of unspecified site [HCC]

I70.74   Atherosclerosis of other type of bypass graft(s) of the left leg with ulceration

Includes: any condition classifiable to I70.712 and I70.722

chronic limb-threatening ischemia of other type of bypass graft(s) of the left leg with ulceration

critical limb ischemia of other type of bypass graft(s) of the left leg with ulceration

Use Additional Code to identify severity of ulcer (L97.-)

I70.741   Atherosclerosis of other type of bypass graft(s) of the left leg with ulceration of thigh [HCC]

I70.742   Atherosclerosis of other type of bypass graft(s) of the left leg with ulceration of calf [HCC]

I70.743   Atherosclerosis of other type of bypass graft(s) of the left leg with ulceration of ankle [HCC]

I70.744   Atherosclerosis of other type of bypass graft(s) of the left leg with ulceration of heel and midfoot [HCC]

Atherosclerosis **of other** type of bypass graft(s) of left leg with ulceration of plantar surface of midfoot

I70.745 **Atherosclerosis of other type of bypass graft(s) of the left leg with ulceration of other part of foot** [HCC]

Atherosclerosis **of other** type of bypass graft(s) of left leg with ulceration of toe

I70.748 **Atherosclerosis of other type of bypass graft(s) of the left leg with ulceration of other part of lower leg** [HCC]

I70.749 **Atherosclerosis of other type of bypass graft(s) of the left leg with ulceration of unspecified site** [HCC]

I70.75 **Atherosclerosis of other type of bypass graft(s) of other extremity with ulceration** [HCC]

Includes: any condition classifiable to I70.718 and I70.728

Use Additional Code to identify severity of ulcer (L98.49)

I70.76 **Atherosclerosis of other type of bypass graft(s) of the extremities with gangrene**

Includes: any condition classifiable to I70.71-, I70.72-, I70.73-, I70.74-, I70.75

chronic limb-threatening ischemia of other type of bypass graft(s) of the extremities with gangrene

critical limb ischemia of other type of bypass graft(s) of the extremities with gangrene

Use Additional Code to identify the severity of any ulcer (L97.-, L98.49-), if applicable

I70.761 **Atherosclerosis of other type of bypass graft(s) of the extremities with gangrene, right leg** [HCC]

I70.762 **Atherosclerosis of other type of bypass graft(s) of the extremities with gangrene, left leg** [HCC]

I70.763 **Atherosclerosis of other type of bypass graft(s) of the extremities with gangrene, bilateral legs** [HCC]

I70.768 **Atherosclerosis of other type of bypass graft(s) of the extremities with gangrene, other extremity** [HCC]

I70.769 **Atherosclerosis of other type of bypass graft(s) of the extremities with gangrene, unspecified extremity** [HCC]

I70.79 **Other atherosclerosis of other type of bypass graft(s) of the extremities** [HCC]

I70.791 **Other atherosclerosis of other type of bypass graft(s) of the extremities, right leg** [HCC]

I70.792 **Other atherosclerosis of other type of bypass graft(s) of the extremities, left leg** [HCC]

I70.793 **Other atherosclerosis of other type of bypass graft(s) of the extremities, bilateral legs** [HCC]

I70.798 **Other atherosclerosis of other type of bypass graft(s) of the extremities, other extremity** [HCC]

I70.799 **Other atherosclerosis of other type of bypass graft(s) of the extremities, unspecified extremity** [HCC]

I70.8 **Atherosclerosis of other arteries**

I70.9 **Other and unspecified atherosclerosis**

I70.90 **Unspecified atherosclerosis**

I70.91 **Generalized atherosclerosis**

I70.92 **Chronic total occlusion of artery of the extremities** [HCC]

Complete occlusion of artery of the extremities

Total occlusion of artery of the extremities

Code first atherosclerosis of arteries of the extremities (I70.2-, I70.3-, I70.4-, I70.5-, I70.6-, I70.7-)

I71 **Aortic aneurysm and dissection**

Definition: Aortic aneurysm and dissection is a localized, abnormal and persistent dilation of a section of the aorta. This usually results from a weakness in the vessel wall. If severe enough, rupture of the aorta with severe hemorrhage is a potential hazard.

Excludes1: aortic ectasia (I77.81-)

syphilitic aortic aneurysm (A52.01)

traumatic aortic aneurysm (S25.09, S35.09)

I71.0 **Dissection of aorta**

I71.00 **Dissection of unspecified site of aorta** [HCC]

I71.01 **Dissection of thoracic aorta** [HCC]

I71.02 **Dissection of abdominal aorta** [HCC]

I71.03 **Dissection of thoracoabdominal aorta** [HCC]

I71.1 **Thoracic aortic aneurysm, ruptured** [HCC]

I71.2 **Thoracic aortic aneurysm, without rupture** [HCC]

I71.3 **Abdominal aortic aneurysm, ruptured** [HCC]

I71.4 **Abdominal aortic aneurysm, without rupture**

I71.5 **Thoracoabdominal aortic aneurysm, ruptured** [HCC]

I71.6 **Thoracoabdominal aortic aneurysm, without rupture** [HCC]

I71.8 **Aortic aneurysm of unspecified site, ruptured** [HCC]

Rupture of aorta NOS

I71.9 **Aortic aneurysm of unspecified site, without rupture** [HCC]

Aneurysm of aorta

Dilatation of aorta

Hyaline necrosis of aorta

I72 **Other aneurysm**

Includes: aneurysm (cirsoid) (false) (ruptured)

Excludes2: acquired aneurysm (I77.0)

aneurysm (of) aorta (I71.-)

aneurysm (of) arteriovenous NOS (Q27.3-)

carotid artery dissection (I77.71)

cerebral (nonruptured) aneurysm (I67.1)

coronary aneurysm (I25.4)

coronary artery dissection (I25.42)

dissection of artery NEC (I77.79)

dissection of precerebral artery, congenital (nonruptured) (Q28.1)

heart aneurysm (I25.3)

iliac artery dissection (I77.72)

pulmonary artery aneurysm (I28.1)

renal artery dissection (I77.73)

retinal aneurysm (H35.0)

ruptured cerebral aneurysm (I60.7)

varicose aneurysm (I77.0)

vertebral artery dissection (I77.74)

I72.0 **Aneurysm of carotid artery** [HCC]

Aneurysm of common carotid artery

Aneurysm of external carotid artery

Aneurysm of internal carotid artery, extracranial portion

Excludes1: aneurysm of internal carotid artery, intracranial portion (I67.1)

aneurysm of internal carotid artery NOS (I67.1)

I72.1   Aneurysm of artery of upper extremity [HCC]

I72.2   Aneurysm of renal artery [HCC]

I72.3   Aneurysm of iliac artery [HCC]

I72.4   Aneurysm of artery of lower extremity [HCC]

I72.5   Aneurysm of other precerebral arteries [HCC]

Aneurysm of basilar artery (trunk)

Excludes2: aneurysm of carotid artery (I72.0)

aneurysm of vertebral artery (I72.6)

dissection of carotid artery (I77.71)

dissection of other precerebral arteries (I77.75)

dissection of vertebral artery (I77.74)

I72.6   Aneurysm of vertebral artery [HCC]

Excludes2: dissection of vertebral artery (I77.74)

I72.8   Aneurysm of other specified arteries [HCC]

I72.9   Aneurysm of unspecified site [HCC]

I73   Other peripheral vascular diseases

Excludes2: chilblains (T69.1)

frostbite (T33-T34)

immersion hand or foot (T69.0-)

spasm of cerebral artery (G45.9)

I73.0   Raynaud's syndrome [HCC]

Raynaud's disease

Raynaud's phenomenon (secondary)

I73.00   Raynaud's syndrome without gangrene [HCC]

I73.01   Raynaud's syndrome with gangrene [HCC]

I73.1   Thromboangiitis obliterans [Buerger's disease] [HCC]

I73.8   Other specified peripheral vascular diseases

Excludes1: diabetic (peripheral) angiopathy (E08-E13 with .51-.52)

I73.81   Erythromelalgia [HCC]

I73.89   Other specified peripheral vascular diseases [HCC]

Acrocyanosis

Erythrocyanosis

Simple acroparesthesia [Schultze's type]

Vasomotor acroparesthesia [Nothnagel's type]

I73.9   Peripheral vascular disease, unspecified [HCC]

Intermittent claudication

Peripheral angiopathy NOS

Spasm of artery

Excludes1: atherosclerosis of the extremities (I70.2--I70.7-)

I74   Arterial embolism and thrombosis

Definition: An embolism is a sudden interruption in arterial blood flow to an organ or body extremity. The blockage is caused by a blood clot or foreign object. A Thrombosis is the formation or presence of a thrombus (a clot of coagulated blood) in a blood [HCC]

Includes: embolic infarction

embolic occlusion thrombotic infarction thrombotic occlusion

Code first embolism and thrombosis complicating abortion or ectopic or molar pregnancy (O00-O07, O08.2)

embolism and thrombosis complicating pregnancy, childbirth and the puerperium (O88.-)

Excludes2: atheroembolism (I75.-)

basilar embolism and thrombosis (I63.0-I63.2, I65.1)

carotid embolism and thrombosis (I63.0-I63.2, I65.2)

cerebral embolism and thrombosis (I63.3-I63.5, I66.-)

coronary embolism and thrombosis (I21-I25)

mesenteric embolism and thrombosis (K55.0-)

ophthalmic embolism and thrombosis (H34.-)

precerebral embolism and thrombosis NOS (I63.0-I63.2, I65.9)

pulmonary embolism and thrombosis (I26.-)

renal embolism and thrombosis (N28.0)

retinal embolism and thrombosis (H34.-)

septic embolism and thrombosis (I76)

vertebral embolism and thrombosis (I63.0-I63.2, I65.0)

I74.0   Embolism and thrombosis of abdominal aorta [HCC]

I74.01   Saddle embolus of abdominal aorta [HCC]

I74.09   Other arterial embolism and thrombosis of abdominal aorta [HCC]

Aortic bifurcation syndrome

Aortoiliac obstruction

Leriche's syndrome

I74.1   Embolism and thrombosis of other and unspecified parts of aorta

I74.10   Embolism and thrombosis of unspecified parts of aorta [HCC]

I74.11   Embolism and thrombosis of thoracic aorta [HCC]

I74.19   Embolism and thrombosis of other parts of aorta [HCC]

I74.2   Embolism and thrombosis of arteries of the upper extremities [HCC]

I74.3   Embolism and thrombosis of arteries of the lower extremities [HCC]

I74.4   Embolism and thrombosis of arteries of extremities, unspecified [HCC]

Peripheral arterial embolism NOS

I74.5   Embolism and thrombosis of iliac artery [HCC]

I74.8   Embolism and thrombosis of other arteries [HCC]

I74.9   Embolism and thrombosis of unspecified artery [HCC]

I75   Atheroembolism [HCC]

Includes: atherothrombotic microembolism

cholesterol embolism

I75.0   Atheroembolism of extremities [HCC]

I75.01   Atheroembolism of upper extremity [HCC]

I75.011   Atheroembolism of right upper extremity [HCC]

I75.012   Atheroembolism of left upper extremity [HCC]

I75.013   Atheroembolism of bilateral upper extremities [HCC]

I75.019   Atheroembolism of unspecified upper extremity [HCC]

I75.02   Atheroembolism of lower extremity [HCC]

I75.021   Atheroembolism of right lower extremity [HCC]

I75.022   Atheroembolism of left lower extremity [HCC]

I75.023   Atheroembolism of bilateral lower extremities [HCC]

I75.029   **Atheroembolism of unspecified lower extremity** [HCC]

I75.8   **Atheroembolism of other sites** [HCC]

    I75.81   **Atheroembolism of kidney** [HCC]

      Use Additional Code for any associated acute kidney failure and chronic kidney disease (N17.-, N18.-)

    I75.89   **Atheroembolism of other site** [HCC]

I76   **Septic arterial embolism** [HCC]

Code first underlying infection, such as:

infective endocarditis (I33.0)

lung abscess (J85.-)

Use Additional Code to identify the site of the embolism (I74.-)

Excludes2: septic pulmonary embolism (I26.01, I26.90)

I77   **Other disorders of arteries and arterioles**

Excludes2: collagen (vascular) diseases (M30-M36)

      hypersensitivity angiitis (M31.0)

      pulmonary artery (I28.-)

I77.0   **Arteriovenous fistula, acquired** [HCC]

Aneurysmal varix

Arteriovenous aneurysm, acquired

Excludes1: arteriovenous aneurysm NOS (Q27.3-)

      presence of arteriovenous shunt (fistula) for dialysis (Z99.2)

      traumatic - see injury of blood vessel by body region

Excludes2: cerebral (I67.1)

      coronary (I25.4)

I77.1   **Stricture of artery** [HCC]

Narrowing of artery

I77.2   **Rupture of artery** [HCC]

Erosion of artery

Fistula of artery

Ulcer of artery

Excludes1: traumatic rupture of artery - see injury of blood vessel by body region

I77.3   **Arterial fibromuscular dysplasia** [HCC]

Fibromuscular hyperplasia (of) carotid artery

Fibromuscular hyperplasia (of) renal artery

I77.4   **Celiac artery compression syndrome** [HCC]

I77.5   **Necrosis of artery** [HCC]

I77.6   **Arteritis, unspecified** [HCC]

Aortitis NOS

Endarteritis NOS

Excludes1: arteritis or endarteritis:

      aortic arch (M31.4)

      cerebral NEC (I67.7)

      coronary (I25.89)

      deformans (I70.-)

      giant cell (M31.5, M31.6)

      obliterans (I70.-)

      senile (I70.-)

I77.7   **Other arterial dissection**

Excludes2: dissection of aorta (I71.0-)

      dissection of coronary artery (I25.42)

    I77.70   **Dissection of unspecified artery** [HCC]

    I77.71   **Dissection of carotid artery** [HCC]

I77.72   **Dissection of iliac artery** [HCC]

I77.73   **Dissection of renal artery** [HCC]

I77.74   **Dissection of vertebral artery** [HCC]

      Excludes2: aneurysm of vertebral artery (I72.6)

I77.75   **Dissection of other precerebral arteries** [HCC]

Dissection of basilar artery (trunk)

      Excludes2: aneurysm of carotid artery (I72.0)

         aneurysm of other precerebral arteries (I72.5)

         aneurysm of vertebral artery (I72.6)

         dissection of carotid artery (I77.71)

         dissection of vertebral artery (I77.74)

I77.76   **Dissection of artery of upper extremity** [HCC]

I77.77   **Dissection of artery of lower extremity** [HCC]

I77.79   **Dissection of other specified artery** [HCC]

I77.8   **Other specified disorders of arteries and arterioles** [HCC]

    I77.81   **Aortic ectasia** [HCC]

Ectasis aorta

      Excludes1: aortic aneurysm and dissection (I71.0-)

    I77.810   **Thoracic aortic ectasia** [HCC]

    I77.811   **Abdominal aortic ectasia** [HCC]

    I77.812   **Thoracoabdominal aortic ectasia** [HCC]

    I77.819   **Aortic ectasia, unspecified site** [HCC]

    I77.89   **Other specified disorders of arteries and arterioles** [HCC]

I77.9   **Disorder of arteries and arterioles, unspecified** [HCC]

I78   **Diseases of capillaries**

I78.0   **Hereditary hemorrhagic telangiectasia** [HCC]

Rendu-Osler-Weber disease

I78.1   **Nevus, non-neoplastic**

Araneus nevus

Senile nevus

Spider nevus

Stellar nevus

Excludes1: nevus NOS (D22.-)

      vascular NOS (Q82.5)

Excludes2: blue nevus (D22.-)

      flammeus nevus (Q82.5)

      hairy nevus (D22.-)

      melanocytic nevus (D22.-)

      pigmented nevus (D22.-)

      port-wine nevus (Q82.5)

      sanguineous nevus (Q82.5)

      strawberry nevus (Q82.5)

      verrucous nevus (Q82.5)

I78.8   **Other diseases of capillaries**

I78.9   **Disease of capillaries, unspecified**

I79   **Disorders of arteries, arterioles and capillaries in diseases classified elsewhere**

I79.0   **Aneurysm of aorta in diseases classified elsewhere** [HCC]

Code first underlying disease

Excludes1: syphilitic aneurysm (A52.01)

I79.1   **Aortitis in diseases classified elsewhere** [HCC]

Code first underlying disease

Excludes1: syphilitic aortitis (A52.02)

   ● New code   ▲ Revised code   **Excludes1:** Not coded here   **Excludes2:** Not included here   ⊗ Placeholder required   ⑦7th digit required

I79.8 **Other disorders of arteries, arterioles and capillaries in diseases classified elsewhere** [HCC]

Code first underlying disease, such as:

amyloidosis (E85.-)

Excludes1: diabetic (peripheral) angiopathy (E08-E13 with .51-.52)

syphilitic endarteritis (A52.09)

tuberculous endarteritis (A18.89)

DISEASES OF VEINS, LYMPHATIC VESSELS AND LYMPH NODES, NOT ELSEWHERE CLASSIFIED (I80-I89)

I80 **Phlebitis and thrombophlebitis**

Includes: endophlebitis

inflammation, vein periphlebitis suppurative phlebitis

Code first phlebitis and thrombophlebitis complicating abortion, ectopic or molar pregnancy (O00-O07, O08.7)

phlebitis and thrombophlebitis complicating pregnancy, childbirth and the puerperium (O22.-, O87.-)

Excludes1: venous embolism and thrombosis of lower extremities (I82.4-, I82.5-, I82.81-)

I80.0 **Phlebitis and thrombophlebitis of superficial vessels of lower extremities**

Phlebitis and thrombophlebitis of femoropopliteal vein

I80.00 **Phlebitis and thrombophlebitis of superficial vessels of unspecified lower extremity**

I80.01 **Phlebitis and thrombophlebitis of superficial vessels of right lower extremity**

I80.02 **Phlebitis and thrombophlebitis of superficial vessels of left lower extremity**

I80.03 **Phlebitis and thrombophlebitis of superficial vessels of lower extremities, bilateral**

I80.1 **Phlebitis and thrombophlebitis of femoral vein** [HCC]

Phlebitis and thrombophlebitis of common femoral vein

Phlebitis and thrombophlebitis of deep femoral vein

I80.10 **Phlebitis and thrombophlebitis of unspecified femoral vein**

I80.11 **Phlebitis and thrombophlebitis of right femoral vein** [HCC]

I80.12 **Phlebitis and thrombophlebitis of left femoral vein** [HCC]

I80.13 **Phlebitis and thrombophlebitis of femoral vein, bilateral** [HCC]

I80.2 **Phlebitis and thrombophlebitis of other and unspecified deep vessels of lower extremities**

I80.20 **Phlebitis and thrombophlebitis of unspecified deep vessels of lower extremities** [HCC]

I80.201 **Phlebitis and thrombophlebitis of unspecified deep vessels of right lower extremity** [HCC]

I80.202 **Phlebitis and thrombophlebitis of unspecified deep vessels of left lower extremity** [HCC]

I80.203 **Phlebitis and thrombophlebitis of unspecified deep vessels of lower extremities, bilateral** [HCC]

I80.209 **Phlebitis and thrombophlebitis of unspecified deep vessels of unspecified lower extremity** [HCC]

I80.21 **Phlebitis and thrombophlebitis of iliac vein**

Phlebitis and thrombophlebitis of common iliac vein

Phlebitis and thrombophlebitis of external iliac vein

Phlebitis and thrombophlebitis of internal iliac vein

I80.211 **Phlebitis and thrombophlebitis of right iliac vein** [HCC]

I80.212 **Phlebitis and thrombophlebitis of left iliac vein** [HCC]

I80.213 **Phlebitis and thrombophlebitis of iliac vein, bilateral** [HCC]

I80.219 **Phlebitis and thrombophlebitis of unspecified iliac vein** [HCC]

I80.22 **Phlebitis and thrombophlebitis of popliteal vein**

I80.221 **Phlebitis and thrombophlebitis of right popliteal vein** [HCC]

I80.222 **Phlebitis and thrombophlebitis of left popliteal vein** [HCC]

I80.223 **Phlebitis and thrombophlebitis of popliteal vein, bilateral** [HCC]

I80.229 **Phlebitis and thrombophlebitis of unspecified popliteal vein** [HCC]

I80.23 **Phlebitis and thrombophlebitis of tibial vein**

Phlebitis and thrombophlebitis of anterior tibial vein

Phlebitis and thrombophlebitis of posterior tibial vein

I80.231 **Phlebitis and thrombophlebitis of right tibial vein** [HCC]

I80.232 **Phlebitis and thrombophlebitis of left tibial vein** [HCC]

I80.233 **Phlebitis and thrombophlebitis of tibial vein, bilateral** [HCC]

I80.239 **Phlebitis and thrombophlebitis of unspecified tibial vein** [HCC]

I80.24 **Phlebitis and thrombophlebitis of peroneal vein**

I80.241 **Phlebitis and thrombophlebitis of right peroneal vein** [HCC]

I80.242 **Phlebitis and thrombophlebitis of left peroneal vein** [HCC]

I80.243 **Phlebitis and thrombophlebitis of peroneal vein, bilateral** [HCC]

I80.249 **Phlebitis and thrombophlebitis of unspecified peroneal vein** [HCC]

I80.25 **Phlebitis and thrombophlebitis of calf muscular vein**

Phlebitis and thrombophlebitis of calf muscular vein, NOS

Phlebitis and thrombophlebitis of gastrocnemial vein

Phlebitis and thrombophlebitis of soleal vein

I80.251 **Phlebitis and thrombophlebitis of right calf muscular vein** [HCC]

I80.252 **Phlebitis and thrombophlebitis of left calf muscular vein** [HCC]

I80.253 **Phlebitis and thrombophlebitis of calf muscular vein, bilateral** [HCC]

I80.259 **Phlebitis and thrombophlebitis of unspecified calf muscular vein** [HCC]

I80.29 **Phlebitis and thrombophlebitis of other deep vessels of lower extremities**

I80.291 **Phlebitis and thrombophlebitis of other deep vessels of right lower extremity** [HCC]

I80.292   **Phlebitis and thrombophlebitis of other deep vessels of left lower extremity** [HCC]

I80.293   **Phlebitis and thrombophlebitis of other deep vessels of lower extremity, bilateral** [HCC]

I80.299   **Phlebitis and thrombophlebitis of other deep vessels of unspecified lower extremity** [HCC]

I80.3   **Phlebitis and thrombophlebitis of lower extremities, unspecified**

I80.8   **Phlebitis and thrombophlebitis of other sites**

I80.9   **Phlebitis and thrombophlebitis of unspecified site**

I81   **Portal vein thrombosis**

Portal (vein) obstruction

Excludes2: hepatic vein thrombosis (I82.0)

phlebitis of portal vein (K75.1)

I82   **Other venous embolism and thrombosis**

Definition: Venous embolism and thrombosis is a mass of clotted blood or other material moved by the blood from one vein and forced into a smaller one.

<u>Code first</u> venous embolism and thrombosis complicating:

abortion, ectopic or molar pregnancy (O00-O07, O08.7)

pregnancy, childbirth and the puerperium (O22.-, O87.-)

Excludes2: venous embolism and thrombosis (of):

cerebral (I63.6, I67.6)

coronary (I21-I25)

intracranial and intraspinal, septic or NOS (G08)

intracranial, nonpyogenic (I67.6)

intraspinal, nonpyogenic (G95.1)

mesenteric (K55.0-)

portal (I81)

pulmonary (I26.-)

I82.0   **Budd-Chiari syndrome** [HCC]

Hepatic vein thrombosis

I82.1   **Thrombophlebitis migrans**

I82.2   **Embolism and thrombosis of vena cava and other thoracic veins**

I82.21   **Embolism and thrombosis of superior vena cava**

I82.210   **Acute embolism and thrombosis of superior vena cava** [HCC]

Embolism and thrombosis of superior vena cava NOS

I82.211   **Chronic embolism and thrombosis of superior vena cava** [HCC]

I82.22   **Embolism and thrombosis of inferior vena cava**

I82.220   **Acute embolism and thrombosis of inferior vena cava** [HCC]

Embolism and thrombosis of inferior vena cava NOS

I82.221   **Chronic embolism and thrombosis of inferior vena cava** [HCC]

I82.29   **Embolism and thrombosis of other thoracic veins**

Embolism and thrombosis of brachiocephalic (innominate) vein

I82.290   **Acute embolism and thrombosis of other thoracic veins** [HCC]

I82.291   **Chronic embolism and thrombosis of other thoracic veins** [HCC]

I82.3   **Embolism and thrombosis of renal vein** [HCC]

I82.4   **Acute embolism and thrombosis of deep veins of lower extremity**

I82.40   **Acute embolism and thrombosis of unspecified deep veins of lower extremity**

Deep vein thrombosis NOS

DVT NOS

Excludes1: acute embolism and thrombosis of unspecified deep veins of distal lower extremity (I82.4Z-)

acute embolism and thrombosis of unspecified deep veins of proximal lower extremity (I82.4Y-)

I82.401   **Acute embolism and thrombosis of unspecified deep veins of right lower extremity**

I82.402   **Acute embolism and thrombosis of unspecified deep veins of left lower extremity** [HCC]

I82.403   **Acute embolism and thrombosis of unspecified deep veins of lower extremity, bilateral** [HCC]

I82.409   **Acute embolism and thrombosis of unspecified deep veins of unspecified lower extremity** [HCC]

I82.41   **Acute embolism and thrombosis of femoral vein**

Acute embolism and thrombosis of common femoral vein

Acute embolism and thrombosis of deep femoral vein

I82.411   **Acute embolism and thrombosis of right femoral vein** [HCC]

I82.412   **Acute embolism and thrombosis of left femoral vein** [HCC]

I82.413   **Acute embolism and thrombosis of femoral vein, bilateral** [HCC]

I82.419   **Acute embolism and thrombosis of unspecified femoral vein** [HCC]

I82.42   **Acute embolism and thrombosis of iliac vein**

Acute embolism and thrombosis of common iliac vein

Acute embolism and thrombosis of external iliac vein

Acute embolism and thrombosis of internal iliac vein

I82.421   **Acute embolism and thrombosis of right iliac vein** [HCC]

I82.422   **Acute embolism and thrombosis of left iliac vein** [HCC]

I82.423   **Acute embolism and thrombosis of iliac vein, bilateral** [HCC]

I82.429   **Acute embolism and thrombosis of unspecified iliac vein** [HCC]

I82.43   **Acute embolism and thrombosis of popliteal vein**

I82.431   **Acute embolism and thrombosis of right popliteal vein** [HCC]

I82.432   **Acute embolism and thrombosis of left popliteal vein** [HCC]

I82.433   **Acute embolism and thrombosis of popliteal vein, bilateral** [HCC]

I82.439   **Acute embolism and thrombosis of unspecified popliteal vein** [HCC]

● New code   ▲ Revised code   Excludes1: Not coded here   Excludes2: Not included here   ⊗ Placeholder required   ⑦7th digit required

I82.44   **Acute embolism and thrombosis of tibial vein**

Acute embolism and thrombosis of anterior tibial vein

Acute embolism and thrombosis of posterior tibial vein

     I82.441   **Acute embolism and thrombosis of right tibial vein** [HCC]

     I82.442   **Acute embolism and thrombosis of left tibial vein** [HCC]

     I82.443   **Acute embolism and thrombosis of tibial vein, bilateral** [HCC]

     I82.449   **Acute embolism and thrombosis of unspecified tibial vein** [HCC]

I82.45   **Acute embolism and thrombosis of peroneal vein**

     I82.451   **Acute embolism and thrombosis of right peroneal vein** [HCC]

     I82.452   **Acute embolism and thrombosis of left peroneal vein** [HCC]

     I82.453   **Acute embolism and thrombosis of peroneal vein, bilateral** [HCC]

     I82.459   **Acute embolism and thrombosis of unspecified peroneal vein** [HCC]

I82.46   **Acute embolism and thrombosis of calf muscular vein**

Acute embolism and thrombosis of calf muscular vein, NOS

Acute embolism and thrombosis of gastrocnemial vein

Acute embolism and thrombosis of soleal vein

     I82.461   **Acute embolism and thrombosis of right calf muscular vein** [HCC]

     I82.462   **Acute embolism and thrombosis of left calf muscular vein** [HCC]

     I82.463   **Acute embolism and thrombosis of calf muscular vein, bilateral** [HCC]

     I82.469   **Acute embolism and thrombosis of unspecified calf muscular vein** [HCC]

I82.49   **Acute embolism and thrombosis of other specified deep vein of lower extremity**

     I82.491   **Acute embolism and thrombosis of other specified deep vein of right lower extremity** [HCC]

     I82.492   **Acute embolism and thrombosis of other specified deep vein of left lower extremity** [HCC]

     I82.493   **Acute embolism and thrombosis of other specified deep vein of lower extremity, bilateral** [HCC]

     I82.499   **Acute embolism and thrombosis of other specified deep vein of unspecified lower extremity** [HCC]

I82.4Y   **Acute embolism and thrombosis of unspecified deep veins of proximal lower extremity**

Acute embolism and thrombosis of deep vein of thigh NOS

Acute embolism and thrombosis of deep vein of upper leg NOS

     I82.4Y1   **Acute embolism and thrombosis of unspecified deep veins of right proximal lower extremity** [HCC]

     I82.4Y2   **Acute embolism and thrombosis of unspecified deep veins of left proximal lower extremity**

     I82.4Y3   **Acute embolism and thrombosis of unspecified deep veins of proximal lower extremity, bilateral** [HCC]

     I82.4Y9   **Acute embolism and thrombosis of unspecified deep veins of unspecified proximal lower extremity** [HCC]

I82.4Z   **Acute embolism and thrombosis of unspecified deep veins of distal lower extremity**

Acute embolism and thrombosis of deep vein of calf NOS

Acute embolism and thrombosis of deep vein of lower leg NOS

     I82.4Z1   **Acute embolism and thrombosis of unspecified deep veins of right distal lower extremity** [HCC]

     I82.4Z2   **Acute embolism and thrombosis of unspecified deep veins of left distal lower extremity** [HCC]

     I82.4Z3   **Acute embolism and thrombosis of unspecified deep veins of distal lower extremity, bilateral** [HCC]

I82.4Z9   **Acute embolism and thrombosis of unspecified deep veins of unspecified distal lower extremity** [HCC]

I82.5   **Chronic embolism and thrombosis of deep veins of lower extremity**

Use Additional Code, if applicable, for associated long-term (current) use of anticoagulants (Z79.01)

Excludes1: personal history of venous embolism and thrombosis (Z86.718)

I82.50   **Chronic embolism and thrombosis of unspecified deep veins of lower extremity**

Excludes1: chronic embolism and thrombosis of unspecified deep veins of distal lower extremity (I82.5Z-)

chronic embolism and thrombosis of unspecified deep veins of proximal lower extremity (I82.5Y-)

     I82.501   **Chronic embolism and thrombosis of unspecified deep veins of right lower extremity** [HCC]

     I82.502   **Chronic embolism and thrombosis of unspecified deep veins of left lower extremity** [HCC]

     I82.503   **Chronic embolism and thrombosis of unspecified deep veins of lower extremity, bilateral** [HCC]

     I82.509   **Chronic embolism and thrombosis of unspecified deep veins of unspecified lower extremity** [HCC]

I82.51   **Chronic embolism and thrombosis of femoral vein**

Chronic embolism and thrombosis of common femoral vein

Chronic embolism and thrombosis of deep femoral vein

     I82.511   **Chronic embolism and thrombosis of right femoral vein** [HCC]

     I82.512   **Chronic embolism and thrombosis of left femoral vein** [HCC]

     I82.513   **Chronic embolism and thrombosis of femoral vein, bilateral** [HCC]

     I82.519   **Chronic embolism and thrombosis of unspecified femoral vein** [HCC]

I82.52   **Chronic embolism and thrombosis of iliac vein** [HCC]

Chronic embolism and thrombosis of common iliac vein

Chronic embolism and thrombosis of external iliac vein

Chronic embolism and thrombosis of internal iliac vein

I82.521 **Chronic embolism and thrombosis of right iliac vein** [HCC]

I82.522 **Chronic embolism and thrombosis of left iliac vein** [HCC]

I82.523 **Chronic embolism and thrombosis of iliac vein, bilateral** [HCC]

I82.529 **Chronic embolism and thrombosis of unspecified iliac vein** [HCC]

I82.53 **Chronic embolism and thrombosis of popliteal vein**

I82.531 **Chronic embolism and thrombosis of right popliteal vein**

I82.532 **Chronic embolism and thrombosis of left popliteal vein** [HCC]

I82.533 **Chronic embolism and thrombosis of popliteal vein, bilateral** [HCC]

I82.539 **Chronic embolism and thrombosis of unspecified popliteal vein** [HCC]

I82.54 **Chronic embolism and thrombosis of tibial vein**

Chronic embolism and thrombosis of anterior tibial vein

Chronic embolism and thrombosis of posterior tibial vein

I82.541 **Chronic embolism and thrombosis of right tibial vein** [HCC]

I82.542 **Chronic embolism and thrombosis of left tibial vein** [HCC]

I82.543 **Chronic embolism and thrombosis of tibial vein, bilateral** [HCC]

I82.549 **Chronic embolism and thrombosis of unspecified tibial vein** [HCC]

I82.55 **Chronic embolism and thrombosis of peroneal vein**

I82.551 **Chronic embolism and thrombosis of right peroneal vein** [HCC]

I82.552 **Chronic embolism and thrombosis of left peroneal vein** [HCC]

I82.553 **Chronic embolism and thrombosis of peroneal vein, bilateral** [HCC]

I82.559 **Chronic embolism and thrombosis of unspecified peroneal vein** [HCC]

I82.56 **Chronic embolism and thrombosis of calf muscular vein**

Chronic embolism and thrombosis of calf muscular vein NOS

Chronic embolism and thrombosis of gastrocnemial vein

Chronic embolism and thrombosis of soleal vein

I82.561 **Chronic embolism and thrombosis of right calf muscular vein** [HCC]

I82.562 **Chronic embolism and thrombosis of left calf muscular vein** [HCC]

I82.563 **Chronic embolism and thrombosis of calf muscular vein, bilateral** [HCC]

I82.569 **Chronic embolism and thrombosis of unspecified calf muscular vein** [HCC]

I82.59 **Chronic embolism and thrombosis of other specified deep vein of lower extremity**

I82.591 **Chronic embolism and thrombosis of other specified deep vein of right lower extremity** [HCC]

I82.592 **Chronic embolism and thrombosis of other specified deep vein of left lower extremity** [HCC]

I82.593 **Chronic embolism and thrombosis of other specified deep vein of lower extremity, bilateral** [HCC]

I82.599 **Chronic embolism and thrombosis of other specified deep vein of unspecified lower extremity** [HCC]

I82.5Y **Chronic embolism and thrombosis of unspecified deep veins of proximal lower extremity**

Chronic embolism and thrombosis of deep veins of thigh NOS

Chronic embolism and thrombosis of deep veins of upper leg NOS

I82.5Y1 **Chronic embolism and thrombosis of unspecified deep veins of right proximal lower extremity** [HCC]

I82.5Y2 **Chronic embolism and thrombosis of unspecified deep veins of left proximal lower extremity** [HCC]

I82.5Y3 **Chronic embolism and thrombosis of unspecified deep veins of proximal lower extremity, bilateral** [HCC]

I82.5Y9 **Chronic embolism and thrombosis of unspecified deep veins of unspecified proximal lower extremity** [HCC]

I82.5Z **Chronic embolism and thrombosis of unspecified deep veins of distal lower extremity**

Chronic embolism and thrombosis of deep veins of calf NOS

Chronic embolism and thrombosis of deep veins of lower leg NOS

I82.5Z1 **Chronic embolism and thrombosis of unspecified deep veins of right distal lower extremity** [HCC]

I82.5Z2 **Chronic embolism and thrombosis of unspecified deep veins of left distal lower extremity** [HCC]

I82.5Z3 **Chronic embolism and thrombosis of unspecified deep veins of distal lower extremity, bilateral** [HCC]

I82.5Z9 **Chronic embolism and thrombosis of unspecified deep veins of unspecified distal lower extremity** [HCC]

I82.6 **Acute embolism and thrombosis of veins of upper extremity**

I82.60 **Acute embolism and thrombosis of unspecified veins of upper extremity** [HCC]

I82.601 **Acute embolism and thrombosis of unspecified veins of right upper extremity** [HCC]

I82.602 **Acute embolism and thrombosis of unspecified veins of left upper extremity**

I82.603 **Acute embolism and thrombosis of unspecified veins of upper extremity, bilateral** [HCC]

I82.609 **Acute embolism and thrombosis of unspecified veins of unspecified upper extremity** [HCC]

I82.61 **Acute embolism and thrombosis of superficial veins of upper extremity**

● New code   ▲ Revised code   **Excludes1:** Not coded here   **Excludes2:** Not included here   ⊗ Placeholder required   ⑦7ᵗʰ digit required

Acute embolism and thrombosis of antecubital vein

Acute embolism and thrombosis of basilic vein

Acute embolism and thrombosis of cephalic vein

I82.611 **Acute embolism and thrombosis of superficial veins of right upper extremity** [HCC]

I82.612 **Acute embolism and thrombosis of superficial veins of left upper extremity** [HCC]

I82.613 **Acute embolism and thrombosis of superficial veins of upper extremity, bilateral** [HCC]

I82.619 **Acute embolism and thrombosis of superficial veins of unspecified upper extremity** [HCC]

I82.62 **Acute embolism and thrombosis of deep veins of upper extremity**

Acute embolism and thrombosis of brachial vein

Acute embolism and thrombosis of radial vein

Acute embolism and thrombosis of ulnar vein

I82.621 **Acute embolism and thrombosis of deep veins of right upper extremity** [HCC]

I82.622 **Acute embolism and thrombosis of deep veins of left upper extremity** [HCC]

I82.623 **Acute embolism and thrombosis of deep veins of upper extremity, bilateral** [HCC]

I82.629 **Acute embolism and thrombosis of deep veins of unspecified upper extremity** [HCC]

I82.7 **Chronic embolism and thrombosis of veins of upper extremity**

Use Additional Code, if applicable, for associated long-term (current) use of anticoagulants (Z79.01)

Excludes1: personal history of venous embolism and thrombosis (Z86.718)

I82.70 **Chronic embolism and thrombosis of unspecified veins of upper extremity**

I82.701 **Chronic embolism and thrombosis of unspecified veins of right upper extremity** [HCC]

I82.702 **Chronic embolism and thrombosis of unspecified veins of left upper extremity** [HCC]

I82.703 **Chronic embolism and thrombosis of unspecified veins of upper extremity, bilateral** [HCC]

I82.709 **Chronic embolism and thrombosis of unspecified veins of unspecified upper extremity** [HCC]

I82.71 **Chronic embolism and thrombosis of superficial veins of upper extremity**

Chronic embolism and thrombosis of antecubital vein

Chronic embolism and thrombosis of basilic vein

Chronic embolism and thrombosis of cephalic vein

I82.711 **Chronic embolism and thrombosis of superficial veins of right upper extremity** [HCC]

I82.712 **Chronic embolism and thrombosis of superficial veins of left upper extremity** [HCC]

I82.713 **Chronic embolism and thrombosis of superficial veins of upper extremity, bilateral** [HCC]

I82.719 **Chronic embolism and thrombosis of superficial veins of unspecified upper extremity** [HCC]

I82.72 **Chronic embolism and thrombosis of deep veins of upper extremity** [HCC]

Chronic embolism and thrombosis of brachial vein

Chronic embolism and thrombosis of radial vein

Chronic embolism and thrombosis of ulnar vein

I82.721 **Chronic embolism and thrombosis of deep veins of right upper extremity** [HCC]

I82.722 **Chronic embolism and thrombosis of deep veins of left upper extremity** [HCC]

I82.723 **Chronic embolism and thrombosis of deep veins of upper extremity, bilateral** [HCC]

I82.729 **Chronic embolism and thrombosis of deep veins of unspecified upper extremity** [HCC]

I82.A **Embolism and thrombosis of axillary vein**

I82.A1 **Acute embolism and thrombosis of axillary vein**

I82.A11 **Acute embolism and thrombosis of right axillary vein** [HCC]

I82.A12 **Acute embolism and thrombosis of left axillary vein** [HCC]

I82.A13 **Acute embolism and thrombosis of axillary vein, bilateral** [HCC]

I82.A19 **Acute embolism and thrombosis of unspecified axillary vein** [HCC]

I82.A2 **Chronic embolism and thrombosis of axillary vein**

I82.A21 **Chronic embolism and thrombosis of right axillary vein** [HCC]

I82.A22 **Chronic embolism and thrombosis of left axillary vein** [HCC]

I82.A23 **Chronic embolism and thrombosis of axillary vein, bilateral** [HCC]

I82.A29 **Chronic embolism and thrombosis of unspecified axillary vein** [HCC]

I82.B **Embolism and thrombosis of subclavian vein**

I82.B1 **Acute embolism and thrombosis of subclavian vein**

I82.B11 **Acute embolism and thrombosis of right subclavian vein** [HCC]

I82.B12 **Acute embolism and thrombosis of left subclavian vein** [HCC]

I82.B13 **Acute embolism and thrombosis of subclavian vein, bilateral** [HCC]

I82.B19 **Acute embolism and thrombosis of unspecified subclavian vein** [HCC]

I82.B2 **Chronic embolism and thrombosis of subclavian vein**

I82.B21 **Chronic embolism and thrombosis of right subclavian vein** [HCC]

I82.B22 **Chronic embolism and thrombosis of left subclavian vein** [HCC]

I82.B23 **Chronic embolism and thrombosis of subclavian vein, bilateral** [HCC]

I82.B29 **Chronic embolism and thrombosis of unspecified subclavian vein** [HCC]

I82.C **Embolism and thrombosis of internal jugular vein**

I82.C1 **Acute embolism and thrombosis of internal jugular vein**

I82.C11 **Acute embolism and thrombosis of right internal jugular vein** [HCC]

I82.C12 **Acute embolism and thrombosis of left internal jugular vein** [HCC]

I82.C13 **Acute embolism and thrombosis of internal jugular vein, bilateral** [HCC]

I82.C19 **Acute embolism and thrombosis of unspecified internal jugular vein** [HCC]

I82.C2 **Chronic embolism and thrombosis of internal jugular vein**

I82.C21 **Chronic embolism and thrombosis of right internal jugular vein** [HCC]

I82.C22 **Chronic embolism and thrombosis of left internal jugular vein** [HCC]

I82.C23 **Chronic embolism and thrombosis of internal jugular vein, bilateral** [HCC]

I82.C29 **Chronic embolism and thrombosis of unspecified internal jugular vein** [HCC]

I82.8 **Embolism and thrombosis of other specified veins**

Use Additional Code, if applicable, for associated long-term (current) use of anticoagulants (Z79.01)

I82.81 **Embolism and thrombosis of superficial veins of lower extremities**

Embolism and thrombosis of saphenous vein (greater) (lesser)

I82.811 **Embolism and thrombosis of superficial veins of right lower extremity** [HCC]

I82.812 **Embolism and thrombosis of superficial veins of left lower extremity** [HCC]

I82.813 **Embolism and thrombosis of superficial veins of lower extremity, bilateral** [HCC]

I82.819 **Embolism and thrombosis of superficial veins of unspecified lower extremity** [HCC]

I82.89 **Embolism and thrombosis of other specified veins**

I82.890 **Acute embolism and thrombosis of other specified veins** [HCC]

I82.891 **Chronic embolism and thrombosis of other specified veins** [HCC]

I82.9 **Embolism and thrombosis of unspecified vein** [HCC]

I82.90 **Acute embolism and thrombosis of unspecified vein** [HCC]

Embolism of vein NOS

Thrombosis (vein) NOS

I82.91 **Chronic embolism and thrombosis of unspecified vein** [HCC]

I83 Varicose veins of lower extremities

Definition: Varicose veins are dilated (widened) tortuous (twisting) veins, usually involving a superficial vein in the leg, often associated with incompetency of the valves in the vein

Excludes2: varicose veins complicating pregnancy (O22.0-)

varicose veins complicating the puerperium (O87.4)

I83.0 **Varicose veins of lower extremities with ulcer** [HCC]

Use Additional Code to identify severity of ulcer (L97.-)

I83.00 **Varicose veins of unspecified lower extremity with ulcer**

I83.001 **Varicose veins of unspecified lower extremity with ulcer of thigh** [HCC]

I83.002 **Varicose veins of unspecified lower extremity with ulcer of calf** [HCC]

I83.003 **Varicose veins of unspecified lower extremity with ulcer of ankle** [HCC]

I83.004 **Varicose veins of unspecified lower extremity with ulcer of heel and midfoot** [HCC]

Varicose veins of unspecified lower extremity with ulcer of plantar surface of midfoot

I83.005 **Varicose veins of unspecified lower extremity with ulcer other part of foot** [HCC]

Varicose veins of unspecified lower extremity with ulcer of toe

I83.008 **Varicose veins of unspecified lower extremity with ulcer other part of lower leg** [HCC]

I83.009 **Varicose veins of unspecified lower extremity with ulcer of unspecified site**

I83.01 **Varicose veins of right lower extremity with ulcer**

I83.011 **Varicose veins of right lower extremity with ulcer of thigh** [HCC]

I83.012 **Varicose veins of right lower extremity with ulcer of calf** [HCC]

I83.013 **Varicose veins of right lower extremity with ulcer of ankle** [HCC]

I83.014 **Varicose veins of right lower extremity with ulcer of heel and midfoot** [HCC]

Varicose veins of right lower extremity with ulcer of plantar surface of midfoot

I83.015 **Varicose veins of right lower extremity with ulcer other part of foot** [HCC]

Varicose veins of right lower extremity with ulcer of toe

I83.018 **Varicose veins of right lower extremity with ulcer other part of lower leg** [HCC]

I83.019 **Varicose veins of right lower extremity with ulcer of unspecified site** [HCC]

I83.02 **Varicose veins of left lower extremity with ulcer**

I83.021 **Varicose veins of left lower extremity with ulcer of thigh** [HCC]

I83.022 **Varicose veins of left lower extremity with ulcer of calf** [HCC]

I83.023 **Varicose veins of left lower extremity with ulcer of ankle** [HCC]

I83.024 **Varicose veins of left lower extremity with ulcer of heel and midfoot** [HCC]

Varicose veins of left lower extremity with ulcer of plantar surface of midfoot

I83.025 **Varicose veins of left lower extremity with ulcer other part of foot** [HCC]

Varicose veins of left lower extremity with ulcer of toe

I83.028 **Varicose veins of left lower extremity with ulcer other part of lower leg** [HCC]

I83.029   Varicose veins of left lower extremity with ulcer of unspecified site [HCC]

I83.1   **Varicose veins of lower extremities with inflammation**

I83.10   **Varicose veins of unspecified lower extremity with inflammation** [HCC]

I83.11   **Varicose veins of right lower extremity with inflammation** [HCC]

I83.12   **Varicose veins of left lower extremity with inflammation** [HCC]

I83.2   **Varicose veins of lower extremities with both ulcer and inflammation**

Use Additional Code to identify severity of ulcer (L97.-)

I83.20   **Varicose veins of unspecified lower extremity with both ulcer and inflammation**

I83.201   **Varicose veins of unspecified lower extremity with both ulcer of thigh and inflammation** [HCC]

I83.202   **Varicose veins of unspecified lower extremity with both ulcer of calf and inflammation** [HCC]

I83.203   **Varicose veins of unspecified lower extremity with both ulcer of ankle and inflammation** [HCC]

I83.204   **Varicose veins of unspecified lower extremity with both ulcer of heel and midfoot and inflammation** [HCC]

Varicose veins of unspecified lower extremity with both ulcer of plantar surface of midfoot and inflammation

I83.205   **Varicose veins of unspecified lower extremity with both ulcer other part of foot and inflammation** [HCC]

Varicose veins of unspecified lower extremity with both ulcer of toe and inflammation

I83.208   **Varicose veins of unspecified lower extremity with both ulcer of other part of lower extremity and inflammation** [HCC]

I83.209   **Varicose veins of unspecified lower extremity with both ulcer of unspecified site and inflammation** [HCC]

I83.21   **Varicose veins of right lower extremity with both ulcer and inflammation**

I83.211   **Varicose veins of right lower extremity with both ulcer of thigh and inflammation** [HCC]

I83.212   **Varicose veins of right lower extremity with both ulcer of calf and inflammation** [HCC]

I83.213   **Varicose veins of right lower extremity with both ulcer of ankle and inflammation** [HCC]

I83.214   **Varicose veins of right lower extremity with both ulcer of heel and midfoot and inflammation** [HCC]

Varicose veins of right lower extremity with both ulcer of plantar surface of midfoot and inflammation

I83.215   **Varicose veins of right lower extremity with both ulcer other part of foot and inflammation** [HCC]

Varicose veins of right lower extremity with both ulcer of toe and inflammation

I83.218   **Varicose veins of right lower extremity with both ulcer of other part of lower extremity and inflammation** [HCC]

I83.219   **Varicose veins of right lower extremity with both ulcer of unspecified site and inflammation** [HCC]

I83.22   **Varicose veins of left lower extremity with both ulcer and inflammation**

I83.221   **Varicose veins of left lower extremity with both ulcer of thigh and inflammation** [HCC]

I83.222   **Varicose veins of left lower extremity with both ulcer of calf and inflammation** [HCC]

I83.223   **Varicose veins of left lower extremity with both ulcer of ankle and inflammation** [HCC]

I83.224   **Varicose veins of left lower extremity with both ulcer of heel and midfoot and inflammation** [HCC]

Varicose veins of left lower extremity with both ulcer of plantar surface of midfoot and inflammation

I83.225   **Varicose veins of left lower extremity with both ulcer other part of foot and inflammation** [HCC]

Varicose veins of left lower extremity with both ulcer of toe and inflammation

I83.228   **Varicose veins of left lower extremity with both ulcer of other part of lower extremity and inflammation** [HCC]

I83.229   **Varicose veins of left lower extremity with both ulcer of unspecified site and inflammation** [HCC]

I83.8   **Varicose veins of lower extremities with other complications**

I83.81   **Varicose veins of lower extremities with pain**

I83.811   **Varicose veins of right lower extremity with pain** [HCC]

I83.812   **Varicose veins of left lower extremity with pain** [HCC]

I83.813   **Varicose veins of bilateral lower extremity with pain** [HCC]

I83.819   **Varicose veins of unspecified lower extremity with pain** [HCC]

I83.89   **Varicose veins of lower extremities with other complications**

Varicose veins of lower extremities with edema

Varicose veins of lower extremity with swelling

I83.891   **Varicose veins of right lower extremity with other complications**

I83.892   **Varicose veins of left lower extremity with other complications** [HCC]

I83.893   **Varicose veins of bilateral lower extremity with other complications** [HCC]

I83.899   **Varicose veins of unspecified lower extremity with other complications** [HCC]

I83.9   **Asymptomatic varicose veins of lower extremities**

Phlebectasia of lower extremities

Varicose veins of lower extremities

Varix of lower extremities

I83.90   **Asymptomatic varicose veins of unspecified lower extremity** [HCC]

Varicose veins NOS

I83.91 **Asymptomatic varicose veins of right lower extremity** [HCC]

I83.92 **Asymptomatic varicose veins of left lower extremity** [HCC]

I83.93 **Asymptomatic varicose veins of bilateral lower extremities** [HCC]

I85 Esophageal varices

Use Additional Code to identify:

alcohol abuse and dependence (F10.-)

I85.0 **Esophageal varices**

Idiopathic esophageal varices

Primary esophageal varices

I85.00 **Esophageal varices without bleeding** [HCC]

Esophageal varices NOS

I85.01 **Esophageal varices with bleeding** [HCC]

I85.1 **Secondary esophageal varices**

Esophageal varices secondary to alcoholic liver disease

Esophageal varices secondary to cirrhosis of liver

Esophageal varices secondary to schistosomiasis

Esophageal varices secondary to toxic liver disease

Code first underlying disease

I85.10 **Secondary esophageal varices without bleeding** [HCC]

I85.11 **Secondary esophageal varices with bleeding** [HCC]

I86 Varicose veins of other sites

Excludes1: varicose veins of unspecified site (I83.9-)

Excludes2: retinal varices (H35.0-)

I86.0 **Sublingual varices** [HCC]

I86.1 **Scrotal varices** [HCC]

Varicocele

I86.2 **Pelvic varices** [HCC]

I86.3 **Vulval varices** [HCC]

Excludes1: vulval varices complicating childbirth and the puerperium (O87.8)

vulval varices complicating pregnancy (O22.1-)

I86.4 **Gastric varices** [HCC]

I86.8 **Varicose veins of other specified sites** [HCC]

Varicose ulcer of nasal septum

I87 Other disorders of veins

I87.0 **Postthrombotic syndrome**

Chronic venous hypertension due to deep vein thrombosis

Postphlebitic syndrome

Excludes1: chronic venous hypertension without deep vein thrombosis (I87.3-)

I87.00 **Postthrombotic syndrome without complications**

Asymptomatic Postthrombotic syndrome

I87.001 **Postthrombotic syndrome without complications of right lower extremity** [HCC]

I87.002 **Postthrombotic syndrome without complications of left lower extremity** [HCC]

I87.003 **Postthrombotic syndrome without complications of bilateral lower extremity** [HCC]

I87.009 **Postthrombotic syndrome without complications of unspecified extremity** [HCC]

Postthrombotic syndrome NOS

I87.01 **Postthrombotic syndrome with ulcer**

Use Additional Code to specify site and severity of ulcer (L97.-)

I87.011 **Postthrombotic syndrome with ulcer of right lower extremity** [HCC]

I87.012 **Postthrombotic syndrome with ulcer of left lower extremity** [HCC]

I87.013 **Postthrombotic syndrome with ulcer of bilateral lower extremity** [HCC]

I87.019 **Postthrombotic syndrome with ulcer of unspecified lower extremity** [HCC]

I87.02 **Postthrombotic syndrome with inflammation**

I87.021 **Postthrombotic syndrome with inflammation of right lower extremity** [HCC]

I87.022 **Postthrombotic syndrome with inflammation of left lower extremity** [HCC]

I87.023 **Postthrombotic syndrome with inflammation of bilateral lower extremity** [HCC]

I87.029 **Postthrombotic syndrome with inflammation of unspecified lower extremity** [HCC]

I87.03 **Postthrombotic syndrome with ulcer and inflammation**

Use Additional Code to specify site and severity of ulcer (L97.-)

I87.031 **Postthrombotic syndrome with ulcer and inflammation of right lower extremity** [HCC]

I87.032 **Postthrombotic syndrome with ulcer and inflammation of left lower extremity** [HCC]

I87.033 **Postthrombotic syndrome with ulcer and inflammation of bilateral lower extremity** [HCC]

I87.039 **Postthrombotic syndrome with ulcer and inflammation of unspecified lower extremity** [HCC]

I87.09 **Postthrombotic syndrome with other complications**

I87.091 **Postthrombotic syndrome with other complications of right lower extremity** [HCC]

I87.092 **Postthrombotic syndrome with other complications of left lower extremity**

I87.093 **Postthrombotic syndrome with other complications of bilateral lower extremity** [HCC]

I87.099 **Postthrombotic syndrome with other complications of unspecified lower extremity** [HCC]

I87.1 **Compression of vein** [HCC]

Stricture of vein

Vena cava syndrome (inferior) (superior)

Excludes2: compression of pulmonary vein (I28.8)

I87.2 **Venous insufficiency (chronic) (peripheral)** [HCC]

Stasis dermatitis

Excludes1: stasis dermatitis with varicose veins of lower extremities (I83.1-, I83.2-)

I87.3 **Chronic venous hypertension (idiopathic)**

Stasis edema

● New code ▲ Revised code Excludes1: Not coded here Excludes2: Not included here ⊗ Placeholder required ⑦7th digit required

Excludes1: chronic venous hypertension due to deep vein thrombosis (I87.0-)

varicose veins of lower extremities (I83.-)

I87.30 Chronic venous hypertension (idiopathic) without complications [HCC]

Asymptomatic chronic venous hypertension (idiopathic)

I87.301 Chronic venous hypertension (idiopathic) without complications of right lower extremity [HCC]

I87.302 Chronic venous hypertension (idiopathic) without complications of left lower extremity [HCC]

I87.303 Chronic venous hypertension (idiopathic) without complications of bilateral lower extremity [HCC]

I87.309 Chronic venous hypertension (idiopathic) without complications of unspecified lower extremity [HCC]

Chronic venous hypertension NOS

I87.31 Chronic venous hypertension (idiopathic) with ulcer

Use Additional Code to specify site and severity of ulcer (L97.-)

I87.311 Chronic venous hypertension (idiopathic) with ulcer of right lower extremity [HCC]

I87.312 Chronic venous hypertension (idiopathic) with ulcer of left lower extremity [HCC]

I87.313 Chronic venous hypertension (idiopathic) with ulcer of bilateral lower extremity [HCC]

I87.319 Chronic venous hypertension (idiopathic) with ulcer of unspecified lower extremity [HCC]

I87.32 Chronic venous hypertension (idiopathic) with inflammation

I87.321 Chronic venous hypertension (idiopathic) with inflammation of right lower extremity [HCC]

I87.322 Chronic venous hypertension (idiopathic) with inflammation of left lower extremity [HCC]

I87.323 Chronic venous hypertension (idiopathic) with inflammation of bilateral lower extremity [HCC]

I87.329 Chronic venous hypertension (idiopathic) with inflammation of unspecified lower extremity [HCC]

I87.33 Chronic venous hypertension (idiopathic) with ulcer and inflammation

Use Additional Code to specify site and severity of ulcer (L97.-)

I87.331 Chronic venous hypertension (idiopathic) with ulcer and inflammation of right lower extremity

I87.332 Chronic venous hypertension (idiopathic) with ulcer and inflammation of left lower extremity [HCC]

I87.333 Chronic venous hypertension (idiopathic) with ulcer and inflammation of bilateral lower extremity [HCC]

I87.339 Chronic venous hypertension (idiopathic) with ulcer and inflammation of unspecified lower extremity [HCC]

I87.39 Chronic venous hypertension (idiopathic) with other complications

I87.391 Chronic venous hypertension (idiopathic) with other complications of right lower extremity

I87.392 Chronic venous hypertension (idiopathic) with other complications of left lower extremity

I87.393 Chronic venous hypertension (idiopathic) with other complications of bilateral lower extremity

I87.399 Chronic venous hypertension (idiopathic) with other complications of unspecified lower extremity

I87.8 Other specified disorders of veins

Phlebosclerosis

Venofibrosis

I87.9 Disorder of vein, unspecified

I88 Nonspecific lymphadenitis

Excludes1: acute lymphadenitis, except mesenteric (L04.-)

enlarged lymph nodes NOS (R59.-)

human immunodeficiency virus [HIV] disease resulting in generalized lymphadenopathy (B20)

I88.0 Nonspecific mesenteric lymphadenitis

Mesenteric lymphadenitis (acute)(chronic)

I88.1 Chronic lymphadenitis, except mesenteric

Adenitis

Lymphadenitis

I88.8 Other nonspecific lymphadenitis

I88.9 Nonspecific lymphadenitis, unspecified

Lymphadenitis NOS

I89 Other noninfective disorders of lymphatic vessels and lymph nodes

Excludes1: chylocele, tunica vaginalis (nonfilarial) NOS (N50.89)

enlarged lymph nodes NOS (R59.-)

filarial chylocele (B74.-)

hereditary lymphedema (Q82.0)

I89.0 Lymphedema, not elsewhere classified

Elephantiasis (nonfilarial) NOS

Lymphangiectasis

Obliteration, lymphatic vessel

Praecox lymphedema

Secondary lymphedema

Excludes1: postmastectomy lymphedema (I97.2)

I89.1 Lymphangitis

Chronic lymphangitis

Lymphangitis NOS

Subacute lymphangitis

Excludes1: acute lymphangitis (L03.-)

I89.8 Other specified noninfective disorders of lymphatic vessels and lymph nodes

Chylocele (nonfilarial)

Chylous ascites

Chylous cyst

Lipomelanotic reticulosis

Lymph node or vessel fistula

Lymph node or vessel infarction

Lymph node or vessel rupture

I89.9 **Noninfective disorder of lymphatic vessels and lymph nodes, unspecified**

Disease of lymphatic vessels NOS

OTHER AND UNSPECIFIED DISORDERS OF THE CIRCULATORY SYSTEM (I95-I99)

I95 **Hypotension**

Excludes1: cardiovascular collapse (R57.9)

maternal hypotension syndrome (O26.5-)

nonspecific low blood pressure reading NOS (R03.1)

I95.0 **Idiopathic hypotension**

I95.1 **Orthostatic hypotension**

Hypotension, postural

Excludes1: neurogenic orthostatic hypotension [Shy-Drager] (G90.3)

orthostatic hypotension due to drugs (I95.2)

I95.2 **Hypotension due to drugs**

Orthostatic hypotension due to drugs

Use Additional Code for adverse effect, if applicable, to identify drug (T36-T50 with fifth or sixth character 5)

I95.3 **Hypotension of hemodialysis**

Intra-dialytic hypotension

I95.8 **Other hypotension**

I95.81 **Postprocedural hypotension**

I95.89 **Other hypotension**

Chronic hypotension

I95.9 **Hypotension, unspecified**

I96 **Gangrene, not elsewhere classified** [HCC]

Gangrenous cellulitis

Excludes2: gangrene in atherosclerosis of native arteries of the extremities (I70.26)

gangrene in diabetes mellitus (E08-E13 with .52)

gangrene in hernia (K40.1, K40.4, K41.1, K41.4, K42.1, K43.1-, K44.1, K45.1, K46.1)

gangrene in other peripheral vascular diseases (I73.-)

gangrene of certain specified sites - see Alphabetical Index gas gangrene (A48.0)

pyoderma gangrenosum (L88)

I97 **Intraoperative and postprocedural complications and disorders of circulatory system, not elsewhere classified**

Excludes2: postprocedural shock (T81.1-)

I97.0 **Postcardiotomy syndrome**

I97.1 **Other postprocedural cardiac functional disturbances**

Excludes2: acute pulmonary insufficiency following thoracic surgery (J95.1)

intraoperative cardiac functional disturbances (I97.7-)

I97.11 **Postprocedural cardiac insufficiency**

I97.110 **Postprocedural cardiac insufficiency following cardiac surgery**

I97.111 **Postprocedural cardiac insufficiency following other surgery**

I97.12 **Postprocedural cardiac arrest**

I97.120 **Postprocedural cardiac arrest following cardiac surgery**

I97.121 **Postprocedural cardiac arrest following other surgery**

I97.13 **Postprocedural heart failure**

Use Additional Code to identify the heart failure (I50.-)

I97.130 **Postprocedural heart failure following cardiac surgery**

I97.131 **Postprocedural heart failure following other surgery**

I97.19 **Other postprocedural cardiac functional disturbances**

Use Additional Code, if applicable, to further specify disorder

I97.190 **Other postprocedural cardiac functional disturbances following cardiac surgery**

Use Additional Code, if applicable, for type 4 or type 5 myocardial infarction, to further specify disorder

I97.191 **Other postprocedural cardiac functional disturbances following other surgery**

I97.2 **Postmastectomy lymphedema syndrome**

Elephantiasis due to mastectomy

Obliteration of lymphatic vessels

I97.3 **Postprocedural hypertension**

I97.4 **Intraoperative hemorrhage and hematoma of a circulatory system organ or structure complicating a procedure**

Excludes1: intraoperative hemorrhage and hematoma of a circulatory system organ or structure due to accidental puncture and laceration during a procedure (I97.5-)

Excludes2: intraoperative cerebrovascular hemorrhage complicating a procedure (G97.3-)

I97.41 **Intraoperative hemorrhage and hematoma of a circulatory system organ or structure complicating a circulatory system procedure**

I97.410 **Intraoperative hemorrhage and hematoma of a circulatory system organ or structure complicating a cardiac catheterization**

I97.411 **Intraoperative hemorrhage and hematoma of a circulatory system organ or structure complicating a cardiac bypass**

I97.418 **Intraoperative hemorrhage and hematoma of a circulatory system organ or structure complicating other circulatory system procedure**

I97.42 **Intraoperative hemorrhage and hematoma of a circulatory system organ or structure complicating other procedure**

I97.5 **Accidental puncture and laceration of a circulatory system organ or structure during a procedure**

Excludes2: accidental puncture and laceration of brain during a procedure (G97.4-)

I97.51 **Accidental puncture and laceration of a circulatory system organ or structure during a circulatory system procedure**

I97.52 **Accidental puncture and laceration of a circulatory system organ or structure during other procedure**

I97.6 **Postprocedural hemorrhage, hematoma and seroma of a circulatory system organ or structure following a procedure**

Excludes2: postprocedural cerebrovascular hemorrhage complicating a procedure (G97.5-)

● New code   ▲ Revised code   **Excludes1:** Not coded here   **Excludes2:** Not included here   ⊗ Placeholder required   ⑦ 7th digit required

I97.61 Postprocedural hemorrhage of a circulatory system organ or structure following a circulatory system procedure

 I97.610 Postprocedural hemorrhage of a circulatory system organ or structure following a cardiac catheterization

 I97.611 Postprocedural hemorrhage of a circulatory system organ or structure following cardiac bypass

 I97.618 Postprocedural hemorrhage of a circulatory system organ or structure following other circulatory system procedure

I97.62 Postprocedural hemorrhage, hematoma and seroma of a circulatory system organ or structure following other procedure

 I97.620 Postprocedural hemorrhage of a circulatory system organ or structure following other procedure

 I97.621 Postprocedural hematoma of a circulatory system organ or structure following other procedure

 I97.622 Postprocedural seroma of a circulatory system organ or structure following other procedure

I97.63 Postprocedural hematoma of a circulatory system organ or structure following a circulatory system procedure

 I97.630 Postprocedural hematoma of a circulatory system organ or structure following a cardiac catheterization

 I97.631 Postprocedural hematoma of a circulatory system organ or structure following cardiac bypass

 I97.638 Postprocedural hematoma of a circulatory system organ or structure following other circulatory system procedure

I97.64 Postprocedural seroma of a circulatory system organ or structure following a circulatory system procedure

 I97.640 Postprocedural seroma of a circulatory system organ or structure following a cardiac catheterization

 I97.641 Postprocedural seroma of a circulatory system organ or structure following cardiac bypass

 I97.648 Postprocedural seroma of a circulatory system organ or structure following other circulatory system procedure

I97.7 Intraoperative cardiac functional disturbances

Excludes2: acute pulmonary insufficiency following thoracic surgery (J95.1)

postprocedural cardiac functional disturbances (I97.1-)

I97.71 Intraoperative cardiac arrest

 I97.710 Intraoperative cardiac arrest during cardiac surgery

 I97.711 Intraoperative cardiac arrest during other surgery

I97.79 Other intraoperative cardiac functional disturbances

Use Additional Code, if applicable, to further specify disorder

 I97.790 Other intraoperative cardiac functional disturbances during cardiac surgery

 I97.791 Other intraoperative cardiac functional disturbances during other surgery

I97.8 Other intraoperative and postprocedural complications and disorders of the circulatory system, not elsewhere classified

Use Additional Code, if applicable, to further specify disorder

I97.81 Intraoperative cerebrovascular infarction

 I97.810 Intraoperative cerebrovascular infarction during cardiac surgery [HCC]

 I97.811 Intraoperative cerebrovascular infarction during other surgery [HCC]

I97.82 Postprocedural cerebrovascular infarction

 I97.820 Postprocedural cerebrovascular infarction following cardiac surgery [HCC]

 I97.821 Postprocedural cerebrovascular infarction following other surgery [HCC]

I97.88 Other intraoperative complications of the circulatory system, not elsewhere classified

I97.89 Other postprocedural complications and disorders of the circulatory system, not elsewhere classified

I99 Other and unspecified disorders of circulatory system

I99.8 Other disorder of circulatory system

I99.9 Unspecified disorder of circulatory system

Chapter 10: Diseases of the Respiratory System (J00-J99)

DEFINITIONS

This chapter includes definitions of selected key words, terms and phrases and coding alerts for adding points to the clinical domain, and references to coding late effects where appropriate. An example from this chapter is as follows:

J01   Acute sinusitis
    Definition: Sinusitis is an infection of the small, air-filled cavities inside the cheekbones and forehead.

MULTIPLE CODING FOR A SINGLE CONDITION

In addition to the etiology/manifestation convention that requires two codes to fully describe a single condition that affects multiple body systems, there are other single conditions that also require more than one code. "**Use Additional Code**" notes are found in the Tabular List at codes that are not part of an etiology/manifestation pair where a secondary code is useful to fully describe a condition. The sequencing rule is the same as the etiology/manifestation pair, "**Use Additional Code**" indicates that a secondary code should be added.

For example, for bacterial infections that are not included in chapter 1, a secondary code from category B95, Streptococcus, Staphylococcus, and Enterococcus, as the cause of diseases classified elsewhere, or B96, Other bacterial agents as the cause of diseases classified elsewhere, may be required to identify the bacterial organism causing the infection. A "**Use Additional Code**" note will normally be found at the infectious disease code, indicating a need for the organism code to be added as a secondary code.

"Code first" notes are also under certain codes that are not specifically manifestation codes but may be due to an underlying cause. When there is a "Code first" note and an underlying condition is present, the underlying condition should be sequenced first.

"Code, if applicable, any causal condition first", notes indicate that this code may be assigned as a principal diagnosis when the causal condition is unknown or not applicable. If a causal condition is known, then the code for that condition should be sequenced as the principal or first-listed diagnosis.

Multiple codes may be needed for sequela, complication codes and obstetric codes to more fully describe a condition. See the specific guidelines for these conditions for further instruction.

COMBINATION CODE

A combination code is a single code used to classify: Two diagnoses, or a diagnosis with an associated secondary process (manifestation) A diagnosis with an associated complication

Combination codes are identified by referring to subterm entries in the Alphabetic Index and by reading the inclusion and exclusion notes in the Tabular List.

Assign only the combination code when that code fully identifies the diagnostic conditions involved or when the Alphabetic Index so directs. Multiple coding should not be used when the classification provides a combination code that clearly identifies all of the elements documented in the diagnosis. When the combination code lacks necessary specificity in describing the manifestation or complication, an additional code should be used as a secondary code.

SEQUELA (LATE EFFECTS)

A sequela is the residual effect (condition produced) after the acute phase of an illness or injury has terminated. There is no time limit on when a sequela code can be used. The residual may be apparent early, such as in cerebral infarction, or it may occur months or years later, such as that due to a previous injury. Coding of sequela generally requires two codes sequenced in the following order: The condition or nature of the sequela is sequenced first.

The sequela code is sequenced second.

An exception to the above guidelines are those instances where the code for the sequela is followed by a manifestation code identified in the Tabular List and title, or the sequela code has been expanded (at the fourth, fifth or sixth character levels) to

J00-J99

include the manifestation(s). The code for the acute phase of an illness or injury that led to the sequela is never used with a code for the late effect.

CHRONIC OBSTRUCTIVE PULMONARY DISEASE [COPD] AND ASTHMA

1)   Acute exacerbation of chronic obstructive bronchitis and asthma

The codes in categories J44 and J45 distinguish between uncomplicated cases and those in acute exacerbation. An acute exacerbation is a worsening or a decompensation of a chronic condition. An acute exacerbation is not equivalent to an infection superimposed on a chronic condition, though an exacerbation may be triggered by an infection.

ACUTE RESPIRATORY FAILURE

1)   Acute respiratory failure as principal diagnosis

A code from subcategory J96.0, Acute respiratory failure, or subcategory J96.2, Acute and chronic respiratory failure, may be assigned as a principal diagnosis when it is the condition established after study to be chiefly responsible for occasioning the admission to the hospital, and the selection is supported by the Alphabetic Index and Tabular List. However, chapter-specific coding guidelines (such as obstetrics, poisoning, HIV, newborn) that provide sequencing direction take precedence.

2)   Acute respiratory failure as secondary diagnosis

Respiratory failure may be listed as a secondary diagnosis if it occurs after admission, or if it is present on admission, but does not meet the definition of principal diagnosis.

3)   Sequencing of acute respiratory failure and another acute condition

When a patient is admitted with respiratory failure and another acute condition, (e.g., myocardial infarction, cerebrovascular accident, aspiration pneumonia), the principal diagnosis will not be the same in every situation. This applies whether the other acute condition is a respiratory or nonrespiratory condition. Selection of the principal diagnosis will be dependent on the circumstances of admission. If both the respiratory failure and the other acute condition are equally responsible for occasioning the admission to the hospital, and there are no chapter-specific sequencing rules, the guideline regarding two or more diagnoses that equally meet the definition for principal diagnosis *(Section II, C.)* may be applied in these situations.

If the documentation is not clear as to whether acute respiratory failure and another condition are equally responsible for occasioning the admission, query the provider for clarification.

INFLUENZA DUE TO CERTAIN IDENTIFIED INFLUENZA VIRUSES

Code only confirmed cases of influenza due to certain identified influenza viruses (category J09), and due to other identified influenza virus (category J10). This is an exception to the hospital inpatient guideline Section II, H. (Uncertain Diagnosis).

In this context, "confirmation" does not require documentation of positive laboratory testing specific for avian or other novel influenza A or other identified influenza virus. However, coding should be based on the provider's diagnostic statement that the patient has avian influenza, or other novel influenza A, for category J09, or has another particular identified strain of influenza, such as H1N1 or H3N2, but not identified as novel or variant, for category J10.

If the provider records "suspected" or "possible" or "probable" avian influenza, or novel influenza, or other identified influenza, then the appropriate influenza code from category J11, Influenza due to unidentified influenza virus, should be assigned. A code from category J09, Influenza due to certain identified influenza viruses, should not be assigned nor should a code from category J10, Influenza due to other identified influenza virus.

VENTILATOR ASSOCIATED PNEUMONIA

1)   Documentation of Ventilator associated Pneumonia

As with all procedural or postprocedural complications, code assignment is based on the provider's documentation of the relationship between the condition and the procedure.

Code J95.851, Ventilator associated pneumonia, should be assigned only when the provider has documented ventilator associated pneumonia (VAP). An additional code to identify the organism (e.g., Pseudomonas aeruginosa, code B96.5) should also be assigned. Do not assign an additional code from categories J12-J18 to identify the type of pneumonia.

Code J95.851 should not be assigned for cases where the patient has pneumonia and is on a mechanical ventilator and the provider has not specifically stated that the pneumonia is ventilator-associated pneumonia. If the documentation is unclear as to whether the patient has a pneumonia that is a complication attributable to the mechanical ventilator, query the provider.

2) **Ventilator associated Pneumonia Develops after Admission**

A patient may be admitted with one type of pneumonia (e.g., code J13, Pneumonia due to Streptococcus pneumonia) and subsequently develop VAP. In this instance, the principal diagnosis would be the appropriate code from categories J12-J18 for the pneumonia diagnosed at the time of admission. Code J95.851, Ventilator associated pneumonia, would be assigned as an additional diagnosis when the provider has also documented the presence of ventilator associated pneumonia.

VAPING-RELATED DISORDERS

For patients presenting with condition(s) related to vaping, assign code U07.0, Vaping-related disorder, as the principal diagnosis. For lung injury due to vaping, assign only code U07.0. Assign additional codes for other manifestations, such as acute respiratory failure (subcategory J96.0-) or pneumonitis (code J68.0).

Associated respiratory signs and symptoms due to vaping, such as cough, shortness of breath, etc., are not coded separately, when a definitive diagnosis has been established. However, it would be appropriate to code separately any gastrointestinal symptoms, such as diarrhea and abdominal pain.

Chapter 10

Diseases of The Respiratory System (J00-J99)

Note: When a respiratory condition is described as occurring in more than one site and is not specifically indexed, it should be classified to the lower anatomic site (e.g., tracheobronchitis to bronchitis in J40).

<u>Use Additional Code</u>, where applicable, to identify:

exposure to environmental tobacco smoke (Z77.22)

exposure to tobacco smoke in the perinatal period (P96.81)

history of tobacco dependence (Z87.891)

occupational exposure to environmental tobacco smoke (Z57.31)

tobacco dependence (F17.-)

tobacco use (Z72.0)

Excludes2: certain conditions originating in the perinatal period (P04-P96)

certain infectious and parasitic diseases (A00-B99)

complications of pregnancy, childbirth and the puerperium (O00-O9A)

congenital malformations, deformations and chromosomal abnormalities (Q00-Q99)

endocrine, nutritional and metabolic diseases (E00-E88)

injury, poisoning and certain other consequences of external causes (S00-T88) neoplasms (C00-D49)

smoke inhalation (T59.81-)

symptoms, signs and abnormal clinical and laboratory findings, not elsewhere classified (R00-R94)

This chapter contains the following blocks:

J00-J06	Acute upper respiratory infections
J09-J18	Influenza and pneumonia
J20-J22	Other acute lower respiratory infections
J30-J39	Other diseases of upper respiratory tract
J40-J47	Chronic lower respiratory diseases
J60-J70	Lung diseases due to external agents
J80-J84	Other respiratory diseases principally affecting the interstitium
J85-J86	Suppurative and necrotic conditions of the lower respiratory tract
J90-J94	Other diseases of the pleura
J95	Intraoperative and postprocedural complications and disorders of respiratory system, not elsewhere classified
J96-J99	Other diseases of the respiratory system

ACUTE UPPER RESPIRATORY INFECTIONS (J00-J06)

Excludes1: chronic obstructive pulmonary disease with acute lower respiratory infection (J44.0)

J00 **Acute nasopharyngitis [common cold]**

Acute rhinitis

Coryza (acute)

Infective nasopharyngitis NOS

Infective rhinitis

Nasal catarrh, acute Nasopharyngitis NOS

Excludes1: acute pharyngitis (J02.-)

acute sore throat NOS (J02.9)

influenza virus with other respiratory manifestations (J09.X2, J10.1, J11.1)

pharyngitis NOS (J02.9)

rhinitis NOS (J31.0)

sore throat NOS (J02.9)

Excludes2: allergic rhinitis (J30.1-J30.9)

chronic pharyngitis (J31.2)

chronic rhinitis (J31.0)

chronic sore throat (J31.2)

nasopharyngitis, chronic (J31.1)

vasomotor rhinitis (J30.0)

J01 **Acute sinusitis**

Includes: acute abscess of sinus

acute empyema of sinus

acute infection of sinus

acute inflammation of sinus

acute suppuration of sinus

Use Additional Code (B95-B97) to identify infectious agent.

Excludes1: sinusitis NOS (J32.9)

Excludes2: chronic sinusitis (J32.0-J32.8)

J01.0 **Acute maxillary sinusitis**

Acute antritis

   J01.00 **Acute maxillary sinusitis, unspecified**

   J01.01 **Acute recurrent maxillary sinusitis**

J01.1 **Acute frontal sinusitis**

   J01.10 **Acute frontal sinusitis, unspecified**

   J01.11 **Acute recurrent frontal sinusitis**

J01.2 **Acute ethmoidal sinusitis**

   J01.20 **Acute ethmoidal sinusitis, unspecified**

   J01.21 **Acute recurrent ethmoidal sinusitis**

J01.3 **Acute sphenoidal sinusitis**

   J01.30 **Acute sphenoidal sinusitis, unspecified**

   J01.31 **Acute recurrent sphenoidal sinusitis**

J01.4 **Acute pansinusitis**

   J01.40 **Acute pansinusitis, unspecified**

   J01.41 **Acute recurrent pansinusitis**

J01.8 **Other acute sinusitis**

   J01.80 **Other acute sinusitis**

Acute sinusitis involving more than one sinus but not pansinusitis

   J01.81 **Other acute recurrent sinusitis**

Acute recurrent sinusitis involving more than one sinus but not pansinusitis

J01.9 **Acute sinusitis, unspecified**

   J01.90 **Acute sinusitis, unspecified**

   J01.91 **Acute recurrent sinusitis, unspecified**

J02 **Acute pharyngitis**

Includes: acute sore throat

Excludes1: acute laryngopharyngitis (J06.0)

influenza virus with other respiratory manifestations (J09.X2, J10.1, J11.1)

peritonsillar abscess (J36)

pharyngeal abscess (J39.1)

retropharyngeal abscess (J39.0)

Excludes2: chronic pharyngitis (J31.2)

J02.0 **Streptococcal pharyngitis**

Septic pharyngitis

Streptococcal sore throat

Excludes2: scarlet fever (A38.-)

J02.8 **Acute pharyngitis due to other specified organisms**

Use Additional Code (B95-B97) to identify infectious agent

Excludes1: acute pharyngitis due to coxsackie virus (B08.5)

acute pharyngitis due to gonococcus (A54.5)

acute pharyngitis due to herpes [simplex] virus (B00.2)

acute pharyngitis due to infectious mononucleosis (B27.-)

enteroviral vesicular pharyngitis (B08.5)

J02.9   Acute pharyngitis, unspecified

> **Excludes1:** influenza virus with other respiratory manifestations (J09.X2, J10.1, J11.1)

Gangrenous pharyngitis (acute)

Infective pharyngitis (acute) NOS

Pharyngitis (acute) NOS

Sore throat (acute) NOS

Suppurative pharyngitis (acute)

Ulcerative pharyngitis (acute)

J03   Acute tonsillitis

> **Excludes1:** acute sore throat (J02.-)

hypertrophy of tonsils (J35.1)

peritonsillar abscess (J36)

sore throat NOS (J02.9)

streptococcal sore throat (J02.0)

> **Excludes2:** chronic tonsillitis (J35.0)

J03.0   Streptococcal tonsillitis

> **J03.00   Acute streptococcal tonsillitis, unspecified**
>
> **J03.01   Acute recurrent streptococcal tonsillitis**

J03.8   Acute tonsillitis due to other specified organisms

> **Use Additional Code** (B95-B97) to identify infectious agent.
>
> **Excludes1:** diphtheritic tonsillitis (A36.0)
>
> herpesviral pharyngotonsillitis (B00.2)
>
> streptococcal tonsillitis (J03.0)
>
> tuberculous tonsillitis (A15.8)
>
> Vincent's tonsillitis (A69.1)
>
> **J03.80   Acute tonsillitis due to other specified organisms**
>
> **J03.81   Acute recurrent tonsillitis due to other specified organisms**

J03.9   Acute tonsillitis, unspecified

> **Excludes1:** influenza virus with other respiratory manifestations (J09.X2, J10.1, J11.1)

Follicular tonsillitis (acute) Gangrenous tonsillitis (acute)

Infective tonsillitis (acute)

Tonsillitis (acute) NOS

Ulcerative tonsillitis (acute)

> **J03.90   Acute tonsillitis, unspecified**
>
> **J03.91   Acute recurrent tonsillitis, unspecified**

J04   Acute laryngitis and tracheitis

> **Use Additional Code** (B95-B97) to identify infectious agent.
>
> **Excludes1:** acute obstructive laryngitis [croup] and epiglottitis (J05.-)
>
> **Excludes2:** laryngismus (stridulus) (J38.5)
>
> **Code also** influenza, if present, such as:
>
> influenza due to identified novel influenza A virus with other respiratory manifestations(J09.X2)
>
> influenza due to other identified influenza virus with other respiratory manifestations (J10.1)
>
> influenza due to unidentified influenza virus with other respiratory manifestations (J11.1)

J04.0   Acute laryngitis

Edematous laryngitis (acute)

Laryngitis (acute) NOS

Subglottic laryngitis (acute)

Suppurative laryngitis (acute)

Ulcerative laryngitis (acute)

> **Excludes1:** acute obstructive laryngitis (J05.0)
>
> **Excludes2:** chronic laryngitis (J37.0)

J04.1   Acute tracheitis

Acute viral tracheitis

Catarrhal tracheitis (acute)

Tracheitis (acute) NOS

> **Excludes2:** chronic tracheitis (J42)
>
> **J04.10   Acute tracheitis without obstruction**
>
> **J04.11   Acute tracheitis with obstruction**

J04.2   Acute laryngotracheitis

Laryngotracheitis NOS

Tracheitis (acute) with laryngitis (acute)

> **Excludes1:** acute obstructive laryngotracheitis (J05.0)
>
> **Excludes2:** chronic laryngotracheitis (J37.1)

J04.3   Supraglottitis, unspecified

> **J04.30   Supraglottitis, unspecified, without obstruction**
>
> **J04.31   Supraglottitis, unspecified, with obstruction**

J05   Acute obstructive laryngitis [croup] and epiglottitis

> **Use Additional Code** (B95-B97) to identify infectious agent.
>
> **Code also**, influenza, if present, such as:
>
> influenza due to identified novel influenza A virus with other respiratory manifestations (J09.X2)
>
> influenza due to other identified influenza virus with other respiratory manifestations (J10.1)
>
> influenza due to unidentified influenza virus with other respiratory manifestations (J11.1)

J05.0   Acute obstructive laryngitis [croup]

Obstructive laryngitis (acute) NOS

Obstructive laryngotracheitis NOS

J05.1   Acute epiglottitis

> **Excludes2:** epiglottitis, chronic (J37.0)
>
> **J05.10   Acute epiglottitis without obstruction**
>
> Epiglottitis NOS
>
> **J05.11   Acute epiglottitis with obstruction**

J06   Acute upper respiratory infections of multiple and unspecified sites

> **Excludes1:** acute respiratory infection NOS (J22)
>
> influenza virus with other respiratory manifestations (J09.X2, J10.1, J11.1)
>
> streptococcal pharyngitis (J02.0)

J06.0   Acute laryngopharyngitis

J06.9   Acute upper respiratory infection, unspecified

Upper respiratory disease, acute

Upper respiratory infection NOS

> **Use Additional Code** (B95-B97) to identify infectious agent, if known, such as:
>
> respiratory syncytial virus (RSV) (B97.4)

INFLUENZA AND PNEUMONIA (J09-J18)

> **Excludes2:** allergic or eosinophilic pneumonia (J82)
>
> aspiration pneumonia NOS (J69.0)

meconium pneumonia (P24.01)

neonatal aspiration pneumonia (P24.-)

pneumonia due to solids and liquids (J69.-)

congenital pneumonia (P23.9)

lipid pneumonia (J69.1)

rheumatic pneumonia (I00)

ventilator associated pneumonia (J95.851)

J09   Influenza due to certain identified influenza viruses

> **Excludes1:** influenza A/H1N1 (J10.-)
>
> influenza due to other identified influenza virus (J10.-)
>
> influenza due to unidentified influenza virus (J11.-)
>
> seasonal influenza due **to other** identified influenza virus (J10.-)
>
> seasonal influenza due to unidentified influenza virus (J11.-)

J09.X   Influenza due to identified novel influenza A virus

Avian influenza

Bird influenza

Influenza A/H5N1

Influenza **of** other animal origin, not bird or swine

Swine influenza virus (viruses that normally cause infections in pigs)

J09.X1   Influenza due to identified novel influenza A virus with pneumonia

> **Code also**, if applicable, associated:
>
> lung abscess (J85.1)
>
> **Other** specified type of pneumonia

J09.X2   Influenza due to identified novel influenza A virus with other respiratory manifestations

Influenza due to identified novel influenza A virus NOS

Influenza due to identified novel influenza A virus with laryngitis

Influenza due to identified novel influenza A virus with pharyngitis

Influenza due to identified novel influenza A virus with upper respiratory symptoms

> **Use Additional Code**, if applicable, for associated:
>
> pleural effusion (J91.8)
>
> sinusitis (J01.-)

J09.X3   Influenza due to identified novel influenza A virus with gastrointestinal manifestations

Influenza due to identified novel influenza A virus gastroenteritis

> **Excludes1:** 'intestinal flu' [viral gastroenteritis] (A08.-)

J09.X9   Influenza due to identified novel influenza A virus with other manifestations

Influenza due to identified novel influenza A virus with encephalopathy

Influenza due to identified novel influenza A virus with myocarditis

Influenza due to identified novel influenza A virus with otitis media

> **Use Additional Code** to identify manifestation

J10   Influenza due to other identified influenza virus

> **Includes:** influenza A (non-novel)

influenza B

influenza C

> **Excludes1:** influenza due to avian influenza virus (J09.X-)
>
> influenza due to swine flu (J09.X-)
>
> influenza due to unidentified influenza virus (J11.-)

J10.0   Influenza due to other identified influenza virus with pneumonia

> **Code also** associated lung abscess, if applicable (J85.1)

J10.00   Influenza due to other identified influenza virus with unspecified type of pneumonia

J10.01   Influenza due to other identified influenza virus with the same other identified influenza virus pneumonia

J10.08   Influenza due to other identified influenza virus with other specified pneumonia

> **Code also** other specified type of pneumonia

J10.1   Influenza due to other identified influenza virus with other respiratory manifestations

Influenza due **to other** identified influenza virus NOS

Influenza due **to** other identified influenza virus with laryngitis

Influenza due to other identified influenza virus with pharyngitis

Influenza due to other identified influenza virus with upper respiratory symptoms

> **Use Additional Code** for associated pleural effusion, if applicable (J91.8)
>
> **Use Additional Code** for associated sinusitis, if applicable (J01.-)

J10.2   Influenza due to other identified influenza virus with gastrointestinal manifestations

Influenza due **to other** identified influenza virus gastroenteritis

> **Excludes1:** 'intestinal flu' [viral gastroenteritis] (A08.-)

J10.8   Influenza due to other identified influenza virus with other manifestations

J10.81   Influenza due to other identified influenza virus with encephalopathy

J10.82   Influenza due to other identified influenza virus with myocarditis

J10.83   Influenza due to other identified influenza virus with otitis media

> **Use Additional Code** for any associated perforated tympanic membrane (H72.-)

J10.89   Influenza due to other identified influenza virus with other manifestations

> **Use Additional Code**s to identify the manifestations

J11   Influenza due to unidentified influenza virus

J11.0   Influenza due to unidentified influenza virus with pneumonia

> **Code also** associated lung abscess, if applicable (J85.1)

J11.00   Influenza due to unidentified influenza virus with unspecified type of pneumonia

Influenza with pneumonia NOS

J11.08   Influenza due to unidentified influenza virus with specified pneumonia

> **Code also** other specified type of pneumonia

J11.1   Influenza due to unidentified influenza virus with other respiratory manifestations

Influenza NOS

Influenzal laryngitis NOS

Influenzal pharyngitis NOS

Influenza with upper respiratory symptoms NOS

Use Additional Code for associated pleural effusion, if applicable (J91.8)

Use Additional Code for associated sinusitis, if applicable (J01.-)

J11.2 **Influenza due to unidentified influenza virus with gastrointestinal manifestations**

Influenza gastroenteritis NOS

Excludes1: 'intestinal flu' [viral gastroenteritis] (A08.-)

J11.8 **Influenza due to unidentified influenza virus with other manifestations**

J11.81 **Influenza due to unidentified influenza virus with encephalopathy**

Influenzal encephalopathy NOS

J11.82 **Influenza due to unidentified influenza virus with myocarditis**

Influenzal myocarditis NOS

J11.83 **Influenza due to unidentified influenza virus with otitis media**

Influenzal otitis media NOS

Use Additional Code for any associated perforated tympanic membrane (H72.-)

J11.89 **Influenza due to unidentified influenza virus with other manifestations**

Use Additional Codes to identify the manifestations

J12 **Viral pneumonia, not elsewhere classified**

Includes: bronchopneumonia due to viruses other than influenza viruses

Code first associated influenza, if applicable (J09.X1, J10.0-, J11.0-)

Code also associated abscess, if applicable (J85.1)

Excludes1: aspiration pneumonia due to anesthesia during labor and delivery (O74.0)

aspiration pneumonia due to anesthesia during pregnancy (O29)

aspiration pneumonia due to anesthesia during puerperium (O89.0)

aspiration pneumonia due to solids and liquids (J69.-)

aspiration pneumonia NOS (J69.0)

congenital pneumonia (P23.0)

congenital rubella pneumonitis (P35.0)

interstitial pneumonia NOS (J84.9)

lipid pneumonia (J69.1)

neonatal aspiration pneumonia (P24.-)

J12.0 **Adenoviral pneumonia**

J12.1 **Respiratory syncytial virus pneumonia**

RSV pneumonia

J12.2 **Parainfluenza virus pneumonia**

J12.3 **Human metapneumovirus pneumonia**

J12.8 **Other viral pneumonia**

J12.81 **Pneumonia due to SARS-associated coronavirus**

Severe acute respiratory syndrome NOS

J12.89 **Other viral pneumonia**

J12.9 **Viral pneumonia, unspecified**

J13 **Pneumonia due to Streptococcus pneumoniae** [HCC]

Bronchopneumonia due to S. pneumoniae

Code first associated influenza, if applicable (J09.X1, J10.0-, J11.0-)

Code also associated abscess, if applicable (J85.1)

Excludes1: congenital pneumonia due to S. pneumoniae (P23.6)

lobar pneumonia, unspecified organism (J18.1)

pneumonia due to other streptococci (J15.3-J15.4)

J14 **Pneumonia due to Hemophilus influenzae** [HCC]

Bronchopneumonia due to H. influenzae

Code first associated influenza, if applicable (J09.X1, J10.0-, J11.0-)

Code also associated abscess, if applicable (J85.1)

Excludes1: congenital pneumonia due to H. influenzae (P23.6)

J15 **Bacterial pneumonia, not elsewhere classified**

Includes: bronchopneumonia due to bacteria other than S. pneumoniae and H. influenzae

Code first associated influenza, if applicable (J09.X1, J10.0-, J11.0-)

Code also associated abscess, if applicable (J85.1)

Excludes1: chlamydial pneumonia (J16.0)

congenital pneumonia (P23.-)

Legionnaires' disease (A48.1)

spirochetal pneumonia (A69.8)

J15.0 **Pneumonia due to Klebsiella pneumoniae** [HCC]

J15.1 **Pneumonia due to Pseudomonas** [HCC]

J15.2 **Pneumonia due to staphylococcus**

J15.20 **Pneumonia due to staphylococcus, unspecified** [HCC]

J15.21 **Pneumonia due to staphylococcus aureus**

J15.211 **Pneumonia due to Methicillin susceptible Staphylococcus aureus** [HCC]

MSSA pneumonia

Pneumonia due to Staphylococcus aureus NOS

J15.212 **Pneumonia due to Methicillin resistant Staphylococcus aureus** [HCC]

J15.29 **Pneumonia due to other staphylococcus** [HCC]

J15.3 **Pneumonia due to streptococcus, group B** [HCC]

J15.4 **Pneumonia due to other streptococci** [HCC]

Excludes1: pneumonia due to streptococcus, group B (J15.3)

pneumonia due to Streptococcus pneumoniae (J13)

J15.5 **Pneumonia due to Escherichia coli** [HCC]

J15.6 **Pneumonia due to other Gram-negative bacteria** [HCC]

Pneumonia due to Serratia marcescens

J15.7 **Pneumonia due to Mycoplasma pneumoniae**

J15.8 **Pneumonia due to other specified bacteria** [HCC]

J15.9 **Unspecified bacterial pneumonia**

Pneumonia due to gram-positive bacteria

J16 **Pneumonia due to other infectious organisms, not elsewhere classified**

Code first associated influenza, if applicable (J09.X1, J10.0-, J11.0-)

Code also associated abscess, if applicable (J85.1)

Excludes1: congenital pneumonia (P23.-)

ornithosis (A70)

pneumocystosis (B59)

pneumonia NOS (J18.9)

J16.0 **Chlamydial pneumonia**

J16.8 **Pneumonia due to other specified infectious organisms**

J17 **Pneumonia in diseases classified elsewhere**

Code first underlying disease, such as:

Q fever (A78) rheumatic fever (I00)

schistosomiasis (B65.0-B65.9)

Excludes1: candidal pneumonia (B37.1)

chlamydial pneumonia (J16.0)

● New code ▲ Revised code **Excludes1:** Not coded here **Excludes2:** Not included here ⊗ Placeholder required ⑦7th digit required

gonorrheal pneumonia (A54.84)

histoplasmosis pneumonia (B39.0-B39.2)

measles pneumonia (B05.2)

nocardiosis pneumonia (A43.0)

pneumocystosis (B59)

pneumonia due to Pneumocystis carinii (B59)

pneumonia due to Pneumocystis jiroveci (B59)

pneumonia in actinomycosis (A42.0)

pneumonia in anthrax (A22.1)

pneumonia in ascariasis (B77.81)

pneumonia in aspergillosis (B44.0-B44.1)

pneumonia in coccidioidomycosis (B38.0-B38.2)

pneumonia in cytomegalovirus disease (B25.0)

pneumonia in toxoplasmosis (B58.3)

rubella pneumonia (B06.81)

salmonella pneumonia (A02.22)

spirochetal infection NEC with pneumonia (A69.8)

tularemia pneumonia (A21.2)

typhoid fever with pneumonia (A01.03)

varicella pneumonia (B01.2)

whooping cough with pneumonia (A37 with fifth-character 1)

J18 **Pneumonia, unspecified organism**

Code first associated influenza, if applicable (J09.X1, J10.0-, J11.0-)

Excludes1: abscess of lung with pneumonia (J85.1)

aspiration pneumonia due to anesthesia during labor and delivery (O74.0)

aspiration pneumonia due to anesthesia during pregnancy (O29)

aspiration pneumonia due to anesthesia during puerperium (O89.0)

aspiration pneumonia due to solids and liquids (J69.-)

aspiration pneumonia NOS (J69.0)

congenital pneumonia (P23.0)

drug-induced interstitial lung disorder (J70.2-J70.4)

interstitial pneumonia NOS (J84.9)

lipid pneumonia (J69.1)

neonatal aspiration pneumonia (P24.-)

pneumonitis due to external agents (J67-J70)

pneumonitis due to fumes and vapors (J68.0)

usual interstitial pneumonia (J84.178)

J18.0 **Bronchopneumonia, unspecified organism**

Definition: Bronchopneumonia is a pneumonia characterized by acute inflammation of the walls of the bronchioles

Excludes1: hypostatic bronchopneumonia (J18.2)

lipid pneumonia (J69.1)

Excludes2: acute bronchiolitis (J21.-)

chronic bronchiolitis (J44.9)

J18.1 **Lobar pneumonia, unspecified organism** [HCC]

J18.2 **Hypostatic pneumonia, unspecified organism**

Hypostatic bronchopneumonia

Passive pneumonia

J18.8 **Other pneumonia, unspecified organism**

J18.9 **Pneumonia, unspecified organism**

OTHER ACUTE LOWER RESPIRATORY INFECTIONS (J20-J22)

Excludes2: chronic obstructive pulmonary disease with acute lower respiratory infection (J44.0)

J20 **Acute bronchitis**

Includes: acute and subacute bronchitis (with) bronchospasm

acute and subacute bronchitis (with) tracheitis

acute and subacute bronchitis (with) tracheobronchitis,

acute and subacute fibrinous bronchitis

acute and subacute membranous bronchitis acute and subacute purulent bronchitis acute and subacute septic bronchitis

Excludes1: bronchitis NOS (J40)

tracheobronchitis NOS (J40)

Excludes2: acute bronchitis with bronchiectasis (J47.0)

acute bronchitis with chronic obstructive asthma (J44.0)

acute bronchitis with chronic obstructive pulmonary disease (J44.0)

allergic bronchitis NOS (J45.909-)

bronchitis due to chemicals, fumes and vapors (J68.0)

chronic bronchitis NOS (J42)

chronic mucopurulent bronchitis (J41.1)

chronic obstructive bronchitis (J44.-)

chronic obstructive tracheobronchitis (J44.-)

chronic simple bronchitis (J41.0)

chronic tracheobronchitis (J42)

J20.0 **Acute bronchitis due to Mycoplasma pneumoniae**

J20.1 **Acute bronchitis due to Hemophilus influenzae**

J20.2 **Acute bronchitis due to streptococcus**

J20.3 **Acute bronchitis due to coxsackievirus**

J20.4 **Acute bronchitis due to parainfluenza virus**

J20.5 **Acute bronchitis due to respiratory syncytial virus**

Acute bronchitis due to RSV

J20.6 **Acute bronchitis due to rhinovirus**

J20.7 **Acute bronchitis due to echovirus**

J20.8 **Acute bronchitis due to other specified organisms**

J20.9 **Acute bronchitis, unspecified**

J21 **Acute bronchiolitis**

Includes: acute bronchiolitis with bronchospasm

Excludes2: respiratory bronchiolitis interstitial lung disease (J84.115)

J21.0 **Acute bronchiolitis due to respiratory syncytial virus**

J21.1 **Acute bronchiolitis due to human metapneumovirus**

J21.8 **Acute bronchiolitis due to other specified organisms**

J21.9 **Acute bronchiolitis, unspecified**

Bronchiolitis (acute)

Excludes1: chronic bronchiolitis (J44.-)

J22 **Unspecified acute lower respiratory infection**

Acute (lower) respiratory (tract) infection NOS

Excludes1: upper respiratory infection (acute) (J06.9)

OTHER DISEASES OF UPPER RESPIRATORY TRACT (J30-J39)

J30 **Vasomotor and allergic rhinitis**

Includes: spasmodic rhinorrhea

Excludes1: allergic rhinitis with asthma (bronchial) (J45.909)

rhinitis NOS (J31.0)

J30.0 **Vasomotor rhinitis**

J30.1 **Allergic rhinitis due to pollen**

Definition: Allergic rhinitis refers to a group of symptoms similar to those of a cold such as runny nose and sore throat, caused by an allergic reaction to an allergen such as dust, plant pollens or animal dander.

Allergy NOS due to pollen

Hay fever

Pollinosis

J30.2 Other seasonal allergic rhinitis

J30.5 Allergic rhinitis due to food

J30.8 Other allergic rhinitis

    J30.81 Allergic rhinitis due to animal (cat) (dog) hair and dander

    J30.89 Other allergic rhinitis

        Perennial allergic rhinitis

J30.9 Allergic rhinitis, unspecified

J31 Chronic rhinitis, nasopharyngitis and pharyngitis

Use Additional Code to identify:

exposure to environmental tobacco smoke (Z77.22)

exposure to tobacco smoke in the perinatal period (P96.81)

history of tobacco dependence (Z87.891)

occupational exposure to environmental tobacco smoke (Z57.31)

tobacco dependence (F17.-)

tobacco use (Z72.0)

J31.0 Chronic rhinitis

    Atrophic rhinitis (chronic)

    Granulomatous rhinitis (chronic)

    Hypertrophic rhinitis (chronic)

    Obstructive rhinitis (chronic)

    Ozena

    Purulent rhinitis (chronic)

    Rhinitis (chronic) NOS

    Ulcerative rhinitis (chronic)

    Excludes1: allergic rhinitis (J30.1-J30.9)

        vasomotor rhinitis (J30.0)

J31.1 Chronic nasopharyngitis

    Excludes2: acute nasopharyngitis (J00)

J31.2 Chronic pharyngitis

    Chronic sore throat

    Atrophic pharyngitis (chronic)

    Granular pharyngitis (chronic)

    Hypertrophic pharyngitis (chronic)

    Excludes2: acute pharyngitis (J02.9)

J32 Chronic sinusitis

Includes: sinus abscess

sinus empyema

sinus infection

sinus suppuration

Use Additional Code to identify:

exposure to environmental tobacco smoke (Z77.22)

exposure to tobacco smoke in the perinatal period (P96.81)

history of tobacco dependence (Z87.891)

infectious agent (B95-B97)

occupational exposure to environmental tobacco smoke (Z57.31)

tobacco dependence (F17.-)

tobacco use (Z72.0)

Excludes2: acute sinusitis (J01.-)

J32.0 Chronic maxillary sinusitis

Antritis (chronic)

Maxillary sinusitis NOS

J32.1 Chronic frontal sinusitis

    Frontal sinusitis NOS

J32.2 Chronic ethmoidal sinusitis

    Ethmoidal sinusitis NOS

    Excludes1: Woakes' ethmoiditis (J33.1)

J32.3 Chronic sphenoidal sinusitis

    Sphenoidal sinusitis NOS

J32.4 Chronic pansinusitis

    Pansinusitis NOS

J32.8 Other chronic sinusitis

    Sinusitis (chronic) involving more than one sinus but not pansinusitis

J32.9 Chronic sinusitis, unspecified

    Sinusitis (chronic) NOS

J33 Nasal polyp

Use Additional Code to identify:

exposure to environmental tobacco smoke (Z77.22)

exposure to tobacco smoke in the perinatal period (P96.81)

history of tobacco dependence (Z87.891)

occupational exposure to environmental tobacco smoke (Z57.31)

tobacco dependence (F17.-)

tobacco use (Z72.0)

Excludes1: adenomatous polyps (D14.0)

J33.0 Polyp of nasal cavity

    Choanal polyp Nasopharyngeal polyp

J33.1 Polypoid sinus degeneration

    Woakes' syndrome or ethmoiditis

J33.8 Other polyp of sinus

    Accessory polyp of sinus

    Ethmoidal polyp of sinus

    Maxillary polyp of sinus

    Sphenoidal polyp of sinus

J33.9 Nasal polyp, unspecified

J34 Other and unspecified disorders of nose and nasal sinuses

Excludes2: varicose ulcer of nasal septum (I86.8)

J34.0 Abscess, furuncle and carbuncle of nose

    Cellulitis of nose

    Necrosis of nose

    Ulceration of nose

J34.1 Cyst and mucocele of nose and nasal sinus

J34.2 Deviated nasal septum

    Deflection or deviation of septum (nasal) (acquired)

    Excludes1: congenital deviated nasal septum (Q67.4)

J34.3 Hypertrophy of nasal turbinates

J34.8 Other specified disorders of nose and nasal sinuses

    J34.81 Nasal mucositis (ulcerative)

        Code also type of associated therapy, such as:

        antineoplastic and immunosuppressive drugs (T45.1X-)

        radiological procedure and radiotherapy (Y84.2)

        Excludes2: gastrointestinal mucositis (ulcerative) (K92.81)

        mucositis (ulcerative) of vagina and vulva (N76.81)

        oral mucositis (ulcerative) (K12.3-)

● New code ▲ Revised code Excludes1: Not coded here Excludes2: Not included here ⊗ Placeholder required ⑦7ᵗʰ digit required

J34.89 Other specified disorders of nose and nasal sinuses

Perforation of nasal septum NOS

Rhinolith

J34.9 Unspecified disorder of nose and nasal sinuses

J35 Chronic diseases of tonsils and adenoids

Use Additional Code to identify:

exposure to environmental tobacco smoke (Z77.22)

exposure to tobacco smoke in the perinatal period (P96.81)

history of tobacco dependence (Z87.891)

occupational exposure to environmental tobacco smoke (Z57.31)

tobacco dependence (F17.-)

tobacco use (Z72.0)

J35.0 Chronic tonsillitis and adenoiditis

Excludes2: acute tonsillitis (J03.-)

J35.01 Chronic tonsillitis

J35.02 Chronic adenoiditis

J35.03 Chronic tonsillitis and adenoiditis

J35.1 Hypertrophy of tonsils

Enlargement of tonsils

Excludes1: hypertrophy of tonsils with tonsillitis (J35.0-)

J35.2 Hypertrophy of adenoids

Enlargement of adenoids

Excludes1: hypertrophy of adenoids with adenoiditis (J35.0-)

J35.3 Hypertrophy of tonsils with hypertrophy of adenoids

Excludes1: hypertrophy of tonsils and adenoids with tonsillitis and adenoiditis (J35.03)

J35.8 Other chronic diseases of tonsils and adenoids

Adenoid vegetations

Amygdalolith

Calculus, tonsil

Cicatrix of tonsil (and adenoid)

Tonsillar tag

Ulcer of tonsil

J35.9 Chronic disease of tonsils and adenoids, unspecified

Disease (chronic) of tonsils and adenoids NOS

J36 Peritonsillar abscess

Definition: A Peritonsillar abscess is an abscess forming in acute tonsillitis around one or both tonsils.

Includes: abscess of tonsil

peritonsillar cellulitis quinsy

Use Additional Code (B95-B97) to identify infectious agent.

Excludes1: acute tonsillitis (J03.-)

chronic tonsillitis (J35.0)

retropharyngeal abscess (J39.0)

tonsillitis NOS (J03.9-)

J37 Chronic laryngitis and laryngotracheitis

Use Additional Code to identify:

exposure to environmental tobacco smoke (Z77.22)

exposure to tobacco smoke in the perinatal period (P96.81)

history of tobacco dependence (Z87.891)

infectious agent (B95-B97)

occupational exposure to environmental tobacco smoke (Z57.31)

tobacco dependence (F17.-)

tobacco use (Z72.0)

J37.0 Chronic laryngitis

Catarrhal laryngitis

Hypertrophic laryngitis

Sicca laryngitis

Excludes2: acute laryngitis (J04.0)

obstructive (acute) laryngitis (J05.0)

J37.1 Chronic laryngotracheitis

Laryngitis, chronic, with tracheitis (chronic)

Tracheitis, chronic, with laryngitis

Excludes1: chronic tracheitis (J42)

Excludes2: acute laryngotracheitis (J04.2)

acute tracheitis (J04.1)

J38 Diseases of vocal cords and larynx, not elsewhere classified

Use Additional Code to identify:

exposure to environmental tobacco smoke (Z77.22)

exposure to tobacco smoke in the perinatal period (P96.81)

history of tobacco dependence (Z87.891)

occupational exposure to environmental tobacco smoke (Z57.31)

tobacco dependence (F17.-)

tobacco use (Z72.0)

Excludes1: congenital laryngeal stridor (P28.89)

obstructive laryngitis (acute) (J05.0)

postprocedural subglottic stenosis (J95.5)

stridor (R06.1)

ulcerative laryngitis (J04.0)

J38.0 Paralysis of vocal cords and larynx

Laryngoplegia

Paralysis of glottis

J38.00 Paralysis of vocal cords and larynx, unspecified

J38.01 Paralysis of vocal cords and larynx, unilateral

J38.02 Paralysis of vocal cords and larynx, bilateral

J38.1 Polyp of vocal cord and larynx

Excludes1: adenomatous polyps (D14.1)

J38.2 Nodules of vocal cords

Chorditis (fibrinous)(nodosa)(tuberosa)

Singer's nodes

Teacher's nodes

J38.3 Other diseases of vocal cords

Abscess of vocal cords

Cellulitis of vocal cords

Granuloma of vocal cords

Leukokeratosis of vocal cords

Leukoplakia of vocal cords

J38.4 Edema of larynx

Edema (of) glottis

Subglottic edema

Supraglottic edema

Excludes1: acute obstructive laryngitis [croup] (J05.0)

edematous laryngitis (J04.0)

J38.5 Laryngeal spasm

Laryngismus (stridulus)

J38.6 Stenosis of larynx

J38.7 Other diseases of larynx

Abscess of larynx

Cellulitis of larynx

Disease of larynx NOS

Necrosis of larynx

Pachyderma of larynx

Perichondritis of larynx

Ulcer of larynx

J39 **Other diseases of upper respiratory tract**

Excludes1: acute respiratory infection NOS (J22)

acute upper respiratory infection (J06.9)

upper respiratory inflammation due to chemicals, gases, fumes or vapors (J68.2)

J39.0 **Retropharyngeal and parapharyngeal abscess**

Peripharyngeal abscess

Excludes1: peritonsillar abscess (J36)

J39.1 **Other abscess of pharynx**

Cellulitis of pharynx Nasopharyngeal abscess

J39.2 **Other diseases of pharynx**

Cyst of pharynx

Edema of pharynx

Excludes2: chronic pharyngitis (J31.2)

ulcerative pharyngitis (J02.9)

J39.3 **Upper respiratory tract hypersensitivity reaction, site unspecified**

Excludes1: hypersensitivity reaction of upper respiratory tract, such as:

extrinsic allergic alveolitis (J67.9)

pneumoconiosis (J60-J67.9)

J39.8 **Other specified diseases of upper respiratory tract**

J39.9 **Disease of upper respiratory tract, unspecified**

CHRONIC LOWER RESPIRATORY DISEASES (J40-J47)

Excludes1: bronchitis due to chemicals, gases, fumes and vapors (J68.0)

Excludes2: cystic fibrosis (E84.-)

J40 **Bronchitis, not specified as acute or chronic**

Bronchitis NOS

Bronchitis with tracheitis NOS

Catarrhal bronchitis

Tracheobronchitis NOS

Use Additional Code to identify:

exposure to environmental tobacco smoke (Z77.22)

exposure to tobacco smoke in the perinatal period (P96.81)

history of tobacco dependence (Z87.891)

occupational exposure to environmental tobacco smoke (Z57.31)

tobacco dependence (F17.-)

tobacco use (Z72.0)

Excludes1: acute bronchitis (J20.-)

allergic bronchitis NOS (J45.909-)

asthmatic bronchitis NOS (J45.9-)

bronchitis due to chemicals, gases, fumes and vapors (J68.0)

J41 **Simple and mucopurulent chronic bronchitis**

Use Additional Code to identify:

exposure to environmental tobacco smoke (Z77.22)

exposure to tobacco smoke in the perinatal period (P96.81)

history of tobacco dependence (Z87.891)

occupational exposure to environmental tobacco smoke (Z57.31)

tobacco dependence (F17.-)

tobacco use (Z72.0)

Excludes1: chronic bronchitis NOS (J42)

chronic obstructive bronchitis (J44.-)

J41.0 **Simple chronic bronchitis** [HCC]

J41.1 **Mucopurulent chronic bronchitis** [HCC]

J41.8 **Mixed simple and mucopurulent chronic bronchitis** [HCC]

J42 **Unspecified chronic bronchitis** [HCC]

Chronic bronchitis NOS

Chronic tracheitis

Chronic tracheobronchitis

Use Additional Code to identify:

exposure to environmental tobacco smoke (Z77.22)

exposure to tobacco smoke in the perinatal period (P96.81)

history of tobacco dependence (Z87.891)

occupational exposure to environmental tobacco smoke (Z57.31)

tobacco dependence (F17.-)

tobacco use (Z72.0)

Excludes1: chronic asthmatic bronchitis (J44.-)

chronic bronchitis with airways obstruction (J44.-)

chronic emphysematous bronchitis (J44.-)

chronic obstructive pulmonary disease NOS (J44.9)

simple and mucopurulent chronic bronchitis (J41.-)

J43 **Emphysema**

Definition: Emphysema is a chronic respiratory disease where there is over-inflation of the air sacs (alveoli) in the lungs, causing a decrease in lung function, and often, breathlessness.

Use Additional Code to identify:

exposure to environmental tobacco smoke (Z77.22)

history of tobacco dependence (Z87.891)

occupational exposure to environmental tobacco smoke (Z57.31)

tobacco dependence (F17.-)

tobacco use (Z72.0)

Excludes1: compensatory emphysema (J98.3)

emphysema due to inhalation of chemicals, gases, fumes or vapors (J68.4)

emphysema with chronic (obstructive)

bronchitis (J44.-)

emphysematous (obstructive) bronchitis (J44.-)

interstitial emphysema (J98.2)

mediastinal emphysema (J98.2)

neonatal interstitial emphysema (P25.0)

surgical (subcutaneous) emphysema (T81.82)

Excludes2: traumatic subcutaneous emphysema (T79.7)

J43.0 **Unilateral pulmonary emphysema [MacLeod's syndrome]** [HCC]

Swyer-James syndrome

Unilateral emphysema

Unilateral hyperlucent lung

Unilateral pulmonary artery functional hypoplasia

Unilateral transparency of lung

J43.1 **Panlobular emphysema** [HCC]

Panacinar emphysema

J43.2 **Centrilobular emphysema** [HCC]

J43.8 **Other emphysema** [HCC]

J43.9 **Emphysema, unspecified** [HCC]

Bullous emphysema (lung)(pulmonary)

Emphysema (lung)(pulmonary) NOS

Emphysematous bleb

Vesicular emphysema (lung)(pulmonary)

J44 **Other chronic obstructive pulmonary disease**

Includes: asthma with chronic obstructive pulmonary disease

chronic asthmatic (obstructive) bronchitis

chronic bronchitis with airways obstruction

chronic bronchitis with emphysema

chronic emphysematous bronchitis

chronic obstructive asthma

chronic obstructive bronchitis

chronic obstructive tracheobronchitis

Code also type of asthma, if applicable (J45.-)

Use Additional Code to identify:

exposure to environmental tobacco smoke (Z77.22) history of tobacco dependence (Z87.891)

occupational exposure to environmental tobacco smoke (Z57.31) tobacco dependence (F17.-)

tobacco use (Z72.0)

Excludes1: bronchiectasis (J47.-)

chronic bronchitis NOS (J42)

chronic simple and mucopurulent bronchitis (J41.-)

chronic tracheitis (J42)

chronic tracheobronchitis (J42)

emphysema without chronic bronchitis (J43.-)

J44.0   **Chronic obstructive pulmonary disease with (acute) lower respiratory infection** [HCC]

Code also to identify the infection

J44.1   **Chronic obstructive pulmonary disease with (acute) exacerbation** [HCC]

Decompensated COPD

Decompensated COPD with (acute) exacerbation

Excludes2: chronic obstructive pulmonary disease [COPD] with acute bronchitis (J44.0)

lung diseases due to external agents (J60-J70)

J44.9   **Chronic obstructive pulmonary disease, unspecified** [HCC]

Chronic obstructive airway disease NOS

Chronic obstructive lung disease NOS

Excludes2: lung diseases due to external agents (J60-J70)

J45   **Asthma**

Use Additional Code eosinophilic asthma (J82.83)

Includes: allergic (predominantly) asthma

allergic bronchitis NOS

allergic rhinitis with asthma

atopic asthma

extrinsic allergic asthma

hay fever with asthma

idiosyncratic asthma

intrinsic nonallergic asthma

nonallergic asthma

Use Additional Code to identify:

exposure to environmental tobacco smoke (Z77.22)

exposure to tobacco smoke in the perinatal period (P96.81)

history of tobacco dependence (Z87.891)

occupational exposure to environmental tobacco smoke (Z57.31)

tobacco dependence (F17.-)

tobacco use (Z72.0)

Excludes1: detergent asthma (J69.8)

eosinophilic asthma (J82)

miner's asthma (J60)

wheezing NOS (R06.2)

wood asthma (J67.8)

Excludes2: asthma with chronic obstructive pulmonary disease (J44.9)

chronic asthmatic (obstructive) bronchitis (J44.9)

chronic obstructive asthma (J44.9)

J45.2   **Mild intermittent asthma**

J45.20   **Mild intermittent asthma, uncomplicated**

Mild intermittent asthma NOS

J45.21   **Mild intermittent asthma with (acute) exacerbation**

J45.22   **Mild intermittent asthma with status asthmaticus**

J45.3   **Mild persistent asthma**

J45.30   **Mild persistent asthma, uncomplicated**

Mild persistent asthma NOS

J45.31   **Mild persistent asthma with (acute) exacerbation**

J45.32   **Mild persistent asthma with status asthmaticus**

J45.4   **Moderate persistent asthma**

J45.40   **Moderate persistent asthma, uncomplicated**

Moderate persistent asthma NOS

J45.41   **Moderate persistent asthma with (acute) exacerbation**

J45.42   **Moderate persistent asthma with status asthmaticus**

J45.5   **Severe persistent asthma**

J45.50   **Severe persistent asthma, uncomplicated**

Severe persistent asthma NOS

J45.51   **Severe persistent asthma with (acute) exacerbation**

J45.52   **Severe persistent asthma with status asthmaticus**

J45.9   **Other and unspecified asthma**

J45.90   **Unspecified asthma**

Asthmatic bronchitis NOS

Childhood asthma NOS

Late onset asthma

J45.901   **Unspecified asthma with (acute) exacerbation**

J45.902   **Unspecified asthma with status asthmaticus**

J45.909   **Unspecified asthma, uncomplicated**

Asthma NOS

Excludes2: lung diseases due to external agents (J60-J70)

J45.99   **Other asthma**

J45.990   **Exercise induced bronchospasm**

J45.991   **Cough variant asthma**

J45.998   **Other asthma**

J47   **Bronchiectasis**

Definition: Bronchiectasis is a condition characterized by abnormal dilatation of the bronchi (airways) and excessive mucus production. The mucus accumulation may obstruct the bronchi. Is often associated with repeated bronchial infections.

Includes: bronchiolectasis

Use Additional Code to identify:

exposure to environmental tobacco smoke (Z77.22)

exposure to tobacco smoke in the perinatal period (P96.81)

history of tobacco dependence (Z87.891)

occupational exposure to environmental tobacco smoke (Z57.31)

tobacco dependence (F17.-)

tobacco use (Z72.0)

Excludes1: congenital bronchiectasis (Q33.4)

tuberculous bronchiectasis (current disease) (A15.0)

J47.0 Bronchiectasis with acute lower respiratory infection [HCC]

Bronchiectasis with acute bronchitis

Code also to identify the infection

J47.1 Bronchiectasis with (acute) exacerbation [HCC]

J47.9 Bronchiectasis, uncomplicated [HCC]

Bronchiectasis NOS

LUNG DISEASES DUE TO EXTERNAL AGENTS (J60-J70)

Excludes2: asthma (J45.-)

malignant neoplasm of bronchus and lung (C34.-)

J60 Coalworker's pneumoconiosis [HCC]

Anthracosilicosis

Anthracosis

Black lung disease

Coalworker's lung

Excludes1: coal worker pneumoconiosis with tuberculosis, any type in A15 (J65)

J61 Pneumoconiosis due to asbestos and other mineral fibers [HCC]

Asbestosis

Excludes1: pleural plaque with asbestosis (J92.0)

pneumoconiosis with tuberculosis, any type in A15 (J65)

J62 Pneumoconiosis due to dust containing silica

Includes: silicotic fibrosis (massive) of lung

Excludes1: pneumoconiosis with tuberculosis, any type in A15 (J65)

J62.0 Pneumoconiosis due to talc dust [HCC]

J62.8 Pneumoconiosis due to other dust containing silica [HCC]

Silicosis NOS

J63 Pneumoconiosis due to other inorganic dusts

Excludes1: pneumoconiosis with tuberculosis, any type in A15 (J65)

J63.0 Aluminosis (of lung) [HCC]

J63.1 Bauxite fibrosis (of lung) [HCC]

J63.2 Berylliosis [HCC]

J63.3 Graphite fibrosis (of lung) [HCC]

J63.4 Siderosis [HCC]

J63.5 Stannosis [HCC]

J63.6 Pneumoconiosis due to other specified inorganic dusts [HCC]

J64 Unspecified pneumoconiosis [HCC]

Excludes1: pneumonoconiosis with tuberculosis, any type in A15 (J65)

J65 Pneumoconiosis associated with tuberculosis [HCC]

Any condition in J60-J64 with tuberculosis, any type in A15

Silicotuberculosis

J66 Airway disease due to specific organic dust

Excludes2: allergic alveolitis (J67.-)

asbestosis (J61)

bagassosis (J67.1)

farmer's lung (J67.0)

hypersensitivity pneumonitis due to organic dust (J67.-)

reactive airways dysfunction syndrome (J68.3)

J66.0 Byssinosis [HCC]

Airway disease due to cotton dust

J66.1 Flax-dressers' disease [HCC]

J66.2 Cannabinosis [HCC]

J66.8 Airway disease due to other specific organic dusts [HCC]

J67 Hypersensitivity pneumonitis due to organic dust

Includes: allergic alveolitis and pneumonitis due to inhaled organic dust and particles of fungal, actinomycetic **or other** origin

Excludes1: pneumonitis due to inhalation of chemicals, gases, fumes or vapors (J68.0)

J67.0 Farmer's lung [HCC]

Harvester's lung

Haymaker's lung

Moldy hay disease

J67.1 Bagassosis [HCC]

Bagasse disease

Bagasse pneumonitis

J67.2 Bird fancier's lung

Budgerigar fancier's disease or lung

Pigeon fancier's disease or lung

J67.3 Suberosis [HCC]

Cork handler's disease or lung

Cork worker's disease or lung

J67.4 Maltworker's lung [HCC]

Alveolitis due to Aspergillus clavatus

J67.5 Mushroom-worker's lung [HCC]

J67.6 Maple-bark-stripper's lung [HCC]

Alveolitis due to

Cryptostroma corticale

Cryptostromosis

J67.7 Air conditioner and humidifier lung [HCC]

Allergic alveolitis due to fungal, thermophilic actinomycetes **and other** organisms growing in ventilation [air conditioning] systems

J67.8 Hypersensitivity pneumonitis due to other organic dusts [HCC]

Cheese-washer's lung

Coffee-worker's lung

Fish-meal worker's lung

Furrier's lung

Sequoiosis

J67.9 Hypersensitivity pneumonitis due to unspecified organic dust [HCC]

Allergic alveolitis (extrinsic) NOS

Hypersensitivity pneumonitis NOS

J68 Respiratory conditions due to inhalation of chemicals, gases, fumes and vapors

Code first (T51-T65) to identify cause

Use Additional Code to identify associated respiratory conditions, such as:

acute respiratory failure (J96.0-)

J68.0 Bronchitis and pneumonitis due to chemicals, gases, fumes and vapors [HCC]

Chemical bronchitis (acute)

J68.1 Pulmonary edema due to chemicals, gases, fumes and vapors [HCC]

Chemical pulmonary edema (acute) (chronic)

> **Excludes1:** pulmonary edema (acute) (chronic) NOS (J81.-)

J68.2 **Upper respiratory inflammation due to chemicals, gases, fumes and vapors, not elsewhere classified** [HCC]

J68.3 **Other acute and subacute respiratory conditions due to chemicals, gases, fumes and vapors** [HCC]

Reactive airways dysfunction syndrome

J68.4 **Chronic respiratory conditions due to chemicals, gases, fumes and vapors** [HCC]

Emphysema (diffuse) (chronic) due to inhalation of chemicals, gases, fumes and vapors

Obliterative bronchiolitis (chronic) (subacute) due to inhalation of chemicals, gases, fumes and vapors

Pulmonary fibrosis (chronic) due to inhalation of chemicals, gases, fumes and vapors

> **Excludes1:** chronic pulmonary edema due to chemicals, gases, fumes and vapors (J68.1)

J68.8 **Other respiratory conditions due to chemicals, gases, fumes and vapors** [HCC]

J68.9 **Unspecified respiratory condition due to chemicals, gases, fumes and vapors** [HCC]

J69 **Pneumonitis due to solids and liquids**

> **Excludes1:** neonatal aspiration syndromes (P24.-)
>
> postprocedural pneumonitis (J95.4)

J69.0 **Pneumonitis due to inhalation of food and vomit** [HCC]

Aspiration pneumonia NOS

Aspiration pneumonia (due to) food (regurgitated)

Aspiration pneumonia (due to) gastric secretions

Aspiration pneumonia (due to) milk

Aspiration pneumonia (due to) vomit

Code also any associated foreign body in respiratory tract (T17.-)

> **Excludes1:** chemical pneumonitis due to anesthesia (J95.4)
>
> obstetric aspiration pneumonitis (O74.0)

J69.1 **Pneumonitis due to inhalation of oils and essences** [HCC]

Exogenous lipoid pneumonia

Lipid pneumonia NOS

Code first (T51-T65) to identify substance

> **Excludes1:** endogenous lipoid pneumonia (J84.89)

J69.8 **Pneumonitis due to inhalation of other solids and liquids** [HCC]

Pneumonitis due to aspiration of blood

Pneumonitis due to aspiration of detergent

Code first (T51-T65) to identify substance

J70 **Respiratory conditions due to other external agents**

J70.0 **Acute pulmonary manifestations due to radiation** [HCC]

Radiation pneumonitis

Use Additional Code (W88-W90, X39.0-) to identify the external cause

J70.1 **Chronic and other pulmonary manifestations due to radiation** [HCC]

Fibrosis of lung following radiation

Use Additional Code (W88-W90, X39.0-) to identify the external cause

J70.2 **Acute drug-induced interstitial lung disorders** [HCC]

Use Additional Code for adverse effect, if applicable, to identify drug (T36-T50 with fifth or sixth character 5)

> **Excludes1:** interstitial pneumonia NOS (J84.9)
>
> lymphoid interstitial pneumonia (J84.2)

J70.3 **Chronic drug-induced interstitial lung disorders** [HCC]

Use Additional Code for adverse effect, if applicable, to identify drug (T36-T50 with fifth or sixth character 5)

> **Excludes1:** interstitial pneumonia NOS (J84.9)
>
> lymphoid interstitial pneumonia (J84.2)

J70.4 **Drug-induced interstitial lung disorders, unspecified** [HCC]

Use Additional Code for adverse effect, if applicable, to identify drug (T36-T50 with fifth or sixth character 5)

> **Excludes1:** interstitial pneumonia NOS (J84.9)
>
> lymphoid interstitial pneumonia (J84.2)

J70.5 **Respiratory conditions due to smoke inhalation**

Code first smoke inhalation (T59.81-)

> **Excludes2:** smoke inhalation due to chemicals, gases, fumes and vapors (J68.9)

J70.8 **Respiratory conditions due to other specified external agents** [HCC]

Code first (T51-T65) to identify the external agent

J70.9 **Respiratory conditions due to unspecified external agent** [HCC]

Code first (T51-T65) to identify the external agent

OTHER RESPIRATORY DISEASES PRINCIPALLY AFFECTING THE INTERSTITIUM (J80-J84)

J80 **Acute respiratory distress syndrome** [HCC]

Acute respiratory distress syndrome in adult or child

Adult hyaline membrane disease

> **Excludes1:** respiratory distress syndrome in newborn (perinatal) (P22.0)

J81 **Pulmonary edema**

Use Additional Code to identify:

exposure to environmental tobacco smoke (Z77.22)

history of tobacco dependence (Z87.891)

occupational exposure to environmental tobacco smoke (Z57.31)

tobacco dependence (F17.-)

tobacco use (Z72.0)

> **Excludes1:** chemical (acute) pulmonary edema (J68.1)
>
> hypostatic pneumonia (J18.2)
>
> passive pneumonia (J18.2)
>
> pulmonary edema due to external agents (J60-J70)
>
> pulmonary edema with heart disease NOS (I50.1)
>
> pulmonary edema with heart failure (I50.1)

J81.0 **Acute pulmonary edema** [HCC]

Acute edema of lung

J81.1 **Chronic pulmonary edema**

Pulmonary congestion (chronic) (passive)

Pulmonary edema NOS

J82 **Pulmonary eosinophilia, not elsewhere classified** [HCC]

> **Excludes2:** pulmonary eosinophilia due to aspergillosis (B44.-)
>
> pulmonary eosinophilia due to drugs (J70.2-J70.4)
>
> pulmonary eosinophilia due to specified parasitic infection (B50-B83)
>
> pulmonary eosinophilia due to systemic connective tissue disorders (M30-M36)
>
> pulmonary infiltrate NOS (R91.8)

J82.8 **Pulmonary eosinophilia, not elsewhere classified**

J82.81 **Chronic eosinophilic pneumonia**

Eosinophilic pneumonia, NOS

J82.82 **Acute eosinophilic pneumonia**

J82.83 **Eosinophilic asthma**

Code first asthma, by type, such as:

mild intermittent asthma (J45.2-)

mild persistent asthma (J45.3-)

moderate persistent asthma (J45.4-)

severe persistent asthma (J45.5-)

J82.89 **Other pulmonary eosinophilia, not elsewhere classified**

Allergic pneumonia

Löffler's pneumonia

Tropical (pulmonary) eosinophilia NOS

J84 **Other interstitial pulmonary diseases**

Excludes1: drug-induced interstitial lung disorders (J70.2-J70.4)

interstitial emphysema (J98.2)

Excludes2: lung diseases due to external agents (J60-J70)

J84.0 **Alveolar and parieto-alveolar conditions**

J84.01 **Alveolar proteinosis** [HCC]

J84.02 **Pulmonary alveolar microlithiasis** [HCC]

J84.03 **Idiopathic pulmonary hemosiderosis** [HCC]

Essential brown induration of lung

Code first underlying disease, such as:

disorders of iron metabolism (E83.1-)

Excludes1: acute idiopathic pulmonary hemorrhage in infants [AIPHI] (R04.81)

J84.09 **Other alveolar and parieto-alveolar conditions** [HCC]

J84.1 **Other interstitial pulmonary diseases with fibrosis** [HCC]

Excludes1: pulmonary fibrosis (chronic) due to inhalation of chemicals, gases, fumes or vapors (J68.4)

pulmonary fibrosis (chronic) following radiation (J70.1)

J84.10 **Pulmonary fibrosis, unspecified** [HCC]

Definition: Pulmonary fibrosis is a condition characterized by deposition of fibrous tissue in the lung. It decreases lung compliance and results in a restrictive ventilatory defect as seen in pulmonary function testing.

Capillary fibrosis of lung

Cirrhosis of lung (chronic) NOS

Fibrosis of lung (atrophic) (chronic) (confluent) (massive) (perialveolar) (peribronchial) NOS

Induration of lung (chronic) NOS

Postinflammatory pulmonary fibrosis

J84.11 **Idiopathic interstitial pneumonia**

Excludes1: lymphoid interstitial pneumonia (J84.2)

pneumocystis pneumonia (B59)

J84.111 **Idiopathic interstitial pneumonia, not otherwise specified** [HCC]

J84.112 **Idiopathic pulmonary fibrosis** [HCC]

Cryptogenic fibrosing alveolitis

Idiopathic fibrosing alveolitis

J84.113 **Idiopathic non-specific interstitial pneumonitis** [HCC]

Excludes1: non-specific interstitial pneumonia NOS, or due to known underlying cause (J84.89)

J84.114 **Acute interstitial pneumonitis** [HCC]

Hamman-Rich syndrome

Excludes1: pneumocystis pneumonia (B59)

J84.115 **Respiratory bronchiolitis interstitial lung disease** [HCC]

J84.116 **Cryptogenic organizing pneumonia** [HCC]

Excludes1: organizing pneumonia NOS, or due to known underlying cause (J84.89)

J84.117 **Desquamative interstitial pneumonia** [HCC]

J84.17 **Other interstitial pulmonary diseases with fibrosis in diseases classified elsewhere** [HCC]

J84.170 **Interstitial lung disease with progressive fibrotic phenotype in diseases classified elsewhere** [HCC]

Progressive fibrotic interstitial lung disease

Code first underlying disease, such as:

lung diseases due to external agents (J60-J70)

rheumatoid arthritis (M05.00-M06.9)

sarcoidosis (D86)

systemic connective tissue disorders (M30-M36)

J84.178 **Other interstitial pulmonary diseases with fibrosis in diseases classified elsewhere** [HCC]

Interstitial pneumonia (nonspecific) (usual) due to collagen vascular disease

Interstitial pneumonia (nonspecific) (usual) in diseases classified elsewhere

Organizing pneumonia due to collagen vascular disease

Organizing pneumonia in diseases classified elsewhere

Code first underlying disease, such as:

progressive systemic sclerosis (M34.0)

rheumatoid arthritis (M05.00-M06.9)

systemic lupus erythematosis (M32.0-M32.9)

J84.2 **Lymphoid interstitial pneumonia** [HCC]

Lymphoid interstitial pneumonitis

J84.8 **Other specified interstitial pulmonary diseases**

Excludes1: exogenous lipoid pneumonia (J69.1)

unspecified lipoid pneumonia (J69.1)

J84.81 **Lymphangioleiomyomatosis** [HCC]

Lymphangiomyomatosis

J84.82 **Adult pulmonary Langerhans cell histiocytosis** [HCC]

Adult PLCH

J84.83 **Surfactant mutations of the lung** [HCC]

J84.84 **Other interstitial lung diseases of childhood**

J84.841 **Neuroendocrine cell hyperplasia of infancy** [HCC]

J84.842 **Pulmonary interstitial glycogenosis** [HCC]

J84.843 **Alveolar capillary dysplasia with vein misalignment** [HCC]

J84.848 **Other interstitial lung diseases of childhood** [HCC]

J84.89 **Other specified interstitial pulmonary diseases** [HCC]

● New code   ▲ Revised code   Excludes1: Not coded here   Excludes2: Not included here   ⊗ Placeholder required   ⑦7th digit required

Endogenous lipoid pneumonia

Interstitial pneumonitis

Non-specific interstitial pneumonitis NOS

Organizing pneumonia NOS

Code first, if applicable:

poisoning due to drug or toxin (T51-T65 with fifth or sixth character to indicate intent), for toxic pneumonopathy

underlying cause of pneumonopathy, if known

Use Additional Code, for adverse effect, to identify drug (T36-T50 with fifth or sixth character 5), if drug-induced

Excludes1: cryptogenic organizing pneumonia (J84.116)

idiopathic non-specific interstitial pneumonitis (J84.113)

lipoid pneumonia, exogenous or unspecified (J69.1)

lymphoid interstitial pneumonia (J84.2)

J84.9   Interstitial pulmonary disease, unspecified [HCC]

Interstitial pneumonia NOS

SUPPURATIVE AND NECROTIC CONDITIONS OF THE LOWER RESPIRATORY TRACT (J85-J86)

J85   Abscess of lung and mediastinum

Use Additional Code (B95-B97) to identify infectious agent.

J85.0   Gangrene and necrosis of lung [HCC]

J85.1   Abscess of lung with pneumonia

Code also the type of pneumonia

J85.2   Abscess of lung without pneumonia [HCC]

Abscess of lung NOS

J85.3   Abscess of mediastinum [HCC]

J86   Pyothorax

Use Additional Code (B95-B97) to identify infectious agent.

Excludes1: abscess of lung (J85.-)

pyothorax due to tuberculosis (A15.6)

J86.0   Pyothorax with fistula [HCC]

Bronchocutaneous fistula

Bronchopleural fistula

Hepatopleural fistula

Mediastinal fistula

Pleural fistula

Thoracic fistula

Any condition classifiable to J86.9 with fistula

J86.9   Pyothorax without fistula [HCC]

Abscess of pleura

Abscess of thorax

Empyema (chest) (lung) (pleura)

Fibrinopurulent pleurisy

Purulent pleurisy

Pyopneumothorax

Septic pleurisy

Seropurulent pleurisy

Suppurative pleurisy

OTHER DISEASES OF THE PLEURA (J90-J94)

J90   Pleural effusion, not elsewhere classified

Definition: Pleurisy is an inflammation of the membrane that surrounds and protects the lungs (the pleura). Inflammation occurs when an infection or damaging agent irritates the pleural surface.

Encysted pleurisy

Pleural effusion NOS

Pleurisy with effusion (exudative) (serous)

Excludes1: chylous (pleural) effusion (J94.0)

malignant pleural effusion (J91.0))

pleurisy NOS (R09.1)

tuberculous pleural effusion (A15.6)

J91   Pleural effusion in conditions classified elsewhere

Excludes2: pleural effusion in heart failure (I50.-)

pleural effusion in systemic lupus erythematosus (M32.13)

J91.0   Malignant pleural effusion

Code first underlying neoplasm

J91.8   Pleural effusion in other conditions classified elsewhere

Code first underlying disease, such as:

filariasis (B74.0-B74.9)

influenza (J09.X2, J10.1, J11.1)

J92   Pleural plaque

Includes: pleural thickening

J92.0   Pleural plaque with presence of asbestos

J92.9   Pleural plaque without asbestos

Pleural plaque NOS

J93   Pneumothorax and air leak

Excludes1: congenital or perinatal pneumothorax (P25.1)

postprocedural air leak (J95.812)

postprocedural pneumothorax (J95.811)

traumatic pneumothorax (S27.0)

tuberculous (current disease)

pneumothorax (A15.-)

pyopneumothorax (J86.-)

J93.0   Spontaneous tension pneumothorax

J93.1   Other spontaneous pneumothorax

J93.11   Primary spontaneous pneumothorax

J93.12   Secondary spontaneous pneumothorax

Code first underlying condition, such as:

catamenial pneumothorax due to endometriosis (N80.8)

cystic fibrosis (E84.-)

eosinophilic pneumonia (J82)

lymphangioleiomyomatosis (J84.81)

malignant neoplasm of bronchus and lung (C34.-)

Marfan's syndrome (Q87.4)

pneumonia due to Pneumocystis carinii (B59)

secondary malignant neoplasm of lung (C78.0-)

spontaneous rupture of the esophagus (K22.3)

J93.8   Other pneumothorax and air leak

J93.81   Chronic pneumothorax

J93.82   Other air leak

Persistent air leak

J93.83   Other pneumothorax

Acute pneumothorax

Spontaneous pneumothorax NOS

J93.9   Pneumothorax, unspecified

Pneumothorax NOS

J94   Other pleural conditions

Excludes1: pleurisy NOS (R09.1)

traumatic hemopneumothorax (S27.2)

traumatic hemothorax (S27.1)

tuberculous pleural conditions (current disease) (A15.-)

J94.0 Chylous effusion

Chyliform effusion

J94.1 Fibrothorax

J94.2 Hemothorax

Hemopneumothorax

J94.8 Other specified pleural conditions

Hydropneumothorax

Hydrothorax

J94.9 Pleural condition, unspecified

INTRAOPERATIVE AND POSTPROCEDURAL COMPLICATIONS AND DISORDERS OF RESPIRATORY SYSTEM, NOT ELSEWHERE CLASSIFIED (J95)

J95 Intraoperative and postprocedural complications and disorders of respiratory system, not elsewhere classified

Excludes2: aspiration pneumonia (J69.-)

emphysema (subcutaneous) resulting from a procedure (T81.82)

hypostatic pneumonia (J18.2)

pulmonary manifestations due to radiation (J70.0-J70.1)

J95.0 Tracheostomy complications

J95.00 Unspecified tracheostomy complication [HCC]

J95.01 Hemorrhage from tracheostomy stoma [HCC]

J95.02 Infection of tracheostomy stoma [HCC]

Use Additional Code to identify type of infection, such as:

cellulitis of neck (L03.221)

sepsis (A40, A41.-)

J95.03 Malfunction of tracheostomy stoma [HCC]

Mechanical complication of tracheostomy stoma

Obstruction of tracheostomy airway

Tracheal stenosis due to tracheostomy

J95.04 Tracheo-esophageal fistula following tracheostomy [HCC]

J95.09 Other tracheostomy complication [HCC]

J95.1 Acute pulmonary insufficiency following thoracic surgery [HCC]

Excludes2: Functional disturbances following cardiac surgery (I97.0, I97.1-)

J95.2 Acute pulmonary insufficiency following nonthoracic surgery [HCC]

Excludes2: Functional disturbances following cardiac surgery (I97.0, I97.1-)

J95.3 Chronic pulmonary insufficiency following surgery [HCC]

Excludes2: Functional disturbances following cardiac surgery (I97.0, I97.1-)

J95.4 Chemical pneumonitis due to anesthesia

Mendelson's syndrome

Postprocedural aspiration pneumonia

Use Additional Code for adverse effect, if applicable, to identify drug (T41.- with fifth or sixth character 5)

Excludes1: aspiration pneumonitis due to anesthesia complicating labor and delivery (O74.0)

aspiration pneumonitis due to anesthesia complicating pregnancy (O29)

aspiration pneumonitis due to anesthesia complicating the puerperium (O89.01)

J95.5 Postprocedural subglottic stenosis

J95.6 Intraoperative hemorrhage and hematoma of a respiratory system organ or structure complicating a procedure

Excludes1: intraoperative hemorrhage and hematoma of a respiratory system organ or structure due to accidental puncture and laceration during procedure (J95.7-)

J95.61 Intraoperative hemorrhage and hematoma of a respiratory system organ or structure complicating a respiratory system procedure

J95.62 Intraoperative hemorrhage and hematoma of a respiratory system organ or structure complicating other procedure

J95.7 Accidental puncture and laceration of a respiratory system organ or structure during a procedure

Excludes2: postprocedural pneumothorax (J95.811)

J95.71 Accidental puncture and laceration of a respiratory system organ or structure during a respiratory system procedure

J95.72 Accidental puncture and laceration of a respiratory system organ or structure during other procedure

J95.8 Other intraoperative and postprocedural complications and disorders of respiratory system, not elsewhere classified

J95.81 Postprocedural pneumothorax and air leak

J95.811 Postprocedural pneumothorax

J95.812 Postprocedural air leak

J95.82 Postprocedural respiratory failure

Excludes1: Respiratory failure in other conditions (J96.-)

J95.821 Acute postprocedural respiratory failure [HCC]

Postprocedural respiratory failure NOS

J95.822 Acute and chronic postprocedural respiratory failure [HCC]

J95.83 Postprocedural hemorrhage of a respiratory system organ or structure following a procedure

J95.830 Postprocedural hemorrhage of a respiratory system organ or structure following a respiratory system procedure

J95.831 Postprocedural hemorrhage of a respiratory system organ or structure following other procedure

J95.84 Transfusion-related acute lung injury (TRALI)

J95.85 Complication of respirator [ventilator]

J95.850 Mechanical complication of respirator [HCC]

Excludes1: encounter for respirator [ventilator] dependence during power failure (Z99.12)

J95.851 Ventilator associated pneumonia [HCC]

Ventilator associated pneumonitis

Use Additional Code to identify the organism, if known (B95.-, B96.-, B97.-)

● New code   ▲ Revised code   **Excludes1:** Not coded here   **Excludes2:** Not included here   ⊗ Placeholder required   ⑦7ᵗʰ digit required

Excludes1: ventilator lung in newborn (P27.8).

J95.859 Other complication of respirator [ventilator] [HCC]

J95.86 Postprocedural hematoma and seroma of a respiratory system organ or structure following a procedure

J95.860 Postprocedural hematoma of a respiratory system organ or structure following a respiratory system procedure

J95.861 Postprocedural hematoma of a respiratory system organ or structure following other procedure

J95.862 Postprocedural seroma of a respiratory system organ or structure following a respiratory system procedure

J95.863 Postprocedural seroma of a respiratory system organ or structure following other procedure

J95.88 Other intraoperative complications of respiratory system, not elsewhere classified

J95.89 Other postprocedural complications and disorders of respiratory system, not elsewhere classified

Use Additional Code to identify disorder, such as:

aspiration pneumonia (J69.-)

bacterial or viral pneumonia (J12-J18)

Excludes2: acute pulmonary insufficiency following thoracic surgery (J95.1)

postprocedural subglottic stenosis (J95.5)

OTHER DISEASES OF THE RESPIRATORY SYSTEM (J96-J99)

J96 **Respiratory failure, not elsewhere classified**

Excludes1: acute respiratory distress syndrome (J80)

cardiorespiratory failure (R09.2)

newborn respiratory distress syndrome (P22.0)

postprocedural respiratory failure (J95.82-)

respiratory arrest (R09.2)

respiratory arrest of newborn (P28.81)

respiratory failure of newborn (P28.5)

J96.0 Acute respiratory failure

J96.00 Acute respiratory failure, unspecified whether with hypoxia or hypercapnia [HCC]

J96.01 Acute respiratory failure with hypoxia [HCC]

J96.02 Acute respiratory failure with hypercapnia [HCC]

J96.1 Chronic respiratory failure

J96.10 Chronic respiratory failure, unspecified whether with hypoxia or hypercapnia [HCC]

J96.11 Chronic respiratory failure with hypoxia [HCC]

J96.12 Chronic respiratory failure with hypercapnia [HCC]

J96.2 Acute and chronic respiratory failure

Acute on chronic respiratory failure

J96.20 Acute and chronic respiratory failure, unspecified whether with hypoxia or hypercapnia [HCC]

J96.21 Acute and chronic respiratory failure with hypoxia [HCC]

J96.22 Acute and chronic respiratory failure with hypercapnia

J96.9 Respiratory failure, unspecified

J96.90 Respiratory failure, unspecified, unspecified whether with hypoxia or hypercapnia [HCC]

J96.91 Respiratory failure, unspecified with hypoxia [HCC]

J96.92 Respiratory failure, unspecified with hypercapnia [HCC]

J98 **Other respiratory disorders**

Use Additional Code to identify:

exposure to environmental tobacco smoke (Z77.22)

exposure to tobacco smoke in the perinatal period (P96.81)

history of tobacco dependence (Z87.891)

occupational exposure to environmental tobacco smoke (Z57.31)

tobacco dependence (F17.-)

tobacco use (Z72.0)

Excludes1: newborn apnea (P28.4)

newborn sleep apnea (P28.3)

Excludes2: apnea NOS (R06.81)

sleep apnea (G47.3-)

J98.0 Diseases of bronchus, not elsewhere classified

J98.01 Acute bronchospasm

Excludes1: acute bronchiolitis with bronchospasm (J21.-)

acute bronchitis with bronchospasm (J20.-)

asthma (J45.-)

exercise induced bronchospasm (J45.990)

J98.09 Other diseases of bronchus, not elsewhere classified

Broncholithiasis

Calcification of bronchus

Stenosis of bronchus

Tracheobronchial collapse

Tracheobronchial dyskinesia

Ulcer of bronchus

J98.1 Pulmonary collapse

Excludes1: therapeutic collapse of lung status (Z98.3)

J98.11 Atelectasis

Excludes1: newborn atelectasis

tuberculous atelectasis (current disease) (A15)

J98.19 Other pulmonary collapse

J98.2 Interstitial emphysema [HCC]

Mediastinal emphysema

Excludes1: emphysema NOS (J43.9)

emphysema in newborn (P25.0)

surgical emphysema (subcutaneous) (T81.82)

traumatic subcutaneous emphysema (T79.7)

J98.3 Compensatory emphysema [HCC]

J98.4 Other disorders of lung

Calcification of lung

Cystic lung disease (acquired)

Lung disease NOS

Pulmolithiasis

Excludes1: acute interstitial pneumonitis (J84.114)

pulmonary insufficiency following surgery (J95.1-J95.2)

J98.5 **Diseases of mediastinum, not elsewhere classified**

Excludes2: abscess of mediastinum (J85.3)

    J98.51 **Mediastinitis**

      Code first underlying condition, if applicable, such as postoperative mediastinitis (T81.-)

    J98.59 **Other diseases of mediastinum, not elsewhere classified**

      Fibrosis of mediastinum

      Hernia of mediastinum

      Retraction of mediastinum

J98.6 **Disorders of diaphragm**

  Diaphragmatitis

  Paralysis of diaphragm

  Relaxation of diaphragm

Excludes1: congenital malformation of diaphragm NEC (Q79.1)

    congenital diaphragmatic hernia (Q79.0)

Excludes2: diaphragmatic hernia (K44.-)

J98.8 **Other specified respiratory disorders**

J98.9 **Respiratory disorder, unspecified**

  Respiratory disease (chronic) NOS

J99 **Respiratory disorders in diseases classified elsewhere** [HCC]

Code first underlying disease, such as:

amyloidosis (E85.-)

ankylosing spondylitis (M45)

congenital syphilis (A50.5)

cryoglobulinemia (D89.1)

early congenital syphilis (A50.0)

plasminogen deficiency (E88.02)

schistosomiasis (B65.0-B65.9)

Excludes1: respiratory disorders in:

    amebiasis (A06.5)

    blastomycosis (B40.0-B40.2)

    candidiasis (B37.1)

    coccidioidomycosis (B38.0-B38.2)

    cystic fibrosis with pulmonary manifestations (E84.0)

    dermatomyositis (M33.01, M33.11)

    histoplasmosis (B39.0-B39.2)

    late syphilis (A52.72, A52.73)

    polymyositis (M33.21)

    Sjögren syndrome (M35.02)

    systemic lupus erythematosus (M32.13)

    systemic sclerosis (M34.81)

    Wegener's granulomatosis (M31.30-M31.31)

Chapter 11: Diseases of the Digestive System (K00-K95)

DEFINITIONS

This chapter includes definitions of selected key words, terms and phrases and coding alerts for adding points to the clinical domain, and references to coding late effects where appropriate. An example from this chapter is as follows:

K04   Diseases of pulp and periapical tissues
Definition: Pulp is the part in the center of a tooth made up of living soft tissue and cells called odontoblasts.

MULTIPLE CODING FOR A SINGLE CONDITION

In addition to the etiology/manifestation convention that requires two codes to fully describe a single condition that affects multiple body systems, there are other single conditions that also require more than one code. "**Use Additional Code**" notes are found in the Tabular List at codes that are not part of an etiology/manifestation pair where a secondary code is useful to fully describe a condition. The sequencing rule is the same as the etiology/manifestation pair, "**Use Additional Code**" indicates that a secondary code should be added.

For example, for bacterial infections that are not included in chapter 1, a secondary code from category B95, Streptococcus, Staphylococcus, and Enterococcus, as the cause of diseases classified elsewhere, or B96, Other bacterial agents as the cause of diseases classified elsewhere, may be required to identify the bacterial organism causing the infection. A "**Use Additional Code**" note will normally be found at the infectious disease code, indicating a need for the organism code to be added as a secondary code.

"Code first" notes are also under certain codes that are not specifically manifestation codes but may be due to an underlying cause. When there is a "Code first" note and an underlying condition is present, the underlying condition should be sequenced first.

"Code, if applicable, any causal condition first", notes indicate that this code may be assigned as a principal diagnosis when the causal condition is unknown or not applicable. If a causal condition is known, then the code for that condition should be sequenced as the principal or first-listed diagnosis.

Multiple codes may be needed for sequela, complication codes and obstetric codes to more fully describe a condition. See the specific guidelines for these conditions for further instruction.

COMBINATION CODE

A combination code is a single code used to classify: Two diagnoses, or a diagnosis with an associated secondary process (manifestation) A diagnosis with an associated complication

Combination codes are identified by referring to subterm entries in the Alphabetic Index and by reading the inclusion and exclusion notes in the Tabular List.

Assign only the combination code when that code fully identifies the diagnostic conditions involved or when the Alphabetic Index so directs. Multiple coding should not be used when the classification provides a combination code that clearly identifies all of the elements documented in the diagnosis. When the combination code lacks necessary specificity in describing the manifestation or complication, an additional code should be used as a secondary code.

SEQUELA (LATE EFFECTS)

A sequela is the residual effect (condition produced) after the acute phase of an illness or injury has terminated. There is no time limit on when a sequela code can be used. The residual may be apparent early, such as in cerebral infarction, or it may occur months or years later, such as that due to a previous injury. Coding of sequela generally requires two codes sequenced in the following order: The condition or nature of the sequela is sequenced first.

The sequela code is sequenced second.

An exception to the above guidelines are those instances where the code for the sequela is followed by a manifestation code identified in the Tabular List and title, or the sequela code has been expanded (at the fourth, fifth or sixth character levels) to include the manifestation(s). The code for the acute phase of an illness or injury that led to the sequela is never used with a code for the late effect.

K00-K95

Chapter 11

Diseases of The Digestive System (K00-K95)

Excludes2: certain conditions originating in the perinatal period (P04-P96)

certain infectious and parasitic diseases (A00-B99)

complications of pregnancy, childbirth and the puerperium (O00-O9A)

congenital malformations, deformations and chromosomal abnormalities (Q00-Q99)

endocrine, nutritional and metabolic diseases (E00-E88)

injury, poisoning and certain other consequences of external causes (S00-T88)

neoplasms (C00-D49)

symptoms, signs and abnormal clinical and laboratory findings, not elsewhere classified (R00-R94)

This chapter contains the following blocks:

K00-K14	Diseases of oral cavity and salivary glands
K20-K31	Diseases of esophagus, stomach and duodenum
K35-K38	Diseases of appendix
K40-K46	Hernia
K50-K52	Noninfective enteritis and colitis
K55-K64	Other diseases of intestines
K65-K68	Diseases of peritoneum and retroperitoneum
K70-K77	Diseases of liver
K80-K87	Disorders of gallbladder, biliary tract and pancreas
K90-K95	Other diseases of the digestive system

DISEASES OF ORAL CAVITY AND SALIVARY GLANDS (K00-K14)

K00 **Disorders of tooth development and eruption**

Excludes2: embedded and impacted teeth (K01.-)

K00.0 **Anodontia**

Hypodontia

Oligodontia

Excludes1: acquired absence of teeth (K08.1-)

K00.1 **Supernumerary teeth**

Distomolar Fourth molar

Mesiodens Paramolar

Supplementary teeth

Excludes2: supernumerary roots (K00.2)

K00.2 **Abnormalities of size and form of teeth**

Concrescence of teeth

Fusion of teeth

Gemination of teeth

Dens evaginatus

Dens in dente

Dens invaginatus

Enamel pearls

Macrodontia

Microdontia

Peg-shaped [conical] teeth

Supernumerary roots

Taurodontism

Tuberculum paramolare

Excludes1: abnormalities of teeth due to congenital syphilis (A50.5)

tuberculum Carabelli, which is regarded as a normal variation and should not be coded

K00.3 **Mottled teeth**

Dental fluorosis

Mottling of enamel

Nonfluoride enamel opacities

Excludes2: deposits [accretions] on teeth (K03.6)

K00.4 **Disturbances in tooth formation**

Aplasia and hypoplasia of cementum

Dilaceration of tooth

Enamel hypoplasia (neonatal) (postnatal) (prenatal)

Regional odontodysplasia

Turner's tooth

Excludes1: Hutchinson's teeth and mulberry molars in congenital syphilis (A50.5)

Excludes2: mottled teeth (K00.3)

K00.5 **Hereditary disturbances in tooth structure, not elsewhere classified**

Amelogenesis imperfecta

Dentinogenesis imperfecta

Odontogenesis imperfecta

Dentinal dysplasia

Shell teeth

K00.6 **Disturbances in tooth eruption**

Dentia praecox Natal tooth Neonatal tooth

Premature eruption of tooth

Premature shedding of primary [deciduous] tooth

Prenatal teeth

Retained [persistent] primary tooth

Excludes2: embedded and impacted teeth (K01.-)

K00.7 **Teething syndrome**

K00.8 **Other disorders of tooth development**

Color changes during tooth formation

Intrinsic staining of teeth NOS

Excludes2: posteruptive color changes (K03.7)

K00.9 **Disorder of tooth development, unspecified**

Disorder of odontogenesis NOS

K01 **Embedded and impacted teeth**

Excludes1: abnormal position of fully erupted teeth (M26.3-)

K01.0 **Embedded teeth**

K01.1 **Impacted teeth**

K02 **Dental caries**

Includes: caries of dentine

dental cavities

early childhood caries

pre-eruptive caries

recurrent caries (dentino enamel junction) (enamel) (to the pulp)

tooth decay

K02.3 **Arrested dental caries**

Arrested coronal and root caries

K02.5 **Dental caries on pit and fissure surface**

Dental caries on chewing surface of tooth

K02.51 **Dental caries on pit and fissure surface limited to enamel**

White spot lesions [initial caries] on pit and fissure surface of tooth

K02.52 Dental caries on pit and fissure surface penetrating into dentin

Primary dental caries, cervical origin

K02.53 Dental caries on pit and fissure surface penetrating into pulp

K02.6 Dental caries on smooth surface

K02.61 Dental caries on smooth surface limited to enamel

White spot lesions [initial caries] on smooth surface of tooth

K02.62 Dental caries on smooth surface penetrating into dentin

K02.63 Dental caries on smooth surface penetrating into pulp

K02.7 Dental root caries

K02.9 Dental caries, unspecified

K03 Other diseases of hard tissues of teeth

Excludes2: bruxism (F45.8)

dental caries (K02.-)

teeth-grinding NOS (F45.8)

K03.0 Excessive attrition of teeth

Approximal wear of teeth

Occlusal wear of teeth

K03.1 Abrasion of teeth

Dentifrice abrasion of teeth

Habitual abrasion of teeth

Occupational abrasion of teeth

Ritual abrasion of teeth

Traditional abrasion of teeth Wedge defect NOS

K03.2 Erosion of teeth

Erosion of teeth due to diet

Erosion of teeth due to drugs and medicaments

Erosion of teeth due to persistent vomiting

Erosion of teeth NOS

Idiopathic erosion of teeth

Occupational erosion of teeth

K03.3 Pathological resorption of teeth

Internal granuloma of pulp

Resorption of teeth (external)

K03.4 Hypercementosis

Cementation hyperplasia

K03.5 Ankylosis of teeth

K03.6 Deposits [accretions] on teeth

Betel deposits [accretions] on teeth

Black deposits [accretions] on teeth

Extrinsic staining of teeth NOS

Green deposits [accretions] on teeth

Materia alba deposits [accretions] on teeth

Orange deposits [accretions] on teeth

Staining of teeth NOS

Subgingival dental calculus

Supragingival dental calculus

Tobacco deposits [accretions] on teeth

K03.7 Posteruptive color changes of dental hard tissues

Excludes2: deposits [accretions] on teeth (K03.6)

K03.8 Other specified diseases of hard tissues of teeth

K03.81 Cracked tooth

Excludes1: asymptomatic craze lines in enamel - omit code

broken or fractured tooth due to trauma (S02.5)

K03.89 Other specified diseases of hard tissues of teeth

K03.9 Disease of hard tissues of teeth, unspecified

K04 Diseases of pulp and periapical tissues

Definition: Pulp is the part in the center of a tooth made up of living soft tissue and cells called odontoblasts.

K04.0 Pulpitis

Acute pulpitis

Chronic (hyperplastic) (ulcerative) pulpitis

K04.01 Reversible pulpitis

K04.02 Irreversible pulpitis

K04.1 Necrosis of pulp

Pulpal gangrene

K04.2 Pulp degeneration

Denticles

Pulpal calcifications

Pulpal stones

K04.3 Abnormal hard tissue formation in pulp

Secondary or irregular dentine

K04.4 Acute apical periodontitis of pulpal origin

Acute apical periodontitis NOS

Excludes1: acute periodontitis (K05.2-)

K04.5 Chronic apical periodontitis

Apical or periapical granuloma

Apical periodontitis NOS

Excludes1: chronic periodontitis (K05.3-)

K04.6 Periapical abscess with sinus

Dental abscess with sinus

Dentoalveolar abscess with sinus

K04.7 Periapical abscess without sinus

Dental abscess without sinus

Dentoalveolar abscess without sinus

K04.8 Radicular cyst

Apical (periodontal) cyst

Periapical cyst

Residual radicular cyst

Excludes2: lateral periodontal cyst (K09.0)

K04.9 Other and unspecified diseases of pulp and periapical tissues

K04.90 Unspecified diseases of pulp and periapical tissues

K04.99 Other diseases of pulp and periapical tissues

K05 Gingivitis and periodontal diseases

Use Additional Code to identify:

alcohol abuse and dependence (F10.-)

exposure to environmental tobacco smoke (Z77.22)

exposure to tobacco smoke in the perinatal period (P96.81)

history of tobacco dependence (Z87.891)

occupational exposure to environmental tobacco smoke (Z57.31)

tobacco dependence (F17.-)

tobacco use (Z72.0)

K05.0 Acute gingivitis

Excludes1: acute necrotizing ulcerative gingivitis (A69.1)

● New code   ▲ Revised code   Excludes1: Not coded here   Excludes2: Not included here   ⊗ Placeholder required   ⑦7th.digit required herpesviral [herpes simplex] gingivostomatitis (B00.2)

K05.00   **Acute gingivitis, plaque induced**

Acute gingivitis NOS

Plaque induced gingival disease

K05.01   **Acute gingivitis, non-plaque induced**

K05.1   **Chronic gingivitis**

Desquamative gingivitis (chronic)

Gingivitis (chronic) NOS

Hyperplastic gingivitis (chronic)

Pregnancy associated gingivitis

Simple marginal gingivitis (chronic)

Ulcerative gingivitis (chronic)

Code first, if applicable, diseases of the digestive system complicating pregnancy (O99.61-)

K05.10   **Chronic gingivitis, plaque induced**

Chronic gingivitis NOS Gingivitis NOS

K05.11   **Chronic gingivitis, non-plaque induced**

K05.2   **Aggressive periodontitis**

Acute pericoronitis

Excludes1: acute apical periodontitis (K04.4)

periapical abscess (K04.7)

periapical abscess with sinus (K04.6)

K05.20   **Aggressive periodontitis, unspecified**

K05.21   **Aggressive periodontitis, localized**

Periodontal abscess

  K05.211   **Aggressive periodontitis, localized, slight**

  K05.212   **Aggressive periodontitis, localized, moderate**

  K05.213   **Aggressive periodontitis, localized, severe**

  K05.219   **Aggressive periodontitis, localized, unspecified severity**

K05.22   **Aggressive periodontitis, generalized**

  K05.221   **Aggressive periodontitis, generalized, slight**

  K05.222   **Aggressive periodontitis, generalized, moderate**

  K05.223   **Aggressive periodontitis, generalized, severe**

  K05.229   **Aggressive periodontitis, generalized, unspecified severity**

K05.3   **Chronic periodontitis**

Chronic pericoronitis

Complex periodontitis

Periodontitis NOS

Simplex periodontitis

Excludes1: chronic apical periodontitis (K04.5)

K05.30   **Chronic periodontitis, unspecified**

K05.31   **Chronic periodontitis, localized**

  K05.311   **Chronic periodontitis, localized, slight**

  K05.312   **Chronic periodontitis, localized, moderate**

  K05.313   **Chronic periodontitis, localized, severe**

  K05.319   **Chronic periodontitis, localized, unspecified severity**

K05.32   **Chronic periodontitis, generalized**

  K05.321   **Chronic periodontitis, generalized, slight**

  K05.322   **Chronic periodontitis, generalized, moderate**

  K05.323   **Chronic periodontitis, generalized, severe**

  K05.329   **Chronic periodontitis, generalized, unspecified severity**

K05.4   **Periodontosis**

Juvenile periodontosis

K05.5   **Other periodontal diseases**

Combined periodontic-endodontic lesion

Narrow gingival width (of periodontal soft tissue)

Excludes2: leukoplakia of gingiva (K13.21)

K05.6   **Periodontal disease, unspecified**

K06   **Other disorders of gingiva and edentulous alveolar ridge**

Excludes2: acute gingivitis (K05.0)

atrophy of edentulous alveolar ridge (K08.2)

chronic gingivitis (K05.1)

gingivitis NOS (K05.1)

K06.0   **Gingival recession**

Gingival recession (postinfective) (postprocedural)

K06.01   **Gingival recession, localized**

  K06.010   **Localized gingival recession, unspecified**

  Localized gingival recession, NOS

  K06.011   **Localized gingival recession, minimal**

  K06.012   **Localized gingival recession, moderate**

  K06.013   **Localized gingival recession, severe**

K06.02   **Gingival recession, generalized**

  K06.020   **Generalized gingival recession, unspecified**

  Generalized gingival recession, NOS

  K06.021   **Generalized gingival recession, minimal**

  K06.022   **Generalized gingival recession, moderate**

  K06.023   **Generalized gingival recession, severe**

K06.1   **Gingival enlargement**

Gingival fibromatosis

K06.2   **Gingival and edentulous alveolar ridge lesions associated with trauma**

Irritative hyperplasia of edentulous ridge [denture hyperplasia]

Use Additional Code (Chapter 20) to identify external cause or denture status (Z97.2)

K06.3   **Horizontal alveolar bone loss**

K06.8   **Other specified disorders of gingiva and edentulous alveolar ridge**

Fibrous epulis

Flabby alveolar ridge

Giant cell epulis

Peripheral giant cell granuloma of gingiva

Pyogenic granuloma of gingiva

Vertical ridge deficiency

Excludes2: gingival cyst (K09.0)

K06.9 Disorder of gingiva and edentulous alveolar ridge, unspecified

K08 Other disorders of teeth and supporting structures

Excludes2: dentofacial anomalies [including malocclusion] (M26.-)

disorders of jaw (M27.-)

K08.0 Exfoliation of teeth due to systemic causes

Code also underlying systemic condition

K08.1 Complete loss of teeth

Acquired loss of teeth, complete

Excludes1: congenital absence of teeth (K00.0)

exfoliation of teeth due to systemic causes (K08.0)

partial loss of teeth (K08.4-)

K08.10 Complete loss of teeth, unspecified cause

K08.101 Complete loss of teeth, unspecified cause, class I

K08.102 Complete loss of teeth, unspecified cause, class II

K08.103 Complete loss of teeth, unspecified cause, class III

K08.104 Complete loss of teeth, unspecified cause, class IV

K08.109 Complete loss of teeth, unspecified cause, unspecified class

Edentulism NOS

K08.11 Complete loss of teeth due to trauma

K08.111 Complete loss of teeth due to trauma, class I

K08.112 Complete loss of teeth due to trauma, class II

K08.113 Complete loss of teeth due to trauma, class III

K08.114 Complete loss of teeth due to trauma, class IV

K08.119 Complete loss of teeth due to trauma, unspecified class

K08.12 Complete loss of teeth due to periodontal diseases

K08.121 Complete loss of teeth due to periodontal diseases, class I

K08.122 Complete loss of teeth due to periodontal diseases, class II

K08.123 Complete loss of teeth due to periodontal diseases, class III

K08.124 Complete loss of teeth due to periodontal diseases, class IV

K08.129 Complete loss of teeth due to periodontal diseases, unspecified class

K08.13 Complete loss of teeth due to caries

K08.131 Complete loss of teeth due to caries, class I

K08.132 Complete loss of teeth due to caries, class II

K08.133 Complete loss of teeth due to caries, class III

K08.134 Complete loss of teeth due to caries, class IV

K08.139 Complete loss of teeth due to caries, unspecified class

K08.19 Complete loss of teeth due to other specified cause

K08.191 Complete loss of teeth due to other specified cause, class I

K08.192 Complete loss of teeth due to other specified cause, class II

K08.193 Complete loss of teeth due to other specified cause, class III

K08.194 Complete loss of teeth due to other specified cause, class IV

K08.199 Complete loss of teeth due to other specified cause, unspecified class

K08.2 Atrophy of edentulous alveolar ridge

K08.20 Unspecified atrophy of edentulous alveolar ridge

Atrophy of the mandible NOS

Atrophy of the maxilla NOS

K08.21 Minimal atrophy of the mandible

Minimal atrophy of the edentulous mandible

K08.22 Moderate atrophy of the mandible

Moderate atrophy of the edentulous mandible

K08.23 Severe atrophy of the mandible

Severe atrophy of the edentulous mandible

K08.24 Minimal atrophy of maxilla

Minimal atrophy of the edentulous maxilla

K08.25 Moderate atrophy of the maxilla

Moderate atrophy of the edentulous maxilla

K08.26 Severe atrophy of the maxilla

Severe atrophy of the edentulous maxilla

K08.3 Retained dental root

K08.4 Partial loss of teeth

Acquired loss of teeth, partial

Excludes1: complete loss of teeth (K08.1-)

congenital absence of teeth (K00.0)

Excludes2: exfoliation of teeth due to systemic causes (K08.0)

K08.40 Partial loss of teeth, unspecified cause

K08.401 Partial loss of teeth, unspecified cause, class I

K08.402 Partial loss of teeth, unspecified cause, class II

K08.403 Partial loss of teeth, unspecified cause, class III

K08.404 Partial loss of teeth, unspecified cause, class IV

K08.409 Partial loss of teeth, unspecified cause, unspecified class

Tooth extraction status NOS

K08.41 Partial loss of teeth due to trauma

K08.411 Partial loss of teeth due to trauma, class I

K08.412 Partial loss of teeth due to trauma, class II

K08.413 Partial loss of teeth due to trauma, class III

K08.414 Partial loss of teeth due to trauma, class IV

K08.419 Partial loss of teeth due to trauma, unspecified class

K08.42 Partial loss of teeth due to periodontal diseases

K08.421 Partial loss of teeth due to periodontal diseases, class I

K08.422 Partial loss of teeth due to periodontal diseases, class II

K08.423 Partial loss of teeth due to periodontal diseases, class III

K08.424 Partial loss of teeth due to periodontal diseases, class IV

K08.429 Partial loss of teeth due to periodontal diseases, unspecified class

K08.43 Partial loss of teeth due to caries

K08.431 Partial loss of teeth due to caries, class I

K08.432 Partial loss of teeth due to caries, class II

K08.433 Partial loss of teeth due to caries, class III

K08.434 Partial loss of teeth due to caries, class IV

K08.439 Partial loss of teeth due to caries, unspecified class

K08.49 Partial loss of teeth due to other specified cause

K08.491 Partial loss of teeth due to other specified cause, class I

K08.492 Partial loss of teeth due to other specified cause, class II

K08.493 Partial loss of teeth due to other specified cause, class III

K08.494 Partial loss of teeth due to other specified cause, class IV

K08.499 Partial loss of teeth due to other specified cause, unspecified class

K08.5 Unsatisfactory restoration of tooth

Defective bridge, crown, filling

Defective dental restoration

Excludes1: dental restoration status (Z98.811)

Excludes2: endosseous dental implant failure (M27.6-)

unsatisfactory endodontic treatment (M27.5-)

K08.50 Unsatisfactory restoration of tooth, unspecified

Defective dental restoration NOS

K08.51 Open restoration margins of tooth

Dental restoration failure of marginal integrity

Open margin on tooth restoration

Poor gingival margin to tooth restoration

K08.52 Unrepairable overhanging of dental restorative materials

Overhanging of tooth restoration

K08.53 Fractured dental restorative material

Excludes1: cracked tooth (K03.81)

traumatic fracture of tooth (S02.5)

K08.530 Fractured dental restorative material without loss of material

K08.531 Fractured dental restorative material with loss of material

K08.539 Fractured dental restorative material, unspecified

K08.54 Contour of existing restoration of tooth biologically incompatible with oral health

Dental restoration failure of periodontal anatomical integrity

Unacceptable contours of existing restoration of tooth

Unacceptable morphology of existing restoration of tooth

K08.55 Allergy to existing dental restorative material

Use Additional Code to identify the specific type of allergy

K08.56 Poor aesthetic of existing restoration of tooth

Dental restoration aesthetically inadequate or displeasing

K08.59 Other unsatisfactory restoration of tooth

Other defective dental restoration

K08.8 Other specified disorders of teeth and supporting structures

K08.81 Primary occlusal trauma

K08.82 Secondary occlusal trauma

K08.89 Other specified disorders of teeth and supporting structures

Enlargement of alveolar ridge NOS

Insufficient anatomic crown height

Insufficient clinical crown length

Irregular alveolar process

Toothache NOS

K08.9 Disorder of teeth and supporting structures, unspecified

K09 Cysts of oral region, not elsewhere classified

Includes: lesions showing histological features both of aneurysmal cyst and of another fibro-osseous lesion

Excludes2: cysts of jaw (M27.0-, M27.4-)

radicular cyst (K04.8)

K09.0 Developmental odontogenic cysts

Dentigerous cyst

Eruption cyst

Follicular cyst

Gingival cyst

Lateral periodontal cyst

Primordial cyst

Excludes2: keratocysts (D16.4, D16.5)

odontogenic keratocystic tumors (D16.4, D16.5)

K09.1 Developmental (nonodontogenic) cysts of oral region

Cyst (of) incisive canal

Cyst (of) palatine of papilla

Globulomaxillary cyst

Median palatal cyst

Nasoalveolar cyst

Nasolabial cyst

Nasopalatine duct cyst

K09.8 Other cysts of oral region, not elsewhere classified

Dermoid cyst

Epidermoid cyst

Lymphoepithelial cyst

Epstein's pearl

K09.9 Cyst of oral region, unspecified

K11 Diseases of salivary glands

Definition: The salivary gland is a gland that secretes saliva, especially any of three pairs of large glands, the parotid, submaxillary, and sublingual, whose secretions enter the mouth and mingle in saliva.

Use Additional Code to identify:

alcohol abuse and dependence (F10.-)

exposure to environmental tobacco smoke (Z77.22)

exposure to tobacco smoke in the perinatal period (P96.81)

history of tobacco dependence (Z87.891)

occupational exposure to environmental tobacco smoke (Z57.31)

tobacco dependence (F17.-)

tobacco use (Z72.0)

K11.0 **Atrophy of salivary gland**

K11.1 **Hypertrophy of salivary gland**

K11.2 **Sialoadenitis**

Parotitis

Excludes1: epidemic parotitis (B26.-)

mumps (B26.-)

uveoparotid fever [Heerfordt] (D86.89)

K11.20 **Sialoadenitis, unspecified**

K11.21 **Acute sialoadenitis**

Excludes1: acute recurrent sialoadenitis (K11.22)

K11.22 **Acute recurrent sialoadenitis**

K11.23 **Chronic sialoadenitis**

K11.3 **Abscess of salivary gland**

K11.4 **Fistula of salivary gland**

Excludes1: congenital fistula of salivary gland (Q38.4)

K11.5 **Sialolithiasis**

Calculus of salivary gland or duct

Stone of salivary gland or duct

K11.6 **Mucocele of salivary gland**

Mucous extravasation cyst of salivary gland

Mucous retention cyst of salivary gland

Ranula

K11.7 **Disturbances of salivary secretion**

Hypoptyalism

Ptyalism

Xerostomia

Excludes2: dry mouth NOS (R68.2)

K11.8 **Other diseases of salivary glands**

Benign lymphoepithelial lesion of salivary gland

Mikulicz' disease

Necrotizing sialometaplasia

Sialectasia

Stenosis of salivary duct

Stricture of salivary duct

Excludes1: Sjögren syndrome (M35.0-)

K11.9 **Disease of salivary gland, unspecified**

Sialadenopathy NOS

K12 **Stomatitis and related lesions**

Use Additional Code to identify:

alcohol abuse and dependence (F10.-)

exposure to environmental tobacco smoke (Z77.22)

exposure to tobacco smoke in the perinatal period (P96.81)

history of tobacco dependence (Z87.891)

occupational exposure to environmental tobacco smoke (Z57.31)

tobacco dependence (F17.-)

tobacco use (Z72.0)

Excludes1: cancrum oris (A69.0)

cheilitis (K13.0)

gangrenous stomatitis (A69.0)

herpesviral [herpes simplex] gingivostomatitis (B00.2)

noma (A69.0)

K12.0 **Recurrent oral aphthae**

Aphthous stomatitis (major) (minor)

Bednar's aphthae

Periadenitis mucosa necrotica recurrens

Recurrent aphthous ulcer

Stomatitis herpetiformis

K12.1 **Other forms of stomatitis**

Stomatitis NOS

Denture stomatitis

Ulcerative stomatitis

Vesicular stomatitis

Excludes1: acute necrotizing ulcerative stomatitis (A69.1)

Vincent's stomatitis (A69.1)

K12.2 **Cellulitis and abscess of mouth**

Cellulitis of mouth (floor)

Submandibular abscess

Excludes2: abscess of salivary gland (K11.3)

abscess of tongue (K14.0)

periapical abscess (K04.6-K04.7)

periodontal abscess (K05.21)

peritonsillar abscess (J36)

K12.3 **Oral mucositis (ulcerative)**

Mucositis (oral) (oropharyngeal)

Excludes2: gastrointestinal mucositis (ulcerative) (K92.81)

mucositis (ulcerative) of vagina and vulva (N76.81)

nasal mucositis (ulcerative) (J34.81)

K12.30 **Oral mucositis (ulcerative), unspecified**

K12.31 **Oral mucositis (ulcerative) due to antineoplastic therapy**

Use Additional Code for adverse effect, if applicable, to identify antineoplastic and immunosuppressive drugs (T45.1X5)

Use Additional Code for other antineoplastic therapy, such as:

radiological procedure and radiotherapy (Y84.2)

K12.32 **Oral mucositis (ulcerative) due to other drugs**

Use Additional Code for adverse effect, if applicable, to identify drug (T36-T50 with fifth or sixth character 5)

K12.33 **Oral mucositis (ulcerative) due to radiation**

Use additional external cause code (W88-W90, X39.0-) to identify cause

K12.39 **Other oral mucositis (ulcerative)**

Viral oral mucositis (ulcerative)

K13 **Other diseases of lip and oral mucosa**

Includes: epithelial disturbances of tongue

Use Additional Code to identify:

alcohol abuse and dependence (F10.-)

exposure to environmental tobacco smoke (Z77.22)

exposure to tobacco smoke in the perinatal period (P96.81)

history of tobacco dependence (Z87.891)

occupational exposure to environmental tobacco smoke (Z57.31)

tobacco dependence (F17.-)

tobacco use (Z72.0)

Excludes2: certain disorders of gingiva and edentulous alveolar ridge (K05-K06)

cysts of oral region (K09.-)

● New code ▲ Revised code Excludes1: Not coded here Excludes2: Not included here ⊗ Placeholder required ⑦ 7th digit required

diseases of tongue (K14.-)

stomatitis and related lesions (K12.-)

K13.0   Diseases of lips

Abscess of lips

Angular cheilitis

Cellulitis of lips

Cheilitis NOS

Cheilodynia

Cheilosis

Exfoliative cheilitis

Fistula of lips

Glandular cheilitis

Hypertrophy of lips

Perlèche NEC

Excludes1: ariboflavinosis (E53.0)

cheilitis due to radiation-related disorders (L55-L59)

congenital fistula of lips (Q38.0)

congenital hypertrophy of lips (Q18.6)

Perlèche due to candidiasis (B37.83)

Perlèche due to riboflavin deficiency (E53.0)

K13.1   Cheek and lip biting

K13.2   Leukoplakia and other disturbances of oral epithelium, including tongue

Excludes1: carcinoma in situ of oral epithelium (D00.0-)

hairy leukoplakia (K13.3)

K13.21   Leukoplakia of oral mucosa, including tongue

Leukokeratosis of oral mucosa

Leukoplakia of gingiva, lips, tongue

Excludes1: hairy leukoplakia (K13.3)

leukokeratosis nicotina palati (K13.24)

K13.22   Minimal keratinized residual ridge mucosa

Minimal keratinization of alveolar ridge mucosa

K13.23   Excessive keratinized residual ridge mucosa

Excessive keratinization of alveolar ridge mucosa

K13.24   Leukokeratosis nicotina palati

Smoker's palate

K13.29   Other disturbances of oral epithelium, including tongue

Erythroplakia of mouth or tongue

Focal epithelial hyperplasia of mouth or tongue

Leukoedema of mouth or tongue

Other oral epithelium disturbances

K13.3   Hairy leukoplakia

K13.4   Granuloma and granuloma-like lesions of oral mucosa

Eosinophilic granuloma pyogenicum

Verrucous xanthoma

K13.5   Oral submucous fibrosis

Submucous fibrosis of tongue

K13.6   Irritative hyperplasia of oral mucosa

Excludes2: irritative hyperplasia of edentulous ridge [denture hyperplasia] (K06.2)

K13.7   Other and unspecified lesions of oral mucosa

K13.70   Unspecified lesions of oral mucosa

K13.79   Other lesions of oral mucosa

Focal oral mucinosis

K14   Diseases of tongue

Use Additional Code to identify:

alcohol abuse and dependence (F10.-)

exposure to environmental tobacco smoke (Z77.22)

history of tobacco dependence (Z87.891)

occupational exposure to environmental tobacco smoke (Z57.31)

tobacco dependence (F17.-)

tobacco use (Z72.0)

Excludes2: erythroplakia (K13.29)

focal epithelial hyperplasia (K13.29)

leukoedema of tongue (K13.29)

leukoplakia of tongue (K13.21)

hairy leukoplakia (K13.3)

macroglossia (congenital) (Q38.2)

submucous fibrosis of tongue (K13.5)

K14.0   Glossitis

Abscess of tongue

Ulceration (traumatic) of tongue

Excludes1: atrophic glossitis (K14.4)

K14.1   Geographic tongue

Benign migratory glossitis

Glossitis areata exfoliativa

K14.2   Median rhomboid glossitis

K14.3   Hypertrophy of tongue papillae

Black hairy tongue

Coated tongue

Hypertrophy of foliate papillae

Lingua villosa nigra

K14.4   Atrophy of tongue papillae

Atrophic glossitis

K14.5   Plicated tongue

Fissured tongue

Furrowed tongue

Scrotal tongue

Excludes1: fissured tongue, congenital (Q38.3)

K14.6   Glossodynia

Glossopyrosis

Painful tongue

K14.8   Other diseases of tongue

Atrophy of tongue

Crenated tongue

Enlargement of tongue

Glossocele

Glossoptosis

Hypertrophy of tongue

K14.9   Disease of tongue, unspecified

Glossopathy NOS

DISEASES OF ESOPHAGUS, STOMACH AND DUODENUM (K20-K31)

Excludes2: hiatus hernia (K44.-)

K20   Esophagitis

Use Additional Code to identify:

alcohol abuse and dependence (F10.-)

Excludes1: erosion of esophagus (K22.1-)

esophagitis with gastro-esophageal reflux disease (K21.0)

reflux esophagitis (K21.0-)

ulcerative esophagitis (K22.1-)

Excludes2: eosinophilic gastritis or gastroenteritis (K52.81)

K20.0 Eosinophilic esophagitis

K20.8 Other esophagitis

    K20.80 Other esophagitis without bleeding

      Abscess of esophagus

      Other esophagitis NOS

    K20.81 Other esophagitis with bleeding

K20.9 Esophagitis, unspecified

    K20.90 Esophagitis, unspecified without bleeding

      Esophagitis NOS

    K20.91 Esophagitis, unspecified with bleeding

K21 Gastro-esophageal reflux disease

Excludes1: newborn esophageal reflux (P78.83)

K21.0 Gastro-esophageal reflux disease with esophagitis

    K21.00 Gastro-esophageal reflux disease with esophagitis, without bleeding

      Reflux esophagitis

    K21.01 Gastro-esophageal reflux disease with esophagitis, with bleeding

K21.9 Gastro-esophageal reflux disease without esophagitis

    Esophageal reflux NOS

K22 Other diseases of esophagus

Excludes2: esophageal varices (I85.-)

K22.0 Achalasia of cardia

    Achalasia NOS

    Cardiospasm

    Excludes1: congenital cardiospasm (Q39.5)

K22.1 Ulcer of esophagus

    Barrett's ulcer

    Erosion of esophagus

    Fungal ulcer of esophagus

    Peptic ulcer of esophagus

    Ulcer of esophagus due to ingestion of chemicals

    Ulcer of esophagus due to ingestion of drugs and medicaments

    Ulcerative esophagitis

    Code first poisoning due to drug or toxin, if applicable (T36-T65 with fifth or sixth character 1-4 or 6)

    Use Additional Code for adverse effect, if applicable, to identify drug (T36-T50 with fifth or sixth character 5)

    Excludes1: Barrett's esophagus (K22.7-)

    K22.10 Ulcer of esophagus without bleeding

      Ulcer of esophagus NOS

    K22.11 Ulcer of esophagus with bleeding

      Excludes2: bleeding esophageal varices (I85.01, I85.11)

K22.2 Esophageal obstruction

    Compression of esophagus

    Constriction of esophagus

    Stenosis of esophagus

    Stricture of esophagus

    Excludes1: congenital stenosis or stricture of esophagus (Q39.3)

K22.3 Perforation of esophagus

    Rupture of esophagus

    Excludes1: traumatic perforation of (thoracic) esophagus (S27.8-)

K22.4 Dyskinesia of esophagus

    Corkscrew esophagus

    Diffuse esophageal spasm

    Spasm of esophagus

    Excludes1: cardiospasm (K22.0)

K22.5 Diverticulum of esophagus, acquired

    Esophageal pouch, acquired

    Excludes1: diverticulum of esophagus (congenital) (Q39.6)

K22.6 Gastro-esophageal laceration-hemorrhage syndrome

    Mallory-Weiss syndrome

K22.7 Barrett's esophagus

    Barrett's disease

    Barrett's syndrome

    Excludes1: Barrett's ulcer (K22.1)

        malignant neoplasm of esophagus (C15.-)

    K22.70 Barrett's esophagus without dysplasia

      Barrett's esophagus NOS

    K22.71 Barrett's esophagus with dysplasia

      K22.710 Barrett's esophagus with low grade dysplasia

      K22.711 Barrett's esophagus with high grade dysplasia

      K22.719 Barrett's esophagus with dysplasia, unspecified

K22.8 Other specified diseases of esophagus

    Excludes2: esophageal varices (I85.-)

      Paterson-Kelly syndrome (D50.1)

    ● **K22.81 Esophageal polyp**

      benign neoplasm of esophagus (D13.0)

    ● **K22.82 Esophagogastric junction polyp**

      benign neoplasm of stomach (D13.1)

    ● **K22.89 Other specified disease of esophagus**

      Hemorrhage of esophagus NOS

K22.9 Disease of esophagus, unspecified

K23 Disorders of esophagus in diseases classified elsewhere

Code first underlying disease, such as:

congenital syphilis (A50.5)

Excludes1: late syphilis (A52.79)

    megaesophagus due to Chagas' disease (B57.31)

    tuberculosis (A18.83)

K25 Gastric ulcer

Definition: A Gastric ulcer is a hole in the lining of the stomach corroded by the acidic digestive juices which are secreted by the stomach cells.

Includes: erosion (acute) of stomach

pylorus ulcer (peptic) stomach ulcer (peptic)

Use Additional Code to identify:

alcohol abuse and dependence (F10.-)

Excludes1: acute gastritis (K29.0-)

    peptic ulcer NOS (K27.-)

K25.0 Acute gastric ulcer with hemorrhage

K25.1 Acute gastric ulcer with perforation [HCC]

K25.2 Acute gastric ulcer with both hemorrhage and perforation [HCC]

K25.3 Acute gastric ulcer without hemorrhage or perforation

K25.4 Chronic or unspecified gastric ulcer with hemorrhage

K25.5 Chronic or unspecified gastric ulcer with perforation [HCC]

● New code   ▲ Revised code   Excludes1: Not coded here   Excludes2: Not included here   ⊗ Placeholder required   ⑦ 7th digit required

K25.6 Chronic or unspecified gastric ulcer with both hemorrhage and perforation [HCC]

K25.7 Chronic gastric ulcer without hemorrhage or perforation

K25.9 Gastric ulcer, unspecified as acute or chronic, without hemorrhage or perforation

K26 Duodenal ulcer

Definition: A Duodenal ulcer is a ulcer in the lining of the first part of the small intestine (duodenum).

Includes: erosion (acute) of duodenum

duodenum ulcer (peptic)

postpyloric ulcer (peptic)

Use Additional Code to identify:

alcohol abuse and dependence (F10.-)

Excludes1: peptic ulcer NOS (K27.-)

K26.0 Acute duodenal ulcer with hemorrhage

K26.1 Acute duodenal ulcer with perforation [HCC]

K26.2 Acute duodenal ulcer with both hemorrhage and perforation [HCC]

K26.3 Acute duodenal ulcer without hemorrhage or perforation

K26.4 Chronic or unspecified duodenal ulcer with hemorrhage

K26.5 Chronic or unspecified duodenal ulcer with perforation [HCC]

K26.6 Chronic or unspecified duodenal ulcer with both hemorrhage and perforation [HCC]

K26.7 Chronic duodenal ulcer without hemorrhage or perforation

K26.9 Duodenal ulcer, unspecified as acute or chronic, without hemorrhage or perforation

K27 Peptic ulcer, site unspecified

Definition: A Peptic ulcer is an ulcer of the mucous membrane lining of the alimentary tract

Includes: gastroduodenal ulcer NOS

peptic ulcer NOS

Use Additional Code to identify:

alcohol abuse and dependence (F10.-)

Excludes1: peptic ulcer of newborn (P78.82)

K27.0 Acute peptic ulcer, site unspecified, with hemorrhage

K27.1 Acute peptic ulcer, site unspecified, with perforation [HCC]

K27.2 Acute peptic ulcer, site unspecified, with both hemorrhage and perforation [HCC]

K27.3 Acute peptic ulcer, site unspecified, without hemorrhage or perforation

K27.4 Chronic or unspecified peptic ulcer, site unspecified, with hemorrhage

K27.5 Chronic or unspecified peptic ulcer, site unspecified, with perforation [HCC]

K27.6 Chronic or unspecified peptic ulcer, site unspecified, with both hemorrhage and perforation [HCC]

K27.7 Chronic peptic ulcer, site unspecified, without hemorrhage or perforation

K27.9 Peptic ulcer, site unspecified, unspecified as acute or chronic, without hemorrhage or perforation

K28 Gastrojejunal ulcer

Definition: A gastrojejunal ulcer is an ulcer that forms in the area between the stomach and the part of the small intestine known as the jejunum.

Includes: anastomotic ulcer (peptic) or erosion

gastrocolic ulcer (peptic) or erosion

gastrointestinal ulcer (peptic) or erosion

gastrojejunal ulcer (peptic) or erosion

jejunal ulcer (peptic) or erosion

marginal ulcer (peptic) or erosion

stomal ulcer (peptic) or erosion

Use Additional Code to identify:

alcohol abuse and dependence (F10.-)

Excludes1: primary ulcer of small intestine (K63.3)

K28.0 Acute gastrojejunal ulcer with hemorrhage

K28.1 Acute gastrojejunal ulcer with perforation [HCC]

K28.2 Acute gastrojejunal ulcer with both hemorrhage and perforation

K28.3 Acute gastrojejunal ulcer without hemorrhage or perforation

K28.4 Chronic or unspecified gastrojejunal ulcer with hemorrhage

K28.5 Chronic or unspecified gastrojejunal ulcer with perforation [HCC]

K28.6 Chronic or unspecified gastrojejunal ulcer with both hemorrhage and perforation [HCC]

K28.7 Chronic gastrojejunal ulcer without hemorrhage or perforation

K28.9 Gastrojejunal ulcer, unspecified as acute or chronic, without hemorrhage or perforation

K29 Gastritis and duodenitis

Excludes1: eosinophilic gastritis or gastroenteritis (K52.81)

Zollinger-Ellison syndrome (E16.4)

K29.0 Acute gastritis

Use Additional Code to identify:

alcohol abuse and dependence (F10.-)

Excludes1: erosion (acute) of stomach (K25.-)

K29.00 Acute gastritis without bleeding

K29.01 Acute gastritis with bleeding

K29.2 Alcoholic gastritis

Use Additional Code to identify:

alcohol abuse and dependence (F10.-)

K29.20 Alcoholic gastritis without bleeding

K29.21 Alcoholic gastritis with bleeding

K29.3 Chronic superficial gastritis

K29.30 Chronic superficial gastritis without bleeding

K29.31 Chronic superficial gastritis with bleeding

K29.4 Chronic atrophic gastritis

Gastric atrophy

K29.40 Chronic atrophic gastritis without bleeding

K29.41 Chronic atrophic gastritis with bleeding

K29.5 Unspecified chronic gastritis

Chronic antral gastritis

Chronic fundal gastritis

K29.50 Unspecified chronic gastritis without bleeding

K29.51 Unspecified chronic gastritis with bleeding

K29.6 Other gastritis

Giant hypertrophic gastritis Granulomatous gastritis

Ménétrier's disease

K29.60 Other gastritis without bleeding

K29.61 Other gastritis with bleeding

K29.7 Gastritis, unspecified

K29.70 Gastritis, unspecified, without bleeding

K29.71 Gastritis, unspecified, with bleeding

K29.8 Duodenitis

K29.80   **Duodenitis without bleeding**

K29.81   **Duodenitis with bleeding**

K29.9   **Gastroduodenitis, unspecified**

   K29.90   **Gastroduodenitis, unspecified, without bleeding**

   K29.91   **Gastroduodenitis, unspecified, with bleeding**

K30   **Functional dyspepsia**

Indigestion

Excludes1: dyspepsia NOS (R10.13)

   heartburn (R12)

   nervous dyspepsia (F45.8)

   neurotic dyspepsia (F45.8)

   psychogenic dyspepsia (F45.8)

K31   **Other diseases of stomach and duodenum**

Includes: functional disorders of stomach

Excludes2: diabetic gastroparesis (E08.43, E09.43, E10.43, E11.43, E13.43)

   diverticulum of duodenum (K57.00-K57.13)

K31.0   **Acute dilatation of stomach**

Acute distention of stomach

K31.1   **Adult hypertrophic pyloric stenosis**

Pyloric stenosis NOS

Excludes1: congenital or infantile pyloric stenosis (Q40.0)

K31.2   **Hourglass stricture and stenosis of stomach**

Excludes1: congenital hourglass stomach (Q40.2)

   hourglass contraction of stomach (K31.89)

K31.3   **Pylorospasm, not elsewhere classified**

Excludes1: congenital or infantile pylorospasm (Q40.0)

   neurotic pylorospasm (F45.8)

   psychogenic pylorospasm (F45.8)

K31.4   **Gastric diverticulum**

Excludes1: congenital diverticulum of stomach (Q40.2)

K31.5   **Obstruction of duodenum**

Constriction of duodenum

Duodenal ileus (chronic)

Stenosis of duodenum

Stricture of duodenum

Volvulus of duodenum

Excludes1: congenital stenosis of duodenum (Q41.0)

K31.6   **Fistula of stomach and duodenum**

Gastrocolic fistula

Gastrojejunocolic fistula

K31.7   **Polyp of stomach and duodenum**

Excludes1: adenomatous polyp of stomach (D13.1)

K31.8   **Other specified diseases of stomach and duodenum**

   K31.81   **Angiodysplasia of stomach and duodenum**

      K31.811   **Angiodysplasia of stomach and duodenum with bleeding**

      K31.819   **Angiodysplasia of stomach and duodenum without bleeding**

      Angiodysplasia of stomach and duodenum NOS

   K31.82   **Dieulafoy lesion (hemorrhagic) of stomach and duodenum**

      Excludes2: Dieulafoy lesion of intestine (K63.81)

   K31.83   **Achlorhydria**

   K31.84   **Gastroparesis**

      Gastroparalysis

Code first underlying disease, if known, such as:

anorexia nervosa (F50.0-)

diabetes mellitus (E08.43, E09.43, E10.43, E11.43, E13.43)

scleroderma (M34.-)

   K31.89   **Other diseases of stomach and duodenum**

K31.9   **Disease of stomach and duodenum, unspecified**

● **K31.A**   **Gastric intestinal metaplasia**

   K31.A0   **Gastric intestinal metaplasia, unspecified**

      Gastric intestinal metaplasia indefinite for dysplasia

      Gastric intestinal metaplasia NOS

   ● **K31.A1**   **Gastric intestinal metaplasia without dysplasia**

      ● **K31.A11**   **Gastric intestinal metaplasia without dysplasia, involving the antrum**

      ● **K31.A12**   **Gastric intestinal metaplasia without dysplasia, involving the body(corpus)**

      ● **K31.A13**   **Gastric intestinal metaplasia without dysplasia, involving the fundus**

      ● **K31.A14**   **Gastric intestinal metaplasia without dysplasia, involving the cardia**

      ● **K31.A15**   **Gastric intestinal metaplasia without dysplasia, involving multiple sites**

      ● **K31.A19**   **Gastric intestinal metaplasia without dysplasia, unspecified site**

   ● **K31.A2**   **Gastric intestinal metaplasia with dysplasia**

      ● **K31.A21**   **Gastric intestinal metaplasia with low grade dysplasia**

      ● **K31.A22**   **Gastric intestinal metaplasia with high grade dysplasia**

      ● **K31.A29**   **Gastric intestinal metaplasia with dysplasia, unspecified**

DISEASES OF APPENDIX (K35-K38)

K35   **Acute appendicitis**

   K35.2   **Acute appendicitis with generalized peritonitis**

      Appendicitis (acute) with generalized (diffuse) peritonitis following rupture or perforation of appendix

      K35.20   **Acute appendicitis with generalized peritonitis, without abscess**

         (Acute) appendicitis with generalized peritonitis NOS

      K35.21   **Acute appendicitis with generalized peritonitis, with abscess**

   K35.3   **Acute appendicitis with localized peritonitis**

      Acute appendicitis with or without perforation or rupture

      K35.30   **Acute appendicitis with localized peritonitis, without perforation or gangrene**

         Acute appendicitis with localized peritonitis NOS

      K35.31   **Acute appendicitis with localized peritonitis and gangrene, without perforation**

      K35.32   **Acute appendicitis with perforation and localized peritonitis, without abscess**

         (Acute) appendicitis with perforation NOS

         Perforated appendix NOS

         Ruptured appendix (with localized peritonitis) NOS

      K35.33   **Acute appendicitis with perforation and localized peritonitis, with abscess**

         (Acute) appendicitis with (peritoneal) abscess NOS

Ruptured appendix with localized peritonitis and abscess

K35.8 **Other and unspecified acute appendicitis**

 K35.80 **Unspecified acute appendicitis**

  Acute appendicitis NOS

  Acute appendicitis without (localized) (generalized) peritonitis

 K35.89 **Other acute appendicitis**

  K35.890 **Other acute appendicitis without perforation or gangrene**

  K35.891 **Other acute appendicitis without perforation, with gangrene**

   (Acute) appendicitis with gangrene NOS

K36 **Other appendicitis**

Chronic appendicitis

Recurrent appendicitis

K37 **Unspecified appendicitis**

Excludes1: unspecified appendicitis with peritonitis (K35.2-, K35.3-)

K38 **Other diseases of appendix**

 K38.0 **Hyperplasia of appendix**

 K38.1 **Appendicular concretions**

  Fecalith of appendix

  Stercolith of appendix

 K38.2 **Diverticulum of appendix**

 K38.3 **Fistula of appendix**

 K38.8 **Other specified diseases of appendix**

  Intussusception of appendix

 K38.9 **Disease of appendix, unspecified**

HERNIA (K40-K46)

Note: Hernia with both gangrene and obstruction is classified to hernia with gangrene.

Includes: acquired hernia

congenital [except diaphragmatic or hiatus] hernia

recurrent hernia

K40 **Inguinal hernia**

Includes: bubonocele

 direct inguinal hernia

 double inguinal hernia

 indirect inguinal hernia

 inguinal hernia NOS

 oblique inguinal hernia

 scrotal hernia

 K40.0 **Bilateral inguinal hernia, with obstruction, without gangrene**

  Inguinal hernia (bilateral) causing obstruction without gangrene

  Incarcerated inguinal hernia (bilateral) without gangrene

  Irreducible inguinal hernia (bilateral) without gangrene

  Strangulated inguinal hernia (bilateral) without gangrene

  K40.00 **Bilateral inguinal hernia, with obstruction, without gangrene, not specified as recurrent**

   Bilateral inguinal hernia, with obstruction, without gangrene NOS

  K40.01 **Bilateral inguinal hernia, with obstruction, without gangrene, recurrent**

 K40.1 **Bilateral inguinal hernia, with gangrene**

  K40.10 **Bilateral inguinal hernia, with gangrene, not specified as recurrent**

   Bilateral inguinal hernia, with gangrene NOS

  K40.11 **Bilateral inguinal hernia, with gangrene, recurrent**

 K40.2 **Bilateral inguinal hernia, without obstruction or gangrene**

  K40.20 **Bilateral inguinal hernia, without obstruction or gangrene, not specified as recurrent**

   Bilateral inguinal hernia NOS

  K40.21 **Bilateral inguinal hernia, without obstruction or gangrene, recurrent**

 K40.3 **Unilateral inguinal hernia, with obstruction, without gangrene**

  Inguinal hernia (unilateral) causing obstruction without gangrene

  Incarcerated inguinal hernia (unilateral) without gangrene

  Irreducible inguinal hernia (unilateral) without gangrene

  Strangulated inguinal hernia (unilateral) without gangrene

  K40.30 **Unilateral inguinal hernia, with obstruction, without gangrene, not specified as recurrent**

   Inguinal hernia, with obstruction NOS

   Unilateral inguinal hernia, with obstruction, without gangrene NOS

  K40.31 **Unilateral inguinal hernia, with obstruction, without gangrene, recurrent**

 K40.4 **Unilateral inguinal hernia, with gangrene**

  K40.40 **Unilateral inguinal hernia, with gangrene, not specified as recurrent**

   Inguinal hernia with gangrene NOS

   Unilateral inguinal hernia with gangrene NOS

  K40.41 **Unilateral inguinal hernia, with gangrene, recurrent**

 K40.9 **Unilateral inguinal hernia, without obstruction or gangrene**

  K40.90 **Unilateral inguinal hernia, without obstruction or gangrene, not specified as recurrent**

   Inguinal hernia NOS

   Unilateral inguinal hernia NOS

  K40.91 **Unilateral inguinal hernia, without obstruction or gangrene, recurrent**

K41 **Femoral hernia**

 K41.0 **Bilateral femoral hernia, with obstruction, without gangrene**

  Femoral hernia (bilateral) causing obstruction, without gangrene

  Incarcerated femoral hernia (bilateral), without gangrene

  Irreducible femoral hernia (bilateral), without gangrene

  Strangulated femoral hernia (bilateral), without gangrene

  K41.00 **Bilateral femoral hernia, with obstruction, without gangrene, not specified as recurrent**

   Bilateral femoral hernia, with obstruction, without gangrene NOS

  K41.01 **Bilateral femoral hernia, with obstruction, without gangrene, recurrent**

 K41.1 **Bilateral femoral hernia, with gangrene**

  K41.10 **Bilateral femoral hernia, with gangrene, not specified as recurrent**

   Bilateral femoral hernia, with gangrene NOS

  K41.11 **Bilateral femoral hernia, with gangrene, recurrent**

K41.2 **Bilateral femoral hernia, without obstruction or gangrene**

    K41.20 **Bilateral femoral hernia, without obstruction or gangrene, not specified as recurrent**

        Bilateral femoral hernia NOS

    K41.21 **Bilateral femoral hernia, without obstruction or gangrene, recurrent**

K41.3 **Unilateral femoral hernia, with obstruction, without gangrene**

    Femoral hernia (unilateral) causing obstruction, without gangrene

    Incarcerated femoral hernia (unilateral), without gangrene

    Irreducible femoral hernia (unilateral), without gangrene

    Strangulated femoral hernia (unilateral), without gangrene

    K41.30 **Unilateral femoral hernia, with obstruction, without gangrene, not specified as recurrent**

        Femoral hernia, with obstruction NOS

        Unilateral femoral hernia, with obstruction NOS

    K41.31 **Unilateral femoral hernia, with obstruction, without gangrene, recurrent**

K41.4 **Unilateral femoral hernia, with gangrene**

    K41.40 **Unilateral femoral hernia, with gangrene, not specified as recurrent**

        Femoral hernia, with gangrene NOS

        Unilateral femoral hernia, with gangrene NOS

    K41.41 **Unilateral femoral hernia, with gangrene, recurrent**

K41.9 **Unilateral femoral hernia, without obstruction or gangrene**

    K41.90 **Unilateral femoral hernia, without obstruction or gangrene, not specified as recurrent**

        Femoral hernia NOS

        Unilateral femoral hernia NOS

    K41.91 **Unilateral femoral hernia, without obstruction or gangrene, recurrent**

K42 **Umbilical hernia**

Includes: paraumbilical hernia

Excludes1: omphalocele (Q79.2)

K42.0 **Umbilical hernia with obstruction, without gangrene**

    Umbilical hernia causing obstruction, without gangrene

    Incarcerated umbilical hernia, without gangrene

    Irreducible umbilical hernia, without gangrene

    Strangulated umbilical hernia, without gangrene

K42.1 **Umbilical hernia with gangrene**

    Gangrenous umbilical hernia

K42.9 **Umbilical hernia without obstruction or gangrene**

    Umbilical hernia NOS

K43 **Ventral hernia**

K43.0 **Incisional hernia with obstruction, without gangrene**

    Incisional hernia causing obstruction, without gangrene

    Incarcerated incisional hernia, without gangrene

    Irreducible incisional hernia, without gangrene

    Strangulated incisional hernia, without gangrene

K43.1 **Incisional hernia with gangrene**

    Gangrenous incisional hernia

K43.2 **Incisional hernia without obstruction or gangrene**

    Incisional hernia NOS

K43.3 **Parastomal hernia with obstruction, without gangrene**

    Incarcerated parastomal hernia, without gangrene

    Irreducible parastomal hernia, without gangrene

    Parastomal hernia causing obstruction, without gangrene

    Strangulated parastomal hernia, without gangrene

K43.4 **Parastomal hernia with gangrene**

    Gangrenous parastomal hernia

K43.5 **Parastomal hernia without obstruction or gangrene**

    Parastomal hernia NOS

K43.6 **Other and unspecified ventral hernia with obstruction, without gangrene**

    Epigastric hernia causing obstruction, without gangrene

    Hypogastric hernia causing obstruction, without gangrene

    Incarcerated epigastric hernia without gangrene

    Incarcerated hypogastric hernia without gangrene

    Incarcerated midline hernia without gangrene

    Incarcerated spigelian hernia without gangrene

    Incarcerated subxiphoid hernia without gangrene

    Irreducible epigastric hernia without gangrene

    Irreducible hypogastric hernia without gangrene

    Irreducible midline hernia without gangrene

    Irreducible spigelian hernia without gangrene

    Irreducible subxiphoid hernia without gangrene

    Midline hernia causing obstruction, without gangrene

    Spigelian hernia causing obstruction, without gangrene

    Strangulated epigastric hernia without gangrene

    Strangulated hypogastric hernia without gangrene

    Strangulated midline hernia without gangrene

    Strangulated spigelian hernia without gangrene

    Strangulated subxiphoid hernia without gangrene

    Subxiphoid hernia causing obstruction, without gangrene

K43.7 **Other and unspecified ventral hernia with gangrene**

    Any condition listed under K43.6 specified as gangrenous

K43.9 **Ventral hernia without obstruction or gangrene**

    Epigastric hernia

    Ventral hernia NOS

K44 **Diaphragmatic hernia**

Includes: hiatus hernia (esophageal) (sliding)

paraesophageal hernia

Excludes1: congenital diaphragmatic hernia (Q79.0)

    congenital hiatus hernia (Q40.1)

K44.0 **Diaphragmatic hernia with obstruction, without gangrene**

    Diaphragmatic hernia causing obstruction

    Incarcerated diaphragmatic hernia

    Irreducible diaphragmatic hernia

    Strangulated diaphragmatic hernia

K44.1 **Diaphragmatic hernia with gangrene**

    Gangrenous diaphragmatic hernia

K44.9 **Diaphragmatic hernia without obstruction or gangrene**

    Diaphragmatic hernia NOS

K45 **Other abdominal hernia**

Includes: abdominal hernia, specified site NEC

lumbar hernia

obturator hernia

pudendal hernia

retroperitoneal hernia

sciatic hernia

K45.0 Other specified abdominal hernia with obstruction, without gangrene

Other specified abdominal hernia causing obstruction

Other specified incarcerated abdominal hernia

Other specified irreducible abdominal hernia

Other specified strangulated abdominal hernia

K45.1 Other specified abdominal hernia with gangrene

Any condition listed under K45 specified as gangrenous

K45.8 Other specified abdominal hernia without obstruction or gangrene

K46 Unspecified abdominal hernia

Includes: enterocele

epiplocele hernia NOS

interstitial hernia

intestinal hernia

intra-abdominal hernia

Excludes1: vaginal enterocele (N81.5)

K46.0 Unspecified abdominal hernia with obstruction, without gangrene

Unspecified abdominal hernia causing obstruction

Unspecified incarcerated abdominal hernia

Unspecified irreducible abdominal hernia

Unspecified strangulated abdominal hernia

K46.1 Unspecified abdominal hernia with gangrene

Any condition listed under K46 specified as gangrenous

K46.9 Unspecified abdominal hernia without obstruction or gangrene

Abdominal hernia NOS

NONINFECTIVE ENTERITIS AND COLITIS (K50-K52)

Includes: noninfective inflammatory bowel disease

Excludes1: irritable bowel syndrome (K58.-)

megacolon (K59.3-)

K50 Crohn's disease [regional enteritis]

Includes: granulomatous enteritis

Use Additional Code to identify manifestations, such as:

pyoderma gangrenosum (L88)

Excludes1: ulcerative colitis (K51.-)

K50.0 Crohn's disease of small intestine

Crohn's disease [regional enteritis] of duodenum

Crohn's disease [regional enteritis] of ileum

Crohn's disease [regional enteritis] of jejunum

Regional ileitis

Terminal ileitis

Excludes1: Crohn's disease of both small and large intestine (K50.8-)

K50.00 Crohn's disease of small intestine without complications [HCC]

K50.01 Crohn's disease of small intestine with complications [HCC]

K50.011 Crohn's disease of small intestine with rectal bleeding

K50.012 Crohn's disease of small intestine with intestinal obstruction [HCC]

K50.013 Crohn's disease of small intestine with fistula [HCC]

K50.014 Crohn's disease of small intestine with abscess [HCC]

K50.018 Crohn's disease of small intestine with other complication [HCC]

K50.019 Crohn's disease of small intestine with unspecified complications [HCC]

K50.1 Crohn's disease of large intestine

Crohn's disease [regional enteritis] of colon

Crohn's disease [regional enteritis] of large bowel

Crohn's disease [regional enteritis] of rectum

Granulomatous colitis

Regional colitis

Excludes1: Crohn's disease of both small and large intestine   (K50.8)

K50.10 Crohn's disease of large intestine without complications [HCC]

K50.11 Crohn's disease of large intestine with complications

K50.111 Crohn's disease of large intestine with rectal bleeding [HCC]

K50.112 Crohn's disease of large intestine with intestinal obstruction [HCC]

K50.113 Crohn's disease of large intestine with fistula [HCC]

K50.114 Crohn's disease of large intestine with abscess [HCC]

K50.118 Crohn's disease of large intestine with other complication [HCC]

K50.119 Crohn's disease of large intestine with unspecified complications [HCC]

K50.8 Crohn's disease of both small and large intestine

K50.80 Crohn's disease of both small and large intestine without complications [HCC]

K50.81 Crohn's disease of both small and large intestine with complications

K50.811 Crohn's disease of both small and large intestine with rectal bleeding [HCC]

K50.812 Crohn's disease of both small and large intestine with intestinal obstruction [HCC]

K50.813 Crohn's disease of both small and large intestine with fistula [HCC]

K50.814 Crohn's disease of both small and large intestine with abscess [HCC]

K50.818 Crohn's disease of both small and large intestine with other complication [HCC]

K50.819 Crohn's disease of both small and large intestine with unspecified complications [HCC]

K50.9 Crohn's disease, unspecified

K50.90 Crohn's disease, unspecified, without complications [HCC]

Crohn's disease NOS

Regional enteritis NOS

K50.91 Crohn's disease, unspecified, with complications [HCC]

K50.911 Crohn's disease, unspecified, with rectal bleeding [HCC]

K50.912 Crohn's disease, unspecified, with intestinal obstruction

K50.913 Crohn's disease, unspecified, with fistula [HCC]

K50.914 Crohn's disease, unspecified, with abscess [HCC]

K50.918 Crohn's disease, unspecified, with other complication [HCC]

K50.919 Crohn's disease, unspecified, with unspecified complications [HCC]

K51 **Ulcerative colitis**

Definition: Ulcerative colitis ulcerative colitis is a form of inflammatory bowel disease (IBD). It causes swelling, ulcerations, and loss of function of the large intestine.

Use Additional Code to identify manifestations, such as:

pyoderma gangrenosum (L88)

Excludes1: Crohn's disease [regional enteritis] (K50.-)

K51.0 **Ulcerative (chronic) pancolitis**

Backwash ileitis

K51.00 Ulcerative (chronic) pancolitis without complications [HCC]

Ulcerative (chronic) pancolitis NOS

K51.01 Ulcerative (chronic) pancolitis with complications

K51.011 Ulcerative (chronic) pancolitis with rectal bleeding [HCC]

K51.012 Ulcerative (chronic) pancolitis with intestinal obstruction [HCC]

K51.013 Ulcerative (chronic) pancolitis with fistula [HCC]

K51.014 Ulcerative (chronic) pancolitis with abscess [HCC]

K51.018 Ulcerative (chronic) pancolitis with other complication [HCC]

K51.019 Ulcerative (chronic) pancolitis with unspecified complications [HCC]

K51.2 **Ulcerative (chronic) proctitis**

K51.20 Ulcerative (chronic) proctitis without complications [HCC]

Ulcerative (chronic) proctitis NOS

K51.21 Ulcerative (chronic) proctitis with complications

K51.211 Ulcerative (chronic) proctitis with rectal bleeding [HCC]

K51.212 Ulcerative (chronic) proctitis with intestinal obstruction [HCC]

K51.213 Ulcerative (chronic) proctitis with fistula [HCC]

K51.214 Ulcerative (chronic) proctitis with abscess [HCC]

K51.218 Ulcerative (chronic) proctitis with other complication [HCC]

K51.219 Ulcerative (chronic) proctitis with unspecified complications [HCC]

K51.3 **Ulcerative (chronic) rectosigmoiditis**

K51.30 Ulcerative (chronic) rectosigmoiditis without complications [HCC]

Ulcerative (chronic) rectosigmoiditis NOS

K51.31 Ulcerative (chronic) rectosigmoiditis with complications

K51.311 Ulcerative (chronic) rectosigmoiditis with rectal bleeding [HCC]

K51.312 Ulcerative (chronic) rectosigmoiditis with intestinal obstruction

K51.313 Ulcerative (chronic) rectosigmoiditis with fistula [HCC]

K51.314 Ulcerative (chronic) rectosigmoiditis with abscess [HCC]

K51.318 Ulcerative (chronic) rectosigmoiditis with other complication [HCC]

K51.319 Ulcerative (chronic) rectosigmoiditis with unspecified complications [HCC]

K51.4 **Inflammatory polyps of colon**

Excludes1: adenomatous polyp of colon (D12.6)

polyposis of colon (D12.6) polyps of colon NOS (K63.5)

K51.40 Inflammatory polyps of colon without complications [HCC]

Inflammatory polyps of colon NOS

K51.41 Inflammatory polyps of colon with complications

K51.411 Inflammatory polyps of colon with rectal bleeding [HCC]

K51.412 Inflammatory polyps of colon with intestinal obstruction [HCC]

K51.413 Inflammatory polyps of colon with fistula [HCC]

K51.414 Inflammatory polyps of colon with abscess [HCC]

K51.418 Inflammatory polyps of colon with other complication [HCC]

K51.419 Inflammatory polyps of colon with unspecified complications [HCC]

K51.5 **Left sided colitis**

Left Hemicolitis

K51.50 Left sided colitis without complications [HCC]

Left sided colitis NOS

K51.51 Left sided colitis with complications

K51.511 Left sided colitis with rectal bleeding [HCC]

K51.512 Left sided colitis with intestinal obstruction [HCC]

K51.513 Left sided colitis with fistula [HCC]

K51.514 Left sided colitis with abscess [HCC]

K51.518 Left sided colitis with other complication [HCC]

K51.519 Left sided colitis with unspecified complications [HCC]

K51.8 **Other ulcerative colitis**

K51.80 Other ulcerative colitis without complications [HCC]

K51.81 Other ulcerative colitis with complications

K51.811 Other ulcerative colitis with rectal bleeding [HCC]

K51.812 Other ulcerative colitis with intestinal obstruction [HCC]

K51.813 Other ulcerative colitis with fistula [HCC]

K51.814 Other ulcerative colitis with abscess

K51.818 Other ulcerative colitis with other complication [HCC]

K51.819 Other ulcerative colitis with unspecified complications [HCC]

K51.9 **Ulcerative colitis, unspecified**

K51.90 Ulcerative colitis, unspecified, without complications [HCC]

K51.91 Ulcerative colitis, unspecified, with complications

K51.911 Ulcerative colitis, unspecified with rectal bleeding [HCC]

K51.912 Ulcerative colitis, unspecified with intestinal obstruction [HCC]

K51.913 Ulcerative colitis, unspecified with fistula [HCC]

K51.914 Ulcerative colitis, unspecified with abscess [HCC]

K51.918 Ulcerative colitis, unspecified with other complication [HCC]

K51.919 Ulcerative colitis, unspecified with unspecified complications [HCC]

K52 **Other and unspecified noninfective gastroenteritis and colitis**

K52.0 **Gastroenteritis and colitis due to radiation**

K52.1 **Toxic gastroenteritis and colitis**

Drug-induced gastroenteritis and colitis

Code first (T51-T65) to identify toxic agent

Use Additional Code for adverse effect, if applicable, to identify drug (T36-T50 with fifth or sixth character 5)

K52.2 **Allergic and dietetic gastroenteritis and colitis**

Food hypersensitivity gastroenteritis or colitis

Use Additional Code to identify type of food allergy (Z91.01-, Z91.02-)

Excludes2: allergic eosinophilic colitis (K52.82)

allergic eosinophilic esophagitis (K20.0)

allergic eosinophilic gastritis (K52.81)

allergic eosinophilic gastroenteritis (K52.81)

K52.21 **Food protein-induced enterocolitis syndrome**

FPIES

Use Additional Code for hypovolemic shock, if present (R57.1)

K52.22 **Food protein-induced enteropathy**

K52.29 **Other allergic and dietetic gastroenteritis and colitis**

Allergic proctocolitis

Food hypersensitivity gastroenteritis or colitis

Food-induced eosinophilic proctocolitis

Food protein-induced proctocolitis

Immediate gastrointestinal hypersensitivity

Milk protein-induced proctocolitis

K52.3 **Indeterminate colitis**

Colonic inflammatory bowel disease unclassified (IBDU)

Excludes1: unspecified colitis (K52.9)

K52.8 **Other specified noninfective gastroenteritis and colitis**

K52.81 **Eosinophilic gastritis or gastroenteritis**

Eosinophilic enteritis

Excludes2: eosinophilic esophagitis (K20.0)

K52.82 **Eosinophilic colitis**

allergic proctocolitis (K52.29)

food-induced eosinophilic proctocolitis (K52.29)

food protein-induced enterocolitis syndrome (FPIES) (K52.21)

food protein-induced proctocolitis (K52.29)

milk protein-induced proctocolitis (K52.29)

K52.83 **Microscopic colitis**

K52.831 **Collagenous colitis**

K52.832 **Lymphocytic colitis**

K52.838 **Other microscopic colitis**

K52.839 **Microscopic colitis, unspecified**

K52.89 **Other specified noninfective gastroenteritis and colitis**

K52.9 **Noninfective gastroenteritis and colitis, unspecified**

Colitis NOS

Enteritis NOS

Gastroenteritis NOS

Ileitis NOS

Jejunitis NOS

Sigmoiditis NOS

Excludes1: diarrhea NOS (R19.7)

functional diarrhea (K59.1)

infectious gastroenteritis and colitis NOS (A09)

neonatal diarrhea (noninfective) (P78.3)

psychogenic diarrhea (F45.8)

OTHER DISEASES OF INTESTINES (K55-K64)

K55 **Vascular disorders of intestine**

Excludes1: necrotizing enterocolitis of newborn (P77.-)

K55.0 **Acute vascular disorders of intestine**

Infarction of appendices epiploicae

Mesenteric (artery) (vein) embolism

Mesenteric (artery) (vein) infarction

Mesenteric (artery) (vein) thrombosis

K55.01 **Acute (reversible) ischemia of small intestine**

K55.011 **Focal (segmental) acute (reversible) ischemia of small intestine** [HCC]

K55.012 **Diffuse acute (reversible) ischemia of small intestine** [HCC]

K55.019 **Acute (reversible) ischemia of small intestine, extent unspecified** [HCC]

K55.02 **Acute infarction of small intestine** [HCC]

Gangrene of small intestine

Necrosis of small intestine

K55.021 **Focal (segmental) acute infarction of small intestine** [HCC]

K55.022 **Diffuse acute infarction of small intestine** [HCC]

K55.029 **Acute infarction of small intestine, extent unspecified**

K55.03 **Acute (reversible) ischemia of large intestine**

Acute fulminant ischemic colitis

Subacute ischemic colitis

K55.031 **Focal (segmental) acute (reversible) ischemia of large intestine** [HCC]

K55.032 **Diffuse acute (reversible) ischemia of large intestine** [HCC]

K55.039 **Acute (reversible) ischemia of large intestine, extent unspecified** [HCC]

K55.04 **Acute infarction of large intestine**

Gangrene of large intestine

Necrosis of large intestine

K55.041 **Focal (segmental) acute infarction of large intestine** [HCC]

K55.042 **Diffuse acute infarction of large intestine** [HCC]

K55.049 **Acute infarction of large intestine, extent unspecified** [HCC]

K55.05 **Acute (reversible) ischemia of intestine, part unspecified**

K55.051 Focal (segmental) acute (reversible) ischemia of intestine, part unspecified [HCC]

K55.052 Diffuse acute (reversible) ischemia of intestine, part unspecified [HCC]

K55.059 Acute (reversible) ischemia of intestine, part and extent unspecified [HCC]

K55.06 Acute infarction of intestine, part unspecified

Acute intestinal infarction

Gangrene of intestine

Necrosis of intestine

K55.061 Focal (segmental) acute infarction of intestine, part unspecified [HCC]

K55.062 Diffuse acute infarction of intestine, part unspecified [HCC]

K55.069 Acute infarction of intestine, part and extent unspecified [HCC]

K55.1 **Chronic vascular disorders of intestine** [HCC]

Chronic ischemic colitis

Chronic ischemic enteritis

Chronic ischemic enterocolitis

Ischemic stricture of intestine

Mesenteric atherosclerosis

Mesenteric vascular insufficiency

K55.2 **Angiodysplasia of colon**

K55.20 Angiodysplasia of colon without hemorrhage

K55.21 Angiodysplasia of colon with hemorrhage

K55.3 **Necrotizing enterocolitis**

Excludes1: necrotizing enterocolitis of newborn (P77.-)

Excludes2: necrotizing enterocolitis due to Clostridium difficile (A04.7-)

K55.30 Necrotizing enterocolitis, unspecified [HCC]

Necrotizing enterocolitis, NOS

K55.31 Stage 1 necrotizing enterocolitis [HCC]

Necrotizing enterocolitis without pneumatosis, without perforation

K55.32 Stage 2 necrotizing enterocolitis [HCC]

Necrotizing enterocolitis with pneumatosis, without perforation

K55.33 Stage 3 necrotizing enterocolitis [HCC]

Necrotizing enterocolitis with perforation

Necrotizing enterocolitis with pneumatosis and perforation

K55.8 **Other vascular disorders of intestine** [HCC]

K55.9 **Vascular disorder of intestine, unspecified** [HCC]

Ischemic colitis Ischemic enteritis

Ischemic enterocolitis

K56 **Paralytic ileus and intestinal obstruction without hernia**

Excludes1: congenital stricture or stenosis of intestine (Q41-Q42)

cystic fibrosis with meconium ileus (E84.11)

ischemic stricture of intestine (K55.1)

meconium ileus NOS (P76.0)

neonatal intestinal obstructions classifiable to P76.-

obstruction of duodenum (K31.5)

postprocedural intestinal obstruction (K91.3-)

stenosis of anus or rectum (K62.4)

K56.0 **Paralytic ileus** [HCC]

Paralysis of bowel

Paralysis of colon

Paralysis of intestine

Excludes1: gallstone ileus (K56.3)

ileus NOS (K56.7)

obstructive ileus NOS (K56.69-)

K56.1 **Intussusception** [HCC]

Intussusception or invagination of bowel

Intussusception or invagination of colon

Intussusception or invagination of intestine

Intussusception or invagination of rectum

Excludes2: intussusception of appendix (K38.8)

K56.2 **Volvulus** [HCC]

Strangulation of colon or intestine

Torsion of colon or intestine

Twist of colon or intestine

Excludes2: volvulus of duodenum (K31.5)

K56.3 **Gallstone ileus** [HCC]

Obstruction of intestine by gallstone

K56.4 **Other impaction of intestine**

K56.41 Fecal impaction [HCC]

Excludes1: constipation (K59.0-)

incomplete defecation (R15.0)

K56.49 Other impaction of intestine [HCC]

K56.5 **Intestinal adhesions [bands] with obstruction (postprocedural) (postinfection)**

Abdominal hernia due to adhesions with obstruction

Peritoneal adhesions [bands] with intestinal obstruction (postinfection)

K56.50 Intestinal adhesions [bands], unspecified as to partial versus complete obstruction [HCC]

Intestinal adhesions with obstruction NOS

K56.51 Intestinal adhesions [bands], with partial obstruction [HCC]

Intestinal adhesions with incomplete obstruction

K56.52 Intestinal adhesions [bands] with complete obstruction [HCC]

K56.6 **Other and unspecified intestinal obstruction**

K56.60 Unspecified intestinal obstruction

K56.600 Partial intestinal obstruction, unspecified as to cause [HCC]

Incomplete intestinal obstruction, NOS

K56.601 Complete intestinal obstruction, unspecified as to cause [HCC]

K56.609 Unspecified intestinal obstruction, unspecified as to partial versus complete obstruction [HCC]

Intestinal obstruction NOS

K56.69 Other intestinal obstruction

Enterostenosis NOS

Obstructive ileus NOS

Occlusión of colon or intestine NOS

Stenosis of colon or intestine NOS

Stricture of colon or intestine NOS

Excludes1: intestinal obstruction due to specified condition-code to condition

K56.690 Other partial intestinal obstruction [HCC]

Other incomplete intestinal obstruction

K56.691 **Other complete intestinal obstruction** [HCC]

K56.699 **Other intestinal obstruction unspecified as to partial versus complete obstruction** [HCC]

Other intestinal obstruction, NEC

K56.7 **Ileus, unspecified** [HCC]

Excludes1: obstructive ileus (K56.69-)

Excludes2: intestinal obstruction with hernia (K40-K46)

K57 **Diverticular disease of intestine**

Definition: Diverticulitis is a common digestive disease which involves the formation of pouches (diverticula) within the bowel wall. This process is known as diverticulosis, and typically occurs within the large intestine, or colon, although it can occasionally occur in the small intestine as well. Diverticulitis results when one of these diverticula becomes inflamed.

Code also if applicable peritonitis K65.-

Excludes1: congenital diverticulum of intestine (Q43.8)

Meckel's diverticulum (Q43.0)

Excludes2: diverticulum of appendix (K38.2)

K57.0 **Diverticulitis of small intestine with perforation and abscess**

Excludes1: diverticulitis of both small and large intestine with perforation and abscess (K57.4-)

K57.00 **Diverticulitis of small intestine with perforation and abscess without bleeding**

K57.01 **Diverticulitis of small intestine with perforation and abscess with bleeding**

K57.1 **Diverticular disease of small intestine without perforation or abscess**

Excludes1: diverticular disease of both small and large intestine without perforation or abscess (K57.5-)

K57.10 **Diverticulosis of small intestine without perforation or abscess without bleeding**

Diverticular disease of small intestine NOS

K57.11 **Diverticulosis of small intestine without perforation or abscess with bleeding**

K57.12 **Diverticulitis of small intestine without perforation or abscess without bleeding**

K57.13 **Diverticulitis of small intestine without perforation or abscess with bleeding**

K57.2 **Diverticulitis of large intestine with perforation and abscess**

Excludes1: diverticulitis of both small and large intestine with perforation and abscess (K57.4-)

K57.20 **Diverticulitis of large intestine with perforation and abscess without bleeding**

K57.21 **Diverticulitis of large intestine with perforation and abscess with bleeding**

K57.3 **Diverticular disease of large intestine without perforation or abscess**

Excludes1: diverticular disease of both small and large intestine without perforation or abscess (K57.5-)

K57.30 **Diverticulosis of large intestine without perforation or abscess without bleeding**

Diverticular disease of colon NOS

K57.31 **Diverticulosis of large intestine without perforation or abscess with bleeding**

K57.32 **Diverticulitis of large intestine without perforation or abscess without bleeding**

K57.33 **Diverticulitis of large intestine without perforation or abscess with bleeding**

K57.4 **Diverticulitis of both small and large intestine with perforation and abscess**

K57.40 **Diverticulitis of both small and large intestine with perforation and abscess without bleeding**

K57.41 **Diverticulitis of both small and large intestine with perforation and abscess with bleeding**

K57.5 **Diverticular disease of both small and large intestine without perforation or abscess**

K57.50 **Diverticulosis of both small and large intestine without perforation or abscess without bleeding**

Diverticular disease of both small and large intestine NOS

K57.51 **Diverticulosis of both small and large intestine without perforation or abscess with bleeding**

K57.52 **Diverticulitis of both small and large intestine without perforation or abscess without bleeding**

K57.53 **Diverticulitis of both small and large intestine without perforation or abscess with bleeding**

K57.8 **Diverticulitis of intestine, part unspecified, with perforation and abscess**

K57.80 **Diverticulitis of intestine, part unspecified, with perforation and abscess without bleeding**

K57.81 **Diverticulitis of intestine, part unspecified, with perforation and abscess with bleeding**

K57.9 **Diverticular disease of intestine, part unspecified, without perforation or abscess**

K57.90 **Diverticulosis of intestine, part unspecified, without perforation or abscess without bleeding**

Diverticular disease of intestine NOS

K57.91 **Diverticulosis of intestine, part unspecified, without perforation or abscess with bleeding**

K57.92 **Diverticulitis of intestine, part unspecified, without perforation or abscess without bleeding**

K57.93 **Diverticulitis of intestine, part unspecified, without perforation or abscess with bleeding**

K58 **Irritable bowel syndrome**

Includes: irritable colon

spastic colon

K58.0 **Irritable bowel syndrome with diarrhea**

K58.1 **Irritable bowel syndrome with constipation**

K58.2 **Mixed irritable bowel syndrome**

K58.8 **Other irritable bowel syndrome**

K58.9 **Irritable bowel syndrome without diarrhea**

Irritable bowel syndrome NOS

K59 **Other functional intestinal disorders**

Excludes1: change in bowel habit NOS (R19.4)

intestinal malabsorption (K90.-)

psychogenic intestinal disorders (F45.8)

Excludes2: functional disorders of stomach (K31.-)

K59.0 **Constipation**

Excludes1: fecal impaction (K56.41)

incomplete defecation (R15.0)

K59.00 **Constipation, unspecified**

K59.01 **Slow transit constipation**

K59.02 **Outlet dysfunction constipation**

K59.03 **Drug induced constipation**

Use Additional Code for adverse effect, if applicable, to identify drug (T36-T50 with fifth or sixth character 5)

K59.04   Chronic idiopathic constipation
Functional constipation

K59.09   Other constipation
Chronic constipation

K59.1   Functional diarrhea
Excludes1: diarrhea NOS (R19.7)
irritable bowel syndrome with diarrhea (K58.0)

K59.2   Neurogenic bowel, not elsewhere classified

K59.3   Megacolon, not elsewhere classified
Dilatation of colon
Code first, if applicable (T51-T65) to identify toxic agent
Excludes1: congenital megacolon (aganglionic) (Q43.1)
megacolon (due to) (in) Chagas' disease (B57.32)
megacolon (due to) (in) Clostridium difficile (A04.7-)
megacolon (due to) (in) Hirschsprung's disease (Q43.1)

K59.31   Toxic megacolon [HCC]

K59.39   Other megacolon
Megacolon NOS

K59.4   Anal spasm
Proctalgia fugax

K59.8   Other specified functional intestinal disorders

K59.81   Ogilvie syndrome
Acute colonic pseudo-obstruction (ACPO)

K59.89   Other specified functional intestinal disorders
Atony of colon
Pseudo-obstruction (acute) (chronic) of intestine

K59.9   Functional intestinal disorder, unspecified

K60   Fissure and fistula of anal and rectal regions
Excludes1: fissure and fistula of anal and rectal regions with abscess or cellulitis (K61.-)
Excludes2: anal sphincter tear (healed) (nontraumatic) (old) (K62.81)

K60.0   Acute anal fissure

K60.1   Chronic anal fissure

K60.2   Anal fissure, unspecified

K60.3   Anal fistula

K60.4   Rectal fistula
Fistula of rectum to skin
Excludes1: rectovaginal fistula (N82.3)
vesicorectal fistula (N32.1)

K60.5   Anorectal fistula

K61   Abscess of anal and rectal regions
Includes: abscess of anal and rectal regions
cellulitis of anal and rectal regions

K61.0   Anal abscess
Perianal abscess
Excludes2: intrasphincteric abscess (K61.4)

K61.1   Rectal abscess
Perirectal abscess
Excludes1: ischiorectal abscess (K61.39)

K61.2   Anorectal abscess

K61.3   Ischiorectal abscess

K61.31   Horseshoe abscess

K61.39   Other ischiorectal abscess

Abscess of ischiorectal fossa
Ischiorectal abscess, NOS

K61.4   Intrasphincteric abscess
Intersphincteric abscess

K61.5   Supralevator abscess

K62   Other diseases of anus and rectum
Includes: anal canal
Excludes2: colostomy and enterostomy malfunction (K94.0-, K94.1-)
fecal incontinence (R15.-)
hemorrhoids (K64.-)

K62.0   Anal polyp

K62.1   Rectal polyp
Excludes1: adenomatous polyp (D12.8)

K62.2   Anal prolapse
Prolapse of anal canal

K62.3   Rectal prolapse
Prolapse of rectal mucosa

K62.4   Stenosis of anus and rectum
Stricture of anus (sphincter)

K62.5   Hemorrhage of anus and rectum
Excludes1: gastrointestinal bleeding NOS (K92.2)
melena (K92.1)
neonatal rectal hemorrhage (P54.2)

K62.6   Ulcer of anus and rectum
Solitary ulcer of anus and rectum
Stercoral ulcer of anus and rectum
Excludes1: fissure and fistula of anus and rectum (K60.-)
ulcerative colitis (K51.-)

K62.7   Radiation proctitis
Use Additional Code to identify the type of radiation (W88.-) or radiation therapy (Y84.2)

K62.8   Other specified diseases of anus and rectum
Excludes2: ulcerative proctitis (K51.2)

K62.81   Anal sphincter tear (healed) (nontraumatic) (old)
Tear of anus, nontraumatic
Use Additional Code for any associated fecal incontinence (R15.-)
Excludes2: anal fissure (K60.-)
anal sphincter tear (healed) (old) complicating delivery (O34.7-)
traumatic tear of anal sphincter (S31.831)

K62.82   Dysplasia of anus
Anal intraepithelial neoplasia I and II (AIN I and II) (histologically confirmed)
Dysplasia of anus NOS
Mild and moderate dysplasia of anus (histologically confirmed)
Excludes1: abnormal results from anal cytologic examination without histologic confirmation (R85.61-)
anal intraepithelial neoplasia III (D01.3)
carcinoma in situ of anus (D01.3)
HGSIL of anus (R85.613)
severe dysplasia of anus (D01.3)

K62.89 Other specified diseases of anus and rectum

Proctitis NOS

Use Additional Code for any associated fecal incontinence (R15.-)

K62.9 Disease of anus and rectum, unspecified

K63 Other diseases of intestine

K63.0 Abscess of intestine

Excludes1: abscess of intestine with Crohn's disease (K50.014, K50.114, K50.814, K50.914,)

abscess of intestine with diverticular disease (K57.0, K57.2, K57.4, K57.8)

abscess of intestine with ulcerative colitis (K51.014, K51.214, K51.314, K51.414, K51.514, K51.814, K51.914)

Excludes2: abscess of anal and rectal regions (K61.-)

abscess of appendix (K35.3-)

K63.1 Perforation of intestine (nontraumatic) [HCC]

Perforation (nontraumatic) of rectum

Excludes1: perforation (nontraumatic) of duodenum (K26.-)

perforation (nontraumatic) of intestine with diverticular disease (K57.0, K57.2, K57.4, K57.8)

Excludes2: perforation (nontraumatic) of appendix (K35.2-, K35.3-)

K63.2 Fistula of intestine

Excludes1: fistula of duodenum (K31.6)

fistula of intestine with Crohn's disease (K50.013, K50.113, K50.813, K50.913,)

fistula of intestine with ulcerative colitis (K51.013, K51.213, K51.313, K51.413, K51.513, K51.813, K51.913)

Excludes2: fistula of anal and rectal regions (K60.-)

fistula of appendix (K38.3)

intestinal-genital fistula, female (N82.2-N82.4)

vesicointestinal fistula (N32.1)

K63.3 Ulcer of intestine

Primary ulcer of small intestine

Excludes1: duodenal ulcer (K26.-)

gastrointestinal ulcer (K28.-)

gastrojejunal ulcer (K28.-)

jejunal ulcer (K28.-)

peptic ulcer, site unspecified (K27.-)

ulcer of intestine with perforation (K63.1)

ulcer of anus or rectum (K62.6)

ulcerative colitis (K51.-)

K63.4 Enteroptosis

K63.5 Polyp of colon

Excludes1: adenomatous polyp of colon (D12.-)

inflammatory polyp of colon (K51.4-)

polyposis of colon (D12.6)

K63.8 Other specified diseases of intestine

K63.81 Dieulafoy lesion of intestine

Excludes2: Dieulafoy lesion of stomach and duodenum (K31.82)

K63.89 Other specified diseases of intestine

K63.9 Disease of intestine, unspecified

K64 Hemorrhoids and perianal venous thrombosis

Includes: piles

Excludes1: hemorrhoids complicating childbirth and the puerperium (O87.2)

hemorrhoids complicating pregnancy (O22.4)

K64.0 First degree hemorrhoids

Grade/stage I hemorrhoids

Hemorrhoids (bleeding) without prolapse outside of anal canal

K64.1 Second degree hemorrhoids

Grade/stage II hemorrhoids

Hemorrhoids (bleeding) that prolapse with straining, but retract spontaneously

K64.2 Third degree hemorrhoids

Grade/stage III hemorrhoids

Hemorrhoids (bleeding) that prolapse with straining and require manual replacement back inside anal canal

K64.3 Fourth degree hemorrhoids

Grade/stage IV hemorrhoids

Hemorrhoids (bleeding) with prolapsed tissue that cannot be manually replaced

K64.4 Residual hemorrhoidal skin tags

External hemorrhoids, NOS

Skin tags of anus

K64.5 Perianal venous thrombosis

External hemorrhoids with thrombosis

Perianal hematoma

Thrombosed hemorrhoids NOS

K64.8 Other hemorrhoids

Internal hemorrhoids, without mention of degree

Prolapsed hemorrhoids, degree not specified

K64.9 Unspecified hemorrhoids

Hemorrhoids (bleeding) NOS

Hemorrhoids (bleeding) without mention of degree

DISEASES OF PERITONEUM AND RETROPERITONEUM (K65-K68)

K65 Peritonitis

Definition: Peritonitis is an inflammation of the membrane which lines the inside of the abdomen and all of the internal organs.

Use Additional Code (B95-B97), to identify infectious agent, if known

Code also if applicable diverticular disease of intestine (K57.-)

Excludes1: acute appendicitis with generalized peritonitis (K35.2-)

aseptic peritonitis (T81.6)

benign paroxysmal peritonitis (E85.0)

chemical peritonitis (T81.6)

gonococcal peritonitis (A54.85)

neonatal peritonitis (P78.0-P78.1)

pelvic peritonitis, female (N73.3-N73.5)

periodic familial peritonitis (E85.0)

peritonitis due to talc or other foreign substance (T81.6)

peritonitis in chlamydia (A74.81)

peritonitis in diphtheria (A36.89)

peritonitis in syphilis (late) (A52.74)

peritonitis in tuberculosis (A18.31)

peritonitis with or following abortion or ectopic or molar pregnancy (O00-O07, O08.0)

peritonitis with or following appendicitis (K35.-)

puerperal peritonitis (O85)

---

retroperitoneal infections (K68.-)

K65.0 **Generalized (acute) peritonitis** [HCC]

Pelvic peritonitis (acute), male

Subphrenic peritonitis (acute)

Suppurative peritonitis (acute)

K65.1 **Peritoneal abscess** [HCC]

Abdominopelvic abscess

Abscess (of) omentum

Abscess (of) peritoneum

Mesenteric abscess

Retrocecal abscess

Subdiaphragmatic abscess

Subhepatic abscess

Subphrenic abscess

K65.2 **Spontaneous bacterial peritonitis** [HCC]

Excludes1: bacterial peritonitis NOS (K65.9)

K65.3 **Choleperitonitis** [HCC]

Peritonitis due to bile

K65.4 **Sclerosing mesenteritis** [HCC]

Fat necrosis of peritoneum (Idiopathic) sclerosing mesenteric fibrosis

Mesenteric lipodystrophy

Mesenteric panniculitis

Retractile mesenteritis

K65.8 **Other peritonitis** [HCC]

Chronic proliferative peritonitis

Peritonitis due to urine

K65.9 **Peritonitis, unspecified** [HCC]

Bacterial peritonitis NOS

K66 **Other disorders of peritoneum**

Excludes2: ascites (R18.-)

peritoneal effusion (chronic) (R18.8)

K66.0 **Peritoneal adhesions (postprocedural) (postinfection)**

Adhesions (of) abdominal (wall)

Adhesions (of) diaphragm

Adhesions (of) intestine

Adhesions (of) male pelvis

Adhesions (of) omentum

Adhesions (of) stomach

Adhesive bands

Mesenteric adhesions

Excludes1: female pelvic adhesions [bands] (N73.6)

peritoneal adhesions with intestinal obstruction (K56.5-)

K66.1 **Hemoperitoneum**

Excludes1: traumatic hemoperitoneum (S36.8-)

K66.8 **Other specified disorders of peritoneum**

K66.9 **Disorder of peritoneum, unspecified**

K67 **Disorders of peritoneum in infectious diseases classified elsewhere** [HCC]

Code first underlying disease, such as:

congenital syphilis (A50.0)

helminthiasis (B65.0 -B83.9)

Excludes1: peritonitis in chlamydia (A74.81)

peritonitis in diphtheria (A36.89)

peritonitis in gonococcal (A54.85)

peritonitis in syphilis (late) (A52.74)

peritonitis in tuberculosis (A18.31)

K68 **Disorders of retroperitoneum**

K68.1 **Retroperitoneal abscess**

K68.11 **Postprocedural retroperitoneal abscess**

Excludes2: infection l (T81.4-)

K68.12 **Psoas muscle abscess** [HCC]

K68.19 **Other retroperitoneal abscess** [HCC]

K68.9 **Other disorders of retroperitoneum**

DISEASES OF LIVER (K70-K77)

Excludes1: jaundice NOS (R17)

Excludes2: hemochromatosis (E83.11-)

Reye's syndrome (G93.7)

viral hepatitis (B15-B19)

Wilson's disease (E83.0)

K70 **Alcoholic liver disease**

Use Additional Code to identify:

alcohol abuse and dependence (F10.-)

K70.0 **Alcoholic fatty liver**

K70.1 **Alcoholic hepatitis**

K70.10 **Alcoholic hepatitis without ascites**

K70.11 **Alcoholic hepatitis with ascites**

K70.2 **Alcoholic fibrosis and sclerosis of liver**

K70.3 **Alcoholic cirrhosis of liver**

Alcoholic cirrhosis NOS

K70.30 **Alcoholic cirrhosis of liver without ascites** [HCC]

K70.31 **Alcoholic cirrhosis of liver with ascites** [HCC]

K70.4 **Alcoholic hepatic failure** [HCC]

Acute alcoholic hepatic failure

Alcoholic hepatic failure NOS

Chronic alcoholic hepatic failure

Subacute alcoholic hepatic failure

K70.40 **Alcoholic hepatic failure without coma** [HCC]

K70.41 **Alcoholic hepatic failure with coma** [HCC]

K70.9 **Alcoholic liver disease, unspecified** [HCC]

K71 **Toxic liver disease**

Includes: drug-induced idiosyncratic (unpredictable) liver disease

drug-induced toxic (predictable) liver disease

Code first poisoning due to drug or toxin, if applicable (T36-T65 with fifth or sixth character 1-4 or 6)

Use Additional Code for adverse effect, if applicable, to identify drug (T36-T50 with fifth or sixth character 5)

Excludes2: alcoholic liver disease (K70.-)

Budd-Chiari syndrome (I82.0)

K71.0 **Toxic liver disease with cholestasis**

Cholestasis with hepatocyte injury 'Pure' cholestasis

K71.1 **Toxic liver disease with hepatic necrosis**

Hepatic failure (acute) (chronic) due to drugs

K71.10 **Toxic liver disease with hepatic necrosis, without coma**

K71.11 **Toxic liver disease with hepatic necrosis, with coma** [HCC]

K71.2 **Toxic liver disease with acute hepatitis**

K71.3 **Toxic liver disease with chronic persistent hepatitis**

K71.4 **Toxic liver disease with chronic lobular hepatitis**

K71.5 **Toxic liver disease with chronic active hepatitis**

Toxic liver disease with lupoid hepatitis

● New code   ▲ Revised code   **Excludes1:** Not coded here   **Excludes2:** Not included here   ⊗ Placeholder required   ⑦7th digit required

K71.50 Toxic liver disease with chronic active hepatitis without ascites

K71.51 Toxic liver disease with chronic active hepatitis with ascites

K71.6 Toxic liver disease with hepatitis, not elsewhere classified

K71.7 Toxic liver disease with fibrosis and cirrhosis of liver

K71.8 Toxic liver disease with other disorders of liver

Toxic liver disease with focal nodular hyperplasia

Toxic liver disease with hepatic granulomas

Toxic liver disease with peliosis hepatis

Toxic liver disease with veno-occlusive disease of liver

K71.9 Toxic liver disease, unspecified

K72 Hepatic failure, not elsewhere classified

Includes: fulminant hepatitis NEC, with hepatic failure

hepatic encephalopathy NOS

liver (cell) necrosis with hepatic failure

malignant hepatitis NEC, with hepatic failure yellow liver atrophy or dystrophy

Excludes1: alcoholic hepatic failure (K70.4)

hepatic failure with toxic liver disease (K71.1-)

icterus of newborn (P55-P59)

postprocedural hepatic failure (K91.82)

Excludes2: hepatic failure complicating abortion or ectopic or molar pregnancy (O00-O07, O08.8)

hepatic failure complicating pregnancy, childbirth and the puerperium (O26.6-)

viral hepatitis with hepatic coma (B15-B19)

K72.0 Acute and subacute hepatic failure

Acute non-viral hepatitis NOS

K72.00 Acute and subacute hepatic failure without coma

K72.01 Acute and subacute hepatic failure with coma

K72.1 Chronic hepatic failure

End stage liver disease

K72.10 Chronic hepatic failure without coma

K72.11 Chronic hepatic failure with coma

K72.9 Hepatic failure, unspecified

K72.90 Hepatic failure, unspecified without coma [HCC]

K72.91 Hepatic failure, unspecified with coma [HCC]

Hepatic coma NOS

K73 Chronic hepatitis, not elsewhere classified

Excludes1: alcoholic hepatitis (chronic) (K70.1-)

drug-induced hepatitis (chronic) (K71.-)

granulomatous hepatitis (chronic) NEC (K75.3)

reactive, nonspecific hepatitis (chronic) (K75.2)

viral hepatitis (chronic) (B15-B19)

K73.0 Chronic persistent hepatitis, not elsewhere classified [HCC]

K73.1 Chronic lobular hepatitis, not elsewhere classified [HCC]

K73.2 Chronic active hepatitis, not elsewhere classified [HCC]

K73.8 Other chronic hepatitis, not elsewhere classified [HCC]

K73.9 Chronic hepatitis, unspecified [HCC]

K74 Fibrosis and cirrhosis of liver

Definition: Cirrhosis is the chronic scarring of the liver, leading to loss of normal liver function.

Code also, if applicable, viral hepatitis (acute) (chronic) (B15-B19)

Excludes1: alcoholic cirrhosis (of liver) (K70.3)

alcoholic fibrosis of liver (K70.2)

cardiac sclerosis of liver (K76.1)

cirrhosis (of liver) with toxic liver disease (K71.7)

congenital cirrhosis (of liver) (P78.81)

pigmentary cirrhosis (of liver) (E83.110)

K74.0 Hepatic fibrosis

Code first underlying liver disease, such as:

nonalcoholic steatohepatitis (NASH) (K75.81)

K74.00 Hepatic fibrosis, unspecified

K74.01 Hepatic fibrosis, early fibrosis

Hepatic fibrosis, stage F1 or stage F2

K74.02 Hepatic fibrosis, advanced fibrosis

Hepatic fibrosis, stage F3

Excludes1: cirrhosis of liver (K74.6-)

hepatic fibrosis, stage F4 (K74.6-)

K74.1 Hepatic sclerosis

K74.2 Hepatic fibrosis with hepatic sclerosis

K74.3 Primary biliary cirrhosis [HCC]

Chronic nonsuppurative destructive cholangitis

Primary biliary cholangitis

Excludes2: primary sclerosing cholangitis (K83.01)

K74.4 Secondary biliary cirrhosis [HCC]

K74.5 Biliary cirrhosis, unspecified [HCC]

K74.6 Other and unspecified cirrhosis of liver [HCC]

K74.60 Unspecified cirrhosis of liver [HCC]

Cirrhosis (of liver) NOS

K74.69 Other cirrhosis of liver [HCC]

Cryptogenic cirrhosis (of liver)

Macronodular cirrhosis (of liver)

Micronodular cirrhosis (of liver)

Mixed type cirrhosis (of liver)

Portal cirrhosis (of liver)

Postnecrotic cirrhosis (of liver)

K75 Other inflammatory liver diseases

Excludes2: toxic liver disease (K71.-)

K75.0 Abscess of liver

Cholangitic hepatic abscess

Hematogenic hepatic abscess

Hepatic abscess NOS

Lymphogenic hepatic abscess

Pylephlebitic hepatic abscess

Excludes1: amebic liver abscess (A06.4)

cholangitis without liver abscess (K83.09)

pylephlebitis without liver abscess (K75.1)

Excludes2: acute or subacute hepatitis NOS (B17.9)

acute or subacute non-viral hepatitis (K72.0)

chronic hepatitis NEC (K73.8)

K75.1 Phlebitis of portal vein

Pylephlebitis

Excludes1: pylephlebitic liver abscess (K75.0)

K75.2 Nonspecific reactive hepatitis

Excludes1: acute or subacute hepatitis (K72.0-)

chronic hepatitis NEC (K73.-)

viral hepatitis (B15-B19)

K75.3 Granulomatous hepatitis, not elsewhere classified

Excludes1: acute or subacute hepatitis (K72.0-)

chronic hepatitis NEC (K73.-)

viral hepatitis (B15-B19)

K75.4   Autoimmune hepatitis [HCC]

Lupoid hepatitis NEC

K75.8   Other specified inflammatory liver diseases

K75.81   Nonalcoholic steatohepatitis (NASH)

<u>Use Additional Code</u>, if applicable, hepatic fibrosis (K74.0-)

K75.89   Other specified inflammatory liver diseases

K75.9   Inflammatory liver disease, unspecified

Hepatitis NOS

Excludes1: acute or subacute hepatitis (K72.0-)

chronic hepatitis NEC (K73.-)

viral hepatitis (B15-B19)

K76   Other diseases of liver

Excludes2: alcoholic liver disease (K70.-)

amyloid degeneration of liver (E85.-)

cystic disease of liver (congenital) (Q44.6)

hepatic vein thrombosis (I82.0)

hepatomegaly NOS (R16.0)

pigmentary cirrhosis (of liver) (E83.110)

portal vein thrombosis (I81)

toxic liver disease (K71.-)

K76.0   Fatty (change of) liver, not elsewhere classified

Nonalcoholic fatty liver disease (NAFLD)

Excludes1: nonalcoholic steatohepatitis (NASH) (K75.81)

K76.1   Chronic passive congestion of liver

Cardiac cirrhosis

Cardiac sclerosis

K76.2   Central hemorrhagic necrosis of liver

Excludes1: liver necrosis with hepatic failure (K72.-)

K76.3   Infarction of liver

K76.4   Peliosis hepatis

Hepatic angiomatosis

K76.5   Hepatic veno-occlusive disease

Excludes1: Budd-Chiari syndrome (I82.0)

K76.6   Portal hypertension [HCC]

<u>Use Additional Code</u> for any associated complications, such as:

portal hypertensive gastropathy (K31.89)

K76.7   Hepatorenal syndrome

Excludes1: hepatorenal syndrome following labor and delivery (O90.4)

postprocedural hepatorenal syndrome (K91.83)

K76.8   Other specified diseases of liver

K76.81   Hepatopulmonary syndrome [HCC]

<u>Code first</u> underlying liver disease, such as:

alcoholic cirrhosis of liver (K70.3-)

cirrhosis of liver without mention of alcohol (K74.6-)

K76.89   Other specified diseases of liver

Cyst (simple) of liver

Focal nodular hyperplasia of liver

Hepatoptosis

K76.9   Liver disease, unspecified

K77   Liver disorders in diseases classified elsewhere

<u>Code first</u> underlying disease, such as:

amyloidosis (E85.-)

congenital syphilis (A50.0, A50.5)

congenital toxoplasmosis (P37.1)

infectious mononucleosis with liver disease (B27.0-B27.9 with .9)

schistosomiasis (B65.0-B65.9)

Excludes1: alcoholic hepatitis (K70.1-)

alcoholic liver disease (K70.-)

cytomegaloviral hepatitis (B25.1)

herpesviral [herpes simplex] hepatitis (B00.81)

mumps hepatitis (B26.81)

sarcoidosis with liver disease (D86.89)

secondary syphilis with liver disease (A51.45)

syphilis (late) with liver disease (A52.74)

toxoplasmosis (acquired) hepatitis (B58.1)

tuberculosis with liver disease (A18.83)

DISORDERS OF GALLBLADDER, BILIARY TRACT AND PANCREAS (K80-K87)

K80   Cholelithiasis

Excludes1: retained cholelithiasis following cholecystectomy (K91.86)

K80.0   Calculus of gallbladder with acute cholecystitis

Any condition listed in K80.2 with acute cholecystitis

<u>Use Additional Code</u> if applicable for associated gangrene of gallbladder (K82.A1), or perforation of gallbladder (K82.A2)

K80.00   Calculus of gallbladder with acute cholecystitis without obstruction

K80.01   Calculus of gallbladder with acute cholecystitis with obstruction

K80.1   Calculus of gallbladder with other cholecystitis

<u>Use Additional Code</u> if applicable for associated gangrene of gallbladder (K82.A1), or perforation of gallbladder (K82.A2)

K80.10   Calculus of gallbladder with chronic cholecystitis without obstruction

Cholelithiasis with cholecystitis NOS

K80.11   Calculus of gallbladder with chronic cholecystitis with obstruction

K80.12   Calculus of gallbladder with acute and chronic cholecystitis without obstruction

K80.13   Calculus of gallbladder with acute and chronic cholecystitis with obstruction

K80.18   Calculus of gallbladder with other cholecystitis without obstruction

K80.19   Calculus of gallbladder with other cholecystitis with obstruction

K80.2   Calculus of gallbladder without cholecystitis

Cholecystolithiasis without cholecystitis

Cholelithiasis (without cholecystitis)

Colic (recurrent) of gallbladder (without cholecystitis)

Gallstone (impacted) of cystic duct (without cholecystitis)

Gallstone (impacted) of gallbladder (without cholecystitis)

K80.20   Calculus of gallbladder without cholecystitis without obstruction

K80.21   Calculus of gallbladder without cholecystitis with obstruction

K80.3   Calculus of bile duct with cholangitis

Any condition listed in K80.5 with cholangitis

K80.30 Calculus of bile duct with cholangitis, unspecified, without obstruction

K80.31 Calculus of bile duct with cholangitis, unspecified, with obstruction

K80.32 Calculus of bile duct with acute cholangitis without obstruction

K80.33 Calculus of bile duct with acute cholangitis with obstruction

K80.34 Calculus of bile duct with chronic cholangitis without obstruction

K80.35 Calculus of bile duct with chronic cholangitis with obstruction

K80.36 Calculus of bile duct with acute and chronic cholangitis without obstruction

K80.37 Calculus of bile duct with acute and chronic cholangitis with obstruction

K80.4 Calculus of bile duct with cholecystitis

Any condition listed in K80.5 with cholecystitis (with cholangitis)

Code also fistula of bile duct (K83.3)

Use Additional Code if applicable for associated gangrene of gallbladder (K82.A1), or perforation of gallbladder (K82.A2)

K80.40 Calculus of bile duct with cholecystitis, unspecified, without obstruction

K80.41 Calculus of bile duct with cholecystitis, unspecified, with obstruction

K80.42 Calculus of bile duct with acute cholecystitis without obstruction

K80.43 Calculus of bile duct with acute cholecystitis with obstruction

K80.44 Calculus of bile duct with chronic cholecystitis without obstruction

K80.45 Calculus of bile duct with chronic cholecystitis with obstruction

K80.46 Calculus of bile duct with acute and chronic cholecystitis without obstruction

K80.47 Calculus of bile duct with acute and chronic cholecystitis with obstruction

K80.5 Calculus of bile duct without cholangitis or cholecystitis

Choledocholithiasis (without cholangitis or cholecystitis)

Gallstone (impacted) of bile duct NOS (without cholangitis or cholecystitis)

Gallstone (impacted) of common duct (without cholangitis or cholecystitis)

Gallstone (impacted) of hepatic duct (without cholangitis or cholecystitis)

Hepatic cholelithiasis (without cholangitis or cholecystitis)

Hepatic colic (recurrent) (without cholangitis or cholecystitis)

K80.50 Calculus of bile duct without cholangitis or cholecystitis without obstruction

K80.51 Calculus of bile duct without cholangitis or cholecystitis with obstruction

K80.6 Calculus of gallbladder and bile duct with cholecystitis

Use Additional Code if applicable for associated gangrene of gallbladder (K82.A1), or perforation of gallbladder (K82.A2)

K80.60 Calculus of gallbladder and bile duct with cholecystitis, unspecified, without obstruction

K80.61 Calculus of gallbladder and bile duct with cholecystitis, unspecified, with obstruction

K80.62 Calculus of gallbladder and bile duct with acute cholecystitis without obstruction

K80.63 Calculus of gallbladder and bile duct with acute cholecystitis with obstruction

K80.64 Calculus of gallbladder and bile duct with chronic cholecystitis without obstruction

K80.65 Calculus of gallbladder and bile duct with chronic cholecystitis with obstruction

K80.66 Calculus of gallbladder and bile duct with acute and chronic cholecystitis without obstruction

K80.67 Calculus of gallbladder and bile duct with acute and chronic cholecystitis with obstruction

K80.7 Calculus of gallbladder and bile duct without cholecystitis

K80.70 Calculus of gallbladder and bile duct without cholecystitis without obstruction

K80.71 Calculus of gallbladder and bile duct without cholecystitis with obstruction

K80.8 Other cholelithiasis

K80.80 Other cholelithiasis without obstruction

K80.81 Other cholelithiasis with obstruction

K81 Cholecystitis

Excludes1: cholecystitis with cholelithiasis (K80.-)

Use Additional Code if applicable for associated gangrene of gallbladder (K82.A1), or perforation of gallbladder (K82.A2)

K81.0 Acute cholecystitis

Abscess of gallbladder

Angiocholecystitis

Emphysematous (acute) cholecystitis

Empyema of gallbladder

Gangrene of gallbladder

Gangrenous cholecystitis

Suppurative cholecystitis

K81.1 Chronic cholecystitis

K81.2 Acute cholecystitis with chronic cholecystitis

K81.9 Cholecystitis, unspecified

K82 Other diseases of gallbladder

Excludes1: nonvisualization of gallbladder (R93.2)

postcholecystectomy syndrome (K91.5)

K82.0 Obstruction of gallbladder

Occlusion of cystic duct or gallbladder without cholelithiasis

Stenosis of cystic duct or gallbladder without cholelithiasis

Stricture of cystic duct or gallbladder without cholelithiasis

Excludes1: obstruction of gallbladder with cholelithiasis (K80.-)

K82.1 Hydrops of gallbladder

Mucocele of gallbladder

K82.2 Perforation of gallbladder

Rupture of cystic duct or gallbladder

Excludes1: Perforation of gallbladder in cholecystitis (K82.A2)

K82.A Disorders of gallbladder in diseases classified elsewhere

Code first the type of cholecystitis (K81.-), or cholelithiasis with cholecystitis (K80.00-K80.19, K80.40-K80.47, K80.60-K80.67)

K82.A1 Gangrene of gallbladder in cholecystitis

K82.A2 Perforation of gallbladder in cholecystitis

K82.3 Fistula of gallbladder

Cholecystocolic fistula

Cholecystoduodenal fistula

K82.4 **Cholesterolosis of gallbladder**

Strawberry gallbladder

Excludes1: cholesterolosis of gallbladder with cholecystitis (K81.-)

cholesterolosis of gallbladder with cholelithiasis (K80.-)

K82.8 **Other specified diseases of gallbladder**

Adhesions of cystic duct or gallbladder

Atrophy of cystic duct or gallbladder

Cyst of cystic duct or gallbladder

Dyskinesia of cystic duct or gallbladder

Hypertrophy of cystic duct or gallbladder

Nonfunctioning of cystic duct or gallbladder

Ulcer of cystic duct or gallbladder

K82.9 **Disease of gallbladder, unspecified**

K83 **Other diseases of biliary tract**

Excludes1: postcholecystectomy syndrome (K91.5)

Excludes2: conditions involving the gallbladder (K81-K82)

conditions involving the cystic duct (K81-K82)

K83.0 **Cholangitis**

Excludes2: chronic nonsuppurative destructive cholangitis (K74.3)

primary biliary cholangitis (K74.3)

primary biliary cirrhosis (K74.3)

K83.01 **Primary sclerosing cholangitis**

K83.09 **Other cholangitis**

Ascending cholangitis

Cholangitis NOS

Primary cholangitis

Recurrent cholangitis

Sclerosing cholangitis

Secondary cholangitis

Stenosing cholangitis

Suppurative cholangitis

K83.1 **Obstruction of bile duct**

Occlusion of bile duct without cholelithiasis

Stenosis of bile duct without cholelithiasis

Stricture of bile duct without cholelithiasis

Excludes1: congenital obstruction of bile duct (Q44.3)

obstruction of bile duct with cholelithiasis (K80.-)

K83.2 **Perforation of bile duct**

Rupture of bile duct

K83.3 **Fistula of bile duct**

Choledochoduodenal fistula

K83.4 **Spasm of sphincter of Oddi**

K83.5 **Biliary cyst**

K83.8 **Other specified diseases of biliary tract**

Adhesions of biliary tract

Atrophy of biliary tract

Hypertrophy of biliary tract

Ulcer of biliary tract

K83.9 **Disease of biliary tract, unspecified**

K85 **Acute pancreatitis**

Includes: acute (recurrent) pancreatitis

subacute pancreatitis

K85.0 **Idiopathic acute pancreatitis**

K85.00 **Idiopathic acute pancreatitis without necrosis or infection**

K85.01 **Idiopathic acute pancreatitis with uninfected necrosis**

K85.02 **Idiopathic acute pancreatitis with infected necrosis**

K85.1 **Biliary acute pancreatitis**

Gallstone pancreatitis

K85.10 **Biliary acute pancreatitis without necrosis or infection**

K85.11 **Biliary acute pancreatitis with uninfected necrosis**

K85.12 **Biliary acute pancreatitis with infected necrosis**

K85.2 **Alcohol induced acute pancreatitis**

Excludes2: alcohol induced chronic pancreatitis (K86.0)

K85.20 **Alcohol induced acute pancreatitis without necrosis or infection**

K85.21 **Alcohol induced acute pancreatitis with uninfected necrosis**

K85.22 **Alcohol induced acute pancreatitis with infected necrosis**

K85.3 **Drug induced acute pancreatitis**

Use Additional Code for adverse effect, if applicable, to identify drug (T36-T50 with fifth or sixth character 5)

Use Additional Code to identify drug abuse and dependence (F11.-F17.-)

K85.30 **Drug induced acute pancreatitis without necrosis or infection**

K85.31 **Drug induced acute pancreatitis with uninfected necrosis**

K85.32 **Drug induced acute pancreatitis with infected necrosis**

K85.8 **Other acute pancreatitis**

K85.80 **Other acute pancreatitis without necrosis or infection**

K85.81 **Other acute pancreatitis with uninfected necrosis**

K85.82 **Other acute pancreatitis with infected necrosis**

K85.9 **Acute pancreatitis, unspecified**

Pancreatitis NOS

K85.90 **Acute pancreatitis without necrosis or infection, unspecified**

K85.91 **Acute pancreatitis with uninfected necrosis, unspecified**

K85.92 **Acute pancreatitis with infected necrosis, unspecified**

K86 **Other diseases of pancreas**

Excludes2: fibrocystic disease of pancreas (E84.-)

islet cell tumor (of pancreas) (D13.7)

pancreatic steatorrhea (K90.3)

K86.0 **Alcohol-induced chronic pancreatitis** [HCC]

Use Additional Code to identify:

alcohol abuse and dependence (F10.-)

Code also exocrine pancreatic insufficiency (K86.81)

Excludes2: alcohol induced acute pancreatitis (K85.2-)

K86.1 **Other chronic pancreatitis** [HCC]

Chronic pancreatitis NOS

Infectious chronic pancreatitis

Recurrent chronic pancreatitis

Relapsing chronic pancreatitis

Code also exocrine pancreatic insufficiency (K86.81)

K86.2   **Cyst of pancreas**

K86.3   **Pseudocyst of pancreas**

K86.8   **Other specified diseases of pancreas**

     K86.81   **Exocrine pancreatic insufficiency**

     K86.89   **Other specified diseases of pancreas**

        Aseptic pancreatic necrosis, unrelated to acute pancreatitis

        Atrophy of pancreas

        Calculus of pancreas

        Cirrhosis of pancreas

        Fibrosis of pancreas

        Pancreatic fat necrosis, unrelated to acute pancreatitis

        Pancreatic infantilism

        Pancreatic necrosis NOS, unrelated to acute pancreatitis

K86.9   **Disease of pancreas, unspecified**

K87   **Disorders of gallbladder, biliary tract and pancreas in diseases classified elsewhere**

   Code first underlying disease

   Excludes1: cytomegaloviral pancreatitis (B25.2)

        mumps pancreatitis (B26.3)

        syphilitic gallbladder (A52.74)

        syphilitic pancreas (A52.74)

        tuberculosis of gallbladder (A18.83)

        tuberculosis of pancreas (A18.83)

OTHER DISEASES OF THE DIGESTIVE SYSTEM (K90-K95)

K90   **Intestinal malabsorption**

   Definition: Intestinal malabsorption is a state arising from abnormality in digestion or absorption of food nutrients across the gastrointestinal(GI) tract.

   Excludes1: intestinal malabsorption following gastrointestinal surgery (K91.2)

K90.0   **Celiac disease**

   Celiac disease with steatorrhea

   Celiac gluten-sensitive enteropathy Nontropical sprue

   Use Additional Code for associated disorders including:

   dermatitis herpetiformis (L13.0)

   gluten ataxia (G32.81)

   Code also exocrine pancreatic insufficiency (K86.81)

K90.1   **Tropical sprue**

   Sprue NOS

   Tropical steatorrhea

K90.2   **Blind loop syndrome, not elsewhere classified**

   Blind loop syndrome NOS

   Excludes1: congenital blind loop syndrome (Q43.8)

        postsurgical blind loop syndrome (K91.2)

K90.3   **Pancreatic steatorrhea**

K90.4   **Other malabsorption due to intolerance**

   Excludes2: celiac gluten-sensitive enteropathy (K90.0)

        lactose intolerance (E73.-)

     K90.41   **Non-celiac gluten sensitivity**

        Gluten sensitivity NOS

        Non-celiac gluten sensitive enteropathy

     K90.49   **Malabsorption due to intolerance, not elsewhere classified**

        Malabsorption due to intolerance to carbohydrate

        Malabsorption due to intolerance to fat

        Malabsorption due to intolerance to protein

        Malabsorption due to intolerance to starch

K90.8   **Other intestinal malabsorption**

     K90.81   **Whipple's disease**

     K90.89   **Other intestinal malabsorption**

K90.9   **Intestinal malabsorption, unspecified**

K91   **Intraoperative and postprocedural complications and disorders of digestive system, not elsewhere classified**

   Excludes2: complications of artificial opening of digestive system (K94.-)

        complications of bariatric procedures (K95.-)

        gastrojejunal ulcer (K28.-)

        postprocedural (radiation) retroperitoneal abscess (K68.11)

        radiation colitis (K52.0)

        radiation gastroenteritis (K52.0)

        radiation proctitis (K62.7)

K91.0   **Vomiting following gastrointestinal surgery**

K91.1   **Postgastric surgery syndromes**

   Dumping syndrome

   Postgastrectomy syndrome

   Postvagotomy syndrome

K91.2   **Postsurgical malabsorption, not elsewhere classified**

   Postsurgical blind loop syndrome

   Excludes1: malabsorption osteomalacia in adults (M83.2)

        malabsorption osteoporosis, postsurgical (M80.8-, M81.8)

K91.3   **Postprocedural intestinal obstruction**

     K91.30   **Postprocedural intestinal obstruction, unspecified as to partial versus complete**

        Postprocedural intestinal obstruction NOS

     K91.31   **Postprocedural partial intestinal obstruction**

        Postprocedural incomplete intestinal obstruction

     K91.32   **Postprocedural complete intestinal obstructionK91.5 Postcholecystectomy syndrome**

K91.6   **Intraoperative hemorrhage and hematoma of a digestive system organ or structure complicating a procedure**

   Excludes1: intraoperative hemorrhage and hematoma of a digestive system organ or structure due to accidental puncture and laceration during a procedure (K91.7-)

     K91.61   **Intraoperative hemorrhage and hematoma of a digestive system organ or structure complicating a digestive system procedure**

     K91.62   **Intraoperative hemorrhage and hematoma of a digestive system organ or structure complicating other procedure**

K91.7   **Accidental puncture and laceration of a digestive system organ or structure during a procedure**

     K91.71   **Accidental puncture and laceration of a digestive system organ or structure during a digestive system procedure**

     K91.72   **Accidental puncture and laceration of a digestive system organ or structure during other procedure**

K91.8   **Other intraoperative and postprocedural complications and disorders of digestive system**

     K91.81   **Other intraoperative complications of digestive system**

     K91.82   **Postprocedural hepatic failure**

K91.83   **Postprocedural hepatorenal syndrome**

K91.84   **Postprocedural hemorrhage of a digestive system organ or structure following a procedure**

    K91.840   **Postprocedural hemorrhage of a digestive system organ or structure following a digestive system procedure**

    K91.841   **Postprocedural hemorrhage of a digestive system organ or structure following other procedure**

K91.85   **Complications of intestinal pouch**

    K91.850   **Pouchitis** [HCC]

        Inflammation of internal ileoanal pouch

    K91.858   **Other complications of intestinal pouch** [HCC]

K91.86   **Retained cholelithiasis following cholecystectomy**

K91.87   **Postprocedural hematoma and seroma of a digestive system organ or structure following a procedure**

    K91.870   **Postprocedural hematoma of a digestive system organ or structure following a digestive system procedure**

    K91.871   **Postprocedural hematoma of a digestive system organ or structure following other procedure**

    K91.872   **Postprocedural seroma of a digestive system organ or structure following a digestive system procedure**

    K91.873   **Postprocedural seroma of a digestive system organ or structure following other procedure**

K91.89   **Other postprocedural complications and disorders of digestive system**

    Use Additional Code, if applicable, to further specify disorder

    Excludes2: postprocedural retroperitoneal abscess (K68.11)

K92   **Other diseases of digestive system**

Excludes1: neonatal gastrointestinal hemorrhage (P54.0-P54.3)

K92.0   **Hematemesis**

K92.1   **Melena**

    Excludes1: occult blood in feces (R19.5)

K92.2   **Gastrointestinal hemorrhage, unspecified**

    Gastric hemorrhage NOS

    Intestinal hemorrhage NOS

    Excludes1: acute hemorrhagic gastritis (K29.01)

    hemorrhage of anus and rectum (K62.5)

    angiodysplasia of stomach with hemorrhage (K31.811)

    diverticular disease with hemorrhage (K57.-)

    gastritis and duodenitis with hemorrhage (K29.-)

    peptic ulcer with hemorrhage (K25-K28)

K92.8   **Other specified diseases of the digestive system**

    K92.81   **Gastrointestinal mucositis (ulcerative)**

        Code also type of associated therapy, such as:

        antineoplastic and immunosuppressive drugs (T45.1X-)

        radiological procedure and radiotherapy (Y84.2)

        Excludes2: mucositis (ulcerative) of vagina and vulva (N76.81)

nasal mucositis (ulcerative) (J34.81)

oral mucositis (ulcerative) (K12.3-)

    K92.89   **Other specified diseases of the digestive system**

K92.9   **Disease of digestive system, unspecified**

K94   **Complications of artificial openings of the digestive system**

K94.0   **Colostomy complications**

    K94.00   **Colostomy complication, unspecified** [HCC]

    K94.01   **Colostomy hemorrhage** [HCC]

    K94.02   **Colostomy infection** [HCC]

        Use Additional Code to specify type of infection, such as:

        cellulitis of abdominal wall (L03.311) sepsis (A40.-, A41.-)

    K94.03   **Colostomy malfunction** [HCC]

        Mechanical complication of colostomy

    K94.09   **Other complications of colostomy** [HCC]

K94.1   **Enterostomy complications** [HCC]

    K94.10   **Enterostomy complication, unspecified** [HCC]

    K94.11   **Enterostomy hemorrhage** [HCC]

    K94.12   **Enterostomy infection** [HCC]

        Use Additional Code to specify type of infection, such as:

        cellulitis of abdominal wall (L03.311) sepsis (A40.-, A41.-)

    K94.13   **Enterostomy malfunction** [HCC]

        Mechanical complication of enterostomy

    K94.19   **Other complications of enterostomy** [HCC]

K94.2   **Gastrostomy complications** [HCC]

    K94.20   **Gastrostomy complication, unspecified** [HCC]

    K94.21   **Gastrostomy hemorrhage** [HCC]

    K94.22   **Gastrostomy infection** [HCC]

        Use Additional Code to specify type of infection, such as:

        cellulitis of abdominal wall (L03.311)

        sepsis (A40.-, A41.-)

    K94.23   **Gastrostomy malfunction** [HCC]

        Mechanical complication of gastrostomy

    K94.29   **Other complications of gastrostomy** [HCC]

K94.3   **Esophagostomy complications** [HCC]

    K94.30   **Esophagostomy complications, unspecified** [HCC]

    K94.31   **Esophagostomy hemorrhage** [HCC]

    K94.32   **Esophagostomy infection** [HCC]

        Use Additional Code to identify the infection

    K94.33   **Esophagostomy malfunction** [HCC]

        Mechanical complication of esophagostomy

    K94.39   **Other complications of esophagostomy** [HCC]

K95   **Complications of bariatric procedures**

K95.0   **Complications of gastric band procedure**

    K95.01   **Infection due to gastric band procedure**

        Use Additional Code to specify type of infection or organism, such as:

        bacterial and viral infectious agents (B95.-, B96.-)

        cellulitis of abdominal wall (L03.311)

        sepsis (A40.-, A41.-)

    K95.09   **Other complications of gastric band procedure**

        Use Additional Code, if applicable, to further specify complication

K95.8 **Complications of other bariatric procedure**

Excludes1: complications of gastric band surgery (K95.0-)

K95.81 **Infection due to other bariatric procedure**

Use Additional Code to specify type of infection or organism, such as:

bacterial and viral infectious agents (B95.-, B96.-)

cellulitis of abdominal wall (L03.311)

sepsis (A40.-, A41.-)

K95.89 **Other complications of other bariatric procedure**

Use Additional Code, if applicable, to further specify complication

● New code ▲ Revised code **Excludes1:** Not coded here **Excludes2:** Not included here ⊗ Placeholder required ⑦7ᵗʰ digit required

Chapter 12: Diseases of the Skin and Subcutaneous Tissue (L00-L99)

DEFINITIONS

This chapter includes definitions of selected key words, terms and phrases and coding alerts for adding points to the clinical domain, and references to coding late effects where appropriate. An example from this chapter is as follows:

L49   Exfoliation due to erythematous conditions according to extent of body surface involved

     Definition: Erythematous conditions refers to conditions causing diffuse or patchy redness of skin.

MULTIPLE CODING FOR A SINGLE CONDITION

In addition to the etiology/manifestation convention that requires two codes to fully describe a single condition that affects multiple body systems, there are other single conditions that also require more than one code. "**Use Additional Code**" notes are found in the Tabular List at codes that are not part of an etiology/manifestation pair where a secondary code is useful to fully describe a condition. The sequencing rule is the same as the etiology/manifestation pair, "**Use Additional Code**" indicates that a secondary code should be added.

For example, for bacterial infections that are not included in chapter 1, a secondary code from category B95, Streptococcus, Staphylococcus, and Enterococcus, as the cause of diseases classified elsewhere, or B96, Other bacterial agents as the cause of diseases classified elsewhere, may be required to identify the bacterial organism causing the infection. A "**Use Additional Code**" note will normally be found at the infectious disease code, indicating a need for the organism code to be added as a secondary code.

"Code first" notes are also under certain codes that are not specifically manifestation codes but may be due to an underlying cause. When there is a "Code first" note and an underlying condition is present, the underlying condition should be sequenced first.

"Code, if applicable, any causal condition first", notes indicate that this code may be assigned as a principal diagnosis when the causal condition is unknown or not applicable. If a causal condition is known, then the code for that condition should be sequenced as the principal or first-listed diagnosis.

Multiple codes may be needed for sequela, complication codes and obstetric codes to more fully describe a condition. See the specific guidelines for these conditions for further instruction.

COMBINATION CODE

A combination code is a single code used to classify: Two diagnoses, or a diagnosis with an associated secondary process (manifestation) A diagnosis with an associated complication

Combination codes are identified by referring to subterm entries in the Alphabetic Index and by reading the inclusion and exclusion notes in the Tabular List.

Assign only the combination code when that code fully identifies the diagnostic conditions involved or when the Alphabetic Index so directs. Multiple coding should not be used when the classification provides a combination code that clearly identifies all of the elements documented in the diagnosis. When the combination code lacks necessary specificity in describing the manifestation or complication, an additional code should be used as a secondary code.

SEQUELA (LATE EFFECTS)

A sequela is the residual effect (condition produced) after the acute phase of an illness or injury has terminated. There is no time limit on when a sequela code can be used. The residual may be apparent early, such as in cerebral infarction, or it may occur months or years later, such as that due to a previous injury. Coding of sequela generally requires two codes sequenced in the following order: The condition or nature of the sequela is sequenced first.

The sequela code is sequenced second.

An exception to the above guidelines are those instances where the code for the sequela is followed by a manifestation code identified in the Tabular List and title, or the sequela code has been expanded (at the fourth, fifth or sixth character levels) to

include the manifestation(s). The code for the acute phase of an illness or injury that led to the sequela is never used with a code for the late effect.

PRESSURE ULCER STAGE CODES

1) Pressure ulcer stages

Codes from category L89, Pressure ulcer, identify the site of the pressure ulcer as well as the stage of the ulcer.

Codes in category L89, Pressure ulcer, identify the site and stage of the pressure ulcer as well.

The ICD-10-CM classifies pressure ulcer stages based on severity, which is designated by stages 1-4, deep tissue pressure injury, unspecified stage and unstageable.

See Section I.B.14 for pressure ulcer stage documentation by clinicians other than patient's provider.

2) Unstageable pressure ulcers

Assignment of the code for unstageable pressure ulcer (L89.--0) should be based on the clinical documentation. These codes are used for pressure ulcers whose stage cannot be clinically determined (e.g., the ulcer is covered by eschar or has been treated with a skin or muscle graft) and pressure ulcers that are documented as deep tissue injury but not documented as due to trauma. This code should not be confused with the codes for unspecified stage (L89.--9). When there is no documentation regarding the stage of the pressure ulcer, assign the appropriate code for unspecified stage (L89.--9).

3) Documented pressure ulcer stage

Assignment of the pressure ulcer stage code should be guided by clinical documentation of the stage or documentation of the terms found in the Alphabetic Index. For clinical terms describing the stage that are not found in the Alphabetic Index, and there is no documentation of the stage, the provider should be queried.

4) Patients admitted with pressure ulcers documented as healed

No code is assigned if the documentation states that the pressure ulcer is completely healed at the time of admission .

5) Patients admitted with pressure ulcers documented as healing

Pressure ulcers described as healing should be assigned the appropriate pressure ulcer stage code based on the documentation in the medical record. If the documentation does not provide information about the stage of the healing pressure ulcer, assign the appropriate code for unspecified stage.

If the documentation is unclear as to whether the patient has a current (new) pressure ulcer or if the patient is being treated for a healing pressure ulcer, query the provider.

For ulcers that were present on admission but healed at the time of discharge, assign the code for the site and stage of the pressure ulcer at the time of admission.

6) Patient admitted with pressure ulcer evolving into another stage during the admission

If a patient is admitted to an inpatient hospital with a pressure ulcer at one stage and it progresses to a higher stage, two separate codes should be assigned: one code for the site and stage of the ulcer on admission and a second code for the same ulcer site and the highest stage reported during the stay.

7) Pressure-induced deep tissue damage

For pressure-induced deep tissue damage or deep tissue pressure injury, assign only the appropriate code for pressure-induced deep tissue damage (L89.--6).

NON-PRESSURE CHRONIC ULCERS

1) Patients admitted with non-pressure ulcers documented as healed

No code is assigned if the documentation states that the non-pressure ulcer is completely healed at the time of admission.

2) **Patients admitted with non-pressure ulcers documented as healing**

Non-pressure ulcers described as healing should be assigned the appropriate non-pressure ulcer code based on the documentation in the medical record. If the documentation does not provide information about the severity of the healing non-pressure ulcer, assign the appropriate code for unspecified severity.

If the documentation is unclear as to whether the patient has a current (new) non-pressure ulcer or if the patient is being treated for a healing non-pressure ulcer, query the provider.

For ulcers that were present on admission but healed at the time of discharge, assign the code for the site and severity of the non-pressure ulcer at the time of admission.

3) **Patient admitted with non-pressure ulcer that progresses to another severity level during the admission**

If a patient is admitted to an inpatient hospital with a non-pressure ulcer at one severity level and it progresses to a higher severity level, two separate codes should be assigned: one code for the site and severity level of the ulcer on admission and a second code for the same ulcer site and the highest severity level reported during the stay.

See Section I.B.14 for pressure ulcer stage documentation by clinicians other than patient's provider

Chapter 12

Diseases of The Skin and Subcutaneous Tissue (L00-L99)

Excludes2: certain conditions originating in the perinatal period (P04-P96)

certain infectious and parasitic diseases (A00-B99)

complications of pregnancy, childbirth and the puerperium (O00-O9A)

congenital malformations, deformations, and chromosomal abnormalities (Q00-Q99)

endocrine, nutritional and metabolic diseases (E00-E88)

lipomelanotic reticulosis (I89.8)

neoplasms (C00-D49)

symptoms, signs and abnormal clinical and laboratory findings, not elsewhere classified (R00-R94)

systemic connective tissue disorders (M30-M36)

viral warts (B07.-)

This chapter contains the following blocks:

L00-L08	Infections of the skin and subcutaneous tissue
L10-L14	Bullous disorders
L20-L30	Dermatitis and eczema
L40-L45	Papulosquamous disorders
L49-L54	Urticaria and erythema
L55-L59	Radiation-related disorders of the skin and subcutaneous tissue
L60-L75	Disorders of skin appendages
L76	Intraoperative and postprocedural complications of skin and subcutaneous tissue
L80-L99	Other disorders of the skin and subcutaneous tissue

INFECTIONS OF THE SKIN AND SUBCUTANEOUS TISSUE (L00-L08)

Use Additional Code (B95-B97) to identify infectious agent.

Excludes2: hordeolum (H00.0)

infective dermatitis (L30.3)

local infections of skin classified in Chapter 1

lupus panniculitis (L93.2)

panniculitis NOS (M79.3)

panniculitis of neck and back (M54.0-)

Perlèche NOS (K13.0)

Perlèche due to candidiasis (B37.0)

Perlèche due to riboflavin deficiency (E53.0)

pyogenic granuloma (L98.0)

relapsing panniculitis [Weber-Christian] (M35.6)

viral warts (B07.-)

zoster (B02.-)

L00   Staphylococcal scalded skin syndrome

Ritter's disease

Use Additional Code to identify percentage of skin exfoliation (L49.-)

Excludes1: bullous impetigo (L01.03)

pemphigus neonatorum (L01.03)

toxic epidermal necrolysis [Lyell] (L51.2)

L01   Impetigo

Excludes1: impetigo herpetiformis (L40.1)

L01.0   Impetigo

Impetigo contagiosa Impetigo vulgaris

L01.00   Impetigo, unspecified

Impetigo NOS

L01.01   Non-bullous impetigo

L01.02   Bockhart's impetigo

Impetigo follicularis

Perifolliculitis NOS

Superficial pustular perifolliculitis

L01.03   Bullous impetigo

Impetigo neonatorum

Pemphigus neonatorum

L01.09   Other impetigo

Ulcerative impetigo

L01.1   Impetiginization of other dermatoses

L02   Cutaneous abscess, furuncle and carbuncle

Definition: A carbuncle is an abscess larger than a boil, usually with one or more openings draining pus onto the skin. It is usually caused by bacterial infection, most commonly staphylococcus aureus. A furuncle is a skin disease caused by the infection of hair follicles, resulting in the localized accumulation of pus and dead tissue.

Use Additional Code to identify organism (B95-B96)

Excludes2: abscess of anus and rectal regions (K61.-)

abscess of female genital organs (external) (N76.4)

abscess of male genital organs (external) (N48.2, N49.-)

L02.0   Cutaneous abscess, furuncle and carbuncle of face

Excludes2: abscess of ear, external (H60.0)

abscess of eyelid (H00.0)

abscess of head [any part, except face] (L02.8)

abscess of lacrimal gland (H04.0)

abscess of lacrimal passages (H04.3)

abscess of mouth (K12.2)

abscess of nose (J34.0)

abscess of orbit (H05.0)

submandibular abscess (K12.2)

L02.01   Cutaneous abscess of face

L02.02   Furuncle of face

Boil of face

Folliculitis of face

L02.03   Carbuncle of face

L02.1   Cutaneous abscess, furuncle and carbuncle of neck

L02.11   Cutaneous abscess of neck

L02.12   Furuncle of neck

Boil of neck

Folliculitis of neck

L02.13   Carbuncle of neck

L02.2   Cutaneous abscess, furuncle and carbuncle of trunk

Excludes1: non-newborn omphalitis (L08.82)

omphalitis of newborn (P38.-)

Excludes2: abscess of breast (N61.1)

abscess of buttocks (L02.3)

abscess of female external genital organs (N76.4)

abscess of male external genital organs (N48.2, N49.-)

abscess of hip (L02.4)

L02.21   Cutaneous abscess of trunk

L02.211   Cutaneous abscess of abdominal wall

L02.212   Cutaneous abscess of back [any part, except buttock]

L02.213   **Cutaneous abscess of chest wall**

L02.214   **Cutaneous abscess of groin**

L02.215   **Cutaneous abscess of perineum**

L02.216   **Cutaneous abscess of umbilicus**

L02.219   **Cutaneous abscess of trunk, unspecified**

L02.22   **Furuncle of trunk**

Boil of trunk

Folliculitis of trunk

L02.221   **Furuncle of abdominal wall**

L02.222   **Furuncle of back [any part, except buttock]**

L02.223   **Furuncle of chest wall**

L02.224   **Furuncle of groin**

L02.225   **Furuncle of perineum**

L02.226   **Furuncle of umbilicus**

L02.229   **Furuncle of trunk, unspecified**

L02.23   **Carbuncle of trunk**

L02.231   **Carbuncle of abdominal wall**

L02.232   **Carbuncle of back [any part, except buttock]**

L02.233   **Carbuncle of chest wall**

L02.234   **Carbuncle of groin**

L02.235   **Carbuncle of perineum**

L02.236   **Carbuncle of umbilicus**

L02.239   **Carbuncle of trunk, unspecified**

L02.3   **Cutaneous abscess, furuncle and carbuncle of buttock**

Excludes1: pilonidal cyst with abscess (L05.01)

L02.31   **Cutaneous abscess of buttock**

Cutaneous abscess of gluteal region

L02.32   **Furuncle of buttock**

Boil of buttock

Folliculitis of buttock

Furuncle of gluteal region

L02.33   **Carbuncle of buttock**

Carbuncle of gluteal region

L02.4   **Cutaneous abscess, furuncle and carbuncle of limb**

Excludes2: Cutaneous abscess, furuncle and carbuncle of groin (L02.214, L02.224, L02.234)

Cutaneous abscess, furuncle and carbuncle of hand (L02.5-)

Cutaneous abscess, furuncle and carbuncle of foot (L02.6-)

L02.41   **Cutaneous abscess of limb**

L02.411   **Cutaneous abscess of right axilla**

L02.412   **Cutaneous abscess of left axilla**

L02.413   **Cutaneous abscess of right upper limb**

L02.414   **Cutaneous abscess of left upper limb**

L02.415   **Cutaneous abscess of right lower limb**

L02.416   **Cutaneous abscess of left lower limb**

L02.419   **Cutaneous abscess of limb, unspecified**

L02.42   **Furuncle of limb**

Boil of limb

Folliculitis of limb

L02.421   **Furuncle of right axilla**

L02.422   **Furuncle of left axilla**

L02.423   **Furuncle of right upper limb**

L02.424   **Furuncle of left upper limb**

L02.425   **Furuncle of right lower limb**

L02.426   **Furuncle of left lower limb**

L02.429   **Furuncle of limb, unspecified**

L02.43   **Carbuncle of limb**

L02.431   **Carbuncle of right axilla**

L02.432   **Carbuncle of left axilla**

L02.433   **Carbuncle of right upper limb**

L02.434   **Carbuncle of left upper limb**

L02.435   **Carbuncle of right lower limb**

L02.436   **Carbuncle of left lower limb**

L02.439   **Carbuncle of limb, unspecified**

L02.5   **Cutaneous abscess, furuncle and carbuncle of hand**

L02.51   **Cutaneous abscess of hand**

L02.511   **Cutaneous abscess of right hand**

L02.512   **Cutaneous abscess of left hand**

L02.519   **Cutaneous abscess of unspecified hand**

L02.52   **Furuncle hand**

Boil of hand

Folliculitis of hand

L02.521   **Furuncle right hand**

L02.522   **Furuncle left hand**

L02.529   **Furuncle unspecified hand**

L02.53   **Carbuncle of hand**

L02.531   **Carbuncle of right hand**

L02.532   **Carbuncle of left hand**

L02.539   **Carbuncle of unspecified hand**

L02.6   **Cutaneous abscess, furuncle and carbuncle of foot**

L02.61   **Cutaneous abscess of foot**

L02.611   **Cutaneous abscess of right foot**

L02.612   **Cutaneous abscess of left foot**

L02.619   **Cutaneous abscess of unspecified foot**

L02.62   **Furuncle of foot**

Boil of foot

Folliculitis of foot

L02.621   **Furuncle of right foot**

L02.622   **Furuncle of left foot**

L02.629   **Furuncle of unspecified foot**

L02.63   **Carbuncle of foot**

L02.631   **Carbuncle of right foot**

L02.632   **Carbuncle of left foot**

L02.639   **Carbuncle of unspecified foot**

L02.8   **Cutaneous abscess, furuncle and carbuncle of other sites**

L02.81   **Cutaneous abscess of other sites**

L02.811   **Cutaneous abscess of head [any part, except face]**

L02.818   **Cutaneous abscess of other sites**

L02.82   **Furuncle of other sites**

Boil of other sites

Folliculitis of other sites

L02.821   **Furuncle of head [any part, except face]**

L02.828   **Furuncle of other sites**

   ● New code   ▲ Revised code   **Excludes1:** Not coded here   **Excludes2:** Not included here   ⊗ Placeholder required   ⑦ 7th digit required

L02.83   **Carbuncle of other sites**

     L02.831   **Carbuncle of head [any part, except face]**

     L02.838   **Carbuncle of other sites**

L02.9   **Cutaneous abscess, furuncle and carbuncle, unspecified**

     L02.91   **Cutaneous abscess, unspecified**

     L02.92   **Furuncle, unspecified**

       Boil NOS

       Furunculosis NOS

     L02.93   **Carbuncle, unspecified**

L03   **Cellulitis and acute lymphangitis**

   Excludes2: cellulitis of anal and rectal region (K61.-)

     cellulitis of external auditory canal (H60.1)

     cellulitis of eyelid (H00.0)

     cellulitis of female external genital organs (N76.4)

     cellulitis of lacrimal apparatus (H04.3)

     cellulitis of male external genital organs (N48.2, N49.-)

     cellulitis of mouth (K12.2)

     cellulitis of nose (J34.0)

     eosinophilic cellulitis [Wells] (L98.3)

     febrile neutrophilic dermatosis [Sweet] (L98.2)

     lymphangitis (chronic) (subacute) (I89.1)

L03.0   **Cellulitis and acute lymphangitis of finger and toe**

     Infection of nail

     Onychia

     Paronychia

     Perionychia

     L03.01   **Cellulitis of finger**

       Felon Whitlow

       Excludes1: herpetic whitlow (B00.89)

       L03.011   **Cellulitis of right finger**

       L03.012   **Cellulitis of left finger**

       L03.019   **Cellulitis of unspecified finger**

     L03.02   **Acute lymphangitis of finger**

       Hangnail with lymphangitis of finger

       L03.021   **Acute lymphangitis of right finger**

       L03.022   **Acute lymphangitis of left finger**

       L03.029   **Acute lymphangitis of unspecified finger**

     L03.03   **Cellulitis of toe**

       L03.031   **Cellulitis of right toe**

       L03.032   **Cellulitis of left toe**

       L03.039   **Cellulitis of unspecified toe**

     L03.04   **Acute lymphangitis of toe**

       Hangnail with lymphangitis of toe

       L03.041   **Acute lymphangitis of right toe**

       L03.042   **Acute lymphangitis of left toe**

       L03.049   **Acute lymphangitis of unspecified toe**

L03.1   **Cellulitis and acute lymphangitis of other parts of limb**

     L03.11   **Cellulitis of other parts of limb**

       Excludes2: cellulitis of fingers (L03.01-)

         cellulitis of toes (L03.03-)

         groin (L03.314)

       L03.111   **Cellulitis of right axilla**

       L03.112   **Cellulitis of left axilla**

       L03.113   **Cellulitis of right upper limb**

       L03.114   **Cellulitis of left upper limb**

       L03.115   **Cellulitis of right lower limb**

       L03.116   **Cellulitis of left lower limb**

       L03.119   **Cellulitis of unspecified part of limb**

     L03.12   **Acute lymphangitis of other parts of limb**

       Excludes2: acute lymphangitis of fingers (L03.2-)

         acute lymphangitis of toes (L03.04-)

         acute lymphangitis of groin (L03.324)

       L03.121   **Acute lymphangitis of right axilla**

       L03.122   **Acute lymphangitis of left axilla**

       L03.123   **Acute lymphangitis of right upper limb**

       L03.124   **Acute lymphangitis of left upper limb**

       L03.125   **Acute lymphangitis of right lower limb**

       L03.126   **Acute lymphangitis of left lower limb**

       L03.129   **Acute lymphangitis of unspecified part of limb**

L03.2   **Cellulitis and acute lymphangitis of face and neck**

     L03.21   **Cellulitis and acute lymphangitis of face**

       L03.211   **Cellulitis of face**

         Excludes2: abscess of orbit (H05.01-)

           cellulitis of ear (H60.1-)

           cellulitis of eyelid (H00.0-)

           cellulitis of head (L03.81)

           cellulitis of lacrimal apparatus (H04.3)

           cellulitis of lip (K13.0)

           cellulitis of mouth (K12.2)

           cellulitis of nose (internal) (J34.0)

           cellulitis of orbit (H05.01-)

           cellulitis of scalp (L03.81)

       L03.212   **Acute lymphangitis of face**

       L03.213   **Periorbital cellulitis**

         Preseptal cellulitis

     L03.22   **Cellulitis and acute lymphangitis of neck**

       L03.221   **Cellulitis of neck**

       L03.222   **Acute lymphangitis of neck**

L03.3   **Cellulitis and acute lymphangitis of trunk**

     L03.31   **Cellulitis of trunk**

       Excludes2: cellulitis of anal and rectal regions (K61.-)

         cellulitis of breast NOS (N61.0)

         cellulitis of female external genital organs (N76.4)

         cellulitis of male external genital organs (N48.2, N49.-)

         omphalitis of newborn (P38.-)

         puerperal cellulitis of breast (O91.2)

       L03.311   **Cellulitis of abdominal wall**

         Excludes2: cellulitis of umbilicus (L03.316)

           cellulitis of groin (L03.314)

L03.312 **Cellulitis of back [any part except buttock]**

L03.313 **Cellulitis of chest wall**

L03.314 **Cellulitis of groin**

L03.315 **Cellulitis of perineum**

L03.316 **Cellulitis of umbilicus**

L03.317 **Cellulitis of buttock**

L03.319 **Cellulitis of trunk, unspecified**

L03.32 **Acute lymphangitis of trunk**

L03.321 **Acute lymphangitis of abdominal wall**

L03.322 **Acute lymphangitis of back [any part except buttock]**

L03.323 **Acute lymphangitis of chest wall**

L03.324 **Acute lymphangitis of groin**

L03.325 **Acute lymphangitis of perineum**

L03.326 **Acute lymphangitis of umbilicus**

L03.327 **Acute lymphangitis of buttock**

L03.329 **Acute lymphangitis of trunk, unspecified**

L03.8 **Cellulitis and acute lymphangitis of other sites**

L03.81 **Cellulitis of other sites**

L03.811 **Cellulitis of head [any part, except face]**

Cellulitis of scalp

Excludes2: cellulitis of face (L03.211)

L03.818 **Cellulitis of other sites**

L03.89 **Acute lymphangitis of other sites**

L03.891 **Acute lymphangitis of head [any part, except face]**

L03.898 **Acute lymphangitis of other sites**

L03.9 **Cellulitis and acute lymphangitis, unspecified**

L03.90 **Cellulitis, unspecified**

L03.91 **Acute lymphangitis, unspecified**

Excludes1: lymphangitis NOS (I89.1)

L04 **Acute lymphadenitis**

Definition: Lymphadenitis is an inflammation of a lymph node. It is often a complication of a bacterial infection of a wound, although it can also be caused by viruses or other disease agents.

Includes: abscess (acute) of lymph nodes, except mesenteric

acute lymphadenitis, except mesenteric

Excludes1: chronic or subacute lymphadenitis, except mesenteric (I88.1)

enlarged lymph nodes (R59.-)

human immunodeficiency virus [HIV] disease resulting in generalized lymphadenopathy (B20)

lymphadenitis NOS (I88.9)

nonspecific mesenteric lymphadenitis (I88.0)

L04.0 **Acute lymphadenitis of face, head and neck**

L04.1 **Acute lymphadenitis of trunk**

L04.2 **Acute lymphadenitis of upper limb**

Acute lymphadenitis of axilla

Acute lymphadenitis of shoulder

L04.3 **Acute lymphadenitis of lower limb**

Acute lymphadenitis of hip

Excludes2: acute lymphadenitis of groin (L04.1)

L04.8 **Acute lymphadenitis of other sites**

L04.9 **Acute lymphadenitis, unspecified**

L05 **Pilonidal cyst and sinus**

L05.0 **Pilonidal cyst and sinus with abscess**

L05.01 **Pilonidal cyst with abscess**

Pilonidal abscess

Pilonidal dimple with abscess

Postanal dimple with abscess

Excludes2: congenital sacral dimple (Q82.6)

parasacral dimple (Q82.6)

L05.02 **Pilonidal sinus with abscess**

Coccygeal fistula with abscess

Coccygeal sinus with abscess

Pilonidal fistula with abscess

L05.9 **Pilonidal cyst and sinus without abscess**

L05.91 **Pilonidal cyst without abscess**

Pilonidal dimple

Postanal dimple

Pilonidal cyst NOS

Excludes2: congenital sacral dimple (Q82.6)

parasacral dimple (Q82.6)

L05.92 **Pilonidal sinus without abscess**

Coccygeal fistula

Coccygeal sinus without abscess

Pilonidal fistula

L08 **Other local infections of skin and subcutaneous tissue**

L08.0 **Pyoderma**

Dermatitis gangrenosa

Purulent dermatitis

Septic dermatitis

Suppurative dermatitis

Excludes1: pyoderma gangrenosum (L88)

pyoderma vegetans (L08.81)

L08.1 **Erythrasma**

L08.8 **Other specified local infections of the skin and subcutaneous tissue**

L08.81 **Pyoderma vegetans**

Excludes1: pyoderma gangrenosum (L88)

pyoderma NOS (L08.0)

L08.82 **Omphalitis not of newborn**

Excludes1: omphalitis of newborn (P38.-)

L08.89 **Other specified local infections of the skin and subcutaneous tissue**

L08.9 **Local infection of the skin and subcutaneous tissue, unspecified**

BULLOUS DISORDERS (L10-L14)

Excludes1: benign familial pemphigus [Hailey-Hailey] (Q82.8)

staphylococcal scalded skin syndrome (L00)

toxic epidermal necrolysis [Lyell] (L51.2)

L10 **Pemphigus**

Excludes1: pemphigus neonatorum (L01.03)

L10.0 **Pemphigus vulgaris**

L10.1 **Pemphigus vegetans**

L10.2 **Pemphigus foliaceous**

L10.3 **Brazilian pemphigus [fogo selvagem]**

L10.4 **Pemphigus erythematosus**

Senear-Usher syndrome

L10.5 **Drug-induced pemphigus**

Use Additional Code for adverse effect, if applicable, to identify drug (T36-T50 with fifth or sixth character 5)

● New code ▲ Revised code **Excludes1:** Not coded here **Excludes2:** Not included here ⊗ Placeholder required ⑦7ᵗʰ digit required

L10.8   **Other pemphigus**

    L10.81   **Paraneoplastic pemphigus**

    L10.89   **Other pemphigus**

L10.9   **Pemphigus, unspecified**

L11   Other acantholytic disorders

    L11.0   **Acquired keratosis follicularis**

    Excludes1: keratosis follicularis (congenital) [Darier-White] (Q82.8)

    L11.1   **Transient acantholytic dermatosis [Grover]**

    L11.8   **Other specified acantholytic disorders**

    L11.9   **Acantholytic disorder, unspecified**

L12   Pemphigoid

    Excludes1: herpes gestationis (O26.4-)

    impetigo herpetiformis (L40.1)

    L12.0   **Bullous pemphigoid**

    L12.1   **Cicatricial pemphigoid**

    Benign mucous membrane pemphigoid

    L12.2   **Chronic bullous disease of childhood**

    Juvenile dermatitis herpetiformis

    L12.3   **Acquired epidermolysis bullosa**

    Excludes1: epidermolysis bullosa (congenital) (Q81.-)

        L12.30   **Acquired epidermolysis bullosa, unspecified** [HCC]

        L12.31   **Epidermolysis bullosa due to drug** [HCC]

        Use Additional Code for adverse effect, if applicable, to identify drug (T36-T50 with fifth or sixth character 5)

        L12.35   **Other acquired epidermolysis bullosa** [HCC]

    L12.8   **Other pemphigoid**

    L12.9   **Pemphigoid, unspecified**

L13   Other bullous disorders

    L13.0   **Dermatitis herpetiformis**

    Duhring's disease

    Hydroa herpetiformis

    Excludes1: juvenile dermatitis herpetiformis (L12.2)

        senile dermatitis herpetiformis (L12.0)

    L13.1   **Subcorneal pustular dermatitis**

    Sneddon-Wilkinson disease

    L13.8   **Other specified bullous disorders**

    L13.9   **Bullous disorder, unspecified**

L14   Bullous disorders in diseases classified elsewhere

    Code first underlying disease

DERMATITIS AND ECZEMA (L20-L30)

Note: In this block the terms dermatitis and eczema are used synonymously and interchangeably.

Excludes2: chronic (childhood) granulomatous disease (D71)

dermatitis gangrenosa (L08.0)

dermatitis herpetiformis (L13.0)

dry skin dermatitis (L85.3)

factitial dermatitis (L98.1)

perioral dermatitis (L71.0)

radiation-related disorders of the skin and subcutaneous tissue (L55-L59)

stasis dermatitis (I87.2)

L20   Atopic dermatitis

Definition: Atopic dermatitis and related conditions, aka eczema, is a chronic, recurring inflammatory skin disorder that usually first

appears in babies or very young children and may last through adulthood. Eczema causes the skin to itch and develop a red, scaly, patchy rash.

L20.0   **Besnier's prurigo**

L20.8   **Other atopic dermatitis**

    Excludes2: circumscribed neurodermatitis (L28.0)

    L20.81   **Atopic neurodermatitis**

    Diffuse neurodermatitis

    L20.82   **Flexural eczema**

    L20.83   **Infantile (acute) (chronic) eczema**

    L20.84   **Intrinsic (allergic) eczema**

    L20.89   **Other atopic dermatitis**

L20.9   **Atopic dermatitis, unspecified**

L21   Seborrheic dermatitis

    Excludes2: infective dermatitis (L30.3)

    seborrheic keratosis (L82.-)

    L21.0   **Seborrhea capitis**

    Cradle cap

    L21.1   **Seborrheic infantile dermatitis**

    L21.8   **Other seborrheic dermatitis**

    L21.9   **Seborrheic dermatitis, unspecified**

    Seborrhea NOS

L22   Diaper dermatitis

Diaper erythema

Diaper rash

Psoriasiform diaper rash

L23   Allergic contact dermatitis

    Excludes1: allergy NOS (T78.40)

    contact dermatitis NOS (L25.9)

    dermatitis NOS (L30.9)

    Excludes2: dermatitis due to substances taken internally (L27.-)

    dermatitis of eyelid (H01.1-)

    diaper dermatitis (L22)

    eczema of external ear (H60.5-)

    irritant contact dermatitis (L24.-)

    perioral dermatitis (L71.0)

    radiation-related disorders of the skin and subcutaneous tissue (L55-L59)

    L23.0   **Allergic contact dermatitis due to metals**

    Allergic contact dermatitis due to chromium

    Allergic contact dermatitis due to nickel

    L23.1   **Allergic contact dermatitis due to adhesives**

    L23.2   **Allergic contact dermatitis due to cosmetics**

    L23.3   **Allergic contact dermatitis due to drugs in contact with skin**

    Use Additional Code for adverse effect, if applicable, to identify drug (T36-T50 with fifth or sixth character 5)

    Excludes2: dermatitis due to ingested drugs and medicaments (L27.0-L27.1)

    L23.4   **Allergic contact dermatitis due to dyes**

    L23.5   **Allergic contact dermatitis due to other chemical products**

    Allergic contact dermatitis due to cement

    Allergic contact dermatitis due to insecticide

    Allergic contact dermatitis due to plastic

    Allergic contact dermatitis due to rubber

    L23.6   **Allergic contact dermatitis due to food in contact with the skin**

Excludes2: dermatitis due to ingested food (L27.2)

L23.7 **Allergic contact dermatitis due to plants, except food**

Excludes2: allergy NOS due to pollen (J30.1)

L23.8 **Allergic contact dermatitis due to other agents**

L23.81 **Allergic contact dermatitis due to animal (cat) (dog) dander**

Allergic contact dermatitis due to animal (cat) (dog) hair

L23.89 **Allergic contact dermatitis due to other agents**

L23.9 **Allergic contact dermatitis, unspecified cause**

Allergic contact eczema NOS

L24 **Irritant contact dermatitis**

Excludes1: allergy NOS (T78.40)

contact dermatitis NOS (L25.9)

dermatitis NOS (L30.9)

Excludes2: allergic contact dermatitis (L23.-)

dermatitis due to substances taken internally (L27.-)

dermatitis of eyelid (H01.1-)

diaper dermatitis (L22)

eczema of external ear (H60.5-)

perioral dermatitis (L71.0)

radiation-related disorders of the skin and subcutaneous tissue (L55-L59)

L24.0 **Irritant contact dermatitis due to detergents**

L24.1 **Irritant contact dermatitis due to oils and greases**

L24.2 **Irritant contact dermatitis due to solvents**

Irritant contact dermatitis due to chlorocompound

Irritant contact dermatitis due to cyclohexane

Irritant contact dermatitis due to ester

Irritant contact dermatitis due to glycol

Irritant contact dermatitis due to hydrocarbon

Irritant contact dermatitis due to ketone

L24.3 **Irritant contact dermatitis due to cosmetics**

L24.4 **Irritant contact dermatitis due to drugs in contact with skin**

Use Additional Code for adverse effect, if applicable, to identify drug (T36-T50 with fifth or sixth character 5)

L24.5 **Irritant contact dermatitis due to other chemical products**

Irritant contact dermatitis due to cement

Irritant contact dermatitis due to insecticide

Irritant contact dermatitis due to plastic

Irritant contact dermatitis due to rubber

L24.6 **Irritant contact dermatitis due to food in contact with skin**

Excludes2: dermatitis due to ingested food (L27.2)

L24.7 **Irritant contact dermatitis due to plants, except food**

Excludes2: allergy NOS to pollen (J30.1)

L24.8 **Irritant contact dermatitis due to other agents**

L24.81 **Irritant contact dermatitis due to metals**

Irritant contact dermatitis due to chromium

Irritant contact dermatitis due to nickel

L24.89 **Irritant contact dermatitis due to other agents**

Irritant contact dermatitis due to dyes

L24.9 **Irritant contact dermatitis, unspecified cause**

Irritant contact eczema NOS

● **L24.A** **Irritant contact dermatitis due to friction or contact with body fluids**

Excludes1: irritant contact dermatitis related to stoma or fistula (L24.B-)

Excludes2: erythema intertrigo (L30.4)

● **L24.A0** **Irritant contact dermatitis due to friction or contact with body fluids, unspecified**

● **L24.A1** **Irritant contact dermatitis due to saliva**

● **L24.A2** **Irritant contact dermatitis due to fecal, urinary or dual incontinence**

Excludes1: diaper dermatitis (L22)

● **L24.A9** **Irritant contact dermatitis due friction or contact with other specified body fluids**

Irritant contact dermatitis related to endotracheal tube

Wound fluids, exudate

● **L24.B** **Irritant contact dermatitis related to stoma or fistula**

Use Additional Code to identify any artificial opening status (Z93.-), if applicable, for contact dermatitis related to stoma secretions

● **L24.B0** **Irritant contact dermatitis related to unspecified stoma or fistula**

Irritant contact dermatitis related to fistula NOS

Irritant contact dermatitis related to stoma NOS

● **L24.B1** **Irritant contact dermatitis related to digestive stoma or fistula**

Irritant contact dermatitis related to gastrostomy

Irritant contact dermatitis related to jejunostomy

Irritant contact dermatitis related to saliva or spit fistula

● **L24.B2** **Irritant contact dermatitis related to respiratory stoma or fistula**

Irritant contact dermatitis related to tracheostomy

● **L24.B3** **Irritant contact dermatitis related to fecal or urinary stoma or fistula**

Irritant contact dermatitis related to colostomy

Irritant contact dermatitis related to enterocutaneous fistula

Irritant contact dermatitis related to ileostomy

L25 **Unspecified contact dermatitis**

Excludes1: allergic contact dermatitis (L23.-)

allergy NOS (T78.40)

dermatitis NOS (L30.9)

irritant contact dermatitis (L24.-)

Excludes2: dermatitis due to ingested substances (L27.-)

dermatitis of eyelid (H01.1-)

eczema of external ear (H60.5-)

perioral dermatitis (L71.0)

radiation-related disorders of the skin and subcutaneous tissue (L55-L59)

L25.0 **Unspecified contact dermatitis due to cosmetics**

L25.1 **Unspecified contact dermatitis due to drugs in contact with skin**

Use Additional Code for adverse effect, if applicable, to identify drug (T36-T50 with fifth or sixth character 5)

Excludes2: dermatitis due to ingested drugs and medicaments (L27.0-L27.1)

L25.2 **Unspecified contact dermatitis due to dyes**

L25.3 **Unspecified contact dermatitis due to other chemical products**

Unspecified contact dermatitis due to cement

● New code ▲ Revised code Excludes1: Not coded here Excludes2: Not included here ⊗ Placeholder required ⑦7th digit required

Unspecified contact dermatitis due to insecticide

L25.4 **Unspecified contact dermatitis due to food in contact with skin**

Excludes2: dermatitis due to ingested food (L27.2)

L25.5 **Unspecified contact dermatitis due to plants, except food**

Excludes1: nettle rash (L50.9)

Excludes2: allergy NOS due to pollen (J30.1)

L25.8 **Unspecified contact dermatitis due to other agents**

L25.9 **Unspecified contact dermatitis, unspecified cause**

Contact dermatitis (occupational) NOS

Contact eczema (occupational) NOS

L26 **Exfoliative dermatitis**

Hebra's pityriasis

Excludes1: Ritter's disease (L00)

L27 **Dermatitis due to substances taken internally**

Excludes1: allergy NOS (T78.40)

Excludes2: adverse food reaction, except dermatitis (T78.0-T78.1)

contact dermatitis (L23-L25)

drug photoallergic response (L56.1)

drug phototoxic response (L56.0)

urticaria (L50.-)

L27.0 **Generalized skin eruption due to drugs and medicaments taken internally**

Use Additional Code for adverse effect, if applicable, to identify drug (T36-T50 with fifth or sixth character 5)

L27.1 **Localized skin eruption due to drugs and medicaments taken internally**

Use Additional Code for adverse effect, if applicable, to identify drug (T36-T50 with fifth or sixth character 5)

L27.2 **Dermatitis due to ingested food**

Excludes2: dermatitis due to food in contact with skin

(L23.6, L24.6, L25.4)

L27.8 **Dermatitis due to other substances taken internally**

L27.9 **Dermatitis due to unspecified substance taken internally**

L28 **Lichen simplex chronicus and prurigo**

L28.0 **Lichen simplex chronicus**

Circumscribed neurodermatitis

Lichen NOS

L28.1 **Prurigo nodularis**

L28.2 **Other prurigo**

Prurigo NOS

Prurigo Hebra

Prurigo mitis

Urticaria papulosa

L29 **Pruritus**

Excludes1: neurotic excoriation (L98.1)

psychogenic pruritus (F45.8)

L29.0 **Pruritus ani**

L29.1 **Pruritus scroti**

L29.2 **Pruritus vulvae**

L29.3 **Anogenital pruritus, unspecified**

L29.8 **Other pruritus**

L29.9 **Pruritus, unspecified**

Itch NOS

L30 **Other and unspecified dermatitis**

Excludes2: contact dermatitis (L23-L25)

dry skin dermatitis (L85.3)

small plaque parapsoriasis (L41.3)

stasis dermatitis (I87.2)

L30.0 **Nummular dermatitis**

L30.1 **Dyshidrosis [pompholyx]**

L30.2 **Cutaneous autosensitization**

Candidid [levurid]

Dermatophytid Eczematid

L30.3 **Infective dermatitis**

Infectious eczematoid dermatitis

L30.4 **Erythema intertrigo**

L30.5 **Pityriasis alba**

L30.8 **Other specified dermatitis**

L30.9 **Dermatitis, unspecified**

Eczema NOS

PAPULOSQUAMOUS DISORDERS (L40-L45)

L40 **Psoriasis**

L40.0 **Psoriasis vulgaris**

Nummular psoriasis

Plaque psoriasis

L40.1 **Generalized pustular psoriasis**

Impetigo herpetiformis

Von Zumbusch's disease

L40.2 **Acrodermatitis continua**

L40.3 **Pustulosis palmaris et plantaris**

L40.4 **Guttate psoriasis**

L40.5 **Arthropathic psoriasis**

L40.50 **Arthropathic psoriasis, unspecified** [HCC]

L40.51 **Distal interphalangeal psoriatic arthropathy** [HCC]

L40.52 **Psoriatic arthritis mutilans** [HCC]

L40.53 **Psoriatic spondylitis** [HCC]

L40.54 **Psoriatic juvenile arthropathy** [HCC]

L40.59 **Other psoriatic arthropathy** [HCC]

L40.8 **Other psoriasis**

Flexural psoriasis

L40.9 **Psoriasis, unspecified**

L41 **Parapsoriasis**

Excludes1: poikiloderma vasculare atrophicans (L94.5)

L41.0 **Pityriasis lichenoides et varioliformis acuta**

Mucha-Habermann disease

L41.1 **Pityriasis lichenoides chronica**

L41.3 **Small plaque parapsoriasis**

L41.4 **Large plaque parapsoriasis**

L41.5 **Retiform parapsoriasis**

L41.8 **Other parapsoriasis**

L41.9 **Parapsoriasis, unspecified**

L42 **Pityriasis rosea**

L43 **Lichen planus**

Excludes1: lichen planopilaris (L66.1)

L43.0 **Hypertrophic lichen planus**

L43.1 **Bullous lichen planus**

L43.2 **Lichenoid drug reaction**

Use Additional Code for adverse effect, if applicable, to identify drug (T36-T50 with fifth or sixth character 5)

L43.3 **Subacute (active) lichen planus**

Lichen planus tropicus

L43.8   **Other lichen planus**

L43.9   **Lichen planus, unspecified**

L44   **Other papulosquamous disorders**

    L44.0   **Pityriasis rubra pilaris**

    L44.1   **Lichen nitidus**

    L44.2   **Lichen striatus**

    L44.3   **Lichen ruber moniliformis**

    L44.4   **Infantile papular acrodermatitis [Gianotti-Crosti]**

    L44.8   **Other specified papulosquamous disorders**

    L44.9   **Papulosquamous disorder, unspecified**

L45   **Papulosquamous disorders in diseases classified elsewhere**

    Code first underlying disease.

URTICARIA AND ERYTHEMA (L49-L54)

Excludes1: Lyme disease (A69.2-)

    rosacea (L71.-)

L49   **Exfoliation due to erythematous conditions according to extent of body surface involved**

    Code first erythematous condition causing exfoliation, such as:

    Ritter's disease (L00)

    (Staphylococcal) scalded skin syndrome (L00)

    Stevens-Johnson syndrome (L51.1)

    Stevens-Johnson syndrome-toxic epidermal necrolysis overlap syndrome (L51.3)

    Toxic epidermal necrolysis (L51.2)

    L49.0   **Exfoliation due to erythematous condition involving less than 10 percent of body surface**

        Exfoliation due to erythematous condition NOS

    L49.1   **Exfoliation due to erythematous condition involving 10-19 percent of body surface**

    L49.2   **Exfoliation due to erythematous condition involving 20-29 percent of body surface**

    L49.3   **Exfoliation due to erythematous condition involving 30-39 percent of body surface**

    L49.4   **Exfoliation due to erythematous condition involving 40-49 percent of body surface**

    L49.5   **Exfoliation due to erythematous condition involving 50-59 percent of body surface**

    L49.6   **Exfoliation due to erythematous condition involving 60-69 percent of body surface**

    L49.7   **Exfoliation due to erythematous condition involving 70-79 percent of body surface**

    L49.8   **Exfoliation due to erythematous condition involving 80-89 percent of body surface**

    L49.9   **Exfoliation due to erythematous condition involving 90 or more percent of body surface**

L50   **Urticaria**

    Excludes1: allergic contact dermatitis (L23.-)

        angioneurotic edema (T78.3)

        giant urticaria (T78.3)

        hereditary angio-edema (D84.1)

        Quincke's edema (T78.3)

        serum urticaria (T80.6-)

        solar urticaria (L56.3)

        urticaria neonatorum (P83.8)

        urticaria papulosa (L28.2)

        urticaria pigmentosa (D47.01)

    L50.0   **Allergic urticaria**

    L50.1   **Idiopathic urticaria**

    L50.2   **Urticaria due to cold and heat**

        Excludes2: familial cold urticaria (M04.2)

    L50.3   **Dermatographic urticaria**

    L50.4   **Vibratory urticaria**

    L50.5   **Cholinergic urticaria**

    L50.6   **Contact urticaria**

    L50.8   **Other urticaria**

        Chronic urticaria

        Recurrent periodic urticaria

    L50.9   **Urticaria, unspecified**

L51   **Erythema multiforme**

    Use Additional Code for adverse effect, if applicable, to identify drug (T36-T50 with fifth or sixth character 5)

    Use Additional Code to identify associated manifestations, such as:

    arthropathy associated with dermatological disorders (M14.8-)

    conjunctival edema (H11.42)

    conjunctivitis (H10.22-)

    corneal scars and opacities (H17.-)

    corneal ulcer (H16.0-)

    edema of eyelid (H02.84-)

    inflammation of eyelid (H01.8)

    keratoconjunctivitis sicca (H16.22-)

    mechanical lagophthalmos (H02.22-)

    stomatitis (K12.-)

    symblepharon (H11.23-)

    Use Additional Code to identify percentage of skin exfoliation (L49.-)

    Excludes1: staphylococcal scalded skin syndrome (L00)

        Ritter's disease (L00)

    L51.0   **Nonbullous erythema multiforme**

    L51.1   **Stevens-Johnson syndrome** [HCC]

    L51.2   **Toxic epidermal necrolysis [Lyell]** [HCC]

    L51.3   **Stevens-Johnson syndrome-toxic epidermal necrolysis overlap syndrome** [HCC]

        SJS-TEN overlap syndrome

    L51.8   **Other erythema multiforme**

    L51.9   **Erythema multiforme, unspecified**

        Erythema iris

        Erythema multiforme major NOS

        Erythema multiforme minor NOS

        Herpes iris

L52   **Erythema nodosum**

    Excludes1: tuberculous erythema nodosum (A18.4)

L53   **Other erythematous conditions**

    Excludes1: erythema ab igne (L59.0)

        erythema due to external agents in contact with skin (L23-L25)

        erythema intertrigo (L30.4)

    L53.0   **Toxic erythema**

        Code first poisoning due to drug or toxin, if applicable (T36-T65 with fifth or sixth character 1-4 or 6)

        Use Additional Code for adverse effect, if applicable, to identify drug (T36-T50 with fifth or sixth character 5)

        Excludes1: neonatal erythema toxicum (P83.1)

    L53.1   **Erythema annulare centrifugum**

    L53.2   **Erythema marginatum**

    L53.3   **Other chronic figurate erythema**

L53.8 Other specified erythematous conditions

L53.9 Erythematous condition, unspecified

Erythema NOS

Erythroderma NOS

L54 Erythema in diseases classified elsewhere

Code first underlying disease.

RADIATION-RELATED DISORDERS OF THE SKIN AND SUBCUTANEOUS TISSUE (L55-L59)

L55 Sunburn

L55.0 Sunburn of first degree

L55.1 Sunburn of second degree

L55.2 Sunburn of third degree

L55.9 Sunburn, unspecified

L56 Other acute skin changes due to ultraviolet radiation

Use Additional Code to identify the source of the ultraviolet radiation (W89, X32)

L56.0 Drug phototoxic response

Use Additional Code for adverse effect, if applicable, to identify drug (T36-T50 with fifth or sixth character 5)

L56.1 Drug photoallergic response

Use Additional Code for adverse effect, if applicable, to identify drug (T36-T50 with fifth or sixth character 5)

L56.2 Photocontact dermatitis [berloque dermatitis]

L56.3 Solar urticaria

L56.4 Polymorphous light eruption

L56.5 Disseminated superficial actinic porokeratosis (DSAP)

L56.8 Other specified acute skin changes due to ultraviolet radiation

L56.9 Acute skin change due to ultraviolet radiation, unspecified

L57 Skin changes due to chronic exposure to nonionizing radiation

Use Additional Code to identify the source of the ultraviolet radiation (W89), or other nonionizing radiation (W90)

L57.0 Actinic keratosis

Keratosis NOS

Senile keratosis

Solar keratosis

L57.1 Actinic reticuloid

L57.2 Cutis rhomboidalis nuchae

L57.3 Poikiloderma of Civatte

L57.4 Cutis laxa senilis

Elastosis senilis

L57.5 Actinic granuloma

L57.8 Other skin changes due to chronic exposure to nonionizing radiation

Farmer's skin

Sailor's skin

Solar dermatitis

L57.9 Skin changes due to chronic exposure to nonionizing radiation, unspecified

L58 Radiodermatitis

Use Additional Code to identify the source of the radiation (W88, W90)

L58.0 Acute radiodermatitis

L58.1 Chronic radiodermatitis

L58.9 Radiodermatitis, unspecified

L59 Other disorders of skin and subcutaneous tissue related to radiation

L59.0 Erythema ab igne [dermatitis ab igne]

L59.8 Other specified disorders of the skin and subcutaneous tissue related to radiation

L59.9 Disorder of the skin and subcutaneous tissue related to radiation, unspecified

DISORDERS OF SKIN APPENDAGES (L60-L75)

Excludes1: congenital malformations of integument (Q84.-)

L60 Nail disorders

Excludes2: clubbing of nails (R68.3)

onychia and paronychia (L03.0-)

L60.0 Ingrowing nail

L60.1 Onycholysis

L60.2 Onychogryphosis

L60.3 Nail dystrophy

L60.4 Beau's lines

L60.5 Yellow nail syndrome

L60.8 Other nail disorders

L60.9 Nail disorder, unspecified

L62 Nail disorders in diseases classified elsewhere

Code first underlying disease, such as:

pachydermoperiostosis (M89.4-)

L63 Alopecia areata

L63.0 Alopecia (capitis) totalis

L63.1 Alopecia universalis

L63.2 Ophiasis

L63.8 Other alopecia areata

L63.9 Alopecia areata, unspecified

L64 Androgenic alopecia

Includes: male-pattern baldness

L64.0 Drug-induced androgenic alopecia

Use Additional Code for adverse effect, if applicable, to identify drug (T36-T50 with fifth or sixth character 5)

L64.8 Other androgenic alopecia

L64.9 Androgenic alopecia, unspecified

L65 Other nonscarring hair loss

Use Additional Code for adverse effect, if applicable, to identify drug (T36-T50 with fifth or sixth character 5)

Excludes1: trichotillomania (F63.3)

L65.0 Telogen effluvium

L65.1 Anagen effluvium

L65.2 Alopecia mucinosa

L65.8 Other specified nonscarring hair loss

L65.9 Nonscarring hair loss, unspecified

Alopecia NOS

L66 Cicatricial alopecia [scarring hair loss]

L66.0 Pseudopelade

L66.1 Lichen planopilaris

Follicular lichen planus

L66.2 Folliculitis decalvans

L66.3 Perifolliculitis capitis abscedens

L66.4 Folliculitis ulerythematosa reticulata

L66.8 Other cicatricial alopecia

L66.9 Cicatricial alopecia, unspecified

L67 Hair color and hair shaft abnormalities

Excludes1: monilethrix (Q84.1)

pili annulati (Q84.1)

telegen effluvium (L65.0)

L67.0   **Trichorrhexis nodosa**

L67.1   **Variations in hair color** Canities

Greyness, hair (premature)

Heterochromia of hair

Poliosis circumscripta, acquired

Poliosis NOS

L67.8   **Other hair color and hair shaft abnormalities**

Fragilitas crinium

L67.9   **Hair color and hair shaft abnormality, unspecified**

L68   **Hypertrichosis**

Includes: excess hair

Excludes1: congenital hypertrichosis (Q84.2)

persistent lanugo (Q84.2)

L68.0   **Hirsutism**

L68.1   **Acquired hypertrichosis lanuginosa**

L68.2   **Localized hypertrichosis**

L68.3   **Polytrichia**

L68.8   **Other hypertrichosis**

L68.9   **Hypertrichosis, unspecified**

L70   **Acne**

Excludes2: acne keloid (L73.0)

L70.0   **Acne vulgaris**

L70.1   **Acne conglobata**

L70.2   **Acne varioliformis**

Acne necrotica miliaris

L70.3   **Acne tropica**

L70.4   **Infantile acne**

L70.5   **Acné excoriée**

Acné excoriée des jeunes filles

Picker's acne

L70.8   **Other acne**

L70.9   **Acne, unspecified**

L71   **Rosacea**

Use Additional Code for adverse effect, if applicable, to identify drug (T36-T50 with fifth or sixth character 5)

L71.0   **Perioral dermatitis**

L71.1   **Rhinophyma**

L71.8   **Other rosacea**

L71.9   **Rosacea, unspecified**

L72   **Follicular cysts of skin and subcutaneous tissue**

L72.0   **Epidermal cyst**

L72.1   **Pilar and trichodermal cyst**

     L72.11   **Pilar cyst**

     L72.12   **Trichodermal cyst**

Trichilemmal (proliferating) cyst

L72.2   **Steatocystoma multiplex**

L72.3   **Sebaceous cyst**

Excludes2: pilar cyst (L72.11)

trichilemmal (proliferating) cyst (L72.12)

L72.8   **Other follicular cysts of the skin and subcutaneous tissue**

L72.9   **Follicular cyst of the skin and subcutaneous tissue, unspecified**

L73   **Other follicular disorders**

L73.0   **Acne keloid**

L73.1   **Pseudofolliculitis barbae**

L73.2   **Hidradenitis suppurativa**

L73.8   **Other specified follicular disorders**

Sycosis barbae

L73.9   **Follicular disorder, unspecified**

L74   **Eccrine sweat disorders**

Excludes2: generalized hyperhidrosis (R61)

L74.0   **Miliaria rubra**

L74.1   **Miliaria crystallina**

L74.2   **Miliaria profunda**

Miliaria tropicalis

L74.3   **Miliaria, unspecified**

L74.4   **Anhidrosis**

Hypohidrosis

L74.5   **Focal hyperhidrosis**

     L74.51   **Primary focal hyperhidrosis**

         L74.510   **Primary focal hyperhidrosis, axilla**

         L74.511   **Primary focal hyperhidrosis, face**

         L74.512   **Primary focal hyperhidrosis, palms**

         L74.513   **Primary focal hyperhidrosis, soles**

         L74.519   **Primary focal hyperhidrosis, unspecified**

     L74.52   **Secondary focal hyperhidrosis**

Frey's syndrome

L74.8   **Other eccrine sweat disorders**

L74.9   **Eccrine sweat disorder, unspecified**

Sweat gland disorder NOS

L75   **Apocrine sweat disorders**

Excludes1: dyshidrosis (L30.1)

hidradenitis suppurativa (L73.2)

L75.0   **Bromhidrosis**

L75.1   **Chromhidrosis**

L75.2   **Apocrine miliaria**

Fox-Fordyce disease

L75.8   **Other apocrine sweat disorders**

L75.9   **Apocrine sweat disorder, unspecified**

INTRAOPERATIVE AND POSTPROCEDURAL COMPLICATIONS OF SKIN AND SUBCUTANEOUS TISSUE (L76)

L76   **Intraoperative and postprocedural complications of skin and subcutaneous tissue**

L76.0   **Intraoperative hemorrhage and hematoma of skin and subcutaneous tissue complicating a procedure**

Excludes1: intraoperative hemorrhage and hematoma of skin and subcutaneous tissue due to accidental puncture and laceration during a procedure (L76.1-)

     L76.01   **Intraoperative hemorrhage and hematoma of skin and subcutaneous tissue complicating a dermatologic procedure**

     L76.02   **Intraoperative hemorrhage and hematoma of skin and subcutaneous tissue complicating other procedure**

L76.1   **Accidental puncture and laceration of skin and subcutaneous tissue during a procedure**

     L76.11   **Accidental puncture and laceration of skin and subcutaneous tissue during a dermatologic procedure**

     L76.12   **Accidental puncture and laceration of skin and subcutaneous tissue during other procedure**

L76.2   **Postprocedural hemorrhage of skin and subcutaneous tissue following a procedure**

L76.21 Postprocedural hemorrhage of skin and subcutaneous tissue following a dermatologic procedure

L76.22 Postprocedural hemorrhage of skin and subcutaneous tissue following other procedure

L76.3 Postprocedural hematoma and seroma of skin and subcutaneous tissue following a procedure

L76.31 Postprocedural hematoma of skin and subcutaneous tissue following a dermatologic procedure

L76.32 Postprocedural hematoma of skin and subcutaneous tissue following other procedure

L76.33 Postprocedural seroma of skin and subcutaneous tissue following a dermatologic procedure

L76.34 Postprocedural seroma of skin and subcutaneous tissue following other procedure

L76.8 Other intraoperative and postprocedural complications of skin and subcutaneous tissue

Use Additional Code, if applicable, to further specify disorder

L76.81 Other intraoperative complications of skin and subcutaneous tissue

L76.82 Other postprocedural complications of skin and subcutaneous tissue

OTHER DISORDERS OF THE SKIN AND SUBCUTANEOUS TISSUE (L80-L99)

L80 Vitiligo

Excludes2: vitiligo of eyelids (H02.73-)

vitiligo of vulva (N90.89)

L81 Other disorders of pigmentation

Excludes1: birthmark NOS (Q82.5)

Peutz-Jeghers syndrome (Q85.8)

Excludes2: nevus - see Alphabetical Index

L81.0 Postinflammatory hyperpigmentation

L81.1 Chloasma

L81.2 Freckles

L81.3 Café au lait spots

L81.4 Other melanin hyperpigmentation

Lentigo

L81.5 Leukoderma, not elsewhere classified

L81.6 Other disorders of diminished melanin formation

L81.7 Pigmented purpuric dermatosis

Angioma serpiginosum

L81.8 Other specified disorders of pigmentation

Iron pigmentation

Tattoo pigmentation

L81.9 Disorder of pigmentation, unspecified

L82 Seborrheic keratosis

Includes: basal cell papilloma

dermatosis papulosa nigra

Leser-Trélat disease

Excludes2: seborrheic dermatitis (L21.-)

L82.0 Inflamed seborrheic keratosis

L82.1 Other seborrheic keratosis

Seborrheic keratosis NOS

L83 Acanthosis nigricans

Confluent and reticulated papillomatosis

L84 Corns and callosities

Callus Clavus

L85 Other epidermal thickening

Excludes2: hypertrophic disorders of the skin (L91.-)

L85.0 Acquired ichthyosis

Excludes1: congenital ichthyosis (Q80.-)

L85.1 Acquired keratosis [keratoderma] palmaris et plantaris

Excludes1: inherited keratosis palmaris et plantaris (Q82.8)

L85.2 Keratosis punctata (palmaris et plantaris)

L85.3 Xerosis cutis

Dry skin dermatitis

L85.8 Other specified epidermal thickening

Cutaneous horn

L85.9 Epidermal thickening, unspecified

L86 Keratoderma in diseases classified elsewhere

Code first underlying disease, such as:

Reiter's disease (M02.3-)

Excludes1: gonococcal keratoderma (A54.89)

gonococcal keratosis (A54.89)

keratoderma due to vitamin A deficiency (E50.8)

keratosis due to vitamin A deficiency (E50.8)

xeroderma due to vitamin A deficiency (E50.8)

L87 Transepidermal elimination disorders

Excludes1: granuloma annulare (perforating) (L92.0)

L87.0 Keratosis follicularis et parafollicularis in cutem penetrans

Kyrle disease

Hyperkeratosis follicularis penetrans

L87.1 Reactive perforating collagenosis

L87.2 Elastosis perforans serpiginosa

L87.8 Other transepidermal elimination disorders

L87.9 Transepidermal elimination disorder, unspecified

L88 Pyoderma gangrenosum

Phagedenic pyoderma

Excludes1: dermatitis gangrenosa (L08.0)

L89 Pressure ulcer

Includes: bed sore

decubitus ulcer

plaster ulcer

pressure area

pressure sore

Code first any associated gangrene (I96)

Excludes2: decubitus (trophic) ulcer of cervix (uteri) (N86)

diabetic ulcers (E08.621, E08.622, E09.621, E09.622, E10.621, E10.622, E11.621, E11.622, E13.621, E13.622)

non-pressure chronic ulcer of skin (L97.-)

skin infections (L00-L08)

varicose ulcer (I83.0, I83.2)

L89.0 Pressure ulcer of elbow

L89.00 Pressure ulcer of unspecified elbow

L89.000 Pressure ulcer of unspecified elbow, unstageable [HCC]

L89.001 Pressure ulcer of unspecified elbow, stage 1 [HCC]

Healing pressure ulcer of unspecified elbow, stage 1

Pressure pre-ulcer skin changes limited to persistent focal edema, unspecified elbow

L89.002 **Pressure ulcer of unspecified elbow, stage 2** [HCC]

Healing pressure ulcer of unspecified elbow, stage 2

Pressure ulcer with abrasion, blister, partial thickness skin loss involving epidermis and/or dermis, unspecified elbow

L89.003 **Pressure ulcer of unspecified elbow, stage 3** [HCC]

Healing pressure ulcer of unspecified elbow, stage 3

Pressure ulcer with full thickness skin loss involving damage or necrosis of subcutaneous tissue, unspecified elbow

L89.004 **Pressure ulcer of unspecified elbow, stage 4**

Healing pressure ulcer of unspecified elbow, stage 4

Pressure ulcer with necrosis of soft tissues through to underlying muscle, tendon, or bone, unspecified elbow

L89.009 **Pressure ulcer of unspecified elbow, unspecified stage** [HCC]

Healing pressure ulcer of elbow NOS

Healing pressure ulcer of unspecified elbow, unspecified stage

L89.01 **Pressure ulcer of right elbow**

L89.010 **Pressure ulcer of right elbow, unstageable** [HCC]

L89.011 **Pressure ulcer of right elbow, stage 1** [HCC]

Healing pressure ulcer of right elbow, stage 1

Pressure pre-ulcer skin changes limited to persistent focal edema, right elbow

L89.012 **Pressure ulcer of right elbow, stage 2** [HCC]

Healing pressure ulcer of right elbow, stage 2

Pressure ulcer with abrasion, blister, partial thickness skin loss involving epidermis and/or dermis, right elbow

L89.013 **Pressure ulcer of right elbow, stage 3** [HCC]

Healing pressure ulcer of right elbow, stage 3

Pressure ulcer with full thickness skin loss involving damage or necrosis of subcutaneous tissue, right elbow

L89.014 **Pressure ulcer of right elbow, stage 4** [HCC]

Healing pressure ulcer of right elbow, stage 4

Pressure ulcer with necrosis of soft tissues through to underlying muscle, tendon, or bone, right elbow

L89.016 **Pressure-induced deep tissue damage of right elbow** [HCC]

L89.019 **Pressure ulcer of right elbow, unspecified stage** [HCC]

Healing pressure of right elbow NOS

Healing pressure ulcer of right elbow, unspecified stage

L89.02 **Pressure ulcer of left elbow**

L89.020 **Pressure ulcer of left elbow, unstageable** [HCC]

L89.021 **Pressure ulcer of left elbow, stage 1** [HCC]

Healing pressure ulcer of left elbow, stage 1

Pressure pre-ulcer skin changes limited to persistent focal edema, left elbow

L89.022 **Pressure ulcer of left elbow, stage 2** [HCC]

Healing pressure ulcer of left elbow, stage 2

Pressure ulcer with abrasion, blister, partial thickness skin loss involving epidermis and/or dermis, left elbow

L89.023 **Pressure ulcer of left elbow, stage 3** [HCC]

Healing pressure ulcer of left elbow, stage 3

Pressure ulcer with full thickness skin loss involving damage or necrosis of subcutaneous tissue, left elbow

L89.024 **Pressure ulcer of left elbow, stage 4** [HCC]

Healing pressure ulcer of left elbow, stage 4

Pressure ulcer with necrosis of soft tissues through to underlying muscle, tendon, or bone, left elbow

L89.026 **Pressure-induced deep tissue damage of left elbow** [HCC]

L89.029 **Pressure ulcer of left elbow, unspecified stage** [HCC]

Healing pressure ulcer of left elbow NOS

Healing pressure ulcer of left elbow, unspecified stage

L89.1 **Pressure ulcer of back**

L89.10 **Pressure ulcer of unspecified part of back**

L89.100 **Pressure ulcer of unspecified part of back, unstageable** [HCC]

L89.101 **Pressure ulcer of unspecified part of back, stage 1** [HCC]

Healing pressure ulcer of unspecified part of back, stage 1

Pressure pre-ulcer skin changes limited to persistent focal edema, unspecified part of back

L89.102 **Pressure ulcer of unspecified part of back, stage 2** [HCC]

Healing pressure ulcer of unspecified part of back, stage 2

Pressure ulcer with abrasion, blister, partial thickness skin loss involving epidermis and/or dermis, unspecified part of back

L89.103 **Pressure ulcer of unspecified part of back, stage 3** [HCC]

Healing pressure ulcer of unspecified part of back, stage 3

Pressure ulcer with full thickness skin loss involving damage or necrosis of

● New code   ▲ Revised code   **Excludes1:** Not coded here   **Excludes2:** Not included here   ⊗ Placeholder required   ⑦7th digit required

subcutaneous tissue, unspecified part of back

L89.104 **Pressure ulcer of unspecified part of back, stage 4** [HCC]

Healing pressure ulcer of unspecified part of back, stage 4

Pressure ulcer with necrosis of soft tissues through to underlying muscle, tendon, or bone, unspecified part of back

L89.106 **Pressure-induced deep tissue damage of unspecified part of back** [HCC]

L89.109 **Pressure ulcer of unspecified part of back, unspecified stage** [HCC]

Healing pressure ulcer of unspecified part of back NOS

Healing pressure ulcer of unspecified part of back, unspecified stage

L89.11 **Pressure ulcer of right upper back**

Pressure ulcer of right shoulder blade

L89.110 **Pressure ulcer of right upper back, unstageable** [HCC]

L89.111 **Pressure ulcer of right upper back, stage 1** [HCC]

Healing pressure ulcer of right upper back, stage 1

Pressure pre-ulcer skin changes limited to persistent focal edema, right upper back

L89.112 **Pressure ulcer of right upper back, stage 2** [HCC]

Healing pressure ulcer of right upper back, stage 2

Pressure ulcer with abrasion, blister, partial thickness skin loss involving epidermis and/or dermis, right upper back

L89.113 **Pressure ulcer of right upper back, stage 3** [HCC]

Healing pressure ulcer of right upper back, stage 3

Pressure ulcer with full thickness skin loss involving damage or necrosis of subcutaneous tissue, right upper back

L89.114 **Pressure ulcer of right upper back, stage 4** [HCC]

Healing pressure ulcer of right upper back, stage 4

Pressure ulcer with necrosis of soft tissues through to underlying muscle, tendon, or bone, right upper back

L89.116 **Pressure-induced deep tissue damage of right upper back** [HCC]

L89.119 **Pressure ulcer of right upper back, unspecified stage** [HCC]

Healing pressure ulcer of right upper back NOS

Healing pressure ulcer of right upper back, unspecified stage

L89.12 **Pressure ulcer of left upper back**

Pressure ulcer of left shoulder blade

L89.120 **Pressure ulcer of left upper back, unstageable**

L89.121 **Pressure ulcer of left upper back, stage 1** [HCC]

Healing pressure ulcer of left upper back, stage 1

Pressure pre-ulcer skin changes limited to persistent focal edema, left upper back

L89.122 **Pressure ulcer of left upper back, stage 2** [HCC]

Healing pressure ulcer of left upper back, stage 2

Pressure ulcer with abrasion, blister, partial thickness skin loss involving epidermis and/or dermis, left upper back

L89.123 **Pressure ulcer of left upper back, stage 3** [HCC]

Healing pressure ulcer of left upper back, stage 3

Pressure ulcer with full thickness skin loss involving damage or necrosis of subcutaneous tissue, left upper back

L89.124 **Pressure ulcer of left upper back, stage 4** [HCC]

Healing pressure ulcer of left upper back, stage 4

Pressure ulcer with necrosis of soft tissues through to underlying muscle, tendon, or bone, left upper back

L89.126 **Pressure-induced deep tissue damage of left upper back** [HCC]

L89.129 **Pressure ulcer of left upper back, unspecified stage** [HCC]

Healing pressure ulcer of left upper back NOS

Healing pressure ulcer of left upper back, unspecified stage

L89.13 **Pressure ulcer of right lower back**

L89.130 **Pressure ulcer of right lower back, unstageable** [HCC]

L89.131 **Pressure ulcer of right lower back, stage 1** [HCC]

Healing pressure ulcer of right lower back, stage 1

Pressure pre-ulcer skin changes limited to persistent focal edema, right lower back

L89.132 **Pressure ulcer of right lower back, stage 2** [HCC]

Healing pressure ulcer of right lower back, stage 2

Pressure ulcer with abrasion, blister, partial thickness skin loss involving epidermis and/or dermis, right lower back

L89.133 **Pressure ulcer of right lower back, stage 3** [HCC]

Healing pressure ulcer of right lower back, stage 3

Pressure ulcer with full thickness skin loss involving damage or necrosis of subcutaneous tissue, right lower back

L89.134 **Pressure ulcer of right lower back, stage 4** [HCC]

Healing pressure ulcer of right lower back, stage 4

Pressure ulcer with necrosis of soft tissues through to underlying muscle, tendon, or bone, right lower back

L89.136 **Pressure-induced deep tissue damage of right lower back** [HCC]

L89.139 **Pressure ulcer of right lower back, unspecified stage** [HCC]

Healing pressure ulcer of right lower back NOS

Healing pressure ulcer of right lower back, unspecified stage

L89.14 **Pressure ulcer of left lower back**

L89.140 **Pressure ulcer of left lower back, unstageable** [HCC]

L89.141 **Pressure ulcer of left lower back, stage 1** [HCC]

Healing pressure ulcer of left lower back, stage 1

Pressure pre-ulcer skin changes limited to persistent focal edema, left lower back

L89.142 **Pressure ulcer of left lower back, stage 2** [HCC]

Healing pressure ulcer of left lower back, stage 2

Pressure ulcer with abrasion, blister, partial thickness skin loss involving epidermis and/or dermis, left lower back

L89.143 **Pressure ulcer of left lower back, stage 3** [HCC]

Healing pressure ulcer of left lower back, stage 3

Pressure ulcer with full thickness skin loss involving damage or necrosis of subcutaneous tissue, left lower back

L89.144 **Pressure ulcer of left lower back, stage 4** [HCC]

Healing pressure ulcer of left lower back, stage 4

Pressure ulcer with necrosis of soft tissues through to underlying muscle, tendon, or bone, left lower back

L89.146 **Pressure-induced deep tissue damage of left lower back** [HCC]

L89.149 **Pressure ulcer of left lower back, unspecified stage** [HCC]

Healing pressure ulcer of left lower back NOS

Healing pressure ulcer of left lower back, unspecified stage

L89.15 **Pressure ulcer of sacral region**

Pressure ulcer of coccyx
Pressure ulcer of tailbone

L89.150 **Pressure ulcer of sacral region, unstageable** [HCC]

L89.151 **Pressure ulcer of sacral region, stage 1** [HCC]

Healing pressure ulcer of sacral region, stage 1

Pressure pre-ulcer skin changes limited to persistent focal edema, sacral region

L89.152 **Pressure ulcer of sacral region, stage 2** [HCC]

Healing pressure ulcer of sacral region, stage 2

Pressure ulcer with abrasion, blister, partial thickness skin loss involving epidermis and/or dermis, sacral region

L89.153 **Pressure ulcer of sacral region, stage 3** [HCC]

Healing pressure ulcer of sacral region, stage 3

Pressure ulcer with full thickness skin loss involving damage or necrosis of subcutaneous tissue, sacral region

L89.154 **Pressure ulcer of sacral region, stage 4** [HCC]

Healing pressure ulcer of sacral region, stage 4

Pressure ulcer with necrosis of soft tissues through to underlying muscle, tendon, or bone, sacral region

L89.156 **Pressure-induced deep tissue damage of sacral region** [HCC]

L89.159 **Pressure ulcer of sacral region, unspecified stage** [HCC]

Healing pressure ulcer of sacral region NOS

Healing pressure ulcer of sacral region, unspecified stage

L89.2 **Pressure ulcer of hip**

L89.20 **Pressure ulcer of unspecified hip**

L89.200 **Pressure ulcer of unspecified hip, unstageable** [HCC]

L89.201 **Pressure ulcer of unspecified hip, stage 1** [HCC]

Healing pressure ulcer of unspecified hip back, stage 1

Pressure pre-ulcer skin changes limited to persistent focal edema, unspecified hip

L89.202 **Pressure ulcer of unspecified hip, stage 2** [HCC]

Healing pressure ulcer of unspecified hip, stage 2

Pressure ulcer with abrasion, blister, partial thickness skin loss involving epidermis and/or dermis, unspecified hip

L89.203 **Pressure ulcer of unspecified hip, stage 3** [HCC]

Healing pressure ulcer of unspecified hip, stage 3

Pressure ulcer with full thickness skin loss involving damage or necrosis of subcutaneous tissue, unspecified hip

L89.204 **Pressure ulcer of unspecified hip, stage 4** [HCC]

Healing pressure ulcer of unspecified hip, stage 4

Pressure ulcer with necrosis of soft tissues through to underlying muscle, tendon, or bone, unspecified hip

L89.206 **Pressure-induced deep tissue damage of unspecified hip** [HCC]

L89.209 **Pressure ulcer of unspecified hip, unspecified stage** [HCC]

Healing pressure ulcer of unspecified hip NOS

Healing pressure ulcer of unspecified hip, unspecified stage

L89.21 **Pressure ulcer of right hip**

L89.210 **Pressure ulcer of right hip, unstageable** [HCC]

L89.211 **Pressure ulcer of right hip, stage 1** [HCC]

Healing pressure ulcer of right hip back, stage 1

Pressure pre-ulcer skin changes limited to persistent focal edema, right hip

L89.212 **Pressure ulcer of right hip, stage 2** [HCC]

Healing pressure ulcer of right hip, stage 2

Pressure ulcer with abrasion, blister, partial thickness skin loss involving epidermis and/or dermis, right hip

L89.213 **Pressure ulcer of right hip, stage 3** [HCC]

Healing pressure ulcer of right hip, stage 3

Pressure ulcer with full thickness skin loss involving damage or necrosis of subcutaneous tissue, right hip

L89.214 **Pressure ulcer of right hip, stage 4** [HCC]

Healing pressure ulcer of right hip, stage 4

Pressure ulcer with necrosis of soft tissues through to underlying muscle, tendon, or bone, right hip

L89.216 **Pressure-induced deep tissue damage of right hip** [HCC]

L89.219 **Pressure ulcer of right hip, unspecified stage** [HCC]

Healing pressure ulcer of right hip NOS

Healing pressure ulcer of right hip, unspecified stage

L89.22 **Pressure ulcer of left hip**

L89.220 **Pressure ulcer of left hip, unstageable** [HCC]

L89.221 **Pressure ulcer of left hip, stage 1** [HCC]

Healing pressure ulcer of left hip back, stage 1

Pressure pre-ulcer skin changes limited to persistent focal edema, left hip

L89.222 **Pressure ulcer of left hip, stage 2** [HCC]

Healing pressure ulcer of left hip, stage 2

Pressure ulcer with abrasion, blister, partial thickness skin loss involving epidermis and/or dermis, left hip

L89.223 **Pressure ulcer of left hip, stage 3** [HCC]

Healing pressure ulcer of left hip, stage 3

Pressure ulcer with full thickness skin loss involving damage or necrosis of subcutaneous tissue, left hip

L89.224 **Pressure ulcer of left hip, stage 4** [HCC]

Healing pressure ulcer of left hip, stage 4

Pressure ulcer with necrosis of soft tissues through to underlying muscle, tendon, or bone, left hip

L89.226 **Pressure-induced deep tissue damage of left hip** [HCC]

L89.229 **Pressure ulcer of left hip, unspecified stage** [HCC]

Healing pressure ulcer of left hip NOS

Healing pressure ulcer of left hip, unspecified stage

L89.3 **Pressure ulcer of buttock**

L89.30 **Pressure ulcer of unspecified buttock**

L89.300 **Pressure ulcer of unspecified buttock, unstageable** [HCC]

L89.301 **Pressure ulcer of unspecified buttock, stage 1** [HCC]

Healing pressure ulcer of unspecified buttock, stage 1

Pressure pre-ulcer skin changes limited to persistent focal edema, unspecified buttock

L89.302 **Pressure ulcer of unspecified buttock, stage 2** [HCC]

Healing pressure ulcer of unspecified buttock, stage 2

Pressure ulcer with abrasion, blister, partial thickness skin loss involving epidermis and/or dermis, unspecified buttock

L89.303 **Pressure ulcer of unspecified buttock, stage 3** [HCC]

Healing pressure ulcer of unspecified buttock, stage 3

Pressure ulcer with full thickness skin loss involving damage or necrosis of subcutaneous tissue, unspecified buttock

L89.304 **Pressure ulcer of unspecified buttock, stage 4** [HCC]

Healing pressure ulcer of unspecified buttock, stage 4

Pressure ulcer with necrosis of soft tissues through to underlying muscle, tendon, or bone, unspecified buttock

L89.306 **Pressure-induced deep tissue damage of unspecified buttock**

L89.309 **Pressure ulcer of unspecified buttock, unspecified stage** [HCC]

Healing pressure ulcer of unspecified buttock NOS

Healing pressure ulcer of unspecified buttock, unspecified stage

L89.31 **Pressure ulcer of right buttock**

L89.310 **Pressure ulcer of right buttock, unstageable** [HCC]

L89.311 **Pressure ulcer of right buttock, stage 1** [HCC]

Healing pressure ulcer of right buttock, stage 1

Pressure pre-ulcer skin changes limited to persistent focal edema, right buttock

L89.312 **Pressure ulcer of right buttock, stage 2** [HCC]

Healing pressure ulcer of right buttock, stage 2

Pressure ulcer with abrasion, blister, partial thickness skin loss involving epidermis and/or dermis, right buttock

L89.313 **Pressure ulcer of right buttock, stage 3** [HCC]

Healing pressure ulcer of right buttock, stage 3

Pressure ulcer with full thickness skin loss involving damage or necrosis of subcutaneous tissue, right buttock

L89.314 **Pressure ulcer of right buttock, stage 4** [HCC]

Healing pressure ulcer of right buttock, stage 4

Pressure ulcer with necrosis of soft tissues through to underlying muscle, tendon, or bone, right buttock

L89.316 **Pressure-induced deep tissue damage of right buttock** [HCC]

L89.319 **Pressure ulcer of right buttock, unspecified stage** [HCC]

Healing pressure ulcer of right buttock NOS

Healing pressure ulcer of right buttock, unspecified stage

L89.32 **Pressure ulcer of left buttock**

L89.320 **Pressure ulcer of left buttock, unstageable** [HCC]

L89.321 **Pressure ulcer of left buttock, stage 1** [HCC]

Healing pressure ulcer of left buttock, stage 1

Pressure pre-ulcer skin changes limited to persistent focal edema, left buttock

L89.322 **Pressure ulcer of left buttock, stage 2** [HCC]

Healing pressure ulcer of left buttock, stage 2

Pressure ulcer with abrasion, blister, partial thickness skin loss involving epidermis and/or dermis, left buttock

L89.323 **Pressure ulcer of left buttock, stage 3** [HCC]

Healing pressure ulcer of left buttock, stage 3

Pressure ulcer with full thickness skin loss involving damage or necrosis of subcutaneous tissue, left buttock

L89.324 **Pressure ulcer of left buttock, stage 4** [HCC]

Healing pressure ulcer of left buttock, stage 4

Pressure ulcer with necrosis of soft tissues through to underlying muscle, tendon, or bone, left buttock

L89.326 **Pressure-induced deep tissue damage of left buttock**

L89.329 **Pressure ulcer of left buttock, unspecified stage** [HCC]

Healing pressure ulcer of left buttock NOS

Healing pressure ulcer of left buttock, unspecified stage

L89.4 **Pressure ulcer of contiguous site of back, buttock and hip**

L89.40 **Pressure ulcer of contiguous site of back, buttock and hip, unspecified stage** [HCC]

Healing pressure ulcer of contiguous site of back, buttock and hip NOS

Healing pressure ulcer of contiguous site of back, buttock and hip, unspecified stage

L89.41 **Pressure ulcer of contiguous site of back, buttock and hip, stage 1** [HCC]

Healing pressure ulcer of contiguous site of back, buttock and hip, stage 1

Pressure pre-ulcer skin changes limited to persistent focal edema, contiguous site of back, buttock and hip

L89.42 **Pressure ulcer of contiguous site of back, buttock and hip, stage 2** [HCC]

Healing pressure ulcer of contiguous site of back, buttock and hip, stage 2

Pressure ulcer with abrasion, blister, partial thickness skin loss involving epidermis and/or dermis, contiguous site of back, buttock and hip

L89.43 **Pressure ulcer of contiguous site of back, buttock and hip, stage 3** [HCC]

Healing pressure ulcer of contiguous site of back, buttock and hip, stage 3

Pressure ulcer with full thickness skin loss involving damage or necrosis of subcutaneous tissue, contiguous site of back, buttock and hip

L89.44 **Pressure ulcer of contiguous site of back, buttock and hip, stage 4** [HCC]

Healing pressure ulcer of contiguous site of back, buttock and hip, stage 4

Pressure ulcer with necrosis of soft tissues through to underlying muscle, tendon, or bone, contiguous site of back, buttock and hip

L89.45 **Pressure ulcer of contiguous site of back, buttock and hip, unstageable** [HCC]

L89.46 **Pressure-induced deep tissue damage of contiguous site of back, buttock and hip**

L89.5 **Pressure ulcer of ankle**

L89.50 **Pressure ulcer of unspecified ankle**

L89.500 **Pressure ulcer of unspecified ankle, unstageable** [HCC]

L89.501 **Pressure ulcer of unspecified ankle, stage 1** [HCC]

Healing pressure ulcer of unspecified ankle, stage 1

Pressure pre-ulcer skin changes limited to persistent focal edema, unspecified ankle

L89.502 **Pressure ulcer of unspecified ankle, stage 2** [HCC]

Healing pressure ulcer of unspecified ankle, stage 2

Pressure ulcer with abrasion, blister, partial thickness skin loss involving epidermis and/or dermis, unspecified ankle

L89.503 **Pressure ulcer of unspecified ankle, stage 3** [HCC]

Healing pressure ulcer of unspecified ankle, stage 3

● New code   ▲ Revised code   **Excludes1:** Not coded here   **Excludes2:** Not included here   ⊗ Placeholder required   ⑦7ᵗʰ digit required

Pressure ulcer with full thickness skin loss involving damage or necrosis of subcutaneous tissue, unspecified ankle

L89.504 **Pressure ulcer of unspecified ankle, stage 4** [HCC]

Healing pressure ulcer of unspecified ankle, stage 4

Pressure ulcer with necrosis of soft tissues through to underlying muscle, tendon, or bone, unspecified ankle

L89.506 **Pressure-induced deep tissue damage of unspecified ankle**

L89.509 **Pressure ulcer of unspecified ankle, unspecified stage** [HCC]

Healing pressure ulcer of unspecified ankle NOS

Healing pressure ulcer of unspecified ankle, unspecified stage

L89.51 **Pressure ulcer of right ankle**

L89.510 **Pressure ulcer of right ankle, unstageable** [HCC]

L89.511 **Pressure ulcer of right ankle, stage 1** [HCC]

Healing pressure ulcer of right ankle, stage 1

Pressure pre-ulcer skin changes limited to persistent focal edema, right ankle

L89.512 **Pressure ulcer of right ankle, stage 2** [HCC]

Healing pressure ulcer of right ankle, stage 2

Pressure ulcer with abrasion, blister, partial thickness skin loss involving epidermis and/or dermis, right ankle

L89.513 **Pressure ulcer of right ankle, stage 3** [HCC]

Healing pressure ulcer of right ankle, stage 3

Pressure ulcer with full thickness skin loss involving damage or necrosis of subcutaneous tissue, right ankle

L89.514 **Pressure ulcer of right ankle, stage 4** [HCC]

Healing pressure ulcer of right ankle, stage 4

Pressure ulcer with necrosis of soft tissues through to underlying muscle, tendon, or bone, right ankle

L89.516 **Pressure-induced deep tissue damage of right ankle**

L89.519 **Pressure ulcer of right ankle, unspecified stage** [HCC]

Healing pressure ulcer of right ankle NOS

Healing pressure ulcer of right ankle, unspecified stage

L89.52 **Pressure ulcer of left ankle**

L89.520 **Pressure ulcer of left ankle, unstageable** [HCC]

L89.521 **Pressure ulcer of left ankle, stage 1** [HCC]

Healing pressure ulcer of left ankle, stage 1

Pressure pre-ulcer skin changes limited to persistent focal edema, left ankle

L89.522 **Pressure ulcer of left ankle, stage 2** [HCC]

Healing pressure ulcer of left ankle, stage 2

Pressure ulcer with abrasion, blister, partial thickness skin loss involving epidermis and/or dermis, left ankle

L89.523 **Pressure ulcer of left ankle, stage 3** [HCC]

Healing pressure ulcer of left ankle, stage 3

Pressure ulcer with full thickness skin loss involving damage or necrosis of subcutaneous tissue, left ankle

L89.524 **Pressure ulcer of left ankle, stage 4**

Healing pressure ulcer of left ankle, stage 4

Pressure ulcer with necrosis of soft tissues through to underlying muscle, tendon, or bone, left ankle

L89.526 **Pressure-induced deep tissue damage of left ankle**

L89.529 **Pressure ulcer of left ankle, unspecified stage** [HCC]

Healing pressure ulcer of left ankle NOS

Healing pressure ulcer of left ankle, unspecified stage

L89.6 **Pressure ulcer of heel**

L89.60 **Pressure ulcer of unspecified heel**

L89.600 **Pressure ulcer of unspecified heel, unstageable** [HCC]

L89.601 **Pressure ulcer of unspecified heel, stage 1** [HCC]

Healing pressure ulcer of unspecified heel, stage 1

Pressure pre-ulcer skin changes limited to persistent focal edema, unspecified heel

L89.602 **Pressure ulcer of unspecified heel, stage 2** [HCC]

Healing pressure ulcer of unspecified heel, stage 2

Pressure ulcer with abrasion, blister, partial thickness skin loss involving epidermis and/or dermis, unspecified heel

L89.603 **Pressure ulcer of unspecified heel, stage 3** [HCC]

Healing pressure ulcer of unspecified heel, stage 3

Pressure ulcer with full thickness skin loss involving damage or necrosis of subcutaneous tissue, unspecified heel

L89.604 **Pressure ulcer of unspecified heel, stage 4** [HCC]

Healing pressure ulcer of unspecified heel, stage 4

Pressure ulcer with necrosis of soft tissues through to underlying muscle, tendon, or bone, unspecified heel

L89.606 **Pressure-induced deep tissue damage of unspecified heel**

L89.609 **Pressure ulcer of unspecified heel, unspecified stage** [HCC]

Add 4th-7th digits   Nonspecific code   Unspecified code   Manifestation code   [HCC] Hierarchical Condition Code   **523**

Healing pressure ulcer of unspecified heel NOS

Healing pressure ulcer of unspecified heel, unspecified stage

L89.61 Pressure ulcer of right heel]

L89.610 Pressure ulcer of right heel, unstageable [HCC]

L89.611 Pressure ulcer of right heel, stage 1 [HCC]

Healing pressure ulcer of right heel, stage 1

Pressure pre-ulcer skin changes limited to persistent focal edema, right heel

L89.612 Pressure ulcer of right heel, stage 2 [HCC]

Healing pressure ulcer of right heel, stage 2

Pressure ulcer with abrasion, blister, partial thickness skin loss involving epidermis and/or dermis, right heel

L89.613 Pressure ulcer of right heel, stage 3 [HCC]

Healing pressure ulcer of right heel, stage 3

Pressure ulcer with full thickness skin loss involving damage or necrosis of subcutaneous tissue, right heel

L89.614 Pressure ulcer of right heel, stage 4 [HCC]

Healing pressure ulcer of right heel, stage 4

Pressure ulcer with necrosis of soft tissues through to underlying muscle, tendon, or bone, right heel

L89.616 Pressure-induced deep tissue damage of right heel [HCC]

L89.619 Pressure ulcer of right heel, unspecified stage [HCC]

Healing pressure ulcer of right heel NOS

Healing pressure ulcer of right heel, unspecified stage

L89.62 Pressure ulcer of left heel

L89.620 Pressure ulcer of left heel, unstageable [HCC]

L89.621 Pressure ulcer of left heel, stage 1 [HCC]

Healing pressure ulcer of left heel, stage 1

Pressure pre-ulcer skin changes limited to persistent focal edema, left heel

L89.622 Pressure ulcer of left heel, stage 2 [HCC]

Healing pressure ulcer of left heel, stage 2

Pressure ulcer with abrasion, blister, partial thickness skin loss involving epidermis and/or dermis, left heel

L89.623 Pressure ulcer of left heel, stage 3 [HCC]

Healing pressure ulcer of left heel, stage 3

Pressure ulcer with full thickness skin loss involving damage or necrosis of subcutaneous tissue, left heel

L89.624 Pressure ulcer of left heel, stage 4 [HCC]

Healing pressure ulcer of left heel, stage 4

Pressure ulcer with necrosis of soft tissues through to underlying muscle, tendon, or bone, left heel

L89.626 Pressure-induced deep tissue damage of left heel [HCC]

L89.629 Pressure ulcer of left heel, unspecified stage [HCC]

Healing pressure ulcer of left heel NOS

Healing pressure ulcer of left heel, unspecified stage

L89.8 Pressure ulcer of other site

L89.81 Pressure ulcer of head

Pressure ulcer of face

L89.810 Pressure ulcer of head, unstageable [HCC]

L89.811 Pressure ulcer of head, stage 1 [HCC]

Healing pressure ulcer of head, stage 1

Pressure pre-ulcer skin changes limited to persistent focal edema, head

L89.812 Pressure ulcer of head, stage 2 [HCC]

Healing pressure ulcer of head, stage 2

Pressure ulcer with abrasion, blister, partial thickness skin loss involving epidermis and/or dermis, head

L89.813 Pressure ulcer of head, stage 3 [HCC]

Healing pressure ulcer of head, stage 3

Pressure ulcer with full thickness skin loss involving damage or necrosis of subcutaneous tissue, head

L89.814 Pressure ulcer of head, stage 4 [HCC]

Healing pressure ulcer of head, stage 4

Pressure ulcer with necrosis of soft tissues through to underlying muscle, tendon, or bone, head

L89.816 Pressure-induced deep tissue damage of head [HCC]

L89.819 Pressure ulcer of head, unspecified stage [HCC]

Healing pressure ulcer of head NOS

Healing pressure ulcer of head, unspecified stage

L89.89 Pressure ulcer of other site

L89.890 Pressure ulcer of other site, unstageable

L89.891 Pressure ulcer of other site, stage 1 [HCC]

Healing pressure ulcer of other site, stage 1

Pressure pre-ulcer skin changes limited to persistent focal edema, **other** site

L89.892 Pressure ulcer of other site, stage 2 [HCC]

Healing pressure ulcer of other site, stage 2

Pressure ulcer with abrasion, blister, partial thickness skin loss involving epidermis and/or dermis, other site

L89.893 Pressure ulcer of other site, stage 3 [HCC]

● New code   ▲ Revised code   **Excludes1:** Not coded here   **Excludes2:** Not included here   ⊗ Placeholder required   ⑦7th digit required

Healing pressure ulcer of other site, stage 3

Pressure ulcer with full thickness skin loss involving damage or necrosis of subcutaneous tissue, other site

L89.894 **Pressure ulcer of other site, stage 4** [HCC]

Healing pressure ulcer of other site, stage 4

Pressure ulcer with necrosis of soft tissues through to underlying muscle, tendon, or bone, other site

L89.899 **Pressure ulcer of other site, unspecified stage** [HCC]

Healing pressure ulcer of other site NOS

Healing pressure ulcer of other site, unspecified stage

L89.9 **Pressure ulcer of unspecified site**

L89.90 **Pressure ulcer of unspecified site, unspecified stage** [HCC]

Healing pressure ulcer of unspecified site NOS

Healing pressure ulcer of unspecified site, unspecified stage

L89.91 **Pressure ulcer of unspecified site, stage 1** [HCC]

Healing pressure ulcer of unspecified site, stage 1

Pressure pre-ulcer skin changes limited to persistent focal edema, unspecified site

L89.92 **Pressure ulcer of unspecified site, stage 2** [HCC]

Healing pressure ulcer of unspecified site, stage 2

Pressure ulcer with abrasion, blister, partial thickness skin loss involving epidermis and/or dermis, unspecified site

L89.93 **Pressure ulcer of unspecified site, stage 3** [HCC]

Healing pressure ulcer of unspecified site, stage 3

Pressure ulcer with full thickness skin loss involving damage or necrosis of subcutaneous tissue, unspecified site

L89.94 **Pressure ulcer of unspecified site, stage 4** [HCC]

Healing pressure ulcer of unspecified site, stage 4

Pressure ulcer with necrosis of soft tissues through to underlying muscle, tendon, or bone, unspecified site

L89.96 **Pressure-induced deep tissue damage of unspecified site** [HCC]

L89.95 **Pressure ulcer of unspecified site, unstageable** [HCC]

L90 **Atrophic disorders of skin**

L90.0 **Lichen sclerosus et atrophicus**

Excludes2: lichen sclerosus of external female genital organs (N90.4)

lichen sclerosus of external male genital organs (N48.0)

L90.1 **Anetoderma of Schweninger-Buzzi**

L90.2 **Anetoderma of Jadassohn-Pellizzari**

L90.3 **Atrophoderma of Pasini and Pierini**

L90.4 **Acrodermatitis chronica atrophicans**

L90.5 **Scar conditions and fibrosis of skin**

Adherent scar (skin)

Cicatrix

Disfigurement of skin due to scar

Fibrosis of skin NOS

Scar NOS

Excludes2: hypertrophic scar (L91.0)

keloid scar (L91.0)

L90.6 **Striae atrophicae**

L90.8 **Other atrophic disorders of skin**

L90.9 **Atrophic disorder of skin, unspecified**

L91 **Hypertrophic disorders of skin**

L91.0 **Hypertrophic scar**

Keloid

Keloid scar

Excludes2: acne keloid (L73.0)

scar NOS (L90.5)

L91.8 **Other hypertrophic disorders of the skin**

L91.9 **Hypertrophic disorder of the skin, unspecified**

L92 **Granulomatous disorders of skin and subcutaneous tissue**

Excludes2: actinic granuloma (L57.5)

L92.0 **Granuloma annulare**

Perforating granuloma annulare

L92.1 **Necrobiosis lipoidica, not elsewhere classified**

Excludes1: necrobiosis lipoidica associated with diabetes mellitus (E08-E13 with .620)

L92.2 **Granuloma faciale [eosinophilic granuloma of skin]**

L92.3 **Foreign body granuloma of the skin and subcutaneous tissue**

Use Additional Code to identify the type of retained foreign body (Z18.-)

L92.8 **Other granulomatous disorders of the skin and subcutaneous tissue**

L92.9 **Granulomatous disorder of the skin and subcutaneous tissue, unspecified**

Excludes2: umbilical granuloma (P83.81)

L93 **Lupus erythematosus**

Use Additional Code for adverse effect, if applicable, to identify drug (T36-T50 with fifth or sixth character 5)

Excludes1: lupus exedens (A18.4)

lupus vulgaris (A18.4)

scleroderma (M34.-)

systemic lupus erythematosus (M32.-)

L93.0 **Discoid lupus erythematosus**

Lupus erythematosus NOS

L93.1 **Subacute cutaneous lupus erythematosus**

L93.2 **Other local lupus erythematosus**

Lupus erythematosus profundus

Lupus panniculitis

L94 **Other localized connective tissue disorders**

Excludes1: systemic connective tissue disorders (M30-M36)

L94.0 **Localized scleroderma [morphea]**

Circumscribed scleroderma

L94.1 **Linear scleroderma**

En coup de sabre lesion

L94.2 **Calcinosis cutis**

L94.3 **Sclerodactyly**

L94.4 **Gottron's papules**

L94.5 **Poikiloderma vasculare atrophicans**

L94.6 **Ainhum**

L94.8 **Other specified localized connective tissue disorders**

L94.9 **Localized connective tissue disorder, unspecified**

L95 **Vasculitis limited to skin, not elsewhere classified**

Excludes1: angioma serpiginosum (L81.7)

Henoch(-Schönlein) purpura (D69.0)

hypersensitivity angiitis (M31.0)

lupus panniculitis (L93.2)

panniculitis NOS (M79.3)

panniculitis of neck and back (M54.0-)

polyarteritis nodosa (M30.0)

relapsing panniculitis (M35.6)

rheumatoid vasculitis (M05.2)

serum sickness (T80.6-)

urticaria (L50.-)

Wegener's granulomatosis (M31.3-)

L95.0 Livedoid vasculitis

Atrophie blanche (en plaque)

L95.1 Erythema elevatum diutinum

L95.8 Other vasculitis limited to the skin

L95.9 Vasculitis limited to the skin, unspecified

L97 Non-pressure chronic ulcer of lower limb, not elsewhere classified

Includes: chronic ulcer of skin of lower limb NOS

non-healing ulcer of skin non-infected sinus of skin trophic ulcer NOS

tropical ulcer NOS

ulcer of skin of lower limb NOS

Code first any associated underlying condition, such as:

any associated gangrene (I96)

atherosclerosis of the lower extremities (I70.23-, I70.24-, I70.33-, I70.34-, I70.43-, I70.44-, I70.53-, I70.54-, I70.63-, I70.64-, I70.73-, I70.74-)

chronic venous hypertension (I87.31-, I87.33-)

diabetic ulcers (E08.621, E08.622, E09.621, E09.622, E10.621, E10.622, E11.621, E11.622, E13.621, E13.622)

postphlebitic syndrome (I87.01-, I87.03-)

postthrombotic syndrome (I87.01-, I87.03-)

varicose ulcer (I83.0-, I83.2-)

Excludes2: pressure ulcer (pressure area) (L89.-)

skin infections (L00-L08)

specific infections classified to A00-B99

L97.1 Non-pressure chronic ulcer of thigh

L97.10 Non-pressure chronic ulcer of unspecified thigh

L97.101 Non-pressure chronic ulcer of unspecified thigh limited to breakdown of skin [HCC]

L97.102 Non-pressure chronic ulcer of unspecified thigh with fat layer exposed [HCC]

L97.103 Non-pressure chronic ulcer of unspecified thigh with necrosis of muscle [HCC]

L97.104 Non-pressure chronic ulcer of unspecified thigh with necrosis of bone [HCC]

L97.105 Non-pressure chronic ulcer of unspecified thigh with muscle involvement without evidence of necrosis [HCC]

L97.106 Non-pressure chronic ulcer of unspecified thigh with bone involvement without evidence of necrosis [HCC]

L97.108 Non-pressure chronic ulcer of unspecified thigh with other specified severity [HCC]

L97.109 Non-pressure chronic ulcer of unspecified thigh with unspecified severity [HCC]

L97.11 Non-pressure chronic ulcer of right thigh

L97.111 Non-pressure chronic ulcer of right thigh limited to breakdown of skin [HCC]

L97.112 Non-pressure chronic ulcer of right thigh with fat layer exposed [HCC]

L97.113 Non-pressure chronic ulcer of right thigh with necrosis of muscle [HCC]

L97.114 Non-pressure chronic ulcer of right thigh with necrosis of bone [HCC]

L97.115 Non-pressure chronic ulcer of right thigh with muscle involvement without evidence of necrosis [HCC]

L97.116 Non-pressure chronic ulcer of right thigh with bone involvement without evidence of necrosis [HCC]

L97.118 Non-pressure chronic ulcer of right thigh with other specified severity [HCC]

L97.119 Non-pressure chronic ulcer of right thigh with unspecified severity [HCC]

L97.12 Non-pressure chronic ulcer of left thigh

L97.121 Non-pressure chronic ulcer of left thigh limited to breakdown of skin [HCC]

L97.122 Non-pressure chronic ulcer of left thigh with fat layer exposed [HCC]

L97.123 Non-pressure chronic ulcer of left thigh with necrosis of muscle [HCC]

L97.124 Non-pressure chronic ulcer of left thigh with necrosis of bone [HCC]

L97.125 Non-pressure chronic ulcer of left thigh with muscle involvement without evidence of necrosis [HCC]

L97.126 Non-pressure chronic ulcer of left thigh with bone involvement without evidence of necrosis [HCC]

L97.128 Non-pressure chronic ulcer of left thigh with other specified severity [HCC]

L97.129 Non-pressure chronic ulcer of left thigh with unspecified severity [HCC]

L97.2 Non-pressure chronic ulcer of calf

L97.20 Non-pressure chronic ulcer of unspecified calf

L97.201 Non-pressure chronic ulcer of unspecified calf limited to breakdown of skin [HCC]

L97.202 Non-pressure chronic ulcer of unspecified calf with fat layer exposed [HCC]

L97.203 Non-pressure chronic ulcer of unspecified calf with necrosis of muscle [HCC]

L97.204 Non-pressure chronic ulcer of unspecified calf with necrosis of bone [HCC]

L97.125 Non-pressure chronic ulcer of left thigh with muscle involvement without evidence of necrosis [HCC]

● New code   ▲ Revised code   **Excludes1:** Not coded here   **Excludes2:** Not included here   ⊗ Placeholder required   ⑦ 7th digit required

L97.126   Non-pressure chronic ulcer of left thigh with bone involvement without evidence of necrosis [HCC]

L97.128   Non-pressure chronic ulcer of left thigh with other specified severity [HCC]

L97.209   Non-pressure chronic ulcer of unspecified calf with unspecified severity [HCC]

L97.21   Non-pressure chronic ulcer of right calf

L97.211   Non-pressure chronic ulcer of right calf limited to breakdown of skin [HCC]

L97.212   Non-pressure chronic ulcer of right calf with fat layer exposed [HCC]

L97.213   Non-pressure chronic ulcer of right calf with necrosis of muscle [HCC]

L97.214   Non-pressure chronic ulcer of right calf with necrosis of bone [HCC]

L97.215   Non-pressure chronic ulcer of right calf with muscle involvement without evidence of necrosis [HCC]

L97.216   Non-pressure chronic ulcer of right calf with bone involvement without evidence of necrosis [HCC]

L97.218   Non-pressure chronic ulcer of right calf with other specified severity [HCC]

L97.219   Non-pressure chronic ulcer of right calf with unspecified severity [HCC]

L97.22   Non-pressure chronic ulcer of left calf

L97.221   Non-pressure chronic ulcer of left calf limited to breakdown of skin [HCC]

L97.222   Non-pressure chronic ulcer of left calf with fat layer exposed [HCC]

L97.223   Non-pressure chronic ulcer of left calf with necrosis of muscle [HCC]

L97.224   Non-pressure chronic ulcer of left calf with necrosis of bone [HCC]

L97.225   Non-pressure chronic ulcer of left calf with muscle involvement without evidence of necrosis [HCC]

L97.226   Non-pressure chronic ulcer of left calf with bone involvement without evidence of necrosis [HCC]

L97.228   Non-pressure chronic ulcer of left calf with other specified severity [HCC]

L97.229   Non-pressure chronic ulcer of left calf with unspecified severity [HCC]

L97.3   Non-pressure chronic ulcer of ankle

L97.30   Non-pressure chronic ulcer of unspecified ankle

L97.301   Non-pressure chronic ulcer of unspecified ankle limited to breakdown of skin [HCC]

L97.302   Non-pressure chronic ulcer of unspecified ankle with fat layer exposed [HCC]

L97.303   Non-pressure chronic ulcer of unspecified ankle with necrosis of muscle [HCC]

L97.304   Non-pressure chronic ulcer of unspecified ankle with necrosis of bone [HCC]

L97.305   Non-pressure chronic ulcer of unspecified ankle with muscle

involvement without evidence of necrosis [HCC]

L97.306   Non-pressure chronic ulcer of unspecified ankle with bone involvement without evidence of necrosis [HCC]

L97.308   Non-pressure chronic ulcer of unspecified ankle with other specified severity [HCC]

L97.309   Non-pressure chronic ulcer of unspecified ankle with unspecified severity [HCC]

L97.31   Non-pressure chronic ulcer of right ankle

L97.311   Non-pressure chronic ulcer of right ankle limited to breakdown of skin [HCC]

L97.312   Non-pressure chronic ulcer of right ankle with fat layer exposed [HCC]

L97.313   Non-pressure chronic ulcer of right ankle with necrosis of muscle [HCC]

L97.314   Non-pressure chronic ulcer of right ankle with necrosis of bone [HCC]

L97.315   Non-pressure chronic ulcer of right ankle with muscle involvement without evidence of necrosis [HCC]

L97.316   Non-pressure chronic ulcer of right ankle with bone involvement without evidence of necrosis [HCC]

L97.318   Non-pressure chronic ulcer of right ankle with other specified severity [HCC]

L97.319   Non-pressure chronic ulcer of right ankle with unspecified severity [HCC]

L97.32   Non-pressure chronic ulcer of left ankle

L97.321   Non-pressure chronic ulcer of left ankle limited to breakdown of skin [HCC]

L97.322   Non-pressure chronic ulcer of left ankle with fat layer exposed [HCC]

L97.323   Non-pressure chronic ulcer of left ankle with necrosis of muscle [HCC]

L97.324   Non-pressure chronic ulcer of left ankle with necrosis of bone [HCC]

L97.325   Non-pressure chronic ulcer of left ankle with muscle involvement without evidence of necrosis [HCC]

L97.326   Non-pressure chronic ulcer of left ankle with bone involvement without evidence of necrosis [HCC]

L97.328   Non-pressure chronic ulcer of left ankle with other specified severity [HCC]

L97.329   Non-pressure chronic ulcer of left ankle with unspecified severity [HCC]

L97.4   Non-pressure chronic ulcer of heel and midfoot

Non-pressure chronic ulcer of plantar surface of midfoot

L97.40   Non-pressure chronic ulcer of unspecified heel and midfoot [HCC]

L97.401   Non-pressure chronic ulcer of unspecified heel and midfoot limited to breakdown of skin [HCC]

L97.402   Non-pressure chronic ulcer of unspecified heel and midfoot with fat layer exposed [HCC]

L97.403   Non-pressure chronic ulcer of unspecified heel and midfoot with necrosis of muscle [HCC]

L97.404 Non-pressure chronic ulcer of unspecified heel and midfoot with necrosis of bone [HCC]

L97.405 Non-pressure chronic ulcer of unspecified heel and midfoot with muscle involvement without evidence of necrosis [HCC]

L97.406 Non-pressure chronic ulcer of unspecified heel and midfoot with bone involvement without evidence of necrosis [HCC]

L97.408 Non-pressure chronic ulcer of unspecified heel and midfoot with other specified severity [HCC]

L97.409 Non-pressure chronic ulcer of unspecified heel and midfoot with unspecified severity [HCC]

L97.41 Non-pressure chronic ulcer of right heel and midfoot

L97.411 Non-pressure chronic ulcer of right heel and midfoot limited to breakdown of skin [HCC]

L97.412 Non-pressure chronic ulcer of right heel and midfoot with fat layer exposed [HCC]

L97.413 Non-pressure chronic ulcer of right heel and midfoot with necrosis of muscle [HCC]

L97.414 Non-pressure chronic ulcer of right heel and midfoot with necrosis of bone [HCC]

L97.415 Non-pressure chronic ulcer of right heel and midfoot with muscle involvement without evidence of necrosis [HCC]

L97.416 Non-pressure chronic ulcer of right heel and midfoot with bone involvement without evidence of necrosis [HCC]

L97.418 Non-pressure chronic ulcer of right heel and midfoot with other specified severity [HCC]

L97.419 Non-pressure chronic ulcer of right heel and midfoot with unspecified severity [HCC]

L97.42 Non-pressure chronic ulcer of left heel and midfoot

L97.421 Non-pressure chronic ulcer of left heel and midfoot limited to breakdown of skin [HCC]

L97.422 Non-pressure chronic ulcer of left heel and midfoot with fat layer exposed [HCC]

L97.423 Non-pressure chronic ulcer of left heel and midfoot with necrosis of muscle [HCC]

L97.424 Non-pressure chronic ulcer of left heel and midfoot with necrosis of bone [HCC]

L97.425 Non-pressure chronic ulcer of left heel and midfoot with muscle involvement without evidence of necrosis [HCC]

L97.426 Non-pressure chronic ulcer of left heel and midfoot with bone involvement without evidence of necrosis [HCC]

L97.428 Non-pressure chronic ulcer of left heel and midfoot with other specified severity [HCC]

L97.429 Non-pressure chronic ulcer of left heel and midfoot with unspecified severity [HCC]

L97.5 Non-pressure chronic ulcer of other part of foot
Non-pressure chronic ulcer of toe

L97.50 Non-pressure chronic ulcer of other part of unspecified foot

L97.501 Non-pressure chronic ulcer of other part of unspecified foot limited to breakdown of skin [HCC]

L97.502 Non-pressure chronic ulcer of other part of unspecified foot with fat layer exposed [HCC]

L97.503 Non-pressure chronic ulcer of other part of unspecified foot with necrosis of muscle [HCC]

L97.504 Non-pressure chronic ulcer of other part of unspecified foot with necrosis of bone [HCC]

L97.505 Non-pressure chronic ulcer of other part of unspecified foot with muscle involvement without evidence of necrosis [HCC]

L97.506 Non-pressure chronic ulcer of other part of unspecified foot with bone involvement without evidence of necrosis [HCC]

L97.508 Non-pressure chronic ulcer of other part of unspecified foot with other specified severity [HCC]

L97.509 Non-pressure chronic ulcer of other part of unspecified foot with unspecified severity [HCC]

L97.51 Non-pressure chronic ulcer of other part of right foot

L97.511 Non-pressure chronic ulcer of other part of right foot limited to breakdown of skin [HCC]

L97.512 Non-pressure chronic ulcer of other part of right foot with fat layer exposed [HCC]

L97.513 Non-pressure chronic ulcer of other part of right foot with necrosis of muscle [HCC]

L97.514 Non-pressure chronic ulcer of other part of right foot with necrosis of bone [HCC]

L97.515 Non-pressure chronic ulcer of other part of right foot with muscle involvement without evidence of necrosis [HCC]

L97.516 Non-pressure chronic ulcer of other part of right foot with bone involvement without evidence of necrosis [HCC]

L97.518 Non-pressure chronic ulcer of other part of right foot with other specified severity [HCC]

L97.519 Non-pressure chronic ulcer of other part of right foot with unspecified severity [HCC]

L97.52 Non-pressure chronic ulcer of other part of left foot

● New code   ▲ Revised code   **Excludes1:** Not coded here   **Excludes2:** Not included here   ⊗ Placeholder required   ⑦7th digit required

L97.521   Non-pressure chronic ulcer of other part of left foot limited to breakdown of skin [HCC]

L97.522   Non-pressure chronic ulcer of other part of left foot with fat layer exposed [HCC]

L97.523   Non-pressure chronic ulcer of other part of left foot with necrosis of muscle [HCC]

L97.524   Non-pressure chronic ulcer of other part of left foot with necrosis of bone [HCC]

L97.525   Non-pressure chronic ulcer of other part of left foot with muscle involvement without evidence of necrosis [HCC]

L97.526   Non-pressure chronic ulcer of other part of left foot with bone involvement without evidence of necrosis [HCC]

L97.528   Non-pressure chronic ulcer of other part of left foot with other specified severity [HCC]

L97.529   Non-pressure chronic ulcer of other part of left foot with unspecified severity [HCC]

L97.8   **Non-pressure chronic ulcer of other part of lower leg**

   L97.80   Non-pressure chronic ulcer of other part of unspecified lower leg [HCC]

L97.801   Non-pressure chronic ulcer of other part of unspecified lower leg limited to breakdown of skin [HCC]

L97.802   Non-pressure chronic ulcer of other part of unspecified lower leg with fat layer exposed [HCC]

L97.803   Non-pressure chronic ulcer of other part of unspecified lower leg with necrosis of muscle [HCC]

L97.804   Non-pressure chronic ulcer of other part of unspecified lower leg with necrosis of bone [HCC]

L97.805   Non-pressure chronic ulcer of other part of unspecified lower leg with muscle involvement without evidence of necrosis [HCC]

L97.806   Non-pressure chronic ulcer of other part of unspecified lower leg with bone involvement without evidence of necrosis [HCC]

L97.808   Non-pressure chronic ulcer of other part of unspecified lower leg with other specified severity [HCC]

L97.809   Non-pressure chronic ulcer of other part of unspecified lower leg with unspecified severity [HCC]

   L97.81   Non-pressure chronic ulcer of other part of right lower leg

L97.811   Non-pressure chronic ulcer of other part of right lower leg limited to breakdown of skin [HCC]

L97.812   Non-pressure chronic ulcer of other part of right lower leg with fat layer exposed [HCC]

L97.813   Non-pressure chronic ulcer of other part of right lower leg with necrosis of muscle [HCC]

L97.814   Non-pressure chronic ulcer of other part of right lower leg with necrosis of bone [HCC]

L97.815   Non-pressure chronic ulcer of other part of right lower leg with muscle involvement without evidence of necrosis [HCC]

L97.816   Non-pressure chronic ulcer of other part of right lower leg with bone involvement without evidence of necrosis [HCC]

L97.818   Non-pressure chronic ulcer of other part of right lower leg with other specified severity [HCC]

L97.819   Non-pressure chronic ulcer of other part of right lower leg with unspecified severity [HCC]

   L97.82   **Non-pressure chronic ulcer of other part of left lower leg**

L97.821   Non-pressure chronic ulcer of other part of left lower leg limited to breakdown of skin [HCC]

L97.822   Non-pressure chronic ulcer of other part of left lower leg with fat layer exposed [HCC]

L97.823   Non-pressure chronic ulcer of other part of left lower leg with necrosis of muscle [HCC]

L97.824   Non-pressure chronic ulcer of other part of left lower leg with necrosis of bone [HCC]

L97.825   Non-pressure chronic ulcer of other part of left lower leg with muscle involvement without evidence of necrosis [HCC]

L97.826   Non-pressure chronic ulcer of other part of left lower leg with bone involvement without evidence of necrosis [HCC]

L97.828   Non-pressure chronic ulcer of other part of left lower leg with other specified severity [HCC]

L97.829   Non-pressure chronic ulcer of other part of left lower leg with unspecified severity [HCC]

L97.9   **Non-pressure chronic ulcer of unspecified part of lower leg**

   L97.90   Non-pressure chronic ulcer of unspecified part of unspecified lower leg

L97.901   Non-pressure chronic ulcer of unspecified part of unspecified lower leg limited to breakdown of skin [HCC]

L97.902   Non-pressure chronic ulcer of unspecified part of unspecified lower leg with fat layer exposed

L97.903   Non-pressure chronic ulcer of unspecified part of unspecified lower leg with necrosis of muscle [HCC]

L97.904   Non-pressure chronic ulcer of unspecified part of unspecified lower leg with necrosis of bone [HCC]

L97.905   Non-pressure chronic ulcer of unspecified part of unspecified lower leg with muscle involvement without evidence of necrosis [HCC]

L97.906   Non-pressure chronic ulcer of unspecified part of unspecified lower

---

leg with bone involvement without
evidence of necrosis [HCC]

L97.908   **Non-pressure chronic ulcer of
unspecified part of unspecified lower
leg with other specified severity** [HCC]

L97.909   **Non-pressure chronic ulcer of
unspecified part of unspecified lower
leg with unspecified severity** [HCC]

L97.91   **Non-pressure chronic ulcer of unspecified part
of right lower leg**

L97.911   **Non-pressure chronic ulcer of
unspecified part of right lower leg
limited to breakdown of skin** [HCC]

L97.912   **Non-pressure chronic ulcer of
unspecified part of right lower leg
with fat layer exposed** [HCC]

L97.913   **Non-pressure chronic ulcer of
unspecified part of right lower leg
with necrosis of muscle** [HCC]

L97.914   **Non-pressure chronic ulcer of
unspecified part of right lower leg
with necrosis of bone** [HCC]

L97.915   **Non-pressure chronic ulcer of
unspecified part of right lower leg
with muscle involvement without
evidence of necrosis** [HCC]

L97.916   **Non-pressure chronic ulcer of
unspecified part of right lower leg
with bone involvement without
evidence of necrosis** [HCC]

L97.918   **Non-pressure chronic ulcer of
unspecified part of right lower leg
with other specified severity** [HCC]

L97.919   **Non-pressure chronic ulcer of
unspecified part of right lower leg
with unspecified severity** [HCC]

L97.92   **Non-pressure chronic ulcer of unspecified part
of left lower leg** [HCC]

L97.921   **Non-pressure chronic ulcer of
unspecified part of left lower leg
limited to breakdown of skin** [HCC]

L97.922   **Non-pressure chronic ulcer of
unspecified part of left lower leg with
fat layer exposed** [HCC]

L97.923   **Non-pressure chronic ulcer of
unspecified part of left lower leg with
necrosis of muscle** [HCC]

L97.924   **Non-pressure chronic ulcer of
unspecified part of left lower leg with
necrosis of bone** [HCC]

L97.925   **Non-pressure chronic ulcer of
unspecified part of left lower leg with
muscle involvement without evidence
of necrosis** [HCC]

L97.926   **Non-pressure chronic ulcer of
unspecified part of left lower leg with
bone involvement without evidence
of necrosis** [HCC]

L97.928   **Non-pressure chronic ulcer of
unspecified part of left lower leg with
other specified severity** [HCC]

L97.929   **Non-pressure chronic ulcer of
unspecified part of left lower leg with
unspecified severity** [HCC]

L98   **Other disorders of skin and subcutaneous tissue, not elsewhere
classified**

L98.0   **Pyogenic granuloma**

Excludes2: pyogenic granuloma of gingiva (K06.8)

pyogenic granuloma of maxillary alveolar ridge (K04.5)

pyogenic granuloma of oral mucosa (K13.4)

L98.1   **Factitial dermatitis**

Neurotic excoriation

Excludes1: Excoriation (skin-picking) disorder (F42.4)

L98.2   **Febrile neutrophilic dermatosis [Sweet]**

L98.3   **Eosinophilic cellulitis [Wells]**

L98.4   **Non-pressure chronic ulcer of skin, not elsewhere
classified**

Chronic ulcer of skin NOS

Tropical ulcer NOS

Ulcer of skin NOS

Excludes2: pressure ulcer (pressure area) (L89.-)

gangrene (I96)

skin infections (L00-L08)

specific infections classified to A00-B99

ulcer of lower limb NEC (L97.-)

varicose ulcer (I83.0-I83.93)

L98.41   **Non-pressure chronic ulcer of buttock**

L98.411   **Non-pressure chronic ulcer of
buttock limited to breakdown of skin**
[HCC]

L98.412   **Non-pressure chronic ulcer of
buttock with fat layer exposed** [HCC]

L98.413   **Non-pressure chronic ulcer of
buttock with necrosis of muscle** [HCC]

L98.414   **Non-pressure chronic ulcer of
buttock with necrosis of bone** [HCC]

L98.415   **Non-pressure chronic ulcer of
buttock with muscle involvement
without evidence of necrosis** [HCC]

L98.416   **Non-pressure chronic ulcer of
buttock with bone involvement
without evidence of necrosis** [HCC]

L98.418   **Non-pressure chronic ulcer of
buttock with other specified severity**
[HCC]

L98.419   **Non-pressure chronic ulcer of
buttock with unspecified severity**
[HCC]

L98.42   **Non-pressure chronic ulcer of back** [HCC]

L98.421   **Non-pressure chronic ulcer of back
limited to breakdown of skin** [HCC]

L98.422   **Non-pressure chronic ulcer of back
with fat layer exposed** [HCC]

L98.423   **Non-pressure chronic ulcer of back
with necrosis of muscle** [HCC]

L98.424   **Non-pressure chronic ulcer of back
with necrosis of bone** [HCC]

L98.425   **Non-pressure chronic ulcer of back
with muscle involvement without
evidence of necrosis** [HCC]

L98.426   **Non-pressure chronic ulcer of back
with bone involvement without
evidence of necrosis** [HCC]

L98.428   **Non-pressure chronic ulcer of back
with other specified severity** [HCC]

L98.429   **Non-pressure chronic ulcer of back
with unspecified severity** [HCC]

L98.49   **Non-pressure chronic ulcer of skin of other sites**

Non-pressure chronic ulcer of skin NOS

    L98.491   **Non-pressure chronic ulcer of skin of other sites limited to breakdown of skin** [HCC]

    L98.492   **Non-pressure chronic ulcer of skin of other sites with fat layer exposed** [HCC]

    L98.493   **Non-pressure chronic ulcer of skin of other sites with necrosis of muscle** [HCC]

    L98.494   **Non-pressure chronic ulcer of skin of other sites with necrosis of bone** [HCC]

    L98.495   **Non-pressure chronic ulcer of skin of other sites with muscle involvement without evidence of necrosis** [HCC]

    L98.496   **Non-pressure chronic ulcer of skin of other sites with bone involvement without evidence of necrosis** [HCC]

    L98.498   **Non-pressure chronic ulcer of skin of other sites with other specified severity** [HCC]

    L98.499   **Non-pressure chronic ulcer of skin of other sites with unspecified severity** [HCC]

L98.5   **Mucinosis of the skin**

    Focal mucinosis

    Lichen myxedematosus

    Reticular erythematous mucinosis

    Excludes1: focal oral mucinosis (K13.79)

        myxedema (E03.9)

    L98.6   **Other infiltrative disorders of the skin and subcutaneous tissue**

    Excludes1: hyalinosis cutis et mucosae (E78.89)

L98.7   **Excessive and redundant skin and subcutaneous tissue**

    Loose or sagging skin following bariatric surgery weight loss

    Loose or sagging skin following dietary weight loss

    Loose or sagging skin, NOS

    Excludes2: acquired excess or redundant skin of eyelid (H02.3-)

        congenital excess or redundant skin of eyelid (Q10.3)

        skin changes due to chronic exposure to nonionizing radiation (L57.-)

L98.8   **Other specified disorders of the skin and subcutaneous tissue**

L98.9   **Disorder of the skin and subcutaneous tissue, unspecified**

L99   **Other disorders of skin and subcutaneous tissue in diseases classified elsewhere**

    <u>Code first</u> underlying disease, such as:

    amyloidosis (E85.-)

    Excludes1: skin disorders in diabetes (E08-E13 with .62-)

        skin disorders in gonorrhea (A54.89)

        skin disorders in syphilis (A51.31, A52.79)

Chapter 13: Diseases of the Musculoskeletal System and Connective Tissue (M00-M99)

DEFINITIONS

This chapter includes definitions of selected key words, terms and phrases and coding alerts for adding points to the clinical domain, and references to coding late effects where appropriate. An example from this chapter is as follows:

M05   Rheumatoid arthritis with rheumatoid factor
   Definition: Rheumatoid arthritis is a chronic, systemic inflammatory disorder that may affect many tissues and organs, but principally attacks the joints producing a inflammatory synovitis that often progresses to destruction of the articular cartilage and ankylosis of the joints.

MULTIPLE CODING FOR A SINGLE CONDITION

In addition to the etiology/manifestation convention that requires two codes to fully describe a single condition that affects multiple body systems, there are other single conditions that also require more than one code. "**Use Additional Code**" notes are found in the Tabular List at codes that are not part of an etiology/manifestation pair where a secondary code is useful to fully describe a condition. The sequencing rule is the same as the etiology/manifestation pair, "**Use Additional Code**" indicates that a secondary code should be added.

For example, for bacterial infections that are not included in chapter 1, a secondary code from category B95, Streptococcus, Staphylococcus, and Enterococcus, as the cause of diseases classified elsewhere, or B96, Other bacterial agents as the cause of diseases classified elsewhere, may be required to identify the bacterial organism causing the infection. A "**Use Additional Code**" note will normally be found at the infectious disease code, indicating a need for the organism code to be added as a secondary code.

 "Code first" notes are also under certain codes that are not specifically manifestation codes but may be due to an underlying cause. When there is a "Code first" note and an underlying condition is present, the underlying condition should be sequenced first.

"Code, if applicable, any causal condition first", notes indicate that this code may be assigned as a principal diagnosis when the causal condition is unknown or not applicable. If a causal condition is known, then the code for that condition should be sequenced as the principal or first-listed diagnosis.

Multiple codes may be needed for sequela, complication codes and obstetric codes to more fully describe a condition. See the specific guidelines for these conditions for further instruction.

COMBINATION CODE

A combination code is a single code used to classify: Two diagnoses, or a diagnosis with an associated secondary process (manifestation) A diagnosis with an associated complication

Combination codes are identified by referring to subterm entries in the Alphabetic Index and by reading the inclusion and exclusion notes in the Tabular List.

Assign only the combination code when that code fully identifies the diagnostic conditions involved or when the Alphabetic Index so directs. Multiple coding should not be used when the classification provides a combination code that clearly identifies all of the elements documented in the diagnosis. When the combination code lacks necessary specificity in describing the manifestation or complication, an additional code should be used as a secondary code.

SEQUELA (LATE EFFECTS)

A sequela is the residual effect (condition produced) after the acute phase of an illness or injury has terminated. There is no time limit on when a sequela code can be used. The residual may be apparent early, such as in cerebral infarction, or it may occur months or years later, such as that due to a previous injury. Coding of sequela generally requires two codes sequenced in the following order: The condition or nature of the sequela is sequenced first.

The sequela code is sequenced second.

An exception to the above guidelines are those instances where the code for the sequela is followed by a manifestation code identified in the Tabular List and title, or the sequela code has been expanded (at the fourth, fifth or sixth character levels) to include the manifestation(s). The code for the acute phase of an illness or injury that led to the sequela is never used with a code for the late effect.

SITE AND LATERALITY

Most of the codes within Chapter 13 have site and laterality designations. The site represents the bone, joint or the muscle involved. For some conditions where more than one bone, joint or muscle is usually involved, such as osteoarthritis, there is a "multiple sites" code available. For categories where no multiple site code is provided and more than one bone, joint or muscle is involved, multiple codes should be used to indicate the different sites involved.

1) **Bone versus joint**

   For certain conditions, the bone may be affected at the upper or lower end, (e.g., avascular necrosis of bone, M87, Osteoporosis, M80, M81). Though the portion of the bone affected may be at the joint, the site designation will be the bone, not the joint.

ACUTE TRAUMATIC VERSUS CHRONIC OR RECURRENT MUSCULOSKELETAL CONDITIONS

Many musculoskeletal conditions are a result of previous injury or trauma to a site or are recurrent conditions. Bone, joint or muscle conditions that are the result of a healed injury are usually found in chapter 13. Recurrent bone, joint or muscle conditions are also usually found in chapter 13. Any current, acute injury should be coded to the appropriate injury code from chapter 19. Chronic or recurrent conditions should generally be coded with a code from chapter 13. If it is difficult to determine from the documentation in the record which code is best to describe a condition, query the provider.

CODING OF PATHOLOGIC FRACTURES

7th character A is for use as long as the patient is receiving active treatment for the fracture. While the patient may be seen by a new or different provider over the course of treatment for a pathological fracture, assignment of the 7th character is based on whether the patient is undergoing active treatment and not whether the provider is seeing the patient for the first time.

7th character D is to be used for encounters after the patient has completed active treatment for the fracture and is receiving routine care for the fracture during the healing or recovery phase. The other 7th characters, listed under each subcategory in the Tabular List, are to be used for subsequent encounters for treatment of problems associated with the healing, such as malunions, nonunions, and sequelae.

Care for complications of surgical treatment for fracture repairs during the healing or recovery phase should be coded with the appropriate complication codes.

See Section I.C.19. Coding of traumatic fractures.

OSTEOPOROSIS

Osteoporosis is a systemic condition, meaning that all bones of the musculoskeletal system are affected. Therefore, site is not a component of the codes under category M81, Osteoporosis without current pathological fracture. The site codes under category M80, Osteoporosis with current pathological fracture, identify the site of the fracture, not the osteoporosis.

1) **Osteoporosis without pathological fracture**

   Category M81, Osteoporosis without current pathological fracture, is for use for patients with osteoporosis who do not currently have a pathologic fracture due to the osteoporosis, even if they have had a fracture in the past For patients with a history of osteoporosis fractures, status code Z87.310, Personal history of (healed) osteoporosis fracture, should follow the code from M81.

2) **Osteoporosis with current pathological fracture** .

   Category M80, Osteoporosis with current pathological fracture, is for patients who have a current pathologic fracture at the time of an encounter. The codes under M80 identify the site of the fracture. A code from category M80, not a traumatic fracture code, should be used for any patient with known osteoporosis who suffers a fracture, even if the patient had a minor fall or trauma, if that fall or trauma would not usually break a normal, healthy bone.

Chapter 13

Diseases of The Musculoskeletal System and Connective Tissue (M00-M99)

Note: Use an external cause code following the code for the musculoskeletal condition, if applicable, to identify the cause of the musculoskeletal condition

Excludes2: arthropathic psoriasis (L40.5-)

certain conditions originating in the perinatal period (P04-P96)

certain infectious and parasitic diseases (A00-B99)

compartment syndrome (traumatic) (T79.A-)

complications of pregnancy, childbirth and the puerperium (O00-O9A)

congenital malformations, deformations, and chromosomal abnormalities (Q00-Q99)

endocrine, nutritional and metabolic diseases (E00-E88)

injury, poisoning and certain other consequences of external causes (S00-T88)

neoplasms (C00-D49)

symptoms, signs and abnormal clinical and laboratory findings, not elsewhere classified (R00-R94)

This chapter contains the following blocks:

M00-M02	Infectious arthropathies
M04	Autoinflammatory syndromes
M97	Periprosthetic fracture around internal prosthetic joint
M05-M14	Inflammatory polyarthropathies
M15-M19	Osteoarthritis
M20-M25	Other joint disorders
M26-M27	Dentofacial anomalies [including malocclusion] and other disorders of jaw
M30-M36	Systemic connective tissue disorders
M40-M43	Deforming dorsopathies
M45-M49	Spondylopathies
M50-M54	Other dorsopathies
M60-M63	Disorders of muscles
M65-M67	Disorders of synovium and tendon
M70-M79	Other soft tissue disorders
M80-M85	Disorders of bone density and structure
M86-M90	Other osteopathies
M91-M94	Chondropathies
M95	Other disorders of the musculoskeletal system and connective tissue
M96	Intraoperative and postprocedural complications and disorders of musculoskeletal system, not elsewhere classified
M99	Biomechanical lesions, not elsewhere classified

ARTHROPATHIES (M00-M25)

Includes: Disorders affecting predominantly peripheral (limb) joints

INFECTIOUS ARTHROPATHIES (M00-M02)

Note: This block comprises arthropathies due to microbiological agents. Distinction is made between the following types of etiological relationship:

a) direct infection of joint, where organisms invade synovial tissue and microbial antigen is present in the joint; b) indirect infection, which may be of two types: a reactive arthropathy, where microbial infection of the body is established but neither organisms nor antigens can be identified in the joint, and a postinfective arthropathy, where microbial antigen is present, but recovery of an organism is inconstant and evidence of local multiplication is lacking.

M00 Pyogenic arthritis

Excludes2: infection and inflammatory reaction due to internal joint prosthesis (T84.5-)

M00.0 **Staphylococcal arthritis and polyarthritis**

Use Additional Code (B95.61-B95.8) to identify bacterial agent

M00.00 **Staphylococcal arthritis, unspecified joint**

M00.01 **Staphylococcal arthritis, shoulder**

M00.011 **Staphylococcal arthritis, right shoulder** [HCC]

M00.012 **Staphylococcal arthritis, left shoulder** [HCC]

M00.019 **Staphylococcal arthritis, unspecified shoulder** [HCC]

M00.02 **Staphylococcal arthritis, elbow]**

M00.021 **Staphylococcal arthritis, right elbow** [HCC]

M00.022 **Staphylococcal arthritis, left elbow** [HCC]

M00.029 **Staphylococcal arthritis, unspecified elbow** [HCC]

M00.03 **Staphylococcal arthritis, wrist**

Staphylococcal arthritis of carpal bones

M00.031 **Staphylococcal arthritis, right wrist** [HCC]

M00.032 **Staphylococcal arthritis, left wrist** [HCC]

M00.039 **Staphylococcal arthritis, unspecified wrist** [HCC]

M00.04 **Staphylococcal arthritis, hand**

Staphylococcal arthritis of metacarpus and phalanges

M00.041 **Staphylococcal arthritis, right hand** [HCC]

M00.042 **Staphylococcal arthritis, left hand** [HCC]

M00.049 **Staphylococcal arthritis, unspecified hand** [HCC]

M00.05 **Staphylococcal arthritis, hip**

M00.051 **Staphylococcal arthritis, right hip** [HCC]

M00.052 **Staphylococcal arthritis, left hip** [HCC]

M00.059 **Staphylococcal arthritis, unspecified hip** [HCC]

M00.06 **Staphylococcal arthritis, knee**

M00.061 **Staphylococcal arthritis, right knee** [HCC]

M00.062 **Staphylococcal arthritis, left knee** [HCC]

M00.069 **Staphylococcal arthritis, unspecified knee** [HCC]

M00.07 **Staphylococcal arthritis, ankle and foot**

Staphylococcal arthritis, tarsus, metatarsus and phalanges

M00.071 **Staphylococcal arthritis, right ankle and foot** [HCC]

M00.072 **Staphylococcal arthritis, left ankle and foot** [HCC]

M00.079 **Staphylococcal arthritis, unspecified ankle and foot** [HCC]

M00.08 **Staphylococcal arthritis, vertebrae** [HCC]

M00.09 **Staphylococcal polyarthritis** [HCC]

M00.1 **Pneumococcal arthritis and polyarthritis**

M00.10 **Pneumococcal arthritis, unspecified joint**

M00.11   **Pneumococcal arthritis, shoulder**

    M00.111 **Pneumococcal arthritis, right shoulder** [HCC]

    M00.112 **Pneumococcal arthritis, left shoulder** [HCC]

    M00.119 **Pneumococcal arthritis, unspecified shoulder** [HCC]

M00.12   **Pneumococcal arthritis, elbow**

    M00.121 **Pneumococcal arthritis, right elbow** [HCC]

    M00.122 **Pneumococcal arthritis, left elbow** [HCC]

    M00.129 **Pneumococcal arthritis, unspecified elbow** [HCC]

M00.13   **Pneumococcal arthritis, wrist**

    Pneumococcal arthritis of carpal bones

    M00.131 **Pneumococcal arthritis, right wrist** [HCC]

    M00.132 **Pneumococcal arthritis, left wrist** [HCC]

    M00.139 **Pneumococcal arthritis, unspecified wrist** [HCC]

M00.14   **Pneumococcal arthritis, hand**

    Pneumococcal arthritis of metacarpus and phalanges

    M00.141 **Pneumococcal arthritis, right hand** [HCC]

    M00.142 **Pneumococcal arthritis, left hand** [HCC]

    M00.149 **Pneumococcal arthritis, unspecified hand** [HCC]

M00.15   **Pneumococcal arthritis, hip**

    M00.151 **Pneumococcal arthritis, right hip** [HCC]

    M00.152 **Pneumococcal arthritis, left hip** [HCC]

    M00.159 **Pneumococcal arthritis, unspecified hip** [HCC]

M00.16   **Pneumococcal arthritis, knee**

    M00.161 **Pneumococcal arthritis, right knee** [HCC]

    M00.162 **Pneumococcal arthritis, left knee** [HCC]

    M00.169 **Pneumococcal arthritis, unspecified knee** [HCC]

M00.17   **Pneumococcal arthritis, ankle and foot**

    Pneumococcal arthritis, tarsus, metatarsus and phalanges

    M00.171 **Pneumococcal arthritis, right ankle and foot** [HCC]

    M00.172 **Pneumococcal arthritis, left ankle and foot** [HCC]

    M00.179 **Pneumococcal arthritis, unspecified ankle and foot**

M00.18   **Pneumococcal arthritis, vertebrae** [HCC]

M00.19   **Pneumococcal polyarthritis** [HCC]

M00.2 **Other streptococcal arthritis and polyarthritis**

   Use Additional Code (B95.0-B95.2, B95.4-B95.5) to identify bacterial agent

M00.20   **Other streptococcal arthritis, unspecified joint** [HCC]

M00.21   **Other streptococcal arthritis, shoulder**

    M00.211 **Other streptococcal arthritis, right shoulder** [HCC]

    M00.212 **Other streptococcal arthritis, left shoulder** [HCC]

    M00.219 **Other streptococcal arthritis, unspecified shoulder** [HCC]

M00.22   **Other streptococcal arthritis, elbow**

    M00.221 **Other streptococcal arthritis, right elbow** [HCC]

    M00.222 **Other streptococcal arthritis, left elbow** [HCC]

    M00.229 **Other streptococcal arthritis, unspecified elbow** [HCC]

M00.23   **Other streptococcal arthritis, wrist**

    Other streptococcal arthritis of carpal bones

    M00.231 **Other streptococcal arthritis, right wrist** [HCC]

    M00.232 **Other streptococcal arthritis, left wrist** [HCC]

    M00.239 **Other streptococcal arthritis, unspecified wrist** [HCC]

M00.24   **Other streptococcal arthritis, hand**

    Other streptococcal arthritis metacarpus and phalanges

    M00.241 **Other streptococcal arthritis, right hand** [HCC]

    M00.242 **Other streptococcal arthritis, left hand** [HCC]

    M00.249 **Other streptococcal arthritis, unspecified hand** [HCC]

M00.25   **Other streptococcal arthritis, hip**

    M00.251 **Other streptococcal arthritis, right hip** [HCC]

    M00.252 **Other streptococcal arthritis, left hip** [HCC]

    M00.259 **Other streptococcal arthritis, unspecified hip** [HCC]

M00.26   **Other streptococcal arthritis, knee**

    M00.261 **Other streptococcal arthritis, right knee** [HCC]

    M00.262 **Other streptococcal arthritis, left knee** [HCC]

    M00.269 **Other streptococcal arthritis, unspecified knee** [HCC]

M00.27   **Other streptococcal arthritis, ankle and foot**

    Other streptococcal arthritis, tarsus, metatarsus and phalanges

    M00.271 **Other streptococcal arthritis, right ankle and foot** [HCC]

    M00.272 **Other streptococcal arthritis, left ankle and foot** [HCC]

    M00.279 **Other streptococcal arthritis, unspecified ankle and foot** [HCC]

M00.28   **Other streptococcal arthritis, vertebrae** [HCC]

M00.29   **Other streptococcal polyarthritis** [HCC]

M00.8 **Arthritis and polyarthritis due to other bacteria**

   Use Additional Code (B96) to identify bacteria

M00.80   **Arthritis due to other bacteria, unspecified joint** [HCC]

M00.81   **Arthritis due to other bacteria, shoulder**

    M00.811 **Arthritis due to other bacteria, right shoulder** [HCC]

    M00.812 **Arthritis due to other bacteria, left shoulder** [HCC]

    M00.819 **Arthritis due to other bacteria, unspecified shoulder** [HCC]

M00.82   **Arthritis due to other bacteria, elbow**

● New code   ▲ Revised code   **Excludes1:** Not coded here   **Excludes2:** Not included here   ⊗ Placeholder required   ⑦7ᵗʰ digit required

M00.821 Arthritis due to other bacteria, right elbow [HCC]

M00.822 Arthritis due to other bacteria, left elbow [HCC]

M00.829 Arthritis due to other bacteria, unspecified elbow [HCC]

M00.83 Arthritis due to other bacteria, wrist

Arthritis due to other bacteria, carpal bones

M00.831 Arthritis due to other bacteria, right wrist [HCC]

M00.832 Arthritis due to other bacteria, left wrist [HCC]

M00.839 Arthritis due to other bacteria, unspecified wrist [HCC]

M00.84 Arthritis due to other bacteria, hand

Arthritis due to other bacteria, metacarpus and phalanges

M00.841 Arthritis due to other bacteria, right hand [HCC]

M00.842 Arthritis due to other bacteria, left hand [HCC]

M00.849 Arthritis due to other bacteria, unspecified hand [HCC]

M00.85 Arthritis due to other bacteria, hip

M00.851 Arthritis due to other bacteria, right hip [HCC]

M00.852 Arthritis due to other bacteria, left hip [HCC]

M00.859 Arthritis due to other bacteria, unspecified hip [HCC]

M00.86 Arthritis due to other bacteria, knee

M00.861 Arthritis due to other bacteria, right knee [HCC]

M00.862 Arthritis due to other bacteria, left knee [HCC]

M00.869 Arthritis due to other bacteria, unspecified knee [HCC]

M00.87 Arthritis due to other bacteria, ankle and foot

Arthritis due to other bacteria, tarsus, metatarsus, and phalanges

M00.871 Arthritis due to other bacteria, right ankle and foot [HCC]

M00.872 Arthritis due to other bacteria, left ankle and foot [HCC]

M00.879 Arthritis due to other bacteria, unspecified ankle and foot [HCC]

M00.88 Arthritis due to other bacteria, vertebrae [HCC]

M00.89 Polyarthritis due to other bacteria [HCC]

M00.9 Pyogenic arthritis, unspecified [HCC]

Infective arthritis NOS

M01 Direct infections of joint in infectious and parasitic diseases classified elsewhere

Code first underlying disease, such as:

leprosy [Hansen's disease] (A30.-)

mycoses (B35-B49)

O'nyong-nyong fever (A92.1)

paratyphoid fever (A01.1-A01.4)

Excludes1: arthropathy in Lyme disease (A69.23)

gonococcal arthritis (A54.42)

meningococcal arthritis (A39.83)

mumps arthritis (B26.85)

postinfective arthropathy (M02.-)

postmeningococcal arthritis (A39.84)

reactive arthritis (M02.3)

rubella arthritis (B06.82)

sarcoidosis arthritis (D86.86)

typhoid fever arthritis (A01.04)

tuberculosis arthritis (A18.01-A18.02)

M01.X Direct infection of joint in infectious and parasitic diseases classified elsewhere

M01.X0 Direct infection of unspecified joint in infectious and parasitic diseases classified elsewhere [HCC]

M01.X1 Direct infection of shoulder joint in infectious and parasitic diseases classified elsewhere

M01.X11 Direct infection of right shoulder in infectious and parasitic diseases classified elsewhere [HCC]

M01.X12 Direct infection of left shoulder in infectious and parasitic diseases classified elsewhere [HCC]

M01.X19 Direct infection of unspecified shoulder in infectious and parasitic diseases classified elsewhere [HCC]

M01.X2 Direct infection of elbow in infectious and parasitic diseases classified elsewhere

M01.X21 Direct infection of right elbow in infectious and parasitic diseases classified elsewhere [HCC]

M01.X22 Direct infection of left elbow in infectious and parasitic diseases classified elsewhere [HCC]

M01.X29 Direct infection of unspecified elbow in infectious and parasitic diseases classified elsewhere [HCC]

M01.X3 Direct infection of wrist in infectious and parasitic diseases classified elsewhere

Direct infection of carpal bones in infectious and parasitic diseases classified elsewhere

M01.X31 Direct infection of right wrist in infectious and parasitic diseases classified elsewhere [HCC]

M01.X32 Direct infection of left wrist in infectious and parasitic diseases classified elsewhere [HCC]

M01.X39 Direct infection of unspecified wrist in infectious and parasitic diseases classified elsewhere [HCC]

M01.X4 Direct infection of hand in infectious and parasitic diseases classified elsewhere

Direct infection of metacarpus and phalanges in infectious and parasitic diseases classified elsewhere

M01.X41 Direct infection of right hand in infectious and parasitic diseases classified elsewhere [HCC]

M01.X42 Direct infection of left hand in infectious and parasitic diseases classified elsewhere [HCC]

M01.X49 Direct infection of unspecified hand in infectious and parasitic diseases classified elsewhere [HCC]

M01.X5 Direct infection of hip in infectious and parasitic diseases classified elsewhere

M01.X51 Direct infection of right hip in infectious and parasitic diseases classified elsewhere [HCC]

M01.X52 Direct infection of left hip in infectious and parasitic diseases classified elsewhere [HCC]

M01.X59 Direct infection of unspecified hip in infectious and parasitic diseases classified elsewhere [HCC]

M01.X6 Direct infection of knee in infectious and parasitic diseases classified elsewhere

M01.X61 Direct infection of right knee in infectious and parasitic diseases classified elsewhere [HCC]

M01.X62 Direct infection of left knee in infectious and parasitic diseases classified elsewhere [HCC]

M01.X69 Direct infection of unspecified knee in infectious and parasitic diseases classified elsewhere [HCC]

M01.X7 Direct infection of ankle and foot in infectious and parasitic diseases classified elsewhere

Direct infection of tarsus, metatarsus and phalanges in infectious and parasitic diseases classified elsewhere

M01.X71 Direct infection of right ankle and foot in infectious and parasitic diseases classified elsewhere [HCC]

M01.X72 Direct infection of left ankle and foot in infectious and parasitic diseases classified elsewhere [HCC]

M01.X79 Direct infection of unspecified ankle and foot in infectious and parasitic diseases [HCC]

classified elsewhere [HCC]

M01.X8 Direct infection of vertebrae in infectious and parasitic diseases classified elsewhere [HCC]

M01.X9 Direct infection of multiple joints in infectious and parasitic diseases classified elsewhere [HCC]

M02 Postinfective and reactive arthropathies

Code first underlying disease, such as:

congenital syphilis [Clutton's joints] (A50.5) enteritis due to Yersinia enterocolitica (A04.6)

infective endocarditis (I33.0)

viral hepatitis (B15-B19)

Excludes1: Behçet's disease (M35.2)

direct infections of joint in infectious and parasitic diseases classified elsewhere (M01.-)

postmeningococcal arthritis (A39.84)

mumps arthritis (B26.85)

rubella arthritis (B06.82)

syphilis arthritis (late) (A52.77)

rheumatic fever (I00)

tabetic arthropathy [Charcôt's] (A52.16)

M02.0 Arthropathy following intestinal bypass

M02.00 Arthropathy following intestinal bypass, unspecified site

M02.01 Arthropathy following intestinal bypass, shoulder

M02.011 Arthropathy following intestinal bypass, right shoulder

M02.012 Arthropathy following intestinal bypass, left shoulder

M02.019 Arthropathy following intestinal bypass, unspecified shoulder

M02.02 Arthropathy following intestinal bypass, elbow

M02.021 Arthropathy following intestinal bypass, right elbow

M02.022 Arthropathy following intestinal bypass, left elbow

M02.029 Arthropathy following intestinal bypass, unspecified elbow

M02.03 Arthropathy following intestinal bypass, wrist

Arthropathy following intestinal bypass, carpal bones

M02.031 Arthropathy following intestinal bypass, right wrist

M02.032 Arthropathy following intestinal bypass, left wrist

M02.039 Arthropathy following intestinal bypass, unspecified wrist

M02.04 Arthropathy following intestinal bypass, hand

Arthropathy following intestinal bypass, metacarpals and phalanges

M02.041 Arthropathy following intestinal bypass, right hand

M02.042 Arthropathy following intestinal bypass, left hand

M02.049 Arthropathy following intestinal bypass, unspecified hand

M02.05 Arthropathy following intestinal bypass, hip

M02.051 Arthropathy following intestinal bypass, right hip

M02.052 Arthropathy following intestinal bypass, left hip

M02.059 Arthropathy following intestinal bypass, unspecified hip

M02.06 Arthropathy following intestinal bypass, knee

M02.061 Arthropathy following intestinal bypass, right knee

M02.062 Arthropathy following intestinal bypass, left knee

M02.069 Arthropathy following intestinal bypass, unspecified knee

M02.07 Arthropathy following intestinal bypass, ankle and foot

Arthropathy following intestinal bypass, tarsus, metatarsus and phalanges

M02.071 Arthropathy following intestinal bypass, right ankle and foot

M02.072 Arthropathy following intestinal bypass, left ankle and foot

M02.079 Arthropathy following intestinal bypass, unspecified ankle and foot

M02.08 Arthropathy following intestinal bypass, vertebrae

M02.09 Arthropathy following intestinal bypass, multiple sites

M02.1 Postdysenteric arthropathy

M02.10 Postdysenteric arthropathy, unspecified site [HCC]

M02.11 Postdysenteric arthropathy, shoulder

M02.111 Postdysenteric arthropathy, right shoulder [HCC]

M02.112 Postdysenteric arthropathy, left shoulder [HCC]

● New code   ▲ Revised code   **Excludes1:** Not coded here   **Excludes2:** Not included here   ⊗ Placeholder required   ⑦ 7th digit required

M02.119 Postdysenteric arthropathy, unspecified shoulder [HCC]

M02.12 Postdysenteric arthropathy, elbow

M02.121 Postdysenteric arthropathy, right elbow [HCC]

M02.122 Postdysenteric arthropathy, left elbow [HCC]

M02.129 Postdysenteric arthropathy, unspecified elbow [HCC]

M02.13 Postdysenteric arthropathy, wrist

Postdysenteric arthropathy, carpal bones

M02.131 Postdysenteric arthropathy, right wrist [HCC]

M02.132 Postdysenteric arthropathy, left wrist [HCC]

M02.139 Postdysenteric arthropathy, unspecified wrist [HCC]

M02.14 Postdysenteric arthropathy, hand

Postdysenteric arthropathy, metacarpus and phalanges

M02.141 Postdysenteric arthropathy, right hand [HCC]

M02.142 Postdysenteric arthropathy, left hand [HCC]

M02.149 Postdysenteric arthropathy, unspecified hand [HCC]

M02.15 Postdysenteric arthropathy, hip

M02.151 Postdysenteric arthropathy, right hip [HCC]

M02.152 Postdysenteric arthropathy, left hip [HCC]

M02.159 Postdysenteric arthropathy, unspecified hip [HCC]

M02.16 Postdysenteric arthropathy, knee

M02.161 Postdysenteric arthropathy, right knee [HCC]

M02.162 Postdysenteric arthropathy, left knee [HCC]

M02.169 Postdysenteric arthropathy, unspecified knee [HCC]

M02.17 Postdysenteric arthropathy, ankle and foot

Postdysenteric arthropathy, tarsus, metatarsus and phalanges

M02.171 Postdysenteric arthropathy, right ankle and foot [HCC]

M02.172 Postdysenteric arthropathy, left ankle and foot [HCC]

M02.179 Postdysenteric arthropathy, unspecified ankle and foot [HCC]

M02.18 Postdysenteric arthropathy, vertebrae [HCC]

M02.19 Postdysenteric arthropathy, multiple sites [HCC]

M02.2 Postimmunization arthropathy

M02.20 Postimmunization arthropathy, unspecified site

M02.21 Postimmunization arthropathy, shoulder

M02.211 Postimmunization arthropathy, right shoulder

M02.212 Postimmunization arthropathy, left shoulder

M02.219 Postimmunization arthropathy, unspecified shoulder

M02.22 Postimmunization arthropathy, elbow

M02.221 Postimmunization arthropathy, right elbow

M02.222 Postimmunization arthropathy, left elbow

M02.229 Postimmunization arthropathy, unspecified elbow

M02.23 Postimmunization arthropathy, wrist

Postimmunization arthropathy, carpal bones

M02.231 Postimmunization arthropathy, right wrist

M02.232 Postimmunization arthropathy, left wrist

M02.239 Postimmunization arthropathy, unspecified wrist

M02.24 Postimmunization arthropathy, hand

Postimmunization arthropathy, metacarpus and phalanges

M02.241 Postimmunization arthropathy, right hand

M02.242 Postimmunization arthropathy, left hand

M02.249 Postimmunization arthropathy, unspecified hand

M02.25 Postimmunization arthropathy, hip

M02.251 Postimmunization arthropathy, right hip

M02.252 Postimmunization arthropathy, left hip

M02.259 Postimmunization arthropathy, unspecified hip

M02.26 Postimmunization arthropathy, knee

M02.261 Postimmunization arthropathy, right knee

M02.262 Postimmunization arthropathy, left knee

M02.269 Postimmunization arthropathy, unspecified knee

M02.27 Postimmunization arthropathy, ankle and foot

Postimmunization arthropathy, tarsus, metatarsus and phalanges

M02.271 Postimmunization arthropathy, right ankle and foot

M02.272 Postimmunization arthropathy, left ankle and foot

M02.279 Postimmunization arthropathy, unspecified ankle and foot

M02.28 Postimmunization arthropathy, vertebrae

M02.29 Postimmunization arthropathy, multiple sites

M02.3 Reiter's disease

Reactive arthritis

M02.30 Reiter's disease, unspecified site [HCC]

M02.31 Reiter's disease, shoulder

M02.311 Reiter's disease, right shoulder [HCC]

M02.312 Reiter's disease, left shoulder [HCC]

M02.319 Reiter's disease, unspecified shoulder [HCC]

M02.32 Reiter's disease, elbow

M02.321 Reiter's disease, right elbow [HCC]

M02.322 Reiter's disease, left elbow [HCC]

M02.329 Reiter's disease, unspecified elbow [HCC]

M02.33 Reiter's disease, wrist

Reiter's disease, carpal bones

M02.331 Reiter's disease, right wrist [HCC]

M02.332 Reiter's disease, left wrist [HCC]

M02.339 Reiter's disease, unspecified wrist [HCC]

M02.34 Reiter's disease, hand

Reiter's disease, metacarpus and phalanges

M02.341 Reiter's disease, right hand [HCC]

M02.342 Reiter's disease, left hand [HCC]

M02.349 Reiter's disease, unspecified hand [HCC]

M02.35 Reiter's disease, hip

M02.351 Reiter's disease, right hip [HCC]

M02.352 Reiter's disease, left hip [HCC]

M02.359 Reiter's disease, unspecified hip [HCC]

M02.36 Reiter's disease, knee

M02.361 Reiter's disease, right knee [HCC]

M02.362 Reiter's disease, left knee

M02.369 Reiter's disease, unspecified knee [HCC]

M02.37 Reiter's disease, ankle and foot

Reiter's disease, tarsus, metatarsus and phalanges

M02.371 Reiter's disease, right ankle and foot [HCC]

M02.372 Reiter's disease, left ankle and foot [HCC]

M02.379 Reiter's disease, unspecified ankle and foot [HCC]

M02.38 Reiter's disease, vertebrae [HCC]

M02.39 Reiter's disease, multiple sites [HCC]

M02.8 Other reactive arthropathies

M02.80 Other reactive arthropathies, unspecified site [HCC]

M02.81 Other reactive arthropathies, shoulder

M02.811 Other reactive arthropathies, right shoulder [HCC]

M02.812 Other reactive arthropathies, left shoulder [HCC]

M02.819 Other reactive arthropathies, unspecified shoulder [HCC]

M02.82 Other reactive arthropathies, elbow

M02.821 Other reactive arthropathies, right elbow [HCC]

M02.822 Other reactive arthropathies, left elbow [HCC]

M02.829 Other reactive arthropathies, unspecified elbow [HCC]

M02.83 Other reactive arthropathies, wrist

Other reactive arthropathies, carpal bones

M02.831 Other reactive arthropathies, right wrist [HCC]

M02.832 Other reactive arthropathies, left wrist [HCC]

M02.839 Other reactive arthropathies, unspecified wrist [HCC]

M02.84 Other reactive arthropathies, hand

Other reactive arthropathies, metacarpus and phalanges

M02.841 Other reactive arthropathies, right hand [HCC]

M02.842 Other reactive arthropathies, left hand [HCC]

M02.849 Other reactive arthropathies, unspecified hand [HCC]

M02.85 Other reactive arthropathies, hip

M02.851 Other reactive arthropathies, right hip [HCC]

M02.852 Other reactive arthropathies, left hip [HCC]

M02.859 Other reactive arthropathies, unspecified hip [HCC]

M02.86 Other reactive arthropathies, knee

M02.861 Other reactive arthropathies, right knee [HCC]

M02.862 Other reactive arthropathies, left knee [HCC]

M02.869 Other reactive arthropathies, unspecified knee [HCC]

M02.87 Other reactive arthropathies, ankle and foot

Other reactive arthropathies, tarsus, metatarsus and phalanges

M02.871 Other reactive arthropathies, right ankle and foot [HCC]

M02.872 Other reactive arthropathies, left ankle and foot [HCC]

M02.879 Other reactive arthropathies, unspecified ankle and foot [HCC]

M02.88 Other reactive arthropathies, vertebrae [HCC]

M02.89 Other reactive arthropathies, multiple sites [HCC]

M02.9 Reactive arthropathy, unspecified [HCC]

AUTOINFLAMMATORY SYNDROMES (M04)

M04 Autoinflammatory syndromes

Excludes2: Crohn's disease (K50.-)

M04.1 Periodic fever syndromes [HCC]

Familial Mediterranean fever

Hyperimmunoglobin D syndrome

Mevalonate kinase deficiency

Tumor necrosis factor receptor associated periodic syndrome [TRAPS]

M04.2 Cryopyrin-associated periodic syndromes [HCC]

Chronic infantile neurological, cutaneous and articular syndrome [CINCA]

Familial cold autoinflammatory syndrome

Familial cold urticaria

Muckle-Wells syndrome

Neonatal onset multisystemic inflammatory disorder [NOMID]

M04.8 Other autoinflammatory syndromes [HCC]

Blau syndrome

Deficiency of interleukin 1 receptor antagonist [DIRA]

Majeed syndrome

Periodic fever, aphthous stomatitis, pharyngitis, and adenopathy syndrome [PFAPA]

Pyogenic arthritis, pyoderma gangrenosum, and acne syndrome [PAPA]

M04.9 Autoinflammatory syndrome, unspecified [HCC]

INFLAMMATORY POLYARTHROPATHIES (M05-M14)

M05 Rheumatoid arthritis with rheumatoid factor

Definition: Rheumatoid arthritis is a chronic, systemic inflammatory disorder that may affect many tissues and organs, but principally attacks the joints producing a inflammatory synovitis that often progresses to destruction of the articular cartilage and ankylosis of the joints.

Excludes1: rheumatic fever (I00)

juvenile rheumatoid arthritis (M08.-)

rheumatoid arthritis of spine (M45.-)

M05.0 Felty's syndrome

Rheumatoid arthritis with splenoadenomegaly and leukopenia

M05.00 Felty's syndrome, unspecified site [HCC]

M05.01 Felty's syndrome, shoulder

M05.011 Felty's syndrome, right shoulder

M05.012 Felty's syndrome, left shoulder [HCC]

M05.019 Felty's syndrome, unspecified shoulder [HCC]

M05.02 Felty's syndrome, elbow

M05.021 Felty's syndrome, right elbow [HCC]

M05.022 Felty's syndrome, left elbow [HCC]

M05.029 Felty's syndrome, unspecified elbow [HCC]

M05.03 Felty's syndrome, wrist

Felty's syndrome, carpal bones

M05.031 Felty's syndrome, right wrist [HCC]

M05.032 Felty's syndrome, left wrist [HCC]

M05.039 Felty's syndrome, unspecified wrist [HCC]

M05.04 Felty's syndrome, hand

Felty's syndrome, metacarpus and phalanges

M05.041 Felty's syndrome, right hand [HCC]

M05.042 Felty's syndrome, left hand [HCC]

M05.049 Felty's syndrome, unspecified hand [HCC]

M05.05 Felty's syndrome, hip

M05.051 Felty's syndrome, right hip [HCC]

M05.052 Felty's syndrome, left hip [HCC]

M05.059 Felty's syndrome, unspecified hip [HCC]

M05.06 Felty's syndrome, knee

M05.061 Felty's syndrome, right knee [HCC]

M05.062 Felty's syndrome, left knee [HCC]

M05.069 Felty's syndrome, unspecified knee [HCC]

M05.07 Felty's syndrome, ankle and foot

Felty's syndrome, tarsus, metatarsus and phalanges

M05.071 Felty's syndrome, right ankle and foot [HCC]

M05.072 Felty's syndrome, left ankle and foot [HCC]

M05.079 Felty's syndrome, unspecified ankle and foot [HCC]

M05.09 Felty's syndrome, multiple sites [HCC]

M05.1 Rheumatoid lung disease with rheumatoid arthritis

M05.10 Rheumatoid lung disease with rheumatoid arthritis of unspecified site [HCC]

M05.11 Rheumatoid lung disease with rheumatoid arthritis of shoulder

M05.111 Rheumatoid lung disease with rheumatoid arthritis of right shoulder

M05.112 Rheumatoid lung disease with rheumatoid arthritis of left shoulder [HCC]

M05.119 Rheumatoid lung disease with rheumatoid arthritis of unspecified shoulder [HCC]

M05.12 Rheumatoid lung disease with rheumatoid arthritis of elbow

M05.121 Rheumatoid lung disease with rheumatoid arthritis of right elbow [HCC]

M05.122 Rheumatoid lung disease with rheumatoid arthritis of left elbow [HCC]

M05.129 Rheumatoid lung disease with rheumatoid arthritis of unspecified elbow [HCC]

M05.13 Rheumatoid lung disease with rheumatoid arthritis of wrist

Rheumatoid lung disease with rheumatoid arthritis, carpal bones

M05.131 Rheumatoid lung disease with rheumatoid arthritis of right wrist [HCC]

M05.132 Rheumatoid lung disease with rheumatoid arthritis of left wrist [HCC]

M05.139 Rheumatoid lung disease with rheumatoid arthritis of unspecified wrist [HCC]

M05.14 Rheumatoid lung disease with rheumatoid arthritis of hand

Rheumatoid lung disease with rheumatoid arthritis, metacarpus and phalanges

M05.141 Rheumatoid lung disease with rheumatoid arthritis of right hand [HCC]

M05.142 Rheumatoid lung disease with rheumatoid arthritis of left hand [HCC]

M05.149 Rheumatoid lung disease with rheumatoid arthritis of unspecified hand [HCC]

M05.15 Rheumatoid lung disease with rheumatoid arthritis of hip

M05.151 Rheumatoid lung disease with rheumatoid arthritis of right hip [HCC]

M05.152 Rheumatoid lung disease with rheumatoid arthritis of left hip [HCC]

M05.159 Rheumatoid lung disease with rheumatoid arthritis of unspecified hip [HCC]

M05.16 Rheumatoid lung disease with rheumatoid arthritis of knee [HCC]

M05.161 Rheumatoid lung disease with rheumatoid arthritis of right knee [HCC]

M05.162 Rheumatoid lung disease with rheumatoid arthritis of left knee [HCC]

M05.169 Rheumatoid lung disease with rheumatoid arthritis of unspecified knee [HCC]

M05.17 Rheumatoid lung disease with rheumatoid arthritis of ankle and foot

Rheumatoid lung disease with rheumatoid arthritis, tarsus, metatarsus and phalanges

M05.171 Rheumatoid lung disease with rheumatoid arthritis of right ankle and foot [HCC]

M05.172 Rheumatoid lung disease with rheumatoid arthritis of left ankle and foot [HCC]

M05.179 Rheumatoid lung disease with rheumatoid arthritis of unspecified ankle and foot [HCC]

M05.19 Rheumatoid lung disease with rheumatoid arthritis of multiple sites [HCC]

M05.2 Rheumatoid vasculitis with rheumatoid arthritis

M05.20 Rheumatoid vasculitis with rheumatoid arthritis of unspecified site [HCC]

M05.21 Rheumatoid vasculitis with rheumatoid arthritis of shoulder

M05.211 Rheumatoid vasculitis with rheumatoid arthritis of right shoulder

M05.212 Rheumatoid vasculitis with rheumatoid arthritis of left shoulder [HCC]

M05.219 Rheumatoid vasculitis with rheumatoid arthritis of unspecified shoulder [HCC]

M05.22 Rheumatoid vasculitis with rheumatoid arthritis of elbow

M05.221 Rheumatoid vasculitis with rheumatoid arthritis of right elbow [HCC]

M05.222 Rheumatoid vasculitis with rheumatoid arthritis of left elbow [HCC]

M05.229 Rheumatoid vasculitis with rheumatoid arthritis of unspecified elbow [HCC]

M05.23 Rheumatoid vasculitis with rheumatoid arthritis of wrist

Rheumatoid vasculitis with rheumatoid arthritis, carpal bones

M05.231 Rheumatoid vasculitis with rheumatoid arthritis of right wrist [HCC]

M05.232 Rheumatoid vasculitis with rheumatoid arthritis of left wrist [HCC]

M05.239 Rheumatoid vasculitis with rheumatoid arthritis of unspecified wrist [HCC]

M05.24 Rheumatoid vasculitis with rheumatoid arthritis of hand

Rheumatoid vasculitis with rheumatoid arthritis, metacarpus and phalanges

M05.241 Rheumatoid vasculitis with rheumatoid arthritis of right hand [HCC]

M05.242 Rheumatoid vasculitis with rheumatoid arthritis of left hand [HCC]

M05.249 Rheumatoid vasculitis with rheumatoid arthritis of unspecified hand [HCC]

M05.25 Rheumatoid vasculitis with rheumatoid arthritis of hip

M05.251 Rheumatoid vasculitis with rheumatoid arthritis of right hip [HCC]

M05.252 Rheumatoid vasculitis with rheumatoid arthritis of left hip [HCC]

M05.259 Rheumatoid vasculitis with rheumatoid arthritis of unspecified hip [HCC]

M05.26 Rheumatoid vasculitis with rheumatoid arthritis of knee

M05.261 Rheumatoid vasculitis with rheumatoid arthritis of right knee [HCC]

M05.262 Rheumatoid vasculitis with rheumatoid arthritis of left knee [HCC]

M05.269 Rheumatoid vasculitis with rheumatoid arthritis of unspecified knee [HCC]

M05.27 Rheumatoid vasculitis with rheumatoid arthritis of ankle and foot

Rheumatoid vasculitis with rheumatoid arthritis, tarsus, metatarsus and phalanges

M05.271 Rheumatoid vasculitis with rheumatoid arthritis of right ankle and foot [HCC]

M05.272 Rheumatoid vasculitis with rheumatoid arthritis of left ankle and foot [HCC]

M05.279 Rheumatoid vasculitis with rheumatoid arthritis of unspecified ankle and foot [HCC]

M05.29 Rheumatoid vasculitis with rheumatoid arthritis of multiple sites [HCC]

M05.3 Rheumatoid heart disease with rheumatoid arthritis

Rheumatoid carditis

Rheumatoid endocarditis

Rheumatoid myocarditis

Rheumatoid pericarditis

M05.30 Rheumatoid heart disease with rheumatoid arthritis of unspecified site

M05.31 Rheumatoid heart disease with rheumatoid arthritis of shoulder

M05.311 Rheumatoid heart disease with rheumatoid arthritis of right shoulder [HCC]

M05.312 Rheumatoid heart disease with rheumatoid arthritis of left shoulder [HCC]

M05.319 Rheumatoid heart disease with rheumatoid arthritis of unspecified shoulder [HCC]

M05.32 Rheumatoid heart disease with rheumatoid arthritis of elbow

M05.321 Rheumatoid heart disease with rheumatoid arthritis of right elbow [HCC]

M05.322 Rheumatoid heart disease with rheumatoid arthritis of left elbow [HCC]

M05.329 Rheumatoid heart disease with rheumatoid arthritis of unspecified elbow [HCC]

M05.33 Rheumatoid heart disease with rheumatoid arthritis of wrist

Rheumatoid heart disease with rheumatoid arthritis, carpal bones

M05.331 Rheumatoid heart disease with rheumatoid arthritis of right wrist [HCC]

● New code　▲ Revised code　Excludes1: Not coded here　Excludes2: Not included here　⊗ Placeholder required　⑦7th digit required

M05.332 Rheumatoid heart disease with rheumatoid arthritis of left wrist [HCC]

M05.339 Rheumatoid heart disease with rheumatoid arthritis of unspecified wrist [HCC]

M05.34 Rheumatoid heart disease with rheumatoid arthritis of hand

Rheumatoid heart disease with rheumatoid arthritis, metacarpus and phalanges

M05.341 Rheumatoid heart disease with rheumatoid arthritis of right hand [HCC]

M05.342 Rheumatoid heart disease with rheumatoid arthritis of left hand [HCC]

M05.349 Rheumatoid heart disease with rheumatoid arthritis of unspecified hand [HCC]

M05.35 Rheumatoid heart disease with rheumatoid arthritis of hip

M05.351 Rheumatoid heart disease with rheumatoid arthritis of right hip [HCC]

M05.352 Rheumatoid heart disease with rheumatoid arthritis of left hip [HCC]

M05.359 Rheumatoid heart disease with rheumatoid arthritis of unspecified hip [HCC]

M05.36 Rheumatoid heart disease with rheumatoid arthritis of knee

M05.361 Rheumatoid heart disease with rheumatoid arthritis of right knee [HCC]

M05.362 Rheumatoid heart disease with rheumatoid arthritis of left knee [HCC]

M05.369 Rheumatoid heart disease with rheumatoid arthritis of unspecified knee [HCC]

M05.37 Rheumatoid heart disease with rheumatoid arthritis of ankle and foot

Rheumatoid heart disease with rheumatoid arthritis, tarsus, metatarsus and phalanges

M05.371 Rheumatoid heart disease with rheumatoid arthritis of right ankle and foot [HCC]

M05.372 Rheumatoid heart disease with rheumatoid arthritis of left ankle and foot [HCC]

M05.379 Rheumatoid heart disease with rheumatoid arthritis of unspecified ankle and foot [HCC]

M05.39 Rheumatoid heart disease with rheumatoid arthritis of multiple sites [HCC]

M05.4 Rheumatoid myopathy with rheumatoid arthritis

M05.40 Rheumatoid myopathy with rheumatoid arthritis of unspecified site

M05.41 Rheumatoid myopathy with rheumatoid arthritis of shoulder

M05.411 Rheumatoid myopathy with rheumatoid arthritis of right shoulder [HCC]

M05.412 Rheumatoid myopathy with rheumatoid arthritis of left shoulder [HCC]

M05.419 Rheumatoid myopathy with rheumatoid arthritis of unspecified shoulder [HCC]

M05.42 Rheumatoid myopathy with rheumatoid arthritis of elbow

M05.421 Rheumatoid myopathy with rheumatoid arthritis of right elbow [HCC]

M05.422 Rheumatoid myopathy with rheumatoid arthritis of left elbow [HCC]

M05.429 Rheumatoid myopathy with rheumatoid arthritis of unspecified elbow [HCC]

M05.43 Rheumatoid myopathy with rheumatoid arthritis of wrist

Rheumatoid myopathy with rheumatoid arthritis, carpal bones

M05.431 Rheumatoid myopathy with rheumatoid arthritis of right wrist [HCC]

M05.432 Rheumatoid myopathy with rheumatoid arthritis of left wrist [HCC]

M05.439 Rheumatoid myopathy with rheumatoid arthritis of unspecified wrist [HCC]

M05.44 Rheumatoid myopathy with rheumatoid arthritis of hand

Rheumatoid myopathy with rheumatoid arthritis, metacarpus and phalanges

M05.441 Rheumatoid myopathy with rheumatoid arthritis of right hand [HCC]

M05.442 Rheumatoid myopathy with rheumatoid arthritis of left hand [HCC]

M05.449 Rheumatoid myopathy with rheumatoid arthritis of unspecified hand [HCC]

M05.45 Rheumatoid myopathy with rheumatoid arthritis of hip

M05.451 Rheumatoid myopathy with rheumatoid arthritis of right hip [HCC]

M05.452 Rheumatoid myopathy with rheumatoid arthritis of left hip [HCC]

M05.459 Rheumatoid myopathy with rheumatoid arthritis of unspecified hip [HCC]

M05.46 Rheumatoid myopathy with rheumatoid arthritis of knee

M05.461 Rheumatoid myopathy with rheumatoid arthritis of right knee [HCC]

M05.462 Rheumatoid myopathy with rheumatoid arthritis of left knee [HCC]

M05.469 Rheumatoid myopathy with rheumatoid arthritis of unspecified knee [HCC]

M05.47 Rheumatoid myopathy with rheumatoid arthritis of ankle and foot

Rheumatoid myopathy with rheumatoid arthritis, tarsus, metatarsus and phalanges

M05.471 Rheumatoid myopathy with rheumatoid arthritis of right ankle and foot [HCC]

M05.472 Rheumatoid myopathy with rheumatoid arthritis of left ankle and foot [HCC]

M05.479 Rheumatoid myopathy with rheumatoid arthritis of unspecified ankle and foot [HCC]

M05.49 Rheumatoid myopathy with rheumatoid arthritis of multiple sites [HCC]

M05.5 Rheumatoid polyneuropathy with rheumatoid arthritis

M05.50 Rheumatoid polyneuropathy with rheumatoid arthritis of unspecified site

M05.51 Rheumatoid polyneuropathy with rheumatoid arthritis of shoulder

M05.511 Rheumatoid polyneuropathy with rheumatoid arthritis of right shoulder [HCC]

M05.512 Rheumatoid polyneuropathy with rheumatoid arthritis of left shoulder [HCC]

M05.519 Rheumatoid polyneuropathy with rheumatoid arthritis of unspecified shoulder [HCC]

M05.52 Rheumatoid polyneuropathy with rheumatoid arthritis of elbow

M05.521 Rheumatoid polyneuropathy with rheumatoid arthritis of right elbow [HCC]

M05.522 Rheumatoid polyneuropathy with rheumatoid arthritis of left elbow [HCC]

M05.529 Rheumatoid polyneuropathy with rheumatoid arthritis of unspecified elbow [HCC]

M05.53 Rheumatoid polyneuropathy with rheumatoid arthritis of wrist

Rheumatoid polyneuropathy with rheumatoid arthritis, carpal bones

M05.531 Rheumatoid polyneuropathy with rheumatoid arthritis of right wrist [HCC]

M05.532 Rheumatoid polyneuropathy with rheumatoid arthritis of left wrist [HCC]

M05.539 Rheumatoid polyneuropathy with rheumatoid arthritis of unspecified wrist [HCC]

M05.54 Rheumatoid polyneuropathy with rheumatoid arthritis of hand

Rheumatoid polyneuropathy with rheumatoid arthritis, metacarpus and phalanges

M05.541 Rheumatoid polyneuropathy with rheumatoid arthritis of right hand [HCC]

M05.542 Rheumatoid polyneuropathy with rheumatoid arthritis of left hand [HCC]

M05.549 Rheumatoid polyneuropathy with rheumatoid arthritis of unspecified hand [HCC]

M05.55 Rheumatoid polyneuropathy with rheumatoid arthritis of hip

M05.551 Rheumatoid polyneuropathy with rheumatoid arthritis of right hip [HCC]

M05.552 Rheumatoid polyneuropathy with rheumatoid arthritis of left hip [HCC]

M05.559 Rheumatoid polyneuropathy with rheumatoid arthritis of unspecified hip [HCC]

M05.56 Rheumatoid polyneuropathy with rheumatoid arthritis of knee

M05.561 Rheumatoid polyneuropathy with rheumatoid arthritis of right knee [HCC]

M05.562 Rheumatoid polyneuropathy with rheumatoid arthritis of left knee [HCC]

M05.569 Rheumatoid polyneuropathy with rheumatoid arthritis of unspecified knee [HCC]

M05.57 Rheumatoid polyneuropathy with rheumatoid arthritis of ankle and foot

Rheumatoid polyneuropathy with rheumatoid arthritis, tarsus, metatarsus and phalanges

M05.571 Rheumatoid polyneuropathy with rheumatoid arthritis of right ankle and foot [HCC]

M05.572 Rheumatoid polyneuropathy with rheumatoid arthritis of left ankle and foot [HCC]

M05.579 Rheumatoid polyneuropathy with rheumatoid arthritis of unspecified ankle and foot [HCC]

M05.59 Rheumatoid polyneuropathy with rheumatoid arthritis of multiple sites [HCC]

M05.6 Rheumatoid arthritis with involvement of other organs and systems

M05.60 Rheumatoid arthritis of unspecified site with involvement of other organs and systems

M05.61 Rheumatoid arthritis of shoulder with involvement of other organs and systems

M05.611 Rheumatoid arthritis of right shoulder with involvement of other organs and systems [HCC]

M05.612 Rheumatoid arthritis of left shoulder with involvement of other organs and systems [HCC]

M05.619 Rheumatoid arthritis of unspecified shoulder with involvement of other organs and systems [HCC]

M05.62 Rheumatoid arthritis of elbow with involvement of other organs and systems

M05.621 Rheumatoid arthritis of right elbow with involvement of other organs and systems [HCC]

M05.622 Rheumatoid arthritis of left elbow with involvement of other organs and systems [HCC]

M05.629 Rheumatoid arthritis of unspecified elbow with involvement of other organs and systems [HCC]

M05.63 Rheumatoid arthritis of wrist with involvement of other organs and systems

Rheumatoid arthritis of carpal bones with involvement of other organs and systems

M05.631 Rheumatoid arthritis of right wrist with involvement of other organs and systems [HCC]

M05.632 Rheumatoid arthritis of left wrist with involvement of other organs and systems [HCC]

● New code ▲ Revised code **Excludes1:** Not coded here **Excludes2:** Not included here ⊗ Placeholder required ⑦7ᵗʰ digit required

M05.639 Rheumatoid arthritis of unspecified wrist with involvement of other organs and systems [HCC]

M05.64 Rheumatoid arthritis of hand with involvement of other organs and systems

Rheumatoid arthritis of metacarpus and phalanges with involvement of other organs and systems

M05.641 Rheumatoid arthritis of right hand with involvement of other organs and systems [HCC]

M05.642 Rheumatoid arthritis of left hand with involvement of other organs and systems [HCC]

M05.649 Rheumatoid arthritis of unspecified hand with involvement of other organs and systems [HCC]

M05.65 Rheumatoid arthritis of hip with involvement of other organs and systems

M05.651 Rheumatoid arthritis of right hip with involvement of other organs and systems [HCC]

M05.652 Rheumatoid arthritis of left hip with involvement of other organs and systems [HCC]

M05.659 Rheumatoid arthritis of unspecified hip with involvement of other organs and systems [HCC]

M05.66 Rheumatoid arthritis of knee with involvement of other organs and systems

M05.661 Rheumatoid arthritis of right knee with involvement of other organs and systems [HCC]

M05.662 Rheumatoid arthritis of left knee with involvement of other organs and systems [HCC]

M05.669 Rheumatoid arthritis of unspecified knee with involvement of other organs and systems [HCC]

M05.67 Rheumatoid arthritis of ankle and foot with involvement of other organs and systems

Rheumatoid arthritis of tarsus, metatarsus and phalanges with involvement of other organs and systems

M05.671 Rheumatoid arthritis of right ankle and foot with involvement of other organs and systems [HCC]

M05.672 Rheumatoid arthritis of left ankle and foot with involvement of other organs and systems

M05.679 Rheumatoid arthritis of unspecified ankle and foot with involvement of other organs and systems [HCC]

M05.69 Rheumatoid arthritis of multiple sites with involvement of other organs and systems [HCC]

M05.7 Rheumatoid arthritis with rheumatoid factor without organ or systems involvement

M05.7A Rheumatoid arthritis with rheumatoid factor of other specified site without organ or systems involvement

M05.70 Rheumatoid arthritis with rheumatoid factor of unspecified site without organ or systems involvement [HCC]

M05.71 Rheumatoid arthritis with rheumatoid factor of shoulder without organ or systems involvement

M05.711 Rheumatoid arthritis with rheumatoid factor of right shoulder without organ or systems involvement [HCC]

M05.712 Rheumatoid arthritis with rheumatoid factor of left shoulder without organ or systems involvement [HCC]

M05.719 Rheumatoid arthritis with rheumatoid factor of unspecified shoulder without organ or systems involvement [HCC]

M05.72 Rheumatoid arthritis with rheumatoid factor of elbow without organ or systems involvement

M05.721 Rheumatoid arthritis with rheumatoid factor of right elbow without organ or systems involvement [HCC]

M05.722 Rheumatoid arthritis with rheumatoid factor of left elbow without organ or systems involvement [HCC]

M05.729 Rheumatoid arthritis with rheumatoid factor of unspecified elbow without organ or systems involvement [HCC]

M05.73 Rheumatoid arthritis with rheumatoid factor of wrist without organ or systems involvement

M05.731 Rheumatoid arthritis with rheumatoid factor of right wrist without organ or systems involvement [HCC]

M05.732 Rheumatoid arthritis with rheumatoid factor of left wrist without organ or systems involvement [HCC]

M05.739 Rheumatoid arthritis with rheumatoid factor of unspecified wrist without organ or systems involvement [HCC]

M05.74 Rheumatoid arthritis with rheumatoid factor of hand without organ or systems involvement

M05.741 Rheumatoid arthritis with rheumatoid factor of right hand without organ or systems involvement [HCC]

M05.742 Rheumatoid arthritis with rheumatoid factor of left hand without organ or systems involvement [HCC]

M05.749 Rheumatoid arthritis with rheumatoid factor of unspecified hand without organ or systems involvement [HCC]

M05.75 Rheumatoid arthritis with rheumatoid factor of hip without organ or systems involvement

M05.751 Rheumatoid arthritis with rheumatoid factor of right hip without organ or systems involvement [HCC]

M05.752 Rheumatoid arthritis with rheumatoid factor of left hip without organ or systems involvement [HCC]

M05.759 Rheumatoid arthritis with rheumatoid factor of unspecified hip without organ or systems involvement [HCC]

M05.76 Rheumatoid arthritis with rheumatoid factor of knee without organ or systems involvement

M05.761   Rheumatoid arthritis with rheumatoid factor of right knee without organ or systems involvement [HCC]

M05.762   Rheumatoid arthritis with rheumatoid factor of left knee without organ or systems involvement [HCC]

M05.769   Rheumatoid arthritis with rheumatoid factor of unspecified knee without organ or systems involvement [HCC]

M05.77   Rheumatoid arthritis with rheumatoid factor of ankle and foot without organ or systems involvement

M05.771   Rheumatoid arthritis with rheumatoid factor of right ankle and foot without organ or systems involvement [HCC]

M05.772   Rheumatoid arthritis with rheumatoid factor of left ankle and foot without organ or systems involvement [HCC]

M05.779   Rheumatoid arthritis with rheumatoid factor of unspecified ankle and foot without organ or systems involvement [HCC]

M05.79   Rheumatoid arthritis with rheumatoid factor of multiple sites without organ or systems involvement [HCC]

M05.8   **Other rheumatoid arthritis with rheumatoid factor**

M05.8A   Other rheumatoid arthritis with rheumatoid factor of other specified site

M05.80   Other rheumatoid arthritis with rheumatoid factor of unspecified site [HCC]

M05.81   Other rheumatoid arthritis with rheumatoid factor of shoulder [HCC]

M05.811   Other rheumatoid arthritis with rheumatoid factor of right shoulder [HCC]

M05.812   Other rheumatoid arthritis with rheumatoid factor of left shoulder [HCC]

M05.819   Other rheumatoid arthritis with rheumatoid factor of unspecified shoulder [HCC]

M05.82   Other rheumatoid arthritis with rheumatoid factor of elbow

M05.821   Other rheumatoid arthritis with rheumatoid factor of right elbow [HCC]

M05.822   Other rheumatoid arthritis with rheumatoid factor of left elbow [HCC]

M05.829   Other rheumatoid arthritis with rheumatoid factor of unspecified elbow [HCC]

M05.83   Other rheumatoid arthritis with rheumatoid factor of wrist

M05.831   Other rheumatoid arthritis with rheumatoid factor of right wrist [HCC]

M05.832   Other rheumatoid arthritis with rheumatoid factor of left wrist [HCC]

M05.839   Other rheumatoid arthritis with rheumatoid factor of unspecified wrist [HCC]

M05.84   Other rheumatoid arthritis with rheumatoid factor of hand

M05.841   Other rheumatoid arthritis with rheumatoid factor of right hand [HCC]

M05.842   Other rheumatoid arthritis with rheumatoid factor of left hand [HCC]

M05.849   Other rheumatoid arthritis with rheumatoid factor of unspecified hand

M05.85   Other rheumatoid arthritis with rheumatoid factor of hip

M05.851   Other rheumatoid arthritis with rheumatoid factor of right hip [HCC]

M05.852   Other rheumatoid arthritis with rheumatoid factor of left hip [HCC]

M05.859   Other rheumatoid arthritis with rheumatoid factor of unspecified hip [HCC]

M05.86   Other rheumatoid arthritis with rheumatoid factor of knee

M05.861   Other rheumatoid arthritis with rheumatoid factor of right knee [HCC]

M05.862   Other rheumatoid arthritis with rheumatoid factor of left knee [HCC]

M05.869   Other rheumatoid arthritis with rheumatoid factor of unspecified knee [HCC]

M05.87   Other rheumatoid arthritis with rheumatoid factor of ankle and foot

M05.871   Other rheumatoid arthritis with rheumatoid factor of right ankle and foot [HCC]

M05.872   Other rheumatoid arthritis with rheumatoid factor of left ankle and foot [HCC]

M05.879   Other rheumatoid arthritis with rheumatoid factor of unspecified ankle and foot [HCC]

M05.89   Other rheumatoid arthritis with rheumatoid factor of multiple sites [HCC]

M05.9   **Rheumatoid arthritis with rheumatoid factor, unspecified** [HCC]

M06   **Other rheumatoid arthritis**

M06.0   **Rheumatoid arthritis without rheumatoid factor**

M06.0A   Rheumatoid arthritis without rheumatoid factor, other specified site

M06.00   Rheumatoid arthritis without rheumatoid factor, unspecified site [HCC]

M06.01   Rheumatoid arthritis without rheumatoid factor, shoulder

M06.011   Rheumatoid arthritis without rheumatoid factor, right shoulder [HCC]

M06.012   Rheumatoid arthritis without rheumatoid factor, left shoulder [HCC]

M06.019   Rheumatoid arthritis without rheumatoid factor, unspecified shoulder

M06.02   Rheumatoid arthritis without rheumatoid factor, elbow [HCC]

M06.021   Rheumatoid arthritis without rheumatoid factor, right elbow [HCC]

M06.022   Rheumatoid arthritis without rheumatoid factor, left elbow [HCC]

● New code   ▲ Revised code   **Excludes1:** Not coded here   **Excludes2:** Not included here   ⊗ Placeholder required   ⑦7th digit required

M06.029   **Rheumatoid arthritis without rheumatoid factor, unspecified elbow** [HCC]

M06.03   **Rheumatoid arthritis without rheumatoid factor, wrist**

   M06.031   **Rheumatoid arthritis without rheumatoid factor, right wrist** [HCC]

   M06.032   **Rheumatoid arthritis without rheumatoid factor, left wrist** [HCC]

   M06.039   **Rheumatoid arthritis without rheumatoid factor, unspecified wrist** [HCC]

M06.04   **Rheumatoid arthritis without rheumatoid factor, hand**

   M06.041   **Rheumatoid arthritis without rheumatoid factor, right hand** [HCC]

   M06.042   **Rheumatoid arthritis without rheumatoid factor, left hand** [HCC]

   M06.049   **Rheumatoid arthritis without rheumatoid factor, unspecified hand**

M06.05   **Rheumatoid arthritis without rheumatoid factor, hip**

   M06.051   **Rheumatoid arthritis without rheumatoid factor, right hip** [HCC]

   M06.052   **Rheumatoid arthritis without rheumatoid factor, left hip** [HCC]

   M06.059   **Rheumatoid arthritis without rheumatoid factor, unspecified hip** [HCC]

M06.06   **Rheumatoid arthritis without rheumatoid factor, knee**

   M06.061   **Rheumatoid arthritis without rheumatoid factor, right knee** [HCC]

   M06.062   **Rheumatoid arthritis without rheumatoid factor, left knee** [HCC]

   M06.069   **Rheumatoid arthritis without rheumatoid factor, unspecified knee** [HCC]

M06.07   **Rheumatoid arthritis without rheumatoid factor, ankle and foot**

   M06.071   **Rheumatoid arthritis without rheumatoid factor, right ankle and foot** [HCC]

   M06.072   **Rheumatoid arthritis without rheumatoid factor, left ankle and foot** [HCC]

   M06.079   **Rheumatoid arthritis without rheumatoid factor, unspecified ankle and foot** [HCC]

M06.08   **Rheumatoid arthritis without rheumatoid factor, vertebrae** [HCC]

M06.09   **Rheumatoid arthritis without rheumatoid factor, multiple sites** [HCC]

M06.1   **Adult-onset Still's disease** [HCC]

   Excludes1: Still's disease NOS (M08.2-)

M06.2   **Rheumatoid bursitis**

   M06.20   **Rheumatoid bursitis, unspecified site** [HCC]

   M06.21   **Rheumatoid bursitis, shoulder**

      M06.211   **Rheumatoid bursitis, right shoulder** [HCC]

      M06.212   **Rheumatoid bursitis, left shoulder** [HCC]

      M06.219   **Rheumatoid bursitis, unspecified shoulder** [HCC]

   M06.22   **Rheumatoid bursitis, elbow**

M06.221   **Rheumatoid bursitis, right elbow** [HCC]

M06.222   **Rheumatoid bursitis, left elbow** [HCC]

M06.229   **Rheumatoid bursitis, unspecified elbow** [HCC]

M06.23   **Rheumatoid bursitis, wrist**

   M06.231   **Rheumatoid bursitis, right wrist** [HCC]

   M06.232   **Rheumatoid bursitis, left wrist** [HCC]

   M06.239   **Rheumatoid bursitis, unspecified wrist** [HCC]

M06.24   **Rheumatoid bursitis, hand** [HCC]

   M06.241   **Rheumatoid bursitis, right hand** [HCC]

   M06.242   **Rheumatoid bursitis, left hand**

   M06.249   **Rheumatoid bursitis, unspecified hand** [HCC]

M06.25   **Rheumatoid bursitis, hip**

   M06.251   **Rheumatoid bursitis, right hip** [HCC]

   M06.252   **Rheumatoid bursitis, left hip** [HCC]

   M06.259   **Rheumatoid bursitis, unspecified hip** [HCC]

M06.26   **Rheumatoid bursitis, knee**

   M06.261   **Rheumatoid bursitis, right knee** [HCC]

   M06.262   **Rheumatoid bursitis, left knee** [HCC]

   M06.269   **Rheumatoid bursitis, unspecified knee** [HCC]

M06.27   **Rheumatoid bursitis, ankle and foot**

   M06.271   **Rheumatoid bursitis, right ankle and foot** [HCC]

   M06.272   **Rheumatoid bursitis, left ankle and foot** [HCC]

   M06.279   **Rheumatoid bursitis, unspecified ankle and foot** [HCC]

M06.28   **Rheumatoid bursitis, vertebrae** [HCC]

M06.29   **Rheumatoid bursitis, multiple sites** [HCC]

M06.3   **Rheumatoid nodule**

   M06.30   **Rheumatoid nodule, unspecified site** [HCC]

   M06.31   **Rheumatoid nodule, shoulder**

      M06.311   **Rheumatoid nodule, right shoulder** [HCC]

      M06.312   **Rheumatoid nodule, left shoulder** [HCC]

      M06.319   **Rheumatoid nodule, unspecified shoulder** [HCC]

   M06.32   **Rheumatoid nodule, elbow**

      M06.321   **Rheumatoid nodule, right elbow** [HCC]

      M06.322   **Rheumatoid nodule, left elbow** [HCC]

      M06.329   **Rheumatoid nodule, unspecified elbow** [HCC]

   M06.33   **Rheumatoid nodule, wrist**

      M06.331   **Rheumatoid nodule, right wrist** [HCC]

      M06.332   **Rheumatoid nodule, left wrist** [HCC]

      M06.339   **Rheumatoid nodule, unspecified wrist** [HCC]

   M06.34   **Rheumatoid nodule, hand**

      M06.341   **Rheumatoid nodule, right hand** [HCC]

      M06.342   **Rheumatoid nodule, left hand** [HCC]

      M06.349   **Rheumatoid nodule, unspecified hand**

   M06.35   **Rheumatoid nodule, hip**

M06.351 Rheumatoid nodule, right hip [HCC]

M06.352 Rheumatoid nodule, left hip [HCC]

M06.359 Rheumatoid nodule, unspecified hip [HCC]

M06.36 Rheumatoid nodule, knee

M06.361 Rheumatoid nodule, right knee [HCC]

M06.362 Rheumatoid nodule, left knee [HCC]

M06.369 Rheumatoid nodule, unspecified knee [HCC]

M06.37 Rheumatoid nodule, ankle and foot

M06.371 Rheumatoid nodule, right ankle and foot [HCC]

M06.372 Rheumatoid nodule, left ankle and foot [HCC]

M06.379 Rheumatoid nodule, unspecified ankle and foot [HCC]

M06.38 Rheumatoid nodule, vertebrae [HCC]

M06.39 Rheumatoid nodule, multiple sites [HCC]

M06.4 Inflammatory polyarthropathy [HCC]

Excludes1: polyarthritis NOS (M13.0)

M06.8 Other specified rheumatoid arthritis

M06.80 Other specified rheumatoid arthritis, unspecified site [HCC]

M06.81 Other specified rheumatoid arthritis, shoulder [HCC]

M06.811 Other specified rheumatoid arthritis, right shoulder [HCC]

M06.812 Other specified rheumatoid arthritis, left shoulder [HCC]

M06.819 Other specified rheumatoid arthritis, unspecified shoulder [HCC]

M06.82 Other specified rheumatoid arthritis, elbow [HCC]

M06.821 Other specified rheumatoid arthritis, right elbow [HCC]

M06.822 Other specified rheumatoid arthritis, left elbow [HCC]

M06.829 Other specified rheumatoid arthritis, unspecified elbow [HCC]

M06.83 Other specified rheumatoid arthritis, wrist [HCC]

M06.831 Other specified rheumatoid arthritis, right wrist [HCC]

M06.832 Other specified rheumatoid arthritis, left wrist [HCC]

M06.839 Other specified rheumatoid arthritis, unspecified wrist [HCC]

M06.84 Other specified rheumatoid arthritis, hand [HCC]

M06.841 Other specified rheumatoid arthritis, right hand [HCC]

M06.842 Other specified rheumatoid arthritis, left hand

M06.849 Other specified rheumatoid arthritis, unspecified hand [HCC]

M06.85 Other specified rheumatoid arthritis, hip [HCC]

M06.851 Other specified rheumatoid arthritis, right hip [HCC]

M06.852 Other specified rheumatoid arthritis, left hip [HCC]

M06.859 Other specified rheumatoid arthritis, unspecified hip [HCC]

M06.86 Other specified rheumatoid arthritis, knee [HCC]

M06.861 Other specified rheumatoid arthritis, right knee [HCC]

M06.862 Other specified rheumatoid arthritis, left knee [HCC]

M06.869 Other specified rheumatoid arthritis, unspecified knee [HCC]

M06.87 Other specified rheumatoid arthritis, ankle and foot [HCC]

M06.871 Other specified rheumatoid arthritis, right ankle and foot [HCC]

M06.872 Other specified rheumatoid arthritis, left ankle and foot [HCC]

M06.879 Other specified rheumatoid arthritis, unspecified ankle and foot [HCC]

M06.88 Other specified rheumatoid arthritis, vertebrae [HCC]

M06.89 Other specified rheumatoid arthritis, multiple sites [HCC]

M06.9 Rheumatoid arthritis, unspecified [HCC]

M07 Enteropathic arthropathies

Code also associated enteropathy, such as:

regional enteritis [Crohn's disease] (K50.-)

ulcerative colitis (K51.-)

Excludes1: psoriatic arthropathies (L40.5-)

M07.6 Enteropathic arthropathies

M07.60 Enteropathic arthropathies, unspecified site

M07.61 Enteropathic arthropathies, shoulder

M07.611 Enteropathic arthropathies, right shoulder

M07.612 Enteropathic arthropathies, left shoulder

M07.619 Enteropathic arthropathies, unspecified shoulder

M07.62 Enteropathic arthropathies, elbow

M07.621 Enteropathic arthropathies, right elbow

M07.622 Enteropathic arthropathies, left elbow

M07.629 Enteropathic arthropathies, unspecified elbow

M07.63 Enteropathic arthropathies, wrist

M07.631 Enteropathic arthropathies, right wrist

M07.632 Enteropathic arthropathies, left wrist

M07.639 Enteropathic arthropathies, unspecified wrist

M07.64 Enteropathic arthropathies, hand

M07.641 Enteropathic arthropathies, right hand

M07.642 Enteropathic arthropathies, left hand

M07.649 Enteropathic arthropathies, unspecified hand

M07.65 Enteropathic arthropathies, hip

M07.651 Enteropathic arthropathies, right hip

M07.652 Enteropathic arthropathies, left hip

M07.659 Enteropathic arthropathies, unspecified hip

M07.66 Enteropathic arthropathies, knee

M07.661 Enteropathic arthropathies, right knee

● New code   ▲ Revised code   Excludes1: Not coded here   Excludes2: Not included here   ⊗ Placeholder required   ⑦7th digit required

M07.662　Enteropathic arthropathies, left knee

M07.669　Enteropathic arthropathies, unspecified knee

M07.67　Enteropathic arthropathies, ankle and foot

M07.671　Enteropathic arthropathies, right ankle and foot

M07.672　Enteropathic arthropathies, left ankle and foot

M07.679　Enteropathic arthropathies, unspecified ankle and foot

M07.68　Enteropathic arthropathies, vertebrae

M07.69　Enteropathic arthropathies, multiple sites

M08　Juvenile arthritis

Code also any associated underlying condition, such as:

regional enteritis [Crohn's disease] (K50.-)

ulcerative colitis (K51.-)

Excludes1: arthropathy in Whipple's disease (M14.8)

Felty's syndrome (M05.0)

juvenile dermatomyositis (M33.0-)

psoriatic juvenile arthropathy (L40.54)

M08.0　Unspecified juvenile rheumatoid arthritis

Juvenile rheumatoid arthritis with or without rheumatoid factor

M08.0A　Unspecified juvenile rheumatoid arthritis, other specified site

M08.00　Unspecified juvenile rheumatoid arthritis of unspecified site [HCC]

M08.01　Unspecified juvenile rheumatoid arthritis, shoulder

M08.011　Unspecified juvenile rheumatoid arthritis, right shoulder [HCC]

M08.012　Unspecified juvenile rheumatoid arthritis, left shoulder [HCC]

M08.019　Unspecified juvenile rheumatoid arthritis, unspecified shoulder [HCC]

M08.02　Unspecified juvenile rheumatoid arthritis of elbow

M08.021　Unspecified juvenile rheumatoid arthritis, right elbow [HCC]

M08.022　Unspecified juvenile rheumatoid arthritis, left elbow [HCC]

M08.029　Unspecified juvenile rheumatoid arthritis, unspecified elbow [HCC]

M08.03　Unspecified juvenile rheumatoid arthritis, wrist

M08.031　Unspecified juvenile rheumatoid arthritis, right wrist [HCC]

M08.032　Unspecified juvenile rheumatoid arthritis, left wrist [HCC]

M08.039　Unspecified juvenile rheumatoid arthritis, unspecified wrist [HCC]

M08.04　Unspecified juvenile rheumatoid arthritis, hand

M08.041　Unspecified juvenile rheumatoid arthritis, right hand [HCC]

M08.042　Unspecified juvenile rheumatoid arthritis, left hand [HCC]

M08.049　Unspecified juvenile rheumatoid arthritis, unspecified hand [HCC]

M08.05　Unspecified juvenile rheumatoid arthritis, hip

M08.051　Unspecified juvenile rheumatoid arthritis, right hip [HCC]

M08.052　Unspecified juvenile rheumatoid arthritis, left hip [HCC]

M08.059　Unspecified juvenile rheumatoid arthritis, unspecified hip [HCC]

M08.06　Unspecified juvenile rheumatoid arthritis, knee

M08.061　Unspecified juvenile rheumatoid arthritis, right knee [HCC]

M08.062　Unspecified juvenile rheumatoid arthritis, left knee [HCC]

M08.069　Unspecified juvenile rheumatoid arthritis, unspecified knee [HCC]

M08.07　Unspecified juvenile rheumatoid arthritis, ankle and foot

M08.071　Unspecified juvenile rheumatoid arthritis, right ankle and foot [HCC]

M08.072　Unspecified juvenile rheumatoid arthritis, left ankle and foot [HCC]

M08.079　Unspecified juvenile rheumatoid arthritis, unspecified ankle and foot [HCC]

M08.08　Unspecified juvenile rheumatoid arthritis, vertebrae [HCC]

M08.09　Unspecified juvenile rheumatoid arthritis, multiple sites [HCC]

M08.1　Juvenile ankylosing spondylitis [HCC]

Excludes1: ankylosing spondylitis in adults (M45.0-)

M08.2　Juvenile rheumatoid arthritis with systemic onset [HCC]

Still's disease NOS

Excludes1: adult-onset Still's disease (M06.1-)

M08.2A　Juvenile rheumatoid arthritis with systemic onset, other specified site

M08.20　Juvenile rheumatoid arthritis with systemic onset, unspecified site [HCC]

M08.21　Juvenile rheumatoid arthritis with systemic onset, shoulder

M08.211　Juvenile rheumatoid arthritis with systemic onset, right shoulder

M08.212　Juvenile rheumatoid arthritis with systemic onset, left shoulder [HCC]

M08.219　Juvenile rheumatoid arthritis with systemic onset, unspecified shoulder [HCC]

M08.22　Juvenile rheumatoid arthritis with systemic onset, elbow

M08.221　Juvenile rheumatoid arthritis with systemic onset, right elbow [HCC]

M08.222　Juvenile rheumatoid arthritis with systemic onset, left elbow [HCC]

M08.229　Juvenile rheumatoid arthritis with systemic onset, unspecified elbow [HCC]

M08.23　Juvenile rheumatoid arthritis with systemic onset, wrist

M08.231　Juvenile rheumatoid arthritis with systemic onset, right wrist [HCC]

M08.232　Juvenile rheumatoid arthritis with systemic onset, left wrist [HCC]

M08.239　Juvenile rheumatoid arthritis with systemic onset, unspecified wrist [HCC]

M08.24　Juvenile rheumatoid arthritis with systemic onset, hand

M08.241　Juvenile rheumatoid arthritis with systemic onset, right hand [HCC]

M08.242　Juvenile rheumatoid arthritis with systemic onset, left hand [HCC]

M08.249 Juvenile rheumatoid arthritis with systemic onset, unspecified hand [HCC]

M08.25 Juvenile rheumatoid arthritis with systemic onset, hip

M08.251 Juvenile rheumatoid arthritis with systemic onset, right hip [HCC]

M08.252 Juvenile rheumatoid arthritis with systemic onset, left hip [HCC]

M08.259 Juvenile rheumatoid arthritis with systemic onset, unspecified hip [HCC]

M08.26 Juvenile rheumatoid arthritis with systemic onset, knee

M08.261 Juvenile rheumatoid arthritis with systemic onset, right knee [HCC]

M08.262 Juvenile rheumatoid arthritis with systemic onset, left knee [HCC]

M08.269 Juvenile rheumatoid arthritis with systemic onset, unspecified knee [HCC]

M08.27 Juvenile rheumatoid arthritis with systemic onset, ankle and foot

M08.271 Juvenile rheumatoid arthritis with systemic onset, right ankle and foot [HCC]

M08.272 Juvenile rheumatoid arthritis with systemic onset, left ankle and foot [HCC]

M08.279 Juvenile rheumatoid arthritis with systemic onset, unspecified ankle and foot [HCC]

M08.28 Juvenile rheumatoid arthritis with systemic onset, vertebrae [HCC]

M08.29 Juvenile rheumatoid arthritis with systemic onset, multiple sites [HCC]

M08.3 Juvenile rheumatoid polyarthritis (seronegative) [HCC]

M08.4 Pauciarticular juvenile rheumatoid arthritis [HCC]

M08.4A Pauciarticular juvenile rheumatoid arthritis, other specified site

M08.40 Pauciarticular juvenile rheumatoid arthritis, unspecified site [HCC]

M08.41 Pauciarticular juvenile rheumatoid arthritis, shoulder

M08.411 Pauciarticular juvenile rheumatoid arthritis, right shoulder

M08.412 Pauciarticular juvenile rheumatoid arthritis, left shoulder [HCC]

M08.419 Pauciarticular juvenile rheumatoid arthritis, unspecified shoulder [HCC]

M08.42 Pauciarticular juvenile rheumatoid arthritis, elbow

M08.421 Pauciarticular juvenile rheumatoid arthritis, right elbow [HCC]

M08.422 Pauciarticular juvenile rheumatoid arthritis, left elbow [HCC]

M08.429 Pauciarticular juvenile rheumatoid arthritis, unspecified elbow [HCC]

M08.43 Pauciarticular juvenile rheumatoid arthritis, wrist

M08.431 Pauciarticular juvenile rheumatoid arthritis, right wrist [HCC]

M08.432 Pauciarticular juvenile rheumatoid arthritis, left wrist [HCC]

M08.439 Pauciarticular juvenile rheumatoid arthritis, unspecified wrist [HCC]

M08.44 Pauciarticular juvenile rheumatoid arthritis, hand

M08.441 Pauciarticular juvenile rheumatoid arthritis, right hand [HCC]

M08.442 Pauciarticular juvenile rheumatoid arthritis, left hand [HCC]

M08.449 Pauciarticular juvenile rheumatoid arthritis, unspecified hand [HCC]

M08.45 Pauciarticular juvenile rheumatoid arthritis, hip

M08.451 Pauciarticular juvenile rheumatoid arthritis, right hip [HCC]

M08.452 Pauciarticular juvenile rheumatoid arthritis, left hip [HCC]

M08.459 Pauciarticular juvenile rheumatoid arthritis, unspecified hip [HCC]

M08.46 Pauciarticular juvenile rheumatoid arthritis, knee

M08.461 Pauciarticular juvenile rheumatoid arthritis, right knee [HCC]

M08.462 Pauciarticular juvenile rheumatoid arthritis, left knee [HCC]

M08.469 Pauciarticular juvenile rheumatoid arthritis, unspecified knee [HCC]

M08.47 Pauciarticular juvenile rheumatoid arthritis, ankle and foot

M08.471 Pauciarticular juvenile rheumatoid arthritis, right ankle and foot [HCC]

M08.472 Pauciarticular juvenile rheumatoid arthritis, left ankle and foot [HCC]

M08.479 Pauciarticular juvenile rheumatoid arthritis, unspecified ankle and foot [HCC]

M08.48 Pauciarticular juvenile rheumatoid arthritis, vertebrae [HCC]

M08.8 Other juvenile arthritis [HCC]

M08.80 Other juvenile arthritis, unspecified site [HCC]

M08.81 Other juvenile arthritis, shoulder [HCC]

M08.811 Other juvenile arthritis, right shoulder [HCC]

M08.812 Other juvenile arthritis, left shoulder [HCC]

M08.819 Other juvenile arthritis, unspecified shoulder

M08.82 Other juvenile arthritis, elbow [HCC]

M08.821 Other juvenile arthritis, right elbow [HCC]

M08.822 Other juvenile arthritis, left elbow [HCC]

M08.829 Other juvenile arthritis, unspecified elbow [HCC]

M08.83 Other juvenile arthritis, wrist [HCC]

M08.831 Other juvenile arthritis, right wrist [HCC]

M08.832 Other juvenile arthritis, left wrist [HCC]

M08.839 Other juvenile arthritis, unspecified wrist [HCC]

M08.84 Other juvenile arthritis, hand [HCC]

M08.841 Other juvenile arthritis, right hand [HCC]

M08.842 Other juvenile arthritis, left hand [HCC]

M08.849 Other juvenile arthritis, unspecified hand [HCC]

M08.85 Other juvenile arthritis, hip [HCC]

● New code   ▲ Revised code   **Excludes1:** Not coded here   **Excludes2:** Not included here   ⊗ Placeholder required   ⑦ 7th digit required

M08.851 Other juvenile arthritis, right hip [HCC]

M08.852 Other juvenile arthritis, left hip [HCC]

M08.859 Other juvenile arthritis, unspecified hip [HCC]

M08.86 Other juvenile arthritis, knee [HCC]

M08.861 Other juvenile arthritis, right knee [HCC]

M08.862 Other juvenile arthritis, left knee [HCC]

M08.869 Other juvenile arthritis, unspecified knee [HCC]

M08.87 Other juvenile arthritis, ankle and foot [HCC]

M08.871 Other juvenile arthritis, right ankle and foot [HCC]

M08.872 Other juvenile arthritis, left ankle and foot [HCC]

M08.879 Other juvenile arthritis, unspecified ankle and foot [HCC]

M08.88 Other juvenile arthritis, other specified site [HCC]

Other juvenile arthritis, vertebrae

M08.89 Other juvenile arthritis, multiple sites [HCC]

M08.9 Juvenile arthritis, unspecified [HCC]

Excludes1: juvenile rheumatoid arthritis, unspecified (M08.0-)

M08.9A Juvenile arthritis, unspecified, other specified site

M08.90 Juvenile arthritis, unspecified, unspecified site [HCC]

M08.91 Juvenile arthritis, unspecified, shoulder

M08.911 Juvenile arthritis, unspecified, right shoulder [HCC]

M08.912 Juvenile arthritis, unspecified, left shoulder

M08.919 Juvenile arthritis, unspecified, unspecified shoulder [HCC]

M08.92 Juvenile arthritis, unspecified, elbow

M08.921 Juvenile arthritis, unspecified, right elbow [HCC]

M08.922 Juvenile arthritis, unspecified, left elbow [HCC]

M08.929 Juvenile arthritis, unspecified, unspecified elbow [HCC]

M08.93 Juvenile arthritis, unspecified, wrist

M08.931 Juvenile arthritis, unspecified, right wrist [HCC]

M08.932 Juvenile arthritis, unspecified, left wrist [HCC]

M08.939 Juvenile arthritis, unspecified, unspecified wrist [HCC]

M08.94 Juvenile arthritis, unspecified, hand

M08.941 Juvenile arthritis, unspecified, right hand [HCC]

M08.942 Juvenile arthritis, unspecified, left hand [HCC]

M08.949 Juvenile arthritis, unspecified, unspecified hand [HCC]

M08.95 Juvenile arthritis, unspecified, hip

M08.951 Juvenile arthritis, unspecified, right hip [HCC]

M08.952 Juvenile arthritis, unspecified, left hip [HCC]

M08.959 Juvenile arthritis, unspecified, unspecified hip [HCC]

M08.96 Juvenile arthritis, unspecified, knee

M08.961 Juvenile arthritis, unspecified, right knee [HCC]

M08.962 Juvenile arthritis, unspecified, left knee [HCC]

M08.969 Juvenile arthritis, unspecified, unspecified knee [HCC]

M08.97 Juvenile arthritis, unspecified, ankle and foot]

M08.971 Juvenile arthritis, unspecified, right ankle and foot [HCC]

M08.972 Juvenile arthritis, unspecified, left ankle and foot [HCC]

M08.979 Juvenile arthritis, unspecified, unspecified ankle and foot [HCC]

M08.98 Juvenile arthritis, unspecified, vertebrae [HCC]

M08.99 Juvenile arthritis, unspecified, multiple sites [HCC]

M1A Chronic gout

Use Additional Code to identify:

Autonomic neuropathy in diseases classified elsewhere (G99.0)

Calculus of urinary tract in diseases classified elsewhere (N22)

Cardiomyopathy in diseases classified elsewhere (I43)

Disorders of external ear in diseases classified elsewhere (H61.1-, H62.8-)

Disorders of iris and ciliary body in diseases classified elsewhere (H22)

Glomerular disorders in diseases classified elsewhere (N08)

Excludes1: gout NOS (M10.-)

Excludes2: acute gout (M10.-)

The appropriate 7th character is to be added to each code from category M1A

0 - without tophus (tophi)

1 - with tophus (tophi)

M1A.0 Idiopathic chronic gout

Chronic gouty bursitis

Primary chronic gout

⊗⑦M1A.00 Idiopathic chronic gout, unspecified site

M1A.01 Idiopathic chronic gout, shoulder

⑦M1A.011 Idiopathic chronic gout, right shoulder

⑦M1A.012 Idiopathic chronic gout, left shoulder

⑦M1A.019 Idiopathic chronic gout, unspecified shoulder

M1A.02 Idiopathic chronic gout, elbow

⑦M1A.021 Idiopathic chronic gout, right elbow

⑦M1A.022 Idiopathic chronic gout, left elbow

⑦M1A.029 Idiopathic chronic gout, unspecified elbow

M1A.03 Idiopathic chronic gout, wrist

⑦M1A.031 Idiopathic chronic gout, right wrist

⑦M1A.032 Idiopathic chronic gout, left wrist

⑦M1A.039 Idiopathic chronic gout, unspecified wrist

M1A.04 Idiopathic chronic gout, hand

⑦M1A.041 Idiopathic chronic gout, right hand

⑦M1A.042 Idiopathic chronic gout, left hand

⑦M1A.049 Idiopathic chronic gout, unspecified hand

M1A.05 Idiopathic chronic gout, hip

⑦**M1A.051 Idiopathic chronic gout, right hip**

⑦**M1A.052 Idiopathic chronic gout, left hip**

⑦**M1A.059 Idiopathic chronic gout, unspecified hip**

M1A.06 Idiopathic chronic gout, knee

⑦**M1A.061 Idiopathic chronic gout, right knee**

⑦**M1A.062 Idiopathic chronic gout, left knee**

⑦**M1A.069 Idiopathic chronic gout, unspecified knee**

M1A.07 Idiopathic chronic gout, ankle and foot

⑦**M1A.071 Idiopathic chronic gout, right ankle and foot**

⑦**M1A.072 Idiopathic chronic gout, left ankle and foot**

⑦**M1A.079 Idiopathic chronic gout, unspecified ankle and foot**

⊗⑦**M1A.08 Idiopathic chronic gout, vertebrae**

⊗⑦**M1A.09 Idiopathic chronic gout, multiple sites**

M1A.1 Lead-induced chronic gout

Code first toxic effects of lead and its compounds (T56.0-)

⊗⑦**M1A.10 Lead-induced chronic gout, unspecified site**

M1A.11 Lead-induced chronic gout, shoulder

⑦**M1A.111 Lead-induced chronic gout, right shoulder**

⑦**M1A.112 Lead-induced chronic gout, left shoulder**

⑦**M1A.119 Lead-induced chronic gout, unspecified shoulder**

M1A.12 Lead-induced chronic gout, elbow

⑦**M1A.121 Lead-induced chronic gout, right elbow**

⑦**M1A.122 Lead-induced chronic gout, left elbow**

⑦**M1A.129 Lead-induced chronic gout, unspecified elbow**

M1A.13 Lead-induced chronic gout, wrist

⑦**M1A.131 Lead-induced chronic gout, right wrist**

⑦**M1A.132 Lead-induced chronic gout, left wrist**

⑦**M1A.139 Lead-induced chronic gout, unspecified wrist**

M1A.14 Lead-induced chronic gout, hand

⑦**M1A.141 Lead-induced chronic gout, right hand**

⑦**M1A.142 Lead-induced chronic gout, left hand**

⑦**M1A.149 Lead-induced chronic gout, unspecified hand**

M1A.15 Lead-induced chronic gout, hip

⑦**M1A.151 Lead-induced chronic gout, right hip**

⑦**M1A.152 Lead-induced chronic gout, left hip**

⑦**M1A.159 Lead-induced chronic gout, unspecified hip**

M1A.16 Lead-induced chronic gout, knee

⑦**M1A.161 Lead-induced chronic gout, right knee**

⑦**M1A.162 Lead-induced chronic gout, left knee**

⑦**M1A.169 Lead-induced chronic gout, unspecified knee**

M1A.17 Lead-induced chronic gout, ankle and foot

⑦**M1A.171 Lead-induced chronic gout, right ankle and foot**

⑦**M1A.172 Lead-induced chronic gout, left ankle and foot**

⑦**M1A.179 Lead-induced chronic gout, unspecified ankle and foot**

⊗⑦**M1A.18 Lead-induced chronic gout, vertebrae**

⊗⑦**M1A.19 Lead-induced chronic gout, multiple sites**

M1A.2 Drug-induced chronic gout

Use Additional Code for adverse effect, if applicable, to identify drug (T36-T50 with fifth or sixth character 5)

⊗⑦**M1A.20 Drug-induced chronic gout, unspecified site**

M1A.21 Drug-induced chronic gout, shoulder

⑦**M1A.211 Drug-induced chronic gout, right shoulder**

⑦**M1A.212 Drug-induced chronic gout, left shoulder**

⑦**M1A.219 Drug-induced chronic gout, unspecified shoulder**

M1A.22 Drug-induced chronic gout, elbow

⑦**M1A.221 Drug-induced chronic gout, right elbow**

⑦**M1A.222 Drug-induced chronic gout, left elbow**

⑦**M1A.229 Drug-induced chronic gout, unspecified elbow**

M1A.23 Drug-induced chronic gout, wrist

⑦**M1A.231 Drug-induced chronic gout, right wrist**

⑦**M1A.232 Drug-induced chronic gout, left wrist**

⑦**M1A.239 Drug-induced chronic gout, unspecified wrist**

M1A.24 Drug-induced chronic gout, hand

⑦**M1A.241 Drug-induced chronic gout, right hand**

⑦**M1A.242 Drug-induced chronic gout, left hand**

⑦**M1A.249 Drug-induced chronic gout, unspecified hand**

M1A.25 Drug-induced chronic gout, hip

⑦**M1A.251 Drug-induced chronic gout, right hip**

⑦**M1A.252 Drug-induced chronic gout, left hip**

⑦**M1A.259 Drug-induced chronic gout, unspecified hip**

M1A.26 Drug-induced chronic gout, knee

⑦**M1A.261 Drug-induced chronic gout, right knee**

⑦**M1A.262 Drug-induced chronic gout, left knee**

⑦**M1A.269 Drug-induced chronic gout, unspecified knee**

M1A.27 Drug-induced chronic gout, ankle and foot

⑦**M1A.271 Drug-induced chronic gout, right ankle and foot**

⑦**M1A.272 Drug-induced chronic gout, left ankle and foot**

⑦**M1A.279 Drug-induced chronic gout, unspecified ankle and foot**

⊗⑦**M1A.28 Drug-induced chronic gout, vertebrae**

⊗⑦**M1A.29 Drug-induced chronic gout, multiple sites**

M1A.3 Chronic gout due to renal impairment

Code first associated renal disease

⊗⑦**M1A.30 Chronic gout due to renal impairment, unspecified site**

● New code   ▲ Revised code   **Excludes1:** Not coded here   **Excludes2:** Not included here   ⊗ Placeholder required   ⑦ 7ᵗʰ digit required

M1A.31 Chronic gout due to renal impairment, shoulder

⑦M1A.311 Chronic gout due to renal impairment, right shoulder

⑦M1A.312 Chronic gout due to renal impairment, left shoulder

⑦M1A.319 Chronic gout due to renal impairment, unspecified shoulder

M1A.32 Chronic gout due to renal impairment, elbow

⑦M1A.321 Chronic gout due to renal impairment, right elbow

⑦M1A.322 Chronic gout due to renal impairment, left elbow

⑦M1A.329 Chronic gout due to renal impairment, unspecified elbow

M1A.33 Chronic gout due to renal impairment, wrist

⑦M1A.331 Chronic gout due to renal impairment, right wrist

⑦M1A.332 Chronic gout due to renal impairment, left wrist

⑦M1A.339 Chronic gout due to renal impairment, unspecified wrist

M1A.34 Chronic gout due to renal impairment, hand

⑦M1A.341 Chronic gout due to renal impairment, right hand

⑦M1A.342 Chronic gout due to renal impairment, left hand

⑦M1A.349 Chronic gout due to renal impairment, unspecified hand

M1A.35 Chronic gout due to renal impairment, hip

⑦M1A.351 Chronic gout due to renal impairment, right hip

⑦M1A.352 Chronic gout due to renal impairment, left hip

⑦M1A.359 Chronic gout due to renal impairment, unspecified hip

M1A.36 Chronic gout due to renal impairment, knee

⑦M1A.361 Chronic gout due to renal impairment, right knee

⑦M1A.362 Chronic gout due to renal impairment, left knee

⑦M1A.369 Chronic gout due to renal impairment, unspecified knee

M1A.37 Chronic gout due to renal impairment, ankle and foot

⑦M1A.371 Chronic gout due to renal impairment, right ankle and foot

⑦M1A.372 Chronic gout due to renal impairment, left ankle and foot

⑦M1A.379 Chronic gout due to renal impairment, unspecified ankle and foot

⊗⑦M1A.38 Chronic gout due to renal impairment, vertebrae

⊗⑦M1A.39 Chronic gout due to renal impairment, multiple sites

M1A.4 Other secondary chronic gout

Code first associated condition

⊗⑦M1A.40 Other secondary chronic gout, unspecified site

M1A.41 Other secondary chronic gout, shoulder

⑦M1A.411 Other secondary chronic gout, right shoulder

⑦M1A.412 Other secondary chronic gout, left shoulder

⑦M1A.419 Other secondary chronic gout, unspecified shoulder

M1A.42 Other secondary chronic gout, elbow

⑦M1A.421 Other secondary chronic gout, right elbow

⑦M1A.422 Other secondary chronic gout, left elbow

⑦M1A.429 Other secondary chronic gout, unspecified elbow

M1A.43 Other secondary chronic gout, wrist

⑦M1A.431 Other secondary chronic gout, right wrist

⑦M1A.432 Other secondary chronic gout, left wrist

⑦M1A.439 Other secondary chronic gout, unspecified wrist

M1A.44 Other secondary chronic gout, hand

⑦M1A.441 Other secondary chronic gout, right hand

⑦M1A.442 Other secondary chronic gout, left hand

⑦M1A.449 Other secondary chronic gout, unspecified hand

M1A.45 Other secondary chronic gout, hip

⑦M1A.451 Other secondary chronic gout, right hip

⑦M1A.452 Other secondary chronic gout, left hip

⑦M1A.459 Other secondary chronic gout, unspecified hip

M1A.46 Other secondary chronic gout, knee

⑦M1A.461 Other secondary chronic gout, right knee

⑦M1A.462 Other secondary chronic gout, left knee

⑦M1A.469 Other secondary chronic gout, unspecified knee

M1A.47 Other secondary chronic gout, ankle and foot

⑦M1A.471 Other secondary chronic gout, right ankle and foot

⑦M1A.472 Other secondary chronic gout, left ankle and foot

⑦M1A.479 Other secondary chronic gout, unspecified ankle and foot

⊗⑦M1A.48 Other secondary chronic gout, vertebrae

⊗⑦M1A.49 Other secondary chronic gout, multiple sites

⊗⑦M1A.9 Chronic gout, unspecified

M10 Gout

Acute gout

Gout attack

Gout flare

Podagra

Use Additional Code to identify:

Autonomic neuropathy in diseases classified elsewhere (G99.0)

Calculus of urinary tract in diseases classified elsewhere (N22)

Cardiomyopathy in diseases classified elsewhere (I43)

Disorders of external ear in diseases classified elsewhere (H61.1-, H62.8-)

Disorders of iris and ciliary body in diseases classified elsewhere (H22)

Glomerular disorders in diseases classified elsewhere (N08)

Excludes2: chronic gout (M1A.-)

M10.0 Idiopathic gout

　　Gouty bursitis

　　Primary gout

　　M10.00 Idiopathic gout, unspecified site

　　M10.01 Idiopathic gout, shoulder

　　　　M10.011 Idiopathic gout, right shoulder

　　　　M10.012 Idiopathic gout, left shoulder

　　　　M10.019 Idiopathic gout, unspecified shoulder

　　M10.02 Idiopathic gout, elbow

　　　　M10.021 Idiopathic gout, right elbow

　　　　M10.022 Idiopathic gout, left elbow

　　　　M10.029 Idiopathic gout, unspecified elbow

　　M10.03 Idiopathic gout, wrist

　　　　M10.031 Idiopathic gout, right wrist

　　　　M10.032 Idiopathic gout, left wrist

　　　　M10.039 Idiopathic gout, unspecified wrist

　　M10.04 Idiopathic gout, hand

　　　　M10.041 Idiopathic gout, right hand

　　　　M10.042 Idiopathic gout, left hand

　　　　M10.049 Idiopathic gout, unspecified hand

　　M10.05 Idiopathic gout, hip

　　　　M10.051 Idiopathic gout, right hip

　　　　M10.052 Idiopathic gout, left hip

　　　　M10.059 Idiopathic gout, unspecified hip

　　M10.06 Idiopathic gout, knee

　　　　M10.061 Idiopathic gout, right knee

　　　　M10.062 Idiopathic gout, left knee

　　　　M10.069 Idiopathic gout, unspecified knee

　　M10.07 Idiopathic gout, ankle and foot

　　　　M10.071 Idiopathic gout, right ankle and foot

　　　　M10.072 Idiopathic gout, left ankle and foot

　　　　M10.079 Idiopathic gout, unspecified ankle and foot

　　M10.08 Idiopathic gout, vertebrae

　　M10.09 Idiopathic gout, multiple sites

M10.1 Lead-induced gout

　　<u>Code first</u> toxic effects of lead and its compounds (T56.0-)

　　M10.10 Lead-induced gout, unspecified site

　　M10.11 Lead-induced gout, shoulder

　　　　M10.111 Lead-induced gout, right shoulder

　　　　M10.112 Lead-induced gout, left shoulder

　　　　M10.119 Lead-induced gout, unspecified shoulder

　　M10.12 Lead-induced gout, elbow

　　　　M10.121 Lead-induced gout, right elbow

　　　　M10.122 Lead-induced gout, left elbow

　　　　M10.129 Lead-induced gout, unspecified elbow

　　M10.13 Lead-induced gout, wrist

　　　　M10.131 Lead-induced gout, right wrist

　　　　M10.132 Lead-induced gout, left wrist

　　　　M10.139 Lead-induced gout, unspecified wrist

　　M10.14 Lead-induced gout, hand

　　　　M10.141 Lead-induced gout, right hand

　　　　M10.142 Lead-induced gout, left hand

　　　　M10.149 Lead-induced gout, unspecified hand

　　M10.15 Lead-induced gout, hip

　　　　M10.151 Lead-induced gout, right hip

　　　　M10.152 Lead-induced gout, left hip

　　　　M10.159 Lead-induced gout, unspecified hip

　　M10.16 Lead-induced gout, knee

　　　　M10.161 Lead-induced gout, right knee

　　　　M10.162 Lead-induced gout, left knee

　　　　M10.169 Lead-induced gout, unspecified knee

　　M10.17 Lead-induced gout, ankle and foot

　　　　M10.171 Lead-induced gout, right ankle and foot

　　　　M10.172 Lead-induced gout, left ankle and foot

　　　　M10.179 Lead-induced gout, unspecified ankle and foot

　　M10.18 Lead-induced gout, vertebrae

　　M10.19 Lead-induced gout, multiple sites

M10.2 Drug-induced gout

　　<u>Use Additional Code</u> for adverse effect, if applicable, to identify drug (T36-T50 with fifth or sixth character 5)

　　M10.20 Drug-induced gout, unspecified site

　　M10.21 Drug-induced gout, shoulder

　　　　M10.211 Drug-induced gout, right shoulder

　　　　M10.212 Drug-induced gout, left shoulder

　　　　M10.219 Drug-induced gout, unspecified shoulder

　　M10.22 Drug-induced gout, elbow

　　　　M10.221 Drug-induced gout, right elbow

　　　　M10.222 Drug-induced gout, left elbow

　　　　M10.229 Drug-induced gout, unspecified elbow

　　M10.23 Drug-induced gout, wrist

　　　　M10.231 Drug-induced gout, right wrist

　　　　M10.232 Drug-induced gout, left wrist

　　　　M10.239 Drug-induced gout, unspecified wrist

　　M10.24 Drug-induced gout, hand

　　　　M10.241 Drug-induced gout, right hand

　　　　M10.242 Drug-induced gout, left hand

　　　　M10.249 Drug-induced gout, unspecified hand

　　M10.25 Drug-induced gout, hip

　　　　M10.251 Drug-induced gout, right hip

　　　　M10.252 Drug-induced gout, left hip

　　　　M10.259 Drug-induced gout, unspecified hip

　　M10.26 Drug-induced gout, knee

　　　　M10.261 Drug-induced gout, right knee

　　　　M10.262 Drug-induced gout, left knee

　　　　M10.269 Drug-induced gout, unspecified knee

　　M10.27 Drug-induced gout, ankle and foot

　　　　M10.271 Drug-induced gout, right ankle and foot

　　　　M10.272 Drug-induced gout, left ankle and foot

　　　　M10.279 Drug-induced gout, unspecified ankle and foot

　　M10.28 Drug-induced gout, vertebrae

　　M10.29 Drug-induced gout, multiple sites

M10.3 Gout due to renal impairment

　　<u>Code first</u> associated renal disease

● New code　　▲ Revised code　　**Excludes1:** Not coded here　　**Excludes2:** Not included here　　⊗ Placeholder required　　⑦7ᵗʰ digit required

M10.30 Gout due to renal impairment, unspecified site

M10.31 Gout due to renal impairment, shoulder

    M10.311 Gout due to renal impairment, right shoulder

    M10.312 Gout due to renal impairment, left shoulder

    M10.319 Gout due to renal impairment, unspecified shoulder

M10.32 Gout due to renal impairment, elbow

    M10.321 Gout due to renal impairment, right elbow

    M10.322 Gout due to renal impairment, left elbow

    M10.329 Gout due to renal impairment, unspecified elbow

M10.33 Gout due to renal impairment, wrist

    M10.331 Gout due to renal impairment, right wrist

    M10.332 Gout due to renal impairment, left wrist

    M10.339 Gout due to renal impairment, unspecified wrist

M10.34 Gout due to renal impairment, hand

    M10.341 Gout due to renal impairment, right hand

    M10.342 Gout due to renal impairment, left hand

    M10.349 Gout due to renal impairment, unspecified hand

M10.35 Gout due to renal impairment, hip

    M10.351 Gout due to renal impairment, right hip

    M10.352 Gout due to renal impairment, left hip

    M10.359 Gout due to renal impairment, unspecified hip

M10.36 Gout due to renal impairment, knee

    M10.361 Gout due to renal impairment, right knee

    M10.362 Gout due to renal impairment, left knee

    M10.369 Gout due to renal impairment, unspecified knee

M10.37 Gout due to renal impairment, ankle and foot

    M10.371 Gout due to renal impairment, right ankle and foot

    M10.372 Gout due to renal impairment, left ankle and foot

    M10.379 Gout due to renal impairment, unspecified ankle and foot

M10.38 Gout due to renal impairment, vertebrae

M10.39 Gout due to renal impairment, multiple sites

M10.4 Other secondary gout

Code first associated condition

M10.40 Other secondary gout, unspecified site

M10.41 Other secondary gout, shoulder

    M10.411 Other secondary gout, right shoulder

    M10.412 Other secondary gout, left shoulder

    M10.419 Other secondary gout, unspecified shoulder

M10.42 Other secondary gout, elbow

    M10.421 Other secondary gout, right elbow

    M10.422 Other secondary gout, left elbow

    M10.429 Other secondary gout, unspecified elbow

M10.43 Other secondary gout, wrist

    M10.431 Other secondary gout, right wrist

    M10.432 Other secondary gout, left wrist

    M10.439 Other secondary gout, unspecified wrist

M10.44 Other secondary gout, hand

    M10.441 Other secondary gout, right hand

    M10.442 Other secondary gout, left hand

    M10.449 Other secondary gout, unspecified hand

M10.45 Other secondary gout, hip

    M10.451 Other secondary gout, right hip

    M10.452 Other secondary gout, left hip

    M10.459 Other secondary gout, unspecified hip

M10.46 Other secondary gout, knee

    M10.461 Other secondary gout, right knee

    M10.462 Other secondary gout, left knee

    M10.469 Other secondary gout, unspecified knee

M10.47 Other secondary gout, ankle and foot

    M10.471 Other secondary gout, right ankle and foot

    M10.472 Other secondary gout, left ankle and foot

    M10.479 Other secondary gout, unspecified ankle and foot

M10.48 Other secondary gout, vertebrae

M10.49 Other secondary gout, multiple sites

M10.9 Gout, unspecified

Gout NOS

M11 Other crystal arthropathies

Definition: Crystal arthropathies refers to a type of arthropathy characterized by accumulation of crystals in joints.

M11.0 Hydroxyapatite deposition disease

M11.00 Hydroxyapatite deposition disease, unspecified site

M11.01 Hydroxyapatite deposition disease, shoulder

    M11.011 Hydroxyapatite deposition disease, right shoulder

    M11.012 Hydroxyapatite deposition disease, left shoulder

    M11.019 Hydroxyapatite deposition disease, unspecified shoulder

M11.02 Hydroxyapatite deposition disease, elbow

    M11.021 Hydroxyapatite deposition disease, right elbow

    M11.022 Hydroxyapatite deposition disease, left elbow

    M11.029 Hydroxyapatite deposition disease, unspecified elbow

M11.03 Hydroxyapatite deposition disease, wrist

    M11.031 Hydroxyapatite deposition disease, right wrist

    M11.032 Hydroxyapatite deposition disease, left wrist

    M11.039 Hydroxyapatite deposition disease, unspecified wrist

M11.04 Hydroxyapatite deposition disease, hand
    M11.041 Hydroxyapatite deposition disease, right hand
    M11.042 Hydroxyapatite deposition disease, left hand
    M11.049 Hydroxyapatite deposition disease, unspecified hand
M11.05 Hydroxyapatite deposition disease, hip
    M11.051 Hydroxyapatite deposition disease, right hip
    M11.052 Hydroxyapatite deposition disease, left hip
    M11.059 Hydroxyapatite deposition disease, unspecified hip
M11.06 Hydroxyapatite deposition disease, knee
    M11.061 Hydroxyapatite deposition disease, right knee
    M11.062 Hydroxyapatite deposition disease, left knee
    M11.069 Hydroxyapatite deposition disease, unspecified knee
M11.07 Hydroxyapatite deposition disease, ankle and foot
    M11.071 Hydroxyapatite deposition disease, right ankle and foot
    M11.072 Hydroxyapatite deposition disease, left ankle and foot
    M11.079 Hydroxyapatite deposition disease, unspecified ankle and foot
M11.08 Hydroxyapatite deposition disease, vertebrae
M11.09 Hydroxyapatite deposition disease, multiple sites
M11.1 Familial chondrocalcinosis
  M11.10 Familial chondrocalcinosis, unspecified site
  M11.11 Familial chondrocalcinosis, shoulder
    M11.111 Familial chondrocalcinosis, right shoulder
    M11.112 Familial chondrocalcinosis, left shoulder
    M11.119 Familial chondrocalcinosis, unspecified shoulder
  M11.12 Familial chondrocalcinosis, elbow
    M11.121 Familial chondrocalcinosis, right elbow
    M11.122 Familial chondrocalcinosis, left elbow
    M11.129 Familial chondrocalcinosis, unspecified elbow
  M11.13 Familial chondrocalcinosis, wrist
    M11.131 Familial chondrocalcinosis, right wrist
    M11.132 Familial chondrocalcinosis, left wrist
    M11.139 Familial chondrocalcinosis, unspecified wrist
  M11.14 Familial chondrocalcinosis, hand
    M11.141 Familial chondrocalcinosis, right hand
    M11.142 Familial chondrocalcinosis, left hand
    M11.149 Familial chondrocalcinosis, unspecified hand
  M11.15 Familial chondrocalcinosis, hip
    M11.151 Familial chondrocalcinosis, right hip

M11.152 Familial chondrocalcinosis, left hip
M11.159 Familial chondrocalcinosis, unspecified hip
M11.16 Familial chondrocalcinosis, knee
    M11.161 Familial chondrocalcinosis, right knee
    M11.162 Familial chondrocalcinosis, left knee
    M11.169 Familial chondrocalcinosis, unspecified knee
M11.17 Familial chondrocalcinosis, ankle and foot
    M11.171 Familial chondrocalcinosis, right ankle and foot
    M11.172 Familial chondrocalcinosis, left ankle and foot
    M11.179 Familial chondrocalcinosis, unspecified ankle and foot
M11.18 Familial chondrocalcinosis, vertebrae
M11.19 Familial chondrocalcinosis, multiple sites
M11.2 Other chondrocalcinosis
  Chondrocalcinosis NOS
  M11.20 Other chondrocalcinosis, unspecified site
  M11.21 Other chondrocalcinosis, shoulder
    M11.211 Other chondrocalcinosis, right shoulder
    M11.212 Other chondrocalcinosis, left shoulder
    M11.219 Other chondrocalcinosis, unspecified shoulder
  M11.22 Other chondrocalcinosis, elbow
    M11.221 Other chondrocalcinosis, right elbow
    M11.222 Other chondrocalcinosis, left elbow
    M11.229 Other chondrocalcinosis, unspecified elbow
  M11.23 Other chondrocalcinosis, wrist
    M11.231 Other chondrocalcinosis, right wrist
    M11.232 Other chondrocalcinosis, left wrist
    M11.239 Other chondrocalcinosis, unspecified wrist
  M11.24 Other chondrocalcinosis, hand
    M11.241 Other chondrocalcinosis, right hand
    M11.242 Other chondrocalcinosis, left hand
    M11.249 Other chondrocalcinosis, unspecified hand
  M11.25 Other chondrocalcinosis, hip
    M11.251 Other chondrocalcinosis, right hip
    M11.252 Other chondrocalcinosis, left hip
    M11.259 Other chondrocalcinosis, unspecified hip
  M11.26 Other chondrocalcinosis, knee
    M11.261 Other chondrocalcinosis, right knee
    M11.262 Other chondrocalcinosis, left knee
    M11.269 Other chondrocalcinosis, unspecified knee
  M11.27 Other chondrocalcinosis, ankle and foot
    M11.271 Other chondrocalcinosis, right ankle and foot
    M11.272 Other chondrocalcinosis, left ankle and foot
    M11.279 Other chondrocalcinosis, unspecified ankle and foot
  M11.28 Other chondrocalcinosis, vertebrae

● New code   ▲ Revised code   **Excludes1:** Not coded here   **Excludes2:** Not included here   ⊗ Placeholder required   ⑦ 7th digit required

M11.29   Other chondrocalcinosis, multiple sites

M11.8   Other specified crystal arthropathies

M11.80   Other specified crystal arthropathies, unspecified site

M11.81   Other specified crystal arthropathies, shoulder

     M11.811   Other specified crystal arthropathies, right shoulder

     M11.812   Other specified crystal arthropathies, left shoulder

     M11.819   Other specified crystal arthropathies, unspecified shoulder

M11.82   Other specified crystal arthropathies, elbow

     M11.821   Other specified crystal arthropathies, right elbow

     M11.822   Other specified crystal arthropathies, left elbow

     M11.829   Other specified crystal arthropathies, unspecified elbow

M11.83   Other specified crystal arthropathies, wrist

     M11.831   Other specified crystal arthropathies, right wrist

     M11.832   Other specified crystal arthropathies, left wrist

     M11.839   Other specified crystal arthropathies, unspecified wrist

M11.84   Other specified crystal arthropathies, hand

     M11.841   Other specified crystal arthropathies, right hand

     M11.842   Other specified crystal arthropathies, left hand

     M11.849   Other specified crystal arthropathies, unspecified hand

M11.85   Other specified crystal arthropathies, hip

     M11.851   Other specified crystal arthropathies, right hip

     M11.852   Other specified crystal arthropathies, left hip

     M11.859   Other specified crystal arthropathies, unspecified hip

M11.86   Other specified crystal arthropathies, knee

     M11.861   Other specified crystal arthropathies, right knee

     M11.862   Other specified crystal arthropathies, left knee

     M11.869   Other specified crystal arthropathies, unspecified knee

M11.87   Other specified crystal arthropathies, ankle and foot

     M11.871   Other specified crystal arthropathies, right ankle and foot

     M11.872   Other specified crystal arthropathies, left ankle and foot

     M11.879   Other specified crystal arthropathies, unspecified ankle and foot

M11.88   Other specified crystal arthropathies, vertebrae

M11.89   Other specified crystal arthropathies, multiple sites

M11.9   Crystal arthropathy, unspecified

M12   Other and unspecified arthropathy

Excludes1: arthrosis (M15-M19)

     cricoarytenoid arthropathy (J38.7)

M12.0   Chronic postrheumatic arthropathy [Jaccoud]

M12.00   Chronic postrheumatic arthropathy [Jaccoud], unspecified site [HCC]

M12.01   Chronic postrheumatic arthropathy [Jaccoud], shoulder

     M12.011   Chronic postrheumatic arthropathy [Jaccoud], right shoulder [HCC]

     M12.012   Chronic postrheumatic arthropathy [Jaccoud], left shoulder [HCC]

     M12.019   Chronic postrheumatic arthropathy [Jaccoud], unspecified shoulder [HCC]

M12.02   Chronic postrheumatic arthropathy [Jaccoud], elbow

     M12.021   Chronic postrheumatic arthropathy [Jaccoud], right elbow [HCC]

     M12.022   Chronic postrheumatic arthropathy [Jaccoud], left elbow [HCC]

     M12.029   Chronic postrheumatic arthropathy [Jaccoud], unspecified elbow [HCC]

M12.03   Chronic postrheumatic arthropathy [Jaccoud], wrist

     M12.031   Chronic postrheumatic arthropathy [Jaccoud], right wrist [HCC]

     M12.032   Chronic postrheumatic arthropathy [Jaccoud], left wrist [HCC]

     M12.039   Chronic postrheumatic arthropathy [Jaccoud], unspecified wrist [HCC]

M12.04   Chronic postrheumatic arthropathy [Jaccoud], hand

     M12.041   Chronic postrheumatic arthropathy [Jaccoud], right hand [HCC]

     M12.042   Chronic postrheumatic arthropathy [Jaccoud], left hand [HCC]

     M12.049   Chronic postrheumatic arthropathy [Jaccoud], unspecified hand [HCC]

M12.05   Chronic postrheumatic arthropathy [Jaccoud], hip

     M12.051   Chronic postrheumatic arthropathy [Jaccoud], right hip [HCC]

     M12.052   Chronic postrheumatic arthropathy [Jaccoud], left hip [HCC]

     M12.059   Chronic postrheumatic arthropathy [Jaccoud], unspecified hip [HCC]

M12.06   Chronic postrheumatic arthropathy [Jaccoud], knee

     M12.061   Chronic postrheumatic arthropathy [Jaccoud], right knee [HCC]

     M12.062   Chronic postrheumatic arthropathy [Jaccoud], left knee [HCC]

     M12.069   Chronic postrheumatic arthropathy [Jaccoud], unspecified knee [HCC]

M12.07   Chronic postrheumatic arthropathy [Jaccoud], ankle and foot

     M12.071   Chronic postrheumatic arthropathy [Jaccoud], right ankle and foot [HCC]

     M12.072   Chronic postrheumatic arthropathy [Jaccoud], left ankle and foot [HCC]

     M12.079   Chronic postrheumatic arthropathy [Jaccoud], unspecified ankle and foot [HCC]

M12.08   Chronic postrheumatic arthropathy [Jaccoud], other specified site [HCC]

     Chronic postrheumatic arthropathy [Jaccoud], vertebrae

M12.09   Chronic postrheumatic arthropathy [Jaccoud], multiple sites [HCC]

M12.1   **Kaschin-Beck disease**

    Osteochondroarthrosis deformans endemica

M12.10   Kaschin-Beck disease, unspecified site

M12.11   Kaschin-Beck disease, shoulder

    M12.111   Kaschin-Beck disease, right shoulder

    M12.112   Kaschin-Beck disease, left shoulder

    M12.119   Kaschin-Beck disease, unspecified shoulder

M12.12   Kaschin-Beck disease, elbow

    M12.121   Kaschin-Beck disease, right elbow

    M12.122   Kaschin-Beck disease, left elbow

    M12.129   Kaschin-Beck disease, unspecified elbow

M12.13   Kaschin-Beck disease, wrist

    M12.131   Kaschin-Beck disease, right wrist

    M12.132   Kaschin-Beck disease, left wrist

    M12.139   Kaschin-Beck disease, unspecified wrist

M12.14   Kaschin-Beck disease, hand

    M12.141   Kaschin-Beck disease, right hand

    M12.142   Kaschin-Beck disease, left hand

    M12.149   Kaschin-Beck disease, unspecified hand

M12.15   Kaschin-Beck disease, hip

    M12.151   Kaschin-Beck disease, right hip

    M12.152   Kaschin-Beck disease, left hip

    M12.159   Kaschin-Beck disease, unspecified hip

M12.16   Kaschin-Beck disease, knee

    M12.161   Kaschin-Beck disease, right knee

    M12.162   Kaschin-Beck disease, left knee

    M12.169   Kaschin-Beck disease, unspecified knee

M12.17   Kaschin-Beck disease, ankle and foot

    M12.171   Kaschin-Beck disease, right ankle and foot

    M12.172   Kaschin-Beck disease, left ankle and foot

    M12.179   Kaschin-Beck disease, unspecified ankle and foot

M12.18   Kaschin-Beck disease, vertebrae

M12.19   Kaschin-Beck disease, multiple sites

M12.2   **Villonodular synovitis (pigmented)**

M12.20   Villonodular synovitis (pigmented), unspecified site

M12.21   Villonodular synovitis (pigmented), shoulder

    M12.211   Villonodular synovitis (pigmented), right shoulder

    M12.212   Villonodular synovitis (pigmented), left shoulder

    M12.219   Villonodular synovitis (pigmented), unspecified shoulder

M12.22   Villonodular synovitis (pigmented), elbow

    M12.221   Villonodular synovitis (pigmented), right elbow

    M12.222   Villonodular synovitis (pigmented), left elbow

    M12.229   Villonodular synovitis (pigmented), unspecified elbow

M12.23   Villonodular synovitis (pigmented), wrist

    M12.231   Villonodular synovitis (pigmented), right wrist

    M12.232   Villonodular synovitis (pigmented), left wrist

    M12.239   Villonodular synovitis (pigmented), unspecified wrist

M12.24   Villonodular synovitis (pigmented), hand

    M12.241   Villonodular synovitis (pigmented), right hand

    M12.242   Villonodular synovitis (pigmented), left hand

    M12.249   Villonodular synovitis (pigmented), unspecified hand

M12.25   Villonodular synovitis (pigmented), hip

    M12.251   Villonodular synovitis (pigmented), right hip

    M12.252   Villonodular synovitis (pigmented), left hip

    M12.259   Villonodular synovitis (pigmented), unspecified hip

M12.26   Villonodular synovitis (pigmented), knee

    M12.261   Villonodular synovitis (pigmented), right knee

    M12.262   Villonodular synovitis (pigmented), left knee

    M12.269   Villonodular synovitis (pigmented), unspecified knee

M12.27   Villonodular synovitis (pigmented), ankle and foot

    M12.271   Villonodular synovitis (pigmented), right ankle and foot

    M12.272   Villonodular synovitis (pigmented), left ankle and foot

    M12.279   Villonodular synovitis (pigmented), unspecified ankle and foot

M12.28   Villonodular synovitis (pigmented), other specified site

    Villonodular synovitis (pigmented), vertebrae

M12.29   Villonodular synovitis (pigmented), multiple sites

M12.3   **Palindromic rheumatism**

M12.30   Palindromic rheumatism, unspecified site

M12.31   Palindromic rheumatism, shoulder

    M12.311   Palindromic rheumatism, right shoulder

    M12.312   Palindromic rheumatism, left shoulder

    M12.319   Palindromic rheumatism, unspecified shoulder

M12.32   Palindromic rheumatism, elbow

    M12.321   Palindromic rheumatism, right elbow

    M12.322   Palindromic rheumatism, left elbow

    M12.329   Palindromic rheumatism, unspecified elbow

M12.33   Palindromic rheumatism, wrist

    M12.331   Palindromic rheumatism, right wrist

    M12.332   Palindromic rheumatism, left wrist

    M12.339   Palindromic rheumatism, unspecified wrist

M12.34   Palindromic rheumatism, hand

  ● New code   ▲ Revised code   **Excludes1:** Not coded here   **Excludes2:** Not included here   ⊗ Placeholder required   ⑦7ᵗʰ digit required

M12.341 Palindromic rheumatism, right hand

M12.342 Palindromic rheumatism, left hand

M12.349 Palindromic rheumatism, unspecified hand

M12.35 Palindromic rheumatism, hip

M12.351 Palindromic rheumatism, right hip

M12.352 Palindromic rheumatism, left hip

M12.359 Palindromic rheumatism, unspecified hip

M12.36 Palindromic rheumatism, knee

M12.361 Palindromic rheumatism, right knee

M12.362 Palindromic rheumatism, left knee

M12.369 Palindromic rheumatism, unspecified knee

M12.37 Palindromic rheumatism, ankle and foot

M12.371 Palindromic rheumatism, right ankle and foot

M12.372 Palindromic rheumatism, left ankle and foot

M12.379 Palindromic rheumatism, unspecified ankle and foot

M12.38 Palindromic rheumatism, other specified site

Palindromic rheumatism, vertebrae

M12.39 Palindromic rheumatism, multiple sites

M12.4 Intermittent hydrarthrosis

M12.40 Intermittent hydrarthrosis, unspecified site

M12.41 Intermittent hydrarthrosis, shoulder

M12.411 Intermittent hydrarthrosis, right shoulder

M12.412 Intermittent hydrarthrosis, left shoulder

M12.419 Intermittent hydrarthrosis, unspecified shoulder

M12.42 Intermittent hydrarthrosis, elbow

M12.421 Intermittent hydrarthrosis, right elbow

M12.422 Intermittent hydrarthrosis, left elbow

M12.429 Intermittent hydrarthrosis, unspecified elbow

M12.43 Intermittent hydrarthrosis, wrist

M12.431 Intermittent hydrarthrosis, right wrist

M12.432 Intermittent hydrarthrosis, left wrist

M12.439 Intermittent hydrarthrosis, unspecified wrist

M12.44 Intermittent hydrarthrosis, hand

M12.441 Intermittent hydrarthrosis, right hand

M12.442 Intermittent hydrarthrosis, left hand

M12.449 Intermittent hydrarthrosis, unspecified hand

M12.45 Intermittent hydrarthrosis, hip

M12.451 Intermittent hydrarthrosis, right hip

M12.452 Intermittent hydrarthrosis, left hip

M12.459 Intermittent hydrarthrosis, unspecified hip

M12.46 Intermittent hydrarthrosis, knee

M12.461 Intermittent hydrarthrosis, right knee

M12.462 Intermittent hydrarthrosis, left knee

M12.469 Intermittent hydrarthrosis, unspecified knee

M12.47 Intermittent hydrarthrosis, ankle and foot

M12.471 Intermittent hydrarthrosis, right ankle and foot

M12.472 Intermittent hydrarthrosis, left ankle and foot

M12.479 Intermittent hydrarthrosis, unspecified ankle and foot

M12.48 Intermittent hydrarthrosis, other site

M12.49 Intermittent hydrarthrosis, multiple sites

M12.5 Traumatic arthropathy

Excludes1: current injury-see Alphabetic Index

post-traumatic osteoarthritis of first carpometacarpal joint (M18.2-M18.3)

post-traumatic osteoarthritis of hip (M16.4-M16.5)

post-traumatic osteoarthritis of knee (M17.2-M17.3)

post-traumatic osteoarthritis NOS (M19.1-)

post-traumatic osteoarthritis of other single joints (M19.1-)

M12.50 Traumatic arthropathy, unspecified site

M12.51 Traumatic arthropathy, shoulder

M12.511 Traumatic arthropathy, right shoulder

M12.512 Traumatic arthropathy, left shoulder

M12.519 Traumatic arthropathy, unspecified shoulder

M12.52 Traumatic arthropathy, elbow

M12.521 Traumatic arthropathy, right elbow

M12.522 Traumatic arthropathy, left elbow

M12.529 Traumatic arthropathy, unspecified elbow

M12.53 Traumatic arthropathy, wrist

M12.531 Traumatic arthropathy, right wrist

M12.532 Traumatic arthropathy, left wrist

M12.539 Traumatic arthropathy, unspecified wrist

M12.54 Traumatic arthropathy, hand

M12.541 Traumatic arthropathy, right hand

M12.542 Traumatic arthropathy, left hand

M12.549 Traumatic arthropathy, unspecified hand

M12.55 Traumatic arthropathy, hip

M12.551 Traumatic arthropathy, right hip

M12.552 Traumatic arthropathy, left hip

M12.559 Traumatic arthropathy, unspecified hip

M12.56 Traumatic arthropathy, knee

M12.561 Traumatic arthropathy, right knee

M12.562 Traumatic arthropathy, left knee

M12.569 Traumatic arthropathy, unspecified knee

M12.57 Traumatic arthropathy, ankle and foot

M12.571 Traumatic arthropathy, right ankle and foot

M12.572 Traumatic arthropathy, left ankle and foot

M12.579 Traumatic arthropathy, unspecified ankle and foot

M12.58 Traumatic arthropathy, other specified site

Traumatic arthropathy, vertebrae

M12.59 Traumatic arthropathy, multiple sites

M12.8 Other specific arthropathies, not elsewhere classified

Transient arthropathy

M12.80 Other specific arthropathies, not elsewhere classified, unspecified site

M12.81 Other specific arthropathies, not elsewhere classified, shoulder

M12.811 Other specific arthropathies, not elsewhere classified, right shoulder

M12.812 Other specific arthropathies, not elsewhere classified, left shoulder

M12.819 Other specific arthropathies, not elsewhere classified, unspecified shoulder

M12.82 Other specific arthropathies, not elsewhere classified, elbow

M12.821 Other specific arthropathies, not elsewhere classified, right elbow

M12.822 Other specific arthropathies, not elsewhere classified, left elbow

M12.829 Other specific arthropathies, not elsewhere classified, unspecified elbow

M12.83 Other specific arthropathies, not elsewhere classified, wrist

M12.831 Other specific arthropathies, not elsewhere classified, right wrist

M12.832 Other specific arthropathies, not elsewhere classified, left wrist

M12.839 Other specific arthropathies, not elsewhere classified, unspecified wrist

M12.84 Other specific arthropathies, not elsewhere classified, hand

M12.841 Other specific arthropathies, not elsewhere classified, right hand

M12.842 Other specific arthropathies, not elsewhere classified, left hand

M12.849 Other specific arthropathies, not elsewhere classified, unspecified hand

M12.85 Other specific arthropathies, not elsewhere classified, hip

M12.851 Other specific arthropathies, not elsewhere classified, right hip

M12.852 Other specific arthropathies, not elsewhere classified, left hip

M12.859 Other specific arthropathies, not elsewhere classified, unspecified hip

M12.86 Other specific arthropathies, not elsewhere classified, knee

M12.861 Other specific arthropathies, not elsewhere classified, right knee

M12.862 Other specific arthropathies, not elsewhere classified, left knee

M12.869 Other specific arthropathies, not elsewhere classified, unspecified knee

M12.87 Other specific arthropathies, not elsewhere classified, ankle and foot

M12.871 Other specific arthropathies, not elsewhere classified, right ankle and foot

M12.872 Other specific arthropathies, not elsewhere classified, left ankle and foot

M12.879 Other specific arthropathies, not elsewhere classified, unspecified ankle and foot

M12.88 Other specific arthropathies, not elsewhere classified, other specified site

Other specific arthropathies, not elsewhere classified, vertebrae

M12.89 Other specific arthropathies, not elsewhere classified, multiple sites

M12.9 Arthropathy, unspecified

M13 Other arthritis

Excludes1: arthrosis (M15-M19)

osteoarthritis (M15-M19)

M13.0 Polyarthritis, unspecified

M13.1 Monoarthritis, not elsewhere classified

M13.10 Monoarthritis, not elsewhere classified, unspecified site

M13.11 Monoarthritis, not elsewhere classified, shoulder

M13.111 Monoarthritis, not elsewhere classified, right shoulder

M13.112 Monoarthritis, not elsewhere classified, left shoulder

M13.119 Monoarthritis, not elsewhere classified, unspecified shoulder

M13.12 Monoarthritis, not elsewhere classified, elbow

M13.121 Monoarthritis, not elsewhere classified, right elbow

M13.122 Monoarthritis, not elsewhere classified, left elbow

M13.129 Monoarthritis, not elsewhere classified, unspecified elbow

M13.13 Monoarthritis, not elsewhere classified, wrist

M13.131 Monoarthritis, not elsewhere classified, right wrist

M13.132 Monoarthritis, not elsewhere classified, left wrist

M13.139 Monoarthritis, not elsewhere classified, unspecified wrist

M13.14 Monoarthritis, not elsewhere classified, hand

M13.141 Monoarthritis, not elsewhere classified, right hand

M13.142 Monoarthritis, not elsewhere classified, left hand

M13.149 Monoarthritis, not elsewhere classified, unspecified hand

M13.15 Monoarthritis, not elsewhere classified, hip

M13.151 Monoarthritis, not elsewhere classified, right hip

M13.152 Monoarthritis, not elsewhere classified, left hip

M13.159 Monoarthritis, not elsewhere classified, unspecified hip

M13.16 Monoarthritis, not elsewhere classified, knee

M13.161 Monoarthritis, not elsewhere classified, right knee

M13.162 Monoarthritis, not elsewhere classified, left knee

M13.169 Monoarthritis, not elsewhere classified, unspecified knee

M13.17 **Monoarthritis, not elsewhere classified, ankle and foot**

 M13.171 **Monoarthritis, not elsewhere classified, right ankle and foot**

 M13.172 **Monoarthritis, not elsewhere classified, left ankle and foot**

 M13.179 **Monoarthritis, not elsewhere classified, unspecified ankle and foot**

M13.8 **Other specified arthritis**

 Allergic arthritis

 Excludes1: osteoarthritis (M15-M19)

 M13.80 **Other specified arthritis, unspecified site**

 M13.81 **Other specified arthritis, shoulder**

 M13.811 **Other specified arthritis, right shoulder**

 M13.812 **Other specified arthritis, left shoulder**

 M13.819 **Other specified arthritis, unspecified shoulder**

 M13.82 **Other specified arthritis, elbow**

 M13.821 **Other specified arthritis, right elbow**

 M13.822 **Other specified arthritis, left elbow**

 M13.829 **Other specified arthritis, unspecified elbow**

 M13.83 **Other specified arthritis, wrist**

 M13.831 **Other specified arthritis, right wrist**

 M13.832 **Other specified arthritis, left wrist**

 M13.839 **Other specified arthritis, unspecified wrist**

 M13.84 **Other specified arthritis, hand**

 M13.841 **Other specified arthritis, right hand**

 M13.842 **Other specified arthritis, left hand**

 M13.849 **Other specified arthritis, unspecified hand**

 M13.85 **Other specified arthritis, hip**

 M13.851 **Other specified arthritis, right hip**

 M13.852 **Other specified arthritis, left hip**

 M13.859 **Other specified arthritis, unspecified hip**

 M13.86 **Other specified arthritis, knee**

 M13.861 **Other specified arthritis, right knee**

 M13.862 **Other specified arthritis, left knee**

 M13.869 **Other specified arthritis, unspecified knee**

 M13.87 **Other specified arthritis, ankle and foot**

 M13.871 **Other specified arthritis, right ankle and foot**

 M13.872 **Other specified arthritis, left ankle and foot**

 M13.879 **Other specified arthritis, unspecified ankle and foot**

 M13.88 **Other specified arthritis, other site**

 M13.89 **Other specified arthritis, multiple sites**

M14 **Arthropathies in other diseases classified elsewhere**

 Excludes1: arthropathy in:

 diabetes mellitus (E08-E13 with .61-)

 hematological disorders (M36.2-M36.3)

 hypersensitivity reactions (M36.4)

 neoplastic disease (M36.1)

 neurosyphillis (A52.16)

 sarcoidosis (D86.86)

 enteropathic arthropathies (M07.-)

 juvenile psoriatic arthropathy (L40.54)

 lipoid dermatoarthritis (E78.81)

M14.6 **Charcôt's joint**

 Neuropathic arthropathy

 Excludes1: Charcôt's joint in diabetes mellitus (E08-E13 with .610)

 Charcôt's joint in tabes dorsalis (A52.16)

 M14.60 **Charcôt's joint, unspecified site**

 M14.61 **Charcôt's joint, shoulder**

 M14.611 **Charcôt's joint, right shoulder**

 M14.612 **Charcôt's joint, left shoulder**

 M14.619 **Charcôt's joint, unspecified shoulder**

 M14.62 **Charcôt's joint, elbow**

 M14.621 **Charcôt's joint, right elbow**

 M14.622 **Charcôt's joint, left elbow**

 M14.629 **Charcôt's joint, unspecified elbow**

 M14.63 **Charcôt's joint, wrist**

 M14.631 **Charcôt's joint, right wrist**

 M14.632 **Charcôt's joint, left wrist**

 M14.639 **Charcôt's joint, unspecified wrist**

 M14.64 **Charcôt's joint, hand**

 M14.641 **Charcôt's joint, right hand**

 M14.642 **Charcôt's joint, left hand**

 M14.649 **Charcôt's joint, unspecified hand**

 M14.65 **Charcôt's joint, hip**

 M14.651 **Charcôt's joint, right hip**

 M14.652 **Charcôt's joint, left hip**

 M14.659 **Charcôt's joint, unspecified hip**

 M14.66 **Charcôt's joint, knee**

 M14.661 **Charcôt's joint, right knee**

 M14.662 **Charcôt's joint, left knee**

 M14.669 **Charcôt's joint, unspecified knee**

 M14.67 **Charcôt's joint, ankle and foot**

 M14.671 **Charcôt's joint, right ankle and foot**

 M14.672 **Charcôt's joint, left ankle and foot**

 M14.679 **Charcôt's joint, unspecified ankle and foot**

 M14.68 **Charcôt's joint, vertebrae**

 M14.69 **Charcôt's joint, multiple sites**

M14.8 **Arthropathies in other specified diseases classified elsewhere**

 Code first underlying disease, such as:

 amyloidosis (E85.-)

 erythema multiforme (L51.-)

 erythema nodosum (L52)

 hemochromatosis (E83.11-)

 hyperparathyroidism (E21.-)

 hypothyroidism (E00-E03)

 sickle-cell disorders (D57.-)

 thyrotoxicosis [hyperthyroidism] (E05.-)

 Whipple's disease (K90.81)

 M14.80 **Arthropathies in other specified diseases classified elsewhere, unspecified site**

 M14.81 **Arthropathies in other specified diseases classified elsewhere, shoulder**

M14.811   Arthropathies in other specified diseases classified elsewhere, right shoulder

M14.812   Arthropathies in other specified diseases classified elsewhere, left shoulder

M14.819   Arthropathies in other specified diseases classified elsewhere, unspecified shoulder

M14.82   Arthropathies in other specified diseases classified elsewhere, elbow

M14.821   Arthropathies in other specified diseases classified elsewhere, right elbow

M14.822   Arthropathies in other specified diseases classified elsewhere, left elbow

M14.829   Arthropathies in other specified diseases classified elsewhere, unspecified elbow

M14.83   Arthropathies in other specified diseases classified elsewhere, wrist

M14.831   Arthropathies in other specified diseases classified elsewhere, right wrist

M14.832   Arthropathies in other specified diseases classified elsewhere, left wrist

M14.839   Arthropathies in other specified diseases classified elsewhere, unspecified wrist

M14.84   Arthropathies in other specified diseases classified elsewhere, hand

M14.841   Arthropathies in other specified diseases classified elsewhere, right hand

M14.842   Arthropathies in other specified diseases classified elsewhere, left hand

M14.849   Arthropathies in other specified diseases classified elsewhere, unspecified hand

M14.85   Arthropathies in other specified diseases classified elsewhere, hip

M14.851   Arthropathies in other specified diseases classified elsewhere, right hip

M14.852   Arthropathies in other specified diseases classified elsewhere, left hip

M14.859   Arthropathies in other specified diseases classified elsewhere, unspecified hip

M14.86   Arthropathies in other specified diseases classified elsewhere, knee

M14.861   Arthropathies in other specified diseases classified elsewhere, right knee

M14.862   Arthropathies in other specified diseases classified elsewhere, left knee

M14.869   Arthropathies in other specified diseases classified elsewhere, unspecified knee

M14.87   Arthropathies in other specified diseases classified elsewhere, ankle and foot

M14.871   Arthropathies in other specified diseases classified elsewhere, right ankle and foot

M14.872   Arthropathies in other specified diseases classified elsewhere, left ankle and foot

M14.879   Arthropathies in other specified diseases classified elsewhere, unspecified ankle and foot

M14.88   Arthropathies in other specified diseases classified elsewhere, vertebrae

M14.89   Arthropathies in other specified diseases classified elsewhere, multiple sites

OSTEOARTHRITIS (M15-M19)

Definition: Osteoarthritis (OA), which is also known as osteoarthrosis or degenerative joint disease (DJD), is a progressive disorder of the joints caused by gradual loss of cartilage and resulting in the development of bony spurs and cysts at the margins of the joints.

Excludes2: osteoarthritis of spine (M47.-)

M15   **Polyosteoarthritis**

Includes: arthritis of multiple sites

Excludes1: bilateral involvement of single joint (M16-M19)

M15.0   Primary generalized (osteo)arthritis

M15.1   Heberden's nodes (with arthropathy)

Interphalangeal distal osteoarthritis

M15.2   Bouchard's nodes (with arthropathy)

Juxtaphalangeal distal osteoarthritis

M15.3   Secondary multiple arthritis

Post-traumatic polyosteoarthritis

M15.4   Erosive (osteo)arthritis

M15.8   Other polyosteoarthritis

M15.9   Polyosteoarthritis, unspecified

Generalized osteoarthritis NOS

M16   **Osteoarthritis of hip**

M16.0   Bilateral primary osteoarthritis of hip

M16.1   Unilateral primary osteoarthritis of hip

Primary osteoarthritis of hip NOS

M16.10   Unilateral primary osteoarthritis, unspecified hip

M16.11   Unilateral primary osteoarthritis, right hip

M16.12   Unilateral primary osteoarthritis, left hip

M16.2   Bilateral osteoarthritis resulting from hip dysplasia

M16.3   Unilateral osteoarthritis resulting from hip dysplasia

Dysplastic osteoarthritis of hip NOS

M16.30   Unilateral osteoarthritis resulting from hip dysplasia, unspecified hip

M16.31   Unilateral osteoarthritis resulting from hip dysplasia, right hip

M16.32   Unilateral osteoarthritis resulting from hip dysplasia, left hip

M16.4   Bilateral post-traumatic osteoarthritis of hip

M16.5   Unilateral post-traumatic osteoarthritis of hip

Post-traumatic osteoarthritis of hip NOS

M16.50   Unilateral post-traumatic osteoarthritis, unspecified hip

M16.51   Unilateral post-traumatic osteoarthritis, right hip

M16.52   Unilateral post-traumatic osteoarthritis, left hip

M16.6   Other bilateral secondary osteoarthritis of hip

M16.7 **Other unilateral secondary osteoarthritis of hip**
Secondary osteoarthritis of hip NOS

M16.9 **Osteoarthritis of hip, unspecified**

M17 **Osteoarthritis of knee**

M17.0 **Bilateral primary osteoarthritis of knee**

M17.1 **Unilateral primary osteoarthritis of knee**
Primary osteoarthritis of knee NOS

  M17.10 **Unilateral primary osteoarthritis, unspecified knee**

  M17.11 **Unilateral primary osteoarthritis, right knee**

  M17.12 **Unilateral primary osteoarthritis, left knee**

M17.2 **Bilateral post-traumatic osteoarthritis of knee**

M17.3 **Unilateral post-traumatic osteoarthritis of knee**
Post-traumatic osteoarthritis of knee NOS

  M17.30 **Unilateral post-traumatic osteoarthritis, unspecified knee**

  M17.31 **Unilateral post-traumatic osteoarthritis, right knee**

  M17.32 **Unilateral post-traumatic osteoarthritis, left knee**

M17.4 **Other bilateral secondary osteoarthritis of knee**

M17.5 **Other unilateral secondary osteoarthritis of knee**
Secondary osteoarthritis of knee NOS

M17.9 **Osteoarthritis of knee, unspecified**

M18 **Osteoarthritis of first carpometacarpal joint**

M18.0 **Bilateral primary osteoarthritis of first carpometacarpal joints**

M18.1 **Unilateral primary osteoarthritis of first carpometacarpal joint**
Primary osteoarthritis of first carpometacarpal joint NOS

  M18.10 **Unilateral primary osteoarthritis of first carpometacarpal joint, unspecified hand**

  M18.11 **Unilateral primary osteoarthritis of first carpometacarpal joint, right hand**

  M18.12 **Unilateral primary osteoarthritis of first carpometacarpal joint, left hand**

M18.2 **Bilateral post-traumatic osteoarthritis of first carpometacarpal joints**

M18.3 **Unilateral post-traumatic osteoarthritis of first carpometacarpal joint**
Post-traumatic osteoarthritis of first carpometacarpal joint NOS

  M18.30 **Unilateral post-traumatic osteoarthritis of first carpometacarpal joint, unspecified hand**

  M18.31 **Unilateral post-traumatic osteoarthritis of first carpometacarpal joint, right hand**

  M18.32 **Unilateral post-traumatic osteoarthritis of first carpometacarpal joint, left hand**

M18.4 **Other bilateral secondary osteoarthritis of first carpometacarpal joints**

M18.5 **Other unilateral secondary osteoarthritis of first carpometacarpal joint**
Secondary osteoarthritis of first carpometacarpal joint NOS

  M18.50 **Other unilateral secondary osteoarthritis of first carpometacarpal joint, unspecified hand**

  M18.51 **Other unilateral secondary osteoarthritis of first carpometacarpal joint, right hand**

  M18.52 **Other unilateral secondary osteoarthritis of first carpometacarpal joint, left hand**

M18.9 **Osteoarthritis of first carpometacarpal joint, unspecified**

M19 **Other and unspecified osteoarthritis**

Excludes1: polyarthritis (M15.-)

Excludes2: arthrosis of spine (M47.-)
hallux rigidus (M20.2)
osteoarthritis of spine (M47.-)

M19.0 **Primary osteoarthritis of other joints**

M19.01 **Primary osteoarthritis, shoulder**

  M19.011 **Primary osteoarthritis, right shoulder**

  M19.012 **Primary osteoarthritis, left shoulder**

  M19.019 **Primary osteoarthritis, unspecified shoulder**

M19.02 **Primary osteoarthritis, elbow**

  M19.021 **Primary osteoarthritis, right elbow**

  M19.022 **Primary osteoarthritis, left elbow**

  M19.029 **Primary osteoarthritis, unspecified elbow**

M19.03 **Primary osteoarthritis, wrist**

  M19.031 **Primary osteoarthritis, right wrist**

  M19.032 **Primary osteoarthritis, left wrist**

  M19.039 **Primary osteoarthritis, unspecified wrist**

M19.04 **Primary osteoarthritis, hand**

  Excludes2: primary osteoarthritis of first carpometacarpal joint (M18.0-, M18.1-)

  M19.041 **Primary osteoarthritis, right hand**

  M19.042 **Primary osteoarthritis, left hand**

  M19.049 **Primary osteoarthritis, unspecified hand**

M19.07 **Primary osteoarthritis ankle and foot**

  M19.071 **Primary osteoarthritis, right ankle and foot**

  M19.072 **Primary osteoarthritis, left ankle and foot**

  M19.079 **Primary osteoarthritis, unspecified ankle and foot**

M19.1 **Post-traumatic osteoarthritis of other joints**

M19.11 **Post-traumatic osteoarthritis, shoulder**

  M19.111 **Post-traumatic osteoarthritis, right shoulder**

  M19.112 **Post-traumatic osteoarthritis, left shoulder**

  M19.119 **Post-traumatic osteoarthritis, unspecified shoulder**

M19.12 **Post-traumatic osteoarthritis, elbow**

  M19.121 **Post-traumatic osteoarthritis, right elbow**

  M19.122 **Post-traumatic osteoarthritis, left elbow**

  M19.129 **Post-traumatic osteoarthritis, unspecified elbow**

M19.13 **Post-traumatic osteoarthritis, wrist**

  M19.131 **Post-traumatic osteoarthritis, right wrist**

  M19.132 **Post-traumatic osteoarthritis, left wrist**

  M19.139 **Post-traumatic osteoarthritis, unspecified wrist**

M19.14 **Post-traumatic osteoarthritis, hand**

  Excludes2: post-traumatic osteoarthritis of first carpometacarpal joint (M18.2-, M18.3-)

■ Add 4th-7th digits   ■ Nonspecific code   ■ Unspecified code   ■ Manifestation code   [HCC] Hierarchical Condition Code   563

M19.141   **Post-traumatic osteoarthritis, right hand**

M19.142   **Post-traumatic osteoarthritis, left hand**

M19.149   **Post-traumatic osteoarthritis, unspecified hand**

M19.17   **Post-traumatic osteoarthritis, ankle and foot**

M19.171   **Post-traumatic osteoarthritis, right ankle and foot**

M19.172   **Post-traumatic osteoarthritis, left ankle and foot**

M19.179   **Post-traumatic osteoarthritis, unspecified ankle and foot**

M19.19   **Post-traumatic osteoarthritis, other specified site**

M19.2   **Secondary osteoarthritis of other joints**

M19.21   **Secondary osteoarthritis, shoulder**

M19.211   **Secondary osteoarthritis, right shoulder**

M19.212   **Secondary osteoarthritis, left shoulder**

M19.219   **Secondary osteoarthritis, unspecified shoulder**

M19.22   **Secondary osteoarthritis, elbow**

M19.221   **Secondary osteoarthritis, right elbow**

M19.222   **Secondary osteoarthritis, left elbow**

M19.229   **Secondary osteoarthritis, unspecified elbow**

M19.23   **Secondary osteoarthritis, wrist**

M19.231   **Secondary osteoarthritis, right wrist**

M19.232   **Secondary osteoarthritis, left wrist**

M19.239   **Secondary osteoarthritis, unspecified wrist**

M19.24   **Secondary osteoarthritis, hand**

M19.241   **Secondary osteoarthritis, right hand**

M19.242   **Secondary osteoarthritis, left hand**

M19.249   **Secondary osteoarthritis, unspecified hand**

M19.27   **Secondary osteoarthritis, ankle and foot**

M19.271   **Secondary osteoarthritis, right ankle and foot**

M19.272   **Secondary osteoarthritis, left ankle and foot**

M19.279   **Secondary osteoarthritis, unspecified ankle and foot**

M19.29   **Secondary osteoarthritis, other specified site**

M19.9   **Osteoarthritis, unspecified site**

M19.90   **Unspecified osteoarthritis, unspecified site**

Arthrosis NOS

Arthritis NOS

Osteoarthritis NOS

M19.91   **Primary osteoarthritis, unspecified site**

Primary osteoarthritis NOS

M19.92   **Post-traumatic osteoarthritis, unspecified site**

Post-traumatic osteoarthritis NOS

M19.93   **Secondary osteoarthritis, unspecified site**

Secondary osteoarthritis NOS

OTHER JOINT DISORDERS (M20-M25)

Excludes2: joints of the spine (M40-M54)

M20   **Acquired deformities of fingers and toes**

Excludes1: acquired absence of fingers and toes (Z89.-)

congenital absence of fingers and toes (Q71.3-, Q72.3-)

congenital deformities and malformations of fingers and toes (Q66.-, Q68-Q70, Q74.-)

M20.0   **Deformity of finger(s)**

Excludes1: clubbing of fingers (R68.3)

palmar fascial fibromatosis [Dupuytren] (M72.0)

trigger finger (M65.3)

M20.00   **Unspecified deformity of finger(s)**

M20.001   **Unspecified deformity of right finger(s)**

M20.002   **Unspecified deformity of left finger(s)**

M20.009   **Unspecified deformity of unspecified finger(s)**

M20.01   **Mallet finger**

M20.011   **Mallet finger of right finger(s)**

M20.012   **Mallet finger of left finger(s)**

M20.019   **Mallet finger of unspecified finger(s)**

M20.02   **Boutonnière deformity**

M20.021   **Boutonnière deformity of right finger(s)**

M20.022   **Boutonnière deformity of left finger(s)**

M20.029   **Boutonnière deformity of unspecified finger(s)**

M20.03   **Swan-neck deformity**

M20.031   **Swan-neck deformity of right finger(s)**

M20.032   **Swan-neck deformity of left finger(s)**

M20.039   **Swan-neck deformity of unspecified finger(s)**

M20.09   **Other deformity of finger(s)**

M20.091   **Other deformity of right finger(s)**

M20.092   **Other deformity of left finger(s)**

M20.099   **Other deformity of finger(s), unspecified finger(s)**

M20.1   **Hallux valgus (acquired)**

Excludes2: bunion (M21.6-)

M20.10   **Hallux valgus (acquired), unspecified foot**

M20.11   **Hallux valgus (acquired), right foot**

M20.12   **Hallux valgus (acquired), left foot**

M20.2   **Hallux rigidus**

M20.20   **Hallux rigidus, unspecified foot**

M20.21   **Hallux rigidus, right foot**

M20.22   **Hallux rigidus, left foot**

M20.3   **Hallux varus (acquired)**

M20.30   **Hallux varus (acquired), unspecified foot**

M20.31   **Hallux varus (acquired), right foot**

M20.32   **Hallux varus (acquired), left foot**

M20.4   **Other hammer toe(s) (acquired)**

M20.40   **Other hammer toe(s) (acquired), unspecified foot**

M20.41   **Other hammer toe(s) (acquired), right foot**

M20.42   **Other hammer toe(s) (acquired), left foot**

M20.5   **Other deformities of toe(s) (acquired)**

M20.5X   **Other deformities of toe(s) (acquired)**

   ● New code   ▲ Revised code   Excludes1: Not coded here   Excludes2: Not included here   ⊗ Placeholder required   ⑦ 7th digit required

M20.5X1 Other deformities of toe(s) (acquired), right foot

M20.5X2 Other deformities of toe(s) (acquired), left foot

M20.5X9 Other deformities of toe(s) (acquired), unspecified foot

M20.6 Acquired deformities of toe(s), unspecified

    M20.60 Acquired deformities of toe(s), unspecified, unspecified foot

    M20.61 Acquired deformities of toe(s), unspecified, right foot

    M20.62 Acquired deformities of toe(s), unspecified, left foot

M21 Other acquired deformities of limbs

Excludes1: acquired absence of limb (Z89.-)

    congenital absence of limbs (Q71-Q73)

    congenital deformities and malformations of limbs (Q65-Q66, Q68-Q74)

Excludes2: acquired deformities of fingers or toes (M20.-)

    coxa plana (M91.2)

M21.0 Valgus deformity, not elsewhere classified

Excludes1: metatarsus valgus (Q66.6)

    talipes calcaneovalgus (Q66.4-)

    M21.00 Valgus deformity, not elsewhere classified, unspecified site

    M21.02 Valgus deformity, not elsewhere classified, elbow

      Cubitus valgus

      M21.021 Valgus deformity, not elsewhere classified, right elbow

      M21.022 Valgus deformity, not elsewhere classified, left elbow

      M21.029 Valgus deformity, not elsewhere classified, unspecified elbow

    M21.05 Valgus deformity, not elsewhere classified, hip

      M21.051 Valgus deformity, not elsewhere classified, right hip

      M21.052 Valgus deformity, not elsewhere classified, left hip

      M21.059 Valgus deformity, not elsewhere classified, unspecified hip

    M21.06 Valgus deformity, not elsewhere classified, knee

      Genu valgum

      Knock knee

      M21.061 Valgus deformity, not elsewhere classified, right knee

      M21.062 Valgus deformity, not elsewhere classified, left knee

      M21.069 Valgus deformity, not elsewhere classified, unspecified knee

    M21.07 Valgus deformity, not elsewhere classified, ankle

      M21.071 Valgus deformity, not elsewhere classified, right ankle

      M21.072 Valgus deformity, not elsewhere classified, left ankle

      M21.079 Valgus deformity, not elsewhere classified, unspecified ankle

M21.1 Varus deformity, not elsewhere classified

Excludes1: metatarsus varus (Q66.22-)

    tibia vara (M92.51-)

M21.10 Varus deformity, not elsewhere classified, unspecified site

M21.12 Varus deformity, not elsewhere classified, elbow

  Cubitus varus, elbow

  M21.121 Varus deformity, not elsewhere classified, right elbow

  M21.122 Varus deformity, not elsewhere classified, left elbow

  M21.129 Varus deformity, not elsewhere classified, unspecified elbow

M21.15 Varus deformity, not elsewhere classified, hip

  M21.151 Varus deformity, not elsewhere classified, right hip

  M21.152 Varus deformity, not elsewhere classified, left hip

  M21.159 Varus deformity, not elsewhere classified, unspecified

M21.16 Varus deformity, not elsewhere classified, knee

  Bow leg Genu varum

  M21.161 Varus deformity, not elsewhere classified, right knee

  M21.162 Varus deformity, not elsewhere classified, left knee

  M21.169 Varus deformity, not elsewhere classified, unspecified knee

M21.17 Varus deformity, not elsewhere classified, ankle

  M21.171 Varus deformity, not elsewhere classified, right ankle

  M21.172 Varus deformity, not elsewhere classified, left ankle

  M21.179 Varus deformity, not elsewhere classified, unspecified ankle

M21.2 Flexion deformity

M21.20 Flexion deformity, unspecified site

M21.21 Flexion deformity, shoulder

  M21.211 Flexion deformity, right shoulder

  M21.212 Flexion deformity, left shoulder

  M21.219 Flexion deformity, unspecified shoulder

M21.22 Flexion deformity, elbow

  M21.221 Flexion deformity, right elbow

  M21.222 Flexion deformity, left elbow

  M21.229 Flexion deformity, unspecified elbow

M21.23 Flexion deformity, wrist

  M21.231 Flexion deformity, right wrist

  M21.232 Flexion deformity, left wrist

  M21.239 Flexion deformity, unspecified wrist

M21.24 Flexion deformity, finger joints

  M21.241 Flexion deformity, right finger joints

  M21.242 Flexion deformity, left finger joints

  M21.249 Flexion deformity, unspecified finger joints

M21.25 Flexion deformity, hip

  M21.251 Flexion deformity, right hip

  M21.252 Flexion deformity, left hip

  M21.259 Flexion deformity, unspecified hip

M21.26 Flexion deformity, knee

  M21.261 Flexion deformity, right knee

  M21.262 Flexion deformity, left knee

M21.269 Flexion deformity, unspecified knee

M21.27 Flexion deformity, ankle and toes

    M21.271 Flexion deformity, right ankle and toes

    M21.272 Flexion deformity, left ankle and toes

    M21.279 Flexion deformity, unspecified ankle and toes

M21.3 Wrist or foot drop (acquired)

M21.33 Wrist drop (acquired)

    M21.331 Wrist drop, right wrist

    M21.332 Wrist drop, left wrist

    M21.339 Wrist drop, unspecified wrist

M21.37 Foot drop (acquired)

    M21.371 Foot drop, right foot

    M21.372 Foot drop, left foot

    M21.379 Foot drop, unspecified foot

M21.4 Flat foot [pes planus] (acquired)

> **Excludes1:** congenital pes planus (Q66.5-)

M21.40 Flat foot [pes planus] (acquired), unspecified foot

M21.41 Flat foot [pes planus] (acquired), right foot

M21.42 Flat foot [pes planus] (acquired), left foot

M21.5 Acquired clawhand, clubhand, clawfoot and clubfoot

> **Excludes1:** clubfoot, not specified as acquired (Q66.89)

M21.51 Acquired clawhand

    M21.511 Acquired clawhand, right hand

    M21.512 Acquired clawhand, left hand

    M21.519 Acquired clawhand, unspecified hand

M21.52 Acquired clubhand

    M21.521 Acquired clubhand, right hand

    M21.522 Acquired clubhand, left hand

    M21.529 Acquired clubhand, unspecified hand

M21.53 Acquired clawfoot

    M21.531 Acquired clawfoot, right foot

    M21.532 Acquired clawfoot, left foot

    M21.539 Acquired clawfoot, unspecified foot

M21.54 Acquired clubfoot

    M21.541 Acquired clubfoot, right foot

    M21.542 Acquired clubfoot, left foot

    M21.549 Acquired clubfoot, unspecified foot

M21.6 Other acquired deformities of foot

> **Excludes2:** deformities of toe (acquired) (M20.1-M20.6-)

M21.61 Bunion

    M21.611 Bunion of right foot

    M21.612 Bunion of left foot

    M21.619 Bunion of unspecified foot

M21.62 Bunionette

    M21.621 Bunionette of right foot

    M21.622 Bunionette of left foot

    M21.629 Bunionette of unspecified foot

M21.6X Other acquired deformities of foot

    M21.6X1 Other acquired deformities of right foot

    M21.6X2 Other acquired deformities of left foot

    M21.6X9 Other acquired deformities of unspecified foot

M21.7 Unequal limb length (acquired)

> **Note:** The site used should correspond to the shorter limb

M21.70 Unequal limb length (acquired), unspecified site

M21.72 Unequal limb length (acquired), humerus

    M21.721 Unequal limb length (acquired), right humerus

    M21.722 Unequal limb length (acquired), left humerus

    M21.729 Unequal limb length (acquired), unspecified humerus

M21.73 Unequal limb length (acquired), ulna and radius

    M21.731 Unequal limb length (acquired), right ulna

    M21.732 Unequal limb length (acquired), left ulna

    M21.733 Unequal limb length (acquired), right radius

    M21.734 Unequal limb length (acquired), left radius

    M21.739 Unequal limb length (acquired), unspecified ulna and radius

M21.75 Unequal limb length (acquired), femur

    M21.751 Unequal limb length (acquired), right femur

    M21.752 Unequal limb length (acquired), left femur

    M21.759 Unequal limb length (acquired), unspecified femur

M21.76 Unequal limb length (acquired), tibia and fibula

    M21.761 Unequal limb length (acquired), right tibia

    M21.762 Unequal limb length (acquired), left tibia

    M21.763 Unequal limb length (acquired), right fibula

    M21.764 Unequal limb length (acquired), left fibula

    M21.769 Unequal limb length (acquired), unspecified tibia and fibula

M21.8 Other specified acquired deformities of limbs

> **Excludes2:** coxa plana (M91.2)

M21.80 Other specified acquired deformities of unspecified limb

M21.82 Other specified acquired deformities of upper arm

    M21.821 Other specified acquired deformities of right upper arm

    M21.822 Other specified acquired deformities of left upper arm

    M21.829 Other specified acquired deformities of unspecified upper arm

M21.83 Other specified acquired deformities of forearm

    M21.831 Other specified acquired deformities of right forearm

    M21.832 Other specified acquired deformities of left forearm

    M21.839 Other specified acquired deformities of unspecified forearm

M21.85 Other specified acquired deformities of thigh

  ● New code ▲ Revised code **Excludes1:** Not coded here **Excludes2:** Not included here ⊗ Placeholder required ⑦ 7th digit required

M21.851   Other specified acquired deformities of right thigh

M21.852   Other specified acquired deformities of left thigh

M21.859   Other specified acquired deformities of unspecified thigh

M21.86   Other specified acquired deformities of lower leg

M21.861   Other specified acquired deformities of right lower leg

M21.862   Other specified acquired deformities of left lower leg

M21.869   Other specified acquired deformities of unspecified lower leg

M21.9   Unspecified acquired deformity of limb and hand

M21.90   Unspecified acquired deformity of unspecified limb

M21.92   Unspecified acquired deformity of upper arm

M21.921   Unspecified acquired deformity of right upper arm

M21.922   Unspecified acquired deformity of left upper arm

M21.929   Unspecified acquired deformity of unspecified upper arm

M21.93   Unspecified acquired deformity of forearm

M21.931   Unspecified acquired deformity of right forearm

M21.932   Unspecified acquired deformity of left forearm

M21.939   Unspecified acquired deformity of unspecified forearm

M21.94   Unspecified acquired deformity of hand

M21.941   Unspecified acquired deformity of hand, right hand

M21.942   Unspecified acquired deformity of hand, left hand

M21.949   Unspecified acquired deformity of hand, unspecified hand

M21.95   Unspecified acquired deformity of thigh

M21.951   Unspecified acquired deformity of right thigh

M21.952   Unspecified acquired deformity of left thigh

M21.959   Unspecified acquired deformity of unspecified thigh

M21.96   Unspecified acquired deformity of lower leg

M21.961   Unspecified acquired deformity of right lower leg

M21.962   Unspecified acquired deformity of left lower leg

M21.969   Unspecified acquired deformity of unspecified lower leg

M22   **Disorder of patella**

Excludes2: traumatic dislocation of patella (S83.0-)

M22.0   Recurrent dislocation of patella

M22.00   Recurrent dislocation of patella, unspecified knee

M22.01   Recurrent dislocation of patella, right knee

M22.02   Recurrent dislocation of patella, left knee

M22.1   Recurrent subluxation of patella

Incomplete dislocation of patella

M22.10   Recurrent subluxation of patella, unspecified knee

M22.11   Recurrent subluxation of patella, right knee

M22.12   Recurrent subluxation of patella, left knee

M22.2   Patellofemoral disorders

M22.2X   Patellofemoral disorders

M22.2X1   Patellofemoral disorders, right knee

M22.2X2   Patellofemoral disorders, left knee

M22.2X9   Patellofemoral disorders, unspecified knee

M22.3   Other derangements of patella

M22.3X   Other derangements of patella

M22.3X1   Other derangements of patella, right knee

M22.3X2   Other derangements of patella, left knee

M22.3X9   Other derangements of patella, unspecified knee

M22.4   Chondromalacia patellae

M22.40   Chondromalacia patellae, unspecified knee

M22.41   Chondromalacia patellae, right knee

M22.42   Chondromalacia patellae, left knee

M22.8   Other disorders of patella

M22.8X   Other disorders of patella

M22.8X1   Other disorders of patella, right knee

M22.8X2   Other disorders of patella, left knee

M22.8X9   Other disorders of patella, unspecified knee

M22.9   Unspecified disorder of patella

M22.90   Unspecified disorder of patella, unspecified knee

M22.91   Unspecified disorder of patella, right knee

M22.92   Unspecified disorder of patella, left knee

M23   **Internal derangement of knee**

Definition: Internal derangement of knee is a term that describes internal damage to the knee joint, generally caused by trauma. It is a nonspecific term that usually must be further refined by history, physical exam, x-rays, and frequently MRI studies.

Excludes1: ankylosis (M24.66)

deformity of knee (M21.-)

osteochondritis dissecans (M93.2)

Excludes2: current injury - see injury of knee and lower leg (S80-S89)

recurrent dislocation or subluxation of joints (M24.4)

recurrent dislocation or subluxation of patella (M22.0-M22.1)

M23.0   Cystic meniscus

M23.00   Cystic meniscus, unspecified meniscus

Cystic meniscus, unspecified lateral meniscus

Cystic meniscus, unspecified medial meniscus

M23.000   Cystic meniscus, unspecified lateral meniscus, right knee

M23.001   Cystic meniscus, unspecified lateral meniscus, left knee

M23.002   Cystic meniscus, unspecified lateral meniscus, unspecified knee

M23.003   Cystic meniscus, unspecified medial meniscus, right knee

M23.004   Cystic meniscus, unspecified medial meniscus, left knee

M23.005 Cystic meniscus, unspecified medial meniscus, unspecified knee

M23.006 Cystic meniscus, unspecified meniscus, right knee

M23.007 Cystic meniscus, unspecified meniscus, left knee

M23.009 Cystic meniscus, unspecified meniscus, unspecified knee

M23.01 Cystic meniscus, anterior horn of medial meniscus

M23.011 Cystic meniscus, anterior horn of medial meniscus, right knee

M23.012 Cystic meniscus, anterior horn of medial meniscus, left knee

M23.019 Cystic meniscus, anterior horn of medial meniscus, unspecified knee

M23.02 Cystic meniscus, posterior horn of medial meniscus

M23.021 Cystic meniscus, posterior horn of medial meniscus, right knee

M23.022 Cystic meniscus, posterior horn of medial meniscus, left knee

M23.029 Cystic meniscus, posterior horn of medial meniscus, unspecified knee

M23.03 Cystic meniscus, other medial meniscus

M23.031 Cystic meniscus, other medial meniscus, right knee

M23.032 Cystic meniscus, other medial meniscus, left knee

M23.039 Cystic meniscus, other medial meniscus, unspecified knee

M23.04 Cystic meniscus, anterior horn of lateral meniscus

M23.041 Cystic meniscus, anterior horn of lateral meniscus, right knee

M23.042 Cystic meniscus, anterior horn of lateral meniscus, left knee

M23.049 Cystic meniscus, anterior horn of lateral meniscus, unspecified knee

M23.05 Cystic meniscus, posterior horn of lateral meniscus

M23.051 Cystic meniscus, posterior horn of lateral meniscus, right knee

M23.052 Cystic meniscus, posterior horn of lateral meniscus, left knee

M23.059 Cystic meniscus, posterior horn of lateral meniscus, unspecified knee

M23.06 Cystic meniscus, other lateral meniscus

M23.061 Cystic meniscus, other lateral meniscus, right knee

M23.062 Cystic meniscus, other lateral meniscus, left knee

M23.069 Cystic meniscus, other lateral meniscus, unspecified knee

M23.2 Derangement of meniscus due to old tear or injury
Old bucket-handle tear

M23.20 Derangement of unspecified meniscus due to old tear or injury
Derangement of unspecified lateral meniscus due to old tear or injury
Derangement of unspecified medial meniscus due to old tear or injury

M23.200 Derangement of unspecified lateral meniscus due to old tear or injury, right knee

M23.201 Derangement of unspecified lateral meniscus due to old tear or injury, left knee

M23.202 Derangement of unspecified lateral meniscus due to old tear or injury, unspecified knee

M23.203 Derangement of unspecified medial meniscus due to old tear or injury, right knee

M23.204 Derangement of unspecified medial meniscus due to old tear or injury, left knee

M23.205 Derangement of unspecified medial meniscus due to old tear or injury, unspecified knee

M23.206 Derangement of unspecified meniscus due to old tear or injury, right knee

M23.207 Derangement of unspecified meniscus due to old tear or injury, left knee

M23.209 Derangement of unspecified meniscus due to old tear or injury, unspecified knee

M23.21 Derangement of anterior horn of medial meniscus due to old tear or injury

M23.211 Derangement of anterior horn of medial meniscus due to old tear or injury, right knee

M23.212 Derangement of anterior horn of medial meniscus due to old tear or injury, left knee

M23.219 Derangement of anterior horn of medial meniscus due to old tear or injury, unspecified knee

M23.22 Derangement of posterior horn of medial meniscus due to old tear or injury

M23.221 Derangement of posterior horn of medial meniscus due to old tear or injury, right knee

M23.222 Derangement of posterior horn of medial meniscus due to old tear or injury, left knee

M23.229 Derangement of posterior horn of medial meniscus due to old tear or injury, unspecified knee

M23.23 Derangement of other medial meniscus due to old tear or injury

M23.231 Derangement of other medial meniscus due to old tear or injury, right knee

M23.232 Derangement of other medial meniscus due to old tear or injury, left knee

M23.239 Derangement of other medial meniscus due to old tear or injury, unspecified knee

M23.24 Derangement of anterior horn of lateral meniscus due to old tear or injury

M23.241 Derangement of anterior horn of lateral meniscus due to old tear or injury, right knee

● New code ▲ Revised code **Excludes1:** Not coded here **Excludes2:** Not included here ⊗ Placeholder required ⑦ 7th digit required

M23.242 Derangement of anterior horn of lateral meniscus due to old tear or injury, left knee

M23.249 Derangement of anterior horn of lateral meniscus due to old tear or injury, unspecified knee

M23.25 Derangement of posterior horn of lateral meniscus due to old tear or injury

M23.251 Derangement of posterior horn of lateral meniscus due to old tear or injury, right knee

M23.252 Derangement of posterior horn of lateral meniscus due to old tear or injury, left knee

M23.259 Derangement of posterior horn of lateral meniscus due to old tear or injury, unspecified knee

M23.26 Derangement of other lateral meniscus due to old tear or injury

M23.261 Derangement of other lateral meniscus due to old tear or injury, right knee

M23.262 Derangement of other lateral meniscus due to old tear or injury, left knee

M23.269 Derangement of other lateral meniscus due to old tear or injury, unspecified knee

M23.3 Other meniscus derangements

Degenerate meniscus

Detached meniscus

Retained meniscus

M23.30 Other meniscus derangements, unspecified meniscus

Other meniscus derangements, unspecified lateral meniscus

Other meniscus derangements, unspecified medial meniscus

M23.300 Other meniscus derangements, unspecified lateral meniscus, right knee

M23.301 Other meniscus derangements, unspecified lateral meniscus, left knee

M23.302 Other meniscus derangements, unspecified lateral meniscus, unspecified knee

M23.303 Other meniscus derangements, unspecified medial meniscus, right knee

M23.304 Other meniscus derangements, unspecified medial meniscus, left knee

M23.305 Other meniscus derangements, unspecified medial meniscus, unspecified knee

M23.306 Other meniscus derangements, unspecified meniscus, right knee

M23.307 Other meniscus derangements, unspecified meniscus, left knee

M23.309 Other meniscus derangements, unspecified meniscus, unspecified knee

M23.31 Other meniscus derangements, anterior horn of medial meniscus

M23.311 Other meniscus derangements, anterior horn of medial meniscus, right knee

M23.312 Other meniscus derangements, anterior horn of medial meniscus, left knee

M23.319 Other meniscus derangements, anterior horn of medial meniscus, unspecified knee

M23.32 Other meniscus derangements, posterior horn of medial meniscus

M23.321 Other meniscus derangements, posterior horn of medial meniscus, right knee

M23.322 Other meniscus derangements, posterior horn of medial meniscus, left knee

M23.329 Other meniscus derangements, posterior horn of medial meniscus, unspecified knee

M23.33 Other meniscus derangements, other medial meniscus

M23.331 Other meniscus derangements, other medial meniscus, right knee

M23.332 Other meniscus derangements, other medial meniscus, left knee

M23.339 Other meniscus derangements, other medial meniscus, unspecified knee

M23.34 Other meniscus derangements, anterior horn of lateral meniscus

M23.341 Other meniscus derangements, anterior horn of lateral meniscus, right knee

M23.342 Other meniscus derangements, anterior horn of lateral meniscus, left knee

M23.349 Other meniscus derangements, anterior horn of lateral meniscus, unspecified knee

M23.35 Other meniscus derangements, posterior horn of lateral meniscus

M23.351 Other meniscus derangements, posterior horn of lateral meniscus, right knee

M23.352 Other meniscus derangements, posterior horn of lateral meniscus, left knee

M23.359 Other meniscus derangements, posterior horn of lateral meniscus, unspecified knee

M23.36 Other meniscus derangements, other lateral meniscus

M23.361 Other meniscus derangements, other lateral meniscus, right knee

M23.362 Other meniscus derangements, other lateral meniscus, left knee

M23.369 Other meniscus derangements, other lateral meniscus, unspecified knee

M23.4 Loose body in knee

M23.40 Loose body in knee, unspecified knee

M23.41 Loose body in knee, right knee

M23.42 Loose body in knee, left knee

M23.5 Chronic instability of knee

M23.50 Chronic instability of knee, unspecified knee

M23.51 Chronic instability of knee, right knee

M23.52   Chronic instability of knee, left knee

M23.6   Other spontaneous disruption of ligament(s) of knee

M23.60   Other spontaneous disruption of unspecified ligament of knee

M23.601   Other spontaneous disruption of unspecified ligament of right knee

M23.602   Other spontaneous disruption of unspecified ligament of left knee

M23.609   Other spontaneous disruption of unspecified ligament of unspecified knee

M23.61   Other spontaneous disruption of anterior cruciate ligament of knee

M23.611   Other spontaneous disruption of anterior cruciate ligament of right knee

M23.612   Other spontaneous disruption of anterior cruciate ligament of left knee

M23.619   Other spontaneous disruption of anterior cruciate ligament of unspecified knee

M23.62   Other spontaneous disruption of posterior cruciate ligament of knee

M23.621   Other spontaneous disruption of posterior cruciate ligament of right knee

M23.622   Other spontaneous disruption of posterior cruciate ligament of left knee

M23.629   Other spontaneous disruption of posterior cruciate ligament of unspecified knee

M23.63   Other spontaneous disruption of medial collateral ligament of knee

M23.631   Other spontaneous disruption of medial collateral ligament of right knee

M23.632   Other spontaneous disruption of medial collateral ligament of left knee

M23.639   Other spontaneous disruption of medial collateral ligament of unspecified knee

M23.64   Other spontaneous disruption of lateral collateral ligament of knee

M23.641   Other spontaneous disruption of lateral collateral ligament of right knee

M23.642   Other spontaneous disruption of lateral collateral ligament of left knee

M23.649   Other spontaneous disruption of lateral collateral ligament of unspecified knee

M23.67   Other spontaneous disruption of capsular ligament of knee

M23.671   Other spontaneous disruption of capsular ligament of right knee

M23.672   Other spontaneous disruption of capsular ligament of left knee

M23.679   Other spontaneous disruption of capsular ligament of unspecified knee

M23.8   Other internal derangements of knee

Laxity of ligament of knee

Snapping knee

M23.8X   Other internal derangements of knee

M23.8X1   Other internal derangements of right knee

M23.8X2   Other internal derangements of left knee

M23.8X9   Other internal derangements of unspecified knee

M23.9   Unspecified internal derangement of knee

M23.90   Unspecified internal derangement of unspecified knee

M23.91   Unspecified internal derangement of right knee

M23.92   Unspecified internal derangement of left knee

M24   **Other specific joint derangements**

Excludes1: current injury - see injury of joint by body region

Excludes2: ganglion (M67.4)

snapping knee (M23.8-)

temporomandibular joint disorders (M26.6-)

M24.0   Loose body in joint

Excludes2: loose body in knee (M23.4)

M24.00   Loose body in unspecified joint

M24.01   Loose body in shoulder

M24.011   Loose body in right shoulder

M24.012   Loose body in left shoulder

M24.019   Loose body in unspecified shoulder

M24.02   Loose body in elbow

M24.021   Loose body in right elbow

M24.022   Loose body in left elbow

M24.029   Loose body in unspecified elbow

M24.03   Loose body in wrist

M24.031   Loose body in right wrist

M24.032   Loose body in left wrist

M24.039   Loose body in unspecified wrist

M24.04   Loose body in finger joints

M24.041   Loose body in right finger joint(s)

M24.042   Loose body in left finger joint(s)

M24.049   Loose body in unspecified finger joint(s)

M24.05   Loose body in hip

M24.051   Loose body in right hip

M24.052   Loose body in left hip

M24.059   Loose body in unspecified hip

M24.07   Loose body in ankle and toe joints

M24.071   Loose body in right ankle

M24.072   Loose body in left ankle

M24.073   Loose body in unspecified ankle

M24.074   Loose body in right toe joint(s)

M24.075   Loose body in left toe joint(s)

M24.076   Loose body in unspecified toe joints

M24.08   Loose body, other site

M24.1   Other articular cartilage disorders

Excludes2: chondrocalcinosis (M11.1, M11.2-)

internal derangement of knee (M23.-)

metastatic calcification (E83.5)

ochronosis (E70.2)

M24.10   Other articular cartilage disorders, unspecified site

● New code   ▲ Revised code   Excludes1: Not coded here   Excludes2: Not included here   ⊗ Placeholder required   ⑦7th digit required

M24.11 Other articular cartilage disorders, shoulder

    M24.111 Other articular cartilage disorders, right shoulder

    M24.112 Other articular cartilage disorders, left shoulder

    M24.119 Other articular cartilage disorders, unspecified shoulder

M24.12 Other articular cartilage disorders, elbow

    M24.121 Other articular cartilage disorders, right elbow

    M24.122 Other articular cartilage disorders, left elbow

    M24.129 Other articular cartilage disorders, unspecified elbow

M24.13 Other articular cartilage disorders, wrist

    M24.131 Other articular cartilage disorders, right wrist

    M24.132 Other articular cartilage disorders, left wrist

    M24.139 Other articular cartilage disorders, unspecified wrist

M24.14 Other articular cartilage disorders, hand

    M24.141 Other articular cartilage disorders, right hand

    M24.142 Other articular cartilage disorders, left hand

    M24.149 Other articular cartilage disorders, unspecified hand

M24.15 Other articular cartilage disorders, hip

    M24.151 Other articular cartilage disorders, right hip

    M24.152 Other articular cartilage disorders, left hip

    M24.159 Other articular cartilage disorders, unspecified hip

M24.17 Other articular cartilage disorders, ankle and foot

    M24.171 Other articular cartilage disorders, right ankle

    M24.172 Other articular cartilage disorders, left ankle

    M24.173 Other articular cartilage disorders, unspecified ankle

    M24.174 Other articular cartilage disorders, right foot

    M24.175 Other articular cartilage disorders, left foot

    M24.176 Other articular cartilage disorders, unspecified foot

M24.19 Other articular cartilage disorders, other specified site

M24.2 **Disorder of ligament**

Instability secondary to old ligament injury

Ligamentous laxity NOS

Excludes1: familial ligamentous laxity (M35.7)

Excludes2: internal derangement of knee (M23.5-M23.8X9)

M24.20 Disorder of ligament, unspecified site

M24.21 Disorder of ligament, shoulder

    M24.211 Disorder of ligament, right shoulder

    M24.212 Disorder of ligament, left shoulder

    M24.219 Disorder of ligament, unspecified shoulder

M24.22 Disorder of ligament, elbow

    M24.221 Disorder of ligament, right elbow

    M24.222 Disorder of ligament, left elbow

    M24.229 Disorder of ligament, unspecified elbow

M24.23 Disorder of ligament, wrist

    M24.231 Disorder of ligament, right wrist

    M24.232 Disorder of ligament, left wrist

    M24.239 Disorder of ligament, unspecified wrist

M24.24 Disorder of ligament, hand

    M24.241 Disorder of ligament, right hand

    M24.242 Disorder of ligament, left hand

    M24.249 Disorder of ligament, unspecified hand

M24.25 Disorder of ligament, hip

    M24.251 Disorder of ligament, right hip

    M24.252 Disorder of ligament, left hip

    M24.259 Disorder of ligament, unspecified hip

M24.27 Disorder of ligament, ankle and foot

    M24.271 Disorder of ligament, right ankle

    M24.272 Disorder of ligament, left ankle

    M24.273 Disorder of ligament, unspecified ankle

    M24.274 Disorder of ligament, right foot

    M24.275 Disorder of ligament, left foot

    M24.276 Disorder of ligament, unspecified foot

M24.28 Disorder of ligament, vertebrae

M24.29 Disorder of ligament, other specified site

M24.3 **Pathological dislocation of joint, not elsewhere classified**

Excludes1: congenital dislocation or displacement of joint-see congenital malformations and deformations of the musculoskeletal system (Q65-Q79)

current injury - see injury of joints and ligaments by body region

recurrent dislocation of joint (M24.4-)

M24.30 Pathological dislocation of unspecified joint, not elsewhere classified

M24.31 Pathological dislocation of shoulder, not elsewhere classified

    M24.311 Pathological dislocation of right shoulder, not elsewhere classified

    M24.312 Pathological dislocation of left shoulder, not elsewhere classified

    M24.319 Pathological dislocation of unspecified shoulder, not elsewhere classified

M24.32 Pathological dislocation of elbow, not elsewhere classified

    M24.321 Pathological dislocation of right elbow, not elsewhere classified

    M24.322 Pathological dislocation of left elbow, not elsewhere classified

    M24.329 Pathological dislocation of unspecified elbow, not elsewhere classified

M24.33 Pathological dislocation of wrist, not elsewhere classified

M24.331 **Pathological dislocation of right wrist, not elsewhere classified**

M24.332 **Pathological dislocation of left wrist, not elsewhere classified**

M24.339 **Pathological dislocation of unspecified wrist, not elsewhere classified**

M24.34 **Pathological dislocation of hand, not elsewhere classified**

M24.341 **Pathological dislocation of right hand, not elsewhere classified**

M24.342 **Pathological dislocation of left hand, not elsewhere classified**

M24.349 **Pathological dislocation of unspecified hand, not elsewhere classified**

M24.35 **Pathological dislocation of hip, not elsewhere classified**

M24.351 **Pathological dislocation of right hip, not elsewhere classified**

M24.352 **Pathological dislocation of left hip, not elsewhere classified**

M24.359 **Pathological dislocation of unspecified hip, not elsewhere classified**

M24.36 **Pathological dislocation of knee, not elsewhere classified**

M24.361 **Pathological dislocation of right knee, not elsewhere classified**

M24.362 **Pathological dislocation of left knee, not elsewhere classified**

M24.369 **Pathological dislocation of unspecified knee, not elsewhere classified**

M24.37 **Pathological dislocation of ankle and foot, not elsewhere classified**

M24.371 **Pathological dislocation of right ankle, not elsewhere classified**

M24.372 **Pathological dislocation of left ankle, not elsewhere classified**

M24.373 **Pathological dislocation of unspecified ankle, not elsewhere classified**

M24.374 **Pathological dislocation of right foot, not elsewhere classified**

M24.375 **Pathological dislocation of left foot, not elsewhere classified**

M24.376 **Pathological dislocation of unspecified foot, not elsewhere classified**

M24.39 **Pathological dislocation of other specified joint, not elsewhere classified**

M24.4 **Recurrent dislocation of joint**

Recurrent subluxation of joint

Excludes2: recurrent dislocation of patella (M22.0-M22.1)

recurrent vertebral dislocation (M43.3-, M43.4, M43.5-)

M24.40 **Recurrent dislocation, unspecified joint**

M24.41 **Recurrent dislocation, shoulder**

M24.411 **Recurrent dislocation, right shoulder**

M24.412 **Recurrent dislocation, left shoulder**

M24.419 **Recurrent dislocation, unspecified shoulder**

M24.42 **Recurrent dislocation, elbow**

M24.421 **Recurrent dislocation, right elbow**

M24.422 **Recurrent dislocation, left elbow**

M24.429 **Recurrent dislocation, unspecified elbow**

M24.43 **Recurrent dislocation, wrist**

M24.431 **Recurrent dislocation, right wrist**

M24.432 **Recurrent dislocation, left wrist**

M24.439 **Recurrent dislocation, unspecified wrist**

M24.44 **Recurrent dislocation, hand and finger(s)**

M24.441 **Recurrent dislocation, right hand**

M24.442 **Recurrent dislocation, left hand**

M24.443 **Recurrent dislocation, unspecified hand**

M24.444 **Recurrent dislocation, right finger**

M24.445 **Recurrent dislocation, left finger**

M24.446 **Recurrent dislocation, unspecified finger**

M24.45 **Recurrent dislocation, hip**

M24.451 **Recurrent dislocation, right hip**

M24.452 **Recurrent dislocation, left hip**

M24.459 **Recurrent dislocation, unspecified hip**

M24.46 **Recurrent dislocation, knee**

M24.461 **Recurrent dislocation, right knee**

M24.462 **Recurrent dislocation, left knee**

M24.469 **Recurrent dislocation, unspecified knee**

M24.47 **Recurrent dislocation, ankle, foot and toes**

M24.471 **Recurrent dislocation, right ankle**

M24.472 **Recurrent dislocation, left ankle**

M24.473 **Recurrent dislocation, unspecified ankle**

M24.474 **Recurrent dislocation, right foot**

M24.475 **Recurrent dislocation, left foot**

M24.476 **Recurrent dislocation, unspecified foot**

M24.477 **Recurrent dislocation, right toe(s)**

M24.478 **Recurrent dislocation, left toe(s)**

M24.479 **Recurrent dislocation, unspecified toe(s)**

M24.49 **Recurrent dislocation, other specified joint**

M24.5 **Contracture of joint**

Excludes1: contracture of muscle without contracture of joint (M62.4-)

contracture of tendon (sheath) without contracture of joint (M62.4-)

Dupuytren's contracture (M72.0)

Excludes2: acquired deformities of limbs (M20-M21)

M24.50 **Contracture, unspecified joint**

M24.51 **Contracture, shoulder**

M24.511 **Contracture, right shoulder**

M24.512 **Contracture, left shoulder**

M24.519 **Contracture, unspecified shoulder**

M24.52 **Contracture, elbow**

M24.521 **Contracture, right elbow**

M24.522 **Contracture, left elbow**

M24.529 **Contracture, unspecified elbow**

M24.53 **Contracture, wrist**

● New code   ▲ Revised code   **Excludes1:** Not coded here   **Excludes2:** Not included here   ⊗ Placeholder required   ⑦7th digit required

M24.531 Contracture, right wrist

M24.532 Contracture, left wrist

M24.539 Contracture, unspecified wrist

M24.54 Contracture, hand

M24.541 Contracture, right hand

M24.542 Contracture, left hand

M24.549 Contracture, unspecified hand

M24.55 Contracture, hip

M24.551 Contracture, right hip

M24.552 Contracture, left hip

M24.559 Contracture, unspecified hip

M24.56 Contracture, knee

M24.561 Contracture, right knee

M24.562 Contracture, left knee

M24.569 Contracture, unspecified knee

M24.57 Contracture, ankle and foot

M24.571 Contracture, right ankle

M24.572 Contracture, left ankle

M24.573 Contracture, unspecified ankle

M24.574 Contracture, right foot

M24.575 Contracture, left foot

M24.576 Contracture, unspecified foot

M24.59 Contracture, other specified joint

M24.6 Ankylosis of joint

Excludes1: stiffness of joint without ankylosis (M25.6-)

Excludes2: spine (M43.2-)

M24.60 Ankylosis, unspecified joint

M24.61 Ankylosis, shoulder

M24.611 Ankylosis, right shoulder

M24.612 Ankylosis, left shoulder

M24.619 Ankylosis, unspecified shoulder

M24.62 Ankylosis, elbow

M24.621 Ankylosis, right elbow

M24.622 Ankylosis, left elbow

M24.629 Ankylosis, unspecified elbow

M24.63 Ankylosis, wrist

M24.631 Ankylosis, right wrist

M24.632 Ankylosis, left wrist

M24.639 Ankylosis, unspecified wrist

M24.64 Ankylosis, hand

M24.641 Ankylosis, right hand

M24.642 Ankylosis, left hand

M24.649 Ankylosis, unspecified hand

M24.65 Ankylosis, hip

M24.651 Ankylosis, right hip

M24.652 Ankylosis, left hip

M24.659 Ankylosis, unspecified hip

M24.66 Ankylosis, knee

M24.661 Ankylosis, right knee

M24.662 Ankylosis, left knee

M24.669 Ankylosis, unspecified knee

M24.67 Ankylosis, ankle and foot

M24.671 Ankylosis, right ankle

M24.672 Ankylosis, left ankle

M24.673 Ankylosis, unspecified ankle

M24.674 Ankylosis, right foot

M24.675 Ankylosis, left foot

M24.676 Ankylosis, unspecified foot

M24.69 Ankylosis, other specified joint

M24.7 Protrusio acetabuli

M24.8 Other specific joint derangements, not elsewhere classified

Excludes2: iliotibial band syndrome (M76.3)

M24.80 Other specific joint derangements of unspecified joint, not elsewhere classified

M24.81 Other specific joint derangements of shoulder, not elsewhere classified

M24.811 Other specific joint derangements of right shoulder, not elsewhere classified

M24.812 Other specific joint derangements of left shoulder, not elsewhere classified

M24.819 Other specific joint derangements of unspecified shoulder, not elsewhere classified

M24.82 Other specific joint derangements of elbow, not elsewhere classified

M24.821 Other specific joint derangements of right elbow, not elsewhere classified

M24.822 Other specific joint derangements of left elbow, not elsewhere classified

M24.829 Other specific joint derangements of unspecified elbow, not elsewhere classified

M24.83 Other specific joint derangements of wrist, not elsewhere classified

M24.831 Other specific joint derangements of right wrist, not elsewhere classified

M24.832 Other specific joint derangements of left wrist, not elsewhere classified

M24.839 Other specific joint derangements of unspecified wrist, not elsewhere classified

M24.84 Other specific joint derangements of hand, not elsewhere classified

M24.841 Other specific joint derangements of right hand, not elsewhere classified

M24.842 Other specific joint derangements of left hand, not elsewhere classified

M24.849 Other specific joint derangements of unspecified hand, not elsewhere classified

M24.85 Other specific joint derangements of hip, not elsewhere classified

Irritable hip

M24.851 Other specific joint derangements of right hip, not elsewhere classified

M24.852 Other specific joint derangements of left hip, not elsewhere classified

M24.859 Other specific joint derangements of unspecified hip, not elsewhere classified

M24.87 Other specific joint derangements of ankle and foot, not elsewhere classified

M24.871 Other specific joint derangements of right ankle, not elsewhere classified

M24.872 Other specific joint derangements of left ankle, not elsewhere classified

---

Add 4th-7th digits   Nonspecific code   Unspecified code   Manifestation code   [HCC] Hierarchical Condition Code

M24.873 **Other specific joint derangements of unspecified ankle, not elsewhere classified**

M24.874 **Other specific joint derangements of right foot, not elsewhere classified**

M24.875 **Other specific joint derangements left foot, not elsewhere classified**

M24.876 **Other specific joint derangements of unspecified foot, not elsewhere**

M24.89 **Other specific joint derangement of other specified joint, not elsewhere classified**

M24.9 **Joint derangement, unspecified**

M25 **Other joint disorder, not elsewhere classified**

Excludes2: abnormality of gait and mobility (R26.-)

acquired deformities of limb (M20-M21)

calcification of bursa (M71.4-)

calcification of shoulder (joint) (M75.3)

calcification of tendon (M65.2-)

difficulty in walking (R26.2)

temporomandibular joint disorder (M26.6-)

M25.0 **Hemarthrosis**

Excludes1: current injury - see injury of joint by body region

hemophilic arthropathy (M36.2)

M25.00 **Hemarthrosis, unspecified joint**

M25.01 **Hemarthrosis, shoulder**

M25.011 **Hemarthrosis, right shoulder**

M25.012 **Hemarthrosis, left shoulder**

M25.019 **Hemarthrosis, unspecified shoulder**

M25.02 **Hemarthrosis, elbow**

M25.021 **Hemarthrosis, right elbow**

M25.022 **Hemarthrosis, left elbow**

M25.029 **Hemarthrosis, unspecified elbow**

M25.03 **Hemarthrosis, wrist**

M25.031 **Hemarthrosis, right wrist**

M25.032 **Hemarthrosis, left wrist**

M25.039 **Hemarthrosis, unspecified wrist**

M25.04 **Hemarthrosis, hand**

M25.041 **Hemarthrosis, right hand**

M25.042 **Hemarthrosis, left hand**

M25.049 **Hemarthrosis, unspecified hand**

M25.05 **Hemarthrosis, hip**

M25.051 **Hemarthrosis, right hip**

M25.052 **Hemarthrosis, left hip**

M25.059 **Hemarthrosis, unspecified hip**

M25.06 **Hemarthrosis, knee**

M25.061 **Hemarthrosis, right knee**

M25.062 **Hemarthrosis, left knee**

M25.069 **Hemarthrosis, unspecified knee**

M25.07 **Hemarthrosis, ankle and foot**

M25.071 **Hemarthrosis, right ankle**

M25.072 **Hemarthrosis, left ankle**

M25.073 **Hemarthrosis, unspecified ankle**

M25.074 **Hemarthrosis, right foot**

M25.075 **Hemarthrosis, left foot**

M25.076 **Hemarthrosis, unspecified foot**

M25.08 **Hemarthrosis, other specified site**

Hemarthrosis, vertebrae

M25.1 **Fistula of joint**

M25.10 **Fistula, unspecified joint**

M25.11 **Fistula, shoulder**

M25.111 **Fistula, right shoulder**

M25.112 **Fistula, left shoulder**

M25.119 **Fistula, unspecified shoulder**

M25.12 **Fistula, elbow**

M25.121 **Fistula, right elbow**

M25.122 **Fistula, left elbow**

M25.129 **Fistula, unspecified elbow**

M25.13 **Fistula, wrist**

M25.131 **Fistula, right wrist**

M25.132 **Fistula, left wrist**

M25.139 **Fistula, unspecified wrist**

M25.14 **Fistula, hand**

M25.141 **Fistula, right hand**

M25.142 **Fistula, left hand**

M25.149 **Fistula, unspecified hand**

M25.15 **Fistula, hip**

M25.151 **Fistula, right hip**

M25.152 **Fistula, left hip**

M25.159 **Fistula, unspecified hip**

M25.16 **Fistula, knee**

M25.161 **Fistula, right knee**

M25.162 **Fistula, left knee**

M25.169 **Fistula, unspecified knee**

M25.17 **Fistula, ankle and foot**

M25.171 **Fistula, right ankle**

M25.172 **Fistula, left ankle**

M25.173 **Fistula, unspecified ankle**

M25.174 **Fistula, right foot**

M25.175 **Fistula, left foot**

M25.176 **Fistula, unspecified foot**

M25.18 **Fistula, other specified site**

Fistula, vertebrae

M25.2 **Flail joint**

M25.20 **Flail joint, unspecified joint**

M25.21 **Flail joint, shoulder**

M25.211 **Flail joint, right shoulder**

M25.212 **Flail joint, left shoulder**

M25.219 **Flail joint, unspecified shoulder**

M25.22 **Flail joint, elbow**

M25.221 **Flail joint, right elbow**

M25.222 **Flail joint, left elbow**

M25.229 **Flail joint, unspecified elbow**

M25.23 **Flail joint, wrist**

M25.231 **Flail joint, right wrist**

M25.232 **Flail joint, left wrist**

M25.239 **Flail joint, unspecified wrist**

M25.24 **Flail joint, hand**

M25.241 **Flail joint, right hand**

M25.242 **Flail joint, left hand**

M25.249 **Flail joint, unspecified hand**

M25.25 **Flail joint, hip**

M25.251 **Flail joint, right hip**

M25.252 **Flail joint, left hip**

M25.259   Flail joint, unspecified hip

M25.26   Flail joint, knee

M25.261   Flail joint, right knee

M25.262   Flail joint, left knee

M25.269   Flail joint, unspecified knee

M25.27   Flail joint, ankle and foot

M25.271   Flail joint, right ankle and foot

M25.272   Flail joint, left ankle and foot

M25.279   Flail joint, unspecified ankle and foot

M25.28   Flail joint, other site

M25.3 Other instability of joint

Excludes1: instability of joint secondary to old ligament injury (M24.2-)

instability of joint secondary to removal of joint prosthesis (M96.8-)

Excludes2: spinal instabilities (M53.2-)

M25.30   Other instability, unspecified joint

M25.31   Other instability, shoulder

M25.311   Other instability, right shoulder

M25.312   Other instability, left shoulder

M25.319   Other instability, unspecified shoulder

M25.32   Other instability, elbow

M25.321   Other instability, right elbow

M25.322   Other instability, left elbow

M25.329   Other instability, unspecified elbow

M25.33   Other instability, wrist

M25.331   Other instability, right wrist

M25.332   Other instability, left wrist

M25.339   Other instability, unspecified wrist

M25.34   Other instability, hand

M25.341   Other instability, right hand

M25.342   Other instability, left hand

M25.349   Other instability, unspecified hand

M25.35   Other instability, hip

M25.351   Other instability, right hip

M25.352   Other instability, left hip

M25.359   Other instability, unspecified hip

M25.36   Other instability, knee

M25.361   Other instability, right knee

M25.362   Other instability, left knee

M25.369   Other instability, unspecified knee

M25.37   Other instability, ankle and foot

M25.371   Other instability, right ankle

M25.372   Other instability, left ankle

M25.373   Other instability, unspecified ankle

M25.374   Other instability, right foot

M25.375   Other instability, left foot

M25.376   Other instability, unspecified foot

M25.39   Other instability, other specified joint

M25.4 Effusion of joint

Excludes1: hydrarthrosis in yaws (A66.6)

intermittent hydrarthrosis (M12.4-)

Other infective (teno)synovitis (M65.1-)

M25.40   Effusion, unspecified joint

M25.41   Effusion, shoulder

M25.411   Effusion, right shoulder

M25.412   Effusion, left shoulder

M25.419   Effusion, unspecified shoulder

M25.42   Effusion, elbow

M25.421   Effusion, right elbow

M25.422   Effusion, left elbow

M25.429   Effusion, unspecified elbow

M25.43   Effusion, wrist

M25.431   Effusion, right wrist

M25.432   Effusion, left wrist

M25.439   Effusion, unspecified wrist

M25.44   Effusion, hand

M25.441   Effusion, right hand

M25.442   Effusion, left hand

M25.449   Effusion, unspecified hand

M25.45   Effusion, hip

M25.451   Effusion, right hip

M25.452   Effusion, left hip

M25.459   Effusion, unspecified hip

M25.46   Effusion, knee

M25.461   Effusion, right knee

M25.462   Effusion, left knee

M25.469   Effusion, unspecified knee

M25.47   Effusion, ankle and foot

M25.471   Effusion, right ankle

M25.472   Effusion, left ankle

M25.473   Effusion, unspecified ankle

M25.474   Effusion, right foot

M25.475   Effusion, left foot

M25.476   Effusion, unspecified foot

M25.48   Effusion, other site

M25.5 Pain in joint

Excludes2: pain in hand (M79.64-)

pain in fingers (M79.64-)

pain in foot (M79.67-)

pain in limb (M79.6-)

pain in toes (M79.67-)

M25.50   Pain in unspecified joint

M25.51   Pain in shoulder

M25.511   Pain in right shoulder

M25.512   Pain in left shoulder

M25.519   Pain in unspecified shoulder

M25.52   Pain in elbow

M25.521   Pain in right elbow

M25.522   Pain in left elbow

M25.529   Pain in unspecified elbow

M25.53   Pain in wrist

M25.531   Pain in right wrist

M25.532   Pain in left wrist

M25.539   Pain in unspecified wrist

M25.54   Pain in joints of hand

M25.541   Pain in joints of right hand

M25.542   Pain in joints of left hand

M25.549   Pain in joints of unspecified hand

Pain in joints of hand NOS

M25.55   Pain in hip

M25.551   Pain in right hip

M25.552 Pain in left hip

M25.559 Pain in unspecified hip

M25.56 Pain in knee

M25.561 Pain in right knee

M25.562 Pain in left knee

M25.569 Pain in unspecified knee

M25.57 Pain in ankle and joints of foot

M25.571 Pain in right ankle and joints of right foot

M25.572 Pain in left ankle and joints of left foot

M25.579 Pain in unspecified ankle and joints of unspecified foot

M25.59 Pain in other specified joint

M25.6 Stiffness of joint, not elsewhere classified

Excludes1: ankylosis of joint (M24.6-)

contracture of joint (M24.5-)

M25.60 Stiffness of unspecified joint, not elsewhere classified

M25.61 Stiffness of shoulder, not elsewhere classified

M25.611 Stiffness of right shoulder, not elsewhere classified

M25.612 Stiffness of left shoulder, not elsewhere classified

M25.619 Stiffness of unspecified shoulder, not elsewhere classified

M25.62 Stiffness of elbow, not elsewhere classified

M25.621 Stiffness of right elbow, not elsewhere classified

M25.622 Stiffness of left elbow, not elsewhere classified

M25.629 Stiffness of unspecified elbow, not elsewhere classified

M25.63 Stiffness of wrist, not elsewhere classified

M25.631 Stiffness of right wrist, not elsewhere classified

M25.632 Stiffness of left wrist, not elsewhere classified

M25.639 Stiffness of unspecified wrist, not elsewhere classified

M25.64 Stiffness of hand, not elsewhere classified

M25.641 Stiffness of right hand, not elsewhere classified

M25.642 Stiffness of left hand, not elsewhere classified

M25.649 Stiffness of unspecified hand, not elsewhere classified

M25.65 Stiffness of hip, not elsewhere classified

M25.651 Stiffness of right hip, not elsewhere classified

M25.652 Stiffness of left hip, not elsewhere classified

M25.659 Stiffness of unspecified hip, not elsewhere classified

M25.66 Stiffness of knee, not elsewhere classified

M25.661 Stiffness of right knee, not elsewhere classified

M25.662 Stiffness of left knee, not elsewhere classified

M25.669 Stiffness of unspecified knee, not elsewhere classified

M25.67 Stiffness of ankle and foot, not elsewhere classified

M25.671 Stiffness of right ankle, not elsewhere classified

M25.672 Stiffness of left ankle, not elsewhere classified

M25.673 Stiffness of unspecified ankle, not elsewhere classified

M25.674 Stiffness of right foot, not elsewhere classified

M25.675 Stiffness of left foot, not elsewhere classified

M25.676 Stiffness of unspecified foot, not elsewhere classified

M25.69 Stiffness of other specified joint, not elsewhere classified

M25.7 Osteophyte

M25.70 Osteophyte, unspecified joint

M25.71 Osteophyte, shoulder

M25.711 Osteophyte, right shoulder

M25.712 Osteophyte, left shoulder

M25.719 Osteophyte, unspecified shoulder

M25.72 Osteophyte, elbow

M25.721 Osteophyte, right elbow

M25.722 Osteophyte, left elbow

M25.729 Osteophyte, unspecified elbow

M25.73 Osteophyte, wrist

M25.731 Osteophyte, right wrist

M25.732 Osteophyte, left wrist

M25.739 Osteophyte, unspecified wrist

M25.74 Osteophyte, hand

M25.741 Osteophyte, right hand

M25.742 Osteophyte, left hand

M25.749 Osteophyte, unspecified hand

M25.75 Osteophyte, hip

M25.751 Osteophyte, right hip

M25.752 Osteophyte, left hip

M25.759 Osteophyte, unspecified hip

M25.76 Osteophyte, knee

M25.761 Osteophyte, right knee

M25.762 Osteophyte, left knee

M25.769 Osteophyte, unspecified knee

M25.77 Osteophyte, ankle and foot

M25.771 Osteophyte, right ankle

M25.772 Osteophyte, left ankle

M25.773 Osteophyte, unspecified ankle

M25.774 Osteophyte, right foot

M25.775 Osteophyte, left foot

M25.776 Osteophyte, unspecified foot

M25.78 Osteophyte, vertebrae

M25.8 Other specified joint disorders

M25.80 Other specified joint disorders, unspecified joint

M25.81 Other specified joint disorders, shoulder

M25.811 Other specified joint disorders, right shoulder

M25.812 Other specified joint disorders, left shoulder

● New code   ▲ Revised code   **Excludes1:** Not coded here   **Excludes2:** Not included here   ⊗ Placeholder required   ⑦7ᵗʰ digit required

M25.819 Other specified joint disorders, unspecified shoulder

M25.82 Other specified joint disorders, elbow

M25.821 Other specified joint disorders, right elbow

M25.822 Other specified joint disorders, left elbow

M25.829 Other specified joint disorders, unspecified elbow

M25.83 Other specified joint disorders, wrist

M25.831 Other specified joint disorders, right wrist

M25.832 Other specified joint disorders, left wrist

M25.839 Other specified joint disorders, unspecified wrist

M25.84 Other specified joint disorders, hand

M25.841 Other specified joint disorders, right hand

M25.842 Other specified joint disorders, left hand

M25.849 Other specified joint disorders, unspecified hand

M25.85 Other specified joint disorders, hip

M25.851 Other specified joint disorders, right hip

M25.852 Other specified joint disorders, left hip

M25.859 Other specified joint disorders, unspecified hip

M25.86 Other specified joint disorders, knee

M25.861 Other specified joint disorders, right knee

M25.862 Other specified joint disorders, left knee

M25.869 Other specified joint disorders, unspecified knee

M25.87 Other specified joint disorders, ankle and foot

M25.871 Other specified joint disorders, right ankle and foot

M25.872 Other specified joint disorders, left ankle and foot

M25.879 Other specified joint disorders, unspecified ankle and foot

M25.9 Joint disorder, unspecified

DENTOFACIAL ANOMALIES [INCLUDING MALOCCLUSION] AND OTHER DISORDERS OF JAW (M26-M27)

Excludes1: hemifacial atrophy or hypertrophy (Q67.4)

unilateral condylar hyperplasia or hypoplasia (M27.8)

M26 Dentofacial anomalies [including malocclusion]

M26.0 Major anomalies of jaw size

Excludes1: acromegaly (E22.0)

Robin's syndrome (Q87.0)

M26.00 Unspecified anomaly of jaw size

M26.01 Maxillary hyperplasia

M26.02 Maxillary hypoplasia

M26.03 Mandibular hyperplasia

M26.04 Mandibular hypoplasia

M26.05 Macrogenia

M26.06 Microgenia

M26.07 Excessive tuberosity of jaw

Entire maxillary tuberosity

M26.09 Other specified anomalies of jaw size

M26.1 Anomalies of jaw-cranial base relationship

M26.10 Unspecified anomaly of jaw-cranial base relationship

M26.11 Maxillary asymmetry

M26.12 Other jaw asymmetry

M26.19 Other specified anomalies of jaw-cranial base relationship

M26.2 Anomalies of dental arch relationship

M26.20 Unspecified anomaly of dental arch relationship

M26.21 Malocclusion, Angle's class

M26.211 Malocclusion, Angle's class I

Neutro-occlusion

M26.212 Malocclusion, Angle's class II

Disto-occlusion Division I

Disto-occlusion Division II

M26.213 Malocclusion, Angle's class III

Mesio-occlusion

M26.219 Malocclusion, Angle's class, unspecified

M26.22 Open occlusal relationship

M26.220 Open anterior occlusal relationship

Anterior open bite

M26.221 Open posterior occlusal relationship

Posterior open bite

M26.23 Excessive horizontal overlap

Excessive horizontal overjet

M26.24 Reverse articulation

Crossbite (anterior) (posterior)

M26.25 Anomalies of interarch distance

M26.29 Other anomalies of dental arch relationship

Midline deviation of dental arch

Overbite (excessive) deep

Overbite (excessive) horizontal

Overbite (excessive) vertical

Posterior lingual occlusion of mandibular teeth

M26.3 Anomalies of tooth position of fully erupted tooth or teeth

Excludes2: embedded and impacted teeth (K01.-)

M26.30 Unspecified anomaly of tooth position of fully erupted tooth or teeth

Abnormal spacing of fully erupted tooth or teeth NOS

Displacement of fully erupted tooth or teeth NOS

Transposition of fully erupted tooth or teeth NOS

M26.31 Crowding of fully erupted teeth

M26.32 Excessive spacing of fully erupted teeth

Diastema of fully erupted tooth or teeth NOS

M26.33 Horizontal displacement of fully erupted tooth or teeth

Tipped tooth or teeth

Tipping of fully erupted tooth

M26.34 Vertical displacement of fully erupted tooth or teeth

Extruded tooth

Infraeruption of tooth or teeth

Supraeruption of tooth or teeth

M26.35 Rotation of fully erupted tooth or teeth

M26.36 Insufficient interocclusal distance of fully erupted teeth (ridge)

Lack of adequate intermaxillary vertical dimension of fully erupted teeth

M26.37 Excessive interocclusal distance of fully erupted teeth

Excessive intermaxillary vertical dimension of fully erupted teeth

Loss of occlusal vertical dimension of fully erupted teeth

M26.39 Other anomalies of tooth position of fully erupted tooth or teeth

M26.4 Malocclusion, unspecified

M26.5 Dentofacial functional abnormalities

Excludes1: bruxism (F45.8)

teeth-grinding NOS (F45.8)

M26.50 Dentofacial functional abnormalities, unspecified

M26.51 Abnormal jaw closure

M26.52 Limited mandibular range of motion

M26.53 Deviation in opening and closing of the mandible

M26.54 Insufficient anterior guidance

Insufficient anterior occlusal guidance

M26.55 Centric occlusion maximum intercuspation discrepancy

Excludes1: centric occlusion NOS (M26.59)

M26.56 Non-working side interference

Balancing side interference

M26.57 Lack of posterior occlusal support

M26.59 Other dentofacial functional abnormalities

Centric occlusion (of teeth) NOS

Malocclusion due to abnormal swallowing

Malocclusion due to mouth breathing

Malocclusion due to tongue, lip or finger habits

M26.6 Temporomandibular joint disorders

Excludes2: current temporomandibular joint dislocation (S03.0)

current temporomandibular joint sprain (S03.4)

M26.60 Temporomandibular joint disorder, unspecified

M26.601 Right temporomandibular joint disorder, unspecified

M26.602 Left temporomandibular joint disorder, unspecified

M26.603 Bilateral temporomandibular joint disorder, unspecified

M26.609 Unspecified temporomandibular joint disorder, unspecified side

Temporomandibular joint disorder NOS

M26.61 Adhesions and ankylosis of temporomandibular joint

M26.611 Adhesions and ankylosis of right temporomandibular joint

M26.612 Adhesions and ankylosis of left temporomandibular joint

M26.613 Adhesions and ankylosis of bilateral temporomandibular joint

M26.619 Adhesions and ankylosis of temporomandibular joint, unspecified side

M26.62 Arthralgia of temporomandibular joint

M26.621 Arthralgia of right temporomandibular joint

M26.622 Arthralgia of left temporomandibular joint

M26.623 Arthralgia of bilateral temporomandibular joint

M26.629 Arthralgia of temporomandibular joint, unspecified side

M26.63 Articular disc disorder of temporomandibular joint

M26.631 Articular disc disorder of right temporomandibular joint

M26.632 Articular disc disorder of left temporomandibular joint

M26.633 Articular disc disorder of bilateral temporomandibular joint

M26.639 Articular disc disorder of temporomandibular joint, unspecified side

M26.64 Arthritis of temporomandibular joint

M26.641 Arthritis of right temporomandibular joint

M26.642 Arthritis of left temporomandibular joint

M26.643 Arthritis of bilateral temporomandibular joint

M26.649 Arthritis of unspecified temporomandibular joint

M26.65 Arthropathy of temporomandibular joint

M26.651 Arthropathy of right temporomandibular joint

M26.652 Arthropathy of left temporomandibular joint

M26.653 Arthropathy of bilateral temporomandibular joint

M26.659 Arthropathy of unspecified temporomandibular joint

M26.69 Other specified disorders of temporomandibular joint

M26.7 Dental alveolar anomalies

M26.70 Unspecified alveolar anomaly

M26.71 Alveolar maxillary hyperplasia

M26.72 Alveolar mandibular hyperplasia

M26.73 Alveolar maxillary hypoplasia

M26.74 Alveolar mandibular hypoplasia

M26.79 Other specified alveolar anomalies

M26.8 Other dentofacial anomalies

M26.81 Anterior soft tissue impingement

Anterior soft tissue impingement on teeth

M26.82 Posterior soft tissue impingement

Posterior soft tissue impingement on teeth

M26.89 Other dentofacial anomalies

M26.9 Dentofacial anomaly, unspecified

M27 Other diseases of jaws

M27.0 Developmental disorders of jaws

Latent bone cyst of jaw

Stafne's cyst

Torus mandibularis

● New code ▲ Revised code Excludes1: Not coded here Excludes2: Not included here ⊗ Placeholder required ⑦ 7th digit required

Torus palatinus

M27.1 Giant cell granuloma, central

Giant cell granuloma NOS

Excludes1: peripheral giant cell granuloma (K06.8)

M27.2 Inflammatory conditions of jaws

Osteitis of jaw(s)

Osteomyelitis (neonatal) jaw(s)

Osteoradionecrosis jaw(s)

Periostitis jaw(s)

Sequestrum of jaw bone

Use Additional Code (W88-W90, X39.0) to identify radiation, if radiation-induced

Excludes2: osteonecrosis of jaw due to drug (M87.180)

M27.3 Alveolitis of jaws

Alveolar osteitis

Dry socket

M27.4 Other and unspecified cysts of jaw

Excludes1: cysts of oral region (K09.-)

latent bone cyst of jaw (M27.0)

Stafne's cyst (M27.0)

M27.40 Unspecified cyst of jaw

Cyst of jaw NOS

M27.49 Other cysts of jaw

Aneurysmal cyst of jaw

Hemorrhagic cyst of jaw

Traumatic cyst of jaw

M27.5 Periradicular pathology associated with previous endodontic treatment

M27.51 Perforation of root canal space due to endodontic treatment

M27.52 Endodontic overfill

M27.53 Endodontic underfill

M27.59 Other periradicular pathology associated with previous endodontic treatment

M27.6 Endosseous dental implant failure

M27.61 Osseointegration failure of dental implant

Hemorrhagic complications of dental implant placement

Iatrogenic osseointegration failure of dental implant

Osseointegration failure of dental implant due to complications of systemic disease

Osseointegration failure of dental implant due to poor bone quality

Pre-integration failure of dental implant NOS

Pre-osseointegration failure of dental implant

M27.62 Post-osseointegration biological failure of dental implant

Failure of dental implant due to lack of attached gingiva

Failure of dental implant due to occlusal trauma (caused by poor prosthetic design)

Failure of dental implant due to parafunctional habits

Failure of dental implant due to periodontal infection (peri-implantitis)

Failure of dental implant due to poor oral hygiene

Iatrogenic post-osseointegration failure of dental implant

Post-osseointegration failure of dental implant due to complications of systemic disease

M27.63 Post-osseointegration mechanical failure of dental implant

Failure of dental prosthesis causing loss of dental implant

Fracture of dental implant

Excludes2: cracked tooth (K03.81)

fractured dental restorative material with loss of material (K08.531)

fractured dental restorative material without loss of material (K08.530)

fractured tooth (S02.5)

M27.69 Other endosseous dental implant failure

Dental implant failure NOS

M27.8 Other specified diseases of jaws

Cherubism

Exostosis

Fibrous dysplasia

Unilateral condylar hyperplasia

Unilateral condylar hypoplasia

Excludes1: jaw pain (R68.84)

M27.9 Disease of jaws, unspecified

SYSTEMIC CONNECTIVE TISSUE DISORDERS (M30-M36)

Includes: autoimmune disease NOS

collagen (vascular) disease NOS

systemic autoimmune disease systemic collagen (vascular) disease

Excludes1: autoimmune disease, single organ or single cell-type -code to relevant condition category

M30 Polyarteritis nodosa and related conditions

Excludes1: microscopic polyarteritis (M31.7)

M30.0 Polyarteritis nodosa [HCC]

M30.1 Polyarteritis with lung involvement [Churg-Strauss] [HCC]

Allergic granulomatous angiitis

Eosinophilic granulomatosis with polyangiitis [EGPA]

M30.2 Juvenile polyarteritis [HCC]

M30.3 Mucocutaneous lymph node syndrome [Kawasaki] [HCC]

M30.8 Other conditions related to polyarteritis nodosa [HCC]

Polyangiitis overlap syndrome

M31 Other necrotizing vasculopathies

M31.0 Hypersensitivity angiitis [HCC]

Goodpasture's syndrome

M31.1 Thrombotic microangiopathy [HCC]

● **M31.10 Thrombotic microangiopathy, unspecified**

● **M31.11 Hematopoietic stem cell transplantation-associated thrombotic microangiopathy [HSCT-TMA]**

Transplant-associated thrombotic microangiopathy [TA-TMA]

Code first if applicable:

complications of bone marrow transplant (T86.0-)

complications of stem cell transplant (T86.5)

Use Additional Code to identify specific organ dysfunction, such as:

acute kidney failure (N17.-)

acute respiratory distress syndrome (J80)

capillary leak syndrome (I78.8)

diffuse alveolar hemorrhage (R04.89)

encephalopathy (metabolic) (septic) (G93.41)

fluid overload, unspecified (E87.70)

graft versus host disease (D89.81-)

hemolytic uremic syndrome (D59.3)

hepatic failure (K72.-)

hepatic veno-occlusive disease (K76.5)

idiopathic interstitial pneumonia (J84.11-)

sinusoidal obstruction syndrome (K76.5)

- **M31.19** **Other thrombotic microangiopathy**

Thrombotic thrombocytopenic purpura

M31.2 **Lethal midline granuloma** [HCC]

M31.3 **Wegener's granulomatosis**

Granulomatosis with polyangiitis

Necrotizing respiratory granulomatosis

M31.30 **Wegener's granulomatosis without renal involvement** [HCC]

Wegener's granulomatosis NOS

M31.31 **Wegener's granulomatosis with renal involvement** [HCC]

M31.4 **Aortic arch syndrome [Takayasu]** [HCC]

M31.5 **Giant cell arteritis with polymyalgia rheumatica** [HCC]

M31.6 **Other giant cell arteritis** [HCC]

M31.7 **Microscopic polyangiitis** [HCC]

Microscopic polyarteritis

Excludes1: polyarteritis nodosa (M30.0)

M31.8 **Other specified necrotizing vasculopathies** [HCC]

Hypocomplementemic vasculitis

Septic vasculitis

M31.9 **Necrotizing vasculopathy, unspecified** [HCC]

M32 **Systemic lupus erythematosus (SLE)**

Excludes1: lupus erythematosus (discoid) (NOS) (L93.0)

M32.0 **Drug-induced systemic lupus erythematosus** [HCC]

Use Additional Code for adverse effect, if applicable, to identify drug (T36-T50 with fifth or sixth character 5)

M32.1 **Systemic lupus erythematosus with organ or system involvement**

M32.10 **Systemic lupus erythematosus, organ or system involvement unspecified**

M32.11 **Endocarditis in systemic lupus erythematosus** [HCC]

Libman-Sacks disease

M32.12 **Pericarditis in systemic lupus erythematosus** [HCC]

Lupus pericarditis

M32.13 **Lung involvement in systemic lupus erythematosus** [HCC]

Pleural effusion due to systemic lupus erythematosus

M32.14 **Glomerular disease in systemic lupus erythematosus** [HCC]

Lupus renal disease NOS

M32.15 **Tubulo-interstitial nephropathy in systemic lupus erythematosus** [HCC]

M32.19 **Other organ or system involvement in systemic lupus erythematosus** [HCC]

M32.8 **Other forms of systemic lupus erythematosus** [HCC]

M32.9 **Systemic lupus erythematosus, unspecified** [HCC]

SLE NOS

Systemic lupus erythematosus NOS

Systemic lupus erythematosus without organ involvement

M33 **Dermatopolymyositis**

M33.0 **Juvenile dermatomyositis**

M33.00 **Juvenile dermatomyositis, organ involvement unspecified** [HCC]

M33.01 **Juvenile dermatomyositis with respiratory involvement** [HCC]

M33.02 **Juvenile dermatomyositis with myopathy** [HCC]

M33.09 **Juvenile dermatomyositis with other organ involvement** [HCC]

M33.1 **Other dermatomyositis**

M33.10 **Other dermatomyositis, organ involvement unspecified** [HCC]

M33.11 **Other dermatomyositis with respiratory involvement** [HCC]

M33.12 **Other dermatomyositis with myopathy** [HCC]

M33.19 **Other dermatomyositis with other organ involvement** [HCC]

M33.2 **Polymyositis**

M33.20 **Polymyositis, organ involvement unspecified** [HCC]

M33.21 **Polymyositis with respiratory involvement** [HCC]

M33.22 **Polymyositis with myopathy** [HCC]

M33.29 **Polymyositis with other organ involvement** [HCC]

M33.9 **Dermatopolymyositis, unspecified**

M33.90 **Dermatopolymyositis, unspecified, organ involvement unspecified** [HCC]

M33.91 **Dermatopolymyositis, unspecified with respiratory involvement** [HCC]

M33.92 **Dermatopolymyositis, unspecified with myopathy** [HCC]

M33.93 **Dermatopolymyositis, unspecified without myopathy** [HCC]

M33.99 **Dermatopolymyositis, unspecified with other organ involvement** [HCC]

M34 **Systemic sclerosis [scleroderma]**

Excludes1: circumscribed scleroderma (L94.0)

neonatal scleroderma (P83.88)

M34.0 **Progressive systemic sclerosis** [HCC]

M34.1 **CR(E)ST syndrome** [HCC]

Combination of calcinosis, Raynaud's phenomenon, esophageal dysfunction, sclerodactyly, telangiectasia

M34.2 **Systemic sclerosis induced by drug and chemical** [HCC]

Code first poisoning due to drug or toxin, if applicable (T36-T65 with fifth or sixth character 1-4 or 6)

Use Additional Code for adverse effect, if applicable, to identify drug (T36-T50 with fifth or sixth character 5)

M34.8 **Other forms of systemic sclerosis**

M34.81 **Systemic sclerosis with lung involvement** [HCC]

Code also if applicable:
other interstitial pulmonary diseases (J84.89)
secondary pulmonary arterial hypertension (I27.21)

M34.82 **Systemic sclerosis with myopathy** [HCC]

M34.83 **Systemic sclerosis with polyneuropathy** [HCC]

M34.89 **Other systemic sclerosis** [HCC]

M34.9 **Systemic sclerosis, unspecified** [HCC]

M35 **Other systemic involvement of connective tissue**

reactive perforating collagenosis (L87.1)

▲ **M35.0** **Sjögren syndrome**

Sicca syndrome

Use **Additional Code** to identify associated manifestations

Excludes1 dry mouth, unspecified (R68.2)

▲ **M35.00 Sjögren syndrome, unspecified** [HCC]

▲ **M35.01 Sjögren syndrome with keratoconjunctivitis** [HCC]

▲ **M35.02 Sjögren syndrome with lung involvement** [HCC]

▲ **M35.03 Sjögren syndrome with myopathy** [HCC]

▲ **M35.04 Sjögren syndrome with tubulo-interstitial nephropathy** [HCC]

Renal tubular acidosis in sicca syndrome

● **M35.05 Sjögren syndrome with inflammatory arthritis**

● **M35.06 Sjögren syndrome with peripheral nervous system involvement**

● **M35.07 Sjögren syndrome with central nervous system involvement**

● **M35.08 Sjögren syndrome with gastrointestinal involvement**

● **M35.0A Sjögren syndrome with glomerular disease**

● **M35.0B Sjögren syndrome with vasculitis**

● **M35.0C Sjögren syndrome with dental involvement**

▲ **M35.09 Sjögren syndrome with other organ involvement** [HCC]

M35.1 Other overlap syndromes [HCC]

Mixed connective tissue disease

Excludes1: polyangiitis overlap syndrome (M30.8)

M35.2 Behçet's disease [HCC]

M35.3 Polymyalgia rheumatica [HCC]

Definition: Polymyalgia rheumatica is a rheumatic disorder that is associated with moderate to severe muscle pain and stiffness in the neck, shoulder and hip areas.

Excludes1: polymyalgia rheumatica with giant cell arteritis (M31.5)

M35.4 Diffuse (eosinophilic) fasciitis

M35.5 Multifocal fibrosclerosis [HCC]

M35.6 Relapsing panniculitis [Weber-Christian]

Excludes1: lupus panniculitis (L93.2)

panniculitis NOS (M79.3-)

M35.7 Hypermobility syndrome

Familial ligamentous laxity

Excludes2: Ehlers-Danlos syndromes (Q79.6-)

ligamentous laxity, NOS (M24.2-)

M35.8 Other specified systemic involvement of connective tissue [HCC]

M35.81 Multisystem inflammatory syndrome

Use **Additional**

post COVID-19 condition (U09.9)

M35.9 Systemic involvement of connective tissue, unspecified [HCC]

Autoimmune disease (systemic) NOS

Collagen (vascular) disease NOS

M36 Systemic disorders of connective tissue in diseases classified elsewhere

Excludes2: arthropathies in diseases classified elsewhere (M14.-)

M36.0 Dermato(poly)myositis in neoplastic disease [HCC]

Code first underlying neoplasm (C00-D49)

M36.1 Arthropathy in neoplastic disease

Code first underlying neoplasm, such as:

leukemia (C91-C95)

malignant histiocytosis (C96.A)

multiple myeloma (C90.0)

M36.2 Hemophilic arthropathy

Hemarthrosis in hemophilic arthropathy

Code first underlying disease, such as:

factor VIII deficiency (D66)

with vascular defect (D68.0)

factor IX deficiency (D67)

hemophilia (classical) (D66)

hemophilia B (D67)

hemophilia C (D68.1)

M36.3 Arthropathy in other blood disorders

M36.4 Arthropathy in hypersensitivity reactions classified elsewhere

Code first underlying disease, such as:

Henoch (-Schönlein) purpura (D69.0)

serum sickness (T80.6-)

M36.8 Systemic disorders of connective tissue in other diseases classified elsewhere [HCC]

Code first underlying disease, such as:

alkaptonuria (E70.2)

hypogammaglobulinemia (D80.-)

ochronosis (E70.2)

DORSOPATHIES (M40-M54)

Deforming dorsopathies (M40-M43)

M40 Kyphosis and lordosis

Code first underlying disease

Excludes1: congenital kyphosis and lordosis (Q76.4)

kyphoscoliosis (M41.-)

postprocedural kyphosis and lordosis (M96.-)

M40.0 Postural kyphosis

Excludes1: osteochondrosis of spine (M42.-)

M40.00 Postural kyphosis, site unspecified

M40.03 Postural kyphosis, cervicothoracic region

M40.04 Posural kyphosis, thoracic region

M40.05 Postural kyphosis, thoracolumbar region

M40.1 Other secondary kyphosis

M40.10 Other secondary kyphosis, site unspecified

M40.12 Other secondary kyphosis, cervical region

M40.13 Other secondary kyphosis, cervicothoracic region

M40.14 Other secondary kyphosis, thoracic region

M40.15 Other secondary kyphosis, thoracolumbar region

M40.2 Other and unspecified kyphosis

M40.20 Unspecified kyphosis

M40.202 Unspecified kyphosis, cervical region

M40.203 Unspecified kyphosis, cervicothoracic region

M40.204 Unspecified kyphosis, thoracic region

M40.205 Unspecified kyphosis, thoracolumbar region

M40.209 Unspecified kyphosis, site unspecified

M40.29 Other kyphosis

M40.292 Other kyphosis, cervical region

M40.293 Other kyphosis, cervicothoracic region

M40.294 Other kyphosis, thoracic region

M40.295　Other kyphosis, thoracolumbar region

M40.299　Other kyphosis, site unspecified

M40.3　Flatback syndrome

M40.30　Flatback syndrome, site unspecified

M40.35　Flatback syndrome, thoracolumbar region

M40.36　Flatback syndrome, lumbar region

M40.37　Flatback syndrome, lumbosacral region

M40.4　Postural lordosis

Acquired lordosis

M40.40　Postural lordosis, site unspecified

M40.45　Postural lordosis, thoracolumbar region

M40.46　Postural lordosis, lumbar region

M40.47　Postural lordosis, lumbosacral region

M40.5　Lordosis, unspecified

M40.50　Lordosis, unspecified, site unspecified

M40.55　Lordosis, unspecified, thoracolumbar region

M40.56　Lordosis, unspecified, lumbar region

M40.57　Lordosis, unspecified, lumbosacral region

M41　Scoliosis

Includes: kyphoscoliosis

Excludes1: congenital scoliosis NOS (Q67.5)

congenital scoliosis due to bony malformation (Q76.3)

postural congenital scoliosis (Q67.5)

kyphoscoliotic heart disease (I27.1)

Excludes2: postprocedural scoliosis (M96.-)

M41.0　Infantile idiopathic scoliosis

M41.00　Infantile idiopathic scoliosis, site unspecified

M41.02　Infantile idiopathic scoliosis, cervical region

M41.03　Infantile idiopathic scoliosis, cervicothoracic region

M41.04　Infantile idiopathic scoliosis, thoracic region

M41.05　Infantile idiopathic scoliosis, thoracolumbar region

M41.06　Infantile idiopathic scoliosis, lumbar region

M41.07　Infantile idiopathic scoliosis, lumbosacral region

M41.08　Infantile idiopathic scoliosis, sacral and sacrococcygeal region

M41.1　Juvenile and adolescent idiopathic scoliosis

M41.11　Juvenile idiopathic scoliosis

M41.112　Juvenile idiopathic scoliosis, cervical region

M41.113　Juvenile idiopathic scoliosis, cervicothoracic region

M41.114　Juvenile idiopathic scoliosis, thoracic region

M41.115　Juvenile idiopathic scoliosis, thoracolumbar region

M41.116　Juvenile idiopathic scoliosis, lumbar region

M41.117　Juvenile idiopathic scoliosis, lumbosacral region

M41.119　Juvenile idiopathic scoliosis, site unspecified

M41.12　Adolescent scoliosis

M41.122　Adolescent idiopathic scoliosis, cervical region

M41.123　Adolescent idiopathic scoliosis, cervicothoracic region

M41.124　Adolescent idiopathic scoliosis, thoracic region

M41.125　Adolescent idiopathic scoliosis, thoracolumbar region

M41.126　Adolescent idiopathic scoliosis, lumbar region

M41.127　Adolescent idiopathic scoliosis, lumbosacral region

M41.129　Adolescent idiopathic scoliosis, site unspecified

M41.2　Other idiopathic scoliosis

M41.20　Other idiopathic scoliosis, site unspecified

M41.22　Other idiopathic scoliosis, cervical region

M41.23　Other idiopathic scoliosis, cervicothoracic region

M41.24　Other idiopathic scoliosis, thoracic region

M41.25　Other idiopathic scoliosis, thoracolumbar region

M41.26　Other idiopathic scoliosis, lumbar region

M41.27　Other idiopathic scoliosis, lumbosacral region

M41.3　Thoracogenic scoliosis

M41.30　Thoracogenic scoliosis, site unspecified

M41.34　Thoracogenic scoliosis, thoracic region

M41.35　Thoracogenic scoliosis, thoracolumbar region

M41.4　Neuromuscular scoliosis

Scoliosis secondary to cerebral palsy, Friedreich's ataxia, poliomyelitis **and other** neuromuscular disorders

Code also underlying condition

M41.40　Neuromuscular scoliosis, site unspecified

M41.41　Neuromuscular scoliosis, occipito-atlanto-axial region

M41.42　Neuromuscular scoliosis, cervical region

M41.43　Neuromuscular scoliosis, cervicothoracic region

M41.44　Neuromuscular scoliosis, thoracic region

M41.45　Neuromuscular scoliosis, thoracolumbar region

M41.46　Neuromuscular scoliosis, lumbar region

M41.47　Neuromuscular scoliosis, lumbosacral region

M41.5　Other secondary scoliosis

Code first underlying disease

M41.50　Other secondary scoliosis, site unspecified

M41.52　Other secondary scoliosis, cervical region

M41.53　Other secondary scoliosis, cervicothoracic region

M41.54　Other secondary scoliosis, thoracic region

M41.55　Other secondary scoliosis, thoracolumbar region

M41.56　Other secondary scoliosis, lumbar region

M41.57　Other secondary scoliosis, lumbosacral region

M41.8　Other forms of scoliosis

M41.80　Other forms of scoliosis, site unspecified

M41.82　Other forms of scoliosis, cervical region

M41.83　Other forms of scoliosis, cervicothoracic region

M41.84　Other forms of scoliosis, thoracic region

M41.85　Other forms of scoliosis, thoracolumbar region

M41.86　Other forms of scoliosis, lumbar region

M41.87　Other forms of scoliosis, lumbosacral region

M41.9　Scoliosis, unspecified

M42　Spinal osteochondrosis

M42.0　Juvenile osteochondrosis of spine

Calvé's disease

Scheuermann's disease

Excludes1: postural kyphosis (M40.0)

M42.00 Juvenile osteochondrosis of spine, site unspecified

M42.01 Juvenile osteochondrosis of spine, occipito-atlanto-axial region

M42.02 Juvenile osteochondrosis of spine, cervical region

M42.03 Juvenile osteochondrosis of spine, cervicothoracic region

M42.04 Juvenile osteochondrosis of spine, thoracic region

M42.05 Juvenile osteochondrosis of spine, thoracolumbar region

M42.06 Juvenile osteochondrosis of spine, lumbar region

M42.07 Juvenile osteochondrosis of spine, lumbosacral region

M42.08 Juvenile osteochondrosis of spine, sacral and sacrococcygeal region

M42.09 Juvenile osteochondrosis of spine, multiple sites in spine

M42.1 Adult osteochondrosis of spine

M42.10 Adult osteochondrosis of spine, site unspecified

M42.11 Adult osteochondrosis of spine, occipito-atlanto-axial region

M42.12 Adult osteochondrosis of spine, cervical region

M42.13 Adult osteochondrosis of spine, cervicothoracic region

M42.14 Adult osteochondrosis of spine, thoracic region

M42.15 Adult osteochondrosis of spine, thoracolumbar region

M42.16 Adult osteochondrosis of spine, lumbar region

M42.17 Adult osteochondrosis of spine, lumbosacral region

M42.18 Adult osteochondrosis of spine, sacral and sacrococcygeal region

M42.19 Adult osteochondrosis of spine, multiple sites in spine

M42.9 Spinal osteochondrosis, unspecified

M43 Other deforming dorsopathies

Excludes1: congenital spondylolysis and spondylolisthesis (Q76.2)

hemivertebra (Q76.3-Q76.4)

Klippel-Feil syndrome (Q76.1)

lumbarization and sacralization (Q76.4)

platyspondylisis (Q76.4)

spina bifida occulta (Q76.0)

spinal curvature in osteoporosis (M80.-)

spinal curvature in

Paget's disease of bone [osteitis deformans] (M88.-)

M43.0 Spondylolysis

Excludes1: congenital spondylolysis (Q76.2)

spondylolisthesis (M43.1)

M43.00 Spondylolysis, site unspecified

M43.01 Spondylolysis, occipito-atlanto-axial region

M43.02 Spondylolysis, cervical region

M43.03 Spondylolysis, cervicothoracic region

M43.04 Spondylolysis, thoracic region

M43.05 Spondylolysis, thoracolumbar region

M43.06 Spondylolysis, lumbar region

M43.07 Spondylolysis, lumbosacral region

M43.08 Spondylolysis, sacral and sacrococcygeal region

M43.09 Spondylolysis, multiple sites in spine

M43.1 Spondylolisthesis

Excludes1: acute traumatic of lumbosacral region (S33.1)

acute traumatic of sites other than lumbosacral-code to Fracture, vertebra, by region congenital spondylolisthesis (Q76.2)

M43.10 Spondylolisthesis, site unspecified

M43.11 Spondylolisthesis, occipito-atlanto-axial region

M43.12 Spondylolisthesis, cervical region

M43.13 Spondylolisthesis, cervicothoracic region

M43.14 Spondylolisthesis, thoracic region

M43.15 Spondylolisthesis, thoracolumbar region

M43.16 Spondylolisthesis, lumbar region

M43.17 Spondylolisthesis, lumbosacral region

M43.18 Spondylolisthesis, sacral and sacrococcygeal region

M43.19 Spondylolisthesis, multiple sites in spine

M43.2 Fusion of spine

Ankylosis of spinal joint

Excludes1: ankylosing spondylitis (M45.0-)

congenital fusion of spine (Q76.4)

Excludes2: arthrodesis status (Z98.1)

pseudoarthrosis after fusion or arthrodesis (M96.0)

M43.20 Fusion of spine, site unspecified

M43.21 Fusion of spine, occipito-atlanto-axial region

M43.22 Fusion of spine, cervical region

M43.23 Fusion of spine, cervicothoracic region

M43.24 Fusion of spine, thoracic region

M43.25 Fusion of spine, thoracolumbar region

M43.26 Fusion of spine, lumbar region

M43.27 Fusion of spine, lumbosacral region

M43.28 Fusion of spine, sacral and sacrococcygeal region

M43.3 Recurrent atlantoaxial dislocation with myelopathy

M43.4 Other recurrent atlantoaxial dislocation

M43.5 Other recurrent vertebral dislocation

Excludes1: biomechanical lesions NEC (M99.-)

M43.5X Other recurrent vertebral dislocation

M43.5X2 Other recurrent vertebral dislocation, cervical region

M43.5X3 Other recurrent vertebral dislocation, cervicothoracic region

M43.5X4 Other recurrent vertebral dislocation, thoracic region

M43.5X5 Other recurrent vertebral dislocation, thoracolumbar region

M43.5X6 Other recurrent vertebral dislocation, lumbar region

M43.5X7 Other recurrent vertebral dislocation, lumbosacral region

M43.5X8 Other recurrent vertebral dislocation, sacral and sacrococcygeal region

M43.5X9 Other recurrent vertebral dislocation, site unspecified

M43.6 Torticollis

Excludes1: congenital (sternomastoid) torticollis (Q68.0)

current injury - see Injury, of spine, by body region ocular torticollis (R29.891)

psychogenic torticollis (F45.8)

spasmodic torticollis (G24.3)

torticollis due to birth injury (P15.2)

M43.8   Other specified deforming dorsopathies

Excludes2: kyphosis and lordosis (M40.-)

scoliosis (M41.-)

M43.8X   Other specified deforming dorsopathies

M43.8X1   Other specified deforming dorsopathies, occipito-atlanto-axial region

M43.8X2   Other specified deforming dorsopathies, cervical region

M43.8X3   Other specified deforming dorsopathies, cervicothoracic region

M43.8X4   Other specified deforming dorsopathies, thoracic region

M43.8X5   Other specified deforming dorsopathies, thoracolumbar region

M43.8X6   Other specified deforming dorsopathies, lumbar region

M43.8X7   Other specified deforming dorsopathies, lumbosacral region

M43.8X8   Other specified deforming dorsopathies, sacral and sacrococcygeal region

M43.8X9   Other specified deforming dorsopathies, site unspecified

M43.9   Deforming dorsopathy, unspecified

Curvature of spine NOS

SPONDYLOPATHIES (M45-M49)

M45   Ankylosing spondylitis

Definition: Ankylosing spondylitis is a long-term disease that causes inflammation of the joints between the spinal bones and the joints between the spine and the pelvis. It eventually causes the affected spinal bones to join together.

Rheumatoid arthritis of spine

Excludes1: arthropathy in Reiter's disease (M02.3-)

juvenile (ankylosing) spondylitis (M08.1)

Excludes2: Behçet's disease (M35.2)

M45.0   Ankylosing spondylitis of multiple sites in spine [HCC]

M45.1   Ankylosing spondylitis of occipito-atlanto-axial region [HCC]

M45.2   Ankylosing spondylitis of cervical region [HCC]

M45.3   Ankylosing spondylitis of cervicothoracic region [HCC]

M45.4   Ankylosing spondylitis of thoracic region [HCC]

M45.5   Ankylosing spondylitis of thoracolumbar region [HCC]

M45.6   Ankylosing spondylitis lumbar region [HCC]

M45.7   Ankylosing spondylitis of lumbosacral region [HCC]

M45.8   Ankylosing spondylitis sacral and sacrococcygeal region

M45.9   Ankylosing spondylitis of unspecified sites in spine [HCC]

● **M45.A   Non-radiographic axial spondyloarthritis**

● **M45.A0   Non-radiographic axial spondyloarthritis of unspecified sites in spine**

● **M45.A1   Non-radiographic axial spondyloarthritis of occipito-atlanto-axial region**

● **M45.A2   Non-radiographic axial spondyloarthritis of cervical region**

● **M45.A3   Non-radiographic axial spondyloarthritis of cervicothoracic region**

● **M45.A4   Non-radiographic axial spondyloarthritis of thoracic region**

● **M45.A5   Non-radiographic axial spondyloarthritis of thoracolumbar region**

● **M45.A6   Non-radiographic axial spondyloarthritis of lumbar region**

● **M45.A7   Non-radiographic axial spondyloarthritis of lumbosacral region**

● **M45.A8   Non-radiographic axial spondyloarthritis of sacral and sacrococcygeal region**

● **M45.AB   Non-radiographic axial spondyloarthritis of multiple sites in spine**

M46   Other inflammatory spondylopathies

M46.0   Spinal enthesopathy

Definition: Enthesopathies are disorders of peripheral ligamentous or muscular attachments, abnormalities in the zones of attachment, for ligaments and tendons to bone.

Disorder of ligamentous or muscular attachments of spine

M46.00   Spinal enthesopathy, site unspecified [HCC]

M46.01   Spinal enthesopathy, occipito-atlanto-axial region [HCC]

M46.02   Spinal enthesopathy, cervical region [HCC]

M46.03   Spinal enthesopathy, cervicothoracic region [HCC]

M46.04   Spinal enthesopathy, thoracic region [HCC]

M46.05   Spinal enthesopathy, thoracolumbar region [HCC]

M46.06   Spinal enthesopathy, lumbar region [HCC]

M46.07   Spinal enthesopathy, lumbosacral region [HCC]

M46.08   Spinal enthesopathy, sacral and sacrococcygeal region [HCC]

M46.09   Spinal enthesopathy, multiple sites in spine [HCC]

M46.1   Sacroiliitis, not elsewhere classified [HCC]

M46.2   Osteomyelitis of vertebra

Definition: Osteomyelitis is an inflammation of bone and bone marrow (usually caused by bacterial infection).

M46.20   Osteomyelitis of vertebra, site unspecified [HCC]

M46.21   Osteomyelitis of vertebra, occipito-atlanto-axial region [HCC]

M46.22   Osteomyelitis of vertebra, cervical region [HCC]

M46.23   Osteomyelitis of vertebra, cervicothoracic region [HCC]

M46.24   Osteomyelitis of vertebra, thoracic region [HCC]

M46.25   Osteomyelitis of vertebra, thoracolumbar region [HCC]

M46.26   Osteomyelitis of vertebra, lumbar region [HCC]

M46.27   Osteomyelitis of vertebra, lumbosacral region [HCC]

M46.28   Osteomyelitis of vertebra, sacral and sacrococcygeal region [HCC]

M46.3   Infection of intervertebral disc (pyogenic)

Use Additional Code (B95-B97) to identify infectious agent.

M46.30   Infection of intervertebral disc (pyogenic), site unspecified [HCC]

M46.31   Infection of intervertebral disc (pyogenic), occipito-atlanto-axial region [HCC]

M46.32   Infection of intervertebral disc (pyogenic), cervical region [HCC]

M46.33 Infection of intervertebral disc (pyogenic), cervicothoracic region [HCC]

M46.34 Infection of intervertebral disc (pyogenic), thoracic region [HCC]

M46.35 Infection of intervertebral disc (pyogenic), thoracolumbar region

M46.36 Infection of intervertebral disc (pyogenic), lumbar region [HCC]

M46.37 Infection of intervertebral disc (pyogenic), lumbosacral region [HCC]

M46.38 Infection of intervertebral disc (pyogenic), sacral and sacrococcygeal region [HCC]

M46.39 Infection of intervertebral disc (pyogenic), multiple sites in spine [HCC]

M46.4 Discitis, unspecified

M46.40 Discitis, unspecified, site unspecified

M46.41 Discitis, unspecified, occipito-atlanto-axial region

M46.42 Discitis, unspecified, cervical region

M46.43 Discitis, unspecified, cervicothoracic region

M46.44 Discitis, unspecified, thoracic region

M46.45 Discitis, unspecified, thoracolumbar region

M46.46 Discitis, unspecified, lumbar region

M46.47 Discitis, unspecified, lumbosacral region

M46.48 Discitis, unspecified, sacral and sacrococcygeal region

M46.49 Discitis, unspecified, multiple sites in spine

M46.5 Other infective spondylopathies

M46.50 Other infective spondylopathies, site unspecified [HCC]

M46.51 Other infective spondylopathies, occipito-atlanto-axial region [HCC]

M46.52 Other infective spondylopathies, cervical region [HCC]

M46.53 Other infective spondylopathies, cervicothoracic region [HCC]

M46.54 Other infective spondylopathies, thoracic region [HCC]

M46.55 Other infective spondylopathies, thoracolumbar region [HCC]

M46.56 Other infective spondylopathies, lumbar region [HCC]

M46.57 Other infective spondylopathies, lumbosacral region [HCC]

M46.58 Other infective spondylopathies, sacral and sacrococcygeal region [HCC]

M46.59 Other infective spondylopathies, multiple sites in spine [HCC]

M46.8 Other specified inflammatory spondylopathies

M46.80 Other specified inflammatory spondylopathies, site unspecified [HCC]

M46.81 Other specified inflammatory spondylopathies, occipito-atlanto-axial region [HCC]

M46.82 Other specified inflammatory spondylopathies, cervical region [HCC]

M46.83 Other specified inflammatory spondylopathies, cervicothoracic region [HCC]

M46.84 Other specified inflammatory spondylopathies, thoracic region [HCC]

M46.85 Other specified inflammatory spondylopathies, thoracolumbar region

M46.86 Other specified inflammatory spondylopathies, lumbar region [HCC]

M46.87 Other specified inflammatory spondylopathies, lumbosacral region [HCC]

M46.88 Other specified inflammatory spondylopathies, sacral and sacrococcygeal region [HCC]

M46.89 Other specified inflammatory spondylopathies, multiple sites in spine [HCC]

M46.9 Unspecified inflammatory spondylopathy

M46.90 Unspecified inflammatory spondylopathy, site unspecified [HCC]

M46.91 Unspecified inflammatory spondylopathy, occipito-atlanto-axial region [HCC]

M46.92 Unspecified inflammatory spondylopathy, cervical region [HCC]

M46.93 Unspecified inflammatory spondylopathy, cervicothoracic region [HCC]

M46.94 Unspecified inflammatory spondylopathy, thoracic region [HCC]

M46.95 Unspecified inflammatory spondylopathy, thoracolumbar region [HCC]

M46.96 Unspecified inflammatory spondylopathy, lumbar region [HCC]

M46.97 Unspecified inflammatory spondylopathy, lumbosacral region [HCC]

M46.98 Unspecified inflammatory spondylopathy, sacral and sacrococcygeal region [HCC]

M46.99 Unspecified inflammatory spondylopathy, multiple sites in spine [HCC]

M47 Spondylosis

Definition: Spondylosis is degenerative arthritis (osteoarthritis) of the spinal vertebra and related tissue.

Includes: arthrosis or osteoarthritis of spine

degeneration of facet joints

M47.0 Anterior spinal and vertebral artery compression syndromes

M47.01 Anterior spinal artery compression syndromes

M47.011 Anterior spinal artery compression syndromes, occipito-atlanto-axial region

M47.012 Anterior spinal artery compression syndromes, cervical region

M47.013 Anterior spinal artery compression syndromes, cervicothoracic region

M47.014 Anterior spinal artery compression syndromes, thoracic region

M47.015 Anterior spinal artery compression syndromes, thoracolumbar region

M47.016 Anterior spinal artery compression syndromes, lumbar region

M47.019 Anterior spinal artery compression syndromes, site unspecified

M47.02 Vertebral artery compression syndromes

M47.021 Vertebral artery compression syndromes, occipito-atlanto-axial region

M47.022 Vertebral artery compression syndromes, cervical region

M47.029 Vertebral artery compression syndromes, site unspecified

M47.1 Other spondylosis with myelopathy

Spondylogenic compression of spinal cord

Excludes1: vertebral subluxation (M43.3-M43.5X9)

M47.10 Other spondylosis with myelopathy, site unspecified

M47.11 Other spondylosis with myelopathy, occipito-atlanto-axial region

M47.12 Other spondylosis with myelopathy, cervical region

M47.13 Other spondylosis with myelopathy, cervicothoracic region

M47.14 Other spondylosis with myelopathy, thoracic region

M47.15 Other spondylosis with myelopathy, thoracolumbar region

M47.16 Other spondylosis with myelopathy, lumbar region

M47.2 Other spondylosis with radiculopathy

M47.20 Other spondylosis with radiculopathy, site unspecified

M47.21 Other spondylosis with radiculopathy, occipito-atlanto-axial region

M47.22 Other spondylosis with radiculopathy, cervical region

M47.23 Other spondylosis with radiculopathy, cervicothoracic region

M47.24 Other spondylosis with radiculopathy, thoracic region

M47.25 Other spondylosis with radiculopathy, thoracolumbar region

M47.26 Other spondylosis with radiculopathy, lumbar region

M47.27 Other spondylosis with radiculopathy, lumbosacral region

M47.28 Other spondylosis with radiculopathy, sacral and sacrococcygeal region

M47.8 Other spondylosis

M47.81 Spondylosis without myelopathy or radiculopathy

M47.811 Spondylosis without myelopathy or radiculopathy, occipito-atlanto-axial region

M47.812 Spondylosis without myelopathy or radiculopathy, cervical region

M47.813 Spondylosis without myelopathy or radiculopathy, cervicothoracic region

M47.814 Spondylosis without myelopathy or radiculopathy, thoracic region

M47.815 Spondylosis without myelopathy or radiculopathy, thoracolumbar region

M47.816 Spondylosis without myelopathy or radiculopathy, lumbar region

M47.817 Spondylosis without myelopathy or radiculopathy, lumbosacral region

M47.818 Spondylosis without myelopathy or radiculopathy, sacral and sacrococcygeal region

M47.819 Spondylosis without myelopathy or radiculopathy, site unspecified

M47.89 Other spondylosis

M47.891 Other spondylosis, occipito-atlanto-axial region

M47.892 Other spondylosis, cervical region

M47.893 Other spondylosis, cervicothoracic region

M47.894 Other spondylosis, thoracic region

M47.895 Other spondylosis, thoracolumbar region

M47.896 Other spondylosis, lumbar region

M47.897 Other spondylosis, lumbosacral region

M47.898 Other spondylosis, sacral and sacrococcygeal region

M47.899 Other spondylosis, site unspecified

M47.9 Spondylosis, unspecified

M48 Other spondylopathies

M48.0 Spinal stenosis

Caudal stenosis

M48.00 Spinal stenosis, site unspecified

M48.01 Spinal stenosis, occipito-atlanto-axial region

M48.02 Spinal stenosis, cervical region

M48.03 Spinal stenosis, cervicothoracic region

M48.04 Spinal stenosis, thoracic region

M48.05 Spinal stenosis, thoracolumbar region

M48.06 Spinal stenosis, lumbar region

M48.061 Spinal stenosis, lumbar region without neurogenic claudication

Spinal stenosis, lumbar region NOS

M48.062 Spinal stenosis, lumbar region with neurogenic claudication

M48.07 Spinal stenosis, lumbosacral region

M48.08 Spinal stenosis, sacral and sacrococcygeal region

M48.1 Ankylosing hyperostosis [Forestier]

Diffuse idiopathic skeletal hyperostosis [DISH]

M48.10 Ankylosing hyperostosis [Forestier], site unspecified

M48.11 Ankylosing hyperostosis [Forestier], occipito-atlanto-axial region

M48.12 Ankylosing hyperostosis [Forestier], cervical region

M48.13 Ankylosing hyperostosis [Forestier], cervicothoracic region

M48.14 Ankylosing hyperostosis [Forestier], thoracic region

M48.15 Ankylosing hyperostosis [Forestier], thoracolumbar region

M48.16 Ankylosing hyperostosis [Forestier], lumbar region

M48.17 Ankylosing hyperostosis [Forestier], lumbosacral region

M48.18 Ankylosing hyperostosis [Forestier], sacral and sacrococcygeal region

M48.19 Ankylosing hyperostosis [Forestier], multiple sites in spine

M48.2 Kissing spine

M48.20 Kissing spine, site unspecified

M48.21 Kissing spine, occipito-atlanto-axial region

M48.22 Kissing spine, cervical region

M48.23 Kissing spine, cervicothoracic region

M48.24 Kissing spine, thoracic region

M48.25 Kissing spine, thoracolumbar region

M48.26 Kissing spine, lumbar region

M48.27 Kissing spine, lumbosacral region

M48.3 Traumatic spondylopathy

M48.30 Traumatic spondylopathy, site unspecified

M48.31 Traumatic spondylopathy, occipito-atlanto-axial region

M48.32 Traumatic spondylopathy, cervical region

M48.33 **Traumatic spondylopathy, cervicothoracic region**

M48.34 **Traumatic spondylopathy, thoracic region**

M48.35 **Traumatic spondylopathy, thoracolumbar region**

M48.36 **Traumatic spondylopathy, lumbar region**

M48.37 **Traumatic spondylopathy, lumbosacral region**

M48.38 **Traumatic spondylopathy, sacral and sacrococcygeal region**

M48.4 **Fatigue fracture of vertebra**

Stress fracture of vertebra

Excludes1: pathological fracture NOS (M84.4-)

pathological fracture of vertebra due to neoplasm (M84.58)

pathological fracture of vertebra due **to other** diagnosis (M84.68)

pathological fracture of vertebra due to osteoporosis (M80.-)

traumatic fracture of vertebrae (S12.0-S12.3-, S22.0-, S32.0-)

The appropriate 7th character is to be added to each code from subcategory M48.4:

A - initial encounter for fracture

D - subsequent encounter for fracture with routine healing

G - subsequent encounter for fracture with delayed healing

S - sequela of fracture

⊗⑦**M48.40 Fatigue fracture of vertebra, site unspecified**

⊗⑦**M48.41 Fatigue fracture of vertebra, occipito-atlanto-axial region**

⊗⑦**M48.42 Fatigue fracture of vertebra, cervical region**

⊗⑦**M48.43 Fatigue fracture of vertebra, cervicothoracic region**

⊗⑦**M48.44 Fatigue fracture of vertebra, thoracic region**

⊗⑦**M48.45 Fatigue fracture of vertebra, thoracolumbar region**

⊗⑦**M48.46 Fatigue fracture of vertebra, lumbar region**

⊗⑦**M48.47 Fatigue fracture of vertebra, lumbosacral region**

⊗⑦**M48.48 Fatigue fracture of vertebra, sacral and sacrococcygeal region**

M48.5 **Collapsed vertebra, not elsewhere classified**

Collapsed vertebra NOS

Compression fracture of vertebra NOS

Wedging of vertebra NOS

Excludes1: current injury - see Injury of spine, by body region

fatigue fracture of vertebra (M48.4)

pathological fracture of vertebra due to neoplasm (M84.58)

pathological fracture of vertebra due **to other** diagnosis (M84.68)

pathological fracture of vertebra due to osteoporosis (M80.-)

pathological fracture NOS (M84.4-)

stress fracture of vertebra (M48.4-)

traumatic fracture of vertebra (S12.-, S22.-, S32.-)

The appropriate 7th character is to be added to each code from subcategory M48.5:

A - initial encounter for fracture

D - subsequent encounter for fracture with routine healing

G - subsequent encounter for fracture with delayed healing

S - sequela of fracture

⊗⑦**M48.50 Collapsed vertebra, not elsewhere classified, site unspecified** [HCC]

⊗⑦**M48.51 Collapsed vertebra, not elsewhere classified, occipito-atlanto-axial region** [HCC]

⊗⑦**M48.52 Collapsed vertebra, not elsewhere classified, cervical region** [HCC]

⊗⑦**M48.53 Collapsed vertebra, not elsewhere classified, cervicothoracic region** [HCC]

⊗⑦**M48.54 Collapsed vertebra, not elsewhere classified, thoracic region** [HCC]

⊗⑦**M48.55 Collapsed vertebra, not elsewhere classified, thoracolumbar region** [HCC]

⊗⑦**M48.56 Collapsed vertebra, not elsewhere classified, lumbar region** [HCC]

⊗⑦**M48.57 Collapsed vertebra, not elsewhere classified, lumbosacral region** [HCC]

⊗⑦**M48.58 Collapsed vertebra, not elsewhere classified, sacral and sacrococcygeal region** [HCC]

M48.8 **Other specified spondylopathies**

Ossification of posterior longitudinal ligament

M48.8X **Other specified spondylopathies**

M48.8X1 **Other specified spondylopathies, occipito-atlanto-axial region** [HCC]

M48.8X2 **Other specified spondylopathies, cervical region** [HCC]

M48.8X3 **Other specified spondylopathies, cervicothoracic region** [HCC]

M48.8X4 **Other specified spondylopathies, thoracic region** [HCC]

M48.8X5 **Other specified spondylopathies, thoracolumbar region** [HCC]

M48.8X6 **Other specified spondylopathies, lumbar region** [HCC]

M48.8X7 **Other specified spondylopathies, lumbosacral region** [HCC]

M48.8X8 **Other specified spondylopathies, sacral and sacrococcygeal region** [HCC]

M48.8X9 **Other specified spondylopathies, site unspecified** [HCC]

M48.9 **Spondylopathy, unspecified**

M49 **Spondylopathies in diseases classified elsewhere**

Includes: curvature of spine in diseases classified elsewhere

deformity of spine in diseases classified elsewhere

kyphosis in diseases classified elsewhere

scoliosis in diseases classified elsewhere

spondylopathy in diseases classified elsewhere

Code first underlying disease, such as:

brucellosis (A23.-)

Charcot-Marie-Tooth disease (G60.0)

enterobacterial infections (A01-A04)

osteitis fibrosa cystica (E21.0)

Excludes1: curvature of spine in tuberculosis [Pott's] (A18.01)

enteropathic arthropathies (M07.-)

gonococcal spondylitis (A54.41)

neuropathic [tabes dorsalis] spondylitis (A52.11)

neuropathic spondylopathy in syringomyelia (G95.0)

neuropathic spondylopathy in tabes dorsalis (A52.11)

nonsyphilitic neuropathic spondylopathy NEC (G98.0)

spondylitis in syphilis (acquired) (A52.77)

tuberculous spondylitis (A18.01)

typhoid fever spondylitis (A01.05)

M49.8 Spondylopathy in diseases classified elsewhere

M49.80 Spondylopathy in diseases classified elsewhere, site unspecified [HCC]

M49.81 Spondylopathy in diseases classified elsewhere, occipito-atlanto-axial region [HCC]

M49.82 Spondylopathy in diseases classified elsewhere, cervical region [HCC]

M49.83 Spondylopathy in diseases classified elsewhere, cervicothoracic region [HCC]

M49.84 Spondylopathy in diseases classified elsewhere, thoracic region [HCC]

M49.85 Spondylopathy in diseases classified elsewhere, thoracolumbar region [HCC]

M49.86 Spondylopathy in diseases classified elsewhere, lumbar region [HCC]

M49.87 Spondylopathy in diseases classified elsewhere, lumbosacral region [HCC]

M49.88 Spondylopathy in diseases classified elsewhere, sacral and sacrococcygeal region [HCC]

M49.89 Spondylopathy in diseases classified elsewhere, multiple sites in spine [HCC]

OTHER DORSOPATHIES (M50-M54)

Excludes1: current injury - see injury of spine by body region

discitis NOS (M46.4-)

M50 Cervical disc disorders

Note: code to the most superior level of disorder

Includes: cervicothoracic disc disorders with cervicalgia

cervicothoracic disc disorders

M50.0 Cervical disc disorder with myelopathy

M50.00 Cervical disc disorder with myelopathy, unspecified cervical region

M50.01 Cervical disc disorder with myelopathy, high cervical region

C2-C3 disc disorder with myelopathy

C3-C4 disc disorder with myelopathy

M50.02 Cervical disc disorder with myelopathy, mid-cervical region

M50.020 Cervical disc disorder with myelopathy, mid-cervical region, unspecified level

M50.021 Cervical disc disorder at C4-C5 level with myelopathy

C4-C5 disc disorder with myelopathy

M50.022 Cervical disc disorder at C5-C6 level with myelopathy

C5-C6 disc disorder with myelopathy

M50.023 Cervical disc disorder at C6-C7 level with myelopathy

C6-C7 disc disorder with myelopathy

M50.03 Cervical disc disorder with myelopathy, cervicothoracic region

C7-T1 disc disorder with myelopathy

M50.1 Cervical disc disorder with radiculopathy

Excludes2: brachial radiculitis NOS (M54.13)

M50.10 Cervical disc disorder with radiculopathy, unspecified cervical region

M50.11 Cervical disc disorder with radiculopathy, high cervical region

C2-C3 disc disorder with radiculopathy

C3 radiculopathy due to disc disorder

C3-C4 disc disorder with radiculopathy

C4 radiculopathy due to disc disorder

M50.12 Cervical disc disorder with radiculopathy, mid-cervical region

M50.120 Mid-cervical disc disorder, unspecified level

M50.121 Cervical disc disorder at C4-C5 level with radiculopathy

C4-C5 disc disorder with radiculopathy

C5 radiculopathy due to disc disorder

M50.122 Cervical disc disorder at C5-C6 level with radiculopathy

C5-C6 disc disorder with radiculopathy

C6 radiculopathy due to disc disorder

M50.123 Cervical disc disorder at C6-C7 level with radiculopathy

C6-C7 disc disorder with radiculopathy

C7 radiculopathy due to disc disorder

M50.13 Cervical disc disorder with radiculopathy, cervicothoracic region

C7-T1 disc disorder with radiculopathy

C8 radiculopathy due to disc disorder

M50.2 Other cervical disc displacement

M50.20 Other cervical disc displacement, unspecified cervical region

M50.21 Other cervical disc displacement, high cervical region

Other C2-C3 cervical disc displacement

Other C3-C4 cervical disc displacement

M50.22 Other cervical disc displacement, mid-cervical region

M50.220 Other cervical disc displacement, mid-cervical region, unspecified level

M50.221 Other cervical disc displacement at C4-C5 level

Other C4-C5 cervical disc displacement

M50.222 Other cervical disc displacement at C5-C6 level

Other C5-C6 cervical disc displacement

M50.223 Other cervical disc displacement at C6-C7 level

Other C6-C7 cervical disc displacement

M50.23 Other cervical disc displacement, cervicothoracic region

Other C7-T1 cervical disc displacement

M50.3 Other cervical disc degeneration

M50.30 Other cervical disc degeneration, unspecified cervical region

M50.31 Other cervical disc degeneration, high cervical region

Other C2-C3 cervical disc degeneration

Other C3-C4 cervical disc degeneration

M50.32 Other cervical disc degeneration, mid-cervical region

M50.320 Other cervical disc degeneration, mid-cervical region, unspecified level

M50.321 Other cervical disc degeneration at C4-C5 level

Other C4-C5 cervical disc degeneration

M50.322 Other cervical disc degeneration at C5-C6 level

Other C5-C6 cervical disc degeneration

M50.323 Other cervical disc degeneration at C6-C7 level

Other C6-C7 cervical disc degeneration

M50.33 Other cervical disc degeneration, cervicothoracic region

Other C7-T1 cervical disc degeneration

M50.8 Other cervical disc disorders

M50.80 Other cervical disc disorders, unspecified cervical region

M50.81 Other cervical disc disorders, high cervical region

Other C2-C3 cervical disc disorders

Other C3-C4 cervical disc disorders

M50.82 Other cervical disc disorders, mid-cervical region

M50.820 Other cervical disc disorders, mid-cervical region, unspecified level

M50.821 Other cervical disc disorders at C4-C5 level

Other C4-C5 cervical disc disorders

M50.822 Other cervical disc disorders at C5-C6 level

Other C5-C6 cervical disc disorders

M50.823 Other cervical disc disorders at C6-C7 level

Other C6-C7 cervical disc disorders

M50.83 Other cervical disc disorders, cervicothoracic region

Other C7-T1 cervical disc disorders

M50.9 Cervical disc disorder, unspecified

M50.90 Cervical disc disorder, unspecified, unspecified cervical region

M50.91 Cervical disc disorder, unspecified, high cervical region

C2-C3 cervical disc disorder, unspecified

C3-C4 cervical disc disorder, unspecified

M50.92 Cervical disc disorder, unspecified, mid-cervical region

M50.920 Unspecified cervical disc disorder, mid-cervical region, unspecified level

M50.921 Unspecified cervical disc disorder at C4-C5 level

Unspecified C4-C5 cervical disc disorder

M50.922 Unspecified cervical disc disorder at C5-C6 level

Unspecified C5-C6 cervical disc disorder

M50.923 Unspecified cervical disc disorder at C6-C7 level

Unspecified C6-C7 cervical disc disorder

M50.93 Cervical disc disorder, unspecified, cervicothoracic region

C7-T1 cervical disc disorder, unspecified

M51 Thoracic, thoracolumbar, and lumbosacral intervertebral disc disorders

Definition: Intervertebral disc disorders result from a protrusion or herniation of one of the gel-like cushions (discs) that separate the vertebrae of the spine.

Excludes2: cervical and cervicothoracic disc disorders (M50.-)

sacral and sacrococcygeal disorders (M53.3)

M51.0 Thoracic, thoracolumbar and lumbosacral intervertebral disc disorders with myelopathy

M51.04 Intervertebral disc disorders with myelopathy, thoracic region

M51.05 Intervertebral disc disorders with myelopathy, thoracolumbar region

M51.06 Intervertebral disc disorders with myelopathy, lumbar region

M51.1 Thoracic, thoracolumbar and lumbosacral intervertebral disc disorders with radiculopathy

Sciatica due to intervertebral disc disorder

Excludes1: lumbar radiculitis NOS (M54.16)

sciatica NOS (M54.3)

M51.14 Intervertebral disc disorders with radiculopathy, thoracic region

M51.15 Intervertebral disc disorders with radiculopathy, thoracolumbar region

M51.16 Intervertebral disc disorders with radiculopathy, lumbar region

M51.17 Intervertebral disc disorders with radiculopathy, lumbosacral region

M51.2 Other thoracic, thoracolumbar and lumbosacral intervertebral disc displacement

Lumbago due to displacement of intervertebral disc

M51.24 Other intervertebral disc displacement, thoracic region

M51.25 Other intervertebral disc displacement, thoracolumbar region

M51.26 Other intervertebral disc displacement, lumbar region

M51.27 Other intervertebral disc displacement, lumbosacral region

M51.3 Other thoracic, thoracolumbar and lumbosacral intervertebral disc degeneration

M51.34 Other intervertebral disc degeneration, thoracic region

M51.35 Other intervertebral disc degeneration, thoracolumbar region

M51.36 Other intervertebral disc degeneration, lumbar region

M51.37 Other intervertebral disc degeneration, lumbosacral region

M51.4 Schmorl's nodes

M51.44 Schmorl's nodes, thoracic region

M51.45 Schmorl's nodes, thoracolumbar region

M51.46 Schmorl's nodes, lumbar region

M51.47 Schmorl's nodes, lumbosacral region

M51.8 Other thoracic, thoracolumbar and lumbosacral intervertebral disc disorders

M51.84 Other intervertebral disc disorders, thoracic region

M51.85 Other intervertebral disc disorders, thoracolumbar region

M51.86 Other intervertebral disc disorders, lumbar region

M51.87 Other intervertebral disc disorders, lumbosacral region

M51.9 Unspecified thoracic, thoracolumbar and lumbosacral intervertebral disc disorder

M53 Other and unspecified dorsopathies, not elsewhere classified

M53.0 Cervicocranial syndrome
Posterior cervical sympathetic syndrome

M53.1 Cervicobrachial syndrome
Excludes2: cervical disc disorder (M50.-)
thoracic outlet syndrome (G54.0)

M53.2 Spinal instabilities

M53.2X Spinal instabilities

M53.2X1 Spinal instabilities, occipito-atlanto-axial region
M53.2X2 Spinal instabilities, cervical region
M53.2X3 Spinal instabilities, cervicothoracic region
M53.2X4 Spinal instabilities, thoracic region
M53.2X5 Spinal instabilities, thoracolumbar region
M53.2X6 Spinal instabilities, lumbar region
M53.2X7 Spinal instabilities, lumbosacral region
M53.2X8 Spinal instabilities, sacral and sacrococcygeal region
M53.2X9 Spinal instabilities, site unspecified

M53.3 Sacrococcygeal disorders, not elsewhere classified
Coccygodynia

M53.8 Other specified dorsopathies
M53.80 Other specified dorsopathies, site unspecified
M53.81 Other specified dorsopathies, occipito-atlanto-axial region
M53.82 Other specified dorsopathies, cervical region
M53.83 Other specified dorsopathies, cervicothoracic region
M53.84 Other specified dorsopathies, thoracic region
M53.85 Other specified dorsopathies, thoracolumbar region
M53.86 Other specified dorsopathies, lumbar region
M53.87 Other specified dorsopathies, lumbosacral region
M53.88 Other specified dorsopathies, sacral and sacrococcygeal region

M53.9 Dorsopathy, unspecified

M54 Dorsalgia
Excludes1: psychogenic dorsalgia (F45.41)

M54.0 Panniculitis affecting regions of neck and back
Excludes1: lupus panniculitis (L93.2)
panniculitis NOS (M79.3)
relapsing [Weber-Christian] panniculitis (M35.6)

M54.00 Panniculitis affecting regions of neck and back, site unspecified
M54.01 Panniculitis affecting regions of neck and back, occipito-atlanto-axial region
M54.02 Panniculitis affecting regions of neck and back, cervical region
M54.03 Panniculitis affecting regions of neck and back, cervicothoracic region
M54.04 Panniculitis affecting regions of neck and back, thoracic region

M54.05 Panniculitis affecting regions of neck and back, thoracolumbar region
M54.06 Panniculitis affecting regions of neck and back, lumbar region
M54.07 Panniculitis affecting regions of neck and back, lumbosacral region
M54.08 Panniculitis affecting regions of neck and back, sacral and sacrococcygeal region
M54.09 Panniculitis affecting regions, neck and back, multiple sites in spine

M54.1 Radiculopathy
Brachial neuritis or radiculitis NOS
Lumbar neuritis or radiculitis NOS
Lumbosacral neuritis or radiculitis NOS
Thoracic neuritis or radiculitis NOS
Radiculitis NOS
Excludes1: neuralgia and neuritis NOS (M79.2)
radiculopathy with cervical disc disorder (M50.1)
radiculopathy with lumbar and other intervertebral disc disorder (M51.1-)
radiculopathy with spondylosis (M47.2-)

M54.10 Radiculopathy, site unspecified
M54.11 Radiculopathy, occipito-atlanto-axial region
M54.12 Radiculopathy, cervical region
M54.13 Radiculopathy, cervicothoracic region
M54.14 Radiculopathy, thoracic region
M54.15 Radiculopathy, thoracolumbar region
M54.16 Radiculopathy, lumbar region
M54.17 Radiculopathy, lumbosacral region
M54.18 Radiculopathy, sacral and sacrococcygeal region

M54.2 Cervicalgia
Excludes1: cervicalgia due to intervertebral cervical disc disorder (M50.-)

M54.3 Sciatica
Excludes1: lesion of sciatic nerve (G57.0)
sciatica due to intervertebral disc disorder (M51.1-)
sciatica with lumbago (M54.4-)

M54.30 Sciatica, unspecified side
M54.31 Sciatica, right side
M54.32 Sciatica, left side

M54.4 Lumbago with sciatica
Excludes1: lumbago with sciatica due to intervertebral disc disorder (M51.1-)

M54.40 Lumbago with sciatica, unspecified side
M54.41 Lumbago with sciatica, right side
M54.42 Lumbago with sciatica, left side

M54.5 Low back pain
Excludes1: low back strain (S39.012)
lumbago due to intervertebral disc displacement (M51.2-)
lumbago with sciatica (M54.4-)

• **M54.50** Low back pain, unspecified
Loin pain
Lumbago NOS
• **M54.51** Vertebrogenic low back pain
Low back vertebral endplate pain
• **M54.59** Other low back pain

M54.6　Pain in thoracic spine

　　　Excludes1: pain in thoracic spine due to intervertebral disc disorder (M51.-)

M54.8　Other dorsalgia

　　　Excludes1: dorsalgia in thoracic region (M54.6)

　　　　　　low back pain (M54.5-)

　　　M54.81　Occipital neuralgia

　　　M54.89　Other dorsalgia

M54.9　Dorsalgia, unspecified

　　　Backache NOS

　　　Back pain NOS

SOFT TISSUE DISORDERS (M60-M79)

DISORDERS OF MUSCLES (M60-M63)

Excludes1: dermatopolymyositis (M33.-)

　　　muscular dystrophies and myopathies (G71-G72)

　　　myopathy in amyloidosis (E85.-)

　　　myopathy in polyarteritis nodosa (M30.0)

　　　myopathy in rheumatoid arthritis (M05.32)

　　　myopathy in scleroderma (M34.-)

　　　myopathy in Sjögren's syndrome (M35.03)

　　　myopathy in systemic lupus erythematosus (M32.-)

M60　Myositis

　　　Excludes2: inclusion body myositis [IBM] (G72.41)

M60.0　Infective myositis

　　　Tropical pyomyositis

　　　Use Additional Code (B95-B97) to identify infectious agent

　　　M60.00　Infective myositis, unspecified site

　　　　　M60.000　Infective myositis, unspecified right arm

　　　　　　　Infective myositis, right upper limb NOS

　　　　　M60.001　Infective myositis, unspecified left arm

　　　　　　　Infective myositis, left upper limb NOS

　　　　　M60.002　Infective myositis, unspecified arm

　　　　　　　Infective myositis, upper limb NOS

　　　　　M60.003　Infective myositis, unspecified right leg

　　　　　　　Infective myositis, right lower limb NOS

　　　　　M60.004　Infective myositis, unspecified left leg

　　　　　　　Infective myositis, left lower limb NOS

　　　　　M60.005　Infective myositis, unspecified leg

　　　　　　　Infective myositis, lower limb NOS

　　　　　M60.009　Infective myositis, unspecified site

　　　M60.01　Infective myositis, shoulder

　　　　　M60.011　Infective myositis, right shoulder

　　　　　M60.012　Infective myositis, left shoulder

　　　　　M60.019　Infective myositis, unspecified shoulder

　　　M60.02　Infective myositis, upper arm

　　　　　M60.021　Infective myositis, right upper arm

　　　　　M60.022　Infective myositis, left upper arm

　　　　　M60.029　Infective myositis, unspecified upper arm

　　　M60.03　Infective myositis, forearm

M60.031　Infective myositis, right forearm

M60.032　Infective myositis, left forearm

M60.039　Infective myositis, unspecified forearm

M60.04　Infective myositis, hand and fingers

　　　M60.041　Infective myositis, right hand

　　　M60.042　Infective myositis, left hand

　　　M60.043　Infective myositis, unspecified hand

　　　M60.044　Infective myositis, right finger(s)

　　　M60.045　Infective myositis, left finger(s)

　　　M60.046　Infective myositis, unspecified finger(s)

M60.05　Infective myositis, thigh

　　　M60.051　Infective myositis, right thigh

　　　M60.052　Infective myositis, left thigh

　　　M60.059　Infective myositis, unspecified thigh

M60.06　Infective myositis, lower leg

　　　M60.061　Infective myositis, right lower leg

　　　M60.062　Infective myositis, left lower leg

　　　M60.069　Infective myositis, unspecified lower leg

M60.07　Infective myositis, ankle, foot and toes

　　　M60.070　Infective myositis, right ankle

　　　M60.071　Infective myositis, left ankle

　　　M60.072　Infective myositis, unspecified ankle

　　　M60.073　Infective myositis, right foot

　　　M60.074　Infective myositis, left foot

　　　M60.075　Infective myositis, unspecified foot

　　　M60.076　Infective myositis, right toe(s)

　　　M60.077　Infective myositis, left toe(s)

　　　M60.078　Infective myositis, unspecified toe(s)

M60.08　Infective myositis, other site

M60.09　Infective myositis, multiple sites

M60.1　Interstitial myositis

M60.10　Interstitial myositis of unspecified site

M60.11　Interstitial myositis, shoulder

　　　M60.111　Interstitial myositis, right shoulder

　　　M60.112　Interstitial myositis, left shoulder

　　　M60.119　Interstitial myositis, unspecified shoulder

M60.12　Interstitial myositis, upper arm

　　　M60.121　Interstitial myositis, right upper arm

　　　M60.122　Interstitial myositis, left upper arm

　　　M60.129　Interstitial myositis, unspecified upper arm

M60.13　Interstitial myositis, forearm

　　　M60.131　Interstitial myositis, right forearm

　　　M60.132　Interstitial myositis, left forearm

　　　M60.139　Interstitial myositis, unspecified forearm

M60.14　Interstitial myositis, hand

　　　M60.141　Interstitial myositis, right hand

　　　M60.142　Interstitial myositis, left hand

　　　M60.149　Interstitial myositis, unspecified hand

M60.15　Interstitial myositis, thigh

　　　M60.151　Interstitial myositis, right thigh

　　　M60.152　Interstitial myositis, left thigh

M60.159 Interstitial myositis, unspecified thigh

M60.16 Interstitial myositis, lower leg

M60.161 Interstitial myositis, right lower leg

M60.162 Interstitial myositis, left lower leg

M60.169 Interstitial myositis, unspecified lower leg

M60.17 Interstitial myositis, ankle and foot

M60.171 Interstitial myositis, right ankle and foot

M60.172 Interstitial myositis, left ankle and foot

M60.179 Interstitial myositis, unspecified ankle and foot

M60.18 Interstitial myositis, other site

M60.19 Interstitial myositis, multiple sites

M60.2 Foreign body granuloma of soft tissue, not elsewhere classified

Use Additional Code to identify the type of retained foreign body (Z18.-)

Excludes1: foreign body granuloma of skin and subcutaneous tissue (L92.3)

M60.20 Foreign body granuloma of soft tissue, not elsewhere classified, unspecified site

M60.21 Foreign body granuloma of soft tissue, not elsewhere classified, shoulder

M60.211 Foreign body granuloma of soft tissue, not elsewhere classified, right shoulder

M60.212 Foreign body granuloma of soft tissue, not elsewhere classified, left shoulder

M60.219 Foreign body granuloma of soft tissue, not elsewhere classified, unspecified shoulder

M60.22 Foreign body granuloma of soft tissue, not elsewhere classified, upper arm

M60.221 Foreign body granuloma of soft tissue, not elsewhere classified, right upper arm

M60.222 Foreign body granuloma of soft tissue, not elsewhere classified, left upper arm

M60.229 Foreign body granuloma of soft tissue, not elsewhere classified, unspecified upper arm

M60.23 Foreign body granuloma of soft tissue, not elsewhere classified, forearm

M60.231 Foreign body granuloma of soft tissue, not elsewhere classified, right forearm

M60.232 Foreign body granuloma of soft tissue, not elsewhere classified, left forearm

M60.239 Foreign body granuloma of soft tissue, not elsewhere classified, unspecified forearm

M60.24 Foreign body granuloma of soft tissue, not elsewhere classified, hand

M60.241 Foreign body granuloma of soft tissue, not elsewhere classified, right hand

M60.242 Foreign body granuloma of soft tissue, not elsewhere classified, left hand

M60.249 Foreign body granuloma of soft tissue, not elsewhere classified, unspecified hand

M60.25 Foreign body granuloma of soft tissue, not elsewhere classified, thigh

M60.251 Foreign body granuloma of soft tissue, not elsewhere classified, right thigh

M60.252 Foreign body granuloma of soft tissue, not elsewhere classified, left thigh

M60.259 Foreign body granuloma of soft tissue, not elsewhere classified, unspecified thigh

M60.26 Foreign body granuloma of soft tissue, not elsewhere classified, lower leg

M60.261 Foreign body granuloma of soft tissue, not elsewhere classified, right lower leg

M60.262 Foreign body granuloma of soft tissue, not elsewhere classified, left lower leg

M60.269 Foreign body granuloma of soft tissue, not elsewhere classified, unspecified lower leg

M60.27 Foreign body granuloma of soft tissue, not elsewhere classified, ankle and foot

M60.271 Foreign body granuloma of soft tissue, not elsewhere classified, right ankle and foot

M60.272 Foreign body granuloma of soft tissue, not elsewhere classified, left ankle and foot

M60.279 Foreign body granuloma of soft tissue, not elsewhere classified, unspecified ankle and foot

M60.28 Foreign body granuloma of soft tissue, not elsewhere classified, other site

M60.8 Other myositis

M60.80 Other myositis, unspecified site

M60.81 Other myositis shoulder

M60.811 Other myositis, right shoulder

M60.812 Other myositis, left shoulder

M60.819 Other myositis, unspecified shoulder

M60.82 Other myositis, upper arm

M60.821 Other myositis, right upper arm

M60.822 Other myositis, left upper arm

M60.829 Other myositis, unspecified upper arm

M60.83 Other myositis, forearm

M60.831 Other myositis, right forearm

M60.832 Other myositis, left forearm

M60.839 Other myositis, unspecified forearm

M60.84 Other myositis, hand

M60.841 Other myositis, right hand

M60.842 Other myositis, left hand

M60.849 Other myositis, unspecified hand

M60.85 Other myositis, thigh

M60.851 Other myositis, right thigh

M60.852 Other myositis, left thigh

M60.859 Other myositis, unspecified thigh

M60.86 Other myositis, lower leg

M60.861 Other myositis, right lower leg

M60.862 Other myositis, left lower leg

M60.869 Other myositis, unspecified lower leg

M60.87 Other myositis, ankle and foot

    M60.871 Other myositis, right ankle and foot

    M60.872 Other myositis, left ankle and foot

    M60.879 Other myositis, unspecified ankle and foot

M60.88 Other myositis, other site

M60.89 Other myositis, multiple sites

M60.9 Myositis, unspecified

M61 Calcification and ossification of muscle

M61.0 Myositis ossificans traumatica

  M61.00 Myositis ossificans traumatica, unspecified site

  M61.01 Myositis ossificans traumatica, shoulder

    M61.011 Myositis ossificans traumatica, right shoulder

    M61.012 Myositis ossificans traumatica, left shoulder

    M61.019 Myositis ossificans traumatica, unspecified shoulder

  M61.02 Myositis ossificans traumatica, upper arm

    M61.021 Myositis ossificans traumatica, right upper arm

    M61.022 Myositis ossificans traumatica, left upper arm

    M61.029 Myositis ossificans traumatica, unspecified upper arm

  M61.03 Myositis ossificans traumatica, forearm

    M61.031 Myositis ossificans traumatica, right forearm

    M61.032 Myositis ossificans traumatica, left forearm

    M61.039 Myositis ossificans traumatica, unspecified forearm

  M61.04 Myositis ossificans traumatica, hand

    M61.041 Myositis ossificans traumatica, right hand

    M61.042 Myositis ossificans traumatica, left hand

    M61.049 Myositis ossificans traumatica, unspecified hand

  M61.05 Myositis ossificans traumatica, thigh

    M61.051 Myositis ossificans traumatica, right thigh

    M61.052 Myositis ossificans traumatica, left thigh

    M61.059 Myositis ossificans traumatica, unspecified thigh

  M61.06 Myositis ossificans traumatica, lower leg

    M61.061 Myositis ossificans traumatica, right lower leg

    M61.062 Myositis ossificans traumatica, left lower leg

    M61.069 Myositis ossificans traumatica, unspecified lower leg

  M61.07 Myositis ossificans traumatica, ankle and foot

    M61.071 Myositis ossificans traumatica, right ankle and foot

    M61.072 Myositis ossificans traumatica, left ankle and foot

    M61.079 Myositis ossificans traumatica, unspecified ankle and foot

M61.08 Myositis ossificans traumatica, other site

M61.09 Myositis ossificans traumatica, multiple sites

M61.1 Myositis ossificans progressiva

Fibrodysplasia ossificans progressiva

  M61.10 Myositis ossificans progressiva, unspecified site

  M61.11 Myositis ossificans progressiva, shoulder

    M61.111 Myositis ossificans progressiva, right shoulder

    M61.112 Myositis ossificans progressiva, left shoulder

    M61.119 Myositis ossificans progressiva, unspecified shoulder

  M61.12 Myositis ossificans progressiva, upper arm

    M61.121 Myositis ossificans progressiva, right upper arm

    M61.122 Myositis ossificans progressiva, left upper arm

    M61.129 Myositis ossificans progressiva, unspecified arm

  M61.13 Myositis ossificans progressiva, forearm

    M61.131 Myositis ossificans progressiva, right forearm

    M61.132 Myositis ossificans progressiva, left forearm

    M61.139 Myositis ossificans progressiva, unspecified forearm

  M61.14 Myositis ossificans progressiva, hand and finger(s)

    M61.141 Myositis ossificans progressiva, right hand

    M61.142 Myositis ossificans progressiva, left hand

    M61.143 Myositis ossificans progressiva, unspecified hand

    M61.144 Myositis ossificans progressiva, right finger(s)

    M61.145 Myositis ossificans progressiva, left finger(s)

    M61.146 Myositis ossificans progressiva, unspecified finger(s)

  M61.15 Myositis ossificans progressiva, thigh

    M61.151 Myositis ossificans progressiva, right thigh

    M61.152 Myositis ossificans progressiva, left thigh

    M61.159 Myositis ossificans progressiva, unspecified thigh

  M61.16 Myositis ossificans progressiva, lower leg

    M61.161 Myositis ossificans progressiva, right lower leg

    M61.162 Myositis ossificans progressiva, left lower leg

    M61.169 Myositis ossificans progressiva, unspecified lower leg

  M61.17 Myositis ossificans progressiva, ankle, foot and toe(s)

    M61.171 Myositis ossificans progressiva, right ankle

    M61.172 Myositis ossificans progressiva, left ankle

    M61.173 Myositis ossificans progressiva, unspecified ankle

M61.174 Myositis ossificans progressiva, right foot

M61.175 Myositis ossificans progressiva, left foot

M61.176 Myositis ossificans progressiva, unspecified foot

M61.177 Myositis ossificans progressiva, right toe(s)

M61.178 Myositis ossificans progressiva, left toe(s)

M61.179 Myositis ossificans progressiva, unspecified toe(s)

M61.18 Myositis ossificans progressiva, other site

M61.19 Myositis ossificans progressiva, multiple sites

M61.2 Paralytic calcification and ossification of muscle

Myositis ossificans associated with quadriplegia or paraplegia

M61.20 Paralytic calcification and ossification of muscle, unspecified site

M61.21 Paralytic calcification and ossification of muscle, shoulder

M61.211 Paralytic calcification and ossification of muscle, right shoulder

M61.212 Paralytic calcification and ossification of muscle, left shoulder

M61.219 Paralytic calcification and ossification of muscle, unspecified shoulder

M61.22 Paralytic calcification and ossification of muscle, upper arm

M61.221 Paralytic calcification and ossification of muscle, right upper arm

M61.222 Paralytic calcification and ossification of muscle, left upper arm

M61.229 Paralytic calcification and ossification of muscle, unspecified upper arm

M61.23 Paralytic calcification and ossification of muscle, forearm

M61.231 Paralytic calcification and ossification of muscle, right forearm

M61.232 Paralytic calcification and ossification of muscle, left forearm

M61.239 Paralytic calcification and ossification of muscle, unspecified forearm

M61.24 Paralytic calcification and ossification of muscle, hand

M61.241 Paralytic calcification and ossification of muscle, right hand

M61.242 Paralytic calcification and ossification of muscle, left hand

M61.249 Paralytic calcification and ossification of muscle, unspecified hand

M61.25 Paralytic calcification and ossification of muscle, thigh

M61.251 Paralytic calcification and ossification of muscle, right thigh

M61.252 Paralytic calcification and ossification of muscle, left thigh

M61.259 Paralytic calcification and ossification of muscle, unspecified thigh

M61.26 Paralytic calcification and ossification of muscle, lower leg

M61.261 Paralytic calcification and ossification of muscle, right lower leg

M61.262 Paralytic calcification and ossification of muscle, left lower leg

M61.269 Paralytic calcification and ossification of muscle, unspecified lower leg

M61.27 Paralytic calcification and ossification of muscle, ankle and foot

M61.271 Paralytic calcification and ossification of muscle, right ankle and foot

M61.272 Paralytic calcification and ossification of muscle, left ankle and foot

M61.279 Paralytic calcification and ossification of muscle, unspecified ankle and foot

M61.28 Paralytic calcification and ossification of muscle, other site

M61.29 Paralytic calcification and ossification of muscle, multiple sites

M61.3 Calcification and ossification of muscles associated with burns

Myositis ossificans associated with burns

M61.30 Calcification and ossification of muscles associated with burns, unspecified site

M61.31 Calcification and ossification of muscles associated with burns, shoulder

M61.311 Calcification and ossification of muscles associated with burns, right shoulder

M61.312 Calcification and ossification of muscles associated with burns, left shoulder

M61.319 Calcification and ossification of muscles associated with burns, unspecified shoulder

M61.32 Calcification and ossification of muscles associated with burns, upper arm

M61.321 Calcification and ossification of muscles associated with burns, right upper arm

M61.322 Calcification and ossification of muscles associated with burns, left upper arm

M61.329 Calcification and ossification of muscles associated with burns, unspecified upper arm

M61.33 Calcification and ossification of muscles associated with burns, forearm

M61.331 Calcification and ossification of muscles associated with burns, right forearm

M61.332 Calcification and ossification of muscles associated with burns, left forearm

M61.339 Calcification and ossification of muscles associated with burns, unspecified forearm

M61.34 Calcification and ossification of muscles associated with burns, hand

● New code   ▲ Revised code   **Excludes1:** Not coded here   **Excludes2:** Not included here   ⊗ Placeholder required   ⑦ 7ᵗʰ digit required

M61.341   Calcification and ossification of muscles associated with burns, right hand

M61.342   Calcification and ossification of muscles associated with burns, left hand

M61.349   Calcification and ossification of muscles associated with burns, unspecified hand

M61.35   Calcification and ossification of muscles associated with burns, thigh

M61.351   Calcification and ossification of muscles associated with burns, right thigh

M61.352   Calcification and ossification of muscles associated with burns, left thigh

M61.359   Calcification and ossification of muscles associated with burns, unspecified thigh

M61.36   Calcification and ossification of muscles associated with burns, lower leg

M61.361   Calcification and ossification of muscles associated with burns, right lower leg

M61.362   Calcification and ossification of muscles associated with burns, left lower leg

M61.369   Calcification and ossification of muscles associated with burns, unspecified lower leg

M61.37   Calcification and ossification of muscles associated with burns, ankle and foot

M61.371   Calcification and ossification of muscles associated with burns, right ankle and foot

M61.372   Calcification and ossification of muscles associated with burns, left ankle and foot

M61.379   Calcification and ossification of muscles associated with burns, unspecified ankle and foot

M61.38   Calcification and ossification of muscles associated with burns, other site

M61.39   Calcification and ossification of muscles associated with burns, multiple sites

M61.4   Other calcification of muscle

Excludes1: calcific tendinitis NOS (M65.2-)

calcific tendinitis of shoulder (M75.3)

M61.40   Other calcification of muscle, unspecified site

M61.41   Other calcification of muscle, shoulder

M61.411   Other calcification of muscle, right shoulder

M61.412   Other calcification of muscle, left shoulder

M61.419   Other calcification of muscle, unspecified shoulder

M61.42   Other calcification of muscle, upper arm

M61.421   Other calcification of muscle, right upper arm

M61.422   Other calcification of muscle, left upper arm

M61.429   Other calcification of muscle, unspecified upper arm

M61.43   Other calcification of muscle, forearm

M61.431   Other calcification of muscle, right forearm

M61.432   Other calcification of muscle, left forearm

M61.439   Other calcification of muscle, unspecified forearm

M61.44   Other calcification of muscle, hand

M61.441   Other calcification of muscle, right hand

M61.442   Other calcification of muscle, left hand

M61.449   Other calcification of muscle, unspecified hand

M61.45   Other calcification of muscle, thigh

M61.451   Other calcification of muscle, right thigh

M61.452   Other calcification of muscle, left thigh

M61.459   Other calcification of muscle, unspecified thigh

M61.46   Other calcification of muscle, lower leg

M61.461   Other calcification of muscle, right lower leg

M61.462   Other calcification of muscle, left lower leg

M61.469   Other calcification of muscle, unspecified lower leg

M61.47   Other calcification of muscle, ankle and foot

M61.471   Other calcification of muscle, right ankle and foot

M61.472   Other calcification of muscle, left ankle and foot

M61.479   Other calcification of muscle, unspecified ankle and foot

M61.48   Other calcification of muscle, other site

M61.49   Other calcification of muscle, multiple sites

M61.5   Other ossification of muscle

M61.50   Other ossification of muscle, unspecified site

M61.51   Other ossification of muscle, shoulder

M61.511   Other ossification of muscle, right shoulder

M61.512   Other ossification of muscle, left shoulder

M61.519   Other ossification of muscle, unspecified shoulder

M61.52   Other ossification of muscle, upper arm

M61.521   Other ossification of muscle, right upper arm

M61.522   Other ossification of muscle, left upper arm

M61.529   Other ossification of muscle, unspecified upper arm

M61.53   Other ossification of muscle, forearm

M61.531   Other ossification of muscle, right forearm

M61.532   Other ossification of muscle, left forearm

M61.539   Other ossification of muscle, unspecified forearm

M61.54   Other ossification of muscle, hand

M61.541   Other ossification of muscle, right hand

M61.542   Other ossification of muscle, left hand

M61.549   Other ossification of muscle, unspecified hand

M61.55   Other ossification of muscle, thigh

    M61.551   Other ossification of muscle, right thigh

    M61.552   Other ossification of muscle, left thigh

    M61.559   Other ossification of muscle, unspecified thigh

M61.56   Other ossification of muscle, lower leg

    M61.561   Other ossification of muscle, right lower leg

    M61.562   Other ossification of muscle, left lower leg

    M61.569   Other ossification of muscle, unspecified lower leg

M61.57   Other ossification of muscle, ankle and foot

    M61.571   Other ossification of muscle, right ankle and foot

    M61.572   Other ossification of muscle, left ankle and foot

    M61.579   Other ossification of muscle, unspecified ankle and foot

M61.58   Other ossification of muscle, other site

M61.59   Other ossification of muscle, multiple sites

M61.9   **Calcification and ossification of muscle, unspecified**

M62   **Other disorders of muscle**

Excludes1: alcoholic myopathy (G72.1)

    cramp and spasm (R25.2)

    drug-induced myopathy (G72.0)

    myalgia (M79.1-)

    stiff-man syndrome (G25.82)

Excludes2: nontraumatic hematoma of muscle (M79.81)

M62.0   **Separation of muscle (nontraumatic)**

    Diastasis of muscle

Excludes1: diastasis recti complicating pregnancy, labor and delivery (O71.8)

    traumatic separation of muscle- see strain of muscle by body region

M62.00   Separation of muscle (nontraumatic), unspecified site

M62.01   Separation of muscle (nontraumatic), shoulder

    M62.011   Separation of muscle (nontraumatic), right shoulder

    M62.012   Separation of muscle (nontraumatic), left shoulder

    M62.019   Separation of muscle (nontraumatic), unspecified shoulder

M62.02   Separation of muscle (nontraumatic), upper arm

    M62.021   Separation of muscle (nontraumatic), right upper arm

    M62.022   Separation of muscle (nontraumatic), left upper arm

    M62.029   Separation of muscle (nontraumatic), unspecified upper arm

M62.03   Separation of muscle (nontraumatic), forearm

    M62.031   Separation of muscle (nontraumatic), right forearm

M62.032   Separation of muscle (nontraumatic), left forearm

M62.039   Separation of muscle (nontraumatic), unspecified forearm

M62.04   Separation of muscle (nontraumatic), hand

    M62.041   Separation of muscle (nontraumatic), right hand

    M62.042   Separation of muscle (nontraumatic), left hand

    M62.049   Separation of muscle (nontraumatic), unspecified hand

M62.05   Separation of muscle (nontraumatic), thigh

    M62.051   Separation of muscle (nontraumatic), right thigh

    M62.052   Separation of muscle (nontraumatic), left thigh

    M62.059   Separation of muscle (nontraumatic), unspecified thigh

M62.06   Separation of muscle (nontraumatic), lower leg

    M62.061   Separation of muscle (nontraumatic), right lower leg

    M62.062   Separation of muscle (nontraumatic), left lower leg

    M62.069   Separation of muscle (nontraumatic), unspecified lower leg

M62.07   Separation of muscle (nontraumatic), ankle and foot

    M62.071   Separation of muscle (nontraumatic), right ankle and foot

    M62.072   Separation of muscle (nontraumatic), left ankle and foot

    M62.079   Separation of muscle (nontraumatic), unspecified ankle and foot

M62.08   Separation of muscle (nontraumatic), other site

M62.1   **Other rupture of muscle (nontraumatic)**

Excludes1: traumatic rupture of muscle - see strain of muscle by body region

Excludes2: rupture of tendon (M66.-)

M62.10   Other rupture of muscle (nontraumatic), unspecified site

M62.11   Other rupture of muscle (nontraumatic), shoulder

    M62.111   Other rupture of muscle (nontraumatic), right shoulder

    M62.112   Other rupture of muscle (nontraumatic), left shoulder

    M62.119   Other rupture of muscle (nontraumatic), unspecified shoulder

M62.12   Other rupture of muscle (nontraumatic), upper arm

    M62.121   Other rupture of muscle (nontraumatic), right upper arm

    M62.122   Other rupture of muscle (nontraumatic), left upper arm

    M62.129   Other rupture of muscle (nontraumatic), unspecified upper arm

M62.13   Other rupture of muscle (nontraumatic), forearm

    M62.131   Other rupture of muscle (nontraumatic), right forearm

    M62.132   Other rupture of muscle (nontraumatic), left forearm

   ● New code   ▲ Revised code   **Excludes1:** Not coded here   **Excludes2:** Not included here   ⊗ Placeholder required   ⑦ 7th digit required

M62.139 Other rupture of muscle (nontraumatic), unspecified forearm

M62.14 Other rupture of muscle (nontraumatic), hand

M62.141 Other rupture of muscle (nontraumatic), right hand

M62.142 Other rupture of muscle (nontraumatic), left hand

M62.149 Other rupture of muscle (nontraumatic), unspecified hand

M62.15 Other rupture of muscle (nontraumatic), thigh

M62.151 Other rupture of muscle (nontraumatic), right thigh

M62.152 Other rupture of muscle (nontraumatic), left thigh

M62.159 Other rupture of muscle (nontraumatic), unspecified thigh

M62.16 Other rupture of muscle (nontraumatic), lower leg

M62.161 Other rupture of muscle (nontraumatic), right lower leg

M62.162 Other rupture of muscle (nontraumatic), left lower leg

M62.169 Other rupture of muscle (nontraumatic), unspecified lower leg

M62.17 Other rupture of muscle (nontraumatic), ankle and foot

M62.171 Other rupture of muscle (nontraumatic), right ankle and foot

M62.172 Other rupture of muscle (nontraumatic), left ankle and foot

M62.179 Other rupture of muscle (nontraumatic), unspecified ankle and foot

M62.18 Other rupture of muscle (nontraumatic), other site

M62.2 Nontraumatic ischemic infarction of muscle

Excludes1: compartment syndrome (traumatic) (T79.A-)

nontraumatic compartment syndrome (M79.A-)

traumatic ischemia of muscle (T79.6)

rhabdomyolysis (M62.82)

Volkmann's ischemic contracture (T79.6)

M62.20 Nontraumatic ischemic infarction of muscle, unspecified site

M62.21 Nontraumatic ischemic infarction of muscle, shoulder

M62.211 Nontraumatic ischemic infarction of muscle, right shoulder

M62.212 Nontraumatic ischemic infarction of muscle, left shoulder

M62.219 Nontraumatic ischemic infarction of muscle, unspecified shoulder

M62.22 Nontraumatic ischemic infarction of muscle, upper arm

M62.221 Nontraumatic ischemic infarction of muscle, right upper arm

M62.222 Nontraumatic ischemic infarction of muscle, left upper arm

M62.229 Nontraumatic ischemic infarction of muscle, unspecified upper arm

M62.23 Nontraumatic ischemic infarction of muscle, forearm

M62.231 Nontraumatic ischemic infarction of muscle, right forearm

M62.232 Nontraumatic ischemic infarction of muscle, left forearm

M62.239 Nontraumatic ischemic infarction of muscle, unspecified forearm

M62.24 Nontraumatic ischemic infarction of muscle, hand

M62.241 Nontraumatic ischemic infarction of muscle, right hand

M62.242 Nontraumatic ischemic infarction of muscle, left hand

M62.249 Nontraumatic ischemic infarction of muscle, unspecified hand

M62.25 Nontraumatic ischemic infarction of muscle, thigh

M62.251 Nontraumatic ischemic infarction of muscle, right thigh

M62.252 Nontraumatic ischemic infarction of muscle, left thigh

M62.259 Nontraumatic ischemic infarction of muscle, unspecified thigh

M62.26 Nontraumatic ischemic infarction of muscle, lower leg

M62.261 Nontraumatic ischemic infarction of muscle, right lower leg

M62.262 Nontraumatic ischemic infarction of muscle, left lower leg

M62.269 Nontraumatic ischemic infarction of muscle, unspecified lower leg

M62.27 Nontraumatic ischemic infarction of muscle, ankle and foot

M62.271 Nontraumatic ischemic infarction of muscle, right ankle and foot

M62.272 Nontraumatic ischemic infarction of muscle, left ankle and foot

M62.279 Nontraumatic ischemic infarction of muscle, unspecified ankle and foot

M62.28 Nontraumatic ischemic infarction of muscle, other site

M62.3 Immobility syndrome (paraplegic)

M62.4 Contracture of muscle

Contracture of tendon (sheath)

Excludes1: contracture of joint (M24.5-)

M62.40 Contracture of muscle, unspecified site

M62.41 Contracture of muscle, shoulder

M62.411 Contracture of muscle, right shoulder

M62.412 Contracture of muscle, left shoulder

M62.419 Contracture of muscle, unspecified shoulder

M62.42 Contracture of muscle, upper arm

M62.421 Contracture of muscle, right upper arm

M62.422 Contracture of muscle, left upper arm

M62.429 Contracture of muscle, unspecified upper arm

M62.43 Contracture of muscle, forearm

M62.431 Contracture of muscle, right forearm

M62.432 Contracture of muscle, left forearm

M62.439 Contracture of muscle, unspecified forearm

M62.44 Contracture of muscle, hand

M62.441   Contracture of muscle, right hand

M62.442   Contracture of muscle, left hand

M62.449   Contracture of muscle, unspecified hand

M62.45   Contracture of muscle, thigh

M62.451   Contracture of muscle, right thigh

M62.452   Contracture of muscle, left thigh

M62.459   Contracture of muscle, unspecified thigh

M62.46   Contracture of muscle, lower leg

M62.461   Contracture of muscle, right lower leg

M62.462   Contracture of muscle, left lower leg

M62.469   Contracture of muscle, unspecified lower leg

M62.47   Contracture of muscle, ankle and foot

M62.471   Contracture of muscle, right ankle and foot

M62.472   Contracture of muscle, left ankle and foot

M62.479   Contracture of muscle, unspecified ankle and foot

M62.48   Contracture of muscle, other site

M62.49   Contracture of muscle, multiple sites

M62.5   **Muscle wasting and atrophy, not elsewhere classified**

Disuse atrophy NEC

Excludes1: neuralgic amyotrophy (G54.5)

progressive muscular atrophy (G12.21)

sarcopenia (M62.84)

Excludes2: pelvic muscle wasting (N81.84)

M62.50   Muscle wasting and atrophy, not elsewhere classified, unspecified site

M62.51   Muscle wasting and atrophy, not elsewhere classified, shoulder

M62.511   Muscle wasting and atrophy, not elsewhere classified, right shoulder

M62.512   Muscle wasting and atrophy, not elsewhere classified, left shoulder

M62.519   Muscle wasting and atrophy, not elsewhere classified, unspecified shoulder

M62.52   Muscle wasting and atrophy, not elsewhere classified, upper arm

M62.521   Muscle wasting and atrophy, not elsewhere classified, right upper arm

M62.522   Muscle wasting and atrophy, not elsewhere classified, left upper arm

M62.529   Muscle wasting and atrophy, not elsewhere classified, unspecified upper arm

M62.53   Muscle wasting and atrophy, not elsewhere classified, forearm

M62.531   Muscle wasting and atrophy, not elsewhere classified, right forearm

M62.532   Muscle wasting and atrophy, not elsewhere classified, left forearm

M62.539   Muscle wasting and atrophy, not elsewhere classified, unspecified forearm

M62.54   Muscle wasting and atrophy, not elsewhere classified, hand

M62.541   Muscle wasting and atrophy, not elsewhere classified, right hand

M62.542   Muscle wasting and atrophy, not elsewhere classified, left hand

M62.549   Muscle wasting and atrophy, not elsewhere classified, unspecified hand

M62.55   Muscle wasting and atrophy, not elsewhere classified, thigh

M62.551   Muscle wasting and atrophy, not elsewhere classified, right thigh

M62.552   Muscle wasting and atrophy, not elsewhere classified, left thigh

M62.559   Muscle wasting and atrophy, not elsewhere classified, unspecified thigh

M62.56   Muscle wasting and atrophy, not elsewhere classified, lower leg

M62.561   Muscle wasting and atrophy, not elsewhere classified, right lower leg

M62.562   Muscle wasting and atrophy, not elsewhere classified, left lower leg

M62.569   Muscle wasting and atrophy, not elsewhere classified, unspecified lower leg

M62.57   Muscle wasting and atrophy, not elsewhere classified, ankle and foot

M62.571   Muscle wasting and atrophy, not elsewhere classified, right ankle and foot

M62.572   Muscle wasting and atrophy, not elsewhere classified, left ankle and foot

M62.579   Muscle wasting and atrophy, not elsewhere classified, unspecified ankle and foot

M62.58   Muscle wasting and atrophy, not elsewhere classified, other site

M62.59   Muscle wasting and atrophy, not elsewhere classified, multiple sites

M62.8   **Other specified disorders of muscle**

Excludes2: nontraumatic hematoma of muscle (M79.81)

M62.81   Muscle weakness (generalized)

Excludes1: muscle weakness in sarcopenia (M62.84)

M62.82   Rhabdomyolysis

Excludes1: traumatic rhabdomyolysis (T79.6)

M62.83   Muscle spasm

M62.830   Muscle spasm of back

M62.831   Muscle spasm of calf

Charley-horse

M62.838   Other muscle spasm

M62.84   Sarcopenia

Age-related sarcopenia

<u>Code first</u> underlying disease, if applicable, such as:

disorders of myoneural junction and muscle disease in diseases classified elsewhere (G73.-)

Other and unspecified myopathies (G72.-)

primary disorders of muscles (G71.-)

M62.89   Other specified disorders of muscle

Muscle (sheath) hernia

   ● New code   ▲ Revised code   **Excludes1:** Not coded here   **Excludes2:** Not included here   ⊗ Placeholder required   ⑦7th digit required

M62.9 Disorder of muscle, unspecified

M63 Disorders of muscle in diseases classified elsewhere

Code first underlying disease, such as:

leprosy (A30.-)

neoplasm (C49.-, C79.89, D21.-, D48.1)

schistosomiasis (B65.-)

trichinellosis (B75)

Excludes1: myopathy in cysticercosis (B69.81)

myopathy in endocrine diseases (G73.7)

myopathy in metabolic diseases (G73.7)

myopathy in sarcoidosis (D86.87)

myopathy in secondary syphilis (A51.49)

myopathy in syphilis (late) (A52.78)

myopathy in toxoplasmosis (B58.82)

myopathy in tuberculosis (A18.09)

M63.8 Disorders of muscle in diseases classified elsewhere

M63.80 Disorders of muscle in diseases classified elsewhere, unspecified site

M63.81 Disorders of muscle in diseases classified elsewhere, shoulder

M63.811 Disorders of muscle in diseases classified elsewhere, right shoulder

M63.812 Disorders of muscle in diseases classified elsewhere, left shoulder

M63.819 Disorders of muscle in diseases classified elsewhere, unspecified shoulder

M63.82 Disorders of muscle in diseases classified elsewhere, upper arm

M63.821 Disorders of muscle in diseases classified elsewhere, right upper arm

M63.822 Disorders of muscle in diseases classified elsewhere, left upper arm

M63.829 Disorders of muscle in diseases classified elsewhere, unspecified upper arm

M63.83 Disorders of muscle in diseases classified elsewhere, forearm

M63.831 Disorders of muscle in diseases classified elsewhere, right forearm

M63.832 Disorders of muscle in diseases classified elsewhere, left forearm

M63.839 Disorders of muscle in diseases classified elsewhere, unspecified forearm

M63.84 Disorders of muscle in diseases classified elsewhere, hand

M63.841 Disorders of muscle in diseases classified elsewhere, right hand

M63.842 Disorders of muscle in diseases classified elsewhere, left hand

M63.849 Disorders of muscle in diseases classified elsewhere, unspecified hand

M63.85 Disorders of muscle in diseases classified elsewhere, thigh

M63.851 Disorders of muscle in diseases classified elsewhere, right thigh

M63.852 Disorders of muscle in diseases classified elsewhere, left thigh

M63.859 Disorders of muscle in diseases classified elsewhere, unspecified thigh

M63.86 Disorders of muscle in diseases classified elsewhere, lower leg

M63.861 Disorders of muscle in diseases classified elsewhere, right lower leg

M63.862 Disorders of muscle in diseases classified elsewhere, left lower leg

M63.869 Disorders of muscle in diseases classified elsewhere, unspecified lower leg

M63.87 Disorders of muscle in diseases classified elsewhere, ankle and foot

M63.871 Disorders of muscle in diseases classified elsewhere, right ankle and foot

M63.872 Disorders of muscle in diseases classified elsewhere, left ankle and foot

M63.879 Disorders of muscle in diseases classified elsewhere, unspecified ankle and foot

M63.88 Disorders of muscle in diseases classified elsewhere, other site

M63.89 Disorders of muscle in diseases classified elsewhere, multiple sites

DISORDERS OF SYNOVIUM AND TENDON (M65-M67)

M65 Synovitis and tenosynovitis

Excludes1: chronic crepitant synovitis of hand and wrist (M70.0-)

current injury - see injury of ligament or tendon by body region soft tissue disorders related to use, overuse and pressure (M70.-)

M65.0 Abscess of tendon sheath

Use Additional Code (B95-B96) to identify bacterial agent.

M65.00 Abscess of tendon sheath, unspecified site

M65.01 Abscess of tendon sheath, shoulder

M65.011 Abscess of tendon sheath, right shoulder

M65.012 Abscess of tendon sheath, left shoulder

M65.019 Abscess of tendon sheath, unspecified shoulder

M65.02 Abscess of tendon sheath, upper arm

M65.021 Abscess of tendon sheath, right upper arm

M65.022 Abscess of tendon sheath, left upper arm

M65.029 Abscess of tendon sheath, unspecified upper arm

M65.03 Abscess of tendon sheath, forearm

M65.031 Abscess of tendon sheath, right forearm

M65.032 Abscess of tendon sheath, left forearm

M65.039 Abscess of tendon sheath, unspecified forearm

M65.04 Abscess of tendon sheath, hand

M65.041 Abscess of tendon sheath, right hand

M65.042 Abscess of tendon sheath, left hand

M65.049 Abscess of tendon sheath, unspecified hand

M65.05 Abscess of tendon sheath, thigh

M65.051 Abscess of tendon sheath, right thigh

M65.052 Abscess of tendon sheath, left thigh

M65.059   Abscess of tendon sheath, unspecified thigh

M65.06 Abscess of tendon sheath, lower leg

M65.061   Abscess of tendon sheath, right lower leg

M65.062   Abscess of tendon sheath, left lower leg

M65.069   Abscess of tendon sheath, unspecified lower leg

M65.07 Abscess of tendon sheath, ankle and foot

M65.071   Abscess of tendon sheath, right ankle and foot

M65.072   Abscess of tendon sheath, left ankle and foot

M65.079   Abscess of tendon sheath, unspecified ankle and foot

M65.08 Abscess of tendon sheath, other site

M65.1 Other infective (teno)synovitis

M65.10   Other infective (teno)synovitis, unspecified site

M65.11   Other infective (teno)synovitis, shoulder

M65.111   Other infective (teno)synovitis, right shoulder

M65.112   Other infective (teno)synovitis, left shoulder

M65.119   Other infective (teno)synovitis, unspecified shoulder

M65.12   Other infective (teno)synovitis, elbow

M65.121   Other infective (teno)synovitis, right elbow

M65.122   Other infective (teno)synovitis, left elbow

M65.129   Other infective (teno)synovitis, unspecified elbow

M65.13   Other infective (teno)synovitis, wrist

M65.131   Other infective (teno)synovitis, right wrist

M65.132   Other infective (teno)synovitis, left wrist

M65.139   Other infective (teno)synovitis, unspecified wrist

M65.14   Other infective (teno)synovitis, hand

M65.141   Other infective (teno)synovitis, right hand

M65.142   Other infective (teno)synovitis, left hand

M65.149   Other infective (teno)synovitis, unspecified hand

M65.15   Other infective (teno)synovitis, hip

M65.151   Other infective (teno)synovitis, right hip

M65.152   Other infective (teno)synovitis, left hip

M65.159   Other infective (teno)synovitis, unspecified hip

M65.16   Other infective (teno)synovitis, knee

M65.161   Other infective (teno)synovitis, right knee

M65.162   Other infective (teno)synovitis, left knee

M65.169   Other infective (teno)synovitis, unspecified knee

M65.17   Other infective (teno)synovitis, ankle and foot

M65.171   Other infective (teno)synovitis, right ankle and foot

M65.172   Other infective (teno)synovitis, left ankle and foot

M65.179   Other infective (teno)synovitis, unspecified ankle and foot

M65.18 Other infective (teno)synovitis, other site

M65.19 Other infective (teno)synovitis, multiple sites

M65.2 Calcific tendinitis

Excludes1: tendinitis as classified in M75-M77

calcified tendinitis of shoulder (M75.3)

M65.20   Calcific tendinitis, unspecified site

M65.22   Calcific tendinitis, upper arm

M65.221   Calcific tendinitis, right upper arm

M65.222   Calcific tendinitis, left upper arm

M65.229   Calcific tendinitis, unspecified upper arm

M65.23   Calcific tendinitis, forearm

M65.231   Calcific tendinitis, right forearm

M65.232   Calcific tendinitis, left forearm

M65.239   Calcific tendinitis, unspecified forearm

M65.24   Calcific tendinitis, hand

M65.241   Calcific tendinitis, right hand

M65.242   Calcific tendinitis, left hand

M65.249   Calcific tendinitis, unspecified hand

M65.25   Calcific tendinitis, thigh

M65.251   Calcific tendinitis, right thigh

M65.252   Calcific tendinitis, left thigh

M65.259   Calcific tendinitis, unspecified thigh

M65.26   Calcific tendinitis, lower leg

M65.261   Calcific tendinitis, right lower leg

M65.262   Calcific tendinitis, left lower leg

M65.269   Calcific tendinitis, unspecified lower leg

M65.27   Calcific tendinitis, ankle and foot

M65.271   Calcific tendinitis, right ankle and foot

M65.272   Calcific tendinitis, left ankle and foot

M65.279   Calcific tendinitis, unspecified ankle and foot

M65.28 Calcific tendinitis, other site

M65.29 Calcific tendinitis, multiple sites

M65.3 Trigger finger

Nodular tendinous disease

M65.30   Trigger finger, unspecified finger

M65.31   Trigger thumb

M65.311   Trigger thumb, right thumb

M65.312   Trigger thumb, left thumb

M65.319   Trigger thumb, unspecified thumb

M65.32   Trigger finger, index finger

M65.321   Trigger finger, right index finger

M65.322   Trigger finger, left index finger

M65.329   Trigger finger, unspecified index finger

M65.33   Trigger finger, middle finger

M65.331   Trigger finger, right middle finger

M65.332   Trigger finger, left middle finger

● New code   ▲ Revised code   Excludes1: Not coded here   Excludes2: Not included here   ⊗ Placeholder required   ⑦7th digit required

M65.339   Trigger finger, unspecified middle finger

M65.34   Trigger finger, ring finger

M65.341   Trigger finger, right ring finger

M65.342   Trigger finger, left ring finger

M65.349   Trigger finger, unspecified ring finger

M65.35   Trigger finger, little finger

M65.351   Trigger finger, right little finger

M65.352   Trigger finger, left little finger

M65.359   Trigger finger, unspecified little finger

M65.4   Radial styloid tenosynovitis [de Quervain]

M65.8   Other synovitis and tenosynovitis

M65.80   Other synovitis and tenosynovitis, unspecified site

M65.81   Other synovitis and tenosynovitis, shoulder

M65.811   Other synovitis and tenosynovitis, right shoulder

M65.812   Other synovitis and tenosynovitis, left shoulder

M65.819   Other synovitis and tenosynovitis, unspecified shoulder

M65.82   Other synovitis and tenosynovitis, upper arm

M65.821   Other synovitis and tenosynovitis, right upper arm

M65.822   Other synovitis and tenosynovitis, left upper arm

M65.829   Other synovitis and tenosynovitis, unspecified upper arm

M65.83   Other synovitis and tenosynovitis, forearm

M65.831   Other synovitis and tenosynovitis, right forearm

M65.832   Other synovitis and tenosynovitis, left forearm

M65.839   Other synovitis and tenosynovitis, unspecified forearm

M65.84   Other synovitis and tenosynovitis, hand

M65.841   Other synovitis and tenosynovitis, right hand

M65.842   Other synovitis and tenosynovitis, left hand

M65.849   Other synovitis and tenosynovitis, unspecified hand

M65.85   Other synovitis and tenosynovitis, thigh

M65.851   Other synovitis and tenosynovitis, right thigh

M65.852   Other synovitis and tenosynovitis, left thigh

M65.859   Other synovitis and tenosynovitis, unspecified thigh

M65.86   Other synovitis and tenosynovitis, lower leg

M65.861   Other synovitis and tenosynovitis, right lower leg

M65.862   Other synovitis and tenosynovitis, left lower leg

M65.869   Other synovitis and tenosynovitis, unspecified lower leg

M65.87   Other synovitis and tenosynovitis, ankle and foot

M65.871   Other synovitis and tenosynovitis, right ankle and foot

M65.872   Other synovitis and tenosynovitis, left ankle and foot

M65.879   Other synovitis and tenosynovitis, unspecified ankle and foot

M65.88   Other synovitis and tenosynovitis, other site

M65.89   Other synovitis and tenosynovitis, multiple sites

M65.9   Synovitis and tenosynovitis, unspecified

M66   Spontaneous rupture of synovium and tendon

Includes: rupture that occurs when a normal force is applied to tissues that are inferred to have less than normal strength

Excludes2: rotator cuff syndrome (M75.1-)

rupture where an abnormal force is applied to normal tissue - see injury of tendon by body region

M66.0   Rupture of popliteal cyst

M66.1   Rupture of synovium

Rupture of synovial cyst

Excludes2: rupture of popliteal cyst (M66.0)

M66.10   Rupture of synovium, unspecified joint

M66.11   Rupture of synovium, shoulder

M66.111   Rupture of synovium, right shoulder

M66.112   Rupture of synovium, left shoulder

M66.119   Rupture of synovium, unspecified shoulder

M66.12   Rupture of synovium, elbow

M66.121   Rupture of synovium, right elbow

M66.122   Rupture of synovium, left elbow

M66.129   Rupture of synovium, unspecified elbow

M66.13   Rupture of synovium, wrist

M66.131   Rupture of synovium, right wrist

M66.132   Rupture of synovium, left wrist

M66.139   Rupture of synovium, unspecified wrist

M66.14   Rupture of synovium, hand and fingers

M66.141   Rupture of synovium, right hand

M66.142   Rupture of synovium, left hand

M66.143   Rupture of synovium, unspecified hand

M66.144   Rupture of synovium, right finger(s)

M66.145   Rupture of synovium, left finger(s)

M66.146   Rupture of synovium, unspecified finger(s)

M66.15   Rupture of synovium, hip

M66.151   Rupture of synovium, right hip

M66.152   Rupture of synovium, left hip

M66.159   Rupture of synovium, unspecified hip

M66.17   Rupture of synovium, ankle, foot and toes

M66.171   Rupture of synovium, right ankle

M66.172   Rupture of synovium, left ankle

M66.173   Rupture of synovium, unspecified ankle

M66.174   Rupture of synovium, right foot

M66.175   Rupture of synovium, left foot

M66.176   Rupture of synovium, unspecified foot

M66.177   Rupture of synovium, right toe(s)

M66.178   Rupture of synovium, left toe(s)

M66.179 Rupture of synovium, unspecified toe(s)

M66.18 Rupture of synovium, other site

M66.2 Spontaneous rupture of extensor tendons

 M66.20 Spontaneous rupture of extensor tendons, unspecified site

 M66.21 Spontaneous rupture of extensor tendons, shoulder

  M66.211 Spontaneous rupture of extensor tendons, right shoulder

  M66.212 Spontaneous rupture of extensor tendons, left shoulder

  M66.219 Spontaneous rupture of extensor tendons, unspecified shoulder

 M66.22 Spontaneous rupture of extensor tendons, upper arm

  M66.221 Spontaneous rupture of extensor tendons, right upper arm

  M66.222 Spontaneous rupture of extensor tendons, left upper arm

  M66.229 Spontaneous rupture of extensor tendons, unspecified upper arm

 M66.23 Spontaneous rupture of extensor tendons, forearm

  M66.231 Spontaneous rupture of extensor tendons, right forearm

  M66.232 Spontaneous rupture of extensor tendons, left forearm

  M66.239 Spontaneous rupture of extensor tendons, unspecified forearm

 M66.24 Spontaneous rupture of extensor tendons, hand

  M66.241 Spontaneous rupture of extensor tendons, right hand

  M66.242 Spontaneous rupture of extensor tendons, left hand

  M66.249 Spontaneous rupture of extensor tendons, unspecified hand

 M66.25 Spontaneous rupture of extensor tendons, thigh

  M66.251 Spontaneous rupture of extensor tendons, right thigh

  M66.252 Spontaneous rupture of extensor tendons, left thigh

  M66.259 Spontaneous rupture of extensor tendons, unspecified thigh

 M66.26 Spontaneous rupture of extensor tendons, lower leg

  M66.261 Spontaneous rupture of extensor tendons, right lower leg

  M66.262 Spontaneous rupture of extensor tendons, left lower leg

  M66.269 Spontaneous rupture of extensor tendons, unspecified lower leg

 M66.27 Spontaneous rupture of extensor tendons, ankle and foot

  M66.271 Spontaneous rupture of extensor tendons, right ankle and foot

  M66.272 Spontaneous rupture of extensor tendons, left ankle and foot

  M66.279 Spontaneous rupture of extensor tendons, unspecified ankle and foot

 M66.28 Spontaneous rupture of extensor tendons, other site

 M66.29 Spontaneous rupture of extensor tendons, multiple sites

M66.3 Spontaneous rupture of flexor tendons

 M66.30 Spontaneous rupture of flexor tendons, unspecified site

 M66.31 Spontaneous rupture of flexor tendons, shoulder

  M66.311 Spontaneous rupture of flexor tendons, right shoulder

  M66.312 Spontaneous rupture of flexor tendons, left shoulder

  M66.319 Spontaneous rupture of flexor tendons, unspecified shoulder

 M66.32 Spontaneous rupture of flexor tendons, upper arm

  M66.321 Spontaneous rupture of flexor tendons, right upper arm

  M66.322 Spontaneous rupture of flexor tendons, left upper arm

  M66.329 Spontaneous rupture of flexor tendons, unspecified upper arm

 M66.33 Spontaneous rupture of flexor tendons, forearm

  M66.331 Spontaneous rupture of flexor tendons, right forearm

  M66.332 Spontaneous rupture of flexor tendons, left forearm

  M66.339 Spontaneous rupture of flexor tendons, unspecified forearm

 M66.34 Spontaneous rupture of flexor tendons, hand

  M66.341 Spontaneous rupture of flexor tendons, right hand

  M66.342 Spontaneous rupture of flexor tendons, left hand

  M66.349 Spontaneous rupture of flexor tendons, unspecified hand

 M66.35 Spontaneous rupture of flexor tendons, thigh

  M66.351 Spontaneous rupture of flexor tendons, right thigh

  M66.352 Spontaneous rupture of flexor tendons, left thigh

  M66.359 Spontaneous rupture of flexor tendons, unspecified thigh

 M66.36 Spontaneous rupture of flexor tendons, lower leg

  M66.361 Spontaneous rupture of flexor tendons, right lower leg

  M66.362 Spontaneous rupture of flexor tendons, left lower leg

  M66.369 Spontaneous rupture of flexor tendons, unspecified lower leg

 M66.37 Spontaneous rupture of flexor tendons, ankle and foot

  M66.371 Spontaneous rupture of flexor tendons, right ankle and foot

  M66.372 Spontaneous rupture of flexor tendons, left ankle and foot

  M66.379 Spontaneous rupture of flexor tendons, unspecified ankle and foot

 M66.38 Spontaneous rupture of flexor tendons, other site

 M66.39 Spontaneous rupture of flexor tendons, multiple sites

M66.8 Spontaneous rupture of other tendons

 M66.80 Spontaneous rupture of other tendons, unspecified site

 M66.81 Spontaneous rupture of other tendons, shoulder

● New code   ▲ Revised code   **Excludes1:** Not coded here   **Excludes2:** Not included here   ⊗ Placeholder required   ⑦ 7th digit required

M66.811   Spontaneous rupture of other tendons, right shoulder

M66.812   Spontaneous rupture of other tendons, left shoulder

M66.819   Spontaneous rupture of other tendons, unspecified shoulder

M66.82   Spontaneous rupture of other tendons, upper arm

M66.821   Spontaneous rupture of other tendons, right upper arm

M66.822   Spontaneous rupture of other tendons, left upper arm

M66.829   Spontaneous rupture of other tendons, unspecified upper arm

M66.83   Spontaneous rupture of other tendons, forearm

M66.831   Spontaneous rupture of other tendons, right forearm

M66.832   Spontaneous rupture of other tendons, left forearm

M66.839   Spontaneous rupture of other tendons, unspecified wrist

M66.84   Spontaneous rupture of other tendons, hand

M66.841   Spontaneous rupture of other tendons, right hand

M66.842   Spontaneous rupture of other tendons, left hand

M66.849   Spontaneous rupture of other tendons, unspecified hand

M66.85   Spontaneous rupture of other tendons, thigh

M66.851   Spontaneous rupture of other tendons, right thigh

M66.852   Spontaneous rupture of other tendons, left thigh

M66.859   Spontaneous rupture of other tendons, unspecified thigh

M66.86   Spontaneous rupture of other tendons, lower leg

M66.861   Spontaneous rupture of other tendons, right lower leg

M66.862   Spontaneous rupture of other tendons, left lower leg

M66.869   Spontaneous rupture of other tendons, unspecified lower leg

M66.87   Spontaneous rupture of other tendons, ankle and foot

M66.871   Spontaneous rupture of other tendons, right ankle and foot

M66.872   Spontaneous rupture of other tendons, left ankle and foot

M66.879   Spontaneous rupture of other tendons, unspecified ankle and foot

M66.88   Spontaneous rupture of other tendons, other sites

M66.89   Spontaneous rupture of other tendons, multiple sites

M66.9   Spontaneous rupture of unspecified tendon

Rupture at musculotendinous junction, nontraumatic

M67   Other disorders of synovium and tendon

Excludes1: palmar fascial fibromatosis [Dupuytren] (M72.0)

tendinitis NOS (M77.9-)

xanthomatosis localized to tendons (E78.2)

M67.0   Short Achilles tendon (acquired)

M67.00   Short Achilles tendon (acquired), unspecified ankle

M67.01   Short Achilles tendon (acquired), right ankle

M67.02   Short Achilles tendon (acquired), left ankle

M67.2   Synovial hypertrophy, not elsewhere classified

Excludes1: villonodular synovitis (pigmented) (M12.2-)

M67.20   Synovial hypertrophy, not elsewhere classified, unspecified site

M67.21   Synovial hypertrophy, not elsewhere classified, shoulder

M67.211   Synovial hypertrophy, not elsewhere classified, right shoulder

M67.212   Synovial hypertrophy, not elsewhere classified, left shoulder

M67.219   Synovial hypertrophy, not elsewhere classified, unspecified shoulder

M67.22   Synovial hypertrophy, not elsewhere classified, upper arm

M67.221   Synovial hypertrophy, not elsewhere classified, right upper arm

M67.222   Synovial hypertrophy, not elsewhere classified, left upper arm

M67.229   Synovial hypertrophy, not elsewhere classified, unspecified upper arm

M67.23   Synovial hypertrophy, not elsewhere classified, forearm

M67.231   Synovial hypertrophy, not elsewhere classified, right forearm

M67.232   Synovial hypertrophy, not elsewhere classified, left forearm

M67.239   Synovial hypertrophy, not elsewhere classified, unspecified forearm

M67.24   Synovial hypertrophy, not elsewhere classified, hand

M67.241   Synovial hypertrophy, not elsewhere classified, right hand

M67.242   Synovial hypertrophy, not elsewhere classified, left hand

M67.249   Synovial hypertrophy, not elsewhere classified, unspecified hand

M67.25   Synovial hypertrophy, not elsewhere classified, thigh

M67.251   Synovial hypertrophy, not elsewhere classified, right thigh

M67.252   Synovial hypertrophy, not elsewhere classified, left thigh

M67.259   Synovial hypertrophy, not elsewhere classified, unspecified thigh

M67.26   Synovial hypertrophy, not elsewhere classified, lower leg

M67.261   Synovial hypertrophy, not elsewhere classified, right lower leg

M67.262   Synovial hypertrophy, not elsewhere classified, left lower leg

M67.269   Synovial hypertrophy, not elsewhere classified, unspecified lower leg

M67.27   Synovial hypertrophy, not elsewhere classified, ankle and foot

M67.271   Synovial hypertrophy, not elsewhere classified, right ankle and foot

M67.272   Synovial hypertrophy, not elsewhere classified, left ankle and foot

M67.279   Synovial hypertrophy, not elsewhere classified, unspecified ankle and foot

M67.28 Synovial hypertrophy, not elsewhere classified, other site

M67.29 Synovial hypertrophy, not elsewhere classified, multiple sites

M67.3 **Transient synovitis**

Toxic synovitis

Excludes1: palindromic rheumatism (M12.3-)

M67.30 Transient synovitis, unspecified site

M67.31 Transient synovitis, shoulder

M67.311 Transient synovitis, right shoulder

M67.312 Transient synovitis, left shoulder

M67.319 Transient synovitis, unspecified shoulder

M67.32 Transient synovitis, elbow

M67.321 Transient synovitis, right elbow

M67.322 Transient synovitis, left elbow

M67.329 Transient synovitis, unspecified elbow

M67.33 Transient synovitis, wrist

M67.331 Transient synovitis, right wrist

M67.332 Transient synovitis, left wrist

M67.339 Transient synovitis, unspecified wrist

M67.34 Transient synovitis, hand

M67.341 Transient synovitis, right hand

M67.342 Transient synovitis, left hand

M67.349 Transient synovitis, unspecified hand

M67.35 Transient synovitis, hip

M67.351 Transient synovitis, right hip

M67.352 Transient synovitis, left hip

M67.359 Transient synovitis, unspecified hip

M67.36 Transient synovitis, knee

M67.361 Transient synovitis, right knee

M67.362 Transient synovitis, left knee

M67.369 Transient synovitis, unspecified knee

M67.37 Transient synovitis, ankle and foot

M67.371 Transient synovitis, right ankle and foot

M67.372 Transient synovitis, left ankle and foot

M67.379 Transient synovitis, unspecified ankle and foot

M67.38 Transient synovitis, other site

M67.39 Transient synovitis, multiple sites

M67.4 **Ganglion**

Ganglion of joint or tendon (sheath)

Excludes1: ganglion in yaws (A66.6)

Excludes2: cyst of bursa (M71.2-M71.3)

cyst of synovium (M71.2-M71.3)

M67.40 Ganglion, unspecified site

M67.41 Ganglion, shoulder

M67.411 Ganglion, right shoulder

M67.412 Ganglion, left shoulder

M67.419 Ganglion, unspecified shoulder

M67.42 Ganglion, elbow

M67.421 Ganglion, right elbow

M67.422 Ganglion, left elbow

M67.429 Ganglion, unspecified elbow

M67.43 Ganglion, wrist

M67.431 Ganglion, right wrist

M67.432 Ganglion, left wrist

M67.439 Ganglion, unspecified wrist

M67.44 Ganglion, hand

M67.441 Ganglion, right hand

M67.442 Ganglion, left hand

M67.449 Ganglion, unspecified hand

M67.45 Ganglion, hip

M67.451 Ganglion, right hip

M67.452 Ganglion, left hip

M67.459 Ganglion, unspecified hip

M67.46 Ganglion, knee

M67.461 Ganglion, right knee

M67.462 Ganglion, left knee

M67.469 Ganglion, unspecified knee

M67.47 Ganglion, ankle and foot

M67.471 Ganglion, right ankle and foot

M67.472 Ganglion, left ankle and foot

M67.479 Ganglion, unspecified ankle and foot

M67.48 Ganglion, other site

M67.49 Ganglion, multiple sites

M67.5 **Plica syndrome**

Plica knee

M67.50 Plica syndrome, unspecified knee

M67.51 Plica syndrome, right knee

M67.52 Plica syndrome, left knee

M67.8 **Other specified disorders of synovium and tendon**

M67.80 Other specified disorders of synovium and tendon, unspecified site

M67.81 Other specified disorders of synovium and tendon, shoulder

M67.811 Other specified disorders of synovium, right shoulder

M67.812 Other specified disorders of synovium, left shoulder

M67.813 Other specified disorders of tendon, right shoulder

M67.814 Other specified disorders of tendon, left shoulder

M67.819 Other specified disorders of synovium and tendon, unspecified shoulder

M67.82 Other specified disorders of synovium and tendon, elbow

M67.821 Other specified disorders of synovium, right elbow

M67.822 Other specified disorders of synovium, left elbow

M67.823 Other specified disorders of tendon, right elbow

M67.824 Other specified disorders of tendon, left elbow

M67.829 Other specified disorders of synovium and tendon, unspecified elbow

M67.83 Other specified disorders of synovium and tendon, wrist

M67.831 Other specified disorders of synovium, right wrist

M67.832 Other specified disorders of synovium, left wrist

M67.833 Other specified disorders of tendon, right wrist

M67.834 Other specified disorders of tendon, left wrist

M67.839 Other specified disorders of synovium and tendon, unspecified wrist

M67.84 Other specified disorders of synovium and tendon, hand

M67.841 Other specified disorders of synovium, right hand

M67.842 Other specified disorders of synovium, left hand

M67.843 Other specified disorders of tendon, right hand

M67.844 Other specified disorders of tendon, left hand

M67.849 Other specified disorders of synovium and tendon, unspecified hand

M67.85 Other specified disorders of synovium and tendon, hip

M67.851 Other specified disorders of synovium, right hip

M67.852 Other specified disorders of synovium, left hip

M67.853 Other specified disorders of tendon, right hip

M67.854 Other specified disorders of tendon, left hip

M67.859 Other specified disorders of synovium and tendon, unspecified hip

M67.86 Other specified disorders of synovium and tendon, knee

M67.861 Other specified disorders of synovium, right knee

M67.862 Other specified disorders of synovium, left knee

M67.863 Other specified disorders of tendon, right knee

M67.864 Other specified disorders of tendon, left knee

M67.869 Other specified disorders of synovium and tendon, unspecified knee

M67.87 Other specified disorders of synovium and tendon, ankle and foot

M67.871 Other specified disorders of synovium, right ankle and foot

M67.872 Other specified disorders of synovium, left ankle and foot

M67.873 Other specified disorders of tendon, right ankle and foot

M67.874 Other specified disorders of tendon, left ankle and foot

M67.879 Other specified disorders of synovium and tendon, unspecified ankle and foot

M67.88 Other specified disorders of synovium and tendon, other site

M67.89 Other specified disorders of synovium and tendon, multiple sites

M67.9 Unspecified disorder of synovium and tendon

M67.90 Unspecified disorder of synovium and tendon, unspecified site

M67.91 Unspecified disorder of synovium and tendon, shoulder

M67.911 Unspecified disorder of synovium and tendon, right shoulder

M67.912 Unspecified disorder of synovium and tendon, left shoulder

M67.919 Unspecified disorder of synovium and tendon, unspecified shoulder

M67.92 Unspecified disorder of synovium and tendon, upper arm

M67.921 Unspecified disorder of synovium and tendon, right upper arm

M67.922 Unspecified disorder of synovium and tendon, left upper arm

M67.929 Unspecified disorder of synovium and tendon, unspecified upper arm

M67.93 Unspecified disorder of synovium and tendon, forearm

M67.931 Unspecified disorder of synovium and tendon, right forearm

M67.932 Unspecified disorder of synovium and tendon, left forearm

M67.939 Unspecified disorder of synovium and tendon, unspecified forearm

M67.94 Unspecified disorder of synovium and tendon, hand

M67.941 Unspecified disorder of synovium and tendon, right hand

M67.942 Unspecified disorder of synovium and tendon, left hand

M67.949 Unspecified disorder of synovium and tendon, unspecified hand

M67.95 Unspecified disorder of synovium and tendon, thigh

M67.951 Unspecified disorder of synovium and tendon, right thigh

M67.952 Unspecified disorder of synovium and tendon, left thigh

M67.959 Unspecified disorder of synovium and tendon, unspecified thigh

M67.96 Unspecified disorder of synovium and tendon, lower leg

M67.961 Unspecified disorder of synovium and tendon, right lower leg

M67.962 Unspecified disorder of synovium and tendon, left lower leg

M67.969 Unspecified disorder of synovium and tendon, unspecified lower leg

M67.97 Unspecified disorder of synovium and tendon, ankle and foot

M67.971 Unspecified disorder of synovium and tendon, right ankle and foot

M67.972 Unspecified disorder of synovium and tendon, left ankle and foot

M67.979 Unspecified disorder of synovium and tendon, unspecified ankle and foot

M67.98 Unspecified disorder of synovium and tendon, other site

M67.99 Unspecified disorder of synovium and tendon, multiple sites

OTHER SOFT TISSUE DISORDERS (M70-M79)

M70 **Soft tissue disorders related to use, overuse and pressure**

Includes: soft tissue disorders of occupational origin

Use additional external cause code to identify activity causing disorder (Y93.-)

Excludes1: bursitis NOS (M71.9-)

Excludes2: bursitis of shoulder (M75.5)

enthesopathies (M76-M77)

pressure ulcer (pressure area) (L89.-)

M70.0 **Crepitant synovitis (acute) (chronic) of hand and wrist**

    M70.03 **Crepitant synovitis (acute) (chronic), wrist**

        M70.031 **Crepitant synovitis (acute) (chronic), right wrist**

        M70.032 **Crepitant synovitis (acute) (chronic), left wrist**

        M70.039 **Crepitant synovitis (acute) (chronic), unspecified wrist**

    M70.04 **Crepitant synovitis (acute) (chronic), hand**

        M70.041 **Crepitant synovitis (acute) (chronic), right hand**

        M70.042 **Crepitant synovitis (acute) (chronic), left hand**

        M70.049 **Crepitant synovitis (acute) (chronic), unspecified hand**

M70.1 **Bursitis of hand**

    M70.10 **Bursitis, unspecified hand**

    M70.11 **Bursitis, right hand**

    M70.12 **Bursitis, left hand**

M70.2 **Olecranon bursitis**

    M70.20 **Olecranon bursitis, unspecified elbow**

    M70.21 **Olecranon bursitis, right elbow**

    M70.22 **Olecranon bursitis, left elbow**

M70.3 **Other bursitis of elbow**

    M70.30 **Other bursitis of elbow, unspecified elbow**

    M70.31 **Other bursitis of elbow, right elbow**

    M70.32 **Other bursitis of elbow, left elbow**

M70.4 **Prepatellar bursitis**

    M70.40 **Prepatellar bursitis, unspecified knee**

    M70.41 **Prepatellar bursitis, right knee**

    M70.42 **Prepatellar bursitis, left knee**

M70.5 **Other bursitis of knee**

    M70.50 **Other bursitis of knee, unspecified knee**

    M70.51 **Other bursitis of knee, right knee**

    M70.52 **Other bursitis of knee, left knee**

M70.6 **Trochanteric bursitis**

Trochanteric tendinitis

    M70.60 **Trochanteric bursitis, unspecified hip**

    M70.61 **Trochanteric bursitis, right hip**

    M70.62 **Trochanteric bursitis, left hip**

M70.7 **Other bursitis of hip**

Ischial bursitis

    M70.70 **Other bursitis of hip, unspecified hip**

    M70.71 **Other bursitis of hip, right hip**

    M70.72 **Other bursitis of hip, left hip**

M70.8 **Other soft tissue disorders related to use, overuse and pressure**

    M70.80 **Other soft tissue disorders related to use, overuse and pressure of unspecified site**

M70.81 **Other soft tissue disorders related to use, overuse and pressure of shoulder**

    M70.811 **Other soft tissue disorders related to use, overuse and pressure, right shoulder**

    M70.812 **Other soft tissue disorders related to use, overuse and pressure, left shoulder**

    M70.819 **Other soft tissue disorders related to use, overuse and pressure, unspecified shoulder**

M70.82 **Other soft tissue disorders related to use, overuse and pressure of upper arm**

    M70.821 **Other soft tissue disorders related to use, overuse and pressure, right upper arm**

    M70.822 **Other soft tissue disorders related to use, overuse and pressure, left upper arm**

    M70.829 **Other soft tissue disorders related to use, overuse and pressure, unspecified upper arms**

M70.83 **Other soft tissue disorders related to use, overuse and pressure of forearm**

    M70.831 **Other soft tissue disorders related to use, overuse and pressure, right forearm**

    M70.832 **Other soft tissue disorders related to use, overuse and pressure, left forearm**

    M70.839 **Other soft tissue disorders related to use, overuse and pressure, unspecified forearm**

M70.84 **Other soft tissue disorders related to use, overuse and pressure of hand**

    M70.841 **Other soft tissue disorders related to use, overuse and pressure, right hand**

    M70.842 **Other soft tissue disorders related to use, overuse and pressure, left hand**

    M70.849 **Other soft tissue disorders related to use, overuse and pressure, unspecified hand**

M70.85 **Other soft tissue disorders related to use, overuse and pressure of thigh**

    M70.851 **Other soft tissue disorders related to use, overuse and pressure, right thigh**

    M70.852 **Other soft tissue disorders related to use, overuse and pressure, left thigh**

    M70.859 **Other soft tissue disorders related to use, overuse and pressure, unspecified thigh**

M70.86 **Other soft tissue disorders related to use, overuse and pressure lower leg**

    M70.861 **Other soft tissue disorders related to use, overuse and pressure, right lower leg**

    M70.862 **Other soft tissue disorders related to use, overuse and pressure, left lower leg**

    M70.869 **Other soft tissue disorders related to use, overuse and pressure, unspecified leg**

M70.87 **Other soft tissue disorders related to use, overuse and pressure of ankle and foot**

M70.871 Other soft tissue disorders related to use, overuse and pressure, right ankle and foot

M70.872 Other soft tissue disorders related to use, overuse and pressure, left ankle and foot

M70.879 Other soft tissue disorders related to use, overuse and pressure, unspecified ankle and foot

M70.88 Other soft tissue disorders related to use, overuse and pressure other site

M70.89 Other soft tissue disorders related to use, overuse and pressure multiple sites

M70.9 Unspecified soft tissue disorder related to use, overuse and pressure

M70.90 Unspecified soft tissue disorder related to use, overuse and pressure of unspecified site

M70.91 Unspecified soft tissue disorder related to use, overuse and pressure of shoulder

M70.911 Unspecified soft tissue disorder related to use, overuse and pressure, right shoulder

M70.912 Unspecified soft tissue disorder related to use, overuse and pressure, left shoulder

M70.919 Unspecified soft tissue disorder related to use, overuse and pressure, unspecified shoulder

M70.92 Unspecified soft tissue disorder related to use, overuse and pressure of upper arm

M70.921 Unspecified soft tissue disorder related to use, overuse and pressure, right upper arm

M70.922 Unspecified soft tissue disorder related to use, overuse and pressure, left upper arm

M70.929 Unspecified soft tissue disorder related to use, overuse and pressure, unspecified upper arm

M70.93 Unspecified soft tissue disorder related to use, overuse and pressure of forearm

M70.931 Unspecified soft tissue disorder related to use, overuse and pressure, right forearm

M70.932 Unspecified soft tissue disorder related to use, overuse and pressure, left forearm

M70.939 Unspecified soft tissue disorder related to use, overuse and pressure, unspecified forearm

M70.94 Unspecified soft tissue disorder related to use, overuse and pressure of hand

M70.941 Unspecified soft tissue disorder related to use, overuse and pressure, right hand

M70.942 Unspecified soft tissue disorder related to use, overuse and pressure, left hand

M70.949 Unspecified soft tissue disorder related to use, overuse and pressure, unspecified hand

M70.95 Unspecified soft tissue disorder related to use, overuse and pressure of thigh

M70.951 Unspecified soft tissue disorder related to use, overuse and pressure, right thigh

M70.952 Unspecified soft tissue disorder related to use, overuse and pressure, left thigh

M70.959 Unspecified soft tissue disorder related to use, overuse and pressure, unspecified thigh

M70.96 Unspecified soft tissue disorder related to use, overuse and pressure lower leg

M70.961 Unspecified soft tissue disorder related to use, overuse and pressure, right lower leg

M70.962 Unspecified soft tissue disorder related to use, overuse and pressure, left lower leg

M70.969 Unspecified soft tissue disorder related to use, overuse and pressure, unspecified lower leg

M70.97 Unspecified soft tissue disorder related to use, overuse and pressure of ankle and foot

M70.971 Unspecified soft tissue disorder related to use, overuse and pressure, right ankle and foot

M70.972 Unspecified soft tissue disorder related to use, overuse and pressure, left ankle and foot

M70.979 Unspecified soft tissue disorder related to use, overuse and pressure, unspecified ankle and foot

M70.98 Unspecified soft tissue disorder related to use, overuse and pressure other

M70.99 Unspecified soft tissue disorder related to use, overuse and pressure multiple sites

M71 **Other bursopathies**

Excludes1: bunion (M20.1)

bursitis related to use, overuse or pressure (M70.-)

enthesopathies (M76-M77)

M71.0 **Abscess of bursa**

Use Additional Code (B95.-, B96.-) to identify causative organism

M71.00 Abscess of bursa, unspecified site

M71.01 Abscess of bursa, shoulder

M71.011 Abscess of bursa, right shoulder

M71.012 Abscess of bursa, left shoulder

M71.019 Abscess of bursa, unspecified shoulder

M71.02 Abscess of bursa, elbow

M71.021 Abscess of bursa, right elbow

M71.022 Abscess of bursa, left elbow

M71.029 Abscess of bursa, unspecified elbow

M71.03 Abscess of bursa, wrist

M71.031 Abscess of bursa, right wrist

M71.032 Abscess of bursa, left wrist

M71.039 Abscess of bursa, unspecified wrist

M71.04 Abscess of bursa, hand

M71.041 Abscess of bursa, right hand

M71.042 Abscess of bursa, left hand

M71.049 Abscess of bursa, unspecified hand

M71.05 Abscess of bursa, hip

M71.051 Abscess of bursa, right hip

M71.052 Abscess of bursa, left hip

M71.059 Abscess of bursa, unspecified hip

M71.06 Abscess of bursa, knee

M71.061   Abscess of bursa, right knee

M71.062   Abscess of bursa, left knee

M71.069   Abscess of bursa, unspecified knee

M71.07 Abscess of bursa, ankle and foot

   M71.071   Abscess of bursa, right ankle and foot

   M71.072   Abscess of bursa, left ankle and foot

   M71.079   Abscess of bursa, unspecified ankle and foot

M71.08 Abscess of bursa, other site

M71.09 Abscess of bursa, multiple sites

M71.1 Other infective bursitis

Use Additional Code (B95.-, B96.-) to identify causative organism

M71.10 Other infective bursitis, unspecified site

M71.11 Other infective bursitis, shoulder

   M71.111   Other infective bursitis, right shoulder

   M71.112   Other infective bursitis, left shoulder

   M71.119   Other infective bursitis, unspecified shoulder

M71.12 Other infective bursitis, elbow

   M71.121   Other infective bursitis, right elbow

   M71.122   Other infective bursitis, left elbow

   M71.129   Other infective bursitis, unspecified elbow

M71.13 Other infective bursitis, wrist

   M71.131   Other infective bursitis, right wrist

   M71.132   Other infective bursitis, left wrist

   M71.139   Other infective bursitis, unspecified wrist

M71.14 Other infective bursitis, hand

   M71.141   Other infective bursitis, right hand

   M71.142   Other infective bursitis, left hand

   M71.149   Other infective bursitis, unspecified hand

M71.15 Other infective bursitis, hip

   M71.151   Other infective bursitis, right hip

   M71.152   Other infective bursitis, left hip

   M71.159   Other infective bursitis, unspecified hip

M71.16 Other infective bursitis, knee

   M71.161   Other infective bursitis, right knee

   M71.162   Other infective bursitis, left knee

   M71.169   Other infective bursitis, unspecified knee

M71.17 Other infective bursitis, ankle and foot

   M71.171   Other infective bursitis, right ankle and foot

   M71.172   Other infective bursitis, left ankle and foot

   M71.179   Other infective bursitis, unspecified ankle and foot

M71.18 Other infective bursitis, other site

M71.19 Other infective bursitis, multiple sites

M71.2 Synovial cyst of popliteal space [Baker]

Excludes1: synovial cyst of popliteal space with rupture (M66.0)

M71.20 Synovial cyst of popliteal space [Baker], unspecified knee

M71.21 Synovial cyst of popliteal space [Baker], right knee

M71.22 Synovial cyst of popliteal space [Baker], left knee

M71.3 Other bursal cyst

Synovial cyst NOS

Excludes1: synovial cyst with rupture (M66.1-)

M71.30 Other bursal cyst, unspecified site

M71.31 Other bursal cyst, shoulder

   M71.311   Other bursal cyst, right shoulder

   M71.312   Other bursal cyst, left shoulder

   M71.319   Other bursal cyst, unspecified shoulder

M71.32 Other bursal cyst, elbow

   M71.321   Other bursal cyst, right elbow

   M71.322   Other bursal cyst, left elbow

   M71.329   Other bursal cyst, unspecified elbow

M71.33 Other bursal cyst, wrist

   M71.331   Other bursal cyst, right wrist

   M71.332   Other bursal cyst, left wrist

   M71.339   Other bursal cyst, unspecified wrist

M71.34 Other bursal cyst, hand

   M71.341   Other bursal cyst, right hand

   M71.342   Other bursal cyst, left hand

   M71.349   Other bursal cyst, unspecified hand

M71.35 Other bursal cyst, hip

   M71.351   Other bursal cyst, right hip

   M71.352   Other bursal cyst, left hip

   M71.359   Other bursal cyst, unspecified hip

M71.37 Other bursal cyst, ankle and foot

   M71.371   Other bursal cyst, right ankle and foot

   M71.372   Other bursal cyst, left ankle and foot

   M71.379   Other bursal cyst, unspecified ankle and foot

M71.38 Other bursal cyst, other site

M71.39 Other bursal cyst, multiple sites

M71.4 Calcium deposit in bursa

Excludes2: calcium deposit in bursa of shoulder (M75.3)

M71.40 Calcium deposit in bursa, unspecified site

M71.42 Calcium deposit in bursa, elbow

   M71.421   Calcium deposit in bursa, right elbow

   M71.422   Calcium deposit in bursa, left elbow

   M71.429   Calcium deposit in bursa, unspecified elbow

M71.43 Calcium deposit in bursa, wrist

   M71.431   Calcium deposit in bursa, right wrist

   M71.432   Calcium deposit in bursa, left wrist

   M71.439   Calcium deposit in bursa, unspecified wrist

M71.44 Calcium deposit in bursa, hand

   M71.441   Calcium deposit in bursa, right hand

   M71.442   Calcium deposit in bursa, left hand

   M71.449   Calcium deposit in bursa, unspecified hand

M71.45 Calcium deposit in bursa, hip

   M71.451   Calcium deposit in bursa, right hip

M71.452   Calcium deposit in bursa, left hip

M71.459   Calcium deposit in bursa, unspecified hip

M71.46   Calcium deposit in bursa, knee

M71.461   Calcium deposit in bursa, right knee

M71.462   Calcium deposit in bursa, left knee

M71.469   Calcium deposit in bursa, unspecified knee

M71.47   Calcium deposit in bursa, ankle and foot

M71.471   Calcium deposit in bursa, right ankle and foot

M71.472   Calcium deposit in bursa, left ankle and foot

M71.479   Calcium deposit in bursa, unspecified ankle and foot

M71.48   Calcium deposit in bursa, other site

M71.49   Calcium deposit in bursa, multiple sites

M71.5   Other bursitis, not elsewhere classified

Excludes1: bursitis NOS (M71.9-)

Excludes2: bursitis of shoulder (M75.5)

bursitis of tibial collateral [Pellegrini-Stieda] (M76.4-)

M71.50   Other bursitis, not elsewhere classified, unspecified site

M71.52   Other bursitis, not elsewhere classified, elbow

M71.521   Other bursitis, not elsewhere classified, right elbow

M71.522   Other bursitis, not elsewhere classified, left elbow

M71.529   Other bursitis, not elsewhere classified, unspecified elbow

M71.53   Other bursitis, not elsewhere classified, wrist

M71.531   Other bursitis, not elsewhere classified, right wrist

M71.532   Other bursitis, not elsewhere classified, left wrist

M71.539   Other bursitis, not elsewhere classified, unspecified wrist

M71.54   Other bursitis, not elsewhere classified, hand

M71.541   Other bursitis, not elsewhere classified, right hand

M71.542   Other bursitis, not elsewhere classified, left hand

M71.549   Other bursitis, not elsewhere classified, unspecified hand

M71.55   Other bursitis, not elsewhere classified, hip

M71.551   Other bursitis, not elsewhere classified, right hip

M71.552   Other bursitis, not elsewhere classified, left hip

M71.559   Other bursitis, not elsewhere classified, unspecified hip

M71.56   Other bursitis, not elsewhere classified, knee

M71.561   Other bursitis, not elsewhere classified, right knee

M71.562   Other bursitis, not elsewhere classified, left knee

M71.569   Other bursitis, not elsewhere classified, unspecified knee

M71.57   Other bursitis, not elsewhere classified, ankle and foot

M71.571   Other bursitis, not elsewhere classified, right ankle and foot

M71.572   Other bursitis, not elsewhere classified, left ankle and foot

M71.579   Other bursitis, not elsewhere classified, unspecified ankle and foot

M71.58   Other bursitis, not elsewhere classified, other site

M71.8   Other specified bursopathies

M71.80   Other specified bursopathies, unspecified site

M71.81   Other specified bursopathies, shoulder

M71.811   Other specified bursopathies, right shoulder

M71.812   Other specified bursopathies, left shoulder

M71.819   Other specified bursopathies, unspecified shoulder

M71.82   Other specified bursopathies, elbow

M71.821   Other specified bursopathies, right elbow

M71.822   Other specified bursopathies, left elbow

M71.829   Other specified bursopathies, unspecified elbow

M71.83   Other specified bursopathies, wrist

M71.831   Other specified bursopathies, right wrist

M71.832   Other specified bursopathies, left wrist

M71.839   Other specified bursopathies, unspecified wrist

M71.84   Other specified bursopathies, hand

M71.841   Other specified bursopathies, right hand

M71.842   Other specified bursopathies, left hand

M71.849   Other specified bursopathies, unspecified hand

M71.85   Other specified bursopathies, hip

M71.851   Other specified bursopathies, right hip

M71.852   Other specified bursopathies, left hip

M71.859   Other specified bursopathies, unspecified hip

M71.86   Other specified bursopathies, knee

M71.861   Other specified bursopathies, right knee

M71.862   Other specified bursopathies, left knee

M71.869   Other specified bursopathies, unspecified knee

M71.87   Other specified bursopathies, ankle and foot

M71.871   Other specified bursopathies, right ankle and foot

M71.872   Other specified bursopathies, left ankle and foot

M71.879   Other specified bursopathies, unspecified ankle and foot

M71.88   Other specified bursopathies, other site

M71.89   Other specified bursopathies, multiple sites

M71.9   Bursopathy, unspecified

Bursitis NOS

M72 **Fibroblastic disorders**

Excludes2: retroperitoneal fibromatosis (D48.3)

M72.0 **Palmar fascial fibromatosis [Dupuytren]**

M72.1 **Knuckle pads**

M72.2 **Plantar fascial fibromatosis**

Plantar fasciitis

M72.4 **Pseudosarcomatous fibromatosis**

Nodular fasciitis

M72.6 **Necrotizing fasciitis** [HCC]

Use Additional Code (B95.-, B96.-) to identify causative organism

M72.8 **Other fibroblastic disorders**

Abscess of fascia

Fasciitis NEC

Other infective fasciitis

Use Additional Code to (B95.-, B96.-) identify causative organism

Excludes1: diffuse (eosinophilic) fasciitis (M35.4)

necrotizing fasciitis (M72.6)

nodular fasciitis (M72.4)

perirenal fasciitis NOS (N13.5)

perirenal fasciitis with infection (N13.6)

plantar fasciitis (M72.2)

M72.9 **Fibroblastic disorder, unspecified**

Fasciitis NOS

Fibromatosis NOS

M75 **Shoulder lesions**

Excludes2: shoulder-hand syndrome (M89.0-)

M75.0 **Adhesive capsulitis of shoulder**

Frozen shoulder

Periarthritis of shoulder

M75.00 **Adhesive capsulitis of unspecified shoulder**

M75.01 **Adhesive capsulitis of right shoulder**

M75.02 **Adhesive capsulitis of left shoulder**

M75.1 **Rotator cuff tear or rupture, not specified as traumatic**

Rotator cuff syndrome

Supraspinatus tear or rupture, not specified as traumatic

Supraspinatus syndrome

Excludes1: tear of rotator cuff, traumatic (S46.01-)

M75.10 **Unspecified rotator cuff tear or rupture, not specified as traumatic**

M75.100 **Unspecified rotator cuff tear or rupture of unspecified shoulder, not specified as traumatic**

M75.101 **Unspecified rotator cuff tear or rupture of right shoulder, not specified as traumatic**

M75.102 **Unspecified rotator cuff tear or rupture of left shoulder, not specified as traumatic**

M75.11 **Incomplete rotator cuff tear or rupture not specified as traumatic**

M75.110 **Incomplete rotator cuff tear or rupture of unspecified shoulder, not specified as traumatic**

M75.111 **Incomplete rotator cuff tear or rupture of right shoulder, not specified as traumatic**

M75.112 **Incomplete rotator cuff tear or rupture of left shoulder, not specified as traumatic**

M75.12 **Complete rotator cuff tear or rupture not specified as traumatic**

M75.120 **Complete rotator cuff tear or rupture of unspecified shoulder, not specified as traumatic**

M75.121 **Complete rotator cuff tear or rupture of right shoulder, not specified as traumatic**

M75.122 **Complete rotator cuff tear or rupture of left shoulder, not specified as traumatic**

M75.2 **Bicipital tendinitis**

M75.20 **Bicipital tendinitis, unspecified shoulder**

M75.21 **Bicipital tendinitis, right shoulder**

M75.22 **Bicipital tendinitis, left shoulder**

M75.3 **Calcific tendinitis of shoulder**

Calcified bursa of shoulder

M75.30 **Calcific tendinitis of unspecified shoulder**

M75.31 **Calcific tendinitis of right shoulder**

M75.32 **Calcific tendinitis of left shoulder**

M75.4 **Impingement syndrome of shoulder**

M75.40 **Impingement syndrome of unspecified shoulder**

M75.41 **Impingement syndrome of right shoulder**

M75.42 **Impingement syndrome of left shoulder**

M75.5 **Bursitis of shoulder**

M75.50 **Bursitis of unspecified shoulder**

M75.51 **Bursitis of right shoulder**

M75.52 **Bursitis of left shoulder**

M75.8 **Other shoulder lesions**

M75.80 **Other shoulder lesions, unspecified shoulder**

M75.81 **Other shoulder lesions, right shoulder**

M75.82 **Other shoulder lesions, left shoulder**

M75.9 **Shoulder lesion, unspecified**

M75.90 **Shoulder lesion, unspecified, unspecified shoulder**

M75.91 **Shoulder lesion, unspecified, right shoulder**

M75.92 **Shoulder lesion, unspecified, left shoulder**

M76 **Enthesopathies, lower limb, excluding foot**

Excludes2: bursitis due to use, overuse and pressure (M70.-)

enthesopathies of ankle and foot (M77.5-)

M76.0 **Gluteal tendinitis**

M76.00 **Gluteal tendinitis, unspecified hip**

M76.01 **Gluteal tendinitis, right hip**

M76.02 **Gluteal tendinitis, left hip**

M76.1 **Psoas tendinitis**

M76.10 **Psoas tendinitis, unspecified hip**

M76.11 **Psoas tendinitis, right hip**

M76.12 **Psoas tendinitis, left hip**

M76.2 **Iliac crest spur**

M76.20 **Iliac crest spur, unspecified hip**

M76.21 **Iliac crest spur, right hip**

M76.22 **Iliac crest spur, left hip**

M76.3 **Iliotibial band syndrome**

M76.30 **Iliotibial band syndrome, unspecified leg**

M76.31 **Iliotibial band syndrome, right leg**

M76.32 **Iliotibial band syndrome, left leg**

M76.4 **Tibial collateral bursitis [Pellegrini-Stieda]**

   M76.40 **Tibial collateral bursitis [Pellegrini-Stieda], unspecified leg**

   M76.41 **Tibial collateral bursitis [Pellegrini-Stieda], right leg**

   M76.42 **Tibial collateral bursitis [Pellegrini-Stieda], left leg**

M76.5 **Patellar tendinitis**

   M76.50 **Patellar tendinitis, unspecified knee**

   M76.51 **Patellar tendinitis, right knee**

   M76.52 **Patellar tendinitis, left knee**

M76.6 **Achilles tendinitis**

   Achilles bursitis

   M76.60 **Achilles tendinitis, unspecified leg**

   M76.61 **Achilles tendinitis, right leg**

   M76.62 **Achilles tendinitis, left leg**

M76.7 **Peroneal tendinitis**

   M76.70 **Peroneal tendinitis, unspecified leg**

   M76.71 **Peroneal tendinitis, right leg**

   M76.72 **Peroneal tendinitis, left leg**

M76.8 **Other specified enthesopathies of lower limb, excluding foot**

   M76.81 **Anterior tibial syndrome**

     M76.811 **Anterior tibial syndrome, right leg**

     M76.812 **Anterior tibial syndrome, left leg**

     M76.819 **Anterior tibial syndrome, unspecified leg**

   M76.82 **Posterior tibial tendinitis**

     M76.821 **Posterior tibial tendinitis, right leg**

     M76.822 **Posterior tibial tendinitis, left leg**

     M76.829 **Posterior tibial tendinitis, unspecified leg**

   M76.89 **Other specified enthesopathies of lower limb, excluding foot**

     M76.891 **Other specified enthesopathies of right lower limb, excluding foot**

     M76.892 **Other specified enthesopathies of left lower limb, excluding foot**

     M76.899 **Other specified enthesopathies of unspecified lower limb, excluding foot**

M76.9 **Unspecified enthesopathy, lower limb, excluding foot**

M77 **Other enthesopathies**

   Excludes1: bursitis NOS (M71.9-)

   Excludes2: bursitis due to use, overuse and pressure (M70.-)

     osteophyte (M25.7)

     spinal enthesopathy (M46.0-)

M77.0 **Medial epicondylitis**

   M77.00 **Medial epicondylitis, unspecified elbow**

   M77.01 **Medial epicondylitis, right elbow**

   M77.02 **Medial epicondylitis, left elbow**

M77.1 **Lateral epicondylitis**

   Tennis elbow

   M77.10 **Lateral epicondylitis, unspecified elbow**

   M77.11 **Lateral epicondylitis, right elbow**

   M77.12 **Lateral epicondylitis, left elbow**

M77.2 **Periarthritis of wrist**

   M77.20 **Periarthritis, unspecified wrist**

   M77.21 **Periarthritis, right wrist**

   M77.22 **Periarthritis, left wrist**

M77.3 **Calcaneal spur**

   M77.30 **Calcaneal spur, unspecified foot**

   M77.31 **Calcaneal spur, right foot**

   M77.32 **Calcaneal spur, left foot**

M77.4 **Metatarsalgia**

   Excludes1: Morton's metatarsalgia (G57.6)

   M77.40 **Metatarsalgia, unspecified foot**

   M77.41 **Metatarsalgia, right foot**

   M77.42 **Metatarsalgia, left foot**

M77.5 **Other enthesopathy of foot and ankle**

   M77.50 **Other enthesopathy of unspecified foot and ankle**

   M77.51 **Other enthesopathy of right foot and ankle**

   M77.52 **Other enthesopathy of left foot and ankle**

M77.8 **Other enthesopathies, not elsewhere classified**

M77.9 **Enthesopathy, unspecified**

   Bone spur NOS

   Capsulitis NOS

   Periarthritis NOS

   Tendinitis NOS

M79 **Other and unspecified soft tissue disorders, not elsewhere classified**

   Excludes1: psychogenic rheumatism (F45.8)

     soft tissue pain, psychogenic (F45.41)

M79.0 **Rheumatism, unspecified**

   Definition: Rheumatism refers to 1) any painful disorder of the joints or muscles or connective tissues or 2) a chronic autoimmune disease with inflammation of the joints and marked deformities.

   Excludes1: fibromyalgia (M79.7)

     palindromic rheumatism (M12.3-)

M79.1 **Myalgia**

   Myofascial pain syndrome

   Excludes1: fibromyalgia (M79.7)

     myositis (M60.-)

   M79.10 **Myalgia, unspecified site**

   M79.11 **Myalgia of mastication muscle**

   M79.12 **Myalgia of auxiliary muscles, head and neck**

   M79.18 **Myalgia, other site**

M79.2 **Neuralgia and neuritis, unspecified**

   Excludes1: brachial radiculitis NOS (M54.1)

     lumbosacral radiculitis NOS (M54.1)

     mononeuropathies (G56-G58)

     radiculitis NOS (M54.1)

     sciatica (M54.3-M54.4)

M79.3 **Panniculitis, unspecified**

   Excludes1: lupus panniculitis (L93.2)

     neck and back panniculitis (M54.0-)

     relapsing [Weber-Christian] panniculitis (M35.6)

M79.4 **Hypertrophy of (infrapatellar) fat pad**

M79.5 **Residual foreign body in soft tissue**

   Excludes1: foreign body granuloma of skin and subcutaneous tissue (L92.3)

     foreign body granuloma of soft tissue (M60.2-)

M79.6 **Pain in limb, hand, foot, fingers and toes**

   Excludes2: pain in joint (M25.5-)

M79.60 **Pain in limb, unspecified**
    M79.601 **Pain in right arm**
        Pain in right upper limb NOS
    M79.602 **Pain in left arm**
        Pain in left upper limb NOS
    M79.603 **Pain in arm, unspecified**
        Pain in upper limb NOS
    M79.604 **Pain in right leg**
        Pain in right lower limb NOS
    M79.605 **Pain in left leg**
        Pain in left lower limb NOS
    M79.606 **Pain in leg, unspecified**
        Pain in lower limb NOS
    M79.609 **Pain in unspecified limb**
        Pain in limb NOS

M79.62 **Pain in upper arm**
    Pain in axillary region
    M79.621 **Pain in right upper arm**
    M79.622 **Pain in left upper arm**
    M79.629 **Pain in unspecified upper arm**

M79.63 **Pain in forearm**
    M79.631 **Pain in right forearm**
    M79.632 **Pain in left forearm**
    M79.639 **Pain in unspecified forearm**

M79.64 **Pain in hand and fingers**
    M79.641 **Pain in right hand**
    M79.642 **Pain in left hand**
    M79.643 **Pain in unspecified hand**
    M79.644 **Pain in right finger(s)**
    M79.645 **Pain in left finger(s)**
    M79.646 **Pain in unspecified finger(s)**

M79.65 **Pain in thigh**
    M79.651 **Pain in right thigh**
    M79.652 **Pain in left thigh**
    M79.659 **Pain in unspecified thigh**

M79.66 **Pain in lower leg**
    M79.661 **Pain in right lower leg**
    M79.662 **Pain in left lower leg**
    M79.669 **Pain in unspecified lower leg**

M79.67 **Pain in foot and toes**
    M79.671 **Pain in right foot**
    M79.672 **Pain in left foot**
    M79.673 **Pain in unspecified foot**
    M79.674 **Pain in right toe(s)**
    M79.675 **Pain in left toe(s)**
    M79.676 **Pain in unspecified toe(s)**

M79.7 Fibromyalgia
    Fibromyositis
    Fibrositis
    Myofibrositis

M79.A Nontraumatic compartment syndrome
    Code first, if applicable, associated postprocedural complication
    Excludes1: compartment syndrome NOS (T79.A-)
        fibromyalgia (M79.7)
        nontraumatic ischemic infarction of muscle (M62.2-)

        traumatic compartment syndrome (T79.A-)
    M79.A1 **Nontraumatic compartment syndrome of upper extremity**
        Nontraumatic compartment syndrome of shoulder, arm, forearm, wrist, hand, and fingers
        M79.A11 **Nontraumatic compartment syndrome of right upper extremity**
        M79.A12 **Nontraumatic compartment syndrome of left upper extremity**
        M79.A19 **Nontraumatic compartment syndrome of unspecified upper extremity**
    M79.A2 **Nontraumatic compartment syndrome of lower extremity**
        Nontraumatic compartment syndrome of hip, buttock, thigh, leg, foot, and toes
        M79.A21 **Nontraumatic compartment syndrome of right lower extremity**
        M79.A22 **Nontraumatic compartment syndrome of left lower extremity**
        M79.A29 **Nontraumatic compartment syndrome of unspecified lower extremity**
    M79.A3 **Nontraumatic compartment syndrome of abdomen**
    M79.A9 **Nontraumatic compartment syndrome of other sites**

M79.8 Other specified soft tissue disorders
    M79.81 **Nontraumatic hematoma of soft tissue**
        Nontraumatic hematoma of muscle
        Nontraumatic seroma of muscle and soft tissue
    M79.89 **Other specified soft tissue disorders**
        Polyalgia

M79.9 Soft tissue disorder, unspecified

OSTEOPATHIES AND CHONDROPATHIES (M80-M94)
DISORDERS OF BONE DENSITY AND STRUCTURE (M80-M85)

M80 **Osteoporosis with current pathological fracture**
    Includes: osteoporosis with current fragility fracture
    Use Additional Code to identify major osseous defect, if applicable (M89.7-)
    Excludes1: collapsed vertebra NOS (M48.5)
        pathological fracture NOS (M84.4)
        wedging of vertebra NOS (M48.5)
    Excludes2: personal history of (healed) osteoporosis fracture (Z87.310)

The appropriate 7th character is to be added to each code from category M80:

A - initial encounter for fracture

D - subsequent encounter for fracture with routine healing

G - subsequent encounter for fracture with delayed healing

K - subsequent encounter for fracture with nonunion

P - subsequent encounter for fracture with malunion

S - sequela

    M80.8A **Other osteoporosis with current pathological fracture, other site**
    M80.0 **Age-related osteoporosis with current pathological fracture**
        Involutional osteoporosis with current pathological fracture
        Osteoporosis NOS with current pathological fracture

● New code ▲ Revised code **Excludes1:** Not coded here **Excludes2:** Not included here ⊗ Placeholder required ⑦ 7th digit required

Postmenopausal osteoporosis with current pathological fracture

Senile osteoporosis with current pathological fracture

⊗⑦**M80.00** **Age-related osteoporosis with current pathological fracture, unspecified site**

M80.01 **Age-related osteoporosis with current pathological fracture, shoulder**

⑦**M80.011** **Age-related osteoporosis with current pathological fracture, right shoulder**

⑦**M80.012** **Age-related osteoporosis with current pathological fracture, left shoulder**

⑦**M80.019** **Age-related osteoporosis with current pathological fracture, unspecified shoulder**

M80.02 **Age-related osteoporosis with current pathological fracture, humerus**

⑦**M80.021** **Age-related osteoporosis with current pathological fracture, right humerus**

⑦**M80.022** **Age-related osteoporosis with current pathological fracture, left humerus**

⑦**M80.029** **Age-related osteoporosis with current pathological fracture, unspecified humerus**

M80.03 **Age-related osteoporosis with current pathological fracture, forearm**

Age-related osteoporosis with current pathological fracture of wrist

⑦**M80.031** **Age-related osteoporosis with current pathological fracture, right forearm**

⑦**M80.032** **Age-related osteoporosis with current pathological fracture, left forearm**

⑦**M80.039** **Age-related osteoporosis with current pathological fracture, unspecified forearm**

M80.04 **Age-related osteoporosis with current pathological fracture, hand**

⑦**M80.041** **Age-related osteoporosis with current pathological fracture, right hand**

⑦**M80.042** **Age-related osteoporosis with current pathological fracture, left hand**

⑦**M80.049** **Age-related osteoporosis with current pathological fracture, unspecified hand**

M80.05 **Age-related osteoporosis with current pathological fracture, femur**

Age-related osteoporosis with current pathological fracture of hip

⑦**M80.051** **Age-related osteoporosis with current pathological fracture, right femur** [HCC]

⑦**M80.052** **Age-related osteoporosis with current pathological fracture, left femur** [HCC]

⑦**M80.059** **Age-related osteoporosis with current pathological fracture, unspecified femur** [HCC]

M80.06 **Age-related osteoporosis with current pathological fracture, lower leg**

⑦**M80.061** **Age-related osteoporosis with current pathological fracture, right lower leg**

⑦**M80.062** **Age-related osteoporosis with current pathological fracture, left lower leg**

⑦**M80.069** **Age-related osteoporosis with current pathological fracture, unspecified lower leg**

M80.07 **Age-related osteoporosis with current pathological fracture, ankle and foot**

⑦**M80.071** **Age-related osteoporosis with current pathological fracture, right ankle and foot**

⑦**M80.072** **Age-related osteoporosis with current pathological fracture, left ankle and foot**

⑦**M80.079** **Age-related osteoporosis with current pathological fracture, unspecified ankle and foot**

⊗⑦**M80.08** **Age-related osteoporosis with current pathological fracture, vertebra(e)** [HCC]

M80.8 **Other osteoporosis with current pathological fracture**

Drug-induced osteoporosis with current pathological fracture

Idiopathic osteoporosis with current pathological fracture

Osteoporosis of disuse with current pathological fracture

Postoophorectomy osteoporosis with current pathological fracture

Postsurgical malabsorption osteoporosis with current pathological fracture

Post-traumatic osteoporosis with current pathological fracture

Use Additional Code for adverse effect, if applicable, to identify drug (T36-T50 with fifth or sixth character 5)

⊗⑦**M80.80** **Other osteoporosis with current pathological fracture, unspecified site**

M80.81 **Other osteoporosis with pathological fracture, shoulder**

⑦**M80.811** **Other osteoporosis with current pathological fracture, right shoulder**

⑦**M80.812** **Other osteoporosis with current pathological fracture, left shoulder**

⑦**M80.819** **Other osteoporosis with current pathological fracture, unspecified shoulder**

M80.82 **Other osteoporosis with current pathological fracture, humerus**

⑦**M80.821** **Other osteoporosis with current pathological fracture, right humerus**

⑦**M80.822** **Other osteoporosis with current pathological fracture, left humerus**

⑦**M80.829** **Other osteoporosis with current pathological fracture, unspecified humerus**

M80.83 **Other osteoporosis with current pathological fracture, forearm**

Other osteoporosis with current pathological fracture of wrist

⑦**M80.831** **Other osteoporosis with current pathological fracture, right forearm**

⑦**M80.832** **Other osteoporosis with current pathological fracture, left forearm**

⑦**M80.839** Other osteoporosis with current pathological fracture, unspecified forearm

M80.84 Other osteoporosis with current pathological fracture, hand

⑦**M80.841** Other osteoporosis with current pathological fracture, right hand

⑦**M80.842** Other osteoporosis with current pathological fracture, left hand

⑦**M80.849** Other osteoporosis with current pathological fracture, unspecified hand

M80.85 Other osteoporosis with current pathological fracture, femur

Other osteoporosis with current pathological fracture of hip

⑦**M80.851** Other osteoporosis with current pathological fracture, right femur [HCC]

⑦**M80.852** Other osteoporosis with current pathological fracture, left femur [HCC]

⑦**M80.859** Other osteoporosis with current pathological fracture, unspecified femur [HCC]

M80.86 Other osteoporosis with current pathological fracture, lower leg

⑦**M80.861** Other osteoporosis with current pathological fracture, right lower leg

⑦**M80.862** Other osteoporosis with current pathological fracture, left lower leg

⑦**M80.869** Other osteoporosis with current pathological fracture, unspecified lower leg

M80.87 Other osteoporosis with current pathological fracture, ankle and foot

⑦**M80.871** Other osteoporosis with current pathological fracture, right ankle and foot

⑦**M80.872** Other osteoporosis with current pathological fracture, left ankle and foot

⑦**M80.879** Other osteoporosis with current pathological fracture, unspecified ankle and foot

⊗⑦**M80.88** Other osteoporosis with current pathological fracture, vertebra(e) [HCC]

M81 **Osteoporosis without current pathological fracture**

Use Additional Code to identify:

major osseous defect, if applicable (M89.7-)

personal history of (healed) osteoporosis fracture, if applicable (Z87.310)

Excludes1: osteoporosis with current pathological fracture (M80.-)

Sudeck's atrophy (M89.0)

M81.0 Age-related osteoporosis without current pathological fracture

Involutional osteoporosis without current pathological fracture

Osteoporosis NOS

Postmenopausal osteoporosis without current pathological fracture

Senile osteoporosis without current pathological fracture

M81.6 Localized osteoporosis [Lequesne]

Excludes1: Sudeck's atrophy (M89.0)

M81.8 Other osteoporosis without current pathological fracture

Drug-induced osteoporosis without current pathological fracture

Idiopathic osteoporosis without current pathological fracture

Osteoporosis of disuse without current pathological fracture

Postoophorectomy osteoporosis without current pathological fracture

Postsurgical malabsorption osteoporosis without current pathological fracture

Post-traumatic osteoporosis without current pathological fracture

Use Additional Code for adverse effect, if applicable, to identify drug (T36-T50 with fifth or sixth character 5)

M83 **Adult osteomalacia**

Excludes1: infantile and juvenile osteomalacia (E55.0)

renal osteodystrophy (N25.0)

rickets (active) (E55.0)

rickets (active) sequelae (E64.3)

vitamin D-resistant osteomalacia (E83.3)

vitamin D-resistant rickets (active) (E83.3)

M83.0 Puerperal osteomalacia

M83.1 Senile osteomalacia

M83.2 Adult osteomalacia due to malabsorption

Postsurgical malabsorption osteomalacia in adults

M83.3 Adult osteomalacia due to malnutrition

M83.4 Aluminum bone disease

M83.5 Other drug-induced osteomalacia in adults

Use Additional Code for adverse effect, if applicable, to identify drug (T36-T50 with fifth or sixth character 5)

M83.8 Other adult osteomalacia

M83.9 Adult osteomalacia, unspecified

M84 **Disorder of continuity of bone**

Excludes2: traumatic fracture of bone-see fracture, by site

M84.3 Stress fracture

Fatigue fracture

March fracture

Stress fracture NOS

Stress reaction

Use additional external cause code(s) to identify the cause of the stress fracture

Excludes1: pathological fracture NOS (M84.4.-)

pathological fracture due to osteoporosis (M80.-)

traumatic fracture (S12.-, S22.-, S32.-, S42.-, S52.-, S62.-, S72.-, S82.-, S92.-)

Excludes2: personal history of (healed) stress (fatigue) fracture (Z87.312)

stress fracture of vertebra (M48.4-)

The appropriate 7th character is to be added to each code from subcategory M84.3:

A - initial encounter for fracture

D - subsequent encounter for fracture with routine healing

G - subsequent encounter for fracture with delayed healing

K - subsequent encounter for fracture with nonunion

P - subsequent encounter for fracture with malunion S - sequela

⊗⑦**M84.30** Stress fracture, unspecified site

M84.31 Stress fracture, shoulder

⑦**M84.311** Stress fracture, right shoulder

● New code   ▲ Revised code   **Excludes1:** Not coded here   **Excludes2:** Not included here   ⊗ Placeholder required   ⑦ 7th digit required

⑦M84.312 Stress fracture, left shoulder

⑦M84.319 Stress fracture, unspecified shoulder

M84.32 Stress fracture, humerus

⑦M84.321 Stress fracture, right humerus

⑦M84.322 Stress fracture, left humerus

⑦M84.329 Stress fracture, unspecified humerus

M84.33 Stress fracture, ulna and radius

⑦M84.331 Stress fracture, right ulna

⑦M84.332 Stress fracture, left ulna

⑦M84.333 Stress fracture, right radius

⑦M84.334 Stress fracture, left radius

⑦M84.339 Stress fracture, unspecified ulna and radius

M84.34 Stress fracture, hand and fingers

⑦M84.341 Stress fracture, right hand

⑦M84.342 Stress fracture, left hand

⑦M84.343 Stress fracture, unspecified hand

⑦M84.344 Stress fracture, right finger(s)

⑦M84.345 Stress fracture, left finger(s)

⑦M84.346 Stress fracture, unspecified finger(s)

M84.35 Stress fracture, pelvis and femur

Stress fracture, hip

⑦M84.350 Stress fracture, pelvis

⑦M84.351 Stress fracture, right femur

⑦M84.352 Stress fracture, left femur

⑦M84.353 Stress fracture, unspecified femur

⑦M84.359 Stress fracture, hip, unspecified

M84.36 Stress fracture, tibia and fibula

⑦M84.361 Stress fracture, right tibia

⑦M84.362 Stress fracture, left tibia

⑦M84.363 Stress fracture, right fibula

⑦M84.364 Stress fracture, left fibula

⑦M84.369 Stress fracture, unspecified tibia and fibula

M84.37 Stress fracture, ankle, foot and toes

⑦M84.371 Stress fracture, right ankle

⑦M84.372 Stress fracture, left ankle

⑦M84.373 Stress fracture, unspecified ankle

⑦M84.374 Stress fracture, right foot

⑦M84.375 Stress fracture, left foot

⑦M84.376 Stress fracture, unspecified foot

⑦M84.377 Stress fracture, right toe(s)

⑦M84.378 Stress fracture, left toe(s)

⑦M84.379 Stress fracture, unspecified toe(s)

⊗⑦M84.38 Stress fracture, other site

Excludes2: stress fracture of vertebra (M48.4-)

M84.4 Pathological fracture, not elsewhere classified

Chronic fracture

Pathological fracture NOS

Excludes1: collapsed vertebra NEC (M48.5)

pathological fracture in neoplastic disease (M84.5-)

pathological fracture in osteoporosis (M80.-)

pathological fracture in other disease (M84.6-)

stress fracture (M84.3-)

traumatic fracture (S12.-, S22.-, S32.-, S42.-, S52.-, S62.-, S72.-, S82.-, S92.-)

Excludes2: personal history of (healed) pathological

fracture (Z87.311)

The appropriate 7th character is to be added to each code from subcategory M84.4:

A - initial encounter for fracture

D - subsequent encounter for fracture with routine healing

G - subsequent encounter for fracture with delayed healing

K - subsequent encounter for fracture with nonunion

P - subsequent encounter for fracture with malunion

S - sequela

⊗⑦M84.40 Pathological fracture, unspecified site

M84.41 Pathological fracture, shoulder

⑦M84.411 Pathological fracture, right shoulder

⑦M84.412 Pathological fracture, left shoulder

⑦M84.419 Pathological fracture, unspecified shoulder

M84.42 Pathological fracture, humerus

⑦M84.421 Pathological fracture, right humerus

⑦M84.422 Pathological fracture, left humerus

⑦M84.429 Pathological fracture, unspecified humerus

M84.43 Pathological fracture, ulna and radius

⑦M84.431 Pathological fracture, right ulna

⑦M84.432 Pathological fracture, left ulna

⑦M84.433 Pathological fracture, right radius

⑦M84.434 Pathological fracture, left radius

⑦M84.439 Pathological fracture, unspecified ulna and radius

M84.44 Pathological fracture, hand and fingers

⑦M84.441 Pathological fracture, right hand

⑦M84.442 Pathological fracture, left hand

⑦M84.443 Pathological fracture, unspecified hand

⑦M84.444 Pathological fracture, right finger(s)

⑦M84.445 Pathological fracture, left finger(s)

⑦M84.446 Pathological fracture, unspecified finger(s)

M84.45 Pathological fracture, femur and pelvis

⑦M84.451 Pathological fracture, right femur [HCC]

⑦M84.452 Pathological fracture, left femur [HCC]

⑦M84.453 Pathological fracture, unspecified femur [HCC]

⑦M84.454 Pathological fracture, pelvis

⑦M84.459 Pathological fracture, hip, unspecified [HCC]

M84.46 Pathological fracture, tibia and fibula

⑦M84.461 Pathological fracture, right tibia

⑦M84.462 Pathological fracture, left tibia

⑦M84.463 Pathological fracture, right fibula

⑦M84.464 Pathological fracture, left fibula

⑦M84.469 Pathological fracture, unspecified tibia and fibula

M84.47 Pathological fracture, ankle, foot and toes

⑦M84.471 Pathological fracture, right ankle

⑦M84.472 Pathological fracture, left ankle

⑦M84.473 Pathological fracture, unspecified ankle

⑦M84.474 Pathological fracture, right foot

⑦M84.475 Pathological fracture, left foot

⑦M84.476   Pathological fracture, unspecified foot

⑦M84.477   Pathological fracture, right toe(s)

⑦M84.478   Pathological fracture, left toe(s)

⑦M84.479   Pathological fracture, unspecified toe(s)

⊗⑦**M84.48**   Pathological fracture, other site

M84.5 Pathological fracture in neoplastic disease

Code also underlying neoplasm

The appropriate 7th character is to be added to each code from subcategory M84.5:

A - initial encounter for fracture

D - subsequent encounter for fracture with routine healing

G - subsequent encounter for fracture with delayed healing

K - subsequent encounter for fracture with nonunion

P - subsequent encounter for fracture with malunion

S - sequela

⊗⑦**M84.50**   Pathological fracture in neoplastic disease, unspecified site

M84.51   Pathological fracture in neoplastic disease, shoulder

⑦M84.511   Pathological fracture in neoplastic disease, right shoulder

⑦M84.512   Pathological fracture in neoplastic disease, left shoulder

⑦M84.519   Pathological fracture in neoplastic disease, unspecified shoulder

M84.52   Pathological fracture in neoplastic disease, humerus

⑦M84.521   Pathological fracture in neoplastic disease, right humerus

⑦M84.522   Pathological fracture in neoplastic disease, left humerus

⑦M84.529   Pathological fracture in neoplastic disease, unspecified humerus

M84.53   Pathological fracture in neoplastic disease, ulna and radius

⑦M84.531   Pathological fracture in neoplastic disease, right ulna

⑦M84.532   Pathological fracture in neoplastic disease, left ulna

⑦M84.533   Pathological fracture in neoplastic disease, right radius

⑦M84.534   Pathological fracture in neoplastic disease, left radius

⑦M84.539   Pathological fracture in neoplastic disease, unspecified ulna and radius

M84.54   Pathological fracture in neoplastic disease, hand

⑦M84.541   Pathological fracture in neoplastic disease, right hand

⑦M84.542   Pathological fracture in neoplastic disease, left hand

⑦M84.549   Pathological fracture in neoplastic disease, unspecified hand

M84.55   Pathological fracture in neoplastic disease, pelvis and femur

⑦M84.550   Pathological fracture in neoplastic disease, pelvis

⑦M84.551   Pathological fracture in neoplastic disease, right femur [HCC]

⑦M84.552   Pathological fracture in neoplastic disease, left femur [HCC]

⑦M84.553   Pathological fracture in neoplastic disease, unspecified femur [HCC]

⑦M84.559   Pathological fracture in neoplastic disease, hip, unspecified [HCC]

M84.56   Pathological fracture in neoplastic disease, tibia and fibula

⑦M84.561   Pathological fracture in neoplastic disease, right tibia

⑦M84.562   Pathological fracture in neoplastic disease, left tibia

⑦M84.563   Pathological fracture in neoplastic disease, right fibula

⑦M84.564   Pathological fracture in neoplastic disease, left fibula

⑦M84.569   Pathological fracture in neoplastic disease, unspecified tibia and fibula

M84.57   Pathological fracture in neoplastic disease, ankle and foot

⑦M84.571   Pathological fracture in neoplastic disease, right ankle

⑦M84.572   Pathological fracture in neoplastic disease, left ankle

⑦M84.573   Pathological fracture in neoplastic disease, unspecified ankle

⑦M84.574   Pathological fracture in neoplastic disease, right foot

⑦M84.575   Pathological fracture in neoplastic disease, left foot

⑦M84.576   Pathological fracture in neoplastic disease, unspecified foot

⊗⑦**M84.58**   Pathological fracture in neoplastic disease, other specified site

Pathological fracture in neoplastic disease, vertebrae

M84.6 Pathological fracture in other disease

Code also underlying condition

Excludes1: pathological fracture in osteoporosis (M80.-)

The appropriate 7th character is to be added to each code from subcategory M84.6:

A - initial encounter for fracture

D - subsequent encounter for fracture with routine healing

G - subsequent encounter for fracture with delayed healing

K - subsequent encounter for fracture with nonunion

P - subsequent encounter for fracture with malunion

S - sequela

⊗⑦**M84.60**   Pathological fracture in other disease, unspecified site

M84.61   Pathological fracture in other disease, shoulder

⑦M84.611   Pathological fracture in other disease, right shoulder

⑦M84.612   Pathological fracture in other disease, left shoulder

⑦M84.619   Pathological fracture in other disease, unspecified shoulder

M84.62   Pathological fracture in other disease, humerus

⑦M84.621   Pathological fracture in other disease, right humerus

⑦M84.622   Pathological fracture in other disease, left humerus

⑦M84.629   Pathological fracture in other disease, unspecified humerus

M84.63   Pathological fracture in other disease, ulna and radius

● New code   ▲ Revised code   **Excludes1:** Not coded here   **Excludes2:** Not included here   ⊗ Placeholder required   ⑦7th digit required

⑦M84.631 **Pathological fracture in other disease, right ulna**

⑦M84.632 **Pathological fracture in other disease, left ulna**

⑦M84.633 **Pathological fracture in other disease, right radius**

⑦M84.634 **Pathological fracture in other disease, left radius**

⑦M84.639 **Pathological fracture in other disease, unspecified ulna and radius**

M84.64 **Pathological fracture in other disease, hand**

⑦M84.641 **Pathological fracture in other disease, right hand**

⑦M84.642 **Pathological fracture in other disease, left hand**

⑦M84.649 **Pathological fracture in other disease, unspecified hand**

M84.65 **Pathological fracture in other disease, pelvis and femur**

⑦M84.650 **Pathological fracture in other disease, pelvis**

⑦M84.651 **Pathological fracture in other disease, right femur** [HCC]

⑦M84.652 **Pathological fracture in other disease, left femur** [HCC]

⑦M84.653 **Pathological fracture in other disease, unspecified femur** [HCC]

⑦M84.659 **Pathological fracture in other disease, hip, unspecified** [HCC]

M84.66 **Pathological fracture in other disease, tibia and fibula**

⑦M84.661 **Pathological fracture in other disease, right tibia**

⑦M84.662 **Pathological fracture in other disease, left tibia**

⑦M84.663 **Pathological fracture in other disease, right fibula**

⑦M84.664 **Pathological fracture in other disease, left fibula**

⑦M84.669 **Pathological fracture in other disease, unspecified tibia and fibula**

M84.67 **Pathological fracture in other disease, ankle and foot**

⑦M84.671 **Pathological fracture in other disease, right ankle**

⑦M84.672 **Pathological fracture in other disease, left ankle**

⑦M84.673 **Pathological fracture in other disease, unspecified ankle**

⑦M84.674 **Pathological fracture in other disease, right foot**

⑦M84.675 **Pathological fracture in other disease, left foot**

⑦M84.676 **Pathological fracture in other disease, unspecified foot**

⊗⑦M84.68 **Pathological fracture in other disease, other site**

M84.7 **Nontraumatic fracture, not elsewhere classified**

M84.75 **Atypical femoral fracture**

The appropriate 7th character is to be added to each code from M84.75:

A - initial encounter for fracture

D - subsequent encounter for fracture with routine healing

G - subsequent encounter for fracture with delayed healing

K - subsequent encounter for fracture with nonunion

P - subsequent encounter for fracture with malunion

S - sequela

⑦M84.750 **Atypical femoral fracture, unspecified**

⑦M84.751 **Incomplete atypical femoral fracture, right leg**

⑦M84.752 **Incomplete atypical femoral fracture, left leg**

⑦M84.753 **Incomplete atypical femoral fracture, unspecified leg**

⑦M84.754 **Complete transverse atypical femoral fracture, right leg** [HCC]

⑦M84.755 **Complete transverse atypical femoral fracture, left leg** [HCC]

⑦M84.756 **Complete transverse atypical femoral fracture, unspecified leg** [HCC]

⑦M84.757 **Complete oblique atypical femoral fracture, right leg** [HCC]

⑦M84.758 **Complete oblique atypical femoral fracture, left leg** [HCC]

⑦M84.759 **Complete oblique atypical femoral fracture, unspecified leg** [HCC]

M84.8 **Other disorders of continuity of bone**

⊗⑦M84.80 **Other disorders of continuity of bone, unspecified site**

M84.81 **Other disorders of continuity of bone, shoulder**

⑦M84.811 **Other disorders of continuity of bone, right shoulder**

⑦M84.812 **Other disorders of continuity of bone, left shoulder**

⑦M84.819 **Other disorders of continuity of bone, unspecified shoulder**

M84.82 **Other disorders of continuity of bone, humerus**

⑦M84.821 **Other disorders of continuity of bone, right humerus**

⑦M84.822 **Other disorders of continuity of bone, left humerus**

⑦M84.829 **Other disorders of continuity of bone, unspecified humerus**

M84.83 **Other disorders of continuity of bone, ulna and radius**

⑦M84.831 **Other disorders of continuity of bone, right ulna**

⑦M84.832 **Other disorders of continuity of bone, left ulna**

⑦M84.833 **Other disorders of continuity of bone, right radius**

⑦M84.834 **Other disorders of continuity of bone, left radius**

⑦M84.839 **Other disorders of continuity of bone, unspecified ulna and radius**

M84.84 **Other disorders of continuity of bone, hand**

⑦M84.841 **Other disorders of continuity of bone, right hand**

⑦M84.842 **Other disorders of continuity of bone, left hand**

⑦M84.849 **Other disorders of continuity of bone, unspecified hand**

M84.85   Other disorders of continuity of bone, pelvic region and thigh

⑦M84.851   Other disorders of continuity of bone, right pelvic region and thigh

⑦M84.852   Other disorders of continuity of bone, left pelvic region and thigh

⑦M84.859   Other disorders of continuity of bone, unspecified pelvic region and thigh

M84.86   Other disorders of continuity of bone, tibia and fibula

⑦M84.861   Other disorders of continuity of bone, right tibia

⑦M84.862   Other disorders of continuity of bone, left tibia

⑦M84.863   Other disorders of continuity of bone, right fibula

⑦M84.864   Other disorders of continuity of bone, left fibula

⑦M84.869   Other disorders of continuity of bone, unspecified tibia and fibula

M84.87   Other disorders of continuity of bone, ankle and foot

⑦M84.871   Other disorders of continuity of bone, right ankle and foot

⑦M84.872   Other disorders of continuity of bone, left ankle and foot

⑦M84.879   Other disorders of continuity of bone, unspecified ankle and foot

⊗⑦M84.88   Other disorders of continuity of bone, other site

⊗M84.9   Disorder of continuity of bone, unspecified

M85   **Other disorders of bone density and structure**

Excludes1: osteogenesis imperfecta (Q78.0)

osteopetrosis (Q78.2)

osteopoikilosis (Q78.8)

polyostotic fibrous dysplasia (Q78.1)

M85.0   Fibrous dysplasia (monostotic)

Excludes2: fibrous dysplasia of jaw (M27.8)

M85.00   Fibrous dysplasia (monostotic), unspecified site

M85.01   Fibrous dysplasia (monostotic), shoulder

M85.011   Fibrous dysplasia (monostotic), right shoulder

M85.012   Fibrous dysplasia (monostotic), left shoulder

M85.019   Fibrous dysplasia (monostotic), unspecified shoulder

M85.02   Fibrous dysplasia (monostotic), upper arm

M85.021   Fibrous dysplasia (monostotic), right upper arm

M85.022   Fibrous dysplasia (monostotic), left upper arm

M85.029   Fibrous dysplasia (monostotic), unspecified upper arm

M85.03   Fibrous dysplasia (monostotic), forearm

M85.031   Fibrous dysplasia (monostotic), right forearm

M85.032   Fibrous dysplasia (monostotic), left forearm

M85.039   Fibrous dysplasia (monostotic), unspecified forearm

M85.04   Fibrous dysplasia (monostotic), hand

M85.041   Fibrous dysplasia (monostotic), right hand

M85.042   Fibrous dysplasia (monostotic), left hand

M85.049   Fibrous dysplasia (monostotic), unspecified hand

M85.05   Fibrous dysplasia (monostotic), thigh

M85.051   Fibrous dysplasia (monostotic), right thigh

M85.052   Fibrous dysplasia (monostotic), left thigh

M85.059   Fibrous dysplasia (monostotic), unspecified thigh

M85.06   Fibrous dysplasia (monostotic), lower leg

M85.061   Fibrous dysplasia (monostotic), right lower leg

M85.062   Fibrous dysplasia (monostotic), left lower leg

M85.069   Fibrous dysplasia (monostotic), unspecified lower leg

M85.07   Fibrous dysplasia (monostotic), ankle and foot

M85.071   Fibrous dysplasia (monostotic), right ankle and foot

M85.072   Fibrous dysplasia (monostotic), left ankle and foot

M85.079   Fibrous dysplasia (monostotic), unspecified ankle and foot

M85.08   Fibrous dysplasia (monostotic), other site

M85.09   Fibrous dysplasia (monostotic), multiple sites

M85.1   Skeletal fluorosis

M85.10   Skeletal fluorosis, unspecified site

M85.11   Skeletal fluorosis, shoulder

M85.111   Skeletal fluorosis, right shoulder

M85.112   Skeletal fluorosis, left shoulder

M85.119   Skeletal fluorosis, unspecified shoulder

M85.12   Skeletal fluorosis, upper arm

M85.121   Skeletal fluorosis, right upper arm

M85.122   Skeletal fluorosis, left upper arm

M85.129   Skeletal fluorosis, unspecified upper arm

M85.13   Skeletal fluorosis, forearm

M85.131   Skeletal fluorosis, right forearm

M85.132   Skeletal fluorosis, left forearm

M85.139   Skeletal fluorosis, unspecified forearm

M85.14   Skeletal fluorosis, hand

M85.141   Skeletal fluorosis, right hand

M85.142   Skeletal fluorosis, left hand

M85.149   Skeletal fluorosis, unspecified hand

M85.15   Skeletal fluorosis, thigh

M85.151   Skeletal fluorosis, right thigh

M85.152   Skeletal fluorosis, left thigh

M85.159   Skeletal fluorosis, unspecified thigh

M85.16   Skeletal fluorosis, lower leg

M85.161   Skeletal fluorosis, right lower leg

M85.162   Skeletal fluorosis, left lower leg

M85.169   Skeletal fluorosis, unspecified lower leg

M85.17   Skeletal fluorosis, ankle and foot

M85.171   Skeletal fluorosis, right ankle and foot

M85.172   Skeletal fluorosis, left ankle and foot

M85.179   Skeletal fluorosis, unspecified ankle and foot

M85.18   Skeletal fluorosis, other site

M85.19   Skeletal fluorosis, multiple sites

M85.2   Hyperostosis of skull

M85.3   Osteitis condensans

   M85.30   Osteitis condensans, unspecified site

   M85.31   Osteitis condensans, shoulder

     M85.311   Osteitis condensans, right shoulder

     M85.312   Osteitis condensans, left shoulder

     M85.319   Osteitis condensans, unspecified shoulder

   M85.32   Osteitis condensans, upper arm

     M85.321   Osteitis condensans, right upper arm

     M85.322   Osteitis condensans, left upper arm

     M85.329   Osteitis condensans, unspecified upper arm

     M85.33   Osteitis condensans, forearm

     M85.331   Osteitis condensans, right forearm

     M85.332   Osteitis condensans, left forearm

     M85.339   Osteitis condensans, unspecified forearm

   M85.34   Osteitis condensans, hand

     M85.341   Osteitis condensans, right hand

     M85.342   Osteitis condensans, left hand

     M85.349   Osteitis condensans, unspecified hand

   M85.35   Osteitis condensans, thigh

     M85.351   Osteitis condensans, right thigh

     M85.352   Osteitis condensans, left thigh

     M85.359   Osteitis condensans, unspecified thigh

   M85.36   Osteitis condensans, lower leg

     M85.361   Osteitis condensans, right lower leg

     M85.362   Osteitis condensans, left lower leg

     M85.369   Osteitis condensans, unspecified lower leg

   M85.37   Osteitis condensans, ankle and foot

     M85.371   Osteitis condensans, right ankle and foot

     M85.372   Osteitis condensans, left ankle and foot

     M85.379   Osteitis condensans, unspecified ankle and foot

   M85.38   Osteitis condensans, other site

   M85.39   Osteitis condensans, multiple sites

M85.4   Solitary bone cyst

   Excludes2: solitary cyst of jaw (M27.4)

   M85.40   Solitary bone cyst, unspecified site

   M85.41   Solitary bone cyst, shoulder

     M85.411   Solitary bone cyst, right shoulder

     M85.412   Solitary bone cyst, left shoulder

     M85.419   Solitary bone cyst, unspecified shoulder

   M85.42   Solitary bone cyst, humerus

     M85.421   Solitary bone cyst, right humerus

M85.422   Solitary bone cyst, left humerus

M85.429   Solitary bone cyst, unspecified humerus

   M85.43   Solitary bone cyst, ulna and radius

     M85.431   Solitary bone cyst, right ulna and radius

     M85.432   Solitary bone cyst, left ulna and radius

     M85.439   Solitary bone cyst, unspecified ulna and radius

   M85.44   Solitary bone cyst, hand

     M85.441   Solitary bone cyst, right hand

     M85.442   Solitary bone cyst, left hand

     M85.449   Solitary bone cyst, unspecified hand

   M85.45   Solitary bone cyst, pelvis

     M85.451   Solitary bone cyst, right pelvis

     M85.452   Solitary bone cyst, left pelvis

     M85.459   Solitary bone cyst, unspecified pelvis

   M85.46   Solitary bone cyst, tibia and fibula

     M85.461   Solitary bone cyst, right tibia and fibula

     M85.462   Solitary bone cyst, left tibia and fibula

     M85.469   Solitary bone cyst, unspecified tibia and fibula

   M85.47   Solitary bone cyst, ankle and foot

     M85.471   Solitary bone cyst, right ankle and foot

     M85.472   Solitary bone cyst, left ankle and foot

     M85.479   Solitary bone cyst, unspecified ankle and foot

   M85.48   Solitary bone cyst, other site

M85.5   Aneurysmal bone cyst

   Excludes2: aneurysmal cyst of jaw (M27.4)

   M85.50   Aneurysmal bone cyst, unspecified site

   M85.51   Aneurysmal bone cyst, shoulder

     M85.511   Aneurysmal bone cyst, right shoulder

     M85.512   Aneurysmal bone cyst, left shoulder

     M85.519   Aneurysmal bone cyst, unspecified shoulder

   M85.52   Aneurysmal bone cyst, upper arm

     M85.521   Aneurysmal bone cyst, right upper arm

     M85.522   Aneurysmal bone cyst, left upper arm

     M85.529   Aneurysmal bone cyst, unspecified upper arm

   M85.53   Aneurysmal bone cyst, forearm

     M85.531   Aneurysmal bone cyst, right forearm

     M85.532   Aneurysmal bone cyst, left forearm

     M85.539   Aneurysmal bone cyst, unspecified forearm

   M85.54   Aneurysmal bone cyst, hand

     M85.541   Aneurysmal bone cyst, right hand

     M85.542   Aneurysmal bone cyst, left hand

     M85.549   Aneurysmal bone cyst, unspecified hand

   M85.55   Aneurysmal bone cyst, thigh

     M85.551   Aneurysmal bone cyst, right thigh

M85.552   Aneurysmal bone cyst, left thigh

M85.559   Aneurysmal bone cyst, unspecified thigh

M85.56   Aneurysmal bone cyst, lower leg

M85.561   Aneurysmal bone cyst, right lower leg

M85.562   Aneurysmal bone cyst, left lower leg

M85.569   Aneurysmal bone cyst, unspecified lower leg

M85.57   Aneurysmal bone cyst, ankle and foot

M85.571   Aneurysmal bone cyst, right ankle and foot

M85.572   Aneurysmal bone cyst, left ankle and foot

M85.579   Aneurysmal bone cyst, unspecified ankle and foot

M85.58   Aneurysmal bone cyst, other site

M85.59   Aneurysmal bone cyst, multiple sites

M85.6   Other cyst of bone

Excludes1: cyst of jaw NEC (M27.4)

osteitis fibrosa cystica generalisata [von Recklinghausen's disease of bone] (E21.0)

M85.60   Other cyst of bone, unspecified site

M85.61   Other cyst of bone, shoulder

M85.611   Other cyst of bone, right shoulder

M85.612   Other cyst of bone, left shoulder

M85.619   Other cyst of bone, unspecified shoulder

M85.62   Other cyst of bone, upper arm

M85.621   Other cyst of bone, right upper arm

M85.622   Other cyst of bone, left upper arm

M85.629   Other cyst of bone, unspecified upper arm

M85.63   Other cyst of bone, forearm

M85.631   Other cyst of bone, right forearm

M85.632   Other cyst of bone, left forearm

M85.639   Other cyst of bone, unspecified forearm

M85.64   Other cyst of bone, hand

M85.641   Other cyst of bone, right hand

M85.642   Other cyst of bone, left hand

M85.649   Other cyst of bone, unspecified hand

M85.65   Other cyst of bone, thigh

M85.651   Other cyst of bone, right thigh

M85.652   Other cyst of bone, left thigh

M85.659   Other cyst of bone, unspecified thigh

M85.66   Other cyst of bone, lower leg

M85.661   Other cyst of bone, right lower leg

M85.662   Other cyst of bone, left lower leg

M85.669   Other cyst of bone, unspecified lower leg

M85.67   Other cyst of bone, ankle and foot

M85.671   Other cyst of bone, right ankle and foot

M85.672   Other cyst of bone, left ankle and foot

M85.679   Other cyst of bone, unspecified ankle and foot

M85.68   Other cyst of bone, other site

M85.69   Other cyst of bone, multiple sites

M85.8   Other specified disorders of bone density and structure

Hyperostosis of bones, except skull

Osteosclerosis, acquired

Excludes1: diffuse idiopathic skeletal hyperostosis [DISH] (M48.1)

osteosclerosis congenita (Q77.4)

osteosclerosis fragilitas (generalisata) (Q78.2)

osteosclerosis myelofibrosis (D75.81)

M85.80   Other specified disorders of bone density and structure, unspecified site

M85.81   Other specified disorders of bone density and structure, shoulder

M85.811   Other specified disorders of bone density and structure, right shoulder

M85.812   Other specified disorders of bone density and structure, left shoulder

M85.819   Other specified disorders of bone density and structure, unspecified shoulder

M85.82   Other specified disorders of bone density and structure, upper arm

M85.821   Other specified disorders of bone density and structure, right upper arm

M85.822   Other specified disorders of bone density and structure, left upper arm

M85.829   Other specified disorders of bone density and structure, unspecified upper arm

M85.83   Other specified disorders of bone density and structure, forearm

M85.831   Other specified disorders of bone density and structure, right forearm

M85.832   Other specified disorders of bone density and structure, left forearm

M85.839   Other specified disorders of bone density and structure, unspecified forearm

M85.84   Other specified disorders of bone density and structure, hand

M85.841   Other specified disorders of bone density and structure, right hand

M85.842   Other specified disorders of bone density and structure, left hand

M85.849   Other specified disorders of bone density and structure, unspecified hand

M85.85   Other specified disorders of bone density and structure, thigh

M85.851   Other specified disorders of bone density and structure, right thigh

M85.852   Other specified disorders of bone density and structure, left thigh

M85.859   Other specified disorders of bone density and structure, unspecified thigh

M85.86   Other specified disorders of bone density and structure, lower leg

M85.861   Other specified disorders of bone density and structure, right lower leg

M85.862   Other specified disorders of bone density and structure, left lower leg

● New code   ▲ Revised code   **Excludes1:** Not coded here   **Excludes2:** Not included here   ⊗ Placeholder required   ⑦7ᵗʰ digit required

M85.869　Other specified disorders of bone density and structure, unspecified lower leg

M85.87　Other specified disorders of bone density and structure, ankle and foot

M85.871　Other specified disorders of bone density and structure, right ankle and foot

M85.872　Other specified disorders of bone density and structure, left ankle and foot

M85.879　Other specified disorders of bone density and structure, unspecified ankle and foot

M85.88　Other specified disorders of bone density and structure, other site

M85.89　Other specified disorders of bone density and structure, multiple sites

M85.9　Disorder of bone density and structure, unspecified

OTHER OSTEOPATHIES (M86-M90)

Excludes1: postprocedural osteopathies (M96.-)

M86　Osteomyelitis

Use Additional Code (B95-B97) to identify infectious agent

Use Additional Code to identify major osseous defect, if applicable (M89.7-)

Excludes1: osteomyelitis due to:

echinococcus (B67.2)

gonococcus (A54.43)

salmonella (A02.24)

Excludes2: osteomyelitis of:

orbit (H05.0-)

petrous bone (H70.2-)

vertebra (M46.2-)

M86.0　Acute hematogenous osteomyelitis

M86.00　Acute hematogenous osteomyelitis, unspecified site [HCC]

M86.01　Acute hematogenous osteomyelitis, shoulder

M86.011　Acute hematogenous osteomyelitis, right shoulder [HCC]

M86.012　Acute hematogenous osteomyelitis, left shoulder [HCC]

M86.019　Acute hematogenous osteomyelitis, unspecified shoulder [HCC]

M86.02　Acute hematogenous osteomyelitis, humerus

M86.021　Acute hematogenous osteomyelitis, right humerus [HCC]

M86.022　Acute hematogenous osteomyelitis, left humerus [HCC]

M86.029　Acute hematogenous osteomyelitis, unspecified humerus [HCC]

M86.03　Acute hematogenous osteomyelitis, radius and ulna

M86.031　Acute hematogenous osteomyelitis, right radius and ulna [HCC]

M86.032　Acute hematogenous osteomyelitis, left radius and ulna [HCC]

M86.039　Acute hematogenous osteomyelitis, unspecified radius and ulna [HCC]

M86.04　Acute hematogenous osteomyelitis, hand

M86.041　Acute hematogenous osteomyelitis, right hand [HCC]

M86.042　Acute hematogenous osteomyelitis, left hand [HCC]

M86.049　Acute hematogenous osteomyelitis, unspecified hand [HCC]

M86.05　Acute hematogenous osteomyelitis, femur

M86.051　Acute hematogenous osteomyelitis, right femur [HCC]

M86.052　Acute hematogenous osteomyelitis, left femur [HCC]

M86.059　Acute hematogenous osteomyelitis, unspecified femur [HCC]

M86.06　Acute hematogenous osteomyelitis, tibia and fibula

M86.061　Acute hematogenous osteomyelitis, right tibia and fibula [HCC]

M86.062　Acute hematogenous osteomyelitis, left tibia and fibula [HCC]

M86.069　Acute hematogenous osteomyelitis, unspecified tibia and fibula [HCC]

M86.07　Acute hematogenous osteomyelitis, ankle and foot

M86.071　Acute hematogenous osteomyelitis, right ankle and foot [HCC]

M86.072　Acute hematogenous osteomyelitis, left ankle and foot [HCC]

M86.079　Acute hematogenous osteomyelitis, unspecified ankle and foot [HCC]

M86.08　Acute hematogenous osteomyelitis, other sites [HCC]

M86.09　Acute hematogenous osteomyelitis, multiple sites [HCC]

M86.1　Other acute osteomyelitis

M86.10　Other acute osteomyelitis, unspecified site

M86.11　Other acute osteomyelitis, shoulder

M86.111　Other acute osteomyelitis, right shoulder [HCC]

M86.112　Other acute osteomyelitis, left shoulder [HCC]

M86.119　Other acute osteomyelitis, unspecified shoulder [HCC]

M86.12　Other acute osteomyelitis, humerus

M86.121　Other acute osteomyelitis, right humerus [HCC]

M86.122　Other acute osteomyelitis, left humerus [HCC]

M86.129　Other acute osteomyelitis, unspecified humerus [HCC]

M86.13　Other acute osteomyelitis, radius and ulna

M86.131　Other acute osteomyelitis, right radius and ulna [HCC]

M86.132　Other acute osteomyelitis, left radius and ulna [HCC]

M86.139　Other acute osteomyelitis, unspecified radius and ulna [HCC]

M86.14　Other acute osteomyelitis, hand

M86.141　Other acute osteomyelitis, right hand [HCC]

M86.142　Other acute osteomyelitis, left hand [HCC]

M86.149　Other acute osteomyelitis, unspecified hand [HCC]

M86.15　Other acute osteomyelitis, femur

M86.151　Other acute osteomyelitis, right femur [HCC]

M86.152 Other acute osteomyelitis, left femur [HCC]

M86.159 Other acute osteomyelitis, unspecified femur [HCC]

M86.16 Other acute osteomyelitis, tibia and fibula

M86.161 Other acute osteomyelitis, right tibia and fibula [HCC]

M86.162 Other acute osteomyelitis, left tibia and fibula [HCC]

M86.169 Other acute osteomyelitis, unspecified tibia and fibula [HCC]

M86.17 Other acute osteomyelitis, ankle and foot

M86.171 Other acute osteomyelitis, right ankle and foot [HCC]

M86.172 Other acute osteomyelitis, left ankle and foot [HCC]

M86.179 Other acute osteomyelitis, unspecified ankle and foot [HCC]

M86.18 Other acute osteomyelitis, other site [HCC]

M86.19 Other acute osteomyelitis, multiple sites [HCC]

M86.2 Subacute osteomyelitis

M86.20 Subacute osteomyelitis, unspecified site [HCC]

M86.21 Subacute osteomyelitis, shoulder

M86.211 Subacute osteomyelitis, right shoulder [HCC]

M86.212 Subacute osteomyelitis, left shoulder [HCC]

M86.219 Subacute osteomyelitis, unspecified shoulder [HCC]

M86.22 Subacute osteomyelitis, humerus

M86.221 Subacute osteomyelitis, right humerus [HCC]

M86.222 Subacute osteomyelitis, left humerus [HCC]

M86.229 Subacute osteomyelitis, unspecified humerus [HCC]

M86.23 Subacute osteomyelitis, radius and ulna

M86.231 Subacute osteomyelitis, right radius and ulna [HCC]

M86.232 Subacute osteomyelitis, left radius and ulna [HCC]

M86.239 Subacute osteomyelitis, unspecified radius and ulna [HCC]

M86.24 Subacute osteomyelitis, hand

M86.241 Subacute osteomyelitis, right hand [HCC]

M86.242 Subacute osteomyelitis, left hand [HCC]

M86.249 Subacute osteomyelitis, unspecified hand [HCC]

M86.25 Subacute osteomyelitis, femur

M86.251 Subacute osteomyelitis, right femur [HCC]

M86.252 Subacute osteomyelitis, left femur [HCC]

M86.259 Subacute osteomyelitis, unspecified femur [HCC]

M86.26 Subacute osteomyelitis, tibia and fibula

M86.261 Subacute osteomyelitis, right tibia and fibula [HCC]

M86.262 Subacute osteomyelitis, left tibia and fibula [HCC]

M86.269 Subacute osteomyelitis, unspecified tibia and fibula [HCC]

M86.27 Subacute osteomyelitis, ankle and foot

M86.271 Subacute osteomyelitis, right ankle and foot [HCC]

M86.272 Subacute osteomyelitis, left ankle and foot [HCC]

M86.279 Subacute osteomyelitis, unspecified ankle and foot [HCC]

M86.28 Subacute osteomyelitis, other site [HCC]

M86.29 Subacute osteomyelitis, multiple sites [HCC]

M86.3 Chronic multifocal osteomyelitis

M86.30 Chronic multifocal osteomyelitis, unspecified site [HCC]

M86.31 Chronic multifocal osteomyelitis, shoulder

M86.311 Chronic multifocal osteomyelitis, right shoulder

M86.312 Chronic multifocal osteomyelitis, left shoulder [HCC]

M86.319 Chronic multifocal osteomyelitis, unspecified shoulder [HCC]

M86.32 Chronic multifocal osteomyelitis, humerus

M86.321 Chronic multifocal osteomyelitis, right humerus [HCC]

M86.322 Chronic multifocal osteomyelitis, left humerus [HCC]

M86.329 Chronic multifocal osteomyelitis, unspecified humerus [HCC]

M86.33 Chronic multifocal osteomyelitis, radius and ulna

M86.331 Chronic multifocal osteomyelitis, right radius and ulna [HCC]

M86.332 Chronic multifocal osteomyelitis, left radius and ulna [HCC]

M86.339 Chronic multifocal osteomyelitis, unspecified radius and ulna [HCC]

M86.34 Chronic multifocal osteomyelitis, hand

M86.341 Chronic multifocal osteomyelitis, right hand [HCC]

M86.342 Chronic multifocal osteomyelitis, left hand [HCC]

M86.349 Chronic multifocal osteomyelitis, unspecified hand [HCC]

M86.35 Chronic multifocal osteomyelitis, femur

M86.351 Chronic multifocal osteomyelitis, right femur [HCC]

M86.352 Chronic multifocal osteomyelitis, left femur [HCC]

M86.359 Chronic multifocal osteomyelitis, unspecified femur [HCC]

M86.36 Chronic multifocal osteomyelitis, tibia and fibula [HCC]

M86.361 Chronic multifocal osteomyelitis, right tibia and fibula [HCC]

M86.362 Chronic multifocal osteomyelitis, left tibia and fibula [HCC]

M86.369 Chronic multifocal osteomyelitis, unspecified tibia and fibula [HCC]

M86.37 Chronic multifocal osteomyelitis, ankle and foot

M86.371 Chronic multifocal osteomyelitis, right ankle and foot [HCC]

M86.372 Chronic multifocal osteomyelitis, left ankle and foot [HCC]

M86.379 Chronic multifocal osteomyelitis, unspecified ankle and foot [HCC]

M86.38 Chronic multifocal osteomyelitis, other site [HCC]

M86.39 Chronic multifocal osteomyelitis, multiple sites [HCC]

M86.4 Chronic osteomyelitis with draining sinus

M86.40 Chronic osteomyelitis with draining sinus, unspecified site [HCC]

M86.41 Chronic osteomyelitis with draining sinus, shoulder

M86.411 Chronic osteomyelitis with draining sinus, right shoulder [HCC]

M86.412 Chronic osteomyelitis with draining sinus, left shoulder

M86.419 Chronic osteomyelitis with draining sinus, unspecified shoulder [HCC]

M86.42 Chronic osteomyelitis with draining sinus, humerus

M86.421 Chronic osteomyelitis with draining sinus, right humerus [HCC]

M86.422 Chronic osteomyelitis with draining sinus, left humerus [HCC]

M86.429 Chronic osteomyelitis with draining sinus, unspecified humerus [HCC]

M86.43 Chronic osteomyelitis with draining sinus, radius and ulna

M86.431 Chronic osteomyelitis with draining sinus, right radius and ulna [HCC]

M86.432 Chronic osteomyelitis with draining sinus, left radius and ulna [HCC]

M86.439 Chronic osteomyelitis with draining sinus, unspecified radius and ulna [HCC]

M86.44 Chronic osteomyelitis with draining sinus, hand

M86.441 Chronic osteomyelitis with draining sinus, right hand [HCC]

M86.442 Chronic osteomyelitis with draining sinus, left hand [HCC]

M86.449 Chronic osteomyelitis with draining sinus, unspecified hand [HCC]

M86.45 Chronic osteomyelitis with draining sinus, femur

M86.451 Chronic osteomyelitis with draining sinus, right femur [HCC]

M86.452 Chronic osteomyelitis with draining sinus, left femur [HCC]

M86.459 Chronic osteomyelitis with draining sinus, unspecified femur [HCC]

M86.46 Chronic osteomyelitis with draining sinus, tibia and fibula

M86.461 Chronic osteomyelitis with draining sinus, right tibia and fibula [HCC]

M86.462 Chronic osteomyelitis with draining sinus, left tibia and fibula [HCC]

M86.469 Chronic osteomyelitis with draining sinus, unspecified tibia and fibula [HCC]

M86.47 Chronic osteomyelitis with draining sinus, ankle and foot

M86.471 Chronic osteomyelitis with draining sinus, right ankle and foot [HCC]

M86.472 Chronic osteomyelitis with draining sinus, left ankle and foot [HCC]

M86.479 Chronic osteomyelitis with draining sinus, unspecified ankle and foot [HCC]

M86.48 Chronic osteomyelitis with draining sinus, other site [HCC]

M86.49 Chronic osteomyelitis with draining sinus, multiple sites [HCC]

M86.5 Other chronic hematogenous osteomyelitis

M86.50 Other chronic hematogenous osteomyelitis, unspecified site [HCC]

M86.51 Other chronic hematogenous osteomyelitis, shoulder

M86.511 Other chronic hematogenous osteomyelitis, right shoulder [HCC]

M86.512 Other chronic hematogenous osteomyelitis, left shoulder [HCC]

M86.519 Other chronic hematogenous osteomyelitis, unspecified shoulder

M86.52 Other chronic hematogenous osteomyelitis, humerus

M86.521 Other chronic hematogenous osteomyelitis, right humerus [HCC]

M86.522 Other chronic hematogenous osteomyelitis, left humerus [HCC]

M86.529 Other chronic hematogenous osteomyelitis, unspecified humerus [HCC]

M86.53 Other chronic hematogenous osteomyelitis, radius and ulna

M86.531 Other chronic hematogenous osteomyelitis, right radius and ulna [HCC]

M86.532 Other chronic hematogenous osteomyelitis, left radius and ulna [HCC]

M86.539 Other chronic hematogenous osteomyelitis, unspecified radius and ulna [HCC]

M86.54 Other chronic hematogenous osteomyelitis, hand

M86.541 Other chronic hematogenous osteomyelitis, right hand [HCC]

M86.542 Other chronic hematogenous osteomyelitis, left hand [HCC]

M86.549 Other chronic hematogenous osteomyelitis, unspecified hand [HCC]

M86.55 Other chronic hematogenous osteomyelitis, femur

M86.551 Other chronic hematogenous osteomyelitis, right femur [HCC]

M86.552 Other chronic hematogenous osteomyelitis, left femur [HCC]

M86.559 Other chronic hematogenous osteomyelitis, unspecified femur [HCC]

M86.56 Other chronic hematogenous osteomyelitis, tibia and fibula

M86.561 Other chronic hematogenous osteomyelitis, right tibia and fibula [HCC]

M86.562 Other chronic hematogenous osteomyelitis, left tibia and fibula [HCC]

M86.569 Other chronic hematogenous osteomyelitis, unspecified tibia and fibula [HCC]

M86.57 Other chronic hematogenous osteomyelitis, ankle and foot

M86.571 Other chronic hematogenous osteomyelitis, right ankle and foot [HCC]

M86.572 Other chronic hematogenous osteomyelitis, left ankle and foot [HCC]

M86.579 Other chronic hematogenous osteomyelitis, unspecified ankle and foot [HCC]

M86.58 Other chronic hematogenous osteomyelitis, other site [HCC]

M86.59 Other chronic hematogenous osteomyelitis, multiple sites [HCC]

M86.6 Other chronic osteomyelitis

M86.60 Other chronic osteomyelitis, unspecified site [HCC]

M86.61 Other chronic osteomyelitis, shoulder

M86.611 Other chronic osteomyelitis, right shoulder [HCC]

M86.612 Other chronic osteomyelitis, left shoulder [HCC]

M86.619 Other chronic osteomyelitis, unspecified shoulder [HCC]

M86.62 Other chronic osteomyelitis, humerus

M86.621 Other chronic osteomyelitis, right humerus [HCC]

M86.622 Other chronic osteomyelitis, left humerus [HCC]

M86.629 Other chronic osteomyelitis, unspecified humerus [HCC]

M86.63 Other chronic osteomyelitis, radius and ulna

M86.631 Other chronic osteomyelitis, right radius and ulna [HCC]

M86.632 Other chronic osteomyelitis, left radius and ulna [HCC]

M86.639 Other chronic osteomyelitis, unspecified radius and ulna [HCC]

M86.64 Other chronic osteomyelitis, hand

M86.641 Other chronic osteomyelitis, right hand [HCC]

M86.642 Other chronic osteomyelitis, left hand [HCC]

M86.649 Other chronic osteomyelitis, unspecified hand [HCC]

M86.65 Other chronic osteomyelitis, thigh

M86.651 Other chronic osteomyelitis, right thigh [HCC]

M86.652 Other chronic osteomyelitis, left thigh [HCC]

M86.659 Other chronic osteomyelitis, unspecified thigh [HCC]

M86.66 Other chronic osteomyelitis, tibia and fibula

M86.661 Other chronic osteomyelitis, right tibia and fibula [HCC]

M86.662 Other chronic osteomyelitis, left tibia and fibula [HCC]

M86.669 Other chronic osteomyelitis, unspecified tibia and fibula [HCC]

M86.67 Other chronic osteomyelitis, ankle and foot

M86.671 Other chronic osteomyelitis, right ankle and foot [HCC]

M86.672 Other chronic osteomyelitis, left ankle and foot [HCC]

M86.679 Other chronic osteomyelitis, unspecified ankle and foot [HCC]

M86.68 Other chronic osteomyelitis, other site [HCC]

M86.69 Other chronic osteomyelitis, multiple sites [HCC]

M86.8 Other osteomyelitis

Brodie's abscess

M86.8X Other osteomyelitis [HCC]

M86.8X0 Other osteomyelitis, multiple sites [HCC]

M86.8X1 Other osteomyelitis, shoulder [HCC]

M86.8X2 Other osteomyelitis, upper arm [HCC]

M86.8X3 Other osteomyelitis, forearm [HCC]

M86.8X4 Other osteomyelitis, hand [HCC]

M86.8X5 Other osteomyelitis, thigh [HCC]

M86.8X6 Other osteomyelitis, lower leg [HCC]

M86.8X7 Other osteomyelitis, ankle and foot [HCC]

M86.8X8 Other osteomyelitis, other site [HCC]

M86.8X9 Other osteomyelitis, unspecified sites [HCC]

M86.9 Osteomyelitis, unspecified [HCC]

Infection of bone NOS

Periostitis without osteomyelitis

M87 Osteonecrosis

Includes: avascular necrosis of bone

Use Additional Code to identify major osseous defect, if applicable (M89.7-)

Excludes1: juvenile osteonecrosis (M91-M92)

osteochondropathies (M90-M93)

M87.0 Idiopathic aseptic necrosis of bone

M87.00 Idiopathic aseptic necrosis of unspecified bone [HCC]

M87.01 Idiopathic aseptic necrosis of shoulder

Idiopathic aseptic necrosis of clavicle and scapula

M87.011 Idiopathic aseptic necrosis of right shoulder [HCC]

M87.012 Idiopathic aseptic necrosis of left shoulder [HCC]

M87.019 Idiopathic aseptic necrosis of unspecified shoulder [HCC]

M87.02 Idiopathic aseptic necrosis of humerus

M87.021 Idiopathic aseptic necrosis of right humerus [HCC]

M87.022 Idiopathic aseptic necrosis of left humerus [HCC]

M87.029 Idiopathic aseptic necrosis of unspecified humerus [HCC]

M87.03 Idiopathic aseptic necrosis of radius, ulna and carpus

M87.031 Idiopathic aseptic necrosis of right radius [HCC]

M87.032 Idiopathic aseptic necrosis of left radius [HCC]

M87.033 Idiopathic aseptic necrosis of unspecified radius [HCC]

M87.034 Idiopathic aseptic necrosis of right ulna [HCC]

M87.035 Idiopathic aseptic necrosis of left ulna [HCC]

M87.036 Idiopathic aseptic necrosis of unspecified ulna [HCC]

M87.037 Idiopathic aseptic necrosis of right carpus [HCC]

M87.038 Idiopathic aseptic necrosis of left carpus [HCC]

M87.039 Idiopathic aseptic necrosis of unspecified carpus [HCC]

M87.04 Idiopathic aseptic necrosis of hand and fingers

Idiopathic aseptic necrosis of metacarpals and phalanges of hands

M87.041 Idiopathic aseptic necrosis of right hand [HCC]

M87.042 Idiopathic aseptic necrosis of left hand [HCC]

M87.043 Idiopathic aseptic necrosis of unspecified hand [HCC]

M87.044 Idiopathic aseptic necrosis of right finger(s) [HCC]

M87.045 Idiopathic aseptic necrosis of left finger(s) [HCC]

M87.046 Idiopathic aseptic necrosis of unspecified finger(s) [HCC]

M87.05 Idiopathic aseptic necrosis of pelvis and femur

M87.050 Idiopathic aseptic necrosis of pelvis [HCC]

M87.051 Idiopathic aseptic necrosis of right femur [HCC]

M87.052 Idiopathic aseptic necrosis of left femur [HCC]

M87.059 Idiopathic aseptic necrosis of unspecified femur [HCC]

Idiopathic aseptic necrosis of hip NOS

M87.06 Idiopathic aseptic necrosis of tibia and fibula

M87.061 Idiopathic aseptic necrosis of right tibia [HCC]

M87.062 Idiopathic aseptic necrosis of left tibia [HCC]

M87.063 Idiopathic aseptic necrosis of unspecified tibia [HCC]

M87.064 Idiopathic aseptic necrosis of right fibula [HCC]

M87.065 Idiopathic aseptic necrosis of left fibula [HCC]

M87.066 Idiopathic aseptic necrosis of unspecified fibula [HCC]

M87.07 Idiopathic aseptic necrosis of ankle, foot and toes

Idiopathic aseptic necrosis of metatarsus, tarsus, and phalanges of toes

M87.071 Idiopathic aseptic necrosis of right ankle [HCC]

M87.072 Idiopathic aseptic necrosis of left ankle [HCC]

M87.073 Idiopathic aseptic necrosis of unspecified ankle [HCC]

M87.074 Idiopathic aseptic necrosis of right foot [HCC]

M87.075 Idiopathic aseptic necrosis of left foot [HCC]

M87.076 Idiopathic aseptic necrosis of unspecified foot [HCC]

M87.077 Idiopathic aseptic necrosis of right toe(s) [HCC]

M87.078 Idiopathic aseptic necrosis of left toe(s) [HCC]

M87.079 Idiopathic aseptic necrosis of unspecified toe(s) [HCC]

M87.08 Idiopathic aseptic necrosis of bone, other site [HCC]

M87.09 Idiopathic aseptic necrosis of bone, multiple sites [HCC]

M87.1 Osteonecrosis due to drugs

<u>Use Additional Code</u> for adverse effect, if applicable, to identify drug (T36-T50 with fifth or sixth character 5)

M87.10 Osteonecrosis due to drugs, unspecified bone [HCC]

M87.11 Osteonecrosis due to drugs, shoulder

M87.111 Osteonecrosis due to drugs, right shoulder [HCC]

M87.112 Osteonecrosis due to drugs, left shoulder [HCC]

M87.119 Osteonecrosis due to drugs, unspecified shoulder [HCC]

M87.12 Osteonecrosis due to drugs, humerus

M87.121 Osteonecrosis due to drugs, right humerus [HCC]

M87.122 Osteonecrosis due to drugs, left humerus [HCC]

M87.129 Osteonecrosis due to drugs, unspecified humerus [HCC]

M87.13 Osteonecrosis due to drugs of radius, ulna and carpus

M87.131 Osteonecrosis due to drugs of right radius [HCC]

M87.132 Osteonecrosis due to drugs of left radius [HCC]

M87.133 Osteonecrosis due to drugs of unspecified radius [HCC]

M87.134 Osteonecrosis due to drugs of right ulna [HCC]

M87.135 Osteonecrosis due to drugs of left ulna [HCC]

M87.136 Osteonecrosis due to drugs of unspecified ulna [HCC]

M87.137 Osteonecrosis due to drugs of right carpus [HCC]

M87.138 Osteonecrosis due to drugs of left carpus [HCC]

M87.139 Osteonecrosis due to drugs of unspecified carpus [HCC]

M87.14 Osteonecrosis due to drugs, hand and fingers]

M87.141 Osteonecrosis due to drugs, right hand [HCC]

M87.142 Osteonecrosis due to drugs, left hand [HCC]

M87.143 Osteonecrosis due to drugs, unspecified hand [HCC]

M87.144 Osteonecrosis due to drugs, right finger(s) [HCC]

M87.145 Osteonecrosis due to drugs, left finger(s) [HCC]

M87.146 Osteonecrosis due to drugs, unspecified finger(s) [HCC]

M87.15 Osteonecrosis due to drugs, pelvis and femur

M87.150 Osteonecrosis due to drugs, pelvis [HCC]

M87.151 Osteonecrosis due to drugs, right femur [HCC]

M87.152 Osteonecrosis due to drugs, left femur [HCC]

M87.159 Osteonecrosis due to drugs, unspecified femur [HCC]

M87.16 Osteonecrosis due to drugs, tibia and fibula

M87.161 Osteonecrosis due to drugs, right tibia [HCC]

M87.162 Osteonecrosis due to drugs, left tibia [HCC]

M87.163 Osteonecrosis due to drugs, unspecified tibia [HCC]

M87.164 Osteonecrosis due to drugs, right fibula [HCC]

M87.165 Osteonecrosis due to drugs, left fibula [HCC]

M87.166 Osteonecrosis due to drugs, unspecified fibula [HCC]

M87.17 Osteonecrosis due to drugs, ankle, foot and toes

M87.171 Osteonecrosis due to drugs, right ankle [HCC]

M87.172 Osteonecrosis due to drugs, left ankle [HCC]

M87.173 Osteonecrosis due to drugs, unspecified ankle [HCC]

M87.174 Osteonecrosis due to drugs, right foot [HCC]

M87.175 Osteonecrosis due to drugs, left foot [HCC]

M87.176 Osteonecrosis due to drugs, unspecified foot [HCC]

M87.177 Osteonecrosis due to drugs, right toe(s) [HCC]

M87.178 Osteonecrosis due to drugs, left toe(s) [HCC]

M87.179 Osteonecrosis due to drugs, unspecified toe(s) [HCC]

M87.18 Osteonecrosis due to drugs, other site

M87.180 Osteonecrosis due to drugs, jaw [HCC]

M87.188 Osteonecrosis due to drugs, other site [HCC]

M87.19 Osteonecrosis due to drugs, multiple sites [HCC]

M87.2 Osteonecrosis due to previous trauma

M87.20 Osteonecrosis due to previous trauma, unspecified bone [HCC]

M87.21 Osteonecrosis due to previous trauma, shoulder

M87.211 Osteonecrosis due to previous trauma, right shoulder [HCC]

M87.212 Osteonecrosis due to previous trauma, left shoulder [HCC]

M87.219 Osteonecrosis due to previous trauma, unspecified shoulder [HCC]

M87.22 Osteonecrosis due to previous trauma, humerus

M87.221 Osteonecrosis due to previous trauma, right humerus [HCC]

M87.222 Osteonecrosis due to previous trauma, left humerus [HCC]

M87.229 Osteonecrosis due to previous trauma, unspecified humerus [HCC]

M87.23 Osteonecrosis due to previous trauma of radius, ulna and carpus

M87.231 Osteonecrosis due to previous trauma of right radius [HCC]

M87.232 Osteonecrosis due to previous trauma of left radius

M87.233 Osteonecrosis due to previous trauma of unspecified radius [HCC]

M87.234 Osteonecrosis due to previous trauma of right ulna [HCC]

M87.235 Osteonecrosis due to previous trauma of left ulna [HCC]

M87.236 Osteonecrosis due to previous trauma of unspecified ulna [HCC]

M87.237 Osteonecrosis due to previous trauma of right carpus [HCC]

M87.238 Osteonecrosis due to previous trauma of left carpus [HCC]

M87.239 Osteonecrosis due to previous trauma of unspecified carpus [HCC]

M87.24 Osteonecrosis due to previous trauma, hand and fingers

M87.241 Osteonecrosis due to previous trauma, right hand [HCC]

M87.242 Osteonecrosis due to previous trauma, left hand [HCC]

M87.243 Osteonecrosis due to previous trauma, unspecified hand [HCC]

M87.244 Osteonecrosis due to previous trauma, right finger(s) [HCC]

M87.245 Osteonecrosis due to previous trauma, left finger(s) [HCC]

M87.246 Osteonecrosis due to previous trauma, unspecified finger(s) [HCC]

M87.25 Osteonecrosis due to previous trauma, pelvis and femur

M87.250 Osteonecrosis due to previous trauma, pelvis [HCC]

M87.251 Osteonecrosis due to previous trauma, right femur [HCC]

M87.252 Osteonecrosis due to previous trauma, left femur [HCC]

M87.256 Osteonecrosis due to previous trauma, unspecified femur [HCC]

M87.26 Osteonecrosis due to previous trauma, tibia and fibula

M87.261 Osteonecrosis due to previous trauma, right tibia [HCC]

M87.262 Osteonecrosis due to previous trauma, left tibia [HCC]

M87.263 Osteonecrosis due to previous trauma, unspecified tibia [HCC]

M87.264 Osteonecrosis due to previous trauma, right fibula [HCC]

M87.265 Osteonecrosis due to previous trauma, left fibula [HCC]

M87.266 Osteonecrosis due to previous trauma, unspecified fibula [HCC]

M87.27 Osteonecrosis due to previous trauma, ankle, foot and toes

M87.271 Osteonecrosis due to previous trauma, right ankle [HCC]

M87.272 Osteonecrosis due to previous trauma, left ankle [HCC]

M87.273 Osteonecrosis due to previous trauma, unspecified ankle [HCC]

M87.274 Osteonecrosis due to previous trauma, right foot [HCC]

M87.275 Osteonecrosis due to previous trauma, left foot [HCC]

M87.276 Osteonecrosis due to previous trauma, unspecified foot

● New code   ▲ Revised code   **Excludes1:** Not coded here   **Excludes2:** Not included here   ⊗ Placeholder required   ⑦7th digit required

M87.277   Osteonecrosis due to previous trauma, right toe(s) [HCC]

M87.278   Osteonecrosis due to previous trauma, left toe(s) [HCC]

M87.279   Osteonecrosis due to previous trauma, unspecified toe(s) [HCC]

M87.28   Osteonecrosis due to previous trauma, other site [HCC]

M87.29   Osteonecrosis due to previous trauma, multiple sites [HCC]

M87.3   Other secondary osteonecrosis

M87.30   Other secondary osteonecrosis, unspecified bone [HCC]

M87.31   Other secondary osteonecrosis, shoulder

M87.311   Other secondary osteonecrosis, right shoulder [HCC]

M87.312   Other secondary osteonecrosis, left shoulder [HCC]

M87.319   Other secondary osteonecrosis, unspecified shoulder [HCC]

M87.32   Other secondary osteonecrosis, humerus

M87.321   Other secondary osteonecrosis, right humerus [HCC]

M87.322   Other secondary osteonecrosis, left humerus [HCC]

M87.329   Other secondary osteonecrosis, unspecified humerus [HCC]

M87.33   Other secondary osteonecrosis of radius, ulna and carpus

M87.331   Other secondary osteonecrosis of right radius [HCC]

M87.332   Other secondary osteonecrosis of left radius [HCC]

M87.333   Other secondary osteonecrosis of unspecified radius [HCC]

M87.334   Other secondary osteonecrosis of right ulna [HCC]

M87.335   Other secondary osteonecrosis of left ulna [HCC]

M87.336   Other secondary osteonecrosis of unspecified ulna [HCC]

M87.337   Other secondary osteonecrosis of right carpus [HCC]

M87.338   Other secondary osteonecrosis of left carpus [HCC]

M87.339   Other secondary osteonecrosis of unspecified carpus [HCC]

M87.34   Other secondary osteonecrosis, hand and fingers

M87.341   Other secondary osteonecrosis, right hand [HCC]

M87.342   Other secondary osteonecrosis, left hand [HCC]

M87.343   Other secondary osteonecrosis, unspecified hand [HCC]

M87.344   Other secondary osteonecrosis, right finger(s) [HCC]

M87.345   Other secondary osteonecrosis, left finger(s) [HCC]

M87.346   Other secondary osteonecrosis, unspecified finger(s) [HCC]

M87.35   Other secondary osteonecrosis, pelvis and femur

M87.350   Other secondary osteonecrosis, pelvis [HCC]

M87.351   Other secondary osteonecrosis, right femur [HCC]

M87.352   Other secondary osteonecrosis, left femur [HCC]

M87.353   Other secondary osteonecrosis, unspecified femur [HCC]

M87.36   Other secondary osteonecrosis, tibia and fibula

M87.361   Other secondary osteonecrosis, right tibia [HCC]

M87.362   Other secondary osteonecrosis, left tibia [HCC]

M87.363   Other secondary osteonecrosis, unspecified tibia [HCC]

M87.364   Other secondary osteonecrosis, right fibula [HCC]

M87.365   Other secondary osteonecrosis, left fibula [HCC]

M87.366   Other secondary osteonecrosis, unspecified fibula [HCC]

M87.37   Other secondary osteonecrosis, ankle and foot

M87.371   Other secondary osteonecrosis, right ankle [HCC]

M87.372   Other secondary osteonecrosis, left ankle [HCC]

M87.373   Other secondary osteonecrosis, unspecified ankle [HCC]

M87.374   Other secondary osteonecrosis, right foot [HCC]

M87.375   Other secondary osteonecrosis, left foot [HCC]

M87.376   Other secondary osteonecrosis, unspecified foot [HCC]

M87.377   Other secondary osteonecrosis, right toe(s) [HCC]

M87.378   Other secondary osteonecrosis, left toe(s) [HCC]

M87.379   Other secondary osteonecrosis, unspecified toe(s) [HCC]

M87.38   Other secondary osteonecrosis, other site [HCC]

M87.39   Other secondary osteonecrosis, multiple sites [HCC]

M87.8   Other osteonecrosis

M87.80   Other osteonecrosis, unspecified bone [HCC]

M87.81   Other osteonecrosis, shoulder [HCC]

M87.811   Other osteonecrosis, right shoulder [HCC]

M87.812   Other osteonecrosis, left shoulder [HCC]

M87.819   Other osteonecrosis, unspecified shoulder [HCC]

M87.82   Other osteonecrosis, humerus

M87.821   Other osteonecrosis, right humerus [HCC]

M87.822   Other osteonecrosis, left humerus [HCC]

M87.829   Other osteonecrosis, unspecified humerus

M87.83   Other osteonecrosis of radius, ulna and carpus

M87.831   Other osteonecrosis of right radius [HCC]

M87.832   Other osteonecrosis of left radius [HCC]

M87.833 Other osteonecrosis of unspecified radius [HCC]

M87.834 Other osteonecrosis of right ulna [HCC]

M87.835 Other osteonecrosis of left ulna [HCC]

M87.836 Other osteonecrosis of unspecified ulna [HCC]

M87.837 Other osteonecrosis of right carpus [HCC]

M87.838 Other osteonecrosis of left carpus [HCC]

M87.839 Other osteonecrosis of unspecified carpus [HCC]

M87.84 Other osteonecrosis, hand and fingers

M87.841 Other osteonecrosis, right hand [HCC]

M87.842 Other osteonecrosis, left hand [HCC]

M87.843 Other osteonecrosis, unspecified hand [HCC]

M87.844 Other osteonecrosis, right finger(s) [HCC]

M87.845 Other osteonecrosis, left finger(s) [HCC]

M87.849 Other osteonecrosis, unspecified finger(s) [HCC]

M87.85 Other osteonecrosis, pelvis and femur

M87.850 Other osteonecrosis, pelvis [HCC]

M87.851 Other osteonecrosis, right femur [HCC]

M87.852 Other osteonecrosis, left femur [HCC]

M87.859 Other osteonecrosis, unspecified femur [HCC]

M87.86 Other osteonecrosis, tibia and fibula

M87.861 Other osteonecrosis, right tibia [HCC]

M87.862 Other osteonecrosis, left tibia [HCC]

M87.863 Other osteonecrosis, unspecified tibia [HCC]

M87.864 Other osteonecrosis, right fibula [HCC]

M87.865 Other osteonecrosis, left fibula [HCC]

M87.869 Other osteonecrosis, unspecified fibula [HCC]

M87.87 Other osteonecrosis, ankle, foot and toes

M87.871 Other osteonecrosis, right ankle [HCC]

M87.872 Other osteonecrosis, left ankle [HCC]

M87.873 Other osteonecrosis, unspecified ankle

M87.874 Other osteonecrosis, right foot [HCC]

M87.875 Other osteonecrosis, left foot [HCC]

M87.876 Other osteonecrosis, unspecified foot [HCC]

M87.877 Other osteonecrosis, right toe(s) [HCC]

M87.878 Other osteonecrosis, left toe(s) [HCC]

M87.879 Other osteonecrosis, unspecified toe(s) [HCC]

M87.88 Other osteonecrosis, other site [HCC]

M87.89 Other osteonecrosis, multiple sites [HCC]

M87.9 **Osteonecrosis, unspecified** [HCC]

Necrosis of bone NOS

M88 **Osteitis deformans [Paget's disease of bone]**

Definition: Osteitis deformans, aka Paget's disease, is a disease of bone occurring in the middle aged and elderly; excessive bone destruction sometimes leading to bone pain and fractures and skeletal deformities.

Excludes1: osteitis deformans in neoplastic disease (M90.6)

M88.0 **Osteitis deformans of skull**

M88.1 **Osteitis deformans of vertebrae**

M88.8 **Osteitis deformans of other bones**

M88.81 Osteitis deformans of shoulder

M88.811 Osteitis deformans of right shoulder

M88.812 Osteitis deformans of left shoulder

M88.819 Osteitis deformans of unspecified shoulder

M88.82 Osteitis deformans of upper arm

M88.821 Osteitis deformans of right upper arm

M88.822 Osteitis deformans of left upper arm

M88.829 Osteitis deformans of unspecified upper arm

M88.83 Osteitis deformans of forearm

M88.831 Osteitis deformans of right forearm

M88.832 Osteitis deformans of left forearm

M88.839 Osteitis deformans of unspecified forearm

M88.84 Osteitis deformans of hand

M88.841 Osteitis deformans of right hand

M88.842 Osteitis deformans of left hand

M88.849 Osteitis deformans of unspecified hand

M88.85 Osteitis deformans of thigh

M88.851 Osteitis deformans of right thigh

M88.852 Osteitis deformans of left thigh

M88.859 Osteitis deformans of unspecified thigh

M88.86 Osteitis deformans of lower leg

M88.861 Osteitis deformans of right lower leg

M88.862 Osteitis deformans of left lower leg

M88.869 Osteitis deformans of unspecified lower leg

M88.87 Osteitis deformans of ankle and foot

M88.871 Osteitis deformans of right ankle and foot

M88.872 Osteitis deformans of left ankle and foot

M88.879 Osteitis deformans of unspecified ankle and foot

M88.88 Osteitis deformans of other bones

Excludes2: osteitis deformans of skull (M88.0)

osteitis deformans of vertebrae (M88.1)

M88.89 Osteitis deformans of multiple sites

M88.9 **Osteitis deformans of unspecified bone**

M89 **Other disorders of bone**

M89.0 **Algoneurodystrophy**

Shoulder-hand syndrome

Sudeck's atrophy

Excludes1: causalgia, lower limb (G57.7-)

causalgia, upper limb (G56.4-)

complex regional pain syndrome II, lower limb (G57.7-)

complex regional pain syndrome II, upper limb (G56.4-)

reflex sympathetic dystrophy (G90.5-)

M89.00 Algoneurodystrophy, unspecified site

● New code ▲ Revised code **Excludes1:** Not coded here **Excludes2:** Not included here ⊗ Placeholder required ⑦7th digit required

M89.01 Algoneurodystrophy, shoulder

   M89.011 Algoneurodystrophy, right shoulder

   M89.012 Algoneurodystrophy, left shoulder

   M89.019 Algoneurodystrophy, unspecified shoulder

M89.02 Algoneurodystrophy, upper arm

   M89.021 Algoneurodystrophy, right upper arm

   M89.022 Algoneurodystrophy, left upper arm

   M89.029 Algoneurodystrophy, unspecified upper arm

M89.03 Algoneurodystrophy, forearm

   M89.031 Algoneurodystrophy, right forearm

   M89.032 Algoneurodystrophy, left forearm

   M89.039 Algoneurodystrophy, unspecified forearm

M89.04 Algoneurodystrophy, hand

   M89.041 Algoneurodystrophy, right hand

   M89.042 Algoneurodystrophy, left hand

   M89.049 Algoneurodystrophy, unspecified hand

M89.05 Algoneurodystrophy, thigh

   M89.051 Algoneurodystrophy, right thigh

   M89.052 Algoneurodystrophy, left thigh

   M89.059 Algoneurodystrophy, unspecified thigh

M89.06 Algoneurodystrophy, lower leg

   M89.061 Algoneurodystrophy, right lower leg

   M89.062 Algoneurodystrophy, left lower leg

   M89.069 Algoneurodystrophy, unspecified lower leg

M89.07 Algoneurodystrophy, ankle and foot

   M89.071 Algoneurodystrophy, right ankle and foot

   M89.072 Algoneurodystrophy, left ankle and foot

   M89.079 Algoneurodystrophy, unspecified ankle and foot

M89.08 Algoneurodystrophy, other site

M89.09 Algoneurodystrophy, multiple sites

M89.1 Physeal arrest

Arrest of growth plate

Epiphyseal arrest

Growth plate arrest

M89.12 Physeal arrest, humerus

   M89.121 Complete physeal arrest, right proximal humerus

   M89.122 Complete physeal arrest, left proximal humerus

   M89.123 Partial physeal arrest, right proximal humerus

   M89.124 Partial physeal arrest, left proximal humerus

   M89.125 Complete physeal arrest, right distal humerus

   M89.126 Complete physeal arrest, left distal humerus

   M89.127 Partial physeal arrest, right distal humerus

   M89.128 Partial physeal arrest, left distal humerus

   M89.129 Physeal arrest, humerus, unspecified

M89.13 Physeal arrest, forearm

   M89.131 Complete physeal arrest, right distal radius

   M89.132 Complete physeal arrest, left distal radius

   M89.133 Partial physeal arrest, right distal radius

   M89.134 Partial physeal arrest, left distal radius

   M89.138 Other physeal arrest of forearm

   M89.139 Physeal arrest, forearm, unspecified

M89.15 Physeal arrest, femur

   M89.151 Complete physeal arrest, right proximal femur

   M89.152 Complete physeal arrest, left proximal femur

   M89.153 Partial physeal arrest, right proximal femur

   M89.154 Partial physeal arrest, left proximal femur

   M89.155 Complete physeal arrest, right distal femur

   M89.156 Complete physeal arrest, left distal femur

   M89.157 Partial physeal arrest, right distal femur

   M89.158 Partial physeal arrest, left distal femur

   M89.159 Physeal arrest, femur, unspecified

M89.16 Physeal arrest, lower leg

   M89.160 Complete physeal arrest, right proximal tibia

   M89.161 Complete physeal arrest, left proximal tibia

   M89.162 Partial physeal arrest, right proximal tibia

   M89.163 Partial physeal arrest, left proximal tibia

   M89.164 Complete physeal arrest, right distal tibia

   M89.165 Complete physeal arrest, left distal tibia

   M89.166 Partial physeal arrest, right distal tibia

   M89.167 Partial physeal arrest, left distal tibia

   M89.168 Other physeal arrest of lower leg

   M89.169 Physeal arrest, lower leg, unspecified

M89.18 Physeal arrest, other site

M89.2 Other disorders of bone development and growth

M89.20 Other disorders of bone development and growth, unspecified site

M89.21 Other disorders of bone development and growth, shoulder

   M89.211 Other disorders of bone development and growth, right shoulder

   M89.212 Other disorders of bone development and growth, left shoulder

   M89.219 Other disorders of bone development and growth, unspecified shoulder

M89.22 Other disorders of bone development and growth, humerus

M89.221 Other disorders of bone development and growth, right humerus

M89.222 Other disorders of bone development and growth, left humerus

M89.229 Other disorders of bone development and growth, unspecified humerus

M89.23 Other disorders of bone development and growth, ulna and radius

M89.231 Other disorders of bone development and growth, right ulna

M89.232 Other disorders of bone development and growth, left ulna

M89.233 Other disorders of bone development and growth, right radius

M89.234 Other disorders of bone development and growth, left radius

M89.239 Other disorders of bone development and growth, unspecified ulna and radius

M89.24 Other disorders of bone development and growth, hand

M89.241 Other disorders of bone development and growth, right hand

M89.242 Other disorders of bone development and growth, left hand

M89.249 Other disorders of bone development and growth, unspecified hand

M89.25 Other disorders of bone development and growth, femur

M89.251 Other disorders of bone development and growth, right femur

M89.252 Other disorders of bone development and growth, left femur

M89.259 Other disorders of bone development and growth, unspecified femur

M89.26 Other disorders of bone development and growth, tibia and fibula

M89.261 Other disorders of bone development and growth, right tibia

M89.262 Other disorders of bone development and growth, left tibia

M89.263 Other disorders of bone development and growth, right fibula

M89.264 Other disorders of bone development and growth, left fibula

M89.269 Other disorders of bone development and growth, unspecified lower leg

M89.27 Other disorders of bone development and growth, ankle and foot

M89.271 Other disorders of bone development and growth, right ankle and foot

M89.272 Other disorders of bone development and growth, left ankle and foot

M89.279 Other disorders of bone development and growth, unspecified ankle and foot

M89.28 Other disorders of bone development and growth, other site

M89.29 Other disorders of bone development and growth, multiple sites

M89.3 Hypertrophy of bone

M89.30 Hypertrophy of bone, unspecified site

M89.31 Hypertrophy of bone, shoulder

M89.311 Hypertrophy of bone, right shoulder

M89.312 Hypertrophy of bone, left shoulder

M89.319 Hypertrophy of bone, unspecified shoulder

M89.32 Hypertrophy of bone, humerus

M89.321 Hypertrophy of bone, right humerus

M89.322 Hypertrophy of bone, left humerus

M89.329 Hypertrophy of bone, unspecified humerus

M89.33 Hypertrophy of bone, ulna and radius

M89.331 Hypertrophy of bone, right ulna

M89.332 Hypertrophy of bone, left ulna

M89.333 Hypertrophy of bone, right radius

M89.334 Hypertrophy of bone, left radius

M89.339 Hypertrophy of bone, unspecified ulna and radius

M89.34 Hypertrophy of bone, hand

M89.341 Hypertrophy of bone, right hand

M89.342 Hypertrophy of bone, left hand

M89.349 Hypertrophy of bone, unspecified hand

M89.35 Hypertrophy of bone, femur

M89.351 Hypertrophy of bone, right femur

M89.352 Hypertrophy of bone, left femur

M89.359 Hypertrophy of bone, unspecified femur

M89.36 Hypertrophy of bone, tibia and fibula

M89.361 Hypertrophy of bone, right tibia

M89.362 Hypertrophy of bone, left tibia

M89.363 Hypertrophy of bone, right fibula

M89.364 Hypertrophy of bone, left fibula

M89.369 Hypertrophy of bone, unspecified tibia and fibula

M89.37 Hypertrophy of bone, ankle and foot

M89.371 Hypertrophy of bone, right ankle and foot

M89.372 Hypertrophy of bone, left ankle and foot

M89.379 Hypertrophy of bone, unspecified ankle and foot

M89.38 Hypertrophy of bone, other site

M89.39 Hypertrophy of bone, multiple sites

M89.4 Other hypertrophic osteoarthropathy

Marie-Bamberger disease

Pachydermoperiostosis

M89.40 Other hypertrophic osteoarthropathy, unspecified site

M89.41 Other hypertrophic osteoarthropathy, shoulder

M89.411 Other hypertrophic osteoarthropathy, right shoulder

M89.412 Other hypertrophic osteoarthropathy, left shoulder

M89.419 Other hypertrophic osteoarthropathy, unspecified shoulder

M89.42 Other hypertrophic osteoarthropathy, upper arm

M89.421 Other hypertrophic osteoarthropathy, right upper arm

M89.422 Other hypertrophic osteoarthropathy, left upper arm

M89.429   Other hypertrophic osteoarthropathy, unspecified upper arm

M89.43   Other hypertrophic osteoarthropathy, forearm

     M89.431   Other hypertrophic osteoarthropathy, right forearm

     M89.432   Other hypertrophic osteoarthropathy, left forearm

     M89.439   Other hypertrophic osteoarthropathy, unspecified forearm

M89.44   Other hypertrophic osteoarthropathy, hand

     M89.441   Other hypertrophic osteoarthropathy, right hand

     M89.442   Other hypertrophic osteoarthropathy, left hand

     M89.449   Other hypertrophic osteoarthropathy, unspecified hand

M89.45   Other hypertrophic osteoarthropathy, thigh

     M89.451   Other hypertrophic osteoarthropathy, right thigh

     M89.452   Other hypertrophic osteoarthropathy, left thigh

     M89.459   Other hypertrophic osteoarthropathy, unspecified thigh

M89.46   Other hypertrophic osteoarthropathy, lower leg

     M89.461   Other hypertrophic osteoarthropathy, right lower leg

     M89.462   Other hypertrophic osteoarthropathy, left lower leg

     M89.469   Other hypertrophic osteoarthropathy, unspecified lower leg

M89.47   Other hypertrophic osteoarthropathy, ankle and foot

     M89.471   Other hypertrophic osteoarthropathy, right ankle and foot

     M89.472   Other hypertrophic osteoarthropathy, left ankle and foot

     M89.479   Other hypertrophic osteoarthropathy, unspecified ankle and foot

M89.48   Other hypertrophic osteoarthropathy, other site

M89.49   Other hypertrophic osteoarthropathy, multiple sites

M89.5   Osteolysis

Use Additional Code to identify major osseous defect, if applicable (M89.7-)

Excludes2: periprosthetic osteolysis of internal prosthetic joint (T84.05-)

M89.50   Osteolysis, unspecified site

M89.51   Osteolysis, shoulder

     M89.511   Osteolysis, right shoulder

     M89.512   Osteolysis, left shoulder

     M89.519   Osteolysis, unspecified shoulder

M89.52   Osteolysis, upper arm

     M89.521   Osteolysis, right upper arm

     M89.522   Osteolysis, left upper arm

     M89.529   Osteolysis, unspecified upper arm

M89.53   Osteolysis, forearm

     M89.531   Osteolysis, right forearm

     M89.532   Osteolysis, left forearm

     M89.539   Osteolysis, unspecified forearm

M89.54   Osteolysis, hand

     M89.541   Osteolysis, right hand

     M89.542   Osteolysis, left hand

     M89.549   Osteolysis, unspecified hand

M89.55   Osteolysis, thigh

     M89.551   Osteolysis, right thigh

     M89.552   Osteolysis, left thigh

     M89.559   Osteolysis, unspecified thigh

M89.56   Osteolysis, lower leg

     M89.561   Osteolysis, right lower leg

     M89.562   Osteolysis, left lower leg

     M89.569   Osteolysis, unspecified lower leg

M89.57   Osteolysis, ankle and foot

     M89.571   Osteolysis, right ankle and foot

     M89.572   Osteolysis, left ankle and foot

     M89.579   Osteolysis, unspecified ankle and foot

M89.58   Osteolysis, other site

M89.59   Osteolysis, multiple sites

M89.6   Osteopathy after poliomyelitis

Use Additional Code (B91) to identify previous poliomyelitis

Excludes1: postpolio syndrome (G14)

M89.60   Osteopathy after poliomyelitis, unspecified site [HCC]

M89.61   Osteopathy after poliomyelitis, shoulder

     M89.611   Osteopathy after poliomyelitis, right shoulder [HCC]

     M89.612   Osteopathy after poliomyelitis, left shoulder [HCC]

     M89.619   Osteopathy after poliomyelitis, unspecified shoulder [HCC]

M89.62   Osteopathy after poliomyelitis, upper arm

     M89.621   Osteopathy after poliomyelitis, right upper arm [HCC]

     M89.622   Osteopathy after poliomyelitis, left upper arm [HCC]

     M89.629   Osteopathy after poliomyelitis, unspecified upper arm [HCC]

M89.63   Osteopathy after poliomyelitis, forearm

     M89.631   Osteopathy after poliomyelitis, right forearm [HCC]

     M89.632   Osteopathy after poliomyelitis, left forearm [HCC]

     M89.639   Osteopathy after poliomyelitis, unspecified forearm [HCC]

M89.64   Osteopathy after poliomyelitis, hand

     M89.641   Osteopathy after poliomyelitis, right hand [HCC]

     M89.642   Osteopathy after poliomyelitis, left hand [HCC]

     M89.649   Osteopathy after poliomyelitis, unspecified hand [HCC]

M89.65   Osteopathy after poliomyelitis, thigh

     M89.651   Osteopathy after poliomyelitis, right thigh [HCC]

     M89.652   Osteopathy after poliomyelitis, left thigh [HCC]

     M89.659   Osteopathy after poliomyelitis, unspecified thigh [HCC]

M89.66   **Osteopathy after poliomyelitis, lower leg**

    M89.661   **Osteopathy after poliomyelitis, right lower leg** [HCC]

    M89.662   **Osteopathy after poliomyelitis, left lower leg** [HCC]

    M89.669   **Osteopathy after poliomyelitis, unspecified lower leg** [HCC]

M89.67   **Osteopathy after poliomyelitis, ankle and foot**

    M89.671   **Osteopathy after poliomyelitis, right ankle and foot** [HCC]

    M89.672   **Osteopathy after poliomyelitis, left ankle and foot**

    M89.679   **Osteopathy after poliomyelitis, unspecified ankle and foot** [HCC]

M89.68   **Osteopathy after poliomyelitis, other site** [HCC]

M89.69   **Osteopathy after poliomyelitis, multiple sites** [HCC]

M89.7   **Major osseous defect**

    <u>Code first</u> underlying disease, if known, such as:

      aseptic necrosis of bone (M87.-)

      malignant neoplasm of bone (C40.-)

      osteolysis (M89.5)

      osteomyelitis (M86.-)

      osteonecrosis (M87.-)

      osteoporosis (M80.-, M81.-)

      periprosthetic osteolysis (T84.05-)

M89.70   **Major osseous defect, unspecified site**

M89.71   **Major osseous defect, shoulder region**

    Major osseous defect clavicle or scapula

    M89.711   **Major osseous defect, right shoulder region**

    M89.712   **Major osseous defect, left shoulder region**

    M89.719   **Major osseous defect, unspecified shoulder region**

M89.72   **Major osseous defect, humerus**

    M89.721   **Major osseous defect, right humerus**

    M89.722   **Major osseous defect, left humerus**

    M89.729   **Major osseous defect, unspecified humerus**

M89.73   **Major osseous defect, forearm**

    Major osseous defect of radius and ulna

    M89.731   **Major osseous defect, right forearm**

    M89.732   **Major osseous defect, left forearm**

    M89.739   **Major osseous defect, unspecified forearm**

M89.74   **Major osseous defect, hand**

    Major osseous defect of carpus, fingers, metacarpus

    M89.741   **Major osseous defect, right hand**

    M89.742   **Major osseous defect, left hand**

    M89.749   **Major osseous defect, unspecified hand**

M89.75   **Major osseous defect, pelvic region and thigh**

    Major osseous defect of femur and pelvis

    M89.751   **Major osseous defect, right pelvic region and thigh**

    M89.752   **Major osseous defect, left pelvic region and thigh**

    M89.759   **Major osseous defect, unspecified pelvic region and thigh**

M89.76   **Major osseous defect, lower leg**

    Major osseous defect of fibula and tibia

    M89.761   **Major osseous defect, right lower leg**

    M89.762   **Major osseous defect, left lower leg**

    M89.769   **Major osseous defect, unspecified lower leg**

M89.77   **Major osseous defect, ankle and foot**

    Major osseous defect of metatarsus, tarsus, toes

    M89.771   **Major osseous defect, right ankle and foot**

    M89.772   **Major osseous defect, left ankle and foot**

    M89.779   **Major osseous defect, unspecified ankle and foot**

M89.78   **Major osseous defect, other site**

M89.79   **Major osseous defect, multiple sites**

M89.8   **Other specified disorders of bone**

    Infantile cortical hyperostoses

    Post-traumatic subperiosteal ossification

M89.8X   **Other specified disorders of bone**

    M89.8X0   **Other specified disorders of bone, multiple sites**

    M89.8X1   **Other specified disorders of bone, shoulder**

    M89.8X2   **Other specified disorders of bone, upper arm**

    M89.8X3   **Other specified disorders of bone, forearm**

    M89.8X4   **Other specified disorders of bone, hand**

    M89.8X5   **Other specified disorders of bone, thigh**

    M89.8X6   **Other specified disorders of bone, lower leg**

    M89.8X7   **Other specified disorders of bone, ankle and foot**

    M89.8X8   **Other specified disorders of bone, other site**

    M89.8X9   **Other specified disorders of bone, unspecified site**

M89.9   **Disorder of bone, unspecified**

M90   **Osteopathies in diseases classified elsewhere**

    Excludes1: osteochondritis, osteomyelitis, and osteopathy (in):

      cryptococcosis (B45.3)

      diabetes mellitus (E08-E13 with .69-)

      gonococcal (A54.43)

      neurogenic syphilis (A52.11)

      renal osteodystrophy (N25.0)

      salmonellosis (A02.24)

      secondary syphilis (A51.46)

      syphilis (late) (A52.77)

M90.5   **Osteonecrosis in diseases classified elsewhere**

    <u>Code first</u> underlying disease, such as:

      caisson disease (T70.3)

      hemoglobinopathy (D50-D64)

    M90.50   **Osteonecrosis in diseases classified elsewhere, unspecified site** [HCC]

    M90.51   **Osteonecrosis in diseases classified elsewhere, shoulder**

M90.511 Osteonecrosis in diseases classified elsewhere, right shoulder [HCC]

M90.512 Osteonecrosis in diseases classified elsewhere, left shoulder [HCC]

M90.519 Osteonecrosis in diseases classified elsewhere, unspecified shoulder [HCC]

M90.52 Osteonecrosis in diseases classified elsewhere, upper arm

M90.521 Osteonecrosis in diseases classified elsewhere, right upper arm [HCC]

M90.522 Osteonecrosis in diseases classified elsewhere, left upper arm [HCC]

M90.529 Osteonecrosis in diseases classified elsewhere, unspecified upper arm [HCC]

M90.53 Osteonecrosis in diseases classified elsewhere, forearm

M90.531 Osteonecrosis in diseases classified elsewhere, right forearm [HCC]

M90.532 Osteonecrosis in diseases classified elsewhere, left forearm [HCC]

M90.539 Osteonecrosis in diseases classified elsewhere, unspecified forearm [HCC]

M90.54 Osteonecrosis in diseases classified elsewhere, hand

M90.541 Osteonecrosis in diseases classified elsewhere, right hand [HCC]

M90.542 Osteonecrosis in diseases classified elsewhere, left hand [HCC]

M90.549 Osteonecrosis in diseases classified elsewhere, unspecified hand [HCC]

M90.55 Osteonecrosis in diseases classified elsewhere, thigh

M90.551 Osteonecrosis in diseases classified elsewhere, right thigh [HCC]

M90.552 Osteonecrosis in diseases classified elsewhere, left thigh [HCC]

M90.559 Osteonecrosis in diseases classified elsewhere, unspecified thigh [HCC]

M90.56 Osteonecrosis in diseases classified elsewhere, lower leg

M90.561 Osteonecrosis in diseases classified elsewhere, right lower leg [HCC]

M90.562 Osteonecrosis in diseases classified elsewhere, left lower leg [HCC]

M90.569 Osteonecrosis in diseases classified elsewhere, unspecified lower leg [HCC]

M90.57 Osteonecrosis in diseases classified elsewhere, ankle and foot

M90.571 Osteonecrosis in diseases classified elsewhere, right ankle and foot [HCC]

M90.572 Osteonecrosis in diseases classified elsewhere, left ankle and foot [HCC]

M90.579 Osteonecrosis in diseases classified elsewhere, unspecified ankle and foot [HCC]

M90.58 Osteonecrosis in diseases classified elsewhere, other site [HCC]

M90.59 Osteonecrosis in diseases classified elsewhere, multiple sites

M90.6 Osteitis deformans in neoplastic diseases

Osteitis deformans in malignant neoplasm of bone

Code first the neoplasm (C40.-, C41.-)

Excludes1: osteitis deformans [Paget's disease of bone] (M88.-)

M90.60 Osteitis deformans in neoplastic diseases, unspecified site

M90.61 Osteitis deformans in neoplastic diseases, shoulder

M90.611 Osteitis deformans in neoplastic diseases, right shoulder

M90.612 Osteitis deformans in neoplastic diseases, left shoulder

M90.619 Osteitis deformans in neoplastic diseases, unspecified shoulder

M90.62 Osteitis deformans in neoplastic diseases, upper arm

M90.621 Osteitis deformans in neoplastic diseases, right upper arm

M90.622 Osteitis deformans in neoplastic diseases, left upper arm

M90.629 Osteitis deformans in neoplastic diseases, unspecified upper arm

M90.63 Osteitis deformans in neoplastic diseases, forearm

M90.631 Osteitis deformans in neoplastic diseases, right forearm

M90.632 Osteitis deformans in neoplastic diseases, left forearm

M90.639 Osteitis deformans in neoplastic diseases, unspecified forearm

M90.64 Osteitis deformans in neoplastic diseases, hand

M90.641 Osteitis deformans in neoplastic diseases, right hand

M90.642 Osteitis deformans in neoplastic diseases, left hand

M90.649 Osteitis deformans in neoplastic diseases, unspecified hand

M90.65 Osteitis deformans in neoplastic diseases, thigh

M90.651 Osteitis deformans in neoplastic diseases, right thigh

M90.652 Osteitis deformans in neoplastic diseases, left thigh

M90.659 Osteitis deformans in neoplastic diseases, unspecified thigh

M90.66 Osteitis deformans in neoplastic diseases, lower leg

M90.661 Osteitis deformans in neoplastic diseases, right lower leg

M90.662 Osteitis deformans in neoplastic diseases, left lower leg

M90.669 Osteitis deformans in neoplastic diseases, unspecified lower leg

M90.67 Osteitis deformans in neoplastic diseases, ankle and foot

M90.671 Osteitis deformans in neoplastic diseases, right ankle and foot

M90.672 Osteitis deformans in neoplastic diseases, left ankle and foot

M90.679 Osteitis deformans in neoplastic diseases, unspecified ankle and foot

M90.68 Osteitis deformans in neoplastic diseases, other site

M90.69 Osteitis deformans in neoplastic diseases, multiple sites

M90.8 Osteopathy in diseases classified elsewhere

Code first underlying disease, such as:

rickets (E55.0)

vitamin-D-resistant rickets (E83.3)

M90.80 Osteopathy in diseases classified elsewhere, unspecified site

M90.81 Osteopathy in diseases classified elsewhere, shoulder

> **M90.811 Osteopathy in diseases classified elsewhere, right shoulder**
>
> **M90.812 Osteopathy in diseases classified elsewhere, left shoulder**
>
> **M90.819 Osteopathy in diseases classified elsewhere, unspecified shoulder**

M90.82 Osteopathy in diseases classified elsewhere, upper arm

> **M90.821 Osteopathy in diseases classified elsewhere, right upper arm**
>
> **M90.822 Osteopathy in diseases classified elsewhere, left upper arm**
>
> **M90.829 Osteopathy in diseases classified elsewhere, unspecified upper arm**

M90.83 Osteopathy in diseases classified elsewhere, forearm

> **M90.831 Osteopathy in diseases classified elsewhere, right forearm**
>
> **M90.832 Osteopathy in diseases classified elsewhere, left forearm**
>
> **M90.839 Osteopathy in diseases classified elsewhere, unspecified forearm**

M90.84 Osteopathy in diseases classified elsewhere, hand

> **M90.841 Osteopathy in diseases classified elsewhere, right hand**
>
> **M90.842 Osteopathy in diseases classified elsewhere, left hand**
>
> **M90.849 Osteopathy in diseases classified elsewhere, unspecified hand**

M90.85 Osteopathy in diseases classified elsewhere, thigh

> **M90.851 Osteopathy in diseases classified elsewhere, right thigh**
>
> **M90.852 Osteopathy in diseases classified elsewhere, left thigh**
>
> **M90.859 Osteopathy in diseases classified elsewhere, unspecified thigh**

M90.86 Osteopathy in diseases classified elsewhere, lower leg

> **M90.861 Osteopathy in diseases classified elsewhere, right lower leg**
>
> **M90.862 Osteopathy in diseases classified elsewhere, left lower leg**
>
> **M90.869 Osteopathy in diseases classified elsewhere, unspecified lower leg**

M90.87 Osteopathy in diseases classified elsewhere, ankle and foot

> **M90.871 Osteopathy in diseases classified elsewhere, right ankle and foot**
>
> **M90.872 Osteopathy in diseases classified elsewhere, left ankle and foot**
>
> **M90.879 Osteopathy in diseases classified elsewhere, unspecified ankle and foot**

M90.88 Osteopathy in diseases classified elsewhere, other site

M90.89 Osteopathy in diseases classified elsewhere, multiple sites

CHONDROPATHIES (M91-M94)

Excludes1: postprocedural chondropathies (M96.-)

M91 Juvenile osteochondrosis of hip and pelvis

> **Excludes1:** slipped upper femoral epiphysis (nontraumatic) (M93.0)

M91.0 Juvenile osteochondrosis of pelvis

Osteochondrosis (juvenile) of acetabulum

Osteochondrosis (juvenile) of iliac crest [Buchanan]

Osteochondrosis (juvenile) of ischiopubic synchondrosis [van Neck]

Osteochondrosis (juvenile) of symphysis pubis [Pierson]

M91.1 Juvenile osteochondrosis of head of femur [Legg-Calvé-Perthes]

> **M91.10 Juvenile osteochondrosis of head of femur [Legg-Calvé-Perthes], unspecified leg**
>
> **M91.11 Juvenile osteochondrosis of head of femur [Legg-Calvé-Perthes], right leg**
>
> **M91.12 Juvenile osteochondrosis of head of femur [Legg-Calvé-Perthes], left leg**

M91.2 Coxa plana

Hip deformity due to previous juvenile osteochondrosis

> **M91.20 Coxa plana, unspecified hip**
>
> **M91.21 Coxa plana, right hip**
>
> **M91.22 Coxa plana, left hip**

M91.3 Pseudocoxalgia

> **M91.30 Pseudocoxalgia, unspecified hip**
>
> **M91.31 Pseudocoxalgia, right hip**
>
> **M91.32 Pseudocoxalgia, left hip**

M91.4 Coxa magna

> **M91.40 Coxa magna, unspecified hip**
>
> **M91.41 Coxa magna, right hip**
>
> **M91.42 Coxa magna, left hip**

M91.8 Other juvenile osteochondrosis of hip and pelvis

Juvenile osteochondrosis after reduction of congenital dislocation of hip

> **M91.80 Other juvenile osteochondrosis of hip and pelvis, unspecified leg**
>
> **M91.81 Other juvenile osteochondrosis of hip and pelvis, right leg**
>
> **M91.82 Other juvenile osteochondrosis of hip and pelvis, left leg**

M91.9 Juvenile osteochondrosis of hip and pelvis, unspecified

> **M91.90 Juvenile osteochondrosis of hip and pelvis, unspecified, unspecified leg**
>
> **M91.91 Juvenile osteochondrosis of hip and pelvis, unspecified, right leg**
>
> **M91.92 Juvenile osteochondrosis of hip and pelvis, unspecified, left leg**

M92 Other juvenile osteochondrosis

M92.0 Juvenile osteochondrosis of humerus

Osteochondrosis (juvenile) of capitulum of humerus [Panner]

Osteochondrosis (juvenile) of head of humerus [Haas]

> **M92.00 Juvenile osteochondrosis of humerus, unspecified arm**
>
> **M92.01 Juvenile osteochondrosis of humerus, right arm**
>
> **M92.02 Juvenile osteochondrosis of humerus, left arm**

M92.1 Juvenile osteochondrosis of radius and ulna

Osteochondrosis (juvenile) of lower ulna [Burns]

Osteochondrosis (juvenile) of radial head [Brailsford]

> **M92.10 Juvenile osteochondrosis of radius and ulna, unspecified arm**

M92.11   Juvenile osteochondrosis of radius and ulna, right arm

M92.12   Juvenile osteochondrosis of radius and ulna, left arm

M92.2   Juvenile osteochondrosis, hand

    M92.20   Unspecified juvenile osteochondrosis, hand

        M92.201   Unspecified juvenile osteochondrosis, right hand

        M92.202   Unspecified juvenile osteochondrosis, left hand

        M92.209   Unspecified juvenile osteochondrosis, unspecified hand

    M92.21   Osteochondrosis (juvenile) of carpal lunate [Kienböck]

        M92.211   Osteochondrosis (juvenile) of carpal lunate [Kienböck], right hand

        M92.212   Osteochondrosis (juvenile) of carpal lunate [Kienböck], left hand

        M92.219   Osteochondrosis (juvenile) of carpal lunate [Kienböck], unspecified hand

    M92.22   Osteochondrosis (juvenile) of metacarpal heads [Mauclaire]

        M92.221   Osteochondrosis (juvenile) of metacarpal heads [Mauclaire], right hand

        M92.222   Osteochondrosis (juvenile) of metacarpal heads [Mauclaire], left hand

        M92.229   Osteochondrosis (juvenile) of metacarpal heads [Mauclaire], unspecified hand

    M92.29   Other juvenile osteochondrosis, hand

        M92.291   Other juvenile osteochondrosis, right hand

        M92.292   Other juvenile osteochondrosis, left hand

        M92.299   Other juvenile osteochondrosis, unspecified hand

M92.3   Other juvenile osteochondrosis, upper limb

    M92.30   Other juvenile osteochondrosis, unspecified upper limb

    M92.31   Other juvenile osteochondrosis, right upper limb

    M92.32   Other juvenile osteochondrosis, left upper limb

M92.4   Juvenile osteochondrosis of patella

Osteochondrosis (juvenile) of primary patellar center [Köhler]

Osteochondrosis (juvenile) of secondary patellar centre [Sinding Larsen]

    M92.40   Juvenile osteochondrosis of patella, unspecified knee

    M92.41   Juvenile osteochondrosis of patella, right knee

    M92.42   Juvenile osteochondrosis of patella, left knee

M92.5   Juvenile osteochondrosis of tibia and fibula

    ▲M92.50   Unspecified juvenile osteochondrosis of tibia and fibula

        M92.501   Unspecified juvenile osteochondrosis, right leg

        M92.502   Unspecified juvenile osteochondrosis, left leg

        M92.503   Unspecified juvenile osteochondrosis, bilateral leg

        M92.509   Unspecified juvenile osteochondrosis, unspecified leg

▲M92.51   Juvenile osteochondrosis of proximal tibia

Blount disease

Tibia vara

        M92.511   Juvenile osteochondrosis of proximal tibia, right leg

        M92.512   Juvenile osteochondrosis of proximal tibia, left leg

        M92.513   Juvenile osteochondrosis of proximal tibia, bilateral

        M92.519   Juvenile osteochondrosis of proximal tibia, unspecified leg

▲M92.52   Juvenile osteochondrosis of tibia tubercle

Osgood-Schlatter disease

        M92.521   Juvenile osteochondrosis of tibia tubercle, right leg

        M92.522   Juvenile osteochondrosis of tibia tubercle, left leg

        M92.523   Juvenile osteochondrosis of tibia tubercle, bilateral

        M92.529   Juvenile osteochondrosis of tibia tubercle, unspecified leg

    M92.59   Other juvenile osteochondrosis of tibia and fibula

        M92.591   Other juvenile osteochondrosis of tibia and fibula, right leg

        M92.592   Other juvenile osteochondrosis of tibia and fibula, left leg

        M92.593   Other juvenile osteochondrosis of tibia and fibula, bilateral

        M92.599   Other juvenile osteochondrosis of tibia and fibula, unspecified leg

M92.6   Juvenile osteochondrosis of tarsus

Osteochondrosis (juvenile) of calcaneum [Sever]

Osteochondrosis (juvenile) of os tibiale externum [Haglund]

Osteochondrosis (juvenile) of talus [Diaz]

Osteochondrosis (juvenile) of tarsal navicular [Köhler]

    M92.60   Juvenile osteochondrosis of tarsus, unspecified ankle

    M92.61   Juvenile osteochondrosis of tarsus, right ankle

    M92.62   Juvenile osteochondrosis of tarsus, left ankle

M92.7   Juvenile osteochondrosis of metatarsus

Osteochondrosis (juvenile) of fifth metatarsus [Iselin]

Osteochondrosis (juvenile) of second metatarsus [Freiberg]

    M92.70   Juvenile osteochondrosis of metatarsus, unspecified foot

    M92.71   Juvenile osteochondrosis of metatarsus, right foot

    M92.72   Juvenile osteochondrosis of metatarsus, left foot

M92.8   Other specified juvenile osteochondrosis

Calcaneal apophysitis

M92.9   Juvenile osteochondrosis, unspecified

Juvenile apophysitis NOS

Juvenile epiphysitis NOS

Juvenile osteochondritis NOS

Juvenile osteochondrosis NOS

M93   **Other osteochondropathies**

Excludes2: osteochondrosis of spine (M42.-)

M93.0   Slipped upper femoral epiphysis (nontraumatic)

Use Additional Code for associated chondrolysis (M94.3)

M93.00 Unspecified slipped upper femoral epiphysis (nontraumatic)

M93.001 Unspecified slipped upper femoral epiphysis (nontraumatic), right hip

M93.002 Unspecified slipped upper femoral epiphysis (nontraumatic), left hip

M93.003 Unspecified slipped upper femoral epiphysis (nontraumatic), unspecified hip

M93.01 Acute slipped upper femoral epiphysis (nontraumatic)

M93.011 Acute slipped upper femoral epiphysis (nontraumatic), right hip

M93.012 Acute slipped upper femoral epiphysis (nontraumatic), left hip

M93.013 Acute slipped upper femoral epiphysis (nontraumatic), unspecified hip

M93.02 Chronic slipped upper femoral epiphysis (nontraumatic)

M93.021 Chronic slipped upper femoral epiphysis (nontraumatic), right hip

M93.022 Chronic slipped upper femoral epiphysis (nontraumatic), left hip

M93.023 Chronic slipped upper femoral epiphysis (nontraumatic), unspecified hip

M93.03 Acute on chronic slipped upper femoral epiphysis (nontraumatic)

M93.031 Acute on chronic slipped upper femoral epiphysis (nontraumatic), right hip

M93.032 Acute on chronic slipped upper femoral epiphysis (nontraumatic), left hip

M93.033 Acute on chronic slipped upper femoral epiphysis (nontraumatic), unspecified hip

M93.1 Kienböck's disease of adults

Adult osteochondrosis of carpal lunates

M93.2 Osteochondritis dissecans

M93.20 Osteochondritis dissecans of unspecified site

M93.21 Osteochondritis dissecans of shoulder

M93.211 Osteochondritis dissecans, right shoulder

M93.212 Osteochondritis dissecans, left shoulder

M93.219 Osteochondritis dissecans, unspecified shoulder

M93.22 Osteochondritis dissecans of elbow

M93.221 Osteochondritis dissecans, right elbow

M93.222 Osteochondritis dissecans, left elbow

M93.229 Osteochondritis dissecans, unspecified elbow

M93.23 Osteochondritis dissecans of wrist

M93.231 Osteochondritis dissecans, right wrist

M93.232 Osteochondritis dissecans, left wrist

M93.239 Osteochondritis dissecans, unspecified wrist

M93.24 Osteochondritis dissecans of joints of hand

M93.241 Osteochondritis dissecans, joints of right hand

M93.242 Osteochondritis dissecans, joints of left hand

M93.249 Osteochondritis dissecans, joints of unspecified hand

M93.25 Osteochondritis dissecans of hip

M93.251 Osteochondritis dissecans, right hip

M93.252 Osteochondritis dissecans, left hip

M93.259 Osteochondritis dissecans, unspecified hip

M93.26 Osteochondritis dissecans knee

M93.261 Osteochondritis dissecans, right knee

M93.262 Osteochondritis dissecans, left knee

M93.269 Osteochondritis dissecans, unspecified knee

M93.27 Osteochondritis dissecans of ankle and joints of foot

M93.271 Osteochondritis dissecans, right ankle and joints of right foot

M93.272 Osteochondritis dissecans, left ankle and joints of left foot

M93.279 Osteochondritis dissecans, unspecified ankle and joints of foot

M93.28 Osteochondritis dissecans other site

M93.29 Osteochondritis dissecans multiple sites

M93.8 Other specified osteochondropathies

M93.80 Other specified osteochondropathies of unspecified site

M93.81 Other specified osteochondropathies of shoulder

M93.811 Other specified osteochondropathies, right shoulder

M93.812 Other specified osteochondropathies, left shoulder

M93.819 Other specified osteochondropathies, unspecified shoulder

M93.82 Other specified osteochondropathies of upper arm

M93.821 Other specified osteochondropathies, right upper arm

M93.822 Other specified osteochondropathies, left upper arm

M93.829 Other specified osteochondropathies, unspecified upper arm

M93.83 Other specified osteochondropathies of forearm

M93.831 Other specified osteochondropathies, right forearm

M93.832 Other specified osteochondropathies, left forearm

M93.839 Other specified osteochondropathies, unspecified forearm

M93.84 Other specified osteochondropathies of hand

M93.841 Other specified osteochondropathies, right hand

M93.842 Other specified osteochondropathies, left hand

M93.849 Other specified osteochondropathies, unspecified hand

M93.85 Other specified osteochondropathies of thigh

M93.851 Other specified osteochondropathies, right thigh

M93.852 Other specified osteochondropathies, left thigh

M93.859   Other specified osteochondropathies, unspecified thigh

M93.86   Other specified osteochondropathies lower leg

     M93.861   Other specified osteochondropathies, right lower leg

     M93.862   Other specified osteochondropathies, left lower leg

     M93.869   Other specified osteochondropathies, unspecified lower leg

M93.87   Other specified osteochondropathies of ankle and foot

     M93.871   Other specified osteochondropathies, right ankle and foot

     M93.872   Other specified osteochondropathies, left ankle and foot

     M93.879   Other specified osteochondropathies, unspecified ankle and foot

M93.88   Other specified osteochondropathies other

M93.89   Other specified osteochondropathies multiple sites

M93.9   Osteochondropathy, unspecified

Apophysitis NOS

Epiphysitis NOS

Osteochondritis NOS

Osteochondrosis NOS

M93.90   Osteochondropathy, unspecified of unspecified site

M93.91   Osteochondropathy, unspecified of shoulder

     M93.911   Osteochondropathy, unspecified, right shoulder

     M93.912   Osteochondropathy, unspecified, left shoulder

     M93.919   Osteochondropathy, unspecified, unspecified shoulder

M93.92   Osteochondropathy, unspecified of upper arm

     M93.921   Osteochondropathy, unspecified, right upper arm

     M93.922   Osteochondropathy, unspecified, left upper arm

     M93.929   Osteochondropathy, unspecified, unspecified upper arm

M93.93   Osteochondropathy, unspecified of forearm

     M93.931   Osteochondropathy, unspecified, right forearm

     M93.932   Osteochondropathy, unspecified, left forearm

     M93.939   Osteochondropathy, unspecified, unspecified forearm

M93.94   Osteochondropathy, unspecified of hand

     M93.941   Osteochondropathy, unspecified, right hand

     M93.942   Osteochondropathy, unspecified, left hand

     M93.949   Osteochondropathy, unspecified, unspecified hand

M93.95   Osteochondropathy, unspecified of thigh

     M93.951   Osteochondropathy, unspecified, right thigh

     M93.952   Osteochondropathy, unspecified, left thigh

     M93.959   Osteochondropathy, unspecified, unspecified thigh

M93.96   Osteochondropathy, unspecified lower leg

M93.961   Osteochondropathy, unspecified, right lower leg

M93.962   Osteochondropathy, unspecified, left lower leg

M93.969   Osteochondropathy, unspecified, unspecified lower leg

M93.97   Osteochondropathy, unspecified of ankle and foot

     M93.971   Osteochondropathy, unspecified, right ankle and foot

     M93.972   Osteochondropathy, unspecified, left ankle and foot

     M93.979   Osteochondropathy, unspecified, unspecified ankle and foot

M93.98   Osteochondropathy, unspecified other

M93.99   Osteochondropathy, unspecified multiple sites

M94   Other disorders of cartilage

M94.0   Chondrocostal junction syndrome [Tietze]

Costochondritis

M94.1   Relapsing polychondritis

M94.2   Chondromalacia

Excludes1: chondromalacia patellae (M22.4)

M94.20   Chondromalacia, unspecified site

M94.21   Chondromalacia, shoulder

     M94.211   Chondromalacia, right shoulder

     M94.212   Chondromalacia, left shoulder

     M94.219   Chondromalacia, unspecified shoulder

M94.22   Chondromalacia, elbow

     M94.221   Chondromalacia, right elbow

     M94.222   Chondromalacia, left elbow

     M94.229   Chondromalacia, unspecified elbow

M94.23   Chondromalacia, wrist

     M94.231   Chondromalacia, right wrist

     M94.232   Chondromalacia, left wrist

     M94.239   Chondromalacia, unspecified wrist

M94.24   Chondromalacia, joints of hand

     M94.241   Chondromalacia, joints of right hand

     M94.242   Chondromalacia, joints of left hand

     M94.249   Chondromalacia, joints of unspecified hand

M94.25   Chondromalacia, hip

     M94.251   Chondromalacia, right hip

     M94.252   Chondromalacia, left hip

     M94.259   Chondromalacia, unspecified hip

M94.26   Chondromalacia, knee

     M94.261   Chondromalacia, right knee

     M94.262   Chondromalacia, left knee

     M94.269   Chondromalacia, unspecified knee

M94.27   Chondromalacia, ankle and joints of foot

     M94.271   Chondromalacia, right ankle and joints of right foot

     M94.272   Chondromalacia, left ankle and joints of left foot

     M94.279   Chondromalacia, unspecified ankle and joints of foot

M94.28   Chondromalacia, other site

M94.29   Chondromalacia, multiple sites

M94.3   Chondrolysis

Code first any associated slipped upper femoral epiphysis (nontraumatic) (M93.0-)

M94.35 **Chondrolysis, hip**

    M94.351 **Chondrolysis, right hip**

    M94.352 **Chondrolysis, left hip**

    M94.359 **Chondrolysis, unspecified hip**

M94.8 **Other specified disorders of cartilage**

  M94.8X **Other specified disorders of cartilage**

    M94.8X0 **Other specified disorders of cartilage, multiple sites**

    M94.8X1 **Other specified disorders of cartilage, shoulder**

    M94.8X2 **Other specified disorders of cartilage, upper arm**

    M94.8X3 **Other specified disorders of cartilage, forearm**

    M94.8X4 **Other specified disorders of cartilage, hand**

    M94.8X5 **Other specified disorders of cartilage, thigh**

    M94.8X6 **Other specified disorders of cartilage, lower leg**

    M94.8X7 **Other specified disorders of cartilage, ankle and foot**

    M94.8X8 **Other specified disorders of cartilage, other site**

    M94.8X9 **Other specified disorders of cartilage, unspecified sites**

M94.9 **Disorder of cartilage, unspecified**

OTHER DISORDERS OF THE MUSCULOSKELETAL SYSTEM AND CONNECTIVE TISSUE (M95)

M95 **Other acquired deformities of musculoskeletal system and connective tissue**

Excludes2: acquired absence of limbs and organs (Z89-Z90)

  acquired deformities of limbs (M20-M21)

  congenital malformations and deformations of the musculoskeletal system (Q65-Q79)

  deforming dorsopathies (M40-M43)

  dentofacial anomalies [including malocclusion] (M26.-)

  postprocedural musculoskeletal disorders (M96.-)

M95.0 **Acquired deformity of nose**

Excludes2: deviated nasal septum (J34.2)

M95.1 **Cauliflower ear**

Excludes2: Other acquired deformities of ear (H61.1)

  M95.10 **Cauliflower ear, unspecified ear**

  M95.11 **Cauliflower ear, right ear**

  M95.12 **Cauliflower ear, left ear**

M95.2 **Other acquired deformity of head**

M95.3 **Acquired deformity of neck**

M95.4 **Acquired deformity of chest and rib**

M95.5 **Acquired deformity of pelvis**

Excludes1: maternal care for known or suspected disproportion (O33.-)

M95.8 **Other specified acquired deformities of musculoskeletal system**

M95.9 **Acquired deformity of musculoskeletal system, unspecified**

INTRAOPERATIVE AND POSTPROCEDURAL COMPLICATIONS AND DISORDERS OF MUSCULOSKELETAL SYSTEM, NOT ELSEWHERE CLASSIFIED (M96)

M96 **Intraoperative and postprocedural complications and disorders of musculoskeletal system, not elsewhere classified**

Excludes2: arthropathy following intestinal bypass (M02.0-)

  complications of internal orthopedic prosthetic devices, implants and grafts (T84.-)

  disorders associated with osteoporosis (M80)

  periprosthetic fracture around internal prosthetic joint (M97.-)

  presence of functional implants and other devices (Z96-Z97)

M96.0 **Pseudarthrosis after fusion or arthrodesis**

M96.1 **Postlaminectomy syndrome, not elsewhere classified**

M96.2 **Postradiation kyphosis**

M96.3 **Postlaminectomy kyphosis**

M96.4 **Postsurgical lordosis**

M96.5 **Postradiation scoliosis**

M96.6 **Fracture of bone following insertion of orthopedic implant, joint prosthesis, or bone plate**

Intraoperative fracture of bone during insertion of orthopedic implant, joint prosthesis, or bone plate

Excludes2: complication of internal orthopedic devices, implants or grafts (T84.-)

M96.62 **Fracture of humerus following insertion of orthopedic implant, joint prosthesis, or bone plate**

  M96.621 **Fracture of humerus following insertion of orthopedic implant, joint prosthesis, or bone plate, right arm** [HCC]

  M96.622 **Fracture of humerus following insertion of orthopedic implant, joint prosthesis, or bone plate, left arm** [HCC]

  M96.629 **Fracture of humerus following insertion of orthopedic implant, joint prosthesis, or bone plate, unspecified arm** [HCC]

M96.63 **Fracture of radius or ulna following insertion of orthopedic implant, joint prosthesis, or bone plate**

  M96.631 **Fracture of radius or ulna following insertion of orthopedic implant, joint prosthesis, or bone plate, right arm** [HCC]

  M96.632 **Fracture of radius or ulna following insertion of orthopedic implant, joint prosthesis, or bone plate, left arm** [HCC]

  M96.639 **Fracture of radius or ulna following insertion of orthopedic implant, joint prosthesis, or bone plate, unspecified arm** [HCC]

M96.65 **Fracture of pelvis following insertion of orthopedic implant, joint prosthesis, or bone plate** [HCC]

M96.66 **Fracture of femur following insertion of orthopedic implant, joint prosthesis, or bone plate**

  M96.661 **Fracture of femur following insertion of orthopedic implant, joint prosthesis, or bone plate, right leg** [HCC]

  M96.662 **Fracture of femur following insertion of orthopedic implant, joint prosthesis, or bone plate, left leg** [HCC]

M96.669   Fracture of femur following insertion of orthopedic implant, joint prosthesis, or bone plate, unspecified leg [HCC]

M96.67   Fracture of tibia or fibula following insertion of orthopedic implant, joint prosthesis, or bone plate

M96.671   Fracture of tibia or fibula following insertion of orthopedic implant, joint prosthesis, or bone plate, right leg [HCC]

M96.672   Fracture of tibia or fibula following insertion of orthopedic implant, joint prosthesis, or bone plate, left leg

M96.679   Fracture of tibia or fibula following insertion of orthopedic implant, joint prosthesis, or bone plate, unspecified leg [HCC]

M96.69   Fracture of other bone following insertion of orthopedic implant, joint prosthesis, or bone plate [HCC]

M96.8   Other intraoperative and postprocedural complications and disorders of musculoskeletal system, not elsewhere classified

M96.81   Intraoperative hemorrhage and hematoma of a musculoskeletal structure complicating a procedure

Excludes1: intraoperative hemorrhage and hematoma of a musculoskeletal structure due to accidental puncture and laceration during a procedure (M96.82-)

M96.810   Intraoperative hemorrhage and hematoma of a musculoskeletal structure complicating a musculoskeletal system procedure

M96.811   Intraoperative hemorrhage and hematoma of a musculoskeletal structure complicating other procedure

M96.82   Accidental puncture and laceration of a musculoskeletal structure during a procedure

M96.820   Accidental puncture and laceration of a musculoskeletal structure during a musculoskeletal system procedure

M96.821   Accidental puncture and laceration of a musculoskeletal structure during other procedure

M96.83   Postprocedural hemorrhage of a musculoskeletal structure following a procedure

M96.830   Postprocedural hemorrhage of a musculoskeletal structure following a musculoskeletal system procedure

M96.831   Postprocedural hemorrhage of a musculoskeletal structure following other procedure

M96.84   Postprocedural hematoma and seroma of a musculoskeletal structure following a procedure

M96.840   Postprocedural hematoma of a musculoskeletal structure following a musculoskeletal system procedure

M96.841   Postprocedural hematoma of a musculoskeletal structure following other procedure

M96.842   Postprocedural seroma of a musculoskeletal structure following a musculoskeletal system procedure

M96.843   Postprocedural seroma of a musculoskeletal structure following other procedure

M96.89   Other intraoperative and postprocedural complications and disorders of the musculoskeletal system

Instability of joint secondary to removal of joint prosthesis

Use Additional Code, if applicable, to further specify disorder

PERIPROSTHETIC FRACTURE AROUND INTERNAL PROSTHETIC JOINT (M97)

M97   Periprosthetic fracture around internal prosthetic joint

Excludes2: fracture of bone following insertion of orthopedic implant, joint prosthesis or bone plate (M96.6-)

breakage (fracture) of prosthetic joint (T84.01-)

The appropriate 7th character is to be added to each code from category M97

A - initial encounter

D - subsequent encounter

S - sequela

M97.0   Periprosthetic fracture around internal prosthetic hip joint

⊗⑦M97.01   Periprosthetic fracture around internal prosthetic right hip joint [HCC]

⊗⑦M97.02   Periprosthetic fracture around internal prosthetic left hip joint [HCC]

M97.1   Periprosthetic fracture around internal prosthetic knee joint

⊗⑦M97.11   Periprosthetic fracture around internal prosthetic right knee joint

⊗⑦M97.12   Periprosthetic fracture around internal prosthetic left knee joint

M97.2   Periprosthetic fracture around internal prosthetic ankle joint

⊗⑦M97.21   Periprosthetic fracture around internal prosthetic right ankle joint

⊗⑦M97.22   Periprosthetic fracture around internal prosthetic left ankle joint

M97.3   Periprosthetic fracture around internal prosthetic shoulder joint

⊗⑦M97.31   Periprosthetic fracture around internal prosthetic right shoulder joint

⊗⑦M97.32   Periprosthetic fracture around internal prosthetic left shoulder joint

M97.4   Periprosthetic fracture around internal prosthetic elbow joint

⊗⑦M97.41   Periprosthetic fracture around internal prosthetic right elbow joint

⊗⑦M97.42   Periprosthetic fracture around internal prosthetic left elbow joint

⊗⑦M97.8   Periprosthetic fracture around other internal prosthetic joint

Periprosthetic fracture around internal prosthetic finger joint

Periprosthetic fracture around internal prosthetic spinal joint

Periprosthetic fracture around internal prosthetic toe joint

Periprosthetic fracture around internal prosthetic wrist joint

Use Additional Code to identify the joint (Z96.6-)

⊗⑦M97.9   Periprosthetic fracture around unspecified internal prosthetic joint

BIOMECHANICAL LESIONS, NOT ELSEWHERE CLASSIFIED (M99)

M99   Biomechanical lesions, not elsewhere classified

Note: This category should not be used if the condition can be classified elsewhere.

M99.0   Segmental and somatic dysfunction

    M99.00   Segmental and somatic dysfunction of head region

    M99.01   Segmental and somatic dysfunction of cervical region

    M99.02   Segmental and somatic dysfunction of thoracic region

    M99.03   Segmental and somatic dysfunction of lumbar region

    M99.04   Segmental and somatic dysfunction of sacral region

    M99.05   Segmental and somatic dysfunction of pelvic region

    M99.06   Segmental and somatic dysfunction of lower extremity

    M99.07   Segmental and somatic dysfunction of upper extremity

    M99.08   Segmental and somatic dysfunction of rib cage

    M99.09   Segmental and somatic dysfunction of abdomen and other regions

M99.1   Subluxation complex (vertebral)

    M99.10   Subluxation complex (vertebral) of head region

    M99.11   Subluxation complex (vertebral) of cervical region

    M99.12   Subluxation complex (vertebral) of thoracic region

    M99.13   Subluxation complex (vertebral) of lumbar region

    M99.14   Subluxation complex (vertebral) of sacral region

    M99.15   Subluxation complex (vertebral) of pelvic region

    M99.16   Subluxation complex (vertebral) of lower extremity

    M99.17   Subluxation complex (vertebral) of upper extremity

    M99.18   Subluxation complex (vertebral) of rib cage

    M99.19   Subluxation complex (vertebral) of abdomen and other regions

M99.2   Subluxation stenosis of neural canal

    M99.20   Subluxation stenosis of neural canal of head region

    M99.21   Subluxation stenosis of neural canal of cervical region

    M99.22   Subluxation stenosis of neural canal of thoracic region

    M99.23   Subluxation stenosis of neural canal of lumbar region

    M99.24   Subluxation stenosis of neural canal of sacral region

    M99.25   Subluxation stenosis of neural canal of pelvic region

    M99.26   Subluxation stenosis of neural canal of lower extremity

    M99.27   Subluxation stenosis of neural canal of upper extremity

    M99.28   Subluxation stenosis of neural canal of rib cage

    M99.29   Subluxation stenosis of neural canal of abdomen and other regions

M99.3   Osseous stenosis of neural canal

    M99.30   Osseous stenosis of neural canal of head region

    M99.31   Osseous stenosis of neural canal of cervical region

    M99.32   Osseous stenosis of neural canal of thoracic region

    M99.33   Osseous stenosis of neural canal of lumbar region

    M99.34   Osseous stenosis of neural canal of sacral region

    M99.35   Osseous stenosis of neural canal of pelvic region

    M99.36   Osseous stenosis of neural canal of lower extremity

    M99.37   Osseous stenosis of neural canal of upper extremity

    M99.38   Osseous stenosis of neural canal of rib cage

    M99.39   Osseous stenosis of neural canal of abdomen and other regions

M99.4   Connective tissue stenosis of neural canal

    M99.40   Connective tissue stenosis of neural canal of head region

    M99.41   Connective tissue stenosis of neural canal of cervical region

    M99.42   Connective tissue stenosis of neural canal of thoracic region

    M99.43   Connective tissue stenosis of neural canal of lumbar region

    M99.44   Connective tissue stenosis of neural canal of sacral region

    M99.45   Connective tissue stenosis of neural canal of pelvic region

    M99.46   Connective tissue stenosis of neural canal of lower extremity

    M99.47   Connective tissue stenosis of neural canal of upper extremity

    M99.48   Connective tissue stenosis of neural canal of rib cage

    M99.49   Connective tissue stenosis of neural canal of abdomen and other regions

M99.5   Intervertebral disc stenosis of neural canal

    M99.50   Intervertebral disc stenosis of neural canal of head region

    M99.51   Intervertebral disc stenosis of neural canal of cervical region

    M99.52   Intervertebral disc stenosis of neural canal of thoracic region

    M99.53   Intervertebral disc stenosis of neural canal of lumbar region

    M99.54   Intervertebral disc stenosis of neural canal of sacral region

    M99.55   Intervertebral disc stenosis of neural canal of pelvic region

    M99.56   Intervertebral disc stenosis of neural canal of lower extremity

    M99.57   Intervertebral disc stenosis of neural canal of upper extremity

    M99.58   Intervertebral disc stenosis of neural canal of rib cage

    M99.59   Intervertebral disc stenosis of neural canal of abdomen and other regions

M99.6   Osseous and subluxation stenosis of intervertebral foramina

    M99.60   Osseous and subluxation stenosis of intervertebral foramina of head region

    M99.61   Osseous and subluxation stenosis of intervertebral foramina of cervical region

   ● New code   ▲ Revised code   **Excludes1:** Not coded here   **Excludes2:** Not included here   ⊗ Placeholder required   ⑦7th digit required

    M99.62 **Osseous and subluxation stenosis of intervertebral foramina of thoracic region**

    M99.63 **Osseous and subluxation stenosis of intervertebral foramina of lumbar region**

    M99.64 **Osseous and subluxation stenosis of intervertebral foramina of sacral region**

    M99.65 **Osseous and subluxation stenosis of intervertebral foramina of pelvic region**

    M99.66 **Osseous and subluxation stenosis of intervertebral foramina of lower extremity**

    M99.67 **Osseous and subluxation stenosis of intervertebral foramina of upper extremity**

    M99.68 **Osseous and subluxation stenosis of intervertebral foramina of rib cage**

    M99.69 **Osseous and subluxation stenosis of intervertebral foramina of abdomen and other regions**

M99.7 **Connective tissue and disc stenosis of intervertebral foramina**

    M99.70 **Connective tissue and disc stenosis of intervertebral foramina of head region**

    M99.71 **Connective tissue and disc stenosis of intervertebral foramina of cervical region**

    M99.72 **Connective tissue and disc stenosis of intervertebral foramina of thoracic region**

    M99.73 **Connective tissue and disc stenosis of intervertebral foramina of lumbar region**

    M99.74 **Connective tissue and disc stenosis of intervertebral foramina of sacral region**

    M99.75 **Connective tissue and disc stenosis of intervertebral foramina of pelvic region**

    M99.76 **Connective tissue and disc stenosis of intervertebral foramina of lower extremity**

    M99.77 **Connective tissue and disc stenosis of intervertebral foramina of upper extremity**

    M99.78 **Connective tissue and disc stenosis of intervertebral foramina of rib cage**

    M99.79 **Connective tissue and disc stenosis of intervertebral foramina of abdomen and other regions**

M99.8 **Other biomechanical lesions**

    M99.80 **Other biomechanical lesions of head region**

    M99.81 **Other biomechanical lesions of cervical region**

    M99.82 **Other biomechanical lesions of thoracic region**

    M99.83 **Other biomechanical lesions of lumbar region**

    M99.84 **Other biomechanical lesions of sacral region**

    M99.85 **Other biomechanical lesions of pelvic region**

    M99.86 **Other biomechanical lesions of lower extremity**

    M99.87 **Other biomechanical lesions of upper extremity**

    M99.88 **Other biomechanical lesions of rib cage**

    M99.89 **Other biomechanical lesions of abdomen and other regions**

M99.9 **Biomechanical lesion, unspecified**

Chapter 14: Diseases of the Genitourinary System (N00-N99)

DEFINITIONS

This chapter includes definitions of selected key words, terms and phrases and coding alerts for adding points to the clinical domain, and references to coding late effects where appropriate. An example from this chapter is as follows:

N03   Chronic nephritic syndrome
     Definition: Nephritic syndrome is a collection of signs associated with disorders affecting the kidneys, more specifically glomerular disorders.

MULTIPLE CODING FOR A SINGLE CONDITION

In addition to the etiology/manifestation convention that requires two codes to fully describe a single condition that affects multiple body systems, there are other single conditions that also require more than one code. "**Use Additional Code**" notes are found in the Tabular List at codes that are not part of an etiology/manifestation pair where a secondary code is useful to fully describe a condition. The sequencing rule is the same as the etiology/manifestation pair, "**Use Additional Code**" indicates that a secondary code should be added.

For example, for bacterial infections that are not included in chapter 1, a secondary code from category B95, Streptococcus, Staphylococcus, and Enterococcus, as the cause of diseases classified elsewhere, or B96, Other bacterial agents as the cause of diseases classified elsewhere, may be required to identify the bacterial organism causing the infection. A "**Use Additional Code**" note will normally be found at the infectious disease code, indicating a need for the organism code to be added as a secondary code.

"Code first" notes are also under certain codes that are not specifically manifestation codes but may be due to an underlying cause. When there is a "Code first" note and an underlying condition is present, the underlying condition should be sequenced first.

"Code, if applicable, any causal condition first", notes indicate that this code may be assigned as a principal diagnosis when the causal condition is unknown or not applicable. If a causal condition is known, then the code for that condition should be sequenced as the principal or first-listed diagnosis.

Multiple codes may be needed for sequela, complication codes and obstetric codes to more fully describe a condition. See the specific guidelines for these conditions for further instruction.

COMBINATION CODE

A combination code is a single code used to classify: Two diagnoses, or a diagnosis with an associated secondary process (manifestation) A diagnosis with an associated complication

Combination codes are identified by referring to subterm entries in the Alphabetic Index and by reading the inclusion and exclusion notes in the Tabular List.

Assign only the combination code when that code fully identifies the diagnostic conditions involved or when the Alphabetic Index so directs. Multiple coding should not be used when the classification provides a combination code that clearly identifies all of the elements documented in the diagnosis. When the combination code lacks necessary specificity in describing the manifestation or complication, an additional code should be used as a secondary code.

SEQUELA (LATE EFFECTS)

A sequela is the residual effect (condition produced) after the acute phase of an illness or injury has terminated. There is no time limit on when a sequela code can be used. The residual may be apparent early, such as in cerebral infarction, or it may occur months or years later, such as that due to a previous injury. Coding of sequela generally requires two codes sequenced in the following order: The condition or nature of the sequela is sequenced first.

The sequela code is sequenced second.

An exception to the above guidelines are those instances where the code for the sequela is followed by a manifestation code identified in the Tabular List and title, or the sequela code has been expanded (at the fourth, fifth or sixth character levels) to

include the manifestation(s). The code for the acute phase of an illness or injury that led to the sequela is never used with a code for the late effect.

CHRONIC KIDNEY DISEASE

1) Stages of chronic kidney disease (CKD)

The ICD-10-CM classifies CKD based on severity. The severity of CKD is designated by stages 1-5. Stage 2, code N18.2, equates to mild CKD; stage 3, code N18.3, equates to moderate CKD; and stage 4, code N18.4, equates to severe CKD. Code N18.6, End stage renal disease (ESRD), is assigned when the provider has documented end-stage-renal disease (ESRD).

If both a stage of CKD and ESRD are documented, assign code N18.6 only.

2) Chronic kidney disease and kidney transplant status

Patients who have undergone kidney transplant may still have some form of chronic kidney disease (CKD) because the kidney transplant may not fully restore kidney function. Therefore, the presence of CKD alone does not constitute a transplant complication. Assign the appropriate N18 code for the patient's stage of CKD and code Z94.0, Kidney transplant status. If a transplant complication such as failure or rejection or other transplant complication is documented, see section I.C.19.g for information on coding complications of a kidney transplant. If the documentation is unclear as to whether the patient has a complication of the transplant, query the provider.

3) Chronic kidney disease with other conditions

Patients with CKD may also suffer from other serious conditions, most commonly diabetes mellitus and hypertension. The sequencing of the CKD code in relationship to codes for other contributing conditions is based on the conventions in the Tabular List.

See I.C.9. Hypertensive chronic kidney disease.

See I.C.19. Chronic kidney disease and kidney transplant complications.

    ● New code   ▲ Revised code   **Excludes1:** Not coded here   **Excludes2:** Not included here   ⊗ Placeholder required   ⑦7th digit required

Chapter 14
Diseases of The Genitourinary System
(N00-N99)

Excludes2: certain conditions originating in the perinatal period (P04-P96)

certain infectious and parasitic diseases (A00-B99)

complications of pregnancy, childbirth and the puerperium (O00-O9A)

congenital malformations, deformations and chromosomal abnormalities (Q00-Q99)

endocrine, nutritional and metabolic diseases (E00-E88)

injury, poisoning and certain other consequences of external causes (S00-T88)

neoplasms (C00-D49)

symptoms, signs and abnormal clinical and laboratory findings, not elsewhere classified (R00-R94)

This chapter contains the following blocks: N00-N08 Glomerular diseases

N10-N16	Renal tubulo-interstitial diseases
N17-N19	Acute kidney failure and chronic kidney disease
N20-N23	Urolithiasis
N25-N29	Other disorders of kidney and ureter
N30-N39	Other diseases of the urinary system
N40-N53	Diseases of male genital organs
N60-N65	Disorders of breast
N70-N77	Inflammatory diseases of female pelvic organs
N80-N98	Noninflammatory disorders of female genital tract
N99	Intraoperative and postprocedural complications and disorders of genitourinary system, not elsewhere classified

GLOMERULAR DISEASES (N00-N08)

Definition: Glomerulonephritis is a form of nephritis with inflammation of the capillary loops in the renal glomeruli. The acute form is characterized by proteinuria, edema, hematuria, renal failure, and hypertension, sometimes preceded by tonsillitis or febrile pharyngitis.

Code also any associated kidney failure (N17-N19).

Excludes1: hypertensive chronic kidney disease (I12.-)

N00 **Acute nephritic syndrome**

Includes: acute glomerular disease

acute glomerulonephritis acute nephritis

Excludes1: acute tubulo-interstitial nephritis (N10)

nephritic syndrome NOS (N05.-)

N00.0 **Acute nephritic syndrome with minor glomerular abnormality**

Acute nephritic syndrome with minimal change lesion

N00.1 **Acute nephritic syndrome with focal and segmental glomerular lesions**

Acute nephritic syndrome with focal and segmental hyalinosis

Acute nephritic syndrome with focal and segmental sclerosis

Acute nephritic syndrome with focal glomerulonephritis

N00.2 **Acute nephritic syndrome with diffuse membranous glomerulonephritis**

N00.3 **Acute nephritic syndrome with diffuse mesangial proliferative glomerulonephritis**

N00.4 **Acute nephritic syndrome with diffuse endocapillary proliferative glomerulonephritis**

N00.5 **Acute nephritic syndrome with diffuse mesangiocapillary glomerulonephritis**

Acute nephritic syndrome with membranoproliferative glomerulonephritis, types 1 and 3, or NOS

Excludes1: Acute nephritic syndrome with C3 glomerulonephritis (N00.A)

Acute nephritic syndrome with C3 glomerulopathy (N00.A)

N00.6 **Acute nephritic syndrome with dense deposit disease**

Acute nephritic syndrome with C3 glomerulopathy, NOS

Acute nephritic syndrome with membranoproliferative glomerulonephritis, type 2

Excludes1: Acute nephritic syndrome (with C3 glomerulopathy) with dense deposit disease(N00.6)

N00.7 **Acute nephritic syndrome with diffuse crescentic glomerulonephritis**

Acute nephritic syndrome with extracapillary glomerulonephritis

N00.8 **Acute nephritic syndrome with other morphologic changes**

Acute nephritic syndrome with proliferative glomerulonephritis NOS

N00.9 **Acute nephritic syndrome with unspecified morphologic changes**

N01 **Rapidly progressive nephritic syndrome**

Includes: rapidly progressive glomerular disease

rapidly progressive glomerulonephritis rapidly progressive nephritis

Excludes1: nephritic syndrome NOS (N05.-)

N01.0 **Rapidly progressive nephritic syndrome with minor glomerular abnormality**

Rapidly progressive nephritic syndrome with minimal change lesion

N01.1 **Rapidly progressive nephritic syndrome with focal and segmental glomerular lesions**

Rapidly progressive nephritic syndrome with focal and segmental hyalinosis

Rapidly progressive nephritic syndrome with focal and segmental sclerosis

Rapidly progressive nephritic syndrome with focal glomerulonephritis

N01.2 **Rapidly progressive nephritic syndrome with diffuse membranous glomerulonephritis**

N01.3 **Rapidly progressive nephritic syndrome with diffuse mesangial proliferative glomerulonephritis**

N01.4 **Rapidly progressive nephritic syndrome with diffuse endocapillary proliferative glomerulonephritis**

N01.5 **Rapidly progressive nephritic syndrome with diffuse mesangiocapillary glomerulonephritis**

Rapidly progressive nephritic syndrome with membranoproliferative glomerulonephritis, types 1 and 3, or NOS

Excludes1: Rapidly progressive nephritic syndrome with C3 glomerulonephritis (N01.A)

Rapidly progressive nephritic syndrome with C3 glomerulopathy (N01.A)

N01.6 **Rapidly progressive nephritic syndrome with dense deposit disease**

Rapidly progressive nephritic syndrome with C3 glomerulopathy with dense deposit disease

Rapidly progressive nephritic syndrome with membranoproliferative glomerulonephritis, type 2

N01.7 **Rapidly progressive nephritic syndrome with diffuse crescentic glomerulonephritis**

Rapidly progressive nephritic syndrome with extracapillary glomerulonephritis

N01.8 **Rapidly progressive nephritic syndrome with other morphologic changes**

Rapidly progressive nephritic syndrome with proliferative glomerulonephritis NOS

N01.9 **Rapidly progressive nephritic syndrome with unspecified morphologic changes**

N01.A **Rapidly progressive nephritic syndrome with C3 glomerulonephritis**

Rapidly progressive nephritic syndrome with C3 glomerulopathy, NOS

Excludes1: Rapidly progressive nephritic syndrome (with C3 glomerulopathy) with dense deposit disease (N01.6)

N02 **Recurrent and persistent hematuria**

Excludes1: acute cystitis with hematuria (N30.01)

hematuria NOS (R31.9)

hematuria not associated with specified morphologic lesions (R31.-)

N02.0 **Recurrent and persistent hematuria with minor glomerular abnormality**

Recurrent and persistent hematuria with minimal change lesion

N02.1 **Recurrent and persistent hematuria with focal and segmental glomerular lesions**

Recurrent and persistent hematuria with focal and segmental hyalinosis

Recurrent and persistent hematuria with focal and segmental sclerosis

Recurrent and persistent hematuria with focal glomerulonephritis

N02.2 **Recurrent and persistent hematuria with diffuse membranous glomerulonephritis**

N02.3 **Recurrent and persistent hematuria with diffuse mesangial proliferative glomerulonephritis**

N02.4 **Recurrent and persistent hematuria with diffuse endocapillary proliferative glomerulonephritis**

N02.5 **Recurrent and persistent hematuria with diffuse mesangiocapillary glomerulonephritis**

Recurrent and persistent hematuria with membranoproliferative glomerulonephritis, types 1 and 3, or NOS

Excludes1: Recurrent and persistent hematuria with C3 glomerulonephritis (N02.A)

Recurrent and persistent hematuria with C3 glomerulopathy (N02.A)

N02.6 **Recurrent and persistent hematuria with dense deposit disease**

Recurrent and persistent hematuria with C3 glomerulopathy with dense deposit disease

Recurrent and persistent hematuria with membranoproliferative glomerulonephritis, type 2

N02.7 **Recurrent and persistent hematuria with diffuse crescentic glomerulonephritis**

Recurrent and persistent hematuria with extracapillary glomerulonephritis

N02.8 **Recurrent and persistent hematuria with other morphologic changes**

Recurrent and persistent hematuria with proliferative glomerulonephritis NOS

N02.9 **Recurrent and persistent hematuria with unspecified morphologic changes**

N03 **Chronic nephritic syndrome**

Definition: Nephritic syndrome is a collection of signs associated with disorders affecting the kidneys, more specifically glomerular disorders.

Includes: chronic glomerular disease

chronic glomerulonephritis chronic nephritis

Excludes1: chronic tubulo-interstitial nephritis (N11.-)

diffuse sclerosing glomerulonephritis (N05.8-)

nephritic syndrome NOS (N05.-)

N03.0 **Chronic nephritic syndrome with minor glomerular abnormality**

Chronic nephritic syndrome with minimal change lesion

N03.1 **Chronic nephritic syndrome with focal and segmental glomerular lesions**

Chronic nephritic syndrome with focal and segmental hyalinosis

Chronic nephritic syndrome with focal and segmental sclerosis

Chronic nephritic syndrome with focal glomerulonephritis

N03.2 **Chronic nephritic syndrome with diffuse membranous glomerulonephritis**

N03.3 **Chronic nephritic syndrome with diffuse mesangial proliferative glomerulonephritis**

N03.4 **Chronic nephritic syndrome with diffuse endocapillary proliferative glomerulonephritis**

N03.5 **Chronic nephritic syndrome with diffuse mesangiocapillary glomerulonephritis**

Chronic nephritic syndrome with membranoproliferative glomerulonephritis, types 1 and 3, or NOS

Excludes1: Chronic nephritic syndrome with C3 glomerulonephritis (N03.A)

Chronic nephritic syndrome with C3 glomerulopathy (N03.A)

N03.6 **Chronic nephritic syndrome with dense deposit disease**

Chronic nephritic syndrome with C3 glomerulopathy with dense deposit disease

Chronic nephritic syndrome with membranoproliferative glomerulonephritis, type 2

N03.7 **Chronic nephritic syndrome with diffuse crescentic glomerulonephritis**

Chronic nephritic syndrome with extracapillary glomerulonephritis

N03.8 **Chronic nephritic syndrome with other morphologic changes**

Chronic nephritic syndrome with proliferative glomerulonephritis NOS

N03.9 **Chronic nephritic syndrome with unspecified morphologic changes**

N03.A **Chronic nephritic syndrome with C3 glomerulonephritis**

Chronic nephritic syndrome with C3 glomerulopathy

Excludes1: Chronic nephritic syndrome (with C3 glomerulopathy) with dense deposit disease(N03.6)

N04 **Nephrotic syndrome**

Definition: Nephrotic syndrome is a collection of symptoms which occur because the glomeruli (tiny blood vessels) in the kidney become leaky. This allows protein, normally never passed out in the urine, to leave the body in large amounts.

Includes: congenital nephrotic syndrome

lipoid nephrosis

N04.0 **Nephrotic syndrome with minor glomerular abnormality**

Nephrotic syndrome with minimal change lesion

N04.1 **Nephrotic syndrome with focal and segmental glomerular lesions**

Nephrotic syndrome with focal and segmental hyalinosis

Nephrotic syndrome with focal and segmental sclerosis

Nephrotic syndrome with focal glomerulonephritis

N04.2 **Nephrotic syndrome with diffuse membranous glomerulonephritis**

N04.3 **Nephrotic syndrome with diffuse mesangial proliferative glomerulonephritis**

N04.4 **Nephrotic syndrome with diffuse endocapillary proliferative glomerulonephritis**

N04.5 **Nephrotic syndrome with diffuse mesangiocapillary glomerulonephritis**

Nephrotic syndrome with membranoproliferative glomerulonephritis, types 1 and 3, or NOS

Excludes1: Nephrotic syndrome with C3 glomerulonephritis (N04.A)

Nephrotic syndrome with C3 glomerulopathy (N04.A)

N04.6 **Nephrotic syndrome with dense deposit disease**

Nephrotic syndrome with C3 glomerulopathy with dense deposit disease

Nephrotic syndrome with membranoproliferative glomerulonephritis, type 2

N04.7 **Nephrotic syndrome with diffuse crescentic glomerulonephritis**

Nephrotic syndrome with extracapillary glomerulonephritis

N04.8 **Nephrotic syndrome with other morphologic changes**

Nephrotic syndrome with proliferative glomerulonephritis NOS

N04.9 **Nephrotic syndrome with unspecified morphologic changes**

N04.A **Nephrotic syndrome with C3 glomerulonephritis**

Nephrotic syndrome with C3 glomerulopathy

Excludes1: Nephrotic syndrome (with C3 glomerulopathy) with dense deposit disease (N04.6)

N05 **Unspecified nephritic syndrome**

Includes: glomerular disease NOS

glomerulonephritis NOS nephritis NOS

nephropathy NOS and renal disease NOS with morphological lesion specified in .0-.8

Excludes1: nephropathy NOS with no stated morphological lesion (N28.9)

renal disease NOS with no stated morphological lesion (N28.9)

tubulo-interstitial nephritis NOS (N12)

N05.0 **Unspecified nephritic syndrome with minor glomerular abnormality**

Unspecified nephritic syndrome with minimal change lesion

N05.1 **Unspecified nephritic syndrome with focal and segmental glomerular lesions**

Unspecified nephritic syndrome with focal and segmental hyalinosis

Unspecified nephritic syndrome with focal and segmental sclerosis

Unspecified nephritic syndrome with focal glomerulonephritis

N05.2 **Unspecified nephritic syndrome with diffuse membranous glomerulonephritis**

N05.3 **Unspecified nephritic syndrome with diffuse mesangial proliferative glomerulonephritis**

N05.4 **Unspecified nephritic syndrome with diffuse endocapillary proliferative glomerulonephritis**

N05.5 **Unspecified nephritic syndrome with diffuse mesangiocapillary glomerulonephritis**

Unspecified nephritic syndrome with membranoproliferative glomerulonephritis, types 1 and 3, or NOS

Excludes1: Unspecified nephritic syndrome with C3 glomerulonephritis (N05.A)

Unspecified nephritic syndrome with C3 glomerulopathy (N05.A)

N05.6 **Unspecified nephritic syndrome with dense deposit disease**

Unspecified nephritic syndrome with C3 glomerulopathy with dense deposit disease

Unspecified nephritic syndrome with membranoproliferative glomerulonephritis, type 2

N05.7 **Unspecified nephritic syndrome with diffuse crescentic glomerulonephritis**

Unspecified nephritic syndrome with extracapillary glomerulonephritis

N05.8 **Unspecified nephritic syndrome with other morphologic changes**

Unspecified nephritic syndrome with proliferative glomerulonephritis NOS

N05.9 **Unspecified nephritic syndrome with unspecified morphologic changes**

N05.A **Unspecified nephritic syndrome with C3 glomerulonephritis**

Unspecified nephritic syndrome with C3 glomerulopathy

Excludes1: Unspecified nephritic syndrome (with C3 glomerulopathy) with dense deposit disease(N05.6)

N06 **Isolated proteinuria with specified morphological lesion**

Excludes1: Proteinuria not associated with specific morphologic lesions (R80.0)

N06.0 **Isolated proteinuria with minor glomerular abnormality**

Isolated proteinuria with minimal change lesion

N06.1 **Isolated proteinuria with focal and segmental glomerular lesions**

Isolated proteinuria with focal and segmental hyalinosis

Isolated proteinuria with focal and segmental sclerosis

Isolated proteinuria with focal glomerulonephritis

N06.2 **Isolated proteinuria with diffuse membranous glomerulonephritis**

N06.3 **Isolated proteinuria with diffuse mesangial proliferative glomerulonephritis**

N06.4 **Isolated proteinuria with diffuse endocapillary proliferative glomerulonephritis**

N06.5 **Isolated proteinuria with diffuse mesangiocapillary glomerulonephritis**

Isolated proteinuria with membranoproliferative glomerulonephritis, types 1 and 3, or NOS

Excludes1: Isolated proteinuria with C3 glomerulonephritis (N06.A)

Isolated proteinuria with C3 glomerulopathy (N06.A)

N06.6 **Isolated proteinuria with dense deposit disease**

Isolated proteinuria with C3 glomerulopathy with dense deposit disease

Isolated proteinuria with membranoproliferative glomerulonephritis, type 2

N06.7 **Isolated proteinuria with diffuse crescentic glomerulonephritis**

Isolated proteinuria with extracapillary glomerulonephritis

N06.8 **Isolated proteinuria with other morphologic lesion**

Isolated proteinuria with proliferative glomerulonephritis NOS

N06.9 **Isolated proteinuria with unspecified morphologic lesion**

N06.A **Isolated proteinuria with C3 glomerulonephritis**

Isolated proteinuria with C3 glomerulopathy

Excludes1: Isolated proteinuria (with C3 glomerulopathy) with dense deposit disease (N06.6)

N07 **Hereditary nephropathy, not elsewhere classified**

Excludes2: Alport's syndrome (Q87.81-)

hereditary amyloid nephropathy (E85.-)

nail patella syndrome (Q87.2)

non-neuropathic heredofamilial amyloidosis (E85.-)

N07.0 **Hereditary nephropathy, not elsewhere classified with minor glomerular abnormality**

Hereditary nephropathy, not elsewhere classified with minimal change lesion

N07.1 **Hereditary nephropathy, not elsewhere classified with focal and segmental glomerular lesions**

Hereditary nephropathy, not elsewhere classified with focal and segmental hyalinosis

Hereditary nephropathy, not elsewhere classified with focal and segmental sclerosis

Hereditary nephropathy, not elsewhere classified with focal glomerulonephritis

N07.2 **Hereditary nephropathy, not elsewhere classified with diffuse membranous glomerulonephritis**

N07.3 **Hereditary nephropathy, not elsewhere classified with diffuse mesangial proliferative glomerulonephritis**

N07.4 **Hereditary nephropathy, not elsewhere classified with diffuse endocapillary proliferative glomerulonephritis**

N07.5 **Hereditary nephropathy, not elsewhere classified with diffuse mesangiocapillary glomerulonephritis**

Hereditary nephropathy, not elsewhere classified with membranoproliferative glomerulonephritis, types 1 and 3, or NOS

Excludes1: Hereditary nephropathy, not elsewhere classified with C3 glomerulonephritis (N07.A)

Hereditary nephropathy, not elsewhere classified with C3 glomerulopathy (N07.A)

N07.6 **Hereditary nephropathy, not elsewhere classified with dense deposit disease**

Hereditary nephropathy, not elsewhere classified with C3 glomerulopathy with dense deposit disease

Hereditary nephropathy, not elsewhere classified with membranoproliferative glomerulonephritis, type 2

N07.7 **Hereditary nephropathy, not elsewhere classified with diffuse crescentic glomerulonephritis**

Hereditary nephropathy, not elsewhere classified with extracapillary glomerulonephritis

N07.8 **Hereditary nephropathy, not elsewhere classified with other morphologic lesions**

Hereditary nephropathy, not elsewhere classified with proliferative glomerulonephritis NOS

N07.9 **Hereditary nephropathy, not elsewhere classified with unspecified morphologic lesions**

N07.A **Hereditary nephropathy, not elsewhere classified with C3 glomerulonephritis**

Hereditary nephropathy, not elsewhere classified with C3 glomerulopathy

Excludes1: Hereditary nephropathy, not elsewhere classified (with C3 glomerulopathy) with dense deposit disease (N07.6)

N08 **Glomerular disorders in diseases classified elsewhere**

Glomerulonephritis Nephritis Nephropathy

Code first underlying disease, such as:

amyloidosis (E85.-)

congenital syphilis (A50.5)

cryoglobulinemia (D89.1)

disseminated intravascular coagulation (D65)

gout (M1A.-, M10.-)

microscopic polyangiitis (M31.7)

multiple myeloma (C90.0-)

sepsis (A40.0-A41.9)

sickle-cell disease (D57.0-D57.8)

Excludes1: glomerulonephritis, nephritis and nephropathy (in):

antiglomerular basement membrane disease (M31.0)

diabetes (E08-E13 with .21)

gonococcal (A54.21)

Goodpasture's syndrome (M31.0)

hemolytic-uremic syndrome (D59.3)

lupus (M32.14)

mumps (B26.83)

syphilis (A52.75)

systemic lupus erythematosus (M32.14)

Wegener's granulomatosis (M31.31)

pyelonephritis in diseases classified elsewhere (N16)

renal tubulo-interstitial disorders classified elsewhere (N16)

RENAL TUBULO-INTERSTITIAL DISEASES (N10-N16)

Includes: pyelonephritis

Excludes1: pyeloureteritis cystica (N28.85)

N10 **Acute pyelonephritis**

Acute infectious interstitial nephritis

Acute pyelitis

Acute tubulo-interstitial nephritis

Hemoglobin nephrosis

Myoglobin nephrosis

Use Additional Code (B95-B97), to identify infectious agent.

N11 **Chronic tubulo-interstitial nephritis**

Includes: chronic infectious interstitial nephritis

chronic pyelitis chronic pyelonephritis

Use Additional Code (B95-B97), to identify infectious agent.

N11.0 **Nonobstructive reflux-associated chronic pyelonephritis**

Pyelonephritis (chronic) associated with (vesicoureteral) reflux

Excludes1: vesicoureteral reflux NOS (N13.70)

N11.1 **Chronic obstructive pyelonephritis**

Pyelonephritis (chronic) associated with anomaly of pelviureteric junction

Pyelonephritis (chronic) associated with anomaly of pyeloureteric junction

Pyelonephritis (chronic) associated with crossing of vessel

Pyelonephritis (chronic) associated with kinking of ureter

Pyelonephritis (chronic) associated with obstruction of ureter

Pyelonephritis (chronic) associated with stricture of pelviureteric junction

Pyelonephritis (chronic) associated with stricture of ureter

Excludes1: calculous pyelonephritis (N20.9)

obstructive uropathy (N13.-)

N11.8 **Other chronic tubulo-interstitial nephritis**

Nonobstructive chronic pyelonephritis NOS

N11.9 **Chronic tubulo-interstitial nephritis, unspecified**

Chronic interstitial nephritis NOS

● New code ▲ Revised code **Excludes1:** Not coded here **Excludes2:** Not included here ⊗ Placeholder required ⑦ 7th digit required

Chronic pyelitis NOS

Chronic pyelonephritis NOS

N12 **Tubulo-interstitial nephritis, not specified as acute or chronic**

Interstitial nephritis NOS

Pyelitis NOS

Pyelonephritis NOS

Excludes1: calculous pyelonephritis (N20.9)

N13 **Obstructive and reflux uropathy**

Excludes2: calculus of kidney and ureter without hydronephrosis (N20.-)

congenital obstructive defects of renal pelvis and ureter (Q62.0-Q62.3)

hydronephrosis with ureteropelvic junction obstruction (Q62.11)

obstructive pyelonephritis (N11.1)

N13.0 **Hydronephrosis with ureteropelvic junction obstruction**

Definition: Hydronephrosis is a condition that occurs as a result of urine accumulation in the upper urinary tract. This usually occurs from a blockage somewhere along the urinary tract.

Hydronephrosis due to acquired occlusion of ureteropelvic junction

Excludes2: Hydronephrosis with ureteropelvic junction obstruction due to calculus (N13.2)

N13.1 **Hydronephrosis with ureteral stricture, not elsewhere classified**

Excludes1: Hydronephrosis with ureteral stricture with infection (N13.6)

N13.2 **Hydronephrosis with renal and ureteral calculous obstruction**

Excludes1: Hydronephrosis with renal and ureteral calculous obstruction with infection (N13.6)

N13.3 **Other and unspecified hydronephrosis**

Excludes1: hydronephrosis with infection (N13.6)

N13.30 **Unspecified hydronephrosis**

N13.39 **Other hydronephrosis**

N13.4 **Hydroureter**

Excludes1: congenital hydroureter (Q62.3-)

hydroureter with infection (N13.6)

vesicoureteral-reflux with hydroureter (N13.73-)

N13.5 **Crossing vessel and stricture of ureter without hydronephrosis**

Kinking and stricture of ureter without hydronephrosis

Excludes1: Crossing vessel and stricture of ureter without hydronephrosis with infection (N13.6)

N13.6 **Pyonephrosis**

Conditions in N13.0-N13.5 with infection

Obstructive uropathy with infection

Use Additional Code (B95-B97), to identify infectious agent.

N13.7 **Vesicoureteral-reflux**

Excludes1: reflux-associated pyelonephritis (N11.0)

N13.70 **Vesicoureteral-reflux, unspecified**

Vesicoureteral-reflux NOS

N13.71 **Vesicoureteral-reflux without reflux nephropathy**

N13.72 **Vesicoureteral-reflux with reflux nephropathy without hydroureter**

N13.721 **Vesicoureteral-reflux with reflux nephropathy without hydroureter, unilateral**

N13.722 **Vesicoureteral-reflux with reflux nephropathy without hydroureter, bilateral**

N13.729 **Vesicoureteral-reflux with reflux nephropathy without hydroureter, unspecified**

N13.731 **Vesicoureteral-reflux with reflux nephropathy with hydroureter, unilateral**

N13.732 **Vesicoureteral-reflux with reflux nephropathy with hydroureter, bilateral**

N13.739 **Vesicoureteral-reflux with reflux nephropathy with hydroureter, unspecified**

N13.8 **Other obstructive and reflux uropathy**

Urinary tract obstruction due to specified cause

Code first, if applicable, any causal condition, such as:

enlarged prostate (N40.1)

N13.9 **Obstructive and reflux uropathy, unspecified**

Urinary tract obstruction NOS

N14 **Drug- and heavy-metal-induced tubulo-interstitial and tubular conditions**

Code first poisoning due to drug or toxin, if applicable (T36-T65 with fifth or sixth character 1-4 or 6)

Use Additional Code for adverse effect, if applicable, to identify drug (T36-T50 with fifth or sixth character 5)

N14.0 **Analgesic nephropathy**

N14.1 **Nephropathy induced by other drugs, medicaments and biological substances**

N14.2 **Nephropathy induced by unspecified drug, medicament or biological substance**

N14.3 **Nephropathy induced by heavy metals**

N14.4 **Toxic nephropathy, not elsewhere classified**

N15 **Other renal tubulo-interstitial diseases**

N15.0 **Balkan nephropathy**

Balkan endemic nephropathy

N15.1 **Renal and perinephric abscess**

N15.8 **Other specified renal tubulo-interstitial diseases**

N15.9 **Renal tubulo-interstitial disease, unspecified**

Infection of kidney NOS

Excludes1: urinary tract infection NOS (N39.0)

N16 **Renal tubulo-interstitial disorders in diseases classified elsewhere**

Pyelonephritis

Tubulo-interstitial nephritis

Code first underlying disease, such as:

brucellosis (A23.0-A23.9)

cryoglobulinemia (D89.1)

glycogen storage disease (E74.0)

leukemia (C91-C95)

lymphoma (C81.0-C85.9, C96.0-C96.9)

multiple myeloma (C90.0-)

sepsis (A40.0-A41.9)

Wilson's disease (E83.0)

Excludes1: diphtheritic pyelonephritis and tubulo-interstitial nephritis (A36.84)

pyelonephritis and tubulo-interstitial nephritis in candidiasis (B37.49) pyelonephritis and tubulo-interstitial nephritis in cystinosis (E72.04)

pyelonephritis and tubulo-interstitial nephritis in salmonella infection (A02.25)

pyelonephritis and tubulo-interstitial nephritis in sarcoidosis (D86.84)

pyelonephritis and tubulo-interstitial nephritis in Sjogren's syndrome (M35.04)

pyelonephritis and tubulo-interstitial nephritis in systemic lupus erythematosus (M32.15)

pyelonephritis and tubulo-interstitial nephritis in toxoplasmosis (B58.83)

renal tubular degeneration in diabetes (E08-E13 with .29)

syphilitic pyelonephritis and tubulo-interstitial nephritis (A52.75)

ACUTE KIDNEY FAILURE AND CHRONIC KIDNEY DISEASE (N17-N19)

Excludes2: congenital renal failure (P96.0)

drug- and heavy-metal-induced tubulo-interstitial and tubular conditions (N14.-)

extrarenal uremia (R39.2)

hemolytic-uremic syndrome (D59.3)

hepatorenal syndrome (K76.7)

postpartum hepatorenal syndrome (O90.4)

posttraumatic renal failure (T79.5)

prerenal uremia (R39.2)

renal failure complicating abortion or ectopic or molar pregnancy (O00-O07, O08.4)

renal failure following labor and delivery (O90.4)

renal failure postprocedural (N99.0)

N17   Acute kidney failure

Code also associated underlying condition

Excludes1: posttraumatic renal failure (T79.5)

N17.0   Acute kidney failure with tubular necrosis [HCC]

Acute tubular necrosis

Renal tubular necrosis

Tubular necrosis NOS

N17.1   Acute kidney failure with acute cortical necrosis [HCC]

Acute cortical necrosis

Cortical necrosis NOS

Renal cortical necrosis

N17.2   Acute kidney failure with medullary necrosis [HCC]

Medullary [papillary] necrosis NOS

Acute medullary [papillary] necrosis

Renal medullary [papillary] necrosis

N17.8   Other acute kidney failure [HCC]

N17.9   Acute kidney failure, unspecified [HCC]

Acute kidney injury (nontraumatic)

Excludes2: traumatic kidney injury (S37.0-)

N18   Chronic kidney disease (CKD)

Definition: Chronic kidney disease (CKD), aka chronic renal disease, is a progressive loss of renal function over a period of months or years.

Code first any associated:

diabetic chronic kidney disease (E08.22, E09.22, E10.22, E11.22, E13.22)

hypertensive chronic kidney disease (I12.-, I13.-)

Use Additional Code to identify kidney transplant status, if applicable, (Z94.0)

N18.1   Chronic kidney disease, stage 1

N18.2   Chronic kidney disease, stage 2 (mild)

N18.3   Chronic kidney disease, stage 3 (moderate) [HCC]

N18.30   Chronic kidney disease, stage 3 unspecified

N18.31   Chronic kidney disease, stage 3a

N18.32   Chronic kidney disease, stage 3b

N18.4   Chronic kidney disease, stage 4 (severe) [HCC]

N18.5   Chronic kidney disease, stage 5 [HCC]

Excludes1: chronic kidney disease, stage 5 requiring chronic dialysis (N18.6)

N18.6   End stage renal disease [HCC]

Chronic kidney disease requiring chronic dialysis

Use Additional Code to identify dialysis status (Z99.2)

N18.9   Chronic kidney disease, unspecified

Chronic renal disease

Chronic renal failure NOS

Chronic renal insufficiency

Chronic uremia NOS

Diffuse sclerosing glomerulonephritis NOS

N19   Unspecified kidney failure

Uremia NOS

Excludes1: acute kidney failure (N17.-)

chronic kidney disease (N18.-)

chronic uremia (N18.9)

extrarenal uremia (R39.2)

prerenal uremia (R39.2)

renal insufficiency (acute) (N28.9)

uremia of newborn (P96.0)

UROLITHIASIS (N20-N23)

N20   Calculus of kidney and ureter

Calculous pyelonephritis

Excludes1: nephrocalcinosis (E83.5)

that with hydronephrosis (N13.2)

N20.0   Calculus of kidney

Nephrolithiasis NOS

Renal calculus

Renal stone

Staghorn calculus

Stone in kidney

Calculus of the ureteropelvic junction

N20.1   Calculus of ureter

Ureteric stone

N20.2   Calculus of kidney with calculus of ureter

N20.9   Urinary calculus, unspecified

N21   Calculus of lower urinary tract

Includes: calculus of lower urinary tract with cystitis and urethritis

N21.0   Calculus in bladder

Calculus in diverticulum of bladder

Urinary bladder stone

Excludes2: staghorn calculus (N20.0)

N21.1   Calculus in urethra

Excludes2: calculus of prostate (N42.0)

N21.8   Other lower urinary tract calculus

N21.9 **Calculus of lower urinary tract, unspecified**

Excludes1: calculus of urinary tract NOS (N20.9)

N22 **Calculus of urinary tract in diseases classified elsewhere**

Code first underlying disease, such as:

gout (M1A.-, M10.-)

schistosomiasis (B65.0-B65.9)

N23 **Unspecified renal colic**

OTHER DISORDERS OF KIDNEY AND URETER (N25-N29)

Excludes2: disorders of kidney and ureter with urolithiasis (N20-N23)

N25 **Disorders resulting from impaired renal tubular function**

N25.0 **Renal osteodystrophy**

Azotemic osteodystrophy

Phosphate-losing tubular disorders

Renal rickets

Renal short stature

Excludes2: metabolic disorders classifiable to E70-E88

N25.1 **Nephrogenic diabetes insipidus** [HCC]

Excludes1: diabetes insipidus NOS (E23.2)

N25.8 **Other disorders resulting from impaired renal tubular function**

N25.81 **Secondary hyperparathyroidism of renal origin** [HCC]

Excludes1: secondary hyperparathyroidism, non-renal (E21.1)

Excludes2: metabolic disorders classifiable to E70-E88

N25.89 **Other disorders resulting from impaired renal tubular function**

Hypokalemic nephropathy

Lightwood-Albright syndrome

Renal tubular acidosis NOS

N25.9 **Disorder resulting from impaired renal tubular function, unspecified**

N26 **Unspecified contracted kidney**

Excludes1: contracted kidney due to hypertension (I12.-)

diffuse sclerosing glomerulonephritis (N05.8.-)

hypertensive nephrosclerosis (arteriolar) (arteriosclerotic) (I12.-)

small kidney of unknown cause (N27.-)

N26.1 **Atrophy of kidney (terminal)**

N26.2 **Page kidney**

N26.9 **Renal sclerosis, unspecified**

N27 **Small kidney of unknown cause**

Includes: oligonephronia

N27.0 **Small kidney, unilateral**

N27.1 **Small kidney, bilateral**

N27.9 **Small kidney, unspecified**

N28 **Other disorders of kidney and ureter, not elsewhere classified**

N28.0 **Ischemia and infarction of kidney** [HCC]

Renal artery embolism

Renal artery obstruction

Renal artery occlusion

Renal artery thrombosis

Renal infarct

Excludes1: atherosclerosis of renal artery (extrarenal part) (I70.1)

congenital stenosis of renal artery (Q27.1)

Goldblatt's kidney (I70.1)

N28.1 **Cyst of kidney, acquired**

Cyst (multiple) (solitary) of kidney, acquired

Excludes1: cystic kidney disease (congenital) (Q61.-)

N28.8 **Other specified disorders of kidney and ureter**

Excludes1: hydroureter (N13.4)

ureteric stricture with hydronephrosis (N13.1)

ureteric stricture without hydronephrosis (N13.5)

N28.81 **Hypertrophy of kidney**

N28.82 **Megaloureter**

N28.83 **Nephroptosis**

N28.84 **Pyelitis cystica**

N28.85 **Pyeloureteritis cystica**

N28.86 **Ureteritis cystica**

N28.89 **Other specified disorders of kidney and ureter**

N28.9 **Disorder of kidney and ureter, unspecified**

Nephropathy NOS

Renal disease (acute) NOS

Renal insufficiency (acute)

Excludes1: chronic renal insufficiency (N18.9)

unspecified nephritic syndrome (N05.-)

N29 **Other disorders of kidney and ureter in diseases classified elsewhere**

Code first underlying disease, such as:

amyloidosis (E85.-)

nephrocalcinosis (E83.5)

schistosomiasis (B65.0-B65.9)

Excludes1: disorders of kidney and ureter in:

cystinosis (E72.0)

gonorrhea (A54.21)

syphilis (A52.75)

tuberculosis (A18.11)

OTHER DISEASES OF THE URINARY SYSTEM (N30-N39)

Excludes2: urinary infection (complicating):

abortion or ectopic or molar pregnancy (O00-O07, O08.8)

pregnancy, childbirth and the puerperium (O23.-, O75.3, O86.2-)

N30 **Cystitis**

Use Additional Code to identify infectious agent (B95-B97)

Excludes1: prostatocystitis (N41.3)

N30.0 **Acute cystitis**

Excludes1: irradiation cystitis (N30.4-)

trigonitis (N30.3-)

N30.00 **Acute cystitis without hematuria**

N30.01 **Acute cystitis with hematuria**

N30.1 **Interstitial cystitis (chronic)**

N30.10 **Interstitial cystitis (chronic) without hematuria**

N30.11 **Interstitial cystitis (chronic) with hematuria**

N30.2 **Other chronic cystitis**

N30.20 **Other chronic cystitis without hematuria**

N30.21 **Other chronic cystitis with hematuria**

N30.3 **Trigonitis**

Urethrotrigonitis

N30.30 **Trigonitis without hematuria**

N30.31 **Trigonitis with hematuria**

N30.4 **Irradiation cystitis**

N30.40   **Irradiation cystitis without hematuria**

N30.41   **Irradiation cystitis with hematuria**

N30.8   **Other cystitis**

Abscess of bladder

N30.80   **Other cystitis without hematuria**

N30.81   **Other cystitis with hematuria**

N30.9   **Cystitis, unspecified**

N30.90   **Cystitis, unspecified without hematuria**

N30.91   **Cystitis, unspecified with hematuria**

N31   **Neuromuscular dysfunction of bladder, not elsewhere classified**

Use Additional Code to identify any associated urinary incontinence (N39.3-N39.4-)

Excludes1: cord bladder NOS (G95.89)

neurogenic bladder due to cauda equina syndrome (G83.4)

neuromuscular dysfunction due to spinal cord lesion (G95.89)

N31.0   **Uninhibited neuropathic bladder, not elsewhere classified**

N31.1   **Reflex neuropathic bladder, not elsewhere classified**

N31.2   **Flaccid neuropathic bladder, not elsewhere classified**

Atonic (motor) (sensory) neuropathic bladder

Autonomous neuropathic bladder

Nonreflex neuropathic bladder

N31.8   **Other neuromuscular dysfunction of bladder**

N31.9   **Neuromuscular dysfunction of bladder, unspecified**

Neurogenic bladder dysfunction NOS

N32   **Other disorders of bladder**

Excludes2: calculus of bladder (N21.0)

cystocele (N81.1-)

hernia or prolapse of bladder, female (N81.1-)

N32.0   **Bladder-neck obstruction**

Bladder-neck stenosis (acquired)

Excludes1: congenital bladder-neck obstruction (Q64.3-)

N32.1   **Vesicointestinal fistula**

Vesicorectal fistula

N32.2   **Vesical fistula, not elsewhere classified**

Excludes1: fistula between bladder and female genital tract (N82.0-N82.1)

N32.3   **Diverticulum of bladder**

Excludes1: congenital diverticulum of bladder (Q64.6)

diverticulitis of bladder (N30.8-)

N32.8   **Other specified disorders of bladder**

N32.81   **Overactive bladder**

Detrusor muscle hyperactivity

Excludes1: frequent urination due to specified bladder condition- code to condition

N32.89   **Other specified disorders of bladder**

Bladder hemorrhage

Bladder hypertrophy

Calcified bladder

Contracted bladder

N32.9   **Bladder disorder, unspecified**

N33   **Bladder disorders in diseases classified elsewhere**

Code first underlying disease, such as:

schistosomiasis (B65.0-B65.9)

Excludes1: bladder disorder in syphilis (A52.76)

bladder disorder in tuberculosis (A18.12)

candidal cystitis (B37.41)

chlamydial cystitis (A56.01)

cystitis in gonorrhea (A54.01)

cystitis in neurogenic bladder (N31.-)

diphtheritic cystitis (A36.85)

syphilitic cystitis (A52.76)

trichomonal cystitis (A59.03)

N34   **Urethritis and urethral syndrome**

Use Additional Code (B95-B97), to identify infectious agent.

Excludes2: Reiter's disease (M02.3-)

urethritis in diseases with a predominantly sexual mode of transmission (A50-A64)

urethrotrigonitis (N30.3-)

N34.0   **Urethral abscess**

Abscess (of) Cowper's gland

Abscess (of) Littre's gland

Abscess (of) urethral (gland)

Periurethral abscess

Excludes1: urethral caruncle (N36.2)

N34.1   **Nonspecific urethritis**

Nongonococcal urethritis Nonvenereal urethritis

N34.2   **Other urethritis**

Meatitis, urethral

Postmenopausal urethritis

Ulcer of urethra (meatus)

Urethritis NOS

N34.3   **Urethral syndrome, unspecified**

N35   **Urethral stricture**

Excludes1: congenital urethral stricture (Q64.3-)

postprocedural urethral stricture (N99.1-)

N35.0   **Post-traumatic urethral stricture**

Urethral stricture due to injury

Excludes1: postprocedural urethral stricture (N99.1-)

N35.01   **Post-traumatic urethral stricture, male**

N35.010   **Post-traumatic urethral stricture, male, meatal**

N35.011   **Post-traumatic bulbous urethral stricture**

N35.012   **Post-traumatic membranous urethral stricture**

N35.013   **Post-traumatic anterior urethral stricture**

N35.014   **Post-traumatic urethral stricture, male, unspecified**

N35.016   **Post-traumatic urethral stricture, male, overlapping sites**

N35.02   **Post-traumatic urethral stricture, female**

N35.021   **Urethral stricture due to childbirth**

N35.028   **Other post-traumatic urethral stricture, female**

N35.1   **Postinfective urethral stricture, not elsewhere classified**

Excludes1: urethral stricture associated with schistosomiasis (B65.-, N29)

gonococcal urethral stricture (A54.01)

syphilitic urethral stricture (A52.76)

N35.11   **Postinfective urethral stricture, not elsewhere classified, male**

N35.111   **Postinfective urethral stricture, not elsewhere classified, male, meatal**

N35.112 **Postinfective bulbous urethral stricture, not elsewhere classified, male**

N35.113 **Postinfective membranous urethral stricture, not elsewhere classified, male**

N35.114 **Postinfective anterior urethral stricture, not elsewhere classified, male**

N35.116 **Postinfective urethral stricture, not elsewhere classified, male, overlapping sites**

N35.119 **Postinfective urethral stricture, not elsewhere classified, male, unspecified**

N35.12 **Postinfective urethral stricture, not elsewhere classified, female**

N35.8 **Other urethral stricture**

Excludes1: postprocedural urethral stricture (N99.1-)

N35.81 **Other urethral stricture, male**

N35.811 **Other urethral stricture, male, meatal**

N35.812 **Other urethral bulbous stricture, male**

N35.813 **Other membranous urethral stricture, male**

N35.814 **Other anterior urethral stricture, male**

N35.816 **Other urethral stricture, male, overlapping sites**

N35.819 **Other urethral stricture, male, unspecified site**

N35.82 **Other urethral stricture, female**

N35.9 **Urethral stricture, unspecified**

N35.91 **Urethral stricture, unspecified, male**

N35.911 **Unspecified urethral stricture, male, meatal**

N35.912 **Unspecified bulbous urethral stricture, male**

N35.913 **Unspecified membranous urethral stricture, male**

N35.914 **Unspecified anterior urethral stricture, male**

N35.916 **Unspecified urethral stricture, male, overlapping sites**

N35.919 **Unspecified urethral stricture, male, unspecified site**

Pinhole meatus NOS

Urethral stricture NOS

N35.92 **Unspecified urethral stricture, female**

N36 **Other disorders of urethra**

N36.0 **Urethral fistula**

Urethroperineal fistula

Urethrorectal fistula

Urinary fistula NOS

Excludes1: urethroscrotal fistula (N50.89)

urethrovaginal fistula (N82.1)

urethrovesicovaginal fistula (N82.1)

N36.1 **Urethral diverticulum**

N36.2 **Urethral caruncle**

N36.4 **Urethral functional and muscular disorders**

Use Additional Code to identify associated urinary stress incontinence (N39.3)

N36.41 **Hypermobility of urethra**

N36.42 **Intrinsic sphincter deficiency (ISD)**

N36.43 **Combined hypermobility of urethra and intrinsic sphincter deficiency**

N36.44 **Muscular disorders of urethra**

Bladder sphincter dyssynergy

N36.5 **Urethral false passage**

N36.8 **Other specified disorders of urethra**

Excludes1: congenital urethrocele (Q64.7)

female urethrocele (N81.0)

N36.9 **Urethral disorder, unspecified**

N37 **Urethral disorders in diseases classified elsewhere**

Code first underlying disease

Excludes1: urethritis (in):

candidal infection (B37.41)

chlamydial (A56.01)

gonorrhea (A54.01)

syphilis (A52.76)

trichomonal infection (A59.03)

tuberculosis (A18.13)

N39 **Other disorders of urinary system**

Excludes1: pyuria (R82.81)

Excludes2: hematuria NOS (R31.-)

recurrent or persistent hematuria (N02.-)

recurrent or persistent hematuria with specified morphological lesion (N02.-)

proteinuria NOS (R80.-)

N39.0 **Urinary tract infection, site not specified**

Use Additional Code (B95-B97), to identify infectious agent.

Excludes1: candidiasis of urinary tract (B37.4-)

neonatal urinary tract infection (P39.3)

urinary tract infection of specified site, such as: cystitis (N30.-)

urethritis (N34.-)

N39.3 **Stress incontinence (female) (male)**

Code also any associated overactive bladder (N32.81)

Excludes1: mixed incontinence (N39.46)

N39.4 **Other specified urinary incontinence**

Code also any associated overactive bladder (N32.81)

Excludes1: enuresis NOS (R32)

functional urinary incontinence (R39.81)

urinary incontinence associated with cognitive impairment (R39.81)

urinary incontinence NOS (R32)

urinary incontinence of nonorganic origin (F98.0)

N39.41 **Urge incontinence**

Excludes1: mixed incontinence (N39.46)

N39.42 **Incontinence without sensory awareness**

Insensible (urinary) incontinence

N39.43 **Post-void dribbling**

N39.44 **Nocturnal enuresis**

N39.45 **Continuous leakage**

Excludes2 nocturnal polyuria (R35.81)

N39.46   Mixed incontinence
Urge and stress incontinence
N39.49   Other specified urinary incontinence
N39.490   Overflow incontinence
N39.491   Coital incontinence
N39.492   Postural (urinary) incontinence
N39.498   Other specified urinary incontinence
Reflex incontinence
Total incontinence
N39.8   Other specified disorders of urinary system
N39.9   Disorder of urinary system, unspecified

DISEASES OF MALE GENITAL ORGANS (N40-N53)

> NOTE: ALL DIAGNOSIS CODES IN THIS SECTION APPLY TO MALE PATIENTS ONLY

N40   Benign prostatic hyperplasia
Includes: adenofibromatous hypertrophy of prostate
benign hypertrophy of the prostate
benign prostatic hypertrophy
BPH
enlarged prostate nodular prostate
polyp of prostate
Excludes1: benign neoplasms of prostate (adenoma, benign)
(fibroadenoma) (fibroma) (myoma) (D29.1)
Excludes2: malignant neoplasm of prostate (C61)
N40.0   Benign prostatic hyperplasia without lower urinary tract symptoms
Enlarged prostate without LUTS
Enlarged prostate NOS
N40.1   Benign prostatic hyperplasia with lower urinary tract symptoms
Enlarged prostate with LUTS
Use Additional Code for associated symptoms, when specified:
incomplete bladder emptying (R39.14)
nocturia (R35.1)
straining on urination (R39.16)
urinary frequency (R35.0)
urinary hesitancy (R39.11)
urinary incontinence (N39.4-)
urinary obstruction (N13.8)
urinary retention (R33.8)
urinary urgency (R39.15)
weak urinary stream (R39.12)
N40.2   Nodular prostate without lower urinary tract symptoms
Nodular prostate without LUTS
N40.3   Nodular prostate with lower urinary tract symptoms
Use Additional Code for associated symptoms, when specified:
incomplete bladder emptying (R39.14)
nocturia (R35.1)
straining on urination (R39.16)
urinary frequency (R35.0)
urinary hesitancy (R39.11)
urinary incontinence (N39.4-)
urinary obstruction (N13.8)

urinary retention (R33.8)
urinary urgency (R39.15)
weak urinary stream (R39.12)
N41   Inflammatory diseases of prostate
Use Additional Code (B95-B97), to identify infectious agent.
N41.0   Acute prostatitis
N41.1   Chronic prostatitis
N41.2   Abscess of prostate
N41.3   Prostatocystitis
N41.4   Granulomatous prostatitis
N41.8   Other inflammatory diseases of prostate
N41.9   Inflammatory disease of prostate, unspecified
Prostatitis NOS
N42   Other and unspecified disorders of prostate
N42.0   Calculus of prostate
Prostatic stone
N42.1   Congestion and hemorrhage of prostate
Excludes1: enlarged prostate (N40.-)
hematuria (R31.-)
hyperplasia of prostate (N40.-)
inflammatory diseases of prostate (N41.-)
N42.3   Dysplasia of prostate
N42.30   Unspecified dysplasia of prostate
N42.31   Prostatic intraepithelial neoplasia
PIN
Prostatic intraepithelial neoplasia I (PIN I)
Prostatic intraepithelial neoplasia II (PIN II)
Excludes1: prostatic intraepithelial neoplasia III
(PIN III) (D07.5)
N42.32   Atypical small acinar proliferation of prostate
N42.39   Other dysplasia of prostate
N42.8   Other specified disorders of prostate
N42.81   Prostatodynia syndrome
Painful prostate syndrome
N42.82   Prostatosis syndrome
N42.83   Cyst of prostate
N42.89   Other specified disorders of prostate
N42.9   Disorder of prostate, unspecified
N43   Hydrocele and spermatocele
Definition: A Hydrocele is a painless swelling of the scrotum, caused by a collection of fluid around the testicle; commonly occurs in middle-aged men.
Includes: hydrocele of spermatic cord, testis or tunica vaginalis
Excludes1: congenital hydrocele (P83.5)
N43.0   Encysted hydrocele
N43.1   Infected hydrocele
Use Additional Code (B95-B97), to identify infectious agent
N43.2   Other hydrocele
N43.3   Hydrocele, unspecified
N43.4   Spermatocele of epididymis
Spermatic cyst
N43.40   Spermatocele of epididymis, unspecified
N43.41   Spermatocele of epididymis, single
N43.42   Spermatocele of epididymis, multiple
N44   Noninflammatory disorders of testis
N44.0   Torsion of testis

N44.00   **Torsion of testis, unspecified**

N44.01   **Extravaginal torsion of spermatic cord**

N44.02   **Intravaginal torsion of spermatic cord**

Torsion of spermatic cord NOS

N44.03   **Torsion of appendix testis**

N44.04   **Torsion of appendix epididymis**

N44.1   **Cyst of tunica albuginea testis**

N44.2   **Benign cyst of testis**

N44.8   **Other noninflammatory disorders of the testis**

N45   **Orchitis and epididymitis**

Definition: Orchitis is the inflammation and swelling of the testes as a result of infection or physical injury. Epididymitis is an inflammation of the epididymis which is located along the posterior aspect of the testicle.

Use Additional Code (B95-B97), to identify infectious agent.

N45.1   **Epididymitis**

N45.2   **Orchitis**

N45.3   **Epididymo-orchitis**

N45.4   **Abscess of epididymis or testis**

N46   **Male infertility**

Excludes1: vasectomy status (Z98.52)

N46.0   **Azoospermia**

Absolute male infertility

Male infertility due to germinal (cell) aplasia

Male infertility due to spermatogenic arrest (complete)

N46.01   **Organic azoospermia**

Azoospermia NOS

N46.02   **Azoospermia due to extratesticular causes**

Code also associated cause

N46.021   **Azoospermia due to drug therapy**

N46.022   **Azoospermia due to infection**

N46.023   **Azoospermia due to obstruction of efferent ducts**

N46.024   **Azoospermia due to radiation**

N46.025   **Azoospermia due to systemic disease**

N46.029   **Azoospermia due to other extratesticular causes**

N46.1   **Oligospermia**

Male infertility due to germinal cell desquamation

Male infertility due to hypospermatogenesis

Male infertility due to incomplete spermatogenic arrest

N46.11   **Organic oligospermia**

Oligospermia NOS

N46.12   **Oligospermia due to extratesticular causes**

Code also associated cause

N46.121   **Oligospermia due to drug therapy**

N46.122   **Oligospermia due to infection**

N46.123   **Oligospermia due to obstruction of efferent ducts**

N46.124   **Oligospermia due to radiation**

N46.125   **Oligospermia due to systemic disease**

N46.129   **Oligospermia due to other extratesticular causes**

N46.8   **Other male infertility**

N46.9   **Male infertility, unspecified**

N47   **Disorders of prepuce**

N47.0   **Adherent prepuce, newborn**

N47.1   **Phimosis**

N47.2   **Paraphimosis**

N47.3   **Deficient foreskin**

N47.4   **Benign cyst of prepuce**

N47.5   **Adhesions of prepuce and glans penis**

N47.6   **Balanoposthitis**

Use Additional Code (B95-B97), to identify infectious agent.

Excludes1: balanitis (N48.1)

N47.7   **Other inflammatory diseases of prepuce**

Use Additional Code (B95-B97), to identify infectious agent.

N47.8   **Other disorders of prepuce**

N48   **Other disorders of penis**

N48.0   **Leukoplakia of penis**

Balanitis xerotica obliterans

Kraurosis of penis

Lichen sclerosus of external male genital organs

Excludes1: carcinoma in situ of penis (D07.4)

N48.1   **Balanitis**

Use Additional Code (B95-B97), to identify infectious agent

Excludes1: amebic balanitis (A06.8)

balanitis xerotica obliterans (N48.0)

candidal balanitis (B37.42)

gonococcal balanitis (A54.23)

herpesviral [herpes simplex] balanitis (A60.01)

N48.2   **Other inflammatory disorders of penis**

Use Additional Code (B95-B97), to identify infectious agent.

Excludes1: balanitis (N48.1)

balanitis xerotica obliterans (N48.0)

balanoposthitis (N47.6)

N48.21   **Abscess of corpus cavernosum and penis**

N48.22   **Cellulitis of corpus cavernosum and penis**

N48.29   **Other inflammatory disorders of penis**

N48.3   **Priapism**

Painful erection

Code first underlying cause

N48.30   **Priapism, unspecified**

N48.31   **Priapism due to trauma**

N48.32   **Priapism due to disease classified elsewhere**

N48.33   **Priapism, drug-induced**

N48.39   **Other priapism**

N48.5   **Ulcer of penis**

N48.6   **Induration penis plastica**

Peyronie's disease

Plastic induration of penis

N48.8   **Other specified disorders of penis**

N48.81   **Thrombosis of superficial vein of penis**

N48.82   **Acquired torsion of penis**

Acquired torsion of penis NOS

Excludes1: congenital torsion of penis (Q55.63)

N48.83   **Acquired buried penis**

Excludes1: congenital hidden penis (Q55.64)

N48.89   **Other specified disorders of penis**

N48.9   **Disorder of penis, unspecified**

N49   **Inflammatory disorders of male genital organs, not elsewhere classified**

Use Additional Code (B95-B97), to identify infectious agent

Excludes1: inflammation of penis (N48.1, N48.2-)

    orchitis and epididymitis (N45.-)

N49.0   **Inflammatory disorders of seminal vesicle**

    Vesiculitis NOS

N49.1   **Inflammatory disorders of spermatic cord, tunica vaginalis and vas deferens**

    Vasitis

N49.2   **Inflammatory disorders of scrotum**

N49.3   **Fournier gangrene**

N49.8   **Inflammatory disorders of other specified male genital organs**

    Inflammation of multiple sites in male genital organs

N49.9   **Inflammatory disorder of unspecified male genital organ**

    Abscess of unspecified male genital organ

    Boil of unspecified male genital organ

    Carbuncle of unspecified male genital organ

    Cellulitis of unspecified male genital organ

N50   **Other and unspecified disorders of male genital organs**

Excludes2: torsion of testis (N44.0-)

N50.0   **Atrophy of testis**

N50.1   **Vascular disorders of male genital organs**

    Hematocele, NOS, of male genital organs

    Hemorrhage of male genital organs

    Thrombosis of male genital organs

N50.3   **Cyst of epididymis**

N50.8   **Other specified disorders of male genital organs**

    N50.81   **Testicular pain**

        N50.811   **Right testicular pain**

        N50.812   **Left testicular pain**

        N50.819   **Testicular pain, unspecified**

    N50.82   **Scrotal pain**

    N50.89   **Other specified disorders of the male genital organs**

        Atrophy of scrotum, seminal vesicle, spermatic cord, tunica vaginalis and vas deferens

        Chylocele, tunica vaginalis (nonfilarial) NOS

        Edema of scrotum, seminal vesicle, spermatic cord, tunica vaginalis and vas deferens

        Hypertrophy of scrotum, seminal vesicle, spermatic cord, tunica vaginalis and vas deferens

        Stricture of spermatic cord, tunica vaginalis, and vas deferens

        Ulcer of scrotum, seminal vesicle, spermatic cord, testis, tunica vaginalis and vas deferens

        Urethroscrotal fistula

N50.9   **Disorder of male genital organs, unspecified**

N51   **Disorders of male genital organs in diseases classified elsewhere**

Code first underlying disease, such as:

filariasis (B74.0-B74.9)

Excludes1: amebic balanitis (A06.8)

    candidal balanitis (B37.42)

    gonococcal balanitis (A54.23)

    gonococcal prostatitis (A54.22)

    herpesviral [herpes simplex] balanitis (A60.01)

    trichomonal prostatitis (A59.02)

    tuberculous prostatitis (A18.14)

N52   **Male erectile dysfunction**

Excludes1: psychogenic impotence (F52.21)

N52.0   **Vasculogenic erectile dysfunction**

    N52.01   **Erectile dysfunction due to arterial insufficiency**

    N52.02   **Corporo-venous occlusive erectile dysfunction**

    N52.03   **Combined arterial insufficiency and corporo-venous occlusive erectile dysfunction**

N52.1   **Erectile dysfunction due to diseases classified elsewhere**

Code first underlying disease

N52.2   **Drug-induced erectile dysfunction**

N52.3   **Postprocedural erectile dysfunction**

    N52.31   **Erectile dysfunction following radical prostatectomy**

    N52.32   **Erectile dysfunction following radical cystectomy**

    N52.33   **Erectile dysfunction following urethral surgery**

    N52.34   **Erectile dysfunction following simple prostatectomy**

    N52.35   **Erectile dysfunction following radiation therapy**

    N52.36   **Erectile dysfunction following interstitial seed therapy**

    N52.37   **Erectile dysfunction following prostate ablative therapy**

        Erectile dysfunction following cryotherapy

        Erectile dysfunction following other prostate ablative therapies

        Erectile dysfunction following ultrasound ablative therapies

    N52.39   **Other and unspecified postprocedural erectile dysfunction**

N52.8   **Other male erectile dysfunction**

N52.9   **Male erectile dysfunction, unspecified**

    Impotence NOS

N53   **Other male sexual dysfunction**

Excludes1: psychogenic sexual dysfunction (F52.-)

N53.1   **Ejaculatory dysfunction**

Excludes1: premature ejaculation (F52.4)

    N53.11   **Retarded ejaculation**

    N53.12   **Painful ejaculation**

    N53.13   **Anejaculatory orgasm**

    N53.14   **Retrograde ejaculation**

    N53.19   **Other ejaculatory dysfunction**

        Ejaculatory dysfunction NOS

N53.8   **Other male sexual dysfunction**

N53.9   **Unspecified male sexual dysfunction**

DISORDERS OF BREAST (N60-N65)

Excludes1: disorders of breast associated with childbirth (O91-O92)

N60   **Benign mammary dysplasia**

Definition: Mammary dysplasia is a common condition marked by benign (noncancerous) changes in breast tissue. These changes may include irregular lumps or cysts, breast discomfort, sensitive nipples, and itching.

Includes: fibrocystic mastopathy

N60.0   **Solitary cyst of breast**

    Cyst of breast

   ● New code   ▲ Revised code   Excludes1: Not coded here   Excludes2: Not included here   ⊗ Placeholder required   ⑦7th digit required

N60.01   **Solitary cyst of right breast**

N60.02   **Solitary cyst of left breast**

N60.09   **Solitary cyst of unspecified breast**

N60.1   **Diffuse cystic mastopathy**

Cystic breast

Fibrocystic disease of breast

Excludes1: diffuse cystic mastopathy with epithelial proliferation (N60.3-)

N60.11   **Diffuse cystic mastopathy of right breast**

N60.12   **Diffuse cystic mastopathy of left breast**

N60.19   **Diffuse cystic mastopathy of unspecified breast**

N60.2   **Fibroadenosis of breast**

Adenofibrosis of breast

Excludes2: fibroadenoma of breast (D24.-)

N60.21   **Fibroadenosis of right breast**

N60.22   **Fibroadenosis of left breast**

N60.29   **Fibroadenosis of unspecified breast**

N60.3   **Fibrosclerosis of breast**

Cystic mastopathy with epithelial proliferation

N60.31   **Fibrosclerosis of right breast**

N60.32   **Fibrosclerosis of left breast**

N60.39   **Fibrosclerosis of unspecified breast**

N60.4   **Mammary duct ectasia**

N60.41   **Mammary duct ectasia of right breast**

N60.42   **Mammary duct ectasia of left breast**

N60.49   **Mammary duct ectasia of unspecified breast**

N60.8   **Other benign mammary dysplasias**

N60.81   **Other benign mammary dysplasias of right breast**

N60.82   **Other benign mammary dysplasias of left breast**

N60.89   **Other benign mammary dysplasias of unspecified breast**

N60.9   **Unspecified benign mammary dysplasia**

N60.91   **Unspecified benign mammary dysplasia of right breast**

N60.92   **Unspecified benign mammary dysplasia of left breast**

N60.99   **Unspecified benign mammary dysplasia of unspecified breast**

N61   **Inflammatory disorders of breast**

Excludes1: inflammatory carcinoma of breast (C50.9)

inflammatory disorder of breast associated with childbirth (O91.-)

neonatal infective mastitis (P39.0)

thrombophlebitis of breast [Mondor's disease] (I80.8)

N61.0   **Mastitis without abscess**

Infective mastitis (acute) (nonpuerperal) (subacute)

Mastitis (acute) (nonpuerperal) (subacute) NOS

Cellulitis (acute) (nonpuerperal) (subacute) of breast NOS

Cellulitis (acute) (nonpuerperal) (subacute) of nipple NOS

N61.1   **Abscess of the breast and nipple**

Abscess (acute) (chronic) (nonpuerperal) of areola

Abscess (acute) (chronic) (nonpuerperal) of breast

Carbuncle of breast

Mastitis with abscess

N61.2   **Granulomatous mastitis**

N61.20   **Granulomatous mastitis, unspecified breast**

N61.21   **Granulomatous mastitis, right breast**

N61.22   **Granulomatous mastitis, left breast**

N61.23   **Granulomatous mastitis, bilateral breast**

N62   **Hypertrophy of breast**

Gynecomastia

Hypertrophy of breast NOS

Massive pubertal hypertrophy of breast

Excludes1: breast engorgement of newborn (P83.4)

disproportion of reconstructed breast (N65.1)

N63   **Unspecified lump in breast**

Nodule(s) NOS in breast

N63.0   **Unspecified lump in unspecified breast**

N63.1   **Unspecified lump in the right breast**

N63.10   **Unspecified lump in the right breast, unspecified quadrant**

N63.11   **Unspecified lump in the right breast, upper outer quadrant**

N63.12   **Unspecified lump in the right breast, upper inner quadrant**

N63.13   **Unspecified lump in the right breast, lower outer quadrant**

N63.14   **Unspecified lump in the right breast, lower inner quadrant**

N63.15   **Unspecified lump in the right breast, overlapping quadrants**

N63.2   **Unspecified lump in the left breast**

N63.20   **Unspecified lump in the left breast, unspecified quadrant**

N63.21   **Unspecified lump in the left breast, upper outer quadrant**

N63.22   **Unspecified lump in the left breast, upper inner quadrant**

N63.23   **Unspecified lump in the left breast, lower outer quadrant**

N63.24   **Unspecified lump in the left breast, lower inner quadrant**

N63.25   **Unspecified lump in the left breast, overlapping quadrants**

N63.3   **Unspecified lump in axillary tail**

N63.31   **Unspecified lump in axillary tail of the right breast**

N63.32   **Unspecified lump in axillary tail of the left breast**

N63.4   **Unspecified lump in breast, subareolar**

N63.41   **Unspecified lump in right breast, subareolar**

N63.42   **Unspecified lump in left breast, subareolar**

N64   **Other disorders of breast**

Excludes2: mechanical complication of breast prosthesis and implant (T85.4-)

N64.0   **Fissure and fistula of nipple**

N64.1   **Fat necrosis of breast**

Fat necrosis (segmental) of breast

Code first breast necrosis due to breast graft (T85.898)

N64.2   **Atrophy of breast**

N64.3   **Galactorrhea not associated with childbirth**

N64.4   **Mastodynia**

N64.5   **Other signs and symptoms in breast**

Excludes2: abnormal findings on diagnostic imaging of breast (R92.-)

N64.51   **Induration of breast**

N64.52 **Nipple discharge**

Excludes1: abnormal findings in nipple discharge (R89.-)

N64.53 **Retraction of nipple**

N64.59 **Other signs and symptoms in breast**

N64.8 **Other specified disorders of breast**

N64.81 **Ptosis of breast**

Excludes1: ptosis of native breast in relation to reconstructed breast (N65.1)

N64.82 **Hypoplasia of breast**

Micromastia

Excludes1: congenital absence of breast (Q83.0)

hypoplasia of native breast in relation to reconstructed breast (N65.1)

N64.89 **Other specified disorders of breast**

Galactocele

Subinvolution of breast (postlactational)

N64.9 **Disorder of breast, unspecified**

N65 **Deformity and disproportion of reconstructed breast**

N65.0 **Deformity of reconstructed breast**

Contour irregularity in reconstructed breast

Excess tissue in reconstructed breast

Misshapen reconstructed breast

N65.1 **Disproportion of reconstructed breast**

Breast asymmetry between native breast and reconstructed breast

Disproportion between native breast and reconstructed breast

INFLAMMATORY DISEASES OF FEMALE PELVIC ORGANS (N70-N77)

NOTE: ALL DIAGNOSIS CODES IN THIS SECTION APPLY TO FEMALE PATIENTS ONLY

Excludes1: inflammatory diseases of female pelvic organs complicating:

abortion or ectopic or molar pregnancy (O00-O07, O08.0)

pregnancy, childbirth and the puerperium (O23.-, O75.3, O85, O86.-)

N70 **Salpingitis and oophoritis**

Includes: abscess (of) fallopian tube

abscess (of) ovary pyosalpinx salpingo-oophoritis

tubo-ovarian abscess

tubo-ovarian inflammatory disease

Use Additional Code (B95-B97), to identify infectious agent

Excludes1: gonococcal infection (A54.24)

tuberculous infection (A18.17)

N70.0 **Acute salpingitis and oophoritis**

N70.01 **Acute salpingitis**

N70.02 **Acute oophoritis**

N70.03 **Acute salpingitis and oophoritis**

N70.1 **Chronic salpingitis and oophoritis**

Hydrosalpinx

N70.11 **Chronic salpingitis**

N70.12 **Chronic oophoritis**

N70.13 **Chronic salpingitis and oophoritis**

N70.9 **Salpingitis and oophoritis, unspecified**

N70.91 **Salpingitis, unspecified**

N70.92 **Oophoritis, unspecified**

N70.93 **Salpingitis and oophoritis, unspecified**

N71 **Inflammatory disease of uterus, except cervix**

Includes: endo (myo) metritis

metritis myometritis pyometra uterine abscess

Use Additional Code (B95-B97), to identify infectious agent

Excludes1: hyperplastic endometritis (N85.0-)

infection of uterus following delivery (O85, O86.-)

N71.0 **Acute inflammatory disease of uterus**

N71.1 **Chronic inflammatory disease of uterus**

N71.9 **Inflammatory disease of uterus, unspecified**

N72 **Inflammatory disease of cervix uteri**

Includes: cervicitis (with or without erosion or ectropion)

endocervicitis (with or without erosion or ectropion)

exocervicitis (with or without erosion or ectropion)

Use Additional Code (B95-B97), to identify infectious agent

Excludes1: erosion and ectropion of cervix without cervicitis (N86)

N73 **Other female pelvic inflammatory diseases**

Use Additional Code (B95-B97), to identify infectious agent.

N73.0 **Acute parametritis and pelvic cellulitis**

Abscess of broad ligament

Abscess of parametrium

Pelvic cellulitis, female

N73.1 **Chronic parametritis and pelvic cellulitis**

Any condition in N73.0 specified as chronic

Excludes1: tuberculous parametritis and pelvic cellulitis (A18.17)

N73.2 **Unspecified parametritis and pelvic cellulitis**

Any condition in N73.0 unspecified whether acute or chronic

N73.3 **Female acute pelvic peritonitis**

N73.4 **Female chronic pelvic peritonitis**

Excludes1: tuberculous pelvic (female) peritonitis (A18.17)

N73.5 **Female pelvic peritonitis, unspecified**

N73.6 **Female pelvic peritoneal adhesions (postinfective)**

Excludes2: postprocedural pelvic peritoneal adhesions (N99.4)

N73.8 **Other specified female pelvic inflammatory diseases**

N73.9 **Female pelvic inflammatory disease, unspecified**

Female pelvic infection or inflammation NOS

N74 **Female pelvic inflammatory disorders in diseases classified elsewhere**

Code first underlying disease

Excludes1: chlamydial cervicitis (A56.02)

chlamydial pelvic inflammatory disease (A56.11)

gonococcal cervicitis (A54.03)

gonococcal pelvic inflammatory disease (A54.24)

herpesviral [herpes simplex] cervicitis (A60.03)

herpesviral [herpes simplex] pelvic inflammatory disease (A60.09)

syphilitic cervicitis (A52.76)

syphilitic pelvic inflammatory disease (A52.76)

trichomonal cervicitis (A59.09)

tuberculous cervicitis (A18.16)

tuberculous pelvic inflammatory disease (A18.17)

N75 **Diseases of Bartholin's gland**

N75.0 **Cyst of Bartholin's gland**

N75.1 **Abscess of Bartholin's gland**

N75.8   **Other diseases of Bartholin's gland**

Bartholinitis

N75.9   **Disease of Bartholin's gland, unspecified**

N76   **Other inflammation of vagina and vulva**

Use Additional Code (B95-B97), to identify infectious agent

Excludes2: senile (atrophic) vaginitis (N95.2)

vulvar vestibulitis (N94.810)

N76.0   **Acute vaginitis**

Acute vulvovaginitis

Vaginitis NOS

Vulvovaginitis NOS

N76.1   **Subacute and chronic vaginitis**

Chronic vulvovaginitis

Subacute vulvovaginitis

N76.2   **Acute vulvitis**

Vulvitis NOS

N76.3   **Subacute and chronic vulvitis**

N76.4   **Abscess of vulva**

Furuncle of vulva

N76.5   **Ulceration of vagina**

N76.6   **Ulceration of vulva**

N76.8   **Other specified inflammation of vagina and vulva**

     N76.81   **Mucositis (ulcerative) of vagina and vulva**

Code also type of associated therapy, such as:

antineoplastic and immunosuppressive drugs (T45.1X-)

radiological procedure and radiotherapy (Y84.2)

Excludes2: gastrointestinal mucositis (ulcerative) (K92.81)

nasal mucositis (ulcerative) (J34.81)

oral mucositis (ulcerative) (K12.3-)

     N76.89   **Other specified inflammation of vagina and vulva**

N77   **Vulvovaginal ulceration and inflammation in diseases classified elsewhere**

N77.0   **Ulceration of vulva in diseases classified elsewhere**

Code first underlying disease, such as:

Behçet's disease (M35.2)

Excludes1: ulceration of vulva in gonococcal infection (A54.02)

ulceration of vulva in herpesviral [herpes simplex] infection (A60.04)

ulceration of vulva in syphilis (A51.0)

ulceration of vulva in tuberculosis (A18.18)

N77.1   **Vaginitis, vulvitis and vulvovaginitis in diseases classified elsewhere**

Code first underlying disease, such as:

pinworm (B80)

Excludes1: candidal vulvovaginitis (B37.3)

chlamydial vulvovaginitis (A56.02)

gonococcal vulvovaginitis (A54.02)

herpesviral [herpes simplex] vulvovaginitis (A60.04)

trichomonal vulvovaginitis (A59.01)

tuberculous vulvovaginitis (A18.18)

vulvovaginitis in early syphilis (A51.0)

vulvovaginitis in late syphilis (A52.76)

NONINFLAMMATORY DISORDERS OF FEMALE GENITAL TRACT (N80-N98)

N80   **Endometriosis**

Definition: Endometriosis is a condition where tissue that normally lines the uterus grows in other areas of the body. This can cause pain, irregular menstrual bleeding, and infertility for some women.

N80.0   **Endometriosis of uterus**

Adenomyosis

Excludes1: stromal endometriosis (D39.0)

N80.1   **Endometriosis of ovary**

N80.2   **Endometriosis of fallopian tube**

N80.3   **Endometriosis of pelvic peritoneum**

N80.4   **Endometriosis of rectovaginal septum and vagina**

N80.5   **Endometriosis of intestine**

N80.6   **Endometriosis in cutaneous scar**

N80.8   **Other endometriosis**

Endometriosis of thorax

N80.9   **Endometriosis, unspecified**

N81   **Female genital prolapse**

Definition: Genital prolapse is a condition in which the vaginal wall or uterus descend below their normal positions; part of the bladder or rectum may protrude from the vagina.

Excludes1: genital prolapse complicating pregnancy, labor or delivery (O34.5-)

prolapse and hernia of ovary and fallopian tube (N83.4-)

prolapse of vaginal vault after hysterectomy (N99.3)

N81.0   **Urethrocele**

Excludes1: urethrocele with cystocele (N81.1-)

urethrocele with prolapse of uterus (N81.2-N81.4)

N81.1   **Cystocele**

Cystocele with urethrocele

Cystourethrocele

Excludes1: cystocele with prolapse of uterus (N81.2-N81.4)

     N81.10   **Cystocele, unspecified**

Prolapse of (anterior) vaginal wall NOS

     N81.11   **Cystocele, midline**

     N81.12   **Cystocele, lateral**

Paravaginal cystocele

N81.2   **Incomplete uterovaginal prolapse**

First degree uterine prolapse

Prolapse of cervix NOS

Second degree uterine prolapse

Excludes1: cervical stump prolapse (N81.85)

N81.3   **Complete uterovaginal prolapse**

Procidentia (uteri) NOS

Third degree uterine prolapse

N81.4   **Uterovaginal prolapse, unspecified**

Prolapse of uterus NOS

N81.5   **Vaginal enterocele**

Excludes1: enterocele with prolapse of uterus (N81.2-N81.4)

N81.6   **Rectocele**

Prolapse of posterior vaginal wall

Use Additional Code for any associated fecal incontinence, if applicable (R15.-)

Excludes2: perineocele (N81.81)

---

rectal prolapse (K62.3)

rectocele with prolapse of uterus (N81.2-N81.4)

N81.8 Other female genital prolapse

N81.81 Perineocele

N81.82 Incompetence or weakening of pubocervical tissue

N81.83 Incompetence or weakening of rectovaginal tissue

N81.84 Pelvic muscle wasting

Disuse atrophy of pelvic muscles and anal sphincter

N81.85 Cervical stump prolapse

N81.89 Other female genital prolapse

Deficient perineum

Old laceration of muscles of pelvic floor

N81.9 Female genital prolapse, unspecified

N82 Fistulae involving female genital tract

Definition: A fistula involving female genital tract is a fistula that has formed in the wall of the vagina. A vaginal fistula may open into the urinary tract, the rectum, the colon, or the small bowel.

Excludes1: vesicointestinal fistulae (N32.1)

N82.0 Vesicovaginal fistula

N82.1 Other female urinary-genital tract fistulae

Cervicovesical fistula

Ureterovaginal fistula

Urethrovaginal fistula

Uteroureteric fistula

Uterovesical fistula

N82.2 Fistula of vagina to small intestine

N82.3 Fistula of vagina to large intestine

Rectovaginal fistula

N82.4 Other female intestinal-genital tract fistulae

Intestinouterine fistula

N82.5 Female genital tract-skin fistulae

Uterus to abdominal wall fistula

Vaginoperineal fistula

N82.8 Other female genital tract fistulae

N82.9 Female genital tract fistula, unspecified

N83 Noninflammatory disorders of ovary, fallopian tube and broad ligament

Excludes2: hydrosalpinx (N70.1-)

N83.0 Follicular cyst of ovary

Cyst of graafian follicle

Hemorrhagic follicular cyst (of ovary)

N83.00 Follicular cyst of ovary, unspecified side

N83.01 Follicular cyst of right ovary

N83.02 Follicular cyst of left ovary

N83.1 Corpus luteum cyst

Hemorrhagic corpus luteum cyst

N83.10 Corpus luteum cyst of ovary, unspecified side

N83.11 Corpus luteum cyst of right ovary

N83.12 Corpus luteum cyst of left ovary

N83.2 Other and unspecified ovarian cysts

Excludes1: developmental ovarian cyst (Q50.1)

neoplastic ovarian cyst (D27.-)

polycystic ovarian syndrome (E28.2)

Stein-Leventhal syndrome (E28.2)

N83.20 Unspecified ovarian cysts

N83.201 Unspecified ovarian cyst, right side

N83.202 Unspecified ovarian cyst, left side

N83.209 Unspecified ovarian cyst, unspecified side

Ovarian cyst, NOS

N83.29 Other ovarian cysts

Retention cyst of ovary

Simple cyst of ovary

N83.291 Other ovarian cyst, right side

N83.292 Other ovarian cyst, left side

N83.299 Other ovarian cyst, unspecified side

N83.3 Acquired atrophy of ovary and fallopian tube

N83.31 Acquired atrophy of ovary

N83.311 Acquired atrophy of right ovary

N83.312 Acquired atrophy of left ovary

N83.319 Acquired atrophy of ovary, unspecified side

Acquired atrophy of ovary, NOS

N83.32 Acquired atrophy of fallopian tube

N83.321 Acquired atrophy of right fallopian tube

N83.322 Acquired atrophy of left fallopian tube

N83.329 Acquired atrophy of fallopian tube, unspecified side

Acquired atrophy of fallopian tube, NOS

N83.33 Acquired atrophy of ovary and fallopian tube

N83.331 Acquired atrophy of right ovary and fallopian tube

N83.332 Acquired atrophy of left ovary and fallopian tube

N83.339 Acquired atrophy of ovary and fallopian tube, unspecified side

Acquired atrophy of ovary and fallopian tube, NOS

N83.4 Prolapse and hernia of ovary and fallopian tube

N83.40 Prolapse and hernia of ovary and fallopian tube, unspecified side

Prolapse and hernia of ovary and fallopian tube, NOS

N83.41 Prolapse and hernia of right ovary and fallopian tube

N83.42 Prolapse and hernia of left ovary and fallopian tube

N83.5 Torsion of ovary, ovarian pedicle and fallopian tube

Torsion of accessory tube

N83.51 Torsion of ovary and ovarian pedicle

N83.511 Torsion of right ovary and ovarian pedicle

N83.512 Torsion of left ovary and ovarian pedicle

N83.519 Torsion of ovary and ovarian pedicle, unspecified side

Torsion of ovary and ovarian pedicle, NOS

N83.52 Torsion of fallopian tube

Torsion of hydatid of Morgagni

N83.521 Torsion of right fallopian tube

N83.522 Torsion of left fallopian tube

N83.529 Torsion of fallopian tube, unspecified side

Torsion of fallopian tube, NOS

N83.53 Torsion of ovary, ovarian pedicle and fallopian tube

N83.6 Hematosalpinx

Excludes1: hematosalpinx (with) (in):

hematocolpos (N89.7)

hematometra (N85.7)

tubal pregnancy (O00.1-)

N83.7 Hematoma of broad ligament

N83.8 Other noninflammatory disorders of ovary, fallopian tube and broad ligament

Broad ligament laceration syndrome [Allen-Masters]

N83.9 Noninflammatory disorder of ovary, fallopian tube and broad ligament, unspecified

N84 Polyp of female genital tract

Excludes1: adenomatous polyp (D28.-)

placental polyp (O90.89)

N84.0 Polyp of corpus uteri

Polyp of endometrium

Polyp of uterus NOS

Excludes1: polypoid endometrial hyperplasia (N85.0-)

N84.1 Polyp of cervix uteri

Mucous polyp of cervix

N84.2 Polyp of vagina

N84.3 Polyp of vulva

Polyp of labia

N84.8 Polyp of other parts of female genital tract

N84.9 Polyp of female genital tract, unspecified

N85 Other noninflammatory disorders of uterus, except cervix

Excludes1: endometriosis (N80.-)

inflammatory diseases of uterus (N71.-)

noninflammatory disorders of cervix, except malposition (N86-N88)

polyp of corpus uteri (N84.0)

uterine prolapse (N81.-)

N85.0 Endometrial hyperplasia

N85.00 Endometrial hyperplasia, unspecified

Hyperplasia (adenomatous) (cystic) (glandular) of endometrium

Hyperplastic endometritis

N85.01 Benign endometrial hyperplasia

Endometrial hyperplasia (complex) (simple) without atypia

N85.02 Endometrial intraepithelial neoplasia [EIN]

Endometrial hyperplasia with atypia

Excludes1: malignant neoplasm of endometrium (with endometrial intraepithelial neoplasia [EIN]) (C54.1)

N85.2 Hypertrophy of uterus

Bulky or enlarged uterus

Excludes1: puerperal hypertrophy of uterus (O90.89)

N85.3 Subinvolution of uterus

Excludes1: puerperal subinvolution of uterus (O90.89)

N85.4 Malposition of uterus

Anteversion of uterus

Retroflexion of uterus

Retroversion of uterus

Excludes1: malposition of uterus complicating pregnancy, labor or delivery (O34.5-, O65.5)

N85.5 Inversion of uterus

Excludes1: current obstetric trauma (O71.2)

postpartum inversion of uterus (O71.2)

N85.6 Intrauterine synechiae

N85.7 Hematometra

Hematosalpinx with hematometra

Excludes1: hematometra with hematocolpos (N89.7)

N85.8 Other specified noninflammatory disorders of uterus

Atrophy of uterus, acquired

Fibrosis of uterus NOS

N85.9 Noninflammatory disorder of uterus, unspecified

Disorder of uterus NOS

N86 Erosion and ectropion of cervix uteri

Decubitus (trophic) ulcer of cervix

Eversion of cervix

Excludes1: erosion and ectropion of cervix with cervicitis (N72)

N87 Dysplasia of cervix uteri

Excludes1: abnormal results from cervical cytologic examination without histologic confirmation (R87.61-)

carcinoma in situ of cervix uteri (D06.-)

cervical intraepithelial neoplasia III [CIN III] (D06.-)

HGSIL of cervix (R87.613)

severe dysplasia of cervix uteri (D06.-)

N87.0 Mild cervical dysplasia

Cervical intraepithelial neoplasia I [CIN I]

N87.1 Moderate cervical dysplasia

Cervical intraepithelial neoplasia II [CIN II]

N87.9 Dysplasia of cervix uteri, unspecified

Anaplasia of cervix

Cervical atypism

Cervical dysplasia NOS

N88 Other noninflammatory disorders of cervix uteri

Excludes2: inflammatory disease of cervix (N72)

polyp of cervix (N84.1)

N88.0 Leukoplakia of cervix uteri

N88.1 Old laceration of cervix uteri

Adhesions of cervix

Excludes1: current obstetric trauma (O71.3)

N88.2 Stricture and stenosis of cervix uteri

Excludes1: stricture and stenosis of cervix uteri complicating labor (O65.5)

N88.3 Incompetence of cervix uteri

Investigation and management of (suspected) cervical incompetence in a nonpregnant woman

Excludes1: cervical incompetence complicating pregnancy (O34.3-)

N88.4 Hypertrophic elongation of cervix uteri

N88.8 Other specified noninflammatory disorders of cervix uteri

Excludes1: current obstetric trauma (O71.3)

N88.9 Noninflammatory disorder of cervix uteri, unspecified

N89 Other noninflammatory disorders of vagina

Excludes1: abnormal results from vaginal cytologic examination without histologic confirmation (R87.62-)

carcinoma in situ of vagina (D07.2)

HGSIL of vagina (R87.623)

inflammation of vagina (N76.-)

senile (atrophic) vaginitis (N95.2)

severe dysplasia of vagina (D07.2)

trichomonal leukorrhea (A59.00)

vaginal intraepithelial neoplasia [VAIN], grade III (D07.2)

N89.0 **Mild vaginal dysplasia**

Vaginal intraepithelial neoplasia [VAIN], grade I

N89.1 **Moderate vaginal dysplasia**

Vaginal intraepithelial neoplasia [VAIN], grade II

N89.3 **Dysplasia of vagina, unspecified**

N89.4 **Leukoplakia of vagina**

N89.5 **Stricture and atresia of vagina**

Vaginal adhesions

Vaginal stenosis

Excludes1: congenital atresia or stricture (Q52.4)

postprocedural adhesions of vagina (N99.2)

N89.6 **Tight hymenal ring**

Rigid hymen

Tight introitus

Excludes1: imperforate hymen (Q52.3)

N89.7 **Hematocolpos**

Hematocolpos with hematometra or hematosalpinx

N89.8 **Other specified noninflammatory disorders of vagina**

Leukorrhea NOS

Old vaginal laceration

Pessary ulcer of vagina

Excludes1: current obstetric trauma (O70.-, O71.4, O71.7-
O71.8)

old laceration involving muscles of pelvic floor
(N81.8)

N89.9 **Noninflammatory disorder of vagina, unspecified**

N90 **Other noninflammatory disorders of vulva and perineum**

Excludes1: anogenital (venereal) warts (A63.0)

carcinoma in situ of vulva (D07.1)

condyloma acuminatum (A63.0)

current obstetric trauma (O70.-, O71.7-O71.8)

inflammation of vulva (N76.-)

severe dysplasia of vulva (D07.1)

vulvar intraepithelial neoplasm III [VIN III] (D07.1)

N90.0 **Mild vulvar dysplasia**

Vulvar intraepithelial neoplasia [VIN], grade I

N90.1 **Moderate vulvar dysplasia**

Vulvar intraepithelial neoplasia [VIN], grade II

N90.3 **Dysplasia of vulva, unspecified**

N90.4 **Leukoplakia of vulva**

Dystrophy of vulva

Kraurosis of vulva

Lichen sclerosus of external female genital organs

N90.5 **Atrophy of vulva**

Stenosis of vulva

N90.6 **Hypertrophy of vulva**

N90.60 **Unspecified hypertrophy of vulva**

Unspecified hypertrophy of labia

N90.61 **Childhood asymmetric labium majus
enlargement**

CALME

N90.69 **Other specified hypertrophy of vulva**

Other specified hypertrophy of labia

N90.7 **Vulvar cyst**

N90.8 **Other specified noninflammatory disorders of vulva and
perineum**

N90.81 **Female genital mutilation status**

Female genital cutting status

N90.810 **Female genital mutilation status,
unspecified**

Female genital cutting status,
unspecified

Female genital mutilation status NOS

N90.811 **Female genital mutilation Type I
status**

Clitorectomy status

Female genital cutting Type I status

N90.812 **Female genital mutilation Type II
status**

Clitorectomy with excision of labia
minora status

Female genital cutting Type II status

N90.813 **Female genital mutilation Type III
status**

Female genital cutting Type III status

Infibulation status

N90.818 **Other female genital mutilation
status**

Female genital cutting Type IV status

Female genital mutilation Type IV
status

Other female genital cutting status

N90.89 **Other specified noninflammatory disorders of
vulva and perineum**

Adhesions of vulva

Hypertrophy of clitoris

N90.9 **Noninflammatory disorder of vulva and perineum,
unspecified**

N91 **Absent, scanty and rare menstruation**

Excludes1: ovarian dysfunction (E28.-)

N91.0 **Primary amenorrhea**

N91.1 **Secondary amenorrhea**

N91.2 **Amenorrhea, unspecified**

N91.3 **Primary oligomenorrhea**

N91.4 **Secondary oligomenorrhea**

N91.5 **Oligomenorrhea, unspecified**

Hypomenorrhea NOS

N92 **Excessive, frequent and irregular menstruation**

Excludes1: postmenopausal bleeding (N95.0)

precocious puberty (menstruation) (E30.1)

N92.0 **Excessive and frequent menstruation with regular cycle**

Heavy periods NOS

Menorrhagia NOS

Polymenorrhea

N92.1 **Excessive and frequent menstruation with irregular
cycle**

Irregular intermenstrual bleeding

Irregular, shortened intervals between menstrual bleeding

Menometrorrhagia

● New code   ▲ Revised code   Excludes1: Not coded here   Excludes2: Not included here   ⊗ Placeholder required   ⑦7th digit required

Metrorrhagia

N92.2 **Excessive menstruation at puberty**

Excessive bleeding associated with onset of menstrual periods

Pubertal menorrhagia

Puberty bleeding

N92.3 **Ovulation bleeding**

Regular intermenstrual bleeding

N92.4 **Excessive bleeding in the premenopausal period**

Climacteric menorrhagia or metrorrhagia

Menopausal menorrhagia or metrorrhagia

Perimenopausal bleeding

Perimenopausal menorrhagia or metrorrhagia

Preclimacteric menorrhagia or metrorrhagia

Premenopausal menorrhagia or metrorrhagia

N92.5 **Other specified irregular menstruation**

N92.6 **Irregular menstruation, unspecified**

Irregular bleeding NOS

Irregular periods NOS

Excludes1: irregular menstruation with:

lengthened intervals or scanty bleeding (N91.3-N91.5)

shortened intervals or excessive bleeding (N92.1)

N93 **Other abnormal uterine and vaginal bleeding**

Excludes1: neonatal vaginal hemorrhage (P54.6)

precocious puberty (menstruation) (E30.1)

pseudomenses (P54.6)

N93.0 **Postcoital and contact bleeding**

N93.1 **Pre-pubertal vaginal bleeding**

N93.8 **Other specified abnormal uterine and vaginal bleeding**

Dysfunctional or functional uterine or vaginal bleeding NOS

N93.9 **Abnormal uterine and vaginal bleeding, unspecified**

N94 **Pain and other conditions associated with female genital organs and menstrual cycle**

N94.0 **Mittelschmerz**

N94.1 **Dyspareunia**

Excludes1: psychogenic dyspareunia (F52.6)

N94.10 **Unspecified dyspareunia**

N94.11 **Superficial (introital) dyspareunia**

N94.12 **Deep dyspareunia**

N94.19 **Other specified dyspareunia**

N94.2 **Vaginismus**

Excludes1: psychogenic vaginismus (F52.5)

N94.3 **Premenstrual tension syndrome**

Code also associated menstrual migraine (G43.82-, G43.83-)

Excludes1: Premenstrual dysphoric disorder (F32.81)

N94.4 **Primary dysmenorrhea**

N94.5 **Secondary dysmenorrhea**

N94.6 **Dysmenorrhea, unspecified**

Excludes1: psychogenic dysmenorrhea (F45.8)

N94.8 **Other specified conditions associated with female genital organs and menstrual cycle**

N94.81 **Vulvodynia**

N94.810 **Vulvar vestibulitis**

N94.818 **Other vulvodynia**

N94.819 **Vulvodynia, unspecified**

Vulvodynia NOS

N94.89 **Other specified conditions associated with female genital organs and menstrual cycle**

N94.9 **Unspecified condition associated with female genital organs and menstrual cycle**

N95 **Menopausal and other perimenopausal disorders**

Menopausal **and other** perimenopausal disorders due to naturally occurring (age-related) menopause and perimenopause

Excludes1: excessive bleeding in the premenopausal period (N92.4)

menopausal and perimenopausal disorders due to artificial or premature menopause (E89.4-, E28.31-)

premature menopause (E28.31-)

Excludes2: postmenopausal osteoporosis (M81.0-)

postmenopausal osteoporosis with current pathological fracture (M80.0-)

postmenopausal urethritis (N34.2)

N95.0 **Postmenopausal bleeding**

N95.1 **Menopausal and female climacteric states**

Symptoms such as flushing, sleeplessness, headache, lack of concentration, associated with natural (age-related) menopause

Use Additional Code for associated symptoms

Excludes1: asymptomatic menopausal state (Z78.0)

symptoms associated with artificial menopause (E89.41)

symptoms associated with premature menopause (E28.310)

N95.2 **Postmenopausal atrophic vaginitis**

Senile (atrophic) vaginitis

N95.8 **Other specified menopausal and perimenopausal disorders**

N95.9 **Unspecified menopausal and perimenopausal disorder**

N96 **Recurrent pregnancy loss**

Investigation or care in a nonpregnant woman with history of recurrent pregnancy loss

Excludes1: recurrent pregnancy loss with current pregnancy (O26.2-)

N97 **Female infertility**

Includes: inability to achieve a pregnancy

sterility, female NOS

Excludes2: female infertility associated with:

hypopituitarism (E23.0)

incompetence of cervix uteri (N88.3)

Stein-Leventhal syndrome (E28.2)

Excludes2: incompetence of cervix uteri (N88.3)

N97.0 **Female infertility associated with anovulation**

N97.1 **Female infertility of tubal origin**

Female infertility associated with congenital anomaly of tube female infertility due to tubal block

Female infertility due to tubal occlusion female infertility due to tubal stenosis

N97.2 **Female infertility of uterine origin**

Female infertility associated with congenital anomaly of uterus female infertility due to nonimplantation of ovum

N97.8 **Female infertility of other origin**

N97.9 **Female infertility, unspecified**

N98 **Complications associated with artificial fertilization**

N98.0 **Infection associated with artificial insemination**

N98.1 **Hyperstimulation of ovaries**

Hyperstimulation of ovaries NOS

Hyperstimulation of ovaries associated with induced ovulation

N98.2 **Complications of attempted introduction of fertilized ovum following in vitro fertilization**

N98.3 **Complications of attempted introduction of embryo in embryo transfer**

N98.8 **Other complications associated with artificial fertilization**

N98.9 **Complication associated with artificial fertilization, unspecified**

INTRAOPERATIVE AND POSTPROCEDURAL COMPLICATIONS AND DISORDERS OF GENITOURINARY SYSTEM, NOT ELSEWHERE CLASSIFIED (N99)

N99 **Intraoperative and postprocedural complications and disorders of genitourinary system, not elsewhere classified**

Excludes2: irradiation cystitis (N30.4-)

postoophorectomy osteoporosis with current pathological fracture (M80.8-)

postoophorectomy osteoporosis without current pathological fracture (M81.8)

N99.0 **Postprocedural (acute) (chronic) kidney failure**

Use Additional Code to type of kidney disease

N99.1 **Postprocedural urethral stricture**

Postcatheterization urethral stricture

N99.11 **Postprocedural urethral stricture, male**

N99.110 **Postprocedural urethral stricture, male, meatal**

N99.111 **Postprocedural bulbous urethral stricture, male**

N99.112 **Postprocedural membranous urethral stricture, male**

N99.113 **Postprocedural anterior bulbous urethral stricture, male**

N99.114 **Postprocedural urethral stricture, male, unspecified**

N99.115 **Postprocedural fossa navicularis urethral stricture**

N99.116 **Postprocedural urethral stricture, male, overlapping sites**

N99.12 **Postprocedural urethral stricture, female**

N99.2 **Postprocedural adhesions of vagina**

N99.3 **Prolapse of vaginal vault after hysterectomy**

N99.4 **Postprocedural pelvic peritoneal adhesions**

Excludes2: pelvic peritoneal adhesions NOS (N73.6)

postinfective pelvic peritoneal adhesions (N73.6)

N99.5 **Complications of stoma of urinary tract**

Excludes2: mechanical complication of urinary catheter (T83.0-)

N99.51 **Complication of cystostomy**

N99.510 **Cystostomy hemorrhage** [HCC]

N99.511 **Cystostomy infection** [HCC]

N99.512 **Cystostomy malfunction** [HCC]

N99.518 **Other cystostomy complication** [HCC]

N99.52 **Complication of incontinent external stoma of urinary tract**

N99.520 **Hemorrhage of incontinent external stoma of urinary tract** [HCC]

N99.521 **Infection of incontinent external stoma of urinary tract** [HCC]

N99.522 **Malfunction of incontinent external stoma of urinary tract** [HCC]

N99.523 **Herniation of incontinent stoma of urinary tract** [HCC]

N99.524 **Stenosis of incontinent stoma of urinary tract** [HCC]

N99.528 **Other complication of incontinent external stoma of urinary tract** [HCC]

N99.53 **Complication of continent stoma of urinary tract**

N99.530 **Hemorrhage of continent stoma of urinary tract** [HCC]

N99.531 **Infection of continent stoma of urinary tract** [HCC]

N99.532 **Malfunction of continent stoma of urinary tract** [HCC]

N99.533 **Herniation of continent stoma of urinary tract** [HCC]

N99.534 **Stenosis of continent stoma of urinary tract** [HCC]

N99.538 **Other complication of continent stoma of urinary tract** [HCC]

N99.6 **Intraoperative hemorrhage and hematoma of a genitourinary system organ or structure complicating a procedure**

Excludes1: intraoperative hemorrhage and hematoma of a genitourinary system organ or structure due to accidental puncture or laceration during a procedure (N99.7-)

N99.61 **Intraoperative hemorrhage and hematoma of a genitourinary system organ or structure complicating a genitourinary system procedure**

N99.62 **Intraoperative hemorrhage and hematoma of a genitourinary system organ or structure complicating other procedure**

N99.7 **Accidental puncture and laceration of a genitourinary system organ or structure during a procedure**

N99.71 **Accidental puncture and laceration of a genitourinary system organ or structure during a genitourinary system procedure**

N99.72 **Accidental puncture and laceration of a genitourinary system organ or structure during other procedure**

N99.8 **Other intraoperative and postprocedural complications and disorders of genitourinary system**

N99.81 **Other intraoperative complications of genitourinary system**

N99.82 **Postprocedural hemorrhage of a genitourinary system organ or structure following a procedure**

N99.820 **Postprocedural hemorrhage of a genitourinary system organ or structure following a genitourinary system procedure**

N99.821 **Postprocedural hemorrhage of a genitourinary system organ or structure following other procedure**

N99.83 **Residual ovary syndrome**

N99.84 **Postprocedural hematoma and seroma of a genitourinary system organ or structure following a procedure**

N99.840 **Postprocedural hematoma of a genitourinary system organ or structure following a genitourinary system procedure**

N99.841   **Postprocedural hematoma of a genitourinary system organ or structure following other procedure**

N99.842   **Postprocedural seroma of a genitourinary system organ or structure following a genitourinary system procedure**

N99.843   **Postprocedural seroma of a genitourinary system organ or structure following other procedure**

N99.85   **Post endometrial ablation syndrome**

N99.89   **Other postprocedural complications and disorders of genitourinary system**

● New code ▲ Revised code **Excludes1:** Not coded here **Excludes2:** Not included here ⊗ Placeholder required ⑦7ᵗʰ digit required

Chapter 15: Pregnancy, Childbirth and the Puerperium (O00-O9A)

DEFINITIONS

This chapter includes definitions of selected key words, terms and phrases and coding alerts for adding points to the clinical domain, and references to coding late effects where appropriate. An example from this chapter is as follows:

O03   Spontaneous abortion

     Definition: *Spontaneous abortion* refers to the loss of pregnancy before 20 weeks of gestation without outside intervention.

MULTIPLE CODING FOR A SINGLE CONDITION

In addition to the etiology/manifestation convention that requires two codes to fully describe a single condition that affects multiple body systems, there are other single conditions that also require more than one code. "**Use Additional Code**" notes are found in the Tabular List at codes that are not part of an etiology/manifestation pair where a secondary code is useful to fully describe a condition. The sequencing rule is the same as the etiology/manifestation pair, "**Use Additional Code**" indicates that a secondary code should be added.

For example, for bacterial infections that are not included in chapter 1, a secondary code from category B95, Streptococcus, Staphylococcus, and Enterococcus, as the cause of diseases classified elsewhere, or B96, Other bacterial agents as the cause of diseases classified elsewhere, may be required to identify the bacterial organism causing the infection. A "**Use Additional Code**" note will normally be found at the infectious disease code, indicating a need for the organism code to be added as a secondary code.

"Code first" notes are also under certain codes that are not specifically manifestation codes but may be due to an underlying cause. When there is a "Code first" note and an underlying condition is present, the underlying condition should be sequenced first.

"Code, if applicable, any causal condition first", notes indicate that this code may be assigned as a principal diagnosis when the causal condition is unknown or not applicable. If a causal condition is known, then the code for that condition should be sequenced as the principal or first-listed diagnosis.

Multiple codes may be needed for sequela, complication codes and obstetric codes to more fully describe a condition. See the specific guidelines for these conditions for further instruction.

COMBINATION CODE

A combination code is a single code used to classify: Two diagnoses, or a diagnosis with an associated secondary process (manifestation) A diagnosis with an associated complication

Combination codes are identified by referring to subterm entries in the Alphabetic Index and by reading the inclusion and exclusion notes in the Tabular List.

Assign only the combination code when that code fully identifies the diagnostic conditions involved or when the Alphabetic Index so directs. Multiple coding should not be used when the classification provides a combination code that clearly identifies all of the elements documented in the diagnosis. When the combination code lacks necessary specificity in describing the manifestation or complication, an additional code should be used as a secondary code.

SEQUELA (LATE EFFECTS)

A sequela is the residual effect (condition produced) after the acute phase of an illness or injury has terminated. There is no time limit on when a sequela code can be used. The residual may be apparent early, such as in cerebral infarction, or it may occur months or years later, such as that due to a previous injury. Coding of sequela generally requires two codes sequenced in the following order: The condition or nature of the sequela is sequenced first.

The sequela code is sequenced second.

An exception to the above guidelines are those instances where the code for the sequela is followed by a manifestation code identified in the Tabular List and title, or the sequela code has been expanded (at the fourth, fifth or sixth character levels) to

include the manifestation(s). The code for the acute phase of an illness or injury that led to the sequela is never used with a code for the late effect.

GENERAL RULES FOR OBSTETRIC CASES

1) Codes from chapter 15 and sequencing priority

Obstetric cases require codes from chapter 15, codes in the range O00-O9A, Pregnancy, Childbirth, and the Puerperium. Chapter 15 codes have sequencing priority over codes from other chapters. Additional codes from other chapters may be used in conjunction with chapter 15 codes to further specify conditions. Should the provider document that the pregnancy is incidental to the encounter, then code Z33.1, Pregnant state, incidental, should be used in place of any chapter 15 codes. It is the provider's responsibility to state that the condition being treated is not affecting the pregnancy.

2) Chapter 15 codes used only on the maternal record

Chapter 15 codes are to be used only on the maternal record, never on the record of the newborn.

3) Final character for trimester

The majority of codes in Chapter 15 have a final character indicating the trimester of pregnancy. The timeframes for the trimesters are indicated at the beginning of the chapter. If trimester is not a component of a code, it is because the condition always occurs in a specific trimester, or the concept of trimester of pregnancy is not applicable. Certain codes have characters for only certain trimesters because the condition does not occur in all trimesters, but it may occur in more than just one.

Assignment of the final character for trimester should be based on the provider's documentation of the trimester (or number of weeks) for the current admission/encounter. This applies to the assignment of trimester for pre-existing conditions as well as those that develop during or are due to the pregnancy. The provider's documentation of the number of weeks may be used to assign the appropriate code identifying the trimester.

Whenever delivery occurs during the current admission, and there is an "in childbirth" option for the obstetric complication being coded, the "in childbirth" code should be assigned. When the classification does not provide an obstetric code with an "in childbirth" option, it is appropriate to assign a code describing the current trimester.

4) Selection of trimester for inpatient admissions that encompass more than one trimester

In instances when a patient is admitted to a hospital for complications of pregnancy during one trimester and remains in the hospital into a subsequent trimester, the trimester character for the antepartum complication code should be assigned on the basis of the trimester when the complication developed, not the trimester of the discharge. If the condition developed prior to the current admission/encounter or represents a pre-existing condition, the trimester character for the trimester at the time of the admission/encounter should be assigned.

5) Unspecified trimester

Each category that includes codes for trimester has a code for "unspecified trimester." The "unspecified trimester" code should rarely be used, such as when the documentation in the record is insufficient to determine the trimester and it is not possible to obtain clarification.

6) 7th character for Fetus Identification

Where applicable, a 7th character is to be assigned for certain categories (O31, O32, O33.3 - O33.6, O35, O36, O40, O41, O60.1, O60.2, O64, and O69) to identify the fetus for which the complication code applies.

Assign 7th character "0":

- For single gestations

- When the documentation in the record is insufficient to determine the fetus affected and it is not possible to obtain clarification.

- When it is not possible to clinically determine which fetus is affected.

SELECTION OF OB PRINCIPAL OR FIRST-LISTED DIAGNOSIS

1) **Routine outpatient prenatal visits**

   For routine outpatient prenatal visits when no complications are present, a code from category Z34, Encounter for supervision of normal pregnancy, should be used as the first-listed diagnosis. These codes should not be used in conjunction with chapter 15 codes.

2) **Supervision of High-Risk Pregnancy**

   Codes from category O09, Supervision of high-risk pregnancy, are intended for use only during the prenatal period. For complications during the labor or delivery episode as a result of a high-risk pregnancy, assign the applicable complication codes from Chapter 15. If there are no complications during the labor or delivery episode, assign code O80, Encounter for full-term uncomplicated delivery.

   For routine prenatal outpatient visits for patients with high-risk pregnancies, a code from category O09, Supervision of high-risk pregnancy, should be used as the first-listed diagnosis. Secondary chapter 15 codes may be used in conjunction with these codes if appropriate.

3) **Episodes when no delivery occurs**

   In episodes when no delivery occurs, the principal diagnosis should correspond to the principal complication of the pregnancy which necessitated the encounter. Should more than one complication exist, all of which are treated or monitored, any of the complications codes may be sequenced first.

4) **When a delivery occurs**

   When an obstetric patient is admitted and delivers during that admission, the condition that prompted the admission should be sequenced as the principal diagnosis. If multiple conditions prompted the admission, sequence the one most related to the delivery as the principal diagnosis. A code for any complication of the delivery should be assigned as an additional diagnosis. In cases of cesarean delivery, if the patient was admitted with a condition that resulted in the performance of a cesarean procedure, that condition should be selected as the principal diagnosis. If the reason for the admission was unrelated to the condition resulting in the cesarean delivery, the condition related to the reason for the admission should be selected as the principal diagnosis.

5) **Outcome of delivery**

   A code from category Z37, Outcome of delivery, should be included on every maternal record when a delivery has occurred. These codes are not to be used on subsequent records or on the newborn record.

PRE-EXISTING CONDITIONS VERSUS CONDITIONS DUE TO THE PREGNANCY

Certain categories in Chapter 15 distinguish between conditions of the mother that existed prior to pregnancy (pre-existing) and those that are a direct result of pregnancy. When assigning codes from Chapter 15, it is important to assess if a condition was pre-existing prior to pregnancy or developed during or due to the pregnancy in order to assign the correct code.

Categories that do not distinguish between pre-existing and pregnancy-related conditions may be used for either. It is acceptable to use codes specifically for the puerperium with codes complicating pregnancy and childbirth if a condition arises postpartum during the delivery encounter.

PRE-EXISTING HYPERTENSION IN PREGNANCY

Category O10, Pre-existing hypertension complicating pregnancy, childbirth and the puerperium, includes codes for hypertensive heart and hypertensive chronic kidney disease. When assigning one of the O10 codes that includes hypertensive heart disease or hypertensive chronic kidney disease, it is necessary to add a secondary code from the appropriate hypertension category to specify the type of heart failure or chronic kidney disease.

See Section I.C.9. Hypertension.

FETAL CONDITIONS AFFECTING THE MANAGEMENT OF THE MOTHER

1) Codes from categories O35 and O36

Codes from categories O35, Maternal care for known or suspected fetal abnormality and damage, and O36, Maternal care for other fetal problems, are assigned only when the fetal condition is actually responsible for modifying the management of the mother, i.e., by requiring diagnostic studies, additional observation, special care, or termination of pregnancy. The fact that the fetal condition exists does not justify assigning a code from this series to the mother's record.

2) In utero surgery

In cases when surgery is performed on the fetus, a diagnosis code from category O35, Maternal care for known or suspected fetal abnormality and damage, should be assigned identifying the fetal condition. Assign the appropriate procedure code for the procedure performed.

No code from Chapter 16, the perinatal codes, should be used on the mother's record to identify fetal conditions. Surgery performed in utero on a fetus is still to be coded as an obstetric encounter.

HIV INFECTION IN PREGNANCY, CHILDBIRTH AND THE PUERPERIUM

During pregnancy, childbirth or the puerperium, a patient admitted because of an HIV-related illness should receive a principal diagnosis from subcategory O98.7-, Human immunodeficiency [HIV] disease complicating pregnancy, childbirth and the puerperium, followed by the code(s) for the HIV-related illness(es).

Patients with asymptomatic HIV infection status admitted during pregnancy, childbirth, or the puerperium should receive codes of O98.7- and Z21, Asymptomatic human immunodeficiency virus [HIV] infection status.

DIABETES MELLITUS IN PREGNANCY

Diabetes mellitus is a significant complicating factor in pregnancy. Pregnant women who are diabetic should be assigned a code from category O24, Diabetes mellitus in pregnancy, childbirth, and the puerperium, first, followed by the appropriate diabetes code(s) (E08-E13) from Chapter 4.

LONG TERM USE OF INSULIN AND ORAL HYPOGLYCEMICS

See section I.C.4.a.3 for information on the long-term use of insulin and oral hypoglycemic.

GESTATIONAL (PREGNANCY INDUCED) DIABETES

Gestational (pregnancy induced) diabetes can occur during the second and thirdtrimester of pregnancy in patients who were not diabetic prior to pregnancy. Gestational diabetes can cause complications in the pregnancy similar to thoseof pre-existing diabetes mellitus. It also puts the patient at greater risk of developing diabetes after the pregnancy.

Codes for gestational diabetes are in subcategory O24.4, Gestational diabetes mellitus. No other code from category O24, Diabetes mellitus in pregnancy, childbirth, and the puerperium, should be used with a code from O24.4.

The codes under subcategory O24.4 include diet controlled, insulin controlled, and controlled by oral hypoglycemic drugs. If a patient with gestational diabetes is treated with both diet and insulin, only the code for insulin-controlled is required. If a patient with gestational diabetes is treated with both diet and oral hypoglycemic medications, only the code for "controlled by oral hypoglycemic drugs" is required. Code Z79.4, Long-term (current) use of insulin or code Z79.84, Long-term (current) use of oral hypoglycemic drugs, should not be assigned with codes from subcategory O24.4.

An abnormal glucose tolerance in pregnancy is assigned a code from subcategory O99.81, Abnormal glucose complicating pregnancy, childbirth, and the puerperium.

SEPSIS AND SEPTIC SHOCK COMPLICATING ABORTION, PREGNANCY, CHILDBIRTH AND THE PUERPERIUM

● New code ▲ Revised code Excludes1: Not coded here Excludes2: Not included here ⊗ Placeholder required ⑦7th digit required

When assigning a chapter 15 code for sepsis complicating abortion, pregnancy, childbirth, and the puerperium, a code for the specific type of infection should be assigned as an additional diagnosis. If severe sepsis is present, a code from subcategory R65.2, Severe sepsis, and code(s) for associated organ dysfunction(s) should also be assigned as additional diagnoses.

PUERPERAL SEPSIS

Code O85, Puerperal sepsis, should be assigned with a secondary code to identify the causal organism (e.g., for a bacterial infection, assign a code from category B95-B96, Bacterial infections in conditions classified elsewhere). A code from category A40, Streptococcal sepsis, or A41, Other sepsis, should not be used for puerperal sepsis. If applicable, **Use Additional Code**s to identify severe sepsis (R65.2-) and any associated acute organ dysfunction.

ALCOHOL, TOBACCO AND DRUG USE DURING PREGNANCY, CHILDBIRTH AND THE PUERPERIUM

1) **Alcohol use during pregnancy, childbirth and the puerperium**

   Codes under subcategory O99.31, Alcohol use complicating pregnancy, childbirth, and the puerperium, should be assigned for any pregnancy case when a patient uses alcohol during the pregnancy or postpartum. A secondary code from category F10, Alcohol related disorders, should also be assigned to identify manifestations of the alcohol use.

2) **Tobacco use during pregnancy, childbirth and the puerperium**

   Codes under subcategory O99.33, Smoking (tobacco) complicating pregnancy, childbirth, and the puerperium, should be assigned for any pregnancy case when a mother uses any type of tobacco product during the pregnancy or postpartum.

   A secondary code from category F17, Nicotine dependence, should also be assigned to identify the type of nicotine dependence.

3) **Drug use during pregnancy, childbirth and the puerperium**

   Codes under subcategory O99.32, Drug use complicating pregnancy, childbirth, and the puerperium, should be assigned for any pregnancy case when a patient uses drugs during the pregnancy or postpartum. This can involve illegal drugs, or inappropriate use or abuse of prescription drugs. Secondary code(s) from categories F11-F16 and F18-F19 should also be assigned to identify manifestations of the drug use.

POISONING, TOXIC EFFECTS, ADVERSE EFFECTS AND UNDERDOSING IN A PREGNANT PATIENT

A code from subcategory O9A.2, Injury, poisoning and certain other consequences of external causes complicating pregnancy, childbirth, and the puerperium, should be sequenced first, followed by the appropriate injury, poisoning, toxic effect, adverse effect or underdosing code, and then the additional code(s) that specifies the condition caused by the poisoning, toxic effect, adverse effect or underdosing.

See Section I.C.19. Adverse effects, poisoning, underdosing and toxic effects.

NORMAL DELIVERY, CODE O80

1) **Encounter for full term uncomplicated delivery**

   Code O80 should be assigned when a patient is admitted for a full-term normal delivery and delivers a single, healthy infant without any complications antepartum, during the delivery, or postpartum during the delivery episode. Code O80 is always a principal diagnosis. It is not to be used if any other code from chapter 15 is needed to describe a current complication of the antenatal, delivery, or postnatal period. Additional codes from other chapters may be used with code O80 if they are not related to or are in any way complicating the pregnancy.

2) **Uncomplicated delivery with resolved antepartum complication**

   Code O80 may be used if the patient had a complication at some point during the pregnancy, but the complication is not present at the time of the admission for delivery.

3) **Outcome of delivery for O80**

Z37.0, Single live birth, is the only outcome of delivery code appropriate for use with O80.

THE PERIPARTUM AND POSTPARTUM PERIODS

1) Peripartum and Postpartum periods

The postpartum period begins immediately after delivery and continues for six weeks following delivery. The peripartum period is defined as the last month of pregnancy to five months postpartum.

2) Peripartum and postpartum complication

A postpartum complication is any complication occurring within the six-week period.

3) Pregnancy-related complications after 6-week period

Chapter 15 codes may also be used to describe pregnancy-related complications after the peripartum or postpartum period if the provider documents that a condition is pregnancy related.

4) Admission for routine postpartum care following delivery outside hospital

When the mother delivers outside the hospital prior to admission and is admitted for routine postpartum care and no complications are noted, code Z39.0, Encounter for care and examination of mother immediately after delivery, should be assigned as the principal diagnosis.

5) Pregnancy associated cardiomyopathy

Pregnancy associated cardiomyopathy, code O90.3, is unique in that it may be diagnosed in the third trimester of pregnancy but may continue to progress months after delivery. For this reason, it is referred to as peripartum cardiomyopathy. Code O90.3 is only for use when the cardiomyopathy develops as a result of pregnancy in a woman who did not have pre-existing heart disease.

CODE O94, SEQUELAE OF COMPLICATION OF PREGNANCY, CHILDBIRTH, AND THE PUERPERIUM

1) Code O94

Code O94, Sequelae of complication of pregnancy, childbirth, and the puerperium, is for use in those cases when an initial complication of a pregnancy develops a sequela or sequelae requiring care or treatment at a future date.

2) After the initial postpartum period

This code may be used at any time after the initial postpartum period.

3) Sequencing of Code O94

This code, like all sequela codes, is to be sequenced following the code describing the sequelae of the complication.

TERMINATION OF PREGNANCY AND SPONTANEOUS ABORTIONS

1) Abortion with Liveborn Fetus

When an attempted termination of pregnancy results in a liveborn fetus, assign code Z33.2, Encounter for elective termination of pregnancy and a code from category Z37, Outcome of Delivery.

2) Retained Products of Conception following an abortion

Subsequent encounters for retained products of conception following a spontaneous abortion or elective termination of pregnancy, without complications are assigned O03.4, Incomplete spontaneous abortion without complication, or code O07.4, Failed attempted termination of pregnancy without complication. This advice is appropriate even when the patient was discharged previously with a discharge diagnosis of complete abortion. If the patient has a specific complication associated with the spontaneous abortion or elective termination of pregnancy in addition to retained products of conception, assign the appropriate complication code (e.g., O03.-, O04.-, O07.-) instead of code O03.4 or O07.4.

3) **Complications leading to abortion**

Codes from Chapter 15 may be used as additional codes to identify any documented complications of the pregnancy in conjunction with codes in categories in O04, O07 and O08.

ABUSE IN A PREGNANT PATIENT

For suspected or confirmed cases of abuse of a pregnant patient, a code(s) from subcategories O9A.3, Physical abuse complicating pregnancy, childbirth, and the puerperium, O9A.4, Sexual abuse complicating pregnancy, childbirth, and the puerperium, and O9A.5, Psychological abuse complicating pregnancy, childbirth, and the puerperium, should be sequenced first, followed by the appropriate codes (if applicable) to identify any associated current injury due to physical abuse, sexual abuse, and the perpetrator of abuse.

See Section I.C.19. Adult and child abuse, neglect and other maltreatment.

COVID-19 INFECTION IN PREGNANCY, CHILDBIRTH, AND THE PUERPERIUM

During pregnancy, childbirth or the puerperium, when COVID-19 is the reason for admission/encounter , code O98.5-, Other viral diseases complicating pregnancy, childbirth and the puerperium, should be sequenced as the principal/first-listed diagnosis, and code U07.1, COVID-19, and the appropriate codes for associated manifestation(s) should be assigned as additional diagnoses. Codes from Chapter 15 always take sequencing priority.

If the reason for admission/encounter is unrelated to COVID-19 but the patient tests positive for COVID-19 during the admission/encounter, the appropriate code for the reason for admission/encounter should be sequenced as the principal/first-listed diagnosis, and codes O98.5- and U07.1, as well as the appropriate codes for associated COVID-19 manifestations, should be assigned as additional diagnoses.

● New code ▲ Revised code **Excludes1:** Not coded here **Excludes2:** Not included here ⊗ Placeholder required ⑦7th digit required

Chapter 15
Pregnancy, Childbirth and The Puerperium (O00-O9A)

NOTE: CODES FROM THIS CHAPTER ARE FOR USE ONLY ON MATERNAL RECORDS, NEVER ON NEWBORN RECORDS

Codes from this chapter are for use for conditions related to or aggravated by the pregnancy, childbirth, or by the puerperium (maternal causes or obstetric causes) trimesters are counted from the first day of the last menstrual period. They are defined as follows:

1st trimester- less than 14 weeks 0 days

2nd trimester- 14 weeks 0 days to less than 28 weeks 0 days

3rd trimester- 28 weeks 0 days until delivery

<u>Use Additional Code</u> from category Z3A, Weeks of gestation, to identify the specific week of the pregnancy, if known.

Excludes1: supervision of normal pregnancy (Z34.-)

Excludes2: mental and behavioral disorders associated with the puerperium (F53-)

    obstetrical tetanus (A34)

    postpartum necrosis of pituitary gland (E23.0)

    puerperal osteomalacia (M83.0)

This chapter contains the following blocks:

O00-O08	Pregnancy with abortive outcome
O09	Supervision of high-risk pregnancy
O10-O16	Edema, proteinuria and hypertensive disorders in pregnancy, childbirth and the puerperium
O20-O29	Other maternal disorders predominantly related to pregnancy
O30-O48	Maternal care related to the fetus and amniotic cavity and possible delivery problems
O60-O77	Complications of labor and delivery
O80-O82	Encounter for delivery
O85-O92	Complications predominantly related to the puerperium
O94-O9A	Other obstetric conditions, not elsewhere classified

PREGNANCY WITH ABORTIVE OUTCOME (O00-O08)

Excludes1: continuing pregnancy in multiple gestation after abortion of one

    fetus or more (O31.1-, O31.3-)

O00   **Ectopic pregnancy**

    Includes: ruptured ectopic pregnancy

    <u>Use Additional Code</u> from category O08 to identify any associated complication

    O00.0   **Abdominal pregnancy**

        Excludes1: maternal care for viable fetus in abdominal pregnancy (O36.7-)

        O00.00   **Abdominal pregnancy without intrauterine pregnancy**

            Abdominal pregnancy NOS

        O00.01   **Abdominal pregnancy with intrauterine pregnancy**

    O00.1   **Tubal pregnancy**

        Fallopian pregnancy

        Rupture of (fallopian) tube due to pregnancy

        Tubal abortion

        O00.10   **Tubal pregnancy without intrauterine pregnancy**

            Tubal pregnancy NOS

        O00.101   **Right tubal pregnancy without intrauterine pregnancy**

        O00.102   **Left tubal pregnancy without intrauterine pregnancy**

        O00.109   **Unspecified tubal pregnancy without intrauterine pregnancy**

        O00.11   **Tubal pregnancy with intrauterine pregnancy**

        O00.111   **Right tubal pregnancy with intrauterine pregnancy**

        O00.112   **Left tubal pregnancy with intrauterine pregnancy**

        O00.119   **Unspecified tubal pregnancy with intrauterine pregnancy**

    O00.2   **Ovarian pregnancy**

        O00.20   **Ovarian pregnancy without intrauterine pregnancy**

            Ovarian pregnancy NOS

        O00.201   **Right ovarian pregnancy without intrauterine pregnancy**

        O00.202   **Left ovarian pregnancy without intrauterine pregnancy**

        O00.209   **Unspecified ovarian pregnancy without intrauterine pregnancy**

        O00.21   **Ovarian pregnancy with intrauterine pregnancy**

        O00.211   **Right ovarian pregnancy with intrauterine pregnancy**

        O00.212   **Left ovarian pregnancy with intrauterine pregnancy**

        O00.219   **Unspecified ovarian pregnancy with intrauterine pregnancy**

    O00.8   **Other ectopic pregnancy**

        Definition: Ectopic pregnancy occurs with the implantation and subsequent development of a fertilized ovum outside the uterus, as in a fallopian tube.

        Cervical pregnancy

        Cornual pregnancy

        Intraligamentous pregnancy

        Mural pregnancy

        O00.80   **Other ectopic pregnancy without intrauterine pregnancy**

            Other ectopic pregnancy NOS

        O00.81   **Other ectopic pregnancy with intrauterine pregnancy**

    O00.9   **Ectopic pregnancy, unspecified**

        O00.90   **Unspecified ectopic pregnancy without intrauterine pregnancy**

            Ectopic pregnancy NOS

        O00.91   **Unspecified ectopic pregnancy with intrauterine pregnancy**

O01   **Hydatidiform mole**

    Definition: A Hydatidiform mole is a rare mass or growth that forms inside the uterus at the beginning of a pregnancy. It is a type of gestational trophoblastic disease (GTD).

    <u>Use Additional Code</u> from category O08 to identify any associated complication.

    Excludes1: chorioadenoma (destruens) (D39.2)

        malignant hydatidiform mole (D39.2)

    O01.0   **Classical hydatidiform mole**

        Complete hydatidiform mole

    O01.1   **Incomplete and partial hydatidiform mole**

O01.9   Hydatidiform mole, unspecified

Trophoblastic disease NOS

Vesicular mole NOS

O02   Other abnormal products of conception

Use Additional Code from category O08 to identify any associated complication.

Excludes1: papyraceous fetus (O31.0-)

O02.0   Blighted ovum and nonhydatidiform mole

Carneous mole

Fleshy mole

Intrauterine mole NOS

Molar pregnancy NEC

Pathological ovum

O02.1   Missed abortion

Definition: A missed abortion is an abortion in which the fetus dies but is retained within the uterus for two months or longer.

Early fetal death, before completion of 20 weeks of gestation, with retention of dead fetus

Excludes1: failed induced abortion (O07.-)

fetal death (intrauterine) (late) (O36.4)

missed abortion with blighted ovum (O02.0)

missed abortion with hydatidiform mole (O01.-)

missed abortion with nonhydatidiform (O02.0)

missed abortion with other abnormal products of conception (O02.8-)

missed delivery (O36.4)

stillbirth (P95)

O02.8   Other specified abnormal products of conception

Excludes1: abnormal products of conception with blighted ovum (O02.0)

abnormal products of conception with hydatidiform mole (O01.-)

abnormal products of conception with nonhydatidiform mole (O02.0)

O02.81   Inappropriate change in quantitative human chorionic gonadotropin (hCG) in early pregnancy

Biochemical pregnancy

Chemical pregnancy

Inappropriate level of quantitative human chorionic gonadotropin (hCG) for gestational age in early pregnancy

O02.89   Other abnormal products of conception

O02.9   Abnormal product of conception, unspecified

O03   Spontaneous abortion

Definition: Spontaneous abortion refers to the loss of pregnancy before 20 weeks of gestation without outside intervention.

Note: Incomplete abortion includes retained products of conception following spontaneous abortion

Includes: miscarriage

O03.0   Genital tract and pelvic infection following incomplete spontaneous abortion

Endometritis following incomplete spontaneous abortion

Oophoritis following incomplete spontaneous abortion

Parametritis following incomplete spontaneous abortion

Pelvic peritonitis following incomplete spontaneous abortion

Salpingitis following incomplete spontaneous abortion

Salpingo-oophoritis following incomplete spontaneous abortion

Excludes1: sepsis following incomplete spontaneous abortion (O03.37)

urinary tract infection following incomplete spontaneous abortion (O03.38)

O03.1   Delayed or excessive hemorrhage following incomplete spontaneous abortion

Afibrinogenemia following incomplete spontaneous abortion

Defibrination syndrome following incomplete spontaneous abortion

Hemolysis following incomplete spontaneous abortion

Intravascular coagulation following incomplete spontaneous abortion

O03.2   Embolism following incomplete spontaneous abortion

Air embolism following incomplete spontaneous abortion

Amniotic fluid embolism following incomplete spontaneous abortion

Blood-clot embolism following incomplete spontaneous abortion

Embolism NOS following incomplete spontaneous abortion

Fat embolism following incomplete spontaneous abortion

Pulmonary embolism following incomplete spontaneous abortion

Pyemic embolism following incomplete spontaneous abortion

Septic or septicopyemic embolism following incomplete spontaneous abortion

Soap embolism following incomplete spontaneous abortion

O03.3   Other and unspecified complications following incomplete spontaneous abortion

O03.30   Unspecified complication following incomplete spontaneous abortion

O03.31   Shock following incomplete spontaneous abortion

Circulatory collapse following incomplete spontaneous abortion

Shock (postprocedural) following incomplete spontaneous abortion

Excludes1: shock due to infection following incomplete spontaneous abortion (O03.37)

O03.32   Renal failure following incomplete spontaneous abortion

Kidney failure (acute) following incomplete spontaneous abortion

Oliguria following incomplete spontaneous abortion

Renal shutdown following incomplete spontaneous abortion

Renal tubular necrosis following incomplete spontaneous abortion

Uremia following incomplete spontaneous abortion

O03.33   Metabolic disorder following incomplete spontaneous abortion

O03.34   Damage to pelvic organs following incomplete spontaneous abortion

Laceration, perforation, tear or chemical damage of bladder following incomplete spontaneous abortion

● New code   ▲ Revised code   **Excludes1:** Not coded here   **Excludes2:** Not included here   ⊗ Placeholder required   ⑦7th digit required

Laceration, perforation, tear or chemical damage of bowel following incomplete spontaneous abortion

Laceration, perforation, tear or chemical damage of broad ligament following incomplete spontaneous abortion

Laceration, perforation, tear or chemical damage of cervix following incomplete spontaneous abortion

Laceration, perforation, tear or chemical damage of periurethral tissue following incomplete spontaneous abortion

Laceration, perforation, tear or chemical damage of uterus following incomplete spontaneous abortion

Laceration, perforation, tear or chemical damage of vagina following incomplete spontaneous abortion

O03.35   Other venous complications following incomplete spontaneous abortion

O03.36   Cardiac arrest following incomplete spontaneous abortion

O03.37   Sepsis following incomplete spontaneous abortion

Use Additional Code to identify infectious agent (B95-B97)

Use Additional Code to identify severe sepsis, if applicable (R65.2-)

Excludes1: septic or septicopyemic embolism following incomplete spontaneous abortion (O03.2)

O03.38   Urinary tract infection following incomplete spontaneous abortion

Cystitis following incomplete spontaneous abortion

O03.39   Incomplete spontaneous abortion with other complications

O03.4   Incomplete spontaneous abortion without complication

O03.5   Genital tract and pelvic infection following complete or unspecified spontaneous abortion

Endometritis following complete or unspecified spontaneous abortion

Oophoritis following complete or unspecified spontaneous abortion

Parametritis following complete or unspecified spontaneous abortion

Pelvic peritonitis following complete or unspecified spontaneous abortion

Salpingitis following complete or unspecified spontaneous abortion

Salpingo-oophoritis following complete or unspecified spontaneous abortion

Excludes1: sepsis following complete or unspecified spontaneous abortion (O03.87)

urinary tract infection following complete or unspecified spontaneous abortion (O03.88)

O03.6   Delayed or excessive hemorrhage following complete or unspecified spontaneous abortion

Afibrinogenemia following complete or unspecified spontaneous abortion

Defibrination syndrome following complete or unspecified spontaneous abortion

Hemolysis following complete or unspecified spontaneous abortion

Intravascular coagulation following complete or unspecified spontaneous abortion

O03.7   Embolism following complete or unspecified spontaneous abortion

Air embolism following complete or unspecified spontaneous abortion

Amniotic fluid embolism following complete or unspecified spontaneous abortion

Blood-clot embolism following complete or unspecified spontaneous abortion

Embolism NOS following complete or unspecified spontaneous abortion

Fat embolism following complete or unspecified spontaneous abortion

Pulmonary embolism following complete or unspecified spontaneous abortion

Pyemic embolism following complete or unspecified spontaneous abortion

Septic or septicopyemic embolism following complete or unspecified spontaneous abortion

Soap embolism following complete or unspecified spontaneous abortion

O03.8   Other and unspecified complications following complete or unspecified spontaneous abortion

O03.80   Unspecified complication following complete or unspecified spontaneous abortion

O03.81   Shock following complete or unspecified spontaneous abortion

Circulatory collapse following complete or unspecified spontaneous abortion

Shock (postprocedural) following complete or unspecified spontaneous abortion

Excludes1: shock due to infection following complete or unspecified spontaneous abortion (O03.87)

O03.82   Renal failure following complete or unspecified spontaneous abortion

Kidney failure (acute) following complete or unspecified spontaneous abortion

Oliguria following complete or unspecified spontaneous abortion

Renal shutdown following complete or unspecified spontaneous abortion

Renal tubular necrosis following complete or unspecified spontaneous abortion

Uremia following complete or unspecified spontaneous abortion

O03.83   Metabolic disorder following complete or unspecified spontaneous abortion

O03.84   Damage to pelvic organs following complete or unspecified spontaneous abortion

Laceration, perforation, tear or chemical damage of bladder following complete or unspecified spontaneous abortion

Laceration, perforation, tear or chemical damage of bowel following complete or unspecified spontaneous abortion

Laceration, perforation, tear or chemical damage of broad ligament following complete or unspecified spontaneous abortion

Laceration, perforation, tear or chemical damage of cervix following complete or unspecified spontaneous abortion

Laceration, perforation, tear or chemical damage of periurethral tissue following complete or unspecified spontaneous abortion

Laceration, perforation, tear or chemical damage of uterus following complete or unspecified spontaneous abortion

Laceration, perforation, tear or chemical damage of vagina following complete or unspecified spontaneous abortion

O03.85 Other venous complications following complete or unspecified spontaneous abortion

O03.86 Cardiac arrest following complete or unspecified spontaneous abortion

O03.87 Sepsis following complete or unspecified spontaneous abortion

<u>Use Additional Code</u> to identify infectious agent (B95-B97)

<u>Use Additional Code</u> to identify severe sepsis, if applicable (R65.2-)

Excludes1: septic or septicopyemic embolism following complete or unspecified spontaneous abortion (O03.7)

O03.88 Urinary tract infection following complete or unspecified spontaneous abortion

Cystitis following complete or unspecified spontaneous abortion

O03.89 Complete or unspecified spontaneous abortion with other complications

O03.9 Complete or unspecified spontaneous abortion without complication

Miscarriage NOS

Spontaneous abortion NOS

O04 Complications following (induced) termination of pregnancy

Includes: complications following (induced) termination of pregnancy

Excludes1: encounter for elective termination of pregnancy, uncomplicated (Z33.2)

failed attempted termination of pregnancy (O07.-)

O04.5 Genital tract and pelvic infection following (induced) termination of pregnancy

Endometritis following (induced) termination of pregnancy

Oophoritis following (induced) termination of pregnancy

Parametritis following (induced) termination of pregnancy

Pelvic peritonitis following (induced) termination of pregnancy

Salpingitis following (induced) termination of pregnancy

Salpingo-oophoritis following (induced) termination of pregnancy

Excludes1: sepsis following (induced) termination of pregnancy (O04.87)

urinary tract infection following (induced) termination of pregnancy (O04.88)

O04.6 Delayed or excessive hemorrhage following (induced) termination of pregnancy

Afibrinogenemia following (induced) termination of pregnancy

Defibrination syndrome following (induced) termination of pregnancy

Hemolysis following (induced) termination of pregnancy

Intravascular coagulation following (induced) termination of pregnancy

O04.7 Embolism following (induced) termination of pregnancy

Air embolism following (induced) termination of pregnancy

Amniotic fluid embolism following (induced) termination of pregnancy

Blood-clot embolism following (induced) termination of pregnancy

Embolism NOS following (induced) termination of pregnancy

Fat embolism following (induced) termination of pregnancy

Pulmonary embolism following (induced) termination of pregnancy

Pyemic embolism following (induced) termination of pregnancy

Septic or septicopyemic embolism following (induced) termination of pregnancy

Soap embolism following (induced) termination of pregnancy

O04.8 (Induced) termination of pregnancy with other and unspecified complications

O04.80 (Induced) termination of pregnancy with unspecified complications

O04.81 Shock following (induced) termination of pregnancy

Circulatory collapse following (induced) termination of pregnancy

Shock (postprocedural) following (induced) termination of pregnancy

Excludes1: shock due to infection following (induced) termination of pregnancy (O04.87)

O04.82 Renal failure following (induced) termination of pregnancy

Kidney failure (acute) following (induced) termination of pregnancy

Oliguria following (induced) termination of pregnancy

Renal shutdown following (induced) termination of pregnancy

Renal tubular necrosis following (induced) termination of pregnancy

Uremia following (induced) termination of pregnancy

O04.83 Metabolic disorder following (induced) termination of pregnancy

O04.84 Damage to pelvic organs following (induced) termination of pregnancy

Laceration, perforation, tear or chemical damage of bladder following (induced) termination of pregnancy

Laceration, perforation, tear or chemical damage of bowel following (induced) termination of pregnancy

Laceration, perforation, tear or chemical damage of broad ligament following (induced) termination of pregnancy

Laceration, perforation, tear or chemical damage of cervix following (induced) termination of pregnancy

Laceration, perforation, tear or chemical damage of periurethral tissue following (induced) termination of pregnancy

Laceration, perforation, tear or chemical damage of uterus following (induced) termination of pregnancy

● New code ▲ Revised code Excludes1: Not coded here Excludes2: Not included here ⊗ Placeholder required ⑦7th digit required

Laceration, perforation, tear or chemical damage of vagina following (induced) termination of pregnancy

O04.85 **Other venous complications following (induced) termination of pregnancy**

O04.86 **Cardiac arrest following (induced) termination of pregnancy**

O04.87 **Sepsis following (induced) termination of pregnancy**

Use Additional Code to identify infectious agent (B95-B97)

Use Additional Code to identify severe sepsis, if applicable (R65.2-)

Excludes1: septic or septicopyemic embolism following (induced) termination of pregnancy (O04.7)

O04.88 **Urinary tract infection following (induced) termination of pregnancy**

Cystitis following (induced) termination of pregnancy

O04.89 **(Induced) termination of pregnancy with other complications**

O07 **Failed attempted termination of pregnancy**

Includes: failure of attempted induction of termination of pregnancy

incomplete elective abortion

Excludes1: incomplete spontaneous abortion (O03.0-)

O07.0 **Genital tract and pelvic infection following failed attempted termination of pregnancy**

Endometritis following failed attempted termination of pregnancy

Oophoritis following failed attempted termination of pregnancy

Parametritis following failed attempted termination of pregnancy

Pelvic peritonitis following failed attempted termination of pregnancy

Salpingitis following failed attempted termination of pregnancy

Salpingo-oophoritis following failed attempted termination of pregnancy

Excludes1: sepsis following failed attempted termination of pregnancy (O07.37)

urinary tract infection following failed attempted termination of pregnancy (O07.38)

O07.1 **Delayed or excessive hemorrhage following failed attempted termination of pregnancy**

Afibrinogenemia following failed attempted termination of pregnancy

Defibrination syndrome following failed attempted termination of pregnancy

Hemolysis following failed attempted termination of pregnancy

Intravascular coagulation following failed attempted termination of pregnancy

O07.2 **Embolism following failed attempted termination of pregnancy**

Air embolism following failed attempted termination of pregnancy

Amniotic fluid embolism following failed attempted termination of pregnancy

Blood-clot embolism following failed attempted termination of pregnancy

Embolism NOS following failed attempted termination of pregnancy

Fat embolism following failed attempted termination of pregnancy

Pulmonary embolism following failed attempted termination of pregnancy

Pyemic embolism following failed attempted termination of pregnancy

Septic or septicopyemic embolism following failed attempted termination of pregnancy

Soap embolism following failed attempted termination of pregnancy

O07.3 **Failed attempted termination of pregnancy with other and unspecified complications**

O07.30 **Failed attempted termination of pregnancy with unspecified complications**

O07.31 **Shock following failed attempted termination of pregnancy**

Circulatory collapse following failed attempted termination of pregnancy

Shock (postprocedural) following failed attempted termination of pregnancy

Excludes1: shock due to infection following failed

attempted termination of pregnancy (O07.37)

O07.32 **Renal failure following failed attempted termination of pregnancy**

Kidney failure (acute) following failed attempted termination of pregnancy

Oliguria following failed attempted termination of pregnancy

Renal shutdown following failed attempted termination of pregnancy

Renal tubular necrosis following failed attempted termination of pregnancy

Uremia following failed attempted termination of pregnancy

O07.33 **Metabolic disorder following failed attempted termination of pregnancy**

O07.34 **Damage to pelvic organs following failed attempted termination of pregnancy**

Laceration, perforation, tear or chemical damage of bladder following failed attempted termination of pregnancy

Laceration, perforation, tear or chemical damage of bowel following failed attempted termination of pregnancy

Laceration, perforation, tear or chemical damage of broad ligament following failed attempted termination of pregnancy

Laceration, perforation, tear or chemical damage of cervix following failed attempted termination of pregnancy

Laceration, perforation, tear or chemical damage of periurethral tissue following failed attempted termination of pregnancy

Laceration, perforation, tear or chemical damage of uterus following failed attempted termination of pregnancy

Laceration, perforation, tear or chemical damage of vagina following failed attempted termination of pregnancy

O07.35 **Other venous complications following failed attempted termination of pregnancy**

O07.36 Cardiac arrest following failed attempted termination of pregnancy

O07.37 Sepsis following failed attempted termination of pregnancy

Use Additional Code (B95-B97), to identify infectious agent

Use Additional Code (R65.2-) to identify severe sepsis, if applicable

Excludes1: septic or septicopyemic embolism following failed attempted termination of pregnancy (O07.2)

O07.38 Urinary tract infection following failed attempted termination of pregnancy

Cystitis following failed attempted termination of pregnancy

O07.39 Failed attempted termination of pregnancy with other complications

O07.4 Failed attempted termination of pregnancy without complication

O08 Complications following ectopic and molar pregnancy

This category is for use with categories O00-O02 to identify any associated complications

O08.0 Genital tract and pelvic infection following ectopic and molar pregnancy

Endometritis following ectopic and molar pregnancy

Oophoritis following ectopic and molar pregnancy

Parametritis following ectopic and molar pregnancy

Pelvic peritonitis following ectopic and molar pregnancy

Salpingitis following ectopic and molar pregnancy

Salpingo-oophoritis following ectopic and molar pregnancy

Excludes1: sepsis following ectopic and molar pregnancy (O08.82)

urinary tract infection (O08.83)

O08.1 Delayed or excessive hemorrhage following ectopic and molar pregnancy

Afibrinogenemia following ectopic and molar pregnancy

Defibrination syndrome following ectopic and molar pregnancy

Hemolysis following ectopic and molar pregnancy

Intravascular coagulation following ectopic and molar pregnancy

Excludes1: delayed or excessive hemorrhage due to incomplete abortion (O03.1)

O08.2 Embolism following ectopic and molar pregnancy

Air embolism following ectopic and molar pregnancy

Amniotic fluid embolism following ectopic and molar pregnancy

Blood-clot embolism following ectopic and molar pregnancy

Embolism NOS following ectopic and molar pregnancy

Fat embolism following ectopic and molar pregnancy

Pulmonary embolism following ectopic and molar pregnancy

Pyemic embolism following ectopic and molar pregnancy

Septic or septicopyemic embolism following ectopic and molar pregnancy

Soap embolism following ectopic and molar pregnancy

O08.3 Shock following ectopic and molar pregnancy

Circulatory collapse following ectopic and molar pregnancy

Shock (postprocedural) following ectopic and molar pregnancy

Excludes1: shock due to infection following ectopic and molar pregnancy (O08.82)

O08.4 Renal failure following ectopic and molar pregnancy

Kidney failure (acute) following ectopic and molar pregnancy

Oliguria following ectopic and molar pregnancy

Renal shutdown following ectopic and molar pregnancy

Renal tubular necrosis following ectopic and molar pregnancy

Uremia following ectopic and molar pregnancy

O08.5 Metabolic disorders following an ectopic and molar pregnancy

O08.6 Damage to pelvic organs and tissues following an ectopic and molar pregnancy

Laceration, perforation, tear or chemical damage of bladder following an ectopic and molar pregnancy

Laceration, perforation, tear or chemical damage of bowel following an ectopic and molar pregnancy

Laceration, perforation, tear or chemical damage of broad ligament following an ectopic and molar pregnancy

Laceration, perforation, tear or chemical damage of cervix following an ectopic and molar pregnancy

Laceration, perforation, tear or chemical damage of periurethral tissue following an ectopic and molar pregnancy

Laceration, perforation, tear or chemical damage of uterus following an ectopic and molar pregnancy

Laceration, perforation, tear or chemical damage of vagina following an ectopic and molar pregnancy

O08.7 Other venous complications following an ectopic and molar pregnancy

O08.8 Other complications following an ectopic and molar pregnancy

O08.81 Cardiac arrest following an ectopic and molar pregnancy

O08.82 Sepsis following ectopic and molar pregnancy

Use Additional Code (B95-B97), to identify infectious agent

Use Additional Code (R65.2-) to identify severe sepsis, if applicable

Excludes1: septic or septicopyemic embolism following ectopic and molar pregnancy (O08.2)

O08.83 Urinary tract infection following an ectopic and molar pregnancy

Cystitis following an ectopic and molar pregnancy

O08.89 Other complications following an ectopic and molar pregnancy

O08.9 Unspecified complication following an ectopic and molar pregnancy

SUPERVISION OF HIGH-RISK PREGNANCY (O09)

O09 Supervision of high-risk pregnancy

O09.0 Supervision of pregnancy with history of infertility

O09.00 Supervision of pregnancy with history of infertility, unspecified trimester

O09.01 Supervision of pregnancy with history of infertility, first trimester

O09.02 Supervision of pregnancy with history of infertility, second trimester

O09.03 Supervision of pregnancy with history of infertility, third trimester

O09.1 **Supervision of pregnancy with history of ectopic pregnancy**

   O09.10 **Supervision of pregnancy with history of ectopic pregnancy, unspecified trimester**

   O09.11 **Supervision of pregnancy with history of ectopic pregnancy, first trimester**

   O09.12 **Supervision of pregnancy with history of ectopic pregnancy, second trimester**

   O09.13 **Supervision of pregnancy with history of ectopic pregnancy, third trimester**

O09.A **Supervision of pregnancy with history of molar pregnancy**

   O09.A0 **Supervision of pregnancy with history of molar pregnancy, unspecified trimester**

   O09.A1 **Supervision of pregnancy with history of molar pregnancy, first trimester**

   O09.A2 **Supervision of pregnancy with history of molar pregnancy, second trimester**

   O09.A3 **Supervision of pregnancy with history of molar pregnancy, third trimester**

O09.2 **Supervision of pregnancy with other poor reproductive or obstetric history**

   Excludes2: pregnancy care for patient with history of recurrent pregnancy loss (O26.2-)

   O09.21 **Supervision of pregnancy with history of pre-term labor**

      O09.211 **Supervision of pregnancy with history of pre-term labor, first trimester**

      O09.212 **Supervision of pregnancy with history of pre-term labor, second trimester**

      O09.213 **Supervision of pregnancy with history of pre-term labor, third trimester**

      O09.219 **Supervision of pregnancy with history of pre-term labor, unspecified trimester**

   O09.29 **Supervision of pregnancy with other poor reproductive or obstetric history**

     Supervision of pregnancy with history of neonatal death

     Supervision of pregnancy with history of stillbirth

      O09.291 **Supervision of pregnancy with other poor reproductive or obstetric history, first trimester**

      O09.292 **Supervision of pregnancy with other poor reproductive or obstetric history, second trimester**

      O09.293 **Supervision of pregnancy with other poor reproductive or obstetric history, third trimester**

      O09.299 **Supervision of pregnancy with other poor reproductive or obstetric history, unspecified trimester**

O09.3 **Supervision of pregnancy with insufficient antenatal care**

   Supervision of concealed pregnancy

   Supervision of hidden pregnancy

   O09.30 **Supervision of pregnancy with insufficient antenatal care, unspecified trimester**

   O09.31 **Supervision of pregnancy with insufficient antenatal care, first trimester**

   O09.32 **Supervision of pregnancy with insufficient antenatal care, second trimester**

   O09.33 **Supervision of pregnancy with insufficient antenatal care, third trimester**

O09.4 **Supervision of pregnancy with grand multiparity**

   O09.40 **Supervision of pregnancy with grand multiparity, unspecified trimester**

   O09.41 **Supervision of pregnancy with grand multiparity, first trimester**

   O09.42 **Supervision of pregnancy with grand multiparity, second trimester**

   O09.43 **Supervision of pregnancy with grand multiparity, third trimester**

O09.5 **Supervision of elderly primigravida and multigravida**

   Pregnancy for a female 35 years and older at expected date of delivery

   O09.51 **Supervision of elderly primigravida**

      O09.511 **Supervision of elderly primigravida, first trimester**

      O09.512 **Supervision of elderly primigravida, second trimester**

      O09.513 **Supervision of elderly primigravida, third trimester**

      O09.519 **Supervision of elderly primigravida, unspecified trimester**

   O09.52 **Supervision of elderly multigravida**

      O09.521 **Supervision of elderly multigravida, first trimester**

      O09.522 **Supervision of elderly multigravida, second trimester**

      O09.523 **Supervision of elderly multigravida, third trimester**

      O09.529 **Supervision of elderly multigravida, unspecified trimester**

O09.6 **Supervision of young primigravida and multigravida**

   Supervision of pregnancy for a female less than 16 years old at expected date of delivery

   O09.61 **Supervision of young primigravida**

      O09.611 **Supervision of young primigravida, first trimester**

      O09.612 **Supervision of young primigravida, second trimester**

      O09.613 **Supervision of young primigravida, third trimester**

      O09.619 **Supervision of young primigravida, unspecified trimester**

   O09.62 **Supervision of young multigravida**

      O09.621 **Supervision of young multigravida, first trimester**

      O09.622 **Supervision of young multigravida, second trimester**

      O09.623 **Supervision of young multigravida, third trimester**

      O09.629 **Supervision of young multigravida, unspecified trimester**

O09.7 **Supervision of high-risk pregnancy due to social problems**

   O09.70 **Supervision of high-risk pregnancy due to social problems, unspecified trimester**

   O09.71 **Supervision of high-risk pregnancy due to social problems, first trimester**

   O09.72 **Supervision of high-risk pregnancy due to social problems, second trimester**

   O09.73 **Supervision of high-risk pregnancy due to social problems, third trimester**

O09.8   Supervision of other high-risk pregnancies

O09.81   Supervision of pregnancy resulting from assisted reproductive technology

Supervision of pregnancy resulting from in-vitro fertilization

Excludes2: gestational carrier status (Z33.3)

O09.811   Supervision of pregnancy resulting from assisted reproductive technology, first trimester

O09.812   Supervision of pregnancy resulting from assisted reproductive technology, second trimester

O09.813   Supervision of pregnancy resulting from assisted reproductive technology, third trimester

O09.819   Supervision of pregnancy resulting from assisted reproductive technology, unspecified trimester

O09.82   Supervision of pregnancy with history of in utero procedure during previous pregnancy

O09.821   Supervision of pregnancy with history of in utero procedure during previous pregnancy, first trimester

O09.822   Supervision of pregnancy with history of in utero procedure during previous pregnancy, second trimester

O09.823   Supervision of pregnancy with history of in utero procedure during previous pregnancy, third trimester

O09.829   Supervision of pregnancy with history of in utero procedure during previous pregnancy, unspecified trimester

Excludes1: supervision of pregnancy affected by in utero procedure during current pregnancy (O35.7)

O09.89   Supervision of other high-risk pregnancies

O09.891   Supervision of other high-risk pregnancies, first trimester

O09.892   Supervision of other high-risk pregnancies, second trimester

O09.893   Supervision of other high-risk pregnancies, third trimester

O09.899   Supervision of other high-risk pregnancies, unspecified trimester

O09.9   Supervision of high-risk pregnancy, unspecified

O09.90   Supervision of high-risk pregnancy, unspecified, unspecified trimester

O09.91   Supervision of high-risk pregnancy, unspecified, first trimester

O09.92   Supervision of high-risk pregnancy, unspecified, second trimester

O09.93   Supervision of high-risk pregnancy, unspecified, third trimester

EDEMA, PROTEINURIA AND HYPERTENSIVE DISORDERS IN PREGNANCY, CHILDBIRTH AND THE PUERPERIUM (O10-O16)

O10   Pre-existing hypertension complicating pregnancy, childbirth and the puerperium

Includes: pre-existing hypertension with pre-existing proteinuria complicating pregnancy, childbirth and the puerperium

Excludes2: pre-existing hypertension with superimposed pre-eclampsia complicating pregnancy, childbirth and the puerperium (O11.-)

O10.0   Pre-existing essential hypertension complicating pregnancy, childbirth and the puerperium

Any condition in I10 specified as a reason for obstetric care during pregnancy, childbirth or the puerperium

O10.01   Pre-existing essential hypertension complicating pregnancy

O10.011   Pre-existing essential hypertension complicating pregnancy, first trimester

O10.012   Pre-existing essential hypertension complicating pregnancy, second trimester

O10.013   Pre-existing essential hypertension complicating pregnancy, third trimester

O10.019   Pre-existing essential hypertension complicating pregnancy, unspecified trimester

O10.02   Pre-existing essential hypertension complicating childbirth

O10.03   Pre-existing essential hypertension complicating the puerperium

O10.1   Pre-existing hypertensive heart disease complicating pregnancy, childbirth and the puerperium

Any condition in I11 specified as a reason for obstetric care during pregnancy, childbirth or the puerperium

Use Additional Code from I11 to identify the type of hypertensive heart disease

O10.11   Pre-existing hypertensive heart disease complicating pregnancy

O10.111   Pre-existing hypertensive heart disease complicating pregnancy, first trimester

O10.112   Pre-existing hypertensive heart disease complicating pregnancy, second trimester

O10.113   Pre-existing hypertensive heart disease complicating pregnancy, third trimester

O10.119   Pre-existing hypertensive heart disease complicating pregnancy, unspecified trimester

O10.12   Pre-existing hypertensive heart disease complicating childbirth

O10.13   Pre-existing hypertensive heart disease complicating the puerperium

O10.2   Pre-existing hypertensive chronic kidney disease complicating pregnancy, childbirth and the puerperium

Any condition in I12 specified as a reason for obstetric care during pregnancy, childbirth or the puerperium

Use Additional Code from I12 to identify the type of hypertensive chronic kidney disease

O10.21   Pre-existing hypertensive chronic kidney disease complicating pregnancy

O10.211   Pre-existing hypertensive chronic kidney disease complicating pregnancy, first trimester

O10.212   Pre-existing hypertensive chronic kidney disease complicating pregnancy, second trimester

O10.213   Pre-existing hypertensive chronic kidney disease complicating pregnancy, third trimester

● New code   ▲ Revised code   Excludes1: Not coded here   Excludes2: Not included here   ⊗ Placeholder required   ⑦7th digit required

O10.219 Pre-existing hypertensive chronic kidney disease complicating pregnancy, unspecified trimester

O10.22 Pre-existing hypertensive chronic kidney disease complicating childbirth

O10.23 Pre-existing hypertensive chronic kidney disease complicating the puerperium

O10.3 Pre-existing hypertensive heart and chronic kidney disease complicating pregnancy, childbirth and the puerperium

Any condition in I13 specified as a reason for obstetric care during pregnancy, childbirth or the puerperium

Use Additional Code from I13 to identify the type of hypertensive heart and chronic kidney disease

O10.31 Pre-existing hypertensive heart and chronic kidney disease complicating pregnancy

O10.311 Pre-existing hypertensive heart and chronic kidney disease complicating pregnancy, first trimester

O10.312 Pre-existing hypertensive heart and chronic kidney disease complicating pregnancy, second trimester

O10.313 Pre-existing hypertensive heart and chronic kidney disease complicating pregnancy, third trimester

O10.319 Pre-existing hypertensive heart and chronic kidney disease complicating pregnancy, unspecified trimester

O10.32 Pre-existing hypertensive heart and chronic kidney disease complicating childbirth

O10.33 Pre-existing hypertensive heart and chronic kidney disease complicating the puerperium

O10.4 Pre-existing secondary hypertension complicating pregnancy, childbirth and the puerperium

Any condition in I15 specified as a reason for obstetric care during pregnancy, childbirth or the puerperium

Use Additional Code from I15 to identify the type of secondary hypertension

O10.41 Pre-existing secondary hypertension complicating pregnancy

O10.411 Pre-existing secondary hypertension complicating pregnancy, first trimester

O10.412 Pre-existing secondary hypertension complicating pregnancy, second trimester

O10.413 Pre-existing secondary hypertension complicating pregnancy, third trimester

O10.419 Pre-existing secondary hypertension complicating pregnancy, unspecified trimester

O10.42 Pre-existing secondary hypertension complicating childbirth

O10.43 Pre-existing secondary hypertension complicating the puerperium

O10.9 Unspecified pre-existing hypertension complicating pregnancy, childbirth and the puerperium

O10.91 Unspecified pre-existing hypertension complicating pregnancy

O10.911 Unspecified pre-existing hypertension complicating pregnancy, first trimester

O10.912 Unspecified pre-existing hypertension complicating pregnancy, second trimester

O10.913 Unspecified pre-existing hypertension complicating pregnancy, third trimester

O10.919 Unspecified pre-existing hypertension complicating pregnancy, unspecified trimester

O10.92 Unspecified pre-existing hypertension complicating childbirth

O10.93 Unspecified pre-existing hypertension complicating the puerperium

O11 Pre-existing hypertension with pre-eclampsia

Includes: conditions in O10 complicated by pre-eclampsia

pre-eclampsia superimposed pre-existing hypertension

Use Additional Code from O10 to identify the type of hypertension

O11.1 Pre-existing hypertension with pre-eclampsia, first trimester

O11.2 Pre-existing hypertension with pre-eclampsia, second trimester

O11.3 Pre-existing hypertension with pre-eclampsia, third trimester

O11.4 Pre-existing hypertension with pre-eclampsia, complicating childbirth

O11.5 Pre-existing hypertension with pre-eclampsia, complicating the puerperium

O11.9 Pre-existing hypertension with pre-eclampsia, unspecified trimester

O12 Gestational [pregnancy-induced] edema and proteinuria without hypertension

O12.0 Gestational edema

O12.00 Gestational edema, unspecified trimester

O12.01 Gestational edema, first trimester

O12.02 Gestational edema, second trimester

O12.03 Gestational edema, third trimester

O12.04 Gestational edema, complicating childbirth

O12.05 Gestational edema, complicating the puerperium

O12.1 Gestational proteinuria

O12.10 Gestational proteinuria, unspecified trimester

O12.11 Gestational proteinuria, first trimester

O12.12 Gestational proteinuria, second trimester

O12.13 Gestational proteinuria, third trimester

O12.14 Gestational proteinuria, complicating childbirth

O12.15 Gestational proteinuria, complicating the puerperium

O12.2 Gestational edema with proteinuria

O12.20 Gestational edema with proteinuria, unspecified trimester

O12.21 Gestational edema with proteinuria, first trimester

O12.22 Gestational edema with proteinuria, second trimester

O12.23 Gestational edema with proteinuria, third trimester

O12.24 Gestational edema with proteinuria, complicating childbirth

O12.25 Gestational edema with proteinuria, complicating the puerperium

O13 Gestational [pregnancy-induced] hypertension without significant proteinuria

Includes: gestational hypertension NOS

transient hypertension of pregnancy

O13.1   Gestational [pregnancy-induced] hypertension without significant proteinuria, first trimester

O13.2   Gestational [pregnancy-induced] hypertension without significant proteinuria, second trimester

O13.3   Gestational [pregnancy-induced] hypertension without significant proteinuria, third trimester

O13.4   Gestational [pregnancy-induced] hypertension without significant proteinuria, complicating childbirth

O13.5   Gestational [pregnancy-induced] hypertension without significant proteinuria, complicating the puerperium

O13.9   Gestational [pregnancy-induced] hypertension without significant proteinuria, unspecified trimester

O14   **Pre-eclampsia**

> **Excludes1:** pre-existing hypertension with pre-eclampsia (O11)

O14.0   Mild to moderate pre-eclampsia

     O14.00   Mild to moderate pre-eclampsia, unspecified trimester

     O14.02   Mild to moderate pre-eclampsia, second trimester

     O14.03   Mild to moderate pre-eclampsia, third trimester

     O14.04   Mild to moderate pre-eclampsia, complicating childbirth

     O14.05   Mild to moderate pre-eclampsia, complicating the puerperium

O14.1   Severe pre-eclampsia

> **Excludes1:** HELLP syndrome (O14.2-)

     O14.10   Severe pre-eclampsia, unspecified trimester

     O14.12   Severe pre-eclampsia, second trimester

     O14.13   Severe pre-eclampsia, third trimester

     O14.14   Severe pre-eclampsia complicating childbirth

     O14.15   Severe pre-eclampsia, complicating the puerperium

O14.2   HELLP syndrome

Severe pre-eclampsia with hemolysis, elevated liver enzymes and low platelet count (HELLP)

     O14.20   HELLP syndrome (HELLP), unspecified trimester

     O14.22   HELLP syndrome (HELLP), second trimester

     O14.23   HELLP syndrome (HELLP), third trimester

     O14.24   HELLP syndrome, complicating childbirth

     O14.25   HELLP syndrome, complicating the puerperium

O14.9   Unspecified pre-eclampsia

     O14.90   Unspecified pre-eclampsia, unspecified trimester

     O14.92   Unspecified pre-eclampsia, second trimester

     O14.93   Unspecified pre-eclampsia, third trimester

     O14.94   Unspecified pre-eclampsia, complicating childbirth

     O14.95   Unspecified pre-eclampsia, complicating the puerperium

O15   **Eclampsia**

> **Includes:** convulsions following conditions in O10-O14 and O16

O15.0   Eclampsia complicating pregnancy

     O15.00   Eclampsia complicating pregnancy, unspecified trimester

     O15.02   Eclampsia complicating pregnancy, second trimester

     O15.03   Eclampsia complicating pregnancy, third trimester

O15.1   Eclampsia complicating labor

O15.2   Eclampsia complicating the puerperium

O15.9   Eclampsia, unspecified as to time period

Eclampsia NOS

O16   **Unspecified maternal hypertension**

O16.1   Unspecified maternal hypertension, first trimester

O16.2   Unspecified maternal hypertension, second trimester

O16.3   Unspecified maternal hypertension, third trimester

O16.4   Unspecified maternal hypertension, complicating childbirth

O16.5   Unspecified maternal hypertension, complicating the puerperium

O16.9   Unspecified maternal hypertension, unspecified trimester

OTHER MATERNAL DISORDERS PREDOMINANTLY RELATED TO PREGNANCY (O20-O29)

> **Excludes2:** maternal care related to the fetus and amniotic cavity and possible delivery problems (O30-O48)
>
> maternal diseases classifiable elsewhere but complicating pregnancy, labor and delivery, and the puerperium (O98-O99)

O20   **Hemorrhage in early pregnancy**

> **Includes:** hemorrhage before completion of 20 weeks gestation

> **Excludes1:** pregnancy with abortive outcome (O00-O08)

O20.0   Threatened abortion

Hemorrhage specified as due to threatened abortion

O20.8   Other hemorrhage in early pregnancy

O20.9   Hemorrhage in early pregnancy, unspecified

O21   **Excessive vomiting in pregnancy**

O21.0   Mild hyperemesis gravidarum

Hyperemesis gravidarum, mild or unspecified, starting before the end of the 20th week of gestation

O21.1   Hyperemesis gravidarum with metabolic disturbance

Hyperemesis gravidarum, starting before the end of the 20th week of gestation, with metabolic disturbance such as carbohydrate depletion

Hyperemesis gravidarum, starting before the end of the 20th week of gestation, with metabolic disturbance such as dehydration

Hyperemesis gravidarum, starting before the end of the 20th week of gestation, with metabolic disturbance such as electrolyte imbalance

O21.2   Late vomiting of pregnancy

Excessive vomiting starting after 20 completed weeks of gestation

O21.8   Other vomiting complicating pregnancy

Vomiting due to diseases classified elsewhere, complicating pregnancy

Use Additional Code, to identify cause.

O21.9   Vomiting of pregnancy, unspecified

O22   **Venous complications and hemorrhoids in pregnancy**

> **Excludes1:** venous complications of:
>
> abortion NOS (O03.9)
>
> ectopic or molar pregnancy (O08.7)
>
> failed attempted abortion (O07.35)
>
> induced abortion (O04.85)
>
> spontaneous abortion (O03.89)

> **Excludes2:** obstetric pulmonary embolism (O88.-)
>
> venous complications and hemorrhoids of childbirth and the puerperium (O87.-)

O22.0 Varicose veins of lower extremity in pregnancy

Varicose veins NOS in pregnancy

O22.00 Varicose veins of lower extremity in pregnancy, unspecified trimester

O22.01 Varicose veins of lower extremity in pregnancy, first trimester

O22.02 Varicose veins of lower extremity in pregnancy, second trimester

O22.03 Varicose veins of lower extremity in pregnancy, third trimester

O22.1 Genital varices in pregnancy

Perineal varices in pregnancy

Vaginal varices in pregnancy

Vulval varices in pregnancy

O22.10 Genital varices in pregnancy, unspecified trimester

O22.11 Genital varices in pregnancy, first trimester

O22.12 Genital varices in pregnancy, second trimester

O22.13 Genital varices in pregnancy, third trimester

O22.2 Superficial thrombophlebitis in pregnancy

Phlebitis in pregnancy NOS

Thrombophlebitis of legs in pregnancy

Thrombosis in pregnancy NOS

<u>Use Additional Code</u> to identify the superficial thrombophlebitis (I80.0-)

O22.20 Superficial thrombophlebitis in pregnancy, unspecified trimester

O22.21 Superficial thrombophlebitis in pregnancy, first trimester

O22.22 Superficial thrombophlebitis in pregnancy, second trimester

O22.23 Superficial thrombophlebitis in pregnancy, third trimester

O22.3 Deep phlebothrombosis in pregnancy

Deep vein thrombosis, antepartum

<u>Use Additional Code</u> to identify the deep vein thrombosis (I82.4-, I82.5-, I82.62-. I82.72-)

<u>Use Additional Code</u>, if applicable, for associated long-term (current) use of anticoagulants (Z79.01)

O22.30 Deep phlebothrombosis in pregnancy, unspecified trimester

O22.31 Deep phlebothrombosis in pregnancy, first trimester

O22.32 Deep phlebothrombosis in pregnancy, second trimester

O22.33 Deep phlebothrombosis in pregnancy, third trimester

O22.4 Hemorrhoids in pregnancy

O22.40 Hemorrhoids in pregnancy, unspecified trimester

O22.41 Hemorrhoids in pregnancy, first trimester

O22.42 Hemorrhoids in pregnancy, second trimester

O22.43 Hemorrhoids in pregnancy, third trimester

O22.5 Cerebral venous thrombosis in pregnancy

Cerebrovenous sinus thrombosis in pregnancy

O22.50 Cerebral venous thrombosis in pregnancy, unspecified trimester

O22.51 Cerebral venous thrombosis in pregnancy, first trimester

O22.52 Cerebral venous thrombosis in pregnancy, second trimester

O22.53 Cerebral venous thrombosis in pregnancy, third trimester

O22.8 Other venous complications in pregnancy

O22.8X Other venous complications in pregnancy

O22.8X1 Other venous complications in pregnancy, first trimester

O22.8X2 Other venous complications in pregnancy, second trimester

O22.8X3 Other venous complications in pregnancy, third trimester

O22.8X9 Other venous complications in pregnancy, unspecified trimester

O22.9 Venous complication in pregnancy, unspecified

Gestational phlebitis NOS

Gestational phlebopathy NOS

Gestational thrombosis NOS

O22.90 Venous complication in pregnancy, unspecified, unspecified trimester

O22.91 Venous complication in pregnancy, unspecified, first trimester

O22.92 Venous complication in pregnancy, unspecified, second trimester

O22.93 Venous complication in pregnancy, unspecified, third trimester

O23 Infections of genitourinary tract in pregnancy

<u>Use Additional Code</u> to identify organism (B95.-, B96.-)

Excludes2: gonococcal infections complicating pregnancy, childbirth
and the puerperium (O98.2)

infections with a predominantly sexual mode of transmission NOS complicating pregnancy, childbirth and the puerperium (O98.3)

syphilis complicating pregnancy, childbirth and the puerperium (O98.1)

tuberculosis of genitourinary system complicating pregnancy, childbirth and the puerperium (O98.0)

venereal disease NOS complicating pregnancy, childbirth and the puerperium (O98.3)

O23.0 Infections of kidney in pregnancy

Pyelonephritis in pregnancy

O23.00 Infections of kidney in pregnancy, unspecified trimester

O23.01 Infections of kidney in pregnancy, first trimester

O23.02 Infections of kidney in pregnancy, second trimester

O23.03 Infections of kidney in pregnancy, third trimester

O23.1 Infections of bladder in pregnancy

O23.10 Infections of bladder in pregnancy, unspecified trimester

O23.11 Infections of bladder in pregnancy, first trimester

O23.12 Infections of bladder in pregnancy, second trimester

O23.13 Infections of bladder in pregnancy, third trimester

O23.2 Infections of urethra in pregnancy

O23.20 Infections of urethra in pregnancy, unspecified trimester

O23.21 Infections of urethra in pregnancy, first trimester

O23.22 Infections of urethra in pregnancy, second trimester

O23.23 Infections of urethra in pregnancy, third trimester

O23.3 Infections of other parts of urinary tract in pregnancy

  O23.30 Infections of other parts of urinary tract in pregnancy, unspecified trimester

  O23.31 Infections of other parts of urinary tract in pregnancy, first trimester

  O23.32 Infections of other parts of urinary tract in pregnancy, second trimester

  O23.33 Infections of other parts of urinary tract in pregnancy, third trimester

O23.4 Unspecified infection of urinary tract in pregnancy

  O23.40 Unspecified infection of urinary tract in pregnancy, unspecified trimester

  O23.41 Unspecified infection of urinary tract in pregnancy, first trimester

  O23.42 Unspecified infection of urinary tract in pregnancy, second trimester

  O23.43 Unspecified infection of urinary tract in pregnancy, third trimester

O23.5 Infections of the genital tract in pregnancy

  O23.51 Infection of cervix in pregnancy

    O23.511 Infections of cervix in pregnancy, first trimester

    O23.512 Infections of cervix in pregnancy, second trimester

    O23.513 Infections of cervix in pregnancy, third trimester

    O23.519 Infections of cervix in pregnancy, unspecified trimester

  O23.52 Salpingo-oophoritis in pregnancy

    Oophoritis in pregnancy

    Salpingitis in pregnancy

    O23.521 Salpingo-oophoritis in pregnancy, first trimester

    O23.522 Salpingo-oophoritis in pregnancy, second trimester

    O23.523 Salpingo-oophoritis in pregnancy, third trimester

    O23.529 Salpingo-oophoritis in pregnancy, unspecified trimester

  O23.59 Infection of other part of genital tract in pregnancy

    O23.591 Infection of other part of genital tract in pregnancy, first trimester

    O23.592 Infection of other part of genital tract in pregnancy, second trimester

    O23.593 Infection of other part of genital tract in pregnancy, third trimester

    O23.599 Infection of other part of genital tract in pregnancy, unspecified trimester

O23.9 Unspecified genitourinary tract infection in pregnancy

    Genitourinary tract infection in pregnancy NOS

  O23.90 Unspecified genitourinary tract infection in pregnancy, unspecified trimester

  O23.91 Unspecified genitourinary tract infection in pregnancy, first trimester

  O23.92 Unspecified genitourinary tract infection in pregnancy, second trimester

O23.93 Unspecified genitourinary tract infection in pregnancy, third trimester

O24 Diabetes mellitus in pregnancy, childbirth, and the puerperium

  O24.0 Pre-existing type 1 diabetes mellitus, in pregnancy, childbirth and the puerperium

    Juvenile onset diabetes mellitus, in pregnancy, childbirth and the puerperium

    Ketosis-prone diabetes mellitus in pregnancy, childbirth and the puerperium

    Use Additional Code from category E10 to further identify any manifestations

    O24.01 Pre-existing type 1 Diabetes mellitus, in pregnancy

      O24.011 Pre-existing type 1 diabetes mellitus, in pregnancy, first trimester

      O24.012 Pre-existing type 1 diabetes mellitus, in pregnancy, second trimester

      O24.013 Pre-existing type 1 diabetes mellitus, in pregnancy, third trimester

      O24.019 Pre-existing type 1 diabetes mellitus, in pregnancy, unspecified trimester

    O24.02 Pre-existing type 1 diabetes mellitus, in childbirth

    O24.03 Pre-existing type 1 diabetes mellitus, in the puerperium

  O24.1 Pre-existing type 2 diabetes mellitus, in pregnancy, childbirth and the puerperium

    Insulin-resistant diabetes mellitus in pregnancy, childbirth and the puerperium

    Use Additional Code (for):

    from category E11 to further identify any manifestations

    long-term (current) use of insulin (Z79.4)

    O24.11 Pre-existing type 2 diabetes mellitus, in pregnancy

      O24.111 Pre-existing type 2 diabetes mellitus, in pregnancy, first trimester

      O24.112 Pre-existing type 2 diabetes mellitus, in pregnancy, second trimester

      O24.113 Pre-existing type 2 diabetes mellitus, in pregnancy, third trimester

      O24.119 Pre-existing type 2 diabetes mellitus, in pregnancy, unspecified trimester

    O24.12 Pre-existing type 2 diabetes mellitus, in childbirth

    O24.13 Pre-existing type 2 diabetes mellitus, in the puerperium

  O24.3 Unspecified pre-existing diabetes mellitus in pregnancy, childbirth and the puerperium

    Use Additional Code (for):

    from category E11 to further identify any manifestation

    long-term (current) use of insulin (Z79.4)

    O24.31 Unspecified pre-existing diabetes mellitus in pregnancy

      O24.311 Unspecified pre-existing diabetes mellitus in pregnancy, first trimester

      O24.312 Unspecified pre-existing diabetes mellitus in pregnancy, second trimester

      O24.313 Unspecified pre-existing diabetes mellitus in pregnancy, third trimester

      O24.319 Unspecified pre-existing diabetes mellitus in pregnancy, unspecified trimester

● New code   ▲ Revised code   **Excludes1:** Not coded here   **Excludes2:** Not included here   ⊗ Placeholder required   ⑦7th digit required

O24.32 Unspecified pre-existing diabetes mellitus in childbirth

O24.33 Unspecified pre-existing diabetes mellitus in the puerperium

O24.4 **Gestational diabetes mellitus**

Diabetes mellitus arising in pregnancy

Gestational diabetes mellitus NOS

O24.41 **Gestational diabetes mellitus in pregnancy**

O24.410 **Gestational diabetes mellitus in pregnancy, diet controlled**

O24.414 **Gestational diabetes mellitus in pregnancy, insulin controlled**

O24.415 **Gestational diabetes mellitus in pregnancy, controlled by oral hypoglycemic drugs**

Gestational diabetes mellitus in pregnancy, controlled by oral antidiabetic drugs

O24.419 **Gestational diabetes mellitus in pregnancy, unspecified control**

O24.42 **Gestational diabetes mellitus in childbirth**

O24.420 **Gestational diabetes mellitus in childbirth, diet controlled**

O24.424 **Gestational diabetes mellitus in childbirth, insulin controlled**

O24.425 **Gestational diabetes mellitus in childbirth, controlled by oral hypoglycemic drugs**

Gestational diabetes mellitus in childbirth, controlled by oral antidiabetic drugs

O24.429 **Gestational diabetes mellitus in childbirth, unspecified control**

O24.43 **Gestational diabetes mellitus in the puerperium**

O24.430 **Gestational diabetes mellitus in the puerperium, diet controlled**

O24.434 **Gestational diabetes mellitus in the puerperium, insulin controlled**

O24.435 **Gestational diabetes mellitus in puerperium, controlled by oral hypoglycemic drugs**

Gestational diabetes mellitus in puerperium, controlled by oral antidiabetic drugs

O24.439 **Gestational diabetes mellitus in the puerperium, unspecified control**

O24.8 **Other pre-existing diabetes mellitus in pregnancy, childbirth, and the puerperium**

Use Additional Code (for):

from categories E08, E09 and E13 to further identify any manifestation long-term (current) use of insulin (Z79.4)

O24.81 **Other pre-existing diabetes mellitus in pregnancy**

O24.811 **Other pre-existing diabetes mellitus in pregnancy, first trimester**

O24.812 **Other pre-existing diabetes mellitus in pregnancy, second trimester**

O24.813 **Other pre-existing diabetes mellitus in pregnancy, third trimester**

O24.819 **Other pre-existing diabetes mellitus in pregnancy, unspecified trimester**

O24.82 **Other pre-existing diabetes mellitus in childbirth**

O24.83 **Other pre-existing diabetes mellitus in the puerperium**

O24.9 **Unspecified diabetes mellitus in pregnancy, childbirth and the puerperium**

Use Additional Code for long-term (current) use of insulin (Z79.4)

O24.91 **Unspecified diabetes mellitus in pregnancy**

O24.911 **Unspecified diabetes mellitus in pregnancy, first trimester**

O24.912 **Unspecified diabetes mellitus in pregnancy, second trimester**

O24.913 **Unspecified diabetes mellitus in pregnancy, third trimester**

O24.919 **Unspecified diabetes mellitus in pregnancy, unspecified trimester**

O24.92 **Unspecified diabetes mellitus in childbirth**

O24.93 **Unspecified diabetes mellitus in the puerperium**

O25 **Malnutrition in pregnancy, childbirth and the puerperium**

O25.1 **Malnutrition in pregnancy**

O25.10 **Malnutrition in pregnancy, unspecified trimester**

O25.11 **Malnutrition in pregnancy, first trimester**

O25.12 **Malnutrition in pregnancy, second trimester**

O25.13 **Malnutrition in pregnancy, third trimester**

O25.2 **Malnutrition in childbirth**

O25.3 **Malnutrition in the puerperium**

O26 **Maternal care for other conditions predominantly related to pregnancy**

O26.0 **Excessive weight gain in pregnancy**

Excludes2: gestational edema (O12.0, O12.2)

O26.00 **Excessive weight gain in pregnancy, unspecified trimester**

O26.01 **Excessive weight gain in pregnancy, first trimester**

O26.02 **Excessive weight gain in pregnancy, second trimester**

O26.03 **Excessive weight gain in pregnancy, third trimester**

O26.1 **Low weight gain in pregnancy**

O26.10 **Low weight gain in pregnancy, unspecified trimester**

O26.11 **Low weight gain in pregnancy, first trimester**

O26.12 **Low weight gain in pregnancy, second trimester**

O26.13 **Low weight gain in pregnancy, third trimester**

O26.2 **Pregnancy care for patient with recurrent pregnancy loss**

O26.20 **Pregnancy care for patient with recurrent pregnancy loss, unspecified trimester**

O26.21 **Pregnancy care for patient with recurrent pregnancy loss, first trimester**

O26.22 **Pregnancy care for patient with recurrent pregnancy loss, second trimester**

O26.23 **Pregnancy care for patient with recurrent pregnancy loss, third trimester**

O26.3 **Retained intrauterine contraceptive device in pregnancy**

O26.30 **Retained intrauterine contraceptive device in pregnancy, unspecified trimester**

O26.31 **Retained intrauterine contraceptive device in pregnancy, first trimester**

O26.32 **Retained intrauterine contraceptive device in pregnancy, second trimester**

O26.33   Retained intrauterine contraceptive device in pregnancy, third trimester

O26.4   Herpes gestationis

     O26.40   Herpes gestationis, unspecified trimester

     O26.41   Herpes gestationis, first trimester

     O26.42   Herpes gestationis, second trimester

     O26.43   Herpes gestationis, third trimester

O26.5   Maternal hypotension syndrome

Supine hypotensive syndrome

     O26.50   Maternal hypotension syndrome, unspecified trimester

     O26.51   Maternal hypotension syndrome, first trimester

     O26.52   Maternal hypotension syndrome, second trimester

     O26.53   Maternal hypotension syndrome, third trimester

O26.6   Liver and biliary tract disorders in pregnancy, childbirth and the puerperium

Use Additional Code to identify the specific disorder

Excludes2: hepatorenal syndrome following labor and delivery (O90.4)

     O26.61   Liver and biliary tract disorders in pregnancy

         O26.611   Liver and biliary tract disorders in pregnancy, first trimester

         O26.612   Liver and biliary tract disorders in pregnancy, second trimester

         O26.613   Liver and biliary tract disorders in pregnancy, third trimester

         O26.619   Liver and biliary tract disorders in pregnancy, unspecified trimester

     O26.62   Liver and biliary tract disorders in childbirth

     O26.63   Liver and biliary tract disorders in the puerperium

O26.7   Subluxation of symphysis (pubis) in pregnancy, childbirth and the puerperium

Excludes1: traumatic separation of symphysis (pubis) during childbirth (O71.6)

     O26.71   Subluxation of symphysis (pubis) in pregnancy

         O26.711   Subluxation of symphysis (pubis) in pregnancy, first trimester

         O26.712   Subluxation of symphysis (pubis) in pregnancy, second trimester

         O26.713   Subluxation of symphysis (pubis) in pregnancy, third trimester

         O26.719   Subluxation of symphysis (pubis) in pregnancy, unspecified trimester

     O26.72   Subluxation of symphysis (pubis) in childbirth

     O26.73   Subluxation of symphysis (pubis) in the puerperium

O26.8   Other specified pregnancy related conditions

     O26.81   Pregnancy related exhaustion and fatigue

         O26.811   Pregnancy related exhaustion and fatigue, first trimester

         O26.812   Pregnancy related exhaustion and fatigue, second trimester

         O26.813   Pregnancy related exhaustion and fatigue, third trimester

         O26.819   Pregnancy related exhaustion and fatigue, unspecified trimester

     O26.82   Pregnancy related peripheral neuritis

         O26.821   Pregnancy related peripheral neuritis, first trimester

         O26.822   Pregnancy related peripheral neuritis, second trimester

         O26.823   Pregnancy related peripheral neuritis, third trimester

         O26.829   Pregnancy related peripheral neuritis, unspecified trimester

     O26.83   Pregnancy related renal disease

Use Additional Code to identify the specific disorder

         O26.831   Pregnancy related renal disease, first trimester

         O26.832   Pregnancy related renal disease, second trimester

         O26.833   Pregnancy related renal disease, third trimester

         O26.839   Pregnancy related renal disease, unspecified trimester

     O26.84   Uterine size-date discrepancy complicating pregnancy

Excludes1: encounter for suspected problem with fetal growth ruled out (Z03.74)

         O26.841   Uterine size-date discrepancy, first trimester

         O26.842   Uterine size-date discrepancy, second trimester

         O26.843   Uterine size-date discrepancy, third trimester

         O26.849   Uterine size-date discrepancy, unspecified trimester

     O26.85   Spotting complicating pregnancy

         O26.851   Spotting complicating pregnancy, first trimester

         O26.852   Spotting complicating pregnancy, second trimester

         O26.853   Spotting complicating pregnancy, third trimester

         O26.859   Spotting complicating pregnancy, unspecified trimester

     O26.86   Pruritic urticarial papules and plaques of pregnancy (PUPPP)

Polymorphic eruption of pregnancy

     O26.87   Cervical shortening

Excludes1: encounter for suspected cervical shortening ruled out (Z03.75)

         O26.872   Cervical shortening, second trimester

         O26.873   Cervical shortening, third trimester

         O26.879   Cervical shortening, unspecified trimester

     O26.89   Other specified pregnancy related conditions

         O26.891   Other specified pregnancy related conditions, first trimester

         O26.892   Other specified pregnancy related conditions, second trimester

         O26.893   Other specified pregnancy related conditions, third trimester

         O26.899   Other specified pregnancy related conditions, unspecified trimester

O26.9   Pregnancy related conditions, unspecified

     O26.90   Pregnancy related conditions, unspecified, unspecified trimester

     O26.91   Pregnancy related conditions, unspecified, first trimester

O26.92 **Pregnancy related conditions, unspecified, second trimester**

O26.93 **Pregnancy related conditions, unspecified, third trimester**

O28 **Abnormal findings on antenatal screening of mother**

Excludes1: diagnostic findings classified elsewhere - see Alphabetical Index

O28.0 **Abnormal hematological finding on antenatal screening of mother**

O28.1 **Abnormal biochemical finding on antenatal screening of mother**

O28.2 **Abnormal cytological finding on antenatal screening of mother**

O28.3 **Abnormal ultrasonic finding on antenatal screening of mother**

O28.4 **Abnormal radiological finding on antenatal screening of mother**

O28.5 **Abnormal chromosomal and genetic finding on antenatal screening of mother**

O28.8 **Other abnormal findings on antenatal screening of mother**

O28.9 **Unspecified abnormal findings on antenatal screening of mother**

O29 **Complications of anesthesia during pregnancy**

Includes: maternal complications arising from the administration of a general, regional or local anesthetic, analgesic **or other** sedation during pregnancy

Use Additional Code, if necessary, to identify the complication

Excludes2: complications of anesthesia during labor and delivery (O74.-)

complications of anesthesia during the puerperium (O89.-)

O29.0 **Pulmonary complications of anesthesia during pregnancy**

O29.01 **Aspiration pneumonitis due to anesthesia during pregnancy**

Inhalation of stomach contents or secretions NOS due to anesthesia during pregnancy

Mendelson's syndrome due to anesthesia during pregnancy

O29.011 **Aspiration pneumonitis due to anesthesia during pregnancy, first trimester**

O29.012 **Aspiration pneumonitis due to anesthesia during pregnancy, second trimester**

O29.013 **Aspiration pneumonitis due to anesthesia during pregnancy, third trimester**

O29.019 **Aspiration pneumonitis due to anesthesia during pregnancy, unspecified trimester**

O29.02 **Pressure collapse of lung due to anesthesia during pregnancy**

O29.021 **Pressure collapse of lung due to anesthesia during pregnancy, first trimester**

O29.022 **Pressure collapse of lung due to anesthesia during pregnancy, second trimester**

O29.023 **Pressure collapse of lung due to anesthesia during pregnancy, third trimester**

O29.029 **Pressure collapse of lung due to anesthesia during pregnancy, unspecified trimester**

O29.09 **Other pulmonary complications of anesthesia during pregnancy**

O29.091 **Other pulmonary complications of anesthesia during pregnancy, first trimester**

O29.092 **Other pulmonary complications of anesthesia during pregnancy, second trimester**

O29.093 **Other pulmonary complications of anesthesia during pregnancy, third trimester**

O29.099 **Other pulmonary complications of anesthesia during pregnancy, unspecified trimester**

O29.1 **Cardiac complications of anesthesia during pregnancy**

O29.11 **Cardiac arrest due to anesthesia during pregnancy**

O29.111 **Cardiac arrest due to anesthesia during pregnancy, first trimester**

O29.112 **Cardiac arrest due to anesthesia during pregnancy, second trimester**

O29.113 **Cardiac arrest due to anesthesia during pregnancy, third trimester**

O29.119 **Cardiac arrest due to anesthesia during pregnancy, unspecified trimester**

O29.12 **Cardiac failure due to anesthesia during pregnancy**

O29.121 **Cardiac failure due to anesthesia during pregnancy, first trimester**

O29.122 **Cardiac failure due to anesthesia during pregnancy, second trimester**

O29.123 **Cardiac failure due to anesthesia during pregnancy, third trimester**

O29.129 **Cardiac failure due to anesthesia during pregnancy, unspecified trimester**

O29.19 **Other cardiac complications of anesthesia during pregnancy**

O29.191 **Other cardiac complications of anesthesia during pregnancy, first trimester**

O29.192 **Other cardiac complications of anesthesia during pregnancy, second trimester**

O29.193 **Other cardiac complications of anesthesia during pregnancy, third trimester**

O29.199 **Other cardiac complications of anesthesia during pregnancy, unspecified trimester**

O29.2 **Central nervous system complications of anesthesia during pregnancy**

O29.21 **Cerebral anoxia due to anesthesia during pregnancy**

O29.211 **Cerebral anoxia due to anesthesia during pregnancy, first trimester**

O29.212 **Cerebral anoxia due to anesthesia during pregnancy, second trimester**

O29.213 **Cerebral anoxia due to anesthesia during pregnancy, third trimester**

O29.219 Cerebral anoxia due to anesthesia during pregnancy, unspecified trimester

O29.29 Other central nervous system complications of anesthesia during pregnancy

   O29.291 Other central nervous system complications of anesthesia during pregnancy, first trimester

   O29.292 Other central nervous system complications of anesthesia during pregnancy, second trimester

   O29.293 Other central nervous system complications of anesthesia during pregnancy, third trimester

   O29.299 Other central nervous system complications of anesthesia during pregnancy, unspecified trimester

O29.3 Toxic reaction to local anesthesia during pregnancy

   O29.3X Toxic reaction to local anesthesia during pregnancy

   O29.3X1 Toxic reaction to local anesthesia during pregnancy, first trimester

   O29.3X2 Toxic reaction to local anesthesia during pregnancy, second trimester

   O29.3X3 Toxic reaction to local anesthesia during pregnancy, third trimester

   O29.3X9 Toxic reaction to local anesthesia during pregnancy, unspecified trimester

O29.4 Spinal and epidural anesthesia induced headache during pregnancy

   O29.40 Spinal and epidural anesthesia induced headache during pregnancy, unspecified trimester

   O29.41 Spinal and epidural anesthesia induced headache during pregnancy, first trimester

   O29.42 Spinal and epidural anesthesia induced headache during pregnancy, second trimester

   O29.43 Spinal and epidural anesthesia induced headache during pregnancy, third trimester

O29.5 Other complications of spinal and epidural anesthesia during pregnancy

   O29.5X Other complications of spinal and epidural anesthesia during pregnancy

   O29.5X1 Other complications of spinal and epidural anesthesia during pregnancy, first trimester

   O29.5X2 Other complications of spinal and epidural anesthesia during pregnancy, second trimester

   O29.5X3 Other complications of spinal and epidural anesthesia during pregnancy, third trimester

   O29.5X9 Other complications of spinal and epidural anesthesia during pregnancy, unspecified trimester

O29.6 Failed or difficult intubation for anesthesia during pregnancy

   O29.60 Failed or difficult intubation for anesthesia during pregnancy, unspecified trimester

   O29.61 Failed or difficult intubation for anesthesia during pregnancy, first trimester

   O29.62 Failed or difficult intubation for anesthesia during pregnancy, second trimester

   O29.63 Failed or difficult intubation for anesthesia during pregnancy, third trimester

O29.8 Other complications of anesthesia during pregnancy

   O29.8X Other complications of anesthesia during pregnancy

   O29.8X1 Other complications of anesthesia during pregnancy, first trimester

   O29.8X2 Other complications of anesthesia during pregnancy, second trimester

   O29.8X3 Other complications of anesthesia during pregnancy, third trimester

   O29.8X9 Other complications of anesthesia during pregnancy, unspecified trimester

O29.9 Unspecified complication of anesthesia during pregnancy

   O29.90 Unspecified complication of anesthesia during pregnancy, unspecified trimester

   O29.91 Unspecified complication of anesthesia during pregnancy, first trimester

   O29.92 Unspecified complication of anesthesia during pregnancy, second trimester

   O29.93 Unspecified complication of anesthesia during pregnancy, third trimester

MATERNAL CARE RELATED TO THE FETUS AND AMNIOTIC CAVITY AND POSSIBLE DELIVERY PROBLEMS (O30-O48)

O30 Multiple gestation

Code also any complications specific to multiple gestation

O30.0 Twin pregnancy

   O30.00 Twin pregnancy, unspecified number of placenta and unspecified number of amniotic sacs

   O30.001 Twin pregnancy, unspecified number of placenta and unspecified number of amniotic sacs, first trimester

   O30.002 Twin pregnancy, unspecified number of placenta and unspecified number of amniotic sacs, second trimester

   O30.003 Twin pregnancy, unspecified number of placenta and unspecified number of amniotic sacs, third trimester

   O30.009 Twin pregnancy, unspecified number of placenta and unspecified number of amniotic sacs, unspecified trimester

   O30.01 Twin pregnancy, monochorionic/monoamniotic

   Twin pregnancy, one placenta, one amniotic sac

   Excludes1: conjoined twins (O30.02-)

   O30.011 Twin pregnancy, monochorionic/monoamniotic, first trimester

   O30.012 Twin pregnancy, monochorionic/monoamniotic, second trimester

   O30.013 Twin pregnancy, monochorionic/monoamniotic, third trimester

   O30.019 Twin pregnancy, monochorionic/monoamniotic, unspecified trimester

   O30.02 Conjoined twin pregnancy

   O30.021 Conjoined twin pregnancy, first trimester

   O30.022 Conjoined twin pregnancy, second trimester

● New code   ▲ Revised code   **Excludes1:** Not coded here   **Excludes2:** Not included here   ⊗ Placeholder required   ⑦7th digit required

O30.023 Conjoined twin pregnancy, third trimester

O30.029 Conjoined twin pregnancy, unspecified trimester

O30.03 Twin pregnancy, monochorionic/ diamniotic
Twin pregnancy, one placenta, two amniotic sacs

O30.031 Twin pregnancy, monochorionic/ diamniotic, first trimester

O30.032 Twin pregnancy, monochorionic/ diamniotic, second trimester

O30.033 Twin pregnancy, monochorionic/ diamniotic, third trimester

O30.039 Twin pregnancy, monochorionic/ diamniotic, unspecified trimester

O30.04 Twin pregnancy, dichorionic/diamniotic Twin pregnancy, two placentae, two amniotic sacs

O30.041 Twin pregnancy, dichorionic/ diamniotic, first trimester

O30.042 Twin pregnancy, dichorionic/ diamniotic, second trimester

O30.043 Twin pregnancy, dichorionic/ diamniotic, third trimester

O30.049 Twin pregnancy, dichorionic/ diamniotic, unspecified trimester

O30.09 Twin pregnancy, unable to determine number of placenta and number of amniotic sacs

O30.091 Twin pregnancy, unable to determine number of placenta and number of amniotic sacs, first trimester

O30.092 Twin pregnancy, unable to determine number of placenta and number of amniotic sacs, second trimester

O30.093 Twin pregnancy, unable to determine number of placenta and number of amniotic sacs, third trimester

O30.099 Twin pregnancy, unable to determine number of placenta and number of amniotic sacs, unspecified trimester

O30.1 Triplet pregnancy

O30.10 Triplet pregnancy, unspecified number of placenta and unspecified number of amniotic sacs

O30.101 Triplet pregnancy, unspecified number of placenta and unspecified number of amniotic sacs, first trimester

O30.102 Triplet pregnancy, unspecified number of placenta and unspecified number of amniotic sacs, second trimester

O30.103 Triplet pregnancy, unspecified number of placenta and unspecified number of amniotic sacs, third trimester

O30.109 Triplet pregnancy, unspecified number of placenta and unspecified number of amniotic sacs, unspecified trimester

O30.11 Triplet pregnancy with two or more monochorionic fetuses

O30.111 Triplet pregnancy with two or more monochorionic fetuses, first trimester

O30.112 Triplet pregnancy with two or more monochorionic fetuses, second trimester

O30.113 Triplet pregnancy with two or more monochorionic fetuses, third trimester

O30.119 Triplet pregnancy with two or more monochorionic fetuses, unspecified trimester

O30.12 Triplet pregnancy with two or more monoamniotic fetuses

O30.121 Triplet pregnancy with two or more monoamniotic fetuses, first trimester

O30.122 Triplet pregnancy with two or more monoamniotic fetuses, second trimester

O30.123 Triplet pregnancy with two or more monoamniotic fetuses, third trimester

O30.129 Triplet pregnancy with two or more monoamniotic fetuses, unspecified trimester

O30.13 Triplet pregnancy, trichorionic/triamniotic

O30.131 Triplet pregnancy, trichorionic/ triamniotic, first trimester

O30.132 Triplet pregnancy, trichorionic/ triamniotic, second trimester

O30.133 Triplet pregnancy, trichorionic/ triamniotic, third trimester

O30.139 Triplet pregnancy, trichorionic/ triamniotic, unspecified trimester

O30.19 Triplet pregnancy, unable to determine number of placenta and number of amniotic sacs

O30.191 Triplet pregnancy, unable to determine number of placenta and number of amniotic sacs, first trimester

O30.192 Triplet pregnancy, unable to determine number of placenta and number of amniotic sacs, second trimester

O30.193 Triplet pregnancy, unable to determine number of placenta and number of amniotic sacs, third trimester

O30.199 Triplet pregnancy, unable to determine number of placenta and number of amniotic sacs, unspecified trimester

O30.2 Quadruplet pregnancy

O30.20 Quadruplet pregnancy, unspecified number of placenta and unspecified number of amniotic sacs

O30.201 Quadruplet pregnancy, unspecified number of placenta and unspecified number of amniotic sacs, first trimester

O30.202 Quadruplet pregnancy, unspecified number of placenta and unspecified number of amniotic sacs, second trimester

O30.203 Quadruplet pregnancy, unspecified number of placenta and unspecified number of amniotic sacs, third trimester

O30.209 Quadruplet pregnancy, unspecified number of placenta and unspecified number of amniotic sacs, unspecified trimester

O30.21   **Quadruplet pregnancy with two or more monochorionic fetuses**

     O30.211   Quadruplet pregnancy with two or more monochorionic fetuses, first trimester

     O30.212   Quadruplet pregnancy with two or more monochorionic fetuses, second trimester

     O30.213   Quadruplet pregnancy with two or more monochorionic fetuses, third trimester

     O30.219   Quadruplet pregnancy with two or more monochorionic fetuses, unspecified trimester

O30.22   **Quadruplet pregnancy with two or more monoamniotic fetuses**

     O30.221   Quadruplet pregnancy with two or more monoamniotic fetuses, first trimester

     O30.222   Quadruplet pregnancy with two or more monoamniotic fetuses, second trimester

     O30.223   Quadruplet pregnancy with two or more monoamniotic fetuses, third trimester

     O30.229   Quadruplet pregnancy with two or more monoamniotic fetuses, unspecified trimester

O30.23   **Quadruplet pregnancy, quadrachorionic/quadra-amniotic**

     O30.231   Quadruplet pregnancy, quadrachorionic/quadra-amniotic, First trimester

     O30.232   Quadruplet pregnancy, quadrachorionic/quadra-amniotic, second trimester

     O30.233   Quadruplet pregnancy, quadrachorionic/quadra-amniotic, third trimester

     O30.239   Quadruplet pregnancy, quadrachorionic/quadra-amniotic, unspecified trimester

O30.29   **Quadruplet pregnancy, unable to determine number of placenta and number of amniotic sacs**

     O30.291   Quadruplet pregnancy, unable to determine number of placenta and number of amniotic sacs, first trimester

     O30.292   Quadruplet pregnancy, unable to determine number of placenta and number of amniotic sacs, second trimester

     O30.293   Quadruplet pregnancy, unable to determine number of placenta and number of amniotic sacs, third trimester

     O30.299   Quadruplet pregnancy, unable to determine number of placenta and number of amniotic sacs, unspecified trimester

O30.8   **Other specified multiple gestation**

Multiple gestation pregnancy greater then quadruplets

O30.80   **Other specified multiple gestation, unspecified number of placenta and unspecified number of amniotic sacs**

     O30.801   Other specified multiple gestation, unspecified number of placenta and unspecified number of amniotic sacs, first trimester

     O30.802   Other specified multiple gestation, unspecified number of placenta and unspecified number of amniotic sacs, second trimester

     O30.803   Other specified multiple gestation, unspecified number of placenta and unspecified number of amniotic sacs, third trimester

     O30.809   Other specified multiple gestation, unspecified number of placenta and unspecified number of amniotic sacs, unspecified trimester

O30.81   **Other specified multiple gestation with two or more monochorionic fetuses**

     O30.811   Other specified multiple gestation with two or more monochorionic fetuses, first trimester

     O30.812   Other specified multiple gestation with two or more monochorionic fetuses, second trimester

     O30.813   Other specified multiple gestation with two or more monochorionic fetuses, third trimester

     O30.819   Other specified multiple gestation with two or more monochorionic fetuses, unspecified trimester

O30.82   **Other specified multiple gestation with two or more monoamniotic fetuses**

     O30.821   Other specified multiple gestation with two or more monoamniotic fetuses, first trimester

     O30.822   Other specified multiple gestation with two or more monoamniotic fetuses, second trimester

     O30.823   Other specified multiple gestation with two or more monoamniotic fetuses, third trimester

     O30.829   Other specified multiple gestation with two or more monoamniotic fetuses, unspecified trimester

O30.83   **Other specified multiple gestation, number of chorions and amnions are both equal to the number of fetuses**

Pentachorionic, penta-amniotic pregnancy (quintuplets)

Hexachorionic, hexa-amniotic pregnancy (sextuplets)

Heptachorionic, hepta-amniotic pregnancy (septuplets)

     O30.831   Other specified multiple gestation, number of chorions and amnions are both equal to the number of fetuses, first trimester

     O30.832   Other specified multiple gestation, number of chorions and amnions are both equal to the number of fetuses, second trimester

     O30.833   Other specified multiple gestation, number of chorions and amnions are both equal to the number of fetuses, third trimester

O30.839   Other specified multiple gestation, number of chorions and amnions are both equal to the number of fetuses, unspecified trimester

O30.89   Other specified multiple gestation, unable to determine number of placenta and number of amniotic sacs

O30.891   Other specified multiple gestation, unable to determine number of placenta and number of amniotic sacs, first trimester

O30.892   Other specified multiple gestation, unable to determine number of placenta and number of amniotic sacs, second trimester

O30.893   Other specified multiple gestation, unable to determine number of placenta and number of amniotic sacs, third trimester

O30.899   Other specified multiple gestation, unable to determine number of placenta and number of amniotic sacs, unspecified trimester

O30.9   **Multiple gestation, unspecified**

Multiple pregnancy NOS

O30.90   **Multiple gestation, unspecified, unspecified trimester**

O30.91   **Multiple gestation, unspecified, first trimester**

O30.92   **Multiple gestation, unspecified, second trimester**

O30.93   **Multiple gestation, unspecified, third trimester**

O31   **Complications specific to multiple gestation**

Excludes2: delayed delivery of second twin, triplet, etc. (O63.2)

malpresentation of one fetus or more (O32.9)

placental transfusion syndromes (O43.0-)

One of the following 7th characters is to be assigned to each code under category O31. 7th character 0 is for single gestations and multiple gestations where the fetus is unspecified. 7th characters 1 through 9 are for cases of multiple gestations to identify the fetus for which the code applies. The appropriate code from category O30, Multiple gestation, must also be assigned when assigning a code from category O31 that has a 7th character of 1 through 9.

0 - not applicable or unspecified

1 - fetus 1

2 - fetus 2

3 - fetus 3

4 - fetus 4

5 - fetus 5

9 - Other fetus

O31.0   **Papyraceous fetus**

Fetus compressus

O31.00   **Papyraceous fetus, unspecified trimester**

O31.01   **Papyraceous fetus, first trimester**

O31.02   **Papyraceous fetus, second trimester**

O31.03   **Papyraceous fetus, third trimester**

O31.1   **Continuing pregnancy after spontaneous abortion of one fetus or more**

O31.10   **Continuing pregnancy after spontaneous abortion of one fetus or more, unspecified trimester**

O31.11   **Continuing pregnancy after spontaneous abortion of one fetus or more, first trimester**

O31.12   **Continuing pregnancy after spontaneous abortion of one fetus or more, second trimester**

O31.13   **Continuing pregnancy after spontaneous abortion of one fetus or more, third trimester**

O31.2   **Continuing pregnancy after intrauterine death of one fetus or more**

O31.20   **Continuing pregnancy after intrauterine death of one fetus or more, unspecified trimester**

O31.21   **Continuing pregnancy after intrauterine death of one fetus or more, first trimester**

O31.22   **Continuing pregnancy after intrauterine death of one fetus or more, second trimester**

O31.23   **Continuing pregnancy after intrauterine death of one fetus or more, third trimester**

O31.3   **Continuing pregnancy after elective fetal reduction of one fetus or more**

Continuing pregnancy after selective termination of one fetus or more

O31.30   **Continuing pregnancy after elective fetal reduction of one fetus or more, unspecified trimester**

O31.31   **Continuing pregnancy after elective fetal reduction of one fetus or more, first trimester**

O31.32   **Continuing pregnancy after elective fetal reduction of one fetus or more, second trimester**

O31.33   **Continuing pregnancy after elective fetal reduction of one fetus or more, third trimester**

O31.8   **Other complications specific to multiple gestation**

O31.8X   **Other complications specific to multiple gestation**

O31.8X1   **Other complications specific to multiple gestation, first trimester**

O31.8X2   **Other complications specific to multiple gestation, second trimester**

O31.8X3   **Other complications specific to multiple gestation, third trimester**

O31.8X9   **Other complications specific to multiple gestation, unspecified trimester**

O32   **Maternal care for malpresentation of fetus**

Includes: the listed conditions as a reason for observation, hospitalization or other obstetric care of the mother, or for cesarean delivery before onset of labor

Excludes1: malpresentation of fetus with obstructed labor (O64.-)

One of the following 7th characters is to be assigned to each code under category O32. 7th character 0 is for single gestations and multiple gestations where the fetus is unspecified. 7th characters 1 through 9 are for cases of multiple gestations to identify the fetus for which the code applies. The appropriate code from category O30, Multiple gestation, must also be assigned when assigning a code from category O32 that has a 7th character of 1 through 9.

0 - not applicable or unspecified

1 - fetus 1

2 - fetus 2

3 - fetus 3

4 - fetus 4

5 - fetus 5

9 - Other fetus

O32.0   **Maternal care for unstable lie**

O32.1   **Maternal care for breech presentation**

Maternal care for buttocks presentation

Maternal care for complete breech

Maternal care for frank breech

Excludes1: footling presentation (O32.8)

incomplete breech (O32.8)

⊗⑦**O32.2** **Maternal care for transverse and oblique lie**

Maternal care for oblique presentation

Maternal care for transverse presentation

⊗⑦**O32.3** **Maternal care for face, brow and chin presentation**

⊗⑦**O32.4** **Maternal care for high head at term**

Maternal care for failure of head to enter pelvic brim

⊗⑦**O32.6** **Maternal care for compound presentation**

⊗⑦**O32.8** **Maternal care for other malpresentation of fetus**

Maternal care for footling presentation

Maternal care for incomplete breech

⊗⑦**O32.9** **Maternal care for malpresentation of fetus, unspecified**

O33 **Maternal care for disproportion**

Includes: the listed conditions as a reason for observation, hospitalization **or other** obstetric care of the mother, or for cesarean delivery before onset of labor

Excludes1: disproportion with obstructed labor (O65-O66)

O33.0 **Maternal care for disproportion due to deformity of maternal pelvic bones**

Maternal care for disproportion due to pelvic deformity causing disproportion NOS

O33.1 **Maternal care for disproportion due to generally contracted pelvis**

Maternal care for disproportion due to contracted pelvis NOS causing disproportion

O33.2 **Maternal care for disproportion due to inlet contraction of pelvis**

Maternal care for disproportion due to inlet contraction (pelvis) causing disproportion

⊗⑦**O33.3** **Maternal care for disproportion due to outlet contraction of pelvis**

Maternal care for disproportion due to mid-cavity contraction (pelvis)

Maternal care for disproportion due to outlet contraction (pelvis)

One of the following 7th characters is to be assigned to code O33.3. 7th character 0 is for single gestations and multiple gestations where the fetus is unspecified. 7th characters 1 through 9 are for cases of multiple gestations to identify the fetus for which the code applies. The appropriate code from category O30, Multiple gestation, must also be assigned when assigning code O33.3 with a 7th character of 1 through 9.

0 - not applicable or unspecified

1 - fetus 1

2 - fetus 2

3 - fetus 3

4 - fetus 4

5 - fetus 5

9 - Other fetus

⊗⑦**O33.4** **Maternal care for disproportion of mixed maternal and fetal origin**

One of the following 7th characters is to be assigned to code O33.4. 7th character 0 is for single gestations and multiple gestations where the fetus is unspecified. 7th characters 1 through 9 are for cases of multiple gestations to identify the fetus for which the code applies. The appropriate code from category O30,

Multiple gestation must also be assigned when assigning code O33.4 with a 7th character of 1 through 9.

0 - not applicable or unspecified

1 - fetus 1

2 - fetus 2

3 - fetus 3

4 - fetus 4

5 - fetus 5

9 - Other fetus

⊗⑦**O33.5** **Maternal care for disproportion due to unusually large fetus**

Maternal care for disproportion due to disproportion of fetal origin with normally formed fetus

Maternal care for disproportion due to fetal disproportion NOS

One of the following 7th characters is to be assigned to code O33.5. 7th character 0 is for single gestations and multiple gestations where the fetus is unspecified. 7th characters 1 through 9 are for cases of multiple gestations to identify the fetus for which the code applies. The appropriate code from category O30,

Multiple gestation must also be assigned when assigning code O33.5 with a 7th character of 1 through 9.

0 - not applicable or unspecified

1 - fetus 1

2 - fetus 2

3 - fetus 3

4 - fetus 4

5 - fetus 5

9 - Other fetus

⊗⑦**O33.6** **Maternal care for disproportion due to hydrocephalic fetus**

One of the following 7th characters is to be assigned to code O33.6. 7th character 0 is for single gestations and multiple gestations where the fetus is unspecified. 7th characters 1 through 9 are for cases of multiple gestations to identify the fetus for which the code applies. The appropriate code from category O30,

Multiple gestation must also be assigned when assigning code O33.6 with a 7th character of 1 through 9.

0 - not applicable or unspecified

1 - fetus 1

2 - fetus 2

3 - fetus 3

4 - fetus 4

5 - fetus 5

9 - Other fetus

⊗⑦**O33.7** **Maternal care for disproportion due to other fetal deformities**

Maternal care for disproportion due to fetal ascites

Maternal care for disproportion due to fetal hydrops

Maternal care for disproportion due to fetal meningomyelocele

Maternal care for disproportion due to fetal sacral teratoma

Maternal care for disproportion due to fetal tumor

One of the following 7th characters is to be assigned to code O33.7. 7th character 0 is for single gestations and multiple gestations where the fetus is unspecified. 7th characters 1 through 9 are for cases of multiple gestations to identify the fetus for which the code applies. The appropriate code from category O30,

Multiple gestation must also be assigned when assigning code O33.7 with a 7th character of 1 through 9.

0 - not applicable or unspecified

1 - fetus 1

2 - fetus 2

3 - fetus 3

4 - fetus 4

5 - fetus 5

9 - Other fetus

Excludes1: obstructed labor due **to other** fetal deformities (O66.3)

O33.8 **Maternal care for disproportion of other origin**

O33.9 **Maternal care for disproportion, unspecified**

Maternal care for disproportion due to cephalopelvic disproportion NOS

Maternal care for disproportion due to fetopelvic disproportion NOS

O34 **Maternal care for abnormality of pelvic organs**

Includes: the listed conditions as a reason for hospitalization or other obstetric care of the mother, or for cesarean

delivery before onset of labor

Code first any associated obstructed labor (O65.5)

Use Additional Code for specific condition

O34.0 **Maternal care for congenital malformation of uterus**

Maternal care for double uterus

Maternal care for uterus bicornis

O34.00 **Maternal care for unspecified congenital malformation of uterus, unspecified trimester**

O34.01 **Maternal care for unspecified congenital malformation of uterus, first trimester**

O34.02 **Maternal care for unspecified congenital malformation of uterus, second trimester**

O34.03 **Maternal care for unspecified congenital malformation of uterus, third trimester**

O34.1 **Maternal care for benign tumor of corpus uteri**

Excludes2: maternal care for benign tumor of cervix (O34.4-)

maternal care for malignant neoplasm of uterus (O9A.1-)

O34.10 **Maternal care for benign tumor of corpus uteri, unspecified trimester**

O34.11 **Maternal care for benign tumor of corpus uteri, first trimester**

O34.12 **Maternal care for benign tumor of corpus uteri, second trimester**

O34.13 **Maternal care for benign tumor of corpus uteri, third trimester**

O34.2 **Maternal care due to uterine scar from previous surgery**

O34.21 **Maternal care for scar from previous cesarean delivery**

O34.211 **Maternal care for low transverse scar from previous cesarean delivery**

O34.212 **Maternal care for vertical scar from previous cesarean delivery**

Maternal care for classical scar from previous cesarean delivery

O34.218 **Maternal care for other type scar from previous cesarean delivery**

Mid-transverse T incision

O34.219 **Maternal care for unspecified type scar from previous cesarean delivery**

O34.22 **Maternal care for cesarean scar defect (isthmocele)**

O34.29 **Maternal care due to uterine scar from other previous surgery**

Maternal care due to uterine scar **from other** transmural uterine incision

O34.3 **Maternal care for cervical incompetence**

Maternal care for cerclage with or without cervical incompetence

Maternal care for Shirodkar suture with or without cervical incompetence

O34.30 **Maternal care for cervical incompetence, unspecified trimester**

O34.31 **Maternal care for cervical incompetence, first trimester**

O34.32 **Maternal care for cervical incompetence, second trimester**

O34.33 **Maternal care for cervical incompetence, third trimester**

O34.4 **Maternal care for other abnormalities of cervix**

O34.40 **Maternal care for other abnormalities of cervix, unspecified trimester**

O34.41 **Maternal care for other abnormalities of cervix, first trimester**

O34.42 **Maternal care for other abnormalities of cervix, second trimester**

O34.43 **Maternal care for other abnormalities of cervix, third trimester**

O34.5 **Maternal care for other abnormalities of gravid uterus**

O34.51 **Maternal care for incarceration of gravid uterus**

O34.511 **Maternal care for incarceration of gravid uterus, first trimester**

O34.512 **Maternal care for incarceration of gravid uterus, second trimester**

O34.513 **Maternal care for incarceration of gravid uterus, third trimester**

O34.519 **Maternal care for incarceration of gravid uterus, unspecified trimester**

O34.52 **Maternal care for prolapse of gravid uterus**

O34.521 **Maternal care for prolapse of gravid uterus, first trimester**

O34.522 **Maternal care for prolapse of gravid uterus, second trimester**

O34.523 **Maternal care for prolapse of gravid uterus, third trimester**

O34.529 **Maternal care for prolapse of gravid uterus, unspecified trimester**

O34.53 **Maternal care for retroversion of gravid uterus**

O34.531 **Maternal care for retroversion of gravid uterus, first trimester**

O34.532 **Maternal care for retroversion of gravid uterus, second trimester**

O34.533 **Maternal care for retroversion of gravid uterus, third trimester**

O34.539 **Maternal care for retroversion of gravid uterus, unspecified trimester**

O34.59 **Maternal care for other abnormalities of gravid uterus**

O34.591 **Maternal care for other abnormalities of gravid uterus, first trimester**

O34.592 **Maternal care for other abnormalities of gravid uterus, second trimester**

O34.593 **Maternal care for other abnormalities of gravid uterus, third trimester**

O34.599 **Maternal care for other abnormalities of gravid uterus, unspecified trimester**

O34.6 **Maternal care for abnormality of vagina**

Excludes2: maternal care for vaginal varices in pregnancy (O22.1-)

O34.60 **Maternal care for abnormality of vagina, unspecified trimester**

O34.61 **Maternal care for abnormality of vagina, first trimester**

O34.62 **Maternal care for abnormality of vagina, second trimester**

O34.63 **Maternal care for abnormality of vagina, third trimester**

O34.7 **Maternal care for abnormality of vulva and perineum**

Excludes2: maternal care for perineal and vulval varices in pregnancy (O22.1-)

O34.70 **Maternal care for abnormality of vulva and perineum, unspecified trimester**

O34.71 **Maternal care for abnormality of vulva and perineum, first trimester**

O34.72 **Maternal care for abnormality of vulva and perineum, second trimester**

O34.73 **Maternal care for abnormality of vulva and perineum, third trimester**

O34.8 **Maternal care for other abnormalities of pelvic organs**

O34.80 **Maternal care for other abnormalities of pelvic organs, unspecified trimester**

O34.81 **Maternal care for other abnormalities of pelvic organs, first trimester**

O34.82 **Maternal care for other abnormalities of pelvic organs, second trimester**

O34.83 **Maternal care for other abnormalities of pelvic organs, third trimester**

O34.9 **Maternal care for abnormality of pelvic organ, unspecified**

O34.90 **Maternal care for abnormality of pelvic organ, unspecified, unspecified trimester**

O34.91 **Maternal care for abnormality of pelvic organ, unspecified, first trimester**

O34.92 **Maternal care for abnormality of pelvic organ, unspecified, second trimester**

O34.93 **Maternal care for abnormality of pelvic organ, unspecified, third trimester**

O35 **Maternal care for known or suspected fetal abnormality and damage**

Includes: the listed conditions in the fetus as a reason for hospitalization or other obstetric care to the mother, or for termination of pregnancy

Code also any associated maternal condition

Excludes1: encounter for suspected maternal and fetal conditions ruled out (Z03.7-)

One of the following 7th characters is to be assigned to each code under category O35. 7th character 0 is for single gestations and multiple gestations where the fetus is unspecified. 7th characters 1 through 9 are for cases of multiple gestations to identify the fetus for which the code applies. The appropriate code from category O30,

Multiple gestation must also be assigned when assigning a code from category O35 that has a 7th character of 1 through 9.

0 - not applicable or unspecified

1 - fetus 1

2 - fetus 2

3 - fetus 3

4 - fetus 4

5 - fetus 5

9 - Other fetus

⊗⑦**O35.0** **Maternal care for (suspected) central nervous system malformation in fetus**

Maternal care for fetal anencephaly

Maternal care for fetal hydrocephalus

Maternal care for fetal spina bifida

Excludes2: chromosomal abnormality in fetus (O35.1)

⊗⑦**O35.1** **Maternal care for (suspected) chromosomal abnormality in fetus**

⊗⑦**O35.2** **Maternal care for (suspected) hereditary disease in fetus**

Excludes2: chromosomal abnormality in fetus (O35.1)

⊗⑦**O35.3** **Maternal care for (suspected) damage to fetus from viral disease in mother**

Maternal care for damage to fetus from maternal cytomegalovirus infection

Maternal care for damage to fetus from maternal rubella

⊗⑦**O35.4** **Maternal care for (suspected) damage to fetus from alcohol**

⊗⑦**O35.5** **Maternal care for (suspected) damage to fetus by drugs**

Maternal care for damage to fetus from drug addiction

⊗⑦**O35.6** **Maternal care for (suspected) damage to fetus by radiation**

⊗⑦**O35.7** **Maternal care for (suspected) damage to fetus by other medical procedures**

Maternal care for damage to fetus by amniocentesis

Maternal care for damage to fetus by biopsy procedures

Maternal care for damage to fetus by hematological investigation

Maternal care for damage to fetus by intrauterine contraceptive device

Maternal care for damage to fetus by intrauterine surgery

⊗⑦**O35.8** **Maternal care for other (suspected) fetal abnormality and damage**

Maternal care for damage to fetus from maternal listeriosis

Maternal care for damage to fetus from maternal toxoplasmosis

⊗⑦**O35.9** **Maternal care for (suspected) fetal abnormality and damage, unspecified**

O36 **Maternal care for other fetal problems**

Includes: the listed conditions in the fetus as a reason for hospitalization or other obstetric care of the mother, or for termination of pregnancy

Excludes1: encounter for suspected maternal and fetal conditions ruled out (Z03.7-)

placental transfusion syndromes (O43.0-)

Excludes2: labor and delivery complicated by fetal stress (O77.-)

One of the following 7th characters is to be assigned to each code under category O36. 7th character 0 is for single gestations and multiple gestations where the fetus is unspecified. 7th characters 1 through 9 are for cases of multiple gestations to identify the fetus for which the code applies. The appropriate code from category O30,

Multiple gestation must also be assigned when assigning a code from category O36 that has a 7th character of 1 through 9.

0 - not applicable or unspecified

1 - fetus 1

2 - fetus 2

3 - fetus 3

4 - fetus 4

5 - fetus 5

9 - Other fetus

O36.0 **Maternal care for rhesus isoimmunization**

● New code ▲ Revised code Excludes1: Not coded here Excludes2: Not included here ⊗ Placeholder required ⑦7th digit required

Maternal care for Rh incompatibility (with hydrops fetalis)

O36.01   Maternal care for anti-D [Rh] antibodies

⑦**O36.011   Maternal care for anti-D [Rh] antibodies, first trimester**

⑦**O36.012   Maternal care for anti-D [Rh] antibodies, second trimester**

⑦**O36.013   Maternal care for anti-D [Rh] antibodies, third trimester**

⑦**O36.019   Maternal care for anti-D [Rh] antibodies, unspecified trimester**

O36.09   Maternal care for other rhesus isoimmunization

⑦**O36.091   Maternal care for other rhesus isoimmunization, first trimester**

⑦**O36.092   Maternal care for other rhesus isoimmunization, second trimester**

⑦**O36.093   Maternal care for other rhesus isoimmunization, third trimester**

⑦**O36.099   Maternal care for other rhesus isoimmunization, unspecified trimester**

O36.1   Maternal care for other isoimmunization

Maternal care for ABO isoimmunization

O36.11   Maternal care for Anti-A sensitization

Maternal care for isoimmunization NOS (with hydrops fetalis)

⑦**O36.111   Maternal care for Anti-A sensitization, first trimester**

⑦**O36.112   Maternal care for Anti-A sensitization, second trimester**

⑦**O36.113   Maternal care for Anti-A sensitization, third trimester**

⑦**O36.119   Maternal care for Anti-A sensitization, unspecified trimester**

O36.19   Maternal care for other isoimmunization

Maternal care for Anti-B sensitization

⑦**O36.191   Maternal care for other isoimmunization, first trimester**

⑦**O36.192   Maternal care for other isoimmunization, second trimester**

⑦**O36.193   Maternal care for other isoimmunization, third trimester**

⑦**O36.199   Maternal care for other isoimmunization, unspecified trimester**

O36.2   Maternal care for hydrops fetalis

Maternal care for hydrops fetalis NOS

Maternal care for hydrops fetalis not associated with isoimmunization

Excludes1: hydrops fetalis associated with ABO isoimmunization (O36.1-)

hydrops fetalis associated with rhesus isoimmunization (O36.0-)

⊗⑦**O36.20   Maternal care for hydrops fetalis, unspecified trimester**

⊗⑦**O36.21   Maternal care for hydrops fetalis, first trimester**

⊗⑦**O36.22   Maternal care for hydrops fetalis, second trimester**

⊗⑦**O36.23   Maternal care for hydrops fetalis, third trimester**

⊗⑦**O36.4   Maternal care for intrauterine death**

Maternal care for intrauterine fetal death NOS

Maternal care for intrauterine fetal death after completion of 20 weeks of gestation

Maternal care for late fetal death

Maternal care for missed delivery

Excludes1: missed abortion (O02.1)

stillbirth (P95)

O36.5   Maternal care for known or suspected poor fetal growth

O36.51   Maternal care for known or suspected placental insufficiency

⑦**O36.511   Maternal care for known or suspected placental insufficiency, first trimester**

⑦**O36.512   Maternal care for known or suspected placental insufficiency, second trimester**

⑦**O36.513   Maternal care for known or suspected placental insufficiency, third trimester**

⑦**O36.519   Maternal care for known or suspected placental insufficiency, unspecified trimester**

O36.59   Maternal care for other known or suspected poor fetal growth

Maternal care for known or suspected light-for-dates NOS

Maternal care for known or suspected small-for-dates NOS

⑦**O36.591   Maternal care for other known or suspected poor fetal growth, first trimester**

⑦**O36.592   Maternal care for other known or suspected poor fetal growth, second trimester**

⑦**O36.593   Maternal care for other known or suspected poor fetal growth, third trimester**

⑦**O36.599   Maternal care for other known or suspected poor fetal growth, unspecified trimester**

O36.6   Maternal care for excessive fetal growth

Maternal care for known or suspected large-for-dates

⊗⑦**O36.60   Maternal care for excessive fetal growth, unspecified trimester**

⊗⑦**O36.61   Maternal care for excessive fetal growth, first trimester**

⊗⑦**O36.62   Maternal care for excessive fetal growth, second trimester**

⊗⑦**O36.63   Maternal care for excessive fetal growth, third trimester**

O36.7   Maternal care for viable fetus in abdominal pregnancy

⊗⑦**O36.70   Maternal care for viable fetus in abdominal pregnancy, unspecified trimester**

⊗⑦**O36.71   Maternal care for viable fetus in abdominal pregnancy, first trimester**

⊗⑦**O36.72   Maternal care for viable fetus in abdominal pregnancy, second trimester**

⊗⑦**O36.73   Maternal care for viable fetus in abdominal pregnancy, third trimester**

O36.8   Maternal care for other specified fetal problems

⊗⑦**O36.80   Pregnancy with inconclusive fetal viability**

Encounter to determine fetal viability of pregnancy

O36.81   Decreased fetal movements

⑦**O36.812**   **Decreased fetal movements, second trimester**

⑦**O36.813**   **Decreased fetal movements, third trimester**

⑦**O36.819**   **Decreased fetal movements, unspecified trimester**

O36.82   **Fetal anemia and thrombocytopenia**

⑦**O36.821**   **Fetal anemia and thrombocytopenia, first trimester**

⑦**O36.822**   **Fetal anemia and thrombocytopenia, second trimester**

⑦**O36.823**   **Fetal anemia and thrombocytopenia, third trimester**

⑦**O36.829**   **Fetal anemia and thrombocytopenia, unspecified trimester**

O36.83   **Maternal care for abnormalities of the fetal heart rate or rhythm**

Maternal care for depressed fetal heart rate tones
Maternal care for fetal bradycardia
Maternal care for fetal heart rate abnormal variability
Maternal care for fetal heart rate decelerations
Maternal care for fetal heart rate irregularity
Maternal care for fetal tachycardia
Maternal care for non-reassuring fetal heart rate or rhythm

⑦**O36.831**   **Maternal care for abnormalities of the fetal heart rate or rhythm, first trimester**

⑦**O36.832**   **Maternal care for abnormalities of the fetal heart rate or rhythm, second trimester**

⑦**O36.833**   **Maternal care for abnormalities of the fetal heart rate or rhythm, third trimester**

⑦**O36.839**   **Maternal care for abnormalities of the fetal heart rate or rhythm, unspecified trimester**

O36.89   **Maternal care for other specified fetal problems**

⑦**O36.891**   **Maternal care for other specified fetal problems, first trimester**

⑦**O36.892**   **Maternal care for other specified fetal problems, second trimester**

⑦**O36.893**   **Maternal care for other specified fetal problems, third trimester**

⑦**O36.899**   **Maternal care for other specified fetal problems, unspecified trimester**

O36.9   **Maternal care for fetal problem, unspecified**

⊗⑦**O36.90**   **Maternal care for fetal problem, unspecified, unspecified trimester**

⊗⑦**O36.91**   **Maternal care for fetal problem, unspecified, first trimester**

⊗⑦**O36.92**   **Maternal care for fetal problem, unspecified, second trimester**

⊗⑦**O36.93**   **Maternal care for fetal problem, unspecified, third trimester**

O40   **Polyhydramnios**

Definition: Polyhydramnios is a condition that exists when there is too much amniotic fluid in the uterus.

Includes: hydramnios

Excludes1: encounter for suspected maternal and fetal conditions
　　　　ruled out (Z03.7-)

One of the following 7th characters is to be assigned to each code under category O40. 7th character 0 is for single gestations and multiple gestations where the fetus is unspecified. 7th characters 1 through 9 are for cases of multiple gestations to identify the fetus for which the code applies. The appropriate code from category O30,

Multiple gestation must also be assigned when assigning a code from category O40 that has a 7th character of 1 through 9.

0 - not applicable or unspecified

1 - fetus 1

2 - fetus 2

3 - fetus 3

4 - fetus 4

5 - fetus 5

9 - Other fetus

⊗⑦**O40.1**   **Polyhydramnios, first trimester**

⊗⑦**O40.2**   **Polyhydramnios, second trimester**

⊗⑦**O40.3**   **Polyhydramnios, third trimester**

⊗⑦**O40.9**   **Polyhydramnios, unspecified trimester**

O41   **Other disorders of amniotic fluid and membranes**

Excludes1: encounter for suspected maternal and fetal conditions
　　　　ruled out (Z03.7-)

One of the following 7th characters is to be assigned to each code under category O41. 7th character 0 is for single gestations and multiple gestations where the fetus is unspecified. 7th characters 1 through 9 are for cases of multiple gestations to identify the fetus for which the code applies. The appropriate code from category O30,

Multiple gestation must also be assigned when assigning a code from category O41 that has a 7th character of 1 through 9.

0 - not applicable or unspecified

1 - fetus 1

2 - fetus 2

3 - fetus 3

4 - fetus 4

5 - fetus 5

9 - Other fetus

O41.0   **Oligohydramnios**

Oligohydramnios without rupture of membranes

⊗⑦**O41.00**   **Oligohydramnios, unspecified trimester**

⊗⑦**O41.01**   **Oligohydramnios, first trimester**

⊗⑦**O41.02**   **Oligohydramnios, second trimester**

⊗⑦**O41.03**   **Oligohydramnios, third trimester**

O41.1   **Infection of amniotic sac and membranes**

O41.10   **Infection of amniotic sac and membranes, unspecified**

⑦**O41.101**   **Infection of amniotic sac and membranes, unspecified, first trimester**

⑦**O41.102**   **Infection of amniotic sac and membranes, unspecified, second trimester**

⑦**O41.103**   **Infection of amniotic sac and membranes, unspecified, third trimester**

⑦**O41.109**   **Infection of amniotic sac and membranes, unspecified, unspecified trimester**

O41.12   **Chorioamnionitis**

⑦**O41.121**   **Chorioamnionitis, first trimester**

⑦**O41.122**   **Chorioamnionitis, second trimester**

⑦**O41.123**   **Chorioamnionitis, third trimester**

⑦**O41.129**   **Chorioamnionitis, unspecified trimester**

O41.14   **Placentitis**

● New code   ▲ Revised code   **Excludes1:** Not coded here   **Excludes2:** Not included here   ⊗ Placeholder required   ⑦ 7th digit required

⑦**O41.141** Placentitis, first trimester

⑦**O41.142** Placentitis, second trimester

⑦**O41.143** Placentitis, third trimester

⑦**O41.149** Placentitis, unspecified trimester

O41.8 Other specified disorders of amniotic fluid and membranes

O41.8X Other specified disorders of amniotic fluid and membranes

⑦**O41.8X1** Other specified disorders of amniotic fluid and membranes, first trimester

⑦**O41.8X2** Other specified disorders of amniotic fluid and membranes, second trimester

⑦**O41.8X3** Other specified disorders of amniotic fluid and membranes, third trimester

⑦**O41.8X9** Other specified disorders of amniotic fluid and membranes, unspecified trimester

O41.9 Disorder of amniotic fluid and membranes, unspecified

⊗⑦**O41.90** Disorder of amniotic fluid and membranes, unspecified, unspecified trimester

⊗⑦**O41.91** Disorder of amniotic fluid and membranes, unspecified, first trimester

⊗⑦**O41.92** Disorder of amniotic fluid and membranes, unspecified, second trimester

⊗⑦**O41.93** Disorder of amniotic fluid and membranes, unspecified, third trimester

O42 **Premature rupture of membranes**

O42.0 Premature rupture of membranes, onset of labor within 24 hours of rupture

O42.00 Premature rupture of membranes, onset of labor within 24 hours of rupture, unspecified weeks of gestation

O42.01 Preterm premature rupture of membranes, onset of labor within 24 hours of rupture

Premature rupture of membranes before 37 completed weeks of gestation

O42.011 Preterm premature rupture of membranes, onset of labor within 24 hours of rupture, first trimester

O42.012 Preterm premature rupture of membranes, onset of labor within 24 hours of rupture, second trimester

O42.013 Preterm premature rupture of membranes, onset of labor within 24 hours of rupture, third trimester

O42.019 Preterm premature rupture of membranes, onset of labor within 24 hours of rupture, unspecified trimester

O42.02 Full-term premature rupture of membranes, onset of labor within 24 hours of rupture

Premature rupture of membranes at or after 37 completed weeks of gestation, onset of labor within 24 hours of rupture

O42.1 Premature rupture of membranes, onset of labor more than 24 hours following rupture

O42.10 Premature rupture of membranes, onset of labor more than 24 hours following rupture, unspecified weeks of gestation

O42.11 Preterm premature rupture of membranes, onset of labor more than 24 hours following rupture

Premature rupture of membranes before 37 completed weeks of gestation

O42.111 Preterm premature rupture of membranes, onset of labor more than 24 hours following rupture, first trimester

O42.112 Preterm premature rupture of membranes, onset of labor more than 24 hours following rupture, second trimester

O42.113 Preterm premature rupture of membranes, onset of labor more than 24 hours following rupture, third trimester

O42.119 Preterm premature rupture of membranes, onset of labor more than 24 hours following rupture, unspecified trimester

O42.12 Full-term premature rupture of membranes, onset of labor more than 24 hours following rupture

Premature rupture of membranes at or after 37 completed weeks of gestation, onset of labor more than 24 hours following rupture

O42.9 Premature rupture of membranes, unspecified as to length of time between rupture and onset of labor

O42.90 Premature rupture of membranes, unspecified as to length of time between rupture and onset of labor, unspecified weeks of gestation

O42.91 Preterm premature rupture of membranes, unspecified as to length of time between rupture and onset of labor

Premature rupture of membranes before 37 completed weeks of gestation

O42.911 Preterm premature rupture of membranes, unspecified as to length of time between rupture and onset of labor, first trimester

O42.912 Preterm premature rupture of membranes, unspecified as to length of time between rupture and onset of labor, second trimester

O42.913 Preterm premature rupture of membranes, unspecified as to length of time between rupture and onset of labor, third trimester

O42.919 Preterm premature rupture of membranes, unspecified as to length of time between rupture and onset of labor, unspecified trimester

O42.92 Full-term premature rupture of membranes, unspecified as to length of time between rupture and onset of labor

Premature rupture of membranes at or after 37 completed weeks of gestation, unspecified as to length of time between rupture and onset of labor

O43 **Placental disorders**

Excludes2: maternal care for poor fetal growth due to placental insufficiency (O36.5-)

placenta previa (O44.-)

placental polyp (O90.89)

placentitis (O41.14-)

premature separation of placenta [abruptio placentae] (O45.-)

O43.0 Placental transfusion syndromes

O43.01 Fetomaternal placental transfusion syndrome

Maternofetal placental transfusion syndrome

O43.011 Fetomaternal placental transfusion syndrome, first trimester

O43.012 **Fetomaternal placental transfusion syndrome, second trimester**

O43.013 **Fetomaternal placental transfusion syndrome, third trimester**

O43.019 **Fetomaternal placental transfusion syndrome, unspecified trimester**

O43.02 **Fetus-to-fetus placental transfusion syndrome**

O43.021 **Fetus-to-fetus placental transfusion syndrome, first trimester**

O43.022 **Fetus-to-fetus placental transfusion syndrome, second trimester**

O43.023 **Fetus-to-fetus placental transfusion syndrome, third trimester**

O43.029 **Fetus-to-fetus placental transfusion syndrome, unspecified trimester**

O43.1 **Malformation of placenta**

O43.10 **Malformation of placenta, unspecified**

Abnormal placenta NOS

O43.101 **Malformation of placenta, unspecified, first trimester**

O43.102 **Malformation of placenta, unspecified, second trimester**

O43.103 **Malformation of placenta, unspecified, third trimester**

O43.109 **Malformation of placenta, unspecified, unspecified trimester**

O43.11 **Circumvallate placenta**

O43.111 **Circumvallate placenta, first trimester**

O43.112 **Circumvallate placenta, second trimester**

O43.113 **Circumvallate placenta, third trimester**

O43.119 **Circumvallate placenta, unspecified trimester**

O43.12 **Velamentous insertion of umbilical cord**

O43.121 **Velamentous insertion of umbilical cord, first trimester**

O43.122 **Velamentous insertion of umbilical cord, second trimester**

O43.123 **Velamentous insertion of umbilical cord, third trimester**

O43.129 **Velamentous insertion of umbilical cord, unspecified trimester**

O43.19 **Other malformation of placenta**

O43.191 **Other malformation of placenta, first trimester**

O43.192 **Other malformation of placenta, second trimester**

O43.193 **Other malformation of placenta, third trimester**

O43.199 **Other malformation of placenta, unspecified trimester**

O43.2 **Morbidly adherent placenta**

Code also associated third stage postpartum hemorrhage, if applicable (O72.0)

Excludes1: retained placenta (O73.-)

O43.21 **Placenta accreta**

O43.211 **Placenta accreta, first trimester**

O43.212 **Placenta accreta, second trimester**

O43.213 **Placenta accreta, third trimester**

O43.219 **Placenta accreta, unspecified trimester**

O43.22 **Placenta increta**

O43.221 **Placenta increta, first trimester**

O43.222 **Placenta increta, second trimester**

O43.223 **Placenta increta, third trimester**

O43.229 **Placenta increta, unspecified trimester**

O43.23 **Placenta percreta**

O43.231 **Placenta percreta, first trimester**

O43.232 **Placenta percreta, second trimester**

O43.233 **Placenta percreta, third trimester**

O43.239 **Placenta percreta, unspecified trimester**

O43.8 **Other placental disorders**

O43.81 **Placental infarction**

O43.811 **Placental infarction, first trimester**

O43.812 **Placental infarction, second trimester**

O43.813 **Placental infarction, third trimester**

O43.819 **Placental infarction, unspecified trimester**

O43.89 **Other placental disorders**

Placental dysfunction

O43.891 **Other placental disorders, first trimester**

O43.892 **Other placental disorders, second trimester**

O43.893 **Other placental disorders, third trimester**

O43.899 **Other placental disorders, unspecified trimester**

O43.9 **Unspecified placental disorder**

O43.90 **Unspecified placental disorder, unspecified trimester**

O43.91 **Unspecified placental disorder, first trimester**

O43.92 **Unspecified placental disorder, second trimester**

O43.93 **Unspecified placental disorder, third trimester**

O44 **Placenta previa**

O44.0 **Complete placenta previa NOS or without hemorrhage**

Placenta previa NOS

O44.00 **Complete placenta previa NOS or without hemorrhage, unspecified trimester**

O44.01 **Complete placenta previa NOS or without hemorrhage, first trimester**

O44.02 **Complete placenta previa NOS or without hemorrhage, second trimester**

O44.03 **Complete placenta previa NOS or without hemorrhage, third trimester**

O44.1 **Complete placenta previa with hemorrhage**

Excludes1: labor and delivery complicated by hemorrhage from vasa previa (O69.4)

O44.10 **Complete placenta previa with hemorrhage, unspecified trimester**

O44.11 **Complete placenta previa with hemorrhage, first trimester**

O44.12 **Complete placenta previa with hemorrhage, second trimester**

O44.13 **Complete placenta previa with hemorrhage, third trimester**

● New code   ▲ Revised code   **Excludes1:** Not coded here   **Excludes2:** Not included here   ⊗ Placeholder required   ⑦7th digit required

O44.2 **Partial placenta previa without hemorrhage**

Marginal placenta previa, NOS or without hemorrhage

    O44.20 Partial placenta previa NOS or without hemorrhage, unspecified trimester

    O44.21 Partial placenta previa NOS or without hemorrhage, first trimester

    O44.22 Partial placenta previa NOS or without hemorrhage, second trimester

    O44.23 Partial placenta previa NOS or without hemorrhage, third trimester

O44.3 **Partial placenta previa with hemorrhage**

Marginal placenta previa with hemorrhage

    O44.30 Partial placenta previa with hemorrhage, unspecified trimester

    O44.31 Partial placenta previa with hemorrhage, first trimester

    O44.32 Partial placenta previa with hemorrhage, second trimester

    O44.33 Partial placenta previa with hemorrhage, third trimester

O44.4 **Low lying placenta NOS or without hemorrhage**

Low implantation of placenta NOS or without hemorrhage

    O44.40 Low lying placenta NOS or without hemorrhage, unspecified trimester

    O44.41 Low lying placenta NOS or without hemorrhage, first trimester

    O44.42 Low lying placenta NOS or without hemorrhage, second trimester

    O44.43 Low lying placenta NOS or without hemorrhage, third trimester

O44.5 **Low lying placenta with hemorrhage**

Low implantation of placenta with hemorrhage

    O44.50 Low lying placenta with hemorrhage, unspecified trimester

    O44.51 Low lying placenta with hemorrhage, first trimester

    O44.52 Low lying placenta with hemorrhage, second trimester

    O44.53 Low lying placenta with hemorrhage, third trimester

O45 **Premature separation of placenta [abruptio placentae]**

O45.0 **Premature separation of placenta with coagulation defect**

    O45.00 Premature separation of placenta with coagulation defect, unspecified

        O45.001 Premature separation of placenta with coagulation defect, unspecified, first trimester

        O45.002 Premature separation of placenta with coagulation defect, unspecified, second trimester

        O45.003 Premature separation of placenta with coagulation defect, unspecified, third trimester

        O45.009 Premature separation of placenta with coagulation defect, unspecified, unspecified trimester

    O45.01 Premature separation of placenta with afibrinogenemia

Premature separation of placenta with hypofibrinogenemia

        O45.011 Premature separation of placenta with afibrinogenemia, first trimester

        O45.012 Premature separation of placenta with afibrinogenemia, second trimester

        O45.013 Premature separation of placenta with afibrinogenemia, third trimester

        O45.019 Premature separation of placenta with afibrinogenemia, unspecified trimester

    O45.02 Premature separation of placenta with disseminated intravascular coagulation

        O45.021 Premature separation of placenta with disseminated intravascular coagulation, first trimester

        O45.022 Premature separation of placenta with disseminated intravascular coagulation, second trimester

        O45.023 Premature separation of placenta with disseminated intravascular coagulation, third trimester

        O45.029 Premature separation of placenta with disseminated intravascular coagulation, unspecified trimester

    O45.09 Premature separation of placenta with other coagulation defect

        O45.091 Premature separation of placenta with other coagulation defect, first trimester

        O45.092 Premature separation of placenta with other coagulation defect, second trimester

        O45.093 Premature separation of placenta with other coagulation defect, third trimester

        O45.099 Premature separation of placenta with other coagulation defect, unspecified trimester

O45.8 **Other premature separation of placenta**

    O45.8X Other premature separation of placenta

        O45.8X1 Other premature separation of placenta, first trimester

        O45.8X2 Other premature separation of placenta, second trimester

        O45.8X3 Other premature separation of placenta, third trimester

        O45.8X9 Other premature separation of placenta, unspecified trimester

O45.9 **Premature separation of placenta, unspecified**

Abruptio placentae NOS

    O45.90 Premature separation of placenta, unspecified, unspecified trimester

    O45.91 Premature separation of placenta, unspecified, first trimester

    O45.92 Premature separation of placenta, unspecified, second trimester

    O45.93 Premature separation of placenta, unspecified, third trimester

O46 **Antepartum hemorrhage, not elsewhere classified**

`Excludes1:` hemorrhage in early pregnancy (O20.-)

intrapartum hemorrhage NEC (O67.-)

placenta previa (O44.-)

premature separation of placenta [abruptio placentae] (O45.-)

O46.0 **Antepartum hemorrhage with coagulation defect**

    O46.00 Antepartum hemorrhage with coagulation defect, unspecified

O46.001 Antepartum hemorrhage with coagulation defect, unspecified, first trimester

O46.002 Antepartum hemorrhage with coagulation defect, unspecified, second trimester

O46.003 Antepartum hemorrhage with coagulation defect, unspecified, third trimester

O46.009 Antepartum hemorrhage with coagulation defect, unspecified, unspecified trimester

O46.01 Antepartum hemorrhage with afibrinogenemia

Antepartum hemorrhage with hypofibrinogenemia

O46.011 Antepartum hemorrhage with afibrinogenemia, first trimester

O46.012 Antepartum hemorrhage with afibrinogenemia, second trimester

O46.013 Antepartum hemorrhage with afibrinogenemia, third trimester

O46.019 Antepartum hemorrhage with afibrinogenemia, unspecified trimester

O46.02 Antepartum hemorrhage with disseminated intravascular coagulation

O46.021 Antepartum hemorrhage with disseminated intravascular coagulation, first trimester

O46.022 Antepartum hemorrhage with disseminated intravascular coagulation, second trimester

O46.023 Antepartum hemorrhage with disseminated intravascular coagulation, third trimester

O46.029 Antepartum hemorrhage with disseminated intravascular coagulation, unspecified trimester

O46.09 Antepartum hemorrhage with other coagulation defect

O46.091 Antepartum hemorrhage with other coagulation defect, first trimester

O46.092 Antepartum hemorrhage with other coagulation defect, second trimester

O46.093 Antepartum hemorrhage with other coagulation defect, third trimester

O46.099 Antepartum hemorrhage with other coagulation defect, unspecified trimester

O46.8 Other antepartum hemorrhage

O46.8X Other antepartum hemorrhage

O46.8X1 Other antepartum hemorrhage, first trimester

O46.8X2 Other antepartum hemorrhage, second trimester

O46.8X3 Other antepartum hemorrhage, third trimester

O46.8X9 Other antepartum hemorrhage, unspecified trimester

O46.9 Antepartum hemorrhage, unspecified

O46.90 Antepartum hemorrhage, unspecified, unspecified trimester

O46.91 Antepartum hemorrhage, unspecified, first trimester

O46.92 Antepartum hemorrhage, unspecified, second trimester

O46.93 Antepartum hemorrhage, unspecified, third trimester

O47 **False labor**

Includes: Braxton Hicks contractions

threatened labor

Excludes1: preterm labor (O60.-)

O47.0 False labor before 37completed weeks of gestation

O47.00 False labor before 37 completed weeks of gestation, unspecified trimester

O47.02 False labor before 37 completed weeks of gestation, second trimester

O47.03 False labor before 37 completed weeks of gestation, third trimester

O47.1 False labor at or after 37completed weeks of gestation

O47.9 False labor, unspecified

O48 **Late pregnancy**

O48.0 Post-term pregnancy

Pregnancy over 40 completed weeks to 42 completed weeks gestation

O48.1 Prolonged pregnancy

Pregnancy which has advanced beyond 42 completed weeks gestation

COMPLICATIONS OF LABOR AND DELIVERY (O60-O77)

O60 **Preterm labor**

Includes: onset (spontaneous) of labor before 37 completed weeks of gestation

Excludes1: false labor (O47.0-)

threatened labor NOS (O47.0-)

O60.0 Preterm labor without delivery

O60.00 Preterm labor without delivery, unspecified trimester

O60.02 Preterm labor without delivery, second trimester

O60.03 Preterm labor without delivery, third trimester

O60.1 Preterm labor with preterm delivery

One of the following 7th characters is to be assigned to each code under subcategory O60.1. 7th character 0 is for single gestations and multiple gestations where the fetus is unspecified. 7th characters 1 through 9 are for cases of multiple gestations to identify the fetus for which the code applies. The appropriate code from category O30, Multiple gestation, must also be assigned when assigning a code from subcategory O60.1 that has a 7th character of 1 through 9.

0 - not applicable or unspecified

1 - fetus 1

2 - fetus 2

3 - fetus 3

4 - fetus 4

5 - fetus 5

9 - Other fetus

⊗⑦**O60.10** Preterm labor with preterm delivery, unspecified trimester

Preterm labor with delivery NOS

⊗⑦**O60.12** Preterm labor second trimester with preterm delivery second trimester

⊗⑦**O60.13** Preterm labor second trimester with preterm delivery third trimester

⊗⑦**O60.14** Preterm labor third trimester with preterm delivery third trimester

O60.2 Term delivery with preterm labor

● New code   ▲ Revised code   **Excludes1:** Not coded here   **Excludes2:** Not included here   ⊗ Placeholder required   ⑦7ᵗʰ digit required

One of the following 7th characters is to be assigned to each code under subcategory O60.2. 7th character 0 is for single gestations and multiple gestations where the fetus is unspecified. 7th characters 1 through 9 are for cases of multiple gestations to identify the fetus for which the code applies. The appropriate code from category O30, Multiple gestation, must also be assigned when assigning a code from subcategory O60.2 that has a 7th character of 1 through 9.

0 - not applicable or unspecified

1 - fetus 1

2 - fetus 2

3 - fetus 3

4 - fetus 4

5 - fetus 5

9 - Other fetus

⊗⑦**O60.20** **Term delivery with preterm labor, unspecified trimester**

⊗⑦**O60.22** **Term delivery with preterm labor, second trimester**

⊗⑦**O60.23** **Term delivery with preterm labor, third trimester**

O61 **Failed induction of labor**

O61.0 **Failed medical induction of labor**

Failed induction (of labor) by oxytocin

Failed induction (of labor) by prostaglandins

O61.1 **Failed instrumental induction of labor**

Failed mechanical induction (of labor)

Failed surgical induction (of labor)

O61.8 **Other failed induction of labor**

O61.9 **Failed induction of labor, unspecified**

O62 **Abnormalities of forces of labor**

O62.0 **Primary inadequate contractions**

Failure of cervical dilatation

Primary hypotonic uterine dysfunction

Uterine inertia during latent phase of labor

O62.1 **Secondary uterine inertia**

Arrested active phase of labor

Secondary hypotonic uterine dysfunction

O62.2 **Other uterine inertia**

Atony of uterus without hemorrhage

Atony of uterus NOS

Desultory labor

Hypotonic uterine dysfunction NOS

Irregular labor

Poor contractions

Slow slope active phase of labor

Uterine inertia NOS

Excludes1: atony of uterus with hemorrhage (postpartum) (O72.1)

postpartum atony of uterus without hemorrhage (O75.89)

O62.3 **Precipitate labor**

O62.4 **Hypertonic, incoordinate, and prolonged uterine contractions**

Cervical spasm

Contraction ring dystocia

Dyscoordinate labor hour-glass contraction of uterus

Hypertonic uterine dysfunction

Incoordinate uterine action

Tetanic contractions

Uterine dystocia NOS

Uterine spasm

Excludes1: dystocia (fetal) (maternal) NOS (O66.9)

O62.8 **Other abnormalities of forces of labor**

O62.9 **Abnormality of forces of labor, unspecified**

O63 **Long labor**

O63.0 **Prolonged first stage (of labor)**

O63.1 **Prolonged second stage (of labor)**

O63.2 **Delayed delivery of second twin, triplet, etc.**

O63.9 **Long labor, unspecified**

Prolonged labor NOS

O64 **Obstructed labor due to malposition and malpresentation of fetus**

Definition: Malposition and malpresentation of fetus refers to presentation of the fetal parts in inappropriate positions for the easiest passage through the cervix, e.g., Retention of the head, breech presentation.

One of the following 7th characters is to be assigned to each code under category O64. 7th character 0 is for single gestations and multiple gestations where the fetus is unspecified. 7th characters 1 through 9 are for cases of multiple gestations to identify the fetus for which the code applies. The appropriate code from category O30, Multiple gestation, must also be assigned when assigning a code from category O64 that has a 7th character of 1 through 9.

0 - not applicable or unspecified

1 - fetus 1

2 - fetus 2

3 - fetus 3

4 - fetus 4

5 - fetus 5

9 - Other fetus

⊗⑦**O64.0** **Obstructed labor due to incomplete rotation of fetal head**

Deep transverse arrest

Obstructed labor due to persistent occipitoiliac (position)

Obstructed labor due to persistent occipitoposterior (position)

Obstructed labor due to persistent occipitosacral (position)

Obstructed labor due to persistent occipitotransverse (position)

⊗⑦**O64.1** **Obstructed labor due to breech presentation**

Obstructed labor due to buttocks presentation

Obstructed labor due to complete breech presentation

Obstructed labor due to frank breech presentation

⊗⑦**O64.2** **Obstructed labor due to face presentation**

Obstructed labor due to chin presentation

⊗⑦**O64.3** **Obstructed labor due to brow presentation**

⊗⑦**O64.4** **Obstructed labor due to shoulder presentation**

Prolapsed arm

Excludes1: impacted shoulders (O66.0)

shoulder dystocia (O66.0)

⊗⑦**O64.5** **Obstructed labor due to compound presentation**

⊗⑦**O64.8** **Obstructed labor due to other malposition and malpresentation**

Obstructed labor due to footling presentation

Obstructed labor due to incomplete breech presentation

⊗⑦**O64.9** **Obstructed labor due to malposition and malpresentation, unspecified**

O65 **Obstructed labor due to maternal pelvic abnormality**

O65.0 **Obstructed labor due to deformed pelvis**

O65.1 **Obstructed labor due to generally contracted pelvis**

O65.2 Obstructed labor due to pelvic inlet contraction

O65.3 Obstructed labor due to pelvic outlet and mid-cavity contraction

O65.4 Obstructed labor due to fetopelvic disproportion, unspecified

> Excludes1: dystocia due to abnormality of fetus (O66.2-O66.3)

O65.5 Obstructed labor due to abnormality of maternal pelvic organs

Obstructed labor due to conditions listed in O34.-

Use Additional Code to identify abnormality of pelvic organs O34.-

O65.8 Obstructed labor due to other maternal pelvic abnormalities

O65.9 Obstructed labor due to maternal pelvic abnormality, unspecified

O66 Other obstructed labor

O66.0 Obstructed labor due to shoulder dystocia

Impacted shoulders

O66.1 Obstructed labor due to locked twins

O66.2 Obstructed labor due to unusually large fetus

O66.3 Obstructed labor due to other abnormalities of fetus

Dystocia due to fetal ascites

Dystocia due to fetal hydrops

Dystocia due to fetal meningomyelocele

Dystocia due to fetal sacral teratoma

Dystocia due to fetal tumor

Dystocia due to hydrocephalic fetus

Use Additional Code to identify cause of obstruction

O66.4 Failed trial of labor O66.40 Failed trial of labor, unspecified

> **O66.40 Failed trial of labor, unspecified**

> **O66.41 Failed attempted vaginal birth after previous cesarean delivery**
>
> Code first rupture of uterus, if applicable (O71.0-O71.1)

O66.5 Attempted application of vacuum extractor and forceps

Attempted application of vacuum or forceps, with subsequent delivery by forceps or cesarean delivery

O66.6 Obstructed labor due to other multiple fetuses

O66.8 Other specified obstructed labor

Use Additional Code to identify cause of obstruction

O66.9 Obstructed labor, unspecified

Dystocia NOS

Fetal dystocia NOS

Maternal dystocia NOS

O67 Labor and delivery complicated by intrapartum hemorrhage, not elsewhere classified

> Excludes1: antepartum hemorrhage NEC (O46.-)
>
> placenta previa (O44.-)
>
> premature separation of placenta [abruptio placentae] (O45.-)

> Excludes2: postpartum hemorrhage (O72.-)

O67.0 Intrapartum hemorrhage with coagulation defect

Intrapartum hemorrhage (excessive) associated with afibrinogenemia

Intrapartum hemorrhage (excessive) associated with disseminated intravascular coagulation

Intrapartum hemorrhage (excessive) associated with hyperfibrinolysis

Intrapartum hemorrhage (excessive) associated with hypofibrinogenemia

O67.8 Other intrapartum hemorrhage

Excessive intrapartum hemorrhage

O67.9 Intrapartum hemorrhage, unspecified

O68 Labor and delivery complicated by abnormality of fetal acid-base balance

Fetal acidemia complicating labor and delivery

Fetal acidosis complicating labor and delivery

Fetal alkalosis complicating labor and delivery

Fetal metabolic acidemia complicating labor and delivery

> Excludes1: fetal stress NOS (O77.9)
>
> labor and delivery complicated by electrocardiographic evidence of fetal stress (O77.8)
>
> labor and delivery complicated by ultrasonic evidence of fetal stress (O77.8)

> Excludes2: abnormality in fetal heart rate or rhythm (O76)
>
> labor and delivery complicated by meconium in amniotic fluid (O77.0)

O69 Labor and delivery complicated by umbilical cord complications

One of the following 7th characters is to be assigned to each code under category O69. 7th character 0 is for single gestations and multiple gestations where the fetus is unspecified. 7th characters 1 through 9 are for cases of multiple gestations to identify the fetus for which the code applies. The appropriate code from category O30, Multiple gestation, must also be assigned when assigning a code from category O69 that has a 7th character of 1 through 9.

0 - not applicable or unspecified

1 - fetus 1

2 - fetus 2

3 - fetus 3

4 - fetus 4

5 - fetus 5

9 - Other fetus

⊗⑦**O69.0 Labor and delivery complicated by prolapse of cord**

⊗⑦**O69.1 Labor and delivery complicated by cord around neck, with compression**

> Excludes1: labor and delivery complicated by cord around neck, without compression (O69.81)

⊗⑦**O69.2 Labor and delivery complicated by other cord entanglement, with compression**

Labor and delivery complicated by compression of cord NOS

Labor and delivery complicated by entanglement of cords of twins in monoamniotic sac

Labor and delivery complicated by knot in cord

> Excludes1: labor and delivery complicated by other cord entanglement, without compression (O69.82)

⊗⑦**O69.3 Labor and delivery complicated by short cord**

⊗⑦**O69.4 Labor and delivery complicated by vasa previa**

Labor and delivery complicated by hemorrhage from vasa previa

⊗⑦**O69.5 Labor and delivery complicated by vascular lesion of cord**

Labor and delivery complicated by cord bruising

Labor and delivery complicated by cord hematoma

Labor and delivery complicated by thrombosis of umbilical vessels

O69.8 Labor and delivery complicated by other cord complications

⊗⑦**O69.81** **Labor and delivery complicated by cord around neck, without compression**

⊗⑦**O69.82** **Labor and delivery complicated by other cord entanglement, without compression**

⊗⑦**O69.89** **Labor and delivery complicated by other cord complications**

⊗⑦**O69.9** **Labor and delivery complicated by cord complication, unspecified**

O70 **Perineal laceration during delivery**

Includes: episiotomy extended by laceration

Excludes1: obstetric high vaginal laceration alone (O71.4)

O70.0 **First degree perineal laceration during delivery**

Perineal laceration, rupture or tear involving fourchette during delivery

Perineal laceration, rupture or tear involving labia during delivery

Perineal laceration, rupture or tear involving skin during delivery

Perineal laceration, rupture or tear involving vagina during delivery

Perineal laceration, rupture or tear involving vulva during delivery

Slight perineal laceration, rupture or tear during delivery

O70.1 **Second degree perineal laceration during delivery**

Perineal laceration, rupture or tear during delivery as in O70.0, also involving pelvic floor

Perineal laceration, rupture or tear during delivery as in O70.0, also involving perineal muscles

Perineal laceration, rupture or tear during delivery as in O70.0, also involving vaginal muscles

Excludes1: perineal laceration involving anal sphincter (O70.2)

O70.2 **Third degree perineal laceration during delivery**

Perineal laceration, rupture or tear during delivery as in O70.1, also involving anal sphincter

Perineal laceration, rupture or tear during delivery as in O70.1, also involving rectovaginal septum

Perineal laceration, rupture or tear during delivery as in O70.1, also involving sphincter NOS

Excludes1: anal sphincter tear during delivery without third degree perineal laceration (O70.4)

perineal laceration involving anal or rectal mucosa (O70.3)

O70.20 **Third degree perineal laceration during delivery, unspecified**

O70.21 **Third degree perineal laceration during delivery, IIIa**

Third degree perineal laceration during delivery with less than 50% of external anal sphincter (EAS) thickness torn

O70.22 **Third degree perineal laceration during delivery, IIIb**

Third degree perineal laceration during delivery with more than 50% external anal sphincter (EAS) thickness torn

O70.23 **Third degree perineal laceration during delivery, IIIC**

Third degree perineal laceration during delivery with both external anal sphincter (EAS) and internal anal sphincter (IAS) torn

O70.3 **Fourth degree perineal laceration during delivery**

Perineal laceration, rupture or tear during delivery as in O70.2, also involving anal mucosa

Perineal laceration, rupture or tear during delivery as in O70.2, also involving rectal mucosa

O70.4 **Anal sphincter tear complicating delivery, not associated with third degree laceration**

Excludes1: anal sphincter tear with third degree perineal laceration (O70.2)

O70.9 **Perineal laceration during delivery, unspecified**

O71 **Other obstetric trauma**

Includes: obstetric damage from instruments

O71.0 **Rupture of uterus (spontaneous) before onset of labor**

Excludes1: disruption of (current) cesarean delivery wound (O90.0)

laceration of uterus, NEC (O71.81)

O71.00 **Rupture of uterus before onset of labor, unspecified trimester**

O71.02 **Rupture of uterus before onset of labor, second trimester**

O71.03 **Rupture of uterus before onset of labor, third trimester**

O71.1 **Rupture of uterus during labor**

Rupture of uterus not stated as occurring before onset of labor

Excludes1: disruption of cesarean delivery wound (O90.0)

laceration of uterus, NEC (O71.81)

O71.2 **Postpartum inversion of uterus**

O71.3 **Obstetric laceration of cervix**

Annular detachment of cervix

O71.4 **Obstetric high vaginal laceration alone**

Laceration of vaginal wall without perineal laceration

Excludes1: obstetric high vaginal laceration with perineal laceration (O70.-)

O71.5 **Other obstetric injury to pelvic organs**

Obstetric injury to bladder

Obstetric injury to urethra

Excludes2: obstetric periurethral trauma (O71.82)

O71.6 **Obstetric damage to pelvic joints and ligaments**

Obstetric avulsion of inner symphyseal cartilage

Obstetric damage to coccyx

Obstetric traumatic separation of symphysis (pubis)

O71.7 **Obstetric hematoma of pelvis**

Obstetric hematoma of perineum

Obstetric hematoma of vagina

Obstetric hematoma of vulva

O71.8 **Other specified obstetric trauma**

O71.81 **Laceration of uterus, not elsewhere classified**

O71.82 **Other specified trauma to perineum and vulva**

Obstetric periurethral trauma

O71.89 **Other specified obstetric trauma**

O71.9 **Obstetric trauma, unspecified**

O72 **Postpartum hemorrhage**

Includes: hemorrhage after delivery of fetus or infant

O72.0 **Third-stage hemorrhage**

Hemorrhage associated with retained, trapped or adherent placenta

Retained placenta NOS

Code also type of adherent placenta (O43.2-)

O72.1 **Other immediate postpartum hemorrhage**

Hemorrhage following delivery of placenta

Postpartum hemorrhage (atonic) NOS

Uterine atony with hemorrhage

Excludes1: uterine atony NOS (O62.2)

uterine atony without hemorrhage (O62.2)

postpartum atony of uterus without hemorrhage (O75.89)

O72.2 **Delayed and secondary postpartum hemorrhage**

Hemorrhage associated with retained portions of placenta or membranes after the first 24 hours following delivery of placenta

Retained products of conception NOS, following delivery

O72.3 **Postpartum coagulation defects**

Postpartum afibrinogenemia

Postpartum fibrinolysis

O73 **Retained placenta and membranes, without hemorrhage**

Excludes1: placenta accreta (O43.21-)

placenta increta (O43.22-)

placenta percreta (O43.23-)

O73.0 **Retained placenta without hemorrhage**

Adherent placenta, without hemorrhage

Trapped placenta without hemorrhage

O73.1 **Retained portions of placenta and membranes, without hemorrhage**

Retained products of conception following delivery, without hemorrhage

O74 **Complications of anesthesia during labor and delivery**

Includes: maternal complications arising from the administration of a general, regional or local anesthetic, analgesic **or other** sedation during labor and delivery

Use Additional Code, if applicable, to identify specific complication

O74.0 **Aspiration pneumonitis due to anesthesia during labor and delivery**

Inhalation of stomach contents or secretions NOS due to anesthesia during labor and delivery

Mendelson's syndrome due to anesthesia during labor and delivery

O74.1 **Other pulmonary complications of anesthesia during labor and delivery**

O74.2 **Cardiac complications of anesthesia during labor and delivery**

O74.3 **Central nervous system complications of anesthesia during labor and delivery**

O74.4 **Toxic reaction to local anesthesia during labor and delivery**

O74.5 **Spinal and epidural anesthesia-induced headache during labor and delivery**

O74.6 **Other complications of spinal and epidural anesthesia during labor and delivery**

O74.7 **Failed or difficult intubation for anesthesia during labor and delivery**

O74.8 **Other complications of anesthesia during labor and delivery**

O74.9 **Complication of anesthesia during labor and delivery, unspecified**

O75 **Other complications of labor and delivery, not elsewhere classified**

Excludes2: puerperal (postpartum) infection (O86.-)

puerperal (postpartum) sepsis (O85)

O75.0 **Maternal distress during labor and delivery**

O75.1 **Shock during or following labor and delivery**

Obstetric shock following labor and delivery

O75.2 **Pyrexia during labor, not elsewhere classified**

O75.3 **Other infection during labor** Sepsis during labor **Use Additional Code** (B95-B97), to identify infectious agent

O75.4 **Other complications of obstetric surgery and procedures**

Cardiac arrest following obstetric surgery or procedures

Cardiac failure following obstetric surgery or procedures

Cerebral anoxia following obstetric surgery or procedures

Pulmonary edema following obstetric surgery or procedures

Use Additional Code to identify specific complication

Excludes2: complications of anesthesia during labor and delivery (O74.-)

disruption of obstetrical (surgical) wound (O90.0-O90.1)

hematoma of obstetrical (surgical) wound (O90.2)

infection of obstetrical (surgical) wound (O86.0-)

O75.5 **Delayed delivery after artificial rupture of membranes**

O75.8 **Other specified complications of labor and delivery**

O75.81 **Maternal exhaustion complicating labor and delivery**

O75.82 **Onset (spontaneous) of labor after 37 completed weeks of gestation but before 39 completed weeks gestation, with delivery by (planned) cesarean section**

Delivery by (planned) cesarean section occurring after 37 completed weeks of gestation but before 39 completed weeks gestation due to (spontaneous) onset of labor

Code first to specify reason for planned cesarean section such as:

cephalopelvic disproportion (normally formed fetus) (O33.9)

previous cesarean delivery (O34.21)

O75.89 **Other specified complications of labor and delivery**

O75.9 **Complication of labor and delivery, unspecified**

O76 **Abnormality in fetal heart rate and rhythm complicating labor and delivery**

Depressed fetal heart rate tones complicating labor and delivery

Fetal bradycardia complicating labor and delivery

Fetal heart rate decelerations complicating labor and delivery

Fetal heart rate irregularity complicating labor and delivery

Fetal heart rate abnormal variability complicating labor and delivery

Fetal tachycardia complicating labor and delivery

Non-reassuring fetal heart rate or rhythm complicating labor and delivery

Excludes1: fetal stress NOS (O77.9)

labor and delivery complicated by electrocardiographic evidence of fetal stress (O77.8)

labor and delivery complicated by ultrasonic evidence of fetal stress (O77.8)

Excludes2: fetal metabolic acidemia (O68)

Other fetal stress (O77.0-O77.1)

O77 **Other fetal stress complicating labor and delivery**

O77.0 **Labor and delivery complicated by meconium in amniotic fluid**

O77.1 **Fetal stress in labor or delivery due to drug administration**

O77.8 **Labor and delivery complicated by other evidence of fetal stress**

Labor and delivery complicated by electrocardiographic evidence of fetal stress

Labor and delivery complicated by ultrasonic evidence of fetal stress

> **Excludes1:** abnormality of fetal acid-base balance (O68)
>
> abnormality in fetal heart rate or rhythm (O76)
>
> fetal metabolic acidemia (O68)

O77.9 Labor and delivery complicated by fetal stress, unspecified

> **Excludes1:** abnormality of fetal acid-base balance (O68)
>
> abnormality in fetal heart rate or rhythm (O76)
>
> fetal metabolic acidemia (O68)

ENCOUNTER FOR DELIVERY (O80-O82)

O80 Encounter for full-term uncomplicated delivery

Delivery requiring minimal or no assistance, with or without episiotomy, without fetal manipulation [e.g., rotation version] or instrumentation [forceps] of a spontaneous, cephalic, vaginal, full-term, single, live-born infant. This code is for use as a single diagnosis code and is not to be used with any other code from chapter 15.

Use Additional Code to indicate outcome of delivery (Z37.0)

O82 Encounter for cesarean delivery without indication

Use Additional Code to indicate outcome of delivery (Z37.0)

COMPLICATIONS PREDOMINANTLY RELATED TO THE PUERPERIUM (O85-O92)

Excludes2: mental and behavioral disorders associated with the puerperium (F53)

> obstetrical tetanus (A34)
>
> puerperal osteomalacia (M83.0)

O85 Puerperal sepsis

Postpartum sepsis

Puerperal peritonitis

Puerperal pyemia

Use Additional Code (B95-B97), to identify infectious agent

Use Additional Code (R65.2-) to identify severe sepsis, if applicable

Excludes1: fever of unknown origin following delivery (O86.4)

> genital tract infection following delivery (O86.1-)
>
> obstetric pyemic and septic embolism (O88.3-)
>
> puerperal septic thrombophlebitis (O86.81)
>
> urinary tract infection following delivery (O86.2-)

Excludes2: sepsis during labor (O75.3)

O86 Other puerperal infections

Use Additional Code (B95-B97), to identify infectious agent

Excludes2: infection during labor (O75.3)

> obstetrical tetanus (A34)

O86.0 Infection of obstetric surgical wound

Infected cesarean delivery wound following delivery

Infected perineal repair following delivery

> **Excludes1:** complications of procedures, not elsewhere classified (T81.4-)

postprocedural fever NOS (R50.82)

postprocedural retroperitoneal abscess (K68.11)

O86.00 Infection of obstetric surgical wound, unspecified

O86.01 Infection of obstetric surgical wound, superficial incisional site

Subcutaneous abscess following an obstetrical procedure

Stitch abscess following an obstetrical procedure

O86.02 Infection of obstetric surgical wound, deep incisional site

Intramuscular abscess following an obstetrical procedure

Sub-fascial abscess following an obstetrical procedure

O86.03 Infection of obstetric surgical wound, organ and space site

Intraabdominal abscess following an obstetrical procedure

Subphrenic abscess following an obstetrical procedure

O86.04 Sepsis following an obstetrical procedure

Use Additional Code to identify the sepsis

O86.09 Infection of obstetric surgical wound, other surgical site

O86.1 Other infection of genital tract following delivery

O86.11 Cervicitis following delivery

O86.12 Endometritis following delivery

O86.13 Vaginitis following delivery

O86.19 Other infection of genital tract following delivery

O86.2 Urinary tract infection following delivery

O86.20 Urinary tract infection following delivery, unspecified

Puerperal urinary tract infection NOS

O86.21 Infection of kidney following delivery

O86.22 Infection of bladder following delivery

Infection of urethra following delivery

O86.29 Other urinary tract infection following delivery

O86.4 Pyrexia of unknown origin following delivery

Puerperal infection NOS following delivery

Puerperal pyrexia NOS following delivery

Excludes2: pyrexia during labor (O75.2)

O86.8 Other specified puerperal infections

O86.81 Puerperal septic thrombophlebitis

O86.89 Other specified puerperal infections

O87 Venous complications and hemorrhoids in the puerperium

Includes: venous complications in labor, delivery and the puerperium

Excludes2: obstetric embolism (O88.-)

> puerperal septic thrombophlebitis (O86.81)
>
> venous complications in pregnancy (O22.-)

O87.0 Superficial thrombophlebitis in the puerperium

Puerperal phlebitis NOS

Puerperal thrombosis NOS

O87.1 Deep phlebothrombosis in the puerperium

Deep vein thrombosis, postpartum

Pelvic thrombophlebitis, postpartum

Use Additional Code to identify the deep vein thrombosis (I82.4-, I82.5-, I82.62-, I82.72-)

Use Additional Code, if applicable, for associated long-term (current) use of anticoagulants (Z79.01)

O87.2 Hemorrhoids in the puerperium

O87.3 Cerebral venous thrombosis in the puerperium

Cerebrovenous sinus thrombosis in the puerperium

O87.4 Varicose veins of lower extremity in the puerperium

O87.8 Other venous complications in the puerperium

Genital varices in the puerperium

O87.9 **Venous complication in the puerperium, unspecified**

Puerperal phlebopathy NOS

O88 **Obstetric embolism**

Excludes1: embolism complicating abortion NOS (O03.2)

embolism complicating ectopic or molar pregnancy (O08.2)

embolism complicating failed attempted abortion (O07.2)

embolism complicating induced abortion (O04.7)

embolism complicating spontaneous abortion (O03.2, O03.7)

O88.0 **Obstetric air embolism**

O88.01 **Obstetric air embolism in pregnancy**

O88.011 **Air embolism in pregnancy, first trimester**

O88.012 **Air embolism in pregnancy, second trimester**

O88.013 **Air embolism in pregnancy, third trimester**

O88.019 **Air embolism in pregnancy, unspecified trimester**

O88.02 **Air embolism in childbirth**

O88.03 **Air embolism in the puerperium**

O88.1 **Amniotic fluid embolism**

Anaphylactoid syndrome in pregnancy

O88.11 **Amniotic fluid embolism in pregnancy**

O88.111 **Amniotic fluid embolism in pregnancy, first trimester**

O88.112 **Amniotic fluid embolism in pregnancy, second trimester**

O88.113 **Amniotic fluid embolism in pregnancy, third trimester**

O88.119 **Amniotic fluid embolism in pregnancy, unspecified trimester**

O88.12 **Amniotic fluid embolism in childbirth**

O88.13 **Amniotic fluid embolism in the puerperium**

O88.2 **Obstetric thromboembolism**

O88.21 **Thromboembolism in pregnancy**

Obstetric (pulmonary) embolism NOS

O88.211 **Thromboembolism in pregnancy, first trimester**

O88.212 **Thromboembolism in pregnancy, second trimester**

O88.213 **Thromboembolism in pregnancy, third trimester**

O88.219 **Thromboembolism in pregnancy, unspecified trimester**

O88.22 **Thromboembolism in childbirth**

O88.23 **Thromboembolism in the puerperium**

Puerperal (pulmonary) embolism NOS

O88.3 **Obstetric pyemic and septic embolism**

O88.31 **Pyemic and septic embolism in pregnancy**

O88.311 **Pyemic and septic embolism in pregnancy, first trimester**

O88.312 **Pyemic and septic embolism in pregnancy, second trimester**

O88.313 **Pyemic and septic embolism in pregnancy, third trimester**

O88.319 **Pyemic and septic embolism in pregnancy, unspecified trimester**

O88.32 **Pyemic and septic embolism in childbirth**

O88.33 **Pyemic and septic embolism in the puerperium**

O88.8 **Other obstetric embolism**

Obstetric fat embolism

O88.81 **Other embolism in pregnancy**

O88.811 **Other embolism in pregnancy, first trimester**

O88.812 **Other embolism in pregnancy, second trimester**

O88.813 **Other embolism in pregnancy, third trimester**

O88.819 **Other embolism in pregnancy, unspecified trimester**

O88.82 **Other embolism in childbirth**

O88.83 **Other embolism in the puerperium**

O89 **Complications of anesthesia during the puerperium**

Includes: maternal complications arising from the administration of a general, regional or local anesthetic, analgesic **or other** sedation during the puerperium

Use Additional Code, if applicable, to identify specific complication

O89.0 **Pulmonary complications of anesthesia during the puerperium**

O89.01 **Aspiration pneumonitis due to anesthesia during the puerperium**

Inhalation of stomach contents or secretions NOS due to anesthesia during the puerperium

Mendelson's syndrome due to anesthesia during the puerperium

O89.09 **Other pulmonary complications of anesthesia during the puerperium**

O89.1 **Cardiac complications of anesthesia during the puerperium**

O89.2 **Central nervous system complications of anesthesia during the puerperium**

O89.3 **Toxic reaction to local anesthesia during the puerperium**

O89.4 **Spinal and epidural anesthesia-induced headache during the puerperium**

O89.5 **Other complications of spinal and epidural anesthesia during the puerperium**

O89.6 **Failed or difficult intubation for anesthesia during the puerperium**

O89.8 **Other complications of anesthesia during the puerperium**

O89.9 **Complication of anesthesia during the puerperium, unspecified**

O90 **Complications of the puerperium, not elsewhere classified**

O90.0 **Disruption of cesarean delivery wound**

Dehiscence of cesarean delivery wound

Excludes1: rupture of uterus (spontaneous) before onset of labor (O71.0-)

rupture of uterus during labor (O71.1)

O90.1 **Disruption of perineal obstetric wound**

Disruption of wound of episiotomy

Disruption of wound of perineal laceration

Secondary perineal tear

O90.2 **Hematoma of obstetric wound**

O90.3 **Peripartum cardiomyopathy**

Conditions in I42.- arising during pregnancy and the puerperium

Excludes1: pre-existing heart disease complicating pregnancy and the puerperium (O99.4-)

O90.4 **Postpartum acute kidney failure**

Hepatorenal syndrome following labor and delivery

O90.5   Postpartum thyroiditis

O90.6   Postpartum mood disturbance

Postpartum blues

Postpartum dysphoria

Postpartum sadness

Excludes1: postpartum depression (F53.0)

puerperal psychosis (F53.1)

O90.8   Other complications of the puerperium, not elsewhere classified

O90.81   Anemia of the puerperium

Postpartum anemia NOS

Excludes1: pre-existing anemia complicating the puerperium (O99.03)

O90.89   Other complications of the puerperium, not elsewhere classified

Placental polyp

O90.9   Complication of the puerperium, unspecified

O91   Infections of breast associated with pregnancy, the puerperium and lactation

Use Additional Code to identify infection

O91.0   Infection of nipple associated with pregnancy, the puerperium and lactation

O91.01   Infection of nipple associated with pregnancy

Gestational abscess of nipple

O91.011   Infection of nipple associated with pregnancy, first trimester

O91.012   Infection of nipple associated with pregnancy, second trimester

O91.013   Infection of nipple associated with pregnancy, third trimester

O91.019   Infection of nipple associated with pregnancy, unspecified trimester

O91.02   Infection of nipple associated with the puerperium

Puerperal abscess of nipple

O91.03   Infection of nipple associated with lactation

Abscess of nipple associated with lactation

O91.1   Abscess of breast associated with pregnancy, the puerperium and lactation

O91.11   Abscess of breast associated with pregnancy

Gestational mammary abscess

Gestational purulent mastitis

Gestational subareolar abscess

O91.111   Abscess of breast associated with pregnancy, first trimester

O91.112   Abscess of breast associated with pregnancy, second trimester

O91.113   Abscess of breast associated with pregnancy, third trimester

O91.119   Abscess of breast associated with pregnancy, unspecified trimester

O91.12   Abscess of breast associated with the puerperium

Puerperal mammary abscess

Puerperal purulent mastitis

Puerperal subareolar abscess

O91.13   Abscess of breast associated with lactation

Mammary abscess associated with lactation

Purulent mastitis associated with lactation

Subareolar abscess associated with lactation

O91.2   Nonpurulent mastitis associated with pregnancy, the puerperium and lactation

O91.21   Nonpurulent mastitis associated with pregnancy

Gestational interstitial mastitis

Gestational lymphangitis of breast

Gestational mastitis NOS

Gestational parenchymatous mastitis

O91.211   Nonpurulent mastitis associated with pregnancy, first trimester

O91.212   Nonpurulent mastitis associated with pregnancy, second trimester

O91.213   Nonpurulent mastitis associated with pregnancy, third trimester

O91.219   Nonpurulent mastitis associated with pregnancy, unspecified trimester

O91.22   Nonpurulent mastitis associated with the puerperium

Puerperal interstitial mastitis

Puerperal lymphangitis of breast

Puerperal mastitis NOS

Puerperal parenchymatous mastitis

O91.23   Nonpurulent mastitis associated with lactation

Interstitial mastitis associated with lactation

Lymphangitis of breast associated with lactation

Mastitis NOS associated with lactation

Parenchymatous mastitis associated with lactation

O92   Other disorders of breast and disorders of lactation associated with pregnancy and the puerperium

O92.0   Retracted nipple associated with pregnancy, the puerperium, and lactation

O92.01   Retracted nipple associated with pregnancy

O92.011   Retracted nipple associated with pregnancy, first trimester

O92.012   Retracted nipple associated with pregnancy, second trimester

O92.013   Retracted nipple associated with pregnancy, third trimester

O92.019   Retracted nipple associated with pregnancy, unspecified trimester

O92.02   Retracted nipple associated with the puerperium

O92.03   Retracted nipple associated with lactation

O92.1   Cracked nipple associated with pregnancy, the puerperium, and lactation

Fissure of nipple, gestational or puerperal

O92.11   Cracked nipple associated with pregnancy

O92.111   Cracked nipple associated with pregnancy, first trimester

O92.112   Cracked nipple associated with pregnancy, second trimester

O92.113   Cracked nipple associated with pregnancy, third trimester

O92.119   Cracked nipple associated with pregnancy, unspecified trimester

O92.12   Cracked nipple associated with the puerperium

O92.13   Cracked nipple associated with lactation

O92.2   Other and unspecified disorders of breast associated with pregnancy and the puerperium

O92.20   Unspecified disorder of breast associated with pregnancy and the puerperium

O92.29 **Other disorders of breast associated with pregnancy and the puerperium**

O92.3 **Agalactia**

Primary agalactia

Excludes1: Elective agalactia (O92.5)

Secondary agalactia (O92.5)

Therapeutic agalactia (O92.5)

O92.4 **Hypogalactia**

O92.5 **Suppressed lactation**

Elective agalactia

Secondary agalactia

Therapeutic agalactia

Excludes1: primary agalactia (O92.3)

O92.6 **Galactorrhea**

O92.7 **Other and unspecified disorders of lactation**

O92.70 **Unspecified disorders of lactation**

O92.79 **Other disorders of lactation**

Puerperal galactocele

OTHER OBSTETRIC CONDITIONS, NOT ELSEWHERE CLASSIFIED (O94-O9A)

O94 **Sequelae of complication of pregnancy, childbirth, and the puerperium**

Note: This category is to be used to indicate conditions in O00-O77.-, O85-O94 and O98-O9A.- as the cause of late effects. The sequelae include conditions specified as such, or as late effects, which may occur at any time after the puerperium

Code first condition resulting from (sequela) of complication of pregnancy, childbirth, and the puerperium

O98 **Maternal infectious and parasitic diseases classifiable elsewhere but complicating pregnancy, childbirth and the puerperium**

Includes: the listed conditions when complicating the pregnant state, when aggravated by the pregnancy, or as a reason for obstetric care

Use Additional Code (Chapter 1), to identify specific infectious or parasitic disease

Excludes2: herpes gestationis (O26.4-)

infectious carrier state (O99.82-, O99.83-)

obstetrical tetanus (A34)

puerperal infection (O86.-)

puerperal sepsis (O85)

when the reason for maternal care is that the disease is known or suspected to have affected the fetus (O35-O36)

O98.0 **Tuberculosis complicating pregnancy, childbirth and the puerperium**

Conditions in A15-A19

O98.01 **Tuberculosis complicating pregnancy**

O98.011 **Tuberculosis complicating pregnancy, first trimester**

O98.012 **Tuberculosis complicating pregnancy, second trimester**

O98.013 **Tuberculosis complicating pregnancy, third trimester**

O98.019 **Tuberculosis complicating pregnancy, unspecified trimester**

O98.02 **Tuberculosis complicating childbirth**

O98.03 **Tuberculosis complicating the puerperium**

O98.1 **Syphilis complicating pregnancy, childbirth and the puerperium**

Conditions in A50-A53

O98.11 **Syphilis complicating pregnancy**

O98.111 **Syphilis complicating pregnancy, first trimester**

O98.112 **Syphilis complicating pregnancy, second trimester**

O98.113 **Syphilis complicating pregnancy, third trimester**

O98.119 **Syphilis complicating pregnancy, unspecified trimester**

O98.12 **Syphilis complicating childbirth**

O98.13 **Syphilis complicating the puerperium**

O98.2 **Gonorrhea complicating pregnancy, childbirth and the puerperium**

Conditions in A54.-

O98.21 **Gonorrhea complicating pregnancy**

O98.211 **Gonorrhea complicating pregnancy, first trimester**

O98.212 **Gonorrhea complicating pregnancy, second trimester**

O98.213 **Gonorrhea complicating pregnancy, third trimester**

O98.219 **Gonorrhea complicating pregnancy, unspecified trimester**

O98.22 **Gonorrhea complicating childbirth**

O98.23 **Gonorrhea complicating the puerperium**

O98.3 **Other infections with a predominantly sexual mode of transmission complicating pregnancy, childbirth and the puerperium**

Conditions in A55-A64

O98.31 **Other infections with a predominantly sexual mode of transmission complicating pregnancy**

O98.311 **Other infections with a predominantly sexual mode of transmission complicating pregnancy, first trimester**

O98.312 **Other infections with a predominantly sexual mode of transmission complicating pregnancy, second trimester**

O98.313 **Other infections with a predominantly sexual mode of transmission complicating pregnancy, third trimester**

O98.319 **Other infections with a predominantly sexual mode of transmission complicating pregnancy, unspecified trimester**

O98.32 **Other infections with a predominantly sexual mode of transmission complicating childbirth**

O98.33 **Other infections with a predominantly sexual mode of transmission complicating the puerperium**

O98.4 **Viral hepatitis complicating pregnancy, childbirth and the puerperium**

Conditions in B15-B19

O98.41 **Viral hepatitis complicating pregnancy**

O98.411 **Viral hepatitis complicating pregnancy, first trimester**

O98.412 **Viral hepatitis complicating pregnancy, second trimester**

O98.413 **Viral hepatitis complicating pregnancy, third trimester**

O98.419 **Viral hepatitis complicating pregnancy, unspecified trimester**

O98.42   Viral hepatitis complicating childbirth

O98.43   Viral hepatitis complicating the puerperium

O98.5   Other viral diseases complicating pregnancy, childbirth and the puerperium

Conditions in A80-B09, B25-B34, R87.81-, R87.82-

Excludes1: human immunodeficiency virus [HIV] disease complicating pregnancy, childbirth and the puerperium (O98.7-)

O98.51   Other viral diseases complicating pregnancy

    O98.511   Other viral diseases complicating pregnancy, first trimester

    O98.512   Other viral diseases complicating pregnancy, second trimester

    O98.513   Other viral diseases complicating pregnancy, third trimester

    O98.519   Other viral diseases complicating pregnancy, unspecified trimester

O98.52   Other viral diseases complicating childbirth

O98.53   Other viral diseases complicating the puerperium

O98.6   Protozoal diseases complicating pregnancy, childbirth and the puerperium

Conditions in B50-B64

O98.61   Protozoal diseases complicating pregnancy

    O98.611   Protozoal diseases complicating pregnancy, first trimester

    O98.612   Protozoal diseases complicating pregnancy, second trimester

    O98.613   Protozoal diseases complicating pregnancy, third trimester

    O98.619   Protozoal diseases complicating pregnancy, unspecified trimester

O98.62   Protozoal diseases complicating childbirth

O98.63   Protozoal diseases complicating the puerperium

O98.7   Human immunodeficiency virus [HIV] disease complicating pregnancy, childbirth and the puerperium

Use Additional Code to identify the type of HIV disease:

Acquired immune deficiency syndrome (AIDS) (B20)

Asymptomatic HIV status (Z21)

HIV positive NOS (Z21)

Symptomatic HIV disease (B20)

O98.71   Human immunodeficiency virus [HIV] disease complicating pregnancy

    O98.711   Human immunodeficiency virus [HIV] disease complicating pregnancy, first trimester

    O98.712   Human immunodeficiency virus [HIV] disease complicating pregnancy, second trimester

    O98.713   Human immunodeficiency virus [HIV] disease complicating pregnancy, third trimester

    O98.719   Human immunodeficiency virus [HIV] disease complicating pregnancy, unspecified trimester

O98.72   Human immunodeficiency virus [HIV] disease complicating childbirth

O98.73   Human immunodeficiency virus [HIV] disease complicating the puerperium

O98.8   Other maternal infectious and parasitic diseases complicating pregnancy, childbirth and the puerperium

O98.81   Other maternal infectious and parasitic diseases complicating pregnancy

    O98.811   Other maternal infectious and parasitic diseases complicating pregnancy, first trimester

    O98.812   Other maternal infectious and parasitic diseases complicating pregnancy, second trimester

    O98.813   Other maternal infectious and parasitic diseases complicating pregnancy, third trimester

    O98.819   Other maternal infectious and parasitic diseases complicating pregnancy, unspecified trimester

O98.82   Other maternal infectious and parasitic diseases complicating childbirth

O98.83   Other maternal infectious and parasitic diseases complicating the puerperium

O98.9   Unspecified maternal infectious and parasitic disease complicating pregnancy, childbirth and the puerperium

O98.91   Unspecified maternal infectious and parasitic disease complicating pregnancy

    O98.911   Unspecified maternal infectious and parasitic disease complicating pregnancy, first trimester

    O98.912   Unspecified maternal infectious and parasitic disease complicating pregnancy, second trimester

    O98.913   Unspecified maternal infectious and parasitic disease complicating pregnancy, third trimester

    O98.919   Unspecified maternal infectious and parasitic disease complicating pregnancy, unspecified trimester

O98.92   Unspecified maternal infectious and parasitic disease complicating childbirth

O98.93   Unspecified maternal infectious and parasitic disease complicating the puerperium

O99   Other maternal diseases classifiable elsewhere but complicating pregnancy, childbirth and the puerperium

Includes: conditions which complicate the pregnant state, are aggravated by the pregnancy or are a main reason for obstetric care

Use Additional Code to identify specific condition

Excludes2: when the reason for maternal care is that the condition is known or suspected to have affected the fetus (O35-O36)

O99.0   Anemia complicating pregnancy, childbirth and the puerperium

Conditions in D50-D64

Excludes1: anemia arising in the puerperium (O90.81)

postpartum anemia NOS (O90.81)

O99.01   Anemia complicating pregnancy

    O99.011   Anemia complicating pregnancy, first trimester

    O99.012   Anemia complicating pregnancy, second trimester

    O99.013   Anemia complicating pregnancy, third trimester

    O99.019   Anemia complicating pregnancy, unspecified trimester

O99.02   Anemia complicating childbirth

O99.03   Anemia complicating the puerperium

Excludes1: postpartum anemia not pre-existing prior to delivery (O90.81)

O99.1   Other diseases of the blood and blood-forming organs and certain disorders involving the immune mechanism complicating pregnancy, childbirth and the puerperium

Conditions in D65-D89

Excludes1: hemorrhage with coagulation defects (O45.-, O46.0-, O67.0, O72.3)

O99.11 **Other diseases of the blood and blood-forming organs and certain disorders involving the immune mechanism complicating pregnancy**

O99.111 Other diseases of the blood and blood-forming organs and certain disorders involving the immune mechanism complicating pregnancy, first trimester

O99.112 Other diseases of the blood and blood-forming organs and certain disorders involving the immune mechanism complicating pregnancy, second trimester

O99.113 Other diseases of the blood and blood-forming organs and certain disorders involving the immune mechanism complicating pregnancy, third trimester

O99.119 Other diseases of the blood and blood-forming organs and certain disorders involving the immune mechanism complicating pregnancy, unspecified trimester

O99.12 **Other diseases of the blood and blood-forming organs and certain disorders involving the immune mechanism complicating childbirth**

O99.13 **Other diseases of the blood and blood-forming organs and certain disorders involving the immune mechanism complicating the puerperium**

O99.2 **Endocrine, nutritional and metabolic diseases complicating pregnancy, childbirth and the puerperium**

Conditions in E00-E89

Excludes2: diabetes mellitus (O24.-)

malnutrition (O25.-)

postpartum thyroiditis (O90.5)

O99.21 **Obesity complicating pregnancy, childbirth, and the puerperium**

Use Additional Code to identify the type of obesity (E66.-)

O99.210 Obesity complicating pregnancy, unspecified trimester

O99.211 Obesity complicating pregnancy, first trimester

O99.212 Obesity complicating pregnancy, second trimester

O99.213 Obesity complicating pregnancy, third trimester

O99.214 Obesity complicating childbirth

O99.215 Obesity complicating the puerperium

O99.28 **Other endocrine, nutritional and metabolic diseases complicating pregnancy, childbirth and the puerperium**

O99.280 Endocrine, nutritional and metabolic diseases complicating pregnancy, unspecified trimester

O99.281 Endocrine, nutritional and metabolic diseases complicating pregnancy, first trimester

O99.282 Endocrine, nutritional and metabolic diseases complicating pregnancy, second trimester

O99.283 Endocrine, nutritional and metabolic diseases complicating pregnancy, third trimester

O99.284 Endocrine, nutritional and metabolic diseases complicating childbirth

O99.285 Endocrine, nutritional and metabolic diseases complicating the puerperium

O99.3 **Mental disorders and diseases of the nervous system complicating pregnancy, childbirth and the puerperium**

O99.31 **Alcohol use complicating pregnancy, childbirth, and the puerperium**

Use Additional Code(s) from F10 to identify manifestations of the alcohol use

O99.310 Alcohol use complicating pregnancy, unspecified trimester

O99.311 Alcohol use complicating pregnancy, first trimester

O99.312 Alcohol use complicating pregnancy, second trimester

O99.313 Alcohol use complicating pregnancy, third trimester

O99.314 Alcohol use complicating childbirth

O99.315 Alcohol use complicating the puerperium

O99.32 **Drug use complicating pregnancy, childbirth, and the puerperium**

Use Additional Code(s) from F11-F16 and F18-F19 to identify manifestations of the drug use

O99.320 Drug use complicating pregnancy, unspecified trimester

O99.321 Drug use complicating pregnancy, first trimester

O99.322 Drug use complicating pregnancy, second trimester

O99.323 Drug use complicating pregnancy, third trimester

O99.324 Drug use complicating childbirth

O99.325 Drug use complicating the puerperium

O99.33 **Tobacco use disorder complicating pregnancy, childbirth, and the puerperium**

Smoking complicating pregnancy, childbirth, and the puerperium

Use Additional Code from category F17 to identify type of tobacco nicotine dependence

O99.330 Smoking (tobacco) complicating pregnancy, unspecified trimester

O99.331 Smoking (tobacco) complicating pregnancy, first trimester

O99.332 Smoking (tobacco) complicating pregnancy, second trimester

O99.333 Smoking (tobacco) complicating pregnancy, third trimester

O99.334 Smoking (tobacco) complicating childbirth

O99.335 Smoking (tobacco) complicating the puerperium

O99.34 **Other mental disorders complicating pregnancy, childbirth, and the puerperium**

Conditions in F01-F09, F20-F52 and F54-F99

Excludes2: postpartum mood disturbance (O90.6)

postnatal psychosis (F53.1)

puerperal psychosis (F53.1)

O99.340 Other mental disorders complicating pregnancy, unspecified trimester

O99.341 Other mental disorders complicating pregnancy, first trimester

O99.342 Other mental disorders complicating pregnancy, second trimester

O99.343 Other mental disorders complicating pregnancy, third trimester

O99.344 Other mental disorders complicating childbirth

O99.345 Other mental disorders complicating the puerperium

O99.35 Diseases of the nervous system complicating pregnancy, childbirth, and the puerperium

Conditions in G00-G99

Excludes2: pregnancy related peripheral neuritis (O26.8-)

O99.350 Diseases of the nervous system complicating pregnancy, unspecified trimester

O99.351 Diseases of the nervous system complicating pregnancy, first trimester

O99.352 Diseases of the nervous system complicating pregnancy, second trimester

O99.353 Diseases of the nervous system complicating pregnancy, third trimester

O99.354 Diseases of the nervous system complicating childbirth

O99.355 Diseases of the nervous system complicating the puerperium

O99.4 Diseases of the circulatory system complicating pregnancy, childbirth and the puerperium

Conditions in I00-I99

Excludes1: peripartum cardiomyopathy (O90.3)

Excludes2: hypertensive disorders (O10-O16)

obstetric embolism (O88.-)

venous complications and cerebrovenous sinus thrombosis in labor, childbirth and the puerperium (O87.-)

venous complications and cerebrovenous sinus thrombosis in pregnancy (O22.-)

O99.41 Diseases of the circulatory system complicating pregnancy

O99.411 Diseases of the circulatory system complicating pregnancy, first trimester

O99.412 Diseases of the circulatory system complicating pregnancy, second trimester

O99.413 Diseases of the circulatory system complicating pregnancy, third trimester

O99.419 Diseases of the circulatory system complicating pregnancy, unspecified trimester

O99.42 Diseases of the circulatory system complicating childbirth

O99.43 Diseases of the circulatory system complicating the puerperium

O99.5 Diseases of the respiratory system complicating pregnancy, childbirth and the puerperium

Conditions in J00-J99

O99.51 Diseases of the respiratory system complicating pregnancy

O99.511 Diseases of the respiratory system complicating pregnancy, first trimester

O99.512 Diseases of the respiratory system complicating pregnancy, second trimester

O99.513 Diseases of the respiratory system complicating pregnancy, third trimester

O99.519 Diseases of the respiratory system complicating pregnancy, unspecified trimester

O99.52 Diseases of the respiratory system complicating childbirth

O99.53 Diseases of the respiratory system complicating the puerperium

O99.6 Diseases of the digestive system complicating pregnancy, childbirth and the puerperium

Conditions in K00-K93

Excludes2: hemorrhoids in pregnancy (O22.4-)

liver and biliary tract disorders in pregnancy, childbirth and the puerperium (O26.6-)

O99.61 Diseases of the digestive system complicating pregnancy

O99.611 Diseases of the digestive system complicating pregnancy, first trimester

O99.612 Diseases of the digestive system complicating pregnancy, second trimester

O99.613 Diseases of the digestive system complicating pregnancy, third trimester

O99.619 Diseases of the digestive system complicating pregnancy, unspecified trimester

O99.62 Diseases of the digestive system complicating childbirth

O99.63 Diseases of the digestive system complicating the puerperium

O99.7 Diseases of the skin and subcutaneous tissue complicating pregnancy, childbirth and the puerperium

Conditions in L00-L99

Excludes2: herpes gestationis (O26.4)

pruritic urticarial papules and plaques of pregnancy (PUPPP) (O26.86)

O99.71 Diseases of the skin and subcutaneous tissue complicating pregnancy

O99.711 Diseases of the skin and subcutaneous tissue complicating pregnancy, first trimester

O99.712 Diseases of the skin and subcutaneous tissue complicating pregnancy, second trimester

O99.713 Diseases of the skin and subcutaneous tissue complicating pregnancy, third trimester

O99.719 Diseases of the skin and subcutaneous tissue complicating pregnancy, unspecified trimester

O99.72 Diseases of the skin and subcutaneous tissue complicating childbirth

O99.73 Diseases of the skin and subcutaneous tissue complicating the puerperium

O99.8 Other specified diseases and conditions complicating pregnancy, childbirth and the puerperium

Conditions in D00-D48, H00-H95, M00-N99, and Q00-Q99

Use Additional Code to identify condition

Excludes2: genitourinary infections in pregnancy (O23.-)

infection of genitourinary tract following delivery (O86.1-O86.4)

malignant neoplasm complicating pregnancy, childbirth and the puerperium (O9A.1-)

maternal care for known or suspected abnormality of maternal pelvic organs (O34.-)

postpartum acute kidney failure (O90.4)

traumatic injuries in pregnancy (O9A.2-)

O99.81 Abnormal glucose complicating pregnancy, childbirth and the puerperium

Excludes1: gestational diabetes (O24.4-)

O99.810 Abnormal glucose complicating pregnancy

O99.814 Abnormal glucose complicating childbirth

O99.815 Abnormal glucose complicating the puerperium

O99.82 Streptococcus B carrier state complicating pregnancy, childbirth and the puerperium

Excludes1: Carrier of streptococcus group B (GBS) in a nonpregnant woman (Z22.330)

O99.820 Streptococcus B carrier state complicating pregnancy

O99.824 Streptococcus B carrier state complicating childbirth

O99.825 Streptococcus B carrier state complicating the puerperium

O99.83 Other infection carrier state complicating pregnancy, childbirth and the puerperium

Use Additional Code to identify the carrier state (Z22.-)

O99.830 Other infection carrier state complicating pregnancy

O99.834 Other infection carrier state complicating childbirth

O99.835 Other infection carrier state complicating the puerperium

O99.84 Bariatric surgery status complicating pregnancy, childbirth and the puerperium

Gastric banding status complicating pregnancy, childbirth and the puerperium

Gastric bypass status for obesity complicating pregnancy, childbirth and the puerperium

Obesity surgery status complicating pregnancy, childbirth and the puerperium

O99.840 Bariatric surgery status complicating pregnancy, unspecified trimester

O99.841 Bariatric surgery status complicating pregnancy, first trimester

O99.842 Bariatric surgery status complicating pregnancy, second trimester

O99.843 Bariatric surgery status complicating pregnancy, third trimester

O99.844 Bariatric surgery status complicating childbirth

O99.845 Bariatric surgery status complicating the puerperium

O99.89 Other specified diseases and conditions complicating pregnancy, childbirth and the puerperium

O99.891 Other specified diseases and conditions complicating pregnancy

O99.892 Other specified diseases and conditions complicating childbirth

O99.893 Other specified diseases and conditions complicating puerperium

O9A Maternal malignant neoplasms, traumatic injuries and abuse classifiable elsewhere but complicating pregnancy, childbirth and the puerperium

O9A.1 Malignant neoplasm complicating pregnancy, childbirth and the puerperium

Conditions in C00-C96

Use Additional Code to identify neoplasm

Excludes2: maternal care for benign tumor of corpus uteri (O34.1-)

maternal care for benign tumor of cervix (O34.4-)

O9A.11 Malignant neoplasm complicating pregnancy

O9A.111 Malignant neoplasm complicating pregnancy, first trimester

O9A.112 Malignant neoplasm complicating pregnancy, second trimester

O9A.113 Malignant neoplasm complicating pregnancy, third trimester

O9A.119 Malignant neoplasm complicating pregnancy, unspecified trimester

O9A.12 Malignant neoplasm complicating childbirth

O9A.13 Malignant neoplasm complicating the puerperium

O9A.2 Injury, poisoning and certain other consequences of external causes complicating pregnancy, childbirth and the puerperium

Conditions in S00-T88, except T74 and T76

Use Additional Code(s) to identify the injury or poisoning

Excludes2: physical, sexual and psychological abuse complicating pregnancy, childbirth and the puerperium (O9A.3-, O9A.4-, O9A.5-)

O9A.21 Injury, poisoning and certain other consequences of external causes complicating pregnancy

O9A.211 Injury, poisoning and certain other consequences of external causes complicating pregnancy, first trimester

O9A.212 Injury, poisoning and certain other consequences of external causes complicating pregnancy, second trimester

O9A.213 Injury, poisoning and certain other consequences of external causes complicating pregnancy, third trimester

O9A.219 Injury, poisoning and certain other consequences of external causes complicating pregnancy, unspecified trimester

O9A.22 Injury, poisoning and certain other consequences of external causes complicating childbirth

O9A.23 **Injury, poisoning and certain other consequences of external causes complicating the puerperium**

O9A.3 **Physical abuse complicating pregnancy, childbirth and the puerperium**

Conditions in T74.11 or T76.11

Use Additional Code (if applicable):

to identify any associated current injury due to physical abuse to identify the perpetrator of abuse (Y07.-)

Excludes2: sexual abuse complicating pregnancy, childbirth

and the puerperium (O9A.4)

O9A.31 **Physical abuse complicating pregnancy**

O9A.311 **Physical abuse complicating pregnancy, first trimester**

O9A.312 **Physical abuse complicating pregnancy, second trimester**

O9A.313 **Physical abuse complicating pregnancy, third trimester**

O9A.319 **Physical abuse complicating pregnancy, unspecified trimester**

O9A.32 **Physical abuse complicating childbirth**

O9A.33 **Physical abuse complicating the puerperium**

O9A.4 **Sexual abuse complicating pregnancy, childbirth and the puerperium**

Conditions in T74.21 or T76.21

Use Additional Code (if applicable):

to identify any associated current injury due to sexual abuse to identify the perpetrator of abuse (Y07.-)

O9A.41 **Sexual abuse complicating pregnancy**

O9A.411 **Sexual abuse complicating pregnancy, first trimester**

O9A.412 **Sexual abuse complicating pregnancy, second trimester**

O9A.413 **Sexual abuse complicating pregnancy, third trimester**

O9A.419 **Sexual abuse complicating pregnancy, unspecified trimester**

O9A.42 **Sexual abuse complicating childbirth**

O9A.43 **Sexual abuse complicating the puerperium**

O9A.5 **Psychological abuse complicating pregnancy, childbirth and the puerperium**

Conditions in T74.31 or T76.31

Use Additional Code to identify the perpetrator of abuse (Y07.-)

O9A.51 **Psychological abuse complicating pregnancy**

O9A.511 **Psychological abuse complicating pregnancy, first trimester**

O9A.512 **Psychological abuse complicating pregnancy, second trimester**

O9A.513 **Psychological abuse complicating pregnancy, third trimester**

O9A.519 **Psychological abuse complicating pregnancy, unspecified trimester**

O9A.52 **Psychological abuse complicating childbirth**

O9A.53 **Psychological abuse complicating the puerperium**

Chapter 16: Certain Conditions Originating in the Perinatal Period (P00-P96)

DEFINITIONS

This chapter includes definitions of selected key words, terms and phrases and coding alerts for adding points to the clinical domain, and references to coding late effects where appropriate. An example from this chapter is as follows:

P36   Bacterial sepsis of newborn
Definition: Neonatal sepsis is a blood infection that occurs in an infant younger than 90 days old. Early-onset sepsis is seen in the first week of life.

MULTIPLE CODING FOR A SINGLE CONDITION

In addition to the etiology/manifestation convention that requires two codes to fully describe a single condition that affects multiple body systems, there are other single conditions that also require more than one code. "**Use Additional Code**" notes are found in the Tabular List at codes that are not part of an etiology/manifestation pair where a secondary code is useful to fully describe a condition. The sequencing rule is the same as the etiology/manifestation pair, "**Use Additional Code**" indicates that a secondary code should be added.

For example, for bacterial infections that are not included in chapter 1, a secondary code from category B95, Streptococcus, Staphylococcus, and Enterococcus, as the cause of diseases classified elsewhere, or B96, Other bacterial agents as the cause of diseases classified elsewhere, may be required to identify the bacterial organism causing the infection. A "**Use Additional Code**" note will normally be found at the infectious disease code, indicating a need for the organism code to be added as a secondary code.

"**Code first**" notes are also under certain codes that are not specifically manifestation codes but may be due to an underlying cause. When there is a "**Code first**" note and an underlying condition is present, the underlying condition should be sequenced first.

"Code, if applicable, any causal condition first", notes indicate that this code may be assigned as a principal diagnosis when the causal condition is unknown or not applicable. If a causal condition is known, then the code for that condition should be sequenced as the principal or first-listed diagnosis.

Multiple codes may be needed for sequela, complication codes and obstetric codes to more fully describe a condition. See the specific guidelines for these conditions for further instruction.

COMBINATION CODE

A combination code is a single code used to classify: Two diagnoses, or a diagnosis with an associated secondary process (manifestation) A diagnosis with an associated complication

Combination codes are identified by referring to subterm entries in the Alphabetic Index and by reading the inclusion and exclusion notes in the Tabular List.

Assign only the combination code when that code fully identifies the diagnostic conditions involved or when the Alphabetic Index so directs. Multiple coding should not be used when the classification provides a combination code that clearly identifies all of the elements documented in the diagnosis. When the combination code lacks necessary specificity in describing the manifestation or complication, an additional code should be used as a secondary code.

SEQUELA (LATE EFFECTS)

A sequela is the residual effect (condition produced) after the acute phase of an illness or injury has terminated. There is no time limit on when a sequela code can be used. The residual may be apparent early, such as in cerebral infarction, or it may occur months or years later, such as that due to a previous injury. Coding of sequela generally requires two codes sequenced in the following order: The condition or nature of the sequela is sequenced first.

The sequela code is sequenced second.

An exception to the above guidelines are those instances where the code for the sequela is followed by a manifestation code identified in the Tabular List and title, or the sequela code has been expanded (at the fourth, fifth or sixth character levels) to

P00-P96

include the manifestation(s). The code for the acute phase of an illness or injury that led to the sequela is never used with a code for the late effect.

GENERAL PERINATAL RULES

1) Use of Chapter 16 Codes

Codes in this chapter are never for use on the maternal record. Codes from Chapter 15, the obstetric chapter, are never permitted on the newborn record. Chapter 16 codes may be used throughout the life of the patient if the condition is still present.

2) Principal Diagnosis for Birth Record

When coding the birth episode in a newborn record, assign a code from category Z38, Liveborn infants according to place of birth and type of delivery, as the principal diagnosis. A code from category Z38 is assigned only once, to a newborn at the time of birth. If a newborn is transferred to another institution, a code from category Z38 should not be used at the receiving hospital.

A code from category Z38 is used only on the newborn record, not on the mother's record.

3) Use of Codes from other Chapters with Codes from Chapter 16

Codes from other chapters may be used with codes from chapter 16 if the codes from the other chapters provide more specific detail. Codes for signs and symptoms may be assigned when a definitive diagnosis has not been established. If the reason for the encounter is a perinatal condition, the code from chapter 16 should be sequenced first.

4) Use of Chapter 16 Codes after the Perinatal Period

Should a condition originate in the perinatal period, and continue throughout the life of the patient, the perinatal code should continue to be used regardless of the patient's age.

5) Birth process or community acquired conditions

If a newborn has a condition that may be either due to the birth process or community acquired and the documentation does not indicate which it is, the default is due to the birth process and the code from Chapter 16 should be used. If the condition is community-acquired, a code from Chapter 16 should not be assigned.

6) Code all clinically significant conditions

All clinically significant conditions noted on routine newborn examination should be coded. A condition is clinically significant if it requires:

§ clinical evaluation; or

§ therapeutic treatment; or

§ diagnostic procedures; or

§ extended length of hospital stay; or

§ increased nursing care and/or monitoring; or

§ has implications for future health care needs

Note: The perinatal guidelines listed above are the same as the general coding guidelines for "additional diagnoses", except for the final point regarding implications for future health care needs. Codes should be assigned for conditions that have been specified by the provider as having implications for future health care needs.

OBSERVATION AND EVALUATION OF NEWBORNS FOR SUSPECTED CONDITIONS NOT FOUND

1) Use of Z05 codes

Assign a code from category Z05, Observation and evaluation of newborns and infants for suspected conditions ruled out, to identify those instances when a healthy newborn is evaluated for a suspected condition that is determined after study not to be present. Do not use a code from category Z05 when the patient has identified signs or symptoms of a suspected problem, in such cases code the sign or symptom.

2) Z05 on Other than the Birth Record

A code from category Z05 may also be assigned as a principal or first-listed code for readmissions or encounters when the code from category Z38 code no longer applies. Codes from category Z05 are for use only for healthy newborns and infants for which no condition after study is found to be present.

3) Z05 on a birth record

A code from category Z05 is to be used as a secondary code after the code from category Z38, Liveborn infants according to place of birth and type of delivery.

CODING ADDITIONAL PERINATAL DIAGNOSES

1) Assigning codes for conditions that require treatment

Assign codes for conditions that require treatment or further investigation, prolong the length of stay, or require resource utilization.

2) Codes for conditions specified as having implications for future health care needs

Assign codes for conditions that have been specified by the provider as having implications for future health care needs.

Note: This guideline should not be used for adult patients.

PREMATURITY AND FETAL GROWTH RETARDATION

Providers utilize different criteria in determining prematurity. A code for prematurity should not be assigned unless it is documented. Assignment of codes in categories P05, Disorders of newborn related to slow fetal growth and fetal malnutrition, and P07, Disorders of newborn related to short gestation and low birth weight, not elsewhere classified, should be based on the recorded birth weight and estimated gestational age.

When both birth weight and gestational age are available, two codes from category P07 should be assigned, with the code for birth weight sequenced before the code for gestational age.

LOW BIRTH WEIGHT AND IMMATURITY STATUS

Codes from category P07, Disorders of newborn related to short gestation and low birth weight, not elsewhere classified, are for use for a child or adult who was premature or had a low birth weight as a newborn and this is affecting the patient's current health status.

See Section I.C.21. Factors influencing health status and contact with health services, Status.

BACTERIAL SEPSIS OF NEWBORN

Category P36, Bacterial sepsis of newborn, includes congenital sepsis. If a perinate is documented as having sepsis without documentation of congenital or community acquired, the default is congenital and a code from category P36 should be assigned. If the P36 code includes the causal organism, an additional code from category B95, Streptococcus, Staphylococcus, and Enterococcus as the cause of diseases classified elsewhere, or B96, Other bacterial agents as the cause of diseases classified elsewhere, should not be assigned. If the P36 code does not include the causal organism, assign an additional code from category B96. If applicable, **Use Additional Code**s to identify severe sepsis (R65.2-) and any associated acute organ dysfunction.

STILLBIRTH

Code P95, Stillbirth, is only for use in institutions that maintain separate records for stillbirths. No other code should be used with P95. Code P95 should not be used on the mother's record.

COVID-19 INFECTION IN NEWBORN

For a newborn that tests positive for COVID-19, assign code U07.1, COVID-19, and the appropriate codes for associated manifestation(s) in neonates/newborns in the absence of documentation indicating a specific type of transmission. For a newborn that tests positive for COVID-19 and the provider documents the condition was contracted in utero or during the birth process, assign codes P35.8, Other congenital viral diseases, and U07.1, COVID-19. When coding the birth episode in a newborn record, the appropriate code from category Z38, Liveborn infants according to place of birth and type of delivery, should be assigned as the principal diagnosis.

● New code   ▲ Revised code   **Excludes1:** Not coded here   **Excludes2:** Not included here   ⊗ Placeholder required   ⑦7ᵗʰ digit required

Chapter 16

Certain Conditions Originating in The Perinatal Period (P00-P96)

NOTE: CODES FROM THIS CHAPTER ARE FOR USE ON NEWBORN RECORDS ONLY, NEVER ON MATERNAL RECORDS

Includes: conditions that have their origin in the fetal or perinatal period (before birth through the first 28 days after birth) even if morbidity occurs later

Excludes2: congenital malformations, deformations and chromosomal abnormalities (Q00-Q99)

endocrine, nutritional and metabolic diseases (E00-E88)

injury, poisoning and certain other consequences of external causes (S00-T88)

neoplasms (C00-D49)

tetanus neonatorum (A33)

This chapter contains the following blocks:

P00-P04	Newborn affected by maternal factors and by complications of pregnancy, labor, and delivery
P05-P08	Disorders of newborn related to length of gestation and fetal growth
P09	Abnormal findings on neonatal screening
P10-P15	Birth trauma
P19-P29	Respiratory and cardiovascular disorders specific to the perinatal period
P35-P39	Infections specific to the perinatal period
P50-P61	Hemorrhagic and hematological disorders of newborn
P70-P74	Transitory endocrine and metabolic disorders specific to newborn
P76-P78	Digestive system disorders of newborn
P80-P83	Conditions involving the integument and temperature regulation of newborn
P84	Other problems with newborn
P90-P96	Other disorders originating in the perinatal period

NEWBORN AFFECTED BY MATERNAL FACTORS AND BY COMPLICATIONS OF PREGNANCY, LABOR, AND DELIVERY (P00-P04)

Note: These codes are for use when the listed maternal conditions are specified as the cause of confirmed morbidity or potential morbidity which have their origin in the perinatal period (before birth through the first 28 days after birth).

P00 **Newborn affected by maternal conditions that may be unrelated to present pregnancy**

Code first any current condition in newborn

Excludes2: encounter for observation of newborn for suspected diseases and conditions ruled out (Z05.-)

newborn affected by maternal complications of pregnancy (P01.-)

newborn affected by maternal endocrine and metabolic disorders (P70-P74)

newborn affected by noxious substances transmitted via placenta or breast milk (P04.-)

P00.0 **Newborn affected by maternal hypertensive disorders**

Newborn affected by maternal conditions classifiable to O10-O11, O13-O16

P00.1 **Newborn affected by maternal renal and urinary tract diseases**

Newborn affected by maternal conditions classifiable to N00-N39

P00.2 **Newborn affected by maternal infectious and parasitic diseases**

Newborn affected by maternal infectious disease classifiable to A00-B99, J09 and J10

Excludes2: infections specific to the perinatal period (P35-P39)

maternal genital tract or other localized infections (P00.8)

newborn affected by (positive) maternal group B streptococcus (GBS) colonization (P00.82)

P00.3 **Newborn affected by other maternal circulatory and respiratory diseases**

Newborn affected by maternal conditions classifiable to I00-I99, J00-J99, Q20-Q34 and not included in P00.0, P00.2

P00.4 **Newborn affected by maternal nutritional disorders**

Newborn affected by maternal disorders classifiable to E40-E64

Maternal malnutrition NOS

P00.5 **Newborn affected by maternal injury**

Newborn affected by maternal conditions classifiable to O9A.2-

P00.6 **Newborn affected by surgical procedure on mother**

Newborn affected by amniocentesis

Excludes1: Cesarean delivery for present delivery (P03.4)

damage to placenta from amniocentesis, Cesarean delivery or surgical induction (P02.1)

previous surgery to uterus or pelvic organs (P03.89)

Excludes2: newborn affected by complication of (fetal) intrauterine procedure (P96.5)

P00.7 **Newborn affected by other medical procedures on mother, not elsewhere classified**

Newborn affected by radiation to mother

Excludes1: damage to placenta from amniocentesis, cesarean delivery or surgical induction (P02.1)

newborn affected by other complications of labor and delivery (P03.-)

P00.8 **Newborn affected by other maternal conditions**

P00.81 **Newborn affected by periodontal disease in mother**

● **P00.82** **Newborn affected by (positive) maternal group B streptococcus (GBS) colonization**

Contact with positive maternal group B streptococcus

P00.89 **Newborn affected by other maternal conditions**

Use Additional Code to identify infectious agent, if known

Newborn affected by conditions classifiable to T80-T88

Newborn affected by maternal genital tract or other localized infections

Newborn affected by maternal systemic lupus erythematosus

P00.9 **Newborn affected by unspecified maternal condition**

P01 **Newborn affected by maternal complications of pregnancy**

Code first any current condition in newborn

Excludes2: encounter for observation of newborn for suspected diseases and conditions ruled out (Z05.-)

P01.0 **Newborn affected by incompetent cervix**

P01.1 **Newborn affected by premature rupture of membranes**

P01.2 **Newborn affected by oligohydramnios**

Excludes1: oligohydramnios due to premature rupture of membranes (P01.1)

P01.3 **Newborn affected by polyhydramnios**

Newborn affected by hydramnios

P01.4 **Newborn affected by ectopic pregnancy**

Newborn affected by abdominal pregnancy

P01.5 **Newborn affected by multiple pregnancy**

Newborn affected by triplet (pregnancy)

Newborn affected by twin (pregnancy)

P01.6 **Newborn affected by maternal death**

P01.7 **Newborn affected by malpresentation before labor**

Newborn affected by breech presentation before labor

Newborn affected by external version before labor

Newborn affected by face presentation before labor

Newborn affected by transverse lie before labor

Newborn affected by unstable lie before labor

P01.8 **Newborn affected by other maternal complications of pregnancy**

P01.9 **Newborn affected by maternal complication of pregnancy, unspecified**

P02 **Newborn affected by complications of placenta, cord and membranes**

Code first any current condition in newborn

Excludes2: encounter for observation of newborn for suspected diseases and conditions ruled out (Z05.-)

P02.0 **Newborn affected by placenta previa**

P02.1 **Newborn affected by other forms of placental separation and hemorrhage**

Newborn affected by abruptio placenta

Newborn affected by accidental hemorrhage

Newborn affected by antepartum hemorrhage

Newborn affected by damage to placenta from amniocentesis, cesarean delivery or surgical induction

Newborn affected by maternal blood loss

Newborn affected by premature separation of placenta

P02.2 **Newborn affected by other and unspecified morphological and functional abnormalities of placenta**

P02.20 **Newborn affected by unspecified morphological and functional abnormalities of placenta**

P02.29 **Newborn affected by other morphological and functional abnormalities of placenta**

Newborn affected by placental dysfunction

Newborn affected by placental infarction

Newborn affected by placental insufficiency

P02.3 **Newborn affected by placental transfusion syndromes**

Newborn affected by placental and cord abnormalities resulting in twin-to-twin or other transplacental transfusion

P02.4 **Newborn affected by prolapsed cord**

P02.5 **Newborn affected by other compression of umbilical cord**

Newborn affected by umbilical cord (tightly) around neck

Newborn affected by entanglement of umbilical cord

Newborn affected by knot in umbilical cord

P02.6 **Newborn affected by other and unspecified conditions of umbilical cord**

P02.60 **Newborn affected by unspecified conditions of umbilical cord**

P02.69 **Newborn affected by other conditions of umbilical cord**

Newborn affected by short umbilical cord

Newborn affected by vasa previa

Excludes1: newborn affected by single umbilical artery (Q27.0)

P02.7 **Newborn affected by chorioamnionitis**

P02.70 **Newborn affected by fetal inflammatory response syndrome**

Newborn affected by FIRS

P02.78 **Newborn affected by other conditions from chorioamnionitis**

Newborn affected by amnionitis

Newborn affected by membranitis

Newborn affected by placentitis

P02.8 **Newborn affected by other abnormalities of membranes**

P02.9 **Newborn affected by abnormality of membranes, unspecified**

P03 **Newborn affected by other complications of labor and delivery**

Code first any current condition in newborn

Excludes2: encounter for observation of newborn for suspected diseases and conditions ruled out (Z05.-)

P03.0 **Newborn affected by breech delivery and extraction**

P03.1 **Newborn affected by other malpresentation, malposition and disproportion during labor and delivery**

Newborn affected by contracted pelvis

Newborn affected by conditions classifiable to O64-O66

Newborn affected by persistent occipitoposterior

Newborn affected by transverse lie

P03.2 **Newborn affected by forceps delivery**

P03.3 **Newborn affected by delivery by vacuum extractor [ventouse]**

P03.4 **Newborn affected by Cesarean delivery**

P03.5 **Newborn affected by precipitate delivery**

Newborn affected by rapid second stage

P03.6 **Newborn affected by abnormal uterine contractions**

Newborn affected by conditions classifiable to O62.-, except O62.3

Newborn affected by hypertonic labor

Newborn affected by uterine inertia

P03.8 **Newborn affected by other specified complications of labor and delivery**

P03.81 **Newborn affected by abnormality in fetal (intrauterine) heart rate or rhythm**

Excludes1: neonatal cardiac dysrhythmia (P29.1-)

P03.810 **Newborn affected by abnormality in fetal (intrauterine) heart rate or rhythm before the onset of labor**

P03.811 **Newborn affected by abnormality in fetal (intrauterine) heart rate or rhythm during labor**

P03.819 **Newborn affected by abnormality in fetal (intrauterine) heart rate or rhythm, unspecified as to time of onset**

P03.82 **Meconium passage during delivery**

Excludes1: meconium aspiration (P24.00, P24.01) meconium staining (P96.83)

P03.89 **Newborn affected by other specified complications of labor and delivery**

Newborn affected by abnormality of maternal soft tissues

Newborn affected by conditions classifiable to O60-O75 and by procedures used in labor and delivery not included in P02.- and P03.0-P03.6

Newborn affected by induction of labor

P03.9 **Newborn affected by complication of labor and delivery, unspecified**

P04 **Newborn affected by noxious substances transmitted via placenta or breast milk**

Code first any current condition in newborn, if applicable

Includes: nonteratogenic effects of substances transmitted via placenta

Excludes2: congenital malformations (Q00-Q99)

encounter for observation of newborn for suspected diseases and conditions ruled out (Z05.-)

neonatal jaundice from excessive hemolysis due to drugs or toxins transmitted from mother (P58.4)

newborn in contact with and (suspected) exposures hazardous to health not transmitted via placenta or breast milk (Z77.-)

P04.0 **Newborn affected by maternal anesthesia and analgesia in pregnancy, labor and delivery**

Newborn affected by reactions and intoxications from maternal opiates and tranquilizers administered for procedures during pregnancy or labor and delivery

Excludes2: newborn affected by other maternal medication (P04.1-)

P04.1 **Newborn affected by other maternal medication**

Code first withdrawal symptoms from maternal use of drugs of addiction, if applicable (P96.1)

Excludes2: maternal anesthesia and analgesia in pregnancy, labor and delivery (P04.0)

maternal use of drugs of Addiction (P04.4-)

P04.11 **Newborn affected by maternal antineoplastic chemotherapy**

P04.12 **Newborn affected by maternal cytotoxic drugs**

P04.13 **Newborn affected by maternal use of anticonvulsants**

P04.14 **Newborn affected by maternal use of opiates**

P04.15 **Newborn affected by maternal use of antidepressants**

P04.16 **Newborn affected by maternal use of amphetamines**

P04.17 **Newborn affected by maternal use of sedative-hypnotics**

P04.1A **Newborn affected by maternal use of anxiolytics**

P04.18 **Newborn affected by other maternal medication**

P04.19 **Newborn affected by maternal use of unspecified medication**

P04.2 **Newborn affected by maternal use of tobacco**

Newborn affected by exposure in utero to tobacco smoke

Excludes2: newborn exposure to environmental tobacco smoke (P96.81)

P04.3 **Newborn affected by maternal use of alcohol**

Excludes1: fetal alcohol syndrome (Q86.0)

P04.4 **Newborn affected by maternal use of drugs of addiction**

P04.40 **Newborn affected by maternal use of unspecified drugs of addiction**

P04.41 **Newborn affected by maternal use of cocaine**

P04.42 **Newborn affected by maternal use of hallucinogens**

Excludes2: newborn affected by other maternal medication (P04.1-)

P04.49 **Newborn affected by maternal use of other drugs of addiction**

Excludes2: newborn affected by maternal anesthesia and analgesia (P04.0)

withdrawal symptoms from maternal use of drugs of addiction (P96.1)

P04.5 **Newborn affected by maternal use of nutritional chemical substances**

P04.6 **Newborn affected by maternal exposure to environmental chemical substances**

P04.8 **Newborn affected by other maternal noxious substances**

P04.81 **Newborn affected by maternal use of cannabis**

P04.89 **Newborn affected by other maternal noxious substances**

P04.9 **Newborn affected by maternal noxious substance, unspecified**

DISORDERS OF NEWBORN RELATED TO LENGTH OF GESTATION AND FETAL GROWTH (P05-P08)

P05 **Disorders of newborn related to slow fetal growth and fetal malnutrition**

P05.0 **Newborn light for gestational age**

Newborn light-for-dates

Weight below but length above 10th percentile for gestational age

P05.00 **Newborn light for gestational age, unspecified weight**

P05.01 **Newborn light for gestational age, less than 500 grams**

P05.02 **Newborn light for gestational age, 500-749 grams**

P05.03 **Newborn light for gestational age, 750-999 grams**

P05.04 **Newborn light for gestational age, 1000-1249 grams**

P05.05 **Newborn light for gestational age, 1250-1499 grams**

P05.06 **Newborn light for gestational age, 1500-1749 grams**

P05.07 **Newborn light for gestational age, 1750-1999 grams**

P05.08 **Newborn light for gestational age, 2000-2499 grams**

P05.09 **Newborn light for gestational age, 2500 grams and over**

Newborn light for gestational age, other

P05.1 **Newborn small for gestational age**

Newborn small-and-light-for-dates

Newborn small-for-dates

Weight and length below 10th percentile for gestational age

P05.10 **Newborn small for gestational age, unspecified weight**

P05.11 **Newborn small for gestational age, less than 500 grams**

P05.12 **Newborn small for gestational age, 500-749 grams**

P05.13 **Newborn small for gestational age, 750-999 grams**

P05.14 **Newborn small for gestational age, 1000-1249 grams**

P05.15   **Newborn small for gestational age, 1250-1499 grams**

P05.16   **Newborn small for gestational age, 1500-1749 grams**

P05.17   **Newborn small for gestational age, 1750-1999 grams**

P05.18   **Newborn small for gestational age, 2000-2499 grams**

P05.19   **Newborn small for gestational age, other**

Newborn small for gestational age, 2500 grams and over

P05.2   Newborn affected by fetal (intrauterine) malnutrition not light or small for gestational age

Infant, not light or small for gestational age, showing signs of fetal malnutrition, such as dry, peeling skin and loss of subcutaneous tissue

Excludes1: newborn affected by fetal malnutrition with light for gestational age (P05.0-)

newborn affected by fetal malnutrition with small for gestational age (P05.1-)

P05.9   Newborn affected by slow intrauterine growth, unspecified

Newborn affected by fetal growth retardation NOS

P07   Disorders of newborn related to short gestation and low birth weight, not elsewhere classified

Note: When both birth weight and gestational age of the newborn are available, both should be coded with birth weight sequenced before gestational age

Includes: the listed conditions, without further specification, as the cause of morbidity or additional care, in newborn

P07.0   Extremely low birth weight newborn

Newborn birth weight 999 g. or less

Excludes1: low birth weight due to slow fetal growth and fetal malnutrition (P05.-)

P07.00   **Extremely low birth weight newborn, unspecified weight**

P07.01   **Extremely low birth weight newborn, less than 500 grams**

P07.02   **Extremely low birth weight newborn, 500-749 grams**

P07.03   **Extremely low birth weight newborn, 750-999 grams**

P07.1   Other low birth weight newborn

Newborn birth weight 1000-2499 g.

Excludes1: low birth weight due to slow fetal growth and fetal malnutrition (P05.-)

P07.10   **Other low birth weight newborn, unspecified weight**

P07.14   **Other low birth weight newborn, 1000-1249 grams**

P07.15   **Other low birth weight newborn, 1250-1499 grams**

P07.16   **Other low birth weight newborn, 1500-1749 grams**

P07.17   **Other low birth weight newborn, 1750-1999 grams**

P07.18   **Other low birth weight newborn, 2000-2499 grams**

P07.2   Extreme immaturity of newborn

Less than 28 completed weeks (less than 196 completed days) of gestation.

P07.20   **Extreme immaturity of newborn, unspecified weeks of gestation**

Gestational age less than 28 completed weeks NOS

P07.21   **Extreme immaturity of newborn, gestational age less than 23 completed weeks**

Extreme immaturity of newborn, gestational age less than 23 weeks, 0 days

P07.22   **Extreme immaturity of newborn, gestational age 23 completed weeks**

Extreme immaturity of newborn, gestational age 23 weeks, 0 days through 23 weeks, 6 days

P07.23   **Extreme immaturity of newborn, gestational age 24completed weeks**

Extreme immaturity of newborn, gestational age 24 weeks, 0 days through 24 weeks, 6 days

P07.24   **Extreme immaturity of newborn, gestational age 25completed weeks**

Extreme immaturity of newborn, gestational age 25 weeks, 0 days through 25 weeks, 6 days

P07.25   **Extreme immaturity of newborn, gestational age 26completed weeks**

Extreme immaturity of newborn, gestational age 26 weeks, 0 days through 26 weeks, 6 days

P07.26   **Extreme immaturity of newborn, gestational age 27completed weeks**

Extreme immaturity of newborn, gestational age 27 weeks, 0 days through 27 weeks, 6 days

P07.3   Preterm [premature] newborn [Other]

28 completed weeks or more but less than 37 completed weeks (196 completed days but less than 259 completed days) of gestation.

Prematurity NOS

P07.30   **Preterm newborn, unspecified weeks of gestation**

P07.31   **Preterm newborn, gestational age 28 completed weeks**

Preterm newborn, gestational age 28 weeks, 0 days through 28 weeks, 6 days

P07.32   **Preterm newborn, gestational age 29 completed weeks**

Preterm newborn, gestational age 29 weeks, 0 days through 29 weeks, 6 days

P07.33   **Preterm newborn, gestational age 30 completed weeks**

Preterm newborn, gestational age 30 weeks, 0 days through 30 weeks, 6 days

P07.34   **Preterm newborn, gestational age 31 completed weeks**

Preterm newborn, gestational age 31 weeks, 0 days through 31 weeks, 6 days

P07.35   **Preterm newborn, gestational age 32 completed weeks**

Preterm newborn, gestational age 32 weeks, 0 days through 32 weeks, 6 days

P07.36   **Preterm newborn, gestational age 33 completed weeks**

Preterm newborn, gestational age 33 weeks, 0 days through 33 weeks, 6 days

P07.37   **Preterm newborn, gestational age 34 completed weeks**

Preterm newborn, gestational age 34 weeks, 0 days through 34 weeks, 6 days

P07.38   **Preterm newborn, gestational age 35 completed weeks**

Preterm newborn, gestational age 35 weeks, 0 days through 35 weeks, 6 days

P07.39   **Preterm newborn, gestational age 36 completed weeks**

Preterm newborn, gestational age 36 weeks, 0 days through 36 weeks, 6 days

P08 **Disorders of newborn related to long gestation and high birth weight**

Note: When both birth weight and gestational age of the newborn are available, priority of assignment should be given to birth weight

`Includes:` the listed conditions, without further specification, as causes of morbidity or additional care, in newborn

P08.0 **Exceptionally large newborn baby**

Usually implies a birth weight of 4500 g. or more

`Excludes1:` syndrome of infant of diabetic mother (P70.1)

syndrome of infant of mother with gestational diabetes (P70.0)

P08.1 **Other heavy for gestational age newborn**

Other newborn heavy- or large-for-dates regardless of period of gestation Usually implies a birth weight of 4000 g. to 4499 g.

`Excludes1:` newborn with a birth weight of 4500 or more (P08.0)

syndrome of infant of diabetic mother (P70.1)

syndrome of infant of mother with gestational diabetes (P70.0).

P08.2 **Late newborn, not heavy for gestational age**

P08.21   **Post-term newborn**

Newborn with gestation period over 40 completed weeks to 42 completed weeks

P08.22   **Prolonged gestation of newborn**

Newborn with gestation period over 42 completed weeks (294 days or more), not heavy- or large-for-dates.

Postmaturity NOS

ABNORMAL FINDINGS ON NEONATAL SCREENING (P09)

P09 **Abnormal findings on neonatal screening**

`Includes` Abnormal findings on state mandated newborn screens

Failed newborn screening

- **P09.1** **Abnormal findings on neonatal screening for inborn errors of metabolism**
- **P09.2** **Abnormal findings on neonatal screening for congenital endocrine disease**

Abnormal findings on neonatal screening for congenital adrenal hyperplasia

Abnormal findings on neonatal screening for hypothyroidism screen

- **P09.3** **Abnormal findings on neonatal screening for congenital hematologic disorders**

Abnormal findings for hemoglobinothies screen

Abnormal findings on red cell membrane defects screen

Abnormal findings on sickle cell screen

- **P09.4** **Abnormal findings on neonatal screening for cystic fibrosis**
- **P09.5** **Abnormal findings on neonatal screening for critical congenital heart disease**

Neonatal congenital heart disease screening failure

- **P09.6** **Abnormal findings on neonatal screening for neonatal hearing loss**

`Excludes2:` encounter for hearing examination following failed hearing screening (Z01.110)

- **P09.8** **Other abnormal findings on neonatal screening**
- **P09.9** **Abnormal findings on neonatal screening, unspecified**

`Excludes2:` nonspecific serologic evidence of human immunodeficiency virus [HIV] (R75)

BIRTH TRAUMA (P10-P15)

`Definition:` Birth trauma refers to: 1) a physical injury sustained by an infant during birth; or 2) the psychological shock said to be experienced by an infant during birth.

P10 **Intracranial laceration and hemorrhage due to birth injury**

`Excludes1:` intracranial hemorrhage of newborn NOS (P52.9)

intracranial hemorrhage of newborn due to anoxia or hypoxia (P52.-)

nontraumatic intracranial hemorrhage of newborn (P52.-)

P10.0 **Subdural hemorrhage due to birth injury**

Subdural hematoma (localized) due to birth injury

`Excludes1:` subdural hemorrhage accompanying tentorial tear (P10.4)

P10.1 **Cerebral hemorrhage due to birth injury**

P10.2 **Intraventricular hemorrhage due to birth injury**

P10.3 **Subarachnoid hemorrhage due to birth injury**

P10.4 **Tentorial tear due to birth injury**

P10.8 **Other intracranial lacerations and hemorrhages due to birth injury**

P10.9 **Unspecified intracranial laceration and hemorrhage due to birth injury**

P11 **Other birth injuries to central nervous system**

P11.0 **Cerebral edema due to birth injury**

P11.1 **Other specified brain damage due to birth injury**

P11.2 **Unspecified brain damage due to birth injury**

P11.3 **Birth injury to facial nerve**

Facial palsy due to birth injury

P11.4 **Birth injury to other cranial nerves**

P11.5 **Birth injury to spine and spinal cord**

Fracture of spine due to birth injury

P11.9 **Birth injury to central nervous system, unspecified**

P12 **Birth injury to scalp**

P12.0 **Cephalhematoma due to birth injury**

P12.1 **Chignon (from vacuum extraction) due to birth injury**

P12.2 **Epicranial subaponeurotic hemorrhage due to birth injury**

Subgaleal hemorrhage

P12.3 **Bruising of scalp due to birth injury**

P12.4 **Injury of scalp of newborn due to monitoring equipment**

Sampling incision of scalp of newborn

Scalp clip (electrode) injury of newborn

P12.8 **Other birth injuries to scalp**

P12.81   **Caput succedaneum**

P12.89   **Other birth injuries to scalp**

P12.9 **Birth injury to scalp, unspecified**

P13 **Birth injury to skeleton**

`Excludes2:` birth injury to spine (P11.5)

P13.0 **Fracture of skull due to birth injury**

P13.1 **Other birth injuries to skull**

`Excludes1:` cephalhematoma (P12.0)

P13.2 **Birth injury to femur**

P13.3   Birth injury to other long bones

P13.4   Fracture of clavicle due to birth injury

P13.8   Birth injuries to other parts of skeleton

P13.9   Birth injury to skeleton, unspecified

P14   Birth injury to peripheral nervous system

P14.0   Erb's paralysis due to birth injury

P14.1   Klumpke's paralysis due to birth injury

P14.2   Phrenic nerve paralysis due to birth injury

P14.3   Other brachial plexus birth injuries

P14.8   Birth injuries to other parts of peripheral nervous system

P14.9   Birth injury to peripheral nervous system, unspecified

P15   Other birth injuries

P15.0   Birth injury to liver

Rupture of liver due to birth injury

P15.1   Birth injury to spleen

Rupture of spleen due to birth injury

P15.2   Sternomastoid injury due to birth injury

P15.3   Birth injury to eye

Subconjunctival hemorrhage due to birth injury

Traumatic glaucoma due to birth injury

P15.4   Birth injury to face

Facial congestion due to birth injury

P15.5   Birth injury to external genitalia

P15.6   Subcutaneous fat necrosis due to birth injury

P15.8   Other specified birth injuries

P15.9   Birth injury, unspecified

RESPIRATORY AND CARDIOVASCULAR DISORDERS SPECIFIC TO THE PERINATAL PERIOD (P19-P29)

P19   Metabolic acidemia in newborn

Includes: metabolic acidemia in newborn

P19.0   Metabolic acidemia in newborn first noted before onset of labor

P19.1   Metabolic acidemia in newborn first noted during labor

P19.2   Metabolic acidemia noted at birth

P19.9   Metabolic acidemia, unspecified

P22   Respiratory distress of newborn

P22.0   Respiratory distress syndrome of newborn

Definition: Respiratory distress syndrome (RDS), formerly known as hyaline membrane disease, is a syndrome of respiratory difficulty in newborn infants caused by a deficiency of a molecule called surfactant.

Cardiorespiratory distress syndrome of newborn

Hyaline membrane disease

Idiopathic respiratory distress syndrome [IRDS or RDS] of newborn

Pulmonary hypoperfusion syndrome

Respiratory distress syndrome, type I

Excludes2: respiratory arrest of newborn (P28.81)

respiratory failure of newborn NOS (P28.5)

P22.1   Transient tachypnea of newborn

Idiopathic tachypnea of newborn

Respiratory distress syndrome, type II

Wet lung syndrome

P22.8   Other

Excludes1: respiratory distress of newborn

Excludes1: respiratory arrest of newborn (P28.81)

respiratory failure of newborn NOS (P28.5)

P22.9   Respiratory distress of newborn, unspecified

Excludes1: respiratory arrest of newborn (P28.81)

respiratory failure of newborn NOS (P28.5)

P23   Congenital pneumonia

Includes: infective pneumonia acquired in utero or during birth

Excludes1: neonatal pneumonia resulting from aspiration (P24.-)

P23.0   Congenital pneumonia due to viral agent

Use Additional Code (B97) to identify organism

Excludes1: congenital rubella pneumonitis (P35.0)

P23.1   Congenital pneumonia due to Chlamydia

P23.2   Congenital pneumonia due to staphylococcus

P23.3   Congenital pneumonia due to streptococcus, group B

P23.4   Congenital pneumonia due to Escherichia coli

P23.5   Congenital pneumonia due to Pseudomonas

P23.6   Congenital pneumonia due to other bacterial agents

Congenital pneumonia due to Hemophilus influenzae

Congenital pneumonia due to Klebsiella pneumoniae

Congenital pneumonia due to Mycoplasma

Congenital pneumonia due to Streptococcus, except group B

Use Additional Code (B95-B96) to identify organism

P23.8   Congenital pneumonia due to other organisms

P23.9   Congenital pneumonia, unspecified

P24   Neonatal aspiration

Includes: aspiration in utero and during delivery

P24.0   Meconium aspiration

Excludes1: meconium passage (without aspiration) during delivery (P03.82)

meconium staining (P96.83)

P24.00   Meconium aspiration without respiratory symptoms

Meconium aspiration NOS

P24.01   Meconium aspiration with respiratory symptoms

Meconium aspiration pneumonia

Meconium aspiration pneumonitis

Meconium aspiration syndrome NOS

Use Additional Code to identify any secondary pulmonary hypertension, if applicable (I27.2-)

P24.1   Neonatal aspiration of (clear) amniotic fluid and mucus

Neonatal aspiration of liquor (amnii)

P24.10   Neonatal aspiration of (clear) amniotic fluid and mucus without respiratory symptoms

Neonatal aspiration of amniotic fluid and mucus NOS

P24.11   Neonatal aspiration of (clear) amniotic fluid and mucus with respiratory symptoms

Neonatal aspiration of amniotic fluid and mucus with pneumonia

Neonatal aspiration of amniotic fluid and mucus with pneumonitis

Use Additional Code to identify any secondary pulmonary hypertension, if applicable (I27.2-)

P24.2   Neonatal aspiration of blood

P24.20   Neonatal aspiration of blood without respiratory symptoms

Neonatal aspiration of blood NOS

● New code   ▲ Revised code   **Excludes1:** Not coded here   **Excludes2:** Not included here   ⊗ Placeholder required   ⑦7th digit required

P24.21 **Neonatal aspiration of blood with respiratory symptoms**

Neonatal aspiration of blood with pneumonia

Neonatal aspiration of blood with pneumonitis

<u>Use Additional Code</u> to identify any secondary pulmonary hypertension, if applicable (I27.2-)

P24.3 **Neonatal aspiration of milk and regurgitated food**

Neonatal aspiration of stomach contents

P24.30 **Neonatal aspiration of milk and regurgitated food without respiratory symptoms**

Neonatal aspiration of milk and regurgitated food NOS

P24.31 **Neonatal aspiration of milk and regurgitated food with respiratory symptoms**

Neonatal aspiration of milk and regurgitated food with pneumonia

Neonatal aspiration of milk and regurgitated food with pneumonitis

<u>Use Additional Code</u> to identify any secondary pulmonary hypertension, if applicable (I27.2-)

P24.8 **Other neonatal aspiration**

P24.80 **Other neonatal aspiration without respiratory symptoms**

Neonatal aspiration NEC

P24.81 **Other neonatal aspiration with respiratory symptoms**

Neonatal aspiration pneumonia NEC

Neonatal aspiration with pneumonitis NEC

Neonatal aspiration with pneumonia NOS

Neonatal aspiration with pneumonitis NOS

<u>Use Additional Code</u> to identify any secondary pulmonary hypertension, if applicable (I27.2-)

P24.9 **Neonatal aspiration, unspecified**

P25 **Interstitial emphysema and related conditions originating in the perinatal period**

P25.0 **Interstitial emphysema originating in the perinatal period**

P25.1 **Pneumothorax originating in the perinatal period**

P25.2 **Pneumomediastinum originating in the perinatal period**

P25.3 **Pneumopericardium originating in the perinatal period**

P25.8 **Other conditions related to interstitial emphysema originating in the perinatal period**

P26 **Pulmonary hemorrhage originating in the perinatal period**

Excludes1: acute idiopathic hemorrhage in infants over 28 days old (R04.81)

P26.0 **Tracheobronchial hemorrhage originating in the perinatal period**

P26.1 **Massive pulmonary hemorrhage originating in the perinatal period**

P26.8 **Other pulmonary hemorrhages originating in the perinatal period**

P26.9 **Unspecified pulmonary hemorrhage originating in the perinatal period**

P27 **Chronic respiratory disease originating in the perinatal period**

Excludes2: respiratory distress of newborn (P22.0-P22.9)

P27.0 **Wilson-Mikity syndrome**

Pulmonary dysmaturity

P27.1 **Bronchopulmonary dysplasia originating in the perinatal period**

P27.8 **Other chronic respiratory diseases originating in the perinatal period**

Congenital pulmonary fibrosis

Ventilator lung in newborn

P27.9 **Unspecified chronic respiratory disease originating in the perinatal period**

P28 **Other respiratory conditions originating in the perinatal period**

Excludes1: congenital malformations of the respiratory system (Q30-Q34)

P28.0 **Primary atelectasis of newborn**

Primary failure to expand terminal respiratory units

Pulmonary hypoplasia associated with short gestation

Pulmonary immaturity NOS

P28.1 **Other and unspecified atelectasis of newborn**

P28.10 **Unspecified atelectasis of newborn**

Atelectasis of newborn NOS

P28.11 **Resorption atelectasis without respiratory distress syndrome**

Excludes1: resorption atelectasis with respiratory distress syndrome (P22.0)

P28.19 **Other atelectasis of newborn**

Partial atelectasis of newborn

Secondary atelectasis of newborn

P28.2 **Cyanotic attacks of newborn**

Excludes1: apnea of newborn (P28.3-P28.4)

P28.3 **Primary sleep apnea of newborn**

Central sleep apnea of newborn

Obstructive sleep apnea of newborn

Sleep apnea of newborn NOS

P28.4 **Other apnea of newborn**

Apnea of prematurity

Obstructive apnea of newborn

Excludes1: obstructive sleep apnea of newborn (P28.3)

P28.5 **Respiratory failure of newborn**

Excludes1: respiratory arrest of newborn (P28.81)

respiratory distress of newborn (P22.0-)

P28.8 **Other specified respiratory conditions of newborn**

P28.81 **Respiratory arrest of newborn**

P28.89 **Other specified respiratory conditions of newborn**

Congenital laryngeal stridor

Sniffles in newborn

Snuffles in newborn

Excludes1: early congenital syphilitic rhinitis A50.05)

P28.9 **Respiratory condition of newborn, unspecified**

Respiratory depression in newborn

P29 **Cardiovascular disorders originating in the perinatal period**

Excludes2: congenital malformations of the circulatory system (Q20-Q28)

P29.0 **Neonatal cardiac failure**

P29.1 **Neonatal cardiac dysrhythmia**

P29.11 **Neonatal tachycardia**

P29.12 **Neonatal bradycardia**

P29.2 **Neonatal hypertension**

P29.3 **Persistent fetal circulation**

P29.30 **Pulmonary hypertension of newborn**

Persistent pulmonary hypertension of newborn

P29.38 **Other persistent fetal circulation**

Delayed closure of ductus arteriosus

P29.4 **Transient myocardial ischemia in newborn**

P29.8 **Other cardiovascular disorders originating in the perinatal period**

P29.81 **Cardiac arrest of newborn**

P29.89 **Other cardiovascular disorders originating in the perinatal period**

P29.9 **Cardiovascular disorder originating in the perinatal period, unspecified**

INFECTIONS SPECIFIC TO THE PERINATAL PERIOD (P35-P39)

Infections acquired in utero, during birth via the umbilicus, or during the first 28 days after birth

Excludes2: asymptomatic human immunodeficiency virus [HIV] infection status (Z21)

congenital gonococcal infection (A54.-)

congenital pneumonia (P23.-)

congenital syphilis (A50.-)

human immunodeficiency virus [HIV] disease (B20)

infant botulism (A48.51)

infectious diseases not specific to the perinatal period (A00-B99, J09, J10.-)

intestinal infectious disease (A00-A09)

laboratory evidence of human immunodeficiency virus [HIV] (R75)

tetanus neonatorum (A33)

P35 **Congenital viral diseases**

Includes: infections acquired in utero or during birth

P35.0 **Congenital rubella syndrome**

Congenital rubella pneumonitis

P35.1 **Congenital cytomegalovirus infection**

P35.2 **Congenital herpesviral [herpes simplex] infection**

P35.3 **Congenital viral hepatitis**

P35.4 **Congenital Zika virus disease**

Use Additional Code to identify manifestations of congenital Zika virus disease

P35.8 **Other congenital viral diseases**

Congenital varicella [chickenpox]

P35.9 **Congenital viral disease, unspecified**

P36 **Bacterial sepsis of newborn**

Definition: Neonatal sepsis is a blood infection that occurs in an infant younger than 90 days old. Early-onset sepsis is seen in the first week of life. Late-onset sepsis occurs between days 8 and 89.

Includes: congenital sepsis

Use Additional Code(s), if applicable, to identify severe sepsis (R652-) and associated acute organ dysfunction(s)

P36.0 **Sepsis of newborn due to streptococcus, group B** [HCC]

P36.1 **Sepsis of newborn due to other and unspecified streptococci**

P36.10 **Sepsis of newborn due to unspecified streptococci** [HCC]

P36.19 **Sepsis of newborn due to other streptococci** [HCC]

P36.2 **Sepsis of newborn due to Staphylococcus aureus** [HCC]

P36.3 **Sepsis of newborn due to other and unspecified staphylococci**

P36.30 **Sepsis of newborn due to unspecified staphylococci** [HCC]

P36.39 **Sepsis of newborn due to other staphylococci** [HCC]

P36.4 **Sepsis of newborn due to Escherichia coli** [HCC]

P36.5 **Sepsis of newborn due to anaerobes** [HCC]

P36.8 **Other bacterial sepsis of newborn** [HCC]

Use Additional Code from category B96 to identify organism

P36.9 **Bacterial sepsis of newborn, unspecified** [HCC]

P37 **Other congenital infectious and parasitic diseases**

Excludes2: congenital syphilis (A50.-)

infectious neonatal diarrhea (A00-A09)

necrotizing enterocolitis in newborn (P77.-)

noninfectious neonatal diarrhea (P78.3)

ophthalmia neonatorum due to gonococcus (A54.31)

tetanus neonatorum (A33)

P37.0 **Congenital tuberculosis**

P37.1 **Congenital toxoplasmosis**

Hydrocephalus due to congenital toxoplasmosis

P37.2 **Neonatal (disseminated) listeriosis**

P37.3 **Congenital falciparum malaria**

P37.4 **Other congenital malaria**

P37.5 **Neonatal candidiasis**

P37.8 **Other specified congenital infectious and parasitic diseases**

P37.9 **Congenital infectious or parasitic disease, unspecified**

P38 **Omphalitis of newborn**

Definition: Omphalitis is the medical term for inflammation of the umbilical cord stump in the neonatal newborn period, most commonly attributed to a bacterial infection.

Excludes1: omphalitis not of newborn (L08.82)

tetanus omphalitis (A33)

umbilical hemorrhage of newborn (P51.-)

P38.1 **Omphalitis with mild hemorrhage**

P38.9 **Omphalitis without hemorrhage**

Omphalitis of newborn NOS

P39 **Other infections specific to the perinatal period**

Use Additional Code to identify organism or specific infection

P39.0 **Neonatal infective mastitis**

Excludes1: breast engorgement of newborn (P83.4)

noninfective mastitis of newborn (P83.4)

P39.1 **Neonatal conjunctivitis and dacryocystitis**

Neonatal chlamydial conjunctivitis

Ophthalmia neonatorum NOS

Excludes1: gonococcal conjunctivitis (A54.31)

P39.2 **Intra-amniotic infection affecting newborn, not elsewhere classified**

P39.3 **Neonatal urinary tract infection**

P39.4 **Neonatal skin infection**

Neonatal pyoderma

Excludes1: pemphigus neonatorum (L00)

staphylococcal scalded skin syndrome (L00)

P39.8 **Other specified infections specific to the perinatal period**

P39.9 **Infection specific to the perinatal period, unspecified**

HEMORRHAGIC AND HEMATOLOGICAL DISORDERS OF NEWBORN (P50-P61)

Excludes1: congenital stenosis and stricture of bile ducts (Q44.3)

Crigler-Najjar syndrome (E80.5)

Dubin-Johnson syndrome (E80.6)

● New code ▲ Revised code **Excludes1:** Not coded here **Excludes2:** Not included here ⊗ Placeholder required ⑦7th digit required

Gilbert syndrome (E80.4)

hereditary hemolytic anemias (D55-D58)

P50 **Newborn affected by intrauterine (fetal) blood loss**

Excludes1: congenital anemia from intrauterine (fetal) blood loss (P61.3)

P50.0 **Newborn affected by intrauterine (fetal) blood loss from vasa previa**

P50.1 **Newborn affected by intrauterine (fetal) blood loss from ruptured cord**

P50.2 **Newborn affected by intrauterine (fetal) blood loss from placenta**

P50.3 **Newborn affected by hemorrhage into co-twin**

P50.4 **Newborn affected by hemorrhage into maternal circulation**

P50.5 **Newborn affected by intrauterine (fetal) blood loss from cut end of co-twin's cord**

P50.8 **Newborn affected by other intrauterine (fetal) blood loss**

P50.9 **Newborn affected by intrauterine (fetal) blood loss, unspecified**

Newborn affected by fetal hemorrhage NOS

P51 **Umbilical hemorrhage of newborn**

Excludes1: omphalitis with mild hemorrhage (P38.1)

umbilical hemorrhage from cut end of co-twins cord (P50.5)

P51.0 **Massive umbilical hemorrhage of newborn**

P51.8 **Other umbilical hemorrhages of newborn**

Slipped umbilical ligature NOS

P51.9 **Umbilical hemorrhage of newborn, unspecified**

P52 **Intracranial nontraumatic hemorrhage of newborn**

Includes: intracranial hemorrhage due to anoxia or hypoxia

Excludes1: intracranial hemorrhage due to birth injury (P10.-)

intracranial hemorrhage due to other injury (S06.-)

P52.0 **Intraventricular (nontraumatic) hemorrhage, grade 1, of newborn**

Subependymal hemorrhage (without intraventricular extension)

Bleeding into germinal matrix

P52.1 **Intraventricular (nontraumatic) hemorrhage, grade 2, of newborn**

Subependymal hemorrhage with intraventricular extension

Bleeding into ventricle

P52.2 **Intraventricular (nontraumatic) hemorrhage, grade 3and grade 4, of newborn**

P52.21 **Intraventricular (nontraumatic) hemorrhage, grade 3, of newborn**

Subependymal hemorrhage with intraventricular extension with enlargement of ventricle

P52.22 **Intraventricular (nontraumatic) hemorrhage, grade 4, of newborn**

Bleeding into cerebral cortex

Subependymal hemorrhage with intracerebral extension

P52.3 **Unspecified intraventricular (nontraumatic) hemorrhage of newborn**

P52.4 **Intracerebral (nontraumatic) hemorrhage of newborn**

P52.5 **Subarachnoid (nontraumatic) hemorrhage of newborn**

P52.6 **Cerebellar (nontraumatic) and posterior fossa hemorrhage of newborn**

P52.8 **Other intracranial (nontraumatic) hemorrhages of newborn**

P52.9 **Intracranial (nontraumatic) hemorrhage of newborn, unspecified**

P53 **Hemorrhagic disease of newborn**

Vitamin K deficiency of newborn

P54 **Other neonatal hemorrhages**

Excludes1: newborn affected by (intrauterine) blood loss (P50.-)

pulmonary hemorrhage originating in the perinatal period (P26.-)

P54.0 **Neonatal hematemesis**

Excludes1: neonatal hematemesis due to swallowed maternal blood (P78.2)

P54.1 **Neonatal melena**

Excludes1: neonatal melena due to swallowed maternal blood (P78.2)

P54.2 **Neonatal rectal hemorrhage**

P54.3 **Other neonatal gastrointestinal hemorrhage**

P54.4 **Neonatal adrenal hemorrhage**

P54.5 **Neonatal cutaneous hemorrhage**

Neonatal bruising

Neonatal ecchymoses

Neonatal petechiae

Neonatal superficial hematomata

Excludes2: bruising of scalp due to birth injury (P12.3)

cephalhematoma due to birth injury (P12.0)

P54.6 **Neonatal vaginal hemorrhage**

Neonatal pseudomenses

P54.8 **Other specified neonatal hemorrhages**

P54.9 **Neonatal hemorrhage, unspecified**

P55 **Hemolytic disease of newborn**

P55.0 **Rh isoimmunization of newborn**

P55.1 **ABO isoimmunization of newborn**

P55.8 **Other hemolytic diseases of newborn**

P55.9 **Hemolytic disease of newborn, unspecified**

P56 **Hydrops fetalis due to hemolytic disease**

Excludes1: hydrops fetalis NOS (P83.2)

P56.0 **Hydrops fetalis due to isoimmunization**

P56.9 **Hydrops fetalis due to other and unspecified hemolytic disease**

P56.90 **Hydrops fetalis due to unspecified hemolytic disease**

P56.99 **Hydrops fetalis due to other hemolytic disease**

P57 **Kernicterus**

Definition: Kernicterus is a disorder that is due to severe jaundice in the newborn, with deposition of the pigment bilirubin in the brain that causes damage to the brain, potentially leading to athetoid cerebral palsy, hearing loss, vision problems, or mental retardation.

P57.0 **Kernicterus due to isoimmunization**

P57.8 **Other specified kernicterus**

Excludes1: Crigler-Najjar syndrome (E80.5)

P57.9 **Kernicterus, unspecified**

P58 **Neonatal jaundice due to other excessive hemolysis**

Excludes1: jaundice due to isoimmunization (P55-P57)

P58.0 **Neonatal jaundice due to bruising**

P58.1 **Neonatal jaundice due to bleeding**

P58.2 **Neonatal jaundice due to infection**

P58.3 **Neonatal jaundice due to polycythemia**

P58.4 **Neonatal jaundice due to drugs or toxins transmitted from mother or given to newborn**

Code first poisoning due to drug or toxin, if applicable (T36-T65 with fifth or sixth character 1-4 or 6)

Use Additional Code for adverse effect, if applicable, to identify drug (T36-T50 with fifth or sixth character 5)

P58.41   **Neonatal jaundice due to drugs or toxins transmitted from mother**

P58.42   **Neonatal jaundice due to drugs or toxins given to newborn**

P58.5   **Neonatal jaundice due to swallowed maternal blood**

P58.8   **Neonatal jaundice due to other specified excessive hemolysis**

P58.9   **Neonatal jaundice due to excessive hemolysis, unspecified**

P59   **Neonatal jaundice from other and unspecified causes**

Excludes1: jaundice due to inborn errors of metabolism (E70-E88)

kernicterus (P57.-)

P59.0   **Neonatal jaundice associated with preterm delivery**

Hyperbilirubinemia of prematurity

Jaundice due to delayed conjugation associated with preterm delivery

P59.1   **Inspissated bile syndrome**

P59.2   **Neonatal jaundice from other and unspecified hepatocellular damage**

Excludes1: congenital viral hepatitis (P35.3)

P59.20   **Neonatal jaundice from unspecified hepatocellular damage**

P59.29   **Neonatal jaundice from other hepatocellular damage**

Neonatal giant cell hepatitis

Neonatal (idiopathic) hepatitis

P59.3   **Neonatal jaundice from breast milk inhibitor**

P59.8   **Neonatal jaundice from other specified causes**

P59.9   **Neonatal jaundice, unspecified**

Neonatal physiological jaundice (intense)(prolonged) NOS

P60   **Disseminated intravascular coagulation of newborn**

Defibrination syndrome of newborn

P61   **Other perinatal hematological disorders**

Excludes1: transient hypogammaglobulinemia of infancy (D80.7)

P61.0   **Transient neonatal thrombocytopenia**

Neonatal thrombocytopenia due to exchange transfusion

Neonatal thrombocytopenia due to idiopathic maternal thrombocytopenia

Neonatal thrombocytopenia due to isoimmunization

P61.1   **Polycythemia neonatorum**

P61.2   **Anemia of prematurity**

P61.3   **Congenital anemia from fetal blood loss**

P61.4   **Other congenital anemias, not elsewhere classified**

Congenital anemia NOS

P61.5   **Transient neonatal neutropenia**

Excludes1: congenital neutropenia (non-transient) (D70.0)

P61.6   **Other transient neonatal disorders of coagulation**

P61.8   **Other specified perinatal hematological disorders**

P61.9   **Perinatal hematological disorder, unspecified**

TRANSITORY ENDOCRINE AND METABOLIC DISORDERS SPECIFIC TO NEWBORN (P70-P74)

Includes: transitory endocrine and metabolic disturbances caused by the infant's response to maternal endocrine and metabolic factors, or its adjustment to extrauterine environment

P70   **Transitory disorders of carbohydrate metabolism specific to newborn**

P70.0   **Syndrome of infant of mother with gestational diabetes**

Newborn (with hypoglycemia) affected by maternal gestational diabetes

Excludes1: newborn (with hypoglycemia) affected by maternal (pre-existing) diabetes mellitus (P70.1)

syndrome of infant of a diabetic mother (P70.1)

P70.1   **Syndrome of infant of a diabetic mother**

Newborn (with hypoglycemia) affected by maternal (pre-existing) diabetes mellitus

Excludes1: newborn (with hypoglycemia) affected by maternal gestational diabetes (P70.0)

syndrome of infant of mother with gestational diabetes (P70.0)

P70.2   **Neonatal diabetes mellitus**

P70.3   **Iatrogenic neonatal hypoglycemia**

P70.4   **Other neonatal hypoglycemia**

Transitory neonatal hypoglycemia

P70.8   **Other transitory disorders of carbohydrate metabolism of newborn**

P70.9   **Transitory disorder of carbohydrate metabolism of newborn, unspecified**

P71   **Transitory neonatal disorders of calcium and magnesium metabolism**

P71.0   **Cow's milk hypocalcemia in newborn**

P71.1   **Other neonatal hypocalcemia**

Excludes1: neonatal hypoparathyroidism (P71.4)

P71.2   **Neonatal hypomagnesemia**

P71.3   **Neonatal tetany without calcium or magnesium deficiency**

Neonatal tetany NOS

P71.4   **Transitory neonatal hypoparathyroidism**

P71.8   **Other transitory neonatal disorders of calcium and magnesium metabolism**

P71.9   **Transitory neonatal disorder of calcium and magnesium metabolism, unspecified**

P72   **Other transitory neonatal endocrine disorders**

Excludes1: congenital hypothyroidism with or without goiter (E03.0-E03.1)

Dyshormonogenetic goiter (E07.1)

Pendred's syndrome (E07.1)

P72.0   **Neonatal goiter, not elsewhere classified**

Transitory congenital goiter with normal functioning

P72.1   **Transitory neonatal hyperthyroidism**

Neonatal thyrotoxicosis

P72.2   **Other transitory neonatal disorders of thyroid function, not elsewhere classified**

Transitory neonatal hypothyroidism

P72.8   **Other specified transitory neonatal endocrine disorders**

P72.9   **Transitory neonatal endocrine disorder, unspecified**

P74   **Other transitory neonatal electrolyte and metabolic disturbances**

P74.0   **Late metabolic acidosis of newborn**

Excludes1: (fetal) metabolic acidosis of newborn (P19)

P74.1   **Dehydration of newborn**

P74.2   **Disturbances of sodium balance of newborn**

P74.21   **Hypernatremia of newborn**

P74.22   **Hyponatremia of newborn**

P74.3   **Disturbances of potassium balance of newborn**

P74.31 **Hyperkalemia of newborn**

P74.32 **Hypokalemia of newborn**

P74.4 **Other transitory electrolyte disturbances of newborn**

P74.41 **Alkalosis of newborn**

Hyperbicarbonatemia

P74.42 **Disturbances of chlorine balance of newborn**

P74.421 **Hyperchloremia of newborn**

Hyperchloremic metabolic acidosis

Excludes2: late metabolic acidosis of the newborn (P74.0)

P74.422 **Hypochloremia of newborn**

P74.49 **Other transitory electrolyte disturbance of newborn**

P74.5 **Transitory tyrosinemia of newborn**

P74.6 **Transitory hyperammonemia of newborn**

P74.8 **Other transitory metabolic disturbances of newborn**

Amino-acid metabolic disorders described as transitory

P74.9 **Transitory metabolic disturbance of newborn, unspecified**

DIGESTIVE SYSTEM DISORDERS OF NEWBORN (P76-P78)

P76 **Other intestinal obstruction of newborn**

P76.0 **Meconium plug syndrome**

Meconium ileus NOS

Excludes1: meconium ileus in cystic fibrosis (E84.11)

P76.1 **Transitory ileus of newborn**

Excludes1: Hirschsprung's disease (Q43.1)

P76.2 **Intestinal obstruction due to inspissated milk**

P76.8 **Other specified intestinal obstruction of newborn**

Excludes1: intestinal obstruction classifiable to K56.-

P76.9 **Intestinal obstruction of newborn, unspecified**

P77 **Necrotizing enterocolitis of newborn**

P77.1 **Stage 1 necrotizing enterocolitis in newborn**

Necrotizing enterocolitis without pneumatosis, without perforation

P77.2 **Stage 2 necrotizing enterocolitis in newborn**

Necrotizing enterocolitis with pneumatosis, without perforation

P77.3 **Stage 3 necrotizing enterocolitis in newborn**

Necrotizing enterocolitis with perforation

Necrotizing enterocolitis with pneumatosis and perforation

P77.9 **Necrotizing enterocolitis in newborn, unspecified**

Necrotizing enterocolitis in newborn, NOS

P78 **Other perinatal digestive system disorders**

Excludes1: cystic fibrosis (E84.0-E84.9)

neonatal gastrointestinal hemorrhages (P54.0-P54.3)

P78.0 **Perinatal intestinal perforation**

Meconium peritonitis

P78.1 **Other neonatal peritonitis**

Neonatal peritonitis NOS

P78.2 **Neonatal hematemesis and melena due to swallowed maternal blood**

P78.3 **Noninfective neonatal diarrhea**

Neonatal diarrhea NOS

P78.8 **Other specified perinatal digestive system disorders**

P78.81 **Congenital cirrhosis (of liver)**

P78.82 **Peptic ulcer of newborn**

P78.83 **Newborn esophageal reflux**

Neonatal esophageal reflux

P78.84 **Gestational alloimmune liver disease**

GALD

Neonatal hemochromatosis

Excludes1: hemochromatosis (E83.11-)

P78.89 **Other specified perinatal digestive system disorders**

P78.9 **Perinatal digestive system disorder, unspecified**

CONDITIONS INVOLVING THE INTEGUMENT AND TEMPERATURE REGULATION OF NEWBORN (P80-P83)

P80 **Hypothermia of newborn**

P80.0 **Cold injury syndrome**

Severe and usually chronic hypothermia associated with a pink flushed appearance, edema and neurological and biochemical abnormalities.

Excludes1: mild hypothermia of newborn (P80.8)

P80.8 **Other hypothermia of newborn**

Mild hypothermia of newborn

P80.9 **Hypothermia of newborn, unspecified**

P81 **Other disturbances of temperature regulation of newborn**

P81.0 **Environmental hyperthermia of newborn**

P81.8 **Other specified disturbances of temperature regulation of newborn**

P81.9 **Disturbance of temperature regulation of newborn, unspecified**

Fever of newborn NOS

P83 **Other conditions of integument specific to newborn**

Excludes1: congenital malformations of skin and integument (Q80-Q84)

hydrops fetalis due to hemolytic disease (P56.-)

neonatal skin infection (P39.4)

staphylococcal scalded skin syndrome (L00)

Excludes2: cradle cap (L21.0)

diaper [napkin] dermatitis (L22)

P83.0 **Sclerema neonatorum**

P83.1 **Neonatal erythema toxicum**

P83.2 **Hydrops fetalis not due to hemolytic disease**

Hydrops fetalis NOS

P83.3 **Other and unspecified edema specific to newborn**

P83.30 **Unspecified edema specific to newborn**

P83.39 **Other edema specific to newborn**

P83.4 **Breast engorgement of newborn**

Noninfective mastitis of newborn

P83.5 **Congenital hydrocele**

P83.6 **Umbilical polyp of newborn**

P83.8 **Other specified conditions of integument specific to newborn**

P83.81 **Umbilical granuloma**

Excludes2: Granulomatous disorder of the skin and subcutaneous tissue, unspecified (L92.9)

P83.88 **Other specified conditions of integument specific to newborn**

Bronze baby syndrome

Neonatal scleroderma

Urticaria neonatorum

P83.9 **Condition of the integument specific to newborn, unspecified**

OTHER PROBLEMS WITH NEWBORN (P84)

P84 **Other problems with newborn**

Acidemia of newborn

Acidosis of newborn

Anoxia of newborn NOS

Asphyxia of newborn NOS

Hypercapnia of newborn

Hypoxemia of newborn

Hypoxia of newborn NOS

Mixed metabolic and respiratory acidosis of newborn

Excludes1: intracranial hemorrhage due to anoxia or hypoxia (P52.-)

hypoxic ischemic encephalopathy [HIE] (P91.6-)

late metabolic acidosis of newborn (P74.0)

OTHER DISORDERS ORIGINATING IN THE PERINATAL PERIOD (P90-P96)

P90 **Convulsions of newborn**

Excludes1: benign myoclonic epilepsy in infancy (G40.3-)

benign neonatal convulsions (familial) (G40.3-)

P91 **Other disturbances of cerebral status of newborn**

P91.0 **Neonatal cerebral ischemia**

P91.1 **Acquired periventricular cysts of newborn**

P91.2 **Neonatal cerebral leukomalacia**

Periventricular leukomalacia

P91.3 **Neonatal cerebral irritability**

P91.4 **Neonatal cerebral depression**

P91.5 **Neonatal coma**

P91.6 **Hypoxic ischemic encephalopathy [HIE]**

Excludes1: Neonatal cerebral depression (P91.4)

Neonatal cerebral irritability (P91.3)

Neonatal coma (P91.5)

P91.60 **Hypoxic ischemic encephalopathy [HIE], unspecified**

P91.61 **Mild hypoxic ischemic encephalopathy [HIE]**

P91.62 **Moderate hypoxic ischemic encephalopathy [HIE]**

P91.63 **Severe hypoxic ischemic encephalopathy [HIE]**

P91.8 **Other specified disturbances of cerebral status of newborn**

P91.81 **Neonatal encephalopathy**

P91.811 **Neonatal encephalopathy in diseases classified elsewhere**

Code first underlying condition, if known, such as:

congenital cirrhosis (of liver) (P78.81)

intracranial nontraumatic hemorrhage of newborn (P52.-)

kernicterus (P57.-)

P91.819 **Neonatal encephalopathy, unspecified**

P91.82 **Neonatal cerebral infarction**

Neonatal stroke

Perinatal arterial ischemic stroke

Perinatal cerebral infarction

Excludes1: cerebral infarction (I63.-)

Excludes2: intracranial hemorrhage of newborn (P52.-)

P91.821 **Neonatal cerebral infarction, right side of brain**

P91.822 **Neonatal cerebral infarction, left side of brain**

P91.823 **Neonatal cerebral infarction, bilateral**

P91.829 **Neonatal cerebral infarction, unspecified side**

P91.88 **Other specified disturbances of cerebral status of newborn**

P91.9 **Disturbance of cerebral status of newborn, unspecified**

P92 **Feeding problems of newborn**

Excludes1: eating disorders (F50.-)

Excludes2: Feeding problems in child over 28 days old (R63.3)

P92.0 **Vomiting of newborn**

Excludes1: vomiting of child over 28 days old (R11.-)

P92.01 **Bilious vomiting of newborn**

Excludes1: bilious vomiting in child over 28 days old (R11.14)

P92.09 **Other vomiting of newborn**

Excludes1: regurgitation of food in newborn (P92.1)

P92.1 **Regurgitation and rumination of newborn**

P92.2 **Slow feeding of newborn**

P92.3 **Underfeeding of newborn**

P92.4 **Overfeeding of newborn**

P92.5 **Neonatal difficulty in feeding at breast**

P92.6 **Failure to thrive in newborn**

Excludes1: failure to thrive in child over 28 days old (R62.51)

P92.8 **Other feeding problems of newborn**

P92.9 **Feeding problem of newborn, unspecified**

P93 **Reactions and intoxications due to drugs administered to newborn**

Includes: reactions and intoxications due to drugs administered to fetus affecting newborn

Excludes1: jaundice due to drugs or toxins transmitted from mother or given to newborn (P58.4-)

reactions and intoxications from maternal opiates, tranquilizers and other medication (P04.0- P04.1, P04.4-)withdrawal symptoms from maternal use of drugs of addiction (P96.1)

withdrawal symptoms from therapeutic use of drugs in newborn (P96.2)

P93.0 **Grey baby syndrome**

Grey syndrome from chloramphenicol administration in newborn

P93.8 **Other reactions and intoxications due to drugs administered to newborn**

Use Additional Code for adverse effect, if applicable, to identify drug (T36-T50 with fifth or sixth character 5)

P94 **Disorders of muscle tone of newborn**

P94.0 **Transient neonatal myasthenia gravis**

Excludes1: myasthenia gravis (G70.0)

P94.1 **Congenital hypertonia**

P94.2 **Congenital hypotonia**

Floppy baby syndrome, unspecified

P94.8 **Other disorders of muscle tone of newborn**

P94.9 **Disorder of muscle tone of newborn, unspecified**

● New code ▲ Revised code **Excludes1:** Not coded here **Excludes2:** Not included here ⊗ Placeholder required ⑦7th digit required

P95 **Stillbirth**

Dead born fetus NOS

Fetal death of unspecified cause

Stillbirth NOS

Excludes1: maternal care for intrauterine death (O36.4)

    missed abortion (O02.1)

    outcome of delivery, stillbirth (Z37.1, Z37.3, Z37.4, Z37.7)

P96 **Other conditions originating in the perinatal period**

P96.0 **Congenital renal failure**

Uremia of newborn

P96.1 **Neonatal withdrawal symptoms from maternal use of drugs of addiction**

Drug withdrawal syndrome in infant of dependent mother

Neonatal abstinence syndrome

Excludes1: reactions and intoxications from maternal opiates and tranquilizers administered during labor and delivery (P04.0)

P96.2 **Withdrawal symptoms from therapeutic use of drugs in newborn**

P96.3 **Wide cranial sutures of newborn**

Neonatal craniotabes

P96.5 **Complication to newborn due to (fetal) intrauterine procedure**

Excludes2: newborn affected by amniocentesis (P00.6)

P96.8 **Other specified conditions originating in the perinatal period**

P96.81 **Exposure to (parental) (environmental) tobacco smoke in the perinatal period**

Excludes2: newborn affected by in utero exposure

to tobacco (P04.2)

exposure to environmental tobacco smoke after the perinatal period (Z77.22)

P96.82 **Delayed separation of umbilical cord**

P96.83 **Meconium staining**

Excludes1: meconium aspiration (P24.00, P24.01)

meconium passage during delivery (P03.82)

P96.89 **Other specified conditions originating in the perinatal period**

Use Additional Code to specify condition

P96.9 **Condition originating in the perinatal period, unspecified**

Congenital debility NOS

Chapter 17: Congenital Malformations, Deformations and Chromosomal Abnormalities (Q00-Q99)

DEFINITIONS

This chapter includes definitions of selected key words, terms and phrases and coding alerts for adding points to the clinical domain, and references to coding late effects where appropriate. An example from this chapter is as follows:

Q11   Anophthalmos, microphthalmos and macrophthalmos
Definition: Anophthalmos is the absence of one or both eyes. Both the globe and the ocular tissue are missing from the orbit.

MULTIPLE CODING FOR A SINGLE CONDITION

In addition to the etiology/manifestation convention that requires two codes to fully describe a single condition that affects multiple body systems, there are other single conditions that also require more than one code. "**Use Additional Code**" notes are found in the Tabular List at codes that are not part of an etiology/manifestation pair where a secondary code is useful to fully describe a condition. The sequencing rule is the same as the etiology/manifestation pair, "**Use Additional Code**" indicates that a secondary code should be added.

For example, for bacterial infections that are not included in chapter 1, a secondary code from category B95, Streptococcus, Staphylococcus, and Enterococcus, as the cause of diseases classified elsewhere, or B96, Other bacterial agents as the cause of diseases classified elsewhere, may be required to identify the bacterial organism causing the infection. A "**Use Additional Code**" note will normally be found at the infectious disease code, indicating a need for the organism code to be added as a secondary code.

 "Code first" notes are also under certain codes that are not specifically manifestation codes but may be due to an underlying cause. When there is a "Code first" note and an underlying condition is present, the underlying condition should be sequenced first.

"Code, if applicable, any causal condition first", notes indicate that this code may be assigned as a principal diagnosis when the causal condition is unknown or not applicable. If a causal condition is known, then the code for that condition should be sequenced as the principal or first-listed diagnosis.

Multiple codes may be needed for sequela, complication codes and obstetric codes to more fully describe a condition. See the specific guidelines for these conditions for further instruction.

COMBINATION CODE

A combination code is a single code used to classify: Two diagnoses, or a diagnosis with an associated secondary process (manifestation) A diagnosis with an associated complication

Combination codes are identified by referring to subterm entries in the Alphabetic Index and by reading the inclusion and exclusion notes in the Tabular List.

Assign only the combination code when that code fully identifies the diagnostic conditions involved or when the Alphabetic Index so directs. Multiple coding should not be used when the classification provides a combination code that clearly identifies all of the elements documented in the diagnosis. When the combination code lacks necessary specificity in describing the manifestation or complication, an additional code should be used as a secondary code.

SEQUELA (LATE EFFECTS)

A sequela is the residual effect (condition produced) after the acute phase of an illness or injury has terminated. There is no time limit on when a sequela code can be used. The residual may be apparent early, such as in cerebral infarction, or it may occur months or years later, such as that due to a previous injury. Coding of sequela generally requires two codes sequenced in the following order: The condition or nature of the sequela is sequenced first.

The sequela code is sequenced second.

Q00-Q99

An exception to the above guidelines are those instances where the code for the sequela is followed by a manifestation code identified in the Tabular List and title, or the sequela code has been expanded (at the fourth, fifth or sixth character levels) to include the manifestation(s). The code for the acute phase of an illness or injury that led to the sequela is never used with a code for the late effect.

Assign an appropriate code(s) from categories Q00-Q99, Congenital malformations, deformations, and chromosomal abnormalities when a malformation/deformation or chromosomal abnormality is documented. A malformation/deformation/or chromosomal abnormality may be the principal/first-listed diagnosis on a record or a secondary diagnosis.

When a malformation/deformation or chromosomal abnormality does not have a unique code assignment, assign additional code(s) for any manifestations that may be present.

When the code assignment specifically identifies the malformation/deformation or chromosomal abnormality, manifestations that are an inherent component of the anomaly should not be coded separately. Additional codes should be assigned for manifestations that are not an inherent component.

Codes from Chapter 17 may be used throughout the life of the patient. If a congenital malformation or deformity has been corrected, a personal history code should be used to identify the history of the malformation or deformity. Although present at birth, a malformation/deformation/or chromosomal abnormality may not be identified until later in life. Whenever the condition is diagnosed by the provider, it is appropriate to assign a code from codes Q00-Q99.For the birth admission, the appropriate code from category Z38, Liveborn infants, according to place of birth and type of delivery, should be sequenced as the principal diagnosis, followed by any congenital anomaly codes, Q00-Q99.

● New code ▲ Revised code **Excludes1:** Not coded here **Excludes2:** Not included here ⊗ Placeholder required ⑦7th digit required

Chapter 17

Congenital Malformations, Deformations and Chromosomal Abnormalities (Q00-Q99)

Note: Codes from this chapter are not for use on maternal or fetal records

Excludes2: inborn errors of metabolism (E70-E88)

This chapter contains the following blocks:

Q00-Q07   Congenital malformations of the nervous system
Q10-Q18   Congenital malformations of eye, ear, face and neck
Q20-Q28   Congenital malformations of the circulatory system
Q30-Q34   Congenital malformations of the respiratory system
Q35-Q37   Cleft lip and cleft palate
Q38-Q45   Other congenital malformations of the digestive system
Q50-Q56   Congenital malformations of genital organs
Q60-Q64   Congenital malformations of the urinary system
Q65-Q79   Congenital malformations and deformations of the musculoskeletal system
Q80-Q89   Other congenital malformations
Q90-Q99   Chromosomal abnormalities, not elsewhere classified

CONGENITAL MALFORMATIONS OF THE NERVOUS SYSTEM (Q00-Q07)

Q00   Anencephaly and similar malformations

Definition: Anencephaly is the absence of a major portion of the brain, skull, and scalp that occurs during embryonic development.

Q00.0   **Anencephaly** [HCC]

Acephaly

Acrania

Amyelencephaly

Hemianencephaly

Hemicephaly

Q00.1   **Craniorachischisis** [HCC]

Q00.2   **Iniencephaly** [HCC]

Q01   Encephalocele

Includes: Arnold-Chiari syndrome, type III

encephalocystocele

encephalomyelocele

hydroencephalocele

hydromeningocele, cranial meningocele, cerebral meningoencephalocele

Excludes1: Meckel-Gruber syndrome (Q61.9)

Q01.0   **Frontal encephalocele** [HCC]

Q01.1   **Nasofrontal encephalocele** [HCC]

Q01.2   **Occipital encephalocele** [HCC]

Q01.8   **Encephalocele of other sites** [HCC]

Q01.9   **Encephalocele, unspecified** [HCC]

Q02   **Microcephaly** [HCC]

Code first, if applicable, congenital Zika virus disease

Includes: hydromicrocephaly

micrencephalon

Excludes1: Meckel-Gruber syndrome (Q61.9)

Q03   Congenital hydrocephalus

Includes: hydrocephalus in newborn

Excludes1: Arnold-Chiari syndrome, type II (Q07.0-)

acquired hydrocephalus (G91.-)

hydrocephalus due to congenital toxoplasmosis (P37.1)

hydrocephalus with spina bifida (Q05.0-Q05.4)

Q03.0   **Malformations of aqueduct of Sylvius** [HCC]

Anomaly of aqueduct of Sylvius

Obstruction of aqueduct of Sylvius, congenital

Stenosis of aqueduct of Sylvius

Q03.1   **Atresia of foramina of Magendie and Luschka** [HCC]

Dandy-Walker syndrome

Q03.8   **Other congenital hydrocephalus** [HCC]

Q03.9   **Congenital hydrocephalus, unspecified** [HCC]

Q04   Other congenital malformations of brain

Excludes1: cyclopia (Q87.0)

macrocephaly (Q75.3)

Q04.0   **Congenital malformations of corpus callosum** [HCC]

Agenesis of corpus callosum

Q04.1   **Arhinencephaly** [HCC]

Q04.2   **Holoprosencephaly** [HCC]

Q04.3   **Other reduction deformities of brain** [HCC]

Absence of part of brain

Agenesis of part of brain

Agyria

Aplasia of part of brain

Hydranencephaly

Hypoplasia of part of brain

Lissencephaly

Microgyria

Pachygyria

Excludes1: congenital malformations of corpus callosum (Q04.0)

Q04.4   **Septo-optic dysplasia of brain** [HCC]

Q04.5   **Megalencephaly** [HCC]

Q04.6   **Congenital cerebral cysts** [HCC]

Porencephaly

Schizencephaly

Excludes1: acquired porencephalic cyst (G93.0)

Q04.8   **Other specified congenital malformations of brain** [HCC]

Arnold-Chiari syndrome, type IV

Macrogyria

Q04.9   **Congenital malformation of brain, unspecified** [HCC]

Congenital anomaly NOS of brain

Congenital deformity NOS of brain

Congenital disease or lesion NOS of brain

Multiple anomalies NOS of brain, congenital

Q05   Spina bifida

Definition: Spina bifida is a serious birth abnormality in which the spinal cord is malformed and lacks its usual protective skeletal and soft tissue coverings.

Includes: hydromeningocele (spinal)

meningocele (spinal)

meningomyelocele

myelocele

myelomeningocele

rachischisis

spina bifida (aperta)(cystica)

syringomyelocele

Use Additional Code for any associated paraplegia (paraparesis) (G82.2-)

Excludes1: Arnold-Chiari syndrome, type II (Q07.0-)

spina bifida occulta (Q76.0)

Q05.0 Cervical spina bifida with hydrocephalus [HCC]

Q05.1 Thoracic spina bifida with hydrocephalus [HCC]

Dorsal spina bifida with hydrocephalus

Thoracolumbar spina bifida with hydrocephalus

Q05.2 Lumbar spina bifida with hydrocephalus [HCC]

Lumbosacral spina bifida with hydrocephalus

Q05.3 Sacral spina bifida with hydrocephalus [HCC]

Q05.4 Unspecified spina bifida with hydrocephalus [HCC]

Q05.5 Cervical spina bifida without hydrocephalus [HCC]

Q05.6 Thoracic spina bifida without hydrocephalus [HCC]

Dorsal spina bifida NOS

Thoracolumbar spina bifida NOS

Q05.7 Lumbar spina bifida without hydrocephalus [HCC]

Lumbosacral spina bifida NOS

Q05.8 Sacral spina bifida without hydrocephalus [HCC]

Q05.9 Spina bifida, unspecified [HCC]

Q06 Other congenital malformations of spinal cord

Q06.0 Amyelia [HCC]

Q06.1 Hypoplasia and dysplasia of spinal cord [HCC]

Atelomyelia

Myelatelia

Myelodysplasia of spinal cord

Q06.2 Diastematomyelia [HCC]

Q06.3 Other congenital cauda equina malformations [HCC]

Q06.4 Hydromyelia [HCC]

Hydrorachis

Q06.8 Other specified congenital malformations of spinal cord [HCC]

Q06.9 Congenital malformation of spinal cord, unspecified [HCC]

Congenital anomaly NOS of spinal cord

Congenital deformity NOS of spinal cord

Congenital disease or lesion NOS of spinal cord

Q07 Other congenital malformations of nervous system

Excludes2: congenital central alveolar hypoventilation syndrome (G47.35)

familial dysautonomia [Riley-Day] (G90.1)

neurofibromatosis (nonmalignant) (Q85.0-)

Q07.0 Arnold-Chiari syndrome

Arnold-Chiari syndrome, type II

Excludes1: Arnold-Chiari syndrome, type III (Q01.-)

Arnold-Chiari syndrome, type IV (Q04.8)

Q07.00 Arnold-Chiari syndrome without spina bifida or hydrocephalus [HCC]

Q07.01 Arnold-Chiari syndrome with spina bifida [HCC]

Q07.02 Arnold-Chiari syndrome with hydrocephalus [HCC]

Q07.03 Arnold-Chiari syndrome with spina bifida and hydrocephalus [HCC]

Q07.8 Other specified congenital malformations of nervous system [HCC]

Agenesis of nerve

Displacement of brachial plexus Jaw-winking syndrome

Marcus Gunn's syndrome

Q07.9 Congenital malformation of nervous system, unspecified [HCC]

Congenital anomaly NOS of nervous system

Congenital deformity NOS of nervous system

Congenital disease or lesion NOS of nervous system

CONGENITAL MALFORMATIONS OF EYE, EAR, FACE AND NECK (Q10-Q18)

Excludes2: cleft lip and cleft palate (Q35-Q37)

congenital malformation of cervical spine (Q05.0, Q05.5, Q67.5, Q76.0-Q76.4)

congenital malformation of larynx (Q31.-)

congenital malformation of lip NEC (Q38.0)

congenital malformation of nose (Q30.-)

congenital malformation of parathyroid gland (Q89.2)

congenital malformation of thyroid gland (Q89.2)

Q10 Congenital malformations of eyelid, lacrimal apparatus and orbit

Excludes1: cryptophthalmos NOS (Q11.2)

cryptophthalmos syndrome (Q87.0)

Q10.0 Congenital ptosis

Q10.1 Congenital ectropion

Q10.2 Congenital entropion

Q10.3 Other congenital malformations of eyelid

Ablepharon

Blepharophimosis, congenital

Coloboma of eyelid

Congenital absence or agenesis of cilia

Congenital absence or agenesis of eyelid

Congenital accessory eyelid

Congenital accessory eye muscle

Congenital malformation of eyelid NOS

Q10.4 Absence and agenesis of lacrimal apparatus

Congenital absence of punctum lacrimale

Q10.5 Congenital stenosis and stricture of lacrimal duct

Q10.6 Other congenital malformations of lacrimal apparatus

Congenital malformation of lacrimal apparatus NOS

Q10.7 Congenital malformation of orbit

Q11 Anophthalmos, microphthalmos and macrophthalmos

Q11.0 Cystic eyeball

Q11.1 Other anophthalmos

Anophthalmos NOS

Agenesis of eye

Aplasia of eye

Q11.2 Microphthalmos

Cryptophthalmos NOS

Dysplasia of eye

Hypoplasia of eye

Rudimentary eye

Excludes1: cryptophthalmos syndrome (Q87.0)

Q11.3 Macrophthalmos

Excludes1: macrophthalmos in congenital glaucoma (Q15.0)

Q12 Congenital lens malformations

Q12.0 Congenital cataract

Q12.1 Congenital displaced lens

Q12.2 Coloboma of lens

Q12.3 Congenital aphakia

Q12.4 Spherophakia

Q12.8   Other congenital lens malformations

Microphakia

Q12.9   Congenital lens malformation, unspecified

Q13   Congenital malformations of anterior segment of eye

Q13.0   Coloboma of iris

Coloboma NOS

Q13.1   Absence of iris

Aniridia

<u>Use Additional Code</u> for associated glaucoma (H42)

Q13.2   Other congenital malformations of iris

Anisocoria, congenital

Atresia of pupil

Congenital malformation of iris NOS

Corectopia

Q13.3   Congenital corneal opacity

Q13.4   Other congenital corneal malformations

Congenital malformation of cornea NOS

Microcornea

Peter's anomaly

Q13.5   Blue sclera

Q13.8   Other congenital malformations of anterior segment of eye

Q13.81   Rieger's anomaly

<u>Use Additional Code</u> for associated glaucoma (H42)

Q13.89   Other congenital malformations of anterior segment of eye

Q13.9   Congenital malformation of anterior segment of eye, unspecified

Q14   Congenital malformations of posterior segment of eye

Excludes2: optic nerve hypoplasia (H47.03-)

Q14.0   Congenital malformation of vitreous humor

Congenital vitreous opacity

Q14.1   Congenital malformation of retina

Congenital retinal aneurysm

Q14.2   Congenital malformation of optic disc

Coloboma of optic disc

Q14.3   Congenital malformation of choroid

Q14.8   Other congenital malformations of posterior segment of eye

Coloboma of the fundus

Q14.9   Congenital malformation of posterior segment of eye, unspecified

Q15   Other congenital malformations of eye

Excludes1: congenital nystagmus (H55.01)

ocular albinism (E70.31-)

optic nerve hypoplasia (H47.03-)

retinitis pigmentosa (H35.52)

Q15.0   Congenital glaucoma

Axenfeld's anomaly

Buphthalmos Glaucoma of childhood Glaucoma of newborn Hydrophthalmos

Keratoglobus, congenital, with glaucoma

Macrocornea with glaucoma

Macrophthalmos in congenital glaucoma

Megalocornea with glaucoma

Q15.8   Other specified congenital malformations of eye

Q15.9   Congenital malformation of eye, unspecified

Congenital anomaly of eye

Congenital deformity of eye

Q16   Congenital malformations of ear causing impairment of hearing

Excludes1: congenital deafness (H90.-)

Q16.0   Congenital absence of (ear) auricle

Q16.1   Congenital absence, atresia and stricture of auditory canal (external)

Congenital atresia or stricture of osseous meatus

Q16.2   Absence of eustachian tube

Q16.3   Congenital malformation of ear ossicles

Congenital fusion of ear ossicles

Q16.4   Other congenital malformations of middle ear

Congenital malformation of middle ear NOS

Q16.5   Congenital malformation of inner ear

Congenital anomaly of membranous labyrinth

Congenital anomaly of organ of Corti

Q16.9   Congenital malformation of ear causing impairment of hearing, unspecified

Congenital absence of ear NOS

Q17   Other congenital malformations of ear

Excludes1: congenital malformations of ear with impairment of hearing (Q16.0-Q16.9)

preauricular sinus (Q18.1)

Q17.0   Accessory auricle

Accessory tragus

Polyotia

Preauricular appendage or tag

Supernumerary ear

Supernumerary lobule

Q17.1   Macrotia

Q17.2   Microtia

Q17.3   Other misshapen ear

Pointed ear

Q17.4   Misplaced ear

Low-set ears

Excludes1: cervical auricle (Q18.2)

Q17.5   Prominent ear

Bat ear

Q17.8   Other specified congenital malformations of ear

Congenital absence of lobe of ear

Q17.9   Congenital malformation of ear, unspecified

Congenital anomaly of ear NOS

Q18   Other congenital malformations of face and neck

Excludes1: cleft lip and cleft palate (Q35-Q37)

conditions classified to Q67.0-Q67.4

congenital malformations of skull and face bones (Q75.-)

cyclopia (Q87.0)

dentofacial anomalies [including malocclusion] (M26.-)

malformation syndromes affecting facial appearance (Q87.0)

persistent thyroglossal duct (Q89.2)

Q18.0   Sinus, fistula and cyst of branchial cleft Branchial vestige

Q18.1   Preauricular sinus and cyst

Fistula of auricle, congenital

Cervicoaural fistula

Q18.2 **Other branchial cleft malformations**
Branchial cleft malformation NOS
Cervical auricle
Otocephaly

Q18.3 **Webbing of neck**
Pterygium colli

Q18.4 **Macrostomia**

Q18.5 **Microstomia**

Q18.6 **Macrocheilia**
Hypertrophy of lip, congenital

Q18.7 **Microcheilia**

Q18.8 **Other specified congenital malformations of face and neck**
Medial cyst of face and neck
Medial fistula of face and neck
Medial sinus of face and neck

Q18.9 **Congenital malformation of face and neck, unspecified**
Congenital anomaly NOS of face and neck

CONGENITAL MALFORMATIONS OF THE CIRCULATORY SYSTEM (Q20-Q28)

Q20 **Congenital malformations of cardiac chambers and connections**
Excludes1: dextrocardia with situs inversus (Q89.3)
mirror-image atrial arrangement with situs inversus (Q89.3)

Q20.0 **Common arterial trunk**
Persistent truncus arteriosus
Excludes1: aortic septal defect (Q21.4)

Q20.1 **Double outlet right ventricle**
Taussig-Bing syndrome

Q20.2 **Double outlet left ventricle**

Q20.3 **Discordant ventriculoarterial connection**
Dextrotransposition of aorta
Transposition of great vessels (complete)

Q20.4 **Double inlet ventricle**
Common ventricle
Cor triloculare biatriatum
Single ventricle

Q20.5 **Discordant atrioventricular connection**
Corrected transposition
Levotransposition
Ventricular inversion

Q20.6 **Isomerism of atrial appendages**
Isomerism of atrial appendages with asplenia or polysplenia

Q20.8 **Other congenital malformations of cardiac chambers and connections**
Cor binoculare

Q20.9 **Congenital malformation of cardiac chambers and connections, unspecified**

Q21 **Congenital malformations of cardiac septa**
Excludes1: acquired cardiac septal defect (I51.0)

Q21.0 **Ventricular septal defect**
Roger's disease

Q21.1 **Atrial septal defect**
Coronary sinus defect
Patent or persistent foramen ovale

Patent or persistent ostium secundum defect (type II)
Patent or persistent sinus venosus defect

Q21.2 **Atrioventricular septal defect**
Common atrioventricular canal
Endocardial cushion defect
Ostium primum atrial septal defect (type I)

Q21.3 **Tetralogy of Fallot**
Definition: Tetralogy of Fallot, which is one of the most common congenital heart disorders, comprises right ventricular (RV) outflow tract obstruction (RVOTO) (infundibular stenosis), ventricular septal defect (VSD), aorta dextroposition, and RV hypertrophy.
Ventricular septal defect with pulmonary stenosis or atresia, dextroposition of aorta and hypertrophy of right ventricle.

Q21.4 **Aortopulmonary septal defect**
Aortic septal defect
Aortopulmonary window

Q21.8 **Other congenital malformations of cardiac septa**
Eisenmenger's defect
Pentalogy of Fallot
Code also , if applicable:
Eisenmenger's complex (I27.83)
Eisenmenger's syndrome (I27.83)

Q21.9 **Congenital malformation of cardiac septum, unspecified**
Septal (heart) defect NOS

Q22 **Congenital malformations of pulmonary and tricuspid valves**

Q22.0 **Pulmonary valve atresia**

Q22.1 **Congenital pulmonary valve stenosis**

Q22.2 **Congenital pulmonary valve insufficiency**
Congenital pulmonary valve regurgitation

Q22.3 **Other congenital malformations of pulmonary valve**
Congenital malformation of pulmonary valve NOS
Supernumerary cusps of pulmonary valve

Q22.4 **Congenital tricuspid stenosis**
Congenital tricuspid atresia

Q22.5 **Ebstein's anomaly**

Q22.6 **Hypoplastic right heart syndrome**

Q22.8 **Other congenital malformations of tricuspid valve**

Q22.9 **Congenital malformation of tricuspid valve, unspecified**

Q23 **Congenital malformations of aortic and mitral valves**

Q23.0 **Congenital stenosis of aortic valve**
Congenital aortic atresia
Congenital aortic stenosis NOS
Excludes1: congenital stenosis of aortic valve in hypoplastic left heart syndrome (Q23.4)
congenital subaortic stenosis (Q24.4)
supravalvular aortic stenosis (congenital) (Q25.3)

Q23.1 **Congenital insufficiency of aortic valve**
Bicuspid aortic valve
Congenital aortic insufficiency

Q23.2 **Congenital mitral stenosis**
Congenital mitral atresia

Q23.3 **Congenital mitral insufficiency**

Q23.4 **Hypoplastic left heart syndrome**

● New code ▲ Revised code Excludes1: Not coded here Excludes2: Not included here ⊗ Placeholder required ⑦7th digit required

Q23.8 **Other congenital malformations of aortic and mitral valves**

Q23.9 **Congenital malformation of aortic and mitral valves, unspecified**

Q24 **Other congenital malformations of heart**

Excludes1: endocardial fibroelastosis (I42.4)

Q24.0 **Dextrocardia**

Excludes1: dextrocardia with situs inversus (Q89.3)

isomerism of atrial appendages (with asplenia or polysplenia) (Q20.6)

mirror-image atrial arrangement with situs inversus (Q89.3)

Q24.1 **Levocardia**

Q24.2 **Cor triatriatum**

Q24.3 **Pulmonary infundibular stenosis**

Subvalvular pulmonic stenosis

Q24.4 **Congenital subaortic stenosis**

Q24.5 **Malformation of coronary vessels**

Congenital coronary (artery) aneurysm

Q24.6 **Congenital heart block**

Q24.8 **Other specified congenital malformations of heart**

Congenital diverticulum of left ventricle

Congenital malformation of myocardium

Congenital malformation of pericardium

Malposition of heart

Uhl's disease

Q24.9 **Congenital malformation of heart, unspecified**

Congenital anomaly of heart

Congenital disease of heart

Q25 **Congenital malformations of great arteries**

Q25.0 **Patent ductus arteriosus**

Patent ductus

Botallo

Persistent ductus arteriosus

Q25.1 **Coarctation of aorta**

Coarctation of aorta (preductal) (postductal)

Stenosis of aorta

Q25.2 **Atresia of aorta**

Q25.21 **Interruption of aortic arch**

Atresia of aortic arch

Q25.29 **Other atresia of aorta**

Atresia of aorta

Q25.3 **Supravalvular aortic stenosis**

Excludes1: congenital aortic stenosis NOS (Q23.0)

congenital stenosis of aortic valve (Q23.0)

Q25.4 **Other congenital malformations of aorta**

Excludes1: hypoplasia of aorta in hypoplastic left heart syndrome (Q23.4)

Q25.40 **Congenital malformation of aorta unspecified**

Q25.41 **Absence and aplasia of aorta**

Q25.42 **Hypoplasia of aorta**

Q25.43 **Congenital aneurysm of aorta**

Congenital aneurysm of aortic root

Congenital aneurysm of aortic sinus

Q25.44 **Congenital dilation of aorta**

Q25.45 **Double aortic arch**

Vascular ring of aorta

Q25.46 **Tortuous aortic arch**

Persistent convolutions of aortic arch

Q25.47 **Right aortic arch**

Persistent right aortic arch

Q25.48 **Anomalous origin of subclavian artery**

Q25.49 **Other congenital malformations of aorta**

Aortic arch

Bovine arch

Q25.5 **Atresia of pulmonary artery**

Q25.6 **Stenosis of pulmonary artery**

Supravalvular pulmonary stenosis

Q25.7 **Other congenital malformations of pulmonary artery**

Q25.71 **Coarctation of pulmonary artery**

Q25.72 **Congenital pulmonary arteriovenous malformation**

Congenital pulmonary arteriovenous aneurysm

Q25.79 **Other congenital malformations of pulmonary artery**

Aberrant pulmonary artery

Agenesis of pulmonary artery

Congenital aneurysm of pulmonary artery

Congenital anomaly of pulmonary artery

Hypoplasia of pulmonary artery

Q25.8 **Other congenital malformations of other great arteries**

Q25.9 **Congenital malformation of great arteries, unspecified**

Q26 **Congenital malformations of great veins**

Q26.0 **Congenital stenosis of vena cava**

Congenital stenosis of vena cava (inferior)(superior)

Q26.1 **Persistent left superior vena cava**

Q26.2 **Total anomalous pulmonary venous connection**

Total anomalous pulmonary venous return [TAPVR], subdiaphragmatic

Total anomalous pulmonary venous return [TAPVR], supradiaphragmatic

Q26.3 **Partial anomalous pulmonary venous connection**

Partial anomalous pulmonary venous return

Q26.4 **Anomalous pulmonary venous connection, unspecified**

Q26.5 **Anomalous portal venous connection**

Q26.6 **Portal vein-hepatic artery fistula**

Q26.8 **Other congenital malformations of great veins**

Absence of vena cava (inferior) (superior)

Azygos continuation of inferior vena cava

Persistent left posterior cardinal vein

Scimitar syndrome

Q26.9 **Congenital malformation of great vein, unspecified**

Congenital anomaly of vena cava (inferior) (superior) NOS

Q27 **Other congenital malformations of peripheral vascular system**

Excludes2: anomalies of cerebral and precerebral vessels (Q28.0-Q28.3)

anomalies of coronary vessels (Q24.5)

anomalies of pulmonary artery (Q25.5-Q25.7)

congenital retinal aneurysm (Q14.1)

hemangioma and lymphangioma (D18.-)

Q27.0 **Congenital absence and hypoplasia of umbilical artery**

Single umbilical artery

Q27.1 **Congenital renal artery stenosis**

Q27.2 **Other congenital malformations of renal artery**

Congenital malformation of renal artery NOS

Multiple renal arteries

Q27.3 **Arteriovenous malformation (peripheral)**

Arteriovenous aneurysm

Excludes1: acquired arteriovenous aneurysm (I77.0)

Excludes2: arteriovenous malformation of cerebral
vessels (Q28.2)

arteriovenous malformation of precerebral
vessels (Q28.0)

Q27.30 **Arteriovenous malformation, site unspecified**

Q27.31 **Arteriovenous malformation of vessel of
upper limb**

Q27.32 **Arteriovenous malformation of vessel of
lower limb**

Q27.33 **Arteriovenous malformation of digestive
system vessel**

Q27.34 **Arteriovenous malformation of renal vessel**

Q27.39 **Arteriovenous malformation, other site**

Q27.4 **Congenital phlebectasia**

Q27.8 **Other specified congenital malformations of
peripheral vascular system**

Absence of peripheral vascular system

Atresia of peripheral vascular system

Congenital aneurysm (peripheral)

Congenital stricture, artery

Congenital varix

Excludes1: arteriovenous malformation (Q27.3-)

Q27.9 **Congenital malformation of peripheral vascular
system, unspecified**

Anomaly of artery or vein NOS

Q28 **Other congenital malformations of circulatory system**

Excludes1: congenital aneurysm NOS (Q27.8)

congenital coronary aneurysm (Q24.5)

ruptured cerebral arteriovenous malformation (I60.8)

ruptured malformation of precerebral vessels (I72.0)

Excludes2: congenital peripheral aneurysm (Q27.8)

congenital pulmonary aneurysm (Q25.79)

congenital retinal aneurysm (Q14.1)

Q28.0 **Arteriovenous malformation of precerebral vessels**

Congenital arteriovenous precerebral aneurysm
(nonruptured)

Q28.1 **Other malformations of precerebral vessels**

Congenital malformation of precerebral vessels NOS

Congenital precerebral aneurysm (nonruptured)

Q28.2 **Arteriovenous malformation of cerebral vessels**

Arteriovenous malformation of brain NOS

Congenital arteriovenous cerebral aneurysm
(nonruptured)

Q28.3 **Other malformations of cerebral vessels**

Congenital cerebral aneurysm (nonruptured)

Congenital malformation of cerebral vessels NOS

Developmental venous anomaly

Q28.8 **Other specified congenital malformations of
circulatory system**

Congenital aneurysm, specified site NEC

Spinal vessel anomaly

Q28.9 **Congenital malformation of circulatory system,
unspecified**

CONGENITAL MALFORMATIONS OF THE RESPIRATORY SYSTEM (Q30-Q34)

Q30 **Congenital malformations of nose**

Excludes1: congenital deviation of nasal septum (Q67.4)

Q30.0 **Choanal atresia**

Atresia of nares (anterior) (posterior)

Congenital stenosis of nares (anterior) (posterior)

Q30.1 **Agenesis and underdevelopment of nose**

Congenital absent of nose

Q30.2 **Fissured, notched and cleft nose**

Q30.3 **Congenital perforated nasal septum**

Q30.8 **Other congenital malformations of nose**

Accessory nose

Congenital anomaly of nasal sinus wall

Q30.9 **Congenital malformation of nose, unspecified**

Q31 **Congenital malformations of larynx**

Excludes1: congenital laryngeal stridor NOS (P28.89)

Q31.0 **Web of larynx**

Glottic web of larynx

Subglottic web of larynx

Web of larynx NOS

Q31.1 **Congenital subglottic stenosis**

Q31.2 **Laryngeal hypoplasia**

Q31.3 **Laryngocele**

Q31.5 **Congenital laryngomalacia**

Q31.8 **Other congenital malformations of larynx**

Absence of larynx

Agenesis of larynx

Atresia of larynx

Congenital cleft thyroid cartilage

Congenital fissure of epiglottis

Congenital stenosis of larynx NEC

Posterior cleft of cricoid cartilage

Q31.9 **Congenital malformation of larynx, unspecified**

Q32 **Congenital malformations of trachea and bronchus**

Excludes1: congenital bronchiectasis (Q33.4)

Q32.0 **Congenital tracheomalacia**

Q32.1 **Other congenital malformations of trachea**

Atresia of trachea

Congenital anomaly of tracheal cartilage

Congenital dilatation of trachea

Congenital malformation of trachea

Congenital stenosis of trachea

Congenital tracheocele

Q32.2 **Congenital bronchomalacia**

Q32.3 **Congenital stenosis of bronchus**

Q32.4 **Other congenital malformations of bronchus**

Absence of bronchus

Agenesis of bronchus

Atresia of bronchus

Congenital diverticulum of bronchus

Congenital malformation of bronchus NOS

Q33 **Congenital malformations of lung**

Q33.0 **Congenital cystic lung**

Congenital cystic lung disease

Congenital honeycomb lung

Congenital polycystic lung disease

Excludes1: cystic fibrosis (E84.0)

cystic lung disease, acquired or unspecified (J98.4)

Q33.1 **Accessory lobe of lung**

Azygos lobe (fissured), lung

Q33.2 **Sequestration of lung**

Q33.3 **Agenesis of lung**

Congenital absence of lung (lobe)

Q33.4 **Congenital bronchiectasis**

Q33.5 **Ectopic tissue in lung**

Q33.6 **Congenital hypoplasia and dysplasia of lung**

Excludes1: pulmonary hypoplasia associated with short gestation (P28.0)

Q33.8 **Other congenital malformations of lung**

Q33.9 **Congenital malformation of lung, unspecified**

Q34 **Other congenital malformations of respiratory system**

Excludes2: congenital central alveolar hypoventilation syndrome (G47.35)

Q34.0 **Anomaly of pleura**

Q34.1 **Congenital cyst of mediastinum**

Q34.8 **Other specified congenital malformations of respiratory system**

Atresia of nasopharynx

Q34.9 **Congenital malformation of respiratory system, unspecified**

Congenital absence of respiratory system

Congenital anomaly of respiratory system NOS

CLEFT LIP AND CLEFT PALATE (Q35-Q37)

Definition: Cleft lip is a congenital deformity characterized by a vertical cleft or pair of clefts in the upper lip, with or without involvement of the palate. Cleft palate is a congenital fissure in the roof of the mouth, resulting from incomplete fusion of the palate during embryonic development.

Use Additional Code to identify associated malformation of the nose (Q30.2)

Excludes2: Robin's syndrome (Q87.0)

Q35 **Cleft palate**

Includes: fissure of palate

palatoschisis

Excludes1: cleft palate with cleft lip (Q37.-)

Q35.1 **Cleft hard palate**

Q35.3 **Cleft soft palate**

Q35.5 **Cleft hard palate with cleft soft palate**

Q35.7 **Cleft uvula**

Q35.9 **Cleft palate, unspecified**

Cleft palate NOS

Q36 **Cleft lip**

Includes: cheiloschisis

congenital fissure of lip harelip

labium leporinum

Excludes1: cleft lip with cleft palate (Q37.-)

Q36.0 **Cleft lip, bilateral**

Q36.1 **Cleft lip, median**

Q36.9 **Cleft lip, unilateral**

Cleft lip NOS

Q37 **Cleft palate with cleft lip**

Includes: cheilopalatoschisis

Q37.0 **Cleft hard palate with bilateral cleft lip**

Q37.1 **Cleft hard palate with unilateral cleft lip**

Cleft hard palate with cleft lip NOS

Q37.2 **Cleft soft palate with bilateral cleft lip**

Q37.3 **Cleft soft palate with unilateral cleft lip**

Cleft soft palate with cleft lip NOS

Q37.4 **Cleft hard and soft palate with bilateral cleft lip**

Q37.5 **Cleft hard and soft palate with unilateral cleft lip**

Cleft hard and soft palate with cleft lip NOS

Q37.8 **Unspecified cleft palate with bilateral cleft lip**

Q37.9 **Unspecified cleft palate with unilateral cleft lip**

Cleft palate with cleft lip NOS

OTHER CONGENITAL MALFORMATIONS OF THE DIGESTIVE SYSTEM (Q38-Q45)

Q38 **Other congenital malformations of tongue, mouth and pharynx**

Excludes1: dentofacial anomalies (M26.-)

macrostomia (Q18.4) microstomia (Q18.5)

Q38.0 **Congenital malformations of lips, not elsewhere classified**

Congenital fistula of lip

Congenital malformation of lip NOS

Van der Woude's syndrome

Excludes1: cleft lip (Q36.-)

cleft lip with cleft palate (Q37.-)

macrocheilia (Q18.6)

microcheilia (Q18.7)

Q38.1 **Ankyloglossia**

Tongue tie

Q38.2 **Macroglossia**

Congenital hypertrophy of tongue

Q38.3 **Other congenital malformations of tongue**

Aglossia

Bifid tongue

Congenital adhesion of tongue

Congenital fissure of tongue

Congenital malformation of tongue NOS

Double tongue

Hypoglossia

Hypoplasia of tongue

Microglossia

Q38.4 **Congenital malformations of salivary glands and ducts**

Atresia of salivary glands and ducts

Congenital absence of salivary glands and ducts

Congenital accessory salivary glands and ducts

Congenital fistula of salivary gland

Q38.5 **Congenital malformations of palate, not elsewhere classified**

Congenital absence of uvula

Congenital malformation of palate NOS

Congenital high arched palate

Excludes1: cleft palate (Q35.-)

cleft palate with cleft lip (Q37.-)

Q38.6 **Other congenital malformations of mouth**

Congenital malformation of mouth NOS

Q38.7 **Congenital pharyngeal pouch**

Add 4th-7th digits   Nonspecific code   Unspecified code   Manifestation code   [HCC] Hierarchical Condition Code   743

Congenital diverticulum of pharynx

Excludes1: pharyngeal pouch syndrome (D82.1)

Q38.8 **Other congenital malformations of pharynx**

Congenital malformation of pharynx NOS

Imperforate pharynx

Q39 **Congenital malformations of esophagus**

Q39.0 **Atresia of esophagus without fistula**

Atresia of esophagus NOS

Q39.1 **Atresia of esophagus with tracheo-esophageal fistula**

Atresia of esophagus with broncho-esophageal fistula

Q39.2 **Congenital tracheo-esophageal fistula without atresia**

Congenital tracheo-esophageal fistula NOS

Q39.3 **Congenital stenosis and stricture of esophagus**

Q39.4 **Esophageal web**

Q39.5 **Congenital dilatation of esophagus**

Congenital cardiospasm

Q39.6 **Congenital diverticulum of esophagus**

Congenital esophageal pouch

Q39.8 **Other congenital malformations of esophagus**

Congenital absence of esophagus

Congenital displacement of esophagus

Congenital duplication of esophagus

Q39.9 **Congenital malformation of esophagus, unspecified**

Q40 **Other congenital malformations of upper alimentary tract**

Q40.0 **Congenital hypertrophic pyloric stenosis**

Congenital or infantile constriction

Congenital or infantile hypertrophy

Congenital or infantile spasm

Congenital or infantile stenosis

Congenital or infantile stricture

Q40.1 **Congenital hiatus hernia**

Congenital displacement of cardia through esophageal hiatus

Excludes1: congenital diaphragmatic hernia (Q79.0)

Q40.2 **Other specified congenital malformations of stomach**

Congenital displacement of stomach

Congenital diverticulum of stomach

Congenital hourglass stomach

Congenital duplication of stomach

Megalogastria

Microgastria

Q40.3 **Congenital malformation of stomach, unspecified**

Q40.8 **Other specified congenital malformations of upper alimentary tract**

Q40.9 **Congenital malformation of upper alimentary tract, unspecified**

Congenital anomaly of upper alimentary tract

Congenital deformity of upper alimentary tract

Q41 **Congenital absence, atresia and stenosis of small intestine**

Includes: congenital obstruction, occlusion or stricture of small intestine or intestine NOS

Excludes1: cystic fibrosis with intestinal manifestation (E84.11)

meconium ileus NOS (without cystic fibrosis) (P76.0)

Q41.0 **Congenital absence, atresia and stenosis of duodenum**

Q41.1 **Congenital absence, atresia and stenosis of jejunum**

Apple peel syndrome

Imperforate jejunum

Q41.2 **Congenital absence, atresia and stenosis of ileum**

Q41.8 **Congenital absence, atresia and stenosis of other specified parts of small intestine**

Q41.9 **Congenital absence, atresia and stenosis of small intestine, part unspecified**

Congenital absence, atresia and stenosis of intestine NOS

Q42 **Congenital absence, atresia and stenosis of large intestine**

Includes: congenital obstruction, occlusion and stricture of large intestine

Q42.0 **Congenital absence, atresia and stenosis of rectum with fistula**

Q42.1 **Congenital absence, atresia and stenosis of rectum without fistula**

Imperforate rectum

Q42.2 **Congenital absence, atresia and stenosis of anus with fistula**

Q42.3 **Congenital absence, atresia and stenosis of anus without fistula**

Imperforate anus

Q42.8 **Congenital absence, atresia and stenosis of other parts of large intestine**

Q42.9 **Congenital absence, atresia and stenosis of large intestine, part unspecified**

Q43 **Other congenital malformations of intestine**

Q43.0 **Meckel's diverticulum (displaced) (hypertrophic)**

Persistent omphalomesenteric duct

Persistent vitelline duct

Q43.1 **Hirschsprung's disease**

Aganglionosis

Congenital (aganglionic) megacolon

Q43.2 **Other congenital functional disorders of colon**

Congenital dilatation of colon

Q43.3 **Congenital malformations of intestinal fixation**

Congenital omental, anomalous adhesions [bands]

Congenital peritoneal adhesions [bands]

Incomplete rotation of cecum and colon

Insufficient rotation of cecum and colon

Jackson's membrane

Malrotation of colon

Rotation failure of cecum and colon

Universal mesentery

Q43.4 **Duplication of intestine**

Q43.5 **Ectopic anus**

Q43.6 **Congenital fistula of rectum and anus**

Excludes1: congenital fistula of anus with absence, atresia and stenosis (Q42.2)

congenital fistula of rectum with absence, atresia and stenosis (Q42.0)

congenital rectovaginal fistula (Q52.2)

congenital urethrorectal fistula (Q64.73)

pilonidal fistula or sinus (L05.-)

Q43.7 **Persistent cloaca**

Cloaca NOS

Q43.8 **Other specified congenital malformations of intestine**

Congenital blind loop syndrome

Congenital diverticulitis, colon

Congenital diverticulum, intestine

Dolichocolon

Megaloappendix

Megaloduodenum

Microcolon

Transposition of appendix

Transposition of colon

Transposition of intestine

Q43.9 Congenital malformation of intestine, unspecified

Q44 Congenital malformations of gallbladder, bile ducts and liver

Q44.0 Agenesis, aplasia and hypoplasia of gallbladder

Congenital absence of gallbladder

Q44.1 Other congenital malformations of gallbladder

Congenital malformation of gallbladder NOS

Intrahepatic gallbladder

Q44.2 Atresia of bile ducts

Q44.3 Congenital stenosis and stricture of bile ducts

Q44.4 Choledochal cyst

Q44.5 Other congenital malformations of bile ducts

Accessory hepatic duct

Biliary duct duplication

Congenital malformation of bile duct NOS

Cystic duct duplication

Q44.6 Cystic disease of liver

Fibrocystic disease of liver

Q44.7 Other congenital malformations of liver

Accessory liver

Alagille's syndrome

Congenital absence of liver

Congenital hepatomegaly

Congenital malformation of liver NOS

Q45 Other congenital malformations of digestive system

Excludes2: congenital diaphragmatic hernia (Q79.0)

congenital hiatus hernia (Q40.1)

Q45.0 Agenesis, aplasia and hypoplasia of pancreas

Congenital absence of pancreas

Q45.1 Annular pancreas

Q45.2 Congenital pancreatic cyst

Q45.3 Other congenital malformations of pancreas and pancreatic duct

Accessory pancreas

Congenital malformation of pancreas or pancreatic duct NOS

Excludes1: congenital diabetes mellitus (E10.-)

cystic fibrosis (E84.0-E84.9)

fibrocystic disease of pancreas (E84.-)

neonatal diabetes mellitus (P70.2)

Q45.8 Other specified congenital malformations of digestive system

Absence (complete) (partial) of alimentary tract NOS

Duplication of digestive system

Malposition, congenital of digestive system

Q45.9 Congenital malformation of digestive system, unspecified

Congenital anomaly of digestive system

Congenital deformity of digestive system

CONGENITAL MALFORMATIONS OF GENITAL ORGANS (Q50-Q56)

Excludes1: androgen insensitivity syndrome (E34.5-)

syndromes associated with anomalies in the number and form of chromosomes (Q90-Q99)

Q50 Congenital malformations of ovaries, fallopian tubes and broad ligaments

Q50.0 Congenital absence of ovary

Excludes1: Turner's syndrome (Q96.-)

Q50.01 Congenital absence of ovary, unilateral

Q50.02 Congenital absence of ovary, bilateral

Q50.1 Developmental ovarian cyst

Q50.2 Congenital torsion of ovary

Q50.3 Other congenital malformations of ovary

Q50.31 Accessory ovary

Q50.32 Ovarian streak

46, XX with streak gonads

Q50.39 Other congenital malformation of ovary

Congenital malformation of ovary NOS

Q50.4 Embryonic cyst of fallopian tube

Fimbrial cyst

Q50.5 Embryonic cyst of broad ligament

Epoophoron cyst

Parovarian cyst

Q50.6 Other congenital malformations of fallopian tube and broad ligament

Absence of fallopian tube and broad ligament

Accessory fallopian tube and broad ligament

Atresia of fallopian tube and broad ligament

Congenital malformation of fallopian tube or broad ligament NOS

Q51 Congenital malformations of uterus and cervix

Q51.0 Agenesis and aplasia of uterus

Congenital absence of uterus

Q51.1 Doubling of uterus with doubling of cervix and vagina

Q51.10 Doubling of uterus with doubling of cervix and vagina without obstruction

Doubling of uterus with doubling of cervix and vagina NOS

Q51.11 Doubling of uterus with doubling of cervix and vagina with obstruction

Q51.2 Other doubling of uterus

Doubling of uterus NOS

Septate uterus

▲**Q51.21 Complete doubling of uterus**

Complete septate uterus

▲**Q51.22 Partial doubling of uterus**

Partial septate uterus

▲**Q51.28 Other and unspecified doubling of uterus**

Septate uterus NOS

Q51.3 Bicornate uterus

Bicornate uterus, complete or partial

Q51.4 Unicornate uterus

Unicornate uterus with or without a separate uterine horn

Uterus with only one functioning horn

Q51.5 Agenesis and aplasia of cervix

Congenital absence of cervix

Q51.6 Embryonic cyst of cervix

Q51.7 Congenital fistulae between uterus and digestive and urinary tracts

Q51.8 Other congenital malformations of uterus and cervix

    Q51.81 Other congenital malformations of uterus

        Q51.810 Arcuate uterus

            Arcuatus uterus

        Q51.811 Hypoplasia of uterus

        Q51.818 Other congenital malformations of uterus

            Müllerian anomaly of uterus NEC

    Q51.82 Other congenital malformations of cervix

        Q51.820 Cervical duplication

        Q51.821 Hypoplasia of cervix

        Q51.828 Other congenital malformations of cervix

Q51.9 Congenital malformation of uterus and cervix, unspecified

Q52 Other congenital malformations of female genitalia

Q52.0 Congenital absence of vagina

    Vaginal agenesis, total or partial

Q52.1 Doubling of vagina

    Excludes1: doubling of vagina with doubling of uterus and cervix (Q51.1-)

    Q52.10 Doubling of vagina, unspecified

        Septate vagina NOS

    Q52.11 Transverse vaginal septum

    Q52.12 Longitudinal vaginal septum

        Q52.120 Longitudinal vaginal septum, nonobstructing

        Q52.121 Longitudinal vaginal septum, obstructing, right side

        Q52.122 Longitudinal vaginal septum, obstructing, left side

        Q52.123 Longitudinal vaginal septum, microperforate, right side

        Q52.124 Longitudinal vaginal septum, microperforate, left side

        Q52.129 Other and unspecified longitudinal vaginal septum

Q52.2 Congenital rectovaginal fistula

    Excludes1: cloaca (Q43.7)

Q52.3 Imperforate hymen

Q52.4 Other congenital malformations of vagina

    Canal of Nuck cyst, congenital

    Congenital malformation of vagina NOS

    Embryonic vaginal cyst

    Gartner's duct cyst

Q52.5 Fusion of labia

Q52.6 Congenital malformation of clitoris

Q52.7 Other and unspecified congenital malformations of vulva

    Q52.70 Unspecified congenital malformations of vulva

        Congenital malformation of vulva NOS

    Q52.71 Congenital absence of vulva

    Q52.79 Other congenital malformations of vulva

        Congenital cyst of vulva

Q52.8 Other specified congenital malformations of female genitalia

Q52.9 Congenital malformation of female genitalia, unspecified

Q53 Undescended and ectopic testicle

Q53.0 Ectopic testis

    Q53.00 Ectopic testis, unspecified

    Q53.01 Ectopic testis, unilateral

    Q53.02 Ectopic testes, bilateral

Q53.1 Undescended testicle, unilateral

    Q53.10 Unspecified undescended testicle, unilateral

    Q53.11 Abdominal testis, unilateral

        Q53.111 Unilateral intraabdominal testis

        Q53.112 Unilateral inguinal testis

    Q53.12 Ectopic perineal testis, unilateral

    Q53.13 Unilateral high scrotal testis

Q53.2 Undescended testicle, bilateral

    Q53.20 Undescended testicle, unspecified, bilateral

    Q53.21 Abdominal testis, bilateral

        Q53.211 Bilateral intraabdominal testes

        Q53.212 Bilateral inguinal testes

    Q53.22 Ectopic perineal testis, bilateral

    Q53.23 Bilateral high scrotal testes

Q53.9 Undescended testicle, unspecified

    Cryptorchism NOS

Q54 Hypospadias

    Excludes1: epispadias (Q64.0)

Q54.0 Hypospadias, balanic

    Hypospadias, coronal

    Hypospadias, glandular

Q54.1 Hypospadias, penile

Q54.2 Hypospadias, penoscrotal

Q54.3 Hypospadias, perineal

Q54.4 Congenital chordee

    Chordee without hypospadias

Q54.8 Other hypospadias

    Hypospadias with intersex state

Q54.9 Hypospadias, unspecified

Q55 Other congenital malformations of male genital organs

    Excludes1: congenital hydrocele (P83.5)

        hypospadias (Q54.-)

Q55.0 Absence and aplasia of testis

    Monorchism

Q55.1 Hypoplasia of testis and scrotum

    Fusion of testes

Q55.2 Other and unspecified congenital malformations of testis and scrotum

    Q55.20 Unspecified congenital malformations of testis and scrotum

        Congenital malformation of testis or scrotum NOS

    Q55.21 Polyorchism

    Q55.22 Retractile testis

    Q55.23 Scrotal transposition

    Q55.29 Other congenital malformations of testis and scrotum

Q55.3 Atresia of vas deferens

    Code first any associated cystic fibrosis (E84.-)

Q55.4 Other congenital malformations of vas deferens, epididymis, seminal vesicles and prostate

Absence or aplasia of prostate

Absence or aplasia of spermatic cord

Congenital malformation of vas deferens, epididymis, seminal vesicles or prostate NOS

Q55.5   **Congenital absence and aplasia of penis**

Q55.6   **Other congenital malformations of penis**

     Q55.61   **Curvature of penis (lateral)**

     Q55.62   **Hypoplasia of penis**

       Micropenis

     Q55.63   **Congenital torsion of penis**

       Excludes1: acquired torsion of penis (N48.82)

     Q55.64   **Hidden penis**

       Buried penis

       Concealed penis

       Excludes1: acquired buried penis (N48.83)

     Q55.69   **Other congenital malformation of penis**

       Congenital malformation of penis NOS

Q55.7   **Congenital vasocutaneous fistula**

Q55.8   **Other specified congenital malformations of male genital organs**

Q55.9   **Congenital malformation of male genital organ, unspecified**

Congenital anomaly of male genital organ

Congenital deformity of male genital organ

Q56   **Indeterminate sex and pseudohermaphroditism**

Excludes1: 46,XX true hermaphrodite (Q99.1)

androgen insensitivity syndrome (E34.5-)

chimera 46,XX/46,XY true hermaphrodite (Q99.0)

female pseudohermaphroditism with adrenocortical disorder (E25.-)

pseudohermaphroditism with specified chromosomal anomaly (Q96-Q99)

pure gonadal dysgenesis (Q99.1)

Q56.0   **Hermaphroditism, not elsewhere classified**

Ovotestis

Q56.1   **Male pseudohermaphroditism, not elsewhere classified**

46, XY with streak gonads

Male pseudohermaphroditism NOS

Q56.2   **Female pseudohermaphroditism, not elsewhere classified**

Female pseudohermaphroditism NOS

Q56.3   **Pseudohermaphroditism, unspecified**

Q56.4   **Indeterminate sex, unspecified**

Ambiguous genitalia

CONGENITAL MALFORMATIONS OF THE URINARY SYSTEM (Q60-Q64)

Q60   **Renal agenesis and other reduction defects of kidney**

Includes: congenital absence of kidney

congenital atrophy of kidney infantile atrophy of kidney

Q60.0   **Renal agenesis, unilateral**

Q60.1   **Renal agenesis, bilateral**

Q60.2   **Renal agenesis, unspecified**

Q60.3   **Renal hypoplasia, unilateral**

Q60.4   **Renal hypoplasia, bilateral**

Q60.5   **Renal hypoplasia, unspecified**

Q60.6   **Potter's syndrome**

Q61   **Cystic kidney disease**

Excludes1: acquired cyst of kidney (N28.1)

Potter's syndrome (Q60.6)

Q61.0   **Congenital renal cyst**

     Q61.00   **Congenital renal cyst, unspecified**

       Cyst of kidney NOS (congenital)

     Q61.01   **Congenital single renal cyst**

     Q61.02   **Congenital multiple renal cysts**

Q61.1   **Polycystic kidney, infantile type**

Polycystic kidney, autosomal recessive

     Q61.11   **Cystic dilatation of collecting ducts**

     Q61.19   **Other polycystic kidney, infantile type**

Q61.2   **Polycystic kidney, adult type**

Polycystic kidney, autosomal dominant

Q61.3   **Polycystic kidney, unspecified**

Q61.4   **Renal dysplasia**

Multicystic dysplastic kidney

Multicystic kidney (development)

Multicystic kidney disease

Multicystic renal dysplasia

Excludes1: polycystic kidney disease (Q61.11-Q61.3)

Q61.5   **Medullary cystic kidney**

Nephronophthisis

Sponge kidney NOS

Q61.8   **Other cystic kidney diseases**

Fibrocystic kidney

Fibrocystic renal degeneration or disease

Q61.9   **Cystic kidney disease, unspecified**

Meckel-Gruber syndrome

Q62   **Congenital obstructive defects of renal pelvis and congenital malformations of ureter**

Q62.0   **Congenital hydronephrosis**

Q62.1   **Congenital occlusion of ureter**

Atresia and stenosis of ureter

     Q62.10   **Congenital occlusion of ureter, unspecified**

     Q62.11   **Congenital occlusion of ureteropelvic junction**

     Q62.12   **Congenital occlusion of ureterovesical orifice**

Q62.2   **Congenital megaureter**

Congenital dilatation of ureter

Q62.3   **Other obstructive defects of renal pelvis and ureter**

     Q62.31   **Congenital ureterocele, orthotopic**

     Q62.32   **Cecoureterocele**

       Ectopic ureterocele

     Q62.39   **Other obstructive defects of renal pelvis and ureter**

       Ureteropelvic junction obstruction NOS

Q62.4   **Agenesis of ureter**

Congenital absence ureter

Q62.5   **Duplication of ureter**

Accessory ureter

Double ureter

Q62.6   **Malposition of ureter**

     Q62.60   **Malposition of ureter, unspecified**

     Q62.61   **Deviation of ureter**

     Q62.62   **Displacement of ureter**

     Q62.63   **Anomalous implantation of ureter**

       Ectopia of ureter

Ectopic ureter

Q62.69   Other malposition of ureter

Q62.7   Congenital vesico-uretero-renal reflux

Q62.8   Other congenital malformations of ureter

Anomaly of ureter NOS

Q63   Other congenital malformations of kidney

Excludes1: congenital nephrotic syndrome (N04.-)

Q63.0   Accessory kidney

Q63.1   Lobulated, fused and horseshoe kidney

Q63.2   Ectopic kidney

Congenital displaced kidney

Malrotation of kidney

Q63.3   Hyperplastic and giant kidney

Compensatory hypertrophy of kidney

Q63.8   Other specified congenital malformations of kidney

Congenital renal calculi

Q63.9   Congenital malformation of kidney, unspecified

Q64   Other congenital malformations of urinary system

Q64.0   Epispadias

Excludes1: hypospadias (Q54.-)

Q64.1   Exstrophy of urinary bladder

Q64.10   Exstrophy of urinary bladder, unspecified

Ectopia vesicae

Q64.11   Supravesical fissure of urinary bladder

Q64.12   Cloacal exstrophy of urinary bladder

Q64.19   Other exstrophy of urinary bladder

Extroversion of bladder

Q64.2   Congenital posterior urethral valves

Q64.3   Other atresia and stenosis of urethra and bladder neck

Q64.31   Congenital bladder neck obstruction

Congenital obstruction of vesicourethral orifice

Q64.32   Congenital stricture of urethra

Q64.33   Congenital stricture of urinary meatus

Q64.39   Other atresia and stenosis of urethra and bladder neck

Atresia and stenosis of urethra and bladder neck NOS

Q64.4   Malformation of urachus

Cyst of urachus

Patent urachus

Prolapse of urachus

Q64.5   Congenital absence of bladder and urethra

Q64.6   Congenital diverticulum of bladder

Q64.7   Other and unspecified congenital malformations of bladder and urethra

Excludes1: congenital prolapse of bladder (mucosa) (Q79.4)

Q64.70   Unspecified congenital malformation of bladder and urethra

Malformation of bladder or urethra NOS

Q64.71   Congenital prolapse of urethra

Q64.72   Congenital prolapse of urinary meatus

Q64.73   Congenital urethrorectal fistula

Q64.74   Double urethra

Q64.75   Double urinary meatus

Q64.79   Other congenital malformations of bladder and urethra

Q64.8   Other specified congenital malformations of urinary system

Q64.9   Congenital malformation of urinary system, unspecified

Congenital anomaly NOS of urinary system

Congenital deformity NOS of urinary system

CONGENITAL MALFORMATIONS AND DEFORMATIONS OF THE MUSCULOSKELETAL SYSTEM (Q65-Q79)

Q65   Congenital deformities of hip

Excludes1: clicking hip (R29.4)

Q65.0   Congenital dislocation of hip, unilateral

Q65.00   Congenital dislocation of unspecified hip, unilateral

Q65.01   Congenital dislocation of right hip, unilateral

Q65.02   Congenital dislocation of left hip, unilateral

Q65.1   Congenital dislocation of hip, bilateral

Q65.2   Congenital dislocation of hip, unspecified

Q65.3   Congenital partial dislocation of hip, unilateral

Q65.30   Congenital partial dislocation of unspecified hip, unilateral

Q65.31   Congenital partial dislocation of right hip, unilateral

Q65.32   Congenital partial dislocation of left hip, unilateral

Q65.4   Congenital partial dislocation of hip, bilateral

Q65.5   Congenital partial dislocation of hip, unspecified

Q65.6   Congenital unstable hip

Congenital dislocatable hip

Q65.8   Other congenital deformities of hip

Q65.81   Congenital coxa valga

Q65.82   Congenital coxa vara

Q65.89   Other specified congenital deformities of hip

Anteversion of femoral neck

Congenital acetabular dysplasia

Q65.9   Congenital deformity of hip, unspecified

Q66   Congenital deformities of feet

Excludes1: reduction defects of feet (Q72.-)

valgus deformities (acquired) (M21.0-)

varus deformities (acquired) (M21.1-)

Q66.0   Congenital talipes equinovarus

Q66.00   Congenital talipes equinovarus, unspecified foot

Q66.01   Congenital talipes equinovarus, right foot

Q66.02   Congenital talipes equinovarus, left foot

Q66.1   Congenital talipes calcaneovarus

Q66.10   Congenital talipes calcaneovarus, unspecified foot

Q66.11   Congenital talipes calcaneovarus, right foot

Q66.12   Congenital talipes calcaneovarus, left foot

Q66.2   Congenital metatarsus (primus) varus

Q66.21   Congenital metatarsus primus varus

Q66.211   Congenital metatarsus primus varus, right foot

Q66.212   Congenital metatarsus primus varus, left foot

Q66.219   Congenital metatarsus primus varus, unspecified foot

Q66.22   Congenital metatarsus adductus

Congenital metatarsus varus

● New code   ▲ Revised code   **Excludes1:** Not coded here   **Excludes2:** Not included here   ⊗ Placeholder required   ⑦7th digit required

Q66.221 Congenital metatarsus adductus, right foot

Q66.222 Congenital metatarsus adductus, left foot

Q66.229 Congenital metatarsus adductus, unspecified foot

Q66.3 Other congenital varus deformities of feet

Hallux varus, congenital

Q66.30 Other congenital varus deformities of feet, unspecified foot

Q66.31 Other congenital varus deformities of feet, right foot

Q66.32 Other congenital varus deformities of feet, left foot

Q66.4 Congenital talipes calcaneovalgus

Q66.40 Congenital talipes calcaneovalgus, unspecified foot

Q66.41 Congenital talipes calcaneovalgus, right foot

Q66.42 Congenital talipes calcaneovalgus, left foot

Q66.5 Congenital pes planus

Congenital flat foot

Congenital rigid flat foot

Congenital spastic (everted) flat foot

Excludes1: pes planus, acquired (M21.4)

Q66.50 Congenital pes planus, unspecified foot

Q66.51 Congenital pes planus, right foot

Q66.52 Congenital pes planus, left foot

Q66.6 Other congenital valgus deformities of feet

Congenital metatarsus valgus

Q66.7 Congenital pes cavus

Q66.70 Congenital pes cavus, unspecified foot

Q66.71 Congenital pes cavus, right foot

Q66.72 Congenital pes cavus, left foot

Q66.8 Other congenital deformities of feet

Q66.80 Congenital vertical talus deformity, unspecified foot

Q66.81 Congenital vertical talus deformity, right foot

Q66.82 Congenital vertical talus deformity, left foot

Q66.89 Other specified congenital deformities of feet

Congenital asymmetric talipes

Congenital clubfoot NOS

Congenital talipes NOS

Congenital tarsal coalition

Hammer toe, congenital

Q66.9 Congenital deformity of feet, unspecified

Q66.90 Congenital deformity of feet, unspecified, unspecified foot

Q66.91 Congenital deformity of feet, unspecified, right foot

Q66.92 Congenital deformity of feet, unspecified, left foot

Q67 Congenital musculoskeletal deformities of head, face, spine and chest

Excludes1: congenital malformation syndromes classified to Q87.-

Potter's syndrome (Q60.6)

Q67.0 Congenital facial asymmetry

Q67.1 Congenital compression facies

Q67.2 Dolichocephaly

Q67.3 Plagiocephaly

Q67.4 Other congenital deformities of skull, face and jaw

Congenital depressions in skull

Congenital hemifacial atrophy or hypertrophy

Deviation of nasal septum, congenital

Squashed or bent nose, congenital

Excludes1: dentofacial anomalies [including malocclusion] (M26.-)

syphilitic saddle nose (A50.5)

Q67.5 Congenital deformity of spine

Congenital postural scoliosis

Congenital scoliosis NOS

Excludes1: infantile idiopathic scoliosis (M41.0)

scoliosis due to congenital bony malformation (Q76.3)

Q67.6 Pectus excavatum

Congenital funnel chest

Q67.7 Pectus carinatum

Congenital pigeon chest

Q67.8 Other congenital deformities of chest

Congenital deformity of chest wall NOS

Q68 Other congenital musculoskeletal deformities

Excludes1: reduction defects of limb(s) (Q71-Q73)

Excludes2: congenital myotonic chondrodystrophy (G71.13)

Q68.0 Congenital deformity of sternocleidomastoid muscle

Congenital contracture of sternocleidomastoid (muscle)

Congenital (sternomastoid) torticollis

Sternomastoid tumor (congenital)

Q68.1 Congenital deformity of finger(s) and hand

Congenital club finger

Spade-like hand (congenital)

Q68.2 Congenital deformity of knee

Congenital dislocation of knee

Congenital genu recurvatum

Q68.3 Congenital bowing of femur

Excludes1: anteversion of femur (neck) (Q65.89)

Q68.4 Congenital bowing of tibia and fibula

Q68.5 Congenital bowing of long bones of leg, unspecified

Q68.6 Discoid meniscus

Q68.8 Other specified congenital musculoskeletal deformities

Congenital deformity of clavicle

Congenital deformity of elbow

Congenital deformity of forearm

Congenital deformity of scapula

Congenital deformity of wrist

Congenital dislocation of elbow

Congenital dislocation of shoulder

Congenital dislocation of wrist

Q69 Polydactyly

Q69.0 Accessory finger(s)

Q69.1 Accessory thumb(s)

Q69.2 Accessory toe(s)

Accessory hallux

Q69.9 Polydactyly, unspecified

Supernumerary digit(s) NOS

Q70 Syndactyly

Q70.0 Fused fingers

Complex syndactyly of fingers with synostosis

Q70.00   **Fused fingers, unspecified hand**

Q70.01   **Fused fingers, right hand**

Q70.02   **Fused fingers, left hand**

Q70.03   **Fused fingers, bilateral**

Q70.1   **Webbed fingers**

Simple syndactyly of fingers without synostosis

Q70.10   **Webbed fingers, unspecified hand**

Q70.11   **Webbed fingers, right hand**

Q70.12   **Webbed fingers, left hand**

Q70.13   **Webbed fingers, bilateral**

Q70.2   **Fused toes**

Complex syndactyly of toes with synostosis

Q70.20   **Fused toes, unspecified foot**

Q70.21   **Fused toes, right foot**

Q70.22   **Fused toes, left foot**

Q70.23   **Fused toes, bilateral**

Q70.3   **Webbed toes**

Simple syndactyly of toes without synostosis

Q70.30   **Webbed toes, unspecified foot**

Q70.31   **Webbed toes, right foot**

Q70.32   **Webbed toes, left foot**

Q70.33   **Webbed toes, bilateral**

Q70.4   **Polysyndactyly, unspecified**

Excludes1: specified syndactyly of hand and feet - code to specified conditions (Q70.0- -Q70.3-)

Q70.9   **Syndactyly, unspecified**

Symphalangy NOS

Q71   **Reduction defects of upper limb**

Q71.0   **Congenital complete absence of upper limb**

Q71.00   **Congenital complete absence of unspecified upper limb**

Q71.01   **Congenital complete absence of right upper limb**

Q71.02   **Congenital complete absence of left upper limb**

Q71.03   **Congenital complete absence of upper limb, bilateral**

Q71.1   **Congenital absence of upper arm and forearm with hand present**

Q71.10   **Congenital absence of unspecified upper arm and forearm with hand present**

Q71.11   **Congenital absence of right upper arm and forearm with hand present**

Q71.12   **Congenital absence of left upper arm and forearm with hand present**

Q71.13   **Congenital absence of upper arm and forearm with hand present, bilateral**

Q71.2   **Congenital absence of both forearm and hand**

Q71.20   **Congenital absence of both forearm and hand, unspecified upper limb**

Q71.21   **Congenital absence of both forearm and hand, right upper limb**

Q71.22   **Congenital absence of both forearm and hand, left upper limb**

Q71.23   **Congenital absence of both forearm and hand, bilateral**

Q71.3   **Congenital absence of hand and finger**

Q71.30   **Congenital absence of unspecified hand and finger**

Q71.31   **Congenital absence of right hand and finger**

Q71.32   **Congenital absence of left hand and finger**

Q71.33   **Congenital absence of hand and finger, bilateral**

Q71.4   **Longitudinal reduction defect of radius**

Clubhand (congenital)

Radial clubhand

Q71.40   **Longitudinal reduction defect of unspecified radius**

Q71.41   **Longitudinal reduction defect of right radius**

Q71.42   **Longitudinal reduction defect of left radius**

Q71.43   **Longitudinal reduction defect of radius, bilateral**

Q71.5   **Longitudinal reduction defect of ulna**

Q71.50   **Longitudinal reduction defect of unspecified ulna**

Q71.51   **Longitudinal reduction defect of right ulna**

Q71.52   **Longitudinal reduction defect of left ulna**

Q71.53   **Longitudinal reduction defect of ulna, bilateral**

Q71.6   **Lobster-claw hand**

Q71.60   **Lobster-claw hand, unspecified hand**

Q71.61   **Lobster-claw right hand**

Q71.62   **Lobster-claw left hand**

Q71.63   **Lobster-claw hand, bilateral**

Q71.8   **Other reduction defects of upper limb**

Q71.81   **Congenital shortening of upper limb**

Q71.811   **Congenital shortening of right upper limb**

Q71.812   **Congenital shortening of left upper limb**

Q71.813   **Congenital shortening of upper limb, bilateral**

Q71.819   **Congenital shortening of unspecified upper limb**

Q71.89   **Other reduction defects of upper limb**

Q71.891   **Other reduction defects of right upper limb**

Q71.892   **Other reduction defects of left upper limb**

Q71.893   **Other reduction defects of upper limb, bilateral**

Q71.899   **Other reduction defects of unspecified upper limb**

Q71.9   **Unspecified reduction defect of upper limb**

Q71.90   **Unspecified reduction defect of unspecified upper limb**

Q71.91   **Unspecified reduction defect of right upper limb**

Q71.92   **Unspecified reduction defect of left upper limb**

Q71.93   **Unspecified reduction defect of upper limb, bilateral**

Q72   **Reduction defects of lower limb**

Q72.0   **Congenital complete absence of lower limb**

Q72.00   **Congenital complete absence of unspecified lower limb**

Q72.01   **Congenital complete absence of right lower limb**

Q72.02   **Congenital complete absence of left lower limb**

Q72.03   Congenital complete absence of lower limb, bilateral

Q72.1   Congenital absence of thigh and lower leg with foot present

Q72.10   Congenital absence of unspecified thigh and lower leg with foot present

Q72.11   Congenital absence of right thigh and lower leg with foot present

Q72.12   Congenital absence of left thigh and lower leg with foot present

Q72.13   Congenital absence of thigh and lower leg with foot present, bilateral

Q72.2   Congenital absence of both lower leg and foot

Q72.20   Congenital absence of both lower leg and foot, unspecified lower limb

Q72.21   Congenital absence of both lower leg and foot, right lower limb

Q72.22   Congenital absence of both lower leg and foot, left lower limb

Q72.23   Congenital absence of both lower leg and foot, bilateral

Q72.3   Congenital absence of foot and toe(s)

Q72.30   Congenital absence of unspecified foot and toe(s)

Q72.31   Congenital absence of right foot and toe(s)

Q72.32   Congenital absence of left foot and toe(s)

Q72.33   Congenital absence of foot and toe(s), bilateral

Q72.4   Longitudinal reduction defect of femur

Proximal femoral focal deficiency

Q72.40   Longitudinal reduction defect of unspecified femur

Q72.41   Longitudinal reduction defect of right femur

Q72.42   Longitudinal reduction defect of left femur

Q72.43   Longitudinal reduction defect of femur, bilateral

Q72.5   Longitudinal reduction defect of tibia

Q72.50   Longitudinal reduction defect of unspecified tibia

Q72.51   Longitudinal reduction defect of right tibia

Q72.52   Longitudinal reduction defect of left tibia

Q72.53   Longitudinal reduction defect of tibia, bilateral

Q72.6   Longitudinal reduction defect of fibula

Q72.60   Longitudinal reduction defect of unspecified fibula

Q72.61   Longitudinal reduction defect of right fibula

Q72.62   Longitudinal reduction defect of left fibula

Q72.63   Longitudinal reduction defect of fibula, bilateral

Q72.7   Split foot

Q72.70   Split foot, unspecified lower limb

Q72.71   Split foot, right lower limb

Q72.72   Split foot, left lower limb

Q72.73   Split foot, bilateral

Q72.8   Other reduction defects of lower limb

Q72.81   Congenital shortening of lower limb

Q72.811   Congenital shortening of right lower limb

Q72.812   Congenital shortening of left lower limb

Q72.813   Congenital shortening of lower limb, bilateral

Q72.819   Congenital shortening of unspecified lower limb

Q72.89   Other reduction defects of lower limb

Q72.891   Other reduction defects of right lower limb

Q72.892   Other reduction defects of left lower limb

Q72.893   Other reduction defects of lower limb, bilateral

Q72.899   Other reduction defects of unspecified lower limb

Q72.9   Unspecified reduction defect of lower limb

Q72.90   Unspecified reduction defect of unspecified lower limb

Q72.91   Unspecified reduction defect of right lower limb

Q72.92   Unspecified reduction defect of left lower limb

Q72.93   Unspecified reduction defect of lower limb, bilateral

Q73   Reduction defects of unspecified limb

Q73.0   Congenital absence of unspecified limb(s)

Amelia NOS

Q73.1   Phocomelia, unspecified limb(s)

Phocomelia NOS

Q73.8   Other reduction defects of unspecified limb(s)

Longitudinal reduction deformity of unspecified limb(s)

Ectromelia of limb NOS

Hemimelia of limb NOS

Reduction defect of limb NOS

Q74   Other congenital malformations of limb(s)

Excludes1: polydactyly (Q69.-)

reduction defect of limb (Q71-Q73)

syndactyly (Q70.-)

Q74.0   Other congenital malformations of upper limb(s), including shoulder girdle

Accessory carpal bones

Cleidocranial dysostosis

Congenital pseudarthrosis of clavicle

Macrodactylia (fingers)

Madelung's deformity

Radioulnar synostosis

Sprengel's deformity

Triphalangeal thumb

Q74.1   Congenital malformation of knee

Congenital absence of patella

Congenital dislocation of patella

Congenital genu valgum

Congenital genu varum

Rudimentary patella

Excludes1: congenital dislocation of knee (Q68.2)

congenital genu recurvatum (Q68.2)

nail patella syndrome (Q87.2)

Q74.2   Other congenital malformations of lower limb(s), including pelvic girdle

Congenital fusion of sacroiliac joint

Congenital malformation of ankle joint

Congenital malformation of sacroiliac joint

Excludes1: anteversion of femur (neck) (Q65.89)

Q74.3   Arthrogryposis multiplex congenita

Q74.8   Other specified congenital malformations of limb(s)

Q74.9   Unspecified congenital malformation of limb(s)

Congenital anomaly of limb(s) NOS

Q75   Other congenital malformations of skull and face bones

Excludes1: congenital malformation of face NOS (Q18.-)

congenital malformation syndromes classified to Q87.-

dentofacial anomalies [including malocclusion] (M26.-)

musculoskeletal deformities of head and face (Q67.0-Q67.4)

skull defects associated with congenital anomalies of brain such as: anencephaly (Q00.0)

encephalocele (Q01.-)

hydrocephalus (Q03.-)

microcephaly (Q02)

Q75.0   Craniosynostosis

Acrocephaly

Imperfect fusion of skull

Oxycephaly

Trigonocephaly

Q75.1   Craniofacial dysostosis

Crouzon's disease

Q75.2   Hypertelorism

Q75.3   Macrocephaly

Q75.4   Mandibulofacial dysostosis

Franceschetti syndrome

Treacher Collins syndrome

Q75.5   Oculomandibular dysostosis

Q75.8   Other specified congenital malformations of skull and face bones

Absence of skull bone, congenital

Congenital deformity of forehead

Platybasia

Q75.9   Congenital malformation of skull and face bones, unspecified

Congenital anomaly of face bones NOS

Congenital anomaly of skull NOS

Q76   Congenital malformations of spine and bony thorax

Excludes1: congenital musculoskeletal deformities of spine and chest (Q67.5-Q67.8)

Q76.0   Spina bifida occulta

Excludes1: meningocele (spinal) (Q05.-)

spina bifida (aperta) (cystica) (Q05.-)

Q76.1   Klippel-Feil syndrome

Cervical fusion syndrome

Q76.2   Congenital spondylolisthesis

Congenital spondylolysis

Excludes1: spondylolisthesis (acquired) (M43.1-)

spondylolysis (acquired) (M43.0-)

Q76.3   Congenital scoliosis due to congenital bony malformation

Hemivertebra fusion or failure of segmentation with scoliosis

Q76.4   Other congenital malformations of spine, not associated with scoliosis

Q76.41   Congenital kyphosis

Q76.411   Congenital kyphosis, occipito-atlanto-axial region

Q76.412   Congenital kyphosis, cervical region

Q76.413   Congenital kyphosis, cervicothoracic region

Q76.414   Congenital kyphosis, thoracic region

Q76.415   Congenital kyphosis, thoracolumbar region

Q76.419   Congenital kyphosis, unspecified region

Q76.42   Congenital lordosis

Q76.425   Congenital lordosis, thoracolumbar region

Q76.426   Congenital lordosis, lumbar region

Q76.427   Congenital lordosis, lumbosacral region

Q76.428   Congenital lordosis, sacral and sacrococcygeal region

Q76.429   Congenital lordosis, unspecified region

Q76.49   Other congenital malformations of spine, not associated with scoliosis

Congenital absence of vertebra NOS

Congenital fusion of spine NOS

Congenital malformation of lumbosacral (joint) (region) NOS

Congenital malformation of spine NOS

Hemivertebra NOS

Malformation of spine NOS

Platyspondylisis NOS

Supernumerary vertebra NOS

Q76.5   Cervical rib

Supernumerary rib in cervical region

Q76.6   Other congenital malformations of ribs

Accessory rib

Congenital absence of rib

Congenital fusion of ribs

Congenital malformation of ribs NOS

Excludes1: short rib syndrome (Q77.2)

Q76.7   Congenital malformation of sternum

Congenital absence of sternum

Sternum bifidum

Q76.8   Other congenital malformations of bony thorax

Q76.9   Congenital malformation of bony thorax, unspecified

Q77   Osteochondrodysplasia with defects of growth of tubular bones and spine

Excludes1: mucopolysaccharidosis (E76.0-E76.3)

Excludes2: congenital myotonic chondrodystrophy (G71.13)

Q77.0   Achondrogenesis

Hypochondrogenesis

Q77.1   Thanatophoric short stature

Q77.2   Short rib syndrome

Asphyxiating thoracic dysplasia [Jeune]

Q77.3   Chondrodysplasia punctata

Excludes1: Rhizomelic chondrodysplasia punctata (E71.43)

Q77.4   Achondroplasia

● New code   ▲ Revised code   **Excludes1:** Not coded here   **Excludes2:** Not included here   ⊗ Placeholder required   ⑦7th digit required

Hypochondroplasia

Osteosclerosis congenita

Q77.5 **Diastrophic dysplasia**

Q77.6 **Chondroectodermal dysplasia**

Ellis-van Creveld syndrome

Q77.7 **Spondyloepiphyseal dysplasia**

Q77.8 **Other osteochondrodysplasia with defects of growth of tubular bones and spine**

Q77.9 **Osteochondrodysplasia with defects of growth of tubular bones and spine, unspecified**

Q78 **Other osteochondrodysplasias**

Excludes2: congenital myotonic chondrodystrophy (G71.13)

Q78.0 **Osteogenesis imperfecta**

Fragilitas ossium

Osteopsathyrosis

Q78.1 **Polyostotic fibrous dysplasia**

Albright(-McCune)(-Sternberg) syndrome

Q78.2 **Osteopetrosis**

Albers-Schönberg syndrome

Osteosclerosis NOS

Q78.3 **Progressive diaphyseal dysplasia**

Camurati-Engelmann syndrome

Q78.4 **Enchondromatosis**

Maffucci's syndrome

Ollier's disease

Q78.5 **Metaphyseal dysplasia**

Pyle's syndrome

Q78.6 **Multiple congenital exostoses**

Diaphyseal aclasis

Q78.8 **Other specified osteochondrodysplasias**

Osteopoikilosis

Q78.9 **Osteochondrodysplasia, unspecified**

Chondrodystrophy NOS

Osteodystrophy NOS

Q79 **Congenital malformations of musculoskeletal system, not elsewhere classified**

Excludes2: congenital (sternomastoid) torticollis (Q68.0)

Q79.0 **Congenital diaphragmatic hernia**

Excludes1: congenital hiatus hernia (Q40.1)

Q79.1 **Other congenital malformations of diaphragm**

Absence of diaphragm

Congenital malformation of diaphragm NOS

Eventration of diaphragm

Q79.2 **Exomphalos**

Omphalocele

Excludes1: umbilical hernia (K42.-)

Q79.3 **Gastroschisis**

Q79.4 **Prune belly syndrome**

Congenital prolapse of bladder mucosa

Eagle-Barrett syndrome

Q79.5 **Other congenital malformations of abdominal wall**

Excludes1: umbilical hernia (K42.-)

Q79.51 **Congenital hernia of bladder**

Q79.59 **Other congenital malformations of abdominal wall**

Q79.6 **Ehlers-Danlos syndromes**

Q79.60 **Ehlers-Danlos syndrome, unspecified**

Q79.61 **Classical Ehlers-Danlos syndrome**

Classical EDS (cEDS)

Q79.62 **Hypermobile Ehlers-Danlos syndrome**

Hypermobile EDS (hEDS)

Q79.63 **Vascular Ehlers-Danlos syndrome**

Vascular EDS (vEDS)

Q79.69 **Other Ehlers-Danlos syndromes**

Q79.8 **Other congenital malformations of musculoskeletal system**

Absence of muscle

Absence of tendon

Accessory muscle

Amyotrophia congenita

Congenital constricting bands

Congenital shortening of tendon

Poland syndrome

Q79.9 **Congenital malformation of musculoskeletal system, unspecified**

Congenital anomaly of musculoskeletal system NOS

Congenital deformity of musculoskeletal system NOS

OTHER CONGENITAL MALFORMATIONS (Q80-Q89)

Q80 **Congenital ichthyosis**

Excludes1: Refsum's disease (G60.1)

Q80.0 **Ichthyosis vulgaris**

Q80.1 **X-linked ichthyosis**

Q80.2 **Lamellar ichthyosis**

Collodion baby

Q80.3 **Congenital bullous ichthyosiform erythroderma**

Q80.4 **Harlequin fetus**

Q80.8 **Other congenital ichthyosis**

Q80.9 **Congenital ichthyosis, unspecified**

Q81 **Epidermolysis bullosa**

Q81.0 **Epidermolysis bullosa simplex**

Excludes1: Cockayne's syndrome (Q87.19)

Q81.1 **Epidermolysis bullosa letalis**

Herlitz' syndrome

Q81.2 **Epidermolysis bullosa dystrophica**

Q81.8 **Other epidermolysis bullosa**

Q81.9 **Epidermolysis bullosa, unspecified**

Q82 **Other congenital malformations of skin**

Excludes1: acrodermatitis enteropathica (E83.2)

congenital erythropoietic porphyria (E80.0)

pilonidal cyst or sinus (L05.-)

Sturge-Weber (-Dimitri) syndrome (Q85.8)

Q82.0 **Hereditary lymphedema**

Q82.1 **Xeroderma pigmentosum**

Q82.2 **Congenital cutaneous mastocytosis**

Congenital diffuse cutaneous mastocytosis

Congenital maculopapular cutaneous mastocytosis

Congenital urticaria pigmentosa

Excludes1: cutaneous mastocytosis NOS (D47.01)

diffuse cutaneous mastocytosis (with onset after newborn period) (D47.01)

malignant mastocytosis (C96.2-)

systemic mastocytosis (D47.02)

urticaria pigmentosa (non-congenital) (with onset after newborn period) (D47.01)

Q82.3 Incontinentia pigmenti

Q82.4 Ectodermal dysplasia (anhidrotic)

Excludes1: Ellis-van Creveld syndrome (Q77.6)

Q82.5 Congenital non-neoplastic nevus

Birthmark NOS

Flammeus Nevus

Port-wine Nevus

Sanguineous Nevus

Strawberry Nevus

Vascular Nevus NOS

Verrucous Nevus

Excludes2: Café au lait spots (L81.3)

lentigo (L81.4)

araneus nevus (I78.1)

melanocytic nevus (D22.-)

nevus NOS (D22.-)

pigmented nevus (D22.-)

spider nevus (I78.1)

stellar nevus (I78.1)

Q82.6 Congenital sacral dimple

Parasacral dimple

Excludes2: pilonidal cyst with abscess (L05.01)

pilonidal cyst without abscess (L05.91)

Q82.8 Other specified congenital malformations of skin

Abnormal palmar creases

Accessory skin tags

Benign familial pemphigus [Hailey-Hailey]

Congenital poikiloderma

Cutis laxa (hyperelastica)

Dermatoglyphic anomalies

Inherited keratosis palmaris et plantaris

Keratosis follicularis [Darier-White]

Excludes1: Ehlers-Danlos syndromes (Q79.6-)

Q82.9 Congenital malformation of skin, unspecified

Q83 Congenital malformations of breast

Excludes2: absence of pectoral muscle (Q79.8)

hypoplasia of breast (N64.82)

micromastia (N64.82)

Q83.0 Congenital absence of breast with absent nipple

Q83.1 Accessory breast

Supernumerary breast

Q83.2 Absent nipple

Q83.3 Accessory nipple

Supernumerary nipple

Q83.8 Other congenital malformations of breast

Q83.9 Congenital malformation of breast, unspecified

Q84 Other congenital malformations of integument

Q84.0 Congenital alopecia

Congenital atrichosis

Q84.1 Congenital morphological disturbances of hair, not elsewhere classified

Beaded hair

Monilethrix

Pili annulati

Excludes1: Menkes' kinky hair syndrome (E83.0)

Q84.2 Other congenital malformations of hair

Congenital hypertrichosis

Congenital malformation of hair NOS

Persistent lanugo

Q84.3 Anonychia

Excludes1: nail patella syndrome (Q87.2)

Q84.4 Congenital leukonychia

Q84.5 Enlarged and hypertrophic nails

Congenital onychauxis

Pachyonychia

Q84.6 Other congenital malformations of nails

Congenital club nail

Congenital koilonychia

Congenital malformation of nail NOS

Q84.8 Other specified congenital malformations of integument

Aplasia cutis congenita

Q84.9 Congenital malformation of integument, unspecified

Congenital anomaly of integument NOS

Congenital deformity of integument NOS

Q85 Phakomatoses, not elsewhere classified

Excludes1: ataxia telangiectasia [Louis-Bar] (G11.3)

familial dysautonomia [Riley-Day] (G90.1)

Q85.0 Neurofibromatosis (nonmalignant)

Q85.00 Neurofibromatosis, unspecified [HCC]

Q85.01 Neurofibromatosis, type 1 [HCC]

Von Recklinghausen disease

Q85.02 Neurofibromatosis, type 2 [HCC]

Acoustic neurofibromatosis

Q85.03 Schwannomatosis [HCC]

Q85.09 Other neurofibromatosis [HCC]

Q85.1 Tuberous sclerosis [HCC]

Bourneville's disease

Epiloia

Q85.8 Other phakomatoses, not elsewhere classified [HCC]

Peutz-Jeghers Syndrome

Sturge-Weber(-Dimitri) syndrome von Hippel-Lindau syndrome

Excludes1: Meckel-Gruber syndrome (Q61.9)

Q85.9 Phakomatosis, unspecified [HCC]

Hamartoses NOS

Q86 Congenital malformation syndromes due to known exogenous causes, not elsewhere classified

Excludes2: iodine-deficiency-related hypothyroidism (E00-E02)

nonteratogenic effects of substances transmitted via placenta or breast milk (P04.-)

Q86.0 Fetal alcohol syndrome (dysmorphic)

Q86.1 Fetal hydantoin syndrome

Meadow's syndrome

Q86.2 Dysmorphism due to warfarin

Q86.8 Other congenital malformation syndromes due to known exogenous causes

Q87 Other specified congenital malformation syndromes affecting multiple systems

Use Additional Code(s) to identify all associated manifestations

Q87.0 Congenital malformation syndromes predominantly affecting facial appearance

● New code　▲ Revised code　Excludes1: Not coded here　Excludes2: Not included here　⊗ Placeholder required　⑦ 7th digit required

Acrocephalopolysyndactyly

Acrocephalosyndactyly [Apert]

Cryptophthalmos syndrome

Cyclopia

Goldenhar syndrome

Moebius syndrome

Oro-facial-digital syndrome

Robin syndrome

Whistling face

Q87.1 Congenital malformation syndromes predominantly associated with short stature

Excludes1: Ellis-van Creveld syndrome (Q77.6)

Smith-Lemli-Opitz syndrome (E78.72)

Q87.11 Prader-Willi syndrome

Q87.19 Other congenital malformation syndromes predominantly associated with short stature

Aarskog syndrome

Cockayne syndrome

De Lange syndrome

Dubowitz syndrome

Noonan syndrome

Robinow-Silverman-Smith syndrome

Russell-Silver syndrome

Seckel syndrome

Q87.2 Congenital malformation syndromes predominantly involving limbs

Holt-Oram syndrome

Klippel-Trenaunay-Weber syndrome

Nail patella syndrome

Rubinstein-Taybi syndrome

Sirenomelia syndrome

Thrombocytopenia with absent radius [TAR] syndrome

VATER syndrome

Q87.3 Congenital malformation syndromes involving early overgrowth

Beckwith-Wiedemann syndrome

Sotos syndrome

Weaver syndrome

Q87.4 Marfan's syndrome

Q87.40 Marfan's syndrome, unspecified

Q87.41 Marfan's syndrome with cardiovascular manifestations

Q87.410 Marfan's syndrome with aortic dilation

Q87.418 Marfan's syndrome with other cardiovascular manifestations

Q87.42 Marfan's syndrome with ocular manifestations

Q87.43 Marfan's syndrome with skeletal manifestation

Q87.5 Other congenital malformation syndromes with other skeletal changes

Q87.8 Other specified congenital malformation syndromes, not elsewhere classified

Excludes1: Zellweger syndrome (E71.510)

Q87.81 Alport syndrome

Use Additional Code to identify stage of chronic kidney disease (N18.1-N18.6)

Q87.82 Arterial tortuosity syndrome

Q87.89 Other specified congenital malformation syndromes, not elsewhere classified

Laurence-Moon (-Bardet)-Biedl syndrome

Q89 Other congenital malformations, not elsewhere classified

Q89.0 Congenital absence and malformations of spleen

Excludes1: isomerism of atrial appendages (with asplenia or polysplenia) (Q20.6)

Q89.01 Asplenia (congenital)

Q89.09 Congenital malformations of spleen

Congenital splenomegaly

Q89.1 Congenital malformations of adrenal gland

Excludes1: adrenogenital disorders (E25.-)

congenital adrenal hyperplasia (E25.0)

Q89.2 Congenital malformations of other endocrine glands

Congenital malformation of parathyroid or thyroid gland

Persistent thyroglossal duct

Thyroglossal cyst

Excludes1: congenital goiter (E03.0)

congenital hypothyroidism (E03.1)

Q89.3 Situs inversus

Dextrocardia with situs inversus

Mirror-image atrial arrangement with situs inversus

Situs inversus or transversus abdominalis

Situs inversus or transversus thoracis

Transposition of abdominal viscera

Transposition of thoracic viscera

Excludes1: dextrocardia NOS (Q24.0)

Q89.4 Conjoined twins

Craniopagus

Dicephaly

Pygopagus

Thoracopagus

Q89.7 Multiple congenital malformations, not elsewhere classified

Multiple congenital anomalies NOS

Multiple congenital deformities NOS

Excludes1: congenital malformation syndromes affecting multiple systems (Q87.-)

Q89.8 Other specified congenital malformations

Use Additional Code(s) to identify all associated manifestations

Q89.9 Congenital malformation, unspecified

Congenital anomaly NOS

Congenital deformity NOS

CHROMOSOMAL ABNORMALITIES, NOT ELSEWHERE CLASSIFIED (Q90-Q99)

Excludes2: mitochondrial metabolic disorders (E88.4-)

Q90 Down syndrome

Use Additional Code(s) to identify any associated physical conditions and degree of intellectual disabilities (F70-F79)

Q90.0 Trisomy 21, nonmosaicism (meiotic nondisjunction)

Q90.1 Trisomy 21, mosaicism (mitotic nondisjunction)

Q90.2 Trisomy 21, translocation

Q90.9 Down syndrome, unspecified

Trisomy 21 NOS

Q91 Trisomy 18 and Trisomy 13

Q91.0 Trisomy 18, nonmosaicism (meiotic nondisjunction)

Q91.1 Trisomy 18, mosaicism (mitotic nondisjunction)

Q91.2 Trisomy 18, translocation

Q91.3 Trisomy 18, unspecified

Q91.4 Trisomy 13, nonmosaicism (meiotic nondisjunction)

Q91.5 Trisomy 13, mosaicism (mitotic nondisjunction)

Q91.6 Trisomy 13, translocation

Q91.7 Trisomy 13, unspecified

Q92 **Other trisomies and partial trisomies of the autosomes, not elsewhere classified**

Includes: unbalanced translocations and insertions

Excludes1: trisomies of chromosomes 13, 18, 21 (Q90-Q91)

Q92.0 Whole chromosome trisomy, nonmosaicism (meiotic nondisjunction)

Q92.1 Whole chromosome trisomy, mosaicism (mitotic nondisjunction)

Q92.2 Partial trisomy

Less than whole arm duplicated Whole arm or more duplicated

Excludes1: partial trisomy due to unbalanced translocation (Q92.5)

Q92.5 Duplications with other complex rearrangements

Partial trisomy due to unbalanced translocations

Code also any associated deletions due to unbalanced translocations, inversions and insertions (Q93.7)

Q92.6 Marker chromosomes

Trisomies due to dicentrics

Trisomies due to extra rings

Trisomies due to isochromosomes

Individual with marker heterochromatin

Q92.61 Marker chromosomes in normal individual

Q92.62 Marker chromosomes in abnormal individual

Q92.7 Triploidy and polyploidy

Q92.8 Other specified trisomies and partial trisomies of autosomes

Duplications identified by fluorescence in situ hybridization (FISH)

Duplications identified by in situ hybridization (ISH)

Duplications seen only at prometaphase

Q92.9 Trisomy and partial trisomy of autosomes, unspecified

Q93 **Monosomies and deletions from the autosomes, not elsewhere classified**

Q93.0 Whole chromosome monosomy, nonmosaicism (meiotic nondisjunction)

Q93.1 Whole chromosome monosomy, mosaicism (mitotic nondisjunction)

Q93.2 Chromosome replaced with ring, dicentric or isochromosome

Q93.3 Deletion of short arm of chromosome 4

Wolff-Hirschorn syndrome

Q93.4 Deletion of short arm of chromosome 5

Cri-du-chat syndrome

Q93.5 Other deletions of part of a chromosome

Q93.51 Angelman syndrome

Q93.59 Other deletions of part of a chromosome

Q93.7 Deletions with other complex rearrangements

Deletions due to unbalanced translocations, inversions and insertions

Code also any associated duplications due to unbalanced translocations, inversions and insertions (Q92.5)

Q93.8 Other deletions from the autosomes

Q93.81 Velo-cardio-facial syndrome

Deletion 22q11.2

Q93.82 Williams syndrome

Q93.88 Other microdeletions

Miller-Dieker syndrome

Smith-Magenis syndrome

Q93.89 Other deletions from the autosomes

Deletions identified by fluorescence in situ hybridization (FISH)

Deletions identified by in situ hybridization (ISH)

Deletions seen only at prometaphase

Q93.9 Deletion from autosomes, unspecified

Q95 **Balanced rearrangements and structural markers, not elsewhere classified**

Includes: Robertsonian and balanced reciprocal translocations and insertions

Q95.0 Balanced translocation and insertion in normal individual

Q95.1 Chromosome inversion in normal individual

Q95.2 Balanced autosomal rearrangement in abnormal individual

Q95.3 Balanced sex/autosomal rearrangement in abnormal individual

Q95.5 Individual with autosomal fragile site

Q95.8 Other balanced rearrangements and structural markers

Q95.9 Balanced rearrangement and structural marker, unspecified

Q96 **Turner's syndrome**

Excludes1: Noonan syndrome (Q87.19)

Q96.0 Karyotype 45, X

Q96.1 Karyotype 46, X iso (Xq)

Karyotype 46, isochromosome Xq

Q96.2 Karyotype 46, X with abnormal sex chromosome, except iso (Xq)

Karyotype 46, X with abnormal sex chromosome, except isochromosome Xq

Q96.3 Mosaicism, 45, X/46, XX or XY

Q96.4 Mosaicism, 45, X/Other cell line(s) with abnormal sex chromosome

Q96.8 Other variants of Turner's syndrome

Q96.9 Turner's syndrome, unspecified

Q97 **Other sex chromosome abnormalities, female phenotype, not elsewhere classified**

Excludes1: Turner's syndrome (Q96.-)

Q97.0 Karyotype 47, XXX

Q97.1 Female with more than three X chromosomes

Q97.2 Mosaicism, lines with various numbers of X chromosomes

Q97.3 Female with 46, XY karyotype

Q97.8 Other specified sex chromosome abnormalities, female phenotype

Q97.9 Sex chromosome abnormality, female phenotype, unspecified

Q98 **Other sex chromosome abnormalities, male phenotype, not elsewhere classified**

Q98.0 Klinefelter syndrome karyotype 47, XXY

Q98.1 Klinefelter syndrome, male with more than two X chromosomes

● New code   ▲ Revised code   Excludes1: Not coded here   Excludes2: Not included here   ⊗ Placeholder required   ⑦7th digit required

Q98.3   Other male with 46, XX karyotype

Q98.4   Klinefelter syndrome, unspecified

Q98.5   Karyotype 47, XYY

Q98.6   Male with structurally abnormal sex chromosome

Q98.7   Male with sex chromosome mosaicism

Q98.8   Other specified sex chromosome abnormalities, male phenotype

Q98.9   Sex chromosome abnormality, male phenotype, unspecified

Q99   **Other chromosome abnormalities, not elsewhere classified**

Q99.0   Chimera 46, XX/46, XY

Chimera 46, XX/46, XY true hermaphrodite

Q99.1   46, XX true hermaphrodite

46, XX with streak gonads

46, XY with streak gonads

Pure gonadal dysgenesis

Q99.2   Fragile X chromosome

Fragile X syndrome

Q99.8   Other specified chromosome abnormalities

Q99.9   Chromosomal abnormality, unspecified

● New code ▲ Revised code **Excludes1:** Not coded here **Excludes2:** Not included here ⊗ Placeholder required ⑦7ᵗʰ digit required

Chapter 18: Symptoms, Signs and Abnormal Clinical and Laboratory Findings, Not Elsewhere Classified (R00-R99)

DEFINITIONS

This chapter includes definitions of selected key words, terms and phrases and coding alerts for adding points to the clinical domain, and references to coding late effects where appropriate. An example from this chapter is as follows:

R16 Hepatomegaly and splenomegaly, not elsewhere classified
Definition: Hepatomegaly refers to abnormal enlargement of the liver. Splenomegaly refers to abnormal enlargement of the spleen.

MULTIPLE CODING FOR A SINGLE CONDITION

In addition to the etiology/manifestation convention that requires two codes to fully describe a single condition that affects multiple body systems, there are other single conditions that also require more than one code. "**Use Additional Code**" notes are found in the Tabular List at codes that are not part of an etiology/manifestation pair where a secondary code is useful to fully describe a condition. The sequencing rule is the same as the etiology/manifestation pair, "**Use Additional Code**" indicates that a secondary code should be added.

For example, for bacterial infections that are not included in chapter 1, a secondary code from category B95, Streptococcus, Staphylococcus, and Enterococcus, as the cause of diseases classified elsewhere, or B96, Other bacterial agents as the cause of diseases classified elsewhere, may be required to identify the bacterial organism causing the infection. A "**Use Additional Code**" note will normally be found at the infectious disease code, indicating a need for the organism code to be added as a secondary code.

"Code first" notes are also under certain codes that are not specifically manifestation codes but may be due to an underlying cause. When there is a "Code first" note and an underlying condition is present, the underlying condition should be sequenced first.

"Code, if applicable, any causal condition first", notes indicate that this code may be assigned as a principal diagnosis when the causal condition is unknown or not applicable. If a causal condition is known, then the code for that condition should be sequenced as the principal or first-listed diagnosis.

Multiple codes may be needed for sequela, complication codes and obstetric codes to more fully describe a condition. See the specific guidelines for these conditions for further instruction.

COMBINATION CODE

A combination code is a single code used to classify: Two diagnoses, or a diagnosis with an associated secondary process (manifestation) A diagnosis with an associated complication

Combination codes are identified by referring to subterm entries in the Alphabetic Index and by reading the inclusion and exclusion notes in the Tabular List.

Assign only the combination code when that code fully identifies the diagnostic conditions involved or when the Alphabetic Index so directs. Multiple coding should not be used when the classification provides a combination code that clearly identifies all of the elements documented in the diagnosis. When the combination code lacks necessary specificity in describing the manifestation or complication, an additional code should be used as a secondary code.

SEQUELA (LATE EFFECTS)

A sequela is the residual effect (condition produced) after the acute phase of an illness or injury has terminated. There is no time limit on when a sequela code can be used. The residual may be apparent early, such as in cerebral infarction, or it may occur months or years later, such as that due to a previous injury. Coding of sequela generally requires two codes sequenced in the following order: The condition or nature of the sequela is sequenced first.

The sequela code is sequenced second.

R00-R99

An exception to the above guidelines are those instances where the code for the sequela is followed by a manifestation code identified in the Tabular List and title, or the sequela code has been expanded (at the fourth, fifth or sixth character levels) to include the manifestation(s). The code for the acute phase of an illness or injury that led to the sequela is never used with a code for the late effect.

Chapter 18 includes symptoms, signs, abnormal results of clinical or other investigative procedures, and ill-defined conditions regarding which no diagnosis classifiable elsewhere is recorded. Signs and symptoms that point to a specific diagnosis have been assigned to a category in other chapters of the classification.

a. Use of symptom codes

Codes that describe symptoms and signs are acceptable for reporting purposes when a related definitive diagnosis has not been established (confirmed) by the provider.

b. Use of a symptom code with a definitive diagnosis code

Codes for signs and symptoms may be reported in addition to a related definitive diagnosis when the sign or symptom is not routinely associated with that diagnosis, such as the various signs and symptoms associated with complex syndromes. The definitive diagnosis code should be sequenced before the symptom code.

Signs or symptoms that are associated routinely with a disease process should not be assigned as additional codes, unless otherwise instructed by the classification.

c. Combination codes that include symptoms

ICD-10-CM contains a number of combination codes that identify both the definitive diagnosis and common symptoms of that diagnosis. When using one of these combination codes, an additional code should not be assigned for the symptom.

d. Repeated falls

Code R29.6, Repeated falls, is for use for encounters when a patient has recently fallen and the reason for the fall is being investigated.

Code Z91.81, History of falling, is for use when a patient has fallen in the past and is at risk for future falls. When appropriate, both codes R29.6 and Z91.81 may be assigned together.

e. Coma scale

Code R40.20, Unspecified coma, may be assigned in conjunction with codes for any medical condition.

Do not report codes for unspecified coma, individual or total Glasgow coma scale scores for a patient with a medically induced coma or a sedated patient.

The coma scale codes (R40.21- to R40.24-) can be used in conjunction with traumatic brain injury codes. These codes are primarily for use by trauma registries, but they may be used in any setting where this information is collected. The coma scale codes should be sequenced after the diagnosis code(s).

These codes, one from each subcategory, are needed to complete the scale. The 7th character indicates when the scale was recorded. The 7th character should match for all three codes.

At a minimum, report the initial score documented on presentation at your facility. This may be a score from the emergency medicine technician (EMT) or in the emergency department. If desired, a facility may choose to capture multiple coma scale scores.

Assign code R40.24-, Glasgow coma scale, total score, when only the total score is documented in the medical record and not the individual score(s).

● New code   ▲ Revised code   **Excludes1:** Not coded here   **Excludes2:** Not included here   ⊗ Placeholder required   ⑦7th digit required

If multiple coma scores are captured within the first 24 hours afterhospital admission, assign only the code for the score at the time ofadmission. ICD-10-CM does not classify coma scores that are reported after admission but less than 24 hours later.

See Section I.B.14 for coma scale documentation by clinicians other thanpatient's provider

f. **Functional quadriplegia**

Guideline deleted effective October 1, 2017

g. **SIRS due to Non-Infectious Process**

The systemic inflammatory response syndrome (SIRS) can develop as a result of certain non-infectious disease processes, such as trauma, malignant neoplasm, or pancreatitis. When SIRS is documented with a noninfectious condition, and no subsequent infection is documented, the code for the underlying condition, such as an injury, should be assigned, followed by code R65.10, Systemic inflammatory response syndrome (SIRS) of non-infectious origin without acute organ dysfunction, or code R65.11, Systemic inflammatory response syndrome (SIRS) of non-infectious origin with acute organ dysfunction. If an associated acute organ dysfunction is documented, the appropriate code(s) for the specific type of organ dysfunction(s) should be assigned in addition to code R65.11. If acute organ dysfunction is documented, but it cannot be determined if the acute organ dysfunction is associated with SIRS or due to another condition (e.g., directly due to the trauma), the provider should be queried.

h. **Death NOS**

Code R99, Ill-defined and unknown cause of mortality, is only for use in the very limited circumstance when a patient who has already died is brought into an emergency department or other healthcare facility and is pronounced dead upon arrival. It does not represent the discharge disposition of death.

i. **NIHSS Stroke Scale**

The NIH stroke scale (NIHSS) codes (R29.7- -) can be used in conjunction with acute stroke codes (I63) to identify the patient's neurological status and the severity of the stroke. The stroke scale codes should be sequenced after the acute stroke diagnosis code(s).

At a minimum, report the initial score documented. If desired, a facility may choose to capture multiple stroke scale scores.

See Section I.B.14 for NIHSS stroke scale documentation by clinicians other than patient's provider

Chapter 18
Symptoms, Signs and Abnormal Clinical and Laboratory Findings, Not Elsewhere Classified (R00-R99)

Note: This chapter includes symptoms, signs, abnormal results of clinical or other investigative procedures, and ill-defined conditions regarding which no diagnosis classifiable elsewhere is recorded.

Signs and symptoms that point rather definitely to a given diagnosis have been assigned to a category in other chapters of the classification. In general, categories in this chapter include the less well-defined conditions and symptoms that, without the necessary study of the case to establish a final diagnosis, point perhaps equally to two or more diseases or to two or more systems of the body. Practically all categories in the chapter could be designated 'not otherwise specified', 'unknown etiology' or 'transient'. The Alphabetical Index should be consulted to determine which symptoms and signs are to be allocated here and which to other chapters. The residual subcategories, numbered .8, are generally provided for other relevant symptoms that cannot be allocated elsewhere in the classification.

The conditions and signs or symptoms included in categories R00-R94 consist of: (a) cases for which no more specific diagnosis can be made even after all the facts bearing on the case have been investigated; (b) signs or symptoms existing at the time of initial encounter that proved to be transient and whose causes could not be determined; (c) provisional diagnosis in a patient who failed to return for further investigation or care; (d) cases referred elsewhere for investigation or treatment before the diagnosis was made; (e) cases in which a more precise diagnosis was not available for any other reason; (f) certain symptoms, for which supplementary information is provided, that represent important problems in medical care in their own right.

Excludes2: abnormal findings on antenatal screening of mother (O28.-)
certain conditions originating in the perinatal period (P04-P96)
signs and symptoms classified in the body system chapters signs and symptoms of breast (N63, N64.5)

This chapter contains the following blocks:

R00-R09	Symptoms and signs involving the circulatory and respiratory systems
R10-R19	Symptoms and signs involving the digestive system and abdomen
R20-R23	Symptoms and signs involving the skin and subcutaneous tissue
R25-R29	Symptoms and signs involving the nervous and musculoskeletal systems
R30-R39	Symptoms and signs involving the genitourinary system
R40-R46	Symptoms and signs involving cognition, perception, emotional state and behavior
R47-R49	Symptoms and signs involving speech and voice
R50-R69	General symptoms and signs
R70-R79	Abnormal findings on examination of blood, without diagnosis
R80-R82	Abnormal findings on examination of urine, without diagnosis
R83-R89	Abnormal findings on examination of other body fluids, substances and tissues, without diagnosis
R90-R94	Abnormal findings on diagnostic imaging and in function studies, without diagnosis
R97	Abnormal tumor markers
R99	Ill-defined and unknown cause of mortality

SYMPTOMS AND SIGNS INVOLVING THE CIRCULATORY AND RESPIRATORY SYSTEMS (R00-R09)

R00 **Abnormalities of heart beat**

Excludes1: abnormalities originating in the perinatal period (P29.1-)

Excludes2: specified arrhythmias (I47-I49)

R00.0 **Tachycardia, unspecified**
Rapid heart beat
Sinoauricular tachycardia NOS
Sinus [sinusal] tachycardia NOS

Excludes1: neonatal tachycardia (P29.11)
paroxysmal tachycardia (I47.-)

R00.1 **Bradycardia, unspecified**
Sinoatrial bradycardia
Sinus bradycardia
Slow heart beat
Vagal bradycardia

Use Additional Code for adverse effect, if applicable, to identify drug (T36-T50 with fifth or sixth character 5)

Excludes1: neonatal bradycardia (P29.12)

R00.2 **Palpitations**
Awareness of heart beat

R00.8 **Other abnormalities of heart beat**

R00.9 **Unspecified abnormalities of heart beat**

R01 **Cardiac murmurs and other cardiac sounds**

Excludes1: cardiac murmurs and sounds originating in the perinatal period (P29.8)

R01.0 **Benign and innocent cardiac murmurs**
Functional cardiac murmur

R01.1 **Cardiac murmur, unspecified**
Cardiac bruit NOS
Heart murmur NOS
Systolic murmur NOS

R01.2 **Other cardiac sounds**
Cardiac dullness, increased or decreased
Precordial friction

R03 **Abnormal blood-pressure reading, without diagnosis**

R03.0 **Elevated blood-pressure reading, without diagnosis of hypertension**
Note: This category is to be used to record an episode of elevated blood pressure in a patient in whom no formal diagnosis of hypertension has been made, or as an isolated incidental finding.

R03.1 **Nonspecific low blood-pressure reading**

Excludes1: hypotension (I95.-)
maternal hypotension syndrome (O26.5-)
neurogenic orthostatic hypotension (G90.3)

R04 **Hemorrhage from respiratory passages**

R04.0 **Epistaxis**
Hemorrhage from nose Nosebleed

R04.1 **Hemorrhage from throat**

Excludes2: hemoptysis (R04.2)

R04.2 **Hemoptysis**
Blood-stained sputum
Cough with hemorrhage

R04.8 **Hemorrhage from other sites in respiratory passages**

R04.81 **Acute idiopathic pulmonary hemorrhage in infants**
AIPHI

Acute idiopathic hemorrhage in infants over 28 days old

> **Excludes1:** perinatal pulmonary hemorrhage (P26.-)
>
> von Willebrand's disease (D68.0)

R04.89 **Hemorrhage from other sites in respiratory passages**

Pulmonary hemorrhage NOS

R04.9 **Hemorrhage from respiratory passages, unspecified**

R05 **Cough**

> **Excludes1:** cough with hemorrhage (R04.2)
>
> paroxysmal cough due to Bordetella pertussis (A37.0-)
>
> smoker's cough (J41.0)

> **Excludes2:** cough with hemorrhage (R04.2)

- **R05.1** **Acute cough**
- **R05.2** **Subacute cough**
- **R05.3** **Chronic cough**

  Persistent cough

  Refractory cough

  Unexplained cough

- **R05.4** **Cough syncope**

  Code first syncope and collapse (R55)

- **R05.8** **Other specified cough**
- **R05.9** **Cough, unspecified**

R06 **Abnormalities of breathing**

> **Excludes1:** acute respiratory distress syndrome (J80)
>
> respiratory arrest (R09.2)
>
> respiratory arrest of newborn (P28.81)
>
> respiratory distress syndrome of newborn (P22.-)
>
> respiratory failure (J96.-)
>
> respiratory failure of newborn (P28.5)

R06.0 **Dyspnea**

> **Excludes1:** tachypnea NOS (R06.82)
>
> transient tachypnea of newborn (P22.1)

R06.00 **Dyspnea, unspecified**

R06.01 **Orthopnea**

R06.02 **Shortness of breath**

R06.03 **Acute respiratory distress**

R06.09 **Other forms of dyspnea**

R06.1 **Stridor**

> **Excludes1:** congenital laryngeal stridor (P28.89)
>
> laryngismus (stridulus) (J38.5)

R06.2 **Wheezing**

> **Excludes1:** Asthma (J45.-)

R06.3 **Periodic breathing**

Cheyne-Stokes breathing

R06.4 **Hyperventilation**

> **Excludes1:** psychogenic hyperventilation (F45.8)

R06.5 **Mouth breathing**

> **Excludes2:** dry mouth NOS (R68.2)

R06.6 **Hiccough**

> **Excludes1:** psychogenic hiccough (F45.8)

R06.7 **Sneezing**

R06.8 **Other abnormalities of breathing**

R06.81 **Apnea, not elsewhere classified**

Apnea NOS

> **Excludes1:** apnea (of) newborn (P28.4)
>
> sleep apnea (G47.3-)
>
> sleep apnea of newborn (primary) (P28.3)

R06.82 **Tachypnea, not elsewhere classified**

Tachypnea NOS

> **Excludes1:** transitory tachypnea of newborn (P22.1)

R06.83 **Snoring**

R06.89 **Other abnormalities of breathing**

Breath-holding (spells)

Sighing

R06.9 **Unspecified abnormalities of breathing**

R07 **Pain in throat and chest**

> **Excludes1:** epidemic myalgia (B33.0)

> **Excludes2:** jaw pain R68.84
>
> pain in breast (N64.4)

R07.0 **Pain in throat**

> **Excludes1:** chronic sore throat (J31.2)
>
> sore throat (acute) NOS (J02.9)

> **Excludes2:** dysphagia (R13.1-)
>
> pain in neck (M54.2)

R07.1 **Chest pain on breathing**

Painful respiration

R07.2 **Precordial pain**

R07.8 **Other chest pain**

R07.81 **Pleurodynia**

Pleurodynia NOS

> **Excludes1:** epidemic pleurodynia (B33.0)

R07.82 **Intercostal pain**

R07.89 **Other chest pain**

Anterior chest-wall pain NOS

R07.9 **Chest pain, unspecified**

R09 **Other symptoms and signs involving the circulatory and respiratory system**

> **Excludes1:** acute respiratory distress syndrome (J80)
>
> respiratory arrest of newborn (P28.81)
>
> respiratory distress syndrome of newborn (P22.0)
>
> respiratory failure (J96.-)
>
> respiratory failure of newborn (P28.5)

R09.0 **Asphyxia and hypoxemia**

> **Excludes1:** asphyxia due to carbon monoxide (T58.-)
>
> asphyxia due to foreign body in respiratory tract (T17.-)
>
> birth (intrauterine) asphyxia (P84)
>
> hyperventilation (R06.4) traumatic asphyxia (T71.-)

> **Excludes2:** hypercapnia (R06.89)

R09.01 **Asphyxia**

R09.02 **Hypoxemia**

R09.1 **Pleurisy**

> **Excludes1:** pleurisy with effusion (J90)

R09.2 **Respiratory arrest** [HCC]

Cardiorespiratory failure

> **Excludes1:** cardiac arrest (I46.-)
>
> respiratory arrest of newborn (P28.81)
>
> respiratory distress of newborn (P22.0)
>
> respiratory failure (J96.-)

respiratory failure of newborn (P28.5)

respiratory insufficiency (R06.89)

respiratory insufficiency of newborn (P28.5)

R09.3 Abnormal sputum

Abnormal amount of sputum

Abnormal color of sputum

Abnormal odor of sputum

Excessive sputum

Excludes1: blood-stained sputum (R04.2)

R09.8 Other specified symptoms and signs involving the circulatory and respiratory systems

R09.81 Nasal congestion

R09.82 Postnasal drip

R09.89 Other specified symptoms and signs involving the circulatory and respiratory systems

Bruit (arterial)

Abnormal chest percussion

Feeling of foreign body in throat

Friction sounds in chest

Chest tympany Choking sensation

Rales

Weak pulse

Excludes2: foreign body in throat (T17.2-)

wheezing (R06.2)

SYMPTOMS AND SIGNS INVOLVING THE DIGESTIVE SYSTEM AND ABDOMEN (R10-R19)

Excludes2: congenital or infantile pylorospasm (Q40.0)

gastrointestinal hemorrhage (K92.0-K92.2)

intestinal obstruction (K56.-)

newborn gastrointestinal hemorrhage (P54.0-P54.3)

newborn intestinal obstruction (P76.-)

pylorospasm (K31.3)

signs and symptoms involving the urinary system (R30-R39)

symptoms referable to female genital organs (N94.-)

symptoms referable to male genital organs (N48-N50)

R10 Abdominal and pelvic pain

Excludes1: renal colic (N23)

Excludes2: dorsalgia (M54.-)

flatulence and related conditions (R14.-)

R10.0 Acute abdomen

Severe abdominal pain (generalized) (with abdominal rigidity)

Excludes1: abdominal rigidity NOS (R19.3)

generalized abdominal pain NOS (R10.84)

localized abdominal pain (R10.1-R10.3-)

R10.1 Pain localized to upper abdomen

R10.10 Upper abdominal pain, unspecified

R10.11 Right upper quadrant pain

R10.12 Left upper quadrant pain

R10.13 Epigastric pain

Dyspepsia

Excludes1: functional dyspepsia (K30)

R10.2 Pelvic and perineal pain

Excludes1: vulvodynia (N94.81)

R10.3 Pain localized to other parts of lower abdomen

R10.30 Lower abdominal pain, unspecified

R10.31 Right lower quadrant pain

R10.32 Left lower quadrant pain

R10.33 Periumbilical pain

R10.8 Other abdominal pain

R10.81 Abdominal tenderness

Abdominal tenderness NOS

R10.811 Right upper quadrant abdominal tenderness

R10.812 Left upper quadrant abdominal tenderness

R10.813 Right lower quadrant abdominal tenderness

R10.814 Left lower quadrant abdominal tenderness

R10.815 Periumbilic abdominal tenderness

R10.816 Epigastric abdominal tenderness

R10.817 Generalized abdominal tenderness

R10.819 Abdominal tenderness, unspecified site

R10.82 Rebound abdominal tenderness

R10.821 Right upper quadrant rebound abdominal tenderness

R10.822 Left upper quadrant rebound abdominal tenderness

R10.823 Right lower quadrant rebound abdominal tenderness

R10.824 Left lower quadrant rebound abdominal tenderness

R10.825 Periumbilic rebound abdominal tenderness

R10.826 Epigastric rebound abdominal tenderness

R10.827 Generalized rebound abdominal tenderness

R10.829 Rebound abdominal tenderness, unspecified site

R10.83 Colic

Colic NOS

Infantile colic

Excludes1: colic in adult and child over 12 months old (R10.84)

R10.84 Generalized abdominal pain

Excludes1: generalized abdominal pain associated

with acute abdomen (R10.0)

R10.9 Unspecified abdominal pain

R11 Nausea and vomiting

Excludes1: cyclical vomiting associated with migraine (G43.A-)

excessive vomiting in pregnancy (O21.-)

hematemesis (K92.0)

neonatal hematemesis (P54.0)

newborn vomiting (P92.0-)

psychogenic vomiting (F50.89)

vomiting associated with bulimia nervosa (F50.2)

vomiting following gastrointestinal surgery (K91.0)

R11.0 Nausea

Nausea NOS

Nausea without vomiting

R11.1 Vomiting

R11.10 Vomiting, unspecified

Vomiting NOS

R11.11   **Vomiting without nausea**

R11.12   **Projectile vomiting**

R11.13   **Vomiting of fecal matter**

R11.14   **Bilious vomiting**

Bilious emesis

R11.15   **Cyclical vomiting syndrome unrelated to migraine**

Cyclic vomiting syndrome NOS

Persistent vomiting

Excludes1: cyclical vomiting in migraine (G43.A-)

bulimia nervosa (F50.2)

Excludes2: diabetes mellitus due to underlying condition (E08.-)

R11.2   **Nausea with vomiting, unspecified**

Persistent nausea with vomiting NOS

R12   **Heartburn**

Excludes1: dyspepsia NOS (R10.13)

functional dyspepsia (K30)

R13   **Aphagia and dysphagia**

R13.0   **Aphagia**

Inability to swallow

Excludes1: psychogenic aphagia (F50.9)

R13.1   **Dysphagia**

Code first, if applicable, dysphagia following cerebrovascular disease (I69. with final characters -91)

Excludes1: psychogenic dysphagia (F45.8)

R13.10   **Dysphagia, unspecified**

Difficulty in swallowing NOS

R13.11   **Dysphagia, oral phase**

R13.12   **Dysphagia, oropharyngeal phase**

R13.13   **Dysphagia, pharyngeal phase**

R13.14   **Dysphagia, pharyngoesophageal phase**

R13.19   **Other dysphagia**

Cervical dysphagia Neurogenic dysphagia

R14   **Flatulence and related conditions**

Excludes1: psychogenic aerophagy (F45.8)

R14.0   **Abdominal distension (gaseous)**

Bloating

Tympanites (abdominal) (intestinal)

R14.1   **Gas pain**

R14.2   **Eructation**

R14.3   **Flatulence**

R15   **Fecal incontinence**

Includes: encopresis NOS

Excludes1: fecal incontinence of nonorganic origin (F98.1)

R15.0   **Incomplete defecation**

Excludes1: constipation (K59.0-)

fecal impaction (K56.41)

R15.1   **Fecal smearing**

Fecal soiling

R15.2   **Fecal urgency**

R15.9   **Full incontinence of feces**

Fecal incontinence NOS

R16   **Hepatomegaly and splenomegaly, not elsewhere classified**

Definition: Cleft lip is a congenital deformity characterized by a vertical cleft or pair of clefts in the upper lip, with or without involvement of the palate. Cleft palate is a congenital fissure in the roof of the mouth, resulting from incomplete fusion of the palate during embryonic development.

R16.0   **Hepatomegaly, not elsewhere classified**

Hepatomegaly NOS

R16.1   **Splenomegaly, not elsewhere classified**

Splenomegaly NOS

R16.2   **Hepatomegaly with splenomegaly, not elsewhere classified**

Hepatosplenomegaly NOS

R17   **Unspecified jaundice**

Excludes1: neonatal jaundice (P55, P57-P59)

R18   **Ascites**

Includes: fluid in peritoneal cavity

Excludes1: ascites in alcoholic cirrhosis (K70.31)

ascites in alcoholic hepatitis (K70.11)

ascites in toxic liver disease with chronic active hepatitis (K71.51)

R18.0   **Malignant ascites**

Code first malignancy, such as:

malignant neoplasm of ovary (C56.-)

secondary malignant neoplasm of retroperitoneum and peritoneum (C78.6)

R18.8   **Other ascites**

Ascites NOS

Peritoneal effusion (chronic)

R19   **Other symptoms and signs involving the digestive system and abdomen**

Excludes1: acute abdomen (R10.0)

R19.0   **Intra-abdominal and pelvic swelling, mass and lump**

Excludes1: abdominal distension (gaseous) (R14.-)

ascites (R18.-)

R19.00   **Intra-abdominal and pelvic swelling, mass and lump, unspecified site**

R19.01   **Right upper quadrant abdominal swelling, mass and lump**

R19.02   **Left upper quadrant abdominal swelling, mass and lump**

R19.03   **Right lower quadrant abdominal swelling, mass and lump**

R19.04   **Left lower quadrant abdominal swelling, mass and lump**

R19.05   **Periumbilic swelling, mass or lump**

Diffuse or generalized umbilical swelling or mass

R19.06   **Epigastric swelling, mass or lump**

R19.07   **Generalized intra-abdominal and pelvic swelling, mass and lump**

Diffuse or generalized intra-abdominal swelling or mass NOS

Diffuse or generalized pelvic swelling or mass NOS

R19.09   **Other intra-abdominal and pelvic swelling, mass and lump**

R19.1   **Abnormal bowel sounds**

R19.11   **Absent bowel sounds**

R19.12   **Hyperactive bowel sounds**

R19.15   **Other abnormal bowel sounds**

Abnormal bowel sounds NOS

   ● New code   ▲ Revised code   Excludes1: Not coded here   Excludes2: Not included here   ⊗ Placeholder required   ⑦ 7th digit required

R19.2   **Visible peristalsis**

Definition: Peristalsis is the involuntary constriction and relaxation of the muscles of the intestine or another canal, creating wavelike movements that push the contents of the canal forward.

Hyperperistalsis

R19.3   **Abdominal rigidity**

Excludes1: abdominal rigidity with severe abdominal pain (R10.0)

  R19.30   **Abdominal rigidity, unspecified site**

  R19.31   **Right upper quadrant abdominal rigidity**

  R19.32   **Left upper quadrant abdominal rigidity**

  R19.33   **Right lower quadrant abdominal rigidity**

  R19.34   **Left lower quadrant abdominal rigidity**

  R19.35   **Periumbilic abdominal rigidity**

  R19.36   **Epigastric abdominal rigidity**

  R19.37   **Generalized abdominal rigidity**

R19.4   **Change in bowel habit**

Excludes1: constipation (K59.0-)

    functional diarrhea (K59.1)

R19.5   **Other fecal abnormalities**

Abnormal stool color

Bulky stools

Mucus in stools

Occult blood in feces

Occult blood in stools

Excludes1: melena (K92.1)

    neonatal melena (P54.1)

R19.6   **Halitosis**

R19.7   **Diarrhea, unspecified**

Diarrhea NOS

Excludes1: functional diarrhea (K59.1)

    neonatal diarrhea (P78.3)

    psychogenic diarrhea (F45.8)

R19.8   **Other specified symptoms and signs involving the digestive system and abdomen**

SYMPTOMS AND SIGNS INVOLVING THE SKIN AND SUBCUTANEOUS TISSUE (R20-R23)

Excludes2: symptoms relating to breast (N64.4-N64.5)

R20   **Disturbances of skin sensation**

Excludes1: dissociative anesthesia and sensory loss (F44.6)

    psychogenic disturbances (F45.8)

R20.0   **Anesthesia of skin**

R20.1   **Hypoesthesia of skin**

R20.2   **Paresthesia of skin**

Formication

Pins and needles

Tingling skin

Excludes1: acroparesthesia (I73.8)

R20.3   **Hyperesthesia**

R20.8   **Other disturbances of skin sensation**

R20.9   **Unspecified disturbances of skin sensation**

R21   **Rash and other nonspecific skin eruption**

Includes: rash NOS

Excludes1: specified type of rash- code to condition

    vesicular eruption (R23.8)

R22   **Localized swelling, mass and lump of skin and subcutaneous tissue**

Includes: subcutaneous nodules (localized)(superficial)

Excludes1: abnormal findings on diagnostic imaging (R90-R93)

    edema (R60.-)

    enlarged lymph nodes (R59.-) \

    localized adiposity (E65)

    swelling of joint (M25.4-)

R22.0   **Localized swelling, mass and lump, head**

R22.1   **Localized swelling, mass and lump, neck**

R22.2   **Localized swelling, mass and lump, trunk**

Excludes1: intra-abdominal or pelvic mass and lump (R19.0-)

    intra-abdominal or pelvic swelling (R19.0-)

Excludes2: breast mass and lump (N63)

R22.3   **Localized swelling, mass and lump, upper limb**

  R22.30   **Localized swelling, mass and lump, unspecified upper limb**

  R22.31   **Localized swelling, mass and lump, right upper limb**

  R22.32   **Localized swelling, mass and lump, left upper limb**

  R22.33   **Localized swelling, mass and lump, upper limb, bilateral**

R22.4   **Localized swelling, mass and lump, lower limb**

  R22.40   **Localized swelling, mass and lump, unspecified lower limb**

  R22.41   **Localized swelling, mass and lump, right lower limb**

  R22.42   **Localized swelling, mass and lump, left lower limb**

  R22.43   **Localized swelling, mass and lump, lower limb, bilateral**

R22.9   **Localized swelling, mass and lump, unspecified**

R23   **Other skin changes**

R23.0   **Cyanosis**

Excludes1: acrocyanosis (I73.8)

    cyanotic attacks of newborn (P28.2)

R23.1   **Pallor** Clammy skin

R23.2   **Flushing**

Excessive blushing

Code first, if applicable, menopausal and female climacteric states (N95.1)

R23.3   **Spontaneous ecchymoses**

Petechiae

Excludes1: ecchymoses of newborn (P54.5)

    purpura (D69.-)

R23.4   **Changes in skin texture**

Desquamation of skin

Induration of skin

Scaling of skin

Excludes1: epidermal thickening NOS (L85.9)

R23.8   **Other skin changes**

R23.9   **Unspecified skin changes**

SYMPTOMS AND SIGNS INVOLVING THE NERVOUS AND MUSCULOSKELETAL SYSTEMS (R25-R29)

R25   **Abnormal involuntary movements**

Excludes1: specific movement disorders (G20-G26)

stereotyped movement disorders (F98.4)

tic disorders (F95.-)

R25.0 Abnormal head movements

R25.1 Tremor, unspecified

Excludes1: chorea NOS (G25.5)

essential tremor (G25.0)

hysterical tremor (F44.4)

intention tremor (G25.2)

R25.2 Cramp and spasm

Excludes2: carpopedal spasm (R29.0)

charley-horse (M62.831)

infantile spasms (G40.4-)

muscle spasm of back (M62.830)

muscle spasm of calf (M62.831)

R25.3 Fasciculation

Twitching NOS

R25.8 Other abnormal involuntary movements

R25.9 Unspecified abnormal involuntary movements

R26 Abnormalities of gait and mobility

Excludes1: ataxia NOS (R27.0)

hereditary ataxia (G11.-)

locomotor (syphilitic) ataxia (A52.11)

immobility syndrome (paraplegic) (M62.3)

R26.0 Ataxic gait

Staggering gait

R26.1 Paralytic gait

Spastic gait

R26.2 Difficulty in walking, not elsewhere classified

Excludes1: falling (R29.6)

unsteadiness on feet (R26.81)

R26.8 Other abnormalities of gait and mobility

R26.81 Unsteadiness on feet

R26.89 Other abnormalities of gait and mobility

R26.9 Unspecified abnormalities of gait and mobility

R27 Other lack of coordination

Excludes1: ataxic gait (R26.0)

hereditary ataxia (G11.-)

vertigo NOS (R42)

R27.0 Ataxia, unspecified

Excludes1: ataxia following cerebrovascular disease (I69. with final characters -93)

R27.8 Other lack of coordination

R27.9 Unspecified lack of coordination

R29 Other symptoms and signs involving the nervous and musculoskeletal systems

R29.0 Tetany Carpopedal spasm

Excludes1: hysterical tetany (F44.5)

neonatal tetany (P71.3)

parathyroid tetany (E20.9)

post-thyroidectomy tetany (E89.2)

R29.1 Meningismus

R29.2 Abnormal reflex

Excludes2: abnormal pupillary reflex (H57.0)

hyperactive gag reflex (J39.2)

vasovagal reaction or syncope (R55)

R29.3 Abnormal posture

R29.4 Clicking hip

Excludes1: congenital deformities of hip (Q65.-)

R29.5 Transient paralysis

Code first any associated spinal cord injury (S14.0, S14.1-, S24.0, S24.1-, S34.0-, S34.1-)

Excludes1: transient ischemic attack (G45.9)

R29.6 Repeated falls

Falling

Tendency to fall

Excludes2: at risk for falling (Z91.81)

history of falling (Z91.81)

R29.7 National Institutes of Health Stroke Scale (NIHSS) score

Code first the type of cerebral infarction (I63.-)

R29.70 NIHSS score 0-9

R29.700 NIHSS score 0

R29.701 NIHSS score 1

R29.702 NIHSS score 2

R29.703 NIHSS score 3

R29.704 NIHSS score 4

R29.705 NIHSS score 5

R29.706 NIHSS score 6

R29.707 NIHSS score 7

R29.708 NIHSS score 8

R29.709 NIHSS score 9

R29.71 NIHSS score 10-19

R29.710 NIHSS score 10

R29.711 NIHSS score 11

R29.712 NIHSS score 12

R29.713 NIHSS score 13

R29.714 NIHSS score 14

R29.715 NIHSS score 15

R29.716 NIHSS score 16

R29.717 NIHSS score 17

R29.718 NIHSS score 18

R29.719 NIHSS score 19

R29.72 NIHSS score 20-29

R29.720 NIHSS score 20

R29.721 NIHSS score 21

R29.722 NIHSS score 22

R29.723 NIHSS score 23

R29.724 NIHSS score 24

R29.725 NIHSS score 25

R29.726 NIHSS score 26

R29.727 NIHSS score 27

R29.728 NIHSS score 28

R29.729 NIHSS score 29

R29.73 NIHSS score 30-39

R29.730 NIHSS score 30

R29.731 NIHSS score 31

R29.732 NIHSS score 32

R29.733 NIHSS score 33

R29.734 NIHSS score 34

R29.735 NIHSS score 35

R29.736 NIHSS score 36

R29.737 NIHSS score 37

R29.738 NIHSS score 38

R29.739 NIHSS score 39

R29.74 NIHSS score 40-42

R29.740 NIHSS score 40

R29.741 NIHSS score 41

R29.742 NIHSS score 42

R29.8 **Other symptoms and signs involving the nervous and musculoskeletal systems**

R29.81 **Other symptoms and signs involving the nervous system**

R29.810 **Facial weakness**

Facial droop

Excludes1: Bell's palsy (G51.0)

facial weakness following cerebrovascular disease (I69. with final characters -92)

R29.818 **Other symptoms and signs involving the nervous system**

R29.89 **Other symptoms and signs involving the musculoskeletal system**

Excludes2: pain in limb (M79.6-)

R29.890 **Loss of height**

Excludes1: osteoporosis (M80-M81)

R29.891 **Ocular torticollis**

Excludes1: congenital (sternomastoid) torticollis Q68.0

psychogenic torticollis (F45.8)

spasmodic torticollis (G24.3)

torticollis due to birth injury (P15.8)

torticollis NOS M43.6

R29.898 **Other symptoms and signs involving the musculoskeletal system**

R29.9 **Unspecified symptoms and signs involving the nervous and musculoskeletal systems**

R29.90 **Unspecified symptoms and signs involving the nervous system**

R29.91 **Unspecified symptoms and signs involving the musculoskeletal system**

SYMPTOMS AND SIGNS INVOLVING THE GENITOURINARY SYSTEM (R30-R39)

R30 **Pain associated with micturition**

Excludes1: psychogenic pain associated with micturition (F45.8)

R30.0 **Dysuria**

Strangury

R30.1 **Vesical tenesmus**

R30.9 **Painful micturition, unspecified**

Painful urination NOS

R31 **Hematuria**

Excludes1: hematuria included with underlying conditions, such as:

acute cystitis with hematuria (N30.01)

recurrent and persistent hematuria in glomerular diseases (N02.-)

R31.0 **Gross hematuria**

R31.1 **Benign essential microscopic hematuria**

R31.2 **Other microscopic hematuria**

R31.21 **Asymptomatic microscopic hematuria**

AMH

R31.29 **Other microscopic hematuria**

R31.9 **Hematuria, unspecified**

R32 **Unspecified urinary incontinence**

Enuresis NOS

Excludes1: functional urinary incontinence (R39.81)

nonorganic enuresis (F98.0)

stress incontinence and other specified urinary incontinence (N39.3-N39.4-)

urinary incontinence associated with cognitive impairment (R39.81)

R33 **Retention of urine**

Excludes1: psychogenic retention of urine (F45.8)

R33.0 **Drug induced retention of urine**

Use Additional Code for adverse effect, if applicable, to identify drug (T36-T50 with fifth or sixth character 5)

R33.8 **Other retention of urine**

Code first, if applicable, any causal condition, such as:

enlarged prostate (N40.1)

R33.9 **Retention of urine, unspecified**

R34 **Anuria and oliguria**

Excludes1: anuria and oliguria complicating abortion or ectopic or molar pregnancy (O00-O07, O08.4)

anuria and oliguria complicating pregnancy (O26.83-)

anuria and oliguria complicating the puerperium (O90.4)

R35 **Polyuria**

Code first, if applicable, any causal condition, such as:

enlarged prostate (N40.1)

Excludes1: psychogenic polyuria (F45.8)

R35.0 **Frequency of micturition**

R35.1 **Nocturia**

R35.8 **Other polyuria**

• R35.81 **Nocturnal polyuria**

Excludes2: nocturnal enuresis (N39.44)

• R35.89 **Other polyuria**

Polyuria NOS

R36 **Urethral discharge**

R36.0 **Urethral discharge without blood**

R36.1 **Hematospermia**

R36.9 **Urethral discharge, unspecified**

Penile discharge NOS

Urethrorrhea

R37 **Sexual dysfunction, unspecified**

R39 **Other and unspecified symptoms and signs involving the genitourinary system**

R39.0 **Extravasation of urine**

R39.1 **Other difficulties with micturition**

Code first, if applicable, any causal condition, such as:

enlarged prostate (N40.1)

R39.11 **Hesitancy of micturition**

R39.12 **Poor urinary stream**

Weak urinary steam

R39.13 **Splitting of urinary stream**

R39.14 **Feeling of incomplete bladder emptying**

R39.15 **Urgency of urination**

Excludes1: urge incontinence (N39.41, N39.46)

R39.16 **Straining to void**

R39.19 **Other difficulties with micturition**

R39.191　　Need to immediately re-void

R39.192　　Position dependent micturition

R39.198　　Other difficulties with micturition

R39.2　Extrarenal uremia

Prerenal uremia

Excludes1: uremia NOS (N19)

R39.8　Other symptoms and signs involving the genitourinary system

R39.81　Functional urinary incontinence

Urinary incontinence due to cognitive impairment, or severe physical disability or immobility

Excludes1: stress incontinence and other specified

urinary incontinence (N39.3-N39.4-)

urinary incontinence NOS (R32)

R39.82　Chronic bladder pain

R39.83　Unilateral non-palpable testicle

R39.84　Bilateral non-palpable testicles

R39.89　Other symptoms and signs involving the genitourinary system

R39.9　Unspecified symptoms and signs involving the genitourinary system

SYMPTOMS AND SIGNS INVOLVING COGNITION, PERCEPTION, EMOTIONAL STATE AND BEHAVIOR (R40-R46)

Excludes2: symptoms and signs constituting part of a pattern of mental disorder (F01-F99)

R40　Somnolence, stupor and coma

Definition: Somnolence (or "drowsiness") is a state of near-sleep, a strong desire for sleep, or sleeping for unusually long periods (cf. hypersomnia).

Excludes1: neonatal coma (P91.5)

somnolence, stupor and coma in diabetes (E08-E13)

somnolence, stupor and coma in hepatic failure (K72.-)

somnolence, stupor and coma in hypoglycemia (nondiabetic) (E15)

R40.0　Somnolence

Drowsiness

Excludes1: coma (R40.2-)

R40.1　Stupor Catatonic stupor

Semicoma

Excludes1: catatonic schizophrenia (F20.2)

coma (R40.2-)

depressive stupor (F31-F33)

dissociative stupor (F44.2)

manic stupor (F30.2)

R40.2　Coma

Code first any associated:

fracture of skull (S02.-)

intracranial injury (S06.-)

Note: One code from each subcategory, R40.21-R40.23, is required to complete the coma scale

R40.20　Unspecified coma [HCC]

Coma NOS

Unconsciousness NOS

R40.21　Coma scale, eyes open

The following appropriate 7th character is to be added to subcategory R40.21-:

0 - unspecified time

1 - in the field [EMT or ambulance]

2 - at arrival to emergency department

3 - at hospital admission

4 - 24 hours or more after hospital admission

⑦**R40.211　Coma scale, eyes open, never** [HCC]

Coma scale eye opening score of 1

⑦**R40.212　Coma scale, eyes open, to pain** [HCC]

Coma scale eye opening score of 2

⑦**R40.213　Coma scale, eyes open, to sound** [HCC]

Coma scale eye opening score of 3

⑦**R40.214　Coma scale, eyes open, spontaneous** [HCC]

Coma scale eye opening score of 4

R40.22　Coma scale, best verbal response

The following appropriate 7th character is to be added to subcategory R40.22-:

0 - unspecified time

1 - in the field [EMT or ambulance]

2 - at arrival to emergency department

3 - at hospital admission

4 - 24 hours or more after hospital admission

⑦**R40.221　Coma scale, best verbal response, none** [HCC]

Coma scale verbal score of 1

⑦**R40.222　Coma scale, best verbal response, incomprehensible words** [HCC]

Coma scale verbal score of 2

Incomprehensible sounds (2-5 years of age)

Moans/grunts to pain; restless (<2 years old)

⑦**R40.223　Coma scale, best verbal response, inappropriate words** [HCC]

Coma scale verbal score of 3

Inappropriate crying or screaming (< 2 years of age)

Screaming (2-5 years of age)

⑦**R40.224　Coma scale, best verbal response, confused conversation** [HCC]

Coma scale verbal score of 4

Inappropriate words (2-5 years of age)

Irritable cries (< 2 years of age)

⑦**R40.225　Coma scale, best verbal response, oriented** [HCC]

Coma scale verbal score of 5

Cooing or babbling or crying appropriately (< 2 years of age)

Uses appropriate words (2- 5 years of age)

R40.23　Coma scale, best motor response

The following appropriate 7th character is to be added to subcategory R40.23-:

0 - unspecified time

1 - in the field [EMT or ambulance]

2 - at arrival to emergency department

3 - at hospital admission

4 - 24 hours or more after hospital admission

⑦**R40.231　Coma scale, best motor response, none** [HCC]

Coma scale motor score of 1

● New code　▲ Revised code　**Excludes1:** Not coded here　**Excludes2:** Not included here　⊗ Placeholder required　⑦7th digit required

⑦**R40.232 Coma scale, best motor response, extension** [HCC]

Abnormal extensor posturing to pain or noxious stimuli (< 2 years of age)

Extensor posturing to pain or noxious stimuli (2-5 years of age)

Coma scale motor score of 2

R40.233 Coma scale, best motor response, abnormal flexion [HCC]

Coma scale motor score of 3

Abnormal flexure posturing to pain or noxious stimuli (2-5 years of age)

Flexion/decorticate posturing (< 2 years of age)

⑦**R40.234 Coma scale, best motor response, flexion withdrawal** [HCC]

Coma scale motor score of 4

Withdraws from pain or noxious stimuli (2-5 years of age)

⑦**R40.235 Coma scale, best motor response, localizes pain** [HCC]

Coma scale motor score of 5

Localizes pain (2-5 years of age)

Withdraws to touch (< 2 years of age)

⑦**R40.236 Coma scale, best motor response, obeys commands** [HCC]

Coma scale motor score of 6

Normal or spontaneous movement (< 2 years of age)

Obeys commands (2-5 years of age)

R40.24 Glasgow coma scale, total score

Note: Assign a code from subcategory R40.24, when only the total coma score is documented

The following appropriate 7th character is to be added to subcategory R40.24-:

0 - unspecified time

1 - in the field [EMT or ambulance]

2 - at arrival to emergency department

3 - at hospital admission

4 - 24 hours or more after hospital admission

⑦**R40.241 Glasgow coma scale score 13-15**

⑦**R40.242 Glasgow coma scale score 9-12**

⑦**R40.243 Glasgow coma scale score 3-8** [HCC]

⑦**R40.244 Other coma, without documented Glasgow coma scale score, or with partial score reported** [HCC]

R40.3 Persistent vegetative state [HCC]

R40.4 Transient alteration of awareness

R41 Other symptoms and signs involving cognitive functions and awareness

Excludes1: dissociative [conversion] disorders (F44.-)

mild cognitive impairment, so stated (G31.84)

R41.0 Disorientation, unspecified

Confusion NOS

Delirium NOS

R41.1 Anterograde amnesia

R41.2 Retrograde amnesia

R41.3 Other amnesia

Amnesia NOS

Memory loss NOS

Excludes1: amnestic disorder due to known physiologic condition (F04)

amnestic syndrome due to psychoactive substance use (F10-F19 with 5th character .6)

mild memory disturbance due to known physiological condition (F06.8)

transient global amnesia (G45.4)

R41.4 Neurologic neglect syndrome

Asomatognosia

Hemi-akinesia

Hemi-inattention

Hemispatial neglect

Left-sided neglect

Sensory neglect

Visuospatial neglect

Excludes1: visuospatial deficit (R41.842)

R41.8 Other symptoms and signs involving cognitive functions and awareness

R41.81 Age-related cognitive decline

Senility NOS

R41.82 Altered mental status, unspecified

Change in mental status NOS

Excludes1: altered level of consciousness (R40.-)

altered mental status due to known condition - code to condition delirium NOS (R41.0)

R41.83 Borderline intellectual functioning

IQ level 71 to 84

Excludes1: intellectual disabilities (F70-F79)

R41.84 Other specified cognitive deficit

Excludes1: cognitive deficits as sequelae of cerebrovascular disease (I69.01-, I69.11-, I69.21-, I69.31-, I69.81-, I69.91-)

R41.840 Attention and concentration deficit

Excludes1: attention-deficit hyperactivity disorders (F90.-)

R41.841 Cognitive communication deficit

R41.842 Visuospatial deficit

R41.843 Psychomotor deficit

R41.844 Frontal lobe and executive function deficit

R41.89 Other symptoms and signs involving cognitive functions and awareness

Anosognosia

R41.9 Unspecified symptoms and signs involving cognitive functions and awareness

Unspecified neurocognitive disorder

R42 Dizziness and giddiness

Light-headedness

Vertigo NOS

Excludes1: vertiginous syndromes (H81.-)

vertigo from infrasound (T75.23)

R43 Disturbances of smell and taste

R43.0 Anosmia

R43.1 Parosmia

R43.2 Parageusia

R43.8 Other disturbances of smell and taste

Mixed disturbance of smell and taste

Add 4th-7th digits   Nonspecific code   Unspecified code   Manifestation code   [HCC] Hierarchical Condition Code

R43.9   **Unspecified disturbances of smell and taste**

R44   **Other symptoms and signs involving general sensations and perceptions**

    Excludes1: alcoholic hallucinations (F10.151, F10.251, F10.951)

        hallucinations in drug psychosis (F11-F19 with fifth to sixth characters 51)

        hallucinations in mood disorders with psychotic symptoms (F30.2, F31.5, F32.3, F33.3)

        hallucinations in schizophrenia, schizotypal and delusional disorders (F20-F29)

    Excludes2: disturbances of skin sensation (R20.-)

R44.0   **Auditory hallucinations**

R44.1   **Visual hallucinations**

R44.2   **Other hallucinations**

R44.3   **Hallucinations, unspecified**

R44.8   **Other symptoms and signs involving general sensations and perceptions**

R44.9   **Unspecified symptoms and signs involving general sensations and perceptions**

R45   **Symptoms and signs involving emotional state**

R45.0   **Nervousness**

    Nervous tension

R45.1   **Restlessness and agitation**

R45.2   **Unhappiness**

R45.3   **Demoralization and apathy**

    Excludes1: anhedonia (R45.84)

R45.4   **Irritability and anger**

R45.5   **Hostility**

R45.6   **Violent behavior**

R45.7   **State of emotional shock and stress, unspecified**

R45.8   **Other symptoms and signs involving emotional state**

    R45.81   **Low self-esteem**

    R45.82   **Worries**

    R45.83   **Excessive crying of child, adolescent or adult**

        Excludes1: excessive crying of infant (baby) R68.11

    R45.84   **Anhedonia**

    R45.85   **Homicidal and suicidal ideations**

        Excludes1: suicide attempt (T14.91)

        R45.850   **Homicidal ideations**

        R45.851   **Suicidal ideations**

    R45.86   **Emotional lability**

    R45.87   **Impulsiveness**

    ● **R45.88**   **Nonsuicidal self-harm**

        Nonsuicidal self-injury

        Nonsuicidal self-mutilation

        Self-inflicted injury without suicidal intent

        Code also injury, if known

    R45.89   **Other symptoms and signs involving emotional state**

R46   **Symptoms and signs involving appearance and behavior**

    Excludes1: appearance and behavior in schizophrenia, schizotypal and delusional disorders (F20-F29)

        mental and behavioral disorders (F01-F99)

R46.0   **Very low level of personal hygiene**

R46.1   **Bizarre personal appearance**

R46.2   **Strange and inexplicable behavior**

R46.3   **Overactivity**

R46.4   **Slowness and poor responsiveness**

    Excludes1: stupor (R40.1)

R46.5   **Suspiciousness and marked evasiveness**

R46.6   **Undue concern and preoccupation with stressful events**

R46.7   **Verbosity and circumstantial detail obscuring reason for contact**

R46.8   **Other symptoms and signs involving appearance and behavior**

    R46.81   **Obsessive-compulsive behavior**

        Excludes1: obsessive-compulsive disorder (F42.-)

    R46.89   **Other symptoms and signs involving appearance and behavior**

SYMPTOMS AND SIGNS INVOLVING SPEECH AND VOICE (R47-R49)

R47   **Speech disturbances, not elsewhere classified**

    Excludes1: autism (F84.0)

        cluttering (F80.81)

        specific developmental disorders of speech and language (F80.-)

        stuttering (F80.81)

R47.0   **Dysphasia and aphasia**

    R47.01   **Aphasia**

        Excludes1: aphasia following cerebrovascular disease (I69. with final characters -20) progressive isolated aphasia (G31.01)

    R47.02   **Dysphasia**

        Excludes1: dysphasia following cerebrovascular disease (I69. with final characters -21)

R47.1   **Dysarthria and anarthria**

    Excludes1: dysarthria following cerebrovascular disease (I69. with final characters -22)

R47.8   **Other speech disturbances**

    Excludes1: dysarthria following cerebrovascular disease (I69. with final characters -28)

    R47.81   **Slurred speech**

    R47.82   **Fluency disorder in conditions classified elsewhere**

        Stuttering in conditions classified elsewhere

        Code first underlying disease or condition, such as:

        Parkinson's disease (G20)

        Excludes1: adult onset fluency disorder (F98.5)

            childhood onset fluency disorder (F80.81)

            fluency disorder (stuttering) following cerebrovascular disease (I69. with final characters -23)

    R47.89   **Other speech disturbances**

R47.9   **Unspecified speech disturbances**

R48   **Dyslexia and other symbolic dysfunctions, not elsewhere classified**

    Definition: Dyslexia is a general term for disorders that involve difficulty in learning to read or interpret words, letters, and other symbols, but that do not affect general intelligence.

    Excludes1: specific developmental disorders of scholastic skills (F81.-)

R48.0   **Dyslexia and alexia**

R48.1   **Agnosia**

Astereognosia (astereognosis)

Autotopagnosia

Excludes1: visual object agnosia (R48.3)

R48.2 Apraxia

Excludes1: apraxia following cerebrovascular disease (I69. with final characters -90)

R48.3 Visual agnosia

Prosopagnosia

Simultanagnosia (asimultagnosia)

R48.8 Other symbolic dysfunctions

Acalculia

Agraphia

R48.9 Unspecified symbolic dysfunctions

R49 Voice and resonance disorders

Excludes1: psychogenic voice and resonance disorders (F44.4)

R49.0 Dysphonia

Hoarseness

R49.1 Aphonia

Loss of voice

R49.2 Hypernasality and hyponasality

R49.21 Hypernasality

R49.22 Hyponasality

R49.8 Other voice and resonance disorders

R49.9 Unspecified voice and resonance disorder

Change in voice NOS Resonance disorder NOS

GENERAL SYMPTOMS AND SIGNS (R50-R69)

R50 Fever of other and unknown origin

Excludes1: chills without fever (R68.83)

febrile convulsions (R56.0-)

fever of unknown origin during labor (O75.2)

fever of unknown origin in newborn (P81.9)

hypothermia due to illness (R68.0)

malignant hyperthermia due to anesthesia (T88.3)

puerperal pyrexia NOS (O86.4)

R50.2 Drug induced fever

Use Additional Code for adverse effect, if applicable, to identify drug (T36-T50 with fifth or sixth character 5)

Excludes1: postvaccination (postimmunization) fever (R50.83)

R50.8 Other specified fever

R50.81 Fever presenting with conditions classified elsewhere

Code first underlying condition when associated fever is present, such as with:

leukemia (C91-C95)

neutropenia (D70.-)

sickle-cell disease (D57.-)

R50.82 Postprocedural fever

Excludes1: postprocedural infection (T81.4-)

posttransfusion fever (R50.84)

postvaccination (postimmunization) fever (R50.83)

R50.83 Postvaccination fever

Postimmunization fever

R50.84 Febrile nonhemolytic transfusion reaction

FNHTR Posttransfusion fever

R50.9 Fever, unspecified

Fever NOS

Fever of unknown origin [FUO]

Fever with chills

Fever with rigors

Hyperpyrexia NOS

Persistent fever

Pyrexia NOS

R51 Headache

Facial pain NOS

Excludes2: atypical face pain (G50.1)

migraine and other headache syndromes (G43-G44)

trigeminal neuralgia (G50.0)

R51.0 Headache with orthostatic component, not elsewhere classified

Headache with positional component, not elsewhere classified

R51.9 Headache, unspecified

Facial pain NOS

R52 Pain, unspecified

Acute pain NOS

Generalized pain NOS

Pain NOS

Excludes1: acute and chronic pain, not elsewhere classified (G89.-)

localized pain, unspecified type - code to pain by site, such as: abdomen pain (R10.-)

back pain (M54.9)

breast pain (N64.4)

chest pain (R07.1-R07.9)

ear pain (H92.0-)

eye pain (H57.1)

headache (R51.9)

joint pain (M25.5-)

limb pain (M79.6-)

lumbar region pain (M54.5-)

pelvic and perineal pain (R10.2)

shoulder pain (M25.51-)

spine pain (M54.-)

throat pain (R07.0)

tongue pain (K14.6)

tooth pain (K08.8)

renal colic (N23)

pain disorders exclusively related to psychological factors (F45.41)

R53 Malaise and fatigue

R53.0 Neoplastic (malignant) related fatigue

Code first associated neoplasm

R53.1 Weakness

Asthenia NOS

Excludes1: age-related weakness (R54)

muscle weakness (generalized) (M62.81)

sarcopenia (M62.84)

senile asthenia (R54)

R53.2 Functional quadriplegia [HCC]

Complete immobility due to severe physical disability or frailty

Excludes1: frailty NOS (R54)

hysterical paralysis (F44.4)

immobility syndrome (M62.3)

neurologic quadriplegia (G82.5-)

quadriplegia (G82.50)

R53.8   Other malaise and fatigue

Excludes1: combat exhaustion and fatigue (F43.0)

congenital debility (P96.9)

exhaustion and fatigue due to excessive exertion (T73.3)

exhaustion and fatigue due to exposure (T73.2)

exhaustion and fatigue due to heat (T67.-)

exhaustion and fatigue due to pregnancy (O26.8-)

exhaustion and fatigue due to recurrent depressive episode (F33)

exhaustion and fatigue due to depressive episode (F32.-)

R53.81   Other malaise

Chronic debility

Debility NOS

General physical deterioration

Malaise NOS

Nervous debility

Excludes1: age-related physical debility (R54)

R53.82   Chronic fatigue, unspecified

Chronic fatigue syndrome NOS

Excludes1: postviral fatigue syndrome (G93.3)

R53.83   Other fatigue

Excludes2: exhaustion and fatigue due to depressive episode (F32.-)

Fatigue NOS

Lack of energy

Lethargy

Tiredness

R54   Age-related physical debility

Frailty

Old age

Senescence

Senile asthenia

Senile debility

Excludes1: age-related cognitive decline (R41.81)

sarcopenia (M62.84)

senile psychosis (F03)

senility NOS (R41.81)

R55   Syncope and collapse

Blackout

Fainting

Vasovagal attack

Excludes1: cardiogenic shock (R57.0)

carotid sinus syncope (G90.01) heat syncope (T67.1)

neurocirculatory asthenia (F45.8)

neurogenic orthostatic hypotension (G90.3)

orthostatic hypotension (I95.1)

postprocedural shock (T81.1-)

psychogenic syncope (F48.8)

shock NOS (R57.9)

shock complicating or following abortion or ectopic or molar pregnancy (O00-O07, O08.3)

shock complicating or following labor and delivery (O75.1)

Stokes-Adams attack (I45.9)

unconsciousness NOS (R40.2-)

R56   Convulsions, not elsewhere classified

Excludes1: dissociative convulsions and seizures (F44.5)

epileptic convulsions and seizures (G40.-)

newborn convulsions and seizures (P90)

R56.0   Febrile convulsions

R56.00   Simple febrile convulsions [HCC]

Febrile convulsion NOS

Febrile seizure NOS

R56.01   Complex febrile convulsions [HCC]

Atypical febrile seizure

Complex febrile seizure

Complicated febrile seizure

Excludes1: status epilepticus (G40.901)

R56.1   Post traumatic seizures [HCC]

Excludes1: post traumatic epilepsy (G40.-)

R56.9   Unspecified convulsions [HCC]

Convulsion disorder

Fit NOS

Recurrent convulsions

Seizure(s) (convulsive) NOS

R57   Shock, not elsewhere classified

Excludes1: anaphylactic shock NOS (T78.2)

anaphylactic reaction or shock due to adverse food reaction (T78.0-)

anaphylactic shock due to adverse effect of correct drug or medicament properly administered (T88.6)

anaphylactic shock due to serum (T80.5-)

electric shock (T75.4)

obstetric shock (O75.1)

postprocedural shock (T81.1-)

psychic shock (F43.0)

shock complicating or following ectopic or molar pregnancy (O00-O07, O08.3)

shock due to anesthesia (T88.2)

shock due to lightning (T75.01)

traumatic shock (T79.4)

toxic shock syndrome (A48.3)

R57.0   Cardiogenic shock [HCC]

Excludes2: septic shock (R65.21)

R57.1   Hypovolemic shock [HCC]

R57.8   Other shock [HCC]

R57.9   Shock, unspecified [HCC]

Failure of peripheral circulation NOS

R58   Hemorrhage, not elsewhere classified

Hemorrhage NOS

Excludes1: hemorrhage included with underlying conditions, such as:

acute duodenal ulcer with hemorrhage (K26.0)

acute gastritis with bleeding (K29.01)

ulcerative enterocolitis with rectal bleeding (K51.01)

R59   Enlarged lymph nodes

Includes: swollen glands

Excludes1: lymphadenitis NOS (I88.9)

acute lymphadenitis (L04.-)

chronic lymphadenitis (I88.1)

mesenteric (acute) (chronic) lymphadenitis (I88.0)

R59.0 Localized enlarged lymph nodes

R59.1 Generalized enlarged lymph nodes

Lymphadenopathy NOS

R59.9 Enlarged lymph nodes, unspecified

R60 Edema, not elsewhere classified

Excludes1: angioneurotic edema (T78.3)

ascites (R18.-)

cerebral edema (G93.6)

cerebral edema due to birth injury (P11.0)

edema of larynx (J38.4)

edema of nasopharynx (J39.2)

edema of pharynx (J39.2)

gestational edema (O12.0-)

hereditary edema (Q82.0)

hydrops fetalis NOS (P83.2)

hydrothorax (J94.8)

hydrops fetalis NOS (P83.2)

newborn edema (P83.3)

pulmonary edema (J81.-)

R60.0 Localized edema

R60.1 Generalized edema

Excludes2: nutritional edema (E40-E46)

R60.9 Edema, unspecified

Fluid retention NOS

R61 Generalized hyperhidrosis

Excessive sweating Night sweats

Secondary hyperhidrosis

Code first, if applicable, menopausal and female climacteric states (N95.1)

Excludes1: focal (primary) (secondary) hyperhidrosis (L74.5-)

Frey's syndrome (L74.52)

localized (primary) (secondary) hyperhidrosis (L74.5-)

R62 Lack of expected normal physiological development in childhood and adults

Excludes1: delayed puberty (E30.0)

gonadal dysgenesis (Q99.1)

hypopituitarism (E23.0)

R62.0 Delayed milestone in childhood

Delayed attainment of expected physiological developmental stage

Late talker

Late walker

R62.5 Other and unspecified lack of expected normal physiological development in childhood

Excludes1: HIV disease resulting in failure to thrive (B20)

physical retardation due to malnutrition (E45)

R62.50 Unspecified lack of expected normal physiological development in childhood

Infantilism NOS

R62.51 Failure to thrive (child)

Failure to gain weight

Excludes1: failure to thrive in child under 28 days old (P92.6)

R62.52 Short stature (child)

Lack of growth

Physical retardation

Short stature NOS

Excludes1: short stature due to endocrine disorder (E34.3)

R62.59 Other lack of expected normal physiological development in childhood

R62.7 Adult failure to thrive

R63 Symptoms and signs concerning food and fluid intake

Excludes1: bulimia NOS (F50.2)

R63.0 Anorexia

Loss of appetite

Excludes1: anorexia nervosa (F50.0-)

loss of appetite of nonorganic origin (F50.89)

R63.1 Polydipsia

Excessive thirst

R63.2 Polyphagia

Excessive eating

Hyperalimentation NOS

R63.3 Feeding difficulties

Excludes2: eating disorders (F50.-)

feeding problems of newborn (P92.-)

infant feeding disorder of nonorganic origin (F98.2-)

- **R63.30 Feeding difficulties, unspecified**

- **R63.31 Pediatric feeding disorder, acute**

Pediatric feeding dysfunction, acute

Code also, if applicable, associated conditions such as:

dysphagia (R13.1-)

gastro-esophageal reflux disease (K21.-)

malnutrition (E40-E46)

- **R63.32 Pediatric feeding disorder, chronic**

Pediatric feeding dysfunction, chronic

Code also, if applicable, associated conditions such as:

aspiration pneumonia (J69.0)

dysphagia (R13.1-)

gastro-esophageal reflux disease (K21.-)

malnutrition (E40-E46)

- **R63.39 Other feeding difficulties**

Feeding problem (elderly) (infant) NOS

Picky eater

R63.4 Abnormal weight loss

R63.5 Abnormal weight gain

Excludes1: excessive weight gain in pregnancy (O26.0-)

obesity (E66.-)

R63.6 Underweight

Use Additional Code to identify body mass index (BMI), if known (Z68.-)

Excludes1: abnormal weight loss (R63.4)

anorexia nervosa (F50.0-)

malnutrition (E40-E46)

R63.8 Other symptoms and signs concerning food and fluid intake

R64 Cachexia [HCC]

Wasting syndrome

Code first underlying condition, if known

Excludes1: abnormal weight loss (R63.4)

nutritional marasmus (E41)

R65 Symptoms and signs specifically associated with systemic inflammation and infection

R65.1 Systemic inflammatory response syndrome (SIRS) of non-infectious origin

Code first underlying condition, such as:

heatstroke (T67.0-)

injury and trauma (S00-T88)

Excludes1: sepsis- code to infection

severe sepsis (R65.2)

R65.10 Systemic inflammatory response syndrome (SIRS) of non-infectious origin without acute organ dysfunction [HCC]

Systemic inflammatory response syndrome (SIRS) NOS

R65.11 Systemic inflammatory response syndrome (SIRS) of non-infectious origin with acute organ dysfunction [HCC]

Use Additional Code to identify specific acute organ dysfunction, such as:

acute kidney failure (N17.-)

acute respiratory failure (J96.0-)

critical illness myopathy (G72.81)

critical illness polyneuropathy (G62.81)

disseminated intravascular coagulopathy [DIC] (D65)

encephalopathy (metabolic) (septic) (G93.41)

hepatic failure (K72.0-)

R65.2 Severe sepsis

Infection with associated acute organ dysfunction

Sepsis with acute organ dysfunction

Sepsis with multiple organ dysfunction

Systemic inflammatory response syndrome due to infectious process with acute organ dysfunction

Code first underlying infection, such as:

infection following a procedure (T81.4-)

infections following infusion, transfusion and therapeutic injection (T80.2-)

puerperal sepsis (O85)

sepsis following complete or unspecified spontaneous abortion (O03.87)

sepsis following ectopic and molar pregnancy (O08.82)

sepsis following incomplete spontaneous abortion (O03.37)

sepsis following (induced) termination of pregnancy (O04.87)

sepsis NOS (A41.9)

Use Additional Code to identify specific acute organ dysfunction, such as:

acute kidney failure (N17.-)

acute respiratory failure (J96.0-)

critical illness myopathy (G72.81)

critical illness polyneuropathy (G62.81)

disseminated intravascular coagulopathy [DIC] (D65)

encephalopathy (metabolic) (septic) (G93.41)

hepatic failure (K72.0-)

R65.20 Severe sepsis without septic shock [HCC]

Severe sepsis NOS

R65.21 Severe sepsis with septic shock [HCC]

R68 Other general symptoms and signs

R68.0 Hypothermia, not associated with low environmental temperature

Excludes1: hypothermia NOS (accidental) (T68)

hypothermia due to anesthesia (T88.51)

hypothermia due to low environmental temperature (T68)

newborn hypothermia (P80.-)

R68.1 Nonspecific symptoms peculiar to infancy

Excludes1: colic, infantile (R10.83)

neonatal cerebral irritability (P91.3)

teething syndrome (K00.7)

R68.11 Excessive crying of infant (baby)

Excludes1: excessive crying of child, adolescent, or adult (R45.83)

R68.12 Fussy infant (baby)

Irritable infant

R68.13 Apparent life-threatening event in infant (ALTE)

Apparent life-threatening event in newborn

Code first confirmed diagnosis, if known

Use Additional Code(s) for associated signs and symptoms if no confirmed diagnosis established, or if signs and symptoms are not associated routinely with confirmed diagnosis, or provide additional information for cause of ALTE

R68.19 Other nonspecific symptoms peculiar to infancy

R68.2 Dry mouth, unspecified

Excludes1: dry mouth due to dehydration (E86.0)

dry mouth due to Sjögren syndrome (M35.0-)

salivary gland hyposecretion (K11.7)

R68.3 Clubbing of fingers

Clubbing of nails

Excludes1: congenital club finger (Q68.1)

R68.8 Other general symptoms and signs

R68.81 Early satiety

R68.82 Decreased libido

Decreased sexual desire

R68.83 Chills (without fever)

Chills NOS

Excludes1: chills with fever (R50.9)

R68.84 Jaw pain

Mandibular pain

Maxilla pain

Excludes1: temporomandibular joint arthralgia (M26.62-)

R68.89 Other general symptoms and signs

R69 Illness, unspecified

Unknown and unspecified cases of morbidity

ABNORMAL FINDINGS ON EXAMINATION OF BLOOD, WITHOUT DIAGNOSIS (R70-R79)

Excludes2: abnormal findings on antenatal screening of mother (O28.-)

abnormalities of lipids (E78.-)

abnormalities of platelets and thrombocytes (D69.-)

abnormalities of white blood cells classified elsewhere (D70-D72)

coagulation hemorrhagic disorders (D65-D68)

diagnostic abnormal findings classified elsewhere - see Alphabetical Index hemorrhagic and hematological disorders of newborn (P50-P61)

R70 **Elevated erythrocyte sedimentation rate and abnormality of plasma viscosity**

    R70.0 **Elevated erythrocyte sedimentation rate**

    R70.1 **Abnormal plasma viscosity**

R71 **Abnormality of red blood cells**

    Excludes1: anemias (D50-D64)

        anemia of premature infant (P61.2)

        benign (familial) polycythemia (D75.0)

        congenital anemias (P61.2-P61.4)

        newborn anemia due to isoimmunization (P55.-)

        polycythemia neonatorum (P61.1)

        polycythemia NOS (D75.1)

        polycythemia vera (D45) secondary polycythemia (D75.1)

    R71.0 **Precipitous drop in hematocrit**

        Drop (precipitous) in hemoglobin

        Drop in hematocrit

    R71.8 **Other abnormality of red blood cells**

        Abnormal red-cell morphology NOS

        Abnormal red-cell volume NOS

        Anisocytosis

        Poikilocytosis

R73 **Elevated blood glucose level**

    Excludes1: diabetes mellitus (E08-E13)

        diabetes mellitus in pregnancy, childbirth and the puerperium (O24.-)

        neonatal disorders (P70.0-P70.2)

        postsurgical hypoinsulinemia (E89.1)

    R73.0 **Abnormal glucose**

        Excludes1: abnormal glucose in pregnancy (O99.81-)

            diabetes mellitus (E08-E13)

            dysmetabolic syndrome X (E88.81)

            gestational diabetes (O24.4-)

            glycosuria (R81)

            hypoglycemia (E16.2)

        R73.01 **Impaired fasting glucose**

            Elevated fasting glucose

        R73.02 **Impaired glucose tolerance (oral)**

            Elevated glucose tolerance

        R73.03 **Prediabetes**

            Latent diabetes

        R73.09 **Other abnormal glucose**

            Abnormal glucose NOS

            Abnormal non-fasting glucose tolerance

    R73.9 **Hyperglycemia, unspecified**

R74 **Abnormal serum enzyme levels**

    R74.0 **Nonspecific elevation of levels of transaminase and lactic acid dehydrogenase [LDH]**

        R74.01 **Elevation of levels of liver transaminase levels**

            Elevation of levels of alanine transaminase (ALT)

            Elevation of levels of aspartate transaminase (AST)

        R74.02 **Elevation of levels of lactic acid dehydrogenase [LDH]**

    R74.8 **Abnormal levels of other serum enzymes**

        Abnormal level of acid phosphatase

        Abnormal level of alkaline phosphatase

        Abnormal level of amylase

        Abnormal level of lipase [triacylglycerol lipase]

    R74.9 **Abnormal serum enzyme level, unspecified**

R75 **Inconclusive laboratory evidence of human immunodeficiency virus [HIV]**

    Nonconclusive HIV-test finding in infants

    Excludes1: asymptomatic human immunodeficiency virus [HIV] infection status (Z21)

        human immunodeficiency virus [HIV] disease (B20)

R76 **Other abnormal immunological findings in serum**

    R76.0 **Raised antibody titer**

        Excludes1: isoimmunization in pregnancy (O36.0-O36.1)

            isoimmunization affecting newborn (P55.-)

    R76.1 **Nonspecific reaction to test for tuberculosis**

        R76.11 **Nonspecific reaction to tuberculin skin test without active tuberculosis**

            Abnormal result of Mantoux test

            PPD positive

            Tuberculin (skin test) positive

            Tuberculin (skin test) reactor

            Excludes1: nonspecific reaction to cell mediated immunity measurement of gamma interferon antigen response without active tuberculosis (R76.12)

        R76.12 **Nonspecific reaction to cell mediated immunity measurement of gamma interferon antigen response without active tuberculosis**

            Nonspecific reaction to QuantiFERON-TB test (QFT) without active tuberculosis

            Excludes1: nonspecific reaction to tuberculin skin test without active tuberculosis (R76.11)

                positive tuberculin skin test (R76.11)

    R76.8 **Other specified abnormal immunological findings in serum**

        Raised level of immunoglobulins NOS

    R76.9 **Abnormal immunological finding in serum, unspecified**

R77 **Other abnormalities of plasma proteins**

    Excludes1: disorders of plasma-protein metabolism (E88.0-)

    R77.0 **Abnormality of albumin**

    R77.1 **Abnormality of globulin**

        Hyperglobulinemia NOS

    R77.2 **Abnormality of alphafetoprotein**

    R77.8 **Other specified abnormalities of plasma proteins**

    R77.9 **Abnormality of plasma protein, unspecified**

R78 **Findings of drugs and other substances, not normally found in blood**

    Use Additional Code to identify the any retained foreign body, if applicable (Z18.-)

    Excludes1: mental or behavioral disorders due to psychoactive substance use (F10-F19)

    R78.0 **Finding of alcohol in blood**

        Use additional external cause code (Y90.-), for detail regarding alcohol level.

    R78.1 **Finding of opiate drug in blood**

    R78.2 **Finding of cocaine in blood**

    R78.3 **Finding of hallucinogen in blood**

R78.4   Finding of other drugs of addictive potential in blood

R78.5   Finding of other psychotropic drug in blood

R78.6   Finding of steroid agent in blood

R78.7   Finding of abnormal level of heavy metals in blood

     R78.71   Abnormal lead level in blood

         Excludes1: lead poisoning (T56.0-)

     R78.79   Finding of abnormal level of heavy metals in blood

R78.8   Finding of other specified substances, not normally found in blood

     R78.81   Bacteremia

         Excludes1: sepsis-code to specified infection

     R78.89   Finding of other specified substances, not normally found in blood

         Finding of abnormal level of lithium in blood

R78.9   Finding of unspecified substance, not normally found in blood

R79   **Other abnormal findings of blood chemistry**

Use Additional Code to identify any retained foreign body, if applicable (Z18.-)

Excludes1: asymptomatic hyperuricemia (E79.0)

     hyperglycemia NOS (R73.9) hypoglycemia NOS (E16.2)

     neonatal hypoglycemia (P70.3-P70.4)

     specific findings indicating disorder of amino-acid metabolism (E70-E72)

     specific findings indicating disorder of carbohydrate metabolism (E73-E74)

     specific findings indicating disorder of lipid metabolism (E75.-)

R79.0   Abnormal level of blood mineral

     Abnormal blood level of cobalt

     Abnormal blood level of copper

     Abnormal blood level of iron

     Abnormal blood level of magnesium

     Abnormal blood level of mineral NEC

     Abnormal blood level of zinc

     Excludes1: abnormal level of lithium (R78.89)

         disorders of mineral metabolism (E83.-)

         neonatal hypomagnesemia (P71.2)

         nutritional mineral deficiency (E58-E61)

R79.1   Abnormal coagulation profile

     Abnormal or prolonged bleeding time

     Abnormal or prolonged coagulation time

     Abnormal or prolonged partial thromboplastin time [PTT]

     Abnormal or prolonged prothrombin time [PT]

     Excludes1: coagulation defects (D68.-)

     Excludes2: abnormality of fluid, electrolyte or acid-base balance (E86-E87)

R79.8   Other specified abnormal findings of blood chemistry

     R79.81   Abnormal blood-gas level

     R79.82   Elevated C-reactive protein (CRP)

     ● **R79.83**   Abnormal findings of blood amino-acid level

     R79.89   Other specified abnormal findings of blood chemistry

R79.9   Abnormal finding of blood chemistry, unspecified

ABNORMAL FINDINGS ON EXAMINATION OF URINE, WITHOUT DIAGNOSIS (R80-R82)

Excludes1: abnormal findings on antenatal screening of mother (O28.-)

     diagnostic abnormal findings classified elsewhere - see Alphabetical Index

     specific findings indicating disorder of amino-acid metabolism (E70-E72)

     specific findings indicating disorder of carbohydrate metabolism (E73-E74)

R80   **Proteinuria**

Excludes1: gestational proteinuria (O12.1-)

R80.0   Isolated proteinuria

     Idiopathic proteinuria

     Excludes1: isolated proteinuria with specific morphological lesion (N06.-)

R80.1   Persistent proteinuria, unspecified

R80.2   Orthostatic proteinuria, unspecified

     Postural proteinuria

R80.3   Bence Jones proteinuria

R80.8   Other proteinuria

R80.9   Proteinuria, unspecified

     Albuminuria NOS

R81   **Glycosuria**

Excludes1: renal glycosuria (E74.818)

R82   **Other and unspecified abnormal findings in urine**

Includes: chromoabnormalities in urine

Use Additional Code to identify any retained foreign body, if applicable (Z18.-)

Excludes2: hematuria (R31.-)

R82.0   Chyluria

     Excludes1: filarial chyluria (B74.-)

R82.1   Myoglobinuria

R82.2   Biliuria

R82.3   Hemoglobinuria

     Excludes1: hemoglobinuria due to hemolysis from external causes NEC (D59.6)

         hemoglobinuria due to paroxysmal nocturnal [Marchiafava-Micheli] (D59.5)

R82.4   Acetonuria

     Ketonuria

R82.5   Elevated urine levels of drugs, medicaments and biological substances

     Elevated urine levels of catecholamines

     Elevated urine levels of indoleacetic acid

     Elevated urine levels of 17-ketosteroids

     Elevated urine levels of steroids

R82.6   Abnormal urine levels of substances chiefly nonmedicinal as to source

     Abnormal urine level of heavy metals

R82.7   Abnormal findings on microbiological examination of urine

     Excludes1: colonization status (Z22.-)

     R82.71   Bacteriuria

     R82.79   Other abnormal findings on microbiological examination of urine

         Positive culture findings of urine

R82.8   Abnormal findings on cytological and histological examination of urine

     R82.81   Pyuria

         Sterile pyuria

   ● New code   ▲ Revised code   **Excludes1:** Not coded here   **Excludes2:** Not included here   ⊗ Placeholder required   ⑦7th digit required

R82.89 **Other abnormal findings on cytological and histological examination of urine**

R82.9 **Other and unspecified abnormal findings in urine**

R82.90 **Unspecified abnormal findings in urine**

R82.91 **Other chromoabnormalities of urine**

Chromoconversion (dipstick)

Idiopathic dipstick converts positive for blood with no cellular forms in sediment

Excludes1: hemoglobinuria (R82.3)

myoglobinuria (R82.1)

R82.99 **Other abnormal findings in urine**

R82.991 **Hypocitraturia**

R82.992 **Hyperoxaluria**

Excludes1: Primary hyperoxaluria (E72.53)

R82.993 **Hyperuricosuria**

R82.994 **Hypercalciuria**

Idiopathic hypercalciuria

R82.998 **Other abnormal findings in urine**

Cells and casts in urine

Crystalluria

Melanuria

ABNORMAL FINDINGS ON EXAMINATION OF OTHER BODY FLUIDS, SUBSTANCES AND TISSUES, WITHOUT DIAGNOSIS (R83-R89)

Excludes1: abnormal findings on antenatal screening of mother (O28.-)

diagnostic abnormal findings classified elsewhere - see Alphabetical Index

Excludes2: abnormal findings on examination of blood, without diagnosis (R70-R79)

abnormal findings on examination of urine, without diagnosis (R80-R82)

abnormal tumor markers (R97.-)

R83 **Abnormal findings in cerebrospinal fluid**

R83.0 **Abnormal level of enzymes in cerebrospinal fluid**

R83.1 **Abnormal level of hormones in cerebrospinal fluid**

R83.2 **Abnormal level of other drugs, medicaments and biological substances in cerebrospinal fluid**

R83.3 **Abnormal level of substances chiefly nonmedicinal as to source in cerebrospinal fluid**

R83.4 **Abnormal immunological findings in cerebrospinal fluid**

R83.5 **Abnormal microbiological findings in cerebrospinal fluid**

Positive culture findings in cerebrospinal fluid

Excludes1: colonization status (Z22.-)

R83.6 **Abnormal cytological findings in cerebrospinal fluid**

R83.8 **Other abnormal findings in cerebrospinal fluid**

Abnormal chromosomal findings in cerebrospinal fluid

R83.9 **Unspecified abnormal finding in cerebrospinal fluid**

R84 **Abnormal findings in specimens from respiratory organs and thorax**

Includes: abnormal findings in bronchial washings

abnormal findings in nasal secretions

abnormal findings in pleural fluid

abnormal findings in sputum

abnormal findings in throat scrapings

Excludes1: blood-stained sputum (R04.2)

R84.0 **Abnormal level of enzymes in specimens from respiratory organs and thorax**

R84.1 **Abnormal level of hormones in specimens from respiratory organs and thorax**

R84.2 **Abnormal level of other drugs, medicaments and biological substances in specimens from respiratory organs and thorax**

R84.3 **Abnormal level of substances chiefly nonmedicinal as to source in specimens from respiratory organs and thorax**

R84.4 **Abnormal immunological findings in specimens from respiratory organs and thorax**

R84.5 **Abnormal microbiological findings in specimens from respiratory organs and thorax**

Positive culture findings in specimens from respiratory organs and thorax

Excludes1: colonization status (Z22.-)

R84.6 **Abnormal cytological findings in specimens from respiratory organs and thorax**

R84.7 **Abnormal histological findings in specimens from respiratory organs and thorax**

R84.8 **Other abnormal findings in specimens from respiratory organs and thorax**

Abnormal chromosomal findings in specimens from respiratory organs and thorax

R84.9 **Unspecified abnormal finding in specimens from respiratory organs and thorax**

R85 **Abnormal findings in specimens from digestive organs and abdominal cavity**

Includes: abnormal findings in peritoneal fluid

abnormal findings in saliva

Excludes1: cloudy peritoneal dialysis effluent (R88.0)

fecal abnormalities (R19.5)

R85.0 **Abnormal level of enzymes in specimens from digestive organs and abdominal cavity**

R85.1 **Abnormal level of hormones in specimens from digestive organs and abdominal cavity**

R85.2 **Abnormal level of other drugs, medicaments and biological substances in specimens from digestive organs and abdominal cavity**

R85.3 **Abnormal level of substances chiefly nonmedicinal as to source in specimens from digestive organs and abdominal cavity**

R85.4 **Abnormal immunological findings in specimens from digestive organs and abdominal cavity**

R85.5 **Abnormal microbiological findings in specimens from digestive organs and abdominal cavity**

Positive culture findings in specimens from digestive organs and abdominal cavity

Excludes1: colonization status (Z22.-)

R85.6 **Abnormal cytological findings in specimens from digestive organs and abdominal cavity**

R85.61 **Abnormal cytologic smear of anus**

Excludes1: abnormal cytological findings in specimens from other digestive organs and abdominal cavity (R85.69)

carcinoma in situ of anus (histologically confirmed) (D01.3)

anal intraepithelial neoplasia I [AIN I] (K62.82)

anal intraepithelial neoplasia II [AIN II] (K62.82)

anal intraepithelial neoplasia III [AIN III] (D01.3)

dysplasia (mild) (moderate) of anus (histologically confirmed) (K62.82)

severe dysplasia of anus (histologically confirmed) (D01.3)

Excludes2: anal high-risk human papillomavirus (HPV) DNA test positive (R85.81)

anal low risk human papillomavirus (HPV) DNA test positive (R85.82)

R85.610   Atypical squamous cells of undetermined significance on cytologic smear of anus (ASC-US)

R85.611   Atypical squamous cells cannot exclude high grade squamous intraepithelial lesion on cytologic smear of anus (ASC-H)

R85.612   Low grade squamous intraepithelial lesion on cytologic smear of anus (LGSIL)

R85.613   High grade squamous intraepithelial lesion on cytologic smear of anus (HGSIL)

R85.614   Cytologic evidence of malignancy on smear of anus

R85.615   Unsatisfactory cytologic smear of anus

Inadequate sample of cytologic smear of anus

R85.616   Satisfactory anal smear but lacking transformation zone

R85.618   Other abnormal cytological findings on specimens from anus

R85.619   Unspecified abnormal cytological findings in specimens from anus

Abnormal anal cytology NOS

Atypical glandular cells of anus NOS

R85.69   Abnormal cytological findings in specimens from other digestive organs and abdominal cavity

R85.7   Abnormal histological findings in specimens from digestive organs and abdominal cavity

R85.8   Other abnormal findings in specimens from digestive organs and abdominal cavity

R85.81   Anal high-risk human papillomavirus (HPV) DNA test positive

Excludes1: anogenital warts due to human papillomavirus (HPV) (A63.0)

condyloma acuminatum (A63.0)

R85.82   Anal low risk human papillomavirus (HPV) DNA test positive

Use Additional Code for associated human papillomavirus (B97.7)

R85.89   Other abnormal findings in specimens from digestive organs and abdominal cavity

Abnormal chromosomal findings in specimens from digestive organs and abdominal cavity

R85.9   Unspecified abnormal finding in specimens from digestive organs and abdominal cavity

R86   Abnormal findings in specimens from male genital organs

Includes: abnormal findings in prostatic secretions

abnormal findings in semen, seminal fluid

abnormal spermatozoa

Excludes1: azoospermia (N46.0-)

oligospermia (N46.1-)

R86.0   Abnormal level of enzymes in specimens from male genital organs

R86.1   Abnormal level of hormones in specimens from male genital organs

R86.2   Abnormal level of other drugs, medicaments and biological substances in specimens from male genital organs

R86.3   Abnormal level of substances chiefly nonmedicinal as to source in specimens from male genital organs

R86.4   Abnormal immunological findings in specimens from male genital organs

R86.5   Abnormal microbiological findings in specimens from male genital organs

Positive culture findings in specimens from male genital organs

Excludes1: colonization status (Z22.-)

R86.6   Abnormal cytological findings in specimens from male genital organs

R86.7   Abnormal histological findings in specimens from male genital organs

R86.8   Other abnormal findings in specimens from male genital organs

Abnormal chromosomal findings in specimens from male genital organs

R86.9   Unspecified abnormal finding in specimens from male genital organs

R87   Abnormal findings in specimens from female genital organs

Includes: abnormal findings in secretion and smears from cervix uteri

abnormal findings in secretion and smears from vagina

abnormal findings in secretion and smears from vulva

R87.0   Abnormal level of enzymes in specimens from female genital organs

R87.1   Abnormal level of hormones in specimens from female genital organs

R87.2   Abnormal level of other drugs, medicaments and biological substances in specimens from female genital organs

R87.3   Abnormal level of substances chiefly nonmedicinal as to source in specimens from female genital organs

R87.4   Abnormal immunological findings in specimens from female genital organs

R87.5   Abnormal microbiological findings in specimens from female genital organs

Positive culture findings in specimens from female genital organs

Excludes1: colonization status (Z22.-)

R87.6   Abnormal cytological findings in specimens from female genital organs

R87.61   Abnormal cytological findings in specimens from cervix uteri

Excludes1: abnormal cytological findings in specimens from other female genital organs (R87.69)

abnormal cytological findings in specimens from vagina (R87.62-)

carcinoma in situ of cervix uteri (histologically confirmed) (D06.-)

cervical intraepithelial neoplasia I [CIN I] (N87.0)

cervical intraepithelial neoplasia II [CIN II] (N87.1)

cervical intraepithelial neoplasia III [CIN III] (D06.-)

dysplasia (mild) (moderate) of cervix uteri (histologically confirmed) (N87.-)

● New code   ▲ Revised code   **Excludes1:** Not coded here   **Excludes2:** Not included here   ⊗ Placeholder required   ⑦7th digit required

severe dysplasia of cervix uteri (histologically confirmed) (D06.-)

Excludes2: cervical high-risk human papillomavirus (HPV) DNA test positive (R87.810)

cervical low risk human papillomavirus (HPV) DNA test positive (R87.820)

R87.610 Atypical squamous cells of undetermined significance on cytologic smear of cervix (ASC-US)

R87.611 Atypical squamous cells cannot exclude high grade squamous intraepithelial lesion on cytologic smear of cervix (ASC-H)

R87.612 Low grade squamous intraepithelial lesion on cytologic smear of cervix (LGSIL)

R87.613 High grade squamous intraepithelial lesion on cytologic smear of cervix (HGSIL)

R87.614 Cytologic evidence of malignancy on smear of cervix

R87.615 Unsatisfactory cytologic smear of cervix

Inadequate sample of cytologic smear of cervix

R87.616 Satisfactory cervical smear but lacking transformation zone

R87.618 Other abnormal cytological findings on specimens from cervix uteri

R87.619 Unspecified abnormal cytological findings in specimens from cervix uteri

Abnormal cervical cytology NOS

Abnormal Papanicolaou smear of cervix NOS

Abnormal thin preparation smear of cervix NOS

Atypical endocervical cells of cervix NOS

Atypical endometrial cells of cervix NOS

Atypical glandular cells of cervix NOS

R87.62 Abnormal cytological findings in specimens from vagina

<u>Use Additional Code</u> to identify acquired absence of uterus and cervix, if applicable (Z90.71-)

Excludes1: abnormal cytological findings in specimens from cervix uteri (R87.61-)

abnormal cytological findings in specimens **from other** female genital organs (R87.69)

carcinoma in situ of vagina (histologically confirmed) (D07.2)

vaginal intraepithelial neoplasia I [VAIN I] (N89.0)

vaginal intraepithelial neoplasia II [VAIN II] (N89.1)

vaginal intraepithelial neoplasia III [VAIN III] (D07.2)

dysplasia (mild) (moderate) of vagina (histologically confirmed) (N89.-)

severe dysplasia of vagina (histologically confirmed) (D07.2)

Excludes2: vaginal high-risk human

papillomavirus (HPV) DNA test positive (R87.811)

vaginal low risk human papillomavirus (HPV) DNA test positive (R87.821)

R87.620 Atypical squamous cells of undetermined significance on cytologic smear of vagina (ASC-US)

R87.621 Atypical squamous cells cannot exclude high grade squamous intraepithelial lesion on cytologic smear of vagina (ASC-H)

R87.622 Low grade squamous intraepithelial lesion on cytologic smear of vagina (LGSIL)

R87.623 High grade squamous intraepithelial lesion on cytologic smear of vagina (HGSIL)

R87.624 Cytologic evidence of malignancy on smear of vagina

R87.625 Unsatisfactory cytologic smear of vagina

Inadequate sample of cytologic smear of vagina

R87.628 Other abnormal cytological findings on specimens from vagina

R87.629 Unspecified abnormal cytological findings in specimens from vagina

Abnormal Papanicolaou smear of vagina NOS

Abnormal thin preparation smear of vagina NOS

Abnormal vaginal cytology NOS

Atypical endocervical cells of vagina NOS

Atypical endometrial cells of vagina NOS

Atypical glandular cells of vagina NOS

R87.69 Abnormal cytological findings in specimens from other female genital organs

Abnormal cytological findings in specimens from female genital organs NOS

Excludes1: dysplasia of vulva (histologically confirmed) (N90.0-N90.3)

R87.7 Abnormal histological findings in specimens from female genital organs

Excludes1: carcinoma in situ (histologically confirmed) of female genital organs (D06-D07.3)

cervical intraepithelial neoplasia I [CIN I] (N87.0)

cervical intraepithelial neoplasia II [CIN II] (N87.1)

cervical intraepithelial neoplasia III [CIN III] (D06.-)

dysplasia (mild) (moderate) of cervix uteri (histologically confirmed) (N87.-)

dysplasia (mild) (moderate) of vagina (histologically confirmed) (N89.-)

vaginal intraepithelial neoplasia I [VAIN I] (N89.0)

vaginal intraepithelial neoplasia II [VAIN II] (N89.1)

vaginal intraepithelial neoplasia III [VAIN III] (D07.2)

severe dysplasia of cervix uteri (histologically confirmed) (D06.-)

severe dysplasia of vagina (histologically confirmed) (D07.2)

R87.8 **Other abnormal findings in specimens from female genital organs**

R87.81 **High risk human papillomavirus (HPV) DNA test positive from female genital organs**

Excludes1: anogenital warts due to human papillomavirus (HPV) (A63.0)

condyloma acuminatum (A63.0)

R87.810 **Cervical high-risk human papillomavirus (HPV) DNA test positive**

R87.811 **Vaginal high-risk human papillomavirus (HPV) DNA test positive**

R87.82 **Low risk human papillomavirus (HPV) DNA test positive from female genital organs**

Use Additional Code for associated human papillomavirus (B97.7)

R87.820 **Cervical low risk human papillomavirus (HPV) DNA test positive**

R87.821 **Vaginal low risk human papillomavirus (HPV) DNA test positive**

R87.89 **Other abnormal findings in specimens from female genital organs**

Abnormal chromosomal findings in specimens from female genital organs

R87.9 **Unspecified abnormal finding in specimens from female genital organs**

R88 **Abnormal findings in other body fluids and substances**

R88.0 **Cloudy (hemodialysis) (peritoneal) dialysis effluent**

R88.8 **Abnormal findings in other body fluids and substances**

R89 **Abnormal findings in specimens from other organs, systems and tissues**

Includes: abnormal findings in nipple discharge

abnormal findings in synovial fluid abnormal findings in wound secretions

R89.0 **Abnormal level of enzymes in specimens from other organs, systems and tissues**

R89.1 **Abnormal level of hormones in specimens from other organs, systems and tissues**

R89.2 **Abnormal level of other drugs, medicaments and biological substances in specimens from other organs, systems and tissues**

R89.3 **Abnormal level of substances chiefly nonmedicinal as to source in specimens from other organs, systems and tissues**

R89.4 **Abnormal immunological findings in specimens from other organs, systems and tissues**

R89.5 **Abnormal microbiological findings in specimens from other organs, systems and tissues**

Positive culture findings in specimens from other organs, systems and tissues

Excludes1: colonization status (Z22.-)

R89.6 **Abnormal cytological findings in specimens from other organs, systems and tissues**

R89.7 **Abnormal histological findings in specimens from other organs, systems and tissues**

R89.8 **Other abnormal findings in specimens from other organs, systems and tissues**

Abnormal chromosomal findings in specimens from other organs, systems and tissues

R89.9 **Unspecified abnormal finding in specimens from other organs, systems and tissues**

ABNORMAL FINDINGS ON DIAGNOSTIC IMAGING AND IN FUNCTION STUDIES, WITHOUT DIAGNOSIS (R90-R94)

Includes: nonspecific abnormal findings on diagnostic imaging by computerized axial tomography [CAT scan]

nonspecific abnormal findings on diagnostic imaging by magnetic resonance imaging [MRI][NMR]

nonspecific abnormal findings on diagnostic imaging by positron emission tomography [PET scan]

nonspecific abnormal findings on diagnostic imaging by thermography

nonspecific abnormal findings on diagnostic imaging by ultrasound [echogram]

nonspecific abnormal findings on diagnostic imaging by X-ray examination

Excludes1: abnormal findings on antenatal screening of mother (O28.-)

diagnostic abnormal findings classified elsewhere - see Alphabetical Index

R90 **Abnormal findings on diagnostic imaging of central nervous system**

R90.0 **Intracranial space-occupying lesion found on diagnostic imaging of central nervous system**

R90.8 **Other abnormal findings on diagnostic imaging of central nervous system**

R90.81 **Abnormal echoencephalogram**

R90.82 **White matter disease, unspecified**

R90.89 **Other abnormal findings on diagnostic imaging of central nervous system**

Other cerebrovascular abnormality found on diagnostic imaging of central nervous system

R91 **Abnormal findings on diagnostic imaging of lung**

R91.1 **Solitary pulmonary nodule**

Coin lesion lung

Solitary pulmonary nodule, subsegmental branch of the bronchial tree

R91.8 **Other nonspecific abnormal finding of lung field**

Lung mass NOS found on diagnostic imaging of lung

Pulmonary infiltrate NOS

Shadow, lung

R92 **Abnormal and inconclusive findings on diagnostic imaging of breast**

R92.0 **Mammographic microcalcification found on diagnostic imaging of breast**

Excludes2: mammographic calcification (calculus) found on diagnostic imaging of breast (R92.1)

R92.1 **Mammographic calcification found on diagnostic imaging of breast**

Mammographic calculus found on diagnostic imaging of breast

R92.2 **Inconclusive mammogram**

Dense breasts NOS

Inconclusive mammogram NEC

Inconclusive mammography due to dense breasts

Inconclusive mammography NEC

R92.8 **Other abnormal and inconclusive findings on diagnostic imaging of breast**

R93 **Abnormal findings on diagnostic imaging of other body structures**

R93.0 **Abnormal findings on diagnostic imaging of skull and head, not elsewhere classified**

Excludes1: intracranial space-occupying lesion found on

● New code ▲ Revised code Excludes1: Not coded here Excludes2: Not included here ⊗ Placeholder required ⑦7th digit required

diagnostic imaging (R90.0)

R93.1 **Abnormal findings on diagnostic imaging of heart and coronary circulation**

Abnormal echocardiogram NOS

Abnormal heart shadow

R93.2 **Abnormal findings on diagnostic imaging of liver and biliary tract**

Nonvisualization of gallbladder

R93.3 **Abnormal findings on diagnostic imaging of other parts of digestive tract**

R93.4 **Abnormal findings on diagnostic imaging of urinary organs**

Excludes2: hypertrophy of kidney (N28.81)

R93.41 **Abnormal radiologic findings on diagnostic imaging of renal pelvis, ureter, or bladder**

Filling defect of bladder found on diagnostic imaging

Filling defect of renal pelvis found on diagnostic imaging

Filling defect of ureter found on diagnostic imaging

R93.42 **Abnormal radiologic findings on diagnostic imaging of kidney**

R93.421 **Abnormal radiologic findings on diagnostic imaging of right kidney**

R93.422 **Abnormal radiologic findings on diagnostic imaging of left kidney**

R93.429 **Abnormal radiologic findings on diagnostic imaging of unspecified kidney**

R93.49 **Abnormal radiologic findings on diagnostic imaging of other urinary organs**

R93.5 **Abnormal findings on diagnostic imaging of other abdominal regions, including retroperitoneum**

R93.6 **Abnormal findings on diagnostic imaging of limbs**

Excludes2: abnormal finding in skin and subcutaneous tissue (R93.8-)

R93.7 **Abnormal findings on diagnostic imaging of other parts of musculoskeletal system**

Excludes2: abnormal findings on diagnostic imaging of skull (R93.0)

R93.8 **Abnormal findings on diagnostic imaging of other specified body structures**

R93.81 **Abnormal radiologic findings on diagnostic imaging of testis**

R93.811 **Abnormal radiologic findings on diagnostic imaging of right testicle**

R93.812 **Abnormal radiologic findings on diagnostic imaging of left testicle**

R93.813 **Abnormal radiologic findings on diagnostic imaging of testicles, bilateral**

R93.819 **Abnormal radiologic findings on diagnostic imaging of unspecified testicle**

R93.89 **Abnormal findings on diagnostic imaging of other specified body structures**

Abnormal finding by radioisotope localization of placenta

Abnormal radiological finding in skin and subcutaneous tissue

Mediastinal shift

R93.9 **Diagnostic imaging inconclusive due to excess body fat of patient**

R94 **Abnormal results of function studies**

Includes: abnormal results of radionuclide [radioisotope] uptake studies

abnormal results of scintigraphy

R94.0 **Abnormal results of function studies of central nervous system**

R94.01 **Abnormal electroencephalogram [EEG]**

R94.02 **Abnormal brain scan**

R94.09 **Abnormal results of other function studies of central nervous system**

R94.1 **Abnormal results of function studies of peripheral nervous system and special senses**

R94.11 **Abnormal results of function studies of eye**

R94.110 **Abnormal electro-oculogram [EOG]**

R94.111 **Abnormal electroretinogram [ERG]**

Abnormal retinal function study

R94.112 **Abnormal visually evoked potential [VEP]**

R94.113 **Abnormal oculomotor study**

R94.118 **Abnormal results of other function studies of eye**

R94.12 **Abnormal results of function studies of ear and other special senses**

R94.120 **Abnormal auditory function study**

R94.121 **Abnormal vestibular function study**

R94.128 **Abnormal results of other function studies of ear and other special senses**

R94.13 **Abnormal results of function studies of peripheral nervous system**

R94.130 **Abnormal response to nerve stimulation, unspecified**

R94.131 **Abnormal electromyogram [EMG]**

Excludes1: electromyogram of eye (R94.113)

R94.138 **Abnormal results of other function studies of peripheral nervous system**

R94.2 **Abnormal results of pulmonary function studies**

Reduced ventilatory capacity Reduced vital capacity

R94.3 **Abnormal results of cardiovascular function studies**

R94.30 **Abnormal result of cardiovascular function study, unspecified**

R94.31 **Abnormal electrocardiogram [ECG] [EKG]**

Excludes1: long QT syndrome (I45.81)

R94.39 **Abnormal result of other cardiovascular function study**

Abnormal electrophysiological intracardiac studies

Abnormal phonocardiogram

Abnormal vectorcardiogram

R94.4 **Abnormal results of kidney function studies**

Abnormal renal function test

R94.5 **Abnormal results of liver function studies**

R94.6 **Abnormal results of thyroid function studies**

R94.7 **Abnormal results of other endocrine function studies**

Excludes2: abnormal glucose (R73.0-)

R94.8 **Abnormal results of function studies of other organs and systems**

Abnormal basal metabolic rate [BMR]

Abnormal bladder function test

Abnormal splenic function test

ABNORMAL TUMOR MARKERS (R97)

Definition: A tumor marker is a biomarker found in the blood, urine, or body tissues that can be elevated in cancer, among other tissue types. There are many different **tumor** markers, each indicative of a particular disease process, and they are used in oncology to help detect the presence of cancer.

R97   **Abnormal tumor markers**

Elevated tumor associated antigens [TAA]

Elevated tumor specific antigens [TSA]

R97.0   **Elevated carcinoembryonic antigen [CEA]**

R97.1   **Elevated cancer antigen 125 [CA 125]**

R97.2   **Elevated prostate specific antigen [PSA]**

   R97.20   **Elevated prostate specific antigen [PSA]**

   R97.21   **Rising PSA following treatment for malignant neoplasm of prostate**

R97.8   **Other abnormal tumor markers**

ILL-DEFINED AND UNKNOWN CAUSE OF MORTALITY (R99)

R99   **Ill-defined and unknown cause of mortality**

Death (unexplained) NOS

Unspecified cause of mortality

Chapter 19: Injury, Poisoning and Certain Other Consequences of External Causes (S00-T88)

DEFINITIONS

This chapter includes definitions of selected key words, terms and phrases and coding alerts for adding points to the clinical domain, and references to coding late effects where appropriate. An example from this chapter is as follows:

S05.7 Avulsion of eye

Traumatic enucleation

Definition: An avulsion is an injury in which a body structure is forcibly detached from its normal point of insertion by either trauma or surgery (from the Latin *avellere*, meaning "to tear off"). The term most commonly refers to a surface trauma where all layers of the skin have been torn away, exposing the underlying structures (i.e., subcutaneous tissue, muscle, tendons, or bone).

MULTIPLE CODING FOR A SINGLE CONDITION

In addition to the etiology/manifestation convention that requires two codes to fully describe a single condition that affects multiple body systems, there are other single conditions that also require more than one code. "**Use Additional Code**" notes are found in the Tabular List at codes that are not part of an etiology/manifestation pair where a secondary code is useful to fully describe a condition. The sequencing rule is the same as the etiology/manifestation pair, "**Use Additional Code**" indicates that a secondary code should be added.

For example, for bacterial infections that are not included in chapter 1, a secondary code from category B95, Streptococcus, Staphylococcus, and Enterococcus, as the cause of diseases classified elsewhere, or B96, Other bacterial agents as the cause of diseases classified elsewhere, may be required to identify the bacterial organism causing the infection. A "**Use Additional Code**" note will normally be found at the infectious disease code, indicating a need for the organism code to be added as a secondary code.

 "**Code first**" notes are also under certain codes that are not specifically manifestation codes but may be due to an underlying cause. When there is a "**Code first**" note and an underlying condition is present, the underlying condition should be sequenced first.

"Code, if applicable, any causal condition first", notes indicate that this code may be assigned as a principal diagnosis when the causal condition is unknown or not applicable. If a causal condition is known, then the code for that condition should be sequenced as the principal or first-listed diagnosis.

Multiple codes may be needed for sequela, complication codes and obstetric codes to more fully describe a condition. See the specific guidelines for these conditions for further instruction.

COMBINATION CODE

A combination code is a single code used to classify: Two diagnoses, or a diagnosis with an associated secondary process (manifestation) A diagnosis with an associated complication

Combination codes are identified by referring to subterm entries in the Alphabetic Index and by reading the inclusion and exclusion notes in the Tabular List.

Assign only the combination code when that code fully identifies the diagnostic conditions involved or when the Alphabetic Index so directs. Multiple coding should not be used when the classification provides a combination code that clearly identifies all of the elements documented in the diagnosis. When the combination code lacks necessary specificity in describing the manifestation or complication, an additional code should be used as a secondary code.

SEQUELA (LATE EFFECTS)

A sequela is the residual effect (condition produced) after the acute phase of an illness or injury has terminated. There is no time limit on when a sequela code can be used. The residual may be apparent early, such as in cerebral infarction, or it may occur months or years later, such as that due to a previous injury. Coding of sequela generally requires two codes sequenced in the following order: The condition or nature of the sequela is sequenced first.

S00-T88

The sequela code is sequenced second.

An exception to the above guidelines are those instances where the code for the sequela is followed by a manifestation code identified in the Tabular List and title, or the sequela code has been expanded (at the fourth, fifth or sixth character levels) to include the manifestation(s). The code for the acute phase of an illness or injury that led to the sequela is never used with a code for the late effect.

APPLICATION OF 7TH CHARACTERS IN CHAPTER 19

Most categories in chapter 19 have a 7th character requirement for each applicable code. Most categories in this chapter have three 7th character values (with the exception of fractures): A, initial encounter, D, subsequent encounter and S, sequela. Categories for traumatic fractures have additional 7th character values. While the patient may be seen by a new or different provider over the course of treatment for an injury, assignment of the 7th character is based on whether the patient is undergoing active treatment and not whether the provider is seeing the patient for the first time.

For complication codes, active treatment refers to treatment for the condition described by the code, even though it may be related to an earlier precipitating problem. For example, code T84.50XA, Infection and inflammatory reaction due to unspecified internal joint prosthesis, initial encounter, is used when active treatment is provided for the infection, even though the condition relates to the prosthetic device, implant or graft that was placed at a previous encounter.

7th character "A", initial encounter is used for each encounter where the patient is receiving active treatment for the condition.

7th character "D" subsequent encounter is used for encounters after the patient has completed active treatment of the condition and is receiving routine care for the condition during the healing or recovery phase.

The aftercare Z codes should not be used for aftercare for conditions such as injuries or poisonings, where 7th characters are provided to identify subsequent care. For example, for aftercare of an injury, assign the acute injury code with the 7th character "D" (subsequent encounter).

7th character "S", sequela, is for use for complications or conditions that arise as a direct result of a condition, such as scar formation after a burn. The scars are sequelae of the burn. When using 7th character "S", it is necessary to use both the injury code that precipitated the sequela and the code for the sequela itself. The "S" is added only to the injury code, not the sequela code. The 7th character "S" identifies the injury responsible for the sequela. The specific type of sequela (e.g., scar) is sequenced first, followed by the injury code.

See Section I.B.10 Sequelae, (Late Effects)

CODING OF INJURIES

When coding injuries, assign separate codes for each injury unless a combination code is provided, in which case the combination code is assigned. Codes from category T07, Unspecified multiple injuries should not be assigned in the inpatient setting unless information for a more specific code is not available. Traumatic injury codes (S00-T14.9) are not to be used for normal, healing surgical wounds or to identify complications of surgical wounds.

The code for the most serious injury, as determined by the provider and the focus of treatment, is sequenced first.

1) Superficial injuries

Superficial injuries such as abrasions or contusions are not coded when associated with more severe injuries of the same site.

2) Primary injury with damage to nerves/blood vessels

When a primary injury results in minor damage to peripheral nerves or blood vessels, the primary injury is sequenced first with additional code(s) for injuries to nerves and spinal cord (such as category S04), and/or injury to blood vessels (such as category S15). When the primary injury is to the blood vessels or nerves, that injury should be sequenced first.

● New code   ▲ Revised code   **Excludes1:** Not coded here   **Excludes2:** Not included here   ⊗ Placeholder required   ⑦7th digit required

3) Iatrogenic injuries

Injury codes from Chapter 19 should not be assigned for injuries that occur during, or as a result of, a medical intervention. Assign the appropriate complication code(s).

CODING OF TRAUMATIC FRACTURES

The principles of multiple coding of injuries should be followed in coding fractures. Fractures of specified sites are coded individually by site in accordance with both the provisions within categories S02, S12, S22, S32, S42, S49, S52, S59, S62, S72, S79, S82, S89, S92 and the level of detail furnished by medical record content.

A fracture not indicated as open or closed should be coded to closed. A fracture not indicated whether displaced or not displaced should be coded to displaced.

More specific guidelines are as follows:

1) Initial vs. Subsequent Encounter for Fractures

Traumatic fractures are coded using the appropriate 7th character for initial encounter (A, B, C) for each encounter where the patient is receiving active treatment for the fracture. The appropriate 7th character for initial encounter should also be assigned for a patient who delayed seeking treatment for the fracture or nonunion.

Fractures are coded using the appropriate 7th character for subsequent care for encounters after the patient has completed active treatment of the fracture and is receiving routine care for the fracture during the healing or recovery phase.

Care for complications of surgical treatment for fracture repairs during the healing or recovery phase should be coded with the appropriate complication codes.

Care of complications of fractures, such as malunion and nonunion, should be reported with the appropriate 7th character for subsequent care with nonunion (K, M, N,) or subsequent care with malunion (P, Q, R).

Malunion/nonunion: The appropriate 7th character for initial encounter should also be assigned for a patient who delayed seeking treatment for the fracture or nonunion.

The open fracture designations in the assignment of the 7th character for fractures of the forearm, femur and lower leg, including ankle are based on the Gustilo open fracture classification. When the Gustilo classification type is not specified for an open fracture, the 7th character for open fracture type I or II should be assigned (B, E, H, M, Q).

A code from category M80, not a traumatic fracture code, should be used for any patient with known osteoporosis who suffers a fracture, even if the patient had a minor fall or trauma, if that fall or trauma would not usually break a normal, healthy bone.

See Section I.C.13. Osteoporosis.

The aftercare Z codes should not be used for aftercare for traumatic fractures. For aftercare of a traumatic fracture, assign the acute fracture code with the appropriate 7th character.

2) Multiple fractures sequencing

Multiple fractures are sequenced in accordance with the severity of the fracture.

3) Physeal fractures

For physeal fractures, assign only the code identifying the type of physeal fracture. Do not assign a separate code to identify the specific bone that is fractured.

CODING OF BURNS AND CORROSIONS

The ICD-10-CM makes a distinction between burns and corrosions. The burn codes are for thermal burns, except sunburns, that come from a heat source, such as a fire or hot appliance. The burn codes are also for burns resulting from electricity and radiation. Corrosions are burns due to chemicals. The guidelines are the same for burns and corrosions.

Current burns (T20-T25) are classified by depth, extent and by agent (X code). Burns are classified by depth as first degree (erythema), second degree (blistering), and third degree (full-thickness involvement). Burns of the eye and internal organs (T26-T28) are classified by site, but not by degree.

1) **Sequencing of burn and related condition codes**

    Sequence first the code that reflects the highest degree of burn when more than one burn is present.

    a. When the reason for the admission or encounter is for treatment of external multiple burns, sequence first the code that reflects the burn of the highest degree.

    b. When a patient has both internal and external burns, the circumstances of admission govern the selection of the principal diagnosis or first-listed diagnosis.

    c. When a patient is admitted for burn injuries and other related conditions such as smoke inhalation and/or respiratory failure, the circumstances of admission govern the selection of the principal or first-listed diagnosis.

2) **Burns of the same *anatomic* site**

    Classify burns of the same anatomic site and on the same side but of different degrees to the subcategory identifying the highest degree recorded in the diagnosis (e.g., for second and third degree burns of right thigh, assign only code T24.311-).

3) **Non-healing burns**

    Non-healing burns are coded as acute burns.

    Necrosis of burned skin should be coded as a non-healed burn.

4) **Infected Burn**

    For any documented infected burn site, use an additional code for the infection.

5) **Assign separate codes for each burn site**

    When coding burns, assign separate codes for each burn site. Category T30, Burn and corrosion, body region unspecified is extremely vague and should rarely be used.

    Codes for burns of "multiple sites" should only be assigned when the medical record documentation does not specify the individual sites.

6) **Burns and Corrosions Classified According to Extent of Body Surface Involved**

    Assign codes from category T31, Burns classified according to extent of body surface involved, or T32, Corrosions classified according to extent of body surface involved, for acute burns or corrosions when the site of the burn or corrosion is not specified or when there is a need for additional data. It is advisable to use category T31 as additional codingwhen needed to provide data for evaluating burn mortality, such as thatneeded by burn units. It is also advisable to use category T31 as an additional code for reporting purposes when there is mention of a third-degree burn involving 20 percent or more of the body surface. Codes from categories T31 and T32 should not be used for sequelae of burns or corrosions.

    Categories T31 and T32 are based on the classic "rule of nines" in estimating body surface involved: head and neck are assigned nine percent, each arm nine percent, each leg 18 percent, the anterior trunk 18 percent, posterior trunk 18 percent, and genitalia one percent. Providers may change these percentage assignments where necessary to accommodate infants

● New code ▲ Revised code **Excludes1:** Not coded here **Excludes2:** Not included here ⊗ Placeholder required ⑦7th digit required

and children who have proportionately larger heads than adults, and patients who have large buttocks, thighs, or abdomen that involve burns.

7)   Encounters for treatment of sequela of burns

Encounters for the treatment of the late effects of burns or corrosions (i.e., scars or joint contractures) should be coded with a burn or corrosion code with the 7ᵗʰ character "S" for sequela.

8)   Sequelae with a late effect code and current burn

When appropriate, both a code for a current burn or corrosion with 7ᵗʰ character "A" or "D" and a burn or corrosion code with 7ᵗʰ character "S" may be assigned on the same record (when both a current burn and sequelae of an old burn exist). Burns and corrosions do not heal at the same rate and a current healing wound may still exist with sequela of a healed burn or corrosion.

See Section I.B.10 Sequela (Late Effects)

9)   Use of an external cause code with burns and corrosions

An external cause code should be used with burns and corrosions to identify the source and intent of the burn, as well as the place where it occurred.

ADVERSE EFFECTS, POISONING, UNDERDOSING AND TOXIC EFFECTS

Codes in categories T36-T65 are combination codes that include the substance that was taken as well as the intent. No additional external cause code is required for poisonings, toxic effects, adverse effects and underdosing codes.

1)   Do not code directly from the Table of Drugs

Do not code directly from the Table of Drugs and Chemicals. Always refer back to the Tabular List.

2)   Use as many codes as necessary to describe

Use as many codes as necessary to describe completely all drugs, medicinal or biological substances.

3)   If the same code would describe the causative agent

If the same code would describe the causative agent for more than one adverse reaction, poisoning, toxic effect or underdosing, assign the code only once.

4)   If two or more drugs, medicinal or biological substances

If two or more drugs, medicinal or biological substances are taken, code each individually unless a combination code is listed in the Table of Drugs and Chemicals.

If multiple unspecified drugs, medicinal or biological substances were taken, assign the appropriate code from subcategory T50.91, Poisoning by adverse effect of and underdosing of multiple unspecified drugs, medicaments and biological substances.

5)   The occurrence of drug toxicity is classified in ICD-10-CM as follows:

(a)   Adverse Effect

When coding an adverse effect of a drug that has been correctly prescribed and properly administered, assign the appropriate code for the nature of the adverse effect followed by the appropriate code for the adverse effect of the drug (T36-T50). The code for the drug should have a 5ᵗʰ or 6ᵗʰ character "5" (for example T36.0X5-) Examples of the nature of an adverse effect are tachycardia, delirium, gastrointestinal hemorrhaging, vomiting, hypokalemia, hepatitis, renal failure, or respiratory failure.

(b)   Poisoning

When coding a poisoning or reaction to the improper use of a medication (e.g., overdose, wrong substance given or taken in error, wrong route of administration), first assign the appropriate code from categories T36-T50. The poisoning codes have an associated intent as their 5th or 6th character (accidental, intentional self-harm, assault and undetermined. If the intent of the poisoning is unknown or unspecified, code the intent as accidental intent. The undetermined intent is only for use if the documentation in the record specifies that the intent cannot be determined. **Use Additional Code**(s) for all manifestations of poisonings.

If there is also a diagnosis of abuse or dependence of the substance, the abuse or dependence is assigned as an additional code.

Examples of poisoning include:

(i) Error was made in drug prescription Errors made in drug prescription or in the administration of the drug by provider, nurse, patient, or other person.

(ii) Overdose of a drug intentionally taken. If an overdose of a drug was intentionally taken or administered and resulted in drug toxicity, it would be coded as a poisoning.

(iii) Nonprescribed drug taken with correctly prescribed and properly administered drug

If a nonprescribed drug or medicinal agent was taken in combination with a correctly prescribed and properly administered drug, any drug toxicity or other reaction resulting from the interaction of the two drugs would be classified as a poisoning.

(iv) Interaction of drug(s) and alcohol

When a reaction results from the interaction of a drug(s) and alcohol, this would be classified as poisoning.

See Section I.C.4. if poisoning is the result of insulin pump malfunctions.

(c) Underdosing

Underdosing refers to taking less of a medication than is prescribed by a provider or a manufacturer's instruction. Discontinuing the use of a prescribed medication on the patient's own initiative (not directed by the patient's provider) is also classified as an underdosing. For underdosing, assign the code from categories T36-T50 (fifth or sixth character "6").

Codes for underdosing should never be assigned as principal or first-listed codes. If a patient has a relapse or exacerbation of the medical condition for which the drug is prescribed because of the reduction in dose, then the medical condition itself should be coded.

Noncompliance (Z91.12-, Z91.13- and Z91.14-) or complication of care (Y63.6-Y63.9) codes are to be used with an underdosing code to indicate intent, if known.

(d) Toxic Effects

When a harmful substance is ingested or comes in contact with a person, this is classified as a toxic effect. The toxic effect codes are in categories T51-T65.

Toxic effect codes have an associated intent: accidental, intentional self-harm, assault and undetermined.

ADULT AND CHILD ABUSE, NEGLECT AND OTHER MALTREATMENT

Sequence first the appropriate code from categories T74, Adult and child abuse, neglect and other maltreatment, confirmed) or T76, Adult and child abuse, neglect and other maltreatment, suspected) for abuse, neglect and other maltreatment, followed by any accompanying mental health or injury code(s).

If the documentation in the medical record states abuse or neglect it is coded as confirmed (T74.-). It is coded as suspected if it is documented as suspected (T76.-).

For cases of confirmed abuse or neglect an external cause code from the assault section (X92-Y09) should be added to identify the cause of any physical injuries. A perpetrator code (Y07) should be added when the perpetrator of the abuse is known. For suspected cases of abuse or neglect, do not report external cause or perpetrator code.

If a suspected case of abuse, neglect or mistreatment is ruled out during an encounter code Z04.71, Encounter for examination and observation following alleged physical adult abuse, ruled out, or code Z04.72, Encounter for examination and observation following alleged child physical abuse, ruled out, should be used, not a code from T76.

If a suspected case of alleged rape or sexual abuse is ruled out during an encounter code Z04.41, Encounter for examination and observation following alleged adult rape or code Z04.42, Encounter for examination and observation following alleged child rape, should be used, not a code from T76.

If a suspected case of forced sexual exploitation or forced labor exploitation is ruled out during an encounter, code Z04.81, Encounter for examination and observation of victim following forced sexual exploitation, or code Z04.82, Encounter for examination and observation of victim following forced labor exploitation, should be used, not a code from T76.

See Section I.C.15. Abuse in a pregnant patient.

COMPLICATIONS OF CARE

1) **General guidelines for complications of care**

   (a) Documentation of complications of care

   See Section I.B.16. for information on documentation of complications of care.

2) **Pain due to medical devices**

   Pain associated with devices, implants or grafts left in a surgical site (for example painful hip prosthesis) is assigned to the appropriate code(s) found in Chapter 19, Injury, poisoning, and certain other consequences of external causes. Specific codes for pain due to medical devices are found in the T code section of the ICD-10-CM. **Use Additional Code**(s) from category G89 to identify acute or chronic pain due to presence of the device, implant or graft (G89.18 or G89.28).

3) **Transplant complications**

   (a) Transplant complications other than kidney

   Codes under category T86, Complications of transplanted organs and tissues, are for use for both complications and rejection of transplanted organs. A transplant complication code is only assigned if the complication affects the function of the transplanted organ. Two codes are required to fully describe a transplant complication: the appropriate code from category T86 and a secondary code that identifies the complication.

   Pre-existing conditions or conditions that develop after the transplant are not coded as complications unless they affect the function of the transplanted organs.

   See I.C.21. for transplant organ removal status See I.C.2. for malignant neoplasm associated with transplanted organ.

   (b) Kidney transplant complications

   Patients who have undergone kidney transplant may still have some form of chronic kidney disease (CKD) because the kidney transplant may not fully restore kidney function. Code T86.1- should be assigned for documented complications of a kidney transplant, such as transplant failure or rejection or other transplant complication. Code T86.1- should not be assigned for post kidney transplant patients who have chronic kidney (CKD) unless a transplant complication such as transplant failure or rejection is documented. If the documentation is unclear as to whether the patient has a complication of the transplant, query the provider.

   Conditions that affect the function of the transplanted kidney, other than CKD, should be assigned a code from subcategory T86.1, Complications of transplanted organ, Kidney, and a secondary code that identifies the complication.

For patients with CKD following a kidney transplant, but who do not have a complication such as failure or rejection, *see section I.C.14. Chronic kidney disease and kidney transplant status.*

4) Complication codes that include the external cause

As with certain other T codes, some of the complications of care codes have the external cause included in the code. The code includes the nature of the complication as well as the type of procedure that caused the complication. No external cause code indicating the type of procedure is necessary for these codes.

5) Complications of care codes within the body system chapters

Intraoperative and postprocedural complication codes are found within the body system chapters with codes specific to the organs and structures of that body system. These codes should be sequenced first, followed by a code(s) for the specific complication, if applicable.

Complication codes from the body system chapters should be assigned for intraoperative and postprocedural complications (e.g., the appropriate complication code from chapter 9 would be assigned for a vascular intraoperative or postprocedural complication) unless the complication is specifically indexed to a T code in chapter 19.

● New code   ▲ Revised code   **Excludes1:** Not coded here   **Excludes2:** Not included here   ⊗ Placeholder required   ⑦7ᵗʰ digit required

Chapter 19

Injury, Poisoning and Certain Other Consequences of External Causes (S00-T88)

Note: Use secondary code(s) from Chapter 20, External causes of morbidity, to indicate cause of injury. Codes within the T section that include the external cause do not require an additional external cause code

Use Additional Code to identify any retained foreign body, if applicable (Z18.-)

Excludes1: birth trauma (P10-P15)

       obstetric trauma (O70-O71)

This chapter contains the following blocks:

S00-S09	Injuries to the head
S10-S19	Injuries to the neck
S20-S29	Injuries to the thorax
S30-S39	Injuries to the abdomen, lower back, lumbar spine, pelvis and external genitals
S40-S49	Injuries to the shoulder and upper arm
S50-S59	Injuries to the elbow and forearm
S60-S69	Injuries to the wrist, hand and fingers
S70-S79	Injuries to the hip and thigh
S80-S89	Injuries to the knee and lower leg
S90-S99	Injuries to the ankle and foot
T07	Injuries involving multiple body regions
T14	Injury of unspecified body region
T15-T19	Effects of foreign body entering through natural orifice
T20-T32	Burns and corrosions
T20-T25	Burns and corrosions of external body surface, specified by site
T26-T28	Burns and corrosions confined to eye and internal organs
T30-T32	Burns and corrosions of multiple and unspecified body regions
T33-T34	Frostbite
T36-T50	Poisoning by adverse effect of and underdosing of drugs, medicaments and biological substances
T51-T65	Toxic effects of substances chiefly nonmedicinal as to source
T66-T78	Other and unspecified effects of external causes
T79	Certain early complications of trauma
T80-T88	Complications of surgical and medical care, not elsewhere classified

Note: The chapter uses the S-section for coding different types of injuries related to single body regions and the T-section to cover injuries to unspecified body regions as well as poisoning and certain other consequences of external causes.

INJURIES TO THE HEAD (S00-S09)

Includes: injuries of ear

injuries of eye

injuries of face [any part] injuries of gum

injuries of jaw injuries of oral cavity injuries of palate

injuries of periocular area injuries of scalp

injuries of temporomandibular joint area injuries of tongue

injuries of tooth

Code also for any associated infection

Excludes2: burns and corrosions (T20-T32)

      effects of foreign body in ear (T16)

      effects of foreign body in larynx (T17.3)

      effects of foreign body in mouth NOS (T18.0)

      effects of foreign body in nose (T17.0-T17.1)

      effects of foreign body in pharynx (T17.2)

      effects of foreign body on external eye (T15.-)

      frostbite (T33-T34)

      insect bite or sting, venomous (T63.4)

S00   **Superficial injury of head**

Excludes1: diffuse cerebral contusion (S06.2-)

      focal cerebral contusion (S06.3-)

      injury of eye and orbit (S05.-)

      open wound of head (S01.-)

The appropriate 7th character is to be added to each code from category S00

A - initial encounter

D - subsequent encounter

S - sequela

S00.0   **Superficial injury of scalp**

  ⊗⑦**S00.00**   **Unspecified superficial injury of scalp**

  ⊗⑦**S00.01**   **Abrasion of scalp**

  ⊗⑦**S00.02**   **Blister (nonthermal) of scalp**

  ⊗⑦**S00.03**   **Contusion of scalp**

        Bruise of scalp

        Hematoma of scalp

  ⊗⑦**S00.04**   **External constriction of part of scalp**

  ⊗⑦**S00.05**   **Superficial foreign body of scalp**

        Splinter in the scalp

  ⊗⑦**S00.06**   **Insect bite (nonvenomous) of scalp**

  ⊗⑦**S00.07**   **Other superficial bite of scalp**

    Excludes1: open bite of scalp (S01.05)

S00.1   **Contusion of eyelid and periocular area**

    Black eye

    Excludes2: contusion of eyeball and orbital tissues (S05.1-)

  ⊗⑦**S00.10**   **Contusion of unspecified eyelid and periocular area**

  ⊗⑦**S00.11**   **Contusion of right eyelid and periocular area**

  ⊗⑦**S00.12**   **Contusion of left eyelid and periocular area**

S00.2   **Other and unspecified superficial injuries of eyelid and periocular area**

    Excludes2: superficial injury of conjunctiva and cornea (S05.0-)

    S00.20   **Unspecified superficial injury of eyelid and periocular area**

      ⑦**S00.201**   **Unspecified superficial injury of right eyelid and periocular area**

      ⑦**S00.202**   **Unspecified superficial injury of left eyelid and periocular area**

      ⑦**S00.209**   **Unspecified superficial injury of unspecified eyelid and periocular area**

    S00.21   **Abrasion of eyelid and periocular area**

      ⑦**S00.211**   **Abrasion of right eyelid and periocular area**

      ⑦**S00.212**   **Abrasion of left eyelid and periocular area**

      ⑦**S00.219**   **Abrasion of unspecified eyelid and periocular area**

    S00.22   **Blister (nonthermal) of eyelid and periocular area**

      ⑦**S00.221**   **Blister (nonthermal) of right eyelid and periocular area**

⑦S00.222 **Blister (nonthermal) of left eyelid and periocular area**

⑦S00.229 **Blister (nonthermal) of unspecified eyelid and periocular area**

S00.24 **External constriction of eyelid and periocular area**

⑦S00.241 **External constriction of right eyelid and periocular area**

⑦S00.242 **External constriction of left eyelid and periocular area**

⑦S00.249 **External constriction of unspecified eyelid and periocular area**

S00.25 **Superficial foreign body of eyelid and periocular area**

Splinter of eyelid and periocular area

Excludes2: retained foreign body in eyelid (H02.81-)

⑦S00.251 **Superficial foreign body of right eyelid and periocular area**

⑦S00.252 **Superficial foreign body of left eyelid and periocular area**

⑦S00.259 **Superficial foreign body of unspecified eyelid and periocular area**

S00.26 **Insect bite (nonvenomous) of eyelid and periocular area**

⑦S00.261 **Insect bite (nonvenomous) of right eyelid and periocular area**

⑦S00.262 **Insect bite (nonvenomous) of left eyelid and periocular area**

⑦S00.269 **Insect bite (nonvenomous) of unspecified eyelid and periocular area**

S00.27 **Other superficial bite of eyelid and periocular area**

Excludes1: open bite of eyelid and periocular area (S01.15)

⑦S00.271 **Other superficial bite of right eyelid and periocular area**

⑦S00.272 **Other superficial bite of left eyelid and periocular area**

⑦S00.279 **Other superficial bite of unspecified eyelid and periocular area**

S00.3 **Superficial injury of nose**

⊗⑦S00.30 **Unspecified superficial injury of nose**

⊗⑦S00.31 **Abrasion of nose**

⊗⑦S00.32 **Blister (nonthermal) of nose**

⊗⑦S00.33 **Contusion of nose**

Bruise of nose

Hematoma of nose

⊗⑦S00.34 **External constriction of nose**

⊗⑦S00.35 **Superficial foreign body of nose**

Splinter in the nose

⊗⑦S00.36 **Insect bite (nonvenomous) of nose**

⊗⑦S00.37 **Other superficial bite of nose**

Excludes1: open bite of nose (S01.25)

S00.4 **Superficial injury of ear**

S00.40 **Unspecified superficial injury of ear**

⑦S00.401 **Unspecified superficial injury of right ear**

⑦S00.402 **Unspecified superficial injury of left ear**

⑦S00.409 **Unspecified superficial injury of unspecified ear**

S00.41 **Abrasion of ear**

⑦S00.411 **Abrasion of right ear**

⑦S00.412 **Abrasion of left ear**

⑦S00.419 **Abrasion of unspecified ear**

S00.42 **Blister (nonthermal) of ear**

⑦S00.421 **Blister (nonthermal) of right ear**

⑦S00.422 **Blister (nonthermal) of left ear**

⑦S00.429 **Blister (nonthermal) of unspecified ear**

S00.43 **Contusion of ear**

Bruise of ear

Hematoma of ear

⑦S00.431 **Contusion of right ear**

⑦S00.432 **Contusion of left ear**

⑦S00.439 **Contusion of unspecified ear**

S00.44 **External constriction of ear**

⑦S00.441 **External constriction of right ear**

⑦S00.442 **External constriction of left ear**

⑦S00.449 **External constriction of unspecified ear**

S00.45 **Superficial foreign body of ear**

Splinter in the ear

⑦S00.451 **Superficial foreign body of right ear**

⑦S00.452 **Superficial foreign body of left ear**

⑦S00.459 **Superficial foreign body of unspecified ear**

S00.46 **Insect bite (nonvenomous) of ear**

⑦S00.461 **Insect bite (nonvenomous) of right ear**

⑦S00.462 **Insect bite (nonvenomous) of left ear**

⑦S00.469 **Insect bite (nonvenomous) of unspecified ear**

S00.47 **Other superficial bite of ear**

Excludes1: open bite of ear (S01.35)

⑦S00.471 **Other superficial bite of right ear**

⑦S00.472 **Other superficial bite of left ear**

⑦S00.479 **Other superficial bite of unspecified ear**

S00.5 **Superficial injury of lip and oral cavity**

S00.50 **Unspecified superficial injury of lip and oral cavity**

⑦S00.501 **Unspecified superficial injury of lip**

⑦S00.502 **Unspecified superficial injury of oral cavity**

S00.51 **Abrasion of lip and oral cavity**

⑦S00.511 **Abrasion of lip**

⑦S00.512 **Abrasion of oral cavity**

S00.52 **Blister (nonthermal) of lip and oral cavity**

⑦S00.521 **Blister (nonthermal) of lip**

⑦S00.522 **Blister (nonthermal) of oral cavity**

S00.53 **Contusion of lip and oral cavity**

⑦S00.531 **Contusion of lip**

Bruise of lip

Hematoma of lip

⑦S00.532 **Contusion of oral cavity**

Bruise of oral cavity

Hematoma of oral cavity

S00.54   **External constriction of lip and oral cavity**

⑦S00.541   **External constriction of lip**

⑦S00.542   **External constriction of oral cavity**

S00.55   **Superficial foreign body of lip and oral cavity**

⑦S00.551   **Superficial foreign body of lip**

Splinter of lip and oral cavity

⑦S00.552   **Superficial foreign body of oral cavity**

Splinter of lip and oral cavity

S00.56   **Insect bite (nonvenomous) of lip and oral cavity**

⑦S00.561   **Insect bite (nonvenomous) of lip**

⑦S00.562   **Insect bite (nonvenomous) of oral cavity**

S00.57   **Other superficial bite of lip and oral cavity**

⑦S00.571   **Other superficial bite of lip**

Excludes1: open bite of lip (S01.551)

⑦S00.572   **Other superficial bite of oral cavity**

Excludes1: open bite of oral cavity (S01.552)

S00.8   **Superficial injury of other parts of head**

Superficial injuries of face [any part]

⊗⑦S00.80   **Unspecified superficial injury of other part of head**

⊗⑦S00.81   **Abrasion of other part of head**

⊗⑦S00.82   **Blister (nonthermal) of other part of head**

⊗⑦S00.83   **Contusion of other part of head**

Bruise of other part of head

Hematoma of other part of head

⊗⑦S00.84   **External constriction of other part of head**

⊗⑦S00.85   **Superficial foreign body of other part of head**

Splinter in other part of head

⊗⑦S00.86   **Insect bite (nonvenomous) of other part of head**

⊗⑦S00.87   **Other superficial bite of other part of head**

Excludes1: open bite of other part of head (S01.85)

S00.9   **Superficial injury of unspecified part of head**

⊗⑦S00.90   **Unspecified superficial injury of unspecified part of head**

⊗⑦S00.91   **Abrasion of unspecified part of head**

⊗⑦S00.92   **Blister (nonthermal) of unspecified part of head**

⊗⑦S00.93   **Contusion of unspecified part of head**

Bruise of head

Hematoma of head

⊗⑦S00.94   **External constriction of unspecified part of head**

⊗⑦S00.95   **Superficial foreign body of unspecified part of head**

Splinter of head

⊗⑦S00.96   **Insect bite (nonvenomous) of unspecified part of head**

⊗⑦S00.97   **Other superficial bite of unspecified part of head**

Excludes1: open bite of head (S01.95)

S01   Open wound of head

Code also any associated:

injury of cranial nerve (S04.-)

injury of muscle and tendon of head (S09.1-)

intracranial injury (S06.-)

wound infection

Excludes1: open skull fracture (S02.- with 7th character B)

Excludes2: injury of eye and orbit (S05.-)

traumatic amputation of part of head (S08.-)

The appropriate 7th character is to be added to each code from category S01

A - initial encounter

D - subsequent encounter

S - sequela

S01.0   **Open wound of scalp**

Excludes1: avulsion of scalp (S08.0)

⊗⑦S01.00   **Unspecified open wound of scalp**

⊗⑦S01.01   **Laceration without foreign body of scalp**

⊗⑦S01.02   **Laceration with foreign body of scalp**

⊗⑦S01.03   **Puncture wound without foreign body of scalp**

⊗⑦S01.04   **Puncture wound with foreign body of scalp**

⊗⑦S01.05   **Open bite of scalp**

Bite of scalp NOS

Excludes1: superficial bite of scalp (S00.06, S00.07-)

S01.1   **Open wound of eyelid and periocular area**

Open wound of eyelid and periocular area with or without involvement of lacrimal passages

S01.10   **Unspecified open wound of eyelid and periocular area**

⑦S01.101   **Unspecified open wound of right eyelid and periocular area**

⑦S01.102   **Unspecified open wound of left eyelid and periocular area**

⑦S01.109   **Unspecified open wound of unspecified eyelid and periocular area**

S01.11   **Laceration without foreign body of eyelid and periocular area**

⑦S01.111   **Laceration without foreign body of right eyelid and periocular area**

⑦S01.112   **Laceration without foreign body of left eyelid and periocular area**

⑦S01.119   **Laceration without foreign body of unspecified eyelid and periocular area**

S01.12   **Laceration with foreign body of eyelid and periocular area**

⑦S01.121   **Laceration with foreign body of right eyelid and periocular area**

⑦S01.122   **Laceration with foreign body of left eyelid and periocular area**

⑦S01.129   **Laceration with foreign body of unspecified eyelid and periocular area**

S01.13   **Puncture wound without foreign body of eyelid and periocular area**

⑦S01.131   **Puncture wound without foreign body of right eyelid and periocular area**

⑦S01.132   **Puncture wound without foreign body of left eyelid and periocular area**

⑦S01.139   **Puncture wound without foreign body of unspecified eyelid and periocular area**

S01.14 Puncture wound with foreign body of eyelid and periocular area

⑦S01.141 Puncture wound with foreign body of right eyelid and periocular area

⑦S01.142 Puncture wound with foreign body of left eyelid and periocular area

⑦S01.149 Puncture wound with foreign body of unspecified eyelid and periocular area

S01.15 Open bite of eyelid and periocular area

Bite of eyelid and periocular area NOS

Excludes1: superficial bite of eyelid and periocular area (S00.26, S00.27)

⑦S01.151 Open bite of right eyelid and periocular area

⑦S01.152 Open bite of left eyelid and periocular area

⑦S01.159 Open bite of unspecified eyelid and periocular area

S01.2 Open wound of nose

⊗⑦S01.20 Unspecified open wound of nose

⊗⑦S01.21 Laceration without foreign body of nose

⊗⑦S01.22 Laceration with foreign body of nose

⊗⑦S01.23 Puncture wound without foreign body of nose

⊗⑦S01.24 Puncture wound with foreign body of nose

⊗⑦S01.25 Open bite of nose

Bite of nose NOS

Excludes1: superficial bite of nose (S00.36, S00.37)

S01.3 Open wound of ear

S01.30 Unspecified open wound of ear

⑦S01.301 Unspecified open wound of right ear

⑦S01.302 Unspecified open wound of left ear

⑦S01.309 Unspecified open wound of unspecified ear

S01.31 Laceration without foreign body of ear

⑦S01.311 Laceration without foreign body of right ear

⑦S01.312 Laceration without foreign body of left ear

⑦S01.319 Laceration without foreign body of unspecified ear

S01.32 Laceration with foreign body of ear

⑦S01.321 Laceration with foreign body of right ear

⑦S01.322 Laceration with foreign body of left ear

⑦S01.329 Laceration with foreign body of unspecified ear

S01.33 Puncture wound without foreign body of ear

⑦S01.331 Puncture wound without foreign body of right ear

⑦S01.332 Puncture wound without foreign body of left ear

⑦S01.339 Puncture wound without foreign body of unspecified ear

S01.34 Puncture wound with foreign body of ear

⑦S01.341 Puncture wound with foreign body of right ear

⑦S01.342 Puncture wound with foreign body of left ear

⑦S01.349 Puncture wound with foreign body of unspecified ear

S01.35 Open bite of ear

Bite of ear NOS

Excludes1: superficial bite of ear (S00.46, S00.47)

⑦S01.351 Open bite of right ear

⑦S01.352 Open bite of left ear

⑦S01.359 Open bite of unspecified ear

S01.4 Open wound of cheek and temporomandibular area

S01.40 Unspecified open wound of cheek and temporomandibular area

⑦S01.401 Unspecified open wound of right cheek and temporomandibular area

⑦S01.402 Unspecified open wound of left cheek and temporomandibular area

⑦S01.409 Unspecified open wound of unspecified cheek and temporomandibular area

S01.41 Laceration without foreign body of cheek and temporomandibular area

⑦S01.411 Laceration without foreign body of right cheek and temporomandibular area

⑦S01.412 Laceration without foreign body of left cheek and temporomandibular area

⑦S01.419 Laceration without foreign body of unspecified cheek and temporomandibular area

S01.42 Laceration with foreign body of cheek and temporomandibular area

⑦S01.421 Laceration with foreign body of right cheek and temporomandibular area

⑦S01.422 Laceration with foreign body of left cheek and temporomandibular area

⑦S01.429 Laceration with foreign body of unspecified cheek and temporomandibular area

S01.43 Puncture wound without foreign body of cheek and temporomandibular area

⑦S01.431 Puncture wound without foreign body of right cheek and temporomandibular area

⑦S01.432 Puncture wound without foreign body of left cheek and temporomandibular area

⑦S01.439 Puncture wound without foreign body of unspecified cheek and temporomandibular area

S01.44 Puncture wound with foreign body of cheek and temporomandibular area

⑦S01.441 Puncture wound with foreign body of right cheek and temporomandibular area

⑦S01.442 Puncture wound with foreign body of left cheek and temporomandibular area

⑦S01.449 Puncture wound with foreign body of unspecified cheek and temporomandibular area

S01.45 Open bite of cheek and temporomandibular area

Bite of cheek and temporomandibular area NOS

Excludes2: superficial bite of cheek and

temporomandibular area (S00.86, S00.87)

⑦**S01.451**   **Open bite of right cheek and temporomandibular area**

⑦**S01.452**   **Open bite of left cheek and temporomandibular area**

⑦**S01.459**   **Open bite of unspecified cheek and temporomandibular area**

S01.5   **Open wound of lip and oral cavity**

Excludes2: tooth dislocation (S03.2)

tooth fracture (S02.5)

S01.50   **Unspecified open wound of lip and oral cavity**

⑦**S01.501**   **Unspecified open wound of lip**

⑦**S01.502**   **Unspecified open wound of oral cavity**

S01.51   **Laceration of lip and oral cavity without foreign body**

⑦**S01.511**   **Laceration without foreign body of lip**

⑦**S01.512**   **Laceration without foreign body of oral cavity**

S01.52   **Laceration of lip and oral cavity with foreign body**

⑦**S01.521**   **Laceration with foreign body of lip**

⑦**S01.522**   **Laceration with foreign body of oral cavity**

S01.53   **Puncture wound of lip and oral cavity without foreign body**

⑦**S01.531**   **Puncture wound without foreign body of lip**

⑦**S01.532**   **Puncture wound without foreign body of oral cavity**

S01.54   **Puncture wound of lip and oral cavity with foreign body**

⑦**S01.541**   **Puncture wound with foreign body of lip**

⑦**S01.542**   **Puncture wound with foreign body of oral cavity**

S01.55   **Open bite of lip and oral cavity**

⑦**S01.551**   **Open bite of lip**

Bite of lip NOS

Excludes1: superficial bite of lip (S00.571)

⑦**S01.552**   **Open bite of oral cavity**

Bite of oral cavity NOS

Excludes1: superficial bite of oral cavity (S00.572)

S01.8   **Open wound of other parts of head**

⊗⑦**S01.80**   **Unspecified open wound of other part of head**

⊗⑦**S01.81**   **Laceration without foreign body of other part of head**

⊗⑦**S01.82**   **Laceration with foreign body of other part of head**

⊗⑦**S01.83**   **Puncture wound without foreign body of other part of head**

⊗⑦**S01.84**   **Puncture wound with foreign body of other part of head**

⊗⑦**S01.85**   **Open bite of other part of head**

Bite of other part of head NOS

Excludes1: superficial bite of other part of head (S00.87)

S01.9   **Open wound of unspecified part of head**

⊗⑦**S01.90**   **Unspecified open wound of unspecified part of head**

⊗⑦**S01.91**   **Laceration without foreign body of unspecified part of head**

⊗⑦**S01.92**   **Laceration with foreign body of unspecified part of head**

⊗⑦**S01.93**   **Puncture wound without foreign body of unspecified part of head**

⊗⑦**S01.94**   **Puncture wound with foreign body of unspecified part of head**

⊗⑦**S01.95**   **Open bite of unspecified part of head**

Bite of head NOS

Excludes1: superficial bite of head NOS (S00.97)

S02   **Fracture of skull and facial bones**

Note: A fracture not indicated as open or closed should be coded to closed

Code also any associated intracranial injury (S06.-)

The appropriate 7th character is to be added to each code from category S02

A - initial encounter for closed fracture

B - initial encounter for open fracture

D - subsequent encounter for fracture with routine healing

G - subsequent encounter for fracture with delayed healing

K - subsequent encounter for fracture with nonunion

S - sequela

⊗⑦**S02.0**   **Fracture of vault of skull** [HCC]

Fracture of frontal bone

Fracture of parietal bone

S02.1   **Fracture of base of skull**

Excludes2: lateral orbital wall (S02.84-)

medial orbital wall (S02.83-)

S02.10   **Unspecified fracture of base of skull**

⑦**S02.101**   **Fracture of base of skull, right side** [HCC]

⑦**S02.102**   **Fracture of base of skull, left side** [HCC]

⑦**S02.109**   **Fracture of base of skull, unspecified side** [HCC]

S02.11   **Fracture of occiput**

⑦**S02.110**   **Type I occipital condyle fracture, unspecified side** [HCC]

⑦**S02.111**   **Type II occipital condyle fracture, unspecified side** [HCC]

⑦**S02.112**   **Type III occipital condyle fracture, unspecified side** [HCC]

⑦**S02.113**   **Unspecified occipital condyle fracture** [HCC]

⑦**S02.118**   **Other fracture of occiput, unspecified side** [HCC]

⑦**S02.119**   **Unspecified fracture of occiput** [HCC]

⑦**S02.11A**   **Type I occipital condyle fracture, right side** [HCC]

⑦**S02.11B**   **Type I occipital condyle fracture, left side** [HCC]

⑦**S02.11C**   **Type II occipital condyle fracture, right side** [HCC]

⑦**S02.11D**   **Type II occipital condyle fracture, left side** [HCC]

⑦**S02.11E**   **Type III occipital condyle fracture, right side** [HCC]

⑦S02.11F   **Type III occipital condyle fracture, left side** [HCC]

⑦S02.11G   **Other fracture of occiput, right side** [HCC]

⑦S02.11H   **Other fracture of occiput, left side** [HCC]

S02.12   **Fracture of orbital roof**

  ⑦S02.121   **Fracture of orbital roof, right side** [HCC]

  ⑦S02.122   **Fracture of orbital roof, left side** [HCC]

  ⑦S02.129   **Fracture of orbital roof, unspecified side** [HCC]

⊗⑦S02.19   **Other fracture of base of skull** [HCC]

Fracture of anterior fossa of base of skull

Fracture of ethmoid sinus

Fracture of frontal sinus

Fracture of middle fossa of base of skull

Fracture of posterior fossa of base of skull

Fracture of sphenoid

Fracture of temporal bone

⊗⑦**S02.2**   **Fracture of nasal bones** [HCC]

⊗⑦**S02.3**   **Fracture of orbital floor** [HCC]

Fracture of inferior orbital wall

Excludes1: orbit NOS (S02.85)

Excludes2: lateral orbital wall (S02.84-)

medial orbital wall (S02.83-)

⊗⑦S02.30   **Fracture of orbital floor, unspecified side** [HCC]

⊗⑦S02.31   **Fracture of orbital floor, right side** [HCC]

⊗⑦S02.32   **Fracture of orbital floor, left side** [HCC]

S02.4   **Fracture of malar, maxillary and zygoma bones** [HCC]

Fracture of superior maxilla

Fracture of upper jaw (bone)

Fracture of zygomatic process of temporal bone

S02.40   **Fracture of malar, maxillary and zygoma bones, unspecified** [HCC]

  ⑦S02.400   **Malar fracture, unspecified side** [HCC]

  ⑦S02.401   **Maxillary fracture, unspecified side** [HCC]

  ⑦S02.402   **Zygomatic fracture, unspecified side**

  ⑦S02.40A   **Malar fracture, right side** [HCC]

  ⑦S02.40B   **Malar fracture, left side** [HCC]

  ⑦S02.40C   **Maxillary fracture, right side** [HCC]

  ⑦S02.40D   **Maxillary fracture, left side** [HCC]

  ⑦S02.40E   **Zygomatic fracture, right side** [HCC]

  ⑦S02.40F   **Zygomatic fracture, left side** [HCC]

S02.41   **LeFort fracture** [HCC]

  ⑦S02.411   **LeFort I fracture** [HCC]

  ⑦S02.412   **LeFort II fracture** [HCC]

  ⑦S02.413   **LeFort III fracture** [HCC]

⊗⑦S02.42   **Fracture of alveolus of maxilla** [HCC]

⊗⑦**S02.5**   **Fracture of tooth (traumatic)** [HCC]

Broken tooth

Excludes1: cracked tooth (nontraumatic) (K03.81)

S02.6   **Fracture of mandible** [HCC]

Fracture of lower jaw (bone)

S02.60   **Fracture of mandible, unspecified** [HCC]

⑦S02.600   **Fracture of unspecified part of body of mandible, unspecified side** [HCC]

⑦S02.601   **Fracture of unspecified part of body of right mandible** [HCC]

⑦S02.602   **Fracture of unspecified part of body of left mandible** [HCC]

⑦S02.609   **Fracture of mandible, unspecified** [HCC]

S02.61   **Fracture of condylar process of mandible** [HCC]

  ⑦S02.610   **Fracture of condylar process of mandible, unspecified side** [HCC]

  ⑦S02.611   **Fracture of condylar process of right mandible** [HCC]

  ⑦S02.612   **Fracture of condylar process of left mandible** [HCC]

S02.62   **Fracture of subcondylar process of mandible** [HCC]

  ⑦S02.620   **Fracture of subcondylar process of mandible, unspecified side** [HCC]

  ⑦S02.621   **Fracture of subcondylar process of right mandible** [HCC]

  ⑦S02.622   **Fracture of subcondylar process of left mandible** [HCC]

S02.63   **Fracture of coronoid process of mandible** [HCC]

  ⑦S02.630   **Fracture of coronoid process of mandible, unspecified side** [HCC]

  ⑦S02.631   **Fracture of coronoid process of right mandible** [HCC]

  ⑦S02.632   **Fracture of coronoid process of left mandible** [HCC]

S02.64   **Fracture of ramus of mandible**

  ⑦S02.640   **Fracture of ramus of mandible, unspecified side** [HCC]

  ⑦S02.641   **Fracture of ramus of right mandible** [HCC]

  ⑦S02.642   **Fracture of ramus of left mandible** [HCC]

S02.65   **Fracture of angle of mandible** [HCC]

  ⑦S02.650   **Fracture of angle of mandible, unspecified side** [HCC]

  ⑦S02.651   **Fracture of angle of right mandible** [HCC]

  ⑦S02.652   **Fracture of angle of left mandible** [HCC]

⊗⑦S02.66   **Fracture of symphysis of mandible** [HCC]

S02.67   **Fracture of alveolus of mandible** [HCC]

  ⑦S02.670   **Fracture of alveolus of mandible, unspecified side** [HCC]

  ⑦S02.671   **Fracture of alveolus of right mandible** [HCC]

  ⑦S02.672   **Fracture of alveolus of left mandible** [HCC]

⊗⑦S02.69   **Fracture of mandible of other specified site** [HCC]

S02.8   **Fractures of other specified skull and facial bones** [HCC]

Fracture of palate

Excludes2: fracture of orbital floor (S02.3-)

fracture of orbital roof (S02.12-)

⊗⑦S02.80   **Fracture of other specified skull and facial bones, unspecified side** [HCC]

⊗⑦S02.81   **Fracture of other specified skull and facial bones, right side** [HCC]

⊗⑦S02.82   **Fracture of other specified skull and facial bones, left side** [HCC]

   ● New code   ▲ Revised code   **Excludes1:** Not coded here   **Excludes2:** Not included here   ⊗ Placeholder required   ⑦7ᵗʰ digit required

⊗⑦S02.83　**Fracture of medial orbital wall** [HCC]

　　Excludes2: orbital floor (S02.3-)

　　　　orbital roof (S02.12-)

　　⑦S02.831　**Fracture of medial orbital wall, right side** [HCC]

　　⑦S02.832　**Fracture of medial orbital wall, left side** [HCC]

　　⑦S02.839　**Fracture of medial orbital wall, unspecified side** [HCC]

　S02.84　**Fracture of lateral orbital wall**

　　orbital floor (S02.3-)

　　orbital roof (S02.12-)

　　⑦S02.841　**Fracture of lateral orbital wall, right side**

　　⑦S02.842　**Fracture of lateral orbital wall, left side**

　　⑦S02.849　**Fracture of lateral orbital wall, unspecified side**

⊗⑦S02.85　**Fracture of orbit, unspecified**

　　Fracture of orbit NOS

　　Fracture of orbit wall NOS

　　lateral orbital wall (S02.84-)

　　medial orbital wall (S02.83-)

　　orbital floor (S02.3-)

　　orbital roof (S02.12-)

　S02.9　**Fracture of unspecified skull and facial bones** [HGC]

　　⊗⑦S02.91　**Unspecified fracture of skull** [HCC]

　　⊗⑦S02.92　**Unspecified fracture of facial bones** [HCC]

S03　**Dislocation and sprain of joints and ligaments of head**

Includes: avulsion of joint (capsule) or ligament of head

laceration of cartilage, joint (capsule) or ligament of head sprain of cartilage, joint (capsule) or ligament of head

traumatic hemarthrosis of joint or ligament of head

traumatic rupture of joint or ligament of head

traumatic subluxation of joint or ligament of head

traumatic tear of joint or ligament of head

Code also any associated open wound

Excludes2: Strain of muscle or tendon of head (S09.1)

The appropriate 7th character is to be added to each code from category S03

A - initial encounter

D - subsequent encounter

S - sequela

　S03.0　**Dislocation of jaw**

　　Dislocation of jaw (cartilage) (meniscus)

　　Dislocation of mandible

　　Dislocation of temporomandibular (joint)

　　⊗⑦S03.00　**Dislocation of jaw, unspecified side**

　　⊗⑦S03.01　**Dislocation of jaw, right side**

　　⊗⑦S03.02　**Dislocation of jaw, left side**

　　⊗⑦S03.03　**Dislocation of jaw, bilateral**

⊗⑦S03.1　**Dislocation of septal cartilage of nose**

⊗⑦S03.2　**Dislocation of tooth**

　S03.4　**Sprain of jaw**

　　Sprain of temporomandibular (joint) (ligament)

　　⊗⑦S03.40　**Sprain of jaw, unspecified side**

　　⊗⑦S03.41　**Sprain of jaw, right side**

　　⊗⑦S03.42　**Sprain of jaw, left side**

　　⊗⑦S03.43　**Sprain of jaw, bilateral**

⊗⑦S03.8　**Sprain of joints and ligaments of other parts of head**

⊗⑦S03.9　**Sprain of joints and ligaments of unspecified parts of head**

S04　**Injury of cranial nerve**

The selection of side should be based on the side of the body being affected

Code first any associated intracranial injury (S06.-)

Code also any associated:

open wound of head (S01.-)

skull fracture (S02.-)

The appropriate 7th character is to be added to each code from category S04

A - initial encounter

D - subsequent encounter

S - sequela

S04.0　**Injury of optic nerve and pathways**

　　Use Additional Code to identify any visual field defect or blindness (H53.4-, H54-)

　S04.01　**Injury of optic nerve**

　　Injury of 2nd cranial nerve

　　⑦S04.011　**Injury of optic nerve, right eye**

　　⑦S04.012　**Injury of optic nerve, left eye**

　　⑦S04.019　**Injury of optic nerve, unspecified eye**

　　　Injury of optic nerve NOS

　⊗⑦S04.02　**Injury of optic chiasm**

　S04.03　**Injury of optic tract and pathways**

　　Injury of optic radiation

　　⑦S04.031　**Injury of optic tract and pathways, right side**

　　⑦S04.032　**Injury of optic tract and pathways, left side**

　　⑦S04.039　**Injury of optic tract and pathways, unspecified side**

　　　Injury of optic tract and pathways NOS

　S04.04　**Injury of visual cortex**

　　⑦S04.041　**Injury of visual cortex, right side**

　　⑦S04.042　**Injury of visual cortex, left side**

　　⑦S04.049　**Injury of visual cortex, unspecified side**

　　　Injury of visual cortex NOS

S04.1　**Injury of oculomotor nerve**

　　Injury of 3rd cranial nerve

　⊗⑦S04.10　**Injury of oculomotor nerve, unspecified side**

　⊗⑦S04.11　**Injury of oculomotor nerve, right side**

　⊗⑦S04.12　**Injury of oculomotor nerve, left side**

S04.2　**Injury of trochlear nerve**

　　Injury of 4th cranial nerve

　⊗⑦S04.20　**Injury of trochlear nerve, unspecified side**

　⊗⑦S04.21　**Injury of trochlear nerve, right side**

　⊗⑦S04.22　**Injury of trochlear nerve, left side**

S04.3　**Injury of trigeminal nerve**

　　Injury of 5th cranial nerve

　⊗⑦S04.30　**Injury of trigeminal nerve, unspecified side**

　⊗⑦S04.31　**Injury of trigeminal nerve, right side**

　⊗⑦S04.32　**Injury of trigeminal nerve, left side**

S04.4　**Injury of abducent nerve**

　　Injury of 6th cranial nerve

⊗⑦S04.40   **Injury of abducent nerve, unspecified side**

⊗⑦S04.41   **Injury of abducent nerve, right side**

⊗⑦S04.42   **Injury of abducent nerve, left side**

S04.5   **Injury of facial nerve**

Injury of 7th cranial nerve

⊗⑦S04.50   **Injury of facial nerve, unspecified side**

⊗⑦S04.51   **Injury of facial nerve, right side**

⊗⑦S04.52   **Injury of facial nerve, left side**

S04.6   **Injury of acoustic nerve**

Injury of auditory nerve Injury of 8th cranial nerve

⊗⑦S04.60   **Injury of acoustic nerve, unspecified side**

⊗⑦S04.61   **Injury of acoustic nerve, right side**

⊗⑦S04.62   **Injury of acoustic nerve, left side**

S04.7   **Injury of accessory nerve**

Injury of 11th cranial nerve

⊗⑦S04.70   **Injury of accessory nerve, unspecified side**

⊗⑦S04.71   **Injury of accessory nerve, right side**

⊗⑦S04.72   **Injury of accessory nerve, left side**

S04.8   **Injury of other cranial nerves**

S04.81   **Injury of olfactory [1st] nerve**

⑦S04.811   **Injury of olfactory [1st] nerve, right side**

⑦S04.812   **Injury of olfactory [1st] nerve, left side**

⑦S04.819   **Injury of olfactory [1st] nerve, unspecified side**

S04.89   **Injury of other cranial nerves**

Injury of vagus [10th] nerve

⑦S04.891   **Injury of other cranial nerves, right side**

⑦S04.892   **Injury of other cranial nerves, left side**

⑦S04.899   **Injury of other cranial nerves, unspecified side**

⊗⑦S04.9   **Injury of unspecified cranial nerve**

S05   **Injury of eye and orbit**

Includes: open wound of eye and orbit

Excludes2: 2nd cranial [optic] nerve injury (S04.0-)

3rd cranial [oculomotor] nerve injury (S04.1-)

open wound of eyelid and periocular area (S01.1-)

orbital bone fracture (S02.1-, S02.3-, S02.8-)

superficial injury of eyelid (S00.1-S00.2)

The appropriate 7th character is to be added to each code from category S05

A - initial encounter

D - subsequent encounter

S - sequela

S05.0   **Injury of conjunctiva and corneal abrasion without foreign body**

Excludes1: foreign body in conjunctival sac (T15.1)

foreign body in cornea (T15.0)

⊗⑦S05.00   **Injury of conjunctiva and corneal abrasion without foreign body, unspecified eye**

⊗⑦S05.01   **Injury of conjunctiva and corneal abrasion without foreign body, right eye**

⊗⑦S05.02   **Injury of conjunctiva and corneal abrasion without foreign body, left eye**

S05.1   **Contusion of eyeball and orbital tissues**

Traumatic hyphema

Excludes2: black eye NOS (S00.1)

contusion of eyelid and periocular area (S00.1)

⊗⑦S05.10   **Contusion of eyeball and orbital tissues, unspecified eye**

⊗⑦S05.11   **Contusion of eyeball and orbital tissues, right eye**

⊗⑦S05.12   **Contusion of eyeball and orbital tissues, left eye**

S05.2   **Ocular laceration and rupture with prolapse or loss of intraocular tissue**

⊗⑦S05.20   **Ocular laceration and rupture with prolapse or loss of intraocular tissue, unspecified eye**

⊗⑦S05.21   **Ocular laceration and rupture with prolapse or loss of intraocular tissue, right eye**

⊗⑦S05.22   **Ocular laceration and rupture with prolapse or loss of intraocular tissue, left eye**

S05.3   **Ocular laceration without prolapse or loss of intraocular tissue**

Laceration of eye NOS

⊗⑦S05.30   **Ocular laceration without prolapse or loss of intraocular tissue, unspecified eye**

⊗⑦S05.31   **Ocular laceration without prolapse or loss of intraocular tissue, right eye**

⊗⑦S05.32   **Ocular laceration without prolapse or loss of intraocular tissue, left eye**

S05.4   **Penetrating wound of orbit with or without foreign body**

Excludes2: retained (old) foreign body following penetrating wound in orbit (H05.5-)

⊗⑦S05.40   **Penetrating wound of orbit with or without foreign body, unspecified eye**

⊗⑦S05.41   **Penetrating wound of orbit with or without foreign body, right eye**

⊗⑦S05.42   **Penetrating wound of orbit with or without foreign body, left eye**

S05.5   **Penetrating wound with foreign body of eyeball**

Excludes2: retained (old) intraocular foreign body (H44.6-, H44.7)

⊗⑦S05.50   **Penetrating wound with foreign body of unspecified eyeball**

⊗⑦S05.51   **Penetrating wound with foreign body of right eyeball**

⊗⑦S05.52   **Penetrating wound with foreign body of left eyeball**

S05.6   **Penetrating wound without foreign body of eyeball**

Ocular penetration NOS

⊗⑦S05.60   **Penetrating wound without foreign body of unspecified eyeball**

⊗⑦S05.61   **Penetrating wound without foreign body of right eyeball**

⊗⑦S05.62   **Penetrating wound without foreign body of left eyeball**

S05.7   **Avulsion of eye**

Definition: An avulsion is an injury in which a body structure is forcibly detached from its normal point of insertion by either trauma or surgery.

Traumatic enucleation

⊗⑦S05.70   **Avulsion of unspecified eye**

⊗⑦S05.71   **Avulsion of right eye**

⊗⑦S05.72   **Avulsion of left eye**

S05.8   **Other injuries of eye and orbit**

Lacrimal duct injury

S05.8X   **Other injuries of eye and orbit**

● New code   ▲ Revised code   **Excludes1:** Not coded here   **Excludes2:** Not included here   ⊗ Placeholder required   ⑦ 7th digit required

⑦**S05.8X1** **Other injuries of right eye and orbit**

⑦**S05.8X2** **Other injuries of left eye and orbit**

⑦**S05.8X9** **Other injuries of unspecified eye and orbit**

S05.9 **Unspecified injury of eye and orbit**

Injury of eye NOS

⊗⑦**S05.90** **Unspecified injury of unspecified eye and orbit**

⊗⑦**S05.91** **Unspecified injury of right eye and orbit**

⊗⑦**S05.92** **Unspecified injury of left eye and orbit**

S06 **Intracranial injury**

Includes: traumatic brain injury

Code also any associated:

open wound of head (S01.-)

skull fracture (S02.-)

Excludes1: head injury NOS (S09.90)

The appropriate 7th character is to be added to each code from category S06

A - initial encounter

D - subsequent encounter

S – sequela

Note: 7th characters D and S do not apply to codes in category S06 with 6th character 7 - death due to brain injury prior to regaining consciousness, or 8 - death due to other cause prior to regaining consciousness.

S06.0 **Concussion**

Commotio cerebri

Excludes1: concussion with other intracranial injuries classified in subcategories S06.1- to S06.6-, S06.81- and S06.82- code to specified intracranial injury

S06.0X **Concussion**

⑦**S06.0X0** **Concussion without loss of consciousness** [HCC]

⑦**S06.0X1** **Concussion with loss of consciousness of 30 minutes or less** [HCC]

⑦**S06.0X9** **Concussion with loss of consciousness of unspecified duration** [HCC]

Concussion NOS

S06.1 **Traumatic cerebral edema**

Diffuse traumatic cerebral edema

Focal traumatic cerebral edema

S06.1X **Traumatic cerebral edema**

⑦**S06.1X0** **Traumatic cerebral edema without loss of consciousness** [HCC]

⑦**S06.1X1** **Traumatic cerebral edema with loss of consciousness of 30 minutes or less** [HCC]

⑦**S06.1X2** **Traumatic cerebral edema with loss of consciousness of 31 minutes to 59 minutes** [HCC]

⑦**S06.1X3** **Traumatic cerebral edema with loss of consciousness of 1hour to 5 hours 59 minutes** [HCC]

⑦**S06.1X4** **Traumatic cerebral edema with loss of consciousness of 6 hours to 24 hours**

⑦**S06.1X5** **Traumatic cerebral edema with loss of consciousness greater than 24 hours with return to pre-existing conscious level** [HCC]

⑦**S06.1X6** **Traumatic cerebral edema with loss of consciousness greater than 24 hours without return to pre-existing conscious level with patient surviving** [HCC]

⑦**S06.1X7** **Traumatic cerebral edema with loss of consciousness of any duration with death due to brain injury prior to regaining consciousness** [HCC]

⑦**S06.1X8** **Traumatic cerebral edema with loss of consciousness of any duration with death due to other cause prior to regaining consciousness** [HCC]

⑦**S06.1X9** **Traumatic cerebral edema with loss of consciousness of unspecified duration** [HCC]

Traumatic cerebral edema NOS

S06.2 **Diffuse traumatic brain injury**

Use Additional Code, if applicable, for traumatic brain compression or herniation (S06.A-)

Diffuse axonal brain injury

Excludes1: traumatic diffuse cerebral edema (S06.1X-)

S06.2X **Diffuse traumatic brain injury**

⑦**S06.2X0** **Diffuse traumatic brain injury without loss of consciousness** [HCC]

⑦**S06.2X1** **Diffuse traumatic brain injury with loss of consciousness of 30 minutes or less** [HCC]

⑦**S06.2X2** **Diffuse traumatic brain injury with loss of consciousness of 31 minutes to 59 minutes** [HCC]

⑦**S06.2X3** **Diffuse traumatic brain injury with loss of consciousness of 1 hour to 5 hours 59 minutes** [HCC]

⑦**S06.2X4** **Diffuse traumatic brain injury with loss of consciousness of 6 hours to 24 hours** [HCC]

⑦**S06.2X5** **Diffuse traumatic brain injury with loss of consciousness greater than 24 hours with return to pre-existing conscious levels** [HCC]

⑦**S06.2X6** **Diffuse traumatic brain injury with loss of consciousness greater than 24 hours without return to pre-existing conscious level with patient surviving** [HCC]

⑦**S06.2X7** **Diffuse traumatic brain injury with loss of consciousness of any duration with death due to brain injury prior to regaining consciousness** [HCC]

⑦**S06.2X8** **Diffuse traumatic brain injury with loss of consciousness of any duration with death due to other cause prior to regaining consciousness** [HCC]

⑦**S06.2X9** **Diffuse traumatic brain injury with loss of consciousness of unspecified duration** [HCC]

Diffuse traumatic brain injury NOS

S06.3 **Focal traumatic brain injury**

Use Additional Code, if applicable, for traumatic brain compression or herniation (S06.A-)

Excludes1: any condition classifiable to S06.4-S06.6

Excludes2: focal cerebral edema (S06.1)

S06.30 **Unspecified focal traumatic brain injury**

---

⑦S06.300   Unspecified focal traumatic brain injury without loss of consciousness [HCC]

⑦S06.301   Unspecified focal traumatic brain injury with loss of consciousness of 30 minutes or less [HCC]

⑦S06.302   Unspecified focal traumatic brain injury with loss of consciousness of 31 minutes to 59 minutes [HCC]

⑦S06.303   Unspecified focal traumatic brain injury with loss of consciousness of 1 hour to 5 hours 59 minutes [HCC]

⑦S06.304   Unspecified focal traumatic brain injury with loss of consciousness of 6 hours to 24 hours [HCC]

⑦S06.305   Unspecified focal traumatic brain injury with loss of consciousness greater than 24 hours with return to pre-existing conscious level [HCC]

⑦S06.306   Unspecified focal traumatic brain injury with loss of consciousness greater than 24 hours without return to pre-existing conscious level with patient surviving [HCC]

⑦S06.307   Unspecified focal traumatic brain injury with loss of consciousness of any duration with death due to brain injury prior to regaining consciousness [HCC]

⑦S06.308   Unspecified focal traumatic brain injury with loss of consciousness of any duration with death due to other cause prior to regaining consciousness [HCC]

⑦S06.309   Unspecified focal traumatic brain injury with loss of consciousness of unspecified duration [HCC]

Unspecified focal traumatic brain injury NOS

S06.31   Contusion and laceration of right cerebrum

⑦S06.310   Contusion and laceration of right cerebrum without loss of consciousness [HCC]

⑦S06.311   Contusion and laceration of right cerebrum with loss of consciousness of 30 minutes or less [HCC]

⑦S06.312   Contusion and laceration of right cerebrum with loss of consciousness of 31 minutes to 59 minutes [HCC]

⑦S06.313   Contusion and laceration of right cerebrum with loss of consciousness of 1 hour to 5 hours 59 minutes [HCC]

⑦S06.314   Contusion and laceration of right cerebrum with loss of consciousness of 6 hours to 24 hours [HCC]

⑦S06.315   Contusion and laceration of right cerebrum with loss of consciousness greater than 24 hours with return to pre-existing conscious level [HCC]

⑦S06.316   Contusion and laceration of right cerebrum with loss of consciousness greater than 24 hours without return to pre-existing conscious level with patient surviving [HCC]

⑦S06.317   Contusion and laceration of right cerebrum with loss of consciousness of any duration with death due to brain injury prior to regaining consciousness [HCC]

⑦S06.318   Contusion and laceration of right cerebrum with loss of consciousness of any duration with death due to other cause prior to regaining consciousness [HCC]

⑦S06.319   Contusion and laceration of right cerebrum with loss of consciousness of unspecified duration [HCC]

Contusion and laceration of right cerebrum NOS

S06.32   Contusion and laceration of left cerebrum

⑦S06.320   Contusion and laceration of left cerebrum without loss of consciousness [HCC]

⑦S06.321   Contusion and laceration of left cerebrum with loss of consciousness of 30 minutes or less [HCC]

⑦S06.322   Contusion and laceration of left cerebrum with loss of consciousness of 31 minutes to59 minutes

⑦S06.323   Contusion and laceration of left cerebrum with loss of consciousness of 1 hour to 5 hours 59 minutes [HCC]

⑦S06.324   Contusion and laceration of left cerebrum with loss of consciousness of 6 hours to 24 hours [HCC]

⑦S06.325   Contusion and laceration of left cerebrum with loss of consciousness greater than 24 hours with return to pre-existing conscious level [HCC]

⑦S06.326   Contusion and laceration of left cerebrum with loss of consciousness greater than 24 hours without return to pre-existing conscious level with patient surviving [HCC]

⑦S06.327   Contusion and laceration of left cerebrum with loss of consciousness of any duration with death due to brain injury prior to regaining consciousness [HCC]

⑦S06.328   Contusion and laceration of left cerebrum with loss of consciousness of any duration with death due to other cause prior to regaining consciousness [HCC]

⑦S06.329   Contusion and laceration of left cerebrum with loss of consciousness of unspecified duration [HCC]

Contusion and laceration of left cerebrum NOS

S06.33   Contusion and laceration of cerebrum, unspecified

⑦S06.330   Contusion and laceration of cerebrum, unspecified, without loss of consciousness [HCC]

⑦S06.331   Contusion and laceration of cerebrum, unspecified, with loss of consciousness of 30 minutes or less [HCC]

⑦S06.332   Contusion and laceration of cerebrum, unspecified, with loss of consciousness of 31 minutes to 59 minutes [HCC]

⑦S06.333   Contusion and laceration of cerebrum, unspecified, with loss of consciousness of 1 hour to 5 hours 59 minutes [HCC]

● New code   ▲ Revised code   **Excludes1:** Not coded here   **Excludes2:** Not included here   ⊗ Placeholder required   ⑦7ᵗʰ digit required

⑦S06.334 **Contusion and laceration of cerebrum, unspecified, with loss of consciousness of 6 hours to 24 hours** [HCC]

⑦S06.335 **Contusion and laceration of cerebrum, unspecified, with loss of consciousness greater than 24 hours with return to pre-existing conscious level** [HCC]

⑦S06.336 **Contusion and laceration of cerebrum, unspecified, with loss of consciousness greater than 24 hours without return to pre-existing conscious level with patient surviving** [HCC]

⑦S06.337 **Contusion and laceration of cerebrum, unspecified, with loss of consciousness of any duration with death due to brain injury prior to regaining consciousness** [HCC]

⑦S06.338 **Contusion and laceration of cerebrum, unspecified, with loss of consciousness of any duration with death due to other cause prior to regaining consciousness** [HCC]

⑦S06.339 **Contusion and laceration of cerebrum, unspecified, with loss of consciousness of unspecified duration** [HCC]

Contusion and laceration of cerebrum NOS

S06.34 **Traumatic hemorrhage of right cerebrum**

Traumatic intracerebral hemorrhage and hematoma of right cerebrum

⑦S06.340 **Traumatic hemorrhage of right cerebrum without loss of consciousness** [HCC]

⑦S06.341 **Traumatic hemorrhage of right cerebrum with loss of consciousness of 30 minutes or less** [HCC]

⑦S06.342 **Traumatic hemorrhage of right cerebrum with loss of consciousness of 31 minutes to 59 minutes** [HCC]

⑦S06.343 **Traumatic hemorrhage of right cerebrum with loss of consciousness of 1 hours to 5 hours 59 minutes** [HCC]

⑦S06.344 **Traumatic hemorrhage of right cerebrum with loss of consciousness of 6 hours to 24 hours** [HCC]

⑦S06.345 **Traumatic hemorrhage of right cerebrum with loss of consciousness greater than 24 hours with return to pre-existing conscious level** [HCC]

⑦S06.346 **Traumatic hemorrhage of right cerebrum with loss of consciousness greater than 24 hours without return to pre-existing conscious level with patient surviving** [HCC]

⑦S06.347 **Traumatic hemorrhage of right cerebrum with loss of consciousness of any duration with death due to brain injury prior to regaining consciousness** [HCC]

⑦S06.348 **Traumatic hemorrhage of right cerebrum with loss of consciousness of any duration with death due to other cause prior to regaining consciousness** [HCC]

⑦S06.349 **Traumatic hemorrhage of right cerebrum with loss of consciousness of unspecified duration** [HCC]

Traumatic hemorrhage of right cerebrum NOS

S06.35 **Traumatic hemorrhage of left cerebrum**

Traumatic intracerebral hemorrhage and hematoma of left cerebrum

⑦S06.350 **Traumatic hemorrhage of left cerebrum without loss of consciousness** [HCC]

⑦S06.351 **Traumatic hemorrhage of left cerebrum with loss of consciousness of 30 minutes or less** [HCC]

⑦S06.352 **Traumatic hemorrhage of left cerebrum with loss of consciousness of 31 minutes to 59 minutes** [HCC]

⑦S06.353 **Traumatic hemorrhage of left cerebrum with loss of consciousness of 1 hours to 5 hours 59 minutes** [HCC]

⑦S06.354 **Traumatic hemorrhage of left cerebrum with loss of consciousness of 6 hours to 24 hours** [HCC]

⑦S06.355 **Traumatic hemorrhage of left cerebrum with loss of consciousness greater than 24 hours with return to pre-existing conscious level** [HCC]

⑦S06.356 **Traumatic hemorrhage of left cerebrum with loss of consciousness greater than 24 hours without return to pre-existing conscious level with patient surviving** [HCC]

⑦S06.357 **Traumatic hemorrhage of left cerebrum with loss of consciousness of any duration with death due to brain injury prior to regaining consciousness** [HCC]

⑦S06.358 **Traumatic hemorrhage of left cerebrum with loss of consciousness of any duration with death due to other cause prior to regaining consciousness** [HCC]

⑦S06.359 **Traumatic hemorrhage of left cerebrum with loss of consciousness of unspecified duration** [HCC]

Traumatic hemorrhage of left cerebrum NOS

S06.36 **Traumatic hemorrhage of cerebrum, unspecified**

Traumatic intracerebral hemorrhage and hematoma, unspecified

⑦S06.360 **Traumatic hemorrhage of cerebrum, unspecified, without loss of consciousness** [HCC]

⑦S06.361 **Traumatic hemorrhage of cerebrum, unspecified, with loss of consciousness of 30 minutes or less** [HCC]

⑦S06.362 **Traumatic hemorrhage of cerebrum, unspecified, with loss of consciousness of 31 minutes to 59 minutes** [HCC]

⑦S06.363 **Traumatic hemorrhage of cerebrum, unspecified, with loss of consciousness of 1 hours to 5 hours 59 minutes** [HCC]

⑦S06.364 **Traumatic hemorrhage of cerebrum, unspecified, with loss of consciousness of 6 hours to 24 hours** [HCC]

⑦S06.365 **Traumatic hemorrhage of cerebrum, unspecified, with loss of consciousness greater than 24 hours with return to pre-existing conscious level** [HCC]

⑦S06.366 **Traumatic hemorrhage of cerebrum, unspecified, with loss of consciousness greater than 24 hours without return to pre-existing conscious level with patient surviving** [HCC]

⑦S06.367 **Traumatic hemorrhage of cerebrum, unspecified, with loss of consciousness of any duration with death due to brain injury prior to regaining consciousness** [HCC]

⑦S06.368 **Traumatic hemorrhage of cerebrum, unspecified, with loss of consciousness of any duration with death due to other cause prior to regaining consciousness** [HCC]

⑦S06.369 **Traumatic hemorrhage of cerebrum, unspecified, with loss of consciousness of unspecified duration** [HCC]

Traumatic hemorrhage of cerebrum NOS

S06.37 **Contusion, laceration, and hemorrhage of cerebellum**

⑦S06.370 **Contusion, laceration, and hemorrhage of cerebellum without loss of consciousness** [HCC]

⑦S06.371 **Contusion, laceration, and hemorrhage of cerebellum with loss of consciousness of 30 minutes or less** [HCC]

⑦S06.372 **Contusion, laceration, and hemorrhage of cerebellum with loss of consciousness of 31 minutes to 59 minutes** [HCC]

⑦S06.373 **Contusion, laceration, and hemorrhage of cerebellum with loss of consciousness of 1 hour to 5 hours 59 minutes** [HCC]

⑦S06.374 **Contusion, laceration, and hemorrhage of cerebellum with loss of consciousness of 6 hours to 24 hours** [HCC]

⑦S06.375 **Contusion, laceration, and hemorrhage of cerebellum with loss of consciousness greater than 24 hours with return to pre-existing conscious level** [HCC]

⑦S06.376 **Contusion, laceration, and hemorrhage of cerebellum with loss of consciousness greater than 24 hours without return to pre-existing conscious level with patient surviving** [HCC]

⑦S06.377 **Contusion, laceration, and hemorrhage of cerebellum with loss of consciousness of any duration with death due to brain injury prior to regaining consciousness** [HCC]

⑦S06.378 **Contusion, laceration, and hemorrhage of cerebellum with loss of consciousness of any duration with**

death due to other cause prior to regaining consciousness [HCC]

⑦S06.379 **Contusion, laceration, and hemorrhage of cerebellum with loss of consciousness of unspecified duration** [HCC]

Contusion, laceration, and hemorrhage of cerebellum NOS

S06.38 **Contusion, laceration, and hemorrhage of brainstem**

⑦S06.380 **Contusion, laceration, and hemorrhage of brainstem without loss of consciousness** [HCC]

⑦S06.381 **Contusion, laceration, and hemorrhage of brainstem with loss of consciousness of 30 minutes or less** [HCC]

⑦S06.382 **Contusion, laceration, and hemorrhage of brainstem with loss of consciousness of 31 minutes to 59 minutes** [HCC]

⑦S06.383 **Contusion, laceration, and hemorrhage of brainstem with loss of consciousness of 1 hour to 5 hours 59 minutes** [HCC]

⑦S06.384 **Contusion, laceration, and hemorrhage of brainstem with loss of consciousness of 6 hours to 24 hours** [HCC]

⑦S06.385 **Contusion, laceration, and hemorrhage of brainstem with loss of consciousness greater than 24 hours with return to pre-existing conscious level** [HCC]

⑦S06.386 **Contusion, laceration, and hemorrhage of brainstem with loss of consciousness greater than 24 hours without return to pre-existing conscious level with patient surviving** [HCC]

⑦S06.387 **Contusion, laceration, and hemorrhage of brainstem with loss of consciousness of any duration with death due to brain injury prior to regaining consciousness** [HCC]

⑦S06.388 **Contusion, laceration, and hemorrhage of brainstem with loss of consciousness of any duration with death due to other cause prior to regaining consciousness** [HCC]

⑦S06.389 **Contusion, laceration, and hemorrhage of brainstem with loss of consciousness of unspecified duration** [HCC]

Contusion, laceration, and hemorrhage of brainstem NOS

S06.4 **Epidural hemorrhage**

Extradural hemorrhage NOS

Extradural hemorrhage (traumatic)

S06.4X **Epidural hemorrhage**

⑦S06.4X0 **Epidural hemorrhage without loss of consciousness** [HCC]

⑦S06.4X1 **Epidural hemorrhage with loss of consciousness of 30 minutes or less** [HCC]

⑦S06.4X2 **Epidural hemorrhage with loss of consciousness of 31 minutes to 59 minutes** [HCC]

⑦S06.4X3   **Epidural hemorrhage with loss of consciousness of 1 hour to 5 hours 59 minutes** [HCC]

⑦S06.4X4   **Epidural hemorrhage with loss of consciousness of 6 hours to 24 hours** [HCC]

⑦S06.4X5   **Epidural hemorrhage with loss of consciousness greater than 24 hours with return to pre-existing conscious level** [HCC]

⑦S06.4X6   **Epidural hemorrhage with loss of consciousness greater than 24 hours without return to pre-existing conscious level with patient surviving** [HCC]

⑦S06.4X7   **Epidural hemorrhage with loss of consciousness of any duration with death due to brain injury prior to regaining consciousness** [HCC]

⑦S06.4X8   **Epidural hemorrhage with loss of consciousness of any duration with death due to other causes prior to regaining consciousness** [HCC]

⑦S06.4X9   **Epidural hemorrhage with loss of consciousness of unspecified duration** [HCC]

     Epidural hemorrhage NOS

S06.5   **Traumatic subdural hemorrhage**

   <u>Use Additional Code</u>, if applicable, for traumatic brain compression or herniation (S06.A-)

   S06.5X   Traumatic subdural hemorrhage

⑦S06.5X0   **Traumatic subdural hemorrhage without loss of consciousness** [HCC]

⑦S06.5X1   **Traumatic subdural hemorrhage with loss of consciousness of 30 minutes or less** [HCC]

⑦S06.5X2   **Traumatic subdural hemorrhage with loss of consciousness of 31 minutes to 59 minutes** [HCC]

⑦S06.5X3   **Traumatic subdural hemorrhage with loss of consciousness of 1 hour to 5 hours 59 minutes** [HCC]

⑦S06.5X4   **Traumatic subdural hemorrhage with loss of consciousness of 6 hours to 24 hours** [HCC]

⑦S06.5X5   **Traumatic subdural hemorrhage with loss of consciousness greater than 24 hours with return to pre-existing conscious level** [HCC]

⑦S06.5X6   **Traumatic subdural hemorrhage with loss of consciousness greater than 24 hours without return to pre-existing conscious level with patient surviving** [HCC]

⑦S06.5X7   **Traumatic subdural hemorrhage with loss of consciousness of any duration with death due to brain injury before regaining consciousness** [HCC]

⑦S06.5X8   **Traumatic subdural hemorrhage with loss of consciousness of any duration with death due to other cause before regaining consciousness** [HCC]

⑦S06.5X9   **Traumatic subdural hemorrhage with loss of consciousness of unspecified duration** [HCC]

     Traumatic subdural hemorrhage NOS

S06.6   **Traumatic subarachnoid hemorrhage**

   <u>Use Additional Code</u>, if applicable, for traumatic brain compression or herniation (S06.A-)

   S06.6X   Traumatic subarachnoid hemorrhage [HCC]

⑦S06.6X0   **Traumatic subarachnoid hemorrhage without loss of consciousness** [HCC]

⑦S06.6X1   **Traumatic subarachnoid hemorrhage with loss of consciousness of 30 minutes or less** [HCC]

⑦S06.6X2   **Traumatic subarachnoid hemorrhage with loss of consciousness of 31 minutes to 59 minutes** [HCC]

⑦S06.6X3   **Traumatic subarachnoid hemorrhage with loss of consciousness of 1 hour to 5 hours 59 minutes** [HCC]

⑦S06.6X4   **Traumatic subarachnoid hemorrhage with loss of consciousness of 6 hours to 24 hours** [HCC]

⑦S06.6X5   **Traumatic subarachnoid hemorrhage with loss of consciousness greater than 24 hours with return to pre-existing conscious level** [HCC]

⑦S06.6X6   **Traumatic subarachnoid hemorrhage with loss of consciousness greater than 24 hours without return to pre-existing conscious level with patient** [HCC]

⑦S06.6X7   **Traumatic subarachnoid hemorrhage with loss of consciousness of any duration with death due to brain injury prior to regaining consciousness** [HCC]

⑦S06.6X8   **Traumatic subarachnoid hemorrhage with loss of consciousness of any duration with death due to other cause prior to regaining consciousness** [HCC]

⑦S06.6X9   **Traumatic subarachnoid hemorrhage with loss of consciousness of unspecified duration** [HCC]

     Traumatic subarachnoid hemorrhage NOS

S06.8   **Other specified intracranial injuries** [HCC]

   S06.81   **Injury of right internal carotid artery, intracranial portion, not elsewhere classified**

⑦S06.810   **Injury of right internal carotid artery, intracranial portion, not elsewhere classified without loss of consciousness** [HCC]

⑦S06.811   **Injury of right internal carotid artery, intracranial portion, not elsewhere classified with loss of consciousness of 30 minutes or less** [HCC]

⑦S06.812   **Injury of right internal carotid artery, intracranial portion, not elsewhere classified with loss of consciousness of 31 minutes to 59 minutes** [HCC]

⑦S06.813   **Injury of right internal carotid artery, intracranial portion, not elsewhere classified with loss of** consciousness of 1 hour to 5 hours 59 minutes [HCC]

⑦S06.814 **Injury of right internal carotid artery, intracranial portion, not elsewhere classified with loss of consciousness of 6 hours to 24 hours** [HCC]

⑦S06.815 **Injury of right internal carotid artery, intracranial portion, not elsewhere classified with loss of consciousness greater than 24 hours with return to pre-existing conscious level** [HCC]

⑦S06.816 **Injury of right internal carotid artery, intracranial portion, not elsewhere classified with loss of consciousness greater than 24 hours without return to pre-existing conscious level with patient surviving** [HCC]

⑦S06.817 **Injury of right internal carotid artery, intracranial portion, not elsewhere classified with loss of consciousness of any duration with death due to brain injury prior to regaining consciousness** [HCC]

⑦S06.818 **Injury of right internal carotid artery, intracranial portion, not elsewhere classified with loss of consciousness of any duration with death due to other cause prior to regaining consciousness** [HCC]

⑦S06.819 **Injury of right internal carotid artery, intracranial portion, not elsewhere classified with loss of consciousness of unspecified duration** [HCC]

Injury of right internal carotid artery, intracranial portion, not elsewhere classified NOS

S06.82 **Injury of left internal carotid artery, intracranial portion, not elsewhere classified**

⑦S06.820 **Injury of left internal carotid artery, intracranial portion, not elsewhere classified without loss of consciousness** [HCC]

⑦S06.821 **Injury of left internal carotid artery, intracranial portion, not elsewhere classified with loss of consciousness of 30 minutes or less** [HCC]

⑦S06.822 **Injury of left internal carotid artery, intracranial portion, not elsewhere classified with loss of consciousness of 31 minutes to 59 minutes** [HCC]

⑦S06.823 **Injury of left internal carotid artery, intracranial portion, not elsewhere classified with loss of consciousness of 1 hour to 5 hours 59 minutes** [HCC]

⑦S06.824 **Injury of left internal carotid artery, intracranial portion, not elsewhere classified with loss of consciousness of 6 hours to 24 hours** [HCC]

⑦S06.825 **Injury of left internal carotid artery, intracranial portion, not elsewhere classified with loss of consciousness greater than 24 hours with return to pre-existing conscious level** [HCC]

⑦S06.826 **Injury of left internal carotid artery, intracranial portion, not elsewhere classified with loss of consciousness**

greater than 24 hours without return to pre-existing conscious level with patient surviving [HCC]

⑦S06.827 **Injury of left internal carotid artery, intracranial portion, not elsewhere classified with loss of consciousness of any duration with death due to brain injury prior to regaining consciousness** [HCC]

⑦S06.828 **Injury of left internal carotid artery, intracranial portion, not elsewhere classified with loss of consciousness of any duration with death due to other cause prior to regaining consciousness** [HCC]

⑦S06.829 **Injury of left internal carotid artery, intracranial portion, not elsewhere classified with loss of consciousness of unspecified duration** [HCC]

Injury of left internal carotid artery, intracranial portion, not elsewhere classified NOS

S06.89 **Other specified intracranial injury**

Excludes1: concussion (S06.0X-)

⑦S06.890 **Other specified intracranial injury without loss of consciousness** [HCC]

⑦S06.891 **Other specified intracranial injury with loss of consciousness of 30 minutes or less** [HCC]

⑦S06.892 **Other specified intracranial injury with loss of consciousness of 31 minutes to 59 minutes** [HCC]

⑦S06.893 **Other specified intracranial injury with loss of consciousness of 1 hour to 5 hours 59 minutes** [HCC]

⑦S06.894 **Other specified intracranial injury with loss of consciousness of 6 hours to 24 hours** [HCC]

⑦S06.895 **Other specified intracranial injury with loss of consciousness greater than 24 hours with return to pre-existing conscious level** [HCC]

⑦S06.896 **Other specified intracranial injury with loss of consciousness greater than 24 hours without return to pre-existing conscious level with patient surviving** [HCC]

⑦S06.897 **Other specified intracranial injury with loss of consciousness of any duration with death due to brain injury prior to regaining consciousness** [HCC]

⑦S06.898 **Other specified intracranial injury with loss of consciousness of any duration with death due to other cause prior to regaining consciousness** [HCC]

⑦S06.899 **Other specified intracranial injury with loss of consciousness of unspecified duration** [HCC]

S06.9 **Unspecified intracranial injury**

Brain injury NOS

Head injury NOS with loss of consciousness

Traumatic brain injury NOS

Excludes1: conditions classifiable to S06.0- to S06.8-code to specified intracranial injury head injury NOS (S09.90)

● New code ▲ Revised code Excludes1: Not coded here Excludes2: Not included here ⊗ Placeholder required ⑦ 7th digit required

S06.9X   Unspecified intracranial injury

⑦**S06.9X0**   Unspecified intracranial injury without loss of consciousness [HCC]

⑦**S06.9X1**   Unspecified intracranial injury with loss of consciousness of 30 minutes or less [HCC]

⑦**S06.9X2**   Unspecified intracranial injury with loss of consciousness of 31 minutes to 59 minutes [HCC]

⑦**S06.9X3**   Unspecified intracranial injury with loss of consciousness of 1 hour to 5 hours 59 minutes [HCC]

⑦**S06.9X4**   Unspecified intracranial injury with loss of consciousness of 6 hours to 24 hours [HCC]

⑦**S06.9X5**   Unspecified intracranial injury with loss of consciousness greater than 24 hours with return to pre-existing conscious level [HCC]

⑦**S06.9X6**   Unspecified intracranial injury with loss of consciousness greater than 24 hours without return to pre-existing conscious level with patient surviving

⑦**S06.9X7**   Unspecified intracranial injury with loss of consciousness of any duration with death due to brain injury prior to regaining consciousness [HCC]

⑦**S06.9X8**   Unspecified intracranial injury with loss of consciousness of any duration with death due to other cause prior to regaining consciousness [HCC]

⑦**S06.9X9**   Unspecified intracranial injury with loss of consciousness of unspecified duration [HCC]

• ⊗⑦ **S06.A**   **Traumatic brain compression and herniation**

Traumatic cerebral compression

<u>Code first</u> the underlying traumatic brain injury, such as:

diffuse traumatic brain injury (S06.2-)

focal traumatic brain injury (S06.3-)

traumatic subdural hemorrhage (S06.5-)

traumatic subarachnoid hemorrhage (S06.6-)

• ⊗⑦**S06.A0**   **Traumatic brain compression without herniation**

Traumatic brain compression NOS

Traumatic cerebral compression NOS

• ⊗⑦ **S06.A1**   **Traumatic brain compression with herniation**

Traumatic brain herniation

Traumatic brainstem compression with herniation

Traumatic cerebellar compression with herniation

Traumatic cerebral compression with herniation

S07   **Crushing injury of head**

<u>Use Additional Code</u> for all associated injuries, such as:

intracranial injuries (S06.-)

skull fractures (S02.-)

The appropriate 7th character is to be added to each code from category S07

A - initial encounter

D - subsequent encounter

S - sequela

⊗⑦**S07.0**   **Crushing injury of face**

⊗⑦**S07.1**   **Crushing injury of skull**

⊗⑦**S07.8**   **Crushing injury of other parts of head**

⊗⑦**S07.9**   **Crushing injury of head, part unspecified**

S08   **Avulsion and traumatic amputation of part of head**

An amputation not identified as partial or complete should be coded to complete

The appropriate 7th character is to be added to each code from category S08

A - initial encounter

D - subsequent encounter

S - sequela

⊗⑦**S08.0**   **Avulsion of scalp**

S08.1   **Traumatic amputation of ear**

S08.11   **Complete traumatic amputation of ear**

⑦**S08.111**   Complete traumatic amputation of right ear

⑦**S08.112**   Complete traumatic amputation of left ear

⑦**S08.119**   Complete traumatic amputation of unspecified ear

S08.12   **Partial traumatic amputation of ear**

⑦**S08.121**   Partial traumatic amputation of right ear

⑦**S08.122**   Partial traumatic amputation of left ear

⑦**S08.129**   Partial traumatic amputation of unspecified ear

S08.8   **Traumatic amputation of other parts of head**

S08.81   **Traumatic amputation of nose**

⑦**S08.811**   Complete traumatic amputation of nose

⑦**S08.812**   Partial traumatic amputation of nose

⊗⑦**S08.89**   **Traumatic amputation of other parts of head**

S09   **Other and unspecified injuries of head**

The appropriate 7th character is to be added to each code from category S09

A - initial encounter

D - subsequent encounter

S - sequela

⊗⑦**S09.0**   **Injury of blood vessels of head, not elsewhere classified**

Excludes1: injury of cerebral blood vessels (S06.-)

injury of precerebral blood vessels (S15.-)

S09.1   **Injury of muscle and tendon of head**

<u>Code also</u> any associated open wound (S01.-)

Excludes2: sprain to joints and ligament of head (S03.9)

⊗⑦**S09.10**   **Unspecified injury of muscle and tendon of head**

Injury of muscle and tendon of head NOS

⊗⑦**S09.11**   **Strain of muscle and tendon of head**

⊗⑦**S09.12**   **Laceration of muscle and tendon of head**

⊗⑦**S09.19**   **Other specified injury of muscle and tendon of head**

S09.2   **Traumatic rupture of ear drum**

Excludes1: traumatic rupture of ear drum due to blast injury (S09.31-)

⊗⑦**S09.20**   **Traumatic rupture of unspecified ear drum**

⊗⑦**S09.21**   **Traumatic rupture of right ear drum**

⊗⑦**S09.22**   **Traumatic rupture of left ear drum**

S09.3   **Other specified and unspecified injury of middle and inner ear**

Excludes1: injury to ear NOS (S09.91-)

Excludes2: injury to external ear (S00.4-, S01.3-, S08.1-)

S09.30   Unspecified injury of middle and inner ear

⑦S09.301   Unspecified injury of right middle and inner ear

⑦S09.302   Unspecified injury of left middle and inner ear

⑦S09.309   Unspecified injury of unspecified middle and inner ear

S09.31   Primary blast injury of ear

Blast injury of ear NOS

⑦S09.311   Primary blast injury of right ear

⑦S09.312   Primary blast injury of left ear

⑦S09.313   Primary blast injury of ear, bilateral

⑦S09.319   Primary blast injury of unspecified ear

S09.39   Other specified injury of middle and inner ear

Secondary blast injury to ear

⑦S09.391   Other specified injury of right middle and inner ear

⑦S09.392   Other specified injury of left middle and inner ear

⑦S09.399   Other specified injury of unspecified middle and inner ear

⊗⑦S09.8   Other specified injuries of head

S09.9   Unspecified injury of face and head

⊗⑦S09.90   Unspecified injury of head

Head injury NOS

Excludes1: brain injury NOS (S06.9-)

head injury NOS with loss of consciousness (S06.9-)

intracranial injury NOS (S06.9-)

⊗⑦S09.91   Unspecified injury of ear

Injury of ear NOS

⊗⑦S09.92   Unspecified injury of nose

Injury of nose NOS

⊗⑦S09.93   Unspecified injury of face

Injury of face NOS

INJURIES TO THE NECK (S10-S19)

Includes: injuries of nape

injuries of supraclavicular region injuries of throat

Excludes2: burns and corrosions (T20-T32)

effects of foreign body in esophagus (T18.1)

effects of foreign body in larynx (T17.3)

effects of foreign body in pharynx (T17.2)

effects of foreign body in trachea (T17.4)

frostbite (T33-T34)

insect bite or sting, venomous (T63.4)

S10   **Superficial injury of neck**

The appropriate 7th character is to be added to each code from category S10

A - initial encounter

D - subsequent encounter

S - sequela

⊗⑦S10.0   **Contusion of throat**

Contusion of cervical esophagus

Contusion of larynx

Contusion of pharynx

Contusion of trachea

S10.1   Other and unspecified superficial injuries of throat

⊗⑦S10.10   Unspecified superficial injuries of throat

⊗⑦S10.11   Abrasion of throat

⊗⑦S10.12   Blister (nonthermal) of throat

⊗⑦S10.14   External constriction of part of throat

⊗⑦S10.15   Superficial foreign body of throat

Splinter in the throat

⊗⑦S10.16   Insect bite (nonvenomous) of throat

⊗⑦S10.17   Other superficial bite of throat

Excludes1: open bite of throat (S11.85)

S10.8   Superficial injury of other specified parts of neck

⊗⑦S10.80   Unspecified superficial injury of other specified part of neck

⊗⑦S10.81   Abrasion of other specified part of neck

⊗⑦S10.82   Blister (nonthermal) of other specified part of neck

⊗⑦S10.83   Contusion of other specified part of neck

⊗⑦S10.84   External constriction of other specified part of neck

⊗⑦S10.85   Superficial foreign body of other specified part of neck

Splinter in other specified part of neck

⊗⑦S10.86   Insect bite of other specified part of neck

⊗⑦S10.87   Other superficial bite of other specified part of neck

Excludes1: open bite of other specified parts of neck (S11.85)

S10.9   Superficial injury of unspecified part of neck

⊗⑦S10.90   Unspecified superficial injury of unspecified part of neck

⊗⑦S10.91   Abrasion of unspecified part of neck

⊗⑦S10.92   Blister (nonthermal) of unspecified part of neck

⊗⑦S10.93   Contusion of unspecified part of neck

⊗⑦S10.94   External constriction of unspecified part of neck

⊗⑦S10.95   Superficial foreign body of unspecified part of neck

⊗⑦S10.96   Insect bite of unspecified part of neck

⊗⑦S10.97   Other superficial bite of unspecified part of neck

S11   **Open wound of neck**

Code also any associated:

spinal cord injury (S14.0, S14.1-)

wound infection

Excludes2: open fracture of vertebra (S12.- with 7th character B)

The appropriate 7th character is to be added to each code from category S11

A - initial encounter

D - subsequent encounter

S - sequela

S11.0   Open wound of larynx and trachea

S11.01   Open wound of larynx

Excludes2: open wound of vocal cord (S11.03)

⑦S11.011   Laceration without foreign body of larynx

⑦S11.012   Laceration with foreign body of larynx

⑦S11.013   Puncture wound without foreign body of larynx

⑦S11.014   **Puncture wound with foreign body of larynx**

⑦S11.015   **Open bite of larynx**

Bite of larynx NOS

⑦S11.019   **Unspecified open wound of larynx**

S11.02   **Open wound of trachea**

Open wound of cervical trachea

Open wound of trachea NOS

Excludes2: open wound of thoracic trachea (S27.5-)

⑦S11.021   **Laceration without foreign body of trachea**

⑦S11.022   **Laceration with foreign body of trachea**

⑦S11.023   **Puncture wound without foreign body of trachea**

⑦S11.024   **Puncture wound with foreign body of trachea**

⑦S11.025   **Open bite of trachea**

Bite of trachea NOS

⑦S11.029   **Unspecified open wound of trachea**

S11.03   **Open wound of vocal cord**

⑦S11.031   **Laceration without foreign body of vocal cord**

⑦S11.032   **Laceration with foreign body of vocal cord**

⑦S11.033   **Puncture wound without foreign body of vocal cord**

⑦S11.034   **Puncture wound with foreign body of vocal cord**

⑦S11.035   **Open bite of vocal cord**

Bite of vocal cord NOS

⑦S11.039   **Unspecified open wound of vocal cord**

S11.1   **Open wound of thyroid gland**

⊗⑦S11.10   **Unspecified open wound of thyroid gland**

⊗⑦S11.11   **Laceration without foreign body of thyroid gland**

⊗⑦S11.12   **Laceration with foreign body of thyroid gland**

⊗⑦S11.13   **Puncture wound without foreign body of thyroid gland**

⊗⑦S11.14   **Puncture wound with foreign body of thyroid gland**

⊗⑦S11.15   **Open bite of thyroid gland**

Bite of thyroid gland NOS

S11.2   **Open wound of pharynx and cervical esophagus**

Excludes1: open wound of esophagus NOS (S27.8-)

⊗⑦S11.20   **Unspecified open wound of pharynx and cervical esophagus**

⊗⑦S11.21   **Laceration without foreign body of pharynx and cervical esophagus**

⊗⑦S11.22   **Laceration with foreign body of pharynx and cervical esophagus**

⊗⑦S11.23   **Puncture wound without foreign body of pharynx and cervical esophagus**

⊗⑦S11.24   **Puncture wound with foreign body of pharynx and cervical esophagus**

⊗⑦S11.25   **Open bite of pharynx and cervical esophagus**

Bite of pharynx and cervical esophagus NOS

S11.8   **Open wound of other specified parts of neck**

⊗⑦S11.80   **Unspecified open wound of other specified part of neck**

⊗⑦S11.81   **Laceration without foreign body of other specified part of neck**

⊗⑦S11.82   **Laceration with foreign body of other specified part of neck**

⊗⑦S11.83   **Puncture wound without foreign body of other specified part of neck**

⊗⑦S11.84   **Puncture wound with foreign body of other specified part of neck**

⊗⑦S11.85   **Open bite of other specified part of neck**

Bite of other specified part of neck NOS

Excludes1: superficial bite of other specified part of neck (S10.87)

⊗⑦S11.89   **Other open wound of other specified part of neck**

S11.9   **Open wound of unspecified part of neck**

⊗⑦S11.90   **Unspecified open wound of unspecified part of neck**

⊗⑦S11.91   **Laceration without foreign body of unspecified part of neck**

⊗⑦S11.92   **Laceration with foreign body of unspecified part of neck**

⊗⑦S11.93   **Puncture wound without foreign body of unspecified part of neck**

⊗⑦S11.94   **Puncture wound with foreign body of unspecified part of neck**

⊗⑦S11.95   **Open bite of unspecified part of neck**

Bite of neck NOS

Excludes1: superficial bite of neck (S10.97)

S12   **Fracture of cervical vertebra and other parts of neck**

Note: A fracture not indicated as displaced or nondisplaced should be coded to displaced

A fracture not indicated as open or closed should be coded to closed

Includes: fracture of cervical neural arch

fracture of cervical spine

fracture of cervical spinous process

fracture of cervical transverse process

fracture of cervical vertebral arch fracture of neck

Code first any associated cervical spinal cord injury (S14.0, S14.1-)

The appropriate 7th character is to be added to all codes from subcategories S12.0-S12.6

A - initial encounter for closed fracture

B - initial encounter for open fracture

D - subsequent encounter for fracture with routine healing

G - subsequent encounter for fracture with delayed healing

K - subsequent encounter for fracture with nonunion

S - sequela

S12.0   **Fracture of first cervical vertebra**

Atlas

S12.00   **Unspecified fracture of first cervical vertebra**

⑦S12.000   **Unspecified displaced fracture of first cervical vertebra** [HCC]

⑦S12.001   **Unspecified nondisplaced fracture of first cervical vertebra** [HCC]

⊗⑦S12.01   **Stable burst fracture of first cervical vertebra** [HCC]

⊗⑦S12.02   **Unstable burst fracture of first cervical vertebra** [HCC]

**S12.03   Posterior arch fracture of first cervical
vertebra**

⑦**S12.030   Displaced posterior arch fracture of
first cervical vertebra** [HCC]

⑦**S12.031   Nondisplaced posterior arch fracture
of first cervical vertebra** [HCC]

S12.04   Lateral mass fracture of first cervical vertebra

⑦**S12.040   Displaced lateral mass fracture of
first cervical vertebra** [HCC]

⑦**S12.041   Nondisplaced lateral mass fracture
of first cervical vertebra** [HCC]

S12.09   Other fracture of first cervical vertebra

⑦**S12.090   Other displaced fracture of first
cervical vertebra** [HCC]

⑦**S12.091   Other nondisplaced fracture of first
cervical vertebra** [HCC]

S12.1   Fracture of second cervical vertebra [HCC]

Axis

S12.10   Unspecified fracture of second cervical vertebra

⑦**S12.100   Unspecified displaced fracture of
second cervical vertebra** [HCC]

⑦**S12.101   Unspecified nondisplaced fracture of
second cervical vertebra** [HCC]

S12.11   Type II dens fracture

⑦**S12.110   Anterior displaced Type II dens
fracture** [HCC]

⑦**S12.111   Posterior displaced Type II dens
fracture** [HCC]

⑦**S12.112   Nondisplaced Type II dens fracture**
[HCC]

S12.12   Other dens fracture

⑦**S12.120   Other displaced dens fracture** [HCC]

⑦**S12.121   Other nondisplaced dens fracture**

**S12.13   Unspecified traumatic spondylolisthesis of
second cervical vertebra**

⑦**S12.130   Unspecified traumatic displaced
spondylolisthesis of second cervical
vertebra** [HCC]

⑦**S12.131   Unspecified traumatic nondisplaced
spondylolisthesis of second cervical
vertebra** [HCC]

⊗⑦**S12.14   Type III traumatic spondylolisthesis of second
cervical vertebra** [HCC]

**S12.15   Other traumatic spondylolisthesis of second
cervical vertebra**

⑦**S12.150   Other traumatic displaced
spondylolisthesis of second cervical
vertebra** [HCC]

⑦**S12.151   Other traumatic nondisplaced
spondylolisthesis of second cervical
vertebra** [HCC]

S12.19   Other fracture of second cervical vertebra

⑦**S12.190   Other displaced fracture of second
cervical vertebra** [HCC]

⑦**S12.191   Other nondisplaced fracture of
second cervical vertebra** [HCC]

S12.2   Fracture of third cervical vertebra [HCC]

S12.20   Unspecified fracture of third cervical vertebra

⑦**S12.200   Unspecified displaced fracture of
third cervical vertebra** [HCC]

⑦**S12.201   Unspecified nondisplaced fracture of
third cervical vertebra** [HCC]

**S12.23   Unspecified traumatic spondylolisthesis of third
cervical vertebra**

⑦**S12.230   Unspecified traumatic displaced
spondylolisthesis of third cervical
vertebra** [HCC]

⑦**S12.231   Unspecified traumatic nondisplaced
spondylolisthesis of third cervical
vertebra** [HCC]

⊗⑦**S12.24   Type III traumatic spondylolisthesis of third
cervical vertebra** [HCC]

**S12.25   Other traumatic spondylolisthesis of third
cervical vertebra**

⑦**S12.250   Other traumatic displaced
spondylolisthesis of third cervical
vertebra** [HCC]

⑦**S12.251   Other traumatic nondisplaced
spondylolisthesis of third cervical
vertebra** [HCC]

S12.29   Other fracture of third cervical vertebra

⑦**S12.290   Other displaced fracture of third
cervical vertebra** [HCC]

⑦**S12.291   Other nondisplaced fracture of third
cervical vertebra** [HCC]

S12.3   Fracture of fourth cervical vertebra [HCC]

S12.30   Unspecified fracture of fourth cervical vertebra

⑦**S12.300   Unspecified displaced fracture of
fourth cervical vertebra** [HCC]

⑦**S12.301   Unspecified nondisplaced fracture of
fourth cervical vertebra** [HCC]

**S12.33   Unspecified traumatic spondylolisthesis of
fourth cervical vertebra**

⑦**S12.330   Unspecified traumatic displaced
spondylolisthesis of fourth cervical
vertebra** [HCC]

⑦**S12.331   Unspecified traumatic nondisplaced
spondylolisthesis of fourth cervical
vertebra** [HCC]

⊗⑦**S12.34   Type III traumatic spondylolisthesis of fourth
cervical vertebra** [HCC]

**S12.35   Other traumatic spondylolisthesis of fourth
cervical vertebra**

⑦**S12.350   Other traumatic displaced
spondylolisthesis of fourth cervical
vertebra** [HCC]

⑦**S12.351   Other traumatic nondisplaced
spondylolisthesis of fourth cervical
vertebra** [HCC]

S12.39   Other fracture of fourth cervical vertebra

⑦**S12.390   Other displaced fracture of fourth
cervical vertebra** [HCC]

⑦**S12.391   Other nondisplaced fracture of
fourth cervical vertebra** [HCC]

S12.4   Fracture of fifth cervical vertebra

S12.40   Unspecified fracture of fifth cervical vertebra

⑦**S12.400   Unspecified displaced fracture of
fifth cervical vertebra** [HCC]

⑦**S12.401   Unspecified nondisplaced fracture of
fifth cervical vertebra** [HCC]

**S12.43   Unspecified traumatic spondylolisthesis of fifth
cervical vertebra**

⑦**S12.430   Unspecified traumatic displaced
spondylolisthesis of fifth cervical
vertebra** [HCC]

● New code   ▲ Revised code   **Excludes1:** Not coded here   **Excludes2:** Not included here   ⊗ Placeholder required   ⑦7ᵗʰ digit required

⑦S12.431   Unspecified traumatic nondisplaced spondylolisthesis of fifth cervical vertebra [HCC]

⊗⑦S12.44   Type III traumatic spondylolisthesis of fifth cervical vertebra [HCC]

S12.45   Other traumatic spondylolisthesis of fifth cervical vertebra [HCC]

⑦S12.450   Other traumatic displaced spondylolisthesis of fifth cervical vertebra [HCC]

⑦S12.451   Other traumatic nondisplaced spondylolisthesis of fifth cervical vertebra [HCC]

S12.49   Other fracture of fifth cervical vertebra

⑦S12.490   Other displaced fracture of fifth cervical vertebra [HCC]

⑦S12.491   Other nondisplaced fracture of fifth cervical vertebra [HCC]

S12.5   Fracture of sixth cervical vertebra

S12.50   Unspecified fracture of sixth cervical vertebra

⑦S12.500   Unspecified displaced fracture of sixth cervical vertebra [HCC]

⑦S12.501   Unspecified nondisplaced fracture of sixth cervical vertebra [HCC]

S12.53   Unspecified traumatic spondylolisthesis of sixth cervical vertebra

⑦S12.530   Unspecified traumatic displaced spondylolisthesis of sixth cervical vertebra [HCC]

⑦S12.531   Unspecified traumatic nondisplaced spondylolisthesis of sixth cervical vertebra [HCC]

⊗⑦S12.54   Type III traumatic spondylolisthesis of sixth cervical vertebra [HCC]

S12.55   Other traumatic spondylolisthesis of sixth cervical vertebra

⑦S12.550   Other traumatic displaced spondylolisthesis of sixth cervical vertebra [HCC]

⑦S12.551   Other traumatic nondisplaced spondylolisthesis of sixth cervical vertebra [HCC]

S12.59   Other fracture of sixth cervical vertebra

⑦S12.590   Other displaced fracture of sixth cervical vertebra [HCC]

⑦S12.591   Other nondisplaced fracture of sixth cervical vertebra

S12.6   Fracture of seventh cervical vertebra

S12.60   Unspecified fracture of seventh cervical vertebra

⑦S12.600   Unspecified displaced fracture of seventh cervical vertebra [HCC]

⑦S12.601   Unspecified nondisplaced fracture of seventh cervical vertebra [HCC]

S12.63   Unspecified traumatic spondylolisthesis of seventh cervical vertebra

⑦S12.630   Unspecified traumatic displaced spondylolisthesis of seventh cervical vertebra [HCC]

⑦S12.631   Unspecified traumatic nondisplaced spondylolisthesis of seventh cervical vertebra [HCC]

⑦S12.64   Type III traumatic spondylolisthesis of seventh cervical vertebra [HCC]

S12.65   Other traumatic spondylolisthesis of seventh cervical vertebra [HCC]

⑦S12.650   Other traumatic displaced spondylolisthesis of seventh cervical vertebra

⑦S12.651   Other traumatic nondisplaced spondylolisthesis of seventh cervical vertebra [HCC]

S12.69   Other fracture of seventh cervical vertebra

⑦S12.690   Other displaced fracture of seventh cervical vertebra [HCC]

⑦S12.691   Other nondisplaced fracture of seventh cervical vertebra [HCC]

⊗⑦S12.8   Fracture of other parts of neck [HCC]

Hyoid bone

Larynx

Thyroid cartilage

Trachea

The appropriate 7th character is to be added to code S12.8

A - initial encounter

D - subsequent encounter

S - sequela

⊗⑦S12.9   Fracture of neck, unspecified [HCC]

Fracture of neck NOS

Fracture of cervical spine NOS

Fracture of cervical vertebra NOS

The appropriate 7th character is to be added to code S12.9

A - initial encounter

D - subsequent encounter

S - sequela

S13   **Dislocation and sprain of joints and ligaments at neck level**

Includes: avulsion of joint or ligament at neck level

laceration of cartilage, joint or ligament at neck level

sprain of cartilage, joint or ligament at neck level

traumatic hemarthrosis of joint or ligament at neck level

traumatic rupture of joint or ligament at neck level

traumatic subluxation of joint or ligament at neck level

traumatic tear of joint or ligament at neck level

Code also any associated open wound

Excludes2: strain of muscle or tendon at neck level (S16.1)

The appropriate 7th character is to be added to each code from category S13

A - initial encounter

D - subsequent encounter

S - sequela

⊗⑦S13.0   **Traumatic rupture of cervical intervertebral disc**

Excludes1: rupture or displacement (nontraumatic) of cervical intervertebral disc NOS (M50.-)

S13.1   **Subluxation and dislocation of cervical vertebrae**

Definition: Subluxation is a condition that occurs when a joint begins to dislocate. Instead of the joint surfaces completely losing contact, a subluxation can be considered a "partial dislocation." A subluxation can be the result of a trauma or acute injury. In these cases, the injury can be quite painful. Subluxations can also occur as a result of loose joints.

Code also any associated:

open wound of neck (S11.-)

spinal cord injury (S14.1-)

Excludes2: fracture of cervical vertebrae (S12.0-S12.3-)

S13.10 **Subluxation and dislocation of unspecified cervical vertebrae**

⑦**S13.100** **Subluxation of unspecified cervical vertebrae**

⑦**S13.101** **Dislocation of unspecified cervical vertebrae**

S13.11 **Subluxation and dislocation of C0/C1 cervical vertebrae**

Subluxation and dislocation of atlantooccipital joint

Subluxation and dislocation of atloido-occipital joint

Subluxation and dislocation of occipitoatloid joint

⑦**S13.110** **Subluxation of C0/C1 cervical vertebrae**

⑦**S13.111** **Dislocation of C0/C1 cervical vertebrae**

S13.12 **Subluxation and dislocation of C1/C2 cervical vertebrae**

Subluxation and dislocation of atlantoaxial joint

⑦**S13.120** **Subluxation of C1/C2 cervical vertebrae**

⑦**S13.121** **Dislocation of C1/C2 cervical vertebrae**

S13.13 **Subluxation and dislocation of C2/C3 cervical vertebrae**

⑦**S13.130** **Subluxation of C2/C3 cervical vertebrae**

⑦**S13.131** **Dislocation of C2/C3 cervical vertebrae**

S13.14 **Subluxation and dislocation of C3/C4 cervical vertebrae**

⑦**S13.140** **Subluxation of C3/C4 cervical vertebrae**

⑦**S13.141** **Dislocation of C3/C4 cervical vertebrae**

S13.15 **Subluxation and dislocation of C4/C5 cervical vertebrae**

⑦**S13.150** **Subluxation of C4/C5 cervical vertebrae**

⑦**S13.151** **Dislocation of C4/C5 cervical vertebrae**

S13.16 **Subluxation and dislocation of C5/C6 cervical vertebrae**

⑦**S13.160** **Subluxation of C5/C6 cervical vertebrae**

⑦**S13.161** **Dislocation of C5/C6 cervical vertebrae**

S13.17 **Subluxation and dislocation of C6/C7 cervical vertebrae**

⑦**S13.170** **Subluxation of C6/C7 cervical vertebrae**

⑦**S13.171** **Dislocation of C6/C7 cervical vertebrae**

S13.18 **Subluxation and dislocation of C7/T1 cervical vertebrae**

⑦**S13.180** **Subluxation of C7/T1 cervical vertebrae**

⑦**S13.181** **Dislocation of C7/T1 cervical vertebrae**

S13.2 **Dislocation of other and unspecified parts of neck**

⊗⑦**S13.20** **Dislocation of unspecified parts of neck**

⊗⑦**S13.29** **Dislocation of other parts of neck**

⊗⑦**S13.4** **Sprain of ligaments of cervical spine**

Sprain of anterior longitudinal (ligament), cervical

Sprain of atlanto-axial (joints)

Sprain of atlanto-occipital (joints)

Whiplash injury of cervical spine

⊗⑦**S13.5** **Sprain of thyroid region**

Sprain of cricoarytenoid (joint) (ligament)

Sprain of cricothyroid (joint) (ligament)

Sprain of thyroid cartilage

⊗⑦**S13.8** **Sprain of joints and ligaments of other parts of neck**

⊗⑦**S13.9** **Sprain of joints and ligaments of unspecified parts of neck**

S14 **Injury of nerves and spinal cord at neck level**

Note: Code to highest level of cervical cord injury

Code also any associated:

fracture of cervical vertebra (S12.0--S12.6.-)

open wound of neck (S11.-)

transient paralysis (R29.5)

The appropriate 7th character is to be added to each code from category S14

A - initial encounter

D - subsequent encounter

S - sequela

⊗⑦**S14.0** **Concussion and edema of cervical spinal cord**

S14.1 **Other and unspecified injuries of cervical spinal cord**

S14.10 **Unspecified injury of cervical spinal cord**

⑦**S14.101** **Unspecified injury at C1 level of cervical spinal cord** [HCC]

⑦**S14.102** **Unspecified injury at C2 level of cervical spinal cord** [HCC]

⑦**S14.103** **Unspecified injury at C3 level of cervical spinal cord** [HCC]

⑦**S14.104** **Unspecified injury at C4 level of cervical spinal cord** [HCC]

⑦**S14.105** **Unspecified injury at C5 level of cervical spinal cord** [HCC]

⑦**S14.106** **Unspecified injury at C6 level of cervical spinal cord** [HCC]

⑦**S14.107** **Unspecified injury at C7 level of cervical spinal cord**

⑦**S14.108** **Unspecified injury at C8 level of cervical spinal cord** [HCC]

⑦**S14.109** **Unspecified injury at unspecified level of cervical spinal cord** [HCC]

Injury of cervical spinal cord NOS

S14.11 **Complete lesion of cervical spinal cord**

⑦**S14.111** **Complete lesion at C1 level of cervical spinal cord** [HCC]

⑦**S14.112** **Complete lesion at C2 level of cervical spinal cord** [HCC]

⑦**S14.113** **Complete lesion at C3 level of cervical spinal cord** [HCC]

⑦**S14.114** **Complete lesion at C4 level of cervical spinal cord** [HCC]

⑦**S14.115** **Complete lesion at C5 level of cervical spinal cord** [HCC]

⑦**S14.116** **Complete lesion at C6 level of cervical spinal cord** [HCC]

⑦**S14.117** **Complete lesion at C7 level of cervical spinal cord** [HCC]

⑦S14.118   Complete lesion at C8 level of cervical spinal cord [HCC]

⑦S14.119   Complete lesion at unspecified level of cervical spinal cord [HCC]

S14.12   **Central cord syndrome of cervical spinal cord**

⑦S14.121   Central cord syndrome at C1 level of cervical spinal cord [HCC]

⑦S14.122   Central cord syndrome at C2 level of cervical spinal cord [HCC]

⑦S14.123   Central cord syndrome at C3 level of cervical spinal cord [HCC]

⑦S14.124   Central cord syndrome at C4 level of cervical spinal cord [HCC]

⑦S14.125   Central cord syndrome at C5 level of cervical spinal cord [HCC]

⑦S14.126   Central cord syndrome at C6 level of cervical spinal cord [HCC]

⑦S14.127   Central cord syndrome at C7 level of cervical spinal cord [HCC]

⑦S14.128   Central cord syndrome at C8 level of cervical spinal cord [HCC]

⑦S14.129   Central cord syndrome at unspecified level of cervical spinal cord [HCC]

S14.13   **Anterior cord syndrome of cervical spinal cord**

⑦S14.131   Anterior cord syndrome at C1 level of cervical spinal cord [HCC]

⑦S14.132   Anterior cord syndrome at C2 level of cervical spinal cord [HCC]

⑦S14.133   Anterior cord syndrome at C3 level of cervical spinal cord [HCC]

⑦S14.134   Anterior cord syndrome at C4 level of cervical spinal cord [HCC]

⑦S14.135   Anterior cord syndrome at C5 level of cervical spinal cord [HCC]

⑦S14.136   Anterior cord syndrome at C6 level of cervical spinal cord [HCC]

⑦S14.137   Anterior cord syndrome at C7 level of cervical spinal cord [HCC]

⑦S14.138   Anterior cord syndrome at C8 level of cervical spinal cord [HCC]

⑦S14.139   Anterior cord syndrome at unspecified level of cervical spinal cord

S14.14   **Brown-Séquard syndrome of cervical spinal cord**

⑦S14.141   Brown-Séquard syndrome at C1 level of cervical spinal cord [HCC]

⑦S14.142   Brown-Séquard syndrome at C2 level of cervical spinal cord [HCC]

⑦S14.143   Brown-Séquard syndrome at C3 level of cervical spinal cord [HCC]

⑦S14.144   Brown-Séquard syndrome at C4 level of cervical spinal cord [HCC]

⑦S14.145   Brown-Séquard syndrome at C5 level of cervical spinal cord [HCC]

⑦S14.146   Brown-Séquard syndrome at C6 level of cervical spinal cord [HCC]

⑦S14.147   Brown-Séquard syndrome at C7 level of cervical spinal cord [HCC]

⑦S14.148   Brown-Séquard syndrome at C8 level of cervical spinal cord [HCC]

⑦S14.149   Brown-Séquard syndrome at unspecified level of cervical spinal cord [HCC]

S14.15   **Other incomplete lesions of cervical spinal cord**

Incomplete lesion of cervical spinal cord NOS

Posterior cord syndrome of cervical spinal cord

⑦S14.151   Other incomplete lesion at C1 level of cervical spinal cord [HCC]

⑦S14.152   Other incomplete lesion at C2 level of cervical spinal cord [HCC]

⑦S14.153   Other incomplete lesion at C3 level of cervical spinal cord [HCC]

⑦S14.154   Other incomplete lesion at C4 level of cervical spinal cord [HCC]

⑦S14.155   Other incomplete lesion at C5 level of cervical spinal cord [HCC]

⑦S14.156   Other incomplete lesion at C6 level of cervical spinal cord [HCC]

⑦S14.157   Other incomplete lesion at C7 level of cervical spinal cord [HCC]

⑦S14.158   Other incomplete lesion at C8 level of cervical spinal cord [HCC]

⑦S14.159   Other incomplete lesion at unspecified level of cervical spinal cord [HCC]

⊗⑦S14.2   **Injury of nerve root of cervical spine**

⊗⑦S14.3   **Injury of brachial plexus**

⊗⑦S14.4   **Injury of peripheral nerves of neck**

⊗⑦S14.5   **Injury of cervical sympathetic nerves**

⊗⑦S14.8   **Injury of other specified nerves of neck**

⊗⑦S14.9   **Injury of unspecified nerves of neck**

S15   **Injury of blood vessels at neck level**

<u>Code also</u> any associated open wound (S11.-)

The appropriate 7th character is to be added to each code from category S15

A - initial encounter

D - subsequent encounter

S - sequela

S15.0   **Injury of carotid artery of neck**

Injury of carotid artery (common) (external) (internal, extracranial portion)

Injury of carotid artery NOS

> **Excludes1:** injury of internal carotid artery, intracranial portion (S06.8)

S15.00   **Unspecified injury of carotid artery**

⑦S15.001   Unspecified injury of right carotid artery

⑦S15.002   Unspecified injury of left carotid artery

⑦S15.009   Unspecified injury of unspecified carotid artery

S15.01   **Minor laceration of carotid artery**

Incomplete transection of carotid artery

Laceration of carotid artery NOS

Superficial laceration of carotid artery

⑦S15.011   Minor laceration of right carotid artery

⑦S15.012   Minor laceration of left carotid artery

⑦S15.019   Minor laceration of unspecified carotid artery

S15.02 **Major laceration of carotid artery**
Complete transection of carotid artery
Traumatic rupture of carotid artery

⑦S15.021 **Major laceration of right carotid artery**

⑦S15.022 **Major laceration of left carotid artery**

⑦S15.029 **Major laceration of unspecified carotid artery**

S15.09 **Other specified injury of carotid artery**

⑦S15.091 **Other specified injury of right carotid artery**

⑦S15.092 **Other specified injury of left carotid artery**

⑦S15.099 **Other specified injury of unspecified carotid artery**

S15.1 **Injury of vertebral artery**

S15.10 **Unspecified injury of vertebral artery**

⑦S15.101 **Unspecified injury of right vertebral artery**

⑦S15.102 **Unspecified injury of left vertebral artery**

⑦S15.109 **Unspecified injury of unspecified vertebral artery**

S15.11 **Minor laceration of vertebral artery**
Incomplete transection of vertebral artery
Laceration of vertebral artery NOS
Superficial laceration of vertebral artery

⑦S15.111 **Minor laceration of right vertebral artery**

⑦S15.112 **Minor laceration of left vertebral artery**

⑦S15.119 **Minor laceration of unspecified vertebral artery**

S15.12 **Major laceration of vertebral artery**
Complete transection of vertebral artery
Traumatic rupture of vertebral artery

⑦S15.121 **Major laceration of right vertebral artery**

⑦S15.122 **Major laceration of left vertebral artery**

⑦S15.129 **Major laceration of unspecified vertebral artery**

S15.19 **Other specified injury of vertebral artery**

⑦S15.191 **Other specified injury of right vertebral artery**

⑦S15.192 **Other specified injury of left vertebral artery**

⑦S15.199 **Other specified injury of unspecified vertebral artery**

S15.2 **Injury of external jugular vein**

S15.20 **Unspecified injury of external jugular vein**

⑦S15.201 **Unspecified injury of right external jugular vein**

⑦S15.202 **Unspecified injury of left external jugular vein**

⑦S15.209 **Unspecified injury of unspecified external jugular vein**

S15.21 **Minor laceration of external jugular vein**
Incomplete transection of external jugular vein
Laceration of external jugular vein NOS
Superficial laceration of external jugular vein

⑦S15.211 **Minor laceration of right external jugular vein**

⑦S15.212 **Minor laceration of left external jugular vein**

⑦S15.219 **Minor laceration of unspecified external jugular vein**

S15.22 **Major laceration of external jugular vein**
Complete transection of external jugular vein
Traumatic rupture of external jugular vein

⑦S15.221 **Major laceration of right external jugular vein**

⑦S15.222 **Major laceration of left external jugular vein**

⑦S15.229 **Major laceration of unspecified external jugular vein**

S15.29 **Other specified injury of external jugular vein**

⑦S15.291 **Other specified injury of right external jugular vein**

⑦S15.292 **Other specified injury of left external jugular vein**

⑦S15.299 **Other specified injury of unspecified external jugular vein**

S15.3 **Injury of internal jugular vein**

S15.30 **Unspecified injury of internal jugular vein**

⑦S15.301 **Unspecified injury of right internal jugular vein**

⑦S15.302 **Unspecified injury of left internal jugular vein**

⑦S15.309 **Unspecified injury of unspecified internal jugular vein**

S15.31 **Minor laceration of internal jugular vein**
Incomplete transection of internal jugular vein
Laceration of internal jugular vein NOS
Superficial laceration of internal jugular vein

⑦S15.311 **Minor laceration of right internal jugular vein**

⑦S15.312 **Minor laceration of left internal jugular vein**

⑦S15.319 **Minor laceration of unspecified internal jugular vein**

⑦S15.32 **Major laceration of internal jugular vein**
Complete transection of internal jugular vein
Traumatic rupture of internal jugular vein

⑦S15.321 **Major laceration of right internal jugular vein**

⑦S15.322 **Major laceration of left internal jugular vein**

⑦S15.329 **Major laceration of unspecified internal jugular vein**

⑦S15.39 **Other specified injury of internal jugular vein**

⑦S15.391 **Other specified injury of right internal jugular vein**

⑦S15.392 **Other specified injury of left internal jugular vein**

⑦S15.399 **Other specified injury of unspecified internal jugular vein**

⊗⑦**S15.8** **Injury of other specified blood vessels at neck level**

⊗⑦**S15.9** **Injury of unspecified blood vessel at neck level**

S16 **Injury of muscle, fascia and tendon at neck level**
Code also any associated open wound (S11.-)
Excludes2: sprain of joint or ligament at neck level (S13.9)

● New code ▲ Revised code Excludes1: Not coded here Excludes2: Not included here ⊗ Placeholder required ⑦7th digit required

The appropriate 7th character is to be added to each code from category S16

A - initial encounter

D - subsequent encounter

S - sequela

⊗⑦**S16.1**   **Strain of muscle, fascia and tendon at neck level**

⊗⑦**S16.2**   **Laceration of muscle, fascia and tendon at neck level**

⊗⑦**S16.8**   **Other specified injury of muscle, fascia and tendon at neck level**

⊗⑦**S16.9**   **Unspecified injury of muscle, fascia and tendon at neck level**

S17   **Crushing injury of neck**

Use Additional Code for all associated injuries, such as:

injury of blood vessels (S15.-)

open wound of neck (S11.-)

spinal cord injury (S14.0, S14.1-)

vertebral fracture (S12.0--S12.3-)

The appropriate 7th character is to be added to each code from category S17

A - initial encounter

D - subsequent encounter

S - sequela

⊗⑦**S17.0**   **Crushing injury of larynx and trachea**

⊗⑦**S17.8**   **Crushing injury of other specified parts of neck**

⊗⑦**S17.9**   **Crushing injury of neck, part unspecified**

S19   **Other specified and unspecified injuries of neck**

The appropriate 7th character is to be added to each code from category S19

A - initial encounter

D - subsequent encounter

S - sequela

S19.8   **Other specified injuries of neck**

⊗⑦**S19.80**   **Other specified injuries of unspecified part of neck**

⊗⑦**S19.81**   **Other specified injuries of larynx**

⊗⑦**S19.82**   **Other specified injuries of cervical trachea**

Excludes2: Other specified injury of thoracic trachea (S27.5-)

⊗⑦**S19.83**   **Other specified injuries of vocal cord**

⊗⑦**S19.84**   **Other specified injuries of thyroid gland**

⊗⑦**S19.85**   **Other specified injuries of pharynx and cervical esophagus**

⊗⑦**S19.89**   **Other specified injuries of other specified part of neck**

⊗⑦**S19.9**   **Unspecified injury of neck**

INJURIES TO THE THORAX (S20-S29)

Includes: injuries of breast

injuries of chest (wall)

injuries of interscapular area

Excludes2: burns and corrosions (T20-T32)

effects of foreign body in bronchus (T17.5)

effects of foreign body in esophagus (T18.1)

effects of foreign body in lung (T17.8)

effects of foreign body in trachea (T17.4)

frostbite (T33-T34)

injuries of axilla injuries of clavicle

injuries of scapular region injuries of shoulder insect bite or sting, venomous (T63.4)

S20   **Superficial injury of thorax**

The appropriate 7th character is to be added to each code from category S20

A - initial encounter

D - subsequent encounter

S - sequela

S20.0   **Contusion of breast**

⊗⑦**S20.00**   **Contusion of breast, unspecified breast**

⊗⑦**S20.01**   **Contusion of right breast**

⊗⑦**S20.02**   **Contusion of left breast**

S20.1   **Other and unspecified superficial injuries of breast**

S20.10   **Unspecified superficial injuries of breast**

⑦**S20.101**   **Unspecified superficial injuries of breast, right breast**

⑦**S20.102**   **Unspecified superficial injuries of breast, left breast**

⑦**S20.109**   **Unspecified superficial injuries of breast, unspecified breast**

S20.11   **Abrasion of breast**

⑦**S20.111**   **Abrasion of breast, right breast**

⑦**S20.112**   **Abrasion of breast, left breast**

⑦**S20.119**   **Abrasion of breast, unspecified breast**

S20.12   **Blister (nonthermal) of breast**

⑦**S20.121**   **Blister (nonthermal) of breast, right breast**

⑦**S20.122**   **Blister (nonthermal) of breast, left breast**

⑦**S20.129**   **Blister (nonthermal) of breast, unspecified breast**

S20.14   **External constriction of part of breast**

⑦**S20.141**   **External constriction of part of breast, right breast**

⑦**S20.142**   **External constriction of part of breast, left breast**

⑦**S20.149**   **External constriction of part of breast, unspecified breast**

S20.15   **Superficial foreign body of breast**

Splinter in the breast

⑦**S20.151**   **Superficial foreign body of breast, right breast**

⑦**S20.152**   **Superficial foreign body of breast, left breast**

⑦**S20.159**   **Superficial foreign body of breast, unspecified breast**

S20.16   **Insect bite (nonvenomous) of breast**

⑦**S20.161**   **Insect bite (nonvenomous) of breast, right breast**

⑦**S20.162**   **Insect bite (nonvenomous) of breast, left breast**

⑦**S20.169**   **Insect bite (nonvenomous) of breast, unspecified breast**

S20.17   **Other superficial bite of breast**

Excludes1: open bite of breast (S21.05-)

⑦**S20.171**   **Other superficial bite of breast, right breast**

⑦**S20.172**   **Other superficial bite of breast, left breast**

⑦**S20.179**   **Other superficial bite of breast, unspecified breast**

S20.2   **Contusion of thorax**

⊗⑦S20.20   Contusion of thorax, unspecified

S20.21   Contusion of front wall of thorax

⑦S20.211   Contusion of right front wall of thorax

⑦S20.212   Contusion of left front wall of thorax

⑦S20.213   Contusion of bilateral front wall of thorax

⑦S20.214   Contusion of middle front wall of thorax

⑦S20.219   Contusion of unspecified front wall of thorax

S20.22   Contusion of back wall of thorax

⑦S20.221   Contusion of right back wall of thorax

⑦S20.222   Contusion of left back wall of thorax

⑦S20.223   Contusion of bilateral back wall of thorax

⑦S20.224   Contusion of middle back wall of thorax

⑦S20.229   Contusion of unspecified back wall of thorax

S20.3   Other and unspecified superficial injuries of front wall of thorax

S20.30   Unspecified superficial injuries of front wall of thorax

⑦S20.301   Unspecified superficial injuries of right front wall of thorax

⑦S20.302   Unspecified superficial injuries of left front wall of thorax

⑦S20.303   Unspecified superficial injuries of bilateral front wall of thorax

⑦S20.304   Unspecified superficial injuries of middle front wall of thorax

⑦S20.309   Unspecified superficial injuries of unspecified front wall of thorax

S20.31   Abrasion of front wall of thorax

⑦S20.311   Abrasion of right front wall of thorax

⑦S20.312   Abrasion of left front wall of thorax

⑦S20.313   Abrasion of bilateral front wall of thorax

⑦S20.314   Abrasion of middle front wall of thorax

⑦S20.319   Abrasion of unspecified front wall of thorax

S20.32   Blister (nonthermal) of front wall of thorax

⑦S20.321   Blister (nonthermal) of right front wall of thorax

⑦S20.322   Blister (nonthermal) of left front wall of thorax

⑦S20.323   Blister (nonthermal) of bilateral front wall of thorax

⑦S20.324   Blister (nonthermal) of middle front wall of thorax

⑦S20.329   Blister (nonthermal) of unspecified front wall of thorax

S20.34   External constriction of front wall of thorax

⑦S20.341   External constriction of right front wall of thorax

⑦S20.342   External constriction of left front wall of thorax

⑦S20.343   External constriction of bilateral front wall of thorax

⑦S20.344   External constriction of middle front wall of thorax

⑦S20.349   External constriction of unspecified front wall of thorax

S20.35   Superficial foreign body of front wall of thorax

Splinter in front wall of thorax

⑦S20.351   Superficial foreign body of right front wall of thorax

⑦S20.352   Superficial foreign body of left front wall of thorax

⑦S20.353   Superficial foreign body of bilateral front wall of thorax

⑦S20.354   Superficial foreign body of middle front wall of thorax

⑦S20.359   Superficial foreign body of unspecified front wall of thorax

S20.36   Insect bite (nonvenomous) of front wall of thorax

⑦S20.361   Insect bite (nonvenomous) of right front wall of thorax

⑦S20.362   Insect bite (nonvenomous) of left front wall of thorax

⑦S20.363   Insect bite (nonvenomous) of bilateral front wall of thorax

⑦S20.364   Insect bite (nonvenomous) of middle front wall of thorax

⑦S20.369   Insect bite (nonvenomous) of unspecified front wall of thorax

S20.37   Other superficial bite of front wall of thorax

Excludes1: open bite of front wall of thorax (S21.14)

⑦S20.371   Other superficial bite of right front wall of thorax

⑦S20.372   Other superficial bite of left front wall of thorax

⑦S20.373   Other superficial bite of bilateral front wall of thorax

⑦S20.374   Other superficial bite of middle front wall of thorax

⑦S20.379   Other superficial bite of unspecified front wall of thorax

S20.4   Other and unspecified superficial injuries of back wall of thorax

S20.40   Unspecified superficial injuries of back wall of thorax

⑦S20.401   Unspecified superficial injuries of right back wall of thorax

⑦S20.402   Unspecified superficial injuries of left back wall of thorax

⑦S20.409   Unspecified superficial injuries of unspecified back wall of thorax

S20.41   Abrasion of back wall of thorax

⑦S20.411   Abrasion of right back wall of thorax

⑦S20.412   Abrasion of left back wall of thorax

⑦S20.419   Abrasion of unspecified back wall of thorax

S20.42   Blister (nonthermal) of back wall of thorax

⑦S20.421   Blister (nonthermal) of right back wall of thorax

⑦S20.422   Blister (nonthermal) of left back wall of thorax

⑦S20.429   Blister (nonthermal) of unspecified back wall of thorax

● New code   ▲ Revised code   Excludes1: Not coded here   Excludes2: Not included here   ⊗ Placeholder required   ⑦7ᵗʰ digit required

S20.44   **External constriction of back wall of thorax**

    ⑦**S20.441**   **External constriction of right back wall of thorax**

    ⑦**S20.442**   **External constriction of left back wall of thorax**

    ⑦**S20.449**   **External constriction of unspecified back wall of thorax**

S20.45   **Superficial foreign body of back wall of thorax**

    Splinter of back wall of thorax

    ⑦**S20.451**   **Superficial foreign body of right back wall of thorax**

    ⑦**S20.452**   **Superficial foreign body of left back wall of thorax**

    ⑦**S20.459**   **Superficial foreign body of unspecified back wall of thorax**

S20.46   **Insect bite (nonvenomous) of back wall of thorax**

    ⑦**S20.461**   **Insect bite (nonvenomous) of right back wall of thorax**

    ⑦**S20.462**   **Insect bite (nonvenomous) of left back wall of thorax**

    ⑦**S20.469**   **Insect bite (nonvenomous) of unspecified back wall of thorax**

S20.47   **Other superficial bite of back wall of thorax**

    `Excludes1:` open bite of back wall of thorax (S21.24)

    ⑦**S20.471**   **Other superficial bite of right back wall of thorax**

    ⑦**S20.472**   **Other superficial bite of left back wall of thorax**

    ⑦**S20.479**   **Other superficial bite of unspecified back wall of thorax**

S20.9   **Superficial injury of unspecified parts of thorax**

    `Excludes1:` contusion of thorax NOS (S20.20)

    ⊗⑦**S20.90**   **Unspecified superficial injury of unspecified parts of thorax**

    Superficial injury of thoracic wall NOS

    ⊗⑦**S20.91**   **Abrasion of unspecified parts of thorax**

    ⊗⑦**S20.92**   **Blister (nonthermal) of unspecified parts of thorax**

    ⊗⑦**S20.94**   **External constriction of unspecified parts of thorax**

    ⊗⑦**S20.95**   **Superficial foreign body of unspecified parts of thorax**

    Splinter in thorax NOS

    ⊗⑦**S20.96**   **Insect bite (nonvenomous) of unspecified parts of thorax**

    ⊗⑦**S20.97**   **Other superficial bite of unspecified parts of thorax**

    `Excludes1:` open bite of thorax NOS (S21.95)

S21   **Open wound of thorax**

Code also any associated injury, such as:

injury of heart (S26.-)

injury of intrathoracic organs (S27.-)

rib fracture (S22.3-, S22.4-)

spinal cord injury (S24.0-, S24.1-)

traumatic hemopneumothorax (S27.3)

traumatic hemothorax (S27.1)

traumatic pneumothorax (S27.0) wound infection

`Excludes1:` traumatic amputation (partial) of thorax (S28.1)

The appropriate 7th character is to be added to each code from category S21

A - initial encounter

D - subsequent encounter

S - sequela

S21.0   **Open wound of breast**

S21.00   **Unspecified open wound of breast**

    ⑦**S21.001**   **Unspecified open wound of right breast**

    ⑦**S21.002**   **Unspecified open wound of left breast**

    ⑦**S21.009**   **Unspecified open wound of unspecified breast**

S21.01   **Laceration without foreign body of breast**

    ⑦**S21.011**   **Laceration without foreign body of right breast**

    ⑦**S21.012**   **Laceration without foreign body of left breast**

    ⑦**S21.019**   **Laceration without foreign body of unspecified breast**

S21.02   **Laceration with foreign body of breast**

    ⑦**S21.021**   **Laceration with foreign body of right breast**

    ⑦**S21.022**   **Laceration with foreign body of left breast**

    ⑦**S21.029**   **Laceration with foreign body of unspecified breast**

S21.03   **Puncture wound without foreign body of breast**

    ⑦**S21.031**   **Puncture wound without foreign body of right breast**

    ⑦**S21.032**   **Puncture wound without foreign body of left breast**

    ⑦**S21.039**   **Puncture wound without foreign body of unspecified breast**

S21.04   **Puncture wound with foreign body of breast**

    ⑦**S21.041**   **Puncture wound with foreign body of right breast**

    ⑦**S21.042**   **Puncture wound with foreign body of left breast**

    ⑦**S21.049**   **Puncture wound with foreign body of unspecified breast**

S21.05   **Open bite of breast**

    Bite of breast NOS

    `Excludes1:` superficial bite of breast (S20.17)

    ⑦**S21.051**   **Open bite of right breast**

    ⑦**S21.052**   **Open bite of left breast**

    ⑦**S21.059**   **Open bite of unspecified breast**

S21.1   **Open wound of front wall of thorax without penetration into thoracic cavity**

    Open wound of chest without penetration into thoracic cavity

S21.10   **Unspecified open wound of front wall of thorax without penetration into thoracic cavity**

    ⑦**S21.101**   **Unspecified open wound of right front wall of thorax without penetration into thoracic cavity**

    ⑦**S21.102**   **Unspecified open wound of left front wall of thorax without penetration into thoracic cavity**

    ⑦**S21.109**   **Unspecified open wound of unspecified front wall of thorax without penetration into thoracic cavity**

S21.11   **Laceration without foreign body of front wall of thorax without penetration into thoracic cavity**

⑦**S21.111**   **Laceration without foreign body of right front wall of thorax without penetration into thoracic cavity**

⑦**S21.112**   **Laceration without foreign body of left front wall of thorax without penetration into thoracic cavity**

⑦**S21.119**   **Laceration without foreign body of unspecified front wall of thorax without penetration into thoracic cavity**

S21.12   **Laceration with foreign body of front wall of thorax without penetration into thoracic cavity**

⑦**S21.121**   **Laceration with foreign body of right front wall of thorax without penetration into thoracic cavity**

⑦**S21.122**   **Laceration with foreign body of left front wall of thorax without penetration into thoracic cavity**

⑦**S21.129**   **Laceration with foreign body of unspecified front wall of thorax without penetration into thoracic cavity**

S21.13   **Puncture wound without foreign body of front wall of thorax without penetration into thoracic cavity**

⑦**S21.131**   **Puncture wound without foreign body of right front wall of thorax without penetration into thoracic cavity**

⑦**S21.132**   **Puncture wound without foreign body of left front wall of thorax without penetration into thoracic cavity**

⑦**S21.139**   **Puncture wound without foreign body of unspecified front wall of thorax without penetration into thoracic cavity**

S21.14   **Puncture wound with foreign body of front wall of thorax without penetration into thoracic cavity**

⑦**S21.141**   **Puncture wound with foreign body of right front wall of thorax without penetration into thoracic cavity**

⑦**S21.142**   **Puncture wound with foreign body of left front wall of thorax without penetration into thoracic cavity**

⑦**S21.149**   **Puncture wound with foreign body of unspecified front wall of thorax without penetration into thoracic cavity**

S21.15   **Open bite of front wall of thorax without penetration into thoracic cavity**

Bite of front wall of thorax NOS

Excludes1: superficial bite of front wall of thorax (S20.37)

⑦**S21.151**   **Open bite of right front wall of thorax without penetration into thoracic cavity**

⑦**S21.152**   **Open bite of left front wall of thorax without penetration into thoracic cavity**

⑦**S21.159**   **Open bite of unspecified front wall of thorax without penetration into thoracic cavity**

S21.2   **Open wound of back wall of thorax without penetration into thoracic cavity**

S21.20   **Unspecified open wound of back wall of thorax without penetration into thoracic cavity**

⑦**S21.201**   **Unspecified open wound of right back wall of thorax without penetration into thoracic cavity**

⑦**S21.202**   **Unspecified open wound of left back wall of thorax without penetration into thoracic cavity**

⑦**S21.209**   **Unspecified open wound of unspecified back wall of thorax without penetration into thoracic cavity**

S21.21   **Laceration without foreign body of back wall of thorax without penetration into thoracic cavity**

⑦**S21.211**   **Laceration without foreign body of right back wall of thorax without penetration into thoracic cavity**

⑦**S21.212**   **Laceration without foreign body of left back wall of thorax without penetration into thoracic cavity**

⑦**S21.219**   **Laceration without foreign body of unspecified back wall of thorax without penetration into thoracic cavity**

S21.22   **Laceration with foreign body of back wall of thorax without penetration into thoracic cavity**

⑦**S21.221**   **Laceration with foreign body of right back wall of thorax without penetration into thoracic cavity**

⑦**S21.222**   **Laceration with foreign body of left back wall of thorax without penetration into thoracic cavity**

⑦**S21.229**   **Laceration with foreign body of unspecified back wall of thorax without penetration into thoracic cavity**

S21.23   **Puncture wound without foreign body of back wall of thorax without penetration into thoracic cavity**

⑦**S21.231**   **Puncture wound without foreign body of right back wall of thorax without penetration into thoracic cavity**

⑦**S21.232**   **Puncture wound without foreign body of left back wall of thorax without penetration into thoracic cavity**

⑦**S21.239**   **Puncture wound without foreign body of unspecified back wall of thorax without penetration into thoracic cavity**

S21.24   **Puncture wound with foreign body of back wall of thorax without penetration into thoracic cavity**

⑦**S21.241**   **Puncture wound with foreign body of right back wall of thorax without penetration into thoracic cavity**

⑦**S21.242**   **Puncture wound with foreign body of left back wall of thorax without penetration into thoracic cavity**

⑦**S21.249**   **Puncture wound with foreign body of unspecified back wall of thorax without penetration into thoracic cavity**

S21.25   **Open bite of back wall of thorax without penetration into thoracic cavity**

   ● New code   ▲ Revised code   **Excludes1:** Not coded here   **Excludes2:** Not included here   ⊗ Placeholder required   ⑦7ᵗʰ digit required

Bite of back wall of thorax NOS

Excludes1: superficial bite of back wall of thorax (S20.47)

⑦S21.251 **Open bite of right back wall of thorax without penetration into thoracic cavity**

⑦S21.252 **Open bite of left back wall of thorax without penetration into thoracic cavity**

⑦S21.259 **Open bite of unspecified back wall of thorax without penetration into thoracic cavity**

S21.3 **Open wound of front wall of thorax with penetration into thoracic cavity**

Open wound of chest with penetration into thoracic cavity

S21.30 **Unspecified open wound of front wall of thorax with penetration into thoracic cavity**

⑦S21.301 **Unspecified open wound of right front wall of thorax with penetration into thoracic cavity**

⑦S21.302 **Unspecified open wound of left front wall of thorax with penetration into thoracic cavity**

⑦S21.309 **Unspecified open wound of unspecified front wall of thorax with penetration into thoracic cavity**

S21.31 **Laceration without foreign body of front wall of thorax with penetration into thoracic cavity**

⑦S21.311 **Laceration without foreign body of right front wall of thorax with penetration into thoracic cavity**

⑦S21.312 **Laceration without foreign body of left front wall of thorax with penetration into thoracic cavity**

⑦S21.319 **Laceration without foreign body of unspecified front wall of thorax with penetration into thoracic cavity**

S21.32 **Laceration with foreign body of front wall of thorax with penetration into thoracic cavity**

⑦S21.321 **Laceration with foreign body of right front wall of thorax with penetration into thoracic cavity**

⑦S21.322 **Laceration with foreign body of left front wall of thorax with penetration into thoracic cavity**

⑦S21.329 **Laceration with foreign body of unspecified front wall of thorax with penetration into thoracic cavity**

S21.33 **Puncture wound without foreign body of front wall of thorax with penetration into thoracic cavity**

⑦S21.331 **Puncture wound without foreign body of right front wall of thorax with penetration into thoracic cavity**

⑦S21.332 **Puncture wound without foreign body of left front wall of thorax with penetration into thoracic cavity**

⑦S21.339 **Puncture wound without foreign body of unspecified front wall of thorax with penetration into thoracic cavity**

S21.34 **Puncture wound with foreign body of front wall of thorax with penetration into thoracic cavity**

⑦S21.341 **Puncture wound with foreign body of right front wall of thorax with penetration into thoracic cavity**

⑦S21.342 **Puncture wound with foreign body of left front wall of thorax with penetration into thoracic cavity**

⑦S21.349 **Puncture wound with foreign body of unspecified front wall of thorax with penetration into thoracic cavity**

S21.35 **Open bite of front wall of thorax with penetration into thoracic cavity**

Excludes1: superficial bite of front wall of thorax (S20.37)

⑦S21.351 **Open bite of right front wall of thorax with penetration into thoracic cavity**

⑦S21.352 **Open bite of left front wall of thorax with penetration into thoracic cavity**

⑦S21.359 **Open bite of unspecified front wall of thorax with penetration into thoracic cavity**

S21.4 **Open wound of back wall of thorax with penetration into thoracic cavity**

S21.40 **Unspecified open wound of back wall of thorax with penetration into thoracic cavity**

⑦S21.401 **Unspecified open wound of right back wall of thorax with penetration into thoracic cavity**

⑦S21.402 **Unspecified open wound of left back wall of thorax with penetration into thoracic cavity**

⑦S21.409 **Unspecified open wound of unspecified back wall of thorax with penetration into thoracic cavity**

S21.41 **Laceration without foreign body of back wall of thorax with penetration into thoracic cavity**

⑦S21.411 **Laceration without foreign body of right back wall of thorax with penetration into thoracic cavity**

⑦S21.412 **Laceration without foreign body of left back wall of thorax with penetration into thoracic cavity**

⑦S21.419 **Laceration without foreign body of unspecified back wall of thorax with penetration into thoracic cavity**

S21.42 **Laceration with foreign body of back wall of thorax with penetration into thoracic cavity**

⑦S21.421 **Laceration with foreign body of right back wall of thorax with penetration into thoracic cavity**

⑦S21.422 **Laceration with foreign body of left back wall of thorax with penetration into thoracic cavity**

⑦S21.429 **Laceration with foreign body of unspecified back wall of thorax with penetration into thoracic cavity**

S21.43 **Puncture wound without foreign body of back wall of thorax with penetration into thoracic cavity**

⑦S21.431 **Puncture wound without foreign body of right back wall of thorax with penetration into thoracic cavity**

⑦S21.432 **Puncture wound without foreign body of left back wall of thorax with penetration into thoracic cavity**

⑦S21.439 **Puncture wound without foreign body of unspecified back wall of thorax with penetration into thoracic cavity**

S21.44   **Puncture wound with foreign body of back wall of thorax with penetration into thoracic cavity**

⑦S21.441   **Puncture wound with foreign body of right back wall of thorax with penetration into thoracic cavity**

⑦S21.442   **Puncture wound with foreign body of left back wall of thorax with penetration into thoracic cavity**

⑦S21.449   **Puncture wound with foreign body of unspecified back wall of thorax with penetration into thoracic cavity**

S21.45   **Open bite of back wall of thorax with penetration into thoracic cavity**

Bite of back wall of thorax NOS

Excludes1: superficial bite of back wall of thorax (S20.47)

⑦S21.451   **Open bite of right back wall of thorax with penetration into thoracic cavity**

⑦S21.452   **Open bite of left back wall of thorax with penetration into thoracic cavity**

⑦S21.459   **Open bite of unspecified back wall of thorax with penetration into thoracic cavity**

S21.9   **Open wound of unspecified part of thorax**

Open wound of thoracic wall NOS

⊗⑦S21.90   **Unspecified open wound of unspecified part of thorax**

⊗⑦S21.91   **Laceration without foreign body of unspecified part of thorax**

⊗⑦S21.92   **Laceration with foreign body of unspecified part of thorax**

⊗⑦S21.93   **Puncture wound without foreign body of unspecified part of thorax**

⊗⑦S21.94   **Puncture wound with foreign body of unspecified part of thorax**

⊗⑦S21.95   **Open bite of unspecified part of thorax**

Excludes1: superficial bite of thorax (S20.97)

S22   **Fracture of rib(s), sternum and thoracic spine**

Note: A fracture not indicated as displaced or nondisplaced should be coded to displaced

A fracture not indicated as open or closed should be coded to closed

Includes: fracture of thoracic neural arch

fracture of thoracic spinous process

fracture of thoracic transverse process

fracture of thoracic vertebra

fracture of thoracic vertebral arch

Code first any associated:

injury of intrathoracic organ (S27.-)

spinal cord injury (S24.0-, S24.1-)

Excludes1: transection of thorax (S28.1)

Excludes2: fracture of clavicle (S42.0-)

fracture of scapula (S42.1-)

The appropriate 7th character is to be added to each code from category S22

A - initial encounter for closed fracture

B - initial encounter for open fracture

D - subsequent encounter for fracture with routine healing

G - subsequent encounter for fracture with delayed healing

K - subsequent encounter for fracture with nonunion

S - sequela

S22.0   **Fracture of thoracic vertebra**

S22.00   **Fracture of unspecified thoracic vertebra**

⑦S22.000   **Wedge compression fracture of unspecified thoracic vertebra** [HCC]

⑦S22.001   **Stable burst fracture of unspecified thoracic vertebra** [HCC]

⑦S22.002   **Unstable burst fracture of unspecified thoracic vertebra** [HCC]

⑦S22.008   **Other fracture of unspecified thoracic vertebra** [HCC]

⑦S22.009   **Unspecified fracture of unspecified thoracic vertebra** [HCC]

S22.01   **Fracture of first thoracic vertebra**

⑦S22.010   **Wedge compression fracture of first thoracic vertebra** [HCC]

⑦S22.011   **Stable burst fracture of first thoracic vertebra**

⑦S22.012   **Unstable burst fracture of first thoracic vertebra** [HCC]

⑦S22.018   **Other fracture of first thoracic vertebra** [HCC]

⑦S22.019   **Unspecified fracture of first thoracic vertebra** [HCC]

S22.02   **Fracture of second thoracic vertebra**

⑦S22.020   **Wedge compression fracture of second thoracic vertebra** [HCC]

⑦S22.021   **Stable burst fracture of second thoracic vertebra** [HCC]

⑦S22.022   **Unstable burst fracture of second thoracic vertebra** [HCC]

⑦S22.028   **Other fracture of second thoracic vertebra** [HCC]

⑦S22.029   **Unspecified fracture of second thoracic vertebra** [HCC]

S22.03   **Fracture of third thoracic vertebra**

⑦S22.030   **Wedge compression fracture of third thoracic vertebra** [HCC]

⑦S22.031   **Stable burst fracture of third thoracic vertebra** [HCC]

⑦S22.032   **Unstable burst fracture of third thoracic vertebra** [HCC]

⑦S22.038   **Other fracture of third thoracic vertebra** [HCC]

⑦S22.039   **Unspecified fracture of third thoracic vertebra** [HCC]

S22.04   **Fracture of fourth thoracic vertebra**

⑦S22.040   **Wedge compression fracture of fourth thoracic vertebra** [HCC]

⑦S22.041   **Stable burst fracture of fourth thoracic vertebra** [HCC]

⑦S22.042   **Unstable burst fracture of fourth thoracic vertebra** [HCC]

⑦S22.048   **Other fracture of fourth thoracic vertebra** [HCC]

⑦S22.049   **Unspecified fracture of fourth thoracic vertebra** [HCC]

S22.05   **Fracture of T5-T6 vertebra**

⑦S22.050   **Wedge compression fracture of T5-T6 vertebra** [HCC]

⑦S22.051   **Stable burst fracture of T5-T6 vertebra** [HCC]

⑦S22.052   **Unstable burst fracture of T5-T6 vertebra** [HCC]

   ● New code   ▲ Revised code   **Excludes1:** Not coded here   **Excludes2:** Not included here   ⊗ Placeholder required   ⑦7th digit required

⑦**S22.058** **Other fracture of T5-T6 vertebra** [HCC]

⑦**S22.059** **Unspecified fracture of T5-T6 vertebra** [HCC]

S22.06 **Fracture of T7-T8 vertebra**

⑦**S22.060** **Wedge compression fracture of T7-T8 vertebra** [HCC]

⑦**S22.061** **Stable burst fracture of T7-T8 vertebra** [HCC]

⑦**S22.062** **Unstable burst fracture of T7-T8 vertebra** [HCC]

⑦**S22.068** **Other fracture of T7-T8 thoracic vertebra** [HCC]

⑦**S22.069** **Unspecified fracture of T7-T8 vertebra**

S22.07 **Fracture of T9-T10 vertebra**

⑦**S22.070** **Wedge compression fracture of T9-T10 vertebra** [HCC]

⑦**S22.071** **Stable burst fracture of T9-T10 vertebra** [HCC]

⑦**S22.072** **Unstable burst fracture of T9-T10 vertebra** [HCC]

⑦**S22.078** **Other fracture of T9-T10 vertebra** [HCC]

⑦**S22.079** **Unspecified fracture of T9-T10 vertebra** [HCC]

S22.08 **Fracture of T11-T12 vertebra**

⑦**S22.080** **Wedge compression fracture of T11-T12 vertebra** [HCC]

⑦**S22.081** **Stable burst fracture of T11-T12 vertebra** [HCC]

⑦**S22.082** **Unstable burst fracture of T11-T12 vertebra** [HCC]

⑦**S22.088** **Other fracture of T11-T12 vertebra** [HCC]

⑦**S22.089** **Unspecified fracture of T11-T12 vertebra** [HCC]

S22.2 **Fracture of sternum**

⊗⑦**S22.20** **Unspecified fracture of sternum**

⊗⑦**S22.21** **Fracture of manubrium**

⊗⑦**S22.22** **Fracture of body of sternum**

⊗⑦**S22.23** **Sternal manubrial dissociation**

⊗⑦**S22.24** **Fracture of xiphoid process**

S22.3 **Fracture of one rib**

⊗⑦**S22.31** **Fracture of one rib, right side**

⊗⑦**S22.32** **Fracture of one rib, left side**

⊗⑦**S22.39** **Fracture of one rib, unspecified side**

S22.4 **Multiple fractures of ribs**

Fractures of two or more ribs

Excludes1: flail chest (S22.5-)

⊗⑦**S22.41** **Multiple fractures of ribs, right side**

⊗⑦**S22.42** **Multiple fractures of ribs, left side**

⊗⑦**S22.43** **Multiple fractures of ribs, bilateral**

⊗⑦**S22.49** **Multiple fractures of ribs, unspecified side**

⊗⑦**S22.5** **Flail chest**

⊗⑦**S22.9** **Fracture of bony thorax, part unspecified**

S23 **Dislocation and sprain of joints and ligaments of thorax**

Includes: avulsion of joint or ligament of thorax

laceration of cartilage, joint or ligament of thorax

sprain of cartilage, joint or ligament of thorax

traumatic hemarthrosis of joint or ligament of thorax

traumatic rupture of joint or ligament of thorax

traumatic subluxation of joint or ligament of thorax

traumatic tear of joint or ligament of thorax

Code also any associated open wound

Excludes2: dislocation, sprain of sternoclavicular joint (S43.2, S43.6)

strain of muscle or tendon of thorax (S29.01-)

The appropriate 7th character is to be added to each code from category S23

A - initial encounter

D - subsequent encounter

S - sequela

⊗⑦**S23.0** **Traumatic rupture of thoracic intervertebral disc**

Excludes1: rupture or displacement (nontraumatic) of thoracic intervertebral disc NOS (M51.- with fifth character 4)

S23.1 **Subluxation and dislocation of thoracic vertebra**

Code also any associated:

open wound of thorax (S21.-)

spinal cord injury (S24.0-, S24.1-)

Excludes2: fracture of thoracic vertebrae (S22.0-)

S23.10 **Subluxation and dislocation of unspecified thoracic vertebra**

⑦**S23.100** **Subluxation of unspecified thoracic vertebra**

⑦**S23.101** **Dislocation of unspecified thoracic vertebra**

S23.11 **Subluxation and dislocation of T1/T2 thoracic vertebra**

⑦**S23.110** **Subluxation of T1/T2 thoracic vertebra**

⑦**S23.111** **Dislocation of T1/T2 thoracic vertebra**

S23.12 **Subluxation and dislocation of T2/T3-T3/T4 thoracic vertebra**

⑦**S23.120** **Subluxation of T2/T3 thoracic vertebra**

⑦**S23.121** **Dislocation of T2/T3 thoracic vertebra**

⑦**S23.122** **Subluxation of T3/T4 thoracic vertebra**

⑦**S23.123** **Dislocation of T3/T4 thoracic vertebra**

S23.13 **Subluxation and dislocation of T4/T5-T5/T6 thoracic vertebra**

⑦**S23.130** **Subluxation of T4/T5 thoracic vertebra**

⑦**S23.131** **Dislocation of T4/T5 thoracic vertebra**

⑦**S23.132** **Subluxation of T5/T6 thoracic vertebra**

⑦**S23.133** **Dislocation of T5/T6 thoracic vertebra**

S23.14 **Subluxation and dislocation of T6/T7-T7/T8 thoracic vertebra**

⑦**S23.140** **Subluxation of T6/T7 thoracic vertebra**

⑦**S23.141** **Dislocation of T6/T7 thoracic vertebra**

⑦**S23.142** **Subluxation of T7/T8 thoracic vertebra**

⑦S23.143   **Dislocation of T7/T8thoracic vertebra**

S23.15   **Subluxation and dislocation of T8/T9-T9/T10 thoracic vertebra**

⑦S23.150   **Subluxation of T8/T9thoracic vertebra**

⑦S23.151   **Dislocation of T8/T9thoracic vertebra**

⑦S23.152   **Subluxation of T9/T10thoracic vertebra**

⑦S23.153   **Dislocation of T9/T10thoracic vertebra**

S23.16   **Subluxation and dislocation of T10/T11-T11/T12 thoracic vertebra**

⑦S23.160   **Subluxation of T10/T11thoracic vertebra**

⑦S23.161   **Dislocation of T10/T11thoracic vertebra**

⑦S23.162   **Subluxation of T11/T12thoracic vertebra**

⑦S23.163   **Dislocation of T11/T12thoracic vertebra**

S23.17   **Subluxation and dislocation of T12/L1 thoracic vertebra**

⑦S23.170   **Subluxation of T12/L1 thoracic vertebra**

⑦S23.171   **Dislocation of T12/L1 thoracic vertebra**

S23.2   **Dislocation of other and unspecified parts of thorax**

⊗⑦S23.20   **Dislocation of unspecified part of thorax**

⊗⑦S23.29   **Dislocation of other parts of thorax**

⊗⑦S23.3   **Sprain of ligaments of thoracic spine**

S23.4   **Sprain of ribs and sternum**

⊗⑦S23.41   **Sprain of ribs**

S23.42   **Sprain of sternum**

⑦S23.420   **Sprain of sternoclavicular (joint) (ligament)**

⑦S23.421   **Sprain of chondrosternal joint**

⑦S23.428   **Other sprain of sternum**

⑦S23.429   **Unspecified sprain of sternum**

⊗⑦S23.8   **Sprain of other specified parts of thorax**

⊗⑦S23.9   **Sprain of unspecified parts of thorax**

S24   **Injury of nerves and spinal cord at thorax level**

Note: Code to highest level of thoracic spinal cord injury

Injuries to the spinal cord (S24.0 and S24.1) refer to the cord level and not bone level injury and can affect nerve roots at and below the level given.

Code also any associated:

fracture of thoracic vertebra (S22.0-)

open wound of thorax (S21.-)

transient paralysis (R29.5)

Excludes2: injury of brachial plexus (S14.3)

The appropriate 7th character is to be added to each code from category S24

A - initial encounter

D - subsequent encounter

S - sequela

⊗⑦S24.0   **Concussion and edema of thoracic spinal cord** [HCC]

S24.1   **Other and unspecified injuries of thoracic spinal cord**

S24.10   **Unspecified injury of thoracic spinal cord**

⑦S24.101   **Unspecified injury at T1 level of thoracic spinal cord** [HCC]

⑦S24.102   **Unspecified injury at T2-T6 level of thoracic spinal cord** [HCC]

⑦S24.103   **Unspecified injury at T7-T10 level of thoracic spinal cord** [HCC]

⑦S24.104   **Unspecified injury at T11-T12 level of thoracic spinal cord** [HCC]

⑦S24.109   **Unspecified injury at unspecified level of thoracic spinal cord** [HCC]

Injury of thoracic spinal cord NOS

S24.11   **Complete lesion of thoracic spinal cord**

⑦S24.111   **Complete lesion at T1 level of thoracic spinal cord** [HCC]

⑦S24.112   **Complete lesion at T2-T6 level of thoracic spinal cord** [HCC]

⑦S24.113   **Complete lesion at T7-T10 level of thoracic spinal cord** [HCC]

⑦S24.114   **Complete lesion at T11-T12 level of thoracic spinal cord** [HCC]

⑦S24.119   **Complete lesion at unspecified level of thoracic spinal cord** [HCC]

S24.13   **Anterior cord syndrome of thoracic spinal cord**

⑦S24.131   **Anterior cord syndrome at T1 level of thoracic spinal cord** [HCC]

⑦S24.132   **Anterior cord syndrome at T2-T6 level of thoracic spinal cord** [HCC]

⑦S24.133   **Anterior cord syndrome at T7-T10 level of thoracic spinal cord** [HCC]

⑦S24.134   **Anterior cord syndrome at T11-T12 level of thoracic spinal cord** [HCC]

⑦S24.139   **Anterior cord syndrome at unspecified level of thoracic spinal cord** [HCC]

S24.14   **Brown-Séquard syndrome of thoracic spinal cord**

⑦S24.141   **Brown-Séquard syndrome at T1 level of thoracic spinal cord** [HCC]

⑦S24.142   **Brown-Séquard syndrome at T2-T6 level of thoracic spinal cord** [HCC]

⑦S24.143   **Brown-Séquard syndrome at T7-T10 level of thoracic spinal cord** [HCC]

⑦S24.144   **Brown-Séquard syndrome at T11-T12 level of thoracic spinal cord** [HCC]

⑦S24.149   **Brown-Séquard syndrome at unspecified level of thoracic spinal cord**

⑦S24.15   **Other incomplete lesions of thoracic spinal cord**

Incomplete lesion of thoracic spinal cord NOS

Posterior cord syndrome of thoracic spinal cord

⑦S24.151   **Other incomplete lesion at T1 level of thoracic spinal cord** [HCC]

⑦S24.152   **Other incomplete lesion at T2-T6 level of thoracic spinal cord** [HCC]

⑦S24.153   **Other incomplete lesion at T7-T10 level of thoracic spinal cord** [HCC]

⑦S24.154   **Other incomplete lesion at T11-T12 level of thoracic spinal cord** [HCC]

⑦S24.159   **Other incomplete lesion at unspecified level of thoracic spinal cord** [HCC]

⊗⑦S24.2   **Injury of nerve root of thoracic spine**

⊗⑦S24.3   **Injury of peripheral nerves of thorax**

   ● New code   ▲ Revised code   **Excludes1:** Not coded here   **Excludes2:** Not included here   ⊗ Placeholder required   ⑦7th digit required

⊗⑦**S24.4** **Injury of thoracic sympathetic nervous system**

Injury of cardiac plexus

Injury of esophageal plexus

Injury of pulmonary plexus

Injury of stellate ganglion

Injury of thoracic sympathetic ganglion

⊗⑦**S24.8** **Injury of other specified nerves of thorax**

⊗⑦**S24.9** **Injury of unspecified nerve of thorax**

S25 **Injury of blood vessels of thorax**

<u>Code also</u> any associated open wound (S21.-)

The appropriate 7th character is to be added to each code from category S25

A - initial encounter

D - subsequent encounter

S - sequela

S25.0 **Injury of thoracic aorta**

Injury of aorta NOS

⊗⑦**S25.00** **Unspecified injury of thoracic aorta**

⊗⑦**S25.01** **Minor laceration of thoracic aorta**

Incomplete transection of thoracic aorta

Laceration of thoracic aorta NOS

Superficial laceration of thoracic aorta

⊗⑦**S25.02** **Major laceration of thoracic aorta**

Complete transection of thoracic aorta

Traumatic rupture of thoracic aorta

⊗⑦**S25.09** **Other specified injury of thoracic aorta**

S25.1 **Injury of innominate or subclavian artery**

S25.10 **Unspecified injury of innominate or subclavian artery**

⑦**S25.101** **Unspecified injury of right innominate or subclavian artery injury of left innominate or subclavian artery**

⑦**S25.109** **Unspecified injury of unspecified innominate or subclavian artery**

S25.11 **Minor laceration of innominate or subclavian artery**

Incomplete transection of innominate or subclavian artery

Laceration of innominate or subclavian artery NOS

Superficial laceration of innominate or subclavian artery

⑦**S25.111** **Minor laceration of right innominate or subclavian artery**

⑦**S25.112** **Minor laceration of left innominate or subclavian artery**

⑦**S25.119** **Minor laceration of unspecified innominate or subclavian artery**

S25.12 **Major laceration of innominate or subclavian artery**

Complete transection of innominate or subclavian artery

Traumatic rupture of innominate or subclavian artery

⑦**S25.121** **Major laceration of right innominate or subclavian artery**

⑦**S25.122** **Major laceration of left innominate or subclavian artery**

⑦**S25.129** **Major laceration of unspecified innominate or subclavian artery**

S25.19 **Other specified injury of innominate or subclavian artery**

⑦**S25.191** **Other specified injury of right innominate or subclavian artery**

⑦**S25.192** **Other specified injury of left innominate or subclavian artery**

⑦**S25.199** **Other specified injury of unspecified innominate or subclavian artery**

S25.2 **Injury of superior vena cava**

Injury of vena cava NOS

⊗⑦**S25.20** **Unspecified injury of superior vena cava**

⊗⑦**S25.21** **Minor laceration of superior vena cava**

Incomplete transection of superior vena cava

Laceration of superior vena cava NOS

Superficial laceration of superior vena cava

⊗⑦**S25.22** **Major laceration of superior vena cava**

Complete transection of superior vena cava

Traumatic rupture of superior vena cava

⊗⑦**S25.29** **Other specified injury of superior vena cava**

S25.3 **Injury of innominate or subclavian vein**

S25.30 **Unspecified injury of innominate or subclavian vein**

⑦**S25.301** **Unspecified injury of right innominate or subclavian vein**

⑦**S25.302** **Unspecified injury of left innominate or subclavian vein**

⑦**S25.309** **Unspecified injury of unspecified innominate or subclavian vein**

S25.31 **Minor laceration of innominate or subclavian vein**

Incomplete transection of innominate or subclavian vein

Laceration of innominate or subclavian vein NOS

Superficial laceration of innominate or subclavian vein

⑦**S25.311** **Minor laceration of right innominate or subclavian vein**

⑦**S25.312** **Minor laceration of left innominate or subclavian vein**

⑦**S25.319** **Minor laceration of unspecified innominate or subclavian vein**

S25.32 **Major laceration of innominate or subclavian vein**

Complete transection of innominate or subclavian vein

Traumatic rupture of innominate or subclavian vein

⑦**S25.321** **Major laceration of right innominate or subclavian vein**

⑦**S25.322** **Major laceration of left innominate or subclavian vein**

⑦**S25.329** **Major laceration of unspecified innominate or subclavian vein**

S25.39 **Other specified injury of innominate or subclavian vein**

⑦**S25.391** **Other specified injury of right innominate or subclavian vein**

⑦**S25.392** **Other specified injury of left innominate or subclavian vein**

⑦**S25.399** **Other specified injury of unspecified innominate or subclavian vein**

S25.4 **Injury of pulmonary blood vessels**

S25.40 Unspecified injury of pulmonary blood vessels

⑦S25.401 Unspecified injury of right pulmonary blood vessels

⑦S25.402 Unspecified injury of left pulmonary blood vessels

⑦S25.409 Unspecified injury of unspecified pulmonary blood vessels

S25.41 Minor laceration of pulmonary blood vessels

Incomplete transection of pulmonary blood vessels

Laceration of pulmonary blood vessels NOS

Superficial laceration of pulmonary blood vessels

⑦S25.411 Minor laceration of right pulmonary blood vessels

⑦S25.412 Minor laceration of left pulmonary blood vessels

⑦S25.419 Minor laceration of unspecified pulmonary blood vessels

S25.42 Major laceration of pulmonary blood vessels

Complete transection of pulmonary blood vessels

Traumatic rupture of pulmonary blood vessels

⑦S25.421 Major laceration of right pulmonary blood vessels

⑦S25.422 Major laceration of left pulmonary blood vessels

⑦S25.429 Major laceration of unspecified pulmonary blood vessels

S25.49 Other specified injury of pulmonary blood vessels

⑦S25.491 Other specified injury of right pulmonary blood vessels

⑦S25.492 Other specified injury of left pulmonary blood vessels

⑦S25.499 Other specified injury of unspecified pulmonary blood vessels

S25.5 Injury of intercostal blood vessels

S25.50 Unspecified injury of intercostal blood vessels

⑦S25.501 Unspecified injury of intercostal blood vessels, right side

⑦S25.502 Unspecified injury of intercostal blood vessels, left side

⑦S25.509 Unspecified injury of intercostal blood vessels, unspecified side

S25.51 Laceration of intercostal blood vessels

⑦S25.511 Laceration of intercostal blood vessels, right side

⑦S25.512 Laceration of intercostal blood vessels, left side

⑦S25.519 Laceration of intercostal blood vessels, unspecified side

S25.59 Other specified injury of intercostal blood vessels

⑦S25.591 Other specified injury of intercostal blood vessels, right side

⑦S25.592 Other specified injury of intercostal blood vessels, left side

⑦S25.599 Other specified injury of intercostal blood vessels, unspecified side

S25.8 Injury of other blood vessels of thorax

Injury of azygos vein

Injury of mammary artery or vein

S25.80 Unspecified injury of other blood vessels of thorax

⑦S25.801 Unspecified injury of other blood vessels of thorax, right side

⑦S25.802 Unspecified injury of other blood vessels of thorax, left side

⑦S25.809 Unspecified injury of other blood vessels of thorax, unspecified side

S25.81 Laceration of other blood vessels of thorax

⑦S25.811 Laceration of other blood vessels of thorax, right side

⑦S25.812 Laceration of other blood vessels of thorax, left side

⑦S25.819 Laceration of other blood vessels of thorax, unspecified side

S25.89 Other specified injury of other blood vessels of thorax

⑦S25.891 Other specified injury of other blood vessels of thorax, right side

⑦S25.892 Other specified injury of other blood vessels of thorax, left side

⑦S25.899 Other specified injury of other blood vessels of thorax, unspecified side

S25.9 Injury of unspecified blood vessel of thorax

⑦S25.90 Unspecified injury of unspecified blood vessel of thorax

⑦S25.91 Laceration of unspecified blood vessel of thorax

⑦S25.99 Other specified injury of unspecified blood vessel of thorax

S26 Injury of heart

<u>Code also</u> any associated:

open wound of thorax (S21.-)

traumatic hemopneumothorax (S27.2)

traumatic hemothorax (S27.1)

traumatic pneumothorax (S27.0)

The appropriate 7th character is to be added to each code from category S26

A - initial encounter

D - subsequent encounter

S - sequela

S26.0 Injury of heart with hemopericardium

⊗⑦S26.00 Unspecified injury of heart with hemopericardium

⊗⑦S26.01 Contusion of heart with hemopericardium

S26.02 Laceration of heart with hemopericardium

⑦S26.020 Mild laceration of heart with hemopericardium

Laceration of heart without penetration of heart chamber

⑦S26.021 Moderate laceration of heart with hemopericardium

Laceration of heart with penetration of heart chamber

⑦S26.022 Major laceration of heart with hemopericardium

Laceration of heart with penetration of multiple heart chambers

⊗⑦S26.09 Other injury of heart with hemopericardium

S26.1 Injury of heart without hemopericardium

⊗⑦S26.10 Unspecified injury of heart without hemopericardium

⊗⑦S26.11 Contusion of heart without hemopericardium

⊗⑦S26.12 Laceration of heart without hemopericardium

● New code   ▲ Revised code   **Excludes1:** Not coded here   **Excludes2:** Not included here   ⊗ Placeholder required   ⑦7th digit required

⊗⑦**S26.19**   **Other injury of heart without hemopericardium**

S26.9   **Injury of heart, unspecified with or without hemopericardium**

⊗⑦**S26.90**   **Unspecified injury of heart, unspecified with or without hemopericardium**

⊗⑦**S26.91**   **Contusion of heart, unspecified with or without hemopericardium**

⊗⑦**S26.92**   **Laceration of heart, unspecified with or without hemopericardium**

Laceration of heart NOS

⊗⑦**S26.99**   **Other injury of heart, unspecified with or without hemopericardium**

S27   **Injury of other and unspecified intrathoracic organs**

Code also any associated open wound of thorax (S21.-)

Excludes2: injury of cervical esophagus (S10-S19)

injury of trachea (cervical) (S10-S19)

The appropriate 7th character is to be added to each code from category S27

A - initial encounter

D - subsequent encounter

S - sequela

⊗⑦**S27.0**   **Traumatic pneumothorax**

Excludes1: spontaneous pneumothorax (J93.-)

⊗⑦**S27.1**   **Traumatic hemothorax**

⊗⑦**S27.2**   **Traumatic hemopneumothorax**

⊗⑦**S27.3**   **Other and unspecified injuries of lung**

S27.30   **Unspecified injury of lung**

⑦**S27.301**   **Unspecified injury of lung, unilateral**

⑦**S27.302**   **Unspecified injury of lung, bilateral**

⑦**S27.309**   **Unspecified injury of lung, unspecified**

S27.31   **Primary blast injury of lung**

Blast injury of lung NOS

⑦**S27.311**   **Primary blast injury of lung, unilateral**

⑦**S27.312**   **Primary blast injury of lung, bilateral**

⑦**S27.319**   **Primary blast injury of lung, unspecified**

S27.32   **Contusion of lung**

⑦**S27.321**   **Contusion of lung, unilateral**

⑦**S27.322**   **Contusion of lung, bilateral**

⑦**S27.329**   **Contusion of lung, unspecified**

S27.33   **Laceration of lung**

⑦**S27.331**   **Laceration of lung, unilateral**

⑦**S27.332**   **Laceration of lung, bilateral**

⑦**S27.339**   **Laceration of lung, unspecified**

S27.39   **Other injuries of lung**

Secondary blast injury of lung

⑦**S27.391**   **Other injuries of lung, unilateral**

⑦**S27.392**   **Other injuries of lung, bilateral**

⑦**S27.399**   **Other injuries of lung, unspecified**

S27.4   **Injury of bronchus**

S27.40   **Unspecified injury of bronchus**

⑦**S27.401**   **Unspecified injury of bronchus, unilateral**

⑦**S27.402**   **Unspecified injury of bronchus, bilateral**

⑦**S27.409**   **Unspecified injury of bronchus, unspecified**

S27.41   **Primary blast injury of bronchus**

Blast injury of bronchus NOS

⑦**S27.411**   **Primary blast injury of bronchus, unilateral**

⑦**S27.412**   **Primary blast injury of bronchus, bilateral**

⑦**S27.419**   **Primary blast injury of bronchus, unspecified**

S27.42   **Contusion of bronchus**

⑦**S27.421**   **Contusion of bronchus, unilateral**

⑦**S27.422**   **Contusion of bronchus, bilateral**

⑦**S27.429**   **Contusion of bronchus, unspecified**

S27.43   **Laceration of bronchus**

⑦**S27.431**   **Laceration of bronchus, unilateral**

⑦**S27.432**   **Laceration of bronchus, bilateral**

⑦**S27.439**   **Laceration of bronchus, unspecified**

S27.49   **Other injury of bronchus**

Secondary blast injury of bronchus

⑦**S27.491**   **Other injury of bronchus, unilateral**

⑦**S27.492**   **Other injury of bronchus, bilateral**

⑦**S27.499**   **Other injury of bronchus, unspecified**

S27.5   **Injury of thoracic trachea**

⊗⑦**S27.50**   **Unspecified injury of thoracic trachea**

⊗⑦**S27.51**   **Primary blast injury of thoracic trachea**

Blast injury of thoracic trachea NOS

⊗⑦**S27.52**   **Contusion of thoracic trachea**

⊗⑦**S27.53**   **Laceration of thoracic trachea**

⊗⑦**S27.59**   **Other injury of thoracic trachea**

Secondary blast injury of thoracic trachea

S27.6   **Injury of pleura**

⊗⑦**S27.60**   **Unspecified injury of pleura**

⊗⑦**S27.63**   **Laceration of pleura**

⊗⑦**S27.69**   **Other injury of pleura**

S27.8   **Injury of other specified intrathoracic organs**

S27.80   **Injury of diaphragm**

⑦**S27.802**   **Contusion of diaphragm**

⑦**S27.803**   **Laceration of diaphragm**

⑦**S27.808**   **Other injury of diaphragm**

⑦**S27.809**   **Unspecified injury of diaphragm**

S27.81   **Injury of esophagus (thoracic part)**

⑦**S27.812**   **Contusion of esophagus (thoracic part)**

⑦**S27.813**   **Laceration of esophagus (thoracic part)**

⑦**S27.818**   **Other injury of esophagus (thoracic part)**

⑦**S27.819**   **Unspecified injury of esophagus (thoracic part)**

S27.89   **Injury of other specified intrathoracic organs**

Injury of lymphatic thoracic duct

Injury of thymus gland

⑦**S27.892**   **Contusion of other specified intrathoracic organs**

⑦**S27.893**   **Laceration of other specified intrathoracic organs**

⑦S27.898   **Other injury of other specified intrathoracic organs**

⑦S27.899   **Unspecified injury of other specified intrathoracic organs**

⊗⑦**S27.9**   **Injury of unspecified intrathoracic organ**

S28   **Crushing injury of thorax, and traumatic amputation of part of thorax**

The appropriate 7th character is to be added to each code from category S28

A - initial encounter

D - subsequent encounter

S - sequela

⊗⑦**S28.0**   **Crushed chest**

     <u>Use Additional Code</u> for all associated injuries

     Excludes1: flail chest (S22.5)

⊗⑦**S28.1**   **Traumatic amputation (partial) of part of thorax, except breast**

S28.2   **Traumatic amputation of breast**

     S28.21   **Complete traumatic amputation of breast**

         Traumatic amputation of breast NOS

         ⑦S28.211   **Complete traumatic amputation of right breast**

         ⑦S28.212   **Complete traumatic amputation of left breast**

         ⑦S28.219   **Complete traumatic amputation of unspecified breast**

     S28.22   **Partial traumatic amputation of breast**

         ⑦S28.221   **Partial traumatic amputation of right breast**

         ⑦S28.222   **Partial traumatic amputation of left breast**

         ⑦S28.229   **Partial traumatic amputation of unspecified breast**

S29   **Other and unspecified injuries of thorax**

<u>Code also</u> any associated open wound (S21.-)

The appropriate 7th character is to be added to each code from category S29

A - initial encounter

D - subsequent encounter

S - sequela

S29.0   **Injury of muscle and tendon at thorax level**

     S29.00   **Unspecified injury of muscle and tendon of thorax**

         ⑦S29.001   **Unspecified injury of muscle and tendon of front wall of thorax**

         ⑦S29.002   **Unspecified injury of muscle and tendon of back wall of thorax**

         ⑦S29.009   **Unspecified injury of muscle and tendon of unspecified wall of thorax**

     S29.01   **Strain of muscle and tendon of thorax**

         ⑦S29.011   **Strain of muscle and tendon of front wall of thorax**

         ⑦S29.012   **Strain of muscle and tendon of back wall of thorax**

         ⑦S29.019   **Strain of muscle and tendon of unspecified wall of thorax**

     S29.02   **Laceration of muscle and tendon of thorax**

         ⑦S29.021   **Laceration of muscle and tendon of front wall of thorax**

         ⑦S29.022   **Laceration of muscle and tendon of back wall of thorax**

⑦S29.029   **Laceration of muscle and tendon of unspecified wall of thorax**

S29.09   **Other injury of muscle and tendon of thorax**

     ⑦S29.091   **Other injury of muscle and tendon of front wall of thorax**

     ⑦S29.092   **Other injury of muscle and tendon of back wall of thorax**

     ⑦S29.099   **Other injury of muscle and tendon of unspecified wall of thorax**

⊗⑦**S29.8**   **Other specified injuries of thorax**

⊗⑦**S29.9**   **Unspecified injury of thorax**

INJURIES TO THE ABDOMEN, LOWER BACK, LUMBAR SPINE, PELVIS AND EXTERNAL GENITALS (S30-S39)

Includes: injuries to the abdominal wall

injuries to the anus injuries to the buttock

injuries to the external genitalia injuries to the flank

injuries to the groin

Excludes2: burns and corrosions (T20-T32)

     effects of foreign body in anus and rectum (T18.5)

     effects of foreign body in genitourinary tract (T19.-)

     effects of foreign body in stomach, small intestine and colon (T18.2-T18.4)

     frostbite (T33-T34)

     insect bite or sting, venomous (T63.4)

S30   **Superficial injury of abdomen, lower back, pelvis and external genitals**

     Excludes2: superficial injury of hip (S70.-)

The appropriate 7th character is to be added to each code from category S30

A - initial encounter

D - subsequent encounter

S - sequela

⊗⑦**S30.0**   **Contusion of lower back and pelvis**

     Contusion of buttock

⊗⑦**S30.1**   **Contusion of abdominal wall**

     Contusion of flank

     Contusion of groin

S30.2   **Contusion of external genital organs**

     S30.20   **Contusion of unspecified external genital organ**

         ⑦S30.201   **Contusion of unspecified external genital organ, male**

         ⑦S30.202   **Contusion of unspecified external genital organ, female**

     ⊗⑦**S30.21**   **Contusion of penis**

     ⊗⑦**S30.22**   **Contusion of scrotum and testes**

     ⊗⑦**S30.23**   **Contusion of vagina and vulva**

S30.3   **Contusion of anus**

S30.8   **Other superficial injuries of abdomen, lower back, pelvis and external genitals**

     S30.81   **Abrasion of abdomen, lower back, pelvis and external genitals**

         ⑦S30.810   **Abrasion of lower back and pelvis**

         ⑦S30.811   **Abrasion of abdominal wall**

         ⑦S30.812   **Abrasion of penis**

         ⑦S30.813   **Abrasion of scrotum and testes**

         ⑦S30.814   **Abrasion of vagina and vulva**

         ⑦S30.815   **Abrasion of unspecified external genital organs, male**

   ● New code   ▲ Revised code   **Excludes1:** Not coded here   **Excludes2:** Not included here   ⊗ Placeholder required   ⑦ 7th digit required

⑦S30.816   **Abrasion of unspecified external genital organs, female**

⑦S30.817   **Abrasion of anus**

S30.82   **Blister (nonthermal) of abdomen, lower back, pelvis and external genitals**

  ⑦S30.820   **Blister (nonthermal) of lower back and pelvis**

  ⑦S30.821   **Blister (nonthermal) of abdominal wall**

  ⑦S30.822   **Blister (nonthermal) of penis**

  ⑦S30.823   **Blister (nonthermal) of scrotum and testes**

  ⑦S30.824   **Blister (nonthermal) of vagina and vulva**

  ⑦S30.825   **Blister (nonthermal) of unspecified external genital organs, male**

  ⑦S30.826   **Blister (nonthermal) of unspecified external genital organs, female**

  ⑦S30.827   **Blister (nonthermal) of anus**

S30.84   **External constriction of abdomen, lower back, pelvis and external genitals**

  ⑦S30.840   **External constriction of lower back and pelvis**

  ⑦S30.841   **External constriction of abdominal wall**

  ⑦S30.842   **External constriction of penis**

    Hair tourniquet syndrome of penis

    Use additional cause code to identify the constricting item (W49.0-)

  ⑦S30.843   **External constriction of scrotum and testes**

  ⑦S30.844   **External constriction of vagina and vulva**

  ⑦S30.845   **External constriction of unspecified external genital organs, male**

  ⑦S30.846   **External constriction of unspecified external genital organs, female**

S30.85   **Superficial foreign body of abdomen, lower back, pelvis and external genitals**

  Splinter in the abdomen, lower back, pelvis and external genitals

  ⑦S30.850   **Superficial foreign body of lower back and pelvis**

  ⑦S30.851   **Superficial foreign body of abdominal wall**

  ⑦S30.852   **Superficial foreign body of penis**

  ⑦S30.853   **Superficial foreign body of scrotum and testes**

  ⑦S30.854   **Superficial foreign body of vagina and vulva**

  ⑦S30.855   **Superficial foreign body of unspecified external genital organs, male**

  ⑦S30.856   **Superficial foreign body of unspecified external genital organs, female**

  ⑦S30.857   **Superficial foreign body of anus**

S30.86   **Insect bite (nonvenomous) of abdomen, lower back, pelvis and external genitals**

  ⑦S30.860   **Insect bite (nonvenomous) of lower back and pelvis**

  ⑦S30.861   **Insect bite (nonvenomous) of abdominal wall**

  ⑦S30.862   **Insect bite (nonvenomous) of penis**

⑦S30.863   **Insect bite (nonvenomous) of scrotum and testes**

⑦S30.864   **Insect bite (nonvenomous) of vagina and vulva**

⑦S30.865   **Insect bite (nonvenomous) of unspecified external genital organs, male**

⑦S30.866   **Insect bite (nonvenomous) of unspecified external genital organs, female**

⑦S30.867   **Insect bite (nonvenomous) of anus**

S30.87   **Other superficial bite of abdomen, lower back, pelvis and external genitals**

  Excludes1: open bite of abdomen, lower back, pelvis and external genitals (S31.05, S31.15, S31.25, S31.35, S31.45, S31.55)

  ⑦S30.870   **Other superficial bite of lower back and pelvis**

  ⑦S30.871   **Other superficial bite of abdominal wall**

  ⑦S30.872   **Other superficial bite of penis**

  ⑦S30.873   **Other superficial bite of scrotum and testes**

  ⑦S30.874   **Other superficial bite of vagina and vulva**

  ⑦S30.875   **Other superficial bite of unspecified external genital organs, male**

  ⑦S30.876   **Other superficial bite of unspecified external genital organs, female**

  ⑦S30.877   **Other superficial bite of anus**

S30.9   **Unspecified superficial injury of abdomen, lower back, pelvis and external genitals**

  ⊗⑦S30.91   **Unspecified superficial injury of lower back and pelvis**

  ⊗⑦S30.92   **Unspecified superficial injury of abdominal wall**

  ⊗⑦S30.93   **Unspecified superficial injury of penis**

  ⊗⑦S30.94   **Unspecified superficial injury of scrotum and testes**

  ⊗⑦S30.95   **Unspecified superficial injury of vagina and vulva**

  ⊗⑦S30.96   **Unspecified superficial injury of unspecified external genital organs, male**

  ⊗⑦S30.97   **Unspecified superficial injury of unspecified external genital organs, female**

  ⊗⑦S30.98   **Unspecified superficial injury of anus**

S31   **Open wound of abdomen, lower back, pelvis and external genitals**

Code also any associated:

spinal cord injury (S24.0, S24.1-, S34.0-, S34.1-)

wound infection

Excludes1: traumatic amputation of part of abdomen, lower back and pelvis (S38.2-, S38.3)

Excludes2: open wound of hip (S71.00-S71.02)

  open fracture of pelvis (S32.1--S32.9 with 7th character B)

The appropriate 7th character is to be added to each code from category S31

A - initial encounter

D - subsequent encounter

S - sequela

S31.0   **Open wound of lower back and pelvis**

S31.00 **Unspecified open wound of lower back and pelvis**

⑦**S31.000** **Unspecified open wound of lower back and pelvis without penetration into retroperitoneum**

Unspecified open wound of lower back and pelvis NOS

⑦**S31.001** **Unspecified open wound of lower back and pelvis with penetration into retroperitoneum**

S31.01 **Laceration without foreign body of lower back and pelvis**

⑦**S31.010** **Laceration without foreign body of lower back and pelvis without penetration into retroperitoneum**

Laceration without foreign body of lower back and pelvis NOS

⑦**S31.011** **Laceration without foreign body of lower back and pelvis with penetration into retroperitoneum**

S31.02 **Laceration with foreign body of lower back and pelvis**

⑦**S31.020** **Laceration with foreign body of lower back and pelvis without penetration into retroperitoneum**

Laceration with foreign body of lower back and pelvis NOS

⑦**S31.021** **Laceration with foreign body of lower back and pelvis with penetration into retroperitoneum**

S31.03 **Puncture wound without foreign body of lower back and pelvis**

⑦**S31.030** **Puncture wound without foreign body of lower back and pelvis without penetration into retroperitoneum**

Puncture wound without foreign body of lower back and pelvis NOS

⑦**S31.031** **Puncture wound without foreign body of lower back and pelvis with penetration into retroperitoneum**

S31.04 **Puncture wound with foreign body of lower back and pelvis**

⑦**S31.040** **Puncture wound with foreign body of lower back and pelvis without penetration into retroperitoneum**

Puncture wound with foreign body of lower back and pelvis NOS

⑦**S31.041** **Puncture wound with foreign body of lower back and pelvis with penetration into retroperitoneum**

S31.05 **Open bite of lower back and pelvis**

Bite of lower back and pelvis NOS

Excludes1: superficial bite of lower back and pelvis (S30.860, S30.870)

⑦**S31.050** **Open bite of lower back and pelvis without penetration into retroperitoneum**

Open bite of lower back and pelvis NOS

⑦**S31.051** **Open bite of lower back and pelvis with penetration into retroperitoneum**

S31.1 **Open wound of abdominal wall without penetration into peritoneal cavity**

Open wound of abdominal wall NOS

Excludes2: open wound of abdominal wall with penetration into peritoneal cavity (S31.6-)

S31.10 **Unspecified open wound of abdominal wall without penetration into peritoneal cavity**

⑦**S31.100** **Unspecified open wound of abdominal wall, right upper quadrant without penetration into peritoneal cavity**

⑦**S31.101** **Unspecified open wound of abdominal wall, left upper quadrant without penetration into peritoneal cavity**

⑦**S31.102** **Unspecified open wound of abdominal wall, epigastric region without penetration into peritoneal cavity**

⑦**S31.103** **Unspecified open wound of abdominal wall, right lower quadrant without penetration into peritoneal cavity**

⑦**S31.104** **Unspecified open wound of abdominal wall, left lower quadrant without penetration into peritoneal cavity**

⑦**S31.105** **Unspecified open wound of abdominal wall, periumbilic region without penetration into peritoneal cavity**

⑦**S31.109** **Unspecified open wound of abdominal wall, unspecified quadrant without penetration into peritoneal cavity**

Unspecified open wound of abdominal wall NOS

⑦**S31.11** **Laceration without foreign body of abdominal wall without penetration into peritoneal cavity**

⑦**S31.110** **Laceration without foreign body of abdominal wall, right upper quadrant without penetration into peritoneal cavity**

⑦**S31.111** **Laceration without foreign body of abdominal wall, left upper quadrant without penetration into peritoneal cavity**

⑦**S31.112** **Laceration without foreign body of abdominal wall, epigastric region without penetration into peritoneal cavity**

⑦**S31.113** **Laceration without foreign body of abdominal wall, right lower quadrant without penetration into peritoneal cavity**

⑦**S31.114** **Laceration without foreign body of abdominal wall, left lower quadrant without penetration into peritoneal cavity**

⑦**S31.115** **Laceration without foreign body of abdominal wall, periumbilic region without penetration into peritoneal cavity**

⑦**S31.119** **Laceration without foreign body of abdominal wall, unspecified quadrant without penetration into peritoneal cavity**

S31.12 **Laceration with foreign body of abdominal wall without penetration into peritoneal cavity**

⑦**S31.120** **Laceration of abdominal wall with foreign body, right upper quadrant**

without penetration into peritoneal cavity

⑦S31.121 **Laceration of abdominal wall with foreign body, left upper quadrant without penetration into peritoneal cavity**

⑦S31.122 **Laceration of abdominal wall with foreign body, epigastric region without penetration into peritoneal cavity**

⑦S31.123 **Laceration of abdominal wall with foreign body, right lower quadrant without penetration into peritoneal cavity**

⑦S31.124 **Laceration of abdominal wall with foreign body, left lower quadrant without penetration into peritoneal cavity**

⑦S31.125 **Laceration of abdominal wall with foreign body, periumbilic region without penetration into peritoneal cavity**

⑦S31.129 **Laceration of abdominal wall with foreign body, unspecified quadrant without penetration into peritoneal cavity**

S31.13 **Puncture wound of abdominal wall without foreign body without penetration into peritoneal cavity**

⑦S31.130 **Puncture wound of abdominal wall without foreign body, right upper quadrant without penetration into peritoneal cavity**

⑦S31.131 **Puncture wound of abdominal wall without foreign body, left upper quadrant without penetration into peritoneal cavity**

⑦S31.132 **Puncture wound of abdominal wall without foreign body, epigastric region without penetration into peritoneal cavity**

⑦S31.133 **Puncture wound of abdominal wall without foreign body, right lower quadrant without penetration into peritoneal cavity**

⑦S31.134 **Puncture wound of abdominal wall without foreign body, left lower quadrant without penetration into peritoneal cavity**

⑦S31.135 **Puncture wound of abdominal wall without foreign body, periumbilic region without penetration into peritoneal cavity**

⑦S31.139 **Puncture wound of abdominal wall without foreign body, unspecified quadrant without penetration into peritoneal cavity**

S31.14 **Puncture wound of abdominal wall with foreign body without penetration into peritoneal cavity**

⑦S31.140 **Puncture wound of abdominal wall with foreign body, right upper quadrant without penetration into peritoneal cavity**

⑦S31.141 **Puncture wound of abdominal wall with foreign body, left upper quadrant without penetration into peritoneal cavity**

⑦S31.142 **Puncture wound of abdominal wall with foreign body, epigastric region**

⑦S31.143 **Puncture wound of abdominal wall with foreign body, right lower quadrant without penetration into peritoneal cavity**

⑦S31.144 **Puncture wound of abdominal wall with foreign body, left lower quadrant without penetration into peritoneal cavity**

⑦S31.145 **Puncture wound of abdominal wall with foreign body, periumbilic region without penetration into peritoneal cavity**

⑦S31.149 **Puncture wound of abdominal wall with foreign body, unspecified quadrant without penetration into peritoneal cavity**

S31.15 **Open bite of abdominal wall without penetration into peritoneal cavity**

Bite of abdominal wall NOS

Excludes1: superficial bite of abdominal wall (S30.871)

⑦S31.150 **Open bite of abdominal wall, right upper quadrant without penetration into peritoneal cavity**

⑦S31.151 **Open bite of abdominal wall, left upper quadrant without penetration into peritoneal cavity**

⑦S31.152 **Open bite of abdominal wall, epigastric region without penetration into peritoneal cavity**

⑦S31.153 **Open bite of abdominal wall, right lower quadrant without penetration into peritoneal cavity**

⑦S31.154 **Open bite of abdominal wall, left lower quadrant without penetration into peritoneal cavity**

⑦S31.155 **Open bite of abdominal wall, periumbilic region without penetration into peritoneal cavity**

⑦S31.159 **Open bite of abdominal wall, unspecified quadrant without penetration into peritoneal cavity**

S31.2 **Open wound of penis**

⊗⑦S31.20 **Unspecified open wound of penis**

⊗⑦S31.21 **Laceration without foreign body of penis**

⊗⑦S31.22 **Laceration with foreign body of penis**

⊗⑦S31.23 **Puncture wound without foreign body of penis**

⊗⑦S31.24 **Puncture wound with foreign body of penis**

⊗⑦S31.25 **Open bite of penis**

Bite of penis NOS

Excludes1: superficial bite of penis (S30.862, S30.872)

S31.3 **Open wound of scrotum and testes**

⊗⑦S31.30 **Unspecified open wound of scrotum and testes**

⊗⑦S31.31 **Laceration without foreign body of scrotum and testes**

⊗⑦S31.32 **Laceration with foreign body of scrotum and testes**

⊗⑦S31.33 **Puncture wound without foreign body of scrotum and testes**

⊗⑦S31.34 **Puncture wound with foreign body of scrotum and testes**

⊗⑦S31.35 **Open bite of scrotum and testes**

Bite of scrotum and testes NOS

> **Excludes1:** superficial bite of scrotum and testes (S30.863, S30.873)

S31.4   **Open wound of vagina and vulva**

> **Excludes1:** injury to vagina and vulva during delivery (O70.-, O71.4)

⊗⑦**S31.40**   **Unspecified open wound of vagina and vulva**

⊗⑦**S31.41**   **Laceration without foreign body of vagina and vulva**

⊗⑦**S31.42**   **Laceration with foreign body of vagina and vulva**

⊗⑦**S31.43**   **Puncture wound without foreign body of vagina and vulva**

⊗⑦**S31.44**   **Puncture wound with foreign body of vagina and vulva**

⊗⑦**S31.45**   **Open bite of vagina and vulva**
Bite of vagina and vulva NOS

> **Excludes1:** superficial bite of vagina and vulva (S30.864, S30.874)

S31.5   **Open wound of unspecified external genital organs**

> **Excludes1:** traumatic amputation of external genital organs (S38.21, S38.22)

S31.50   **Unspecified open wound of unspecified external genital organs**

⑦**S31.501**   **Unspecified open wound of unspecified external genital organs, male**

⑦**S31.502**   **Unspecified open wound of unspecified external genital organs, female**

S31.51   **Laceration without foreign body of unspecified external genital organs**

⑦**S31.511**   **Laceration without foreign body of unspecified external genital organs, male**

⑦**S31.512**   **Laceration without foreign body of unspecified external genital organs, female**

S31.52   **Laceration with foreign body of unspecified external genital organs**

⑦**S31.521**   **Laceration with foreign body of unspecified external genital organs, male**

⑦**S31.522**   **Laceration with foreign body of unspecified external genital organs, female**

S31.53   **Puncture wound without foreign body of unspecified external genital organs**

⑦**S31.531**   **Puncture wound without foreign body of unspecified external genital organs, male**

⑦**S31.532**   **Puncture wound without foreign body of unspecified external genital organs, female**

S31.54   **Puncture wound with foreign body of unspecified external genital organs**

⑦**S31.541**   **Puncture wound with foreign body of unspecified external genital organs, male**

⑦**S31.542**   **Puncture wound with foreign body of unspecified external genital organs, female**

S31.55   **Open bite of unspecified external genital organs**

Bite of unspecified external genital organs NOS

> **Excludes1:** superficial bite of unspecified external genital organs (S30.865, S30.866, S30.875, S30.876)

⑦**S31.551**   **Open bite of unspecified external genital organs, male**

⑦**S31.552**   **Open bite of unspecified external genital organs, female**

S31.6   **Open wound of abdominal wall with penetration into peritoneal cavity**

S31.60   **Unspecified open wound of abdominal wall with penetration into peritoneal cavity**

⑦**S31.600**   **Unspecified open wound of abdominal wall, right upper quadrant with penetration into peritoneal cavity**

⑦**S31.601**   **Unspecified open wound of abdominal wall, left upper quadrant with penetration into peritoneal cavity**

⑦**S31.602**   **Unspecified open wound of abdominal wall, epigastric region with penetration into peritoneal cavity**

⑦**S31.603**   **Unspecified open wound of abdominal wall, right lower quadrant with penetration into peritoneal cavity**

⑦**S31.604**   **Unspecified open wound of abdominal wall, left lower quadrant with penetration into peritoneal cavity**

⑦**S31.605**   **Unspecified open wound of abdominal wall, periumbilic region with penetration into peritoneal cavity**

⑦**S31.609**   **Unspecified open wound of abdominal wall, unspecified quadrant with penetration into peritoneal cavity**

S31.61   **Laceration without foreign body of abdominal wall with penetration into peritoneal cavity**

⑦**S31.610**   **Laceration without foreign body of abdominal wall, right upper quadrant with penetration into peritoneal cavity**

⑦**S31.611**   **Laceration without foreign body of abdominal wall, left upper quadrant with penetration into peritoneal cavity**

⑦**S31.612**   **Laceration without foreign body of abdominal wall, epigastric region with penetration into peritoneal cavity**

⑦**S31.613**   **Laceration without foreign body of abdominal wall, right lower quadrant with penetration into peritoneal cavity**

⑦**S31.614**   **Laceration without foreign body of abdominal wall, left lower quadrant with penetration into peritoneal cavity**

⑦**S31.615**   **Laceration without foreign body of abdominal wall, periumbilic region with penetration into peritoneal cavity**

⑦**S31.619**   **Laceration without foreign body of abdominal wall, unspecified**

● New code   ▲ Revised code   **Excludes1:** Not coded here   **Excludes2:** Not included here   ⊗ Placeholder required   ⑦ 7ᵗʰ digit required

quadrant with penetration into peritoneal cavity

S31.62 **Laceration with foreign body of abdominal wall with penetration into peritoneal cavity**

⑦S31.620 **Laceration with foreign body of abdominal wall, right upper quadrant with penetration** into peritoneal cavity

⑦S31.621 **Laceration with foreign body of abdominal wall, left upper quadrant with penetration into peritoneal cavity**

⑦S31.622 **Laceration with foreign body of abdominal wall, epigastric region with penetration into peritoneal cavity**

⑦S31.623 **Laceration with foreign body of abdominal wall, right lower quadrant with penetration into peritoneal cavity**

⑦S31.624 **Laceration with foreign body of abdominal wall, left lower quadrant with penetration into peritoneal cavity**

⑦S31.625 **Laceration with foreign body of abdominal wall, periumbilic region with penetration into peritoneal cavity**

⑦S31.629 **Laceration with foreign body of abdominal wall, unspecified quadrant with penetration into peritoneal cavity**

S31.63 **Puncture wound without foreign body of abdominal wall with penetration into peritoneal cavity**

⑦S31.630 **Puncture wound without foreign body of abdominal wall, right upper quadrant with penetration into peritoneal cavity**

⑦S31.631 **Puncture wound without foreign body of abdominal wall, left upper quadrant with penetration into peritoneal cavity**

⑦S31.632 **Puncture wound without foreign body of abdominal wall, epigastric region with penetration into peritoneal cavity**

⑦S31.633 **Puncture wound without foreign body of abdominal wall, right lower quadrant with penetration into peritoneal cavity**

⑦S31.634 **Puncture wound without foreign body of abdominal wall, left lower quadrant with penetration into peritoneal cavity**

⑦S31.635 **Puncture wound without foreign body of abdominal wall, periumbilic region with penetration into peritoneal cavity**

⑦S31.639 **Puncture wound without foreign body of abdominal wall, unspecified quadrant with penetration into peritoneal cavity**

S31.64 **Puncture wound with foreign body of abdominal wall with penetration into peritoneal cavity**

⑦S31.640 **Puncture wound with foreign body of abdominal wall, right upper**

⑦S31.641 **Puncture wound with foreign body of abdominal wall, left upper quadrant with penetration into peritoneal cavity**

⑦S31.642 **Puncture wound with foreign body of abdominal wall, epigastric region with penetration into peritoneal cavity**

⑦S31.643 **Puncture wound with foreign body of abdominal wall, right lower quadrant with penetration into peritoneal cavity**

⑦S31.644 **Puncture wound with foreign body of abdominal wall, left lower quadrant with penetration into peritoneal cavity**

⑦S31.645 **Puncture wound with foreign body of abdominal wall, periumbilic region with penetration into peritoneal cavity**

⑦S31.649 **Puncture wound with foreign body of abdominal wall, unspecified quadrant with penetration into peritoneal cavity**

S31.65 **Open bite of abdominal wall with penetration into peritoneal cavity**

Excludes1: superficial bite of abdominal wall (S30.861, S30.871)

⑦S31.650 **Open bite of abdominal wall, right upper quadrant with penetration into peritoneal cavity**

⑦S31.651 **Open bite of abdominal wall, left upper quadrant with penetration into peritoneal cavity**

⑦S31.652 **Open bite of abdominal wall, epigastric region with penetration into peritoneal cavity**

⑦S31.653 **Open bite of abdominal wall, right lower quadrant with penetration into peritoneal cavity**

⑦S31.654 **Open bite of abdominal wall, left lower quadrant with penetration into peritoneal cavity**

⑦S31.655 **Open bite of abdominal wall, periumbilic region with penetration into peritoneal cavity**

⑦S31.659 **Open bite of abdominal wall, unspecified quadrant with penetration into peritoneal cavity**

S31.8 **Open wound of other parts of abdomen, lower back and pelvis**

S31.80 **Open wound of unspecified buttock**

⑦S31.801 **Laceration without foreign body of unspecified buttock**

⑦S31.802 **Laceration with foreign body of unspecified buttock**

⑦S31.803 **Puncture wound without foreign body of unspecified buttock**

⑦S31.804 **Puncture wound with foreign body of unspecified buttock**

⑦S31.805 **Open bite of unspecified buttock**

Bite of buttock NOS

Excludes1: superficial bite of buttock (S30.870)

⑦S31.809   **Unspecified open wound of unspecified buttock**

S31.81   **Open wound of right buttock**

⑦S31.811   **Laceration without foreign body of right buttock**

⑦S31.812   **Laceration with foreign body of right buttock**

⑦S31.813   **Puncture wound without foreign body of right buttock**

⑦S31.814   **Puncture wound with foreign body of right buttock**

⑦S31.815   **Open bite of right buttock**

Bite of right buttock NOS

Excludes1: superficial bite of buttock (S30.870)

⑦S31.819   **Unspecified open wound of right buttock**

S31.82   **Open wound of left buttock**

⑦S31.821   **Laceration without foreign body of left buttock**

⑦S31.822   **Laceration with foreign body of left buttock**

⑦S31.823   **Puncture wound without foreign body of left buttock**

⑦S31.824   **Puncture wound with foreign body of left buttock**

⑦S31.825   **Open bite of left buttock**

Bite of left buttock NOS

Excludes1: superficial bite of buttock (S30.870)

⑦S31.829   **Unspecified open wound of left buttock**

⑦S31.83   **Open wound of anus**

⑦S31.831   **Laceration without foreign body of anus**

⑦S31.832   **Laceration with foreign body of anus**

⑦S31.833   **Puncture wound without foreign body of anus**

⑦S31.834   **Puncture wound with foreign body of anus**

⑦S31.835   **Open bite of anus**

Bite of anus NOS

Excludes1: superficial bite of anus (S30.877)

⑦S31.839   **Unspecified open wound of anus**

S32   **Fracture of lumbar spine and pelvis**

Note: A fracture not indicated as displaced or nondisplaced should be coded to displaced

A fracture not indicated as opened or closed should be coded to closed

Includes: fracture of lumbosacral neural arch

fracture of lumbosacral spinous process

fracture of lumbosacral transverse process

fracture of lumbosacral vertebra

fracture of lumbosacral vertebral arch

Code first any associated spinal cord and spinal nerve injury (S34.-)

Excludes1: transection of abdomen (S38.3)

Excludes2: fracture of hip NOS (S72.0-)

The appropriate 7th character is to be added to each code from category S32

A - initial encounter for closed fracture

B - initial encounter for open fracture

D - subsequent encounter for fracture with routine healing

G - subsequent encounter for fracture with delayed healing

K - subsequent encounter for fracture with nonunion

S - sequela

S32.0   **Fracture of lumbar vertebra**

Fracture of lumbar spine NOS

S32.00   **Fracture of unspecified lumbar vertebra**

⑦S32.000   **Wedge compression fracture of unspecified lumbar vertebra** [HCC]

⑦S32.001   **Stable burst fracture of unspecified lumbar vertebra** [HCC]

⑦S32.002   **Unstable burst fracture of unspecified lumbar vertebra**

⑦S32.008   **Other fracture of unspecified lumbar vertebra** [HCC]

⑦S32.009   **Unspecified fracture of unspecified lumbar vertebra** [HCC]

S32.01   **Fracture of first lumbar vertebra** [HCC]

⑦S32.010   **Wedge compression fracture of first lumbar vertebra** [HCC]

⑦S32.011   **Stable burst fracture of first lumbar vertebra** [HCC]

⑦S32.012   **Unstable burst fracture of first lumbar vertebra** [HCC]

⑦S32.018   **Other fracture of first lumbar vertebra** [HCC]

⑦S32.019   **Unspecified fracture of first lumbar vertebra** [HCC]

S32.02   **Fracture of second lumbar vertebra** [HCC]

⑦S32.020   **Wedge compression fracture of second lumbar vertebra** [HCC]

⑦S32.021   **Stable burst fracture of second lumbar vertebra** [HCC]

⑦S32.022   **Unstable burst fracture of second lumbar vertebra** [HCC]

⑦S32.028   **Other fracture of second lumbar vertebra** [HCC]

⑦S32.029   **Unspecified fracture of second lumbar vertebra** [HCC]

S32.03   **Fracture of third lumbar vertebra**

⑦S32.030   **Wedge compression fracture of third lumbar vertebra** [HCC]

⑦S32.031   **Stable burst fracture of third lumbar vertebra** [HCC]

⑦S32.032   **Unstable burst fracture of third lumbar vertebra** [HCC]

⑦S32.038   **Other fracture of third lumbar vertebra** [HCC]

⑦S32.039   **Unspecified fracture of third lumbar vertebra** [HCC]

S32.04   **Fracture of fourth lumbar vertebra** [HCC]

⑦S32.040   **Wedge compression fracture of fourth lumbar vertebra** [HCC]

⑦S32.041   **Stable burst fracture of fourth lumbar vertebra** [HCC]

⑦S32.042   **Unstable burst fracture of fourth lumbar vertebra** [HCC]

⑦S32.048   **Other fracture of fourth lumbar vertebra** [HCC]

⑦S32.049   **Unspecified fracture of fourth lumbar vertebra** [HCC]

S32.05 **Fracture of fifth lumbar vertebra** [HCC]

⑦**S32.050** **Wedge compression fracture of fifth lumbar vertebra** [HCC]

⑦**S32.051** **Stable burst fracture of fifth lumbar vertebra** [HCC]

⑦**S32.052** **Unstable burst fracture of fifth lumbar vertebra** [HCC]

⑦**S32.058** **Other fracture of fifth lumbar vertebra** [HCC]

⑦**S32.059** **Unspecified fracture of fifth lumbar vertebra** [HCC]

S32.1 **Fracture of sacrum**

For vertical fractures, code to most medial fracture extension

Use two codes if both a vertical and transverse fracture are present

<u>Code also</u> any associated fracture of pelvic ring (S32.8-)

⊗⑦**S32.10** **Unspecified fracture of sacrum** [HCC]

S32.11 **Zone I fracture of sacrum** [HCC]

Vertical sacral ala fracture of sacrum

⑦**S32.110** **Nondisplaced Zone I fracture of sacrum** [HCC]

⑦**S32.111** **Minimally displaced Zone I fracture of sacrum** [HCC]

⑦**S32.112** **Severely displaced Zone I fracture of sacrum** [HCC]

⑦**S32.119** **Unspecified Zone I fracture of sacrum** [HCC]

S32.12 **Zone II fracture of sacrum** [HCC]

Vertical foraminal region fracture of sacrum

⑦**S32.120** **Nondisplaced Zone II fracture of sacrum** [HCC]

⑦**S32.121** **Minimally displaced Zone II fracture of sacrum** [HCC]

⑦**S32.122** **Severely displaced Zone II fracture of sacrum** [HCC]

⑦**S32.129** **Unspecified Zone II fracture of sacrum** [HCC]

S32.13 **Zone III fracture of sacrum** [HCC]

Vertical fracture into spinal canal region of sacrum

⑦**S32.130** **Nondisplaced Zone III fracture of sacrum** [HCC]

⑦**S32.131** **Minimally displaced Zone III fracture of sacrum** [HCC]

⑦**S32.132** **Severely displaced Zone III fracture of sacrum** [HCC]

⑦**S32.139** **Unspecified Zone III fracture of sacrum** [HCC]

⊗⑦**S32.14** **Type 1 fracture of sacrum** [HCC]

Transverse flexion fracture of sacrum without displacement

⊗⑦**S32.15** **Type 2 fracture of sacrum** [HCC]

Transverse flexion fracture of sacrum with posterior displacement

⊗⑦**S32.16** **Type 3 fracture of sacrum** [HCC]

Transverse extension fracture of sacrum with anterior displacement

⊗⑦**S32.17** **Type 4 fracture of sacrum** [HCC]

Transverse segmental comminution of upper sacrum

⊗⑦**S32.19** **Other fracture of sacrum** [HCC]

⊗⑦**S32.2** **Fracture of coccyx** [HCC]

S32.3 **Fracture of ilium**

Excludes1: fracture of ilium with associated disruption of pelvic ring (S32.8-)

S32.30 **Unspecified fracture of ilium**

⑦**S32.301** **Unspecified fracture of right ilium**

⑦**S32.302** **Unspecified fracture of left ilium** [HCC]

⑦**S32.309** **Unspecified fracture of unspecified ilium** [HCC]

S32.31 **Avulsion fracture of ilium**

⑦**S32.311** **Displaced avulsion fracture of right ilium** [HCC]

⑦**S32.312** **Displaced avulsion fracture of left ilium** [HCC]

⑦**S32.313** **Displaced avulsion fracture of unspecified ilium** [HCC]

⑦**S32.314** **Nondisplaced avulsion fracture of right ilium** [HCC]

⑦**S32.315** **Nondisplaced avulsion fracture of left ilium** [HCC]

⑦**S32.316** **Nondisplaced avulsion fracture of unspecified ilium** [HCC]

S32.39 **Other fracture of ilium**

⑦**S32.391** **Other fracture of right ilium** [HCC]

⑦**S32.392** **Other fracture of left ilium** [HCC]

⑦**S32.399** **Other fracture of unspecified ilium** [HCC]

S32.4 **Fracture of acetabulum**

<u>Code also</u> any associated fracture of pelvic ring (S32.8-)

S32.40 **Unspecified fracture of acetabulum**

⑦**S32.401** **Unspecified fracture of right acetabulum** [HCC]

⑦**S32.402** **Unspecified fracture of left acetabulum** [HCC]

⑦**S32.409** **Unspecified fracture of unspecified acetabulum** [HCC]

S32.41 **Fracture of anterior wall of acetabulum** [HCC]

⑦**S32.411** **Displaced fracture of anterior wall of right acetabulum** [HCC]

⑦**S32.412** **Displaced fracture of anterior wall of left acetabulum** [HCC]

⑦**S32.413** **Displaced fracture of anterior wall of unspecified acetabulum** [HCC]

⑦**S32.414** **Nondisplaced fracture of anterior wall of right acetabulum** [HCC]

⑦**S32.415** **Nondisplaced fracture of anterior wall of left acetabulum** [HCC]

⑦**S32.416** **Nondisplaced fracture of anterior wall of unspecified acetabulum** [HCC]

S32.42 **Fracture of posterior wall of acetabulum**

⑦**S32.421** **Displaced fracture of posterior wall of right acetabulum** [HCC]

⑦**S32.422** **Displaced fracture of posterior wall of left acetabulum** [HCC]

⑦**S32.423** **Displaced fracture of posterior wall of unspecified acetabulum** [HCC]

⑦**S32.424** **Nondisplaced fracture of posterior wall of right acetabulum** [HCC]

⑦**S32.425** **Nondisplaced fracture of posterior wall of left acetabulum** [HCC]

⑦**S32.426** **Nondisplaced fracture of posterior wall of unspecified acetabulum**

S32.43 **Fracture of anterior column [iliopubic] of acetabulum**

---

⑦S32.431 Displaced fracture of anterior column [iliopubic] of right acetabulum [HCC]

⑦S32.432 Displaced fracture of anterior column [iliopubic] of left acetabulum [HCC]

⑦S32.433 Displaced fracture of anterior column [iliopubic] of unspecified acetabulum [HCC]

⑦S32.434 Nondisplaced fracture of anterior column [iliopubic] of right acetabulum [HCC]

⑦S32.435 Nondisplaced fracture of anterior column [iliopubic] of left acetabulum [HCC]

⑦S32.436 Nondisplaced fracture of anterior column [iliopubic] of unspecified acetabulum [HCC]

S32.44 Fracture of posterior column [ilioischial] of acetabulum

⑦S32.441 Displaced fracture of posterior column [ilioischial] of right acetabulum [HCC]

⑦S32.442 Displaced fracture of posterior column [ilioischial] of left acetabulum [HCC]

⑦S32.443 Displaced fracture of posterior column [ilioischial] of unspecified acetabulum [HCC]

⑦S32.444 Nondisplaced fracture of posterior column [ilioischial] of right acetabulum [HCC]

⑦S32.445 Nondisplaced fracture of posterior column [ilioischial] of left acetabulum [HCC]

⑦S32.446 Nondisplaced fracture of posterior column [ilioischial] of unspecified acetabulum [HCC]

S32.45 Transverse fracture of acetabulum

⑦S32.451 Displaced transverse fracture of right acetabulum [HCC]

⑦S32.452 Displaced transverse fracture of left acetabulum [HCC]

⑦S32.453 Displaced transverse fracture of unspecified acetabulum [HCC]

⑦S32.454 Nondisplaced transverse fracture of right acetabulum [HCC]

⑦S32.455 Nondisplaced transverse fracture of left acetabulum [HCC]

⑦S32.456 Nondisplaced transverse fracture of unspecified acetabulum [HCC]

S32.46 Associated transverse-posterior fracture of acetabulum

⑦S32.461 Displaced associated transverse-posterior fracture of right acetabulum [HCC]

⑦S32.462 Displaced associated transverse-posterior fracture of left acetabulum [HCC]

⑦S32.463 Displaced associated transverse-posterior fracture of unspecified acetabulum [HCC]

⑦S32.464 Nondisplaced associated transverse-posterior fracture of right acetabulum [HCC]

⑦S32.465 Nondisplaced associated transverse-posterior fracture of left acetabulum [HCC]

⑦S32.466 Nondisplaced associated transverse-posterior fracture of unspecified acetabulum [HCC]

S32.47 Fracture of medial wall of acetabulum

⑦S32.471 Displaced fracture of medial wall of right acetabulum [HCC]

⑦S32.472 Displaced fracture of medial wall of left acetabulum [HCC]

⑦S32.473 Displaced fracture of medial wall of unspecified acetabulum [HCC]

⑦S32.474 Nondisplaced fracture of medial wall of right acetabulum

⑦S32.475 Nondisplaced fracture of medial wall of left acetabulum [HCC]

⑦S32.476 Nondisplaced fracture of medial wall of unspecified acetabulum [HCC]

S32.48 Dome fracture of acetabulum]

⑦S32.481 Displaced dome fracture of right acetabulum [HCC]

⑦S32.482 Displaced dome fracture of left acetabulum [HCC]

⑦S32.483 Displaced dome fracture of unspecified acetabulum [HCC]

⑦S32.484 Nondisplaced dome fracture of right acetabulum [HCC]

⑦S32.485 Nondisplaced dome fracture of left acetabulum [HCC]

⑦S32.486 Nondisplaced dome fracture of unspecified acetabulum [HCC]

S32.49 Other specified fracture of acetabulum

⑦S32.491 Other specified fracture of right acetabulum [HCC]

⑦S32.492 Other specified fracture of left acetabulum [HCC]

⑦S32.499 Other specified fracture of unspecified acetabulum [HCC]

S32.5 Fracture of pubis

Excludes1: fracture of pubis with associated disruption of pelvic ring (S32.8-)

S32.50 Unspecified fracture of pubis [HCC]

⑦S32.501 Unspecified fracture of right pubis [HCC]

⑦S32.502 Unspecified fracture of left pubis [HCC]

⑦S32.509 Unspecified fracture of unspecified pubis [HCC]

S32.51 Fracture of superior rim of pubis

⑦S32.511 Fracture of superior rim of right pubis [HCC]

⑦S32.512 Fracture of superior rim of left pubis [HCC]

⑦S32.519 Fracture of superior rim of unspecified pubis [HCC]

S32.59 Other specified fracture of pubis

⑦S32.591 Other specified fracture of right pubis [HCC]

⑦S32.592 Other specified fracture of left pubis [HCC]

⑦S32.599 Other specified fracture of unspecified pubis [HCC]

S32.6 Fracture of ischium

● New code ▲ Revised code **Excludes1:** Not coded here **Excludes2:** Not included here ⊗ Placeholder required ⑦7th digit required

Excludes1: fracture of ischium with associated disruption of pelvic ring (S32.8-)

  S32.60 **Unspecified fracture of ischium**

    ⑦**S32.601** **Unspecified fracture of right ischium** [HCC]

    ⑦**S32.602** **Unspecified fracture of left ischium** [HCC]

    ⑦**S32.609** **Unspecified fracture of unspecified ischium**

  S32.61 **Avulsion fracture of ischium**

    ⑦**S32.611** **Displaced avulsion fracture of right ischium** [HCC]

    ⑦**S32.612** **Displaced avulsion fracture of left ischium** [HCC]

    ⑦**S32.613** **Displaced avulsion fracture of unspecified ischium** [HCC]

    ⑦**S32.614** **Nondisplaced avulsion fracture of right ischium** [HCC]

    ⑦**S32.615** **Nondisplaced avulsion fracture of left ischium** [HCC]

    ⑦**S32.616** **Nondisplaced avulsion fracture of unspecified ischium** [HCC]

  S32.69 **Other specified fracture of ischium**

    ⑦**S32.691** **Other specified fracture of right ischium** [HCC]

    ⑦**S32.692** **Other specified fracture of left ischium** [HCC]

    ⑦**S32.699** **Other specified fracture of unspecified ischium** [HCC]

S32.8 **Fracture of other parts of pelvis**

  <u>Code also</u> any associated:

  fracture of acetabulum (S32.4-)

  sacral fracture (S32.1-)

  S32.81 **Multiple fractures of pelvis with disruption of pelvic ring**

    Multiple pelvic fractures with disruption of pelvic circle

    ⑦**S32.810** **Multiple fractures of pelvis with stable disruption of pelvic ring** [HCC]

    ⑦**S32.811** **Multiple fractures of pelvis with unstable disruption of pelvic ring** [HCC]

  ⊗⑦**S32.82** **Multiple fractures of pelvis without disruption of pelvic ring** [HCC]

    Multiple pelvic fractures without disruption of pelvic circle

  ⊗⑦**S32.89** **Fracture of other parts of pelvis** [HCC]

S32.9 **Fracture of unspecified parts of lumbosacral spine and pelvis** [HCC]

  Fracture of lumbosacral spine NOS

  Fracture of pelvis NOS

S33 **Dislocation and sprain of joints and ligaments of lumbar spine and pelvis**

Includes: avulsion of joint or ligament of lumbar spine and pelvis

laceration of cartilage, joint or ligament of lumbar spine and pelvis

sprain of cartilage, joint or ligament of lumbar spine and pelvis

traumatic hemarthrosis of joint or ligament of lumbar spine and pelvis

traumatic rupture of joint or ligament of lumbar spine and pelvis

traumatic subluxation of joint or ligament of lumbar spine and pelvis

traumatic tear of joint or ligament of lumbar spine and pelvis

<u>Code also</u> any associated open wound

Excludes1: nontraumatic rupture or displacement of lumbar intervertebral disc NOS (M51.-)

obstetric damage to pelvic joints and ligaments (O71.6)

Excludes2: dislocation and sprain of joints and ligaments of hip (S73.-)

strain of muscle of lower back and pelvis (S39.01-)

The appropriate 7th character is to be added to each code from category S33

  A - initial encounter

  D - subsequent encounter

  S - sequela

⊗⑦**S33.0** **Traumatic rupture of lumbar intervertebral disc**

  Excludes1: rupture or displacement (nontraumatic) of lumbar intervertebral disc NOS (M51.- with fifth character 6)

S33.1 **Subluxation and dislocation of lumbar vertebra**

  <u>Code also</u> any associated:

  open wound of abdomen, lower back and pelvis (S31)

  spinal cord injury (S24.0, S24.1-, S34.0-, S34.1-)

  Excludes2: fracture of lumbar vertebrae (S32.0-)

  S33.10 **Subluxation and dislocation of unspecified lumbar vertebra**

    ⑦**S33.100** **Subluxation of unspecified lumbar vertebra**

    ⑦**S33.101** **Dislocation of unspecified lumbar vertebra**

  S33.11 **Subluxation and dislocation of L1/L2 lumbar vertebra**

    ⑦**S33.110** **Subluxation of L1/L2 lumbar vertebra**

    ⑦**S33.111** **Dislocation of L1/L2 lumbar vertebra**

  S33.12 **Subluxation and dislocation of L2/L3 lumbar vertebra**

    ⑦**S33.120** **Subluxation of L2/L3 lumbar vertebra**

    ⑦**S33.121** **Dislocation of L2/L3 lumbar vertebra**

  S33.13 **Subluxation and dislocation of L3/L4 lumbar vertebra**

    ⑦**S33.130** **Subluxation of L3/L4 lumbar vertebra**

    ⑦**S33.131** **Dislocation of L3/L4 lumbar vertebra**

    ⑦**S33.14** **Subluxation and dislocation of L4/L5 lumbar vertebra**

    ⑦**S33.140** **Subluxation of L4/L5 lumbar vertebra**

    ⑦**S33.141** **Dislocation of L4/L5 lumbar vertebra**

⊗⑦**S33.2** **Dislocation of sacroiliac and sacrococcygeal joint**

  S33.3 **Dislocation of other and unspecified parts of lumbar spine and pelvis**

    ⊗⑦**S33.30** **Dislocation of unspecified parts of lumbar spine and pelvis**

    ⊗⑦**S33.39** **Dislocation of other parts of lumbar spine and pelvis**

⊗⑦**S33.4** **Traumatic rupture of symphysis pubis**

⊗⑦**S33.5** **Sprain of ligaments of lumbar spine**

⊗⑦**S33.6** **Sprain of sacroiliac joint**

⊗⑦**S33.8** **Sprain of other parts of lumbar spine and pelvis**

⊗⑦**S33.9**   **Sprain of unspecified parts of lumbar spine and pelvis**

S34   **Injury of lumbar and sacral spinal cord and nerves at abdomen, lower back and pelvis level**

Note: Code to highest level of lumbar cord injury

Injuries to the spinal cord (S34.0 and S34.1) refer to the cord level and not bone level injury and can affect nerve roots at and below the level given.

<u>Code also</u> any associated:

fracture of vertebra (S22.0-, S32.0-)

open wound of abdomen, lower back and pelvis (S31.-)

transient paralysis (R29.5)

The appropriate 7th character is to be added to each code from category S34

A - initial encounter

D - subsequent encounter

S - sequela

S34.0   **Concussion and edema of lumbar and sacral spinal cord**

　⊗⑦**S34.01**   **Concussion and edema of lumbar spinal cord**

　⊗⑦**S34.02**   **Concussion and edema of sacral spinal cord**

　　　Concussion and edema of conus medullaris

S34.1   **Other and unspecified injury of lumbar and sacral spinal cord**

　S34.10   **Unspecified injury to lumbar spinal cord**

　　⑦**S34.101**   **Unspecified injury to L1 level of lumbar spinal cord** [HCC]

　　　　Unspecified injury to lumbar spinal cord level 1

　　⑦**S34.102**   **Unspecified injury to L2 level of lumbar spinal cord** [HCC]

　　　　Unspecified injury to lumbar spinal cord level 2

　　⑦**S34.103**   **Unspecified injury to L3 level of lumbar spinal cord** [HCC]

　　　　Unspecified injury to lumbar spinal cord level 3

　　⑦**S34.104**   **Unspecified injury to L4 level of lumbar spinal cord** [HCC]

　　　　Unspecified injury to lumbar spinal cord level 4

　　⑦**S34.105**   **Unspecified injury to L5 level of lumbar spinal cord** [HCC]

　　　　Unspecified injury to lumbar spinal cord level 5

　　⑦**S34.109**   **Unspecified injury to unspecified level of lumbar spinal cord** [HCC]

　S34.11   **Complete lesion of lumbar spinal cord**

　　⑦**S34.111**   **Complete lesion of L1 level of lumbar spinal cord** [HCC]

　　　　Complete lesion of lumbar spinal cord level 1

　　⑦**S34.112**   **Complete lesion of L2 level of lumbar spinal cord** [HCC]

　　　　Complete lesion of lumbar spinal cord level 2

　　⑦**S34.113**   **Complete lesion of L3 level of lumbar spinal cord** [HCC]

　　　　Complete lesion of lumbar spinal cord level 3

　　⑦**S34.114**   **Complete lesion of L4 level of lumbar spinal cord** [HCC]

　　　　Complete lesion of lumbar spinal cord level 4

　　⑦**S34.115**   **Complete lesion of L5 level of lumbar spinal cord** [HCC]

　　　　Complete lesion of lumbar spinal cord level 5

　　⑦**S34.119**   **Complete lesion of unspecified level of lumbar spinal cord** [HCC]

　S34.12   **Incomplete lesion of lumbar spinal cord**

　　⑦**S34.121**   **Incomplete lesion of L1 level of lumbar spinal cord** [HCC]

　　　　Incomplete lesion of lumbar spinal cord level 1

　　⑦**S34.122**   **Incomplete lesion of L2 level of lumbar spinal cord** [HCC]

　　　　Incomplete lesion of lumbar spinal cord level 2

　　⑦**S34.123**   **Incomplete lesion of L3 level of lumbar spinal cord** [HCC]

　　　　Incomplete lesion of lumbar spinal cord level 3

　　⑦**S34.124**   **Incomplete lesion of L4 level of lumbar spinal cord** [HCC]

　　　　Incomplete lesion of lumbar spinal cord level 4

　　⑦**S34.125**   **Incomplete lesion of L5 level of lumbar spinal cord** [HCC]

　　　　Incomplete lesion of lumbar spinal cord level 5

　　⑦**S34.129**   **Incomplete lesion of unspecified level of lumbar spinal cord** [HCC]

　S34.13   **Other and unspecified injury to sacral spinal cord**

　　　Other injury to conus medullaris

　　⑦**S34.131**   **Complete lesion of sacral spinal cord** [HCC]

　　　　Complete lesion of conus medullaris

　　⑦**S34.132**   **Incomplete lesion of sacral spinal cord** [HCC]

　　　　Incomplete lesion of conus medullaris

　　⑦**S34.139**   **Unspecified injury to sacral spinal cord** [HCC]

　　　　Unspecified injury of conus medullaris

S34.2   **Injury of nerve root of lumbar and sacral spine**

　⊗⑦**S34.21**   **Injury of nerve root of lumbar spine**

　⊗⑦**S34.22**   **Injury of nerve root of sacral spine**

⊗⑦**S34.3**   **Injury of cauda equina**

⊗⑦**S34.4**   **Injury of lumbosacral plexus**

⊗⑦**S34.5**   **Injury of lumbar, sacral and pelvic sympathetic nerves**

　　Injury of celiac ganglion or plexus

　　Injury of hypogastric plexus

　　Injury of mesenteric plexus (inferior) (superior)

　　Injury of splanchnic nerve

⊗⑦**S34.6**   **Injury of peripheral nerve(s) at abdomen, lower back and pelvis level**

⊗⑦**S34.8**   **Injury of other nerves at abdomen, lower back and pelvis level**

⊗⑦**S34.9**   **Injury of unspecified nerves at abdomen, lower back and pelvis level**

S35   **Injury of blood vessels at abdomen, lower back and pelvis level**

　<u>Code also</u> any associated open wound (S31.-)

The appropriate 7th character is to be added to each code from category S35

A - initial encounter

D - subsequent encounter

S - sequela

S35.0 Injury of abdominal aorta

Excludes1: injury of aorta NOS (S25.0)

⊗⑦**S35.00 Unspecified injury of abdominal aorta**

⊗⑦**S35.01 Minor laceration of abdominal aorta**

Incomplete transection of abdominal aorta

Laceration of abdominal aorta NOS

Superficial laceration of abdominal aorta

⊗⑦**S35.02 Major laceration of abdominal aorta**

Complete transection of abdominal aorta

Traumatic rupture of abdominal aorta

⊗⑦**S35.09 Other injury of abdominal aorta**

S35.1 Injury of inferior vena cava

Injury of hepatic vein

Excludes1: injury of vena cava NOS (S25.2)

⊗⑦**S35.10 Unspecified injury of inferior vena cava**

⊗⑦**S35.11 Minor laceration of inferior vena cava**

Incomplete transection of inferior vena cava

Laceration of inferior vena cava NOS

Superficial laceration of inferior vena cava

⊗⑦**S35.12 Major laceration of inferior vena cava**

Complete transection of inferior vena cava

Traumatic rupture of inferior vena cava

⊗⑦**S35.19 Other injury of inferior vena cava**

S35.2 Injury of celiac or mesenteric artery and branches

S35.21 Injury of celiac artery

⑦**S35.211 Minor laceration of celiac artery**

Incomplete transection of celiac artery

Laceration of celiac artery NOS

Superficial laceration of celiac artery

⑦**S35.212 Major laceration of celiac artery**

Complete transection of celiac artery

Traumatic rupture of celiac artery

⑦**S35.218 Other injury of celiac artery**

⑦**S35.219 Unspecified injury of celiac artery**

S35.22 Injury of superior mesenteric artery

⑦**S35.221 Minor laceration of superior mesenteric artery**

Incomplete transection of superior mesenteric artery

Laceration of superior mesenteric artery NOS

Superficial laceration of superior mesenteric artery

⑦**S35.222 Major laceration of superior mesenteric artery**

Complete transection of superior mesenteric artery

Traumatic rupture of superior mesenteric artery

⑦**S35.228 Other injury of superior mesenteric artery**

⑦**S35.229 Unspecified injury of superior mesenteric artery**

S35.23 Injury of inferior mesenteric artery

⑦**S35.231 Minor laceration of inferior mesenteric artery**

Incomplete transection of inferior mesenteric artery

Laceration of inferior mesenteric artery NOS

Superficial laceration of inferior mesenteric artery

⑦**S35.232 Major laceration of inferior mesenteric artery**

Complete transection of inferior mesenteric artery

Traumatic rupture of inferior mesenteric artery

⑦**S35.238 Other injury of inferior mesenteric artery**

⑦**S35.239 Unspecified injury of inferior mesenteric artery**

S35.29 Injury of branches of celiac and mesenteric artery

Injury of gastric artery

Injury of gastroduodenal artery

Injury of hepatic artery

Injury of splenic artery

⑦**S35.291 Minor laceration of branches of celiac and mesenteric artery**

Incomplete transection of branches of celiac and mesenteric artery

Laceration of branches of celiac and mesenteric artery NOS

Superficial laceration of branches of celiac and mesenteric artery

⑦**S35.292 Major laceration of branches of celiac and mesenteric artery**

Complete transection of branches of celiac and mesenteric artery

Traumatic rupture of branches of celiac and mesenteric artery

⑦**S35.298 Other injury of branches of celiac and mesenteric artery**

⑦**S35.299 Unspecified injury of branches of celiac and mesenteric artery**

S35.3 Injury of portal or splenic vein and branches

S35.31 Injury of portal vein

⑦**S35.311 Laceration of portal vein**

⑦**S35.318 Other specified injury of portal vein**

⑦**S35.319 Unspecified injury of portal vein**

S35.32 Injury of splenic vein

⑦**S35.321 Laceration of splenic vein**

⑦**S35.328 Other specified injury of splenic vein**

⑦**S35.329 Unspecified injury of splenic vein**

S35.33 Injury of superior mesenteric vein

⑦**S35.331 Laceration of superior mesenteric vein**

⑦**S35.338 Other specified injury of superior mesenteric vein**

⑦**S35.339 Unspecified injury of superior mesenteric vein**

S35.34 Injury of inferior mesenteric vein

⑦**S35.341 Laceration of inferior mesenteric vein**

⑦**S35.348 Other specified injury of inferior mesenteric vein**

⑦S35.349 **Unspecified injury of inferior mesenteric vein**

S35.4 Injury of renal blood vessels

S35.40 Unspecified injury of renal blood vessel

⑦S35.401 **Unspecified injury of right renal artery**

⑦S35.402 **Unspecified injury of left renal artery**

⑦S35.403 **Unspecified injury of unspecified renal artery**

⑦S35.404 **Unspecified injury of right renal vein**

⑦S35.405 **Unspecified injury of left renal vein**

⑦S35.406 **Unspecified injury of unspecified renal vein**

S35.41 Laceration of renal blood vessel

⑦S35.411 **Laceration of right renal artery**

⑦S35.412 **Laceration of left renal artery**

⑦S35.413 **Laceration of unspecified renal artery**

⑦S35.414 **Laceration of right renal vein**

⑦S35.415 **Laceration of left renal vein**

⑦S35.416 **Laceration of unspecified renal vein**

S35.49 Other specified injury of renal blood vessel

⑦S35.491 **Other specified injury of right renal artery**

⑦S35.492 **Other specified injury of left renal artery**

⑦S35.493 **Other specified injury of unspecified renal artery**

⑦S35.494 **Other specified injury of right renal vein**

⑦S35.495 **Other specified injury of left renal vein**

⑦S35.496 **Other specified injury of unspecified renal vein**

S35.5 Injury of iliac blood vessels

⊗⑦S35.50 **Injury of unspecified iliac blood vessel(s)**

S35.51 Injury of iliac artery or vein

Injury of hypogastric artery or vein

⑦S35.511 **Injury of right iliac artery**

⑦S35.512 **Injury of left iliac artery**

⑦S35.513 **Injury of unspecified iliac artery**

⑦S35.514 **Injury of right iliac vein**

⑦S35.515 **Injury of left iliac vein**

⑦S35.516 **Injury of unspecified iliac vein**

S35.53 Injury of uterine artery or vein

⑦S35.531 **Injury of right uterine artery**

⑦S35.532 **Injury of left uterine artery**

⑦S35.533 **Injury of unspecified uterine artery**

⑦S35.534 **Injury of right uterine vein**

⑦S35.535 **Injury of left uterine vein**

⑦S35.536 **Injury of unspecified uterine vein**

⊗⑦S35.59 **Injury of other iliac blood vessels**

S35.8 Injury of other blood vessels at abdomen, lower back and pelvis level

Injury of ovarian artery or vein

S35.8X Injury of other blood vessels at abdomen, lower back and pelvis level

⑦S35.8X1 **Laceration of other blood vessels at abdomen, lower back and pelvis level**

⑦S35.8X8 **Other specified injury of other blood vessels at abdomen, lower back and pelvis level**

⑦S35.8X9 **Unspecified injury of other blood vessels at abdomen, lower back and pelvis level**

S35.9 Injury of unspecified blood vessel at abdomen, lower back and pelvis level

⊗⑦S35.90 **Unspecified injury of unspecified blood vessel at abdomen, lower back and pelvis level**

⊗⑦S35.91 **Laceration of unspecified blood vessel at abdomen, lower back and pelvis level**

⊗⑦S35.99 **Other specified injury of unspecified blood vessel at abdomen, lower back and pelvis level**

S36 Injury of intra-abdominal organs

Code also any associated open wound (S31.-)

The appropriate 7th character is to be added to each code from category S36

A - initial encounter

D - subsequent encounter

S - sequela

S36.0 Injury of spleen

⊗⑦S36.00 **Unspecified injury of spleen**

S36.02 Contusion of spleen

⑦S36.020 **Minor contusion of spleen**

Contusion of spleen less than 2 cm

⑦S36.021 **Major contusion of spleen**

Contusion of spleen greater than 2 cm

⑦S36.029 **Unspecified contusion of spleen**

S36.03 Laceration of spleen

⑦S36.030 **Superficial (capsular) laceration of spleen**

Laceration of spleen less than 1 cm

Minor laceration of spleen

⑦S36.031 **Moderate laceration of spleen**

Laceration of spleen 1 to 3 cm

⑦S36.032 **Major laceration of spleen**

Avulsion of spleen

Laceration of spleen greater than 3 cm

Massive laceration of spleen

Multiple moderate lacerations of spleen

Stellate laceration of spleen

⑦S36.039 **Unspecified laceration of spleen**

S36.09 Other injury of spleen

S36.1 Injury of liver and gallbladder and bile duct

S36.11 Injury of liver

⑦S36.112 **Contusion of liver**

⑦S36.113 **Laceration of liver, unspecified degree**

⑦S36.114 **Minor laceration of liver**

Laceration involving capsule only, or, without significant involvement of hepatic parenchyma [i.e., less than 1 cm deep]

⑦S36.115 **Moderate laceration of liver**

Laceration involving parenchyma but without major disruption of parenchyma [i.e., less than 10 cm long and less than 3 cm deep]

⑦S36.116 **Major laceration of liver**

● New code　▲ Revised code　**Excludes1:** Not coded here　**Excludes2:** Not included here　⊗ Placeholder required　⑦7th digit required

Laceration with significant disruption of hepatic parenchyma [i.e., greater than 10 cm long and 3 cm deep]

Multiple moderate lacerations, with or without hematoma

Stellate laceration of liver

⑦S36.118　　Other injury of liver

⑦S36.119　　Unspecified injury of liver

S36.12　Injury of gallbladder

⑦S36.122　　Contusion of gallbladder

⑦S36.123　　Laceration of gallbladder

⑦S36.128　　Other injury of gallbladder

⑦S36.129　　Unspecified injury of gallbladder

⊗⑦S36.13　Injury of bile duct

S36.2　Injury of pancreas

S36.20　Unspecified injury of pancreas

⑦S36.200　　Unspecified injury of head of pancreas

⑦S36.201　　Unspecified injury of body of pancreas

⑦S36.202　　Unspecified injury of tail of pancreas

⑦S36.209　　Unspecified injury of unspecified part of pancreas

S36.22　Contusion of pancreas

⑦S36.220　　Contusion of head of pancreas

⑦S36.221　　Contusion of body of pancreas

⑦S36.222　　Contusion of tail of pancreas

⑦S36.229　　Contusion of unspecified part of pancreas

S36.23　Laceration of pancreas, unspecified degree

⑦S36.230　　Laceration of head of pancreas, unspecified degree

⑦S36.231　　Laceration of body of pancreas, unspecified degree

⑦S36.232　　Laceration of tail of pancreas, unspecified degree

⑦S36.239　　Laceration of unspecified part of pancreas, unspecified degree

S36.24　Minor laceration of pancreas

⑦S36.240　　Minor laceration of head of pancreas

⑦S36.241　　Minor laceration of body of pancreas

⑦S36.242　　Minor laceration of tail of pancreas

⑦S36.249　　Minor laceration of unspecified part of pancreas

S36.25　Moderate laceration of pancreas

⑦S36.250　　Moderate laceration of head of pancreas

⑦S36.251　　Moderate laceration of body of pancreas

⑦S36.252　　Moderate laceration of tail of pancreas

⑦S36.259　　Moderate laceration of unspecified part of pancreas

S36.26　Major laceration of pancreas

⑦S36.260　　Major laceration of head of pancreas

⑦S36.261　　Major laceration of body of pancreas

⑦S36.262　　Major laceration of tail of pancreas

⑦S36.269　　Major laceration of unspecified part of pancreas

S36.29　Other injury of pancreas

⑦S36.290　　Other injury of head of pancreas

⑦S36.291　　Other injury of body of pancreas

⑦S36.292　　Other injury of tail of pancreas

⑦S36.299　　Other injury of unspecified part of pancreas

S36.3　Injury of stomach

⊗⑦S36.30　Unspecified injury of stomach

⊗⑦S36.32　Contusion of stomach

⊗⑦S36.33　Laceration of stomach

⊗⑦S36.39　Other injury of stomach

S36.4　Injury of small intestine

S36.40　Unspecified injury of small intestine

⑦S36.400　　Unspecified injury of duodenum

⑦S36.408　　Unspecified injury of other part of small intestine

⑦S36.409　　Unspecified injury of unspecified part of small intestine

S36.41　Primary blast injury of small intestine

Blast injury of small intestine NOS

⑦S36.410　　Primary blast injury of duodenum

⑦S36.418　　Primary blast injury of other part of small intestine

⑦S36.419　　Primary blast injury of unspecified part of small intestine

S36.42　Contusion of small intestine

⑦S36.420　　Contusion of duodenum

⑦S36.428　　Contusion of other part of small intestine

⑦S36.429　　Contusion of unspecified part of small intestine

S36.43　Laceration of small intestine

⑦S36.430　　Laceration of duodenum

⑦S36.438　　Laceration of other part of small intestine

⑦S36.439　　Laceration of unspecified part of small intestine

S36.49　Other injury of small intestine

⑦S36.490　　Other injury of duodenum

⑦S36.498　　Other injury of other part of small intestine

⑦S36.499　　Other injury of unspecified part of small intestine

S36.5　Injury of colon

Excludes2: injury of rectum (S36.6-)

S36.50　Unspecified injury of colon

⑦S36.500　　Unspecified injury of ascending [right] colon

⑦S36.501　　Unspecified injury of transverse colon

⑦S36.502　　Unspecified injury of descending [left] colon

⑦S36.503　　Unspecified injury of sigmoid colon

⑦S36.508　　Unspecified injury of other part of colon

⑦S36.509　　Unspecified injury of unspecified part of colon

S36.51　Primary blast injury of colon

Blast injury of colon NOS

⑦S36.510　　Primary blast injury of ascending [right] colon

⑦S36.511　　Primary blast injury of transverse colon

⑦S36.512   **Primary blast injury of descending [left] colon**

⑦S36.513   **Primary blast injury of sigmoid colon**

⑦S36.518   **Primary blast injury of other part of colon**

⑦S36.519   **Primary blast injury of unspecified part of colon**

S36.52   **Contusion of colon**

⑦S36.520   **Contusion of ascending [right] colon**

⑦S36.521   **Contusion of transverse colon**

⑦S36.522   **Contusion of descending [left] colon**

⑦S36.523   **Contusion of sigmoid colon**

⑦S36.528   **Contusion of other part of colon**

⑦S36.529   **Contusion of unspecified part of colon**

S36.53   **Laceration of colon**

⑦S36.530   **Laceration of ascending [right] colon**

⑦S36.531   **Laceration of transverse colon**

⑦S36.532   **Laceration of descending [left] colon**

⑦S36.533   **Laceration of sigmoid colon**

⑦S36.538   **Laceration of other part of colon**

⑦S36.539   **Laceration of unspecified part of colon**

S36.59   **Other injury of colon**

Secondary blast injury of colon

⑦S36.590   **Other injury of ascending [right] colon**

⑦S36.591   **Other injury of transverse colon**

⑦S36.592   **Other injury of descending [left] colon**

⑦S36.593   **Other injury of sigmoid colon**

⑦S36.598   **Other injury of other part of colon**

⑦S36.599   **Other injury of unspecified part of colon**

S36.6   **Injury of rectum**

⊗⑦S36.60   **Unspecified injury of rectum**

⊗⑦S36.61   **Primary blast injury of rectum**

Blast injury of rectum NOS

⊗⑦S36.62   **Contusion of rectum**

⊗⑦S36.63   **Laceration of rectum**

⊗⑦S36.69   **Other injury of rectum**

Secondary blast injury of rectum

S36.8   **Injury of other intra-abdominal organs**

⊗⑦S36.81   **Injury of peritoneum**

S36.89   **Injury of other intra-abdominal organs**

Injury of retroperitoneum

⑦S36.892   **Contusion of other intra-abdominal organs**

⑦S36.893   **Laceration of other intra-abdominal organs**

⑦S36.898   **Other injury of other intra-abdominal organs**

⑦S36.899   **Unspecified injury of other intra-abdominal organs**

S36.9   **Injury of unspecified intra-abdominal organ**

⊗⑦S36.90   **Unspecified injury of unspecified intra-abdominal organ**

⊗⑦S36.92   **Contusion of unspecified intra-abdominal organ**

⊗⑦S36.93   **Laceration of unspecified intra-abdominal organ**

⊗⑦S36.99   **Other injury of unspecified intra-abdominal organ**

S37   **Injury of urinary and pelvic organs**

Code also any associated open wound (S31.-)

Excludes1: obstetric trauma to pelvic organs (O71.-)

Excludes2: injury of peritoneum (S36.81)

injury of retroperitoneum (S36.89-)

The appropriate 7th character is to be added to each code from category S37

A - initial encounter

D - subsequent encounter

S - sequela

S37.0   **Injury of kidney**

Excludes2: acute kidney injury (nontraumatic) (N17.9)

S37.00   **Unspecified injury of kidney**

⑦S37.001   **Unspecified injury of right kidney**

⑦S37.002   **Unspecified injury of left kidney**

⑦S37.009   **Unspecified injury of unspecified kidney**

S37.01   **Minor contusion of kidney**

Contusion of kidney less than 2 cm

Contusion of kidney NOS

⑦S37.011   **Minor contusion of right kidney**

⑦S37.012   **Minor contusion of left kidney**

⑦S37.019   **Minor contusion of unspecified kidney**

S37.02   **Major contusion of kidney**

Contusion of kidney greater than 2 cm

⑦S37.021   **Major contusion of right kidney**

⑦S37.022   **Major contusion of left kidney**

⑦S37.029   **Major contusion of unspecified kidney**

S37.03   **Laceration of kidney, unspecified degree**

⑦S37.031   **Laceration of right kidney, unspecified degree**

⑦S37.032   **Laceration of left kidney, unspecified degree**

⑦S37.039   **Laceration of unspecified kidney, unspecified degree**

S37.04   **Minor laceration of kidney**

Laceration of kidney less than 1 cm

⑦S37.041   **Minor laceration of right kidney**

⑦S37.042   **Minor laceration of left kidney**

⑦S37.049   **Minor laceration of unspecified kidney**

S37.05   **Moderate laceration of kidney**

Laceration of kidney 1 to 3 cm

⑦S37.051   **Moderate laceration of right kidney**

⑦S37.052   **Moderate laceration of left kidney**

⑦S37.059   **Moderate laceration of unspecified kidney**

S37.06   **Major laceration of kidney**

Avulsion of kidney

Laceration of kidney greater than 3 cm

Massive laceration of kidney

Multiple moderate lacerations of kidney

Stellate laceration of kidney

⑦S37.061   Major laceration of right kidney

⑦S37.062   Major laceration of left kidney

⑦S37.069   Major laceration of unspecified kidney

S37.09   Other injury of kidney

⑦S37.091   Other injury of right kidney

⑦S37.092   Other injury of left kidney

⑦S37.099   Other injury of unspecified kidney

S37.1   Injury of ureter

⊗⑦S37.10   Unspecified injury of ureter

⊗⑦S37.12   Contusion of ureter

⊗⑦S37.13   Laceration of ureter

⊗⑦S37.19   Other injury of ureter

S37.2   Injury of bladder

⊗⑦S37.20   Unspecified injury of bladder

⊗⑦S37.22   Contusion of bladder

⊗⑦S37.23   Laceration of bladder

⊗⑦S37.29   Other injury of bladder

S37.3   Injury of urethra

⊗⑦S37.30   Unspecified injury of urethra

⊗⑦S37.32   Contusion of urethra

⊗⑦S37.33   Laceration of urethra

⊗⑦S37.39   Other injury of urethra

S37.4   Injury of ovary

S37.40   Unspecified injury of ovary

⑦S37.401   Unspecified injury of ovary, unilateral

⑦S37.402   Unspecified injury of ovary, bilateral

⑦S37.409   Unspecified injury of ovary, unspecified

S37.42   Contusion of ovary

⑦S37.421   Contusion of ovary, unilateral

⑦S37.422   Contusion of ovary, bilateral

⑦S37.429   Contusion of ovary, unspecified

S37.43   Laceration of ovary

⑦S37.431   Laceration of ovary, unilateral

⑦S37.432   Laceration of ovary, bilateral

⑦S37.439   Laceration of ovary, unspecified

S37.49   Other injury of ovary

⑦S37.491   Other injury of ovary, unilateral

⑦S37.492   Other injury of ovary, bilateral

⑦S37.499   Other injury of ovary, unspecified

S37.5   Injury of fallopian tube

S37.50   Unspecified injury of fallopian tube

⑦S37.501   Unspecified injury of fallopian tube, unilateral

⑦S37.502   Unspecified injury of fallopian tube, bilateral

⑦S37.509   Unspecified injury of fallopian tube, unspecified

S37.51   Primary blast injury of fallopian tube

Blast injury of fallopian tube NOS

⑦S37.511   Primary blast injury of fallopian tube, unilateral

⑦S37.512   Primary blast injury of fallopian tube, bilateral

⑦S37.519   Primary blast injury of fallopian tube, unspecified

S37.52   Contusion of fallopian tube

⑦S37.521   Contusion of fallopian tube, unilateral

⑦S37.522   Contusion of fallopian tube, bilateral

⑦S37.529   Contusion of fallopian tube, unspecified

S37.53   Laceration of fallopian tube

⑦S37.531   Laceration of fallopian tube, unilateral

⑦S37.532   Laceration of fallopian tube, bilateral

⑦S37.539   Laceration of fallopian tube, unspecified

S37.59   Other injury of fallopian tube

Secondary blast injury of fallopian tube

⑦S37.591   Other injury of fallopian tube, unilateral

⑦S37.592   Other injury of fallopian tube, bilateral

⑦S37.599   Other injury of fallopian tube, unspecified

S37.6   Injury of uterus

Excludes1: injury to gravid uterus (O9A.2-)

injury to uterus during delivery (O71.-)

⊗⑦S37.60   Unspecified injury of uterus

⊗⑦S37.62   Contusion of uterus

⊗⑦S37.63   Laceration of uterus

⊗⑦S37.69   Other injury of uterus

S37.8   Injury of other urinary and pelvic organs

S37.81   Injury of adrenal gland

⑦S37.812   Contusion of adrenal gland

⑦S37.813   Laceration of adrenal gland

⑦S37.818   Other injury of adrenal gland

⑦S37.819   Unspecified injury of adrenal gland

S37.82   Injury of prostate

⑦S37.822   Contusion of prostate

⑦S37.823   Laceration of prostate

⑦S37.828   Other injury of prostate

⑦S37.829   Unspecified injury of prostate

S37.89   Injury of other urinary and pelvic organ

⑦S37.892   Contusion of other urinary and pelvic organ

⑦S37.893   Laceration of other urinary and pelvic organ

⑦S37.898   Other injury of other urinary and pelvic organ

⑦S37.899   Unspecified injury of other urinary and pelvic organ

S37.9   Injury of unspecified urinary and pelvic organ

⊗⑦S37.90   Unspecified injury of unspecified urinary and pelvic organ

⊗⑦S37.92   Contusion of unspecified urinary and pelvic organ

⊗⑦S37.93   Laceration of unspecified urinary and pelvic organ

⊗⑦S37.99   Other injury of unspecified urinary and pelvic organ

S38   **Crushing injury and traumatic amputation of abdomen, lower back, pelvis and external genitals**

An amputation not identified as partial or complete should be coded to complete

---

The appropriate 7th character is to be added to each code from category S38

A - initial encounter

D - subsequent encounter

S - sequela

S38.0   Crushing injury of external genital organs

    <u>Use Additional Code</u> for any associated injuries

    S38.00   Crushing injury of unspecified external genital organs

        ⑦**S38.001   Crushing injury of unspecified external genital organs, male**

        ⑦**S38.002   Crushing injury of unspecified external genital organs, female**

    ⊗⑦**S38.01   Crushing injury of penis**

    ⊗⑦**S38.02   Crushing injury of scrotum and testis**

    ⊗⑦**S38.03   Crushing injury of vulva**

S38.1   Crushing injury of abdomen, lower back, and pelvis

    <u>Use Additional Code</u> for all associated injuries, such as:

    fracture of thoracic or lumbar spine and pelvis (S22.0-, S32.-)

    injury to intra-abdominal organs (S36.-)

    injury to urinary and pelvic organs (S37.-)

    open wound of abdominal wall (S31.-)

    spinal cord injury (S34.0, S34.1-)

    Excludes2: crushing injury of external genital organs (S38.0-)

S38.2   Traumatic amputation of external genital organs

    S38.21   Traumatic amputation of female external genital organs

        Traumatic amputation of clitoris

        Traumatic amputation of labium (majus) (minus)

        Traumatic amputation of vulva

        ⑦**S38.211   Complete traumatic amputation of female external genital organs**

        ⑦**S38.212   Partial traumatic amputation of female external genital organs**

    S38.22   Traumatic amputation of penis

        ⑦**S38.221   Complete traumatic amputation of penis**

        ⑦**S38.222   Partial traumatic amputation of penis**

    S38.23   Traumatic amputation of scrotum and testis

        ⑦**S38.231   Complete traumatic amputation of scrotum and testis**

        ⑦**S38.232   Partial traumatic amputation of scrotum and testis**

⊗⑦**S38.3   Transection (partial) of abdomen**

S39   Other and unspecified injuries of abdomen, lower back, pelvis and external genitals

    <u>Code also</u> any associated open wound (S31.-)

    Excludes2: sprain of joints and ligaments of lumbar spine and pelvis (S33.-)

    The appropriate 7th character is to be added to each code from category S39

    A - initial encounter

    D - subsequent encounter

    S - sequela

    S39.0   Injury of muscle, fascia and tendon of abdomen, lower back and pelvis

        S39.00   Unspecified injury of muscle, fascia and tendon of abdomen, lower back and pelvis

        ⑦**S39.001   Unspecified injury of muscle, fascia and tendon of abdomen**

        ⑦**S39.002   Unspecified injury of muscle, fascia and tendon of lower back**

        ⑦**S39.003   Unspecified injury of muscle, fascia and tendon of pelvis**

    S39.01   Strain of muscle, fascia and tendon of abdomen, lower back and pelvis

        ⑦**S39.011   Strain of muscle, fascia and tendon of abdomen**

        ⑦**S39.012   Strain of muscle, fascia and tendon of lower back**

        ⑦**S39.013   Strain of muscle, fascia and tendon of pelvis**

    S39.02   Laceration of muscle, fascia and tendon of abdomen, lower back and pelvis

        ⑦**S39.021   Laceration of muscle, fascia and tendon of abdomen**

        ⑦**S39.022   Laceration of muscle, fascia and tendon of lower back**

        ⑦**S39.023   Laceration of muscle, fascia and tendon of pelvis**

    S39.09   Other injury of muscle, fascia and tendon of abdomen, lower back and pelvis

        ⑦**S39.091   Other injury of muscle, fascia and tendon of abdomen**

        ⑦**S39.092   Other injury of muscle, fascia and tendon of lower back**

        ⑦**S39.093   Other injury of muscle, fascia and tendon of pelvis**

    S39.8   Other specified injuries of abdomen, lower back, pelvis and external genitals

        ⊗⑦**S39.81   Other specified injuries of abdomen**

        ⊗⑦**S39.82   Other specified injuries of lower back**

        ⊗⑦**S39.83   Other specified injuries of pelvis**

        S39.84   Other specified injuries of external genitals

        ⑦**S39.840   Fracture of corpus cavernosum penis**

        ⑦**S39.848   Other specified injuries of external genitals**

    S39.9   Unspecified injury of abdomen, lower back, pelvis and external genitals

        ⊗⑦**S39.91   Unspecified injury of abdomen**

        ⊗⑦**S39.92   Unspecified injury of lower back**

        ⊗⑦**S39.93   Unspecified injury of pelvis**

        ⊗⑦**S39.94   Unspecified injury of external genitals**

INJURIES TO THE SHOULDER AND UPPER ARM (S40-S49)

Includes: injuries of axilla

injuries of scapular region

Excludes2: burns and corrosions (T20-T32)

    frostbite (T33-T34)

    injuries of elbow (S50-S59)

    insect bite or sting, venomous (T63.4)

S40   Superficial injury of shoulder and upper arm

    The appropriate 7th character is to be added to each code from category S40

    A - initial encounter

    D - subsequent encounter

    S - sequela

    S40.0   Contusion of shoulder and upper arm

        S40.01   Contusion of shoulder

● New code   ▲ Revised code   **Excludes1:** Not coded here   **Excludes2:** Not included here   ⊗ Placeholder required   ⑦7th digit required

⑦S40.011 **Contusion of right shoulder**

⑦S40.012 **Contusion of left shoulder**

⑦S40.019 **Contusion of unspecified shoulder**

S40.02 **Contusion of upper arm**

⑦S40.021 **Contusion of right upper arm**

⑦S40.022 **Contusion of left upper arm**

⑦S40.029 **Contusion of unspecified upper arm**

S40.2 **Other superficial injuries of shoulder**

S40.21 **Abrasion of shoulder**

⑦S40.211 **Abrasion of right shoulder**

⑦S40.212 **Abrasion of left shoulder**

⑦S40.219 **Abrasion of unspecified shoulder**

S40.22 **Blister (nonthermal) of shoulder**

⑦S40.221 **Blister (nonthermal) of right shoulder**

⑦S40.222 **Blister (nonthermal) of left shoulder**

⑦S40.229 **Blister (nonthermal) of unspecified shoulder**

S40.24 **External constriction of shoulder**

⑦S40.241 **External constriction of right shoulder**

⑦S40.242 **External constriction of left shoulder**

⑦S40.249 **External constriction of unspecified shoulder**

S40.25 **Superficial foreign body of shoulder**

Splinter in the shoulder

⑦S40.251 **Superficial foreign body of right shoulder**

⑦S40.252 **Superficial foreign body of left shoulder**

⑦S40.259 **Superficial foreign body of unspecified shoulder**

S40.26 **Insect bite (nonvenomous) of shoulder**

⑦S40.261 **Insect bite (nonvenomous) of right shoulder**

⑦S40.262 **Insect bite (nonvenomous) of left shoulder**

⑦S40.269 **Insect bite (nonvenomous) of unspecified shoulder**

S40.27 **Other superficial bite of shoulder**

Excludes1: open bite of shoulder (S41.05)

⑦S40.271 **Other superficial bite of right shoulder**

⑦S40.272 **Other superficial bite of left shoulder**

⑦S40.279 **Other superficial bite of unspecified shoulder**

S40.8 **Other superficial injuries of upper arm**

S40.81 **Abrasion of upper arm**

⑦S40.811 **Abrasion of right upper arm**

⑦S40.812 **Abrasion of left upper arm**

⑦S40.819 **Abrasion of unspecified upper arm**

S40.82 **Blister (nonthermal) of upper arm**

⑦S40.821 **Blister (nonthermal) of right upper arm**

⑦S40.822 **Blister (nonthermal) of left upper arm**

⑦S40.829 **Blister (nonthermal) of unspecified upper arm**

S40.84 **External constriction of upper arm**

⑦S40.841 **External constriction of right upper arm**

⑦S40.842 **External constriction of left upper arm**

⑦S40.849 **External constriction of unspecified upper arm**

S40.85 **Superficial foreign body of upper arm**

Splinter in the upper arm

⑦S40.851 **Superficial foreign body of right upper arm**

⑦S40.852 **Superficial foreign body of left upper arm**

⑦S40.859 **Superficial foreign body of unspecified upper arm**

S40.86 **Insect bite (nonvenomous) of upper arm**

⑦S40.861 **Insect bite (nonvenomous) of right upper arm**

⑦S40.862 **Insect bite (nonvenomous) of left upper arm**

⑦S40.869 **Insect bite (nonvenomous) of unspecified upper arm**

S40.87 **Other superficial bite of upper arm**

Excludes1: open bite of upper arm (S41.14)

Excludes2: Other superficial bite of shoulder (S40.27-)

⑦S40.871 **Other superficial bite of right upper arm**

⑦S40.872 **Other superficial bite of left upper arm**

⑦S40.879 **Other superficial bite of unspecified upper arm**

S40.9 **Unspecified superficial injury of shoulder and upper arm**

S40.91 **Unspecified superficial injury of shoulder**

⑦S40.911 **Unspecified superficial injury of right shoulder**

⑦S40.912 **Unspecified superficial injury of left shoulder**

⑦S40.919 **Unspecified superficial injury of unspecified shoulder**

S40.92 **Unspecified superficial injury of upper arm**

⑦S40.921 **Unspecified superficial injury of right upper arm**

⑦S40.922 **Unspecified superficial injury of left upper arm**

⑦S40.929 **Unspecified superficial injury of unspecified upper arm**

S41 **Open wound of shoulder and upper arm**

Code also any associated wound infection

Excludes1: traumatic amputation of shoulder and upper arm (S48.-)

Excludes2: open fracture of shoulder and upper arm (S42.- with 7th character B or C)

The appropriate 7th character is to be added to each code from category S41

A - initial encounter

D - subsequent encounter

S - sequela

S41.0 **Open wound of shoulder**

S41.00 **Unspecified open wound of shoulder**

⑦S41.001 **Unspecified open wound of right shoulder**

⑦S41.002   **Unspecified open wound of left shoulder**

⑦S41.009   **Unspecified open wound of unspecified shoulder**

S41.01   **Laceration without foreign body of shoulder**

⑦S41.011   **Laceration without foreign body of right shoulder**

⑦S41.012   **Laceration without foreign body of left shoulder**

⑦S41.019   **Laceration without foreign body of unspecified shoulder**

S41.02   **Laceration with foreign body of shoulder**

⑦S41.021   **Laceration with foreign body of right shoulder**

⑦S41.022   **Laceration with foreign body of left shoulder**

⑦S41.029   **Laceration with foreign body of unspecified shoulder**

S41.03   **Puncture wound without foreign body of shoulder**

⑦S41.031   **Puncture wound without foreign body of right shoulder**

⑦S41.032   **Puncture wound without foreign body of left shoulder**

⑦S41.039   **Puncture wound without foreign body of unspecified shoulder**

S41.04   **Puncture wound with foreign body of shoulder**

⑦S41.041   **Puncture wound with foreign body of right shoulder**

⑦S41.042   **Puncture wound with foreign body of left shoulder**

⑦S41.049   **Puncture wound with foreign body of unspecified shoulder**

S41.05   **Open bite of shoulder**

Bite of shoulder NOS

Excludes1: superficial bite of shoulder (S40.27)

⑦S41.051   **Open bite of right shoulder**

⑦S41.052   **Open bite of left shoulder**

⑦S41.059   **Open bite of unspecified shoulder**

S41.1   **Open wound of upper arm**

S41.10   **Unspecified open wound of upper arm**

⑦S41.101   **Unspecified open wound of right upper arm**

⑦S41.102   **Unspecified open wound of left upper arm**

⑦S41.109   **Unspecified open wound of unspecified upper arm**

S41.11   **Laceration without foreign body of upper arm**

⑦S41.111   **Laceration without foreign body of right upper arm**

⑦S41.112   **Laceration without foreign body of left upper arm**

⑦S41.119   **Laceration without foreign body of unspecified upper arm**

S41.12   **Laceration with foreign body of upper arm**

⑦S41.121   **Laceration with foreign body of right upper arm**

⑦S41.122   **Laceration with foreign body of left upper arm**

⑦S41.129   **Laceration with foreign body of unspecified upper arm**

S41.13   **Puncture wound without foreign body of upper arm**

⑦S41.131   **Puncture wound without foreign body of right upper arm**

⑦S41.132   **Puncture wound without foreign body of left upper arm**

⑦S41.139   **Puncture wound without foreign body of unspecified upper arm**

S41.14   **Puncture wound with foreign body of upper arm**

⑦S41.141   **Puncture wound with foreign body of right upper arm**

⑦S41.142   **Puncture wound with foreign body of left upper arm**

⑦S41.149   **Puncture wound with foreign body of unspecified upper arm**

S41.15   **Open bite of upper arm**

Bite of upper arm NOS

Excludes1: superficial bite of upper arm (S40.87)

⑦S41.151   **Open bite of right upper arm**

⑦S41.152   **Open bite of left upper arm**

⑦S41.159   **Open bite of unspecified upper arm**

S42   **Fracture of shoulder and upper arm**

Note: A fracture not indicated as displaced or nondisplaced should be coded to displaced

A fracture not indicated as open or closed should be coded to closed

Excludes1: traumatic amputation of shoulder and upper arm (S48.-)

The appropriate 7th character is to be added to all codes from category S42

A - initial encounter for closed fracture

B - initial encounter for open fracture

D - subsequent encounter for fracture with routine healing

G - subsequent encounter for fracture with delayed healing

K - subsequent encounter for fracture with nonunion

P - subsequent encounter for fracture with malunion

S - sequela

S42.0   **Fracture of clavicle**

S42.00   **Fracture of unspecified part of clavicle**

⑦S42.001   **Fracture of unspecified part of right clavicle**

⑦S42.002   **Fracture of unspecified part of left clavicle**

⑦S42.009   **Fracture of unspecified part of unspecified clavicle**

S42.01   **Fracture of sternal end of clavicle**

⑦S42.011   **Anterior displaced fracture of sternal end of right clavicle**

⑦S42.012   **Anterior displaced fracture of sternal end of left clavicle**

⑦S42.013   **Anterior displaced fracture of sternal end of unspecified clavicle**

Displaced fracture of sternal end of clavicle NOS

⑦S42.014   **Posterior displaced fracture of sternal end of right clavicle**

⑦S42.015   **Posterior displaced fracture of sternal end of left clavicle**

⑦S42.016   **Posterior displaced fracture of sternal end of unspecified clavicle**

⑦S42.017   **Nondisplaced fracture of sternal end of right clavicle**

⑦S42.018   Nondisplaced fracture of sternal end of left clavicle

⑦S42.019   Nondisplaced fracture of sternal end of unspecified clavicle

S42.02   **Fracture of shaft of clavicle**

⑦S42.021   Displaced fracture of shaft of right clavicle

⑦S42.022   Displaced fracture of shaft of left clavicle

⑦S42.023   Displaced fracture of shaft of unspecified clavicle

⑦S42.024   Nondisplaced fracture of shaft of right clavicle

⑦S42.025   Nondisplaced fracture of shaft of left clavicle

⑦S42.026   Nondisplaced fracture of shaft of unspecified clavicle

S42.03   **Fracture of lateral end of clavicle**

Fracture of acromial end of clavicle

⑦S42.031   Displaced fracture of lateral end of right clavicle

⑦S42.032   Displaced fracture of lateral end of left clavicle

⑦S42.033   Displaced fracture of lateral end of unspecified clavicle

⑦S42.034   Nondisplaced fracture of lateral end of right clavicle

⑦S42.035   Nondisplaced fracture of lateral end of left clavicle

⑦S42.036   Nondisplaced fracture of lateral end of unspecified clavicle

S42.1   **Fracture of scapula**

S42.10   **Fracture of unspecified part of scapula**

⑦S42.101   Fracture of unspecified part of scapula, right shoulder

⑦S42.102   Fracture of unspecified part of scapula, left shoulder

⑦S42.109   Fracture of unspecified part of scapula, unspecified shoulder

S42.11   **Fracture of body of scapula**

⑦S42.111   Displaced fracture of body of scapula, right shoulder

⑦S42.112   Displaced fracture of body of scapula, left shoulder

⑦S42.113   Displaced fracture of body of scapula, unspecified shoulder

⑦S42.114   Nondisplaced fracture of body of scapula, right shoulder

⑦S42.115   Nondisplaced fracture of body of scapula, left shoulder

⑦S42.116   Nondisplaced fracture of body of scapula, unspecified shoulder

S42.12   **Fracture of acromial process**

⑦S42.121   Displaced fracture of acromial process, right shoulder

⑦S42.122   Displaced fracture of acromial process, left shoulder

⑦S42.123   Displaced fracture of acromial process, unspecified shoulder

⑦S42.124   Nondisplaced fracture of acromial process, right shoulder

⑦S42.125   Nondisplaced fracture of acromial process, left shoulder

⑦S42.126   Nondisplaced fracture of acromial process, unspecified shoulder

S42.13   **Fracture of coracoid process**

⑦S42.131   Displaced fracture of coracoid process, right shoulder

⑦S42.132   Displaced fracture of coracoid process, left shoulder

⑦S42.133   Displaced fracture of coracoid process, unspecified shoulder

⑦S42.134   Nondisplaced fracture of coracoid process, right shoulder

⑦S42.135   Nondisplaced fracture of coracoid process, left shoulder

⑦S42.136   Nondisplaced fracture of coracoid process, unspecified shoulder

S42.14   **Fracture of glenoid cavity of scapula**

⑦S42.141   Displaced fracture of glenoid cavity of scapula, right shoulder

⑦S42.142   Displaced fracture of glenoid cavity of scapula, left shoulder

⑦S42.143   Displaced fracture of glenoid cavity of scapula, unspecified shoulder

⑦S42.144   Nondisplaced fracture of glenoid cavity of scapula, right shoulder

⑦S42.145   Nondisplaced fracture of glenoid cavity of scapula, left shoulder

⑦S42.146   Nondisplaced fracture of glenoid cavity of scapula, unspecified shoulder

S42.15   **Fracture of neck of scapula**

⑦S42.151   Displaced fracture of neck of scapula, right shoulder

⑦S42.152   Displaced fracture of neck of scapula, left shoulder

⑦S42.153   Displaced fracture of neck of scapula, unspecified shoulder

⑦S42.154   Nondisplaced fracture of neck of scapula, right shoulder

⑦S42.155   Nondisplaced fracture of neck of scapula, left shoulder

⑦S42.156   Nondisplaced fracture of neck of scapula, unspecified shoulder

S42.19   **Fracture of other part of scapula**

⑦S42.191   Fracture of other part of scapula, right shoulder

⑦S42.192   Fracture of other part of scapula, left shoulder

⑦S42.199   Fracture of other part of scapula, unspecified shoulder

S42.2   **Fracture of upper end of humerus**

Fracture of proximal end of humerus

Excludes2: fracture of shaft of humerus (S42.3-)

physeal fracture of upper end of humerus (S49.0-)

S42.20   **Unspecified fracture of upper end of humerus**

⑦S42.201   Unspecified fracture of upper end of right humerus

⑦S42.202   Unspecified fracture of upper end of left humerus

⑦S42.209   Unspecified fracture of upper end of unspecified humerus

S42.21   **Unspecified fracture of surgical neck of humerus**

Fracture of neck of humerus NOS

⑦S42.211   **Unspecified displaced fracture of surgical neck of right humerus**

⑦S42.212   **Unspecified displaced fracture of surgical neck of left humerus**

⑦S42.213   **Unspecified displaced fracture of surgical neck of unspecified humerus**

⑦S42.214   **Unspecified nondisplaced fracture of surgical neck of right humerus**

⑦S42.215   **Unspecified nondisplaced fracture of surgical neck of left humerus**

⑦S42.216   **Unspecified nondisplaced fracture of surgical neck of unspecified humerus**

S42.22   2-part fracture of surgical neck of humerus

⑦S42.221   **2-part displaced fracture of surgical neck of right humerus**

⑦S42.222   **2-part displaced fracture of surgical neck of left humerus**

⑦S42.223   **2-part displaced fracture of surgical neck of unspecified humerus**

⑦S42.224   **2-part nondisplaced fracture of surgical neck of right humerus**

⑦S42.225   **2-part nondisplaced fracture of surgical neck of left humerus**

⑦S42.226   **2-part nondisplaced fracture of surgical neck of unspecified humerus**

S42.23   3-part fracture of surgical neck of humerus

⑦S42.231   **3-part fracture of surgical neck of right humerus**

⑦S42.232   **3-part fracture of surgical neck of left humerus**

⑦S42.239   **3-part fracture of surgical neck of unspecified humerus**

S42.24   4-part fracture of surgical neck of humerus

⑦S42.241   **4-part fracture of surgical neck of right humerus**

⑦S42.242   **4-part fracture of surgical neck of left humerus**

⑦S42.249   **4-part fracture of surgical neck of unspecified humerus**

S42.25   Fracture of greater tuberosity of humerus

⑦S42.251   **Displaced fracture of greater tuberosity of right humerus**

⑦S42.252   **Displaced fracture of greater tuberosity of left humerus**

⑦S42.253   **Displaced fracture of greater tuberosity of unspecified humerus**

⑦S42.254   **Nondisplaced fracture of greater tuberosity of right humerus**

⑦S42.255   **Nondisplaced fracture of greater tuberosity of left humerus**

⑦S42.256   **Nondisplaced fracture of greater tuberosity of unspecified humerus**

S42.26   Fracture of lesser tuberosity of humerus

⑦S42.261   **Displaced fracture of lesser tuberosity of right humerus**

⑦S42.262   **Displaced fracture of lesser tuberosity of left humerus**

⑦S42.263   **Displaced fracture of lesser tuberosity of unspecified humerus**

⑦S42.264   **Nondisplaced fracture of lesser tuberosity of right humerus**

⑦S42.265   **Nondisplaced fracture of lesser tuberosity of left humerus**

⑦S42.266   **Nondisplaced fracture of lesser tuberosity of unspecified humerus**

S42.27   Torus fracture of upper end of humerus

The appropriate 7th character is to be added to all codes in subcategory S42.27

A - initial encounter for closed fracture

D - subsequent encounter for fracture with routine healing

G - subsequent encounter for fracture with delayed healing

K - subsequent encounter for fracture with nonunion

P - subsequent encounter for fracture with malunion S - sequela

⑦S42.271   **Torus fracture of upper end of right humerus**

⑦S42.272   **Torus fracture of upper end of left humerus**

⑦S42.279   **Torus fracture of upper end of unspecified humerus**

S42.29   Other fracture of upper end of humerus

Fracture of anatomical neck of humerus

Fracture of articular head of humerus

⑦S42.291   **Other displaced fracture of upper end of right humerus**

⑦S42.292   **Other displaced fracture of upper end of left humerus**

⑦S42.293   **Other displaced fracture of upper end of unspecified humerus**

⑦S42.294   **Other nondisplaced fracture of upper end of right humerus**

⑦S42.295   **Other nondisplaced fracture of upper end of left humerus**

⑦S42.296   **Other nondisplaced fracture of upper end of unspecified humerus**

S42.3   Fracture of shaft of humerus

Fracture of humerus NOS

Fracture of upper arm NOS

Excludes2: physeal fractures of upper end of humerus (S49.0-)

physeal fractures of lower end of humerus (S49.1-)

S42.30   Unspecified fracture of shaft of humerus

⑦S42.301   **Unspecified fracture of shaft of humerus, right arm**

⑦S42.302   **Unspecified fracture of shaft of humerus, left arm**

⑦S42.309   **Unspecified fracture of shaft of humerus, unspecified arm**

S42.31   Greenstick fracture of shaft of humerus

The appropriate 7th character is to be added to all codes in subcategory S42.31

A - initial encounter for closed fracture

D - subsequent encounter for fracture with routine healing

G - subsequent encounter for fracture with delayed healing

K - subsequent encounter for fracture with nonunion

P - subsequent encounter for fracture with malunion S - sequela

⑦S42.311   **Greenstick fracture of shaft of humerus, right arm**

● New code   ▲ Revised code   Excludes1: Not coded here   Excludes2: Not included here   ⊗ Placeholder required   ⑦7th digit required

⑦S42.312   Greenstick fracture of shaft of humerus, left arm

⑦S42.319   Greenstick fracture of shaft of humerus, unspecified arm

S42.32   Transverse fracture of shaft of humerus

⑦S42.321   Displaced transverse fracture of shaft of humerus, right arm

⑦S42.322   Displaced transverse fracture of shaft of humerus, left arm

⑦S42.323   Displaced transverse fracture of shaft of humerus, unspecified arm

⑦S42.324   Nondisplaced transverse fracture of shaft of humerus, right arm

⑦S42.325   Nondisplaced transverse fracture of shaft of humerus, left arm

⑦S42.326   Nondisplaced transverse fracture of shaft of humerus, unspecified arm

S42.33   Oblique fracture of shaft of humerus

⑦S42.331   Displaced oblique fracture of shaft of humerus, right arm

⑦S42.332   Displaced oblique fracture of shaft of humerus, left arm

⑦S42.333   Displaced oblique fracture of shaft of humerus, unspecified arm

⑦S42.334   Nondisplaced oblique fracture of shaft of humerus, right arm

⑦S42.335   Nondisplaced oblique fracture of shaft of humerus, left arm

⑦S42.336   Nondisplaced oblique fracture of shaft of humerus, unspecified arm

S42.34   ⑦Spiral fracture of shaft of humerus

⑦S42.341   Displaced spiral fracture of shaft of humerus, right arm

⑦S42.342   Displaced spiral fracture of shaft of humerus, left arm

⑦S42.343   Displaced spiral fracture of shaft of humerus, unspecified arm

⑦S42.344   Nondisplaced spiral fracture of shaft of humerus, right arm

⑦S42.345   Nondisplaced spiral fracture of shaft of humerus, left arm

⑦S42.346   Nondisplaced spiral fracture of shaft of humerus, unspecified arm

S42.35   Comminuted fracture of shaft of humerus

⑦S42.351   Displaced comminuted fracture of shaft of humerus, right arm

⑦S42.352   Displaced comminuted fracture of shaft of humerus, left arm

⑦S42.353   Displaced comminuted fracture of shaft of humerus, unspecified arm

⑦S42.354   Nondisplaced comminuted fracture of shaft of humerus, right arm

⑦S42.355   Nondisplaced comminuted fracture of shaft of humerus, left arm

⑦S42.356   Nondisplaced comminuted fracture of shaft of humerus, unspecified arm

S42.36   Segmental fracture of shaft of humerus

⑦S42.361   Displaced segmental fracture of shaft of humerus, right arm

⑦S42.362   Displaced segmental fracture of shaft of humerus, left arm

⑦S42.363   Displaced segmental fracture of shaft of humerus, unspecified arm

⑦S42.364   Nondisplaced segmental fracture of shaft of humerus, right arm

⑦S42.365   Nondisplaced segmental fracture of shaft of humerus, left arm

⑦S42.366   Nondisplaced segmental fracture of shaft of humerus, unspecified arm

S42.39   Other fracture of shaft of humerus

⑦S42.391   Other fracture of shaft of right humerus

⑦S42.392   Other fracture of shaft of left humerus

⑦S42.399   Other fracture of shaft of unspecified humerus

S42.4   Fracture of lower end of humerus

Fracture of distal end of humerus

Excludes2: fracture of shaft of humerus (S42.3-)

physeal fracture of lower end of humerus (S49.1-)

S42.40   Unspecified fracture of lower end of humerus

Fracture of elbow NOS

⑦S42.401   Unspecified fracture of lower end of right humerus

⑦S42.402   Unspecified fracture of lower end of left humerus

⑦S42.409   Unspecified fracture of lower end of unspecified humerus

S42.41   Simple supracondylar fracture without intercondylar fracture of humerus

⑦S42.411   Displaced simple supracondylar fracture without intercondylar fracture of right humerus

⑦S42.412   Displaced simple supracondylar fracture without intercondylar fracture of left humerus

⑦S42.413   Displaced simple supracondylar fracture without intercondylar fracture of unspecified humerus

⑦S42.414   Nondisplaced simple supracondylar fracture without intercondylar fracture of right humerus

⑦S42.415   Nondisplaced simple supracondylar fracture without intercondylar fracture of left humerus

⑦S42.416   Nondisplaced simple supracondylar fracture without intercondylar fracture of unspecified humerus

S42.42   Comminuted supracondylar fracture without intercondylar fracture of humerus

⑦S42.421   Displaced comminuted supracondylar fracture without intercondylar fracture of right humerus

⑦S42.422   Displaced comminuted supracondylar fracture without intercondylar fracture of left humerus

⑦S42.423   Displaced comminuted supracondylar fracture without intercondylar fracture of unspecified humerus

⑦S42.424   Nondisplaced comminuted supracondylar fracture without intercondylar fracture of right humerus

S42.425 Nondisplaced comminuted supracondylar fracture without intercondylar fracture of left humerus

S42.426 Nondisplaced comminuted supracondylar fracture without intercondylar fracture of unspecified humerus

S42.43 Fracture (avulsion) of lateral epicondyle of humerus

⑦**S42.431** Displaced fracture (avulsion) of lateral epicondyle of right humerus

⑦**S42.432** Displaced fracture (avulsion) of lateral epicondyle of left humerus

⑦**S42.433** Displaced fracture (avulsion) of lateral epicondyle of unspecified humerus

⑦**S42.434** Nondisplaced fracture (avulsion) of lateral epicondyle of right humerus

⑦**S42.435** Nondisplaced fracture (avulsion) of lateral epicondyle of left humerus

⑦**S42.436** Nondisplaced fracture (avulsion) of lateral epicondyle of unspecified humerus

S42.44 Fracture (avulsion) of medial epicondyle of humerus

⑦**S42.441** Displaced fracture (avulsion) of medial epicondyle of right humerus

⑦**S42.442** Displaced fracture (avulsion) of medial epicondyle of left humerus

⑦**S42.443** Displaced fracture (avulsion) of medial epicondyle of unspecified humerus

⑦**S42.444** Nondisplaced fracture (avulsion) of medial epicondyle of right humerus

⑦**S42.445** Nondisplaced fracture (avulsion) of medial epicondyle of left humerus

⑦**S42.446** Nondisplaced fracture (avulsion) of medial epicondyle of unspecified humerus

⑦**S42.447** Incarcerated fracture (avulsion) of medial epicondyle of right humerus

⑦**S42.448** Incarcerated fracture (avulsion) of medial epicondyle of left humerus

⑦**S42.449** Incarcerated fracture (avulsion) of medial epicondyle of unspecified humerus

S42.45 Fracture of lateral condyle of humerus

Fracture of capitellum of humerus

⑦**S42.451** Displaced fracture of lateral condyle of right humerus

⑦**S42.452** Displaced fracture of lateral condyle of left humerus

⑦**S42.453** Displaced fracture of lateral condyle of unspecified humerus

⑦**S42.454** Nondisplaced fracture of lateral condyle of right humerus

⑦**S42.455** Nondisplaced fracture of lateral condyle of left humerus

⑦**S42.456** Nondisplaced fracture of lateral condyle of unspecified humerus

S42.46 Fracture of medial condyle of humerus

Trochlea fracture of humerus

⑦**S42.461** Displaced fracture of medial condyle of right humerus

⑦**S42.462** Displaced fracture of medial condyle of left humerus

⑦**S42.463** Displaced fracture of medial condyle of unspecified humerus

⑦**S42.464** Nondisplaced fracture of medial condyle of right humerus

⑦**S42.465** Nondisplaced fracture of medial condyle of left humerus

⑦**S42.466** Nondisplaced fracture of medial condyle of unspecified humerus

S42.47 Transcondylar fracture of humerus

⑦**S42.471** Displaced transcondylar fracture of right humerus

⑦**S42.472** Displaced transcondylar fracture of left humerus

⑦**S42.473** Displaced transcondylar fracture of unspecified humerus

⑦**S42.474** Nondisplaced transcondylar fracture of right humerus

⑦**S42.475** Nondisplaced transcondylar fracture of left humerus

⑦**S42.476** Nondisplaced transcondylar fracture of unspecified humerus

S42.48 Torus fracture of lower end of humerus

The appropriate 7th character is to be added to all codes in subcategory S42.48

A - initial encounter for closed fracture

D - subsequent encounter for fracture with routine healing

G - subsequent encounter for fracture with delayed healing

K - subsequent encounter for fracture with nonunion

P - subsequent encounter for fracture with malunion

S - sequela

⑦**S42.481** Torus fracture of lower end of right humerus

⑦**S42.482** Torus fracture of lower end of left humerus

⑦**S42.489** Torus fracture of lower end of unspecified humerus

S42.49 Other fracture of lower end of humerus

⑦**S42.491** Other displaced fracture of lower end of right humerus

⑦**S42.492** Other displaced fracture of lower end of left humerus

⑦**S42.493** Other displaced fracture of lower end of unspecified humerus

⑦**S42.494** Other nondisplaced fracture of lower end of right humerus

⑦**S42.495** Other nondisplaced fracture of lower end of left humerus

⑦**S42.496** Other nondisplaced fracture of lower end of unspecified humerus

S42.9 Fracture of shoulder girdle, part unspecified

Fracture of shoulder NOS

⊗**S42.90** Fracture of unspecified shoulder girdle, part unspecified

⊗**S42.91** Fracture of right shoulder girdle, part unspecified

⊗**S42.92** Fracture of left shoulder girdle, part unspecified

● New code ▲ Revised code **Excludes1:** Not coded here **Excludes2:** Not included here ⊗ Placeholder required ⑦7th digit required

S43 **Dislocation and sprain of joints and ligaments of shoulder girdle**

Includes: avulsion of joint or ligament of shoulder girdle

laceration of cartilage, joint or ligament of shoulder girdle

sprain of cartilage, joint or ligament of shoulder girdle

traumatic hemarthrosis of joint or ligament of shoulder girdle

traumatic rupture of joint or ligament of shoulder girdle

traumatic subluxation of joint or ligament of shoulder girdle

traumatic tear of joint or ligament of shoulder girdle

Code also any associated open wound

Excludes2: strain of muscle, fascia and tendon of shoulder and upper arm (S46.-)

The appropriate 7th character is to be added to each code from category S43

A - initial encounter

D - subsequent encounter

S - sequela

S43.0 **Subluxation and dislocation of shoulder joint**

Dislocation of glenohumeral joint

Subluxation of glenohumeral joint

S43.00 **Unspecified subluxation and dislocation of shoulder joint**

Dislocation of humerus NOS

Subluxation of humerus NOS

⑦**S43.001** **Unspecified subluxation of right shoulder joint**

⑦**S43.002** **Unspecified subluxation of left shoulder joint**

⑦**S43.003** **Unspecified subluxation of unspecified shoulder joint**

⑦**S43.004** **Unspecified dislocation of right shoulder joint**

⑦**S43.005** **Unspecified dislocation of left shoulder joint**

⑦**S43.006** **Unspecified dislocation of unspecified shoulder joint**

S43.01 **Anterior subluxation and dislocation of humerus**

⑦**S43.011** **Anterior subluxation of right humerus**

⑦**S43.012** **Anterior subluxation of left humerus**

⑦**S43.013** **Anterior subluxation of unspecified humerus**

⑦**S43.014** **Anterior dislocation of right humerus**

⑦**S43.015** **Anterior dislocation of left humerus**

⑦**S43.016** **Anterior dislocation of unspecified humerus**

S43.02 **Posterior subluxation and dislocation of humerus**

⑦**S43.021** **Posterior subluxation of right humerus**

⑦**S43.022** **Posterior subluxation of left humerus**

⑦**S43.023** **Posterior subluxation of unspecified humerus**

⑦**S43.024** **Posterior dislocation of right humerus**

⑦**S43.025** **Posterior dislocation of left humerus**

⑦**S43.026** **Posterior dislocation of unspecified humerus**

S43.03 **Inferior subluxation and dislocation of humerus**

⑦**S43.031** **Inferior subluxation of right humerus**

⑦**S43.032** **Inferior subluxation of left humerus**

⑦**S43.033** **Inferior subluxation of unspecified humerus**

⑦**S43.034** **Inferior dislocation of right humerus**

⑦**S43.035** **Inferior dislocation of left humerus**

⑦**S43.036** **Inferior dislocation of unspecified humerus**

S43.08 **Other subluxation and dislocation of shoulder joint**

⑦**S43.081** **Other subluxation of right shoulder joint**

⑦**S43.082** **Other subluxation of left shoulder joint**

⑦**S43.083** **Other subluxation of unspecified shoulder joint**

⑦**S43.084** **Other dislocation of right shoulder joint**

⑦**S43.085** **Other dislocation of left shoulder joint**

⑦**S43.086** **Other dislocation of unspecified shoulder joint**

S43.1 **Subluxation and dislocation of acromioclavicular joint**

S43.10 **Unspecified dislocation of acromioclavicular joint**

⑦**S43.101** **Unspecified dislocation of right acromioclavicular joint**

⑦**S43.102** **Unspecified dislocation of left acromioclavicular joint**

⑦**S43.109** **Unspecified dislocation of unspecified acromioclavicular joint**

S43.11 **Subluxation of acromioclavicular joint**

⑦**S43.111** **Subluxation of right acromioclavicular joint**

⑦**S43.112** **Subluxation of left acromioclavicular joint**

⑦**S43.119** **Subluxation of unspecified acromioclavicular joint**

S43.12 **Dislocation of acromioclavicular joint, 100%-200% displacement**

⑦**S43.121** **Dislocation of right acromioclavicular joint, 100%-200% displacement**

⑦**S43.122** **Dislocation of left acromioclavicular joint, 100%-200% displacement**

⑦**S43.129** **Dislocation of unspecified acromioclavicular joint, 100%-200% displacement**

S43.13 **Dislocation of acromioclavicular joint, greater than 200% displacement**

⑦**S43.131** **Dislocation of right acromioclavicular joint, greater than 200% displacement**

⑦**S43.132** **Dislocation of left acromioclavicular joint, greater than 200% displacement**

⑦**S43.139** **Dislocation of unspecified acromioclavicular joint, greater than 200% displacement**

S43.14 **Inferior dislocation of acromioclavicular joint**

⑦**S43.141** **Inferior dislocation of right acromioclavicular joint**

⑦S43.142   **Inferior dislocation of left acromioclavicular joint**

⑦S43.149   **Inferior dislocation of unspecified acromioclavicular joint**

S43.15   **Posterior dislocation of acromioclavicular joint**

⑦S43.151   **Posterior dislocation of right acromioclavicular joint**

⑦S43.152   **Posterior dislocation of left acromioclavicular joint**

⑦S43.159   **Posterior dislocation of unspecified acromioclavicular joint**

S43.2   **Subluxation and dislocation of sternoclavicular joint**

S43.20   **Unspecified subluxation and dislocation of sternoclavicular joint**

⑦S43.201   **Unspecified subluxation of right sternoclavicular joint**

⑦S43.202   **Unspecified subluxation of left sternoclavicular joint**

⑦S43.203   **Unspecified subluxation of unspecified sternoclavicular joint**

⑦S43.204   **Unspecified dislocation of right sternoclavicular joint**

⑦S43.205   **Unspecified dislocation of left sternoclavicular joint**

⑦S43.206   **Unspecified dislocation of unspecified sternoclavicular joint**

S43.21   **Anterior subluxation and dislocation of sternoclavicular joint**

⑦S43.211   **Anterior subluxation of right sternoclavicular joint**

⑦S43.212   **Anterior subluxation of left sternoclavicular joint**

⑦S43.213   **Anterior subluxation of unspecified sternoclavicular joint**

⑦S43.214   **Anterior dislocation of right sternoclavicular joint**

⑦S43.215   **Anterior dislocation of left sternoclavicular joint**

⑦S43.216   **Anterior dislocation of unspecified sternoclavicular joint**

S43.22   **Posterior subluxation and dislocation of sternoclavicular joint**

⑦S43.221   **Posterior subluxation of right sternoclavicular joint**

⑦S43.222   **Posterior subluxation of left sternoclavicular joint**

⑦S43.223   **Posterior subluxation of unspecified sternoclavicular joint**

⑦S43.224   **Posterior dislocation of right sternoclavicular joint**

⑦S43.225   **Posterior dislocation of left sternoclavicular joint**

⑦S43.226   **Posterior dislocation of unspecified sternoclavicular joint**

S43.3   **Subluxation and dislocation of other and unspecified parts of shoulder girdle**

S43.30   **Subluxation and dislocation of unspecified parts of shoulder girdle**

Dislocation of shoulder girdle NOS

Subluxation of shoulder girdle NOS

⑦S43.301   **Subluxation of unspecified parts of right shoulder girdle**

⑦S43.302   **Subluxation of unspecified parts of left shoulder girdle**

⑦S43.303   **Subluxation of unspecified parts of unspecified shoulder girdle**

⑦S43.304   **Dislocation of unspecified parts of right shoulder girdle**

⑦S43.305   **Dislocation of unspecified parts of left shoulder girdle**

⑦S43.306   **Dislocation of unspecified parts of unspecified shoulder girdle**

S43.31   **Subluxation and dislocation of scapula**

⑦S43.311   **Subluxation of right scapula**

⑦S43.312   **Subluxation of left scapula**

⑦S43.313   **Subluxation of unspecified scapula**

⑦S43.314   **Dislocation of right scapula**

⑦S43.315   **Dislocation of left scapula**

⑦S43.316   **Dislocation of unspecified scapula**

S43.39   **Subluxation and dislocation of other parts of shoulder girdle**

⑦S43.391   **Subluxation of other parts of right shoulder girdle**

⑦S43.392   **Subluxation of other parts of left shoulder girdle**

⑦S43.393   **Subluxation of other parts of unspecified shoulder girdle**

⑦S43.394   **Dislocation of other parts of right shoulder girdle**

⑦S43.395   **Dislocation of other parts of left shoulder girdle**

⑦S43.396   **Dislocation of other parts of unspecified shoulder girdle**

S43.4   **Sprain of shoulder joint**

S43.40   **Unspecified sprain of shoulder joint**

⑦S43.401   **Unspecified sprain of right shoulder joint**

⑦S43.402   **Unspecified sprain of left shoulder joint**

⑦S43.409   **Unspecified sprain of unspecified shoulder joint**

S43.41   **Sprain of coracohumeral (ligament)**

⑦S43.411   **Sprain of right coracohumeral (ligament)**

⑦S43.412   **Sprain of left coracohumeral (ligament)**

⑦S43.419   **Sprain of unspecified coracohumeral (ligament)**

S43.42   **Sprain of rotator cuff capsule**

Excludes1: rotator cuff syndrome (complete)(incomplete), not specified as traumatic (M75.1-)

Excludes2: injury of tendon of rotator cuff (S46.0-)

⑦S43.421   **Sprain of right rotator cuff capsule**

⑦S43.422   **Sprain of left rotator cuff capsule**

⑦S43.429   **Sprain of unspecified rotator cuff capsule**

S43.43   **Superior glenoid labrum lesion**

SLAP lesion

⑦S43.431   **Superior glenoid labrum lesion of right shoulder**

⑦S43.432   **Superior glenoid labrum lesion of left shoulder**

⑦S43.439   **Superior glenoid labrum lesion of unspecified shoulder**

● New code   ▲ Revised code   **Excludes1:** Not coded here   **Excludes2:** Not included here   ⊗ Placeholder required   ⑦ 7th digit required

S43.49   **Other sprain of shoulder joint**

⑦**S43.491**   Other sprain of right shoulder joint

⑦**S43.492**   Other sprain of left shoulder joint

⑦**S43.499**   Other sprain of unspecified shoulder joint

S43.5   **Sprain of acromioclavicular joint**

Sprain of acromioclavicular ligament

⊗⑦**S43.50**   Sprain of unspecified acromioclavicular joint

⊗⑦**S43.51**   Sprain of right acromioclavicular joint

⊗⑦**S43.52**   Sprain of left acromioclavicular joint

S43.6   **Sprain of sternoclavicular joint**

⊗⑦**S43.60**   Sprain of unspecified sternoclavicular joint

⊗⑦**S43.61**   Sprain of right sternoclavicular joint

⊗⑦**S43.62**   Sprain of left sternoclavicular joint

S43.8   **Sprain of other specified parts of shoulder girdle**

⊗⑦**S43.80**   Sprain of other specified parts of unspecified shoulder girdle

⊗⑦**S43.81**   Sprain of other specified parts of right shoulder girdle

⊗⑦**S43.82**   Sprain of other specified parts of left shoulder girdle

S43.9   **Sprain of unspecified parts of shoulder girdle**

⊗⑦**S43.90**   Sprain of unspecified parts of unspecified shoulder girdle

Sprain of shoulder girdle NOS

⊗⑦**S43.91**   Sprain of unspecified parts of right shoulder girdle

⊗⑦**S43.92**   Sprain of unspecified parts of left shoulder girdle

S44   **Injury of nerves at shoulder and upper arm level**

Code also any associated open wound (S41.-)

Excludes2: injury of brachial plexus (S14.3-)

The appropriate 7th character is to be added to each code from category S44

A - initial encounter

D - subsequent encounter

S - sequela

S44.0   **Injury of ulnar nerve at upper arm level**

Excludes1: ulnar nerve NOS (S54.0)

⊗⑦**S44.00**   Injury of ulnar nerve at upper arm level, unspecified arm

⊗⑦**S44.01**   Injury of ulnar nerve at upper arm level, right arm

⊗⑦**S44.02**   Injury of ulnar nerve at upper arm level, left arm

S44.1   **Injury of median nerve at upper arm level**

Excludes1: median nerve NOS (S54.1)

⊗⑦**S44.10**   Injury of median nerve at upper arm level, unspecified arm

⊗⑦**S44.11**   Injury of median nerve at upper arm level, right arm

⊗⑦**S44.12**   Injury of median nerve at upper arm level, left arm

S44.2   **Injury of radial nerve at upper arm level**

Excludes1: radial nerve NOS (S54.2)

⊗⑦**S44.20**   Injury of radial nerve at upper arm level, unspecified arm

⊗⑦**S44.21**   Injury of radial nerve at upper arm level, right arm

⊗⑦**S44.22**   Injury of radial nerve at upper arm level, left arm

S44.3   **Injury of axillary nerve**

⊗⑦**S44.30**   Injury of axillary nerve, unspecified arm

⊗⑦**S44.31**   Injury of axillary nerve, right arm

⊗⑦**S44.32**   Injury of axillary nerve, left arm

S44.4   **Injury of musculocutaneous nerve**

⊗⑦**S44.40**   Injury of musculocutaneous nerve, unspecified arm

⊗⑦**S44.41**   Injury of musculocutaneous nerve, right arm

⊗⑦**S44.42**   Injury of musculocutaneous nerve, left arm

S44.5   **Injury of cutaneous sensory nerve at shoulder and upper arm level**

⊗⑦**S44.50**   Injury of cutaneous sensory nerve at shoulder and upper arm level, unspecified arm

⊗⑦**S44.51**   Injury of cutaneous sensory nerve at shoulder and upper arm level, right arm

⊗⑦**S44.52**   Injury of cutaneous sensory nerve at shoulder and upper arm level, left arm

S44.8   **Injury of other nerves at shoulder and upper arm level**

S44.8X   **Injury of other nerves at shoulder and upper arm level**

⑦**S44.8X1**   Injury of other nerves at shoulder and upper arm level, right arm

⑦**S44.8X2**   Injury of other nerves at shoulder and upper arm level, left arm

⑦**S44.8X9**   Injury of other nerves at shoulder and upper arm level, unspecified arm

S44.9   **Injury of unspecified nerve at shoulder and upper arm level**

⊗⑦**S44.90**   Injury of unspecified nerve at shoulder and upper arm level, unspecified arm

⊗⑦**S44.91**   Injury of unspecified nerve at shoulder and upper arm level, right arm

⊗⑦**S44.92**   Injury of unspecified nerve at shoulder and upper arm level, left arm

S45   **Injury of blood vessels at shoulder and upper arm level**

Code also any associated open wound (S41.-)

Excludes2: injury of subclavian artery (S25.1)

injury of subclavian vein (S25.3)

The appropriate 7th character is to be added to each code from category S45

A - initial encounter

D - subsequent encounter

S - sequela

S45.0   **Injury of axillary artery**

S45.00   **Unspecified injury of axillary artery**

⑦**S45.001**   Unspecified injury of axillary artery, right side

⑦**S45.002**   Unspecified injury of axillary artery, left side

⑦**S45.009**   Unspecified injury of axillary artery, unspecified side

S45.01   **Laceration of axillary artery**

⑦**S45.011**   Laceration of axillary artery, right side

⑦**S45.012**   Laceration of axillary artery, left side

⑦**S45.019**   Laceration of axillary artery, unspecified side

S45.09   **Other specified injury of axillary artery**

⑦S45.091   **Other specified injury of axillary artery, right side**

⑦S45.092   **Other specified injury of axillary artery, left side**

⑦S45.099   **Other specified injury of axillary artery, unspecified side**

S45.1   **Injury of brachial artery**

    S45.10   **Unspecified injury of brachial artery**

        ⑦S45.101   **Unspecified injury of brachial artery, right side**

        ⑦S45.102   **Unspecified injury of brachial artery, left side**

        ⑦S45.109   **Unspecified injury of brachial artery, unspecified side**

    S45.11   **Laceration of brachial artery**

        ⑦S45.111   **Laceration of brachial artery, right side**

        ⑦S45.112   **Laceration of brachial artery, left side**

        ⑦S45.119   **Laceration of brachial artery, unspecified side**

    S45.19   **Other specified injury of brachial artery**

        ⑦S45.191   **Other specified injury of brachial artery, right side**

        ⑦S45.192   **Other specified injury of brachial artery, left side**

        ⑦S45.199   **Other specified injury of brachial artery, unspecified side**

S45.2   **Injury of axillary or brachial vein**

    S45.20   **Unspecified injury of axillary or brachial vein**

        ⑦S45.201   **Unspecified injury of axillary or brachial vein, right side**

        ⑦S45.202   **Unspecified injury of axillary or brachial vein, left side**

        ⑦S45.209   **Unspecified injury of axillary or brachial vein, unspecified side**

    S45.21   **Laceration of axillary or brachial vein**

        ⑦S45.211   **Laceration of axillary or brachial vein, right side**

        ⑦S45.212   **Laceration of axillary or brachial vein, left side**

        ⑦S45.219   **Laceration of axillary or brachial vein, unspecified side**

    S45.29   **Other specified injury of axillary or brachial vein**

        ⑦S45.291   **Other specified injury of axillary or brachial vein, right side**

        ⑦S45.292   **Other specified injury of axillary or brachial vein, left side**

        ⑦S45.299   **Other specified injury of axillary or brachial vein, unspecified side**

S45.3   **Injury of superficial vein at shoulder and upper arm level**

    S45.30   **Unspecified injury of superficial vein at shoulder and upper arm level**

        ⑦S45.301   **Unspecified injury of superficial vein at shoulder and upper arm level, right arm**

        ⑦S45.302   **Unspecified injury of superficial vein at shoulder and upper arm level, left arm**

        ⑦S45.309   **Unspecified injury of superficial vein at shoulder and upper arm level, unspecified arm**

S45.31   **Laceration of superficial vein at shoulder and upper arm level**

    ⑦S45.311   **Laceration of superficial vein at shoulder and upper arm level, right arm**

    ⑦S45.312   **Laceration of superficial vein at shoulder and upper arm level, left arm**

    ⑦S45.319   **Laceration of superficial vein at shoulder and upper arm level, unspecified arm**

    S45.39   **Other specified injury of superficial vein at shoulder and upper arm level**

        ⑦S45.391   **Other specified injury of superficial vein at shoulder and upper arm level, right arm**

        ⑦S45.392   **Other specified injury of superficial vein at shoulder and upper arm level, left arm**

        ⑦S45.399   **Other specified injury of superficial vein at shoulder and upper arm level, unspecified arm**

S45.8   **Injury of other specified blood vessels at shoulder and upper arm level**

    S45.80   **Unspecified injury of other specified blood vessels at shoulder and upper arm level**

        ⑦S45.801   **Unspecified injury of other specified blood vessels at shoulder and upper arm level, right arm**

        ⑦S45.802   **Unspecified injury of other specified blood vessels at shoulder and upper arm level, left arm**

        ⑦S45.809   **Unspecified injury of other specified blood vessels at shoulder and upper arm level, unspecified arm**

    S45.81   **Laceration of other specified blood vessels at shoulder and upper arm level**

        ⑦S45.811   **Laceration of other specified blood vessels at shoulder and upper arm level, right arm**

        ⑦S45.812   **Laceration of other specified blood vessels at shoulder and upper arm level, left arm**

        ⑦S45.819   **Laceration of other specified blood vessels at shoulder and upper arm level, unspecified arm**

    S45.89   **Other specified injury of other specified blood vessels at shoulder and upper arm level**

        ⑦S45.891   **Other specified injury of other specified blood vessels at shoulder and upper arm level, right arm**

        ⑦S45.892   **Other specified injury of other specified blood vessels at shoulder and upper arm level, left arm**

        ⑦S45.899   **Other specified injury of other specified blood vessels at shoulder and upper arm level, unspecified arm**

S45.9   **Injury of unspecified blood vessel at shoulder and upper arm level**

    S45.90   **Unspecified injury of unspecified blood vessel at shoulder and upper arm level**

        ⑦S45.901   **Unspecified injury of unspecified blood vessel at shoulder and upper arm level, right arm**

● New code   ▲ Revised code   **Excludes1:** Not coded here   **Excludes2:** Not included here   ⊗ Placeholder required   ⑦ 7th digit required

⑦S45.902 Unspecified injury of unspecified blood vessel at shoulder and upper arm level, left arm

⑦S45.909 Unspecified injury of unspecified blood vessel at shoulder and upper arm level, unspecified arm

S45.91 Laceration of unspecified blood vessel at shoulder and upper arm level

⑦S45.911 Laceration of unspecified blood vessel at shoulder and upper arm level, right arm

⑦S45.912 Laceration of unspecified blood vessel at shoulder and upper arm level, left arm

⑦S45.919 Laceration of unspecified blood vessel at shoulder and upper arm level, unspecified arm

S45.99 Other specified injury of unspecified blood vessel at shoulder and upper arm level

⑦S45.991 Other specified injury of unspecified blood vessel at shoulder and upper arm level, right arm

⑦S45.992 Other specified injury of unspecified blood vessel at shoulder and upper arm level, left arm

⑦S45.999 Other specified injury of unspecified blood vessel at shoulder and upper arm level, unspecified arm

S46 Injury of muscle, fascia and tendon at shoulder and upper arm level

Code also any associated open wound (S41.-)

Excludes2: injury of muscle, fascia and tendon at elbow (S56.-)
sprain of joints and ligaments of shoulder girdle (S43.9)

The appropriate 7th character is to be added to each code from category S46

A - initial encounter

D - subsequent encounter

S - sequela

S46.0 Injury of muscle(s) and tendon(s) of the rotator cuff of shoulder

S46.00 Unspecified injury of muscle(s) and tendon(s) of the rotator cuff of shoulder

⑦S46.001 Unspecified injury of muscle(s) and tendon(s) of the rotator cuff of right shoulder

⑦S46.002 Unspecified injury of muscle(s) and tendon(s) of the rotator cuff of left shoulder

⑦S46.009 Unspecified injury of muscle(s) and tendon(s) of the rotator cuff of unspecified shoulder

S46.01 Strain of muscle(s) and tendon(s) of the rotator cuff of shoulder

⑦S46.011 Strain of muscle(s) and tendon(s) of the rotator cuff of right shoulder

⑦S46.012 Strain of muscle(s) and tendon(s) of the rotator cuff of left shoulder

⑦S46.019 Strain of muscle(s) and tendon(s) of the rotator cuff of unspecified shoulder

S46.02 Laceration of muscle(s) and tendon(s) of the rotator cuff of shoulder

⑦S46.021 Laceration of muscle(s) and tendon(s) of the rotator cuff of right shoulder

⑦S46.022 Laceration of muscle(s) and tendon(s) of the rotator cuff of left shoulder

⑦S46.029 Laceration of muscle(s) and tendon(s) of the rotator cuff of unspecified shoulder

S46.09 Other injury of muscle(s) and tendon(s) of the rotator cuff of shoulder

⑦S46.091 Other injury of muscle(s) and tendon(s) of the rotator cuff of right shoulder

⑦S46.092 Other injury of muscle(s) and tendon(s) of the rotator cuff of left shoulder

⑦S46.099 Other injury of muscle(s) and tendon(s) of the rotator cuff of unspecified shoulder

S46.1 Injury of muscle, fascia and tendon of long head of biceps

S46.10 Unspecified injury of muscle, fascia and tendon of long head of biceps

⑦S46.101 Unspecified injury of muscle, fascia and tendon of long head of biceps, right arm

⑦S46.102 Unspecified injury of muscle, fascia and tendon of long head of biceps, left arm

⑦S46.109 Unspecified injury of muscle, fascia and tendon of long head of biceps, unspecified arm

S46.11 Strain of muscle, fascia and tendon of long head of biceps

⑦S46.111 Strain of muscle, fascia and tendon of long head of biceps, right arm

⑦S46.112 Strain of muscle, fascia and tendon of long head of biceps, left arm

⑦S46.119 Strain of muscle, fascia and tendon of long head of biceps, unspecified arm

S46.12 Laceration of muscle, fascia and tendon of long head of biceps

⑦S46.121 Laceration of muscle, fascia and tendon of long head of biceps, right arm

⑦S46.122 Laceration of muscle, fascia and tendon of long head of biceps, left arm

⑦S46.129 Laceration of muscle, fascia and tendon of long head of biceps, unspecified arm

S46.19 Other injury of muscle, fascia and tendon of long head of biceps

⑦S46.191 Other injury of muscle, fascia and tendon of long head of biceps, right arm

⑦S46.192 Other injury of muscle, fascia and tendon of long head of biceps, left arm

⑦S46.199 Other injury of muscle, fascia and tendon of long head of biceps, unspecified arm

S46.2 Injury of muscle, fascia and tendon of other parts of biceps

S46.20 Unspecified injury of muscle, fascia and tendon of other parts of biceps

⑦S46.201 Unspecified injury of muscle, fascia and tendon of other parts of biceps, right arm

⑦S46.202 Unspecified injury of muscle, fascia and tendon of other parts of biceps, left arm

⑦S46.209 Unspecified injury of muscle, fascia and tendon of other parts of biceps, unspecified arm

S46.21 Strain of muscle, fascia and tendon of other parts of biceps

⑦S46.211 Strain of muscle, fascia and tendon of other parts of biceps, right arm

⑦S46.212 Strain of muscle, fascia and tendon of other parts of biceps, left arm

⑦S46.219 Strain of muscle, fascia and tendon of other parts of biceps, unspecified arm

S46.22 Laceration of muscle, fascia and tendon of other parts of biceps

⑦S46.221 Laceration of muscle, fascia and tendon of other parts of biceps, right arm

⑦S46.222 Laceration of muscle, fascia and tendon of other parts of biceps, left arm

⑦S46.229 Laceration of muscle, fascia and tendon of other parts of biceps, unspecified arm

S46.29 Other injury of muscle, fascia and tendon of other parts of biceps

⑦S46.291 Other injury of muscle, fascia and tendon of other parts of biceps, right arm

⑦S46.292 Other injury of muscle, fascia and tendon of other parts of biceps, left arm

⑦S46.299 Other injury of muscle, fascia and tendon of other parts of biceps, unspecified arm

S46.3 Injury of muscle, fascia and tendon of triceps

S46.30 Unspecified injury of muscle, fascia and tendon of triceps

⑦S46.301 Unspecified injury of muscle, fascia and tendon of triceps, right arm

⑦S46.302 Unspecified injury of muscle, fascia and tendon of triceps, left arm

⑦S46.309 Unspecified injury of muscle, fascia and tendon of triceps, unspecified arm

S46.31 Strain of muscle, fascia and tendon of triceps

⑦S46.311 Strain of muscle, fascia and tendon of triceps, right arm

⑦S46.312 Strain of muscle, fascia and tendon of triceps, left arm

⑦S46.319 Strain of muscle, fascia and tendon of triceps, unspecified arm

S46.32 Laceration of muscle, fascia and tendon of triceps

⑦S46.321 Laceration of muscle, fascia and tendon of triceps, right arm

⑦S46.322 Laceration of muscle, fascia and tendon of triceps, left arm

⑦S46.329 Laceration of muscle, fascia and tendon of triceps, unspecified arm

S46.39 Other injury of muscle, fascia and tendon of triceps

⑦S46.391 Other injury of muscle, fascia and tendon of triceps, right arm

⑦S46.392 Other injury of muscle, fascia and tendon of triceps, left arm

⑦S46.399 Other injury of muscle, fascia and tendon of triceps, unspecified arm

S46.8 Injury of other muscles, fascia and tendons at shoulder and upper arm level

S46.80 Unspecified injury of other muscles, fascia and tendons at shoulder and upper arm level

⑦S46.801 Unspecified injury of other muscles, fascia and tendons at shoulder and upper arm level, right arm

⑦S46.802 Unspecified injury of other muscles, fascia and tendons at shoulder and upper arm level, left arm

⑦S46.809 Unspecified injury of other muscles, fascia and tendons at shoulder and upper arm level, unspecified arm

S46.81 Strain of other muscles, fascia and tendons at shoulder and upper arm level

⑦S46.811 Strain of other muscles, fascia and tendons at shoulder and upper arm level, right arm

⑦S46.812 Strain of other muscles, fascia and tendons at shoulder and upper arm level, left arm

⑦S46.819 Strain of other muscles, fascia and tendons at shoulder and upper arm level, unspecified arm

S46.82 Laceration of other muscles, fascia and tendons at shoulder and upper arm level

⑦S46.821 Laceration of other muscles, fascia and tendons at shoulder and upper arm level, right arm

⑦S46.822 Laceration of other muscles, fascia and tendons at shoulder and upper arm level, left arm

⑦S46.829 Laceration of other muscles, fascia and tendons at shoulder and upper arm level, unspecified arm

S46.89 Other injury of other muscles, fascia and tendons at shoulder and upper arm level

⑦S46.891 Other injury of other muscles, fascia and tendons at shoulder and upper arm level, right arm

⑦S46.892 Other injury of other muscles, fascia and tendons at shoulder and upper arm level, left arm

⑦S46.899 Other injury of other muscles, fascia and tendons at shoulder and upper arm level, unspecified arm

S46.9 Injury of unspecified muscle, fascia and tendon at shoulder and upper arm level

S46.90 Unspecified injury of unspecified muscle, fascia and tendon at shoulder and upper arm level

⑦S46.901 Unspecified injury of unspecified muscle, fascia and tendon at shoulder and upper arm level, right arm

⑦S46.902 Unspecified injury of unspecified muscle, fascia and tendon at shoulder and upper arm level, left arm

● New code   ▲ Revised code   **Excludes1:** Not coded here   **Excludes2:** Not included here   ⊗ Placeholder required   ⑦7th digit required

⑦S46.909　Unspecified injury of unspecified muscle, fascia and tendon at shoulder and upper arm level, unspecified arm

S46.91　Strain of unspecified muscle, fascia and tendon at shoulder and upper arm level

⑦S46.911　Strain of unspecified muscle, fascia and tendon at shoulder and upper arm level, right arm

⑦S46.912　Strain of unspecified muscle, fascia and tendon at shoulder and upper arm level, left arm

⑦S46.919　Strain of unspecified muscle, fascia and tendon at shoulder and upper arm level, unspecified arm

S46.92　Laceration of unspecified muscle, fascia and tendon at shoulder and upper arm level

⑦S46.921　Laceration of unspecified muscle, fascia and tendon at shoulder and upper arm level, right arm

⑦S46.922　Laceration of unspecified muscle, fascia and tendon at shoulder and upper arm level, left arm

⑦S46.929　Laceration of unspecified muscle, fascia and tendon at shoulder and upper arm level, unspecified arm

S46.99　Other injury of unspecified muscle, fascia and tendon at shoulder and upper arm level

⑦S46.991　Other injury of unspecified muscle, fascia and tendon at shoulder and upper arm level, right arm

⑦S46.992　Other injury of unspecified muscle, fascia and tendon at shoulder and upper arm level, left arm

⑦S46.999　Other injury of unspecified muscle, fascia and tendon at shoulder and upper arm level, unspecified arm

S47　Crushing injury of shoulder and upper arm

Use Additional Code for all associated injuries

Excludes2: crushing injury of elbow (S57.0-)

The appropriate 7th character is to be added to each code from category S47

A - initial encounter

D - subsequent encounter

S - sequela

⊗⑦S47.1　Crushing injury of right shoulder and upper arm

⊗⑦S47.2　Crushing injury of left shoulder and upper arm

⊗⑦S47.9　Crushing injury of shoulder and upper arm, unspecified arm

S48　Traumatic amputation of shoulder and upper arm

An amputation not identified as partial or complete should be coded to complete

Excludes1: traumatic amputation at elbow level (S58.0)

The appropriate 7th character is to be added to each code from category S48

A - initial encounter

D - subsequent encounter

S - sequela

S48.0　Traumatic amputation at shoulder joint

S48.01　Complete traumatic amputation at shoulder joint

⑦S48.011　Complete traumatic amputation at right shoulder joint [HCC]

⑦S48.012　Complete traumatic amputation at left shoulder joint [HCC]

⑦S48.019　Complete traumatic amputation at unspecified shoulder joint [HCC]

S48.02　Partial traumatic amputation at shoulder joint [HCC]

⑦S48.021　Partial traumatic amputation at right shoulder joint [HCC]

⑦S48.022　Partial traumatic amputation at left shoulder joint [HCC]

⑦S48.029　Partial traumatic amputation at unspecified shoulder joint [HCC]

S48.1　Traumatic amputation at level between shoulder and elbow

S48.11　Complete traumatic amputation at level between shoulder and elbow

⑦S48.111　Complete traumatic amputation at level between right shoulder and elbow [HCC]

⑦S48.112　Complete traumatic amputation at level between left shoulder and elbow [HCC]

⑦S48.119　Complete traumatic amputation at level between unspecified shoulder and elbow [HCC]

S48.12　Partial traumatic amputation at level between shoulder and elbow

⑦S48.121　Partial traumatic amputation at level between right shoulder and elbow [HCC]

⑦S48.122　Partial traumatic amputation at level between left shoulder and elbow [HCC]

⑦S48.129　Partial traumatic amputation at level between unspecified shoulder and elbow [HCC]

S48.9　Traumatic amputation of shoulder and upper arm, level unspecified

S48.91　Complete traumatic amputation of shoulder and upper arm, level unspecified

⑦S48.911　Complete traumatic amputation of right shoulder and upper arm, level unspecified [HCC]

⑦S48.912　Complete traumatic amputation of left shoulder and upper arm, level unspecified [HCC]

⑦S48.919　Complete traumatic amputation of unspecified shoulder and upper arm, level unspecified [HCC]

S48.92　Partial traumatic amputation of shoulder and upper arm, level unspecified

⑦S48.921　Partial traumatic amputation of right shoulder and upper arm, level unspecified [HCC]

⑦S48.922　Partial traumatic amputation of left shoulder and upper arm, level unspecified [HCC]

⑦S48.929　Partial traumatic amputation of unspecified shoulder and upper arm, level unspecified [HCC]

S49　Other and unspecified injuries of shoulder and upper arm

The appropriate 7th character is to be added to each code from subcategories S49.0 and S49.1

A - initial encounter for closed fracture

D - subsequent encounter for fracture with routine healing

G - subsequent encounter for fracture with delayed healing

K - subsequent encounter for fracture with nonunion

P - subsequent encounter for fracture with malunion

S - sequela

S49.0   Physeal fracture of upper end of humerus

    S49.00   Unspecified physeal fracture of upper end of humerus

        ⑦**S49.001   Unspecified physeal fracture of upper end of humerus, right arm**

        ⑦**S49.002   Unspecified physeal fracture of upper end of humerus, left arm**

        ⑦**S49.009   Unspecified physeal fracture of upper end of humerus, unspecified arm**

    S49.01   Salter-Harris Type I physeal fracture of upper end of humerus

        ⑦**S49.011   Salter-Harris Type I physeal fracture of upper end of humerus, right arm**

        ⑦**S49.012   Salter-Harris Type I physeal fracture of upper end of humerus, left arm**

        ⑦**S49.019   Salter-Harris Type I physeal fracture of upper end of humerus, unspecified arm**

    S49.02   Salter-Harris Type II physeal fracture of upper end of humerus

        ⑦**S49.021   Salter-Harris Type II physeal fracture of upper end of humerus, right arm**

        ⑦**S49.022   Salter-Harris Type II physeal fracture of upper end of humerus, left arm**

        ⑦**S49.029   Salter-Harris Type II physeal fracture of upper end of humerus, unspecified arm**

    S49.03   Salter-Harris Type III physeal fracture of upper end of humerus

        ⑦**S49.031   Salter-Harris Type III physeal fracture of upper end of humerus, right arm**

        ⑦**S49.032   Salter-Harris Type III physeal fracture of upper end of humerus, left arm**

        ⑦**S49.039   Salter-Harris Type III physeal fracture of upper end of humerus, unspecified arm**

    S49.04   Salter-Harris Type IV physeal fracture of upper end of humerus

        ⑦**S49.041   Salter-Harris Type IV physeal fracture of upper end of humerus, right arm**

        ⑦**S49.042   Salter-Harris Type IV physeal fracture of upper end of humerus, left arm**

        ⑦**S49.049   Salter-Harris Type IV physeal fracture of upper end of humerus, unspecified arm**

    S49.09   Other physeal fracture of upper end of humerus

        ⑦**S49.091   Other physeal fracture of upper end of humerus, right arm**

        ⑦**S49.092   Other physeal fracture of upper end of humerus, left arm**

        ⑦**S49.099   Other physeal fracture of upper end of humerus, unspecified arm**

S49.1   Physeal fracture of lower end of humerus

    S49.10   Unspecified physeal fracture of lower end of humerus

        ⑦**S49.101   Unspecified physeal fracture of lower end of humerus, right arm**

        ⑦**S49.102   Unspecified physeal fracture of lower end of humerus, left arm**

        ⑦**S49.109   Unspecified physeal fracture of lower end of humerus, unspecified arm**

    S49.11   Salter-Harris Type I physeal fracture of lower end of humerus

        ⑦**S49.111   Salter-Harris Type I physeal fracture of lower end of humerus, right arm**

        ⑦**S49.112   Salter-Harris Type I physeal fracture of lower end of humerus, left arm**

        ⑦**S49.119   Salter-Harris Type I physeal fracture of lower end of humerus, unspecified arm**

    S49.12   Salter-Harris Type II physeal fracture of lower end of humerus

        ⑦**S49.121   Salter-Harris Type II physeal fracture of lower end of humerus, right arm**

        ⑦**S49.122   Salter-Harris Type II physeal fracture of lower end of humerus, left arm**

        ⑦**S49.129   Salter-Harris Type II physeal fracture of lower end of humerus, unspecified arm**

    S49.13   Salter-Harris Type III physeal fracture of lower end of humerus

        ⑦**S49.131   Salter-Harris Type III physeal fracture of lower end of humerus, right arm**

        ⑦**S49.132   Salter-Harris Type III physeal fracture of lower end of humerus, left arm**

        ⑦**S49.139   Salter-Harris Type III physeal fracture of lower end of humerus, unspecified arm**

    S49.14   Salter-Harris Type IV physeal fracture of lower end of humerus

        ⑦**S49.141   Salter-Harris Type IV physeal fracture of lower end of humerus, right arm**

        ⑦**S49.142   Salter-Harris Type IV physeal fracture of lower end of humerus, left arm**

        ⑦**S49.149   Salter-Harris Type IV physeal fracture of lower end of humerus, unspecified arm**

    S49.19   Other physeal fracture of lower end of humerus

        ⑦**S49.191   Other physeal fracture of lower end of humerus, right arm**

        ⑦**S49.192   Other physeal fracture of lower end of humerus, left arm**

        ⑦**S49.199   Other physeal fracture of lower end of humerus, unspecified arm**

S49.8   Other specified injuries of shoulder and upper arm

The appropriate 7th character is to be added to each code in subcategory S49.8

A - initial encounter

D - subsequent encounter

● New code   ▲ Revised code   **Excludes1:** Not coded here   **Excludes2:** Not included here   ⊗ Placeholder required   ⑦ 7th digit required

S - sequela

⊗ **S49.80** **Other specified injuries of shoulder and upper arm, unspecified arm**

⊗ **S49.81** **Other specified injuries of right shoulder and upper arm**

⊗ **S49.82** **Other specified injuries of left shoulder and upper arm**

S49.9 **Unspecified injury of shoulder and upper arm**

The appropriate 7th character is to be added to each code in subcategory S49.9

A - initial encounter

D - subsequent encounter

S - sequela

⊗⑦ **S49.90** **Unspecified injury of shoulder and upper arm, unspecified arm**

⊗⑦ **S49.91** **Unspecified injury of right shoulder and upper arm**

⊗⑦ **S49.92** **Unspecified injury of left shoulder and upper arm**

INJURIES TO THE ELBOW AND FOREARM (S50-S59)

Excludes2: burns and corrosions (T20-T32)

frostbite (T33-T34)

injuries of wrist and hand (S60-S69)

insect bite or sting, venomous (T63.4)

S50 **Superficial injury of elbow and forearm**

Excludes2: superficial injury of wrist and hand (S60.-)

The appropriate 7th character is to be added to each code from category S50

A - initial encounter

D - subsequent encounter

S - sequela

S50.0 **Contusion of elbow**

⊗⑦ **S50.00** **Contusion of unspecified elbow**

⊗⑦ **S50.01** **Contusion of right elbow**

⊗⑦ **S50.02** **Contusion of left elbow**

S50.1 **Contusion of forearm**

⊗⑦ **S50.10** **Contusion of unspecified forearm**

⊗⑦ **S50.11** **Contusion of right forearm**

⊗⑦ **S50.12** **Contusion of left forearm**

S50.3 **Other superficial injuries of elbow**

S50.31 **Abrasion of elbow**

⑦ **S50.311** **Abrasion of right elbow**

⑦ **S50.312** **Abrasion of left elbow**

⑦ **S50.319** **Abrasion of unspecified elbow**

S50.32 **Blister (nonthermal) of elbow**

⑦ **S50.321** **Blister (nonthermal) of right elbow**

⑦ **S50.322** **Blister (nonthermal) of left elbow**

⑦ **S50.329** **Blister (nonthermal) of unspecified elbow**

S50.34 **External constriction of elbow**

⑦ **S50.341** **External constriction of right elbow**

⑦ **S50.342** **External constriction of left elbow**

⑦ **S50.349** **External constriction of unspecified elbow**

S50.35 **Superficial foreign body of elbow**

Splinter in the elbow

⑦ **S50.351** **Superficial foreign body of right elbow**

⑦ **S50.352** **Superficial foreign body of left elbow**

⑦ **S50.359** **Superficial foreign body of unspecified elbow**

S50.36 **Insect bite (nonvenomous) of elbow**

⑦ **S50.361** **Insect bite (nonvenomous) of right elbow**

⑦ **S50.362** **Insect bite (nonvenomous) of left elbow**

⑦ **S50.369** **Insect bite (nonvenomous) of unspecified elbow**

S50.37 **Other superficial bite of elbow**

Excludes1: open bite of elbow (S51.04)

⑦ **S50.371** **Other superficial bite of right elbow**

⑦ **S50.372** **Other superficial bite of left elbow**

⑦ **S50.379** **Other superficial bite of unspecified elbow**

S50.8 **Other superficial injuries of forearm**

S50.81 **Abrasion of forearm**

⑦ **S50.811** **Abrasion of right forearm**

⑦ **S50.812** **Abrasion of left forearm**

⑦ **S50.819** **Abrasion of unspecified forearm**

S50.82 **Blister (nonthermal) of forearm**

⑦ **S50.821** **Blister (nonthermal) of right forearm**

⑦ **S50.822** **Blister (nonthermal) of left forearm**

⑦ **S50.829** **Blister (nonthermal) of unspecified forearm**

S50.84 **External constriction of forearm**

⑦ **S50.841** **External constriction of right forearm**

⑦ **S50.842** **External constriction of left forearm**

⑦ **S50.849** **External constriction of unspecified forearm**

S50.85 **Superficial foreign body of forearm**

Splinter in the forearm

⑦ **S50.851** **Superficial foreign body of right forearm**

⑦ **S50.852** **Superficial foreign body of left forearm**

⑦ **S50.859** **Superficial foreign body of unspecified forearm**

S50.86 **Insect bite (nonvenomous) of forearm**

⑦ **S50.861** **Insect bite (nonvenomous) of right forearm**

⑦ **S50.862** **Insect bite (nonvenomous) of left forearm**

⑦ **S50.869** **Insect bite (nonvenomous) of unspecified forearm**

S50.87 **Other superficial bite of forearm**

Excludes1: open bite of forearm (S51.84)

⑦ **S50.871** **Other superficial bite of right forearm**

⑦ **S50.872** **Other superficial bite of left forearm**

⑦ **S50.879** **Other superficial bite of unspecified forearm**

S50.9 **Unspecified superficial injury of elbow and forearm**

S50.90 **Unspecified superficial injury of elbow**

⑦ **S50.901** **Unspecified superficial injury of right elbow**

⑦ **S50.902** **Unspecified superficial injury of left elbow**

⑦S50.909 **Unspecified superficial injury of unspecified elbow**

S50.91 **Unspecified superficial injury of forearm**

⑦S50.911 **Unspecified superficial injury of right forearm**

⑦S50.912 **Unspecified superficial injury of left forearm**

⑦S50.919 **Unspecified superficial injury of unspecified forearm**

S51 **Open wound of elbow and forearm**

<u>Code also</u> any associated wound infection

Excludes1: open fracture of elbow and forearm (S52.- with open fracture 7th character)

traumatic amputation of elbow and forearm (S58.-)

Excludes2: open wound of wrist and hand (S61.-)

The appropriate 7th character is to be added to each code from category S51

A - initial encounter

D - subsequent encounter

S - sequela

S51.0 **Open wound of elbow**

S51.00 **Unspecified open wound of elbow**

⑦S51.001 **Unspecified open wound of right elbow**

⑦S51.002 **Unspecified open wound of left elbow**

⑦S51.009 **Unspecified open wound of unspecified elbow**

Open wound of elbow NOS

S51.01 **Laceration without foreign body of elbow**

⑦S51.011 **Laceration without foreign body of right elbow**

⑦S51.012 **Laceration without foreign body of left elbow**

⑦S51.019 **Laceration without foreign body of unspecified elbow**

S51.02 **Laceration with foreign body of elbow**

⑦S51.021 **Laceration with foreign body of right elbow**

⑦S51.022 **Laceration with foreign body of left elbow**

⑦S51.029 **Laceration with foreign body of unspecified elbow**

S51.03 **Puncture wound without foreign body of elbow**

⑦S51.031 **Puncture wound without foreign body of right elbow**

⑦S51.032 **Puncture wound without foreign body of left elbow**

⑦S51.039 **Puncture wound without foreign body of unspecified elbow**

S51.04 **Puncture wound with foreign body of elbow**

⑦S51.041 **Puncture wound with foreign body of right elbow**

⑦S51.042 **Puncture wound with foreign body of left elbow**

⑦S51.049 **Puncture wound with foreign body of unspecified elbow**

S51.05 **Open bite of elbow**

Bite of elbow NOS

Excludes1: superficial bite of elbow (S50.36, S50.37)

⑦S51.051 **Open bite, right elbow**

⑦S51.052 **Open bite, left elbow**

⑦S51.059 **Open bite, unspecified elbow**

S51.8 **Open wound of forearm**

Excludes2: open wound of elbow (S51.0-)

S51.80 **Unspecified open wound of forearm**

⑦S51.801 **Unspecified open wound of right forearm**

⑦S51.802 **Unspecified open wound of left forearm**

⑦S51.809 **Unspecified open wound of unspecified forearm**

Open wound of forearm NOS

S51.81 **Laceration without foreign body of forearm**

⑦S51.811 **Laceration without foreign body of right forearm**

⑦S51.812 **Laceration without foreign body of left forearm**

⑦S51.819 **Laceration without foreign body of unspecified forearm**

S51.82 **Laceration with foreign body of forearm**

⑦S51.821 **Laceration with foreign body of right forearm**

⑦S51.822 **Laceration with foreign body of left forearm**

⑦S51.829 **Laceration with foreign body of unspecified forearm**

S51.83 **Puncture wound without foreign body of forearm**

⑦S51.831 **Puncture wound without foreign body of right forearm**

⑦S51.832 **Puncture wound without foreign body of left forearm**

⑦S51.839 **Puncture wound without foreign body of unspecified forearm**

S51.84 **Puncture wound with foreign body of forearm**

⑦S51.841 **Puncture wound with foreign body of right forearm**

⑦S51.842 **Puncture wound with foreign body of left forearm**

⑦S51.849 **Puncture wound with foreign body of unspecified forearm**

S51.85 **Open bite of forearm**

Bite of forearm NOS

Excludes1: superficial bite of forearm (S50.86, S50.87)

⑦S51.851 **Open bite of right forearm**

⑦S51.852 **Open bite of left forearm**

⑦S51.859 **Open bite of unspecified forearm**

S52 **Fracture of forearm**

Note: A fracture not indicated as displaced or nondisplaced should be coded to displaced

A fracture not indicated as open or closed should be coded to closed

The open fracture designations are based on the Gustilo open fracture classification

Excludes1: traumatic amputation of forearm (S58.-)

Excludes2: fracture at wrist and hand level (S62.-)

The appropriate 7th character is to be added to all codes from category S52

A - initial encounter for closed fracture

B - initial encounter for open fracture type I or II initial encounter for open fracture NOS

● New code ▲ Revised code Excludes1: Not coded here Excludes2: Not included here ⊗ Placeholder required ⑦7th digit required

C - initial encounter for open fracture type IIIA, IIIB, or IIIC

D - subsequent encounter for closed fracture with routine healing

E - subsequent encounter for open fracture type I or II with routine healing

F - subsequent encounter for open fracture type IIIA, IIIB, or IIIC with routine healing

G - subsequent encounter for closed fracture with delayed healing

H - subsequent encounter for open fracture type I or II with delayed healing

J - subsequent encounter for open fracture type IIIA, IIIB, or IIIC with delayed healing

K - subsequent encounter for closed fracture with nonunion

M - subsequent encounter for open fracture type I or II with nonunion

N - subsequent encounter for open fracture type IIIA, IIIB, or IIIC with nonunion P - subsequent encounter for closed fracture with malunion

Q - subsequent encounter for open fracture type I or II with malunion

R - subsequent encounter for open fracture type IIIA, IIIB, or IIIC with malunion

S - sequela

S52.0   Fracture of upper end of ulna

Fracture of proximal end of ulna

Excludes2: fracture of elbow NOS (S42.40-)

fractures of shaft of ulna (S52.2-)

S52.00   Unspecified fracture of upper end of ulna

⑦S52.001   **Unspecified fracture of upper end of right ulna**

⑦S52.002   **Unspecified fracture of upper end of left ulna**

⑦S52.009   **Unspecified fracture of upper end of unspecified ulna**

S52.01   Torus fracture of upper end of ulna

The appropriate 7th character is to be added to all codes in subcategory S52.01

A - initial encounter for closed fracture

D - subsequent encounter for fracture with routine healing

G - subsequent encounter for fracture with delayed healing

K - subsequent encounter for fracture with nonunion

P - subsequent encounter for fracture with malunion

S - sequela

⑦S52.011   **Torus fracture of upper end of right ulna**

⑦S52.012   **Torus fracture of upper end of left ulna**

⑦S52.019   **Torus fracture of upper end of unspecified ulna**

S52.02   Fracture of olecranon process without intraarticular extension of ulna

⑦S52.021   **Displaced fracture of olecranon process without intraarticular extension of right ulna**

⑦S52.022   **Displaced fracture of olecranon process without intraarticular extension of left ulna**

⑦S52.023   **Displaced fracture of olecranon process without intraarticular extension of unspecified ulna**

⑦S52.024   **Nondisplaced fracture of olecranon process without intraarticular extension of right ulna**

⑦S52.025   **Nondisplaced fracture of olecranon process without intraarticular extension of left ulna**

⑦S52.026   **Nondisplaced fracture of olecranon process without intraarticular extension of unspecified ulna**

S52.03   Fracture of olecranon process with intraarticular extension of ulna

⑦S52.031   **Displaced fracture of olecranon process with intraarticular extension of right ulna**

⑦S52.032   **Displaced fracture of olecranon process with intraarticular extension of left ulna**

⑦S52.033   **Displaced fracture of olecranon process with intraarticular extension of unspecified ulna**

⑦S52.034   **Nondisplaced fracture of olecranon process with intraarticular extension of right ulna**

⑦S52.035   **Nondisplaced fracture of olecranon process with intraarticular extension of left ulna**

⑦S52.036   **Nondisplaced fracture of olecranon process with intraarticular extension of unspecified ulna**

S52.04   Fracture of coronoid process of ulna

⑦S52.041   **Displaced fracture of coronoid process of right ulna**

⑦S52.042   **Displaced fracture of coronoid process of left ulna**

⑦S52.043   **Displaced fracture of coronoid process of unspecified ulna**

⑦S52.044   **Nondisplaced fracture of coronoid process of right ulna**

⑦S52.045   **Nondisplaced fracture of coronoid process of left ulna**

⑦S52.046   **Nondisplaced fracture of coronoid process of unspecified ulna**

S52.09   Other fracture of upper end of ulna

⑦S52.091   **Other fracture of upper end of right ulna**

⑦S52.092   **Other fracture of upper end of left ulna**

⑦S52.099   **Other fracture of upper end of unspecified ulna**

S52.1   Fracture of upper end of radius

Fracture of proximal end of radius

Excludes2: physeal fractures of upper end of radius (S59.2-)

fracture of shaft of radius (S52.3-)

S52.10   Unspecified fracture of upper end of radius

⑦S52.101   **Unspecified fracture of upper end of right radius**

⑦S52.102   **Unspecified fracture of upper end of left radius**

⑦S52.109   **Unspecified fracture of upper end of unspecified radius**

S52.11   Torus fracture of upper end of radius

The appropriate 7th character is to be added to all codes in subcategory S52.11

A - initial encounter for closed fracture

D - subsequent encounter for fracture with routine healing

G - subsequent encounter for fracture with delayed healing

K - subsequent encounter for fracture with nonunion

P - subsequent encounter for fracture with malunion

S - sequela

⑦**S52.111** **Torus fracture of upper end of right radius**

⑦**S52.112** **Torus fracture of upper end of left radius**

⑦**S52.119** **Torus fracture of upper end of unspecified radius**

S52.12 **Fracture of head of radius**

⑦**S52.121** **Displaced fracture of head of right radius**

⑦**S52.122** **Displaced fracture of head of left radius**

⑦**S52.123** **Displaced fracture of head of unspecified radius**

⑦**S52.124** **Nondisplaced fracture of head of right radius**

⑦**S52.125** **Nondisplaced fracture of head of left radius**

⑦**S52.126** **Nondisplaced fracture of head of unspecified radius**

S52.13 **Fracture of neck of radius**

⑦**S52.131** **Displaced fracture of neck of right radius**

⑦**S52.132** **Displaced fracture of neck of left radius**

⑦**S52.133** **Displaced fracture of neck of unspecified radius**

⑦**S52.134** **Nondisplaced fracture of neck of right radius**

⑦**S52.135** **Nondisplaced fracture of neck of left radius**

⑦**S52.136** **Nondisplaced fracture of neck of unspecified radius**

S52.18 **Other fracture of upper end of radius**

⑦**S52.181** **Other fracture of upper end of right radius**

⑦**S52.182** **Other fracture of upper end of left radius**

⑦**S52.189** **Other fracture of upper end of unspecified radius**

S52.2 **Fracture of shaft of ulna**

S52.20 **Unspecified fracture of shaft of ulna**

Fracture of ulna NOS

⑦**S52.201** **Unspecified fracture of shaft of right ulna**

⑦**S52.202** **Unspecified fracture of shaft of left ulna**

⑦**S52.209** **Unspecified fracture of shaft of unspecified ulna**

S52.21 **Greenstick fracture of shaft of ulna**

The appropriate 7th character is to be added to all codes in subcategory S52.21

A - initial encounter for closed fracture

D - subsequent encounter for fracture with routine healing

G - subsequent encounter for fracture with delayed healing

K - subsequent encounter for fracture with nonunion

P - subsequent encounter for fracture with malunion

S - sequela

⑦**S52.211** **Greenstick fracture of shaft of right ulna**

⑦**S52.212** **Greenstick fracture of shaft of left ulna**

⑦**S52.219** **Greenstick fracture of shaft of unspecified ulna**

S52.22 **Transverse fracture of shaft of ulna**

⑦**S52.221** **Displaced transverse fracture of shaft of right ulna**

⑦**S52.222** **Displaced transverse fracture of shaft of left ulna**

⑦**S52.223** **Displaced transverse fracture of shaft of unspecified ulna**

⑦**S52.224** **Nondisplaced transverse fracture of shaft of right ulna**

⑦**S52.225** **Nondisplaced transverse fracture of shaft of left ulna**

⑦**S52.226** **Nondisplaced transverse fracture of shaft of unspecified ulna**

S52.23 **Oblique fracture of shaft of ulna**

⑦**S52.231** **Displaced oblique fracture of shaft of right ulna**

⑦**S52.232** **Displaced oblique fracture of shaft of left ulna**

⑦**S52.233** **Displaced oblique fracture of shaft of unspecified ulna**

⑦**S52.234** **Nondisplaced oblique fracture of shaft of right ulna**

⑦**S52.235** **Nondisplaced oblique fracture of shaft of left ulna**

⑦**S52.236** **Nondisplaced oblique fracture of shaft of unspecified ulna**

S52.24 **Spiral fracture of shaft of ulna**

⑦**S52.241** **Displaced spiral fracture of shaft of ulna, right arm**

⑦**S52.242** **Displaced spiral fracture of shaft of ulna, left arm**

⑦**S52.243** **Displaced spiral fracture of shaft of ulna, unspecified arm**

⑦**S52.244** **Nondisplaced spiral fracture of shaft of ulna, right arm**

⑦**S52.245** **Nondisplaced spiral fracture of shaft of ulna, left arm**

⑦**S52.246** **Nondisplaced spiral fracture of shaft of ulna, unspecified arm**

S52.25 **Comminuted fracture of shaft of ulna**

⑦**S52.251** **Displaced comminuted fracture of shaft of ulna, right arm**

⑦**S52.252** **Displaced comminuted fracture of shaft of ulna, left arm**

⑦**S52.253** **Displaced comminuted fracture of shaft of ulna, unspecified arm**

⑦**S52.254** **Nondisplaced comminuted fracture of shaft of ulna, right arm**

⑦S52.255   **Nondisplaced comminuted fracture of shaft of ulna, left arm**

⑦S52.256   **Nondisplaced comminuted fracture of shaft of ulna, unspecified arm**

S52.26   **Segmental fracture of shaft of ulna**

⑦S52.261   **Displaced segmental fracture of shaft of ulna, right arm**

⑦S52.262   **Displaced segmental fracture of shaft of ulna, left arm**

⑦S52.263   **Displaced segmental fracture of shaft of ulna, unspecified arm**

⑦S52.264   **Nondisplaced segmental fracture of shaft of ulna, right arm**

⑦S52.265   **Nondisplaced segmental fracture of shaft of ulna, left arm**

⑦S52.266   **Nondisplaced segmental fracture of shaft of ulna, unspecified arm**

S52.27   **Monteggia's fracture of ulna**

Fracture of upper shaft of ulna with dislocation of radial head

⑦S52.271   **Monteggia's fracture of right ulna**

⑦S52.272   **Monteggia's fracture of left ulna**

⑦S52.279   **Monteggia's fracture of unspecified ulna**

S52.28   **Bent bone of ulna**

⑦S52.281   **Bent bone of right ulna**

⑦S52.282   **Bent bone of left ulna**

⑦S52.283   **Bent bone of unspecified ulna**

S52.29   **Other fracture of shaft of ulna**

⑦S52.291   **Other fracture of shaft of right ulna**

⑦S52.292   **Other fracture of shaft of left ulna**

⑦S52.299   **Other fracture of shaft of unspecified ulna**

S52.3   **Fracture of shaft of radius**

S52.30   **Unspecified fracture of shaft of radius**

⑦S52.301   **Unspecified fracture of shaft of right radius**

⑦S52.302   **Unspecified fracture of shaft of left radius**

⑦S52.309   **Unspecified fracture of shaft of unspecified radius**

S52.31   **Greenstick fracture of shaft of radius**

The appropriate 7th character is to be added to all codes in subcategory S52.31

A - initial encounter for closed fracture

D - subsequent encounter for fracture with routine healing

G - subsequent encounter for fracture with delayed healing

K - subsequent encounter for fracture with nonunion

P - subsequent encounter for fracture with malunion

S - sequela

⑦S52.311   **Greenstick fracture of shaft of radius, right arm**

⑦S52.312   **Greenstick fracture of shaft of radius, left arm**

⑦S52.319   **Greenstick fracture of shaft of radius, unspecified arm**

S52.32   **Transverse fracture of shaft of radius**

⑦S52.321   **Displaced transverse fracture of shaft of right radius**

⑦S52.322   **Displaced transverse fracture of shaft of left radius**

⑦S52.323   **Displaced transverse fracture of shaft of unspecified radius**

⑦S52.324   **Nondisplaced transverse fracture of shaft of right radius**

⑦S52.325   **Nondisplaced transverse fracture of shaft of left radius**

⑦S52.326   **Nondisplaced transverse fracture of shaft of unspecified radius**

S52.33   **Oblique fracture of shaft of radius**

⑦S52.331   **Displaced oblique fracture of shaft of right radius**

⑦S52.332   **Displaced oblique fracture of shaft of left radius**

⑦S52.333   **Displaced oblique fracture of shaft of unspecified radius**

⑦S52.334   **Nondisplaced oblique fracture of shaft of right radius**

⑦S52.335   **Nondisplaced oblique fracture of shaft of left radius**

⑦S52.336   **Nondisplaced oblique fracture of shaft of unspecified radius**

S52.34   **Spiral fracture of shaft of radius**

⑦S52.341   **Displaced spiral fracture of shaft of radius, right arm**

⑦S52.342   **Displaced spiral fracture of shaft of radius, left arm**

⑦S52.343   **Displaced spiral fracture of shaft of radius, unspecified arm**

⑦S52.344   **Nondisplaced spiral fracture of shaft of radius, right arm**

⑦S52.345   **Nondisplaced spiral fracture of shaft of radius, left arm**

⑦S52.346   **Nondisplaced spiral fracture of shaft of radius, unspecified arm**

S52.35   **Comminuted fracture of shaft of radius**

⑦S52.351   **Displaced comminuted fracture of shaft of radius, right arm**

⑦S52.352   **Displaced comminuted fracture of shaft of radius, left arm**

⑦S52.353   **Displaced comminuted fracture of shaft of radius, unspecified arm**

⑦S52.354   **Nondisplaced comminuted fracture of shaft of radius, right arm**

⑦S52.355   **Nondisplaced comminuted fracture of shaft of radius, left arm**

⑦S52.356   **Nondisplaced comminuted fracture of shaft of radius, unspecified arm**

S52.36   **Segmental fracture of shaft of radius**

⑦S52.361   **Displaced segmental fracture of shaft of radius, right arm**

⑦S52.362   **Displaced segmental fracture of shaft of radius, left arm**

⑦S52.363   **Displaced segmental fracture of shaft of radius, unspecified arm**

⑦S52.364   **Nondisplaced segmental fracture of shaft of radius, right arm**

⑦S52.365   **Nondisplaced segmental fracture of shaft of radius, left arm**

⑦S52.366   **Nondisplaced segmental fracture of shaft of radius, unspecified arm**

S52.37   Galeazzi's fracture

Fracture of lower shaft of radius with radioulnar joint dislocation

⑦S52.371   Galeazzi's fracture of right radius

⑦S52.372   Galeazzi's fracture of left radius

⑦S52.379   Galeazzi's fracture of unspecified radius

S52.38   Bent bone of radius

⑦S52.381   Bent bone of right radius

⑦S52.382   Bent bone of left radius

⑦S52.389   Bent bone of unspecified radius

S52.39   Other fracture of shaft of radius

⑦S52.391   Other fracture of shaft of radius, right arm

⑦S52.392   Other fracture of shaft of radius, left arm

⑦S52.399   Other fracture of shaft of radius, unspecified arm

S52.5   Fracture of lower end of radius

Fracture of distal end of radius

Excludes2: physeal fractures of lower end of radius (S59.2-)

S52.50   Unspecified fracture of the lower end of radius

⑦S52.501   Unspecified fracture of the lower end of right radius

⑦S52.502   Unspecified fracture of the lower end of left radius

⑦S52.509   Unspecified fracture of the lower end of unspecified radius

S52.51   Fracture of radial styloid process

⑦S52.511   Displaced fracture of right radial styloid process

⑦S52.512   Displaced fracture of left radial styloid process

⑦S52.513   Displaced fracture of unspecified radial styloid process

⑦S52.514   Nondisplaced fracture of right radial styloid process

⑦S52.515   Nondisplaced fracture of left radial styloid process

⑦S52.516   Nondisplaced fracture of unspecified radial styloid process

S52.52   Torus fracture of lower end of radius

The appropriate 7th character is to be added to all codes in subcategory S52.52

A - initial encounter for closed fracture

D - subsequent encounter for fracture with routine healing

G - subsequent encounter for fracture with delayed healing

K - subsequent encounter for fracture with nonunion

P - subsequent encounter for fracture with malunion

S - sequela

⑦S52.521   Torus fracture of lower end of right radius

⑦S52.522   Torus fracture of lower end of left radius

⑦S52.529   Torus fracture of lower end of unspecified radius

S52.53   Colles' fracture

⑦S52.531   Colles' fracture of right radius

⑦S52.532   Colles' fracture of left radius

⑦S52.539   Colles' fracture of unspecified radius

S52.54   Smith's fracture

⑦S52.541   Smith's fracture of right radius

⑦S52.542   Smith's fracture of left radius

⑦S52.549   Smith's fracture of unspecified radius

S52.55   Other extraarticular fracture of lower end of radius

⑦S52.551   Other extraarticular fracture of lower end of right radius

⑦S52.552   Other extraarticular fracture of lower end of left radius

⑦S52.559   Other extraarticular fracture of lower end of unspecified radius

S52.56   Barton's fracture

⑦S52.561   Barton's fracture of right radius

⑦S52.562   Barton's fracture of left radius

⑦S52.569   Barton's fracture of unspecified radius

S52.57   Other intraarticular fracture of lower end of radius

⑦S52.571   Other intraarticular fracture of lower end of right radius .

⑦S52.572   Other intraarticular fracture of lower end of left radius

⑦S52.579   Other intraarticular fracture of lower end of unspecified radius

S52.59   Other fractures of lower end of radius

⑦S52.591   Other fractures of lower end of right radius

⑦S52.592   Other fractures of lower end of left radius

⑦S52.599   Other fractures of lower end of unspecified radius

S52.6   Fracture of lower end of ulna

S52.60   Unspecified fracture of lower end of ulna

⑦S52.601   Unspecified fracture of lower end of right ulna

⑦S52.602   Unspecified fracture of lower end of left ulna

⑦S52.609   Unspecified fracture of lower end of unspecified ulna

S52.61   Fracture of ulna styloid process

⑦S52.611   Displaced fracture of right ulna styloid process

⑦S52.612   Displaced fracture of left ulna styloid process

⑦S52.613   Displaced fracture of unspecified ulna styloid process

⑦S52.614   Nondisplaced fracture of right ulna styloid process

⑦S52.615   Nondisplaced fracture of left ulna styloid process

⑦S52.616   Nondisplaced fracture of unspecified ulna styloid process

S52.62   Torus fracture of lower end of ulna

The appropriate 7th character is to be added to all codes in subcategory S52.62

A - initial encounter for closed fracture

D - subsequent encounter for fracture with routine healing

● New code   ▲ Revised code   Excludes1: Not coded here   Excludes2: Not included here   ⊗ Placeholder required   ⑦7th digit required

G - subsequent encounter for fracture with delayed healing

K - subsequent encounter for fracture with nonunion

P - subsequent encounter for fracture with malunion

S - sequela

⑦S52.621 **Torus fracture of lower end of right ulna**

⑦S52.622 **Torus fracture of lower end of left ulna**

⑦S52.629 **Torus fracture of lower end of unspecified ulna**

S52.69 **Other fracture of lower end of ulna**

⑦S52.691 **Other fracture of lower end of right ulna**

⑦S52.692 **Other fracture of lower end of left ulna**

⑦S52.699 **Other fracture of lower end of unspecified ulna**

S52.9 **Unspecified fracture of forearm**

⊗⑦S52.90 **Unspecified fracture of unspecified forearm**

⊗⑦S52.91 **Unspecified fracture of right forearm**

⊗⑦S52.92 **Unspecified fracture of left forearm**

S53 **Dislocation and sprain of joints and ligaments of elbow**

Includes: avulsion of joint or ligament of elbow

laceration of cartilage, joint or ligament of elbow sprain of cartilage, joint or ligament of elbow

traumatic hemarthrosis of joint or ligament of elbow

traumatic rupture of joint or ligament of elbow

traumatic subluxation of joint or ligament of elbow

traumatic tear of joint or ligament of elbow

Code also any associated open wound

Excludes2: strain of muscle, fascia and tendon at forearm level (S56.-)

The appropriate 7th character is to be added to each code from category S53

A - initial encounter

D - subsequent encounter

S - sequela

S53.0 **Subluxation and dislocation of radial head**

Dislocation of radiohumeral joint

Subluxation of radiohumeral joint

Excludes1: Monteggia's fracture-dislocation (S52.27-)

S53.00 **Unspecified subluxation and dislocation of radial head**

⑦S53.001 **Unspecified subluxation of right radial head**

⑦S53.002 **Unspecified subluxation of left radial head**

⑦S53.003 **Unspecified subluxation of unspecified radial head**

⑦S53.004 **Unspecified dislocation of right radial head**

⑦S53.005 **Unspecified dislocation of left radial head**

⑦S53.006 **Unspecified dislocation of unspecified radial head**

S53.01 **Anterior subluxation and dislocation of radial head**

Anteromedial subluxation and dislocation of radial head

⑦S53.011 **Anterior subluxation of right radial head**

⑦S53.012 **Anterior subluxation of left radial head**

⑦S53.013 **Anterior subluxation of unspecified radial head**

⑦S53.014 **Anterior dislocation of right radial head**

⑦S53.015 **Anterior dislocation of left radial head**

⑦S53.016 **Anterior dislocation of unspecified radial head**

S53.02 **Posterior subluxation and dislocation of radial head**

Posterolateral subluxation and dislocation of radial head

⑦S53.021 **Posterior subluxation of right radial head**

⑦S53.022 **Posterior subluxation of left radial head**

⑦S53.023 **Posterior subluxation of unspecified radial head**

⑦S53.024 **Posterior dislocation of right radial head**

⑦S53.025 **Posterior dislocation of left radial head**

⑦S53.026 **Posterior dislocation of unspecified radial head**

S53.03 **Nursemaid's elbow**

⑦S53.031 **Nursemaid's elbow, right elbow**

⑦S53.032 **Nursemaid's elbow, left elbow**

⑦S53.033 **Nursemaid's elbow, unspecified elbow**

S53.09 **Other subluxation and dislocation of radial head**

⑦S53.091 **Other subluxation of right radial head**

⑦S53.092 **Other subluxation of left radial head**

⑦S53.093 **Other subluxation of unspecified radial head**

⑦S53.094 **Other dislocation of right radial head**

⑦S53.095 **Other dislocation of left radial head**

⑦S53.096 **Other dislocation of unspecified radial head**

S53.1 **Subluxation and dislocation of ulnohumeral joint**

Subluxation and dislocation of elbow NOS

Excludes1: dislocation of radial head alone (S53.0-)

S53.10 **Unspecified subluxation and dislocation of ulnohumeral joint**

⑦S53.101 **Unspecified subluxation of right ulnohumeral joint**

⑦S53.102 **Unspecified subluxation of left ulnohumeral joint**

⑦S53.103 **Unspecified subluxation of unspecified ulnohumeral joint**

⑦S53.104 **Unspecified dislocation of right ulnohumeral joint**

⑦S53.105 **Unspecified dislocation of left ulnohumeral joint**

⑦S53.106 **Unspecified dislocation of unspecified ulnohumeral joint**

S53.11   **Anterior subluxation and dislocation of ulnohumeral joint**

⑦S53.111   **Anterior subluxation of right ulnohumeral joint**

⑦S53.112   **Anterior subluxation of left ulnohumeral joint**

⑦S53.113   **Anterior subluxation of unspecified ulnohumeral joint**

⑦S53.114   **Anterior dislocation of right ulnohumeral joint**

⑦S53.115   **Anterior dislocation of left ulnohumeral joint**

⑦S53.116   **Anterior dislocation of unspecified ulnohumeral joint**

S53.12   **Posterior subluxation and dislocation of ulnohumeral joint**

⑦S53.121   **Posterior subluxation of right ulnohumeral joint**

⑦S53.122   **Posterior subluxation of left ulnohumeral joint**

⑦S53.123   **Posterior subluxation of unspecified ulnohumeral joint**

⑦S53.124   **Posterior dislocation of right ulnohumeral joint**

⑦S53.125   **Posterior dislocation of left ulnohumeral joint**

⑦S53.126   **Posterior dislocation of unspecified ulnohumeral joint**

S53.13   **Medial subluxation and dislocation of ulnohumeral joint**

⑦S53.131   **Medial subluxation of right ulnohumeral joint**

⑦S53.132   **Medial subluxation of left ulnohumeral joint**

⑦S53.133   **Medial subluxation of unspecified ulnohumeral joint**

⑦S53.134   **Medial dislocation of right ulnohumeral joint**

⑦S53.135   **Medial dislocation of left ulnohumeral joint**

⑦S53.136   **Medial dislocation of unspecified ulnohumeral joint**

S53.14   **Lateral subluxation and dislocation of ulnohumeral joint**

⑦S53.141   **Lateral subluxation of right ulnohumeral joint**

⑦S53.142   **Lateral subluxation of left ulnohumeral joint**

⑦S53.143   **Lateral subluxation of unspecified ulnohumeral joint**

⑦S53.144   **Lateral dislocation of right ulnohumeral joint**

⑦S53.145   **Lateral dislocation of left ulnohumeral joint**

⑦S53.146   **Lateral dislocation of unspecified ulnohumeral joint**

S53.19   **Other subluxation and dislocation of ulnohumeral joint**

⑦S53.191   **Other subluxation of right ulnohumeral joint**

⑦S53.192   **Other subluxation of left ulnohumeral joint**

⑦S53.193   **Other subluxation of unspecified ulnohumeral joint**

⑦S53.194   **Other dislocation of right ulnohumeral joint**

⑦S53.195   **Other dislocation of left ulnohumeral joint**

⑦S53.196   **Other dislocation of unspecified ulnohumeral joint**

S53.2   **Traumatic rupture of radial collateral ligament**

> **Excludes1:** sprain of radial collateral ligament NOS (S53.43-)

⊗⑦S53.20   **Traumatic rupture of unspecified radial collateral ligament**

⊗⑦S53.21   **Traumatic rupture of right radial collateral ligament**

⊗⑦S53.22   **Traumatic rupture of left radial collateral ligament**

S53.3   **Traumatic rupture of ulnar collateral ligament**

> **Excludes1:** sprain of ulnar collateral ligament (S53.44-)

⊗⑦S53.30   **Traumatic rupture of unspecified ulnar collateral ligament**

⊗⑦S53.31   **Traumatic rupture of right ulnar collateral ligament**

⊗⑦S53.32   **Traumatic rupture of left ulnar collateral ligament**

S53.4   **Sprain of elbow**

> **Excludes2:** traumatic rupture of radial collateral ligament (S53.2-)
>
> traumatic rupture of ulnar collateral ligament (S53.3-)

S53.40   **Unspecified sprain of elbow**

⑦S53.401   **Unspecified sprain of right elbow**

⑦S53.402   **Unspecified sprain of left elbow**

⑦S53.409   **Unspecified sprain of unspecified elbow**

Sprain of elbow NOS

S53.41   **Radiohumeral (joint) sprain**

⑦S53.411   **Radiohumeral (joint) sprain of right elbow**

⑦S53.412   **Radiohumeral (joint) sprain of left elbow**

⑦S53.419   **Radiohumeral (joint) sprain of unspecified elbow**

S53.42   **Ulnohumeral (joint) sprain**

⑦S53.421   **Ulnohumeral (joint) sprain of right elbow**

⑦S53.422   **Ulnohumeral (joint) sprain of left elbow**

⑦S53.429   **Ulnohumeral (joint) sprain of unspecified elbow**

S53.43   **Radial collateral ligament sprain**

⑦S53.431   **Radial collateral ligament sprain of right elbow**

⑦S53.432   **Radial collateral ligament sprain of left elbow**

⑦S53.439   **Radial collateral ligament sprain of unspecified elbow**

S53.44   **Ulnar collateral ligament sprain**

⑦S53.441   **Ulnar collateral ligament sprain of right elbow**

⑦S53.442   **Ulnar collateral ligament sprain of left elbow**

⑦S53.449   **Ulnar collateral ligament sprain of unspecified elbow**

S53.49   Other sprain of elbow

⑦S53.491   Other sprain of right elbow

⑦S53.492   Other sprain of left elbow

⑦S53.499   Other sprain of unspecified elbow

S54   **Injury of nerves at forearm level**

Code also any associated open wound (S51.-)

Excludes2: injury of nerves at wrist and hand level (S64.-)

The appropriate 7th character is to be added to each code from category S54

A - initial encounter

D - subsequent encounter

S - sequela

S54.0   **Injury of ulnar nerve at forearm level**

Injury of ulnar nerve NOS

⊗⑦S54.00   Injury of ulnar nerve at forearm level, unspecified arm

⊗⑦S54.01   Injury of ulnar nerve at forearm level, right arm

⊗⑦S54.02   Injury of ulnar nerve at forearm level, left arm

S54.1   **Injury of median nerve at forearm level**

Injury of median nerve NOS

⊗⑦S54.10   Injury of median nerve at forearm level, unspecified arm

⊗⑦S54.11   Injury of median nerve at forearm level, right arm

⊗⑦S54.12   Injury of median nerve at forearm level, left arm

S54.2   **Injury of radial nerve at forearm level**

Injury of radial nerve NOS

⊗⑦S54.20   Injury of radial nerve at forearm level, unspecified arm

⊗⑦S54.21   Injury of radial nerve at forearm level, right arm

⊗⑦S54.22   Injury of radial nerve at forearm level, left arm

S54.3   **Injury of cutaneous sensory nerve at forearm level**

⊗⑦S54.30   Injury of cutaneous sensory nerve at forearm level, unspecified arm

⊗⑦S54.31   Injury of cutaneous sensory nerve at forearm level, right arm

⊗⑦S54.32   Injury of cutaneous sensory nerve at forearm level, left arm

S54.8   **Injury of other nerves at forearm level**

S54.8X   **Injury of other nerves at forearm level**

⑦S54.8X1   Injury of other nerves at forearm level, right arm

⑦S54.8X2   Injury of other nerves at forearm level, left arm

⑦S54.8X9   Injury of other nerves at forearm level, unspecified arm

S54.9   **Injury of unspecified nerve at forearm level**

⊗⑦S54.90   Injury of unspecified nerve at forearm level, unspecified arm

⊗⑦S54.91   Injury of unspecified nerve at forearm level, right arm

⊗⑦S54.92   Injury of unspecified nerve at forearm level, left arm

S55   **Injury of blood vessels at forearm level**

Code also any associated open wound (S51.-)

Excludes2: injury of blood vessels at wrist and hand level (S65.-)

injury of brachial vessels (S45.1-S45.2)

The appropriate 7th character is to be added to each code from category S55

A - initial encounter

D - subsequent encounter

S - sequela

S55.0   **Injury of ulnar artery at forearm level**

S55.00   **Unspecified injury of ulnar artery at forearm level**

⑦S55.001   Unspecified injury of ulnar artery at forearm level, right arm

⑦S55.002   Unspecified injury of ulnar artery at forearm level, left arm

⑦S55.009   Unspecified injury of ulnar artery at forearm level, unspecified arm

S55.01   **Laceration of ulnar artery at forearm level**

⑦S55.011   Laceration of ulnar artery at forearm level, right arm

⑦S55.012   Laceration of ulnar artery at forearm level, left arm

⑦S55.019   Laceration of ulnar artery at forearm level, unspecified arm

S55.09   **Other specified injury of ulnar artery at forearm level**

⑦S55.091   Other specified injury of ulnar artery at forearm level, right arm

⑦S55.092   Other specified injury of ulnar artery at forearm level, left arm

⑦S55.099   Other specified injury of ulnar artery at forearm level, unspecified arm

S55.1   **Injury of radial artery at forearm level**

S55.10   **Unspecified injury of radial artery at forearm level**

⑦S55.101   Unspecified injury of radial artery at forearm level, right arm

⑦S55.102   Unspecified injury of radial artery at forearm level, left arm

⑦S55.109   Unspecified injury of radial artery at forearm level, unspecified arm

S55.11   **Laceration of radial artery at forearm level**

⑦S55.111   Laceration of radial artery at forearm level, right arm

⑦S55.112   Laceration of radial artery at forearm level, left arm

⑦S55.119   Laceration of radial artery at forearm level, unspecified arm

S55.19   **Other specified injury of radial artery at forearm level**

⑦S55.191   Other specified injury of radial artery at forearm level, right arm

⑦S55.192   Other specified injury of radial artery at forearm level, left arm

⑦S55.199   Other specified injury of radial artery at forearm level, unspecified arm

S55.2   **Injury of vein at forearm level**

S55.20   **Unspecified injury of vein at forearm level**

⑦S55.201   Unspecified injury of vein at forearm level, right arm

⑦S55.202   Unspecified injury of vein at forearm level, left arm

⑦S55.209   Unspecified injury of vein at forearm level, unspecified arm

S55.21   Laceration of vein at forearm level

⑦S55.211   Laceration of vein at forearm level, right arm

⑦S55.212   Laceration of vein at forearm level, left arm

⑦S55.219   Laceration of vein at forearm level, unspecified arm

S55.29   Other specified injury of vein at forearm level

⑦S55.291   Other specified injury of vein at forearm level, right arm

⑦S55.292   Other specified injury of vein at forearm level, left arm

⑦S55.299   Other specified injury of vein at forearm level, unspecified arm

S55.8   Injury of other blood vessels at forearm level

S55.80   Unspecified injury of other blood vessels at forearm level

⑦S55.801   Unspecified injury of other blood vessels at forearm level, right arm

⑦S55.802   Unspecified injury of other blood vessels at forearm level, left arm

⑦S55.809   Unspecified injury of other blood vessels at forearm level, unspecified arm

S55.81   Laceration of other blood vessels at forearm level

⑦S55.811   Laceration of other blood vessels at forearm level, right arm

⑦S55.812   Laceration of other blood vessels at forearm level, left arm

⑦S55.819   Laceration of other blood vessels at forearm level, unspecified arm

S55.89   Other specified injury of other blood vessels at forearm level

⑦S55.891   Other specified injury of other blood vessels at forearm level, right arm

⑦S55.892   Other specified injury of other blood vessels at forearm level, left arm

⑦S55.899   Other specified injury of other blood vessels at forearm level, unspecified arm

S55.9   Injury of unspecified blood vessel at forearm level

S55.90   Unspecified injury of unspecified blood vessel at forearm level

⑦S55.901   Unspecified injury of unspecified blood vessel at forearm level, right arm

⑦S55.902   Unspecified injury of unspecified blood vessel at forearm level, left arm

⑦S55.909   Unspecified injury of unspecified blood vessel at forearm level, unspecified arm

S55.91   Laceration of unspecified blood vessel at forearm level

⑦S55.911   Laceration of unspecified blood vessel at forearm level, right arm

⑦S55.912   Laceration of unspecified blood vessel at forearm level, left arm

⑦S55.919   Laceration of unspecified blood vessel at forearm level, unspecified arm

S55.99   Other specified injury of unspecified blood vessel at forearm level

⑦S55.991   Other specified injury of unspecified blood vessel at forearm level, right arm

⑦S55.992   Other specified injury of unspecified blood vessel at forearm level, left arm

⑦S55.999   Other specified injury of unspecified blood vessel at forearm level, unspecified arm

S56   **Injury of muscle, fascia and tendon at forearm level**

Code also any associated open wound (S51.-)

Excludes2: injury of muscle, fascia and tendon at or below wrist (S66.-)

sprain of joints and ligaments of elbow (S53.4-)

The appropriate 7th character is to be added to each code from category S56

A - initial encounter

D - subsequent encounter

S - sequela

S56.0   Injury of flexor muscle, fascia and tendon of thumb at forearm level

S56.00   Unspecified injury of flexor muscle, fascia and tendon of thumb at forearm level

⑦S56.001   Unspecified injury of flexor muscle, fascia and tendon of right thumb at forearm level

⑦S56.002   Unspecified injury of flexor muscle, fascia and tendon of left thumb at forearm level

⑦S56.009   Unspecified injury of flexor muscle, fascia and tendon of unspecified thumb at forearm level

S56.01   Strain of flexor muscle, fascia and tendon of thumb at forearm level

⑦S56.011   Strain of flexor muscle, fascia and tendon of right thumb at forearm level

⑦S56.012   Strain of flexor muscle, fascia and tendon of left thumb at forearm level

⑦S56.019   Strain of flexor muscle, fascia and tendon of unspecified thumb at forearm level

S56.02   Laceration of flexor muscle, fascia and tendon of thumb at forearm level

⑦S56.021   Laceration of flexor muscle, fascia and tendon of right thumb at forearm level

⑦S56.022   Laceration of flexor muscle, fascia and tendon of left thumb at forearm level

⑦S56.029   Laceration of flexor muscle, fascia and tendon of unspecified thumb at forearm level

S56.09   Other injury of flexor muscle, fascia and tendon of thumb at forearm level

⑦S56.091   Other injury of flexor muscle, fascia and tendon of right thumb at forearm level

⑦S56.092   Other injury of flexor muscle, fascia and tendon of left thumb at forearm level

⑦S56.099   Other injury of flexor muscle, fascia and tendon of unspecified thumb at forearm level

S56.1   Injury of flexor muscle, fascia and tendon of other and unspecified finger at forearm level

S56.10   Unspecified injury of flexor muscle, fascia and tendon of other and unspecified finger at forearm level

⑦S56.101   Unspecified injury of flexor muscle, fascia and tendon of right index finger at forearm level

⑦S56.102   Unspecified injury of flexor muscle, fascia and tendon of left index finger at forearm level

⑦S56.103   Unspecified injury of flexor muscle, fascia and tendon of right middle finger at forearm level

⑦S56.104   Unspecified injury of flexor muscle, fascia and tendon of left middle finger at forearm level

⑦S56.105   Unspecified injury of flexor muscle, fascia and tendon of right ring finger at forearm level

⑦S56.106   Unspecified injury of flexor muscle, fascia and tendon of left ring finger at forearm level

⑦S56.107   Unspecified injury of flexor muscle, fascia and tendon of right little finger at forearm level

⑦S56.108   Unspecified injury of flexor muscle, fascia and tendon of left little finger at forearm level

⑦S56.109   Unspecified injury of flexor muscle, fascia and tendon of unspecified finger at forearm level

S56.11   Strain of flexor muscle, fascia and tendon of other and unspecified finger at forearm level

⑦S56.111   Strain of flexor muscle, fascia and tendon of right index finger at forearm level

⑦S56.112   Strain of flexor muscle, fascia and tendon of left index finger at forearm level

⑦S56.113   Strain of flexor muscle, fascia and tendon of right middle finger at forearm level

⑦S56.114   Strain of flexor muscle, fascia and tendon of left middle finger at forearm level

⑦S56.115   Strain of flexor muscle, fascia and tendon of right ring finger at forearm level

⑦S56.116   Strain of flexor muscle, fascia and tendon of left ring finger at forearm level

⑦S56.117   Strain of flexor muscle, fascia and tendon of right little finger at forearm level

⑦S56.118   Strain of flexor muscle, fascia and tendon of left little finger at forearm level

⑦S56.119   Strain of flexor muscle, fascia and tendon of finger of unspecified finger at forearm level

S56.12   Laceration of flexor muscle, fascia and tendon of other and unspecified finger at forearm level

⑦S56.121   Laceration of flexor muscle, fascia and tendon of right index finger at forearm level

⑦S56.122   Laceration of flexor muscle, fascia and tendon of left index finger at forearm level

⑦S56.123   Laceration of flexor muscle, fascia and tendon of right middle finger at forearm level

⑦S56.124   Laceration of flexor muscle, fascia and tendon of left middle finger at forearm level

⑦S56.125   Laceration of flexor muscle, fascia and tendon of right ring finger at forearm level

⑦S56.126   Laceration of flexor muscle, fascia and tendon of left ring finger at forearm level

⑦S56.127   Laceration of flexor muscle, fascia and tendon of right little finger at forearm level

⑦S56.128   Laceration of flexor muscle, fascia and tendon of left little finger at forearm level

⑦S56.129   Laceration of flexor muscle, fascia and tendon of unspecified finger at forearm level

S56.19   Other injury of flexor muscle, fascia and tendon of other and unspecified finger at forearm level

⑦S56.191   Other injury of flexor muscle, fascia and tendon of right index finger at forearm level

⑦S56.192   Other injury of flexor muscle, fascia and tendon of left index finger at forearm level

⑦S56.193   Other injury of flexor muscle, fascia and tendon of right middle finger at forearm level

⑦S56.194   Other injury of flexor muscle, fascia and tendon of left middle finger at forearm level

⑦S56.195   Other injury of flexor muscle, fascia and tendon of right ring finger at forearm level

⑦S56.196   Other injury of flexor muscle, fascia and tendon of left ring finger at forearm level

⑦S56.197   Other injury of flexor muscle, fascia and tendon of right little finger at forearm level

⑦S56.198   Other injury of flexor muscle, fascia and tendon of left little finger at forearm level

⑦S56.199   Other injury of flexor muscle, fascia and tendon of unspecified finger at forearm level

S56.2   Injury of other flexor muscle, fascia and tendon at forearm level

S56.20   Unspecified injury of other flexor muscle, fascia and tendon at forearm level

⑦S56.201   Unspecified injury of other flexor muscle, fascia and tendon at forearm level, right arm

⑦S56.202   Unspecified injury of other flexor muscle, fascia and tendon at forearm level, left arm

⑦S56.209   Unspecified injury of other flexor muscle, fascia and tendon at forearm level, unspecified arm

S56.21   Strain of other flexor muscle, fascia and tendon at forearm level

⑦ **S56.211   Strain of other flexor muscle, fascia and tendon at forearm level, right arm**

⑦ **S56.212   Strain of other flexor muscle, fascia and tendon at forearm level, left arm**

⑦ **S56.219   Strain of other flexor muscle, fascia and tendon at forearm level, unspecified arm**

S56.22   Laceration of other flexor muscle, fascia and tendon at forearm level

⑦ **S56.221   Laceration of other flexor muscle, fascia and tendon at forearm level, right arm**

⑦ **S56.222   Laceration of other flexor muscle, fascia and tendon at forearm level, left arm**

⑦ **S56.229   Laceration of other flexor muscle, fascia and tendon at forearm level, unspecified arm**

S56.29   Other injury of other flexor muscle, fascia and tendon at forearm level

⑦ **S56.291   Other injury of other flexor muscle, fascia and tendon at forearm level, right arm**

⑦ **S56.292   Other injury of other flexor muscle, fascia and tendon at forearm level, left arm**

⑦ **S56.299   Other injury of other flexor muscle, fascia and tendon at forearm level, unspecified arm**

S56.3   Injury of extensor or abductor muscles, fascia and tendons of thumb at forearm level

S56.30   Unspecified injury of extensor or abductor muscles, fascia and tendons of thumb at forearm level

⑦ **S56.301   Unspecified injury of extensor or abductor muscles, fascia and tendons of right thumb at forearm level**

⑦ **S56.302   Unspecified injury of extensor or abductor muscles, fascia and tendons of left thumb at forearm level**

⑦ **S56.309   Unspecified injury of extensor or abductor muscles, fascia and tendons of unspecified thumb at forearm level**

S56.31   Strain of extensor or abductor muscles, fascia and tendons of thumb at forearm level

⑦ **S56.311   Strain of extensor or abductor muscles, fascia and tendons of right thumb at forearm level**

⑦ **S56.312   Strain of extensor or abductor muscles, fascia and tendons of left thumb at forearm level**

⑦ **S56.319   Strain of extensor or abductor muscles, fascia and tendons of unspecified thumb at forearm level**

S56.32   Laceration of extensor or abductor muscles, fascia and tendons of thumb at forearm level

⑦ **S56.321   Laceration of extensor or abductor muscles, fascia and tendons of right thumb at forearm level**

⑦ **S56.322   Laceration of extensor or abductor muscles, fascia and tendons of left thumb at forearm level**

⑦ **S56.329   Laceration of extensor or abductor muscles, fascia and tendons of unspecified thumb at forearm level**

S56.39   Other injury of extensor or abductor muscles, fascia and tendons of thumb at forearm level

⑦ **S56.391   Other injury of extensor or abductor muscles, fascia and tendons of right thumb at forearm level**

⑦ **S56.392   Other injury of extensor or abductor muscles, fascia and tendons of left thumb at forearm level**

⑦ **S56.399   Other injury of extensor or abductor muscles, fascia and tendons of unspecified thumb at forearm level**

S56.4   Injury of extensor muscle, fascia and tendon of other and unspecified finger at forearm level

S56.40   Unspecified injury of extensor muscle, fascia and tendon of other and unspecified finger at forearm level

⑦ **S56.401   Unspecified injury of extensor muscle, fascia and tendon of right index finger at forearm level**

⑦ **S56.402   Unspecified injury of extensor muscle, fascia and tendon of left index finger at forearm level**

⑦ **S56.403   Unspecified injury of extensor muscle, fascia and tendon of right middle finger at forearm level**

⑦ **S56.404   Unspecified injury of extensor muscle, fascia and tendon of left middle finger at forearm level**

⑦ **S56.405   Unspecified injury of extensor muscle, fascia and tendon of right ring finger at forearm level**

⑦ **S56.406   Unspecified injury of extensor muscle, fascia and tendon of left ring finger at forearm level**

⑦ **S56.407   Unspecified injury of extensor muscle, fascia and tendon of right little finger at forearm level**

⑦ **S56.408   Unspecified injury of extensor muscle, fascia and tendon of left little finger at forearm level**

⑦ **S56.409   Unspecified injury of extensor muscle, fascia and tendon of unspecified finger at forearm level**

S56.41   Strain of extensor muscle, fascia and tendon of other and unspecified finger at forearm level

⑦ **S56.411   Strain of extensor muscle, fascia and tendon of right index finger at forearm level**

⑦ **S56.412   Strain of extensor muscle, fascia and tendon of left index finger at forearm level**

⑦ **S56.413   Strain of extensor muscle, fascia and tendon of right middle finger at forearm level**

⑦ **S56.414   Strain of extensor muscle, fascia and tendon of left middle finger at forearm level**

⑦ **S56.415   Strain of extensor muscle, fascia and tendon of right ring finger at forearm level**

⑦ **S56.416   Strain of extensor muscle, fascia and tendon of left ring finger at forearm level**

● New code   ▲ Revised code   **Excludes1:** Not coded here   **Excludes2:** Not included here   ⊗ Placeholder required   ⑦ 7th digit required

⑦S56.417 **Strain of extensor muscle, fascia and tendon of right little finger at forearm level**

⑦S56.418 **Strain of extensor muscle, fascia and tendon of left little finger at forearm level**

⑦S56.419 **Strain of extensor muscle, fascia and tendon of finger, unspecified finger at forearm level**

S56.42 **Laceration of extensor muscle, fascia and tendon of other and unspecified finger at forearm level**

⑦S56.421 **Laceration of extensor muscle, fascia and tendon of right index finger at forearm level**

⑦S56.422 **Laceration of extensor muscle, fascia and tendon of left index finger at forearm level**

⑦S56.423 **Laceration of extensor muscle, fascia and tendon of right middle finger at forearm level**

⑦S56.424 **Laceration of extensor muscle, fascia and tendon of left middle finger at forearm level**

⑦S56.425 **Laceration of extensor muscle, fascia and tendon of right ring finger at forearm level**

⑦S56.426 **Laceration of extensor muscle, fascia and tendon of left ring finger at forearm level**

⑦S56.427 **Laceration of extensor muscle, fascia and tendon of right little finger at forearm level**

⑦S56.428 **Laceration of extensor muscle, fascia and tendon of left little finger at forearm level**

⑦S56.429 **Laceration of extensor muscle, fascia and tendon of unspecified finger at forearm level**

S56.49 **Other injury of extensor muscle, fascia and tendon of other and unspecified finger at forearm level**

⑦S56.491 **Other injury of extensor muscle, fascia and tendon of right index finger at forearm level**

⑦S56.492 **Other injury of extensor muscle, fascia and tendon of left index finger at forearm level**

⑦S56.493 **Other injury of extensor muscle, fascia and tendon of right middle finger at forearm level**

⑦S56.494 **Other injury of extensor muscle, fascia and tendon of left middle finger at forearm level**

⑦S56.495 **Other injury of extensor muscle, fascia and tendon of right ring finger at forearm level**

⑦S56.496 **Other injury of extensor muscle, fascia and tendon of left ring finger at forearm level**

⑦S56.497 **Other injury of extensor muscle, fascia and tendon of right little finger at forearm level**

⑦S56.498 **Other injury of extensor muscle, fascia and tendon of left little finger at forearm level**

⑦S56.499 **Other injury of extensor muscle, fascia and tendon of unspecified finger at forearm level**

S56.5 **Injury of other extensor muscle, fascia and tendon at forearm level**

S56.50 **Unspecified injury of other extensor muscle, fascia and tendon at forearm level**

⑦S56.501 **Unspecified injury of other extensor muscle, fascia and tendon at forearm level, right arm**

⑦S56.502 **Unspecified injury of other extensor muscle, fascia and tendon at forearm level, left arm**

⑦S56.509 **Unspecified injury of other extensor muscle, fascia and tendon at forearm level, unspecified arm**

S56.51 **Strain of other extensor muscle, fascia and tendon at forearm level**

⑦S56.511 **Strain of other extensor muscle, fascia and tendon at forearm level, right arm**

⑦S56.512 **Strain of other extensor muscle, fascia and tendon at forearm level, left arm**

⑦S56.519 **Strain of other extensor muscle, fascia and tendon at forearm level, unspecified arm**

S56.52 **Laceration of other extensor muscle, fascia and tendon at forearm level**

⑦S56.521 **Laceration of other extensor muscle, fascia and tendon at forearm level, right arm**

⑦S56.522 **Laceration of other extensor muscle, fascia and tendon at forearm level, left arm**

⑦S56.529 **Laceration of other extensor muscle, fascia and tendon at forearm level, unspecified arm**

S56.59 **Other injury of other extensor muscle, fascia and tendon at forearm level**

⑦S56.591 **Other injury of other extensor muscle, fascia and tendon at forearm level, right arm**

⑦S56.592 **Other injury of other extensor muscle, fascia and tendon at forearm level, left arm**

⑦S56.599 **Other injury of other extensor muscle, fascia and tendon at forearm level, unspecified arm**

S56.8 **Injury of other muscles, fascia and tendons at forearm level**

S56.80 **Unspecified injury of other muscles, fascia and tendons at forearm level**

⑦S56.801 **Unspecified injury of other muscles, fascia and tendons at forearm level, right arm**

⑦S56.802 **Unspecified injury of other muscles, fascia and tendons at forearm level, left arm**

⑦S56.809 **Unspecified injury of other muscles, fascia and tendons at forearm level, unspecified arm**

S56.81 **Strain of other muscles, fascia and tendons at forearm level**

⑦S56.811 **Strain of other muscles, fascia and tendons at forearm level, right arm**

⑦S56.812   **Strain of other muscles, fascia and tendons at forearm level, left arm**

⑦S56.819   **Strain of other muscles, fascia and tendons at forearm level, unspecified arm**

S56.82   **Laceration of other muscles, fascia and tendons at forearm level**

⑦S56.821   **Laceration of other muscles, fascia and tendons at forearm level, right arm**

⑦S56.822   **Laceration of other muscles, fascia and tendons at forearm level, left arm**

⑦S56.829   **Laceration of other muscles, fascia and tendons at forearm level, unspecified arm**

S56.89   **Other injury of other muscles, fascia and tendons at forearm level**

⑦S56.891   **Other injury of other muscles, fascia and tendons at forearm level, right arm**

⑦S56.892   **Other injury of other muscles, fascia and tendons at forearm level, left arm**

⑦S56.899   **Other injury of other muscles, fascia and tendons at forearm level, unspecified arm**

S56.9   **Injury of unspecified muscles, fascia and tendons at forearm level**

S56.90   **Unspecified injury of unspecified muscles, fascia and tendons at forearm level**

⑦S56.901   **Unspecified injury of unspecified muscles, fascia and tendons at forearm level, right arm**

⑦S56.902   **Unspecified injury of unspecified muscles, fascia and tendons at forearm level, left arm**

⑦S56.909   **Unspecified injury of unspecified muscles, fascia and tendons at forearm level, unspecified arm**

S56.91   **Strain of unspecified muscles, fascia and tendons at forearm level**

⑦S56.911   **Strain of unspecified muscles, fascia and tendons at forearm level, right arm**

⑦S56.912   **Strain of unspecified muscles, fascia and tendons at forearm level, left arm**

⑦S56.919   **Strain of unspecified muscles, fascia and tendons at forearm level, unspecified arm**

S56.92   **Laceration of unspecified muscles, fascia and tendons at forearm level**

⑦S56.921   **Laceration of unspecified muscles, fascia and tendons at forearm level, right arm**

⑦S56.922   **Laceration of unspecified muscles, fascia and tendons at forearm level, left arm**

⑦S56.929   **Laceration of unspecified muscles, fascia and tendons at forearm level, unspecified arm**

S56.99   **Other injury of unspecified muscles, fascia and tendons at forearm level**

⑦S56.991   **Other injury of unspecified muscles, fascia and tendons at forearm level, right arm**

⑦S56.992   **Other injury of unspecified muscles, fascia and tendons at forearm level, left arm**

⑦S56.999   **Other injury of unspecified muscles, fascia and tendons at forearm level, unspecified arm**

S57   **Crushing injury of elbow and forearm**

Use Additional Code(s) for all associated injuries

Excludes2: crushing injury of wrist and hand (S67.-)

The appropriate 7th character is to be added to each code from category S57

A - initial encounter

D - subsequent encounter

S - sequela

S57.0   **Crushing injury of elbow**

⊗⑦S57.00   **Crushing injury of unspecified elbow**

⊗⑦S57.01   **Crushing injury of right elbow**

⊗⑦S57.02   **Crushing injury of left elbow**

S57.8   **Crushing injury of forearm**

⊗⑦S57.80   **Crushing injury of unspecified forearm**

⊗⑦S57.81   **Crushing injury of right forearm**

⊗⑦S57.82   **Crushing injury of left forearm**

S58   **Traumatic amputation of elbow and forearm**

An amputation not identified as partial or complete should be coded to complete

Excludes1: traumatic amputation of wrist and hand (S68.-)

The appropriate 7th character is to be added to each code from category S58

A - initial encounter

D - subsequent encounter

S - sequela

S58.0   **Traumatic amputation at elbow level**

S58.01   **Complete traumatic amputation at elbow level**

⑦S58.011   **Complete traumatic amputation at elbow level, right arm** [HCC]

⑦S58.012   **Complete traumatic amputation at elbow level, left arm** [HCC]

⑦S58.019   **Complete traumatic amputation at elbow level, unspecified arm** [HCC]

S58.02   **Partial traumatic amputation at elbow level**

⑦S58.021   **Partial traumatic amputation at elbow level, right arm** [HCC]

⑦S58.022   **Partial traumatic amputation at elbow level, left arm** [HCC]

⑦S58.029   **Partial traumatic amputation at elbow level, unspecified arm** [HCC]

S58.1   **Traumatic amputation at level between elbow and wrist**

S58.11   **Complete traumatic amputation at level between elbow and wrist**

⑦S58.111   **Complete traumatic amputation at level between elbow and wrist, right arm** [HCC]

⑦S58.112   **Complete traumatic amputation at level between elbow and wrist, left arm** [HCC]

⑦S58.119   **Complete traumatic amputation at level between elbow and wrist, unspecified arm** [HCC]

S58.12   **Partial traumatic amputation at level between elbow and wrist**

⑦**S58.121**   **Partial traumatic amputation at level between elbow and wrist, right arm** [HCC]

⑦**S58.122**   **Partial traumatic amputation at level between elbow and wrist, left arm** [HCC]

⑦**S58.129**   **Partial traumatic amputation at level between elbow and wrist, unspecified arm** [HCC]

S58.9   **Traumatic amputation of forearm, level unspecified**

> **Excludes1:** traumatic amputation of wrist (S68.-)

S58.91   **Complete traumatic amputation of forearm, level unspecified**

⑦**S58.911**   **Complete traumatic amputation of right forearm, level unspecified** [HCC]

⑦**S58.912**   **Complete traumatic amputation of left forearm, level unspecified** [HCC]

⑦**S58.919**   **Complete traumatic amputation of unspecified forearm, level unspecified** [HCC]

S58.92   **Partial traumatic amputation of forearm, level unspecified**

⑦**S58.921**   **Partial traumatic amputation of right forearm, level unspecified** [HCC]

⑦**S58.922**   **Partial traumatic amputation of left forearm, level unspecified** [HCC]

⑦**S58.929**   **Partial traumatic amputation of unspecified forearm, level unspecified** [HCC]

S59   **Other and unspecified injuries of elbow and forearm**

> **Excludes2:** Other and unspecified injuries of wrist and hand (S69.-)

The appropriate 7th character is to be added to each code from subcategories S59.0, S59.1, and S59.2

A - initial encounter for closed fracture

D - subsequent encounter for fracture with routine healing

G - subsequent encounter for fracture with delayed healing

K - subsequent encounter for fracture with nonunion

P - subsequent encounter for fracture with malunion

S - sequela

S59.0   **Physeal fracture of lower end of ulna**

S59.00   **Unspecified physeal fracture of lower end of ulna**

⑦**S59.001**   **Unspecified physeal fracture of lower end of ulna, right arm**

⑦**S59.002**   **Unspecified physeal fracture of lower end of ulna, left arm**

⑦**S59.009**   **Unspecified physeal fracture of lower end of ulna, unspecified arm**

S59.01   **Salter-Harris Type I physeal fracture of lower end of ulna**

⑦**S59.011**   **Salter-Harris Type I physeal fracture of lower end of ulna, right arm**

⑦**S59.012**   **Salter-Harris Type I physeal fracture of lower end of ulna, left arm**

⑦**S59.019**   **Salter-Harris Type I physeal fracture of lower end of ulna, unspecified arm**

S59.02   **Salter-Harris Type II physeal fracture of lower end of ulna**

⑦**S59.021**   **Salter-Harris Type II physeal fracture of lower end of ulna, right arm**

⑦**S59.022**   **Salter-Harris Type II physeal fracture of lower end of ulna, left arm**

⑦**S59.029**   **Salter-Harris Type II physeal fracture of lower end of ulna, unspecified arm**

S59.03   **Salter-Harris Type III physeal fracture of lower end of ulna**

⑦**S59.031**   **Salter-Harris Type III physeal fracture of lower end of ulna, right arm**

⑦**S59.032**   **Salter-Harris Type III physeal fracture of lower end of ulna, left arm**

⑦**S59.039**   **Salter-Harris Type III physeal fracture of lower end of ulna, unspecified arm**

S59.04   **Salter-Harris Type IV physeal fracture of lower end of ulna**

⑦**S59.041**   **Salter-Harris Type IV physeal fracture of lower end of ulna, right arm**

⑦**S59.042**   **Salter-Harris Type IV physeal fracture of lower end of ulna, left arm**

⑦**S59.049**   **Salter-Harris Type IV physeal fracture of lower end of ulna, unspecified arm**

S59.09   **Other physeal fracture of lower end of ulna**

⑦**S59.091**   **Other physeal fracture of lower end of ulna, right arm**

⑦**S59.092**   **Other physeal fracture of lower end of ulna, left arm**

⑦**S59.099**   **Other physeal fracture of lower end of ulna, unspecified arm**

S59.1   **Physeal fracture of upper end of radius**

S59.10   **Unspecified physeal fracture of upper end of radius**

⑦**S59.101**   **Unspecified physeal fracture of upper end of radius, right arm**

⑦**S59.102**   **Unspecified physeal fracture of upper end of radius, left arm**

⑦**S59.109**   **Unspecified physeal fracture of upper end of radius, unspecified arm**

S59.11   **Salter-Harris Type I physeal fracture of upper end of radius**

⑦**S59.111**   **Salter-Harris Type I physeal fracture of upper end of radius, right arm**

⑦**S59.112**   **Salter-Harris Type I physeal fracture of upper end of radius, left arm**

⑦**S59.119**   **Salter-Harris Type I physeal fracture of upper end of radius, unspecified arm**

S59.12   **Salter-Harris Type II physeal fracture of upper end of radius**

⑦**S59.121**   **Salter-Harris Type II physeal fracture of upper end of radius, right arm**

⑦**S59.122**   **Salter-Harris Type II physeal fracture of upper end of radius, left arm**

⑦S59.129   Salter-Harris Type II physeal fracture of upper end of radius, unspecified arm

S59.13   Salter-Harris Type III physeal fracture of upper end of radius

⑦S59.131   Salter-Harris Type III physeal fracture of upper end of radius, right arm

⑦S59.132   Salter-Harris Type III physeal fracture of upper end of radius, left arm

⑦S59.139   Salter-Harris Type III physeal fracture of upper end of radius, unspecified arm

S59.14   Salter-Harris Type IV physeal fracture of upper end of radius

⑦S59.141   Salter-Harris Type IV physeal fracture of upper end of radius, right arm

⑦S59.142   Salter-Harris Type IV physeal fracture of upper end of radius, left arm

⑦S59.149   Salter-Harris Type IV physeal fracture of upper end of radius, unspecified arm

S59.19   Other physeal fracture of upper end of radius

S59.191   Other physeal fracture of upper end of radius, right arm

⑦S59.192   Other physeal fracture of upper end of radius, left arm

⑦S59.199   Other physeal fracture of upper end of radius, unspecified arm

S59.2   Physeal fracture of lower end of radius

S59.20   Unspecified physeal fracture of lower end of radius

⑦S59.201   Unspecified physeal fracture of lower end of radius, right arm

⑦S59.202   Unspecified physeal fracture of lower end of radius, left arm

⑦S59.209   Unspecified physeal fracture of lower end of radius, unspecified arm

S59.21   Salter-Harris Type I physeal fracture of lower end of radius

⑦S59.211   Salter-Harris Type I physeal fracture of lower end of radius, right arm

⑦S59.212   Salter-Harris Type I physeal fracture of lower end of radius, left arm

⑦S59.219   Salter-Harris Type I physeal fracture of lower end of radius, unspecified arm

S59.22   Salter-Harris Type II physeal fracture of lower end of radius

⑦S59.221   Salter-Harris Type II physeal fracture of lower end of radius, right arm

⑦S59.222   Salter-Harris Type II physeal fracture of lower end of radius, left arm

⑦S59.229   Salter-Harris Type II physeal fracture of lower end of radius, unspecified arm

S59.23   Salter-Harris Type III physeal fracture of lower end of radius

⑦S59.231   Salter-Harris Type III physeal fracture of lower end of radius, right arm

⑦S59.232   Salter-Harris Type III physeal fracture of lower end of radius, left arm

⑦S59.239   Salter-Harris Type III physeal fracture of lower end of radius, unspecified arm

S59.24   Salter-Harris Type IV physeal fracture of lower end of radius

⑦S59.241   Salter-Harris Type IV physeal fracture of lower end of radius, right arm

⑦S59.242   Salter-Harris Type IV physeal fracture of lower end of radius, left arm

⑦S59.249   Salter-Harris Type IV physeal fracture of lower end of radius, unspecified arm

S59.29   Other physeal fracture of lower end of radius

⑦S59.291   Other physeal fracture of lower end of radius, right arm

⑦S59.292   Other physeal fracture of lower end of radius, left arm

⑦S59.299   Other physeal fracture of lower end of radius, unspecified arm

S59.8   Other specified injuries of elbow and forearm

The appropriate 7th character is to be added to each code in subcategory S59.8

A - initial encounter

D - subsequent encounter

S - sequela

S59.80   Other specified injuries of elbow

⑦S59.801   Other specified injuries of right elbow

⑦S59.802   Other specified injuries of left elbow

⑦S59.809   Other specified injuries of unspecified elbow

S59.81   Other specified injuries of forearm

⑦S59.811   Other specified injuries right forearm

⑦S59.812   Other specified injuries left forearm

⑦S59.819   Other specified injuries unspecified forearm

S59.9   Unspecified injury of elbow and forearm

The appropriate 7th character is to be added to each code in subcategory S59.9

A - initial encounter

D - subsequent encounter

S - sequela

S59.90   Unspecified injury of elbow

⑦S59.901   Unspecified injury of right elbow

⑦S59.902   Unspecified injury of left elbow

⑦S59.909   Unspecified injury of unspecified elbow

S59.91   Unspecified injury of forearm

⑦S59.911   Unspecified injury of right forearm

⑦S59.912   Unspecified injury of left forearm

⑦S59.919   Unspecified injury of unspecified forearm

    ● New code   ▲ Revised code   **Excludes1:** Not coded here   **Excludes2:** Not included here   ⊗ Placeholder required   ⑦7ᵗʰ digit required

INJURIES TO THE WRIST, HAND AND FINGERS (S60-S69)

Excludes2: burns and corrosions (T20-T32)

frostbite (T33-T34)

insect bite or sting, venomous (T63.4)

S60 Superficial injury of wrist, hand and fingers

The appropriate 7th character is to be added to each code from category S60 .

A - initial encounter

D - subsequent encounter

S - sequela

S60.0 Contusion of finger without damage to nail

Excludes1: contusion involving nail (matrix) (S60.1)

⊗⑦**S60.00 Contusion of unspecified finger without damage to nail**

Contusion of finger(s) NOS

S60.01 Contusion of thumb without damage to nail

⑦S60.011 Contusion of right thumb without damage to nail

⑦S60.012 Contusion of left thumb without damage to nail

⑦S60.019 Contusion of unspecified thumb without damage to nail

S60.02 Contusion of index finger without damage to nail

⑦S60.021 Contusion of right index finger without damage to nail

⑦S60.022 Contusion of left index finger without damage to nail

⑦S60.029 Contusion of unspecified index finger without damage to nail

S60.03 Contusion of middle finger without damage to nail

⑦S60.031 Contusion of right middle finger without damage to nail

⑦S60.032 Contusion of left middle finger without damage to nail

⑦S60.039 Contusion of unspecified middle finger without damage to nail

S60.04 Contusion of ring finger without damage to nail

⑦S60.041 Contusion of right ring finger without damage to nail

⑦S60.042 Contusion of left ring finger without damage to nail

⑦S60.049 Contusion of unspecified ring finger without damage to nail

S60.05 Contusion of little finger without damage to nail

⑦S60.051 Contusion of right little finger without damage to nail

⑦S60.052 Contusion of left little finger without damage to nail

⑦S60.059 Contusion of unspecified little finger without damage to nail

S60.1 Contusion of finger with damage to nail

⊗⑦**S60.10 Contusion of unspecified finger with damage to nail**

S60.11 Contusion of thumb with damage to nail

⑦S60.111 Contusion of right thumb with damage to nail

⑦S60.112 Contusion of left thumb with damage to nail

⑦S60.119 Contusion of unspecified thumb with damage to nail

S60.12 Contusion of index finger with damage to nail

⑦S60.121 Contusion of right index finger with damage to nail

⑦S60.122 Contusion of left index finger with damage to nail

⑦S60.129 Contusion of unspecified index finger with damage to nail

S60.13 Contusion of middle finger with damage to nail

⑦S60.131 Contusion of right middle finger with damage to nail

⑦S60.132 Contusion of left middle finger with damage to nail

⑦S60.139 Contusion of unspecified middle finger with damage to nail

S60.14 Contusion of ring finger with damage to nail

⑦S60.141 Contusion of right ring finger with damage to nail

⑦S60.142 Contusion of left ring finger with damage to nail

⑦S60.149 Contusion of unspecified ring finger with damage to nail

S60.15 Contusion of little finger with damage to nail

⑦S60.151 Contusion of right little finger with damage to nail

⑦S60.152 Contusion of left little finger with damage to nail

⑦S60.159 Contusion of unspecified little finger with damage to nail

S60.2 Contusion of wrist and hand

Excludes2: contusion of fingers (S60.0-, S60.1-)

S60.21 Contusion of wrist

⑦S60.211 Contusion of right wrist

⑦S60.212 Contusion of left wrist

⑦S60.219 Contusion of unspecified wrist

S60.22 Contusion of hand

⑦S60.221 Contusion of right hand

⑦S60.222 Contusion of left hand

⑦S60.229 Contusion of unspecified hand

S60.3 Other superficial injuries of thumb

S60.31 Abrasion of thumb

⑦S60.311 Abrasion of right thumb

⑦S60.312 Abrasion of left thumb

⑦S60.319 Abrasion of unspecified thumb

S60.32 Blister (nonthermal) of thumb

⑦S60.321 Blister (nonthermal) of right thumb

⑦S60.322 Blister (nonthermal) of left thumb

⑦S60.329 Blister (nonthermal) of unspecified thumb

S60.34 External constriction of thumb

Hair tourniquet syndrome of thumb

Use additional cause code to identify the constricting item (W49.0-)

⑦S60.341 External constriction of right thumb

⑦S60.342 External constriction of left thumb

⑦S60.349 External constriction of unspecified thumb

S60.35 Superficial foreign body of thumb

Splinter in the thumb

---

⑦S60.351 **Superficial foreign body of right thumb**

⑦S60.352 **Superficial foreign body of left thumb**

⑦S60.359 **Superficial foreign body of unspecified thumb**

S60.36 **Insect bite (nonvenomous) of thumb**

⑦S60.361 **Insect bite (nonvenomous) of right thumb**

⑦S60.362 **Insect bite (nonvenomous) of left thumb**

⑦S60.369 **Insect bite (nonvenomous) of unspecified thumb**

S60.37 **Other superficial bite of thumb**

Excludes1: open bite of thumb (S61.05-, S61.15-)

⑦S60.371 **Other superficial bite of right thumb**

⑦S60.372 **Other superficial bite of left thumb**

⑦S60.379 **Other superficial bite of unspecified thumb**

S60.39 **Other superficial injuries of thumb**

⑦S60.391 **Other superficial injuries of right thumb**

⑦S60.392 **Other superficial injuries of left thumb**

⑦S60.399 **Other superficial injuries of unspecified thumb**

S60.4 **Other superficial injuries of other fingers**

S60.41 **Abrasion of fingers**

⑦S60.410 **Abrasion of right index finger**

⑦S60.411 **Abrasion of left index finger**

⑦S60.412 **Abrasion of right middle finger**

⑦S60.413 **Abrasion of left middle finger**

⑦S60.414 **Abrasion of right ring finger**

⑦S60.415 **Abrasion of left ring finger**

⑦S60.416 **Abrasion of right little finger**

⑦S60.417 **Abrasion of left little finger**

⑦S60.418 **Abrasion of other finger**

Abrasion of specified finger with unspecified laterality

⑦S60.419 **Abrasion of unspecified finger**

S60.42 **Blister (nonthermal) of fingers**

⑦S60.420 **Blister (nonthermal) of right index finger**

⑦S60.421 **Blister (nonthermal) of left index finger**

⑦S60.422 **Blister (nonthermal) of right middle finger**

⑦S60.423 **Blister (nonthermal) of left middle finger**

⑦S60.424 **Blister (nonthermal) of right ring finger**

⑦S60.425 **Blister (nonthermal) of left ring finger**

⑦S60.426 **Blister (nonthermal) of right little finger**

⑦S60.427 **Blister (nonthermal) of left little finger**

⑦S60.428 **Blister (nonthermal) of other finger**

Blister (nonthermal) of specified finger with unspecified laterality

⑦S60.429 **Blister (nonthermal) of unspecified finger**

S60.44 **External constriction of fingers**

Hair tourniquet syndrome of finger

Use additional cause code to identify the constricting item (W49.0-)

⑦S60.440 **External constriction of right index finger**

⑦S60.441 **External constriction of left index finger**

⑦S60.442 **External constriction of right middle finger**

⑦S60.443 **External constriction of left middle finger**

⑦S60.444 **External constriction of right ring finger**

⑦S60.445 **External constriction of left ring finger**

⑦S60.446 **External constriction of right little finger**

⑦S60.447 **External constriction of left little finger**

⑦S60.448 **External constriction of other finger**

External constriction of specified finger with unspecified laterality

⑦S60.449 **External constriction of unspecified finger**

S60.45 **Superficial foreign body of fingers**

Splinter in the finger(s)

⑦S60.450 **Superficial foreign body of right index finger**

⑦S60.451 **Superficial foreign body of left index finger**

⑦S60.452 **Superficial foreign body of right middle finger**

⑦S60.453 **Superficial foreign body of left middle finger**

⑦S60.454 **Superficial foreign body of right ring finger**

⑦S60.455 **Superficial foreign body of left ring finger**

⑦S60.456 **Superficial foreign body of right little finger**

⑦S60.457 **Superficial foreign body of left little finger**

⑦S60.458 **Superficial foreign body of other finger**

Superficial foreign body of specified finger with unspecified laterality

⑦S60.459 **Superficial foreign body of unspecified finger**

S60.46 **Insect bite (nonvenomous) of fingers**

⑦S60.460 **Insect bite (nonvenomous) of right index finger**

⑦S60.461 **Insect bite (nonvenomous) of left index finger**

⑦S60.462 **Insect bite (nonvenomous) of right middle finger**

⑦S60.463 **Insect bite (nonvenomous) of left middle finger**

⑦S60.464 **Insect bite (nonvenomous) of right ring finger**

⑦S60.465 **Insect bite (nonvenomous) of left ring finger**

● New code ▲ Revised code Excludes1: Not coded here Excludes2: Not included here ⊗ Placeholder required ⑦7th digit required

⑦S60.466　Insect bite (nonvenomous) of right little finger

⑦S60.467　Insect bite (nonvenomous) of left little finger

⑦S60.468　Insect bite (nonvenomous) of other finger

Insect bite (nonvenomous) of specified finger with unspecified laterality

⑦S60.469　Insect bite (nonvenomous) of unspecified finger

S60.47　Other superficial bite of fingers

Excludes1: open bite of fingers (S61.25-, S61.35-)

⑦S60.470　Other superficial bite of right index finger

⑦S60.471　Other superficial bite of left index finger

⑦S60.472　Other superficial bite of right middle finger

⑦S60.473　Other superficial bite of left middle finger

⑦S60.474　Other superficial bite of right ring finger

⑦S60.475　Other superficial bite of left ring finger

⑦S60.476　Other superficial bite of right little finger

⑦S60.477　Other superficial bite of left little finger

⑦S60.478　Other superficial bite of other finger

Other superficial bite of specified finger with unspecified laterality

⑦S60.479　Other superficial bite of unspecified finger

S60.5　Other superficial injuries of hand

Excludes2: superficial injuries of fingers (S60.3-, S60.4-)

S60.51　Abrasion of hand

⑦S60.511　Abrasion of right hand

⑦S60.512　Abrasion of left hand

⑦S60.519　Abrasion of unspecified hand

S60.52　Blister (nonthermal) of hand

⑦S60.521　Blister (nonthermal) of right hand

⑦S60.522　Blister (nonthermal) of left hand

⑦S60.529　Blister (nonthermal) of unspecified hand

S60.54　External constriction of hand

⑦S60.541　External constriction of right hand

⑦S60.542　External constriction of left hand

⑦S60.549　External constriction of unspecified hand

S60.55　Superficial foreign body of hand

Splinter in the hand

⑦S60.551　Superficial foreign body of right hand

⑦S60.552　Superficial foreign body of left hand

⑦S60.559　Superficial foreign body of unspecified hand

S60.56　Insect bite (nonvenomous) of hand

⑦S60.561　Insect bite (nonvenomous) of right hand

⑦S60.562　Insect bite (nonvenomous) of left hand

⑦S60.569　Insect bite (nonvenomous) of unspecified hand

S60.57　Other superficial bite of hand

Excludes1: open bite of hand (S61.45-)

⑦S60.571　Other superficial bite of hand of right hand

⑦S60.572　Other superficial bite of hand of left hand

⑦S60.579　Other superficial bite of hand of unspecified hand

S60.8　Other superficial injuries of wrist

S60.81　Abrasion of wrist

⑦S60.811　Abrasion of right wrist

⑦S60.812　Abrasion of left wrist

⑦S60.819　Abrasion of unspecified wrist

S60.82　Blister (nonthermal) of wrist

⑦S60.821　Blister (nonthermal) of right wrist

⑦S60.822　Blister (nonthermal) of left wrist

⑦S60.829　Blister (nonthermal) of unspecified wrist

S60.84　External constriction of wrist

⑦S60.841　External constriction of right wrist

⑦S60.842　External constriction of left wrist

⑦S60.849　External constriction of unspecified wrist

S60.85　Superficial foreign body of wrist

Splinter in the wrist

⑦S60.851　Superficial foreign body of right wrist

⑦S60.852　Superficial foreign body of left wrist

⑦S60.859　Superficial foreign body of unspecified wrist

S60.86　Insect bite (nonvenomous) of wrist

⑦S60.861　Insect bite (nonvenomous) of right wrist

⑦S60.862　Insect bite (nonvenomous) of left wrist

⑦S60.869　Insect bite (nonvenomous) of unspecified wrist

S60.87　Other superficial bite of wrist

Excludes1: open bite of wrist (S61.55)

⑦S60.871　Other superficial bite of right wrist

⑦S60.872　Other superficial bite of left wrist

⑦S60.879　Other superficial bite of unspecified wrist

S60.9　Unspecified superficial injury of wrist, hand and fingers

S60.91　Unspecified superficial injury of wrist

⑦S60.911　Unspecified superficial injury of right wrist

⑦S60.912　Unspecified superficial injury of left wrist

⑦S60.919　Unspecified superficial injury of unspecified wrist

S60.92　Unspecified superficial injury of hand

⑦S60.921　Unspecified superficial injury of right hand

⑦S60.922　Unspecified superficial injury of left hand

⑦S60.929　Unspecified superficial injury of unspecified hand

S60.93　Unspecified superficial injury of thumb

⑦S60.931 Unspecified superficial injury of right thumb

⑦S60.932 Unspecified superficial injury of left thumb

⑦S60.939 Unspecified superficial injury of unspecified thumb

S60.94 Unspecified superficial injury of other fingers

⑦S60.940 Unspecified superficial injury of right index finger

⑦S60.941 Unspecified superficial injury of left index finger

⑦S60.942 Unspecified superficial injury of right middle finger

⑦S60.943 Unspecified superficial injury of left middle finger

⑦S60.944 Unspecified superficial injury of right ring finger

⑦S60.945 Unspecified superficial injury of left ring finger

⑦S60.946 Unspecified superficial injury of right little finger

⑦S60.947 Unspecified superficial injury of left little finger

⑦S60.948 Unspecified superficial injury of other finger

Unspecified superficial injury of specified finger with unspecified laterality

⑦S60.949 Unspecified superficial injury of unspecified finger

S61 **Open wound of wrist, hand and fingers**

<u>Code also</u> any associated wound infection

Excludes1: open fracture of wrist, hand and finger (S62.- with 7th character B)

traumatic amputation of wrist and hand (S68.-)

The appropriate 7th character is to be added to each code from category S61

A - initial encounter

D - subsequent encounter

S - sequela

S61.0 Open wound of thumb without damage to nail

Excludes1: open wound of thumb with damage to nail (S61.1-)

S61.00 Unspecified open wound of thumb without damage to nail

⑦S61.001 Unspecified open wound of right thumb without damage to nail

⑦S61.002 Unspecified open wound of left thumb without damage to nail

⑦S61.009 Unspecified open wound of unspecified thumb without damage to nail

⑦S61.01 Laceration without foreign body of thumb without damage to nail

⑦S61.011 Laceration without foreign body of right thumb without damage to nail

⑦S61.012 Laceration without foreign body of left thumb without damage to nail

⑦S61.019 Laceration without foreign body of unspecified thumb without damage to nail

S61.02 Laceration with foreign body of thumb without damage to nail

⑦S61.021 Laceration with foreign body of right thumb without damage to nail

⑦S61.022 Laceration with foreign body of left thumb without damage to nail

⑦S61.029 Laceration with foreign body of unspecified thumb without damage to nail

S61.03 Puncture wound without foreign body of thumb without damage to nail

⑦S61.031 Puncture wound without foreign body of right thumb without damage to nail

⑦S61.032 Puncture wound without foreign body of left thumb without damage to nail

⑦S61.039 Puncture wound without foreign body of unspecified thumb without damage to nail

S61.04 Puncture wound with foreign body of thumb without damage to nail

⑦S61.041 Puncture wound with foreign body of right thumb without damage to nail

⑦S61.042 Puncture wound with foreign body of left thumb without damage to nail

⑦S61.049 Puncture wound with foreign body of unspecified thumb without damage to nail

S61.05 Open bite of thumb without damage to nail

Bite of thumb NOS

Excludes1: superficial bite of thumb (S60.36-, S60.37-)

⑦S61.051 Open bite of right thumb without damage to nail

⑦S61.052 Open bite of left thumb without damage to nail

⑦S61.059 Open bite of unspecified thumb without damage to nail

S61.1 Open wound of thumb with damage to nail

S61.10 Unspecified open wound of thumb with damage to nail

⑦S61.101 Unspecified open wound of right thumb with damage to nail

⑦S61.102 Unspecified open wound of left thumb with damage to nail

⑦S61.109 Unspecified open wound of unspecified thumb with damage to nail

S61.11 Laceration without foreign body of thumb with damage to nail

⑦S61.111 Laceration without foreign body of right thumb with damage to nail

⑦S61.112 Laceration without foreign body of left thumb with damage to nail

⑦S61.119 Laceration without foreign body of unspecified thumb with damage to nail

S61.12 Laceration with foreign body of thumb with damage to nail

⑦S61.121 Laceration with foreign body of right thumb with damage to nail

⑦S61.122 Laceration with foreign body of left thumb with damage to nail

⑦S61.129 Laceration with foreign body of unspecified thumb with damage to nail

● New code   ▲ Revised code   Excludes1: Not coded here   Excludes2: Not included here   ⊗ Placeholder required   ⑦7th digit required

S61.13 **Puncture wound without foreign body of thumb with damage to nail**

⑦S61.131 Puncture wound without foreign body of right thumb with damage to nail

⑦S61.132 Puncture wound without foreign body of left thumb with damage to nail

⑦S61.139 Puncture wound without foreign body of unspecified thumb with damage to nail

S61.14 **Puncture wound with foreign body of thumb with damage to nail**

⑦S61.141 Puncture wound with foreign body of right thumb with damage to nail

⑦S61.142 Puncture wound with foreign body of left thumb with damage to nail

⑦S61.149 Puncture wound with foreign body of unspecified thumb with damage to nail

S61.15 **Open bite of thumb with damage to nail**

Bite of thumb with damage to nail NOS

Excludes1: superficial bite of thumb (S60.36-, S60.37-)

⑦S61.151 Open bite of right thumb with damage to nail

⑦S61.152 Open bite of left thumb with damage to nail

⑦S61.159 Open bite of unspecified thumb with damage to nail

S61.2 **Open wound of other finger without damage to nail**

Excludes1: open wound of finger involving nail (matrix) (S61.3-)

Excludes2: open wound of thumb without damage to nail (S61.0-)

S61.20 **Unspecified open wound of other finger without damage to nail**

⑦S61.200 Unspecified open wound of right index finger without damage to nail

⑦S61.201 Unspecified open wound of left index finger without damage to nail

⑦S61.202 Unspecified open wound of right middle finger without damage to nail

⑦S61.203 Unspecified open wound of left middle finger without damage to nail

⑦S61.204 Unspecified open wound of right ring finger without damage to nail

⑦S61.205 Unspecified open wound of left ring finger without damage to nail

⑦S61.206 Unspecified open wound of right little finger without damage to nail

⑦S61.207 Unspecified open wound of left little finger without damage to nail

⑦S61.208 Unspecified open wound of other finger without damage to nail

Unspecified open wound of specified finger with unspecified laterality without damage to nail

⑦S61.209 Unspecified open wound of unspecified finger without damage to nail

S61.21 **Laceration without foreign body of finger without damage to nail**

⑦S61.210 Laceration without foreign body of right index finger without damage to nail

⑦S61.211 Laceration without foreign body of left index finger without damage to nail

⑦S61.212 Laceration without foreign body of right middle finger without damage to nail

⑦S61.213 Laceration without foreign body of left middle finger without damage to nail

⑦S61.214 Laceration without foreign body of right ring finger without damage to nail

⑦S61.215 Laceration without foreign body of left ring finger without damage to nail

⑦S61.216 Laceration without foreign body of right little finger without damage to nail

⑦S61.217 Laceration without foreign body of left little finger without damage to nail

⑦S61.218 Laceration without foreign body of other finger without damage to nail

Laceration without foreign body of specified finger with unspecified laterality without damage to nail

⑦S61.219 Laceration without foreign body of unspecified finger without damage to nail

S61.22 **Laceration with foreign body of finger without damage to nail**

⑦S61.220 Laceration with foreign body of right index finger without damage to nail

⑦S61.221 Laceration with foreign body of left index finger without damage to nail

⑦S61.222 Laceration with foreign body of right middle finger without damage to nail

⑦S61.223 Laceration with foreign body of left middle finger without damage to nail

⑦S61.224 Laceration with foreign body of right ring finger without damage to nail

⑦S61.225 Laceration with foreign body of left ring finger without damage to nail

⑦S61.226 Laceration with foreign body of right little finger without damage to nail

⑦S61.227 Laceration with foreign body of left little finger without damage to nail

⑦S61.228 Laceration with foreign body of other finger without damage to nail

Laceration with foreign body of specified finger with unspecified laterality without damage to nail

⑦S61.229 Laceration with foreign body of unspecified finger without damage to nail

S61.23 **Puncture wound without foreign body of finger without damage to nail**

⑦S61.230 Puncture wound without foreign body of right index finger without damage to nail

⑦S61.231 Puncture wound without foreign body of left index finger without damage to nail

⑦S61.232 Puncture wound without foreign body of right middle finger without damage to nail

⑦S61.233 Puncture wound without foreign body of left middle finger without damage to nail

⑦S61.234 Puncture wound without foreign body of right ring finger without damage to nail

⑦S61.235 Puncture wound without foreign body of left ring finger without damage to nail

⑦S61.236 Puncture wound without foreign body of right little finger without damage to nail

⑦S61.237 Puncture wound without foreign body of left little finger without damage to nail

⑦S61.238 Puncture wound without foreign body of other finger without damage to nail

Puncture wound without foreign body of specified finger with unspecified laterality without damage to nail

⑦S61.239 Puncture wound without foreign body of unspecified finger without damage to nail

S61.24 Puncture wound with foreign body of finger without damage to nail

⑦S61.240 Puncture wound with foreign body of right index finger without damage to nail

⑦S61.241 Puncture wound with foreign body of left index finger without damage to nail

⑦S61.242 Puncture wound with foreign body of right middle finger without damage to nail

⑦S61.243 Puncture wound with foreign body of left middle finger without damage to nail

⑦S61.244 Puncture wound with foreign body of right ring finger without damage to nail

⑦S61.245 Puncture wound with foreign body of left ring finger without damage to nail

⑦S61.246 Puncture wound with foreign body of right little finger without damage to nail

⑦S61.247 Puncture wound with foreign body of left little finger without damage to nail

⑦S61.248 Puncture wound with foreign body of other finger without damage to nail

Puncture wound with foreign body of specified finger with unspecified laterality without damage to nail

⑦S61.249 Puncture wound with foreign body of unspecified finger without damage to nail

S61.25 Open bite of finger without damage to nail

Bite of finger without damage to nail NOS

Excludes1: superficial bite of finger (S60.46-, S60.47-)

⑦S61.250 Open bite of right index finger without damage to nail

⑦S61.251 Open bite of left index finger without damage to nail

⑦S61.252 Open bite of right middle finger without damage to nail

⑦S61.253 Open bite of left middle finger without damage to nail

⑦S61.254 Open bite of right ring finger without damage to nail

⑦S61.255 Open bite of left ring finger without damage to nail

⑦S61.256 Open bite of right little finger without damage to nail

⑦S61.257 Open bite of left little finger without damage to nail

⑦S61.258 Open bite of other finger without damage to nail

Open bite of specified finger with unspecified laterality without damage to nail

⑦S61.259 Open bite of unspecified finger without damage to nail

S61.3 Open wound of other finger with damage to nail

S61.30 Unspecified open wound of finger with damage to nail

⑦S61.300 Unspecified open wound of right index finger with damage to nail

⑦S61.301 Unspecified open wound of left index finger with damage to nail

⑦S61.302 Unspecified open wound of right middle finger with damage to nail

⑦S61.303 Unspecified open wound of left middle finger with damage to nail

⑦S61.304 Unspecified open wound of right ring finger with damage to nail

⑦S61.305 Unspecified open wound of left ring finger with damage to nail

⑦S61.306 Unspecified open wound of right little finger with damage to nail

⑦S61.307 Unspecified open wound of left little finger with damage to nail

⑦S61.308 Unspecified open wound of other finger with damage to nail

Unspecified open wound of specified finger with unspecified laterality with damage to nail

⑦S61.309 Unspecified open wound of unspecified finger with damage to nail

S61.31 Laceration without foreign body of finger with damage to nail

⑦S61.310 Laceration without foreign body of right index finger with damage to nail

⑦S61.311 Laceration without foreign body of left index finger with damage to nail

⑦S61.312 Laceration without foreign body of right middle finger with damage to nail

⑦S61.313 Laceration without foreign body of left middle finger with damage to nail

⑦S61.314 Laceration without foreign body of right ring finger with damage to nail

● New code   ▲ Revised code   **Excludes1:** Not coded here   **Excludes2:** Not included here   ⊗ Placeholder required   ⑦7th digit required

⑦S61.315 Laceration without foreign body of left ring finger with damage to nail

⑦S61.316 Laceration without foreign body of right little finger with damage to nail

⑦S61.317 Laceration without foreign body of left little finger with damage to nail

⑦S61.318 Laceration without foreign body of other finger with damage to nail

Laceration without foreign body of specified finger with unspecified laterality with damage to nail

⑦S61.319 Laceration without foreign body of unspecified finger with damage to nail

S61.32 Laceration with foreign body of finger with damage to nail

⑦S61.320 Laceration with foreign body of right index finger with damage to nail

⑦S61.321 Laceration with foreign body of left index finger with damage to nail

⑦S61.322 Laceration with foreign body of right middle finger with damage to nail

⑦S61.323 Laceration with foreign body of left middle finger with damage to nail

⑦S61.324 Laceration with foreign body of right ring finger with damage to nail

⑦S61.325 Laceration with foreign body of left ring finger with damage to nail

⑦S61.326 Laceration with foreign body of right little finger with damage to nail

⑦S61.327 Laceration with foreign body of left little finger with damage to nail

⑦S61.328 Laceration with foreign body of other finger with damage to nail

Laceration with foreign body of specified finger with unspecified laterality with damage to nail

⑦S61.329 Laceration with foreign body of unspecified finger with damage to nail

S61.33 Puncture wound without foreign body of finger with damage to nail

⑦S61.330 Puncture wound without foreign body of right index finger with damage to nail

⑦S61.331 Puncture wound without foreign body of left index finger with damage to nail

⑦S61.332 Puncture wound without foreign body of right middle finger with damage to nail

⑦S61.333 Puncture wound without foreign body of left middle finger with damage to nail

⑦S61.334 Puncture wound without foreign body of right ring finger with damage to nail

⑦S61.335 Puncture wound without foreign body of left ring finger with damage to nail

⑦S61.336 Puncture wound without foreign body of right little finger with damage to nail

⑦S61.337 Puncture wound without foreign body of left little finger with damage to nail

⑦S61.338 Puncture wound without foreign body of other finger with damage to nail

Puncture wound without foreign body of specified finger with unspecified laterality with damage to nail

⑦S61.339 Puncture wound without foreign body of unspecified finger with damage to nail

S61.34 Puncture wound with foreign body of finger with damage to nail

⑦S61.340 Puncture wound with foreign body of right index finger with damage to nail

⑦S61.341 Puncture wound with foreign body of left index finger with damage to nail

⑦S61.342 Puncture wound with foreign body of right middle finger with damage to nail

⑦S61.343 Puncture wound with foreign body of left middle finger with damage to nail

⑦S61.344 Puncture wound with foreign body of right ring finger with damage to nail

⑦S61.345 Puncture wound with foreign body of left ring finger with damage to nail

⑦S61.346 Puncture wound with foreign body of right little finger with damage to nail

⑦S61.347 Puncture wound with foreign body of left little finger with damage to nail

⑦S61.348 Puncture wound with foreign body of other finger with damage to nail

Puncture wound with foreign body of specified finger with unspecified laterality with damage to nail

⑦S61.349 Puncture wound with foreign body of unspecified finger with damage to nail

S61.35 Open bite of finger with damage to nail

Bite of finger with damage to nail NOS

Excludes1: superficial bite of finger (S60.46-, S60.47-)

⑦S61.350 Open bite of right index finger with damage to nail

⑦S61.351 Open bite of left index finger with damage to nail

⑦S61.352 Open bite of right middle finger with damage to nail

⑦S61.353 Open bite of left middle finger with damage to nail

⑦S61.354 Open bite of right ring finger with damage to nail

⑦S61.355 Open bite of left ring finger with damage to nail

⑦S61.356 Open bite of right little finger with damage to nail

⑦S61.357 Open bite of left little finger with damage to nail

⑦S61.358 Open bite of other finger with damage to nail

Open bite of specified finger with unspecified laterality with damage to nail

⑦S61.359 Open bite of unspecified finger with damage to nail

S61.4   Open wound of hand

S61.40   Unspecified open wound of hand

⑦S61.401   Unspecified open wound of right hand

⑦S61.402   Unspecified open wound of left hand

⑦S61.409   Unspecified open wound of unspecified hand

S61.41   Laceration without foreign body of hand

⑦S61.411   Laceration without foreign body of right hand

⑦S61.412   Laceration without foreign body of left hand

⑦S61.419   Laceration without foreign body of unspecified hand

S61.42   Laceration with foreign body of hand

⑦S61.421   Laceration with foreign body of right hand

⑦S61.422   Laceration with foreign body of left hand

⑦S61.429   Laceration with foreign body of unspecified hand

S61.43   Puncture wound without foreign body of hand

S61.431   Puncture wound without foreign body of right hand

⑦S61.432   Puncture wound without foreign body of left hand

⑦S61.439   Puncture wound without foreign body of unspecified hand

S61.44   Puncture wound with foreign body of hand

⑦S61.441   Puncture wound with foreign body of right hand

⑦S61.442   Puncture wound with foreign body of left hand

S61.449   Puncture wound with foreign body of unspecified hand

S61.45   Open bite of hand

Bite of hand NOS

Excludes1: superficial bite of hand (S60.56-, S60.57-)

⑦S61.451   Open bite of right hand

⑦S61.452   Open bite of left hand

⑦S61.459   Open bite of unspecified hand

S61.5   Open wound of wrist

S61.50   Unspecified open wound of wrist

⑦S61.501   Unspecified open wound of right wrist

⑦S61.502   Unspecified open wound of left wrist

⑦S61.509   Unspecified open wound of unspecified wrist

S61.51   Laceration without foreign body of wrist

⑦S61.511   Laceration without foreign body of right wrist

⑦S61.512   Laceration without foreign body of left wrist

⑦S61.519   Laceration without foreign body of unspecified wrist

S61.52   Laceration with foreign body of wrist

⑦S61.521   Laceration with foreign body of right wrist

⑦S61.522   Laceration with foreign body of left wrist

⑦S61.529   Laceration with foreign body of unspecified wrist

S61.53   Puncture wound without foreign body of wrist

⑦S61.531   Puncture wound without foreign body of right wrist

⑦S61.532   Puncture wound without foreign body of left wrist

⑦S61.539   Puncture wound without foreign body of unspecified wrist

S61.54   Puncture wound with foreign body of wrist

⑦S61.541   Puncture wound with foreign body of right wrist

⑦S61.542   Puncture wound with foreign body of left wrist

⑦S61.549   Puncture wound with foreign body of unspecified wrist

S61.55   Open bite of wrist

Bite of wrist NOS

Excludes1: superficial bite of wrist (S60.86-, S60.87-)

⑦S61.551   Open bite of right wrist

⑦S61.552   Open bite of left wrist

⑦S61.559   Open bite of unspecified wrist

S62   Fracture at wrist and hand level

Note: A fracture not indicated as displaced or nondisplaced should be coded to displaced

A fracture not indicated as open or closed should be coded to closed

Excludes1: traumatic amputation of wrist and hand (S68.-)

Excludes2: fracture of distal parts of ulna and radius (S52.-)

The appropriate 7th character is to be added to each code from category S62

A - initial encounter for closed fracture

B - initial encounter for open fracture

D - subsequent encounter for fracture with routine healing

G - subsequent encounter for fracture with delayed healing

K - subsequent encounter for fracture with nonunion

P - subsequent encounter for fracture with malunion

S - sequela

S62.0   Fracture of navicular [scaphoid] bone of wrist

S62.00   Unspecified fracture of navicular [scaphoid] bone of wrist

⑦S62.001   Unspecified fracture of navicular [scaphoid] bone of right wrist

⑦S62.002   Unspecified fracture of navicular [scaphoid] bone of left wrist

⑦S62.009   Unspecified fracture of navicular [scaphoid] bone of unspecified wrist

S62.01   Fracture of distal pole of navicular [scaphoid] bone of wrist

Fracture of volar tuberosity of navicular [scaphoid] bone of wrist

⑦S62.011   Displaced fracture of distal pole of navicular [scaphoid] bone of right wrist

⑦S62.012   Displaced fracture of distal pole of navicular [scaphoid] bone of left wrist

⑦S62.013   Displaced fracture of distal pole of navicular [scaphoid] bone of unspecified wrist

● New code   ▲ Revised code   Excludes1: Not coded here   Excludes2: Not included here   ⊗ Placeholder required   ⑦7th digit required

⑦S62.014   Nondisplaced fracture of distal pole of navicular [scaphoid] bone of right wrist

⑦S62.015   Nondisplaced fracture of distal pole of navicular [scaphoid] bone of left wrist

⑦S62.016   Nondisplaced fracture of distal pole of navicular [scaphoid] bone of unspecified wrist

S62.02   **Fracture of middle third of navicular [scaphoid] bone of wrist**

⑦S62.021   Displaced fracture of middle third of navicular [scaphoid] bone of right wrist

⑦S62.022   Displaced fracture of middle third of navicular [scaphoid] bone of left wrist

⑦S62.023   Displaced fracture of middle third of navicular [scaphoid] bone of unspecified wrist

⑦S62.024   Nondisplaced fracture of middle third of navicular [scaphoid] bone of right wrist

⑦S62.025   Nondisplaced fracture of middle third of navicular [scaphoid] bone of left wrist

⑦S62.026   Nondisplaced fracture of middle third of navicular [scaphoid] bone of unspecified wrist

S62.03   **Fracture of proximal third of navicular [scaphoid] bone of wrist**

⑦S62.031   Displaced fracture of proximal third of navicular [scaphoid] bone of right wrist

⑦S62.032   Displaced fracture of proximal third of navicular [scaphoid] bone of left wrist

⑦S62.033   Displaced fracture of proximal third of navicular [scaphoid] bone of unspecified wrist

⑦S62.034   Nondisplaced fracture of proximal third of navicular [scaphoid] bone of right wrist

⑦S62.035   Nondisplaced fracture of proximal third of navicular [scaphoid] bone of left wrist

⑦S62.036   Nondisplaced fracture of proximal third of navicular [scaphoid] bone of unspecified wrist

S62.1   **Fracture of other and unspecified carpal bone(s)**

Excludes2: fracture of scaphoid of wrist (S62.0-)

S62.10   **Fracture of unspecified carpal bone**

Fracture of wrist NOS

⑦S62.101   Fracture of unspecified carpal bone, right wrist

⑦S62.102   Fracture of unspecified carpal bone, left wrist

⑦S62.109   Fracture of unspecified carpal bone, unspecified wrist

S62.11   **Fracture of triquetrum [cuneiform] bone of wrist**

⑦S62.111   Displaced fracture of triquetrum [cuneiform] bone, right wrist

⑦S62.112   Displaced fracture of triquetrum [cuneiform] bone, left wrist

⑦S62.113   Displaced fracture of triquetrum [cuneiform] bone, unspecified wrist

⑦S62.114   Nondisplaced fracture of triquetrum [cuneiform] bone, right wrist

⑦S62.115   Nondisplaced fracture of triquetrum [cuneiform] bone, left wrist

⑦S62.116   Nondisplaced fracture of triquetrum [cuneiform] bone, unspecified wrist

S62.12   **Fracture of lunate [semilunar]**

⑦S62.121   Displaced fracture of lunate [semilunar], right wrist

⑦S62.122   Displaced fracture of lunate [semilunar], left wrist

⑦S62.123   Displaced fracture of lunate [semilunar], unspecified wrist

⑦S62.124   Nondisplaced fracture of lunate [semilunar], right wrist

⑦S62.125   Nondisplaced fracture of lunate [semilunar], left wrist

⑦S62.126   Nondisplaced fracture of lunate [semilunar], unspecified wrist

S62.13   **Fracture of capitate [os magnum] bone**

⑦S62.131   Displaced fracture of capitate [os magnum] bone, right wrist

⑦S62.132   Displaced fracture of capitate [os magnum] bone, left wrist

⑦S62.133   Displaced fracture of capitate [os magnum] bone, unspecified wrist

⑦S62.134   Nondisplaced fracture of capitate [os magnum] bone, right wrist

⑦S62.135   Nondisplaced fracture of capitate [os magnum] bone, left wrist

⑦S62.136   Nondisplaced fracture of capitate [os magnum] bone, unspecified wrist

S62.14   **Fracture of body of hamate [unciform] bone**

Fracture of hamate [unciform] bone NOS

⑦S62.141   Displaced fracture of body of hamate [unciform] bone, right wrist

⑦S62.142   Displaced fracture of body of hamate [unciform] bone, left wrist

⑦S62.143   Displaced fracture of body of hamate [unciform] bone, unspecified wrist

⑦S62.144   Nondisplaced fracture of body of hamate [unciform] bone, right wrist

⑦S62.145   Nondisplaced fracture of body of hamate [unciform] bone, left wrist

⑦S62.146   Nondisplaced fracture of body of hamate [unciform] bone, unspecified wrist

S62.15   **Fracture of hook process of hamate [unciform] bone**

Fracture of unciform process of hamate [unciform] bone

⑦S62.151   Displaced fracture of hook process of hamate [unciform] bone, right wrist

⑦S62.152   Displaced fracture of hook process of hamate [unciform] bone, left wrist

⑦S62.153   Displaced fracture of hook process of hamate [unciform] bone, unspecified wrist

⑦S62.154   Nondisplaced fracture of hook process of hamate [unciform] bone, right wrist

⑦S62.155   Nondisplaced fracture of hook process of hamate [unciform] bone, left wrist

⑦S62.156   Nondisplaced fracture of hook process of hamate [unciform] bone, unspecified wrist

S62.16   Fracture of pisiform

⑦S62.161   Displaced fracture of pisiform, right wrist

⑦S62.162   Displaced fracture of pisiform, left wrist

⑦S62.163   Displaced fracture of pisiform, unspecified wrist

⑦S62.164   Nondisplaced fracture of pisiform, right wrist

⑦S62.165   Nondisplaced fracture of pisiform, left wrist

⑦S62.166   Nondisplaced fracture of pisiform, unspecified wrist

S62.17   Fracture of trapezium [larger multangular]

⑦S62.171   Displaced fracture of trapezium [larger multangular], right wrist

⑦S62.172   Displaced fracture of trapezium [larger multangular], left wrist

⑦S62.173   Displaced fracture of trapezium [larger multangular], unspecified wrist

⑦S62.174   Nondisplaced fracture of trapezium [larger multangular], right wrist

⑦S62.175   Nondisplaced fracture of trapezium [larger multangular], left wrist

⑦S62.176   Nondisplaced fracture of trapezium [larger multangular], unspecified wrist

S62.18   Fracture of trapezoid [smaller multangular]

⑦S62.181   Displaced fracture of trapezoid [smaller multangular], right wrist

⑦S62.182   Displaced fracture of trapezoid [smaller multangular], left wrist

⑦S62.183   Displaced fracture of trapezoid [smaller multangular], unspecified wrist

⑦S62.184   Nondisplaced fracture of trapezoid [smaller multangular], right wrist

⑦S62.185   Nondisplaced fracture of trapezoid [smaller multangular], left wrist

⑦S62.186   Nondisplaced fracture of trapezoid [smaller multangular], unspecified wrist

S62.2   Fracture of first metacarpal bone

S62.20   Unspecified fracture of first metacarpal bone

⑦S62.201   Unspecified fracture of first metacarpal bone, right hand

⑦S62.202   Unspecified fracture of first metacarpal bone, left hand

⑦S62.209   Unspecified fracture of first metacarpal bone, unspecified hand

S62.21   Bennett's fracture

⑦S62.211   Bennett's fracture, right hand

⑦S62.212   Bennett's fracture, left hand

⑦S62.213   Bennett's fracture, unspecified hand

S62.22   Rolando's fracture

⑦S62.221   Displaced Rolando's fracture, right hand

⑦S62.222   Displaced Rolando's fracture, left hand

⑦S62.223   Displaced Rolando's fracture, unspecified hand

⑦S62.224   Nondisplaced Rolando's fracture, right hand

⑦S62.225   Nondisplaced Rolando's fracture, left hand

⑦S62.226   Nondisplaced Rolando's fracture, unspecified hand

S62.23   Other fracture of base of first metacarpal bone

⑦S62.231   Other displaced fracture of base of first metacarpal bone, right hand

⑦S62.232   Other displaced fracture of base of first metacarpal bone, left hand

⑦S62.233   Other displaced fracture of base of first metacarpal bone, unspecified hand

⑦S62.234   Other nondisplaced fracture of base of first metacarpal bone, right hand

⑦S62.235   Other nondisplaced fracture of base of first metacarpal bone, left hand

⑦S62.236   Other nondisplaced fracture of base of first metacarpal bone, unspecified hand

S62.24   Fracture of shaft of first metacarpal bone

⑦S62.241   Displaced fracture of shaft of first metacarpal bone, right hand

⑦S62.242   Displaced fracture of shaft of first metacarpal bone, left hand

⑦S62.243   Displaced fracture of shaft of first metacarpal bone, unspecified hand

⑦S62.244   Nondisplaced fracture of shaft of first metacarpal bone, right hand

⑦S62.245   Nondisplaced fracture of shaft of first metacarpal bone, left hand

⑦S62.246   Nondisplaced fracture of shaft of first metacarpal bone, unspecified hand

S62.25   Fracture of neck of first metacarpal bone

⑦S62.251   Displaced fracture of neck of first metacarpal bone, right hand

⑦S62.252   Displaced fracture of neck of first metacarpal bone, left hand

⑦S62.253   Displaced fracture of neck of first metacarpal bone, unspecified hand

⑦S62.254   Nondisplaced fracture of neck of first metacarpal bone, right hand

⑦S62.255   Nondisplaced fracture of neck of first metacarpal bone, left hand

⑦S62.256   Nondisplaced fracture of neck of first metacarpal bone, unspecified hand

S62.29   Other fracture of first metacarpal bone

⑦S62.291   Other fracture of first metacarpal bone, right hand

⑦S62.292   Other fracture of first metacarpal bone, left hand

⑦S62.299   Other fracture of first metacarpal bone, unspecified hand

S62.3   Fracture of other and unspecified metacarpal bone

Excludes2: fracture of first metacarpal bone (S62.2-)

S62.30   Unspecified fracture of other metacarpal bone

⑦S62.300   Unspecified fracture of second metacarpal bone, right hand

   ● New code   ▲ Revised code   Excludes1: Not coded here   Excludes2: Not included here   ⊗ Placeholder required   ⑦7th digit required

⑦S62.301 **Unspecified fracture of second metacarpal bone, left hand**

⑦S62.302 **Unspecified fracture of third metacarpal bone, right hand**

⑦S62.303 **Unspecified fracture of third metacarpal bone, left hand**

⑦S62.304 **Unspecified fracture of fourth metacarpal bone, right hand**

⑦S62.305 **Unspecified fracture of fourth metacarpal bone, left hand**

⑦S62.306 **Unspecified fracture of fifth metacarpal bone, right hand**

⑦S62.307 **Unspecified fracture of fifth metacarpal bone, left hand**

⑦S62.308 **Unspecified fracture of other metacarpal bone**

Unspecified fracture of specified metacarpal bone with unspecified laterality

⑦S62.309 **Unspecified fracture of unspecified metacarpal bone**

S62.31 **Displaced fracture of base of other metacarpal bone**

⑦S62.310 **Displaced fracture of base of second metacarpal bone, right hand**

⑦S62.311 **Displaced fracture of base of second metacarpal bone, left hand**

⑦S62.312 **Displaced fracture of base of third metacarpal bone, right hand**

⑦S62.313 **Displaced fracture of base of third metacarpal bone, left hand**

⑦S62.314 **Displaced fracture of base of fourth metacarpal bone, right hand**

⑦S62.315 **Displaced fracture of base of fourth metacarpal bone, left hand**

⑦S62.316 **Displaced fracture of base of fifth metacarpal bone, right hand**

⑦S62.317 **Displaced fracture of base of fifth metacarpal bone. left hand**

⑦S62.318 **Displaced fracture of base of other metacarpal bone**

Displaced fracture of base of specified metacarpal bone with unspecified laterality

⑦S62.319 **Displaced fracture of base of unspecified metacarpal bone**

S62.32 **Displaced fracture of shaft of other metacarpal bone**

⑦S62.320 **Displaced fracture of shaft of second metacarpal bone, right hand**

⑦S62.321 **Displaced fracture of shaft of second metacarpal bone, left hand**

⑦S62.322 **Displaced fracture of shaft of third metacarpal bone, right hand**

⑦S62.323 **Displaced fracture of shaft of third metacarpal bone, left hand**

⑦S62.324 **Displaced fracture of shaft of fourth metacarpal bone, right hand**

⑦S62.325 **Displaced fracture of shaft of fourth metacarpal bone, left hand**

⑦S62.326 **Displaced fracture of shaft of fifth metacarpal bone, right hand**

⑦S62.327 **Displaced fracture of shaft of fifth metacarpal bone, left hand**

⑦S62.328 **Displaced fracture of shaft of other metacarpal bone**

Displaced fracture of shaft of specified metacarpal bone with unspecified laterality

⑦S62.329 **Displaced fracture of shaft of unspecified metacarpal bone**

S62.33 **Displaced fracture of neck of other metacarpal bone**

⑦S62.330 **Displaced fracture of neck of second metacarpal bone, right hand**

⑦S62.331 **Displaced fracture of neck of second metacarpal bone, left hand**

⑦S62.332 **Displaced fracture of neck of third metacarpal bone, right hand**

⑦S62.333 **Displaced fracture of neck of third metacarpal bone, left hand**

⑦S62.334 **Displaced fracture of neck of fourth metacarpal bone, right hand**

⑦S62.335 **Displaced fracture of neck of fourth metacarpal bone, left hand**

⑦S62.336 **Displaced fracture of neck of fifth metacarpal bone, right hand**

⑦S62.337 **Displaced fracture of neck of fifth metacarpal bone, left hand**

⑦S62.338 **Displaced fracture of neck of other metacarpal bone**

Displaced fracture of neck of specified metacarpal bone with unspecified laterality

⑦S62.339 **Displaced fracture of neck of unspecified metacarpal bone**

S62.34 **Nondisplaced fracture of base of other metacarpal bone**

⑦S62.340 **Nondisplaced fracture of base of second metacarpal bone, right hand**

⑦S62.341 **Nondisplaced fracture of base of second metacarpal bone, left hand**

⑦S62.342 **Nondisplaced fracture of base of third metacarpal bone, right hand**

⑦S62.343 **Nondisplaced fracture of base of third metacarpal bone, left hand**

⑦S62.344 **Nondisplaced fracture of base of fourth metacarpal bone, right hand**

⑦S62.345 **Nondisplaced fracture of base of fourth metacarpal bone, left hand**

⑦S62.346 **Nondisplaced fracture of base of fifth metacarpal bone, right hand**

⑦S62.347 **Nondisplaced fracture of base of fifth metacarpal bone, left hand**

⑦S62.348 **Nondisplaced fracture of base of other metacarpal bone**

Nondisplaced fracture of base of specified metacarpal bone with unspecified laterality

⑦S62.349 **Nondisplaced fracture of base of unspecified metacarpal bone**

S62.35 **Nondisplaced fracture of shaft of other metacarpal bone**

⑦S62.350 **Nondisplaced fracture of shaft of second metacarpal bone, right hand**

⑦S62.351 **Nondisplaced fracture of shaft of second metacarpal bone, left hand**

⑦S62.352 **Nondisplaced fracture of shaft of third metacarpal bone, right hand**

⑦S62.353 **Nondisplaced fracture of shaft of third metacarpal bone, left hand**

⑦S62.354 **Nondisplaced fracture of shaft of fourth metacarpal bone, right hand**

⑦S62.355 **Nondisplaced fracture of shaft of fourth metacarpal bone, left hand**

⑦S62.356 **Nondisplaced fracture of shaft of fifth metacarpal bone, right hand**

⑦S62.357 **Nondisplaced fracture of shaft of fifth metacarpal bone, left hand**

⑦S62.358 **Nondisplaced fracture of shaft of other metacarpal bone**

Nondisplaced fracture of shaft of specified metacarpal bone with unspecified laterality

⑦S62.359 **Nondisplaced fracture of shaft of unspecified metacarpal bone**

S62.36 **Nondisplaced fracture of neck of other metacarpal bone**

⑦S62.360 **Nondisplaced fracture of neck of second metacarpal bone, right hand**

⑦S62.361 **Nondisplaced fracture of neck of second metacarpal bone, left hand**

⑦S62.362 **Nondisplaced fracture of neck of third metacarpal bone, right hand**

⑦S62.363 **Nondisplaced fracture of neck of third metacarpal bone, left hand**

⑦S62.364 **Nondisplaced fracture of neck of fourth metacarpal bone, right hand**

⑦S62.365 **Nondisplaced fracture of neck of fourth metacarpal bone, left hand**

⑦S62.366 **Nondisplaced fracture of neck of fifth metacarpal bone, right hand**

⑦S62.367 **Nondisplaced fracture of neck of fifth metacarpal bone, left hand**

⑦S62.368 **Nondisplaced fracture of neck of other metacarpal bone**

Nondisplaced fracture of neck of specified metacarpal bone with unspecified laterality

⑦S62.369 **Nondisplaced fracture of neck of unspecified metacarpal bone**

S62.39 **Other fracture of other metacarpal bone**

⑦S62.390 **Other fracture of second metacarpal bone, right hand**

⑦S62.391 **Other fracture of second metacarpal bone, left hand**

⑦S62.392 **Other fracture of third metacarpal bone, right hand**

⑦S62.393 **Other fracture of third metacarpal bone, left hand**

⑦S62.394 **Other fracture of fourth metacarpal bone, right hand**

⑦S62.395 **Other fracture of fourth metacarpal bone, left hand**

⑦S62.396 **Other fracture of fifth metacarpal bone, right hand**

⑦S62.397 **Other fracture of fifth metacarpal bone, left hand**

⑦S62.398 **Other fracture of other metacarpal bone**

Other fracture of specified metacarpal bone with unspecified laterality

⑦S62.399 **Other fracture of unspecified metacarpal bone**

S62.5 **Fracture of thumb**

S62.50 **Fracture of unspecified phalanx of thumb**

⑦S62.501 **Fracture of unspecified phalanx of right thumb**

⑦S62.502 **Fracture of unspecified phalanx of left thumb**

⑦S62.509 **Fracture of unspecified phalanx of unspecified thumb**

S62.51 **Fracture of proximal phalanx of thumb**

⑦S62.511 **Displaced fracture of proximal phalanx of right thumb**

⑦S62.512 **Displaced fracture of proximal phalanx of left thumb**

⑦S62.513 **Displaced fracture of proximal phalanx of unspecified thumb**

⑦S62.514 **Nondisplaced fracture of proximal phalanx of right thumb**

⑦S62.515 **Nondisplaced fracture of proximal phalanx of left thumb**

⑦S62.516 **Nondisplaced fracture of proximal phalanx of unspecified thumb**

S62.52 **Fracture of distal phalanx of thumb**

⑦S62.521 **Displaced fracture of distal phalanx of right thumb**

⑦S62.522 **Displaced fracture of distal phalanx of left thumb**

⑦S62.523 **Displaced fracture of distal phalanx of unspecified thumb**

⑦S62.524 **Nondisplaced fracture of distal phalanx of right thumb**

⑦S62.525 **Nondisplaced fracture of distal phalanx of left thumb**

⑦S62.526 **Nondisplaced fracture of distal phalanx of unspecified thumb**

S62.6 **Fracture of other and unspecified finger(s)**

Excludes2: fracture of thumb (S62.5-)

S62.60 **Fracture of unspecified phalanx of finger**

⑦S62.600 **Fracture of unspecified phalanx of right index finger**

⑦S62.601 **Fracture of unspecified phalanx of left index finger**

⑦S62.602 **Fracture of unspecified phalanx of right middle finger**

⑦S62.603 **Fracture of unspecified phalanx of left middle finger**

⑦S62.604 **Fracture of unspecified phalanx of right ring finger**

⑦S62.605 **Fracture of unspecified phalanx of left ring finger**

⑦S62.606 **Fracture of unspecified phalanx of right little finger**

⑦S62.607 **Fracture of unspecified phalanx of left little finger**

⑦S62.608 **Fracture of unspecified phalanx of other finger**

Fracture of unspecified phalanx of specified finger with unspecified laterality

⑦S62.609 **Fracture of unspecified phalanx of unspecified finger**

● New code   ▲ Revised code   Excludes1: Not coded here   Excludes2: Not included here   ⊗ Placeholder required   ⑦7th digit required

S62.61   **Displaced fracture of proximal phalanx of finger**

⑦**S62.610**   **Displaced fracture of proximal phalanx of right index finger**

⑦**S62.611**   **Displaced fracture of proximal phalanx of left index finger**

⑦**S62.612**   **Displaced fracture of proximal phalanx of right middle finger**

⑦**S62.613**   **Displaced fracture of proximal phalanx of left middle finger**

⑦**S62.614**   **Displaced fracture of proximal phalanx of right ring finger**

⑦**S62.615**   **Displaced fracture of proximal phalanx of left ring finger**

⑦**S62.616**   **Displaced fracture of proximal phalanx of right little finger**

⑦**S62.617**   **Displaced fracture of proximal phalanx of left little finger**

⑦**S62.618**   **Displaced fracture of proximal phalanx of other finger**

Displaced fracture of proximal phalanx of specified finger with unspecified laterality

⑦**S62.619**   **Displaced fracture of proximal phalanx of unspecified finger**

S62.62   **Displaced fracture of middle phalanx of finger**

⑦**S62.620**   **Displaced fracture of middle phalanx of right index finger**

⑦**S62.621**   **Displaced fracture of middle phalanx of left index finger**

⑦**S62.622**   **Displaced fracture of middle phalanx of right middle finger**

⑦**S62.623**   **Displaced fracture of middle phalanx of left middle finger**

⑦**S62.624**   **Displaced fracture of middle phalanx of right ring finger**

⑦**S62.625**   **Displaced fracture of middle phalanx of left ring finger**

⑦**S62.626**   **Displaced fracture of middle phalanx of right little finger**

⑦**S62.627**   **Displaced fracture of middle phalanx of right little finger**

⑦**S62.628**   **Displaced fracture of middle phalanx of other finger**

Displaced fracture of middle phalanx of specified finger with unspecified laterality

⑦**S62.629**   **Displaced fracture of middle phalanx of unspecified finger**

S62.63   **Displaced fracture of distal phalanx of finger**

⑦**S62.630**   **Displaced fracture of distal phalanx of right index finger**

⑦**S62.631**   **Displaced fracture of distal phalanx of left index finger**

⑦**S62.632**   **Displaced fracture of distal phalanx of right middle finger**

⑦**S62.633**   **Displaced fracture of distal phalanx of left middle finger**

⑦**S62.634**   **Displaced fracture of distal phalanx of right ring finger**

⑦**S62.635**   **Displaced fracture of distal phalanx of left ring finger**

⑦**S62.636**   **Displaced fracture of distal phalanx of right little finger**

⑦**S62.637**   **Displaced fracture of distal phalanx of left little finger**

⑦**S62.638**   **Displaced fracture of distal phalanx of other finger**

Displaced fracture of distal phalanx of specified finger with unspecified laterality

⑦**S62.639**   **Displaced fracture of distal phalanx of unspecified finger**

S62.64   **Nondisplaced fracture of proximal phalanx of finger**

⑦**S62.640**   **Nondisplaced fracture of proximal phalanx of right index finger**

⑦**S62.641**   **Nondisplaced fracture of proximal phalanx of left index finger**

⑦**S62.642**   **Nondisplaced fracture of proximal phalanx of right middle finger**

⑦**S62.643**   **Nondisplaced fracture of proximal phalanx of left middle finger**

⑦**S62.644**   **Nondisplaced fracture of proximal phalanx of right ring finger**

⑦**S62.645**   **Nondisplaced fracture of proximal phalanx of left ring finger**

⑦**S62.646**   **Nondisplaced fracture of proximal phalanx of right little finger**

⑦**S62.647**   **Nondisplaced fracture of proximal phalanx of left little finger**

⑦**S62.648**   **Nondisplaced fracture of proximal phalanx of other finger**

Nondisplaced fracture of proximal phalanx of specified finger with unspecified laterality

⑦**S62.649**   **Nondisplaced fracture of proximal phalanx of unspecified finger**

S62.65   **Nondisplaced fracture of middle phalanx of finger**

⑦**S62.650**   **Nondisplaced fracture of middle phalanx of right index finger**

⑦**S62.651**   **Nondisplaced fracture of middle phalanx of left index finger**

⑦**S62.652**   **Nondisplaced fracture of middle phalanx of right middle finger**

⑦**S62.653**   **Nondisplaced fracture of middle phalanx of left middle finger**

⑦**S62.654**   **Nondisplaced fracture of middle phalanx of right ring finger**

⑦**S62.655**   **Nondisplaced fracture of middle phalanx of left ring finger**

⑦**S62.656**   **Nondisplaced fracture of middle phalanx of right little finger**

⑦**S62.657**   **Nondisplaced fracture of middle phalanx of left little finger**

⑦**S62.658**   **Nondisplaced fracture of middle phalanx of other finger**

Nondisplaced fracture of middle phalanx of specified finger with unspecified laterality

⑦**S62.659**   **Nondisplaced fracture of middle phalanx of unspecified finger**

S62.66   **Nondisplaced fracture of distal phalanx of finger**

⑦**S62.660**   **Nondisplaced fracture of distal phalanx of right index finger**

⑦**S62.661**   **Nondisplaced fracture of distal phalanx of left index finger**

⑦S62.662   **Nondisplaced fracture of distal phalanx of right middle finger**

⑦S62.663   **Nondisplaced fracture of distal phalanx of left middle finger**

⑦S62.664   **Nondisplaced fracture of distal phalanx of right ring finger**

⑦S62.665   **Nondisplaced fracture of distal phalanx of left ring finger**

⑦S62.666   **Nondisplaced fracture of distal phalanx of right little finger**

⑦S62.667   **Nondisplaced fracture of distal phalanx of left little finger**

⑦S62.668   **Nondisplaced fracture of distal phalanx of other finger**

     Nondisplaced fracture of distal phalanx of specified finger with unspecified laterality

⑦S62.669   **Nondisplaced fracture of distal phalanx of unspecified finger**

S62.9   **Unspecified fracture of wrist and hand**

⊗⑦S62.90   **Unspecified fracture of unspecified wrist and hand**

⊗⑦S62.91   **Unspecified fracture of right wrist and hand**

⊗⑦S62.92   **Unspecified fracture of left wrist and hand**

S63   **Dislocation and sprain of joints and ligaments at wrist and hand level**

Includes: avulsion of joint or ligament at wrist and hand level

laceration of cartilage, joint or ligament at wrist and hand level

sprain of cartilage, joint or ligament at wrist and hand level

traumatic hemarthrosis of joint or ligament at wrist and hand level

traumatic rupture of joint or ligament at wrist and hand level

traumatic subluxation of joint or ligament at wrist and hand level

traumatic tear of joint or ligament at wrist and hand level

Code also any associated open wound

Excludes2: strain of muscle, fascia and tendon of wrist and hand (S66.-)

The appropriate 7th character is to be added to each code from category S63

A - initial encounter

D - subsequent encounter

S - sequela

S63.0   **Subluxation and dislocation of wrist and hand joints**

S63.00   **Unspecified subluxation and dislocation of wrist and hand**

     Dislocation of carpal bone NOS

     Dislocation of distal end of radius NOS

     Subluxation of carpal bone NOS

     Subluxation of distal end of radius NOS

⑦S63.001   **Unspecified subluxation of right wrist and hand**

⑦S63.002   **Unspecified subluxation of left wrist and hand**

⑦S63.003   **Unspecified subluxation of unspecified wrist and hand**

⑦S63.004   **Unspecified dislocation of right wrist and hand**

⑦S63.005   **Unspecified dislocation of left wrist and hand**

⑦S63.006   **Unspecified dislocation of unspecified wrist and hand**

S63.01   **Subluxation and dislocation of distal radioulnar joint**

⑦S63.011   **Subluxation of distal radioulnar joint of right wrist**

⑦S63.012   **Subluxation of distal radioulnar joint of left wrist**

⑦S63.013   **Subluxation of distal radioulnar joint of unspecified wrist**

⑦S63.014   **Dislocation of distal radioulnar joint of right wrist**

⑦S63.015   **Dislocation of distal radioulnar joint of left wrist**

⑦S63.016   **Dislocation of distal radioulnar joint of unspecified wrist**

S63.02   **Subluxation and dislocation of radiocarpal joint**

⑦S63.021   **Subluxation of radiocarpal joint of right wrist**

⑦S63.022   **Subluxation of radiocarpal joint of left wrist**

⑦S63.023   **Subluxation of radiocarpal joint of unspecified wrist**

⑦S63.024   **Dislocation of radiocarpal joint of right wrist**

⑦S63.025   **Dislocation of radiocarpal joint of left wrist**

⑦S63.026   **Dislocation of radiocarpal joint of unspecified wrist**

S63.03   **Subluxation and dislocation of midcarpal joint**

⑦S63.031   **Subluxation of midcarpal joint of right wrist**

⑦S63.032   **Subluxation of midcarpal joint of left wrist**

⑦S63.033   **Subluxation of midcarpal joint of unspecified wrist**

⑦S63.034   **Dislocation of midcarpal joint of right wrist**

⑦S63.035   **Dislocation of midcarpal joint of left wrist**

⑦S63.036   **Dislocation of midcarpal joint of unspecified wrist**

S63.04   **Subluxation and dislocation of carpometacarpal joint of thumb**

Excludes2: interphalangeal subluxation and dislocation of thumb (S63.1-)

⑦S63.041   **Subluxation of carpometacarpal joint of right thumb**

⑦S63.042   **Subluxation of carpometacarpal joint of left thumb**

⑦S63.043   **Subluxation of carpometacarpal joint of unspecified thumb**

⑦S63.044   **Dislocation of carpometacarpal joint of right thumb**

⑦S63.045   **Dislocation of carpometacarpal joint of left thumb**

⑦S63.046   **Dislocation of carpometacarpal joint of unspecified thumb**

S63.05   **Subluxation and dislocation of other carpometacarpal joint**

Excludes2: subluxation and dislocation of carpometacarpal joint of thumb (S63.04-)

⑦S63.051   **Subluxation of other carpometacarpal joint of right hand**

⑦S63.052   **Subluxation of other carpometacarpal joint of left hand**

⑦**S63.053** Subluxation of other carpometacarpal joint of unspecified hand

⑦**S63.054** Dislocation of other carpometacarpal joint of right hand

⑦**S63.055** Dislocation of other carpometacarpal joint of left hand

⑦**S63.056** Dislocation of other carpometacarpal joint of unspecified hand

S63.06 Subluxation and dislocation of metacarpal (bone), proximal end

⑦**S63.061** Subluxation of metacarpal (bone), proximal end of right hand

⑦**S63.062** Subluxation of metacarpal (bone), proximal end of left hand

⑦**S63.063** Subluxation of metacarpal (bone), proximal end of unspecified hand

⑦**S63.064** Dislocation of metacarpal (bone), proximal end of right hand

⑦**S63.065** Dislocation of metacarpal (bone), proximal end of left hand

⑦**S63.066** Dislocation of metacarpal (bone), proximal end of unspecified hand

S63.07 Subluxation and dislocation of distal end of ulna

⑦**S63.071** Subluxation of distal end of right ulna

⑦**S63.072** Subluxation of distal end of left ulna

⑦**S63.073** Subluxation of distal end of unspecified ulna

⑦**S63.074** Dislocation of distal end of right ulna

⑦**S63.075** Dislocation of distal end of left ulna

⑦**S63.076** Dislocation of distal end of unspecified ulna

S63.09 Other subluxation and dislocation of wrist and hand

⑦**S63.091** Other subluxation of right wrist and hand

⑦**S63.092** Other subluxation of left wrist and hand

⑦**S63.093** Other subluxation of unspecified wrist and hand

⑦**S63.094** Other dislocation of right wrist and hand

⑦**S63.095** Other dislocation of left wrist and hand

⑦**S63.096** Other dislocation of unspecified wrist and hand

S63.1 Subluxation and dislocation of thumb

S63.10 Unspecified subluxation and dislocation of thumb

⑦**S63.101** Unspecified subluxation of right thumb

⑦**S63.102** Unspecified subluxation of left thumb

⑦**S63.103** Unspecified subluxation of unspecified thumb

⑦**S63.104** Unspecified dislocation of right thumb

⑦**S63.105** Unspecified dislocation of left thumb

⑦**S63.106** Unspecified dislocation of unspecified thumb

S63.11 Subluxation and dislocation of metacarpophalangeal joint of thumb

⑦**S63.111** Subluxation of metacarpophalangeal joint of right thumb

⑦**S63.112** Subluxation of metacarpophalangeal joint of left thumb

⑦**S63.113** Subluxation of metacarpophalangeal joint of unspecified thumb

⑦**S63.114** Dislocation of metacarpophalangeal joint of right thumb

⑦**S63.115** Dislocation of metacarpophalangeal joint of left thumb

⑦**S63.116** Dislocation of metacarpophalangeal joint of unspecified thumb

S63.12 Subluxation and dislocation of interphalangeal joint of thumb

⑦**S63.121** Subluxation of interphalangeal joint of right thumb

⑦**S63.122** Subluxation of interphalangeal joint of left thumb

⑦**S63.123** Subluxation of interphalangeal joint of unspecified thumb

⑦**S63.124** Dislocation of interphalangeal joint of right thumb

⑦**S63.125** Dislocation of interphalangeal joint of left thumb

⑦**S63.126** Dislocation of interphalangeal joint of unspecified thumb

S63.2 Subluxation and dislocation of other finger(s)

Excludes2: subluxation and dislocation of thumb (S63.1-)

S63.20 Unspecified subluxation of other finger

⑦**S63.200** Unspecified subluxation of right index finger

⑦**S63.201** Unspecified subluxation of left index finger

⑦**S63.202** Unspecified subluxation of right middle finger

⑦**S63.203** Unspecified subluxation of left middle finger

⑦**S63.204** Unspecified subluxation of right ring finger

⑦**S63.205** Unspecified subluxation of left ring finger

⑦**S63.206** Unspecified subluxation of right little finger

⑦**S63.207** Unspecified subluxation of left little finger

⑦**S63.208** Unspecified subluxation of other finger

Unspecified subluxation of specified finger with unspecified laterality

⑦**S63.209** Unspecified subluxation of unspecified finger

S63.21 Subluxation of metacarpophalangeal joint of finger

⑦**S63.210** Subluxation of metacarpophalangeal joint of right index finger

⑦**S63.211** Subluxation of metacarpophalangeal joint of left index finger

⑦**S63.212** Subluxation of metacarpophalangeal joint of right middle finger

⑦**S63.213** Subluxation of metacarpophalangeal joint of left middle finger

⑦**S63.214** Subluxation of metacarpophalangeal joint of right ring finger

⑦S63.215　Subluxation of metacarpophalangeal joint of left ring finger

⑦S63.216　Subluxation of metacarpophalangeal joint of right little finger

⑦S63.217　Subluxation of metacarpophalangeal joint of left little finger

⑦S63.218　Subluxation of metacarpophalangeal joint of other finger

Subluxation of metacarpophalangeal joint of specified finger with unspecified laterality

⑦S63.219　Subluxation of metacarpophalangeal joint of unspecified finger

S63.22　Subluxation of unspecified interphalangeal joint of finger

⑦S63.220　Subluxation of unspecified interphalangeal joint of right index finger

⑦S63.221　Subluxation of unspecified interphalangeal joint of left index finger

⑦S63.222　Subluxation of unspecified interphalangeal joint of right middle finger

⑦S63.223　Subluxation of unspecified interphalangeal joint of left middle finger

⑦S63.224　Subluxation of unspecified interphalangeal joint of right ring finger

⑦S63.225　Subluxation of unspecified interphalangeal joint of left ring finger

⑦S63.226　Subluxation of unspecified interphalangeal joint of right little finger

⑦S63.227　Subluxation of unspecified interphalangeal joint of left little finger

⑦S63.228　Subluxation of unspecified interphalangeal joint of other finger

Subluxation of unspecified interphalangeal joint of specified finger with unspecified laterality

⑦S63.229　Subluxation of unspecified interphalangeal joint of unspecified finger

S63.23　Subluxation of proximal interphalangeal joint of finger

⑦S63.230　Subluxation of proximal interphalangeal joint of right index finger

⑦S63.231　Subluxation of proximal interphalangeal joint of left index finger

⑦S63.232　Subluxation of proximal interphalangeal joint of right middle finger

⑦S63.233　Subluxation of proximal interphalangeal joint of left middle finger

⑦S63.234　Subluxation of proximal interphalangeal joint of right ring finger

⑦S63.235　Subluxation of proximal interphalangeal joint of left ring finger

⑦S63.236　Subluxation of proximal interphalangeal joint of right little finger

⑦S63.237　Subluxation of proximal interphalangeal joint of left little finger

⑦S63.238　Subluxation of proximal interphalangeal joint of other finger

Subluxation of proximal interphalangeal joint of specified finger with unspecified laterality

⑦S63.239　Subluxation of proximal interphalangeal joint of unspecified finger

S63.24　Subluxation of distal interphalangeal joint of finger

⑦S63.240　Subluxation of distal interphalangeal joint of right index finger

⑦S63.241　Subluxation of distal interphalangeal joint of left index finger

⑦S63.242　Subluxation of distal interphalangeal joint of right middle finger

⑦S63.243　Subluxation of distal interphalangeal joint of left middle finger

⑦S63.244　Subluxation of distal interphalangeal joint of right ring finger

⑦S63.245　Subluxation of distal interphalangeal joint of left ring finger

⑦S63.246　Subluxation of distal interphalangeal joint of right little finger

⑦S63.247　Subluxation of distal interphalangeal joint of left little finger

⑦S63.248　Subluxation of distal interphalangeal joint of other finger

Subluxation of distal interphalangeal joint of specified finger with unspecified laterality

⑦S63.249　Subluxation of distal interphalangeal joint of unspecified finger

S63.25　Unspecified dislocation of other finger

⑦S63.250　Unspecified dislocation of right index finger

⑦S63.251　Unspecified dislocation of left index finger

⑦S63.252　Unspecified dislocation of right middle finger

⑦S63.253　Unspecified dislocation of left middle finger

⑦S63.254　Unspecified dislocation of right ring finger

⑦S63.255　Unspecified dislocation of left ring finger

⑦S63.256　Unspecified dislocation of right little finger

⑦S63.257　Unspecified dislocation of left little finger

⑦S63.258　Unspecified dislocation of other finger

Unspecified dislocation of specified finger with unspecified laterality

⑦S63.259　Unspecified dislocation of unspecified finger

Unspecified dislocation of unspecified finger with unspecified laterality

　● New code　▲ Revised code　Excludes1: Not coded here　Excludes2: Not included here　⊗ Placeholder required　⑦ 7th digit required

S63.26   Dislocation of metacarpophalangeal joint of finger

⑦S63.260   Dislocation of metacarpophalangeal joint of right index finger

⑦S63.261   Dislocation of metacarpophalangeal joint of left index finger

⑦S63.262   Dislocation of metacarpophalangeal joint of right middle finger

⑦S63.263   Dislocation of metacarpophalangeal joint of left middle finger

⑦S63.264   Dislocation of metacarpophalangeal joint of right ring finger

⑦S63.265   Dislocation of metacarpophalangeal joint of left ring finger

⑦S63.266   Dislocation of metacarpophalangeal joint of right little finger

⑦S63.267   Dislocation of metacarpophalangeal joint of left little finger

⑦S63.268   Dislocation of metacarpophalangeal joint of other finger

Dislocation of metacarpophalangeal joint of specified finger with unspecified laterality

⑦S63.269   Dislocation of metacarpophalangeal joint of unspecified finger

S63.27   Dislocation of unspecified interphalangeal joint of finger

⑦S63.270   Dislocation of unspecified interphalangeal joint of right index finger

⑦S63.271   Dislocation of unspecified interphalangeal joint of left index finger

⑦S63.272   Dislocation of unspecified interphalangeal joint of right middle finger

⑦S63.273   Dislocation of unspecified interphalangeal joint of left middle finger

⑦S63.274   Dislocation of unspecified interphalangeal joint of right ring finger

⑦S63.275   Dislocation of unspecified interphalangeal joint of left ring finger

⑦S63.276   Dislocation of unspecified interphalangeal joint of right little finger

⑦S63.277   Dislocation of unspecified interphalangeal joint of left little finger

⑦S63.278   Dislocation of unspecified interphalangeal joint of other finger

Dislocation of unspecified interphalangeal joint of specified finger with unspecified laterality

⑦S63.279   Dislocation of unspecified interphalangeal joint of unspecified finger

Dislocation of unspecified interphalangeal joint of unspecified finger without specified laterality

S63.28   Dislocation of proximal interphalangeal joint of finger

⑦S63.280   Dislocation of proximal interphalangeal joint of right index finger

⑦S63.281   Dislocation of proximal interphalangeal joint of left index finger

⑦S63.282   Dislocation of proximal interphalangeal joint of right middle finger

⑦S63.283   Dislocation of proximal interphalangeal joint of left middle finger

⑦S63.284   Dislocation of proximal interphalangeal joint of right ring finger

⑦S63.285   Dislocation of proximal interphalangeal joint of left ring finger

⑦S63.286   Dislocation of proximal interphalangeal joint of right little finger

⑦S63.287   Dislocation of proximal interphalangeal joint of left little finger

⑦S63.288   Dislocation of proximal interphalangeal joint of other finger

Dislocation of proximal interphalangeal joint of specified finger with unspecified laterality

⑦S63.289   Dislocation of proximal interphalangeal joint of unspecified finger

S63.29   Dislocation of distal interphalangeal joint of finger

⑦S63.290   Dislocation of distal interphalangeal joint of right index finger

⑦S63.291   Dislocation of distal interphalangeal joint of left index finger

⑦S63.292   Dislocation of distal interphalangeal joint of right middle finger

⑦S63.293   Dislocation of distal interphalangeal joint of left middle finger

⑦S63.294   Dislocation of distal interphalangeal joint of right ring finger

⑦S63.295   Dislocation of distal interphalangeal joint of left ring finger

⑦S63.296   Dislocation of distal interphalangeal joint of right little finger

⑦S63.297   Dislocation of distal interphalangeal joint of left little finger

⑦S63.298   Dislocation of distal interphalangeal joint of other finger

Dislocation of distal interphalangeal joint of specified finger with unspecified laterality

⑦S63.299   Dislocation of distal interphalangeal joint of unspecified finger

S63.3   Traumatic rupture of ligament of wrist

S63.30   Traumatic rupture of unspecified ligament of wrist

⑦S63.301   Traumatic rupture of unspecified ligament of right wrist

⑦S63.302   Traumatic rupture of unspecified ligament of left wrist

⑦S63.309   Traumatic rupture of unspecified ligament of unspecified wrist

S63.31 **Traumatic rupture of collateral ligament of wrist**

⑦**S63.311** **Traumatic rupture of collateral ligament of right wrist**

⑦**S63.312** **Traumatic rupture of collateral ligament of left wrist**

⑦**S63.319** **Traumatic rupture of collateral ligament of unspecified wrist**

S63.32 **Traumatic rupture of radiocarpal ligament**

⑦**S63.321** **Traumatic rupture of right radiocarpal ligament**

⑦**S63.322** **Traumatic rupture of left radiocarpal ligament**

⑦**S63.329** **Traumatic rupture of unspecified radiocarpal ligament**

S63.33 **Traumatic rupture of ulnocarpal (palmar) ligament**

⑦**S63.331** **Traumatic rupture of right ulnocarpal (palmar) ligament**

⑦**S63.332** **Traumatic rupture of left ulnocarpal (palmar) ligament**

⑦**S63.339** **Traumatic rupture of unspecified ulnocarpal (palmar) ligament**

S63.39 **Traumatic rupture of other ligament of wrist**

⑦**S63.391** **Traumatic rupture of other ligament of right wrist**

⑦**S63.392** **Traumatic rupture of other ligament of left wrist**

⑦**S63.399** **Traumatic rupture of other ligament of unspecified wrist**

S63.4 **Traumatic rupture of ligament of finger at metacarpophalangeal and interphalangeal joint(s)**

S63.40 **Traumatic rupture of unspecified ligament of finger at metacarpophalangeal and interphalangeal joint**

⑦**S63.400** **Traumatic rupture of unspecified ligament of right index finger at metacarpophalangeal and interphalangeal joint**

⑦**S63.401** **Traumatic rupture of unspecified ligament of left index finger at metacarpophalangeal and interphalangeal joint**

⑦**S63.402** **Traumatic rupture of unspecified ligament of right middle finger at metacarpophalangeal and interphalangeal joint**

⑦**S63.403** **Traumatic rupture of unspecified ligament of left middle finger at metacarpophalangeal and interphalangeal joint**

⑦**S63.404** **Traumatic rupture of unspecified ligament of right ring finger at metacarpophalangeal and interphalangeal joint**

⑦**S63.405** **Traumatic rupture of unspecified ligament of left ring finger at metacarpophalangeal and interphalangeal joint**

⑦**S63.406** **Traumatic rupture of unspecified ligament of right little finger at metacarpophalangeal and interphalangeal joint**

⑦**S63.407** **Traumatic rupture of unspecified ligament of left little finger at**

metacarpophalangeal and interphalangeal joint

⑦**S63.408** **Traumatic rupture of unspecified ligament of other finger at metacarpophalangeal and interphalangeal joint**

Traumatic rupture of unspecified ligament of specified finger with unspecified laterality at metacarpophalangeal and interphalangeal joint

⑦**S63.409** **Traumatic rupture of unspecified ligament of unspecified finger at metacarpophalangeal and interphalangeal joint**

S63.41 **Traumatic rupture of collateral ligament of finger at metacarpophalangeal and interphalangeal joint**

⑦**S63.410** **Traumatic rupture of collateral ligament of right index finger at metacarpophalangeal and interphalangeal joint**

⑦**S63.411** **Traumatic rupture of collateral ligament of left index finger at metacarpophalangeal and interphalangeal joint**

⑦**S63.412** **Traumatic rupture of collateral ligament of right middle finger at metacarpophalangeal and interphalangeal joint**

⑦**S63.413** **Traumatic rupture of collateral ligament of left middle finger at metacarpophalangeal and interphalangeal joint**

⑦**S63.414** **Traumatic rupture of collateral ligament of right ring finger at metacarpophalangeal and interphalangeal joint**

⑦**S63.415** **Traumatic rupture of collateral ligament of left ring finger at metacarpophalangeal and interphalangeal joint**

⑦**S63.416** **Traumatic rupture of collateral ligament of right little finger at metacarpophalangeal and interphalangeal joint**

⑦**S63.417** **Traumatic rupture of collateral ligament of left little finger at metacarpophalangeal and interphalangeal joint**

⑦**S63.418** **Traumatic rupture of collateral ligament of other finger at metacarpophalangeal and interphalangeal joint**

Traumatic rupture of collateral ligament of specified finger with unspecified laterality at metacarpophalangeal and interphalangeal joint

⑦**S63.419** **Traumatic rupture of collateral ligament of unspecified finger at metacarpophalangeal and interphalangeal joint**

S63.42 **Traumatic rupture of palmar ligament of finger at metacarpophalangeal and interphalangeal joint**

⑦**S63.420** **Traumatic rupture of palmar ligament of right index finger at**

● New code ▲ Revised code **Excludes1:** Not coded here **Excludes2:** Not included here ⊗ Placeholder required ⑦7th digit required

metacarpophalangeal and interphalangeal joint

⑦S63.421 **Traumatic rupture of palmar ligament of left index finger at metacarpophalangeal and interphalangeal joint**

⑦S63.422 **Traumatic rupture of palmar ligament of right middle finger at metacarpophalangeal and interphalangeal joint**

⑦S63.423 **Traumatic rupture of palmar ligament of left middle finger at metacarpophalangeal and interphalangeal joint**

⑦S63.424 **Traumatic rupture of palmar ligament of right ring finger at metacarpophalangeal and interphalangeal joint**

⑦S63.425 **Traumatic rupture of palmar ligament of left ring finger at metacarpophalangeal and interphalangeal joint**

⑦S63.426 **Traumatic rupture of palmar ligament of right little finger at metacarpophalangeal and interphalangeal joint**

⑦S63.427 **Traumatic rupture of palmar ligament of left little finger at metacarpophalangeal and interphalangeal joint**

⑦S63.428 **Traumatic rupture of palmar ligament of other finger at metacarpophalangeal and interphalangeal joint**

Traumatic rupture of palmar ligament of specified finger with unspecified laterality at metacarpophalangeal and interphalangeal joint

⑦S63.429 **Traumatic rupture of palmar ligament of unspecified finger at metacarpophalangeal and interphalangeal joint**

S63.43 **Traumatic rupture of volar plate of finger at metacarpophalangeal and interphalangeal joint**

⑦S63.430 **Traumatic rupture of volar plate of right index finger at metacarpophalangeal and interphalangeal joint**

⑦S63.431 **Traumatic rupture of volar plate of left index finger at metacarpophalangeal and interphalangeal joint**

⑦S63.432 **Traumatic rupture of volar plate of right middle finger at metacarpophalangeal and interphalangeal joint**

⑦S63.433 **Traumatic rupture of volar plate of left middle finger at metacarpophalangeal and interphalangeal joint**

⑦S63.434 **Traumatic rupture of volar plate of right ring finger at metacarpophalangeal and interphalangeal joint**

⑦S63.435 **Traumatic rupture of volar plate of left ring finger at metacarpophalangeal and interphalangeal joint**

⑦S63.436 **Traumatic rupture of volar plate of right little finger at metacarpophalangeal and interphalangeal joint**

⑦S63.437 **Traumatic rupture of volar plate of left little finger at metacarpophalangeal and interphalangeal joint**

⑦S63.438 **Traumatic rupture of volar plate of other finger at metacarpophalangeal and interphalangeal joint**

Traumatic rupture of volar plate of specified finger with unspecified laterality at metacarpophalangeal and interphalangeal joint

⑦S63.439 **Traumatic rupture of volar plate of unspecified finger at metacarpophalangeal and interphalangeal joint**

S63.49 **Traumatic rupture of other ligament of finger at metacarpophalangeal and interphalangeal joint**

⑦S63.490 **Traumatic rupture of other ligament of right index finger at metacarpophalangeal and interphalangeal joint**

⑦S63.491 **Traumatic rupture of other ligament of left index finger at metacarpophalangeal and interphalangeal joint**

⑦S63.492 **Traumatic rupture of other ligament of right middle finger at metacarpophalangeal and interphalangeal joint**

⑦S63.493 **Traumatic rupture of other ligament of left middle finger at metacarpophalangeal and interphalangeal joint**

⑦S63.494 **Traumatic rupture of other ligament of right ring finger at metacarpophalangeal and interphalangeal joint**

⑦S63.495 **Traumatic rupture of other ligament of left ring finger at metacarpophalangeal and interphalangeal joint**

⑦S63.496 **Traumatic rupture of other ligament of right little finger at metacarpophalangeal and interphalangeal joint**

⑦S63.497 **Traumatic rupture of other ligament of left little finger at metacarpophalangeal and interphalangeal joint**

⑦S63.498 **Traumatic rupture of other ligament of other finger at metacarpophalangeal and interphalangeal joint**

Traumatic rupture of ligament of specified finger with unspecified laterality at metacarpophalangeal and interphalangeal joint

⑦S63.499 **Traumatic rupture of other ligament of unspecified finger at metacarpophalangeal and interphalangeal joint**

S63.5 **Other and unspecified sprain of wrist**

S63.50 **Unspecified sprain of wrist**

⑦S63.501 Unspecified sprain of right wrist

⑦S63.502 Unspecified sprain of left wrist

⑦S63.509 Unspecified sprain of unspecified wrist

S63.51 Sprain of carpal (joint)

⑦S63.511 Sprain of carpal joint of right wrist

⑦S63.512 Sprain of carpal joint of left wrist

⑦S63.519 Sprain of carpal joint of unspecified wrist

S63.52 Sprain of radiocarpal joint

Excludes1: traumatic rupture of radiocarpal ligament (S63.32-)

⑦S63.521 Sprain of radiocarpal joint of right wrist

⑦S63.522 Sprain of radiocarpal joint of left wrist

⑦S63.529 Sprain of radiocarpal joint of unspecified wrist

S63.59 Other specified sprain of wrist

⑦S63.591 Other specified sprain of right wrist

⑦S63.592 Other specified sprain of left wrist

⑦S63.599 Other specified sprain of unspecified wrist

S63.6 Other and unspecified sprain of finger(s)

Excludes1: traumatic rupture of ligament of finger at metacarpophalangeal and interphalangeal joint(s) (S63.4-)

S63.60 Unspecified sprain of thumb

⑦S63.601 Unspecified sprain of right thumb

⑦S63.602 Unspecified sprain of left thumb

⑦S63.609 Unspecified sprain of unspecified thumb

S63.61 Unspecified sprain of other and unspecified finger(s)

⑦S63.610 Unspecified sprain of right index finger

⑦S63.611 Unspecified sprain of left index finger

⑦S63.612 Unspecified sprain of right middle finger

⑦S63.613 Unspecified sprain of left middle finger

⑦S63.614 Unspecified sprain of right ring finger

⑦S63.615 Unspecified sprain of left ring finger

⑦S63.616 Unspecified sprain of right little finger

⑦S63.617 Unspecified sprain of left little finger

⑦S63.618 Unspecified sprain of other finger

Unspecified sprain of specified finger with unspecified laterality

⑦S63.619 Unspecified sprain of unspecified finger

S63.62 Sprain of interphalangeal joint of thumb

⑦S63.621 Sprain of interphalangeal joint of right thumb

⑦S63.622 Sprain of interphalangeal joint of left thumb

⑦S63.629 Sprain of interphalangeal joint of unspecified thumb

S63.63 Sprain of interphalangeal joint of other and unspecified finger(s)

⑦S63.630 Sprain of interphalangeal joint of right index finger

⑦S63.631 Sprain of interphalangeal joint of left index finger

⑦S63.632 Sprain of interphalangeal joint of right middle finger

⑦S63.633 Sprain of interphalangeal joint of left middle finger

⑦S63.634 Sprain of interphalangeal joint of right ring finger

⑦S63.635 Sprain of interphalangeal joint of left ring finger

⑦S63.636 Sprain of interphalangeal joint of right little finger

⑦S63.637 Sprain of interphalangeal joint of left little finger

⑦S63.638 Sprain of interphalangeal joint of other finger

⑦S63.639 Sprain of interphalangeal joint of unspecified finger

S63.64 Sprain of metacarpophalangeal joint of thumb

⑦S63.641 Sprain of metacarpophalangeal joint of right thumb

⑦S63.642 Sprain of metacarpophalangeal joint of left thumb

S63.649 Sprain of metacarpophalangeal joint of unspecified thumb

S63.65 Sprain of metacarpophalangeal joint of other and unspecified finger(s)

⑦S63.650 Sprain of metacarpophalangeal joint of right index finger

⑦S63.651 Sprain of metacarpophalangeal joint of left index finger

⑦S63.652 Sprain of metacarpophalangeal joint of right middle finger

⑦S63.653 Sprain of metacarpophalangeal joint of left middle finger

⑦S63.654 Sprain of metacarpophalangeal joint of right ring finger

⑦S63.655 Sprain of metacarpophalangeal joint of left ring finger

⑦S63.656 Sprain of metacarpophalangeal joint of right little finger

⑦S63.657 Sprain of metacarpophalangeal joint of left little finger

⑦S63.658 Sprain of metacarpophalangeal joint of other finger

Sprain of metacarpophalangeal joint of specified finger with unspecified laterality

⑦S63.659 Sprain of metacarpophalangeal joint of unspecified finger

S63.68 Other sprain of thumb

⑦S63.681 Other sprain of right thumb

⑦S63.682 Other sprain of left thumb

⑦S63.689 Other sprain of unspecified thumb

S63.69 Other sprain of other and unspecified finger(s)

⑦S63.690 Other sprain of right index finger

⑦S63.691 Other sprain of left index finger

⑦S63.692 Other sprain of right middle finger

⑦S63.693 Other sprain of left middle finger

⑦S63.694 Other sprain of right ring finger

⑦S63.695 Other sprain of left ring finger

● New code ▲ Revised code **Excludes1:** Not coded here **Excludes2:** Not included here ⊗ Placeholder required ⑦ 7th digit required

⑦**S63.696** Other sprain of right little finger

⑦**S63.697** Other sprain of left little finger

⑦**S63.698** Other sprain of other finger

Other sprain of specified finger with unspecified laterality

⑦**S63.699** Other sprain of unspecified finger

S63.8 Sprain of other part of wrist and hand

S63.8X Sprain of other part of wrist and hand

⑦**S63.8X1** Sprain of other part of right wrist and hand

⑦**S63.8X2** Sprain of other part of left wrist and hand

⑦**S63.8X9** Sprain of other part of unspecified wrist and hand

S63.9 Sprain of unspecified part of wrist and hand

⊗⑦**S63.90** Sprain of unspecified part of unspecified wrist and hand

⊗⑦**S63.91** Sprain of unspecified part of right wrist and hand

⊗⑦**S63.92** Sprain of unspecified part of left wrist and hand

S64 **Injury of nerves at wrist and hand level**

Code also any associated open wound (S61.-)

The appropriate 7th character is to be added to each code from category S64

A - initial encounter

D - subsequent encounter

S - sequela

S64.0 Injury of ulnar nerve at wrist and hand level

⊗⑦**S64.00** Injury of ulnar nerve at wrist and hand level of unspecified arm

⊗⑦**S64.01** Injury of ulnar nerve at wrist and hand level of right arm

⊗⑦**S64.02** Injury of ulnar nerve at wrist and hand level of left arm

S64.1 Injury of median nerve at wrist and hand level

⊗⑦**S64.10** Injury of median nerve at wrist and hand level of unspecified arm

⊗⑦**S64.11** Injury of median nerve at wrist and hand level of right arm

⊗⑦**S64.12** Injury of median nerve at wrist and hand level of left arm

S64.2 Injury of radial nerve at wrist and hand level

⊗⑦**S64.20** Injury of radial nerve at wrist and hand level of unspecified arm

⊗⑦**S64.21** Injury of radial nerve at wrist and hand level of right arm

⊗⑦**S64.22** Injury of radial nerve at wrist and hand level of left arm

S64.3 Injury of digital nerve of thumb

⊗⑦**S64.30** Injury of digital nerve of unspecified thumb

⊗⑦**S64.31** Injury of digital nerve of right thumb

⊗⑦**S64.32** Injury of digital nerve of left thumb

S64.4 Injury of digital nerve of other and unspecified finger

⊗⑦**S64.40** Injury of digital nerve of unspecified finger

S64.49 Injury of digital nerve of other finger

⑦**S64.490** Injury of digital nerve of right index finger

⑦**S64.491** Injury of digital nerve of left index finger

⑦**S64.492** Injury of digital nerve of right middle finger

⑦**S64.493** Injury of digital nerve of left middle finger

⑦**S64.494** Injury of digital nerve of right ring finger

⑦**S64.495** Injury of digital nerve of left ring finger

⑦**S64.496** Injury of digital nerve of right little finger

⑦**S64.497** Injury of digital nerve of left little finger

⑦**S64.498** Injury of digital nerve of other finger

Injury of digital nerve of specified finger with unspecified laterality

S64.8 Injury of other nerves at wrist and hand level

S64.8X Injury of other nerves at wrist and hand level

⑦**S64.8X1** Injury of other nerves at wrist and hand level of right arm

⑦**S64.8X2** Injury of other nerves at wrist and hand level of left arm

⑦**S64.8X9** Injury of other nerves at wrist and hand level of unspecified arm

S64.9 Injury of unspecified nerve at wrist and hand level

⊗⑦**S64.90** Injury of unspecified nerve at wrist and hand level of unspecified arm

⊗⑦**S64.91** Injury of unspecified nerve at wrist and hand level of right arm

⊗⑦**S64.92** Injury of unspecified nerve at wrist and hand level of left arm

S65 **Injury of blood vessels at wrist and hand level**

Code also any associated open wound (S61.-)

The appropriate 7th character is to be added to each code from category S65

A - initial encounter

D - subsequent encounter

S - sequela

S65.0 Injury of ulnar artery at wrist and hand level

S65.00 Unspecified injury of ulnar artery at wrist and hand level

⑦**S65.001** Unspecified injury of ulnar artery at wrist and hand level of right arm

⑦**S65.002** Unspecified injury of ulnar artery at wrist and hand level of left arm

⑦**S65.009** Unspecified injury of ulnar artery at wrist and hand level of unspecified arm

S65.01 Laceration of ulnar artery at wrist and hand level

⑦**S65.011** Laceration of ulnar artery at wrist and hand level of right arm

⑦**S65.012** Laceration of ulnar artery at wrist and hand level of left arm

⑦**S65.019** Laceration of ulnar artery at wrist and hand level of unspecified arm

S65.09 Other specified injury of ulnar artery at wrist and hand level

⑦**S65.091** Other specified injury of ulnar artery at wrist and hand level of right arm

⑦**S65.092** Other specified injury of ulnar artery at wrist and hand level of left arm

⑦S65.099   Other specified injury of ulnar artery at wrist and hand level of unspecified arm

S65.1   **Injury of radial artery at wrist and hand level**

   S65.10   Unspecified injury of radial artery at wrist and hand level

     ⑦S65.101   Unspecified injury of radial artery at wrist and hand level of right arm

     ⑦S65.102   Unspecified injury of radial artery at wrist and hand level of left arm

     ⑦S65.109   Unspecified injury of radial artery at wrist and hand level of unspecified arm

   S65.11   Laceration of radial artery at wrist and hand level

     ⑦S65.111   Laceration of radial artery at wrist and hand level of right arm

     ⑦S65.112   Laceration of radial artery at wrist and hand level of left arm

     ⑦S65.119   Laceration of radial artery at wrist and hand level of unspecified arm

   S65.19   Other specified injury of radial artery at wrist and hand level

     ⑦S65.191   Other specified injury of radial artery at wrist and hand level of right arm

     ⑦S65.192   Other specified injury of radial artery at wrist and hand level of left arm

     ⑦S65.199   Other specified injury of radial artery at wrist and hand level of unspecified arm

S65.2   **Injury of superficial palmar arch**

   S65.20   Unspecified injury of superficial palmar arch

     ⑦S65.201   Unspecified injury of superficial palmar arch of right hand

     ⑦S65.202   Unspecified injury of superficial palmar arch of left hand

     ⑦S65.209   Unspecified injury of superficial palmar arch of unspecified hand

   S65.21   Laceration of superficial palmar arch

     ⑦S65.211   Laceration of superficial palmar arch of right hand

     ⑦S65.212   Laceration of superficial palmar arch of left hand

     ⑦S65.219   Laceration of superficial palmar arch of unspecified hand

   S65.29   Other specified injury of superficial palmar arch

     ⑦S65.291   Other specified injury of superficial palmar arch of right hand

     ⑦S65.292   Other specified injury of superficial palmar arch of left hand

     ⑦S65.299   Other specified injury of superficial palmar arch of unspecified hand

S65.3   **Injury of deep palmar arch**

   S65.30   Unspecified injury of deep palmar arch

     ⑦S65.301   Unspecified injury of deep palmar arch of right hand

     ⑦S65.302   Unspecified injury of deep palmar arch of left hand

     ⑦S65.309   Unspecified injury of deep palmar arch of unspecified hand

   S65.31   Laceration of deep palmar arch

     ⑦S65.311   Laceration of deep palmar arch of right hand

     ⑦S65.312   Laceration of deep palmar arch of left hand

     ⑦S65.319   Laceration of deep palmar arch of unspecified hand

   S65.39   Other specified injury of deep palmar arch

     ⑦S65.391   Other specified injury of deep palmar arch of right hand

     ⑦S65.392   Other specified injury of deep palmar arch of left hand

     ⑦S65.399   Other specified injury of deep palmar arch of unspecified hand

S65.4   **Injury of blood vessel of thumb**

   S65.40   Unspecified injury of blood vessel of thumb

     ⑦S65.401   Unspecified injury of blood vessel of right thumb

     ⑦S65.402   Unspecified injury of blood vessel of left thumb

     ⑦S65.409   Unspecified injury of blood vessel of unspecified thumb

   S65.41   Laceration of blood vessel of thumb

     ⑦S65.411   Laceration of blood vessel of right thumb

     ⑦S65.412   Laceration of blood vessel of left thumb

     ⑦S65.419   Laceration of blood vessel of unspecified thumb

   S65.49   Other specified injury of blood vessel of thumb

     ⑦S65.491   Other specified injury of blood vessel of right thumb

     ⑦S65.492   Other specified injury of blood vessel of left thumb

     ⑦S65.499   Other specified injury of blood vessel of unspecified thumb

S65.5   **Injury of blood vessel of other and unspecified finger**

   S65.50   Unspecified injury of blood vessel of other and unspecified finger

     ⑦S65.500   Unspecified injury of blood vessel of right index finger

     ⑦S65.501   Unspecified injury of blood vessel of left index finger

     ⑦S65.502   Unspecified injury of blood vessel of right middle finger

     ⑦S65.503   Unspecified injury of blood vessel of left middle finger

     ⑦S65.504   Unspecified injury of blood vessel of right ring finger

     ⑦S65.505   Unspecified injury of blood vessel of left ring finger

     ⑦S65.506   Unspecified injury of blood vessel of right little finger

     ⑦S65.507   Unspecified injury of blood vessel of left little finger

     ⑦S65.508   Unspecified injury of blood vessel of other finger

            Unspecified injury of blood vessel of specified finger with unspecified laterality

     ⑦S65.509   Unspecified injury of blood vessel of unspecified finger

   S65.51   Laceration of blood vessel of other and unspecified finger

● New code   ▲ Revised code   **Excludes1:** Not coded here   **Excludes2:** Not included here   ⊗ Placeholder required   ⑦7ᵗʰ digit required

⑦S65.510 **Laceration of blood vessel of right index finger**

⑦S65.511 **Laceration of blood vessel of left index finger**

⑦S65.512 **Laceration of blood vessel of right middle finger**

⑦S65.513 **Laceration of blood vessel of left middle finger**

⑦S65.514 **Laceration of blood vessel of right ring finger**

⑦S65.515 **Laceration of blood vessel of left ring finger**

⑦S65.516 **Laceration of blood vessel of right little finger**

⑦S65.517 **Laceration of blood vessel of left little finger**

⑦S65.518 **Laceration of blood vessel of other finger**

Laceration of blood vessel of specified finger with unspecified laterality

⑦S65.519 **Laceration of blood vessel of unspecified finger**

S65.59 **Other specified injury of blood vessel of other and unspecified finger**

⑦S65.590 **Other specified injury of blood vessel of right index finger**

⑦S65.591 **Other specified injury of blood vessel of left index finger**

⑦S65.592 **Other specified injury of blood vessel of right middle finger**

⑦S65.593 **Other specified injury of blood vessel of left middle finger**

⑦S65.594 **Other specified injury of blood vessel of right ring finger**

⑦S65.595 **Other specified injury of blood vessel of left ring finger**

⑦S65.596 **Other specified injury of blood vessel of right little finger**

⑦S65.597 **Other specified injury of blood vessel of left little finger**

⑦S65.598 **Other specified injury of blood vessel of other finger**

Other specified injury of blood vessel of specified finger with unspecified laterality

⑦S65.599 **Other specified injury of blood vessel of unspecified finger**

S65.8 **Injury of other blood vessels at wrist and hand level**

S65.80 **Unspecified injury of other blood vessels at wrist and hand level**

⑦S65.801 **Unspecified injury of other blood vessels at wrist and hand level of right arm**

⑦S65.802 **Unspecified injury of other blood vessels at wrist and hand level of left arm**

⑦S65.809 **Unspecified injury of other blood vessels at wrist and hand level of unspecified arm**

S65.81 **Laceration of other blood vessels at wrist and hand level**

⑦S65.811 **Laceration of other blood vessels at wrist and hand level of right arm**

⑦S65.812 **Laceration of other blood vessels at wrist and hand level of left arm**

⑦S65.819 **Laceration of other blood vessels at wrist and hand level of unspecified arm**

S65.89 **Other specified injury of other blood vessels at wrist and hand level**

⑦S65.891 **Other specified injury of other blood vessels at wrist and hand level of right arm**

⑦S65.892 **Other specified injury of other blood vessels at wrist and hand level of left arm**

⑦S65.899 **Other specified injury of other blood vessels at wrist and hand level of unspecified arm**

S65.9 **Injury of unspecified blood vessel at wrist and hand level**

S65.90 **Unspecified injury of unspecified blood vessel at wrist and hand level**

⑦S65.901 **Unspecified injury of unspecified blood vessel at wrist and hand level of right arm**

⑦S65.902 **Unspecified injury of unspecified blood vessel at wrist and hand level of left arm**

⑦S65.909 **Unspecified injury of unspecified blood vessel at wrist and hand level of unspecified arm**

S65.91 **Laceration of unspecified blood vessel at wrist and hand level**

⑦S65.911 **Laceration of unspecified blood vessel at wrist and hand level of right arm**

⑦S65.912 **Laceration of unspecified blood vessel at wrist and hand level of left arm**

⑦S65.919 **Laceration of unspecified blood vessel at wrist and hand level of unspecified arm**

S65.99 **Other specified injury of unspecified blood vessel at wrist and hand level**

⑦S65.991 **Other specified injury of unspecified blood vessel at wrist and hand of right arm**

⑦S65.992 **Other specified injury of unspecified blood vessel at wrist and hand of left arm**

⑦S65.999 **Other specified injury of unspecified blood vessel at wrist and hand of unspecified arm**

S66 **Injury of muscle, fascia and tendon at wrist and hand level**

Code also any associated open wound (S61.-)

Excludes2: sprain of joints and ligaments of wrist and hand (S63.-)

The appropriate 7th character is to be added to each code from category S66

A - initial encounter

D - subsequent encounter

S - sequela

S66.0 **Injury of long flexor muscle, fascia and tendon of thumb at wrist and hand level**

S66.00 **Unspecified injury of long flexor muscle, fascia and tendon of thumb at wrist and hand level**

⑦S66.001 **Unspecified injury of long flexor muscle, fascia and tendon of right thumb at wrist and hand level**

⑦S66.002 Unspecified injury of long flexor muscle, fascia and tendon of left thumb at wrist and hand level

⑦S66.009 Unspecified injury of long flexor muscle, fascia and tendon of unspecified thumb at wrist and hand level

S66.01 Strain of long flexor muscle, fascia and tendon of thumb at wrist and hand level

⑦S66.011 Strain of long flexor muscle, fascia and tendon of right thumb at wrist and hand level

⑦S66.012 Strain of long flexor muscle, fascia and tendon of left thumb at wrist and hand level

⑦S66.019 Strain of long flexor muscle, fascia and tendon of unspecified thumb at wrist and hand level

S66.02 Laceration of long flexor muscle, fascia and tendon of thumb at wrist and hand level

⑦S66.021 Laceration of long flexor muscle, fascia and tendon of right thumb at wrist and hand level

⑦S66.022 Laceration of long flexor muscle, fascia and tendon of left thumb at wrist and hand level

⑦S66.029 Laceration of long flexor muscle, fascia and tendon of unspecified thumb at wrist and hand level

S66.09 Other specified injury of long flexor muscle, fascia and tendon of thumb at wrist and hand level

⑦S66.091 Other specified injury of long flexor muscle, fascia and tendon of right thumb at wrist and hand level

⑦S66.092 Other specified injury of long flexor muscle, fascia and tendon of left thumb at wrist and hand level

⑦S66.099 Other specified injury of long flexor muscle, fascia and tendon of unspecified thumb at wrist and hand level

S66.1 Injury of flexor muscle, fascia and tendon of other and unspecified finger at wrist and hand level

Excludes2: Injury of long flexor muscle, fascia and tendon of thumb at wrist and hand level (S66.0-)

S66.10 Unspecified injury of flexor muscle, fascia and tendon of other and unspecified finger at wrist and hand level

⑦S66.100 Unspecified injury of flexor muscle, fascia and tendon of right index finger at wrist and hand level

⑦S66.101 Unspecified injury of flexor muscle, fascia and tendon of left index finger at wrist and hand level

⑦S66.102 Unspecified injury of flexor muscle, fascia and tendon of right middle finger at wrist and hand level

⑦S66.103 Unspecified injury of flexor muscle, fascia and tendon of left middle finger at wrist and hand level

⑦S66.104 Unspecified injury of flexor muscle, fascia and tendon of right ring finger at wrist and hand level

⑦S66.105 Unspecified injury of flexor muscle, fascia and tendon of left ring finger at wrist and hand level

⑦S66.106 Unspecified injury of flexor muscle, fascia and tendon of right little finger at wrist and hand level

⑦S66.107 Unspecified injury of flexor muscle, fascia and tendon of left little finger at wrist and hand level

⑦S66.108 Unspecified injury of flexor muscle, fascia and tendon of other finger at wrist and hand level

Unspecified injury of flexor muscle, fascia and tendon of specified finger with unspecified laterality at wrist and hand level

⑦S66.109 Unspecified injury of flexor muscle, fascia and tendon of unspecified finger at wrist and hand level

S66.11 Strain of flexor muscle, fascia and tendon of other and unspecified finger at wrist and hand level

⑦S66.110 Strain of flexor muscle, fascia and tendon of right index finger at wrist and hand level

⑦S66.111 Strain of flexor muscle, fascia and tendon of left index finger at wrist and hand level

⑦S66.112 Strain of flexor muscle, fascia and tendon of right middle finger at wrist and hand level

⑦S66.113 Strain of flexor muscle, fascia and tendon of left middle finger at wrist and hand level

⑦S66.114 Strain of flexor muscle, fascia and tendon of right ring finger at wrist and hand level

⑦S66.115 Strain of flexor muscle, fascia and tendon of left ring finger at wrist and hand level

⑦S66.116 Strain of flexor muscle, fascia and tendon of right little finger at wrist and hand level

⑦S66.117 Strain of flexor muscle, fascia and tendon of left little finger at wrist and hand level

⑦S66.118 Strain of flexor muscle, fascia and tendon of other finger at wrist and hand level

Strain of flexor muscle, fascia and tendon of specified finger with unspecified laterality at wrist and hand level

⑦S66.119 Strain of flexor muscle, fascia and tendon of unspecified finger at wrist and hand level

S66.12 Laceration of flexor muscle, fascia and tendon of other and unspecified finger at wrist and hand level

⑦S66.120 Laceration of flexor muscle, fascia and tendon of right index finger at wrist and hand level

⑦S66.121 Laceration of flexor muscle, fascia and tendon of left index finger at wrist and hand level

⑦S66.122 Laceration of flexor muscle, fascia and tendon of right middle finger at wrist and hand level

⑦S66.123 Laceration of flexor muscle, fascia and tendon of left middle finger at wrist and hand level

● New code ▲ Revised code **Excludes1:** Not coded here **Excludes2:** Not included here ⊗ Placeholder required ⑦7th digit required

⑦S66.124 **Laceration of flexor muscle, fascia and tendon of right ring finger at wrist and hand level**

⑦S66.125 **Laceration of flexor muscle, fascia and tendon of left ring finger at wrist and hand level**

⑦S66.126 **Laceration of flexor muscle, fascia and tendon of right little finger at wrist and hand level**

⑦S66.127 **Laceration of flexor muscle, fascia and tendon of left little finger at wrist and hand level**

⑦S66.128 **Laceration of flexor muscle, fascia and tendon of other finger at wrist and hand level**

Laceration of flexor muscle, fascia and tendon of specified finger with unspecified laterality at wrist and hand level

⑦S66.129 **Laceration of flexor muscle, fascia and tendon of unspecified finger at wrist and hand level**

S66.19 **Other injury of flexor muscle, fascia and tendon of other and unspecified finger at wrist and hand level**

⑦S66.190 **Other injury of flexor muscle, fascia and tendon of right index finger at wrist and hand level**

⑦S66.191 **Other injury of flexor muscle, fascia and tendon of left index finger at wrist and hand level**

⑦S66.192 **Other injury of flexor muscle, fascia and tendon of right middle finger at wrist and hand level**

⑦S66.193 **Other injury of flexor muscle, fascia and tendon of left middle finger at wrist and hand level**

⑦S66.194 **Other injury of flexor muscle, fascia and tendon of right ring finger at wrist and hand level**

⑦S66.195 **Other injury of flexor muscle, fascia and tendon of left ring finger at wrist and hand level**

⑦S66.196 **Other injury of flexor muscle, fascia and tendon of right little finger at wrist and hand level**

⑦S66.197 **Other injury of flexor muscle, fascia and tendon of left little finger at wrist and hand level**

⑦S66.198 **Other injury of flexor muscle, fascia and tendon of other finger at wrist and hand level**

Other injury of flexor muscle, fascia and tendon of specified finger with unspecified laterality at wrist and hand level

⑦S66.199 **Other injury of flexor muscle, fascia and tendon of unspecified finger at wrist and hand level**

S66.2 **Injury of extensor muscle, fascia and tendon of thumb at wrist and hand level**

S66.20 **Unspecified injury of extensor muscle, fascia and tendon of thumb at wrist and hand level**

⑦S66.201 **Unspecified injury of extensor muscle, fascia and tendon of right thumb at wrist and hand level**

⑦S66.202 **Unspecified injury of extensor muscle, fascia and tendon of left thumb at wrist and hand level**

⑦S66.209 **Unspecified injury of extensor muscle, fascia and tendon of unspecified thumb at wrist and hand level**

S66.21 **Strain of extensor muscle, fascia and tendon of thumb at wrist and hand level**

⑦S66.211 **Strain of extensor muscle, fascia and tendon of right thumb at wrist and hand level**

⑦S66.212 **Strain of extensor muscle, fascia and tendon of left thumb at wrist and hand level**

⑦S66.219 **Strain of extensor muscle, fascia and tendon of unspecified thumb at wrist and hand level**

S66.22 **Laceration of extensor muscle, fascia and tendon of thumb at wrist and hand level**

⑦S66.221 **Laceration of extensor muscle, fascia and tendon of right thumb at wrist and hand level**

⑦S66.222 **Laceration of extensor muscle, fascia and tendon of left thumb at wrist and hand level**

⑦S66.229 **Laceration of extensor muscle, fascia and tendon of unspecified thumb at wrist and hand level**

S66.29 **Other specified injury of extensor muscle, fascia and tendon of thumb at wrist and hand level**

⑦S66.291 **Other specified injury of extensor muscle, fascia and tendon of right thumb at wrist and hand level**

⑦S66.292 **Other specified injury of extensor muscle, fascia and tendon of left thumb at wrist and hand level**

⑦S66.299 **Other specified injury of extensor muscle, fascia and tendon of unspecified thumb at wrist and hand level**

S66.3 **Injury of extensor muscle, fascia and tendon of other and unspecified finger at wrist and hand level**

Excludes2: Injury of extensor muscle, fascia and tendon of thumb at wrist and hand level (S66.2-)

S66.30 **Unspecified injury of extensor muscle, fascia and tendon of other and unspecified finger at wrist and hand level**

⑦S66.300 **Unspecified injury of extensor muscle, fascia and tendon of right index finger at wrist and hand level**

⑦S66.301 **Unspecified injury of extensor muscle, fascia and tendon of left index finger at wrist and hand level**

⑦S66.302 **Unspecified injury of extensor muscle, fascia and tendon of right middle finger at wrist and hand level**

⑦S66.303 **Unspecified injury of extensor muscle, fascia and tendon of left middle finger at wrist and hand level**

⑦S66.304 **Unspecified injury of extensor muscle, fascia and tendon of right ring finger at wrist and hand level**

⑦S66.305 **Unspecified injury of extensor muscle, fascia and tendon of left ring finger at wrist and hand level**

⑦S66.306 Unspecified injury of extensor muscle, fascia and tendon of right little finger at wrist and hand level

⑦S66.307 Unspecified injury of extensor muscle, fascia and tendon of left little finger at wrist and hand level

⑦S66.308 Unspecified injury of extensor muscle, fascia and tendon of other finger at wrist and hand level

Unspecified injury of extensor muscle, fascia and tendon of specified finger with unspecified laterality at wrist and hand level

⑦S66.309 Unspecified injury of extensor muscle, fascia and tendon of unspecified finger at wrist and hand level

S66.31 Strain of extensor muscle, fascia and tendon of other and unspecified finger at wrist and hand level

⑦S66.310 Strain of extensor muscle, fascia and tendon of right index finger at wrist and hand level

⑦S66.311 Strain of extensor muscle, fascia and tendon of left index finger at wrist and hand level

⑦S66.312 Strain of extensor muscle, fascia and tendon of right middle finger at wrist and hand level

⑦S66.313 Strain of extensor muscle, fascia and tendon of left middle finger at wrist and hand level

⑦S66.314 Strain of extensor muscle, fascia and tendon of right ring finger at wrist and hand level

⑦S66.315 Strain of extensor muscle, fascia and tendon of left ring finger at wrist and hand level

⑦S66.316 Strain of extensor muscle, fascia and tendon of right little finger at wrist and hand level

⑦S66.317 Strain of extensor muscle, fascia and tendon of left little finger at wrist and hand level

⑦S66.318 Strain of extensor muscle, fascia and tendon of other finger at wrist and hand level

Strain of extensor muscle, fascia and tendon of specified finger with unspecified laterality at wrist and hand level

⑦S66.319 Strain of extensor muscle, fascia and tendon of unspecified finger at wrist and hand level

S66.32 Laceration of extensor muscle, fascia and tendon of other and unspecified finger at wrist and hand level

⑦S66.320 Laceration of extensor muscle, fascia and tendon of right index finger at wrist and hand level

⑦S66.321 Laceration of extensor muscle, fascia and tendon of left index finger at wrist and hand level

⑦S66.322 Laceration of extensor muscle, fascia and tendon of right middle finger at wrist and hand level

⑦S66.323 Laceration of extensor muscle, fascia and tendon of left middle finger at wrist and hand level

⑦S66.324 Laceration of extensor muscle, fascia and tendon of right ring finger at wrist and hand level

⑦S66.325 Laceration of extensor muscle, fascia and tendon of left ring finger at wrist and hand level

⑦S66.326 Laceration of extensor muscle, fascia and tendon of right little finger at wrist and hand level

⑦S66.327 Laceration of extensor muscle, fascia and tendon of left little finger at wrist and hand level

⑦S66.328 Laceration of extensor muscle, fascia and tendon of other finger at wrist and hand level

Laceration of extensor muscle, fascia and tendon of specified finger with unspecified laterality at wrist and hand level

⑦S66.329 Laceration of extensor muscle, fascia and tendon of unspecified finger at wrist and hand level

S66.39 Other injury of extensor muscle, fascia and tendon of other and unspecified finger at wrist and hand level

⑦S66.390 Other injury of extensor muscle, fascia and tendon of right index finger at wrist and hand level

⑦S66.391 Other injury of extensor muscle, fascia and tendon of left index finger at wrist and hand level

⑦S66.392 Other injury of extensor muscle, fascia and tendon of right middle finger at wrist and hand level

⑦S66.393 Other injury of extensor muscle, fascia and tendon of left middle finger at wrist and hand level

⑦S66.394 Other injury of extensor muscle, fascia and tendon of right ring finger at wrist and hand level

⑦S66.395 Other injury of extensor muscle, fascia and tendon of left ring finger at wrist and hand level

⑦S66.396 Other injury of extensor muscle, fascia and tendon of right little finger at wrist and hand level

⑦S66.397 Other injury of extensor muscle, fascia and tendon of left little finger at wrist and hand level

⑦S66.398 Other injury of extensor muscle, fascia and tendon of other finger at wrist and hand level

Other injury of extensor muscle, fascia and tendon of specified finger with unspecified laterality at wrist and hand level

⑦S66.399 Other injury of extensor muscle, fascia and tendon of unspecified finger at wrist and hand level

S66.4 Injury of intrinsic muscle, fascia and tendon of thumb at wrist and hand level

S66.40 Unspecified injury of intrinsic muscle, fascia and tendon of thumb at wrist and hand level

⑦S66.401 Unspecified injury of intrinsic muscle, fascia and tendon of right thumb at wrist and hand level

⑦S66.402 Unspecified injury of intrinsic muscle, fascia and tendon of left thumb at wrist and hand level

⑦S66.409 Unspecified injury of intrinsic muscle, fascia and tendon of unspecified thumb at wrist and hand level

S66.41 Strain of intrinsic muscle, fascia and tendon of thumb at wrist and hand level

⑦S66.411 Strain of intrinsic muscle, fascia and tendon of right thumb at wrist and hand level

⑦S66.412 Strain of intrinsic muscle, fascia and tendon of left thumb at wrist and hand level

⑦S66.419 Strain of intrinsic muscle, fascia and tendon of unspecified thumb at wrist and hand level

S66.42 Laceration of intrinsic muscle, fascia and tendon of thumb at wrist and hand level

⑦S66.421 Laceration of intrinsic muscle, fascia and tendon of right thumb at wrist and hand level

⑦S66.422 Laceration of intrinsic muscle, fascia and tendon of left thumb at wrist and hand level

⑦S66.429 Laceration of intrinsic muscle, fascia and tendon of unspecified thumb at wrist and hand level

S66.49 Other specified injury of intrinsic muscle, fascia and tendon of thumb at wrist and hand level

⑦S66.491 Other specified injury of intrinsic muscle, fascia and tendon of right thumb at wrist and hand level

⑦S66.492 Other specified injury of intrinsic muscle, fascia and tendon of left thumb at wrist and hand level

⑦S66.499 Other specified injury of intrinsic muscle, fascia and tendon of unspecified thumb at wrist and hand level

S66.5 Injury of intrinsic muscle, fascia and tendon of other and unspecified finger at wrist and hand level

Excludes2: injury of intrinsic muscle, fascia and tendon of thumb at wrist and hand level (S66.4-)

S66.50 Unspecified injury of intrinsic muscle, fascia and tendon of other and unspecified finger at wrist and hand level

⑦S66.500 Unspecified injury of intrinsic muscle, fascia and tendon of right index finger at wrist and hand level

⑦S66.501 Unspecified injury of intrinsic muscle, fascia and tendon of left index finger at wrist and hand level

⑦S66.502 Unspecified injury of intrinsic muscle, fascia and tendon of right middle finger at wrist and hand level

⑦S66.503 Unspecified injury of intrinsic muscle, fascia and tendon of left middle finger at wrist and hand level

⑦S66.504 Unspecified injury of intrinsic muscle, fascia and tendon of right ring finger at wrist and hand level

⑦S66.505 Unspecified injury of intrinsic muscle, fascia and tendon of left ring finger at wrist and hand level

⑦S66.506 Unspecified injury of intrinsic muscle, fascia and tendon of right little finger at wrist and hand level

⑦S66.507 Unspecified injury of intrinsic muscle, fascia and tendon of left little finger at wrist and hand level

⑦S66.508 Unspecified injury of intrinsic muscle, fascia and tendon of other finger at wrist and hand level

Unspecified injury of intrinsic muscle, fascia and tendon of specified finger with unspecified laterality at wrist and hand level

⑦S66.509 Unspecified injury of intrinsic muscle, fascia and tendon of unspecified finger at wrist and hand level

S66.51 Strain of intrinsic muscle, fascia and tendon of other and unspecified finger at wrist and hand level

⑦S66.510 Strain of intrinsic muscle, fascia and tendon of right index finger at wrist and hand level

⑦S66.511 Strain of intrinsic muscle, fascia and tendon of left index finger at wrist and hand level

⑦S66.512 Strain of intrinsic muscle, fascia and tendon of right middle finger at wrist and hand level

⑦S66.513 Strain of intrinsic muscle, fascia and tendon of left middle finger at wrist and hand level

⑦S66.514 Strain of intrinsic muscle, fascia and tendon of right ring finger at wrist and hand level

⑦S66.515 Strain of intrinsic muscle, fascia and tendon of left ring finger at wrist and hand level

⑦S66.516 Strain of intrinsic muscle, fascia and tendon of right little finger at wrist and hand level

⑦S66.517 Strain of intrinsic muscle, fascia and tendon of left little finger at wrist and hand level

⑦S66.518 Strain of intrinsic muscle, fascia and tendon of other finger at wrist and hand level

Strain of intrinsic muscle, fascia and tendon of specified finger with unspecified laterality at wrist and hand level

⑦S66.519 Strain of intrinsic muscle, fascia and tendon of unspecified finger at wrist and hand level

S66.52 Laceration of intrinsic muscle, fascia and tendon of other and unspecified finger at wrist and hand level

⑦S66.520 Laceration of intrinsic muscle, fascia and tendon of right index finger at wrist and hand level

⑦S66.521 Laceration of intrinsic muscle, fascia and tendon of left index finger at wrist and hand level

⑦S66.522 **Laceration of intrinsic muscle, fascia and tendon of right middle finger at wrist and hand level**

⑦S66.523 **Laceration of intrinsic muscle, fascia and tendon of left middle finger at wrist and hand level**

⑦S66.524 **Laceration of intrinsic muscle, fascia and tendon of right ring finger at wrist and hand level**

⑦S66.525 **Laceration of intrinsic muscle, fascia and tendon of left ring finger at wrist and hand level**

⑦S66.526 **Laceration of intrinsic muscle, fascia and tendon of right little finger at wrist and hand level**

⑦S66.527 **Laceration of intrinsic muscle, fascia and tendon of left little finger at wrist and hand level**

⑦S66.528 **Laceration of intrinsic muscle, fascia and tendon of other finger at wrist and hand level**

Laceration of intrinsic muscle, fascia and tendon of specified finger with unspecified laterality at wrist and hand level

⑦S66.529 **Laceration of intrinsic muscle, fascia and tendon of unspecified finger at wrist and hand level**

S66.59 **Other injury of intrinsic muscle, fascia and tendon of other and unspecified finger at wrist and hand level**

⑦S66.590 **Other injury of intrinsic muscle, fascia and tendon of right index finger at wrist and hand level**

⑦S66.591 **Other injury of intrinsic muscle, fascia and tendon of left index finger at wrist and hand level**

⑦S66.592 **Other injury of intrinsic muscle, fascia and tendon of right middle finger at wrist and hand level**

⑦S66.593 **Other injury of intrinsic muscle, fascia and tendon of left middle finger at wrist and hand level**

⑦S66.594 **Other injury of intrinsic muscle, fascia and tendon of right ring finger at wrist and hand level**

⑦S66.595 **Other injury of intrinsic muscle, fascia and tendon of left ring finger at wrist and hand level**

⑦S66.596 **Other injury of intrinsic muscle, fascia and tendon of right little finger at wrist and hand level**

⑦S66.597 **Other injury of intrinsic muscle, fascia and tendon of left little finger at wrist and hand level**

⑦S66.598 **Other injury of intrinsic muscle, fascia and tendon of other finger at wrist and hand level**

Other injury of intrinsic muscle, fascia and tendon of specified finger with unspecified laterality at wrist and hand level

⑦S66.599 **Other injury of intrinsic muscle, fascia and tendon of unspecified finger at wrist and hand level**

S66.8 **Injury of other specified muscles, fascia and tendons at wrist and hand level**

S66.80 **Unspecified injury of other specified muscles, fascia and tendons at wrist and hand level**

⑦S66.801 **Unspecified injury of other specified muscles, fascia and tendons at wrist and hand level, right hand**

⑦S66.802 **Unspecified injury of other specified muscles, fascia and tendons at wrist and hand level, left hand**

⑦S66.809 **Unspecified injury of other specified muscles, fascia and tendons at wrist and hand level, unspecified hand**

S66.81 **Strain of other specified muscles, fascia and tendons at wrist and hand level**

⑦S66.811 **Strain of other specified muscles, fascia and tendons at wrist and hand level, right hand**

⑦S66.812 **Strain of other specified muscles, fascia and tendons at wrist and hand level, left hand**

⑦S66.819 **Strain of other specified muscles, fascia and tendons at wrist and hand level, unspecified hand**

S66.82 **Laceration of other specified muscles, fascia and tendons at wrist and hand level**

⑦S66.821 **Laceration of other specified muscles, fascia and tendons at wrist and hand level, right hand**

⑦S66.822 **Laceration of other specified muscles, fascia and tendons at wrist and hand level, left hand**

⑦S66.829 **Laceration of other specified muscles, fascia and tendons at wrist and hand level, unspecified hand**

S66.89 **Other injury of other specified muscles, fascia and tendons at wrist and hand level**

⑦S66.891 **Other injury of other specified muscles, fascia and tendons at wrist and hand level, right hand**

⑦S66.892 **Other injury of other specified muscles, fascia and tendons at wrist and hand level, left hand**

⑦S66.899 **Other injury of other specified muscles, fascia and tendons at wrist and hand level, unspecified hand**

S66.9 **Injury of unspecified muscle, fascia and tendon at wrist and hand level**

S66.90 **Unspecified injury of unspecified muscle, fascia and tendon at wrist and hand level**

⑦S66.901 **Unspecified injury of unspecified muscle, fascia and tendon at wrist and hand level, right hand**

⑦S66.902 **Unspecified injury of unspecified muscle, fascia and tendon at wrist and hand level, left hand**

⑦S66.909 **Unspecified injury of unspecified muscle, fascia and tendon at wrist and hand level, unspecified hand**

S66.91 **Strain of unspecified muscle, fascia and tendon at wrist and hand level**

⑦S66.911 **Strain of unspecified muscle, fascia and tendon at wrist and hand level, right hand**

⑦S66.912 **Strain of unspecified muscle, fascia and tendon at wrist and hand level, left hand**

● New code ▲ Revised code **Excludes1:** Not coded here **Excludes2:** Not included here ⊗ Placeholder required ⑦7th digit required

⑦S66.919   Strain of unspecified muscle, fascia and tendon at wrist and hand level, unspecified hand

S66.92   Laceration of unspecified muscle, fascia and tendon at wrist and hand level

⑦S66.921   Laceration of unspecified muscle, fascia and tendon at wrist and hand level, right hand

⑦S66.922   Laceration of unspecified muscle, fascia and tendon at wrist and hand level, left hand

⑦S66.929   Laceration of unspecified muscle, fascia and tendon at wrist and hand level, unspecified hand

S66.99   Other injury of unspecified muscle, fascia and tendon at wrist and hand level

⑦S66.991   Other injury of unspecified muscle, fascia and tendon at wrist and hand level, right hand

⑦S66.992   Other injury of unspecified muscle, fascia and tendon at wrist and hand level, left hand

⑦S66.999   Other injury of unspecified muscle, fascia and tendon at wrist and hand level, unspecified hand

S67   Crushing injury of wrist, hand and fingers

Use Additional Code for all associated injuries, such as:

fracture of wrist and hand (S62.-) open wound of wrist and hand (S61.-)

The appropriate 7th character is to be added to each code from category S67

A - initial encounter

D - subsequent encounter

S - sequela

S67.0   Crushing injury of thumb

⊗⑦S67.00   Crushing injury of unspecified thumb

⊗⑦S67.01   Crushing injury of right thumb

⊗⑦S67.02   Crushing injury of left thumb

S67.1   Crushing injury of other and unspecified finger(s)

Excludes2: crushing injury of thumb (S67.0-)

⊗⑦S67.10   Crushing injury of unspecified finger(s)

S67.19   Crushing injury of other finger(s)

⑦S67.190   Crushing injury of right index finger

⑦S67.191   Crushing injury of left index finger

⑦S67.192   Crushing injury of right middle finger

⑦S67.193   Crushing injury of left middle finger

⑦S67.194   Crushing injury of right ring finger

⑦S67.195   Crushing injury of left ring finger

⑦S67.196   Crushing injury of right little finger

⑦S67.197   Crushing injury of left little finger

⑦S67.198   Crushing injury of other finger

Crushing injury of specified finger with unspecified laterality

S67.2   Crushing injury of hand

Excludes2: crushing injury of fingers (S67.1-)

crushing injury of thumb (S67.0-)

⊗⑦S67.20   Crushing injury of unspecified hand

⊗⑦S67.21   Crushing injury of right hand

⊗⑦S67.22   Crushing injury of left hand

S67.3   Crushing injury of wrist

⊗⑦S67.30   Crushing injury of unspecified wrist

⊗⑦S67.31   Crushing injury of right wrist

⊗⑦S67.32   Crushing injury of left wrist

S67.4   Crushing injury of wrist and hand

Excludes1: crushing injury of hand alone (S67.2-)

crushing injury of wrist alone (S67.3-)

Excludes2: crushing injury of fingers (S67.1-)

crushing injury of thumb (S67.0-)

⊗⑦S67.40   Crushing injury of unspecified wrist and hand

⊗⑦S67.41   Crushing injury of right wrist and hand

⊗⑦S67.42   Crushing injury of left wrist and hand

S67.9   Crushing injury of unspecified part(s) of wrist, hand and fingers

⊗⑦S67.90   Crushing injury of unspecified part(s) of unspecified wrist, hand and fingers

⊗⑦S67.91   Crushing injury of unspecified part(s) of right wrist, hand and fingers

⊗⑦S67.92   Crushing injury of unspecified part(s) of left wrist, hand and fingers

S68   Traumatic amputation of wrist, hand and fingers

An amputation not identified as partial or complete should be coded to complete

The appropriate 7th character is to be added to each code from category S68

A - initial encounter

D - subsequent encounter

S - sequela

S68.0   Traumatic metacarpophalangeal amputation of thumb

Traumatic amputation of thumb NOS

S68.01   Complete traumatic metacarpophalangeal amputation of thumb

⑦S68.011   Complete traumatic metacarpophalangeal amputation of right thumb [HCC]

⑦S68.012   Complete traumatic metacarpophalangeal amputation of left thumb [HCC]

⑦S68.019   Complete traumatic metacarpophalangeal amputation of unspecified thumb [HCC]

S68.02   Partial traumatic metacarpophalangeal amputation of thumb

⑦S68.021   Partial traumatic metacarpophalangeal amputation of right thumb [HCC]

⑦S68.022   Partial traumatic metacarpophalangeal amputation of left thumb [HCC]

⑦S68.029   Partial traumatic metacarpophalangeal amputation of unspecified thumb [HCC]

S68.1   Traumatic metacarpophalangeal amputation of other and unspecified finger

Traumatic amputation of finger NOS

Excludes2: traumatic metacarpophalangeal amputation of thumb (S68.0-)

S68.11   Complete traumatic metacarpophalangeal amputation of other and unspecified finger

⑦S68.110   Complete traumatic metacarpophalangeal amputation of right index finger [HCC]

⑦S68.111 **Complete traumatic metacarpophalangeal amputation of left index finger** [HCC]

⑦S68.112 **Complete traumatic metacarpophalangeal amputation of right middle finger** [HCC]

⑦S68.113 **Complete traumatic metacarpophalangeal amputation of left middle finger** [HCC]

⑦S68.114 **Complete traumatic metacarpophalangeal amputation of right ring finger**

⑦S68.115 **Complete traumatic metacarpophalangeal amputation of left ring finger** [HCC]

⑦S68.116 **Complete traumatic metacarpophalangeal amputation of right little finger** [HCC]

⑦S68.117 **Complete traumatic metacarpophalangeal amputation of left little finger** [HCC]

⑦S68.118 **Complete traumatic metacarpophalangeal amputation of other finger** [HCC]

Complete traumatic metacarpophalangeal amputation of specified finger with unspecified laterality

⑦S68.119 **Complete traumatic metacarpophalangeal amputation of unspecified finger** [HCC]

S68.12 **Partial traumatic metacarpophalangeal amputation of other and unspecified finger**

⑦S68.120 **Partial traumatic metacarpophalangeal amputation of right index finger** [HCC]

⑦S68.121 **Partial traumatic metacarpophalangeal amputation of left index finger** [HCC]

⑦S68.122 **Partial traumatic metacarpophalangeal amputation of right middle finger** [HCC]

⑦S68.123 **Partial traumatic metacarpophalangeal amputation of left middle finger** [HCC]

⑦S68.124 **Partial traumatic metacarpophalangeal amputation of right ring finger** [HCC]

⑦S68.125 **Partial traumatic metacarpophalangeal amputation of left ring finger** [HCC]

⑦S68.126 **Partial traumatic metacarpophalangeal amputation of right little finger** [HCC]

⑦S68.127 **Partial traumatic metacarpophalangeal amputation of left little finger** [HCC]

⑦S68.128 **Partial traumatic metacarpophalangeal amputation of other finger** [HCC]

Partial traumatic metacarpophalangeal amputation of specified finger with unspecified laterality

⑦S68.129 **Partial traumatic metacarpophalangeal amputation of unspecified finger** [HCC]

S68.4 **Traumatic amputation of hand at wrist level**

Traumatic amputation of hand NOS

Traumatic amputation of wrist

S68.41 **Complete traumatic amputation of hand at wrist level**

⑦S68.411 **Complete traumatic amputation of right hand at wrist level** [HCC]

⑦S68.412 **Complete traumatic amputation of left hand at wrist level** [HCC]

⑦S68.419 **Complete traumatic amputation of unspecified hand at wrist level** [HCC]

S68.42 **Partial traumatic amputation of hand at wrist level**

⑦S68.421 **Partial traumatic amputation of right hand at wrist level** [HCC]

⑦S68.422 **Partial traumatic amputation of left hand at wrist level** [HCC]

⑦S68.429 **Partial traumatic amputation of unspecified hand at wrist level** [HCC]

S68.5 **Traumatic transphalangeal amputation of thumb** [HCC]

Traumatic interphalangeal joint amputation of thumb

S68.51 **Complete traumatic transphalangeal amputation of thumb** [HCC]

⑦S68.511 **Complete traumatic transphalangeal amputation of right thumb** [HCC]

⑦S68.512 **Complete traumatic transphalangeal amputation of left thumb**

⑦S68.519 **Complete traumatic transphalangeal amputation of unspecified thumb** [HCC]

S68.52 **Partial traumatic transphalangeal amputation of thumb**

⑦S68.521 **Partial traumatic transphalangeal amputation of right thumb** [HCC]

⑦S68.522 **Partial traumatic transphalangeal amputation of left thumb** [HCC]

⑦S68.529 **Partial traumatic transphalangeal amputation of unspecified thumb** [HCC]

S68.6 **Traumatic transphalangeal amputation of other and unspecified finger**

S68.61 **Complete traumatic transphalangeal amputation of other and unspecified finger(s)**

⑦S68.610 **Complete traumatic transphalangeal amputation of right index finger** [HCC]

⑦S68.611 **Complete traumatic transphalangeal amputation of left index finger** [HCC]

⑦S68.612 **Complete traumatic transphalangeal amputation of right middle finger** [HCC]

⑦S68.613 **Complete traumatic transphalangeal amputation of left middle finger** [HCC]

⑦S68.614 **Complete traumatic transphalangeal amputation of right ring finger** [HCC]

⑦S68.615 **Complete traumatic transphalangeal amputation of left ring finger** [HCC]

⑦S68.616 **Complete traumatic transphalangeal amputation of right little finger** [HCC]

⑦S68.617 **Complete traumatic transphalangeal amputation of left little finger** [HCC]

⑦S68.618 **Complete traumatic transphalangeal amputation of other finger** [HCC]

Complete traumatic transphalangeal amputation of specified finger with unspecified laterality

● New code ▲ Revised code **Excludes1:** Not coded here **Excludes2:** Not included here ⊗ Placeholder required ⑦7th digit required

⑦S68.619 **Complete traumatic transphalangeal amputation of unspecified finger** [HCC]

S68.62 **Partial traumatic transphalangeal amputation of other and unspecified finger**

⑦S68.620 **Partial traumatic transphalangeal amputation of right index finger** [HCC]

⑦S68.621 **Partial traumatic transphalangeal amputation of left index finger** [HCC]

⑦S68.622 **Partial traumatic transphalangeal amputation of right middle finger** [HCC]

⑦S68.623 **Partial traumatic transphalangeal amputation of left middle finger** [HCC]

⑦S68.624 **Partial traumatic transphalangeal amputation of right ring finger** [HCC]

⑦S68.625 **Partial traumatic transphalangeal amputation of left ring finger** [HCC]

⑦S68.626 **Partial traumatic transphalangeal amputation of right little finger** [HCC]

⑦S68.627 **Partial traumatic transphalangeal amputation of left little finger** [HCC]

⑦S68.628 **Partial traumatic transphalangeal amputation of other finger** [HCC]

Partial traumatic transphalangeal amputation of specified finger with unspecified laterality

⑦S68.629 **Partial traumatic transphalangeal amputation of unspecified finger** [HCC]

S68.7 **Traumatic transmetacarpal amputation of hand**

S68.71 **Complete traumatic transmetacarpal amputation of hand**

⑦S68.711 **Complete traumatic transmetacarpal amputation of right hand** [HCC]

⑦S68.712 **Complete traumatic transmetacarpal amputation of left hand**

⑦S68.719 **Complete traumatic transmetacarpal amputation of unspecified hand** [HCC]

S68.72 **Partial traumatic transmetacarpal amputation of hand**

⑦S68.721 **Partial traumatic transmetacarpal amputation of right hand** [HCC]

⑦S68.722 **Partial traumatic transmetacarpal amputation of left hand** [HCC]

⑦S68.729 **Partial traumatic transmetacarpal amputation of unspecified hand** [HCC]

S69 **Other and unspecified injuries of wrist, hand and finger(s)**

The appropriate 7th character is to be added to each code from category S69

A - initial encounter

D - subsequent encounter

S - sequela

S69.8 **Other specified injuries of wrist, hand and finger(s)**

⊗⑦S69.80 **Other specified injuries of unspecified wrist, hand and finger(s)**

⊗⑦S69.81 **Other specified injuries of right wrist, hand and finger(s)**

⊗⑦S69.82 **Other specified injuries of left wrist, hand and finger(s)**

S69.9 **Unspecified injury of wrist, hand and finger(s)**

⊗⑦S69.90 **Unspecified injury of unspecified wrist, hand and finger(s)**

⊗⑦S69.91 **Unspecified injury of right wrist, hand and finger(s)**

⊗⑦S69.92 **Unspecified injury of left wrist, hand and finger(s)**

INJURIES TO THE HIP AND THIGH (S70-S79)

Excludes2: burns and corrosions (T20-T32)

frostbite (T33-T34) snake bite (T63.0-)

venomous insect bite or sting (T63.4-)

S70 **Superficial injury of hip and thigh**

The appropriate 7th character is to be added to each code from category S70

A - initial encounter

D - subsequent encounter

S - sequela

S70.0 **Contusion of hip**

⊗⑦S70.00 **Contusion of unspecified hip**

⊗⑦S70.01 **Contusion of right hip**

⊗⑦S70.02 **Contusion of left hip**

S70.1 **Contusion of thigh**

⊗⑦S70.10 **Contusion of unspecified thigh**

⊗⑦S70.11 **Contusion of right thigh**

⊗⑦S70.12 **Contusion of left thigh**

S70.2 **Other superficial injuries of hip**

S70.21 **Abrasion of hip**

⑦S70.211 **Abrasion, right hip**

⑦S70.212 **Abrasion, left hip**

⑦S70.219 **Abrasion, unspecified hip**

S70.22 **Blister (nonthermal) of hip**

⑦S70.221 **Blister (nonthermal), right hip**

⑦S70.222 **Blister (nonthermal), left hip**

⑦S70.229 **Blister (nonthermal), unspecified hip**

S70.24 **External constriction of hip**

⑦S70.241 **External constriction, right hip**

⑦S70.242 **External constriction, left hip**

⑦S70.249 **External constriction, unspecified hip**

S70.25 **Superficial foreign body of hip**

Splinter in the hip

⑦S70.251 **Superficial foreign body, right hip**

⑦S70.252 **Superficial foreign body, left hip**

⑦S70.259 **Superficial foreign body, unspecified hip**

S70.26 **Insect bite (nonvenomous) of hip**

⑦S70.261 **Insect bite (nonvenomous), right hip**

⑦S70.262 **Insect bite (nonvenomous), left hip**

⑦S70.269 **Insect bite (nonvenomous), unspecified hip**

S70.27 **Other superficial bite of hip**

Excludes1: open bite of hip (S71.05-)

⑦S70.271 **Other superficial bite of hip, right hip**

⑦S70.272 **Other superficial bite of hip, left hip**

⑦S70.279 **Other superficial bite of hip, unspecified hip**

S70.3 **Other superficial injuries of thigh**

S70.31 **Abrasion of thigh**

⑦S70.311 **Abrasion, right thigh**

⑦S70.312   **Abrasion, left thigh**

⑦S70.319   **Abrasion, unspecified thigh**

S70.32   **Blister (nonthermal) of thigh**

    ⑦S70.321   **Blister (nonthermal), right thigh**

    ⑦S70.322   **Blister (nonthermal), left thigh**

    ⑦S70.329   **Blister (nonthermal), unspecified thigh**

S70.34   **External constriction of thigh**

    ⑦S70.341   **External constriction, right thigh**

    ⑦S70.342   **External constriction, left thigh**

    ⑦S70.349   **External constriction, unspecified thigh**

S70.35   **Superficial foreign body of thigh**

    Splinter in the thigh

    ⑦S70.351   **Superficial foreign body, right thigh**

    ⑦S70.352   **Superficial foreign body, left thigh**

    ⑦S70.359   **Superficial foreign body, unspecified thigh**

S70.36   **Insect bite (nonvenomous) of thigh**

    ⑦S70.361   **Insect bite (nonvenomous), right thigh**

    ⑦S70.362   **Insect bite (nonvenomous), left thigh**

    ⑦S70.369   **Insect bite (nonvenomous), unspecified thigh**

S70.37   **Other superficial bite of thigh**

    Excludes1: open bite of thigh (S71.15)

    ⑦S70.371   **Other superficial bite of right thigh**

    ⑦S70.372   **Other superficial bite of left thigh**

    ⑦S70.379   **Other superficial bite of unspecified thigh**

S70.9   **Unspecified superficial injury of hip and thigh**

S70.91   **Unspecified superficial injury of hip**

    ⑦S70.911   **Unspecified superficial injury of right hip**

    ⑦S70.912   **Unspecified superficial injury of left hip**

    ⑦S70.919   **Unspecified superficial injury of unspecified hip**

S70.92   **Unspecified superficial injury of thigh**

    ⑦S70.921   **Unspecified superficial injury of right thigh**

    ⑦S70.922   **Unspecified superficial injury of left thigh**

    ⑦S70.929   **Unspecified superficial injury of unspecified thigh**

S71   **Open wound of hip and thigh**

<u>Code also</u> any associated wound infection

Excludes1: open fracture of hip and thigh (S72.-)

    traumatic amputation of hip and thigh (S78.-)

Excludes2: bite of venomous animal (T63.-)

    open wound of ankle, foot and toes (S91.-)

    open wound of knee and lower leg (S81.-)

The appropriate 7th character is to be added to each code from category S71

A - initial encounter

D - subsequent encounter

S - sequela

S71.0   **Open wound of hip**

S71.00   **Unspecified open wound of hip**

⑦S71.001   **Unspecified open wound, right hip**

⑦S71.002   **Unspecified open wound, left hip**

⑦S71.009   **Unspecified open wound, unspecified hip**

S71.01   **Laceration without foreign body of hip**

    ⑦S71.011   **Laceration without foreign body, right hip**

    ⑦S71.012   **Laceration without foreign body, left hip**

    ⑦S71.019   **Laceration without foreign body, unspecified hip**

S71.02   **Laceration with foreign body of hip**

    ⑦S71.021   **Laceration with foreign body, right hip**

    ⑦S71.022   **Laceration with foreign body, left hip**

    ⑦S71.029   **Laceration with foreign body, unspecified hip**

S71.03   **Puncture wound without foreign body of hip**

    ⑦S71.031   **Puncture wound without foreign body, right hip**

    ⑦S71.032   **Puncture wound without foreign body, left hip**

    ⑦S71.039   **Puncture wound without foreign body, unspecified hip**

S71.04   **Puncture wound with foreign body of hip**

    ⑦S71.041   **Puncture wound with foreign body, right hip**

    ⑦S71.042   **Puncture wound with foreign body, left hip**

    ⑦S71.049   **Puncture wound with foreign body, unspecified hip**

S71.05   **Open bite of hip**

    Bite of hip NOS

    Excludes1: superficial bite of hip (S70.26, S70.27)

    ⑦S71.051   **Open bite, right hip**

    ⑦S71.052   **Open bite, left hip**

    ⑦S71.059   **Open bite, unspecified hip**

S71.1   **Open wound of thigh**

S71.10   **Unspecified open wound of thigh**

    ⑦S71.101   **Unspecified open wound, right thigh**

    ⑦S71.102   **Unspecified open wound, left thigh**

    ⑦S71.109   **Unspecified open wound, unspecified thigh**

S71.11   **Laceration without foreign body of thigh**

    ⑦S71.111   **Laceration without foreign body, right thigh**

    ⑦S71.112   **Laceration without foreign body, left thigh**

    ⑦S71.119   **Laceration without foreign body, unspecified thigh**

S71.12   **Laceration with foreign body of thigh**

    ⑦S71.121   **Laceration with foreign body, right thigh**

    ⑦S71.122   **Laceration with foreign body, left thigh**

    ⑦S71.129   **Laceration with foreign body, unspecified thigh**

S71.13   **Puncture wound without foreign body of thigh**

    ⑦S71.131   **Puncture wound without foreign body, right thigh**

    ● New code   ▲ Revised code   **Excludes1:** Not coded here   **Excludes2:** Not included here   ⊗ Placeholder required   ⑦7th digit required

⑦**S71.132** **Puncture wound without foreign body, left thigh**

⑦**S71.139** **Puncture wound without foreign body, unspecified thigh**

S71.14 **Puncture wound with foreign body of thigh**

⑦**S71.141** **Puncture wound with foreign body, right thigh**

⑦**S71.142** **Puncture wound with foreign body, left thigh**

⑦**S71.149** **Puncture wound with foreign body, unspecified thigh**

S71.15 **Open bite of thigh**

Bite of thigh NOS

Excludes1: superficial bite of thigh (S70.37-)

⑦**S71.151** **Open bite, right thigh**

⑦**S71.152** **Open bite, left thigh**

⑦**S71.159** **Open bite, unspecified thigh**

S72 **Fracture of femur**

Note: A fracture not indicated as displaced or nondisplaced should be coded to displaced

A fracture not indicated as open or closed should be coded to closed

The open fracture designations are based on the Gustilo open fracture classification

Excludes1: traumatic amputation of hip and thigh (S78.-)

Excludes2: fracture of lower leg and ankle (S82.-)

fracture of foot (S92.-)

periprosthetic fracture of prosthetic implant of hip (M97.0-)

The appropriate 7th character is to be added to all codes from category S72

A - initial encounter for closed fracture

B - initial encounter for open fracture type I or II initial encounter for open fracture NOS

C - initial encounter for open fracture type IIIA, IIIB, or IIIC

D - subsequent encounter for closed fracture with routine healing

E - subsequent encounter for open fracture type I or II with routine healing

F - subsequent encounter for open fracture type IIIA, IIIB, or IIIC with routine healing

G - subsequent encounter for closed fracture with delayed healing

H - subsequent encounter for open fracture type I or II with delayed healing

J - subsequent encounter for open fracture type IIIA, IIIB, or IIIC with delayed healing

K - subsequent encounter for closed fracture with nonunion

M - subsequent encounter for open fracture type I or II with nonunion

N - subsequent encounter for open fracture type IIIA, IIIB, or IIIC with nonunion

P - subsequent encounter for closed fracture with malunion

Q - subsequent encounter for open fracture type I or II with malunion

R - subsequent encounter for open fracture type IIIA, IIIB, or IIIC with malunion

S - sequela

S72.0 **Fracture of head and neck of femur**

Excludes2: physeal fracture of upper end of femur (S79.0-)

S72.00 **Fracture of unspecified part of neck of femur**

Fracture of hip NOS

Fracture of neck of femur NOS

⑦**S72.001** **Fracture of unspecified part of neck of right femur** [HCC]

⑦**S72.002** **Fracture of unspecified part of neck of left femur** [HCC]

⑦**S72.009** **Fracture of unspecified part of neck of unspecified femur** [HCC]

S72.01 **Unspecified intracapsular fracture of femur**

Subcapital fracture of femur

⑦**S72.011** **Unspecified intracapsular fracture of right femur** [HCC]

⑦**S72.012** **Unspecified intracapsular fracture of left femur** [HCC]

⑦**S72.019** **Unspecified intracapsular fracture of unspecified femur** [HCC]

S72.02 **Fracture of epiphysis (separation) (upper) of femur**

Transepiphyseal fracture of femur

Excludes1: capital femoral epiphyseal fracture (pediatric) of femur (S79.01-)

Salter-Harris Type I physeal fracture of upper end of femur (S79.01-)

⑦**S72.021** **Displaced fracture of epiphysis (separation) (upper) of right femur** [HCC]

⑦**S72.022** **Displaced fracture of epiphysis (separation) (upper) of left femur** [HCC]

⑦**S72.023** **Displaced fracture of epiphysis (separation) (upper) of unspecified femur** [HCC]

⑦**S72.024** **Nondisplaced fracture of epiphysis (separation) (upper) of right femur** [HCC]

⑦**S72.025** **Nondisplaced fracture of epiphysis (separation) (upper) of left femur** [HCC]

⑦**S72.026** **Nondisplaced fracture of epiphysis (separation) (upper) of unspecified femur** [HCC]

S72.03 **Midcervical fracture of femur**

Transcervical fracture of femur NOS

⑦**S72.031** **Displaced midcervical fracture of right femur** [HCC]

⑦**S72.032** **Displaced midcervical fracture of left femur**

⑦**S72.033** **Displaced midcervical fracture of unspecified femur** [HCC]

⑦**S72.034** **Nondisplaced midcervical fracture of right femur** [HCC]

⑦**S72.035** **Nondisplaced midcervical fracture of left femur** [HCC]

⑦**S72.036** **Nondisplaced midcervical fracture of unspecified femur** [HCC]

S72.04 **Fracture of base of neck of femur**

Cervicotrochanteric fracture of femur

⑦**S72.041** **Displaced fracture of base of neck of right femur** [HCC]

⑦**S72.042** **Displaced fracture of base of neck of left femur** [HCC]

⑦**S72.043** **Displaced fracture of base of neck of unspecified femur** [HCC]

⑦**S72.044** **Nondisplaced fracture of base of neck of right femur** [HCC]

⑦**S72.045** **Nondisplaced fracture of base of neck of left femur** [HCC]

⑦**S72.046** **Nondisplaced fracture of base of neck of unspecified femur** [HCC]

S72.05   Unspecified fracture of head of femur
Fracture of head of femur NOS

⑦**S72.051   Unspecified fracture of head of right femur** [HCC]

⑦**S72.052   Unspecified fracture of head of left femur** [HCC]

⑦**S72.059   Unspecified fracture of head of unspecified femur** [HCC]

S72.06   Articular fracture of head of femur

⑦**S72.061   Displaced articular fracture of head of right femur** [HCC]

⑦**S72.062   Displaced articular fracture of head of left femur** [HCC]

⑦**S72.063   Displaced articular fracture of head of unspecified femur** [HCC]

⑦**S72.064   Nondisplaced articular fracture of head of right femur** [HCC]

⑦**S72.065   Nondisplaced articular fracture of head of left femur** [HCC]

⑦**S72.066   Nondisplaced articular fracture of head of unspecified femur** [HCC]

S72.09   Other fracture of head and neck of femur

⑦**S72.091   Other fracture of head and neck of right femur** [HCC]

⑦**S72.092   Other fracture of head and neck of left femur** [HCC]

⑦**S72.099   Other fracture of head and neck of unspecified femur** [HCC]

S72.1   Pertrochanteric fracture

S72.10   Unspecified trochanteric fracture of femur
Fracture of trochanter NOS

⑦**S72.101   Unspecified trochanteric fracture of right femur** [HCC]

⑦**S72.102   Unspecified trochanteric fracture of left femur** [HCC]

⑦**S72.109   Unspecified trochanteric fracture of unspecified femur**

S72.11   Fracture of greater trochanter of femur

⑦**S72.111   Displaced fracture of greater trochanter of right femur** [HCC]

⑦**S72.112   Displaced fracture of greater trochanter of left femur** [HCC]

⑦**S72.113   Displaced fracture of greater trochanter of unspecified femur** [HCC]

⑦**S72.114   Nondisplaced fracture of greater trochanter of right femur** [HCC]

⑦**S72.115   Nondisplaced fracture of greater trochanter of left femur** [HCC]

⑦**S72.116   Nondisplaced fracture of greater trochanter of unspecified femur** [HCC]

S72.12   Fracture of lesser trochanter of femur

⑦**S72.121   Displaced fracture of lesser trochanter of right femur** [HCC]

⑦**S72.122   Displaced fracture of lesser trochanter of left femur** [HCC]

⑦**S72.123   Displaced fracture of lesser trochanter of unspecified femur** [HCC]

⑦**S72.124   Nondisplaced fracture of lesser trochanter of right femur** [HCC]

⑦**S72.125   Nondisplaced fracture of lesser trochanter of left femur** [HCC]

⑦**S72.126   Nondisplaced fracture of lesser trochanter of unspecified femur** [HCC]

S72.13   Apophyseal fracture of femur

Excludes1: chronic (nontraumatic) slipped upper femoral epiphysis (M93.0-)

⑦**S72.131   Displaced apophyseal fracture of right femur** [HCC]

⑦**S72.132   Displaced apophyseal fracture of left femur** [HCC]

⑦**S72.133   Displaced apophyseal fracture of unspecified femur** [HCC]

⑦**S72.134   Nondisplaced apophyseal fracture of right femur** [HCC]

⑦**S72.135   Nondisplaced apophyseal fracture of left femur** [HCC]

⑦**S72.136   Nondisplaced apophyseal fracture of unspecified femur** [HCC]

S72.14   Intertrochanteric fracture of femur

⑦**S72.141   Displaced intertrochanteric fracture of right femur** [HCC]

⑦**S72.142   Displaced intertrochanteric fracture of left femur** [HCC]

⑦**S72.143   Displaced intertrochanteric fracture of unspecified femur** [HCC]

⑦**S72.144   Nondisplaced intertrochanteric fracture of right femur** [HCC]

⑦**S72.145   Nondisplaced intertrochanteric fracture of left femur** [HCC]

⑦**S72.146   Nondisplaced intertrochanteric fracture of unspecified femur** [HCC]

S72.2   Subtrochanteric fracture of femur

⊗⑦**S72.21   Displaced subtrochanteric fracture of right femur** [HCC]

⊗⑦**S72.22   Displaced subtrochanteric fracture of left femur** [HCC]

⊗⑦**S72.23   Displaced subtrochanteric fracture of unspecified femur**

⊗⑦**S72.24   Nondisplaced subtrochanteric fracture of right femur** [HCC]

⊗⑦**S72.25   Nondisplaced subtrochanteric fracture of left femur** [HCC]

⊗⑦**S72.26   Nondisplaced subtrochanteric fracture of unspecified femur** [HCC]

S72.3   Fracture of shaft of femur

S72.30   Unspecified fracture of shaft of femur

⑦**S72.301   Unspecified fracture of shaft of right femur** [HCC]

⑦**S72.302   Unspecified fracture of shaft of left femur** [HCC]

⑦**S72.309   Unspecified fracture of shaft of unspecified femur** [HCC]

S72.32   Transverse fracture of shaft of femur

⑦**S72.321   Displaced transverse fracture of shaft of right femur** [HCC]

⑦**S72.322   Displaced transverse fracture of shaft of left femur** [HCC]

⑦**S72.323   Displaced transverse fracture of shaft of unspecified femur** [HCC]

⑦**S72.324   Nondisplaced transverse fracture of shaft of right femur** [HCC]

⑦**S72.325   Nondisplaced transverse fracture of shaft of left femur** [HCC]

⑦**S72.326   Nondisplaced transverse fracture of shaft of unspecified femur** [HCC]

S72.33   Oblique fracture of shaft of femur

● New code   ▲ Revised code   **Excludes1:** Not coded here   **Excludes2:** Not included here   ⊗ Placeholder required   ⑦7th digit required

⑦S72.331 **Displaced oblique fracture of shaft of right femur** [HCC]

⑦S72.332 **Displaced oblique fracture of shaft of left femur** [HCC]

⑦S72.333 **Displaced oblique fracture of shaft of unspecified femur** [HCC]

⑦S72.334 **Nondisplaced oblique fracture of shaft of right femur** [HCC]

⑦S72.335 **Nondisplaced oblique fracture of shaft of left femur** [HCC]

⑦S72.336 **Nondisplaced oblique fracture of shaft of unspecified femur** [HCC]

S72.34 **Spiral fracture of shaft of femur**

⑦S72.341 **Displaced spiral fracture of shaft of right femur** [HCC]

⑦S72.342 **Displaced spiral fracture of shaft of left femur** [HCC]

⑦S72.343 **Displaced spiral fracture of shaft of unspecified femur** [HCC]

⑦S72.344 **Nondisplaced spiral fracture of shaft of right femur** [HCC]

⑦S72.345 **Nondisplaced spiral fracture of shaft of left femur** [HCC]

⑦S72.346 **Nondisplaced spiral fracture of shaft of unspecified femur** [HCC]

S72.35 **Comminuted fracture of shaft of femur**

⑦S72.351 **Displaced comminuted fracture of shaft of right femur** [HCC]

⑦S72.352 **Displaced comminuted fracture of shaft of left femur** [HCC]

⑦S72.353 **Displaced comminuted fracture of shaft of unspecified femur**

⑦S72.354 **Nondisplaced comminuted fracture of shaft of right femur** [HCC]

⑦S72.355 **Nondisplaced comminuted fracture of shaft of left femur** [HCC]

⑦S72.356 **Nondisplaced comminuted fracture of shaft of unspecified femur** [HCC]

S72.36 **Segmental fracture of shaft of femur**

⑦S72.361 **Displaced segmental fracture of shaft of right femur** [HCC]

⑦S72.362 **Displaced segmental fracture of shaft of left femur** [HCC]

⑦S72.363 **Displaced segmental fracture of shaft of unspecified femur** [HCC]

⑦S72.364 **Nondisplaced segmental fracture of shaft of right femur** [HCC]

⑦S72.365 **Nondisplaced segmental fracture of shaft of left femur** [HCC]

⑦S72.366 **Nondisplaced segmental fracture of shaft of unspecified femur** [HCC]

S72.39 **Other fracture of shaft of femur**

⑦S72.391 **Other fracture of shaft of right femur** [HCC]

⑦S72.392 **Other fracture of shaft of left femur** [HCC]

⑦S72.399 **Other fracture of shaft of unspecified femur** [HCC]

S72.4 **Fracture of lower end of femur**

Fracture of distal end of femur

Excludes2: fracture of shaft of femur (S72.3-)

physeal fracture of lower end of femur (S79.1-)

S72.40 **Unspecified fracture of lower end of femur**

⑦S72.401 **Unspecified fracture of lower end of right femur** [HCC]

⑦S72.402 **Unspecified fracture of lower end of left femur** [HCC]

⑦S72.409 **Unspecified fracture of lower end of unspecified femur** [HCC]

S72.41 **Unspecified condyle fracture of lower end of femur**

Condyle fracture of femur NOS

⑦S72.411 **Displaced unspecified condyle fracture of lower end of right femur** [HCC]

⑦S72.412 **Displaced unspecified condyle fracture of lower end of left femur** [HCC]

⑦S72.413 **Displaced unspecified condyle fracture of lower end of unspecified femur** [HCC]

⑦S72.414 **Nondisplaced unspecified condyle fracture of lower end of right femur** [HCC]

⑦S72.415 **Nondisplaced unspecified condyle fracture of lower end of left femur** [HCC]

⑦S72.416 **Nondisplaced unspecified condyle fracture of lower end of unspecified femur** [HCC]

S72.42 **Fracture of lateral condyle of femur**

⑦S72.421 **Displaced fracture of lateral condyle of right femur** [HCC]

⑦S72.422 **Displaced fracture of lateral condyle of left femur** [HCC]

⑦S72.423 **Displaced fracture of lateral condyle of unspecified femur**

⑦S72.424 **Nondisplaced fracture of lateral condyle of right femur** [HCC]

⑦S72.425 **Nondisplaced fracture of lateral condyle of left femur** [HCC]

⑦S72.426 **Nondisplaced fracture of lateral condyle of unspecified femur** [HCC]

S72.43 **Fracture of medial condyle of femur**

⑦S72.431 **Displaced fracture of medial condyle of right femur** [HCC]

⑦S72.432 **Displaced fracture of medial condyle of left femur** [HCC]

⑦S72.433 **Displaced fracture of medial condyle of unspecified femur** [HCC]

⑦S72.434 **Nondisplaced fracture of medial condyle of right femur** [HCC]

⑦S72.435 **Nondisplaced fracture of medial condyle of left femur** [HCC]

⑦S72.436 **Nondisplaced fracture of medial condyle of unspecified femur** [HCC]

S72.44 **Fracture of lower epiphysis (separation) of femur**

Excludes1: Salter-Harris Type I physeal fracture of lower end of femur (S79.11-)

⑦S72.441 **Displaced fracture of lower epiphysis (separation) of right femur** [HCC]

⑦S72.442 **Displaced fracture of lower epiphysis (separation) of left femur** [HCC]

⑦S72.443 **Displaced fracture of lower epiphysis (separation) of unspecified femur** [HCC]

⑦S72.444　**Nondisplaced fracture of lower epiphysis (separation) of right femur** [HCC]

⑦S72.445　**Nondisplaced fracture of lower epiphysis (separation) of left femur** [HCC]

⑦S72.446　**Nondisplaced fracture of lower epiphysis (separation) of unspecified femur** [HCC]

S72.45　**Supracondylar fracture without intracondylar extension of lower end of femur**

Supracondylar fracture of lower end of femur NOS

Excludes1: supracondylar fracture with intracondylar extension of lower end of femur (S72.46-)

⑦S72.451　**Displaced supracondylar fracture without intracondylar extension of lower end of right femur** [HCC]

⑦S72.452　**Displaced supracondylar fracture without intracondylar extension of lower end of left femur** [HCC]

⑦S72.453　**Displaced supracondylar fracture without intracondylar extension of lower end of unspecified femur** [HCC]

⑦S72.454　**Nondisplaced supracondylar fracture without intracondylar extension of lower end of right femur** [HCC]

⑦S72.455　**Nondisplaced supracondylar fracture without intracondylar extension of lower end of left femur** [HCC]

⑦S72.456　**Nondisplaced supracondylar fracture without intracondylar extension of lower end of unspecified femur** [HCC]

S72.46　**Supracondylar fracture with intracondylar extension of lower end of femur**

Excludes1: supracondylar fracture without intracondylar extension of lower end of femur (S72.45-)

⑦S72.461　**Displaced supracondylar fracture with intracondylar extension of lower end of right femur** [HCC]

⑦S72.462　**Displaced supracondylar fracture with intracondylar extension of lower end of left femur** [HCC]

⑦S72.463　**Displaced supracondylar fracture with intracondylar extension of lower end of unspecified femur** [HCC]

⑦S72.464　**Nondisplaced supracondylar fracture with intracondylar extension of lower end of right femur** [HCC]

⑦S72.465　**Nondisplaced supracondylar fracture with intracondylar extension of lower end of left femur** [HCC]

⑦S72.466　**Nondisplaced supracondylar fracture with intracondylar extension of lower end of unspecified femur** [HCC]

S72.47　**Torus fracture of lower end of femur**]

The appropriate 7th character is to be added to all codes in subcategory S72.47

A - initial encounter for closed fracture

D - subsequent encounter for fracture with routine healing

G - subsequent encounter for fracture with delayed healing

K - subsequent encounter for fracture with nonunion

P - subsequent encounter for fracture with malunion

S - sequela

⑦S72.471　**Torus fracture of lower end of right femur** [HCC]

⑦S72.472　**Torus fracture of lower end of left femur** [HCC]

⑦S72.479　**Torus fracture of lower end of unspecified femur** [HCC]

S72.49　**Other fracture of lower end of femur**

⑦S72.491　**Other fracture of lower end of right femur** [HCC]

⑦S72.492　**Other fracture of lower end of left femur** [HCC]

⑦S72.499　**Other fracture of lower end of unspecified femur** [HCC]

S72.8　**Other fracture of femur]**

S72.8X　**Other fracture of femur**

⑦S72.8X1　**Other fracture of right femur** [HCC]

⑦S72.8X2　**Other fracture of left femur** [HCC]

⑦S72.8X9　**Other fracture of unspecified femur** [HCC]

S72.9　**Unspecified fracture of femur**

Fracture of thigh NOS

Fracture of upper leg NOS

Excludes1: fracture of hip NOS (S72.00-, S72.01-)

⊗⑦S72.90　**Unspecified fracture of unspecified femur** [HCC]

⊗⑦S72.91　**Unspecified fracture of right femur** [HCC]

⊗⑦S72.92　**Unspecified fracture of left femur** [HCC]

S73　**Dislocation and sprain of joint and ligaments of hip**

Includes: avulsion of joint or ligament of hip

laceration of cartilage, joint or ligament of hip sprain of cartilage, joint or ligament of hip

traumatic hemarthrosis of joint or ligament of hip

traumatic rupture of joint or ligament of hip

traumatic subluxation of joint or ligament of hip

traumatic tear of joint or ligament of hip

Code also any associated open wound

Excludes2: strain of muscle, fascia and tendon of hip and thigh (S76.-)

The appropriate 7th character is to be added to each code from category S73

A - initial encounter

D - subsequent encounter

S - sequela

S73.0　**Subluxation and dislocation of hip**

Excludes2: dislocation and subluxation of hip prosthesis (T84.020, T84.021)

S73.00　**Unspecified subluxation and dislocation of hip**

Dislocation of hip NOS Subluxation of hip NOS

⑦S73.001　**Unspecified subluxation of right hip** [HCC]

⑦S73.002　**Unspecified subluxation of left hip** [HCC]

⑦S73.003　**Unspecified subluxation of unspecified hip** [HCC]

　● New code　▲ Revised code　Excludes1: Not coded here　Excludes2: Not included here　⊗ Placeholder required　⑦ 7th digit required

⑦**S73.004** **Unspecified dislocation of right hip** [HCC]

⑦**S73.005** **Unspecified dislocation of left hip** [HCC]

⑦**S73.006** **Unspecified dislocation of unspecified hip** [HCC]

S73.01 **Posterior subluxation and dislocation of hip**

⑦**S73.011** **Posterior subluxation of right hip** [HCC]

⑦**S73.012** **Posterior subluxation of left hip** [HCC]

⑦**S73.013** **Posterior subluxation of unspecified hip** [HCC]

⑦**S73.014** **Posterior dislocation of right hip** [HCC]

⑦**S73.015** **Posterior dislocation of left hip** [HCC]

⑦**S73.016** **Posterior dislocation of unspecified hip** [HCC]

S73.02 **Obturator subluxation and dislocation of hip**

⑦**S73.021** **Obturator subluxation of right hip** [HCC]

⑦**S73.022** **Obturator subluxation of left hip** [HCC]

⑦**S73.023** **Obturator subluxation of unspecified hip** [HCC]

⑦**S73.024** **Obturator dislocation of right hip** [HCC]

⑦**S73.025** **Obturator dislocation of left hip** [HCC]

⑦**S73.026** **Obturator dislocation of unspecified hip**

S73.03 **Other anterior subluxation and dislocation of hip**

⑦**S73.031** **Other anterior subluxation of right hip** [HCC]

⑦**S73.032** **Other anterior subluxation of left hip** [HCC]

⑦**S73.033** **Other anterior subluxation of unspecified hip** [HCC]

⑦**S73.034** **Other anterior dislocation of right hip** [HCC]

⑦**S73.035** **Other anterior dislocation of left hip** [HCC]

⑦**S73.036** **Other anterior dislocation of unspecified hip** [HCC]

S73.04 **Central subluxation and dislocation of hip**

⑦**S73.041** **Central subluxation of right hip** [HCC]

⑦**S73.042** **Central subluxation of left hip** [HCC]

⑦**S73.043** **Central subluxation of unspecified hip** [HCC]

⑦**S73.044** **Central dislocation of right hip** [HCC]

⑦**S73.045** **Central dislocation of left hip** [HCC]

⑦**S73.046** **Central dislocation of unspecified hip** [HCC]

S73.1 **Sprain of hip**

S73.10 **Unspecified sprain of hip**

⑦**S73.101** **Unspecified sprain of right hip**

⑦**S73.102** **Unspecified sprain of left hip**

⑦**S73.109** **Unspecified sprain of unspecified hip**

S73.11 **Iliofemoral ligament sprain of hip**

⑦**S73.111** **Iliofemoral ligament sprain of right hip**

⑦**S73.112** **Iliofemoral ligament sprain of left hip**

⑦**S73.119** **Iliofemoral ligament sprain of unspecified hip**

S73.12 **Ischiocapsular (ligament) sprain of hip**

⑦**S73.121** **Ischiocapsular ligament sprain of right hip**

⑦**S73.122** **Ischiocapsular ligament sprain of left hip**

⑦**S73.129** **Ischiocapsular ligament sprain of unspecified hip**

S73.19 **Other sprain of hip**

⑦**S73.191** **Other sprain of right hip**

⑦**S73.192** **Other sprain of left hip**

⑦**S73.199** **Other sprain of unspecified hip**

S74 **Injury of nerves at hip and thigh level**

Code also any associated open wound (S71.-)

Excludes2: injury of nerves at ankle and foot level (S94.-)

injury of nerves at lower leg level (S84.-)

The appropriate 7th character is to be added to each code from category S74

A - initial encounter

D - subsequent encounter

S - sequela

S74.0 **Injury of sciatic nerve at hip and thigh level**

⊗⑦**S74.00** **Injury of sciatic nerve at hip and thigh level, unspecified leg**

⊗⑦**S74.01** **Injury of sciatic nerve at hip and thigh level, right leg**

⊗⑦**S74.02** **Injury of sciatic nerve at hip and thigh level, left leg**

S74.1 **Injury of femoral nerve at hip and thigh level**

⊗⑦**S74.10** **Injury of femoral nerve at hip and thigh level, unspecified leg**

⊗⑦**S74.11** **Injury of femoral nerve at hip and thigh level, right leg**

⊗⑦**S74.12** **Injury of femoral nerve at hip and thigh level, left leg**

S74.2 **Injury of cutaneous sensory nerve at hip and thigh level**

⊗⑦**S74.20** **Injury of cutaneous sensory nerve at hip and thigh level, unspecified leg**

⊗⑦**S74.21** **Injury of cutaneous sensory nerve at hip and high level, right leg**

⊗⑦**S74.22** **Injury of cutaneous sensory nerve at hip and thigh level, left leg**

S74.8 **Injury of other nerves at hip and thigh level**

S74.8X **Injury of other nerves at hip and thigh level**

⑦**S74.8X1** **Injury of other nerves at hip and thigh level, right leg**

⑦**S74.8X2** **Injury of other nerves at hip and thigh level, left leg**

⑦**S74.8X9** **Injury of other nerves at hip and thigh level, unspecified leg**

S74.9 **Injury of unspecified nerve at hip and thigh level**

⊗⑦**S74.90** **Injury of unspecified nerve at hip and thigh level, unspecified leg**

⊗⑦**S74.91** **Injury of unspecified nerve at hip and thigh level, right leg**

⊗⑦**S74.92** **Injury of unspecified nerve at hip and thigh level, left leg**

S75 **Injury of blood vessels at hip and thigh level**

Code also any associated open wound (S71.-)

Excludes2: injury of blood vessels at lower leg level (S85.-)

injury of popliteal artery (S85.0)

The appropriate 7th character is to be added to each code from category S75

A - initial encounter

D - subsequent encounter

S - sequela

S75.0   Injury of femoral artery

S75.00   Unspecified injury of femoral artery

⑦S75.001   Unspecified injury of femoral artery, right leg

⑦S75.002   Unspecified injury of femoral artery, left leg

⑦S75.009   Unspecified injury of femoral artery, unspecified leg

S75.01   Minor laceration of femoral artery

Incomplete transection of femoral artery

Laceration of femoral artery NOS

Superficial laceration of femoral artery

⑦S75.011   Minor laceration of femoral artery, right leg

⑦S75.012   Minor laceration of femoral artery, left leg

⑦S75.019   Minor laceration of femoral artery, unspecified leg

S75.02   Major laceration of femoral artery

Complete transection of femoral artery

Traumatic rupture of femoral artery

⑦S75.021   Major laceration of femoral artery, right leg

⑦S75.022   Major laceration of femoral artery, left leg

⑦S75.029   Major laceration of femoral artery, unspecified leg

S75.09   Other specified injury of femoral artery

⑦S75.091   Other specified injury of femoral artery, right leg

⑦S75.092   Other specified injury of femoral artery, left leg

⑦S75.099   Other specified injury of femoral artery, unspecified leg

S75.1   Injury of femoral vein at hip and thigh level

S75.10   Unspecified injury of femoral vein at hip and thigh level

⑦S75.101   Unspecified injury of femoral vein at hip and thigh level, right leg

⑦S75.102   Unspecified injury of femoral vein at hip and thigh level, left leg

⑦S75.109   Unspecified injury of femoral vein at hip and thigh level, unspecified leg

S75.11   Minor laceration of femoral vein at hip and thigh level

Incomplete transection of femoral vein at hip and thigh level

Laceration of femoral vein at hip and thigh level NOS

Superficial laceration of femoral vein at hip and thigh level

⑦S75.111   Minor laceration of femoral vein at hip and thigh level, right leg

⑦S75.112   Minor laceration of femoral vein at hip and thigh level, left leg

⑦S75.119   Minor laceration of femoral vein at hip and thigh level, unspecified leg

S75.12   Major laceration of femoral vein at hip and thigh level

Complete transection of femoral vein at hip and thigh level

Traumatic rupture of femoral vein at hip and thigh level

⑦S75.121   Major laceration of femoral vein at hip and thigh level, right leg

⑦S75.122   Major laceration of femoral vein at hip and thigh level, left leg

⑦S75.129   Major laceration of femoral vein at hip and thigh level, unspecified leg

S75.19   Other specified injury of femoral vein at hip and thigh level

⑦S75.191   Other specified injury of femoral vein at hip and thigh level, right leg

⑦S75.192   Other specified injury of femoral vein at hip and thigh level, left leg

⑦S75.199   Other specified injury of femoral vein at hip and thigh level, unspecified leg

S75.2   Injury of greater saphenous vein at hip and thigh level

Excludes1: greater saphenous vein NOS (S85.3)

S75.20   Unspecified injury of greater saphenous vein at hip and thigh level

⑦S75.201   Unspecified injury of greater saphenous vein at hip and thigh level, right leg

⑦S75.202   Unspecified injury of greater saphenous vein at hip and thigh level, left leg

⑦S75.209   Unspecified injury of greater saphenous vein at hip and thigh level, unspecified leg

S75.21   Minor laceration of greater saphenous vein at hip and thigh level

Incomplete transection of greater saphenous vein at hip and thigh level

Laceration of greater saphenous vein at hip and thigh level NOS

Superficial laceration of greater saphenous vein at hip and thigh level

⑦S75.211   Minor laceration of greater saphenous vein at hip and thigh level, right leg

⑦S75.212   Minor laceration of greater saphenous vein at hip and thigh level, left leg

⑦S75.219   Minor laceration of greater saphenous vein at hip and thigh level, unspecified leg

S75.22   Major laceration of greater saphenous vein at hip and thigh level

Complete transection of greater saphenous vein at hip and thigh level

Traumatic rupture of greater saphenous vein at hip and thigh level

⑦S75.221   Major laceration of greater saphenous vein at hip and thigh level, right leg

⑦S75.222   Major laceration of greater saphenous vein at hip and thigh level, left leg

⑦S75.229 Major laceration of greater saphenous vein at hip and thigh level, unspecified leg

S75.29 Other specified injury of greater saphenous vein at hip and thigh level

⑦S75.291 Other specified injury of greater saphenous vein at hip and thigh level, right leg

⑦S75.292 Other specified injury of greater saphenous vein at hip and thigh level, left leg

⑦S75.299 Other specified injury of greater saphenous vein at hip and thigh level, unspecified leg

S75.8 Injury of other blood vessels at hip and thigh level

S75.80 Unspecified injury of other blood vessels at hip and thigh level

⑦S75.801 Unspecified injury of other blood vessels at hip and thigh level, right leg

⑦S75.802 Unspecified injury of other blood vessels at hip and thigh level, left leg

⑦S75.809 Unspecified injury of other blood vessels at hip and thigh level, unspecified leg

S75.81 Laceration of other blood vessels at hip and thigh level

⑦S75.811 Laceration of other blood vessels at hip and thigh level, right leg

⑦S75.812 Laceration of other blood vessels at hip and thigh level, left leg

⑦S75.819 Laceration of other blood vessels at hip and thigh level, unspecified leg

S75.89 Other specified injury of other blood vessels at hip and thigh level

⑦S75.891 Other specified injury of other blood vessels at hip and thigh level, right leg

⑦S75.892 Other specified injury of other blood vessels at hip and thigh level, left leg

⑦S75.899 Other specified injury of other blood vessels at hip and thigh level, unspecified leg

S75.9 Injury of unspecified blood vessel at hip and thigh level

S75.90 Unspecified injury of unspecified blood vessel at hip and thigh level

⑦S75.901 Unspecified injury of unspecified blood vessel at hip and thigh level, right leg

⑦S75.902 Unspecified injury of unspecified blood vessel at hip and thigh level, left leg

⑦S75.909 Unspecified injury of unspecified blood vessel at hip and thigh level, unspecified leg

S75.91 Laceration of unspecified blood vessel at hip and thigh level

⑦S75.911 Laceration of unspecified blood vessel at hip and thigh level, right leg

⑦S75.912 Laceration of unspecified blood vessel at hip and thigh level, left leg

⑦S75.919 Laceration of unspecified blood vessel at hip and thigh level, unspecified leg

S75.99 Other specified injury of unspecified blood vessel at hip and thigh level

⑦S75.991 Other specified injury of unspecified blood vessel at hip and thigh level, right leg

⑦S75.992 Other specified injury of unspecified blood vessel at hip and thigh level, left leg

⑦S75.999 Other specified injury of unspecified blood vessel at hip and thigh level, unspecified leg

S76 Injury of muscle, fascia and tendon at hip and thigh level

Code also any associated open wound (S71.-)

Excludes2: injury of muscle, fascia and tendon at lower leg level (S86)

sprain of joint and ligament of hip (S73.1)

The appropriate 7th character is to be added to each code from category S76

A - initial encounter

D - subsequent encounter

S - sequela

S76.0 Injury of muscle, fascia and tendon of hip

S76.00 Unspecified injury of muscle, fascia and tendon of hip

⑦S76.001 Unspecified injury of muscle, fascia and tendon of right hip

⑦S76.002 Unspecified injury of muscle, fascia and tendon of left hip

⑦S76.009 Unspecified injury of muscle, fascia and tendon of unspecified hip

S76.01 Strain of muscle, fascia and tendon of hip

⑦S76.011 Strain of muscle, fascia and tendon of right hip

⑦S76.012 Strain of muscle, fascia and tendon of left hip

⑦S76.019 Strain of muscle, fascia and tendon of unspecified hip

S76.02 Laceration of muscle, fascia and tendon of hip

⑦S76.021 Laceration of muscle, fascia and tendon of right hip

⑦S76.022 Laceration of muscle, fascia and tendon of left hip

⑦S76.029 Laceration of muscle, fascia and tendon of unspecified hip

S76.09 Other specified injury of muscle, fascia and tendon of hip

⑦S76.091 Other specified injury of muscle, fascia and tendon of right hip

⑦S76.092 Other specified injury of muscle, fascia and tendon of left hip

⑦S76.099 Other specified injury of muscle, fascia and tendon of unspecified hip

S76.1 Injury of quadriceps muscle, fascia and tendon

Injury of patellar ligament (tendon)

S76.10 Unspecified injury of quadriceps muscle, fascia and tendon

⑦S76.101 Unspecified injury of right quadriceps muscle, fascia and tendon

⑦S76.102 Unspecified injury of left quadriceps muscle, fascia and tendon

⑦S76.109 Unspecified injury of unspecified quadriceps muscle, fascia and tendon

S76.11 Strain of quadriceps muscle, fascia and tendon

⑦S76.111 Strain of right quadriceps muscle, fascia and tendon

⑦S76.112 Strain of left quadriceps muscle, fascia and tendon

⑦S76.119 Strain of unspecified quadriceps muscle, fascia and tendon

S76.12 Laceration of quadriceps muscle, fascia and tendon

⑦S76.121 Laceration of right quadriceps muscle, fascia and tendon

⑦S76.122 Laceration of left quadriceps muscle, fascia and tendon

⑦S76.129 Laceration of unspecified quadriceps muscle, fascia and tendon

S76.19 Other specified injury of quadriceps muscle, fascia and tendon

⑦S76.191 Other specified injury of right quadriceps muscle, fascia and tendon

⑦S76.192 Other specified injury of left quadriceps muscle, fascia and tendon

⑦S76.199 Other specified injury of unspecified quadriceps muscle, fascia and tendon

S76.2 Injury of adductor muscle, fascia and tendon of thigh

S76.20 Unspecified injury of adductor muscle, fascia and tendon of thigh

⑦S76.201 Unspecified injury of adductor muscle, fascia and tendon of right thigh

⑦S76.202 Unspecified injury of adductor muscle, fascia and tendon of left thigh

⑦S76.209 Unspecified injury of adductor muscle, fascia and tendon of unspecified thigh

S76.21 Strain of adductor muscle, fascia and tendon of thigh

⑦S76.211 Strain of adductor muscle, fascia and tendon of right thigh

⑦S76.212 Strain of adductor muscle, fascia and tendon of left thigh

⑦S76.219 Strain of adductor muscle, fascia and tendon of unspecified thigh

S76.22 Laceration of adductor muscle, fascia and tendon of thigh

⑦S76.221 Laceration of adductor muscle, fascia and tendon of right thigh

⑦S76.222 Laceration of adductor muscle, fascia and tendon of left thigh

⑦S76.229 Laceration of adductor muscle, fascia and tendon of unspecified thigh

S76.29 Other injury of adductor muscle, fascia and tendon of thigh

⑦S76.291 Other injury of adductor muscle, fascia and tendon of right thigh

⑦S76.292 Other injury of adductor muscle, fascia and tendon of left thigh

⑦S76.299 Other injury of adductor muscle, fascia and tendon of unspecified thigh

S76.3 Injury of muscle, fascia and tendon of the posterior muscle group at thigh level

S76.30 Unspecified injury of muscle, fascia and tendon of the posterior muscle group at thigh level

⑦S76.301 Unspecified injury of muscle, fascia and tendon of the posterior muscle group at thigh level, right thigh

⑦S76.302 Unspecified injury of muscle, fascia and tendon of the posterior muscle group at thigh level, left thigh

⑦S76.309 Unspecified injury of muscle, fascia and tendon of the posterior muscle group at thigh level, unspecified thigh

S76.31 Strain of muscle, fascia and tendon of the posterior muscle group at thigh level

⑦S76.311 Strain of muscle, fascia and tendon of the posterior muscle group at thigh level, right thigh

⑦S76.312 Strain of muscle, fascia and tendon of the posterior muscle group at thigh level, left thigh

⑦S76.319 Strain of muscle, fascia and tendon of the posterior muscle group at thigh level, unspecified thigh

S76.32 Laceration of muscle, fascia and tendon of the posterior muscle group at thigh level

⑦S76.321 Laceration of muscle, fascia and tendon of the posterior muscle group at thigh level, right thigh

⑦S76.322 Laceration of muscle, fascia and tendon of the posterior muscle group at thigh level, left thigh

⑦S76.329 Laceration of muscle, fascia and tendon of the posterior muscle group at thigh level, unspecified thigh

S76.39 Other specified injury of muscle, fascia and tendon of the posterior muscle group at thigh level

⑦S76.391 Other specified injury of muscle, fascia and tendon of the posterior muscle group at thigh level, right thigh

⑦S76.392 Other specified injury of muscle, fascia and tendon of the posterior muscle group at thigh level, left thigh

⑦S76.399 Other specified injury of muscle, fascia and tendon of the posterior muscle group at thigh level, unspecified thigh

S76.8 Injury of other specified muscles, fascia and tendons at thigh level

S76.80 Unspecified injury of other specified muscles, fascia and tendons at thigh level

⑦S76.801 Unspecified injury of other specified muscles, fascia and tendons at thigh level, right thigh

⑦S76.802 Unspecified injury of other specified muscles, fascia and tendons at thigh level, left thigh

⑦S76.809 Unspecified injury of other specified muscles, fascia and tendons at thigh level, unspecified thigh

S76.81 Strain of other specified muscles, fascia and tendons at thigh level

⑦S76.811 Strain of other specified muscles, fascia and tendons at thigh level, right thigh

⑦S76.812 Strain of other specified muscles, fascia and tendons at thigh level, left thigh

⑦S76.819 Strain of other specified muscles, fascia and tendons at thigh level, unspecified thigh

● New code ▲ Revised code **Excludes1:** Not coded here **Excludes2:** Not included here ⊗ Placeholder required ⑦7th digit required

S76.82 **Laceration of other specified muscles, fascia and tendons at thigh level**

⑦S76.821 **Laceration of other specified muscles, fascia and tendons at thigh level, right thigh**

⑦S76.822 **Laceration of other specified muscles, fascia and tendons at thigh level, left thigh**

⑦S76.829 **Laceration of other specified muscles, fascia and tendons at thigh level, unspecified thigh**

S76.89 **Other injury of other specified muscles, fascia and tendons at thigh level**

⑦S76.891 **Other injury of other specified muscles, fascia and tendons at thigh level, right thigh**

⑦S76.892 **Other injury of other specified muscles, fascia and tendons at thigh level, left thigh**

⑦S76.899 **Other injury of other specified muscles, fascia and tendons at thigh level, unspecified thigh**

S76.9 **Injury of unspecified muscles, fascia and tendons at thigh level**

S76.90 **Unspecified injury of unspecified muscles, fascia and tendons at thigh level**

⑦S76.901 **Unspecified injury of unspecified muscles, fascia and tendons at thigh level, right thigh**

⑦S76.902 **Unspecified injury of unspecified muscles, fascia and tendons at thigh level, left thigh**

⑦S76.909 **Unspecified injury of unspecified muscles, fascia and tendons at thigh level, unspecified thigh**

S76.91 **Strain of unspecified muscles, fascia and tendons at thigh level**

⑦S76.911 **Strain of unspecified muscles, fascia and tendons at thigh level, right thigh**

⑦S76.912 **Strain of unspecified muscles, fascia and tendons at thigh level, left thigh**

⑦S76.919 **Strain of unspecified muscles, fascia and tendons at thigh level, unspecified thigh**

S76.92 **Laceration of unspecified muscles, fascia and tendons at thigh level**

⑦S76.921 **Laceration of unspecified muscles, fascia and tendons at thigh level, right thigh**

⑦S76.922 **Laceration of unspecified muscles, fascia and tendons at thigh level, left thigh**

⑦S76.929 **Laceration of unspecified muscles, fascia and tendons at thigh level, unspecified thigh**

S76.99 **Other specified injury of unspecified muscles, fascia and tendons at thigh level**

⑦S76.991 **Other specified injury of unspecified muscles, fascia and tendons at thigh level, right thigh**

⑦S76.992 **Other specified injury of unspecified muscles, fascia and tendons at thigh level, left thigh**

⑦S76.999 **Other specified injury of unspecified muscles, fascia and tendons at thigh level, unspecified thigh**

S77 **Crushing injury of hip and thigh**

Use Additional Code(s) for all associated injuries

Excludes2: crushing injury of ankle and foot (S97.-)

crushing injury of lower leg (S87.-)

The appropriate 7th character is to be added to each code from category S77

A - initial encounter

D - subsequent encounter

S - sequela

S77.0 **Crushing injury of hip**

⊗⑦S77.00 **Crushing injury of unspecified hip**

⊗⑦S77.01 **Crushing injury of right hip**

⊗⑦S77.02 **Crushing injury of left hip**

S77.1 **Crushing injury of thigh**

⊗⑦S77.10 **Crushing injury of unspecified thigh**

⊗⑦S77.11 **Crushing injury of right thigh**

⊗⑦S77.12 **Crushing injury of left thigh**

S77.2 **Crushing injury of hip with thigh**

⊗⑦S77.20 **Crushing injury of unspecified hip with thigh**

⊗⑦S77.21 **Crushing injury of right hip with thigh**

⊗⑦S77.22 **Crushing injury of left hip with thigh**

S78 **Traumatic amputation of hip and thigh**

An amputation not identified as partial or complete should be coded to complete

Excludes1: traumatic amputation of knee (S88.0-)

The appropriate 7th character is to be added to each code from category S78

A - initial encounter

D - subsequent encounter

S - sequela

S78.0 **Traumatic amputation at hip joint**

S78.01 **Complete traumatic amputation at hip joint**

⑦S78.011 **Complete traumatic amputation at right hip joint** [HCC]

⑦S78.012 **Complete traumatic amputation at left hip joint** [HCC]

⑦S78.019 **Complete traumatic amputation at unspecified hip joint** [HCC]

S78.02 **Partial traumatic amputation at hip joint**

⑦S78.021 **Partial traumatic amputation at right hip joint** [HCC]

⑦S78.022 **Partial traumatic amputation at left hip joint** [HCC]

⑦S78.029 **Partial traumatic amputation at unspecified hip joint** [HCC]

S78.1 **Traumatic amputation at level between hip and knee**

Excludes1: traumatic amputation of knee (S88.0-)

S78.11 **Complete traumatic amputation at level between hip and knee**

⑦S78.111 **Complete traumatic amputation at level between right hip and knee** [HCC]

⑦S78.112 **Complete traumatic amputation at level between left hip and knee** [HCC]

⑦S78.119 **Complete traumatic amputation at level between unspecified hip and knee** [HCC]

S78.12 **Partial traumatic amputation at level between hip and knee**

⑦S78.121 **Partial traumatic amputation at level between right hip and knee** [HCC]

⑦S78.122 **Partial traumatic amputation at level between left hip and knee** [HCC]

⑦S78.129 **Partial traumatic amputation at level between unspecified hip and knee** [HCC]

S78.9 **Traumatic amputation of hip and thigh, level unspecified**

S78.91 **Complete traumatic amputation of hip and thigh, level unspecified**

⑦S78.911 **Complete traumatic amputation of right hip and thigh, level unspecified** [HCC]

⑦S78.912 **Complete traumatic amputation of left hip and thigh, level unspecified** [HCC]

⑦S78.919 **Complete traumatic amputation of unspecified hip and thigh, level unspecified** [HCC]

S78.92 **Partial traumatic amputation of hip and thigh, level unspecified**

⑦S78.921 **Partial traumatic amputation of right hip and thigh, level unspecified** [HCC]

⑦S78.922 **Partial traumatic amputation of left hip and thigh, level unspecified** [HCC]

⑦S78.929 **Partial traumatic amputation of unspecified hip and thigh, level unspecified** [HCC]

S79 **Other and unspecified injuries of hip and thigh**

Note: A fracture not indicated as open or closed should be coded to closed

The appropriate 7th character is to be added to each code from subcategories S79.0 and S79.1

A - initial encounter for closed fracture

D - subsequent encounter for fracture with routine healing

G - subsequent encounter for fracture with delayed healing

K - subsequent encounter for fracture with nonunion

P - subsequent encounter for fracture with malunion

S - sequela

S79.0 **Physeal fracture of upper end of femur**

Excludes1: apophyseal fracture of upper end of femur (S72.13-)

nontraumatic slipped upper femoral epiphysis (M93.0-)

S79.00 **Unspecified physeal fracture of upper end of femur**

⑦S79.001 **Unspecified physeal fracture of upper end of right femur** [HCC]

⑦S79.002 **Unspecified physeal fracture of upper end of left femur** [HCC]

⑦S79.009 **Unspecified physeal fracture of upper end of unspecified femur** [HCC]

S79.01 **Salter-Harris Type I physeal fracture of upper end of femur**

Acute on chronic slipped capital femoral epiphysis (traumatic)

Acute slipped capital femoral epiphysis (traumatic)

Capital femoral epiphyseal fracture

Excludes1: chronic slipped upper femoral epiphysis (nontraumatic) (M93.02-)

⑦S79.011 **Salter-Harris Type I physeal fracture of upper end of right femur** [HCC]

⑦S79.012 **Salter-Harris Type I physeal fracture of upper end of left femur** [HCC]

⑦S79.019 **Salter-Harris Type I physeal fracture of upper end of unspecified femur** [HCC]

S79.09 **Other physeal fracture of upper end of femur**

⑦S79.091 **Other physeal fracture of upper end of right femur** [HCC]

⑦S79.092 **Other physeal fracture of upper end of left femur** [HCC]

⑦S79.099 **Other physeal fracture of upper end of unspecified femur** [HCC]

S79.1 **Physeal fracture of lower end of femur**

S79.10 **Unspecified physeal fracture of lower end of femur**

⑦S79.101 **Unspecified physeal fracture of lower end of right femur** [HCC]

⑦S79.102 **Unspecified physeal fracture of lower end of left femur** [HCC]

⑦S79.109 **Unspecified physeal fracture of lower end of unspecified femur** [HCC]

S79.11 **Salter-Harris Type I physeal fracture of lower end of femur**

⑦S79.111 **Salter-Harris Type I physeal fracture of lower end of right femur** [HCC]

⑦S79.112 **Salter-Harris Type I physeal fracture of lower end of left femur** [HCC]

⑦S79.119 **Salter-Harris Type I physeal fracture of lower end of unspecified femur** [HCC]

S79.12 **Salter-Harris Type II physeal fracture of lower end of femur**

⑦S79.121 **Salter-Harris Type II physeal fracture of lower end of right femur** [HCC]

⑦S79.122 **Salter-Harris Type II physeal fracture of lower end of left femur** [HCC]

⑦S79.129 **Salter-Harris Type II physeal fracture of lower end of unspecified femur** [HCC]

S79.13 **Salter-Harris Type III physeal fracture of lower end of femur**

⑦S79.131 **Salter-Harris Type III physeal fracture of lower end of right femur** [HCC]

⑦S79.132 **Salter-Harris Type III physeal fracture of lower end of left femur** [HCC]

⑦S79.139 **Salter-Harris Type III physeal fracture of lower end of unspecified femur** [HCC]

S79.14 **Salter-Harris Type IV physeal fracture of lower end of femur**

⑦S79.141 **Salter-Harris Type IV physeal fracture of lower end of right femur** [HCC]

⑦S79.142 **Salter-Harris Type IV physeal fracture of lower end of left femur** [HCC]

● New code　　▲ Revised code　　**Excludes1:** Not coded here　　**Excludes2:** Not included here　　⊗ Placeholder required　　⑦7th digit required

⑦S79.149   **Salter-Harris Type IV physeal fracture of lower end of unspecified femur** [HCC]

S79.19   **Other physeal fracture of lower end of femur**

⑦S79.191   **Other physeal fracture of lower end of right femur** [HCC]

⑦S79.192   **Other physeal fracture of lower end of left femur** [HCC]

⑦S79.199   **Other physeal fracture of lower end of unspecified femur** [HCC]

S79.8   **Other specified injuries of hip and thigh**

The appropriate 7th character is to be added to each code in subcategory S79.8

A - initial encounter

D - subsequent encounter

S - sequela

S79.81   **Other specified injuries of hip**

⑦S79.811   **Other specified injuries of right hip**

⑦S79.812   **Other specified injuries of left hip**

⑦S79.819   **Other specified injuries of unspecified hip**

S79.82   **Other specified injuries of thigh**

⑦S79.821   **Other specified injuries of right thigh**

⑦S79.822   **Other specified injuries of left thigh**

⑦S79.829   **Other specified injuries of unspecified thigh**

S79.9   **Unspecified injury of hip and thigh**

The appropriate 7th character is to be added to each code in subcategory S79.9

A - initial encounter

D - subsequent encounter

S - sequela

S79.91   **Unspecified injury of hip**

⑦S79.911   **Unspecified injury of right hip**

⑦S79.912   **Unspecified injury of left hip**

⑦S79.919   **Unspecified injury of unspecified hip**

S79.92   **Unspecified injury of thigh**

⑦S79.921   **Unspecified injury of right thigh**

⑦S79.922   **Unspecified injury of left thigh**

⑦S79.929   **Unspecified injury of unspecified thigh**

INJURIES TO THE KNEE AND LOWER LEG (S80-S89)

Excludes2: burns and corrosions (T20-T32)

frostbite (T33-T34)

injuries of ankle and foot, except fracture of ankle and malleolus (S90-S99)

insect bite or sting, venomous (T63.4)

S80   **Superficial injury of knee and lower leg**

Excludes2: superficial injury of ankle and foot (S90.-)

The appropriate 7th character is to be added to each code from category S80

A - initial encounter

D - subsequent encounter

S - sequela

S80.0   **Contusion of knee**

⊗⑦S80.00   **Contusion of unspecified knee**

⊗⑦S80.01   **Contusion of right knee**

⊗⑦S80.02   **Contusion of left knee**

S80.1   **Contusion of lower leg**

⊗⑦S80.10   **Contusion of unspecified lower leg**

⊗⑦S80.11   **Contusion of right lower leg**

⊗⑦S80.12   **Contusion of left lower leg**

S80.2   **Other superficial injuries of knee**

S80.21   **Abrasion of knee**

⑦S80.211   **Abrasion, right knee**

⑦S80.212   **Abrasion, left knee**

⑦S80.219   **Abrasion, unspecified knee**

S80.22   **Blister (nonthermal) of knee**

⑦S80.221   **Blister (nonthermal), right knee**

⑦S80.222   **Blister (nonthermal), left knee**

⑦S80.229   **Blister (nonthermal), unspecified knee**

S80.24   **External constriction of knee**

⑦S80.241   **External constriction, right knee**

⑦S80.242   **External constriction, left knee**

⑦S80.249   **External constriction, unspecified knee**

S80.25   **Superficial foreign body of knee**

Splinter in the knee

⑦S80.251   **Superficial foreign body, right knee**

⑦S80.252   **Superficial foreign body, left knee**

⑦S80.259   **Superficial foreign body, unspecified knee**

S80.26   **Insect bite (nonvenomous) of knee**

⑦S80.261   **Insect bite (nonvenomous), right knee**

⑦S80.262   **Insect bite (nonvenomous), left knee**

⑦S80.269   **Insect bite (nonvenomous), unspecified knee**

S80.27   **Other superficial bite of knee**

Excludes1: open bite of knee (S81.05-)

⑦S80.271   **Other superficial bite of right knee**

⑦S80.272   **Other superficial bite of left knee**

⑦S80.279   **Other superficial bite of unspecified knee**

S80.8   **Other superficial injuries of lower leg**

S80.81   **Abrasion of lower leg**

⑦S80.811   **Abrasion, right lower leg**

⑦S80.812   **Abrasion, left lower leg**

⑦S80.819   **Abrasion, unspecified lower leg**

S80.82   **Blister (nonthermal) of lower leg**

⑦S80.821   **Blister (nonthermal), right lower leg**

⑦S80.822   **Blister (nonthermal), left lower leg**

⑦S80.829   **Blister (nonthermal), unspecified lower leg**

S80.84   **External constriction of lower leg**

⑦S80.841   **External constriction, right lower leg**

⑦S80.842   **External constriction, left lower leg**

⑦S80.849   **External constriction, unspecified lower leg**

S80.85   **Superficial foreign body of lower leg**

Splinter in the lower leg

⑦S80.851   **Superficial foreign body, right lower leg**

⑦S80.852   **Superficial foreign body, left lower leg**

⑦S80.859   **Superficial foreign body, unspecified lower leg**

S80.86   **Insect bite (nonvenomous) of lower leg**

⑦S80.861   **Insect bite (nonvenomous), right lower leg**

⑦S80.862   **Insect bite (nonvenomous), left lower leg**

⑦S80.869   **Insect bite (nonvenomous), unspecified lower leg**

S80.87   **Other superficial bite of lower leg**

Excludes1: open bite of lower leg (S81.85-)

⑦S80.871   **Other superficial bite, right lower leg**

⑦S80.872   **Other superficial bite, left lower leg**

⑦S80.879   **Other superficial bite, unspecified lower leg**

S80.9   **Unspecified superficial injury of knee and lower leg**

S80.91   **Unspecified superficial injury of knee**

⑦S80.911   **Unspecified superficial injury of right knee**

⑦S80.912   **Unspecified superficial injury of left knee**

⑦S80.919   **Unspecified superficial injury of unspecified knee**

S80.92   **Unspecified superficial injury of lower leg**

⑦S80.921   **Unspecified superficial injury of right lower leg**

⑦S80.922   **Unspecified superficial injury of left lower leg**

⑦S80.929   **Unspecified superficial injury of unspecified lower leg**

S81   **Open wound of knee and lower leg**

Code also any associated wound infection

Excludes1: open fracture of knee and lower leg (S82.-)

traumatic amputation of lower leg (S88.-)

Excludes2: open wound of ankle and foot (S91.-)

The appropriate 7th character is to be added to each code from category S81

A - initial encounter

D - subsequent encounter

S - sequela

S81.0   **Open wound of knee**

S81.00   **Unspecified open wound of knee**

⑦S81.001   **Unspecified open wound, right knee**

⑦S81.002   **Unspecified open wound, left knee**

⑦S81.009   **Unspecified open wound, unspecified knee**

S81.01   **Laceration without foreign body of knee**

⑦S81.011   **Laceration without foreign body, right knee**

⑦S81.012   **Laceration without foreign body, left knee**

⑦S81.019   **Laceration without foreign body, unspecified knee**

S81.02   **Laceration with foreign body of knee**

⑦S81.021   **Laceration with foreign body, right knee**

⑦S81.022   **Laceration with foreign body, left knee**

⑦S81.029   **Laceration with foreign body, unspecified knee**

S81.03   **Puncture wound without foreign body of knee**

⑦S81.031   **Puncture wound without foreign body, right knee**

⑦S81.032   **Puncture wound without foreign body, left knee**

⑦S81.039   **Puncture wound without foreign body, unspecified knee**

S81.04   **Puncture wound with foreign body of knee**

⑦S81.041   **Puncture wound with foreign body, right knee**

⑦S81.042   **Puncture wound with foreign body, left knee**

⑦S81.049   **Puncture wound with foreign body, unspecified knee**

S81.05   **Open bite of knee**

Bite of knee NOS

Excludes1: superficial bite of knee (S80.27-)

⑦S81.051   **Open bite, right knee**

⑦S81.052   **Open bite, left knee**

⑦S81.059   **Open bite, unspecified knee**

S81.8   **Open wound of lower leg**

S81.80   **Unspecified open wound of lower leg**

⑦S81.801   **Unspecified open wound, right lower leg**

⑦S81.802   **Unspecified open wound, left lower leg**

⑦S81.809   **Unspecified open wound, unspecified lower leg**

S81.81   **Laceration without foreign body of lower leg**

⑦S81.811   **Laceration without foreign body, right lower leg**

⑦S81.812   **Laceration without foreign body, left lower leg**

⑦S81.819   **Laceration without foreign body, unspecified lower leg**

S81.82   **Laceration with foreign body of lower leg**

⑦S81.821   **Laceration with foreign body, right lower leg**

⑦S81.822   **Laceration with foreign body, left lower leg**

⑦S81.829   **Laceration with foreign body, unspecified lower leg**

S81.83   **Puncture wound without foreign body of lower leg**

⑦S81.831   **Puncture wound without foreign body, right lower leg**

⑦S81.832   **Puncture wound without foreign body, left lower leg**

⑦S81.839   **Puncture wound without foreign body, unspecified lower leg**

S81.84   **Puncture wound with foreign body of lower leg**

⑦S81.841   **Puncture wound with foreign body, right lower leg**

⑦S81.842   **Puncture wound with foreign body, left lower leg**

⑦S81.849   **Puncture wound with foreign body, unspecified lower leg**

S81.85   **Open bite of lower leg**

Bite of lower leg NOS

Excludes1: superficial bite of lower leg (S80.86-S80.87-)

⑦S81.851   **Open bite, right lower leg**

   ● New code   ▲ Revised code   Excludes1: Not coded here   Excludes2: Not included here   ⊗ Placeholder required   ⑦7th digit required

⑦**S81.852   Open bite, left lower leg**

⑦**S81.859   Open bite, unspecified lower leg**

S82   Fracture of lower leg, including ankle

Note: A fracture not indicated as displaced or nondisplaced should be coded to displaced

A fracture not indicated as open or closed should be coded to closed

The open fracture designations are based on the Gustilo open fracture classification

Includes: fracture of malleolus

Excludes1: traumatic amputation of lower leg (S88.-)

Excludes2: fracture of foot, except ankle (S92.-)

periprosthetic fracture of prosthetic implant of knee (M97.0-)

The appropriate 7th character is to be added to all codes from category S82

A - initial encounter for closed fracture

B - initial encounter for open fracture type I or II initial encounter for open fracture NOS

C - initial encounter for open fracture type IIIA, IIIB, or IIIC

D - subsequent encounter for closed fracture with routine healing

E - subsequent encounter for open fracture type I or II with routine healing

F - subsequent encounter for open fracture type IIIA, IIIB, or IIIC with routine healing

G - subsequent encounter for closed fracture with delayed healing

H - subsequent encounter for open fracture type I or II with delayed healing

J - subsequent encounter for open fracture type IIIA, IIIB, or IIIC with delayed healing

K - subsequent encounter for closed fracture with nonunion

M - subsequent encounter for open fracture type I or II with nonunion

N - subsequent encounter for open fracture type IIIA, IIIB, or IIIC with nonunion

P - subsequent encounter for closed fracture with malunion

Q - subsequent encounter for open fracture type I or II with malunion

R - subsequent encounter for open fracture type IIIA, IIIB, or IIIC with malunion

S - sequela

S82.0   Fracture of patella

Knee cap

S82.00   Unspecified fracture of patella

⑦**S82.001   Unspecified fracture of right patella**

⑦**S82.002   Unspecified fracture of left patella**

⑦**S82.009   Unspecified fracture of unspecified patella**

S82.01   Osteochondral fracture of patella

⑦**S82.011   Displaced osteochondral fracture of right patella**

⑦**S82.012   Displaced osteochondral fracture of left patella**

⑦**S82.013   Displaced osteochondral fracture of unspecified patella**

⑦**S82.014   Nondisplaced osteochondral fracture of right patella**

⑦**S82.015   Nondisplaced osteochondral fracture of left patella**

⑦**S82.016   Nondisplaced osteochondral fracture of unspecified patella**

S82.02   Longitudinal fracture of patella

⑦**S82.021   Displaced longitudinal fracture of right patella**

⑦**S82.022   Displaced longitudinal fracture of left patella**

⑦**S82.023   Displaced longitudinal fracture of unspecified patella**

⑦**S82.024   Nondisplaced longitudinal fracture of right patella**

⑦**S82.025   Nondisplaced longitudinal fracture of left patella**

⑦**S82.026   Nondisplaced longitudinal fracture of unspecified patella**

S82.03   Transverse fracture of patella

⑦**S82.031   Displaced transverse fracture of right patella**

⑦**S82.032   Displaced transverse fracture of left patella**

⑦**S82.033   Displaced transverse fracture of unspecified patella**

⑦**S82.034   Nondisplaced transverse fracture of right patella**

⑦**S82.035   Nondisplaced transverse fracture of left patella**

⑦**S82.036   Nondisplaced transverse fracture of unspecified patella**

S82.04   Comminuted fracture of patella

⑦**S82.041   Displaced comminuted fracture of right patella**

⑦**S82.042   Displaced comminuted fracture of left patella**

⑦**S82.043   Displaced comminuted fracture of unspecified patella**

⑦**S82.044   Nondisplaced comminuted fracture of right patella**

⑦**S82.045   Nondisplaced comminuted fracture of left patella**

⑦**S82.046   Nondisplaced comminuted fracture of unspecified patella**

S82.09   Other fracture of patella

⑦**S82.091   Other fracture of right patella**

⑦**S82.092   Other fracture of left patella**

⑦**S82.099   Other fracture of unspecified patella**

S82.1   Fracture of upper end of tibia

Fracture of proximal end of tibia

Excludes2: fracture of shaft of tibia (S82.2-)

physeal fracture of upper end of tibia (S89.0-)

S82.10   Unspecified fracture of upper end of tibia

⑦**S82.101   Unspecified fracture of upper end of right tibia**

⑦**S82.102   Unspecified fracture of upper end of left tibia**

⑦**S82.109   Unspecified fracture of upper end of unspecified tibia**

S82.11   Fracture of tibial spine

⑦**S82.111   Displaced fracture of right tibial spine**

⑦**S82.112   Displaced fracture of left tibial spine**

⑦**S82.113   Displaced fracture of unspecified tibial spine**

⑦**S82.114   Nondisplaced fracture of right tibial spine**

⑦**S82.115   Nondisplaced fracture of left tibial spine**

⑦S82.116   **Nondisplaced fracture of unspecified tibial spine**

S82.12   **Fracture of lateral condyle of tibia**

⑦S82.121   **Displaced fracture of lateral condyle of right tibia**

⑦S82.122   **Displaced fracture of lateral condyle of left tibia**

⑦S82.123   **Displaced fracture of lateral condyle of unspecified tibia**

⑦S82.124   **Nondisplaced fracture of lateral condyle of right tibia**

⑦S82.125   **Nondisplaced fracture of lateral condyle of left tibia**

⑦S82.126   **Nondisplaced fracture of lateral condyle of unspecified tibia**

S82.13   **Fracture of medial condyle of tibia**

⑦S82.131   **Displaced fracture of medial condyle of right tibia**

⑦S82.132   **Displaced fracture of medial condyle of left tibia**

⑦S82.133   **Displaced fracture of medial condyle of unspecified tibia**

⑦S82.134   **Nondisplaced fracture of medial condyle of right tibia**

⑦S82.135   **Nondisplaced fracture of medial condyle of left tibia**

⑦S82.136   **Nondisplaced fracture of medial condyle of unspecified tibia**

S82.14   **Bicondylar fracture of tibia**

Fracture of tibial plateau NOS

⑦S82.141   **Displaced bicondylar fracture of right tibia**

⑦S82.142   **Displaced bicondylar fracture of left tibia**

⑦S82.143   **Displaced bicondylar fracture of unspecified tibia**

⑦S82.144   **Nondisplaced bicondylar fracture of right tibia**

⑦S82.145   **Nondisplaced bicondylar fracture of left tibia**

⑦S82.146   **Nondisplaced bicondylar fracture of unspecified tibia**

S82.15   **Fracture of tibial tuberosity**

⑦S82.151   **Displaced fracture of right tibial tuberosity**

⑦82.152   **Displaced fracture of left tibial tuberosity**

⑦S82.153   **Displaced fracture of unspecified tibial tuberosity**

⑦S82.154   **Nondisplaced fracture of right tibial tuberosity**

⑦S82.155   **Nondisplaced fracture of left tibial tuberosity**

⑦S82.156   **Nondisplaced fracture of unspecified tibial tuberosity**

S82.16   **Torus fracture of upper end of tibia**

The appropriate 7th character is to be added to all codes in subcategory S82.16

A - initial encounter for closed fracture

D - subsequent encounter for fracture with routine healing

G - subsequent encounter for fracture with delayed healing

K - subsequent encounter for fracture with nonunion

P - subsequent encounter for fracture with malunion

S - sequela

⑦S82.161   **Torus fracture of upper end of right tibia**

⑦S82.162   **Torus fracture of upper end of left tibia**

⑦S82.169   **Torus fracture of upper end of unspecified tibia**

S82.19   **Other fracture of upper end of tibia**

⑦S82.191   **Other fracture of upper end of right tibia**

⑦S82.192   **Other fracture of upper end of left tibia**

⑦S82.199   **Other fracture of upper end of unspecified tibia**

S82.2   **Fracture of shaft of tibia**

S82.20   **Unspecified fracture of shaft of tibia**

Fracture of tibia NOS

⑦S82.201   **Unspecified fracture of shaft of right tibia**

⑦S82.202   **Unspecified fracture of shaft of left tibia**

⑦S82.209   **Unspecified fracture of shaft of unspecified tibia**

S82.22   **Transverse fracture of shaft of tibia**

⑦S82.221   **Displaced transverse fracture of shaft of right tibia**

⑦S82.222   **Displaced transverse fracture of shaft of left tibia**

⑦S82.223   **Displaced transverse fracture of shaft of unspecified tibia**

⑦S82.224   **Nondisplaced transverse fracture of shaft of right tibia**

⑦S82.225   **Nondisplaced transverse fracture of shaft of left tibia**

⑦S82.226   **Nondisplaced transverse fracture of shaft of unspecified tibia**

S82.23   **Oblique fracture of shaft of tibia**

⑦S82.231   **Displaced oblique fracture of shaft of right tibia**

⑦S82.232   **Displaced oblique fracture of shaft of left tibia**

⑦S82.233   **Displaced oblique fracture of shaft of unspecified tibia**

⑦S82.234   **Nondisplaced oblique fracture of shaft of right tibia**

⑦S82.235   **Nondisplaced oblique fracture of shaft of left tibia**

⑦S82.236   **Nondisplaced oblique fracture of shaft of unspecified tibia**

S82.24   **Spiral fracture of shaft of tibia**

Toddler fracture

⑦S82.241   **Displaced spiral fracture of shaft of right tibia**

⑦S82.242   **Displaced spiral fracture of shaft of left tibia**

⑦S82.243   **Displaced spiral fracture of shaft of unspecified tibia**

⑦S82.244   **Nondisplaced spiral fracture of shaft of right tibia**

   ● New code   ▲ Revised code   **Excludes1:** Not coded here   **Excludes2:** Not included here   ⊗ Placeholder required   ⑦7th digit required

⑦S82.245　Nondisplaced spiral fracture of shaft of left tibia

⑦S82.246　Nondisplaced spiral fracture of shaft of unspecified tibia

S82.25　Comminuted fracture of shaft of tibia

⑦S82.251　Displaced comminuted fracture of shaft of right tibia

⑦S82.252　Displaced comminuted fracture of shaft of left tibia

⑦S82.253　Displaced comminuted fracture of shaft of unspecified tibia

⑦S82.254　Nondisplaced comminuted fracture of shaft of right tibia

⑦S82.255　Nondisplaced comminuted fracture of shaft of left tibia

⑦S82.256　Nondisplaced comminuted fracture of shaft of unspecified tibia

S82.26　Segmental fracture of shaft of tibia

⑦S82.261　Displaced segmental fracture of shaft of right tibia

⑦S82.262　Displaced segmental fracture of shaft of left tibia

⑦S82.263　Displaced segmental fracture of shaft of unspecified tibia

⑦S82.264　Nondisplaced segmental fracture of shaft of right tibia

⑦S82.265　Nondisplaced segmental fracture of shaft of left tibia

⑦S82.266　Nondisplaced segmental fracture of shaft of unspecified tibia

S82.29　Other fracture of shaft of tibia

⑦S82.291　Other fracture of shaft of right tibia

⑦S82.292　Other fracture of shaft of left tibia

⑦S82.299　Other fracture of shaft of unspecified tibia

S82.3　Fracture of lower end of tibia

Excludes1: bimalleolar fracture of lower leg (S82.84-)

fracture of medial malleolus alone (S82.5-)

Maisonneuve's fracture (S82.86-)

pilon fracture of distal tibia (S82.87-)

trimalleolar fractures of lower leg (S82.85-)

S82.30　Unspecified fracture of lower end of tibia

⑦S82.301　Unspecified fracture of lower end of right tibia

⑦S82.302　Unspecified fracture of lower end of left tibia

⑦S82.309　Unspecified fracture of lower end of unspecified tibia

S82.31　Torus fracture of lower end of tibia

The appropriate 7th character is to be added to all codes in subcategory S82.31

A - initial encounter for closed fracture

D - subsequent encounter for fracture with routine healing

G - subsequent encounter for fracture with delayed healing

K - subsequent encounter for fracture with nonunion

P - subsequent encounter for fracture with malunion

S - sequela

⑦S82.311　Torus fracture of lower end of right tibia

⑦S82.312　Torus fracture of lower end of left tibia

⑦S82.319　Torus fracture of lower end of unspecified tibia

S82.39　Other fracture of lower end of tibia

⑦S82.391　Other fracture of lower end of right tibia

⑦S82.392　Other fracture of lower end of left tibia

⑦S82.399　Other fracture of lower end of unspecified tibia

S82.4　Fracture of shaft of fibula

Excludes2: fracture of lateral malleolus alone (S82.6-)

S82.40　Unspecified fracture of shaft of fibula

⑦S82.401　Unspecified fracture of shaft of right fibula

⑦S82.402　Unspecified fracture of shaft of left fibula

⑦S82.409　Unspecified fracture of shaft of unspecified fibula

S82.42　Transverse fracture of shaft of fibula

⑦S82.421　Displaced transverse fracture of shaft of right fibula

⑦S82.422　Displaced transverse fracture of shaft of left fibula

⑦S82.423　Displaced transverse fracture of shaft of unspecified fibula

⑦S82.424　Nondisplaced transverse fracture of shaft of right fibula

⑦S82.425　Nondisplaced transverse fracture of shaft of left fibula

⑦S82.426　Nondisplaced transverse fracture of shaft of unspecified fibula

S82.43　Oblique fracture of shaft of fibula

⑦S82.431　Displaced oblique fracture of shaft of right fibula

⑦S82.432　Displaced oblique fracture of shaft of left fibula

⑦S82.433　Displaced oblique fracture of shaft of unspecified fibula

⑦S82.434　Nondisplaced oblique fracture of shaft of right fibula

⑦S82.435　Nondisplaced oblique fracture of shaft of left fibula

⑦S82.436　Nondisplaced oblique fracture of shaft of unspecified fibula

S82.44　Spiral fracture of shaft of fibula

⑦S82.441　Displaced spiral fracture of shaft of right fibula

⑦S82.442　Displaced spiral fracture of shaft of left fibula

⑦S82.443　Displaced spiral fracture of shaft of unspecified fibula

⑦S82.444　Nondisplaced spiral fracture of shaft of right fibula

⑦S82.445　Nondisplaced spiral fracture of shaft of left fibula

⑦S82.446　Nondisplaced spiral fracture of shaft of unspecified fibula

S82.45　Comminuted fracture of shaft of fibula

⑦S82.451 **Displaced comminuted fracture of shaft of right fibula**

⑦S82.452 **Displaced comminuted fracture of shaft of left fibula**

⑦S82.453 **Displaced comminuted fracture of shaft of unspecified fibula**

⑦S82.454 **Nondisplaced comminuted fracture of shaft of right fibula**

⑦S82.455 **Nondisplaced comminuted fracture of shaft of left fibula**

⑦S82.456 **Nondisplaced comminuted fracture of shaft of unspecified fibula**

S82.46 **Segmental fracture of shaft of fibula**

⑦S82.461 **Displaced segmental fracture of shaft of right fibula**

⑦S82.462 **Displaced segmental fracture of shaft of left fibula**

⑦S82.463 **Displaced segmental fracture of shaft of unspecified fibula**

⑦S82.464 **Nondisplaced segmental fracture of shaft of right fibula**

⑦S82.465 **Nondisplaced segmental fracture of shaft of left fibula**

⑦S82.466 **Nondisplaced segmental fracture of shaft of unspecified fibula**

S82.49 **Other fracture of shaft of fibula**

⑦S82.491 **Other fracture of shaft of right fibula**

⑦S82.492 **Other fracture of shaft of left fibula**

⑦S82.499 **Other fracture of shaft of unspecified fibula**

S82.5 **Fracture of medial malleolus**

Excludes1: pilon fracture of distal tibia (S82.87-)

Salter-Harris type III of lower end of tibia (S89.13-)

Salter-Harris type IV of lower end of tibia (S89.14-)

⊗⑦S82.51 **Displaced fracture of medial malleolus of right tibia**

⊗⑦S82.52 **Displaced fracture of medial malleolus of left tibia**

⊗⑦S82.53 **Displaced fracture of medial malleolus of unspecified tibia**

⊗⑦S82.54 **Nondisplaced fracture of medial malleolus of right tibia**

⊗⑦S82.55 **Nondisplaced fracture of medial malleolus of left tibia**

⊗⑦S82.56 **Nondisplaced fracture of medial malleolus of unspecified tibia**

S82.6 **Fracture of lateral malleolus**

Excludes1: pilon fracture of distal tibia (S82.87-)

⊗⑦S82.61 **Displaced fracture of lateral malleolus of right fibula**

⊗⑦S82.62 **Displaced fracture of lateral malleolus of left fibula**

⊗⑦S82.63 **Displaced fracture of lateral malleolus of unspecified fibula**

⊗⑦S82.64 **Nondisplaced fracture of lateral malleolus of right fibula**

⊗⑦S82.65 **Nondisplaced fracture of lateral malleolus of left fibula**

⊗⑦S82.66 **Nondisplaced fracture of lateral malleolus of unspecified fibula**

S82.8 **Other fractures of lower leg**

S82.81 **Torus fracture of upper end of fibula**

The appropriate 7th character is to be added to all codes in subcategory S82.81

A - initial encounter for closed fracture

D - subsequent encounter for fracture with routine healing

G - subsequent encounter for fracture with delayed healing

K - subsequent encounter for fracture with nonunion

P - subsequent encounter for fracture with malunion

S - sequela

⑦S82.811 **Torus fracture of upper end of right fibula**

⑦S82.812 **Torus fracture of upper end of left fibula**

⑦S82.819 **Torus fracture of upper end of unspecified fibula**

S82.82 **Torus fracture of lower end of fibula**

The appropriate 7th character is to be added to all codes in subcategory S82.82

A - initial encounter for closed fracture

D - subsequent encounter for fracture with routine healing

G - subsequent encounter for fracture with delayed healing

K - subsequent encounter for fracture with nonunion

P - subsequent encounter for fracture with malunion

S - sequela

⑦S82.821 **Torus fracture of lower end of right fibula**

⑦S82.822 **Torus fracture of lower end of left fibula**

⑦S82.829 **Torus fracture of lower end of unspecified fibula**

S82.83 **Other fracture of upper and lower end of fibula**

⑦S82.831 **Other fracture of upper and lower end of right fibula**

⑦S82.832 **Other fracture of upper and lower end of left fibula**

⑦S82.839 **Other fracture of upper and lower end of unspecified fibula**

S82.84 **Bimalleolar fracture of lower leg**

⑦S82.841 **Displaced bimalleolar fracture of right lower leg**

⑦S82.842 **Displaced bimalleolar fracture of left lower leg**

⑦S82.843 **Displaced bimalleolar fracture of unspecified lower leg**

⑦S82.844 **Nondisplaced bimalleolar fracture of right lower leg**

⑦S82.845 **Nondisplaced bimalleolar fracture of left lower leg**

⑦S82.846 **Nondisplaced bimalleolar fracture of unspecified lower leg**

S82.85 **Trimalleolar fracture of lower leg**

⑦S82.851 **Displaced trimalleolar fracture of right lower leg**

⑦S82.852 **Displaced trimalleolar fracture of left lower leg**

● New code ▲ Revised code Excludes1: Not coded here Excludes2: Not included here ⊗ Placeholder required ⑦ 7th digit required

⑦S82.853 **Displaced trimalleolar fracture of unspecified lower leg**

⑦S82.854 **Nondisplaced trimalleolar fracture of right lower leg**

⑦S82.855 **Nondisplaced trimalleolar fracture of left lower leg**

⑦S82.856 **Nondisplaced trimalleolar fracture of unspecified lower leg**

S82.86 **Maisonneuve's fracture**

⑦S82.861 **Displaced Maisonneuve's fracture of right leg**

⑦S82.862 **Displaced Maisonneuve's fracture of left leg**

⑦S82.863 **Displaced Maisonneuve's fracture of unspecified leg**

⑦S82.864 **Nondisplaced Maisonneuve's fracture of right leg**

⑦S82.865 **Nondisplaced Maisonneuve's fracture of left leg**

⑦S82.866 **Nondisplaced Maisonneuve's fracture of unspecified leg**

S82.87 **Pilon fracture of tibia**

⑦S82.871 **Displaced pilon fracture of right tibia**

⑦S82.872 **Displaced pilon fracture of left tibia**

⑦S82.873 **Displaced pilon fracture of unspecified tibia**

⑦S82.874 **Nondisplaced pilon fracture of right tibia**

⑦S82.875 **Nondisplaced pilon fracture of left tibia**

⑦S82.876 **Nondisplaced pilon fracture of unspecified tibia**

S82.89 **Other fractures of lower leg**

Fracture of ankle NOS

⑦S82.891 **Other fracture of right lower leg**

⑦S82.892 **Other fracture of left lower leg**

⑦S82.899 **Other fracture of unspecified lower leg**

S82.9 **Unspecified fracture of lower leg**

⊗⑦S82.90 **Unspecified fracture of unspecified lower leg**

⊗⑦S82.91 **Unspecified fracture of right lower leg**

⊗⑦S82.92 **Unspecified fracture of left lower leg**

S83 **Dislocation and sprain of joints and ligaments of knee**

Includes: avulsion of joint or ligament of knee

laceration of cartilage, joint or ligament of knee

sprain of cartilage, joint or ligament of knee

traumatic hemarthrosis of joint or ligament of knee

traumatic rupture of joint or ligament of knee

traumatic subluxation of joint or ligament of knee

traumatic tear of joint or ligament of knee

Code also any associated open wound

Excludes2: derangement of patella (M22.0-M22.3)

injury of patellar ligament (tendon) (S76.1-)

internal derangement of knee (M23.-)

old dislocation of knee (M24.36)

pathological dislocation of knee (M24.36)

recurrent dislocation of knee (M22.0)

strain of muscle, fascia and tendon of lower leg (S86.-)

The appropriate 7th character is to be added to each code from category S83

A - initial encounter

D - subsequent encounter

S - sequela

S83.0 **Subluxation and dislocation of patella**

S83.00 **Unspecified subluxation and dislocation of patella**

⑦S83.001 **Unspecified subluxation of right patella**

⑦S83.002 **Unspecified subluxation of left patella**

⑦S83.003 **Unspecified subluxation of unspecified patella**

⑦S83.004 **Unspecified dislocation of right patella**

⑦S83.005 **Unspecified dislocation of left patella**

⑦S83.006 **Unspecified dislocation of unspecified patella**

S83.01 **Lateral subluxation and dislocation of patella**

⑦S83.011 **Lateral subluxation of right patella**

⑦S83.012 **Lateral subluxation of left patella**

⑦S83.013 **Lateral subluxation of unspecified patella**

⑦S83.014 **Lateral dislocation of right patella**

⑦S83.015 **Lateral dislocation of left patella**

⑦S83.016 **Lateral dislocation of unspecified patella**

S83.09 **Other subluxation and dislocation of patella**

⑦S83.091 **Other subluxation of right patella**

⑦S83.092 **Other subluxation of left patella**

⑦S83.093 **Other subluxation of unspecified patella**

⑦S83.094 **Other dislocation of right patella**

⑦S83.095 **Other dislocation of left patella**

⑦S83.096 **Other dislocation of unspecified patella**

S83.1 **Subluxation and dislocation of knee**

Excludes2: instability of knee prosthesis (T84.022, T84.023)

S83.10 **Unspecified subluxation and dislocation of knee**

⑦S83.101 **Unspecified subluxation of right knee**

⑦S83.102 **Unspecified subluxation of left knee**

⑦S83.103 **Unspecified subluxation of unspecified knee**

⑦S83.104 **Unspecified dislocation of right knee**

⑦S83.105 **Unspecified dislocation of left knee**

⑦S83.106 **Unspecified dislocation of unspecified knee**

S83.11 **Anterior subluxation and dislocation of proximal end of tibia**

Posterior subluxation and dislocation of distal end of femur

⑦S83.111 **Anterior subluxation of proximal end of tibia, right knee**

⑦S83.112 **Anterior subluxation of proximal end of tibia, left knee**

⑦S83.113 **Anterior subluxation of proximal end of tibia, unspecified knee**

⑦S83.114 **Anterior dislocation of proximal end of tibia, right knee**

⑦S83.115 **Anterior dislocation of proximal end of tibia, left knee**

⑦S83.116　Anterior dislocation of proximal end of tibia, unspecified knee

S83.12　Posterior subluxation and dislocation of proximal end of tibia

Anterior dislocation of distal end of femur

⑦S83.121　Posterior subluxation of proximal end of tibia, right knee

⑦S83.122　Posterior subluxation of proximal end of tibia, left knee

⑦S83.123　Posterior subluxation of proximal end of tibia, unspecified knee

⑦S83.124　Posterior dislocation of proximal end of tibia, right knee

⑦S83.125　Posterior dislocation of proximal end of tibia, left knee

⑦S83.126　Posterior dislocation of proximal end of tibia, unspecified knee

S83.13　Medial subluxation and dislocation of proximal end of tibia

⑦S83.131　Medial subluxation of proximal end of tibia, right knee

⑦S83.132　Medial subluxation of proximal end of tibia, left knee

⑦S83.133　Medial subluxation of proximal end of tibia, unspecified knee

⑦S83.134　Medial dislocation of proximal end of tibia, right knee

⑦S83.135　Medial dislocation of proximal end of tibia, left knee

⑦S83.136　Medial dislocation of proximal end of tibia, unspecified knee

S83.14　Lateral subluxation and dislocation of proximal end of tibia

⑦S83.141　Lateral subluxation of proximal end of tibia, right knee

⑦S83.142　Lateral subluxation of proximal end of tibia, left knee

⑦S83.143　Lateral subluxation of proximal end of tibia, unspecified knee

⑦S83.144　Lateral dislocation of proximal end of tibia, right knee

⑦S83.145　Lateral dislocation of proximal end of tibia, left knee

⑦S83.146　Lateral dislocation of proximal end of tibia, unspecified knee

S83.19　Other subluxation and dislocation of knee

⑦S83.191　Other subluxation of right knee

⑦S83.192　Other subluxation of left knee

⑦S83.193　Other subluxation of unspecified knee

⑦S83.194　Other dislocation of right knee

⑦S83.195　Other dislocation of left knee

⑦S83.196　Other dislocation of unspecified knee

S83.2　Tear of meniscus, current injury

Excludes1: old bucket-handle tear (M23.2)

S83.20　Tear of unspecified meniscus, current injury

Tear of meniscus of knee NOS

⑦S83.200　Bucket-handle tear of unspecified meniscus, current injury, right knee

⑦S83.201　Bucket-handle tear of unspecified meniscus, current injury, left knee

⑦S83.202　Bucket-handle tear of unspecified meniscus, current injury, unspecified knee

⑦S83.203　Other tear of unspecified meniscus, current injury, right knee

⑦S83.204　Other tear of unspecified meniscus, current injury, left knee

⑦S83.205　Other tear of unspecified meniscus, current injury, unspecified knee

⑦S83.206　Unspecified tear of unspecified meniscus, current injury, right knee

⑦S83.207　Unspecified tear of unspecified meniscus, current injury, left knee

⑦S83.209　Unspecified tear of unspecified meniscus, current injury, unspecified knee

S83.21　Bucket-handle tear of medial meniscus, current injury

⑦S83.211　Bucket-handle tear of medial meniscus, current injury, right knee

⑦S83.212　Bucket-handle tear of medial meniscus, current injury, left knee

⑦S83.219　Bucket-handle tear of medial meniscus, current injury, unspecified knee

S83.22　Peripheral tear of medial meniscus, current injury

⑦S83.221　Peripheral tear of medial meniscus, current injury, right knee

⑦S83.222　Peripheral tear of medial meniscus, current injury, left knee

⑦S83.229　Peripheral tear of medial meniscus, current injury, unspecified knee

S83.23　Complex tear of medial meniscus, current injury

⑦S83.231　Complex tear of medial meniscus, current injury, right knee

⑦S83.232　Complex tear of medial meniscus, current injury, left knee

⑦S83.239　Complex tear of medial meniscus, current injury, unspecified knee

S83.24　Other tear of medial meniscus, current injury

⑦S83.241　Other tear of medial meniscus, current injury, right knee

⑦S83.242　Other tear of medial meniscus, current injury, left knee

⑦S83.249　Other tear of medial meniscus, current injury, unspecified knee

S83.25　Bucket-handle tear of lateral meniscus, current injury

⑦S83.251　Bucket-handle tear of lateral meniscus, current injury, right knee

⑦S83.252　Bucket-handle tear of lateral meniscus, current injury, left knee

⑦S83.259　Bucket-handle tear of lateral meniscus, current injury, unspecified knee

S83.26　Peripheral tear of lateral meniscus, current injury

⑦S83.261　Peripheral tear of lateral meniscus, current injury, right knee

⑦S83.262　Peripheral tear of lateral meniscus, current injury, left knee

⑦S83.269　Peripheral tear of lateral meniscus, current injury, unspecified knee

　● New code　▲ Revised code　Excludes1: Not coded here　Excludes2: Not included here　⊗ Placeholder required　⑦7th digit required

S83.27   **Complex tear of lateral meniscus, current injury**

⑦ S83.271   Complex tear of lateral meniscus, current injury, right knee

⑦ S83.272   Complex tear of lateral meniscus, current injury, left knee

⑦ S83.279   Complex tear of lateral meniscus, current injury, unspecified knee

S83.28   **Other tear of lateral meniscus, current injury**

⑦ S83.281   Other tear of lateral meniscus, current injury, right knee

⑦ S83.282   Other tear of lateral meniscus, current injury, left knee

⑦ S83.289   Other tear of lateral meniscus, current injury, unspecified knee

S83.3   **Tear of articular cartilage of knee, current**

⊗⑦ S83.30   Tear of articular cartilage of unspecified knee, current

⊗⑦ S83.31   Tear of articular cartilage of right knee, current

⊗⑦ S83.32   Tear of articular cartilage of left knee, current

S83.4   **Sprain of collateral ligament of knee**

S83.40   Sprain of unspecified collateral ligament of knee

⑦ S83.401   Sprain of unspecified collateral ligament of right knee

⑦ S83.402   Sprain of unspecified collateral ligament of left knee

⑦ S83.409   Sprain of unspecified collateral ligament of unspecified knee

S83.41   Sprain of medial collateral ligament of knee

Sprain of tibial collateral ligament

⑦ S83.411   Sprain of medial collateral ligament of right knee

⑦ S83.412   Sprain of medial collateral ligament of left knee

⑦ S83.419   Sprain of medial collateral ligament of unspecified knee

S83.42   Sprain of lateral collateral ligament of knee

Sprain of fibular collateral ligament

⑦ S83.421   Sprain of lateral collateral ligament of right knee

⑦ S83.422   Sprain of lateral collateral ligament of left knee

⑦ S83.429   Sprain of lateral collateral ligament of unspecified knee

S83.5   **Sprain of cruciate ligament of knee**

S83.50   Sprain of unspecified cruciate ligament of knee

⑦ S83.501   Sprain of unspecified cruciate ligament of right knee

⑦ S83.502   Sprain of unspecified cruciate ligament of left knee

⑦ S83.509   Sprain of unspecified cruciate ligament of unspecified knee

S83.51   Sprain of anterior cruciate ligament of knee

⑦ S83.511   Sprain of anterior cruciate ligament of right knee

⑦ S83.512   Sprain of anterior cruciate ligament of left knee

⑦ S83.519   Sprain of anterior cruciate ligament of unspecified knee

S83.52   Sprain of posterior cruciate ligament of knee

⑦ S83.521   Sprain of posterior cruciate ligament of right knee

⑦ S83.522   Sprain of posterior cruciate ligament of left knee

⑦ S83.529   Sprain of posterior cruciate ligament of unspecified knee

S83.6   **Sprain of the superior tibiofibular joint and ligament**

⊗⑦ S83.60   Sprain of the superior tibiofibular joint and ligament, unspecified knee

⊗⑦ S83.61   Sprain of the superior tibiofibular joint and ligament, right knee

⊗⑦ S83.62   Sprain of the superior tibiofibular joint and ligament, left knee

S83.8   **Sprain of other specified parts of knee**

S83.8X   Sprain of other specified parts of knee

⑦ S83.8X1   Sprain of other specified parts of right knee

⑦ S83.8X2   Sprain of other specified parts of left knee

⑦ S83.8X9   Sprain of other specified parts of unspecified knee

S83.9   **Sprain of unspecified site of knee**

⊗⑦ S83.90   Sprain of unspecified site of unspecified knee

⊗⑦ S83.91   Sprain of unspecified site of right knee

⊗⑦ S83.92   Sprain of unspecified site of left knee

S84   **Injury of nerves at lower leg level**

Code also any associated open wound (S81.-)

Excludes2: injury of nerves at ankle and foot level (S94.-)

The appropriate 7th character is to be added to each code from category S84

A - initial encounter

D - subsequent encounter

. S - sequela

S84.0   **Injury of tibial nerve at lower leg level**

⊗⑦ S84.00   Injury of tibial nerve at lower leg level, unspecified leg

⊗⑦ S84.01   Injury of tibial nerve at lower leg level, right leg

⊗⑦ S84.02   Injury of tibial nerve at lower leg level, left leg

S84.1   **Injury of peroneal nerve at lower leg level**

⊗⑦ S84.10   Injury of peroneal nerve at lower leg level, unspecified leg

⊗⑦ S84.11   Injury of peroneal nerve at lower leg level, right leg

⊗⑦ S84.12   Injury of peroneal nerve at lower leg level, left leg

S84.2   **Injury of cutaneous sensory nerve at lower leg level**

⊗⑦ S84.20   Injury of cutaneous sensory nerve at lower leg level, unspecified leg

⊗⑦ S84.21   Injury of cutaneous sensory nerve at lower leg level, right leg

⊗⑦ S84.22   Injury of cutaneous sensory nerve at lower leg level, left leg

S84.8   **Injury of other nerves at lower leg level**

S84.80   Injury of other nerves at lower leg level

⑦ S84.801   Injury of other nerves at lower leg level, right leg

⑦ S84.802   Injury of other nerves at lower leg level, left leg

⑦ S84.809   Injury of other nerves at lower leg level, unspecified leg

S84.9   **Injury of unspecified nerve at lower leg level**

⊗⑦S84.90   **Injury of unspecified nerve at lower leg level, unspecified leg**

⊗⑦S84.91   **Injury of unspecified nerve at lower leg level, right leg**

⊗⑦S84.92   **Injury of unspecified nerve at lower leg level, left leg**

S85   **Injury of blood vessels at lower leg level**

> Code also any associated open wound (S81.-)

> Excludes2: injury of blood vessels at ankle and foot level (S95.-)

The appropriate 7th character is to be added to each code from category S85

A - initial encounter

D - subsequent encounter

S - sequela

S85.0   **Injury of popliteal artery**

    S85.00   **Unspecified injury of popliteal artery**

      ⑦S85.001   **Unspecified injury of popliteal artery, right leg**

      ⑦S85.002   **Unspecified injury of popliteal artery, left leg**

      ⑦S85.009   **Unspecified injury of popliteal artery, unspecified leg**

    S85.01   **Laceration of popliteal artery**

      ⑦S85.011   **Laceration of popliteal artery, right leg**

      ⑦S85.012   **Laceration of popliteal artery, left leg**

      ⑦S85.019   **Laceration of popliteal artery, unspecified leg**

    S85.09   **Other specified injury of popliteal artery**

      ⑦S85.091   **Other specified injury of popliteal artery, right leg**

      ⑦S85.092   **Other specified injury of popliteal artery, left leg**

      ⑦S85.099   **Other specified injury of popliteal artery, unspecified leg**

S85.1   **Injury of tibial artery**

    S85.10   **Unspecified injury of unspecified tibial artery**

        Injury of tibial artery NOS

      ⑦S85.101   **Unspecified injury of unspecified tibial artery, right leg**

      ⑦S85.102   **Unspecified injury of unspecified tibial artery, left leg**

      ⑦S85.109   **Unspecified injury of unspecified tibial artery, unspecified leg**

    S85.11   **Laceration of unspecified tibial artery**

      ⑦S85.111   **Laceration of unspecified tibial artery, right leg**

      ⑦S85.112   **Laceration of unspecified tibial artery, left leg**

      ⑦S85.119   **Laceration of unspecified tibial artery, unspecified leg**

    S85.12   **Other specified injury of unspecified tibial artery**

      ⑦S85.121   **Other specified injury of unspecified tibial artery, right leg**

      ⑦S85.122   **Other specified injury of unspecified tibial artery, left leg**

      ⑦S85.129   **Other specified injury of unspecified tibial artery, unspecified leg**

    S85.13   **Unspecified injury of anterior tibial artery**

      ⑦S85.131   **Unspecified injury of anterior tibial artery, right leg**

      ⑦S85.132   **Unspecified injury of anterior tibial artery, left leg**

      ⑦S85.139   **Unspecified injury of anterior tibial artery, unspecified leg**

    S85.14   **Laceration of anterior tibial artery**

      ⑦S85.141   **Laceration of anterior tibial artery, right leg**

      ⑦S85.142   **Laceration of anterior tibial artery, left leg**

      ⑦S85.149   **Laceration of anterior tibial artery, unspecified leg**

    S85.15   **Other specified injury of anterior tibial artery**

      ⑦S85.151   **Other specified injury of anterior tibial artery, right leg**

      ⑦S85.152   **Other specified injury of anterior tibial artery, left leg**

      ⑦S85.159   **Other specified injury of anterior tibial artery, unspecified leg**

    S85.16   **Unspecified injury of posterior tibial artery**

      ⑦S85.161   **Unspecified injury of posterior tibial artery, right leg**

      ⑦S85.162   **Unspecified injury of posterior tibial artery, left leg**

      ⑦S85.169   **Unspecified injury of posterior tibial artery, unspecified leg**

    S85.17   **Laceration of posterior tibial artery**

      ⑦S85.171   **Laceration of posterior tibial artery, right leg**

      ⑦S85.172   **Laceration of posterior tibial artery, left leg**

      ⑦S85.179   **Laceration of posterior tibial artery, unspecified leg**

    S85.18   **Other specified injury of posterior tibial artery**

      ⑦S85.181   **Other specified injury of posterior tibial artery, right leg**

      ⑦S85.182   **Other specified injury of posterior tibial artery, left leg**

      ⑦S85.189   **Other specified injury of posterior tibial artery, unspecified leg**

S85.2   **Injury of peroneal artery**

    S85.20   **Unspecified injury of peroneal artery**

      ⑦S85.201   **Unspecified injury of peroneal artery, right leg**

      ⑦S85.202   **Unspecified injury of peroneal artery, left leg**

      ⑦S85.209   **Unspecified injury of peroneal artery, unspecified leg**

    S85.21   **Laceration of peroneal artery**

      ⑦S85.211   **Laceration of peroneal artery, right leg**

      ⑦S85.212   **Laceration of peroneal artery, left leg**

      ⑦S85.219   **Laceration of peroneal artery, unspecified leg**

    S85.29   **Other specified injury of peroneal artery**

      ⑦S85.291   **Other specified injury of peroneal artery, right leg**

      ⑦S85.292   **Other specified injury of peroneal artery, left leg**

      ⑦S85.299   **Other specified injury of peroneal artery, unspecified leg**

● New code   ▲ Revised code   **Excludes1:** Not coded here   **Excludes2:** Not included here   ⊗ Placeholder required   ⑦ 7th digit required

S85.3 Injury of greater saphenous vein at lower leg level

Injury of greater saphenous vein NOS

Injury of saphenous vein NOS

S85.30 Unspecified injury of greater saphenous vein at lower leg level

⑦S85.301 Unspecified injury of greater saphenous vein at lower leg level, right leg

⑦S85.302 Unspecified injury of greater saphenous vein at lower leg level, left leg

⑦S85.309 Unspecified injury of greater saphenous vein at lower leg level, unspecified leg

S85.31 Laceration of greater saphenous vein at lower leg level

⑦S85.311 Laceration of greater saphenous vein at lower leg level, right leg

⑦S85.312 Laceration of greater saphenous vein at lower leg level, left leg

⑦S85.319 Laceration of greater saphenous vein at lower leg level, unspecified leg

S85.39 Other specified injury of greater saphenous vein at lower leg level

⑦S85.391 Other specified injury of greater saphenous vein at lower leg level, right leg

⑦S85.392 Other specified injury of greater saphenous vein at lower leg level, left leg

⑦S85.399 Other specified injury of greater saphenous vein at lower leg level, unspecified leg

S85.4 Injury of lesser saphenous vein at lower leg level

S85.40 Unspecified injury of lesser saphenous vein at lower leg level

⑦S85.401 Unspecified injury of lesser saphenous vein at lower leg level, right leg

⑦S85.402 Unspecified injury of lesser saphenous vein at lower leg level, left leg

⑦S85.409 Unspecified injury of lesser saphenous vein at lower leg level, unspecified leg

S85.41 Laceration of lesser saphenous vein at lower leg level

⑦S85.411 Laceration of lesser saphenous vein at lower leg level, right leg

⑦S85.412 Laceration of lesser saphenous vein at lower leg level, left leg

⑦S85.419 Laceration of lesser saphenous vein at lower leg level, unspecified leg

S85.49 Other specified injury of lesser saphenous vein at lower leg level

⑦S85.491 Other specified injury of lesser saphenous vein at lower leg level, right leg

⑦S85.492 Other specified injury of lesser saphenous vein at lower leg level, left leg

⑦S85.499 Other specified injury of lesser saphenous vein at lower leg level, unspecified leg

S85.5 Injury of popliteal vein

S85.50 Unspecified injury of popliteal vein

⑦S85.501 Unspecified injury of popliteal vein, right leg

⑦S85.502 Unspecified injury of popliteal vein, left leg

⑦S85.509 Unspecified injury of popliteal vein, unspecified leg

S85.51 Laceration of popliteal vein

⑦S85.511 Laceration of popliteal vein, right leg

⑦S85.512 Laceration of popliteal vein, left leg

⑦S85.519 Laceration of popliteal vein, unspecified leg

S85.59 Other specified injury of popliteal vein

⑦S85.591 Other specified injury of popliteal vein, right leg

⑦S85.592 Other specified injury of popliteal vein, left leg

⑦S85.599 Other specified injury of popliteal vein, unspecified leg

S85.8 Injury of other blood vessels at lower leg level

S85.80 Unspecified injury of other blood vessels at lower leg level

⑦S85.801 Unspecified injury of other blood vessels at lower leg level, right leg

⑦S85.802 Unspecified injury of other blood vessels at lower leg level, left leg

⑦S85.809 Unspecified injury of other blood vessels at lower leg level, unspecified leg

S85.81 Laceration of other blood vessels at lower leg level

⑦S85.811 Laceration of other blood vessels at lower leg level, right leg

⑦S85.812 Laceration of other blood vessels at lower leg level, left leg

⑦S85.819 Laceration of other blood vessels at lower leg level, unspecified leg

S85.89 Other specified injury of other blood vessels at lower leg level

⑦S85.891 Other specified injury of other blood vessels at lower leg level, right leg

⑦S85.892 Other specified injury of other blood vessels at lower leg level, left leg

⑦S85.899 Other specified injury of other blood vessels at lower leg level, unspecified leg

S85.9 Injury of unspecified blood vessel at lower leg level

S85.90 Unspecified injury of unspecified blood vessel at lower leg level

⑦S85.901 Unspecified injury of unspecified blood vessel at lower leg level, right leg

⑦S85.902 Unspecified injury of unspecified blood vessel at lower leg level, left leg

⑦S85.909 Unspecified injury of unspecified blood vessel at lower leg level, unspecified leg

S85.91 Laceration of unspecified blood vessel at lower leg level

⑦S85.911 Laceration of unspecified blood vessel at lower leg level, right leg

⑦S85.912 Laceration of unspecified blood vessel at lower leg level, left leg

---

⑦S85.919 **Laceration of unspecified blood vessel at lower leg level, unspecified leg**

S85.99 **Other specified injury of unspecified blood vessel at lower leg level**

⑦S85.991 **Other specified injury of unspecified blood vessel at lower leg level, right leg**

⑦S85.992 **Other specified injury of unspecified blood vessel at lower leg level, left leg**

⑦S85.999 **Other specified injury of unspecified blood vessel at lower leg level, unspecified leg**

S86 **Injury of muscle, fascia and tendon at lower leg level**

Code also any associated open wound (S81.-)

Excludes2: injury of muscle, fascia and tendon at ankle (S96.-)

injury of patellar ligament (tendon) (S76.1-)

sprain of joints and ligaments of knee (S83.-)

The appropriate 7th character is to be added to each code from category S86

A - initial encounter

D - subsequent encounter

S - sequela

S86.0 **Injury of Achilles tendon**

S86.00 **Unspecified injury of Achilles tendon**

⑦S86.001 **Unspecified injury of right Achilles tendon**

⑦S86.002 **Unspecified injury of left Achilles tendon**

⑦S86.009 **Unspecified injury of unspecified Achilles tendon**

S86.01 **Strain of Achilles tendon**

⑦S86.011 **Strain of right Achilles tendon**

⑦S86.012 **Strain of left Achilles tendon**

⑦S86.019 **Strain of unspecified Achilles tendon**

S86.02 **Laceration of Achilles tendon**

⑦S86.021 **Laceration of right Achilles tendon**

⑦S86.022 **Laceration of left Achilles tendon**

⑦S86.029 **Laceration of unspecified Achilles tendon**

S86.09 **Other specified injury of Achilles tendon**

⑦S86.091 **Other specified injury of right Achilles tendon**

⑦S86.092 **Other specified injury of left Achilles tendon**

⑦S86.099 **Other specified injury of unspecified Achilles tendon**

S86.1 **Injury of other muscle(s) and tendon(s) of posterior muscle group at lower leg level**

S86.10 **Unspecified injury of other muscle(s) and tendon(s) of posterior muscle group at lower leg level**

⑦S86.101 **Unspecified injury of other muscle(s) and tendon(s) of posterior muscle group at lower leg level, right leg**

⑦S86.102 **Unspecified injury of other muscle(s) and tendon(s) of posterior muscle group at lower leg level, left leg**

⑦S86.109 **Unspecified injury of other muscle(s) and tendon(s) of posterior muscle group at lower leg level, unspecified leg**

S86.11 **Strain of other muscle(s) and tendon(s) of posterior muscle group at lower leg level**

⑦S86.111 **Strain of other muscle(s) and tendon(s) of posterior muscle group at lower leg level, right leg**

⑦S86.112 **Strain of other muscle(s) and tendon(s) of posterior muscle group at lower leg level, left leg**

⑦S86.119 **Strain of other muscle(s) and tendon(s) of posterior muscle group at lower leg level, unspecified leg**

S86.12 **Laceration of other muscle(s) and tendon(s) of posterior muscle group at lower leg level**

⑦S86.121 **Laceration of other muscle(s) and tendon(s) of posterior muscle group at lower leg level, right leg**

⑦S86.122 **Laceration of other muscle(s) and tendon(s) of posterior muscle group at lower leg level, left leg**

⑦S86.129 **Laceration of other muscle(s) and tendon(s) of posterior muscle group at lower leg level, unspecified leg**

S86.19 **Other injury of other muscle(s) and tendon(s) of posterior muscle group at lower leg level**

⑦S86.191 **Other injury of other muscle(s) and tendon(s) of posterior muscle group at lower leg level, right leg**

⑦S86.192 **Other injury of other muscle(s) and tendon(s) of posterior muscle group at lower leg level, left leg**

⑦S86.199 **Other injury of other muscle(s) and tendon(s) of posterior muscle group at lower leg level, unspecified leg**

S86.2 **Injury of muscle(s) and tendon(s) of anterior muscle group at lower leg level**

S86.20 **Unspecified injury of muscle(s) and tendon(s) of anterior muscle group at lower leg level**

⑦S86.201 **Unspecified injury of muscle(s) and tendon(s) of anterior muscle group at lower leg level, right leg**

⑦S86.202 **Unspecified injury of muscle(s) and tendon(s) of anterior muscle group at lower leg level, left leg**

⑦S86.209 **Unspecified injury of muscle(s) and tendon(s) of anterior muscle group at lower leg level, unspecified leg**

S86.21 **Strain of muscle(s) and tendon(s) of anterior muscle group at lower leg level**

⑦S86.211 **Strain of muscle(s) and tendon(s) of anterior muscle group at lower leg level, right leg**

⑦S86.212 **Strain of muscle(s) and tendon(s) of anterior muscle group at lower leg level, left leg**

⑦S86.219 **Strain of muscle(s) and tendon(s) of anterior muscle group at lower leg level, unspecified leg**

S86.22 **Laceration of muscle(s) and tendon(s) of anterior muscle group at lower leg level**

⑦S86.221 **Laceration of muscle(s) and tendon(s) of anterior muscle group at lower leg level, right leg**

⑦S86.222 **Laceration of muscle(s) and tendon(s) of anterior muscle group at lower leg level, left leg**

⑦S86.229 Laceration of muscle(s) and tendon(s) of anterior muscle group at lower leg level, unspecified leg

S86.29 Other injury of muscle(s) and tendon(s) of anterior muscle group at lower leg level

⑦S86.291 Other injury of muscle(s) and tendon(s) of anterior muscle group at lower leg level, right leg

⑦S86.292 Other injury of muscle(s) and tendon(s) of anterior muscle group at lower leg level, left leg

⑦S86.299 Other injury of muscle(s) and tendon(s) of anterior muscle group at lower leg level, unspecified leg

S86.3 Injury of muscle(s) and tendon(s) of peroneal muscle group at lower leg level

S86.30 Unspecified injury of muscle(s) and tendon(s) of peroneal muscle group at lower leg level

⑦S86.301 Unspecified injury of muscle(s) and tendon(s) of peroneal muscle group at lower leg level, right leg

⑦S86.302 Unspecified injury of muscle(s) and tendon(s) of peroneal muscle group at lower leg level, left leg

⑦S86.309 Unspecified injury of muscle(s) and tendon(s) of peroneal muscle group at lower leg level, unspecified leg

S86.31 Strain of muscle(s) and tendon(s) of peroneal muscle group at lower leg level

⑦S86.311 Strain of muscle(s) and tendon(s) of peroneal muscle group at lower leg level, right leg

⑦S86.312 Strain of muscle(s) and tendon(s) of peroneal muscle group at lower leg level, left leg

⑦S86.319 Strain of muscle(s) and tendon(s) of peroneal muscle group at lower leg level, unspecified leg

S86.32 Laceration of muscle(s) and tendon(s) of peroneal muscle group at lower leg level

⑦S86.321 Laceration of muscle(s) and tendon(s) of peroneal muscle group at lower leg level, right leg

⑦S86.322 Laceration of muscle(s) and tendon(s) of peroneal muscle group at lower leg level, left leg

⑦S86.329 Laceration of muscle(s) and tendon(s) of peroneal muscle group at lower leg level, unspecified leg

S86.39 Other injury of muscle(s) and tendon(s) of peroneal muscle group at lower leg level

⑦S86.391 Other injury of muscle(s) and tendon(s) of peroneal muscle group at lower leg level, right leg

⑦S86.392 Other injury of muscle(s) and tendon(s) of peroneal muscle group at lower leg level, left leg

⑦S86.399 Other injury of muscle(s) and tendon(s) of peroneal muscle group at lower leg level, unspecified leg

S86.8 Injury of other muscles and tendons at lower leg level

S86.80 Unspecified injury of other muscles and tendons at lower leg level

⑦S86.801 Unspecified injury of other muscle(s) and tendon(s) at lower leg level, right leg

⑦S86.802 Unspecified injury of other muscle(s) and tendon(s) at lower leg level, left leg

⑦S86.809 Unspecified injury of other muscle(s) and tendon(s) at lower leg level, unspecified leg

S86.81 Strain of other muscles and tendons at lower leg level

⑦S86.811 Strain of other muscle(s) and tendon(s) at lower leg level, right leg

⑦S86.812 Strain of other muscle(s) and tendon(s) at lower leg level, left leg

⑦S86.819 Strain of other muscle(s) and tendon(s) at lower leg level, unspecified leg

S86.82 Laceration of other muscles and tendons at lower leg level

⑦S86.821 Laceration of other muscle(s) and tendon(s) at lower leg level, right leg

⑦S86.822 Laceration of other muscle(s) and tendon(s) at lower leg level, left leg

⑦S86.829 Laceration of other muscle(s) and tendon(s) at lower leg level, unspecified leg

S86.89 Other injury of other muscles and tendons at lower leg level

⑦S86.891 Other injury of other muscle(s) and tendon(s) at lower leg level, right leg

⑦S86.892 Other injury of other muscle(s) and tendon(s) at lower leg level, left leg

⑦S86.899 Other injury of other muscle(s) and tendon(s) at lower leg level, unspecified leg

S86.9 Injury of unspecified muscle and tendon at lower leg level

S86.90 Unspecified injury of unspecified muscle and tendon at lower leg level

⑦S86.901 Unspecified injury of unspecified muscle(s) and tendon(s) at lower leg level, right leg

⑦S86.902 Unspecified injury of unspecified muscle(s) and tendon(s) at lower leg level, left leg

⑦S86.909 Unspecified injury of unspecified muscle(s) and tendon(s) at lower leg level, unspecified leg

S86.91 Strain of unspecified muscle and tendon at lower leg level

⑦S86.911 Strain of unspecified muscle(s) and tendon(s) at lower leg level, right leg

⑦S86.912 Strain of unspecified muscle(s) and tendon(s) at lower leg level, left leg

⑦S86.919 Strain of unspecified muscle(s) and tendon(s) at lower leg level, unspecified leg

S86.92 Laceration of unspecified muscle and tendon at lower leg level

⑦S86.921 Laceration of unspecified muscle(s) and tendon(s) at lower leg level, right leg

⑦S86.922 Laceration of unspecified muscle(s) and tendon(s) at lower leg level, left leg

⑦S86.929 Laceration of unspecified muscle(s) and tendon(s) at lower leg level, unspecified leg

S86.99 Other injury of unspecified muscle and tendon at lower leg level

⑦S86.991 Other injury of unspecified muscle(s) and tendon(s) at lower leg level, right leg

⑦S86.992 Other injury of unspecified muscle(s) and tendon(s) at lower leg level, left leg

⑦S86.999 Other injury of unspecified muscle(s) and tendon(s) at lower leg level, unspecified leg

S87 **Crushing injury of lower leg**

Use Additional Code(s) for all associated injuries

Excludes2: crushing injury of ankle and foot (S97.-)

The appropriate 7th character is to be added to each code from category S87

A - initial encounter

D - subsequent encounter

S - sequela

S87.0 **Crushing injury of knee**

⊗⑦S87.00 Crushing injury of unspecified knee

⊗⑦S87.01 Crushing injury of right knee

⊗⑦S87.02 Crushing injury of left knee

S87.8 **Crushing injury of lower leg**

⊗⑦S87.80 Crushing injury of unspecified lower leg

⊗⑦S87.81 Crushing injury of right lower leg

⊗⑦S87.82 Crushing injury of left lower leg

S88 **Traumatic amputation of lower leg**

An amputation not identified as partial or complete should be coded to complete

Excludes1: traumatic amputation of ankle and foot (S98.-)

The appropriate 7th character is to be added to each code from category S88

A - initial encounter

D - subsequent encounter

S - sequela

S88.0 **Traumatic amputation at knee level**

S88.01 **Complete traumatic amputation at knee level**

⑦S88.011 Complete traumatic amputation at knee level, right lower leg [HCC]

⑦S88.012 Complete traumatic amputation at knee level, left lower leg [HCC]

⑦S88.019 Complete traumatic amputation at knee level, unspecified lower leg [HCC]

S88.02 **Partial traumatic amputation at knee level** [HCC]

⑦S88.021 Partial traumatic amputation at knee level, right lower leg [HCC]

⑦S88.022 Partial traumatic amputation at knee level, left lower leg

⑦S88.029 Partial traumatic amputation at knee level, unspecified lower leg [HCC]

S88.1 **Traumatic amputation at level between knee and ankle**

S88.11 **Complete traumatic amputation at level between knee and ankle** [HCC]

⑦S88.111 Complete traumatic amputation at level between knee and ankle, right lower leg [HCC]

⑦S88.112 Complete traumatic amputation at level between knee and ankle, left lower leg [HCC]

⑦S88.119 Complete traumatic amputation at level between knee and ankle, unspecified lower leg [HCC]

S88.12 **Partial traumatic amputation at level between knee and ankle**

⑦S88.121 Partial traumatic amputation at level between knee and ankle, right lower leg [HCC]

⑦S88.122 Partial traumatic amputation at level between knee and ankle, left lower leg [HCC]

⑦S88.129 Partial traumatic amputation at level between knee and ankle, unspecified lower leg [HCC]

S88.9 **Traumatic amputation of lower leg, level unspecified** [HCC]

S88.91 **Complete traumatic amputation of lower leg, level unspecified** [HCC]

⑦S88.911 Complete traumatic amputation of right lower leg, level unspecified [HCC]

⑦S88.912 Complete traumatic amputation of left lower leg, level unspecified [HCC]

⑦S88.919 Complete traumatic amputation of unspecified lower leg, level unspecified [HCC]

S88.92 **Partial traumatic amputation of lower leg, level unspecified** [HCC]

⑦S88.921 Partial traumatic amputation of right lower leg, level unspecified [HCC]

⑦S88.922 Partial traumatic amputation of left lower leg, level unspecified [HCC]

⑦S88.929 Partial traumatic amputation of unspecified lower leg, level unspecified [HCC]

S89 **Other and unspecified injuries of lower leg**

Note: A fracture not indicated as open or closed should be coded to closed

Excludes2: Other and unspecified injuries of ankle and foot (S99.-)

The appropriate 7th character is to be added to each code from subcategories S89.0, S89.1, S89.2, and S89.3

A - initial encounter for closed fracture

D - subsequent encounter for fracture with routine healing

G - subsequent encounter for fracture with delayed healing

K - subsequent encounter for fracture with nonunion

P - subsequent encounter for fracture with malunion

S - sequela

S89.0 **Physeal fracture of upper end of tibia**

S89.00 **Unspecified physeal fracture of upper end of tibia**

⑦S89.001 Unspecified physeal fracture of upper end of right tibia

⑦S89.002 Unspecified physeal fracture of upper end of left tibia

⑦S89.009 Unspecified physeal fracture of upper end of unspecified tibia

S89.01 **Salter-Harris Type I physeal fracture of upper end of tibia**

⑦S89.011 Salter-Harris Type I physeal fracture of upper end of right tibia

⑦S89.012 Salter-Harris Type I physeal fracture of upper end of left tibia

⑦S89.019   Salter-Harris Type I physeal fracture of upper end of unspecified tibia

S89.02   Salter-Harris Type II physeal fracture of upper end of tibia

⑦S89.021   Salter-Harris Type II physeal fracture of upper end of right tibia

⑦S89.022   Salter-Harris Type II physeal fracture of upper end of left tibia

⑦S89.029   Salter-Harris Type II physeal fracture of upper end of unspecified tibia

S89.03   Salter-Harris Type III physeal fracture of upper end of tibia

⑦S89.031   Salter-Harris Type III physeal fracture of upper end of right tibia

⑦S89.032   Salter-Harris Type III physeal fracture of upper end of left tibia

⑦S89.039   Salter-Harris Type III physeal fracture of upper end of unspecified tibia

S89.04   Salter-Harris Type IV physeal fracture of upper end of tibia

⑦S89.041   Salter-Harris Type IV physeal fracture of upper end of right tibia

⑦S89.042   Salter-Harris Type IV physeal fracture of upper end of left tibia

⑦S89.049   Salter-Harris Type IV physeal fracture of upper end of unspecified tibia

S89.09   Other physeal fracture of upper end of tibia

⑦S89.091   Other physeal fracture of upper end of right tibia

⑦S89.092   Other physeal fracture of upper end of left tibia

⑦S89.099   Other physeal fracture of upper end of unspecified tibia

S89.1   Physeal fracture of lower end of tibia

S89.10   Unspecified physeal fracture of lower end of tibia

⑦S89.101   Unspecified physeal fracture of lower end of right tibia

⑦S89.102   Unspecified physeal fracture of lower end of left tibia

⑦S89.109   Unspecified physeal fracture of lower end of unspecified tibia

S89.11   Salter-Harris Type I physeal fracture of lower end of tibia

⑦S89.111   Salter-Harris Type I physeal fracture of lower end of right tibia

⑦S89.112   Salter-Harris Type I physeal fracture of lower end of left tibia

⑦S89.119   Salter-Harris Type I physeal fracture of lower end of unspecified tibia

S89.12   Salter-Harris Type II physeal fracture of lower end of tibia

⑦S89.121   Salter-Harris Type II physeal fracture of lower end of right tibia

⑦S89.122   Salter-Harris Type II physeal fracture of lower end of left tibia

⑦S89.129   Salter-Harris Type II physeal fracture of lower end of unspecified tibia

S89.13   Salter-Harris Type III physeal fracture of lower end of tibia

Excludes1: fracture of medial malleolus (adult) (S82.5-)

⑦S89.131   Salter-Harris Type III physeal fracture of lower end of right tibia

⑦S89.132   Salter-Harris Type III physeal fracture of lower end of left tibia

⑦S89.139   Salter-Harris Type III physeal fracture of lower end of unspecified tibia

S89.14   Salter-Harris Type IV physeal fracture of lower end of tibia

Excludes1: fracture of medial malleolus (adult) (S82.5-)

⑦S89.141   Salter-Harris Type IV physeal fracture of lower end of right tibia

⑦S89.142   Salter-Harris Type IV physeal fracture of lower end of left tibia

⑦S89.149   Salter-Harris Type IV physeal fracture of lower end of unspecified tibia

S89.19   Other physeal fracture of lower end of tibia

⑦S89.191   Other physeal fracture of lower end of right tibia

⑦S89.192   Other physeal fracture of lower end of left tibia

⑦S89.199   Other physeal fracture of lower end of unspecified tibia

S89.2   Physeal fracture of upper end of fibula

S89.20   Unspecified physeal fracture of upper end of fibula

⑦S89.201   Unspecified physeal fracture of upper end of right fibula

⑦S89.202   Unspecified physeal fracture of upper end of left fibula

⑦S89.209   Unspecified physeal fracture of upper end of unspecified fibula

S89.21   Salter-Harris Type I physeal fracture of upper end of fibula

⑦S89.211   Salter-Harris Type I physeal fracture of upper end of right fibula

⑦S89.212   Salter-Harris Type I physeal fracture of upper end of left fibula

⑦S89.219   Salter-Harris Type I physeal fracture of upper end of unspecified fibula

S89.22   Salter-Harris Type II physeal fracture of upper end of fibula

⑦S89.221   Salter-Harris Type II physeal fracture of upper end of right fibula

⑦S89.222   Salter-Harris Type II physeal fracture of upper end of left fibula

⑦S89.229   Salter-Harris Type II physeal fracture of upper end of unspecified fibula

S89.29   Other physeal fracture of upper end of fibula

⑦S89.291   Other physeal fracture of upper end of right fibula

⑦S89.292   Other physeal fracture of upper end of left fibula

⑦S89.299   Other physeal fracture of upper end of unspecified fibula

S89.3   Physeal fracture of lower end of fibula

S89.30 Unspecified physeal fracture of lower end of fibula

⑦S89.301 Unspecified physeal fracture of lower end of right fibula

⑦S89.302 Unspecified physeal fracture of lower end of left fibula

⑦S89.309 Unspecified physeal fracture of lower end of unspecified fibula

S89.31 Salter-Harris Type I physeal fracture of lower end of fibula

⑦S89.311 Salter-Harris Type I physeal fracture of lower end of right fibula

⑦S89.312 Salter-Harris Type I physeal fracture of lower end of left fibula

⑦S89.319 Salter-Harris Type I physeal fracture of lower end of unspecified fibula

S89.32 Salter-Harris Type II physeal fracture of lower end of fibula

⑦S89.321 Salter-Harris Type II physeal fracture of lower end of right fibula

⑦S89.322 Salter-Harris Type II physeal fracture of lower end of left fibula

⑦S89.329 Salter-Harris Type II physeal fracture of lower end of unspecified fibula

S89.39 Other physeal fracture of lower end of fibula

⑦S89.391 Other physeal fracture of lower end of right fibula

⑦S89.392 Other physeal fracture of lower end of left fibula

⑦S89.399 Other physeal fracture of lower end of unspecified fibula

S89.8 Other specified injuries of lower leg

The appropriate 7th character is to be added to each code in subcategory S89.8

A - initial encounter

D - subsequent encounter

S - sequela

⊗⑦S89.80 Other specified injuries of unspecified lower leg

⊗⑦S89.81 Other specified injuries of right lower leg

⊗⑦S89.82 Other specified injuries of left lower leg

S89.9 Unspecified injury of lower leg

The appropriate 7th character is to be added to each code in subcategory S89.9

A - initial encounter

D - subsequent encounter

S - sequela

⊗⑦S89.90 Unspecified injury of unspecified lower leg

⊗⑦S89.91 Unspecified injury of right lower leg

⊗⑦S89.92 Unspecified injury of left lower leg

INJURIES TO THE ANKLE AND FOOT (S90-S99)

Excludes2: burns and corrosions (T20-T32)

fracture of ankle and malleolus (S82.-)

frostbite (T33-T34)

insect bite or sting, venomous (T63.4)

S90 Superficial injury of ankle, foot and toes

The appropriate 7th character is to be added to each code from category S90

A - initial encounter

D - subsequent encounter

S - sequela

S90.0 Contusion of ankle

⊗⑦S90.00 Contusion of unspecified ankle

⊗⑦S90.01 Contusion of right ankle

⊗⑦S90.02 Contusion of left ankle

S90.1 Contusion of toe without damage to nail

S90.11 Contusion of great toe without damage to nail

⑦S90.111 Contusion of right great toe without damage to nail

⑦S90.112 Contusion of left great toe without damage to nail

⑦S90.119 Contusion of unspecified great toe without damage to nail

S90.12 Contusion of lesser toe without damage to nail

⑦S90.121 Contusion of right lesser toe(s) without damage to nail

⑦S90.122 Contusion of left lesser toe(s) without damage to nail

⑦S90.129 Contusion of unspecified lesser toe(s) without damage to nail

Contusion of toe NOS

S90.2 Contusion of toe with damage to nail

S90.21 Contusion of great toe with damage to nail

⑦S90.211 Contusion of right great toe with damage to nail

⑦S90.212 Contusion of left great toe with damage to nail

⑦S90.219 Contusion of unspecified great toe with damage to nail

S90.22 Contusion of lesser toe with damage to nail

⑦S90.221 Contusion of right lesser toe(s) with damage to nail

⑦S90.222 Contusion of left lesser toe(s) with damage to nail

⑦S90.229 Contusion of unspecified lesser toe(s) with damage to nail

S90.3 Contusion of foot

Excludes2: contusion of toes (S90.1-, S90.2-)

⊗⑦S90.30 Contusion of unspecified foot

Contusion of foot NOS

⊗⑦S90.31 Contusion of right foot

⊗⑦S90.32 Contusion of left foot

S90.4 Other superficial injuries of toe

S90.41 Abrasion of toe

⑦S90.411 Abrasion, right great toe

⑦S90.412 Abrasion, left great toe

⑦S90.413 Abrasion, unspecified great toe

⑦S90.414 Abrasion, right lesser toe(s)

⑦S90.415 Abrasion, left lesser toe(s)

⑦S90.416 Abrasion, unspecified lesser toe(s)

S90.42 Blister (nonthermal) of toe

⑦S90.421 Blister (nonthermal), right great toe

⑦S90.422 Blister (nonthermal), left great toe

⑦S90.423 Blister (nonthermal), unspecified great toe

⑦S90.424 Blister (nonthermal), right lesser toe(s)

⑦S90.425 Blister (nonthermal), left lesser toe(s)

⑦S90.426　Blister (nonthermal), unspecified lesser toe(s)

S90.44　External constriction of toe

Hair tourniquet syndrome of toe

⑦S90.441　External constriction, right great toe

⑦S90.442　External constriction, left great toe

⑦S90.443　External constriction, unspecified great toe

⑦S90.444　External constriction, right lesser toe(s)

⑦S90.445　External constriction, left lesser toe(s)

⑦S90.446　External constriction, unspecified lesser toe(s)

S90.45　Superficial foreign body of toe

Splinter in the toe

⑦S90.451　Superficial foreign body, right great toe

⑦S90.452　Superficial foreign body, left great toe

⑦S90.453　Superficial foreign body, unspecified great toe

⑦S90.454　Superficial foreign body, right lesser toe(s)

⑦S90.455　Superficial foreign body, left lesser toe(s)

⑦S90.456　Superficial foreign body, unspecified lesser toe(s)

S90.46　Insect bite (nonvenomous) of toe

⑦S90.461　Insect bite (nonvenomous), right great toe

⑦S90.462　Insect bite (nonvenomous), left great toe

⑦S90.463　Insect bite (nonvenomous), unspecified great toe

⑦S90.464　Insect bite (nonvenomous), right lesser toe(s)

⑦S90.465　Insect bite (nonvenomous), left lesser toe(s)

⑦S90.466　Insect bite (nonvenomous), unspecified lesser toe(s)

S90.47　Other superficial bite of toe

Excludes1: open bite of toe (S91.15-, S91.25-)

⑦S90.471　Other superficial bite of right great toe

⑦S90.472　Other superficial bite of left great toe

⑦S90.473　Other superficial bite of unspecified great toe

⑦S90.474　Other superficial bite of right lesser toe(s)

⑦S90.475　Other superficial bite of left lesser toe(s)

⑦S90.476　Other superficial bite of unspecified lesser toe(s)

S90.5　Other superficial injuries of ankle

S90.51　Abrasion of ankle

⑦S90.511　Abrasion, right ankle

⑦S90.512　Abrasion, left ankle

⑦S90.519　Abrasion, unspecified ankle

S90.52　Blister (nonthermal) of ankle

⑦S90.521　Blister (nonthermal), right ankle

⑦S90.522　Blister (nonthermal), left ankle

⑦S90.529　Blister (nonthermal), unspecified ankle

S90.54　External constriction of ankle

⑦S90.541　External constriction, right ankle

⑦S90.542　External constriction, left ankle

⑦S90.549　External constriction, unspecified ankle

S90.55　Superficial foreign body of ankle

Splinter in the ankle

⑦S90.551　Superficial foreign body, right ankle

⑦S90.552　Superficial foreign body, left ankle

⑦S90.559　Superficial foreign body, unspecified ankle

S90.56　Insect bite (nonvenomous) of ankle

⑦S90.561　Insect bite (nonvenomous), right ankle

⑦S90.562　Insect bite (nonvenomous), left ankle

⑦S90.569　Insect bite (nonvenomous), unspecified ankle

S90.57　Other superficial bite of ankle

Excludes1: open bite of ankle (S91.05-)

⑦S90.571　Other superficial bite of ankle, right ankle

⑦S90.572　Other superficial bite of ankle, left ankle

⑦S90.579　Other superficial bite of ankle, unspecified ankle

S90.8　Other superficial injuries of foot

S90.81　Abrasion of foot

⑦S90.811　Abrasion, right foot

⑦S90.812　Abrasion, left foot

⑦S90.819　Abrasion, unspecified foot

S90.82　Blister (nonthermal) of foot

⑦S90.821　Blister (nonthermal), right foot

⑦S90.822　Blister (nonthermal), left foot

⑦S90.829　Blister (nonthermal), unspecified foot

S90.84　External constriction of foot

⑦S90.841　External constriction, right foot

⑦S90.842　External constriction, left foot

⑦S90.849　External constriction, unspecified foot

S90.85　Superficial foreign body of foot

Splinter in the foot

⑦S90.851　Superficial foreign body, right foot

⑦S90.852　Superficial foreign body, left foot

⑦S90.859　Superficial foreign body, unspecified foot

S90.86　Insect bite (nonvenomous) of foot

⑦S90.861　Insect bite (nonvenomous), right foot

⑦S90.862　Insect bite (nonvenomous), left foot

⑦S90.869　Insect bite (nonvenomous), unspecified foot

S90.87　Other superficial bite of foot

Excludes1: open bite of foot (S91.35-)

⑦S90.871　Other superficial bite of right foot

⑦S90.872　Other superficial bite of left foot

⑦S90.879　Other superficial bite of unspecified foot

S90.9   Unspecified superficial injury of ankle, foot and toe

S90.91   Unspecified superficial injury of ankle

⑦S90.911   Unspecified superficial injury of right ankle

⑦S90.912   Unspecified superficial injury of left ankle

⑦S90.919   Unspecified superficial injury of unspecified ankle

S90.92   Unspecified superficial injury of foot

⑦S90.921   Unspecified superficial injury of right foot

⑦S90.922   Unspecified superficial injury of left foot

⑦S90.929   Unspecified superficial injury of unspecified foot

S90.93   Unspecified superficial injury of toes

⑦S90.931   Unspecified superficial injury of right great toe

⑦S90.932   Unspecified superficial injury of left great toe

⑦S90.933   Unspecified superficial injury of unspecified great toe

⑦S90.934   Unspecified superficial injury of right lesser toe(s)

⑦S90.935   Unspecified superficial injury of left lesser toe(s)

⑦S90.936   Unspecified superficial injury of unspecified lesser toe(s)

S91   **Open wound of ankle, foot and toes**

Code also any associated wound infection

Excludes1: open fracture of ankle, foot and toes (S92.-with 7th character B)

traumatic amputation of ankle and foot (S98.-)

The appropriate 7th character is to be added to each code from category S91

A - initial encounter

D - subsequent encounter

S - sequela

S91.0   Open wound of ankle

S91.00   Unspecified open wound of ankle

⑦S91.001   Unspecified open wound, right ankle

⑦S91.002   Unspecified open wound, left ankle

⑦S91.009   Unspecified open wound, unspecified ankle

S91.01   Laceration without foreign body of ankle

⑦S91.011   Laceration without foreign body, right ankle

⑦S91.012   Laceration without foreign body, left ankle

⑦S91.019   Laceration without foreign body, unspecified ankle

S91.02   Laceration with foreign body of ankle

⑦S91.021   Laceration with foreign body, right ankle

⑦S91.022   Laceration with foreign body, left ankle

⑦S91.029   Laceration with foreign body, unspecified ankle

S91.03   Puncture wound without foreign body of ankle

⑦S91.031   Puncture wound without foreign body, right ankle

⑦S91.032   Puncture wound without foreign body, left ankle

⑦S91.039   Puncture wound without foreign body, unspecified ankle

S91.04   Puncture wound with foreign body of ankle

⑦S91.041   Puncture wound with foreign body, right ankle

⑦S91.042   Puncture wound with foreign body, left ankle

⑦S91.049   Puncture wound with foreign body, unspecified ankle

S91.05   Open bite of ankle

Excludes1: superficial bite of ankle (S90.56-, S90.57-)

⑦S91.051   Open bite, right ankle

⑦S91.052   Open bite, left ankle

⑦S91.059   Open bite, unspecified ankle

S91.1   Open wound of toe without damage to nail

S91.10   Unspecified open wound of toe without damage to nail

⑦S91.101   Unspecified open wound of right great toe without damage to nail

⑦S91.102   Unspecified open wound of left great toe without damage to nail

⑦S91.103   Unspecified open wound of unspecified great toe without damage to nail

⑦S91.104   Unspecified open wound of right lesser toe(s) without damage to nail

⑦S91.105   Unspecified open wound of left lesser toe(s) without damage to nail

⑦S91.106   Unspecified open wound of unspecified lesser toe(s) without damage to nail

⑦S91.109   Unspecified open wound of unspecified toe(s) without damage to nail

S91.11   Laceration without foreign body of toe without damage to nail

⑦S91.111   Laceration without foreign body of right great toe without damage to nail

⑦S91.112   Laceration without foreign body of left great toe without damage to nail

⑦S91.113   Laceration without foreign body of unspecified great toe without damage to nail

⑦S91.114   Laceration without foreign body of right lesser toe(s) without damage to nail

⑦S91.115   Laceration without foreign body of left lesser toe(s) without damage to nail

⑦S91.116   Laceration without foreign body of unspecified lesser toe(s) without damage to nail

⑦S91.119   Laceration without foreign body of unspecified toe without damage to nail

S91.12   Laceration with foreign body of toe without damage to nail

⑦S91.121   Laceration with foreign body of right great toe without damage to nail

⑦S91.122   Laceration with foreign body of left great toe without damage to nail

⑦S91.123 **Laceration with foreign body of unspecified great toe without damage to nail**

⑦S91.124 **Laceration with foreign body of right lesser toe(s) without damage to nail**

⑦S91.125 **Laceration with foreign body of left lesser toe(s) without damage to nail**

⑦S91.126 **Laceration with foreign body of unspecified lesser toe(s) without damage to nail**

⑦S91.129 **Laceration with foreign body of unspecified toe(s) without damage to nail**

S91.13 **Puncture wound without foreign body of toe without damage to nail**

⑦S91.131 **Puncture wound without foreign body of right great toe without damage to nail**

⑦S91.132 **Puncture wound without foreign body of left great toe without damage to nail**

⑦S91.133 **Puncture wound without foreign body of unspecified great toe without damage to nail**

⑦S91.134 **Puncture wound without foreign body of right lesser toe(s) without damage to nail**

⑦S91.135 **Puncture wound without foreign body of left lesser toe(s) without damage to nail**

⑦S91.136 **Puncture wound without foreign body of unspecified lesser toe(s) without damage to nail**

⑦S91.139 **Puncture wound without foreign body of unspecified toe(s) without damage to nail**

S91.14 **Puncture wound with foreign body of toe without damage to nail**

⑦S91.141 **Puncture wound with foreign body of right great toe without damage to nail**

⑦S91.142 **Puncture wound with foreign body of left great toe without damage to nail**

⑦S91.143 **Puncture wound with foreign body of unspecified great toe without damage to nail**

⑦S91.144 **Puncture wound with foreign body of right lesser toe(s) without damage to nail**

⑦S91.145 **Puncture wound with foreign body of left lesser toe(s) without damage to nail**

⑦S91.146 **Puncture wound with foreign body of unspecified lesser toe(s) without damage to nail**

⑦S91.149 **Puncture wound with foreign body of unspecified toe(s) without damage to nail**

S91.15 **Open bite of toe without damage to nail**

Bite of toe NOS

Excludes1: superficial bite of toe (S90.46-, S90.47-)

⑦S91.151 **Open bite of right great toe without damage to nail**

⑦S91.152 **Open bite of left great toe without damage to nail**

⑦S91.153 **Open bite of unspecified great toe without damage to nail**

⑦S91.154 **Open bite of right lesser toe(s) without damage to nail**

⑦S91.155 **Open bite of left lesser toe(s) without damage to nail**

⑦S91.156 **Open bite of unspecified lesser toe(s) without damage to nail**

⑦S91.159 **Open bite of unspecified toe(s) without damage to nail**

S91.2 **Open wound of toe with damage to nail**

S91.20 **Unspecified open wound of toe with damage to nail**

⑦S91.201 **Unspecified open wound of right great toe with damage to nail**

⑦S91.202 **Unspecified open wound of left great toe with damage to nail**

⑦S91.203 **Unspecified open wound of unspecified great toe with damage to nail**

⑦S91.204 **Unspecified open wound of right lesser toe(s) with damage to nail**

⑦S91.205 **Unspecified open wound of left lesser toe(s) with damage to nail**

⑦S91.206 **Unspecified open wound of unspecified lesser toe(s) with damage to nail**

⑦S91.209 **Unspecified open wound of unspecified toe(s) with damage to nail**

S91.21 **Laceration without foreign body of toe with damage to nail**

⑦S91.211 **Laceration without foreign body of right great toe with damage to nail**

⑦S91.212 **Laceration without foreign body of left great toe with damage to nail**

⑦S91.213 **Laceration without foreign body of unspecified great toe with damage to nail**

⑦S91.214 **Laceration without foreign body of right lesser toe(s) with damage to nail**

⑦S91.215 **Laceration without foreign body of left lesser toe(s) with damage to nail**

⑦S91.216 **Laceration without foreign body of unspecified lesser toe(s) with damage to nail**

⑦S91.219 **Laceration without foreign body of unspecified toe(s) with damage to nail**

S91.22 **Laceration with foreign body of toe with damage to nail**

⑦S91.221 **Laceration with foreign body of right great toe with damage to nail**

⑦S91.222 **Laceration with foreign body of left great toe with damage to nail**

⑦S91.223 **Laceration with foreign body of unspecified great toe with damage to nail**

⑦S91.224 **Laceration with foreign body of right lesser toe(s) with damage to nail**

⑦S91.225 **Laceration with foreign body of left lesser toe(s) with damage to nail**

⑦S91.226 Laceration with foreign body of unspecified lesser toe(s) with damage to nail

⑦S91.229 Laceration with foreign body of unspecified toe(s) with damage to nail

S91.23 Puncture wound without foreign body of toe with damage to nail

⑦S91.231 Puncture wound without foreign body of right great toe with damage to nail

⑦S91.232 Puncture wound without foreign body of left great toe with damage to nail

⑦S91.233 Puncture wound without foreign body of unspecified great toe with damage to nail

⑦S91.234 Puncture wound without foreign body of right lesser toe(s) with damage to nail

⑦S91.235 Puncture wound without foreign body of left lesser toe(s) with damage to nail

⑦S91.236 Puncture wound without foreign body of unspecified lesser toe(s) with damage to nail

⑦S91.239 Puncture wound without foreign body of unspecified toe(s) with damage to nail

S91.24 Puncture wound with foreign body of toe with damage to nail

⑦S91.241 Puncture wound with foreign body of right great toe with damage to nail

⑦S91.242 Puncture wound with foreign body of left great toe with damage to nail

⑦S91.243 Puncture wound with foreign body of unspecified great toe with damage to nail

⑦S91.244 Puncture wound with foreign body of right lesser toe(s) with damage to nail

⑦S91.245 Puncture wound with foreign body of left lesser toe(s) with damage to nail

⑦S91.246 Puncture wound with foreign body of unspecified lesser toe(s) with damage to nail

⑦S91.249 Puncture wound with foreign body of unspecified toe(s) with damage to nail

S91.25 Open bite of toe with damage to nail

Bite of toe with damage to nail NOS

Excludes1: superficial bite of toe (S90.46-, S90.47-)

⑦S91.251 Open bite of right great toe with damage to nail

⑦S91.252 Open bite of left great toe with damage to nail

⑦S91.253 Open bite of unspecified great toe with damage to nail

⑦S91.254 Open bite of right lesser toe(s) with damage to nail

⑦S91.255 Open bite of left lesser toe(s) with damage to nail

⑦S91.256 Open bite of unspecified lesser toe(s) with damage to nail

⑦S91.259 Open bite of unspecified toe(s) with damage to nail

S91.3 Open wound of foot

S91.30 Unspecified open wound of foot

⑦S91.301 Unspecified open wound, right foot

⑦S91.302 Unspecified open wound, left foot

⑦S91.309 Unspecified open wound, unspecified foot

S91.31 Laceration without foreign body of foot

⑦S91.311 Laceration without foreign body, right foot

⑦S91.312 Laceration without foreign body, left foot

⑦S91.319 Laceration without foreign body, unspecified foot

S91.32 Laceration with foreign body of foot

⑦S91.321 Laceration with foreign body, right foot

⑦S91.322 Laceration with foreign body, left foot

⑦S91.329 Laceration with foreign body, unspecified foot

S91.33 Puncture wound without foreign body of foot

⑦S91.331 Puncture wound without foreign body, right foot

⑦S91.332 Puncture wound without foreign body, left foot

⑦S91.339 Puncture wound without foreign body, unspecified foot

S91.34 Puncture wound with foreign body of foot

⑦S91.341 Puncture wound with foreign body, right foot

⑦S91.342 Puncture wound with foreign body, left foot

⑦S91.349 Puncture wound with foreign body, unspecified foot

S91.35 Open bite of foot

Excludes1: superficial bite of foot (S90.86-, S90.87-)

⑦S91.351 Open bite, right foot

⑦S91.352 Open bite, left foot

⑦S91.359 Open bite, unspecified foot

S92 Fracture of foot and toe, except ankle

Note: A fracture not indicated as displaced or nondisplaced should be coded to displaced

A fracture not indicated as open or closed should be coded to closed

Excludes1: traumatic amputation of ankle and foot (S98.-)

Excludes2: fracture of ankle (S82.-)

fracture of malleolus (S82.-)

traumatic amputation of ankle and foot (S98.-)

The appropriate 7th character is to be added to each code from category S92

A - initial encounter for closed fracture

B - initial encounter for open fracture

D - subsequent encounter for fracture with routine healing

G - subsequent encounter for fracture with delayed healing

K - subsequent encounter for fracture with nonunion

P - subsequent encounter for fracture with malunion

S - sequela

S92.0 Fracture of calcaneus

● New code ▲ Revised code **Excludes1:** Not coded here **Excludes2:** Not included here ⊗ Placeholder required ⑦7th digit required

Heel bone Os calcis

Excludes2: Physeal fracture of calcaneus (S99.0-)

S92.00   Unspecified fracture of calcaneus

⑦S92.001   Unspecified fracture of right calcaneus

⑦S92.002   Unspecified fracture of left calcaneus

⑦S92.009   Unspecified fracture of unspecified calcaneus

S92.01   Fracture of body of calcaneus

⑦S92.011   Displaced fracture of body of right calcaneus

⑦S92.012   Displaced fracture of body of left calcaneus

⑦S92.013   Displaced fracture of body of unspecified calcaneus

⑦S92.014   Nondisplaced fracture of body of right calcaneus

⑦S92.015   Nondisplaced fracture of body of left calcaneus

⑦S92.016   Nondisplaced fracture of body of unspecified calcaneus

S92.02   Fracture of anterior process of calcaneus

⑦S92.021   Displaced fracture of anterior process of right calcaneus

⑦S92.022   Displaced fracture of anterior process of left calcaneus

⑦S92.023   Displaced fracture of anterior process of unspecified calcaneus

⑦S92.024   Nondisplaced fracture of anterior process of right calcaneus

⑦S92.025   Nondisplaced fracture of anterior process of left calcaneus

⑦S92.026   Nondisplaced fracture of anterior process of unspecified calcaneus

S92.03   Avulsion fracture of tuberosity of calcaneus

⑦S92.031   Displaced avulsion fracture of tuberosity of right calcaneus

⑦S92.032   Displaced avulsion fracture of tuberosity of left calcaneus

⑦S92.033   Displaced avulsion fracture of tuberosity of unspecified calcaneus

⑦S92.034   Nondisplaced avulsion fracture of tuberosity of right calcaneus

⑦S92.035   Nondisplaced avulsion fracture of tuberosity of left calcaneus

⑦S92.036   Nondisplaced avulsion fracture of tuberosity of unspecified calcaneus

S92.04   Other fracture of tuberosity of calcaneus

⑦S92.041   Displaced other fracture of tuberosity of right calcaneus

⑦S92.042   Displaced other fracture of tuberosity of left calcaneus

⑦S92.043   Displaced other fracture of tuberosity of unspecified calcaneus

⑦S92.044   Nondisplaced other fracture of tuberosity of right calcaneus

⑦S92.045   Nondisplaced other fracture of tuberosity of left calcaneus

⑦S92.046   Nondisplaced other fracture of tuberosity of unspecified calcaneus

S92.05   Other extraarticular fracture of calcaneus

⑦S92.051   Displaced other extraarticular fracture of right calcaneus

⑦S92.052   Displaced other extraarticular fracture of left calcaneus

⑦S92.053   Displaced other extraarticular fracture of unspecified calcaneus

⑦S92.054   Nondisplaced other extraarticular fracture of right calcaneus

⑦S92.055   Nondisplaced other extraarticular fracture of left calcaneus

⑦S92.056   Nondisplaced other extraarticular fracture of unspecified calcaneus

S92.06   Intraarticular fracture of calcaneus

⑦S92.061   Displaced intraarticular fracture of right calcaneus

⑦S92.062   Displaced intraarticular fracture of left calcaneus

⑦S92.063   Displaced intraarticular fracture of unspecified calcaneus

⑦S92.064   Nondisplaced intraarticular fracture of right calcaneus

⑦S92.065   Nondisplaced intraarticular fracture of left calcaneus

⑦S92.066   Nondisplaced intraarticular fracture of unspecified calcaneus

S92.1   Fracture of talus

Astragalus

S92.10   Unspecified fracture of talus

⑦S92.101   Unspecified fracture of right talus

⑦S92.102   Unspecified fracture of left talus

⑦S92.109   Unspecified fracture of unspecified talus

S92.11   Fracture of neck of talus

⑦S92.111   Displaced fracture of neck of right talus

⑦S92.112   Displaced fracture of neck of left talus

⑦S92.113   Displaced fracture of neck of unspecified talus

⑦S92.114   Nondisplaced fracture of neck of right talus

⑦S92.115   Nondisplaced fracture of neck of left talus

⑦S92.116   Nondisplaced fracture of neck of unspecified talus

S92.12   Fracture of body of talus

⑦S92.121   Displaced fracture of body of right talus

⑦S92.122   Displaced fracture of body of left talus

⑦S92.123   Displaced fracture of body of unspecified talus

⑦S92.124   Nondisplaced fracture of body of right talus

⑦S92.125   Nondisplaced fracture of body of left talus

⑦S92.126   Nondisplaced fracture of body of unspecified talus

S92.13   Fracture of posterior process of talus

⑦S92.131   Displaced fracture of posterior process of right talus

⑦S92.132   Displaced fracture of posterior process of left talus

⑦S92.133   Displaced fracture of posterior process of unspecified talus

⑦S92.134   Nondisplaced fracture of posterior process of right talus

⑦S92.135   Nondisplaced fracture of posterior process of left talus

⑦S92.136   Nondisplaced fracture of posterior process of unspecified talus

S92.14   Dome fracture of talus

Excludes1: osteochondritis dissecans (M93.2)

⑦S92.141   Displaced dome fracture of right talus

⑦S92.142   Displaced dome fracture of left talus

⑦S92.143   Displaced dome fracture of unspecified talus

⑦S92.144   Nondisplaced dome fracture of right talus

⑦S92.145   Nondisplaced dome fracture of left talus

⑦S92.146   Nondisplaced dome fracture of unspecified talus

S92.15   Avulsion fracture (chip fracture) of talus

⑦S92.151   Displaced avulsion fracture (chip fracture) of right talus

⑦S92.152   Displaced avulsion fracture (chip fracture) of left talus

⑦S92.153   Displaced avulsion fracture (chip fracture) of unspecified talus

⑦S92.154   Nondisplaced avulsion fracture (chip fracture) of right talus

⑦S92.155   Nondisplaced avulsion fracture (chip fracture) of left talus

⑦S92.156   Nondisplaced avulsion fracture (chip fracture) of unspecified talus

S92.19   Other fracture of talus

⑦S92.191   Other fracture of right talus

⑦S92.192   Other fracture of left talus

⑦S92.199   Other fracture of unspecified talus

S92.2   Fracture of other and unspecified tarsal bone(s)

S92.20   Fracture of unspecified tarsal bone(s)

⑦S92.201   Fracture of unspecified tarsal bone(s) of right foot

⑦S92.202   Fracture of unspecified tarsal bone(s) of left foot

⑦S92.209   Fracture of unspecified tarsal bone(s) of unspecified foot

S92.21   Fracture of cuboid bone

⑦S92.211   Displaced fracture of cuboid bone of right foot

⑦S92.212   Displaced fracture of cuboid bone of left foot

⑦S92.213   Displaced fracture of cuboid bone of unspecified foot

⑦S92.214   Nondisplaced fracture of cuboid bone of right foot

⑦S92.215   Nondisplaced fracture of cuboid bone of left foot

⑦S92.216   Nondisplaced fracture of cuboid bone of unspecified foot

S92.22   Fracture of lateral cuneiform

⑦S92.221   Displaced fracture of lateral cuneiform of right foot

⑦S92.222   Displaced fracture of lateral cuneiform of left foot

⑦S92.223   Displaced fracture of lateral cuneiform of unspecified foot

⑦S92.224   Nondisplaced fracture of lateral cuneiform of right foot

⑦S92.225   Nondisplaced fracture of lateral cuneiform of left foot

⑦S92.226   Nondisplaced fracture of lateral cuneiform of unspecified foot

S92.23   Fracture of intermediate cuneiform

⑦S92.231   Displaced fracture of intermediate cuneiform of right foot

⑦S92.232   Displaced fracture of intermediate cuneiform of left foot

⑦S92.233   Displaced fracture of intermediate cuneiform of unspecified foot

⑦S92.234   Nondisplaced fracture of intermediate cuneiform of right foot

⑦S92.235   Nondisplaced fracture of intermediate cuneiform of left foot

⑦S92.236   Nondisplaced fracture of intermediate cuneiform of unspecified foot

S92.24   Fracture of medial cuneiform

⑦S92.241   Displaced fracture of medial cuneiform of right foot

⑦S92.242   Displaced fracture of medial cuneiform of left foot

⑦S92.243   Displaced fracture of medial cuneiform of unspecified foot

⑦S92.244   Nondisplaced fracture of medial cuneiform of right foot

⑦S92.245   Nondisplaced fracture of medial cuneiform of left foot

⑦S92.246   Nondisplaced fracture of medial cuneiform of unspecified foot

S92.25   Fracture of navicular [scaphoid] of foot

⑦S92.251   Displaced fracture of navicular [scaphoid] of right foot

⑦S92.252   Displaced fracture of navicular [scaphoid] of left foot

⑦S92.253   Displaced fracture of navicular [scaphoid] of unspecified foot

⑦S92.254   Nondisplaced fracture of navicular [scaphoid] of right foot

⑦S92.255   Nondisplaced fracture of navicular [scaphoid] of left foot

⑦S92.256   Nondisplaced fracture of navicular [scaphoid] of unspecified foot

S92.3   Fracture of metatarsal bone(s)

Excludes2: Physeal fracture of metatarsal (S99.1-)

S92.30   Fracture of unspecified metatarsal bone(s)

⑦S92.301   Fracture of unspecified metatarsal bone(s), right foot

⑦S92.302   Fracture of unspecified metatarsal bone(s), left foot

⑦S92.309   Fracture of unspecified metatarsal bone(s), unspecified foot

S92.31   Fracture of first metatarsal bone

⑦S92.311   Displaced fracture of first metatarsal bone, right foot

⑦S92.312   Displaced fracture of first metatarsal bone, left foot

● New code   ▲ Revised code   **Excludes1:** Not coded here   **Excludes2:** Not included here   ⊗ Placeholder required   ⑦7ᵗʰ digit required

⑦S92.313　**Displaced fracture of first metatarsal bone, unspecified foot**

⑦S92.314　**Nondisplaced fracture of first metatarsal bone, right foot**

⑦S92.315　**Nondisplaced fracture of first metatarsal bone, left foot**

⑦S92.316　**Nondisplaced fracture of first metatarsal bone, unspecified foot**

S92.32　**Fracture of second metatarsal bone**

⑦S92.321　**Displaced fracture of second metatarsal bone, right foot**

⑦S92.322　**Displaced fracture of second metatarsal bone, left foot**

⑦S92.323　**Displaced fracture of second metatarsal bone, unspecified foot**

⑦S92.324　**Nondisplaced fracture of second metatarsal bone, right foot**

⑦S92.325　**Nondisplaced fracture of second metatarsal bone, left foot**

⑦S92.326　**Nondisplaced fracture of second metatarsal bone, unspecified foot**

S92.33　**Fracture of third metatarsal bone**

⑦S92.331　**Displaced fracture of third metatarsal bone, right foot**

⑦S92.332　**Displaced fracture of third metatarsal bone, left foot**

⑦S92.333　**Displaced fracture of third metatarsal bone, unspecified foot**

⑦S92.334　**Nondisplaced fracture of third metatarsal bone, right foot**

⑦S92.335　**Nondisplaced fracture of third metatarsal bone, left foot**

⑦S92.336　**Nondisplaced fracture of third metatarsal bone, unspecified foot**

S92.34　**Fracture of fourth metatarsal bone**

⑦S92.341　**Displaced fracture of fourth metatarsal bone, right foot**

⑦S92.342　**Displaced fracture of fourth metatarsal bone, left foot**

⑦S92.343　**Displaced fracture of fourth metatarsal bone, unspecified foot**

⑦S92.344　**Nondisplaced fracture of fourth metatarsal bone, right foot**

⑦S92.345　**Nondisplaced fracture of fourth metatarsal bone, left foot**

⑦S92.346　**Nondisplaced fracture of fourth metatarsal bone, unspecified foot**

S92.35　**Fracture of fifth metatarsal bone**

⑦S92.351　**Displaced fracture of fifth metatarsal bone, right foot**

⑦S92.352　**Displaced fracture of fifth metatarsal bone, left foot**

⑦S92.353　**Displaced fracture of fifth metatarsal bone, unspecified foot**

⑦S92.354　**Nondisplaced fracture of fifth metatarsal bone, right foot**

⑦S92.355　**Nondisplaced fracture of fifth metatarsal bone, left foot**

⑦S92.356　**Nondisplaced fracture of fifth metatarsal bone, unspecified foot**

S92.4　**Fracture of great toe**

Excludes2: Physeal fracture of phalanx of toe (S99.2-)

S92.40　**Unspecified fracture of great toe**

⑦S92.401　**Displaced unspecified fracture of right great toe**

⑦S92.402　**Displaced unspecified fracture of left great toe**

⑦S92.403　**Displaced unspecified fracture of unspecified great toe**

⑦S92.404　**Nondisplaced unspecified fracture of right great toe**

⑦S92.405　**Nondisplaced unspecified fracture of left great toe**

⑦S92.406　**Nondisplaced unspecified fracture of unspecified great toe**

S92.41　**Fracture of proximal phalanx of great toe**

⑦S92.411　**Displaced fracture of proximal phalanx of right great toe**

⑦S92.412　**Displaced fracture of proximal phalanx of left great toe**

⑦S92.413　**Displaced fracture of proximal phalanx of unspecified great toe**

⑦S92.414　**Nondisplaced fracture of proximal phalanx of right great toe**

⑦S92.415　**Nondisplaced fracture of proximal phalanx of left great toe**

⑦S92.416　**Nondisplaced fracture of proximal phalanx of unspecified great toe**

S92.42　**Fracture of distal phalanx of great toe**

⑦S92.421　**Displaced fracture of distal phalanx of right great toe**

⑦S92.422　**Displaced fracture of distal phalanx of left great toe**

⑦S92.423　**Displaced fracture of distal phalanx of unspecified great toe**

⑦S92.424　**Nondisplaced fracture of distal phalanx of right great toe**

⑦S92.425　**Nondisplaced fracture of distal phalanx of left great toe**

⑦S92.426　**Nondisplaced fracture of distal phalanx of unspecified great toe**

S92.49　**Other fracture of great toe**

⑦S92.491　**Other fracture of right great toe**

⑦S92.492　**Other fracture of left great toe**

⑦S92.499　**Other fracture of unspecified great toe**

S92.5　**Fracture of lesser toe(s)**

Excludes2: Physeal fracture of phalanx of toe (S99.2-)

S92.50　**Unspecified fracture of lesser toe(s)**

⑦S92.501　**Displaced unspecified fracture of right lesser toe(s)**

⑦S92.502　**Displaced unspecified fracture of left lesser toe(s)**

⑦S92.503　**Displaced unspecified fracture of unspecified lesser toe(s)**

⑦S92.504　**Nondisplaced unspecified fracture of right lesser toe(s)**

⑦S92.505　**Nondisplaced unspecified fracture of left lesser toe(s)**

⑦S92.506　**Nondisplaced unspecified fracture of unspecified lesser toe(s)**

S92.51　**Fracture of proximal phalanx of lesser toe(s)**

⑦S92.511　**Displaced fracture of proximal phalanx of right lesser toe(s)**

⑦S92.512　**Displaced fracture of proximal phalanx of left lesser toe(s)**

⑦S92.513   **Displaced fracture of proximal phalanx of unspecified lesser toe(s)**

⑦S92.514   **Nondisplaced fracture of proximal phalanx of right lesser toe(s)**

⑦S92.515   **Nondisplaced fracture of proximal phalanx of left lesser toe(s)**

⑦S92.516   **Nondisplaced fracture of proximal phalanx of unspecified lesser toe(s)**

S92.52   **Fracture of middle phalanx of lesser toe(s)**

⑦S92.521   **Displaced fracture of middle phalanx of right lesser toe(s)**

⑦S92.522   **Displaced fracture of middle phalanx of left lesser toe(s)**

⑦S92.523   **Displaced fracture of middle phalanx of unspecified lesser toe(s)**

⑦S92.524   **Nondisplaced fracture of middle phalanx of right lesser toe(s)**

⑦S92.525   **Nondisplaced fracture of middle phalanx of left lesser toe(s)**

⑦S92.526   **Nondisplaced fracture of middle phalanx of unspecified lesser toe(s)**

S92.53   **Fracture of distal phalanx of lesser toe(s)**

⑦S92.531   **Displaced fracture of distal phalanx of right lesser toe(s)**

⑦S92.532   **Displaced fracture of distal phalanx of left lesser toe(s)**

⑦S92.533   **Displaced fracture of distal phalanx of unspecified lesser toe(s)**

⑦S92.534   **Nondisplaced fracture of distal phalanx of right lesser toe(s)**

⑦S92.535   **Nondisplaced fracture of distal phalanx of left lesser toe(s)**

⑦S92.536   **Nondisplaced fracture of distal phalanx of unspecified lesser toe(s)**

S92.59   **Other fracture of lesser toe(s)**

⑦S92.591   **Other fracture of right lesser toe(s)**

⑦S92.592   **Other fracture of left lesser toe(s)**

⑦S92.599   **Other fracture of unspecified lesser toe(s)**

S92.8   **Other fracture of foot, except ankle**

S92.81   **Other fracture of foot**

Sesamoid fracture of foot

⑦S92.811   **Other fracture of right foot**

⑦S92.812   **Other fracture of left foot**

⑦S92.819   **Other fracture of unspecified foot**

S92.9   **Unspecified fracture of foot and toe**

S92.90   **Unspecified fracture of foot**

⑦S92.901   **Unspecified fracture of right foot**

⑦S92.902   **Unspecified fracture of left foot**

⑦S92.909   **Unspecified fracture of unspecified foot**

S92.91   **Unspecified fracture of toe**

⑦S92.911   **Unspecified fracture of right toe(s)**

⑦S92.912   **Unspecified fracture of left toe(s)**

⑦S92.919   **Unspecified fracture of unspecified toe(s)**

S93   **Dislocation and sprain of joints and ligaments at ankle, foot and toe level**

Includes: avulsion of joint or ligament of ankle, foot and toe

laceration of cartilage, joint or ligament of ankle, foot and toe

sprain of cartilage, joint or ligament of ankle, foot and toe

traumatic hemarthrosis of joint or ligament of ankle, foot and toe

traumatic rupture of joint or ligament of ankle, foot and toe

traumatic subluxation of joint or ligament of ankle, foot and toe

traumatic tear of joint or ligament of ankle, foot and toe

Code also any associated open wound

Excludes2: strain of muscle and tendon of ankle and foot (S96.-)

The appropriate 7th character is to be added to each code from category S93

A - initial encounter

D - subsequent encounter

S - sequela

S93.0   **Subluxation and dislocation of ankle joint**

Subluxation and dislocation of astragalus Subluxation and dislocation of fibula, lower end Subluxation and dislocation of talus Subluxation and dislocation of tibia, lower end

⊗⑦S93.01   **Subluxation of right ankle joint**

⊗⑦S93.02   **Subluxation of left ankle joint**

⊗⑦S93.03   **Subluxation of unspecified ankle joint**

⊗⑦S93.04   **Dislocation of right ankle joint**

⊗⑦S93.05   **Dislocation of left ankle joint**

⊗⑦S93.06   **Dislocation of unspecified ankle joint**

S93.1   **Subluxation and dislocation of toe**

S93.10   **Unspecified subluxation and dislocation of toe**

Dislocation of toe NOS Subluxation of toe NOS

⑦S93.101   **Unspecified subluxation of right toe(s)**

⑦S93.102   **Unspecified subluxation of left toe(s)**

⑦S93.103   **Unspecified subluxation of unspecified toe(s)**

⑦S93.104   **Unspecified dislocation of right toe(s)**

⑦S93.105   **Unspecified dislocation of left toe(s)**

⑦S93.106   **Unspecified dislocation of unspecified toe(s)**

S93.11   **Dislocation of interphalangeal joint**

⑦S93.111   **Dislocation of interphalangeal joint of right great toe**

⑦S93.112   **Dislocation of interphalangeal joint of left great toe**

⑦S93.113   **Dislocation of interphalangeal joint of unspecified great toe**

⑦S93.114   **Dislocation of interphalangeal joint of right lesser toe(s)**

⑦S93.115   **Dislocation of interphalangeal joint of left lesser toe(s)**

⑦S93.116   **Dislocation of interphalangeal joint of unspecified lesser toe(s)**

⑦S93.119   **Dislocation of interphalangeal joint of unspecified toe(s)**

⑦S93.12   **Dislocation of metatarsophalangeal joint**

⑦S93.121   **Dislocation of metatarsophalangeal joint of right great toe**

⑦S93.122   **Dislocation of metatarsophalangeal joint of left great toe**

⑦S93.123   **Dislocation of metatarsophalangeal joint of unspecified great toe**

⑦S93.124   **Dislocation of metatarsophalangeal joint of right lesser toe(s)**

⑦S93.125   **Dislocation of metatarsophalangeal joint of left lesser toe(s)**

⑦S93.126   **Dislocation of metatarsophalangeal joint of unspecified lesser toe(s)**

● New code   ▲ Revised code   **Excludes1:** Not coded here   **Excludes2:** Not included here   ⊗ Placeholder required   ⑦7th digit required

⑦S93.129   **Dislocation of metatarsophalangeal joint of unspecified toe(s)**

S93.13   **Subluxation of interphalangeal joint**

⑦S93.131   **Subluxation of interphalangeal joint of right great toe**

⑦S93.132   **Subluxation of interphalangeal joint of left great toe**

⑦S93.133   **Subluxation of interphalangeal joint of unspecified great toe**

⑦S93.134   **Subluxation of interphalangeal joint of right lesser toe(s)**

⑦S93.135   **Subluxation of interphalangeal joint of left lesser toe(s)**

⑦S93.136   **Subluxation of interphalangeal joint of unspecified lesser toe(s)**

⑦S93.139   **Subluxation of interphalangeal joint of unspecified toe(s)**

S93.14   **Subluxation of metatarsophalangeal joint**

⑦S93.141   **Subluxation of metatarsophalangeal joint of right great toe**

⑦S93.142   **Subluxation of metatarsophalangeal joint of left great toe**

⑦S93.143   **Subluxation of metatarsophalangeal joint of unspecified great toe**

⑦S93.144   **Subluxation of metatarsophalangeal joint of right lesser toe(s)**

⑦S93.145   **Subluxation of metatarsophalangeal joint of left lesser toe(s)**

⑦S93.146   **Subluxation of metatarsophalangeal joint of unspecified lesser toe(s)**

⑦S93.149   **Subluxation of metatarsophalangeal joint of unspecified toe(s)**

S93.3   **Subluxation and dislocation of foot**

Excludes2: dislocation of toe (S93.1-)

S93.30   **Unspecified subluxation and dislocation of foot**

Dislocation of foot NOS

Subluxation of foot NOS

⑦S93.301   **Unspecified subluxation of right foot**

⑦S93.302   **Unspecified subluxation of left foot**

⑦S93.303   **Unspecified subluxation of unspecified foot**

⑦S93.304   **Unspecified dislocation of right foot**

⑦S93.305   **Unspecified dislocation of left foot**

⑦S93.306   **Unspecified dislocation of unspecified foot**

S93.31   **Subluxation and dislocation of tarsal joint**

⑦S93.311   **Subluxation of tarsal joint of right foot**

⑦S93.312   **Subluxation of tarsal joint of left foot**

⑦S93.313   **Subluxation of tarsal joint of unspecified foot**

⑦S93.314   **Dislocation of tarsal joint of right foot**

⑦S93.315   **Dislocation of tarsal joint of left foot**

⑦S93.316   **Dislocation of tarsal joint of unspecified foot**

S93.32   **Subluxation and dislocation of tarsometatarsal joint**

⑦S93.321   **Subluxation of tarsometatarsal joint of right foot**

⑦S93.322   **Subluxation of tarsometatarsal joint of left foot**

⑦S93.323   **Subluxation of tarsometatarsal joint of unspecified foot**

⑦S93.324   **Dislocation of tarsometatarsal joint of right foot**

⑦S93.325   **Dislocation of tarsometatarsal joint of left foot**

⑦S93.326   **Dislocation of tarsometatarsal joint of unspecified foot**

S93.33   **Other subluxation and dislocation of foot**

⑦S93.331   **Other subluxation of right foot**

⑦S93.332   **Other subluxation of left foot**

⑦S93.333   **Other subluxation of unspecified foot**

⑦S93.334   **Other dislocation of right foot**

⑦S93.335   **Other dislocation of left foot**

⑦S93.336   **Other dislocation of unspecified foot**

S93.4   **Sprain of ankle**

Excludes2: injury of Achilles tendon (S86.0-)

S93.40   **Sprain of unspecified ligament of ankle**

Sprain of ankle NOS

Sprained ankle NOS

⑦S93.401   **Sprain of unspecified ligament of right ankle**

⑦S93.402   **Sprain of unspecified ligament of left ankle**

⑦S93.409   **Sprain of unspecified ligament of unspecified ankle**

S93.41   **Sprain of calcaneofibular ligament**

⑦S93.411   **Sprain of calcaneofibular ligament of right ankle**

⑦S93.412   **Sprain of calcaneofibular ligament of left ankle**

⑦S93.419   **Sprain of calcaneofibular ligament of unspecified ankle**

S93.42   **Sprain of deltoid ligament**

⑦S93.421   **Sprain of deltoid ligament of right ankle**

⑦S93.422   **Sprain of deltoid ligament of left ankle**

⑦S93.429   **Sprain of deltoid ligament of unspecified ankle**

S93.43   **Sprain of tibiofibular ligament**

⑦S93.431   **Sprain of tibiofibular ligament of right ankle**

⑦S93.432   **Sprain of tibiofibular ligament of left ankle**

⑦S93.439   **Sprain of tibiofibular ligament of unspecified ankle**

S93.49   **Sprain of other ligament of ankle**

Sprain of internal collateral ligament

Sprain of talofibular ligament

⑦S93.491   **Sprain of other ligament of right ankle**

⑦S93.492   **Sprain of other ligament of left ankle**

⑦S93.499   **Sprain of other ligament of unspecified ankle**

S93.5   **Sprain of toe**

S93.50   **Unspecified sprain of toe**

⑦S93.501   **Unspecified sprain of right great toe**

⑦S93.502   **Unspecified sprain of left great toe**

⑦S93.503   **Unspecified sprain of unspecified great toe**

⑦S93.504   **Unspecified sprain of right lesser toe(s)**

⑦S93.505   **Unspecified sprain of left lesser toe(s)**

⑦S93.506   **Unspecified sprain of unspecified lesser toe(s)**

⑦S93.509   **Unspecified sprain of unspecified toe(s)**

S93.51   Sprain of interphalangeal joint of toe

⑦S93.511   **Sprain of interphalangeal joint of right great toe**

⑦S93.512   **Sprain of interphalangeal joint of left great toe**

⑦S93.513   **Sprain of interphalangeal joint of unspecified great toe**

⑦S93.514   **Sprain of interphalangeal joint of right lesser toe(s)**

⑦S93.515   **Sprain of interphalangeal joint of left lesser toe(s)**

⑦S93.516   **Sprain of interphalangeal joint of unspecified lesser toe(s)**

⑦S93.519   **Sprain of interphalangeal joint of unspecified toe(s)**

S93.52   Sprain of metatarsophalangeal joint of toe

⑦S93.521   **Sprain of metatarsophalangeal joint of right great toe**

⑦S93.522   **Sprain of metatarsophalangeal joint of left great toe**

⑦S93.523   **Sprain of metatarsophalangeal joint of unspecified great toe**

⑦S93.524   **Sprain of metatarsophalangeal joint of right lesser toe(s)**

⑦S93.525   **Sprain of metatarsophalangeal joint of left lesser toe(s)**

⑦S93.526   **Sprain of metatarsophalangeal joint of unspecified lesser toe(s)**

⑦S93.529   **Sprain of metatarsophalangeal joint of unspecified toe(s)**

S93.6   **Sprain of foot**

Excludes2: sprain of metatarsophalangeal joint of toe (S93.52-)

sprain of toe (S93.5-)

S93.60   **Unspecified sprain of foot**

⑦S93.601   **Unspecified sprain of right foot**

⑦S93.602   **Unspecified sprain of left foot**

⑦S93.609   **Unspecified sprain of unspecified foot**

S93.61   **Sprain of tarsal ligament of foot**

⑦S93.611   **Sprain of tarsal ligament of right foot**

⑦S93.612   **Sprain of tarsal ligament of left foot**

⑦S93.619   **Sprain of tarsal ligament of unspecified foot**

S93.62   **Sprain of tarsometatarsal ligament of foot**

⑦S93.621   **Sprain of tarsometatarsal ligament of right foot**

⑦S93.622   **Sprain of tarsometatarsal ligament of left foot**

⑦S93.629   **Sprain of tarsometatarsal ligament of unspecified foot**

S93.69   **Other sprain of foot**

⑦S93.691   **Other sprain of right foot**

⑦S93.692   **Other sprain of left foot**

⑦S93.699   **Other sprain of unspecified foot**

S94   **Injury of nerves at ankle and foot level**

Code also any associated open wound (S91.-)

The appropriate 7th character is to be added to each code from category S94

A - initial encounter

D - subsequent encounter

S - sequela

S94.0   **Injury of lateral plantar nerve**

⊗⑦S94.00   **Injury of lateral plantar nerve, unspecified leg**

⊗⑦S94.01   **Injury of lateral plantar nerve, right leg**

⊗⑦S94.02   **Injury of lateral plantar nerve, left leg**

S94.1   **Injury of medial plantar nerve**

⊗⑦S94.10   **Injury of medial plantar nerve, unspecified leg**

⊗⑦S94.11   **Injury of medial plantar nerve, right leg**

⊗⑦S94.12   **Injury of medial plantar nerve, left leg**

S94.2   **Injury of deep peroneal nerve at ankle and foot level**

Injury of terminal, lateral branch of deep peroneal nerve

⊗⑦S94.20   **Injury of deep peroneal nerve at ankle and foot level, unspecified leg**

⊗⑦S94.21   **Injury of deep peroneal nerve at ankle and foot level, right leg**

⊗⑦S94.22   **Injury of deep peroneal nerve at ankle and foot level, left leg**

S94.3   **Injury of cutaneous sensory nerve at ankle and foot level**

⊗⑦S94.30   **Injury of cutaneous sensory nerve at ankle and foot level, unspecified leg**

⊗⑦S94.31   **Injury of cutaneous sensory nerve at ankle and foot level, right leg**

⊗⑦S94.32   **Injury of cutaneous sensory nerve at ankle and foot level, left leg**

S94.8   **Injury of other nerves at ankle and foot level**

S94.8X   **Injury of other nerves at ankle and foot level**

⑦S94.8X1   **Injury of other nerves at ankle and foot level, right leg**

⑦S94.8X2   **Injury of other nerves at ankle and foot level, left leg**

⑦S94.8X9   **Injury of other nerves at ankle and foot level, unspecified leg**

S94.9   **Injury of unspecified nerve at ankle and foot level**

⊗⑦S94.90   **Injury of unspecified nerve at ankle and foot level, unspecified leg**

⊗⑦S94.91   **Injury of unspecified nerve at ankle and foot level, right leg**

⊗⑦S94.92   **Injury of unspecified nerve at ankle and foot level, left leg**

S95   **Injury of blood vessels at ankle and foot level**

Code also any associated open wound (S91.-)

Excludes2: injury of posterior tibial artery and vein (S85.1-, S85.8-)

The appropriate 7th character is to be added to each code from category S95

A - initial encounter

D - subsequent encounter

S - sequela

S95.0   **Injury of dorsal artery of foot**

S95.00   **Unspecified injury of dorsal artery of foot**

⑦S95.001   **Unspecified injury of dorsal artery of right foot**

● New code   ▲ Revised code   **Excludes1:** Not coded here   **Excludes2:** Not included here   ⊗ Placeholder required   ⑦7th digit required

⑦S95.002 **Unspecified injury of dorsal artery of left foot**

⑦S95.009 **Unspecified injury of dorsal artery of unspecified foot**

S95.01 **Laceration of dorsal artery of foot**

⑦S95.011 **Laceration of dorsal artery of right foot**

⑦S95.012 **Laceration of dorsal artery of left foot**

⑦S95.019 **Laceration of dorsal artery of unspecified foot**

S95.09 **Other specified injury of dorsal artery of foot**

⑦S95.091 **Other specified injury of dorsal artery of right foot**

⑦S95.092 **Other specified injury of dorsal artery of left foot**

⑦S95.099 **Other specified injury of dorsal artery of unspecified foot**

S95.1 **Injury of plantar artery of foot**

S95.10 **Unspecified injury of plantar artery of foot**

⑦S95.101 **Unspecified injury of plantar artery of right foot**

⑦S95.102 **Unspecified injury of plantar artery of left foot**

⑦S95.109 **Unspecified injury of plantar artery of unspecified foot**

S95.11 **Laceration of plantar artery of foot**

⑦S95.111 **Laceration of plantar artery of right foot**

⑦S95.112 **Laceration of plantar artery of left foot**

⑦S95.119 **Laceration of plantar artery of unspecified foot**

S95.19 **Other specified injury of plantar artery of foot**

⑦S95.191 **Other specified injury of plantar artery of right foot**

⑦S95.192 **Other specified injury of plantar artery of left foot**

⑦S95.199 **Other specified injury of plantar artery of unspecified foot**

S95.2 **Injury of dorsal vein of foot**

S95.20 **Unspecified injury of dorsal vein of foot**

⑦S95.201 **Unspecified injury of dorsal vein of right foot**

⑦S95.202 **Unspecified injury of dorsal vein of left foot**

⑦S95.209 **Unspecified injury of dorsal vein of unspecified foot**

S95.21 **Laceration of dorsal vein of foot**

⑦S95.211 **Laceration of dorsal vein of right foot**

⑦S95.212 **Laceration of dorsal vein of left foot**

⑦S95.219 **Laceration of dorsal vein of unspecified foot**

S95.29 **Other specified injury of dorsal vein of foot**

⑦S95.291 **Other specified injury of dorsal vein of right foot**

⑦S95.292 **Other specified injury of dorsal vein of left foot**

⑦S95.299 **Other specified injury of dorsal vein of unspecified foot**

S95.8 **Injury of other blood vessels at ankle and foot level**

S95.80 **Unspecified injury of other blood vessels at ankle and foot level**

⑦S95.801 **Unspecified injury of other blood vessels at ankle and foot level, right leg**

⑦S95.802 **Unspecified injury of other blood vessels at ankle and foot level, left leg**

⑦S95.809 **Unspecified injury of other blood vessels at ankle and foot level, unspecified leg**

S95.81 **Laceration of other blood vessels at ankle and foot level**

⑦S95.811 **Laceration of other blood vessels at ankle and foot level, right leg**

⑦S95.812 **Laceration of other blood vessels at ankle and foot level, left leg**

⑦S95.819 **Laceration of other blood vessels at ankle and foot level, unspecified leg**

S95.89 **Other specified injury of other blood vessels at ankle and foot level**

⑦S95.891 **Other specified injury of other blood vessels at ankle and foot level, right leg**

⑦S95.892 **Other specified injury of other blood vessels at ankle and foot level, left leg**

⑦S95.899 **Other specified injury of other blood vessels at ankle and foot level, unspecified leg**

S95.9 **Injury of unspecified blood vessel at ankle and foot level**

S95.90 **Unspecified injury of unspecified blood vessel at ankle and foot level**

⑦S95.901 **Unspecified injury of unspecified blood vessel at ankle and foot level, right leg**

⑦S95.902 **Unspecified injury of unspecified blood vessel at ankle and foot level, left leg**

⑦S95.909 **Unspecified injury of unspecified blood vessel at ankle and foot level, unspecified leg**

S95.91 **Laceration of unspecified blood vessel at ankle and foot level**

⑦S95.911 **Laceration of unspecified blood vessel at ankle and foot level, right leg**

⑦S95.912 **Laceration of unspecified blood vessel at ankle and foot level, left leg**

⑦S95.919 **Laceration of unspecified blood vessel at ankle and foot level, unspecified leg**

S95.99 **Other specified injury of unspecified blood vessel at ankle and foot level**

⑦S95.991 **Other specified injury of unspecified blood vessel at ankle and foot level, right leg**

⑦S95.992 **Other specified injury of unspecified blood vessel at ankle and foot level, left leg**

⑦S95.999 **Other specified injury of unspecified blood vessel at ankle and foot level, unspecified leg**

S96 **Injury of muscle and tendon at ankle and foot level**

Code also any associated open wound (S91.-)

Excludes2: injury of Achilles tendon (S86.0-)

sprain of joints and ligaments of ankle and foot (S93.-)

Add 4th-7th digits   Nonspecific code   Unspecified code   Manifestation code   [HCC] Hierarchical Condition Code

The appropriate 7th character is to be added to each code from category S96

A - initial encounter

D - subsequent encounter

S - sequela

S96.0 **Injury of muscle and tendon of long flexor muscle of toe at ankle and foot level**

    S96.00 **Unspecified injury of muscle and tendon of long flexor muscle of toe at ankle and foot level**

        ⑦**S96.001** **Unspecified injury of muscle and tendon of long flexor muscle of toe at ankle and foot level, right foot**

        ⑦**S96.002** **Unspecified injury of muscle and tendon of long flexor muscle of toe at ankle and foot level, left foot**

        ⑦**S96.009** **Unspecified injury of muscle and tendon of long flexor muscle of toe at ankle and foot level, unspecified foot**

    S96.01 **Strain of muscle and tendon of long flexor muscle of toe at ankle and foot level**

        ⑦**S96.011** **Strain of muscle and tendon of long flexor muscle of toe at ankle and foot level, right foot**

        ⑦**S96.012** **Strain of muscle and tendon of long flexor muscle of toe at ankle and foot level, left foot**

        ⑦**S96.019** **Strain of muscle and tendon of long flexor muscle of toe at ankle and foot level, unspecified foot**

    S96.02 **Laceration of muscle and tendon of long flexor muscle of toe at ankle and foot level**

        ⑦**S96.021** **Laceration of muscle and tendon of long flexor muscle of toe at ankle and foot level, right foot**

        ⑦**S96.022** **Laceration of muscle and tendon of long flexor muscle of toe at ankle and foot level, left foot**

        ⑦**S96.029** **Laceration of muscle and tendon of long flexor muscle of toe at ankle and foot level, unspecified foot**

    S96.09 **Other injury of muscle and tendon of long flexor muscle of toe at ankle and foot level**

        ⑦**S96.091** **Other injury of muscle and tendon of long flexor muscle of toe at ankle and foot level, right foot**

        ⑦**S96.092** **Other injury of muscle and tendon of long flexor muscle of toe at ankle and foot level, left foot**

        ⑦**S96.099** **Other injury of muscle and tendon of long flexor muscle of toe at ankle and foot level, unspecified foot**

S96.1 **Injury of muscle and tendon of long extensor muscle of toe at ankle and foot level**

    S96.10 **Unspecified injury of muscle and tendon of long extensor muscle of toe at ankle and foot level**

        ⑦**S96.101** **Unspecified injury of muscle and tendon of long extensor muscle of toe at ankle and foot level, right foot**

        ⑦**S96.102** **Unspecified injury of muscle and tendon of long extensor muscle of toe at ankle and foot level, left foot**

        ⑦**S96.109** **Unspecified injury of muscle and tendon of long extensor muscle of toe at ankle and foot level, unspecified foot**

    S96.11 **Strain of muscle and tendon of long extensor muscle of toe at ankle and foot level**

        ⑦**S96.111** **Strain of muscle and tendon of long extensor muscle of toe at ankle and foot level, right foot**

        ⑦**S96.112** **Strain of muscle and tendon of long extensor muscle of toe at ankle and foot level, left foot**

        ⑦**S96.119** **Strain of muscle and tendon of long extensor muscle of toe at ankle and foot level, unspecified foot**

    S96.12 **Laceration of muscle and tendon of long extensor muscle of toe at ankle and foot level**

        ⑦**S96.121** **Laceration of muscle and tendon of long extensor muscle of toe at ankle and foot level, right foot**

        ⑦**S96.122** **Laceration of muscle and tendon of long extensor muscle of toe at ankle and foot level, left foot**

        ⑦**S96.129** **Laceration of muscle and tendon of long extensor muscle of toe at ankle and foot level, unspecified foot**

    S96.19 **Other specified injury of muscle and tendon of long extensor muscle of toe at ankle and foot level**

        ⑦**S96.191** **Other specified injury of muscle and tendon of long extensor muscle of toe at ankle and foot level, right foot**

        ⑦**S96.192** **Other specified injury of muscle and tendon of long extensor muscle of toe at ankle and foot level, left foot**

        ⑦**S96.199** **Other specified injury of muscle and tendon of long extensor muscle of toe at ankle and foot level, unspecified foot**

S96.2 **Injury of intrinsic muscle and tendon at ankle and foot level**

    S96.20 **Unspecified injury of intrinsic muscle and tendon at ankle and foot level**

        ⑦**S96.201** **Unspecified injury of intrinsic muscle and tendon at ankle and foot level, right foot**

        ⑦**S96.202** **Unspecified injury of intrinsic muscle and tendon at ankle and foot level, left foot**

        ⑦**S96.209** **Unspecified injury of intrinsic muscle and tendon at ankle and foot level, unspecified foot**

    S96.21 **Strain of intrinsic muscle and tendon at ankle and foot level**

        ⑦**S96.211** **Strain of intrinsic muscle and tendon at ankle and foot level, right foot**

        ⑦**S96.212** **Strain of intrinsic muscle and tendon at ankle and foot level, left foot**

        ⑦**S96.219** **Strain of intrinsic muscle and tendon at ankle and foot level, unspecified foot**

    S96.22 **Laceration of intrinsic muscle and tendon at ankle and foot level**

        ⑦**S96.221** **Laceration of intrinsic muscle and tendon at ankle and foot level, right foot**

        ⑦**S96.222** **Laceration of intrinsic muscle and tendon at ankle and foot level, left foot**

● New code   ▲ Revised code   **Excludes1:** Not coded here   **Excludes2:** Not included here   ⊗ Placeholder required   ⑦7th digit required

⑦S96.229 Laceration of intrinsic muscle and tendon at ankle and foot level, unspecified foot

S96.29 Other specified injury of intrinsic muscle and tendon at ankle and foot level

⑦S96.291 Other specified injury of intrinsic muscle and tendon at ankle and foot level, right foot

⑦S96.292 Other specified injury of intrinsic muscle and tendon at ankle and foot level, left foot

⑦S96.299 Other specified injury of intrinsic muscle and tendon at ankle and foot level, unspecified foot

S96.8 Injury of other specified muscles and tendons at ankle and foot level

S96.80 Unspecified injury of other specified muscles and tendons at ankle and foot level

⑦S96.801 Unspecified injury of other specified muscles and tendons at ankle and foot level, right foot

⑦S96.802 Unspecified injury of other specified muscles and tendons at ankle and foot level, left foot

⑦S96.809 Unspecified injury of other specified muscles and tendons at ankle and foot level, unspecified foot

S96.81 Strain of other specified muscles and tendons at ankle and foot level

⑦S96.811 Strain of other specified muscles and tendons at ankle and foot level, right foot

⑦S96.812 Strain of other specified muscles and tendons at ankle and foot level, left foot

⑦S96.819 Strain of other specified muscles and tendons at ankle and foot level, unspecified foot

S96.82 Laceration of other specified muscles and tendons at ankle and foot level

⑦S96.821 Laceration of other specified muscles and tendons at ankle and foot level, right foot

⑦S96.822 Laceration of other specified muscles and tendons at ankle and foot level, left foot

⑦S96.829 Laceration of other specified muscles and tendons at ankle and foot level, unspecified foot

S96.89 Other specified injury of other specified muscles and tendons at ankle and foot level

⑦S96.891 Other specified injury of other specified muscles and tendons at ankle and foot level, right foot

⑦S96.892 Other specified injury of other specified muscles and tendons at ankle and foot level, left foot

⑦S96.899 Other specified injury of other specified muscles and tendons at ankle and foot level, unspecified foot

S96.9 Injury of unspecified muscle and tendon at ankle and foot level

S96.90 Unspecified injury of unspecified muscle and tendon at ankle and foot level

⑦S96.901 Unspecified injury of unspecified muscle and tendon at ankle and foot level, right foot

⑦S96.902 Unspecified injury of unspecified muscle and tendon at ankle and foot level, left foot

⑦S96.909 Unspecified injury of unspecified muscle and tendon at ankle and foot level, unspecified foot

S96.91 Strain of unspecified muscle and tendon at ankle and foot level

⑦S96.911 Strain of unspecified muscle and tendon at ankle and foot level, right foot

⑦S96.912 Strain of unspecified muscle and tendon at ankle and foot level, left foot

⑦S96.919 Strain of unspecified muscle and tendon at ankle and foot level, unspecified foot

S96.92 Laceration of unspecified muscle and tendon at ankle and foot level

⑦S96.921 Laceration of unspecified muscle and tendon at ankle and foot level, right foot

⑦S96.922 Laceration of unspecified muscle and tendon at ankle and foot level, left foot

⑦S96.929 Laceration of unspecified muscle and tendon at ankle and foot level, unspecified foot

S96.99 Other specified injury of unspecified muscle and tendon at ankle and foot level

⑦S96.991 Other specified injury of unspecified muscle and tendon at ankle and foot level, right foot

⑦S96.992 Other specified injury of unspecified muscle and tendon at ankle and foot level, left foot

⑦S96.999 Other specified injury of unspecified muscle and tendon at ankle and foot level, unspecified foot

S97 Crushing injury of ankle and foot

Use Additional Code(s) for all associated injuries

The appropriate 7th character is to be added to each code from category S97

A - initial encounter

D - subsequent encounter

S - sequela

S97.0 Crushing injury of ankle

⊗⑦S97.00 Crushing injury of unspecified ankle

⊗⑦S97.01 Crushing injury of right ankle

⊗⑦S97.02 Crushing injury of left ankle

S97.1 Crushing injury of toe

S97.10 Crushing injury of unspecified toe(s)

⑦S97.101 Crushing injury of unspecified right toe(s)

⑦S97.102 Crushing injury of unspecified left toe(s)

⑦S97.109 Crushing injury of unspecified toe(s)
Crushing injury of toe NOS

S97.11 Crushing injury of great toe

⑦S97.111 Crushing injury of right great toe

⑦S97.112 Crushing injury of left great toe

⑦S97.119 Crushing injury of unspecified great toe

S97.12 Crushing injury of lesser toe(s)

⑦**S97.121**   **Crushing injury of right lesser toe(s)**

⑦**S97.122**   **Crushing injury of left lesser toe(s)**

⑦**S97.129**   **Crushing injury of unspecified lesser toe(s)**

S97.8   **Crushing injury of foot**

⊗⑦**S97.80**   **Crushing injury of unspecified foot**

Crushing injury of foot NOS

⊗⑦**S97.81**   **Crushing injury of right foot**

⊗⑦**S97.82**   **Crushing injury of left foot**

S98   **Traumatic amputation of ankle and foot**

An amputation not identified as partial or complete should be coded to complete

The appropriate 7th character is to be added to each code from category S98

A - initial encounter

D - subsequent encounter

S - sequela

S98.0   **Traumatic amputation of foot at ankle level**

S98.01   **Complete traumatic amputation of foot at ankle level**

⑦**S98.011**   **Complete traumatic amputation of right foot at ankle level** [HCC]

⑦**S98.012**   **Complete traumatic amputation of left foot at ankle level** [HCC]

⑦**S98.019**   **Complete traumatic amputation of unspecified foot at ankle level** [HCC]

S98.02   **Partial traumatic amputation of foot at ankle level**

⑦**S98.021**   **Partial traumatic amputation of right foot at ankle level** [HCC]

⑦**S98.022**   **Partial traumatic amputation of left foot at ankle level** [HCC]

⑦**S98.029**   **Partial traumatic amputation of unspecified foot at ankle level** [HCC]

S98.1   **Traumatic amputation of one toe** [HCC]

S98.11   **Complete traumatic amputation of great toe**

⑦**S98.111**   **Complete traumatic amputation of right great toe** [HCC]

⑦**S98.112**   **Complete traumatic amputation of left great toe** [HCC]

⑦**S98.119**   **Complete traumatic amputation of unspecified great toe** [HCC]

S98.12   **Partial traumatic amputation of great toe**

⑦**S98.121**   **Partial traumatic amputation of right great toe** [HCC]

⑦**S98.122**   **Partial traumatic amputation of left great toe** [HCC]

⑦**S98.129**   **Partial traumatic amputation of unspecified great toe** [HCC]

S98.13   **Complete traumatic amputation of one lesser toe**

Traumatic amputation of toe NOS

⑦**S98.131**   **Complete traumatic amputation of one right lesser toe** [HCC]

⑦**S98.132**   **Complete traumatic amputation of one left lesser toe** [HCC]

⑦**S98.139**   **Complete traumatic amputation of one unspecified lesser toe** [HCC]

S98.14   **Partial traumatic amputation of one lesser toe**

⑦**S98.141**   **Partial traumatic amputation of one right lesser toe** [HCC]

⑦**S98.142**   **Partial traumatic amputation of one left lesser toe** [HCC]

⑦**S98.149**   **Partial traumatic amputation of one unspecified lesser toe** [HCC]

S98.2   **Traumatic amputation of two or more lesser toes**

S98.21   **Complete traumatic amputation of two or more lesser toes**

⑦**S98.211**   **Complete traumatic amputation of two or more right lesser toes** [HCC]

⑦**S98.212**   **Complete traumatic amputation of two or more left lesser toes** [HCC]

⑦**S98.219**   **Complete traumatic amputation of two or more unspecified lesser toes** [HCC]

S98.22   **Partial traumatic amputation of two or more lesser toes**

⑦**S98.221**   **Partial traumatic amputation of two or more right lesser toes** [HCC]

⑦**S98.222**   **Partial traumatic amputation of two or more left lesser toes** [HCC]

⑦**S98.229**   **Partial traumatic amputation of two or more unspecified lesser toes** [HCC]

S98.3   **Traumatic amputation of midfoot**

S98.31   **Complete traumatic amputation of midfoot**

⑦**S98.311**   **Complete traumatic amputation of right midfoot** [HCC]

⑦**S98.312**   **Complete traumatic amputation of left midfoot** [HCC]

⑦**S98.319**   **Complete traumatic amputation of unspecified midfoot** [HCC]

S98.32   **Partial traumatic amputation of midfoot**

⑦**S98.321**   **Partial traumatic amputation of right midfoot** [HCC]

⑦**S98.322**   **Partial traumatic amputation of left midfoot** [HCC]

⑦**S98.329**   **Partial traumatic amputation of unspecified midfoot** [HCC]

S98.9   **Traumatic amputation of foot, level unspecified**

S98.91   **Complete traumatic amputation of foot, level unspecified**

⑦**S98.911**   **Complete traumatic amputation of right foot, level unspecified** [HCC]

⑦**S98.912**   **Complete traumatic amputation of left foot, level unspecified** [HCC]

⑦**S98.919**   **Complete traumatic amputation of unspecified foot, level unspecified** [HCC]

S98.92   **Partial traumatic amputation of foot, level unspecified**

⑦**S98.921**   **Partial traumatic amputation of right foot, level unspecified**

⑦**S98.922**   **Partial traumatic amputation of left foot, level unspecified** [HCC]

⑦**S98.929**   **Partial traumatic amputation of unspecified foot, level unspecified** [HCC]

S99   **Other and unspecified injuries of ankle and foot**

S99.0   **Physeal fracture of calcaneus**

The appropriate 7th character is to be added to each code from subcategories S99.0

A - initial encounter for closed fracture

B - initial encounter for open fracture

D - subsequent encounter for fracture with routine healing

G - subsequent encounter for fracture with delayed healing

   ● New code   ▲ Revised code   **Excludes1:** Not coded here   **Excludes2:** Not included here   ⊗ Placeholder required   ⑦7th digit required

K - subsequent encounter for fracture with nonunion

P - subsequent encounter for fracture with malunion

S - sequela

S99.00   Unspecified physeal fracture of calcaneus

⑦S99.001   Unspecified physeal fracture of right calcaneus

⑦S99.002   Unspecified physeal fracture of left calcaneus

⑦S99.009   Unspecified physeal fracture of unspecified calcaneus

S99.01   Salter-Harris Type I physeal fracture of calcaneus

⑦S99.011   Salter-Harris Type I physeal fracture of right calcaneus

⑦S99.012   Salter-Harris Type I physeal fracture of left calcaneus

⑦S99.019   Salter-Harris Type I physeal fracture of unspecified calcaneus

S99.02   Salter-Harris Type II physeal fracture of calcaneus

⑦S99.021   Salter-Harris Type II physeal fracture of right calcaneus

⑦S99.022   Salter-Harris Type II physeal fracture of left calcaneus

⑦S99.029   Salter-Harris Type II physeal fracture of unspecified calcaneus

S99.03   Salter-Harris Type III physeal fracture of calcaneus

⑦S99.031   Salter-Harris Type III physeal fracture of right calcaneus

⑦S99.032   Salter-Harris Type III physeal fracture of left calcaneus

⑦S99.039   Salter-Harris Type III physeal fracture of unspecified calcaneus

S99.04   Salter-Harris Type IV physeal fracture of calcaneus

⑦S99.041   Salter-Harris Type IV physeal fracture of right calcaneus

⑦S99.042   Salter-Harris Type IV physeal fracture of left calcaneus

⑦S99.049   Salter-Harris Type IV physeal fracture of unspecified calcaneus

S99.09   Other physeal fracture of calcaneus

⑦S99.091   Other physeal fracture of right calcaneus

⑦S99.092   Other physeal fracture of left calcaneus

⑦S99.099   Other physeal fracture of unspecified calcaneus

S99.1   Physeal fracture of metatarsal

The appropriate 7th character is to be added to each code from subcategories S99.1

A - initial encounter for closed fracture

B - initial encounter for open fracture

D - subsequent encounter for fracture with routine healing

G - subsequent encounter for fracture with delayed healing

K - subsequent encounter for fracture with nonunion

P - subsequent encounter for fracture with malunion

S - sequela

S99.10   Unspecified physeal fracture of metatarsal

⑦S99.101   Unspecified physeal fracture of right metatarsal

⑦S99.102   Unspecified physeal fracture of left metatarsal

⑦S99.109   Unspecified physeal fracture of unspecified metatarsal

S99.11   Salter-Harris Type I physeal fracture of metatarsal

⑦S99.111   Salter-Harris Type I physeal fracture of right metatarsal

⑦S99.112   Salter-Harris Type I physeal fracture of left metatarsal

⑦S99.119   Salter-Harris Type I physeal fracture of unspecified metatarsal

S99.12   Salter-Harris Type II physeal fracture of metatarsal

⑦S99.121   Salter-Harris Type II physeal fracture of right metatarsal

⑦S99.122   Salter-Harris Type II physeal fracture of left metatarsal

⑦S99.129   Salter-Harris Type II physeal fracture of unspecified metatarsal

S99.13   Salter-Harris Type III physeal fracture of metatarsal

⑦S99.131   Salter-Harris Type III physeal fracture of right metatarsal

⑦S99.132   Salter-Harris Type III physeal fracture of left metatarsal

⑦S99.139   Salter-Harris Type III physeal fracture of unspecified metatarsal

S99.14   Salter-Harris Type IV physeal fracture of metatarsal

⑦S99.141   Salter-Harris Type IV physeal fracture of right metatarsal

⑦S99.142   Salter-Harris Type IV physeal fracture of left metatarsal

⑦S99.149   Salter-Harris Type IV physeal fracture of unspecified metatarsal

S99.19   Other physeal fracture of metatarsal

⑦S99.191   Other physeal fracture of right metatarsal

⑦S99.192   Other physeal fracture of left metatarsal

⑦S99.199   Other physeal fracture of unspecified metatarsal

S99.2   Physeal fracture of phalanx of toe

The appropriate 7th character is to be added to each code from subcategories S99.2

A - initial encounter for closed fracture

B - initial encounter for open fracture

D - subsequent encounter for fracture with routine healing

G - subsequent encounter for fracture with delayed healing

K - subsequent encounter for fracture with nonunion

P - subsequent encounter for fracture with malunion

S - sequela

S99.20   Unspecified physeal fracture of phalanx of toe

⑦S99.201   Unspecified physeal fracture of phalanx of right toe

⑦S99.202   Unspecified physeal fracture of phalanx of left toe

⑦S99.209   Unspecified physeal fracture of phalanx of unspecified toe

S99.21   Salter-Harris Type I physeal fracture of phalanx of toe

⑦S99.211 Salter-Harris Type I physeal fracture of phalanx of right toe

⑦S99.212 Salter-Harris Type I physeal fracture of phalanx of left toe

⑦S99.219 Salter-Harris Type I physeal fracture of phalanx of unspecified toe

S99.22 Salter-Harris Type II physeal fracture of phalanx of toe

⑦S99.221 Salter-Harris Type II physeal fracture of phalanx of right toe

⑦S99.222 Salter-Harris Type II physeal fracture of phalanx of left toe

⑦S99.229 Salter-Harris Type II physeal fracture of phalanx of unspecified toe

S99.23 Salter-Harris Type III physeal fracture of phalanx of toe

⑦S99.231 Salter-Harris Type III physeal fracture of phalanx of right toe

⑦S99.232 Salter-Harris Type III physeal fracture of phalanx of left toe

⑦S99.239 Salter-Harris Type III physeal fracture of phalanx of unspecified toe

S99.24 Salter-Harris Type IV physeal fracture of phalanx of toe

⑦S99.241 Salter-Harris Type IV physeal fracture of phalanx of right toe

⑦S99.242 Salter-Harris Type IV physeal fracture of phalanx of left toe

⑦S99.249 Salter-Harris Type IV physeal fracture of phalanx of unspecified toe

S99.29 Other physeal fracture of phalanx of toe

⑦S99.291 Other physeal fracture of phalanx of right toe

⑦S99.292 Other physeal fracture of phalanx of left toe

⑦S99.299 Other physeal fracture of phalanx of unspecified toe

S99.8 Other specified injuries of ankle and foot

The appropriate 7th character is to be added to each code from subcategory S99.8

A - initial encounter

D - subsequent encounter

S - sequela

S99.81 Other specified injuries of ankle

⑦S99.811 Other specified injuries of right ankle

⑦S99.812 Other specified injuries of left ankle

⑦S99.819 Other specified injuries of unspecified ankle

S99.82 Other specified injuries of foot

⑦S99.821 Other specified injuries of right foot

⑦S99.822 Other specified injuries of left foot

⑦S99.829 Other specified injuries of unspecified foot

S99.9 Unspecified injury of ankle and foot

The appropriate 7th character is to be added to each code from subcategory S99.9

A - initial encounter

D - subsequent encounter

S - sequela

S99.91 Unspecified injury of ankle

⑦S99.911 Unspecified injury of right ankle

⑦S99.912 Unspecified injury of left ankle

⑦S99.919 Unspecified injury of unspecified ankle

S99.92 Unspecified injury of foot

⑦S99.921 Unspecified injury of right foot

⑦S99.922 Unspecified injury of left foot

⑦S99.929 Unspecified injury of unspecified foot

INJURY, POISONING AND CERTAIN OTHER CONSEQUENCES OF EXTERNAL CAUSES (T07-T88)

INJURIES INVOLVING MULTIPLE BODY REGIONS (T07)

Excludes1: burns and corrosions (T20-T32)

frostbite (T33-T34)

insect bite or sting, venomous (T63.4)

sunburn (L55.-)

⊗⑦T07 Unspecified multiple injuries

Excludes1: injury NOS (T14.90)

The appropriate 7th character is to be added to code T07

A initial encounter

D subsequent encounter

S sequela

INJURY OF UNSPECIFIED BODY REGION (T14)

T14 Injury of unspecified body region

The appropriate 7th character is to be added to each code from category T14

A initial encounter

D subsequent encounter

S sequela

Excludes1: multiple unspecified injuries (T07)

⊗⑦T14.8 Other injury of unspecified body region

Abrasion NOS

Contusion NOS

Crush injury NOS

Fracture NOS

Skin injury NOS

Vascular injury NOS

Wound NOS

T14.9 Unspecified injury

⊗⑦T14.90 Injury, unspecified

Injury NOS

⊗⑦T14.91 Suicide attempt [HCC]

Attempted suicide NOS

EFFECTS OF FOREIGN BODY ENTERING THROUGH NATURAL ORIFICE (T15-T19)

Excludes2: foreign body accidentally left in operation wound (T81.5-)

foreign body in penetrating wound - See open wound by body region residual foreign body in soft tissue (M79.5)

splinter, without open wound - See superficial injury by body region

T15 Foreign body on external eye

Excludes2: foreign body in penetrating wound of orbit and eye ball (S05.4-, S05.5-)

open wound of eyelid and periocular area (S01.1-)

retained foreign body in eyelid (H02.8-)

retained (old) foreign body in penetrating wound of orbit and eye ball (H05.5-, H44.6-, H44.7-)

superficial foreign body of eyelid and periocular area (S00.25-)

The appropriate 7th character is to be added to each code from category T15

A - initial encounter

D - subsequent encounter

S - sequela

T15.0 **Foreign body in cornea**

⊗⑦T15.00 **Foreign body in cornea, unspecified eye**

⊗⑦T15.01 **Foreign body in cornea, right eye**

⊗⑦T15.02 **Foreign body in cornea, left eye**

T15.1 **Foreign body in conjunctival sac**

⊗⑦T15.10 **Foreign body in conjunctival sac, unspecified eye**

⊗⑦T15.11 **Foreign body in conjunctival sac, right eye**

⊗⑦T15.12 **Foreign body in conjunctival sac, left eye**

T15.8 **Foreign body in other and multiple parts of external eye**

Foreign body in lacrimal punctum

⊗⑦T15.80 **Foreign body in other and multiple parts of external eye, unspecified eye**

⊗⑦T15.81 **Foreign body in other and multiple parts of external eye, right eye**

⊗⑦T15.82 **Foreign body in other and multiple parts of external eye, left eye**

T15.9 **Foreign body on external eye, part unspecified**

⊗⑦T15.90 **Foreign body on external eye, part unspecified, unspecified eye**

⊗⑦T15.91 **Foreign body on external eye, part unspecified, right eye**

⊗⑦T15.92 **Foreign body on external eye, part unspecified, left eye**

T16 **Foreign body in ear**

Includes: foreign body in auditory canal

The appropriate 7th character is to be added to each code from category T16

A - initial encounter

D - subsequent encounter

S - sequela

⊗⑦T16.1 **Foreign body in right ear**

⊗⑦T16.2 **Foreign body in left ear**

⊗⑦T16.9 **Foreign body in ear, unspecified ear**

T17 **Foreign body in respiratory tract**

The appropriate 7th character is to be added to each code from category T17

A - initial encounter

D - subsequent encounter

S - sequela

⊗⑦T17.0 **Foreign body in nasal sinus**

⊗⑦T17.1 **Foreign body in nostril**

Foreign body in nose NOS

T17.2 **Foreign body in pharynx**

Foreign body in nasopharynx

Foreign body in throat NOS

T17.20 **Unspecified foreign body in pharynx**

⑦T17.200 **Unspecified foreign body in pharynx causing asphyxiation**

⑦T17.208 **Unspecified foreign body in pharynx causing other injury**

T17.21 **Gastric contents in pharynx**

Aspiration of gastric contents into pharynx

Vomitus in pharynx

⑦T17.210 **Gastric contents in pharynx causing asphyxiation**

⑦T17.218 **Gastric contents in pharynx causing other injury**

T17.22 **Food in pharynx**

Bones in pharynx

Seeds in pharynx

⑦T17.220 **Food in pharynx causing asphyxiation**

⑦T17.228 **Food in pharynx causing other injury**

T17.29 **Other foreign object in pharynx**

⑦T17.290 **Other foreign object in pharynx causing asphyxiation**

⑦T17.298 **Other foreign object in pharynx causing other injury**

T17.3 **Foreign body in larynx**

T17.30 **Unspecified foreign body in larynx**

⑦T17.300 **Unspecified foreign body in larynx causing asphyxiation**

⑦T17.308 **Unspecified foreign body in larynx causing other injury**

T17.31 **Gastric contents in larynx**

Aspiration of gastric contents into larynx

Vomitus in larynx

⑦T17.310 **Gastric contents in larynx causing asphyxiation**

⑦T17.318 **Gastric contents in larynx causing other injury**

T17.32 **Food in larynx**

Bones in larynx

Seeds in larynx

⑦T17.320 **Food in larynx causing asphyxiation**

⑦T17.328 **Food in larynx causing other injury**

T17.39 **Other foreign object in larynx**

⑦T17.390 **Other foreign object in larynx causing asphyxiation**

⑦T17.398 **Other foreign object in larynx causing other injury**

T17.4 **Foreign body in trachea**

T17.40 **Unspecified foreign body in trachea**

⑦T17.400 **Unspecified foreign body in trachea causing asphyxiation**

⑦T17.408 **Unspecified foreign body in trachea causing other injury**

T17.41 **Gastric contents in trachea**

Aspiration of gastric contents into trachea

Vomitus in trachea

⑦T17.410 **Gastric contents in trachea causing asphyxiation**

⑦T17.418 **Gastric contents in trachea causing other injury**

T17.42 **Food in trachea**

Bones in trachea

Seeds in trachea

⑦T17.420 **Food in trachea causing asphyxiation**

⑦T17.428 **Food in trachea causing other injury**

T17.49 **Other foreign object in trachea**

⑦ **T17.490**   **Other foreign object in trachea causing asphyxiation**

⑦ **T17.498**   **Other foreign object in trachea causing other injury**

T17.5   **Foreign body in bronchus**

   T17.50   **Unspecified foreign body in bronchus**

     ⑦ **T17.500**   **Unspecified foreign body in bronchus causing asphyxiation**

     ⑦ **T17.508**   **Unspecified foreign body in bronchus causing other injury**

   T17.51   **Gastric contents in bronchus**

     Aspiration of gastric contents into bronchus

     Vomitus in bronchus

     ⑦ **T17.510**   **Gastric contents in bronchus causing asphyxiation**

     ⑦ **T17.518**   **Gastric contents in bronchus causing other injury**

   T17.52   **Food in bronchus**

     Bones in bronchus

     Seeds in bronchus

     ⑦ **T17.520**   **Food in bronchus causing asphyxiation**

     ⑦ **T17.528**   **Food in bronchus causing other injury**

   T17.59   **Other foreign object in bronchus**

     ⑦ **T17.590**   **Other foreign object in bronchus causing asphyxiation**

     ⑦ **T17.598**   **Other foreign object in bronchus causing other injury**

T17.8   **Foreign body in other parts of respiratory tract**

   Foreign body in bronchioles

   Foreign body in lung

   T17.80   **Unspecified foreign body in other parts of respiratory tract**

     ⑦ **T17.800**   **Unspecified foreign body in other parts of respiratory tract causing asphyxiation**

     ⑦ **T17.808**   **Unspecified foreign body in other parts of respiratory tract causing other injury**

   T17.81   **Gastric contents in other parts of respiratory tract**

     Aspiration of gastric contents into other parts of respiratory tract

     Vomitus in other parts of respiratory tract

     ⑦ **T17.810**   **Gastric contents in other parts of respiratory tract causing asphyxiation**

     ⑦ **T17.818**   **Gastric contents in other parts of respiratory tract causing other injury**

   T17.82   **Food in other parts of respiratory tract**

     Bones in other parts of respiratory tract

     Seeds in other parts of respiratory tract

     ⑦ **T17.820**   **Food in other parts of respiratory tract causing asphyxiation**

     ⑦ **T17.828**   **Food in other parts of respiratory tract causing other injury**

   T17.89   **Other foreign object in other parts of respiratory tract**

     ⑦ **T17.890**   **Other foreign object in other parts of respiratory tract causing asphyxiation**

     ⑦ **T17.898**   **Other foreign object in other parts of respiratory tract causing other injury**

T17.9   **Foreign body in respiratory tract, part unspecified**

   T17.90   **Unspecified foreign body in respiratory tract, part unspecified**

     ⑦ **T17.900**   **Unspecified foreign body in respiratory tract, part unspecified causing asphyxiation**

     ⑦ **T17.908**   **Unspecified foreign body in respiratory tract, part unspecified causing other injury**

   T17.91   **Gastric contents in respiratory tract, part unspecified**

     Aspiration of gastric contents into respiratory tract, part unspecified

     Vomitus in trachea respiratory tract, part unspecified

     ⑦ **T17.910**   **Gastric contents in respiratory tract, part unspecified causing asphyxiation**

     ⑦ **T17.918**   **Gastric contents in respiratory tract, part unspecified causing other injury**

   T17.92   **Food in respiratory tract, part unspecified**

     Bones in respiratory tract, part unspecified

     Seeds in respiratory tract, part unspecified

     ⑦ **T17.920**   **Food in respiratory tract, part unspecified causing asphyxiation**

     ⑦ **T17.928**   **Food in respiratory tract, part unspecified causing other injury**

   T17.99   **Other foreign object in respiratory tract, part unspecified**

     ⑦ **T17.990**   **Other foreign object in respiratory tract, part unspecified in causing asphyxiation**

     ⑦ **T17.998**   **Other foreign object in respiratory tract, part unspecified causing other injury**

T18   **Foreign body in alimentary tract**

   Excludes2: foreign body in pharynx (T17.2-)

   The appropriate 7th character is to be added to each code from category T18

   A - initial encounter

   D - subsequent encounter

   S - sequela

⊗⑦ **T18.0**   **Foreign body in mouth**

T18.1   **Foreign body in esophagus**

   Excludes2: foreign body in respiratory tract (T17.-)

   T18.10   **Unspecified foreign body in esophagus**

     ⑦ **T18.100**   **Unspecified foreign body in esophagus causing compression of trachea**

       Unspecified foreign body in esophagus causing obstruction of respiration

     ⑦ **T18.108**   **Unspecified foreign body in esophagus causing other injury**

   T18.11   **Gastric contents in esophagus**

     Vomitus in esophagus

     ⑦ **T18.110**   **Gastric contents in esophagus causing compression of trachea**

       Gastric contents in esophagus causing obstruction of respiration

   ● New code   ▲ Revised code   **Excludes1:** Not coded here   **Excludes2:** Not included here   ⊗ Placeholder required   ⑦ 7th digit required

⑦**T18.118** **Gastric contents in esophagus causing other injury**

T18.12 **Food in esophagus**

Bones in esophagus

Seeds in esophagus

⑦**T18.120** **Food in esophagus causing compression of trachea**

Food in esophagus causing obstruction of respiration

⑦**T18.128** **Food in esophagus causing other injury**

T18.19 **Other foreign object in esophagus**

⑦**T18.190** **Other foreign object in esophagus causing compression of trachea**

Other foreign body in esophagus causing obstruction of respiration

⑦**T18.198** **Other foreign object in esophagus causing other injury**

⊗⑦**T18.2** **Foreign body in stomach**

⊗⑦**T18.3** **Foreign body in small intestine**

⊗⑦**T18.4** **Foreign body in colon**

⊗⑦**T18.5** **Foreign body in anus and rectum**

Foreign body in rectosigmoid (junction)

⊗⑦**T18.8** **Foreign body in other parts of alimentary tract**

⊗⑦**T18.9** **Foreign body of alimentary tract, part unspecified**

Foreign body in digestive system NOS

Swallowed foreign body NOS

T19 **Foreign body in genitourinary tract**

Excludes2: complications due to implanted mesh (T83.7-)

mechanical complications of contraceptive device (intrauterine) (vaginal) (T83.3-)

presence of contraceptive device (intrauterine) (vaginal) (Z97.5)

The appropriate 7th character is to be added to each code from category T19

A - initial encounter

D - subsequent encounter

S - sequela

⊗⑦**T19.0** **Foreign body in urethra**

⊗⑦**T19.1** **Foreign body in bladder**

⊗⑦**T19.2** **Foreign body in vulva and vagina**

⊗⑦**T19.3** **Foreign body in uterus**

⊗⑦**T19.4** **Foreign body in penis**

⊗⑦**T19.8** **Foreign body in other parts of genitourinary tract**

⊗⑦**T19.9** **Foreign body in genitourinary tract, part unspecified**

BURNS AND CORROSIONS (T20-T32)

Includes: burns (thermal) from electrical heating appliances

burns (thermal) from electricity

burns (thermal) from flame

burns (thermal) from friction

burns (thermal) from hot air and hot gases

burns (thermal) from hot objects

burns (thermal) from lightning

burns (thermal) from radiation

chemical burn [corrosion] (external) (internal) scalds

Excludes2: erythema [dermatitis] ab igne (L59.0)

radiation-related disorders of the skin and subcutaneous tissue (L55-L59)

sunburn (L55.-)

BURNS AND CORROSIONS OF EXTERNAL BODY SURFACE, SPECIFIED BY SITE (T20-T25)

Includes: burns and corrosions of first degree [erythema]

burns and corrosions of second degree [blisters][epidermal loss]

burns and corrosions of third degree [deep necrosis of underlying tissue] [full- thickness skin loss]

Use Additional Code from category T31 or T32 to identify extent of body surface involved

T20 **Burn and corrosion of head, face, and neck**

Excludes2: burn and corrosion of ear drum (T28.41, T28.91)

burn and corrosion of eye and adnexa (T26.-)

burn and corrosion of mouth and pharynx (T28.0)

The appropriate 7th character is to be added to each code from category T20

A - initial encounter

D - subsequent encounter

S - sequela

T20.0 **Burn of unspecified degree of head, face, and neck**

Use additional external cause code to identify the source, place and intent of the burn (X00-X19, X75-X77, X96-X98, Y92)

⊗⑦**T20.00** **Burn of unspecified degree of head, face, and neck, unspecified site**

T20.01 **Burn of unspecified degree of ear [any part, except ear drum]**

Excludes2: burn of ear drum (T28.41-)

⑦**T20.011** **Burn of unspecified degree of right ear [any part, except ear drum]**

⑦**T20.012** **Burn of unspecified degree of left ear [any part, except ear drum]**

⑦**T20.019** **Burn of unspecified degree of unspecified ear [any part, except ear drum]**

⊗⑦**T20.02** **Burn of unspecified degree of lip(s)**

⊗⑦**T20.03** **Burn of unspecified degree of chin**

⊗⑦**T20.04** **Burn of unspecified degree of nose (septum)**

⊗⑦**T20.05** **Burn of unspecified degree of scalp [any part]**

⊗⑦**T20.06** **Burn of unspecified degree of forehead and cheek**

⊗⑦**T20.07** **Burn of unspecified degree of neck**

⊗⑦**T20.09** **Burn of unspecified degree of multiple sites of head, face, and neck**

T20.1 **Burn of first degree of head, face, and neck**

Use additional external cause code to identify the source, place and intent of the burn (X00-X19, X75-X77, X96-X98, Y92)

⊗⑦**T20.10** **Burn of first degree of head, face, and neck, unspecified site**

T20.11 **Burn of first degree of ear [any part, except ear drum]**

Excludes2: burn of ear drum (T28.41-)

⑦**T20.111** **Burn of first degree of right ear [any part, except ear drum]**

⑦**T20.112** **Burn of first degree of left ear [any part, except ear drum]**

⑦**T20.119** **Burn of first degree of unspecified ear [any part, except ear drum]**

⊗⑦**T20.12** **Burn of first degree of lip(s)**

⊗⑦**T20.13** **Burn of first degree of chin**

⊗⑦**T20.14** **Burn of first degree of nose (septum)**

⊗⑦**T20.15** **Burn of first degree of scalp [any part]**

⊗⑦T20.16   Burn of first degree of forehead and cheek

⊗⑦T20.17   Burn of first degree of neck

⊗⑦T20.19   Burn of first degree of multiple sites of head, face, and neck

T20.2   **Burn of second degree of head, face, and neck**

Use additional external cause code to identify the source, place and intent of the burn (X00-X19, X75-X77, X96-X98, Y92)

⊗⑦T20.20   Burn of second degree of head, face, and neck, unspecified site

T20.21   Burn of second degree of ear [any part, except ear drum]

Excludes2: burn of ear drum (T28.41-)

⑦T20.211   Burn of second degree of right ear [any part, except ear drum]

⑦T20.212   Burn of second degree of left ear [any part, except ear drum]

⑦T20.219   Burn of second degree of unspecified ear [any part, except ear drum]

⊗⑦T20.22   Burn of second degree of lip(s)

⊗⑦T20.23   Burn of second degree of chin

⊗⑦T20.24   Burn of second degree of nose (septum)

⊗⑦T20.25   Burn of second degree of scalp [any part]

⊗⑦T20.26   Burn of second degree of forehead and cheek

⊗⑦T20.27   Burn of second degree of neck

⊗⑦T20.29   Burn of second degree of multiple sites of head, face, and neck

T20.3   **Burn of third degree of head, face, and neck**

Use additional external cause code to identify the source, place and intent of the burn (X00-X19, X75-X77, X96-X98, Y92)

⊗⑦T20.30   Burn of third degree of head, face, and neck, unspecified site

T20.31   Burn of third degree of ear [any part, except ear drum]

Excludes2: burn of ear drum (T28.41-)

⑦T20.311   Burn of third degree of right ear [any part, except ear drum]

⑦T20.312   Burn of third degree of left ear [any part, except ear drum]

⑦T20.319   Burn of third degree of unspecified ear [any part, except ear drum]

⊗⑦T20.32   Burn of third degree of lip(s)

⊗⑦T20.33   Burn of third degree of chin

⊗⑦T20.34   Burn of third degree of nose (septum)

⊗⑦T20.35   Burn of third degree of scalp [any part]

⊗⑦T20.36   Burn of third degree of forehead and cheek

⊗⑦T20.37   Burn of third degree of neck

⊗⑦T20.39   Burn of third degree of multiple sites of head, face, and neck

T20.4   **Corrosion of unspecified degree of head, face, and neck**

Code first (T51-T65) to identify chemical and intent

Use additional external cause code to identify place (Y92)

⊗⑦T20.40   Corrosion of unspecified degree of head, face, and neck, unspecified site

T20.41   Corrosion of unspecified degree of ear [any part, except ear drum]

Excludes2: corrosion of ear drum (T28.91-)

⑦T20.411   Corrosion of unspecified degree of right ear [any part, except ear drum]

⑦T20.412   Corrosion of unspecified degree of left ear [any part, except ear drum]

⑦T20.419   Corrosion of unspecified degree of unspecified ear [any part, except ear drum]

⊗⑦T20.42   Corrosion of unspecified degree of lip(s)

⊗⑦T20.43   Corrosion of unspecified degree of chin

⊗⑦T20.44   Corrosion of unspecified degree of nose (septum)

⊗⑦T20.45   Corrosion of unspecified degree of scalp [any part]

⊗⑦T20.46   Corrosion of unspecified degree of forehead and cheek

⊗⑦T20.47   Corrosion of unspecified degree of neck

⊗⑦T20.49   Corrosion of unspecified degree of multiple sites of head, face, and neck

T20.5   **Corrosion of first degree of head, face, and neck**

Code first (T51-T65) to identify chemical and intent

Use additional external cause code to identify place (Y92)

⊗⑦T20.50   Corrosion of first degree of head, face, and neck, unspecified site

T20.51   Corrosion of first degree of ear [any part, except ear drum]

Excludes2: corrosion of ear drum (T28.91-)

⑦T20.511   Corrosion of first degree of right ear [any part, except ear drum]

⑦T20.512   Corrosion of first degree of left ear [any part, except ear drum]

⑦T20.519   Corrosion of first degree of unspecified ear [any part, except ear drum]

⊗⑦T20.52   Corrosion of first degree of lip(s)

⊗⑦T20.53   Corrosion of first degree of chin

⊗⑦T20.54   Corrosion of first degree of nose (septum)

⊗⑦T20.55   Corrosion of first degree of scalp [any part]

⊗⑦T20.56   Corrosion of first degree of forehead and cheek

⊗⑦T20.57   Corrosion of first degree of neck

⊗⑦T20.59   Corrosion of first degree of multiple sites of head, face, and neck

T20.6   **Corrosion of second degree of head, face, and neck**

Code first (T51-T65) to identify chemical and intent

Use additional external cause code to identify place (Y92)

⊗⑦T20.60   Corrosion of second degree of head, face, and neck, unspecified site

T20.61   Corrosion of second degree of ear [any part, except ear drum]

Excludes2: corrosion of ear drum (T28.91-)

⑦T20.611   Corrosion of second degree of right ear [any part, except ear drum]

⑦T20.612   Corrosion of second degree of left ear [any part, except ear drum]

⑦T20.619   Corrosion of second degree of unspecified ear [any part, except ear drum]

⊗⑦T20.62   Corrosion of second degree of lip(s)

⊗⑦T20.63   Corrosion of second degree of chin

⊗⑦T20.64   Corrosion of second degree of nose (septum)

⊗⑦T20.65   Corrosion of second degree of scalp [any part]

⊗⑦T20.66   Corrosion of second degree of forehead and cheek

⊗⑦T20.67   Corrosion of second degree of neck

⊗⑦T20.69 **Corrosion of second degree of multiple sites of head, face, and neck**

T20.7 **Corrosion of third degree of head, face, and neck**

Code first (T51-T65) to identify chemical and intent

Use additional external cause code to identify place (Y92)

⊗⑦T20.70 **Corrosion of third degree of head, face, and neck, unspecified site**

T20.71 **Corrosion of third degree of ear [any part, except ear drum]**

Excludes2: corrosion of ear drum (T28.91-)

⑦T20.711 **Corrosion of third degree of right ear [any part, except ear drum]**

⑦T20.712 **Corrosion of third degree of left ear [any part, except ear drum]**

⑦T20.719 **Corrosion of third degree of unspecified ear [any part, except ear drum]**

⊗⑦T20.72 **Corrosion of third degree of lip(s)**

⊗⑦T20.73 **Corrosion of third degree of chin**

⊗⑦T20.74 **Corrosion of third degree of nose (septum)**

⊗⑦T20.75 **Corrosion of third degree of scalp [any part]**

⊗⑦T20.76 **Corrosion of third degree of forehead and cheek**

⊗⑦T20.77 **Corrosion of third degree of neck**

⊗⑦T20.79 **Corrosion of third degree of multiple sites of head, face, and neck**

T21 **Burn and corrosion of trunk**

Includes: burns and corrosion of hip region

Excludes2: burns and corrosion of axilla (T22.- with fifth character 4)

burns and corrosion of scapular region (T22.- with fifth character 6)

burns and corrosion of shoulder (T22.- with fifth character 5)

The appropriate 7th character is to be added to each code from category T21

A - initial encounter

D - subsequent encounter

S - sequela

T21.0 **Burn of unspecified degree of trunk**

Use additional external cause code to identify the source, place and intent of the burn (X00-X19, X75-X77, X96-X98, Y92)

⊗⑦T21.00 **Burn of unspecified degree of trunk, unspecified site**

⊗⑦T21.01 **Burn of unspecified degree of chest wall**

Burn of unspecified degree of breast

⊗⑦T21.02 **Burn of unspecified degree of abdominal wall**

Burn of unspecified degree of flank

Burn of unspecified degree of groin

⊗⑦T21.03 **Burn of unspecified degree of upper back**

Burn of unspecified degree of interscapular region

⊗⑦T21.04 **Burn of unspecified degree of lower back**

⊗⑦T21.05 **Burn of unspecified degree of buttock**

Burn of unspecified degree of anus

⊗⑦T21.06 **Burn of unspecified degree of male genital region**

Burn of unspecified degree of penis

Burn of unspecified degree of scrotum

Burn of unspecified degree of testis

⊗⑦T21.07 **Burn of unspecified degree of female genital region**

Burn of unspecified degree of labium (majus) (minus)

Burn of unspecified degree of perineum

Burn of unspecified degree of vulva

Excludes2: burn of vagina (T28.3)

⊗⑦T21.09 **Burn of unspecified degree of other site of trunk**

T21.1 **Burn of first degree of trunk**

Use additional external cause code to identify the source, place and intent of the burn (X00-X19, X75-X77, X96-X98, Y92)

⊗⑦T21.10 **Burn of first degree of trunk, unspecified site**

⊗⑦T21.11 **Burn of first degree of chest wall**

Burn of first degree of breast

⊗⑦T21.12 **Burn of first degree of abdominal wall**

Burn of first degree of flank

Burn of first degree of groin

⊗⑦T21.13 **Burn of first degree of upper back**

Burn of first degree of interscapular region

⊗⑦T21.14 **Burn of first degree of lower back**

⊗⑦T21.15 **Burn of first degree of buttock**

Burn of first degree of anus

⊗⑦T21.16 **Burn of first degree of male genital region**

Burn of first degree of penis

Burn of first degree of scrotum

Burn of first degree of testis

⊗⑦T21.17 **Burn of first degree of female genital region**

Burn of first degree of labium (majus) (minus)

Burn of first degree of perineum

Burn of first degree of vulva

Excludes2: burn of vagina (T28.3)

⊗⑦T21.19 **Burn of first degree of other site of trunk**

T21.2 **Burn of second degree of trunk**

Use additional external cause code to identify the source, place and intent of the burn (X00-X19, X75-X77, X96-X98, Y92)

⊗⑦T21.20 **Burn of second degree of trunk, unspecified site**

⊗⑦T21.21 **Burn of second degree of chest wall**

Burn of second degree of breast

⊗⑦T21.22 **Burn of second degree of abdominal wall**

Burn of second degree of flank

Burn of second degree of groin

⊗⑦T21.23 **Burn of second degree of upper back**

Burn of second degree of interscapular region

⊗⑦T21.24 **Burn of second degree of lower back**

⊗⑦T21.25 **Burn of second degree of buttock**

Burn of second degree of anus

⊗⑦T21.26 **Burn of second degree of male genital region**

Burn of second degree of penis

Burn of second degree of scrotum

Burn of second degree of testis

⊗⑦T21.27 **Burn of second degree of female genital region**

Burn of second degree of labium (majus) (minus)

Burn of second degree of perineum

Burn of second degree of vulva

Excludes2: burn of vagina (T28.3)

⊗⑦T21.29   **Burn of second degree of other site of trunk**

T21.3   **Burn of third degree of trunk**

    Use additional external cause code to identify the source, place and intent of the burn (X00-X19, X75-X77, X96-X98, Y92)

⊗⑦T21.30   **Burn of third degree of trunk, unspecified site**

⊗⑦T21.31   **Burn of third degree of chest wall**

    Burn of third degree of breast

⊗⑦T21.32   **Burn of third degree of abdominal wall**

    Burn of third degree of flank

    Burn of third degree of groin

⊗⑦T21.33   **Burn of third degree of upper back**

    Burn of third degree of interscapular region

⊗⑦T21.34   **Burn of third degree of lower back**

⊗⑦T21.35   **Burn of third degree of buttock**

    Burn of third degree of anus

⊗⑦T21.36   **Burn of third degree of male genital region**

    Burn of third degree of penis

    Burn of third degree of scrotum

    Burn of third degree of testis

⊗⑦T21.37   **Burn of third degree of female genital region**

    Burn of third degree of labium (majus) (minus)

    Burn of third degree of perineum

    Burn of third degree of vulva

    Excludes2: burn of vagina (T28.3)

⊗⑦T21.39   **Burn of third degree of other site of trunk**

T21.4   **Corrosion of unspecified degree of trunk**

    Code first (T51-T65) to identify chemical and intent

    Use additional external cause code to identify place (Y92)

⊗⑦T21.40   **Corrosion of unspecified degree of trunk, unspecified site**

⊗⑦T21.41   **Corrosion of unspecified degree of chest wall**

    Corrosion of unspecified degree of breast

⊗⑦T21.42   **Corrosion of unspecified degree of abdominal wall**

    Corrosion of unspecified degree of flank

    Corrosion of unspecified degree of groin

⊗⑦T21.43   **Corrosion of unspecified degree of upper back**

    Corrosion of unspecified degree of interscapular region

⊗⑦T21.44   **Corrosion of unspecified degree of lower back**

⊗⑦T21.45   **Corrosion of unspecified degree of buttock**

    Corrosion of unspecified degree of anus

⊗⑦T21.46   **Corrosion of unspecified degree of male genital region**

    Corrosion of unspecified degree of penis

    Corrosion of unspecified degree of scrotum

    Corrosion of unspecified degree of testis

⊗⑦T21.47   **Corrosion of unspecified degree of female genital region**

    Corrosion of unspecified degree of labium (majus) (minus)

    Corrosion of unspecified degree of perineum

    Corrosion of unspecified degree of vulva

    Excludes2: corrosion of vagina (T28.8)

⊗⑦T21.49   **Corrosion of unspecified degree of other site of trunk**

T21.5   **Corrosion of first degree of trunk**

    Code first (T51-T65) to identify chemical and intent

    Use additional external cause code to identify place (Y92)

⊗⑦T21.50   **Corrosion of first degree of trunk, unspecified site**

⊗⑦T21.51   **Corrosion of first degree of chest wall**

    Corrosion of first degree of breast

⊗⑦T21.52   **Corrosion of first degree of abdominal wall**

    Corrosion of first degree of flank

    Corrosion of first degree of groin

⊗⑦T21.53   **Corrosion of first degree of upper back**

    Corrosion of first degree of interscapular region

⊗⑦T21.54   **Corrosion of first degree of lower back**

⊗⑦T21.55   **Corrosion of first degree of buttock**

    Corrosion of first degree of anus

⊗⑦T21.56   **Corrosion of first degree of male genital region**

    Corrosion of first degree of penis

    Corrosion of first degree of scrotum

    Corrosion of first degree of testis

⊗⑦T21.57   **Corrosion of first degree of female genital region**

    Corrosion of first degree of labium (majus) (minus)

    Corrosion of first degree of perineum

    Corrosion of first degree of vulva

    Excludes2: corrosion of vagina (T28.8)

⊗⑦T21.59   **Corrosion of first degree of other site of trunk**

T21.6   **Corrosion of second degree of trunk**

    Code first (T51-T65) to identify chemical and intent

    Use additional external cause code to identify place (Y92)

⊗⑦T21.60   **Corrosion of second degree of trunk, unspecified site**

⊗⑦T21.61   **Corrosion of second degree of chest wall**

    Corrosion of second degree of breast

⊗⑦T21.62   **Corrosion of second degree of abdominal wall**

    Corrosion of second degree of flank

    Corrosion of second degree of groin

⊗⑦T21.63   **Corrosion of second degree of upper back**

    Corrosion of second degree of interscapular region

⊗⑦T21.64   **Corrosion of second degree of lower back**

⊗⑦T21.65   **Corrosion of second degree of buttock**

    Corrosion of second degree of anus

⊗⑦T21.66   **Corrosion of second degree of male genital region**

    Corrosion of second degree of penis

    Corrosion of second degree of scrotum

    Corrosion of second degree of testis

⊗⑦T21.67   **Corrosion of second degree of female genital region**

    Corrosion of second degree of labium (majus) (minus)

    Corrosion of second degree of perineum

    Corrosion of second degree of vulva

    Excludes2: corrosion of vagina (T28.8)

⊗⑦T21.69   **Corrosion of second degree of other site of trunk**

T21.7   **Corrosion of third degree of trunk**

    Code first (T51-T65) to identify chemical and intent

    Use additional external cause code to identify place (Y92)

  ● New code   ▲ Revised code   **Excludes1:** Not coded here   **Excludes2:** Not included here   ⊗ Placeholder required   ⑦7th digit required

⊗⑦**T21.70** **Corrosion of third degree of trunk, unspecified site**

⊗⑦**T21.71** **Corrosion of third degree of chest wall**
Corrosion of third degree of breast

⊗⑦**T21.72** **Corrosion of third degree of abdominal wall**
Corrosion of third degree of flank
Corrosion of third degree of groin

⊗⑦**T21.73** **Corrosion of third degree of upper back**
Corrosion of third degree of interscapular region

⊗⑦**T21.74** **Corrosion of third degree of lower back**

⊗⑦**T21.75** **Corrosion of third degree of buttock**
Corrosion of third degree of anus

⊗⑦**T21.76** **Corrosion of third degree of male genital region**
Corrosion of third degree of penis
Corrosion of third degree of scrotum
Corrosion of third degree of testis

⊗⑦**T21.77** **Corrosion of third degree of female genital region**
Corrosion of third degree of labium (majus) (minus)
Corrosion of third degree of perineum
Corrosion of third degree of vulva
Excludes2: corrosion of vagina (T28.8)

⊗⑦**T21.79** **Corrosion of third degree of other site of trunk**

T22 **Burn and corrosion of shoulder and upper limb, except wrist and hand**

Excludes2: burn and corrosion of interscapular region (T21.-)
burn and corrosion of wrist and hand (T23.-)

The appropriate 7th character is to be added to each code from category T22

A - initial encounter

D - subsequent encounter

S - sequela

T22.0 **Burn of unspecified degree of shoulder and upper limb, except wrist and hand**

Use additional external cause code to identify the source, place and intent of the burn (X00-X19, X75-X77, X96-X98, Y92)

⊗⑦**T22.00** **Burn of unspecified degree of shoulder and upper limb, except wrist and hand, unspecified site**

T22.01 **Burn of unspecified degree of forearm**
⑦**T22.011** **Burn of unspecified degree of right forearm**
⑦**T22.012** **Burn of unspecified degree of left forearm**
⑦**T22.019** **Burn of unspecified degree of unspecified forearm**

T22.02 **Burn of unspecified degree of elbow**
⑦**T22.021** **Burn of unspecified degree of right elbow**
⑦**T22.022** **Burn of unspecified degree of left elbow**
⑦**T22.029** **Burn of unspecified degree of unspecified elbow**

T22.03 **Burn of unspecified degree of upper arm**
⑦**T22.031** **Burn of unspecified degree of right upper arm**
⑦**T22.032** **Burn of unspecified degree of left upper arm**

⑦**T22.039** **Burn of unspecified degree of unspecified upper arm**

T22.04 **Burn of unspecified degree of axilla**
⑦**T22.041** **Burn of unspecified degree of right axilla**
⑦**T22.042** **Burn of unspecified degree of left axilla**
⑦**T22.049** **Burn of unspecified degree of unspecified axilla**

T22.05 **Burn of unspecified degree of shoulder**
⑦**T22.051** **Burn of unspecified degree of right shoulder**
⑦**T22.052** **Burn of unspecified degree of left shoulder**
⑦**T22.059** **Burn of unspecified degree of unspecified shoulder**

T22.06 **Burn of unspecified degree of scapular region**
⑦**T22.061** **Burn of unspecified degree of right scapular region**
⑦**T22.062** **Burn of unspecified degree of left scapular region**
⑦**T22.069** **Burn of unspecified degree of unspecified scapular region**

T22.09 **Burn of unspecified degree of multiple sites of shoulder and upper limb, except wrist and hand**
⑦**T22.091** **Burn of unspecified degree of multiple sites of right shoulder and upper limb, except wrist and hand**
⑦**T22.092** **Burn of unspecified degree of multiple sites of left shoulder and upper limb, except wrist and hand**
⑦**T22.099** **Burn of unspecified degree of multiple sites of unspecified shoulder and upper limb, except wrist and hand**

T22.1 **Burn of first degree of shoulder and upper limb, except wrist and hand**

Use additional external cause code to identify the source, place and intent of the burn (X00-X19, X75-X77, X96-X98, Y92)

⊗⑦**T22.10** **Burn of first degree of shoulder and upper limb, except wrist and hand, unspecified site**

T22.11 **Burn of first degree of forearm**
⑦**T22.111** **Burn of first degree of right forearm**
⑦**T22.112** **Burn of first degree of left forearm**
⑦**T22.119** **Burn of first degree of unspecified forearm**

T22.12 **Burn of first degree of elbow**
⑦**T22.121** **Burn of first degree of right elbow**
⑦**T22.122** **Burn of first degree of left elbow**
⑦**T22.129** **Burn of first degree of unspecified elbow**

T22.13 **Burn of first degree of upper arm**
⑦**T22.131** **Burn of first degree of right upper arm**
⑦**T22.132** **Burn of first degree of left upper arm**
⑦**T22.139** **Burn of first degree of unspecified upper arm**

T22.14 **Burn of first degree of axilla**
⑦**T22.141** **Burn of first degree of right axilla**
⑦**T22.142** **Burn of first degree of left axilla**

⑦T22.149   **Burn of first degree of unspecified axilla**

T22.15   **Burn of first degree of shoulder**

⑦T22.151   **Burn of first degree of right shoulder**

⑦T22.152   **Burn of first degree of left shoulder**

⑦T22.159   **Burn of first degree of unspecified shoulder**

T22.16   **Burn of first degree of scapular region**

⑦T22.161   **Burn of first degree of right scapular region**

⑦T22.162   **Burn of first degree of left scapular region**

⑦T22.169   **Burn of first degree of unspecified scapular region**

T22.19   **Burn of first degree of multiple sites of shoulder and upper limb, except wrist and hand**

⑦T22.191   **Burn of first degree of multiple sites of right shoulder and upper limb, except wrist and hand**

⑦T22.192   **Burn of first degree of multiple sites of left shoulder and upper limb, except wrist and hand**

⑦T22.199   **Burn of first degree of multiple sites of unspecified shoulder and upper limb, except wrist and hand**

T22.2   **Burn of second degree of shoulder and upper limb, except wrist and hand**

Use additional external cause code to identify the source, place and intent of the burn (X00-X19, X75-X77, X96-X98, Y92)

⊗⑦T22.20   **Burn of second degree of shoulder and upper limb, except wrist and hand, unspecified site**

T22.21   **Burn of second degree of forearm**

⑦T22.211   **Burn of second degree of right forearm**

⑦T22.212   **Burn of second degree of left forearm**

⑦T22.219   **Burn of second degree of unspecified forearm**

T22.22   **Burn of second degree of elbow**

⑦T22.221   **Burn of second degree of right elbow**

⑦T22.222   **Burn of second degree of left elbow**

⑦T22.229   **Burn of second degree of unspecified elbow**

T22.23   **Burn of second degree of upper arm**

⑦T22.231   **Burn of second degree of right upper arm**

⑦T22.232   **Burn of second degree of left upper arm**

⑦T22.239   **Burn of second degree of unspecified upper arm**

T22.24   **Burn of second degree of axilla**

⑦T22.241   **Burn of second degree of right axilla**

⑦T22.242   **Burn of second degree of left axilla**

⑦T22.249   **Burn of second degree of unspecified axilla**

T22.25   **Burn of second degree of shoulder**

⑦T22.251   **Burn of second degree of right shoulder**

⑦T22.252   **Burn of second degree of left shoulder**

⑦T22.259   **Burn of second degree of unspecified shoulder**

T22.26   **Burn of second degree of scapular region**

⑦T22.261   **Burn of second degree of right scapular region**

⑦T22.262   **Burn of second degree of left scapular region**

⑦T22.269   **Burn of second degree of unspecified scapular region**

T22.29   **Burn of second degree of multiple sites of shoulder and upper limb, except wrist and hand**

⑦T22.291   **Burn of second degree of multiple sites of right shoulder and upper limb, except wrist and hand**

⑦T22.292   **Burn of second degree of multiple sites of left shoulder and upper limb, except wrist and hand**

⑦T22.299   **Burn of second degree of multiple sites of unspecified shoulder and upper limb, except wrist and hand**

T22.3   **Burn of third degree of shoulder and upper limb, except wrist and hand**

Use additional external cause code to identify the source, place and intent of the burn (X00-X19, X75-X77, X96-X98, Y92)

⊗⑦T22.30   **Burn of third degree of shoulder and upper limb, except wrist and hand, unspecified site**

T22.31   **Burn of third degree of forearm**

⑦T22.311   **Burn of third degree of right forearm**

⑦T22.312   **Burn of third degree of left forearm**

⑦T22.319   **Burn of third degree of unspecified forearm**

T22.32   **Burn of third degree of elbow**

⑦T22.321   **Burn of third degree of right elbow**

⑦T22.322   **Burn of third degree of left elbow**

⑦T22.329   **Burn of third degree of unspecified elbow**

T22.33   **Burn of third degree of upper arm**

⑦T22.331   **Burn of third degree of right upper arm**

⑦T22.332   **Burn of third degree of left upper arm**

⑦T22.339   **Burn of third degree of unspecified upper arm**

T22.34   **Burn of third degree of axilla**

⑦T22.341   **Burn of third degree of right axilla**

⑦T22.342   **Burn of third degree of left axilla**

⑦T22.349   **Burn of third degree of unspecified axilla**

T22.35   **Burn of third degree of shoulder**

⑦T22.351   **Burn of third degree of right shoulder**

⑦T22.352   **Burn of third degree of left shoulder**

⑦T22.359   **Burn of third degree of unspecified shoulder**

T22.36   **Burn of third degree of scapular region**

⑦T22.361   **Burn of third degree of right scapular region**

⑦T22.362   **Burn of third degree of left scapular region**

⑦T22.369   **Burn of third degree of unspecified scapular region**

   ● New code   ▲ Revised code   **Excludes1:** Not coded here   **Excludes2:** Not included here   ⊗ Placeholder required   ⑦ 7th digit required

T22.39 Burn of third degree of multiple sites of shoulder and upper limb, except wrist and hand

⑦**T22.391** Burn of third degree of multiple sites of right shoulder and upper limb, except wrist and hand

⑦**T22.392** Burn of third degree of multiple sites of left shoulder and upper limb, except wrist and hand

⑦**T22.399** Burn of third degree of multiple sites of unspecified shoulder and upper limb, except wrist and hand

T22.4 Corrosion of unspecified degree of shoulder and upper limb, except wrist and hand

Code first (T51-T65) to identify chemical and intent

Use additional external cause code to identify place (Y92)

⊗⑦**T22.40** Corrosion of unspecified degree of shoulder and upper limb, except wrist and hand, unspecified site

T22.41 Corrosion of unspecified degree of forearm

⑦**T22.411** Corrosion of unspecified degree of right forearm

⑦**T22.412** Corrosion of unspecified degree of left forearm

⑦**T22.419** Corrosion of unspecified degree of unspecified forearm

T22.42 Corrosion of unspecified degree of elbow

⑦**T22.421** Corrosion of unspecified degree of right elbow

⑦**T22.422** Corrosion of unspecified degree of left elbow

⑦**T22.429** Corrosion of unspecified degree of unspecified elbow

T22.43 Corrosion of unspecified degree of upper arm

⑦**T22.431** Corrosion of unspecified degree of right upper arm

⑦**T22.432** Corrosion of unspecified degree of left upper arm

⑦**T22.439** Corrosion of unspecified degree of unspecified upper arm

T22.44 Corrosion of unspecified degree of axilla

⑦**T22.441** Corrosion of unspecified degree of right axilla

⑦**T22.442** Corrosion of unspecified degree of left axilla

⑦**T22.449** Corrosion of unspecified degree of unspecified axilla

T22.45 Corrosion of unspecified degree of shoulder

⑦**T22.451** Corrosion of unspecified degree of right shoulder

⑦**T22.452** Corrosion of unspecified degree of left shoulder

⑦**T22.459** Corrosion of unspecified degree of unspecified shoulder

T22.46 Corrosion of unspecified degree of scapular region

⑦**T22.461** Corrosion of unspecified degree of right scapular region

⑦**T22.462** Corrosion of unspecified degree of left scapular region

⑦**T22.469** Corrosion of unspecified degree of unspecified scapular region

T22.49 Corrosion of unspecified degree of multiple sites of shoulder and upper limb, except wrist and hand

⑦**T22.491** Corrosion of unspecified degree of multiple sites of right shoulder and upper limb, except wrist and hand

⑦**T22.492** Corrosion of unspecified degree of multiple sites of left shoulder and upper limb, except wrist and hand

⑦**T22.499** Corrosion of unspecified degree of multiple sites of unspecified shoulder and upper limb, except wrist and hand

T22.5 Corrosion of first degree of shoulder and upper limb, except wrist and hand

Code first (T51-T65) to identify chemical and intent

Use additional external cause code to identify place (Y92)

⊗⑦**T22.50** Corrosion of first degree of shoulder and upper limb, except wrist and hand unspecified site

T22.51 Corrosion of first degree of forearm

⑦**T22.511** Corrosion of first degree of right forearm

⑦**T22.512** Corrosion of first degree of left forearm

⑦**T22.519** Corrosion of first degree of unspecified forearm

T22.52 Corrosion of first degree of elbow

⑦**T22.521** Corrosion of first degree of right elbow

⑦**T22.522** Corrosion of first degree of left elbow

⑦**T22.529** Corrosion of first degree of unspecified elbow

T22.53 Corrosion of first degree of upper arm

⑦**T22.531** Corrosion of first degree of right upper arm

⑦**T22.532** Corrosion of first degree of left upper arm

⑦**T22.539** Corrosion of first degree of unspecified upper arm

T22.54 Corrosion of first degree of axilla

⑦**T22.541** Corrosion of first degree of right axilla

⑦**T22.542** Corrosion of first degree of left axilla

⑦**T22.549** Corrosion of first degree of unspecified axilla

T22.55 Corrosion of first degree of shoulder

⑦**T22.551** Corrosion of first degree of right shoulder

⑦**T22.552** Corrosion of first degree of left shoulder

⑦**T22.559** Corrosion of first degree of unspecified shoulder

T22.56 Corrosion of first degree of scapular region

⑦**T22.561** Corrosion of first degree of right scapular region

⑦**T22.562** Corrosion of first degree of left scapular region

⑦**T22.569** Corrosion of first degree of unspecified scapular region

T22.59 Corrosion of first degree of multiple sites of shoulder and upper limb, except wrist and hand

⑦**T22.591** Corrosion of first degree of multiple sites of right shoulder and upper limb, except wrist and hand

⑦**T22.592** Corrosion of first degree of multiple sites of left shoulder and upper limb, except wrist and hand

⑦**T22.599** Corrosion of first degree of multiple sites of unspecified shoulder and upper limb, except wrist and hand

T22.6 **Corrosion of second degree of shoulder and upper limb, except wrist and hand**

Code first (T51-T65) to identify chemical and intent

Use additional external cause code to identify place (Y92)

⊗⑦**T22.60** Corrosion of second degree of shoulder and upper limb, except wrist and hand, unspecified site

T22.61 Corrosion of second degree of forearm

⑦**T22.611** Corrosion of second degree of right forearm

⑦**T22.612** Corrosion of second degree of left forearm

⑦**T22.619** Corrosion of second degree of unspecified forearm

T22.62 Corrosion of second degree of elbow

⑦**T22.621** Corrosion of second degree of right elbow

⑦**T22.622** Corrosion of second degree of left elbow

⑦**T22.629** Corrosion of second degree of unspecified elbow

T22.63 Corrosion of second degree of upper arm

⑦**T22.631** Corrosion of second degree of right upper arm

⑦**T22.632** Corrosion of second degree of left upper arm

⑦**T22.639** Corrosion of second degree of unspecified upper arm

T22.64 Corrosion of second degree of axilla

⑦**T22.641** Corrosion of second degree of right axilla

⑦**T22.642** Corrosion of second degree of left axilla

⑦**T22.649** Corrosion of second degree of unspecified axilla

T22.65 Corrosion of second degree of shoulder

⑦**T22.651** Corrosion of second degree of right shoulder

⑦**T22.652** Corrosion of second degree of left shoulder

⑦**T22.659** Corrosion of second degree of unspecified shoulder

T22.66 Corrosion of second degree of scapular region

⑦**T22.661** Corrosion of second degree of right scapular region

⑦**T22.662** Corrosion of second degree of left scapular region

⑦**T22.669** Corrosion of second degree of unspecified scapular region

T22.69 Corrosion of second degree of multiple sites of shoulder and upper limb, except wrist and hand

⑦**T22.691** Corrosion of second degree of multiple sites of right shoulder and upper limb, except wrist and hand

⑦**T22.692** Corrosion of second degree of multiple sites of left shoulder and upper limb, except wrist and hand

⑦**T22.699** Corrosion of second degree of multiple sites of unspecified shoulder and upper limb, except wrist and hand

T22.7 **Corrosion of third degree of shoulder and upper limb, except wrist and hand**

Code first (T51-T65) to identify chemical and intent

Use additional external cause code to identify place (Y92)

⊗⑦**T22.70** Corrosion of third degree of shoulder and upper limb, except wrist and hand, unspecified site

T22.71 Corrosion of third degree of forearm

⑦**T22.711** Corrosion of third degree of right forearm

⑦**T22.712** Corrosion of third degree of left forearm

⑦**T22.719** Corrosion of third degree of unspecified forearm

T22.72 Corrosion of third degree of elbow

⑦**T22.721** Corrosion of third degree of right elbow

⑦**T22.722** Corrosion of third degree of left elbow

⑦**T22.729** Corrosion of third degree of unspecified elbow

T22.73 Corrosion of third degree of upper arm

⑦**T22.731** Corrosion of third degree of right upper arm

⑦**T22.732** Corrosion of third degree of left upper arm

⑦**T22.739** Corrosion of third degree of unspecified upper arm

T22.74 Corrosion of third degree of axilla

⑦**T22.741** Corrosion of third degree of right axilla

⑦**T22.742** Corrosion of third degree of left axilla

⑦**T22.749** Corrosion of third degree of unspecified axilla

T22.75 Corrosion of third degree of shoulder

⑦**T22.751** Corrosion of third degree of right shoulder

⑦**T22.752** Corrosion of third degree of left shoulder

⑦**T22.759** Corrosion of third degree of unspecified shoulder

T22.76 Corrosion of third degree of scapular region

⑦**T22.761** Corrosion of third degree of right scapular region

⑦**T22.762** Corrosion of third degree of left scapular region

⑦**T22.769** Corrosion of third degree of unspecified scapular region

T22.79 Corrosion of third degree of multiple sites of shoulder and upper limb, except wrist and hand

⑦**T22.791** Corrosion of third degree of multiple sites of right shoulder and upper limb, except wrist and hand

● New code　▲ Revised code　**Excludes1:** Not coded here　**Excludes2:** Not included here　⊗ Placeholder required　⑦ 7th digit required

⑦**T22.792** **Corrosion of third degree of multiple sites of left shoulder and upper limb, except wrist and hand**

⑦**T22.799** **Corrosion of third degree of multiple sites of unspecified shoulder and upper limb, except wrist and hand**

T23 **Burn and corrosion of wrist and hand**

The appropriate 7th character is to be added to each code from category T23

A - initial encounter

D - subsequent encounter

S - sequela

T23.0 **Burn of unspecified degree of wrist and hand**

Use additional external cause code to identify the source, place and intent of the burn (X00-X19, X75-X77, X96-X98, Y92)

T23.00 **Burn of unspecified degree of hand, unspecified site**

⑦**T23.001** **Burn of unspecified degree of right hand, unspecified site**

⑦**T23.002** **Burn of unspecified degree of left hand, unspecified site**

⑦**T23.009** **Burn of unspecified degree of unspecified hand, unspecified site**

T23.01 **Burn of unspecified degree of thumb (nail)**

⑦**T23.011** **Burn of unspecified degree of right thumb (nail)**

⑦**T23.012** **Burn of unspecified degree of left thumb (nail)**

⑦**T23.019** **Burn of unspecified degree of unspecified thumb (nail)**

T23.02 **Burn of unspecified degree of single finger (nail) except thumb**

⑦**T23.021** **Burn of unspecified degree of single right finger (nail) except thumb**

⑦**T23.022** **Burn of unspecified degree of single left finger (nail) except thumb**

⑦**T23.029** **Burn of unspecified degree of unspecified single finger (nail) except thumb**

T23.03 **Burn of unspecified degree of multiple fingers (nail), not including thumb**

⑦**T23.031** **Burn of unspecified degree of multiple right fingers (nail), not including thumb**

⑦**T23.032** **Burn of unspecified degree of multiple left fingers (nail), not including thumb**

⑦**T23.039** **Burn of unspecified degree of unspecified multiple fingers (nail), not including thumb**

T23.04 **Burn of unspecified degree of multiple fingers (nail), including thumb**

⑦**T23.041** **Burn of unspecified degree of multiple right fingers (nail), including thumb**

⑦**T23.042** **Burn of unspecified degree of multiple left fingers (nail), including thumb**

⑦**T23.049** **Burn of unspecified degree of unspecified multiple fingers (nail), including thumb**

T23.05 **Burn of unspecified degree of palm**

⑦**T23.051** **Burn of unspecified degree of right palm**

⑦**T23.052** **Burn of unspecified degree of left palm**

⑦**T23.059** **Burn of unspecified degree of unspecified palm**

T23.06 **Burn of unspecified degree of back of hand**

⑦**T23.061** **Burn of unspecified degree of back of right hand**

⑦**T23.062** **Burn of unspecified degree of back of left hand**

⑦**T23.069** **Burn of unspecified degree of back of unspecified hand**

T23.07 **Burn of unspecified degree of wrist**

⑦**T23.071** **Burn of unspecified degree of right wrist**

⑦**T23.072** **Burn of unspecified degree of left wrist**

⑦**T23.079** **Burn of unspecified degree of unspecified wrist**

T23.09 **Burn of unspecified degree of multiple sites of wrist and hand**

⑦**T23.091** **Burn of unspecified degree of multiple sites of right wrist and hand**

⑦**T23.092** **Burn of unspecified degree of multiple sites of left wrist and hand**

⑦**T23.099** **Burn of unspecified degree of multiple sites of unspecified wrist and hand**

T23.1 **Burn of first degree of wrist and hand**

Use additional external cause code to identify the source, place and intent of the burn (X00-X19, X75-X77, X96-X98, Y92)

T23.10 **Burn of first degree of hand, unspecified site**

⑦**T23.101** **Burn of first degree of right hand, unspecified site**

⑦**T23.102** **Burn of first degree of left hand, unspecified site**

⑦**T23.109** **Burn of first degree of unspecified hand, unspecified site**

T23.11 **Burn of first degree of thumb (nail)**

⑦**T23.111** **Burn of first degree of right thumb (nail)**

⑦**T23.112** **Burn of first degree of left thumb (nail)**

⑦**T23.119** **Burn of first degree of unspecified thumb (nail)**

T23.12 **Burn of first degree of single finger (nail) except thumb**

⑦**T23.121** **Burn of first degree of single right finger (nail) except thumb**

⑦**T23.122** **Burn of first degree of single left finger (nail) except thumb**

⑦**T23.129** **Burn of first degree of unspecified single finger (nail) except thumb**

T23.13 **Burn of first degree of multiple fingers (nail), not including thumb**

⑦**T23.131** **Burn of first degree of multiple right fingers (nail), not including thumb**

⑦**T23.132** **Burn of first degree of multiple left fingers (nail), not including thumb**

⑦**T23.139** **Burn of first degree of unspecified multiple fingers (nail), not including thumb**

T23.14 **Burn of first degree of multiple fingers (nail), including thumb**

⑦T23.141 **Burn of first degree of multiple right fingers (nail), including thumb**

⑦T23.142 **Burn of first degree of multiple left fingers (nail), including thumb**

⑦T23.149 **Burn of first degree of unspecified multiple fingers (nail), including thumb**

T23.15 **Burn of first degree of palm**

⑦T23.151 **Burn of first degree of right palm**

⑦T23.152 **Burn of first degree of left palm**

⑦T23.159 **Burn of first degree of unspecified palm**

T23.16 **Burn of first degree of back of hand**

⑦T23.161 **Burn of first degree of back of right hand**

⑦T23.162 **Burn of first degree of back of left hand**

⑦T23.169 **Burn of first degree of back of unspecified hand**

⑦T23.17 **Burn of first degree of wrist**

⑦T23.171 **Burn of first degree of right wrist**

⑦T23.172 **Burn of first degree of left wrist**

⑦T23.179 **Burn of first degree of unspecified wrist**

⑦T23.19 **Burn of first degree of multiple sites of wrist and hand**

⑦T23.191 **Burn of first degree of multiple sites of right wrist and hand**

⑦T23.192 **Burn of first degree of multiple sites of left wrist and hand**

⑦T23.199 **Burn of first degree of multiple sites of unspecified wrist and hand**

T23.2 **Burn of second degree of wrist and hand**

Use additional external cause code to identify the source, place and intent of the burn (X00-X19, X75-X77, X96-X98, Y92)

T23.20 **Burn of second degree of hand, unspecified site**

⑦T23.201 **Burn of second degree of right hand, unspecified site**

⑦T23.202 **Burn of second degree of left hand, unspecified site**

⑦T23.209 **Burn of second degree of unspecified hand, unspecified site**

T23.21 **Burn of second degree of thumb (nail)**

⑦T23.211 **Burn of second degree of right thumb (nail)**

⑦T23.212 **Burn of second degree of left thumb (nail)**

⑦T23.219 **Burn of second degree of unspecified thumb (nail)**

T23.22 **Burn of second degree of single finger (nail) except thumb**

⑦T23.221 **Burn of second degree of single right finger (nail) except thumb**

⑦T23.222 **Burn of second degree of single left finger (nail) except thumb**

⑦T23.229 **Burn of second degree of unspecified single finger (nail) except thumb**

T23.23 **Burn of second degree of multiple fingers (nail), not including thumb**

⑦T23.231 **Burn of second degree of multiple right fingers (nail), not including thumb**

⑦T23.232 **Burn of second degree of multiple left fingers (nail), not including thumb**

⑦T23.239 **Burn of second degree of unspecified multiple fingers (nail), not including thumb**

T23.24 **Burn of second degree of multiple fingers (nail), including thumb**

⑦T23.241 **Burn of second degree of multiple right fingers (nail), including thumb**

⑦T23.242 **Burn of second degree of multiple left fingers (nail), including thumb**

⑦T23.249 **Burn of second degree of unspecified multiple fingers (nail), including thumb**

T23.25 **Burn of second degree of palm**

⑦T23.251 **Burn of second degree of right palm**

⑦T23.252 **Burn of second degree of left palm**

⑦T23.259 **Burn of second degree of unspecified palm**

T23.26 **Burn of second degree of back of hand**

⑦T23.261 **Burn of second degree of back of right hand**

⑦T23.262 **Burn of second degree of back of left hand**

⑦T23.269 **Burn of second degree of back of unspecified hand**

T23.27 **Burn of second degree of wrist**

⑦T23.271 **Burn of second degree of right wrist**

⑦T23.272 **Burn of second degree of left wrist**

⑦T23.279 **Burn of second degree of unspecified wrist**

T23.29 **Burn of second degree of multiple sites of wrist and hand**

⑦T23.291 **Burn of second degree of multiple sites of right wrist and hand**

⑦T23.292 **Burn of second degree of multiple sites of left wrist and hand**

⑦T23.299 **Burn of second degree of multiple sites of unspecified wrist and hand**

T23.3 **Burn of third degree of wrist and hand**

Use additional external cause code to identify the source, place and intent of the burn (X00-X19, X75-X77, X96-X98, Y92)

T23.30 **Burn of third degree of hand, unspecified site**

⑦T23.301 **Burn of third degree of right hand, unspecified site**

⑦T23.302 **Burn of third degree of left hand, unspecified site**

⑦T23.309 **Burn of third degree of unspecified hand, unspecified site**

T23.31 **Burn of third degree of thumb (nail)**

⑦T23.311 **Burn of third degree of right thumb (nail)**

⑦T23.312 **Burn of third degree of left thumb (nail)**

⑦T23.319 **Burn of third degree of unspecified thumb (nail)**

T23.32 **Burn of third degree of single finger (nail) except thumb**

⑦T23.321 **Burn of third degree of single right finger (nail) except thumb**

⑦T23.322 **Burn of third degree of single left finger (nail) except thumb**

● New code   ▲ Revised code   **Excludes1:** Not coded here   **Excludes2:** Not included here   ⊗ Placeholder required   ⑦7th digit required

⑦**T23.329** Burn of third degree of unspecified single finger (nail) except thumb

T23.33 Burn of third degree of multiple fingers (nail), not including thumb

⑦**T23.331** Burn of third degree of multiple right fingers (nail), not including thumb

⑦**T23.332** Burn of third degree of multiple left fingers (nail), not including thumb

⑦**T23.339** Burn of third degree of unspecified multiple fingers (nail), not including thumb

T23.34 Burn of third degree of multiple fingers (nail), including thumb

⑦**T23.341** Burn of third degree of multiple right fingers (nail), including thumb

⑦**T23.342** Burn of third degree of multiple left fingers (nail), including thumb

⑦**T23.349** Burn of third degree of unspecified multiple fingers (nail), including thumb

T23.35 Burn of third degree of palm

⑦**T23.351** Burn of third degree of right palm

⑦**T23.352** Burn of third degree of left palm

⑦**T23.359** Burn of third degree of unspecified palm

T23.36 Burn of third degree of back of hand

⑦**T23.361** Burn of third degree of back of right hand

⑦**T23.362** Burn of third degree of back of left hand

⑦**T23.369** Burn of third degree of back of unspecified hand

T23.37 Burn of third degree of wrist

⑦**T23.371** Burn of third degree of right wrist

⑦**T23.372** Burn of third degree of left wrist

⑦**T23.379** Burn of third degree of unspecified wrist

T23.39 Burn of third degree of multiple sites of wrist and hand

⑦**T23.391** Burn of third degree of multiple sites of right wrist and hand

⑦**T23.392** Burn of third degree of multiple sites of left wrist and hand

⑦**T23.399** Burn of third degree of multiple sites of unspecified wrist and hand

T23.4 Corrosion of unspecified degree of wrist and hand

Code first (T51-T65) to identify chemical and intent

Use additional external cause code to identify place (Y92)

T23.40 Corrosion of unspecified degree of hand, unspecified site

⑦**T23.401** Corrosion of unspecified degree of right hand, unspecified site

⑦**T23.402** Corrosion of unspecified degree of left hand, unspecified site

⑦**T23.409** Corrosion of unspecified degree of unspecified hand, unspecified site

T23.41 Corrosion of unspecified degree of thumb (nail)

⑦**T23.411** Corrosion of unspecified degree of right thumb (nail)

⑦**T23.412** Corrosion of unspecified degree of left thumb (nail)

⑦**T23.419** Corrosion of unspecified degree of unspecified thumb (nail)

T23.42 Corrosion of unspecified degree of single finger (nail) except thumb

⑦**T23.421** Corrosion of unspecified degree of single right finger (nail) except thumb

⑦**T23.422** Corrosion of unspecified degree of single left finger (nail) except thumb

⑦**T23.429** Corrosion of unspecified degree of unspecified single finger (nail) except thumb

T23.43 Corrosion of unspecified degree of multiple fingers (nail), not including thumb

⑦**T23.431** Corrosion of unspecified degree of multiple right fingers (nail), not including thumb

⑦**T23.432** Corrosion of unspecified degree of multiple left fingers (nail), not including thumb

⑦**T23.439** Corrosion of unspecified degree of unspecified multiple fingers (nail), not including thumb

T23.44 Corrosion of unspecified degree of multiple fingers (nail), including thumb

⑦**T23.441** Corrosion of unspecified degree of multiple right fingers (nail), including thumb

⑦**T23.442** Corrosion of unspecified degree of multiple left fingers (nail), including thumb

⑦**T23.449** Corrosion of unspecified degree of unspecified multiple fingers (nail), including thumb

T23.45 Corrosion of unspecified degree of palm

⑦**T23.451** Corrosion of unspecified degree of right palm

⑦**T23.452** Corrosion of unspecified degree of left palm

⑦**T23.459** Corrosion of unspecified degree of unspecified palm

T23.46 Corrosion of unspecified degree of back of hand

⑦**T23.461** Corrosion of unspecified degree of back of right hand

⑦**T23.462** Corrosion of unspecified degree of back of left hand

⑦**T23.469** Corrosion of unspecified degree of back of unspecified hand

T23.47 Corrosion of unspecified degree of wrist

⑦**T23.471** Corrosion of unspecified degree of right wrist

⑦**T23.472** Corrosion of unspecified degree of left wrist

⑦**T23.479** Corrosion of unspecified degree of unspecified wrist

T23.49 Corrosion of unspecified degree of multiple sites of wrist and hand

⑦**T23.491** Corrosion of unspecified degree of multiple sites of right wrist and hand

⑦**T23.492** Corrosion of unspecified degree of multiple sites of left wrist and hand

⑦**T23.499** Corrosion of unspecified degree of multiple sites of unspecified wrist and hand

T23.5 Corrosion of first degree of wrist and hand

Code first (T51-T65) to identify chemical and intent

Use additional external cause code to identify place (Y92)

T23.50 Corrosion of first degree of hand, unspecified site

⑦**T23.501** Corrosion of first degree of right hand, unspecified site

⑦**T23.502** Corrosion of first degree of left hand, unspecified site

⑦**T23.509** Corrosion of first degree of unspecified hand, unspecified site

T23.51 Corrosion of first degree of thumb (nail)

⑦**T23.511** Corrosion of first degree of right thumb (nail)

⑦**T23.512** Corrosion of first degree of left thumb (nail)

⑦**T23.519** Corrosion of first degree of unspecified thumb (nail)

T23.52 Corrosion of first degree of single finger (nail) except thumb

⑦**T23.521** Corrosion of first degree of single right finger (nail) except thumb

⑦**T23.522** Corrosion of first degree of single left finger (nail) except thumb

⑦**T23.529** Corrosion of first degree of unspecified single finger (nail) except thumb

T23.53 Corrosion of first degree of multiple fingers (nail), not including thumb

⑦**T23.531** Corrosion of first degree of multiple right fingers (nail), not including thumb

⑦**T23.532** Corrosion of first degree of multiple left fingers (nail), not including thumb

⑦**T23.539** Corrosion of first degree of unspecified multiple fingers (nail), not including thumb

T23.54 Corrosion of first degree of multiple fingers (nail), including thumb

⑦**T23.541** Corrosion of first degree of multiple right fingers (nail), including thumb

⑦**T23.542** Corrosion of first degree of multiple left fingers (nail), including thumb

⑦**T23.549** Corrosion of first degree of unspecified multiple fingers (nail), including thumb

T23.55 Corrosion of first degree of palm

⑦**T23.551** Corrosion of first degree of right palm

⑦**T23.552** Corrosion of first degree of left palm

⑦**T23.559** Corrosion of first degree of unspecified palm

T23.56 Corrosion of first degree of back of hand

⑦**T23.561** Corrosion of first degree of back of right hand

⑦**T23.562** Corrosion of first degree of back of left hand

⑦**T23.569** Corrosion of first degree of back of unspecified hand

T23.57 Corrosion of first degree of wrist

⑦**T23.571** Corrosion of first degree of right wrist

⑦**T23.572** Corrosion of first degree of left wrist

⑦**T23.579** Corrosion of first degree of unspecified wrist

T23.59 Corrosion of first degree of multiple sites of wrist and hand

⑦**T23.591** Corrosion of first degree of multiple sites of right wrist and hand

⑦**T23.592** Corrosion of first degree of multiple sites of left wrist and hand

⑦**T23.599** Corrosion of first degree of multiple sites of unspecified wrist and hand

T23.6 Corrosion of second degree of wrist and hand

Code first (T51-T65) to identify chemical and intent

Use additional external cause code to identify place (Y92)

T23.60 Corrosion of second degree of hand, unspecified site

⑦**T23.601** Corrosion of second degree of right hand, unspecified site

⑦**T23.602** Corrosion of second degree of left hand, unspecified site

⑦**T23.609** Corrosion of second degree of unspecified hand, unspecified site

T23.61 Corrosion of second degree of thumb (nail)

⑦**T23.611** Corrosion of second degree of right thumb (nail)

⑦**T23.612** Corrosion of second degree of left thumb (nail)

⑦**T23.619** Corrosion of second degree of unspecified thumb (nail)

T23.62 Corrosion of second degree of single finger (nail) except thumb

⑦**T23.621** Corrosion of second degree of single right finger (nail) except thumb

⑦**T23.622** Corrosion of second degree of single left finger (nail) except thumb

⑦**T23.629** Corrosion of second degree of unspecified single finger (nail) except thumb

T23.63 Corrosion of second degree of multiple fingers (nail), not including thumb

⑦**T23.631** Corrosion of second degree of multiple right fingers (nail), not including thumb

⑦**T23.632** Corrosion of second degree of multiple left fingers (nail), not including thumb

⑦**T23.639** Corrosion of second degree of unspecified multiple fingers (nail), not including thumb

T23.64 Corrosion of second degree of multiple fingers (nail), including thumb

⑦**T23.641** Corrosion of second degree of multiple right fingers (nail), including thumb

⑦**T23.642** Corrosion of second degree of multiple left fingers (nail), including thumb

⑦**T23.649** Corrosion of second degree of unspecified multiple fingers (nail), including thumb

T23.65 Corrosion of second degree of palm

⑦**T23.651** Corrosion of second degree of right palm

⑦**T23.652** Corrosion of second degree of left palm

● New code ▲ Revised code **Excludes1:** Not coded here **Excludes2:** Not included here ⊗ Placeholder required ⑦ 7th digit required

⑦T23.659   Corrosion of second degree of unspecified palm

T23.66   Corrosion of second degree of back of hand

⑦T23.661   Corrosion of second degree back of right hand

⑦T23.662   Corrosion of second degree back of left hand

⑦T23.669   Corrosion of second degree back of unspecified hand

T23.67   Corrosion of second degree of wrist

⑦T23.671   Corrosion of second degree of right wrist

⑦T23.672   Corrosion of second degree of left wrist

⑦T23.679   Corrosion of second degree of unspecified wrist

T23.69   Corrosion of second degree of multiple sites of wrist and hand

⑦T23.691   Corrosion of second degree of multiple sites of right wrist and hand

⑦T23.692   Corrosion of second degree of multiple sites of left wrist and hand

⑦T23.699   Corrosion of second degree of multiple sites of unspecified wrist and hand

T23.7   Corrosion of third degree of wrist and hand

Code first (T51-T65) to identify chemical and intent

Use additional external cause code to identify place (Y92)

T23.70   Corrosion of third degree of hand, unspecified site

⑦T23.701   Corrosion of third degree of right hand, unspecified site

⑦T23.702   Corrosion of third degree of left hand, unspecified site

⑦T23.709   Corrosion of third degree of unspecified hand, unspecified site

T23.71   Corrosion of third degree of thumb (nail)

⑦T23.711   Corrosion of third degree of right thumb (nail)

⑦T23.712   Corrosion of third degree of left thumb (nail)

⑦T23.719   Corrosion of third degree of unspecified thumb (nail)

T23.72   Corrosion of third degree of single finger (nail) except thumb

⑦T23.721   Corrosion of third degree of single right finger (nail) except thumb

⑦T23.722   Corrosion of third degree of single left finger (nail) except thumb

⑦T23.729   Corrosion of third degree of unspecified single finger (nail) except thumb

T23.73   Corrosion of third degree of multiple fingers (nail), not including thumb

⑦T23.731   Corrosion of third degree of multiple right fingers (nail), not including thumb

⑦T23.732   Corrosion of third degree of multiple left fingers (nail), not including thumb

⑦T23.739   Corrosion of third degree of unspecified multiple fingers (nail), not including thumb

T23.74   Corrosion of third degree of multiple fingers (nail), including thumb

⑦T23.741   Corrosion of third degree of multiple right fingers (nail), including thumb

⑦T23.742   Corrosion of third degree of multiple left fingers (nail), including thumb

⑦T23.749   Corrosion of third degree of unspecified multiple fingers (nail), including thumb

T23.75   Corrosion of third degree of palm

⑦T23.751   Corrosion of third degree of right palm

⑦T23.752   Corrosion of third degree of left palm

⑦T23.759   Corrosion of third degree of unspecified palm

T23.76   Corrosion of third degree of back of hand

⑦T23.761   Corrosion of third degree of back of right hand

⑦T23.762   Corrosion of third degree of back of left hand

⑦T23.769   Corrosion of third degree back of unspecified hand

T23.77   Corrosion of third degree of wrist

⑦T23.771   Corrosion of third degree of right wrist

⑦T23.772   Corrosion of third degree of left wrist

⑦T23.779   Corrosion of third degree of unspecified wrist

T23.79   Corrosion of third degree of multiple sites of wrist and hand

⑦T23.791   Corrosion of third degree of multiple sites of right wrist and hand

⑦T23.792   Corrosion of third degree of multiple sites of left wrist and hand

⑦T23.799   Corrosion of third degree of multiple sites of unspecified wrist and hand

T24   Burn and corrosion of lower limb, except ankle and foot

Excludes2: burn and corrosion of ankle and foot (T25.-)

burn and corrosion of hip region (T21.-)

The appropriate 7th character is to be added to each code from category T24

A - initial encounter

D - subsequent encounter

S - sequela

T24.0   Burn of unspecified degree of lower limb, except ankle and foot

Use additional external cause code to identify the source, place and intent of the burn (X00-X19, X75-X77, X96-X98, Y92)

T24.00   Burn of unspecified degree of unspecified site of lower limb, except ankle and foot

⑦T24.001   Burn of unspecified degree of unspecified site of right lower limb, except ankle and foot

⑦T24.002   Burn of unspecified degree of unspecified site of left lower limb, except ankle and foot

⑦T24.009   Burn of unspecified degree of unspecified site of unspecified lower limb, except ankle and foot

T24.01   Burn of unspecified degree of thigh

⑦**T24.011**   Burn of unspecified degree of right thigh

⑦**T24.012**   Burn of unspecified degree of left thigh

⑦**T24.019**   Burn of unspecified degree of unspecified thigh

T24.02   Burn of unspecified degree of knee

⑦**T24.021**   Burn of unspecified degree of right knee

⑦**T24.022**   Burn of unspecified degree of left knee

⑦**T24.029**   Burn of unspecified degree of unspecified knee

T24.03   Burn of unspecified degree of lower leg

⑦**T24.031**   Burn of unspecified degree of right lower leg

⑦**T24.032**   Burn of unspecified degree of left lower leg

⑦**T24.039**   Burn of unspecified degree of unspecified lower leg

T24.09   Burn of unspecified degree of multiple sites of lower limb, except ankle and foot

⑦**T24.091**   Burn of unspecified degree of multiple sites of right lower limb, except ankle and foot

⑦**T24.092**   Burn of unspecified degree of multiple sites of left lower limb, except ankle and foot

⑦**T24.099**   Burn of unspecified degree of multiple sites of unspecified lower limb, except ankle and foot

T24.1   Burn of first degree of lower limb, except ankle and foot

Use additional external cause code to identify the source, place and intent of the burn (X00-X19, X75-X77, X96-X98, Y92)

T24.10   Burn of first degree of unspecified site of lower limb, except ankle and foot

⑦**T24.101**   Burn of first degree of unspecified site of right lower limb, except ankle and foot

⑦**T24.102**   Burn of first degree of unspecified site of left lower limb, except ankle and foot

⑦**T24.109**   Burn of first degree of unspecified site of unspecified lower limb, except ankle and foot

T24.11   Burn of first degree of thigh

⑦**T24.111**   Burn of first degree of right thigh

⑦**T24.112**   Burn of first degree of left thigh

⑦**T24.119**   Burn of first degree of unspecified thigh

T24.12   Burn of first degree of knee

⑦**T24.121**   Burn of first degree of right knee

⑦**T24.122**   Burn of first degree of left knee

⑦**T24.129**   Burn of first degree of unspecified knee

T24.13   Burn of first degree of lower leg

⑦**T24.131**   Burn of first degree of right lower leg

⑦**T24.132**   Burn of first degree of left lower leg

⑦**T24.139**   Burn of first degree of unspecified lower leg

T24.19   Burn of first degree of multiple sites of lower limb, except ankle and foot

⑦**T24.191**   Burn of first degree of multiple sites of right lower limb, except ankle and foot

⑦**T24.192**   Burn of first degree of multiple sites of left lower limb, except ankle and foot

⑦**T24.199**   Burn of first degree of multiple sites of unspecified lower limb, except ankle and foot

T24.2   Burn of second degree of lower limb, except ankle and foot

Use additional external cause code to identify the source, place and intent of the burn (X00-X19, X75-X77, X96-X98, Y92)

T24.20   Burn of second degree of unspecified site of lower limb, except ankle and foot

⑦**T24.201**   Burn of second degree of unspecified site of right lower limb, except ankle and foot

⑦**T24.202**   Burn of second degree of unspecified site of left lower limb, except ankle and foot

⑦**T24.209**   Burn of second degree of unspecified site of unspecified lower limb, except ankle and foot

T24.21   Burn of second degree of thigh

⑦**T24.211**   Burn of second degree of right thigh

⑦**T24.212**   Burn of second degree of left thigh

⑦**T24.219**   Burn of second degree of unspecified thigh

T24.22   Burn of second degree of knee

⑦**T24.221**   Burn of second degree of right knee

⑦**T24.222**   Burn of second degree of left knee

⑦**T24.229**   Burn of second degree of unspecified knee

T24.23   Burn of second degree of lower leg

⑦**T24.231**   Burn of second degree of right lower leg

⑦**T24.232**   Burn of second degree of left lower leg

⑦**T24.239**   Burn of second degree of unspecified lower leg

T24.29   Burn of second degree of multiple sites of lower limb, except ankle and foot

⑦**T24.291**   Burn of second degree of multiple sites of right lower limb, except ankle and foot

⑦**T24.292**   Burn of second degree of multiple sites of left lower limb, except ankle and foot

⑦**T24.299**   Burn of second degree of multiple sites of unspecified lower limb, except ankle and foot

T24.3   Burn of third degree of lower limb, except ankle and foot

Use additional external cause code to identify the source, place and intent of the burn (X00-X19, X75-X77, X96-X98, Y92)

T24.30   Burn of third degree of unspecified site of lower limb, except ankle and foot

⑦**T24.301**   Burn of third degree of unspecified site of right lower limb, except ankle and foot

⑦**T24.302**   Burn of third degree of unspecified site of left lower limb, except ankle and foot

● New code   ▲ Revised code   **Excludes1:** Not coded here   **Excludes2:** Not included here   ⊗ Placeholder required   ⑦7ᵗʰ digit required

⑦T24.309 Burn of third degree of unspecified site of unspecified lower limb, except ankle and foot

T24.31 Burn of third degree of thigh

⑦T24.311 Burn of third degree of right thigh

⑦T24.312 Burn of third degree of left thigh

⑦T24.319 Burn of third degree of unspecified thigh

T24.32 Burn of third degree of knee

⑦T24.321 Burn of third degree of right knee

⑦T24.322 Burn of third degree of left knee

⑦T24.329 Burn of third degree of unspecified knee

T24.33 Burn of third degree of lower leg

⑦T24.331 Burn of third degree of right lower leg

⑦T24.332 Burn of third degree of left lower leg

⑦T24.339 Burn of third degree of unspecified lower leg

T24.39 Burn of third degree of multiple sites of lower limb, except ankle and foot

⑦T24.391 Burn of third degree of multiple sites of right lower limb, except ankle and foot

⑦T24.392 Burn of third degree of multiple sites of left lower limb, except ankle and foot

⑦T24.399 Burn of third degree of multiple sites of unspecified lower limb, except ankle and foot

T24.4 Corrosion of unspecified degree of lower limb, except ankle and foot

Code first (T51-T65) to identify chemical and intent

Use additional external cause code to identify place (Y92)

T24.40 Corrosion of unspecified degree of unspecified site of lower limb, except ankle and foot

⑦T24.401 Corrosion of unspecified degree of unspecified site of right lower limb, except ankle and foot

⑦T24.402 Corrosion of unspecified degree of unspecified site of left lower limb, except ankle and foot

⑦T24.409 Corrosion of unspecified degree of unspecified site of unspecified lower limb, except ankle and foot

T24.41 Corrosion of unspecified degree of thigh

⑦T24.411 Corrosion of unspecified degree of right thigh

⑦T24.412 Corrosion of unspecified degree of left thigh

⑦T24.419 Corrosion of unspecified degree of unspecified thigh

T24.42 Corrosion of unspecified degree of knee

⑦T24.421 Corrosion of unspecified degree of right knee

⑦T24.422 Corrosion of unspecified degree of left knee

⑦T24.429 Corrosion of unspecified degree of unspecified knee

T24.43 Corrosion of unspecified degree of lower leg

⑦T24.431 Corrosion of unspecified degree of right lower leg

⑦T24.432 Corrosion of unspecified degree of left lower leg

⑦T24.439 Corrosion of unspecified degree of unspecified lower leg

T24.49 Corrosion of unspecified degree of multiple sites of lower limb, except ankle and foot

⑦T24.491 Corrosion of unspecified degree of multiple sites of right lower limb, except ankle and foot

⑦T24.492 Corrosion of unspecified degree of multiple sites of left lower limb, except ankle and foot

⑦T24.499 Corrosion of unspecified degree of multiple sites of unspecified lower limb, except ankle and foot

T24.5 Corrosion of first degree of lower limb, except ankle and foot

Code first (T51-T65) to identify chemical and intent

Use additional external cause code to identify place (Y92)

T24.50 Corrosion of first degree of unspecified site of lower limb, except ankle and foot

⑦T24.501 Corrosion of first degree of unspecified site of right lower limb, except ankle and foot

⑦T24.502 Corrosion of first degree of unspecified site of left lower limb, except ankle and foot

⑦T24.509 Corrosion of first degree of unspecified site of unspecified lower limb, except ankle and foot

T24.51 Corrosion of first degree of thigh

⑦T24.511 Corrosion of first degree of right thigh

⑦T24.512 Corrosion of first degree of left thigh

⑦T24.519 Corrosion of first degree of unspecified thigh

T24.52 Corrosion of first degree of knee

⑦T24.521 Corrosion of first degree of right knee

⑦T24.522 Corrosion of first degree of left knee

⑦T24.529 Corrosion of first degree of unspecified knee

T24.53 Corrosion of first degree of lower leg

⑦T24.531 Corrosion of first degree of right lower leg

⑦T24.532 Corrosion of first degree of left lower leg

⑦T24.539 Corrosion of first degree of unspecified lower leg

T24.59 Corrosion of first degree of multiple sites of lower limb, except ankle and foot

⑦T24.591 Corrosion of first degree of multiple sites of right lower limb, except ankle and foot

⑦T24.592 Corrosion of first degree of multiple sites of left lower limb, except ankle and foot

⑦T24.599 Corrosion of first degree of multiple sites of unspecified lower limb, except ankle and foot

T24.6 Corrosion of second degree of lower limb, except ankle and foot

Code first (T51-T65) to identify chemical and intent

Use additional external cause code to identify place (Y92)

T24.60 Corrosion of second degree of unspecified site of lower limb, except ankle and foot

⑦T24.601 Corrosion of second degree of unspecified site of right lower limb, except ankle and foot

⑦T24.602 Corrosion of second degree of unspecified site of left lower limb, except ankle and foot

⑦T24.609 Corrosion of second degree of unspecified site of unspecified lower limb, except ankle and foot

T24.61 Corrosion of second degree of thigh

⑦T24.611 Corrosion of second degree of right thigh

⑦T24.612 Corrosion of second degree of left thigh

⑦T24.619 Corrosion of second degree of unspecified thigh

T24.62 Corrosion of second degree of knee

⑦T24.621 Corrosion of second degree of right knee

⑦T24.622 Corrosion of second degree of left knee

⑦T24.629 Corrosion of second degree of unspecified knee

T24.63 Corrosion of second degree of lower leg

⑦T24.631 Corrosion of second degree of right lower leg

⑦T24.632 Corrosion of second degree of left lower leg

⑦T24.639 Corrosion of second degree of unspecified lower leg

T24.69 Corrosion of second degree of multiple sites of lower limb, except ankle and foot

⑦T24.691 Corrosion of second degree of multiple sites of right lower limb, except ankle and foot

⑦T24.692 Corrosion of second degree of multiple sites of left lower limb, except ankle and foot

⑦T24.699 Corrosion of second degree of multiple sites of unspecified lower limb, except ankle and foot

T24.7 Corrosion of third degree of lower limb, except ankle and foot

Code first (T51-T65) to identify chemical and intent

Use additional external cause code to identify place (Y92)

T24.70 Corrosion of third degree of unspecified site of lower limb, except ankle and foot

⑦T24.701 Corrosion of third degree of unspecified site of right lower limb, except ankle and foot

⑦T24.702 Corrosion of third degree of unspecified site of left lower limb, except ankle and foot

⑦T24.709 Corrosion of third degree of unspecified site of unspecified lower limb, except ankle and foot

T24.71 Corrosion of third degree of thigh

⑦T24.711 Corrosion of third degree of right thigh

⑦T24.712 Corrosion of third degree of left thigh

⑦T24.719 Corrosion of third degree of unspecified thigh

T24.72 Corrosion of third degree of knee

⑦T24.721 Corrosion of third degree of right knee

⑦T24.722 Corrosion of third degree of left knee

⑦T24.729 Corrosion of third degree of unspecified knee

T24.73 Corrosion of third degree of lower leg

⑦T24.731 Corrosion of third degree of right lower leg

⑦T24.732 Corrosion of third degree of left lower leg

⑦T24.739 Corrosion of third degree of unspecified lower leg

T24.79 Corrosion of third degree of multiple sites of lower limb, except ankle and foot

⑦T24.791 Corrosion of third degree of multiple sites of right lower limb, except ankle and foot

⑦T24.792 Corrosion of third degree of multiple sites of left lower limb, except ankle and foot

⑦T24.799 Corrosion of third degree of multiple sites of unspecified lower limb, except ankle and foot

T25 **Burn and corrosion of ankle and foot**

The appropriate 7th character is to be added to each code from category T25

A - initial encounter

D - subsequent encounter

S - sequela

T25.0 Burn of unspecified degree of ankle and foot

Use additional external cause code to identify the source, place and intent of the burn (X00-X19, X75-X77, X96-X98, Y92)

T25.01 Burn of unspecified degree of ankle

⑦T25.011 Burn of unspecified degree of right ankle

⑦T25.012 Burn of unspecified degree of left ankle

⑦T25.019 Burn of unspecified degree of unspecified ankle

T25.02 Burn of unspecified degree of foot

Excludes2: burn of unspecified degree of toe(s) (nail) (T25.03-)

⑦T25.021 Burn of unspecified degree of right foot

⑦T25.022 Burn of unspecified degree of left foot

⑦T25.029 Burn of unspecified degree of unspecified foot

T25.03 Burn of unspecified degree of toe(s) (nail)

⑦T25.031 Burn of unspecified degree of right toe(s) (nail)

⑦T25.032 Burn of unspecified degree of left toe(s) (nail)

⑦T25.039 Burn of unspecified degree of unspecified toe(s) (nail)

T25.09 Burn of unspecified degree of multiple sites of ankle and foot

⑦T25.091 Burn of unspecified degree of multiple sites of right ankle and foot

⑦T25.092 Burn of unspecified degree of multiple sites of left ankle and foot

● New code   ▲ Revised code   **Excludes1:** Not coded here   **Excludes2:** Not included here   ⊗ Placeholder required   ⑦ 7th digit required

⑦T25.099   Burn of unspecified degree of multiple sites of unspecified ankle and foot

T25.1   **Burn of first degree of ankle and foot**

Use additional external cause code to identify the source, place and intent of the burn (X00-X19, X75-X77, X96-X98, Y92)

T25.11   **Burn of first degree of ankle**

⑦T25.111   **Burn of first degree of right ankle**

⑦T25.112   **Burn of first degree of left ankle**

⑦T25.119   **Burn of first degree of unspecified ankle**

T25.12   **Burn of first degree of foot**

> Excludes2: burn of first degree of toe(s) (nail) (T25.13-)

⑦T25.121   **Burn of first degree of right foot**

⑦T25.122   **Burn of first degree of left foot**

⑦T25.129   **Burn of first degree of unspecified foot**

T25.13   **Burn of first degree of toe(s) (nail)**

⑦T25.131   **Burn of first degree of right toe(s) (nail)**

⑦T25.132   **Burn of first degree of left toe(s) (nail)**

⑦T25.139   **Burn of first degree of unspecified toe(s) (nail)**

T25.19   **Burn of first degree of multiple sites of ankle and foot**

⑦T25.191   **Burn of first degree of multiple sites of right ankle and foot**

⑦T25.192   **Burn of first degree of multiple sites of left ankle and foot**

⑦T25.199   **Burn of first degree of multiple sites of unspecified ankle and foot**

T25.2   **Burn of second degree of ankle and foot**

Use additional external cause code to identify the source, place and intent of the burn (X00-X19, X75-X77, X96-X98, Y92)

T25.21   **Burn of second degree of ankle**

⑦T25.211   **Burn of second degree of right ankle**

⑦T25.212   **Burn of second degree of left ankle**

⑦T25.219   **Burn of second degree of unspecified ankle**

T25.22   **Burn of second degree of foot**

> Excludes2: burn of second degree of toe(s) (nail) (T25.23-)

⑦T25.221   **Burn of second degree of right foot**

⑦T25.222   **Burn of second degree of left foot**

⑦T25.229   **Burn of second degree of unspecified foot**

T25.23   **Burn of second degree of toe(s) (nail)**

⑦T25.231   **Burn of second degree of right toe(s) (nail)**

⑦T25.232   **Burn of second degree of left toe(s) (nail)**

⑦T25.239   **Burn of second degree of unspecified toe(s) (nail)**

T25.29   **Burn of second degree of multiple sites of ankle and foot**

⑦T25.291   **Burn of second degree of multiple sites of right ankle and foot**

⑦T25.292   **Burn of second degree of multiple sites of left ankle and foot**

⑦T25.299   **Burn of second degree of multiple sites of unspecified ankle and foot**

T25.3   **Burn of third degree of ankle and foot**

Use additional external cause code to identify the source, place and intent of the burn (X00-X19, X75-X77, X96-X98, Y92)

T25.31   **Burn of third degree of ankle**

⑦T25.311   **Burn of third degree of right ankle**

⑦T25.312   **Burn of third degree of left ankle**

⑦T25.319   **Burn of third degree of unspecified ankle**

T25.32   **Burn of third degree of foot**

> Excludes2: burn of third degree of toe(s) (nail) (T25.33-)

⑦T25.321   **Burn of third degree of right foot**

⑦T25.322   **Burn of third degree of left foot**

⑦T25.329   **Burn of third degree of unspecified foot**

T25.33   **Burn of third degree of toe(s) (nail)**

⑦T25.331   **Burn of third degree of right toe(s) (nail)**

⑦T25.332   **Burn of third degree of left toe(s) (nail)**

⑦T25.339   **Burn of third degree of unspecified toe(s) (nail)**

T25.39   **Burn of third degree of multiple sites of ankle and foot**

⑦T25.391   **Burn of third degree of multiple sites of right ankle and foot**

⑦T25.392   **Burn of third degree of multiple sites of left ankle and foot**

⑦T25.399   **Burn of third degree of multiple sites of unspecified ankle and foot**

T25.4   **Corrosion of unspecified degree of ankle and foot**

Code first (T51-T65) to identify chemical and intent

Use additional external cause code to identify place (Y92)

T25.41   **Corrosion of unspecified degree of ankle**

⑦T25.411   **Corrosion of unspecified degree of right ankle**

⑦T25.412   **Corrosion of unspecified degree of left ankle**

⑦T25.419   **Corrosion of unspecified degree of unspecified ankle**

T25.42   **Corrosion of unspecified degree of foot**

> Excludes2: corrosion of unspecified degree of toe(s) (nail) (T25.43-)

⑦T25.421   **Corrosion of unspecified degree of right foot**

⑦T25.422   **Corrosion of unspecified degree of left foot**

⑦T25.429   **Corrosion of unspecified degree of unspecified foot**

T25.43   **Corrosion of unspecified degree of toe(s) (nail)**

⑦T25.431   **Corrosion of unspecified degree of right toe(s) (nail)**

⑦T25.432   **Corrosion of unspecified degree of left toe(s) (nail)**

⑦T25.439   **Corrosion of unspecified degree of unspecified toe(s) (nail)**

T25.49 Corrosion of unspecified degree of multiple sites of ankle and foot

⑦T25.491 Corrosion of unspecified degree of multiple sites of right ankle and foot

⑦T25.492 Corrosion of unspecified degree of multiple sites of left ankle and foot

⑦T25.499 Corrosion of unspecified degree of multiple sites of unspecified ankle and foot

T25.5 Corrosion of first degree of ankle and foot

Code first (T51-T65) to identify chemical and intent

Use additional external cause code to identify place (Y92)

T25.51 Corrosion of first degree of ankle

⑦T25.511 Corrosion of first degree of right ankle

⑦T25.512 Corrosion of first degree of left ankle

⑦T25.519 Corrosion of first degree of unspecified ankle

T25.52 Corrosion of first degree of foot

Excludes2: corrosion of first degree of toe(s) (nail) (T25.53-)

⑦T25.521 Corrosion of first degree of right foot

⑦T25.522 Corrosion of first degree of left foot

⑦T25.529 Corrosion of first degree of unspecified foot

T25.53 Corrosion of first degree of toe(s) (nail)

⑦T25.531 Corrosion of first degree of right toe(s) (nail)

⑦T25.532 Corrosion of first degree of left toe(s) (nail)

⑦T25.539 Corrosion of first degree of unspecified toe(s) (nail)

T25.59 Corrosion of first degree of multiple sites of ankle and foot

⑦T25.591 Corrosion of first degree of multiple sites of right ankle and foot

⑦T25.592 Corrosion of first degree of multiple sites of left ankle and foot

⑦T25.599 Corrosion of first degree of multiple sites of unspecified ankle and foot

T25.6 Corrosion of second degree of ankle and foot

Code first (T51-T65) to identify chemical and intent

Use additional external cause code to identify place (Y92)

T25.61 Corrosion of second degree of ankle

⑦T25.611 Corrosion of second degree of right ankle

⑦T25.612 Corrosion of second degree of left ankle

⑦T25.619 Corrosion of second degree of unspecified ankle

T25.62 Corrosion of second degree of foot

Excludes2: corrosion of second degree of toe(s) (nail) (T25.63-)

⑦T25.621 Corrosion of second degree of right foot

⑦T25.622 Corrosion of second degree of left foot

⑦T25.629 Corrosion of second degree of unspecified foot

T25.63 Corrosion of second degree of toe(s) (nail)

⑦T25.631 Corrosion of second degree of right toe(s) (nail)

⑦T25.632 Corrosion of second degree of left toe(s) (nail)

⑦T25.639 Corrosion of second degree of unspecified toe(s) (nail)

⑦T25.69 Corrosion of second degree of multiple sites of ankle and foot

⑦T25.691 Corrosion of second degree of right ankle and foot

⑦T25.692 Corrosion of second degree of left ankle and foot

⑦T25.699 Corrosion of second degree of unspecified ankle and foot

T25.7 Corrosion of third degree of ankle and foot

Code first (T51-T65) to identify chemical and intent

Use additional external cause code to identify place (Y92)

T25.71 Corrosion of third degree of ankle

⑦T25.711 Corrosion of third degree of right ankle

⑦T25.712 Corrosion of third degree of left ankle

⑦T25.719 Corrosion of third degree of unspecified ankle

T25.72 Corrosion of third degree of foot

Excludes2: corrosion of third degree of toe(s) (nail) (T25.73-)

⑦T25.721 Corrosion of third degree of right foot

⑦T25.722 Corrosion of third degree of left foot

⑦T25.729 Corrosion of third degree of unspecified foot

⑦T25.73 Corrosion of third degree of toe(s) (nail)

⑦T25.731 Corrosion of third degree of right toe(s) (nail)

⑦T25.732 Corrosion of third degree of left toe(s) (nail)

⑦T25.739 Corrosion of third degree of unspecified toe(s) (nail)

T25.79 Corrosion of third degree of multiple sites of ankle and foot

⑦T25.791 Corrosion of third degree of multiple sites of right ankle and foot

⑦T25.792 Corrosion of third degree of multiple sites of left ankle and foot

⑦T25.799 Corrosion of third degree of multiple sites of unspecified ankle and foot

BURNS AND CORROSIONS CONFINED TO EYE AND INTERNAL ORGANS (T26-T28)

T26 Burn and corrosion confined to eye and adnexa

The appropriate 7th character is to be added to each code from category T26

A - initial encounter

D - subsequent encounter

S - sequela

T26.0 Burn of eyelid and periocular area

Use additional external cause code to identify the source, place and intent of the burn (X00-X19, X75-X77, X96-X98, Y92)

⊗⑦T26.00 Burn of unspecified eyelid and periocular area

⊗⑦T26.01 Burn of right eyelid and periocular area

⊗⑦T26.02 Burn of left eyelid and periocular area

T26.1 Burn of cornea and conjunctival sac

● New code ▲ Revised code **Excludes1:** Not coded here **Excludes2:** Not included here ⊗ Placeholder required ⑦7th digit required

Use **additional** external cause code to identify the source, place and intent of the burn (X00-X19, X75-X77, X96-X98, Y92)

⊗⑦**T26.10**   **Burn of cornea and conjunctival sac, unspecified eye**

⊗⑦**T26.11**   **Burn of cornea and conjunctival sac, right eye**

⊗⑦**T26.12**   **Burn of cornea and conjunctival sac, left eye**

T26.2   **Burn with resulting rupture and destruction of eyeball**

Use **additional** external cause code to identify the source, place and intent of the burn (X00-X19, X75-X77, X96-X98, Y92)

⊗⑦**T26.20**   **Burn with resulting rupture and destruction of unspecified eyeball**

⊗⑦**T26.21**   **Burn with resulting rupture and destruction of right eyeball**

⊗⑦**T26.22**   **Burn with resulting rupture and destruction of left eyeball**

T26.3   **Burns of other specified parts of eye and adnexa**

Use **additional** external cause code to identify the source, place and intent of the burn (X00-X19, X75-X77, X96-X98, Y92)

⊗⑦**T26.30**   **Burns of other specified parts of unspecified eye and adnexa**

⊗⑦**T26.31**   **Burns of other specified parts of right eye and adnexa**

⊗⑦**T26.32**   **Burns of other specified parts of left eye and adnexa**

T26.4   **Burn of eye and adnexa, part unspecified**

Use **additional** external cause code to identify the source, place and intent of the burn (X00-X19, X75-X77, X96-X98, Y92)

⊗⑦**T26.40**   **Burn of unspecified eye and adnexa, part unspecified**

⊗⑦**T26.41**   **Burn of right eye and adnexa, part unspecified**

⊗⑦**T26.42**   **Burn of left eye and adnexa, part unspecified**

T26.5   **Corrosion of eyelid and periocular area**

Code first (T51-T65) to identify chemical and intent

Use **additional** external cause code to identify place (Y92)

⊗⑦**T26.50**   **Corrosion of unspecified eyelid and periocular area**

⊗⑦**T26.51**   **Corrosion of right eyelid and periocular area**

⊗⑦**T26.52**   **Corrosion of left eyelid and periocular area**

T26.6   **Corrosion of cornea and conjunctival sac**

Code first (T51-T65) to identify chemical and intent

Use **additional** external cause code to identify place (Y92)

⊗⑦**T26.60**   **Corrosion of cornea and conjunctival sac, unspecified eye**

⊗⑦**T26.61**   **Corrosion of cornea and conjunctival sac, right eye**

⊗⑦**T26.62**   **Corrosion of cornea and conjunctival sac, left eye**

T26.7   **Corrosion with resulting rupture and destruction of eyeball**

Code first (T51-T65) to identify chemical and intent

Use **additional** external cause code to identify place (Y92)

⊗⑦**T26.70**   **Corrosion with resulting rupture and destruction of unspecified eyeball**

⊗⑦**T26.71**   **Corrosion with resulting rupture and destruction of right eyeball**

⊗⑦**T26.72**   **Corrosion with resulting rupture and destruction of left eyeball**

T26.8   **Corrosions of other specified parts of eye and adnexa**

Code first (T51-T65) to identify chemical and intent

Use **additional** external cause code to identify place (Y92)

⊗⑦**T26.80**   **Corrosions of other specified parts of unspecified eye and adnexa**

⊗⑦**T26.81**   **Corrosions of other specified parts of right eye and adnexa**

⊗⑦**T26.82**   **Corrosions of other specified parts of left eye and adnexa**

⑦**T26.9**   **Corrosion of eye and adnexa, part unspecified**

Code first (T51-T65) to identify chemical and intent

Use **additional** external cause code to identify place (Y92)

⊗⑦**T26.90**   **Corrosion of unspecified eye and adnexa, part unspecified**

⊗⑦**T26.91**   **Corrosion of right eye and adnexa, part unspecified**

⊗⑦**T26.92**   **Corrosion of left eye and adnexa, part unspecified**

T27   **Burn and corrosion of respiratory tract**

Use **additional** external cause code to identify the source and intent of the burn (X00-X19, X75-X77, X96-X98)

Use **additional** external cause code to identify place (Y92)

The appropriate 7th character is to be added to each code from category T27

A - initial encounter

D - subsequent encounter

S - sequela

⊗⑦**T27.0**   **Burn of larynx and trachea**

⊗⑦**T27.1**   **Burn involving larynx and trachea with lung**

⊗⑦**T27.2**   **Burn of other parts of respiratory tract**

Burn of thoracic cavity

⊗⑦**T27.3**   **Burn of respiratory tract, part unspecified**

⊗⑦**T27.4**   **Corrosion of larynx and trachea**

Code first (T51-T65) to identify chemical and intent

⊗⑦**T27.5**   **Corrosion involving larynx and trachea with lung**

Code first (T51-T65) to identify chemical and intent

⊗⑦**T27.6**   **Corrosion of other parts of respiratory tract**

Code first (T51-T65) to identify chemical and intent

⊗⑦**T27.7**   **Corrosion of respiratory tract, part unspecified**

Code first (T51-T65) to identify chemical and intent

T28   **Burn and corrosion of other internal organs**

Use **additional** external cause code to identify the source and intent of the burn (X00-X19, X75-X77, X96-X98)

Use **additional** external cause code to identify place (Y92)

The appropriate 7th character is to be added to each code from category T28

A - initial encounter

D - subsequent encounter

S - sequela

⊗⑦**T28.0**   **Burn of mouth and pharynx**

⊗⑦**T28.1**   **Burn of esophagus**

⊗⑦**T28.2**   **Burn of other parts of alimentary tract**

⊗⑦**T28.3**   **Burn of internal genitourinary organs**

T28.4   **Burns of other and unspecified internal organs**

Code first (T51-T65) to identify chemical and intent

⊗⑦**T28.40**   **Burn of unspecified internal organ**

T28.41   **Burn of ear drum**

⑦**T28.411**   **Burn of right ear drum**

⑦**T28.412**   **Burn of left ear drum**

⑦**T28.419**   **Burn of unspecified ear drum**

⊗⑦**T28.49**   **Burn of other internal organ**

⊗⑦**T28.5**   **Corrosion of mouth and pharynx**

<u>Code first</u> (T51-T65) to identify chemical and intent

⊗⑦**T28.6**   **Corrosion of esophagus**

<u>Code first</u> (T51-T65) to identify chemical and intent

⊗⑦**T28.7**   **Corrosion of other parts of alimentary tract**

<u>Code first</u> (T51-T65) to identify chemical and intent

⊗⑦**T28.8**   **Corrosion of internal genitourinary organs**

<u>Code first</u> (T51-T65) to identify chemical and intent

T28.9   **Corrosions of other and unspecified internal organs**

<u>Code first</u> (T51-T65) to identify chemical and intent

⊗⑦**T28.90**   **Corrosions of unspecified internal organs**

T28.91   **Corrosions of ear drum**

⑦**T28.911**   **Corrosions of right ear drum**

⑦**T28.912**   **Corrosions of left ear drum**

⑦**T28.919**   **Corrosions of unspecified ear drum**

⊗⑦**T28.99**   **Corrosions of other internal organs**

BURNS AND CORROSIONS OF MULTIPLE AND UNSPECIFIED BODY REGIONS (T30-T32)

T30   **Burn and corrosion, body region unspecified**

T30.0   **Burn of unspecified body region, unspecified degree**

This code is not for inpatient use. Code to specified site and degree of burns

Burn NOS

Multiple burns NOS

T30.4   **Corrosion of unspecified body region, unspecified degree**

This code is not for inpatient use. Code to specified site and degree of corrosion

Corrosion NOS

Multiple corrosion NOS

T31   **Burns classified according to extent of body surface involved**

Note: This category is to be used as the primary code only when the site of the burn is unspecified. It should be used as a supplementary code with categories T20-T25 when the site is specified.

T31.0   **Burns involving less than 10% of body surface**

T31.1   **Burns involving 10-19% of body surface**

T31.10   **Burns involving 10-19% of body surface with 0% to 9% third degree burns**

Burns involving 10-19% of body surface NOS

T31.11   **Burns involving 10-19% of body surface with 10-19% third degree burns** [HCC]

T31.2   **Burns involving 20-29% of body surface**

T31.20   **Burns involving 20-29% of body surface with 0% to 9% third degree burns**

Burns involving 20-29% of body surface NOS

T31.21   **Burns involving 20-29% of body surface with 10-19% third degree burns** [HCC]

T31.22   **Burns involving 20-29% of body surface with 20-29% third degree burns** [HCC]

T31.3   **Burns involving 30-39% of body surface**

T31.30   **Burns involving 30-39% of body surface with 0% to 9% third degree burns**

Burns involving 30-39% of body surface NOS

T31.31   **Burns involving 30-39% of body surface with 10-19% third degree burns** [HCC]

T31.32   **Burns involving 30-39% of body surface with 20-29% third degree burns** [HCC]

T31.33   **Burns involving 30-39% of body surface with 30-39% third degree burns** [HCC]

T31.4   **Burns involving 40-49% of body surface**

T31.40   **Burns involving 40-49% of body surface with 0% to 9% third degree burns**

Burns involving 40-49% of body surface NOS

T31.41   **Burns involving 40-49% of body surface with 10-19% third degree burns** [HCC]

T31.42   **Burns involving 40-49% of body surface with 20-29% third degree burns** [HCC]

T31.43   **Burns involving 40-49% of body surface with 30-39% third degree burns** [HCC]

T31.44   **Burns involving 40-49% of body surface with 40-49% third degree burns** [HCC]

T31.5   **Burns involving 50-59% of body surface**

T31.50   **Burns involving 50-59% of body surface with 0% to 9% third degree burns**

Burns involving 50-59% of body surface NOS

T31.51   **Burns involving 50-59% of body surface with 10-19% third degree burns** [HCC]

T31.52   **Burns involving 50-59% of body surface with 20-29% third degree burns** [HCC]

T31.53   **Burns involving 50-59% of body surface with 30-39% third degree burns** [HCC]

T31.54   **Burns involving 50-59% of body surface with 40-49% third degree burns** [HCC]

T31.55   **Burns involving 50-59% of body surface with 50-59% third degree burns** [HCC]

T31.6   **Burns involving 60-69% of body surface**

T31.60   **Burns involving 60-69% of body surface with 0% to 9% third degree burns**

Burns involving 60-69% of body surface NOS

T31.61   **Burns involving 60-69% of body surface with 10-19% third degree burns** [HCC]

T31.62   **Burns involving 60-69% of body surface with 20-29% third degree burns** [HCC]

T31.63   **Burns involving 60-69% of body surface with 30-39% third degree burns** [HCC]

T31.64   **Burns involving 60-69% of body surface with 40-49% third degree burns** [HCC]

T31.65   **Burns involving 60-69% of body surface with 50-59% third degree burns** [HCC]

T31.66   **Burns involving 60-69% of body surface with 60-69% third degree burns** [HCC]

T31.7   **Burns involving 70-79% of body surface**

T31.70   **Burns involving 70-79% of body surface with 0% to 9% third degree burns**

Burns involving 70-79% of body surface NOS

T31.71   **Burns involving 70-79% of body surface with 10-19% third degree burns** [HCC]

T31.72   **Burns involving 70-79% of body surface with 20-29% third degree burns** [HCC]

T31.73   **Burns involving 70-79% of body surface with 30-39% third degree burns** [HCC]

T31.74   **Burns involving 70-79% of body surface with 40-49% third degree burns** [HCC]

T31.75   **Burns involving 70-79% of body surface with 50-59% third degree burns** [HCC]

T31.76   **Burns involving 70-79% of body surface with 60-69% third degree burns** [HCC]

T31.77   **Burns involving 70-79% of body surface with 70-79% third degree burns** [HCC]

T31.8   **Burns involving 80-89% of body surface**

T31.80   **Burns involving 80-89% of body surface with 0% to 9% third degree burns**

Burns involving 80-89% of body surface NOS

T31.81 **Burns involving 80-89% of body surface with 10-19% third degree burns** [HCC]

T31.82 **Burns involving 80-89% of body surface with 20-29% third degree burns** [HCC]

T31.83 **Burns involving 80-89% of body surface with 30-39% third degree burns** [HCC]

T31.84 **Burns involving 80-89% of body surface with 40-49% third degree burns** [HCC]

T31.85 **Burns involving 80-89% of body surface with 50-59% third degree burns** [HCC]

T31.86 **Burns involving 80-89% of body surface with 60-69% third degree burns** [HCC]

T31.87 **Burns involving 80-89% of body surface with 70-79% third degree burns** [HCC]

T31.88 **Burns involving 80-89% of body surface with 80-89% third degree burns** [HCC]

T31.9 **Burns involving 90% or more of body surface**

T31.90 **Burns involving 90% or more of body surface with 0% to 9% third degree burns**

Burns involving 90% or more of body surface NOS

T31.91 **Burns involving 90% or more of body surface with 10-19% third degree burns** [HCC]

T31.92 **Burns involving 90% or more of body surface with 20-29% third degree burns**

T31.93 **Burns involving 90% or more of body surface with 30-39% third degree burns** [HCC]

T31.94 **Burns involving 90% or more of body surface with 40-49% third degree burns** [HCC]

T31.95 **Burns involving 90% or more of body surface with 50-59% third degree burns** [HCC]

T31.96 **Burns involving 90% or more of body surface with 60-69% third degree burns** [HCC]

T31.97 **Burns involving 90% or more of body surface with 70-79% third degree burns** [HCC]

T31.98 **Burns involving 90% or more of body surface with 80-89% third degree burns** [HCC]

T31.99 **Burns involving 90% or more of body surface with 90% or more third degree burns** [HCC]

T32 **Corrosions classified according to extent of body surface involved**

Note: This category is to be used as the primary code only when the site of the corrosion is unspecified. It may be used as a supplementary code with categories T20-T25 when the site is specified.

T32.0 **Corrosions involving less than 10% of body surface**

T32.1 **Corrosions involving 10-19% of body surface**

T32.10 **Corrosions involving 10-19% of body surface with 0% to 9% third degree corrosion**

Corrosions involving 10-19% of body surface NOS

T32.11 **Corrosions involving 10-19% of body surface with 10-19% third degree corrosion** [HCC]

T32.2 **Corrosions involving 20-29% of body surface**

T32.20 **Corrosions involving 20-29% of body surface with 0% to 9% third degree corrosion**

T32.21 **Corrosions involving 20-29% of body surface with 10-19% third degree corrosion** [HCC]

T32.22 **Corrosions involving 20-29% of body surface with 20-29% third degree corrosion** [HCC]

T32.3 **Corrosions involving 30-39% of body surface**

T32.30 **Corrosions involving 30-39% of body surface with 0% to 9% third degree corrosion**

T32.31 **Corrosions involving 30-39% of body surface with 10-19% third degree corrosion** [HCC]

T32.32 **Corrosions involving 30-39% of body surface with 20-29% third degree corrosion** [HCC]

T32.33 **Corrosions involving 30-39% of body surface with 30-39% third degree corrosion** [HCC]

T32.4 **Corrosions involving 40-49% of body surface**

T32.40 **Corrosions involving 40-49% of body surface with 0% to 9% third degree corrosion**

T32.41 **Corrosions involving 40-49% of body surface with 10-19% third degree corrosion** [HCC]

T32.42 **Corrosions involving 40-49% of body surface with 20-29% third degree corrosion** [HCC]

T32.43 **Corrosions involving 40-49% of body surface with 30-39% third degree corrosion** [HCC]

T32.44 **Corrosions involving 40-49% of body surface with 40-49% third degree corrosion** [HCC]

T32.5 **Corrosions involving 50-59% of body surface**

T32.50 **Corrosions involving 50-59% of body surface with 0% to 9% third degree corrosion**

T32.51 **Corrosions involving 50-59% of body surface with 10-19% third degree corrosion** [HCC]

T32.52 **Corrosions involving 50-59% of body surface with 20-29% third degree corrosion**

T32.53 **Corrosions involving 50-59% of body surface with 30-39% third degree corrosion** [HCC]

T32.54 **Corrosions involving 50-59% of body surface with 40-49% third degree corrosion** [HCC]

T32.55 **Corrosions involving 50-59% of body surface with 50-59% third degree corrosion** [HCC]

T32.6 **Corrosions involving 60-69% of body surface**

T32.60 **Corrosions involving 60-69% of body surface with 0% to 9% third degree corrosion**

T32.61 **Corrosions involving 60-69% of body surface with 10-19% third degree corrosion** [HCC]

T32.62 **Corrosions involving 60-69% of body surface with 20-29% third degree corrosion** [HCC]

T32.63 **Corrosions involving 60-69% of body surface with 30-39% third degree corrosion** [HCC]

T32.64 **Corrosions involving 60-69% of body surface with 40-49% third degree corrosion** [HCC]

T32.65 **Corrosions involving 60-69% of body surface with 50-59% third degree corrosion** [HCC]

T32.66 **Corrosions involving 60-69% of body surface with 60-69% third degree corrosion** [HCC]

T32.7 **Corrosions involving 70-79% of body surface**

T32.70 **Corrosions involving 70-79% of body surface with 0% to 9% third degree corrosion**

T32.71 **Corrosions involving 70-79% of body surface with 10-19% third degree corrosion** [HCC]

T32.72 **Corrosions involving 70-79% of body surface with 20-29% third degree corrosion** [HCC]

T32.73 **Corrosions involving 70-79% of body surface with 30-39% third degree corrosion** [HCC]

T32.74 **Corrosions involving 70-79% of body surface with 40-49% third degree corrosion** [HCC]

T32.75 **Corrosions involving 70-79% of body surface with 50-59% third degree corrosion** [HCC]

T32.76 **Corrosions involving 70-79% of body surface with 60-69% third degree corrosion** [HCC]

T32.77 **Corrosions involving 70-79% of body surface with 70-79% third degree corrosion** [HCC]

T32.8 **Corrosions involving 80-89% of body surface**

T32.80 Corrosions involving 80-89% of body surface with 0% to 9% third degree corrosion

T32.81 Corrosions involving 80-89% of body surface with 10-19% third degree corrosion [HCC]

T32.82 Corrosions involving 80-89% of body surface with 20-29% third degree corrosion [HCC]

T32.83 Corrosions involving 80-89% of body surface with 30-39% third degree corrosion [HCC]

T32.84 Corrosions involving 80-89% of body surface with 40-49% third degree corrosion [HCC]

T32.85 Corrosions involving 80-89% of body surface with 50-59% third degree corrosion [HCC]

T32.86 Corrosions involving 80-89% of body surface with 60-69% third degree corrosion [HCC]

T32.87 Corrosions involving 80-89% of body surface with 70-79% third degree corrosion [HCC]

T32.88 Corrosions involving 80-89% of body surface with 80-89% third degree corrosion [HCC]

T32.9 **Corrosions involving 90% or more of body surface**

T32.90 Corrosions involving 90% or more of body surface with 0% to 9% third degree corrosion

T32.91 Corrosions involving 90% or more of body surface with 10-19% third degree corrosion [HCC]

T32.92 Corrosions involving 90% or more of body surface with 20-29% third degree corrosion [HCC]

T32.93 Corrosions involving 90% or more of body surface with 30-39% third degree corrosion [HCC]

T32.94 Corrosions involving 90% or more of body surface with 40-49% third degree corrosion [HCC]

T32.95 Corrosions involving 90% or more of body surface with 50-59% third degree corrosion [HCC]

T32.96 Corrosions involving 90% or more of body surface with 60-69% third degree corrosion [HCC]

T32.97 Corrosions involving 90% or more of body surface with 70-79% third degree corrosion [HCC]

T32.98 Corrosions involving 90% or more of body surface with 80-89% third degree corrosion [HCC]

T32.99 Corrosions involving 90% or more of body surface with 90% or more third degree corrosion [HCC]

FROSTBITE (T33-T34)

Excludes2: hypothermia and other effects of reduced temperature (T68, T69.-)

⬛ **T33** **Superficial frostbite**

Includes: frostbite with partial thickness skin loss

The appropriate 7th character is to be added to each code from category T33

A - initial encounter

D - subsequent encounter

S - sequela

T33.0 **Superficial frostbite of head**

T33.01 Superficial frostbite of ear

⑦T33.011 Superficial frostbite of right ear

⑦T33.012 Superficial frostbite of left ear

⑦T33.019 Superficial frostbite of unspecified ear

⊗⑦**T33.02** Superficial frostbite of nose

⊗⑦**T33.09** Superficial frostbite of other part of head

⊗⑦**T33.1** **Superficial frostbite of neck**

⊗⑦**T33.2** **Superficial frostbite of thorax**

⊗⑦**T33.3** **Superficial frostbite of abdominal wall, lower back and pelvis**

T33.4 **Superficial frostbite of arm**

Excludes2: superficial frostbite of wrist and hand (T33.5-)

⊗⑦**T33.40** Superficial frostbite of unspecified arm

⊗⑦**T33.41** Superficial frostbite of right arm

⊗⑦**T33.42** Superficial frostbite of left arm

T33.5 **Superficial frostbite of wrist, hand, and fingers**

T33.51 Superficial frostbite of wrist

⑦T33.511 Superficial frostbite of right wrist

⑦T33.512 Superficial frostbite of left wrist

⑦T33.519 Superficial frostbite of unspecified wrist

T33.52 Superficial frostbite of hand

Excludes2: superficial frostbite of fingers (T33.53-)

⑦T33.521 Superficial frostbite of right hand

⑦T33.522 Superficial frostbite of left hand

⑦T33.529 Superficial frostbite of unspecified hand

T33.53 Superficial frostbite of finger(s)

⑦T33.531 Superficial frostbite of right finger(s)

⑦T33.532 Superficial frostbite of left finger(s)

⑦T33.539 Superficial frostbite of unspecified finger(s)

T33.6 **Superficial frostbite of hip and thigh**

⊗⑦**T33.60** Superficial frostbite of unspecified hip and thigh

⊗⑦**T33.61** Superficial frostbite of right hip and thigh

⊗⑦**T33.62** Superficial frostbite of left hip and thigh

T33.7 **Superficial frostbite of knee and lower leg**

Excludes2: superficial frostbite of ankle and foot (T33.8-)

⊗⑦**T33.70** Superficial frostbite of unspecified knee and lower leg

⊗⑦**T33.71** Superficial frostbite of right knee and lower leg

⊗⑦**T33.72** Superficial frostbite of left knee and lower leg

T33.8 **Superficial frostbite of ankle, foot, and toe(s)**

T33.81 Superficial frostbite of ankle

⑦T33.811 Superficial frostbite of right ankle

⑦T33.812 Superficial frostbite of left ankle

⑦T33.819 Superficial frostbite of unspecified ankle

T33.82 Superficial frostbite of foot

⑦T33.821 Superficial frostbite of right foot

⑦T33.822 Superficial frostbite of left foot

⑦T33.829 Superficial frostbite of unspecified foot

T33.83 Superficial frostbite of toe(s)

⑦T33.831 Superficial frostbite of right toe(s)

⑦T33.832 Superficial frostbite of left toe(s)

⑦T33.839 Superficial frostbite of unspecified toe(s)

T33.9 **Superficial frostbite of other and unspecified sites**

⊗⑦**T33.90** Superficial frostbite of unspecified sites

Superficial frostbite NOS

● New code ▲ Revised code **Excludes1:** Not coded here **Excludes2:** Not included here ⊗ Placeholder required ⑦7th digit required

⊗⑦**T33.99** **Superficial frostbite of other sites**
Superficial frostbite of leg NOS
Superficial frostbite of trunk NOS

T34 **Frostbite with tissue necrosis**

The appropriate 7th character is to be added to each code from category T34

A - initial encounter

D - subsequent encounter

S - sequela

T34.0 **Frostbite with tissue necrosis of head**

T34.01 **Frostbite with tissue necrosis of ear**

⑦**T34.011** **Frostbite with tissue necrosis of right ear**

⑦**T34.012** **Frostbite with tissue necrosis of left ear**

⑦**T34.019** **Frostbite with tissue necrosis of unspecified ear**

⊗⑦**T34.02** **Frostbite with tissue necrosis of nose**

⊗⑦**T34.09** **Frostbite with tissue necrosis of other part of head**

⊗⑦**T34.1** **Frostbite with tissue necrosis of neck**

⊗⑦**T34.2** **Frostbite with tissue necrosis of thorax**

⊗⑦**T34.3** **Frostbite with tissue necrosis of abdominal wall, lower back and pelvis**

T34.4 **Frostbite with tissue necrosis of arm**

Excludes2: frostbite with tissue necrosis of wrist and hand (T34.5-)

⊗⑦**T34.40** **Frostbite with tissue necrosis of unspecified arm**

⊗⑦**T34.41** **Frostbite with tissue necrosis of right arm**

⊗⑦**T34.42** **Frostbite with tissue necrosis of left arm**

T34.5 **Frostbite with tissue necrosis of wrist, hand, and finger(s)**

T34.51 **Frostbite with tissue necrosis of wrist**

⑦**T34.511** **Frostbite with tissue necrosis of right wrist**

⑦**T34.512** **Frostbite with tissue necrosis of left wrist**

⑦**T34.519** **Frostbite with tissue necrosis of unspecified wrist**

T34.52 **Frostbite with tissue necrosis of hand**

Excludes2: frostbite with tissue necrosis of finger(s) (T34.53-)

⑦**T34.521** **Frostbite with tissue necrosis of right hand**

⑦**T34.522** **Frostbite with tissue necrosis of left hand**

⑦**T34.529** **Frostbite with tissue necrosis of unspecified hand**

T34.53 **Frostbite with tissue necrosis of finger(s)**

⑦**T34.531** **Frostbite with tissue necrosis of right finger(s)**

⑦**T34.532** **Frostbite with tissue necrosis of left finger(s)**

⑦**T34.539** **Frostbite with tissue necrosis of unspecified finger(s)**

T34.6 **Frostbite with tissue necrosis of hip and thigh**

⊗⑦**T34.60** **Frostbite with tissue necrosis of unspecified hip and thigh**

⊗⑦**T34.61** **Frostbite with tissue necrosis of right hip and thigh**

⊗⑦**T34.62** **Frostbite with tissue necrosis of left hip and thigh**

T34.7 **Frostbite with tissue necrosis of knee and lower leg**

Excludes2: frostbite with tissue necrosis of ankle and foot (T34.8-)

⊗⑦**T34.70** **Frostbite with tissue necrosis of unspecified knee and lower leg**

⊗⑦**T34.71** **Frostbite with tissue necrosis of right knee and lower leg**

⊗⑦**T34.72** **Frostbite with tissue necrosis of left knee and lower leg**

T34.8 **Frostbite with tissue necrosis of ankle, foot, and toe(s)**

T34.81 **Frostbite with tissue necrosis of ankle**

⑦**T34.811** **Frostbite with tissue necrosis of right ankle**

⑦**T34.812** **Frostbite with tissue necrosis of left ankle**

⑦**T34.819** **Frostbite with tissue necrosis of unspecified ankle**

T34.82 **Frostbite with tissue necrosis of foot**

⑦**T34.821** **Frostbite with tissue necrosis of right foot**

⑦**T34.822** **Frostbite with tissue necrosis of left foot**

⑦**T34.829** **Frostbite with tissue necrosis of unspecified foot**

T34.83 **Frostbite with tissue necrosis of toe(s)**

⑦**T34.831** **Frostbite with tissue necrosis of right toe(s)**

⑦**T34.832** **Frostbite with tissue necrosis of left toe(s)**

⑦**T34.839** **Frostbite with tissue necrosis of unspecified toe(s)**

T34.9 **Frostbite with tissue necrosis of other and unspecified sites**

⊗⑦**T34.90** **Frostbite with tissue necrosis of unspecified sites**
Frostbite with tissue necrosis NOS

⊗⑦**T34.99** **Frostbite with tissue necrosis of other sites**
Frostbite with tissue necrosis of leg NOS
Frostbite with tissue necrosis of trunk NOS

POISONING BY ADVERSE EFFECTS OF AND UNDERDOSING OF DRUGS, MEDICAMENTS AND BIOLOGICAL SUBSTANCES (T36-T50)

Includes: adverse effect of correct substance properly administered

poisoning by overdose of substance

poisoning by wrong substance given or taken in error underdosing by (inadvertently) (deliberately) taking less substance than prescribed or instructed

Code first, for adverse effects, the nature of the adverse effect, such as:

adverse effect NOS (T88.7)

aspirin gastritis (K29.-)

blood disorders (D56-D76)

contact dermatitis (L23-L25)

dermatitis due to substances taken internally (L27.-)

nephropathy (N14.0-N14.2)

Note: The drug giving rise to the adverse effect should be identified by use of codes from categories T36-T50 with fifth or sixth character 5.

Use Additional Code(s) to specify:

manifestations of poisoning

underdosing or failure in dosage during medical and surgical care (Y63.6, Y63.8-Y63.9)

underdosing of medication regimen (Z91.12-, Z91.13-)

Excludes1: toxic reaction to local anesthesia in pregnancy (O29.3-)

Excludes2: abuse and dependence of psychoactive substances (F10-F19)

abuse of non-dependence-producing substances (F55.-)

drug reaction and poisoning affecting newborn (P00-P96)

immunodeficiency due to drugs (D84.821)

pathological drug intoxication (inebriation) (F10-F19)

T36   **Poisoning by adverse effect of and underdosing of systemic antibiotics**

     Excludes1: antineoplastic antibiotics (T45.1-)

         locally applied antibiotic NEC (T49.0)

         topically used antibiotic for ear, nose and throat (T49.6)

         topically used antibiotic for eye (T49.5)

The appropriate 7th character is to be added to each code from category T36

A - initial encounter

D - subsequent encounter

S - sequela

    T36.0   **Poisoning by adverse effect of and underdosing of penicillins**

       T36.0X   **Poisoning by adverse effect of and underdosing of penicillins**

          ⑦**T36.0X1**   **Poisoning by penicillins, accidental (unintentional)**

              Poisoning by penicillins NOS

          ⑦**T36.0X2**   **Poisoning by penicillins, intentional self-harm** [HCC]

          ⑦**T36.0X3**   **Poisoning by penicillins, assault**

          ⑦**T36.0X4**   **Poisoning by penicillins, undetermined**

          ⑦**T36.0X5**   **Adverse effect of penicillins**

          ⑦**T36.0X6**   **Underdosing of penicillins**

    T36.1   **Poisoning by adverse effect of and underdosing of cephalosporins and other beta-lactam antibiotics**

       T36.1X   **Poisoning by adverse effect of and underdosing of cephalosporins and other beta-lactam antibiotics**

          ⑦**T36.1X1**   **Poisoning by cephalosporins and other beta-lactam antibiotics, accidental (unintentional)**

              Poisoning by cephalosporins and other beta-lactam antibiotics NOS

          ⑦**T36.1X2**   **Poisoning by cephalosporins and other beta-lactam antibiotics, intentional self-harm** [HCC]

          ⑦**T36.1X3**   **Poisoning by cephalosporins and other beta-lactam antibiotics, assault**

          ⑦**T36.1X4**   **Poisoning by cephalosporins and other beta-lactam antibiotics, undetermined**

          ⑦**T36.1X5**   **Adverse effect of cephalosporins and other beta-lactam antibiotics**

          ⑦**T36.1X6**   **Underdosing of cephalosporins and other beta-lactam antibiotics**

    T36.2   **Poisoning by adverse effect of and underdosing of chloramphenicol group**

       T36.2X   **Poisoning by adverse effect of and underdosing of chloramphenicol group**

          ⑦**T36.2X1**   **Poisoning by chloramphenicol group, accidental (unintentional)**

              Poisoning by chloramphenicol group NOS

          ⑦**T36.2X2**   **Poisoning by chloramphenicol group, intentional self-harm** [HCC]

          ⑦**T36.2X3**   **Poisoning by chloramphenicol group, assault**

          ⑦**T36.2X4**   **Poisoning by chloramphenicol group, undetermined**

          ⑦**T36.2X5**   **Adverse effect of chloramphenicol group**

          ⑦**T36.2X6**   **Underdosing of chloramphenicol group**

    T36.3   **Poisoning by adverse effect of and underdosing of macrolides**

       T36.3X   **Poisoning by adverse effect of and underdosing of macrolides**

          ⑦**T36.3X1**   **Poisoning by macrolides, accidental (unintentional)**

              Poisoning by macrolides NOS

          ⑦**T36.3X2**   **Poisoning by macrolides, intentional self-harm** [HCC]

          ⑦**T36.3X3**   **Poisoning by macrolides, assault**

          ⑦**T36.3X4**   **Poisoning by macrolides, undetermined**

          ⑦**T36.3X5**   **Adverse effect of macrolides**

          ⑦**T36.3X6**   **Underdosing of macrolides**

    T36.4   **Poisoning by adverse effect of and underdosing of tetracyclines**

       T36.4X   **Poisoning by adverse effect of and underdosing of tetracyclines**

          ⑦**T36.4X1**   **Poisoning by tetracyclines, accidental (unintentional)**

              Poisoning by tetracyclines NOS

          ⑦**T36.4X2**   **Poisoning by tetracyclines, intentional self-harm** [HCC]

          ⑦**T36.4X3**   **Poisoning by tetracyclines, assault**

          ⑦**T36.4X4**   **Poisoning by tetracyclines, undetermined**

          ⑦**T36.4X5**   **Adverse effect of tetracyclines**

          ⑦**T36.4X6**   **Underdosing of tetracyclines**

    T36.5   **Poisoning by adverse effect of and underdosing of aminoglycosides**

       Poisoning by adverse effect of and underdosing of streptomycin

       T36.5X   **Poisoning by adverse effect of and underdosing of aminoglycosides**

          ⑦**T36.5X1**   **Poisoning by aminoglycosides, accidental (unintentional)**

              Poisoning by aminoglycosides NOS

          ⑦**T36.5X2**   **Poisoning by aminoglycosides, intentional self-harm** [HCC]

          ⑦**T36.5X3**   **Poisoning by aminoglycosides, assault**

          ⑦**T36.5X4**   **Poisoning by aminoglycosides, undetermined**

          ⑦**T36.5X5**   **Adverse effect of aminoglycosides**

          ⑦**T36.5X6**   **Underdosing of aminoglycosides**

    T36.6   **Poisoning by adverse effect of and underdosing of rifampicins**

       T36.6X   **Poisoning by adverse effect of and underdosing of rifampicins**

   ● New code   ▲ Revised code   **Excludes1:** Not coded here   **Excludes2:** Not included here   ⊗ Placeholder required   ⑦7th digit required

⑦**T36.6X1** **Poisoning by rifampicins, accidental (unintentional)**

Poisoning by rifampicins NOS

⑦**T36.6X2** **Poisoning by rifampicins, intentional self-harm** [HCC]

⑦**T36.6X3** **Poisoning by rifampicins, assault**

⑦**T36.6X4** **Poisoning by rifampicins, undetermined**

⑦**T36.6X5** **Adverse effect of rifampicins**

⑦**T36.6X6** **Underdosing of rifampicins**

T36.7 **Poisoning by adverse effect of and underdosing of antifungal antibiotics, systemically used**

T36.7X **Poisoning by adverse effect of and underdosing of antifungal antibiotics, systemically used**

⑦**T36.7X1** **Poisoning by antifungal antibiotics, systemically used, accidental (unintentional)**

Poisoning by antifungal antibiotics, systemically used NOS

⑦**T36.7X2** **Poisoning by antifungal antibiotics, systemically used, intentional self-harm** [HCC]

⑦**T36.7X3** **Poisoning by antifungal antibiotics, systemically used, assault**

⑦**T36.7X4** **Poisoning by antifungal antibiotics, systemically used, undetermined**

⑦**T36.7X5** **Adverse effect of antifungal antibiotics, systemically used**

⑦**T36.7X6** **Underdosing of antifungal antibiotics, systemically used**

T36.8 **Poisoning by adverse effect of and underdosing of other systemic antibiotics**

T36.8X **Poisoning by adverse effect of and underdosing of other systemic antibiotics**

⑦**T36.8X1** **Poisoning by other systemic antibiotics, accidental (unintentional)**

Poisoning by other systemic antibiotics NOS

⑦**T36.8X2** **Poisoning by other systemic antibiotics, intentional self-harm** [HCC]

⑦**T36.8X3** **Poisoning by other systemic antibiotics, assault**

⑦**T36.8X4** **Poisoning by other systemic antibiotics, undetermined**

⑦**T36.8X5** **Adverse effect of other systemic antibiotics**

⑦**T36.8X6** **Underdosing of other systemic antibiotics**

T36.9 **Poisoning by adverse effect of and underdosing of unspecified systemic antibiotic**

⊗⑦**T36.91** **Poisoning by unspecified systemic antibiotic, accidental (unintentional)**

Poisoning by systemic antibiotic NOS

⊗⑦**T36.92** **Poisoning by unspecified systemic antibiotic, intentional self-harm** [HCC]

⊗⑦**T36.93** **Poisoning by unspecified systemic antibiotic, assault**

⊗⑦**T36.94** **Poisoning by unspecified systemic antibiotic, undetermined**

⊗⑦**T36.95** **Adverse effect of unspecified systemic antibiotic**

⊗⑦**T36.96** **Underdosing of unspecified systemic antibiotic**

T37 **Poisoning by adverse effect of and underdosing of other systemic anti-infectives and antiparasitics**

Excludes1: anti-infectives topically used for ear, nose and throat (T49.6-)

anti-infectives topically used for eye (T49.5-)

locally applied anti-infectives NEC (T49.0-)

The appropriate 7th character is to be added to each code from category T37

A - initial encounter

D - subsequent encounter

S - sequela

T37.0 **Poisoning by adverse effect of and underdosing of sulfonamides**

T37.0X **Poisoning by adverse effect of and underdosing of sulfonamides**

⑦**T37.0X1** **Poisoning by sulfonamides, accidental (unintentional)**

Poisoning by sulfonamides NOS

⑦**T37.0X2** **Poisoning by sulfonamides, intentional self-harm** [HCC]

⑦**T37.0X3** **Poisoning by sulfonamides, assault**

⑦**T37.0X4** **Poisoning by sulfonamides, undetermined**

⑦**T37.0X5** **Adverse effect of sulfonamides**

⑦**T37.0X6** **Underdosing of sulfonamides**

T37.1 **Poisoning by adverse effect of and underdosing of antimycobacterial drugs**

Excludes1: rifampicins (T36.6-)

streptomycin (T36.5-)

T37.1X **Poisoning by adverse effect of and underdosing of antimycobacterial drugs**

⑦**T37.1X1** **Poisoning by antimycobacterial drugs, accidental (unintentional)**

Poisoning by antimycobacterial drugs NOS

⑦**T37.1X2** **Poisoning by antimycobacterial drugs, intentional self-harm** [HCC]

⑦**T37.1X3** **Poisoning by antimycobacterial drugs, assault**

⑦**T37.1X4** **Poisoning by antimycobacterial drugs, undetermined**

⑦**T37.1X5** **Adverse effect of antimycobacterial drugs**

⑦**T37.1X6** **Underdosing of antimycobacterial drugs**

T37.2 **Poisoning by adverse effect of and underdosing of antimalarials and drugs acting on other blood protozoa**

Excludes1: hydroxyquinoline derivatives (T37.8-)

T37.2X **Poisoning by adverse effect of and underdosing of antimalarials and drugs acting on other blood protozoa**

⑦**T37.2X1** **Poisoning by antimalarials and drugs acting on other blood protozoa, accidental (unintentional)**

Poisoning by antimalarials and drugs acting on other blood protozoa NOS

⑦**T37.2X2** **Poisoning by antimalarials and drugs acting on other blood protozoa, intentional self-harm** [HCC]

⑦**T37.2X3** **Poisoning by antimalarials and drugs acting on other blood protozoa, assault**

⑦**T37.2X4** **Poisoning by antimalarials and drugs acting on other blood protozoa, undetermined**

⑦**T37.2X5** **Adverse effect of antimalarials and drugs acting on other blood protozoa**

⑦**T37.2X6** **Underdosing of antimalarials and drugs acting on other blood protozoa**

T37.3 **Poisoning by adverse effect of and underdosing of other antiprotozoal drugs**

    T37.3X **Poisoning by adverse effect of and underdosing of other antiprotozoal drugs**

      ⑦**T37.3X1** **Poisoning by other antiprotozoal drugs, accidental (unintentional)**

          Poisoning by other antiprotozoal drugs NOS

      ⑦**T37.3X2** **Poisoning by other antiprotozoal drugs, intentional self-harm** [HCC]

      ⑦**T37.3X3** **Poisoning by other antiprotozoal drugs, assault**

      ⑦**T37.3X4** **Poisoning by other antiprotozoal drugs, undetermined**

      ⑦**T37.3X5** **Adverse effect of other antiprotozoal drugs**

      ⑦**T37.3X6** **Underdosing of other antiprotozoal drugs**

T37.4 **Poisoning by adverse effect of and underdosing of anthelminthics**

    T37.4X **Poisoning by adverse effect of and underdosing of anthelminthics**

      ⑦**T37.4X1** **Poisoning by anthelminthics, accidental (unintentional)**

          Poisoning by anthelminthics NOS

      ⑦**T37.4X2** **Poisoning by anthelminthics, intentional self-harm** [HCC]

      ⑦**T37.4X3** **Poisoning by anthelminthics, assault**

      ⑦**T37.4X4** **Poisoning by anthelminthics, undetermined**

      ⑦**T37.4X5** **Adverse effect of anthelminthics**

      ⑦**T37.4X6** **Underdosing of anthelminthics**

T37.5 **Poisoning by adverse effect of and underdosing of antiviral drugs**

    Excludes1: amantadine (T42.8-)

          cytarabine (T45.1-)

    T37.5X **Poisoning by adverse effect of and underdosing of antiviral drugs**

      ⑦**T37.5X1** **Poisoning by antiviral drugs, accidental (unintentional)**

          Poisoning by antiviral drugs NOS

      ⑦**T37.5X2** **Poisoning by antiviral drugs, intentional self-harm** [HCC]

      ⑦**T37.5X3** **Poisoning by antiviral drugs, assault**

      ⑦**T37.5X4** **Poisoning by antiviral drugs, undetermined**

      ⑦**T37.5X5** **Adverse effect of antiviral drugs**

      ⑦**T37.5X6** **Underdosing of antiviral drugs**

T37.8 **Poisoning by adverse effect of and underdosing of other specified systemic anti-infectives and antiparasitics**

    Poisoning by adverse effect of and underdosing of hydroxyquinoline derivatives

    Excludes1: antimalarial drugs (T37.2-)

    T37.8X **Poisoning by adverse effect of and underdosing of other specified systemic anti-infectives and antiparasitics**

      ⑦**T37.8X1** **Poisoning by other specified systemic anti-infectives and antiparasitics, accidental (unintentional)**

          Poisoning by other specified systemic anti-infectives and antiparasitics NOS

      ⑦**T37.8X2** **Poisoning by other specified systemic anti-infectives and antiparasitics, intentional self-harm**

      ⑦**T37.8X3** **Poisoning by other specified systemic anti-infectives and antiparasitics, assault**

      ⑦**T37.8X4** **Poisoning by other specified systemic anti-infectives and antiparasitics, undetermined**

      ⑦**T37.8X5** **Adverse effect of other specified systemic anti-infectives and antiparasitics**

      ⑦**T37.8X6** **Underdosing of other specified systemic anti-infectives and antiparasitics**

⑦**T37.9** **Poisoning by adverse effect of and underdosing of unspecified systemic anti-infective and antiparasitics**

    ⊗⑦**T37.91** **Poisoning by unspecified systemic anti-infective and antiparasitics, accidental (unintentional)**

      Poisoning by adverse effect of and underdosing of systemic anti-infective and antiparasitics NOS

    ⊗⑦**T37.92** **Poisoning by unspecified systemic anti-infective and antiparasitics, intentional self-harm** [HCC]

    ⊗⑦**T37.93** **Poisoning by unspecified systemic anti-infective and antiparasitics, assault**

    ⊗⑦**T37.94** **Poisoning by unspecified systemic anti-infective and antiparasitics, undetermined**

    ⊗⑦**T37.95** **Adverse effect of unspecified systemic anti-infective and antiparasitic**

    ⊗⑦**T37.96** **Underdosing of unspecified systemic anti-infectives and antiparasitics**

T38 **Poisoning by adverse effect of and underdosing of hormones and their synthetic substitutes and antagonists, not elsewhere classified**

    Excludes1: mineralocorticoids and their antagonists (T50.0-)

          oxytocic hormones (T48.0-)

          parathyroid hormones and derivatives (T50.9-)

The appropriate 7th character is to be added to each code from category T38

A - initial encounter

D - subsequent encounter

S - sequela

T38.0 **Poisoning by adverse effect of and underdosing of glucocorticoids and synthetic analogues**

    Excludes1: glucocorticoids, topically used (T49.-)

    T38.0X **Poisoning by adverse effect of and underdosing of glucocorticoids and synthetic analogues**

      ⑦**T38.0X1** **Poisoning by glucocorticoids and synthetic analogues, accidental (unintentional)**

          Poisoning by glucocorticoids and synthetic analogues NOS

      ⑦**T38.0X2** **Poisoning by glucocorticoids and synthetic analogues, intentional self-harm** [HCC]

      ⑦**T38.0X3** **Poisoning by glucocorticoids and synthetic analogues, assault**

      ⑦**T38.0X4** **Poisoning by glucocorticoids and synthetic analogues, undetermined**

      ⑦**T38.0X5** **Adverse effect of glucocorticoids and synthetic analogues**

● New code   ▲ Revised code   **Excludes1:** Not coded here   **Excludes2:** Not included here   ⊗ Placeholder required   ⑦7th digit required

⑦**T38.0X6** Underdosing of glucocorticoids and synthetic analogues

T38.1 Poisoning by adverse effect of and underdosing of thyroid hormones and substitutes

    T38.1X Poisoning by adverse effect of and underdosing of thyroid hormones and substitutes

      ⑦**T38.1X1** Poisoning by thyroid hormones and substitutes, accidental (unintentional)

        Poisoning by thyroid hormones and substitutes NOS

      ⑦**T38.1X2** Poisoning by thyroid hormones and substitutes, intentional self-harm [HCC]

      ⑦**T38.1X3** Poisoning by thyroid hormones and substitutes, assault

      ⑦**T38.1X4** Poisoning by thyroid hormones and substitutes, undetermined

      ⑦**T38.1X5** Adverse effect of thyroid hormones and substitutes

      ⑦**T38.1X6** Underdosing of thyroid hormones and substitutes

T38.2 Poisoning by adverse effect of and underdosing of antithyroid drugs

    T38.2X Poisoning by adverse effect of and underdosing of antithyroid drugs

      ⑦**T38.2X1** Poisoning by antithyroid drugs, accidental (unintentional)

        Poisoning by antithyroid drugs NOS

      ⑦**T38.2X2** Poisoning by antithyroid drugs, intentional self-harm [HCC]

      ⑦**T38.2X3** Poisoning by antithyroid drugs, assault

      ⑦**T38.2X4** Poisoning by antithyroid drugs, undetermined

      ⑦**T38.2X5** Adverse effect of antithyroid drugs

      ⑦**T38.2X6** Underdosing of antithyroid drugs

T38.3 Poisoning by adverse effect of and underdosing of insulin and oral hypoglycemic [antidiabetic] drugs

    T38.3X Poisoning by adverse effect of and underdosing of insulin and oral hypoglycemic [antidiabetic] drugs

      ⑦**T38.3X1** Poisoning by insulin and oral hypoglycemic [antidiabetic] drugs, accidental (unintentional)

        Poisoning by insulin and oral hypoglycemic [antidiabetic] drugs NOS

      ⑦**T38.3X2** Poisoning by insulin and oral hypoglycemic [antidiabetic] drugs, intentional self-harm [HCC]

      ⑦**T38.3X3** Poisoning by insulin and oral hypoglycemic [antidiabetic] drugs, assault

      ⑦**T38.3X4** Poisoning by insulin and oral hypoglycemic [antidiabetic] drugs, undetermined

      ⑦**T38.3X5** Adverse effect of insulin and oral hypoglycemic [antidiabetic] drugs

      ⑦**T38.3X6** Underdosing of insulin and oral hypoglycemic [antidiabetic] drugs

T38.4 Poisoning by adverse effect of and underdosing of oral contraceptives

    Poisoning by adverse effect of and underdosing of multiple- and single-ingredient oral contraceptive preparations

T38.4X Poisoning by adverse effect of and underdosing of oral contraceptives

    ⑦**T38.4X1** Poisoning by oral contraceptives, accidental (unintentional)

      Poisoning by oral contraceptives NOS

    ⑦**T38.4X2** Poisoning by oral contraceptives, intentional self-harm [HCC]

    ⑦**T38.4X3** Poisoning by oral contraceptives, assault

    ⑦**T38.4X4** Poisoning by oral contraceptives, undetermined

    ⑦**T38.4X5** Adverse effect of oral contraceptives

    ⑦**T38.4X6** Underdosing of oral contraceptives

T38.5 Poisoning by adverse effect of and underdosing of other estrogens and progestogens

    Poisoning by adverse effect of and underdosing of estrogens and progestogens mixtures and substitutes

T38.5X Poisoning by adverse effect of and underdosing of other estrogens and progestogens

    ⑦**T38.5X1** Poisoning by other estrogens and progestogens, accidental (unintentional)

      Poisoning by other estrogens and progestogens NOS

    ⑦**T38.5X2** Poisoning by other estrogens and progestogens, intentional self-harm [HCC]

    ⑦**T38.5X3** Poisoning by other estrogens and progestogens, assault

    ⑦**T38.5X4** Poisoning by other estrogens and progestogens, undetermined

    ⑦**T38.5X5** Adverse effect of other estrogens and progestogens

    ⑦**T38.5X6** Underdosing of other estrogens and progestogens

T38.6 Poisoning by adverse effect of and underdosing of antigonadotrophins, antiestrogens, antiandrogens, not elsewhere classified

    Poisoning by adverse effect of and underdosing of tamoxifen

T38.6X Poisoning by adverse effect of and underdosing of antigonadotrophins, antiestrogens, antiandrogens, not elsewhere classified

    ⑦**T38.6X1** Poisoning by antigonadotrophins, antiestrogens, antiandrogens, not elsewhere classified, accidental (unintentional)

      Poisoning by antigonadotrophins, antiestrogens, antiandrogens, not elsewhere classified NOS

    ⑦**T38.6X2** Poisoning by antigonadotrophins, antiestrogens, antiandrogens, not elsewhere classified, intentional self-harm [HCC]

    ⑦**T38.6X3** Poisoning by antigonadotrophins, antiestrogens, antiandrogens, not elsewhere classified, assault

    ⑦**T38.6X4** Poisoning by antigonadotrophins, antiestrogens, antiandrogens, not elsewhere classified, undetermined

    ⑦**T38.6X5** Adverse effect of antigonadotrophins, antiestrogens, antiandrogens, not elsewhere classified

---

■ Add 4th-7th digits   Nonspecific code   Unspecified code   Manifestation code   [HCC] Hierarchical Condition Code

⑦T38.6X6 **Underdosing of antigonadotrophins, antiestrogens, antiandrogens, not elsewhere classified**

T38.7 **Poisoning by adverse effect of and underdosing of androgens and anabolic congeners**

T38.7X **Poisoning by adverse effect of and underdosing of androgens and anabolic congeners**

⑦T38.7X1 **Poisoning by androgens and anabolic congeners, accidental (unintentional)**

Poisoning by androgens and anabolic congeners NOS

⑦T38.7X2 **Poisoning by androgens and anabolic congeners, intentional self-harm** [HCC]

⑦T38.7X3 **Poisoning by androgens and anabolic congeners, assault**

⑦T38.7X4 **Poisoning by androgens and anabolic congeners, undetermined**

⑦T38.7X5 **Adverse effect of androgens and anabolic congeners**

⑦T38.7X6 **Underdosing of androgens and anabolic congeners**

T38.8 **Poisoning by adverse effect of and underdosing of other and unspecified hormones and synthetic substitutes**

T38.80 **Poisoning by adverse effect of and underdosing of unspecified hormones and synthetic substitutes**

⑦T38.801 **Poisoning by unspecified hormones and synthetic substitutes, accidental (unintentional)**

Poisoning by unspecified hormones and synthetic substitutes NOS

⑦T38.802 **Poisoning by unspecified hormones and synthetic substitutes, intentional self-harm** [HCC]

⑦T38.803 **Poisoning by unspecified hormones and synthetic substitutes, assault**

⑦T38.804 **Poisoning by unspecified hormones and synthetic substitutes, undetermined**

⑦T38.805 **Adverse effect of unspecified hormones and synthetic substitutes**

⑦T38.806 **Underdosing of unspecified hormones and synthetic substitutes**

T38.81 **Poisoning by adverse effect of and underdosing of anterior pituitary [adenohypophyseal] hormones**

⑦T38.811 **Poisoning by anterior pituitary [adenohypophyseal] hormones, accidental (unintentional)**

Poisoning by anterior pituitary [adenohypophyseal] hormones NOS

⑦T38.812 **Poisoning by anterior pituitary [adenohypophyseal] hormones, intentional self-harm** [HCC]

⑦T38.813 **Poisoning by anterior pituitary [adenohypophyseal] hormones, assault**

⑦T38.814 **Poisoning by anterior pituitary [adenohypophyseal] hormones, undetermined**

⑦T38.815 **Adverse effect of anterior pituitary [adenohypophyseal] hormones**

⑦T38.816 **Underdosing of anterior pituitary [adenohypophyseal] hormones**

T38.89 **Poisoning by adverse effect of and underdosing of other hormones and synthetic substitutes**

⑦T38.891 **Poisoning by other hormones and synthetic substitutes, accidental (unintentional)**

Poisoning by other hormones and synthetic substitutes NOS

⑦T38.892 **Poisoning by other hormones and synthetic substitutes, intentional self-harm** [HCC]

⑦T38.893 **Poisoning by other hormones and synthetic substitutes, assault**

⑦T38.894 **Poisoning by other hormones and synthetic substitutes, undetermined**

⑦T38.895 **Adverse effect of other hormones and synthetic substitutes**

⑦T38.896 **Underdosing of other hormones and synthetic substitutes**

T38.9 **Poisoning by adverse effect of and underdosing of other and unspecified hormone antagonists**

T38.90 **Poisoning by adverse effect of and underdosing of unspecified hormone antagonists**

⑦T38.901 **Poisoning by unspecified hormone antagonists, accidental (unintentional)**

Poisoning by unspecified hormone antagonists NOS

⑦T38.902 **Poisoning by unspecified hormone antagonists, intentional self-harm** [HCC]

⑦T38.903 **Poisoning by unspecified hormone antagonists, assault**

⑦T38.904 **Poisoning by unspecified hormone antagonists, undetermined**

⑦T38.905 **Adverse effect of unspecified hormone antagonists**

⑦T38.906 **Underdosing of unspecified hormone antagonists**

T38.99 **Poisoning by adverse effect of and underdosing of other hormone antagonists**

⑦T38.991 **Poisoning by other hormone antagonists, accidental (unintentional)**

Poisoning by other hormone antagonists NOS

⑦T38.992 **Poisoning by other hormone antagonists, intentional self-harm** [HCC]

⑦T38.993 **Poisoning by other hormone antagonists, assault**

⑦T38.994 **Poisoning by other hormone antagonists, undetermined**

⑦T38.995 **Adverse effect of other hormone antagonists**

⑦T38.996 **Underdosing of other hormone antagonists**

T39 **Poisoning by adverse effect of and underdosing of nonopioid analgesics, antipyretics and antirheumatics**

The appropriate 7th character is to be added to each code from category T39

A - initial encounter

D - subsequent encounter

S - sequela

T39.0 **Poisoning by adverse effect of and underdosing of salicylates**

● New code   ▲ Revised code   **Excludes1:** Not coded here   **Excludes2:** Not included here   ⊗ Placeholder required   ⑦7ᵗʰ digit required

T39.01 **Poisoning by adverse effect of and underdosing of aspirin**

Poisoning by adverse effect of and underdosing of acetylsalicylic acid

⑦ **T39.011** **Poisoning by aspirin, accidental (unintentional)**

⑦ **T39.012** **Poisoning by aspirin, intentional self-harm** [HCC]

⑦ **T39.013** **Poisoning by aspirin, assault**

⑦ **T39.014** **Poisoning by aspirin, undetermined**

⑦ **T39.015** **Adverse effect of aspirin**

⑦ **T39.016** **Underdosing of aspirin**

T39.09 **Poisoning by adverse effect of and underdosing of other salicylates**

⑦ **T39.091** **Poisoning by salicylates, accidental (unintentional)**

Poisoning by salicylates NOS

⑦ **T39.092** **Poisoning by salicylates, intentional self-harm** [HCC]

⑦ **T39.093** **Poisoning by salicylates, assault**

⑦ **T39.094** **Poisoning by salicylates, undetermined**

⑦ **T39.095** **Adverse effect of salicylates**

⑦ **T39.096** **Underdosing of salicylates**

T39.1 **Poisoning by adverse effect of and underdosing of 4-Aminophenol derivatives**

T39.1X **Poisoning by adverse effect of and underdosing of 4-Aminophenol derivatives**

⑦ **T39.1X1** **Poisoning by 4-Aminophenol derivatives, accidental (unintentional)**

Poisoning by 4-Aminophenol derivatives NOS

⑦ **T39.1X2** **Poisoning by 4-Aminophenol derivatives, intentional self-harm** [HCC]

⑦ **T39.1X3** **Poisoning by 4-Aminophenol derivatives, assault**

⑦ **T39.1X4** **Poisoning by 4-Aminophenol derivatives, undetermined**

⑦ **T39.1X5** **Adverse effect of 4-Aminophenol derivatives**

⑦ **T39.1X6** **Underdosing of 4-Aminophenol derivatives**

T39.2 **Poisoning by adverse effect of and underdosing of pyrazolone derivatives**

T39.2X **Poisoning by adverse effect of and underdosing of pyrazolone derivatives**

⑦ **T39.2X1** **Poisoning by pyrazolone derivatives, accidental (unintentional)**

Poisoning by pyrazolone derivatives NOS

⑦ **T39.2X2** **Poisoning by pyrazolone derivatives, intentional self-harm** [HCC]

⑦ **T39.2X3** **Poisoning by pyrazolone derivatives, assault**

⑦ **T39.2X4** **Poisoning by pyrazolone derivatives, undetermined**

⑦ **T39.2X5** **Adverse effect of pyrazolone derivatives**

⑦ **T39.2X6** **Underdosing of pyrazolone derivatives**

T39.3 **Poisoning by adverse effect of and underdosing of other nonsteroidal anti-inflammatory drugs [NSAID]**

T39.31 **Poisoning by adverse effect of and underdosing of propionic acid derivatives**

Poisoning by adverse effect of and underdosing of fenoprofen

Poisoning by adverse effect of and underdosing of flurbiprofen

Poisoning by adverse effect of and underdosing of ibuprofen

Poisoning by adverse effect of and underdosing of ketoprofen

Poisoning by adverse effect of and underdosing of naproxen

Poisoning by adverse effect of and underdosing of oxaprozin

⑦ **T39.311** **Poisoning by propionic acid derivatives, accidental (unintentional)**

⑦ **T39.312** **Poisoning by propionic acid derivatives, intentional self-harm** [HCC]

⑦ **T39.313** **Poisoning by propionic acid derivatives, assault**

⑦ **T39.314** **Poisoning by propionic acid derivatives, undetermined**

⑦ **T39.315** **Adverse effect of propionic acid derivatives**

⑦ **T39.316** **Underdosing of propionic acid derivatives**

T39.39 **Poisoning by adverse effect of and underdosing of other nonsteroidal anti-inflammatory drugs [NSAID]**

⑦ **T39.391** **Poisoning by other nonsteroidal anti-inflammatory drugs [NSAID], accidental (unintentional)**

Poisoning by other nonsteroidal anti-inflammatory drugs NOS

⑦ **T39.392** **Poisoning by other nonsteroidal anti-inflammatory drugs [NSAID], intentional self-harm** [HCC]

⑦ **T39.393** **Poisoning by other nonsteroidal anti-inflammatory drugs [NSAID], assault**

⑦ **T39.394** **Poisoning by other nonsteroidal anti-inflammatory drugs [NSAID], undetermined**

⑦ **T39.395** **Adverse effect of other nonsteroidal anti-inflammatory drugs [NSAID]**

⑦ **T39.396** **Underdosing of other nonsteroidal anti-inflammatory drugs [NSAID]**

T39.4 **Poisoning by adverse effect of and underdosing of antirheumatics, not elsewhere classified**

Excludes1: poisoning by adverse effect of and underdosing of glucocorticoids (T38.0-)

poisoning by adverse effect of and underdosing of salicylates (T39.0-)

T39.4X **Poisoning by adverse effect of and underdosing of antirheumatics, not elsewhere classified**

⑦ **T39.4X1** **Poisoning by antirheumatics, not elsewhere classified, accidental (unintentional)**

Poisoning by antirheumatics, not elsewhere classified NOS

⑦ **T39.4X2** **Poisoning by antirheumatics, not elsewhere classified, intentional self-harm** [HCC]

⑦**T39.4X3**   **Poisoning by antirheumatics, not elsewhere classified, assault**

⑦**T39.4X4**   **Poisoning by antirheumatics, not elsewhere classified, undetermined**

⑦**T39.4X5**   **Adverse effect of antirheumatics, not elsewhere classified**

⑦**T39.4X6**   **Underdosing of antirheumatics, not elsewhere classified**

T39.8   **Poisoning by adverse effect of and underdosing of other nonopioid analgesics and antipyretics, not elsewhere classified**

     T39.8X   **Poisoning by adverse effect of and underdosing of other nonopioid analgesics and antipyretics, not elsewhere classified**

       ⑦**T39.8X1**   **Poisoning by other nonopioid analgesics and antipyretics, not elsewhere classified, accidental (unintentional)**

           Poisoning by other nonopioid analgesics and antipyretics, not elsewhere classified NOS

       ⑦**T39.8X2**   **Poisoning by other nonopioid analgesics and antipyretics, not elsewhere classified, intentional self-harm** [HCC]

       ⑦**T39.8X3**   **Poisoning by other nonopioid analgesics and antipyretics, not elsewhere classified, assault**

       ⑦**T39.8X4**   **Poisoning by other nonopioid analgesics and antipyretics, not elsewhere classified, undetermined**

       ⑦**T39.8X5**   **Adverse effect of other nonopioid analgesics and antipyretics, not elsewhere classified**

       ⑦**T39.8X6**   **Underdosing of other nonopioid analgesics and antipyretics, not elsewhere classified**

T39.9   **Poisoning by adverse effect of and underdosing of unspecified nonopioid analgesic, antipyretic and antirheumatic**

     ⊗⑦**T39.91**   **Poisoning by unspecified nonopioid analgesic, antipyretic and antirheumatic, accidental (unintentional)**

         Poisoning by nonopioid analgesic, antipyretic and antirheumatic NOS

     ⊗⑦**T39.92**   **Poisoning by unspecified nonopioid analgesic, antipyretic and antirheumatic, intentional self-harm** [HCC]

     ⊗⑦**T39.93**   **Poisoning by unspecified nonopioid analgesic, antipyretic and antirheumatic, assault**

     ⊗⑦**T39.94**   **Poisoning by unspecified nonopioid analgesic, antipyretic and antirheumatic, undetermined**

     ⊗⑦**T39.95**   **Adverse effect of unspecified nonopioid analgesic, antipyretic and antirheumatic**

     ⊗⑦**T39.96**   **Underdosing of unspecified nonopioid analgesic, antipyretic and antirheumatic**

T40   **Poisoning by adverse effect of and underdosing of narcotics and psychodysleptics [hallucinogens]**

   Excludes2: drug dependence and related mental and behavioral disorders due to psychoactive substance use (F10.-F19.-)

The appropriate 7th character is to be added to each code from category T40

A - initial encounter

D - subsequent encounter

S - sequela

T40.0   **Poisoning by adverse effect of and underdosing of opium**

     T40.0X   **Poisoning by adverse effect of and underdosing of opium**

       ⑦**T40.0X1**   **Poisoning by opium, accidental (unintentional)** [HCC]

           Poisoning by opium NOS

       ⑦**T40.0X2**   **Poisoning by opium, intentional self-harm** [HCC]

       ⑦**T40.0X3**   **Poisoning by opium, assault**

       ⑦**T40.0X4**   **Poisoning by opium, undetermined** [HCC]

       ⑦**T40.0X5**   **Adverse effect of opium**

       ⑦**T40.0X6**   **Underdosing of opium**

T40.1   **Poisoning by and adverse effect of heroin**

     T40.1X   **Poisoning by and adverse effect of heroin**

       ⑦**T40.1X1**   **Poisoning by heroin, accidental (unintentional)** [HCC]

           Poisoning by heroin NOS

       ⑦**T40.1X2**   **Poisoning by heroin, intentional self-harm** [HCC]

       ⑦**T40.1X3**   **Poisoning by heroin, assault**

       ⑦**T40.1X4**   **Poisoning by heroin, undetermined** [HCC]

T40.2   **Poisoning by adverse effect of and underdosing of other opioids**

     T40.2X   **Poisoning by adverse effect of and underdosing of other opioids**

       ⑦**T40.2X1**   **Poisoning by other opioids, accidental (unintentional)** [HCC]

           Poisoning by other opioids NOS

       ⑦**T40.2X2**   **Poisoning by other opioids, intentional self-harm** [HCC]

       ⑦**T40.2X3**   **Poisoning by other opioids, assault**

       ⑦**T40.2X4**   **Poisoning by other opioids, undetermined** [HCC]

       ⑦**T40.2X5**   **Adverse effect of other opioids**

       ⑦**T40.2X6**   **Underdosing of other opioids**

T40.3   **Poisoning by adverse effect of and underdosing of methadone**

     T40.3X   **Poisoning by adverse effect of and underdosing of methadone**

       ⑦**T40.3X1**   **Poisoning by methadone, accidental (unintentional)** [HCC]

           Poisoning by methadone NOS

       ⑦**T40.3X2**   **Poisoning by methadone, intentional self-harm** [HCC]

       ⑦**T40.3X3**   **Poisoning by methadone, assault**

       ⑦**T40.3X4**   **Poisoning by methadone, undetermined** [HCC]

       ⑦**T40.3X5**   **Adverse effect of methadone**

       ⑦**T40.3X6**   **Underdosing of methadone**

T40.4   **Poisoning by adverse effect of and underdosing of other synthetic narcotics**

     T40.41   **Poisoning by adverse effect of and underdosing of fentanyl or fentanyl analogs**

       ⑦**T40.411**   **Poisoning by fentanyl or fentanyl analogs, accidental (unintentional)**

       ⑦**T40.412**   **Poisoning by fentanyl or fentanyl analogs, intentional self-harm**

       ⑦**T40.413**   **Poisoning by fentanyl or fentanyl analogs, assault**

⑦T40.414 **Poisoning by fentanyl or fentanyl analogs, undetermined**

⑦T40.415 **Adverse effect of fentanyl or fentanyl analogs**

⑦T40.416 **Underdosing of fentanyl or fentanyl analogs**

T40.42 **Poisoning by adverse effect of and underdosing of tramadol**

⑦T40.421 **Poisoning by tramadol, accidental (unintentional)**

⑦T40.422 **Poisoning by tramadol, intentional self-harm**

⑦T40.423 **Poisoning by tramadol, assault**

⑦T40.424 **Poisoning by tramadol, undetermined**

⑦T40.425 **Adverse effect of tramadol**

⑦T40.426 **Underdosing of tramadol**

T40.49 **Poisoning by adverse effect of and underdosing of other synthetic narcotics**

⑦T40.491 **Poisoning by other synthetic narcotics, accidental (unintentional)**

⑦T40.492 **Poisoning by other synthetic narcotics, intentional self-harm**

⑦T40.493 **Poisoning by other synthetic narcotics, assault**

⑦T40.494 **Poisoning by other synthetic narcotics, undetermined**

⑦T40.495 **Adverse effect of other synthetic narcotics**

⑦T40.496 **Underdosing of other synthetic narcotics**

T40.5 **Poisoning by adverse effect of and underdosing of cocaine**

T40.5X **Poisoning by adverse effect of and underdosing of cocaine**

⑦T40.5X1 **Poisoning by cocaine, accidental (unintentional)** [HCC]

Poisoning by cocaine NOS

⑦T40.5X2 **Poisoning by cocaine, intentional self-harm** [HCC]

⑦T40.5X3 **Poisoning by cocaine, assault**

⑦T40.5X4 **Poisoning by cocaine, undetermined** [HCC]

⑦T40.5X5 **Adverse effect of cocaine**

⑦T40.5X6 **Underdosing of cocaine**

T40.6 **Poisoning by adverse effect of and underdosing of other and unspecified narcotics**

T40.60 **Poisoning by adverse effect of and underdosing of unspecified narcotics**

⑦T40.601 **Poisoning by unspecified narcotics, accidental (unintentional)** [HCC]

Poisoning by narcotics NOS

⑦T40.602 **Poisoning by unspecified narcotics, intentional self-harm** [HCC]

⑦T40.603 **Poisoning by unspecified narcotics, assault**

⑦T40.604 **Poisoning by unspecified narcotics, undetermined** [HCC]

⑦T40.605 **Adverse effect of unspecified narcotics**

⑦T40.606 **Underdosing of unspecified narcotics**

T40.69 **Poisoning by adverse effect of and underdosing of other narcotics**

⑦T40.691 **Poisoning by other narcotics, accidental (unintentional)** [HCC]

Poisoning by other narcotics NOS

⑦T40.692 **Poisoning by other narcotics, intentional self-harm** [HCC]

⑦T40.693 **Poisoning by other narcotics, assault**

⑦T40.694 **Poisoning by other narcotics, undetermined** [HCC]

⑦T40.695 **Adverse effect of other narcotics**

⑦T40.696 **Underdosing of other narcotics**

T40.7 **Poisoning by adverse effect of and underdosing of cannabis (derivatives)**

• T40.71 **Poisoning by adverse effect of and underdosing of cannabisderivatives)**

• T40.711 **Poisoning by cannabis, accidental (unintentional)**

• T40.712 **Poisoning by cannabis, intentional self-harm**

• T40.713 **Poisoning by cannabis, assault**

• T40.714 **Poisoning by cannabis, undetermined**

• T40.715 **Adverse effect of cannabis**

• T40.716 **Underdosing of cannabis**

• T40.72 **Poisoning by adverse effect of and underdosing of synthetic cannabinoids**

• T40.721 **Poisoning by synthetic cannabinoids, accidental (unintentional)**

• T40.722 **Poisoning by synthetic cannabinoids, intentional self-harm**

• T40.723 **Poisoning by synthetic cannabinoids, assault**

• T40.724 **Poisoning by synthetic cannabinoids, undetermined**

• T40.725 **Adverse effect of synthetic cannabinoids**

• T40.726 **Underdosing of synthetic cannabinoids**

T40.8 **Poisoning by and adverse effect of lysergide [LSD]**

T40.8X **Poisoning by and adverse effect of lysergide [LSD]**

⑦T40.8X1 **Poisoning by lysergide [LSD], accidental (unintentional)** [HCC]

Poisoning by lysergide [LSD] NOS

⑦T40.8X2 **Poisoning by lysergide [LSD], intentional self-harm**

⑦T40.8X3 **Poisoning by lysergide [LSD], assault**

⑦T40.8X4 **Poisoning by lysergide [LSD], undetermined**

T40.9 **Poisoning by adverse effect of and underdosing of other and unspecified psychodysleptics [hallucinogens]**

T40.90 **Poisoning by adverse effect of and underdosing of unspecified psychodysleptics [hallucinogens]**

⑦T40.901 **Poisoning by unspecified psychodysleptics [hallucinogens], accidental (unintentional)** [HCC]

⑦T40.902 **Poisoning by unspecified psychodysleptics [hallucinogens], intentional self-harm** [HCC]

⑦T40.903 **Poisoning by unspecified psychodysleptics [hallucinogens], assault**

⑦T40.904 **Poisoning by unspecified psychodysleptics [hallucinogens], undetermined** [HCC]

⑦**T40.905** **Adverse effect of unspecified**
psychodysleptics [hallucinogens]

⑦**T40.906** **Underdosing of unspecified**
psychodysleptics [hallucinogens]

T40.99 **Poisoning by adverse effect of and underdosing**
of other psychodysleptics [hallucinogens]

⑦**T40.991** **Poisoning by other psychodysleptics**
[hallucinogens], accidental
(unintentional) [HCC]

Poisoning by other psychodysleptics
[hallucinogens] NOS

⑦**T40.992** **Poisoning by other psychodysleptics**
[hallucinogens], intentional self-harm
[HCC]

⑦**T40.993** **Poisoning by other psychodysleptics**
[hallucinogens], assault

⑦**T40.994** **Poisoning by other psychodysleptics**
[hallucinogens], undetermined [HCC]

⑦**T40.995** **Adverse effect of other**
psychodysleptics [hallucinogens]

⑦**T40.996** **Underdosing of other**
psychodysleptics[hallucinogens]

T41 **Poisoning by adverse effect of and underdosing of anesthetics**
and therapeutic gases

Excludes1: benzodiazepines (T42.4-)

cocaine (T40.5-)

complications of anesthesia during pregnancy (O29.-)

complications of anesthesia during labor and delivery (O74.-)

complications of anesthesia during the puerperium (O89.-)

opioids (T40.0-T40.2-)

The appropriate 7th character is to be added to each code from
category T41

A - initial encounter

D - subsequent encounter

S - sequela

T41.0 **Poisoning by adverse effect of and underdosing of**
inhaled anesthetics

Excludes1: oxygen (T41.5-)

T41.0X **Poisoning by adverse effect of and underdosing**
of inhaled anesthetics

⑦**T41.0X1** **Poisoning by inhaled anesthetics,**
accidental (unintentional)

Poisoning by inhaled anesthetics NOS

⑦**T41.0X2** **Poisoning by inhaled anesthetics,**
intentional self-harm [HCC]

⑦**T41.0X3** **Poisoning by inhaled anesthetics,**
assault

⑦**T41.0X4** **Poisoning by inhaled anesthetics,**
undetermined

⑦**T41.0X5** **Adverse effect of inhaled anesthetics**

⑦**T41.0X6** **Underdosing of inhaled anesthetics**

T41.1 **Poisoning by adverse effect of and underdosing of**
intravenous anesthetics

Poisoning by adverse effect of and underdosing of
thiobarbiturates

T41.1X **Poisoning by adverse effect of and underdosing**
of intravenous anesthetics

⑦**T41.1X1** **Poisoning by intravenous anesthetics,**
accidental (unintentional)

Poisoning by intravenous anesthetics
NOS

⑦**T41.1X2** **Poisoning by intravenous anesthetics,**
intentional self-harm [HCC]

⑦**T41.1X3** **Poisoning by intravenous anesthetics,**
assault

⑦**T41.1X4** **Poisoning by intravenous anesthetics,**
undetermined

⑦**T41.1X5** **Adverse effect of intravenous**
anesthetics

⑦**T41.1X6** **Underdosing of intravenous**
anesthetics

T41.2 **Poisoning by adverse effect of and underdosing of other**
and unspecified general anesthetics

T41.20 **Poisoning by adverse effect of and underdosing**
of unspecified general anesthetics

⑦**T41.201** **Poisoning by unspecified general**
anesthetics, accidental
(unintentional)

Poisoning by general anesthetics NOS

⑦**T41.202** **Poisoning by unspecified general**
anesthetics, intentional self-harm
[HCC]

⑦**T41.203** **Poisoning by unspecified general**
anesthetics, assault

⑦**T41.204** **Poisoning by unspecified general**
anesthetics, undetermined

⑦**T41.205** **Adverse effect of unspecified general**
anesthetics

⑦**T41.206** **Underdosing of unspecified general**
anesthetics

T41.29 **Poisoning by adverse effect of and underdosing**
of other general anesthetics

⑦**T41.291** **Poisoning by other general**
anesthetics, accidental
(unintentional)

Poisoning by other general anesthetics
NOS

⑦**T41.292** **Poisoning by other general**
anesthetics, intentional self-harm
[HCC]

⑦**T41.293** **Poisoning by other general**
anesthetics, assault

⑦**T41.294** **Poisoning by other general**
anesthetics, undetermined

⑦**T41.295** **Adverse effect of other general**
anesthetics

⑦**T41.296** **Underdosing of other general**
anesthetics

T41.3 **Poisoning by adverse effect of and underdosing of local**
anesthetics

Cocaine (topical)

Excludes2: poisoning by cocaine used as a central nervous
system stimulant (T40.5X1-T40.5X4)

T41.3X **Poisoning by adverse effect of and underdosing**
of local anesthetics

⑦**T41.3X1** **Poisoning by local anesthetics,**
accidental (unintentional)

Poisoning by local anesthetics NOS

⑦**T41.3X2** **Poisoning by local anesthetics,**
intentional self-harm [HCC]

⑦**T41.3X3** **Poisoning by local anesthetics,**
assault

⑦**T41.3X4** **Poisoning by local anesthetics,**
undetermined

⑦**T41.3X5** **Adverse effect of local anesthetics**

⑦**T41.3X6** **Underdosing of local anesthetics**

● New code ▲ Revised code **Excludes1:** Not coded here **Excludes2:** Not included here ⊗ Placeholder required ⑦7th digit required

T41.4   Poisoning by adverse effect of and underdosing of unspecified anesthetic

⊗⑦**T41.41   Poisoning by unspecified anesthetic, accidental (unintentional)**

Poisoning by anesthetic NOS

⊗⑦**T41.42   Poisoning by unspecified anesthetic, intentional self-harm** [HCC]

⊗⑦**T41.43   Poisoning by unspecified anesthetic, assault**

⊗⑦**T41.44   Poisoning by unspecified anesthetic, undetermined**

⊗⑦**T41.45   Adverse effect of unspecified anesthetic**

⊗⑦**T41.46   Underdosing of unspecified anesthetics**

T41.5   Poisoning by adverse effect of and underdosing of therapeutic gases

T41.5X   Poisoning by adverse effect of and underdosing of therapeutic gases

⑦**T41.5X1   Poisoning by therapeutic gases, accidental (unintentional)**

Poisoning by therapeutic gases NOS

⑦**T41.5X2   Poisoning by therapeutic gases, intentional self-harm** [HCC]

⑦**T41.5X3   Poisoning by therapeutic gases, assault**

⑦**T41.5X4   Poisoning by therapeutic gases, undetermined**

⑦**T41.5X5   Adverse effect of therapeutic gases**

⑦**T41.5X6   Underdosing of therapeutic gases**

T42   Poisoning by adverse effect of and underdosing of antiepileptic, sedative- hypnotic and antiparkinsonism drugs

Excludes2: drug dependence and related mental and behavioral disorders due to psychoactive substance use (F10.--F19.-)

The appropriate 7th character is to be added to each code from category T42

A - initial encounter

D - subsequent encounter

S - sequela

T42.0   Poisoning by adverse effect of and underdosing of hydantoin derivatives

T42.0X   Poisoning by adverse effect of and underdosing of hydantoin derivatives

⑦**T42.0X1   Poisoning by hydantoin derivatives, accidental (unintentional)**

Poisoning by hydantoin derivatives NOS

⑦**T42.0X2   Poisoning by hydantoin derivatives, intentional self-harm** [HCC]

⑦**T42.0X3   Poisoning by hydantoin derivatives, assault**

⑦**T42.0X4   Poisoning by hydantoin derivatives, undetermined**

⑦**T42.0X5   Adverse effect of hydantoin derivatives**

⑦**T42.0X6   Underdosing of hydantoin derivatives**

T42.1   Poisoning by adverse effect of and underdosing of iminostilbenes

Poisoning by adverse effect of and underdosing of carbamazepine

T42.1X   Poisoning by adverse effect of and underdosing of iminostilbenes

⑦**T42.1X1   Poisoning by iminostilbenes, accidental (unintentional)**

Poisoning by iminostilbenes NOS

⑦**T42.1X2   Poisoning by iminostilbenes, intentional self-harm** [HCC]

⑦**T42.1X3   Poisoning by iminostilbenes, assault**

⑦**T42.1X4   Poisoning by iminostilbenes, undetermined**

⑦**T42.1X5   Adverse effect of iminostilbenes**

⑦**T42.1X6   Underdosing of iminostilbenes**

T42.2   Poisoning by adverse effect of and underdosing of succinimides and oxazolidinediones

T42.2X   Poisoning by adverse effect of and underdosing of succinimides and oxazolidinediones

⑦**T42.2X1   Poisoning by succinimides and oxazolidinediones, accidental (unintentional)**

Poisoning by succinimides and oxazolidinediones NOS

⑦**T42.2X2   Poisoning by succinimides and oxazolidinediones, intentional self-harm** [HCC]

⑦**T42.2X3   Poisoning by succinimides and oxazolidinediones, assault**

⑦**T42.2X4   Poisoning by succinimides and oxazolidinediones, undetermined**

⑦**T42.2X5   Adverse effect of succinimides and oxazolidinediones**

⑦**T42.2X6   Underdosing of succinimides and oxazolidinediones**

T42.3   Poisoning by adverse effect of and underdosing of barbiturates

Excludes1: poisoning by adverse effect of and underdosing of thiobarbiturates (T41.1-)

T42.3X   Poisoning by adverse effect of and underdosing of barbiturates

⑦**T42.3X1   Poisoning by barbiturates, accidental (unintentional)**

Poisoning by barbiturates NOS

⑦**T42.3X2   Poisoning by barbiturates, intentional self-harm** [HCC]

⑦**T42.3X3   Poisoning by barbiturates, assault**

⑦**T42.3X4   Poisoning by barbiturates, undetermined**

⑦**T42.3X5   Adverse effect of barbiturates**

⑦**T42.3X6   Underdosing of barbiturates**

T42.4   Poisoning by adverse effect of and underdosing of benzodiazepines

T42.4X   Poisoning by adverse effect of and underdosing of benzodiazepines

⑦**T42.4X1   Poisoning by benzodiazepines, accidental (unintentional)**

Poisoning by benzodiazepines NOS

⑦**T42.4X2   Poisoning by benzodiazepines, intentional self-harm** [HCC]

⑦**T42.4X3   Poisoning by benzodiazepines, assault**

⑦**T42.4X4   Poisoning by benzodiazepines, undetermined**

⑦**T42.4X5   Adverse effect of benzodiazepines**

⑦**T42.4X6   Underdosing of benzodiazepines**

T42.5   Poisoning by adverse effect of and underdosing of mixed antiepileptics

T42.5X   Poisoning by adverse effect of and underdosing of antiepileptics

⑦T42.5X1 **Poisoning by mixed antiepileptics, accidental (unintentional)**

Poisoning by mixed antiepileptics NOS

⑦T42.5X2 **Poisoning by mixed antiepileptics, intentional self-harm** [HCC]

⑦T42.5X3 **Poisoning by mixed antiepileptics, assault**

⑦T42.5X4 **Poisoning by mixed antiepileptics, undetermined**

⑦T42.5X5 **Adverse effect of mixed antiepileptics**

⑦T42.5X6 **Underdosing of mixed antiepileptics**

T42.6 **Poisoning by adverse effect of and underdosing of other antiepileptic and sedative-hypnotic drugs**

Poisoning by adverse effect of and underdosing of methaqualone

Poisoning by adverse effect of and underdosing of valproic acid

Excludes1: poisoning by adverse effect of and underdosing of carbamazepine (T42.1-)

T42.6X **Poisoning by adverse effect of and underdosing of other antiepileptic and sedative-hypnotic drugs**

⑦T42.6X1 **Poisoning by other antiepileptic and sedative-hypnotic drugs, accidental (unintentional)**

Poisoning by other antiepileptic and sedative-hypnotic drugs NOS

⑦T42.6X2 **Poisoning by other antiepileptic and sedative-hypnotic drugs, intentional self-harm** [HCC]

⑦T42.6X3 **Poisoning by other antiepileptic and sedative-hypnotic drugs, assault**

⑦T42.6X4 **Poisoning by other antiepileptic and sedative-hypnotic drugs, undetermined**

⑦T42.6X5 **Adverse effect of other antiepileptic and sedative-hypnotic drugs**

⑦T42.6X6 **Underdosing of other antiepileptic and sedative-hypnotic drugs**

T42.7 **Poisoning by adverse effect of and underdosing of unspecified antiepileptic and sedative-hypnotic drugs**

⊗⑦T42.71 **Poisoning by unspecified antiepileptic and sedative-hypnotic drugs, accidental (unintentional)**

Poisoning by antiepileptic and sedative-hypnotic drugs NOS

⊗⑦T42.72 **Poisoning by unspecified antiepileptic and sedative-hypnotic drugs, intentional self-harm** [HCC]

⊗⑦T42.73 **Poisoning by unspecified antiepileptic and sedative-hypnotic drugs, assault**

⊗⑦T42.74 **Poisoning by unspecified antiepileptic and sedative-hypnotic drugs, undetermined**

⊗⑦T42.75 **Adverse effect of unspecified antiepileptic and sedative-hypnotic drugs**

⊗⑦T42.76 **Underdosing of unspecified antiepileptic and sedative-hypnotic drugs**

T42.8 **Poisoning by adverse effect of and underdosing of antiparkinsonism drugs and other central muscle-tone depressants**

Poisoning by adverse effect of and underdosing of amantadine

T42.8X **Poisoning by adverse effect of and underdosing of antiparkinsonism drugs and other central muscle-tone depressants**

⑦T42.8X1 **Poisoning by antiparkinsonism drugs and other central muscle-tone depressants, accidental (unintentional)**

Poisoning by antiparkinsonism drugs and other central muscle-tone depressants NOS

⑦T42.8X2 **Poisoning by antiparkinsonism drugs and other central muscle-tone depressants, intentional self-harm** [HCC]

⑦T42.8X3 **Poisoning by antiparkinsonism drugs and other central muscle-tone depressants, assault**

⑦T42.8X4 **Poisoning by antiparkinsonism drugs and other central muscle-tone depressants, undetermined**

⑦T42.8X5 **Adverse effect of antiparkinsonism drugs and other central muscle-tone depressants**

⑦T42.8X6 **Underdosing of antiparkinsonism drugs and other central muscle-tone depressants**

T43 **Poisoning by adverse effect of and underdosing of psychotropic drugs, not elsewhere classified**

Excludes1: appetite depressants (T50.5-)

barbiturates (T42.3-)

benzodiazepines (T42.4-)

methaqualone (T42.6-)

psychodysleptics [hallucinogens] (T40.7-T40.9-)

Excludes2: drug dependence and related mental and behavioral disorders due to psychoactive substance use (F10.--F19.-)

The appropriate 7th character is to be added to each code from category T43

A - initial encounter

D - subsequent encounter

S - sequela

T43.0 **Poisoning by adverse effect of and underdosing of tricyclic and tetracyclic antidepressants**

T43.01 **Poisoning by adverse effect of and underdosing of tricyclic antidepressants**

⑦T43.011 **Poisoning by tricyclic antidepressants, accidental (unintentional)**

Poisoning by tricyclic antidepressants NOS

⑦T43.012 **Poisoning by tricyclic antidepressants, intentional self-harm** [HCC]

⑦T43.013 **Poisoning by tricyclic antidepressants, assault**

⑦T43.014 **Poisoning by tricyclic antidepressants, undetermined**

⑦T43.015 **Adverse effect of tricyclic antidepressants**

⑦T43.016 **Underdosing of tricyclic antidepressants**

T43.02 **Poisoning by adverse effect of and underdosing of tetracyclic antidepressants**

⑦T43.021 **Poisoning by tetracyclic antidepressants, accidental (unintentional)**

Poisoning by tetracyclic antidepressants NOS

⑦T43.022 Poisoning by tetracyclic antidepressants, intentional self-harm [HCC]

⑦T43.023 Poisoning by tetracyclic antidepressants, assault

⑦T43.024 Poisoning by tetracyclic antidepressants, undetermined

⑦T43.025 Adverse effect of tetracyclic antidepressants

⑦T43.026 Underdosing of tetracyclic antidepressants

T43.1 **Poisoning by adverse effect of and underdosing of monoamine-oxidase-inhibitor antidepressants**

  T43.1X **Poisoning by adverse effect of and underdosing of monoamine-oxidase-inhibitor antidepressants**

⑦T43.1X1 Poisoning by monoamine-oxidase-inhibitor antidepressants, accidental (unintentional)

  Poisoning by monoamine-oxidase-inhibitor antidepressants NOS

⑦T43.1X2 Poisoning by monoamine-oxidase-inhibitor antidepressants, intentional self-harm [HCC]

⑦T43.1X3 Poisoning by monoamine-oxidase-inhibitor antidepressants, assault

⑦T43.1X4 Poisoning by monoamine-oxidase-inhibitor antidepressants, undetermined

⑦T43.1X5 Adverse effect of monoamine-oxidase-inhibitor antidepressants

⑦T43.1X6 Underdosing of monoamine-oxidase-inhibitor antidepressants

T43.2 **Poisoning by adverse effect of and underdosing of other and unspecified antidepressants**

  T43.20 **Poisoning by adverse effect of and underdosing of unspecified antidepressants**

⑦T43.201 Poisoning by unspecified antidepressants, accidental (unintentional)

  Poisoning by antidepressants NOS

⑦T43.202 Poisoning by unspecified antidepressants, intentional self-harm [HCC]

⑦T43.203 Poisoning by unspecified antidepressants, assault

⑦T43.204 Poisoning by unspecified antidepressants, undetermined

⑦T43.205 Adverse effect of unspecified antidepressants

  Antidepressant discontinuation syndrome

⑦T43.206 Underdosing of unspecified antidepressants

  T43.21 **Poisoning by adverse effect of and underdosing of selective serotonin and norepinephrine reuptake inhibitors**

  Poisoning by adverse effect of and underdosing of SSNRI antidepressants

⑦T43.211 Poisoning by selective serotonin and norepinephrine reuptake inhibitors, accidental (unintentional)

⑦T43.212 Poisoning by selective serotonin and norepinephrine reuptake inhibitors, intentional self-harm [HCC]

⑦T43.213 Poisoning by selective serotonin and norepinephrine reuptake inhibitors, assault

⑦T43.214 Poisoning by selective serotonin and norepinephrine reuptake inhibitors, undetermined

⑦T43.215 Adverse effect of selective serotonin and norepinephrine reuptake inhibitors

⑦T43.216 Underdosing of selective serotonin and norepinephrine reuptake inhibitors

  T43.22 **Poisoning by adverse effect of and underdosing of selective serotonin reuptake inhibitors**

  Poisoning by adverse effect of and underdosing of SSRI antidepressants

⑦T43.221 Poisoning by selective serotonin reuptake inhibitors, accidental (unintentional)

⑦T43.222 Poisoning by selective serotonin reuptake inhibitors, intentional self-harm [HCC]

⑦T43.223 Poisoning by selective serotonin reuptake inhibitors, assault

⑦T43.224 Poisoning by selective serotonin reuptake inhibitors, undetermined

⑦T43.225 Adverse effect of selective serotonin reuptake inhibitors

⑦T43.226 Underdosing of selective serotonin reuptake inhibitors

  T43.29 **Poisoning by adverse effect of and underdosing of other antidepressants**

⑦T43.291 Poisoning by other antidepressants, accidental (unintentional)

  Poisoning by other antidepressants NOS

⑦T43.292 Poisoning by other antidepressants, intentional self-harm [HCC]

⑦T43.293 Poisoning by other antidepressants, assault

⑦T43.294 Poisoning by other antidepressants, undetermined

⑦T43.295 Adverse effect of other antidepressants

⑦T43.296 Underdosing of other antidepressants

T43.3 **Poisoning by adverse effect of and underdosing of phenothiazine antipsychotics and neuroleptics**

  T43.3X **Poisoning by adverse effect of and underdosing of phenothiazine antipsychotics and neuroleptics**

⑦T43.3X1 Poisoning by phenothiazine antipsychotics and neuroleptics, accidental (unintentional)

  Poisoning by phenothiazine antipsychotics and neuroleptics NOS

⑦T43.3X2 Poisoning by phenothiazine antipsychotics and neuroleptics, intentional self-harm [HCC]

⑦T43.3X3 Poisoning by phenothiazine antipsychotics and neuroleptics, assault

⑦T43.3X4 Poisoning by phenothiazine antipsychotics and neuroleptics, undetermined

⑦**T43.3X5** Adverse effect of phenothiazine antipsychotics and neuroleptics

⑦**T43.3X6** Underdosing of phenothiazine antipsychotics and neuroleptics

T43.4 **Poisoning by adverse effect of and underdosing of butyrophenone and thiothixene neuroleptics**

T43.4X **Poisoning by adverse effect of and underdosing of butyrophenone and thiothixene neuroleptics**

⑦**T43.4X1** Poisoning by butyrophenone and thiothixene neuroleptics, accidental (unintentional)

Poisoning by butyrophenone and thiothixene neuroleptics NOS

⑦**T43.4X2** Poisoning by butyrophenone and thiothixene neuroleptics, intentional self-harm [HCC]

⑦**T43.4X3** Poisoning by butyrophenone and thiothixene neuroleptics, assault

⑦**T43.4X4** Poisoning by butyrophenone and thiothixene neuroleptics, undetermined

⑦**T43.4X5** Adverse effect of butyrophenone and thiothixene neuroleptics

⑦**T43.4X6** Underdosing of butyrophenone and thiothixene neuroleptics

T43.5 **Poisoning by adverse effect of and underdosing of other and unspecified antipsychotics and neuroleptics**

Excludes1: poisoning by adverse effect of and underdosing of rauwolfia (T46.5-)

T43.50 **Poisoning by adverse effect of and underdosing of unspecified antipsychotics and neuroleptics**

⑦**T43.501** Poisoning by unspecified antipsychotics and neuroleptics, accidental (unintentional)

Poisoning by antipsychotics and neuroleptics NOS

⑦**T43.502** Poisoning by unspecified antipsychotics and neuroleptics, intentional self-harm [HCC]

⑦**T43.503** Poisoning by unspecified antipsychotics and neuroleptics, assault

⑦**T43.504** Poisoning by unspecified antipsychotics and neuroleptics, undetermined

⑦**T43.505** Adverse effect of unspecified antipsychotics and neuroleptics

⑦**T43.506** Underdosing of unspecified antipsychotics and neuroleptics

T43.59 **Poisoning by adverse effect of and underdosing of other antipsychotics and neuroleptics**

⑦**T43.591** Poisoning by other antipsychotics and neuroleptics, accidental (unintentional)

Poisoning by other antipsychotics and neuroleptics NOS

⑦**T43.592** Poisoning by other antipsychotics and neuroleptics, intentional self-harm [HCC]

⑦**T43.593** Poisoning by other antipsychotics and neuroleptics, assault

⑦**T43.594** Poisoning by other antipsychotics and neuroleptics, undetermined

⑦**T43.595** Adverse effect of other antipsychotics and neuroleptics

⑦**T43.596** Underdosing of other antipsychotics and neuroleptics

T43.6 **Poisoning by adverse effect of and underdosing of psychostimulants**

Excludes1: poisoning by adverse effect of and underdosing of cocaine (T40.5-)

T43.60 **Poisoning by adverse effect of and underdosing of unspecified psychostimulant**

⑦**T43.601** Poisoning by unspecified psychostimulants, accidental (unintentional) [HCC]

Poisoning by psychostimulants NOS

⑦**T43.602** Poisoning by unspecified psychostimulants, intentional self-harm [HCC]

⑦**T43.603** Poisoning by unspecified psychostimulants, assault

⑦**T43.604** Poisoning by unspecified psychostimulants, undetermined [HCC]

⑦**T43.605** Adverse effect of unspecified psychostimulants

⑦**T43.606** Underdosing of unspecified psychostimulants

T43.61 **Poisoning by adverse effect of and underdosing of caffeine**

⑦**T43.611** Poisoning by caffeine, accidental (unintentional) [HCC]

Poisoning by caffeine NOS

⑦**T43.612** Poisoning by caffeine, intentional self-harm [HCC]

⑦**T43.613** Poisoning by caffeine, assault

⑦**T43.614** Poisoning by caffeine, undetermined [HCC]

⑦**T43.615** Adverse effect of caffeine

⑦**T43.616** Underdosing of caffeine

T43.62 **Poisoning by adverse effect of and underdosing of amphetamines**

Poisoning by adverse effect of and underdosing of methamphetamines

⑦**T43.621** Poisoning by amphetamines, accidental (unintentional) [HCC]

Poisoning by amphetamines NOS

⑦**T43.622** Poisoning by amphetamines, intentional self-harm [HCC]

⑦**T43.623** Poisoning by amphetamines, assault

⑦**T43.624** Poisoning by amphetamines, undetermined [HCC]

⑦**T43.625** Adverse effect of amphetamines

⑦**T43.626** Underdosing of amphetamines

T43.63 **Poisoning by adverse effect of and underdosing of methylphenidate**

⑦**T43.631** Poisoning by methylphenidate, accidental (unintentional) [HCC]

Poisoning by methylphenidate NOS

⑦**T43.632** Poisoning by methylphenidate, intentional self-harm [HCC]

⑦**T43.633** Poisoning by methylphenidate, assault

⑦**T43.634** Poisoning by methylphenidate, undetermined [HCC]

⑦**T43.635** Adverse effect of methylphenidate

⑦**T43.636** Underdosing of methylphenidate

T43.64 **Poisoning by ecstasy**

Poisoning by MDMA

Poisoning by 3,4-ethylenedioxymethamphetamine

T43.641 **Poisoning by ecstasy, accidental (unintentional)**

Poisoning by ecstasy NOS

T43.642 **Poisoning by ecstasy, intentional self-harm**

T43.643 **Poisoning by ecstasy, assault**

T43.644 **Poisoning by ecstasy, undetermined**

T43.69 **Poisoning by adverse effect of and underdosing of other psychostimulants**

⑦T43.691 **Poisoning by other psychostimulants, accidental (unintentional)** [HCC]

Poisoning by other psychostimulants NOS

⑦T43.692 **Poisoning by other psychostimulants, intentional self-harm** [HCC]

⑦T43.693 **Poisoning by other psychostimulants, assault**

⑦T43.694 **Poisoning by other psychostimulants, undetermined** [HCC]

⑦T43.695 **Adverse effect of other psychostimulants**

⑦T43.696 **Underdosing of other psychostimulants**

T43.8 **Poisoning by adverse effect of and underdosing of other psychotropic drugs**

T43.8X **Poisoning by adverse effect of and underdosing of other psychotropic drugs**

⑦T43.8X1 **Poisoning by other psychotropic drugs, accidental (unintentional)**

Poisoning by other psychotropic drugs NOS

⑦T43.8X2 **Poisoning by other psychotropic drugs, intentional self-harm** [HCC]

⑦T43.8X3 **Poisoning by other psychotropic drugs, assault**

⑦T43.8X4 **Poisoning by other psychotropic drugs, undetermined**

⑦T43.8X5 **Adverse effect of other psychotropic drugs**

⑦T43.8X6 **Underdosing of other psychotropic drugs**

T43.9 **Poisoning by adverse effect of and underdosing of unspecified psychotropic drug**

⊗⑦T43.91 **Poisoning by unspecified psychotropic drug, accidental (unintentional)**

Poisoning by psychotropic drug NOS

⊗⑦T43.92 **Poisoning by unspecified psychotropic drug, intentional self-harm** [HCC]

⊗⑦T43.93 **Poisoning by unspecified psychotropic drug, assault**

⊗⑦T43.94 **Poisoning by unspecified psychotropic drug, undetermined**

⊗⑦T43.95 **Adverse effect of unspecified psychotropic drug**

⊗⑦T43.96 **Underdosing of unspecified psychotropic drug**

T44 **Poisoning by adverse effect of and underdosing of drugs primarily affecting the autonomic nervous system**

The appropriate 7th character is to be added to each code from category T44

A - initial encounter

D - subsequent encounter

S - sequela

T44.0 **Poisoning by adverse effect of and underdosing of anticholinesterase agents**

T44.0X **Poisoning by adverse effect of and underdosing of anticholinesterase agents**

⑦T44.0X1 **Poisoning by anticholinesterase agents, accidental (unintentional)**

poisoning by anticholinesterase agents NOS

⑦T44.0X2 **Poisoning by anticholinesterase agents, intentional self-harm** [HCC]

⑦T44.0X3 **Poisoning by anticholinesterase agents, assault**

⑦T44.0X4 **Poisoning by anticholinesterase agents, undetermined**

⑦T44.0X5 **Adverse effect of anticholinesterase agents**

⑦T44.0X6 **Underdosing of anticholinesterase agents**

T44.1 **Poisoning by adverse effect of and underdosing of other parasympathomimetics [cholinergics]**

T44.1X **Poisoning by adverse effect of and underdosing of other parasympathomimetics [cholinergics]**

⑦T44.1X1 **Poisoning by other parasympathomimetics [cholinergics], accidental (unintentional)**

Poisoning by other parasympatho-mimetics [cholinergics] NOS

⑦T44.1X2 **Poisoning by other parasympathomimetics [cholinergics], intentional self-harm** [HCC]

⑦T44.1X3 **Poisoning by other parasympathomimetics [cholinergics], assault**

⑦T44.1X4 **Poisoning by other parasympathomimetics [cholinergics], undetermined**

⑦T44.1X5 **Adverse effect of other parasympathomimetics [cholinergics]**

⑦T44.1X6 **Underdosing of other parasympathomimetics [cholinergics]**

T44.2 **Poisoning by adverse effect of and underdosing of ganglionic blocking drugs**

T44.2X **Poisoning by adverse effect of and underdosing of ganglionic blocking drugs**

⑦T44.2X1 **Poisoning by ganglionic blocking drugs, accidental (unintentional)**

Poisoning by ganglionic blocking drugs NOS

⑦T44.2X2 **Poisoning by ganglionic blocking drugs, intentional self-harm** [HCC]

⑦T44.2X3 **Poisoning by ganglionic blocking drugs, assault**

⑦T44.2X4 **Poisoning by ganglionic blocking drugs, undetermined**

⑦T44.2X5 **Adverse effect of ganglionic blocking drugs**

⑦T44.2X6 **Underdosing of ganglionic blocking drugs**

T44.3 **Poisoning by adverse effect of and underdosing of other parasympatholytics [anticholinergics and antimuscarinics] and spasmolytics**

Poisoning by adverse effect of and underdosing of papaverine

T44.3X Poisoning by adverse effect of and underdosing of other parasympatholytics [anticholinergics and antimuscarinics] and spasmolytics

⑦ **T44.3X1 Poisoning by other parasympatholytics [anticholinergics and antimuscarinics] and spasmolytics, accidental (unintentional)**

Poisoning by other parasympatholytics [anticholinergics and antimuscarinics] and spasmolytics NOS

⑦ **T44.3X2 Poisoning by other parasympatholytics [anticholinergics and antimuscarinics] and spasmolytics, intentional self-harm** [HCC]

⑦ **T44.3X3 Poisoning by other parasympatholytics [anticholinergics and antimuscarinics] and spasmolytics, assault**

⑦ **T44.3X4 Poisoning by other parasympatholytics [anticholinergics and antimuscarinics] and spasmolytics, undetermined**

⑦ **T44.3X5 Adverse effect of other parasympatholytics [anticholinergics and antimuscarinics] and spasmolytics**

⑦ **T44.3X6 Underdosing of other parasympatholytics [anticholinergics and antimuscarinics] and spasmolytics**

T44.4 Poisoning by adverse effect of and underdosing of predominantly alpha-adrenoreceptor agonists

Poisoning by adverse effect of and underdosing of metaraminol

T44.4X Poisoning by adverse effect of and underdosing of predominantly alpha-adrenoreceptor agonists

⑦ **T44.4X1 Poisoning by predominantly alpha-adrenoreceptor agonists, accidental (unintentional)**

Poisoning by predominantly alpha-adrenoreceptor agonists NOS

⑦ **T44.4X2 Poisoning by predominantly alpha-adrenoreceptor agonists, intentional self-harm** [HCC]

⑦ **T44.4X3 Poisoning by predominantly alpha-adrenoreceptor agonists, assault**

⑦ **T44.4X4 Poisoning by predominantly alpha-adrenoreceptor agonists, undetermined**

⑦ **T44.4X5 Adverse effect of predominantly alpha-adrenoreceptor agonists**

⑦ **T44.4X6 Underdosing of predominantly alpha-adrenoreceptor agonists**

T44.5 Poisoning by adverse effect of and underdosing of predominantly beta-adrenoreceptor agonists

Excludes1: poisoning by adverse effect of and underdosing of beta-adrenoreceptor agonists used in asthma therapy (T48.6-)

T44.5X Poisoning by adverse effect of and underdosing of predominantly beta-adrenoreceptor agonists

⑦ **T44.5X1 Poisoning by predominantly beta-adrenoreceptor agonists, accidental (unintentional)**

Poisoning by predominantly beta-adrenoreceptor agonists NOS

⑦ **T44.5X2 Poisoning by predominantly beta-adrenoreceptor agonists, intentional self-harm** [HCC]

⑦ **T44.5X3 Poisoning by predominantly beta-adrenoreceptor agonists, assault**

⑦ **T44.5X4 Poisoning by predominantly beta-adrenoreceptor agonists, undetermined**

⑦ **T44.5X5 Adverse effect of predominantly beta-adrenoreceptor agonists**

⑦ **T44.5X6 Underdosing of predominantly beta-adrenoreceptor agonists**

T44.6 Poisoning by adverse effect of and underdosing of alpha-adrenoreceptor antagonists

Excludes1: poisoning by adverse effect of and underdosing of ergot alkaloids (T48.0)

T44.6X Poisoning by adverse effect of and underdosing of alpha-adrenoreceptor antagonists

⑦ **T44.6X1 Poisoning by alpha-adrenoreceptor antagonists, accidental (unintentional)**

Poisoning by alpha-adrenoreceptor antagonists NOS

⑦ **T44.6X2 Poisoning by alpha-adrenoreceptor antagonists, intentional self-harm** [HCC]

⑦ **T44.6X3 Poisoning by alpha-adrenoreceptor antagonists, assault**

⑦ **T44.6X4 Poisoning by alpha-adrenoreceptor antagonists, undetermined**

⑦ **T44.6X5 Adverse effect of alpha-adrenoreceptor antagonists**

⑦ **T44.6X6 Underdosing of alpha-adrenoreceptor antagonists**

T44.7 Poisoning by adverse effect of and underdosing of beta-adrenoreceptor antagonists

T44.7X Poisoning by adverse effect of and underdosing of beta-adrenoreceptor antagonists

⑦ **T44.7X1 Poisoning by beta-adrenoreceptor antagonists, accidental (unintentional)**

Poisoning by beta-adrenoreceptor antagonists NOS

⑦ **T44.7X2 Poisoning by beta-adrenoreceptor antagonists, intentional self-harm** [HCC]

⑦ **T44.7X3 Poisoning by beta-adrenoreceptor antagonists, assault**

⑦ **T44.7X4 Poisoning by beta-adrenoreceptor antagonists, undetermined**

⑦ **T44.7X5 Adverse effect of beta-adrenoreceptor antagonists**

⑦ **T44.7X6 Underdosing of beta-adrenoreceptor antagonists**

T44.8 Poisoning by adverse effect of and underdosing of centrally-acting and adrenergic-neuron- blocking agents

Excludes2: poisoning by adverse effect of and underdosing of clonidine (T46.5)

poisoning by adverse effect of and underdosing of guanethidine (T46.5)

T44.8X   **Poisoning by adverse effect of and underdosing of centrally-acting and adrenergic- neuron-blocking agents**

⑦T44.8X1   **Poisoning by centrally-acting and adrenergic-neuron-blocking agents, accidental (unintentional)**

Poisoning by centrally-acting and adrenergic-neuron-blocking agents NOS

⑦T44.8X2   **Poisoning by centrally-acting and adrenergic-neuron-blocking agents, intentional self-harm** [HCC]

⑦T44.8X3   **Poisoning by centrally-acting and adrenergic-neuron-blocking agents, assault**

⑦T44.8X4   **Poisoning by centrally-acting and adrenergic-neuron-blocking agents, undetermined**

⑦T44.8X5   **Adverse effect of centrally-acting and adrenergic-neuron-blocking agents**

⑦T44.8X6   **Underdosing of centrally-acting and adrenergic-neuron-blocking agents**

T44.9   **Poisoning by adverse effect of and underdosing of other and unspecified drugs primarily affecting the autonomic nervous system**

Poisoning by adverse effect of and underdosing of drug stimulating both alpha and beta-adrenoreceptors

T44.90   **Poisoning by adverse effect of and underdosing of unspecified drugs primarily affecting the autonomic nervous system**

⑦T44.901   **Poisoning by unspecified drugs primarily affecting the autonomic nervous system, accidental (unintentional)**

Poisoning by unspecified drugs primarily affecting the autonomic nervous system NOS

⑦T44.902   **Poisoning by unspecified drugs primarily affecting the autonomic nervous system, intentional self-harm** [HCC]

⑦T44.903   **Poisoning by unspecified drugs primarily affecting the autonomic nervous system, assault**

⑦T44.904   **Poisoning by unspecified drugs primarily affecting the autonomic nervous system, undetermined**

⑦T44.905   **Adverse effect of unspecified drugs primarily affecting the autonomic nervous system**

⑦T44.906   **Underdosing of unspecified drugs primarily affecting the autonomic nervous system**

T44.99   **Poisoning by adverse effect of and underdosing of other drugs primarily affecting the autonomic nervous system**

⑦T44.991   **Poisoning by other drug primarily affecting the autonomic nervous system, accidental (unintentional)**

Poisoning by other drugs primarily affecting the autonomic nervous system NOS

⑦T44.992   **Poisoning by other drug primarily affecting the autonomic nervous system, intentional self-harm** [HCC]

⑦T44.993   **Poisoning by other drug primarily affecting the autonomic nervous system, assault**

⑦T44.994   **Poisoning by other drug primarily affecting the autonomic nervous system, undetermined**

⑦T44.995   **Adverse effect of other drug primarily affecting the autonomic nervous system**

⑦T44.996   **Underdosing of other drug primarily affecting the autonomic nervous system**

T45   **Poisoning by adverse effect of and underdosing of primarily systemic and hematological agents, not elsewhere classified**

The appropriate 7th character is to be added to each code from category T45

A - initial encounter

D - subsequent encounter

S - sequela

T45.0   **Poisoning by adverse effect of and underdosing of antiallergic and antiemetic drugs**

Excludes1: poisoning by adverse effect of and underdosing of phenothiazine-based neuroleptics (T43.3)

T45.0X   **Poisoning by adverse effect of and underdosing of antiallergic and antiemetic drugs**

⑦T45.0X1   **Poisoning by antiallergic and antiemetic drugs, accidental (unintentional)**

Poisoning by antiallergic and antiemetic drugs NOS

⑦T45.0X2   **Poisoning by antiallergic and antiemetic drugs, intentional self-harm** [HCC]

⑦T45.0X3   **Poisoning by antiallergic and antiemetic drugs, assault**

⑦T45.0X4   **Poisoning by antiallergic and antiemetic drugs, undetermined**

⑦T45.0X5   **Adverse effect of antiallergic and antiemetic drugs**

⑦T45.0X6   **Underdosing of antiallergic and antiemetic drugs**

T45.1   **Poisoning by adverse effect of and underdosing of antineoplastic and immunosuppressive drugs**

Excludes1: poisoning by adverse effect of and underdosing of tamoxifen (T38.6)

T45.1X   **Poisoning by adverse effect of and underdosing of antineoplastic and immunosuppressive drugs**

⑦T45.1X1   **Poisoning by antineoplastic and immunosuppressive drugs, accidental (unintentional)**

Poisoning by antineoplastic and immunosuppressive drugs NOS

⑦T45.1X2   **Poisoning by antineoplastic and immunosuppressive drugs, intentional self-harm** [HCC]

⑦T45.1X3   **Poisoning by antineoplastic and immunosuppressive drugs, assault**

⑦T45.1X4   **Poisoning by antineoplastic and immunosuppressive drugs, undetermined**

⑦T45.1X5   **Adverse effect of antineoplastic and immunosuppressive drugs**

⑦T45.1X6   **Underdosing of antineoplastic and immunosuppressive drugs**

T45.2   **Poisoning by adverse effect of and underdosing of vitamins**

> **Excludes2:** poisoning by adverse effect of and underdosing of nicotinic acid (derivatives) (T46.7)
>
> poisoning by adverse effect of and underdosing of iron (T45.4)
>
> poisoning by adverse effect of and underdosing of vitamin K (T45.7)

T45.2X   **Poisoning by adverse effect of and underdosing of vitamins**

⑦**T45.2X1**   **Poisoning by vitamins, accidental (unintentional)**

Poisoning by vitamins NOS

⑦**T45.2X2**   **Poisoning by vitamins, intentional self-harm** [HCC]

⑦**T45.2X3**   **Poisoning by vitamins, assault**

⑦**T45.2X4**   **Poisoning by vitamins, undetermined**

⑦**T45.2X5**   **Adverse effect of vitamins**

⑦**T45.2X6**   **Underdosing of vitamins**

> **Excludes1:** vitamin deficiencies (E50-E56)

T45.3   **Poisoning by adverse effect of and underdosing of enzymes**

T45.3X   **Poisoning by adverse effect of and underdosing of enzymes**

⑦**T45.3X1**   **Poisoning by enzymes, accidental (unintentional)**

Poisoning by enzymes NOS

⑦**T45.3X2**   **Poisoning by enzymes, intentional self-harm** [HCC]

⑦**T45.3X3**   **Poisoning by enzymes, assault**

⑦**T45.3X4**   **Poisoning by enzymes, undetermined**

⑦**T45.3X5**   **Adverse effect of enzymes**

⑦**T45.3X6**   **Underdosing of enzymes**

T45.4   **Poisoning by adverse effect of and underdosing of iron and its compounds**

T45.4X   **Poisoning by adverse effect of and underdosing of iron and its compounds**

⑦**T45.4X1**   **Poisoning by iron and its compounds, accidental (unintentional)**

Poisoning by iron and its compounds NOS

⑦**T45.4X2**   **Poisoning by iron and its compounds, intentional self-harm** [HCC]

⑦**T45.4X3**   **Poisoning by iron and its compounds, assault**

⑦**T45.4X4**   **Poisoning by iron and its compounds, undetermined**

⑦**T45.4X5**   **Adverse effect of iron and its compounds**

⑦**T45.4X6**   **Underdosing of iron and its compounds**

> **Excludes1:** iron deficiency (E61.1)

T45.5   **Poisoning by adverse effect of and underdosing of anticoagulants and antithrombotic drugs**

T45.51   **Poisoning by adverse effect of and underdosing of anticoagulants**

⑦**T45.511**   **Poisoning by anticoagulants, accidental (unintentional)**

Poisoning by anticoagulants NOS

⑦**T45.512**   **Poisoning by anticoagulants, intentional self-harm** [HCC]

⑦**T45.513**   **Poisoning by anticoagulants, assault**

⑦**T45.514**   **Poisoning by anticoagulants, undetermined**

⑦**T45.515**   **Adverse effect of anticoagulants**

⑦**T45.516**   **Underdosing of anticoagulants**

T45.52   **Poisoning by adverse effect of and underdosing of antithrombotic drugs**

Poisoning by adverse effect of and underdosing of antiplatelet drugs

> **Excludes2:** poisoning by adverse effect of and underdosing of aspirin (T39.01-)
>
> poisoning by adverse effect of and underdosing of acetylsalicylic acid (T39.01-)

⑦**T45.521**   **Poisoning by antithrombotic drugs, accidental (unintentional)**

Poisoning by antithrombotic drug NOS

⑦**T45.522**   **Poisoning by antithrombotic drugs, intentional self-harm** [HCC]

⑦**T45.523**   **Poisoning by antithrombotic drugs, assault**

⑦**T45.524**   **Poisoning by antithrombotic drugs, undetermined**

⑦**T45.525**   **Adverse effect of antithrombotic drugs**

⑦**T45.526**   **Underdosing of antithrombotic drugs**

T45.6   **Poisoning by adverse effect of and underdosing of fibrinolysis-affecting drugs**

T45.60   **Poisoning by adverse effect of and underdosing of unspecified fibrinolysis-affecting drugs**

⑦**T45.601**   **Poisoning by unspecified fibrinolysis-affecting drugs, accidental (unintentional)**

Poisoning by fibrinolysis-affecting drug NOS

⑦**T45.602**   **Poisoning by unspecified fibrinolysis-affecting drugs, intentional self-harm** [HCC]

⑦**T45.603**   **Poisoning by unspecified fibrinolysis-affecting drugs, assault**

⑦**T45.604**   **Poisoning by unspecified fibrinolysis-affecting drugs, undetermined**

⑦**T45.605**   **Adverse effect of unspecified fibrinolysis-affecting drugs**

⑦**T45.606**   **Underdosing of unspecified fibrinolysis-affecting drugs**

T45.61   **Poisoning by adverse effect of and underdosing of thrombolytic drugs**

⑦**T45.611**   **Poisoning by thrombolytic drug, accidental (unintentional)**

Poisoning by thrombolytic drug NOS

⑦**T45.612**   **Poisoning by thrombolytic drug, intentional self-harm** [HCC]

⑦**T45.613**   **Poisoning by thrombolytic drug, assault**

⑦**T45.614**   **Poisoning by thrombolytic drug, undetermined**

⑦**T45.615**   **Adverse effect of thrombolytic drugs**

⑦**T45.616**   **Underdosing of thrombolytic drugs**

T45.62   **Poisoning by adverse effect of and underdosing of hemostatic drugs**

● New code   ▲ Revised code   **Excludes1:** Not coded here   **Excludes2:** Not included here   ⊗ Placeholder required   ⑦7ᵗʰ digit required

⑦T45.621 **Poisoning by hemostatic drug, accidental (unintentional)**

Poisoning by hemostatic drug NOS

⑦T45.622 **Poisoning by hemostatic drug, intentional self-harm** [HCC]

⑦T45.623 **Poisoning by hemostatic drug, assault**

⑦T45.624 **Poisoning by hemostatic drug, undetermined**

⑦T45.625 **Adverse effect of hemostatic drug**

⑦T45.626 **Underdosing of hemostatic drugs**

T45.69 **Poisoning by adverse effect of and underdosing of other fibrinolysis-affecting drugs**

⑦T45.691 **Poisoning by other fibrinolysis-affecting drugs, accidental (unintentional)**

Poisoning by other fibrinolysis-affecting drug NOS

⑦T45.692 **Poisoning by other fibrinolysis-affecting drugs, intentional self-harm** [HCC]

⑦T45.693 **Poisoning by other fibrinolysis-affecting drugs, assault**

⑦T45.694 **Poisoning by other fibrinolysis-affecting drugs, undetermined**

⑦T45.695 **Adverse effect of other fibrinolysis-affecting drugs**

⑦T45.696 **Underdosing of other fibrinolysis-affecting drugs**

T45.7 **Poisoning by adverse effect of and underdosing of anticoagulant antagonists, vitamin K and other coagulants**

T45.7X **Poisoning by adverse effect of and underdosing of anticoagulant antagonists, vitamin K and other coagulants**

⑦T45.7X1 **Poisoning by anticoagulant antagonists, vitamin K and other coagulants, accidental (unintentional)**

Poisoning by anticoagulant antagonists, vitamin K and other coagulants NOS

⑦T45.7X2 **Poisoning by anticoagulant antagonists, vitamin K and other coagulants, intentional self-harm** [HCC]

⑦T45.7X3 **Poisoning by anticoagulant antagonists, vitamin K and other coagulants, assault**

⑦T45.7X4 **Poisoning by anticoagulant antagonists, vitamin K and other coagulants, undetermined**

⑦T45.7X5 **Adverse effect of anticoagulant antagonists, vitamin K and other coagulants**

⑦T45.7X6 **Underdosing of anticoagulant antagonist, vitamin K and other coagulants**

Excludes1: vitamin K deficiency (E56.1)

T45.8 **Poisoning by adverse effect of and underdosing of other primarily systemic and hematological agents**

Poisoning by adverse effect of and underdosing of liver preparations **and other** antianemic agents

Poisoning by adverse effect of and underdosing of natural blood and blood products

Poisoning by adverse effect of and underdosing of plasma substitute

Excludes2: poisoning by adverse effect of and underdosing of immunoglobulin (T50.Z1)

poisoning by adverse effect of and underdosing of iron (T45.4) transfusion reactions (T80.-)

T45.8X **Poisoning by adverse effect of and underdosing of other primarily systemic and hematological agents**

⑦T45.8X1 **Poisoning by other primarily systemic and hematological agents, accidental (unintentional)**

Poisoning by other primarily systemic and hematological agents NOS

⑦T45.8X2 **Poisoning by other primarily systemic and hematological agents, intentional self-harm** [HCC]

⑦T45.8X3 **Poisoning by other primarily systemic and hematological agents, assault**

⑦T45.8X4 **Poisoning by other primarily systemic and hematological agents, undetermined**

⑦T45.8X5 **Adverse effect of other primarily systemic and hematological agents**

⑦T45.8X6 **Underdosing of other primarily systemic and hematological agents**

T45.9 **Poisoning by adverse effect of and underdosing of unspecified primarily systemic and hematological agent**

T45.91 **Poisoning by unspecified primarily systemic and hematological agent, accidental (unintentional)**

Poisoning by primarily systemic and hematological agent NOS

T45.92 **Poisoning by unspecified primarily systemic and hematological agent, intentional self-harm** [HCC]

T45.93 **Poisoning by unspecified primarily systemic and hematological agent, assault**

T45.94 **Poisoning by unspecified primarily systemic and hematological agent, undetermined**

T45.95 **Adverse effect of unspecified primarily systemic and hematological agent**

T45.96 **Underdosing of unspecified primarily systemic and hematological agent**

T46 **Poisoning by adverse effect of and underdosing of agents primarily affecting the cardiovascular system**

Excludes1: poisoning by adverse effect of and underdosing of metaraminol (T44.4)

The appropriate 7th character is to be added to each code from category T46

A - initial encounter

D - subsequent encounter

S - sequela

T46.0 **Poisoning by adverse effect of and underdosing of cardiac-stimulant glycosides and drugs of similar action**

T46.0X **Poisoning by adverse effect of and underdosing of cardiac-stimulant glycosides and drugs of similar action**

⑦T46.0X1 **Poisoning by cardiac-stimulant glycosides and drugs of similar action, accidental (unintentional)**

Poisoning by cardiac-stimulant glycosides and drugs of similar action NOS

⑦ T46.0X2 **Poisoning by cardiac-stimulant glycosides and drugs of similar action, intentional self-harm** [HCC]

⑦ T46.0X3 **Poisoning by cardiac-stimulant glycosides and drugs of similar action, assault**

⑦ T46.0X4 **Poisoning by cardiac-stimulant glycosides and drugs of similar action, undetermined**

⑦ T46.0X5 **Adverse effect of cardiac-stimulant glycosides and drugs of similar action**

⑦ T46.0X6 **Underdosing of cardiac-stimulant glycosides and drugs of similar action**

T46.1 **Poisoning by adverse effect of and underdosing of calcium-channel blockers**

T46.1X **Poisoning by adverse effect of and underdosing of calcium-channel blockers**

⑦ T46.1X1 **Poisoning by calcium-channel blockers, accidental (unintentional)**

Poisoning by calcium-channel blockers NOS

⑦ T46.1X2 **Poisoning by calcium-channel blockers, intentional self-harm** [HCC]

⑦ T46.1X3 **Poisoning by calcium-channel blockers, assault**

⑦ T46.1X4 **Poisoning by calcium-channel blockers, undetermined**

⑦ T46.1X5 **Adverse effect of calcium-channel blockers**

⑦ T46.1X6 **Underdosing of calcium-channel blockers**

T46.2 **Poisoning by adverse effect of and underdosing of other antidysrhythmic drugs, not elsewhere classified**

Excludes1: poisoning by adverse effect of and underdosing of beta-adrenoreceptor antagonists (T44.7-)

T46.2X **Poisoning by adverse effect of and underdosing of other antidysrhythmic drugs**

⑦ T46.2X1 **Poisoning by other antidysrhythmic drugs, accidental (unintentional)**

Poisoning by other antidysrhythmic drugs NOS

⑦ T46.2X2 **Poisoning by other antidysrhythmic drugs, intentional self-harm** [HCC]

⑦ T46.2X3 **Poisoning by other antidysrhythmic drugs, assault**

⑦ T46.2X4 **Poisoning by other antidysrhythmic drugs, undetermined**

⑦ T46.2X5 **Adverse effect of other antidysrhythmic drugs**

⑦ T46.2X6 **Underdosing of other antidysrhythmic drugs**

T46.3 **Poisoning by adverse effect of and underdosing of coronary vasodilators**

Poisoning by adverse effect of and underdosing of dipyridamole

Excludes1: poisoning by adverse effect of and underdosing of calcium-channel blockers (T46.1)

T46.3X **Poisoning by adverse effect of and underdosing of coronary vasodilators**

⑦ T46.3X1 **Poisoning by coronary vasodilators, accidental (unintentional)**

Poisoning by coronary vasodilators NOS

⑦ T46.3X2 **Poisoning by coronary vasodilators, intentional self-harm** [HCC]

⑦ T46.3X3 **Poisoning by coronary vasodilators, assault**

⑦ T46.3X4 **Poisoning by coronary vasodilators, undetermined**

⑦ T46.3X5 **Adverse effect of coronary vasodilators**

⑦ T46.3X6 **Underdosing of coronary vasodilators**

T46.4 **Poisoning by adverse effect of and underdosing of angiotensin-converting-enzyme inhibitors**

T46.4X **Poisoning by adverse effect of and underdosing of angiotensin-converting-enzyme inhibitors**

⑦ T46.4X1 **Poisoning by angiotensin-converting-enzyme inhibitors, accidental (unintentional)**

Poisoning by angiotensin-converting-enzyme inhibitors NOS

⑦ T46.4X2 **Poisoning by angiotensin-converting-enzyme inhibitors, intentional self-harm** [HCC]

⑦ T46.4X3 **Poisoning by angiotensin-converting-enzyme inhibitors, assault**

⑦ T46.4X4 **Poisoning by angiotensin-converting-enzyme inhibitors, undetermined**

⑦ T46.4X5 **Adverse effect of angiotensin-converting-enzyme inhibitors**

⑦ T46.4X6 **Underdosing of angiotensin-converting-enzyme inhibitors**

T46.5 **Poisoning by adverse effect of and underdosing of other antihypertensive drugs**

Excludes2: poisoning by adverse effect of and underdosing of beta-adrenoreceptor antagonists (T44.7)

poisoning by adverse effect of and underdosing of calcium-channel blockers (T46.1) \

poisoning by adverse effect of and underdosing of diuretics (T50.0-T50.2)

T46.5X **Poisoning by adverse effect of and underdosing of other antihypertensive drugs**

⑦ T46.5X1 **Poisoning by other antihypertensive drugs, accidental (unintentional)**

Poisoning by other antihypertensive drugs NOS

⑦ T46.5X2 **Poisoning by other antihypertensive drugs, intentional self-harm** [HCC]

⑦ T46.5X3 **Poisoning by other antihypertensive drugs, assault**

⑦ T46.5X4 **Poisoning by other antihypertensive drugs, undetermined**

⑦ T46.5X5 **Adverse effect of other antihypertensive drugs**

⑦ T46.5X6 **Underdosing of other antihypertensive drugs**

T46.6 **Poisoning by adverse effect of and underdosing of antihyperlipidemic and antiarteriosclerotic drugs**

T46.6X **Poisoning by adverse effect of and underdosing of antihyperlipidemic and antiarteriosclerotic drugs**

⑦ T46.6X1 **Poisoning by antihyperlipidemic and antiarteriosclerotic drugs, accidental (unintentional)**

Poisoning by antihyperlipidemic and antiarteriosclerotic drugs NOS

⑦**T46.6X2** **Poisoning by antihyperlipidemic and antiarteriosclerotic drugs, intentional self-harm** [HCC]

⑦**T46.6X3** **Poisoning by antihyperlipidemic and antiarteriosclerotic drugs, assault**

⑦**T46.6X4** **Poisoning by antihyperlipidemic and antiarteriosclerotic drugs, undetermined**

⑦**T46.6X5** **Adverse effect of antihyperlipidemic and antiarteriosclerotic drugs**

⑦**T46.6X6** **Underdosing of antihyperlipidemic and antiarteriosclerotic drugs**

T46.7 **Poisoning by adverse effect of and underdosing of peripheral vasodilators**

Poisoning by adverse effect of and underdosing of nicotinic acid (derivatives)

Excludes1: poisoning by adverse effect of and underdosing of papaverine (T44.3)

T46.7X **Poisoning by adverse effect of and underdosing of peripheral vasodilators**

⑦**T46.7X1** **Poisoning by peripheral vasodilators, accidental (unintentional)**

Poisoning by peripheral vasodilators NOS

⑦**T46.7X2** **Poisoning by peripheral vasodilators, intentional self-harm** [HCC]

⑦**T46.7X3** **Poisoning by peripheral vasodilators, assault**

⑦**T46.7X4** **Poisoning by peripheral vasodilators, undetermined**

⑦**T46.7X5** **Adverse effect of peripheral vasodilators**

⑦**T46.7X6** **Underdosing of peripheral vasodilators**

T46.8 **Poisoning by adverse effect of and underdosing of antivaricose drugs, including sclerosing agents**

T46.8X **Poisoning by adverse effect of and underdosing of antivaricose drugs, including sclerosing agents**

⑦**T46.8X1** **Poisoning by antivaricose drugs, including sclerosing agents, accidental (unintentional)**

Poisoning by antivaricose drugs, including sclerosing agents NOS

⑦**T46.8X2** **Poisoning by antivaricose drugs, including sclerosing agents, intentional self-harm** [HCC]

⑦**T46.8X3** **Poisoning by antivaricose drugs, including sclerosing agents, assault**

⑦**T46.8X4** **Poisoning by antivaricose drugs, including sclerosing agents, undetermined**

⑦**T46.8X5** **Adverse effect of antivaricose drugs, including sclerosing agents**

⑦**T46.8X6** **Underdosing of antivaricose drugs, including sclerosing agents**

T46.9 **Poisoning by adverse effect of and underdosing of other and unspecified agents primarily affecting the cardiovascular system**

T46.90 **Poisoning by adverse effect of and underdosing of unspecified agents primarily affecting the cardiovascular system**

⑦**T46.901** **Poisoning by unspecified agents primarily affecting the cardiovascular system, accidental (unintentional)**

⑦**T46.902** **Poisoning by unspecified agents primarily affecting the cardiovascular system, intentional self-harm** [HCC]

⑦**T46.903** **Poisoning by unspecified agents primarily affecting the cardiovascular system, assault**

⑦**T46.904** **Poisoning by unspecified agents primarily affecting the cardiovascular system, undetermined**

⑦**T46.905** **Adverse effect of unspecified agents primarily affecting the cardiovascular system**

⑦**T46.906** **Underdosing of unspecified agents primarily affecting the cardiovascular system**

T46.99 **Poisoning by adverse effect of and underdosing of other agents primarily affecting the cardiovascular system**

⑦**T46.991** **Poisoning by other agents primarily affecting the cardiovascular system, accidental (unintentional)**

⑦**T46.992** **Poisoning by other agents primarily affecting the cardiovascular system, intentional self-harm** [HCC]

⑦**T46.993** **Poisoning by other agents primarily affecting the cardiovascular system, assault**

⑦**T46.994** **Poisoning by other agents primarily affecting the cardiovascular system, undetermined**

⑦**T46.995** **Adverse effect of other agents primarily affecting the cardiovascular system**

⑦**T46.996** **Underdosing of other agents primarily affecting the cardiovascular system**

T47 **Poisoning by adverse effect of and underdosing of agents primarily affecting the gastrointestinal system**

The appropriate 7th character is to be added to each code from category T47

A - initial encounter

D - subsequent encounter

S - sequela

T47.0 **Poisoning by adverse effect of and underdosing of histamine H2-receptor blockers**

T47.0X **Poisoning by adverse effect of and underdosing of histamine H2-receptor blockers**

⑦**T47.0X1** **Poisoning by histamine H2-receptor blockers, accidental (unintentional)**

Poisoning by histamine H2-receptor blockers NOS

⑦**T47.0X2** **Poisoning by histamine H2-receptor blockers, intentional self-harm** [HCC]

⑦**T47.0X3** **Poisoning by histamine H2-receptor blockers, assault**

⑦**T47.0X4** **Poisoning by histamine H2-receptor blockers, undetermined**

⑦**T47.0X5** **Adverse effect of histamine H2-receptor blockers**

⑦**T47.0X6** **Underdosing of histamine H2-receptor blockers**

T47.1 **Poisoning by adverse effect of and underdosing of other antacids and anti-gastric-secretion drugs**

    T47.1X **Poisoning by adverse effect of and underdosing of other antacids and anti-gastric-secretion drugs**

        ⑦**T47.1X1** **Poisoning by other antacids and anti-gastric-secretion drugs, accidental (unintentional)**

            Poisoning by other antacids and anti-gastric-secretion drugs NOS

        ⑦**T47.1X2** **Poisoning by other antacids and anti-gastric-secretion drugs, intentional self-harm** [HCC]

        ⑦**T47.1X3** **Poisoning by other antacids and anti-gastric-secretion drugs, assault**

        ⑦**T47.1X4** **Poisoning by other antacids and anti-gastric-secretion drugs, undetermined**

        ⑦**T47.1X5** **Adverse effect of other antacids and anti-gastric-secretion drugs**

        ⑦**T47.1X6** **Underdosing of other antacids and anti-gastric-secretion drugs**

T47.2 **Poisoning by adverse effect of and underdosing of stimulant laxatives**

    T47.2X **Poisoning by adverse effect of and underdosing of stimulant laxatives**

        ⑦**T47.2X1** **Poisoning by stimulant laxatives, accidental (unintentional)**

            Poisoning by stimulant laxatives NOS

        ⑦**T47.2X2** **Poisoning by stimulant laxatives, intentional self-harm** [HCC]

        ⑦**T47.2X3** **Poisoning by stimulant laxatives, assault**

        ⑦**T47.2X4** **Poisoning by stimulant laxatives, undetermined**

        ⑦**T47.2X5** **Adverse effect of stimulant laxatives**

        ⑦**T47.2X6** **Underdosing of stimulant laxatives**

T47.3 **Poisoning by adverse effect of and underdosing of saline and osmotic laxatives**

    T47.3X **Poisoning by and adverse effect of saline and osmotic laxatives**

        ⑦**T47.3X1** **Poisoning by saline and osmotic laxatives, accidental (unintentional)**

            Poisoning by saline and osmotic laxatives NOS

        ⑦**T47.3X2** **Poisoning by saline and osmotic laxatives, intentional self-harm** [HCC]

        ⑦**T47.3X3** **Poisoning by saline and osmotic laxatives, assault**

        ⑦**T47.3X4** **Poisoning by saline and osmotic laxatives, undetermined**

        ⑦**T47.3X5** **Adverse effect of saline and osmotic laxatives**

        ⑦**T47.3X6** **Underdosing of saline and osmotic laxatives**

T47.4 **Poisoning by adverse effect of and underdosing of other laxatives**

    T47.4X **Poisoning by adverse effect of and underdosing of other laxatives**

        ⑦**T47.4X1** **Poisoning by other laxatives, accidental (unintentional)**

            Poisoning by other laxatives NOS

        ⑦**T47.4X2** **Poisoning by other laxatives, intentional self-harm** [HCC]

        ⑦**T47.4X3** **Poisoning by other laxatives, assault**

        ⑦**T47.4X4** **Poisoning by other laxatives, undetermined**

        ⑦**T47.4X5** **Adverse effect of other laxatives**

        ⑦**T47.4X6** **Underdosing of other laxatives**

T47.5 **Poisoning by adverse effect of and underdosing of digestants**

    T47.5X **Poisoning by adverse effect of and underdosing of digestants**

        ⑦**T47.5X1** **Poisoning by digestants, accidental (unintentional)**

            Poisoning by digestants NOS

        ⑦**T47.5X2** **Poisoning by digestants, intentional self-harm** [HCC]

        ⑦**T47.5X3** **Poisoning by digestants, assault**

        ⑦**T47.5X4** **Poisoning by digestants, undetermined**

        ⑦**T47.5X5** **Adverse effect of digestants**

        ⑦**T47.5X6** **Underdosing of digestants**

T47.6 **Poisoning by adverse effect of and underdosing of antidiarrheal drugs**

    Excludes2: poisoning by adverse effect of and underdosing of systemic antibiotics and other anti-infectives (T36-T37)

    T47.6X **Poisoning by adverse effect of and underdosing of antidiarrheal drugs**

        ⑦**T47.6X1** **Poisoning by antidiarrheal drugs, accidental (unintentional)**

            Poisoning by antidiarrheal drugs NOS

        ⑦**T47.6X2** **Poisoning by antidiarrheal drugs, intentional self-harm** [HCC]

        ⑦**T47.6X3** **Poisoning by antidiarrheal drugs, assault**

        ⑦**T47.6X4** **Poisoning by antidiarrheal drugs, undetermined**

        ⑦**T47.6X5** **Adverse effect of antidiarrheal drugs**

        ⑦**T47.6X6** **Underdosing of antidiarrheal drugs**

T47.7 **Poisoning by adverse effect of and underdosing of emetics**

    T47.7X **Poisoning by adverse effect of and underdosing of emetics**

        ⑦**T47.7X1** **Poisoning by emetics, accidental (unintentional)**

            Poisoning by emetics NOS

        ⑦**T47.7X2** **Poisoning by emetics, intentional self-harm** [HCC]

        ⑦**T47.7X3** **Poisoning by emetics, assault**

        ⑦**T47.7X4** **Poisoning by emetics, undetermined**

        ⑦**T47.7X5** **Adverse effect of emetics**

        ⑦**T47.7X6** **Underdosing of emetics**

T47.8 **Poisoning by adverse effect of and underdosing of other agents primarily affecting gastrointestinal system**

    T47.8X **Poisoning by adverse effect of and underdosing of other agents primarily affecting gastrointestinal system**

        ⑦**T47.8X1** **Poisoning by other agents primarily affecting gastrointestinal system, accidental (unintentional)**

            Poisoning by other agents primarily affecting gastrointestinal system NOS

    ● New code   ▲ Revised code   Excludes1: Not coded here   Excludes2: Not included here   ⊗ Placeholder required   ⑦7th digit required

⑦T47.8X2 **Poisoning by other agents primarily affecting gastrointestinal system, intentional self-harm** [HCC]

⑦T47.8X3 **Poisoning by other agents primarily affecting gastrointestinal system, assault**

⑦T47.8X4 **Poisoning by other agents primarily affecting gastrointestinal system, undetermined**

⑦T47.8X5 **Adverse effect of other agents primarily affecting gastrointestinal system**

⑦T47.8X6 **Underdosing of other agents primarily affecting gastrointestinal system**

T47.9 **Poisoning by adverse effect of and underdosing of unspecified agents primarily affecting the gastrointestinal system**

⊗⑦T47.91 **Poisoning by unspecified agents primarily affecting the gastrointestinal system, accidental (unintentional)**

Poisoning by agents primarily affecting the gastrointestinal system NOS

⊗⑦T47.92 **Poisoning by unspecified agents primarily affecting the gastrointestinal system, intentional self-harm** [HCC]

⊗⑦T47.93 **Poisoning by unspecified agents primarily affecting the gastrointestinal system, assault**

⊗⑦T47.94 **Poisoning by unspecified agents primarily affecting the gastrointestinal system, undetermined**

⊗⑦T47.95 **Adverse effect of unspecified agents primarily affecting the gastrointestinal system**

⊗⑦T47.96 **Underdosing of unspecified agents primarily affecting the gastrointestinal system**

T48 **Poisoning by adverse effect of and underdosing of agents primarily acting on smooth and skeletal muscles and the respiratory system**

The appropriate 7th character is to be added to each code from category T48

A - initial encounter

D - subsequent encounter

S - sequela

T48.0 **Poisoning by adverse effect of and underdosing of oxytocic drugs**

Excludes1: poisoning by adverse effect of and underdosing of estrogens, progestogens and antagonists (T38.4-T38.6)

T48.0X **Poisoning by adverse effect of and underdosing of oxytocic drugs**

⑦T48.0X1 **Poisoning by oxytocic drugs, accidental (unintentional)**

Poisoning by oxytocic drugs NOS

⑦T48.0X2 **Poisoning by oxytocic drugs, intentional self-harm** [HCC]

⑦T48.0X3 **Poisoning by oxytocic drugs, assault**

⑦T48.0X4 **Poisoning by oxytocic drugs, undetermined**

⑦T48.0X5 **Adverse effect of oxytocic drugs**

⑦T48.0X6 **Underdosing of oxytocic drugs**

T48.1 **Poisoning by adverse effect of and underdosing of skeletal muscle relaxants [neuromuscular blocking agents]**

T48.1X **Poisoning by adverse effect of and underdosing of skeletal muscle relaxants [neuromuscular blocking agents]**

⑦T48.1X1 **Poisoning by skeletal muscle relaxants [neuromuscular blocking agents], accidental (unintentional)**

Poisoning by skeletal muscle relaxants [neuromuscular blocking agents] NOS

⑦T48.1X2 **Poisoning by skeletal muscle relaxants [neuromuscular blocking agents], intentional self-harm** [HCC]

⑦T48.1X3 **Poisoning by skeletal muscle relaxants [neuromuscular blocking agents], assault**

⑦T48.1X4 **Poisoning by skeletal muscle relaxants [neuromuscular blocking agents], undetermined**

⑦T48.1X5 **Adverse effect of skeletal muscle relaxants [neuromuscular blocking agents]**

⑦T48.1X6 **Underdosing of skeletal muscle relaxants [neuromuscular blocking agents]**

T48.2 **Poisoning by adverse effect of and underdosing of other and unspecified drugs acting on muscles**

T48.20 **Poisoning by adverse effect of and underdosing of unspecified drugs acting on muscles**

⑦T48.201 **Poisoning by unspecified drugs acting on muscles, accidental (unintentional)**

Poisoning by unspecified drugs acting on muscles NOS

⑦T48.202 **Poisoning by unspecified drugs acting on muscles, intentional self-harm** [HCC]

⑦T48.203 **Poisoning by unspecified drugs acting on muscles, assault**

⑦T48.204 **Poisoning by unspecified drugs acting on muscles, undetermined**

⑦T48.205 **Adverse effect of unspecified drugs acting on muscles**

⑦T48.206 **Underdosing of unspecified drugs acting on muscles**

T48.29 **Poisoning by adverse effect of and underdosing of other drugs acting on muscles**

⑦T48.291 **Poisoning by other drugs acting on muscles, accidental (unintentional)**

Poisoning by other drugs acting on muscles NOS

⑦T48.292 **Poisoning by other drugs acting on muscles, intentional self-harm** [HCC]

⑦T48.293 **Poisoning by other drugs acting on muscles, assault**

⑦T48.294 **Poisoning by other drugs acting on muscles, undetermined**

⑦T48.295 **Adverse effect of other drugs acting on muscles**

⑦T48.296 **Underdosing of other drugs acting on muscles**

T48.3 **Poisoning by adverse effect of and underdosing of antitussives**

T48.3X **Poisoning by adverse effect of and underdosing of antitussives**

⑦T48.3X1 **Poisoning by antitussives, accidental (unintentional)**

Poisoning by antitussives NOS

⑦**T48.3X2** **Poisoning by antitussives, intentional self-harm** [HCC]

⑦**T48.3X3** **Poisoning by antitussives, assault**

⑦**T48.3X4** **Poisoning by antitussives, undetermined**

⑦**T48.3X5** **Adverse effect of antitussives**

⑦**T48.3X6** **Underdosing of antitussives**

T48.4 **Poisoning by adverse effect of and underdosing of expectorants**

T48.4X **Poisoning by adverse effect of and underdosing of expectorants**

⑦**T48.4X1** **Poisoning by expectorants, accidental (unintentional)**

Poisoning by expectorants NOS

⑦**T48.4X2** **Poisoning by expectorants, intentional self-harm** [HCC]

⑦**T48.4X3** **Poisoning by expectorants, assault**

⑦**T48.4X4** **Poisoning by expectorants, undetermined**

⑦**T48.4X5** **Adverse effect of expectorants**

⑦**T48.4X6** **Underdosing of expectorants**

T48.5 **Poisoning by adverse effect of and underdosing of other anti-common-cold drugs**

Poisoning by adverse effect of and underdosing of decongestants

Excludes2: poisoning by adverse effect of and underdosing of antipyretics, NEC (T39.9-)

poisoning by adverse effect of and underdosing of non-steroidal antiinflammatory drugs (T39.3-)

poisoning by adverse effect of and underdosing of salicylates (T39.0-)

T48.5X **Poisoning by adverse effect of and underdosing of other anti-common-cold drugs**

⑦**T48.5X1** **Poisoning by other anti-common-cold drugs, accidental (unintentional)**

Poisoning by other anti-common-cold drugs NOS

⑦**T48.5X2** **Poisoning by other anti-common-cold drugs, intentional self-harm** [HCC]

⑦**T48.5X3** **Poisoning by other anti-common-cold drugs, assault**

⑦**T48.5X4** **Poisoning by other anti-common-cold drugs, undetermined**

⑦**T48.5X5** **Adverse effect of other anti-common-cold drugs**

⑦**T48.5X6** **Underdosing of other anti-common-cold drugs**

T48.6 **Poisoning by adverse effect of and underdosing of antiasthmatics, not elsewhere classified**

Poisoning by adverse effect of and underdosing of beta-adrenoreceptor agonists used in asthma therapy

Excludes1: poisoning by adverse effect of and underdosing of beta-adrenoreceptor agonists not used in asthma therapy (T44.5)

poisoning by adverse effect of and underdosing of anterior pituitary [adenohypophyseal] hormones (T38.8)

T48.6X **Poisoning by adverse effect of and underdosing of antiasthmatics**

⑦**T48.6X1** **Poisoning by antiasthmatics, accidental (unintentional)**

Poisoning by antiasthmatics NOS

⑦**T48.6X2** **Poisoning by antiasthmatics, intentional self-harm** [HCC]

⑦**T48.6X3** **Poisoning by antiasthmatics, assault**

⑦**T48.6X4** **Poisoning by antiasthmatics, undetermined**

⑦**T48.6X5** **Adverse effect of antiasthmatics**

⑦**T48.6X6** **Underdosing of antiasthmatics**

T48.9 **Poisoning by adverse effect of and underdosing of other and unspecified agents primarily acting on the respiratory system**

T48.90 **Poisoning by adverse effect of and underdosing of unspecified agents primarily acting on the respiratory system**

⑦**T48.901** **Poisoning by unspecified agents primarily acting on the respiratory system, accidental (unintentional)**

⑦**T48.902** **Poisoning by unspecified agents primarily acting on the respiratory system, intentional self-harm** [HCC]

⑦**T48.903** **Poisoning by unspecified agents primarily acting on the respiratory system, assault**

⑦**T48.904** **Poisoning by unspecified agents primarily acting on the respiratory system, undetermined**

⑦**T48.905** **Adverse effect of unspecified agents primarily acting on the respiratory system**

⑦**T48.906** **Underdosing of unspecified agents primarily acting on the respiratory system**

T48.99 **Poisoning by adverse effect of and underdosing of other agents primarily acting on the respiratory system**

⑦**T48.991** **Poisoning by other agents primarily acting on the respiratory system, accidental (unintentional)**

⑦**T48.992** **Poisoning by other agents primarily acting on the respiratory system, intentional self-harm** [HCC]

⑦**T48.993** **Poisoning by other agents primarily acting on the respiratory system, assault**

⑦**T48.994** **Poisoning by other agents primarily acting on the respiratory system, undetermined**

⑦**T48.995** **Adverse effect of other agents primarily acting on the respiratory system**

⑦**T48.996** **Underdosing of other agents primarily acting on the respiratory system**

T49 **Poisoning by adverse effect of and underdosing of topical agents primarily affecting skin and mucous membrane and by ophthalmological, otorhinolaryngological and dental drugs**

Includes: poisoning by adverse effect of and underdosing of glucocorticoids, topically used

The appropriate 7th character is to be added to each code from category T49

A - initial encounter

D - subsequent encounter

S - sequela

T49.0 **Poisoning by adverse effect of and underdosing of local antifungal, anti-infective and anti-inflammatory drugs**

T49.0X **Poisoning by adverse effect of and underdosing of local antifungal, anti-infective and anti-inflammatory drugs**

⑦**T49.0X1** Poisoning by local antifungal, anti-infective and anti-inflammatory drugs, accidental (unintentional)

Poisoning by local antifungal, anti-infective and anti-inflammatory drugs NOS

⑦**T49.0X2** Poisoning by local antifungal, anti-infective and anti-inflammatory drugs, intentional self-harm [HCC]

⑦**T49.0X3** Poisoning by local antifungal, anti-infective and anti-inflammatory drugs, assault

⑦**T49.0X4** Poisoning by local antifungal, anti-infective and anti-inflammatory drugs, undetermined

⑦**T49.0X5** Adverse effect of local antifungal, anti-infective and anti-inflammatory drugs

⑦**T49.0X6** Underdosing of local antifungal, anti-infective and anti-inflammatory drugs

T49.1 **Poisoning by adverse effect of and underdosing of antipruritics**

T49.1X **Poisoning by adverse effect of and underdosing of antipruritics**

⑦**T49.1X1** Poisoning by antipruritics, accidental (unintentional)

Poisoning by antipruritics NOS

⑦**T49.1X2** Poisoning by antipruritics, intentional self-harm [HCC]

⑦**T49.1X3** Poisoning by antipruritics, assault

⑦**T49.1X4** Poisoning by antipruritics, undetermined

⑦**T49.1X5** Adverse effect of antipruritics

⑦**T49.1X6** Underdosing of antipruritics

T49.2 **Poisoning by adverse effect of and underdosing of local astringents and local detergents**

T49.2X **Poisoning by adverse effect of and underdosing of local astringents and local detergents**

⑦**T49.2X1** Poisoning by local astringents and local detergents, accidental (unintentional)

Poisoning by local astringents and local detergents NOS

⑦**T49.2X2** Poisoning by local astringents and local detergents, intentional self-harm [HCC]

⑦**T49.2X3** Poisoning by local astringents and local detergents, assault

⑦**T49.2X4** Poisoning by local astringents and local detergents, undetermined

⑦**T49.2X5** Adverse effect of local astringents and local detergents

⑦**T49.2X6** Underdosing of local astringents and local detergents

T49.3 **Poisoning by adverse effect of and underdosing of emollients, demulcents and protectants**

T49.3X **Poisoning by adverse effect of and underdosing of emollients, demulcents and protectants**

⑦**T49.3X1** Poisoning by emollients, demulcents and protectants, accidental (unintentional)

Poisoning by emollients, demulcents and protectants NOS

⑦**T49.3X2** Poisoning by emollients, demulcents and protectants, intentional self-harm [HCC]

⑦**T49.3X3** Poisoning by emollients, demulcents and protectants, assault

⑦**T49.3X4** Poisoning by emollients, demulcents and protectants, undetermined

⑦**T49.3X5** Adverse effect of emollients, demulcents and protectants

⑦**T49.3X6** Underdosing of emollients, demulcents and protectants

T49.4 **Poisoning by adverse effect of and underdosing of keratolytics, keratoplastics, and other hair treatment drugs and preparations**

T49.4X **Poisoning by adverse effect of and underdosing of keratolytics, keratoplastics, and other hair treatment drugs and preparations**

⑦**T49.4X1** Poisoning by keratolytics, keratoplastics, and other hair treatment drugs and preparations, accidental (unintentional)

Poisoning by keratolytics, keratoplastics, and other hair treatment drugs and preparations NOS

⑦**T49.4X2** Poisoning by keratolytics, keratoplastics, and other hair treatment drugs and preparations, intentional self-harm [HCC]

⑦**T49.4X3** Poisoning by keratolytics, keratoplastics, and other hair treatment drugs and preparations, assault

⑦**T49.4X4** Poisoning by keratolytics, keratoplastics, and other hair treatment drugs and preparations, undetermined

⑦**T49.4X5** Adverse effect of keratolytics, keratoplastics, and other hair treatment drugs and preparations

⑦**T49.4X6** Underdosing of keratolytics, keratoplastics, and other hair treatment drugs and preparations

T49.5 **Poisoning by adverse effect of and underdosing of ophthalmological drugs and preparations**

T49.5X **Poisoning by adverse effect of and underdosing of ophthalmological drugs and preparations**

⑦**T49.5X1** Poisoning by ophthalmological drugs and preparations, accidental (unintentional)

Poisoning by ophthalmological drugs and preparations NOS

⑦**T49.5X2** Poisoning by ophthalmological drugs and preparations, intentional self-harm [HCC]

⑦**T49.5X3** Poisoning by ophthalmological drugs and preparations, assault

⑦**T49.5X4** Poisoning by ophthalmological drugs and preparations, undetermined

⑦**T49.5X5** Adverse effect of ophthalmological drugs and preparations

⑦**T49.5X6** Underdosing of ophthalmological drugs and preparations

T49.6 **Poisoning by adverse effect of and underdosing of otorhinolaryngological drugs and preparations**

T49.6X Poisoning by adverse effect of and underdosing of otorhinolaryngological drugs and preparations

⑦**T49.6X1** Poisoning by otorhinolaryngological drugs and preparations, accidental (unintentional)

Poisoning by otorhinolaryngological drugs and preparations NOS

⑦**T49.6X2** Poisoning by otorhinolaryngological drugs and preparations, intentional self-harm [HCC]

⑦**T49.6X3** Poisoning by otorhinolaryngological drugs and preparations, assault

⑦**T49.6X4** Poisoning by otorhinolaryngological drugs and preparations, undetermined

⑦**T49.6X5** Adverse effect of otorhinolaryngological drugs and preparations

⑦**T49.6X6** Underdosing of otorhinolaryngological drugs and preparations

T49.7 Poisoning by adverse effect of and underdosing of dental drugs, topically applied

T49.7X Poisoning by adverse effect of and underdosing of dental drugs, topically applied

⑦**T49.7X1** Poisoning by dental drugs, topically applied, accidental (unintentional)

Poisoning by dental drugs, topically applied NOS

⑦**T49.7X2** Poisoning by dental drugs, topically applied, intentional self-harm [HCC]

⑦**T49.7X3** Poisoning by dental drugs, topically applied, assault

⑦**T49.7X4** Poisoning by dental drugs, topically applied, undetermined

⑦**T49.7X5** Adverse effect of dental drugs, topically applied

⑦**T49.7X6** Underdosing of dental drugs, topically applied

T49.8 Poisoning by adverse effect of and underdosing of other topical agents

Poisoning by adverse effect of and underdosing of spermicides

T49.8X Poisoning by adverse effect of and underdosing of other topical agents

⑦**T49.8X1** Poisoning by other topical agents, accidental (unintentional)

Poisoning by other topical agents NOS

⑦**T49.8X2** Poisoning by other topical agents, intentional self-harm [HCC]

⑦**T49.8X3** Poisoning by other topical agents, assault

⑦**T49.8X4** Poisoning by other topical agents, undetermined

⑦**T49.8X5** Adverse effect of other topical agents

⑦**T49.8X6** Underdosing of other topical agents

T49.9 Poisoning by adverse effect of and underdosing of unspecified topical agent

⊗⑦**T49.91** Poisoning by unspecified topical agent, accidental (unintentional)

⊗⑦**T49.92** Poisoning by unspecified topical agent, intentional self-harm [HCC]

⊗⑦**T49.93** Poisoning by unspecified topical agent, assault

⊗⑦**T49.94** Poisoning by unspecified topical agent, undetermined

⊗⑦**T49.95** Adverse effect of unspecified topical agent

⊗⑦**T49.96** Underdosing of unspecified topical agent

T50 Poisoning by adverse effect of and underdosing of diuretics and other and unspecified drugs, medicaments and biological substances

The appropriate 7th character is to be added to each code from category T50

A - initial encounter

D - subsequent encounter

S - sequela

T50.0 Poisoning by adverse effect of and underdosing of mineralocorticoids and their antagonists

T50.0X Poisoning by adverse effect of and underdosing of mineralocorticoids and their antagonists

⑦**T50.0X1** Poisoning by mineralocorticoids and their antagonists, accidental (unintentional)

Poisoning by mineralocorticoids and their antagonists NOS

⑦**T50.0X2** Poisoning by mineralocorticoids and their antagonists, intentional self-harm [HCC]

⑦**T50.0X3** Poisoning by mineralocorticoids and their antagonists, assault

⑦**T50.0X4** Poisoning by mineralocorticoids and their antagonists, undetermined

⑦**T50.0X5** Adverse effect of mineralocorticoids and their antagonists

⑦**T50.0X6** Underdosing of mineralocorticoids and their antagonists

T50.1 Poisoning by adverse effect of and underdosing of loop [high-ceiling] diuretics

T50.1X Poisoning by adverse effect of and underdosing of loop [high-ceiling] diuretics

⑦**T50.1X1** Poisoning by loop [high-ceiling] diuretics, accidental (unintentional)

Poisoning by loop [high-ceiling] diuretics NOS

⑦**T50.1X2** Poisoning by loop [high-ceiling] diuretics, intentional self-harm [HCC]

⑦**T50.1X3** Poisoning by loop [high-ceiling] diuretics, assault

⑦**T50.1X4** Poisoning by loop [high-ceiling] diuretics, undetermined

⑦**T50.1X5** Adverse effect of loop [high-ceiling] diuretics

⑦**T50.1X6** Underdosing of loop [high-ceiling] diuretics

T50.2 Poisoning by adverse effect of and underdosing of carbonic-anhydrase inhibitors, benzothiadiazides and other diuretics

Poisoning by adverse effect of and underdosing of acetazolamide

T50.2X Poisoning by adverse effect of and underdosing of carbonic-anhydrase inhibitors, benzothiadiazides and other diuretics

⑦**T50.2X1** Poisoning by carbonic-anhydrase inhibitors, benzothiadiazides and other diuretics, accidental (unintentional)

Poisoning by carbonic-anhydrase inhibitors, benzothiadiazides and other diuretics NOS

● New code ▲ Revised code **Excludes1:** Not coded here **Excludes2:** Not included here ⊗ Placeholder required ⑦ 7th digit required

⑦**T50.2X2** Poisoning by carbonic-anhydrase inhibitors, benzothiadiazides and other diuretics, intentional self-harm [HCC]

⑦**T50.2X3** Poisoning by carbonic-anhydrase inhibitors, benzothiadiazides and other diuretics, assault

⑦**T50.2X4** Poisoning by carbonic-anhydrase inhibitors, benzothiadiazides and other diuretics, undetermined

⑦**T50.2X5** Adverse effect of carbonic-anhydrase inhibitors, benzothiadiazides and other diuretics

⑦**T50.2X6** Underdosing of carbonic-anhydrase inhibitors, benzothiadiazides and other diuretics

T50.3 Poisoning by adverse effect of and underdosing of electrolytic, caloric and water-balance agents

Poisoning by adverse effect of and underdosing of oral rehydration salts

T50.3X Poisoning by adverse effect of and underdosing of electrolytic, caloric and water-balance agents

⑦**T50.3X1** Poisoning by electrolytic, caloric and water-balance agents, accidental (unintentional)

Poisoning by electrolytic, caloric and water-balance agents NOS

⑦**T50.3X2** Poisoning by electrolytic, caloric and water-balance agents, intentional self-harm [HCC]

⑦**T50.3X3** Poisoning by electrolytic, caloric and water-balance agents, assault

⑦**T50.3X4** Poisoning by electrolytic, caloric and water-balance agents, undetermined

⑦**T50.3X5** Adverse effect of electrolytic, caloric and water-balance agents

⑦**T50.3X6** Underdosing of electrolytic, caloric and water-balance agents

T50.4 Poisoning by adverse effect of and underdosing of drugs affecting uric acid metabolism

T50.4X Poisoning by adverse effect of and underdosing of drugs affecting uric acid metabolism

⑦**T50.4X1** Poisoning by drugs affecting uric acid metabolism, accidental (unintentional)

Poisoning by drugs affecting uric acid metabolism NOS

⑦**T50.4X2** Poisoning by drugs affecting uric acid metabolism, intentional self-harm [HCC]

⑦**T50.4X3** Poisoning by drugs affecting uric acid metabolism, assault

⑦**T50.4X4** Poisoning by drugs affecting uric acid metabolism, undetermined

⑦**T50.4X5** Adverse effect of drugs affecting uric acid metabolism

⑦**T50.4X6** Underdosing of drugs affecting uric acid metabolism

T50.5 Poisoning by adverse effect of and underdosing of appetite depressants

T50.5X Poisoning by adverse effect of and underdosing of appetite depressants

⑦**T50.5X1** Poisoning by appetite depressants, accidental (unintentional)

Poisoning by appetite depressants NOS

⑦**T50.5X2** Poisoning by appetite depressants, intentional self-harm [HCC]

⑦**T50.5X3** Poisoning by appetite depressants, assault

⑦**T50.5X4** Poisoning by appetite depressants, undetermined

⑦**T50.5X5** Adverse effect of appetite depressants

⑦**T50.5X6** Underdosing of appetite depressants

T50.6 Poisoning by adverse effect of and underdosing of antidotes and chelating agents

Poisoning by adverse effect of and underdosing of alcohol deterrents

T50.6X Poisoning by adverse effect of and underdosing of antidotes and chelating agents

⑦**T50.6X1** Poisoning by antidotes and chelating agents, accidental (unintentional)

Poisoning by antidotes and chelating agents NOS

⑦**T50.6X2** Poisoning by antidotes and chelating agents, intentional self-harm [HCC]

⑦**T50.6X3** Poisoning by antidotes and chelating agents, assault

⑦**T50.6X4** Poisoning by antidotes and chelating agents, undetermined

⑦**T50.6X5** Adverse effect of antidotes and chelating agents

⑦**T50.6X6** Underdosing of antidotes and chelating agents

T50.7 Poisoning by adverse effect of and underdosing of analeptics and opioid receptor antagonists

T50.7X Poisoning by adverse effect of and underdosing of analeptics and opioid receptor antagonists

⑦**T50.7X1** Poisoning by analeptics and opioid receptor antagonists, accidental (unintentional)

Poisoning by analeptics and opioid receptor antagonists NOS

⑦**T50.7X2** Poisoning by analeptics and opioid receptor antagonists, intentional self-harm [HCC]

⑦**T50.7X3** Poisoning by analeptics and opioid receptor antagonists, assault

⑦**T50.7X4** Poisoning by analeptics and opioid receptor antagonists, undetermined

⑦**T50.7X5** Adverse effect of analeptics and opioid receptor antagonists

⑦**T50.7X6** Underdosing of analeptics and opioid receptor antagonists

T50.8 Poisoning by adverse effect of and underdosing of diagnostic agents

T50.8X Poisoning by adverse effect of and underdosing of diagnostic agents

⑦**T50.8X1** Poisoning by diagnostic agents, accidental (unintentional)

Poisoning by diagnostic agents NOS

⑦**T50.8X2** Poisoning by diagnostic agents, intentional self-harm [HCC]

⑦**T50.8X3** Poisoning by diagnostic agents, assault

⑦**T50.8X4** Poisoning by diagnostic agents, undetermined

⑦**T50.8X5** Adverse effect of diagnostic agents

⑦**T50.8X6** Underdosing of diagnostic agents

■ Add 4th-7th digits   ■ Nonspecific code   ■ Unspecified code   ■ Manifestation code   [HCC] Hierarchical Condition Code

T50.A Poisoning by adverse effect of and underdosing of bacterial vaccines

    T50.A1 Poisoning by adverse effect of and underdosing of pertussis vaccine, including combinations with a pertussis component

        ⑦**T50.A11 Poisoning by pertussis vaccine, including combinations with a pertussis component, accidental (unintentional)**

        ⑦**T50.A12 Poisoning by pertussis vaccine, including combinations with a pertussis component, intentional self-harm** [HCC]

        ⑦**T50.A13 Poisoning by pertussis vaccine, including combinations with a pertussis component, assault**

        ⑦**T50.A14 Poisoning by pertussis vaccine, including combinations with a pertussis component, undetermined**

        ⑦**T50.A15 Adverse effect of pertussis vaccine, including combinations with a pertussis component**

        ⑦**T50.A16 Underdosing of pertussis vaccine, including combinations with a pertussis component**

    T50.A2 Poisoning by adverse effect of and underdosing of mixed bacterial vaccines without a pertussis component

        ⑦**T50.A21 Poisoning by mixed bacterial vaccines without a pertussis component, accidental (unintentional)**

        ⑦**T50.A22 Poisoning by mixed bacterial vaccines without a pertussis component, intentional self-harm** [HCC]

        ⑦**T50.A23 Poisoning by mixed bacterial vaccines without a pertussis component, assault**

        ⑦**T50.A24 Poisoning by mixed bacterial vaccines without a pertussis component, undetermined**

        ⑦**T50.A25 Adverse effect of mixed bacterial vaccines without a pertussis component**

        ⑦**T50.A26 Underdosing of mixed bacterial vaccines without a pertussis component**

    T50.A9 Poisoning by adverse effect of and underdosing of other bacterial vaccines

        ⑦**T50.A91 Poisoning by other bacterial vaccines, accidental (unintentional)**

        ⑦**T50.A92 Poisoning by other bacterial vaccines, intentional self-harm** [HCC]

        ⑦**T50.A93 Poisoning by other bacterial vaccines, assault**

        ⑦**T50.A94 Poisoning by other bacterial vaccines, undetermined**

        ⑦**T50.A95 Adverse effect of other bacterial vaccines**

        ⑦**T50.A96 Underdosing of other bacterial vaccines**

T50.B Poisoning by adverse effect of and underdosing of viral vaccines

    T50.B1 Poisoning by adverse effect of and underdosing of smallpox vaccines

        ⑦**T50.B11 Poisoning by smallpox vaccines, accidental (unintentional)**

        ⑦**T50.B12 Poisoning by smallpox vaccines, intentional self-harm** [HCC]

        ⑦**T50.B13 Poisoning by smallpox vaccines, assault**

        ⑦**T50.B14 Poisoning by smallpox vaccines, undetermined**

        ⑦**T50.B15 Adverse effect of smallpox vaccines**

        ⑦**T50.B16 Underdosing of smallpox vaccines**

    T50.B9 Poisoning by adverse effect of and underdosing of other viral vaccines

        ⑦**T50.B91 Poisoning by other viral vaccines, accidental (unintentional)**

        ⑦**T50.B92 Poisoning by other viral vaccines, intentional self-harm** [HCC]

        ⑦**T50.B93 Poisoning by other viral vaccines, assault**

        ⑦**T50.B94 Poisoning by other viral vaccines, undetermined**

        ⑦**T50.B95 Adverse effect of other viral vaccines**

        ⑦**T50.B96 Underdosing of other viral vaccines**

T50.Z Poisoning by adverse effect of and underdosing of other vaccines and biological substances

    T50.Z1 Poisoning by adverse effect of and underdosing of immunoglobulin

        ⑦**T50.Z11 Poisoning by immunoglobulin, accidental (unintentional)**

        ⑦**T50.Z12 Poisoning by immunoglobulin, intentional self-harm** [HCC]

        ⑦**T50.Z13 Poisoning by immunoglobulin, assault**

        ⑦**T50.Z14 Poisoning by immunoglobulin, undetermined**

        ⑦**T50.Z15 Adverse effect of immunoglobulin**

        ⑦**T50.Z16 Underdosing of immunoglobulin**

    T50.Z9 Poisoning by adverse effect of and underdosing of other vaccines and biological substances

        ⑦**T50.Z91 Poisoning by other vaccines and biological substances, accidental (unintentional)**

        ⑦**T50.Z92 Poisoning by other vaccines and biological substances, intentional self-harm** [HCC]

        ⑦**T50.Z93 Poisoning by other vaccines and biological substances, assault**

        ⑦**T50.Z94 Poisoning by other vaccines and biological substances, undetermined**

        ⑦**T50.Z95 Adverse effect of other vaccines and biological substances**

        ⑦**T50.Z96 Underdosing of other vaccines and biological substances**

T50.9 Poisoning by adverse effect of and underdosing of other and unspecified drugs, medicaments and biological substances

    T50.90 Poisoning by adverse effect of and underdosing of unspecified drugs, medicaments and biological substances

        ⑦**T50.901 Poisoning by unspecified drugs, medicaments and biological substances, accidental (unintentional)**

        ⑦**T50.902 Poisoning by unspecified drugs, medicaments and biological**

● New code ▲ Revised code **Excludes1:** Not coded here **Excludes2:** Not included here ⊗ Placeholder required ⑦ 7ᵗʰ digit required

substances, intentional self-harm [HCC]

⑦**T50.903** Poisoning by unspecified drugs, medicaments and biological substances, assault

⑦**T50.904** Poisoning by unspecified drugs, medicaments and biological substances, undetermined

⑦**T50.905** Adverse effect of unspecified drugs, medicaments and biological substances

⑦**T50.906** Underdosing of unspecified drugs, medicaments and biological substances

T50.91 Poisoning by adverse effect of and underdosing of multiple unspecified drugs, medicaments and biological substances

Multiple drug ingestion NOS

Code also any specific drugs, medicaments and biological substances

⑦**T50.911** Poisoning by multiple unspecified drugs, medicaments and biological substances, accidental (unintentional)

⑦**T50.912** Poisoning by multiple unspecified drugs, medicaments and biological substances, intentional self-harm

⑦**T50.913** Poisoning by multiple unspecified drugs, medicaments and biological substances, assault

⑦**T50.914** Poisoning by multiple unspecified drugs, medicaments and biological substances, undetermined

⑦**T50.915** Adverse effect of multiple unspecified drugs, medicaments and biological substances

⑦**T50.916** Underdosing of multiple unspecified drugs, medicaments and biological substances

T50.99 Poisoning by adverse effect of and underdosing of other drugs, medicaments and biological substances

⑦**T50.991** Poisoning by other drugs, medicaments and biological substances, accidental (unintentional)

⑦**T50.992** Poisoning by other drugs, medicaments and biological substances, intentional self-harm [HCC]

⑦**T50.993** Poisoning by other drugs, medicaments and biological substances, assault

⑦**T50.994** Poisoning by other drugs, medicaments and biological substances, undetermined

⑦**T50.995** Adverse effect of other drugs, medicaments and biological substances

⑦**T50.996** Underdosing of other drugs, medicaments and biological substances

TOXIC EFFECTS OF SUBSTANCES CHIEFLY NONMEDICINAL AS TO SOURCE (T51-T65)

Note: When no intent is indicated code to accidental. Undetermined intent is only for use when there is specific documentation in the record that the intent of the toxic effect cannot be determined.

Use Additional Code(s):

for all associated manifestations of toxic effect, such as: respiratory conditions due to external agents (J60-J70)

personal history of foreign body fully removed (Z87.821)

to identify any retained foreign body, if applicable (Z18.-)

Excludes1: contact with and (suspected) exposure to toxic substances (Z77.-)

T51 Toxic effect of alcohol

The appropriate 7th character is to be added to each code from category T51

A - initial encounter

D - subsequent encounter

S - sequela

T51.0 Toxic effect of ethanol

Toxic effect of ethyl alcohol

Excludes2: acute alcohol intoxication or 'hangover' effects (F10.129, F10.229, F10.929)

drunkenness (F10.129, F10.229, F10.929)

pathological alcohol intoxication (F10.129, F10.229, F10.929)

T51.0X Toxic effect of ethanol

⑦**T51.0X1** Toxic effect of ethanol, accidental (unintentional)

Toxic effect of ethanol NOS

⑦**T51.0X2** Toxic effect of ethanol, intentional self-harm [HCC]

⑦**T51.0X3** Toxic effect of ethanol, assault

⑦**T51.0X4** Toxic effect of ethanol, undetermined

T51.1 Toxic effect of methanol

Toxic effect of methyl alcohol

T51.1X Toxic effect of methanol

⑦**T51.1X1** Toxic effect of methanol, accidental (unintentional)

Toxic effect of methanol NOS

⑦**T51.1X2** Toxic effect of methanol, intentional self-harm [HCC]

⑦**T51.1X3** Toxic effect of methanol, assault

⑦**T51.1X4** Toxic effect of methanol, undetermined

T51.2 Toxic effect of 2-Propanol

Toxic effect of isopropyl alcohol

T51.2X Toxic effect of 2-Propanol

⑦**T51.2X1** Toxic effect of 2-Propanol, accidental (unintentional)

Toxic effect of 2-Propanol NOS

⑦**T51.2X2** Toxic effect of 2-Propanol, intentional self-harm [HCC]

⑦**T51.2X3** Toxic effect of 2-Propanol, assault

⑦**T51.2X4** Toxic effect of 2-Propanol, undetermined

T51.3 Toxic effect of fusel oil

Toxic effect of amyl alcohol

Toxic effect of butyl [1-butanol] alcohol

Toxic effect of propyl [1-propanol] alcohol

T51.3X Toxic effect of fusel oil

⑦**T51.3X1** Toxic effect of fusel oil, accidental (unintentional)

Toxic effect of fusel oil NOS

⑦**T51.3X2** Toxic effect of fusel oil, intentional self-harm [HCC]

⑦**T51.3X3** Toxic effect of fusel oil, assault

⑦**T51.3X4** Toxic effect of fusel oil, undetermined

T51.8 **Toxic effect of other alcohols**

T51.8X **Toxic effect of other alcohols**

⑦**T51.8X1** Toxic effect of other alcohols, accidental (unintentional)

Toxic effect of other alcohols NOS

⑦**T51.8X2** Toxic effect of other alcohols, intentional self-harm [HCC]

⑦**T51.8X3** Toxic effect of other alcohols, assault

⑦**T51.8X4** Toxic effect of other alcohols, undetermined

T51.9 **Toxic effect of unspecified alcohol**

⊗⑦**T51.91** Toxic effect of unspecified alcohol, accidental (unintentional)

⊗⑦**T51.92** Toxic effect of unspecified alcohol, intentional self-harm [HCC]

⊗⑦**T51.93** Toxic effect of unspecified alcohol, assault

⊗⑦**T51.94** Toxic effect of unspecified alcohol, undetermined

T52 **Toxic effect of organic solvents**

Excludes1: halogen derivatives of aliphatic and aromatic hydrocarbons (T53.-)

The appropriate 7th character is to be added to each code from category T52

A - initial encounter

D - subsequent encounter

S - sequela

⑦**T52.0** **Toxic effects of petroleum products**

Toxic effects of gasoline [petrol]

Toxic effects of kerosene [paraffin oil]

Toxic effects of paraffin wax

Toxic effects of ether petroleum

Toxic effects of naphtha petroleum

Toxic effects of spirit petroleum

T52.0X **Toxic effects of petroleum products**

⑦**T52.0X1** Toxic effect of petroleum products, accidental (unintentional)

Toxic effects of petroleum products NOS

⑦**T52.0X2** Toxic effect of petroleum products, intentional self-harm [HCC]

⑦**T52.0X3** Toxic effect of petroleum products, assault

⑦**T52.0X4** Toxic effect of petroleum products, undetermined

T52.1 **Toxic effects of benzene**

Excludes1: homologues of benzene (T52.2)

nitroderivatives and aminoderivatives of benzene and its homologues (T65.3)

T52.1X **Toxic effects of benzene**

⑦**T52.1X1** Toxic effect of benzene, accidental (unintentional)

Toxic effects of benzene NOS

⑦**T52.1X2** Toxic effect of benzene, intentional self-harm [HCC]

⑦**T52.1X3** Toxic effect of benzene, assault

⑦**T52.1X4** Toxic effect of benzene, undetermined

T52.2 **Toxic effects of homologues of benzene**

Toxic effects of toluene [methylbenzene]

Toxic effects of xylene [dimethylbenzene]

T52.2X **Toxic effects of homologues of benzene**

⑦**T52.2X1** Toxic effect of homologues of benzene, accidental (unintentional)

Toxic effects of homologues of benzene NOS

⑦**T52.2X2** Toxic effect of homologues of benzene, intentional self-harm [HCC]

⑦**T52.2X3** Toxic effect of homologues of benzene, assault

⑦**T52.2X4** Toxic effect of homologues of benzene, undetermined

T52.3 **Toxic effects of glycols**

T52.3X **Toxic effects of glycols**

⑦**T52.3X1** Toxic effect of glycols, accidental (unintentional)

Toxic effects of glycols NOS

⑦**T52.3X2** Toxic effect of glycols, intentional self-harm [HCC]

⑦**T52.3X3** Toxic effect of glycols, assault

⑦**T52.3X4** Toxic effect of glycols, undetermined

T52.4 **Toxic effects of ketones**

T52.4X **Toxic effects of ketones**

⑦**T52.4X1** Toxic effect of ketones, accidental (unintentional)

Toxic effects of ketones NOS

⑦**T52.4X2** Toxic effect of ketones, intentional self-harm [HCC]

⑦**T52.4X3** Toxic effect of ketones, assault

⑦**T52.4X4** Toxic effect of ketones, undetermined

T52.8 **Toxic effects of other organic solvents**

T52.8X **Toxic effects of other organic solvents**

⑦**T52.8X1** Toxic effect of other organic solvents, accidental (unintentional)

Toxic effects of other organic solvents NOS

⑦**T52.8X2** Toxic effect of other organic solvents, intentional self-harm [HCC]

⑦**T52.8X3** Toxic effect of other organic solvents, assault

⑦**T52.8X4** Toxic effect of other organic solvents, undetermined

T52.9 **Toxic effects of unspecified organic solvent**

⊗⑦**T52.91** Toxic effect of unspecified organic solvent, accidental (unintentional)

⊗⑦**T52.92** Toxic effect of unspecified organic solvent, intentional self-harm [HCC]

⊗⑦**T52.93** Toxic effect of unspecified organic solvent, assault

⊗⑦**T52.94** Toxic effect of unspecified organic solvent, undetermined

T53 **Toxic effect of halogen derivatives of aliphatic and aromatic hydrocarbons**

The appropriate 7th character is to be added to each code from category T53

A - initial encounter

D - subsequent encounter

S - sequela

T53.0 **Toxic effects of carbon tetrachloride**

● New code　▲ Revised code　**Excludes1:** Not coded here　**Excludes2:** Not included here　⊗ Placeholder required　⑦ 7th digit required

Toxic effects of tetrachloromethane

T53.0X **Toxic effects of carbon tetrachloride**

⑦**T53.0X1** **Toxic effect of carbon tetrachloride, accidental (unintentional)**

Toxic effects of carbon tetrachloride NOS

⑦**T53.0X2** **Toxic effect of carbon tetrachloride, intentional self-harm** [HCC]

⑦**T53.0X3** **Toxic effect of carbon tetrachloride, assault**

⑦**T53.0X4** **Toxic effect of carbon tetrachloride, undetermined**

T53.1 **Toxic effects of chloroform**

Toxic effects of trichloromethane

T53.1X **Toxic effects of chloroform**

⑦**T53.1X1** **Toxic effect of chloroform, accidental (unintentional)**

Toxic effects of chloroform NOS

⑦**T53.1X2** **Toxic effect of chloroform, intentional self-harm** [HCC]

⑦**T53.1X3** **Toxic effect of chloroform, assault**

⑦**T53.1X4** **Toxic effect of chloroform, undetermined**

T53.2 **Toxic effects of trichloroethylene**

Toxic effects of trichloroethene

T53.2X **Toxic effects of trichloroethylene**

⑦**T53.2X1** **Toxic effect of trichloroethylene, accidental (unintentional)**

Toxic effects of trichloroethylene NOS

⑦**T53.2X2** **Toxic effect of trichloroethylene, intentional self-harm** [HCC]

⑦**T53.2X3** **Toxic effect of trichloroethylene, assault**

⑦**T53.2X4** **Toxic effect of trichloroethylene, undetermined**

T53.3 **Toxic effects of tetrachloroethylene**

Toxic effects of perchloroethylene

Toxic effect of tetrachloroethane

T53.3X **Toxic effects of tetrachloroethylene**

⑦**T53.3X1** **Toxic effect of tetrachloroethylene, accidental (unintentional)**

toxic effects of tetrachloroethylene NOS

⑦**T53.3X2** **Toxic effect of tetrachloroethylene, intentional self-harm** [HCC]

⑦**T53.3X3** **Toxic effect of tetrachloroethylene, assault**

⑦**T53.3X4** **Toxic effect of tetrachloroethylene, undetermined**

T53.4 **Toxic effects of dichloromethane**

Toxic effects of methylene chloride

T53.4X **Toxic effects of dichloromethane**

⑦**T53.4X1** **Toxic effect of dichloromethane, accidental (unintentional)**

Toxic effects of dichloromethane NOS

⑦**T53.4X2** **Toxic effect of dichloromethane, intentional self-harm** [HCC]

⑦**T53.4X3** **Toxic effect of dichloromethane, assault**

⑦**T53.4X4** **Toxic effect of dichloromethane, undetermined**

T53.5 **Toxic effects of chlorofluorocarbons**

T53.5X **Toxic effects of chlorofluorocarbons**

⑦**T53.5X1** **Toxic effect of chlorofluorocarbons, accidental (unintentional)**

Toxic effects of chlorofluorocarbons NOS

⑦**T53.5X2** **Toxic effect of chlorofluorocarbons, intentional self-harm** [HCC]

⑦**T53.5X3** **Toxic effect of chlorofluorocarbons, assault**

⑦**T53.5X4** **Toxic effect of chlorofluorocarbons, undetermined**

T53.6 **Toxic effects of other halogen derivatives of aliphatic hydrocarbons**

T53.6X **Toxic effects of other halogen derivatives of aliphatic hydrocarbons**

⑦**T53.6X1** **Toxic effect of other halogen derivatives of aliphatic hydrocarbons, accidental (unintentional)**

Toxic effects of other halogen derivatives of aliphatic hydrocarbons NOS

⑦**T53.6X2** **Toxic effect of other halogen derivatives of aliphatic hydrocarbons, intentional self-harm** [HCC]

⑦**T53.6X3** **Toxic effect of other halogen derivatives of aliphatic hydrocarbons, assault**

⑦**T53.6X4** **Toxic effect of other halogen derivatives of aliphatic hydrocarbons, undetermined**

T53.7 **Toxic effects of other halogen derivatives of aromatic hydrocarbons**

T53.7X **Toxic effects of other halogen derivatives of aromatic hydrocarbons**

⑦**T53.7X1** **Toxic effect of other halogen derivatives of aromatic hydrocarbons, accidental (unintentional)**

Toxic effects of other halogen derivatives of aromatic hydrocarbons NOS

⑦**T53.7X2** **Toxic effect of other halogen derivatives of aromatic hydrocarbons, intentional self-harm** [HCC]

⑦**T53.7X3** **Toxic effect of other halogen derivatives of aromatic hydrocarbons, assault**

⑦**T53.7X4** **Toxic effect of other halogen derivatives of aromatic hydrocarbons, undetermined**

T53.9 **Toxic effects of unspecified halogen derivatives of aliphatic and aromatic hydrocarbons**

⊗⑦**T53.91** **Toxic effect of unspecified halogen derivatives of aliphatic and aromatic hydrocarbons, accidental (unintentional)**

⊗⑦**T53.92** **Toxic effect of unspecified halogen derivatives of aliphatic and aromatic hydrocarbons, intentional self-harm** [HCC]

⊗⑦**T53.93** **Toxic effect of unspecified halogen derivatives of aliphatic and aromatic hydrocarbons, assault**

⊗⑦**T53.94** **Toxic effect of unspecified halogen derivatives of aliphatic and aromatic hydrocarbons, undetermined**

T54 **Toxic effect of corrosive substances**

Add 4th-7th digits　　Nonspecific code　　Unspecified code　　Manifestation code　　[HCC] Hierarchical Condition Code

The appropriate 7th character is to be added to each code from category T54

A - initial encounter

D - subsequent encounter

S - sequela

T54.0   Toxic effects of phenol and phenol homologues

T54.0X   Toxic effects of phenol and phenol homologues

⑦T54.0X1   **Toxic effect of phenol and phenol homologues, accidental (unintentional)**

Toxic effects of phenol and phenol homologues NOS

⑦T54.0X2   **Toxic effect of phenol and phenol homologues, intentional self-harm** [HCC]

⑦T54.0X3   **Toxic effect of phenol and phenol homologues, assault**

⑦T54.0X4   **Toxic effect of phenol and phenol homologues, undetermined**

T54.1   Toxic effects of other corrosive organic compounds

T54.1X   Toxic effects of other corrosive organic compounds

⑦T54.1X1   **Toxic effect of other corrosive organic compounds, accidental (unintentional)**

Toxic effects of other corrosive organic compounds NOS

⑦T54.1X2   **Toxic effect of other corrosive organic compounds, intentional self-harm** [HCC]

⑦T54.1X3   **Toxic effect of other corrosive organic compounds, assault**

⑦T54.1X4   **Toxic effect of other corrosive organic compounds, undetermined**

T54.2   Toxic effects of corrosive acids and acid-like substances

Toxic effects of hydrochloric acid

Toxic effects of sulfuric acid

T54.2X   Toxic effects of corrosive acids and acid-like substances

⑦T54.2X1   **Toxic effect of corrosive acids and acid-like substances, accidental (unintentional)**

Toxic effects of corrosive acids and acid-like substances NOS

⑦T54.2X2   **Toxic effect of corrosive acids and acid-like substances, intentional self-harm** [HCC]

⑦T54.2X3   **Toxic effect of corrosive acids and acid-like substances, assault**

⑦T54.2X4   **Toxic effect of corrosive acids and acid-like substances, undetermined**

T54.3   Toxic effects of corrosive alkalis and alkali-like substances

Toxic effects of potassium hydroxide

Toxic effects of sodium hydroxide

T54.3X   Toxic effects of corrosive alkalis and alkali-like substances

⑦T54.3X1   **Toxic effect of corrosive alkalis and alkali-like substances, accidental (unintentional)**

Toxic effects of corrosive alkalis and alkali-like substances NOS

⑦T54.3X2   **Toxic effect of corrosive alkalis and alkali-like substances, intentional self-harm** [HCC]

⑦T54.3X3   **Toxic effect of corrosive alkalis and alkali-like substances, assault**

⑦T54.3X4   **Toxic effect of corrosive alkalis and alkali-like substances, undetermined**

T54.9   Toxic effects of unspecified corrosive substance

⊗⑦**T54.91**   **Toxic effect of unspecified corrosive substance, accidental (unintentional)**

⊗⑦**T54.92**   **Toxic effect of unspecified corrosive substance, intentional self-harm** [HCC]

⊗⑦**T54.93**   **Toxic effect of unspecified corrosive substance, assault**

⊗⑦**T54.94**   **Toxic effect of unspecified corrosive substance, undetermined**

T55   Toxic effect of soaps and detergents

The appropriate 7th character is to be added to each code from category T55

A - initial encounter

D - subsequent encounter

S - sequela

T55.0   Toxic effect of soaps

T55.0X   Toxic effect of soaps

⑦T55.0X1   **Toxic effect of soaps, accidental (unintentional)**

Toxic effect of soaps NOS

⑦T55.0X2   **Toxic effect of soaps, intentional self-harm** [HCC]

⑦T55.0X3   **Toxic effect of soaps, assault**

⑦T55.0X4   **Toxic effect of soaps, undetermined**

T55.1   Toxic effect of detergents

T55.1X   Toxic effect of detergents

⑦T55.1X1   **Toxic effect of detergents, accidental (unintentional)**

Toxic effect of detergents NOS

⑦T55.1X2   **Toxic effect of detergents, intentional self-harm** [HCC]

⑦T55.1X3   **Toxic effect of detergents, assault**

⑦T55.1X4   **Toxic effect of detergents, undetermined**

T56   Toxic effect of metals

Includes: toxic effects of fumes and vapors of metals

toxic effects of metals from all sources, except medicinal substances

Use Additional Code to identify any retained metal foreign body, if applicable (Z18.0-, T18.1-)

Excludes1: arsenic and its compounds (T57.0)

manganese and its compounds (T57.2)

The appropriate 7th character is to be added to each code from category T56

A - initial encounter

D - subsequent encounter

S - sequela

T56.0   Toxic effects of lead and its compounds

T56.0X   Toxic effects of lead and its compounds

⑦T56.0X1   **Toxic effect of lead and its compounds, accidental (unintentional)**

Toxic effects of lead and its compounds NOS

⑦T56.0X2 Toxic effect of lead and its compounds, intentional self-harm [HCC]

⑦T56.0X3 Toxic effect of lead and its compounds, assault

⑦T56.0X4 Toxic effect of lead and its compounds, undetermined

T56.1 Toxic effects of mercury and its compounds

⑦T56.1X Toxic effects of mercury and its compounds

⑦T56.1X1 Toxic effect of mercury and its compounds, accidental (unintentional)

Toxic effects of mercury and its compounds NOS

⑦T56.1X2 Toxic effect of mercury and its compounds, intentional self-harm [HCC]

⑦T56.1X3 Toxic effect of mercury and its compounds, assault

⑦T56.1X4 Toxic effect of mercury and its compounds, undetermined

T56.2 Toxic effects of chromium and its compounds

T56.2X Toxic effects of chromium and its compounds

⑦T56.2X1 Toxic effect of chromium and its compounds, accidental (unintentional)

Toxic effects of chromium and its compounds NOS

⑦T56.2X2 Toxic effect of chromium and its compounds, intentional self-harm [HCC]

⑦T56.2X3 Toxic effect of chromium and its compounds, assault

⑦T56.2X4 Toxic effect of chromium and its compounds, undetermined

T56.3 Toxic effects of cadmium and its compounds

T56.3X Toxic effects of cadmium and its compounds

⑦T56.3X1 Toxic effect of cadmium and its compounds, accidental (unintentional)

Toxic effects of cadmium and its compounds NOS

⑦T56.3X2 Toxic effect of cadmium and its compounds, intentional self-harm [HCC]

⑦T56.3X3 Toxic effect of cadmium and its compounds, assault

⑦T56.3X4 Toxic effect of cadmium and its compounds, undetermined

T56.4 Toxic effects of copper and its compounds

T56.4X Toxic effects of copper and its compounds

⑦T56.4X1 Toxic effect of copper and its compounds, accidental (unintentional)

Toxic effects of copper and its compounds NOS

⑦T56.4X2 Toxic effect of copper and its compounds, intentional self-harm [HCC]

⑦T56.4X3 Toxic effect of copper and its compounds, assault

⑦T56.4X4 Toxic effect of copper and its compounds, undetermined

T56.5 Toxic effects of zinc and its compounds

T56.5X Toxic effects of zinc and its compounds

⑦T56.5X1 Toxic effect of zinc and its compounds, accidental (unintentional)

Toxic effects of zinc and its compounds NOS

⑦T56.5X2 Toxic effect of zinc and its compounds, intentional self-harm [HCC]

⑦T56.5X3 Toxic effect of zinc and its compounds, assault

⑦T56.5X4 Toxic effect of zinc and its compounds, undetermined

T56.6 Toxic effects of tin and its compounds

T56.6X Toxic effects of tin and its compounds

⑦T56.6X1 Toxic effect of tin and its compounds, accidental (unintentional)

Toxic effects of tin and its compounds NOS

⑦T56.6X2 Toxic effect of tin and its compounds, intentional self-harm [HCC]

⑦T56.6X3 Toxic effect of tin and its compounds, assault

⑦T56.6X4 Toxic effect of tin and its compounds, undetermined

T56.7 Toxic effects of beryllium and its compounds

T56.7X Toxic effects of beryllium and its compounds

⑦T56.7X1 Toxic effect of beryllium and its compounds, accidental (unintentional)

Toxic effects of beryllium and its compounds NOS

⑦T56.7X2 Toxic effect of beryllium and its compounds, intentional self-harm [HCC]

⑦T56.7X3 Toxic effect of beryllium and its compounds, assault

⑦T56.7X4 Toxic effect of beryllium and its compounds, undetermined

T56.8 Toxic effects of other metals

T56.81 Toxic effect of thallium

⑦T56.811 Toxic effect of thallium, accidental (unintentional)

Toxic effect of thallium NOS

⑦T56.812 Toxic effect of thallium, intentional self-harm [HCC]

⑦T56.813 Toxic effect of thallium, assault

⑦T56.814 Toxic effect of thallium, undetermined

T56.89 Toxic effects of other metals

⑦T56.891 Toxic effect of other metals, accidental (unintentional)

Toxic effects of other metals NOS

⑦T56.892 Toxic effect of other metals, intentional self-harm [HCC]

⑦T56.893 Toxic effect of other metals, assault

⑦T56.894 Toxic effect of other metals, undetermined

T56.9 Toxic effects of unspecified metal

⊗⑦T56.91 Toxic effect of unspecified metal, accidental (unintentional)

⊗⑦T56.92 Toxic effect of unspecified metal, intentional self-harm [HCC]

⊗⑦T56.93 Toxic effect of unspecified metal, assault

⊗⑦**T56.94**   **Toxic effect of unspecified metal, undetermined**

T57   **Toxic effect of other inorganic substances**

The appropriate 7th character is to be added to each code from category T57

A - initial encounter

D - subsequent encounter

S - sequela

T57.0   **Toxic effect of arsenic and its compounds**

T57.0X   **Toxic effect of arsenic and its compounds**

⑦**T57.0X1**   **Toxic effect of arsenic and its compounds, accidental (unintentional)**

Toxic effect of arsenic and its compounds NOS

⑦**T57.0X2**   **Toxic effect of arsenic and its compounds, intentional self-harm** [HCC]

⑦**T57.0X3**   **Toxic effect of arsenic and its compounds, assault**

⑦**T57.0X4**   **Toxic effect of arsenic and its compounds, undetermined**

T57.1   **Toxic effect of phosphorus and its compounds**

Excludes1: organophosphate insecticides (T60.0)

T57.1X   **Toxic effect of phosphorus and its compounds**

⑦**T57.1X1**   **Toxic effect of phosphorus and its compounds, accidental (unintentional)**

Toxic effect of phosphorus and its compounds NOS

⑦**T57.1X2**   **Toxic effect of phosphorus and its compounds, intentional self-harm** [HCC]

⑦**T57.1X3**   **Toxic effect of phosphorus and its compounds, assault**

⑦**T57.1X4**   **Toxic effect of phosphorus and its compounds, undetermined**

T57.2   **Toxic effect of manganese and its compounds**

T57.2X   **Toxic effect of manganese and its compounds**

⑦**T57.2X1**   **Toxic effect of manganese and its compounds, accidental (unintentional)**

Toxic effect of manganese and its compounds NOS

⑦**T57.2X2**   **Toxic effect of manganese and its compounds, intentional self-harm** [HCC]

⑦**T57.2X3**   **Toxic effect of manganese and its compounds, assault**

⑦**T57.2X4**   **Toxic effect of manganese and its compounds, undetermined**

T57.3   **Toxic effect of hydrogen cyanide**

T57.3X   **Toxic effect of hydrogen cyanide**

⑦**T57.3X1**   **Toxic effect of hydrogen cyanide, accidental (unintentional)**

Toxic effect of hydrogen cyanide NOS

⑦**T57.3X2**   **Toxic effect of hydrogen cyanide, intentional self-harm**

⑦**T57.3X3**   **Toxic effect of hydrogen cyanide, assault**

⑦**T57.3X4**   **Toxic effect of hydrogen cyanide, undetermined**

T57.8   **Toxic effect of other specified inorganic substances**

T57.8X   **Toxic effect of other specified inorganic substances**

⑦**T57.8X1**   **Toxic effect of other specified inorganic substances, accidental (unintentional)**

Toxic effect of other specified inorganic substances NOS

⑦**T57.8X2**   **Toxic effect of other specified inorganic substances, intentional self-harm** [HCC]

⑦**T57.8X3**   **Toxic effect of other specified inorganic substances, assault**

⑦**T57.8X4**   **Toxic effect of other specified inorganic substances, undetermined**

T57.9   **Toxic effect of unspecified inorganic substance**

⊗⑦**T57.91**   **Toxic effect of unspecified inorganic substance, accidental (unintentional)**

⊗⑦**T57.92**   **Toxic effect of unspecified inorganic substance, intentional self-harm** [HCC]

⊗⑦**T57.93**   **Toxic effect of unspecified inorganic substance, assault**

⊗⑦**T57.94**   **Toxic effect of unspecified inorganic substance, undetermined**

T58   **Toxic effect of carbon monoxide**

Includes: asphyxiation from carbon monoxide

toxic effect of carbon monoxide from all sources

The appropriate 7th character is to be added to each code from category T58

A - initial encounter

D - subsequent encounter

S - sequela

T58.0   **Toxic effect of carbon monoxide from motor vehicle exhaust**

Toxic effect of exhaust gas from gas engine

Toxic effect of exhaust gas from motor pump

⊗⑦**T58.01**   **Toxic effect of carbon monoxide from motor vehicle exhaust, accidental (unintentional)**

⊗⑦**T58.02**   **Toxic effect of carbon monoxide from motor vehicle exhaust, intentional self-harm** [HCC]

⊗⑦**T58.03**   **Toxic effect of carbon monoxide from motor vehicle exhaust, assault**

⊗⑦**T58.04**   **Toxic effect of carbon monoxide from motor vehicle exhaust, undetermined**

T58.1   **Toxic effect of carbon monoxide from utility gas**

Toxic effect of acetylene

Toxic effect of gas NOS used for lighting, heating, cooking

Toxic effect of water gas

⊗⑦**T58.11**   **Toxic effect of carbon monoxide from utility gas, accidental (unintentional)**

⊗⑦**T58.12**   **Toxic effect of carbon monoxide from utility gas, intentional self-harm** [HCC]

⊗⑦**T58.13**   **Toxic effect of carbon monoxide from utility gas, assault**

⊗⑦**T58.14**   **Toxic effect of carbon monoxide from utility gas, undetermined**

T58.2   **Toxic effect of carbon monoxide from incomplete combustion of other domestic fuels**

Toxic effect of carbon monoxide from incomplete combustion of coal, coke, kerosene, wood

T58.2X   **Toxic effect of carbon monoxide from incomplete combustion of other domestic fuels**

⑦**T58.2X1**   **Toxic effect of carbon monoxide from incomplete combustion of other** domestic fuels, accidental (unintentional)

⑦**T58.2X2** **Toxic effect of carbon monoxide from incomplete combustion of other domestic fuels, intentional self-harm** [HCC]

⑦**T58.2X3** **Toxic effect of carbon monoxide from incomplete combustion of other domestic fuels, assault**

⑦**T58.2X4** **Toxic effect of carbon monoxide from incomplete combustion of other domestic fuels, undetermined**

T58.8 **Toxic effect of carbon monoxide from other source**

Toxic effect of carbon monoxide from blast furnace gas

Toxic effect of carbon monoxide from fuels in industrial use

Toxic effect of carbon monoxide from kiln vapor

T58.8X **Toxic effect of carbon monoxide from other source**

⑦**T58.8X1** **Toxic effect of carbon monoxide from other source, accidental (unintentional)**

⑦**T58.8X2** **Toxic effect of carbon monoxide from other source, intentional self-harm** [HCC]

⑦**T58.8X3** **Toxic effect of carbon monoxide from other source, assault**

⑦**T58.8X4** **Toxic effect of carbon monoxide from other source, undetermined**

T58.9 **Toxic effect of carbon monoxide from unspecified source**

⊗⑦**T58.91** **Toxic effect of carbon monoxide from unspecified source, accidental (unintentional)**

⊗⑦**T58.92** **Toxic effect of carbon monoxide from unspecified source, intentional self-harm** [HCC]

⊗⑦**T58.93** **Toxic effect of carbon monoxide from unspecified source, assault**

⊗⑦**T58.94** **Toxic effect of carbon monoxide from unspecified source, undetermined**

T59 **Toxic effect of other gases, fumes and vapors**

Includes: aerosol propellants

Excludes1: chlorofluorocarbons (T53.5)

The appropriate 7th character is to be added to each code from category T59

A - initial encounter

D - subsequent encounter

S - sequela

T59.0 **Toxic effect of nitrogen oxides**

T59.0X **Toxic effect of nitrogen oxides**

⑦**T59.0X1** **Toxic effect of nitrogen oxides, accidental (unintentional)**

Toxic effect of nitrogen oxides NOS

⑦**T59.0X2** **Toxic effect of nitrogen oxides, intentional self-harm** [HCC]

⑦**T59.0X3** **Toxic effect of nitrogen oxides, assault**

⑦**T59.0X4** **Toxic effect of nitrogen oxides, undetermined**

T59.1 **Toxic effect of sulfur dioxide**

T59.1X **Toxic effect of sulfur dioxide**

⑦**T59.1X1** **Toxic effect of sulfur dioxide, accidental (unintentional)**

Toxic effect of sulfur dioxide NOS

⑦**T59.1X2** **Toxic effect of sulfur dioxide, intentional self-harm** [HCC]

⑦**T59.1X3** **Toxic effect of sulfur dioxide, assault**

⑦**T59.1X4** **Toxic effect of sulfur dioxide, undetermined**

T59.2 **Toxic effect of formaldehyde**

T59.2X **Toxic effect of formaldehyde**

⑦**T59.2X1** **Toxic effect of formaldehyde, accidental (unintentional)**

Toxic effect of formaldehyde NOS

⑦**T59.2X2** **Toxic effect of formaldehyde, intentional self-harm** [HCC]

⑦**T59.2X3** **Toxic effect of formaldehyde, assault**

⑦**T59.2X4** **Toxic effect of formaldehyde, undetermined**

T59.3 **Toxic effect of lacrimogenic gas**

Toxic effect of tear gas

T59.3X **Toxic effect of lacrimogenic gas**

⑦**T59.3X1** **Toxic effect of lacrimogenic gas, accidental (unintentional)**

Toxic effect of lacrimogenic gas NOS

⑦**T59.3X2** **Toxic effect of lacrimogenic gas, intentional self-harm** [HCC]

⑦**T59.3X3** **Toxic effect of lacrimogenic gas, assault**

⑦**T59.3X4** **Toxic effect of lacrimogenic gas, undetermined**

T59.4 **Toxic effect of chlorine gas**

T59.4X **Toxic effect of chlorine gas**

⑦**T59.4X1** **Toxic effect of chlorine gas, accidental (unintentional)**

Toxic effect of chlorine gas NOS

⑦**T59.4X2** **Toxic effect of chlorine gas, intentional self-harm** [HCC]

⑦**T59.4X3** **Toxic effect of chlorine gas, assault**

⑦**T59.4X4** **Toxic effect of chlorine gas, undetermined**

T59.5 **Toxic effect of fluorine gas and hydrogen fluoride**

T59.5X **Toxic effect of fluorine gas and hydrogen fluoride**

⑦**T59.5X1** **Toxic effect of fluorine gas and hydrogen fluoride, accidental (unintentional)**

Toxic effect of fluorine gas and hydrogen fluoride NOS

⑦**T59.5X2** **Toxic effect of fluorine gas and hydrogen fluoride, intentional self-harm** [HCC]

⑦**T59.5X3** **Toxic effect of fluorine gas and hydrogen fluoride, assault**

⑦**T59.5X4** **Toxic effect of fluorine gas and hydrogen fluoride, undetermined**

T59.6 **Toxic effect of hydrogen sulfide**

T59.6X **Toxic effect of hydrogen sulfide**

⑦**T59.6X1** **Toxic effect of hydrogen sulfide, accidental (unintentional)**

Toxic effect of hydrogen sulfide NOS

⑦**T59.6X2** **Toxic effect of hydrogen sulfide, intentional self-harm** [HCC]

⑦**T59.6X3** **Toxic effect of hydrogen sulfide, assault**

⑦**T59.6X4** **Toxic effect of hydrogen sulfide, undetermined**

T59.7 **Toxic effect of carbon dioxide**

T59.7X Toxic effect of carbon dioxide

⑦**T59.7X1** Toxic effect of carbon dioxide, accidental (unintentional)

Toxic effect of carbon dioxide NOS

⑦**T59.7X2** Toxic effect of carbon dioxide, intentional self-harm [HCC]

⑦**T59.7X3** Toxic effect of carbon dioxide, assault

⑦**T59.7X4** Toxic effect of carbon dioxide, undetermined

T59.8 Toxic effect of other specified gases, fumes and vapors

T59.81 Toxic effect of smoke

Smoke inhalation

Excludes2: toxic effect of cigarette (tobacco) smoke (T65.22-)

⑦**T59.811** Toxic effect of smoke, accidental (unintentional)

Toxic effect of smoke NOS

⑦**T59.812** Toxic effect of smoke, intentional self-harm [HCC]

⑦**T59.813** Toxic effect of smoke, assault

⑦**T59.814** Toxic effect of smoke, undetermined

T59.89 Toxic effect of other specified gases, fumes and vapors

⑦**T59.891** Toxic effect of other specified gases, fumes and vapors, accidental (unintentional)

⑦**T59.892** Toxic effect of other specified gases, fumes and vapors, intentional self-harm [HCC]

⑦**T59.893** Toxic effect of other specified gases, fumes and vapors, assault

⑦**T59.894** Toxic effect of other specified gases, fumes and vapors, undetermined

T59.9 Toxic effect of unspecified gases, fumes and vapors

⊗⑦**T59.91** Toxic effect of unspecified gases, fumes and vapors, accidental (unintentional)

⊗⑦**T59.92** Toxic effect of unspecified gases, fumes and vapors, intentional self-harm [HCC]

⊗⑦**T59.93** Toxic effect of unspecified gases, fumes and vapors, assault

⊗⑦**T59.94** Toxic effect of unspecified gases, fumes and vapors, undetermined

T60 **Toxic effect of pesticides**

Includes: toxic effect of wood preservatives

The appropriate 7th character is to be added to each code from category T60

A - initial encounter

D - subsequent encounter

S - sequela

T60.0 Toxic effect of organophosphate and carbamate insecticides

T60.0X Toxic effect of organophosphate and carbamate insecticides

⑦**T60.0X1** Toxic effect of organophosphate and carbamate insecticides, accidental (unintentional)

Toxic effect of organophosphate and carbamate insecticides NOS

⑦**T60.0X2** Toxic effect of organophosphate and carbamate insecticides, intentional self-harm [HCC]

⑦**T60.0X3** Toxic effect of organophosphate and carbamate insecticides, assault

⑦**T60.0X4** Toxic effect of organophosphate and carbamate insecticides, undetermined

T60.1 Toxic effect of halogenated insecticides

Excludes1: chlorinated hydrocarbon (T53.-)

T60.1X Toxic effect of halogenated insecticides

⑦**T60.1X1** Toxic effect of halogenated insecticides, accidental (unintentional)

Toxic effect of halogenated insecticides NOS

⑦**T60.1X2** Toxic effect of halogenated insecticides, intentional self-harm [HCC]

⑦**T60.1X3** Toxic effect of halogenated insecticides, assault

⑦**T60.1X4** Toxic effect of halogenated insecticides, undetermined

T60.2 Toxic effect of other insecticides

T60.2X Toxic effect of other insecticides

⑦**T60.2X1** Toxic effect of other insecticides, accidental (unintentional)

Toxic effect of other insecticides NOS

⑦**T60.2X2** Toxic effect of other insecticides, intentional self-harm [HCC]

⑦**T60.2X3** Toxic effect of other insecticides, assault

⑦**T60.2X4** Toxic effect of other insecticides, undetermined

T60.3 Toxic effect of herbicides and fungicides

T60.3X Toxic effect of herbicides and fungicides

⑦**T60.3X1** Toxic effect of herbicides and fungicides, accidental (unintentional)

Toxic effect of herbicides and fungicides NOS

⑦**T60.3X2** Toxic effect of herbicides and fungicides, intentional self-harm [HCC]

⑦**T60.3X3** Toxic effect of herbicides and fungicides, assault

⑦**T60.3X4** Toxic effect of herbicides and fungicides, undetermined

T60.4 Toxic effect of rodenticides

Excludes1: strychnine and its salts (T65.1)

thallium (T56.81-)

T60.4X Toxic effect of rodenticides

⑦**T60.4X1** Toxic effect of rodenticides, accidental (unintentional)

Toxic effect of rodenticides NOS

⑦**T60.4X2** Toxic effect of rodenticides, intentional self-harm [HCC]

⑦**T60.4X3** Toxic effect of rodenticides, assault

⑦**T60.4X4** Toxic effect of rodenticides, undetermined

T60.8 Toxic effect of other pesticides

T60.8X Toxic effect of other pesticides

⑦**T60.8X1** Toxic effect of other pesticides, accidental (unintentional)

Toxic effect of other pesticides NOS

⑦**T60.8X2** Toxic effect of other pesticides, intentional self-harm [HCC]

● New code   ▲ Revised code   Excludes1: Not coded here   Excludes2: Not included here   ⊗ Placeholder required   ⑦7th digit required

⑦**T60.8X3**   **Toxic effect of other pesticides, assault**

⑦**T60.8X4**   **Toxic effect of other pesticides, undetermined**

T60.9   **Toxic effect of unspecified pesticide**

⊗⑦**T60.91**   **Toxic effect of unspecified pesticide, accidental (unintentional)**

⊗⑦**T60.92**   **Toxic effect of unspecified pesticide, intentional self-harm** [HCC]

⊗⑦**T60.93**   **Toxic effect of unspecified pesticide, assault**

⊗⑦**T60.94**   **Toxic effect of unspecified pesticide, undetermined**

T61   **Toxic effect of noxious substances eaten as seafood**

Excludes1: allergic reaction to food, such as:

anaphylactic reaction or shock due to adverse food reaction (T78.0-)

bacterial foodborne intoxications (A05.-)

dermatitis (L23.6, L25.4, L27.2)

food protein-induced enterocolitis syndrome (K52.21)

food protein-induced enteropathy (K52.22)

gastroenteritis (noninfective) (K52.29)

toxic effect of aflatoxin **and other** mycotoxins (T64)

toxic effect of cyanides (T65.0-)

toxic effect of harmful algae bloom (T65.82-)

toxic effect of hydrogen cyanide (T57.3-)

toxic effect of mercury (T56.1-)

toxic effect of red tide (T65.82-)

The appropriate 7th character is to be added to each code from category T61

A - initial encounter

D - subsequent encounter

S - sequela

T61.0   **Ciguatera fish poisoning**

⊗⑦**T61.01**   **Ciguatera fish poisoning, accidental (unintentional)**

⊗⑦**T61.02**   **Ciguatera fish poisoning, intentional self-harm** [HCC]

⊗⑦**T61.03**   **Ciguatera fish poisoning, assault**

⊗⑦**T61.04**   **Ciguatera fish poisoning, undetermined**

T61.1   **Scombroid fish poisoning**

Histamine-like syndrome

⊗⑦**T61.11**   **Scombroid fish poisoning, accidental (unintentional)**

⊗⑦**T61.12**   **Scombroid fish poisoning, intentional self-harm** [HCC]

⊗⑦**T61.13**   **Scombroid fish poisoning, assault**

⊗⑦**T61.14**   **Scombroid fish poisoning, undetermined**

T61.7   **Other fish and shellfish poisoning**

T61.77   **Other fish poisoning**

⑦**T61.771**   **Other fish poisoning, accidental (unintentional)**

⑦**T61.772**   **Other fish poisoning, intentional self-harm** [HCC]

⑦**T61.773**   **Other fish poisoning, assault**

⑦**T61.774**   **Other fish poisoning, undetermined**

T61.78   **Other shellfish poisoning**

⑦**T61.781**   **Other shellfish poisoning, accidental (unintentional)**

⑦**T61.782**   **Other shellfish poisoning, intentional self-harm** [HCC]

⑦**T61.783**   **Other shellfish poisoning, assault**

⑦**T61.784**   **Other shellfish poisoning, undetermined**

T61.8   **Toxic effect of other seafood**

T61.8X   **Toxic effect of other seafood**

⑦**T61.8X1**   **Toxic effect of other seafood, accidental (unintentional)**

⑦**T61.8X2**   **Toxic effect of other seafood, intentional self-harm** [HCC]

⑦**T61.8X3**   **Toxic effect of other seafood, assault**

⑦**T61.8X4**   **Toxic effect of other seafood, undetermined**

T61.9   **Toxic effect of unspecified seafood**

⊗⑦**T61.91**   **Toxic effect of unspecified seafood, accidental (unintentional)**

⊗⑦**T61.92**   **Toxic effect of unspecified seafood, intentional self-harm** [HCC]

⊗⑦**T61.93**   **Toxic effect of unspecified seafood, assault**

⊗⑦**T61.94**   **Toxic effect of unspecified seafood, undetermined**

T62   **Toxic effect of other noxious substances eaten as food**

Excludes1: allergic reaction to food, such as:

anaphylactic shock (reaction) due to adverse food reaction (T78.0-)

bacterial food borne intoxications (A05.-)

dermatitis (L23.6, L25.4, L27.2)

food protein-induced enterocolitis syndrome (K52.21)

food protein-induced enteropathy (K52.22)

gastroenteritis (noninfective) (K52.29)

toxic effect of aflatoxin **and other** mycotoxins (T64)

toxic effect of cyanides (T65.0-)

toxic effect of hydrogen cyanide (T57.3-)

toxic effect of mercury (T56.1-)

The appropriate 7th character is to be added to each code from category T62

A - initial encounter

D - subsequent encounter

S - sequela

T62.0   **Toxic effect of ingested mushrooms**

T62.0X   **Toxic effect of ingested mushrooms**

⑦**T62.0X1**   **Toxic effect of ingested mushrooms, accidental (unintentional)**

Toxic effect of ingested mushrooms NOS

⑦**T62.0X2**   **Toxic effect of ingested mushrooms, intentional self-harm** [HCC]

⑦**T62.0X3**   **Toxic effect of ingested mushrooms, assault**

⑦**T62.0X4**   **Toxic effect of ingested mushrooms, undetermined**

T62.1   **Toxic effect of ingested berries**

T62.1X   **Toxic effect of ingested berries**

⑦**T62.1X1**   **Toxic effect of ingested berries, accidental (unintentional)**

Toxic effect of ingested berries NOS

⑦**T62.1X2**   **Toxic effect of ingested berries, intentional self-harm** [HCC]

⑦**T62.1X3**   **Toxic effect of ingested berries, assault**

⑦T62.1X4　Toxic effect of ingested berries, undetermined

T62.2　Toxic effect of other ingested (parts of) plant(s)

　　T62.2X　Toxic effect of other ingested (parts of) plant(s)

　　　⑦T62.2X1　Toxic effect of other ingested (parts of) plant(s), accidental (unintentional)

　　　　Toxic effect of other ingested (parts of) plant(s) NOS

　　　⑦T62.2X2　Toxic effect of other ingested (parts of) plant(s), intentional self-harm [HCC]

　　　⑦T62.2X3　Toxic effect of other ingested (parts of) plant(s), assault

　　　⑦T62.2X4　Toxic effect of other ingested (parts of) plant(s), undetermined

T62.8　Toxic effect of other specified noxious substances eaten as food

　　T62.8X　Toxic effect of other specified noxious substances eaten as food

　　　⑦T62.8X1　Toxic effect of other specified noxious substances eaten as food, accidental (unintentional)

　　　　Toxic effect of other specified noxious substances eaten as food NOS

　　　⑦T62.8X2　Toxic effect of other specified noxious substances eaten as food, intentional self-harm [HCC]

　　　⑦T62.8X3　Toxic effect of other specified noxious substances eaten as food, assault

　　　⑦T62.8X4　Toxic effect of other specified noxious substances eaten as food, undetermined

T62.9　Toxic effect of unspecified noxious substance eaten as food

　　⊗⑦T62.91　Toxic effect of unspecified noxious substance eaten as food, accidental (unintentional)

　　　　Toxic effect of unspecified noxious substance eaten as food NOS

　　⊗⑦T62.92　Toxic effect of unspecified noxious substance eaten as food, intentional self-harm [HCC]

　　⊗⑦T62.93　Toxic effect of unspecified noxious substance eaten as food, assault

　　⊗⑦T62.94　Toxic effect of unspecified noxious substance eaten as food, undetermined

T63　**Toxic effect of contact with venomous animals and plants**

Includes: bite or touch of venomous animal

pricked or stuck by thorn or leaf

Excludes2: ingestion of toxic animal or plant (T61.-, T62.-)

The appropriate 7th character is to be added to each code from category T63

A - initial encounter

D - subsequent encounter

S - sequela

T63.0　Toxic effect of snake venom

　　T63.00　Toxic effect of unspecified snake venom

　　　⑦T63.001　Toxic effect of unspecified snake venom, accidental (unintentional)

　　　　Toxic effect of unspecified snake venom NOS

　　　⑦T63.002　Toxic effect of unspecified snake venom, intentional self-harm [HCC]

⑦T63.003　Toxic effect of unspecified snake venom, assault

⑦T63.004　Toxic effect of unspecified snake venom, undetermined

T63.01　Toxic effect of rattlesnake venom

　　⑦T63.011　Toxic effect of rattlesnake venom, accidental (unintentional)

　　　Toxic effect of rattlesnake venom NOS

　　⑦T63.012　Toxic effect of rattlesnake venom, intentional self-harm [HCC]

　　⑦T63.013　Toxic effect of rattlesnake venom, assault

　　⑦T63.014　Toxic effect of rattlesnake venom, undetermined

T63.02　Toxic effect of coral snake venom

　　⑦T63.021　Toxic effect of coral snake venom, accidental (unintentional)

　　　Toxic effect of coral snake venom NOS

　　⑦T63.022　Toxic effect of coral snake venom, intentional self-harm [HCC]

　　⑦T63.023　Toxic effect of coral snake venom, assault

　　⑦T63.024　Toxic effect of coral snake venom, undetermined

T63.03　Toxic effect of taipan venom

　　⑦T63.031　Toxic effect of taipan venom, accidental (unintentional)

　　　Toxic effect of taipan venom NOS

　　⑦T63.032　Toxic effect of taipan venom, intentional self-harm [HCC]

　　⑦T63.033　Toxic effect of taipan venom, assault

　　⑦T63.034　Toxic effect of taipan venom, undetermined

T63.04　Toxic effect of cobra venom

　　⑦T63.041　Toxic effect of cobra venom, accidental (unintentional)

　　　Toxic effect of cobra venom NOS

　　⑦T63.042　Toxic effect of cobra venom, intentional self-harm [HCC]

　　⑦T63.043　Toxic effect of cobra venom, assault

　　⑦T63.044　Toxic effect of cobra venom, undetermined

T63.06　Toxic effect of venom of other North and South American snake

　　⑦T63.061　Toxic effect of venom of other North and South American snake, accidental (unintentional)

　　　Toxic effect of venom of other North and South American snake NOS

　　⑦T63.062　Toxic effect of venom of other North and South American snake, intentional self-harm [HCC]

　　⑦T63.063　Toxic effect of venom of other North and South American snake, assault

　　⑦T63.064　Toxic effect of venom of other North and South American snake, undetermined

T63.07　Toxic effect of venom of other Australian snake

　　⑦T63.071　Toxic effect of venom of other Australian snake, accidental (unintentional)

　　　Toxic effect of venom of other Australian snake NOS

　● New code　▲ Revised code　Excludes1: Not coded here　Excludes2: Not included here　⊗ Placeholder required　⑦7th digit required

⑦ **T63.072** Toxic effect of venom of other Australian snake, intentional self-harm [HCC]

⑦ **T63.073** Toxic effect of venom of other Australian snake, assault

⑦ **T63.074** Toxic effect of venom of other Australian snake, undetermined

T63.08 **Toxic effect of venom of other African and Asian snake**

⑦ **T63.081** Toxic effect of venom of other African and Asian snake, accidental (unintentional)

Toxic effect of venom of other African and Asian snake NOS

⑦ **T63.082** Toxic effect of venom of other African and Asian snake, intentional self-harm [HCC]

⑦ **T63.083** Toxic effect of venom of other African and Asian snake, assault

⑦ **T63.084** Toxic effect of venom of other African and Asian snake, undetermined

T63.09 **Toxic effect of venom of other snake**

⑦ **T63.091** Toxic effect of venom of other snake, accidental (unintentional)

Toxic effect of venom of other snake NOS

⑦ **T63.092** Toxic effect of venom of other snake, intentional self-harm [HCC]

⑦ **T63.093** Toxic effect of venom of other snake, assault

⑦ **T63.094** Toxic effect of venom of other snake, undetermined

T63.1 **Toxic effect of venom of other reptiles**

T63.11 **Toxic effect of venom of gila monster**

⑦ **T63.111** Toxic effect of venom of gila monster, accidental (unintentional)

Toxic effect of venom of gila monster NOS

⑦ **T63.112** Toxic effect of venom of gila monster, intentional self-harm [HCC]

⑦ **T63.113** Toxic effect of venom of gila monster, assault

⑦ **T63.114** Toxic effect of venom of gila monster, undetermined

T63.12 **Toxic effect of venom of other venomous lizard**

⑦ **T63.121** Toxic effect of venom of other venomous lizard, accidental (unintentional)

Toxic effect of venom of other venomous lizard NOS

⑦ **T63.122** Toxic effect of venom of other venomous lizard, intentional self-harm [HCC]

⑦ **T63.123** Toxic effect of venom of other venomous lizard, assault

⑦ **T63.124** Toxic effect of venom of other venomous lizard, undetermined

T63.19 **Toxic effect of venom of other reptiles**

⑦ **T63.191** Toxic effect of venom of other reptiles, accidental (unintentional)

Toxic effect of venom of other reptiles NOS

⑦ **T63.192** Toxic effect of venom of other reptiles, intentional self-harm [HCC]

⑦ **T63.193** Toxic effect of venom of other reptiles, assault

⑦ **T63.194** Toxic effect of venom of other reptiles, undetermined

T63.2 **Toxic effect of venom of scorpion**

T63.2X **Toxic effect of venom of scorpion**

⑦ **T63.2X1** Toxic effect of venom of scorpion, accidental (unintentional)

Toxic effect of venom of scorpion NOS

⑦ **T63.2X2** Toxic effect of venom of scorpion, intentional self-harm [HCC]

⑦ **T63.2X3** Toxic effect of venom of scorpion, assault

⑦ **T63.2X4** Toxic effect of venom of scorpion, undetermined

T63.3 **Toxic effect of venom of spider**

T63.30 **Toxic effect of unspecified spider venom**

⑦ **T63.301** Toxic effect of unspecified spider venom, accidental (unintentional)

⑦ **T63.302** Toxic effect of unspecified spider venom, intentional self-harm [HCC]

⑦ **T63.303** Toxic effect of unspecified spider venom, assault

⑦ **T63.304** Toxic effect of unspecified spider venom, undetermined

T63.31 **Toxic effect of venom of black widow spider**

⑦ **T63.311** Toxic effect of venom of black widow spider, accidental (unintentional)

⑦ **T63.312** Toxic effect of venom of black widow spider, intentional self-harm [HCC]

⑦ **T63.313** Toxic effect of venom of black widow spider, assault

⑦ **T63.314** Toxic effect of venom of black widow spider, undetermined

T63.32 **Toxic effect of venom of tarantula**

⑦ **T63.321** Toxic effect of venom of tarantula, accidental (unintentional)

⑦ **T63.322** Toxic effect of venom of tarantula, intentional self-harm [HCC]

⑦ **T63.323** Toxic effect of venom of tarantula, assault

⑦ **T63.324** Toxic effect of venom of tarantula, undetermined

T63.33 **Toxic effect of venom of brown recluse spider**

⑦ **T63.331** Toxic effect of venom of brown recluse spider, accidental (unintentional)

⑦ **T63.332** Toxic effect of venom of brown recluse spider, intentional self-harm [HCC]

⑦ **T63.333** Toxic effect of venom of brown recluse spider, assault

⑦ **T63.334** Toxic effect of venom of brown recluse spider, undetermined

T63.39 **Toxic effect of venom of other spider**

⑦ **T63.391** Toxic effect of venom of other spider, accidental (unintentional)

⑦ **T63.392** Toxic effect of venom of other spider, intentional self-harm [HCC]

⑦ **T63.393** Toxic effect of venom of other spider, assault

⑦**T63.394** Toxic effect of venom of other spider, undetermined

T63.4 **Toxic effect of venom of other arthropods**

   T63.41 **Toxic effect of venom of centipedes and venomous millipedes**

      ⑦**T63.411** Toxic effect of venom of centipedes and venomous millipedes, accidental (unintentional)

      ⑦**T63.412** Toxic effect of venom of centipedes and venomous millipedes, intentional self-harm [HCC]

      ⑦**T63.413** Toxic effect of venom of centipedes and venomous millipedes, assault

      ⑦**T63.414** Toxic effect of venom of centipedes and venomous millipedes, undetermined

   T63.42 **Toxic effect of venom of ants**

      ⑦**T63.421** Toxic effect of venom of ants, accidental (unintentional)

      ⑦**T63.422** Toxic effect of venom of ants, intentional self-harm [HCC]

      ⑦**T63.423** Toxic effect of venom of ants, assault

      ⑦**T63.424** Toxic effect of venom of ants, undetermined

   T63.43 **Toxic effect of venom of caterpillars**

      ⑦**T63.431** Toxic effect of venom of caterpillars, accidental (unintentional)

      ⑦**T63.432** Toxic effect of venom of caterpillars, intentional self-harm [HCC]

      ⑦**T63.433** Toxic effect of venom of caterpillars, assault

      ⑦**T63.434** Toxic effect of venom of caterpillars, undetermined

   T63.44 **Toxic effect of venom of bees**

      ⑦**T63.441** Toxic effect of venom of bees, accidental (unintentional)

      ⑦**T63.442** Toxic effect of venom of bees, intentional self-harm [HCC]

      ⑦**T63.443** Toxic effect of venom of bees, assault

      ⑦**T63.444** Toxic effect of venom of bees, undetermined

   T63.45 **Toxic effect of venom of hornets**

      ⑦**T63.451** Toxic effect of venom of hornets, accidental (unintentional)

      ⑦**T63.452** Toxic effect of venom of hornets, intentional self-harm [HCC]

      ⑦**T63.453** Toxic effect of venom of hornets, assault

      ⑦**T63.454** Toxic effect of venom of hornets, undetermined

   T63.46 **Toxic effect of venom of wasps**

      Toxic effect of yellow jacket

      ⑦**T63.461** Toxic effect of venom of wasps, accidental (unintentional)

      ⑦**T63.462** Toxic effect of venom of wasps, intentional self-harm [HCC]

      ⑦**T63.463** Toxic effect of venom of wasps, assault

      ⑦**T63.464** Toxic effect of venom of wasps, undetermined

   T63.48 **Toxic effect of venom of other arthropod**

      ⑦**T63.481** Toxic effect of venom of other arthropod, accidental (unintentional)

⑦**T63.482** Toxic effect of venom of other arthropod, intentional self-harm [HCC]

⑦**T63.483** Toxic effect of venom of other arthropod, assault

⑦**T63.484** Toxic effect of venom of other arthropod, undetermined

T63.5 **Toxic effect of contact with venomous fish**

   Excludes2: poisoning by ingestion of fish (T61.-)

   T63.51 **Toxic effect of contact with stingray**

      ⑦**T63.511** Toxic effect of contact with stingray, accidental (unintentional)

      ⑦**T63.512** Toxic effect of contact with stingray, intentional self-harm [HCC]

      ⑦**T63.513** Toxic effect of contact with stingray, assault

      ⑦**T63.514** Toxic effect of contact with stingray, undetermined

   T63.59 **Toxic effect of contact with other venomous fish**

      ⑦**T63.591** Toxic effect of contact with other venomous fish, accidental (unintentional)

      ⑦**T63.592** Toxic effect of contact with other venomous fish, intentional self-harm [HCC]

      ⑦**T63.593** Toxic effect of contact with other venomous fish, assault

      ⑦**T63.594** Toxic effect of contact with other venomous fish, undetermined

T63.6 **Toxic effect of contact with other venomous marine animals**

   Excludes1: sea-snake venom (T63.09)

   Excludes2: poisoning by ingestion of shellfish (T61.78-)

  ▲ **T63.61** **Toxic effect of contact with Portuguese Man-o-war**

      Toxic effect of contact with bluebottle

    ▲ ⑦**T63.611** Toxic effect of contact with Portuguese Man-o-war, accidental (unintentional)

    ▲ ⑦**T63.612** Toxic effect of contact with Portuguese Man-o-war, intentional self-harm [HCC]

    ▲ ⑦**T63.613** Toxic effect of contact with Portuguese Man-o-war, assault

    ▲ ⑦**T63.614** Toxic effect of contact with Portuguese Man-o-war, undetermined

   T63.62 **Toxic effect of contact with other jellyfish**

      ⑦**T63.621** Toxic effect of contact with other jellyfish, accidental (unintentional)

      ⑦**T63.622** Toxic effect of contact with other jellyfish, intentional self-harm [HCC]

      ⑦**T63.623** Toxic effect of contact with other jellyfish, assault

      ⑦**T63.624** Toxic effect of contact with other jellyfish, undetermined

   T63.63 **Toxic effect of contact with sea anemone**

      ⑦**T63.631** Toxic effect of contact with sea anemone, accidental (unintentional)

      ⑦**T63.632** Toxic effect of contact with sea anemone, intentional self-harm [HCC]

      ⑦**T63.633** Toxic effect of contact with sea anemone, assault

⑦T63.634 Toxic effect of contact with sea anemone, undetermined

T63.69 Toxic effect of contact with other venomous marine animals

⑦T63.691 Toxic effect of contact with other venomous marine animals, accidental (unintentional)

⑦T63.692 Toxic effect of contact with other venomous marine animals, intentional self-harm [HCC]

⑦T63.693 Toxic effect of contact with other venomous marine animals, assault

⑦T63.694 Toxic effect of contact with other venomous marine animals, undetermined

T63.7 Toxic effect of contact with venomous plant

T63.71 Toxic effect of contact with venomous marine plant

⑦T63.711 Toxic effect of contact with venomous marine plant, accidental (unintentional)

⑦T63.712 Toxic effect of contact with venomous marine plant, intentional self-harm [HCC]

⑦T63.713 Toxic effect of contact with venomous marine plant, assault

⑦T63.714 Toxic effect of contact with venomous marine plant, undetermined

T63.79 Toxic effect of contact with other venomous plant

⑦T63.791 Toxic effect of contact with other venomous plant, accidental (unintentional)

⑦T63.792 Toxic effect of contact with other venomous plant, intentional self-harm [HCC]

⑦T63.793 Toxic effect of contact with other venomous plant, assault

⑦T63.794 Toxic effect of contact with other venomous plant, undetermined

T63.8 Toxic effect of contact with other venomous animals

T63.81 Toxic effect of contact with venomous frog

Excludes1: contact with nonvenomous frog (W62.0)

⑦T63.811 Toxic effect of contact with venomous frog, accidental (unintentional)

⑦T63.812 Toxic effect of contact with venomous frog, intentional self-harm [HCC]

⑦T63.813 Toxic effect of contact with venomous frog, assault

⑦T63.814 Toxic effect of contact with venomous frog, undetermined

T63.82 Toxic effect of contact with venomous toad

Excludes1: contact with nonvenomous toad (W62.1)

⑦T63.821 Toxic effect of contact with venomous toad, accidental (unintentional)

⑦T63.822 Toxic effect of contact with venomous toad, intentional self-harm [HCC]

⑦T63.823 Toxic effect of contact with venomous toad, assault

⑦T63.824 Toxic effect of contact with venomous toad, undetermined

T63.83 Toxic effect of contact with other venomous amphibian

Excludes1: contact with nonvenomous amphibian (W62.9)

⑦T63.831 Toxic effect of contact with other venomous amphibian, accidental (unintentional)

⑦T63.832 Toxic effect of contact with other venomous amphibian, intentional self-harm [HCC]

⑦T63.833 Toxic effect of contact with other venomous amphibian, assault

⑦T63.834 Toxic effect of contact with other venomous amphibian, undetermined

T63.89 Toxic effect of contact with other venomous animals

⑦T63.891 Toxic effect of contact with other venomous animals, accidental (unintentional)

⑦T63.892 Toxic effect of contact with other venomous animals, intentional self-harm [HCC]

⑦T63.893 Toxic effect of contact with other venomous animals, assault

⑦T63.894 Toxic effect of contact with other venomous animals, undetermined

T63.9 Toxic effect of contact with unspecified venomous animal

⊗⑦T63.91 Toxic effect of contact with unspecified venomous animal, accidental (unintentional)

⊗⑦T63.92 Toxic effect of contact with unspecified venomous animal, intentional self-harm [HCC]

⊗⑦T63.93 Toxic effect of contact with unspecified venomous animal, assault

⊗⑦T63.94 Toxic effect of contact with unspecified venomous animal, undetermined

T64 Toxic effect of aflatoxin and other mycotoxin food contaminants

The appropriate 7th character is to be added to each code from category T64

A - initial encounter

D - subsequent encounter

S - sequela

T64.0 Toxic effect of aflatoxin

⊗⑦T64.01 Toxic effect of aflatoxin, accidental (unintentional)

⊗⑦T64.02 Toxic effect of aflatoxin, intentional self-harm [HCC]

⊗⑦T64.03 Toxic effect of aflatoxin, assault

⊗⑦T64.04 Toxic effect of aflatoxin, undetermined

T64.8 Toxic effect of other mycotoxin food contaminants

⊗⑦T64.81 Toxic effect of other mycotoxin food contaminants, accidental (unintentional)

⊗⑦T64.82 Toxic effect of other mycotoxin food contaminants, intentional self-harm [HCC]

⊗⑦T64.83 Toxic effect of other mycotoxin food contaminants, assault

⊗⑦T64.84 Toxic effect of other mycotoxin food contaminants, undetermined

T65 Toxic effect of other and unspecified substances

The appropriate 7th character is to be added to each code from category T65

A - initial encounter
D - subsequent encounter
S - sequela

T65.0   Toxic effect of cyanides

> Excludes1: hydrogen cyanide (T57.3-)

T65.0X   Toxic effect of cyanides

⑦ **T65.0X1   Toxic effect of cyanides, accidental (unintentional)**

Toxic effect of cyanides NOS

⑦ **T65.0X2   Toxic effect of cyanides, intentional self-harm**

⑦ **T65.0X3   Toxic effect of cyanides, assault**

⑦ **T65.0X4   Toxic effect of cyanides, undetermined**

T65.1   Toxic effect of strychnine and its salts

T65.1X   Toxic effect of strychnine and its salts

⑦ **T65.1X1   Toxic effect of strychnine and its salts, accidental (unintentional)**

Toxic effect of strychnine and its salts NOS

⑦ **T65.1X2   Toxic effect of strychnine and its salts, intentional self-harm** [HCC]

⑦ **T65.1X3   Toxic effect of strychnine and its salts, assault**

⑦ **T65.1X4   Toxic effect of strychnine and its salts, undetermined**

T65.2   Toxic effect of tobacco and nicotine

> Excludes2: nicotine dependence (F17.-)

T65.21   Toxic effect of chewing tobacco

⑦ **T65.211   Toxic effect of chewing tobacco, accidental (unintentional)**

Toxic effect of chewing tobacco NOS

⑦ **T65.212   Toxic effect of chewing tobacco, intentional self-harm** [HCC]

⑦ **T65.213   Toxic effect of chewing tobacco, assault**

⑦ **T65.214   Toxic effect of chewing tobacco, undetermined**

T65.22   Toxic effect of tobacco cigarettes

Toxic effect of tobacco smoke

Use Additional Code for exposure to second hand tobacco smoke (Z57.31, Z77.22)

⑦ **T65.221   Toxic effect of tobacco cigarettes, accidental (unintentional)**

Toxic effect of tobacco cigarettes NOS

⑦ **T65.222   Toxic effect of tobacco cigarettes, intentional self-harm** [HCC]

⑦ **T65.223   Toxic effect of tobacco cigarettes, assault**

⑦ **T65.224   Toxic effect of tobacco cigarettes, undetermined**

T65.29   Toxic effect of other tobacco and nicotine

⑦ **T65.291   Toxic effect of other tobacco and nicotine, accidental (unintentional)**

Toxic effect of other tobacco and nicotine NOS

⑦ **T65.292   Toxic effect of other tobacco and nicotine, intentional self-harm** [HCC]

⑦ **T65.293   Toxic effect of other tobacco and nicotine, assault**

⑦ **T65.294   Toxic effect of other tobacco and nicotine, undetermined**

T65.3   Toxic effect of nitroderivatives and aminoderivatives of benzene and its homologues

Toxic effect of anilin [benzeneamine]

Toxic effect of nitrobenzene

Toxic effect of trinitrotoluene

T65.3X   Toxic effect of nitroderivatives and aminoderivatives of benzene and its homologues

⑦ **T65.3X1   Toxic effect of nitroderivatives and aminoderivatives of benzene and its homologues, accidental (unintentional)**

Toxic effect of nitroderivatives and aminoderivatives of benzene and its homologues NOS

⑦ **T65.3X2   Toxic effect of nitroderivatives and aminoderivatives of benzene and its homologues, intentional self-harm** [HCC]

⑦ **T65.3X3   Toxic effect of nitroderivatives and aminoderivatives of benzene and its homologues, assault**

⑦ **T65.3X4   Toxic effect of nitroderivatives and aminoderivatives of benzene and its homologues, undetermined**

T65.4   Toxic effect of carbon disulfide

T65.4X   Toxic effect of carbon disulfide

⑦ **T65.4X1   Toxic effect of carbon disulfide, accidental (unintentional)**

Toxic effect of carbon disulfide NOS

⑦ **T65.4X2   Toxic effect of carbon disulfide, intentional self-harm** [HCC]

⑦ **T65.4X3   Toxic effect of carbon disulfide, assault**

⑦ **T65.4X4   Toxic effect of carbon disulfide, undetermined**

T65.5   Toxic effect of nitroglycerin and other nitric acids and esters

Toxic effect of 1,2,3-Propanetriol trinitrate

T65.5X   Toxic effect of nitroglycerin and other nitric acids and esters

⑦ **T65.5X1   Toxic effect of nitroglycerin and other nitric acids and esters, accidental (unintentional)**

Toxic effect of nitroglycerin and other nitric acids and esters NOS

⑦ **T65.5X2   Toxic effect of nitroglycerin and other nitric acids and esters, intentional self-harm** [HCC]

⑦ **T65.5X3   Toxic effect of nitroglycerin and other nitric acids and esters, assault**

⑦ **T65.5X4   Toxic effect of nitroglycerin and other nitric acids and esters, undetermined**

T65.6   Toxic effect of paints and dyes, not elsewhere classified

T65.6X   Toxic effect of paints and dyes, not elsewhere classified

⑦ **T65.6X1   Toxic effect of paints and dyes, not elsewhere classified, accidental (unintentional)**

Toxic effect of paints and dyes NOS

⑦ **T65.6X2   Toxic effect of paints and dyes, not elsewhere classified, intentional self-harm** [HCC]

● New code   ▲ Revised code   **Excludes1:** Not coded here   **Excludes2:** Not included here   ⊗ Placeholder required   ⑦7ᵗʰ digit required

⑦**T65.6X3** Toxic effect of paints and dyes, not elsewhere classified, assault

⑦**T65.6X4** Toxic effect of paints and dyes, not elsewhere classified, undetermined

T65.8 Toxic effect of other specified substances

T65.81 Toxic effect of latex

⑦**T65.811** **Toxic effect of latex, accidental (unintentional)**

Toxic effect of latex NOS

⑦**T65.812** **Toxic effect of latex, intentional self-harm** [HCC]

⑦**T65.813** **Toxic effect of latex, assault**

⑦**T65.814** **Toxic effect of latex, undetermined**

T65.82 Toxic effect of harmful algae and algae toxins

Toxic effect of (harmful) algae bloom NOS

Toxic effect of blue-green algae bloom

Toxic effect of brown tide

Toxic effect of cyanobacteria bloom

Toxic effect of Florida red tide

Toxic effect of pfiesteria piscicida

Toxic effect of red tide

⑦**T65.821** **Toxic effect of harmful algae and algae toxins, accidental (unintentional)**

Toxic effect of harmful algae and algae toxins NOS

⑦**T65.822** **Toxic effect of harmful algae and algae toxins, intentional self-harm** [HCC]

⑦**T65.823** **Toxic effect of harmful algae and algae toxins, assault**

⑦**T65.824** **Toxic effect of harmful algae and algae toxins, undetermined**

T65.83 Toxic effect of fiberglass

⑦**T65.831** **Toxic effect of fiberglass, accidental (unintentional)**

Toxic effect of fiberglass NOS

⑦**T65.832** **Toxic effect of fiberglass, intentional self-harm** [HCC]

⑦**T65.833** **Toxic effect of fiberglass, assault**

⑦**T65.834** **Toxic effect of fiberglass, undetermined**

T65.89 Toxic effect of other specified substances

⑦**T65.891** **Toxic effect of other specified substances, accidental (unintentional)**

Toxic effect of other specified substances NOS

⑦**T65.892** **Toxic effect of other specified substances, intentional self-harm** [HCC]

⑦**T65.893** **Toxic effect of other specified substances, assault**

⑦**T65.894** **Toxic effect of other specified substances, undetermined**

T65.9 Toxic effect of unspecified substance

⊗⑦**T65.91** **Toxic effect of unspecified substance, accidental (unintentional)**

Poisoning NOS

⊗⑦**T65.92** **Toxic effect of unspecified substance, intentional self-harm** [HCC]

⊗⑦**T65.93** **Toxic effect of unspecified substance, assault**

⊗⑦**T65.94** **Toxic effect of unspecified substance, undetermined**

OTHER AND UNSPECIFIED EFFECTS OF EXTERNAL CAUSES (T66-T78)

⊗⑦**T66 Radiation sickness, unspecified**

Excludes1: specified adverse effects of radiation, such as:

burns (T20-T31)

leukemia (C91-C95)

radiation gastroenteritis and colitis (K52.0)

radiation pneumonitis (J70.0)

radiation related disorders of the skin and subcutaneous tissue (L55-L59)

sunburn (L55.-)

The appropriate 7th character is to be added to code T66

A - initial encounter

D - subsequent encounter

S - sequela

T67 Effects of heat and light

Excludes1: erythema [dermatitis] ab igne (L59.0)

malignant hyperpyrexia due to anesthesia (T88.3)

radiation-related disorders of the skin and subcutaneous tissue (L55-L59)

Excludes2: burns (T20-T31)

sunburn (L55.-)

sweat disorder due to heat (L74-L75)

The appropriate 7th character is to be added to each code from category T67

A - initial encounter

D - subsequent encounter

S - sequela

T67.0 Heatstroke and sunstroke

Use Additional rhabdomyolysis (M62.82)

Use Additional Code(s) to identify any associated complications of heatstroke, such as:

coma and stupor (R40.-)

systemic inflammatory response syndrome (R65.1-)

⊗⑦**T67.01** **Heatstroke and sunstroke**

Heat apoplexy

Heat pyrexia

Siriasis

Thermoplegia

⊗⑦**T67.02** **Exertional heatstroke**

⊗⑦**T67.09** **Other heatstroke and sunstroke**

⊗⑦**T67.1 Heat syncope**

Heat collapse

⊗⑦**T67.2 Heat cramp**

⊗⑦**T67.3 Heat exhaustion, anhydrotic**

Heat prostration due to water depletion

Excludes1: heat exhaustion due to salt depletion (T67.4)

⊗⑦**T67.4 Heat exhaustion due to salt depletion**

Heat prostration due to salt (and water) depletion

⊗⑦**T67.5 Heat exhaustion, unspecified**

Heat prostration NOS

⊗⑦**T67.6 Heat fatigue, transient**

⊗⑦**T67.7 Heat edema**

⊗⑦**T67.8 Other effects of heat and light**

⊗⑦**T67.9 Effect of heat and light, unspecified**

⊗⑦**T68** **Hypothermia**

Accidental hypothermia

Hypothermia NOS

Use Additional Code to identify source of exposure:

Exposure to excessive cold of man-made origin (W93)

Exposure to excessive cold of natural origin (X31)

Excludes1: hypothermia following anesthesia (T88.51)

hypothermia not associated with low environmental temperature (R68.0)

hypothermia of newborn (P80.-)

Excludes2: frostbite (T33-T34)

The appropriate 7th character is to be added to code T68

A - initial encounter

D - subsequent encounter

S - sequela

T69 **Other effects of reduced temperature**

Use Additional Code to identify source of exposure:

Exposure to excessive cold of man-made origin (W93)

Exposure to excessive cold of natural origin (X31)

Excludes2: frostbite (T33-T34)

The appropriate 7th character is to be added to each code from category T69

A - initial encounter

D - subsequent encounter

S - sequela

T69.0 **Immersion hand and foot**

T69.01 **Immersion hand**

⑦**T69.011** **Immersion hand, right hand**

⑦**T69.012** **Immersion hand, left hand**

⑦**T69.019** **Immersion hand, unspecified hand**

T69.02 **Immersion foot**

Trench foot

⑦**T69.021** **Immersion foot, right foot**

⑦**T69.022** **Immersion foot, left foot**

⑦**T69.029** **Immersion foot, unspecified foot**

⊗⑦**T69.1** **Chilblains**

⊗⑦**T69.8** **Other specified effects of reduced temperature**

⊗⑦**T69.9** **Effect of reduced temperature, unspecified**

T70 **Effects of air pressure and water pressure**

The appropriate 7th character is to be added to each code from category T70

A - initial encounter

D - subsequent encounter

S - sequela

⊗⑦**T70.0** **Otitic barotrauma**

Aero-otitis media

Effects of change in ambient atmospheric pressure or water pressure on ears

⊗⑦**T70.1** **Sinus barotrauma**

Aerosinusitis

Effects of change in ambient atmospheric pressure on sinuses

T70.2 **Other and unspecified effects of high altitude**

Excludes2: polycythemia due to high altitude (D75.1)

⊗⑦**T70.20** **Unspecified effects of high altitude**

⊗⑦**T70.29** **Other effects of high altitude**

Alpine sickness

Anoxia due to high altitude

Barotrauma NOS

Hypobaropathy

Mountain sickness

⊗⑦**T70.3** **Caisson disease [decompression sickness]**

Compressed-air disease

Diver's palsy or paralysis

⊗⑦**T70.4** **Effects of high-pressure fluids**

Hydraulic jet injection (industrial)

Pneumatic jet injection (industrial)

Traumatic jet injection (industrial)

⊗⑦**T70.8** **Other effects of air pressure and water pressure**

⊗⑦**T70.9** **Effect of air pressure and water pressure, unspecified**

T71 **Asphyxiation**

Mechanical suffocation

Traumatic suffocation

Excludes1: acute respiratory distress (syndrome) (J80)

anoxia due to high altitude (T70.2) asphyxia NOS (R09.01)

asphyxia from carbon monoxide (T58.-)

asphyxia from inhalation of food or foreign body (T17.-)

asphyxia from other gases, fumes and vapors (T59.-)

respiratory distress (syndrome) in newborn (P22.-)

The appropriate 7th character is to be added to each code from category T71

A - initial encounter

D - subsequent encounter

S - sequela

T71.1 **Asphyxiation due to mechanical threat to breathing**

Suffocation due to mechanical threat to breathing

T71.11 **Asphyxiation due to smothering under pillow**

⑦**T71.111** **Asphyxiation due to smothering under pillow, accidental**

Asphyxiation due to smothering under pillow NOS

⑦**T71.112** **Asphyxiation due to smothering under pillow, intentional self-harm** [HCC]

⑦**T71.113** **Asphyxiation due to smothering under pillow, assault**

⑦**T71.114** **Asphyxiation due to smothering under pillow, undetermined**

T71.12 **Asphyxiation due to plastic bag**

⑦**T71.121** **Asphyxiation due to plastic bag, accidental**

Asphyxiation due to plastic bag NOS

⑦**T71.122** **Asphyxiation due to plastic bag, intentional self-harm** [HCC]

⑦**T71.123** **Asphyxiation due to plastic bag, assault**

⑦**T71.124** **Asphyxiation due to plastic bag, undetermined**

T71.13 **Asphyxiation due to being trapped in bed linens**

⑦**T71.131** **Asphyxiation due to being trapped in bed linens, accidental**

Asphyxiation due to being trapped in bed linens NOS

⑦**T71.132** **Asphyxiation due to being trapped in bed linens, intentional self-harm** [HCC]

● New code ▲ Revised code **Excludes1:** Not coded here **Excludes2:** Not included here ⊗ Placeholder required ⑦ 7th digit required

⑦T71.133 **Asphyxiation due to being trapped in bed linens, assault**

⑦T71.134 **Asphyxiation due to being trapped in bed linens, undetermined**

T71.14 **Asphyxiation due to smothering under another person's body (in bed)**

⑦T71.141 **Asphyxiation due to smothering under another person's body (in bed), accidental**

Asphyxiation due to smothering under another person's body (in bed) NOS

⑦T71.143 **Asphyxiation due to smothering under another person's body (in bed), assault**

⑦T71.144 **Asphyxiation due to smothering under another person's body (in bed), undetermined**

T71.15 **Asphyxiation due to smothering in furniture**

⑦T71.151 **Asphyxiation due to smothering in furniture, accidental**

Asphyxiation due to smothering in furniture NOS

⑦T71.152 **Asphyxiation due to smothering in furniture, intentional self-harm** [HCC]

⑦T71.153 **Asphyxiation due to smothering in furniture, assault**

⑦T71.154 **Asphyxiation due to smothering in furniture, undetermined**

T71.16 **Asphyxiation due to hanging**

Hanging by window shade cord

Use Additional Code for any associated injuries, such as:

crushing injury of neck (S17.-)

fracture of cervical vertebrae (S12.0-S12.2-)

open wound of neck (S11.-)

⑦T71.161 **Asphyxiation due to hanging, accidental**

Asphyxiation due to hanging NOS

Hanging NOS

⑦T71.162 **Asphyxiation due to hanging, intentional self-harm** [HCC]

⑦T71.163 **Asphyxiation due to hanging, assault**

⑦T71.164 **Asphyxiation due to hanging, undetermined**

T71.19 **Asphyxiation due to mechanical threat to breathing due to other causes**

⑦T71.191 **Asphyxiation due to mechanical threat to breathing due to other causes, accidental**

Asphyxiation due to other causes NOS

⑦T71.192 **Asphyxiation due to mechanical threat to breathing due to other causes, intentional self-harm** [HCC]

⑦T71.193 **Asphyxiation due to mechanical threat to breathing due to other causes, assault**

⑦T71.194 **Asphyxiation due to mechanical threat to breathing due to other causes, undetermined**

T71.2 **Asphyxiation due to systemic oxygen deficiency due to low oxygen content in ambient air**

Suffocation due to systemic oxygen deficiency due to low oxygen content in ambient air

⊗⑦T71.20 **Asphyxiation due to systemic oxygen deficiency due to low oxygen content in ambient air due to unspecified cause**

⊗⑦T71.21 **Asphyxiation due to cave-in or falling earth**

Use Additional Code for any associated cataclysm (X34-X38)

T71.22 **Asphyxiation due to being trapped in a car trunk**

⑦T71.221 **Asphyxiation due to being trapped in a car trunk, accidental**

⑦T71.222 **Asphyxiation due to being trapped in a car trunk, intentional self-harm** [HCC]

⑦T71.223 **Asphyxiation due to being trapped in a car trunk, assault**

⑦T71.224 **Asphyxiation due to being trapped in a car trunk, undetermined**

T71.23 **Asphyxiation due to being trapped in a (discarded) refrigerator**

⑦T71.231 **Asphyxiation due to being trapped in a (discarded) refrigerator, accidental**

⑦T71.232 **Asphyxiation due to being trapped in a (discarded) refrigerator, intentional self-harm** [HCC]

⑦T71.233 **Asphyxiation due to being trapped in a (discarded) refrigerator, assault**

⑦T71.234 **Asphyxiation due to being trapped in a (discarded) refrigerator, undetermined**

⊗⑦T71.29 **Asphyxiation due to being trapped in other low oxygen environment**

⊗⑦T71.9 **Asphyxiation due to unspecified cause**

Suffocation (by strangulation) due to unspecified cause

Suffocation NOS

Systemic oxygen deficiency due to low oxygen content in ambient air due to unspecified cause

Systemic oxygen deficiency due to mechanical threat to breathing due to unspecified cause

Traumatic asphyxia NOS

T73 **Effects of other deprivation**

The appropriate 7th character is to be added to each code from category T73

A - initial encounter

D - subsequent encounter

S - sequela

⊗⑦T73.0 **Starvation**

Deprivation of food

⊗⑦T73.1 **Deprivation of water**

⊗⑦T73.2 **Exhaustion due to exposure**

⊗⑦T73.3 **Exhaustion due to excessive exertion**

Exhaustion due to overexertion

⊗⑦T73.8 **Other effects of deprivation**

⊗⑦T73.9 **Effect of deprivation, unspecified**

T74 **Adult and child abuse, neglect and other maltreatment, confirmed**

Use Additional Code, if applicable, to identify any associated current injury

Use additional external cause code to identify perpetrator, if known (Y07.-)

Excludes1: abuse and maltreatment in pregnancy (O9A.3-, O9A.4-, O9A.5-)

adult and child maltreatment, suspected (T76.-)

The appropriate 7th character is to be added to each code from category T74

A - initial encounter

D - subsequent encounter

S - sequela

T74.0 Neglect or abandonment, confirmed

⊗⑦T74.01 Adult neglect or abandonment, confirmed

⊗⑦T74.02 Child neglect or abandonment, confirmed

T74.1 Physical abuse, confirmed

Excludes2: sexual abuse (T74.2-)

⊗⑦T74.11 Adult physical abuse, confirmed

⊗⑦T74.12 Child physical abuse, confirmed

Excludes2: shaken infant syndrome (T74.4)

T74.2 Sexual abuse, confirmed

Rape, confirmed

Sexual assault, confirmed

⊗⑦T74.21 Adult sexual abuse, confirmed

⊗⑦T74.22 Child sexual abuse, confirmed

T74.3 Psychological abuse, confirmed

Bullying and intimidation, confirmed

Intimidation through social media, confirmed

⊗⑦T74.31 Adult psychological abuse, confirmed

⊗⑦T74.32 Child psychological abuse, confirmed

T74.4 Shaken infant syndrome

T74.5 Forced sexual exploitation, confirmed

⊗⑦T74.51 Adult forced sexual exploitation, confirmed

⊗⑦T74.52 Child sexual exploitation, confirmed

T74.6 Forced labor exploitation, confirmed

⊗⑦T74.61 Adult forced labor exploitation, confirmed

⊗⑦T74.62 Child forced labor exploitation, confirmed

T74.9 Unspecified maltreatment, confirmed

⊗⑦T74.91 Unspecified adult maltreatment, confirmed

⊗⑦T74.92 Unspecified child maltreatment, confirmed

T75 Other and unspecified effects of other external causes

Excludes1: adverse effects NEC (T78.-)

Excludes2: burns (electric) (T20-T31)

The appropriate 7th character is to be added to each code from category T75

A - initial encounter

D - subsequent encounter

S - sequela

T75.0 Effects of lightning

Struck by lightning

⊗⑦T75.00 Unspecified effects of lightning

Struck by lightning NOS

⊗⑦T75.01 Shock due to being struck by lightning

⊗⑦T75.09 Other effects of lightning

Use Additional Code for other effects of lightning

⊗⑦T75.1 Unspecified effects of drowning and nonfatal submersion

Immersion

Excludes1: specified effects of drowning- code to effects

T75.2 Effects of vibration

⊗⑦T75.20 Unspecified effects of vibration

⊗⑦T75.21 Pneumatic hammer syndrome

⊗⑦T75.22 Traumatic vasospastic syndrome

⊗⑦T75.23 Vertigo from infrasound

Excludes1: vertigo NOS (R42)

⊗⑦T75.29 Other effects of vibration

⊗⑦T75.3 Motion sickness

Airsickness

Seasickness

Travel sickness

Use additional external cause code to identify vehicle or type of motion (Y92.81-, Y93.5-)

⊗⑦T75.4 Electrocution

Shock from electric current

Shock from electroshock gun (taser)

T75.8 Other specified effects of external causes

⊗⑦T75.81 Effects of abnormal gravitation [G] forces

⊗⑦T75.82 Effects of weightlessness

⊗⑦T75.89 Other specified effects of external causes

T76 Adult and child abuse, neglect and other maltreatment, suspected

Use Additional Code, if applicable, to identify any associated current injury

Excludes1: adult and child maltreatment, confirmed (T74.-)

suspected abuse and maltreatment in pregnancy (O9A.3-, O9A.4-, O9A.5-)

suspected adult physical abuse, ruled out (Z04.71)

suspected adult sexual abuse, ruled out (Z04.41)

suspected child physical abuse, ruled out (Z04.72)

suspected child sexual abuse, ruled out (Z04.42)

The appropriate 7th character is to be added to each code from category T76

A - initial encounter

D - subsequent encounter

S - sequela

T76.0 Neglect or abandonment, suspected

⊗⑦T76.01 Adult neglect or abandonment, suspected

⊗⑦T76.02 Child neglect or abandonment, suspected

T76.1 Physical abuse, suspected

⊗⑦T76.11 Adult physical abuse, suspected

⊗⑦T76.12 Child physical abuse, suspected

T76.2 Sexual abuse, suspected

Rape, suspected

Excludes1: alleged abuse, ruled out (Z04.7)

⊗⑦T76.21 Adult sexual abuse, suspected

⊗⑦T76.22 Child sexual abuse, suspected

T76.3 Psychological abuse, suspected

Bullying and intimidation, suspected

Intimidation through social media, suspected

⊗⑦T76.31 Adult psychological abuse, suspected

⊗⑦T76.32 Child psychological abuse, suspected

T76.5 Forced sexual exploitation, suspected

T76.51 Adult forced sexual exploitation, suspected

T76.52 Child sexual exploitation, suspected

T76.6 Forced labor exploitation, suspected

T76.61 Adult forced labor exploitation, suspected

T76.62 Child forced labor exploitation, suspected

T76.9 Unspecified maltreatment, suspected

⊗⑦T76.91 Unspecified adult maltreatment, suspected

⊗⑦T76.92 Unspecified child maltreatment, suspected

T78 Adverse effects, not elsewhere classified

● New code ▲ Revised code Excludes1: Not coded here Excludes2: Not included here ⊗ Placeholder required ⑦ 7th digit required

Excludes2: complications of surgical and medical care NEC (T80-T88)

The appropriate 7th character is to be added to each code from category T78

A - initial encounter

D - subsequent encounter

S - sequela

T78.0 Anaphylactic reaction due to food

Anaphylactic reaction due to adverse food reaction

Anaphylactic shock or reaction due to nonpoisonous foods

Anaphylactoid reaction due to food

⊗⑦**T78.00 Anaphylactic reaction due to unspecified food**

⊗⑦**T78.01 Anaphylactic reaction due to peanuts**

⊗⑦**T78.02 Anaphylactic reaction due to shellfish (crustaceans)**

⊗⑦**T78.03 Anaphylactic reaction due to other fish**

⊗⑦**T78.04 Anaphylactic reaction due to fruits and vegetables**

⊗⑦**T78.05 Anaphylactic reaction due to tree nuts and seeds**

Excludes2: anaphylactic reaction due to peanuts (T78.01)

⊗⑦**T78.06 Anaphylactic reaction due to food additives**

⊗⑦**T78.07 Anaphylactic reaction due to milk and dairy products**

⊗⑦**T78.08 Anaphylactic reaction due to eggs**

⊗⑦**T78.09 Anaphylactic reaction due to other food products**

⊗⑦**T78.1 Other adverse food reactions, not elsewhere classified**

Use Additional Code to identify the type of reaction, if applicable

Excludes1: anaphylactic reaction or shock due to adverse food reaction (T78.0-)

anaphylactic reaction due to food (T78.0-)

bacterial food borne intoxications (A05.-)

Excludes2: allergic and dietetic gastroenteritis and colitis (K52.29)

allergic rhinitis due to food (J30.5)

dermatitis due to food in contact with skin (L23.6, L24.6, L25.4)

dermatitis due to ingested food (L27.2)

food protein-induced enterocolitis syndrome (K52.21)

food protein-induced enteropathy (K52.22)

⊗⑦**T78.2 Anaphylactic shock, unspecified**

Allergic shock

Anaphylactic reaction

Anaphylaxis

Excludes1: anaphylactic reaction or shock due to adverse effect of correct medicinal substance properly administered (T88.6)

anaphylactic reaction or shock due to adverse food reaction (T78.0-)

anaphylactic reaction or shock due to serum (T80.5-)

⊗⑦**T78.3 Angioneurotic edema**

Allergic angioedema Giant urticaria Quincke's edema

Excludes1: serum urticaria (T80.6-)

urticaria (L50.-)

T78.4 Other and unspecified allergy

Excludes1: specified types of allergic reaction such as:

allergic diarrhea (K52.29)

allergic gastroenteritis and colitis (K52.29)

dermatitis (L23-L25, L27.-)

food protein-induced enterocolitis syndrome (K52.21)

food protein-induced enteropathy (K52.22)

hay fever (J30.1)

⊗⑦**T78.40 Allergy, unspecified**

Allergic reaction NOS

Hypersensitivity NOS

⊗⑦**T78.41 Arthus phenomenon**

Arthus reaction

⊗⑦**T78.49 Other allergy**

⊗⑦**T78.8 Other adverse effects, not elsewhere classified**

CERTAIN EARLY COMPLICATIONS OF TRAUMA (T79)

T79 Certain early complications of trauma, not elsewhere classified

Excludes2: acute respiratory distress syndrome (J80)

complications occurring during or following medical procedures (T80-T88)

complications of surgical and medical care NEC (T80-T88)

newborn respiratory distress syndrome (P22.0)

The appropriate 7th character is to be added to each code from category T79

A - initial encounter

D - subsequent encounter

S - sequela

⊗⑦**T79.0 Air embolism (traumatic)** [HCC]

Excludes1: air embolism complicating abortion or ectopic or molar pregnancy (O00-O07, O08.2)

air embolism complicating pregnancy, childbirth and the puerperium (O88.0)

air embolism following infusion, transfusion, and therapeutic injection (T80.0)

air embolism following procedure NEC (T81.7-)

⊗⑦**T79.1 Fat embolism (traumatic)** [HCC]

Excludes1: fat embolism complicating:

abortion or ectopic or molar pregnancy (O00-O07, O08.2)

pregnancy, childbirth and the puerperium (O88.8)

⊗⑦**T79.2 Traumatic secondary and recurrent hemorrhage and seroma** [HCC]

⊗⑦**T79.4 Traumatic shock** [HCC]

Shock (immediate) (delayed) following injury

Excludes1: anaphylactic shock due to adverse food reaction (T78.0-)

anaphylactic shock due to correct medicinal substance properly administered (T88.6)

anaphylactic shock due to serum (T80.5-)

anaphylactic shock NOS (T78.2)

electric shock (T75.4)

nontraumatic shock NEC (R57.-)

obstetric shock (O75.1)

postprocedural shock (T81.1-)

septic shock (R65.21)

shock complicating abortion or ectopic or molar pregnancy (O00-O07, O08.3)

shock due to anesthesia (T88.2)

shock due to lightning (T75.01)

shock NOS (R57.9)

⊗⑦**T79.5** **Traumatic anuria** [HCC]

Crush syndrome

Renal failure following crushing

⊗⑦**T79.6** **Traumatic ischemia of muscle** [HCC]

Traumatic rhabdomyolysis

Volkmann's ischemic contracture

Excludes2: anterior tibial syndrome (M76.8)

compartment syndrome (traumatic) (T79.A-)

nontraumatic ischemia of muscle (M62.2-)

⊗⑦**T79.7** **Traumatic subcutaneous emphysema**

Excludes2: emphysema NOS (J43)

emphysema (subcutaneous) resulting from a procedure (T81.82)

T79.A **Traumatic compartment syndrome** [HCC]

Excludes1: fibromyalgia (M79.7)

nontraumatic compartment syndrome (M79.A-)

Excludes2 traumatic ischemic infarction of muscle (T79.6)

⊗⑦**T79.A0** **Compartment syndrome, unspecified** [HCC]

Compartment syndrome NOS

T79.A1 **Traumatic compartment syndrome of upper extremity** [HCC]

Traumatic compartment syndrome of shoulder, arm, forearm, wrist, hand, and fingers

⑦**T79.A11** **Traumatic compartment syndrome of right upper extremity** [HCC]

⑦**T79.A12** **Traumatic compartment syndrome of left upper extremity** [HCC]

⑦**T79.A19** **Traumatic compartment syndrome of unspecified upper extremity** [HCC]

T79.A2 **Traumatic compartment syndrome of lower extremity** [HCC]

Traumatic compartment syndrome of hip, buttock, thigh, leg, foot, and toes

⑦**T79.A21** **Traumatic compartment syndrome of right lower extremity** [HCC]

⑦**T79.A22** **Traumatic compartment syndrome of left lower extremity** [HCC]

⑦**T79.A29** **Traumatic compartment syndrome of unspecified lower extremity** [HCC]

⊗⑦**T79.A3** **Traumatic compartment syndrome of abdomen** [HCC]

⊗⑦**T79.A9** **Traumatic compartment syndrome of other sites** [HCC]

⊗⑦**T79.8** **Other early complications of trauma**

⊗⑦**T79.9** **Unspecified early complication of trauma**

COMPLICATIONS OF SURGICAL AND MEDICAL CARE, NOT ELSEWHERE CLASSIFIED (T80-T88)

Use Additional Code for adverse effect, if applicable, to identify drug (T36-T50 with fifth or sixth character 5)

Use Additional Code(s) to identify the specified condition resulting from the complication

Use Additional Code to identify devices involved and details of circumstances (Y62-Y82)

Excludes2: any encounters with medical care for postprocedural conditions

in which no complications are present, such as:

artificial opening status (Z93.-) closure of external stoma (Z43.-)

fitting and adjustment of external prosthetic device (Z44.-)

burns and corrosions from local applications and irradiation (T20-T32)

complications of surgical procedures during pregnancy, childbirth and the puerperium (O00-O9A)

mechanical complication of respirator [ventilator] (J95.850)

poisoning and toxic effects of drugs and chemicals (T36-T65 with fifth or sixth character 1-4 or 6)

postprocedural fever (R50.82)

specified complications classified elsewhere, such as: cerebrospinal fluid leak from spinal puncture (G97.0)

colostomy malfunction (K94.0-)

disorders of fluid and electrolyte imbalance (E86-E87) f

functional disturbances following cardiac surgery (I97.0-I97.1)

intraoperative and postprocedural complications of specified body systems (D78.-, E36.-, E89.-, G97.3-, G97.4, H59.3-, H59.-, H95.2-, H95.3, I97.4-, I97.5, J95.6-, J95.7, K91.6-, L76.-, M96.-, N99.-)

ostomy complications (J95.0-, K94.-, N99.5-)

postgastric surgery syndromes (K91.1)

postlaminectomy syndrome NEC (M96.1)

postmastectomy lymphedema syndrome (I97.2)

postsurgical blind-loop syndrome (K91.2)

ventilator associated pneumonia (J95.851)

T80 **Complications following infusion, transfusion and therapeutic injection**

Includes: complications following perfusion

Excludes2: bone marrow transplant rejection (T86.01)

febrile nonhemolytic transfusion reaction (R50.84)

fluid overload due to transfusion (E87.71)

posttransfusion purpura (D69.51)

transfusion associated circulatory overload (TACO) (E87.71)

transfusion (red blood cell) associated hemochromatosis (E83.111)

transfusion related acute lung injury (TRALI) (J95.84)

The appropriate 7th character is to be added to each code from category T80

A - initial encounter

D - subsequent encounter

S - sequela

⊗⑦**T80.0** **Air embolism following infusion, transfusion and therapeutic injection**

⊗⑦**T80.1** **Vascular complications following infusion, transfusion and therapeutic injection**

Use Additional Code to identify the vascular complication

Excludes2: extravasation of vesicant agent (T80.81-)

infiltration of vesicant agent (T80.81-)

vascular complications specified as due to prosthetic devices, implants and grafts (T82.8-, T83.8-, T84.8-, T85.8-)

postprocedural vascular complications (T81.7-)

T80.2 **Infections following infusion, transfusion and therapeutic injection**

Use Additional Code to identify the specific infection, such as:

sepsis (A41.9)

Use Additional Code (R65.2-) to identify severe sepsis, if applicable

Excludes2: infections specified as due to prosthetic devices, implants and grafts (T82.6-T82.7, T83.5-T83.6, T84.5-T84.7, T85.7)

postprocedural infections (T81.4-)

T80.21   Infection due to central venous catheter

Infection due to pulmonary artery catheter (Swan-Ganz catheter)

⑦**T80.211   Bloodstream infection due to central venous catheter**

Catheter-related bloodstream infection (CRBSI) NOS

Central line-associated bloodstream infection (CLABSI)

Bloodstream infection due to Hickman catheter

Bloodstream infection due to peripherally inserted central catheter (PICC)

Bloodstream infection due to portacath (port-a-cath)

Bloodstream infection due to pulmonary artery catheter

Bloodstream infection due to triple lumen catheter

Bloodstream infection due to umbilical venous catheter

⑦**T80.212   Local infection due to central venous catheter**

Exit or insertion site infection

Local infection due to Hickman catheter

Local infection due to peripherally inserted central catheter (PICC)

Local infection due to portacath (port-a-cath)

Local infection due to pulmonary artery catheter

Local infection due to triple lumen catheter

Local infection due to umbilical venous catheter

Port or reservoir infection

Tunnel infection

⑦**T80.218   Other infection due to central venous catheter**

Other central line-associated infection

Other infection due to Hickman catheter

Other infection due to peripherally inserted central catheter (PICC)

Other infection due to portacath (port-a-cath)

Other infection due to pulmonary artery catheter

Other infection due to triple lumen catheter

Other infection due to umbilical venous catheter

⑦**T80.219   Unspecified infection due to central venous catheter**

Central line-associated infection NOS

Unspecified infection due to Hickman catheter

Unspecified infection due to peripherally inserted central catheter (PICC)

Unspecified infection due to portacath (port-a-cath)

Unspecified infection due to pulmonary artery catheter

Unspecified infection due to triple lumen catheter

Unspecified infection due to umbilical venous catheter

⊗⑦**T80.22   Acute infection following transfusion, infusion, or injection of blood and blood products**

⊗⑦**T80.29   Infection following other infusion, transfusion and therapeutic inject ion**

T80.3   ABO incompatibility reaction due to transfusion of blood or blood products

Excludes1: minor blood group antigens reactions (Duffy) (E) (K) (Kell) (Kidd) (Lewis) (M) (N) (P) (S) (T80.A-)

⊗⑦**T80.30   ABO incompatibility reaction due to transfusion of blood or blood products, unspecified**

ABO incompatibility blood transfusion NOS

Reaction to ABO incompatibility from transfusion NOS

T80.31   ABO incompatibility with hemolytic transfusion reaction

⑦**T80.310   ABO incompatibility with acute hemolytic transfusion reaction**

ABO incompatibility with hemolytic transfusion reaction less than 24 hours after transfusion

Acute hemolytic transfusion reaction (AHTR) due to ABO incompatibility

⑦**T80.311   ABO incompatibility with delayed hemolytic transfusion reaction**

ABO incompatibility with hemolytic transfusion reaction 24 hours or more after transfusion

Delayed hemolytic transfusion reaction (DHTR) due to ABO incompatibility

⑦**T80.319   ABO incompatibility with hemolytic transfusion reaction, unspecified**

ABO incompatibility with hemolytic transfusion reaction at unspecified time after transfusion

Hemolytic transfusion reaction (HTR) due to ABO incompatibility NOS

⑦**T80.39   Other ABO incompatibility reaction due to transfusion of blood or blood products**

Delayed serologic transfusion reaction (DSTR) from ABO incompatibility

Other ABO incompatible blood transfusion

Other reaction to ABO incompatible blood transfusion

T80.4   Rh incompatibility reaction due to transfusion of blood or blood products

Reaction due to incompatibility of Rh antigens (C) (c) (D) (E) (e)

⊗⑦**T80.40   Rh incompatibility reaction due to transfusion of blood or blood products, unspecified**

Reaction due to Rh factor in transfusion NOS

Rh incompatible blood transfusion NOS

T80.41   Rh incompatibility with hemolytic transfusion reaction

⑦**T80.410   Rh incompatibility with acute hemolytic transfusion reaction**

Acute hemolytic transfusion reaction (AHTR) due to Rh incompatibility

Rh incompatibility with hemolytic transfusion reaction less than 24 hours after transfusion

⑦**T80.411   Rh incompatibility with delayed hemolytic transfusion reaction**

Delayed hemolytic transfusion reaction (DHTR) due to Rh incompatibility

Rh incompatibility with hemolytic transfusion reaction 24 hours or more after transfusion

⑦**T80.419   Rh incompatibility with hemolytic transfusion reaction, unspecified**

Rh incompatibility with hemolytic transfusion reaction at unspecified time after transfusion

Hemolytic transfusion reaction (HTR) due to Rh incompatibility NOS

⊗⑦**T80.49   Other Rh incompatibility reaction due to transfusion of blood or blood products**

Delayed serologic transfusion reaction (DSTR) from Rh incompatibility

Other reaction to Rh incompatible blood transfusion

T80.A   Non-ABO incompatibility reaction due to transfusion of blood or blood products

Reaction due to incompatibility of minor antigens (Duffy) (Kell) (Kidd) (Lewis) (M) (N) (P) (S)

⊗⑦**T80.A0   Non-ABO incompatibility reaction due to transfusion of blood or blood products, unspecified**

Non-ABO antigen incompatibility reaction from transfusion NOS

T80.A1   Non-ABO incompatibility with hemolytic transfusion reaction

⑦**T80.A10   Non-ABO incompatibility with acute hemolytic transfusion reaction**

Acute hemolytic transfusion reaction (AHTR) due to non-ABO incompatibility

Non-ABO incompatibility with hemolytic transfusion reaction less than 24 hours after transfusion

⑦**T80.A11   Non-ABO incompatibility with delayed hemolytic transfusion reaction**

Delayed hemolytic transfusion reaction (DHTR) due to non-ABO incompatibility

Non-ABO incompatibility with hemolytic transfusion reaction 24 or more hours after transfusion

⑦**T80.A19   Non-ABO incompatibility with hemolytic transfusion reaction, unspecified**

Hemolytic transfusion reaction (HTR) due to non-ABO incompatibility NOS

Non-ABO incompatibility with hemolytic transfusion reaction at unspecified time after transfusion

⊗⑦**T80.A9   Other non-ABO incompatibility reaction due to transfusion of blood or blood products**

Delayed serologic transfusion reaction (DSTR) from non-ABO incompatibility

Other reaction to non-ABO incompatible blood transfusion

T80.5   Anaphylactic reaction due to serum

Allergic shock due to serum

Anaphylactic shock due to serum

Anaphylactoid reaction due to serum

Anaphylaxis due to serum

Excludes1: ABO incompatibility reaction due to transfusion of blood or blood products (T80.3-)

allergic reaction or shock NOS (T78.2) anaphylactic reaction or shock NOS (T78.2)

anaphylactic reaction or shock due to adverse effect of correct medicinal substance properly administered (T88.6) **Other** serum reaction (T80.6-)

⊗⑦**T80.51   Anaphylactic reaction due to administration of blood and blood products**

⊗⑦**T80.52   Anaphylactic reaction due to vaccination**

⊗⑦**T80.59   Anaphylactic reaction due to other serum**

T80.6   Other serum reactions intoxication by serum

Protein sickness

Serum rash

Serum sickness

Serum urticaria

Excludes2: serum hepatitis (B16-B19)

⊗⑦**T80.61   Other serum reaction due to administration of blood and blood products**

⊗⑦**T80.62   Other serum reaction due to vaccination**

⊗⑦**T80.69   Other serum reaction due to other serum**

Code also, if applicable, arthropathy in hypersensitivity reactions classified elsewhere (M36.4)

T80.8   Other complications following infusion, transfusion and therapeutic injection

T80.81   Extravasation of vesicant agent

Infiltration of vesicant agent

⑦**T80.810   Extravasation of vesicant antineoplastic chemotherapy**

Infiltration of vesicant antineoplastic chemotherapy

⑦**T80.818   Extravasation of other vesicant agent**

Infiltration of other vesicant agent

● ⊗⑦ **T80.82   Complication of immune effector cellular therapy**

Complication of chimeric antigen receptor (CAR-T) cell therapy Complication of IEC therapy

Excludes2 complication of bone marrow transplant (T86.0) complication of stem cell transplant (T86.5)

Use Additional Code to identify the specific complication, such as:

cytokine release syndrome (D89.83-)

immune effector cell-associated neurotoxicity syndrome (G92.0-)

⊗⑦**T80.89   Other complications following infusion, transfusion and therapeutic injection**

Delayed serologic transfusion reaction (DSTR), unspecified incompatibility

Use Additional Code to identify graft-versus-host reaction, if applicable, (D89.81-)

T80.9   Unspecified complication following infusion, transfusion and therapeutic injection

⊗⑦**T80.90** **Unspecified complication following infusion and therapeutic injection**

T80.91 **Hemolytic transfusion reaction, unspecified incompatibility**

Excludes1: ABO incompatibility with hemolytic transfusion reaction (T80.31-)

Non-ABO incompatibility with hemolytic transfusion reaction (T80.A1-)

Rh incompatibility with hemolytic transfusion reaction (T80.41-)

⑦**T80.910** **Acute hemolytic transfusion reaction, unspecified incompatibility**

⑦**T80.911** **Delayed hemolytic transfusion reaction, unspecified incompatibility**

⑦**T80.919** **Hemolytic transfusion reaction, unspecified incompatibility, unspecified as acute or delayed**

Hemolytic transfusion reaction NOS

⊗⑦**T80.92** **Unspecified transfusion reaction**

Transfusion reaction NOS

T81 **Complications of procedures, not elsewhere classified**

Use Additional Code for adverse effect, if applicable, to identify drug (T36-T50 with fifth or sixth character 5)

Excludes2: complications following immunization (T88.0-T88.1)

complications following infusion, transfusion and therapeutic injection (T80.-)

complications of transplanted organs and tissue (T86.-)

specified complications classified elsewhere, such as: complication of prosthetic devices, implants and grafts (T82-T85)

dermatitis due to drugs and medicaments (L23.3, L24.4, L25.1, L27.0-L27.1)

endosseous dental implant failure (M27.6-)

floppy iris syndrome (IFIS) (intraoperative) H21.81

intraoperative and postprocedural complications of specific body system (D78.-, E36.-, E89.-, G97.3-, G97.4, H59.3-, H59.-, H95.2-, H95.3, I97.4-, I97.5, J95, K91.-, L76.-, M96.-, N99.-)

ostomy complications (J95.0-, K94.-, N99.5-)

plateau iris syndrome (post-iridectomy) (postprocedural) H21.82

poisoning and toxic effects of drugs and chemicals (T36-T65 with fifth or sixth character 1-4 or 6)

The appropriate 7th character is to be added to each code from category T81

A - initial encounter

D - subsequent encounter

S - sequela

T81.1 **Postprocedural shock**

Shock during or resulting from a procedure, not elsewhere classified

Excludes1: anaphylactic shock NOS (T78.2)

anaphylactic shock due to correct substance properly administered (T88.6)

anaphylactic shock due to serum (T80.5-)

electric shock (T75.4)

obstetric shock (O75.1)

septic shock (R65.21)

shock due to anesthesia (T88.2)

shock following abortion or ectopic or molar pregnancy (O00-O07, O08.3)

traumatic shock (T79.4)

⊗⑦**T81.10** **Postprocedural shock unspecified**

Collapse NOS during or resulting from a procedure, not elsewhere classified

Postprocedural failure of peripheral circulation

Postprocedural shock NOS

⊗⑦**T81.11** **Postprocedural cardiogenic shock** [HCC]

⊗⑦**T81.12** **Postprocedural septic shock** [HCC]

Postprocedural endotoxic shock resulting from a procedure, not elsewhere classified

Postprocedural gram-negative shock resulting from a procedure, not elsewhere classified

Code first underlying infection

Use Additional Code, to identify any associated acute organ dysfunction, if applicable

⊗⑦**T81.19** **Other postprocedural shock**

Postprocedural hypovolemic shock

T81.3 **Disruption of wound, not elsewhere classified**

Disruption of any suture materials or other closure methods

Excludes1: breakdown (mechanical) of permanent sutures (T85.612)

displacement of permanent sutures (T85.622)

disruption of cesarean delivery wound (O90.0)

disruption of perineal obstetric wound (O90.1)

mechanical complication of permanent sutures NEC (T85.692)

⊗⑦**T81.30** **Disruption of wound, unspecified**

Disruption of wound NOS

⊗⑦**T81.31** **Disruption of external operation (surgical) wound, not elsewhere classified**

Dehiscence of operation wound NOS

Disruption of operation wound NOS

Disruption or dehiscence of closure of cornea

Disruption or dehiscence of closure of mucosa

Disruption or dehiscence of closure of skin and subcutaneous tissue

Full-thickness skin disruption or dehiscence

Superficial disruption or dehiscence of operation wound

Excludes1: dehiscence of amputation stump (T87.81)

⊗⑦**T81.32** **Disruption of internal operation (surgical) wound, not elsewhere classified**

Deep disruption or dehiscence of operation wound NOS

Disruption or dehiscence of closure of internal organ or other internal tissue

Disruption or dehiscence of closure of muscle or muscle flap

Disruption or dehiscence of closure of ribs or rib cage

Disruption or dehiscence of closure of skull or craniotomy

Disruption or dehiscence of closure of sternum or sternotomy

Disruption or dehiscence of closure of tendon or ligament

Disruption or dehiscence of closure of superficial or muscular fascia

⊗⑦**T81.33** **Disruption of traumatic injury wound repair**

Disruption or dehiscence of closure of traumatic laceration (external) (internal)

⊗⑦**T81.4** **Infection following a procedure**

Excludes2: obstetric surgical wound infection (O86.0-)

postprocedural fever NOS (R50.82)

postprocedural retroperitoneal abscess (K68.11)

⊗⑦**T81.40** **Infection following a procedure, unspecified**

⊗⑦**T81.41** **Infection following a procedure, superficial incisional surgical site**

Subcutaneous abscess following a procedure

Stitch abscess following a procedure

⊗⑦**T81.42** **Infection following a procedure, deep incisional surgical site**

Intra-muscular abscess following a procedure

⊗⑦**T81.43** **Infection following a procedure, organ and space surgical site**

Intra-abdominal abscess following a procedure

Subphrenic abscess following a procedure

⊗⑦**T81.44** **Sepsis following a procedure**

<u>Use Additional Code</u> to identify the sepsis

⊗⑦**T81.49** **Infection following a procedure, other surgical site**

T81.5 **Complications of foreign body accidentally left in body following procedure**

T81.50 **Unspecified complication of foreign body accidentally left in body following procedure**

⑦**T81.500** **Unspecified complication of foreign body accidentally left in body following surgical operation**

⑦**T81.501** **Unspecified complication of foreign body accidentally left in body following infusion or transfusion**

⑦**T81.502** **Unspecified complication of foreign body accidentally left in body following kidney dialysis** [HCC]

⑦**T81.503** **Unspecified complication of foreign body accidentally left in body following injection or immunization**

⑦**T81.504** **Unspecified complication of foreign body accidentally left in body following endoscopic examination**

⑦**T81.505** **Unspecified complication of foreign body accidentally left in body following heart catheterization**

⑦**T81.506** **Unspecified complication of foreign body accidentally left in body following aspiration, puncture or other catheterization**

⑦**T81.507** **Unspecified complication of foreign body accidentally left in body following removal of catheter or packing**

⑦**T81.508** **Unspecified complication of foreign body accidentally left in body following other procedure**

⑦**T81.509** **Unspecified complication of foreign body accidentally left in body following unspecified procedure**

T81.51 **Adhesions due to foreign body accidentally left in body following procedure**

⑦**T81.510** **Adhesions due to foreign body accidentally left in body following surgical operation**

⑦**T81.511** **Adhesions due to foreign body accidentally left in body following infusion or transfusion**

⑦**T81.512** **Adhesions due to foreign body accidentally left in body following kidney dialysis** [HCC]

⑦**T81.513** **Adhesions due to foreign body accidentally left in body following injection or immunization**

⑦**T81.514** **Adhesions due to foreign body accidentally left in body following endoscopic examination**

⑦**T81.515** **Adhesions due to foreign body accidentally left in body following heart catheterization**

⑦**T81.516** **Adhesions due to foreign body accidentally left in body following aspiration, puncture or other catheterization**

⑦**T81.517** **Adhesions due to foreign body accidentally left in body following removal of catheter or packing**

⑦**T81.518** **Adhesions due to foreign body accidentally left in body following other procedure**

⑦**T81.519** **Adhesions due to foreign body accidentally left in body following unspecified procedure**

T81.52 **Obstruction due to foreign body accidentally left in body following procedure**

⑦**T81.520** **Obstruction due to foreign body accidentally left in body following surgical operation**

⑦**T81.521** **Obstruction due to foreign body accidentally left in body following infusion or transfusion**

⑦**T81.522** **Obstruction due to foreign body accidentally left in body following kidney dialysis** [HCC]

⑦**T81.523** **Obstruction due to foreign body accidentally left in body following injection or immunization**

⑦**T81.524** **Obstruction due to foreign body accidentally left in body following endoscopic examination**

⑦**T81.525** **Obstruction due to foreign body accidentally left in body following heart catheterization**

⑦**T81.526** **Obstruction due to foreign body accidentally left in body following aspiration, puncture or other catheterization**

⑦**T81.527** **Obstruction due to foreign body accidentally left in body following removal of catheter or packing**

⑦**T81.528** **Obstruction due to foreign body accidentally left in body following other procedure**

⑦**T81.529** **Obstruction due to foreign body accidentally left in body following unspecified procedure**

T81.53 **Perforation due to foreign body accidentally left in body following procedure**

⑦**T81.530** **Perforation due to foreign body accidentally left in body following surgical operation**

● New code ▲ Revised code Excludes1: Not coded here Excludes2: Not included here ⊗ Placeholder required ⑦7th digit required

⑦ **T81.531** **Perforation due to foreign body accidentally left in body following infusion or transfusion**

⑦ **T81.532** **Perforation due to foreign body accidentally left in body following kidney dialysis** [HCC]

⑦ **T81.533** **Perforation due to foreign body accidentally left in body following injection or immunization**

⑦ **T81.534** **Perforation due to foreign body accidentally left in body following endoscopic examination**

⑦ **T81.535** **Perforation due to foreign body accidentally left in body following heart catheterization**

⑦ **T81.536** **Perforation due to foreign body accidentally left in body following aspiration, puncture or other catheterization**

⑦ **T81.537** **Perforation due to foreign body accidentally left in body following removal of catheter or packing**

⑦ **T81.538** **Perforation due to foreign body accidentally left in body following other procedure**

⑦ **T81.539** **Perforation due to foreign body accidentally left in body following unspecified procedure**

T81.59 **Other complications of foreign body accidentally left in body following procedure**

Excludes2: obstruction or perforation due to prosthetic devices and implants intentionally left in body (T82.0-T82.5, T83.0-T83.4, T83.7, T84.0-T84.4, T85.0-T85.6)

⑦ **T81.590** **Other complications of foreign body accidentally left in body following surgical operation**

⑦ **T81.591** **Other complications of foreign body accidentally left in body following infusion or transfusion**

⑦ **T81.592** **Other complications of foreign body accidentally left in body following kidney dialysis** [HCC]

⑦ **T81.593** **Other complications of foreign body accidentally left in body following injection or immunization**

⑦ **T81.594** **Other complications of foreign body accidentally left in body following endoscopic examination**

⑦ **T81.595** **Other complications of foreign body accidentally left in body following heart catheterization**

⑦ **T81.596** **Other complications of foreign body accidentally left in body following aspiration, puncture or other catheterization**

⑦ **T81.597** **Other complications of foreign body accidentally left in body following removal of catheter or packing**

⑦ **T81.598** **Other complications of foreign body accidentally left in body following other procedure**

⑦ **T81.599** **Other complications of foreign body accidentally left in body following unspecified procedure**

T81.6 **Acute reaction to foreign substance accidentally left during a procedure**

Excludes2: complications of foreign body accidentally left in body cavity or operation wound following procedure (T81.5-)

⊗⑦ **T81.60** **Unspecified acute reaction to foreign substance accidentally left during a procedure**

⊗⑦ **T81.61** **Aseptic peritonitis due to foreign substance accidentally left during a procedure**

Chemical peritonitis

⊗⑦ **T81.69** **Other acute reaction to foreign substance accidentally left during a procedure**

T81.7 **Vascular complications following a procedure, not elsewhere classified**

Air embolism following procedure NEC

Phlebitis or thrombophlebitis resulting from a procedure

Excludes1: embolism complicating abortion or ectopic or molar pregnancy (O00-O07, O08.2)

embolism complicating pregnancy, childbirth and the puerperium (O88.-)

traumatic embolism (T79.0)

Excludes2: embolism due to prosthetic devices, implants and grafts (T82.8-, T83.81, T84.8-, T85.81-)

embolism following infusion, transfusion and therapeutic injection (T80.0)

T81.71 **Complication of artery following a procedure, not elsewhere classified**

⑦ **T81.710** **Complication of mesenteric artery following a procedure, not elsewhere classified**

⑦ **T81.711** **Complication of renal artery following a procedure, not elsewhere classified**

⑦ **T81.718** **Complication of other artery following a procedure, not elsewhere classified**

⑦ **T81.719** **Complication of unspecified artery following a procedure, not elsewhere classified**

⊗⑦ **T81.72** **Complication of vein following a procedure, not elsewhere classified**

T81.8 **Other complications of procedures, not elsewhere classified**

Excludes2: hypothermia following anesthesia (T88.51)

malignant hyperpyrexia due to anesthesia (T88.3)

⊗⑦ **T81.81** **Complication of inhalation therapy**

⊗⑦ **T81.82** **Emphysema (subcutaneous) resulting from a procedure**

⊗⑦ **T81.83** **Persistent postprocedural fistula**

⊗⑦ **T81.89** **Other complications of procedures, not elsewhere classified**

Use Additional Code to specify complication, such as:

postprocedural delirium (F05)

⊗⑦ **T81.9** **Unspecified complication of procedure**

T82 **Complications of cardiac and vascular prosthetic devices, implants and grafts**

Excludes2: failure and rejection of transplanted organs and tissue (T86.-)

The appropriate 7th character is to be added to each code from category T82

A - initial encounter

D - subsequent encounter

S - sequela

T82.0 **Mechanical complication of heart valve prosthesis**

Mechanical complication of artificial heart valve

Excludes1: mechanical complication of biological heart valve graft (T82.22-)

⊗⑦**T82.01** **Breakdown (mechanical) of heart valve prosthesis**

⊗⑦**T82.02** **Displacement of heart valve prosthesis**

Malposition of heart valve prosthesis

⊗⑦**T82.03** **Leakage of heart valve prosthesis**

⊗⑦**T82.09** **Other mechanical complication of heart valve prosthesis**

Obstruction (mechanical) of heart valve prosthesis

Perforation of heart valve prosthesis

Protrusion of heart valve prosthesis

T82.1 **Mechanical complication of cardiac electronic device**

T82.11 **Breakdown (mechanical) of cardiac electronic device**

⑦**T82.110** **Breakdown (mechanical) of cardiac electrode**

⑦**T82.111** **Breakdown (mechanical) of cardiac pulse generator (battery)**

⑦**T82.118** **Breakdown (mechanical) of other cardiac electronic device**

⑦**T82.119** **Breakdown (mechanical) of unspecified cardiac electronic device**

T82.12 **Displacement of cardiac electronic device**

Malposition of cardiac electronic device

⑦**T82.120** **Displacement of cardiac electrode**

⑦**T82.121** **Displacement of cardiac pulse generator (battery)**

⑦**T82.128** **Displacement of other cardiac electronic device**

⑦**T82.129** **Displacement of unspecified cardiac electronic device**

T82.19 **Other mechanical complication of cardiac electronic device**

Leakage of cardiac electronic device

Obstruction of cardiac electronic device

Perforation of cardiac electronic device

Protrusion of cardiac electronic device

⑦**T82.190** **Other mechanical complication of cardiac electrode**

⑦**T82.191** **Other mechanical complication of cardiac pulse generator (battery)**

⑦**T82.198** **Other mechanical complication of other cardiac electronic device**

⑦**T82.199** **Other mechanical complication of unspecified cardiac device**

T82.2 **Mechanical complication of coronary artery bypass graft and biological heart valve graft**

Excludes1: mechanical complication of artificial heart valve

prosthesis (T82.0-)

T82.21 **Mechanical complication of coronary artery bypass graft**

⑦**T82.211** **Breakdown (mechanical) of coronary artery bypass graft**

⑦**T82.212** **Displacement of coronary artery bypass graft**

Malposition of coronary artery bypass graft

⑦**T82.213** **Leakage of coronary artery bypass graft**

⑦**T82.218** **Other mechanical complication of coronary artery bypass graft**

Obstruction, mechanical of coronary artery bypass graft

Perforation of coronary artery bypass graft

Protrusion of coronary artery bypass graft

T82.22 **Mechanical complication of biological heart valve graft**

⑦**T82.221** **Breakdown (mechanical) of biological heart valve graft**

⑦**T82.222** **Displacement of biological heart valve graft**

Malposition of biological heart valve graft

⑦**T82.223** **Leakage of biological heart valve graft**

⑦**T82.228** **Other mechanical complication of biological heart valve graft**

Obstruction of biological heart valve graft

Perforation of biological heart valve graft

Protrusion of biological heart valve graft

T82.3 **Mechanical complication of other vascular grafts**

T82.31 **Breakdown (mechanical) of other vascular grafts**

⑦**T82.310** **Breakdown (mechanical) of aortic (bifurcation) graft (replacement)** [HCC]

⑦**T82.311** **Breakdown (mechanical) of carotid arterial graft (bypass)** [HCC]

⑦**T82.312** **Breakdown (mechanical) of femoral arterial graft (bypass)** [HCC]

⑦**T82.318** **Breakdown (mechanical) of other vascular grafts** [HCC]

⑦**T82.319** **Breakdown (mechanical) of unspecified vascular grafts** [HCC]

T82.32 **Displacement of other vascular grafts**

Malposition of other vascular grafts

⑦**T82.320** **Displacement of aortic (bifurcation) graft (replacement)**

⑦**T82.321** **Displacement of carotid arterial graft (bypass)** [HCC]

⑦**T82.322** **Displacement of femoral arterial graft (bypass)** [HCC]

⑦**T82.328** **Displacement of other vascular grafts** [HCC]

⑦**T82.329** **Displacement of unspecified vascular grafts** [HCC]

T82.33 **Leakage of other vascular grafts** [HCC]

⑦**T82.330** **Leakage of aortic (bifurcation) graft (replacement)** [HCC]

⑦**T82.331** **Leakage of carotid arterial graft (bypass)** [HCC]

⑦**T82.332** **Leakage of femoral arterial graft (bypass)** [HCC]

⑦**T82.338** **Leakage of other vascular grafts** [HCC]

⑦T82.339 Leakage of unspecified vascular graft [HCC]

T82.39 Other mechanical complication of other vascular grafts

Obstruction (mechanical) of other vascular grafts

Perforation of other vascular grafts

Protrusion of other vascular grafts

⑦T82.390 Other mechanical complication of aortic (bifurcation) graft (replacement) [HCC]

⑦T82.391 Other mechanical complication of carotid arterial graft (bypass) [HCC]

⑦T82.392 Other mechanical complication of femoral arterial graft (bypass) [HCC]

⑦T82.398 Other mechanical complication of other vascular grafts [HCC]

⑦T82.399 Other mechanical complication of unspecified vascular grafts [HCC]

T82.4 Mechanical complication of vascular dialysis catheter

Mechanical complication of hemodialysis catheter

Excludes1: mechanical complication of intraperitoneal dialysis catheter (T85.62)

⊗⑦T82.41 Breakdown (mechanical) of vascular dialysis catheter [HCC]

⊗⑦T82.42 Displacement of vascular dialysis catheter [HCC]

Malposition of vascular dialysis catheter

⊗⑦T82.43 Leakage of vascular dialysis catheter [HCC]

⊗⑦T82.49 Other complication of vascular dialysis catheter [HCC]

Obstruction (mechanical) of vascular dialysis catheter

Perforation of vascular dialysis catheter

Protrusion of vascular dialysis catheter

T82.5 Mechanical complication of other cardiac and vascular devices and implants

Excludes2: mechanical complication of epidural and subdural infusion catheter (T85.61)

T82.51 Breakdown (mechanical) of other cardiac and vascular devices and implants

⑦T82.510 Breakdown (mechanical) of surgically created arteriovenous fistula [HCC]

⑦T82.511 Breakdown (mechanical) of surgically created arteriovenous shunt [HCC]

⑦T82.512 Breakdown (mechanical) of artificial heart

⑦T82.513 Breakdown (mechanical) of balloon (counterpulsation) device [HCC]

⑦T82.514 Breakdown (mechanical) of infusion catheter [HCC]

⑦T82.515 Breakdown (mechanical) of umbrella device [HCC]

⑦T82.518 Breakdown (mechanical) of other cardiac and vascular devices and implants [HCC]

⑦T82.519 Breakdown (mechanical) of unspecified cardiac and vascular devices and implants

T82.52 Displacement of other cardiac and vascular devices and implants

Malposition of other cardiac and vascular devices and implants

⑦T82.520 Displacement of surgically created arteriovenous fistula [HCC]

⑦T82.521 Displacement of surgically created arteriovenous shunt [HCC]

⑦T82.522 Displacement of artificial heart

⑦T82.523 Displacement of balloon (counterpulsation) device [HCC]

⑦T82.524 Displacement of infusion catheter [HCC]

⑦T82.525 Displacement of umbrella device [HCC]

⑦T82.528 Displacement of other cardiac and vascular devices and implants [HCC]

⑦T82.529 Displacement of unspecified cardiac and vascular devices and implants

T82.53 Leakage of other cardiac and vascular devices and implants

⑦T82.530 Leakage of surgically created arteriovenous fistula [HCC]

⑦T82.531 Leakage of surgically created arteriovenous shunt [HCC]

⑦T82.532 Leakage of artificial heart

⑦T82.533 Leakage of balloon (counterpulsation) device [HCC]

⑦T82.534 Leakage of infusion catheter [HCC]

⑦T82.535 Leakage of umbrella device [HCC]

⑦T82.538 Leakage of other cardiac and vascular devices and implants [HCC]

⑦T82.539 Leakage of unspecified cardiac and vascular devices and implants

T82.59 Other mechanical complication of other cardiac and vascular devices and implants

Obstruction (mechanical) of other cardiac and vascular devices and implants

Perforation of other cardiac and vascular devices and implants

Protrusion of other cardiac and vascular devices and implants

⑦T82.590 Other mechanical complication of surgically created arteriovenous fistula [HCC]

⑦T82.591 Other mechanical complication of surgically created arteriovenous shunt [HCC]

⑦T82.592 Other mechanical complication of artificial heart

⑦T82.593 Other mechanical complication of balloon (counterpulsation) device [HCC]

⑦T82.594 Other mechanical complication of infusion catheter [HCC]

⑦T82.595 Other mechanical complication of umbrella device [HCC]

⑦T82.598 Other mechanical complication of other cardiac and vascular devices and implants [HCC]

⑦T82.599 Other mechanical complication of unspecified cardiac and vascular devices and implants

⊗⑦T82.6 Infection and inflammatory reaction due to cardiac valve prosthesis [HCC]

Use Additional Code to identify infection

⊗⑦T82.7 Infection and inflammatory reaction due to other cardiac and vascular devices, implants and grafts [HCC]

Use Additional Code to identify infection

T82.8   **Other specified complications of cardiac and vascular prosthetic devices, implants and grafts**

    T82.81   **Embolism due to cardiac and vascular prosthetic devices, implants and grafts**

      ⑦**T82.817**   **Embolism due to cardiac prosthetic devices, implants and grafts**

      ⑦**T82.818**   **Embolism due to vascular prosthetic devices, implants and grafts** [HCC]

    T82.82   **Fibrosis due to cardiac and vascular prosthetic devices, implants and grafts**

      ⑦**T82.827**   **Fibrosis due to cardiac prosthetic devices, implants and grafts** [HCC]

      ⑦**T82.828**   **Fibrosis due to vascular prosthetic devices, implants and grafts**

    T82.83   **Hemorrhage due to cardiac and vascular prosthetic devices, implants and grafts**

      ⑦**T82.837**   **Hemorrhage due to cardiac prosthetic devices, implants and grafts**

      ⑦**T82.838**   **Hemorrhage due to vascular prosthetic devices, implants and grafts** [HCC]

    T82.84   **Pain due to cardiac and vascular prosthetic devices, implants and grafts**

      ⑦**T82.847**   **Pain due to cardiac prosthetic devices, implants and grafts**

      ⑦**T82.848**   **Pain due to vascular prosthetic devices, implants and grafts** [HCC]

    T82.85   **Stenosis due to cardiac and vascular prosthetic devices, implants and grafts**

      ⑦**T82.855**   **Stenosis of coronary artery stent**

          In-stent stenosis (restenosis) of coronary artery stent

          Restenosis of coronary artery stent

      ⑦**T82.856**   **Stenosis of peripheral vascular stent** [HCC]

          In-stent stenosis (restenosis) of peripheral vascular stent

          Restenosis of peripheral vascular stent

      ⑦**T82.857**   **Stenosis of other cardiac prosthetic devices, implants and grafts**

      ⑦**T82.858**   **Stenosis of other vascular prosthetic devices, implants and grafts** [HCC]

    T82.86   **Thrombosis of cardiac and vascular prosthetic devices, implants and grafts**

      ⑦**T82.867**   **Thrombosis due to cardiac prosthetic devices, implants and grafts**

      ⑦**T82.868**   **Thrombosis due to vascular prosthetic devices, implants and grafts** [HCC]

    T82.89   **Other specified complication of cardiac and vascular prosthetic devices, implants and grafts**

      ⑦**T82.897**   **Other specified complication of cardiac prosthetic devices, implants and grafts**

      ⑦**T82.898**   **Other specified complication of vascular prosthetic devices, implants and grafts** [HCC]

⊗⑦**T82.9**   **Unspecified complication of cardiac and vascular prosthetic device, implant and graft**

T83   **Complications of genitourinary prosthetic devices, implants and grafts**

    Excludes2: failure and rejection of transplanted organs and tissue (T86.-)

The appropriate 7th character is to be added to each code from category T83

A - initial encounter

D - subsequent encounter

S - sequela

T83.0   **Mechanical complication of urinary catheter**

    Excludes2: complications of stoma of urinary tract (N99.5-)

    T83.01   **Breakdown (mechanical) of urinary catheter**

      ⑦**T83.010**   **Breakdown (mechanical) of cystostomy catheter** [HCC]

      ⑦**T83.011**   **Breakdown (mechanical) of indwelling urethral catheter** [HCC]

      ⑦**T83.012**   **Breakdown (mechanical) of nephrostomy catheter** [HCC]

      ⑦**T83.018**   **Breakdown (mechanical) of other urinary catheter** [HCC]

          Breakdown (mechanical) of Hopkins catheter

          Breakdown (mechanical) of ileostomy catheter

          Breakdown (mechanical) urostomy catheter

    ⑦**T83.02**   **Displacement of urinary catheter**

          Malposition of urinary catheter

      ⑦**T83.020**   **Displacement of cystostomy catheter** [HCC]

      ⑦**T83.021**   **Displacement of indwelling urethral catheter** [HCC]

      ⑦**T83.022**   **Displacement of nephrostomy catheter** [HCC]

      ⑦**T83.028**   **Displacement of other urinary catheter** [HCC]

          Displacement of Hopkins catheter

          Displacement of ileostomy catheter

          Displacement of urostomy catheter

    T83.03   **Leakage of urinary catheter**

      ⑦**T83.030**   **Leakage of cystostomy catheter** [HCC]

      ⑦**T83.031**   **Leakage of indwelling urethral catheter** [HCC]

      ⑦**T83.032**   **Leakage of nephrostomy catheter** [HCC]

      ⑦**T83.038**   **Leakage of other urinary catheter** [HCC]

          Leakage of Hopkins catheter

          Leakage of ileostomy catheter

          Leakage of urostomy catheter

    T83.09   **Other mechanical complication of urinary catheter**

          Obstruction (mechanical) of urinary catheter

          Perforation of urinary catheter

          Protrusion of urinary catheter

      ⑦**T83.090**   **Other mechanical complication of cystostomy catheter** [HCC]

      ⑦**T83.091**   **Other mechanical complication of indwelling urethral catheter** [HCC]

      ⑦**T83.092**   **Other mechanical complication of nephrostomy catheter** [HCC]

      ⑦**T83.098**   **Other mechanical complication of other urinary catheter** [HCC]

          Other mechanical complication of Hopkins catheter

Other mechanical complication of
ileostomy catheter

Other mechanical complication of
urostomy catheter

**T83.1   Mechanical complication of other urinary devices and
implants**

**T83.11   Breakdown (mechanical) of other urinary
devices and implants**

⑦**T83.110   Breakdown (mechanical) of urinary
electronic stimulator device** [HCC]

Excludes2: Breakdown (mechanical)
of electrode (lead) for sacral
nerve neurostimulator
(T85.111)

Breakdown mechanical) of
implanted electronic sacral
neurostimulator, pulse
generator or receiver
(T85.113)

⑦**T83.111   Breakdown (mechanical) of
implanted urinary sphincter** [HCC]

⑦**T83.112   Breakdown (mechanical) of
indwelling ureteral stent** [HCC]

⑦**T83.113   Breakdown (mechanical) of other
urinary stents** [HCC]

Breakdown (mechanical) of ileal
conduit stent

Breakdown (mechanical) of
nephroureteral stent

⑦**T83.118   Breakdown (mechanical) of other
urinary devices and implants** [HCC]

**T83.12   Displacement of other urinary devices and
implants**

Malposition of other urinary devices and implants

⑦**T83.120   Displacement of urinary electronic
stimulator device** [HCC]

Excludes2: Displacement of electrode
(lead) for sacral nerve
neurostimulator (T85.121)

Displacement of implanted
electronic sacral
neurostimulator, pulse
generator or receiver
(T85.123)

⑦**T83.121   Displacement of implanted urinary
sphincter** [HCC]

⑦**T83.122   Displacement of indwelling ureteral
stent** [HCC]

⑦**T83.123   Displacement of other urinary stents**
[HCC]

Displacement of ileal conduit stent

Displacement of nephroureteral stent

⑦**T83.128   Displacement of other urinary
devices and implants** [HCC]

⑦**T83.19   Other mechanical complication of other
urinary devices and implants**

Leakage of other urinary devices and implants

Obstruction (mechanical) of other urinary devices
and implants

Perforation of other urinary devices and implants

Protrusion of other urinary devices and implants

⑦**T83.190   Other mechanical complication of
urinary electronic stimulator device**
[HCC]

Excludes2: Other mechanical
complication of electrode
(lead) for sacral nerve
neurostimulator (T85.191)

Other mechanical
complication of implanted
electronic sacral
neurostimulator, pulse
generator or receiver
(T85.193)

⑦**T83.191   Other mechanical complication of
implanted urinary sphincter** [HCC]

⑦**T83.192   Other mechanical complication of
indwelling ureteral stent** [HCC]

⑦**T83.193   Other mechanical complication of
other urinary stent** [HCC]

Other mechanical complication of ileal
conduit stent

Other mechanical complication of
nephroureteral stent

⑦**T83.198   Other mechanical complication of
other urinary devices and implants**
[HCC]

T83.2   Mechanical complication of graft of urinary organ

⊗⑦**T83.21   Breakdown (mechanical) of graft of urinary
organ** [HCC]

⊗⑦**T83.22   Displacement of graft of urinary organ** [HCC]

Malposition of graft of urinary organ

⊗⑦**T83.23   Leakage of graft of urinary organ** [HCC]

⊗⑦**T83.24   Erosion of graft of urinary organ** [HCC]

⊗⑦**T83.25   Exposure of graft of urinary organ** [HCC]

⊗⑦**T83.29   Other mechanical complication of graft of
urinary organ** [HCC]

Obstruction (mechanical) of graft of urinary organ

Perforation of graft of urinary organ

Protrusion of graft of urinary organ

**T83.3   Mechanical complication of intrauterine contraceptive
device**

⊗⑦**T83.31   Breakdown (mechanical) of intrauterine
contraceptive device**

⊗⑦**T83.32   Displacement of intrauterine contraceptive
device**

Malposition of intrauterine contraceptive device

Missing string of intrauterine contraceptive device

⊗⑦**T83.39   Other mechanical complication of intrauterine
contraceptive device**

Leakage of intrauterine contraceptive device

Obstruction (mechanical) of intrauterine
contraceptive device

Perforation of intrauterine contraceptive device

Protrusion of intrauterine contraceptive device

**T83.4   Mechanical complication of other prosthetic devices,
implants and grafts of genital tract**

**T83.41   Breakdown (mechanical) of other prosthetic
devices, implants and grafts of genital tract**

⑦**T83.410   Breakdown (mechanical) of
implanted penile prosthesis** [HCC]

Breakdown (mechanical) of penile
prosthesis cylinder

Breakdown (mechanical) of penile
prosthesis pump

Breakdown (mechanical) of penile
prosthesis reservoir

⑦T83.411   **Breakdown (mechanical) of implanted testicular prosthesis** [HCC]

⑦T83.418   **Breakdown (mechanical) of other prosthetic devices, implants and grafts of genital tract** [HCC]

T83.42   **Displacement of other prosthetic devices, implants and grafts of genital tract**

Malposition of other prosthetic devices, implants and grafts of genital tract

⑦T83.420   **Displacement of implanted penile prosthesis** [HCC]

Displacement of penile prosthesis cylinder

Displacement of penile prosthesis pump

Displacement of penile prosthesis reservoir

⑦T83.421   **Displacement of implanted testicular prosthesis** [HCC]

⑦T83.428   **Displacement of other prosthetic devices, implants and grafts of genital tract** [HCC]

T83.49   **Other mechanical complication of other prosthetic devices, implants and grafts of genital tract**

Leakage of other prosthetic devices, implants and grafts of genital tract

Obstruction, mechanical of other prosthetic devices, implants and grafts of genital tract

Perforation of other prosthetic devices, implants and grafts of genital tract

Protrusion of other prosthetic devices, implants and grafts of genital tract

⑦T83.490   **Other mechanical complication of implanted penile prosthesis** [HCC]

Other mechanical complication of penile prosthesis cylinder

Other mechanical complication of penile prosthesis pump

Other mechanical complication of penile prosthesis reservoir

⑦T83.491   **Other mechanical complication of implanted testicular prosthesis** [HCC]

⑦T83.498   **Other mechanical complication of other prosthetic devices, implants and grafts of genital tract** [HCC]

T83.5   **Infection and inflammatory reaction due to prosthetic device, implant and graft in urinary system** [HCC]

Use Additional Code to identify infection

T83.51   **Infection and inflammatory reaction due to urinary catheter**

Excludes2: complications of stoma of urinary tract (N99.5-)

⑦T83.510   **Infection and inflammatory reaction due to cystostomy catheter**

⑦T83.511   **Infection and inflammatory reaction due to indwelling urethral catheter** [HCC]

⑦T83.512   **Infection and inflammatory reaction due to nephrostomy catheter** [HCC]

⑦T83.518   **Infection and inflammatory reaction due to other urinary catheter** [HCC]

Infection and inflammatory reaction due to Hopkins catheter

Infection and inflammatory reaction due to ileostomy catheter

Infection and inflammatory reaction due to urostomy catheter

T83.59   **Infection and inflammatory reaction due to prosthetic device, implant and graft in urinary system**

⑦T83.590   **Infection and inflammatory reaction due to implanted urinary neurostimulation device** [HCC]

Excludes2: Infection and inflammatory reaction due to electrode lead of sacral nerve neurostimulator (T85.732)

Infection and inflammatory reaction due to pulse generator or receiver of sacral nerve neurostimulator (T85.734)

⑦T83.591   **Infection and inflammatory reaction due to implanted urinary sphincter** [HCC]

⑦T83.592   **Infection and inflammatory reaction due to indwelling ureteral stent** [HCC]

⑦T83.593   **Infection and inflammatory reaction due to other urinary stents** [HCC]

Infection and inflammatory reaction due to ileal conduit stents

Infection and inflammatory reaction due to nephroureteral stent

⑦T83.598   **Infection and inflammatory reaction due to other prosthetic device, implant and graft in urinary system** [HCC]

T83.6   **Infection and inflammatory reaction due to prosthetic device, implant and graft in genital tract**

Use Additional Code to identify infection

⊗⑦T83.61   **Infection and inflammatory reaction due to implanted penile prosthesis** [HCC]

Infection and inflammatory reaction due to penile prosthesis cylinder

Infection and inflammatory reaction due to penile prosthesis pump

Infection and inflammatory reaction due to penile prosthesis reservoir

⊗⑦T83.62   **Infection and inflammatory reaction due to implanted testicular prosthesis** [HCC]

⊗⑦T83.69   **Infection and inflammatory reaction due to other prosthetic device, implant and graft in genital tract** [HCC]

T83.7   **Complications due to implanted mesh and other prosthetic materials**

T83.71   **Erosion of implanted mesh and other prosthetic materials to surrounding organ or tissue**

⑦T83.711   **Erosion of implanted vaginal mesh to surrounding organ or tissue** [HCC]

Erosion of implanted vaginal mesh into pelvic floor muscles

⑦T83.712   **Erosion of implanted urethral mesh to surrounding organ or tissue** [HCC]

Erosion of implanted female urethral sling

Erosion of implanted male urethral sling

● New code   ▲ Revised code   **Excludes1:** Not coded here   **Excludes2:** Not included here   ⊗ Placeholder required   ⑦7th digit required

    Erosion of implanted urethral mesh into pelvic floor muscles

⑦**T83.713** **Erosion of implanted urethral bulking agent to surrounding organ or tissue** [HCC]

⑦**T83.714** **Erosion of implanted ureteral bulking agent to surrounding organ or tissue** [HCC]

⑦**T83.718** **Erosion of other implanted mesh to organ or tissue** [HCC]

⑦**T83.719** **Erosion of other prosthetic materials to surrounding organ or tissue** [HCC]

 T83.72 **Exposure of implanted mesh and other prosthetic materials into surrounding organ or tissue**

  Extrusion of implanted mesh

⑦**T83.721** **Exposure of implanted vaginal mesh into vagina** [HCC]

  Exposure of implanted vaginal mesh through vaginal wall

⑦**T83.722** **Exposure of implanted urethral mesh into urethra**

  Exposure of implanted female urethral sling

  Exposure of implanted male urethral sling

  Exposure of implanted urethral mesh through urethral wall

⑦**T83.723** **Exposure of implanted urethral bulking agent into urethra** [HCC]

⑦**T83.724** **Exposure of implanted ureteral bulking agent into ureter** [HCC]

⑦**T83.728** **Exposure of other implanted mesh into organ or tissue** [HCC]

⑦**T83.729** **Exposure of other prosthetic materials into organ or tissue** [HCC]

⊗⑦**T83.79** **Other specified complications due to other genitourinary prosthetic materials** [HCC]

 T83.8 **Other specified complications of genitourinary prosthetic devices, implants and grafts**

⊗⑦**T83.81** **Embolism due to genitourinary prosthetic devices, implants and grafts** [HCC]

⊗⑦**T83.82** **Fibrosis due to genitourinary prosthetic devices, implants and grafts** [HCC]

⊗⑦**T83.83** **Hemorrhage due to genitourinary prosthetic devices, implants and grafts** [HCC]

⊗⑦**T83.84** **Pain due to genitourinary prosthetic devices, implants and grafts** [HCC]

⊗⑦**T83.85** **Stenosis due to genitourinary prosthetic devices, implants and grafts** [HCC]

⊗⑦**T83.86** **Thrombosis due to genitourinary prosthetic devices, implants and grafts** [HCC]

⊗⑦**T83.89** **Other specified complication of genitourinary prosthetic devices, implants and grafts** [HCC]

⑦**T83.9** **Unspecified complication of genitourinary prosthetic device, implant and graft** [HCC]

T84 **Complications of internal orthopedic prosthetic devices, implants and grafts**

 Excludes2: failure and rejection of transplanted organs and tissues (T86.-)

  fracture of bone following insertion of orthopedic implant, joint prosthesis or bone plate (M96.6)

 The appropriate 7th character is to be added to each code from category T84

A - initial encounter

D - subsequent encounter

S - sequela

 T84.0 **Mechanical complication of internal joint prosthesis**

  T84.01 **Broken internal joint prosthesis**

   Breakage (fracture) of prosthetic joint

   Broken prosthetic joint implant

   Excludes1: periprosthetic joint implant fracture (M97.-)

⑦**T84.010** **Broken internal right hip prosthesis** [HCC]

⑦**T84.011** **Broken internal left hip prosthesis** [HCC]

⑦**T84.012** **Broken internal right knee prosthesis** [HCC]

⑦**T84.013** **Broken internal left knee prosthesis** [HCC]

⑦**T84.018** **Broken internal joint prosthesis, other site** [HCC]

  Use Additional Code to identify the joint (Z96.6-)

⑦**T84.019** **Broken internal joint prosthesis, unspecified site** [HCC]

  T84.02 **Dislocation of internal joint prosthesis**

   Instability of internal joint prosthesis

   Subluxation of internal joint prosthesis

⑦**T84.020** **Dislocation of internal right hip prosthesis** [HCC]

⑦**T84.021** **Dislocation of internal left hip prosthesis** [HCC]

⑦**T84.022** **Instability of internal right knee prosthesis** [HCC]

⑦**T84.023** **Instability of internal left knee prosthesis** [HCC]

⑦**T84.028** **Dislocation of other internal joint prosthesis** [HCC]

  Use Additional Code to identify the joint (Z96.6-)

⑦**T84.029** **Dislocation of unspecified internal joint prosthesis** [HCC]

  T84.03 **Mechanical loosening of internal prosthetic joint** [HCC]

   Aseptic loosening of prosthetic joint

⑦**T84.030** **Mechanical loosening of internal right hip prosthetic joint** [HCC]

⑦**T84.031** **Mechanical loosening of internal left hip prosthetic joint** [HCC]

⑦**T84.032** **Mechanical loosening of internal right knee prosthetic joint** [HCC]

⑦**T84.033** **Mechanical loosening of internal left knee prosthetic joint** [HCC]

⑦**T84.038** **Mechanical loosening of other internal prosthetic joint** [HCC]

  Use Additional Code to identify the joint (Z96.6-)

⑦**T84.039** **Mechanical loosening of unspecified internal prosthetic joint** [HCC]

  T84.05 **Periprosthetic osteolysis of internal prosthetic joint**

   Use Additional Code to identify major osseous defect, if applicable (M89.7-)

⑦**T84.050** **Periprosthetic osteolysis of internal prosthetic right hip joint** [HCC]

⑦T84.051 **Periprosthetic osteolysis of internal prosthetic left hip joint** [HCC]

⑦T84.052 **Periprosthetic osteolysis of internal prosthetic right knee joint** [HCC]

⑦T84.053 **Periprosthetic osteolysis of internal prosthetic left knee joint** [HCC]

⑦T84.058 **Periprosthetic osteolysis of other internal prosthetic joint** [HCC]

Use Additional Code to identify the joint (Z96.6-)

⑦T84.059 **Periprosthetic osteolysis of unspecified internal prosthetic joint** [HCC]

T84.06 **Wear of articular bearing surface of internal prosthetic joint**

⑦T84.060 **Wear of articular bearing surface of internal prosthetic right hip joint** [HCC]

⑦T84.061 **Wear of articular bearing surface of internal prosthetic left hip joint** [HCC]

⑦T84.062 **Wear of articular bearing surface of internal prosthetic right knee joint** [HCC]

⑦T84.063 **Wear of articular bearing surface of internal prosthetic left knee joint** [HCC]

⑦T84.068 **Wear of articular bearing surface of other internal prosthetic joint** [HCC]

Use Additional Code to identify the joint (Z96.6-)

⑦T84.069 **Wear of articular bearing surface of unspecified internal prosthetic joint** [HCC]

T84.09 **Other mechanical complication of internal joint prosthesis**

Prosthetic joint implant failure NOS

⑦T84.090 **Other mechanical complication of internal right hip prosthesis** [HCC]

⑦T84.091 **Other mechanical complication of internal left hip prosthesis** [HCC]

⑦T84.092 **Other mechanical complication of internal right knee prosthesis** [HCC]

⑦T84.093 **Other mechanical complication of internal left knee prosthesis** [HCC]

⑦T84.098 **Other mechanical complication of other internal joint prosthesis** [HCC]

Use Additional Code to identify the joint (Z96.6-)

⑦T84.099 **Other mechanical complication of unspecified internal joint prosthesis** [HCC]

T84.1 **Mechanical complication of internal fixation device of bones of limb**

Excludes2: mechanical complication of internal fixation device of bones of feet (T84.2-)

mechanical complication of internal fixation device of bones of fingers (T84.2-)

mechanical complication of internal fixation device of bones of hands (T84.2-)

mechanical complication of internal fixation device of bones of toes (T84.2-)

T84.11 **Breakdown (mechanical) of internal fixation device of bones of limb**

⑦T84.110 **Breakdown (mechanical) of internal fixation device of right humerus** [HCC]

⑦T84.111 **Breakdown (mechanical) of internal fixation device of left humerus** [HCC]

⑦T84.112 **Breakdown (mechanical) of internal fixation device of bone of right forearm** [HCC]

⑦T84.113 **Breakdown (mechanical) of internal fixation device of bone of left forearm** [HCC]

⑦T84.114 **Breakdown (mechanical) of internal fixation device of right femur** [HCC]

⑦T84.115 **Breakdown (mechanical) of internal fixation device of left femur** [HCC]

⑦T84.116 **Breakdown (mechanical) of internal fixation device of bone of right lower leg** [HCC]

⑦T84.117 **Breakdown (mechanical) of internal fixation device of bone of left lower leg** [HCC]

⑦T84.119 **Breakdown (mechanical) of internal fixation device of unspecified bone of limb** [HCC]

T84.12 **Displacement of internal fixation device of bones of limb**

Malposition of internal fixation device of bones of limb

⑦T84.120 **Displacement of internal fixation device of right humerus** [HCC]

⑦T84.121 **Displacement of internal fixation device of left humerus** [HCC]

⑦T84.122 **Displacement of internal fixation device of bone of right forearm** [HCC]

⑦T84.123 **Displacement of internal fixation device of bone of left forearm**

⑦T84.124 **Displacement of internal fixation device of right femur** [HCC]

⑦T84.125 **Displacement of internal fixation device of left femur** [HCC]

⑦T84.126 **Displacement of internal fixation device of bone of right lower leg** [HCC]

⑦T84.127 **Displacement of internal fixation device of bone of left lower leg** [HCC]

⑦T84.129 **Displacement of internal fixation device of unspecified bone of limb** [HCC]

T84.19 **Other mechanical complication of internal fixation device of bones of limb**

Obstruction (mechanical) of internal fixation device of bones of limb

Perforation of internal fixation device of bones of limb

Protrusion of internal fixation device of bones of limb

⑦T84.190 **Other mechanical complication of internal fixation device of right humerus** [HCC]

⑦T84.191 **Other mechanical complication of internal fixation device of left humerus** [HCC]

⑦T84.192 **Other mechanical complication of internal fixation device of bone of right forearm** [HCC]

⑦T84.193 **Other mechanical complication of internal fixation device of bone of left forearm** [HCC]

⑦**T84.194** **Other mechanical complication of internal fixation device of right femur** [HCC]

⑦**T84.195** **Other mechanical complication of internal fixation device of left femur** [HCC]

⑦**T84.196** **Other mechanical complication of internal fixation device of bone of right lower leg** [HCC]

⑦**T84.197** **Other mechanical complication of internal fixation device of bone of left lower leg** [HCC]

⑦**T84.199** **Other mechanical complication of internal fixation device of unspecified bone of limb** [HCC]

T84.2 **Mechanical complication of internal fixation device of other bones**

   T84.21 **Breakdown (mechanical) of internal fixation device of other bones** [HCC]

      ⑦**T84.210** **Breakdown (mechanical) of internal fixation device of bones of hand and fingers** [HCC]

      ⑦**T84.213** **Breakdown (mechanical) of internal fixation device of bones of foot and toes** [HCC]

      ⑦**T84.216** **Breakdown (mechanical) of internal fixation device of vertebrae** [HCC]

      ⑦**T84.218** **Breakdown (mechanical) of internal fixation device of other bones** [HCC]

   T84.22 **Displacement of internal fixation device of other bones**

      Malposition of internal fixation device of other bones

      ⑦**T84.220** **Displacement of internal fixation device of bones of hand and fingers** [HCC]

      ⑦**T84.223** **Displacement of internal fixation device of bones of foot and toes** [HCC]

      ⑦**T84.226** **Displacement of internal fixation device of vertebrae** [HCC]

      ⑦**T84.228** **Displacement of internal fixation device of other bones** [HCC]

   T84.29 **Other mechanical complication of internal fixation device of other bones**

      Obstruction (mechanical) of internal fixation device of other bones

      Perforation of internal fixation device of other bones

      Protrusion of internal fixation device of other bones

      ⑦**T84.290** **Other mechanical complication of internal fixation device of bones of hand and fingers** [HCC]

      ⑦**T84.293** **Other mechanical complication of internal fixation device of bones of foot and toes**

      ⑦**T84.296** **Other mechanical complication of internal fixation device of vertebrae** [HCC]

      ⑦**T84.298** **Other mechanical complication of internal fixation device of other bones** [HCC]

T84.3 **Mechanical complication of other bone devices, implants and grafts**

    Excludes2: Other complications of bone graft (T86.83-)

T84.31 **Breakdown (mechanical) of other bone devices, implants and grafts**

   ⑦**T84.310** **Breakdown (mechanical) of electronic bone stimulator** [HCC]

   ⑦**T84.318** **Breakdown (mechanical) of other bone devices, implants and grafts** [HCC]

T84.32 **Displacement of other bone devices, implants and grafts** [HCC]

   Malposition **of other** bone devices, implants and grafts

   ⑦**T84.320** **Displacement of electronic bone stimulator** [HCC]

   ⑦**T84.328** **Displacement of other bone devices, implants and grafts** [HCC]

T84.39 **Other mechanical complication of other bone devices, implants and grafts** [HCC]

   Obstruction (mechanical) **of other** bone devices, implants and grafts

   Perforation **of other** bone devices, implants and grafts

   Protrusion **of other** bone devices, implants and grafts

   ⑦**T84.390** **Other mechanical complication of electronic bone stimulator** [HCC]

   ⑦**T84.398** **Other mechanical complication of other bone devices, implants and grafts** [HCC]

T84.4 **Mechanical complication of other internal orthopedic devices, implants and grafts**

   T84.41 **Breakdown (mechanical) of other internal orthopedic devices, implants and grafts** [HCC]

      ⑦**T84.410** **Breakdown (mechanical) of muscle and tendon graft** [HCC]

      ⑦**T84.418** **Breakdown (mechanical) of other internal orthopedic devices, implants and grafts** [HCC]

   T84.42 **Displacement of other internal orthopedic devices, implants and grafts**

      Malposition **of other** internal orthopedic devices, implants and grafts

      ⑦**T84.420** **Displacement of muscle and tendon graft** [HCC]

      ⑦**T84.428** **Displacement of other internal orthopedic devices, implants and grafts** [HCC]

   T84.49 **Other mechanical complication of other internal orthopedic devices, implants and grafts**

      Mechanical complication of other internal orthopedic devices, implants and grafts NOS

      Obstruction (mechanical) of other internal orthopedic devices, implants and grafts

      Perforation of other internal orthopedic devices, implants and grafts

      Protrusion of other internal orthopedic devices, implants and grafts

      ⑦**T84.490** **Other mechanical complication of muscle and tendon graft** [HCC]

      ⑦**T84.498** **Other mechanical complication of other internal orthopedic devices, implants and grafts** [HCC]

T84.5 **Infection and inflammatory reaction due to internal joint prosthesis**

   Use Additional Code to identify infection

⊗Ⓣ**T84.50** Infection and inflammatory reaction due to unspecified internal joint prosthesis [HCC]

⊗Ⓣ**T84.51** Infection and inflammatory reaction due to internal right hip prosthesis [HCC]

⊗Ⓣ**T84.52** Infection and inflammatory reaction due to internal left hip prosthesis

⊗Ⓣ**T84.53** Infection and inflammatory reaction due to internal right knee prosthesis [HCC]

⊗Ⓣ**T84.54** Infection and inflammatory reaction due to internal left knee prosthesis [HCC]

⊗Ⓣ**T84.59** Infection and inflammatory reaction due to other internal joint prosthesis [HCC]

T84.6 Infection and inflammatory reaction due to internal fixation device

Use Additional Code to identify infection

⊗Ⓣ**T84.60** Infection and inflammatory reaction due to internal fixation device of unspecified site [HCC]

T84.61 Infection and inflammatory reaction due to internal fixation device of arm [HCC]

Ⓣ**T84.610** Infection and inflammatory reaction due to internal fixation device of right humerus [HCC]

Ⓣ**T84.611** Infection and inflammatory reaction due to internal fixation device of left humerus [HCC]

Ⓣ**T84.612** Infection and inflammatory reaction due to internal fixation device of right radius [HCC]

Ⓣ**T84.613** Infection and inflammatory reaction due to internal fixation device of left radius [HCC]

Ⓣ**T84.614** Infection and inflammatory reaction due to internal fixation device of right ulna [HCC]

Ⓣ**T84.615** Infection and inflammatory reaction due to internal fixation device of left ulna [HCC]

Ⓣ**T84.619** Infection and inflammatory reaction due to internal fixation device of unspecified bone of arm [HCC]

T84.62 Infection and inflammatory reaction due to internal fixation device of leg

Ⓣ**T84.620** Infection and inflammatory reaction due to internal fixation device of right femur [HCC]

Ⓣ**T84.621** Infection and inflammatory reaction due to internal fixation device of left femur [HCC]

Ⓣ**T84.622** Infection and inflammatory reaction due to internal fixation device of right tibia [HCC]

Ⓣ**T84.623** Infection and inflammatory reaction due to internal fixation device of left tibia [HCC]

Ⓣ**T84.624** Infection and inflammatory reaction due to internal fixation device of right fibula [HCC]

Ⓣ**T84.625** Infection and inflammatory reaction due to internal fixation device of left fibula [HCC]

Ⓣ**T84.629** Infection and inflammatory reaction due to internal fixation device of unspecified bone of leg [HCC]

⊗Ⓣ**T84.63** Infection and inflammatory reaction due to internal fixation device of spine [HCC]

⊗Ⓣ**T84.69** Infection and inflammatory reaction due to internal fixation device of other site [HCC]

⊗Ⓣ**T84.7** Infection and inflammatory reaction due to other internal orthopedic prosthetic devices, implants and grafts

Use Additional Code to identify infection

T84.8 Other specified complications of internal orthopedic prosthetic devices, implants and grafts [HCC]

⊗Ⓣ**T84.81** Embolism due to internal orthopedic prosthetic devices, implants and grafts [HCC]

⊗Ⓣ**T84.82** Fibrosis due to internal orthopedic prosthetic devices, implants and grafts [HCC]

⊗Ⓣ**T84.83** Hemorrhage due to internal orthopedic prosthetic devices, implants and grafts [HCC]

⊗Ⓣ**T84.84** Pain due to internal orthopedic prosthetic devices, implants and grafts

⊗Ⓣ**T84.85** Stenosis due to internal orthopedic prosthetic devices, implants and grafts [HCC]

⊗Ⓣ**T84.86** Thrombosis due to internal orthopedic prosthetic devices, implants and grafts [HCC]

⊗Ⓣ**T84.89** Other specified complication of internal orthopedic prosthetic devices, implants and grafts [HCC]

⊗Ⓣ**T84.9** Unspecified complication of internal orthopedic prosthetic device, implant and graft [HCC]

T85 **Complications of other internal prosthetic devices, implants and grafts**

Excludes2: failure and rejection of transplanted organs and tissue (T86.-)

The appropriate 7th character is to be added to each code from category T85

A - initial encounter

D - subsequent encounter

S - sequela

T85.0 Mechanical complication of ventricular intracranial (communicating) shunt

⊗Ⓣ**T85.01** Breakdown (mechanical) of ventricular intracranial (communicating) shunt [HCC]

⊗Ⓣ**T85.02** Displacement of ventricular intracranial (communicating) shunt [HCC]

Malposition of ventricular intracranial (communicating) shunt

⊗Ⓣ**T85.03** Leakage of ventricular intracranial (communicating) shunt [HCC]

⊗Ⓣ**T85.09** Other mechanical complication of ventricular intracranial (communicating) shunt [HCC]

Obstruction (mechanical) of ventricular intracranial (communicating) shunt

Perforation of ventricular intracranial (communicating) shunt

Protrusion of ventricular intracranial (communicating) shunt

T85.1 Mechanical complication of implanted electronic stimulator of nervous system

T85.11 Breakdown (mechanical) of implanted electronic stimulator of nervous system [HCC]

Ⓣ**T85.110** Breakdown (mechanical) of implanted electronic neurostimulator of brain electrode (lead) [HCC]

Ⓣ**T85.111** Breakdown (mechanical) of implanted electronic neurostimulator of peripheral nerve electrode (lead) [HCC]

Breakdown of electrode (lead) for cranial nerve neurostimulators

Breakdown of electrode (lead) for gastric neurostimulator

Breakdown of electrode (lead) for sacral nerve neurostimulator

Breakdown of electrode (lead) for vagal nerve neurostimulators

⑦T85.112 **Breakdown (mechanical) of implanted electronic neurostimulator of spinal cord electrode (lead)** [HCC]

⑦T85.113 **Breakdown (mechanical) of implanted electronic neurostimulator, generator** [HCC]

Breakdown (mechanical) of implanted electronic neurostimulator generator, brain, peripheral, gastric, spinal

Breakdown (mechanical) of implanted electronic sacral neurostimulator, pulse generator or receiver

⑦T85.118 **Breakdown (mechanical) of other implanted electronic stimulator of nervous system** [HCC]

T85.12 **Displacement of implanted electronic stimulator of nervous system** [HCC]

Malposition of implanted electronic stimulator of nervous system

⑦T85.120 **Displacement of implanted electronic neurostimulator of brain electrode (lead)** [HCC]

⑦T85.121 **Displacement of implanted electronic neurostimulator of peripheral nerve electrode (lead)**

Displacement of electrode (lead) for cranial nerve neurostimulators

Displacement of electrode (lead) for gastric neurostimulator

Displacement of electrode (lead) for sacral nerve neurostimulator

Displacement of electrode (lead) for vagal nerve neurostimulators

⑦T85.122 **Displacement of implanted electronic neurostimulator of spinal cord electrode (lead)** [HCC]

⑦T85.123 **Displacement of implanted electronic neurostimulator, generator** [HCC]

Displacement of implanted electronic neurostimulator generator, brain, peripheral, gastric, spinal

Displacement of implanted electronic sacral neurostimulator, pulse generator or receiver

⑦T85.128 **Displacement of other implanted electronic stimulator of nervous system** [HCC]

T85.19 **Other mechanical complication of implanted electronic stimulator of nervous system** [HCC]

Leakage of implanted electronic stimulator of nervous system

Obstruction (mechanical) of implanted electronic stimulator of nervous system

Perforation of implanted electronic stimulator of nervous system

Protrusion of implanted electronic stimulator of nervous system

⑦T85.190 **Other mechanical complication of implanted electronic neurostimulator of brain electrode (lead)** [HCC]

⑦T85.191 **Other mechanical complication of implanted electronic neurostimulator of peripheral nerve electrode (lead)** [HCC]

Other mechanical complication of electrode (lead) for cranial nerve neurostimulators

Other mechanical complication of electrode (lead) for gastric neurostimulator

Other mechanical complication of electrode (lead) for sacral nerve neurostimulator

Other mechanical complication of electrode (lead) for vagal nerve neurostimulators

⑦T85.192 **Other mechanical complication of implanted electronic neurostimulator of spinal cord electrode (lead)** [HCC]

⑦T85.193 **Other mechanical complication of implanted electronic neurostimulator, generator** [HCC]

Other mechanical complication of implanted electronic neurostimulator generator, brain, peripheral, gastric, spinal

Other mechanical complication of implanted electronic sacral neurostimulator, pulse generator or receiver

⑦T85.199 **Other mechanical complication of other implanted electronic stimulator of nervous system** [HCC]

T85.2 **Mechanical complication of intraocular lens**

⊗⑦T85.21 **Breakdown (mechanical) of intraocular lens** [HCC]

⊗⑦T85.22 **Displacement of intraocular lens** [HCC]

Malposition of intraocular lens

⊗⑦T85.29 **Other mechanical complication of intraocular lens** [HCC]

Obstruction (mechanical) of intraocular lens

Perforation of intraocular lens

Protrusion of intraocular lens

T85.3 **Mechanical complication of other ocular prosthetic devices, implants and grafts**

Excludes2: Other complications of corneal graft (T86.84-)

T85.31 **Breakdown (mechanical) of other ocular prosthetic devices, implants and grafts** [HCC]

⑦T85.310 **Breakdown (mechanical) of prosthetic orbit of right eye** [HCC]

⑦T85.311 **Breakdown (mechanical) of prosthetic orbit of left eye**

⑦T85.318 **Breakdown (mechanical) of other ocular prosthetic devices, implants and grafts** [HCC]

T85.32 **Displacement of other ocular prosthetic devices, implants and grafts**

Malposition of other ocular prosthetic devices, implants and grafts

⑦T85.320 **Displacement of prosthetic orbit of right eye** [HCC]

⑦T85.321 **Displacement of prosthetic orbit of left eye** [HCC]

⑦T85.328 **Displacement of other ocular prosthetic devices, implants and grafts** [HCC]

T85.39 **Other mechanical complication of other ocular prosthetic devices, implants and grafts** [HCC]

Obstruction (mechanical) of other ocular prosthetic devices, implants and grafts

Perforation of other ocular prosthetic devices, implants and grafts

Protrusion of other ocular prosthetic devices, implants and grafts

⑦T85.390 **Other mechanical complication of prosthetic orbit of right eye** [HCC]

⑦T85.391 **Other mechanical complication of prosthetic orbit of left eye** [HCC]

⑦T85.398 **Other mechanical complication of other ocular prosthetic devices, implants and grafts** [HCC]

T85.4 **Mechanical complication of breast prosthesis and implant** [HCC]

⊗⑦T85.41 **Breakdown (mechanical) of breast prosthesis and implant** [HCC]

⊗⑦T85.42 **Displacement of breast prosthesis and implant** [HCC]

Malposition of breast prosthesis and implant

⊗⑦T85.43 **Leakage of breast prosthesis and implant** [HCC]

⊗⑦T85.44 **Capsular contracture of breast implant** [HCC]

⊗⑦T85.49 **Other mechanical complication of breast prosthesis and implant** [HCC]

Obstruction (mechanical) of breast prosthesis and implant

Perforation of breast prosthesis and implant

Protrusion of breast prosthesis and implant

T85.5 **Mechanical complication of gastrointestinal prosthetic devices, implants and grafts**

T85.51 **Breakdown (mechanical) of gastrointestinal prosthetic devices, implants and grafts**

⑦T85.510 **Breakdown (mechanical) of bile duct prosthesis** [HCC]

⑦T85.511 **Breakdown (mechanical) of esophageal anti-reflux device** [HCC]

⑦T85.518 **Breakdown (mechanical) of other gastrointestinal prosthetic devices, implants and grafts** [HCC]

T85.52 **Displacement of gastrointestinal prosthetic devices, implants and grafts**

Malposition of gastrointestinal prosthetic devices, implants and grafts

⑦T85.520 **Displacement of bile duct prosthesis** [HCC]

⑦T85.521 **Displacement of esophageal anti-reflux device** [HCC]

⑦T85.528 **Displacement of other gastrointestinal prosthetic devices, implants and grafts** [HCC]

T85.59 **Other mechanical complication of gastrointestinal prosthetic devices, implants and grafts**

Obstruction, mechanical of gastrointestinal prosthetic devices, implants and grafts

Perforation of gastrointestinal prosthetic devices, implants and grafts

Protrusion of gastrointestinal prosthetic devices, implants and grafts

⑦T85.590 **Other mechanical complication of bile duct prosthesis**

⑦T85.591 **Other mechanical complication of esophageal anti-reflux device** [HCC]

⑦T85.598 **Other mechanical complication of other gastrointestinal prosthetic devices, implants and grafts** [HCC]

T85.6 **Mechanical complication of other specified internal and external prosthetic devices, implants and grafts**

T85.61 **Breakdown (mechanical) of other specified internal prosthetic devices, implants and grafts**

⑦T85.610 **Breakdown (mechanical) of cranial or spinal infusion catheter** [HCC]

Breakdown (mechanical) of epidural infusion catheter

Breakdown (mechanical) of intrathecal infusion catheter

Breakdown (mechanical) of subarachnoid infusion catheter

Breakdown (mechanical) of subdural infusion catheter

⑦T85.611 **Breakdown (mechanical) of intraperitoneal dialysis catheter** [HCC]

Excludes1: mechanical complication of vascular dialysis catheter (T82.4-)

⑦T85.612 **Breakdown (mechanical) of permanent sutures** [HCC]

Excludes1: mechanical complication of permanent (wire) suture used in bone repair (T84.1-T84.2)

⑦T85.613 **Breakdown (mechanical) of artificial skin graft and decellularized allodermis** [HCC]

Failure of artificial skin graft and decellularized allodermis

Non-adherence of artificial skin graft and decellularized allodermis

Poor incorporation of artificial skin graft and decellularized allodermis

Shearing of artificial skin graft and decellularized allodermis

⑦T85.614 **Breakdown (mechanical) of insulin pump** [HCC]

⑦T85.615 **Breakdown (mechanical) of other nervous system device, implant or graft** [HCC]

Breakdown (mechanical) of intrathecal infusion pump

⑦T85.618 **Breakdown (mechanical) of other specified internal prosthetic devices, implants and grafts** [HCC]

T85.62 **Displacement of other specified internal prosthetic devices, implants and grafts**

Malposition of other specified internal prosthetic devices, implants and grafts

⑦T85.620 **Displacement of cranial or spinal infusion catheter** [HCC]

Displacement of epidural infusion catheter

Displacement of intrathecal infusion catheter

Displacement of subarachnoid infusion catheter

● New code ▲ Revised code **Excludes1:** Not coded here **Excludes2:** Not included here ⊗ Placeholder required ⑦7th digit required

Displacement of subdural infusion catheter

⑦ **T85.621** **Displacement of intraperitoneal dialysis catheter** [HCC]

Excludes1: mechanical complication of vascular dialysis catheter (T82.4-)

⑦ **T85.622** **Displacement of permanent sutures** [HCC]

Excludes1: mechanical complication of permanent (wire) suture used in bone repair (T84.1-T84.2)

⑦ **T85.623** **Displacement of artificial skin graft and decellularized allodermis** [HCC]

Dislodgement of artificial skin graft and decellularized allodermis

⑦ **T85.624** **Displacement of insulin pump**

⑦ **T85.625** **Displacement of other nervous system device, implant or graft** [HCC]

Displacement of intrathecal infusion pump

⑦ **T85.628** **Displacement of other specified internal prosthetic devices, implants and grafts** [HCC]

T85.63 **Leakage of other specified internal prosthetic devices, implants and grafts**

⑦ **T85.630** **Leakage of cranial or spinal infusion catheter** [HCC]

Leakage of epidural infusion catheter

Leakage of intrathecal infusion catheter infusion catheter

Leakage of subdural infusion catheter

Leakage of subarachnoid infusion catheter

⑦ **T85.631** **Leakage of intraperitoneal dialysis catheter** [HCC]

Excludes1: mechanical complication of vascular dialysis catheter (T82.4)

⑦ **T85.633** **Leakage of insulin pump** [HCC]

⑦ **T85.635** **Leakage of other nervous system device, implant or graft** [HCC]

Leakage of intrathecal infusion pump

⑦ **T85.638** **Leakage of other specified internal prosthetic devices, implants and grafts** [HCC]

T85.69 **Other mechanical complication of other specified internal prosthetic devices, implants and grafts**

Obstruction, mechanical of other specified internal prosthetic devices, implants and grafts

Perforation of other specified internal prosthetic devices, implants and grafts

Protrusion of other specified internal prosthetic devices, implants and grafts

⑦ **T85.690** **Other mechanical complication of cranial or spinal infusion catheter** [HCC]

Other mechanical complication of epidural infusion catheter

Other mechanical complication of intrathecal infusion catheter

Other mechanical complication of subarachnoid infusion catheter

Other mechanical complication of subdural infusion catheter

⑦ **T85.691** **Other mechanical complication of intraperitoneal dialysis catheter** [HCC]

Excludes1: mechanical complication of vascular dialysis catheter (T82.4)

⑦ **T85.692** **Other mechanical complication of permanent sutures** [HCC]

Excludes1: mechanical complication of permanent (wire) suture used in bone repair (T84.1-T84.2)

⑦ **T85.693** **Other mechanical complication of artificial skin graft and decellularized allodermis** [HCC]

⑦ **T85.694** **Other mechanical complication of insulin pump** [HCC]

⑦ **T85.695** **Other mechanical complication of other nervous system device, implant or graft** [HCC]

Other mechanical complication of intrathecal infusion pump

⑦ **T85.698** **Other mechanical complication of other specified internal prosthetic devices, implants and grafts** [HCC]

Mechanical complication of nonabsorbable surgical material NOS

T85.7 **Infection and inflammatory reaction due to other internal prosthetic devices, implants and grafts**

Use Additional Code to identify infection

⊗⑦ **T85.71** **Infection and inflammatory reaction due to peritoneal dialysis catheter** [HCC]

⊗⑦ **T85.72** **Infection and inflammatory reaction due to insulin pump**

T85.73 **Infection and inflammatory reaction due to nervous system devices, implants and graft**

⑦ **T85.730** **Infection and inflammatory reaction due to ventricular intracranial (communicating) shunt** [HCC]

⑦ **T85.731** **Infection and inflammatory reaction due to implanted electronic neurostimulator of brain, electrode (lead)** [HCC]

⑦ **T85.732** **Infection and inflammatory reaction due to implanted electronic neurostimulator of peripheral nerve, electrode (lead)** [HCC]

Infection and inflammatory reaction due to electrode (lead) for cranial nerve neurostimulators

Infection and inflammatory reaction due to electrode (lead) for gastric neurostimulator

Infection and inflammatory reaction due to electrode (lead) for sacral nerve neurostimulator

Infection and inflammatory reaction due to electrode (lead) for vagal nerve neurostimulators

⑦ **T85.733** **Infection and inflammatory reaction due to implanted electronic neurostimulator of spinal cord, electrode (lead)** [HCC]

⑦ **T85.734** **Infection and inflammatory reaction due to implanted electronic**

neurostimulator, generator pocket
infection

⑦ **T85.735** **Infection and inflammatory reaction
due to cranial or spinal infusion
catheter** [HCC]

Infection and inflammatory reaction
due to epidural catheter

Infection and inflammatory reaction
due to intrathecal infusion catheter

Infection and inflammatory reaction
due to subarachnoid catheter

Infection and inflammatory reaction
due to subdural catheter

⑦ **T85.738** **Infection and inflammatory reaction
due to other nervous system device,
implant or graft** [HCC]

Infection and inflammatory reaction
due to intrathecal infusion pump

⊗⑦ **T85.79** **Infection and inflammatory reaction due to
other internal prosthetic devices, implants and
grafts** [HCC]

T85.8 **Other specified complications of internal prosthetic
devices, implants and grafts, not elsewhere classified**

T85.81 **Embolism due to internal prosthetic devices,
implants and grafts, not elsewhere classified**
[HCC]

⑦ **T85.810** **Embolism due to nervous system
prosthetic devices, implants and
grafts** [HCC]

⑦ **T85.818** **Embolism due to other internal
prosthetic devices, implants and
grafts** [HCC]

T85.82 **Fibrosis due to internal prosthetic devices,
implants and grafts, not elsewhere classified**

⑦ **T85.820** **Fibrosis due to nervous system
prosthetic devices, implants and
grafts** [HCC]

⑦ **T85.828** **Fibrosis due to other internal
prosthetic devices, implants and
grafts** [HCC]

T85.83 **Hemorrhage due to internal prosthetic devices,
implants and grafts, not elsewhere classified**

⑦ **T85.830** **Hemorrhage due to nervous system
prosthetic devices, implants and
grafts** [HCC]

⑦ **T85.838** **Hemorrhage due to other internal
prosthetic devices, implants and
grafts** [HCC]

T85.84 **Pain due to internal prosthetic devices,
implants and grafts, not elsewhere classified**

⑦ **T85.840** **Pain due to nervous system
prosthetic devices, implants and
grafts** [HCC]

⑦ **T85.848** **Pain due to other internal prosthetic
devices, implants and grafts** [HCC]

T85.85 **Stenosis due to internal prosthetic devices,
implants and grafts, not elsewhere classified**

⑦ **T85.850** **Stenosis due to nervous system
prosthetic devices, implants and
grafts** [HCC]

⑦ **T85.858** **Stenosis due to other internal
prosthetic devices, implants and
grafts** [HCC]

T85.86 **Thrombosis due to internal prosthetic devices,
implants and grafts, not elsewhere classified**

⑦ **T85.860** **Thrombosis due to nervous system
prosthetic devices, implants and
grafts** [HCC]

⑦ **T85.868** **Thrombosis due to other internal
prosthetic devices, implants and
grafts** [HCC]

T85.89 **Other specified complication of internal
prosthetic devices, implants and grafts, not
elsewhere classified**

Erosion or breakdown of subcutaneous device
pocket

⑦ **T85.890** **Other specified complication of
nervous system prosthetic devices,
implants and grafts** [HCC]

⑦ **T85.898** **Other specified complication of other
internal prosthetic devices, implants
and grafts** [HCC]

⑦ **T85.9** **Unspecified complication of internal prosthetic device,
implant and graft**

Complication of internal prosthetic device, implant and graft
NOS

T86 **Complications of transplanted organs and tissue**

Use Additional Code to identify **Other** transplant complications,
such as:

graft-versus-host disease (D89.81-)

malignancy associated with organ transplant (C80.2)

post-transplant lymphoproliferative disorders (PTLD) (D47.Z1)

T86.0 **Complications of bone marrow transplant**

T86.00 **Unspecified complication of bone marrow
transplant** [HCC]

T86.01 **Bone marrow transplant rejection** [HCC]

T86.02 **Bone marrow transplant failure** [HCC]

T86.03 **Bone marrow transplant infection** [HCC]

T86.09 **Other complications of bone marrow transplant**

T86.1 **Complications of kidney transplant**

T86.10 **Unspecified complication of kidney transplant**

T86.11 **Kidney transplant rejection**

T86.12 **Kidney transplant failure**

T86.13 **Kidney transplant infection**

Use Additional Code to specify infection

T86.19 **Other complication of kidney transplant**

T86.2 **Complications of heart transplant**

Excludes1: complication of artificial heart device (T82.5-)

heart-lung transplant (T86.3-)

T86.20 **Unspecified complication of heart transplant**
[HCC]

T86.21 **Heart transplant rejection**

T86.22 **Heart transplant failure** [HCC]

T86.23 **Heart transplant infection** [HCC]

Use Additional Code to specify infection

T86.29 **Other complications of heart transplant** [HCC]

T86.290 **Cardiac allograft vasculopathy** [HCC]

Excludes1: atherosclerosis of coronary
arteries (I25.75-, I25.76-,
I25.81-)

T86.298 **Other complications of heart
transplant** [HCC]

T86.3 **Complications of heart-lung transplant**

T86.30 **Unspecified complication of heart-lung
transplant** [HCC]

T86.31 **Heart-lung transplant rejection** [HCC]

T86.32   **Heart-lung transplant failure** [HCC]

T86.33   **Heart-lung transplant infection** [HCC]

     <u>Use Additional Code</u> to specify infection

T86.39   **Other complications of heart-lung transplant** [HCC]

T86.4   **Complications of liver transplant**

T86.40   **Unspecified complication of liver transplant** [HCC]

T86.41   **Liver transplant rejection** [HCC]

T86.42   **Liver transplant failure** [HCC]

T86.43   **Liver transplant infection** [HCC]

     <u>Use Additional Code</u> to identify infection, such as:

     Cytomegalovirus (CMV) infection (B25.-)

T86.49   **Other complications of liver transplant** [HCC]

T86.5   **Complications of stem cell transplant** [HCC]

Complications from stem cells from peripheral blood

Complications from stem cells from umbilical cord

T86.8   **Complications of other transplanted organs and tissues**

T86.81   **Complications of lung transplant**

     Excludes1: complication of heart-lung transplant (T86.3-)

T86.810   **Lung transplant rejection** [HCC]

T86.811   **Lung transplant failure** [HCC]

T86.812   **Lung transplant infection** [HCC]

     <u>Use Additional Code</u> to specify infection

T86.818   **Other complications of lung transplant** [HCC]

T86.819   **Unspecified complication of lung transplant**

T86.82   **Complications of skin graft (allograft) (autograft)**

     Excludes2: complication of artificial skin graft (T85.693)

T86.820   **Skin graft (allograft) rejection**

T86.821   **Skin graft (allograft) (autograft) failure**

T86.822   **Skin graft (allograft) (autograft) infection**

     <u>Use Additional Code</u> to specify infection

T86.828   **Other complications of skin graft (allograft) (autograft)**

T86.829   **Unspecified complication of skin graft (allograft) (autograft)**

T86.83   **Complications of bone graft**

     Excludes2: mechanical complications of bone graft (T84.3-)

T86.830   **Bone graft rejection**

T86.831   **Bone graft failure**

T86.832   **Bone graft infection**

     <u>Use Additional Code</u> to specify infection

T86.838   **Other complications of bone graft**

T86.839   **Unspecified complication of bone graft**

T86.84   **Complications of corneal transplant**

     Excludes2: mechanical complications of corneal graft (T85.3-)

T86.840   **Corneal transplant rejection**

T86.8401   **Corneal transplant rejection, right eye**

T86.8402   **Corneal transplant rejection, left eye**

T86.8403   **Corneal transplant rejection, bilateral**

T86.8409   **Corneal transplant rejection, unspecified eye**

T86.841   **Corneal transplant failure**

T86.8411   **Corneal transplant failure, right eye**

T86.8412   **Corneal transplant failure, left eye**

T86.8413   **Corneal transplant failure, bilateral**

T86.8419   **Corneal transplant failure, unspecified eye**

T86.842   **Corneal transplant infection** [HCC]

     <u>Use Additional Code</u> to specify infection

T86.8421   **Corneal transplant infection, right eye**

T86.8422   **Corneal transplant infection, left eye**

T86.8423   **Corneal transplant infection, bilateral**

T86.8429   **Corneal transplant infection, unspecified eye**

T86.848   **Other complications of corneal transplant**

T86.8481   **Other complications of corneal transplant, right eye**

T86.8482   **Other complications of corneal transplant, left eye**

T86.8483   **Other complications of corneal transplant, bilateral**

T86.8489   **Other complications of corneal transplant, unspecified e**

T86.849   **Unspecified complication of corneal transplant**

T86.8491   **Unspecified complication of corneal transplant, right eye**

T86.8492   **Unspecified complication of corneal transplant, left eye**

T86.8493   **Unspecified complication of corneal transplant, bilateral**

T86.8499   **Unspecified complication of corneal transplant, unspecified eye**

T86.85   **Complication of intestine transplant**

T86.850   **Intestine transplant rejection** [HCC]

T86.851   **Intestine transplant failure** [HCC]

T86.852   **Intestine transplant infection** [HCC]

     <u>Use Additional Code</u> to specify infection

T86.858   **Other complications of intestine transplant** [HCC]

T86.859 Unspecified complication of intestine transplant [HCC]

T86.89 Complications of other transplanted tissue

Transplant failure or rejection of pancreas

T86.890 Other transplanted tissue rejection

T86.891 Other transplanted tissue failure

T86.892 Other transplanted tissue infection

Use Additional Code to specify infection

T86.898 Other complications of other transplanted tissue

T86.899 Unspecified complication of other transplanted tissue

T86.9 Complication of unspecified transplanted organ and tissue

T86.90 Unspecified complication of unspecified transplanted organ and tissue

T86.91 Unspecified transplanted organ and tissue rejection

T86.92 Unspecified transplanted organ and tissue failure

T86.93 Unspecified transplanted organ and tissue infection

Use Additional Code to specify infection

T86.99 Other complications of unspecified transplanted organ and tissue

T87 Complications peculiar to reattachment and amputation

T87.0 Complications of reattached (part of) upper extremity

T87.0X Complications of reattached (part of) upper extremity

T87.0X1 Complications of reattached (part of) right upper extremity [HCC]

T87.0X2 Complications of reattached (part of) left upper extremity [HCC]

T87.0X9 Complications of reattached (part of) unspecified upper extremity [HCC]

T87.1 Complications of reattached (part of) lower extremity

T87.1X Complications of reattached (part of) lower extremity

T87.1X1 Complications of reattached (part of) right lower extremity [HCC]

T87.1X2 Complications of reattached (part of) left lower extremity [HCC]

T87.1X9 Complications of reattached (part of) unspecified lower extremity [HCC]

T87.2 Complications of other reattached body part [HCC]

T87.3 Neuroma of amputation stump

T87.30 Neuroma of amputation stump, unspecified extremity [HCC]

T87.31 Neuroma of amputation stump, right upper extremity [HCC]

T87.32 Neuroma of amputation stump, left upper extremity [HCC]

T87.33 Neuroma of amputation stump, right lower extremity [HCC]

T87.34 Neuroma of amputation stump, left lower extremity [HCC]

T87.4 Infection of amputation stump

T87.40 Infection of amputation stump, unspecified extremity

T87.41 Infection of amputation stump, right upper extremity [HCC]

T87.42 Infection of amputation stump, left upper extremity [HCC]

T87.43 Infection of amputation stump, right lower extremity [HCC]

T87.44 Infection of amputation stump, left lower extremity [HCC]

T87.5 Necrosis of amputation stump

T87.50 Necrosis of amputation stump, unspecified extremity [HCC]

T87.51 Necrosis of amputation stump, right upper extremity [HCC]

T87.52 Necrosis of amputation stump, left upper extremity [HCC]

T87.53 Necrosis of amputation stump, right lower extremity [HCC]

T87.54 Necrosis of amputation stump, left lower extremity [HCC]

T87.8 Other complications of amputation stump

T87.81 Dehiscence of amputation stump [HCC]

T87.89 Other complications of amputation stump [HCC]

Amputation stump contracture

Amputation stump contracture of next proximal joint

Amputation stump flexion

Amputation stump edema

Amputation stump hematoma

Excludes2: phantom limb syndrome (G54.6-G54.7)

T87.9 Unspecified complications of amputation stump [HCC]

T88 Other complications of surgical and medical care, not elsewhere classified

Excludes2: complication following infusion, transfusion and therapeutic injection (T80.-)

complication following procedure NEC (T81.-)

complications of anesthesia in labor and delivery (O74.-)

complications of anesthesia in pregnancy (O29.-)

complications of anesthesia in puerperium (O89.-)

complications of devices, implants and grafts (T82-T85)

complications of obstetric surgery and procedure (O75.4)

dermatitis due to drugs and medicaments (L23.3, L24.4, L25.1, L27.0-L27.1)

poisoning and toxic effects of drugs and chemicals (T36-T65 with fifth or sixth character 1-4 or 6) specified complications classified elsewhere

The appropriate 7th character is to be added to each code from category T88

A - initial encounter

D - subsequent encounter

S - sequela

⊗⑦**T88.0** Infection following immunization

Sepsis following immunization

⊗⑦**T88.1** Other complications following immunization, not elsewhere classified

Generalized vaccinia

Rash following immunization

Excludes1: vaccinia not from vaccine (B08.011)

Excludes2: anaphylactic shock due to serum (T80.5-)

Other serum reactions (T80.6-)

postimmunization arthropathy (M02.2)

postimmunization encephalitis (G04.02)

● New code   ▲ Revised code   Excludes1: Not coded here   Excludes2: Not included here   ⊗ Placeholder required   ⑦ 7th digit required

postimmunization fever (R50.83)

⊗⑦**T88.2   Shock due to anesthesia**

Use Additional Code for adverse effect, if applicable, to identify drug (T41.- with fifth or sixth character 5)

Excludes1: complications of anesthesia (in):

> labor and delivery (O74.-)
>
> pregnancy (O29.-)
>
> puerperium (O89.-)
>
> postprocedural shock NOS (T81.1-)

⊗⑦**T88.3   Malignant hyperthermia due to anesthesia**

Use Additional Code for adverse effect, if applicable, to identify drug (T41.- with fifth or sixth character 5)

⊗⑦**T88.4   Failed or difficult intubation**

T88.5   Other complications of anesthesia

Use Additional Code for adverse effect, if applicable, to identify drug (T41.- with fifth or sixth character 5)

⊗⑦**T88.51   Hypothermia following anesthesia**

⊗⑦**T88.52   Failed moderate sedation during procedure**

Failed conscious sedation during procedure

Excludes2: personal history of failed moderate sedation (Z92.83)

⊗⑦**T88.53   Unintended awareness under general anesthesia during procedure**

Excludes2: personal history of unintended awareness under general anesthesia (Z92.84)

⊗⑦**T88.59   Other complications of anesthesia**

⊗⑦**T88.6   Anaphylactic reaction due to adverse effect of correct drug or medicament properly administered**

Anaphylactic shock due to adverse effect of correct drug or medicament properly administered

Anaphylactoid reaction NOS

Use Additional Code for adverse effect, if applicable, to identify drug (T36-T50 with fifth or sixth character 5)

Excludes1: anaphylactic reaction due to serum (T80.5-)

> anaphylactic shock or reaction due to adverse food reaction (T78.0-)

⊗⑦**T88.7   Unspecified adverse effect of drug or medicament**

Drug hypersensitivity NOS

Drug reaction NOS

Use Additional Code for adverse effect, if applicable, to identify drug (T36-T50 with fifth or sixth character 5)

Excludes1: specified adverse effects of drugs and medicaments (A00-R94 and T80-T88.6, T88.8)

⊗⑦**T88.8   Other specified complications of surgical and medical care, not elsewhere classified**

Use Additional Code to identify the complication

⊗⑦**T88.9   Complication of surgical and medical care, unspecified**

Chapter 20: External Causes of Morbidity (V00-Y99)

MULTIPLE CODING FOR A SINGLE CONDITION

In addition to the etiology/manifestation convention that requires two codes to fully describe a single condition that affects multiple body systems, there are other single conditions that also require more than one code. "**Use Additional Code**" notes are found in the Tabular List at codes that are not part of an etiology/manifestation pair where a secondary code is useful to fully describe a condition. The sequencing rule is the same as the etiology/manifestation pair, "**Use Additional Code**" indicates that a secondary code should be added.

For example, for bacterial infections that are not included in chapter 1, a secondary code from category B95, Streptococcus, Staphylococcus, and Enterococcus, as the cause of diseases classified elsewhere, or B96, Other bacterial agents as the cause of diseases classified elsewhere, may be required to identify the bacterial organism causing the infection. A "**Use Additional Code**" note will normally be found at the infectious disease code, indicating a need for the organism code to be added as a secondary code.

"Code first" notes are also under certain codes that are not specifically manifestation codes but may be due to an underlying cause. When there is a "Code first" note and an underlying condition is present, the underlying condition should be sequenced first.

"Code, if applicable, any causal condition first", notes indicate that this code may be assigned as a principal diagnosis when the causal condition is unknown or not applicable. If a causal condition is known, then the code for that condition should be sequenced as the principal or first-listed diagnosis.

Multiple codes may be needed for sequela, complication codes and obstetric codes to more fully describe a condition. See the specific guidelines for these conditions for further instruction.

COMBINATION CODE

A combination code is a single code used to classify: Two diagnoses, or a diagnosis with an associated secondary process (manifestation) A diagnosis with an associated complication

Combination codes are identified by referring to subterm entries in the Alphabetic Index and by reading the inclusion and exclusion notes in the Tabular List.

Assign only the combination code when that code fully identifies the diagnostic conditions involved or when the Alphabetic Index so directs. Multiple coding should not be used when the classification provides a combination code that clearly identifies all of the elements documented in the diagnosis. When the combination code lacks necessary specificity in describing the manifestation or complication, an additional code should be used as a secondary code.

SEQUELA (LATE EFFECTS)

A sequela is the residual effect (condition produced) after the acute phase of an illness or injury has terminated. There is no time limit on when a sequela code can be used. The residual may be apparent early, such as in cerebral infarction, or it may occur months or years later, such as that due to a previous injury. Coding of sequela generally requires two codes sequenced in the following order: The condition or nature of the sequela is sequenced first.

The sequela code is sequenced second.

An exception to the above guidelines are those instances where the code for the sequela is followed by a manifestation code identified in the Tabular List and title, or the sequela code has been expanded (at the fourth, fifth or sixth character levels) to include the manifestation(s). The code for the acute phase of an illness or injury that led to the sequela is never used with a code for the late effect.

The external causes of morbidity codes should never be sequenced as the first-listed or principal diagnosis.

External cause codes are intended to provide data for injury research and evaluation of injury prevention strategies. These codes capture how the injury or health condition happened (cause), the intent (unintentional or accidental; or intentional, such

V00-Y99

as suicide or assault), the place where the event occurred the activity of the patient at the time of the event, and the person's status (e.g., civilian, military).

There is no national requirement for mandatory ICD-10-CM external cause code reporting. Unless a provider is subject to a state-based external cause code reporting mandate or these codes are required by a particular payer, reporting of ICD-10-CM codes in Chapter 20, External Causes of Morbidity, is not required. In the absence of a mandatory reporting requirement, providers are encouraged to voluntarily report external cause codes, as they provide valuable data for injury research and evaluation of injury prevention strategies.

GENERAL EXTERNAL CAUSE CODING GUIDELINES

1)   Used with any code in the range of A00.0-T88.9 Z00-Z99

An external cause code may be used with any code in the range of A00.0-T88.9, Z00-Z99, classification that represents a health condition due to an external cause. Though they are most applicable to injuries, they are also valid for use with such things as infections or diseases due to an external source, and other health conditions, such as a heart attack that occurs during strenuous physical activity.

2)   External cause code used for length of treatment

Assign the external cause code, with the appropriate 7th character (initial encounter, subsequent encounter or sequela) for each encounter for which the injury or condition is being treated.

Most categories in chapter 20 have a 7th character requirement for each applicable code. Most categories in this chapter have three 7th character values: A, initial encounter, D, subsequent encounter and S, sequela. While the patient may be seen by a new or different provider over the course of treatment for an injury or condition, assignment of the 7th character for external cause should match the 7th character of the code assigned for the associated injury or condition for the encounter.

3)   Use the full range of external cause codes

Use the full range of external cause codes to completely describe the cause, the intent, the place of occurrence, and if applicable, the activity of the patient at the time of the event, and the patient's status, for all injuries, and other health conditions due to an external cause.

4)   Assign as many external cause codes as necessary

Assign as many external cause codes as necessary to fully explain each cause. If only one external code can be recorded, assign the code most related to the principal diagnosis.

5)   The selection of the appropriate external cause code

The selection of the appropriate external cause code is guided by the Alphabetic Index of External Causes and by Inclusion and Exclusion notes in the Tabular List.

6)   External cause code can never be a principal diagnosis

An external cause code can never be a principal (first-listed) diagnosis.

7)   Combination external cause codes

Certain of the external cause codes are combination codes that identify sequential events that result in an injury, such as a fall which results in striking against an object. The injury may be due to either event or both. The combination external cause code used should correspond to the sequence of events regardless of which caused the most serious injury.

8)   No external cause code needed in certain circumstances

No external cause code from Chapter 20 is needed if the external cause and intent are included in a code from another chapter (e.g. T36.0X1- Poisoning by penicillins, accidental (unintentional)).

PLACE OF OCCURRENCE GUIDELINE

Codes from category Y92, Place of occurrence of the external cause, are secondary codes for use after other external cause codes to identify the location of the patient at the time of injury or other condition.

Generally, a place of occurrence code is assigned only once, at the initial encounter for treatment. However, in the rare instance that a new injury occurs during hospitalization, an additional place of occurrence code may be assigned. No 7th characters are used for Y92.

Do not use place of occurrence code Y92.9 if the place is not stated or is not applicable.

ACTIVITY CODE

Assign a code from category Y93, Activity code, to describe the activity of the patient at the time the injury or other health condition occurred.

An activity code is used only once, at the initial encounter for treatment. Only one code from Y93 should be recorded on a medical record.

The activity codes are not applicable to poisonings, adverse effects, misadventures or sequela.

Do not assign Y93.9, Unspecified activity, if the activity is not stated.

A code from category Y93 is appropriate for use with external cause and intent codes if identifying the activity provides additional information about the event.

PLACE OF OCCURRENCE, ACTIVITY, AND STATUS CODES USED WITH OTHER EXTERNAL CAUSE CODE

When applicable, place of occurrence, activity, and external cause status codes are sequenced after the main external cause code(s). Regardless of the number of external cause codes assigned, generally there should be only one place of occurrence code, one activity code, and one external cause status code assigned to an encounter. However, in the rare instance that a new injury occurs during hospitalization, an additional place of occurrence code may be assigned.

IF THE REPORTING FORMAT LIMITS THE NUMBER OF EXTERNAL CAUSE CODES

If the reporting format limits the number of external cause codes that can be used in reporting clinical data, report the code for the cause/intent most related to the principal diagnosis. If the format permits capture of additional external cause codes, the cause/intent, including medical misadventures, of the additional events should be reported rather than the codes for place, activity, or external status.

MULTIPLE EXTERNAL CAUSE CODING GUIDELINES

More than one external cause code is required to fully describe the external cause of an illness or injury. The assignment of external cause codes should be sequenced in the following priority:

If two or more events cause separate injuries, an external cause code should be assigned for each cause. The first-listed external cause code will be selected in the following order:

External codes for child and adult abuse take priority over all other external cause codes.

See Section I.C.19., Child and Adult abuse guidelines.

External cause codes for terrorism events take priority over all other external cause codes except child and adult abuse.

External cause codes for cataclysmic events take priority over all other external cause codes except child and adult abuse and terrorism.

External cause codes for transport accidents take priority over all other external cause codes except cataclysmic events, child and adult abuse and terrorism.

Activity and external cause status codes are assigned following all causal (intent) external cause codes.

The first-listed external cause code should correspond to the cause of the most serious diagnosis due to an assault, accident, or self-harm, following the order of hierarchy listed above.

CHILD AND ADULT ABUSE GUIDELINE

Adult and child abuse, neglect and maltreatment are classified as assault. Any of the assault codes may be used to indicate the external cause of any injury resulting from the confirmed abuse.

For confirmed cases of abuse, neglect and maltreatment, when the perpetrator is known, a code from Y07, Perpetrator of maltreatment and neglect, should accompany any other assault codes.

See Section I.C.19. Adult and child abuse, neglect and other maltreatment

UNKNOWN OR UNDETERMINED INTENT GUIDELINE

If the intent (accident, self-harm, assault) of the cause of an injury or other condition is unknown or unspecified, code the intent as accidental intent. All transport accident categories assume accidental intent.

1) **Use of undetermined intent**

   External cause codes for events of undetermined intent are only for use if the documentation in the record specifies that the intent cannot be determined.

SEQUELAE (LATE EFFECTS) OF EXTERNAL CAUSE GUIDELINES

1) **Sequelae external cause codes**

   Sequela are reported using the external cause code with the 7th character "S" for sequela. These codes should be used with any report of a late effect or sequela resulting from a previous injury.

   See Section I.B.10 Sequela (Late Effects)

2) **Sequela external cause code with a related current injury**

   A sequela external cause code should never be used with a related current nature of injury code.

3) **Use of sequela external cause codes for subsequent visits**

   Use a late effect external cause code for subsequent visits when a late effect of the initial injury is being treated. Do not use a late effect external cause code for subsequent visits for follow-up care (e.g., to assess healing, to receive rehabilitative therapy) of the injury when no late effect of the injury has been documented.

TERRORISM GUIDELINES

1) **Cause of injury identified by the Federal Government (FBI) as terrorism**

   When the cause of an injury is identified by the Federal Government (FBI) as terrorism, the first-listed external cause code should be a code from category Y38, Terrorism. The definition of terrorism employed by the FBI is found at the inclusion note at the beginning of category Y38. <u>Use Additional Code</u> for place of occurrence (Y92.-). More than one Y38 code may be assigned if the injury is the result of more than one mechanism of terrorism.

2) **Cause of an injury is suspected to be the result of terrorism**

   When the cause of an injury is suspected to be the result of terrorism a code from category Y38 should not be assigned. Suspected cases should be classified as assault.

3) **Code Y38.9, Terrorism, secondary effects**

Assign code Y38.9, Terrorism, secondary effects, for conditions occurring subsequent to the terrorist event. This code should not be assigned for conditions that are due to the initial terrorist act.

It is acceptable to assign code Y38.9 with another code from Y38 if there is an injury due to the initial terrorist event and an injury that is a subsequent result of the terrorist event.

EXTERNAL CAUSE STATUS

A code from category Y99, External cause status, should be assigned whenever any other external cause code is assigned for an encounter, including an Activity code, except for the events noted below. Assign a code from category Y99, External cause status, to indicate the work status of the person at the time the event occurred. The status code indicates whether the event occurred during military activity, whether a non-military person was at work, whether an individual including a student or volunteer was involved in a non-work activity at the time of the causal event.

A code from Y99, External cause status, should be assigned, when applicable, with other external cause codes, such as transport accidents and falls. The external cause status codes are not applicable to poisonings, adverse effects, misadventures or late effects.

Do not assign a code from category Y99 if no other external cause codes (cause, activity) are applicable for the encounter.

An external cause status code is used only once, at the initial encounter for treatment. Only one code from Y99 should be recorded on a medical record.

Do not assign code Y99.9, Unspecified external cause status, if the status is not stated.

● New code   ▲ Revised code   **Excludes1:** Not coded here   **Excludes2:** Not included here   ⊗ Placeholder required   ⑦7th digit required

Chapter 20
External Causes of Morbidity (V00-Y99)

Note: This chapter permits the classification of environmental events and circumstances as the cause of injury, and other adverse effects. Where a code from this section is applicable, it is intended that it shall be used secondary to a code from another chapter of the Classification indicating the nature of the condition.

Most often, the condition will be classifiable to Chapter 19, Injury, poisoning and certain other consequences of external causes (S00-T88). Other conditions that may be stated to be due to external causes are classified in Chapters I to XVIII. For these conditions, codes from Chapter 20 should be used to provide additional information as to the cause of the condition.

This chapter contains the following blocks: V00-X58 Accidents

V00-V99	Transport accidents
V00-V09	Pedestrian injured in transport accident
V10-V19	Pedal cycle rider injured in transport accident
V20-V29	Motorcycle rider injured in transport accident
V30-V39	Occupant of three-wheeled motor vehicle injured in transport accident
V40-V49	Car occupant injured in transport accident
V50-V59	Occupant of pick-up truck or van injured in transport accident
V60-V69	Occupant of heavy transport vehicle injured in transport accident
V70-V79	Bus occupant injured in transport accident
V80-V89	Other land transport accidents
V90-V94	Water transport accidents
V95-V97	Air and space transport accidents
V98-V99	Other and unspecified transport accidents
W00-X58	Other external causes of accidental injury
W00-W19	Slipping, tripping, stumbling and falls
W20-W49	Exposure to inanimate mechanical forces
W50-W64	Exposure to animate mechanical forces
W65-W74	Accidental non-transport drowning and submersion
W85-W99	Exposure to electric current, radiation and extreme ambient air temperature and pressure
X00-X08	Exposure to smoke, fire and flames
X10-X19	Contact with heat and hot substances
X30-X39	Exposure to forces of nature
X52-X58	Accidental exposure **to other** specified factors
X71-X83	Intentional self-harm
X92-Y09	Assault
Y21-Y33	Event of undetermined intent
Y35-Y38	Legal intervention, operations of war, military operations, and terrorism
Y62-Y84	Complications of medical and surgical care
Y62-Y69	Misadventures to patients during surgical and medical care
Y70-Y82	Medical devices associated with adverse incidents in diagnostic and therapeutic use
Y83-Y84	Surgical and other medical procedures as the cause of abnormal reaction of the patient, or of later complication, without mention of misadventure at the time of the procedure
Y90-Y99	Supplementary factors related to causes of morbidity classified elsewhere

ACCIDENTS (V00-X58)
TRANSPORT ACCIDENTS (V00-V99)

Note: This section is structured in 12 groups. Those relating to land transport accidents (V00-V89) reflect the victim's mode of transport and are subdivided to identify the victim's 'counterpart' or the type of event. The vehicle of which the injured person is an occupant is identified in the first two characters since it is seen as the most important factor to identify for prevention purposes. A transport accident is one in which the vehicle involved must be moving or running or in use for transport purposes at the time of the accident.

Use Additional Code to identify:

Airbag injury (W22.1)

Type of street or road (Y92.4-)

Use of cellular telephone and other electronic equipment at the time of the transport accident (Y93.C-)

Excludes1: agricultural vehicles in stationary use or maintenance (W31.-)

assault by crashing of motor vehicle (Y03.-)

automobile or motor cycle in stationary use or maintenance- code to type of accident crashing of motor vehicle, undetermined intent (Y32)

intentional self-harm by crashing of motor vehicle (X82)

Excludes2: transport accidents due to cataclysm (X34-X38)

Note: Definitions related to transport accidents:

a) A transport accident (V00-V99) is any accident involving a device designed primarily for, or used at the time primarily for, conveying persons or good from one place to another.

b) A public highway [traffic way] or street is the entire width between property lines (or other boundary lines) of land open to the public as a matter of right or custom for purposes of moving persons or property from one place to another. A roadway is that part of the public highway designed, improved and customarily used for vehicular traffic.

c) A traffic accident is any vehicle accident occurring on the public highway [i.e. originating on, terminating on, or involving a vehicle partially on the highway]. A vehicle accident is assumed to have occurred on the public highway unless another place is specified, except in the case of accidents involving only off-road motor vehicles, which are classified as nontraffic accidents unless the contrary is stated.

d) A nontraffic accident is any vehicle accident that occurs entirely in any place other than a public highway.

e) A pedestrian is any person involved in an accident who was not at the time of the accident riding in or on a motor vehicle, railway train, streetcar or animal-drawn or other vehicle, or on a pedal cycle or animal. This includes, a person changing a tire, working on a parked car, or a person on foot. It also includes the user of a pedestrian conveyance such as a baby stroller, ice-skates, skis, sled, roller skates, a skateboard, nonmotorized or motorized wheelchair, motorized mobility scooter, or nonmotorized scooter.

f) A driver is an occupant of a transport vehicle who is operating or intending to operate it.

g) A passenger is any occupant of a transport vehicle other than the driver, except a person traveling on the outside of the vehicle.

h) A person on the outside of a vehicle is any person being transported by a vehicle but not occupying the space normally reserved for the driver or passengers, or the space intended for the transport of property. This includes a person travelling on the bodywork, bumper, fender, roof, running board or step of a vehicle, as well as, hanging on the outside of the vehicle.

i) A pedal cycle is any land transport vehicle operated solely by nonmotorized pedals including a bicycle or tricycle.

j) A pedal cyclist is any person riding a pedal cycle or in a sidecar or trailer attached to a pedal cycle.

k) A motorcycle is a two-wheeled motor vehicle with one or two riding saddles and sometimes with a third wheel for the support of a sidecar. The sidecar is considered part of the motorcycle. This includes a moped, motor scooter, or motorized bicycle.

l) A motorcycle rider is any person riding a motorcycle or in a sidecar or trailer attached to the motorcycle.

m) A three-wheeled motor vehicle is a motorized tricycle designed primarily for on-road use. This includes a motor-driven tricycle, a motorized rickshaw, or a three-wheeled motor car.

n) A car [automobile] is a four-wheeled motor vehicle designed primarily for carrying up to 7 persons. A trailer being towed by the car is considered part of the car. It does not include a van or minivan - see definition

o) A pick-up truck or van is a four or six-wheeled motor vehicle designed for carrying passengers as well as property or cargo weighing less than the local limit for classification as a heavy goods vehicle, and not requiring a special driver's license. This includes a minivan and a sport-utility vehicle (SUV).

p) A heavy transport vehicle is a motor vehicle designed primarily for carrying property, meeting local criteria for classification as a heavy goods vehicle in terms of weight and requiring a special driver's license.

q) A bus (coach) is a motor vehicle designed or adapted primarily for carrying more than 10 passengers and requiring a special driver's license.

r) A railway train or railway vehicle is any device, with or without freight or passenger cars couple to it, designed for traffic on a railway track. This includes subterranean (subways) or elevated trains.

s) A streetcar, is a device designed and used primarily for transporting passengers within a municipality, running on rails, usually subject to normal traffic control signals, and operated principally on a right-of-way that forms part of the roadway. This includes a tram or trolley that runs on rails. A trailer being towed by a streetcar is considered part of the streetcar.

t) A special vehicle mainly used on industrial premises is a motor vehicle designed primarily for use within the buildings and premises of industrial or commercial establishments. This includes battery-powered airport passenger vehicles or baggage/mail trucks, forklifts, coal-cars in a coal mine, logging cars and trucks used in mines or quarries.

u) A special vehicle mainly used in agriculture is a motor vehicle designed specifically for use in farming and agriculture (horticulture), to work the land, tend and harvest crops and transport materials on the farm. This includes harvesters, farm machinery and tractor and trailers.

v) A special construction vehicle is a motor vehicle designed specifically for use on construction and demolition sites. This includes bulldozers, diggers, earth levellers, dump trucks. backhoes, front-end loaders, pavers, and mechanical shovels.

w) A special all-terrain vehicle is a motor vehicle of special design to enable it to negotiate over rough or soft terrain, snow or sand. Examples of special design are high construction, special wheels and tires, tracks, and support on a cushion of air. This includes snow mobiles, All-terrain vehicles (ATV), and dune buggies. It does not include passenger vehicle designated as Sport Utility Vehicles. (SUV)

x) A watercraft is any device designed for transporting passengers or goods on water. This includes motor or sail boats, ships, and hovercraft.

y) An aircraft is any device for transporting passengers or goods in the air. This includes hot-air balloons, gliders, helicopters and airplanes. (z) A military vehicle is any motorized vehicle operating on a public roadway owned by the military and being operated by a member of the military.

PEDESTRIAN INJURED IN TRANSPORT ACCIDENT (V00-V09)

Includes: person changing tire on transport vehicle

person examining engine of vehicle broken down in (on side of) road

Excludes1: fall due to non-transport collision with other person (W03)

pedestrian on foot falling (slipping) on ice and snow (W00.-)

struck or bumped by another person (W51)

V00 **Pedestrian conveyance accident**

Use additional place of occurrence and activity external cause codes, if known (Y92.-, Y93.-)

Excludes1: collision with another person without fall (W51)

fall due to person on foot colliding with another person on foot (W03)

fall from non-moving wheelchair, nonmotorized scooter and motorized mobility scooter without collision (W05.-)

pedestrian (conveyance) collision with other land transport vehicle (V01-V09)

pedestrian on foot falling (slipping) on ice and snow (W00.-)

The appropriate 7th character is to be added to each code from category V00

A - initial encounter

D - subsequent encounter

S - sequela

V00.0 **Pedestrian on foot injured in collision with pedestrian conveyance**

⊗⑦**V00.01** **Pedestrian on foot injured in collision with roller-skater**

⊗⑦**V00.02** **Pedestrian on foot injured in collision with skateboarder**

⊗⑦**V00.03** **Pedestrian on foot injured in collision with standing micro-mobility pedestrian conveyance**

⑦**V00.031** **Pedestrian on foot injured in collision with rider of standing electric scooter**

⑦**V00.038** **Pedestrian on foot injured in collision with rider of other standing micro-mobility pedestrian conveyance**

Pedestrian on foot injured in collision with rider of hoverboard

Pedestrian on foot injured in collision with rider of Segway

⊗⑦**V00.09** **Pedestrian on foot injured in collision with other pedestrian conveyance**

V00.1 **Rolling-type pedestrian conveyance accident**

Excludes1: accident with baby stroller (V00.82-)

accident with wheelchair (powered) (V00.81-)

accident with motorized mobility scooter (V00.83-)

V00.11 **In-line roller-skate accident**

⑦**V00.111** **Fall from in-line roller-skates**

⑦**V00.112** **In-line roller-skater colliding with stationary object**

⑦**V00.118** **Other in-line roller-skate accident**

Excludes1: roller-skater collision with other land transport vehicle (V01-V09 with 5th character 1)

V00.12 **Non-in- line roller-skate accident**

⑦**V00.121** **Fall from non-in-line roller-skates**

⑦**V00.122** **Non-in-line roller-skater colliding with stationary object**

⑦**V00.128** **Other non-in-line roller-skating accident**

Excludes1: roller-skater collision with other land transport vehicle (V01-V09 with 5th character 1)

V00.13 **Skateboard accident**

⑦**V00.131** **Fall from skateboard**

⑦**V00.132** **Skateboarder colliding with stationary object**

⑦**V00.138** **Other skateboard accident**

Excludes1: skateboarder collision with other land transport

● New code ▲ Revised code **Excludes1:** Not coded here **Excludes2:** Not included here ⊗ Placeholder required ⑦7th digit required

vehicle (V01-V09 with 5th character 2)

V00.14 Scooter (nonmotorized) accident

Excludes1: motor scooter accident (V20-V29)

⑦ **V00.141 Fall from scooter (nonmotorized)**

⑦ **V00.142 Scooter (nonmotorized) colliding with stationary object**

⑦ **V00.148 Other scooter (nonmotorized) accident**

Excludes1: scooter (nonmotorized) collision with other land transport vehicle (V01-V09 with fifth character 9)

V00.15 Heelies accident

Rolling shoe Wheeled shoe Wheelies accident

⑦ **V00.151 Fall from heelies**

⑦ **V00.152 Heelies colliding with stationary object**

⑦ **V00.158 Other heelies accident**

V00.18 Accident on other rolling-type pedestrian conveyance

⑦ **V00.181 Fall from other rolling-type pedestrian conveyance**

⑦ **V00.182 Pedestrian on other rolling-type pedestrian conveyance colliding with stationary object**

⑦ **V00.188 Other accident on other rolling-type pedestrian conveyance**

V00.2 Gliding-type pedestrian conveyance accident

V00.21 Ice-skates accident

⑦ **V00.211 Fall from ice-skates**

⑦ **V00.212 Ice-skater colliding with stationary object**

⑦ **V00.218 Other ice-skates accident**

Excludes1: ice-skater collision with other land transport vehicle (V01-V09 with 5th character 9)

V00.22 Sled accident

⑦ **V00.221 Fall from sled**

⑦ **V00.222 Sledder colliding with stationary object**

⑦ **V00.228 Other sled accident**

Excludes1: sled collision with other land transport vehicle (V01-V09 with 5th character 9)

V00.28 Other gliding-type pedestrian conveyance accident

⑦ **V00.281 Fall from other gliding-type pedestrian conveyance**

⑦ **V00.282 Pedestrian on other gliding-type pedestrian conveyance colliding with stationary object**

⑦ **V00.288 Other accident on other gliding-type pedestrian conveyance**

Excludes1: gliding-type pedestrian conveyance collision with other land transport vehicle (V01-V09 with 5th character 9)

V00.3 Flat-bottomed pedestrian conveyance accident

V00.31 Snowboard accident

⑦ **V00.311 Fall from snowboard**

⑦ **V00.312 Snowboarder colliding with stationary object**

⑦ **V00.318 Other snowboard accident**

Excludes1: snowboarder collision with other land transport vehicle (V01-V09 with 5th character 9)

V00.32 Snow-ski accident

⑦ **V00.321 Fall from snow-skis**

⑦ **V00.322 Snow-skier colliding with stationary object**

⑦ **V00.328 Other snow-ski accident**

Excludes1: snow-skier collision with other land transport vehicle (V01-V09 with 5th character 9)

V00.38 Other flat-bottomed pedestrian conveyance accident

⑦ **V00.381 Fall from other flat-bottomed pedestrian conveyance**

⑦ **V00.382 Pedestrian on other flat-bottomed pedestrian conveyance colliding with stationary object**

⑦ **V00.388 Other accident on other flat-bottomed pedestrian conveyance**

V00.8 Accident on other pedestrian conveyance

V00.81 Accident with wheelchair (powered)

⑦ **V00.811 Fall from moving wheelchair (powered)**

Excludes1: fall from non-moving wheelchair (W05.0)

⑦ **V00.812 Wheelchair (powered) colliding with stationary object**

⑦ **V00.818 Other accident with wheelchair (powered)**

V00.82 Accident with baby stroller

⑦ **V00.821 Fall from baby stroller**

⑦ **V00.822 Baby stroller colliding with stationary object**

⑦ **V00.828 Other accident with baby stroller**

V00.83 Accident with motorized mobility scooter

⑦ **V00.831 Fall from motorized mobility scooter**

Excludes1: fall from non-moving motorized mobility scooter (W05.2)

⑦ **V00.832 Motorized mobility scooter colliding with stationary object**

⑦ **V00.838 Other accident with motorized mobility scooter**

V00.84 Accident with standing micro-mobility pedestrian conveyance

⑦ **V00.841 Fall from standing electric scooter**

⑦ **V00.842 Pedestrian on standing electric scooter colliding with stationary object**

⑦ **V00.848 Other accident with standing micro-mobility pedestrian conveyance**

Accident with hoverboard

Accident with Segway

V00.89 Accident on other pedestrian conveyance

⑦ **V00.891 Fall from other pedestrian conveyance**

⑦**V00.892** **Pedestrian on other pedestrian conveyance colliding with stationary object**

⑦**V00.898** **Other accident on other pedestrian conveyance**

Excludes1: Other pedestrian (conveyance) collision with other land transport vehicle (V01-V09 with 5th character 9)

V01 **Pedestrian injured in collision with pedal cycle**

The appropriate 7th character is to be added to each code from category V01

A - initial encounter

D - subsequent encounter

S - sequela

V01.0 **Pedestrian injured in collision with pedal cycle in nontraffic accident**

⊗⑦**V01.00** **Pedestrian on foot injured in collision with pedal cycle in nontraffic accident**

Pedestrian NOS injured in collision with pedal cycle in nontraffic accident

⊗⑦**V01.01** **Pedestrian on roller-skates injured in collision with pedal cycle in nontraffic accident**

⊗⑦**V01.02** **Pedestrian on skateboard injured in collision with pedal cycle in nontraffic accident**

V01.03 **Pedestrian on standing micro-mobility pedestrian conveyance injured in collision with pedal cycle in nontraffic accident**

⑦**V01.031** **Pedestrian on standing electric scooter injured in collision with pedal cycle in nontraffic accident**

⑦**V01.038** **Pedestrian on other standing micro-mobility pedestrian conveyance injured in collision with pedal cycle in nontraffic accident**

Pedestrian on hoverboard injured in collision with pedal cycle in nontraffic accident

Pedestrian on Segway injured in collision with pedal cycle in nontraffic accident

⊗⑦**V01.09** **Pedestrian with other conveyance injured in collision with pedal cycle in nontraffic accident**

Pedestrian with baby stroller injured in collision with pedal cycle in nontraffic accident

Pedestrian on ice-skates injured in collision with pedal cycle in nontraffic accident

Pedestrian on nonmotorized scooter injured in collision with pedal cycle in nontraffic accident

Pedestrian on sled injured in collision with pedal cycle in nontraffic accident

Pedestrian on snowboard injured in collision with pedal cycle in nontraffic accident

Pedestrian on snow-skis injured in collision with pedal cycle in nontraffic accident

Pedestrian in wheelchair (powered) injured in collision with pedal cycle in nontraffic accident

Pedestrian in motorized mobility scooter injured in collision with pedal cycle in nontraffic accident

V01.1 **Pedestrian injured in collision with pedal cycle in traffic accident**

⊗⑦**V01.10** **Pedestrian on foot injured in collision with pedal cycle in traffic accident**

Pedestrian NOS injured in collision with pedal cycle in traffic accident

⊗⑦**V01.11** **Pedestrian on roller-skates injured in collision with pedal cycle in traffic accident**

⊗⑦**V01.12** **Pedestrian on skateboard injured in collision with pedal cycle in traffic accident**

V01.13 **Pedestrian on standing micro-mobility pedestrian conveyance injured in collision with pedal cycle in traffic accident**

⑦**V01.131** **Pedestrian on standing electric scooter injured in collision with pedal cycle in traffic accident**

⑦**V01.138** **Pedestrian on other standing micro-mobility pedestrian conveyance injured in collision with pedal cycle in traffic accident**

Pedestrian on hoverboard injured in collision with pedal cycle in traffic accident

Pedestrian on Segway injured in collision with pedal cycle in traffic accident

⊗⑦**V01.19** **Pedestrian with other conveyance injured in collision with pedal cycle in traffic accident**

Pedestrian with baby stroller injured in collision with pedal cycle in traffic accident

Pedestrian on ice-skates injured in collision with pedal cycle in traffic accident

Pedestrian on nonmotorized scooter injured in collision with pedal cycle in traffic accident

Pedestrian on sled injured in collision with pedal cycle in traffic accident

Pedestrian on snowboard injured in collision with pedal cycle in traffic accident

Pedestrian on snow-skis injured in collision with pedal cycle in traffic accident

Pedestrian in wheelchair (powered) injured in collision with pedal cycle in traffic accident

Pedestrian in motorized mobility scooter injured in collision with pedal cycle in traffic accident

V01.9 **Pedestrian injured in collision with pedal cycle, unspecified whether traffic or nontraffic accident**

⊗⑦**V01.90** **Pedestrian on foot injured in collision with pedal cycle, unspecified whether traffic or nontraffic accident**

Pedestrian NOS injured in collision with pedal cycle, unspecified whether traffic or nontraffic accident

⊗⑦**V01.91** **Pedestrian on roller-skates injured in collision with pedal cycle, unspecified whether traffic or nontraffic accident**

⊗⑦**V01.92** **Pedestrian on skateboard injured in collision with pedal cycle, unspecified whether traffic or nontraffic accident**

V01.93 **Pedestrian on standing micro-mobility pedestrian conveyance injured in collision with pedal cycle, unspecified whether traffic or nontraffic accident**

⑦**V01.931** **Pedestrian on standing electric scooter injured in collision with pedal cycle, unspecified whether traffic or nontraffic accident**

⑦**V01.938** **Pedestrian on other standing micro-mobility pedestrian conveyance injured in collision with pedal cycle, unspecified whether traffic or nontraffic accident**

Pedestrian on hoverboard injured in collision with pedal cycle, unspecified whether traffic or nontraffic accident

Pedestrian on Segway injured in collision with pedal cycle, unspecified whether traffic or nontraffic accident

⊗⑦**V01.99** **Pedestrian with other conveyance injured in collision with pedal cycle, unspecified whether traffic or nontraffic accident**

Pedestrian with baby stroller injured in collision with pedal cycle, unspecified whether traffic or nontraffic accident

Pedestrian on ice-skates injured in collision with pedal cycle unspecified, whether traffic or nontraffic accident

Pedestrian on nonmotorized scooter injured in collision with pedal cycle, unspecified whether traffic or nontraffic accident

Pedestrian on sled injured in collision with pedal cycle unspecified, whether traffic or nontraffic accident

Pedestrian on snowboard injured in collision with pedal cycle, unspecified whether traffic or nontraffic accident

Pedestrian on snow-skis injured in collision with pedal cycle, unspecified whether traffic or nontraffic accident

Pedestrian in wheelchair (powered) injured in collision with pedal cycle, unspecified whether traffic or nontraffic accident

Pedestrian in motorized mobility scooter injured in collision with pedal cycle, unspecified whether traffic or nontraffic accident

V02 **Pedestrian injured in collision with two- or three-wheeled motor vehicle**

The appropriate 7th character is to be added to each code from category V02

A - initial encounter

D - subsequent encounter

S - sequela

V02.0 **Pedestrian injured in collision with two- or three-wheeled motor vehicle in nontraffic accident**

⊗⑦**V02.00** **Pedestrian on foot injured in collision with two- or three-wheeled motor vehicle in nontraffic accident**

Pedestrian NOS injured in collision with two- or three-wheeled motor vehicle in nontraffic accident

⊗⑦**V02.01** **Pedestrian on roller-skates injured in collision with two- or three-wheeled motor vehicle in nontraffic accident**

⊗⑦**V02.02** **Pedestrian on skateboard injured in collision with two- or three-wheeled motor vehicle in nontraffic accident**

V02.03 **Pedestrian on standing micro-mobility pedestrian conveyance injured in collision with two- or three-wheeled motor vehicle in nontraffic accident**

⑦**V02.031** **Pedestrian on standing electric scooter injured in collision with two- or three-wheeled motor vehicle in nontraffic accident**

⑦**V02.038** **Pedestrian on other standing micro-mobility pedestrian conveyance injured in collision with two- or three-wheeled motor vehicle in nontraffic accident**

Pedestrian on hoverboard injured in collision with two- or three wheeled motor vehicle in nontraffic accident

Pedestrian on Segway injured in collision with two- or three-wheeled motor vehicle in nontraffic accident

⊗⑦**V02.09** **Pedestrian with other conveyance injured in collision with two- or three-wheeled motor vehicle in nontraffic accident**

Pedestrian with baby stroller injured in collision with two- or three-wheeled motor vehicle in nontraffic accident

Pedestrian on ice-skates injured in collision with two- or three-wheeled motor vehicle in nontraffic accident

Pedestrian on nonmotorized scooter injured in collision with two- or three-wheeled motor vehicle in nontraffic accident

Pedestrian on sled injured in collision with two- or three-wheeled motor vehicle in nontraffic accident

Pedestrian on snowboard injured in collision with two- or three-wheeled motor vehicle in nontraffic accident

Pedestrian on snow-skis injured in collision with two- or three-wheeled motor vehicle in nontraffic accident

Pedestrian in wheelchair (powered) injured in collision with two- or three-wheeled motor vehicle in nontraffic accident

Pedestrian in motorized mobility scooter injured in collision with two- or three-wheeled motor vehicle in nontraffic accident

V02.1 **Pedestrian injured in collision with two- or three-wheeled motor vehicle in traffic accident**

⊗⑦**V02.10** **Pedestrian on foot injured in collision with two- or three-wheeled motor vehicle in traffic accident**

Pedestrian NOS injured in collision with two- or three-wheeled motor vehicle in traffic accident

⊗⑦**V02.11** **Pedestrian on roller-skates injured in collision with two- or three-wheeled motor vehicle in traffic accident**

⊗⑦**V02.12** **Pedestrian on skateboard injured in collision with two- or three-wheeled motor vehicle in traffic accident**

V02.13 **Pedestrian on standing micro-mobility pedestrian conveyance injured in collision with two- or three-wheeled motor vehicle in traffic accident**

⑦**V02.131** **Pedestrian on standing electric scooter injured in collision with two- or three-wheeled motor vehicle in traffic accident**

⑦**V02.138** **Pedestrian on other standing micro-mobility pedestrian conveyance injured in collision with two- or three-wheeled motor vehicle in traffic accident**

Pedestrian on hoverboard injured in collision with two- or three wheeled motor vehicle in traffic accident
Pedestrian on Segway injured in collision with two- or three-wheeled motor vehicle in traffic accident

⊗⑦**V02.19** **Pedestrian with other conveyance injured in collision with two- or three-wheeled motor vehicle in traffic accident**

Pedestrian with baby stroller injured in collision with two- or three-wheeled motor vehicle in traffic accident

Pedestrian on ice-skates injured in collision with two- or three-wheeled motor vehicle in traffic accident

Pedestrian on nonmotorized scooter injured in collision with two- or three-wheeled motor vehicle in traffic accident

Pedestrian on sled injured in collision with two- or three-wheeled motor vehicle in traffic accident

Pedestrian on snowboard injured in collision with two- or three-wheeled motor vehicle in traffic accident

Pedestrian on snow-skis injured in collision with two- or three-wheeled motor vehicle in traffic accident

Pedestrian in wheelchair (powered) injured in collision with two- or three-wheeled motor vehicle in traffic accident

Pedestrian in motorized mobility scooter injured in collision with two- or three-wheeled motor vehicle in traffic accident

V02.9 Pedestrian injured in collision with two- or three-wheeled motor vehicle, unspecified whether traffic or nontraffic accident

⊗⑦**V02.90 Pedestrian on foot injured in collision with two- or three-wheeled motor vehicle, unspecified whether traffic or nontraffic accident**

Pedestrian NOS injured in collision with two- or three-wheeled motor vehicle, unspecified whether traffic or nontraffic accident

⊗⑦**V02.91 Pedestrian on roller-skates injured in collision with two- or three-wheeled motor vehicle, unspecified whether traffic or nontraffic accident**

⊗⑦**V02.92 Pedestrian on skateboard injured in collision with two- or three-wheeled motor vehicle, unspecified whether traffic or nontraffic accident**

V02.93 Pedestrian on standing micro-mobility pedestrian conveyance injured in collision with two- or three-wheeled motor vehicle, unspecified whether traffic or nontraffic accident

⑦**V02.931 Pedestrian on standing electric scooter injured in collision with two- or three wheeled motor vehicle, unspecified whether traffic or nontraffic accident**

⑦**V02.938 Pedestrian on other standing micro-mobility pedestrian conveyance injured in collision with two- or three wheeled motor vehicle, unspecified whether traffic or nontraffic accident**

Pedestrian on hoverboard injured in collision with two-three-wheeled motor vehicle, unspecified whether traffic or nontraffic accident

Pedestrian on Segway injured in collision with two- or three wheeled motor vehicle, unspecified whether traffic or nontraffic accident

⊗⑦**V02.99 Pedestrian with other conveyance injured in collision with two- or three-wheeled motor vehicle, unspecified whether traffic or nontraffic accident**

Pedestrian with baby stroller injured in collision with two- or three-wheeled motor vehicle, unspecified whether traffic or nontraffic accident

Pedestrian on ice-skates injured in collision with two- or three-wheeled motor vehicle, unspecified whether traffic or nontraffic accident

Pedestrian on nonmotorized scooter injured in collision with two- or three-wheeled motor vehicle, unspecified whether traffic or nontraffic accident

Pedestrian on sled injured in collision with two- or three-wheeled motor vehicle, unspecified whether traffic or nontraffic accident

Pedestrian on snowboard injured in collision with two- or three-wheeled motor vehicle, unspecified whether traffic or nontraffic accident

Pedestrian on snow-skis injured in collision with two- or three-wheeled motor vehicle, unspecified whether traffic or nontraffic accident

Pedestrian in wheelchair (powered) injured in collision with two- or three-wheeled motor vehicle, unspecified whether traffic or nontraffic accident

Pedestrian in motorized mobility scooter injured in collision with two- or three-wheeled motor vehicle, unspecified whether traffic or nontraffic accident

V03 Pedestrian injured in collision with car, pick-up truck or van

The appropriate 7th character is to be added to each code from category V03

A - initial encounter

D - subsequent encounter

S - sequela

V03.0 Pedestrian injured in collision with car, pick-up truck or van in nontraffic accident

⊗⑦**V03.00 Pedestrian on foot injured in collision with car, pick-up truck or van in nontraffic accident**

Pedestrian NOS injured in collision with car, pick-up truck or van in nontraffic accident

⊗⑦**V03.01 Pedestrian on roller-skates injured in collision with car, pick-up truck or van in nontraffic accident**

⊗⑦**V03.02 Pedestrian on skateboard injured in collision with car, pick-up truck or van in nontraffic accident**

V03.03 Pedestrian on standing micro-mobility pedestrian conveyance injured in collision with car, pick-up or van in nontraffic accident

⑦**V03.031 Pedestrian on standing electric scooter injured in collision with car, pick-up or van in nontraffic accident**

⑦**V03.038 Pedestrian on other standing micro-mobility pedestrian conveyance injured in collision with car, pick-up or van in nontraffic accident**

Pedestrian on hoverboard injured in collision with car, pick-up or van in nontraffic accident

Pedestrian on Segway injured in collision with car, pick-up or van in nontraffic accident

⊗⑦**V03.09 Pedestrian with other conveyance injured in collision with car, pick-up truck or van in nontraffic accident**

Pedestrian with baby stroller injured in collision with car, pick-up truck or van in nontraffic accident

● New code ▲ Revised code **Excludes1:** Not coded here **Excludes2:** Not included here ⊗ Placeholder required ⑦ 7th digit required

Pedestrian on ice-skates injured in collision with car, pick-up truck or van in nontraffic accident

Pedestrian on nonmotorized scooter injured in collision with car, pick-up truck or van in nontraffic accident

Pedestrian on sled injured in collision with car, pick-up truck or van in nontraffic accident

Pedestrian on snowboard injured in collision with car, pick-up truck or van in nontraffic accident

Pedestrian on snow-skis injured in collision with car, pick-up truck or van in nontraffic accident

Pedestrian in wheelchair (powered) injured in collision with car, pick-up truck or van in nontraffic accident

Pedestrian in motorized mobility scooter injured in collision with car, pick-up truck or van in nontraffic accident

V03.1 Pedestrian injured in collision with car, pick-up truck or van in traffic accident

⊗7**V03.10 Pedestrian on foot injured in collision with car, pick-up truck or van in traffic accident**

Pedestrian NOS injured in collision with car, pick-up truck or van in traffic accident

⊗7**V03.11 Pedestrian on roller-skates injured in collision with car, pick-up truck or van in traffic accident**

⊗7**V03.12 Pedestrian on skateboard injured in collision with car, pick-up truck or van in traffic accident**

V03.13 Pedestrian on standing micro-mobility pedestrian conveyance injured in collision with car, pick-up or van in traffic accident

7**V03.131 Pedestrian on standing electric scooter injured in collision with car, pick-up or van in traffic accident**

7**V03.138 Pedestrian on other standing micro-mobility pedestrian conveyance injured in collision with car, pick-up or van in traffic accident**

Pedestrian on hoverboard injured in collision with car, pick-up or van in traffic accident

Pedestrian on Segway injured in collision with car, pick-up or van in traffic accident

⊗7**V03.19 Pedestrian with other conveyance injured in collision with car, pick-up truck or van in traffic accident**

Pedestrian with baby stroller injured in collision with car, pick-up truck or van in traffic accident

Pedestrian on ice-skates injured in collision with car, pick-up truck or van in traffic accident

Pedestrian on nonmotorized scooter injured in collision with car, pick-up truck or van in traffic accident

Pedestrian on sled injured in collision with car, pick-up truck or van in traffic accident

Pedestrian on snowboard injured in collision with car, pick-up truck or van in traffic accident

Pedestrian on snow-skis injured in collision with car, pick-up truck or van in traffic accident

Pedestrian in wheelchair (powered) injured in collision with car, pick-up truck or van in traffic accident

Pedestrian in motorized mobility scooter injured in collision with car, pick-up truck or van in traffic accident

V03.9 Pedestrian injured in collision with car, pick-up truck or van, unspecified whether traffic or nontraffic accident

⊗7**V03.90 Pedestrian on foot injured in collision with car, pick-up truck or van, unspecified whether traffic or nontraffic accident**

Pedestrian NOS injured in collision with car, pick-up truck or van, unspecified whether traffic or nontraffic accident

⊗7**V03.91 Pedestrian on roller-skates injured in collision with car, pick-up truck or van, unspecified whether traffic or nontraffic accident**

⊗7**V03.92 Pedestrian on skateboard injured in collision with car, pick-up truck or van, unspecified whether traffic or nontraffic accident**

V03.93 Pedestrian on standing micro-mobility pedestrian conveyance injured in collision with car, pick-up or van, unspecified whether traffic or nontraffic accident

7**V03.931 Pedestrian on standing electric scooter injured in collision with car, pick-up or van, unspecified whether traffic or nontraffic accident**

7**V03.938 Pedestrian on other standing micro-mobility pedestrian conveyance injured in collision with car, pick-up or van, unspecified whether traffic or nontraffic accident**

Pedestrian on hoverboard injured in collision with car, pick-up or van, unspecified whether traffic or nontraffic accident

Pedestrian on Segway injured in collision with car, pick-up or van, unspecified whether traffic or nontraffic accident

⊗7**V03.99 Pedestrian with other conveyance injured in collision with car, pick-up truck or van, unspecified whether traffic or nontraffic accident**

Pedestrian with baby stroller injured in collision with car, pick-up truck or van, unspecified whether traffic or nontraffic accident

Pedestrian on ice-skates injured in collision with car, pick-up truck or van, unspecified whether traffic or nontraffic accident

Pedestrian on nonmotorized scooter injured in collision with car, pick-up truck or van, unspecified whether traffic or nontraffic accident

Pedestrian on sled injured in collision with car, pick-up truck or van in nontraffic accident

Pedestrian on snowboard injured in collision with car, pick-up truck or van, unspecified whether traffic or nontraffic accident

Pedestrian on snow-skis injured in collision with car, pick-up truck or van, unspecified whether traffic or nontraffic accident

Pedestrian in wheelchair (powered) injured in collision with car, pick-up truck or van, unspecified whether traffic or nontraffic accident

Pedestrian in motorized mobility scooter injured in collision with car, pick-up truck or van, unspecified whether traffic or nontraffic accident

V04 Pedestrian injured in collision with heavy transport vehicle or bus

Excludes1: pedestrian injured in collision with military vehicle

(V09.01, V09.21)

The appropriate 7th character is to be added to each code from category V04

A - initial encounter

D - subsequent encounter

S - sequela

V04.0 **Pedestrian injured in collision with heavy transport vehicle or bus in nontraffic accident**

⊗⑦**V04.00** **Pedestrian on foot injured in collision with heavy transport vehicle or bus in nontraffic accident**

Pedestrian NOS injured in collision with heavy transport vehicle or bus in nontraffic accident

⊗⑦**V04.01** **Pedestrian on roller-skates injured in collision with heavy transport vehicle or bus in nontraffic accident**

⊗⑦**V04.02** **Pedestrian on skateboard injured in collision with heavy transport vehicle or bus in nontraffic accident**

⑦**V04.03** **Pedestrian on standing micro-mobility pedestrian conveyance injured in collision with heavy transport vehicle or bus in nontraffic accident**

⑦**V04.031** **Pedestrian on standing electric scooter injured in collision with heavy transport vehicle or bus in nontraffic accident**

⑦**V04.038** **Pedestrian on other standing micro-mobility pedestrian conveyance injured in collision with heavy transport vehicle or bus in nontraffic accident**

Pedestrian on hoverboard injured in collision with heavy transport vehicle or bus in nontraffic accident

Pedestrian on Segway injured in collision with heavy transport vehicle or bus in nontraffic accident

⑦**V04.09** **Pedestrian with other conveyance injured in collision with heavy transport vehicle or bus in nontraffic accident**

Pedestrian with baby stroller injured in collision with heavy transport vehicle or bus in nontraffic accident

Pedestrian on ice-skates injured in collision with heavy transport vehicle or bus in nontraffic accident

Pedestrian on nonmotorized scooter injured in collision with heavy transport vehicle or bus in nontraffic accident

Pedestrian on sled injured in collision with heavy transport vehicle or bus in nontraffic accident

Pedestrian on snowboard injured in collision with heavy transport vehicle or bus in nontraffic accident

Pedestrian on snow-skis injured in collision with heavy transport vehicle or bus in nontraffic accident

Pedestrian in wheelchair (powered) injured in collision with heavy transport vehicle or bus in nontraffic accident

Pedestrian in motorized mobility scooter injured in collision with heavy transport vehicle or bus in nontraffic accident

V04.1 **Pedestrian injured in collision with heavy transport vehicle or bus in traffic accident**

⊗⑦**V04.10** **Pedestrian on foot injured in collision with heavy transport vehicle or bus in traffic accident**

Pedestrian NOS injured in collision with heavy transport vehicle or bus in traffic accident

⊗⑦**V04.11** **Pedestrian on roller-skates injured in collision with heavy transport vehicle or bus in traffic accident**

⊗⑦**V04.12** **Pedestrian on skateboard injured in collision with heavy transport vehicle or bus in traffic**

V04.13 **Pedestrian on standing micro-mobility pedestrian conveyance injured in collision with heavy transport vehicle or bus in traffic accident**

⑦**V04.131** **Pedestrian on standing electric scooter injured in collision with heavy transport vehicle or bus in traffic accident**

⑦**V04.138** **Pedestrian on other standing micro-mobility pedestrian conveyance injured in collision with heavy transport vehicle or bus in traffic accident**

Pedestrian on hoverboard injured in collision with heavy transport vehicle or bus in traffic accident

Pedestrian on Segway injured in collision with heavy transport vehicle or bus in traffic accident

⊗⑦**V04.19** **Pedestrian with other conveyance injured in collision with heavy transport vehicle or bus in traffic accident**

Pedestrian with baby stroller injured in collision with heavy transport vehicle or bus in traffic accident

Pedestrian on ice-skates injured in collision with heavy transport vehicle or bus in traffic accident

Pedestrian on nonmotorized scooter injured in collision with heavy transport vehicle or bus in traffic accident

Pedestrian on sled injured in collision with heavy transport vehicle or bus in traffic accident

Pedestrian on snowboard injured in collision with heavy transport vehicle or bus in traffic accident

Pedestrian on snow-skis injured in collision with heavy transport vehicle or bus in traffic accident

Pedestrian in wheelchair (powered) injured in collision with heavy transport vehicle or bus in traffic accident

Pedestrian in motorized mobility scooter injured in collision with heavy transport vehicle or bus in traffic accident

V04.9 **Pedestrian injured in collision with heavy transport vehicle or bus, unspecified whether traffic or nontraffic accident**

⊗⑦**V04.90** **Pedestrian on foot injured in collision with heavy transport vehicle or bus, unspecified whether traffic or nontraffic accident**

Pedestrian NOS injured in collision with heavy transport vehicle or bus, unspecified whether traffic or nontraffic accident

⊗⑦**V04.91** **Pedestrian on roller-skates injured in collision with heavy transport vehicle or bus, unspecified whether traffic or nontraffic accident**

⊗⑦**V04.92** **Pedestrian on skateboard injured in collision with heavy transport vehicle or bus, unspecified whether traffic or nontraffic accident**

● New code ▲ Revised code **Excludes1:** Not coded here **Excludes2:** Not included here ⊗ Placeholder required ⑦ 7th digit required

V04.93 Pedestrian on standing micro-mobility pedestrian conveyance injured in collision with heavy transport vehicle or bus, unspecified whether traffic or nontraffic accident

⑦**V04.931 Pedestrian on standing electric scooter injured in collision with heavy transport vehicle or bus, unspecified whether traffic or nontraffic accident**

⑦**V04.938 Pedestrian on other standing micro-mobility pedestrian conveyance injured in collision with heavy transport vehicle or bus, unspecified whether traffic or nontraffic accident**

Pedestrian on hoverboard injured in collision with heavy transport vehicle or bus, unspecified whether traffic or nontraffic accident

Pedestrian on Segway injured in collision with heavy transport vehicle or bus, unspecified whether traffic or nontraffic accident

⊗⑦**V04.99 Pedestrian with other conveyance injured in collision with heavy transport vehicle or bus, unspecified whether traffic or nontraffic accident**

Pedestrian with baby stroller injured in collision with heavy transport vehicle or bus, unspecified whether traffic or nontraffic accident

Pedestrian on ice-skates injured in collision with heavy transport vehicle or bus, unspecified whether traffic or nontraffic accident

Pedestrian on nonmotorized scooter injured in collision with heavy transport vehicle or bus, unspecified whether traffic or nontraffic accident

Pedestrian on sled injured in collision with heavy transport vehicle or bus, unspecified whether traffic or nontraffic accident

Pedestrian on snowboard injured in collision with heavy transport vehicle or bus, unspecified whether traffic or nontraffic accident

Pedestrian on snow-skis injured in collision with heavy transport vehicle or bus, unspecified whether traffic or nontraffic accident

Pedestrian in wheelchair (powered) injured in collision with heavy transport vehicle or bus, unspecified whether traffic or nontraffic accident

Pedestrian in motorized mobility scooter injured in collision with heavy transport vehicle or bus, unspecified whether traffic or nontraffic accident

V05 Pedestrian injured in collision with railway train or railway vehicle

The appropriate 7th character is to be added to each code from category V05

A - initial encounter

D - subsequent encounter

S - sequela

V05.0 Pedestrian injured in collision with railway train or railway vehicle in nontraffic accident

⊗⑦**V05.00 Pedestrian on foot injured in collision with railway train or railway vehicle in nontraffic accident**

Pedestrian NOS injured in collision with railway train or railway vehicle in nontraffic accident

⊗⑦**V05.01 Pedestrian on roller-skates injured in collision with railway train or railway vehicle in nontraffic accident**

⊗⑦**V05.02 Pedestrian on skateboard injured in collision with railway train or railway vehicle in nontraffic accident**

V05.03 Pedestrian on standing micro-mobility pedestrian conveyance injured in collision with railway train or railway vehicle in nontraffic accident

⑦**V05.031 Pedestrian on standing electric scooter injured in collision with railway train or railway vehicle in nontraffic accident**

⑦**V05.038 Pedestrian on other standing micro-mobility pedestrian conveyance injured in collision with railway train or railway vehicle in nontraffic accident**

Pedestrian on hoverboard injured in collision with railway train or railway vehicle in nontraffic accident

Pedestrian on Segway injured in collision with railway train or railway vehicle in nontraffic accident

⊗⑦**V05.09 Pedestrian with other conveyance injured in collision with railway train or railway vehicle in nontraffic accident**

Pedestrian with baby stroller injured in collision with railway train or railway vehicle in nontraffic accident

Pedestrian on ice-skates injured in collision with railway train or railway vehicle in nontraffic accident

Pedestrian on nonmotorized scooter injured in collision with railway train or railway vehicle in nontraffic accident

Pedestrian on sled injured in collision with railway train or railway vehicle in nontraffic accident

Pedestrian on snowboard injured in collision with railway train or railway vehicle in nontraffic accident

Pedestrian on snow-skis injured in collision with railway train or railway vehicle in nontraffic accident

Pedestrian in wheelchair (powered) injured in collision with railway train or railway vehicle in nontraffic accident

Pedestrian in motorized mobility scooter injured in collision with railway train or railway vehicle in nontraffic accident

V05.1 Pedestrian injured in collision with railway train or railway vehicle in traffic accident

⊗⑦**V05.10 Pedestrian on foot injured in collision with railway train or railway vehicle in traffic accident**

Pedestrian NOS injured in collision with railway train or railway vehicle in traffic accident

⊗⑦**V05.11 Pedestrian on roller-skates injured in collision with railway train or railway vehicle in traffic accident**

⊗⑦**V05.12 Pedestrian on skateboard injured in collision with railway train or railway vehicle in traffic accident**

V05.13 Pedestrian on standing micro-mobility pedestrian conveyance injured in collision with railway train or railway vehicle in traffic accident

⑦**V05.131 Pedestrian on standing electric scooter injured in collision with** railway train or railway vehicle in traffic accident

⑦V05.138 **Pedestrian on other standing micro-mobility pedestrian conveyance injured in collision with railway train or railway vehicle in traffic accident**

Pedestrian on hoverboard injured in collision with railway train or railway vehicle in traffic accident

Pedestrian on Segway injured in collision with railway train or railway vehicle in traffic accident

⊗⑦V05.19 **Pedestrian with other conveyance injured in collision with railway train or railway vehicle in traffic accident**

Pedestrian with baby stroller injured in collision with railway train or railway vehicle in traffic accident

Pedestrian on ice-skates injured in collision with railway train or railway vehicle in traffic accident

Pedestrian on nonmotorized scooter injured in collision with railway train or railway vehicle in traffic accident

Pedestrian on sled injured in collision with railway train or railway vehicle in traffic accident

Pedestrian on snowboard injured in collision with railway train or railway vehicle in traffic accident

Pedestrian on snow-skis injured in collision with railway train or railway vehicle in traffic accident

Pedestrian in wheelchair (powered) injured in collision with railway train or railway vehicle in traffic accident

Pedestrian in motorized mobility scooter injured in collision with railway train or railway vehicle in traffic accident

V05.9 **Pedestrian injured in collision with railway train or railway vehicle, unspecified whether traffic or nontraffic accident**

⊗⑦V05.90 **Pedestrian on foot injured in collision with railway train or railway vehicle, unspecified whether traffic or nontraffic accident**

Pedestrian NOS injured in collision with railway train or railway vehicle, unspecified whether traffic or nontraffic accident

⊗⑦V05.91 **Pedestrian on roller-skates injured in collision with railway train or railway vehicle, unspecified whether traffic or nontraffic accident**

⊗⑦V05.92 **Pedestrian on skateboard injured in collision with railway train or railway vehicle, unspecified whether traffic or nontraffic accident**

V05.93 **Pedestrian on standing micro-mobility pedestrian conveyance injured in collision with railway train or railway vehicle, unspecified whether traffic or nontraffic accident**

⑦V05.931 **Pedestrian on standing electric scooter injured in collision with railway train or railway vehicle, unspecified whether traffic or nontraffic accident**

⑦V05.938 **Pedestrian on other standing micro-mobility pedestrian conveyance injured in collision with railway train or railway vehicle, unspecified whether traffic or nontraffic accident**

Pedestrian on hoverboard injured in collision with railway train or railway vehicle, unspecified whether traffic or nontraffic accident

Pedestrian on Segway injured in collision with railway train or railway vehicle, unspecified whether traffic or nontraffic accident

⊗⑦V05.99 **Pedestrian with other conveyance injured in collision with railway train or railway vehicle, unspecified whether traffic or nontraffic accident**

Pedestrian with baby stroller injured in collision with railway train or railway vehicle, unspecified whether traffic or nontraffic

Pedestrian on ice-skates injured in collision with railway train or railway vehicle, unspecified whether traffic or nontraffic

Pedestrian on nonmotorized scooter injured in collision with railway train or railway vehicle, unspecified whether traffic or nontraffic

Pedestrian on sled injured in collision with railway train or railway vehicle, unspecified whether traffic or nontraffic

Pedestrian on snowboard injured in collision with railway train or railway vehicle, unspecified whether traffic or nontraffic

Pedestrian on snow-skis injured in collision with railway train or railway vehicle, unspecified whether traffic or nontraffic

Pedestrian in wheelchair (powered) injured in collision with railway train or railway vehicle, unspecified whether traffic or nontraffic

Pedestrian in motorized mobility scooter injured in collision with railway train or railway vehicle, unspecified whether traffic or nontraffic

V06 **Pedestrian injured in collision with other nonmotor vehicle**

Includes: collision with animal-drawn vehicle, animal being ridden, nonpowered streetcar

Excludes1: pedestrian injured in collision with pedestrian conveyance (V00.0-)

The appropriate 7th character is to be added to each code from category V06

A - initial encounter

D - subsequent encounter

S - sequela

V06.0 **Pedestrian injured in collision with other nonmotor vehicle in nontraffic accident**

⊗⑦V06.00 **Pedestrian on foot injured in collision with other nonmotor vehicle in nontraffic accident**

Pedestrian NOS injured in collision with other nonmotor vehicle in nontraffic accident

⊗⑦V06.01 **Pedestrian on roller-skates injured in collision with other nonmotor vehicle in nontraffic accident**

⊗⑦V06.02 **Pedestrian on skateboard injured in collision with other nonmotor vehicle in nontraffic accident**

V06.03 **Pedestrian on standing micro-mobility pedestrian conveyance injured in collision with other nonmotor vehicle in nontraffic accident**

⑦V06.031 **Pedestrian on standing electric scooter injured in collision with other nonmotor vehicle in nontraffic accident**

● New code ▲ Revised code **Excludes1:** Not coded here **Excludes2:** Not included here ⊗ Placeholder required ⑦ 7ᵗʰ digit required

⑦**V06.038** **Pedestrian on other standing micro-mobility pedestrian conveyance injured in collision with other nonmotor vehicle in nontraffic accident**

Pedestrian on hoverboard injured in collision with other nonmotor vehicle in nontraffic accident

Pedestrian on Segway injured in collision with other nonmotor vehicle in nontraffic accident

⊗⑦**V06.09** **Pedestrian with other conveyance injured in collision with other nonmotor vehicle in nontraffic accident**

Pedestrian with baby stroller injured in collision with other nonmotor vehicle in nontraffic accident

Pedestrian on ice-skates injured in collision with other nonmotor vehicle in nontraffic accident

Pedestrian on nonmotorized scooter injured in collision with other nonmotor vehicle in nontraffic accident

Pedestrian on sled injured in collision with other nonmotor vehicle in nontraffic accident

Pedestrian on snowboard injured in collision with other nonmotor vehicle in nontraffic accident

Pedestrian on snow-skis injured in collision with other nonmotor vehicle in nontraffic accident

Pedestrian in wheelchair (powered) injured in collision with other nonmotor vehicle in nontraffic accident

Pedestrian in motorized mobility scooter injured in collision with other nonmotor vehicle in nontraffic accident

V06.1 **Pedestrian injured in collision with other nonmotor vehicle in traffic accident**

⊗⑦**V06.10** **Pedestrian on foot injured in collision with other nonmotor vehicle in traffic accident**

Pedestrian NOS injured in collision with other nonmotor vehicle in traffic accident

⊗⑦**V06.11** **Pedestrian on roller-skates injured in collision with other nonmotor vehicle in traffic accident**

⊗⑦**V06.12** **Pedestrian on skateboard injured in collision with other nonmotor vehicle in traffic accident**

V06.13 **Pedestrian on standing micro-mobility pedestrian conveyance injured in collision with other nonmotor vehicle in traffic accident**

⑦**V06.131** **Pedestrian on standing electric scooter injured in collision with other nonmotor vehicle in traffic accident**

⑦**V06.138** **Pedestrian on other standing micro-mobility pedestrian conveyance injured in collision with other nonmotor vehicle in traffic accident**

Pedestrian on hoverboard injured in collision with other nonmotor vehicle in traffic accident

Pedestrian on Segway injured in collision with other nonmotor vehicle in traffic accident

⊗⑦**V06.19** **Pedestrian with other conveyance injured in collision with other nonmotor vehicle in traffic accident**

Pedestrian with baby stroller injured in collision with other nonmotor vehicle in nontraffic accident

Pedestrian on ice-skates injured in collision with other nonmotor vehicle in traffic accident

Pedestrian on nonmotorized scooter injured in collision with other nonmotor vehicle in traffic accident

Pedestrian on sled injured in collision with other nonmotor vehicle in traffic accident

Pedestrian on snowboard injured in collision with other nonmotor vehicle in traffic accident

Pedestrian on snow-skis injured in collision with other nonmotor vehicle in traffic accident

Pedestrian in wheelchair (powered) injured in collision with other nonmotor vehicle in traffic accident

Pedestrian in motorized mobility scooter injured in collision with other nonmotor vehicle in traffic accident

V06.9 **Pedestrian injured in collision with other nonmotor vehicle, unspecified whether traffic or nontraffic accident**

⊗⑦**V06.90** **Pedestrian on foot injured in collision with other nonmotor vehicle, unspecified whether traffic or nontraffic accident**

Pedestrian NOS injured in collision with other nonmotor vehicle, unspecified whether traffic or nontraffic accident

⊗⑦**V06.91** **Pedestrian on roller-skates injured in collision with other nonmotor vehicle, unspecified whether traffic or nontraffic accident**

⊗⑦**V06.92** **Pedestrian on skateboard injured in collision with other nonmotor vehicle, unspecified whether traffic or nontraffic accident**

V06.93 **Pedestrian on standing micro-mobility pedestrian conveyance injured in collision with other nonmotor vehicle, unspecified whether traffic or nontraffic accident**

⑦**V06.931** **Pedestrian on standing electric scooter injured in collision with other nonmotor vehicle, unspecified whether traffic or nontraffic accident**

⑦**V06.938** **Pedestrian on other standing micro-mobility pedestrian conveyance injured in collision with other nonmotor vehicle, unspecified whether traffic or nontraffic accident**

Pedestrian on hoverboard injured in collision with other nonmotor, unspecified whether traffic or nontraffic accident

Pedestrian on Segway injured in collision with other nonmotor vehicle, unspecified whether traffic or nontraffic accident

⊗⑦**V06.99** **Pedestrian with other conveyance injured in collision with other nonmotor vehicle, unspecified whether traffic or nontraffic accident**

Pedestrian with baby stroller injured in collision with other nonmotor vehicle, unspecified whether traffic or nontraffic accident

Pedestrian on ice-skates injured in collision with other nonmotor vehicle, unspecified whether traffic or nontraffic accident

Pedestrian on nonmotorized scooter injured in collision with other nonmotor vehicle, unspecified whether traffic or nontraffic accident

Pedestrian on sled injured in collision with other nonmotor vehicle, unspecified whether traffic or nontraffic accident

Pedestrian on snowboard injured in collision with other nonmotor vehicle, unspecified whether traffic or nontraffic accident

Pedestrian on snow-skis injured in collision with other nonmotor vehicle, unspecified whether traffic or nontraffic accident

Pedestrian in wheelchair (powered) injured in collision with other nonmotor vehicle, unspecified whether traffic or nontraffic accident

Pedestrian in motorized mobility scooter injured in collision with other nonmotor vehicle, unspecified whether traffic or nontraffic accident

V09 **Pedestrian injured in other and unspecified transport accidents**

The appropriate 7th character is to be added to each code from category V09

A - initial encounter

D - subsequent encounter

S - sequela

V09.0 **Pedestrian injured in nontraffic accident involving other and unspecified motor vehicles**

⊗⑦**V09.00** Pedestrian injured in nontraffic accident involving unspecified motor vehicles

⊗⑦**V09.01** Pedestrian injured in nontraffic accident involving military vehicle

⊗⑦**V09.09** Pedestrian injured in nontraffic accident involving other motor vehicles

Pedestrian injured in nontraffic accident by special vehicle

⊗⑦**V09.1** **Pedestrian injured in unspecified nontraffic accident**

V09.2 **Pedestrian injured in traffic accident involving other and unspecified motor vehicles**

⊗⑦**V09.20** Pedestrian injured in traffic accident involving unspecified motor vehicles

⊗⑦**V09.21** Pedestrian injured in traffic accident involving military vehicle

⊗⑦**V09.29** Pedestrian injured in traffic accident involving other motor vehicles

⊗⑦**V09.3** **Pedestrian injured in unspecified traffic accident**

⊗⑦**V09.9** **Pedestrian injured in unspecified transport accident**

PEDAL CYCLE RIDER INJURED IN TRANSPORT ACCIDENT (V10-V19)

Includes: any non-motorized vehicle, excluding an animal-drawn vehicle, or a sidecar or trailer attached to the pedal cycle

Excludes2: rupture of pedal cycle tire (W37.0)

V10 **Pedal cycle rider injured in collision with pedestrian or animal**

Excludes1: pedal cycle rider collision with animal-drawn vehicle or animal being ridden (V16.-)

The appropriate 7th character is to be added to each code from category V10

A - initial encounter

D - subsequent encounter

S - sequela

⊗⑦**V10.0** **Pedal cycle driver injured in collision with pedestrian or animal in nontraffic accident**

⊗⑦**V10.1** **Pedal cycle passenger injured in collision with pedestrian or animal in nontraffic accident**

⊗⑦**V10.2** **Unspecified pedal cyclist injured in collision with pedestrian or animal in nontraffic accident**

⊗⑦**V10.3** **Person boarding or alighting a pedal cycle injured in collision with pedestrian or animal**

⊗⑦**V10.4** **Pedal cycle driver injured in collision with pedestrian or animal in traffic accident**

⊗⑦**V10.5** **Pedal cycle passenger injured in collision with pedestrian or animal in traffic accident**

⊗⑦**V10.9** **Unspecified pedal cyclist injured in collision with pedestrian or animal in traffic accident**

V11 **Pedal cycle rider injured in collision with other pedal cycle**

The appropriate 7th character is to be added to each code from category V11

A - initial encounter

D - subsequent encounter

S - sequela

⊗⑦**V11.0** **Pedal cycle driver injured in collision with other pedal cycle in nontraffic accident**

⊗⑦**V11.1** **Pedal cycle passenger injured in collision with other pedal cycle in nontraffic accident**

⊗⑦**V11.2** **Unspecified pedal cyclist injured in collision with other pedal cycle in nontraffic accident**

⊗⑦**V11.3** **Person boarding or alighting a pedal cycle injured in collision with other pedal cycle**

⊗⑦**V11.4** **Pedal cycle driver injured in collision with other pedal cycle in traffic accident**

⊗⑦**V11.5** **Pedal cycle passenger injured in collision with other pedal cycle in traffic accident**

⊗⑦**V11.9** **Unspecified pedal cyclist injured in collision with other pedal cycle in traffic accident**

V12 **Pedal cycle rider injured in collision with two- or three-wheeled motor vehicle**

The appropriate 7th character is to be added to each code from category V12

A - initial encounter

D - subsequent encounter

S - sequela

⊗⑦**V12.0** **Pedal cycle driver injured in collision with two- or three-wheeled motor vehicle in nontraffic accident**

⊗⑦**V12.1** **Pedal cycle passenger injured in collision with two- or three-wheeled motor vehicle in nontraffic accident**

⊗⑦**V12.2** **Unspecified pedal cyclist injured in collision with two- or three-wheeled motor vehicle in nontraffic accident**

⊗⑦**V12.3** **Person boarding or alighting a pedal cycle injured in collision with two- or three-wheeled motor vehicle**

⊗⑦**V12.4** **Pedal cycle driver injured in collision with two- or three-wheeled motor vehicle in traffic accident**

⊗⑦**V12.5** **Pedal cycle passenger injured in collision with two- or three-wheeled motor vehicle in traffic accident**

⊗⑦**V12.9** **Unspecified pedal cyclist injured in collision with two- or three-wheeled motor vehicle in traffic accident**

V13 **Pedal cycle rider injured in collision with car, pick-up truck or van**

The appropriate 7th character is to be added to each code from category V13

A - initial encounter

D - subsequent encounter

S - sequela

⊗⑦**V13.0** **Pedal cycle driver injured in collision with car, pick-up truck or van in nontraffic accident**

⊗⑦**V13.1** **Pedal cycle passenger injured in collision with car, pick-up truck or van in nontraffic accident**

⊗⑦**V13.2** **Unspecified pedal cyclist injured in collision with car, pick-up truck or van in nontraffic accident**

⊗⑦**V13.3** **Person boarding or alighting a pedal cycle injured in collision with car, pick-up truck or van**

⊗⑦**V13.4** **Pedal cycle driver injured in collision with car, pick-up truck or van in traffic accident**

⊗⑦**V13.5** **Pedal cycle passenger injured in collision with car, pick-up truck or van in traffic accident**

⊗⑦**V13.9** **Unspecified pedal cyclist injured in collision with car, pick-up truck or van in traffic accident**

V14 **Pedal cycle rider injured in collision with heavy transport vehicle or bus**

Excludes1: pedal cycle rider injured in collision with military vehicle (V19.81)

The appropriate 7th character is to be added to each code from category V14

A - initial encounter

D - subsequent encounter

S - sequela

⊗⑦**V14.0** **Pedal cycle driver injured in collision with heavy transport vehicle or bus in nontraffic accident**

⊗⑦**V14.1** **Pedal cycle passenger injured in collision with heavy transport vehicle or bus in nontraffic accident**

⊗⑦**V14.2** **Unspecified pedal cyclist injured in collision with heavy transport vehicle or bus in nontraffic accident**

⊗⑦**V14.3** **Person boarding or alighting a pedal cycle injured in collision with heavy transport vehicle or bus**

⊗⑦**V14.4** **Pedal cycle driver injured in collision with heavy transport vehicle or bus in traffic accident**

⊗⑦**V14.5** **Pedal cycle passenger injured in collision with heavy transport vehicle or bus in traffic accident**

⊗⑦**V14.9** **Unspecified pedal cyclist injured in collision with heavy transport vehicle or bus in traffic accident**

V15 **Pedal cycle rider injured in collision with railway train or railway vehicle**

The appropriate 7th character is to be added to each code from category V15

A - initial encounter

D - subsequent encounter

S - sequela

⊗⑦**V15.0** **Pedal cycle driver injured in collision with railway train or railway vehicle in nontraffic accident**

⊗⑦**V15.1** **Pedal cycle passenger injured in collision with railway train or railway vehicle in nontraffic accident**

⊗⑦**V15.2** **Unspecified pedal cyclist injured in collision with railway train or railway vehicle in nontraffic accident**

⊗⑦**V15.3** **Person boarding or alighting a pedal cycle injured in collision with railway train or railway vehicle**

⊗⑦**V15.4** **Pedal cycle driver injured in collision with railway train or railway vehicle in traffic accident**

⊗⑦**V15.5** **Pedal cycle passenger injured in collision with railway train or railway vehicle in traffic accident**

⊗⑦**V15.9** **Unspecified pedal cyclist injured in collision with railway train or railway vehicle in traffic accident**

V16 **Pedal cycle rider injured in collision with other nonmotor vehicle**

Includes: collision with animal-drawn vehicle, animal being ridden, streetcar

The appropriate 7th character is to be added to each code from category V16

A - initial encounter

D - subsequent encounter

S - sequela

⊗⑦**V16.0** **Pedal cycle driver injured in collision with other nonmotor vehicle in nontraffic accident**

⊗⑦**V16.1** **Pedal cycle passenger injured in collision with other nonmotor vehicle in nontraffic accident**

⊗⑦**V16.2** **Unspecified pedal cyclist injured in collision with other nonmotor vehicle in nontraffic accident**

⊗⑦**V16.3** **Person boarding or alighting a pedal cycle injured in collision with other nonmotor vehicle in nontraffic accident**

⊗⑦**V16.4** **Pedal cycle driver injured in collision with other nonmotor vehicle in traffic accident**

⊗⑦**V16.5** **Pedal cycle passenger injured in collision with other nonmotor vehicle in traffic accident**

⊗⑦**V16.9** **Unspecified pedal cyclist injured in collision with other nonmotor vehicle in traffic accident**

V17 **Pedal cycle rider injured in collision with fixed or stationary object**

The appropriate 7th character is to be added to each code from category V17

A - initial encounter

D - subsequent encounter

S - sequela

⊗⑦**V17.0** **Pedal cycle driver injured in collision with fixed or stationary object in nontraffic accident**

⊗⑦**V17.1** **Pedal cycle passenger injured in collision with fixed or stationary object in nontraffic accident**

⊗⑦**V17.2** **Unspecified pedal cyclist injured in collision with fixed or stationary object in nontraffic accident**

⊗⑦**V17.3** **Person boarding or alighting a pedal cycle injured in collision with fixed or stationary object**

⊗⑦**V17.4** **Pedal cycle driver injured in collision with fixed or stationary object in traffic accident**

⊗⑦**V17.5** **Pedal cycle passenger injured in collision with fixed or stationary object in traffic accident**

⊗⑦**V17.9** **Unspecified pedal cyclist injured in collision with fixed or stationary object in traffic accident**

V18 **Pedal cycle rider injured in Non collision transport accident**

Includes: fall or thrown from pedal cycle (without antecedent collision)

overturning pedal cycle NOS overturning pedal cycle without collision

The appropriate 7th character is to be added to each code from category V18

A - initial encounter

D - subsequent encounter

S - sequela

⊗⑦**V18.0** **Pedal cycle driver injured in Non collision transport accident in nontraffic accident**

⊗⑦**V18.1** **Pedal cycle passenger injured in Non collision transport accident in nontraffic accident**

⊗⑦**V18.2** **Unspecified pedal cyclist injured in Non collision transport accident in nontraffic accident**

⊗⑦**V18.3** **Person boarding or alighting a pedal cycle injured in Non collision transport accident**

⊗⑦**V18.4** **Pedal cycle driver injured in Non collision transport accident in traffic accident**

⊗⑦**V18.5** **Pedal cycle passenger injured in Non collision transport accident in traffic accident**

⊗⑦**V18.9** **Unspecified pedal cyclist injured in Non collision transport accident in traffic accident**

V19 **Pedal cycle rider injured in other and unspecified transport accidents**

The appropriate 7th character is to be added to each code from category V19

A - initial encounter

D - subsequent encounter

S - sequela

V19.0 Pedal cycle driver injured in collision with other and unspecified motor vehicles in nontraffic accident

⊗⑦**V19.00** Pedal cycle driver injured in collision with unspecified motor vehicles in nontraffic accident

⊗⑦**V19.09** Pedal cycle driver injured in collision with other motor vehicles in nontraffic accident

V19.1 Pedal cycle passenger injured in collision with other and unspecified motor vehicles in nontraffic accident

⊗⑦**V19.10** Pedal cycle passenger injured in collision with unspecified motor vehicles in nontraffic accident

⊗⑦**V19.19** Pedal cycle passenger injured in collision with other motor vehicles in nontraffic accident

V19.2 Unspecified pedal cyclist injured in collision with other and unspecified motor vehicles in nontraffic accident

⊗⑦**V19.20** Unspecified pedal cyclist injured in collision with unspecified motor vehicles in nontraffic accident

Pedal cycle collision NOS, nontraffic

⊗⑦**V19.29** Unspecified pedal cyclist injured in collision with other motor vehicles in nontraffic accident

⊗⑦**V19.3** Pedal cyclist (driver) (passenger) injured in unspecified nontraffic accident

Pedal cycle accident NOS, nontraffic

Pedal cyclist injured in nontraffic accident NOS

V19.4 Pedal cycle driver injured in collision with other and unspecified motor vehicles in traffic accident

⊗⑦**V19.40** Pedal cycle driver injured in collision with unspecified motor vehicles in traffic accident

⊗⑦**V19.49** Pedal cycle driver injured in collision with other motor vehicles in traffic accident

V19.5 Pedal cycle passenger injured in collision with other and unspecified motor vehicles in traffic accident

⊗⑦**V19.50** Pedal cycle passenger injured in collision with unspecified motor vehicles in traffic accident

⊗⑦**V19.59** Pedal cycle passenger injured in collision with other motor vehicles in traffic accident

V19.6 Unspecified pedal cyclist injured in collision with other and unspecified motor vehicles in traffic accident

⊗⑦**V19.60** Unspecified pedal cyclist injured in collision with unspecified motor vehicles in traffic accident

Pedal cycle collision NOS (traffic)

⊗⑦**V19.69** Unspecified pedal cyclist injured in collision with other motor vehicles in traffic accident

V19.8 Pedal cyclist (driver) (passenger) injured in other specified transport accidents

⊗⑦**V19.81** Pedal cyclist (driver) (passenger) injured in transport accident with military vehicle

⊗⑦**V19.88** Pedal cyclist (driver) (passenger) injured in other specified transport accidents

⊗⑦**V19.9** Pedal cyclist (driver) (passenger) injured in unspecified traffic accident

Pedal cycle accident NOS

MOTORCYCLE RIDER INJURED IN TRANSPORT ACCIDENT (V20-V29)

Includes: moped

motorcycle with sidecar motorized bicycle motor scooter

Excludes1: three-wheeled motor vehicle (V30-V39)

V20 Motorcycle rider injured in collision with pedestrian or animal

Excludes1: motorcycle rider collision with animal-drawn vehicle or animal being ridden (V26.-)

The appropriate 7th character is to be added to each code from category V20

A - initial encounter

D - subsequent encounter

S - sequela

⊗⑦**V20.0** Motorcycle driver injured in collision with pedestrian or animal in nontraffic accident

⊗⑦**V20.1** Motorcycle passenger injured in collision with pedestrian or animal in nontraffic accident

⊗⑦**V20.2** Unspecified motorcycle rider injured in collision with pedestrian or animal in nontraffic accident

⊗⑦**V20.3** Person boarding or alighting a motorcycle injured in collision with pedestrian or animal

⊗⑦**V20.4** Motorcycle driver injured in collision with pedestrian or animal in traffic accident

⊗⑦**V20.5** Motorcycle passenger injured in collision with pedestrian or animal in traffic accident

⊗⑦**V20.9** Unspecified motorcycle rider injured in collision with pedestrian or animal in traffic accident

V21 Motorcycle rider injured in collision with pedal cycle

The appropriate 7th character is to be added to each code from category V21

A - initial encounter

D - subsequent encounter

S - sequela

⊗⑦**V21.0** Motorcycle driver injured in collision with pedal cycle in nontraffic accident

⊗⑦**V21.1** Motorcycle passenger injured in collision with pedal cycle in nontraffic accident

⊗⑦**V21.2** Unspecified motorcycle rider injured in collision with pedal cycle in nontraffic accident

⊗⑦**V21.3** Person boarding or alighting a motorcycle injured in collision with pedal cycle

⊗⑦**V21.4** Motorcycle driver injured in collision with pedal cycle in traffic accident

⊗⑦**V21.5** Motorcycle passenger injured in collision with pedal cycle in traffic accident

⊗⑦**V21.9** Unspecified motorcycle rider injured in collision with pedal cycle in traffic accident

V22 Motorcycle rider injured in collision with two- or three-wheeled motor vehicle

The appropriate 7th character is to be added to each code from category V22

A - initial encounter

D - subsequent encounter

S - sequela

⊗⑦**V22.0** Motorcycle driver injured in collision with two- or three-wheeled motor vehicle in nontraffic accident

⊗⑦**V22.1** Motorcycle passenger injured in collision with two- or three-wheeled motor vehicle in nontraffic accident

⊗⑦**V22.2** Unspecified motorcycle rider injured in collision with two- or three-wheeled motor vehicle in nontraffic accident

⊗⑦**V22.3** Person boarding or alighting a motorcycle injured in collision with two- or three-wheeled motor vehicle

⊗⑦**V22.4** Motorcycle driver injured in collision with two- or three-wheeled motor vehicle in traffic accident

⊗⑦**V22.5** Motorcycle passenger injured in collision with two- or three-wheeled motor vehicle in traffic accident

⊗⑦**V22.9** Unspecified motorcycle rider injured in collision with two- or three-wheeled motor vehicle in traffic accident

● New code ▲ Revised code Excludes1: Not coded here Excludes2: Not included here ⊗ Placeholder required ⑦ 7th digit required

V23 Motorcycle rider injured in collision with car, pick-up truck or van

The appropriate 7th character is to be added to each code from category V23

A - initial encounter

D - subsequent encounter

S - sequela

⊗⑦**V23.0** Motorcycle driver injured in collision with car, pick-up truck or van in nontraffic accident

⊗⑦**V23.1** Motorcycle passenger injured in collision with car, pick-up truck or van in nontraffic accident

⊗⑦**V23.2** Unspecified motorcycle rider injured in collision with car, pick-up truck or van in nontraffic accident

⊗⑦**V23.3** Person boarding or alighting a motorcycle injured in collision with car, pick-up truck or van

⊗⑦**V23.4** Motorcycle driver injured in collision with car, pick-up truck or van in traffic accident

⊗⑦**V23.5** Motorcycle passenger injured in collision with car, pick-up truck or van in traffic accident

⊗⑦**V23.9** Unspecified motorcycle rider injured in collision with car, pick-up truck or van in traffic accident

V24 Motorcycle rider injured in collision with heavy transport vehicle or bus

Excludes1: motorcycle rider injured in collision with military vehicle (V29.81)

The appropriate 7th character is to be added to each code from category V24

A - initial encounter

D - subsequent encounter

S - sequela

⊗⑦**V24.0** Motorcycle driver injured in collision with heavy transport vehicle or bus in nontraffic accident

⊗⑦**V24.1** Motorcycle passenger injured in collision with heavy transport vehicle or bus in nontraffic accident

⊗⑦**V24.2** Unspecified motorcycle rider injured in collision with heavy transport vehicle or bus in nontraffic accident

⊗⑦**V24.3** Person boarding or alighting a motorcycle injured in collision with heavy transport vehicle or bus

⊗⑦**V24.4** Motorcycle driver injured in collision with heavy transport vehicle or bus in traffic accident

⊗⑦**V24.5** Motorcycle passenger injured in collision with heavy transport vehicle or bus in traffic accident

⊗⑦**V24.9** Unspecified motorcycle rider injured in collision with heavy transport vehicle or bus in traffic accident

V25 Motorcycle rider injured in collision with railway train or railway vehicle

The appropriate 7th character is to be added to each code from category V25

A - initial encounter

D - subsequent encounter

S - sequela

⊗⑦**V25.0** Motorcycle driver injured in collision with railway train or railway vehicle in nontraffic accident

⊗⑦**V25.1** Motorcycle passenger injured in collision with railway train or railway vehicle in nontraffic accident

⊗⑦**V25.2** Unspecified motorcycle rider injured in collision with railway train or railway vehicle in nontraffic accident

⊗⑦**V25.3** Person boarding or alighting a motorcycle injured in collision with railway train or railway vehicle

⊗⑦**V25.4** Motorcycle driver injured in collision with railway train or railway vehicle in traffic accident

⊗⑦**V25.5** Motorcycle passenger injured in collision with railway train or railway vehicle in traffic accident

⊗⑦**V25.9** Unspecified motorcycle rider injured in collision with railway train or railway vehicle in traffic accident

V26 Motorcycle rider injured in collision with other nonmotor vehicle

Includes: collision with animal-drawn vehicle, animal being ridden, streetcar

The appropriate 7th character is to be added to each code from category V26

A - initial encounter

D - subsequent encounter

S - sequela

⊗⑦**V26.0** Motorcycle driver injured in collision with other nonmotor vehicle in nontraffic accident

⊗⑦**V26.1** Motorcycle passenger injured in collision with other nonmotor vehicle in nontraffic accident

⊗⑦**V26.2** Unspecified motorcycle rider injured in collision with other nonmotor vehicle in nontraffic accident

⊗⑦**V26.3** Person boarding or alighting a motorcycle injured in collision with other nonmotor vehicle

⊗⑦**V26.4** Motorcycle driver injured in collision with other nonmotor vehicle in traffic accident

⊗⑦**V26.5** Motorcycle passenger injured in collision with other nonmotor vehicle in traffic accident

⊗⑦**V26.9** Unspecified motorcycle rider injured in collision with other nonmotor vehicle in traffic accident

V27 Motorcycle rider injured in collision with fixed or stationary object

The appropriate 7th character is to be added to each code from category V27

A - initial encounter

D - subsequent encounter

S - sequela

⊗⑦**V27.0** Motorcycle driver injured in collision with fixed or stationary object in nontraffic accident

⊗⑦**V27.1** Motorcycle passenger injured in collision with fixed or stationary object in nontraffic accident

⊗⑦**V27.2** Unspecified motorcycle rider injured in collision with fixed or stationary object in nontraffic accident

⊗⑦**V27.3** Person boarding or alighting a motorcycle injured in collision with fixed or stationary object

⊗⑦**V27.4** Motorcycle driver injured in collision with fixed or stationary object in traffic accident

⊗⑦**V27.5** Motorcycle passenger injured in collision with fixed or stationary object in traffic accident

⊗⑦**V27.9** Unspecified motorcycle rider injured in collision with fixed or stationary object in traffic accident

V28 Motorcycle rider injured in Non collision transport accident

Includes: fall or thrown from motorcycle (without antecedent collision)

overturning motorcycle NOS overturning motorcycle without collision

The appropriate 7th character is to be added to each code from category V28

A - initial encounter

D - subsequent encounter

S - sequela

⊗⑦**V28.0** Motorcycle driver injured in Non collision transport accident in nontraffic accident

⊗⑦**V28.1** Motorcycle passenger injured in Non collision transport accident in nontraffic accident

⊗⑦**V28.2** Unspecified motorcycle rider injured in Non collision transport accident in nontraffic accident

⊗⑦V28.3   Person boarding or alighting a motorcycle injured in Non collision transport accident

⊗⑦V28.4   Motorcycle driver injured in Non collision transport accident in traffic accident

⊗⑦V28.5   Motorcycle passenger injured in Non collision transport accident in traffic accident

⊗⑦V28.9   Unspecified motorcycle rider injured in Non collision transport accident in traffic accident

V29   Motorcycle rider injured in other and unspecified transport accidents

The appropriate 7th character is to be added to each code from category V29

A - initial encounter

D - subsequent encounter

S - sequela

V29.0   Motorcycle driver injured in collision with other and unspecified motor vehicles in nontraffic accident

⊗⑦V29.00   Motorcycle driver injured in collision with unspecified motor vehicles in nontraffic accident

⊗⑦V29.09   Motorcycle driver injured in collision with other motor vehicles in nontraffic accident

V29.1   Motorcycle passenger injured in collision with other and unspecified motor vehicles in nontraffic accident

⊗⑦V29.10   Motorcycle passenger injured in collision with unspecified motor vehicles in nontraffic accident

⊗⑦V29.19   Motorcycle passenger injured in collision with other motor vehicles in nontraffic accident

V29.2   Unspecified motorcycle rider injured in collision with other and unspecified motor vehicles in nontraffic accident

⊗⑦V29.20   Unspecified motorcycle rider injured in collision with unspecified motor vehicles in nontraffic accident

Motorcycle collision NOS, nontraffic

⊗⑦V29.29   Unspecified motorcycle rider injured in collision with other motor vehicles in nontraffic accident

⊗⑦V29.3   Motorcycle rider (driver) (passenger) injured in unspecified nontraffic accident

Motorcycle accident NOS, nontraffic

Motorcycle rider injured in nontraffic accident NOS

V29.4   Motorcycle driver injured in collision with other and unspecified motor vehicles in traffic accident

⊗⑦V29.40   Motorcycle driver injured in collision with unspecified motor vehicles in traffic accident

⊗⑦V29.49   Motorcycle driver injured in collision with other motor vehicles in traffic accident

V29.5   Motorcycle passenger injured in collision with other and unspecified motor vehicles in traffic accident

⊗⑦V29.50   Motorcycle passenger injured in collision with unspecified motor vehicles in traffic accident

⊗⑦V29.59   Motorcycle passenger injured in collision with other motor vehicles in traffic accident

V29.6   Unspecified motorcycle rider injured in collision with other and unspecified motor vehicles in traffic accident

⊗⑦V29.60   Unspecified motorcycle rider injured in collision with unspecified motor vehicles in traffic accident

Motorcycle collision NOS (traffic)

⊗⑦V29.69   Unspecified motorcycle rider injured in collision with other motor vehicles in traffic accident

V29.8   Motorcycle rider (driver) (passenger) injured in other specified transport accidents

⊗⑦V29.81   Motorcycle rider (driver) (passenger) injured in transport accident with military vehicle

⊗⑦V29.88   Motorcycle rider (driver) (passenger) injured in other specified transport accidents

⊗⑦V29.9   Motorcycle rider (driver) (passenger) injured in unspecified traffic accident

Motorcycle accident NOS

OCCUPANT OF THREE-WHEELED MOTOR VEHICLE INJURED IN TRANSPORT ACCIDENT (V30-V39)

Includes: motorized tricycle

motorized rickshaw three-wheeled motor car

Excludes1: all-terrain vehicles (V86.-)

motorcycle with sidecar (V20-V29)

vehicle designed primarily for off-road use (V86.-)

V30   Occupant of three-wheeled motor vehicle injured in collision with pedestrian or animal

Excludes1: three-wheeled motor vehicle collision with animal-drawn vehicle or animal being ridden (V36.-)

The appropriate 7th character is to be added to each code from category V30

A - initial encounter

D - subsequent encounter

S - sequela

⊗⑦V30.0   Driver of three-wheeled motor vehicle injured in collision with pedestrian or animal in nontraffic accident

⊗⑦V30.1   Passenger in three-wheeled motor vehicle injured in collision with pedestrian or animal in nontraffic accident

⊗⑦V30.2   Person on outside of three-wheeled motor vehicle injured in collision with pedestrian or animal in nontraffic accident

⊗⑦V30.3   Unspecified occupant of three-wheeled motor vehicle injured in collision with pedestrian or animal in nontraffic accident

⊗⑦V30.4   Person boarding or alighting a three-wheeled motor vehicle injured in collision with pedestrian or animal

⊗⑦V30.5   Driver of three-wheeled motor vehicle injured in collision with pedestrian or animal in traffic accident

⊗⑦V30.6   Passenger in three-wheeled motor vehicle injured in collision with pedestrian or animal in traffic accident

⊗⑦V30.7   Person on outside of three-wheeled motor vehicle injured in collision with pedestrian or animal in traffic accident

⊗⑦V30.9   Unspecified occupant of three-wheeled motor vehicle injured in collision with pedestrian or animal in traffic accident

V31   Occupant of three-wheeled motor vehicle injured in collision with pedal cycle

The appropriate 7th character is to be added to each code from category V31

A - initial encounter

D - subsequent encounter

S - sequela

⊗⑦V31.0   Driver of three-wheeled motor vehicle injured in collision with pedal cycle in nontraffic accident

⊗⑦V31.1   Passenger in three-wheeled motor vehicle injured in collision with pedal cycle in nontraffic accident

⊗⑦V31.2   Person on outside of three-wheeled motor vehicle injured in collision with pedal cycle in nontraffic accident

⊗⑦**V31.3** **Unspecified occupant of three-wheeled motor vehicle injured in collision with pedal cycle in nontraffic accident**

⊗⑦**V31.4** **Person boarding or alighting a three-wheeled motor vehicle injured in collision with pedal cycle**

⊗⑦**V31.5** **Driver of three-wheeled motor vehicle injured in collision with pedal cycle in traffic accident**

⊗⑦**V31.6** **Passenger in three-wheeled motor vehicle injured in collision with pedal cycle in traffic accident**

⊗⑦**V31.7** **Person on outside of three-wheeled motor vehicle injured in collision with pedal cycle in traffic accident**

⊗⑦**V31.9** **Unspecified occupant of three-wheeled motor vehicle injured in collision with pedal cycle in traffic accident**

V32 **Occupant of three-wheeled motor vehicle injured in collision with two- or three-wheeled motor vehicle**

The appropriate 7th character is to be added to each code from category V32

A - initial encounter

D - subsequent encounter

S - sequela

⊗⑦**V32.0** **Driver of three-wheeled motor vehicle injured in collision with two- or three-wheeled motor vehicle in nontraffic accident**

⊗⑦**V32.1** **Passenger in three-wheeled motor vehicle injured in collision with two- or three-wheeled motor vehicle in nontraffic accident**

⊗⑦**V32.2** **Person on outside of three-wheeled motor vehicle injured in collision with two- or three-wheeled motor vehicle in nontraffic accident**

⊗⑦**V32.3** **Unspecified occupant of three-wheeled motor vehicle injured in collision with two- or three-wheeled motor vehicle in nontraffic accident**

⊗⑦**V32.4** **Person boarding or alighting a three-wheeled motor vehicle injured in collision with two- or three-wheeled motor vehicle**

⊗⑦**V32.5** **Driver of three-wheeled motor vehicle injured in collision with two- or three-wheeled motor vehicle in traffic accident**

⊗⑦**V32.6** **Passenger in three-wheeled motor vehicle injured in collision with two- or three-wheeled motor vehicle in traffic accident**

⊗⑦**V32.7** **Person on outside of three-wheeled motor vehicle injured in collision with two- or three-wheeled motor vehicle in traffic accident**

⊗⑦**V32.9** **Unspecified occupant of three-wheeled motor vehicle injured in collision with two- or three-wheeled motor vehicle in traffic accident**

V33 **Occupant of three-wheeled motor vehicle injured in collision with car, pick-up truck or van**

The appropriate 7th character is to be added to each code from category V33

A - initial encounter

D - subsequent encounter

S - sequela

⊗⑦**V33.0** **Driver of three-wheeled motor vehicle injured in collision with car, pick-up truck or van in nontraffic accident**

⊗⑦**V33.1** **Passenger in three-wheeled motor vehicle injured in collision with car, pick-up truck or van in nontraffic accident**

⊗⑦**V33.2** **Person on outside of three-wheeled motor vehicle injured in collision with car, pick-up truck or van in nontraffic accident**

⊗⑦**V33.3** **Unspecified occupant of three-wheeled motor vehicle injured in collision with car, pick-up truck or van in nontraffic accident**

⊗⑦**V33.4** **Person boarding or alighting a three-wheeled motor vehicle injured in collision with car, pick-up truck or van**

⊗⑦**V33.5** **Driver of three-wheeled motor vehicle injured in collision with car, pick-up truck or van in traffic accident**

⊗⑦**V33.6** **Passenger in three-wheeled motor vehicle injured in collision with car, pick-up truck or van in traffic accident**

⊗⑦**V33.7** **Person on outside of three-wheeled motor vehicle injured in collision with car, pick-up truck or van in traffic accident**

⊗⑦**V33.9** **Unspecified occupant of three-wheeled motor vehicle injured in collision with car, pick-up truck or van in traffic accident**

V34 **Occupant of three-wheeled motor vehicle injured in collision with heavy transport vehicle or bus**

> **Excludes1:** occupant of three-wheeled motor vehicle injured in collision with military vehicle (V39.81)

The appropriate 7th character is to be added to each code from category V34

A - initial encounter

D - subsequent encounter

S - sequela

⊗⑦**V34.0** **Driver of three-wheeled motor vehicle injured in collision with heavy transport vehicle or bus in nontraffic accident**

⊗⑦**V34.1** **Passenger in three-wheeled motor vehicle injured in collision with heavy transport vehicle or bus in nontraffic accident**

⊗⑦**V34.2** **Person on outside of three-wheeled motor vehicle injured in collision with heavy transport vehicle or bus in nontraffic accident**

⊗⑦**V34.3** **Unspecified occupant of three-wheeled motor vehicle injured in collision with heavy transport vehicle or bus in nontraffic accident**

⊗⑦**V34.4** **Person boarding or alighting a three-wheeled motor vehicle injured in collision with heavy transport vehicle or bus**

⊗⑦**V34.5** **Driver of three-wheeled motor vehicle injured in collision with heavy transport vehicle or bus in traffic accident**

⊗⑦**V34.6** **Passenger in three-wheeled motor vehicle injured in collision with heavy transport vehicle or bus in traffic accident**

⊗⑦**V34.7** **Person on outside of three-wheeled motor vehicle injured in collision with heavy transport vehicle or bus in traffic accident**

⊗⑦**V34.9** **Unspecified occupant of three-wheeled motor vehicle injured in collision with heavy transport vehicle or bus in traffic accident**

V35 **Occupant of three-wheeled motor vehicle injured in collision with railway train or railway vehicle**

The appropriate 7th character is to be added to each code from category V35

A - initial encounter

D - subsequent encounter

S - sequela

⊗⑦**V35.0** **Driver of three-wheeled motor vehicle injured in collision with railway train or railway vehicle in nontraffic accident**

⊗⑦V35.1 **Passenger in three-wheeled motor vehicle injured in collision with railway train or railway vehicle in nontraffic accident**

⊗⑦V35.2 **Person on outside of three-wheeled motor vehicle injured in collision with railway train or railway vehicle in nontraffic accident**

⊗⑦V35.3 **Unspecified occupant of three-wheeled motor vehicle injured in collision with railway train or railway vehicle in nontraffic accident**

⊗⑦V35.4 **Person boarding or alighting a three-wheeled motor vehicle injured in collision with railway train or railway vehicle**

⊗⑦V35.5 **Driver of three-wheeled motor vehicle injured in collision with railway train or railway vehicle in traffic accident**

⊗⑦V35.6 **Passenger in three-wheeled motor vehicle injured in collision with railway train or railway vehicle in traffic accident**

⊗⑦V35.7 **Person on outside of three-wheeled motor vehicle injured in collision with railway train or railway vehicle in traffic accident**

⊗⑦V35.9 **Unspecified occupant of three-wheeled motor vehicle injured in collision with railway train or railway vehicle in traffic accident**

V36 **Occupant of three-wheeled motor vehicle injured in collision with other nonmotor vehicle**

Includes: collision with animal-drawn vehicle, animal being ridden, streetcar

The appropriate 7th character is to be added to each code from category V36

A - initial encounter

D - subsequent encounter

S - sequela

⊗⑦V36.0 **Driver of three-wheeled motor vehicle injured in collision with other nonmotor vehicle in nontraffic accident**

⊗⑦V36.1 **Passenger in three-wheeled motor vehicle injured in collision with other nonmotor vehicle in nontraffic accident**

⊗⑦V36.2 **Person on outside of three-wheeled motor vehicle injured in collision with other nonmotor vehicle in nontraffic accident**

⊗⑦V36.3 **Unspecified occupant of three-wheeled motor vehicle injured in collision with other nonmotor vehicle in nontraffic accident**

⊗⑦V36.4 **Person boarding or alighting a three-wheeled motor vehicle injured in collision with other nonmotor vehicle**

⊗⑦V36.5 **Driver of three-wheeled motor vehicle injured in collision with other nonmotor vehicle in traffic accident**

⊗⑦V36.6 **Passenger in three-wheeled motor vehicle injured in collision with other nonmotor vehicle in traffic accident**

⊗⑦V36.7 **Person on outside of three-wheeled motor vehicle injured in collision with other nonmotor vehicle in traffic accident**

⊗⑦V36.9 **Unspecified occupant of three-wheeled motor vehicle injured in collision with other nonmotor vehicle in traffic accident**

V37 **Occupant of three-wheeled motor vehicle injured in collision with fixed or stationary object**

The appropriate 7th character is to be added to each code from category V37

A - initial encounter

D - subsequent encounter

S - sequela

⊗⑦V37.0 **Driver of three-wheeled motor vehicle injured in collision with fixed or stationary object in nontraffic accident**

⊗⑦V37.1 **Passenger in three-wheeled motor vehicle injured in collision with fixed or stationary object in nontraffic accident**

⊗⑦V37.2 **Person on outside of three-wheeled motor vehicle injured in collision with fixed or stationary object in nontraffic accident**

⊗⑦V37.3 **Unspecified occupant of three-wheeled motor vehicle injured in collision with fixed or stationary object in nontraffic accident**

⊗⑦V37.4 **Person boarding or alighting a three-wheeled motor vehicle injured in collision with fixed or stationary object**

⊗⑦V37.5 **Driver of three-wheeled motor vehicle injured in collision with fixed or stationary object in traffic accident**

⊗⑦V37.6 **Passenger in three-wheeled motor vehicle injured in collision with fixed or stationary object in traffic accident**

⊗⑦V37.7 **Person on outside of three-wheeled motor vehicle injured in collision with fixed or stationary object in traffic accident**

⊗⑦V37.9 **Unspecified occupant of three-wheeled motor vehicle injured in collision with fixed or stationary object in traffic accident**

V38 **Occupant of three-wheeled motor vehicle injured in Non collision transport accident**

Includes: fall or thrown from three-wheeled motor vehicle

overturning of three-wheeled motor vehicle NOS

overturning of three-wheeled motor vehicle without collision

The appropriate 7th character is to be added to each code from category V38

A - initial encounter

D - subsequent encounter

S - sequela

⊗⑦V38.0 **Driver of three-wheeled motor vehicle injured in Non collision transport accident in nontraffic accident**

⊗⑦V38.1 **Passenger in three-wheeled motor vehicle injured in Non collision transport accident in nontraffic accident**

⊗⑦V38.2 **Person on outside of three-wheeled motor vehicle injured in Non collision transport accident in nontraffic accident**

⊗⑦V38.3 **Unspecified occupant of three-wheeled motor vehicle injured in Non collision transport accident in nontraffic accident**

⊗⑦V38.4 **Person boarding or alighting a three-wheeled motor vehicle injured in Non collision transport accident**

⊗⑦V38.5 **Driver of three-wheeled motor vehicle injured in Non collision transport accident in traffic accident**

⊗⑦V38.6 **Passenger in three-wheeled motor vehicle injured in Non collision transport accident in traffic accident**

⊗⑦V38.7 **Person on outside of three-wheeled motor vehicle injured in Non collision transport accident in traffic accident**

⊗⑦V38.9 **Unspecified occupant of three-wheeled motor vehicle injured in Non collision transport accident in traffic accident**

V39 **Occupant of three-wheeled motor vehicle injured in other and unspecified transport accidents**

The appropriate 7th character is to be added to each code from category V39

A - initial encounter

D - subsequent encounter

S - sequela

● New code   ▲ Revised code   Excludes1: Not coded here   Excludes2: Not included here   ⊗ Placeholder required   ⑦7th digit required

V39.0 Driver of three-wheeled motor vehicle injured in collision with other and unspecified motor vehicles in nontraffic accident

⊗⑦**V39.00** Driver of three-wheeled motor vehicle injured in collision with unspecified motor vehicles in nontraffic accident

⊗⑦**V39.09** Driver of three-wheeled motor vehicle injured in collision with other motor vehicles in nontraffic accident

V39.1 Passenger in three-wheeled motor vehicle injured in collision with other and unspecified motor vehicles in nontraffic accident

⊗⑦**V39.10** Passenger in three-wheeled motor vehicle injured in collision with unspecified motor vehicles in nontraffic accident

⊗⑦**V39.19** Passenger in three-wheeled motor vehicle injured in collision with other motor vehicles in nontraffic accident

V39.2 Unspecified occupant of three-wheeled motor vehicle injured in collision with other and unspecified motor vehicles in nontraffic accident

⊗⑦**V39.20** Unspecified occupant of three-wheeled motor vehicle injured in collision with unspecified motor vehicles in nontraffic accident

Collision NOS involving three-wheeled motor vehicle, nontraffic

⊗⑦**V39.29** Unspecified occupant of three-wheeled motor vehicle injured in collision with other motor vehicles in nontraffic accident

⊗⑦**V39.3** Occupant (driver) (passenger) of three-wheeled motor vehicle injured in unspecified nontraffic accident

Accident NOS involving three-wheeled motor vehicle, nontraffic

Occupant of three-wheeled motor vehicle injured in nontraffic accident NOS

V39.4 Driver of three-wheeled motor vehicle injured in collision with other and unspecified motor vehicles in traffic accident

⊗⑦**V39.40** Driver of three-wheeled motor vehicle injured in collision with unspecified motor vehicles in traffic accident

⊗⑦**V39.49** Driver of three-wheeled motor vehicle injured in collision with other motor vehicles in traffic accident

V39.5 Passenger in three-wheeled motor vehicle injured in collision with other and unspecified motor vehicles in traffic accident

⊗⑦**V39.50** Passenger in three-wheeled motor vehicle injured in collision with unspecified motor vehicles in traffic accident

⊗⑦**V39.59** Passenger in three-wheeled motor vehicle injured in collision with other motor vehicles in traffic accident

V39.6 Unspecified occupant of three-wheeled motor vehicle injured in collision with other and unspecified motor vehicles in traffic accident

⊗⑦**V39.60** Unspecified occupant of three-wheeled motor vehicle injured in collision with unspecified motor vehicles in traffic accident

Collision NOS involving three-wheeled motor vehicle (traffic)

⊗⑦**V39.69** Unspecified occupant of three-wheeled motor vehicle injured in collision with other motor vehicles in traffic accident

V39.8 Occupant (driver) (passenger) of three-wheeled motor vehicle injured in other specified transport accidents

⊗⑦**V39.81** Occupant (driver) (passenger) of three-wheeled motor vehicle injured in transport accident with military vehicle

⊗⑦**V39.89** Occupant (driver) (passenger) of three-wheeled motor vehicle injured in other specified transport accidents

⊗⑦**V39.9** Occupant (driver) (passenger) of three-wheeled motor vehicle injured in unspecified traffic accident

Accident NOS involving three-wheeled motor vehicle

CAR OCCUPANT INJURED IN TRANSPORT ACCIDENT (V40-V49)

Includes: a four-wheeled motor vehicle designed primarily for carrying passengers

automobile (pulling a trailer or camper)

Excludes1: bus (V50-V59)

minibus (V50-V59)

minivan (V50-V59)

motorcoach (V70-V79)

pick-up truck (V50-V59)

sport utility vehicle (SUV) (V50-V59)

V40 Car occupant injured in collision with pedestrian or animal

Excludes1: car collision with animal-drawn vehicle or animal being ridden (V46.-)

The appropriate 7th character is to be added to each code from category V40

A - initial encounter

D - subsequent encounter

S - sequela

⊗⑦**V40.0** Car driver injured in collision with pedestrian or animal in nontraffic accident

⊗⑦**V40.1** Car passenger injured in collision with pedestrian or animal in nontraffic accident

⊗⑦**V40.2** Person on outside of car injured in collision with pedestrian or animal in nontraffic accident

⊗⑦**V40.3** Unspecified car occupant injured in collision with pedestrian or animal in nontraffic accident

⊗⑦**V40.4** Person boarding or alighting a car injured in collision with pedestrian or animal

⊗⑦**V40.5** Car driver injured in collision with pedestrian or animal in traffic accident

⊗⑦**V40.6** Car passenger injured in collision with pedestrian or animal in traffic accident

⊗⑦**V40.7** Person on outside of car injured in collision with pedestrian or animal in traffic accident

⊗⑦**V40.9** Unspecified car occupant injured in collision with pedestrian or animal in traffic accident

V41 Car occupant injured in collision with pedal cycle

The appropriate 7th character is to be added to each code from category V41

A - initial encounter

D - subsequent encounter

S - sequela

⊗⑦**V41.0** Car driver injured in collision with pedal cycle in nontraffic accident

⊗⑦**V41.1** Car passenger injured in collision with pedal cycle in nontraffic accident

⊗⑦**V41.2** Person on outside of car injured in collision with pedal cycle in nontraffic accident

⊗⑦**V41.3** Unspecified car occupant injured in collision with pedal cycle in nontraffic accident

⊗⑦**V41.4** Person boarding or alighting a car injured in collision with pedal cycle

⊗⑦**V41.5** Car driver injured in collision with pedal cycle in traffic accident

⊗⑦**V41.6** Car passenger injured in collision with pedal cycle in traffic accident

⊗⑦**V41.7** Person on outside of car injured in collision with pedal cycle in traffic accident

⊗⑦**V41.9** Unspecified car occupant injured in collision with pedal cycle in traffic accident

V42 Car occupant injured in collision with two- or three-wheeled motor vehicle

The appropriate 7th character is to be added to each code from category V42

A - initial encounter

D - subsequent encounter

S - sequela

⊗⑦**V42.0** Car driver injured in collision with two- or three-wheeled motor vehicle in nontraffic accident

⊗⑦**V42.1** Car passenger injured in collision with two- or three-wheeled motor vehicle in nontraffic accident

⊗⑦**V42.2** Person on outside of car injured in collision with two- or three-wheeled motor vehicle in nontraffic accident

⊗⑦**V42.3** Unspecified car occupant injured in collision with two- or three-wheeled motor vehicle in nontraffic accident

⊗⑦**V42.4** Person boarding or alighting a car injured in collision with two- or three-wheeled motor vehicle

⊗⑦**V42.5** Car driver injured in collision with two- or three-wheeled motor vehicle in traffic accident

⊗⑦**V42.6** Car passenger injured in collision with two- or three-wheeled motor vehicle in traffic accident

⊗⑦**V42.7** Person on outside of car injured in collision with two- or three-wheeled motor vehicle in traffic accident

⊗⑦**V42.9** Unspecified car occupant injured in collision with two- or three-wheeled motor vehicle in traffic accident

V43 Car occupant injured in collision with car, pick-up truck or van

The appropriate 7th character is to be added to each code from category V43

A - initial encounter

D - subsequent encounter

S - sequela

V43.0 Car driver injured in collision with car, pick-up truck or van in nontraffic accident

⊗⑦**V43.01** Car driver injured in collision with sport utility vehicle in nontraffic accident

⊗⑦**V43.02** Car driver injured in collision with other type car in nontraffic accident

⊗⑦**V43.03** Car driver injured in collision with pick-up truck in nontraffic accident

⊗⑦**V43.04** Car driver injured in collision with van in nontraffic accident

V43.1 Car passenger injured in collision with car, pick-up truck or van in nontraffic accident

⊗⑦**V43.11** Car passenger injured in collision with sport utility vehicle in nontraffic accident

⊗⑦**V43.12** Car passenger injured in collision with other type car in nontraffic accident

⊗⑦**V43.13** Car passenger injured in collision with pick-up truck in nontraffic accident

⊗⑦**V43.14** Car passenger injured in collision with van in nontraffic accident

V43.2 Person on outside of car injured in collision with car, pick-up truck or van in nontraffic accident

⊗⑦**V43.21** Person on outside of car injured in collision with sport utility vehicle in nontraffic accident

⊗⑦**V43.22** Person on outside of car injured in collision with other type car in nontraffic accident

⊗⑦**V43.23** Person on outside of car injured in collision with pick-up truck in nontraffic accident

⊗⑦**V43.24** Person on outside of car injured in collision with van in nontraffic accident

V43.3 Unspecified car occupant injured in collision with car, pick-up truck or van in nontraffic accident

⊗⑦**V43.31** Unspecified car occupant injured in collision with sport utility vehicle in nontraffic accident

⊗⑦**V43.32** Unspecified car occupant injured in collision with other type car in nontraffic accident

⊗⑦**V43.33** Unspecified car occupant injured in collision with pick-up truck in nontraffic accident

⊗⑦**V43.34** Unspecified car occupant injured in collision with van in nontraffic accident

V43.4 Person boarding or alighting a car injured in collision with car, pick-up truck or van

⊗⑦**V43.41** Person boarding or alighting a car injured in collision with sport utility vehicle

⊗⑦**V43.42** Person boarding or alighting a car injured in collision with other type car

⊗⑦**V43.43** Person boarding or alighting a car injured in collision with pick-up truck

⊗⑦**V43.44** Person boarding or alighting a car injured in collision with van

V43.5 Car driver injured in collision with car, pick-up truck or van in traffic accident

⊗⑦**V43.51** Car driver injured in collision with sport utility vehicle in traffic accident

⊗⑦**V43.52** Car driver injured in collision with other type car in traffic accident

⊗⑦**V43.53** Car driver injured in collision with pick-up truck in traffic accident

⊗⑦**V43.54** Car driver injured in collision with van in traffic accident

V43.6 Car passenger injured in collision with car, pick-up truck or van in traffic accident

⊗⑦**V43.61** Car passenger injured in collision with sport utility vehicle in traffic accident

⊗⑦**V43.62** Car passenger injured in collision with other type car in traffic accident

⊗⑦**V43.63** Car passenger injured in collision with pick-up truck in traffic accident

⊗⑦**V43.64** Car passenger injured in collision with van in traffic accident

V43.7 Person on outside of car injured in collision with car, pick-up truck or van in traffic accident

⊗⑦**V43.71** Person on outside of car injured in collision with sport utility vehicle in traffic accident

⊗⑦**V43.72** Person on outside of car injured in collision with other type car in traffic accident

⊗⑦**V43.73** Person on outside of car injured in collision with pick-up truck in traffic accident

⊗⑦**V43.74** Person on outside of car injured in collision with van in traffic accident

V43.9 Unspecified car occupant injured in collision with car, pick-up truck or van in traffic accident

⊗⑦**V43.91** Unspecified car occupant injured in collision with sport utility vehicle in traffic accident

● New code   ▲ Revised code   **Excludes1:** Not coded here   **Excludes2:** Not included here   ⊗ Placeholder required   ⑦ 7th digit required

⊗⑦**V43.92** **Unspecified car occupant injured in collision with other type car in traffic accident**

⊗⑦**V43.93** **Unspecified car occupant injured in collision with pick-up truck in traffic accident**

⊗⑦**V43.94** **Unspecified car occupant injured in collision with van in traffic accident**

V44 **Car occupant injured in collision with heavy transport vehicle or bus**

Excludes1: car occupant injured in collision with military vehicle (V49.81)

The appropriate 7th character is to be added to each code from category V44

A - initial encounter

D - subsequent encounter

S - sequela

⊗⑦**V44.0** **Car driver injured in collision with heavy transport vehicle or bus in nontraffic accident**

⊗⑦**V44.1** **Car passenger injured in collision with heavy transport vehicle or bus in nontraffic accident**

⊗⑦**V44.2** **Person on outside of car injured in collision with heavy transport vehicle or bus in nontraffic accident**

⊗⑦**V44.3** **Unspecified car occupant injured in collision with heavy transport vehicle or bus in nontraffic accident**

⊗⑦**V44.4** **Person boarding or alighting a car injured in collision with heavy transport vehicle or bus**

⊗⑦**V44.5** **Car driver injured in collision with heavy transport vehicle or bus in traffic accident**

⊗⑦**V44.6** **Car passenger injured in collision with heavy transport vehicle or bus in traffic accident**

⊗⑦**V44.7** **Person on outside of car injured in collision with heavy transport vehicle or bus in traffic accident**

⊗⑦**V44.9** **Unspecified car occupant injured in collision with heavy transport vehicle or bus in traffic accident**

V45 **Car occupant injured in collision with railway train or railway vehicle**

The appropriate 7th character is to be added to each code from category V45

A - initial encounter

D - subsequent encounter

S - sequela

⊗⑦**V45.0** **Car driver injured in collision with railway train or railway vehicle in nontraffic accident**

⊗⑦**V45.1** **Car passenger injured in collision with railway train or railway vehicle in nontraffic accident**

⊗⑦**V45.2** **Person on outside of car injured in collision with railway train or railway vehicle in nontraffic accident**

⊗⑦**V45.3** **Unspecified car occupant injured in collision with railway train or railway vehicle in nontraffic accident**

⊗⑦**V45.4** **Person boarding or alighting a car injured in collision with railway train or railway vehicle**

⊗⑦**V45.5** **Car driver injured in collision with railway train or railway vehicle in traffic accident**

⊗⑦**V45.6** **Car passenger injured in collision with railway train or railway vehicle in traffic accident**

⊗⑦**V45.7** **Person on outside of car injured in collision with railway train or railway vehicle in traffic accident**

⊗⑦**V45.9** **Unspecified car occupant injured in collision with railway train or railway vehicle in traffic accident**

V46 **Car occupant injured in collision with other nonmotor vehicle**

Includes: collision with animal-drawn vehicle, animal being ridden, streetcar

The appropriate 7th character is to be added to each code from category V46

A - initial encounter

D - subsequent encounter

S - sequela

⊗⑦**V46.0** **Car driver injured in collision with other nonmotor vehicle in nontraffic accident**

⊗⑦**V46.1** **Car passenger injured in collision with other nonmotor vehicle in nontraffic accident**

⊗⑦**V46.2** **Person on outside of car injured in collision with other nonmotor vehicle in nontraffic accident**

⊗⑦**V46.3** **Unspecified car occupant injured in collision with other nonmotor vehicle in nontraffic accident**

⊗⑦**V46.4** **Person boarding or alighting a car injured in collision with other nonmotor vehicle**

⊗⑦**V46.5** **Car driver injured in collision with other nonmotor vehicle in traffic accident**

⊗⑦**V46.6** **Car passenger injured in collision with other nonmotor vehicle in traffic accident**

⊗⑦**V46.7** **Person on outside of car injured in collision with other nonmotor vehicle in traffic accident**

⊗⑦**V46.9** **Unspecified car occupant injured in collision with other nonmotor vehicle in traffic accident**

V47 **Car occupant injured in collision with fixed or stationary object**

The appropriate 7th character is to be added to each code from category V47

A - initial encounter

D - subsequent encounter

S - sequela

⊗⑦**V47.0** **Car driver injured in collision with fixed or stationary object in nontraffic accident**

⊗⑦**V47.1** **Car passenger injured in collision with fixed or stationary object in nontraffic accident**

⊗⑦**V47.2** **Person on outside of car injured in collision with fixed or stationary object in nontraffic accident**

⊗⑦**V47.3** **Unspecified car occupant injured in collision with fixed or stationary object in nontraffic accident**

⊗⑦**V47.4** **Person boarding or alighting a car injured in collision with fixed or stationary object**

⊗⑦**V47.5** **Car driver injured in collision with fixed or stationary object in traffic accident**

⊗⑦**V47.6** **Car passenger injured in collision with fixed or stationary object in traffic accident**

⊗⑦**V47.7** **Person on outside of car injured in collision with fixed or stationary object in traffic accident**

⊗⑦**V47.9** **Unspecified car occupant injured in collision with fixed or stationary object in traffic accident**

V48 **Car occupant injured in Non collision transport accident**

Includes: overturning car NOS

overturning car without collision

The appropriate 7th character is to be added to each code from category V48

A - initial encounter

D - subsequent encounter

S - sequela

⊗⑦**V48.0** **Car driver injured in Non collision transport accident in nontraffic accident**

⊗⑦**V48.1** **Car passenger injured in Non collision transport accident in nontraffic accident**

⊗⑦**V48.2** **Person on outside of car injured in Non collision transport accident in nontraffic accident**

⊗⑦**V48.3** **Unspecified car occupant injured in Non collision transport accident in nontraffic accident**

⊗⑦**V48.4** Person boarding or alighting a car injured in Non collision transport accident

⊗⑦**V48.5** Car driver injured in Non collision transport accident in traffic accident

⊗⑦**V48.6** Car passenger injured in Non collision transport accident in traffic accident

⊗⑦**V48.7** Person on outside of car injured in Non collision transport accident in traffic accident

⊗⑦**V48.9** Unspecified car occupant injured in Non collision transport accident in traffic accident

V49 Car occupant injured in other and unspecified transport accidents

The appropriate 7th character is to be added to each code from category V49

A - initial encounter

D - subsequent encounter

S - sequela

V49.0 Driver injured in collision with other and unspecified motor vehicles in nontraffic accident

⊗⑦**V49.00** Driver injured in collision with unspecified motor vehicles in nontraffic accident

⊗⑦**V49.09** Driver injured in collision with other motor vehicles in nontraffic accident

V49.1 Passenger injured in collision with other and unspecified motor vehicles in nontraffic accident

⊗⑦**V49.10** Passenger injured in collision with unspecified motor vehicles in nontraffic accident

⊗⑦**V49.19** Passenger injured in collision with other motor vehicles in nontraffic accident

V49.2 Unspecified car occupant injured in collision with other and unspecified motor vehicles in nontraffic accident

⊗⑦**V49.20** Unspecified car occupant injured in collision with unspecified motor vehicles in nontraffic accident

Car collision NOS, nontraffic

⊗⑦**V49.29** Unspecified car occupant injured in collision with other motor vehicles in nontraffic accident

⊗⑦**V49.3** Car occupant (driver) (passenger) injured in unspecified nontraffic accident

Car accident NOS, nontraffic

Car occupant injured in nontraffic accident NOS

V49.4 Driver injured in collision with other and unspecified motor vehicles in traffic accident

⊗⑦**V49.40** Driver injured in collision with unspecified motor vehicles in traffic accident

⊗⑦**V49.49** Driver injured in collision with other motor vehicles in traffic accident

V49.5 Passenger injured in collision with other and unspecified motor vehicles in traffic accident

⊗⑦**V49.50** Passenger injured in collision with unspecified motor vehicles in traffic accident

⊗⑦**V49.59** Passenger injured in collision with other motor vehicles in traffic accident

V49.6 Unspecified car occupant injured in collision with other and unspecified motor vehicles in traffic accident

⊗⑦**V49.60** Unspecified car occupant injured in collision with unspecified motor vehicles in traffic accident

Car collision NOS (traffic)

⊗⑦**V49.69** Unspecified car occupant injured in collision with other motor vehicles in traffic accident

V49.8 Car occupant (driver) (passenger) injured in other specified transport accidents

⊗⑦**V49.81** Car occupant (driver) (passenger) injured in transport accident with military vehicle

⊗⑦**V49.88** Car occupant (driver) (passenger) injured in other specified transport accidents

⊗⑦**V49.9** Car occupant (driver) (passenger) injured in unspecified traffic accident

Car accident NOS

OCCUPANT OF PICK-UP TRUCK OR VAN INJURED IN TRANSPORT ACCIDENT (V50-V59)

Includes: a four- or six-wheel motor vehicle designed primarily for carrying passengers and property but weighing less than the local limit for classification as a heavy goods vehicle

minibus

minivan

sport utility vehicle (SUV)

truck

van

Excludes1: heavy transport vehicle (V60-V69)

V50 Occupant of pick-up truck or van injured in collision with pedestrian or animal

Excludes1: pick-up truck or van collision with animal-drawn vehicle or animal being ridden (V56.-)

The appropriate 7th character is to be added to each code from category V50

A - initial encounter

D - subsequent encounter

S - sequela

⊗⑦**V50.0** Driver of pick-up truck or van injured in collision with pedestrian or animal in nontraffic accident

⊗⑦**V50.1** Passenger in pick-up truck or van injured in collision with pedestrian or animal in nontraffic accident

⊗⑦**V50.2** Person on outside of pick-up truck or van injured in collision with pedestrian or animal in nontraffic accident

⊗⑦**V50.3** Unspecified occupant of pick-up truck or van injured in collision with pedestrian or animal in nontraffic accident

⊗⑦**V50.4** Person boarding or alighting a pick-up truck or van injured in collision with pedestrian or animal

⊗⑦**V50.5** Driver of pick-up truck or van injured in collision with pedestrian or animal in traffic accident

⊗⑦**V50.6** Passenger in pick-up truck or van injured in collision with pedestrian or animal in traffic accident

⊗⑦**V50.7** Person on outside of pick-up truck or van injured in collision with pedestrian or animal in traffic accident

⊗⑦**V50.9** Unspecified occupant of pick-up truck or van injured in collision with pedestrian or animal in traffic accident

V51 Occupant of pick-up truck or van injured in collision with pedal cycle

The appropriate 7th character is to be added to each code from category V51

A - initial encounter

D - subsequent encounter

S - sequela

⊗⑦**V51.0** Driver of pick-up truck or van injured in collision with pedal cycle in nontraffic accident

⊗⑦**V51.1** Passenger in pick-up truck or van injured in collision with pedal cycle in nontraffic accident

⊗⑦**V51.2** Person on outside of pick-up truck or van injured in collision with pedal cycle in nontraffic accident

⊗⑦**V51.3** Unspecified occupant of pick-up truck or van injured in collision with pedal cycle in nontraffic accident

● New code   ▲ Revised code   **Excludes1:** Not coded here   **Excludes2:** Not included here   ⊗ Placeholder required   ⑦ 7th digit required

⊗⑦**V51.4** Person boarding or alighting a pick-up truck or van injured in collision with pedal cycle

⊗⑦**V51.5** Driver of pick-up truck or van injured in collision with pedal cycle in traffic accident

⊗⑦**V51.6** Passenger in pick-up truck or van injured in collision with pedal cycle in traffic accident

⊗⑦**V51.7** Person on outside of pick-up truck or van injured in collision with pedal cycle in traffic accident

⊗⑦**V51.9** Unspecified occupant of pick-up truck or van injured in collision with pedal cycle in traffic accident

V52 Occupant of pick-up truck or van injured in collision with two- or three-wheeled motor vehicle

The appropriate 7th character is to be added to each code from category V52

A - initial encounter

D - subsequent encounter

S - sequela

⊗⑦**V52.0** Driver of pick-up truck or van injured in collision with two- or three-wheeled motor vehicle in nontraffic accident

⊗⑦**V52.1** Passenger in pick-up truck or van injured in collision with two- or three-wheeled motor vehicle in nontraffic accident

⊗⑦**V52.2** Person on outside of pick-up truck or van injured in collision with two- or three-wheeled motor vehicle in nontraffic accident

⊗⑦**V52.3** Unspecified occupant of pick-up truck or van injured in collision with two- or three-wheeled motor vehicle in nontraffic accident

⊗⑦**V52.4** Person boarding or alighting a pick-up truck or van injured in collision with two- or three-wheeled motor vehicle

⊗⑦**V52.5** Driver of pick-up truck or van injured in collision with two- or three-wheeled motor vehicle in traffic accident

⊗⑦**V52.6** Passenger in pick-up truck or van injured in collision with two- or three-wheeled motor vehicle in traffic accident

⊗⑦**V52.7** Person on outside of pick-up truck or van injured in collision with two- or three-wheeled motor vehicle in traffic accident

⊗⑦**V52.9** Unspecified occupant of pick-up truck or van injured in collision with two- or three-wheeled motor vehicle in traffic accident

V53 Occupant of pick-up truck or van injured in collision with car, pick-up truck or van

The appropriate 7th character is to be added to each code from category V53

A - initial encounter

D - subsequent encounter

S - sequela

⊗⑦**V53.0** Driver of pick-up truck or van injured in collision with car, pick-up truck or van in nontraffic accident

⊗⑦**V53.1** Passenger in pick-up truck or van injured in collision with car, pick-up truck or van in nontraffic accident

⊗⑦**V53.2** Person on outside of pick-up truck or van injured in collision with car, pick-up truck or van in nontraffic accident

⊗⑦**V53.3** Unspecified occupant of pick-up truck or van injured in collision with car, pick-up truck or van in nontraffic accident

⊗⑦**V53.4** Person boarding or alighting a pick-up truck or van injured in collision with car, pick-up truck or van

⊗⑦**V53.5** Driver of pick-up truck or van injured in collision with car, pick-up truck or van in traffic accident

⊗⑦**V53.6** Passenger in pick-up truck or van injured in collision with car, pick-up truck or van in traffic accident

⊗⑦**V53.7** Person on outside of pick-up truck or van injured in collision with car, pick-up truck or van in traffic accident

⊗⑦**V53.9** Unspecified occupant of pick-up truck or van injured in collision with car, pick-up truck or van in traffic accident

V54 Occupant of pick-up truck or van injured in collision with heavy transport vehicle or bus

Excludes1: occupant of pick-up truck or van injured in collision with military vehicle (V59.81)

The appropriate 7th character is to be added to each code from category V54

A - initial encounter

D - subsequent encounter

S - sequela

⊗⑦**V54.0** Driver of pick-up truck or van injured in collision with heavy transport vehicle or bus in nontraffic accident

⊗⑦**V54.1** Passenger in pick-up truck or van injured in collision with heavy transport vehicle or bus in nontraffic accident

⊗⑦**V54.2** Person on outside of pick-up truck or van injured in collision with heavy transport vehicle or bus in nontraffic accident

⊗⑦**V54.3** Unspecified occupant of pick-up truck or van injured in collision with heavy transport vehicle or bus in nontraffic accident

⊗⑦**V54.4** Person boarding or alighting a pick-up truck or van injured in collision with heavy transport vehicle or bus

⊗⑦**V54.5** Driver of pick-up truck or van injured in collision with heavy transport vehicle or bus in traffic accident

⊗⑦**V54.6** Passenger in pick-up truck or van injured in collision with heavy transport vehicle or bus in traffic accident

⊗⑦**V54.7** Person on outside of pick-up truck or van injured in collision with heavy transport vehicle or bus in traffic accident

⊗⑦**V54.9** Unspecified occupant of pick-up truck or van injured in collision with heavy transport vehicle or bus in traffic accident

V55 Occupant of pick-up truck or van injured in collision with railway train or railway vehicle

The appropriate 7th character is to be added to each code from category V55

A - initial encounter

D - subsequent encounter

S - sequela

⊗⑦**V55.0** Driver of pick-up truck or van injured in collision with railway train or railway vehicle in nontraffic accident

⊗⑦**V55.1** Passenger in pick-up truck or van injured in collision with railway train or railway vehicle in nontraffic accident

⊗⑦**V55.2** Person on outside of pick-up truck or van injured in collision with railway train or railway vehicle in nontraffic accident

⊗⑦**V55.3** Unspecified occupant of pick-up truck or van injured in collision with railway train or railway vehicle in nontraffic accident

⊗⑦**V55.4** Person boarding or alighting a pick-up truck or van injured in collision with railway train or railway vehicle

⊗⑦**V55.5** Driver of pick-up truck or van injured in collision with railway train or railway vehicle in traffic accident

⊗⑦**V55.6** Passenger in pick-up truck or van injured in collision with railway train or railway vehicle in traffic accident

⊗⑦V55.7 Person on outside of pick-up truck or van injured in collision with railway train or railway vehicle in traffic accident

⊗⑦V55.9 Unspecified occupant of pick-up truck or van injured in collision with railway train or railway vehicle in traffic accident

V56 Occupant of pick-up truck or van injured in collision with other nonmotor vehicle

Includes: collision with animal-drawn vehicle, animal being ridden, streetcar

The appropriate 7th character is to be added to each code from category V56

A - initial encounter

D - subsequent encounter

S - sequela

⊗⑦V56.0 Driver of pick-up truck or van injured in collision with other nonmotor vehicle in nontraffic accident

⊗⑦V56.1 Passenger in pick-up truck or van injured in collision with other nonmotor vehicle in nontraffic accident

⊗⑦V56.2 Person on outside of pick-up truck or van injured in collision with other nonmotor vehicle in nontraffic accident

⊗⑦V56.3 Unspecified occupant of pick-up truck or van injured in collision with other nonmotor vehicle in nontraffic accident

⊗⑦V56.4 Person boarding or alighting a pick-up truck or van injured in collision with other nonmotor vehicle

⊗⑦V56.5 Driver of pick-up truck or van injured in collision with other nonmotor vehicle in traffic accident

⊗⑦V56.6 Passenger in pick-up truck or van injured in collision with other nonmotor vehicle in traffic accident

⊗⑦V56.7 Person on outside of pick-up truck or van injured in collision with other nonmotor vehicle in traffic accident

⊗⑦V56.9 Unspecified occupant of pick-up truck or van injured in collision with other nonmotor vehicle in traffic accident

V57 Occupant of pick-up truck or van injured in collision with fixed or stationary object

The appropriate 7th character is to be added to each code from category V57

A - initial encounter

D - subsequent encounter

S - sequela

⊗⑦V57.0 Driver of pick-up truck or van injured in collision with fixed or stationary object in nontraffic accident

⊗⑦V57.1 Passenger in pick-up truck or van injured in collision with fixed or stationary object in nontraffic accident

⊗⑦V57.2 Person on outside of pick-up truck or van injured in collision with fixed or stationary object in nontraffic accident

⊗⑦V57.3 Unspecified occupant of pick-up truck or van injured in collision with fixed or stationary object in nontraffic accident

⊗⑦V57.4 Person boarding or alighting a pick-up truck or van injured in collision with fixed or stationary object

⊗⑦V57.5 Driver of pick-up truck or van injured in collision with fixed or stationary object in traffic accident

⊗⑦V57.6 Passenger in pick-up truck or van injured in collision with fixed or stationary object in traffic accident

⊗⑦V57.7 Person on outside of pick-up truck or van injured in collision with fixed or stationary object in traffic accident

⊗⑦V57.9 Unspecified occupant of pick-up truck or van injured in collision with fixed or stationary object in traffic accident

V58 Occupant of pick-up truck or van injured in Non collision transport accident

Includes: overturning pick-up truck or van NOS

overturning pick-up truck or van without collision

The appropriate 7th character is to be added to each code from category V58

A - initial encounter

D - subsequent encounter

S - sequela

⊗⑦V58.0 Driver of pick-up truck or van injured in Non collision transport accident in nontraffic accident

⊗⑦V58.1 Passenger in pick-up truck or van injured in Non collision transport accident in nontraffic accident

⊗⑦V58.2 Person on outside of pick-up truck or van injured in Non collision transport accident in nontraffic accident

⊗⑦V58.3 Unspecified occupant of pick-up truck or van injured in Non collision transport accident in nontraffic accident

⊗⑦V58.4 Person boarding or alighting a pick-up truck or van injured in Non collision transport accident

⊗⑦V58.5 Driver of pick-up truck or van injured in Non collision transport accident in traffic accident

⊗⑦V58.6 Passenger in pick-up truck or van injured in Non collision transport accident in traffic accident

⊗⑦V58.7 Person on outside of pick-up truck or van injured in Non collision transport accident in traffic accident

⊗⑦V58.9 Unspecified occupant of pick-up truck or van injured in Non collision transport accident in traffic accident

V59 Occupant of pick-up truck or van injured in other and unspecified transport accidents

The appropriate 7th character is to be added to each code from category V59

A - initial encounter

D - subsequent encounter

S - sequela

V59.0 Driver of pick-up truck or van injured in collision with other and unspecified motor vehicles in nontraffic accident

⊗⑦V59.00 Driver of pick-up truck or van injured in collision with unspecified motor vehicles in nontraffic accident

⊗⑦V59.09 Driver of pick-up truck or van injured in collision with other motor vehicles in nontraffic accident

V59.1 Passenger in pick-up truck or van injured in collision with other and unspecified motor vehicles in nontraffic accident

⊗⑦V59.10 Passenger in pick-up truck or van injured in collision with unspecified motor vehicles in nontraffic accident

⊗⑦V59.19 Passenger in pick-up truck or van injured in collision with other motor vehicles in nontraffic accident

V59.2 Unspecified occupant of pick-up truck or van injured in collision with other and unspecified motor vehicles in nontraffic accident

⊗⑦V59.20 Unspecified occupant of pick-up truck or van injured in collision with unspecified motor vehicles in nontraffic accident

Collision NOS involving pick-up truck or van, nontraffic

⊗⑦V59.29 Unspecified occupant of pick-up truck or van injured in collision with other motor vehicles in nontraffic accident

● New code ▲ Revised code **Excludes1:** Not coded here **Excludes2:** Not included here ⊗ Placeholder required ⑦ 7th digit required

⊗⑦V59.3　**Occupant (driver) (passenger) of pick-up truck or van injured in unspecified nontraffic accident**

　　Accident NOS involving pick-up truck or van, nontraffic

　　Occupant of pick-up truck or van injured in nontraffic accident NOS

V59.4　**Driver of pick-up truck or van injured in collision with other and unspecified motor vehicles in traffic accident**

　⊗⑦V59.40　**Driver of pick-up truck or van injured in collision with unspecified motor vehicles in traffic accident**

　⊗⑦V59.49　**Driver of pick-up truck or van injured in collision with other motor vehicles in traffic accident**

V59.5　**Passenger in pick-up truck or van injured in collision with other and unspecified motor vehicles in traffic accident**

　⊗⑦V59.50　**Passenger in pick-up truck or van injured in collision with unspecified motor vehicles in traffic accident**

　⊗⑦V59.59　**Passenger in pick-up truck or van injured in collision with other motor vehicles in traffic accident**

V59.6　**Unspecified occupant of pick-up truck or van injured in collision with other and unspecified motor vehicles in traffic accident**

　⊗⑦V59.60　**Unspecified occupant of pick-up truck or van injured in collision with unspecified motor vehicles in traffic accident**

　　　Collision NOS involving pick-up truck or van (traffic)

　⊗⑦V59.69　**Unspecified occupant of pick-up truck or van injured in collision with other motor vehicles in traffic accident**

V59.8　**Occupant (driver) (passenger) of pick-up truck or van injured in other specified transport accidents**

　⊗⑦V59.81　**Occupant (driver) (passenger) of pick-up truck or van injured in transport accident with military vehicle**

　⊗⑦V59.88　**Occupant (driver) (passenger) of pick-up truck or van injured in other specified transport accidents**

⊗⑦V59.9　**Occupant (driver) (passenger) of pick-up truck or van injured in unspecified traffic accident**

　　Accident NOS involving pick-up truck or van

OCCUPANT OF HEAVY TRANSPORT VEHICLE INJURED IN TRANSPORT ACCIDENT (V60-V69)

Includes: 18-wheeler

armored car panel truck

Excludes1: bus

motorcoach

V60　**Occupant of heavy transport vehicle injured in collision with pedestrian or animal**

　Excludes1: heavy transport vehicle collision with animal-drawn vehicle or animal being ridden (V66.-)

The appropriate 7th character is to be added to each code from category V60

A - initial encounter

D - subsequent encounter

S - sequela

⊗⑦V60.0　**Driver of heavy transport vehicle injured in collision with pedestrian or animal in nontraffic accident**

⊗⑦V60.1　**Passenger in heavy transport vehicle injured in collision with pedestrian or animal in nontraffic accident**

⊗⑦V60.2　**Person on outside of heavy transport vehicle injured in collision with pedestrian or animal in nontraffic accident**

⊗⑦V60.3　**Unspecified occupant of heavy transport vehicle injured in collision with pedestrian or animal in nontraffic accident**

⊗⑦V60.4　**Person boarding or alighting a heavy transport vehicle injured in collision with pedestrian or animal**

⊗⑦V60.5　**Driver of heavy transport vehicle injured in collision with pedestrian or animal in traffic accident**

⊗⑦V60.6　**Passenger in heavy transport vehicle injured in collision with pedestrian or animal in traffic accident**

⊗⑦V60.7　**Person on outside of heavy transport vehicle injured in collision with pedestrian or animal in traffic accident**

⊗⑦V60.9　**Unspecified occupant of heavy transport vehicle injured in collision with pedestrian or animal in traffic accident**

V61　**Occupant of heavy transport vehicle injured in collision with pedal cycle**

The appropriate 7th character is to be added to each code from category V61

A - initial encounter

D - subsequent encounter

S - sequela

⊗⑦V61.0　**Driver of heavy transport vehicle injured in collision with pedal cycle in nontraffic accident**

⊗⑦V61.1　**Passenger in heavy transport vehicle injured in collision with pedal cycle in nontraffic accident**

⊗⑦V61.2　**Person on outside of heavy transport vehicle injured in collision with pedal cycle in nontraffic accident**

⊗⑦V61.3　**Unspecified occupant of heavy transport vehicle injured in collision with pedal cycle in nontraffic accident**

⊗⑦V61.4　**Person boarding or alighting a heavy transport vehicle injured in collision with pedal cycle while boarding or alighting**

⊗⑦V61.5　**Driver of heavy transport vehicle injured in collision with pedal cycle in traffic accident**

⊗⑦V61.6　**Passenger in heavy transport vehicle injured in collision with pedal cycle in traffic accident**

⊗⑦V61.7　**Person on outside of heavy transport vehicle injured in collision with pedal cycle in traffic accident**

⊗⑦V61.9　**Unspecified occupant of heavy transport vehicle injured in collision with pedal cycle in traffic accident**

V62　**Occupant of heavy transport vehicle injured in collision with two- or three-wheeled motor vehicle**

The appropriate 7th character is to be added to each code from category V62

A - initial encounter

D - subsequent encounter

S - sequela

⊗⑦V62.0　**Driver of heavy transport vehicle injured in collision with two- or three-wheeled motor vehicle in nontraffic accident**

⊗⑦V62.1　**Passenger in heavy transport vehicle injured in collision with two- or three-wheeled motor vehicle in nontraffic accident**

⊗⑦V62.2　**Person on outside of heavy transport vehicle injured in collision with two- or three-wheeled motor vehicle in nontraffic accident**

⊗⑦V62.3　**Unspecified occupant of heavy transport vehicle injured in collision with two- or three-wheeled motor vehicle in nontraffic accident**

⊗⑦V62.4　**Person boarding or alighting a heavy transport vehicle injured in collision with two- or three-way vehicle**

⊗⑦**V62.5** Driver of heavy transport vehicle injured in collision with two- or three-wheeled motor vehicle in traffic accident

⊗⑦**V62.6** Passenger in heavy transport vehicle injured in collision with two- or three-wheeled motor vehicle in traffic accident

⊗⑦**V62.7** Person on outside of heavy transport vehicle injured in collision with two- or three-wheeled motor vehicle in traffic accident

⊗⑦**V62.9** Unspecified occupant of heavy transport vehicle injured in collision with two- or three-wheeled motor vehicle in traffic accident

V63 Occupant of heavy transport vehicle injured in collision with car, pick-up truck or van

The appropriate 7th character is to be added to each code from category V63

A - initial encounter

D - subsequent encounter

S - sequela

⊗⑦**V63.0** Driver of heavy transport vehicle injured in collision with car, pick-up truck or van in nontraffic accident

⊗⑦**V63.1** Passenger in heavy transport vehicle injured in collision with car, pick-up truck or van in nontraffic accident

⊗⑦**V63.2** Person on outside of heavy transport vehicle injured in collision with car, pick-up truck or van in nontraffic accident

⊗⑦**V63.3** Unspecified occupant of heavy transport vehicle injured in collision with car, pick-up truck or van in nontraffic accident

⊗⑦**V63.4** Person boarding or alighting a heavy transport vehicle injured in collision with car, pick-up truck or van

⊗⑦**V63.5** Driver of heavy transport vehicle injured in collision with car, pick-up truck or van in traffic accident

⊗⑦**V63.6** Passenger in heavy transport vehicle injured in collision with car, pick-up truck or van in traffic accident

⊗⑦**V63.7** Person on outside of heavy transport vehicle injured in collision with car, pick-up truck or van in traffic accident

⊗⑦**V63.9** Unspecified occupant of heavy transport vehicle injured in collision with car, pick-up truck or van in traffic accident

V64 Occupant of heavy transport vehicle injured in collision with heavy transport vehicle or bus

Excludes1: occupant of heavy transport vehicle injured in collision with military vehicle (V69.81)

The appropriate 7th character is to be added to each code from category V64

A - initial encounter

D - subsequent encounter

S - sequela

⊗⑦**V64.0** Driver of heavy transport vehicle injured in collision with heavy transport vehicle or bus in nontraffic accident

⊗⑦**V64.1** Passenger in heavy transport vehicle injured in collision with heavy transport vehicle or bus in nontraffic accident

⊗⑦**V64.2** Person on outside of heavy transport vehicle injured in collision with heavy transport vehicle or bus in nontraffic accident

⊗⑦**V64.3** Unspecified occupant of heavy transport vehicle injured in collision with heavy transport vehicle or bus in nontraffic accident

⊗⑦**V64.4** Person boarding or alighting a heavy transport vehicle injured in collision with heavy transport vehicle or bus while boarding or alighting

⊗⑦**V64.5** Driver of heavy transport vehicle injured in collision with heavy transport vehicle or bus in traffic accident

⊗⑦**V64.6** Passenger in heavy transport vehicle injured in collision with heavy transport vehicle or bus in traffic accident

⊗⑦**V64.7** Person on outside of heavy transport vehicle injured in collision with heavy transport vehicle or bus in traffic accident

⊗⑦**V64.9** Unspecified occupant of heavy transport vehicle injured in collision with heavy transport vehicle or bus in traffic accident

V65 Occupant of heavy transport vehicle injured in collision with railway train or railway vehicle

The appropriate 7th character is to be added to each code from category V65

A - initial encounter

D - subsequent encounter

S - sequela

⊗⑦**V65.0** Driver of heavy transport vehicle injured in collision with railway train or railway vehicle in nontraffic accident

⊗⑦**V65.1** Passenger in heavy transport vehicle injured in collision with railway train or railway vehicle in nontraffic accident

⊗⑦**V65.2** Person on outside of heavy transport vehicle injured in collision with railway train or railway vehicle in nontraffic accident

⊗⑦**V65.3** Unspecified occupant of heavy transport vehicle injured in collision with railway train or railway vehicle in nontraffic accident

⊗⑦**V65.4** Person boarding or alighting a heavy transport vehicle injured in collision with railway train or railway vehicle

⊗⑦**V65.5** Driver of heavy transport vehicle injured in collision with railway train or railway vehicle in traffic accident

⊗⑦**V65.6** Passenger in heavy transport vehicle injured in collision with railway train or railway vehicle in traffic accident

⊗⑦**V65.7** Person on outside of heavy transport vehicle injured in collision with railway train or railway vehicle in traffic accident

⊗⑦**V65.9** Unspecified occupant of heavy transport vehicle injured in collision with railway train or railway vehicle in traffic accident

V66 Occupant of heavy transport vehicle injured in collision with other nonmotor vehicle

Includes: collision with animal-drawn vehicle, animal being ridden, streetcar

The appropriate 7th character is to be added to each code from category V66

A - initial encounter

D - subsequent encounter

S - sequela

⊗⑦**V66.0** Driver of heavy transport vehicle injured in collision with other nonmotor vehicle in nontraffic accident

⊗⑦**V66.1** Passenger in heavy transport vehicle injured in collision with other nonmotor vehicle in nontraffic accident

⊗⑦**V66.2** Person on outside of heavy transport vehicle injured in collision with other nonmotor vehicle in nontraffic accident

⊗⑦**V66.3** Unspecified occupant of heavy transport vehicle injured in collision with other nonmotor vehicle in nontraffic accident

⊗⑦**V66.4** Person boarding or alighting a heavy transport vehicle injured in collision with other nonmotor vehicle

⊗⑦**V66.5** Driver of heavy transport vehicle injured in collision with other nonmotor vehicle in traffic accident

⊗⑦V66.6 **Passenger in heavy transport vehicle injured in collision with other nonmotor vehicle in traffic accident**

⊗⑦V66.7 **Person on outside of heavy transport vehicle injured in collision with other nonmotor vehicle in traffic accident**

⊗⑦V66.9 **Unspecified occupant of heavy transport vehicle injured in collision with other nonmotor vehicle in traffic accident**

V67 **Occupant of heavy transport vehicle injured in collision with fixed or stationary object**

The appropriate 7th character is to be added to each code from category V67

A - initial encounter

D - subsequent encounter

S - sequela

⊗⑦V67.0 **Driver of heavy transport vehicle injured in collision with fixed or stationary object in nontraffic accident**

⊗⑦V67.1 **Passenger in heavy transport vehicle injured in collision with fixed or stationary object in nontraffic accident**

⊗⑦V67.2 **Person on outside of heavy transport vehicle injured in collision with fixed or stationary object in nontraffic accident**

⊗⑦V67.3 **Unspecified occupant of heavy transport vehicle injured in collision with fixed or stationary object in nontraffic accident**

⊗⑦V67.4 **Person boarding or alighting a heavy transport vehicle injured in collision with fixed or stationary object vehicle injured in collision with other motor vehicles in nontraffic accident**

V69.2 **Unspecified occupant of heavy transport vehicle injured in collision with other and unspecified motor vehicles in nontraffic accident**

⊗⑦V69.20 **Unspecified occupant of heavy transport vehicle injured in collision with unspecified motor vehicles in nontraffic accident**

Collision NOS involving heavy transport vehicle, nontraffic

⊗⑦V69.29 **Unspecified occupant of heavy transport vehicle injured in collision with other motor vehicles in nontraffic accident**

⊗⑦V69.3 **Occupant (driver) (passenger) of heavy transport vehicle injured in unspecified nontraffic accident**

Accident NOS involving heavy transport vehicle, nontraffic

Occupant of heavy transport vehicle injured in nontraffic accident NOS

V69.4 **Driver of heavy transport vehicle injured in collision with other and unspecified motor vehicles in traffic accident**

⊗⑦V69.40 **Driver of heavy transport vehicle injured in collision with unspecified motor vehicles in traffic accident**

⊗⑦V69.49 **Driver of heavy transport vehicle injured in collision with other motor vehicles in traffic accident**

V69.5 **Passenger in heavy transport vehicle injured in collision with other and unspecified motor vehicles in traffic accident**

⊗⑦V69.50 **Passenger in heavy transport vehicle injured in collision with unspecified motor vehicles in traffic accident**

⊗⑦V69.59 **Passenger in heavy transport vehicle injured in collision with other motor vehicles in traffic accident**

V69.6 **Unspecified occupant of heavy transport vehicle injured in collision with other and unspecified motor vehicles in traffic accident**

⊗⑦V69.60 **Unspecified occupant of heavy transport vehicle injured in collision with unspecified motor vehicles in traffic accident**

Collision NOS involving heavy transport vehicle (traffic)

⊗⑦V69.69 **Unspecified occupant of heavy transport vehicle injured in collision with other motor vehicles in traffic accident**

V69.8 **Occupant (driver) (passenger) of heavy transport vehicle injured in other specified transport accidents**

⊗⑦V69.81 **Occupant (driver) (passenger) of heavy transport vehicle injured in transport accidents with military vehicle**

⊗⑦V69.88 **Occupant (driver) (passenger) of heavy transport vehicle injured in other specified transport accidents**

⊗⑦V69.9 **Occupant (driver) (passenger) of heavy transport vehicle injured in unspecified traffic accident**

Accident NOS involving heavy transport vehicle

BUS OCCUPANT INJURED IN TRANSPORT ACCIDENT (V70-V79)

Includes: motorcoach

Excludes1: minibus (V50-V59)

V70 **Bus occupant injured in collision with pedestrian or animal**

The appropriate 7th character is to be added to each code from category V70

A - initial encounter

D - subsequent encounter

S - sequela

Excludes1: bus collision with animal-drawn vehicle or animal being ridden (V76.-)

⊗⑦V70.0 **Driver of bus injured in collision with pedestrian or animal in nontraffic accident**

⊗⑦V70.1 **Passenger on bus injured in collision with pedestrian or animal in nontraffic accident**

⊗⑦V70.2 **Person on outside of bus injured in collision with pedestrian or animal in nontraffic accident**

⊗⑦V70.3 **Unspecified occupant of bus injured in collision with pedestrian or animal in nontraffic accident**

⊗⑦V70.4 **Person boarding or alighting from bus injured in collision with pedestrian or animal**

⊗⑦V70.5 **Driver of bus injured in collision with pedestrian or animal in traffic accident**

⊗⑦V70.6 **Passenger on bus injured in collision with pedestrian or animal in traffic accident**

⊗⑦V70.7 **Person on outside of bus injured in collision with pedestrian or animal in traffic accident**

⊗⑦V70.9 **Unspecified occupant of bus injured in collision with pedestrian or animal in traffic accident**

V71 **Bus occupant injured in collision with pedal cycle**

The appropriate 7th character is to be added to each code from category V71

A - initial encounter

D - subsequent encounter

S - sequela

⊗⑦V71.0 **Driver of bus injured in collision with pedal cycle in nontraffic accident**

⊗⑦V71.1 **Passenger on bus injured in collision with pedal cycle in nontraffic accident**

⊗⑦V71.2 **Person on outside of bus injured in collision with pedal cycle in nontraffic accident**

⊗⑦**V71.3** Unspecified occupant of bus injured in collision with pedal cycle in nontraffic accident

⊗⑦**V71.4** Person boarding or alighting from bus injured in collision with pedal cycle

⊗⑦**V71.5** Driver of bus injured in collision with pedal cycle in traffic accident

⊗⑦**V71.6** Passenger on bus injured in collision with pedal cycle in traffic accident

⊗⑦**V71.7** Person on outside of bus injured in collision with pedal cycle in traffic accident

⊗⑦**V71.9** Unspecified occupant of bus injured in collision with pedal cycle in traffic accident

V72 Bus occupant injured in collision with two- or three-wheeled motor vehicle

The appropriate 7th character is to be added to each code from category V72

A - initial encounter

D - subsequent encounter

S - sequela

⊗⑦**V72.0** Driver of bus injured in collision with two- or three-wheeled motor vehicle in nontraffic accident

⊗⑦**V72.1** Passenger on bus injured in collision with two- or three-wheeled motor vehicle in nontraffic accident

⊗⑦**V72.2** Person on outside of bus injured in collision with two- or three-wheeled motor vehicle in nontraffic accident

⊗⑦**V72.3** Unspecified occupant of bus injured in collision with two- or three-wheeled motor vehicle in nontraffic accident

⊗⑦**V72.4** Person boarding or alighting from bus injured in collision with two- or three-wheeled motor vehicle

⊗⑦**V72.5** Driver of bus injured in collision with two- or three-wheeled motor vehicle in traffic accident

⊗⑦**V72.6** Passenger on bus injured in collision with two- or three-wheeled motor vehicle in traffic accident

⊗⑦**V72.7** Person on outside of bus injured in collision with two- or three-wheeled motor vehicle in traffic accident

⊗⑦**V72.9** Unspecified occupant of bus injured in collision with two- or three-wheeled motor vehicle in traffic accident

V73 Bus occupant injured in collision with car, pick-up truck or van

The appropriate 7th character is to be added to each code from category V73

A - initial encounter

D - subsequent encounter

S - sequela

⊗⑦**V73.0** Driver of bus injured in collision with car, pick-up truck or van in nontraffic accident

⊗⑦**V73.1** Passenger on bus injured in collision with car, pick-up truck or van in nontraffic accident

⊗⑦**V73.2** Person on outside of bus injured in collision with car, pick-up truck or van in nontraffic accident

⊗⑦**V73.3** Unspecified occupant of bus injured in collision with car, pick-up truck or van in nontraffic accident

⊗⑦**V73.4** Person boarding or alighting from bus injured in collision with car, pick-up truck or van

⊗⑦**V73.5** Driver of bus injured in collision with car, pick-up truck or van in traffic accident

⊗⑦**V73.6** Passenger on bus injured in collision with car, pick-up truck or van in traffic accident

⊗⑦**V73.7** Person on outside of bus injured in collision with car, pick-up truck or van in traffic accident

⊗⑦**V73.9** Unspecified occupant of bus injured in collision with car, pick-up truck or van in traffic accident

V74 Bus occupant injured in collision with heavy transport vehicle or bus

Excludes1: bus occupant injured in collision with military vehicle (V79.81)

The appropriate 7th character is to be added to each code from category V74

A - initial encounter

D - subsequent encounter

S - sequela

⊗⑦**V74.0** Driver of bus injured in collision with heavy transport vehicle or bus in nontraffic accident

⊗⑦**V74.1** Passenger on bus injured in collision with heavy transport vehicle or bus in nontraffic accident

⊗⑦**V74.2** Person on outside of bus injured in collision with heavy transport vehicle or bus in nontraffic accident

⊗⑦**V74.3** Unspecified occupant of bus injured in collision with heavy transport vehicle or bus in nontraffic accident

⊗⑦**V74.4** Person boarding or alighting from bus injured in collision with heavy transport vehicle or bus

⊗⑦**V74.5** Driver of bus injured in collision with heavy transport vehicle or bus in traffic accident

⊗⑦**V74.6** Passenger on bus injured in collision with heavy transport vehicle or bus in traffic accident

⊗⑦**V74.7** Person on outside of bus injured in collision with heavy transport vehicle or bus in traffic accident

⊗⑦**V74.9** Unspecified occupant of bus injured in collision with heavy transport vehicle or bus in traffic accident

V75 Bus occupant injured in collision with railway train or railway vehicle

The appropriate 7th character is to be added to each code from category V75

A - initial encounter

D - subsequent encounter

S - sequela

⊗⑦**V75.0** Driver of bus injured in collision with railway train or railway vehicle in nontraffic accident

⊗⑦**V75.1** Passenger on bus injured in collision with railway train or railway vehicle in nontraffic accident

⊗⑦**V75.2** Person on outside of bus injured in collision with railway train or railway vehicle in nontraffic accident

⊗⑦**V75.3** Unspecified occupant of bus injured in collision with railway train or railway vehicle in nontraffic accident

⊗⑦**V75.4** Person boarding or alighting from bus injured in collision with railway train or railway vehicle

⊗⑦**V75.5** Driver of bus injured in collision with railway train or railway vehicle in traffic accident

⊗⑦**V75.6** Passenger on bus injured in collision with railway train or railway vehicle in traffic accident

⊗⑦**V75.7** Person on outside of bus injured in collision with railway train or railway vehicle in traffic accident

⊗⑦**V75.9** Unspecified occupant of bus injured in collision with railway train or railway vehicle in traffic accident

V76 Bus occupant injured in collision with other nonmotor vehicle

Includes: collision with animal-drawn vehicle, animal being ridden, streetcar

The appropriate 7th character is to be added to each code from category V76

A - initial encounter

D - subsequent encounter

S - sequela

⊗⑦**V76.0** Driver of bus injured in collision with other nonmotor vehicle in nontraffic accident

⊗⑦**V76.1** Passenger on bus injured in collision with other nonmotor vehicle in nontraffic accident

● New code ▲ Revised code **Excludes1:** Not coded here **Excludes2:** Not included here ⊗ Placeholder required ⑦ 7th digit required

⊗⑦**V76.2** Person on outside of bus injured in collision with other nonmotor vehicle in nontraffic accident

⊗⑦**V76.3** Unspecified occupant of bus injured in collision with other nonmotor vehicle in nontraffic accident

⊗⑦**V76.4** Person boarding or alighting from bus injured in collision with other nonmotor vehicle

⊗⑦**V76.5** Driver of bus injured in collision with other nonmotor vehicle in traffic accident

⊗⑦**V76.6** Passenger on bus injured in collision with other nonmotor vehicle in traffic accident

⊗⑦**V76.7** Person on outside of bus injured in collision with other nonmotor vehicle in traffic accident

⊗⑦**V76.9** Unspecified occupant of bus injured in collision with other nonmotor vehicle in traffic accident

V77 Bus occupant injured in collision with fixed or stationary object

The appropriate 7th character is to be added to each code from category V77

A - initial encounter

D - subsequent encounter

S - sequela

⊗⑦**V77.0** Driver of bus injured in collision with fixed or stationary object in nontraffic accident

⊗⑦**V77.1** Passenger on bus injured in collision with fixed or stationary object in nontraffic accident

⊗⑦**V77.2** Person on outside of bus injured in collision with fixed or stationary object in nontraffic accident

⊗⑦**V77.3** Unspecified occupant of bus injured in collision with fixed or stationary object in nontraffic accident

⊗⑦**V77.4** Person boarding or alighting from bus injured in collision with fixed or stationary object

⊗⑦**V77.5** Driver of bus injured in collision with fixed or stationary object in traffic accident

⊗⑦**V77.6** Passenger on bus injured in collision with fixed or stationary object in traffic accident

⊗⑦**V77.7** Person on outside of bus injured in collision with fixed or stationary object in traffic accident

⊗⑦**V77.9** Unspecified occupant of bus injured in collision with fixed or stationary object in traffic accident

V78 Bus occupant injured in Non collision transport accident

Includes: overturning bus NOS

overturning bus without collision

The appropriate 7th character is to be added to each code from category V78

A - initial encounter

D - subsequent encounter

S - sequela

⊗⑦**V78.0** Driver of bus injured in Non collision transport accident in nontraffic accident

⊗⑦**V78.1** Passenger on bus injured in Non collision transport accident in nontraffic accident

⊗⑦**V78.2** Person on outside of bus injured in Non collision transport accident in nontraffic accident

⊗⑦**V78.3** Unspecified occupant of bus injured in Non collision transport accident in nontraffic accident

⊗⑦**V78.4** Person boarding or alighting from bus injured in Non collision transport accident

⊗⑦**V78.5** Driver of bus injured in Non collision transport accident in traffic accident

⊗⑦**V78.6** Passenger on bus injured in Non collision transport accident in traffic accident

⊗⑦**V78.7** Person on outside of bus injured in Non collision transport accident in traffic accident

⊗⑦**V78.9** Unspecified occupant of bus injured in Non collision transport accident in traffic accident

V79 Bus occupant injured in other and unspecified transport accidents

The appropriate 7th character is to be added to each code from category V79

A - initial encounter

D - subsequent encounter

S - sequela

V79.0 Driver of bus injured in collision with other and unspecified motor vehicles in nontraffic accident

⊗⑦**V79.00** Driver of bus injured in collision with unspecified motor vehicles in nontraffic accident

⊗⑦**V79.09** Driver of bus injured in collision with other motor vehicles in nontraffic accident

V79.1 Passenger on bus injured in collision with other and unspecified motor vehicles in nontraffic accident

⊗⑦**V79.10** Passenger on bus injured in collision with unspecified motor vehicles in nontraffic accident

⊗⑦**V79.19** Passenger on bus injured in collision with other motor vehicles in nontraffic accident

V79.2 Unspecified bus occupant injured in collision with other and unspecified motor vehicles in nontraffic accident

⊗⑦**V79.20** Unspecified bus occupant injured in collision with unspecified motor vehicles in nontraffic accident

Bus collision NOS, nontraffic

⊗⑦**V79.29** Unspecified bus occupant injured in collision with other motor vehicles in nontraffic accident

V79.3 Bus occupant (driver) (passenger) injured in unspecified nontraffic accident

Bus accident NOS, nontraffic

Bus occupant injured in nontraffic accident NOS

V79.4 Driver of bus injured in collision with other and unspecified motor vehicles in traffic accident

⊗⑦**V79.40** Driver of bus injured in collision with unspecified motor vehicles in traffic accident

⊗⑦**V79.49** Driver of bus injured in collision with other motor vehicles in traffic accident

V79.5 Passenger on bus injured in collision with other and unspecified motor vehicles in traffic accident

⊗⑦**V79.50** Passenger on bus injured in collision with unspecified motor vehicles in traffic accident

⊗⑦**V79.59** Passenger on bus injured in collision with other motor vehicles in traffic accident

V79.6 Unspecified bus occupant injured in collision with other and unspecified motor vehicles in traffic accident

⊗⑦**V79.60** Unspecified bus occupant injured in collision with unspecified motor vehicles in traffic accident

Bus collision NOS (traffic)

⊗⑦**V79.69** Unspecified bus occupant injured in collision with other motor vehicles in traffic accident

V79.8 Bus occupant (driver) (passenger) injured in other specified transport accidents

⊗⑦**V79.81** Bus occupant (driver) (passenger) injured in transport accidents with military vehicle

⊗⑦**V79.88** Bus occupant (driver) (passenger) injured in other specified transport accidents

⊗⑦**V79.9** Bus occupant (driver) (passenger) injured in unspecified traffic accident

Bus accident NOS

OTHER LAND TRANSPORT ACCIDENTS (V80-V89)

V80 **Animal-rider or occupant of animal-drawn vehicle injured in transport accident**

The appropriate 7th character is to be added to each code from category V80

A - initial encounter

D - subsequent encounter

S - sequela

V80.0 **Animal-rider or occupant of animal drawn vehicle injured by fall from or being thrown from animal or animal-drawn vehicle in Non collision accident**

  V80.01 **Animal-rider injured by fall from or being thrown from animal in Non collision accident**

  ⑦**V80.010** **Animal-rider injured by fall from or being thrown from horse in Non collision accident**

  ⑦**V80.018** **Animal-rider injured by fall from or being thrown from other animal in Non collision accident**

  ⊗⑦**V80.02** **Occupant of animal-drawn vehicle injured by fall from or being thrown from animal-drawn vehicle in Non collision accident**

  Overturning animal-drawn vehicle NOS

  Overturning animal-drawn vehicle without collision

V80.1 **Animal-rider or occupant of animal-drawn vehicle injured in collision with pedestrian or animal**

  Excludes1: animal-rider or animal-drawn vehicle collision with animal-drawn vehicle or animal being ridden (V80.7)

  ⊗⑦**V80.11** **Animal-rider injured in collision with pedestrian or animal**

  ⊗⑦**V80.12** **Occupant of animal-drawn vehicle injured in collision with pedestrian or animal**

V80.2 **Animal-rider or occupant of animal-drawn vehicle injured in collision with pedal cycle**

  ⊗⑦**V80.21** **Animal-rider injured in collision with pedal cycle**

  ⊗⑦**V80.22** **Occupant of animal-drawn vehicle injured in collision with pedal cycle**

V80.3 **Animal-rider or occupant of animal-drawn vehicle injured in collision with two- or three-wheeled motor vehicle**

  ⊗⑦**V80.31** **Animal-rider injured in collision with two- or three-wheeled motor vehicle**

  ⊗⑦**V80.32** **Occupant of animal-drawn vehicle injured in collision with two- or three-wheeled motor vehicle**

V80.4 **Animal-rider or occupant of animal-drawn vehicle injured in collision with car, pick-up truck, van, heavy transport vehicle or bus**

  Excludes1: animal-rider injured in collision with military vehicle (V80.910)

  occupant of animal-drawn vehicle injured in collision with military vehicle (V80.920)

  ⊗⑦**V80.41** **Animal-rider injured in collision with car, pick-up truck, van, heavy transport vehicle or bus**

  ⊗⑦**V80.42** **Occupant of animal-drawn vehicle injured in collision with car, pick-up truck, van, heavy transport vehicle or bus**

V80.5 **Animal-rider or occupant of animal-drawn vehicle injured in collision with other specified motor vehicle**

  ⊗⑦**V80.51** **Animal-rider injured in collision with other specified motor vehicle**

  ⊗⑦**V80.52** **Occupant of animal-drawn vehicle injured in collision with other specified motor vehicle**

V80.6 **Animal-rider or occupant of animal-drawn vehicle injured in collision with railway train or railway vehicle**

  ⊗⑦**V80.61** **Animal-rider injured in collision with railway train or railway vehicle**

  ⊗⑦**V80.62** **Occupant of animal-drawn vehicle injured in collision with railway train or railway vehicle**

V80.7 **Animal-rider or occupant of animal-drawn vehicle injured in collision with other nonmotor vehicles**

  V80.71 **Animal-rider or occupant of animal-drawn vehicle injured in collision with animal being ridden**

  ⑦**V80.710** **Animal-rider injured in collision with other animal being ridden**

  ⑦**V80.711** **Occupant of animal-drawn vehicle injured in collision with animal being ridden**

  V80.72 **Animal-rider or occupant of animal-drawn vehicle injured in collision with other animal-drawn vehicle**

  ⑦**V80.720** **Animal-rider injured in collision with animal-drawn vehicle**

  ⑦**V80.721** **Occupant of animal-drawn vehicle injured in collision with other animal-drawn vehicle**

  V80.73 **Animal-rider or occupant of animal-drawn vehicle injured in collision with streetcar**

  ⑦**V80.730** **Animal-rider injured in collision with streetcar**

  ⑦**V80.731** **Occupant of animal-drawn vehicle injured in collision with streetcar**

  V80.79 **Animal-rider or occupant of animal-drawn vehicle injured in collision with other nonmotor vehicles**

  ⑦**V80.790** **Animal-rider injured in collision with other nonmotor vehicles**

  ⑦**V80.791** **Occupant of animal-drawn vehicle injured in collision with other nonmotor vehicles**

V80.8 **Animal-rider or occupant of animal-drawn vehicle injured in collision with fixed or stationary object**

  ⊗⑦**V80.81** **Animal-rider injured in collision with fixed or stationary object**

  ⊗⑦**V80.82** **Occupant of animal-drawn vehicle injured in collision with fixed or stationary object**

V80.9 **Animal-rider or occupant of animal-drawn vehicle injured in other and unspecified transport accidents**

  V80.91 **Animal-rider injured in other and unspecified transport accidents**

  ⑦**V80.910** **Animal-rider injured in transport accident with military vehicle**

  ⑦**V80.918** **Animal-rider injured in other transport accident**

  ⑦**V80.919** **Animal-rider injured in unspecified transport accident**

  Animal rider accident NOS

  V80.92 **Occupant of animal-drawn vehicle injured in other and unspecified transport accidents**

  ⑦**V80.920** **Occupant of animal-drawn vehicle injured in transport accident with military vehicle**

⑦**V80.928** **Occupant of animal-drawn vehicle injured in other transport accident**

⑦**V80.929** **Occupant of animal-drawn vehicle injured in unspecified transport accident**

Animal-drawn vehicle accident NOS

V81 **Occupant of railway train or railway vehicle injured in transport accident**

Includes: derailment of railway train or railway vehicle

person on outside of train

Excludes1: streetcar (V82.-)

The appropriate 7th character is to be added to each code from category V81

A - initial encounter

D - subsequent encounter

S - sequela

⊗⑦**V81.0** **Occupant of railway train or railway vehicle injured in collision with motor vehicle in nontraffic accident**

Excludes1: Occupant of railway train or railway vehicle injured due to collision with military vehicle (V81.83)

⊗⑦**V81.1** **Occupant of railway train or railway vehicle injured in collision with motor vehicle in traffic accident**

Excludes1: Occupant of railway train or railway vehicle injured due to collision with military vehicle (V81.83)

⊗⑦**V81.2** **Occupant of railway train or railway vehicle injured in collision with or hit by rolling stock**

⊗⑦**V81.3** **Occupant of railway train or railway vehicle injured in collision with other object**

Railway collision NOS

⊗⑦**V81.4** **Person injured while boarding or alighting from railway train or railway vehicle**

⊗⑦**V81.5** **Occupant of railway train or railway vehicle injured by fall in railway train or railway vehicle**

⊗⑦**V81.6** **Occupant of railway train or railway vehicle injured by fall from railway train or railway vehicle**

⊗⑦**V81.7** **Occupant of railway train or railway vehicle injured in derailment without antecedent collision**

V81.8 **Occupant of railway train or railway vehicle injured in other specified railway accidents**

⊗⑦**V81.81** **Occupant of railway train or railway vehicle injured due to explosion or fire on train**

⊗⑦**V81.82** **Occupant of railway train or railway vehicle injured due to object falling onto train**

Occupant of railway train or railway vehicle injured due to falling earth onto train

Occupant of railway train or railway vehicle injured due to falling rocks onto train

Occupant of railway train or railway vehicle injured due to falling snow onto train

Occupant of railway train or railway vehicle injured due to falling trees onto train

⊗⑦**V81.83** **Occupant of railway train or railway vehicle injured due to collision with military vehicle**

⊗⑦**V81.89** **Occupant of railway train or railway vehicle injured due to other specified railway accident**

⊗⑦**V81.9** **Occupant of railway train or railway vehicle injured in unspecified railway accident**

Railway accident NOS

V82 **Occupant of powered streetcar injured in transport accident**

Includes: interurban electric car

person on outside of streetcar tram (car)

trolley (car)

Excludes1: bus (V70-V79)

motorcoach (V70-V79)

nonpowered streetcar (V76.-) train (V81.-)

The appropriate 7th character is to be added to each code from category V82

A - initial encounter

D - subsequent encounter

S - sequela

⊗⑦**V82.0** **Occupant of streetcar injured in collision with motor vehicle in nontraffic accident**

⊗⑦**V82.1** **Occupant of streetcar injured in collision with motor vehicle in traffic accident**

⊗⑦**V82.2** **Occupant of streetcar injured in collision with or hit by rolling stock**

⊗⑦**V82.3** **Occupant of streetcar injured in collision with other object**

Excludes1: collision with animal-drawn vehicle or animal being ridden (V82.8)

⊗⑦**V82.4** **Person injured while boarding or alighting from streetcar**

⊗⑦**V82.5** **Occupant of streetcar injured by fall in streetcar**

Excludes1: fall in streetcar:

while boarding or alighting (V82.4)

with antecedent collision (V82.0-V82.3)

⊗⑦**V82.6** **Occupant of streetcar injured by fall from streetcar**

Excludes1: fall from streetcar:

while boarding or alighting (V82.4)

with antecedent collision (V82.0-V82.3)

⊗⑦**V82.7** **Occupant of streetcar injured in derailment without antecedent collision**

Excludes1: occupant of streetcar injured in derailment with antecedent collision (V82.0-V82.3)

⊗⑦**V82.8** **Occupant of streetcar injured in other specified transport accidents**

Streetcar collision with military vehicle

Streetcar collision with train or nonmotor vehicles

⊗⑦**V82.9** **Occupant of streetcar injured in unspecified traffic accident**

Streetcar accident NOS

V83 **Occupant of special vehicle mainly used on industrial premises injured in transport accident**

Includes: battery-powered airport passenger vehicle

battery-powered truck (baggage) (mail)

coal-car in mine

forklift (truck)

logging car

self-propelled industrial truck

station baggage truck (powered)

tram, truck, or tub (powered) in mine or quarry

Excludes1: special construction vehicles (V85.-)

special industrial vehicle in stationary use or maintenance (W31.-)

The appropriate 7th character is to be added to each code from category V83

A - initial encounter

D - subsequent encounter

S - sequela

⊗⑦**V83.0** Driver of special industrial vehicle injured in traffic accident

⊗⑦**V83.1** Passenger of special industrial vehicle injured in traffic accident

⊗⑦**V83.2** Person on outside of special industrial vehicle injured in traffic accident

⊗⑦**V83.3** Unspecified occupant of special industrial vehicle injured in traffic accident

⊗⑦**V83.4** Person injured while boarding or alighting from special industrial vehicle

⊗⑦**V83.5** Driver of special industrial vehicle injured in nontraffic accident

⊗⑦**V83.6** Passenger of special industrial vehicle injured in nontraffic accident

⊗⑦**V83.7** Person on outside of special industrial vehicle injured in nontraffic accident

⊗⑦**V83.9** Unspecified occupant of special industrial vehicle injured in nontraffic accident

Special-industrial-vehicle accident NOS

V84 Occupant of special vehicle mainly used in agriculture injured in transport accident

Includes: self-propelled farm machinery

tractor (and trailer)

Excludes1: animal-powered farm machinery accident (W30.8-)

contact with combine harvester (W30.0)

special agricultural vehicle in stationary use or maintenance (W30.-)

The appropriate 7th character is to be added to each code from category V84

A - initial encounter

D - subsequent encounter

S - sequela

⊗⑦**V84.0** Driver of special agricultural vehicle injured in traffic accident

⊗⑦**V84.1** Passenger of special agricultural vehicle injured in traffic accident

⊗⑦**V84.2** Person on outside of special agricultural vehicle injured in traffic accident

⊗⑦**V84.3** Unspecified occupant of special agricultural vehicle injured in traffic accident

⊗⑦**V84.4** Person injured while boarding or alighting from special agricultural vehicle

⊗⑦**V84.5** Driver of special agricultural vehicle injured in nontraffic accident

⊗⑦**V84.6** Passenger of special agricultural vehicle injured in nontraffic accident

⊗⑦**V84.7** Person on outside of special agricultural vehicle injured in nontraffic accident

⊗⑦**V84.9** Unspecified occupant of special agricultural vehicle injured in nontraffic accident

Special-agricultural vehicle accident NOS

V85 Occupant of special construction vehicle injured in transport accident

Includes: bulldozer

digger dump truck

earth-leveller mechanical shovel road-roller

Excludes1: special industrial vehicle (V83.-)

special construction vehicle in stationary use or maintenance (W31.-)

The appropriate 7th character is to be added to each code from category V85

A - initial encounter

D - subsequent encounter

S - sequela

⊗⑦**V85.0** Driver of special construction vehicle injured in traffic accident

⊗⑦**V85.1** Passenger of special construction vehicle injured in traffic accident

⊗⑦**V85.2** Person on outside of special construction vehicle injured in traffic accident

⊗⑦**V85.3** Unspecified occupant of special construction vehicle injured in traffic accident

⊗⑦**V85.4** Person injured while boarding or alighting from special construction vehicle

⊗⑦**V85.5** Driver of special construction vehicle injured in nontraffic accident

⊗⑦**V85.6** Passenger of special construction vehicle injured in nontraffic accident

⊗⑦**V85.7** Person on outside of special construction vehicle injured in nontraffic accident

⊗⑦**V85.9** Unspecified occupant of special construction vehicle injured in nontraffic accident

Special-construction-vehicle accident NOS

V86 Occupant of special all-terrain or other off-road motor vehicle, injured in transport accident

Excludes1: special all-terrain vehicle in stationary use or maintenance (W31.-)

sport-utility vehicle (V50-V59)

three-wheeled motor vehicle designed for on-road use (V30-V39)

The appropriate 7th character is to be added to each code from category V86

A - initial encounter

D - subsequent encounter

S - sequela

V86.0 Driver of special all-terrain or other off-road motor vehicle injured in traffic accident

⊗⑦**V86.01** Driver of ambulance or fire engine injured in traffic accident

⊗⑦**V86.02** Driver of snowmobile injured in traffic accident

⊗⑦**V86.03** Driver of dune buggy injured in traffic accident

⊗⑦**V86.04** Driver of military vehicle injured in traffic accident

⊗⑦**V86.05** Driver of 3- or 4- wheeled all-terrain vehicle (ATV) injured in traffic accident

⊗⑦**V86.06** Driver of dirt bike or motor/cross bike injured in traffic accident

⊗⑦**V86.09** Driver of other special all-terrain or other off-road motor vehicle injured in traffic accident

Driver of go cart injured in traffic accident

Driver of golf cart injured in traffic accident

V86.1 Passenger of special all-terrain or other off-road motor vehicle injured in traffic accident

⊗⑦**V86.11** Passenger of ambulance or fire engine injured in traffic accident

⊗⑦**V86.12** Passenger of snowmobile injured in traffic accident

⊗⑦**V86.13** Passenger of dune buggy injured in traffic accident

⊗⑦**V86.14** Passenger of military vehicle injured in traffic accident

⊗⑦**V86.15** Passenger of 3- or 4- wheeled all-terrain vehicle (ATV) injured in traffic accident

⊗⑦**V86.16** Passenger of dirt bike or motor/cross bike injured in traffic accident

⊗⑦**V86.19** **Passenger of other special all-terrain or other off-road motor vehicle injured in traffic accident**

Passenger of go cart injured in traffic accident

Passenger of golf cart injured in traffic accident

V86.2 **Person on outside of special all-terrain or other off-road motor vehicle injured in traffic accident**

⊗⑦**V86.21** **Person on outside of ambulance or fire engine injured in traffic accident**

⊗⑦**V86.22** **Person on outside of snowmobile injured in traffic accident**

⊗⑦**V86.23** **Person on outside of dune buggy injured in traffic accident**

⊗⑦**V86.24** **Person on outside of military vehicle injured in traffic accident**

⊗⑦**V86.25 Person on outside of 3- or 4- wheeled all-terrain vehicle (ATV) injured in traffic accident**

⊗⑦**V86.26 Person on outside of dirt bike or motor/cross bike injured in traffic accident**

⊗⑦**V86.29** **Person on outside of other special all-terrain or other off-road motor vehicle injured in traffic accident**

Person on outside of go cart in traffic accident

Person on outside of golf cart injured in traffic accident

V86.3 **Unspecified occupant of special all-terrain or other off-road motor vehicle injured in traffic accident**

⊗⑦**V86.31** **Unspecified occupant of ambulance or fire engine injured in traffic accident**

⊗⑦**V86.32** **Unspecified occupant of snowmobile injured in traffic accident**

⊗⑦**V86.33** **Unspecified occupant of dune buggy injured in traffic accident**

⊗⑦**V86.34** **Unspecified occupant of military vehicle injured in traffic accident**

⊗⑦**V86.35** **Unspecified occupant of 3- or 4- wheeled all-terrain vehicle (ATV) injured in traffic accident**

⊗⑦**V86.36** **Unspecified occupant of dirt bike or motor/cross bike injured in traffic accident**

⊗⑦**V86.39** **Unspecified occupant of other special all-terrain or other off-road motor vehicle injured in traffic accident**

Unspecified occupant of go cart injured in traffic accident

Unspecified occupant of golf cart injured in traffic accident

V86.4 **Person injured while boarding or alighting from special all-terrain or other off-road motor vehicle**

⊗⑦**V86.41** **Person injured while boarding or alighting from ambulance or fire engine**

⊗⑦**V86.42** **Person injured while boarding or alighting from snowmobile**

⊗⑦**V86.43** **Person injured while boarding or alighting from dune buggy**

⊗⑦**V86.44** **Person injured while boarding or alighting from military vehicle**

⊗⑦**V86.45** **Person injured while boarding or alighting from a 3- or 4- wheeled all-terrain vehicle (ATV)**

⊗⑦**V86.46** **Person injured while boarding or alighting from a dirt bike or motor/cross bike**

⊗⑦**V86.49** **Person injured while boarding or alighting from other special all-terrain or other off-road motor vehicle**

Person injured while boarding or alighting from go cart

Person injured while boarding or alighting from golf cart

V86.5 **Driver of special all-terrain or other off-road motor vehicle injured in nontraffic accident**

⊗⑦**V86.51** **Driver of ambulance or fire engine injured in nontraffic accident**

⊗⑦**V86.52** **Driver of snowmobile injured in nontraffic accident**

⊗⑦**V86.53** **Driver of dune buggy injured in nontraffic accident**

⊗⑦**V86.54** **Driver of military vehicle injured in nontraffic accident**

⊗⑦**V86.55** **Driver of 3- or 4- wheeled all-terrain vehicle (ATV) injured in nontraffic accident**

⊗⑦**V86.56** **Driver of dirt bike or motor/cross bike injured in nontraffic accident**

⊗⑦**V86.59** **Driver of other special all-terrain or other off-road motor vehicle injured in nontraffic accident**

Driver of go cart injured in nontraffic accident

Driver of golf cart injured in nontraffic accident

V86.6 **Passenger of special all-terrain or other off-road motor vehicle injured in nontraffic accident**

⊗⑦**V86.61** **Passenger of ambulance or fire engine injured in nontraffic accident**

⊗⑦**V86.62** **Passenger of snowmobile injured in nontraffic accident**

⊗⑦**V86.63** **Passenger of dune buggy injured in nontraffic accident**

⊗⑦**V86.64** **Passenger of military vehicle injured in nontraffic accident**

⊗⑦**V86.65** **Passenger of 3- or 4- wheeled all-terrain vehicle (ATV) injured in nontraffic accident**

⊗⑦**V86.66** **Passenger of dirt bike or motor/cross bike injured in nontraffic accident**

⊗⑦**V86.69** **Passenger of other special all-terrain or other off-road motor vehicle injured in nontraffic accident**

Passenger of go cart injured in nontraffic accident

Passenger of golf cart injured in nontraffic accident

V86.7 **Person on outside of special all-terrain or other off-road motor vehicle injured in nontraffic accident**

⊗⑦**V86.71** **Person on outside of ambulance or fire engine injured in nontraffic accident**

⊗⑦**V86.72** **Person on outside of snowmobile injured in nontraffic accident**

⊗⑦**V86.73** **Person on outside of dune buggy injured in nontraffic accident**

⊗⑦**V86.74** **Person on outside of military vehicle injured in nontraffic accident**

⊗⑦**V86.75** **Person on outside of 3- or 4- wheeled all-terrain vehicle (ATV) injured in nontraffic accident**

⊗⑦**V86.76** **Person on outside of dirt bike or motor/cross bike injured in nontraffic accident**

⊗⑦**V86.79** **Person on outside of other special all-terrain or other off-road motor vehicles injured in nontraffic accident**

Person on outside of go cart injured in nontraffic accident

Person on outside of golf cart injured in nontraffic accident

V86.9 Unspecified occupant of special all-terrain or other off-road motor vehicle injured in nontraffic accident

⊗⑦**V86.91** Unspecified occupant of ambulance or fire engine injured in nontraffic accident

⊗⑦**V86.92** Unspecified occupant of snowmobile injured in nontraffic accident

⊗⑦**V86.93** Unspecified occupant of dune buggy injured in nontraffic accident

⊗⑦**V86.94** Unspecified occupant of military vehicle injured in nontraffic accident

⊗⑦**V86.95** Unspecified occupant of 3- or 4- wheeled all-terrain vehicle (ATV) injured in nontraffic accident

⊗⑦**V86.96** Unspecified occupant of dirt bike or motor/cross bike injured in nontraffic accident

⊗⑦**V86.99** Unspecified occupant of other special all-terrain or other off-road motor vehicle injured in nontraffic accident

Off-road motor-vehicle accident NOS

Other motor-vehicle accident NOS

Unspecified occupant of go cart injured in nontraffic accident

Unspecified occupant of golf cart injured in nontraffic accident

V87 Traffic accident of specified type but victim's mode of transport unknown

Excludes1: collision involving:

pedal cycle (V10-V19)

pedestrian (V01-V09)

The appropriate 7th character is to be added to each code from category V87

A - initial encounter

D - subsequent encounter

S - sequela

⊗⑦**V87.0** Person injured in collision between car and two- or three-wheeled powered vehicle (traffic)

⊗⑦**V87.1** Person injured in collision between other motor vehicle and two- or three-wheeled motor vehicle (traffic)

⊗⑦**V87.2** Person injured in collision between car and pick-up truck or van (traffic)

⊗⑦**V87.3** Person injured in collision between car and bus (traffic)

⊗⑦**V87.4** Person injured in collision between car and heavy transport vehicle (traffic)

⊗⑦**V87.5** Person injured in collision between heavy transport vehicle and bus (traffic)

⊗⑦**V87.6** Person injured in collision between railway train or railway vehicle and car (traffic)

⊗⑦**V87.7** Person injured in collision between other specified motor vehicles (traffic)

⊗⑦**V87.8** Person injured in other specified Non collision transport accidents involving motor vehicle (traffic)

⊗⑦**V87.9** Person injured in other specified (collision)(Non collision) transport accidents involving nonmotor vehicle (traffic)

V88 Nontraffic accident of specified type but victim's mode of transport unknown

Excludes1: collision involving:

pedal cycle (V10-V19)

pedestrian (V01-V09)

The appropriate 7th character is to be added to each code from category V88

A - initial encounter

D - subsequent encounter

S - sequela

⊗⑦**V88.0** Person injured in collision between car and two- or three-wheeled motor vehicle, nontraffic

⊗⑦**V88.1** Person injured in collision between other motor vehicle and two- or three-wheeled motor vehicle, nontraffic

⊗⑦**V88.2** Person injured in collision between car and pick-up truck or van, nontraffic

⊗⑦**V88.3** Person injured in collision between car and bus, nontraffic

⊗⑦**V88.4** Person injured in collision between car and heavy transport vehicle, nontraffic

⊗⑦**V88.5** Person injured in collision between heavy transport vehicle and bus, nontraffic

⊗⑦**V88.6** Person injured in collision between railway train or railway vehicle and car, nontraffic

⊗⑦**V88.7** Person injured in collision between other specified motor vehicle, nontraffic

⊗⑦**V88.8** Person injured in other specified Non collision transport accidents involving motor vehicle, nontraffic

⊗⑦**V88.9** Person injured in other specified (collision)(Non collision) transport accidents involving nonmotor vehicle, nontraffic

V89 Motor- or nonmotor-vehicle accident, type of vehicle unspecified

The appropriate 7th character is to be added to each code from category V89

A - initial encounter

D - subsequent encounter

S - sequela

⊗⑦**V89.0** Person injured in unspecified motor-vehicle accident, nontraffic

Motor-vehicle accident NOS, nontraffic

⊗⑦**V89.1** Person injured in unspecified nonmotor-vehicle accident, nontraffic

Nonmotor-vehicle accident NOS (nontraffic)

⊗⑦**V89.2** Person injured in unspecified motor-vehicle accident, traffic

Motor-vehicle accident [MVA] NOS

Road (traffic) accident [RTA] NOS

⊗⑦**V89.3** Person injured in unspecified nonmotor-vehicle accident, traffic

Nonmotor-vehicle traffic accident NOS

⊗⑦**V89.9** Person injured in unspecified vehicle accident

Collision NOS

WATER TRANSPORT ACCIDENTS (V90-V94)

V90 Drowning and submersion due to accident to watercraft

Excludes1: civilian water transport accident involving military watercraft (V94.81-)

fall into water not from watercraft (W16.-)

military watercraft accident in military or war operations (Y36.0-, Y37.0-)

water-transport-related drowning or submersion without accident to watercraft (V92.-)

The appropriate 7th character is to be added to each code from category V90

A - initial encounter

D - subsequent encounter

S - sequela

V90.0 Drowning and submersion due to watercraft overturning

⊗⑦**V90.00** Drowning and submersion due to merchant ship overturning

● New code ▲ Revised code **Excludes1:** Not coded here **Excludes2:** Not included here ⊗ Placeholder required ⑦ 7th digit required

⊗⑦**V90.01 Drowning and submersion due to passenger ship overturning**

Drowning and submersion due to Ferry-boat overturning

Drowning and submersion due to Liner overturning

⊗⑦**V90.02 Drowning and submersion due to fishing boat overturning**

⊗⑦**V90.03 Drowning and submersion due to other powered watercraft overturning**

Drowning and submersion due to Hovercraft (on open water) overturning

Drowning and submersion due to Jet ski overturning

⊗⑦**V90.04 Drowning and submersion due to sailboat overturning**

⊗⑦**V90.05 Drowning and submersion due to canoe or kayak overturning**

⊗⑦**V90.06 Drowning and submersion due to (nonpowered) inflatable craft overturning**

⊗⑦**V90.08 Drowning and submersion due to other unpowered watercraft overturning**

Drowning and submersion due to windsurfer overturning

⊗⑦**V90.09 Drowning and submersion due to unspecified watercraft overturning**

Drowning and submersion due to boat NOS overturning

Drowning and submersion due to ship NOS overturning

Drowning and submersion due to watercraft NOS overturning

V90.1 Drowning and submersion due to watercraft sinking

⊗⑦**V90.10 Drowning and submersion due to merchant ship sinking**

⊗⑦**V90.11 Drowning and submersion due to passenger ship sinking**

Drowning and submersion due to Ferry-boat sinking

Drowning and submersion due to Liner sinking

⊗⑦**V90.12 Drowning and submersion due to fishing boat sinking**

⊗⑦**V90.13 Drowning and submersion due to other powered watercraft sinking**

Drowning and submersion due to Hovercraft (on open water) sinking

Drowning and submersion due to Jet ski sinking

⊗⑦**V90.14 Drowning and submersion due to sailboat sinking**

⊗⑦**V90.15 Drowning and submersion due to canoe or kayak sinking**

⊗⑦**V90.16 Drowning and submersion due to (nonpowered) inflatable craft sinking**

⊗⑦**V90.18 Drowning and submersion due to other unpowered watercraft sinking**

⊗⑦**V90.19 Drowning and submersion due to unspecified watercraft sinking**

Drowning and submersion due to boat NOS sinking

Drowning and submersion due to ship NOS sinking

Drowning and submersion due to watercraft NOS sinking

V90.2 Drowning and submersion due to falling or jumping from burning watercraft

⊗⑦**V90.20 Drowning and submersion due to falling or jumping from burning merchant ship**

⊗⑦**V90.21 Drowning and submersion due to falling or jumping from burning passenger ship**

Drowning and submersion due to falling or jumping from burning Ferry-boat

Drowning and submersion due to falling or jumping from burning Liner

⊗⑦**V90.22 Drowning and submersion due to falling or jumping from burning fishing boat**

⊗⑦**V90.23 Drowning and submersion due to falling or jumping from other burning powered watercraft**

Drowning and submersion due to falling and jumping from burning Hovercraft (on open water)

Drowning and submersion due to falling and jumping from burning Jet ski

⊗⑦**V90.24 Drowning and submersion due to falling or jumping from burning sailboat**

⊗⑦**V90.25 Drowning and submersion due to falling or jumping from burning canoe or kayak**

⊗⑦**V90.26 Drowning and submersion due to falling or jumping from burning (nonpowered) inflatable craft**

⊗⑦**V90.27 Drowning and submersion due to falling or jumping from burning water-skis**

⊗⑦**V90.28 Drowning and submersion due to falling or jumping from other burning unpowered watercraft**

Drowning and submersion due to falling and jumping from burning surf-board

Drowning and submersion due to falling and jumping from burning windsurfer

⊗⑦**V90.29 Drowning and submersion due to falling or jumping from unspecified burning watercraft**

Drowning and submersion due to falling or jumping from burning boat NOS

Drowning and submersion due to falling or jumping from burning ship NOS

Drowning and submersion due to falling or jumping from burning watercraft NOS

V90.3 Drowning and submersion due to falling or jumping from crushed watercraft

⊗⑦**V90.30 Drowning and submersion due to falling or jumping from crushed merchant ship**

⊗⑦**V90.31 Drowning and submersion due to falling or jumping from crushed passenger ship**

Drowning and submersion due to falling and jumping from crushed Ferry boat

Drowning and submersion due to falling and jumping from crushed Liner

⊗⑦**V90.32 Drowning and submersion due to falling or jumping from crushed fishing boat**

⊗⑦**V90.33 Drowning and submersion due to falling or jumping from other crushed powered watercraft**

Drowning and submersion due to falling and jumping from crushed Hovercraft

Drowning and submersion due to falling and jumping from crushed Jet ski

⊗⑦**V90.34 Drowning and submersion due to falling or jumping from crushed sailboat**

| | Add 4th-7th digits | | Nonspecific code | | Unspecified code | | Manifestation code | [HCC] Hierarchical Condition Code | 1081 |

⊗⑦**V90.35** **Drowning and submersion due to falling or jumping from crushed canoe or kayak**

⊗⑦**V90.36** **Drowning and submersion due to falling or jumping from crushed (nonpowered) inflatable craft**

⊗⑦**V90.37** **Drowning and submersion due to falling or jumping from crushed water-skis**

⊗⑦**V90.38** **Drowning and submersion due to falling or jumping from other crushed unpowered watercraft**

Drowning and submersion due to falling and jumping from crushed surf-board

Drowning and submersion due to falling and jumping from crushed windsurfer

⊗⑦**V90.39** **Drowning and submersion due to falling or jumping from crushed unspecified watercraft**

Drowning and submersion due to falling and jumping from crushed boat NOS

Drowning and submersion due to falling and jumping from crushed ship NOS

Drowning and submersion due to falling and jumping from crushed watercraft NOS

V90.8 **Drowning and submersion due to other accident to watercraft**

⊗⑦**V90.80** **Drowning and submersion due to other accident to merchant ship**

⊗⑦**V90.81** **Drowning and submersion due to other accident to passenger ship**

Drowning and submersion due to other accident to Ferry-boat

Drowning and submersion due to other accident to Liner

⊗⑦**V90.82** **Drowning and submersion due to other accident to fishing boat**

⊗⑦**V90.83** **Drowning and submersion due to other accident to other powered watercraft**

Drowning and submersion due to other accident to Hovercraft (on open water)

Drowning and submersion due to other accident to Jet ski

⊗⑦**V90.84** **Drowning and submersion due to other accident to sailboat**

⊗⑦**V90.85** **Drowning and submersion due to other accident to canoe or kayak**

⊗⑦**V90.86** **Drowning and submersion due to other accident to (nonpowered) inflatable craft**

⊗⑦**V90.87** **Drowning and submersion due to other accident to water-skis**

⊗⑦**V90.88** **Drowning and submersion due to other accident to other unpowered watercraft**

Drowning and submersion due to other accident to surf-board

Drowning and submersion due to other accident to windsurfer

⊗⑦**V90.89** **Drowning and submersion due to other accident to unspecified watercraft**

Drowning and submersion due to other accident to boat NOS

Drowning and submersion due to other accident to ship NOS

Drowning and submersion due to other accident to watercraft NOS

V91 **Other injury due to accident to watercraft**

Includes: any injury except drowning and submersion as a result of an accident to watercraft

Excludes1: civilian water transport accident involving military watercraft (V94.81-)

military watercraft accident in military or war operations (Y36, Y37.-)

Excludes2: drowning and submersion due to accident to watercraft (V90.-)

The appropriate 7th character is to be added to each code from category V91

A - initial encounter

D - subsequent encounter

S - sequela

V91.0 **Burn due to watercraft on fire**

Excludes1: burn from localized fire or explosion on board ship without accident to watercraft (V93.-)

⊗⑦**V91.00** **Burn due to merchant ship on fire**

⊗⑦**V91.01** **Burn due to passenger ship on fire**

Burn due to Ferry-boat on fire

Burn due to Liner on fire

⊗⑦**V91.02** **Burn due to fishing boat on fire**

⊗⑦**V91.03** **Burn due to other powered watercraft on fire**

Burn due to Hovercraft (on open water) on fire

Burn due to Jet ski on fire

⊗⑦**V91.04** **Burn due to sailboat on fire**

⊗⑦**V91.05** **Burn due to canoe or kayak on fire**

⊗⑦**V91.06** **Burn due to (nonpowered) inflatable craft on fire**

⊗⑦**V91.07** **Burn due to water-skis on fire**

⊗⑦**V91.08** **Burn due to other unpowered watercraft on fire**

⊗⑦**V91.09** **Burn due to unspecified watercraft on fire**

Burn due to boat NOS on fire

Burn due to ship NOS on fire

Burn due to watercraft NOS on fire

V91.1 **Crushed between watercraft and other watercraft or other object due to collision**

Crushed by lifeboat after abandoning ship in a collision

Note: select the specified type of watercraft that the victim was on at the time of the collision

⊗⑦**V91.10** **Crushed between merchant ship and other watercraft or other object due to collision**

⊗⑦**V91.11** **Crushed between passenger ship and other watercraft or other object due to collision**

Crushed between Ferry-boat and other watercraft or other object due to collision

Crushed between Liner and other watercraft or other object due to collision

⊗⑦**V91.12** **Crushed between fishing boat and other watercraft or other object due to collision**

⊗⑦**V91.13** **Crushed between other powered watercraft and other watercraft or other object due to collision**

Crushed between Hovercraft (on open water) and other watercraft or other object due to collision

Crushed between Jet ski and other watercraft or other object due to collision

⊗⑦**V91.14** **Crushed between sailboat and other watercraft or other object due to collision**

⊗⑦**V91.15** **Crushed between canoe or kayak and other watercraft or other object due to collision**

● New code ▲ Revised code **Excludes1:** Not coded here **Excludes2:** Not included here ⊗ Placeholder required ⑦7th digit required

⊗⑦**V91.16** **Crushed between (nonpowered) inflatable craft and other watercraft or other object due to collision**

⊗⑦**V91.18** **Crushed between other unpowered watercraft and other watercraft or other object due to collision**

Crushed between surfboard and other watercraft or other object due to collision

Crushed between windsurfer and other watercraft or other object due to collision

⊗⑦**V91.19** **Crushed between unspecified watercraft and other watercraft or other object due to collision**

Crushed between boat NOS and other watercraft or other object due to collision

Crushed between ship NOS and other watercraft or other object due to collision

Crushed between watercraft NOS and other watercraft or other object due to collision

V91.2 **Fall due to collision between watercraft and other watercraft or other object**

Fall while remaining on watercraft after collision

Note: select the specified type of watercraft that the victim was on at the time of the collision

Excludes1: crushed between watercraft and other watercraft and other object due to collision (V91.1-)

drowning and submersion due to falling from crushed watercraft (V90.3-)

⊗⑦**V91.20** **Fall due to collision between merchant ship and other watercraft or other object**

⊗⑦**V91.21** **Fall due to collision between passenger ship and other watercraft or other object**

Fall due to collision between Ferry-boat and other watercraft or other object

Fall due to collision between Liner and other watercraft or other object

⊗⑦**V91.22** **Fall due to collision between fishing boat and other watercraft or other object**

⊗⑦**V91.23** **Fall due to collision between other powered watercraft and other watercraft or other object**

Fall due to collision between Hovercraft (on open water) and other watercraft or other object

Fall due to collision between Jet ski and other watercraft or other object

⊗⑦**V91.24** **Fall due to collision between sailboat and other watercraft or other object**

⊗⑦**V91.25** **Fall due to collision between canoe or kayak and other watercraft or other object**

⊗⑦**V91.26** **Fall due to collision between (nonpowered) inflatable craft and other watercraft or other object**

⊗⑦**V91.29** **Fall due to collision between unspecified watercraft and other watercraft or other object**

Fall due to collision between boat NOS and other watercraft or other object

Fall due to collision between ship NOS and other watercraft or other object

Fall due to collision between watercraft NOS and other watercraft or other object

V91.3 **Hit or struck by falling object due to accident to watercraft**

Hit or struck by falling object (part of damaged watercraft or other object) after falling or jumping from damaged watercraft

Excludes2: drowning or submersion due to fall or jumping from damaged watercraft (V90.2-, V90.3-)

⊗⑦**V91.30** **Hit or struck by falling object due to accident to merchant ship**

⊗⑦**V91.31** **Hit or struck by falling object due to accident to passenger ship**

Hit or struck by falling object due to accident to Ferry-boat

Hit or struck by falling object due to accident to Liner

⊗⑦**V91.32** **Hit or struck by falling object due to accident to fishing boat**

⊗⑦**V91.33** **Hit or struck by falling object due to accident to other powered watercraft**

Hit or struck by falling object due to accident to Hovercraft (on open water)

Hit or struck by falling object due to accident to Jet ski

⊗⑦**V91.34** **Hit or struck by falling object due to accident to sailboat**

⊗⑦**V91.35** **Hit or struck by falling object due to accident to canoe or kayak**

⊗⑦**V91.36** **Hit or struck by falling object due to accident to (nonpowered) inflatable craft**

⊗⑦**V91.37** **Hit or struck by falling object due to accident to water-skis**

Hit by water-skis after jumping off of water skis

⊗⑦**V91.38** **Hit or struck by falling object due to accident to other unpowered watercraft**

Hit or struck by surf-board after falling off damaged surf-board

Hit or struck by object after falling off damaged windsurfer

⊗⑦**V91.39** **Hit or struck by falling object due to accident to unspecified watercraft**

Hit or struck by falling object due to accident to boat NOS

Hit or struck by falling object due to accident to ship NOS

Hit or struck by falling object due to accident to watercraft NOS

V91.8 **Other injury due to other accident to watercraft**

⊗⑦**V91.80** **Other injury due to other accident to merchant ship**

⊗⑦**V91.81** **Other injury due to other accident to passenger ship**

Other injury due to other accident to Ferry-boat

Other injury due to other accident to Liner

⊗⑦**V91.82** **Other injury due to other accident to fishing boat**

⊗⑦**V91.83** **Other injury due to other accident to other powered watercraft**

Other injury due to other accident to Hovercraft (on open water)

Other injury due to other accident to Jet ski

⊗⑦**V91.84** **Other injury due to other accident to sailboat**

⊗⑦**V91.85** **Other injury due to other accident to canoe or kayak**

⊗⑦**V91.86** **Other injury due to other accident to (nonpowered) inflatable craft**

⊗⑦**V91.87** **Other injury due to other accident to water-skis**

⊗⑦**V91.88** **Other injury due to other accident to other unpowered watercraft**

Other injury due to other accident to surf-board

Other injury due to other accident to windsurfer

⊗⑦**V91.89** **Other injury due to other accident to unspecified watercraft**

Other injury due to other accident to boat NOS

Other injury due to other accident to ship NOS

Other injury due to other accident to watercraft NOS

V92 **Drowning and submersion due to accident on board watercraft, without accident to watercraft**

Excludes1: civilian water transport accident involving military watercraft (V94.81-)

drowning or submersion due to accident to watercraft (V90-V91)

drowning or submersion of diver who voluntarily jumps from boat not involved in an accident (W16.711, W16.721)

fall into water without watercraft (W16.-)

military watercraft accident in military or war operations (Y36, Y37)

The appropriate 7th character is to be added to each code from category V92

A - initial encounter

D - subsequent encounter

S - sequela

V92.0 **Drowning and submersion due to fall off watercraft**

Drowning and submersion due to fall from gangplank of watercraft

Drowning and submersion due to fall overboard watercraft

Excludes2: hitting head on object or bottom of body of water due to fall from watercraft (V94.0-)

⊗⑦**V92.00** **Drowning and submersion due to fall off merchant ship**

⊗⑦**V92.01** **Drowning and submersion due to fall off passenger ship**

Drowning and submersion due to fall off Ferry-boat

Drowning and submersion due to fall off Liner

⊗⑦**V92.02** **Drowning and submersion due to fall off fishing boat**

⊗⑦**V92.03** **Drowning and submersion due to fall off other powered watercraft**

Drowning and submersion due to fall off Hovercraft (on open water)

Drowning and submersion due to fall off Jet ski

⊗⑦**V92.04** **Drowning and submersion due to fall off sailboat**

⊗⑦**V92.05** **Drowning and submersion due to fall off canoe or kayak**

⊗⑦**V92.06** **Drowning and submersion due to fall off (nonpowered) inflatable craft**

⊗⑦**V92.07** **Drowning and submersion due to fall off water-skis**

Excludes1: drowning and submersion due to falling off burning water-skis (V90.27)

drowning and submersion due to falling off crushed water-skis (V90.37)

hit by boat while water-skiing NOS (V94.X)

⊗⑦**V92.08** **Drowning and submersion due to fall off other unpowered watercraft**

Drowning and submersion due to fall off surf-board

Drowning and submersion due to fall off windsurfer

Excludes1: drowning and submersion due to fall off burning unpowered watercraft (V90.28)

drowning and submersion due to fall off crushed unpowered watercraft (V90.38)

drowning and submersion due to fall off damaged unpowered watercraft (V90.88)

drowning and submersion due to rider of nonpowered watercraft being hit by other watercraft (V94.-)

Other injury due to rider of nonpowered watercraft being hit by other watercraft (V94.-)

⊗⑦**V92.09** **Drowning and submersion due to fall off unspecified watercraft**

Drowning and submersion due to fall off boat NOS

Drowning and submersion due to fall off ship

Drowning and submersion due to fall off watercraft NOS

V92.1 **Drowning and submersion due to being thrown overboard by motion of watercraft**

Excludes1: drowning and submersion due to fall off surf-board (V92.08)

drowning and submersion due to fall off water-skis (V92.07)

drowning and submersion due to fall off windsurfer (V92.08)

⊗⑦**V92.10** **Drowning and submersion due to being thrown overboard by motion of merchant ship**

⊗⑦**V92.11** **Drowning and submersion due to being thrown overboard by motion of passenger ship**

Drowning and submersion due to being thrown overboard by motion of Ferry-boat

Drowning and submersion due to being thrown overboard by motion of Liner

⊗⑦**V92.12** **Drowning and submersion due to being thrown overboard by motion of fishing boat**

⊗⑦**V92.13** **Drowning and submersion due to being thrown overboard by motion of other powered watercraft**

Drowning and submersion due to being thrown overboard by motion of Hovercraft

⊗⑦**V92.14** **Drowning and submersion due to being thrown overboard by motion of sailboat**

⊗⑦**V92.15** **Drowning and submersion due to being thrown overboard by motion of canoe or kayak**

⊗⑦**V92.16** **Drowning and submersion due to being thrown overboard by motion of (nonpowered) inflatable craft**

⊗⑦**V92.19** **Drowning and submersion due to being thrown overboard by motion of unspecified watercraft**

Drowning and submersion due to being thrown overboard by motion of boat NOS

Drowning and submersion due to being thrown overboard by motion of ship NOS

Drowning and submersion due to being thrown overboard by motion of watercraft NOS

V92.2 **Drowning and submersion due to being washed overboard from watercraft**

Code first any associated cataclysm (X37.0-)

⊗⑦**V92.20** **Drowning and submersion due to being washed overboard from merchant ship**

⊗⑦**V92.21** **Drowning and submersion due to being washed overboard from passenger ship**

Drowning and submersion due to being washed overboard from Ferry-boat

Drowning and submersion due to being washed overboard from Liner

⊗⑦**V92.22** **Drowning and submersion due to being washed overboard from fishing boat**

⊗⑦**V92.23** **Drowning and submersion due to being washed overboard from other powered watercraft**

Drowning and submersion due to being washed overboard from Hovercraft (on open water)

Drowning and submersion due to being washed overboard from Jet ski

⊗⑦**V92.24** **Drowning and submersion due to being washed overboard from sailboat**

⊗⑦**V92.25** **Drowning and submersion due to being washed overboard from canoe or kayak**

⊗⑦**V92.26** **Drowning and submersion due to being washed overboard from (nonpowered) inflatable craft**

⊗⑦**V92.27** **Drowning and submersion due to being washed overboard from water-skis**

Excludes1: drowning and submersion due to fall off water-skis (V92.07)

⊗⑦**V92.28** **Drowning and submersion due to being washed overboard from other unpowered watercraft**

Drowning and submersion due to being washed overboard from surf-board

Drowning and submersion due to being washed overboard from windsurfer

⊗⑦**V92.29** **Drowning and submersion due to being washed overboard from unspecified watercraft**

Drowning and submersion due to being washed overboard from boat NOS

Drowning and submersion due to being washed overboard from ship NOS

Drowning and submersion due to being washed overboard from watercraft NOS

V93 **Other injury due to accident on board watercraft, without accident to watercraft**

Excludes1: civilian water transport accident involving military watercraft (V94.81-)

Other injury due to accident to watercraft (V91.-)

military watercraft accident in military or war operations (Y36, Y37.-)

Excludes2: drowning and submersion due to accident on board watercraft, without accident to watercraft (V92.-)

The appropriate 7th character is to be added to each code from category V93

A - initial encounter

D - subsequent encounter

S - sequela

V93.0 **Burn due to localized fire on board watercraft**

Excludes1: burn due to watercraft on fire (V91.0-)

⊗⑦**V93.00** **Burn due to localized fire on board merchant vessel**

⊗⑦**V93.01** **Burn due to localized fire on board passenger vessel**

Burn due to localized fire on board Ferry-boat

Burn due to localized fire on board Liner

⊗⑦**V93.02** **Burn due to localized fire on board fishing boat**

⊗⑦**V93.03** **Burn due to localized fire on board other powered watercraft**

Burn due to localized fire on board Hovercraft

Burn due to localized fire on board Jet ski

⊗⑦**V93.04** **Burn due to localized fire on board sailboat**

⊗⑦**V93.09** **Burn due to localized fire on board unspecified watercraft**

Burn due to localized fire on board boat NOS

Burn due to localized fire on board ship NOS

Burn due to localized fire on board watercraft NOS

V93.1 **Other burn on board watercraft**

Burn due to source **Other** than fire on board watercraft

Excludes1: burn due to watercraft on fire (V91.0-)

⊗⑦**V93.10** **Other burn on board merchant vessel**

⊗⑦**V93.11** **Other burn on board passenger vessel**

Other burn on board Ferry-boat

Other burn on board Liner

⊗⑦**V93.12** **Other burn on board fishing boat**

⊗⑦**V93.13** **Other burn on board other powered watercraft**

Other burn on board Hovercraft

Other burn on board Jet ski

⊗⑦**V93.14** **Other burn on board sailboat**

⊗⑦**V93.19** **Other burn on board unspecified watercraft**

Other burn on board boat NOS

Other burn on board ship NOS

Other burn on board watercraft NOS

V93.2 **Heat exposure on board watercraft**

Excludes1: exposure to man-made heat not aboard watercraft (W92)

exposure to natural heat while on board watercraft (X30)

exposure to sunlight while on board watercraft (X32)

Excludes2: burn due to fire on board watercraft (V93.0-)

⊗⑦**V93.20** **Heat exposure on board merchant ship**

⊗⑦**V93.21** **Heat exposure on board passenger ship**

Heat exposure on board Ferry-boat

Heat exposure on board Liner

⊗⑦**V93.22** **Heat exposure on board fishing boat**

⊗⑦**V93.23** **Heat exposure on board other powered watercraft**

Heat exposure on board hovercraft

⊗⑦**V93.24** **Heat exposure on board sailboat**

⊗⑦**V93.29** **Heat exposure on board unspecified watercraft**

Heat exposure on board boat NOS

Heat exposure on board ship NOS

Heat exposure on board watercraft NOS

V93.3 **Fall on board watercraft**

Excludes1: fall due to collision of watercraft (V91.2-)

⊗⑦**V93.30** **Fall on board merchant ship**

⊗⑦**V93.31** **Fall on board passenger ship**

Fall on board Ferry-boat Fall on board Liner

⊗⑦**V93.32** **Fall on board fishing boat**

⊗⑦**V93.33** **Fall on board other powered watercraft**

Fall on board Hovercraft (on open water)

Fall on board Jet ski

⊗⑦**V93.34** **Fall on board sailboat**

⊗⑦**V93.35** **Fall on board canoe or kayak**

⊗⑦**V93.36** **Fall on board (nonpowered) inflatable craft**

⊗⑦**V93.38** **Fall on board other unpowered watercraft**

⊗⑦**V93.39** **Fall on board unspecified watercraft**

Fall on board boat NOS Fall on board ship NOS

Fall on board watercraft NOS

V93.4 **Struck by falling object on board watercraft**

Hit by falling object on board watercraft

Excludes1: struck by falling object due to accident to watercraft (V91.3)

⊗⑦**V93.40** **Struck by falling object on merchant ship**

⊗⑦**V93.41** **Struck by falling object on passenger ship**

Struck by falling object on Ferry-boat

Struck by falling object on Liner

⊗⑦**V93.42** **Struck by falling object on fishing boat**

⊗⑦**V93.43** **Struck by falling object on other powered watercraft**

Struck by falling object on Hovercraft

⊗⑦**V93.44** **Struck by falling object on sailboat**

⊗⑦**V93.48** **Struck by falling object on other unpowered watercraft**

⊗⑦**V93.49** **Struck by falling object on unspecified watercraft**

V93.5 **Explosion on board watercraft**

Boiler explosion on steamship

Excludes2: fire on board watercraft (V93.0-)

⊗⑦**V93.50** **Explosion on board merchant ship**

⊗⑦**V93.51** **Explosion on board passenger ship**

Explosion on board Ferry-boat

Explosion on board Liner

⊗⑦**V93.52** **Explosion on board fishing boat**

⊗⑦**V93.53** **Explosion on board other powered watercraft**

Explosion on board Hovercraft

Explosion on board Jet ski

⊗⑦**V93.54** **Explosion on board sailboat**

⊗⑦**V93.59** **Explosion on board unspecified watercraft**

Explosion on board boat NOS

Explosion on board ship NOS

Explosion on board watercraft NOS

V93.6 **Machinery accident on board watercraft**

Excludes1: machinery explosion on board watercraft (V93.4-)

machinery fire on board watercraft (V93.0-)

⊗⑦**V93.60** **Machinery accident on board merchant ship**

⊗⑦**V93.61** **Machinery accident on board passenger ship**

Machinery accident on board Ferry-boat

Machinery accident on board Liner

⊗⑦**V93.62** **Machinery accident on board fishing boat**

⊗⑦**V93.63** **Machinery accident on board other powered watercraft**

Machinery accident on board Hovercraft

⊗⑦**V93.64** **Machinery accident on board sailboat**

⊗⑦**V93.69** **Machinery accident on board unspecified watercraft**

Machinery accident on board boat NOS

Machinery accident on board ship NOS

Machinery accident on board watercraft NOS

V93.8 **Other injury due to other accident on board watercraft**

Accidental poisoning by gases or fumes on watercraft

⊗⑦**V93.80** **Other injury due to other accident on board merchant ship**

⊗⑦**V93.81** **Other injury due to other accident on board passenger ship**

Other injury due to other accident on board Ferry-boat

Other injury due to other accident on board Liner

⊗⑦**V93.82** **Other injury due to other accident on board fishing boat**

⊗⑦**V93.83** **Other injury due to other accident on board other powered watercraft**

Other injury due to other accident on board Hovercraft

Other injury due to other accident on board Jet ski

⊗⑦**V93.84** **Other injury due to other accident on board sailboat**

⊗⑦**V93.85** **Other injury due to other accident on board canoe or kayak**

⊗⑦**V93.86** **Other injury due to other accident on board (nonpowered) inflatable craft**

⊗⑦**V93.87** **Other injury due to other accident on board water-skis**

Hit or struck by object while waterskiing

⊗⑦**V93.88** **Other injury due to other accident on board other unpowered watercraft**

Hit or struck by object while surfing

Hit or struck by object while on board windsurfer

⊗⑦**V93.89** **Other injury due to other accident on board unspecified watercraft**

Other injury due to other accident on board boat NOS

Other injury due to other accident on board ship NOS

Other injury due to other accident on board watercraft NOS

V94 **Other and unspecified water transport accidents**

Excludes1: military watercraft accidents in military or war operations (Y36, Y37)

The appropriate 7th character is to be added to each code from category V94

A - initial encounter

D - subsequent encounter

S - sequela

⊗⑦**V94.0** **Hitting object or bottom of body of water due to fall from watercraft**

Excludes2: drowning and submersion due to fall from watercraft (V92.0-)

⊗⑦**V94.1** **Bather struck by watercraft**

Swimmer hit by watercraft

⊗⑦**V94.11** **Bather struck by powered watercraft**

⊗⑦**V94.12** **Bather struck by nonpowered watercraft**

V94.2 **Rider of nonpowered watercraft struck by other watercraft**

⊗⑦**V94.21** **Rider of nonpowered watercraft struck by other nonpowered watercraft**

Canoer hit by other nonpowered watercraft

Surfer hit by other nonpowered watercraft

Windsurfer hit by other nonpowered watercraft

⊗⑦**V94.22** **Rider of nonpowered watercraft struck by powered watercraft**

Canoer hit by motorboat

Surfer hit by motorboat

Windsurfer hit by motorboat

V94.3 **Injury to rider of (inflatable) watercraft being pulled behind other watercraft**

⊗⑦**V94.31** **Injury to rider of (inflatable) recreational watercraft being pulled behind other watercraft**

Injury to rider of inner-tube pulled behind motor boat

⊗⑦**V94.32** **Injury to rider of non-recreational watercraft being pulled behind other watercraft**

Injury to occupant of dingy being pulled behind boat or ship

Injury to occupant of life-raft being pulled behind boat or ship

⊗⑦**V94.4** **Injury to barefoot water-skier**

Injury to person being pulled behind boat or ship

V94.8 **Other water transport accident**

V94.81 **Water transport accident involving military watercraft**

⑦**V94.810** **Civilian watercraft involved in water transport accident with military watercraft**

Passenger on civilian watercraft injured due to accident with military watercraft

⑦**V94.811** **Civilian in water injured by military watercraft**

⑦**V94.818** **Other water transport accident involving military watercraft**

⊗⑦**V94.89** **Other water transport accident**

⊗⑦**V94.9** **Unspecified water transport accident**

Water transport accident NOS

AIR AND SPACE TRANSPORT ACCIDENTS (V95-V97)

Excludes1: military aircraft accidents in military or war operations (Y36, Y37)

V95 **Accident to powered aircraft causing injury to occupant**

The appropriate 7th character is to be added to each code from category V95

A - initial encounter

D - subsequent encounter

S - sequela

V95.0 **Helicopter accident injuring occupant**

⊗⑦**V95.00** **Unspecified helicopter accident injuring occupant**

⊗⑦**V95.01** **Helicopter crash injuring occupant**

⊗⑦**V95.02** **Forced landing of helicopter injuring occupant**

⊗⑦**V95.03** **Helicopter collision injuring occupant**

Helicopter collision with any object, fixed, movable or moving

⊗⑦**V95.04** **Helicopter fire injuring occupant**

⊗⑦**V95.05** **Helicopter explosion injuring occupant**

⊗⑦**V95.09** **Other helicopter accident injuring occupant**

V95.1 **Ultralight, microlight or powered-glider accident injuring occupant**

⊗⑦**V95.10** **Unspecified ultralight, microlight or powered-glider accident injuring occupant**

⊗⑦**V95.11** **Ultralight, microlight or powered-glider crash injuring occupant**

⊗⑦**V95.12** **Forced landing of ultralight, microlight or powered-glider injuring occupant**

⊗⑦**V95.13** **Ultralight, microlight or powered-glider collision injuring occupant**

Ultralight, microlight or powered-glider collision with any object, fixed, movable or moving

⊗⑦**V95.14** **Ultralight, microlight or powered-glider fire injuring occupant**

⊗⑦**V95.15** **Ultralight, microlight or powered-glider explosion injuring occupant**

⊗⑦**V95.19** **Other ultralight, microlight or powered-glider accident injuring occupant**

V95.2 **Other private fixed-wing aircraft accident injuring occupant**

⊗⑦**V95.20** **Unspecified accident to other private fixed-wing aircraft, injuring occupant**

⊗⑦**V95.21** **Other private fixed-wing aircraft crash injuring occupant**

⊗⑦**V95.22** **Forced landing of other private fixed-wing aircraft injuring occupant**

⊗⑦**V95.23** **Other private fixed-wing aircraft collision injuring occupant**

Other private fixed-wing aircraft collision with any object, fixed, movable or moving

⊗⑦**V95.24** **Other private fixed-wing aircraft fire injuring occupant**

⊗⑦**V95.25** **Other private fixed-wing aircraft explosion injuring occupant**

⊗⑦**V95.29** **Other accident to other private fixed-wing aircraft injuring occupant**

V95.3 **Commercial fixed-wing aircraft accident injuring occupant**

⊗⑦**V95.30** **Unspecified accident to commercial fixed-wing aircraft injuring occupant**

⊗⑦**V95.31** **Commercial fixed-wing aircraft crash injuring occupant**

⊗⑦**V95.32** **Forced landing of commercial fixed-wing aircraft injuring occupant**

⊗⑦**V95.33** **Commercial fixed-wing aircraft collision injuring occupant**

Commercial fixed-wing aircraft collision with any object, fixed, movable or moving

⊗⑦**V95.34** **Commercial fixed-wing aircraft fire injuring occupant**

⊗⑦**V95.35** **Commercial fixed-wing aircraft explosion injuring occupant**

⊗⑦**V95.39** **Other accident to commercial fixed-wing aircraft injuring occupant**

V95.4 **Spacecraft accident injuring occupant**

⊗⑦**V95.40** **Unspecified spacecraft accident injuring occupant**

⊗⑦**V95.41** **Spacecraft crash injuring occupant**

⊗⑦**V95.42** **Forced landing of spacecraft injuring occupant**

⊗⑦**V95.43** **Spacecraft collision injuring occupant**

Spacecraft collision with any object, fixed, moveable or moving

⊗⑦**V95.44** **Spacecraft fire injuring occupant**

⊗⑦**V95.45** **Spacecraft explosion injuring occupant**

⊗⑦**V95.49** **Other spacecraft accident injuring occupant**

⊗⑦**V95.8** **Other powered aircraft accidents injuring occupant**

⊗⑦**V95.9** **Unspecified aircraft accident injuring occupant**

Aircraft accident NOS

Air transport accident NOS

■ Add 4th-7th digits   ■ Nonspecific code   ■ Unspecified code   ■ Manifestation code   [HCC] Hierarchical Condition Code   1087

V96 **Accident to nonpowered aircraft causing injury to occupant**

The appropriate 7th character is to be added to each code from category V96

A - initial encounter

D - subsequent encounter

S - sequela

V96.0 **Balloon accident injuring occupant**

⊗⑦**V96.00** **Unspecified balloon accident injuring occupant**

⊗⑦**V96.01** **Balloon crash injuring occupant**

⊗⑦**V96.02** **Forced landing of balloon injuring occupant**

⊗⑦**V96.03** **Balloon collision injuring occupant**

Balloon collision with any object, fixed, moveable or moving

⊗⑦**V96.04** **Balloon fire injuring occupant**

⊗⑦**V96.05** **Balloon explosion injuring occupant**

⊗⑦**V96.09** **Other balloon accident injuring occupant**

V96.1 **Hang-glider accident injuring occupant**

⊗⑦**V96.10** **Unspecified hang-glider accident injuring occupant**

⊗⑦**V96.11** **Hang-glider crash injuring occupant**

⊗⑦**V96.12** **Forced landing of hang-glider injuring occupant**

⊗⑦**V96.13** **Hang-glider collision injuring occupant**

Hang-glider collision with any object, fixed, moveable or moving

⊗⑦**V96.14** **Hang-glider fire injuring occupant**

⊗⑦**V96.15** **Hang-glider explosion injuring occupant**

⊗⑦**V96.19** **Other hang-glider accident injuring occupant**

V96.2 **Glider (nonpowered) accident injuring occupant**

⊗⑦**V96.20** **Unspecified glider (nonpowered) accident injuring occupant**

⊗⑦**V96.21** **Glider (nonpowered) crash injuring occupant**

⊗⑦**V96.22** **Forced landing of glider (nonpowered) injuring occupant**

⊗⑦**V96.23** **Glider (nonpowered) collision injuring occupant**

Glider (nonpowered) collision with any object, fixed, moveable or moving

⊗⑦**V96.24** **Glider (nonpowered) fire injuring occupant**

⊗⑦**V96.25** **Glider (nonpowered) explosion injuring occupant**

⊗⑦**V96.29** **Other glider (nonpowered) accident injuring occupant**

⊗⑦**V96.8** **Other nonpowered-aircraft accidents injuring occupant**

Kite carrying a person accident injuring occupant

⊗⑦**V96.9** **Unspecified nonpowered-aircraft accident injuring occupant**

Nonpowered-aircraft accident NOS

V97 **Other specified air transport accidents**

The appropriate 7th character is to be added to each code from category V97

A - initial encounter

D - subsequent encounter

S - sequela

⊗⑦**V97.0** **Occupant of aircraft injured in other specified air transport accidents**

Fall in, on or from aircraft in air transport accident

Excludes1: accident while boarding or alighting aircraft (V97.1)

⊗⑦**V97.1** **Person injured while boarding or alighting from aircraft**

V97.2 **Parachutist accident**

⊗⑦**V97.21** **Parachutist entangled in object**

Parachutist landing in tree

⊗⑦**V97.22** **Parachutist injured on landing**

⊗⑦**V97.29** **Other parachutist accident**

V97.3 **Person on ground injured in air transport accident**

⊗⑦**V97.31** **Hit by object falling from aircraft**

Hit by crashing aircraft

Injured by aircraft hitting house

Injured by aircraft hitting car

⊗⑦**V97.32** **Injured by rotating propeller**

⊗⑦**V97.33** **Sucked into jet engine**

⊗⑦**V97.39** **Other injury to person on ground due to air transport accident**

⊗⑦**V97.8** **Other air transport accidents, not elsewhere classified**

Excludes1: aircraft accident NOS (V95.9)

exposure to changes in air pressure during ascent or descent (W94.-)

V97.81 **Air transport accident involving military aircraft**

⑦**V97.810** **Civilian aircraft involved in air transport accident with military aircraft**

Passenger in civilian aircraft injured due to accident with military aircraft

⑦**V97.811** **Civilian injured by military aircraft**

⑦**V97.818** **Other air transport accident involving military aircraft**

⊗⑦**V97.89** **Other air transport accidents, not elsewhere classified**

Injury from machinery on aircraft

OTHER AND UNSPECIFIED TRANSPORT ACCIDENTS (V98-V99)

Excludes1: vehicle accident, type of vehicle unspecified (V89.-)

V98 **Other specified transport accidents**

The appropriate 7th character is to be added to each code from category V98

A - initial encounter

D - subsequent encounter

S - sequela

⊗⑦**V98.0** **Accident to, on or involving cable-car, not on rails**

Caught or dragged by cable-car, not on rails

Fall or jump from cable-car, not on rails

Object thrown from or in cable-car, not on rails

⊗⑦**V98.1** **Accident to, on or involving land-yacht**

⊗⑦**V98.2** **Accident to, on or involving ice yacht**

⊗⑦**V98.3** **Accident to, on or involving ski lift**

Accident to, on or involving ski chair-lift

Accident to, on or involving ski-lift with gondola

⊗⑦**V98.8** **Other specified transport accidents**

⊗⑦**V99** **Unspecified transport accident**

The appropriate 7th character is to be added to code V99

A - initial encounter

D - subsequent encounter

S - sequela

OTHER EXTERNAL CAUSES OF ACCIDENTAL INJURY (W00-X58)

SLIPPING, TRIPPING, STUMBLING AND FALLS (W00-W19)

Excludes1: assault involving a fall (Y01-Y02)

> fall from animal (V80.-)
>
> fall (in) (from) machinery (in operation) (W28-W31)
>
> fall (in) (from) transport vehicle (V01-V99)
>
> intentional self-harm involving a fall (X80-X81)

Excludes2: at risk for fall (history of fall) Z91.81

> fall (in) (from) burning building (X00.-)
>
> fall into fire (X00-X04, X08)

W00 Fall due to ice and snow

> **Includes:** pedestrian on foot falling (slipping) on ice and snow
>
> **Excludes1:** fall on (from) ice and snow involving pedestrian conveyance (V00.-)
>
> > fall from stairs and steps not due to ice and snow (W10.-)

The appropriate 7th character is to be added to each code from category W00

A - initial encounter

D - subsequent encounter

S - sequela

⊗⑦**W00.0 Fall on same level due to ice and snow**

⊗⑦**W00.1 Fall from stairs and steps due to ice and snow**

⊗⑦**W00.2 Other fall from one level to another due to ice and snow**

⊗⑦**W00.9 Unspecified fall due to ice and snow**

W01 Fall on same level from slipping, tripping and stumbling

> **Includes:** fall on moving sidewalk
>
> **Excludes1:** fall due to bumping (striking) against object (W18.0-)
>
> > fall in shower or bathtub (W18.2-)
> >
> > fall on same level NOS (W18.30)
> >
> > fall on same level from slipping, tripping and stumbling due to ice or snow (W00.0)
> >
> > fall off or from toilet (W18.1-)
> >
> > slipping, tripping and stumbling NOS (W18.40)
> >
> > slipping, tripping and stumbling without falling (W18.4-)

The appropriate 7th character is to be added to each code from category W01

A - initial encounter

D - subsequent encounter

S - sequela

⊗⑦**W01.0 Fall on same level from slipping, tripping and stumbling without subsequent striking against object**

> Falling over animal

W01.1 Fall on same level from slipping, tripping and stumbling with subsequent striking against object

> ⊗⑦**W01.10 Fall on same level from slipping, tripping and stumbling with subsequent striking against unspecified object**
>
> **W01.11 Fall on same level from slipping, tripping and stumbling with subsequent striking against sharp object**
>
> > ⑦**W01.110 Fall on same level from slipping, tripping and stumbling with subsequent striking against sharp glass**
> >
> > ⑦**W01.111 Fall on same level from slipping, tripping and stumbling with subsequent striking against power tool or machine**
> >
> > ⑦**W01.118 Fall on same level from slipping, tripping and stumbling with**

subsequent striking against other sharp object

> > ⑦**W01.119 Fall on same level from slipping, tripping and stumbling with subsequent striking against unspecified sharp object**
>
> **W01.19 Fall on same level from slipping, tripping and stumbling with subsequent striking against other object**
>
> > ⑦**W01.190 Fall on same level from slipping, tripping and stumbling with subsequent striking against furniture**
> >
> > ⑦**W01.198 Fall on same level from slipping, tripping and stumbling with subsequent striking against other object**

⊗⑦**W03 Other fall on same level due to collision with another person**

Fall due to non-transport collision **with other** person

> **Excludes1:** collision with another person without fall (W51)
>
> > crushed or pushed by a crowd or human stampede (W52)
> >
> > fall involving pedestrian conveyance (V00-V.09)
> >
> > fall due to ice or snow (W00)
> >
> > fall on same level NOS (W18.30)

The appropriate 7th character is to be added to code W03

A - initial encounter

D - subsequent encounter

S – sequela

⊗⑦**W04 Fall while being carried or supported by other persons**

Accidentally dropped while being carried

The appropriate 7th character is to be added to code W04

A - initial encounter

D - subsequent encounter

S - sequela

W05 Fall from non-moving wheelchair, nonmotorized scooter and motorized mobility scooter

> **Excludes1:** fall from moving wheelchair (powered) (V00.811)
>
> > fall from moving motorized mobility scooter (V00.831)
> >
> > fall from nonmotorized scooter (V00.141)

The appropriate 7th character is to be added to each code from category W05

A - initial encounter

D - subsequent encounter

S - sequela

⊗⑦**W05.0 Fall from non-moving wheelchair**

⊗⑦**W05.1 Fall from non-moving nonmotorized scooter**

⊗⑦**W05.2 Fall from non-moving motorized mobility scooter**

⊗⑦**W06 Fall from bed**

The appropriate 7th character is to be added to code W06

A - initial encounter

D - subsequent encounter

S – sequela

⊗⑦**W07 Fall from chair**

The appropriate 7th character is to be added to code W07

A - initial encounter

D - subsequent encounter

S – sequela

⊗⑦**W08 Fall from other furniture**

The appropriate 7th character is to be added to code W08

A - initial encounter

D - subsequent encounter

S - sequela

W09 **Fall on and from playground equipment**

> **Excludes1:** fall involving recreational machinery (W31)

The appropriate 7th character is to be added to each code from category W09

A - initial encounter

D - subsequent encounter

S - sequela

⊗⑦**W09.0** **Fall on or from playground slide**

⊗⑦**W09.1** **Fall from playground swing**

⊗⑦**W09.2** **Fall on or from jungle gym**

⊗⑦**W09.8** **Fall on or from other playground equipment**

W10 **Fall on and from stairs and steps**

> **Excludes1:** Fall from stairs and steps due to ice and snow (W00.1)

The appropriate 7th character is to be added to each code from category W10

A - initial encounter

D - subsequent encounter

S - sequela

⊗⑦**W10.0** **Fall (on)(from) escalator**

⊗⑦**W10.1** **Fall (on)(from) sidewalk curb**

⊗⑦**W10.2** **Fall (on)(from) incline**

> Fall (on) (from) ramp

⊗⑦**W10.8** **Fall (on) (from) other stairs and steps**

⊗⑦**W10.9** **Fall (on) (from) unspecified stairs and steps**

⊗⑦**W11** **Fall on and from ladder**

The appropriate 7th character is to be added to code W11

A - initial encounter

D - subsequent encounter

S - sequela

⊗⑦**W12** **Fall on and from scaffolding**

The appropriate 7th character is to be added to code W12

A - initial encounter

D - subsequent encounter

S - sequela

W13 **Fall from, out of or through building or structure**

The appropriate 7th character is to be added to each code from category W13

A - initial encounter

D - subsequent encounter

S - sequela

⊗⑦**W13.0** **Fall from, out of or through balcony**

> Fall from, out of or through railing

⊗⑦**W13.1** **Fall from, out of or through bridge**

⊗⑦**W13.2** **Fall from, out of or through roof**

⊗⑦**W13.3** **Fall through floor**

⊗⑦**W13.4** **Fall from, out of or through window**

> **Excludes2:** fall with subsequent striking against sharp glass (W01.110-)

⊗⑦**W13.8** **Fall from, out of or through other building or structure**

> Fall from, out of or through viaduct

> Fall from, out of or through wall

> Fall from, out of or through flag-pole

⊗⑦**W13.9** **Fall from, out of or through building, not otherwise specified**

> **Excludes1:** collapse of a building or structure (W20.-)

fall or jump from burning building or structure (X00.-)

⊗⑦**W14** **Fall from tree**

The appropriate 7th character is to be added to code W14

A - initial encounter

D - subsequent encounter

S - sequela

⊗⑦**W15** **Fall from cliff**

The appropriate 7th character is to be added to code W15

A - initial encounter

D - subsequent encounter

S - sequela

W16 **Fall, jump or diving into water**

> **Excludes1:** accidental non-watercraft drowning and submersion not involving fall (W65-W74)
>
> effects of air pressure from diving (W94.-)
>
> fall into water from watercraft (V90-V94)
>
> hitting an object or against bottom when falling from watercraft (V94.0)

> **Excludes2:** striking or hitting diving board (W21.4)

The appropriate 7th character is to be added to each code from category W16

A - initial encounter

D - subsequent encounter

S - sequela

W16.0 **Fall into swimming pool**

> Fall into swimming pool NOS

> **Excludes1:** fall into empty swimming pool (W17.3)

W16.01 **Fall into swimming pool striking water surface**

⑦**W16.011** **Fall into swimming pool striking water surface causing drowning and submersion**

> **Excludes1:** drowning and submersion while in swimming pool without fall (W67)

⑦**W16.012** **Fall into swimming pool striking water surface causing other injury**

W16.02 **Fall into swimming pool striking bottom**

⑦**W16.021** **Fall into swimming pool striking bottom causing drowning and submersion**

> **Excludes1:** drowning and submersion while in swimming pool without fall (W67)

⑦**W16.022** **Fall into swimming pool striking bottom causing other injury**

W16.03 **Fall into swimming pool striking wall**

⑦**W16.031** **Fall into swimming pool striking wall causing drowning and submersion**

> **Excludes1:** drowning and submersion while in swimming pool without fall (W67)

⑦**W16.032** **Fall into swimming pool striking wall causing other injury**

W16.1 **Fall into natural body of water**

> Fall into lake

> Fall into open sea Fall into river

> Fall into stream

W16.11 **Fall into natural body of water striking water surface**

⑦W16.111　**Fall into natural body of water striking water surface causing drowning and submersion**

　　Excludes1: drowning and submersion while in natural body of water without fall (W69)

⑦W16.112　**Fall into natural body of water striking water surface causing other injury**

W16.12　**Fall into natural body of water striking bottom**

⑦W16.121　**Fall into natural body of water striking bottom causing drowning and submersion**

　　Excludes1: drowning and submersion while in natural body of water without fall (W69)

⑦W16.122　**Fall into natural body of water striking bottom causing other injury**

W16.13　**Fall into natural body of water striking side**

⑦W16.131　**Fall into natural body of water striking side causing drowning and submersion**

　　Excludes1: drowning and submersion while in natural body of water without fall (W69)

⑦W16.132　**Fall into natural body of water striking side causing other injury**

W16.2　**Fall in (into) filled bathtub or bucket of water**

W16.21　**Fall in (into) filled bathtub**

　　Excludes1: fall into empty bathtub (W18.2)

⑦W16.211　**Fall in (into) filled bathtub causing drowning and submersion**

　　Excludes1: drowning and submersion while in filled bathtub without fall (W65)

⑦W16.212　**Fall in (into) filled bathtub causing other injury**

W16.22　**Fall in (into) bucket of water**

⑦W16.221　**Fall in (into) bucket of water causing drowning and submersion**

⑦W16.222　**Fall in (into) bucket of water causing other injury**

W16.3　**Fall into other water**

Fall into fountain Fall into reservoir

W16.31　**Fall into other water striking water surface**

⑦W16.311　**Fall into other water striking water surface causing drowning and submersion**

　　Excludes1: drowning and submersion while **in other** water without fall (W73)

⑦W16.312　**Fall into other water striking water surface causing other injury**

W16.32　**Fall into other water striking bottom**

⑦W16.321　**Fall into other water striking bottom causing drowning and submersion**

　　Excludes1: drowning and submersion while **in other** water without fall (W73)

⑦W16.322　**Fall into other water striking bottom causing other injury**

W16.33　**Fall into other water striking wall**

⑦W16.331　**Fall into other water striking wall causing drowning and submersion**

　　Excludes1: drowning and submersion while **in other** water without fall (W73)

⑦W16.332　**Fall into other water striking wall causing other injury**

W16.4　**Fall into unspecified water**

⊗⑦W16.41　**Fall into unspecified water causing drowning and submersion**

⊗⑦W16.42　**Fall into unspecified water causing other injury**

W16.5　**Jumping or diving into swimming pool**

⊗⑦W16.51　**Jumping or diving into swimming pool striking water surface**

⑦W16.511　**Jumping or diving into swimming pool striking water surface causing drowning and submersion**

　　Excludes1: drowning and submersion while in swimming pool without jumping or diving (W67)

⑦W16.512　**Jumping or diving into swimming pool striking water surface causing other injury**

W16.52　**Jumping or diving into swimming pool striking bottom**

⑦W16.521　**Jumping or diving into swimming pool striking bottom causing drowning and submersion**

　　Excludes1: drowning and submersion while in swimming pool without jumping or diving (W67)

⑦W16.522　**Jumping or diving into swimming pool striking bottom causing other injury**

W16.53　**Jumping or diving into swimming pool striking wall**

⑦W16.531　**Jumping or diving into swimming pool striking wall causing drowning and submersion**

　　Excludes1: drowning and submersion while in swimming pool without jumping or diving (W67)

⑦W16.532　**Jumping or diving into swimming pool striking wall causing other injury**

W16.6　**Jumping or diving into natural body of water**

Jumping or diving into lake

Jumping or diving into open sea

Jumping or diving into river

Jumping or diving into stream

W16.61　**Jumping or diving into natural body of water striking water surface**

⑦W16.611　**Jumping or diving into natural body of water striking water surface causing drowning and submersion**

　　Excludes1: drowning and submersion while in natural body of water without jumping or diving (W69)

⑦W16.612　**Jumping or diving into natural body of water striking water surface causing other injury**

W16.62　**Jumping or diving into natural body of water striking bottom**

⑦**W16.621 Jumping or diving into natural body of water striking bottom causing drowning and submersion**

　　Excludes1: drowning and submersion while in natural body of water without jumping or diving (W69)

⑦**W16.622 Jumping or diving into natural body of water striking bottom causing other injury**

W16.7 Jumping or diving from boat

　Excludes1: Fall from boat into water -see watercraft accident (V90-V94)

W16.71 Jumping or diving from boat striking water surface

⑦**W16.711 Jumping or diving from boat striking water surface causing drowning and submersion**

⑦**W16.712 Jumping or diving from boat striking water surface causing other injury**

W16.72 Jumping or diving from boat striking bottom

⑦**W16.721 Jumping or diving from boat striking bottom causing drowning and submersion**

⑦**W16.722 Jumping or diving from boat striking bottom causing other injury**

W16.8 Jumping or diving into other water

　Jumping or diving into fountain

　Jumping or diving into reservoir

W16.81 Jumping or diving into other water striking water surface

⑦**W16.811 Jumping or diving into other water striking water surface causing drowning and submersion**

　　Excludes1: drowning and submersion while in other water without jumping or diving (W73)

⑦**W16.812 Jumping or diving into other water striking water surface causing other injury**

W16.82 Jumping or diving into other water striking bottom

⑦**W16.821 Jumping or diving into other water striking bottom causing drowning and submersion**

　　Excludes1: drowning and submersion while in other water without jumping or diving (W73)

⑦**W16.822 Jumping or diving into other water striking bottom causing other injury**

W16.83 Jumping or diving into other water striking wall

⑦**W16.831 Jumping or diving into other water striking wall causing drowning and submersion**

　　Excludes1: drowning and submersion while in other water without jumping or diving (W73)

⑦**W16.832 Jumping or diving into other water striking wall causing other injury**

W16.9 Jumping or diving into unspecified water

⊗⑦**W16.91 Jumping or diving into unspecified water causing drowning and submersion**

⊗⑦**W16.92 Jumping or diving into unspecified water causing other injury**

W17 **Other fall from one level to another**

The appropriate 7th character is to be added to each code from category W17

A - initial encounter

D - subsequent encounter

S - sequela

⊗⑦**W17.0 Fall into well**

⊗⑦**W17.1 Fall into storm drain or manhole**

⊗⑦**W17.2 Fall into hole**

　Fall into pit

⊗⑦**W17.3 Fall into empty swimming pool**

　Excludes1: fall into filled swimming pool (W16.0-)

⊗⑦**W17.4 Fall from dock**

W17.8 Other fall from one level to another

⊗⑦**W17.81 Fall down embankment (hill)**

⊗⑦**W17.82 Fall from (out of) grocery cart**

　Fall due to grocery cart tipping over

⊗⑦**W17.89 Other fall from one level to another**

　Fall from cherry picker Fall from lifting device

　Fall from mobile elevated work platform [MEWP]

　Fall from sky lift

W18 **Other slipping, tripping and stumbling and falls**

The appropriate 7th character is to be added to each code from category W18

A - initial encounter

D - subsequent encounter

S - sequela

W18.0 Fall due to bumping against object

　Striking against object with subsequent fall

　Excludes1: fall on same level due to slipping, tripping, or stumbling with subsequent striking against object (W01.1-)

⊗⑦**W18.00 Striking against unspecified object with subsequent fall**

⊗⑦**W18.01 Striking against sports equipment with subsequent fall**

⊗⑦**W18.02 Striking against glass with subsequent fall**

⊗⑦**W18.09 Striking against other object with subsequent fall**

W18.1 Fall from or off toilet

⊗⑦**W18.11 Fall from or off toilet without subsequent striking against object**

　Fall from (off) toilet NOS

⊗⑦**W18.12 Fall from or off toilet with subsequent striking against object**

⊗⑦**W18.2 Fall in (into) shower or empty bathtub**

　Excludes1: fall in full bathtub causing drowning or submersion (W16.21-)

W18.3 Other and unspecified fall on same level

⊗⑦**W18.30 Fall on same level, unspecified**

⊗⑦**W18.31 Fall on same level due to stepping on an object**

　Fall on same level due to stepping on an animal

　　Excludes1: slipping, tripping and stumbling without fall due to stepping on animal (W18.41)

⊗⑦**W18.39 Other fall on same level**

W18.4 Slipping, tripping and stumbling without falling

　Excludes1: collision with another person without fall (W51)

⊗⑦**W18.40** **Slipping, tripping and stumbling without falling, unspecified**

⊗⑦**W18.41** **Slipping, tripping and stumbling without falling due to stepping on object**

Slipping, tripping and stumbling without falling due to stepping on animal

Excludes1: slipping, tripping and stumbling with fall due to stepping on animal (W18.31)

⊗⑦**W18.42** **Slipping, tripping and stumbling without falling due to stepping into hole or opening**

⊗⑦**W18.43** **Slipping, tripping and stumbling without falling due to stepping from one level to another**

⊗⑦**W18.49** **Other slipping, tripping and stumbling without falling**

⊗⑦**W19** **Unspecified fall**

Accidental fall NOS

The appropriate 7th character is to be added to code W19

A - initial encounter

D - subsequent encounter

S - sequela

EXPOSURE TO INANIMATE MECHANICAL FORCES (W20-W49)

Excludes1: assault (X92-Y09)

contact or collision with animals or persons (W50-W64)

exposure to inanimate mechanical forces involving military or war operations (Y36.-, Y37.-)

intentional self-harm (X71-X83)

W20 **Struck by thrown, projected or falling object**

Code first any associated:

cataclysm (X34-X39)

lightning strike (T75.00)

Excludes1: falling object in machinery accident (W24, W28-W31)

falling object in transport accident (V01-V99)

object set in motion by explosion (W35-W40)

object set in motion by firearm (W32-W34)

struck by thrown sports equipment (W21.-)

The appropriate 7th character is to be added to each code from category W20

A - initial encounter

D - subsequent encounter

S - sequela

⊗⑦**W20.0** **Struck by falling object in cave-in**

Excludes2: asphyxiation due to cave-in (T71.21)

⊗⑦**W20.1** **Struck by object due to collapse of building**

Excludes1: struck by object due to collapse of burning building (X00.2, X02.2)

⊗⑦**W20.8** **Other cause of strike by thrown, projected or falling object**

Excludes1: struck by thrown sports equipment (W21.-)

W21 **Striking against or struck by sports equipment**

Excludes1: assault with sports equipment (Y08.0-)

striking against or struck by sports equipment with subsequent fall (W18.01)

The appropriate 7th character is to be added to each code from category W21

A - initial encounter

D - subsequent encounter

S - sequela

W21.0 **Struck by hit or thrown ball**

⊗⑦**W21.00** **Struck by hit or thrown ball, unspecified type**

⊗⑦**W21.01** **Struck by football**

⊗⑦**W21.02** **Struck by soccer ball**

⊗⑦**W21.03** **Struck by baseball**

⊗⑦**W21.04** **Struck by golf ball**

⊗⑦**W21.05** **Struck by basketball**

⊗⑦**W21.06** **Struck by volleyball**

⊗⑦**W21.07** **Struck by softball**

⊗⑦**W21.09** **Struck by other hit or thrown ball**

W21.1 **Struck by bat, racquet or club**

⊗⑦**W21.11** **Struck by baseball bat**

⊗⑦**W21.12** **Struck by tennis racquet**

⊗⑦**W21.13** **Struck by golf club**

⊗⑦**W21.19** **Struck by other bat, racquet or club**

W21.2 **Struck by hockey stick or puck**

W21.21 **Struck by hockey stick**

⑦**W21.210** **Struck by ice hockey stick**

⑦**W21.211** **Struck by field hockey stick**

W21.22 **Struck by hockey puck**

⑦**W21.220** **Struck by ice hockey puck**

⑦**W21.221** **Struck by field hockey puck**

W21.3 **Struck by sports foot wear**

⊗⑦**W21.31** **Struck by shoe cleats**

Stepped on by shoe cleats

⊗⑦**W21.32** **Struck by skate blades**

Skated over by skate blades

⊗⑦**W21.39** **Struck by other sports foot wear**

⊗⑦**W21.4** **Striking against diving board**

Use Additional Code for subsequent falling into water, if applicable (W16.-)

W21.8 **Striking against or struck by other sports equipment**

⊗⑦**W21.81** **Striking against or struck by football helmet**

⊗⑦**W21.89** **Striking against or struck by other sports equipment**

⊗⑦**W21.9** **Striking against or struck by unspecified sports equipment**

W22 **Striking against or struck by other objects**

Excludes1: striking against or struck by object with subsequent fall (W18.09)

The appropriate 7th character is to be added to each code from category W22

A - initial encounter

D - subsequent encounter

S - sequela

W22.0 **Striking against stationary object**

Excludes1: striking against stationary sports equipment (W21.8)

⊗⑦**W22.01** **Walked into wall**

⊗⑦**W22.02** **Walked into lamppost**

⊗⑦**W22.03** **Walked into furniture**

W22.04 **Striking against wall of swimming pool**

⑦**W22.041** **Striking against wall of swimming pool causing drowning and submersion**

Excludes1: drowning and submersion while swimming without striking against wall (W67)

⑦**W22.042** **Striking against wall of swimming pool causing other injury**

⊗⑦**W22.09** **Striking against other stationary object**

W22.1 **Striking against or struck by automobile airbag**

⊗⑦**W22.10** **Striking against or struck by unspecified automobile airbag**

⊗⑦**W22.11** **Striking against or struck by driver side automobile airbag**

⊗⑦**W22.12** **Striking against or struck by front passenger side automobile airbag**

⊗⑦**W22.19** **Striking against or struck by other automobile airbag**

⊗⑦**W22.8** **Striking against or struck by other objects**

Striking against or struck by object NOS

Excludes1: struck by thrown, projected or falling object (W20.-)

W23 **Caught, crushed, jammed or pinched in or between objects**

Excludes1: injury caused by cutting or piercing instruments (W25-W27)

injury caused by firearms malfunction (W32.1, W33.1-, W34.1-)

injury caused by lifting and transmission devices (W24.-)

injury caused by machinery (W28-W31)

injury caused by nonpowered hand tools (W27.-)

injury caused by transport vehicle being used as a means of transportation (V01-V99)

injury caused by struck by thrown, projected or falling object (W20.-)

The appropriate 7th character is to be added to each code from category W23

A - initial encounter

D - subsequent encounter

S - sequela

⊗⑦**W23.0** **Caught, crushed, jammed, or pinched between moving objects**

⊗⑦**W23.1** **Caught, crushed, jammed, or pinched between stationary objects**

W24 **Contact with lifting and transmission devices, not elsewhere classified**

Excludes1: transport accidents (V01-V99)

The appropriate 7th character is to be added to each code from category W24

A - initial encounter

D - subsequent encounter

S - sequela

⊗⑦**W24.0** **Contact with lifting devices, not elsewhere classified**

Contact with chain hoist

Contact with drive belt

Contact with pulley (block)

⊗⑦**W24.1** **Contact with transmission devices, not elsewhere classified**

Contact with transmission belt or cable

⊗⑦**W25** **Contact with sharp glass**

Code first any associated:

injury due to flying glass from explosion or firearm discharge (W32-W40)

transport accident (V00-V99)

Excludes1: fall on same level due to slipping, tripping and stumbling with subsequent striking against sharp glass (W01.110-)

striking against sharp glass with subsequent fall (W18.02-)

Excludes2: glass embedded in skin (W45-)

The appropriate 7th character is to be added to code W25

A - initial encounter

D - subsequent encounter

S - sequela

W26 **Contact with other sharp objects**

Excludes2: sharp object(s) embedded in skin (W45-)

The appropriate 7th character is to be added to each code from category W26

A - initial encounter

D - subsequent encounter

S - sequela

⊗⑦**W26.0** **Contact with knife**

Excludes1: contact with electric knife (W29.1)

⊗⑦**W26.1** **Contact with sword or dagger**

⊗⑦**W26.2** **Contact with edge of stiff paper**

Paper cut

⊗⑦**W26.8** **Contact with other sharp object(s), not elsewhere classified**

Contact with tin can lid

⊗⑦**W26.9** **Contact with unspecified sharp object(s)**

W27 **Contact with nonpowered hand tool**

The appropriate 7th character is to be added to each code from category W27

A - initial encounter

D - subsequent encounter

S - sequela

⊗⑦**W27.0** **Contact with workbench tool**

Contact with auger

Contact with axe

Contact with chisel

Contact with handsaw

Contact with screwdriver

⊗⑦**W27.1** **Contact with garden tool**

Contact with hoe

Contact with nonpowered lawn mower

Contact with pitchfork

Contact with rake

⊗⑦**W27.2** **Contact with scissors**

⊗⑦**W27.3** **Contact with needle (sewing)**

Excludes1: contact with hypodermic needle (W46.-)

⊗⑦**W27.4** **Contact with kitchen utensil**

Contact with fork

Contact with icepick

Contact with can-opener NOS

⊗⑦**W27.5** **Contact with paper-cutter**

⊗⑦**W27.8** **Contact with other nonpowered hand tool**

Contact with nonpowered sewing machine

Contact with shovel

⊗⑦**W28** **Contact with powered lawn mower**

Powered lawn mower (commercial) (residential)

Excludes1: contact with nonpowered lawn mower (W27.1)

Excludes2: exposure to electric current (W86.-)

The appropriate 7th character is to be added to code W28

A - initial encounter

D - subsequent encounter

S - sequela

W29 **Contact with other powered hand tools and household machinery**

> **Excludes1:** contact with commercial machinery (W31.82)
>> contact with hot household appliance (X15)
>> contact with nonpowered hand tool (W27.-)
>> exposure to electric current (W86)

The appropriate 7th character is to be added to each code from category W29

A - initial encounter

D - subsequent encounter

S - sequela

⊗⑦**W29.0** **Contact with powered kitchen appliance**

> Contact with blender
> Contact with can-opener
> Contact with garbage disposal
> Contact with mixer

⊗⑦**W29.1** **Contact with electric knife**

⊗⑦**W29.2** **Contact with other powered household machinery**

> Contact with electric fan
> Contact with powered dryer (clothes) (powered) (spin)
> Contact with washing-machine
> Contact with sewing machine

⊗⑦**W29.3** **Contact with powered garden and outdoor hand tools and machinery**

> Contact with chainsaw
> Contact with edger
> Contact with garden cultivator (tiller)
> Contact with hedge trimmer
> Contact with other powered garden tool

> **Excludes1:** contact with powered lawn mower (W28)

⊗⑦**W29.4** **Contact with nail gun**

⊗⑦**W29.8** **Contact with other powered hand tools and household machinery**

> Contact with do-it-yourself tool NOS

W30 **Contact with agricultural machinery**

> **Includes:** animal-powered farm machine

> **Excludes1:** agricultural transport vehicle accident (V01-V99)
>> explosion of grain store (W40.8)
>> exposure to electric current (W86.-)

The appropriate 7th character is to be added to each code from category W30

A - initial encounter

D - subsequent encounter

S - sequela

⊗⑦**W30.0** **Contact with combine harvester**

> Contact with reaper
> Contact with thresher

⊗⑦**W30.1** **Contact with power take-off devices (PTO)**

⊗⑦**W30.2** **Contact with hay derrick**

⊗⑦**W30.3** **Contact with grain storage elevator**

> **Excludes1:** explosion of grain store (W40.8)

W30.8 **Contact with other specified agricultural machinery**

⊗⑦**W30.81** **Contact with agricultural transport vehicle in stationary use**

> Contact with agricultural transport vehicle under repair, not on public roadway

> **Excludes1:** agricultural transport vehicle accident (V01-V99)

⊗⑦**W30.89** **Contact with other specified agricultural machinery**

⊗⑦**W30.9** **Contact with unspecified agricultural machinery**

> Contact with farm machinery NOS

W31 **Contact with other and unspecified machinery**

> **Excludes1:** contact with agricultural machinery (W30.-)
>> contact with machinery in transport under own power or being towed by a vehicle (V01-V99)
>> exposure to electric current (W86)

The appropriate 7th character is to be added to each code from category W31

A - initial encounter

D - subsequent encounter

S - sequela

⊗⑦**W31.0** **Contact with mining and earth-drilling machinery**

> Contact with bore or drill (land) (seabed)
> Contact with shaft hoist
> Contact with shaft lift
> Contact with under cutter

⊗⑦**W31.1** **Contact with metalworking machines**

> Contact with abrasive wheel
> Contact with forging machine
> Contact with lathe
> Contact with mechanical shears
> Contact with metal drilling machine
> Contact with milling machine
> Contact with power press
> Contact with rolling-mill
> Contact with metal sawing machine

⊗⑦**W31.2** **Contact with powered woodworking and forming machines**

> Contact with band saw
> Contact with bench saw
> Contact with circular saw
> Contact with molding machine
> Contact with overhead plane
> Contact with powered saw
> Contact with radial saw
> Contact with sander

> **Excludes1:** nonpowered woodworking tools (W27.0)

⊗⑦**W31.3** **Contact with prime movers**

> Contact with gas turbine
> Contact with internal combustion engine
> Contact with steam engine
> Contact with water driven turbine

W31.8 **Contact with other specified machinery**

⊗⑦**W31.81** **Contact with recreational machinery**

> Contact with roller coaster

⊗⑦**W31.82** **Contact with other commercial machinery**

> Contact with commercial electric fan
> Contact with commercial kitchen appliances
> Contact with commercial powered dryer (clothes) (powered) (spin)
> Contact with commercial washing-machine
> Contact with commercial sewing machine

> **Excludes1:** contact with household machinery (W29.-)
>> contact with powered lawn mower (W28)

⊗⑦**W31.83** **Contact with special construction vehicle in stationary use**

Contact with special construction vehicle under repair, not on public roadway

Excludes1: special construction vehicle accident (V01-V99)

⊗⑦**W31.89** **Contact with other specified machinery**

⊗⑦**W31.9** **Contact with unspecified machinery**

Contact with machinery NOS

W32 **Accidental handgun discharge and malfunction**

Includes: accidental discharge and malfunction of gun for single hand use

accidental discharge and malfunction of pistol accidental discharge and malfunction of revolver

Handgun discharge and malfunction NOS

Excludes1: accidental air gun discharge and malfunction (W34.010, W34.110)

accidental BB gun discharge and malfunction (W34.010, W34.110)

accidental pellet gun discharge and malfunction (W34.010, W34.110)

accidental shotgun discharge and malfunction (W33.01, W33.11)

assault by handgun discharge (X93)

handgun discharge involving legal intervention (Y35.0-)

handgun discharge involving military or war operations (Y36.4-)

intentional self-harm by handgun discharge (X72)

Very pistol discharge and malfunction (W34.09, W34.19)

The appropriate 7th character is to be added to each code from category W32

A - initial encounter

D - subsequent encounter

S - sequela

⊗⑦**W32.0** **Accidental handgun discharge**

⊗⑦**W32.1** **Accidental handgun malfunction**

Injury due to explosion of handgun (parts)

Injury due to malfunction of mechanism or component of handgun

Injury due to recoil of handgun

Powder burn from handgun

W33 **Accidental rifle, shotgun and larger firearm discharge and malfunction**

Includes: rifle, shotgun and larger firearm discharge and malfunction NOS

Excludes1: accidental air gun discharge and malfunction (W34.010, W34.110)

accidental BB gun discharge and malfunction (W34.010, W34.110)

accidental handgun discharge and malfunction (W32.-)

accidental pellet gun discharge and malfunction (W34.010, W34.110)

assault by rifle, shotgun and larger firearm discharge (X94)

firearm discharge involving legal intervention (Y35.0-)

firearm discharge involving military or war operations (Y36.4-)

intentional self-harm by rifle, shotgun and larger firearm discharge (X73)

The appropriate 7th character is to be added to each code from category W33

A - initial encounter

D - subsequent encounter

S - sequela

W33.0 **Accidental rifle, shotgun and larger firearm discharge**

⊗⑦**W33.00** **Accidental discharge of unspecified larger firearm**

Discharge of unspecified larger firearm NOS

⊗⑦**W33.01** **Accidental discharge of shotgun**

Discharge of shotgun NOS

⊗⑦**W33.02** **Accidental discharge of hunting rifle**

Discharge of hunting rifle NOS

⊗⑦**W33.03** **Accidental discharge of machine gun**

Discharge of machine gun NOS

⊗⑦**W33.09** **Accidental discharge of other larger firearm**

Discharge of other larger firearm NOS

W33.1 **Accidental rifle, shotgun and larger firearm malfunction**

Injury due to explosion of rifle, shotgun and larger firearm (parts)

Injury due to malfunction of mechanism or component of rifle, shotgun and larger firearm

Injury due to piercing, cutting, crushing or pinching due to (by) slide trigger mechanism, scope or other gun part

Injury due to recoil of rifle, shotgun and larger firearm

Powder burn from rifle, shotgun and larger firearm

⊗⑦**W33.10** **Accidental malfunction of unspecified larger firearm**

Malfunction of unspecified larger firearm NOS

⊗⑦**W33.11** **Accidental malfunction of shotgun**

Malfunction of shotgun NOS

⊗⑦**W33.12** **Accidental malfunction of hunting rifle**

Malfunction of hunting rifle NOS

⊗⑦**W33.13** **Accidental malfunction of machine gun**

Malfunction of machine gun NOS

⊗⑦**W33.19** **Accidental malfunction of other larger firearm**

Malfunction of other larger firearm NOS

W34 **Accidental discharge and malfunction from other and unspecified firearms and guns**

The appropriate 7th character is to be added to each code from category W34

A - initial encounter

D - subsequent encounter

S - sequela

W34.0 **Accidental discharge from other and unspecified firearms and guns**

⊗⑦**W34.00** **Accidental discharge from unspecified firearms or gun**

Discharge from firearm NOS

Gunshot wound NOS

Shot NOS

W34.01 **Accidental discharge of gas, air or spring-operated guns**

⑦**W34.010** **Accidental discharge of air gun**

Accidental discharge of BB gun

Accidental discharge of pellet gun

⑦**W34.011** **Accidental discharge of paintball gun**

Accidental injury due to paintball discharge

⑦**W34.018** **Accidental discharge of other gas, air or spring-operated gun**

⊗⑦**W34.09** **Accidental discharge from other specified firearms**

● New code ▲ Revised code Excludes1: Not coded here Excludes2: Not included here ⊗ Placeholder required ⑦7th digit required

Accidental discharge from Very pistol [flare]

W34.1 Accidental malfunction from other and unspecified firearms and guns

⊗⑦**W34.10 Accidental malfunction from unspecified firearms or gun**

Firearm malfunction NOS

W34.11 Accidental malfunction of gas, air or spring-operated guns

⑦**W34.110 Accidental malfunction of air gun**

Accidental malfunction of BB gun

Accidental malfunction of pellet gun

⑦**W34.111 Accidental malfunction of paintball gun**

Accidental injury due to paintball gun malfunction

⑦**W34.118 Accidental malfunction of other gas, air or spring-operated gun**

⊗⑦**W34.19 Accidental malfunction from other specified firearms**

Accidental malfunction from Very pistol [flare]

⊗⑦**W35 Explosion and rupture of boiler**

Excludes1: explosion and rupture of boiler on watercraft (V93.4)

The appropriate 7th character is to be added to code W35

A - initial encounter

D - subsequent encounter

S - sequela

W36 Explosion and rupture of gas cylinder

The appropriate 7th character is to be added to each code from category W36

A - initial encounter

D - subsequent encounter

S - sequela

⊗⑦**W36.1 Explosion and rupture of aerosol can**

⊗⑦**W36.2 Explosion and rupture of air tank**

⊗⑦**W36.3 Explosion and rupture of pressurized-gas tank**

⊗⑦**W36.8 Explosion and rupture of other gas cylinder**

⊗⑦**W36.9 Explosion and rupture of unspecified gas cylinder**

W37 Explosion and rupture of pressurized tire, pipe or hose

The appropriate 7th character is to be added to each code from category W37

A - initial encounter

D - subsequent encounter

S - sequela

⊗⑦**W37.0 Explosion of bicycle tire**

⊗⑦**W37.8 Explosion and rupture of other pressurized tire, pipe or hose**

⊗⑦**W38 Explosion and rupture of other specified pressurized devices**

The appropriate 7th character is to be added to code W38

A - initial encounter

D - subsequent encounter

S - sequela

⊗⑦**W39 Discharge of firework**

The appropriate 7th character is to be added to code W39

A - initial encounter

D - subsequent encounter

S - sequela

W40 Explosion of other materials

Excludes1: assault by explosive material (X96)

explosion involving legal intervention (Y35.1-)

explosion involving military or war operations (Y36.0-, Y36.2-)

intentional self-harm by explosive material (X75)

The appropriate 7th character is to be added to each code from category W40

A - initial encounter

D - subsequent encounter

S - sequela

⊗⑦**W40.0 Explosion of blasting material**

Explosion of blasting cap

Explosion of detonator

Explosion of dynamite

Explosion of explosive (any) used in blasting operations

⊗⑦**W40.1 Explosion of explosive gases**

Explosion of acetylene

Explosion of butane

Explosion of coal gas

Explosion in mine NOS

Explosion of explosive gas

Explosion of fire damp

Explosion of gasoline fumes

Explosion of methane

Explosion of propane

⊗⑦**W40.8 Explosion of other specified explosive materials**

Explosion in dump NOS

Explosion in factory NOS

Explosion in grain store

Explosion in munitions

Excludes1: explosion involving legal intervention (Y35.1-)

explosion involving military or war operations (Y36.0-, Y36.2-)

⊗⑦**W40.9 Explosion of unspecified explosive materials**

Explosion NOS

W42 Exposure to noise

The appropriate 7th character is to be added to each code from category W42

A - initial encounter

D - subsequent encounter

S - sequela

⊗⑦**W42.0 Exposure to supersonic waves**

⊗⑦**W42.9 Exposure to other noise**

Exposure to sound waves NOS

W45 Foreign body or object entering through skin

Includes: foreign body or object embedded in skin

nail embedded in skin

Excludes2: contact with hand tools (nonpowered) (powered) (W27-W29)

contact with other sharp object(s) (W26.-)

contact with sharp glass (W25.-)

struck by objects (W20-W22)

The appropriate 7th character is to be added to each code from category W45

A - initial encounter

D - subsequent encounter

S - sequela

⊗⑦**W45.0 Nail entering through skin**

⊗⑦**W45.8 Other foreign body or object entering through skin**

Splinter in skin NOS

W46 **Contact with hypodermic needle**

The appropriate 7th character is to be added to each code from category W46

A - initial encounter

D - subsequent encounter

S - sequela

⊗⑦**W46.0** **Contact with hypodermic needle**

Hypodermic needle stick NOS

⊗⑦**W46.1** **Contact with contaminated hypodermic needle**

W49 **Exposure to other inanimate mechanical forces**

Includes: exposure to abnormal gravitational [G] forces

exposure to inanimate mechanical forces NEC

Excludes1: exposure to inanimate mechanical forces involving military or war operations (Y36.-, Y37.-)

The appropriate 7th character is to be added to each code from category W49

A - initial encounter

D - subsequent encounter

S - sequela

W49.0 **Item causing external constriction**

⊗⑦**W49.01** **Hair causing external constriction**

⊗⑦**W49.02** **String or thread causing external constriction**

⊗⑦**W49.03** **Rubber band causing external constriction**

⊗⑦**W49.04** **Ring or other jewelry causing external constriction**

⊗⑦**W49.09** **Other specified item causing external constriction**

⊗⑦**W49.9** **Exposure to other inanimate mechanical forces**

EXPOSURE TO ANIMATE MECHANICAL FORCES (W50-W64)

Excludes1: Toxic effect of contact with venomous animals and plants (T63.-)

W50 **Accidental hit, strike, kick, twist, bite or scratch by another person**

Includes: hit, strike, kick, twist, bite, or scratch by another person NOS

Excludes1: assault by bodily force (Y04)

struck by objects (W20-22)

The appropriate 7th character is to be added to each code from category W50

A - initial encounter

D - subsequent encounter

S - sequela

⊗⑦**W50.0** **Accidental hit or strike by another person**

Hit or strike by another person NOS

⊗⑦**W50.1** **Accidental kick by another person**

Kick by another person NOS

⊗⑦**W50.2** **Accidental twist by another person**

Twist by another person NOS

⊗⑦**W50.3** **Accidental bite by another person**

Human bite

Bite by another person NOS

⊗⑦**W50.4** **Accidental scratch by another person**

Scratch by another person NOS

⑦**W51** **Accidental striking against or bumped into by another person**

Excludes1: assault by striking against or bumping into by another person (Y04.2)

fall due to collision with another person (W03)

The appropriate 7th character is to be added to code W51

A - initial encounter

D - subsequent encounter

S - sequela

⊗⑦**W52** **Crushed, pushed or stepped on by crowd or human stampede**

Crushed, pushed or stepped on by crowd or human stampede with or without fall

The appropriate 7th character is to be added to code W52

A - initial encounter

D - subsequent encounter

S - sequela

W53 **Contact with rodent**

Includes: contact with saliva, feces or urine of rodent

The appropriate 7th character is to be added to each code from category W53

A - initial encounter

D - subsequent encounter

S - sequela

W53.0 **Contact with mouse**

⊗⑦**W53.01** **Bitten by mouse**

⊗⑦**W53.09** **Other contact with mouse**

W53.1 **Contact with rat**

⊗⑦**W53.11** **Bitten by rat**

⊗⑦**W53.19** **Other contact with rat**

W53.2 **Contact with squirrel**

⊗⑦**W53.21** **Bitten by squirrel**

⊗⑦**W53.29** **Other contact with squirrel**

W53.8 **Contact with other rodent**

⊗⑦**W53.81** **Bitten by other rodent**

⊗⑦**W53.89** **Other contact with other rodent**

W54 **Contact with dog**

Includes: contact with saliva, feces or urine of dog

The appropriate 7th character is to be added to each code from category W54

A - initial encounter

D - subsequent encounter

S - sequela

⊗⑦**W54.0** **Bitten by dog**

⊗⑦**W54.1** **Struck by dog**

Knocked over by dog

⊗⑦**W54.8** **Other contact with dog**

W55 **Contact with other mammals**

Includes: contact with saliva, feces or urine of mammal

Excludes1: animal being ridden- see transport accidents

bitten or struck by dog (W54)

bitten or struck by rodent (W53.-)

contact with marine mammals (W56.-)

The appropriate 7th character is to be added to each code from category W55

A - initial encounter

D - subsequent encounter

S - sequela

W55.0 **Contact with cat**

⊗⑦**W55.01** **Bitten by cat**

⊗⑦**W55.03** **Scratched by cat**

⊗⑦**W55.09** **Other contact with cat**

W55.1 **Contact with horse**

● New code ▲ Revised code Excludes1: Not coded here Excludes2: Not included here ⊗ Placeholder required ⑦ 7th digit required

⊗⑦W55.11   **Bitten by horse**

⊗⑦W55.12   **Struck by horse**

⊗⑦W55.19   **Other contact with horse**

W55.2   **Contact with cow**

Contact with bull

⊗⑦W55.21   **Bitten by cow**

⊗⑦W55.22   **Struck by cow**

Gored by bull

⊗⑦W55.29   **Other contact with cow**

W55.3   **Contact with other hoof stock**

Contact with goats

Contact with sheep

⊗⑦W55.31   **Bitten by other hoof stock**

⊗⑦W55.32   **Struck by other hoof stock**

Gored by goat

Gored by ram

⊗⑦W55.39   **Other contact with other hoof stock**

W55.4   **Contact with pig**

⊗⑦W55.41   **Bitten by pig**

⊗⑦W55.42   **Struck by pig**

⊗⑦W55.49   **Other contact with pig**

W55.5   **Contact with raccoon**

⊗⑦W55.51   **Bitten by raccoon**

⊗⑦W55.52   **Struck by raccoon**

⊗⑦W55.59   **Other contact with raccoon**

W55.8   **Contact with other mammals**

⊗⑦W55.81   **Bitten by other mammals**

⊗⑦W55.82   **Struck by other mammals**

⊗⑦W55.89   **Other contact with other mammals**

W56   **Contact with nonvenomous marine animal**

Excludes1: contact with venomous marine animal (T63.-)

The appropriate 7th character is to be added to each code from category W56

A - initial encounter

D - subsequent encounter

S - sequela

W56.0   **Contact with dolphin**

⊗⑦W56.01   **Bitten by dolphin**

⊗⑦W56.02   **Struck by dolphin**

⊗⑦W56.09   **Other contact with dolphin**

W56.1   **Contact with sea lion**

⊗⑦W56.11   **Bitten by sea lion**

⊗⑦W56.12   **Struck by sea lion**

⊗⑦W56.19   **Other contact with sea lion**

W56.2   **Contact with orca**

Contact with killer whale

⊗⑦W56.21   **Bitten by orca**

⊗⑦W56.22   **Struck by orca**

⊗⑦W56.29   **Other contact with orca**

W56.3   **Contact with other marine mammals**

⊗⑦W56.31   **Bitten by other marine mammals**

⊗⑦W56.32   **Struck by other marine mammals**

⊗⑦W56.39   **Other contact with other marine mammals**

W56.4   **Contact with shark**

⊗⑦W56.41   **Bitten by shark**

⊗⑦W56.42   **Struck by shark**

⊗⑦W56.49   **Other contact with shark**

W56.5   **Contact with other fish**

⊗⑦W56.51   **Bitten by other fish**

⊗⑦W56.52   **Struck by other fish**

⊗⑦W56.59   **Other contact with other fish**

W56.8   **Contact with other nonvenomous marine animals**

⊗⑦W56.81   **Bitten by other nonvenomous marine animals**

⊗⑦W56.82   **Struck by other nonvenomous marine animals**

⊗⑦W56.89   **Other contact with other nonvenomous marine animals**

⊗⑦W57   **Bitten or stung by nonvenomous insect and other nonvenomous arthropods**

Excludes1: contact with venomous insects and arthropods (T63.2-, T63.3-, T63.4-)

The appropriate 7th character is to be added to code W57

A - initial encounter

D - subsequent encounter

S - sequela

W58   **Contact with crocodile or alligator**

The appropriate 7th character is to be added to each code from category W58

A - initial encounter

D - subsequent encounter

S - sequela

W58.0   **Contact with alligator**

⊗⑦W58.01   **Bitten by alligator**

⊗⑦W58.02   **Struck by alligator**

⊗⑦W58.03   **Crushed by alligator**

⊗⑦W58.09   **Other contact with alligator**

W58.1   **Contact with crocodile**

⊗⑦W58.11   **Bitten by crocodile**

⊗⑦W58.12   **Struck by crocodile**

⊗⑦W58.13   **Crushed by crocodile**

⊗⑦W58.19   **Other contact with crocodile**

W59   **Contact with other nonvenomous reptiles**

Excludes1: contact with venomous reptile (T63.0-, T63.1-)

The appropriate 7th character is to be added to each code from category W59

A - initial encounter

D - subsequent encounter

S - sequela

W59.0   **Contact with nonvenomous lizards**

⊗⑦W59.01   **Bitten by nonvenomous lizards**

⊗⑦W59.02   **Struck by nonvenomous lizards**

⊗⑦W59.09   **Other contact with nonvenomous lizards**

Exposure to nonvenomous lizards

W59.1   **Contact with nonvenomous snakes**

⊗⑦W59.11   **Bitten by nonvenomous snake**

⊗⑦W59.12   **Struck by nonvenomous snake**

⊗⑦W59.13   **Crushed by nonvenomous snake**

⊗⑦W59.19   **Other contact with nonvenomous snake**

W59.2   **Contact with turtles**

Excludes1: contact with tortoises (W59.8-)

⊗⑦W59.21   **Bitten by turtle**

⊗⑦W59.22   **Struck by turtle**

⊗⑦W59.29   **Other contact with turtle**

Exposure to turtles

W59.8   **Contact with other nonvenomous reptiles**

⊗⑦**W59.81** Bitten by other nonvenomous reptiles

⊗⑦**W59.82** Struck by other nonvenomous reptiles

⊗⑦**W59.83** Crushed by other nonvenomous reptiles

⊗⑦**W59.89** Other contact with other nonvenomous reptiles

⊗⑦**W60** **Contact with nonvenomous plant thorns and spines and sharp leaves**

Excludes1: Contact with venomous plants (T63.7-)

The appropriate 7th character is to be added to code W60

A - initial encounter

D - subsequent encounter

S - sequela

W61 **Contact with birds (domestic) (wild)**

Includes: contact with excreta of birds

The appropriate 7th character is to be added to each code from category W61

A - initial encounter

D - subsequent encounter

S - sequela

W61.0 Contact with parrot

⊗⑦**W61.01** Bitten by parrot

⊗⑦**W61.02** Struck by parrot

⊗⑦**W61.09** Other contact with parrot

Exposure to parrots

W61.1 Contact with macaw

⊗⑦**W61.11** Bitten by macaw

⊗⑦**W61.12** Struck by macaw

⊗⑦**W61.19** Other contact with macaw

Exposure to macaws

W61.2 Contact with other psittacines

⊗⑦**W61.21** Bitten by other psittacines

⊗⑦**W61.22** Struck by other psittacines

⊗⑦**W61.29** Other contact with other psittacines

Exposure to other psittacines

W61.3 Contact with chicken

⊗⑦**W61.32** Struck by chicken

⊗⑦**W61.33** Pecked by chicken

⊗⑦**W61.39** Other contact with chicken

Exposure to chickens

W61.4 Contact with turkey

⊗⑦**W61.42** Struck by turkey

⊗⑦**W61.43** Pecked by turkey

⊗⑦**W61.49** Other contact with turkey

W61.5 Contact with goose

⊗⑦**W61.51** Bitten by goose

⊗⑦**W61.52** Struck by goose

⊗⑦**W61.59** Other contact with goose

W61.6 Contact with duck

⊗⑦**W61.61** Bitten by duck

⊗⑦**W61.62** Struck by duck

⊗⑦**W61.69** Other contact with duck

W61.9 Contact with other birds

⊗⑦**W61.91** Bitten by other birds

⊗⑦**W61.92** Struck by other birds

⊗⑦**W61.99** Other contact with other birds

Contact with bird NOS

W62 **Contact with nonvenomous amphibians**

Excludes1: contact with venomous amphibians (T63.81-R63.83)

The appropriate 7th character is to be added to each code from category W62

A - initial encounter

D - subsequent encounter

S - sequela

⊗⑦**W62.0** **Contact with nonvenomous frogs**

⊗⑦**W62.1** **Contact with nonvenomous toads**

⊗⑦**W62.9** **Contact with other nonvenomous amphibians**

⊗⑦**W64** **Exposure to other animate mechanical forces**

Includes: exposure to nonvenomous animal NOS

Excludes1: contact with venomous animal (T63.-)

The appropriate 7th character is to be added to code W64

A - initial encounter

D - subsequent encounter

S - sequela

ACCIDENTAL NON-TRANSPORT DROWNING AND SUBMERSION (W65-W74)

Excludes1: accidental drowning and submersion due to fall into water (W16.-)

accidental drowning and submersion due to water transport accident (V90.-, V92.-)

Excludes2: accidental drowning and submersion due to cataclysm (X34-X39)

⊗⑦**W65** **Accidental drowning and submersion while in bath-tub**

Excludes1: accidental drowning and submersion due to fall in (into) bathtub (W16.211)

The appropriate 7th character is to be added to code W65

A - initial encounter

D - subsequent encounter

S – sequela

⊗⑦**W67** **Accidental drowning and submersion while in swimming-pool**

Excludes1: accidental drowning and submersion due to fall into swimming pool (W16.011, W16.021, W16.031)

accidental drowning and submersion due to striking into wall of swimming pool (W22.041)

The appropriate 7th character is to be added to code W67

A - initial encounter

D - subsequent encounter

S – sequela

⊗⑦**W69** **Accidental drowning and submersion while in natural water**

Accidental drowning and submersion while in lake

Accidental drowning and submersion while in open sea

Accidental drowning and submersion while in river

Accidental drowning and submersion while in stream

Excludes1: accidental drowning and submersion due to fall into natural body of water (W16.111, W16.121, W16.131)

The appropriate 7th character is to be added to code W69

A - initial encounter

D - subsequent encounter

S – sequela

⊗⑦**W73** **Other specified cause of accidental non-transport drowning and submersion**

Accidental drowning and submersion while in quenching tank

Accidental drowning and submersion while in reservoir

Excludes1: accidental drowning and submersion due to fall into other water (W16.311, W16.321, W16.331)

The appropriate 7th character is to be added to code W73

A - initial encounter

D - subsequent encounter

● New code ▲ Revised code Excludes1: Not coded here Excludes2: Not included here ⊗ Placeholder required ⑦7th digit required

S - sequela

⊗⑦**W74** **Unspecified cause of accidental drowning and submersion**

Drowning NOS

The appropriate 7th character is to be added to code W74

A - initial encounter

D - subsequent encounter

S - sequela

EXPOSURE TO ELECTRIC CURRENT, RADIATION AND EXTREME AMBIENT AIR TEMPERATURE AND PRESSURE (W85-W99)

Excludes1: exposure to:

failure in dosage of radiation or temperature during surgical and medical care (Y63.2-Y63.5)

lightning (T75.0-)

natural cold (X31)

natural heat (X30)

natural radiation NOS (X39)

radiological procedure and radiotherapy (Y84.2)

sunlight (X32)

⊗⑦**W85** **Exposure to electric transmission lines**

Broken power line

The appropriate 7th character is to be added to code W85

A - initial encounter

D - subsequent encounter

S - sequela

W86 **Exposure to other specified electric current**

The appropriate 7th character is to be added to each code from category W86

A - initial encounter

D - subsequent encounter

S - sequela

⊗⑦**W86.0** **Exposure to domestic wiring and appliances**

⊗⑦**W86.1** **Exposure to industrial wiring, appliances and electrical machinery**

Exposure to conductors

Exposure to control apparatus

Exposure to electrical equipment and machinery

Exposure to transformers

⊗⑦**W86.8** **Exposure to other electric current**

Exposure to wiring and appliances in or on farm (not farmhouse)

Exposure to wiring and appliances outdoors

Exposure to wiring and appliances in or on public building

Exposure to wiring and appliances in or on residential institutions

Exposure to wiring and appliances in or on schools

W88 **Exposure to ionizing radiation**

Excludes1: exposure to sunlight (X32)

The appropriate 7th character is to be added to each code from category W88

A - initial encounter

D - subsequent encounter

S - sequela

⊗⑦**W88.0** **Exposure to X-rays**

⊗⑦**W88.1** **Exposure to radioactive isotopes**

⊗⑦**W88.8** **Exposure to other ionizing radiation**

W89 **Exposure to man-made visible and ultraviolet light**

Includes: exposure to welding light (arc)

Excludes2: exposure to sunlight (X32)

The appropriate 7th character is to be added to each code from category W89

A - initial encounter

D - subsequent encounter

S - sequela

⊗⑦**W89.0** **Exposure to welding light (arc)**

⊗⑦**W89.1** **Exposure to tanning bed**

⊗⑦**W89.8** **Exposure to other man-made visible and ultraviolet light**

⊗⑦**W89.9** **Exposure to unspecified man-made visible and ultraviolet light**

W90 **Exposure to other nonionizing radiation**

Excludes2: exposure to sunlight (X32)

The appropriate 7th character is to be added to each code from category W90

A - initial encounter

D - subsequent encounter

S - sequela

⊗⑦**W90.0** **Exposure to radiofrequency**

⊗⑦**W90.1** **Exposure to infrared radiation**

⊗⑦**W90.2** **Exposure to laser radiation**

⊗⑦**W90.8** **Exposure to other nonionizing radiation**

⊗⑦**W92** **Exposure to excessive heat of man-made origin**

The appropriate 7th character is to be added to code W92

A - initial encounter

D - subsequent encounter

S - sequela

W93 **Exposure to excessive cold of man-made origin**

The appropriate 7th character is to be added to each code from category W93

A - initial encounter

D - subsequent encounter

S - sequela

W93.0 **Contact with or inhalation of dry ice**

⊗⑦**W93.01** **Contact with dry ice**

⊗⑦**W93.02** **Inhalation of dry ice**

W93.1 **Contact with or inhalation of liquid air**

⊗⑦**W93.11** **Contact with liquid air**

Contact with liquid hydrogen

Contact with liquid nitrogen

⊗⑦**W93.12** **Inhalation of liquid air**

Inhalation of liquid hydrogen

Inhalation of liquid nitrogen

⊗⑦**W93.2** **Prolonged exposure in deep freeze unit or refrigerator**

⊗⑦**W93.8** **Exposure to other excessive cold of man-made origin**

⊗⑦**W94** **Exposure to high and low air pressure and changes in air pressure**

The appropriate 7th character is to be added to each code from category W94

A - initial encounter

D - subsequent encounter

S - sequela

⊗⑦**W94.0** **Exposure to prolonged high air pressure**

W94.1 **Exposure to prolonged low air pressure**

⊗⑦**W94.11** **Exposure to residence or prolonged visit at high altitude**

⊗⑦**W94.12** **Exposure to other prolonged low air pressure**

W94.2 Exposure to rapid changes in air pressure during ascent

⊗⑦W94.21 Exposure to reduction in atmospheric pressure while surfacing from deep-water diving

⊗⑦W94.22 Exposure to reduction in atmospheric pressure while surfacing from underground

⊗⑦W94.23 Exposure to sudden change in air pressure in aircraft during ascent

⊗⑦W94.29 Exposure to other rapid changes in air pressure during ascent

W94.3 Exposure to rapid changes in air pressure during descent

⊗⑦W94.31 Exposure to sudden change in air pressure in aircraft during descent

⊗⑦W94.32 Exposure to high air pressure from rapid descent in water

⊗⑦W94.39 Exposure to other rapid changes in air pressure during descent

⊗⑦**W99   Exposure to other man-made environmental factors**

The appropriate 7th character is to be added to code W99

A - initial encounter

D - subsequent encounter

S - sequela

EXPOSURE TO SMOKE, FIRE AND FLAMES (X00-X08)

Excludes1: arson (X97)

Excludes2: explosions (W35-W40)

lightning (T75.0-)

transport accident (V01-V99)

X00   Exposure to uncontrolled fire in building or structure

Includes: conflagration in building or structure

Code first any associated cataclysm

Excludes2: Exposure to ignition or melting of nightwear (X05)

Exposure to ignition or melting of other clothing and apparel (X06.-)

Exposure to other specified smoke, fire and flames (X08.-)

The appropriate 7th character is to be added to each code from category X00

A - initial encounter

D - subsequent encounter

S - sequela

⊗⑦**X00.0   Exposure to flames in uncontrolled fire in building or structure**

⊗⑦**X00.1   Exposure to smoke in uncontrolled fire in building or structure**

⊗⑦**X00.2   Injury due to collapse of burning building or structure in uncontrolled fire**

Excludes1: injury due to collapse of building not on fire (W20.1)

⊗⑦**X00.3   Fall from burning building or structure in uncontrolled fire**

⊗⑦**X00.4   Hit by object from burning building or structure in uncontrolled fire**

⊗⑦**X00.5   Jump from burning building or structure in uncontrolled fire**

⊗⑦**X00.8   Other exposure to uncontrolled fire in building or structure**

X01   Exposure to uncontrolled fire, not in building or structure

Includes: exposure to forest fire

The appropriate 7th character is to be added to each code from category X01

A - initial encounter

D - subsequent encounter

S - sequela

⊗⑦**X01.0   Exposure to flames in uncontrolled fire, not in building or structure**

⊗⑦**X01.1   Exposure to smoke in uncontrolled fire, not in building or structure**

⊗⑦**X01.3   Fall due to uncontrolled fire, not in building or structure**

⊗⑦**X01.4   Hit by object due to uncontrolled fire, not in building or structure**

⊗⑦**X01.8   Other exposure to uncontrolled fire, not in building or structure**

X02   Exposure to controlled fire in building or structure

Includes: exposure to fire in fireplace

exposure to fire in stove

The appropriate 7th character is to be added to each code from category X02

A - initial encounter

D - subsequent encounter

S - sequela

⊗⑦**X02.0   Exposure to flames in controlled fire in building or structure**

⊗⑦**X02.1   Exposure to smoke in controlled fire in building or structure**

⊗⑦**X02.2   Injury due to collapse of burning building or structure in controlled fire**

Excludes1: injury due to collapse of building not on fire (W20.1)

⊗⑦**X02.3   Fall from burning building or structure in controlled fire**

⊗⑦**X02.4   Hit by object from burning building or structure in controlled fire**

⊗⑦**X02.5   Jump from burning building or structure in controlled fire**

⊗⑦**X02.8   Other exposure to controlled fire in building or structure**

X03   Exposure to controlled fire, not in building or structure

Includes: exposure to bon fire

exposure to camp-fire

exposure to trash fire

The appropriate 7th character is to be added to each code from category X03

A - initial encounter

D - subsequent encounter

S - sequela

⊗⑦**X03.0   Exposure to flames in controlled fire, not in building or structure**

⊗⑦**X03.1   Exposure to smoke in controlled fire, not in building or structure**

⊗⑦**X03.3   Fall due to controlled fire, not in building or structure**

⊗⑦**X03.4   Hit by object due to controlled fire, not in building or structure**

⊗⑦**X03.8   Other exposure to controlled fire, not in building or structure**

X04   Exposure to ignition of highly flammable material

Exposure to ignition of gasoline

Exposure to ignition of kerosene

Exposure to ignition of petrol

Excludes2: exposure to ignition or melting of nightwear (X05)

exposure to ignition or melting of other clothing and apparel (X06)

The appropriate 7th character is to be added to code X04

A - initial encounter

● New code   ▲ Revised code   **Excludes1:** Not coded here   **Excludes2:** Not included here   ⊗ Placeholder required   ⑦7th digit required

D - subsequent encounter

S - sequela

⊗⑦**X05** **Exposure to ignition or melting of nightwear**

Excludes2: exposure to uncontrolled fire in building or structure (X00.-)

exposure to uncontrolled fire, not in building or structure (X01.-)

exposure to controlled fire in building or structure (X02.-)

exposure to controlled fire, not in building or structure (X03.-)

exposure to ignition of highly flammable materials (X04.-)

The appropriate 7th character is to be added to code X05

A - initial encounter

D - subsequent encounter

S - sequela

X06 **Exposure to ignition or melting of other clothing and apparel**

Excludes2: exposure to uncontrolled fire in building or structure (X00.-)

exposure to uncontrolled fire, not in building or structure (X01.-)

exposure to controlled fire in building or structure (X02.-)

exposure to controlled fire, not in building or structure (X03.-)

exposure to ignition of highly flammable materials (X04.-)

The appropriate 7th character is to be added to each code from category X06

A - initial encounter

D - subsequent encounter

S - sequela

⊗⑦**X06.0** **Exposure to ignition of plastic jewelry**

⊗⑦**X06.1** **Exposure to melting of plastic jewelry**

⊗⑦**X06.2** **Exposure to ignition of other clothing and apparel**

⊗⑦**X06.3** **Exposure to melting of other clothing and apparel**

X08 **Exposure to other specified smoke, fire and flames**

The appropriate 7th character is to be added to each code from category X08

A - initial encounter

D - subsequent encounter

S - sequela

X08.0 **Exposure to bed fire**

Exposure to mattress fire

⊗⑦**X08.00** **Exposure to bed fire due to unspecified burning material**

⊗⑦**X08.01** **Exposure to bed fire due to burning cigarette**

⊗⑦**X08.09** **Exposure to bed fire due to other burning material**

X08.1 **Exposure to sofa fire**

⊗⑦**X08.10** **Exposure to sofa fire due to unspecified burning material**

⊗⑦**X08.11** **Exposure to sofa fire due to burning cigarette**

⊗⑦**X08.19** **Exposure to sofa fire due to other burning material**

X08.2 **Exposure to other furniture fire**

⊗⑦**X08.20** **Exposure to other furniture fire due to unspecified burning material**

⊗⑦**X08.21** **Exposure to other furniture fire due to burning cigarette**

⊗⑦**X08.29** **Exposure to other furniture fire due to other burning material**

⊗⑦**X08.8** **Exposure to other specified smoke, fire and flames**

CONTACT WITH HEAT AND HOT SUBSTANCES (X10-X19)

Excludes1: exposure to excessive natural heat (X30)

exposure to fire and flames (X00-X08)

X10 **Contact with hot drinks, food, fats and cooking oils**

The appropriate 7th character is to be added to each code from category X10

A - initial encounter

D - subsequent encounter

S - sequela

⊗⑦**X10.0** **Contact with hot drinks**

⊗⑦**X10.1** **Contact with hot food**

⊗⑦**X10.2** **Contact with fats and cooking oils**

X11 **Contact with hot tap-water**

Includes: contact with boiling tap-water

contact with boiling water NOS

Excludes1: contact with water heated on stove (X12)

The appropriate 7th character is to be added to each code from category X11

A - initial encounter

D - subsequent encounter

S - sequela

⊗⑦**X11.0** **Contact with hot water in bath or tub**

Excludes1: contact with running hot water in bath or tub (X11.1)

⊗⑦**X11.1** **Contact with running hot water**

Contact with hot water running out of hose

Contact with hot water running out of tap

⊗⑦**X11.8** **Contact with other hot tap-water**

Contact with hot water in bucket

Contact with hot tap-water NOS

⊗⑦**X12** **Contact with other hot fluids**

Contact with water heated on stove

Excludes1: hot (liquid) metals (X18)

The appropriate 7th character is to be added to code X12

A - initial encounter

D - subsequent encounter

S - sequela

X13 **Contact with steam and other hot vapors**

The appropriate 7th character is to be added to each code from category X13

A - initial encounter

D - subsequent encounter

S - sequela

⊗⑦**X13.0** **Inhalation of steam and other hot vapors**

⊗⑦**X13.1** **Other contact with steam and other hot vapors**

X14 **Contact with hot air and other hot gases**

The appropriate 7th character is to be added to each code from category X14

A - initial encounter

D - subsequent encounter

S - sequela

⊗⑦**X14.0** **Inhalation of hot air and gases**

⊗⑦**X14.1** **Other contact with hot air and other hot gases**

X15 **Contact with hot household appliances**

Excludes1: contact with heating appliances (X16)

contact with powered household appliances (W29.-)

exposure to controlled fire in building or structure due to household appliance (X02.8)

exposure to household appliances electrical current (W86.0)

The appropriate 7th character is to be added to each code from category X15

A - initial encounter

D - subsequent encounter

S - sequela

⊗⑦**X15.0** **Contact with hot stove (kitchen)**

⊗⑦**X15.1** **Contact with hot toaster**

⊗⑦**X15.2** **Contact with hotplate**

⊗⑦**X15.3** **Contact with hot saucepan or skillet**

⊗⑦**X15.8** **Contact with other hot household appliances**

Contact with cooker

Contact with kettle

Contact with light bulbs

⊗⑦**X16** **Contact with hot heating appliances, radiators and pipes**

Excludes1: contact with powered appliances (W29.-)

exposure to controlled fire in building or structure due to appliance (X02.8)

exposure to industrial appliances electrical current (W86.1)

The appropriate 7th character is to be added to code X16

A - initial encounter

D - subsequent encounter

S - sequela

⊗⑦**X17** **Contact with hot engines, machinery and tools**

Excludes1: contact with hot heating appliances, radiators and pipes (X16)

contact with hot household appliances (X15)

The appropriate 7th character is to be added to code X17

A - initial encounter

D - subsequent encounter

S - sequela

⊗⑦**X18** **Contact with other hot metals**

Contact with liquid metal

The appropriate 7th character is to be added to code X18

A - initial encounter

D - subsequent encounter

S - sequela

⊗⑦**X19** **Contact with other heat and hot substances**

Excludes1: objects that are not normally hot, e.g., an object made hot by a house fire (X00-X08)

The appropriate 7th character is to be added to code X19

A - initial encounter

D - subsequent encounter

S - sequela

EXPOSURE TO FORCES OF NATURE (X30-X39)

⊗⑦**X30** **Exposure to excessive natural heat**

Exposure to excessive heat as the cause of sunstroke

Exposure to heat NOS

Excludes1: excessive heat of man-made origin (W92)

exposure to man-made radiation (W89)

exposure to sunlight (X32)

exposure to tanning bed (W89)

The appropriate 7th character is to be added to code X30

A - initial encounter

D - subsequent encounter

S - sequela

⊗⑦**X31** **Exposure to excessive natural cold**

Excessive cold as the cause of chilblains NOS

Excessive cold as the cause of immersion foot or hand

Exposure to cold NOS

Exposure to weather conditions

Excludes1: cold of man-made origin (W93.-)

contact with or inhalation of dry ice (W93.-)

contact with or inhalation of liquefied gas (W93.-)

The appropriate 7th character is to be added to code X31

A - initial encounter

D - subsequent encounter

S - sequela

⊗⑦**X32** **Exposure to sunlight**

Excludes1: man-made radiation (tanning bed) (W89)

Excludes2: radiation-related disorders of the skin and subcutaneous tissue (L55-L59)

The appropriate 7th character is to be added to code X32

A - initial encounter

D - subsequent encounter

S – sequela

⊗⑦**X34** **Earthquake**

Excludes2: tidal wave (tsunami) due to earthquake (X37.41)

The appropriate 7th character is to be added to code X34

A - initial encounter

D - subsequent encounter

S – sequela

⊗⑦**X35** **Volcanic eruption**

Excludes2: tidal wave (tsunami) due to volcanic eruption (X37.41)

The appropriate 7th character is to be added to code X35

A - initial encounter

D - subsequent encounter

S - sequela

X36 **Avalanche, landslide and other earth movements**

Includes: victim of mudslide of cataclysmic nature

Excludes1: earthquake (X34)

Excludes2: transport accident involving collision with avalanche or landslide not in motion (V01-V99)

The appropriate 7th character is to be added to each code from category X36

A - initial encounter

D - subsequent encounter

S - sequela

⊗⑦**X36.0** **Collapse of dam or man-made structure causing earth movement**

⊗⑦**X36.1** **Avalanche, landslide, or mudslide**

X37 **Cataclysmic storm**

The appropriate 7th character is to be added to each code from category X37

A - initial encounter

D - subsequent encounter

S - sequela

⊗⑦**X37.0** **Hurricane**

Storm surge

Typhoon

● New code ▲ Revised code **Excludes1:** Not coded here **Excludes2:** Not included here ⊗ Placeholder required ⑦7th digit required

⊗⑦**X37.1** **Tornado**
Cyclone
Twister

⊗⑦**X37.2** **Blizzard (snow)(ice)**

⊗⑦**X37.3** **Dust storm**

X37.4 **Tidal wave**

⊗⑦**X37.41** **Tidal wave due to earthquake or volcanic eruption**
Tidal wave NOS
Tsunami

⊗⑦**X37.42** **Tidal wave due to storm**

⊗⑦**X37.43** **Tidal wave due to landslide**

⊗⑦**X37.8** **Other cataclysmic storms**
Cloudburst
Torrential rain

Excludes2: flood (X38)

⊗⑦**X37.9** **Unspecified cataclysmic storm**
Storm NOS

Excludes1: collapse of dam or man-made structure causing earth movement (X36.0)

⊗⑦**X38** **Flood**
Flood arising from remote storm
Flood of cataclysmic nature arising from melting snow
Flood resulting directly from storm

Excludes1: collapse of dam or man-made structure causing earth movement (X36.0)
tidal wave NOS (X37.2)
tidal wave caused by storm (X37.42)

The appropriate 7th character is to be added to code X38
A - initial encounter
D - subsequent encounter
S - sequela

X39 **Exposure to other forces of nature**
The appropriate 7th character is to be added to each code from category X39
A - initial encounter
D - subsequent encounter
S - sequela

⊗⑦**X39.0** **Exposure to natural radiation**

Excludes1: contact with and (suspected) exposure to radon and other naturally occurring radiation (Z77.123)
exposure to man-made radiation (W88-W90)
exposure to sunlight (X32)

⊗⑦**X39.01** **Exposure to radon**

⊗⑦**X39.08** **Exposure to other natural radiation**

⊗⑦**X39.8** **Other exposure to forces of nature**

OVEREXERTION AND STRENUOUS OR REPETITIVE MOVEMENTS (X50)

X50 **Overexertion and strenuous or repetitive movements**
The appropriate 7th character is to be added to each code from category X50
A - initial encounter
D - subsequent encounter
S - sequela

⊗⑦**X50.0** **Overexertion from strenuous movement or load**
Lifting heavy objects

Lifting weights

⊗⑦**X50.1** **Overexertion from prolonged static or awkward postures**
Prolonged bending
Prolonged kneeling
Prolonged reaching
Prolonged sitting
Prolonged standing
Prolonged twisting
Static bending
Static kneeling
Static reaching
Static sitting
Static standing
Static twisting

⊗⑦**X50.3** **Overexertion from repetitive movements**
Use of hand as hammer

Excludes2: Overuse from prolonged static or awkward postures (X50.1)

⊗⑦**X50.9** **Other and unspecified overexertion or strenuous movements or postures**
Contact pressure
Contact stress

ACCIDENTAL EXPOSURE TO OTHER SPECIFIED FACTORS (X52-X58)

⊗⑦**X52** **Prolonged stay in weightless environment**
Weightlessness in spacecraft (simulator)

The appropriate 7th character is to be added to code X52
A - initial encounter
D - subsequent encounter
S – sequela

⊗⑦**X58** **Exposure to other specified factors**
Accident NOS
Exposure NOS

The appropriate 7th character is to be added to code X58
A - initial encounter
D - subsequent encounter
S - sequela

INTENTIONAL SELF-HARM (X71-X83)

Purposely self-inflicted injury Suicide (attempted)

X71 **Intentional self-harm by drowning and submersion**
The appropriate 7th character is to be added to each code from category X71
A - initial encounter
D - subsequent encounter
S - sequela

⊗⑦**X71.0** **Intentional self-harm by drowning and submersion while in bathtub** [HCC]

⊗⑦**X71.1** **Intentional self-harm by drowning and submersion while in swimming pool** [HCC]

⊗⑦**X71.2** **Intentional self-harm by drowning and submersion after jump into swimming pool** [HCC]

⊗⑦**X71.3** **Intentional self-harm by drowning and submersion in natural water**

⊗⑦**X71.8** **Other intentional self-harm by drowning and submersion** [HCC]

⊗⑦**X71.9** **Intentional self-harm by drowning and submersion, unspecified** [HCC]

⊗⑦**X72** **Intentional self-harm by handgun discharge** [HCC]

Intentional self-harm by gun for single hand use

Intentional self-harm by pistol

Intentional self-harm by revolver

Excludes1: Very pistol (X74.8)

The appropriate 7th character is to be added to code X72

A - initial encounter

D - subsequent encounter

S - sequela

X73 **Intentional self-harm by rifle, shotgun and larger firearm discharge**

Excludes1: air gun (X74.01)

The appropriate 7th character is to be added to each code from category X73

A - initial encounter

D - subsequent encounter

S - sequela

⊗⑦**X73.0** **Intentional self-harm by shotgun discharge** [HCC]

⊗⑦**X73.1** **Intentional self-harm by hunting rifle discharge** [HCC]

⊗⑦**X73.2** **Intentional self-harm by machine gun discharge** [HCC]

⊗⑦**X73.8** **Intentional self-harm by other larger firearm discharge** [HCC]

⊗⑦**X73.9** **Intentional self-harm by unspecified larger firearm discharge** [HCC]

X74 **Intentional self-harm by other and unspecified firearm and gun discharge**

The appropriate 7th character is to be added to each code from category X74

A - initial encounter

D - subsequent encounter

S - sequela

X74.0 **Intentional self-harm by gas, air or spring-operated guns**

⊗⑦**X74.01** **Intentional self-harm by air gun** [HCC]

Intentional self-harm by BB gun discharge

Intentional self-harm by pellet gun discharge

⊗⑦**X74.02** **Intentional self-harm by paintball gun** [HCC]

⊗⑦**X74.09** **Intentional self-harm by other gas, air or spring-operated gun** [HCC]

⊗⑦**X74.8** **Intentional self-harm by other firearm discharge** [HCC]

Intentional self-harm by Very pistol [flare] discharge

⊗⑦**X74.9** **Intentional self-harm by unspecified firearm discharge** [HCC]

⊗⑦**X75** **Intentional self-harm by explosive material** [HCC]

The appropriate 7th character is to be added to code X75

A - initial encounter

D - subsequent encounter

S - sequela

⊗⑦**X76** **Intentional self-harm by smoke, fire and flames** [HCC]

The appropriate 7th character is to be added to code X76

A - initial encounter

D - subsequent encounter

S - sequela

X77 **Intentional self-harm by steam, hot vapors and hot objects**

The appropriate 7th character is to be added to each code from category X77

A - initial encounter

D - subsequent encounter

S - sequela

⊗⑦**X77.0** **Intentional self-harm by steam or hot vapors** [HCC]

⊗⑦**X77.1** **Intentional self-harm by hot tap water** [HCC]

⊗⑦**X77.2** **Intentional self-harm by other hot fluids** [HCC]

⊗⑦**X77.3** **Intentional self-harm by hot household appliances** [HCC]

⊗⑦**X77.8** **Intentional self-harm by other hot objects** [HCC]

⊗⑦**X77.9** **Intentional self-harm by unspecified hot objects** [HCC]

X78 **Intentional self-harm by sharp object**

The appropriate 7th character is to be added to each code from category X78

A - initial encounter

D - subsequent encounter

S - sequela

⊗⑦**X78.0** **Intentional self-harm by sharp glass** [HCC]

⊗⑦**X78.1** **Intentional self-harm by knife** [HCC]

⊗⑦**X78.2** **Intentional self-harm by sword or dagger** [HCC]

⊗⑦**X78.8** **Intentional self-harm by other sharp object** [HCC]

⊗⑦**X78.9** **Intentional self-harm by unspecified sharp object** [HCC]

⊗⑦**X79** **Intentional self-harm by blunt object** [HCC]

The appropriate 7th character is to be added to code X79

A - initial encounter

D - subsequent encounter

S – sequela

⊗⑦**X80** **Intentional self-harm by jumping from a high place** [HCC]

Intentional fall from one level to another

The appropriate 7th character is to be added to code X80

A - initial encounter

D - subsequent encounter

S - sequela

X81 **Intentional self-harm by jumping or lying in front of moving object**

The appropriate 7th character is to be added to each code from category X81

A - initial encounter

D - subsequent encounter

S - sequela

⊗⑦**X81.0** **Intentional self-harm by jumping or lying in front of motor vehicle** [HCC]

⊗⑦**X81.1** **Intentional self-harm by jumping or lying in front of (subway) train** [HCC]

⊗⑦**X81.8** **Intentional self-harm by jumping or lying in front of other moving object** [HCC]

X82 **Intentional self-harm by crashing of motor vehicle**

The appropriate 7th character is to be added to each code from category X82

A - initial encounter

D - subsequent encounter

S - sequela

⊗⑦**X82.0** **Intentional collision of motor vehicle with other motor vehicle** [HCC]

⊗⑦**X82.1** **Intentional collision of motor vehicle with train** [HCC]

⊗⑦**X82.2** **Intentional collision of motor vehicle with tree** [HCC]

⊗⑦**X82.8** **Other intentional self-harm by crashing of motor vehicle** [HCC]

X83 **Intentional self-harm by other specified means**

Excludes1: intentional self-harm by poisoning or contact with toxic substance- See Table of Drugs and Chemicals

The appropriate 7th character is to be added to each code from category X83

A - initial encounter

D - subsequent encounter

S - sequela

⊗⑦**X83.0 Intentional self-harm by crashing of aircraft** [HCC]

⊗⑦**X83.1 Intentional self-harm by electrocution** [HCC]

⊗⑦**X83.2 Intentional self-harm by exposure to extremes of cold** [HCC]

⊗⑦**X83.8 Intentional self-harm by other specified means** [HCC]

ASSAULT (X92-Y09)

Includes: homicide

injuries inflicted by another person with intent to injure or kill, by any means

Excludes1: injuries due to legal intervention (Y35.-)

injuries due to operations of war (Y36.-)

injuries due to terrorism (Y38.-)

X92 **Assault by drowning and submersion**

The appropriate 7th character is to be added to each code from category X92

A - initial encounter

D - subsequent encounter

S - sequela

⊗⑦**X92.0 Assault by drowning and submersion while in bathtub**

⊗⑦**X92.1 Assault by drowning and submersion while in swimming pool**

⊗⑦**X92.2 Assault by drowning and submersion after push into swimming pool**

⊗⑦**X92.3 Assault by drowning and submersion in natural water**

⊗⑦**X92.8 Other assault by drowning and submersion**

⊗⑦**X92.9 Assault by drowning and submersion, unspecified**

⊗⑦**X93 Assault by handgun discharge**

Assault by discharge of gun for single hand use

Assault by discharge of pistol

Assault by discharge of revolver

Excludes1: Very pistol (X95.8)

The appropriate 7th character is to be added to code X93

A - initial encounter

D - subsequent encounter

S - sequela

X94 **Assault by rifle, shotgun and larger firearm discharge**

Excludes1: air gun (X95.01)

The appropriate 7th character is to be added to each code from category X94

A - initial encounter

D - subsequent encounter

S - sequela

⊗⑦**X94.0 Assault by shotgun**

⊗⑦**X94.1 Assault by hunting rifle**

⊗⑦**X94.2 Assault by machine gun**

⊗⑦**X94.8 Assault by other larger firearm discharge**

⊗⑦**X94.9 Assault by unspecified larger firearm discharge**

X95 **Assault by other and unspecified firearm and gun discharge**

The appropriate 7th character is to be added to each code from category X95

A - initial encounter

D - subsequent encounter

S - sequela

X95.0 Assault by gas, air or spring-operated guns

⊗⑦**X95.01 Assault by air gun discharge**

Assault by BB gun discharge

Assault by pellet gun discharge

⊗⑦**X95.02 Assault by paintball gun discharge**

⊗⑦**X95.09 Assault by other gas, air or spring-operated gun**

⊗⑦**X95.8 Assault by other firearm discharge**

Assault by very pistol [flare] discharge

⊗⑦**X95.9 Assault by unspecified firearm discharge**

X96 **Assault by explosive material**

Excludes1: incendiary device (X97)

terrorism involving explosive material (Y38.2-)

The appropriate 7th character is to be added to each code from category X96

A - initial encounter

D - subsequent encounter

S - sequela

⊗⑦**X96.0 Assault by antipersonnel bomb**

Excludes1: antipersonnel bomb use in military or war (Y36.2-)

⊗⑦**X96.1 Assault by gasoline bomb**

⊗⑦**X96.2 Assault by letter bomb**

⊗⑦**X96.3 Assault by fertilizer bomb**

⊗⑦**X96.4 Assault by pipe bomb**

⊗⑦**X96.8 Assault by other specified explosive**

⊗⑦**X96.9 Assault by unspecified explosive**

⊗⑦**X97 Assault by smoke, fire and flames**

Assault by arson

Assault by cigarettes

Assault by incendiary device

The appropriate 7th character is to be added to code X97

A - initial encounter

D - subsequent encounter

S - sequela

X98 **Assault by steam, hot vapors and hot objects**

The appropriate 7th character is to be added to each code from category X98

A - initial encounter

D - subsequent encounter

S - sequela

⊗⑦**X98.0 Assault by steam or hot vapors**

⊗⑦**X98.1 Assault by hot tap water**

⊗⑦**X98.2 Assault by hot fluids**

⊗⑦**X98.3 Assault by hot household appliances**

⊗⑦**X98.8 Assault by other hot objects**

⊗⑦**X98.9 Assault by unspecified hot objects**

X99 **Assault by sharp object**

Excludes1: assault by strike by sports equipment (Y08.0-)

The appropriate 7th character is to be added to each code from category X99

A - initial encounter

D - subsequent encounter

S - sequela

⊗⑦**X99.0 Assault by sharp glass**

⊗⑦**X99.1 Assault by knife**

⊗⑦**X99.2 Assault by sword or dagger**

⊗⑦**X99.8 Assault by other sharp object**

⊗⑦**X99.9 Assault by unspecified sharp object**
　　Assault by stabbing NOS

⊗⑦**Y00 Assault by blunt object**

　Excludes1: assault by strike by sports equipment (Y08.0-)

　The appropriate 7th character is to be added to code Y00

　A - initial encounter

　D - subsequent encounter

　S - sequela

⊗⑦**Y01 Assault by pushing from high place**

　The appropriate 7th character is to be added to code Y01

　A - initial encounter

　D - subsequent encounter

　S - sequela

Y02 Assault by pushing or placing victim in front of moving object

　The appropriate 7th character is to be added to each code from category Y02

　A - initial encounter

　D - subsequent encounter

　S - sequela

⊗⑦**Y02.0 Assault by pushing or placing victim in front of motor vehicle**

⊗⑦**Y02.1 Assault by pushing or placing victim in front of (subway) train**

⊗⑦**Y02.8 Assault by pushing or placing victim in front of other moving object**

Y03 Assault by crashing of motor vehicle

　The appropriate 7th character is to be added to each code from category Y03

　A - initial encounter

　D - subsequent encounter

　S - sequela

⊗⑦**Y03.0 Assault by being hit or run over by motor vehicle**

⊗⑦**Y03.8 Other assault by crashing of motor vehicle**

Y04 Assault by bodily force

　Excludes1: assault by:

　　submersion (X92.-)

　　use of weapon (X93-X95, X99, Y00)

　The appropriate 7th character is to be added to each code from category Y04

　A - initial encounter

　D - subsequent encounter

　S - sequela

⊗⑦**Y04.0 Assault by unarmed brawl or fight**

⊗⑦**Y04.1 Assault by human bite**

⊗⑦**Y04.2 Assault by strike against or bumped into by another person**

⊗⑦**Y04.8 Assault by other bodily force**

　Assault by bodily force NOS

Y07 Perpetrator of assault, maltreatment and neglect

　Note: Codes from this category are for use only in cases of confirmed abuse (T74.-)

　Selection of the correct perpetrator code is based on the relationship between the perpetrator and the victim

　Includes: perpetrator of abandonment

　perpetrator of emotional neglect perpetrator of mental cruelty

　perpetrator of physical abuse perpetrator of physical neglect

　perpetrator of sexual abuse perpetrator of torture

　Y07.0 Spouse or partner, perpetrator of maltreatment and neglect

Spouse or partner, perpetrator of maltreatment and neglect against spouse or partner

　Y07.01 Husband, perpetrator of maltreatment and neglect

　Y07.02 Wife, perpetrator of maltreatment and neglect

　Y07.03 Male partner, perpetrator of maltreatment and neglect

　Y07.04 Female partner, perpetrator of maltreatment and neglect

Y07.1 Parent (adoptive) (biological), perpetrator of maltreatment and neglect

　Y07.11 Biological father, perpetrator of maltreatment and neglect

　Y07.12 Biological mother, perpetrator of maltreatment and neglect

　Y07.13 Adoptive father, perpetrator of maltreatment and neglect

　Y07.14 Adoptive mother, perpetrator of maltreatment and neglect

Y07.4 Other family member, perpetrator of maltreatment and neglect

　Y07.41 Sibling, perpetrator of maltreatment and neglect

　　Excludes1: stepsibling, perpetrator of maltreatment and neglect (Y07.435, Y07.436)

　　Y07.410 Brother, perpetrator of maltreatment and neglect

　　Y07.411 Sister, perpetrator of maltreatment and neglect

　Y07.42 Foster parent, perpetrator of maltreatment and neglect

　　Y07.420 Foster father, perpetrator of maltreatment and neglect

　　Y07.421 Foster mother, perpetrator of maltreatment and neglect

　Y07.43 Stepparent or stepsibling, perpetrator of maltreatment and neglect

　　Y07.430 Stepfather, perpetrator of maltreatment and neglect

　　Y07.432 Male friend of parent (co-residing in household), perpetrator of maltreatment and neglect

　　Y07.433 Stepmother, perpetrator of maltreatment and neglect

　　Y07.434 Female friend of parent (co-residing in household), perpetrator of maltreatment and neglect

　　Y07.435 Stepbrother, perpetrator or maltreatment and neglect

　　Y07.436 Stepsister, perpetrator of maltreatment and neglect

　Y07.49 Other family member, perpetrator of maltreatment and neglect

　　Y07.490 Male cousin, perpetrator of maltreatment and neglect

　　Y07.491 Female cousin, perpetrator of maltreatment and neglect

　　Y07.499 Other family member, perpetrator of maltreatment and neglect

Y07.5 Non-family member, perpetrator of maltreatment and neglect

　Y07.50 Unspecified non-family member, perpetrator of maltreatment and neglect

Y07.51 **Daycare provider, perpetrator of maltreatment and neglect**

    Y07.510 **At-home childcare provider, perpetrator of maltreatment and neglect**

    Y07.511 **Daycare center childcare provider, perpetrator of maltreatment and neglect**

    Y07.512 **At-home adult care provider, perpetrator of maltreatment and neglect**

    Y07.513 **Adult care center provider, perpetrator of maltreatment and neglect**

    Y07.519 **Unspecified daycare provider, perpetrator of maltreatment and neglect**

Y07.52 **Healthcare provider, perpetrator of maltreatment and neglect**

    Y07.521 **Mental health provider, perpetrator of maltreatment and neglect**

    Y07.528 **Other therapist or healthcare provider, perpetrator of maltreatment and neglect**

    Nurse perpetrator of maltreatment and neglect

    Occupational therapist perpetrator of maltreatment and neglect

    Physical therapist perpetrator of maltreatment and neglect

    Speech therapist perpetrator of maltreatment and neglect

    Y07.529 **Unspecified healthcare provider, perpetrator of maltreatment and neglect**

Y07.53 **Teacher or instructor, perpetrator of maltreatment and neglect**

    Coach, perpetrator of maltreatment and neglect

Y07.59 **Other non-family member, perpetrator of maltreatment and neglect**

Y07.6 **Multiple perpetrators of maltreatment and neglect**

Y07.9 **Unspecified perpetrator of maltreatment and neglect**

Y08 **Assault by other specified means**

The appropriate 7th character is to be added to each code from category Y08

A - initial encounter

D - subsequent encounter

S - sequela

Y08.0 **Assault by strike by sport equipment**

    ⊗⑦Y08.01 **Assault by strike by hockey stick**

    ⊗⑦Y08.02 **Assault by strike by baseball bat**

    ⊗⑦Y08.09 **Assault by strike by other specified type of sport equipment**

Y08.8 **Assault by other specified means**

    ⊗⑦Y08.81 **Assault by crashing of aircraft**

    ⊗⑦Y08.89 **Assault by other specified means**

Y09 **Assault by unspecified means**

Assassination (attempted) NOS

Homicide (attempted) NOS

Manslaughter (attempted) NOS

Murder (attempted) NOS

EVENT OF UNDETERMINED INTENT (Y21-Y33)

Undetermined intent is only for use when there is specific documentation in the record that the intent of the injury cannot be determined. If no such documentation is present, code to accidental (unintentional)

Y21 **Drowning and submersion, undetermined intent**

The appropriate 7th character is to be added to each code from category Y21

A - initial encounter

D - subsequent encounter

S - sequela

    ⊗⑦Y21.0 **Drowning and submersion while in bathtub, undetermined intent**

    ⊗⑦Y21.1 **Drowning and submersion after fall into bathtub, undetermined intent**

    ⊗⑦Y21.2 **Drowning and submersion while in swimming pool, undetermined intent**

    ⊗⑦Y21.3 **Drowning and submersion after fall into swimming pool, undetermined intent**

    ⊗⑦Y21.4 **Drowning and submersion in natural water, undetermined intent**

    ⊗⑦Y21.8 **Other drowning and submersion, undetermined intent**

    ⊗⑦Y21.9 **Unspecified drowning and submersion, undetermined intent**

⊗⑦Y22 **Handgun discharge, undetermined intent**

Discharge of gun for single hand use, undetermined intent

Discharge of pistol, undetermined intent

Discharge of revolver, undetermined intent

Excludes2: very pistol (Y24.8)

The appropriate 7th character is to be added to code Y22

A - initial encounter

D - subsequent encounter

S - sequela

Y23 **Rifle, shotgun and larger firearm discharge, undetermined intent**

Excludes2: air gun (Y24.0)

The appropriate 7th character is to be added to each code from category Y23

A - initial encounter

D - subsequent encounter

S - sequela

    ⊗⑦Y23.0 **Shotgun discharge, undetermined intent**

    ⊗⑦Y23.1 **Hunting rifle discharge, undetermined intent**

    ⊗⑦Y23.2 **Military firearm discharge, undetermined intent**

    ⊗⑦Y23.3 **Machine gun discharge, undetermined intent**

    ⊗⑦Y23.8 **Other larger firearm discharge, undetermined intent**

    ⊗⑦Y23.9 **Unspecified larger firearm discharge, undetermined intent**

Y24 **Other and unspecified firearm discharge, undetermined intent**

The appropriate 7th character is to be added to each code from category Y24

A - initial encounter

D - subsequent encounter

S - sequela

    ⊗⑦Y24.0 **Air gun discharge, undetermined intent**

    BB gun discharge, undetermined intent

    Pellet gun discharge, undetermined intent

    ⊗⑦Y24.8 **Other firearm discharge, undetermined intent**

    Paintball gun discharge, undetermined intent

    Very pistol [flare] discharge, undetermined intent

    ⊗⑦Y24.9 **Unspecified firearm discharge, undetermined intent**

⊗⑦**Y25** Contact with explosive material, undetermined intent

The appropriate 7th character is to be added to code Y25

A - initial encounter

D - subsequent encounter

S - sequela

⊗⑦**Y26** Exposure to smoke, fire and flames, undetermined intent

The appropriate 7th character is to be added to code Y26

A - initial encounter

D - subsequent encounter

S - sequela

Y27 Contact with steam, hot vapors and hot objects, undetermined intent

The appropriate 7th character is to be added to each code from category Y27

A - initial encounter

D - subsequent encounter

S - sequela

⊗⑦**Y27.0** Contact with steam and hot vapors, undetermined intent

⊗⑦**Y27.1** Contact with hot tap water, undetermined intent

⊗⑦**Y27.2** Contact with hot fluids, undetermined intent

⊗⑦**Y27.3** Contact with hot household appliance, undetermined intent

⊗⑦**Y27.8** Contact with other hot objects, undetermined intent

⊗⑦**Y27.9** Contact with unspecified hot objects, undetermined intent

Y28 Contact with sharp object, undetermined intent

The appropriate 7th character is to be added to each code from category Y28

A - initial encounter

D - subsequent encounter

S - sequela

⊗⑦**Y28.0** Contact with sharp glass, undetermined intent

⊗⑦**Y28.1** Contact with knife, undetermined intent

⊗⑦**Y28.2** Contact with sword or dagger, undetermined intent

⊗⑦**Y28.8** Contact with other sharp object, undetermined intent

⊗⑦**Y28.9** Contact with unspecified sharp object, undetermined intent

⊗⑦**Y29** Contact with blunt object, undetermined intent

The appropriate 7th character is to be added to code Y29

A - initial encounter

D - subsequent encounter

S - sequela

⊗⑦**Y30** Falling, jumping or pushed from a high place, undetermined intent

Victim falling from one level to another, undetermined intent

The appropriate 7th character is to be added to code Y30

A - initial encounter

D - subsequent encounter

S - sequela

⊗⑦**Y31** Falling, lying or running before or into moving object, undetermined intent

The appropriate 7th character is to be added to code Y31

A - initial encounter

D - subsequent encounter

S - sequela

⊗⑦**Y32** Crashing of motor vehicle, undetermined intent

The appropriate 7th character is to be added to code Y32

A - initial encounter

D - subsequent encounter

S - sequela

⊗⑦**Y33** Other specified events, undetermined intent

The appropriate 7th character is to be added to code Y33

A - initial encounter

D - subsequent encounter

S - sequela

LEGAL INTERVENTION, OPERATIONS OF WAR, MILITARY OPERATIONS, AND TERRORISM (Y35-Y38)

Y35 Legal intervention

Includes: any injury sustained as a result of an encounter with any law enforcement official, serving in any capacity at the time of the encounter, whether on-duty or off-duty

Includes: injury to law enforcement official, suspect and bystander

The appropriate 7th character is to be added to each code from category Y35

A - initial encounter

D - subsequent encounter

S - sequela

Y35.0 Legal intervention involving firearm discharge

Y35.00 Legal intervention involving unspecified firearm discharge

Legal intervention involving gunshot wound

Legal intervention involving shot NOS

⑦**Y35.001** Legal intervention involving unspecified firearm discharge, law enforcement official injured

⑦**Y35.002** Legal intervention involving unspecified firearm discharge, bystander injured

⑦**Y35.003** Legal intervention involving unspecified firearm discharge, suspect injured

⑦**Y35.009** Legal intervention involving unspecified firearm discharge, unspecified person injured

Y35.01 Legal intervention involving injury by machine gun

⑦**Y35.011** Legal intervention involving injury by machine gun, law enforcement official injured

⑦**Y35.012** Legal intervention involving injury by machine gun, bystander injured

⑦**Y35.013** Legal intervention involving injury by machine gun, suspect injured

⑦**Y35.019** Legal intervention involving injury by machine gun, unspecified person injured

Y35.02 Legal intervention involving injury by handgun

⑦**Y35.021** Legal intervention involving injury by handgun, law enforcement official injured

⑦**Y35.022** Legal intervention involving injury by handgun, bystander injured

⑦**Y35.023** Legal intervention involving injury by handgun, suspect

⑦**Y35.029** Legal intervention involving injury by handgun, unspecified person injured

Y35.03 Legal intervention involving injury by rifle pellet

⑦**Y35.031** Legal intervention involving injury by rifle pellet, law enforcement official injured

⑦**Y35.032** Legal intervention involving injury by rifle pellet, bystander injured

⑦**Y35.033** Legal intervention involving injury by rifle pellet, suspect injured

⑦**Y35.039** Legal intervention involving injury by rifle pellet, unspecified person injured

Y35.04 Legal intervention involving injury by rubber bullet

⑦**Y35.041** Legal intervention involving injury by rubber bullet, law enforcement official injured

⑦**Y35.042** Legal intervention involving injury by rubber bullet, bystander injured

⑦**Y35.043** Legal intervention involving injury by rubber bullet, suspect injured

⑦**Y35.049** Legal intervention involving injury by rubber bullet, unspecified person injured

Y35.09 Legal intervention involving other firearm discharge

⑦**Y35.091** Legal intervention involving other firearm discharge, law enforcement official injured

⑦**Y35.092** Legal intervention involving other firearm discharge, bystander injured

⑦**Y35.093** Legal intervention involving other firearm discharge, suspect injured

⑦**Y35.099** Legal intervention involving other firearm discharge, unspecified person injured

Y35.1 Legal intervention involving explosives

Y35.10 Legal intervention involving unspecified explosives

⑦**Y35.101** Legal intervention involving unspecified explosives, law enforcement official injured

⑦**Y35.102** Legal intervention involving unspecified explosives, bystander injured

⑦**Y35.103** Legal intervention involving unspecified explosives, suspect injured

⑦**Y35.109** Legal intervention involving unspecified explosives, unspecified person injured

Y35.11 Legal intervention involving injury by dynamite

⑦**Y35.111** Legal intervention involving injury by dynamite, law enforcement official injured

⑦**Y35.112** Legal intervention involving injury by dynamite, bystander injured

⑦**Y35.113** Legal intervention involving injury by dynamite, suspect injured

⑦**Y35.119** Legal intervention involving injury by dynamite, unspecified person injured

Y35.12 Legal intervention involving injury by explosive shell

⑦**Y35.121** Legal intervention involving injury by explosive shell, law enforcement official injured

⑦**Y35.122** Legal intervention involving injury by explosive shell, bystander injured

⑦**Y35.123** Legal intervention involving injury by explosive shell, suspect injured

⑦**Y35.129** Legal intervention involving injury by explosive shell, unspecified person injured

Y35.19 Legal intervention involving other explosives

Legal intervention involving injury by grenade
Legal intervention involving injury by mortar bomb

⑦**Y35.191** Legal intervention involving other explosives, law enforcement official injured

⑦**Y35.192** Legal intervention involving other explosives, bystander injured

⑦**Y35.193** Legal intervention involving other explosives, suspect injured

⑦**Y35.199** Legal intervention involving other explosives, unspecified person injured

Y35.2 Legal intervention involving gas

Legal intervention involving asphyxiation by gas
Legal intervention involving poisoning by gas

Y35.20 Legal intervention involving unspecified gas

⑦**Y35.201** Legal intervention involving unspecified gas, law enforcement official injured

⑦**Y35.202** Legal intervention involving unspecified gas, bystander injured

⑦**Y35.203** Legal intervention involving unspecified gas, suspect injured

⑦**Y35.209** Legal intervention involving unspecified gas, unspecified person injured

Y35.21 Legal intervention involving injury by tear gas

⑦**Y35.211** Legal intervention involving injury by tear gas, law enforcement official injured

⑦**Y35.212** Legal intervention involving injury by tear gas, bystander injured

⑦**Y35.213** Legal intervention involving injury by tear gas, suspect injured

⑦**Y35.219** Legal intervention involving injury by tear gas, unspecified person injured

Y35.29 Legal intervention involving other gas

⑦**Y35.291** Legal intervention involving other gas, law enforcement official injured

⑦**Y35.292** Legal intervention involving other gas, bystander injured

⑦**Y35.293** Legal intervention involving other gas, suspect injured

⑦**Y35.299** Legal intervention involving other gas, unspecified person injured

Y35.3 Legal intervention involving blunt objects

Legal intervention involving being hit or struck by blunt object

Y35.30 Legal intervention involving unspecified blunt objects

⑦**Y35.301** Legal intervention involving unspecified blunt objects, law enforcement official injured

⑦**Y35.302** Legal intervention involving unspecified blunt objects, bystander injured

⑦**Y35.303** Legal intervention involving unspecified blunt objects, suspect injured

⑦**Y35.309** Legal intervention involving unspecified blunt objects, unspecified person injured

Y35.31 Legal intervention involving baton

⑦**Y35.311** Legal intervention involving baton, law enforcement official injured

⑦**Y35.312** Legal intervention involving baton, bystander injured

⑦**Y35.313** Legal intervention involving baton, suspect injured

⑦**Y35.319** Legal intervention involving baton, unspecified person injured

Y35.39 Legal intervention involving other blunt objects

⑦**Y35.391** Legal intervention involving other blunt objects, law enforcement official injured

⑦**Y35.392** Legal intervention involving other blunt objects, bystander injured

⑦**Y35.393** Legal intervention involving other blunt objects, suspect injured

⑦**Y35.399** Legal intervention involving other blunt objects, unspecified person injured

Y35.4 Legal intervention involving sharp objects

Legal intervention involving being cut by sharp objects

Legal intervention involving being stabbed by sharp objects

Y35.40 Legal intervention involving unspecified sharp objects

⑦**Y35.401** Legal intervention involving unspecified sharp objects, law enforcement official injured

⑦**Y35.402** Legal intervention involving unspecified sharp objects, bystander injured

⑦**Y35.403** Legal intervention involving unspecified sharp objects, suspect injured

⑦**Y35.409** Legal intervention involving unspecified sharp objects, unspecified person injured

Y35.41 Legal intervention involving bayonet

⑦**Y35.411** Legal intervention involving bayonet, law enforcement official injured

⑦**Y35.412** Legal intervention involving bayonet, bystander injured

⑦**Y35.413** Legal intervention involving bayonet, suspect injured

⑦**Y35.419** Legal intervention involving bayonet, unspecified person injured

Y35.49 Legal intervention involving other sharp objects

⑦**Y35.491** Legal intervention involving other sharp objects, law enforcement official injured

⑦**Y35.492** Legal intervention involving other sharp objects, bystander injured

⑦**Y35.493** Legal intervention involving other sharp objects, suspect injured

⑦**Y35.499** Legal intervention involving other sharp objects, unspecified person injured

Y35.8 Legal intervention involving other specified means

Y35.81 Legal intervention involving manhandling

⑦**Y35.811** Legal intervention involving manhandling, law enforcement official injured

⑦**Y35.812** Legal intervention involving manhandling, bystander injured

⑦**Y35.813** Legal intervention involving manhandling, suspect injured

⑦**Y35.819** Legal intervention involving manhandling, unspecified person injured

Y35.83 Legal intervention involving a conducted energy device

Electroshock device (taser)

Stun gun

⑦**Y35.831** Legal intervention involving a conducted energy device, law enforcement official injured

⑦**Y35.832** Legal intervention involving a conducted energy device, bystander injured

⑦**Y35.833** Legal intervention involving a conducted energy device, suspect injured

⑦**Y35.839** Legal intervention involving a conducted energy device, unspecified person injured

Y35.89 Legal intervention involving other specified means

⑦**Y35.891** Legal intervention involving other specified means, law enforcement official injured

⑦**Y35.892** Legal intervention involving other specified means, bystander injured

⑦**Y35.893** Legal intervention involving other specified means, suspect injured

●⑦**Y35.899** Legal intervention involving other specified means, unspecified person injured

Y35.9 Legal intervention, means unspecified

⊗⑦**Y35.91** Legal intervention, means unspecified, law enforcement official injured

⊗⑦**Y35.92** Legal intervention, means unspecified, bystander injured

⊗⑦**Y35.93** Legal intervention, means unspecified, suspect injured

⊗⑦**Y35.99** Legal intervention, means unspecified, unspecified person injured

Y36 **Operations of war**

Includes: injuries to military personnel and civilians caused by war, civil insurrection, and peacekeeping missions

Excludes1: injury to military personnel occurring during peacetime military operations (Y37.-)

military vehicles involved in transport accidents with non-military vehicle during peacetime (V09.01, V09.21, V19.81, V29.81, V39.81, V49.81, V59.81, V69.81, V79.81)

The appropriate 7th character is to be added to each code from category Y36

A - initial encounter

D - subsequent encounter

S - sequela

Y36.0 **War operations involving explosion of marine weapons**

  Y36.00 **War operations involving explosion of unspecified marine weapon**

  War operations involving underwater blast NOS

  ⑦**Y36.000** **War operations involving explosion of unspecified marine weapon, military personnel**

  ⑦**Y36.001** **War operations involving explosion of unspecified marine weapon, civilian**

  Y36.01 **War operations involving explosion of depth-charge**

  ⑦**Y36.010** **War operations involving explosion of depth-charge, military personnel**

  ⑦**Y36.011** **War operations involving explosion of depth-charge, civilian**

  Y36.02 **War operations involving explosion of marine mine**

  War operations involving explosion of marine mine, at sea or in harbor

  ⑦**Y36.020** **War operations involving explosion of marine mine, military personnel**

  ⑦**Y36.021** **War operations involving explosion of marine mine, civilian**

  Y36.03 **War operations involving explosion of sea-based artillery shell**

  ⑦**Y36.030** **War operations involving explosion of sea-based artillery shell, military personnel**

  ⑦**Y36.031** **War operations involving explosion of sea-based artillery shell, civilian**

  Y36.04 **War operations involving explosion of torpedo**

  ⑦**Y36.040** **War operations involving explosion of torpedo, military personnel**

  ⑦**Y36.041** **War operations involving explosion of torpedo, civilian**

  Y36.05 **War operations involving accidental detonation of onboard marine weapons**

  ⑦**Y36.050** **War operations involving accidental detonation of onboard marine weapons, military personnel**

  ⑦**Y36.051** **War operations involving accidental detonation of onboard marine weapons, civilian**

  Y36.09 **War operations involving explosion of other marine weapons**

  ⑦**Y36.090** **War operations involving explosion of other marine weapons, military personnel**

  ⑦**Y36.091** **War operations involving explosion of other marine weapons, civilian**

Y36.1 **War operations involving destruction of aircraft**

  Y36.10 **War operations involving unspecified destruction of aircraft**

  ⑦**Y36.100** **War operations involving unspecified destruction of aircraft, military personnel**

  ⑦**Y36.101** **War operations involving unspecified destruction of aircraft, civilian**

  Y36.11 **War operations involving destruction of aircraft due to enemy fire or explosives**

  War operations involving destruction of aircraft due to air to air missile

  War operations involving destruction of aircraft due to explosive placed on aircraft

  War operations involving destruction of aircraft due to rocket propelled grenade [RPG]

  War operations involving destruction of aircraft due to small arms fire

  War operations involving destruction of aircraft due to surface to air missile

  ⑦**Y36.110** **War operations involving destruction of aircraft due to enemy fire or explosives, military personnel**

  ⑦**Y36.111** **War operations involving destruction of aircraft due to enemy fire or explosives, civilian**

  Y36.12 **War operations involving destruction of aircraft due to collision with other aircraft**

  ⑦**Y36.120** **War operations involving destruction of aircraft due to collision with other aircraft, military personnel**

  ⑦**Y36.121** **War operations involving destruction of aircraft due to collision with other aircraft, civilian**

  Y36.13 **War operations involving destruction of aircraft due to onboard fire**

  ⑦**Y36.130** **War operations involving destruction of aircraft due to onboard fire, military personnel**

  ⑦**Y36.131** **War operations involving destruction of aircraft due to onboard fire, civilian**

  Y36.14 **War operations involving destruction of aircraft due to accidental detonation of onboard munitions and explosives**

  ⑦**Y36.140** **War operations involving destruction of aircraft due to accidental detonation of onboard munitions and explosives, military personnel**

  ⑦**Y36.141** **War operations involving destruction of aircraft due to accidental detonation of onboard munitions and explosives, civilian**

  Y36.19 **War operations involving other destruction of aircraft**

  ⑦**Y36.190** **War operations involving other destruction of aircraft, military personnel**

  ⑦**Y36.191** **War operations involving other destruction of aircraft, civilian**

Y36.2 **War operations involving other explosions and fragments**

  Excludes1: war operations involving explosion of aircraft (Y36.1-)

  war operations involving explosion of marine weapons (Y36.0-)

  war operations involving explosion of nuclear weapons (Y36.5-)

  war operations involving explosion occurring after cessation of hostilities (Y36.8-)

  Y36.20 **War operations involving unspecified explosion and fragments**

  War operations involving air blast NOS

  War operations involving blast NOS

  War operations involving blast fragments NOS

War operations involving blast wave NOS

War operations involving blast wind NOS

War operations involving explosion NOS

War operations involving explosion of bomb NOS

⑦**Y36.200** **War operations involving unspecified explosion and fragments, military personnel**

⑦**Y36.201** **War operations involving unspecified explosion and fragments, civilian**

Y36.21 **War operations involving explosion of aerial bomb**

⑦**Y36.210** **War operations involving explosion of aerial bomb, military personnel**

⑦**Y36.211** **War operations involving explosion of aerial bomb, civilian**

Y36.22 **War operations involving explosion of guided missile**

⑦**Y36.220** **War operations involving explosion of guided missile, military personnel**

⑦**Y36.221** **War operations involving explosion of guided missile, civilian**

Y36.23 **War operations involving explosion of improvised explosive device [IED]**

War operations involving explosion of person-borne improvised explosive device [IED]

War operations involving explosion of vehicle-borne improvised explosive device [IED]

War operations involving explosion of roadside improvised explosive device [IED]

⑦**Y36.230** **War operations involving explosion of improvised explosive device [IED], military personnel**

⑦**Y36.231** **War operations involving explosion of improvised explosive device [IED], civilian**

Y36.24 **War operations involving explosion due to accidental detonation and discharge of own munitions or munitions launch device**

⑦**Y36.240** **War operations involving explosion due to accidental detonation and discharge of own munitions or munitions launch device, military personnel**

⑦**Y36.241** **War operations involving explosion due to accidental detonation and discharge of own munitions or munitions launch device, civilian**

Y36.25 **War operations involving fragments from munitions**

⑦**Y36.250** **War operations involving fragments from munitions, military personnel**

⑦**Y36.251** **War operations involving fragments from munitions, civilian**

Y36.26 **War operations involving fragments of improvised explosive device [IED]**

War operations involving fragments of person-borne improvised explosive device [IED]

War operations involving fragments of vehicle-borne improvised explosive device [IED]

War operations involving fragments of roadside improvised explosive device [IED]

⑦**Y36.260** **War operations involving fragments of improvised explosive device [IED], military personnel**

⑦**Y36.261** **War operations involving fragments of improvised explosive device [IED], civilian**

Y36.27 **War operations involving fragments from weapons**

⑦**Y36.270** **War operations involving fragments from weapons, military personnel**

⑦**Y36.271** **War operations involving fragments from weapons, civilian**

Y36.29 **War operations involving other explosions and fragments**

War operations involving explosion of grenade

War operations involving explosions of land mine

War operations involving shrapnel NOS

⑦**Y36.290** **War operations involving other explosions and fragments, military personnel**

⑦**Y36.291** **War operations involving other explosions and fragments, civilian**

Y36.3 **War operations involving fires, conflagrations and hot substances**

War operations involving smoke, fumes, and heat from fires, conflagrations and hot substances

Excludes1: war operations involving fires and conflagrations aboard military aircraft (Y36.1-)

war operations involving fires and conflagrations aboard military watercraft (Y36.0-)

war operations involving fires and conflagrations caused indirectly by conventional weapons (Y36.2-)

war operations involving fires and thermal effects of nuclear weapons (Y36.53-)

Y36.30 **War operations involving unspecified fire, conflagration and hot substance**

⑦**Y36.300** **War operations involving unspecified fire, conflagration and hot substance, military personnel**

⑦**Y36.301** **War operations involving unspecified fire, conflagration and hot substance, civilian**

Y36.31 **War operations involving gasoline bomb**

War operations involving incendiary bomb

War operations involving petrol bomb

⑦**Y36.310** **War operations involving gasoline bomb, military personnel**

⑦**Y36.311** **War operations involving gasoline bomb, civilian**

Y36.32 **War operations involving incendiary bullet**

⑦**Y36.320** **War operations involving incendiary bullet, military personnel**

⑦**Y36.321** **War operations involving incendiary bullet, civilian**

Y36.33 **War operations involving flamethrower**

⑦**Y36.330** **War operations involving flamethrower, military personnel**

⑦**Y36.331** **War operations involving flamethrower, civilian**

Y36.39 **War operations involving other fires, conflagrations and hot substances**

⑦**Y36.390** **War operations involving other fires, conflagrations and hot substances, military personnel**

⑦**Y36.391** **War operations involving other fires, conflagrations and hot substances, civilian**

Y36.4   War operations involving firearm discharge and other forms of conventional warfare

    Y36.41   War operations involving rubber bullets

       ⑦Y36.410   War operations involving rubber bullets, military personnel

       ⑦Y36.411   War operations involving rubber bullets, civilian

    Y36.42   War operations involving firearms pellets

       ⑦Y36.420   War operations involving firearms pellets, military personnel

       ⑦Y36.421   War operations involving firearms pellets, civilian

    Y36.43   War operations involving other firearms discharge

       War operations involving bullets NOS

       Excludes1: war operations involving munitions fragments (Y36.25-)

             war operations involving incendiary bullets (Y36.32-)

       ⑦Y36.430   War operations involving other firearms discharge, military personnel

       ⑦Y36.431   War operations involving other firearms discharge, civilian

    Y36.44   War operations involving unarmed hand to hand combat

       Excludes1: war operations involving combat using blunt or piercing object (Y36.45-)

             war operations involving intentional restriction of air and airway (Y36.46-)

             war operations involving unintentional restriction of air and airway (Y36.47-)

       ⑦Y36.440   War operations involving unarmed hand to hand combat, military personnel

       ⑦Y36.441   War operations involving unarmed hand to hand combat, civilian

    Y36.45   War operations involving combat using blunt or piercing object

       ⑦Y36.450   War operations involving combat using blunt or piercing object, military personnel

       ⑦Y36.451   War operations involving combat using blunt or piercing object, civilian

    Y36.46   War operations involving intentional restriction of air and airway

       ⑦Y36.460   War operations involving intentional restriction of air and airway, military personnel

       ⑦Y36.461   War operations involving intentional restriction of air and airway, civilian

    Y36.47   War operations involving unintentional restriction of air and airway

       ⑦Y36.470   War operations involving unintentional restriction of air and airway, military personnel

       ⑦Y36.471   War operations involving unintentional restriction of air and airway, civilian

    Y36.49   War operations involving other forms of conventional warfare

       ⑦Y36.490   War operations involving other forms of conventional warfare, military personnel

       ⑦Y36.491   War operations involving other forms of conventional warfare, civilian

Y36.5   War operations involving nuclear weapons

    War operations involving dirty bomb NOS

    Y36.50   War operations involving unspecified effect of nuclear weapon

       ⑦Y36.500   War operations involving unspecified effect of nuclear weapon, military personnel

       ⑦Y36.501   War operations involving unspecified effect of nuclear weapon, civilian

    Y36.51   War operations involving direct blast effect of nuclear weapon

       War operations involving blast pressure of nuclear weapon

       ⑦Y36.510   War operations involving direct blast effect of nuclear weapon, military personnel

       ⑦Y36.511   War operations involving direct blast effect of nuclear weapon, civilian

    Y36.52   War operations involving indirect blast effect of nuclear weapon

       War operations involving being thrown by blast of nuclear weapon

       War operations involving being struck or crushed by blast debris of nuclear weapon

       ⑦Y36.520   War operations involving indirect blast effect of nuclear weapon, military personnel

       ⑦Y36.521   War operations involving indirect blast effect of nuclear weapon, civilian

    Y36.53   War operations involving thermal radiation effect of nuclear weapon

       War operations involving direct heat from nuclear weapon

       War operation involving fireball effects from nuclear weapon

       ⑦Y36.530   War operations involving thermal radiation effect of nuclear weapon, military personnel

       ⑦Y36.531   War operations involving thermal radiation effect of nuclear weapon, civilian

    Y36.54   War operation involving nuclear radiation effects of nuclear weapon

       War operation involving acute radiation exposure from nuclear weapon

       War operation involving exposure to immediate ionizing radiation from nuclear weapon

       War operation involving fallout exposure from nuclear weapon

       War operation involving secondary effects of nuclear weapons

       ⑦Y36.540   War operation involving nuclear radiation effects of nuclear weapon, military personnel

       ⑦Y36.541   War operation involving nuclear radiation effects of nuclear weapon, civilian

    Y36.59   War operation involving other effects of nuclear weapons

---

⑦**Y36.590**   War operation involving other effects of nuclear weapons, military personnel

⑦**Y36.591**   War operation involving other effects of nuclear weapons, civilian

Y36.6   War operations involving biological weapons

     Y36.6X War operations involving biological weapons

⑦**Y36.6X0**   War operations involving biological weapons, military personnel

⑦**Y36.6X1**   War operations involving biological weapons, civilian

Y36.7   War operations involving chemical weapons and other forms of unconventional warfare

     Excludes1: war operations involving incendiary devices (Y36.3-, Y36.5-)

     Y36.7X War operations involving chemical weapons and other forms of unconventional warfare

⑦**Y36.7X0**   War operations involving chemical weapons and other forms of unconventional warfare, military personnel

⑦**Y36.7X1**   War operations involving chemical weapons and other forms of unconventional warfare, civilian

Y36.8   War operations occurring after cessation of hostilities

War operations classifiable to categories Y36.0-Y36.8 but occurring after cessation of hostilities

     Y36.81   Explosion of mine placed during war operations but exploding after cessation of hostilities

⑦**Y36.810**   Explosion of mine placed during war operations but exploding after cessation of hostilities, military personnel

⑦**Y36.811**   Explosion of mine placed during war operations but exploding after cessation of hostilities, civilian

     Y36.82   Explosion of bomb placed during war operations but exploding after cessation of hostilities

⑦**Y36.820**   Explosion of bomb placed during war operations but exploding after cessation of hostilities, military personnel

⑦**Y36.821**   Explosion of bomb placed during war operations but exploding after cessation of hostilities, civilian

     Y36.88   Other war operations occurring after cessation of hostilities

⑦**Y36.880**   Other war operations occurring after cessation of hostilities, military personnel

⑦**Y36.881**   Other war operations occurring after cessation of hostilities, civilian

     Y36.89   Unspecified war operations occurring after cessation of hostilities

⑦**Y36.890**   Unspecified war operations occurring after cessation of hostilities, military personnel

⑦**Y36.891**   Unspecified war operations occurring after cessation of hostilities, civilian

Y36.9   Other and unspecified war operations

   ⊗⑦**Y36.90**   War operations, unspecified

   ⊗⑦**Y36.91**   War operations involving unspecified weapon of mass destruction [WMD]

   ⊗⑦**Y36.92**   War operations involving friendly fire

Y37   **Military operations**

Includes: injuries to military personnel and civilians occurring during peacetime on military property and during routine military exercises and operations

Excludes1: military aircraft involved in aircraft accident with civilian aircraft (V97.81-)

     military vehicles involved in transport accident with civilian vehicle (V09.01, V09.21, V19.81, V29.81, V39.81, V49.81, V59.81, V69.81, V79.81)

     military watercraft involved in water transport accident with civilian watercraft (V94.81-) war operations (Y36.-)

The appropriate 7th character is to be added to each code from category Y37

A - initial encounter

D - subsequent encounter

S - sequela

Y37.0   Military operations involving explosion of marine weapons

     Y37.00   Military operations involving explosion of unspecified marine weapon

Military operations involving underwater blast NOS

⑦**Y37.000**   Military operations involving explosion of unspecified marine weapon, military personnel

⑦**Y37.001**   Military operations involving explosion of unspecified marine weapon, civilian

     Y37.01   Military operations involving explosion of depth-charge

⑦**Y37.010**   Military operations involving explosion of depth-charge, military personnel

⑦**Y37.011**   Military operations involving explosion of depth-charge, civilian

     Y37.02   Military operations involving explosion of marine mine

Military operations involving explosion of marine mine, at sea or in harbor

⑦**Y37.020**   Military operations involving explosion of marine mine, military personnel

⑦**Y37.021**   Military operations involving explosion of marine mine, civilian

     Y37.03   Military operations involving explosion of sea-based artillery shell

⑦**Y37.030**   Military operations involving explosion of sea-based artillery shell, military personnel

⑦**Y37.031**   Military operations involving explosion of sea-based artillery shell, civilian

     Y37.04   Military operations involving explosion of torpedo

⑦**Y37.040**   Military operations involving explosion of torpedo, military personnel

⑦**Y37.041**   Military operations involving explosion of torpedo, civilian

     Y37.05   Military operations involving accidental detonation of onboard marine weapons

⑦**Y37.050**   Military operations involving accidental detonation of onboard marine weapons, military personnel

⑦Y37.051　**Military operations involving accidental detonation of onboard marine weapons, civilian**

Y37.09　Military operations involving explosion of other marine weapons

⑦**Y37.090**　**Military operations involving explosion of other marine weapons, military personnel**

⑦**Y37.091**　**Military operations involving explosion of other marine weapons, civilian**

Y37.1　Military operations involving destruction of aircraft

Y37.10　Military operations involving unspecified destruction of aircraft

⑦**Y37.100**　**Military operations involving unspecified destruction of aircraft, military personnel**

⑦**Y37.101**　**Military operations involving unspecified destruction of aircraft, civilian**

Y37.11　Military operations involving destruction of aircraft due to enemy fire or explosives

Military operations involving destruction of aircraft due to air to air missile

Military operations involving destruction of aircraft due to explosive placed on aircraft

Military operations involving destruction of aircraft due to rocket propelled grenade [RPG]

Military operations involving destruction of aircraft due to small arms fire

Military operations involving destruction of aircraft due to surface to air missile

⑦**Y37.110**　**Military operations involving destruction of aircraft due to enemy fire or explosives, military personnel**

⑦**Y37.111**　**Military operations involving destruction of aircraft due to enemy fire or explosives, civilian**

Y37.12　Military operations involving destruction of aircraft due to collision with other aircraft

⑦**Y37.120**　**Military operations involving destruction of aircraft due to collision with other aircraft, military personnel**

⑦**Y37.121**　**Military operations involving destruction of aircraft due to collision with other aircraft, civilian**

Y37.13　Military operations involving destruction of aircraft due to onboard fire

⑦**Y37.130**　**Military operations involving destruction of aircraft due to onboard fire, military personnel**

⑦**Y37.131**　**Military operations involving destruction of aircraft due to onboard fire, civilian**

Y37.14　Military operations involving destruction of aircraft due to accidental detonation of onboard munitions and explosives

⑦**Y37.140**　**Military operations involving destruction of aircraft due to accidental detonation of onboard munitions and explosives, military personnel**

⑦**Y37.141**　**Military operations involving destruction of aircraft due to accidental detonation of onboard munitions and explosives, civilian**

Y37.19　Military operations involving other destruction of aircraft

⑦**Y37.190**　**Military operations involving other destruction of aircraft, military personnel**

⑦**Y37.191**　**Military operations involving other destruction of aircraft, civilian**

Y37.2　Military operations involving other explosions and fragments

Excludes1: military operations involving explosion of aircraft (Y37.1-)

military operations involving explosion of marine weapons (Y37.0-)

military operations involving explosion of nuclear weapons (Y37.5-)

Y37.20　Military operations involving unspecified explosion and fragments

Military operations involving air blast NOS

Military operations involving blast NOS

Military operations involving blast fragments NOS

Military operations involving blast wave NOS

Military operations involving blast wind NOS

Military operations involving explosion NOS

Military operations involving explosion of bomb NOS

⑦**Y37.200**　**Military operations involving unspecified explosion and fragments, military personnel**

⑦**Y37.201**　**Military operations involving unspecified explosion and fragments, civilian**

Y37.21　Military operations involving explosion of aerial bomb

⑦**Y37.210**　**Military operations involving explosion of aerial bomb, military personnel**

⑦**Y37.211**　**Military operations involving explosion of aerial bomb, civilian**

Y37.22　Military operations involving explosion of guided missile

⑦**Y37.220**　**Military operations involving explosion of guided missile, military personnel**

⑦**Y37.221**　**Military operations involving explosion of guided missile, civilian**

Y37.23　Military operations involving explosion of improvised explosive device [IED]

Military operations involving explosion of person-borne improvised explosive device [IED]

Military operations involving explosion of vehicle-borne improvised explosive device [IED]

Military operations involving explosion of roadside improvised explosive device [IED]

⑦**Y37.230**　**Military operations involving explosion of improvised explosive device [IED], military personnel**

⑦**Y37.231**　**Military operations involving explosion of improvised explosive device [IED], civilian**

Y37.24　Military operations involving explosion due to accidental detonation and discharge of own munitions or munitions launch device

⑦**Y37.240**　**Military operations involving explosion due to accidental detonation and discharge of own** munitions or munitions launch device, military personnel

⑦**Y37.241** **Military operations involving explosion due to accidental detonation and discharge of own munitions or munitions launch device, civilian**

Y37.25 **Military operations involving fragments from munitions**

⑦**Y37.250** **Military operations involving fragments from munitions, military personnel**

⑦**Y37.251** **Military operations involving fragments from munitions, civilian**

Y37.26 **Military operations involving fragments of improvised explosive device [IED]**

Military operations involving fragments of person-borne improvised explosive device [IED]

Military operations involving fragments of vehicle-borne improvised explosive device [IED]

Military operations involving fragments of roadside improvised explosive device [IED]

⑦**Y37.260** **Military operations involving fragments of improvised explosive device [IED], military personnel**

⑦**Y37.261** **Military operations involving fragments of improvised explosive device [IED], civilian**

Y37.27 **Military operations involving fragments from weapons**

⑦**Y37.270** **Military operations involving fragments from weapons, military personnel**

⑦**Y37.271** **Military operations involving fragments from weapons, civilian**

Y37.29 **Military operations involving other explosions and fragments**

Military operations involving explosion of grenade

Military operations involving explosions of land mine

Military operations involving shrapnel NOS

⑦**Y37.290** **Military operations involving other explosions and fragments, military personnel**

⑦**Y37.291** **Military operations involving other explosions and fragments, civilian**

Y37.3 **Military operations involving fires, conflagrations and hot substances**

Military operations involving smoke, fumes, and heat from fires, conflagrations and hot substances

Excludes1: military operations involving fires and conflagrations aboard military aircraft (Y37.1-)

military operations involving fires and conflagrations aboard military watercraft (Y37.0-)

military operations involving fires and conflagrations caused indirectly by conventional weapons (Y37.2-)

military operations involving fires and thermal effects of nuclear weapons (Y36.53-)

Y37.30 **Military operations involving unspecified fire, conflagration and hot substance**

⑦**Y37.300** **Military operations involving unspecified fire, conflagration and hot substance, military personnel**

⑦**Y37.301** **Military operations involving unspecified fire, conflagration and hot substance, civilian**

Y37.31 **Military operations involving gasoline bomb**

Military operations involving incendiary bomb

Military operations involving petrol bomb

⑦**Y37.310** **Military operations involving gasoline bomb, military personnel**

⑦**Y37.311** **Military operations involving gasoline bomb, civilian**

Y37.32 **Military operations involving incendiary bullet**

⑦**Y37.320** **Military operations involving incendiary bullet, military personnel**

⑦**Y37.321** **Military operations involving incendiary bullet, civilian**

Y37.33 **Military operations involving flamethrower**

⑦**Y37.330** **Military operations involving flamethrower, military personnel**

⑦**Y37.331** **Military operations involving flamethrower, civilian**

Y37.39 **Military operations involving other fires, conflagrations and hot substances**

⑦**Y37.390** **Military operations involving other fires, conflagrations and hot substances, military personnel**

⑦**Y37.391** **Military operations involving other fires, conflagrations and hot substances, civilian**

Y37.4 **Military operations involving firearm discharge and other forms of conventional warfare**

Y37.41 **Military operations involving rubber bullets**

⑦**Y37.410** **Military operations involving rubber bullets, military personnel**

⑦**Y37.411** **Military operations involving rubber bullets, civilian**

Y37.42 **Military operations involving firearms pellets**

⑦**Y37.420** **Military operations involving firearms pellets, military personnel**

⑦**Y37.421** **Military operations involving firearms pellets, civilian**

Y37.43 **Military operations involving other firearms discharge**

Military operations involving bullets NOS

Excludes1: military operations involving munitions fragments (Y37.25-)

military operations involving incendiary bullets (Y37.32-)

⑦**Y37.430** **Military operations involving other firearms discharge, military personnel**

⑦**Y37.431** **Military operations involving other firearms discharge, civilian**

Y37.44 **Military operations involving unarmed hand to hand combat**

Excludes1: military operations involving combat using blunt or piercing object (Y37.45-)

military operations involving intentional restriction of air and airway (Y37.46-)

military operations involving unintentional restriction of air and airway (Y37.47-)

⑦Y37.440 **Military operations involving unarmed hand to hand combat, military personnel**

⑦Y37.441 **Military operations involving unarmed hand to hand combat, civilian**

Y37.45 **Military operations involving combat using blunt or piercing object**

⑦Y37.450 **Military operations involving combat using blunt or piercing object, military personnel**

⑦Y37.451 **Military operations involving combat using blunt or piercing object, civilian**

Y37.46 **Military operations involving intentional restriction of air and airway**

⑦Y37.460 **Military operations involving intentional restriction of air and airway, military personnel**

⑦Y37.461 **Military operations involving intentional restriction of air and airway, civilian**

Y37.47 **Military operations involving unintentional restriction of air and airway**

⑦Y37.470 **Military operations involving unintentional restriction of air and airway, military personnel**

⑦Y37.471 **Military operations involving unintentional restriction of air and airway, civilian**

Y37.49 **Military operations involving other forms of conventional warfare**

⑦Y37.490 **Military operations involving other forms of conventional warfare, military personnel**

⑦Y37.491 **Military operations involving other forms of conventional warfare, civilian**

Y37.5 **Military operations involving nuclear weapons**

Military operation involving dirty bomb NOS

Y37.50 **Military operations involving unspecified effect of nuclear weapon**

⑦Y37.500 **Military operations involving unspecified effect of nuclear weapon, military personnel**

⑦Y37.501 **Military operations involving unspecified effect of nuclear weapon, civilian**

Y37.51 **Military operations involving direct blast effect of nuclear weapon**

Military operations involving blast pressure of nuclear weapon

⑦Y37.510 **Military operations involving direct blast effect of nuclear weapon, military personnel**

⑦Y37.511 **Military operations involving direct blast effect of nuclear weapon, civilian**

Y37.52 **Military operations involving indirect blast effect of nuclear weapon**

Military operations involving being thrown by blast of nuclear weapon

Military operations involving being struck or crushed by blast debris of nuclear weapon

⑦Y37.520 **Military operations involving indirect blast effect of nuclear weapon, military personnel**

⑦Y37.521 **Military operations involving indirect blast effect of nuclear weapon, civilian**

Y37.53 **Military operations involving thermal radiation effect of nuclear weapon**

Military operations involving direct heat from nuclear weapon

Military operation involving fireball effects from nuclear weapon

⑦Y37.530 **Military operations involving thermal radiation effect of nuclear weapon, military personnel**

⑦Y37.531 **Military operations involving thermal radiation effect of nuclear weapon, civilian**

Y37.54 **Military operation involving nuclear radiation effects of nuclear weapon**

Military operation involving acute radiation exposure from nuclear weapon

Military operation involving exposure to immediate ionizing radiation from nuclear weapon

Military operation involving fallout exposure from nuclear weapon

Military operation involving secondary effects of nuclear weapons

⑦Y37.540 **Military operation involving nuclear radiation effects of nuclear weapon, military personnel**

⑦Y37.541 **Military operation involving nuclear radiation effects of nuclear weapon, civilian**

Y37.59 **Military operation involving other effects of nuclear weapons**

⑦Y37.590 **Military operation involving other effects of nuclear weapons, military personnel**

⑦Y37.591 **Military operation involving other effects of nuclear weapons, civilian**

Y37.6 **Military operations involving biological weapons**

Y37.6X **Military operations involving biological weapons**

⑦Y37.6X0 **Military operations involving biological weapons, military personnel**

⑦Y37.6X1 **Military operations involving biological weapons, civilian**

Y37.7 **Military operations involving chemical weapons and other forms of unconventional warfare**

Excludes1: military operations involving incendiary devices (Y36.3-, Y36.5-)

Y37.7X **Military operations involving chemical weapons and other forms of unconventional warfare**

⑦Y37.7X0 **Military operations involving chemical weapons and other forms of unconventional warfare, military personnel**

⑦Y37.7X1 **Military operations involving chemical weapons and other forms of unconventional warfare, civilian**

Y37.9 **Other and unspecified military operations**

⊗⑦Y37.90 **Military operations, unspecified**

⊗⑦**Y37.91** **Military operations involving unspecified weapon of mass destruction [WMD]**

⊗⑦**Y37.92** **Military operations involving friendly fire**

Y38 **Terrorism**

These codes are for use to identify injuries resulting from the unlawful use of force or violence against persons or property to intimidate or coerce a Government, the civilian population, or any segment thereof, in furtherance of political or social objective

<u>Use Additional Code</u> for place of occurrence (Y92.-)

The appropriate 7th character is to be added to each code from category Y38

A - initial encounter

D - subsequent encounter

S - sequela

Y38.0 **Terrorism involving explosion of marine weapons**

Terrorism involving depth-charge

Terrorism involving marine mine

Terrorism involving mine NOS, at sea or in harbor

Terrorism involving sea-based artillery shell

Terrorism involving torpedo

Terrorism involving underwater blast

Y38.0X **Terrorism involving explosion of marine weapons**

⑦**Y38.0X1** **Terrorism involving explosion of marine weapons, public safety official injured**

⑦**Y38.0X2** **Terrorism involving explosion of marine weapons, civilian injured**

⑦**Y38.0X3** **Terrorism involving explosion of marine weapons, terrorist injured**

Y38.1 **Terrorism involving destruction of aircraft**

Terrorism involving aircraft burned

Terrorism involving aircraft exploded

Terrorism involving aircraft being shot down

Terrorism involving aircraft used as a weapon

Y38.1X **Terrorism involving destruction of aircraft**

⑦**Y38.1X1** **Terrorism involving destruction of aircraft, public safety official injured**

⑦**Y38.1X2** **Terrorism involving destruction of aircraft, civilian injured**

⑦**Y38.1X3** **Terrorism involving destruction of aircraft, terrorist injured**

Y38.2 **Terrorism involving other explosions and fragments**

Terrorism involving antipersonnel (fragments) bomb

Terrorism involving blast NOS

Terrorism involving explosion NOS

Terrorism involving explosion of breech block

Terrorism involving explosion of cannon block

Terrorism involving explosion (fragments) of artillery shell

Terrorism involving explosion (fragments) of bomb

Terrorism involving explosion (fragments) of grenade

Terrorism involving explosion (fragments) of guided missile

Terrorism involving explosion (fragments) of land mine

Terrorism involving explosion of mortar bomb

Terrorism involving explosion of munitions

Terrorism involving explosion (fragments) of rocket

Terrorism involving explosion (fragments) of shell

Terrorism involving shrapnel

Terrorism involving mine NOS, on land

Excludes1: terrorism involving explosion of nuclear weapon (Y38.5)

terrorism involving suicide bomber (Y38.81)

Y38.2X **Terrorism involving other explosions and fragments**

⑦**Y38.2X1** **Terrorism involving other explosions and fragments, public safety official injured**

⑦**Y38.2X2** **Terrorism involving other explosions and fragments, civilian injured**

⑦**Y38.2X3** **Terrorism involving other explosions and fragments, terrorist injured**

Y38.3 **Terrorism involving fires, conflagration and hot substances**

Terrorism involving conflagration NOS

Terrorism involving fire NOS

Terrorism involving petrol bomb

Excludes1: terrorism involving fire or heat of nuclear weapon (Y38.5)

Y38.3X **Terrorism involving fires, conflagration and hot substances**

⑦**Y38.3X1** **Terrorism involving fires, conflagration and hot substances, public safety official injured**

⑦**Y38.3X2** **Terrorism involving fires, conflagration and hot substances, civilian injured**

⑦**Y38.3X3** **Terrorism involving fires, conflagration and hot substances, terrorist injured**

Y38.4 **Terrorism involving firearms**

Terrorism involving carbine bullet

Terrorism involving machine gun bullet

Terrorism involving pellets (shotgun)

Terrorism involving pistol bullet

Terrorism involving rifle bullet

Terrorism involving rubber (rifle) bullet

Y38.4X **Terrorism involving firearms**

⑦**Y38.4X1** **Terrorism involving firearms, public safety official injured**

⑦**Y38.4X2** **Terrorism involving firearms, civilian injured**

⑦**Y38.4X3** **Terrorism involving firearms, terrorist injured**

Y38.5 **Terrorism involving nuclear weapons**

Terrorism involving blast effects of nuclear weapon

Terrorism involving exposure to ionizing radiation from nuclear weapon

Terrorism involving fireball effect of nuclear weapon

Terrorism involving heat from nuclear weapon

Y38.5X **Terrorism involving nuclear weapons**

⑦**Y38.5X1** **Terrorism involving nuclear weapons, public safety official injured**

⑦**Y38.5X2** **Terrorism involving nuclear weapons, civilian injured**

⑦**Y38.5X3** **Terrorism involving nuclear weapons, terrorist injured**

Y38.6 **Terrorism involving biological weapons**

Terrorism involving anthrax

Terrorism involving cholera

Terrorism involving smallpox

● New code ▲ Revised code **Excludes1:** Not coded here **Excludes2:** Not included here ⊗ Placeholder required ⑦ 7th digit required

Y38.6X **Terrorism involving biological weapons**

⑦Y38.6X1 **Terrorism involving biological weapons, public safety official injured**

⑦Y38.6X2 **Terrorism involving biological weapons, civilian injured**

⑦Y38.6X3 **Terrorism involving biological weapons, terrorist injured**

Y38.7 **Terrorism involving chemical weapons**

Terrorism involving gases, fumes, chemicals

Terrorism involving hydrogen cyanide

Terrorism involving phosgene

Terrorism involving sarin

Y38.7X **Terrorism involving chemical weapons**

⑦Y38.7X1 **Terrorism involving chemical weapons, public safety official injured**

⑦Y38.7X2 **Terrorism involving chemical weapons, civilian injured**

⑦Y38.7X3 **Terrorism involving chemical weapons, terrorist injured**

Y38.8 **Terrorism involving other and unspecified means**

⊗⑦Y38.80 **Terrorism involving unspecified means**

Terrorism NOS

Y38.81 **Terrorism involving suicide bomber**

⑦Y38.811 **Terrorism involving suicide bomber, public safety official injured**

⑦Y38.812 **Terrorism involving suicide bomber, civilian injured**

Y38.89 **Terrorism involving other means**

Terrorism involving drowning and submersion

Terrorism involving lasers

Terrorism involving piercing or stabbing instruments

⑦Y38.891 **Terrorism involving other means, public safety official injured**

⑦Y38.892 **Terrorism involving other means, civilian injured**

⑦Y38.893 **Terrorism involving other means, terrorist injured**

Y38.9 **Terrorism, secondary effects**

Note: This code is for use to identify conditions occurring subsequent to a terrorist attack not those that are due to the initial terrorist attack

Y38.9X **Terrorism, secondary effects**

⑦Y38.9X1 **Terrorism, secondary effects, public safety official injured**

⑦Y38.9X2 **Terrorism, secondary effects, civilian injured**

COMPLICATIONS OF MEDICAL AND SURGICAL CARE (Y62-Y84)

Includes: complications of medical devices

surgical and medical procedures as the cause of abnormal reaction of the patient, or of later complication, without mention of misadventure at the time of the procedure

MISADVENTURES TO PATIENTS DURING SURGICAL AND MEDICAL CARE (Y62-Y69)

Excludes1: surgical and medical procedures as the cause of abnormal reaction of the patient, without mention of misadventure at the time of the procedure (Y83-Y84)

Excludes2: breakdown or malfunctioning of medical device (during procedure) (after implantation) (ongoing use) (Y70-Y82)

Y62 **Failure of sterile precautions during surgical and medical care**

Y62.0 **Failure of sterile precautions during surgical operation**

Y62.1 **Failure of sterile precautions during infusion or transfusion**

Y62.2 **Failure of sterile precautions during kidney dialysis and other perfusion** [HCC]

Y62.3 **Failure of sterile precautions during injection or immunization**

Y62.4 **Failure of sterile precautions during endoscopic examination**

Y62.5 **Failure of sterile precautions during heart catheterization**

Y62.6 **Failure of sterile precautions during aspiration, puncture and other catheterization**

Y62.8 **Failure of sterile precautions during other surgical and medical care**

Y62.9 **Failure of sterile precautions during unspecified surgical and medical care**

Y63 **Failure in dosage during surgical and medical care**

Excludes2: accidental overdose of drug or wrong drug given in error (T36-T50)

Y63.0 **Excessive amount of blood or other fluid given during transfusion or infusion**

Y63.1 **Incorrect dilution of fluid used during infusion**

Y63.2 **Overdose of radiation given during therapy**

Y63.3 **Inadvertent exposure of patient to radiation during medical care**

Y63.4 **Failure in dosage in electroshock or insulin-shock therapy**

Y63.5 **Inappropriate temperature in local application and packing**

Y63.6 **Underdosing and nonadministration of necessary drug, medicament or biological substance**

Y63.8 **Failure in dosage during other surgical and medical care**

Y63.9 **Failure in dosage during unspecified surgical and medical care**

Y64 **Contaminated medical or biological substances**

Y64.0 **Contaminated medical or biological substance, transfused or infused**

Y64.1 **Contaminated medical or biological substance, injected or used for immunization**

Y64.8 **Contaminated medical or biological substance administered by other means**

Y64.9 **Contaminated medical or biological substance administered by unspecified means**

Administered contaminated medical or biological substance NOS

Y65 **Other misadventures during surgical and medical care**

Y65.0 **Mismatched blood in transfusion**

Y65.1 **Wrong fluid used in infusion**

Y65.2 **Failure in suture or ligature during surgical operation**

Y65.3 **Endotracheal tube wrongly placed during anesthetic procedure**

Y65.4 **Failure to introduce or to remove other tube or instrument**

Y65.5 **Performance of wrong procedure (operation)**

Y65.51 **Performance of wrong procedure (operation) on correct patient**

Wrong device implanted into correct surgical site

█ Add 4th-7th digits   ▒ Nonspecific code   ░ Unspecified code   Manifestation code   [HCC] Hierarchical Condition Code   **1121**

Excludes1: performance of correct procedure (operation) on wrong side or body part (Y65.53)

Y65.52 Performance of procedure (operation) on patient not scheduled for surgery

Performance of procedure (operation) intended for another patient

Performance of procedure (operation) on wrong patient

Y65.53 Performance of correct procedure (operation) on wrong side or body part

Performance of correct procedure (operation) on wrong side

Performance of correct procedure (operation) on wrong site

Y65.8 Other specified misadventures during surgical and medical care

Y66 Nonadministration of surgical and medical care

Premature cessation of surgical and medical care

Excludes1: DNR status (Z66)

palliative care (Z51.5)

Y69 Unspecified misadventure during surgical and medical care

MEDICAL DEVICES ASSOCIATED WITH ADVERSE INCIDENTS IN DIAGNOSTIC AND THERAPEUTIC USE (Y70-Y82)

Includes: breakdown or malfunction of medical devices (during use) (after implantation) (ongoing use)

Excludes2: later complications following use of medical devices without breakdown or malfunctioning of device (Y83-Y84)

misadventure to patients during surgical and medical care, classifiable to (Y62-Y69)

surgical and other medical procedures as the cause of abnormal reaction of the patient, or of later complication, without mention of misadventure at the time of the procedure (Y83-Y84)

Y70 Anesthesiology devices associated with adverse incidents

Y70.0 Diagnostic and monitoring anesthesiology devices associated with adverse incidents

Y70.1 Therapeutic (nonsurgical) and rehabilitative anesthesiology devices associated with adverse incidents

Y70.2 Prosthetic and other implants, materials and accessory anesthesiology devices associated with adverse incidents

Y70.3 Surgical instruments, materials and anesthesiology devices (including sutures) associated with adverse incidents

Y70.8 Miscellaneous anesthesiology devices associated with adverse incidents, not elsewhere classified

Y71 Cardiovascular devices associated with adverse incidents

Y71.0 Diagnostic and monitoring cardiovascular devices associated with adverse incidents

Y71.1 Therapeutic (nonsurgical) and rehabilitative cardiovascular devices associated with adverse incidents

Y71.2 Prosthetic and other implants, materials and accessory cardiovascular devices associated with adverse incidents

Y71.3 Surgical instruments, materials and cardiovascular devices (including sutures) associated with adverse incidents

Y71.8 Miscellaneous cardiovascular devices associated with adverse incidents, not elsewhere classified

Y72 Otorhinolaryngological devices associated with adverse incidents

Y72.0 Diagnostic and monitoring otorhinolaryngological devices associated with adverse incidents

Y72.1 Therapeutic (nonsurgical) and rehabilitative otorhinolaryngological devices associated with adverse incidents

Y72.2 Prosthetic and other implants, materials and accessory otorhinolaryngological devices associated with adverse incidents

Y72.3 Surgical instruments, materials and otorhinolaryngological devices (including sutures) associated with adverse incidents

Y72.8 Miscellaneous otorhinolaryngological devices associated with adverse incidents, not elsewhere classified

Y73 Gastroenterology and urology devices associated with adverse incidents

Y73.0 Diagnostic and monitoring gastroenterology and urology devices associated with adverse incidents

Y73.1 Therapeutic (nonsurgical) and rehabilitative gastroenterology and urology devices associated with adverse incidents

Y73.2 Prosthetic and other implants, materials and accessory gastroenterology and urology devices associated with adverse incidents

Y73.3 Surgical instruments, materials and gastroenterology and urology devices (including sutures) associated with adverse incidents

Y73.8 Miscellaneous gastroenterology and urology devices associated with adverse incidents, not elsewhere classified

Y74 General hospital and personal-use devices associated with adverse incidents

Y74.0 Diagnostic and monitoring general hospital and personal-use devices associated with adverse incidents

Y74.1 Therapeutic (nonsurgical) and rehabilitative general hospital and personal-use devices associated with adverse incidents

Y74.2 Prosthetic and other implants, materials and accessory general hospital and personal-use devices associated with adverse incidents

Y74.3 Surgical instruments, materials and general hospital and personal-use devices (including sutures) associated with adverse incidents

Y74.8 Miscellaneous general hospital and personal-use devices associated with adverse incidents, not elsewhere classified

Y75 Neurological devices associated with adverse incidents

Y75.0 Diagnostic and monitoring neurological devices associated with adverse incidents

Y75.1 Therapeutic (nonsurgical) and rehabilitative neurological devices associated with adverse incidents

Y75.2 Prosthetic and other implants, materials and neurological devices associated with adverse incidents

Y75.3 Surgical instruments, materials and neurological devices (including sutures) associated with adverse incidents

Y75.8 Miscellaneous neurological devices associated with adverse incidents, not elsewhere classified

Y76 Obstetric and gynecological devices associated with adverse incidents

Y76.0 Diagnostic and monitoring obstetric and gynecological devices associated with adverse incidents

Y76.1 Therapeutic (nonsurgical) and rehabilitative obstetric and gynecological devices associated with adverse incidents

Y76.2 Prosthetic and other implants, materials and accessory obstetric and gynecological devices associated with adverse incidents

Y76.3 Surgical instruments, materials and obstetric and gynecological devices (including sutures) associated with adverse incidents

Y76.8 Miscellaneous obstetric and gynecological devices associated with adverse incidents, not elsewhere classified

Y77 Ophthalmic devices associated with adverse incidents

Y77.0 Diagnostic and monitoring ophthalmic devices associated with adverse incidents

Y77.1 Therapeutic (nonsurgical) and rehabilitative ophthalmic devices associated with adverse incidents

Y77.11 Contact lens associated with adverse incidents

Rigid gas permeable contact lens associated with adverse incidents

Soft (hydrophilic) contact lens associated with adverse incidents

Y77.19 Other therapeutic (nonsurgical) and rehabilitative ophthalmic devices associated with adverse incidents

Y77.2 Prosthetic and other implants, materials and accessory ophthalmic devices associated with adverse incidents

Y77.3 Surgical instruments, materials and ophthalmic devices (including sutures) associated with adverse incidents

Y77.8 Miscellaneous ophthalmic devices associated with adverse incidents, not elsewhere classified

Y78 Radiological devices associated with adverse incidents

Y78.0 Diagnostic and monitoring radiological devices associated with adverse incidents

Y78.1 Therapeutic (nonsurgical) and rehabilitative radiological devices associated with adverse incidents

Y78.2 Prosthetic and other implants, materials and accessory radiological devices associated with adverse incidents

Y78.3 Surgical instruments, materials and radiological devices (including sutures) associated with adverse incidents

Y78.8 Miscellaneous radiological devices associated with adverse incidents, not elsewhere classified

Y79 Orthopedic devices associated with adverse incidents

Y79.0 Diagnostic and monitoring orthopedic devices associated with adverse incidents

Y79.1 Therapeutic (nonsurgical) and rehabilitative orthopedic devices associated with adverse incidents

Y79.2 Prosthetic and other implants, materials and accessory orthopedic devices associated with adverse incidents

Y79.3 Surgical instruments, materials and orthopedic devices (including sutures) associated with adverse incidents

Y79.8 Miscellaneous orthopedic devices associated with adverse incidents, not elsewhere classified

Y80 Physical medicine devices associated with adverse incidents

Y80.0 Diagnostic and monitoring physical medicine devices associated with adverse incidents

Y80.1 Therapeutic (nonsurgical) and rehabilitative physical medicine devices associated with adverse incidents

Y80.2 Prosthetic and other implants, materials and accessory physical medicine devices associated with adverse incidents

Y80.3 Surgical instruments, materials and physical medicine devices (including sutures) associated with adverse incidents

Y80.8 Miscellaneous physical medicine devices associated with adverse incidents, not elsewhere classified

Y81 General- and plastic-surgery devices associated with adverse incidents

Y81.0 Diagnostic and monitoring general- and plastic-surgery devices associated with adverse incidents

Y81.1 Therapeutic (nonsurgical) and rehabilitative general- and plastic-surgery devices associated with adverse incidents

Y81.2 Prosthetic and other implants, materials and accessory general- and plastic-surgery devices associated with adverse incidents

Y81.3 Surgical instruments, materials and general- and plastic-surgery devices (including sutures) associated with adverse incidents

Y81.8 Miscellaneous general- and plastic-surgery devices associated with adverse incidents, not elsewhere classified

Y82 Other and unspecified medical devices associated with adverse incidents

Y82.8 Other medical devices associated with adverse incidents

Y82.9 Unspecified medical devices associated with adverse incidents

SURGICAL AND OTHER MEDICAL PROCEDURES AS THE CAUSE OF ABNORMAL REACTION OF THE PATIENT, OR OF LATER COMPLICATION, WITHOUT MENTION OF MISADVENTURE AT THE TIME OF THE PROCEDURE (Y83-Y84)

Excludes1: misadventures to patients during surgical and medical care, classifiable to (Y62-Y69)

Excludes2: breakdown or malfunctioning of medical device (after implantation) (during procedure) (ongoing use) (Y70-Y82)

Y83 Surgical operation and other surgical procedures as the cause of abnormal reaction of the patient, or of later complication, without mention of misadventure at the time of the procedure

Y83.0 Surgical operation with transplant of whole organ as the cause of abnormal reaction of the patient, or of later complication, without mention of misadventure at the time of the procedure

Y83.1 Surgical operation with implant of artificial internal device as the cause of abnormal reaction of the patient, or of later complication, without mention of misadventure at the time of the procedure

Y83.2 Surgical operation with anastomosis, bypass or graft as the cause of abnormal reaction of the patient, or of later complication, without mention of misadventure at the time of the procedure

Y83.3 Surgical operation with formation of external stoma as the cause of abnormal reaction of the patient, or of later complication, without mention of misadventure at the time of the procedure

Y83.4 Other reconstructive surgery as the cause of abnormal reaction of the patient, or of later complication, without mention of misadventure at the time of the procedure

Y83.5 Amputation of limb(s) as the cause of abnormal reaction of the patient, or of later complication, without mention of misadventure at the time of the procedure

Y83.6 Removal of other organ (partial) (total) as the cause of abnormal reaction of the patient, or of later complication, without mention of misadventure at the time of the procedure

Y83.8 Other surgical procedures as the cause of abnormal reaction of the patient, or of later complication, without mention of misadventure at the time of the procedure

Y83.9 Surgical procedure, unspecified as the cause of abnormal reaction of the patient, or of later complication, without mention of misadventure at the time of the procedure

Y84 Other medical procedures as the cause of abnormal reaction of the patient, or of later complication, without mention of misadventure at the time of the procedure

Y84.0 Cardiac catheterization as the cause of abnormal reaction of the patient, or of later complication, without mention of misadventure at the time of the procedure

Y84.1 Kidney dialysis as the cause of abnormal reaction of the patient, or of later complication, without mention of misadventure at the time of the procedure

Y84.2 Radiological procedure and radiotherapy as the cause of abnormal reaction of the patient, or of later complication, without mention of misadventure at the time of the procedure

Y84.3 Shock therapy as the cause of abnormal reaction of the patient, or of later complication, without mention of misadventure at the time of the procedure

Y84.4 Aspiration of fluid as the cause of abnormal reaction of the patient, or of later complication, without mention of misadventure at the time of the procedure

Y84.5 Insertion of gastric or duodenal sound as the cause of abnormal reaction of the patient, or of later complication, without mention of misadventure at the time of the procedure

Y84.6 Urinary catheterization as the cause of abnormal reaction of the patient, or of later complication, without mention of misadventure at the time of the procedure

Y84.7 Blood-sampling as the cause of abnormal reaction of the patient, or of later complication, without mention of misadventure at the time of the procedure

Y84.8 Other medical procedures as the cause of abnormal reaction of the patient, or of later complication, without mention of misadventure at the time of the procedure

Y84.9 Medical procedure, unspecified as the cause of abnormal reaction of the patient, or of later complication, without mention of misadventure at the time of the procedure

SUPPLEMENTARY FACTORS RELATED TO CAUSES OF MORBIDITY CLASSIFIED ELSEWHERE (Y90-Y99)

Note: These categories may be used to provide supplementary information concerning causes of morbidity. They are not to be used for single-condition coding.

Y90 Evidence of alcohol involvement determined by blood alcohol level

Code first any associated alcohol related disorders (F10)

Y90.0 Blood alcohol level of less than 20 mg/100 ml

Y90.1 Blood alcohol level of 20-39 mg/100 ml

Y90.2 Blood alcohol level of 40-59 mg/100 ml

Y90.3 Blood alcohol level of 60-79 mg/100 ml

Y90.4 Blood alcohol level of 80-99 mg/100 ml

Y90.5 Blood alcohol level of 100-119 mg/100 ml

Y90.6 Blood alcohol level of 120-199 mg/100 ml

Y90.7 Blood alcohol level of 200-239 mg/100 ml

Y90.8 Blood alcohol level of 240 mg/100 ml or more

Y90.9 Presence of alcohol in blood, level not specified

Y92 Place of occurrence of the external cause

The following category is for use, when relevant, to identify the place of occurrence of the external cause. Use in conjunction with an activity code.

Place of occurrence should be recorded only at the initial encounter for treatment

Y92.0 Non-institutional (private) residence as the place of occurrence of the external cause

Excludes1: abandoned or derelict house (Y92.89)

home under construction but not yet occupied (Y92.6-)

institutional place of residence (Y92.1-)

Y92.00 Unspecified non-institutional (private) residence as the place of occurrence of the external cause

Y92.000 Kitchen of unspecified non-institutional (private) residence as the place of occurrence of the external cause

Y92.001 Dining room of unspecified non-institutional (private) residence as the place of occurrence of the external cause

▲Y92.002 Bathroom of unspecified non-institutional (private) residence as the place of occurrence of the external cause

Y92.003 Bedroom of unspecified non-institutional (private) residence as the place of occurrence of the external cause

Y92.007 Garden or yard of unspecified non-institutional (private) residence as the place of occurrence of the external cause

Y92.008 Other place in unspecified non-institutional (private) residence as the place of occurrence of the external cause

Y92.009 Unspecified place in unspecified non-institutional (private) residence as the place of occurrence of the external cause

Home (NOS) as the place of occurrence of the external cause

Y92.01 Single-family non-institutional (private) house as the place of occurrence of the external cause

Farmhouse as the place of occurrence of the external cause

Excludes1: barn (Y92.71)

chicken coop or hen house (Y92.72)

farm field (Y92.73)

orchard (Y92.74)

single family mobile home or trailer (Y92.02-)

slaughter house (Y92.86)

Y92.010 Kitchen of single-family (private) house as the place of occurrence of the external cause

Y92.011 Dining room of single-family (private) house as the place of occurrence of the external cause

Y92.012 Bathroom of single-family (private) house as the place of occurrence of the external cause

Y92.013 Bedroom of single-family (private) house as the place of occurrence of the external cause

Y92.014 Private driveway to single-family (private) house as the place of occurrence of the external cause

Y92.015 Private garage of single-family (private) house as the place of occurrence of the external cause

Y92.016 Swimming-pool in single-family (private) house or garden as the place of occurrence of the external cause

Y92.017 Garden or yard in single-family (private) house as the place of occurrence of the external cause

● New code   ▲ Revised code   **Excludes1:** Not coded here   **Excludes2:** Not included here   ⊗ Placeholder required   ⑦7th digit required

Y92.018 Other place in single-family (private) house as the place of occurrence of the external cause

Y92.019 Unspecified place in single-family (private) house as the place of occurrence of the external cause

Y92.02 Mobile home as the place of occurrence of the external cause

Y92.020 Kitchen in mobile home as the place of occurrence of the external cause

Y92.021 Dining room in mobile home as the place of occurrence of the external cause

Y92.022 Bathroom in mobile home as the place of occurrence of the external cause

Y92.023 Bedroom in mobile home as the place of occurrence of the external cause

Y92.024 Driveway of mobile home as the place of occurrence of the external cause

Y92.025 Garage of mobile home as the place of occurrence of the external cause

Y92.026 Swimming-pool of mobile home as the place of occurrence of the external cause

Y92.027 Garden or yard of mobile home as the place of occurrence of the external cause

Y92.028 Other place in mobile home as the place of occurrence of the external cause

Y92.029 Unspecified place in mobile home as the place of occurrence of the external cause

Y92.03 Apartment as the place of occurrence of the external cause

Condominium as the place of occurrence of the external cause

Co-op apartment as the place of occurrence of the external cause

Y92.030 Kitchen in apartment as the place of occurrence of the external cause

Y92.031 Bathroom in apartment as the place of occurrence of the external cause

Y92.032 Bedroom in apartment as the place of occurrence of the external cause

Y92.038 Other place in apartment as the place of occurrence of the external cause

Y92.039 Unspecified place in apartment as the place of occurrence of the external cause

Y92.04 Boarding-house as the place of occurrence of the external cause

Y92.040 Kitchen in boarding-house as the place of occurrence of the external cause

Y92.041 Bathroom in boarding-house as the place of occurrence of the external cause

Y92.042 Bedroom in boarding-house as the place of occurrence of the external cause

Y92.043 Driveway of boarding-house as the place of occurrence of the external cause

Y92.044 Garage of boarding-house as the place of occurrence of the external cause

Y92.045 Swimming-pool of boarding-house as the place of occurrence of the external cause

Y92.046 Garden or yard of boarding-house as the place of occurrence of the external cause

Y92.048 Other place in boarding-house as the place of occurrence of the external cause

Y92.049 Unspecified place in boarding-house as the place of occurrence of the external cause

Y92.09 Other non-institutional residence as the place of occurrence of the external cause

Y92.090 Kitchen in other non-institutional residence as the place of occurrence of the external cause

Y92.091 Bathroom in other non-institutional residence as the place of occurrence of the external cause

Y92.092 Bedroom in other non-institutional residence as the place of occurrence of the external cause

Y92.093 Driveway of other non-institutional residence as the place of occurrence of the external cause

Y92.094 Garage of other non-institutional residence as the place of occurrence of the external cause

Y92.095 Swimming-pool of other non-institutional residence as the place of occurrence of the external cause

Y92.096 Garden or yard of other non-institutional residence as the place of occurrence of the external cause

Y92.098 Other place in other non-institutional residence as the place of occurrence of the external cause

Y92.099 Unspecified place in other non-institutional residence as the place of occurrence of the external cause

Y92.1 Institutional (nonprivate) residence as the place of occurrence of the external cause

Y92.10 Unspecified residential institution as the place of occurrence of the external cause

Y92.11 Children's home and orphanage as the place of occurrence of the external cause

Y92.110 Kitchen in children's home and orphanage as the place of occurrence of the external cause

Y92.111 Bathroom in children's home and orphanage as the place of occurrence of the external cause

Y92.112 Bedroom in children's home and orphanage as the place of occurrence of the external cause

Y92.113 Driveway of children's home and orphanage as the place of occurrence of the external cause

Y92.114 Garage of children's home and orphanage as the place of occurrence of the external cause

Y92.115 Swimming-pool of children's home and orphanage as the place of occurrence of the external cause

Y92.116 Garden or yard of children's home and orphanage as the place of occurrence of the external cause

Y92.118 Other place in children's home and orphanage as the place of occurrence of the external cause

Y92.119 Unspecified place in children's home and orphanage as the place of occurrence of the external cause

Y92.12 Nursing home as the place of occurrence of the external cause

Home for the sick as the place of occurrence of the external cause

Hospice as the place of occurrence of the external cause

Y92.120 Kitchen in nursing home as the place of occurrence of the external cause

Y92.121 Bathroom in nursing home as the place of occurrence of the external cause

Y92.122 Bedroom in nursing home as the place of occurrence of the external cause

Y92.123 Driveway of nursing home as the place of occurrence of the external cause

Y92.124 Garage of nursing home as the place of occurrence of the external cause

Y92.125 Swimming-pool of nursing home as the place of occurrence of the external cause

Y92.126 Garden or yard of nursing home as the place of occurrence of the external cause

Y92.128 Other place in nursing home as the place of occurrence of the external cause

Y92.129 Unspecified place in nursing home as the place of occurrence of the external cause

Y92.13 Military base as the place of occurrence of the external cause

Excludes1: military training grounds (Y92.83)

Y92.130 Kitchen on military base as the place of occurrence of the external cause

Y92.131 Mess hall on military base as the place of occurrence of the external cause

Y92.133 Barracks on military base as the place of occurrence of the external cause

Y92.135 Garage on military base as the place of occurrence of the external cause

Y92.136 Swimming-pool on military base as the place of occurrence of the external cause

Y92.137 Garden or yard on military base as the place of occurrence of the external cause

Y92.138 Other place on military base as the place of occurrence of the external cause

Y92.139 Unspecified place military base as the place of occurrence of the external cause

Y92.14 Prison as the place of occurrence of the external cause

Y92.140 Kitchen in prison as the place of occurrence of the external cause

Y92.141 Dining room in prison as the place of occurrence of the external cause

Y92.142 Bathroom in prison as the place of occurrence of the external cause

Y92.143 Cell of prison as the place of occurrence of the external cause

Y92.146 Swimming-pool of prison as the place of occurrence of the external cause

Y92.147 Courtyard of prison as the place of occurrence of the external cause

Y92.148 Other place in prison as the place of occurrence of the external cause

Y92.149 Unspecified place in prison as the place of occurrence of the external cause

Y92.15 Reform school as the place of occurrence of the external cause

Y92.150 Kitchen in reform school as the place of occurrence of the external cause

Y92.151 Dining room in reform school as the place of occurrence of the external cause

Y92.152 Bathroom in reform school as the place of occurrence of the external cause

Y92.153 Bedroom in reform school as the place of occurrence of the external cause

Y92.154 Driveway of reform school as the place of occurrence of the external cause

Y92.155 Garage of reform school as the place of occurrence of the external cause

Y92.156 Swimming-pool of reform school as the place of occurrence of the external cause

Y92.157 Garden or yard of reform school as the place of occurrence of the external cause

Y92.158 Other place in reform school as the place of occurrence of the external cause

Y92.159 Unspecified place in reform school as the place of occurrence of the external cause

Y92.16 School dormitory as the place of occurrence of the external cause

Excludes1: reform school as the place of occurrence of the external cause (Y92.15-)

school buildings and grounds as the place of occurrence of the external cause (Y92.2-)

school sports and athletic areas as the place of occurrence of the external cause (Y92.3-)

Y92.160 Kitchen in school dormitory as the place of occurrence of the external cause

Y92.161 Dining room in school dormitory as the place of occurrence of the external cause

Y92.162 Bathroom in school dormitory as the place of occurrence of the external cause

Y92.163 Bedroom in school dormitory as the place of occurrence of the external cause

Y92.168 Other place in school dormitory as the place of occurrence of the external cause

Y92.169 Unspecified place in school dormitory as the place of occurrence of the external cause

Y92.19 Other specified residential institution as the place of occurrence of the external cause

Y92.190 Kitchen in other specified residential institution as the place of occurrence of the external cause

Y92.191 Dining room in other specified residential institution as the place of occurrence of the external cause

Y92.192 Bathroom in other specified residential institution as the place of occurrence of the external cause

Y92.193 Bedroom in other specified residential institution as the place of occurrence of the external cause

Y92.194 Driveway of other specified residential institution as the place of occurrence of the external cause

Y92.195 Garage of other specified residential institution as the place of occurrence of the external cause

Y92.196 Pool of other specified residential institution as the place of occurrence of the external cause

Y92.197 Garden or yard of other specified residential institution as the place of occurrence of the external cause

Y92.198 Other place in other specified residential institution as the place of occurrence of the external cause

Y92.199 Unspecified place in other specified residential institution as the place of occurrence of the external cause

Y92.2 School, other institution and public administrative area as the place of occurrence of the external cause

Building and adjacent grounds used by the general public or by a particular group of the public

Excludes1: building under construction as the place of occurrence of the external cause (Y92.6)

residential institution as the place of occurrence of the external cause (Y92.1)

school dormitory as the place of occurrence of the external cause (Y92.16-)

sports and athletics area of schools as the place of occurrence of the external cause (Y92.3-)

Y92.21 School (private) (public) (state) as the place of occurrence of the external cause

Y92.210 Daycare center as the place of occurrence of the external cause

Y92.211 Elementary school as the place of occurrence of the external cause

Kindergarten as the place of occurrence of the external cause

Y92.212 Middle school as the place of occurrence of the external cause

Y92.213 High school as the place of occurrence of the external cause

Y92.214 College as the place of occurrence of the external cause

University as the place of occurrence of the external cause

Y92.215 Trade school as the place of occurrence of the external cause

Y92.218 Other school as the place of occurrence of the external cause

Y92.219 Unspecified school as the place of occurrence of the external cause

Y92.22 Religious institution as the place of occurrence of the external cause

Church as the place of occurrence of the external cause

Mosque as the place of occurrence of the external cause

Synagogue as the place of occurrence of the external cause

Y92.23 Hospital as the place of occurrence of the external cause

Excludes1: ambulatory (outpatient) health services establishments (Y92.53-)

home for the sick as the place of occurrence of the external cause (Y92.12-)

hospice as the place of occurrence of the external cause (Y92.12-)

nursing home as the place of occurrence of the external cause (Y92.12-)

Y92.230 Patient room in hospital as the place of occurrence of the external cause

Y92.231 Patient bathroom in hospital as the place of occurrence of the external cause

Y92.232 Corridor of hospital as the place of occurrence of the external cause

Y92.233 Cafeteria of hospital as the place of occurrence of the external cause

Y92.234 Operating room of hospital as the place of occurrence of the external cause

Y92.238 Other place in hospital as the place of occurrence of the external cause

Y92.239 Unspecified place in hospital as the place of occurrence of the external cause

Y92.24 Public administrative building as the place of occurrence of the external cause

Y92.240 Courthouse as the place of occurrence of the external cause

Y92.241 Library as the place of occurrence of the external cause

Y92.242 Post office as the place of occurrence of the external cause

Y92.243 City hall as the place of occurrence of the external cause

Y92.248 Other public administrative building as the place of occurrence of the external cause

Y92.25 Cultural building as the place of occurrence of the external cause

Y92.250 Art Gallery as the place of occurrence of the external cause

Y92.251 Museum as the place of occurrence of the external cause

Y92.252 Music hall as the place of occurrence of the external cause

Y92.253 Opera house as the place of occurrence of the external cause

Y92.254 Theater (live) as the place of occurrence of the external cause

Y92.258 Other cultural public building as the place of occurrence of the external cause

Y92.26 Movie house or cinema as the place of occurrence of the external cause

Y92.29 Other specified public building as the place of occurrence of the external cause

Assembly hall as the place of occurrence of the external cause

Clubhouse as the place of occurrence of the external cause

Y92.3 Sports and athletics area as the place of occurrence of the external cause

Y92.31 Athletic court as the place of occurrence of the external cause

Excludes1: tennis court in private home or garden (Y92.09)

Y92.310 Basketball court as the place of occurrence of the external cause

Y92.311 Squash court as the place of occurrence of the external cause

Y92.312 Tennis court as the place of occurrence of the external cause

Y92.318 Other athletic court as the place of occurrence of the external cause

Y92.32 Athletic field as the place of occurrence of the external cause

Y92.320 Baseball field as the place of occurrence of the external cause

Y92.321 Football field as the place of occurrence of the external cause

Y92.322 Soccer field as the place of occurrence of the external cause

Y92.328 Other athletic field as the place of occurrence of the external cause

Cricket field as the place of occurrence of the external cause

Hockey field as the place of occurrence of the external cause

Y92.33 Skating rink as the place of occurrence of the external cause

Y92.330 Ice skating rink (indoor) (outdoor) as the place of occurrence of the external cause

Y92.331 Roller skating rink as the place of occurrence of the external cause

Y92.34 Swimming pool (public) as the place of occurrence of the external cause

Excludes1: swimming pool in private home or garden (Y92.016)

Y92.39 Other specified sports and athletic area as the place of occurrence of the external cause

Golf-course as the place of occurrence of the external cause

Gymnasium as the place of occurrence of the external cause

Riding-school as the place of occurrence of the external cause

Stadium as the place of occurrence of the external cause

Y92.4 Street, highway and other paved roadways as the place of occurrence of the external cause

Excludes1: private driveway of residence (Y92.014, Y92.024, Y92.043, Y92.093, Y92.113, Y92.123, Y92.154, Y92.194)

Y92.41 Street and highway as the place of occurrence of the external cause

Y92.410 Unspecified street and highway as the place of occurrence of the external cause

Road NOS as the place of occurrence of the external cause

Y92.411 Interstate highway as the place of occurrence of the external cause

Freeway as the place of occurrence of the external cause

Motorway as the place of occurrence of the external cause

Y92.412 Parkway as the place of occurrence of the external cause

Y92.413 State road as the place of occurrence of the external cause

Y92.414 Local residential or business street as the place of occurrence of the external cause

Y92.415 Exit ramp or entrance ramp of street or highway as the place of occurrence of the external cause

Y92.48 Other paved roadways as the place of occurrence of the external cause

Y92.480 Sidewalk as the place of occurrence of the external cause

Y92.481 Parking lot as the place of occurrence of the external cause

Y92.482 Bike path as the place of occurrence of the external cause

Y92.488 Other paved roadways as the place of occurrence of the external cause

Y92.5 Trade and service area as the place of occurrence of the external cause

Excludes1: garage in private home (Y92.015)

schools and other public administration buildings (Y92.2-)

Y92.51 Private commercial establishments as the place of occurrence of the external cause

Y92.510 Bank as the place of occurrence of the external cause

Y92.511 Restaurant or café as the place of occurrence of the external cause

Y92.512 Supermarket, store or market as the place of occurrence of the external cause

Y92.513 Shop (commercial) as the place of occurrence of the external cause

● New code ▲ Revised code Excludes1: Not coded here Excludes2: Not included here ⊗ Placeholder required ⑦7th digit required

Y92.52 **Service areas as the place of occurrence of the external cause**

    Y92.520 **Airport as the place of occurrence of the external cause**

    Y92.521 **Bus station as the place of occurrence of the external cause**

    Y92.522 **Railway station as the place of occurrence of the external cause**

    Y92.523 **Highway rest stop as the place of occurrence of the external cause**

    Y92.524 **Gas station as the place of occurrence of the external cause**

        Petroleum station as the place of occurrence of the external cause

        Service station as the place of occurrence of the external cause

Y92.53 **Ambulatory health services establishments as the place of occurrence of the external cause**

    Y92.530 **Ambulatory surgery center as the place of occurrence of the external cause**

        Outpatient surgery center, including that connected with a hospital as the place of occurrence of the external cause

        Same day surgery center, including that connected with a hospital as the place of occurrence of the external cause

    Y92.531 **Health care provider office as the place of occurrence of the external cause**

        Physician office as the place of occurrence of the external cause

    Y92.532 **Urgent care center as the place of occurrence of the external cause**

    Y92.538 **Other ambulatory health services establishments as the place of occurrence of the external cause**

Y92.59 **Other trade areas as the place of occurrence of the external cause**

    Office building as the place of occurrence of the external cause

    Casino as the place of occurrence of the external cause

    Garage (commercial) as the place of occurrence of the external cause

    Hotel as the place of occurrence of the external cause

    Radio or television station as the place of occurrence of the external cause

    Shopping mall as the place of occurrence of the external cause

    Warehouse as the place of occurrence of the external cause

Y92.6 **Industrial and construction area as the place of occurrence of the external cause**

    Y92.61 **Building [any] under construction as the place of occurrence of the external cause**

    Y92.62 **Dock or shipyard as the place of occurrence of the external cause**

        Dockyard as the place of occurrence of the external cause

        Dry dock as the place of occurrence of the external cause

        Shipyard as the place of occurrence of the external cause

Y92.63 **Factory as the place of occurrence of the external cause**

    Factory building as the place of occurrence of the external cause

    Factory premises as the place of occurrence of the external cause

    Industrial yard as the place of occurrence of the external cause

Y92.64 **Mine or pit as the place of occurrence of the external cause**

    Mine as the place of occurrence of the external cause

Y92.65 **Oil rig as the place of occurrence of the external cause**

    Pit (coal) (gravel) (sand) as the place of occurrence of the external cause

Y92.69 **Other specified industrial and construction area as the place of occurrence of the external cause**

    Gasworks as the place of occurrence of the external cause

    Power-station (coal) (nuclear) (oil) as the place of occurrence of the external cause

    Tunnel under construction as the place of occurrence of the external cause

    Workshop as the place of occurrence of the external cause

Y92.7 **Farm as the place of occurrence of the external cause**

Ranch as the place of occurrence of the external cause

Excludes1: farmhouse and home premises of farm (Y92.01-)

    Y92.71 **Barn as the place of occurrence of the external cause**

    Y92.72 **Chicken coop as the place of occurrence of the external cause**

        Hen house as the place of occurrence of the external cause

    Y92.73 **Farm field as the place of occurrence of the external cause**

    Y92.74 **Orchard as the place of occurrence of the external cause**

    Y92.79 **Other farm location as the place of occurrence of the external cause**

Y92.8 **Other places as the place of occurrence of the external cause**

    Y92.81 **Transport vehicle as the place of occurrence of the external cause**

    Excludes1: transport accidents (V00-V99)

    Y92.810 **Car as the place of occurrence of the external cause**

    Y92.811 **Bus as the place of occurrence of the external cause**

    Y92.812 **Truck as the place of occurrence of the external cause**

    Y92.813 **Airplane as the place of occurrence of the external cause**

    Y92.814 **Boat as the place of occurrence of the external cause**

    Y92.815 **Train as the place of occurrence of the external cause**

    Y92.816 **Subway car as the place of occurrence of the external cause**

Y92.818 Other transport vehicle as the place of occurrence of the external cause

Y92.82 **Wilderness area**

Y92.820 Desert as the place of occurrence of the external cause

Y92.821 Forest as the place of occurrence of the external cause

Y92.828 Other wilderness area as the place of occurrence of the external cause

Swamp as the place of occurrence of the external cause

Mountain as the place of occurrence of the external cause

Marsh as the place of occurrence of the external cause

Prairie as the place of occurrence of the external cause

Y92.83 **Recreation area as the place of occurrence of the external cause**

Y92.830 Public park as the place of occurrence of the external cause

Y92.831 Amusement park as the place of occurrence of the external cause

Y92.832 Beach as the place of occurrence of the external cause

Seashore as the place of occurrence of the external cause

Y92.833 Campsite as the place of occurrence of the external cause

Y92.834 Zoological garden (Zoo) as the place of occurrence of the external cause

Y92.838 Other recreation area as the place of occurrence of the external cause

Y92.84 **Military training ground as the place of occurrence of the external cause**

Y92.85 **Railroad track as the place of occurrence of the external cause**

Y92.86 **Slaughter house as the place of occurrence of the external cause**

Y92.89 **Other specified places as the place of occurrence of the external cause**

Derelict house as the place of occurrence of the external cause

Y92.9 **Unspecified place or not applicable**

Y93 **Activity codes**

Note: Category Y93 is provided for use to indicate the activity of the person seeking healthcare for an injury or health condition, such as a heart attack while shoveling snow, which resulted from, or was contributed to, by the activity. These codes are appropriate for use for both acute injuries, such as those from chapter 19, and conditions that are due to the long-term, cumulative effects of an activity, such as those from chapter 13. They are also appropriate for use with external cause codes for cause and intent if identifying the activity provides additional information on the event. These codes should be used in conjunction with codes for external cause status (Y99) and place of occurrence (Y92).

This section contains the following broad activity categories: Y93.0

Activities involving walking and running Y93.1

Activities involving water and water craft Y93.2

Activities involving ice and snow Y93.3

Activities involving climbing, rappelling, and jumping off Y93.4

Activities involving dancing and other rhythmic movement Y93.5

Activities involving other sports and athletics played individually Y93.6

Activities involving other sports and athletics played as a team or group Y93.7

Activities involving other specified sports and athletics Y93.A

Activities involving other cardiorespiratory exercise Y93.B

Activities involving other muscle strengthening exercises Y93.C

Activities involving computer technology and electronic devices Y93.D

Activities involving arts and handcrafts Y93.E

Activities involving personal hygiene and interior property and clothing maintenance Y93.F

Activities involving caregiving Y93.G

Activities involving food preparation, cooking and grilling Y93.H

Activities involving exterior property and land maintenance, building and construction Y93.I

Activities involving roller coasters and other types of external motion Y93.J

Activities involving playing musical instrument Y93.K

Activities involving animal care Y93.8

Activities, other specified Y93.9

Activity, unspecified

Y93.0 **Activities involving walking and running**

Excludes1: activity, walking an animal (Y93.K1)

activity, walking or running on a treadmill (Y93.A1)

Y93.01 **Activity, walking, marching and hiking**

Activity, walking, marching and hiking on level or elevated terrain

Excludes1: activity, mountain climbing (Y93.31)

Y93.02 **Activity, running**

Y93.1 **Activities involving water and water craft**

Excludes1: activities involving ice (Y93.2-)

Y93.11 **Activity, swimming**

Y93.12 **Activity, springboard and platform diving**

Y93.13 **Activity, water polo**

Y93.14 **Activity, water aerobics and water exercise**

Y93.15 **Activity, underwater diving and snorkeling**

Activity, SCUBA diving

Y93.16 **Activity, rowing, canoeing, kayaking, rafting and tubing**

Activity, canoeing, kayaking, rafting and tubing in calm and turbulent water

Y93.17 **Activity, water skiing and wake boarding**

Y93.18 **Activity, surfing, windsurfing and boogie boarding**

Activity, water sliding

Y93.19 **Activity, other involving water and watercraft**

Activity involving water NOS

Activity, parasailing

Activity, water survival training and testing

Y93.2 **Activities involving ice and snow**

Excludes1: activity, shoveling ice and snow (Y93.H1)

Y93.21 **Activity, ice skating**

Activity, figure skating (singles) (pairs)

Activity, ice dancing

Excludes1: activity, ice hockey (Y93.22)

Y93.22 **Activity, ice hockey**

Y93.23 **Activity, snow (alpine) (downhill) skiing, snowboarding, sledding, tobogganing and snow tubing**

Excludes1: activity, cross country skiing (Y93.24)

Y93.24 **Activity, cross country skiing**
Activity, Nordic skiing

Y93.29 **Activity, other involving ice and snow**
Activity involving ice and snow NOS

Y93.3 **Activities involving climbing, rappelling and jumping off**

Excludes1: activity, hiking on level or elevated terrain (Y93.01)
activity, jumping rope (Y93.56)
activity, trampoline jumping (Y93.44)

Y93.31 **Activity, mountain climbing, rock climbing and wall climbing**

Y93.32 **Activity, rappelling**

Y93.33 **Activity, BASE jumping**
Activity, Building, Antenna, Span, Earth jumping

Y93.34 **Activity, bungee jumping**

Y93.35 **Activity, hang gliding**

Y93.39 **Activity, other involving climbing, rappelling and jumping off**

Y93.4 **Activities involving dancing and other rhythmic movement**

Excludes1: activity, martial arts (Y93.75)

Y93.41 **Activity, dancing**

Y93.42 **Activity, yoga**

Y93.43 **Activity, gymnastics**
Activity, rhythmic gymnastics
Excludes1: activity, trampolining (Y93.44)

Y93.44 **Activity, trampolining**

Y93.45 **Activity, cheerleading**

Y93.49 **Activity, other involving dancing and other rhythmic movements**

Y93.5 **Activities involving other sports and athletics played individually**

Excludes1: activity, dancing (Y93.41)
activity, gymnastic (Y93.43)
activity, trampolining (Y93.44)
activity, yoga (Y93.42)

Y93.51 **Activity, roller skating (inline) and skateboarding**

Y93.52 **Activity, horseback riding**

Y93.53 **Activity, golf**

Y93.54 **Activity, bowling**

Y93.55 **Activity, bike riding**

Y93.56 **Activity, jumping rope**

Y93.57 **Activity, non-running track and field events**
Excludes1: activity, running (any form) (Y93.02)

Y93.59 **Activity, other involving other sports and athletics played individually**
Excludes1: activities involving climbing, rappelling, and jumping (Y93.3-)
activities involving ice and snow (Y93.2-)
activities involving walking and running (Y93.0-)
activities involving water and watercraft (Y93.1-)

Y93.6 **Activities involving other sports and athletics played as a team or group**

Excludes1: activity, ice hockey (Y93.22)
activity, water polo (Y93.13)

Y93.61 **Activity, American tackle football**
Activity, football NOS

Y93.62 **Activity, American flag or touch football**

Y93.63 **Activity, rugby**

Y93.64 **Activity, baseball**
Activity, softball

Y93.65 **Activity, lacrosse and field hockey**

Y93.66 **Activity, soccer**

Y93.67 **Activity, basketball**

Y93.68 **Activity, volleyball (beach) (court)**

Y93.6A **Activity, physical games generally associated with school recess, summer camp and children**
Activity, capture the flag
Activity, dodge ball
Activity, four square
Activity, kickball

Y93.69 **Activity, other involving other sports and athletics played as a team or group**
Activity, cricket

Y93.7 **Activities involving other specified sports and athletics**

Y93.71 **Activity, boxing**

Y93.72 **Activity, wrestling**

Y93.73 **Activity, racquet and hand sports**
Activity, handball
Activity, racquetball
Activity, squash
Activity, tennis

Y93.74 **Activity, frisbee**
Activity, ultimate frisbee

Y93.75 **Activity, martial arts**
Activity, combatives

Y93.79 **Activity, other specified sports and athletics**
Excludes1: sports and athletics activities specified in categories Y93.0-Y93.6

Y93.A **Activities involving other cardiorespiratory exercise**
Activities involving physical training

Y93.A1 **Activity, exercise machines primarily for cardiorespiratory conditioning**
Activity, elliptical and stepper machines
Activity, stationary bike
Activity, treadmill

Y93.A2 **Activity, calisthenics**
Activity, jumping jacks
Activity, warm up and cool down

Y93.A3 **Activity, aerobic and step exercise**

Y93.A4 **Activity, circuit training**

Y93.A5 **Activity, obstacle course**
Activity, challenge course
Activity, confidence course

Y93.A6 **Activity, grass drills**
Activity, guerilla drills

Y93.A9 **Activity, other involving cardiorespiratory exercise**

Excludes1: activities involving cardiorespiratory exercise specified in categories Y93.0-Y93.7

Y93.B Activities involving other muscle strengthening exercises

Y93.B1 Activity, exercise machines primarily for muscle strengthening

Y93.B2 Activity, push-ups, pull-ups, sit-ups

Y93.B3 Activity, free weights

Activity, barbells

Activity, dumbbells

Y93.B4 Activity, pilates

Y93.B9 Activity, other involving muscle strengthening exercises

Excludes1: activities involving muscle strengthening specified in categories Y93.0-Y93.A

Y93.C Activities involving computer technology and electronic devices

Excludes1: activity, electronic musical keyboard or instruments (Y93.J-)

Y93.C1 Activity, computer keyboarding

Activity, electronic game playing using keyboard or other stationary device

Y93.C2 Activity, hand held interactive electronic device

Activity, cellular telephone and communication device

Activity, electronic game playing using interactive device

Excludes1: activity, electronic game playing using keyboard or other stationary device (Y93.C1)

Y93.C9 Activity, other involving computer technology and electronic devices

Y93.D Activities involving arts and handcrafts

Excludes1: activities involving playing musical instrument (Y93.J-)

Y93.D1 Activity, knitting and crocheting

Y93.D2 Activity, sewing

Y93.D3 Activity, furniture building and finishing

Activity, furniture repair

Y93.D9 Activity, other involving arts and handcrafts

Y93.E Activities involving personal hygiene and interior property and clothing maintenance

Excludes1: activities involving cooking and grilling (Y93.G-)

activities involving exterior property and land maintenance, building and construction (Y93.H-)

activities involving caregiving (Y93.F-)

activity, dishwashing (Y93.G1)

activity, food preparation (Y93.G1)

activity, gardening (Y93.H2)

Y93.E1 Activity, personal bathing and showering

Y93.E2 Activity, laundry

Y93.E3 Activity, vacuuming

Y93.E4 Activity, ironing

Y93.E5 Activity, floor mopping and cleaning

Y93.E6 Activity, residential relocation

Activity, packing up and unpacking involved in moving to a new residence

Y93.E8 Activity, other personal hygiene

Y93.E9 Activity, other interior property and clothing maintenance

Y93.F Activities involving caregiving

Activity involving the provider of caregiving

Y93.F1 Activity, caregiving, bathing

Y93.F2 Activity, caregiving, lifting

Y93.F9 Activity, other caregiving

Y93.G Activities involving food preparation, cooking and grilling

Y93.G1 Activity, food preparation and clean up

Activity, dishwashing

Y93.G2 Activity, grilling and smoking food

Y93.G3 Activity, cooking and baking

Activity, use of stove, oven and microwave oven

Y93.G9 Activity, other involving cooking and grilling

Y93.H Activities involving exterior property and land maintenance, building and construction

Y93.H1 Activity, digging, shoveling and raking

Activity, dirt digging

Activity, raking leaves

Activity, snow shoveling

Y93.H2 Activity, gardening and landscaping

Activity, pruning, trimming shrubs, weeding

Y93.H3 Activity, building and construction

Y93.H9 Activity, other involving exterior property and land maintenance, building and construction

Y93.I Activities involving roller coasters and other types of external motion

Y93.I1 Activity, roller coaster riding

Y93.I9 Activity, other involving external motion

Y93.J Activities involving playing musical instrument

Activity involving playing electric musical instrument

Y93.J1 Activity, piano playing

Activity, musical keyboard (electronic) playing

Y93.J2 Activity, drum and other percussion instrument playing

Y93.J3 Activity, string instrument playing

Y93.J4 Activity, winds and brass instrument playing

Y93.K Activities involving animal care

Excludes1: activity, horseback riding (Y93.52)

Y93.K1 Activity, walking an animal

Y93.K2 Activity, milking an animal

Y93.K3 Activity, grooming and shearing an animal

Y93.K9 Activity, other involving animal care

Y93.8 Activities, other specified

Y93.81 Activity, refereeing a sports activity

Y93.82 Activity, spectator at an event

Y93.83 Activity, rough housing and horseplay

Y93.84 Activity, sleeping

Y93.85 Activity, choking game

Activity, blackout game

Activity, fainting game

Activity, pass out game

Y93.89 Activity, other specified

Y93.9 Activity, unspecified

Y95 Nosocomial condition

Y99 External cause status

● New code   ▲ Revised code   Excludes1: Not coded here   Excludes2: Not included here   ⊗ Placeholder required   ⑦7th digit required

Note: A single code from category Y99 should be used in conjunction with the external cause code(s) assigned to a record to indicate the status of the person at the time the event occurred.

Y99.0   Civilian activity done for income or pay

Civilian activity done for financial or other compensation

Excludes1: military activity (Y99.1)

volunteer activity (Y99.2)

Y99.1   Military activity

Excludes1: activity of off duty military personnel (Y99.8)

Y99.2   Volunteer activity

Excludes1: activity of child or other family member assisting in compensated work **of other** family member (Y99.8)

Y99.8   Other external cause status

Activity NEC

Activity of child or other family member assisting in compensated work of other family member

Hobby not done for income

Leisure activity

Off-duty activity of military personnel

Recreation or sport not for income or while a student

Student activity

Excludes1: civilian activity done for income or compensation (Y99.0)

military activity (Y99.1)

Y99.9   Unspecified external cause status

Chapter 21: Factors Influencing Health Status and Contact with Health Services (Z00-Z99)

DEFINITIONS

This chapter includes definitions of selected key words, terms and phrases and coding alerts for adding points to the clinical domain, and references to coding late effects where appropriate. An example from this chapter is as follows:

 Z14   Genetic carrier

Definition: A genetic carrier (or just carrier), is a person who has inherited a genetic trait or mutation but does not display that trait or show symptoms of the disease. Carriers are, however, able to pass the gene onto their offspring, who may then express the gene.

MULTIPLE CODING FOR A SINGLE CONDITION

In addition to the etiology/manifestation convention that requires two codes to fully describe a single condition that affects multiple body systems, there are other single conditions that also require more than one code. "**Use Additional Code**" notes are found in the Tabular List at codes that are not part of an etiology/manifestation pair where a secondary code is useful to fully describe a condition. The sequencing rule is the same as the etiology/manifestation pair, "**Use Additional Code**" indicates that a secondary code should be added.

For example, for bacterial infections that are not included in chapter 1, a secondary code from category B95, Streptococcus, Staphylococcus, and Enterococcus, as the cause of diseases classified elsewhere, or B96, Other bacterial agents as the cause of diseases classified elsewhere, may be required to identify the bacterial organism causing the infection. A "**Use Additional Code**" note will normally be found at the infectious disease code, indicating a need for the organism code to be added as a secondary code.

"Code first" notes are also under certain codes that are not specifically manifestation codes but may be due to an underlying cause. When there is a "Code first" note and an underlying condition is present, the underlying condition should be sequenced first.

"Code, if applicable, any causal condition first", notes indicate that this code may be assigned as a principal diagnosis when the causal condition is unknown or not applicable. If a causal condition is known, then the code for that condition should be sequenced as the principal or first-listed diagnosis.

Multiple codes may be needed for sequela, complication codes and obstetric codes to more fully describe a condition. See the specific guidelines for these conditions for further instruction.

COMBINATION CODE

A combination code is a single code used to classify: Two diagnoses, or a diagnosis with an associated secondary process (manifestation) A diagnosis with an associated complication

Combination codes are identified by referring to subterm entries in the Alphabetic Index and by reading the inclusion and exclusion notes in the Tabular List.

Assign only the combination code when that code fully identifies the diagnostic conditions involved or when the Alphabetic Index so directs. Multiple coding should not be used when the classification provides a combination code that clearly identifies all of the elements documented in the diagnosis. When the combination code lacks necessary specificity in describing the manifestation or complication, an additional code should be used as a secondary code.

SEQUELA (LATE EFFECTS)

A sequela is the residual effect (condition produced) after the acute phase of an illness or injury has terminated. There is no time limit on when a sequela code can be used. The residual may be apparent early, such as in cerebral infarction, or it may occur months or years later, such as that due to a previous injury. Coding of sequela generally requires two codes sequenced in the following order: The condition or nature of the sequela is sequenced first.

The sequela code is sequenced second.

Z00-Z99

An exception to the above guidelines are those instances where the code for the sequela is followed by a manifestation code identified in the Tabular List and title, or the sequela code has been expanded (at the fourth, fifth or sixth character levels) to include the manifestation(s). The code for the acute phase of an illness or injury that led to the sequela is never used with a code for the late effect.

Note: The chapter specific guidelines provide additional information about the use of Z codes for specified encounters.

USE OF Z CODES IN ANY HEALTHCARE SETTING

Z codes are for use in any healthcare setting. Z codes may be used as either a first-listed (principal diagnosis code in the inpatient setting) or secondary code, depending on the circumstances of the encounter. Certain Z codes may only be used as first-listed or principal diagnosis.

Z CODES INDICATE A REASON FOR AN ENCOUNTER

Z codes are not procedure codes. A corresponding procedure code must accompany a Z code to describe any procedure performed.

CATEGORIES OF Z CODES

1) Contact/Exposure

Category Z20 indicates contact with, and suspected exposure to, communicable diseases. These codes are for patients who do not show any sign or symptom of a disease but are suspected to have been exposed to it by close personal contact with an infected individual or are in an area where a disease is epidemic.

Category Z77, Other contact with and (suspected) exposures hazardous to health, indicates contact with and suspected exposures hazardous to health.

Contact/exposure codes may be used as a first-listed code to explain an encounter for testing, or, more commonly, as a secondary code to identify a potential risk.

2) Inoculations and vaccinations

Code Z23 is for encounters for inoculations and vaccinations. It indicates that a patient is being seen to receive a prophylactic inoculation against a disease. Procedure codes are required to identify the actual administration of the injection and the type(s) of immunizations given. Code Z23 may be used as a secondary code if the inoculation is given as a routine part of preventive health care, such as a well-baby visit.

3) Status

Status codes indicate that a patient is either a carrier of a disease or has the sequelae or residual of a past disease or condition. This includes such things as the presence of prosthetic or mechanical devices resulting from past treatment. A status code is informative, because the status may affect the course of treatment and its outcome. A status code is distinct from a history code. The history code indicates that the patient no longer has the condition.

A status code should not be used with a diagnosis code from one of the body system chapters, if the diagnosis code includes the information provided by the status code. For example, code Z94.1, Heart transplant status, should not be used with a code from subcategory T86.2, Complications of heart transplant. The status code does not provide additional information. The complication code indicates that the patient is a heart transplant patient.

For encounters for weaning from a mechanical ventilator, assign a code from subcategory J96.1, Chronic respiratory failure, followed by code Z99.11, Dependence on respirator [ventilator] status.

The status Z codes/categories are:

Z14   Genetic carrier

Genetic carrier status indicates that a person carries a gene, associated with a particular disease, which may be passed to offspring who may develop that disease. The person does not have the disease and is not at risk of developing the disease.

Z15   Genetic susceptibility to disease

Genetic susceptibility indicates that a person has a gene that increases the risk of that person developing the disease.

Codes from category Z15 should not be used as principal or first-listed codes. If the patient has the condition to which he/she is susceptible, and that condition is the reason for the encounter, the code for the current condition should be sequenced first. If the patient is being seen for follow-up after completed treatment for this condition, and the condition no longer exists, a follow-up code should be sequenced first, followed by the appropriate personal history and genetic susceptibility codes. If the purpose of the encounter is genetic counseling associated with procreative management, code Z31.5, Encounter for genetic counseling, should be assigned as the first-listed code, followed by a code from category Z15. Additional codes should be assigned for any applicable family or personal history.

Z16   Resistance to antimicrobial drugs

This code indicates that a patient has a condition that is resistant to antimicrobial drug treatment. Sequence the infection Code first.

Z17   Estrogen receptor status

Z18   Retained foreign body fragments

Z19   Hormone sensitivity malignancy status

Z21   Asymptomatic HIV infection status

This code indicates that a patient has tested positive for HIV but has manifested no signs or symptoms of the disease.

Z22   Carrier of infectious disease

Carrier status indicates that a person harbors the specific organisms of a disease without manifest symptoms and is capable of transmitting the infection.

Z28.3   Underimmunization status

Z33.1   Pregnant state, incidental

This code is a secondary code only for use when the pregnancy is in no way complicating the reason for visit. Otherwise, a code from the obstetric chapter is required.

Z66   Do not resuscitate

This code may be used when it is documented by the provider that a patient is on do not resuscitate status at any time during the stay.

Z67   Blood type

Z68   Body mass index (BMI)

BMI codes should only be assigned when there is an associated, reportable diagnosis (such as obesity). Do not assign BMI codes during pregnancy.

See Section I.B.14 for BMI documentation by clinicians other than the patient's provider.

Z74.01   Bed confinement status

Z76.82   Awaiting organ transplant status

Z78   Other specified health status

Code Z78.1, Physical restraint status, may be used when it is documented by the provider that a patient has been put in restraints during the current encounter. Please note that this code should not be reported when it is documented by the provider that a patient is temporarily restrained during a procedure.

Z79   Long-term (current) drug therapy

Codes from this category indicate a patient's continuous use of a prescribed drug (including such things as aspirin therapy) for the long-term treatment of a condition or for prophylactic use. It is not for use for patients who have addictions to drugs. This subcategory is not for use of medications for detoxification or maintenance programs to prevent withdrawal symptoms in patients with drug dependence (e.g., methadone maintenance for opiate dependence). Assign the appropriate code for the drug dependence instead.

Assign a code from Z79 if the patient is receiving a medication for an extended period as a prophylactic measure (such as for the prevention of deep vein thrombosis) or as treatment of a chronic condition (such as arthritis) or a disease requiring a lengthy course of treatment (such as cancer). Do not assign a code from category Z79 for medication being administered for a brief period of time to treat an acute illness or injury (such as a course of antibiotics to treat acute bronchitis).

Z88   Allergy status to drugs, medicaments and biological substances

Except: Z88.9, Allergy status to unspecified drugs, medicaments and biological substances status

Z89   Acquired absence of limb

Z90   Acquired absence of organs, not elsewhere classified

Z91.0-   Allergy status, other than to drugs and biological substances

Z92.82   Status post administration of tPA (rtPA) in a different facility within the last 24 hours prior to admission to a current facility

Assign code Z92.82, Status post administration of tPA (rtPA) in a different facility within the last 24 hours prior to admission to current facility, as a secondary diagnosis when a patient is received by transfer into a facility and documentation indicates they were administered tissue plasminogen activator (tPA) within the last 24 hours prior to admission to the current facility.

This guideline applies even if the patient is still receiving the tPA at the time they are received into the current facility.

The appropriate code for the condition for which the tPA was administered (such as cerebrovascular disease or myocardial infarction) should be assigned first.

Code Z92.82 is only applicable to the receiving facility record and not to the transferring facility record.

Z93   Artificial opening status

Z94   Transplanted organ and tissue status

Z95   Presence of cardiac and vascular implants and grafts

Z96   Presence of other functional implants

Z97   Presence of other devices

Z98   Other postprocedural states

Assign code Z98.85, Transplanted organ removal status, to indicate that a transplanted organ has been previously removed. This code should not be assigned for the encounter in which the transplanted organ is removed. The complication necessitating removal of the transplant organ should be assigned for that encounter.
See section I.C19. for information on the coding of organ transplant complications.

Z99   Dependence on enabling machines and devices, not elsewhere classified

Note: Categories Z89-Z90 and Z93-Z99 are for use only if there are no complications or malfunctions of the organ or tissue replaced, the amputation site or the equipment on which the patient is dependent.

4)   History (of)

There are two types of history Z codes, personal and family. Personal history codes explain a patient's past medical condition that no longer exists and is not receiving any treatment, but that has the potential for recurrence, and therefore may require continued monitoring.

Family history codes are for use when a patient has a family member(s) who has had a particular disease that causes the patient to be at higher risk of also contracting the disease.

Personal history codes may be used in conjunction with follow-up codes and family history codes may be used in conjunction with screening codes to explain the need for a test or procedure. History codes are also acceptable on any medical record regardless of the reason for visit. A history of an illness, even if no longer present, is important information that may alter the type of treatment ordered.

The reason for the encounter (for example, screening or counseling)should be sequenced first and the appropriate personal and/or family history code(s) should be assigned as additional diagnos(es).

The history Z code categories are:

Z80   Family history of primary malignant neoplasm

Z81   Family history of mental and behavioral disorders

Z82   Family history of certain disabilities and chronic diseases (leading to disablement)

Z83   Family history of other specific disorders

Z84   Family history of other conditions

Z85   Personal history of malignant neoplasm

Z86   Personal history of certain other diseases

Z87   Personal history of other diseases and conditions

Z91.4-   Personal history of psychological trauma, not elsewhere classified

Z91.5   Personal history of self-harm

Z91.81   History of falling

Z91.82   Personal history of military deployment

Z92   Personal history of medical treatment

Except: Z92.0, Personal history of contraception Except: Z92.82, Status post administration of tPA (rtPA) in a different facility within the last 24 hours prior to admission to a current facility

5) Screening

Screening is the testing for disease or disease precursors in seemingly well individuals so that early detection and treatment can be provided for those who test positive for the disease (e.g., screening mammogram).

The testing of a person to rule out or confirm a suspected diagnosis because the patient has some sign or symptom is a diagnostic examination, not a screening. In these cases, the sign or symptom is used to explain the reason for the test.

A screening code may be a first-listed code if the reason for the visit is specifically the screening exam. It may also be used as an additional code if the screening is done during an office visit for other health problems. A screening code is not necessary if the screening is inherent to a routine examination, such as a pap smear done during a routine pelvic examination.

Should a condition be discovered during the screening then the code for the condition may be assigned as an additional diagnosis.

The Z code indicates that a screening exam is planned. A procedure code is required to confirm that the screening was performed.

The screening Z codes/categories:

Z11   Encounter for screening for infectious and parasitic diseases

Z12   Encounter for screening for malignant neoplasms

Z13   Encounter for screening for other diseases and disorders

        Except: Z13.9, Encounter for screening, unspecified

Z36   Encounter for antenatal screening for mother

6) Observation

There are three observation Z code categories. They are for use in very limited circumstances when a person is being observed for a suspected condition that is ruled out. The observation codes are not for use if an injury or illness or any signs or symptoms related to the suspected condition are present. In such cases the diagnosis/symptom code is used with the corresponding external cause code.

The observation codes are primarily to be used as a principal/first-listed diagnosis. An observation code may be assigned as a secondary diagnosis code when the patient is being observed for a condition that is ruled out and is unrelated to the principal/first-listed diagnosis (e.g., patient presents for treatment following injuries sustained in a motor vehicle accident and is also observed for suspected COVID-19 infection that is subsequently ruled out). Also, when the principal diagnosis is required to be a code from category Z38, Liveborn infants according to place of birth and type of delivery, then a code from category Z05, Encounter for observation and evaluation of newborn for suspected diseases and conditions ruled out, is sequenced after the Z38 code. Additional codes may be used in addition to the observation code, but only if they are unrelated to the suspected condition being observed.

Codes from subcategory Z03.7, Encounter for suspected maternal and fetal conditions ruled out, may either be used as a first-listed or as an additional code assignment depending on the case. They are for use in very limited circumstances on a maternal record when an encounter is for a suspected maternal or fetal condition that is ruled out during that encounter (for example, a maternal or fetal condition may be suspected due to an abnormal test result). These codes should not be used when the condition is confirmed. In those cases, the confirmed condition should be coded. In addition, these codes are not for use if an illness or any signs or symptoms related to the suspected condition or problem are present. In such cases the diagnosis/symptom code is used.

Additional codes may be used in addition to the code from subcategory Z03.7, but only if they are unrelated to the suspected condition being evaluated.

Codes from subcategory Z03.7 may not be used for encounters for antenatal screening of mother. *See Section I.C.21. Screening.*

● New code   ▲ Revised code   **Excludes1:** Not coded here   **Excludes2:** Not included here   ⊗ Placeholder required   ⑦7th digit required

For encounters for suspected fetal condition that are inconclusive following testing and evaluation, assign the appropriate code from category O35, O36, O40 or O41.

The observation Z code categories:

Z03   Encounter for medical observation for suspected diseases and conditions ruled out

Z04   Encounter for examination and observation for other reasons

          Except: Z04.9, Encounter for examination and observation for unspecified reason

Z05   Encounter for observation and evaluation of newborn for suspected diseases and conditions ruled out

7) Aftercare

Aftercare visit codes cover situations when the initial treatment of a disease has been performed and the patient requires continued care during the healing or recovery phase, or for the long-term consequences of the disease. The aftercare Z code should not be used if treatment is directed at a current, acute disease. The diagnosis code is to be used in these cases. Exceptions to this rule are codes Z51.0, Encounter for antineoplastic radiation therapy, and codes from subcategory Z51.1, Encounter for antineoplastic chemotherapy and immunotherapy. These codes are to be first-listed, followed by the diagnosis code when a patient's encounter is solely to receive radiation therapy, chemotherapy, or immunotherapy for the treatment of a neoplasm. If the reason for the encounter is more than one type of antineoplastic therapy, code Z51.0 and a code from subcategory Z51.1 may be assigned together, in which case one of these codes would be reported as a secondary diagnosis.

The aftercare Z codes should also not be used for aftercare for injuries. For aftercare of an injury, assign the acute injury code with the appropriate 7th character (for subsequent encounter).

The aftercare codes are generally first-listed to explain the specific reason for the encounter. An aftercare code may be used as an additional code when some type of aftercare is provided in addition to the reason for admission and no diagnosis code is applicable. An example of this would be the closure of a colostomy during an encounter for treatment of another condition.

Aftercare codes should be used in conjunction with other aftercare codes or diagnosis codes to provide better detail on the specifics of an aftercare encounter visit, unless otherwise directed by the classification. Should a patient receive multiple types of antineoplastic therapy during the same encounter, code Z51.0, Encounter for antineoplastic radiation therapy, and codes from subcategory Z51.1, Encounter for antineoplastic chemotherapy and immunotherapy, may be used together on a record. The sequencing of multiple aftercare codes depends on the circumstances of the encounter.

Certain aftercare Z code categories need a secondary diagnosis code to describe the resolving condition or sequelae. For others, the condition is included in the code title.

Additional Z code aftercare category terms include fitting and adjustment, and attention to artificial openings.

Status Z codes may be used with aftercare Z codes to indicate the nature of the aftercare. For example, code Z95.1, Presence of aortocoronary bypass graft, may be used with code Z48.812, Encounter for surgical aftercare following surgery on the circulatory system, to indicate the surgery for which the aftercare is being performed. A status code should not be used when the aftercare code indicates the type of status, such as using Z43.0, Encounter for attention to tracheostomy, with Z93.0, Tracheostomy status.

The aftercare Z category/codes:

Z42   Encounter for plastic and reconstructive surgery following medical procedure or healed injury

Z43   Encounter for attention to artificial openings

Z44   Encounter for fitting and adjustment of external prosthetic device

Z45   Encounter for adjustment and management of implanted device

Z46   Encounter for fitting and adjustment of other devices

Z47   Orthopedic aftercare

Z48   Encounter for other postprocedural aftercare

Z49   Encounter for care involving renal dialysis

Z51   Encounter for other aftercare and medical care

8) Follow-up

The follow-up codes are used to explain continuing surveillance following completed treatment of a disease, condition, or injury. They imply that the condition has been fully treated and no longer exists. They should not be confused with aftercare codes, or injury codes with a 7th character for subsequent encounter, that explain ongoing care of a healing condition or its sequelae. Follow-up codes may be used in conjunction with history codes to provide the full picture of the healed condition and its treatment. The follow-up code is sequenced first, followed by the history code.

A follow-up code may be used to explain multiple visits. Should a condition be found to have recurred on the follow-up visit, then the diagnosis code for the condition should be assigned in place of the follow-up code.

The follow-up Z code categories:

Z08   Encounter for follow-up examination after completed treatment for malignant neoplasm

Z09   Encounter for follow-up examination after completed treatment for conditions other than malignant neoplasm

Z39   Encounter for maternal postpartum care and examination

9) Donor

Codes in category Z52, Donors of organs and tissues, are used for living individuals who are donating blood or other body tissue. These codes are only for individuals donating for others, not for self-donations. They are not used to identify cadaveric donations.

10) Counseling

Counseling Z codes are used when a patient or family member receives assistance in the aftermath of an illness or injury, or when support is required in coping with family or social problems.

The counseling Z codes/categories:

Z30.0-   Encounter for general counseling and advice on contraception

Z31.5   Encounter for procreative genetic counseling

Z31.6-   Encounter for general counseling and advice on procreation

Z32.2   Encounter for childbirth instruction

Z32.3   Encounter for childcare instruction

Z69   Encounter for mental health services for victim and perpetrator of abuse

Z70   Counseling related to sexual attitude, behavior and orientation

Z71   Persons encountering health services for other counseling and medical advice, not elsewhere classified

Note: Code Z71.84, Encounter for health counseling related to travel, is to be used for health risk and safety counseling for future travel purposes.

Code Z71.85, Encounter for immunization safety counseling, is to be used for counseling of the patient or caregiver regarding the safety of a vaccine. This code should not be used for the provision of general information regarding risks and potential side effects during routine encounters for the administration of vaccines.

Z76.81   Expectant mother prebirth pediatrician visit

11) Encounters for Obstetrical and Reproductive Services

See Section I.C.15. Pregnancy, Childbirth, and the Puerperium, for further instruction on the use of these codes.
Z codes for pregnancy are for use in those circumstances when none of the problems or complications included in the codes from the Obstetrics chapter exist (a routine prenatal visit or postpartum care). Codes in category Z34, Encounter for supervision of normal pregnancy, are always first-listed and are not to be used with any other code from the OB chapter.

Codes in category Z3A, Weeks of gestation, may be assigned to provide additional information about the pregnancy. Category Z3A codes should not be assigned for pregnancies with abortive outcomes (categories O00-O08), elective termination of pregnancy (code Z33.2), nor for postpartum conditions, as category Z3A is not applicable to these conditions. The date of the admission should be used to determine weeks of gestation for inpatient admissions that encompass more than one gestational week.

The outcome of delivery, category Z37, should be included on all maternal delivery records. It is always a secondary code. Codes in category Z37 should not be used on the newborn record.

Z codes for family planning (contraceptive) or procreative management and counseling should be included on an obstetric record either during the pregnancy or the postpartum stage, if applicable.

Z codes/categories for obstetrical and reproductive services:

Z30   Encounter for contraceptive management

Z31   Encounter for procreative management

Z32.2   Encounter for childbirth instruction

Z32.3   Encounter for childcare instruction

Z33   Pregnant state

Z34   Encounter for supervision of normal pregnancy

Z36   Encounter for antenatal screening of mother

Z3A   Weeks of gestation

Z37   Outcome of delivery

Z39   Encounter for maternal postpartum care and examination

Z76.81   Expectant mother prebirth pediatrician visit

12) Newborns and Infants

See Section I.C.16. Newborn (Perinatal) Guidelines, for further instruction on the use of these codes.

Newborn Z codes/categories:

Z76.1   Encounter for health supervision and care of foundling

Z00.1-   Encounter for routine child health examination

Z38   Liveborn infants according to place of birth and type of delivery

13) Routine and administrative examinations

The Z codes allow for the description of encounters for routine examinations, such as, a general check-up, or examinations for administrative purposes, such as, a pre-employment physical. The codes are not to be used if the examination is for diagnosis of a suspected condition or for treatment purposes. In such cases the diagnosis code is used. During a routine exam, should a diagnosis or condition be discovered, it should be coded as an additional code. Pre-existing and chronic conditions and history codes may also be included as additional codes as long as the examination is for administrative purposes and not focused on any particular condition.

Some of the codes for routine health examinations distinguish between "with" and "without" abnormal findings. Code assignment depends on the information that is known at the time the encounter is being coded. For example, if no abnormal findings were found during the examination, but the encounter is being coded before test results are back, it is acceptable to assign the code for "without abnormal findings." When assigning a code for "with abnormal findings," additional code(s) should be assigned to identify the specific abnormal finding(s).

Pre-operative examination and pre-procedural laboratory examination Z codes are for use only in those situations when a patient is being cleared for a procedure or surgery and no treatment is given.

The Z codes/categories for routine and administrative examinations:

Z00   Encounter for general examination without complaint, suspected or reported diagnosis

Z01   Encounter for other special examination without complaint, suspected or reported diagnosis

Z02   Encounter for administrative examination

       Except: Z02.9, Encounter for administrative examinations, unspecified

Z32.0-   Encounter for pregnancy test

14) Miscellaneous Z codes

The miscellaneous Z codes capture a number of other health care encounters that do not fall into one of the other categories. Certain of these codes identify the reason for the encounter; others are for use as additional codes that provide useful information on circumstances that may affect a patient's care and treatment.

Prophylactic Organ Removal

For encounters specifically for prophylactic removal of an organ (such as prophylactic removal of breasts due to a genetic susceptibility to cancer or a family history of cancer), the principal or first-listed code should be a code from category Z40, Encounter for prophylactic surgery, followed by the appropriate codes to identify the associated risk factor (such as genetic susceptibility or family history).

If the patient has a malignancy of one site and is having prophylactic removal at another site to prevent either a new primary malignancy or metastatic disease, a code for the malignancy should also be assigned in addition to a code from subcategory Z40.0, Encounter for prophylactic surgery for risk factors related to malignant neoplasms. A Z40.0 code should not be assigned if the patient is having organ removal for treatment of a malignancy, such as the removal of the testes for the treatment of prostate cancer.

Miscellaneous Z codes/categories:

Z28   Immunization not carried out

       Except: Z28.3, Underimmunization status

Z29   Encounter for other prophylactic measures

Z40   Encounter for prophylactic surgery

● New code   ▲ Revised code   **Excludes1:** Not coded here   **Excludes2:** Not included here   ⊗ Placeholder required   ⑦7th digit required

Z41   Encounter for procedures for purposes other than remedying health state

        Except: Z41.9, Encounter for procedure for purposes other than remedying health state, unspecified

Z53   Persons encountering health services for specific procedures and treatment, not carried out

Z55   Problems related to education and literacy

Z56   Problems related to employment and unemployment

Z57   Occupational exposure to risk factors

Z58   Problems related to physical environment

Z59   Problems related to housing and economic circumstances

Z60   Problems related to social environment

Z62   Problems related to upbringing

Z63   Other problems related to primary support group, including family circumstances

Z64   Problems related to certain psychosocial circumstances

Z65   Problems related to other psychosocial circumstances

Z72   Problems related to lifestyle

        Note: These codes should be assigned only when the documentation specifies that the patient has an associated problem

Z73   Problems related to life management difficulty

Z74   Problems related to care provider dependency

        Except: Z74.01, Bed confinement status

Z75   Problems related to medical facilities and other health care

Z76.0   Encounter for issue of repeat prescription

Z76.3   Healthy person accompanying sick person

Z76.4   Other boarder to healthcare facility

Z76.5   Malingerer [conscious simulation]

Z91.1- Patient's noncompliance with medical treatment and regimen

Z91.83 Wandering in diseases classified elsewhere

Z91.84- Oral health risk factors

Z91.89 Other specified personal risk factors, not elsewhere classified

See Section I.B.14 for Z55-Z65 Persons with potential health hazards related to socioeconomic and psychosocial circumstances, documentation by clinicians other than the patient's provider

15) Nonspecific Z codes

Certain Z codes are so non-specific, or potentially redundant with other codes in the classification, that there can be little justification for their use in the inpatient setting. Their use in the outpatient setting should be limited to those instances when there is no further documentation to permit more precise coding. Otherwise, any sign or symptom or any other reason for visit that is captured in another code should be used.

Nonspecific Z codes/categories:

Z02.9   Encounter for administrative examinations, unspecified

Z04.9   Encounter for examination and observation for unspecified reason

Z13.9   Encounter for screening, unspecified

Z41.9   Encounter for procedure for purposes other than remedying health state, unspecified

Z52.9   Donor of unspecified organ or tissue

Z86.59   Personal history of other mental and behavioral disorders

Z88.9   Allergy status to unspecified drugs, medicaments and biological substances status

Z92.0   Personal history of contraception

16) Z Codes That May Only be Principal/First-Listed Diagnosis

The following Z codes/categories may only be reported as the principal/first-listed diagnosis, except when there are multiple encounters on the same day and the medical records for the encounters are combined:

Z00   Encounter for general examination without complaint, suspected or reported diagnosis Except: Z00.6

Z01   Encounter for other special examination without complaint, suspected or reported diagnosis

Z02   Encounter for administrative examination

Z03   Encounter for medical observation for suspected diseases and conditions ruled out

Z04   Encounter for examination and observation for other reasons

Z33.2   Encounter for elective termination of pregnancy

Z31.81   Encounter for male factor infertility in female patient

Z31.83   Encounter for assisted reproductive fertility procedure cycle

Z31.84   Encounter for fertility preservation procedure

Z34   Encounter for supervision of normal pregnancy

Z39   Encounter for maternal postpartum care and examination

Z38   Liveborn infants according to place of birth and type of delivery

Z40   Encounter for prophylactic surgery

Z42   Encounter for plastic and reconstructive surgery following medical procedure or healed injury

Z51.0   Encounter for antineoplastic radiation therapy

Z51.1-   Encounter for antineoplastic chemotherapy and immunotherapy

Z52   Donors of organs and tissues

Except: Z52.9, Donor of unspecified organ or tissue

Z76.1   Encounter for health supervision and care of foundling

Z76.2   Encounter for health supervision and care of other healthy infant and child

Z99.12   Encounter for respirator [ventilator] dependence during power failure

17) Social Determinants of Health

Codes describing social determinants of health (SDOH) should beassigned when this information is documented.

For social determinants of health, such as information found in categories Z55-Z65, Persons with potential health hazards related to socioeconomic and psychosocial circumstances, code assignment may bebased on medical record documentation from clinicians involved in the care of the patient who are not the patient's provider since this information represents social information, rather than medical diagnoses.For example, coding professionals may utilize documentation of social information from social workers, community health workers, case managers, or nurses, if their documentation is included in the official medical record.

Patient self-reported documentation may be used to assign codes for social determinants of health, as long as the patient self-reported information is signed-off by and incorporated into the medical record byeither a clinician or provider.

Social determinants of health codes are located primarily in these Z code categories:

Z55   Problems related to education and literacy

Z56   Problems related to employment and unemployment

Z57   Occupational exposure to risk factors

Z58   Problems related to physical environment

Z59   Problems related to housing and economic circumstances

Z60   Problems related to social environment

Z62   Problems related to upbringing

Z63   Other problems related to primary support group,including family circumstances

Z64   Problems related to certain psychosocial circumstances

Z65   Problems related to other psychosocial circumstances

See Section I.B.14. Documentation by Clinicians Other than thePatient's Provider.

Chapter 21

Factors Influencing Health Status and Contact with Health Services (Z00-Z99)

Note: Z codes represent reasons for encounters. A corresponding procedure code must accompany a Z code if a procedure is performed. Categories Z00-Z99 are provided for occasions when circumstances other than a disease, injury or external cause classifiable to categories A00-Y89 are recorded as 'diagnoses' or 'problems'. This can arise in two main ways: (a) When a person who may or may not be sick encounters the health services for some specific purpose, such as to receive limited care or service for a current condition, to donate an organ or tissue, to receive prophylactic vaccination (immunization), or to discuss a problem which is in itself not a disease or injury. (b) When some circumstance or problem is present which influences the person's health status but is not in itself a current illness or injury.

This chapter contains the following blocks:

Z00-Z13	Persons encountering health services for examinations
Z14-Z15	Genetic carrier and genetic susceptibility to disease
Z16	Resistance to antimicrobial drugs
Z17	Estrogen receptor status
Z18	Retained foreign body fragments
Z19	Hormone sensitivity malignancy status
Z20-Z29	Persons with potential health hazards related to communicable diseases
Z30-Z39	Persons encountering health services in circumstances related to reproduction
Z40-Z53	Encounters for other specific health care
Z55-Z65	Persons with potential health hazards related to socioeconomic and psychosocial circumstances
Z66	Do not resuscitate status
Z67	Blood type
Z68	Body mass index (BMI)
Z69-Z76	Persons encountering health services **in other** circumstances
Z77-Z99	Persons with potential health hazards related to family and personal history and certain conditions influencing health status

PERSONS ENCOUNTERING HEALTH SERVICES FOR EXAMINATIONS (Z00-Z13)

Note: Nonspecific abnormal findings disclosed at the time of these examinations are classified to categories R70-R94.

`Excludes1:` examinations related to pregnancy and reproduction (Z30-Z36, Z39.-)

`Z00` **Encounter for general examination without complaint, suspected or reported diagnosis**

`Excludes1:` encounter for examination for administrative purposes (Z02.-)

`Excludes2:` encounter for pre-procedural examinations (Z01.81-)

special screening examinations (Z11-Z13)

Z00.0 **Encounter for general adult medical examination**

Encounter for adult periodic examination (annual) (physical) and any associated laboratory and radiologic examinations

`Excludes1:` encounter for examination of sign or symptom-code to sign or symptom

general health check-up of infant or child (Z00.12.-)

Z00.00 **Encounter for general adult medical examination without abnormal findings**

Encounter for adult health check-up NOS

Z00.01 **Encounter for general adult medical examination with abnormal findings**

Use Additional Code to identify abnormal findings

Z00.1 **Encounter for newborn, infant and child health examinations**

Z00.11 **Newborn health examination**

Health check for child under 29 days old

Use Additional Code to identify any abnormal findings

`Excludes1:` health check for child over 28 days old (Z00.12-)

Z00.110 **Health examination for newborn under 8 days old**

Health check for newborn under 8 days old

Z00.111 **Health examination for newborn 8 to 28 days old**

Health check for newborn 8 to 28 days old Newborn weight check

Z00.12 **Encounter for routine child health examination**

Health check (routine) for child over 28 days old

Immunizations appropriate for age

Routine developmental screening of infant or child

Routine vision and hearing testing

`Excludes1:` health check for child under 29 days old (Z00.11-)

health supervision of foundling or other healthy infant or child (Z76.1-Z76.2)

newborn examination (Z00.11-)

Z00.121 **Encounter for routine child health examination with abnormal findings**

Use Additional Code to identify abnormal findings

Z00.129 **Encounter for routine child health examination without abnormal findings**

Encounter for routine child health examination NOS

Z00.2 **Encounter for examination for period of rapid growth in childhood**

Z00.3 **Encounter for examination for adolescent development state**

Encounter for puberty development state

Z00.5 **Encounter for examination of potential donor of organ and tissue**

Z00.6 **Encounter for examination for normal comparison and control in clinical research program**

Examination of participant or control in clinical research program

Z00.7 **Encounter for examination for period of delayed growth in childhood**

Z00.70 **Encounter for examination for period of delayed growth in childhood without abnormal findings**

Z00.71 **Encounter for examination for period of delayed growth in childhood with abnormal findings**

Use Additional Code to identify abnormal findings

Z00.8 **Encounter for other general examination**

Encounter for health examination in population surveys

`Z01` **Encounter for other special examination without complaint, suspected or reported diagnosis**

`Includes:` routine examination of specific system

Note: Codes from category Z01 represent the reason for the encounter. A separate procedure code is required to identify any examinations or procedures performed

Excludes1: encounter for examination for administrative purposes (Z02.-)

encounter for examination for suspected conditions, proven not to exist (Z03.-)

encounter for laboratory and radiologic examinations as a component of general medical examinations (Z00.0-)

encounter for laboratory, radiologic and imaging examinations for sign(s) and symptom(s) - code to the sign(s) or symptom(s)

Excludes2: screening examinations (Z11-Z13)

Z01.0   Encounter for examination of eyes and vision

Excludes1: examination for driving license (Z02.4)

Z01.00   Encounter for examination of eyes and vision without abnormal findings

Encounter for examination of eyes and vision NOS

Z01.01   Encounter for examination of eyes and vision with abnormal findings

Use Additional Code to identify abnormal findings

Z01.02 Encounter for examination of eyes and vision following failed vision screening

Excludes1: encounter for examination of eyes and vision with abnormal findings(Z01.01)

encounter for examination of eyes and vision without abnormal findings(Z01.00)

Z01.020 Encounter for examination of eyes and vision following failed vision screening without abnormal findings

Z01.021 Encounter for examination of eyes and vision following failed vision screening with abnormal findings

Use Additional Code to identify abnormal findings

Z01.1   Encounter for examination of ears and hearing

Z01.10   Encounter for examination of ears and hearing without abnormal findings

Encounter for examination of ears and hearing NOS

Z01.11   Encounter for examination of ears and hearing with abnormal findings

Z01.110   Encounter for hearing examination following failed hearing screening

Z01.118   Encounter for examination of ears and hearing with other abnormal findings

Use Additional Code to identify abnormal findings

Z01.12   Encounter for hearing conservation and treatment

Z01.2   Encounter for dental examination and cleaning

Z01.20   Encounter for dental examination and cleaning without abnormal findings

Encounter for dental examination and cleaning NOS

Z01.21   Encounter for dental examination and cleaning with abnormal findings

Use Additional Code to identify abnormal findings

Z01.3   Encounter for examination of blood pressure

Z01.30   Encounter for examination of blood pressure without abnormal findings

Encounter for examination of blood pressure NOS

Z01.31   Encounter for examination of blood pressure with abnormal findings

Use Additional Code to identify abnormal findings

Z01.4   Encounter for gynecological examination

Excludes2: pregnancy examination or test (Z32.0-)

routine examination for contraceptive maintenance (Z30.4-)

Z01.41   Encounter for routine gynecological examination

Encounter for general gynecological examination with or without cervical smear

Encounter for gynecological examination (general) (routine) NOS

Encounter for pelvic examination (annual) (periodic)

Use Additional Code:

for screening for human papillomavirus, if applicable, (Z11.51)

for screening vaginal pap smear, if applicable (Z12.72)

to identify acquired absence of uterus, if applicable (Z90.71-)

Excludes1: gynecologic examination status-post hysterectomy for malignant condition (Z08)

screening cervical pap smear not a part of a routine gynecological examination (Z12.4)

Z01.411   Encounter for gynecological examination (general) (routine) with abnormal findings

Use Additional Code to identify abnormal findings

Z01.419   Encounter for gynecological examination (general) (routine) without abnormal findings

Z01.42   Encounter for cervical smear to confirm findings of recent normal smear following initial abnormal smear

Z01.8   Encounter for other specified special examinations

Z01.81   Encounter for preprocedural examinations

Encounter for preoperative examinations

Encounter for radiological and imaging examinations as part of preprocedural examination

Z01.810   Encounter for preprocedural cardiovascular examination

Z01.811   Encounter for preprocedural respiratory examination

Z01.812   Encounter for preprocedural laboratory examination

Blood and urine tests prior to treatment or procedure

Z01.818   Encounter for other preprocedural examination

Encounter for preprocedural examination NOS

Encounter for examinations prior to antineoplastic chemotherapy

Z01.82   Encounter for allergy testing

Excludes1: encounter for antibody response examination (Z01.84)

Z01.83   Encounter for blood typing

Encounter for Rh typing

Z01.84   Encounter for antibody response examination

Encounter for immunity status testing

● New code   ▲ Revised code   **Excludes1:** Not coded here   **Excludes2:** Not included here   ⊗ Placeholder required   ⑦7th digit required

Excludes1: encounter for allergy testing (Z01.82)

Z01.89 **Encounter for other specified special examinations**

Z02 **Encounter for administrative examination**

Z02.0 **Encounter for examination for admission to educational institution**

Encounter for examination for admission to preschool (education)

Encounter for examination for re-admission to school following illness or medical treatment

Z02.1 **Encounter for pre-employment examination**

Z02.2 **Encounter for examination for admission to residential institution**

Excludes1: examination for admission to prison (Z02.89)

Z02.3 **Encounter for examination for recruitment to armed forces**

Z02.4 **Encounter for examination for driving license**

Z02.5 **Encounter for examination for participation in sport**

Excludes1: blood-alcohol and blood-drug test (Z02.83)

Z02.6 **Encounter for examination for insurance purposes**

Z02.7 **Encounter for issue of medical certificate**

Excludes1: encounter for general medical examination (Z00-Z01, Z02.0-Z02.6, Z02.8-Z02.9)

Z02.71 **Encounter for disability determination**

Encounter for issue of medical certificate of incapacity

Encounter for issue of medical certificate of invalidity

Z02.79 **Encounter for issue of other medical certificate**

Z02.8 **Encounter for other administrative examinations**

Z02.81 **Encounter for paternity testing**

Z02.82 **Encounter for adoption services**

Z02.83 **Encounter for blood-alcohol and blood-drug test**

Use Additional Code for findings of alcohol or drugs in blood (R78.-)

Z02.89 **Encounter for other administrative examinations**

Encounter for examination for admission to prison

Encounter for examination for admission to summer camp

Encounter for immigration examination

Encounter for naturalization examination

Encounter for premarital examination

Excludes1: health supervision of foundling or other healthy infant or child (Z76.1-Z76.2)

Z02.9 **Encounter for administrative examinations, unspecified**

Z03 **Encounter for medical observation for suspected diseases and conditions ruled out**

This category is to be used when a person without a diagnosis is suspected of having an abnormal condition, without signs or symptoms, which requires study, but after examination and observation, is ruled out. This category is also for use for administrative and legal observation status.

Excludes1: contact with and (suspected) exposures hazardous to health (Z77.-)

encounter for observation and evaluation of newborn for suspected diseases and conditions ruled out (Z05-)

person with feared complaint in whom no diagnosis is made (Z71.1) signs or symptoms under study- code to signs or symptoms

Z03.6 **Encounter for observation for suspected toxic effect from ingested substance ruled out**

Encounter for observation for suspected adverse effect from drug

Encounter for observation for suspected poisoning

Z03.7 **Encounter for suspected maternal and fetal conditions ruled out**

Encounter for suspected maternal and fetal conditions not found

Excludes1: known or suspected fetal anomalies affecting management of mother, not ruled out (O26.-, O35.-, O36.-, O40.-, O41.-)

Z03.71 **Encounter for suspected problem with amniotic cavity and membrane ruled out**

Encounter for suspected oligohydramnios ruled out

Encounter for suspected polyhydramnios ruled out

Z03.72 **Encounter for suspected placental problem ruled out**

Z03.73 **Encounter for suspected fetal anomaly ruled out**

Z03.74 **Encounter for suspected problem with fetal growth ruled out**

Z03.75 **Encounter for suspected cervical shortening ruled out**

Z03.79 **Encounter for other suspected maternal and fetal conditions ruled out**

Z03.8 **Encounter for observation for other suspected diseases and conditions ruled out**

Z03.81 **Encounter for observation for suspected exposure to biological agents ruled out**

Z03.810 **Encounter for observation for suspected exposure to anthrax ruled out**

Z03.818 **Encounter for observation for suspected exposure to other biological agents ruled out**

Z03.82 **Encounter for observation for suspected foreign body ruled out**

Excludes1: retained foreign body (Z18.-)

retained foreign body in eyelid (H02.81)

residual foreign body in soft tissue (M79.5)

Excludes2: confirmed foreign body ingestion or aspiration including:

foreign body in alimentary tract (T18)

foreign body in ear (T16)

foreign body on external eye (T15)

foreign body in respiratory tract (T17)

Z03.821 **Encounter for observation for suspected ingested foreign body ruled out**

Z03.822 **Encounter for observation for suspected aspirated (inhaled) foreign body ruled out**

Z03.823 **Encounter for observation for suspected inserted (injected) foreign body ruled out**

Encounter for observation for suspected inserted (injected) foreign body in eye ruled out

Encounter for observation for suspected inserted (injected) foreign body in orifice ruled out

Encounter for observation for suspected inserted (injected) foreign body in skin ruled out

Z03.89 **Encounter for observation for other suspected diseases and conditions ruled out**

Z04 **Encounter for examination and observation for other reasons**

Includes: encounter for examination for medicolegal reasons

This category is to be used when a person without a diagnosis is suspected of having an abnormal condition, without signs or symptoms, which requires study, but after examination and observation, is ruled-out. This category is also for use for administrative and legal observation status.

Z04.1 **Encounter for examination and observation following transport accident**

Excludes1: encounter for examination and observation following work accident (Z04.2)

Z04.2 **Encounter for examination and observation following work accident**

Z04.3 **Encounter for examination and observation following other accident**

Z04.4 **Encounter for examination and observation following alleged rape**

Encounter for examination and observation of victim following alleged rape

Encounter for examination and observation of victim following alleged sexual abuse

Z04.41 **Encounter for examination and observation following alleged adult rape**

Suspected adult rape, ruled out

Suspected adult sexual abuse, ruled out

Z04.42 **Encounter for examination and observation following alleged child rape**

Suspected child rape, ruled out

Suspected child sexual abuse, ruled out

Z04.6 **Encounter for general psychiatric examination, requested by authority**

Z04.7 **Encounter for examination and observation following alleged physical abuse**

Z04.71 **Encounter for examination and observation following alleged adult physical abuse**

Suspected adult physical abuse, ruled out

Excludes1: confirmed case of adult physical abuse (T74.-)

encounter for examination and observation following alleged adult sexual abuse (Z04.41)

suspected case of adult physical abuse, not ruled out (T76.-)

Z04.72 **Encounter for examination and observation following alleged child physical abuse**

Suspected child physical abuse, ruled out

Excludes1: confirmed case of child physical abuse (T74.-)

encounter for examination and observation following alleged child sexual abuse (Z04.42)

suspected case of child physical abuse, not ruled out (T76.-)

Z04.8 **Encounter for examination and observation for other specified reasons**

Encounter for examination and observation for request for expert evidence

Z04.81 **Encounter for examination and observation of victim following forced sexual exploitation**

Z04.82 **Encounter for examination and observation of victim following forced labor exploitation**

Z04.89 **Encounter for examination and observation for other specified reasons**

Z04.9 **Encounter for examination and observation for unspecified reason**

Encounter for observation NOS

Z05 **Encounter for observation and evaluation of newborn for suspected diseases and conditions ruled out**

This category is to be used for newborns, within the neonatal period (the first 28 days of life), who are suspected of having an abnormal condition, but without signs or symptoms, and which, after examination and observation, is ruled out.

Z05.0 **Observation and evaluation of newborn for suspected cardiac condition ruled out**

Z05.1 **Observation and evaluation of newborn for suspected infectious condition ruled out**

Z05.2 **Observation and evaluation of newborn for suspected neurological condition ruled out**

Z05.3 **Observation and evaluation of newborn for suspected respiratory condition ruled out**

Z05.4 **Observation and evaluation of newborn for suspected genetic, metabolic or immunologic condition ruled out**

Z05.41 **Observation and evaluation of newborn for suspected genetic condition ruled out**

Z05.42 **Observation and evaluation of newborn for suspected metabolic condition ruled out**

Z05.43 **Observation and evaluation of newborn for suspected immunologic condition ruled out**

Z05.5 **Observation and evaluation of newborn for suspected gastrointestinal condition ruled out**

Z05.6 **Observation and evaluation of newborn for suspected genitourinary condition ruled out**

Z05.7 **Observation and evaluation of newborn for suspected skin, subcutaneous, musculoskeletal and connective tissue condition ruled out**

Z05.71 **Observation and evaluation of newborn for suspected skin and subcutaneous tissue condition ruled out**

Z05.72 **Observation and evaluation of newborn for suspected musculoskeletal condition ruled out**

Z05.73 **Observation and evaluation of newborn for suspected connective tissue condition ruled out**

Z05.8 **Observation and evaluation of newborn for other specified suspected condition ruled out**

Z05.9 **Observation and evaluation of newborn for unspecified suspected condition ruled out**

Z08 **Encounter for follow-up examination after completed treatment for malignant neoplasm**

Medical surveillance following completed treatment

Use Additional Code to identify any acquired absence of organs (Z90.-)

Use Additional Code to identify the personal history of malignant neoplasm (Z85.-)

Excludes1: aftercare following medical care (Z43-Z49, Z51)

Z09 **Encounter for follow-up examination after completed treatment for conditions other than malignant neoplasm**

Medical surveillance following completed treatment

Use Additional Code to identify any applicable history of disease code (Z86.-. Z87.-)

Excludes1: aftercare following medical care (Z43-Z49, Z51)

surveillance of contraception (Z30.4-)

surveillance of prosthetic and other medical devices (Z44-Z46)

Z11 **Encounter for screening for infectious and parasitic diseases**

Screening is the testing for disease or disease precursors in asymptomatic individuals so that early detection and

treatment can be provided for those who test positive for the disease.

Excludes1: encounter for diagnostic examination-code to sign or symptom

Z11.0 **Encounter for screening for intestinal infectious diseases**

Z11.1 **Encounter for screening for respiratory tuberculosis**

Encounter for screening for active tuberculosis disease

Z11.2 **Encounter for screening for other bacterial diseases**

Z11.3 **Encounter for screening for infections with a predominantly sexual mode of transmission**

Excludes2: encounter for screening for human immunodeficiency virus [HIV] (Z11.4)

encounter for screening for human papillomavirus (Z11.51)

Z11.4 **Encounter for screening for human immunodeficiency virus [HIV]**

Z11.5 **Encounter for screening for other viral diseases**

Excludes2: encounter for screening for viral intestinal disease (Z11.0)

Z11.51 **Encounter for screening for human papillomavirus (HPV)**

Z11.59 **Encounter for screening for other viral diseases**

Z11.6 **Encounter for screening for other protozoal diseases and helminthiases**

Excludes2: encounter for screening for protozoal intestinal disease (Z11.0)

Z11.7 **Encounter for testing for latent tuberculosis infection**

Z11.8 **Encounter for screening for other infectious and parasitic diseases**

Encounter for screening for chlamydia

Encounter for screening for rickettsial

Encounter for screening for spirochetal

Encounter for screening for mycoses

Z11.9 **Encounter for screening for infectious and parasitic diseases, unspecified**

Z12 **Encounter for screening for malignant neoplasms**

Screening is the testing for disease or disease precursors in asymptomatic individuals so that early detection and

treatment can be provided for those who test positive for the disease.

Use Additional Code to identify any family history of malignant neoplasm (Z80.-)

Excludes1: encounter for diagnostic examination-code to sign or symptom

Z12.0 **Encounter for screening for malignant neoplasm of stomach**

Z12.1 **Encounter for screening for malignant neoplasm of intestinal tract**

Z12.10 **Encounter for screening for malignant neoplasm of intestinal tract, unspecified**

Z12.11 **Encounter for screening for malignant neoplasm of colon**

Encounter for screening colonoscopy NOS

Z12.12 **Encounter for screening for malignant neoplasm of rectum**

Z12.13 **Encounter for screening for malignant neoplasm of small intestine**

Z12.2 **Encounter for screening for malignant neoplasm of respiratory organs**

Z12.3 **Encounter for screening for malignant neoplasm of breast**

Z12.31 **Encounter for screening mammogram for malignant neoplasm of breast**

Excludes1: inconclusive mammogram (R92.2)

Z12.39 **Encounter for other screening for malignant neoplasm of breast**

Z12.4 **Encounter for screening for malignant neoplasm of cervix**

Encounter for screening pap smear for malignant neoplasm of cervix

Excludes1: when screening is part of general gynecological examination (Z01.4-)

Excludes2: encounter for screening for human papillomavirus (Z11.51)

Z12.5 **Encounter for screening for malignant neoplasm of prostate**

Z12.6 **Encounter for screening for malignant neoplasm of bladder**

Z12.7 **Encounter for screening for malignant neoplasm of other genitourinary organs**

Z12.71 **Encounter for screening for malignant neoplasm of testis**

Z12.72 **Encounter for screening for malignant neoplasm of vagina**

Vaginal pap smear status-post hysterectomy for non-malignant condition

Use Additional Code to identify acquired absence of uterus (Z90.71-)

Excludes1: vaginal pap smear status-post hysterectomy for malignant conditions (Z08)

Z12.73 **Encounter for screening for malignant neoplasm of ovary**

Z12.79 **Encounter for screening for malignant neoplasm of other genitourinary organs**

Z12.8 **Encounter for screening for malignant neoplasm of other sites**

Z12.81 **Encounter for screening for malignant neoplasm of oral cavity**

Z12.82 **Encounter for screening for malignant neoplasm of nervous system**

Z12.83 **Encounter for screening for malignant neoplasm of skin**

Z12.89 **Encounter for screening for malignant neoplasm of other sites**

Z12.9 **Encounter for screening for malignant neoplasm, site unspecified**

Z13 **Encounter for screening for other diseases and disorders**

Screening is the testing for disease or disease precursors in asymptomatic individuals so that early detection and treatment can be provided for those who test positive for the disease.

Excludes1: encounter for diagnostic examination-code to sign or symptom

Z13.0 **Encounter for screening for diseases of the blood and blood-forming organs and certain disorders involving the immune mechanism**

Z13.1 **Encounter for screening for diabetes mellitus**

Z13.2 **Encounter for screening for nutritional, metabolic and other endocrine disorders**

Z13.21 **Encounter for screening for nutritional disorder**

Z13.22 **Encounter for screening for metabolic disorder**

Z13.220 **Encounter for screening for lipoid disorders**

Encounter for screening for cholesterol level

Encounter for screening for hypercholesterolemia

Encounter for screening for hyperlipidemia

Z13.228 Encounter for screening for other metabolic disorders

Z13.29 Encounter for screening for other suspected endocrine disorder

Excludes2: encounter for screening for diabetes mellitus (Z13.1)

Z13.3 Encounter for screening examination for mental health and behavioral disorders

Z13.30 Encounter for screening examination for mental health and behavioral disorders, unspecified

Z13.31 Encounter for screening for depression

Encounter for screening for depression, adult

Encounter for screening for depression for child or adolescent

Z13.32 Encounter for screening for maternal depression

Encounter for screening for perinatal depression

Z13.39 Encounter for screening examination for other mental health and behavioral disorders

Encounter for screening for alcoholism

Encounter for screening for intellectual disabilities

Z13.4 Encounter for screening for certain developmental disorders in childhood

Encounter for screening for developmental handicaps in early childhood

Excludes2: encounter for routine child health examination (Z00.12-)

Z13.40 Encounter for screening for unspecified developmental delays

Z13.41 Encounter for autism screening

Z13.42 Encounter for screening for global developmental delays (milestones)

Encounter for screening for developmental handicaps in early childhood

Z13.49 Encounter for screening for other developmental delays

Z13.5 Encounter for screening for eye and ear disorders

Excludes2: encounter for general hearing examination (Z01.1-)

encounter for general vision examination (Z01.0-)

Z13.6 Encounter for screening for cardiovascular disorders

Z13.7 Encounter for screening for genetic and chromosomal anomalies

Excludes1: genetic testing for procreative management (Z31.4-)

Z13.71 Encounter for nonprocreative screening for genetic disease carrier status

Z13.79 Encounter for other screening for genetic and chromosomal anomalies

Z13.8 Encounter for screening for other specified diseases and disorders

Excludes2: screening for malignant neoplasms (Z12.-)

Z13.81 Encounter for screening for digestive system disorders

Z13.810 Encounter for screening for upper gastrointestinal disorder

Z13.811 Encounter for screening for lower gastrointestinal disorder

Excludes1: encounter for screening for intestinal infectious disease (Z11.0)

Z13.818 Encounter for screening for other digestive system disorders

Z13.82 Encounter for screening for musculoskeletal disorder

Z13.820 Encounter for screening for osteoporosis

Z13.828 Encounter for screening for other musculoskeletal disorder

Z13.83 Encounter for screening for respiratory disorder NEC

Excludes1: encounter for screening for respiratory tuberculosis (Z11.1)

Z13.84 Encounter for screening for dental disorders

Z13.85 Encounter for screening for nervous system disorders

Z13.850 Encounter for screening for traumatic brain injury

Z13.858 Encounter for screening for other nervous system disorders

Z13.88 Encounter for screening for disorder due to exposure to contaminants

Excludes1: those exposed to contaminants without suspected disorders (Z57.-, Z77.-)

Z13.89 Encounter for screening for other disorder

Encounter for screening for genitourinary disorders

Z13.9 Encounter for screening, unspecified

GENETIC CARRIER AND GENETIC SUSCEPTIBILITY TO DISEASE (Z14-Z15)

Z14 Genetic carrier

Definition: A genetic carrier is a person who has inherited a genetic trait or mutation but does not display that trait or show symptoms of the disease. Genetic carriers are, however, able to pass the gene onto their offspring, who may then express the gene.

Z14.0 Hemophilia A carrier

Z14.01 Asymptomatic hemophilia A carrier

Z14.02 Symptomatic hemophilia A carrier

Z14.1 Cystic fibrosis carrier

Z14.8 Genetic carrier of other disease

Z15 Genetic susceptibility to disease

Includes: confirmed abnormal gene

Use Additional Code, if applicable, for any associated family history of the disease (Z80-Z84)

Excludes1: chromosomal anomalies (Q90-Q99)

Z15.0 Genetic susceptibility to malignant neoplasm

Code first, if applicable, any current malignant neoplasm (C00-C75, C81-C96)

Use Additional Code, if applicable, for any personal history of malignant neoplasm (Z85.-)

Z15.01 Genetic susceptibility to malignant neoplasm of breast

Z15.02 Genetic susceptibility to malignant neoplasm of ovary

Z15.03 Genetic susceptibility to malignant neoplasm of prostate

Z15.04 Genetic susceptibility to malignant neoplasm of endometrium

Z15.09   Genetic susceptibility to other malignant neoplasm

Z15.8   **Genetic susceptibility to other disease**

Z15.81   Genetic susceptibility to multiple endocrine neoplasia [MEN]

Excludes1: multiple endocrine neoplasia [MEN] syndromes (E31.2-)

Z15.89   Genetic susceptibility to other disease

RESISTANCE TO ANTIMICROBIAL DRUGS (Z16)

Definition: An antimicrobial is an agent that kills microorganisms or inhibits their growth. Antimicrobial drugs can be grouped according to the microorganisms they act primarily against.

Z16   **Resistance to antimicrobial drugs**

Note: The codes in this category are provided for use as additional codes to identify the resistance and non-responsiveness of a condition to antimicrobial drugs.

Code first the infection

Excludes1: Methicillin resistant Staphylococcus aureus infection (A49.02)

Methicillin resistant Staphylococcus aureus infection in diseases classified elsewhere (B95.62)

Methicillin resistant Staphylococcus aureus pneumonia (J15.212)

Sepsis due to Methicillin resistant Staphylococcus aureus (A41.02)

Z16.1   **Resistance to beta lactam antibiotics**

Z16.10   Resistance to unspecified beta lactam antibiotics

Z16.11   Resistance to penicillins

Resistance to amoxicillin

Resistance to ampicillin

Z16.12   Extended spectrum beta lactamase (ESBL) resistance

Excludes2: Methicillin resistant Staphylococcus aureus infection in diseases classified elsewhere (B95.62)

Z16.19   Resistance to other specified beta lactam antibiotics

Resistance to cephalosporins

Z16.2   **Resistance to other antibiotics**

Z16.20   Resistance to unspecified antibiotic

Resistance to antibiotics NOS

Z16.21   Resistance to vancomycin

Z16.22   Resistance to vancomycin related antibiotics

Z16.23   Resistance to quinolones and fluoroquinolones

Z16.24   Resistance to multiple antibiotics

Z16.29   Resistance to other single specified antibiotic

Resistance to aminoglycosides

Resistance to macrolides

Resistance to sulfonamides

Resistance to tetracyclines

Z16.3   **Resistance to other antimicrobial drugs**

Excludes1: resistance to antibiotics (Z16.1-, Z16.2-)

Z16.30   Resistance to unspecified antimicrobial drugs

Drug resistance NOS

Z16.31   Resistance to antiparasitic drug(s)

Resistance to quinine and related compounds

Z16.32   Resistance to antifungal drug(s)

Z16.33   Resistance to antiviral drug(s)

Z16.34   Resistance to antimycobacterial drug(s)

Resistance to tuberculostatics

Z16.341   Resistance to single antimycobacterial drug

Resistance to antimycobacterial drug NOS

Z16.342   Resistance to multiple antimycobacterial drugs

Z16.35   Resistance to multiple antimicrobial drugs

Excludes1: Resistance to multiple antibiotics only (Z16.24)

Z16.39   Resistance to other specified antimicrobial drug

ESTROGEN RECEPTOR STATUS (Z17)

Z17   **Estrogen receptor status**

Code first malignant neoplasm of breast (C50.-)

Z17.0   **Estrogen receptor positive status [ER+]**

Z17.1   **Estrogen receptor negative status [ER-]**

RETAINED FOREIGN BODY FRAGMENTS (Z18)

Z18   **Retained foreign body fragments**

Includes: embedded fragment (status)

embedded splinter (status) retained foreign body status

Excludes1: artificial joint prosthesis status (Z96.6-)

foreign body accidentally left during a procedure (T81.5-)

foreign body entering through orifice (T15-T19)

in situ cardiac device (Z95.-)

organ or tissue replaced by means other than transplant (Z96.-, Z97.-)

organ or tissue replaced by transplant (Z94.-)

personal history of retained foreign body fully removed Z87.821

superficial foreign body (non-embedded splinter) - code to superficial foreign body, by site

Z18.0   **Retained radioactive fragments**

Z18.01   Retained depleted uranium fragments

Z18.09   Other retained radioactive fragments

Other retained depleted isotope fragments

Retained nontherapeutic radioactive fragments

Z18.1   **Retained metal fragments**

Excludes1: retained radioactive metal fragments (Z18.01-Z18.09)

Z18.10   Retained metal fragments, unspecified

Retained metal fragment NOS

Z18.11   Retained magnetic metal fragments

Z18.12   Retained nonmagnetic metal fragments

Z18.2   **Retained plastic fragments**

Acrylics fragments

Diethylhexyl phthalates fragments

Isocyanate fragments

Z18.3   Retained organic fragments

Z18.31   Retained animal quills or spines

Z18.32   Retained tooth

Z18.33   Retained wood fragments

Z18.39   Other retained organic fragments

Z18.8   **Other specified retained foreign body**

Z18.81   Retained glass fragments

Z18.83   Retained stone or crystalline fragments

Retained concrete or cement fragments

Z18.89   Other specified retained foreign body fragments

Z18.9   Retained foreign body fragments, unspecified material

HORMONE SENSITIVITY MALIGNANCY STATUS (Z19)

Z19   **Hormone sensitivity malignancy status**

Code first malignant neoplasm - see Table of Neoplasms, by site, malignant

Z19.1   **Hormone sensitive malignancy status**

Z19.2   **Hormone resistant malignancy status**

Castrate resistant prostate malignancy status

PERSONS WITH POTENTIAL HEALTH HAZARDS RELATED TO COMMUNICABLE DISEASES (Z20-Z29)

Z20   **Contact with and (suspected) exposure to communicable diseases**

Excludes1: carrier of infectious disease (Z22.-)

diagnosed current infectious or parasitic disease -see Alphabetic Index

Excludes2: personal history of infectious and parasitic diseases (Z86.1-)

Z20.0   **Contact with and (suspected) exposure to intestinal infectious diseases**

Z20.01   **Contact with and (suspected) exposure to intestinal infectious diseases due to Escherichia coli (E. coli)**

Z20.09   **Contact with and (suspected) exposure to other intestinal infectious diseases**

Z20.1   **Contact with and (suspected) exposure to tuberculosis**

Z20.2   **Contact with and (suspected) exposure to infections with a predominantly sexual mode of transmission**

Z20.3   **Contact with and (suspected) exposure to rabies**

Z20.4   **Contact with and (suspected) exposure to rubella**

Z20.5   **Contact with and (suspected) exposure to viral hepatitis**

Z20.6   **Contact with and (suspected) exposure to human immunodeficiency virus [HIV]**

Excludes1: asymptomatic human immunodeficiency virus [HIV]

HIV infection status (Z21)

Z20.7   **Contact with and (suspected) exposure to pediculosis, acariasis and other infestations**

Z20.8   **Contact with and (suspected) exposure to other communicable diseases**

Z20.81   **Contact with and (suspected) exposure to other bacterial communicable diseases**

Z20.810   **Contact with and (suspected) exposure to anthrax**

Z20.811   **Contact with and (suspected) exposure to meningococcus**

Z20.818   **Contact with and (suspected) exposure to other bacterial communicable diseases**

Z20.82   **Contact with and (suspected) exposure to other viral communicable diseases**

Z20.820   **Contact with and (suspected) exposure to varicella**

Z20.821   **Contact with and (suspected) exposure to Zika virus**

Z20.828   **Contact with and (suspected) exposure to other viral communicable diseases**

Z20.89   **Contact with and (suspected) exposure to other communicable diseases**

Z20.9   **Contact with and (suspected) exposure to unspecified communicable disease**

Z21   **Asymptomatic human immunodeficiency virus [HIV] infection status** [HCC]

HIV positive NOS

Code first Human immunodeficiency virus [HIV] disease complicating pregnancy, childbirth and the puerperium, if applicable (O98.7-)

Excludes1: acquired immunodeficiency syndrome (B20)

contact with human immunodeficiency virus [HIV] (Z20.6)

exposure to human immunodeficiency virus [HIV] (Z20.6)

human immunodeficiency virus [HIV] disease (B20)

inconclusive laboratory evidence of human immunodeficiency virus [HIV] (R75)

Z22   **Carrier of infectious disease**

Includes: colonization status

suspected carrier

Excludes2: carrier of viral hepatitis (B18.-)

Z22.0   **Carrier of typhoid**

Z22.1   **Carrier of other intestinal infectious diseases**

Z22.2   **Carrier of diphtheria**

Z22.3   **Carrier of other specified bacterial diseases**

Z22.31   **Carrier of bacterial disease due to meningococci**

Z22.32   **Carrier of bacterial disease due to staphylococci**

Z22.321   **Carrier or suspected carrier of Methicillin susceptible Staphylococcus aureus**

MSSA colonization

Z22.322   **Carrier or suspected carrier of Methicillin resistant Staphylococcus aureus**

MRSA colonization

Z22.33   **Carrier of bacterial disease due to streptococci**

Z22.330   **Carrier of Group B streptococcus**

Excludes1: Carrier of streptococcus group B (GBS) complicating pregnancy, childbirth and the puerperium (O99.82-)

Z22.338   **Carrier of other streptococcus**

Z22.39   **Carrier of other specified bacterial diseases**

Z22.4   **Carrier of infections with a predominantly sexual mode of transmission**

Z22.6   **Carrier of human T-lymphotropic virus type-1 [HTLV-1] infection**

Z22.7   **Latent tuberculosis**

Latent tuberculosis infection (LTBI)

Excludes1: nonspecific reaction to cell mediated immunity measurement of gamma interferon antigen response without active tuberculosis (R76.12)

nonspecific reaction to tuberculin skin test without active tuberculosis (R76.11)

Z22.8   **Carrier of other infectious diseases**

Z22.9   **Carrier of infectious disease, unspecified**

Z23   **Encounter for immunization**

Code first any routine childhood examination

Code also, if applicable, encounter for immunization safety counseling (Z71.85)

Note: procedure codes are required to identify the types of immunizations given

Z28   **Immunization not carried out and underimmunization status**

Code also, if applicable, encounter for immunization safety counseling (Z71.85)

Includes: vaccination not carried out

Z28.0 **Immunization not carried out because of contraindication**

Z28.01 **Immunization not carried out because of acute illness of patient**

Z28.02 **Immunization not carried out because of chronic illness or condition of patient**

Z28.03 **Immunization not carried out because of immune compromised state of patient**

Z28.04 **Immunization not carried out because of patient allergy to vaccine or component**

Z28.09 **Immunization not carried out because of other contraindication**

Z28.1 **Immunization not carried out because of patient decision for reasons of belief or group pressure**

Immunization not carried out because of religious belief

Z28.2 **Immunization not carried out because of patient decision for other and unspecified reason**

Z28.20 **Immunization not carried out because of patient decision for unspecified reason**

Z28.21 **Immunization not carried out because of patient refusal**

Z28.29 **Immunization not carried out because of patient decision for other reason**

Z28.3 **Underimmunization status**

Delinquent immunization status Lapsed immunization schedule status

Z28.8 **Immunization not carried out for other reason**

Z28.81 **Immunization not carried out due to patient having had the disease**

Z28.82 **Immunization not carried out because of caregiver refusal**

Immunization not carried out because of guardian refusal

Immunization not carried out because of parent refusal

Excludes1: immunization not carried out because of caregiver refusal because of religious belief (Z28.1)

Z28.83 **Immunization not carried out due to unavailability of vaccine**

Delay in delivery of vaccine

Lack of availability of vaccine

Manufacturer delay of vaccine

Z28.89 **Immunization not carried out for other reason**

Z28.9 **Immunization not carried out for unspecified reason**

Z29 **Encounter for other prophylactic measures**

Excludes1: desensitization to allergens (Z51.6)

prophylactic surgery (Z40.-)

Z29.1 **Encounter for prophylactic immunotherapy**

Encounter for administration of immunoglobulin

Z29.11 **Encounter for prophylactic immunotherapy for respiratory syncytial virus (RSV)**

Z29.12 **Encounter for prophylactic antivenin**

Z29.13 **Encounter for prophylactic Rho(D) immune globulin**

Z29.14 **Encounter for prophylactic rabies immune globin**

Z29.3 **Encounter for prophylactic fluoride administration**

Z29.8 **Encounter for other specified prophylactic measures**

Z29.9 **Encounter for prophylactic measures, unspecified**

PERSONS ENCOUNTERING HEALTH SERVICES IN CIRCUMSTANCES RELATED TO REPRODUCTION (Z30-Z39)

Z30 **Encounter for contraceptive management**

Z30.0 **Encounter for general counseling and advice on contraception**

Z30.01 **Encounter for initial prescription of contraceptives**

Excludes1: encounter for surveillance of contraceptives (Z30.4-)

Z30.011 **Encounter for initial prescription of contraceptive pills**

Z30.012 **Encounter for prescription of emergency contraception**

Encounter for postcoital contraception

Z30.013 **Encounter for initial prescription of injectable contraceptive**

Z30.014 **Encounter for initial prescription of intrauterine contraceptive device**

Excludes1: encounter for insertion of intrauterine contraceptive device (Z30.430, Z30.432)

Z30.015 **Encounter for initial prescription of vaginal ring hormonal contraceptive**

Z30.016 **Encounter for initial prescription of transdermal patch hormonal contraceptive device**

Z30.017 **Encounter for initial prescription of implantable subdermal contraceptive**

Z30.018 **Encounter for initial prescription of other contraceptives**

Encounter for initial prescription of barrier contraception

Encounter for initial prescription of diaphragm

Z30.019 **Encounter for initial prescription of contraceptives, unspecified**

Z30.02 **Counseling and instruction in natural family planning to avoid pregnancy**

Z30.09 **Encounter for other general counseling and advice on contraception**

Encounter for family planning advice NOS

Z30.2 **Encounter for sterilization**

Z30.4 **Encounter for surveillance of contraceptives**

Z30.40 **Encounter for surveillance of contraceptives, unspecified**

Z30.41 **Encounter for surveillance of contraceptive pills**

Encounter for repeat prescription for contraceptive pill

Z30.42 **Encounter for surveillance of injectable contraceptive**

Z30.43 **Encounter for surveillance of intrauterine contraceptive device**

Z30.430 **Encounter for insertion of intrauterine contraceptive device**

Z30.431 **Encounter for routine checking of intrauterine contraceptive device**

Z30.432 **Encounter for removal of intrauterine contraceptive device**

Z30.433 **Encounter for removal and reinsertion of intrauterine contraceptive device**

Encounter for replacement of intrauterine contraceptive device

Z30.44 Encounter for surveillance of vaginal ring hormonal contraceptive device

Z30.45 Encounter for surveillance of transdermal patch hormonal contraceptive device

Z30.46 Encounter for surveillance of implantable subdermal contraceptive

Encounter for checking, reinsertion or removal of implantable subdermal contraceptive

Z30.49 Encounter for surveillance of other contraceptives

Encounter for surveillance of barrier contraception

Encounter for surveillance of diaphragm

Z30.8 Encounter for other contraceptive management

Encounter for postvasectomy sperm count

Encounter for routine examination for contraceptive maintenance

Excludes1: sperm count following sterilization reversal (Z31.42)

sperm count for fertility testing (Z31.41)

Z30.9 Encounter for contraceptive management, unspecified

Z31 Encounter for procreative management

Excludes2: complications associated with artificial fertilization (N98.-)

female infertility (N97.-)

male infertility (N46.-)

Z31.0 Encounter for reversal of previous sterilization

Z31.4 Encounter for procreative investigation and testing

Excludes1: postvasectomy sperm count (Z30.8)

Z31.41 Encounter for fertility testing

Encounter for fallopian tube patency testing

Encounter for sperm count for fertility testing

Z31.42 Aftercare following sterilization reversal

Sperm count following sterilization reversal

Z31.43 Encounter for genetic testing of female for procreative management

Use Additional Code for recurrent pregnancy loss, if applicable (N96, O26.2-)

Excludes1: nonprocreative genetic testing (Z13.7-)

Z31.430 Encounter of female for testing for genetic disease carrier status for procreative management

Z31.438 Encounter for other genetic testing of female for procreative management

Z31.44 Encounter for genetic testing of male for procreative management

Excludes1: nonprocreative genetic testing (Z13.7-)

Z31.440 Encounter of male for testing for genetic disease carrier status for procreative management

Z31.441 Encounter for testing of male partner of patient with recurrent pregnancy loss

Z31.448 Encounter for other genetic testing of male for procreative management

Z31.49 Encounter for other procreative investigation and testing

Z31.5 Encounter for procreative genetic counseling

Z31.6 Encounter for general counseling and advice on procreation

Z31.61 Procreative counseling and advice using natural family planning

Z31.62 Encounter for fertility preservation counseling

Encounter for fertility preservation counseling prior to cancer therapy

Encounter for fertility preservation counseling prior to surgical removal of gonads

Z31.69 Encounter for other general counseling and advice on procreation

Z31.7 Encounter for procreative management and counseling for gestational carrier

Excludes1: pregnant state, gestational carrier (Z33.3)

Z31.8 Encounter for other procreative management

Z31.81 Encounter for male factor infertility in female patient

Z31.82 Encounter for Rh incompatibility status

Z31.83 Encounter for assisted reproductive fertility procedure cycle

Patient undergoing in vitro fertilization cycle

Use Additional Code to identify the type of infertility

Excludes1: pre-cycle diagnosis and testing - code to reason for encounter

Z31.84 Encounter for fertility preservation procedure

Encounter for fertility preservation procedure prior to cancer therapy

Encounter for fertility preservation procedure prior to surgical removal of gonads

Z31.89 Encounter for other procreative management

Z31.9 Encounter for procreative management, unspecified

Z32 Encounter for pregnancy test and childbirth and childcare instruction

Z32.0 Encounter for pregnancy test

Z32.00 Encounter for pregnancy test, result unknown

Encounter for pregnancy test NOS

Z32.01 Encounter for pregnancy test, result positive

Z32.02 Encounter for pregnancy test, result negative

Z32.2 Encounter for childbirth instruction

Z32.3 Encounter for childcare instruction

Encounter for prenatal or postpartum childcare instruction

Z33 Pregnant state

Z33.1 Pregnant state, incidental

Pregnancy NOS

Pregnant state NOS

Excludes1: complications of pregnancy (O00-O9A)

pregnant state, gestational carrier (Z33.3)

Z33.2 Encounter for elective termination of pregnancy

Excludes1: early fetal death with retention of dead fetus (O02.1)

late fetal death (O36.4) spontaneous abortion (O03)

Z33.3 Pregnant state, gestational carrier

Excludes1: encounter for procreative management and counseling for gestational carrier (Z31.7)

Z34 Encounter for supervision of normal pregnancy

Excludes1: any complication of pregnancy (O00-O9A)

encounter for pregnancy test (Z32.0-)

encounter for supervision of high-risk pregnancy (O09.-)

Z34.0 Encounter for supervision of normal first pregnancy

Z34.00 Encounter for supervision of normal first pregnancy, unspecified trimester

Z34.01 Encounter for supervision of normal first pregnancy, first trimester

Z34.02 Encounter for supervision of normal first pregnancy, second trimester

Z34.03 Encounter for supervision of normal first pregnancy, third trimester

Z34.8 Encounter for supervision of other normal pregnancy

    Z34.80 Encounter for supervision of other normal pregnancy, unspecified trimester

    Z34.81 Encounter for supervision of other normal pregnancy, first trimester

    Z34.82 Encounter for supervision of other normal pregnancy, second trimester

    Z34.83 Encounter for supervision of other normal pregnancy, third trimester

Z34.9 Encounter for supervision of normal pregnancy, unspecified

    Z34.90 Encounter for supervision of normal pregnancy, unspecified, unspecified trimester

    Z34.91 Encounter for supervision of normal pregnancy, unspecified, first trimester

    Z34.92 Encounter for supervision of normal pregnancy, unspecified, second trimester

    Z34.93 Encounter for supervision of normal pregnancy, unspecified, third trimester

Z36 Encounter for antenatal screening of mother

Includes: Encounter for placental sample (taken vaginally)

Screening is the testing for disease or disease precursors in asymptomatic individuals so that early detection and treatment can be provided for those who test positive for the disease.

Excludes1: diagnostic examination- code to sign or symptom

    encounter for suspected maternal and fetal conditions ruled out (Z03.7-)

    suspected fetal condition affecting management of pregnancy - code to condition in Chapter 15

Excludes2: abnormal findings on antenatal screening of mother (O28.-)

    genetic counseling and testing (Z31.43-, Z31.5)

    routine prenatal care (Z34)

Z36.0 Encounter for antenatal screening for chromosomal anomalies

Z36.1 Encounter for antenatal screening for raised alphafetoprotein level

    Encounter for antenatal screening for elevated maternal serum alphafetoprotein level

Z36.2 Encounter for other antenatal screening follow-up

    Non-visualized anatomy on a previous scan

Z36.3 Encounter for antenatal screening for malformations

    Screening for a suspected anomaly

Z36.4 Encounter for antenatal screening for fetal growth retardation

    Intrauterine growth restriction (IUGR)/small-for-dates

Z36.5 Encounter for antenatal screening for isoimmunization

Z36.8 Encounter for other antenatal screening

    Z36.81 Encounter for antenatal screening for hydrops fetalis

    Z36.82 Encounter for antenatal screening for nuchal translucency

    Z36.83 Encounter for fetal screening for congenital cardiac abnormalities

    Z36.84 Encounter for antenatal screening for fetal lung maturity

    Z36.85 Encounter for antenatal screening for Streptococcus B

    Z36.86 Encounter for antenatal screening for cervical length

        Screening for risk of pre-term labor

    Z36.87 Encounter for antenatal screening for uncertain dates

    Z36.88 Encounter for antenatal screening for fetal macrosomia

        Screening for large-for-dates

    Z36.89 Encounter for other specified antenatal screening

    Z36.8A Encounter for antenatal screening for other genetic defects

Z36.9 Encounter for antenatal screening, unspecified

Z3A Weeks of gestation

Note: Codes from category Z3A are for use, only on the maternal record, to indicate the weeks of gestation of the pregnancy, if known.

Code first obstetric condition or encounter for delivery (O09-O60, O80-O82)

Z3A.0 Weeks of gestation of pregnancy, unspecified or less than 10 weeks

    Z3A.00 Weeks of gestation of pregnancy not specified

    Z3A.01 Less than 8 weeks gestation of pregnancy

    Z3A.08 8 weeks gestation of pregnancy

    Z3A.09 9 weeks gestation of pregnancy

Z3A.1 Weeks of gestation of pregnancy, weeks 10-19

    Z3A.10 10 weeks gestation of pregnancy

    Z3A.11 11 weeks gestation of pregnancy

    Z3A.12 12 weeks gestation of pregnancy

    Z3A.13 13 weeks gestation of pregnancy

    Z3A.14 14 weeks gestation of pregnancy

    Z3A.15 15 weeks gestation of pregnancy

    Z3A.16 16 weeks gestation of pregnancy

    Z3A.17 17 weeks gestation of pregnancy

    Z3A.18 18 weeks gestation of pregnancy

    Z3A.19 19 weeks gestation of pregnancy

Z3A.2 Weeks of gestation of pregnancy, weeks 20-29

    Z3A.20 20 weeks gestation of pregnancy

    Z3A.21 21 weeks gestation of pregnancy

    Z3A.22 22 weeks gestation of pregnancy

    Z3A.23 23 weeks gestation of pregnancy

    Z3A.24 24 weeks gestation of pregnancy

    Z3A.25 25 weeks gestation of pregnancy

    Z3A.26 26 weeks gestation of pregnancy

    Z3A.27 27 weeks gestation of pregnancy

    Z3A.28 28 weeks gestation of pregnancy

    Z3A.29 29 weeks gestation of pregnancy

Z3A.3 Weeks of gestation of pregnancy, weeks 30-39

    Z3A.30 30 weeks gestation of pregnancy

    Z3A.31 31 weeks gestation of pregnancy

    Z3A.32 32 weeks gestation of pregnancy

    Z3A.33 33 weeks gestation of pregnancy

    Z3A.34 34 weeks gestation of pregnancy

    Z3A.35 35 weeks gestation of pregnancy

    Z3A.36 36 weeks gestation of pregnancy

    Z3A.37 37 weeks gestation of pregnancy

    Z3A.38 38 weeks gestation of pregnancy

    Z3A.39 39 weeks gestation of pregnancy

Z3A.4 Weeks of gestation of pregnancy, weeks 40 or greater

Z3A.40   **40 weeks gestation of pregnancy**

Z3A.41   **41 weeks gestation of pregnancy**

Z3A.42   **42 weeks gestation of pregnancy**

Z3A.49   **Greater than 42 weeks gestation of pregnancy**

Z37   **Outcome of delivery**

This category is intended for use as an additional code to identify the outcome of delivery on the mother's record. It is not for use on the newborn record.

Excludes1: stillbirth (P95)

Z37.0   **Single live birth**

Z37.1   **Single stillbirth**

Z37.2   **Twins, both liveborn**

Z37.3   **Twins, one liveborn and one stillborn**

Z37.4   **Twins, both stillborn**

Z37.5   **Other multiple births, all liveborn**

    Z37.50   **Multiple births, unspecified, all liveborn**

    Z37.51   **Triplets, all liveborn**

    Z37.52   **Quadruplets, all liveborn**

    Z37.53   **Quintuplets, all liveborn**

    Z37.54   **Sextuplets, all liveborn**

    Z37.59   **Other multiple births, all liveborn**

Z37.6   **Other multiple births, some liveborn**

    Z37.60   **Multiple births, unspecified, some liveborn**

    Z37.61   **Triplets, some liveborn**

    Z37.62   **Quadruplets, some liveborn**

    Z37.63   **Quintuplets, some liveborn**

    Z37.64   **Sextuplets, some liveborn**

    Z37.69   **Other multiple births, some liveborn**

Z37.7   **Other multiple births, all stillborn**

Z37.9   **Outcome of delivery, unspecified**

    Multiple birth NOS

Single birth NOS

Z38   **Liveborn infants according to place of birth and type of delivery**

This category is for use as the principal code on the initial record of a newborn baby. It is to be used for the initial birth record only. It is not to be used on the mother's record.

Z38.0   **Single liveborn infant, born in hospital**

    Single liveborn infant, born in birthing center **or other** health care facility

    Z38.00   **Single liveborn infant, delivered vaginally**

    Z38.01   **Single liveborn infant, delivered by cesarean**

Z38.1   **Single liveborn infant, born outside hospital**

Z38.2   **Single liveborn infant, unspecified as to place of birth**

    Single liveborn infant NOS

Z38.3   **Twin liveborn infant, born in hospital**

    Z38.30   **Twin liveborn infant, delivered vaginally**

    Z38.31   **Twin liveborn infant, delivered by cesarean**

Z38.4   **Twin liveborn infant, born outside hospital**

Z38.5   **Twin liveborn infant, unspecified as to place of birth**

Z38.6   **Other multiple liveborn infant, born in hospital**

    Z38.61   **Triplet liveborn infant, delivered vaginally**

    Z38.62   **Triplet liveborn infant, delivered by cesarean**

    Z38.63   **Quadruplet liveborn infant, delivered vaginally**

    Z38.64   **Quadruplet liveborn infant, delivered by cesarean**

    Z38.65   **Quintuplet liveborn infant, delivered vaginally**

    Z38.66   **Quintuplet liveborn infant, delivered by cesarean**

    Z38.68   **Other multiple liveborn infant, delivered vaginally**

    Z38.69   **Other multiple liveborn infant, delivered by cesarean**

Z38.7   **Other multiple liveborn infant, born outside hospital**

Z38.8   **Other multiple liveborn infant, unspecified as to place of birth**

Z39   **Encounter for maternal postpartum care and examination**

Z39.0   **Encounter for care and examination of mother immediately after delivery**

    Care and observation in uncomplicated cases when the delivery occurs outside a healthcare facility

    Excludes1: care for postpartum complication- see Alphabetic index

Z39.1   **Encounter for care and examination of lactating mother**

    Encounter for supervision of lactation

    Excludes1: disorders of lactation (O92.-)

Z39.2   **Encounter for routine postpartum follow-up**

ENCOUNTERS FOR OTHER SPECIFIC HEALTH CARE (Z40-Z53)

Categories Z40-Z53 are intended for use to indicate a reason for care. They may be used for patients who have already been treated for a disease or injury, but who are receiving aftercare or prophylactic care, or care to consolidate the treatment, or to deal with a residual state

Excludes2: follow-up examination for medical surveillance after treatment (Z08-Z09)

Z40   **Encounter for prophylactic surgery**

Excludes1: organ donations (Z52.-)

    therapeutic organ removal-code to condition

Z40.0   **Encounter for prophylactic surgery for risk factors related to malignant neoplasms**

    Admission for prophylactic organ removal

    Use Additional Code to identify risk factor

    Z40.00   **Encounter for prophylactic removal of unspecified organ**

    Z40.01   **Encounter for prophylactic removal of breast**

    Z40.02   **Encounter for prophylactic removal of ovary(s)**

      Encounter for prophylactic removal of ovary(s) and fallopian tube(s)

    Z40.03   **Encounter for prophylactic removal of Fallopian tube(s)**

    Z40.09   **Encounter for prophylactic removal of other organ**

Z40.8   **Encounter for other prophylactic surgery**

Z40.9   **Encounter for prophylactic surgery, unspecified**

Z41   **Encounter for procedures for purposes other than remedying health state**

Z41.1   **Encounter for cosmetic surgery**

    Encounter for cosmetic breast implant

    Encounter for cosmetic procedure

    Excludes1: encounter for plastic and reconstructive surgery following medical procedure or healed injury (Z42.-)

    encounter for post-mastectomy breast implantation (Z42.1)

Z41.2   **Encounter for routine and ritual male circumcision**

Z41.3   **Encounter for ear piercing**

Z41.8   **Encounter for other procedures for purposes other than remedying health state**

Z41.9   **Encounter for procedure for purposes other than remedying health state, unspecified**

Z42 **Encounter for plastic and reconstructive surgery following medical procedure or healed injury**

Excludes1: encounter for cosmetic plastic surgery (Z41.1)

encounter for plastic surgery for treatment of current injury - code to relevant injury

Z42.1 **Encounter for breast reconstruction following mastectomy**

Excludes1: deformity and disproportion of reconstructed breast (N65.1-)

Z42.8 **Encounter for other plastic and reconstructive surgery following medical procedure or healed injury**

Z43 **Encounter for attention to artificial openings**

Includes: closure of artificial openings

passage of sounds or bougies through artificial openings

reforming artificial openings

removal of catheter from artificial openings toilet or cleansing of artificial openings

Excludes1: complications of external stoma (J95.0-, K94.-, N99.5-)

Excludes2: artificial opening status only, without need for care (Z93.-)

fitting and adjustment of prosthetic and other devices (Z44-Z46)

Z43.0 **Encounter for attention to tracheostomy** [HCC]

Z43.1 **Encounter for attention to gastrostomy** [HCC]

Z43.2 **Encounter for attention to ileostomy**

Z43.3 **Encounter for attention to colostomy** [HCC]

Z43.4 **Encounter for attention to other artificial openings of digestive tract** [HCC]

Z43.5 **Encounter for attention to cystostomy** [HCC]

Z43.6 **Encounter for attention to other artificial openings of urinary tract** [HCC]

Encounter for attention to nephrostomy

Encounter for attention to ureterostomy

Encounter for attention to urethrostomy

Z43.7 **Encounter for attention to artificial vagina** [HCC]

Z43.8 **Encounter for attention to other artificial openings** [HCC]

Z43.9 **Encounter for attention to unspecified artificial opening** [HCC]

Z44 **Encounter for fitting and adjustment of external prosthetic device**

Includes: removal or replacement of external prosthetic device

Excludes1: malfunction **or other** complications of device - see Alphabetical Index

presence of prosthetic device (Z97.-)

Z44.0 **Encounter for fitting and adjustment of artificial arm**

Z44.00 **Encounter for fitting and adjustment of unspecified artificial arm**

Z44.001 **Encounter for fitting and adjustment of unspecified right artificial arm**

Z44.002 **Encounter for fitting and adjustment of unspecified left artificial arm**

Z44.009 **Encounter for fitting and adjustment of unspecified artificial arm, unspecified arm**

Z44.01 **Encounter for fitting and adjustment of complete artificial arm**

Z44.011 **Encounter for fitting and adjustment of complete right artificial arm**

Z44.012 **Encounter for fitting and adjustment of complete left artificial arm**

Z44.019 **Encounter for fitting and adjustment of complete artificial arm, unspecified arm**

Z44.02 **Encounter for fitting and adjustment of partial artificial arm**

Z44.021 **Encounter for fitting and adjustment of partial artificial right arm**

Z44.022 **Encounter for fitting and adjustment of partial artificial left arm**

Z44.029 **Encounter for fitting and adjustment of partial artificial arm, unspecified arm**

Z44.1 **Encounter for fitting and adjustment of artificial leg**

Z44.10 **Encounter for fitting and adjustment of unspecified artificial leg**

Z44.101 **Encounter for fitting and adjustment of unspecified right artificial leg** [HCC]

Z44.102 **Encounter for fitting and adjustment of unspecified left artificial leg** [HCC]

Z44.109 **Encounter for fitting and adjustment of unspecified artificial leg, unspecified leg** [HCC]

Z44.11 **Encounter for fitting and adjustment of complete artificial leg** [HCC],

Z44.111 **Encounter for fitting and adjustment of complete right artificial leg** [HCC]

Z44.112 **Encounter for fitting and adjustment of complete left artificial leg**

Z44.119 **Encounter for fitting and adjustment of complete artificial leg, unspecified leg** [HCC]

Z44.12 **Encounter for fitting and adjustment of partial artificial leg** [HCC]

Z44.121 **Encounter for fitting and adjustment of partial artificial right leg** [HCC]

Z44.122 **Encounter for fitting and adjustment of partial artificial left leg** [HCC]

Z44.129 **Encounter for fitting and adjustment of partial artificial leg, unspecified leg** [HCC]

Z44.2 **Encounter for fitting and adjustment of artificial eye**

Excludes1: mechanical complication of ocular prosthesis (T85.3)

Z44.20 **Encounter for fitting and adjustment of artificial eye, unspecified**

Z44.21 **Encounter for fitting and adjustment of artificial right eye**

Z44.22 **Encounter for fitting and adjustment of artificial left eye**

Z44.3 **Encounter for fitting and adjustment of external breast prosthesis**

Excludes1: complications of breast implant (T85.4-)

encounter for adjustment or removal of breast implant (Z45.81-)

encounter for initial breast implant insertion for cosmetic breast augmentation (Z41.1)

encounter for breast reconstruction following mastectomy (Z42.1)

Z44.30 **Encounter for fitting and adjustment of external breast prosthesis, unspecified breast**

Z44.31 **Encounter for fitting and adjustment of external right breast prosthesis**

Z44.32 **Encounter for fitting and adjustment of external left breast prosthesis**

Z44.8   Encounter for fitting and adjustment of other external prosthetic devices

Z44.9   Encounter for fitting and adjustment of unspecified external prosthetic device

Z45   Encounter for adjustment and management of implanted device

Includes: removal or replacement of implanted device

Excludes1: malfunction or other complications of device - see Alphabetical Index

Excludes2: encounter for fitting and adjustment of non-implanted device (Z46.-)

Z45.0   Encounter for adjustment and management of cardiac device

Z45.01   Encounter for adjustment and management of cardiac pacemaker

Encounter for adjustment and management of cardiac resynchronization therapy pacemaker (CRT-P)

Excludes1: encounter for adjustment and management of automatic implantable cardiac defibrillator with synchronous cardiac pacemaker (Z45.02)

Z45.010   Encounter for checking and testing of cardiac pacemaker pulse generator [battery]

Encounter for replacing cardiac pacemaker pulse generator [battery]

Z45.018   Encounter for adjustment and management of other part of cardiac pacemaker

Excludes1: presence of other part of cardiac pacemaker (Z95.0)

Excludes2: presence of prosthetic and other devices (Z95.1-Z95.5, Z95.811-Z97)

Z45.02   Encounter for adjustment and management of automatic implantable cardiac defibrillator

Encounter for adjustment and management of automatic implantable cardiac defibrillator with synchronous cardiac pacemaker

Encounter for adjustment and management of cardiac resynchronization therapy defibrillator (CRT-D)

Z45.09   Encounter for adjustment and management of other cardiac device

Z45.1   Encounter for adjustment and management of infusion pump

Z45.2   Encounter for adjustment and management of vascular access device

Encounter for adjustment and management of vascular catheters

Excludes1: encounter for adjustment and management of renal dialysis catheter (Z49.01)

Z45.3   Encounter for adjustment and management of implanted devices of the special senses

Z45.31   Encounter for adjustment and management of implanted visual substitution device

Z45.32   Encounter for adjustment and management of implanted hearing device

Excludes1: Encounter for fitting and adjustment of hearing aid (Z46.1)

Z45.320   Encounter for adjustment and management of bone conduction device

Z45.321   Encounter for adjustment and management of cochlear device

Z45.328   Encounter for adjustment and management of other implanted hearing device

Z45.4   Encounter for adjustment and management of implanted nervous system device

Z45.41   Encounter for adjustment and management of cerebrospinal fluid drainage device

Encounter for adjustment and management of cerebral ventricular (communicating) shunt

Z45.42   Encounter for adjustment and management of neurostimulator

Encounter for adjustment and management of brain neurostimulator

Encounter for adjustment and management of gastric neurostimulator

Encounter for adjustment and management of peripheral nerve neurostimulator

Encounter for adjustment and management of sacral nerve neurostimulator

Encounter for adjustment and management of spinal cord neurostimulator

Encounter for adjustment and management of vagus nerve neurostimulator

Z45.49   Encounter for adjustment and management of other implanted nervous system device

Z45.8   Encounter for adjustment and management of other implanted devices

Z45.81   Encounter for adjustment or removal of breast implant

Encounter for elective implant exchange (different material) (different size)

Encounter for removal of tissue expander with or without synchronous insertion of permanent implant

Excludes1: complications of breast implant (T85.4-)

encounter for initial breast implant insertion for cosmetic breast augmentation (Z41.1)

encounter for breast reconstruction following mastectomy (Z42.1)

Z45.811   Encounter for adjustment or removal of right breast implant

Z45.812   Encounter for adjustment or removal of left breast implant

Z45.819   Encounter for adjustment or removal of unspecified breast implant

Z45.82   Encounter for adjustment or removal of myringotomy device (stent) (tube)

Z45.89   Encounter for adjustment and management of other implanted devices

Z45.9   Encounter for adjustment and management of unspecified implanted device

Z46   Encounter for fitting and adjustment of other devices

Includes: removal or replacement of other device

Excludes1: malfunction or other complications of device - see Alphabetical Index

Excludes2: encounter for fitting and management of implanted devices (Z45.-)

issue of repeat prescription only (Z76.0)

presence of prosthetic and other devices (Z95-Z97)

Z46.0   Encounter for fitting and adjustment of spectacles and contact lenses

Z46.1   Encounter for fitting and adjustment of hearing aid

Excludes1: encounter for adjustment and management of implanted hearing device (Z45.32-)

Z46.2 Encounter for fitting and adjustment of other devices related to nervous system and special senses

> **Excludes2:** encounter for adjustment and management of implanted nervous system device (Z45.4-)
>
> encounter for adjustment and management of implanted visual substitution device (Z45.31)

Z46.3 Encounter for fitting and adjustment of dental prosthetic device

Encounter for fitting and adjustment of dentures

Z46.4 Encounter for fitting and adjustment of orthodontic device

Z46.5 Encounter for fitting and adjustment of other gastrointestinal appliance and device

> **Excludes1:** encounter for attention to artificial openings of digestive tract (Z43.1-Z43.4)

    Z46.51 Encounter for fitting and adjustment of gastric lap band

    Z46.59 Encounter for fitting and adjustment of other gastrointestinal appliance and device

Z46.6 Encounter for fitting and adjustment of urinary device

> **Excludes2:** attention to artificial openings of urinary tract (Z43.5, Z43.6)

Z46.8 Encounter for fitting and adjustment of other specified devices

    Z46.81 Encounter for fitting and adjustment of insulin pump

    Encounter for insulin pump instruction and training

    Encounter for insulin pump titration

    Z46.82 Encounter for fitting and adjustment of non-vascular catheter

    Z46.89 Encounter for fitting and adjustment of other specified devices

    Encounter for fitting and adjustment of wheelchair

Z46.9 Encounter for fitting and adjustment of unspecified device

Z47 Orthopedic aftercare

Excludes1: aftercare for healing fracture-code to fracture with 7th character D

Z47.1 Aftercare following joint replacement surgery

Use Additional Code to identify the joint (Z96.6-)

Z47.2 Encounter for removal of internal fixation device

> **Excludes1:** encounter for adjustment of internal fixation device for fracture treatment- code to fracture with appropriate 7th character
>
> encounter for removal of external fixation device- code to fracture with 7th character D infection or inflammatory reaction to internal fixation device (T84.6-)
>
> mechanical complication of internal fixation device (T84.1-)

Z47.3 Aftercare following explantation of joint prosthesis

Aftercare following explantation of joint prosthesis, staged procedure

Encounter for joint prosthesis insertion following prior explantation of joint prosthesis

    Z47.31 Aftercare following explantation of shoulder joint prosthesis

>   **Excludes1:** acquired absence of shoulder joint following prior explantation of shoulder joint prosthesis (Z89.23-)

shoulder joint prosthesis explantation status (Z89.23-)

    Z47.32 Aftercare following explantation of hip joint prosthesis

>   **Excludes1:** acquired absence of hip joint following prior explantation of hip joint prosthesis (Z89.62-)
>
>   hip joint prosthesis explantation status (Z89.62-)

    Z47.33 Aftercare following explantation of knee joint prosthesis

>   **Excludes1:** acquired absence of knee joint following prior explantation of knee prosthesis (Z89.52-
>
>   knee joint prosthesis explantation status (Z89.52-)

Z47.8 Encounter for other orthopedic aftercare

    Z47.81 Encounter for orthopedic aftercare following surgical amputation

    Use Additional Code to identify the limb amputated (Z89.-)

    Z47.82 Encounter for orthopedic aftercare following scoliosis surgery

    Z47.89 Encounter for other orthopedic aftercare

Z48 Encounter for other postprocedural aftercare

Excludes1: encounter for follow-up examination after completed treatment (Z08-Z09)

Excludes2: encounter for attention to artificial openings (Z43.-)

encounter for fitting and adjustment of prosthetic **and** other devices (Z44-Z46)

Z48.0 Encounter for attention to dressings, sutures and drains

> **Excludes1:** encounter for aftercare following injury - code to Injury, by site, with appropriate 7th character for subsequent encounter
>
> encounter for planned postprocedural wound closure (Z48.1)

    Z48.00 Encounter for change or removal of nonsurgical wound dressing

    Encounter for change or removal of wound dressing NOS

    Z48.01 Encounter for change or removal of surgical wound dressing

    Z48.02 Encounter for removal of sutures

    Encounter for removal of staples

    Z48.03 Encounter for change or removal of drains

Z48.1 Encounter for planned postprocedural wound closure

> **Excludes1:** encounter for attention to dressings and sutures (Z48.0-)

Z48.2 Encounter for aftercare following organ transplant

    Z48.21 Encounter for aftercare following heart transplant [HCC]

    Z48.22 Encounter for aftercare following kidney transplant

    Z48.23 Encounter for aftercare following liver transplant [HCC]

    Z48.24 Encounter for aftercare following lung transplant [HCC]

    Z48.28 Encounter for aftercare following multiple organ transplant

      Z48.280 Encounter for aftercare following heart-lung transplant [HCC]

Z48.288 Encounter for aftercare following multiple organ transplant

Z48.29 Encounter for aftercare following other organ transplant

Z48.290 Encounter for aftercare following bone marrow transplant [HCC]

Z48.298 Encounter for aftercare following other organ transplant

Z48.3 Aftercare following surgery for neoplasm

Use Additional Code to identify the neoplasm

Z48.8 Encounter for other specified postprocedural aftercare

Z48.81 Encounter for surgical aftercare following surgery on specified body systems

These codes identify the body system requiring aftercare. They are for use in conjunction with other aftercare codes to fully explain the aftercare encounter. The condition treated should also be coded if still present.

Excludes1: aftercare for injury- code the injury with 7th character D

aftercare following surgery for neoplasm (Z48.3)

Excludes2: aftercare following organ transplant (Z48.2-)

orthopedic aftercare (Z47.-)

Z48.810 Encounter for surgical aftercare following surgery on the sense organs

Z48.811 Encounter for surgical aftercare following surgery on the nervous system

Excludes2: encounter for surgical aftercare following surgery on the sense organs (Z48.810)

Z48.812 Encounter for surgical aftercare following surgery on the circulatory system

Z48.813 Encounter for surgical aftercare following surgery on the respiratory system

Z48.814 Encounter for surgical aftercare following surgery on the teeth or oral cavity

Z48.815 Encounter for surgical aftercare following surgery on the digestive system

Z48.816 Encounter for surgical aftercare following surgery on the genitourinary system

Excludes1: encounter for aftercare following sterilization reversal (Z31.42)

Z48.817 Encounter for surgical aftercare following surgery on the skin and subcutaneous tissue

Z48.89 Encounter for other specified surgical aftercare

Z49 Encounter for care involving renal dialysis

Code also associated end stage renal disease (N18.6)

Z49.0 Preparatory care for renal dialysis

Encounter for dialysis instruction and training

Z49.01 Encounter for fitting and adjustment of extracorporeal dialysis catheter [HCC]

Removal or replacement of renal dialysis catheter

Toilet or cleansing of renal dialysis catheter

Z49.02 Encounter for fitting and adjustment of peritoneal dialysis catheter [HCC]

Z49.3 Encounter for adequacy testing for dialysis

Z49.31 Encounter for adequacy testing for hemodialysis [HCC]

Z49.32 Encounter for adequacy testing for peritoneal dialysis [HCC]

Encounter for peritoneal equilibration test

Z51 Encounter for other aftercare and medical care

Code also condition requiring care

Excludes1: follow-up examination after treatment (Z08-Z09)

Z51.0 Encounter for antineoplastic radiation therapy

Z51.1 Encounter for antineoplastic chemotherapy and immunotherapy

Excludes2: encounter for chemotherapy and immunotherapy for nonneoplastic condition - code to condition

Z51.11 Encounter for antineoplastic chemotherapy

Z51.12 Encounter for antineoplastic immunotherapy

Z51.5 Encounter for palliative care

Z51.6 Encounter for desensitization to allergens

Z51.8 Encounter for other specified aftercare

Excludes1: holiday relief care (Z75.5)

Z51.81 Encounter for therapeutic drug level monitoring

Code also any long-term (current) drug therapy (Z79.-)

Excludes1: encounter for blood-drug test for administrative or medicolegal reasons (Z02.83)

Z51.89 Encounter for other specified aftercare

Z52 Donors of organs and tissues

Includes: autologous and other living donors

Excludes1: cadaveric donor - omit code

examination of potential donor (Z00.5)

Z52.0 Blood donor

Z52.00 Unspecified blood donor

Z52.000 Unspecified donor, whole blood

Z52.001 Unspecified donor, stem cells

Z52.008 Unspecified donor, other blood

Z52.01 Autologous blood donor

Z52.010 Autologous donor, whole blood

Z52.011 Autologous donor, stem cells

Z52.018 Autologous donor, other blood

Z52.09 Other blood donor Volunteer donor

Z52.090 Other blood donor, whole blood

Z52.091 Other blood donor, stem cells

Z52.098 Other blood donor, other blood

Z52.1 Skin donor

Z52.10 Skin donor, unspecified

Z52.11 Skin donor, autologous

Z52.19 Skin donor, other

Z52.2 Bone donor

Z52.20 Bone donor, unspecified

Z52.21 Bone donor, autologous

Z52.29 Bone donor, other

Z52.3 Bone marrow donor

Z52.4 Kidney donor

Z52.5 Cornea donor

Z52.6 Liver donor

Z52.8   **Donor of other specified organs or tissues**

     Z52.81   **Egg (Oocyte) donor**

        Z52.810   **Egg (Oocyte) donor under age 35, anonymous recipient**

           Egg donor under age 35 NOS

        Z52.811   **Egg (Oocyte) donor under age 35, designated recipient**

        Z52.812   **Egg (Oocyte) donor age 35 and over, anonymous recipient**

           Egg donor age 35 and over NOS

        Z52.813   **Egg (Oocyte) donor age 35 and over, designated recipient**

        Z52.819   **Egg (Oocyte) donor, unspecified**

     Z52.89   **Donor of other specified organs or tissues**

Z52.9   **Donor of unspecified organ or tissue**

     Donor NOS

Z53   **Persons encountering health services for specific procedures and treatment, not carried out**

Z53.0   **Procedure and treatment not carried out because of contraindication**

     Z53.01   **Procedure and treatment not carried out due to patient smoking**

     Z53.09   **Procedure and treatment not carried out because of other contraindication**

Z53.1   **Procedure and treatment not carried out because of patient's decision for reasons of belief and group pressure**

Z53.2   **Procedure and treatment not carried out because of patient's decision for other and unspecified reasons**

     Z53.20   **Procedure and treatment not carried out because of patient's decision for unspecified reasons**

     Z53.21   **Procedure and treatment not carried out due to patient leaving prior to being seen by health care provider**

     Z53.29   **Procedure and treatment not carried out because of patient's decision for other reasons**

Z53.3   **Procedure converted to open procedure**

     Z53.31   **Laparoscopic surgical procedure converted to open procedure**

     Z53.32   **Thoracoscopic surgical procedure converted to open procedure**

     Z53.33   **Arthroscopic surgical procedure converted to open procedure**

     Z53.39   **Other specified procedure converted to open procedure**

Z53.8   **Procedure and treatment not carried out for other reasons**

Z53.9   **Procedure and treatment not carried out, unspecified reason**

PERSONS WITH POTENTIAL HEALTH HAZARDS RELATED TO SOCIOECONOMIC AND PSYCHOSOCIAL CIRCUMSTANCES (Z55-Z65)

Z55   **Problems related to education and literacy**

     Excludes1: disorders of psychological development (F80-F89)

Z55.0   **Illiteracy and low-level literacy**

Z55.1   **Schooling unavailable and unattainable**

Z55.2   **Failed school examinations**

Z55.3   **Underachievement in school**

Z55.4   **Educational maladjustment and discord with teachers and classmates**

• Z55.5   **Less than a high school diploma**

     No general equivalence degree (GED)

Z55.8   **Other problems related to education and literacy**

     Problems related to inadequate teaching

Z55.9   **Problems related to education and literacy, unspecified**

     Academic problems NOS

Z56   **Problems related to employment and unemployment**

     occupational exposure to risk factors (Z57.-)

     problems related to housing and economic circumstances (Z59.-)

Z56.0   **Unemployment, unspecified**

Z56.1   **Change of job**

Z56.2   **Threat of job loss**

Z56.3   **Stressful work schedule**

Z56.4   **Discord with boss and workmates**

Z56.5   **Uncongenial work environment**

     Difficult conditions at work

Z56.6   **Other physical and mental strain related to work**

Z56.8   **Other problems related to employment**

     Z56.81   **Sexual harassment on the job**

     Z56.82   **Military deployment status**

        Individual (civilian or military) currently deployed in theater or in support of military war, peacekeeping and humanitarian operations

     Z56.89   **Other problems related to employment**

Z56.9   **Unspecified problems related to employment**

     Occupational problems NOS

Z57   **Occupational exposure to risk factors**

Z57.0   **Occupational exposure to noise**

Z57.1   **Occupational exposure to radiation**

Z57.2   **Occupational exposure to dust**

Z57.3   **Occupational exposure to other air contaminants**

     Z57.31   **Occupational exposure to environmental tobacco smoke**

        exposure to environmental tobacco smoke (Z77.22)

     Z57.39   **Occupational exposure to other air contaminants**

Z57.4   **Occupational exposure to toxic agents in agriculture**

     Occupational exposure to solids, liquids, gases or vapors in agriculture

Z57.5   **Occupational exposure to toxic agents in other industries**

     Occupational exposure to solids, liquids, gases or vapors in other industries

Z57.6   **Occupational exposure to extreme temperature**

Z57.7   **Occupational exposure to vibration**

Z57.8   **Occupational exposure to other risk factors**

Z57.9   **Occupational exposure to unspecified risk factor**

• **Z58**   **Problems related to physical environment**

     occupational exposure (Z57.-)

• Z58.6   **Inadequate drinking-water supply**

     Lack of safe drinking water

        deprivation of water (T73.1)

Z59   **Problems related to housing and economic circumstances**

     problems related to upbringing (Z62.-)

• Z59.0   **Homelessness**

     • Z59.00   **Homelessness unspecified**

     • Z59.01   **Sheltered homelessness**

        Doubled up

Living in a shelter such as: motel, scattered site housing, temporary or transitional living situation

- **Z59.02 Unsheltered homelessness**

    Residing in place not meant for human habitation such as: abandoned buildings, cars, parks, sidewalk

    Residing on the street

Z59.1 Inadequate housing

Lack of heating

Restriction of space

Technical defects in home preventing adequate care

Unsatisfactory surroundings

Excludes1: problems related to the natural and physical environment (Z77.1-)

Z59.2 Discord with neighbors, lodgers and landlord

Z59.3 Problems related to living in residential institution

Boarding-school resident

Excludes1: institutional upbringing (Z62.2)

Z59.4 Lack of adequate food

Excludes2: deprivation of food (T73.0)

    effects of hunger (T73.0)

    inappropriate diet or eating habits (Z72.4)

    malnutrition (E40-E46)

- **Z59.41 Food insecurity**

- **Z59.48 Other specified lack of adequate food**

    Inadequate food

    Lack of food

Z59.5 Extreme poverty

Z59.6 Low income

Z59.7 Insufficient social insurance and welfare support

Z59.8 Other problems related to housing and economic circumstances

- **Z59.81 Housing instability, housed**

    Foreclosure on home loan

    Past due on rent or mortgage

    Unwanted multiple moves in the last 12 months

    - **Z59.811 Housing instability, housed, with risk of homelessness**

        Imminent risk of homelessness

    - **Z59.812 Housing instability, housed, homelessness in past 12 months**

    - **Z59.819 Housing instability, housed unspecified**

- **Z59.89 Other problems related to housing and economic circumstances**

    Foreclosure on loan

    Isolated dwelling

    Problems with creditors

Z59.9 Problem related to housing and economic circumstances, unspecified

Z60 Problems related to social environment

Z60.0 Problems of adjustment to life-cycle transitions

Empty nest syndrome

Phase of life problem

Problem with adjustment to retirement [pension]

Z60.2 Problems related to living alone

Z60.3 Acculturation difficulty

Problem with migration

Problem with social transplantation

Z60.4 Social exclusion and rejection

Exclusion and rejection on the basis of personal characteristics, such as unusual physical appearance, illness or behavior.

Excludes1: target of adverse discrimination such as for racial or religious reasons (Z60.5)

Z60.5 Target of (perceived) adverse discrimination and persecution

Excludes1: social exclusion and rejection (Z60.4)

Z60.8 Other problems related to social environment

Z60.9 Problem related to social environment, unspecified

Z62 Problems related to upbringing

Includes: current and past negative life events in childhood

current and past problems of a child related to upbringing

Excludes2: maltreatment syndrome (T74.-)

    problems related to housing and economic circumstances (Z59.-)

Z62.0 Inadequate parental supervision and control

Z62.1 Parental overprotection

Z62.2 Upbringing away from parents

Excludes1: problems with boarding school (Z59.3)

- **Z62.21 Child in welfare custody**

    Child in care of non-parental family member

    Child in foster care

    Excludes2: problem for parent due to child in welfare custody (Z63.5)

- **Z62.22 Institutional upbringing**

    Child living in orphanage or group home

- **Z62.29 Other upbringing away from parents**

Z62.3 Hostility towards and scapegoating of child

Z62.6 Inappropriate (excessive) parental pressure

Z62.8 Other specified problems related to upbringing

- **Z62.81 Personal history of abuse in childhood**

    - **Z62.810 Personal history of physical and sexual abuse in childhood**

        Excludes1: current child physical abuse (T74.12, T76.12)

        current child sexual abuse (T74.22, T76.22)

    - **Z62.811 Personal history of psychological abuse in childhood**

        Excludes1: current child psychological abuse (T74.32, T76.32)

    - **Z62.812 Personal history of neglect in childhood**

        Excludes1: current child neglect (T74.02, T76.02)

    - **Z62.813 Personal history of forced labor or sexual exploitation in childhood**

    - **Z62.819 Personal history of unspecified abuse in childhood**

        Excludes1: current child abuse NOS (T74.92, T76.92)

- **Z62.82 Parent-child conflict**

    - **Z62.820 Parent-biological child conflict**

        Parent-child problem NOS

    - **Z62.821 Parent-adopted child conflict**

    - **Z62.822 Parent-foster child conflict**

● New code ▲ Revised code **Excludes1:** Not coded here **Excludes2:** Not included here ⊗ Placeholder required ⑦ 7th digit required

Z62.89   Other specified problems related to upbringing

    Z62.890   Parent-child estrangement NEC

    Z62.891   Sibling rivalry

    Z62.898   Other specified problems related to upbringing

Z62.9   Problem related to upbringing, unspecified

Z63   Other problems related to primary support group, including family circumstances

Excludes2: maltreatment syndrome (T74.-, T76)

parent-child problems (Z62.-)

problems related to negative life events in childhood (Z62.-)

problems related to upbringing (Z62.-)

Z63.0   **Problems in relationship with spouse or partner**

Relationship distress with spouse or intimate partner

Excludes1: counseling for spousal or partner abuse problems (Z69.1)

counseling related to sexual attitude, behavior, and orientation (Z70.-)

Z63.1   **Problems in relationship with in-laws**

Z63.3   **Absence of family member**

Excludes1: absence of family member due to disappearance and death (Z63.4)

absence of family member due to separation and divorce (Z63.5)

    Z63.31   **Absence of family member due to military deployment**

Individual or family affected by other family member being on military deployment

Excludes1: family disruption due to return of family member from military deployment (Z63.71)

    Z63.32   **Other absence of family member**

Z63.4   **Disappearance and death of family member**

Assumed death of family member

Bereavement

Z63.5   **Disruption of family by separation and divorce**

Marital estrangement

Z63.6   **Dependent relative needing care at home**

Z63.7   **Other stressful life events affecting family and household**

    Z63.71   **Stress on family due to return of family member from military deployment**

Individual or family affected by family member having returned from military deployment (current or past conflict)

    Z63.72   **Alcoholism and drug addiction in family**

    Z63.79   **Other stressful life events affecting family and household**

Anxiety (normal) about sick person in family

Health problems within family

Ill or disturbed family member

Isolated family

Z63.8   **Other specified problems related to primary support group**

Family discord NOS Family estrangement NOS

High expressed emotional level within family

Inadequate family support NOS

Inadequate or distorted communication within family

Z63.9   **Problem related to primary support group, unspecified**

Relationship disorder NOS

Z64   Problems related to certain psychosocial circumstances

Z64.0   **Problems related to unwanted pregnancy**

Z64.1   **Problems related to multiparity**

Z64.4   **Discord with counselors**

Discord with probation officer

Discord with social worker

Z65   Problems related to other psychosocial circumstances

Z65.0   **Conviction in civil and criminal proceedings without imprisonment**

Z65.1   **Imprisonment and other incarceration**

Z65.2   **Problems related to release from prison**

Z65.3   **Problems related to other legal circumstances**

Arrest

Child custody or support proceedings Litigation

Prosecution

Z65.4   **Victim of crime and terrorism**

Victim of torture

Z65.5   **Exposure to disaster, war and other hostilities**

Excludes1: target of perceived discrimination or persecution (Z60.5)

Z65.8   **Other specified problems related to psychosocial circumstances**

Religious or spiritual problem

Z65.9   **Problem related to unspecified psychosocial circumstances**

DO NOT RESUSCITATE STATUS (Z66)

Z66   Do not resuscitate

DNR status

BLOOD TYPE (Z67)

Z67   Blood type

Z67.1   **Type A blood**

    Z67.10   **Type A blood, Rh positive**

    Z67.11   **Type A blood, Rh negative**

Z67.2   **Type B blood**

    Z67.20   **Type B blood, Rh positive**

    Z67.21   **Type B blood, Rh negative**

Z67.3   **Type AB blood**

    Z67.30   **Type AB blood, Rh positive**

    Z67.31   **Type AB blood, Rh negative**

Z67.4   **Type O blood**

    Z67.40   **Type O blood, Rh positive**

    Z67.41   **Type O blood, Rh negative**

Z67.9   **Unspecified blood type**

    Z67.90   **Unspecified blood type, Rh positive**

    Z67.91   **Unspecified blood type, Rh negative**

BODY MASS INDEX [BMI] (Z68)

Definition: Body Mass Index is a measure of body fat that is the ratio of the weight of the body in kilograms to the square of its height in meters.

Z68   Body mass index [BMI]

Kilograms per meters squared

Note: BMI adult codes are for use for persons 20 years of age or older

BMI pediatric codes are for use for persons 2-19 years of age. These percentiles are based on the growth charts published by the Centers for Disease Control and Prevention (CDC)

These percentiles are based on the growth charts published by the Centers for Disease Control and Prevention (CDC)

Z68.1 **Body mass index [BMI] 19.9 or less, adult**

Z68.2 **Body mass index [BMI] 20-29, adult**

Z68.20 Body mass index [BMI] 20.0-20.9, adult

Z68.21 Body mass index [BMI] 21.0-21.9, adult

Z68.22 Body mass index [BMI] 22.0-22.9, adult

Z68.23 Body mass index [BMI] 23.0-23.9, adult

Z68.24 Body mass index [BMI] 24.0-24.9, adult

Z68.25 Body mass index [BMI] 25.0-25.9, adult

Z68.26 Body mass index [BMI] 26.0-26.9, adult

Z68.27 Body mass index [BMI] 27.0-27.9, adult

Z68.28 Body mass index [BMI] 28.0-28.9, adult

Z68.29 Body mass index [BMI] 29.0-29.9, adult

Z68.3 **Body mass index [BMI] 30-39, adult**

Z68.30 Body mass index [BMI] 30.0-30.9, adult

Z68.31 Body mass index [BMI] 31.0-31.9, adult

Z68.32 Body mass index [BMI] 32.0-32.9, adult

Z68.33 Body mass index [BMI] 33.0-33.9, adult

Z68.34 Body mass index [BMI] 34.0-34.9, adult

Z68.35 Body mass index [BMI] 35.0-35.9, adult

Z68.36 Body mass index [BMI] 36.0-36.9, adult

Z68.37 Body mass index [BMI] 37.0-37.9, adult

Z68.38 Body mass index [BMI] 38.0-38.9, adult

Z68.39 Body mass index [BMI] 39.0-39.9, adult

Z68.4 **Body mass index [BMI] 40 or greater, adult**

Z68.41 Body mass index [BMI] 40.0-44.9, adult [HCC]

Z68.42 Body mass index [BMI] 45.0-49.9, adult [HCC]

Z68.43 Body mass index [BMI] 50.0-59.9, adult [HCC]

Z68.44 Body mass index [BMI] 60.0-69.9, adult [HCC]

Z68.45 Body mass index [BMI] 70 or greater, adult [HCC]

Z68.5 **Body mass index [BMI] pediatric**

Z68.51 Body mass index [BMI] pediatric, less than 5th percentile for age

Z68.52 Body mass index [BMI] pediatric, 5th percentile to less than 85th percentile for age

Z68.53 Body mass index [BMI] pediatric, 85th percentile to less than 95th percentile for age

Z68.54 Body mass index [BMI] pediatric, greater than or equal to 95th percentile for age

PERSONS ENCOUNTERING HEALTH SERVICES IN OTHER CIRCUMSTANCES (Z69-Z76)

Z69 **Encounter for mental health services for victim and perpetrator of abuse**

Includes: counseling for victims and perpetrators of abuse

Z69.0 **Encounter for mental health services for child abuse problems**

Z69.01 **Encounter for mental health services for parental child abuse**

Z69.010 **Encounter for mental health services for victim of parental child abuse**

Encounter for mental health services for victim of child abuse by parent

Encounter for mental health services for victim of child neglect by parent

Encounter for mental health services for victim of child psychological abuse by parent

Encounter for mental health services for victim of child sexual abuse by parent

Z69.011 **Encounter for mental health services for perpetrator of parental child abuse**

Encounter for mental health services for perpetrator of parental child neglect

Encounter for mental health services for perpetrator of parental child psychological abuse

Encounter for mental health services for perpetrator of parental child sexual abuse

Excludes1: encounter for mental health services for non-parental child abuse (Z69.02-)

Z69.02 **Encounter for mental health services for non-parental child abuse**

Z69.020 **Encounter for mental health services for victim of non-parental child abuse**

Encounter for mental health services for victim of non-parental child neglect

Encounter for mental health services for victim of non-parental child psychological abuse

Encounter for mental health services for victim of non-parental child sexual abuse

Z69.021 **Encounter for mental health services for perpetrator of non-parental child abuse**

Encounter for mental health services for perpetrator of non-parental child neglect

Encounter for mental health services for perpetrator of non-parental child psychological abuse

Encounter for mental health services for perpetrator of non-parental child sexual abuse

Z69.1 **Encounter for mental health services for spousal or partner abuse problems**

Z69.11 **Encounter for mental health services for victim of spousal or partner abuse**

Encounter for mental health services for victim of spouse or partner neglect

Encounter for mental health services for victim of spouse or partner psychological abuse

Encounter for mental health services for victim of spouse or partner violence, physical

Z69.12 **Encounter for mental health services for perpetrator of spousal or partner abuse**

Encounter for mental health services for perpetrator of spouse or partner neglect

Encounter for mental health services for perpetrator of spouse or partner psychological abuse

Encounter for mental health services for perpetrator of spouse or partner violence, physical

Encounter for mental health services for perpetrator of spouse or partner violence, sexual

Z69.8 **Encounter for mental health services for victim or perpetrator of other abuse**

Z69.81 **Encounter for mental health services for victim of other abuse**

Encounter for mental health services for victim of non-spousal adult abuse

● New code ▲ Revised code Excludes1: Not coded here Excludes2: Not included here ⊗ Placeholder required ⑦7th digit required

Encounter for mental health services for victim of spouse or partner violence, sexual

Encounter for rape victim counseling

Z69.82 **Encounter for mental health services for perpetrator of other abuse**

Encounter for mental health services for perpetrator of non-spousal adult abuse

Z70 **Counseling related to sexual attitude, behavior and orientation**

Includes: encounter for mental health services for sexual attitude, behavior and orientation

Excludes2: contraceptive or procreative counseling (Z30-Z31)

Z70.0 **Counseling related to sexual attitude**

Z70.1 **Counseling related to patient's sexual behavior and orientation**

Patient concerned regarding impotence

Patient concerned regarding non-responsiveness

Patient concerned regarding promiscuity

Patient concerned regarding sexual orientation

Z70.2 **Counseling related to sexual behavior and orientation of third party**

Advice sought regarding sexual behavior and orientation of child

Advice sought regarding sexual behavior and orientation of partner

Advice sought regarding sexual behavior and orientation of spouse

Z70.3 **Counseling related to combined concerns regarding sexual attitude, behavior and orientation**

Z70.8 **Other sex counseling**

Encounter for sex education

Z70.9 **Sex counseling, unspecified**

Z71 **Persons encountering health services for other counseling and medical advice, not elsewhere classified**

Excludes2: contraceptive or procreation counseling (Z30-Z31)

sex counseling (Z70.-)

Z71.0 **Person encountering health services to consult on behalf of another person**

Person encountering health services to seek advice or treatment for non-attending third party

Excludes2: anxiety (normal) about sick person in family (Z63.7)

expectant (adoptive) parent(s) pre-birth pediatrician visit (Z76.81)

Z71.1 **Person with feared health complaint in whom no diagnosis is made**

Person encountering health services with feared condition which was not demonstrated

Person encountering health services in which problem was normal state

'Worried well'

Excludes1: medical observation for suspected diseases and conditions proven not to exist (Z03.-)

Z71.2 **Person consulting for explanation of examination or test findings**

Z71.3 **Dietary counseling and surveillance**

Use Additional Code for any associated underlying medical condition

Use Additional Code to identify body mass index (BMI), if known (Z68.-)

Z71.4 **Alcohol abuse counseling and surveillance**

Use Additional Code for alcohol abuse or dependence (F10.-)

Z71.41 **Alcohol abuse counseling and surveillance of alcoholic**

Z71.42 **Counseling for family member of alcoholic**

Counseling for significant other, partner, or friend of alcoholic

Z71.5 **Drug abuse counseling and surveillance**

Use Additional Code for drug abuse or dependence (F11-F16, F18-F19)

Z71.51 **Drug abuse counseling and surveillance of drug abuser**

Z71.52 **Counseling for family member of drug abuser**

Counseling for significant **Other**, partner, or friend of drug abuser

Z71.6 **Tobacco abuse counseling**

Use Additional Code for nicotine dependence (F17.-)

Z71.7 **Human immunodeficiency virus [HIV] counseling**

Z71.8 **Other specified counseling**

Excludes2: counseling for contraception (Z30.0-)

Z71.81 **Spiritual or religious counseling**

Z71.82 **Exercise counseling**

Z71.83 **Encounter for nonprocreative genetic counseling**

Excludes1: counseling for procreative genetics (Z31.5)

counseling for procreative management (Z31.6)

Z71.84 **Encounter for health counseling related to travel**

Encounter for health risk and safety counseling for (international) travel

Code also, if applicable, encounter for immunization (Z23)

Excludes2: encounter for administrative examination (Z02.-)

encounter for other special examination without complaint, suspected or reported diagnosis (Z01.-)

• **Z71.85** **Encounter for immunization safety counseling**

Code also, if applicable, encounter for immunization (Z23)

Code also, if applicable, immunization not carried out (Z28.-)

Excludes1: encounter for health counseling related to travel (Z71.84)

Z71.89 **Other specified counseling**

Z71.9 **Counseling, unspecified**

Encounter for medical advice NOS

Z72 **Problems related to lifestyle**

Excludes2: problems related to life-management difficulty (Z73.-)

problems related to socioeconomic and psychosocial circumstances (Z55-Z65)

Z72.0 **Tobacco use**

Tobacco use NOS

Excludes1: history of tobacco dependence (Z87.891)

nicotine dependence (F17.2-)

tobacco dependence (F17.2-)

tobacco use during pregnancy (O99.33-)

Z72.3 **Lack of physical exercise**

Z72.4 **Inappropriate diet and eating habits**

Excludes1: behavioral eating disorders of infancy or childhood (F98.2.-F98.3)

eating disorders (F50.-)

lack of adequate food (Z59.48)

malnutrition and other nutritional deficiencies (E40-E64)

Z72.5 **High risk sexual behavior**

Promiscuity

Excludes1: paraphilias (F65)

Z72.51 **High risk heterosexual behavior**

Z72.52 **High risk homosexual behavior**

Z72.53 **High risk bisexual behavior**

Z72.6 **Gambling and betting**

Excludes1: compulsive or pathological gambling (F63.0)

Z72.8 **Other problems related to lifestyle**

Z72.81 **Antisocial behavior**

Excludes1: conduct disorders (F91.-)

Z72.810 **Child and adolescent antisocial behavior** Antisocial behavior (child) (adolescent) without manifest psychiatric disorder

Delinquency NOS

Group delinquency

Offenses in the context of gang membership

Stealing in company with others

Truancy from school

Z72.811 **Adult antisocial behavior** Adult antisocial behavior without manifest psychiatric disorder

Z72.82 **Problems related to sleep**

Z72.820 **Sleep deprivation**

Lack of adequate sleep

Excludes1: insomnia (G47.0-)

Z72.821 **Inadequate sleep hygiene**

Bad sleep habits

Irregular sleep habits

Unhealthy sleep wake schedule

Excludes1: insomnia (F51.0-, G47.0-)

Z72.89 **Other problems related to lifestyle**

Self-damaging behavior

Z72.9 **Problem related to lifestyle, unspecified**

Z73 **Problems related to life management difficulty**

Excludes2: problems related to socioeconomic and psychosocial circumstances (Z55-Z65)

Z73.0 **Burn-out**

Z73.1 **Type A behavior pattern**

Z73.2 **Lack of relaxation and leisure**

Z73.3 **Stress, not elsewhere classified**

Physical and mental strain NOS

Excludes1: stress related to employment or unemployment (Z56.-)

Z73.4 **Inadequate social skills, not elsewhere classified**

Z73.5 **Social role conflict, not elsewhere classified**

Z73.6 **Limitation of activities due to disability**

Excludes1: care-provider dependency (Z74.-)

Z73.8 **Other problems related to life management difficulty**

Z73.81 **Behavioral insomnia of childhood**

Z73.810 **Behavioral insomnia of childhood, sleep-onset association type**

Z73.811 **Behavioral insomnia of childhood, limit setting type**

Z73.812 **Behavioral insomnia of childhood, combined type**

Z73.819 **Behavioral insomnia of childhood, unspecified type**

Z73.82 **Dual sensory impairment**

Z73.89 **Other problems related to life management difficulty**

Z73.9 **Problem related to life management difficulty, unspecified**

Z74 **Problems related to care provider dependency**

Excludes2: dependence on enabling machines or devices NEC0 (Z99.-)

Z74.0 **Reduced mobility**

Z74.01 **Bed confinement status**

Bedridden

Z74.09 **Other reduced mobility**

Chair ridden

Reduced mobility NOS

Excludes2: wheelchair dependence (Z99.3)

Z74.1 **Need for assistance with personal care**

Z74.2 **Need for assistance at home and no other household member able to render care**

Z74.3 **Need for continuous supervision**

Z74.8 **Other problems related to care provider dependency**

Z74.9 **Problem related to care provider dependency, unspecified**

Z75 **Problems related to medical facilities and other health care**

Z75.0 **Medical services not available in home**

Excludes1: no other household member able to render care (Z74.2)

Z75.1 **Person awaiting admission to adequate facility elsewhere**

Z75.2 **Other waiting period for investigation and treatment**

Z75.3 **Unavailability and inaccessibility of health-care facilities**

Excludes1: bed unavailable (Z75.1)

Z75.4 **Unavailability and inaccessibility of other helping agencies**

Z75.5 **Holiday relief care**

Z75.8 **Other problems related to medical facilities and other health care**

Z75.9 **Unspecified problem related to medical facilities and other health care**

Z76 **Persons encountering health services in other circumstances**

Z76.0 **Encounter for issue of repeat prescription**

Encounter for issue of repeat prescription for appliance

Encounter for issue of repeat prescription for medicaments

Encounter for issue of repeat prescription for spectacles

Excludes2: issue of medical certificate (Z02.7)

repeat prescription for contraceptive (Z30.4-)

Z76.1 **Encounter for health supervision and care of foundling**

Z76.2 **Encounter for health supervision and care of other healthy infant and child**

Encounter for medical or nursing care or supervision of healthy infant under circumstances such as adverse socioeconomic conditions at home

Encounter for medical or nursing care or supervision of healthy infant under circumstances such as awaiting foster or adoptive placement

● New code ▲ Revised code Excludes1: Not coded here Excludes2: Not included here ⊗ Placeholder required ⑦7th digit required

Encounter for medical or nursing care or supervision of healthy infant under circumstances such as maternal illness

Encounter for medical or nursing care or supervision of healthy infant under circumstances such as number of children at home preventing or interfering with normal care

Z76.3 **Healthy person accompanying sick person**

Z76.4 **Other boarder to healthcare facility**

Excludes1: homelessness (Z59.0-)

Z76.5 **Malingerer [conscious simulation]**

Person feigning illness (with obvious motivation)

Excludes1: factitious disorder (F68.1-, F68.A)

peregrinating patient (F68.1-)

Z76.8 **Persons encountering health services in other specified circumstances**

Z76.81 **Expectant parent(s) prebirth pediatrician visit**

Pre-adoption pediatrician visit for adoptive parent(s)

Z76.82 **Awaiting organ transplant status**

Patient waiting for organ availability

Z76.89 **Persons encountering health services in other specified circumstances**

Persons encountering health services NOS

PERSONS WITH POTENTIAL HEALTH HAZARDS RELATED TO FAMILY AND PERSONAL HISTORY AND CERTAIN CONDITIONS INFLUENCING HEALTH STATUS (Z77-Z99)

Code also any follow-up examination (Z08-Z09)

Z77 **Other contact with and (suspected) exposures hazardous to health**

Includes: contact with and (suspected) exposures to potential hazards to health

Excludes2: contact with and (suspected) exposure to communicable diseases (Z20.-)

exposure to (parental) (environmental) tobacco smoke in the perinatal period (P96.81)

newborn affected by noxious substances transmitted via placenta or breast milk (P04.-)

occupational exposure to risk factors (Z57.-)

retained foreign body (Z18.-)

retained foreign body fully removed (Z87.821)

toxic effects of substances chiefly nonmedicinal as to source (T51-T65)

Z77.0 **Contact with and (suspected) exposure to hazardous, chiefly nonmedicinal, chemicals**

Z77.01 **Contact with and (suspected) exposure to hazardous metals**

Z77.010 **Contact with and (suspected) exposure to arsenic**

Z77.011 **Contact with and (suspected) exposure to lead**

Z77.012 **Contact with and (suspected) exposure to uranium**

Excludes1: retained depleted uranium fragments (Z18.01)

Z77.018 **Contact with and (suspected) exposure to other hazardous metals**

Contact with and (suspected) exposure to chromium compounds

Contact with and (suspected) exposure to nickel dust

Z77.02 **Contact with and (suspected) exposure to hazardous aromatic compounds**

Z77.020 **Contact with and (suspected) exposure to aromatic amines**

Z77.021 **Contact with and (suspected) exposure to benzene**

Z77.028 **Contact with and (suspected) exposure to other hazardous aromatic compounds**

Aromatic dyes NOS

Polycyclic aromatic hydrocarbons

Z77.09 **Contact with and (suspected) exposure to other hazardous, chiefly nonmedicinal, chemicals**

Z77.090 **Contact with and (suspected) exposure to asbestos**

Z77.098 **Contact with and (suspected) exposure to other hazardous, chiefly nonmedicinal, chemicals Dyes NOS**

Z77.1 **Contact with and (suspected) exposure to environmental pollution and hazards in the physical environment**

Z77.11 **Contact with and (suspected) exposure to environmental pollution**

Z77.110 **Contact with and (suspected) exposure to air pollution**

Z77.111 **Contact with and (suspected) exposure to water pollution**

Z77.112 **Contact with and (suspected) exposure to soil pollution**

Z77.118 **Contact with and (suspected) exposure to other environmental pollution**

Z77.12 **Contact with and (suspected) exposure to hazards in the physical environment**

Z77.120 **Contact with and (suspected) exposure to mold (toxic)**

Z77.121 **Contact with and (suspected) exposure to harmful algae and algae toxins**

Contact with and (suspected) exposure to (harmful) algae bloom NOS

Contact with and (suspected) exposure to blue-green algae bloom

Contact with and (suspected) exposure to brown tide

Contact with and (suspected) exposure to cyanobacteria bloom

Contact with and (suspected) exposure to Florida red tide

Contact with and (suspected) exposure to pfiesteria piscicida

Contact with and (suspected) exposure to red tide

Z77.122 **Contact with and (suspected) exposure to noise**

Z77.123 **Contact with and (suspected) exposure to radon and other naturally occurring radiation**

Excludes2: radiation exposure as the cause of a confirmed condition (W88-W90, X39.0-)

radiation sickness NOS (T66)

Z77.128 **Contact with and (suspected) exposure to other hazards in the physical environment**

Z77.2 **Contact with and (suspected) exposure to other hazardous substances**

Z77.21   **Contact with and (suspected) exposure to potentially hazardous body fluids**

Z77.22   **Contact with and (suspected) exposure to environmental tobacco smoke (acute) (chronic)**

Exposure to second hand tobacco smoke (acute) (chronic)

Passive smoking (acute) (chronic)

Excludes1: nicotine dependence (F17.-)

tobacco use (Z72.0)

Excludes2: occupational exposure to environmental tobacco smoke (Z57.31)

Z77.29   **Contact with and (suspected) exposure to other hazardous substances**

Z77.9   **Other contact with and (suspected) exposures hazardous to health**

Z78   **Other specified health status**

Excludes2: asymptomatic human immunodeficiency virus [HIV] infection status (Z21)

postprocedural status (Z93-Z99)

sex reassignment status (Z87.890)

Z78.0   **Asymptomatic menopausal state**

Menopausal state NOS

Postmenopausal status NOS

Excludes2: symptomatic menopausal state (N95.1)

Z78.1   **Physical restraint status**

Excludes1: physical restraint due to a procedure - omit code

Z78.9   **Other specified health status**

Z79   **Long term (current) drug therapy**

Includes: long term (current) drug use for prophylactic purposes

Code also any therapeutic drug level monitoring (Z51.81)

Excludes2: drug abuse and dependence (F11-F19)

drug use complicating pregnancy, childbirth, and the puerperium (O99.32-)

Z79.0   **Long term (current) use of anticoagulants and antithrombotics/antiplatelets**

Excludes2: long term (current) use of aspirin (Z79.82)

Z79.01   **Long term (current) use of anticoagulants**

Z79.02   **Long term (current) use of antithrombotics/antiplatelets**

Z79.1   **Long term (current) use of non-steroidal anti-inflammatories (NSAID)**

Excludes2: long term (current) use of aspirin (Z79.82)

Z79.2   **Long term (current) use of antibiotics**

Z79.3   **Long term (current) use of hormonal contraceptives**

Long term (current) use of birth control pill or patch

Z79.4   **Long term (current) use of insulin** [HCC]

Excludes2: long term (current) use of oral antidiabetic drugs (Z79.84)

long term (current) use of oral hypoglycemic drugs (Z79.84)

Z79.5   **Long term (current) use of steroids**

Z79.51   **Long term (current) use of inhaled steroids**

Z79.52   **Long term (current) use of systemic steroids**

Z79.8   **Other long term (current) drug therapy**

Z79.81   **Long term (current) use of agents affecting estrogen receptors and estrogen levels**

Code first, if applicable:

malignant neoplasm of breast (C50.-)

malignant neoplasm of prostate (C61)

Use Additional Code, if applicable, to identify:

estrogen receptor positive status (Z17.0)

family history of breast cancer (Z80.3)

genetic susceptibility to malignant neoplasm (cancer) (Z15.0-)

personal history of breast cancer (Z85.3)

personal history of prostate cancer (Z85.46)

postmenopausal status (Z78.0)

Excludes1: hormone replacement therapy (Z79.890)

Z79.810   **Long term (current) use of selective estrogen receptor modulators (SERMs)**

Long term (current) use of raloxifene (Evista)

Long term (current) use of tamoxifen (Nolvadex)

Long term (current) use of toremifene (Fareston)

Z79.811   **Long term (current) use of aromatase inhibitors**

Long term (current) use of anastrozole (Arimidex)

Long term (current) use of exemestane (Aromasin)

Long term (current) use of letrozole (Femara)

Z79.818   **Long term (current) use of other agents affecting estrogen receptors and estrogen levels**

Long term (current) use of estrogen receptor down regulators

Long term (current) use of fulvestrant (Faslodex)

Long term (current) use of gonadotropin-releasing hormone (GnRH) agonist

Long term (current) use of goserelin acetate (Zoladex)

Long term (current) use of leuprolide acetate (leuprorelin) (Lupron)

Long term (current) use of megestrol acetate (Megace)

Z79.82   **Long term (current) use of aspirin**

Z79.83   **Long term (current) use of bisphosphonates**

Z79.84   **Long term (current) use of oral hypoglycemic drugs**

Long term (current) use of oral antidiabetic drugs

Excludes2: long term (current) use of insulin (Z79.4)

Z79.89   **Other long term (current) drug therapy**

Z79.890   **Hormone replacement therapy**

Z79.891   **Long term (current) use of opiate analgesic**

Long term (current) use of methadone for pain management

Excludes1: methadone use NOS (F11.9-)

use of methadone for treatment of heroin addiction (F11.2-)

Z79.899   **Other long term (current) drug therapy**

 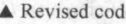

Z80 **Family history of primary malignant neoplasm**

Z80.0 **Family history of malignant neoplasm of digestive organs**
Conditions classifiable to C15-C26

Z80.1 **Family history of malignant neoplasm of trachea, bronchus and lung**
Conditions classifiable to C33-C34

Z80.2 **Family history of malignant neoplasm of other respiratory and intrathoracic organs**
Conditions classifiable to C30-C32, C37-C39

Z80.3 **Family history of malignant neoplasm of breast**
Conditions classifiable to C50.-

Z80.4 **Family history of malignant neoplasm of genital organs**
Conditions classifiable to C51-C63

Z80.41 **Family history of malignant neoplasm of ovary**

Z80.42 **Family history of malignant neoplasm of prostate**

Z80.43 **Family history of malignant neoplasm of testis**

Z80.49 **Family history of malignant neoplasm of other genital organs**

Z80.5 **Family history of malignant neoplasm of urinary tract**
Conditions classifiable to C64-C68

Z80.51 **Family history of malignant neoplasm of kidney**

Z80.52 **Family history of malignant neoplasm of bladder**

Z80.59 **Family history of malignant neoplasm of other urinary tract organ**

Z80.6 **Family history of leukemia**
Conditions classifiable to C91-C95

Z80.7 **Family history of other malignant neoplasms of lymphoid, hematopoietic and related tissues**
Conditions classifiable to C81-C90, C96.-

Z80.8 **Family history of malignant neoplasm of other organs or systems**
Conditions classifiable to C00-C14, C40-C49, C69-C79

Z80.9 **Family history of malignant neoplasm, unspecified**
Conditions classifiable to C80.1

Z81 **Family history of mental and behavioral disorders**

Z81.0 **Family history of intellectual disabilities**
Conditions classifiable to F70-F79

Z81.1 **Family history of alcohol abuse and dependence**
Conditions classifiable to F10.-

Z81.2 **Family history of tobacco abuse and dependence**
Conditions classifiable to F17.-

Z81.3 **Family history of other psychoactive substance abuse and dependence**
Conditions classifiable to F11-F16, F18-F19

Z81.4 **Family history of other substance abuse and dependence**
Conditions classifiable to F55

Z81.8 **Family history of other mental and behavioral disorders**
Conditions classifiable elsewhere in F01-F99

Z82 **Family history of certain disabilities and chronic diseases (leading to disablement)**

Z82.0 **Family history of epilepsy and other diseases of the nervous system**
Conditions classifiable to G00-G99

Z82.1 **Family history of blindness and visual loss**
Conditions classifiable to H54.-

Z82.2 **Family history of deafness and hearing loss**
Conditions classifiable to H90-H91

Z82.3 **Family history of stroke**
Conditions classifiable to I60-I64

Z82.4 **Family history of ischemic heart disease and other diseases of the circulatory system**
Conditions classifiable to I00-I5A, I65-I99

Z82.41 **Family history of sudden cardiac death**

Z82.49 **Family history of ischemic heart disease and other diseases of the circulatory system**

Z82.5 **Family history of asthma and other chronic lower respiratory diseases**
Conditions classifiable to J40-J47

Excludes2: family history of other diseases of the respiratory system (Z83.6)

Z82.6 **Family history of arthritis and other diseases of the musculoskeletal system and connective tissue**
Conditions classifiable to M00-M99

Z82.61 **Family history of arthritis**

Z82.62 **Family history of osteoporosis**

Z82.69 **Family history of other diseases of the musculoskeletal system and connective tissue**

Z82.7 **Family history of congenital malformations, deformations and chromosomal abnormalities**
Conditions classifiable to Q00-Q99

Z82.71 **Family history of polycystic kidney**

Z82.79 **Family history of other congenital malformations, deformations and chromosomal abnormalities**

Z82.8 **Family history of other disabilities and chronic diseases leading to disablement, not elsewhere classified**

Z83 **Family history of other specific disorders**

Excludes2: contact with and (suspected) exposure to communicable disease in the family (Z20.-)

Z83.0 **Family history of human immunodeficiency virus [HIV] disease**
Conditions classifiable to B20

Z83.1 **Family history of other infectious and parasitic diseases**
Conditions classifiable to A00-B19, B25-B94, B99

Z83.2 **Family history of diseases of the blood and blood-forming organs and certain disorders involving the immune mechanism**
Conditions classifiable to D50-D89

Z83.3 **Family history of diabetes mellitus**
Conditions classifiable to E08-E13

Z83.4 **Family history of other endocrine, nutritional and metabolic diseases**
Conditions classifiable to E00-E07, E15-E88

Z83.41 **Family history of multiple endocrine neoplasia [MEN] syndrome**

Z83.42 **Family history of familial hypercholesterolemia**

Z83.43 **Family history of other disorder of lipoprotein metabolism and other lipidemias**

Z83.430 **Family history of elevated lipoprotein(a)**
Family history of elevated Lp(a)

Z83.438 **Family history of other disorder of lipoprotein metabolism and other lipidemia**
Family history of familial combined hyperlipidemia

Z83.49 **Family history of other endocrine, nutritional and metabolic diseases**

Z83.5 **Family history of eye and ear disorders**

Z83.51 **Family history of eye disorders**

Conditions classifiable to H00-H53, H55-H59

Excludes2: family history of blindness and visual loss (Z82.1)

Z83.511 **Family history of glaucoma**

Z83.518 **Family history of other specified eye disorder**

Z83.52 **Family history of ear disorders**

Conditions classifiable to H60-H83, H92-H95

Excludes2: family history of deafness and hearing loss (Z82.2)

Z83.6 **Family history of other diseases of the respiratory system**

Conditions classifiable to J00-J39, J60-J99

Excludes2: family history of asthma and other chronic lower respiratory diseases (Z82.5)

Z83.7 **Family history of diseases of the digestive system**

Conditions classifiable to K00-K93

Z83.71 **Family history of colonic polyps**

Excludes2: family history of malignant neoplasm of digestive organs (Z80.0)

Z83.79 **Family history of other diseases of the digestive system**

Z84 **Family history of other conditions**

Z84.0 **Family history of diseases of the skin and subcutaneous tissue**

Conditions classifiable to L00-L99

Z84.1 **Family history of disorders of kidney and ureter**

Conditions classifiable to N00-N29

Z84.2 **Family history of other diseases of the genitourinary system**

Conditions classifiable to N30-N99

Z84.3 **Family history of consanguinity**

Z84.8 **Family history of other specified conditions**

Z84.81 **Family history of carrier of genetic disease**

Z84.82 **Family history of sudden infant death syndrome**

Family history of SIDS

Z84.89 **Family history of other specified conditions**

Z85 **Personal history of malignant neoplasm**

Code first any follow-up examination after treatment of malignant neoplasm (Z08)

Use Additional Code to identify:

alcohol use and dependence (F10.-)

exposure to environmental tobacco smoke (Z77.22)

history of tobacco dependence (Z87.891)

occupational exposure to environmental tobacco smoke (Z57.31)

tobacco dependence (F17.-)

tobacco use (Z72.0)

Excludes2: personal history of benign neoplasm (Z86.01-)

personal history of carcinoma-in-situ (Z86.00-)

Z85.0 **Personal history of malignant neoplasm of digestive organs**

Z85.00 **Personal history of malignant neoplasm of unspecified digestive organ**

Z85.01 **Personal history of malignant neoplasm of esophagus**

Conditions classifiable to C15

Z85.02 **Personal history of malignant neoplasm of stomach**

Z85.020 **Personal history of malignant carcinoid tumor of stomach**

Conditions classifiable to C7A.092

Z85.028 **Personal history of other malignant neoplasm of stomach**

Conditions classifiable to C16

Z85.03 **Personal history of malignant neoplasm of large intestine**

Z85.030 **Personal history of malignant carcinoid tumor of large intestine**

Conditions classifiable to C7A.022-C7A.025, C7A.029

Z85.038 **Personal history of other malignant neoplasm of large intestine**

Conditions classifiable to C18

Z85.04 **Personal history of malignant neoplasm of rectum, rectosigmoid junction, and anus**

Z85.040 **Personal history of malignant carcinoid tumor of rectum**

Conditions classifiable to C7A.026

Z85.048 **Personal history of other malignant neoplasm of rectum, rectosigmoid junction, and anus**

Conditions classifiable to C19-C21

Z85.05 **Personal history of malignant neoplasm of liver**

Conditions classifiable to C22

Z85.06 **Personal history of malignant neoplasm of small intestine**

Z85.060 **Personal history of malignant carcinoid tumor of small intestine**

Conditions classifiable to C7A.01-

Z85.068 **Personal history of other malignant neoplasm of small intestine**

Conditions classifiable to C17

Z85.07 **Personal history of malignant neoplasm of pancreas**

Conditions classifiable to C25

Z85.09 **Personal history of malignant neoplasm of other digestive organs**

Z85.1 **Personal history of malignant neoplasm of trachea, bronchus and lung**

Z85.11 **Personal history of malignant neoplasm of bronchus and lung**

Z85.110 **Personal history of malignant carcinoid tumor of bronchus and lung**

Conditions classifiable to C7A.090

Z85.118 **Personal history of other malignant neoplasm of bronchus and lung**

Conditions classifiable to C34

Z85.12 **Personal history of malignant neoplasm of trachea**

Conditions classifiable to C33

Z85.2 **Personal history of malignant neoplasm of other respiratory and intrathoracic organs**

Z85.20 **Personal history of malignant neoplasm of unspecified respiratory organ**

Z85.21 **Personal history of malignant neoplasm of larynx**

Conditions classifiable to C32

Z85.22 **Personal history of malignant neoplasm of nasal cavities, middle ear, and accessory sinuses**

● New code ▲ Revised code Excludes1: Not coded here Excludes2: Not included here ⊗ Placeholder required ⑦7th digit required

Conditions classifiable to C30-C31

Z85.23 **Personal history of malignant neoplasm of thymus**

Z85.230 **Personal history of malignant carcinoid tumor of thymus**

Conditions classifiable to C7A.091

Z85.238 **Personal history of other malignant neoplasm of thymus**

Conditions classifiable to C37

Z85.29 **Personal history of malignant neoplasm of other respiratory and intrathoracic organs**

Z85.3 **Personal history of malignant neoplasm of breast**

Conditions classifiable to C50.-

Z85.4 **Personal history of malignant neoplasm of genital organs**

Conditions classifiable to C51-C63

Z85.40 **Personal history of malignant neoplasm of unspecified female genital organ**

Z85.41 **Personal history of malignant neoplasm of cervix uteri**

Z85.42 **Personal history of malignant neoplasm of other parts of uterus**

Z85.43 **Personal history of malignant neoplasm of ovary**

Z85.44 **Personal history of malignant neoplasm of other female genital organs**

Z85.45 **Personal history of malignant neoplasm of unspecified male genital organ**

Z85.46 **Personal history of malignant neoplasm of prostate**

Z85.47 **Personal history of malignant neoplasm of testis**

Z85.48 **Personal history of malignant neoplasm of epididymis**

Z85.49 **Personal history of malignant neoplasm of other male genital organs**

Z85.5 **Personal history of malignant neoplasm of urinary tract**

Conditions classifiable to C64-C68

Z85.50 **Personal history of malignant neoplasm of unspecified urinary tract organ**

Z85.51 **Personal history of malignant neoplasm of bladder**

Z85.52 **Personal history of malignant neoplasm of kidney**

Excludes1: personal history of malignant neoplasm of renal pelvis (Z85.53)

Z85.520 **Personal history of malignant carcinoid tumor of kidney**

Conditions classifiable to C7A.093

Z85.528 **Personal history of other malignant neoplasm of kidney**

Conditions classifiable to C64

Z85.53 **Personal history of malignant neoplasm of renal pelvis**

Z85.54 **Personal history of malignant neoplasm of ureter**

Z85.59 **Personal history of malignant neoplasm of other urinary tract organ**

Z85.6 **Personal history of leukemia**

Conditions classifiable to C91-C95

Excludes1: leukemia in remission C91.0-C95.9 with 5th character 1

Z85.7 **Personal history of other malignant neoplasms of lymphoid, hematopoietic and related tissues**

Z85.71 **Personal history of Hodgkin lymphoma**

Conditions classifiable to C81

Z85.72 **Personal history of non-Hodgkin lymphomas**

Conditions classifiable to C82-C85

Z85.79 **Personal history of other malignant neoplasms of lymphoid, hematopoietic and related tissues**

Conditions classifiable to C88-C90, C96

Excludes1: multiple myeloma in remission (C90.01)

plasma cell leukemia in remission (C90.11)

plasmacytoma in remission (C90.21)

Z85.8 **Personal history of malignant neoplasms of other organs and systems**

Conditions classifiable to C00-C14, C40-C49, C69-C75, C7A.098, C76-C79

Z85.81 **Personal history of malignant neoplasm of lip, oral cavity, and pharynx**

Conditions classifiable to C00-C14

Z85.810 **Personal history of malignant neoplasm of tongue**

Z85.818 **Personal history of malignant neoplasm of other sites of lip, oral cavity, and pharynx**

Z85.819 **Personal history of malignant neoplasm of unspecified site of lip, oral cavity, and pharynx**

Z85.82 **Personal history of malignant neoplasm of skin**

Z85.820 **Personal history of malignant melanoma of skin**

Conditions classifiable to C43

Z85.821 **Personal history of Merkel cell carcinoma**

Conditions classifiable to C4A

Z85.828 **Personal history of other malignant neoplasm of skin**

Conditions classifiable to C44

Z85.83 **Personal history of malignant neoplasm of bone and soft tissue**

Conditions classifiable to C40-C41; C45-C49

Z85.830 **Personal history of malignant neoplasm of bone**

Z85.831 **Personal history of malignant neoplasm of soft tissue**

Excludes2: personal history of malignant neoplasm of skin (Z85.82-)

Z85.84 **Personal history of malignant neoplasm of eye and nervous tissue**

Conditions classifiable to C69-C72

Z85.840 **Personal history of malignant neoplasm of eye**

Z85.841 **Personal history of malignant neoplasm of brain**

Z85.848 **Personal history of malignant neoplasm of other parts of nervous tissue**

Z85.85 **Personal history of malignant neoplasm of endocrine glands**

Conditions classifiable to C73-C75

Z85.850 **Personal history of malignant neoplasm of thyroid**

Z85.858 **Personal history of malignant neoplasm of other endocrine glands**

Z85.89 **Personal history of malignant neoplasm of other organs and systems**

Conditions classifiable to C7A.098, C76, C77-C79

Z85.9 **Personal history of malignant neoplasm, unspecified**

Conditions classifiable to C7A.00, C80.1

Z86 **Personal history of certain other diseases**

Code first any follow-up examination after treatment (Z09)

Z86.0 **Personal history of in-situ and benign neoplasms and neoplasms of uncertain behavior**

Excludes2: personal history of malignant neoplasms (Z85.-)

Z86.00 **Personal history of in-situ neoplasm**

Conditions classifiable to D00-D09

Z86.000 **Personal history of in-situ neoplasm of breast**

Conditions classifiable to D06

Z86.001 **Personal history of in-situ neoplasm of cervix uteri**

Personal history of cervical intraepithelial neoplasia III [CIN III]

Z86.002 **Personal history of in-situ neoplasm of other and unspecified genital organs**

Conditions classifiable to D07

Personal history of high-grade prostatic intraepithelial neoplasia III [HGPIN III]

Personal history of vaginal intraepithelial neoplasia III [VAIN III]

Personal history of vulvar intraepithelial neoplasia III [VIN III]

Z86.003 **Personal history of in-situ neoplasm of oral cavity, esophagus and stomach**

Conditions classifiable to D00

Z86.004 **Personal history of in-situ neoplasm of other and unspecified digestive organs**

Conditions classifiable to D01

Personal history of anal intraepithelial neoplasia (AIN III)

Z86.005 **Personal history of in-situ neoplasm of middle ear and respiratory system**

Conditions classifiable to D02

Z86.006 **Personal history of melanoma in-situ**

Conditions classifiable to D03

Excludes2: sites other than skin - code to personal history of in-situ neoplasm other site

Z86.007 **Personal history of in-situ neoplasm of skin**

Conditions classifiable to D04

Personal history of carcinoma in situ of skin

Z86.008 **Personal history of in-situ neoplasm of other site**

Conditions classifiable to D09

Z86.01 **Personal history of benign neoplasm**

Z86.010 **Personal history of colonic polyps**

Z86.011 **Personal history of benign neoplasm of the brain**

Z86.012 **Personal history of benign carcinoid tumor**

Z86.018 **Personal history of other benign neoplasm**

Z86.03 **Personal history of neoplasm of uncertain behavior**

Z86.1 **Personal history of infectious and parasitic diseases**

Conditions classifiable to A00-B89, B99

Excludes1: personal history of infectious diseases specific to a body system

sequelae of infectious and parasitic diseases (B90-B94)

Z86.11 **Personal history of tuberculosis**

Z86.12 **Personal history of poliomyelitis**

Z86.13 **Personal history of malaria**

Z86.14 **Personal history of Methicillin resistant Staphylococcus aureus infection**

Personal history of MRSA infection

Z86.15 **Personal history of latent tuberculosis infection**

Z86.16 **Personal history of COVID-19**

Excludes1 post COVID-19 condition (U09.9)

Z86.19 **Personal history of other infectious and parasitic diseases**

Z86.2 **Personal history of diseases of the blood and blood-forming organs and certain disorders involving the immune mechanism**

Conditions classifiable to D50-D89

Z86.3 **Personal history of endocrine, nutritional and metabolic diseases**

Conditions classifiable to E00-E88

Z86.31 **Personal history of diabetic foot ulcer**

Excludes2: current diabetic foot ulcer (E08.621, E09.621, E10.621, E11.621, E13.621)

Z86.32 **Personal history of gestational diabetes**

Personal history of conditions classifiable to O24.4-

Excludes1: gestational diabetes mellitus in current pregnancy (O24.4-)

Z86.39 **Personal history of other endocrine, nutritional and metabolic disease**

Z86.5 **Personal history of mental and behavioral disorders**

Conditions classifiable to F40-F59

Z86.51 **Personal history of combat and operational stress reaction**

Z86.59 **Personal history of other mental and behavioral disorders**

Z86.6 **Personal history of diseases of the nervous system and sense organs**

Conditions classifiable to G00-G99, H00-H95

Z86.61 **Personal history of infections of the central nervous system**

Personal history of encephalitis

Personal history of meningitis

Z86.69 **Personal history of other diseases of the nervous system and sense organs**

Z86.7 **Personal history of diseases of the circulatory system**

Conditions classifiable to I00-I99

Excludes2: old myocardial infarction (I25.2)

personal history of anaphylactic shock (Z87.892)

postmyocardial infarction syndrome (I24.1)

● New code ▲ Revised code Excludes1: Not coded here Excludes2: Not included here ⊗ Placeholder required ⑦7th digit required

Z86.71 **Personal history of venous thrombosis and embolism**

    Z86.711 **Personal history of pulmonary embolism**

    Z86.718 **Personal history of other venous thrombosis and embolism**

Z86.72 **Personal history of thrombophlebitis**

Z86.73 **Personal history of transient ischemic attack (TIA), and cerebral infarction without residual deficits**

Personal history of prolonged reversible ischemic neurological deficit (PRIND)

Personal history of stroke NOS without residual deficits

    Excludes1: personal history of traumatic brain injury (Z87.820)

        sequelae of cerebrovascular disease (I69.-)

Z86.74 **Personal history of sudden cardiac arrest**

Personal history of sudden cardiac death successfully resuscitated

Z86.79 **Personal history of other diseases of the circulatory system**

Z87 **Personal history of other diseases and conditions**

Code first any follow-up examination after treatment (Z09)

Z87.0 **Personal history of diseases of the respiratory system**

Conditions classifiable to J00-J99

    Z87.01 **Personal history of pneumonia (recurrent)**

    Z87.09 **Personal history of other diseases of the respiratory system**

Z87.1 **Personal history of diseases of the digestive system**

Conditions classifiable to K00-K93

    Z87.11 **Personal history of peptic ulcer disease**

    Z87.19 **Personal history of other diseases of the digestive system**

Z87.2 **Personal history of diseases of the skin and subcutaneous tissue**

Conditions classifiable to L00-L99

    Excludes2: personal history of diabetic foot ulcer (Z86.31)

Z87.3 **Personal history of diseases of the musculoskeletal system and connective tissue**

Conditions classifiable to M00-M99

    Excludes2: personal history of (healed) traumatic fracture (Z87.81)

    Z87.31 **Personal history of (healed) nontraumatic fracture**

        Z87.310 **Personal history of (healed) osteoporosis fracture**

        Personal history of (healed) fragility fracture

        Personal history of (healed) collapsed vertebra due to osteoporosis

        Z87.311 **Personal history of (healed) other pathological fracture**

        Personal history of (healed) collapsed vertebra NOS

        Excludes2: personal history of osteoporosis fracture (Z87.310)

        Z87.312 **Personal history of (healed) stress fracture**

Personal history of (healed) fatigue fracture

Z87.39 **Personal history of other diseases of the musculoskeletal system and connective tissue**

Z87.4 **Personal history of diseases of genitourinary system**

Conditions classifiable to N00-N99

    Z87.41 **Personal history of dysplasia of the female genital tract**

    Excludes1: personal history of intraepithelial neoplasia III of female genital tract (Z86.001, Z87.008)

        personal history of malignant neoplasm of female genital tract (Z85.40-Z85.44)

        Z87.410 **Personal history of cervical dysplasia**

        Z87.411 **Personal history of vaginal dysplasia**

        Z87.412 **Personal history of vulvar dysplasia**

    Z87.42 **Personal history of other diseases of the female genital tract**

    Z87.43 **Personal history of diseases of male genital organs**

        Z87.430 **Personal history of prostatic dysplasia**

        Excludes1: personal history of malignant neoplasm of prostate (Z85.46)

        Z87.438 **Personal history of other diseases of male genital organs**

    Z87.44 **Personal history of diseases of urinary system**

    Excludes1: personal history of malignant neoplasm

        of cervix uteri (Z85.41)

        Z87.440 **Personal history of urinary (tract) infections**

        Z87.441 **Personal history of nephrotic syndrome**

        Z87.442 **Personal history of urinary calculi**

        Personal history of kidney stones

        Z87.448 **Personal history of other diseases of urinary system**

Z87.5 **Personal history of complications of pregnancy, childbirth and the puerperium**

Conditions classifiable to O00-O9A

    Excludes2: recurrent pregnancy loss (N96)

    Z87.51 **Personal history of pre-term labor**

    Excludes1: current pregnancy with history of pre-term labor (O09.21-)

    Z87.59 **Personal history of other complications of pregnancy, childbirth and the puerperium**

    Personal history of trophoblastic disease

Z87.7 **Personal history of (corrected) congenital malformations**

Conditions classifiable to Q00-Q89 that have been repaired or corrected

    Excludes1: congenital malformations that have been partially corrected or repaired but which still require medical treatment - code to condition

    Excludes2: Other postprocedural states (Z98.-)

    personal history of medical treatment (Z92.-)

    presence of cardiac and vascular implants and grafts (Z95.-) presence of other devices (Z97.-)

    presence of other functional implants (Z96.-) transplanted organ and tissue status (Z94.-)

    Z87.71 **Personal history of (corrected) congenital malformations of genitourinary system**

Z87.710 Personal history of (corrected) hypospadias

Z87.718 Personal history of other specified (corrected) congenital malformations of genitourinary system

Z87.72 Personal history of (corrected) congenital malformations of nervous system and sense organs

Z87.720 Personal history of (corrected) congenital malformations of eye

Z87.721 Personal history of (corrected) congenital malformations of ear

Z87.728 Personal history of other specified (corrected) congenital malformations of nervous system and sense organs

Z87.73 Personal history of (corrected) congenital malformations of digestive system

Z87.730 Personal history of (corrected) cleft lip and palate

Z87.738 Personal history of other specified (corrected) congenital malformations of digestive system

Z87.74 Personal history of (corrected) congenital malformations of heart and circulatory system

Z87.75 Personal history of (corrected) congenital malformations of respiratory system

Z87.76 Personal history of (corrected) congenital malformations of integument, limbs and musculoskeletal system

Z87.79 Personal history of other (corrected) congenital malformations

Z87.790 Personal history of (corrected) congenital malformations of face and neck

Z87.798 Personal history of other (corrected) congenital malformations

Z87.8 Personal history of other specified conditions

Excludes2: personal history of self harm (Z91.5-)

Z87.81 Personal history of (healed) traumatic fracture

Excludes2: personal history of (healed) nontraumatic fracture (Z87.31-)

Z87.82 Personal history of other (healed) physical injury and trauma

Conditions classifiable to S00-T88, except traumatic fractures

Z87.820 Personal history of traumatic brain injury

Excludes1: personal history of transient ischemic attack (TIA), and cerebral infarction without residual deficits (Z86.73)

Z87.821 Personal history of retained foreign body fully removed

Z87.828 Personal history of other (healed) physical injury and trauma

Z87.89 Personal history of other specified conditions

Z87.890 Personal history of sex reassignment

Z87.891 Personal history of nicotine dependence

Excludes1: current nicotine dependence (F17.2-)

Z87.892 Personal history of anaphylaxis

Code also allergy status such as:

allergy status to drugs, medicaments and biological substances (Z88.-)

allergy status, other than to drugs and biological substances (Z91.0-)

Z87.898 Personal history of other specified conditions

Z88 Allergy status to drugs, medicaments and biological substances

Excludes2: Allergy status, other than to drugs and biological substances (Z91.0-)

Z88.0 Allergy status to penicillin

Z88.1 Allergy status to other antibiotic agents

Z88.2 Allergy status to sulfonamides

Z88.3 Allergy status to other anti-infective agents

Z88.4 Allergy status to anesthetic agent

Z88.5 Allergy status to narcotic agent

Z88.6 Allergy status to analgesic agent

Z88.7 Allergy status to serum and vaccine

Z88.8 Allergy status to other drugs, medicaments and biological substances

Z88.9 Allergy status to unspecified drugs, medicaments and biological substances

Z89 Acquired absence of limb

Includes: amputation status

postprocedural loss of limb

post-traumatic loss of limb

Excludes1: acquired deformities of limbs (M20-M21)

congenital absence of limbs (Q71-Q73)

Z89.0 Acquired absence of thumb and other finger(s)

Z89.01 Acquired absence of thumb

Z89.011 Acquired absence of right thumb

Z89.012 Acquired absence of left thumb

Z89.019 Acquired absence of unspecified thumb

Z89.02 Acquired absence of other finger(s)

Excludes2: acquired absence of thumb (Z89.01-)

Z89.021 Acquired absence of right finger(s)

Z89.022 Acquired absence of left finger(s)

Z89.029 Acquired absence of unspecified finger(s)

Z89.1 Acquired absence of hand and wrist

Z89.11 Acquired absence of hand

Z89.111 Acquired absence of right hand

Z89.112 Acquired absence of left hand

Z89.119 Acquired absence of unspecified hand

Z89.12 Acquired absence of wrist

Disarticulation at wrist

Z89.121 Acquired absence of right wrist

Z89.122 Acquired absence of left wrist

Z89.129 Acquired absence of unspecified wrist

Z89.2 Acquired absence of upper limb above wrist

Z89.20 Acquired absence of upper limb, unspecified level

Z89.201 Acquired absence of right upper limb, unspecified level

Z89.202 Acquired absence of left upper limb, unspecified level

Z89.209 Acquired absence of unspecified upper limb, unspecified level

Acquired absence of arm NOS

Z89.21 Acquired absence of upper limb below elbow

● New code   ▲ Revised code   **Excludes1:** Not coded here   **Excludes2:** Not included here   ⊗ Placeholder required   ⑦7th digit required

Z89.211 **Acquired absence of right upper limb below elbow**

Z89.212 **Acquired absence of left upper limb below elbow**

Z89.219 **Acquired absence of unspecified upper limb below elbow**

Z89.22 **Acquired absence of upper limb above elbow**

Disarticulation at elbow

Z89.221 **Acquired absence of right upper limb above elbow**

Z89.222 **Acquired absence of left upper limb above elbow**

Z89.229 **Acquired absence of unspecified upper limb above elbow**

Z89.23 **Acquired absence of shoulder**

Acquired absence of shoulder joint following explantation of shoulder joint prosthesis, with or without presence of antibiotic-impregnated cement spacer

Z89.231 **Acquired absence of right shoulder**

Z89.232 **Acquired absence of left shoulder**

Z89.239 **Acquired absence of unspecified shoulder**

Z89.4 **Acquired absence of toe(s), foot, and ankle**

Z89.41 **Acquired absence of great toe**

Z89.411 **Acquired absence of right great toe**

Z89.412 **Acquired absence of left great toe** [HCC]

Z89.419 **Acquired absence of unspecified great toe** [HCC]

Z89.42 **Acquired absence of other toe(s)**

Excludes2: acquired absence of great toe (Z89.41-)

Z89.421 **Acquired absence of other right toe(s)** [HCC]

Z89.422 **Acquired absence of other left toe(s)** [HCC]

Z89.429 **Acquired absence of other toe(s), unspecified side** [HCC]

Z89.43 **Acquired absence of foot** [HCC]

Z89.431 **Acquired absence of right foot** [HCC]

Z89.432 **Acquired absence of left foot** [HCC]

Z89.439 **Acquired absence of unspecified foot** [HCC]

Z89.44 **Acquired absence of ankle**

Disarticulation of ankle

Z89.441 **Acquired absence of right ankle** [HCC]

Z89.442 **Acquired absence of left ankle** [HCC]

Z89.449 **Acquired absence of unspecified ankle** [HCC]

Z89.5 **Acquired absence of leg below knee**

Z89.51 **Acquired absence of leg below knee**

Z89.511 **Acquired absence of right leg below knee** [HCC]

Z89.512 **Acquired absence of left leg below knee** [HCC]

Z89.519 **Acquired absence of unspecified leg below knee** [HCC]

Z89.52 **Acquired absence of knee**

Acquired absence of knee joint following explantation of knee joint prosthesis, with or without presence of antibiotic-impregnated cement spacer

Z89.521 **Acquired absence of right knee**

Z89.522 **Acquired absence of left knee**

Z89.529 **Acquired absence of unspecified knee**

Z89.6 **Acquired absence of leg above knee**

Z89.61 **Acquired absence of leg above knee**

Acquired absence of leg NOS

Disarticulation at knee

Z89.611 **Acquired absence of right leg above knee** [HCC]

Z89.612 **Acquired absence of left leg above knee** [HCC]

Z89.619 **Acquired absence of unspecified leg above knee** [HCC]

Z89.62 **Acquired absence of hip**

Acquired absence of hip joint following explantation of hip joint prosthesis, with or without presence of antibiotic-impregnated cement spacer

Disarticulation at hip

Z89.621 **Acquired absence of right hip joint**

Z89.622 **Acquired absence of left hip joint**

Z89.629 **Acquired absence of unspecified hip joint**

Z89.9 **Acquired absence of limb, unspecified**

Z90 **Acquired absence of organs, not elsewhere classified**

Includes: postprocedural or post-traumatic loss of body part NEC

Excludes1: congenital absence - see Alphabetical Index

Excludes2: postprocedural absence of endocrine glands (E89.-)

Z90.0 **Acquired absence of part of head and neck**

Z90.01 **Acquired absence of eye**

Z90.02 **Acquired absence of larynx**

Z90.09 **Acquired absence of other part of head and neck**

Acquired absence of nose

Excludes2: teeth (K08.1)

Z90.1 **Acquired absence of breast and nipple**

Z90.10 **Acquired absence of unspecified breast and nipple**

Z90.11 **Acquired absence of right breast and nipple**

Z90.12 **Acquired absence of left breast and nipple**

Z90.13 **Acquired absence of bilateral breasts and nipples**

Z90.2 **Acquired absence of lung [part of]**

Z90.3 **Acquired absence of stomach [part of]**

Z90.4 **Acquired absence of other specified parts of digestive tract**

Z90.41 **Acquired absence of pancreas**

Code also exocrine pancreatic insufficiency (K86.81)

Use Additional Code to identify any associated:

diabetes mellitus, postpancreatectomy (E13.-)

insulin use (Z79.4)

Z90.410 **Acquired total absence of pancreas**

Acquired absence of pancreas NOS

Z90.411 **Acquired partial absence of pancreas**

Z90.49 **Acquired absence of other specified parts of digestive tract**

Z90.5 **Acquired absence of kidney**

Z90.6 **Acquired absence of other parts of urinary tract**

Acquired absence of bladder

Z90.7 **Acquired absence of genital organ(s)**

Excludes1: personal history of sex reassignment (Z87.890)

Excludes2: female genital mutilation status (N90.81-)

Z90.71 **Acquired absence of cervix and uterus**

    Z90.710 **Acquired absence of both cervix and uterus**

        Acquired absence of uterus NOS

        Status post total hysterectomy

    Z90.711 **Acquired absence of uterus with remaining cervical stump**

        Status post partial hysterectomy with remaining cervical stump

    Z90.712 **Acquired absence of cervix with remaining uterus**

Z90.72 **Acquired absence of ovaries**

    Z90.721 **Acquired absence of ovaries, unilateral**

    Z90.722 **Acquired absence of ovaries, bilateral**

Z90.79 **Acquired absence of other genital organ(s)**

Z90.8 **Acquired absence of other organs**

  Z90.81 **Acquired absence of spleen**

  Z90.89 **Acquired absence of other organs**

Z91 **Personal risk factors, not elsewhere classified**

Excludes2: contact with and (suspected) exposures hazardous to health (Z77.-)

exposure to pollution and other problems related to physical environment (Z77.1-)

female genital mutilation status (N90.81-)

personal history of physical injury and trauma (Z87.81, Z87.82-)

occupational exposure to risk factors (Z57.-)

Z91.0 **Allergy status, other than to drugs and biological substances**

Excludes2: Allergy status to drugs, medicaments, and biological substances (Z88.-)

Z91.01 **Food allergy status**

Excludes2: food additives allergy status (Z91.02)

  Z91.010 **Allergy to peanuts**

  Z91.011 **Allergy to milk products**

    Excludes1: lactose intolerance (E73.-)

  Z91.012 **Allergy to eggs**

  Z91.013 **Allergy to seafood**

    Allergy to shellfish

    Allergy to octopus or squid ink

  • **Z91.014** **Allergy to mammalian meats**

    Allergy to beef

    Allergy to lamb

    Allergy to pork

    Allergy to red meats

  Z91.018 **Allergy to other foods**

    Allergy to nuts other than peanuts

Z91.02 **Food additives allergy status**

Z91.03 **Insect allergy status**

  Z91.030 **Bee allergy status**

  Z91.038 **Other insect allergy status**

Z91.04 **Nonmedicinal substance allergy status**

  Z91.040 **Latex allergy status**

    Latex sensitivity status

  Z91.041 **Radiographic dye allergy status**

    Allergy status to contrast media used for diagnostic X-ray procedure

  Z91.048 **Other nonmedicinal substance allergy status**

Z91.09 **Other allergy status, other than to drugs and biological substances**

Z91.1 **Patient's noncompliance with medical treatment and regimen**

Z91.11 **Patient's noncompliance with dietary regimen**

Z91.12 **Patient's intentional underdosing of medication regimen**

Code first underdosing of medication (T36-T50) with fifth or sixth character 6

Excludes1: adverse effect of prescribed drug taken as directed- code to adverse effect poisoning (overdose) -code to poisoning

  Z91.120 **Patient's intentional underdosing of medication regimen due to financial hardship**

  Z91.128 **Patient's intentional underdosing of medication regimen for other reason**

Z91.13 **Patient's unintentional underdosing of medication regimen**

Code first underdosing of medication (T36-T50) with fifth or sixth character 6

Excludes1: adverse effect of prescribed drug taken as directed- code to adverse effect poisoning (overdose) -code to poisoning

  Z91.130 **Patient's unintentional underdosing of medication regimen due to age-related debility**

  Z91.138 **Patient's unintentional underdosing of medication regimen for other reason**

Z91.14 **Patient's other noncompliance with medication regimen**

Patient's underdosing of medication NOS

Z91.15 **Patient's noncompliance with renal dialysis** [HCC]

Z91.19 **Patient's noncompliance with other medical treatment and regimen**

Nonadherence to medical treatment

Z91.4 **Personal history of psychological trauma, not elsewhere classified**

Z91.41 **Personal history of adult abuse**

Excludes2: personal history of abuse in childhood (Z62.81-)

  Z91.410 **Personal history of adult physical and sexual abuse**

    Excludes1: current adult physical abuse (T74.11, T76.11)

        current adult sexual abuse (T74.21, T76.11)

  Z91.411 **Personal history of adult psychological abuse**

  Z91.412 **Personal history of adult neglect**

    Excludes1: current adult neglect (T74.01, T76.01)

  Z91.419 **Personal history of unspecified adult abuse**

Z91.42 **Personal history of forced labor or sexual exploitation**

Z91.49 **Other personal history of psychological trauma, not elsewhere classified**

Z91.5 **Personal history of self-harm**

Code also mental health disorder, if known

- **Z91.51** **Personal history of suicidal behavior**

  Personal history of parasuicide

  Personal history of self-poisoning

  Personal history of suicide attempt

- **Z91.52** **Personal history of nonsuicidal self-harm**

  Personal history of nonsuicidal self-injury

  Personal history of self-inflicted injury without suicidal intent

  Personal history of self-mutilation

Z91.8 **Other specified personal risk factors, not elsewhere classified**

  Z91.81 **History of falling**

  At risk for falling

  Z91.82 **Personal history of military deployment**

  Individual (civilian or military) with past history of military war, peacekeeping and humanitarian deployment (current or past conflict)

  Returned from military deployment

  Z91.83 **Wandering in diseases classified elsewhere**

  Code first underlying disorder such as:

  Alzheimer's disease (G30.-)

  autism or pervasive developmental disorder (F84.-)

  intellectual disabilities (F70-F79)

  unspecified dementia with behavioral disturbance (F03.9-)

  Z91.84 **Oral health risk factors**

  Z91.841 **Risk for dental caries, low**

  Z91.842 **Risk for dental caries, moderate**

  Z91.843 **Risk for dental caries, high**

  Z91.849 **Unspecified risk for dental caries**

  Z91.89 **Other specified personal risk factors, not elsewhere classified**

Z92 **Personal history of medical treatment**

Excludes2: postprocedural states (Z98.-)

Z92.0 **Personal history of contraception**

Excludes1: counseling or management of current contraceptive practices (Z30.-)

  long term (current) use of contraception (Z79.3)

  presence of (intrauterine) contraceptive device (Z97.5)

Z92.2 **Personal history of drug therapy**

Excludes2: long term (current) drug therapy (Z79.-)

  Z92.21 **Personal history of antineoplastic chemotherapy**

  Z92.22 **Personal history of monoclonal drug therapy**

  Z92.23 **Personal history of estrogen therapy**

  Z92.24 **Personal history of steroid therapy**

  Z92.240 **Personal history of inhaled steroid therapy**

  Z92.241 **Personal history of systemic steroid therapy**

  Personal history of steroid therapy NOS

  ▲ **Z92.25** **Personal history of immunosuppression therapy**

  Excludes2: personal history of steroid therapy (Z92.24)

  Z92.29 **Personal history of other drug therapy**

Z92.3 **Personal history of irradiation**

  Personal history of exposure to therapeutic radiation

Excludes1: exposure to radiation in the physical environment (Z77.12)

  occupational exposure to radiation (Z57.1)

Z92.8 **Personal history of other medical treatment**

  Z92.81 **Personal history of extracorporeal membrane oxygenation (ECMO)**

  Z92.82 **Status post administration of tPA (rtPA) in a different facility within the last 24 hours prior to admission to current facility**

  Code first condition requiring tPA administration, such as:

  acute cerebral infarction (I63.-)

  acute myocardial infarction (I21.-, I22.-)

  Z92.83 **Personal history of failed moderate sedation**

  Personal history of failed conscious sedation

  Excludes2: failed moderate sedation during procedure (T88.52)

  Z92.84 **Personal history of unintended awareness under general anesthesia**

  Excludes2: unintended awareness under general anesthesia during procedure (T88.53)

- **Z92.85** **Personal history of cellular therapy**

  - **Z92.850** **Personal history of Chimeric Antigen Receptor T-cell therapy**

    Personal history of CAR T-cell therapy

  - **Z92.858** **Personal history of other cellular therapy**

  - **Z92.859** **Personal history of cellular therapy, unspecified**

- **Z92.86** **Personal history of gene therapy**

  Z92.89 **Personal history of other medical treatment**

Z93 **Artificial opening status**

Excludes1: artificial openings requiring attention or management (Z43.-)

  complications of external stoma (J95.0-, K94.-, N99.5-)

Z93.0 **Tracheostomy status** [HCC]

Z93.1 **Gastrostomy status** [HCC]

Z93.2 **Ileostomy status** [HCC]

Z93.3 **Colostomy status** [HCC]

Z93.4 **Other artificial openings of gastrointestinal tract status** [HCC]

Z93.5 **Cystostomy status**

  Z93.50 **Unspecified cystostomy status** [HCC]

  Z93.51 **Cutaneous-vesicostomy status** [HCC]

  Z93.52 **Appendico-vesicostomy status** [HCC]

  Z93.59 **Other cystostomy status** [HCC]

Z93.6 **Other artificial openings of urinary tract statu** [HCC]**s**

  Nephrostomy status

  Ureterostomy status

  Urethrostomy status

Z93.8 **Other artificial opening status** [HCC]

Z93.9 **Artificial opening status, unspecified** [HCC]

Z94 **Transplanted organ and tissue status**

Includes: organ or tissue replaced by heterogenous or homogenous transplant

Excludes1: complications of transplanted organ or tissue - see Alphabetical Index

Excludes2: presence of vascular grafts (Z95.-)

Z94.0 **Kidney transplant status**

Z94.1 **Heart transplant status** [HCC]

    Excludes1: artificial heart status (Z95.812)

        heart-valve replacement status (Z95.2-Z95.4)

Z94.2 **Lung transplant status** [HCC]

Z94.3 **Heart and lungs transplant status** [HCC]

Z94.4 **Liver transplant status** [HCC]

Z94.5 **Skin transplant status**

    Autogenous skin transplant status

Z94.6 **Bone transplant status**

Z94.7 **Corneal transplant status**

Z94.8 **Other transplanted organ and tissue status**

    Z94.81 **Bone marrow transplant status** [HCC]

    Z94.82 **Intestine transplant status** [HCC]

    Z94.83 **Pancreas transplant status** [HCC]

    Z94.84 **Stem cells transplant status** [HCC]

    Z94.89 **Other transplanted organ and tissue status**

Z94.9 **Transplanted organ and tissue status, unspecified**

Z95 **Presence of cardiac and vascular implants and grafts**

    Excludes2: complications of cardiac and vascular devices, implants and grafts (T82.-)

Z95.0 **Presence of cardiac pacemaker**

    Presence of cardiac resynchronization therapy (CRT-P) pacemaker

    Excludes1: adjustment or management of cardiac device (Z45.0-)

        adjustment or management of cardiac pacemaker (Z45.0)

        presence of automatic (implantable) cardiac defibrillator with synchronous cardiac pacemaker (Z95.810)

Z95.1 **Presence of aortocoronary bypass graft**

    Presence of coronary artery bypass graft

Z95.2 **Presence of prosthetic heart valve**

    Presence of heart valve NOS

Z95.3 **Presence of xenogenic heart valve**

Z95.4 **Presence of other heart-valve replacement**

Z95.5 **Presence of coronary angioplasty implant and graft**

    Excludes1: coronary angioplasty status without implant and graft (Z98.61)

Z95.8 **Presence of other cardiac and vascular implants and grafts**

    Z95.81 **Presence of other cardiac implants and grafts**

        Z95.810 **Presence of automatic (implantable) cardiac defibrillator**

            Presence of automatic (implantable) cardiac defibrillator with synchronous cardiac pacemaker

            Presence of cardiac resynchronization therapy defibrillator (CRT-D)

            Presence of cardioverter-defibrillator (ICD)

        Z95.811 **Presence of heart assist device** [HCC]

        Z95.812 **Presence of fully implantable artificial heart** [HCC]

        Z95.818 **Presence of other cardiac implants and grafts**

    Z95.82 **Presence of other vascular implants and grafts**

        Z95.820 **Peripheral vascular angioplasty status with implants and grafts**

            Excludes1: peripheral vascular angioplasty without implant and graft (Z98.62)

        Z95.828 **Presence of other vascular implants and grafts**

            Presence of intravascular prosthesis NEC

Z95.9 **Presence of cardiac and vascular implant and graft, unspecified**

Z96 **Presence of other functional implants**

    Excludes2: complications of internal prosthetic devices, implants and grafts (T82-T85)

        fitting and adjustment of prosthetic and other devices (Z44-Z46)

Z96.0 **Presence of urogenital implants**

Z96.1 **Presence of intraocular lens**

    Presence of pseudophakia

Z96.2 **Presence of otological and audiological implants**

    Z96.20 **Presence of otological and audiological implant, unspecified**

    Z96.21 **Cochlear implant status**

    Z96.22 **Myringotomy tube(s) status**

    Z96.29 **Presence of other otological and audiological implants**

        Presence of bone-conduction hearing device

        Presence of eustachian tube stent

        Stapes replacement

Z96.3 **Presence of artificial larynx**

Z96.4 **Presence of endocrine implants**

    Z96.41 **Presence of insulin pump (external) (internal)**

    Z96.49 **Presence of other endocrine implants**

Z96.5 **Presence of tooth-root and mandibular implants**

Z96.6 **Presence of orthopedic joint implants**

    Z96.60 **Presence of unspecified orthopedic joint implant**

    Z96.61 **Presence of artificial shoulder joint**

        Z96.611 **Presence of right artificial shoulder joint**

        Z96.612 **Presence of left artificial shoulder joint**

        Z96.619 **Presence of unspecified artificial shoulder joint**

    Z96.62 **Presence of artificial elbow joint**

        Z96.621 **Presence of right artificial elbow joint**

        Z96.622 **Presence of left artificial elbow joint**

        Z96.629 **Presence of unspecified artificial elbow joint**

    Z96.63 **Presence of artificial wrist joint**

        Z96.631 **Presence of right artificial wrist joint**

        Z96.632 **Presence of left artificial wrist joint**

        Z96.639 **Presence of unspecified artificial wrist joint**

    Z96.64 **Presence of artificial hip joint**

        Hip-joint replacement (partial) (total)

        Z96.641 **Presence of right artificial hip joint**

        Z96.642 **Presence of left artificial hip joint**

        Z96.643 **Presence of artificial hip joint, bilateral**

        Z96.649 **Presence of unspecified artificial hip joint**

    Z96.65 **Presence of artificial knee joint**

        Z96.651 **Presence of right artificial knee joint**

        Z96.652 **Presence of left artificial knee joint**

        Z96.653 **Presence of artificial knee joint, bilateral**

● New code ▲ Revised code **Excludes1:** Not coded here **Excludes2:** Not included here ⊗ Placeholder required ⑦7th digit required

Z96.659   Presence of unspecified artificial knee joint

Z96.66   Presence of artificial ankle joint

Z96.661   Presence of right artificial ankle joint

Z96.662   Presence of left artificial ankle joint

Z96.669   Presence of unspecified artificial ankle joint

Z96.69   Presence of other orthopedic joint implants

Z96.691   Finger-joint replacement of right hand

Z96.692   Finger-joint replacement of left hand

Z96.693   Finger-joint replacement, bilateral

Z96.698   Presence of other orthopedic joint implants

Z96.7   Presence of other bone and tendon implants

Presence of skull plate

Z96.8   Presence of other specified functional implants

Z96.81   Presence of artificial skin

Z96.82   Presence of neurostimulator

Presence of brain neurostimulator

Presence of gastric neurostimulator

Presence of peripheral nerve neurostimulator

Presence of sacral nerve neurostimulator

Presence of spinal cord neurostimulator

Presence of vagus nerve neurostimulator

Z96.89   Presence of other specified functional implants

Z96.9   Presence of functional implant, unspecified

Z97   Presence of other devices

Excludes1: complications of internal prosthetic devices, implants and grafts (T82-T85)

Excludes2: fitting and adjustment of prosthetic and other devices (Z44-Z46)

presence of cerebrospinal fluid drainage device (Z98.2)

Z97.0   Presence of artificial eye

Z97.1   Presence of artificial limb (complete) (partial)

Z97.10   Presence of artificial limb (complete) (partial), unspecified

Z97.11   Presence of artificial right arm (complete) (partial)

Z97.12   Presence of artificial left arm (complete) (partial)

Z97.13   Presence of artificial right leg (complete) (partial)

Z97.14   Presence of artificial left leg (complete) (partial)

Z97.15   Presence of artificial arms, bilateral (complete) (partial)

Z97.16   Presence of artificial legs, bilateral (complete) (partial)

Z97.2   Presence of dental prosthetic device (complete) (partial)

Presence of dentures (complete) (partial)

Z97.3   Presence of spectacles and contact lenses

Z97.4   Presence of external hearing-aid

Z97.5   Presence of (intrauterine) contraceptive device

Excludes1: checking, reinsertion or removal of implantable subdermal contraceptive (Z30.46)

checking, reinsertion or removal of intrauterine contraceptive device (Z30.43-)

Z97.8   Presence of other specified devices

Z98   Other postprocedural states

Excludes2: aftercare (Z43-Z49, Z51)

follow-up medical care (Z08-Z09)

postprocedural complication - see Alphabetical Index

Z98.0   Intestinal bypass and anastomosis status

Excludes2: bariatric surgery status (Z98.84)

gastric bypass status (Z98.84)

obesity surgery status (Z98.84)

Z98.1   Arthrodesis status

Z98.2   Presence of cerebrospinal fluid drainage device

Presence of CSF shunt

Z98.3   Post therapeutic collapse of lung status

Code first underlying disease

Z98.4   Cataract extraction status

Use Additional Code to identify intraocular lens implant status (Z96.1)

Excludes1: aphakia (H27.0)

Z98.41   Cataract extraction status, right eye

Z98.42   Cataract extraction status, left eye

Z98.49   Cataract extraction status, unspecified eye

Z98.5   Sterilization status

Excludes1: female infertility (N97.-)

male infertility (N46.-)

Z98.51   Tubal ligation status

Z98.52   Vasectomy status

Z98.6   Angioplasty status

Z98.61   Coronary angioplasty status

Excludes1: coronary angioplasty status with implant and graft (Z95.5)

Z98.62   Peripheral vascular angioplasty status

Excludes1: peripheral vascular angioplasty status with implant and graft (Z95.820)

Z98.8   Other specified postprocedural states

Z98.81   Dental procedure status

Z98.810   Dental sealant status

Z98.811   Dental restoration status

Dental crown status

Dental fillings status

Z98.818   Other dental procedure status

Z98.82   Breast implant status

Excludes1: breast implant removal status (Z98.86)

Z98.83   Filtering (vitreous) bleb after glaucoma surgery status

Excludes1: Inflammation (infection) of postprocedural bleb (H59.4-)

Z98.84   Bariatric surgery status

Gastric banding status

Gastric bypass status for obesity

Obesity surgery status

Excludes1: bariatric surgery status complicating pregnancy, childbirth, or the puerperium (O99.84)

Excludes2: intestinal bypass and anastomosis status (Z98.0)

Z98.85   Transplanted organ removal status

Transplanted organ previously removed due to complication, failure, rejection or infection

Excludes1: encounter for removal of transplanted organ -code to complication of transplanted organ (T86.-)

Z98.86 **Personal history of breast implant removal**

Z98.87 **Personal history of in utero procedure**

Z98.870 **Personal history of in utero procedure during pregnancy**

Excludes2: complications from in utero procedure for current pregnancy (O35.7)

supervision of current pregnancy with history of in utero procedure during previous pregnancy (O09.82-)

Z98.871 **Personal history of in utero procedure while a fetus**

Z98.89 **Other specified postprocedural states**

Z98.890 **Other specified postprocedural states**

Personal history of surgery, not elsewhere classified

Z98.891 **History of uterine scar from previous surgery**

Excludes1: Maternal care due to uterine scar from previous surgery (O34.2-)

Z99 **Dependence on enabling machines and devices, not elsewhere classified**

Z99.0 **Dependence on aspirator**

Z99.1 **Dependence on respirator** Dependence on ventilator

Z99.11 **Dependence on respirator [ventilator] status**
[HCC]

Z99.12 **Encounter for respirator [ventilator] dependence during power failure**

Excludes1: mechanical complication of respirator [ventilator] (J95.850) [HCC]

Z99.2 **Dependence on renal dialysis** [HCC]

Hemodialysis status

Peritoneal dialysis status

Presence of arteriovenous shunt for dialysis

Renal dialysis status NOS

Excludes1: encounter for fitting and adjustment of dialysis catheter (Z49.0-)

Excludes2: noncompliance with renal dialysis (Z91.15)

Z99.3 **Dependence on wheelchair**

Wheelchair confinement status

Code first cause of dependence, such as:

muscular dystrophy (G71.0-)

obesity (E66.-)

Z99.8 **Dependence on other enabling machines and devices**

Z99.81 **Dependence on supplemental oxygen**

Dependence on long-term oxygen

Z99.89 **Dependence on other enabling machines and devices**

Dependence on machine or device NOS

Chapter 22
Codes for special purposes (U00-U85)

This chapter contains the following blocks:

U00-U49 Provisional assignment of new diseases of uncertain etiology or emergency use

Provisional assignment of new diseases of uncertain etiology or emergency use (U00-U49)

U07 **Emergency use of U07**

    U07.0 **Vaping-related disorder**

Dabbing related lung damage

Dabbing related lung injury

E-cigarette, or vaping, product use associated lung injury [EVALI]

Electronic cigarette related lung damage

Electronic cigarette related lung injury

Use Additional Code to identify manifestations, such as:

abdominal pain (R10.84)

acute respiratory distress syndrome (J80)

diarrhea (R19.7)

drug-induced interstitial lung disorder (J70.4)

lipoid pneumonia (J69.1)

weight loss (R63.4)

    U07.1 **COVID-19**

Use Additional Code to identify pneumonia or other manifestations

Excludes1: coronavirus infection, unspecified (B34.2)

coronavirus as the cause of diseases classified elsewhere (B97.2-)

pneumonia due to SARS-associated coronavirus (J12.81)

• **U09** **Post COVID-19 condition**

    • **U09.9** **Post COVID-19 condition, unspecified**

Note: This code enables establishment of a link with COVID-19.

This code is not to be used in cases that are still presenting with active COVID-19.

However, an exception is made in cases of re-infection with COVID-19, occurring with a condition related to prior COVID-19.

Post-acute sequela of COVID-19

Code first the specific condition related to COVID-19 if known, such as:

        chronic respiratory failure (J96.1-)

        loss of smell (R43.8)

        loss of taste (R43.8)

        multisystem inflammatory syndrome (M35.81)

        pulmonary embolism (I26.-)

        pulmonary fibrosis (J84.10)

● New code   ▲ Revised code   **Excludes1:** Not coded here   **Excludes2:** Not included here   ⊗ Placeholder required   ⑦7ᵗʰ digit required

VOL 2
ABC

A

Aarskog's syndrome Q87.1
Abandonment see Maltreatment
Abasia (-Astasia) (hysterical) F44.4
Abderhalden-Kaufmann-Lignac syndrome (cystinosis) E72.04
Abdomen, abdominal see also condition
| acute R10.0
| angina K55.1
| muscle deficiency syndrome Q79.4
Abdominalgia see Pain, abdominal
Abduction contracture, hip or other joint see Contraction, joint
Aberrant (congenital) see also Malposition, congenital
| adrenal gland Q89.1
| artery (peripheral) Q27.8
| | basilar NEC Q28.1
| | cerebral Q28.3
| | coronary Q24.5
| | digestive system Q27.8
| | eye Q15.8
| | lower limb Q27.8
| | precerebral Q28.1
| | pulmonary Q25.79
| | renal Q27.2
| | retina Q14.1
| | specified site NEC Q27.8
| | subclavian Q27.8
| | upper limb Q27.8
| | vertebral Q28.1
| breast Q83.8
| endocrine gland NEC Q89.2
| hepatic duct Q44.5
| pancreas Q45.3
| parathyroid gland Q89.2
| pituitary gland Q89.2
| sebaceous glands, mucous membrane, mouth, congenital Q38.6
| spleen Q89.09
| subclavian artery Q27.8
| thymus (gland) Q89.2
| thyroid gland Q89.2
| vein (peripheral) NEC Q27.8
| | cerebral Q28.3
| | digestive system Q27.8
| | lower limb Q27.8
| | precerebral Q28.1
| | specified site NEC Q27.8
| | upper limb Q27.8
Aberration
| distantial see Disturbance, visual
| mental F99
Abetalipoproteinemia E78.6
Abiotrophy R68.89
Ablatio, ablation
| retinae see Detachment, retina
Ablepharia, ablepharon Q10.3
Abnormal, abnormality, abnormalities see also Anomaly
| acid-base balance (mixed) E87.4
| albumin R77.0
| alphafetoprotein R77.2
| alveolar ridge K08.9
| anatomical relationship Q89.9
| apertures, congenital, diaphragm Q79.1
| auditory perception H93.29-
| | diplacusis see Diplacusis
| | hyperacusis see Hyperacusis
| | recruitment see Recruitment, auditory
| | threshold shift see Shift, auditory threshold
| autosomes Q99.9
| | fragile site Q95.5

Abnormal, abnormality, abnormalities - continued

| basal metabolic rate R94.8
| biosynthesis, testicular androgen E29.1
| bleeding time R79.1
| blood amino-acid level R79.83
| blood-gas level R79.81
| blood level (of)
| | cobalt R79.0
| | copper R79.0
| | iron R79.0
| | lithium R78.89
| | magnesium R79.0
| | mineral NEC R79.0
| | zinc R79.0
| blood pressure
| | elevated R03.0
| | low reading (nonspecific) R03.1
| blood sugar R73.09
| bowel sounds R19.15
| | absent R19.11
| | hyperactive R19.12
| brain scan R94.02
| breathing R06.9
| caloric test R94.138
| cerebrospinal fluid R83.9
| | cytology R83.6
| | drug level R83.2
| | enzyme level R83.0
| | hormones R83.1
| | immunology R83.4
| | microbiology R83.5
| | nonmedicinal level R83.3
| | specified type NEC R83.8
| chemistry, blood R79.9
| | C-reactive protein R79.82
| | drugs see Findings, abnormal, in blood
| | gas level R79.81
| | minerals R79.0
| | pancytopenia D61.818
| | PTT R79.1
| | specified NEC R79.89
| | toxins see Findings, abnormal, in blood
| chest sounds (friction) (rales) R09.89
| chromosome, chromosomal Q99.9
| | with more than three X chromosomes, female Q97.1
| | analysis result R89.8
| | | bronchial washings R84.8
| | | cerebrospinal fluid R83.8
| | | cervix uteri NEC R87.89
| | | nasal secretions R84.8
| | | nipple discharge R89.8
| | | peritoneal fluid R85.89
| | | pleural fluid R84.8
| | | prostatic secretions R86.8
| | | saliva R85.89
| | | seminal fluid R86.8
| | | sputum R84.8
| | | synovial fluid R89.8
| | | throat scrapings R84.8
| | | vagina R87.89
| | | vulva R87.89
| | | wound secretions R89.8
| | dicentric replacement Q93.2
| | ring replacement Q93.2
| | sex Q99.8
| | | female phenotype Q97.9
| | | | specified NEC Q97.8
| | | male phenotype Q98.9
| | | | specified NEC Q98.8
| | | structural male Q98.6
| | specified NEC Q99.8
| clinical findings NEC R68.89
| coagulation D68.9

Abnormal, abnormality, abnormalities - continued

| newborn, transient P61.6
| time R79.1
| communication see Fistula
| conjunctiva, vascular H11.41-
| | profile R79.1
| | time R79.1
| communication see Fistula
| conjunctiva, vascular H11.41-
| coronary artery Q24.5
| cortisol-binding globulin E27.8
| course, eustachian tube Q17.8
| creatinine clearance R94.4
| cytology
| | anus R85.619
| | | atypical squamous cells cannot exclude high grade squamous intraepithelial lesion (ASC-H) R85.611
| | | atypical squamous cells of undetermined significance (ASC-US) R85.610
| | | cytologic evidence of malignancy R85.614
| | | high grade squamous intraepithelial lesion (HGSIL) R85.613
| | | human papillomavirus (HPV) DNA test
| | | | high risk positive R85.81
| | | | low risk positive R85.82
| | | inadequate smear R85.615
| | | low grade squamous intraepithelial lesion (LGSIL) R85.612
| | | satisfactory anal smear but lacking transformation zone R85.616
| | | specified NEC R85.618
| | | unsatisfactory smear R85.615
| | female genital organs see Abnormal, Papanicolaou (smear)
| dark adaptation curve H53.61
| dentofacial NEC see Anomaly, dentofacial
| development, developmental Q89.9
| | central nervous system Q07.9
| diagnostic imaging
| | abdomen, abdominal region NEC R93.5
| | biliary tract R93.2
| | bladder R93.41
| | breast R92.8
| | central nervous system NEC R90.89
| | cerebrovascular NEC R90.89
| | coronary circulation R93.1
| | digestive tract NEC R93.3
| | gastrointestinal (tract) R93.3
| | genitourinary organs R93.89
| | head R93.0
| | heart R93.1
| | intrathoracic organ NEC R93.89
| | kidney R93.42-
| | limbs R93.6
| | liver R93.2
| | lung (field) R91.8
| | musculoskeletal system NEC R93.7
| | renal pelvis R93.41
| | retroperitoneum R93.5
| | site specified NEC R93.89
| | skin and subcutaneous tissue R93.89
| | skull R93.0
| | testis R93.81-
| | urinary organs specified NEC R93.49
| | ureter R93.41
| direction, teeth, fully erupted M26.30
| ear ossicles, acquired NEC H74.39
| | ankylosis see Ankylosis, ear ossicles
| | discontinuity see Discontinuity, ossicles, ear
| | partial loss see Loss, ossicles, ear (partial)
| | | Ebstein Q22.5

Abnormal, abnormality, abnormalities -
continued
  |echocardiogram R93.1
  |echoencephalogram R90.81
  |echogram *see* Abnormal, diagnostic imaging
  |electrocardiogram [ECG] [EKG] R94.31
  |electrocardiogram [ECG] [EKG] R94.31
  |electroencephalogram [EEG] R94.01
  |electrolyte *see* Imbalance, electrolyte
  |electromyogram [EMG] R94.131
  |electro-oculogram [EOG] R94.110
  |electrophysiological intracardiac studies
    R94.39
  |electroretinogram [ERG] R94.111
  |erythrocytes
    |congenital, with perinatal jaundice D58.9
  |feces (color) (contents) (mucus) R19.5
  |finding *see* Findings, abnormal, without
    diagnosis
  |fluid
    |amniotic *see* Abnormal, specimen, specified
    |cerebrospinal *see* Abnormal, cerebrospinal
      fluid
    |peritoneal *see* Abnormal, specimen,
      digestive organs
    |pleural *see* Abnormal, specimen, respiratory
      organs
    |synovial *see* Abnormal, specimen, specified
    |thorax (bronchial washings) (pleural fluid)
      see Abnormal, specimen, respiratory
      organs
    |vaginal *see* Abnormal, specimen, female
      genital organs
  |form
    |teeth K00.2
    |uterus *see* Anomaly, uterus
  |function studies
    |auditory R94.120
    |bladder R94.8
    |brain R94.09
    |cardiovascular R94.30
    |ear R94.128
    |endocrine NEC R94.7
    |eye NEC R94.118
    |kidney R94.4
    |liver R94.5
    |nervous system
      |central NEC R94.09
      |peripheral NEC R94.138
    |pancreas R94.8
    |placenta R94.8
    |pulmonary R94.2
    |special senses NEC R94.128
    |spleen R94.8
    |thyroid R94.6
    |vestibular R94.121
  |gait *see* Gait
    |hysterical F44.4
  |gastrin secretion E16.4
  |globulin R77.1
    |cortisol-binding E27.8
    |thyroid-binding E07.89
  |glomerular, minor *see also* N00-N07 with
    fourth character .0 N05.0
  |glucagon secretion E16.3
  |glucose tolerance (test) (non-fasting) R73.09
  |gravitational (G) forces or states (effect of)
    T75.81
  |hair (color) (shaft) L67.9
    |specified NEC L67.8
  |hard tissue formation in pulp (dental) K04.3
  |head movement R25.0
  |heart
    |rate R00.9
      |specified NEC R00.8

Abnormal, abnormality, abnormalities -
continued
  |shadow R93.1
  |sounds NEC R01.2
  |hemoglobin (disease) *see also* Disease,
    hemoglobin D58.2
    |trait *see* Trait, hemoglobin, abnormal
  |histology NEC R89.7
  |immunological findings R89.4
    |in serum R76.9
      |specified NEC R76.8
  |increase in appetite R63.2
  |involuntary movement *see* Abnormal,
    movement, involuntary
  |jaw closure M26.51
  |karyotype R89.8
  |kidney function test R94.4
  |knee jerk R29.2
  |leukocyte (cell) (differential) NEC D72.9
  |liver function test (see also Elevated, liver
    function, test) R79.89
  |loss of
    |height R29.890
    |weight R63.4
  |mammogram NEC R92.8
    |calcification (calculus) R92.1
    |microcalcification R92.0
  |Mantoux test R76.11
  |movement (disorder) *see also* Disorder,
    movement
    |head R25.0
    |involuntary R25.9
      |fasciculation R25.3
      |of head R25.0
      |spasm R25.2
      |specified type NEC R25.8
      |tremor R25.1
  |myoglobin (Aberdeen) (Annapolis) R89.7
  |neonatal screening P09.9
    |for
      |congenital adrenal hyperplasia P09.2
      |congenital endocrine disease P09.2
      |congenital hematologic disorders P09.3
      |critical congenital heart disease P09.5
      |cystic fibrosis P09.4
      |hemoglobinothies P09.3
    |hypothyroidism P09.2
    |inborn errors of metabolism P09.1
    |neonatal hearing loss P09.6
    |red cell membrane defects P09.3
    |sickle cell P09.3
    |specified NEC P09.8
  |oculomotor study R94.113
  |palmar creases Q82.8
  |Papanicolaou (smear)
    |anus R85.619
      |atypical squamous cells cannot exclude
        high grade squamous intraepithelial
        lesion (ASC-H) R85.611
      |atypical squamous cells of undetermined
        significance (ASC-US) R85.610
      |cytologic evidence of malignancy
        R85.614
      |high grade squamous intraepithelial lesion
        (HGSIL) R85.613
      |human papillomavirus (HPV) DNA test
        |high risk positive R85.81
        |low risk positive R85.82
      |inadequate smear R85.615
      |low grade squamous intraepithelial lesion
        (LGSIL) R85.612
      |satisfactory anal smear but lacking
        transformation zone R85.616
      |specified NEC R85.618

Abnormal, abnormality, abnormalities -
continued
    |unsatisfactory smear R85.615
  |bronchial washings R84.6
  |cerebrospinal fluid R83.6
  |cervix R87.619
    |atypical squamous cells cannot exclude
      high grade squamous intraepithelial
      lesion (ASC-H) R87.611
    |atypical squamous cells of undetermined
      significance (ASC-US) R87.610
    |cytologic evidence of malignancy
      R87.614
    |high grade squamous intraepithelial lesion
      (HGSIL) R87.613
    |inadequate smear R87.615
    |low grade squamous intraepithelial lesion
      (LGSIL) R87.612
    |non-atypical endometrial cells R87.618
    |satisfactory cervical smear but lacking
      transformation zone R87.616
    |specified NEC R87.618
    |thin preparation R87.619
    |unsatisfactory smear R87.615
  |nasal secretions R84.6
  |nipple discharge R89.6
  |peritoneal fluid R85.69
  |pleural fluid R84.6
  |prostatic secretions R86.6
  |saliva R85.69
  |seminal fluid R86.6
  |sites NEC R89.6
  |sputum R84.6
  |synovial fluid R89.6
  |throat scrapings R84.6
  |vagina R87.629
    |atypical squamous cells cannot exclude
      high grade squamous intraepithelial
      lesion (ASC-H) R87.621
    |atypical squamous cells of undetermined
      significance (ASC-US) R87.620
    |cytologic evidence of malignancy
      R87.624
    |high grade squamous intraepithelial lesion
      (HGSIL) R87.623
    |inadequate smear R87.625
    |low grade squamous intraepithelial lesion
      (LGSIL) R87.622
    |specified NEC R87.628
    |thin preparation R87.629
    |unsatisfactory smear R87.625
  |vulva R87.69
  |wound secretions R89.6
  |partial thromboplastin time (PTT) R79.1
  |pelvis (bony) *see* Deformity, pelvis
  |percussion, chest (tympany) R09.89
  |periods (grossly) *see* Menstruation
  |phonocardiogram R94.39
  |plantar reflex R29.2
  |plasma
    |protein R77.9
      |specified NEC R77.8
    |viscosity R70.1
  |pleural (folds) Q34.0
  |posture R29.3
  |product of conception O02.9
    |specified type NEC O02.89
  |prothrombin time (PT) R79.1
  |pulmonary
    |artery, congenital Q25.79
    |function, newborn P28.89
    |test results R94.2
  |pulsations in neck R00.2
  |pupillary H21.56-
    |function (reaction) (reflex) *see* Anomaly,
      pupil, function

Abnormal, abnormality, abnormalities -
continued
  |radiological examination *see* Abnormal,
    diagnostic imaging
  |red blood cell(s) (morphology) (volume)
    R71.8
  |reflex *see* Reflex
  |renal function test R94.4
  |response to nerve stimulation R94.130
  |retinal correspondence H53.31
  |retinal function study R94.111
  |rhythm, heart *see also* Arrhythmia
  |saliva *see* Abnormal, specimen, digestive
    organs
  |scan
    |kidney R94.4
    |liver R93.2
    |thyroid R94.6
  |secretion
    |gastrin E16.4
    |glucagon E16.3
  |serum level (of)
    |acid phosphatase R74.8
    |alkaline phosphatase R74.8
    |amylase R74.8
    |enzymes R74.9
      |specified NEC R74.8
    |lipase R74.8
    |triacylglycerol lipase R74.8
  |shape
    |gravid uterus *see* Anomaly, uterus
  |sinus venosus Q21.1
  |size, tooth, teeth K00.2
  |spacing, tooth, teeth, fully erupted M26.30
  |specimen
    |digestive organs (peritoneal fluid) (saliva)
      R85.9
      |cytology R85.69
      |drug level R85.2
      |enzyme level R85.0
      |histology R85.7
      |hormones R85.1
      |immunology R85.4
      |microbiology R85.5
      |nonmedicinal level R85.3
      |specified type NEC R85.89
    |female genital organs (secretions) (smears)
      R87.9
      |cytology R87.69
        |cervix R87.619
          |human papillomavirus (HPV) DNA
            test
            |high risk positive R87.810
            |low risk positive R87.820
          |inadequate (unsatisfactory) smear
            R87.615
         |non-atypical endometrial cells
            R87.618
         |specified NEC R87.618
        |vagina R87.629
          |human papillomavirus (HPV) DNA
            test
            |high risk positive R87.811
            |low risk positive R87.821
          |inadequate (unsatisfactory) smear
            R87.625
        |vulva R87.69
      |drug level R87.2
      |enzyme level R87.0
      |histological R87.7
      |hormones R87.1
      |immunology R87.4
      |microbiology R87.5 .
      |nonmedicinal level R87.3
      |specified type NEC R87.89

Abnormal, abnormality, abnormalities -
continued
  |male genital organs (prostatic secretions)
    (semen) R86.9
    |cytology R86.6
    |drug level R86.2
    |enzyme level R86.0
    |histological R86.7
    |hormones R86.1
    |immunology R86.4
    |microbiology R86.5
    |nonmedicinal level R86.3
    |specified type NEC R86.8
  |nipple discharge *see* Abnormal, specimen,
    specified
  |respiratory organs (bronchial washings)
    (nasal secretions) (pleural fluid) (sputum)
    R84.9
    |cytology R84.6
    |drug level R84.2
    |enzyme level R84.0
    |histology R84.7
    |hormones R84.1
    |immunology R84.4
    |microbiology R84.5
    |nonmedicinal level R84.3
    |specified type NEC R84.8
  |specified organ, system and tissue NOS
    R89.9
    |cytology R89.6
    |drug level R89.2
    |enzyme level R89.0
    |histology R89.7
    |hormones R89.1
    |immunology R89.4
    |microbiology R89.5
    |nonmedicinal level R89.3
    |specified type NEC R89.8
  |synovial fluid *see* Abnormal, specimen,
    specified
  |thorax (bronchial washings) (pleural fluids)
    see Abnormal, specimen, respiratory
    organs
    |vagina (secretion) (smear) R87.629
    |vulva (secretion) (smear) R87.69
    |wound secretion *see* Abnormal, specimen,
      specified
  |spermatozoa *see* Abnormal, specimen, male
    genital organs
  |sputum (amount) (color) (odor) R09.3
  |stool (color) (contents) (mucus) R19.5
    |bloody K92.1
    |guaiac positive R19.5
  |synchondrosis Q78.8
  |thermography *see also* Abnormal, diagnostic
    imaging R93.89
  |thyroid-binding globulin E07.89
  |tooth, teeth (form) (size) K00.2
  |toxicology (findings) R78.9
  |transport protein E88.09
  |tumor marker NEC R97.8
  |ultrasound results *see* Abnormal, diagnostic
    imaging
  |umbilical cord complicating delivery O69.9
  |urination NEC R39.198
  |urine (constituents) R82.90
    |bile R82.2
    |cytological examination R82.8
    |drugs R82.5
    |fat R82.0
    |glucose R81
    |heavy metals R82.6
    |hemoglobin R82.3
    |histological examination R82.8
    |ketones R82.4

Abnormal, abnormality, abnormalities -
continued
  |microbiological examination (culture)
    R82.79
  |myoglobin R82.1
  |positive culture R82.79
  |protein *see* Proteinuria
  |specified substance NEC R82.998
    |chromoabnormality NEC R82.91
  |substances nonmedical R82.6
  |uterine hemorrhage *see* Hemorrhage, uterus
  |vectorcardiogram R94.39
  |visually evoked potential (VEP) R94.112
  |white blood cells D72.9
    |specified NEC D72.89
  |X-ray examination *see* Abnormal, diagnostic
    imaging
Abnormity (any organ or part) *see* Anomaly
Abocclusion M26.29
  |hemolytic disease (newborn) P55.1
  |incompatibility reaction ABO *see*
    Complication(s), transfusion, incompatibility
    reaction, ABO
Abolition, language R48.8
Aborter, habitual or recurrent *see* Loss (of),
  pregnancy, recurrent
Abortion (complete) (spontaneous) O03.9
  |with
    |retained products of conception *see*
      Abortion, incomplete
  |attempted (elective) (failed) O07.4
    |complicated by O07.30
      |afibrinogenemia O07.1
      |cardiac arrest O07.36
      |chemical damage of pelvic organ(s)
        O07.34
      |circulatory collapse O07.31
      |cystitis O07.38
      |defibrination syndrome O07.1
      |electrolyte imbalance O07.33
      |embolism (air) (amniotic fluid) (blood
        clot) (fat) (pulmonary) (septic) (soap)
        O07.2
      |endometritis O07.0
      |genital tract and pelvic infection O07.0
      |hemolysis O07.1
      |hemorrhage (delayed) (excessive) O07.1
      |infection
        |genital tract or pelvic O07.0
        |urinary tract O07.38
      |intravascular coagulation O07.1
      |laceration of pelvic organ(s) O07.34
      |metabolic disorder O07.33
      |oliguria O07.32
      |oophoritis O07.0
      |parametritis O07.0
      |pelvic peritonitis O07.0
      |perforation of pelvic organ(s) O07.34
      |renal failure or shutdown O07.32
      |salpingitis or salpingo-oophoritis O07.0
      |sepsis O07.37
      |shock O07.31
      |specified condition NEC O07.39
      |tubular necrosis (renal) O07.32
      |uremia O07.32
      |urinary tract infection O07.38
      |venous complication NEC O07.35
        |embolism (air) (amniotic fluid) (blood
          clot) (fat) (pulmonary) (septic) (soap)
          O07.2
  |complicated (by) (following) O03.80
    |afibrinogenemia O03.6
    |cardiac arrest O03.86
    |chemical damage of pelvic organ(s) O03.84
    |circulatory collapse O03.81
    |cystitis O03.88

Abortion (complete) (spontaneous) - *continued*
|defibrination syndrome O03.6
|electrolyte imbalance O03.83
|embolism (air) (amniotic fluid) (blood clot)
   (fat) (pulmonary) (septic) (soap) O03.7
|endometritis O03.5
|genital tract and pelvic infection O03.5
|hemolysis O03.6
|hemorrhage (delayed) (excessive) O03.6
|infection
   |genital tract or pelvic O03.5
   |urinary tract O03.88
|intravascular coagulation O03.6
|laceration of pelvic organ(s) O03.84
|metabolic disorder O03.83
|oliguria O03.82
|oophoritis O03.5
|parametritis O03.5
|pelvic peritonitis O03.5
|perforation of pelvic organ(s) O03.84
|renal failure or shutdown O03.82
|salpingitis or salpingo-oophoritis O03.5
|sepsis O03.87
|shock O03.81
|specified condition NEC O03.89
|tubular necrosis (renal) O03.82
|uremia O03.82
|urinary tract infection O03.88
|venous complication NEC O03.85
   |embolism (air) (amniotic fluid) (blood
     clot) (fat) (pulmonary) (septic) (soap)
     O03.7
|failed *see* Abortion, attempted
|habitual or recurrent N96
|with current abortion *see* categories O03-
   O04
|without current pregnancy N96
|care in current pregnancy O26.2-
|incomplete (spontaneous) O03.4
|complicated (by) (following) O03.30
   |afibrinogenemia O03.1
   |cardiac arrest O03.36
   |chemical damage of pelvic organ(s)
     O03.34
   |circulatory collapse O03.31
   |cystitis O03.38
   |defibrination syndrome O03.1
   |electrolyte imbalance O03.33
   |embolism (air) (amniotic fluid) (blood
     clot) (fat) (pulmonary) (septic) (soap)
     O03.2
   |endometritis O03.0
   |genital tract and pelvic infection O03.0
   |hemolysis O03.1
   |hemorrhage (delayed) (excessive) O03.1
   |infection
     |genital tract or pelvic O03.0
     |urinary tract O03.38
   |intravascular coagulation O03.1
   |laceration of pelvic organ(s) O03.34
   |metabolic disorder O03.33
   |oliguria O03.32
   |oophoritis O03.0
   |parametritis O03.0
   |pelvic peritonitis O03.0
   |perforation of pelvic organ(s) O03.34
   |renal failure or shutdown O03.32
   |salpingitis or salpingo-oophoritis O03.0
   |sepsis O03.37
   |shock O03.31
   |specified condition NEC O03.39
   |tubular necrosis (renal) O03.32
   |uremia O03.32
   |urinary infection O03.38
   |venous complication NEC O03.35
     |embolism (air) (amniotic fluid) (blood
       clot) (fat) (pulmonary) (septic) (soap)
       O03.2

Abortion (complete) (spontaneous) - *continued*
|induced (encounter for) Z33.2
|complicated by O04.80
   |afibrinogenemia O04.6
   |cardiac arrest O04.86
   |chemical damage of pelvic organ(s)
     O04.84
   |circulatory collapse O04.81
   |cystitis O04.88
   |defibrination syndrome O04.6
   |electrolyte imbalance O04.83
   |embolism (air) (amniotic fluid) (blood
     clot) (fat) (pulmonary) (septic) (soap)
     O04.7
   |endometritis O04.5
   |genital tract and pelvic infection O04.5
   |hemolysis O04.6
   |hemorrhage (delayed) (excessive) O04.6
   |infection
     |genital tract or pelvic O04.5
     |urinary tract O04.88
   |intravascular coagulation O04.6
   |laceration of pelvic organ(s) O04.84
   |metabolic disorder O04.83
   |oliguria O04.82
   |oophoritis O04.5
   |parametritis O04.5
   |pelvic peritonitis O04.5
   |perforation of pelvic organ(s) O04.84
   |renal failure or shutdown O04.82
   |salpingitis or salpingo-oophoritis O04.5
   |sepsis O04.87
   |shock O04.81
   |specified condition NEC O04.89
   |tubular necrosis (renal) O04.82
   |uremia O04.82
   |urinary tract infection O04.88
   |venous complication NEC O04.85
     |embolism (air) (amniotic fluid) (blood
       clot) (fat) (pulmonary) (septic)
       (soap) O04.7
|inevitable O03.4
|missed O02.1
|spontaneous *see* Abortion (complete)
   (spontaneous)
   |threatened O20.0
|threatened (spontaneous) O20.0
|tubal O00.10-
|with intrauterine pregnancy O00.11-
Abortus fever A23.1
Aboulomania F60.7
Abrami's disease D59.8
Abramov-Fiedler myocarditis (acute isolated
  myocarditis) I40.1
Abrasion T14.8
|abdomen, abdominal (wall) S30.811
|alveolar process S00.512
|ankle S90.51-
|antecubital space *see* Abrasion, elbow
|anus S30.817
|arm (upper) S40.81-
|auditory canal *see* Abrasion, ear
|auricle *see* Abrasion, ear
|axilla *see* Abrasion, arm
|back, lower S30.810
|breast S20.11-
|brow S00.81
|buttock S30.810
|calf *see* Abrasion, leg
|canthus *see* Abrasion, eyelid
|cheek S00.81
   |internal S00.512
|chest wall *see* Abrasion, thorax
|chin S00.81
|clitoris S30.814
|cornea S05.0-
|costal region *see* Abrasion, thorax

Abrasion - *continued*
|dental K03.1
|digit(s)
   |foot *see* Abrasion, toe
   |hand *see* Abrasion, finger
|ear S00.41-
|elbow S50.31-
|epididymis S30.813
|epigastric region S30.811
|epiglottis S10.11
|esophagus (thoracic) S27.818
   |cervical S10.11
|eyebrow *see* Abrasion, eyelid
|eyelid S00.21-
|face S00.81
|finger(s) S60.41-
   |index S60.41-
   |little S60.41-
   |middle S60.41-
   |ring S60.41-
|flank S30.811
|foot (except toe(s) alone) S90.81-
   |toe *see* Abrasion, toe
|forearm S50.81-
   |elbow only *see* Abrasion, elbow
|forehead S00.81
|genital organs, external
   |female S30.816
   |male S30.815
|groin S30.811
|gum S00.512
|hand S60.51-
|head S00.91
   |ear *see* Abrasion, ear
   |eyelid *see* Abrasion, eyelid
   |lip S00.511
   |nose S00.31
   |oral cavity S00.512
   |scalp S00.01
   |specified site NEC S00.81
|heel *see* Abrasion, foot
|hip S70.21-
|inguinal region S30.811
|interscapular region S20.419
|jaw S00.81
|knee S80.21-
|labium (majus) (minus) S30.814
|larynx S10.11
|leg (lower) S80.81-
   |knee *see* Abrasion, knee
   |upper *see* Abrasion, thigh
|lip S00.511
|lower back S30.810
|lumbar region S30.810
|malar region S00.81
|mammary *see* Abrasion, breast
|mastoid region S00.81
|mouth S00.512
|nail
   |finger *see* Abrasion, finger
   |toe *see* Abrasion, toe
|nape S10.81
|nasal S00.31
|neck S10.91
   |specified site NEC S10.81
   |throat S10.11
|nose S00.31
|occipital region S00.01
|oral cavity S00.512
|orbital region *see* Abrasion, eyelid
|palate S00.512
|palm *see* Abrasion, hand
|parietal region S00.01
|pelvis S30.810
|penis S30.812
|perineum

Abrasion - *continued*
|female S30.814
|male S30.810
|periocular area *see* Abrasion, eyelid
|phalanges
  |finger *see* Abrasion, finger
  |toe *see* Abrasion, toe
|pharynx S10.11
|pinna *see* Abrasion, ear
|popliteal space *see* Abrasion, knee
|prepuce S30.812
|pubic region S30.810
|pudendum
  |female S30.816
  |male S30.815
|sacral region S30.810
|scalp S00.01
|scapular region *see* Abrasion, shoulder
|scrotum S30.813
|shin *see* Abrasion, leg
|shoulder S40.21-
|skin NEC T14.8
|sternal region S20.319
|submaxillary region S00.81
|submental region S00.81
|subungual
  |finger(s) *see* Abrasion, finger
  |toe(s) *see* Abrasion, toe
|supraclavicular fossa S10.81
|supraorbital S00.81
|temple S00.81
|temporal region S00.81
|testis S30.813
|thigh S70.31-
|thorax, thoracic (wall) S20.91
  |back S20.41-
  |front S20.31-
|throat S10.11
|thumb S60.31
|toe(s) (lesser) S90.416
  |great S90.41-
|tongue S00.512
|tooth, teeth (dentifrice) (habitual) (hard
  tissues) (occupational) (ritual) (traditional)
  K03.1
|trachea S10.11
|tunica vaginalis S30.813
|tympanum, tympanic membrane *see* Abrasion,
  ear
|uvula S00.512
|vagina S30.814
|vocal cords S10.11
|vulva S30.814
|wrist S60.81-
Abrism *see* Poisoning, food, noxious, plant
Abruptio placentae O45.9-
|with
  |afibrinogenemia O45.01-
  |coagulation defect O45.00-
    |specified NEC O45.09-
  |disseminated intravascular coagulation
    O45.02-
  |hypofibrinogenemia O45.01-
|specified NEC O45.8-
Abruption, placenta *see* Abruptio placentae
Abscess (connective tissue) (embolic) (fistulous)
  (infective) (metastatic) (multiple) (pernicious)
  (pyogenic) (septic) L02.91
|with
  |diverticular disease (intestine) K57.80
    |with bleeding K57.81
    |large intestine K57.20
      |with
        |bleeding K57.21
        |small intestine K57.40
          |with bleeding K57.41

Abscess - *continued*
  |small intestine K57.00
    |with
      |bleeding K57.01
      |large intestine K57.40
        |with bleeding K57.41
  |lymphangitis   code by site under Abscess
|abdomen, abdominal
  |cavity K65.1
  |wall L02.211
|abdominopelvic K65.1
|accessory sinus *see* Sinusitis
|adrenal (capsule) (gland) E27.8
|alveolar K04.7
  |with sinus K04.6
|ambic A06.4
  |brain (and liver or lung abscess) A06.6
  |genitourinary tract A06.82
  |liver (without mention of brain or lung
    abscess) A06.4
  |lung (and liver) (without mention of brain
    abscess) A06.5
  |specified site NEC A06.89
  |spleen A06.89
|anaerobic A48.0
|ankle *see* Abscess, lower limb
|anorectal K61.2
|antecubital space *see* Abscess, upper limb
|antrum (chronic) (Highmore) *see* Sinusitis,
  maxillary
|anus K61.0
|apical (tooth) K04.7
  |with sinus (alveolar) K04.6
|appendix K35.33
|areola (acute) (chronic) (nonpuerperal) N61.1
  |puerperal, postpartum or gestational *see*
    Infection, nipple
|arm (any part) *see* Abscess, upper limb
|artery (wall) I77.89
|atheromatous I77.2
|auricle, ear *see* Abscess, ear, external
|axilla (region) L02.41-
  |lymph gland or node L04.2
|back (any part, except buttock) L02.212
|Bartholin's gland N75.1
  |with
    |abortion *see* Abortion, by type
      complicated by, sepsis
    |ectopic or molar pregnancy O08.0
  |following ectopic or molar pregnancy O08.0
|Bezold's *see* Mastoiditis, acute
|bilharziasis B65.1
|bladder (wall) *see* Cystitis, specified type
  NEC
|bone (subperiosteal) *see also* Osteomyelitis,
  specified type NEC
  |accessory sinus (chronic) *see* Sinusitis
  |chronic or old *see* Osteomyelitis, chronic
  |jaw (lower) (upper) M27.2
  |mastoid *see* Mastoiditis, acute, subperiosteal
  |petrous *see* Petrositis
  |spinal (tuberculous) A18.01
    |nontuberculous *see* Osteomyelitis,
      vertebra
|bowel K63.0
|brain (any part) (cystic) (otogenic) G06.0
  |amebic (with abscess of any other site)
    A06.6
  |gonococcal A54.82
  |pheomycotic (chromomycotic) B43.1
  |tuberculous A17.81
|breast (acute) (chronic) (nonpuerperal) N61.1
  |newborn P39.0
  |puerperal, postpartum, gestational *see*
    Mastitis, obstetric, purulent

Abscess - *continued*
|broad ligament N73.2
  |acute N73.0
  |chronic N73.1
|Brodie's (localized) (chronic) M86.8X-
|bronchi J98.09
|buccal cavity K12.2
|bulbourethral gland N34.0
|bursa M71.00
  |ankle M71.07-
  |elbow M71.02-
  |foot M71.07-
  |hand M71.04-
  |hip M71.05-
  |knee M71.06-
  |multiple sites M71.09
  |pharyngeal J39.1
  |shoulder M71.01-
  |specified site NEC M71.08
  |wrist M71.03-
|buttock L02.31
|canthus *see* Blepharoconjunctivitis
|cartilage *see* Disorder, cartilage, specified type
  NEC
|cecum K35.33
|cerebellum, cerebellar G06.0
  |sequelae G09
|cerebral (embolic) G06.0
  |sequelae G09
|cervical (meaning neck) L02.11
  |lymph gland or node L04.0
|cervix (stump) (uteri) *see* Cervicitis
|cheek (external) L02.01
  |inner K12.2
|chest J86.9
  |with fistula J86.0
  |wall L02.213
|chin L02.01
|choroid *see* Inflammation, chorioretinal
|circumtonsillar J36
|cold (lung) (tuberculous) *see also*
  Tuberculosis, abscess, lung
  |articular *see* Tuberculosis, joint
|colon (wall) K63.0
|colostomy K94.02
|conjunctiva *see* Conjunctivitis, acute
|cornea H16.31-
|corpus
  |cavernosum N48.21
  |luteum *see* Oophoritis
|Cowper's gland N34.0
|cranium G06.0
|cul-de-sac (Douglas') (posterior) *see*
  Peritonitis, pelvic, female
|cutaneous *see* Abscess, by site
|dental K04.7
  |with sinus (alveolar) K04.6
|dentoalveolar K04.7
  |with sinus K04.6
|diaphragm, diaphragmatic K65.1
|Douglas' cul-de-sac or pouch *see* Peritonitis,
  pelvic, female
|Dubois A50.59
|ear (middle) *see also* Otitis, media,
  suppurative
  |acute *see* Otitis, media, suppurative, acute
  |external H60.0-
|entamebic *see* Abscess, amebic
|enterostomy K94.12
|epididymis N45.4
|epidural G06.2
  |brain G06.0
  |spinal cord G06.1
|epiglottis J38.7
|epiploon, epiploic K65.1
|erysipelatous *see* Erysipelas

Abscess - *continued*

|esophagus K20.80
|ethmoid (bone) (chronic) (sinus) J32.2
|external auditory canal *see* Abscess, ear, external
|extradural G06.2
  |brain G06.0
    |sequelae G09
  |spinal cord G06.1
|extraperitoneal K68.19
|eye *see* Endophthalmitis, purulent
|eyelid H00.03-
|face (any part, except ear, eye and nose) L02.01
|fallopian tube *see* Salpingitis
|fascia M72.8
|fauces J39.1
|fecal K63.0
|femoral (region) *see* Abscess, lower limb
|filaria, filarial *see* Infestation, filarial
|finger (any) *see also* Abscess, hand
  |nail *see* Cellulitis, finger
|foot L02.61-
|forehead L02.01
|frontal sinus (chronic) J32.1
|gallbladder K81.0
|genital organ or tract
  |female (external) N76.4
  |male N49.9
    |multiple sites N49.8
    |specified NEC N49.8
|gestational mammary O91.11-
|gestational subareolar O91.11-
|gingival *see* Periodontitis, localized
|gland, glandular (lymph) (acute) *see* Lymphadenitis, acute
|gluteal (region) L02.31
|gonorrheal *see* Gonococcus
|groin L02.214
|gum *see* Periodontitis, localized
|hand L02.51-
|head NEC L02.811
  |face (any part, except ear, eye and nose) L02.01
|heart *see* Carditis
|heel *see* Abscess, foot
|helminthic *see* Infestation, helminth
|hepatic (cholangitic) (hematogenic) (lymphogenic) (pylephlebitic) K75.0
  |amebic A06.4
|hip (region) *see* Abscess, lower limb
|horseshoe K61.31
|ileocecal K35.33
|ileostomy (bud) K94.12
|iliac (region) L02.214
  |fossa K35.33
|infraclavicular (fossa) *see* Abscess, upper limb
|inguinal (region) L02.214
  |lymph gland or node L04.1
|intersphincteric K61.4
|intestine, intestinal NEC K63.0
  |rectal K61.1
|intra-abdominal *see also* Abscess, peritoneum K65.1
  |following procedure T81.43
    |obstetrical O86.03
  |postprocedural T81.43
    |retroperitoneal K68.11
|intracranial G06.0
|intramammary *see* Abscess, breast
|intramuscular, following procedure T81.42
  |obstetrical O86.02
|intraorbital *see* Abscess, orbit
|intraperitoneal K65.1
|intrasphincteric (anus) K61.4
|intraspinal G06.1

Abscess - *continued*

|intratonsillar J36
|ischiorectal (fossa) (specified NEC) K61.39
|jaw (bone) (lower) (upper) M27.2
|joint *see* Arthritis, pyogenic or pyemic
  |spine (tuberculous) A18.01
    |nontuberculous *see* Spondylopathy, infective
|kidney N15.1
  |with calculus N20.0
    |with hydronephrosis N13.6
  |puerperal (postpartum) O86.21
|knee *see also* Abscess, lower limb
  |joint M00.9
|labium (majus) (minus) N76.4
|lacrimal
  |caruncle *see* Inflammation, lacrimal, passages, acute
  |gland *see* Dacryoadenitis
  |passages (duct) (sac) *see* Inflammation, lacrimal, passages, acute
|lacunar N34.0
|larynx J38.7
|lateral (alveolar) K04.7
  |with sinus K04.6
|leg (any part) *see* Abscess, lower limb
|lens H27.8
|lingual K14.0
  |tonsil J36
|lip K13.0
|Littre's gland N34.0
|liver (cholangitic) (hematogenic) (lymphogenic) (pylephlebitic) (pyogenic) K75.0
  |amebic (due to Entamoeba histolytica) (dysenteric) (tropical) A06.4
    |with
      |brain abscess (and liver or lung abscess) A06.6
      |lung abscess A06.5
|loin (region) L02.211
|lower limb L02.41-
|lumbar (tuberculous) A18.01
  |nontuberculous L02.212
|lung (miliary) (putrid) J85.2
  |with pneumonia J85.1
    |due to specified organism (*see* Pneumonia, in (due to))
  |amebic (with liver abscess) A06.5
    |with
      |brain abscess A06.6
      |pneumonia A06.5
|lymph, lymphatic, gland or node (acute) *see also* Lymphadenitis, acute
  |mesentery I88.0
|malar M27.2
|mammary gland *see* Abscess, breast
|marginal, anus K61.0
|mastoid *see* Mastoiditis, acute
|maxilla, maxillary M27.2
  |molar (tooth) K04.7
    |with sinus K04.6
  |premolar K04.7
  |sinus (chronic) J32.0
|mediastinum J85.3
|meibomian gland *see* Hordeolum
|meninges G06.2
|mesentery, mesenteric K65.1
|mesosalpinx *see* Salpingitis
|mons pubis L02.215
|mouth (floor) K12.2
|muscle *see* Myositis, infective
|myocardium I40.0
|nabothian (follicle) *see* Cervicitis
|nasal J32.9
|nasopharyngeal J39.1

Abscess - *continued*

|navel L02.216
  |newborn P38.9
    |with mild hemorrhage P38.1
    |without hemorrhage P38.9
|neck (region) L02.11
  |lymph gland or node L04.0
|nephritic *see* Abscess, kidney
|nipple N61.1
  |associated with
    |lactation *see* Pregnancy, complicated by
    |pregnancy *see* Pregnancy, complicated by
|nose (external) (fossa) (septum) J34.0
  |sinus (chronic) *see* Sinusitis
|omentum K65.1
|operative wound T81.49
|orbit, orbital *see* Cellulitis, orbit
|otogenic G06.0
|ovary, ovarian (corpus luteum) *see* Oophoritis
|oviduct *see* Oophoritis
|palate (soft) K12.2
  |hard M27.2
|palmar (space) *see* Abscess, hand
|pancreas (duct) *see* Pancreatitis, acute
|parafrenal N48.21
|parametric, parametrium N73.2
  |acute N73.0
  |chronic N73.1
|paranephric N15.1
|parapancreatic *see* Pancreatitis, acute
|parapharyngeal J39.0
|pararectal K61.1
|parasinus *see* Sinusitis
|parauterine *see also* Disease, pelvis, inflammatory N73.2
|paravaginal *see* Vaginitis
|parietal region (scalp) L02.811
|parodontal *see* Periodontitis, aggressive, localized
|parotid (duct) (gland) K11.3
  |region K12.2
|pectoral (region) L02.213
|pelvis, pelvic
  |female *see* Disease, pelvis, inflammatory
  |male, peritoneal K65.1
|penis N48.21
  |gonococcal (accessory gland) (periurethral) A54.1
|perianal K61.0
|periapical K04.7
  |with sinus (alveolar) K04.6
|periappendicular K35.33
|pericardial I30.1
|pericecal K35.33
|pericemental *see* Periodontitis, aggressive, localized
|pericholecystic *see* Cholecystitis, acute
|pericoronal *see* Periodontitis, aggressive, localized
|peridental *see* Periodontitis, aggressive, localized
|perimetric *see also* Disease, pelvis, inflammatory N73.2
|perinephric, perinephritic *see* Abscess, kidney
|perineum, perineal (superficial) L02.215
  |urethra N34.0
|periodontal (parietal) *see* Periodontitis, aggressive, localized
  |apical K04.7
|periosteum, periosteal *see also* Osteomyelitis, specified type NEC
  |with osteomyelitis *see also* Osteomyelitis, specified type NEC
    |acute *see* Osteomyelitis, acute
    |chronic *see* Osteomyelitis, chronic
|peripharyngeal J39.0

Abscess - *continued*
|peripleuritic J86.9
  |with fistula J86.0
|periprostatic N41.2
|perirectal K61.1
|perirenal (tissue) *see* Abscess, kidney
|perisinuous (nose) *see* Sinusitis
|peritoneum, peritoneal (perforated) (ruptured)
  K65.1
  |with appendicitis (*see also* Appendicitis)
    K35.33
  |pelvic
    |female *see* Peritonitis, pelvic, female
    |male K65.1
  |postoperative T81.49
  |puerperal, postpartum, childbirth O85
  |tuberculous A18.31
|peritonsillar J36
|perityphlic K35.33
|periureteral N28.89
|periurethral N34.0
  |gonococcal (accessory gland) (periurethral)
    A54.1
|periuterine *see also* Disease, pelvis,
  inflammatory N73.2
|perivesical *see* Cystitis, specified type NEC
|petrous bone *see* Petrositis
|phagedenic NOS L02.91
  |chancroid A57
|pharynx, pharyngeal (lateral) J39.1
|pilonidal L05.01
|pituitary (gland) E23.6
|pleura J86.9
  |with fistula J86.0
|popliteal *see* Abscess, lower limb
|postcecal K35.33
|postlaryngeal J38.7
|postnasal J34.0
|postoperative (any site) (*see also* Infection,
  postoperative wound) T81.49
  |retroperitoneal K68.11
|postpharyngeal J39.0
|posttonsillar J36
|post-typhoid A01.09
|pouch of Douglas *see* Peritonitis, pelvic,
  female
|premammary *see* Abscess, breast
|prepatellar *see* Abscess, lower limb
- presacral K68.19
|prostate N41.2
  |gonococcal (acute) (chronic) A54.22
|psoas muscle K68.12
|puerperal   code by site under Puerperal,
  abscess
|pulmonary *see* Abscess, lung
|pulp, pulpal (dental) K04.01
  |irreversible K04.02
  |reversible K04.01
|rectovaginal septum K63.0
|rectovesical *see* Cystitis, specified type NEC
|rectum K61.1
|renal *see* Abscess, kidney
|retina *see* Inflammation, chorioretinal
|retrobulbar *see* Abscess, orbit
|retrocecal K65.1
|retrolaryngeal J38.7
|retromammary *see* Abscess, breast
|retroperitoneal NEC K68.19
  |postprocedural K68.11
|retropharyngeal J39.0
|retrouterine *see* Peritonitis, pelvic, female
|retrovesical *see* Cystitis, specified type NEC
|root, tooth K04.7
  |with sinus (alveolar) K04.6
|round ligament *see also* Disease, pelvis,
  inflammatory N73.2

Abscess - *continued*
|rupture (spontaneous) NOS L02.91
|sacrum (tuberculous) A18.01
  |nontuberculous M46.28
|salivary (duct) (gland) K11.3
|scalp (any part) L02.811
|scapular *see* Osteomyelitis, specified type
  NEC
|sclera *see* Scleritis
|scrofulous (tuberculous) A18.2
|scrotum N49.2
|seminal vesicle N49.0
|septal, dental K04.7
  |with sinus (alveolar) K04.6
|serous *see* Periostitis
|shoulder (region) *see* Abscess, upper limb
|sigmoid K63.0
|sinus (accessory) (chronic) (nasal) *see also*
  Sinusitis
  |intracranial venous (any) G06.0
|Skene's duct or gland N34.0
|skin *see* Abscess, by site
|specified site NEC L02.818
|spermatic cord N49.1
|sphenoidal (sinus) (chronic) J32.3
|spinal cord (any part) (staphylococcal) G06.1
  |tuberculous A17.81
|spine (column) (tuberculous) A18.01
  |epidural G06.1
  |nontuberculous *see* Osteomyelitis, vertebra
|spleen D73.3
  |amebic A06.89
|stitch T81.41
  |following an obstetrical procedure O86.01
|subarachnoid G06.2
  |brain G06.0
  |spinal cord G06.1
|subareolar *see* Abscess, breast
|subcecal K35.33
|subcutaneous *see also* Abscess, by site
  |pheomycotic (chromomycotic) B43.2
  |following procedure T81.41
    |obstetrical O86.01
|subdiaphragmatic K65.1
|subdural G06.2
  |brain G06.0
    |sequelae G09
  |spinal cord G06.1
|sub-fascial, following an obstetrical procedure
  O86.02
|subgaleal L02.811
|subhepatic K65.1
|sublingual K12.2
  |gland K11.3
|submammary *see* Abscess, breast
|submandibular (region) (space) (triangle)
  K12.2
  |gland K11.3
|submaxillary (region) L02.01
  |gland K11.3
|submental L02.01
  |gland K11.3
|subperiosteal *see* Osteomyelitis, specified type
  NEC
|subphrenic K65.1
  |following an obstetrical procedure O86.03
  |postoperative T81.43
|supralevator K61.5
|suburethral N34.0
|sudoriparous L75.8
|supraclavicular (fossa) *see* Abscess, upper
  limb
|suprapelvic, acute N73.0
|suprarenal (capsule) (gland) E27.8
|sweat gland L74.8

Abscess - *continued*
|tear duct *see* Inflammation, lacrimal, passages,
  acute
|temple L02.01
|temporal region L02.01
|temporosphenoidal G06.0
|tendon (sheath) M65.00
  |ankle M65.07-
  |foot M65.07-
  |forearm M65.03-
  |hand M65.04-
  |lower leg M65.06-
  |pelvic region M65.05-
  |shoulder region M65.01-
  |specified site NEC M65.08
  |thigh M65.05-
  |upper arm M65.02-
|testis N45.4
|thigh *see* Abscess, lower limb
|thorax J86.9
  |with fistula J86.0
|throat J39.1
|thumb *see also* Abscess, hand
  |nail *see* Cellulitis, finger
|thymus (gland) E32.1
|thyroid (gland) E06.0
|toe (any) *see also* Abscess, foot
  |nail *see* Cellulitis, toe
|tongue (staphylococcal) K14.0
|tonsil(s) (lingual) J36
|tonsillopharyngeal J36
|tooth, teeth (root) K04.7
  |with sinus (alveolar) K04.6
  |supporting structures NEC *see* Periodontitis,
    aggressive, localized
|trachea J39.8
|trunk L02.219
  |abdominal wall L02.211
  |back L02.212
  |chest wall L02.213
  |groin L02.214
  |perineum L02.215
  |umbilicus L02.216
|tubal *see* Salpingitis
|tuberculous *see* Tuberculosis, abscess
|tubo-ovarian *see* Salpingo-oophoritis
|tunica vaginalis N49.1
|umbilicus L02.216
|upper
  |limb L02.41-
  |respiratory J39.8
|urethral (gland) N34.0
|urinary N34.0
|uterus, uterine (wall) *see also* Endometritis
  |ligament *see also* Disease, pelvis,
    inflammatory N73.2
  |neck *see* Cervicitis
|uvula K12.2
|vagina (wall) *see* Vaginitis
|vaginorectal *see* Vaginitis
|vas deferens N49.1
|vermiform appendix K35.33
|vertebra (column) (tuberculous) A18.01
  |nontuberculous *see* Osteomyelitis, vertebra
|vesical *see* Cystitis, specified type NEC
|vesico-uterine pouch *see* Peritonitis, pelvic,
  female
|vitreous (humor) *see* Endophthalmitis,
  purulent
|vocal cord J38.3
|von Bezold's *see* Mastoiditis, acute
|vulva N76.4
|vulvovaginal gland N75.1
|web space *see* Abscess, hand
|wound T81.49
|wrist *see* Abscess, upper limb

Absence (of) (organ or part) (complete or partial)
- adrenal (gland) (congenital) Q89.1
  - acquired E89.6
- albumin in blood E88.09
- alimentary tract (congenital) Q45.8
  - upper Q40.8
- alveolar process (acquired) *see* Anomaly, alveolar
- ankle (acquired) Z89.44-
- anus (congenital) Q42.3
- aorta (congenital) Q25.41
- appendix, congenital Q42.8
- arm (acquired) Z89.20-
  - above elbow Z89.22-
    - congenital (with hand present) *see* Agenesis, arm, with hand present
      - and hand *see* Agenesis, forearm, and hand
  - below elbow Z89.21-
    - congenital (with hand present) *see* Agenesis, arm, with hand present
      - and hand *see* Agenesis, forearm, and hand
  - congenital *see* Defect, reduction, upper limb
  - shoulder (following explanation of shoulder joint prosthesis) (joint) (with or without presence of antibiotic-impregnated cement spacer) Z89.23-
    - congenital (with hand present) *see* Agenesis, arm, with hand present
- artery (congenital) (peripheral) Q27.8
  - brain Q28.3
  - coronary Q24.5
  - pulmonary Q25.79
  - specified NEC Q27.8
  - umbilical Q27.0
- atrial septum (congenital) Q21.1
- auditory canal (congenital) (external) Q16.1
- auricle (ear), congenital Q16.0
- bile, biliary duct, congenital Q44.5
- bladder (acquired) Z90.6
  - congenital Q64.5
- bowel sounds R19.11
- brain Q00.0
  - part of Q04.3
- breast(s) (and nipple(s)) (acquired) Z90.1-
  - congenital Q83.8
- broad ligament Q50.6
- bronchus (congenital) Q32.4
- canaliculus lacrimalis, congenital Q10.4
- cerebellum (vermis) Q04.3
- cervix (acquired) (with uterus) Z90.710
  - with remaining uterus Z90.712
  - congenital Q51.5
- chin, congenital Q18.8
- cilia (congenital) Q10.3
  - acquired *see* Madarosis
- clitoris (congenital) Q52.6
- coccyx, congenital Q76.49
- cold sense R20.8
- congenital
  - lumen *see* Atresia
  - organ or site NEC *see* Agenesis
  - septum *see* Imperfect, closure
- corpus callosum Q04.0
- cricoid cartilage, congenital Q31.8
- diaphragm (with hernia), congenital Q79.1
- digestive organ(s) or tract, congenital Q45.8
  - acquired NEC Z90.49
  - upper Q40.8
- ductus arteriosus Q28.8
- duodenum (acquired) Z90.49
  - congenital Q41.0
- ear, congenital Q16.9
  - acquired H93.8-

Absence (of) (organ or part) (complete or partial) - *continued*
- auricle Q16.0
  - external Q16.0
  - inner Q16.5
  - lobe, lobule Q17.8
  - middle, except ossicles Q16.4
    - ossicles Q16.3
  - ossicles Q16.3
- ejaculatory duct (congenital) Q55.4
- endocrine gland (congenital) NEC Q89.2
  - acquired E89.89
- epididymis (congenital) Q55.4
  - acquired Z90.79
- epiglottis, congenital Q31.8
- esophagus (congenital) Q39.8
  - acquired (partial) Z90.49
- eustachian tube (congenital) Q16.2
- extremity (acquired) Z89.9
  - congenital Q73.0
  - knee (following explantation of knee joint prosthesis) (joint) (with or without presence of antibiotic-impregnated cement spacer) Z89.52-
  - lower (above knee) Z89.619
    - below knee Z89.51-
  - upper *see* Absence, arm
- eye (acquired) Z90.01
  - congenital Q11.1
  - muscle (congenital) Q10.3
- eyeball (acquired) Z90.01
- eyelid (fold) (congenital) Q10.3
  - acquired Z90.01
- face, specified part NEC Q18.8
- fallopian tube(s) (acquired) Z90.79
  - congenital Q50.6
- family member (causing problem in home) NEC *see also* Disruption, family Z63.32
- femur, congenital *see* Defect, reduction, lower limb, longitudinal, femur
- fibrinogen (congenital) D68.2
  - acquired D65
- finger(s) (acquired) Z89.02-
  - congenital *see* Agenesis, hand
- foot (acquired) Z89.43-
  - congenital *see* Agenesis, foot
- forearm (acquired) *see* Absence, arm, below elbow
- gallbladder (acquired) Z90.49
  - congenital Q44.0
- gamma globulin in blood D80.1
  - hereditary D80.0
- genital organs
  - acquired (female) (male) Z90.79
  - female, congenital Q52.8
    - external Q52.71
    - internal NEC Q52.8
  - male, congenital Q55.8
- genitourinary organs, congenital NEC
  - female Q52.8
  - male Q55.8
- globe (acquired) Z90.01
  - congenital Q11.1
- glottis, congenital Q31.8
- hand and wrist (acquired) Z89.11-
  - congenital *see* Agenesis, hand
- head, part (acquired) NEC Z90.09
- heat sense R20.8
- hip (following explantation of hip joint prosthesis) (joint) (with or without presence of antibiotic-impregnated cement spacer) Z89.62-
- hymen (congenital) Q52.4
- ileum (acquired) Z90.49
  - congenital Q41.2
- immunoglobulin, isolated NEC D80.3

Absence (of) (organ or part) (complete or partial) - *continued*
- IgA D80.2
- IgG D80.3
- IgM D80.4
- incus (acquired) *see* Loss, ossicles, ear
  - congenital Q16.3
- inner ear, congenital Q16.5
- intestine (acquired) (small) Z90.49
  - congenital Q41.9
    - specified NEC Q41.8
  - large Z90.49
    - congenital Q42.9
      - specified NEC Q42.8
- iris, congenital Q13.1
- jejunum (acquired) Z90.49
  - congenital Q41.1
- joint
  - acquired
    - hip (following explantation of hip joint prosthesis) (with or without presence of antibiotic-impregnated cement spacer) Z89.62-
    - knee (following explantation of knee joint prosthesis) (with or without presence of antibiotic-impregnated cement spacer) Z89.52-
    - shoulder (following explantation of shoulder joint prosthesis) (with or without presence of antibiotic-impregnated cement spacer) Z89.23-
  - congenital NEC Q74.8
- kidney(s) (acquired) Z90.5
  - congenital Q60.2
    - bilateral Q60.1
    - unilateral Q60.0
- knee (following explantation of knee joint prosthesis) (joint) (with or without presence of antibiotic-impregnated cement spacer) Z89.52-
- labyrinth, membranous Q16.5
- larynx (congenital) Q31.8
  - acquired Z90.02
- leg (acquired) (above knee) Z89.61-
  - below knee (acquired) Z89.51-
  - congenital *see* Defect, reduction, lower limb
- lens (acquired) *see also* Aphakia
  - congenital Q12.3
  - post cataract extraction Z98.4-
- limb (acquired) *see* Absence, extremity
- lip Q38.6
- liver (congenital) Q44.7
- lung (fissure) (lobe) (bilateral) (unilateral) (congenital) Q33.3
  - acquired (any part) Z90.2
- menstruation *see* Amenorrhea
- muscle (congenital) (pectoral) Q79.8
  - ocular Q10.3
- neck, part Q18.8
- neutrophil *see* Agranulocytosis
- nipple(s) (with breast(s)) (acquired) Z90.1-
  - congenital Q83.2
- nose (congenital) Q30.1
  - acquired Z90.09
- organ
  - of Corti, congenital Q16.5
  - or site, congenital NEC Q89.8
    - acquired NEC Z90.89
- osseous meatus (ear) Q16.4
- ovary (acquired)
  - bilateral Z90.722
  - congenital
    - bilateral Q50.02
    - unilateral Q50.01
  - unilateral Z90.721
- oviduct (acquired)

Absence (of) (organ or part) (complete or partial) - *continued*
|bilateral Z90.722
|congenital Q50.6
|unilateral Z90.721
|pancreas (congenital) Q45.0
|acquired Z90.410
|complete Z90.410
|partial Z90.411
|total Z90.410
|parathyroid gland (acquired) E89.2
|congenital Q89.2
|patella, congenital Q74.1
|penis (congenital) Q55.5
|acquired Z90.79
|pericardium (congenital) Q24.8
|pituitary gland (congenital) Q89.2
|acquired E89.3
|prostate (acquired) Z90.79
|congenital Q55.4
|pulmonary valve Q22.0
|punctum lacrimale (congenital) Q10.4
|radius, congenital *see* Defect, reduction, upper limb, longitudinal, radius
|rectum (congenital) Q42.1
|with fistula Q42.0
|acquired Z90.49
|respiratory organ NOS Q34.9
|rib (acquired) Z90.89
|congenital Q76.6
|sacrum, congenital Q76.49
|salivary gland(s), congenital Q38.4
|scrotum, congenital Q55.29
|seminal vesicles (congenital) Q55.4
|acquired Z90.79
|septum
|atrial (congenital) Q21.1
|between aorta and pulmonary artery Q21.4
|ventricular (congenital) Q20.4
|sex chromosome
|female phenotype Q97.8
|male phenotype Q98.8
|skull bone (congenital) Q75.8
|with
|anencephaly Q00.0
|encephalocele *see* Encephalocele
|hydrocephalus Q03.9
|with spina bifida *see* Spina bifida, by site, with hydrocephalus
|microcephaly Q02
|spermatic cord, congenital Q55.4
|spine, congenital Q76.49
|spleen (congenital) Q89.01
|acquired Z90.81
|sternum, congenital Q76.7
|stomach (acquired) (partial) Z90.3
|congenital Q40.2
|superior vena cava, congenital Q26.8
|teeth, tooth (congenital) K00.0
|acquired (complete) K08.109
|class I K08.101
|class II K08.102
|class III K08.103
|class IV K08.104
|due to
|caries K08.139
|class I K08.131
|class II K08.132
|class III K08.133
|class IV K08.134
|periodontal disease K08.129
|class I K08.121
|class II K08.122
|class III K08.123
|class IV K08.124
|specified NEC K08.199

Absence (of) (organ or part) (complete or partial) - *continued*
|class I K08.191
|class II K08.192
|class III K08.193
|class IV K08.194
|trauma K08.119
|class I K08.111
|class II K08.112
|class III K08.113
|class IV K08.114
|partial K08.409
|class I K08.401
|class II K08.402
|class III K08.403
|class IV K08.404
|due to
|caries K08.439
|class I K08.431
|class II K08.432
|class III K08.433
|class IV K08.434
|periodontal disease K08.429
|class I K08.421
|class II K08.422
|class III K08.423
|class IV K08.424
|specified NEC K08.499
|class I K08.491
|class II K08.492
|class III K08.493
|class IV K08.494
|trauma K08.419
|class I K08.411
|class II K08.412
|class III K08.413
|class IV K08.414
|tendon (congenital) Q79.8
|testis (congenital) Q55.0
|acquired Z90.79
|thumb (acquired) Z89.01-
|congenital *see* Agenesis, hand
|thymus gland Q89.2
|thyroid (gland) (acquired) E89.0
|cartilage, congenital Q31.8
|congenital E03.1
|toe(s) (acquired) Z89.42-
|with foot *see* Absence, foot and ankle
|congenital *see* Agenesis, foot
|great Z89.41-
|tongue, congenital Q38.3
|trachea (cartilage), congenital Q32.1
|transverse aortic arch, congenital Q25.49
|tricuspid valve Q22.4
|umbilical artery, congenital Q27.0
|upper arm and forearm with hand present, congenital *see* Agenesis, arm, with hand present
|ureter (congenital) Q62.4
|acquired Z90.6
|urethra, congenital Q64.5
|uterus (acquired) Z90.710
|with cervix Z90.710
|with remaining cervical stump Z90.711
|congenital Q51.0
|uvula, congenital Q38.5
|vagina, congenital Q52.0
|vas deferens (congenital) Q55.4
|acquired Z90.79
|vein (peripheral) congenital NEC Q27.8
|cerebral Q28.3
|digestive system Q27.8
|great Q26.8
|lower limb Q27.8
|portal Q26.5
|precerebral Q28.1

Absence (of) (organ or part) (complete or partial) - *continued*
|specified site NEC Q27.8
|upper limb Q27.8
|vena cava (inferior) (superior), congenital Q26.8
|ventricular septum Q20.4
|vertebra, congenital Q76.49
|vulva, congenital Q52.71
|wrist (acquired) Z89.12-
Absorbent system disease I87.8
Absorption
|carbohydrate, disturbance K90.49
|chemical *see* Table of Drugs and Chemicals
|through placenta (newborn) P04.9
|environmental substance P04.6
|nutritional substance P04.5
|obstetric anesthetic or analgesic drug P04.0
|drug NEC *see* Table of Drugs and Chemicals
|addictive
|through placenta (newborn) (*see also* Newborn, affected by, maternal, use of) P04.40
|cocaine P04.41
|hallucinogens P04.42
|specified drug NEC P04.49
|medicinal
|through placenta (newborn) P04.19
|through placenta (newborn) P04.19
|obstetric anesthetic or analgesic drug P04.0
|fat, disturbance K90.49
|pancreatic K90.3
|noxious substance *see* Table of Drugs and Chemicals
|protein, disturbance K90.49
|starch, disturbance K90.49
|toxic substance *see* Table of Drugs and Chemicals
|uremic *see* Uremia
Abstinence symptoms, syndrome
|alcohol F10.239
|with delirium F10.231
|cocaine F14.23
|neonatal P96.1
|nicotine *see* Dependence, drug, nicotine, with, withdrawal
|opioid F11.93
|with dependence F11.23
|psychoactive NEC F19.939
|with
|delirium F19.931
|dependence F19.239
|with
|delirium F19.231
|perceptual disturbance F19.232
|uncomplicated F19.230
|perceptual disturbance F19.932
|uncomplicated F19.930
|sedative F13.939
|with
|delirium F13.931
|dependence F13.239
|with
|delirium F13.231
|perceptual disturbance F13.232
|uncomplicated F13.230
|perceptual disturbance F13.932
|uncomplicated F13.930
|stimulant NEC F15.93
|with dependence F15.23
Abulia R68.89
Abulomania F60.7

Abuse
|adult *see* Maltreatment, adult
|as reason for
|couple seeking advice (including
offender) Z63.0
|alcohol (non-Dependent) F10.10
|in remission (early) (sustained) F10.11
|with
|anxiety disorder F10.180
|intoxication F10.129
|with delirium F10.121
|uncomplicated F10.120
|mood disorder F10.14
|other specified disorder F10.188
|psychosis F10.159
|delusions F10.150
|hallucinations F10.151
|sexual dysfunction F10.181
|sleep disorder F10.182
|unspecified disorder F10.19
|withdrawal F10.139
|with
|perceptual disturbance F10.132
|delirium F10.131
|uncomplicated F10.130
|counseling and surveillance Z71.41
|amphetamine (or related substance) *see also*
Abuse, drug, stimulant NEC
|stimulant NEC F15.10
|with
|withdrawal F15.13
|analgesics (non-prescribed) (over the counter)
F55.8
|antacids F55.0
|antidepressants *see* Abuse, drug, psychoactive
NEC
|anxiolytic *see* Abuse, drug, sedative
|barbiturates *see* Abuse, drug, sedative
|caffeine *see* Abuse, drug, stimulant NEC
|cannabis, cannabinoids *see* Abuse, drug,
cannabis
|child *see* Maltreatment, child
|cocaine *see* Abuse, drug, cocaine
|drug NEC (non-Dependent) F19.10
|with sleep disorder F19.182
|amphetamine type *see* Abuse, drug,
stimulant NEC
|analgesics (non-prescribed) (over the
counter) F55.8
|antacids F55.0
|antidepressants *see* Abuse, drug,
psychoactive NEC
|anxiolytics *see* Abuse, drug, sedative
|barbiturates *see* Abuse, drug, sedative
|caffeine *see* Abuse, drug, stimulant NEC
|cannabis F12.10
|in remission (early) (sustained) F12.11
|with
|anxiety disorder F12.180
|intoxication F12.129
|with
|delirium F12.121
|perceptual disturbance F12.122
-|withdrawal F12.13
|uncomplicated F12.120
|other specified disorder F12.188
|psychosis F12.159
|delusions F12.150
|hallucinations F12.151
|unspecified disorder F12.19
|cocaine F14.10
|in remission (early) (sustained) F14.11
|with
|anxiety disorder F14.180
|intoxication F14.129
|with
|delirium F14.121

Abuse - *continued*
|perceptual disturbance F14.122
|withdrawal F14.13
|uncomplicated F14.120
|mood disorder F14.14
|other specified disorder F14.188
|psychosis F14.159
|delusions F14.150
|hallucinations F14.151
|sexual dysfunction F14.181
|sleep disorder F14.182
|unspecified disorder F14.19
|counseling and surveillance Z71.51
|hallucinogen F16.10
|with
|anxiety disorder F16.180
|flashbacks F16.183
|intoxication F16.129
|with
|delirium F16.121
|perceptual disturbance F16.122
|uncomplicated F16.120
|mood disorder F16.14
|other specified disorder F16.188
|perception disorder, persisting F16.183
|psychosis F16.159
|delusions F16.150
|hallucinations F16.151
|unspecified disorder F16.19
|in remission (early) (sustained) F16.11
|hashish *see* Abuse, drug, cannabis
|herbal or folk remedies F55.1
|hormones F55.3
|hypnotics *see* Abuse, drug, sedative
|inhalant F18.10
|with
|anxiety disorder F18.180
|dementia, persisting F18.17
|intoxication F18.129
|with delirium F18.121
|uncomplicated F18.120
|mood disorder F18.14
|other specified disorder F18.188
|psychosis F18.159
|delusions F18.150
|hallucinations F18.151
|unspecified disorder F18.19
|in remission (early) (sustained) F18.11
|in remission (early) (sustained) F19.11
|laxatives F55.2
|LSD *see* Abuse, drug, hallucinogen
|marihuana *see* Abuse, drug, cannabis
|morphine type (opioids) *see* Abuse, drug,
opioid
|opioid F11.10
|with
|intoxication F11.129
|with
|delirium F11.121
|perceptual disturbance F11.122
|withdrawal F11.13
|uncomplicated F11.120
|mood disorder F11.14
|other specified disorder F11.188
|psychosis F11.159
|delusions F11.150
|hallucinations F11.151
|sexual dysfunction F11.181
|sleep disorder F11.182
|unspecified disorder F11.19
|in remission (early) (sustained) F11.11
|PCP (phencyclidine) (or related substance)
see Abuse, drug, hallucinogen
|psychoactive NEC F19.10
|with
|amnestic disorder F19.16

Abuse - *continued*
|anxiety disorder F19.180
|dementia F19.17
|intoxication F19.129
|with
|delirium F19.121
|perceptual disturbance F19.122
|withdrawal F19.139
|with
|perceptual disturbance F19.132
|delirium F19.131
|uncomplicated F19.130
|uncomplicated F19.120
|mood disorder F19.14
|other specified disorder F19.188
|psychosis F19.159
|delusions F19.150
|hallucinations F19.151
|sexual dysfunction F19.181
|sleep disorder F19.182
|unspecified disorder F19.19
|sedative, hypnotic or anxiolytic F13.10
|with
|anxiety disorder F13.180
|intoxication F13.129
|with delirium F13.121
|uncomplicated F13.120
|mood disorder F13.14
|other specified disorder F13.188
|psychosis F13.159
|delusions F13.150
|hallucinations F13.151
|sexual dysfunction F13.181
|sleep disorder F13.182
|unspecified disorder F13.19
|withdrawal F13.139
|with
|perceptual disturbance F13.132
|delirium F13.131
|uncomplicated F13.130
|in remission (early) (sustained) F13.11
|solvent *see* Abuse, drug, inhalant
|steroids F55.3
|stimulant NEC F15.10
|with
|anxiety disorder F15.180
|intoxication F15.129
|with
|delirium F15.121
|perceptual disturbance F15.122
|withdrawal F15.13
|uncomplicated F15.120
|mood disorder F15.14
|other specified disorder F15.188
|psychosis F15.159
|delusions F15.150
|hallucinations F15.151
|sexual dysfunction F15.181
|sleep disorder F15.182
|unspecified disorder F15.19
|in remission (early) (sustained) F15.11
|tranquilizers *see* Abuse, drug, sedative
|vitamins F55.4
|hallucinogens *see* Abuse, drug, hallucinogen
|hashish *see* Abuse, drug, cannabis
|herbal or folk remedies F55.1
|hormones F55.3
|hypnotic *see* Abuse, drug, sedative
|inhalant *see* Abuse, drug, inhalant
|laxatives F55.2
|LSD *see* Abuse, drug, hallucinogen
|marihuana *see* Abuse, drug, cannabis
|morphine type (opioids) *see* Abuse, drug,
opioid
|non-psychoactive substance NEC F55.8

Abuse - *continued*
|antacids F55.0
|folk remedies F55.1
|herbal remedies F55.1
|hormones F55.3
|laxatives F55.2
|steroids F55.3
|vitamins F55.4
|opioids *see* Abuse, drug, opioid
|PCP (phencyclidine) (or related substance) *see*
　　Abuse, drug, hallucinogen
|physical (adult) (child) *see* Maltreatment
|psychoactive substance *see* Abuse, drug,
　　psychoactive NEC
|psychological (adult) (child) *see* Maltreatment
|sedative *see* Abuse, drug, sedative
|sexual *see* Maltreatment
|solvent *see* Abuse, drug, inhalant
|steroids F55.3
|vitamins F55.4
Acalculia R48.8
|developmental F81.2
Acanthamebiasis (with) B60.10
|conjunctiva B60.12
|keratoconjunctivitis B60.13
|meningoencephalitis B60.11
|other specified B60.19
Acanthocephaliasis B83.8
Acanthocheilonemiasis B74.4
Acanthocytosis E78.6
Acantholysis L11.9
Acanthosis (acquired) (nigricans) L83
|benign Q82.8
|congenital Q82.8
|seborrheic L82.1
　|inflamed L82.0
|tongue K14.3
Acapnia E87.3
Acarbia E87.2
Acardia, acardius Q89.8
Acardiacus amorphus Q89.8
Acardiotrophia I51.4
Acariasis B88.0
|scabies B86
Acarodermatitis (urticarioides) B88.0
Acarophobia F40.218
Acatalasemia, acatalasia E80.3
Acathisia (drug induced) G25.71
Accelerated atrioventricular conduction I45.6
Accentuation of personality traits (type A)
　　Z73.1
Accessory (congenital)
|adrenal gland Q89.1
|anus Q43.4
|appendix Q43.4
|atrioventricular conduction I45.6
|auditory ossicles Q16.3
|auricle (ear) Q17.0
|biliary duct or passage Q44.5
|bladder Q64.79
|blood vessels NEC Q27.9
　|coronary Q24.5
|bone NEC Q79.8
|breast tissue, axilla Q83.1
|carpal bones Q74.0
|cecum Q43.4
|chromosome(s) NEC (nonsex) Q92.9
　|with complex rearrangements NEC Q92.5
　　|seen only at prometaphase Q92.8
　|partial Q92.9
　|sex
　　|female phenotype Q97.8
|13 *see* Trisomy, 13
|18 *see* Trisomy, 18
|21 *see* Trisomy, 21
|coronary artery Q24.5

Accessory (congenital) - *continued*
|cusp(s), heart valve NEC Q24.8
　|pulmonary Q22.3
|cystic duct Q44.5
|digit(s) Q69.9
|ear (auricle) (lobe) Q17.0
|endocrine gland NEC Q89.2
|eye muscle Q10.3
|eyelid Q10.3
|face bone(s) Q75.8
|fallopian tube (fimbria) (ostium) Q50.6
|finger(s) Q69.0
|foreskin N47.8
|frontonasal process Q75.8
|gallbladder Q44.1
|genital organ(s)
　|female Q52.8
　　|external Q52.79
　　|internal NEC Q52.8
　|male Q55.8
|genitourinary organs NEC Q89.8
　|female Q52.8
　|male Q55.8
|hallux Q69.2
|heart Q24.8
　|valve NEC Q24.8
　　|pulmonary Q22.3
|hepatic ducts Q44.5
|hymen Q52.4
|intestine (large) (small) Q43.4
|kidney Q63.0
|lacrimal canal Q10.6
|leaflet, heart valve NEC Q24.8
|ligament, broad Q50.6
|liver Q44.7
　|duct Q44.5
|lobule (ear) Q17.0
|lung (lobe) Q33.1
|muscle Q79.8
|navicular of carpus Q74.0
|nervous system, part NEC Q07.8
|nipple Q83.3
|nose Q30.8
|organ or site not listed *see* Anomaly, by site
|ovary Q50.31
|oviduct Q50.6
|pancreas Q45.3
|parathyroid gland Q89.2
|parotid gland (and duct) Q38.4
|pituitary gland Q89.2
|preauricular appendage Q17.0
|prepuce N47.8
|renal arteries (multiple) Q27.2
|rib Q76.6
　|cervical Q76.5
|roots (teeth) K00.2
|salivary gland Q38.4
|sesamoid bones Q74.8
　|foot Q74.2
　|hand Q74.0
|skin tags Q82.8
|spleen Q89.09
|sternum Q76.7
|submaxillary gland Q38.4
|tarsal bones Q74.2
|teeth, tooth K00.1
|tendon Q79.8
|thumb Q69.1
|thymus gland Q89.2
|thyroid gland Q89.2
|toes Q69.2
|tongue Q38.3
|tooth, teeth K00.1
|tragus Q17.0
|ureter Q62.5

Accessory (congenital) - *continued*
|urethra Q64.79
|urinary organ or tract NEC Q64.8
|uterus Q51.28
|vagina Q52.10
|valve, heart NEC Q24.8
　|pulmonary Q22.3
|vertebra Q76.49
|vocal cords Q31.8
|vulva Q52.79
Accident
|birth *see* Birth, injury
|cardiac *see* Infarct, myocardium
|cerebral I63.9
|cerebrovascular (embolic) (ischemic)
　　(thrombotic) I63.9
　|aborted I63.9
　|hemorrhagic *see* Hemorrhage, intracranial,
　　intracerebral
　|old (without sequelae) Z86.73
　　|with sequelae (of) *see* Sequelae,
　　infarction, cerebral
|coronary *see* Infarct, myocardium
|craniovascular I63.9
|vascular, brain I63.9
Accidental *see* condition
Accommodation (disorder) *see also* condition
|hysterical paralysis of F44.89
|insufficiency of H52.4
|paresis *see* Paresis, of accommodation
|spasm *see* Spasm, of accommodation
Accouchement *see* Delivery
Accreta placenta O43.21-
Accretio cordis (nonrheumatic) I31.0
Accretions, tooth, teeth K03.6
Acculturation difficulty Z60.3
Accumulation secretion, prostate N42.89
Acephalia, acephalism, acephalus, acephaly
　　Q00.0
Acephalobrachia monster Q89.8
Acephalochirus monster Q89.8
Acephalogaster Q89.8
Acephalostomus monster Q89.8
Acephalothorax Q89.8
Acerophobia F40.298
Acetonemia R79.89
|in Type 1 diabetes E10.10
　|with coma E10.11
Acetonuria R82.4
Achalasia (cardia) (esophagus) K22.0
|congenital Q39.5
|pylorus Q40.0
|sphincteral NEC K59.89
Ache(s) *see* Pain
Acheilia Q38.6
Achillobursitis *see* Tendinitis, Achilles
Achillodynia *see* Tendinitis, Achilles
Achlorhydria, achlorhydric (neurogenic)
　　K31.83
|anemia D50.8
|diarrhea K31.83
|psychogenic F45.8
|secondary to vagotomy K91.1
Achluophobia F40.228
Acholia K82.8
Acholuric jaundice (familial) (splenomegalic)
　　see also Spherocytosis
|acquired D59.8
Achondrogenesis Q77.0
Achondroplasia (osteosclerosis congenita)
　　Q77.4
Achroma, cutis L80
Achromat (ism), achromatopsia (acquired)
　　(congenital) H53.51
Achromia, congenital *see* Albinism
Achromia parasitica B36.0
Achylia gastrica K31.89
|psychogenic F45.8

Acid
| burn *see* Corrosion
| deficiency
| | amide nicotinic E52
| | ascorbic E54
| | folic E53.8
| | nicotinic E52
| | pantothenic E53.8
| intoxication E87.2
| peptic disease K30
| phosphatase deficiency E83.39
| stomach K30
| | psychogenic F45.8**Acidemia** E87.2
| argininosuccinic E72.22
| isovaleric E71.110
| metabolic (newborn) P19.9
| | first noted before onset of labor P19.0
| | first noted during labor P19.1
| | noted at birth P19.2
| methylmalonic E71.120
| pipecolic E72.3
| propionic E71.121
Acidity, gastric (high) K30
| psychogenic F45.8
Acidocytopenia *see* Agranulocytosis
Acidocytosis D72.10
Acidopenia *see* Agranulocytosis
Acidosis (lactic) (respiratory) E87.2
| in Type 1 diabetes E10.10
| | with coma E10.11
| kidney, tubular N25.89
| lactic E87.2
| metabolic NEC E87.2
| | with respiratory acidosis E87.4
| | hyperchloremic, of newborn P74.421
| | late, of newborn P74.0
| mixed metabolic and respiratory, newborn P84
| newborn P84
Acephalothorax renal (hyperchloremic) (tubular) N25.89
| respiratory E87.2
| | complicated by
| | | metabolic
| | | | acidosis E87.4
| | | | alkalosis E87.4
Aciduria
| 4-hydroxybutyric E72.81
| argininosuccinic E72.22
| gamma-hydroxybutyric E72.81
| glutaric (type I) E72.3
| | type II E71.313
| | type III E71.5-
| orotic (congenital) (hereditary) (pyrimidine deficiency) E79.8
| | anemia D53.0
Acladiosis (skin) B36.0
Aclasis, diaphyseal Q78.6
Acleistocardia Q21.1
Aclusion *see* Anomaly, dentofacial, malocclusion
Acne L70.9
| artificialis L70.8
| atrophica L70.2
| cachecticorum (Hebra) L70.8
| conglobata L70.1
| cystic L70.0
| decalvans L66.2
| excoriée (des jeunes filles) L70.5
| frontalis L70.2
| indurata L70.0
| infantile L70.4
| keloid L73.0
| lupoid L70.2
| necrotic, necrotica (miliaris) L70.2
| neonatal L70.4
| nodular L70.0

Acne - *continued*
| occupational L70.8
| picker's L70.5
| pustular L70.0
| rodens L70.2
| rosacea L71.9
| specified NEC L70.8
| tropica L70.3
| varioliformis L70.2
| vulgaris L70.0
Acnitis (primary) A18.4
Acosta's disease T70.29
Acoustic *see* condition
Acousticophobia F40.298
ACPO (acute colonic pseudo-obstruction) K59.81
Acquired *see also* condition
| immunodeficiency syndrome (AIDS) B20
Acrania Q00.0
Acroangiodermatitis I78.9
Acroasphyxia, chronic I73.89
Acrobystitis N47.7
Acrocephalopolysyndactyly Q87.0
Acrocephalosyndactyly Q87.0
Acrocephaly Q75.0
Acrochondrohyperplasia *see* Syndrome, Marfan's
Acrocyanosis I73.8
| newborn P28.2
| | meaning transient blue hands and feet
| omit code
Acrodermatitis L30.8
| atrophicans (chronica) L90.4
| continua (Hallopeau) L40.2
| enteropathica (hereditary) E83.2
| Hallopeau's L40.2
| infantile papular L44.4
| perstans L40.2
| pustulosa continua L40.2
| recalcitrant pustular L40.2
Acrodynia *see* Poisoning, mercury
Acromegaly, acromegalia E22.0
Acromelalgia I73.81
Acromicria, acromicria Q79.8
Acronyx L60.0
Acropachy, thyroid *see* Thyrotoxicosis
Acroparesthesia (simple) (vasomotor) I73.89
Acropathy, thyroid *see* Thyrotoxicosis
Acrophobia F40.241
Acroposthitis N47.7
Acroscleriasis, acroscleroderma, acrosclerosis *see* Sclerosis, systemic
Acrosphacelus I96
Acrospiroma, eccrine *see* Neoplasm, skin, benign
Acrostealgia *see* Osteochondropathy
Acrotrophodynia *see* Immersion
ACTH ectopic syndrome E24.3
Actinic *see* condition
Actinobacillosis, actinobacillus A28.8
| mallei A24.0
| muris A25.1
Actinomyces israelii (infection) *see* Actinomycosis
Actinomycetoma (foot) B47.1
Actinomycosis, actinomycotic A42.9
| with pneumonia A42.0
| abdominal A42.1
| cervicofacial A42.2
| cutaneous A42.89
| gastrointestinal A42.1
| pulmonary A42.0
| sepsis A42.7
| specified site NEC A42.89
Actinoneuritis G62.82

Action, heart
| disorder I49.9
| irregular I49.9
| | psychogenic F45.8
Activated protein C resistance D68.51
Activation
| mast cell (disorder) (syndrome) D89.40
| | idiopathic D89.42
| | monoclonal D89.41
| | secondary D89.43
| | specified type NEC D89.49
Active *see* condition
Acute *see also* condition
| abdomen R10.0
| gallbladder *see* Cholecystitis, acute
Acyanotic heart disease (congenital) Q24.9
Acystia Q64.5
Adair-Dighton syndrome (brittle bones and blue sclera, deafness) Q78.0
Adamantinoblastoma *see* Ameloblastoma
Adamantinoma *see also* Cyst, calcifying odontogenic
| long bones C40.90
| | lower limb C40.2-
| | upper limb C40.0-
| malignant C41.1
| | jaw (bone) (lower) C41.1
| | | upper C41.0
| tibial C40.2-
Adamantoblastoma *see* Ameloblastoma
Adams-Stokes (-Morgagni) disease or syndrome I45.9
Adaption reaction *see* Disorder, adjustment
Addiction *see also* Dependence F19.20
| alcohol, alcoholic (ethyl) (methyl) (wood) (without remission) F10.20
| | with remission F10.21
| drug *see* Dependence, drug
| ethyl alcohol (without remission) F10.20
| | with remission F10.21
| heroin *see* Dependence, drug, opioid
| methyl alcohol (without remission) F10.20
| | with remission F10.21
| methylated spirit (without remission) F10.20
| | with remission F10.21
| morphine (-like substances) *see* Dependence, drug, opioid
| nicotine *see* Dependence, drug, nicotine
| opium and opioids *see* Dependence, drug, opioid
| tobacco *see* Dependence, drug, nicotine
Addisonian crisis E27.2
Addison's
| anemia (pernicious) D51.0
| disease (bronze) or syndrome E27.1
| | tuberculous A18.7
| keloid L94.0
Addison-Biermer anemia (pernicious) D51.0
Addison-Schilder complex E71.528
Additional *see also* Accessory
| chromosome(s) Q99.8
| | sex *see* Abnormal, chromosome, sex
| | 21 *see* Trisomy, 21
Adduction contracture, hip or other joint *see* Contraction, joint
Adenitis *see also* Lymphadenitis
| acute, unspecified site L04.9
| axillary I88.9
| | acute L04.2
| | chronic or subacute I88.1
| Bartholin's gland N75.8
| bulbourethral gland *see* Urethritis
| cervical I88.9
| | acute L04.0
| | chronic or subacute I88.1
| chancroid (Hemophilus ducreyi) A57

Adenitis - *continued*
|chronic, unspecified site I88.1
|Cowper's gland *see* Urethritis
|due to Pasteurella multocida (P. septica)
    A28.0
|epidemic, acute B27.09
|gangrenous L04.9
|gonorrheal NEC A54.89
|groin I88.9
    |acute L04.1
    |chronic or subacute I88.1
|in
|infectious (acute) (epidemic) B27.09
|inguinal I88.9
    |acute L04.1
    |chronic or subacute I88.1
|lymph gland or node, except mesenteric I88.9
    |acute *see* Lymphadenitis, acute
    |chronic or subacute I88.1
|mesenteric (acute) (chronic) (nonspecific)
    (subacute) I88.0
|parotid gland (suppurative) *see* Sialoadenitis
|salivary gland (any) (suppurative) *see*
    Sialoadenitis
|scrofulous (tuberculous) A18.2
|Skene's duct or gland *see* Urethritis
|strumous, tuberculous A18.2
|subacute, unspecified site I88.1
|sublingual gland (suppurative) *see*
    Sialoadenitis
|submandibular gland (suppurative) *see*
    Sialoadenitis
|submaxillary gland (suppurative) *see*
    Sialoadenitis
|tuberculous *see* Tuberculosis, lymph gland
|urethral gland *see* Urethritis
|Wharton's duct (suppurative) *see* Sialoadenitis
Adenoacanthoma *see* Neoplasm, malignant, by
    site
Adenoameloblastoma *see* Cyst, calcifying
    odontogenic
Adenocarcinoid (tumor) *see* Neoplasm,
    malignant, by site
Adenocarcinoma *see also* Neoplasm, malignant,
    by site
|acidophil
    |specified site *see* Neoplasm, malignant, by
        site
    |unspecified site C75.1
|adrenal cortical C74.0-
|alveolar *see* Neoplasm, lung, malignant
|apocrine
    |breast *see* Neoplasm, breast, malignant
    |in situ
        |breast D05.8-
        |specified site NEC *see* Neoplasm, skin, in
            situ
        |unspecified site D04.9
    |specified site NEC *see* Neoplasm, skin,
        malignant
    |unspecified site C44.99
|basal cell
    |specified site *see* Neoplasm, skin, malignant
    |unspecified site C08.9
|basophil
    |specified site *see* Neoplasm, malignant, by
        site
    |unspecified site C75.1
|bile duct type C22.1
    |liver C22.1
    |specified site NEC *see* Neoplasm,
        malignant, by site
    |unspecified site C22.1
|bronchiolar *see* Neoplasm, lung, malignant
|bronchioloalveolar *see* Neoplasm, lung,
    malignant

Adenocarcinoma - *continued*
|ceruminous C44.29-
|cervix, in situ *see also* Carcinoma, cervix
    uteri, in situ D06.9
|chromophobe
    |specified site *see* Neoplasm, malignant, by
        site
    |unspecified site C75.1
|diffuse type
    |specified site *see* Neoplasm, malignant, by
        site
    |unspecified site C16.9
|duct
    |infiltrating
        |with Paget's disease *see* Neoplasm, breast,
            malignant
        |specified site *see* Neoplasm, malignant, by
            site
        |unspecified site (female) C50.91-
            |male C50.92-
    |specified site *see* Neoplasm, malignant, by
        site
    |unspecified site
        |female C56.9
        |male C61
|eosinophil
    |specified site *see* Neoplasm, malignant, by
        site
    |unspecified site C75.1
|follicular
    |with papillary C73
    |moderately differentiated C73
    |specified site *see* Neoplasm, malignant, by
        site
    |trabecular C73
    |unspecified site C73
    |well differentiated C73
|Hürthle cell C73
|in
    |adenomatous
        |polyposis coli C18.9
|infiltrating duct
    |with Paget's disease *see* Neoplasm, breast,
        malignant
    |specified site *see* Neoplasm, by site,
        malignant
    |unspecified site (female) C50.91-
        |male C50.92-
|inflammatory
    |specified site *see* Neoplasm, by site,
        malignant
    |unspecified site (female) C50.91-
        |male C50.92-
|intestinal type
    |specified site *see* Neoplasm, by site,
        malignant
    |unspecified site C16.9
|intracystic papillary
|intraductal
    |breast D05.1-
    |noninfiltrating
        |breast D05.1-
        |papillary
            |with invasion
                |specified site *see* Neoplasm, by site,
                    malignant
                |unspecified site (female) C50.91-
                    |male C50.92-
            |breast D05.1-
            |specified site NEC *see* Neoplasm, in
                situ, by site
            |unspecified site D05.1-
    |specified site NEC *see* Neoplasm, in situ,
        by site
    |unspecified site D05.1-

Adenocarcinoma - *continued*
|papillary
    |with invasion
        |specified site *see* Neoplasm, malignant,
            by site
        |unspecified site (female) C50.91-
            |male C50.92-
    |breast D05.1-
    |specified site *see* Neoplasm, in situ, by
        site
    |unspecified site D05.1-
|specified site NEC *see* Neoplasm, in situ, by
    site
|unspecified site D05.1-
|islet cell
    |with exocrine, mixed
        |specified site *see* Neoplasm, malignant, by
            site
        |unspecified site C25.9
    |pancreas C25.4
    |specified site NEC *see* Neoplasm,
        malignant, by site
    |unspecified site C25.4
|lobular
    |in situ
        |breast D05.0-
        |specified site NEC *see* Neoplasm, in situ,
            by site
        |unspecified site D05.0-
    |specified site *see* Neoplasm, malignant, by
        site
    |unspecified site (female) C50.91-
        |male C50.92-
|mucoid *see also* Neoplasm, malignant, by site
    |cell
        |specified site *see* Neoplasm, malignant, by
            site
        |unspecified site C75.1
|nonencapsulated sclerosing C73
|papillary
    |with follicular C73
    |follicular variant C73
    |intraductal (noninfiltrating)
        |with invasion
            |specified site *see* Neoplasm, malignant,
                by site
            |unspecified site (female) C50.91-
                |male C50.92-
        |breast D05.1-
        |specified site NEC *see* Neoplasm, in situ,
            by site
        |unspecified site D05.1-
    |serous
        |specified site *see* Neoplasm, malignant, by
            site
        |unspecified site C56.9
|papillocystic
    |specified site *see* Neoplasm, malignant, by
        site
    |unspecified site C56.9
|pseudomucinous
    |specified site *see* Neoplasm, malignant, by
        site
    |unspecified site C56.9
|renal cell C64-
|sebaceous *see* Neoplasm, skin, malignant
|serous *see also* Neoplasm, malignant, by site
    |papillary
        |specified site *see* Neoplasm, malignant, by
            site
        |unspecified site C56.9
|sweat gland *see* Neoplasm, skin, malignant
|water-clear cell C75.0

Adenocarcinoma-In-Situ *see also* Neoplasm, in situ, by site
 |breast D05.9-
Adenofibroma
 |clear cell *see* Neoplasm, benign, by site
 |endometrioid D27.9
  |borderline malignancy D39.10
  |malignant C56-
 |mucinous
  |specified site *see* Neoplasm, benign, by site
  |unspecified site D27.9
 |papillary
  |specified site *see* Neoplasm, benign, by site
  |unspecified site D27.9
 |prostate *see* Enlargement, enlarged, prostate
 |serous
  |specified site *see* Neoplasm, benign, by site
  |unspecified site D27.9
 |specified site *see* Neoplasm, benign, by site
 |unspecified site D27.9
Adenofibrosis
 |breast *see* Fibroadenosis, breast
 |endometrioid N80.0
Adenoiditis (chronic) J35.02
 |with tonsillitis J35.03
 |acute J03.90
  |recurrent J03.91
  |specified organism NEC J03.80
   |recurrent J03.81
  |staphylococcal J03.80
   |recurrent J03.81
  |streptococcal J03.00
   |recurrent J03.01
Adenoids *see* condition
Adenolipoma *see* Neoplasm, benign, by site
Adenolipomatosis, Launois-Bensaude E88.89
Adenolymphoma
 |specified site *see* Neoplasm, benign, by site
 |unspecified site D11.9
Adenoma *see also* Neoplasm, benign, by site
 |acidophil
  |specified site *see* Neoplasm, benign, by site
  |unspecified site D35.2
 |acidophil-basophil, mixed
  |specified site *see* Neoplasm, benign, by site
  |unspecified site D35.2
 |adrenal (cortical) D35.00
  |clear cell D35.00
  |compact cell D35.00
  |glomerulosa cell D35.00
  |heavily pigmented variant D35.00
  |mixed cell D35.00
 |alpha-cell
  |pancreas D13.7
  |specified site NEC *see* Neoplasm, benign, by site
  |unspecified site D13.7
 |alveolar D14.30
 |apocrine
  |breast D24-
  |specified site NEC *see* Neoplasm, skin, benign, by site
  |unspecified site D23.9
 |basal cell D11.9
 |basophil
  |specified site *see* Neoplasm, benign, by site
  |unspecified site D35.2
 |basophil-acidophil, mixed
  |specified site *see* Neoplasm, benign, by site
  |unspecified site D35.2
 |beta-cell
  |pancreas D13.7
  |specified site NEC *see* Neoplasm, benign, by site
  |unspecified site D13.7
 |bile duct D13.4

Adenoma - *continued*
 |common D13.5
  |extrahepatic D13.5
  |intrahepatic D13.4
  |specified site NEC *see* Neoplasm, benign, by site
  |unspecified site D13.4
 |black D35.00
 |bronchial D38.1
  |cylindroid type *see* Neoplasm, lung, malignant
 |ceruminous D23.2-
 |chief cell D35.1
 |chromophobe
  |specified site *see* Neoplasm, benign, by site
  |unspecified site D35.2
 |colloid
  |specified site *see* Neoplasm, benign, by site
  |unspecified site D34
 |eccrine, papillary *see* Neoplasm, skin, benign
 |endocrine, multiple
  |single specified site *see* Neoplasm, uncertain behavior, by site
  |two or more specified sites D44-
  |unspecified site D44.9
 |endometrioid *see also* Neoplasm, benign
  |borderline malignancy *see* Neoplasm, uncertain behavior, by site
 |eosinophil
  |specified site *see* Neoplasm, benign, by site
  |unspecified site D35.2
 |fetal
  |specified site *see* Neoplasm, benign, by site
  |unspecified site D34
 |follicular
  |specified site *see* Neoplasm, benign, by site
  |unspecified site D34
 |hepatocellular D13.4
 |Hürthle cell D34
 |islet cell
  |pancreas D13.7
  |specified site NEC *see* Neoplasm, benign, by site
  |unspecified site D13.7
 |liver cell D13.4
 |macrofollicular
  |specified site *see* Neoplasm, benign, by site
  |unspecified site D34
 |malignant, malignum *see* Neoplasm, malignant, by site
 |microcystic
  |pancreas D13.6
  |specified site NEC *see* Neoplasm, benign, by site
  |unspecified site D13.6
 |microfollicular
  |specified site *see* Neoplasm, benign, by site
  |unspecified site D34
 |mucoid cell
  |specified site *see* Neoplasm, benign, by site
  |unspecified site D35.2
 |multiple endocrine
  |single specified site *see* Neoplasm, uncertain behavior, by site
  |two or more specified sites D44-
  |unspecified site D44.9
 |nipple D24-
 |papillary *see also* Neoplasm, benign, by site
  |eccrine *see* Neoplasm, skin, benign, by site
 |Pick's tubular
  |specified site *see* Neoplasm, benign, by site
  |unspecified site
   |female D27.9
   |male D29.20

Adenoma - *continued*
 |pleomorphic
  |carcinoma in *see* Neoplasm, salivary gland, malignant
   |specified site *see* Neoplasm, malignant, by site
   |unspecified site C08.9
 |polypoid *see also* Neoplasm, benign
  |adenocarcinoma in *see* Neoplasm, malignant, by site
  |adenocarcinoma in situ *see* Neoplasm, in situ, by site
 |prostate *see* Neoplasm, benign, prostate
 |rete cell D29.20
 |sebaceous *see* Neoplasm, skin, benign
 |Sertoli cell
  |specified site *see* Neoplasm, benign, by site
  |unspecified site
   |female D27.9
   |male D29.20
 |skin appendage *see* Neoplasm, skin, benign
 |sudoriferous gland *see* Neoplasm, skin, benign
 |sweat gland *see* Neoplasm, skin, benign
 |testicular
  |specified site *see* Neoplasm, benign, by site
  |unspecified site
   |female D27.9
   |male D29.20
 |tubular *see also* Neoplasm, benign, by site
  |adenocarcinoma in *see* Neoplasm, malignant, by site
  |adenocarcinoma in situ *see* Neoplasm, in situ, by site
  |Pick's
   |specified site *see* Neoplasm, benign, by site
   |unspecified site
    |female D27.9
    |male D29.20
 |tubulovillous *see also* Neoplasm, benign, by site
  |adenocarcinoma in *see* Neoplasm, malignant, by site
  |adenocarcinoma in situ *see* Neoplasm, in situ, by site
 |villous *see* Neoplasm, uncertain behavior, by site
  |adenocarcinoma in *see* Neoplasm, malignant, by site
  |adenocarcinoma in situ *see* Neoplasm, in situ, by site
 |water-clear cell D35.1
Adenomatosis
 |endocrine (multiple) E31.20
  |single specified site *see* Neoplasm, uncertain behavior, by site
 |erosive of nipple D24-
 |pluriendocrine *see* Adenomatosis, endocrine
 |pulmonary D38.1
  |malignant *see* Neoplasm, lung, malignant
 |specified site *see* Neoplasm, benign, by site
 |unspecified site D12.6
Adenomatous
 |goiter (nontoxic) E04.9
  |with hyperthyroidism *see* Hyperthyroidism, with, goiter, nodular
  |toxic *see* Hyperthyroidism, with, goiter, nodular
Adenomyoma *see also* Neoplasm, benign, by site
 |prostate *see* Enlarged, prostate
Adenomyometritis N80.0
Adenomyosis N80.0

Adenopathy (lymph gland) R59.9
|generalized R59.1
|inguinal R59.0
|localized R59.0
|mediastinal R59.0
|mesentery R59.0
|syphilitic (secondary) A51.49
|tracheobronchial R59.0
  |tuberculous A15.4
    |primary (progressive) A15.7
|tuberculous see also Tuberculosis, lymph
  gland
  |tracheobronchial A15.4
    |primary (progressive) A15.7
Adenosalpingitis see Salpingitis
Adenosarcoma see Neoplasm, malignant, by
  site
Adenosclerosis I88.8
Adenosis (sclerosing) breast see Fibroadenosis,
  breast
**Adenovirus, as cause of disease classified
  elsewhere** B97.0
Adentia (complete) (partial) see Absence, teeth
Adherent see also Adhesions
|labia (minora) N90.89
|pericardium (nonrheumatic) I31.0
  |rheumatic I09.2
|placenta (with hemorrhage) O72.0
  |without hemorrhage O73.0
|prepuce, newborn N47.0
|scar (skin) L90.5
|tendon in scar L90.5
Adhesions, adhesive (postinfective) K66.0
|with intestinal obstruction K56.50
  |complete K56.52
  |incomplete K56.51
  |partial K56.51
|abdominal (wall) see Adhesions, peritoneum
|appendix K38.8
|bile duct (common) (hepatic) K83.8
|bladder (sphincter) N32.89
|bowel see Adhesions, peritoneum
|cardiac I31.0
  |rheumatic I09.2
|cecum see Adhesions, peritoneum
|cervicovaginal N88.1
  |congenital Q52.8
  |postpartal O90.89
    |old N88.1
|cervix N88.1
|ciliary body NEC see Adhesions, iris
|clitoris N90.89
|colon see Adhesions, peritoneum
|common duct K83.8
|congenital see also Anomaly, by site
  |fingers see Syndactylism, complex, fingers
  |omental, anomalous Q43.3
  |peritoneal Q43.3
  |tongue (to gum or roof of mouth) Q38.3
|conjunctiva (acquired) H11.21-
  |congenital Q15.8
|cystic duct K82.8
|diaphragm see Adhesions, peritoneum
|due to foreign body see Foreign body
|duodenum see Adhesions, peritoneum
|ear
  |middle H74.1-
|epididymis N50.89
|epidural see Adhesions, meninges
|epiglottis J38.7
|eyelid H02.59
|female pelvis N73.6
|gallbladder K82.8
|globe H44.89
|heart I31.0
  |rheumatic I09.2
|ileocecal (coil) see Adhesions, peritoneum

Adhesions, adhesive (postinfective) -
  continued
|ileum see Adhesions, peritoneum
|intestine see also Adhesions, peritoneum
  |with obstruction K56.50
    |complete K56.52
    |incomplete K56.51
    |partial K56.51
|intra-abdominal see Adhesions, peritoneum
|iris H21.50-
  |anterior H21.51-
  |goniosynechiae H21.52-
  |posterior H21.54-
  |to corneal graft T85.898
|joint see Ankylosis
  |knee M23.8X
  |temporomandibular M26.61-
|labium (majus) (minus), congenital Q52.5
|liver see Adhesions, peritoneum
|lung J98.4
|mediastinum J98.59
|meninges (cerebral) (spinal) G96.12
  |congenital Q07.8
  |tuberculous (cerebral) (spinal) A17.0
|mesenteric see Adhesions, peritoneum
|nasal (septum) (to turbinates) J34.89
|ocular muscle see Strabismus, mechanical
|omentum see Adhesions, peritoneum
|ovary N73.6
  |congenital (to cecum, kidney or omentum)
    Q50.39
|paraovarian N73.6
|pelvic (peritoneal)
  |female N73.6
    |postprocedural N99.4
  |male see Adhesions, peritoneum
  |postpartal (old) N73.6
  |tuberculous A18.17
|penis to scrotum (congenital) Q55.8
|periappendiceal see also Adhesions,
  peritoneum
|pericardium (nonrheumatic) I31.0
  |focal I31.8
  |rheumatic I09.2
  |tuberculous A18.84
|pericholecystic K82.8
|perigastric see Adhesions, peritoneum
|periovarian N73.6
|periprostatic N42.89
|perirectal see Adhesions, peritoneum
|perirenal N28.89
|peritoneum, peritoneal (postinfective)
  |with obstruction (intestinal) K56.50
    |complete K56.52
    |incomplete K56.51
    |partial K56.51
  |congenital Q43.3
  |pelvic, female N73.6
    |postprocedural N99.4
  |postpartal, pelvic N73.6
  |postprocedural K66.0
  |to uterus N73.6
|peritubal N73.6
|periureteral N28.89
|periuterine N73.6
|perivesical N32.89
|perivesicular (seminal vesicle) N50.89
|pleura, pleuritic J94.8
  |tuberculous NEC A15.6
|pleuropericardial J94.8
|postoperative (gastrointestinal tract) K66.0
  |due to foreign body accidentally left in
    wound see Foreign body, accidentally
    left during a procedure
  |pelvic peritoneal N99.4

Adhesions, adhesive (postinfective) -
  continued
  |urethra see Stricture, urethra, postprocedural
  |vagina N99.2
  |with obstruction (see also Obstruction,
    intestine, postoperative) K91.30
|postpartal, old (vulva or perineum) N90.89
|preputial, prepuce N47.5
|pulmonary J98.4
|pylorus see Adhesions, peritoneum
|sciatic nerve see Lesion, nerve, sciatic
|seminal vesicle N50.89
|shoulder (joint) see Capsulitis, adhesive
|sigmoid flexure see Adhesions, peritoneum
|spermatic cord (acquired) N50.89
  |congenital Q55.4
|spinal canal G96.12
|stomach see Adhesions, peritoneum
|subscapular see Capsulitis, adhesive
|temporomandibular M26.61-
|tendinitis see also Tenosynovitis, specified
    type NEC
  |shoulder see Capsulitis, adhesive
|testis N44.8
|tongue, congenital (to gum or roof of mouth)
    Q38.3
  |acquired K14.8
|trachea J39.8
|tubo-ovarian N73.6
|tunica vaginalis N44.8
|uterus N73.6
  |internal N85.6
  |to abdominal wall N73.6
|vagina (chronic) N89.5
  |postoperative N99.2
|vitreomacular H43.82-
|vitreous H43.89
|vulva N90.89
Adiaspiromycosis B48.8
Adie (-Holmes) pupil or syndrome see
  Anomaly, pupil, function, tonic pupil
Adiponecrosis neonatorum P83.88
Adiposis see also Obesity |cerebralis E23.6
|dolorosa E88.2
Adiposity see also Obesity
|heart see Degeneration, myocardial
|localized E65
Adiposogenital dystrophy E23.6
Adjustment
|disorder see Disorder, adjustment
|implanted device see Encounter (for),
    adjustment (of)
|prosthesis, external see Fitting
|reaction see Disorder, adjustment
**Administration of tPA (rtPA) in a different
  facility within the last 24 hours prior to
  admission to current facility** Z92.82
Admission (for) see also Encounter (for)
|adjustment (of)
  |artificial
    |arm Z44.00-
      |complete Z44.01-
      |partial Z44.02-
    |eye Z44.2
    |leg Z44.10-
      |complete Z44.11-
      |partial Z44.12-
  |brain neuropacemaker Z46.2
    |implanted Z45.42
  |breast
    |implant Z45.81
    |prosthesis (external) Z44.3
  |colostomy belt Z46.89
  |contact lenses Z46.0
  |cystostomy device Z46.6
  |dental prosthesis Z46.3

Admission (for) - *continued*
|device NEC
  |abdominal Z46.89
  |implanted Z45.89
  |cardiac Z45.09
    |defibrillator (with synchronous cardiac pacemaker) Z45.02
    |pacemaker (cardiac resynchronization therapy (CRT-P)) Z45.018
      |pulse generator Z45.010
    |resynchronization therapy defibrillator (CRT-D) Z45.02
  |hearing device Z45.328
    |bone conduction Z45.320
    |cochlear Z45.321
  |infusion pump Z45.1
  |nervous system Z45.49
    |CSF drainage Z45.41
    |hearing device *see* Admission, adjustment, device, implanted, hearing device
    |neuropacemaker Z45.42
    |visual substitution Z45.31
  |specified NEC Z45.89
  |vascular access Z45.2
  |visual substitution Z45.31
|nervous system Z46.2
  |implanted *see* Admission, adjustment, device, implanted, nervous system
|orthodontic Z46.4
|prosthetic Z44.9
  |arm *see* Admission, adjustment, artificial, arm
  |breast Z44.3
  |dental Z46.3
  |eye Z44.2
  |leg *see* Admission, adjustment, artificial, leg
  |specified type NEC Z44.8
|substitution
  |auditory Z46.2
    |implanted *see* Admission, adjustment, device, implanted, hearing device
  |nervous system Z46.2
    |implanted *see* Admission, adjustment, device, implanted, nervous system
  |visual Z46.2
    |implanted Z45.31
  |urinary Z46.6
|hearing aid Z46.1
  |implanted *see* Admission, adjustment, device, implanted, hearing device
|ileostomy device Z46.89
|intestinal appliance or device NEC Z46.89
|neuropacemaker (brain) (peripheral nerve) (spinal cord) Z46.2
  |implanted Z45.42
|orthodontic device Z46.4
|orthopedic (brace) (cast) (device) (shoes) Z46.89
|pacemaker (cardiac resynchronization therapy (CRT-P))
  |cardiac Z45.018
    |pulse generator Z45.010
  |nervous system Z46.2
    |implanted Z45.42
|portacath (port-a-cath) Z45.2
|prosthesis Z44.9
  |arm *see* Admission, adjustment, artificial, arm
  |breast Z44.3
  |dental Z46.3
  |eye Z44.2
  |leg *see* Admission, adjustment, artificial, leg
  |specified NEC Z44.8

Admission (for) - *continued*
|spectacles Z46.0
|aftercare *see also* Aftercare Z51.89
  |postpartum
    |immediately after delivery Z39.0
    |routine follow-up Z39.2
  |radiation therapy (antineoplastic) Z51.0
|attention to artificial opening (of) Z43.9
  |artificial vagina Z43.7
  |colostomy Z43.3
  |cystostomy Z43.5
  |enterostomy Z43.4
  |gastrostomy Z43.1
  |ileostomy Z43.2
  |jejunostomy Z43.4
  |nephrostomy Z43.6
  |specified site NEC Z43.8
    |intestinal tract Z43.4
    |urinary tract Z43.6
  |tracheostomy Z43.0
  |ureterostomy Z43.6
  |urethrostomy Z43.6
|breast augmentation or reduction Z41.1
|breast reconstruction following mastectomy Z42.1
|change of
  |dressing (nonsurgical) Z48.00
  |neuropacemaker device (brain) (peripheral nerve) (spinal cord) Z46.2
    |implanted Z45.42
  |surgical dressing Z48.01
|circumcision, ritual or routine (in absence of diagnosis) Z41.2
|clinical research investigation (control) (normal comparison) (participant) Z00.6
|contraceptive management Z30.9
|cosmetic surgery NEC Z41.1
|counseling *see also* Counseling
  |dietary Z71.3
  |gestational carrier Z31.7
  |HIV Z71.7
  |human immunodeficiency virus Z71.7
  |nonattending third party Z71.0
  |procreative management NEC Z31.69
|delivery, full-term, uncomplicated O80
  |cesarean, without indication O82
|desensitization to allergens Z51.6
|dietary surveillance and counseling Z71.3
|ear piercing Z41.3
|examination at health care facility (adult) *see also* Examination Z00.00
  |with abnormal findings Z00.01
  |clinical research investigation (control) (normal comparison) (participant) Z00.6
  |dental Z01.20
    |with abnormal findings Z01.21
  |donor (potential) Z00.5
  |ear Z01.10
    |with abnormal findings NEC Z01.118
  |eye Z01.00
    |with abnormal findings Z01.01
  |general, specified reason NEC Z00.8
  |hearing Z01.10
    |with abnormal findings NEC Z01.118
    |infant or child (over 28 days old) Z00.129
      |with abnormal findings Z00.121
  |postpartum checkup Z39.2
  |psychiatric (general) Z00.8
    |requested by authority Z04.6
  |vision Z01.00
    |with abnormal findings Z01.01
|fitting (of)
  |artificial
    |arm *see* Admission, adjustment, artificial, arm

Admission (for) - *continued*
|eye Z44.2
|leg *see* Admission, adjustment, artificial, leg
|brain neuropacemaker Z46.2
  |implanted Z45.42
|breast prosthesis (external) Z44.3
|colostomy belt Z46.89
|contact lenses Z46.0
|cystostomy device Z46.6
|dental prosthesis Z46.3
|dentures Z46.3
|device NEC
  |abdominal Z46.89
  |nervous system Z46.2
    |implanted *see* Admission, adjustment, device, implanted, nervous system
  |orthodontic Z46.4
  |prosthetic Z44.9
    |breast Z44.3
    |dental Z46.3
    |eye Z44.2
  |substitution
    |auditory Z46.2
      |implanted *see* Admission, adjustment, device, implanted, hearing device
    |nervous system Z46.2
      |implanted *see* Admission, adjustment, device, implanted, nervous system
    |visual Z46.2
      |implanted Z45.31
|hearing aid Z46.1
|ileostomy device Z46.89
|intestinal appliance or device NEC Z46.89
|neuropacemaker (brain) (peripheral nerve) (spinal cord) Z46.2
  |implanted Z45.42
|orthodontic device Z46.4
|orthopedic device (brace) (cast) (shoes) Z46.89
|prosthesis Z44.9
  |arm *see* Admission, adjustment, artificial, arm
  |breast Z44.3
  |dental Z46.3
  |eye Z44.2
  |leg *see* Admission, adjustment, artificial, leg
  |specified type NEC Z44.8
|spectacles Z46.0
|follow-up examination Z09
|intrauterine device management Z30.431
  |initial prescription Z30.014
|mental health evaluation Z00.8
  |requested by authority Z04.6
|observation *see* Observation
|Papanicolaou smear, cervix Z12.4
  |for suspected malignant neoplasm Z12.4
|plastic and reconstructive surgery following medical procedure or healed injury NEC Z42.8
|plastic surgery, cosmetic NEC Z41.1
|postpartum observation
  |immediately after delivery Z39.0
  |routine follow-up Z39.2
|poststerilization (for restoration) Z31.0
  |aftercare Z31.42
|procreative management Z31.9
|prophylactic (measure) *see also* Encounter, prophylactic measures
  |organ removal Z40.00
    |breast Z40.01
    |fallopian tube(s) Z40.03
      |with ovary(s) Z40.02

Admission (for) - *continued*
|ovary(s) Z40.02
|specified organ NEC Z40.09
|testes Z40.09
|vaccination Z23
|psychiatric examination (general) Z00.8
|requested by authority Z04.6
|radiation therapy (antineoplastic) Z51.0
|reconstructive surgery following medical
procedure or healed injury NEC Z42.8
|removal of
|cystostomy catheter Z43.5
|drains Z48.03
|dressing (nonsurgical) Z48.00
|implantable subdermal contraceptive Z30.46
|intrauterine contraceptive device Z30.432
|neuropacemaker (brain) (peripheral nerve)
(spinal cord) Z46.2
|implanted Z45.42
|staples Z48.02
|surgical dressing Z48.01
|sutures Z48.02
|ureteral stent Z46.6
|respirator [ventilator] use during power failure
Z99.12
|restoration of organ continuity
(poststerilization) Z31.0
|aftercare Z31.42
|sensitivity test *see also* Test, skin
|allergy NEC Z01.82
|Mantoux Z11.1
|tuboplasty following previous sterilization
Z31.0
|aftercare Z31.42
|vasoplasty following previous sterilization
Z31.0
|aftercare Z31.42
|vision examination Z01.00
|infant or child (over 28 days old) Z00.129
|with abnormal findings Z00.121
|with abnormal findings Z01.01
|waiting period for admission to other facility
Z75.1
Adnexitis (suppurative) *see* Salpingo-
oophoritis
Adolescent X-Linked adrenoleukodystrophy
E71.521
Adrenal (gland) *see* condition
Adrenalism, tuberculous A18.7
Adrenalitis, adrenitis E27.8
|autoimmune E27.1
|meningococcal, hemorrhagic A39.1
Adrenarche, premature E27.0
Adrenocortical syndrome *see* Cushing's,
syndrome
Adrenogenital syndrome E25.9
|acquired E25.8
|congenital E25.0
|salt loss E25.0
Adrenogenitalism, congenital E25.0
Adrenoleukodystrophy E71.529
|neonatal E71.511
|X-linked E71.529
|Addison only phenotype E71.528
|Addison-Schilder E71.528
|adolescent E71.521
|adrenomyeloneuropathy E71.522
|childhood cerebral E71.520
|other specified E71.528
Adrenomyeloneuropathy E71.522
Adventitious bursa *see* Bursopathy, specified
type NEC
Adverse effect *see* Table of Drugs and
Chemicals, categories T36-T50, with 6th
character 5

Advice *see* Counseling
Adynamia (episodica) (hereditary) (periodic)
G72.3
Aeration lung imperfect, newborn *see*
Atelectasis
Aerobullosis T70.3
Aerocele *see* Embolism, air
Aerodermectasia
|subcutaneous (traumatic) T79.7
Aerodontalgia T70.29
Aeroembolism T70.3
Aerogenes capsulatus infection A48.0
Aero-Otitis media T70.0
Aerophagy, aerophagia (psychogenic) F45.8
Aerophobia F40.228
Aerosinusitis T70.1
Aerotitis T70.0
Affection *see* Disease
Afibrinogenemia *see also* Defect, coagulation
D68.8
|acquired D65
|congenital D68.2
|following ectopic or molar pregnancy O08.1
|in abortion *see* Abortion, by type, complicated
by, afibrinogenemia
|puerperal O72.3
African
|sleeping sickness B56.9
|tick fever A68.1
|trypanosomiasis B56.9
|Gambian B56.0
|Rhodesian B56.1
Aftercare *see also* Care Z51.89
|following surgery (for) (on)
|amputation Z47.81
|attention to
|drains Z48.03
|dressings (nonsurgical) Z48.00
|surgical Z48.01
|sutures Z48.02
|circulatory system Z48.812
|delayed (planned) wound closure Z48.1
|digestive system Z48.815
|explantation of joint prosthesis (staged
procedure)
|hip Z47.32
|knee Z47.33
|shoulder Z47.31
|genitourinary system Z48.816
|joint replacement Z47.1
|neoplasm Z48.3
|nervous system Z48.811
|oral cavity Z48.814
|organ transplant
|bone marrow Z48.290
|heart Z48.21
|heart-lung Z48.280
|kidney Z48.22
|liver Z48.23
|lung Z48.24
|multiple organs NEC Z48.288
|specified NEC Z48.298
|orthopedic NEC Z47.89
|planned wound closure Z48.1
|removal of internal fixation device Z47.2
|respiratory system Z48.813
|scoliosis Z47.82
|sense organs Z48.810
|skin and subcutaneous tissue Z48.817
|specified body system
|circulatory Z48.812
|digestive Z48.815
|genitourinary Z48.816
|nervous Z48.811
|oral cavity Z48.814
|respiratory Z48.813

Aftercare - *continued*
|sense organs Z48.810
|skin and subcutaneous tissue Z48.817
|teeth Z48.814
|specified NEC Z48.89
|spinal Z47.89
|teeth Z48.814
|fracture   code to fracture with seventh
character D
|involving
|removal of
|drains Z48.03
|dressings (nonsurgical) Z48.00
|staples Z48.02
|surgical dressings Z48.01
|sutures Z48.02
|neuropacemaker (brain) (peripheral nerve)
(spinal cord) Z46.2
|implanted Z45.42
|orthopedic NEC Z47.89
|postprocedural *see* Aftercare, following
surgery
After-Cataract *see* Cataract, secondary
Agalactia (primary) O92.3
|elective, secondary or therapeutic O92.5
Agammaglobulinemia (acquired (secondary))
(nonfamilial) D80.1
|with
|immunoglobulin-bearing B-lymphocytes
D80.1
|lymphopenia D81.9
|autosomal recessive (Swiss type) D80.0
|Bruton's X-linked D80.0
|common variable (CVA gamma) D80.1
|congenital sex-linked D80.0
|hereditary D80.0
|lymphopenic D81.9
|Swiss type (autosomal recessive) D80.0
|X-linked (with growth hormone deficiency)
(Bruton) D80.0
Aganglionosis (bowel) (colon) Q43.1
Age (old) *see* Senility
Agenesis
|adrenal (gland) Q89.1
|alimentary tract (complete) (partial) NEC
Q45.8
|upper Q40.8
|anus, anal (canal) Q42.3
|with fistula Q42.2
|aorta Q25.41
|appendix Q42.8
|arm (complete) Q71.0-
|with hand present Q71.1-
|artery (peripheral) Q27.9
|brain Q28.3
|coronary Q24.5
|pulmonary Q25.79
|specified NEC Q27.8
|umbilical Q27.0
|auditory (canal) (external) Q16.1
|auricle (ear) Q16.0
|bile duct or passage Q44.5
|bladder Q64.5
|bone Q79.9
|brain Q00.0
|part of Q04.3
|breast (with nipple present) Q83.8
|with absent nipple Q83.0
|bronchus Q32.4
|canaliculus lacrimalis Q10.4
|carpus *see* Agenesis, hand
|cartilage Q79.9
|cecum Q42.8
|cerebellum Q04.3
|cervix Q51.5

Agenesis - *continued*
|chin Q18.8
|cilia Q10.3
|circulatory system, part NOS Q28.9
|clavicle Q74.0
|clitoris Q52.6
|coccyx Q76.49
|colon Q42.9
||specified NEC Q42.8
|corpus callosum Q04.0
|cricoid cartilage Q31.8
|diaphragm (with hernia) Q79.1
|digestive organ(s) or tract (complete) (partial)
|| NEC Q45.8
||upper Q40.8
|ductus arteriosus Q28.8
|duodenum Q41.0
|ear Q16.9
||auricle Q16.0
||lobe Q17.8
|ejaculatory duct Q55.4
|endocrine (gland) NEC Q89.2
|epiglottis Q31.8
|esophagus Q39.8
|eustachian tube Q16.2
|eye Q11.1
||adnexa Q15.8
|eyelid (fold) Q10.3
|face
||bones NEC Q75.8
||specified part NEC Q18.8
|fallopian tube Q50.6
|femur *see* Defect, reduction, lower limb,
|| longitudinal, femur
|fibula *see* Defect, reduction, lower limb,
|| longitudinal, fibula
|finger (complete) (partial) *see* Agenesis, hand
|foot (and toes) (complete) (partial) Q72.3-
|forearm (with hand present) *see* Agenesis,
|| arm, with hand present
||and hand Q71.2-
|gallbladder Q44.0
|gastric Q40.2
|genitalia, genital (organ(s))
||female Q52.8
|||external Q52.71
|||internal NEC Q52.8
||male Q55.8
|glottis Q31.8
|hair Q84.0
|hand (and fingers) (complete) (partial) Q71.3-
|heart Q24.8
||valve NEC Q24.8
||pulmonary Q22.0
|hepatic Q44.7
|humerus *see* Defect, reduction, upper limb
|hymen Q52.4
|ileum Q41.2
|incus Q16.3
|intestine (small) Q41.9
||large Q42.9
|||specified NEC Q42.8
|iris (dilator fibers) Q13.1
|jaw M26.09
|jejunum Q41.1
|kidney(s) (partial) Q60.2
||bilateral Q60.1
||unilateral Q60.0
|labium (majus) (minus) Q52.71
|labyrinth, membranous Q16.5
|lacrimal apparatus Q10.4
|larynx Q31.8
|leg (complete) Q72.0-
||with foot present Q72.1-
||lower leg (with foot present) *see* Agenesis,
||| leg, with foot present
|||and foot Q72.2-

Agenesis - *continued*
|lens Q12.3
|limb (complete) Q73.0
||lower *see* Agenesis, leg
||upper *see* Agenesis, arm
|lip Q38.0
|liver Q44.7
|lung (fissure) (lobe) (bilateral) (unilateral)
|| Q33.3
|mandible, maxilla M26.09
|metacarpus *see* Agenesis, hand
|metatarsus *see* Agenesis, foot
|muscle Q79.8
||eyelid Q10.3
||ocular Q15.8
|musculoskeletal system NEC Q79.8
|nail(s) Q84.3
|neck, part Q18.8
|nerve Q07.8
|nervous system, part NEC Q07.8
|nipple Q83.2
|nose Q30.1
|nuclear Q07.8
|organ
||of Corti Q16.5
||or site not listed *see* Anomaly, by site
|osseous meatus (ear) Q16.1
|ovary
||bilateral Q50.02
||unilateral Q50.01
|oviduct Q50.6
|pancreas Q45.0
|parathyroid (gland) Q89.2
|parotid gland(s) Q38.4
|patella Q74.1
|pelvic girdle (complete) (partial) Q74.2
|penis Q55.5
|pericardium Q24.8
|pituitary (gland) Q89.2
|prostate Q55.4
|punctum lacrimale Q10.4
|radioulnar *see* Defect, reduction, upper limb
|radius *see* Defect, reduction, upper limb,
|| longitudinal, radius
|rectum Q42.1
||with fistula Q42.0
|renal Q60.2
||bilateral Q60.1
||unilateral Q60.0
|respiratory organ NEC Q34.8
|rib Q76.6
|roof of orbit Q75.8
|round ligament Q52.8
|sacrum Q76.49
|salivary gland Q38.4
|scapula Q74.0
|scrotum Q55.29
|seminal vesicles Q55.4
|septum
||atrial Q21.1
||between aorta and pulmonary artery Q21.4
||ventricular Q20.4
|shoulder girdle (complete) (partial) Q74.0
|skull (bone) Q75.8
||with
|||anencephaly Q00.0
|||encephalocele *see* Encephalocele
|||hydrocephalus Q03.9
||||with spina bifida *see* Spina bifida, by
|||| site, with hydrocephalus
|||microcephaly Q02
|spermatic cord Q55.4
|spinal cord Q06.0
|spine Q76.49
|spleen Q89.01

Agenesis - *continued*
|sternum Q76.7
|stomach Q40.2
|submaxillary gland(s) (congenital) Q38.4
|tarsus *see* Agenesis, foot
|tendon Q79.8
|testicle Q55.0
|thymus (gland) Q89.2
|thyroid (gland) E03.1
||cartilage Q31.8
|tibia *see* Defect, reduction, lower limb,
|| longitudinal, tibia
|tibiofibular *see* Defect, reduction, lower limb,
|| specified type NEC
|toe (and foot) (complete) (partial) *see*
|| Agenesis, foot
|tongue Q38.3
|trachea (cartilage) Q32.1
|ulna *see* Defect, reduction, upper limb,
|| longitudinal, ulna
|upper limb *see* Agenesis, arm
|ureter Q62.4
|urethra Q64.5
|urinary tract NEC Q64.8
|uterus Q51.0
|uvula Q38.5
|vagina Q52.0
|vas deferens Q55.4
|vein(s) (peripheral) Q27.9
||brain Q28.3
||great NEC Q26.8
||portal Q26.5
|vena cava (inferior) (superior) Q26.8
|vermis of cerebellum Q04.3
|vertebra Q76.49
|vulva Q52.71
Ageusia R43.2
Agitated *see* condition **Agitation** R45.1
Aglossia (congenital) Q38.3
Aglossia-Adactylia syndrome Q87.0
Aglycogenosis E74.00
Agnosia (body image) (other senses) (tactile)
| R48.1
|developmental F88
|verbal R48.1
||auditory R48.1
|||developmental F80.2
||developmental F80.2
|visual (object) R48.3
Agoraphobia F40.00
|with panic disorder F40.01
|without panic disorder F40.02
Agrammatism R48.8
Agranulocytopenia *see* Agranulocytosis
Agranulocytosis (chronic) (cyclical) (genetic)
| (infantile) (periodic) (pernicious) *see also*
| Neutropenia D70.9
|congenital D70.0
|cytoreductive cancer chemotherapy sequela
|| D70.1
|drug-induced D70.2
||due to cytoreductive cancer chemotherapy
||| D70.1
|due to infection D70.3
|secondary D70.4
||drug-induced D70.2
|||due to cytoreductive cancer chemotherapy
|||| D70.1
Agraphia (absolute) R48.8
|with alexia R48.0
|developmental F81.81
Ague (dumb) *see* Malaria
Agyria Q04.3

Ahumada-Del Castillo syndrome E23.0
Aichmophobia F40.298
AIDS (related complex) B20
Ailment heart see Disease, heart
Ailurophobia F40.218
Ainhum (disease) L94.6
AIN see Neoplasia, intraepithelial, anal
AIPHI (acute idiopathic pulmonary hemorrhage in infants (over 28 days old)) R04.81
Air
|anterior mediastinum J98.2
|compressed, disease T70.3
|conditioner lung or pneumonitis J67.7
|embolism (artery) (cerebral) (any site) T79.0
  |with ectopic or molar pregnancy O08.2
  |due to implanted device NEC see Complications, by site and type, specified NEC
  |following
    |abortion see Abortion by type, complicated by, embolism
    |ectopic or molar pregnancy O08.2
    |infusion, therapeutic injection or transfusion T80.0
  |in pregnancy, childbirth or puerperium see Embolism, obstetric
  |traumatic T79.0
|hunger, psychogenic F45.8
|rarefied, effects of see Effect, adverse, high altitude
|sickness T75.3
Airplane sickness T75.3
Akathisia (drug-Induced) (treatment-Induced) G25.71
|neuroleptic induced (acute) G25.71
|tardive G25.71
Akinesia R29.898
Akinetic mutism R41.89
Akureyri's disease G93.3
Alactasia, congenital E73.0
Alagille's syndrome Q44.7
Alastrim B03
Albers-Schonberg syndrome Q78.2
Albert's syndrome see Tendinitis, Achilles
Albinism, albino E70.30
|with hematologic abnormality E70.339
  |Chédiak-Higashi syndrome E70.330
  |Hermansky-Pudlak syndrome E70.331
  |other specified E70.338
|I E70.320
|II E70.321
|ocular E70.319
  |autosomal recessive E70.311
  |other specified E70.318
  |X-linked E70.310
|oculocutaneous E70.329
  |other specified E70.328
  |tyrosinase (ty) negative E70.320
  |tyrosinase (ty) positive E70.321
|other specified E70.39
Albinismus E70.30
Albright (-McCune)(-Sternberg) syndrome Q78.1
Albuminous see condition
Albuminuria, albuminuric (acute) (chronic) (subacute) see also Proteinuria R80.9
|complicating pregnancy see Proteinuria, gestational
|with
  |gestational hypertension see Pre-eclampsia
  |pre-existing hypertension see Hypertension, complicating pregnancy, pre-existing, with, pre-eclampsia

Albuminuria - continued
|gestational see Proteinuria, gestational
|with
  |gestational hypertension see Pre-eclampsia
  |pre-existing hypertension see Hypertension, complicating pregnancy, pre-existing, with, pre-eclampsia
|orthostatic R80.2
|postural R80.2
|pre-eclamptic see Pre-eclampsia
|scarlatinal A38.8
Albuminurophobia F40.298
Alcaptonuria E70.29
Alcohol, alcoholic, alcohol-Induced
|addiction (without remission) F10.20
  |with remission F10.21
|amnestic disorder, persisting F10.96
  |with dependence F10.26
|anxiety disorder F10.980
|bipolar and related disorder F10.94
|depressive disorder F10.94
|major neurocognitive disorder, amnestic-confabulatory type F10.96
|major neurocognitive disorder, non-amnestic-confabulatory type F10.97
|mild neurocognitive disorder F10.988
|psychotic disorder F10.959
|sexual dysfunction F10.981
|sleep disorder F10.982
|brain syndrome, chronic F10.97
  |with dependence F10.27
|cardiopathy I42.6
|counseling and surveillance Z71.41
  |family member Z71.42
|delirium (acute) (tremens) (withdrawal) F10.231
  |with intoxication F10.921
  |in
    |abuse F10.121
    |dependence F10.221
|dementia F10.97
  |with dependence F10.27
|deterioration F10.97
  |with dependence F10.27
|hallucinosis (acute) F10.951
  |in
    |abuse F10.151
    |dependence F10.251
|insanity F10.959
|intoxication (acute) (without dependence) F10.129
  |with
    |delirium F10.121
    |dependence F10.229
      |with delirium F10.221
      |uncomplicated F10.220
    |uncomplicated F10.120
|jealousy F10.988
|Korsakoff's, Korsakov's, Korsakow's F10.26
|liver K70.9
  |acute see Disease, liver, alcoholic, hepatitis
|mania (acute) (chronic) F10.959
|paranoia, paranoid (type) psychosis F10.950
|pellagra E52
|poisoning, accidental (acute) NEC see Table of Drugs and Chemicals, alcohol, poisoning
|psychosis see Psychosis, alcoholic
|withdrawal (without convulsions) F10.239
  |with delirium F10.231

Alcoholism (chronic) (without remission) F10.20
|with
  |psychosis see Psychosis, alcoholic
  |remission F10.21
|Korsakov's F10.96
  |with dependence F10.26
Alder (-Reilly) anomaly or syndrome (leukocyte granulation) D72.0
Aldosteronism E26.9
|familial (type I) E26.02
|glucocorticoid-remediable E26.02
|primary (due to (bilateral) adrenal hyperplasia) E26.09
|primary NEC E26.09
|secondary E26.1
|specified NEC E26.89
Aldosteronoma D44.10
Aldrich (-Wiskott) syndrome (eczema-Thrombocytopenia) D82.0
Alektorophobia F40.218
Aleppo boil B55.1
Aleukemic see condition
Aleukia
|congenital D70.0
|hemorrhagica D61.9
  |congenital D61.09
|splenica D73.1
Alexia R48.0
|developmental F81.0
|secondary to organic lesion R48.0
Algoneurodystrophy M89.00
|ankle M89.07-
|foot M89.07-
|forearm M89.03-
|hand M89.04-
|lower leg M89.06-
|multiple sites M89.0-
|shoulder M89.01-
|specified site NEC M89.08
|thigh M89.05-
|upper arm M89.02-
Algophobia F40.298
Alienation, mental see Psychosis
Alkalemia E87.3
Alkalosis E87.3
|metabolic E87.3
  |of newborn P74.41
  |with respiratory acidosis E87.4
|respiratory E87.3
Alkaptonuria E70.29
Allen-Masters syndrome N83.8
Allergy, allergic (reaction) (to) T78.40
|air-borne substance NEC (rhinitis) J30.89
|alveolitis (extrinsic) J67.9
  |due to
    |Aspergillus clavatus J67.4
    |Cryptostroma corticale J67.6
    |organisms (fungal, thermophilic actinomycete) growing in ventilation (air conditioning) systems J67.7
  |specified type NEC J67.8
|anaphylactic reaction or shock T78.2
|angioneurotic edema T78.3
|animal (dander) (epidermal) (hair) (rhinitis) J30.81
|bee sting (anaphylactic shock) see Toxicity, venom, arthropod, bee
|biological see Allergy, drug
|colitis see also Colitis, allergic K52.29
|dander (animal) (rhinitis) J30.81
|dandruff (rhinitis) J30.81
|dental restorative material (existing) K08.55
|dermatitis see Dermatitis, contact, allergic

Allergy, allergic (reaction) (to) - *continued*
|diathesis *see* History, allergy
|drug, medicament & biological (any) (external) (internal) T78.40
   |correct substance properly administered *see* Table of Drugs and Chemicals, by drug, adverse effect
   |wrong substance given or taken NEC (by accident) *see* Table of Drugs and Chemicals, by drug, poisoning
|due to pollen J30.1
|dust (house) (stock) (rhinitis) J30.89
   |with asthma *see* Asthma, allergic extrinsic
|eczema *see* Dermatitis, contact, allergic
|epidermal (animal) (rhinitis) J30.81
|feathers (rhinitis) J30.89
|food (any) (ingested) NEC T78.1
   |anaphylactic shock *see* Shock, anaphylactic, due to food
   |dermatitis *see* Dermatitis, due to, food
   |dietary counseling and surveillance Z71.3
   |in contact with skin L23.6
   |rhinitis J30.5
   |status (without reaction) Z91.018
      |beef Z91.014
      |eggs Z91.012
      |lamb Z91.014
      |mammalian meats Z91.014
      |milk products Z91.011
      |peanuts Z91.010
      |pork Z91.014
      |red meats Z91.014
      |seafood Z91.013
      |specified NEC Z91.018
|gastrointestinal *see also* specific type of allergic reaction
   |meaning colitis *see also* Colitis, allergic K52.29
   |meaning gastroenteritis *see also* Gastroenteritis, allergic K52.29
   |meaning other adverse food reaction not elsewhere classified T78.1
|grain J30.1
|grass (hay fever) (pollen) J30.1
   |asthma *see* Asthma, allergic extrinsic
|hair (animal) (rhinitis) J30.81
|history (of) *see* History, allergy
|horse serum *see* Allergy, serum
|inhalant (rhinitis) J30.89
   |pollen J30.1
|kapok (rhinitis) J30.89
|medicine *see* Allergy, drug
|milk protein *see also* Allergy, food Z91.011
   |anaphylactic reaction T78.07
   |dermatitis L27.2
   |enterocolitis syndrome K52.21
   |enteropathy K52.22
   |gastroenteritis K52.29
   |gastroesophageal reflux *see also* Reaction, adverse, food K21.9
      |with esophagitis (without bleeding) K21.00
      |with bleeding K21.01
   |proctocolitis K52.29
|nasal, seasonal due to pollen J30.1
|pneumonia J82.89
|pollen (any) (hay fever) J30.1
   |asthma *see* Asthma, allergic extrinsic
|primrose J30.1
|primula J30.1
|proctocolitis K52.29
|purpura D69.0
|ragweed (hay fever) (pollen) J30.1
   |asthma *see* Asthma, allergic extrinsic
|rose (pollen) J30.1
|seasonal NEC J30.2

Allergy, allergic (reaction) (to) - *continued*
|Senecio jacobae (pollen) J30.1
|serum *see also* Reaction, serum T80.69
   |anaphylactic shock T80.59
|shock (anaphylactic) T78.2
   |due to
      |administration of blood and blood products T80.51
      |adverse effect of correct medicinal substance properly administered T88.6
         |immunization T80.52
         |serum NEC T80.59
         |vaccination T80.52
   |specific NEC T78.49
|tree (any) (hay fever) (pollen) J30.1
   |asthma *see* Asthma, allergic extrinsic
|upper respiratory J30.9
|urticaria L50.0
|vaccine *see* Allergy, serum
|wheat *see* Allergy, food
Allescheriasis B48.2
Alligator skin disease Q80.9
Allocheiria, allochiria R20.8
Almeida's disease *see* Paracoccidioidomycosis
Alopecia (hereditaria) (seborrheica) L65.9
|androgenic L64.9
   |drug-induced L64.0
   |specified NEC L64.8
|areata L63.9
   |ophiasis L63.2
   |specified NEC L63.8
   |totalis L63.0
   |universalis L63.1
|cicatricial L66.9
   |specified NEC L66.8
|circumscripta L63.9
|congenital, congenitalis Q84.0
|due to cytotoxic drugs NEC L65.8
|mucinosa L65.2
|postinfective NEC L65.8
|postpartum L65.0
|premature L64.8
|specific (syphilitic) A51.32
|specified NEC L65.8
|syphilitic (secondary) A51.32
|totalis (capitis) L63.0
|universalis (entire body) L63.1
|X-ray L58.1
Alpers' disease G31.81
Alpine sickness T70.29
Alport syndrome Q87.81
ALTE (apparent life threatening event) in newborn and infant R68.13
Alteration (of), Altered
|awareness
   |transient R40.4
   |unintended under general anesthesia, during procedure T88.53
|mental status R41.82
|pattern of family relationships affecting child Z62.898
|sensation
|following
   |cerebrovascular disease I69.998
      |cerebral infarction I69.398
      |intracerebral hemorrhage I69.198
      |nontraumatic intracranial hemorrhage NEC I69.298
      |specified disease NEC I69.898
      |subarachnoid hemorrhage I69.098
Alternating *see* condition
Altitude, high (effects) *see* Effect, adverse, high altitude
Aluminosis (of lung) J63.0

Alveolitis
|allergic (extrinsic) *see* Pneumonitis, hypersensitivity |due to
   |Aspergillus clavatus J67.4
   |Cryptostroma corticale J67.6
|fibrosing (cryptogenic) (idiopathic) J84.112
|jaw M27.3
|sicca dolorosa M27.3
Alveolus, alveolar *see* condition
Alymphocytosis D72.810
|thymic (with immunodeficiency) D82.1
Alymphoplasia, thymic D82.1
Alzheimer's disease or sclerosis *see* Disease, Alzheimer's
Amastia (with nipple present) Q83.8
|with absent nipple Q83.0
Amathophobia F40.228
Amaurosis (acquired) (congenital) *see also* Blindness
|fugax G45.3
|hysterical F44.6
|Leber's congenital H35.50
|uremic *see* Uremia
Amaurotic idiocy (infantile) (juvenile) (late) E75.4
Amaxophobia F40.248
Ambiguous genitalia Q56.4
Amblyopia (congenital) (ex anopsia) (partial) (suppression) H53.00-
|anisometropic *see* Amblyopia, refractive
|deprivation H53.01-
|hysterical F44.6
|nocturnal *see also* Blindness, night
   |vitamin A deficiency E50.5
|refractive H53.02-
|strabismic H53.03-
|suspect H53.04-
|tobacco H53.8
|toxic NEC H53.8
|uremic *see* Uremia
Ameba, amebic (histolytica) *see also* Amebiasis
|abscess (liver) A06.4
Amebiasis A06.9
|with abscess *see* Abscess, amebic
|acute A06.0
|chronic (intestine) A06.1
   |with abscess *see* Abscess, amebic
|cutaneous A06.7
|cutis A06.7
|cystitis A06.81
|genitourinary tract NEC A06.82
|hepatic *see* Abscess, liver, amebic
|intestine A06.0
|nondysenteric colitis A06.2
|skin A06.7
|specified site NEC A06.89
Ameboma (of intestine) A06.3
Amelia Q73.0
|lower limb *see* Agenesis, leg
|upper limb *see* Agenesis, arm
Ameloblastoma *see also* Cyst, calcifying odontogenic
|long bones C40.9-
   |lower limb C40.2-
   |upper limb C40.0-
|malignant C41.1
   |jaw (bone) (lower) C41.1
      |upper C41.0
|tibial C40.2-
Amelogenesis imperfecta K00.5
|nonhereditaria (segmentalis) K00.4

Amenorrhea N91.2
|hyperhormonal E28.8
|primary N91.0
|secondary N91.1
Amentia *see* Disability, intellectual
|Meynert's (nonalcoholic) F04
American
|leishmaniasis B55.2
|mountain tick fever A93.2
Ametropia *see* Disorder, refraction
AMH (asymptomatic microscopic hematuria)
   R31.21
Amianthosis J61
Amimia R48.8
Amino-Acid disorder E72.9
|anemia D53.0
Aminoacidopathy E72.9
Aminoaciduria E72.9
Amnes (t)ic syndrome (post-Traumatic) F04
|induced by
  |alcohol F10.96
    |with dependence F10.26
  |psychoactive NEC F19.96
    |with
      |abuse F19.16
      |dependence F19.26
  |sedative F13.96
    |with dependence F13.26
Amnesia R41.3
|anterograde R41.1
|auditory R48.8
|dissociative F44.0
  |with dissociative fugue F44.1
|hysterical F44.0
|postictal in epilepsy *see* Epilepsy
|psychogenic F44.0
|retrograde R41.2
|transient global G45.4
Amnion, amniotic *see* condition
Amnionitis *see* Pregnancy, complicated by
Amok F68.8
Amoral traits F60.89
Amphetamine (or other stimulant) –induced
|anxiety disorder F15.980
|bipolar and related disorder F15.94
|delirium F15.921
|depressive disorder F15.94
|obsessive-compulsive and related disorder
  F15.988
|psychotic disorder F15.959
|sexual dysfunction F15.981
|sleep disorder F15.982
|stimulant withdrawal F15.23
Ampulla
|lower esophagus K22.89
|phrenic K22.89
Amputation *see also* Absence, by site, acquired
|neuroma (postoperative) (traumatic) *see*
  Complications, amputation stump, neuroma
|stump (surgical)
  |abnormal, painful, or with complication
    (late) *see* Complications, amputation stump
  |healed or old NOS Z89.9
|traumatic (complete) (partial)
  |arm (upper) (complete) S48.91-
    |at
      |elbow S58.01-
        |partial S58.02-
      |shoulder joint (complete) S48.01-
        |partial S48.02-
    |between
      |elbow and wrist (complete) S58.11-
        |partial S58.12-
      |shoulder and elbow (complete) S48.11-

Amputation - *continued*
    |partial S48.12-
  |partial S48.92-
|breast (complete) S28.21-
  |partial S28.22-
|clitoris (complete) S38.211
  |partial S38.212
|ear (complete) S08.11-
  |partial S08.12-
|finger (complete) (metacarpophalangeal)
  S68.11-
  |index S68.11-
  |little S68.11-
  |middle S68.11-
  |partial S68.12-
    |index S68.12-
    |little S68.12-
    |middle S68.12-
    |ring S68.12-
  |ring S68.11-
  |thumb *see* Amputation, traumatic, thumb
  |transphalangeal (complete) S68.61-
    |index S68.61-
    |little S68.61-
    |middle S68.61-
    |partial S68.62-
      |index S68.62-
      |little S68.62-
      |middle S68.62-
      |ring S68.62-
    |ring S68.61-
|foot (complete) S98.91-
  |at ankle level S98.01-
    |partial S98.02-
  |midfoot S98.31-
    |partial S98.32-
  |partial S98.92-
|forearm (complete) S58.91-
  |at elbow level (complete) S58.01-
    |partial S58.02-
  |between elbow and wrist (complete)
    S58.11-
    |partial S58.12-
  |partial S58.92-
|genital organ(s) (external)
  |female (complete) S38.211
    |partial S38.212
  |male
    |penis (complete) S38.221
      |partial S38.222
    |scrotum (complete) S38.231
      |partial S38.232
    |testes (complete) S38.231
      |partial S38.232
|hand (complete) (wrist level) S68.41-
  |finger(s) alone *see* Amputation, traumatic,
  finger
  |partial S68.42-
  |thumb alone *see* Amputation, traumatic,
  thumb
  |transmetacarpal (complete) S68.71-
    |partial S68.72-
|head
  |ear *see* Amputation, traumatic, ear
  |nose (partial) S08.812
    |complete S08.811
  |part S08.89
    |scalp S08.0
|hip (and thigh) (complete) S78.91-
  |at hip joint (complete) S78.01-
    |partial S78.02-
  |between hip and knee (complete) S78.11-
    |partial S78.12-
  |partial S78.92-
|labium (majus) (minus) (complete) S38.21-
  |partial S38.21-
|leg (lower) S88.91-

Amputation - *continued*
  |at knee level S88.01-
    |partial S88.02-
  |between knee and ankle S88.11-
    |partial S88.12-
  |partial S88.92-
|nose (partial) S08.812
  |complete S08.811
|penis (complete) S38.221
  |partial S38.222
|scrotum (complete) S38.231
  |partial S38.232
|shoulder *see* Amputation, traumatic, arm
  |at shoulder joint *see* Amputation,
    traumatic, arm, at shoulder joint
|testes (complete) S38.231
  |partial S38.232
|thigh *see* Amputation, traumatic, hip
|thorax, part of S28.1
  |breast *see* Amputation, traumatic, breast
|thumb (complete) (metacarpophalangeal)
  S68.01-
  |partial S68.02-
  |transphalangeal (complete) S68.51-
    |partial S68.52-
|toe (lesser) S98.13-
  |great S98.11-
    |partial S98.12-
  |more than one S98.21-
    |partial S98.22-
  |partial S98.14-
|vulva (complete) S38.211
  |partial S38.212
Amputee (bilateral) (old) Z89.9
Amsterdam dwarfism Q87.1
Amusia R48.8
|developmental F80.89
Amyelencephalus, amyelencephaly Q00.0
Amyelia Q06.0
Amygdalitis *see* Tonsillitis
Amygdalolith J35.8
Amyloid heart (disease) E85.4 [*I43*]
Amyloidosis (generalized) (primary) E85.9
|with lung involvement E85.4 [*J99*]
|familial E85.2
|genetic E85.2
|heart E85.4 [*I43*]
|hemodialysis-associated E85.3
|light chain (AL) E85.81
|liver E85.4 [*K77*]
|localized E85.4
|neuropathic heredofamilial E85.1
|non-neuropathic heredofamilial E85.0
|organ limited E85.4
|Portuguese E85.1
|pulmonary E85.4 [*J99*]
|secondary systemic E85.3
|senile systemic (SSA) E85.82
|skin (lichen) (macular) E85.4 [*L99*]
|specified NEC E85.89
|subglottic E85.4 [*J99*]
|wild-type transthyretin-related (ATTR)
  E85.82
Amylopectinosis (brancher enzyme
  deficiency) E74.03
Amylophagia *see* Pica
Amyoplasia congenita Q79.8
Amyotonia M62.89
|congenita G70.2
Amyotrophia, amyotrophy, amyotrophic
  G71.8
|congenita Q79.8
|diabetic *see* Diabetes, amyotrophy
|lateral sclerosis G12.21
|neuralgic G54.5
|spinal progressive G12.25

Anacidity, gastric K31.83
|psychogenic F45.8
Anaerosis of newborn P28.89
Analbuminemia E88.09
Analgesia *see* Anesthesia
Analphalipoproteinemia E78.6
Anaphylactic
|purpura D69.0
|shock or reaction *see* Shock, anaphylactic
Anaphylactoid shock or reaction *see* Shock, anaphylactic
Anaphylactoid syndrome of pregnancy O88.01-
Anaphylaxis *see* Shock, anaphylactic
Anaplasia cervix *see also* Dysplasia, cervix N87.9
Anaplasmosis [A. phagocytophilum] (transfusion transmitted) A79.82
- human A77.49
Anarthria R47.1
Anasarca R60.1
|cardiac *see* Failure, heart, congestive
|lung J18.2
|newborn P83.2
|nutritional E43
|pulmonary J18.2
|renal N04.9
Anastomosis
|aneurysmal *see* Aneurysm
|arteriovenous ruptured brain I60.8
|intestinal K63.89
|complicated NEC K91.89
|involving urinary tract N99.89
|retinal and choroidal vessels (congenital) Q14.8
Anatomical narrow angle H40.03-
Ancylostoma, ancylostomiasis (braziliense) (caninum) (ceylanicum) (duodenale) B76.0
|Necator americanus B76.1
Andersen's disease (glycogen storage) E74.09
Anderson-Fabry disease E75.21
Andes disease T70.29
Andrews' disease (bacterid) L08.89
Androblastoma
|benign
|specified site *see* Neoplasm, benign, by site
|unspecified site
|female D27.9
|male D29.20
|malignant
|specified site *see* Neoplasm, malignant, by site
|unspecified site
|female C56.9
|male C62.90
|specified site *see* Neoplasm, uncertain behavior, by site
|tubular
|with lipid storage
|specified site *see* Neoplasm, benign, by site
|unspecified site
|female D27.9
|male D29.20
|specified site *see* Neoplasm, benign, by site
|unspecified site
|female D27.9
|male D29.20
|unspecified site
|female D39.10
|male D40.10
Androgen insensitivity syndrome *see also* Syndrome, androgen insensitivity E34.50

Androgen resistance syndrome *see also* Syndrome, androgen insensitivity E34.50
Android pelvis Q74.2
|with disproportion (fetopelvic) O33.3
|causing obstructed labor O65.3
Androphobia F40.290
Anectasis, pulmonary (newborn) *see* Atelectasis
Anemia (essential) (general) (hemoglobin deficiency) (infantile) (primary) (profound) D64.9
|with (due to) (in)
|disorder of
|anaerobic glycolysis D55.29
|pentose phosphate pathway D55.1
|koilonychia D50.9
|achlorhydric D50.8
|achrestic D53.1
|Addison (-Biermer) (pernicious) D51.0
|agranulocytic *see* Agranulocytosis
|amino-acid-Deficiency D53.0
|aplastic D61.9
|congenital D61.09
|drug-induced D61.1
|due to
|drugs D61.1
|external agents NEC D61.2
|infection D61.2
|radiation D61.2
|idiopathic D61.3
|red cell (pure) D60.9
|chronic D60.0
|congenital D61.01
|specified type NEC D60.8
|transient D60.1
|specified type NEC D61.89
|toxic D61.2
|aregenerative
|congenital D61.09
|asiderotic D50.9
|atypical (primary) D64.9
|Baghdad spring D55.0
|Balantidium coli A07.0
|Biermer's (pernicious) D51.0
|blood loss (chronic) D50.0
|acute D62
|bothriocephalus B70.0 [*D63.8*]
|brickmaker's B76.9 [*D63.8*]
|cerebral I67.89
|childhood D58.9
|chlorotic D50.8
|chronic
|blood loss D50.0
|hemolytic D58.9
|idiopathic D59.9
|simple D53.9
|chronica congenita aregenerativa D61.09
|combined system disease NEC D51.0 [*G32.0*]
|due to dietary vitamin B12 deficiency D51.3 [*G32.0*]
|complicating pregnancy, childbirth or puerperium *see* Pregnancy, complicated by (management affected by), anemia
|congenital P61.4
|aplastic D61.09
|due to isoimmunization NOS P55.9
|dyserythropoietic, dyshematopoietic D64.4
|following fetal blood loss P61.3
|Heinz body D58.2
|hereditary hemolytic NOS D58.9
|pernicious D51.0
|spherocytic D58.0
|Cooley's (erythroblastic) D56.1
|cytogenic D51.0
|deficiency D53.9
|2, 3 diphosphoglycerate mutase D55.29

Anemia - *continued*
|2, 3 PG D55.29
|6 phosphogluconate dehydrogenase D55.1
|6-PGD D55.1
|amino-acid D53.0
|combined B12 and folate D53.1
|enzyme D55.9
|drug-induced (hemolytic) D59.2
|glucose 6-phosphate dehydrogenase (G6PD) D55.0
|glycolytic D55.29
|nucleotide metabolism D55.3
|related to hexose monophosphate (HMP) shunt pathway NEC D55.1
|specified type NEC D55.8
|erythrocytic glutathione D55.1
|folate D52.9
|dietary D52.0
|drug-induced D52.1
|folic acid D52.9
|dietary D52.0
|drug-induced D52.1
|G SH D55.1
|GGS-R D55.1
|glucose 6-phosphate dehydrogenase D55.0
|glutathione reductase D55.1
|glyceraldehyde phosphate dehydrogenase D55.29
|G6PD D55.0
|hexokinase D55.29
|iron D50.9
|secondary to blood loss (chronic) D50.0
|nutritional D53.9
|with
|poor iron absorption D50.8
|specified deficiency NEC D53.8
|phosphofructo-aldolase D55.29
|phosphoglycerate kinase D55.29
|PK D55.21
|protein D53.0
|pyruvate kinase D55.29
|transcobalamin II D51.2
|triose-phosphate isomerase D55.29
|vitamin B12 NOS D51.9
|dietary D51.3
|due to
|intrinsic factor deficiency D51.0
|selective vitamin B12 malabsorption with proteinuria D51.1
|pernicious D51.0
|specified type NEC D51.8
|Diamond-Blackfan (congenital hypoplastic) D61.01
|Dibothriocephalus B70.0 [*D63.8*]
|dimorphic D53.1
|diphasic D53.1
|Diphyllobothrium (Dibothriocephalus) B70.0 [*D63.8*]
|due to (in) (with)
|antineoplastic chemotherapy D64.81
|blood loss (chronic) D50.0
|acute D62
|chemotherapy, antineoplastic D64.81
|chronic disease classified elsewhere NEC D63.8
|chronic kidney disease D63.1
|deficiency
|amino-acid D53.0
|copper D53.8
|folate (folic acid) D52.9
|dietary D52.0
|drug-induced D52.1
|molybdenum D53.8
|protein D53.0
|zinc D53.8
|dietary vitamin B12 deficiency D51.3

Anemia - *continued*
  |disorder of
    |glutathione metabolism D55.1
    |nucleotide metabolism D55.3
  |drug *see* Anemia, by type *see also* Table of
    Drugs and Chemicals
  |end stage renal disease D63.1
  |enzyme disorder D55.9
  |fetal blood loss P61.3
  |fish tapeworm (D. Latum) infestation B70.0
    [*D63.8*]
  |hemorrhage (chronic) D50.0
    |acute D62
  |impaired absorption D50.9
  |loss of blood (chronic) D50.0
    |acute D62
  |myxedema E03.9 [*D63.8*]
  |Necator americanus B76.1 [*D63.8*]
  |prematurity P61.2
  |selective vitamin B12 malabsorption with
    proteinuria D51.1
  |transcobalamin II deficiency D51.2
  |Dyke-Young type (secondary) (symptomatic)
    D59.19
  |dyserythropoietic (congenital) D64.4
  |dyshematopoietic (congenital) D64.4
  |Egyptian B76.9 [*D63.8*]
  |elliptocytosis *see* Elliptocytosis
  |enzyme-Deficiency, drug-induced D59.2
  |epidemic *see also* Ancylostomiasis B76.9
    [*D63.8*]
  |erythroblastic
    |familial D56.1
    |newborn *see also* Disease, hemolytic P55.9
    |of childhood D56.1
  |erythrocytic glutathione deficiency D55.1
  |erythropoietin-resistant anemia (EPO resistant
    anemia) D63.1
  |Faber's (achlorhydric anemia) D50.9
  |factitious (self-induced blood letting) D50.0
  |familial erythroblastic D56.1
  |Fanconi's (congenital pancytopenia) D61.09
  |favism D55.0
  |fish tapeworm (D. latum) infestation B70.0
    [*D63.8*]
  |folate (folic acid) deficiency D52.9
  |glucose 6-phosphate dehydrogenase (G6PD)
    deficiency D55.0
  |glutathione-reductase deficiency D55.1
  |goat's milk D52.0
  |granulocytic *see* Agranulocytosis
  |Heinz body, congenital D58.2
  |hemolytic D58.9
    |acquired D59.9
      |with hemoglobinuria NEC D59.6
      |autoimmune NEC D59.19
      |infectious D59.4
      |specified type NEC D59.8
      |toxic D59.4
    |acute D59.9
      |due to enzyme deficiency specified type
        NEC D55.8
      |Lederer's D59.19
    |autoimmune D59.10
    -|cold D59.12
      |drug-induced D59.0
      |mixed D59.13
      |warm D59.11
    |chronic D58.9
      |idiopathic D59.9
    |cold type (secondary) (symptomatic) D59.12
    |congenital (spherocytic) *see* Spherocytosis
    |due to
      |cardiac conditions D59.4
      |drugs (nonautoimmune) D59.2
        |autoimmune D59.0

Anemia - *continued*
    |enzyme disorder D55.9
      |drug-induced D59.2
    |presence of shunt or other internal
      prosthetic device D59.4
    |familial D58.9
    |hereditary D58.9
      |due to enzyme disorder D55.9
        |specified type NEC D55.8
      |specified type NEC D58.8
    |idiopathic (chronic) D59.9
    |mechanical D59.4
    |microangiopathic D59.4
    |mixed type (primary) (secondary)
      (symptomatic) D59.13
    |primary
      |autoimmune
        |cold type D59.12
        |mixed type D59.13
        |warm type D59.11
    |nonautoimmune D59.4
      |drug-induced D59.2
    |nonspherocytic
      |congenital or hereditary NEC D55.8
        |glucose 6-phosphate dehydrogenase
          deficiency D55.0
        |pyruvate kinase deficiency D55.21
        |type
          |I D55.1
          |II D55.29
      |type
        |I D55.1
        |II D55.29
    |secondary D59.4
      |autoimmune
        |cold type D59.12
        |mixed type D59.13
        |warm type D59.11
    |specified (hereditary) type NEC D58.8
    |Stransky-Regala type *see also*
      Hemoglobinopathy D58.8
    |symptomatic D59.4
      |autoimmune
        |cold type D59.12
        |mixed type D59.13
        |warm type D59.11
    |toxic D59.4
    |warm type (primary)(secondary)
      (symptomatic) D59.11
  |hemorrhagic (chronic) D50.0
    |acute D62
  |Herrick's D57.1
  |hexokinase deficiency D55.29
  |hookworm B76.9 [*D63.8*]
  |hypochromic (idiopathic) (microcytic)
    (normoblastic) D50.9
    |due to blood loss (chronic) D50.0
      |acute D62
    |familial sex-linked D64.0
    |pyridoxine-responsive D64.3
    |sideroblastic, sex-linked D64.0
  |hypoplasia, red blood cells D61.9
    |congenital or familial D61.01
  |hypoplastic (idiopathic) D61.9
    |congenital or familial (of childhood) D61.01
  |hypoproliferative (refractive) D61.9
  |idiopathic D64.9
    |aplastic D61.3
    |hemolytic, chronic D59.9
  |in (due to) (with)
    |chronic kidney disease D63.1
    |end stage renal disease D63.1
    |failure, kidney (renal) D63.1
    |neoplastic disease *see also* Neoplasm D63.0
  |intertropical *see also* Ancylostomiasis D63.8

Anemia - *continued*
  |iron deficiency D50.9
    |secondary to blood loss (chronic) D50.0
      |acute D62
    |specified type NEC D50.8
  |Joseph-Diamond-Blackfan (congenital
    hypoplastic) D61.01
  |Lederer's (hemolytic) D59.19
  |leukoerythroblastic D61.82
  |macrocytic D53.9
    |nutritional D52.0
    |tropical D52.8
  |malarial *see also* Malaria B54 [*D63.8*]
  |malignant (progressive) D51.0
  |malnutrition D53.9
  |marsh *see also* Malaria B54 [*D63.8*]
  |Mediterranean (with other hemoglobinopathy)
    D56.9
  |megaloblastic D53.1
    |combined B12 and folate deficiency D53.1
    |hereditary D51.1
    |nutritional D52.0
    |orotic aciduria D53.0
    |refractory D53.1
    |specified type NEC D53.1
  |megalocytic D53.1
  |microcytic (hypochromic) D50.9
    |due to blood loss (chronic) D50.0
      |acute D62
    |familial D56.8
  |microdrepanocytosis D57.40
  |microelliptopoikilocytic (Rietti-Grippe-
    Micheli) D56.9
  |miner's B76.9 [*D63.8*]
  |myelodysplastic D46.9
  |myelofibrosis D75.81
  |myelogenous D64.89
  |myelopathic D64.89
  |myelophthisic D61.82
  |myeloproliferative D47.Z9
  |newborn P61.4
    |due to
      |ABO (antibodies, isoimmunization,
        maternal/fetal incompatibility) P55.1
      |Rh (antibodies, isoimmunization,
        maternal/fetal incompatibility) P55.0
    |following fetal blood loss P61.3
    |posthemorrhagic (fetal) P61.3
  |nonspherocytic hemolytic *see* Anemia,
    hemolytic, nonspherocytic
  |normocytic (infectional) D64.9
    |due to blood loss (chronic) D50.0
      |acute D62
    |myelophthisic D61.82
  |nutritional (deficiency) D53.9
    |with
      |poor iron absorption D50.8
      |specified deficiency NEC D53.8
    |megaloblastic D52.0
  |of prematurity P61.2
  |orotaciduric (congenital) (hereditary) D53.0
  |osteosclerotic D64.89
  |ovalocytosis (hereditary) *see* Elliptocytosis
  |paludal *see also* Malaria B54 [*D63.8*]
  |pernicious (congenital) (malignant)
    (progressive) D51.0
  |pleochromic D64.89
    |of sprue D52.8
  |posthemorrhagic (chronic) D50.0
    |acute D62
    |newborn P61.3
  |postoperative (postprocedural)
    |due to (acute) blood loss D62
      |chronic blood loss D50.0
    |specified NEC D64.89
  |postpartum O90.81

Anemia - *continued*
|pressure D64.89
|progressive D64.9
||malignant D51.0
||pernicious D51.0
|protein-deficiency D53.0
|pseudoleukemica infantum D64.89
|pure red cell D60.9
||congenital D61.01
|pyridoxine-responsive D64.3
|pyruvate kinase deficiency D55.21
|refractory D46.4
||with
|||excess of blasts D46.20
||||1 (RAEB 1) D46.21
||||2 (RAEB 2) D46.22
||||in transformation (RAEB T) *see*
|||||Leukemia, acute myeloblastic
|||hemochromatosis D46.1
|||sideroblasts (ring) (RARS) D46.1
||megaloblastic D53.1
||sideroblastic D46.1
||sideropenic D50.9
||without ring sideroblasts, so stated D46.0
||without sideroblasts without excess of blasts
|||D46.0
|Rietti-Greppe-Micheli D56.9
|scorbutic D53.2
|secondary to
||blood loss (chronic) D50.0
|||acute D62
||hemorrhage (chronic) D50.0
|||acute D62
|semiplastic D61.89
|sickle-cell *see* Disease, sickle-cell
|sideroblastic D64.3
||hereditary D64.0
||hypochromic, sex-linked D64.0
||pyridoxine-responsive NEC D64.3
||refractory D46.1
||secondary (due to)
|||disease D64.1
|||drugs and toxins D64.2
||specified type NEC D64.3
|sideropenic (refractory) D50.9
||due to blood loss (chronic) D50.0
|||acute D62
|simple chronic D53.9
|specified type NEC D64.89
|spherocytic (hereditary) *see* Spherocytosis
|splenic D64.89
|splenomegalic D64.89
|stomatocytosis D58.8
|syphilitic (acquired) (late) A52.79 [*D63.8*]
|target cell D64.89
|thalassemia D56.9
|thrombocytopenic *see* Thrombocytopenia
|toxic D61.2
|tropical B76.9 [*D63.8*]
||macrocytic D52.8
|tuberculous A18.89 [*D63.8*]
|vegan D51.3
|vitamin
||B6-responsive D64.3
||B12 deficiency (dietary) pernicious D51.0
|von Jaksch's D64.89
|Witts' (achlorhydric anemia) D50.8
Anemophobia F40.228
Anencephalus, anencephaly Q00.0
Anergasia *see* Psychosis, organic
Anesthesia, anesthetic R20.0
|complication or reaction NEC *see also*
||Complications, anesthesia T88.59
|due to

Anesthesia, anesthetic - *continued*
||correct substance properly administered
|||*see* Table of Drugs and Chemicals, by
|||drug, adverse effect
||overdose or wrong substance given *see*
|||Table of Drugs and Chemicals, by drug,
|||poisoning
|unintended awareness under general
||anesthesia during procedure T88.53
|||personal history of Z92.84
|cornea H18.81-
|dissociative F44.6
|functional (hysterical) F44.6
|hyperesthetic, thalamic G89.0
|hysterical F44.6
|local skin lesion R20.0
|sexual (psychogenic) F52.1
|shock (due to) T88.2
|skin R20.0
|testicular N50.9
Anetoderma (maculosum) (of) L90.8
|Jadassohn-Pellizzari L90.2
|Schweniger-Buzzi L90.1
Aneurin deficiency E51.9
Aneurysm (anastomotic) (artery) (cirsoid)
|(diffuse) (false) (fusiform) (multiple)
|(saccular) I72.9
|abdominal (aorta) I71.4
||ruptured I71.3
||syphilitic A52.01
|aorta, aortic (nonsyphilitic) I71.9
||abdominal I71.4
|||ruptured I71.3
||arch I71.2
|||ruptured I71.1
||arteriosclerotic I71.9
|||ruptured I71.8
||ascending I71.2
|||ruptured I71.1
||congenital Q25.43
||descending I71.9
|||abdominal I71.4
||||ruptured I71.3
|||ruptured I71.8
|||thoracic I71.2
||||ruptured I71.1
||root Q25.43
||ruptured I71.8
||sinus, congenital Q25.43
||syphilitic A52.01
||thoracic I71.2
|||ruptured I71.1
||thoracoabdominal I71.6
|||ruptured I71.5
||thorax, thoracic (arch) I71.2
|||ruptured I71.1
||transverse I71.2
|||ruptured I71.1
||valve (heart) *see also* Endocarditis, aortic
|||I35.8
|arteriosclerotic I72.9
||cerebral I67.1
|||ruptured *see* Hemorrhage, intracranial,
||||subarachnoid
|arteriovenous (congenital) *see also*
||Malformation, arteriovenous
|acquired I77.0
||brain I67.1
||coronary I25.41
||pulmonary I28.0
|brain Q28.2
||ruptured I60.8
|peripheral *see* Malformation, arteriovenous,
||peripheral
|precerebral vessels Q28.0

Aneurysm - *continued*
|specified site NEC *see also* Malformation,
||arteriovenous
|acquired I77.0
|basal *see* Aneurysm, brain
|basilar (trunk) I72.5
|berry (congenital) (nonruptured) I67.1
||ruptured I60.7
|brain I67.1
||arteriosclerotic I67.1
|||ruptured *see* Hemorrhage, intracranial,
||||subarachnoid
||arteriovenous (congenital) (nonruptured)
|||Q28.2
||acquired I67.1
|||ruptured I60.8-
|||ruptured I60.8-
||berry (congenital) (nonruptured) I67.1
|||ruptured *see also* Hemorrhage,
||||intracranial, subarachnoid I60.7
||congenital Q28.3
|||ruptured I60.7
||meninges I67.1
|||ruptured I60.8
||miliary (congenital) (nonruptured) I67.1
|||ruptured *see also* Hemorrhage,
||||intracranial, subarachnoid I60.7
||mycotic I33.0
||ruptured *see* Hemorrhage, intracranial,
|||subarachnoid
||syphilitic (hemorrhage) A52.05
|cardiac (false) *see also* Aneurysm, heart I25.3
|carotid artery (common) (external) I72.0
||internal (intracranial) I67.1
|||extracranial portion I72.0
||ruptured into brain I60.0-
||syphilitic A52.09
|||intracranial A52.05
|cavernous sinus I67.1
||arteriovenous (congenital) (nonruptured)
|||Q28.3
||ruptured I60.8
|celiac I72.8
|central nervous system, syphilitic A52.05
|cerebral *see* Aneurysm, brain
|chest *see* Aneurysm, thorax |circle of Willis
|I67.1
||congenital Q28.3
|||ruptured I60.6
||ruptured I60.6
|common iliac artery I72.3
|congenital (peripheral) Q27.8
||aorta (root) (sinus) Q25.43
||brain Q28.3
|||ruptured I60.7
||coronary Q24.5
||digestive system Q27.8
||lower limb Q27.8
||pulmonary Q25.79
||retina Q14.1
||specified site NEC Q27.8
||upper limb Q27.8
|conjunctiva *see* Abnormality, conjunctiva,
||vascular
|conus arteriosus *see* Aneurysm, heart
|coronary (arteriosclerotic) (artery) I25.41
||arteriovenous, congenital Q24.5
||congenital Q24.5
||ruptured *see* Infarct, myocardium
||syphilitic A52.06
||vein I25.89
|cylindroid (aorta) I71.9
||ruptured I71.8
||syphilitic A52.01
|ductus arteriosus Q25.0
|endocardial, infective (any valve) I33.0

Aneurysm - *continued*
| femoral (artery) (ruptured) I72.4
| gastroduodenal I72.8
| gastroepiploic I72.8
| heart (wall) (chronic or with a stated duration
    of over 4 weeks) I25.3
    | valve *see* Endocarditis
| hepatic I72.8
| iliac (common) (artery) (ruptured) I72.3
| infective I72.9
    | endocardial (any valve) I33.0
| innominate (nonsyphilitic) I72.8
    | syphilitic A52.09
| interauricular septum *see* Aneurysm, heart
| interventricular septum *see* Aneurysm, heart
| intrathoracic (nonsyphilitic) I71.2
    | ruptured I71.1
    | syphilitic A52.01
| lower limb I72.4
| lung (pulmonary artery) I28.1
| mediastinal (nonsyphilitic) I72.8
    | syphilitic A52.09
| miliary (congenital) I67.1
    | ruptured *see* Hemorrhage, intracerebral,
       subarachnoid, intracranial
| mitral (heart) (valve) I34.8
| mural *see* Aneurysm, heart
| mycotic I72.9
    | endocardial (any valve) I33.0
    | ruptured, brain *see* Hemorrhage,
       intracerebral, subarachnoid
| myocardium *see* Aneurysm, heart
| neck I72.0
| pancreaticoduodenal I72.8
| patent ductus arteriosus Q25.0
| peripheral NEC I72.8
    | congenital Q27.8
       | digestive system Q27.8
       | lower limb Q27.8
       | specified site NEC Q27.8
       | upper limb Q27.8
| popliteal (artery) (ruptured) I72.4
| precerebral
    | congenital (nonruptured) Q28.1
    | specified site, NEC I72.5
| pulmonary I28.1
    | arteriovenous Q25.72
       | acquired I28.0
    | syphilitic A52.09
    | valve (heart) *see* Endocarditis, pulmonary
| racemose (peripheral) I72.9
    | congenital *see* Aneurysm, congenital
| radial I72.1
| Rasmussen NEC A15.0
| renal (artery) I72.2
| retina *see also* Disorder, retina,
    microaneurysms
    | congenital Q14.1
    | diabetic *see* Diabetes, microaneurysms,
    retinal
| sinus of Valsalva Q25.49
| specified NEC I72.8
| spinal (cord) I72.8
    | syphilitic (hemorrhage) A52.09
| splenic I72.8
| subclavian (artery) (ruptured) I72.8
    | syphilitic A52.09
| superior mesenteric I72.8
| syphilitic (aorta) A52.01
    | central nervous system A52.05
    | congenital (late) A50.54 *[I79.0]*
    spine, spinal A52.09
| thoracoabdominal (aorta) I71.6
    | ruptured I71.5
    | syphilitic A52.01

Aneurysm - *continued*
| thorax, thoracic (aorta) (arch) (nonsyphilitic)
    I71.2
    | ruptured I71.1
    | syphilitic A52.01
| traumatic (complication) (early), specified site
    see Injury, blood vessel
| tricuspid (heart) (valve) I07.8
| ulnar I72.1
| upper limb (ruptured) I72.1
| valve, valvular *see* Endocarditis
| venous *see also* Varix I86.8
    | congenital Q27.8
       | digestive system Q27.8
       | lower limb Q27.8
       | specified site NEC Q27.8
       | upper limb Q27.8
| ventricle *see* Aneurysm, heart
| vertebral artery I72.6
| visceral NEC I72.8
Angelman syndrome Q93.51
Anger R45.4
Angiectasis, angiectopia I99.8
Angiitis I77.6
| allergic granulomatous M30.1
| hypersensitivity M31.0
| necrotizing M31.9
    | specified NEC M31.8
| nervous system, granulomatous I67.7
Angina (attack) (cardiac) (chest) (heart)
    (pectoris) (syndrome) (vasomotor) I20.9
| with
    | atherosclerotic heart disease *see*
       Arteriosclerosis, coronary (artery),
    | documented spasm I20.1
| abdominal K55.1
| accelerated *see* Angina, unstable
| agranulocytic *see* Agranulocytosis
| angiospastic *see* Angina, with documented
    spasm
| aphthous B08.5
| crescendo *see* Angina, unstable
| croupous J05.0
| cruris I73.9
| de novo effort *see* Angina, unstable
| diphtheritic, membranous A36.0
| equivalent I20.8
| exudative, chronic J37.0
| following acute myocardial infarction I23.7
| gangrenous diphtheritic A36.0
| intestinal K55.1
| Ludovici K12.2
| Ludwig's K12.2
| malignant diphtheritic A36.0
| membranous J05.0
    | diphtheritic A36.0
    | Vincent's A69.1
| mesenteric K55.1
| monocytic *see* Mononucleosis, infectious
| of effort *see* Angina, specified NEC
| phlegmonous J36
    | diphtheritic A36.0
| post-infarctional I23.7
| pre-infarctional *see* Angina, unstable
| Prinzmetal *see* Angina, with documented
    spasm
| progressive *see* Angina, unstable
| pseudomembranous A69.1
| pultaceous, diphtheritic A36.0
| spasm-induced *see* Angina, with documented
    spasm
| specified NEC I20.8
| stable I20.8
| stenocardia *see* Angina, specified NEC
| stridulous, diphtheritic A36.2

Angina - *continued*
| tonsil J36
| trachealis J05.0
| unstable I20.0
| variant *see* Angina, with documented spasm
| Vincent's A69.1
| worsening effort *see* Angina, unstable
Angioblastoma *see* Neoplasm, connective
    tissue, uncertain behavior
Angiocholecystitis *see* Cholecystitis, acute
Angiocholitis *see also* Cholecystitis, acute
    K83.09
Angiodysgenesis spinalis G95.19
Angiodysplasia (cecum) (colon) K55.20
| with bleeding K55.21
| duodenum (and stomach) K31.819
    | with bleeding K31.811
| stomach (and duodenum) K31.819
    | with bleeding K31.811
Angioedema (allergic) (any site) (with
    urticaria) T78.3
| episodic, with eosinophilia D72.118
| hereditary D84.1
Angioendothelioma *see* Neoplasm, uncertain
    behavior, by site
| benign D18.00
    | intra-abdominal D18.03
    | intracranial D18.02
    | skin D18.01
    | specified site NEC D18.09
| bone *see* Neoplasm, bone, malignant
| Ewing's *see* Neoplasm, bone, malignant
Angioendotheliomatosis C85.8-
Angiofibroma *see also* Neoplasm, benign, by
    site
| juvenile
    | specified site *see* Neoplasm, benign, by site
    | unspecified site D10.6
Angiohemophilia (A) (B) D68.0
Angioid streaks (choroid) (macula) (retina)
    H35.33
Angiokeratoma *see* Neoplasm, skin, benign
| corporis diffusum E75.21
Angioleiomyoma *see* Neoplasm, connective
    tissue, benign
Angiolipoma *see also* Lipoma
| infiltrating *see* Lipoma
Angioma *see also* Hemangioma, by site
| capillary I78.1
| hemorrhagicum hereditaria I78.0
| intra-abdominal D18.03
| intracranial D18.02
| malignant *see* Neoplasm, connective tissue,
    malignant
| plexiform D18.00
    | intra-abdominal D18.03
    | intracranial D18.02
    | skin D18.01
    | specified site NEC D18.09
| senile I78.1
| serpiginosum L81.7
| skin D18.01
| specified site NEC D18.09
| spider I78.1
| stellate I78.1
| venous Q28.3
Angiomatosis Q82.8
| bacillary A79.89
| encephalotrigeminal Q85.8
| hemorrhagic familial I78.0
| hereditary familial I78.0
| liver K76.4
Angiomyolipoma *see* Lipoma
Angiomyoliposarcoma *see* Neoplasm,
    connective tissue, malignant

Angiomyoma *see* Neoplasm, connective tissue, benign
Angiomyosarcoma *see* Neoplasm, connective tissue, malignant
Angiomyxoma *see* Neoplasm, connective tissue, uncertain behavior
Angioneurosis F45.8
Angioneurotic edema (allergic) (any site) (with urticaria) T78.3
|hereditary D84.1
Angiopathia, angiopathy I99.9
|cerebral I67.9
|amyloid E85.4 [I68.0]
|diabetic (peripheral) *see* Diabetes, angiopathy
|peripheral I73.9
|diabetic *see* Diabetes, angiopathy
|specified type NEC I73.89
|retinae syphilitica A52.05
|retinalis (juvenilis)
|diabetic *see* Diabetes, retinopathy
|proliferative *see* Retinopathy, proliferative
Angiosarcoma *see also* Neoplasm, connective tissue, malignant
|liver C22.3
Angiosclerosis *see* Arteriosclerosis
Angiospasm (peripheral) (traumatic) (vessel) I73.9
|brachial plexus G54.0
|cerebral G45.9
|cervical plexus G54.2
|nerve
|arm *see* Mononeuropathy, upper limb
|axillary G54.0
|median *see* Lesion, nerve, median
|ulnar *see* Lesion, nerve, ulnar
|axillary G54.0
|leg *see* Mononeuropathy, lower limb
|median *see* Lesion, nerve, median
|plantar *see* Lesion, nerve, plantar
|ulnar *see* Lesion, nerve, ulnar
Angiospastic disease or edema I73.9
Angiostrongyliasis
|due to
|Parastrongylus
|cantonensis B83.2
|costaricensis B81.3
|intestinal B81.3
Anguillulosis *see* Strongyloidiasis
Angulation
|cecum *see* Obstruction, intestine
|coccyx (acquired) *see also* subcategory M43.8
|congenital NEC Q76.49
|femur (acquired) *see also* Deformity, limb, specified type NEC, thigh
|congenital Q74.2
|intestine (large) (small) *see* Obstruction, intestine
|sacrum (acquired) *see also* subcategory M43.8
|congenital NEC Q76.49
|sigmoid (flexure) *see* Obstruction, intestine
|spine *see* Dorsopathy, deforming, specified NEC
|tibia (acquired) *see also* Deformity, limb, specified type NEC, lower leg
|congenital Q74.2
|ureter N13.5
|with infection N13.6
|wrist (acquired) *see also* Deformity, limb, specified type NEC, forearm
|congenital Q74.0
Angulus infectiosus (lips) K13.0
Anhedonia R45.84
|sexual F52.0
Anhidrosis L74.4
Anhydration E86.0

Anhydremia E86.0
Anidrosis L74.4
Aniridia (congenital) Q13.1
Anisakiasis (infection) (infestation) B81.0
Anisakis larvae infestation B81.0
Aniseikonia H52.32
Anisocoria (pupil) H57.02
|congenital Q13.2
Anisocytosis R71.8
Anisometropia (congenital) H52.31
Ankle *see* condition
Ankyloblepharon (eyelid) (acquired) *see also* Blepharophimosis
|filiforme (adnatum) (congenital) Q10.3
|total Q10.3
Ankyloglossia Q38.1
Ankylosis (fibrous) (osseous) (joint) M24.60
|ankle M24.67-
|arthrodesis status Z98.1
|cricoarytenoid (cartilage) (joint) (larynx) J38.7
|dental K03.5
|ear ossicles H74.31-
|elbow M24.62-
|foot M24.67-
|hand M24.64-
|hip M24.65-
|incostapedial joint (infectional) *see* Ankylosis, ear ossicles
|jaw (temporomandibular) M26.61-
|knee M24.66-
|lumbosacral (joint) M43.27
|postoperative (status) Z98.1
|produced by surgical fusion, status Z98.1
|sacro-iliac (joint) M43.28
|shoulder M24.61-
|specified site NEC M24.69
|spine (joint) *see also* Fusion, spine
|spondylitic *see* Spondylitis, ankylosing
|surgical Z98.1
|temporomandibular M26.61-
|tooth, teeth (hard tissues) K03.5
|wrist M24.63-
Ankylostoma *see* Ancylostoma
Ankylostomiasis *see* Ancylostomiasis
Ankylurethria *see* Stricture, urethra
Annular *see also* condition
|detachment, cervix N88.8
|organ or site, congenital NEC *see* Distortion
|pancreas (congenital) Q45.1
Anodontia (complete) (partial) (vera) K00.0
|acquired K08.10
Anomaly, anomalous (congenital) (unspecified type) Q89.9
|abdominal wall NEC Q79.59
|acoustic nerve Q07.8
|adrenal (gland) Q89.1
|Alder (-Reilly) (leukocyte granulation) D72.0
|alimentary tract Q45.9
|upper Q40.9
|alveolar M26.70
|hyperplasia M26.79
|mandibular M26.72
|maxillary M26.71
|hypoplasia M26.79
|mandibular M26.74
|maxillary M26.73
|ridge (process) M26.79
|specified NEC M26.79
|ankle (joint) Q74.2
|anus Q43.9
|aorta (arch) NEC Q25.40
|coarctation (preductal) (postductal) Q25.1
|aortic cusp or valve Q23.9
|appendix Q43.8
|apple peel syndrome Q41.1
|aqueduct of Sylvius Q03.0

Anomaly, anomalous - *continued*
|with spina bifida *see* Spina bifida, with hydrocephalus
|arm Q74.0
|arteriovenous NEC
|coronary Q24.5
|gastrointestinal Q27.33
|acquired *see* Angiodysplasia
|artery (peripheral) Q27.9
|basilar NEC Q28.1
|cerebral Q28.3
|coronary Q24.5
|digestive system Q27.8
|eye Q15.8
|great Q25.9
|specified NEC Q25.8
|lower limb Q27.8
|peripheral Q27.9
|specified NEC Q27.8
|pulmonary NEC Q25.79
|renal Q27.2
|retina Q14.1
|specified site NEC Q27.8
|subclavian Q27.8
|origin Q25.48
|umbilical Q27.0
|upper limb Q27.8
|vertebral NEC Q28.1
|aryteno-epiglottic folds Q31.8
|atrial
|bands or folds Q20.8
|septa Q21.1
|atrioventricular
|excitation I45.6
|septum Q21.0
|auditory canal Q17.8
|auricle
|ear Q17.8
|causing impairment of hearing Q16.9
|heart Q20.8
|Axenfeld's Q15.0
|back Q89.9
|band
|atrial Q20.8
|heart Q24.8
|ventricular Q24.8
|Bartholin's duct Q38.4
|biliary duct or passage Q44.5
|bladder Q64.70
|absence Q64.5
|diverticulum Q64.6
|exstrophy Q64.10
|cloacal Q64.12
|extroversion Q64.19
|specified type NEC Q64.19
|supravesical fissure Q64.11
|neck obstruction Q64.31
|specified type NEC Q64.79
|bone Q79.9
|arm Q74.0
|face Q75.9
|leg Q74.2
|pelvic girdle Q74.2
|shoulder girdle Q74.0
|skull Q75.9
|with
|anencephaly Q00.0
|encephalocele *see* Encephalocele
|hydrocephalus Q03.9
|with spina bifida *see* Spina bifida, by site, with hydrocephalus
|microcephaly Q02
|brain (multiple) Q04.9
|vessel Q28.3
|breast Q83.9
|broad ligament Q50.6

Anomaly, anomalous - *continued*

|bronchus Q32.4
|bulbus cordis Q21.9
|bursa Q79.9
|canal of Nuck Q52.4
|canthus Q10.3
|capillary Q27.9
|cardiac Q24.9
  |chambers Q20.9
    |specified NEC Q20.8
  |septal closure Q21.9
    |specified NEC Q21.8
  |valve NEC Q24.8
    |pulmonary Q22.3
|cardiovascular system Q28.8
|carpus Q74.0
|caruncle, lacrimal Q10.6
|cascade stomach Q40.2
|cauda equina Q06.3
|cecum Q43.9
|cerebral Q04.9
  |vessels Q28.3
|cervix Q51.9
|Chédiak-Higashi (-Steinbrinck) (congenital
  gigantism of peroxidase granules) E70.330
|cheek Q18.9
|chest wall Q67.8
  |bones Q76.9
|chin Q18.9
|chordae tendineae Q24.8
|choroid Q14.3
  |plexus Q07.8
|chromosomes, chromosomal Q99.9
  |D (1) *see* condition, chromosome 13
  |E (3) *see* condition, chromosome 18
  |G *see* condition, chromosome 21
  |sex
    |female phenotype Q97.8
    |gonadal dysgenesis (pure) Q99.1
    |Klinefelter's Q98.4
    |male phenotype Q98.9
    |Turner's Q96.9
  |specified NEC Q99.8
|cilia Q10.3
|circulatory system Q28.9
|clavicle Q74.0
|clitoris Q52.6
|coccyx Q76.49
|colon Q43.9
|common duct Q44.5
|communication
  |coronary artery Q24.5
  |left ventricle with right atrium Q21.0
|concha (ear) Q17.3
|connection
  |portal vein Q26.5
  |pulmonary venous Q26.4
    |partial Q26.3
    |total Q26.2
  |renal artery with kidney Q27.2
|cornea (shape) Q13.4
|coronary artery or vein Q24.5
|cranium *see* Anomaly, skull
|cricoid cartilage Q31.8
|cystic duct Q44.5
|dental
  |alveolar *see* Anomaly, alveolar
  |arch relationship M26.20
    |specified NEC M26.29
|dentofacial M26.9
  |alveolar *see* Anomaly, alveolar
  |dental arch relationship M26.20
    |specified NEC M26.29
  |functional M26.50
    |specified NEC M26.59
  |jaw-cranial base relationship M26.10

Anomaly, anomalous - *continued*

|asymmetry M26.12
  |maxillary M26.11
|specified type NEC M26.19
|jaw size M26.00
  |macrogenia M26.05
  |mandibular
    |hyperplasia M26.03
    |hypoplasia M26.04
  |maxillary
    |hyperplasia M26.01
    |hypoplasia M26.02
  |microgenia M26.06
  |specified type NEC M26.09
|malocclusion M26.4
  |dental arch relationship NEC M26.29
  |jaw-cranial base relationship *see*
    Anomaly, dentofacial, jaw-cranial base
    relationship
  |jaw size *see* Anomaly, dentofacial, jaw
    size
  |specified type NEC M26.89
  |temporomandibular joint M26.60-
    |adhesions M26.61-
    |ankylosis M26.61-
    |arthralgia M26.62-
    |articular disc M26.63-
    |specified type NEC M26.69
  |tooth position, fully erupted M26.30
    |specified NEC M26.39
|dermatoglyphic Q82.8
|diaphragm (apertures) NEC Q79.1
|digestive organ(s) or tract Q45.9
  |lower Q43.9
  |upper Q40.9
|distance, interarch (excessive) (inadequate)
  M26.25
|distribution, coronary artery Q24.5
|ductus
  |arteriosus Q25.0
  |botalli Q25.0
|duodenum Q43.9
|dura (brain) Q04.9
  |spinal cord Q06.9
|ear (external) Q17.9
  |causing impairment of hearing Q16.9
  |inner Q16.5
  |middle (causing impairment of hearing)
    Q16.4
  |ossicles Q16.3
|Ebstein's (heart) (tricuspid valve) Q22.5
|ectodermal Q82.9
|Eisenmenger's (ventricular septal defect)
  Q21.8
|ejaculatory duct Q55.4
|elbow Q74.0
|endocrine gland NEC Q89.2
|epididymis Q55.4
|epiglottis Q31.8
|esophagus Q39.9
|eustachian tube Q17.8
|eye Q15.9
  |anterior segment Q13.9
    |specified NEC Q13.89
  |posterior segment Q14.9
    |specified NEC Q14.8
  |ptosis (eyelid) Q10.0
  |specified NEC Q15.8
|eyebrow Q18.8
|eyelid Q10.3
  |ptosis Q10.0
|face Q18.9
  |bone(s) Q75.9
|fallopian tube Q50.6
|fascia Q79.9
|femur NEC Q74.2

Anomaly, anomalous - *continued*

|fibula NEC Q74.2
|finger Q74.0
|fixation, intestine Q43.3
|flexion (joint) NOS Q74.9
  |hip or thigh Q65.89
|foot NEC Q74.2
  |varus (congenital) Q66.3
|foramen
  |Botalli Q21.1
  |ovale Q21.1
|forearm Q74.0
|forehead Q75.8
|form, teeth K00.2
|fovea centralis Q14.1
|frontal bone *see* Anomaly, skull
|gallbladder (position) (shape) (size) Q44.1
|Gartner's duct Q52.4
|gastrointestinal tract Q45.9
|genitalia, genital organ(s) or system
  |female Q52.9
    |external Q52.70
    |internal NOS Q52.9
  |male Q55.9
    |hydrocele P83.5
    |specified NEC Q55.8
|genitourinary NEC
  |female Q52.9
  |male Q55.9
|Gerbode Q21.0
|glottis Q31.8
|granulation or granulocyte, genetic
  (constitutional) (leukocyte) D72.0
|gum Q38.6
|gyri Q07.9
|hair Q84.2
|hand Q74.0
|hard tissue formation in pulp K04.3
|head *see* Anomaly, skull
|heart Q24.9
  |auricle Q20.8
  |bands or folds Q24.8
  |fibroelastosis cordis I42.4
  |obstructive NEC Q22.6
  |patent ductus arteriosus (Botalli) Q25.0
  |septum Q21.9
    |auricular Q21.1
    |interatrial Q21.1
    |interventricular Q21.0
      |with pulmonary stenosis or atresia,
        dextroposition of aorta and
        hypertrophy of right ventricle Q21.3
    |specified NEC Q21.8
    |ventricular Q21.0
      |with pulmonary stenosis or atresia,
        dextroposition of aorta and
        hypertrophy of right ventricle Q21.3
  |tetralogy of Fallot Q21.3
  |valve NEC Q24.8
    |aortic
      |bicuspid valve Q23.1
      |insufficiency Q23.1
      |stenosis Q23.0
        |subaortic Q24.4
    |mitral
      |insufficiency Q23.3
      |stenosis Q23.2
    |pulmonary Q22.3
      |atresia Q22.0
      |insufficiency Q22.2
      |stenosis Q22.1
        |infundibular Q24.3
        |subvalvular Q24.3
    |tricuspid
      |atresia Q22.4
      |stenosis Q22.4

Anomaly, anomalous - *continued*

|ventricle Q20.8
|heel NEC Q74.2
|Hegglin's D72.0
|hemianencephaly Q00.0
|hemicephaly Q00.0
|hemicrania Q00.0
|hepatic duct Q44.5
|hip NEC Q74.2
|hourglass stomach Q40.2
|humerus Q74.0
|hydatid of Morgagni
  |female Q50.5
  |male (epididymal) Q55.4
    |testicular Q55.29
|hymen Q52.4
|hypersegmentation of neutrophils, hereditary
  D72.0
|hypophyseal Q89.2
|ileocecal (coil) (valve) Q43.9
|ileum Q43.9
|ilium NEC Q74.2
|integument Q84.9
  |specified NEC Q84.8
|interarch distance (excessive) (inadequate)
  M26.25
|intervertebral cartilage or disc Q76.49
|intestine (large) (small) Q43.9
  |with anomalous adhesions, fixation or
    malrotation Q43.3
|iris Q13.2
|ischium NEC Q74.2
|jaw *see* Anomaly, dentofacial
  |alveolar *see* Anomaly, alveolar
|jaw-cranial base relationship *see* Anomaly,
  dentofacial, jaw-cranial base relationship
|jejunum Q43.8
|joint Q74.9
  |specified NEC Q74.8
|Jordan's D72.0
|kidney(s) (calyx) (pelvis) Q63.9
  |artery Q27.2
  |specified NEC Q63.8
|Klippel-Feil (brevicollis) Q76.1
|knee Q74.1
|labium (majus) (minus) Q52.70
|labyrinth, membranous Q16.5
|lacrimal apparatus or duct Q10.6
|larynx, laryngeal (muscle) Q31.9
  |web (bed) Q31.0
|lens Q12.9
|leukocytes, genetic D72.0
  |granulation (constitutional) D72.0
|lid (fold) Q10.3
|ligament Q79.9
  |broad Q50.6
  |round Q52.8
|limb Q74.9
  |lower NEC Q74.2
    |reduction deformity *see* Defect, reduction,
      lower limb
  |upper Q74.0
|lip Q38.0
|liver Q44.7
  |duct Q44.5
|lower limb NEC Q74.2
|lumbosacral (joint) (region) Q76.49
  |kyphosis *see* Kyphosis, congenital
  |lordosis *see* Lordosis, congenital
|lung (fissure) (lobe) Q33.9
|mandible *see* Anomaly, dentofacial
|maxilla *see* Anomaly, dentofacial
|May (-Hegglin) D72.0
|meatus urinarius NEC Q64.79
|meningeal bands or folds Q07.9

Anomaly, anomalous - *continued*

|constriction of Q07.8
  |spinal Q06.9
|meninges Q07.9
  |cerebral Q04.8
  |spinal Q06.9
|meningocele Q05.9
|mesentery Q45.9
|metacarpus Q74.0
|metatarsus NEC Q74.2
|middle ear Q16.4
  |ossicles Q16.3
|mitral (leaflets) (valve) Q23.9
  |insufficiency Q23.3
  |specified NEC Q23.8
  |stenosis Q23.2
|mouth Q38.6
|Müllerian *see also* Anomaly, by site
  |uterus NEC Q51.818
|multiple NEC Q89.7
|muscle Q79.9
  |eyelid Q10.3
|musculoskeletal system, except limbs Q79.9
|myocardium Q24.8
|nail Q84.6
|narrowness, eyelid Q10.3
|nasal sinus (wall) Q30.8
|neck (any part) Q18.9
|nerve Q07.9
  |acoustic Q07.8
  |optic Q07.8
|nervous system (central) Q07.9
|nipple Q83.9
|nose, nasal (bones) (cartilage) (septum)
  (sinus) Q30.9
  |specified NEC Q30.8
|ocular muscle Q15.8
|omphalomesenteric duct Q43.0
|opening, pulmonary veins Q26.4
|optic
  |disc Q14.2
  |nerve Q07.8
|opticociliary vessels Q13.2
|orbit (eye) Q10.7
|organ Q89.9
  |of Corti Q16.5
|origin
  |artery
    |innominate Q25.8
    |pulmonary Q25.79
    |renal Q27.2
    |subclavian Q25.48
|osseous meatus (ear) Q16.1
|ovary Q50.39
|oviduct Q50.6
|palate (hard) (soft) NEC Q38.5
|pancreas or pancreatic duct Q45.3
|papillary muscles Q24.8
|parathyroid gland Q89.2
|paraurethral ducts Q64.79
|parotid (gland) Q38.4
|patella Q74.1
|Pelger-Huët (hereditary hyposegmentation)
  D72.0
|pelvic girdle NEC Q74.2
|pelvis (bony) NEC Q74.2
  |rachitic E64.3
|penis (glans) Q55.69
|pericardium Q24.8
|peripheral vascular system Q27.9
|Peter's Q13.4
|pharynx Q38.8
|pigmentation L81.9
  |congenital Q82.8
|pituitary (gland) Q89.2
|pleural (folds) Q34.0

Anomaly, anomalous - *continued*

|portal vein Q26.5
  |connection Q26.5
|position, tooth, teeth, fully erupted M26.30
  |specified NEC M26.39
|precerebral vessel Q28.1
|prepuce Q55.69
|prostate Q55.4
|pulmonary Q33.9
  |artery NEC Q25.79
  |valve Q22.3
    |atresia Q22.0
    |insufficiency Q22.2
    |specified type NEC Q22.3
    |stenosis Q22.1
      |infundibular Q24.3
      |subvalvular Q24.3
  |venous connection Q26.4
    |partial Q26.3
    |total Q26.2
|pupil Q13.2
  |function H57.00
    |anisocoria H57.02
    |Argyll Robertson pupil H57.01
    |miosis H57.03
    |mydriasis H57.04
    |specified type NEC H57.09
    |tonic pupil H57.05-
|pylorus Q40.3
|radius Q74.0
|rectum Q43.9
|reduction (extremity) (limb)
  |femur (longitudinal) *see* Defect, reduction,
    lower limb, longitudinal, femur
  |fibula (longitudinal) *see* Defect, reduction,
    lower limb, longitudinal, fibula
  |lower limb *see* Defect, reduction, lower
    limb
  |radius (longitudinal) *see* Defect, reduction,
    upper limb, longitudinal, radius
  |tibia (longitudinal) *see* Defect, reduction,
    lower limb, longitudinal, tibia
  |ulna (longitudinal) *see* Defect, reduction,
    upper limb, longitudinal, ulna
  |upper limb *see* Defect, reduction, upper
    limb
|refraction *see* Disorder, refraction
|renal Q63.9
  |artery Q27.2
  |pelvis Q63.9
    |specified NEC Q63.8
|respiratory system Q34.9
  |specified NEC Q34.8
|retina Q14.1
|rib Q76.6
  |cervical Q76.5
|Rieger's Q13.81
|rotation *see* Malrotation
  |hip or thigh Q65.89
|round ligament Q52.8
|sacroiliac (joint) NEC Q74.2
|sacrum NEC Q76.49
  |kyphosis *see* Kyphosis, congenital
  |lordosis *see* Lordosis, congenital
|saddle nose, syphilitic A50.57
|salivary duct or gland Q38.4
|scapula Q74.0
|scrotum *see* Malformation, testis and scrotum
|sebaceous gland Q82.9
|seminal vesicles Q55.4
|sense organs NEC Q07.8
|sex chromosomes NEC *see also* Anomaly,
  chromosomes
  |female phenotype Q97.8
  |male phenotype Q98.9
|shoulder (girdle) (joint) Q74.0

Anomaly, anomalous - *continued*
|sigmoid (flexure) Q43.9
|simian crease Q82.8
|sinus of Valsalva Q25.49
|skeleton generalized Q78.9
|skin (appendage) Q82.9
|skull Q75.9
| |with
| | |anencephaly Q00.0
| | |encephalocele *see* Encephalocele
| | |hydrocephalus Q03.9
| | | |with spina bifida *see* Spina bifida, by
| | | | site, with hydrocephalus
| | |microcephaly Q02
|specified organ or site NEC Q89.8
|spermatic cord Q55.4
|spine, spinal NEC Q76.49
| |column NEC Q76.49
| | |kyphosis *see* Kyphosis, congenital
| | |lordosis *see* Lordosis, congenital
| |cord Q06.9
| |nerve root Q07.8
|spleen Q89.09
| |agenesis Q89.01
|stenonian duct Q38.4
|sternum NEC Q76.7
|stomach Q40.3
|submaxillary gland Q38.4
|tarsus NEC Q74.2
|tendon Q79.9
|testis *see* Malformation, testis and scrotum
|thigh NEC Q74.2
|thorax (wall) Q67.8
| |bony Q76.9
|throat Q38.8
|thumb Q74.0
|thymus gland Q89.2
|thyroid (gland) Q89.2
| |cartilage Q31.8
|tibia NEC Q74.2
| |saber A50.56
|toe Q74.2
|tongue Q38.3
|tooth, teeth K00.9
| |eruption K00.6
| |position, fully erupted M26.30
| |spacing, fully erupted M26.30
|trachea (cartilage) Q32.1
|tragus Q17.9
|tricuspid (leaflet) (valve) Q22.9
| |atresia or stenosis Q22.4
| |Ebstein's Q22.5
|Uhl's (hypoplasia of myocardium, right
| ventricle) Q24.8
|ulna Q74.0
|umbilical artery Q27.0
|union
| |cricoid cartilage and thyroid cartilage Q31.8
| |thyroid cartilage and hyoid bone Q31.8
| |trachea with larynx Q31.8
|upper limb Q74.0
|urachus Q64.4
|ureter Q62.8
| |obstructive NEC Q62.39
| | |cecoureterocele Q62.32
| | |orthotopic ureterocele Q62.31
|urethra Q64.70
| |absence Q64.5
| |double Q64.74
| |fistula to rectum Q64.73
| |obstructive Q64.39
| | |stricture Q64.32
| |prolapse Q64.71
| |specified type NEC Q64.79
|urinary tract Q64.9
|uterus Q51.9

Anomaly, anomalous - *continued*
| |with only one functioning horn Q51.4
|uvula Q38.5
|vagina Q52.4
|valleculae Q31.8
|valve (heart) NEC Q24.8
| |coronary sinus Q24.5
| |inferior vena cava Q24.8
| |pulmonary Q22.3
| |sinus coronario Q24.5
| |venae cavae inferioris Q24.8
|vas deferens Q55.4
|vascular Q27.9
| |brain Q28.3
| |ring Q25.45
|vein(s) (peripheral) Q27.9
| |brain Q28.3
| |cerebral Q28.3
| |coronary Q24.5
| |developmental Q28.3
| |great Q26.9
| | |specified NEC Q26.8
|vena cava (inferior) (superior) Q26.9
|venous *see* Anomaly, vein(s)
|venous return Q26.8
|ventricular
| |bands or folds Q24.8
| |septa Q21.0
|vertebra Q76.49
| |kyphosis *see* Kyphosis, congenital
| |lordosis *see* Lordosis, congenital
|vesicourethral orifice Q64.79
|vessel(s) Q27.9
| |optic papilla Q14.2
| |precerebral Q28.1
|vitelline duct Q43.0
|vitreous body or humor Q14.0
|vulva Q52.70
|wrist (joint) Q74.0
Anomia R48.8
Anonychia (congenital) Q84.3
|acquired L60.8
Anophthalmos, anophthalmus (congenital)
| **(globe)** Q11.1
|acquired Z90.01
Anopia, anopsia H53.46-
|quadrant H53.46-
Anorchia, anorchism, anorchidism Q55.0
Anorexia R63.0
|hysterical F44.89
|nervosa F50.00
| |atypical F50.9
| |binge-eating type F50.2
| | |with purging F50.02
| |restricting type F50.01
Anorgasmy, psychogenic (female) F52.31
|male F52.32
Anosmia R43.0
|hysterical F44.6
|postinfectional J39.8
Anosognosia R41.89
Anosteoplasia Q78.9
Anovulatory cycle N97.0
Anoxemia R09.02
|newborn P84
Anoxia (pathological) R09.02
|altitude T70.29
|cerebral G93.1
| |complicating
| | |anesthesia (general) (local) or other
| | | sedation T88.59
| | |in labor and delivery O74.3
| | |in pregnancy O29.21-
| | |postpartum, puerperal O89.2
| |delivery (cesarean) (instrumental) O75.4

Anoxia (pathological) - *continued*
| |during a procedure G97.81
| |newborn P84
| |resulting from a procedure G97.82
|due to
| |drowning T75.1
| |high altitude T70.29
|heart *see* Insufficiency, coronary
|intrauterine P84
|myocardial *see* Insufficiency, coronary
|newborn P84
|spinal cord G95.11
|systemic (by suffocation) (low content in
| atmosphere) *see* Asphyxia, traumatic
Anteflexion *see* Anteversion
Antenatal
|care (normal pregnancy) Z34.90
|screening (encounter for) of mother (*see also*
| Encounter, antenatal screening) Z36.9
Antepartum *see* condition
Anterior *see* condition
Antero-Occlusion M26.220
Anteversion
|cervix *see* Anteversion, uterus
|femur (neck), congenital Q65.89
|uterus, uterine (cervix) (postinfectional)
| (postpartal, old) N85.4
| |congenital Q51.818
| |in pregnancy or childbirth *see* Pregnancy,
| complicated by
Anthophobia F40.228
Anthracosilicosis J60
Anthracosis (lung) (occupational) J60
|lingua K14.3
Anthrax A22.9
|with pneumonia A22.1
|cerebral A22.8
|colitis A22.2
|cutaneous A22.0
|gastrointestinal A22.2
|inhalation A22.1
|intestinal A22.2
|meningitis A22.8
|pulmonary A22.1
|respiratory A22.1
|sepsis A22.7
|specified manifestation NEC A22.8
Anthropoid pelvis Q74.2
|with disproportion (fetopelvic) O33.0
Anthropophobia F40.10
|generalized F40.11
Antibodies, maternal (blood group) *see*
| Isoimmunization, affecting management of
| pregnancy
|anti-D *see* Isoimmunization, affecting
| management of pregnancy, Rh
|newborn P55.0
Antibody
|anticardiolipin R76.0
| |with
| | |hemorrhagic disorder D68.312
| | |hypercoagulable state D68.61
|antiphosphatidylglycerol R76.0
| |with
| | |hemorrhagic disorder D68.312
| | |hypercoagulable state D68.61
|antiphosphatidylinositol R76.0
| |with
| | |hemorrhagic disorder D68.312
| | |hypercoagulable state D68.61
|antiphosphatidylserine R76.0
| |with
| | |hemorrhagic disorder D68.312
| | |hypercoagulable state D68.61

Antibody - *continued*
|antiphospholipid R76.0
|with
|hemorrhagic disorder D68.312
|hypercoagulable state D68.61
Anticardiolipin syndrome D68.61
Anticoagulant, circulating (intrinsic) *see also*
|*Disorder, hemorrhagic* D68.318
|drug-induced (extrinsic) *see also* |*Disorder,*
hemorrhagic D68.32
|iatrogenic D68.32
Antidiuretic hormone syndrome E22.2
Antimonial cholera *see* Poisoning, antimony
Antiphospholipid
|antibody
|with hemorrhagic disorder D68.312
|syndrome D68.61
Antisocial personality F60.2
Antithrombinemia *see* Circulating
anticoagulants
Antithromboplastinemia D68.318
Antithromboplastinogenemia D68.318
Antitoxin complication or reaction *see*
Complications, vaccination
Antlophobia F40.228
Antritis J32.0
|maxilla J32.0
|acute J01.00
|recurrent J01.01
|stomach K29.60
|with bleeding K29.61
Antrum, antral *see* condition
Anuria R34
|calculus (impacted) (recurrent) *see also*
Calculus, urinary N20.9
|following
|abortion *see* Abortion by type complicated
by, renal failure
|ectopic or molar pregnancy O08.4
|newborn P96.0
|postprocedural N99.0
|postrenal N13.8
|traumatic (following crushing) T79.5
Anus, anal *see* condition
Anusitis K62.89
Anxiety F41.9
|depression F41.8
|episodic paroxysmal F41.0
|generalized F41.1
|hysteria F41.8
|neurosis F41.1
|panic type F41.0
|reaction F41.1
|separation, abnormal (of childhood) F93.0
|specified NEC F41.8
|state F41.1
Aorta, aortic *see* condition
Aortectasia *see* Ectasia, aorta
|with aneurysm *see* Aneurysm, aorta
Aortitis (nonsyphilitic) (calcific) I77.6
|arteriosclerotic I70.0
|Doehle-Heller A52.02
|luetic A52.02
|rheumatic *see* Endocarditis, acute, rheumatic
|specific (syphilitic) A52.02
|syphilitic A52.02
|congenital A50.54 [*I79.1*]
Apathetic thyroid storm *see* Thyrotoxicosis
Apathy R45.3
Apeirophobia F40.228
Apepsia K30
|psychogenic F45.8
Aperistalsis, esophagus K22.0
Apertognathia M26.29
Apert's syndrome Q87.0

Aphagia R13.0
|psychogenic F50.9
Aphakia (acquired) (postoperative) H27.0-
|congenital Q12.3
Aphasia (amnestic) (global) (nominal)
(semantic) (syntactic) R47.01
|acquired, with epilepsy (Landau-Kleffner
syndrome) *see* Epilepsy, specified NEC
|auditory (developmental) F80.2
|developmental (receptive type) F80.2
|expressive type F80.1
|Wernicke's F80.2
|following
|cerebrovascular disease I69.920
|cerebral infarction I69.320
|intracerebral hemorrhage I69.120
|nontraumatic intracranial hemorrhage
NEC I69.220
|specified disease NEC I69.820
|subarachnoid hemorrhage I69.020
|primary progressive G31.01 [*F02.80*]
|with behavioral disturbance G31.01
[*F02.81*]
|progressive isolated G31.01 [*F02.80*]
|with behavioral disturbance G31.01
[*F02.81*]
|sensory F80.2
|syphilis, tertiary A52.19
|Wernicke's (developmental) F80.2
Aphonia (organic) R49.1
|hysterical F44.4
|psychogenic F44.4
|Bednar's K12.0
|cachectic K14.0
|epizootic B08.8
|fever B08.8
|oral (recurrent) K12.0
|stomatitis (major) (minor) K12.0
|thrush B37.0
|ulcer (oral) (recurrent) K12.0
|genital organ(s) NEC
|female N76.6
|male N50.89
|larynx J38.7
Apical *see* condition
Apiphobia F40.218
Aplasia *see also* Agenesis
|abdominal muscle syndrome Q79.4
|alveolar process (acquired) *see* Anomaly,
alveolar
|congenital Q38.6
|aorta (congenital) Q25.41
|axialis extracorticalis (congenita) E75.29
|bone marrow (myeloid) D61.9
|congenital D61.01
|brain Q00.0
|part of Q04.3
|bronchus Q32.4
|cementum K00.4
|cerebellum Q04.3
|cervix (congenital) Q51.5
|congenital pure red cell D61.01
|corpus callosum Q04.0
|cutis congenita Q84.8
|erythrocyte congenital D61.01
|extracortical axial E75.29
|eye Q11.1
|fovea centralis (congenital) Q14.1
|gallbladder, congenital Q44.0
|iris Q13.1
|labyrinth, membranous Q16.5
|limb (congenital) Q73.8
|lower *see* Defect, reduction, lower limb
|upper *see* Agenesis, arm
|lung, congenital (bilateral) (unilateral) Q33.3
|pancreas Q45.0

Aplasia - *continued*
|parathyroid-thymic D82.1
|Pelizaeus-Merzbacher E75.29
|penis Q55.5
|prostate Q55.4
|red cell (with thymoma) D60.9
|acquired D60.9
|due to drugs D60.9
|adult D60.9
|chronic D60.0
|congenital D61.01
|constitutional D61.01
|due to drugs D60.9
|hereditary D61.01
|of infants D61.01
|primary D61.01
|pure D61.01
|due to drugs D60.9
|specified type NEC D60.8
|transient D60.1
|round ligament Q52.8
|skin Q84.8
|spermatic cord Q55.4
|spleen Q89.01
|testicle Q55.0
|thymic, with immunodeficiency D82.1
|thyroid (congenital) (with myxedema) E03.1
|uterus Q51.0
|ventral horn cell Q06.1
Apnea, apneic (of) (spells) R06.81
|newborn NEC P28.4
|obstructive P28.4
|sleep (central) (obstructive) (primary) P28.3
|prematurity P28.4
|sleep G47.30
|central (primary) G47.31
|idiopathic G47.31
|in conditions classified elsewhere G47.37
|obstructive (adult) (pediatric) G47.33
|hypopnea G47.33
|primary central G47.31
|specified NEC G47.39
Apneumatosis, newborn P28.0
Apocrine metaplasia (breast) *see* Dysplasia,
mammary, specified type NEC
Apophysitis (bone) *see also* Osteochondropathy
|calcaneus M92.8
|juvenile M92.9
Apoplectiform convulsions (cerebral ischemia)
I67.82
Apoplexia, apoplexy, apoplectic
|adrenal A39.1
|heart (auricle) (ventricle) *see* Infarct,
myocardium
|heat T67.0
|hemorrhagic (stroke) *see* Hemorrhage,
intracranial
|meninges, hemorrhagic *see* Hemorrhage,
intracranial, subarachnoid
|uremic N18.9 [*I68.8*]
Appearance
|bizarre R46.1
|specified NEC R46.89
|very low level of personal hygiene R46.0
Appendage
|epididymal (organ of Morgagni) Q55.4
|intestine (epiploic) Q43.8
|preauricular Q17.0
|testicular (organ of Morgagni) Q55.29
Appendicitis (pneumococcal) (retrocecal) K37
|with
|gangrene K35.891
|perforation NOS K35.32
|peritoneal abscess K35.33
|peritonitis NEC K35.33

Appendicitis - *continued*
    |generalized (with perforation or rupture)
        K35.20
      |with abscess K35.21
    |localized (with perforation or rupture)
        K35.30
      |with
        |gangrene K35.31
        |perforation K35.32
          |and abscess K35.33
    |rupture (with localized peritonitis) K35.32
  |acute (catarrhal) (fulminating) (gangrenous)
      (obstructive) (retrocecal) (suppurative)
      K35.80
    |with
      |peritoneal abscess K35.33
      |peritonitis NEC K35.33
        |generalized (with perforation or rupture)
          K35.20
          |with abscess K35.21
        |localized (with perforation or rupture)
          K35.30
          |with
            |gangrene K35.31
            |perforation K35.32
              |and abscess K35.33
    |specified NEC K35.890
      |with gangrene K35.891
  |ruptured NOS (with localized peritonitis)
      K35.32
  |amebic A06.89
  |chronic (recurrent) K36
  |exacerbation *see* Appendicitis, acute
  |gangrenous *see* Appendicitis, acute
  |healed (obliterative) K36
  |interval K36
  |neurogenic K36
  |obstructive K36
  |recurrent K36
  |relapsing K36
  |subacute (adhesive) K36
  |subsiding K36
  |suppurative *see* Appendicitis, acute
  |tuberculous A18.32
Appendicopathia oxyurica B80
Appendix, appendicular *see also* condition
  |epididymis Q55.4
  |Morgagni
    |female Q50.5
    |male (epididymal) Q55.4
      |testicular Q55.29
  |testis Q55.29
Appetite
  |depraved *see* Pica
  |excessive R63.2
  |lack or loss *see also* Anorexia R63.0
    |nonorganic origin F50.89
    |psychogenic F50.89
  |perverted (hysterical) *see* Pica
Apple peel syndrome Q41.1
Apprehension state F41.1
Apprehensiveness, abnormal F41.9
Approximal wear K03.0
Apraxia (classic) (ideational) (ideokinetic)
  (ideomotor) (motor) (verbal) R48.2
  |following
    |cerebrovascular disease I69.990
      |cerebral infarction I69.390
      |intracerebral hemorrhage I69.190
      |nontraumatic intracranial hemorrhage
      NEC I69.290
      |specified disease NEC I69.890
      |subarachnoid hemorrhage I69.090
  |oculomotor, congenital H51.8
Aptyalism K11.7

Apudoma *see* Neoplasm, uncertain behavior, by
  site
Aqueous misdirection H40.83-
Arabicum elephantiasis *see* Infestation, filarial
Arachnitis *see* Meningitis
Arachnodactyly *see* Syndrome, Marfan's
Arachnoiditis (acute) (adhesive) (basal)
  (brain) (cerebrospinal) *see* Meningitis
Arachnophobia F40.210
Arboencephalitis, Australian A83.4
Arborization block (heart) I45.5
ARC (AIDS-Related complex) B20
Arch
  |aortic Q25.49
  |bovine Q25.49
Arches *see* condition
Arcuate uterus Q51.810
Arcuatus uterus Q51.810
Arcus (cornea) senilis *see* Degeneration, cornea,
  senile
Arc-Welder's lung J63.4
Areflexia R29.2
Areola *see* condition
Argentaffinoma *see also* Neoplasm, uncertain
  behavior, by site
  |malignant *see* Neoplasm, malignant, by site
  |syndrome E34.0
Argininemia E72.21
Arginosuccinic aciduria E72.22
Argyll Robertson phenomenon, pupil or
  syndrome (syphilitic) A52.19
  |atypical H57.09
  |nonsyphilitic H57.09
Argyria, argyriasis
  |conjunctival H11.13-
Argyria, argyriasis
  |from drug or medicament *see* Table of Drugs
    and Chemicals, by substance
Argyrosis, conjunctival H11.13-
Arhinencephaly Q04.1
Ariboflavinosis E53.0
Arm *see* condition
Arnold-Chiari disease, obstruction or
  syndrome (type II) Q07.00
  |with
    |hydrocephalus Q07.02
      |with spina bifida Q07.03
    |spina bifida Q07.01
      |with hydrocephalus Q07.03
  |type III *see* Encephalocele
  |type IV Q04.8
Aromatic amino-Acid metabolism disorder
  E70.9
  |specified NEC E70.89
Arousals, confusional G47.51
Arrest, arrested
  |cardiac I46.9
    |complicating
      |abortion *see* Abortion, by type,
        complicated by, cardiac arrest
      |anesthesia (general) (local) or other
        sedation *see* Table of Drugs and
        Chemicals, by drug,
        |in labor and delivery O74.2
        |in pregnancy O29.11-
        |postpartum, puerperal O89.1
      |delivery (cesarean) (instrumental) O75.4
    |due to
      |cardiac condition I46.2
      |specified condition NEC I46.8
    |intraoperative I97.71-
    |newborn P29.81
    |postprocedural I97.12-
      |obstetric procedure O75.4
  |cardiorespiratory *see* Arrest, cardiac
  |circulatory *see* Arrest, cardiac

Arrest, arrested - *continued*
  |deep transverse O64.0
  |development or growth
    |bone *see* Disorder, bone, development or
      growth
    |child R62.50
    |tracheal rings Q32.1
  |epiphyseal
    |complete
      |femur M89.15-
      |humerus M89.12-
      |tibia M89.16-
      |ulna M89.13-
    |forearm M89.13-
      |specified NEC M89.13-
      |ulna *see* Arrest, epiphyseal, by type, ulna
    |lower leg M89.16-
      |specified NEC M89.168
      |tibia *see* Arrest, epiphyseal, by type, tibia
    |partial
      |femur M89.15-
      |humerus M89.12-
      |tibia M89.16-
      |ulna M89.13-
    |personal history, successfully resuscitated
      Z86.74
    |specified NEC M89.18
  |granulopoiesis *see* Agranulocytosis
  |growth plate *see* Arrest, epiphyseal
  |heart *see* Arrest, cardiac
  |legal, anxiety concerning Z65.3
  |physeal *see* Arrest, epiphyseal
  |respiratory R09.2
    |newborn P28.81
  |sinus I45.5
  |spermatogenesis (complete) *see* Azoospermia
    |incomplete *see* Oligospermia
  |transverse (deep) O64.0
Arrhenoblastoma
  |benign
    |specified site *see* Neoplasm, benign, by site
    |unspecified site
      |female D27.9
      |male D29.20
  |malignant
    |specified site *see* Neoplasm, malignant, by
      site
    |unspecified site
      |female C56.9
      |male C62.90
  |specified site *see* Neoplasm, uncertain
    behavior, by site
  |unspecified site
    |female D39.10
    |male D40.10
Arrhythmia (auricle) (cardiac)
  (juvenile)(nodal) (reflex) (sinus)
  (supraventricular) (transitory)(ventricle)
  I49.8
  |block I45.9
  |extrasystolic I49.49
  |newborn
    |bradycardia P29.12
    |occurring before birth P03.819
      |before onset of labor P03.810
      |during labor P03.811
    |tachycardia P29.11
  |psychogenic F45.8
  |specified NEC I49.8
  |vagal R55
  |ventricular re-entry I47.0
Arrillaga-Ayerza syndrome (pulmonary
  sclerosis with pulmonary hypertension)
  I27.0

Arsenical pigmentation L81.8
  |from drug or medicament *see* Table of Drugs
    and Chemicals
Arsenism *see* Poisoning, arsenic
Arterial *see* condition
Arteriofibrosis *see* Arteriosclerosis
Arteriolar sclerosis *see* Arteriosclerosis
Arteriolith *see* Arteriosclerosis
Arteriolitis I77.6
  |necrotizing, kidney I77.5
  |renal *see* Hypertension, kidney
Arteriolosclerosis *see* Arteriosclerosis
Arterionephrosclerosis *see* Hypertension,
  kidney
Arteriopathy I77.9
  |cerebral autosomal dominant, with subcortical
    infarcts and leukoencephalopathy
    (CADASIL) I67.850
Arteriosclerosis, arteriosclerotic (diffuse)
  (obliterans) (of) (senile) (with calcification)
  I70.90
  |aorta I70.0
  |arteries of extremities *see* Arteriosclerosis,
    extremities
    |with
      |chronic limb-threatening ischemia *see*
        Arteriosclerosis, with critical limb
        ischemia
      |critical limb ischemia *see*
        Arteriosclerosis, with critical limb
        ischemia
  |brain I67.2
  |bypass graft
    |coronary *see* Arteriosclerosis, coronary,
      bypass graft
    |extremities *see* Arteriosclerosis, extremities,
      bypass graft
    |with
      |chronic limb-threatening ischemia *see*
        Arteriosclerosis, with critical limb
        ischemia
      |critical limb ischemia *see*
        Arteriosclerosis, with critical limb
        ischemia
  |cardiac *see* Disease, heart, ischemic,
    atherosclerotic
  |cardiopathy *see* Disease, heart, ischemic,
    atherosclerotic
  |cardiorenal *see* Hypertension, cardiorenal
  |cardiovascular *see* Disease, heart, ischemic,
    atherosclerotic
  |carotid *see also* Occlusion, artery, carotid
    I65.2-
  |central nervous system I67.2
  |cerebral I67.2
  |cerebrovascular I67.2
  |coronary (artery) I25.10
    |due to
      |calcified coronary lesion (severely) I25.84
      |lipid rich plaque I25.83
    |bypass graft I25.810
      |with
        |angina pectoris I25.709
          |with documented spasm I25.701
          |specified type NEC I25.708
          |unstable I25.700
        |ischemic chest pain I25.709
      |autologous artery I25.810
        |with
          |angina pectoris I25.729
            |with documented spasm I25.721
            |specified type I25.728
            |unstable I25.720
          |ischemic chest pain I25.729
      |autologous vein I25.810
        |with
          |angina pectoris I25.719

Arteriosclerosis, arteriosclerotic - *continued*
          |with documented spasm I25.711
          |specified type I25.718
          |unstable I25.710
        |ischemic chest pain I25.719
      |nonautologous biological I25.810
        |with
          |angina pectoris I25.739
            |with documented spasm I25.731
            |specified type I25.738
            |unstable I25.730
          |ischemic chest pain I25.739
    |specified type NEC I25.810
      |with
        |angina pectoris I25.799
          |with documented spasm I25.791
          |specified type I25.798
          |unstable I25.790
        |ischemic chest pain I25.799
    |native vessel
      |with
        |angina pectoris I25.119
          |with documented spasm I25.111
          |specified type NEC I25.118
          |unstable I25.110
        |ischemic chest pain I25.119
    |transplanted heart I25.811
      |bypass graft I25.812
        |with
          |angina pectoris I25.769
            |with documented spasm I25.761
            |specified type I25.768
            |unstable I25.760
          |ischemic chest pain I25.769
      |native coronary artery I25.811
        |with
          |angina pectoris I25.759
            |with documented spasm I25.751
            |specified type I25.758
            |unstable I25.750
          |ischemic chest pain I25.759
  |extremities (native arteries) I70.209
    |with
      |chronic limb-threatening ischemia *see*
        Arteriosclerosis, with critical limb
        ischemia
      |critical limb ischemia *see*
        Arteriosclerosis, with critical limb
        ischemia
    |bypass graft I70.309
      |with
        |chronic limb-threatening ischemia *see*
          Arteriosclerosis, with critical limb
          ischemia
        |critical limb ischemia *see*
          Arteriosclerosis, with critical limb
          ischemia
      |autologous vein graft I70.409
        |leg I70.409
          |with
            |gangrene (and intermittent
              claudication, rest pain and ulcer)
              I70.469
            |intermittent claudication I70.419
            |rest pain (and intermittent
              claudication) I70.429
            |bilateral I70.403
              |with
                |gangrene (and intermittent
                  claudication, rest pain and
                  ulcer) I70.463
                |intermittent claudication I70.413
                |rest pain (and intermittent
                  claudication) I70.423
              |specified type NEC I70.493

Arteriosclerosis, arteriosclerotic - *continued*
  |left I70.402
    |with
      |gangrene (and intermittent
        claudication, rest pain and
        ulcer) I70.462
      |intermittent claudication I70.412
      |rest pain (and intermittent
        claudication) I70.422
      |ulceration (and intermittent
        claudication and rest pain)
        I70.449
        |ankle I70.443
        |calf I70.442
        |foot site NEC I70.445
        |heel I70.444
        |lower leg NEC I70.448
        |midfoot I70.444
        |thigh I70.441
    |specified type NEC I70.492
    |right I70.401
      |with
        |gangrene (and intermittent
          claudication, rest pain and
          ulcer) I70.461
        |intermittent claudication I70.411
        |rest pain (and intermittent
          claudication) I70.421
        |ulceration (and intermittent
          claudication and rest pain)
          I70.439
          |ankle I70.433
          |calf I70.432
          |foot site NEC I70.435
          |heel I70.434
          |lower leg NEC I70.438
          |midfoot I70.434
          |thigh I70.431
      |specified type NEC I70.491
    |specified type NEC I70.499
    |specified NEC I70.408
      |with
        |gangrene (and intermittent
          claudication, rest pain and
          ulcer) I70.468
        |intermittent claudication I70.418
        |rest pain (and intermittent
          claudication) I70.428
        |ulceration (and intermittent
          claudication and rest pain) I70.45
    |specified type NEC I70.498
    |leg I70.309
      |with
        |gangrene (and intermittent
          claudication, rest pain and ulcer)
          I70.369
        |intermittent claudication I70.319
        |rest pain (and intermittent
          claudication) I70.329
      |bilateral I70.303
        |with
          |gangrene (and intermittent
            claudication, rest pain and
            ulcer) I70.363
          |intermittent claudication I70.313
          |rest pain (and intermittent
            claudication) I70.323
      |specified type NEC I70.393
    |left I70.302
      |with
        |gangrene (and intermittent
          claudication, rest pain and
          ulcer) I70.362
        |intermittent claudication I70.312

Arteriosclerosis, arteriosclerotic - *continued*
- rest pain (and intermittent claudication) I70.322
- ulceration (and intermittent claudication and rest pain) I70.349
  - ankle I70.343
  - calf I70.342
  - foot site NEC I70.345
  - heel I70.344
  - lower leg NEC I70.348
  - midfoot I70.344
  - thigh I70.341
- specified type NEC I70.392
- right I70.301
  - with
    - gangrene (and intermittent claudication, rest pain and ulcer) I70.361
    - intermittent claudication I70.311
    - rest pain (and intermittent claudication) I70.321
    - ulceration (and intermittent claudication and rest pain) I70.339
      - ankle I70.333
      - calf I70.332
      - foot site NEC I70.335
      - heel I70.334
      - lower leg NEC I70.338
      - midfoot I70.334
      - thigh I70.331
    - specified type NEC I70.391
  - specified type NEC I70.399
- nonautologous biological graft I70.509
  - leg I70.509
    - with
      - gangrene (and intermittent claudication, rest pain and ulcer) I70.569
      - intermittent claudication I70.519
      - rest pain (and intermittent claudication) I70.529
    - bilateral I70.503
      - with
        - gangrene (and intermittent claudication, rest pain and ulcer) I70.563
        - intermittent claudication I70.513
        - rest pain (and intermittent claudication) I70.523
      - specified type NEC I70.593
    - left I70.502
      - with
        - gangrene (and intermittent claudication, rest pain and ulcer) I70.562
        - intermittent claudication I70.512
        - rest pain (and intermittent claudication) I70.522
        - ulceration (and intermittent claudication and rest pain) I70.549
          - ankle I70.543
          - calf I70.542
          - foot site NEC I70.545
          - heel I70.544
          - lower leg NEC I70.548
          - midfoot I70.544
          - thigh I70.541
      - specified type NEC I70.592
    - right I70.501
      - with

Arteriosclerosis, arteriosclerotic - *continued*
- gangrene (and intermittent claudication, rest pain and ulcer) I70.561
- intermittent claudication I70.511
- rest pain (and intermittent claudication) I70.521
- ulceration (and intermittent claudication and rest pain) I70.539
  - ankle I70.533
  - calf I70.532
  - foot site NEC I70.535
  - heel I70.534
  - lower leg NEC I70.538
  - midfoot I70.534
  - thigh I70.531
- specified type NEC I70.591
- specified type NEC I70.599
- specified NEC I70.508
  - with
    - gangrene (and intermittent claudication, rest pain and ulcer) I70.568
    - intermittent claudication I70.518
    - rest pain (and intermittent claudication) I70.528
    - ulceration (and intermittent claudication and rest pain) I70.55
  - specified type NEC I70.598
- nonbiological graft I70.609
  - leg I70.609
    - with
      - gangrene (and intermittent claudication, rest pain and ulcer) I70.669
      - intermittent claudication I70.619
      - rest pain (and intermittent claudication) I70.629
    - bilateral I70.603
      - with
        - gangrene (and intermittent claudication, rest pain and ulcer) I70.663
        - intermittent claudication I70.613
        - rest pain (and intermittent claudication) I70.623
      - specified type NEC I70.693
    - left I70.602
      - with
        - gangrene (and intermittent claudication, rest pain and ulcer) I70.662
        - intermittent claudication I70.612
        - rest pain (and intermittent claudication) I70.622
        - ulceration (and intermittent claudication and rest pain) I70.649
          - ankle I70.643
          - calf I70.642
          - foot site NEC I70.645
          - heel I70.644
          - lower leg NEC I70.648
          - midfoot I70.644
          - thigh I70.641
      - specified type NEC I70.692
    - right I70.601
      - with
        - gangrene (and intermittent claudication, rest pain and ulcer) I70.661
        - intermittent claudication I70.611
        - rest pain (and intermittent claudication) I70.621

Arteriosclerosis, arteriosclerotic - *continued*
- ulceration (and intermittent claudication and rest pain) I70.639
  - ankle I70.633
  - calf I70.632
  - foot site NEC I70.635
  - heel I70.634
  - lower leg NEC I70.638
  - midfoot I70.634
  - thigh I70.631
- specified type NEC I70.691
- specified type NEC I70.699
- specified NEC I70.608
  - with
    - gangrene (and intermittent claudication, rest pain and ulcer) I70.668
    - intermittent claudication I70.618
    - rest pain (and intermittent claudication) I70.628
    - ulceration (and intermittent claudication and rest pain) I70.65
  - specified type NEC I70.698
- specified graft NEC I70.709
  - leg I70.709
    - with
      - gangrene (and intermittent claudication, rest pain and ulcer) I70.769
      - intermittent claudication I70.719
      - rest pain (and intermittent claudication) I70.729
    - bilateral I70.703
      - with
        - gangrene (and intermittent claudication, rest pain and ulcer) I70.763
        - intermittent claudication I70.713
        - rest pain (and intermittent claudication) I70.723
      - specified type NEC I70.793
    - left I70.702
      - with
        - gangrene (and intermittent claudication, rest pain and ulcer) I70.762
        - intermittent claudication I70.712
        - rest pain (and intermittent claudication) I70.722
        - ulceration (and intermittent claudication and rest pain) I70.749
          - ankle I70.743
          - calf I70.742
          - foot site NEC I70.745
          - heel I70.744
          - lower leg NEC I70.748
          - midfoot I70.744
          - thigh I70.741
      - specified type NEC I70.792
    - right I70.701
      - with
        - gangrene (and intermittent claudication, rest pain and ulcer) I70.761
        - intermittent claudication I70.711
        - rest pain (and intermittent claudication) I70.721
        - ulceration (and intermittent claudication and rest pain) I70.739
          - ankle I70.733
          - calf I70.732
          - foot site NEC I70.735

Arteriosclerosis, arteriosclerotic - *continued*

    |heel I70.734
     |lower leg NEC I70.738
     |midfoot I70.734
     |thigh I70.731
    |specified type NEC I70.791
   |specified type NEC I70.799
  |specified NEC I70.708
   |with
    |gangrene (and intermittent
     claudication, rest pain and ulcer)
     I70.768
    |intermittent claudication I70.718
    |rest pain (and intermittent
     claudication) I70.728
    |ulceration (and intermittent
     claudication and rest pain) I70.75
   |specified type NEC I70.798
  |specified NEC I70.308
   |with
    |gangrene (and intermittent
     claudication, rest pain and ulcer)
     I70.368
    |intermittent claudication I70.318
    |rest pain (and intermittent
     claudication) I70.328
    |ulceration (and intermittent
     claudication and rest pain) I70.35
   |specified type NEC I70.398
 |leg I70.209
  |with
   |gangrene (and intermittent claudication,
    rest pain and ulcer) I70.269
   |intermittent claudication I70.219
   |rest pain (and intermittent claudication)
    I70.229
  |bilateral I70.203
   |with
    |gangrene (and intermittent
     claudication, rest pain and ulcer)
     I70.263
    |intermittent claudication I70.213
    |rest pain (and intermittent
     claudication) I70.223
   |specified type NEC I70.293
  |left I70.202
   |with
    |gangrene (and intermittent
     claudication, rest pain and ulcer)
     I70.262
    |intermittent claudication I70.212
    |rest pain (and intermittent
     claudication) I70.222
    |ulceration (and intermittent
     claudication and rest pain) I70.249
    |ankle I70.243
    |calf I70.242
    |foot site NEC I70.245
    |heel I70.244
    |lower leg NEC I70.248
    |midfoot I70.244
    |thigh I70.241
   |specified type NEC I70.292
  |right I70.201
   |with
    |gangrene (and intermittent
     claudication, rest pain and ulcer)
     I70.261
    |intermittent claudication I70.211
    |rest pain (and intermittent
     claudication) I70.221
    |ulceration (and intermittent
     claudication and rest pain) I70.239
    |ankle I70.233
    |calf I70.232

Arteriosclerosis, arteriosclerotic - *continued*

    |foot site NEC I70.235
    |heel I70.234
    |lower leg NEC I70.238
    |midfoot I70.234
    |thigh I70.231
   |specified type NEC I70.291
  |specified type NEC I70.299
 |specified site NEC I70.208
  |with
   |gangrene (and intermittent claudication,
    rest pain and ulcer) I70.268
   |intermittent claudication I70.218
   |rest pain (and intermittent claudication)
    I70.228
   |ulceration (and intermittent claudication
  and rest pain) I70.25
   |specified type NEC I70.298
 |generalized I70.91
 |heart (disease) *see* Arteriosclerosis, coronary
  (artery),
 |kidney *see* Hypertension, kidney
 |medial *see* Arteriosclerosis, extremities
 |mesenteric (artery) K55.1
 |Mönckeberg's *see* Arteriosclerosis, extremities
 |myocarditis I51.4
 |peripheral (of extremities) *see*
  Arteriosclerosis, extremities
 |pulmonary (idiopathic) I27.0
 |renal (arterioles) *see also* Hypertension,
  kidney
  |artery I70.1
 |retina (vascular) I70.8 [*H35.0*]
 |specified artery NEC I70.8
 |spinal (cord) G95.19
 |vertebral (artery) I67.2
 |with
  |chronic limb-threatening ischemia *see*
   Arteriosclerosis, with critical limb
   ischemia
  |critical limb ischemia
   |bypass graft I70.329
    |autologous vein graft I70.429
     |leg I70.429
      |with
       |gangrene (and intermittent
        claudication, rest pain, and
        ulcer) I70.469
       |rest pain (and intermittent
        claudication) I70.429
     |bilateral I70.423
      |with
       |gangrene (and intermittent
        claudication, rest pain, and
        ulcer) I70.463
       |rest pain (and intermittent
        claudication) I70.423
     |left I70.422
      |with
       |gangrene (and intermittent
        claudication, rest pain, and
        ulcer) I70.462
       |rest pain (and intermittent
        claudication) I70.422
       |ulceration (and intermittent
        claudication and rest pain)
        I70.449
       |ankle I70.443
       |calf I70.442
       |foot site NEC I70.445
       |heel I70.444
       |lower leg NEC I70.448
       |mid foot I70.444
       |thigh I70.441
     |right I70.421

Arteriosclerosis, arteriosclerotic - *continued*

      |with
       |gangrene (and intermittent
        claudication, rest pain, and
        ulcer) I70.461
       |rest pain (and intermittent
        claudication) I70.421
       |ulceration (and intermittent
        claudication and rest pain)
        I70.439
       |ankle I70.433
       |calf I70.432
       |foot site NEC I70.435
       |heel I70.434
       |lower leg NEC I70.438
       |midfoot I70.434
       |thigh I70.431
    |leg I70.329
     |with
      |gangrene (and intermittent
       claudication, rest pain, and
       ulcer) I70.369
      |rest pain (and intermittent
       claudication) I70.329
     |bilateral I70.323
      |with
       |gangrene (and intermittent
        claudication, rest pain, and
        ulcer) I70.363
       |rest pain (and intermittent
        claudication) I70.323
     |left I70.322
      |with
       |gangrene (and intermittent
        claudication, rest pain, and
        ulcer) I70.362
       |rest pain (and intermittent
        claudication) I70.322
       |ulceration (and intermittent
        claudication and rest pain)
        I70.349
       |ankle I70.343
       |calf I70.342
       |foot site NEC I70.345
       |heel I70.344
       |lower leg NEC I70.348
       |midfoot I70.344
       |thigh I70.341
     |right I70.321
      |with
       |gangrene (and intermittent
        claudication, rest pain, and
        ulcer) I70.361
       |rest pain (and intermittent
        claudication) I70.321
       |ulceration (and intermittent
        claudication and rest pain)
        I70.339
       |ankle I70.333
        |calf I70.332
        |foot site NEC I70.335
        |heel I70.334
        |lower leg NEC I70.338
        |midfoot I70.334
        |thigh I70.331
    |nonautologous biological graft I70.529
     |leg I70.529
      |with
       |gangrene (and intermittent
        claudication, rest pain, and ulcer)
        I70.569
       |rest pain (and intermittent
        claudication) I70.529
     |bilateral I70.523
      |with

Arteriosclerosis, arteriosclerotic - *continued*
- |gangrene (and intermittent claudication, rest pain, and ulcer) I70.563
- |rest pain (and intermittent claudication) I70.523
- |left I70.522
- |with
  - |gangrene (and intermittent claudication, rest pain, and ulcer) I70.562
  - |rest pain (and intermittent claudication) I70.522
  - |ulceration (and intermittent claudication and rest pain) I70.549
    - |ankle I70.543
    - |calf I70.542
    - |foot site NEC I70.545
    - |heel I70.544
    - |lower leg NEC I70.548
    - |midfoot I70.544
    - |thigh I70.541
- |right I70.521
- |with
  - |gangrene (and intermittent claudication, rest pain, and ulcer) I70.561
  - |rest pain (and intermittent claudication) I70.521
  - |ulceration (and intermittent claudication and rest pain) I70.539
    - |ankle I70.533
    - |calf I70.532
    - |foot site NEC I70.535
    - |heel I70.534
    - |lower leg NEC I70.538
    - |midfoot I70.534
    - |thigh I70.531
- |nonbiological graft I70.629
- |leg I70.629
- |with
  - |gangrene (and intermittent claudication, rest pain, and ulcer) I70.669
  - |rest pain (and intermittent claudication) I70.629
- |bilateral I70.623
  - |with
  - |with
    - |gangrene (and intermittent claudication, rest pain, and ulcer) I70.663
    - |rest pain (and intermittent claudication) I70.623
- |left I70.622
  - |with
    - |gangrene (and intermittent claudication, rest pain, and ulcer) I70.662
    - |rest pain (and intermittent claudication) I70.622
    - |ulceration (and intermittent claudication and rest pain) I70.649
      - |ankle I70.643
      - |calf I70.642
      - |foot site NEC I70.645
      - |heel I70.644
      - |lower leg NEC I70.648
      - |midfoot I70.644
      - |thigh I70.641
- |right I70.621
  - |with

Arteriosclerosis, arteriosclerotic - *continued*
- |gangrene (and intermittent claudication, rest pain, and ulcer) I70.661
- |rest pain (and intermittent claudication) I70.621
- |ulceration (and intermittent claudication and rest pain) I70.639
  - |ankle I70.633
  - |calf I70.632
  - |foot site NEC I70.635
  - |heel I70.634
  - |lower leg NEC I70.638
  - |midfoot I70.634
  - |thigh I70.631
- |specified graft NEC I70.729
- |leg I70.729
  - |with
    - |gangrene (and intermittent claudication, rest pain, and ulcer) I70.769
    - |rest pain (and intermittent claudication) I70.729
- |bilateral I70.723
  - |with
    - |gangrene (and intermittent claudication, rest pain, and ulcer) I70.763
    - |rest pain (and intermittent claudication) I70.723
- |left I70.722
  - |with
    - |gangrene (and intermittent claudication, rest pain, and ulcer) I70.762
    - |rest pain (and intermittent claudication) I70.722
    - |ulceration (and intermittent claudication and rest pain) I70.749
      - |ankle I70.743
      - |calf I70.742
      - |foot site NEC I70.745
      - |heel I70.744
      - |lower leg NEC I70.748
      - |midfoot I70.744
      - |thigh I70.741
- |right I70.721
  - |with
    - |gangrene (and intermittent claudication, rest pain, and ulcer) I70.761
    - |rest pain (and intermittent claudication) I70.721
    - |ulceration (and intermittent claudication and rest pain) I70.739
      - |ankle I70.733
      - |calf I70.732
      - |foot site NEC I70.735
      - |heel I70.734
      - |lower leg NEC I70.738
      - |midfoot I70.734
      - |thigh I70.731
- |leg I70.229
  - |with
    - |gangrene (and intermittent claudication, rest pain, and ulcer) I70.269
    - |rest pain (and intermittent claudication) I70.229
- |bilateral I70.223
  - |with

Arteriosclerosis, arteriosclerotic - *continued*
- |gangrene (and intermittent claudication, rest pain, and ulcer) I70.263
- |rest pain (and intermittent claudication) I70.223
- |left I70.222
  - |with
    - |gangrene (and intermittent claudication, rest pain, and ulcer) I70.262
    - |rest pain (and intermittent claudication) I70.222
    - |ulceration (and intermittent claudication and rest pain) I70.249
      - |ankle I70.243
      - |calf I70.242
      - |foot site NEC I70.245
      - |heel I70.244
      - |lower leg NEC I70.248
      - |midfoot I70.244
      - |thigh I70.241
- |right I70.221
  - |with
    - |gangrene (and intermittent claudication, rest pain, and ulcer) I70.261
    - |rest pain (and intermittent claudication) I70.221
    - |ulceration (and intermittent claudication and rest pain) I70.239
      - |ankle I70.233
      - |calf I70.232
      - |foot site NEC I70.235
      - |heel I70.234
      - |lower leg NEC I70.238
      - |midfoot I70.234
      - |thigh I70.231

Arteriospasm I73.9
Arteriovenous *see* condition
Arteritis I77.6
- |allergic M31.0
- |aorta (nonsyphilitic) I77.6
  - |syphilitic A52.02
- |aortic arch M31.4
- |brachiocephalic M31.4
- |brain I67.7
  - |syphilitic A52.04
- |cerebral I67.7
  - |in
    - |diseases classified elsewhere I68.2
    - |systemic lupus erythematosus M32.19
  - |listerial A32.89
  - |syphilitic A52.04
  - |tuberculous A18.89
- |coronary (artery) I25.89
  - |rheumatic I01.8
    - |chronic I09.89
  - |syphilitic A52.06
- |cranial (left) (right), giant cell M31.6
- |deformans *see* Arteriosclerosis
- |giant cell NEC M31.6
  - |with polymyalgia rheumatica M31.5
- |necrosing or necrotizing M31.9
  - |specified NEC M31.8
- |nodosa M30.0
- |obliterans *see* Arteriosclerosis
- |pulmonary I28.8
- |rheumatic *see* Fever, rheumatic
- |senile *see* Arteriosclerosis
- |suppurative I77.2
- |syphilitic (general) A52.09
  - |brain A52.04

Arteritis - *continued*

coronary A52.06
spinal A52.09
temporal, giant cell M31.6
young female aortic arch syndrome M31.4

Artery, arterial *see also* condition

abscess I77.89
single umbilical Q27.0

Arthralgia (allergic) *see also* Pain, joint

in caisson disease T70.3
temporomandibular M26.62-

Arthritis, arthritic (acute) (chronic) (nonpyogenic) (subacute) M19.90

allergic *see* Arthritis, specified form NEC
ankylosing (crippling) (spine) *see also*
 Spondylitis, ankylosing
 sites other than spine *see* Arthritis, specified
  form NEC
atrophic *see* Osteoarthritis
 spine *see* Spondylitis, ankylosing
back *see* Spondylopathy, inflammatory
blennorrhagic (gonococcal) A54.42
Charcot's *see* Arthropathy, neuropathic
diabetic *see* Diabetes, arthropathy,
 neuropathic
syringomyelic G95.0
chylous (filarial) *see also* category M01 B74.9
climacteric (any site) NEC *see* Arthritis,
 specified form NEC
crystal (-induced) *see* Arthritis, in, crystals
deformans *see* Osteoarthritis
degenerative *see* Osteoarthritis
due to or associated with
 acromegaly E22.0
 brucellosis *see* Brucellosis
 caisson disease T70.3
 diabetes *see* Diabetes, arthropathy
 dracontiasis *see also* category M01 B72
 enteritis NEC
  regional *see* Enteritis, regional
 erysipelas *see also* category M01 A46
 erythema
  epidemic A25.1
  nodosum L52
 filariasis NOS B74.9
 glanders A24.0
 helminthiasis *see also* category M01 B83.9
 hemophilia D66 *[M36.2]*
 Henoch (Schönlein) purpura D69.0
  [M36.4]
 human parvovirus *see also* category M01
  B97.6
 infectious disease NEC *see* category M01
 leprosy (*see also* category M01) *see also*
  Leprosy A30.9
 Lyme disease A69.23
 mycobacteria *see also* category M01 A31.8
 parasitic disease NEC *see also* category
  M01 B89
 paratyphoid fever (*see also* category M01)
  see also Fever, paratyphoid A01.4
 rat bite fever *see also* category M01 A25.1
 regional enteritis *see* Enteritis, regional
 respiratory disorder NOS J98.9
 serum sickness *see also* Reaction, serum
  T80.69
 syringomyelia G95.0
 typhoid fever A01.04
epidemic erythema A25.1
- facet joint (see also Spondylosis) M47.819
febrile *see* Fever, rheumatic
gonococcal A54.42
gouty (acute) *see* Gout
in (due to)
 acromegaly *see also* subcategory M14.8
  E22.0

Arthritis, arthritic - *continued*

amyloidosis *see also* subcategory M14.8
 E85.4
bacterial disease *see also* subcategory M01
 A49.9
Behçet's syndrome M35.2
caisson disease *see also* subcategory M14.8
 T70.3
coliform bacilli (Escherichia coli) *see*
 Arthritis, in, pyogenic organism NEC
crystals M11.9
 dicalcium phosphate *see* Arthritis, in,
 crystals, specified type NEC
  hydroxyapatite M11.0-
  pyrophosphate *see* Arthritis, in, crystals,
 specified type NEC
  specified type NEC M11.80
   ankle M11.87-
   elbow M11.82-
   foot joint M11.87-
   hand joint M11.84-
   hip M11.85-
   knee M11.86-
   multiple sites M11.8-
   shoulder M11.81-
   vertebrae M11.88
   wrist M11.83-
dermatoarthritis, lipoid E78.81
dracontiasis (dracunculiasis) *see also*
 category M01 B72
endocrine disorder NEC *see also*
 subcategory M14.8 E34.9
enteritis, infectious NEC *see also* category
 M01 A09
 specified organism NEC *see also* category
  M01 A08.8
erythema
 multiforme *see also* subcategory M14.8
  L51.9
 nodosum *see also* subcategory M14.8
  L52
gout *see* Gout
helminthiasis NEC *see also* category M01
 B83.9
hemochromatosis *see also* subcategory
 M14.8 E83.118
hemoglobinopathy NEC D58.2 *[M36.3]*
hemophilia NEC D66 *[M36.2]*
Hemophilus influenzae M00.8 *[B96.3]*
Henoch (-Schönlein) purpura D69.0
 [M36.4]
hyperparathyroidism NEC *see also*
 subcategory M14.8 E21.3
hypersensitivity reaction NEC T78.49
 [M36.4]
hypogammaglobulinemia *see also*
 subcategory M14.8 D80.1
hypothyroidism NEC *see also* subcategory
 M14.8- E03.9
infection *see* Arthritis, pyogenic or pyemic
 spine *see* Spondylopathy, infective
infectious disease NEC *see* category M01
leprosy *see also* category M01 A30.9
leukemia NEC C95.9 *[M36.1]*
lipoid dermatoarthritis E78.81
Lyme disease A69.23
Mediterranean fever, familial *see also*
 subcategory M14.8 M04.1
Meningococcus A39.83
metabolic disorder NEC *see also*
 subcategory M14.8- E88.9
multiple myelomatosis C90.0 *[M36.1]*
mumps B26.85
mycosis NEC *see also* category M01 B49
myelomatosis (multiple) C90.0 *[M36.1]*
neurological disorder NEC G98.0

Arthritis, arthritic - *continued*

ochronosis *see also* subcategory M14.8
 E70.29
O'nyong-Nyong *see also* category M01
 A92.1
parasitic disease NEC *see also* category
 M01 B89
paratyphoid fever *see also* category M01
 A01.4
Pseudomonas *see* Arthritis, pyogenic,
 bacterial NEC
psoriasis L40.50
pyogenic organism NEC *see* Arthritis,
 pyogenic, bacterial NEC
Reiter's disease *see* Reiter's disease
respiratory disorder NEC *see also*
 subcategory M14.8- J98.9
reticulosis, malignant *see also* subcategory
 M14.8 C86.0
rubella B06.82
Salmonella (arizonae) (cholerae-suis)
 (enteritidis) (typhimurium) A02.23
sarcoidosis D86.86
specified bacteria NEC *see* Arthritis,
 pyogenic, bacterial NEC
sporotrichosis B42.82
syringomyelia G95.0
thalassemia NEC D56.9 *[M36.3]*
tuberculosis *see* Tuberculosis, arthritis
typhoid fever A01.04
urethritis, Reiter's *see* Reiter's disease
viral disease NEC *see also* category M01
 B34.9
infectious or infective *see also* Arthritis,
 pyogenic or pyemic
spine *see* Spondylopathy, infective
juvenile M08.90
 with systemic onset *see* Still's disease
 ankle M08.97-
 elbow M08.92-
 foot joint M08.97-
 hand joint M08.94-
 hip M08.95-
 knee M08.96-
 multiple site M08.99
 pauciarticular M08.40
  ankle M08.47-
  elbow M08.42-
  foot joint M08.47-
  hand joint M08.44-
  hip M08.45-
  knee M08.46-
  shoulder M08.41-
  specified site NEC M08.4A
  vertebrae M08.48
  wrist M08.43-
 psoriatic L40.54
 rheumatoid *see* Arthritis, rheumatoid,
  juvenile
 shoulder M08.91
 vertebra M08.98
 specified site NEC M08.9A
 specified type NEC M08.80
  ankle M08.87-
  elbow M08.82-
  foot joint M08.87-
  hand joint M08.84-
  hip M08.85-
  knee M08.86-
  multiple site M08.89
  shoulder M08.81-
  specified joint NEC M08.88
  vertebrae M08.88
  wrist M08.83-
 wrist M08.93-

Arthritis, arthritic - *continued*
|meaning osteoarthritis *see* Osteoarthritis
|meningococcal A39.83
|menopausal (any site) NEC *see* Arthritis, specified form NEC
|mutilans (psoriatic) L40.52
|mycotic NEC *see also* category M01 B49
|neuropathic (Charcot) *see* Arthropathy, neuropathic
|diabetic *see* Diabetes, arthropathy, neuropathic
|nonsyphilitic NEC G98.0
|syringomyelic G95.0
|ochronotic *see also* subcategory M14.8- E70.29
|palindromic (any site) *see* Rheumatism, palindromic
|pneumococcal M00.10
|ankle M00.17-
|elbow M00.12-
|foot joint *see* Arthritis, pneumococcal, ankle
|hand joint M00.14-
|hip M00.15-
|knee M00.16-
|multiple site M00.19
|shoulder M00.11-
|vertebra M00.18
|wrist M00.13-
|postdysenteric *see* Arthropathy, postdysenteric
|postmeningococcal A39.84
|postrheumatic, chronic *see* Arthropathy, postrheumatic, chronic
|primary progressive *see also* Arthritis, specified form NEC
|spine *see* Spondylitis, ankylosing
|psoriatic L40.50
|purulent (any site except spine) *see* Arthritis, pyogenic or pyemic
|spine *see* Spondylopathy, infective
|pyogenic or pyemic (any site except spine) M00.9
|bacterial NEC M00.80
|ankle M00.87-
|elbow M00.82-
|foot joint *see* Arthritis, pyogenic, bacterial NEC, ankle
|hand joint M00.84-
|hip M00.85-
|knee M00.86-
|multiple site M00.89
|shoulder M00.81-
|vertebra M00.88
|wrist M00.83-
|pneumococcal *see* Arthritis, pneumococcal
|spine *see* Spondylopathy, infective
|staphylococcal *see* Arthritis, staphylococcal
|streptococcal *see* Arthritis, streptococcal NEC
|pneumococcal *see* Arthritis, pneumococcal
|reactive *see* Reiter's disease
|rheumatic *see also* Arthritis, rheumatoid
|acute or subacute *see* Fever, rheumatic
|rheumatoid M06.9
|with
|carditis *see* Rheumatoid, carditis
|endocarditis *see* Rheumatoid, carditis
|heart involvement NEC *see* Rheumatoid, carditis
|lung involvement *see* Rheumatoid, lung
|myocarditis *see* Rheumatoid, carditis
|myopathy *see* Rheumatoid, myopathy
|pericarditis *see* Rheumatoid, carditis
|polyneuropathy *see* Rheumatoid, polyneuropathy

Arthritis, arthritic - *continued*
|rheumatoid factor *see* Arthritis, rheumatoid, seropositive
|splenoadenomegaly and leukopenia *see* Felty's syndrome
|vasculitis *see* Rheumatoid, vasculitis
|visceral involvement NEC *see* Rheumatoid, arthritis, with involvement of organs NEC
|juvenile (with or without rheumatoid factor) M08.00
|ankle M08.07-
|elbow M08.02-
|foot joint M08.07-
|hand joint M08.04-
|hip M08.05-
|knee M08.06-
|multiple site M08.09
|shoulder M08.01-
|vertebra M08.08
|wrist M08.03-
|with systemic onset   *see* Still's disease
|specified site NEC M08.0A
|seronegative M06.00
|ankle M06.07-
|elbow M06.02-
|foot joint M06.07-
|hand joint M06.04-
|hip M06.05-
|knee M06.06-
|multiple site M06.09
|shoulder M06.01-
|specified site NEC M06.0A
|vertebra M06.08
|wrist M06.03-
|seropositive M05.9
|specified NEC M05.80
|ankle M05.87-
|elbow M05.82-
|foot joint M05.87-
|hand joint M05.84-
|hip M05.85-
|knee M05.86-
|multiple sites M05.89
|shoulder M05.81-
|specified site NEC M05.8A
|vertebra *see* Spondylitis, ankylosing
|wrist M05.83-
|without organ involvement M05.70
|ankle M05.77-
|elbow M05.72-
|foot joint M05.77-
|hand joint M05.74-
|hip M05.75-
|knee M05.76-
|multiple sites M05.79
|shoulder M05.71-
|specified site NEC M05.8A
|vertebra *see* Spondylitis, ankylosing
|wrist M05.73-
|specified site NEC M05.7A
|specified type NEC M06.80
|ankle M06.87-
|elbow M06.82-
|foot joint M06.87-
|hand joint M06.84-
|hip M06.85-
|knee M06.86-
|multiple site M06.89
|shoulder M06.81-
|specified site NEC M06.8A
|vertebra M06.88
|wrist M06.83-
|spine *see* Spondylitis, ankylosing
|rubella B06.82
|scorbutic *see also* subcategory M14.8- E54
|senile or senescent *see* Osteoarthritis

Arthritis, arthritic - *continued*
|septic (any site except spine) *see* Arthritis, pyogenic or pyemic
|spine *see* Spondylopathy, infective
|serum (nontherapeutic) (therapeutic) *see* Arthropathy, postimmunization
|specified form NEC M13.80
|ankle M13.87-
|elbow M13.82-
|foot joint M13.87-
|hand joint M13.84-
|hip M13.85-
|knee M13.86-
|multiple site M13.89
|shoulder M13.81-
|specified joint NEC M13.88
|wrist M13.83-
|spine *see also* Spondylosis
|infectious or infective NEC *see* Spondylopathy, infective
|Marie-Strumpell *see* Spondylitis, ankylosing
|pyogenic *see* Spondylopathy, infective
|rheumatoid *see* Spondylitis, ankylosing
|traumatic (old) *see* Spondylopathy, traumatic
|tuberculous A18.01
|staphylococcal M00.00
|ankle M00.07-
|elbow M00.02-
|foot joint *see* Arthritis, staphylococcal, ankle
|hand joint M00.04-
|hip M00.05-
|knee M00.06-
|multiple site M00.09
|shoulder M00.01-
|vertebra M00.08
|wrist M00.03-
|streptococcal NEC M00.20
|ankle M00.27-
|elbow M00.22-
|foot joint *see* Arthritis, streptococcal, ankle
|hand joint M00.24-
|hip M00.25-
|knee M00.26-
|multiple site M00.29
|shoulder M00.21-
|vertebra M00.28
|wrist M00.23-
|suppurative *see* Arthritis, pyogenic or pyemic
|syphilitic (late) A52.16
|congenital A50.55 *[M12.80]*
|syphilitica deformans (Charcot) A52.16
|temporomandibular joint M26.64-
|toxic of menopause (any site) *see* Arthritis, specified form NEC
|transient *see* Arthropathy, specified form NEC
|traumatic (chronic) *see* Arthropathy, traumatic
|tuberculous A18.02
|spine A18.01
|uratic *see* Gout
|urethritica (Reiter's) *see* Reiter's disease
|vertebral *see* Spondylopathy, inflammatory
|villous (any site) *see* Arthropathy, specified form NEC
Arthrocele *see* Effusion, joint
Arthrodesis status Z98.1
Arthrodynia *see also* Pain, joint
Arthrodysplasia Q74.9
Arthrofibrosis, joint *see* Ankylosis
Arthrogryposis (congenital) Q68.8
|multiplex congenita Q74.3
Arthrokatadysis M24.7

Arthropathy see also Arthritis M12.9
- |Charcot's see Arthropathy, neuropathic
  - |diabetic see Diabetes, arthropathy, neuropathic
  - |syringomyelic G95.0
- |cricoarytenoid J38.7
- |crystal (-induced) see Arthritis, in, crystals
- |diabetic NEC see Diabetes, arthropathy
- |distal interphalangeal, psoriatic L40.51
- |enteropathic M07.60
  - |ankle M07.67-
  - |elbow M07.62-
  - |foot joint M07.67-
  - |hand joint M07.64-
  - |hip M07.65-
  - |knee M07.66-
  - |multiple site M07.69
  - |shoulder M07.61-
  - |vertebra M07.68
  - |wrist M07.63-
- - facet joint (see also Spondylosis) M47.819
- |following intestinal bypass M02.00
  - |ankle M02.07-
  - |elbow M02.02-
  - |foot joint M02.07-
  - |hand joint M02.04-
  - |hip M02.05-
  - |knee M02.06-
  - |multiple site M02.09
  - |shoulder M02.01-
  - |vertebra M02.08
  - |wrist M02.03-
- |gouty see also Gout
  - |in (due to)
    - |Lesch-Nyhan syndrome E79.1 [M14.8]
    - |sickle-cell disorders D57 [M14.8]
- |hemophilic NEC D66 [M36.2]
  - in (due to)
    - |hyperparathyroidism NEC E21.3 [M14.8]
    - |metabolic disease NOS E88.9 [M14.8]
- |in (due to)
  - |acromegaly E22.0 [M14.8]
  - |amyloidosis E85.4 [M14.8]
  - |blood disorder NOS D75.9 [M36.3]
  - |diabetes see Diabetes, arthropathy
  - |endocrine disease NOS E34.9 [M14.8]
  - |erythema
    - |multiforme L51.9 [M14.8]
    - |nodosum L52 [M14.8]
  - |hemochromatosis E83.118 [M14.8]
  - |hemoglobinopathy NEC D58.2 [M36.3]
  - |hemophilia NEC D66 [M36.2]
  - |Henoch-Schönlein purpura D69.0 [M36.4]
  - |hyperthyroidism E05.90 [M14.8]
  - |hypothyroidism E03.9 [M14.8]
  - |infective endocarditis I33.0 [M12.80]
  - |leukemia NEC C95.9 [M36.1]
  - |malignant histiocytosis C96.A [M36.1]
  - |metabolic disease NOS E88.9 [M14.8]
  - |multiple myeloma C90.0 [M36.1]
  - |neoplastic disease NOS (see also Neoplasm) D49.9 [M36.1]
  - |nutritional deficiency see also subcategory M14.8- E63.9
  - |psoriasis NOS L40.50
  - |sarcoidosis D86.86
  - |syphilis (late) A52.77
    - |congenital A50.55 [M12.80]
  - |thyrotoxicosis see also subcategory M14.8- E05.90
  - |ulcerative colitis K51.90 [M07.60]
  - |viral hepatitis (postinfectious) NEC B19.9 [M12.80]
  - |Whipple's disease see also subcategory M14.8- K90.81

Arthropathy - continued
- |Jaccoud see Arthropathy, postrheumatic, chronic
- |juvenile see Arthritis, juvenile
  - |psoriatic L40.54
- |mutilans (psoriatic) L40.52
- |neuropathic (Charcot) M14.60
  - |ankle M14.67-
  - |diabetic see Diabetes, arthropathy, neuropathic
  - |elbow M14.62-
  - |foot joint M14.67-
  - |hand joint M14.64-
  - |hip M14.65-
  - |knee M14.66-
  - |multiple site M14.69
  - |nonsyphilitic NEC G98.0
  - |shoulder M14.61-
  - |syringomyelic G95.0
  - |vertebra M14.68
  - |wrist M14.63-
- |osteopulmonary see Osteoarthropathy, hypertrophic, specified NEC
- |postdysenteric M02.10
  - |ankle M02.17-
  - |elbow M02.12-
  - |foot joint M02.17-
  - |hand joint M02.14-
  - |hip M02.15-
  - |knee M02.16-
  - |multiple site M02.19
  - |shoulder M02.11-
  - |vertebra M02.18
  - |wrist M02.13-
- |postimmunization M02.20
  - |ankle M02.27-
  - |elbow M02.22-
  - |foot joint M02.27-
  - |hand joint M02.24-
  - |hip M02.25-
  - |knee M02.26-
  - |multiple site M02.29
  - |shoulder M02.21-
  - |vertebra M02.28
  - |wrist M02.23-
- |postinfectious NEC B99 [M12.80]
  - in (due to)
    - |enteritis due to Yersinia enterocolitica A04.6 [M12.80]
    - |syphilis A52.77
    - |viral hepatitis NEC B19.9 [M12.80]
- |postrheumatic, chronic (Jaccoud) M12.00
  - |ankle M12.07-
  - |elbow M12.02-
  - |foot joint M12.07-
  - |hand joint M12.04-
  - |hip M12.05-
  - |knee M12.06-
  - |multiple site M12.09
  - |shoulder M12.01-
  - |specified joint NEC M12.08
  - |vertebrae M12.08
  - |wrist M12.03-
- |psoriatic NEC L40.59
  - |interphalangeal, distal L40.51
- |reactive M02.9
  - |in (due to)
    - |infective endocarditis I33.0 [M02.9]
  - |specified type NEC M02.80
    - |ankle M02.87-
    - |elbow M02.82-
    - |foot joint M02.87-
    - |hand joint M02.84-
    - |hip M02.85-
    - |knee M02.86-
    - |multiple site M02.89

Arthropathy - continued
- |shoulder M02.81-
- |vertebra M02.88
- |wrist M02.83-
- |specified form NEC M12.80
  - |ankle M12.87-
  - |elbow M12.82-
  - |foot joint M12.87-
  - |hand joint M12.84-
  - |hip M12.85-
  - |knee M12.86-
  - |multiple site M12.89
  - |shoulder M12.81-
  - |specified joint NEC M12.88
  - |vertebrae M12.88
  - |wrist M12.83-
- |syringomyelic G95.0
- |tabes dorsalis A52.16
- |tabetic A52.16
- |temporomandibular joint M26.65-
- |transient see Arthropathy, specified form NEC
- |traumatic M12.50
  - |ankle M12.57-
  - |elbow M12.52-
  - |foot joint M12.57-
  - |hand joint M12.54-
  - |hip M12.55-
  - |knee M12.56-
  - |multiple site M12.59
  - |shoulder M12.51-
  - |specified joint NEC M12.58
  - |vertebrae M12.58
  - |wrist M12.53-
Arthropyosis see Arthritis, pyogenic or pyemic
Arthrosis (deformans) (degenerative) (localized) see also Osteoarthritis M19.90
- |spine see Spondylosis
Arthus' phenomenon or reaction T78.41
- |due to
  - |drug see Table of Drugs and Chemicals, by drug
Articular see condition
Articulation, reverse (teeth) M26.24
Artificial
- |insemination complication see Complications, artificial, fertilization
- |opening status (functioning) (without complication) Z93.9
  - |anus (colostomy) Z93.3
  - |colostomy Z93.3
  - |cystostomy Z93.50
    - |appendico-vesicostomy Z93.52
    - |cutaneous Z93.51
    - |specified NEC Z93.59
  - |enterostomy Z93.4
  - |gastrostomy Z93.1
  - |ileostomy Z93.2
  - |intestinal tract NEC Z93.4
  - |jejunostomy Z93.4
  - |nephrostomy Z93.6
  - |specified site NEC Z93.8
  - |tracheostomy Z93.0
  - |ureterostomy Z93.6
  - |urethrostomy Z93.6
  - |urinary tract NEC Z93.6
  - |vagina Z93.8
- |vagina status Z93.8
Arytenoid see condition
Asbestosis (occupational) J61
ASC-H (atypical squamous cells cannot exclude high grade squamous intraepithelial lesion on cytologic smear)
- |anus R85.611
- |cervix R87.611
- |vagina R87.621

ASC-US (atypical squamous cells of undetermined significance on cytologic smear)
|anus R85.610
|cervix R87.610
|vagina R87.620
Ascariasis B77.9
|with
|complications NEC B77.89
|intestinal complications B77.0
|pneumonia, pneumonitis B77.81
Ascaridosis, ascaridiasis see Ascariasis
Ascaris (infection) (infestation) (lumbricoides) see Ascariasis
Ascending see condition
Aschoff's bodies see Myocarditis, rheumatic
Ascites (abdominal) R18.8
|cardiac (see also Failure, heart, right) I50.810
|chylous (nonfilarial) I89.8
|filarial see Infestation, filarial
|due to
|cirrhosis, alcoholic K70.31
|hepatitis
|alcoholic K70.11
|chronic active K71.51
|S. japonicum B65.2
|heart (see also Failure, heart, right) I50.810
|malignant R18.0
|pseudochylous R18.8
|syphilitic A52.74
|tuberculous A18.31
Aseptic see condition
Asherman's syndrome N85.6
Asialia K11.7
Asiatic cholera see Cholera
Asimultagnosia (simultanagnosia) R48.3
Askin's tumor see Neoplasm, connective tissue, malignant
Asocial personality F60.2
Asomatognosia R41.4
Aspartylglucosaminuria E77.1
Asperger's disease or syndrome F84.5
Aspergilloma see Aspergillosis
Aspergillosis (with pneumonia) B44.9
|bronchopulmonary, allergic B44.81
|disseminated B44.7
|generalized B44.7
|pulmonary NEC B44.1
|allergic B44.81
|invasive B44.0
|specified NEC B44.89
|tonsillar B44.2
Aspergillus (flavus) (fumigatus) (infection) (terreus) see Aspergillosis
Aspermatogenesis see Azoospermia
Aspermia (testis) see Azoospermia
Asphyxia, asphyxiation (by) R09.01
|antenatal P84
|birth P84
|bunny bag see Asphyxia, due to, mechanical threat to breathing, trapped in bed clothes
|crushing S28.0
|drowning T75.1
|gas, fumes, or vapor see Table of Drugs and Chemicals
|inhalation see Inhalation
|intrauterine P84
|local I73.00
|with gangrene I73.01
|mucus see also Foreign body, respiratory tract, causing asphyxia
|newborn P84
|pathological R09.01
|postnatal P84

Asphyxia, asphyxiation - continued
|mechanical see Asphyxia, due to, mechanical threat to breathing
|prenatal P84
|reticularis R23.1
|strangulation see Asphyxia, due to, mechanical threat to breathing
|submersion T75.1
|traumatic T71.9
|due to
|crushed chest S28.0
|foreign body (in) see Foreign body, respiratory tract, causing asphyxia
|low oxygen content of ambient air T71.20
|due to
|being trapped in
|low oxygen environment T71.29
|in car trunk T71.221
|circumstances undetermined T71.224
|done with intent to harm by
|another person T71.223
|self T71.222
|in refrigerator T71.231
|circumstances undetermined T71.234
|done with intent to harm by
|another person T71.233
|self T71.232
|cave-in T71.21
|mechanical threat to breathing (accidental) T71.191
|circumstances undetermined T71.194
|done with intent to harm by
|another person T71.193
|self T71.192
|hanging T71.161
|circumstances undetermined T71.164
|done with intent to harm by
|another person T71.163
|self T71.162
|plastic bag T71.121
|circumstances undetermined T71.124
|done with intent to harm by
|another person T71.123
|self T71.122
|smothering
|in furniture T71.151
|circumstances undetermined T71.154
|done with intent to harm by
|another person T71.153
|self T71.152
|under
|another person's body T71.141
|circumstances undetermined T71.144
|done with intent to harm T71.143
|pillow T71.111
|circumstances undetermined T71.114
|done with intent to harm by
|another person T71.113
|self T71.112
|trapped in bed clothes T71.131
|circumstances undetermined T71.134
|done with intent to harm by
|another person T71.133
|self T71.132
|vomiting, vomitus see Foreign body, respiratory tract, causing asphyxia
Aspiration
|amniotic (clear) fluid (newborn) P24.10
|with
|pneumonia (pneumonitis) P24.11
|respiratory symptoms P24.11
|blood

Aspiration - continued
|newborn (without respiratory symptoms) P24.20
|with
|pneumonia (pneumonitis) P24.21
|respiratory symptoms P24.21
|specified age NEC see Foreign body, respiratory tract
|bronchitis J69.0
|food or foreign body - see Foreign body, by site |liquor (amnii) (newborn) P24.10
|with
|pneumonia (pneumonitis) P24.11
|respiratory symptoms P24.11
|meconium (newborn) (without respiratory symptoms) P24.00
|with
|pneumonitis (pneumonitis) P24.01
|respiratory symptoms P24.01
|milk (newborn) (without respiratory symptoms) P24.30
|with
|pneumonia (pneumonitis) P24.31
|respiratory symptoms P24.31
|specified age NEC see Foreign body, respiratory tract
|mucus see also Foreign body, by site, causing asphyxia
|newborn P24.10
|with
|pneumonia (pneumonitis) P24.11
|respiratory symptoms P24.11
|neonatal P24.9
|specific NEC (without respiratory symptoms) P24.80
|with
|pneumonia (pneumonitis) P24.81
|respiratory symptoms P24.81
|newborn P24.9
|specific NEC (without respiratory symptoms) P24.80
|with
|pneumonia (pneumonitis) P24.81
|respiratory symptoms P24.81
|pneumonia J69.0
|pneumonitis J69.0
|syndrome of newborn see Aspiration, by substance, with pneumonia
|vernix caseosa (newborn) P24.80
|with
|pneumonia (pneumonitis) P24.81
-|respiratory symptoms P24.81
|vomitus see also Foreign body, respiratory tract
|newborn (without respiratory symptoms) P24.30
|with
|pneumonia (pneumonitis) P24.31
|respiratory symptoms P24.31
Asplenia (congenital) Q89.01
|postsurgical Z90.81
Assam fever B55.0
Assault, sexual see Maltreatment
Assmann's focus NEC A15.0
Astasia (-Abasia) (hysterical) F44.4
Asteatosis cutis L85.3
Astereognosia, astereognosis R48.1
Asterixis R27.8
|in liver disease K71.3
Asteroid hyalitis see Deposit, crystalline
Asthenia, asthenic R53.1
|cardiac see also Failure, heart I50.9
|psychogenic F45.8
|cardiovascular see also Failure, heart I50.9
|psychogenic F45.8

Asthenia, asthenic - *continued*
|heart *see also* Failure, heart I50.9
  |psychogenic F45.8
|hysterical F44.4
|myocardial *see also* Failure, heart I50.9
  |psychogenic F45.8
|nervous F48.8
|neurocirculatory F45.8
|neurotic F48.8
|psychogenic F48.8
|psychoneurotic F48.8
|psychophysiologic F48.8
|reaction (psychophysiologic) F48.8
|senile R54
Asthenopia *see also* Discomfort, visual
|hysterical F44.6
|psychogenic F44.6
Asthenospermia *see* Abnormal, specimen, male
  genital organs
Asthma, asthmatic (bronchial) (catarrh)
  (spasmodic) J45.909
|with
  |chronic obstructive bronchitis J44.9
    |with
      |acute lower respiratory infection J44.0
      |exacerbation (acute) J44.1
  |chronic obstructive pulmonary disease J44.9
    |with
      |acute lower respiratory infection J44.0
      |exacerbation (acute) J44.1
  |exacerbation (acute) J45.901
  |hay fever *see* Asthma, allergic extrinsic
  |rhinitis, allergic *see* Asthma, allergic
    extrinsic
  |status asthmaticus J45.902
|allergic extrinsic J45.909
  |with
    |exacerbation (acute) J45.901
    |status asthmaticus J45.902
|atopic *see* Asthma, allergic extrinsic
|cardiac *see* Failure, ventricular, left
|cardiobronchial I50.1
|childhood J45.909
  |with
    |exacerbation (acute) J45.901
    |status asthmaticus J45.902
|chronic obstructive J44.9
  |with
    |acute lower respiratory infection J44.0
    |exacerbation (acute) J44.1
|collier's J60
|cough variant J45.991
|detergent J69.8
|due to
  |detergent J69.8
  |inhalation of fumes J68.3
|eosinophilic J82.83
|extrinsic, allergic *see* Asthma, allergic
  extrinsic
|grinder's J62.8
|hay *see* Asthma, allergic extrinsic
|heart I50.1
|idiosyncratic *see* Asthma, nonallergic
|intermittent (mild) J45.20
  |with
    |exacerbation (acute) J45.21
    |status asthmaticus J45.22
|intrinsic, nonallergic *see* Asthma, nonallergic
|Kopp's E32.8
|late-onset J45.909
  |with
    |exacerbation (acute) J45.901
    |status asthmaticus J45.902
|mild intermittent J45.20
  |with

Asthma, asthmatic - *continued*
    |exacerbation (acute) J45.21
    |status asthmaticus J45.22
|mild persistent J45.30
  |with
    |exacerbation (acute) J45.31
    |status asthmaticus J45.32
|Millar's (laryngismus stridulus) J38.5
|miner's J60
|mixed J45.909
  |with
    |exacerbation (acute) J45.901
    |status asthmaticus J45.902
|moderate persistent J45.40
  |with
    |exacerbation (acute) J45.41
    |status asthmaticus J45.42
|nervous *see* Asthma, nonallergic
|nonallergic (intrinsic) J45.909
  |with
    |exacerbation (acute) J45.901
    |status asthmaticus J45.902
|persistent
  |mild J45.30
    |with
      |exacerbation (acute) J45.31
      |status asthmaticus J45.32
  |moderate J45.40
    |with
      |exacerbation (acute) J45.41
      |status asthmaticus J45.42
  |severe J45.50
    |with
      |exacerbation (acute) J45.51
      |status asthmaticus J45.52
|platinum J45.998
|pneumoconiotic NEC J64
|potter's J62.8
|predominantly allergic J45.909
|psychogenic F54
|pulmonary eosinophilic J82
|red cedar J67.8
|Rostan's I50.1
|sandblaster's J62.8
|sequoiosis J67.8
|severe persistent J45.50
  |with
    |exacerbation (acute) J45.51
    |status asthmaticus J45.52
|specified NEC J45.998
|stonemason's J62.8
|thymic E32.8
|tuberculous *see* Tuberculosis, pulmonary
|Wichmann's (laryngismus stridulus) J38.5
|wood J67.8
Astigmatism (compound) (congenital) H52.20-
|irregular H52.21-
|regular H52.22-
Astraphobia F40.220
Astroblastoma
|specified site *see* Neoplasm, malignant, by site
|unspecified site C71.9
Astrocytoma (cystic)
|anaplastic
  |specified site *see* Neoplasm, malignant, by
    site
  |unspecified site C71.9
|fibrillary
  |specified site *see* Neoplasm, malignant, by
    site
  |unspecified site C71.9
|fibrous
  |specified site *see* Neoplasm, malignant, by
    site
  |unspecified site C71.9

Astrocytoma (cystic) - *continued*
|gemistocytic
  |specified site *see* Neoplasm, malignant, by
    site
  |unspecified site C71.9
|juvenile
  |specified site *see* Neoplasm, malignant, by
    site
  |unspecified site C71.9
|pilocytic
  |specified site *see* Neoplasm, malignant, by
    site
  |unspecified site C71.9
|piloid
  |specified site *see* Neoplasm, malignant, by
    site
  |unspecified site C71.9
|protoplasmic
  |specified site *see* Neoplasm, malignant, by
    site
  |unspecified site C71.9
|specified site NEC *see* Neoplasm, malignant,
  by site
|subependymal D43.2
  |giant cell
    |specified site *see* Neoplasm, uncertain
      behavior, by site
    |unspecified site D43.2
  |specified site *see* Neoplasm, uncertain
    behavior, by site
  |unspecified site D43.2
|unspecified site C71.9
Astroglioma
|specified site *see* Neoplasm, malignant, by site
|unspecified site C71.9
Asymbolia R48.8
Asymmetry *see also* Distortion
|between native and reconstructed breast N65.1
|face Q67.0
|jaw (lower) *see* Anomaly, dentofacial, jaw-
  cranial base relationship, asymmetry
Asynergia, asynergy R27.8
|ventricular I51.89
Asystole (heart) *see* Arrest, cardiac
At risk
|for
  |dental caries Z91.849
    |high Z91.843
    |low Z91.841
    |moderate Z91.842
  |falling Z91.81
Ataxia, ataxy, ataxic R27.0
|acute R27.8
|autosomal recessive Friedreich G11.11
|brain (hereditary) G11.9
|cerebellar (hereditary) G11.9
  |with defective DNA repair G11.3
  |alcoholic G31.2
  |early-onset G11.10
  |in
    |alcoholism G31.2
    |myxedema E03.9 [*G13.2*]
    |neoplastic disease *see also* Neoplasm
      D49.9 [*G32.81*]
    |specified disease NEC G32.81
  |late-onset (Marie's) G11.2
  |with
    |essential tremor G11.19
    |myoclonus [Hunt's ataxia] G11.19
    |retained tendon reflexes G11.19
|cerebral (hereditary) G11.9
|congenital nonprogressive G11.0
|family, familial *see* Ataxia, hereditary
|following
  |cerebrovascular disease I69.993
    |cerebral infarction I69.393
    |intracerebral hemorrhage I69.193

Ataxia, ataxy, ataxic - *continued*
  |nontraumatic intracranial hemorrhage
    NEC I69.293
    |specified disease NEC I69.893
    |subarachnoid hemorrhage I69.093
  |Friedreich's (heredofamilial) (cerebellar)
    (spinal) (with retained reflexes) G11.1
  |gait R26.0
    |hysterical F44.4
  |general R27.8
  |gluten M35.9 [*G32.81*]
    |with celiac disease K90.0 [*G32.81*]
  |hereditary G11.9
    |with neuropathy G60.2
    |cerebellar *see* Ataxia, cerebellar
    |spastic G11.4
    |specified NEC G11.8
    |spinal (Friedreich's) G11.11
  |heredofamilial *see* Ataxia, hereditary
  |Hunt's G11.19
  |hysterical F44.4
  |locomotor (progressive) (syphilitic) (partial)
    (spastic) A52.11
    |diabetic *see* Diabetes, ataxia
  |Marie's (cerebellar) (heredofamilial) (late
    |onset) G11.2
  |nonorganic origin F44.4
  |nonprogressive, congenital G11.0
  |psychogenic F44.4
  |Roussy-Lévy G60.0
  |Sanger-Brown's (hereditary) G11.2
  |spastic hereditary G11.4
  |spinal
    |hereditary (Friedreich's) G11.11
    |progressive (syphilitic) A52.11
  |spinocerebellar, X-linked recessive G11.19
  |telangiectasia (Louis-Bar) G11.3
Ataxia-Telangiectasia (Louis-Bar) G11.3
Atelectasis (massive) (partial) (pressure)
  (pulmonary) J98.11
  |newborn P28.10
    |due to resorption P28.11
    |partial P28.19
    |primary P28.0
    |secondary P28.19
  |primary (newborn) P28.0
  |tuberculous *see* Tuberculosis, pulmonary
Atelocardia Q24.9
Atelomyelia Q06.1
Atheroembolism
  |of
    |extremities
      |lower I75.02-
      |upper I75.01-
    |kidney I75.81
    |specified NEC I75.89
Atheroma, atheromatous *see also*
  Arteriosclerosis I70.90
  |aorta, aortic I70.0
    |valve *see also* Endocarditis, aortic I35.8
  |aorto-iliac I70.0
  |artery *see* Arteriosclerosis
  |basilar (artery) I67.2
  |carotid (artery) (common) (internal) I67.2
  |cerebral (arteries) I67.2
  |coronary (artery) I25.10
    |with angina pectoris *see* Arteriosclerosis,
      coronary (artery),
  |degeneration *see* Arteriosclerosis
  |heart, cardiac *see* Disease, heart, ischemic,
    atherosclerotic
  |mitral (valve) I34.8

Atheroma - *continued*
  |myocardium, myocardial *see* Disease, heart,
    ischemic, atherosclerotic pulmonary valve
    (heart) *see also* Endocarditis, pulmonary
    I37.8
  |tricuspid (heart) (valve) I36.8
  |valve, valvular *see* Endocarditis
  |vertebral (artery) I67.2
Atheromatosis *see* Arteriosclerosis
Atherosclerosis *see also* Arteriosclerosis
  |coronary
    |artery I25.10
      |with angina pectoris *see* Arteriosclerosis,
      coronary (artery),
      |due to
        |calcified coronary lesion (severely)
          I25.84
        |lipid rich plaque I25.83
    |transplanted heart I25.811
      |bypass graft I25.812
        |with angina pectoris *see* Arteriosclerosis,
          coronary (artery),
      |native coronary artery I25.811
        |with angina pectoris *see* Arteriosclerosis,
          coronary (artery),
Athetosis (acquired) R25.8
  |bilateral (congenital) G80.3
  |congenital (bilateral) (double) G80.3
  |double (congenital) G80.3
  |unilateral R25.8
Athlete's
  |foot B35.3
  |heart I51.7
Athrepsia E41
Athyrea (acquired) *see also* Hypothyroidism
  |congenital E03.1
Atonia, atony, atonic
  |bladder (sphincter) (neurogenic) N31.2
  |capillary I78.8
  |cecum K59.89
    |psychogenic F45.8
  |colon *see* Atony, intestine
  |congenital P94.2
  |esophagus K22.89
  |intestine K59.89
    |psychogenic F45.8
  |stomach K31.89
    |neurotic or psychogenic F45.8
  |uterus (during labor) O62.2
    |with hemorrhage (postpartum) O72.1
    |postpartum (with hemorrhage) O72.1
      |without hemorrhage O75.89
Atopy *see* History, allergy
Atransferrinemia, congenital E88.09
Atresia, atretic
  |alimentary organ or tract NEC Q45.8
    |upper Q40.8
  |ani, anus, anal (canal) Q42.3
    |with fistula Q42.2
  |aorta (ring) Q25.29
  |aortic (orifice) (valve) Q23.0
    |arch Q25.21
    |congenital with hypoplasia of ascending
      aorta and defective development of left
      ventricle (with mitral stenosis) Q23.4
    |in hypoplastic left heart syndrome Q23.4
  |aqueduct of Sylvius Q03.0
    |with spina bifida *see* Spina bifida, with
      hydrocephalus
  |artery NEC Q27.8
    |cerebral Q28.3
    |coronary Q24.5
    |digestive system Q27.8
    |eye Q15.8
    |lower limb Q27.8
    |pulmonary Q25.5
    |specified site NEC Q27.8

Atresia, atretic - *continued*
  |umbilical Q27.0
  |upper limb Q27.8
  |auditory canal (external) Q16.1
  |bile duct (common) (congenital) (hepatic)
    Q44.2
    |acquired *see* Obstruction, bile duct
  |bladder (neck) Q64.39
    |obstruction Q64.31
  |bronchus Q32.4
  |cecum Q42.8
  |cervix (acquired) N88.2
    |congenital Q51.828
    |in pregnancy or childbirth *see* Anomaly,
      cervix, in pregnancy or childbirth
      |causing obstructed labor O65.5
  |choana Q30.0
  |colon Q42.9
    |specified NEC Q42.8
  |common duct Q44.2
  |cricoid cartilage Q31.8
  |cystic duct Q44.2
    |acquired K82.8
      |with obstruction K82.0
  |digestive organs NEC Q45.8
  |duodenum Q41.0
  |ear canal Q16.1
  |ejaculatory duct Q55.4
  |epiglottis Q31.8
  |esophagus Q39.0
    |with tracheoesophageal fistula Q39.1
  |eustachian tube Q17.8
  |fallopian tube (congenital) Q50.6
    |acquired N97.1
  |follicular cyst N83.0-
  |foramen of
    |Luschka Q03.1
      |with spina bifida *see* Spina bifida, with
        hydrocephalus
    |Magendie Q03.1
      |with spina bifida *see* Spina bifida, with
        hydrocephalus
  |gallbladder Q44.1
  |genital organ
    |external
      |female Q52.79
      |male Q55.8
    |internal
      |female Q52.8
      |male Q55.8
  |glottis Q31.8
  |gullet Q39.0
    |with tracheoesophageal fistula Q39.1
  |heart valve NEC Q24.8
    |pulmonary Q22.0
    |tricuspid Q22.4
  |hymen Q52.3
    |acquired (postinfective) N89.6
  |ileum Q41.2
  |intestine (small) Q41.9
    |large Q42.9
      |specified NEC Q42.8
  |iris, filtration angle Q15.0
  |jejunum Q41.1
  |lacrimal apparatus Q10.4
  |larynx Q31.8
  |meatus urinarius Q64.33
  |mitral valve Q23.2
    |in hypoplastic left heart syndrome Q23.4
  |nares (anterior) (posterior) Q30.0
  |nasopharynx Q34.8
  |nose, nostril Q30.0
    |acquired J34.89
  |organ or site NEC Q89.8
  |osseous meatus (ear) Q16.1
  |oviduct (congenital) Q50.6
    |acquired N97.1

Atresia, atretic - *continued*
| parotid duct Q38.4
|| acquired K11.8
| pulmonary (artery) Q25.5
|| valve Q22.0
| pulmonic Q22.0
| pupil Q13.2
| rectum Q42.1
|| with fistula Q42.0
| salivary duct Q38.4
|| acquired K11.8
| sublingual duct Q38.4
|| acquired K11.8
| submandibular duct Q38.4
|| acquired K11.8
| submaxillary duct Q38.4
|| acquired K11.8
| thyroid cartilage Q31.8
| trachea Q32.1
| tricuspid valve Q22.4
| ureter Q62.10
|| pelvic junction Q62.11
|| vesical orifice Q62.12
| ureteropelvic junction Q62.11
| ureterovesical orifice Q62.12
| urethra (valvular) Q64.39
|| stricture Q64.32
| urinary tract NEC Q64.8
| uterus Q51.818
|| acquired N85.8
| vagina (congenital) Q52.4
|| acquired (postinfectional) (senile) N89.5
| vas deferens Q55.3
| vascular NEC Q27.8
|| cerebral Q28.3
|| digestive system Q27.8
|| lower limb Q27.8
|| specified site NEC Q27.8
|| upper limb Q27.8
| vein NEC Q27.8
|| digestive system Q27.8
|| great Q26.8
|| lower limb Q27.8
|| portal Q26.5
|| pulmonary Q26.4
||| partial Q26.3
||| total Q26.2
|| specified site NEC Q27.8
|| upper limb Q27.8
| vena cava (inferior) (superior) Q26.8
| vesicourethral orifice Q64.31
| vulva Q52.79
|| acquired N90.5
Atrichia, atrichosis *see* Alopecia
Atrophia *see also* Atrophy
| cutis senilis L90.8
|| due to radiation L57.8
| gyrata of choroid and retina H31.23
| senilis R54
|| dermatological L90.8
||| due to radiation (nonionizing) (solar) L57.8
| unguium L60.3
|| congenita Q84.6
Atrophie blanche (en plaque) (de Milian) L95.0
Atrophoderma, atrophoderma (of) L90.9
| diffusum (idiopathic) L90.4
| maculatum L90.8
|| et striatum L90.8
||| due to syphilis A52.79
|| syphilitic A51.39
| neuriticum L90.8
| Pasini and Pierini L90.3
| pigmentosum Q82.1
| reticulatum symmetricum faciei L66.4

Atrophoderma - *continued*
| senile L90.8
|| due to radiation (nonionizing) (solar) L57.8
| vermiculata (cheeks) L66.4
Atrophy, atrophic (of)
| adrenal (capsule) (gland) E27.49
|| primary (autoimmune) E27.1
| alveolar process or ridge (edentulous) K08.20
| anal sphincter (disuse) N81.84
| appendix K38.8
| arteriosclerotic *see* Arteriosclerosis
| bile duct (common) (hepatic) K83.8
| bladder N32.89
|| neurogenic N31.8
| blanche (en plaque) (of Milian) L95.0
| bone (senile) NEC *see also* Disorder, bone, specified type NEC
|| due to
||| tabes dorsalis (neurogenic) A52.11
| brain (cortex) (progressive) G31.9
|| frontotemporal circumscribed G31.01 *[F02.80]*
||| with behavioral disturbance G31.01 *[F02.81]*
|| senile NEC G31.1
| breast N64.2
|| obstetric *see* Disorder, breast, specified type NEC
| buccal cavity K13.79
| cardiac *see* Degeneration, myocardial
| cartilage (infectional) (joint) *see* Disorder, cartilage, specified NEC
| cerebellar *see* Atrophy, brain
| cerebral *see* Atrophy, brain
| cervix (mucosa) (senile) (uteri) N88.8
|| menopausal N95.8
| Charcot-Marie-Tooth G60.0
| choroid (central) (macular) (myopic) (retina) H31.10-
|| diffuse secondary H31.12-
|| gyrate H31.23
|| senile H31.11-
| ciliary body *see* Atrophy, iris
| conjunctiva (senile) H11.89
| corpus cavernosum N48.89
| cortical *see* Atrophy, brain
| cystic duct K82.8
| Déjérine-Thomas G23.8
| disuse NEC *see* Atrophy, muscle
| Duchenne-Aran G12.21
| ear H93.8-
| edentulous alveolar ridge K08.20
| endometrium (senile) N85.8
|| cervix N88.8
| enteric K63.89
| epididymis N50.89
| eyeball *see* Disorder, globe, degenerated condition, atrophy
| eyelid (senile) *see* Disorder, eyelid, degenerative
| facial (skin) L90.9
| fallopian tube (senile) N83.32-
|| with ovary N83.33-
| fascioscapulohumeral (Landouzy | Déjérine) G71.02
| fatty, thymus (gland) E32.8
| gallbladder K82.8
| gastric K29.40
|| with bleeding K29.41
| gastrointestinal K63.89
| glandular I89.8
| globe H44.52-
| gum *see* Recession, gingival
| hair L67.8
| heart (brown) *see* Degeneration, myocardial
| hemifacial Q67.4

Atrophy, atrophic (of) - *continued*
| Romberg G51.8
| infantile E41
|| paralysis, acute *see* Poliomyelitis, paralytic
| intestine K63.89
| iris (essential) (progressive) H21.26-
|| specified NEC H21.29
| kidney (senile) (terminal) *see also* Sclerosis, renal N26.1
|| congenital or infantile Q60.5
||| bilateral Q60.4
||| unilateral Q60.3
|| hydronephrotic *see* Hydronephrosis
| lacrimal gland (primary) H04.14-
|| secondary H04.15-
| Landouzy-Dejerine G71.02
| laryngitis, infective J37.0
| larynx J38.7
| Leber's optic (hereditary) H47.22
| lip K13.0
| liver (yellow) K72.90
|| with coma K72.91
|| acute, subacute K72.00
||| with coma K72.01
|| chronic K72.10
||| with coma K72.11
| lung (senile) J98.4
| macular (dermatological) L90.8
|| syphilitic, skin A51.39
||| striated A52.79
| mandible (edentulous) K08.20
|| minimal K08.21
|| moderate K08.22
|| severe K08.23
| maxilla K08.20
|| minimal K08.24
|| moderate K08.25
|| severe K08.26
| muscle, muscular (diffuse) (general) (idiopathic) (primary) M62.50
|| ankle M62.57-
|| Duchenne-Aran G12.21
|| foot M62.57-
|| forearm M62.53-
|| hand M62.54-
|| infantile spinal G12.0
|| lower leg M62.56-
|| multiple sites M62.59
|| myelopathic *see* Atrophy, muscle, spinal
|| myotonic G71.11
|| neuritic G58.9
|| neuropathic (peroneal) (progressive) G60.0
|| pelvic (disuse) N81.84
|| peroneal G60.0
|| progressive (bulbar) G12.25
||| adult G12.1
||| infantile (spinal) G12.0
||| spinal G12.25
|||| adult G12.1
|||| infantile G12.0
|| pseudohypertrophic G71.02
|| shoulder region M62.51-
|| specified site NEC M62.58
|| spinal G12.9
||| adult form G12.1
||| Aran-Duchenne G12.21
||| childhood form, type II G12.1
||| distal G12.1
||| hereditary NEC G12.1
||| infantile, type I (Werdnig-Hoffmann) G12.0
||| juvenile form, type III (Kugelberg | Welander) G12.1
||| progressive G12.21
||| scapuloperoneal form G12.1
||| specified NEC G12.8

Atrophy, atrophic (of) - *continued*
|syphilitic A52.78
|thigh M62.55-
|upper arm M62.52-
|myocardium *see* Degeneration, myocardial
|myometrium (senile) N85.8
|cervix N88.8
|myopathic NEC *see* Atrophy, muscle
|myotonia G71.11
|nail L60.3
|nasopharynx J31.1
|nerve *see also* Disorder, nerve
|abducens *see* Strabismus, paralytic, sixth
nerve
|accessory G52.8
|acoustic or auditory *see* subcategory H93.3
|cranial G52.9
|eighth (auditory) *see* subcategory H93.3
|eleventh (accessory) G52.8
|fifth (trigeminal) G50.8
|first (olfactory) G52.0
|fourth (trochlear) *see* Strabismus,
paralytic, fourth nerve
|second (optic) H47.20
|sixth (abducens) *see* Strabismus, paralytic,
sixth nerve
|tenth (pneumogastric) (vagus) G52.2
|third (oculomotor) *see* Strabismus,
paralytic, third nerve
|twelfth (hypoglossal) G52.3
|hypoglossal G52.3
|oculomotor *see* Strabismus, paralytic, third
nerve
|olfactory G52.0
|optic (papillomacular bundle)
|syphilitic (late) A52.15
|congenital A50.44
|pneumogastric G52.2
|trigeminal G50.8
|trochlear *see* Strabismus, paralytic, fourth
nerve
|vagus (pneumogastric) G52.2
|neurogenic, bone, tabetic A52.11
|nutritional E43
with marasmus E41
|old age R54
|olivopontocerebellar G23.8
|optic (nerve) H47.20
|glaucomatous H47.23-
|hereditary H47.22
|primary H47.21-
|specified type NEC H47.29-
|syphilitic (late) A52.15
|congenital A50.44
|orbit H05.31-
|ovary (senile) N83.31-
|with fallopian tube N83.33-
|oviduct (senile) *see* Atrophy, fallopian tube
|palsy, diffuse (progressive) G12.22
|pancreas (duct) (senile) K86.89
|parotid gland K11.0
|pelvic muscle N81.84
|penis N48.89
|pharynx J39.2
|pluriglandular E31.8
|autoimmune E31.0
|polyarthritis M15.9
|prostate N42.89
|pseudohypertrophic (muscle) G71.02
|renal *see also* Sclerosis, renal N26.1
|retina, retinal (postinfectional) H35.89
|rhinitis J31.0
|salivary gland K11.0
|scar L90.5
|sclerosis, lobar (of brain) G31.09 *[F02.80]*
|with behavioral disturbance G31.09
[F02.81]
|scrotum N50.89

Atrophy, atrophic (of) - *continued*
|seminal vesicle N50.89
|senile R54
|due to radiation (nonionizing) (solar) L57.8
|skin (patches) (spots) L90.9
|degenerative (senile) L90.8
|due to radiation (nonionizing) (solar) L57.8
|senile L90.8
|spermatic cord N50.89
|spinal (acute) (cord) G95.89
|muscular *see* Atrophy, muscle, spinal
|paralysis G12.20
|acute *see* Poliomyelitis, paralytic
|meaning progressive muscular atrophy
G12.21
|spine (column) *see* Spondylopathy, specified
NEC
|spleen (senile) D73.0
|stomach K29.40
|with bleeding K29.41
|striate (skin) L90.6
|syphilitic A52.79
|subcutaneous L90.9
|sublingual gland K11.0
|submandibular gland K11.0
|submaxillary gland K11.0
|Sudeck's *see* Algoneurodystrophy
|suprarenal (capsule) (gland) E27.49
|primary E27.1
|systemic affecting central nervous system
|in
|myxedema E03.9 *[G13.2]*
|neoplastic disease *see also* Neoplasm
D49.9 *[G13.1]*
|specified disease NEC G13.8
|tarso-orbital fascia, congenital Q10.3
|testis N50.0
|thenar, partial *see* Syndrome, carpal tunnel
|thymus (fatty) E32.8
|thyroid (gland) (acquired) E03.4
|with cretinism E03.1
|congenital (with myxedema) E03.1
|tongue (senile) K14.8
|papillae K14.4
|trachea J39.8
|tunica vaginalis N50.89
|turbinate J34.89
|tympanic membrane (nonflaccid) H73.82-
|flaccid H73.81-
|upper respiratory tract J39.8
|uterus, uterine (senile) N85.8
|cervix N88.8
|due to radiation (intended effect) N85.8
|adverse effect or misadventure N99.89
|vagina (senile) N95.2
|vas deferens N50.89
|vascular I99.8
|vertebra (senile) *see* Spondylopathy, specified
NEC
|vulva (senile) N90.5
|Werdnig-Hoffmann G12.0
|yellow *see* Failure, hepatic
Attack, attacks
|with alteration of consciousness (with
automatisms) *see* Epilepsy, localization-
related, symptomatic, with complex partial
seizures
|Adams-Stokes I45.9
|akinetic *see* Epilepsy, generalized, specified
NEC
|angina *see* Angina
|atonic *see* Epilepsy, generalized, specified
NEC
|benign shuddering G25.83
|cataleptic *see* Catalepsy
|coronary *see* Infarct, myocardium
|cyanotic, newborn P28.2

Attack, attacks - *continued*
|drop NEC R55
|epileptic *see* Epilepsy
|heart *see* infarct, myocardium
|hysterical F44.9
|jacksonian *see* Epilepsy, localization-related,
symptomatic, with simple partial seizures
|myocardium, myocardial *see* Infarct,
myocardium
|myoclonic *see* Epilepsy, generalized, specified
NEC
|panic F41.0
|psychomotor *see* Epilepsy, localization-
related, symptomatic, with complex partial
seizures
|salaam *see* Epilepsy, spasms
|schizophreniform, brief F23
|shuddering, benign G25.83
|Stokes-Adams I45.9
|syncope R55
|transient ischemic (TIA) G45.9
|specified NEC G45.8
|unconsciousness R55
|hysterical F44.89
|vasomotor R55
|vasovagal (paroxysmal) (idiopathic) R55
|without alteration of consciousness *see*
Epilepsy, localization-related, symptomatic,
with simple partial seizures
Attention (to)
|artificial
|opening (of) Z43.9
|digestive tract NEC Z43.4
|colon Z43.3
|ilium Z43.2
|stomach Z43.1
|specified NEC Z43.8
|trachea Z43.0
|urinary tract NEC Z43.6
|cystostomy Z43.5
|nephrostomy Z43.6
|ureterostomy Z43.6
|urethrostomy Z43.6
|vagina Z43.7
|colostomy Z43.3
|cystostomy Z43.5
|deficit disorder or syndrome F98.8
|with hyperactivity *see* Disorder, attention-
deficit hyperactivity
|gastrostomy Z43.1
|ileostomy Z43.2
|jejunostomy Z43.4
|nephrostomy Z43.6
|surgical dressings Z48.01
|sutures Z48.02
|tracheostomy Z43.0
|ureterostomy Z43.6
|urethrostomy Z43.6
Attrition
|gum *see* Recession, gingival
|tooth, teeth (excessive) (hard tissues) K03.0
Atypical, atypism *see also* condition
|cells (on cytological smear) (endocervical)
(endometrial) (glandular)
|cervix R87.619
|vagina R87.629
|cervical N87.9
|endometrium N85.9
|hyperplasia N85.00
|parenting situation Z62.9
Auditory *see* condition
Aujeszky's disease B33.8
Aurantiasis, cutis E67.1
Auricle, auricular *see also* condition
|cervical Q18.2
Auriculotemporal syndrome G50.8

Austin Flint murmur (aortic insufficiency)
  I35.1
Australian
  |Q fever A78
  |X disease A83.4
Autism, autistic (childhood) (infantile) F84.0
  |atypical F84.9
  |spectrum disorder F84.0
Autodigestion R68.89
Autoerythrocyte sensitization (syndrome)
  D69.2
Autographism L50.3
Autoimmune
  |disease (systemic) M35.9
  |inhibitors to clotting factors D68.311
  |lymphoproliferative syndrome [ALPS]
    D89.82
  |thyroiditis E06.3
Autointoxication R68.89
Automatism G93.89
  |with temporal sclerosis G93.81
  |epileptic *see* Epilepsy, localization-related,
    symptomatic, with complex partial seizures
  |paroxysmal, idiopathic *see* Epilepsy,
    localization-related, symptomatic, with
    complex partial seizures
Autonomic, autonomous
  |bladder (neurogenic) N31.2
  |hysteria seizure F44.5
Autosensitivity, erythrocyte D69.2
Autosensitization, cutaneous L30.2
Autosome *see* condition by chromosome
  involved
Autotopagnosia R48.1
Autotoxemia R68.89
Autumn *see* condition
Avellis' syndrome G46.8
Aversion
  |oral R63.39
    |newborn P92.-
    |nonorganic origin F98.2
  |sexual F52.1
Aviator's
  |disease or sickness *see* Effect, adverse, high
    altitude
  |ear T70.0
Avitaminosis (multiple) *see also* Deficiency,
  vitamin E56.9
  |B E53.9
    |with
      |beriberi E51.11
      |pellagra E52
  |B2 E53.0
  |B6 E53.1
  |B12 E53.8
  |D E55.9
    |with rickets E55.0
  |G E53.0
  |K E56.1
  |nicotinic acid E52
AVNRT (atrioventricular nodal re-Entrant
  tachycardia) I47.1
AVRT (atrioventricular nodal re-Entrant
  tachycardia) I47.1
Avulsion (traumatic)
  |blood vessel *see* Injury, blood vessel
  |bone *see* Fracture, by site
  |cartilage *see also* Dislocation, by site
    |symphyseal (inner), complicating delivery
      O71.6
  |external site other than limb *see* Wound, open,
    by site
  |eye S05.7-
  |head (intracranial)
    |external site NEC S08.89
    |scalp S08.0
  |internal organ or site *see* Injury, by site
  |joint *see also* Dislocation, by site
    |capsule *see* Sprain, by site

Avulsion (traumatic) - *continued*
  |kidney S37.06-
  |ligament *see* Sprain, by site
  |limb *see also* Amputation, traumatic, by site
    |skin and subcutaneous tissue *see* Wound,
      open, by site
  |muscle *see* Injury, muscle
  |nerve (root) *see* Injury, nerve
  |scalp S08.0
  |skin and subcutaneous tissue *see* Wound,
    open, by site
  |spleen S36.032
  |symphyseal cartilage (inner), complicating
    delivery O71.6
  |tendon *see* Injury, muscle
  |tooth S03.2
Awareness of heart beat R00.2
Axenfeld's
  |anomaly or syndrome Q15.0
  |degeneration (calcareous) Q13.4
Axilla, axillary *see also* condition
  |breast Q83.1
Axonotmesis *see* Injury, nerve
Ayerza's disease or syndrome (pulmonary
  artery sclerosis with pulmonary
  hypertension) I27.0
Azoospermia (organic) N46.01
  |due to
    |drug therapy N46.021
    |efferent duct obstruction N46.023
    |infection N46.022
    |radiation N46.024
    |specified cause NEC N46.029
    |systemic disease N46.025
Azotemia R79.89
  |meaning uremia N19
Aztec ear Q17.3
Azygos
  |continuation inferior vena cava Q26.8
  |lobe (lung) Q33.1

B

Baastrup's disease *see* Kissing spine
Babesiosis B60.00
  |due to
    |Babesia
      |divergens B60.03
      |duncani B60.02
      |KO-1 B60.09
      |microti B60.01
      |MO-1 B60.03
      |species
        |unspecified B60.00
      |venatorum B60.09
    |specified NEC B60.09
Babington's disease (familial hemorrhagic
  telangiectasia) I78.0
Babinski's syndrome A52.79
Baby
  |crying constantly R68.11
  |floppy (syndrome) P94.2
Bacillary *see* condition
Bacilluria R82.71
Bacillus *see also* Infection, bacillus
  |abortus infection A23.1
  |anthracis infection A22.9
  |coli infection *see also* Escherichia coli B96.20
  |Flexner's A03.1
  |mallei infection A24.0
  |Shiga's A03.0
  |suipestifer infection *see* Infection, salmonella

Back *see* condition
Backache (postural) M54.9
  |sacroiliac M53.3
  |specified NEC M54.89
Backflow *see* Reflux
Backward reading (dyslexia) F81.0
Bacteremia R78.81
  |with sepsis *see* Sepsis
Bactericholia *see* Cholecystitis, acute
Bacterid, bacteride (pustular) L40.3
Bacterium, bacteria, bacterial
  |agent NEC, as cause of disease classified
    elsewhere B96.89
  |in blood *see* Bacteremia
  |in urine *see* Bacteriuria
Bacteriuria, bacteruria R82.71
  |asymptomatic R82.71
Bacteroides
  |fragilis, as cause of disease classified
    elsewhere B96.6
Bad
  |heart *see* Disease, heart
  |trip
    |due to drug abuse *see* Abuse, drug,
      hallucinogen
    |due to drug dependence *see* Dependence,
      drug, hallucinogen
Baelz's disease (cheilitis glandularis
  apostematosa) K13.0
Baerensprung's disease (eczema marginatum)
  B35.6
Bagasse disease or pneumonitis J67.1
Bagassosis J67.1
Baker's cyst *see* Cyst, Baker's
Bakwin-Krida syndrome (metaphyseal
  dysplasia) Q78.5
Balancing side interference M26.56
Balanitis (circinata) (erosiva) (gangrenosa)
  (phagedenic) (vulgaris) N48.1
  |amebic A06.82
  |candidal B37.42
  |due to Haemophilus ducreyi A57
  |gonococcal (acute) (chronic) A54.23
  |xerotica obliterans N48.0
Balanoposthitis N47.6
  |gonococcal (acute) (chronic) A54.23
  |ulcerative (specific) A63.8
Balanorrhagia *see* Balanitis
Balantidiasis, balantidiosis A07.0
Bald tongue K14.4
Baldness *see also* Alopecia
  |male-pattern *see* Alopecia, androgenic
Balkan grippe A78
Balloon disease *see* Effect, adverse, high
  altitude
Balo's disease (concentric sclerosis) G37.5
Bamberger-Marie disease *see*
  Osteoarthropathy, hypertrophic, specified
  type NEC
Bancroft's filariasis B74.0
Band(s)
  |adhesive *see* Adhesions, peritoneum
  |anomalous or congenital *see also* Anomaly, by
    site
    |heart (atrial) (ventricular) Q24.8
    |intestine Q43.3
    |omentum Q43.3
  |cervix N88.1
  |constricting, congenital Q79.8
  |gallbladder (congenital) Q44.1
  |intestinal (adhesive) *see* Adhesions,
    peritoneum
  |obstructive
    |intestine K56.50
      |complete K56.52

Band(s) - *continued*
|incomplete K56.51
|partial K56.51
|peritoneum K56.50
|complete K56.52
|incomplete K56.51
|partial K56.51
|periappendiceal, congenital Q43.3
|peritoneal (adhesive) *see* Adhesions, peritoneum
|uterus N73.6
|internal N85.6
|vagina N89.5
Bandemia D72.825
Bandl's ring (contraction), complicating delivery O62.4
Bangkok hemorrhagic fever A91
Bang's disease (brucella abortus) A23.1
Bankruptcy, anxiety concerning Z59.89
Bannister's disease T78.3
|hereditary D84.1
Banti's disease or syndrome (with cirrhosis) (with portal hypertension) K76.6
Bar, median, prostate *see* Enlargement, enlarged, prostate
Barcoo disease or rot *see* Ulcer, skin
Barlow's disease E54
Barodontalgia T70.29
Baron Münchausen syndrome *see* Disorder, factitious
Barosinusitis T70.1
Barotitis T70.0
Barotrauma T70.29
|odontalgia T70.29
|otitic T70.0
|sinus T70.1
Barraquer (-Simons) disease or syndrome (progressive lipodystrophy) E88.1
Barré-Guillain disease or syndrome G61.0
Barré-Liéou syndrome (posterior cervical sympathetic) M53.0
Barrel chest M95.4
Barrett's
|disease *see* Barrett's, esophagus
|esophagus K22.70
|with dysplasia K22.719
|high grade K22.711
|low grade K22.710
|without dysplasia K22.70
|syndrome *see* Barrett's, esophagus
|ulcer K22.10
|with bleeding K22.11
|without bleeding K22.10
Bársony (-Polgár) (-Teschendorf) syndrome (corkscrew esophagus) K22.4
Bartholinitis (suppurating) N75.8
|gonococcal (acute) (chronic) (with abscess) A54.1
Barth syndrome E78.71
Bartonellosis A44.9
|cutaneous A44.1
|mucocutaneous A44.1
|specified NEC A44.8
|systemic A44.0
Barton's fracture S52.56-
Bartter's syndrome E26.81
Basal *see* condition
Basan's (hidrotic) ectodermal dysplasia Q82.4
Baseball finger *see* Dislocation, finger
Basedow's disease (exophthalmic goiter) *see* Hyperthyroidism, with, goiter
Basic *see* condition

Basilar *see* condition
Bason's (hidrotic) ectodermal dysplasia Q82.4
Basopenia *see* Agranulocytosis
Basophilia D72.824
Basophilism (cortico-Adrenal) (Cushing's) (pituitary) E24.0
Bassen-Kornzweig disease or syndrome E78.6
Bat ear Q17.5
Bateman's
|disease B08.1
|purpura (senile) D69.2
Bathing cramp T75.1
Bathophobia F40.248
Batten (-Mayou) disease E75.4
|retina E75.4 [*H36*]
Batten-Steinert syndrome G71.11
Battered *see* Maltreatment
Battey Mycobacterium infection A31.0
Battle exhaustion F43.0
Battledore placenta O43.19-
Baumgarten-Cruveilhier cirrhosis, disease or syndrome K74.69
Bauxite fibrosis (of lung) J63.1
Bayle's disease (general paresis) A52.17
Bazin's disease (primary) (tuberculous) A18.4
Beach ear *see* Swimmer's, ear
Beaded hair (congenital) Q84.1
Béal conjunctivitis or syndrome B30.2
Beard's disease (neurasthenia) F48.8
Beat(s)
|atrial, premature I49.1
|ectopic I49.49
|elbow *see* Bursitis, elbow
|escaped, heart I49.49
|hand *see* Bursitis, hand
|knee *see* Bursitis, knee
|premature I49.40
|atrial I49.1
|auricular I49.1
|supraventricular I49.1
Beau's
|disease or syndrome *see* Degeneration, myocardial
|lines (transverse furrows on fingernails) L60.4
Beck's syndrome (anterior spinal artery occlusion) I65.8
Becker's
|cardiomyopathy I42.8
|disease
|idiopathic mural endomyocardial disease I42.3
|myotonia congenita, recessive form G71.12
|dystrophy G71.01
|pigmented hairy nevus D22.5
Beckwith-Wiedemann syndrome Q87.3
Bed confinement status Z74.01
Bed sore *see* Ulcer, pressure, by site
Bedbug bite(s) *see* Bite(s), by site, superficial, insect
Bedclothes, asphyxiation or suffocation by *see* Asphyxia, traumatic, due to, mechanical, trapped
Bednar's
|aphthae K12.0
|tumor *see* Neoplasm, malignant, by site
Bedridden Z74.01
Bedsore *see* Ulcer, pressure, by site
Bedwetting *see* Enuresis
Bee sting (with allergic or anaphylactic shock) *see* Toxicity, venom, arthropod, bee
Beer drinker's heart (disease) I42.6
Begbie's disease (exophthalmic goiter) *see* Hyperthyroidism, with, goiter

Behavior
|antisocial
|adult Z72.811
|child or adolescent Z72.810
|disorder, disturbance *see* Disorder, conduct
|disruptive *see* Disorder, conduct
|drug seeking Z76.5
|inexplicable R46.2
|marked evasiveness R46.5
|obsessive-compulsive R46.81
|overactivity R46.3
|poor responsiveness R46.4
|self-damaging (life-style) Z72.89
|sleep-incompatible Z72.821
|slowness R46.4
|specified NEC R46.89
|strange (and inexplicable) R46.2
|suspiciousness R46.5
|type A pattern Z73.1
|undue concern or preoccupation with stressful events R46.6
|verbosity and circumstantial detail obscuring reason for contact R46.7
Behçet's disease or syndrome M35.2
Behr's disease *see* Degeneration, macula
Beigel's disease or morbus (white piedra) B36.2
Bejel A65
Bekhterev's syndrome *see* Spondylitis, ankylosing
Belching *see* Eructation
Bell's
|mania F30.8
|palsy, paralysis G51.0
|infant or newborn P11.3
|spasm G51.3-
Bence Jones albuminuria or proteinuria NEC R80.3
Bends T70.3
Benedikt's paralysis or syndrome G46.3
Benign *see also* condition
|prostatic hyperplasia *see* Hyperplasia, prostate
Bennett's fracture (displaced) S62.21-
Benson's disease *see* Deposit, crystalline
Bent
|back (hysterical) F44.4
|nose M95.0
|congenital Q67.4
Bereavement (uncomplicated) Z63.4
Bergeron's disease (hysterical chorea) F44.4
Berger's disease *see* Nephropathy, IgA
Beriberi (dry) E51.11
|heart (disease) E51.12
|polyneuropathy E51.11
|wet E51.12
|involving circulatory system E51.11
Berlin's disease or edema (traumatic) S05.8X-
Berlock (berloque) dermatitis L56.2
Bernard-Horner syndrome G90.2
Bernard-Soulier disease or thrombopathia D69.1
Bernhardt (-Roth) disease *see* Mononeuropathy, lower limb, meralgia paresthetica
Bernheim's syndrome *see* Failure, heart, right
Bertielliasis B71.8
Berylliosis (lung) J63.2
Besnier-Boeck (-Schaumann) disease *see* Sarcoidosis
Besnier's
|lupus pernio D86.3
|prurigo L20.0
Bestiality F65.89
Best's disease H35.50
Beta-Mercaptolactate-Cysteine disulfiduria E72.09
Betalipoproteinemia, broad or floating E78.2

Betting and gambling Z72.6
  |pathological (compulsive) F63.0
Bezoar T18.9
  |intestine T18.3
  |stomach T18.2
Bezold's abscess *see* Mastoiditis, acute
Bianchi's syndrome R48.8
Bicornate or bicornis uterus Q51.3
  |in pregnancy or childbirth O34.00
    |causing obstructed labor O65.5
Bicuspid aortic valve Q23.1
Biedl-Bardet syndrome Q87.89
Bielschowsky (-Jansky) disease E75.4
Biermer's (pernicious) anemia or disease
  D51.0
Biett's disease L93.0
Bifid (congenital)
  |apex, heart Q24.8
  |clitoris Q52.6
  |kidney Q63.8
  |nose Q30.2
  |patella Q74.1
  |scrotum Q55.29
  |toe NEC Q74.2
  |tongue Q38.3
  |ureter Q62.8
  |uterus Q51.3
  |uvula Q35.7
Biforis uterus (suprasimplex) Q51.3
Bifurcation (congenital)
  |gallbladder Q44.1
  |kidney pelvis Q63.8
  |renal pelvis Q63.8
  |rib Q76.6
  |tongue, congenital Q38.3
  |trachea Q32.1
  |ureter Q62.8
  |urethra Q64.74
  |vertebra Q76.49
Big spleen syndrome D73.1
Bigeminal pulse R00.8
Bilateral *see* condition
Bile
  |duct *see* condition
  |pigments in urine R82.2
Bilharziasis *see also* Schistosomiasis
  |chyluria B65.0
  |cutaneous B65.3
  |galacturia B65.0
  |hematochyluria B65.0
  |intestinal B65.1
  |lipemia B65.9
  |lipuria B65.0
  |oriental B65.2
  |piarhemia B65.9
  |pulmonary NOS B65.9 [*J99*]
    pneumonia B65.9 [*J17*]
  |tropical hematuria B65.0
  |vesical B65.0
Biliary *see* condition
Bilirubin metabolism disorder E80.7
  |specified NEC E80.6
Bilirubinemia, familial nonhemolytic E80.4
Bilirubinuria R82.2
Biliuria R82.2
Bilocular stomach K31.2
Binswanger's disease I67.3
Biparta, bipartite
  |carpal scaphoid Q74.0
  |patella Q74.1
  |vagina Q52.10
Bird
  |face Q75.8
  |fancier's disease or lung J67.2
Birt-Hogg-Dube syndrome Q87.89

Birth
  |complications in mother *see* Delivery,
    complicated
  |compression during NOS P15.9
  |defect *see* Anomaly
  |immature (less than 37 completed weeks) *see*
    Preterm, newborn
    |extremely (less than 28 completed weeks)
      see Immaturity, extreme
  |inattention, at or after *see* Maltreatment, child,
    neglect
  |injury NOS P15.9
    |basal ganglia P11.1
    |brachial plexus NEC P14.3
    |brain (compression) (pressure) P11.2
    |central nervous system NOS P11.9
    |cerebellum P11.1
    |cerebral hemorrhage P10.1
    |external genitalia P15.5
    |eye P15.3
    |face P15.4
    |fracture
      |bone P13.9
        |specified NEC P13.8
      |clavicle P13.4
      |femur P13.2
      |humerus P13.3
      |long bone, except femur P13.3
      |radius and ulna P13.3
      |skull P13.0
      |spine P11.5
      |tibia and fibula P13.3
    |intracranial P11.2
      |laceration or hemorrhage P10.9
        |specified NEC P10.8
    |intraventricular hemorrhage P10.2
    |laceration
      |brain P10.1
      |by scalpel P15.8
      |peripheral nerve P14.9
    |liver P15.0
    |meninges
      |brain P11.1
      |spinal cord P11.5
    |nerve
      |brachial plexus P14.3
      |cranial NEC (except facial) P11.4
      |facial P11.3
      |peripheral P14.9
      |phrenic (paralysis) P14.2
    |paralysis
      |facial nerve P11.3
      |spinal P11.5
    |penis P15.5
    |rupture
      |spinal cord P11.5
    |scalp P12.9
    |scalpel wound P15.8
    |scrotum P15.5
    |skull NEC P13.1
      |fracture P13.0
    |specified type NEC P15.8
    |spinal cord P11.5
    |spine P11.5
    |spleen P15.1
    |sternomastoid (hematoma) P15.2
    |subarachnoid hemorrhage P10.3
    |subcutaneous fat necrosis P15.6
    |subdural hemorrhage P10.0
    |tentorial tear P10.4
    |testes P15.5
    |vulva P15.5
  |lack of care, at or after *see* Maltreatment,
    child, neglect

Birth - *continued*
  |neglect, at or after *see* Maltreatment, child,
    neglect
  |palsy or paralysis, newborn, NOS (birth
    injury) P14.9
  |premature (infant) *see* Preterm, newborn
  |shock, newborn P96.89
  |trauma *see* Birth, injury
  |weight
    |low (2499 grams or less) *see* Low,
      birthweight
    |extremely (999 grams or less) *see* Low,
      birthweight, extreme
    |4000 grams to 4499 grams P08.1
    |4500 grams or more P08.0
Birthmark Q82.5
Bisalbuminemia E88.09
Biskra's button B55.1
Bite(s) (animal) (human)
  |abdomen, abdominal
    |wall S31.159
      |with penetration into peritoneal cavity
        S31.659
      |epigastric region S31.152
        |with penetration into peritoneal cavity
          S31.652
      |left
        |lower quadrant S31.154
          |with penetration into peritoneal cavity
            S31.654
        |upper quadrant S31.151
          |with penetration into peritoneal cavity
            S31.651
      |periumbilic region S31.155
        |with penetration into peritoneal cavity
          S31.655
      |right
        |lower quadrant S31.153
          |with penetration into peritoneal cavity
            S31.653
        |upper quadrant S31.150
          |with penetration into peritoneal cavity
            S31.650
      |superficial NEC S30.871
        |insect S30.861
  |alveolar (process) *see* Bite, oral cavity
  |amphibian (venomous) *see* Venom, bite,
    amphibian
  |animal *see also* Bite, by site
    |venomous *see* Venom
  |ankle S91.05-
    |superficial NEC S90.57-
      |insect S90.56-
  |antecubital space *see* Bite, elbow
  |anus S31.835
    |superficial NEC S30.877
      |insect S30.867
  |arm (upper) S41.15-
    |lower *see* Bite, forearm
    |superficial NEC S40.87-
      |insect S40.86-
  |arthropod NEC *see* Venom, bite, arthropod
  |auditory canal (external) (meatus) *see* Bite, ear
  |auricle, ear *see* Bite, ear
  |axilla *see* Bite, arm
  |back *see also* Bite, thorax, back
    |lower S31.050
      |with penetration into retroperitoneal space
        S31.051
      |superficial NEC S30.870
        |insect S30.860
  |bedbug *see* Bite(s), by site, superficial, insect
  |breast S21.05-
    |superficial NEC S20.17-
      |insect S20.16-
  |brow *see* Bite, head, specified site NEC
  |buttock S31.805

Bite(s) (animal) (human) - *continued*
- |left S31.825
- |right S31.815
- |superficial NEC S30.870
  - |insect S30.860
- |calf *see* Bite, leg
- |canaliculus lacrimalis *see* Bite, eyelid
- |canthus, eye *see* Bite, eyelid
- |centipede *see* Toxicity, venom, arthropod, centipede
- |cheek (external) S01.45-
  - |superficial NEC S00.87
    - |insect S00.86
  - |internal *see* Bite, oral cavity |chest wall *see* Bite, thorax
- |chigger B88.0
- |chin *see* Bite, head, specified site NEC
- |clitoris *see* Bite, vulva
- |costal region *see* Bite, thorax
- |digit(s)
  - |hand *see* Bite, finger
  - |toe *see* Bite, toe
- |ear (canal) (external) S01.35-
  - |superficial NEC S00.47-
    - |insect S00.46-
- |elbow S51.05-
  - |superficial NEC S50.37-
    - |insect S50.36-
- |epididymis *see* Bite, testis
- |epigastric region *see* Bite, abdomen
- |epiglottis *see* Bite, neck, specified site NEC
- |esophagus, cervical S11.25
  - |superficial NEC S10.17
    - |insect S10.16
- |eyebrow *see* Bite, eyelid
- |eyelid S01.15-
  - |superficial NEC S00.27-
    - |insect S00.26-
- |face NEC *see* Bite, head, specified site NEC
- |finger(s) S61.259
  - |with
    - |damage to nail S61.359
  - |index S61.258
    - |with
      - |damage to nail S61.358
    - |left S61.251
      - |with
        - |damage to nail S61.351
    - |right S61.250
      - |with
        - |damage to nail S61.350
    - |superficial NEC S60.478
      - |insect S60.46-
  - |little S61.25-
    - |with
      - |damage to nail S61.35-
    - |superficial NEC S60.47-
      - |insect S60.46-
  - |middle S61.25-
    - |with
      - |damage to nail S61.35-
    - |superficial NEC S60.47-
      - |insect S60.46-
  - |ring S61.25-
    - |with
      - |damage to nail S61.35-
    - |superficial NEC S60.47-
      - |insect S60.46-
  - |superficial NEC S60.479
    - |insect S60.469
  - |thumb *see* Bite, thumb
- |flank *see* Bite, abdomen, wall
- |flea *see* Bite, by site, superficial, insect
- |foot (except toe(s) alone) S91.35-
  - |superficial NEC S90.87-
    - |insect S90.86-
  - |toe *see* Bite, toe |forearm S51.85-

- |elbow only *see* Bite, elbow
  - |superficial NEC S50.87-
    - |insect S50.86-
- |forehead *see* Bite, head, specified site NEC
- |genital organs, external
  - |female S31.552
    - |superficial NEC S30.876
      - |insect S30.866
    - |vagina and vulva *see* Bite, vulva
  - |male S31.551
    - |penis *see* Bite, penis
    - |scrotum *see* Bite, scrotum
    - |superficial NEC S30.875
      - |insect S30.865
    - |testes *see* Bite, testis
- |groin *see* Bite, abdomen, wall
- |gum *see* Bite, oral cavity
- |hand S61.45-
  - |finger *see* Bite, finger
  - |superficial NEC S60.57-
    - |insect S60.56-
  - |thumb *see* Bite, thumb
- |head S01.95
  - |cheek *see* Bite, cheek
  - |ear *see* Bite, ear
  - |eyelid *see* Bite, eyelid
  - |lip *see* Bite, lip
  - |nose *see* Bite, nose
  - |oral cavity *see* Bite, oral cavity
  - |scalp *see* Bite, scalp
  - |specified site NEC S01.85
    - |superficial NEC S00.87
      - |insect S00.86
  - |superficial NEC S00.97
    - |insect S00.96
  - |temporomandibular area *see* Bite, cheek
- |heel *see* Bite, foot
- |hip S71.05-
  - |superficial NEC S70.27-
    - |insect S70.26-
- |hymen S31.45
- |hypochondrium *see* Bite, abdomen, wall
- |hypogastric region *see* Bite, abdomen, wall
- |inguinal region *see* Bite, abdomen, wall
- |insect *see* Bite, by site, superficial, insect
- |instep *see* Bite, foot
- |interscapular region *see* Bite, thorax, back
- |jaw *see* Bite, head, specified site NEC
- |knee S81.05-
  - |superficial NEC S80.27-
    - |insect S80.26-
- |labium (majus) (minus) *see* Bite, vulva
- |lacrimal duct *see* Bite, eyelid
- |larynx S11.015
  - |superficial NEC S10.17
    - |insect S10.16
- |leg (lower) S81.85-
  - |ankle *see* Bite, ankle
  - |foot *see* Bite, foot
  - |knee *see* Bite, knee
  - |superficial NEC S80.87-
    - |insect S80.86-
  - |toe *see* Bite, toe
  - |upper *see* Bite, thigh
- |lip S01.551
  - |superficial NEC S00.571
    - |insect S00.561
- |lizard (venomous) *see* Venom, bite, reptile
- |loin *see* Bite, abdomen, wall
- |lower back *see* Bite, back, lower
- |lumbar region *see* Bite, back, lower
- |malar region *see* Bite, head, specified site NEC
- |mammary *see* Bite, breast
- |marine animals (venomous) *see* Toxicity, venom, marine animal

- |mastoid region *see* Bite, head, specified site NEC
- |mouth *see* Bite, oral cavity |nail
  - |finger *see* Bite, finger
  - |toe *see* Bite, toe
- |nape *see* Bite, neck, specified site NEC
- |nasal (septum) (sinus) *see* Bite, nose
- |nasopharynx *see* Bite, head, specified site NEC
- |neck S11.95
  - |involving
    - |cervical esophagus *see* Bite, esophagus, cervical
    - |larynx *see* Bite, larynx
    - |pharynx *see* Bite, pharynx
    - |thyroid gland S11.15
    - |trachea *see* Bite, trachea
  - |specified site NEC S11.85
    - |superficial NEC S10.87
      - |insect S10.86
  - |superficial NEC S10.97
    - |insect S10.96
  - |throat S11.85
    - |superficial NEC S10.17
      - |insect S10.16
- |nose (septum) (sinus) S01.25
  - |superficial NEC S00.37
    - |insect S00.36
- |occipital region *see* Bite, scalp
- |oral cavity S01.552
  - |superficial NEC S00.572
    - |insect S00.562
- |orbital region *see* Bite, eyelid
- |palate *see* Bite, oral cavity
- |palm *see* Bite, hand
- |parietal region *see* Bite, scalp
- |pelvis S31.050
  - |with penetration into retroperitoneal space S31.051
  - |superficial NEC S30.870
    - |insect S30.860
- |penis S31.25
  - |superficial NEC S30.872
    - |insect S30.862
- |perineum
  - |female *see* Bite, vulva
  - |male *see* Bite, pelvis
- |periocular area (with or without lacrimal passages) *see* Bite, eyelid
- |phalanges
  - |finger *see* Bite, finger
  - |toe *see* Bite, toe
- |pharynx S11.25
  - |superficial NEC S10.17
    - |insect S10.16
- |pinna *see* Bite, ear
- |poisonous *see* Venom
- |popliteal space *see* Bite, knee |prepuce *see* Bite, penis
- |pubic region *see* Bite, abdomen, wall
- |rectovaginal septum *see* Bite, vulva
- |red bug B88.0
- |reptile NEC *see also* Venom, bite, reptile
  - |nonvenomous *see* Bite, by site
  - |snake *see* Venom, bite, snake
- |sacral region *see* Bite, back, lower
- |sacroiliac region *see* Bite, back, lower
- |salivary gland *see* Bite, oral cavity
- |scalp S01.05
  - |superficial NEC S00.07
    - |insect S00.06
- |scapular region *see* Bite, shoulder
- |scrotum S31.35
  - |superficial NEC S30.873
    - |insect S30.863
- |sea-snake (venomous) *see* Toxicity, venom, snake, sea snake |shin *see* Bite, leg

Bite(s) (animal) (human) - *continued*
|shoulder S41.05-
| |superficial NEC S40.27-
| | |insect S40.26-
|snake *see also* Venom, bite, snake
| |nonvenomous *see* Bite, by site
|spermatic cord *see* Bite, testis
|spider (venomous) *see* Toxicity, venom,
| spider
| |nonvenomous *see* Bite, by site, superficial,
| insect
|sternal region *see* Bite, thorax, front
|submaxillary region *see* Bite, head, specified
| site NEC
|submental region *see* Bite, head, specified site
| NEC
|subungual
| |finger(s) *see* Bite, finger
| |toe *see* Bite, toe
|superficial *see* Bite, by site, superficial
|supraclavicular fossa S11.85
|supraorbital *see* Bite, head, specified site NEC
|temple, temporal region *see* Bite, head,
| specified site NEC
|temporomandibular area *see* Bite, cheek
|testis S31.35
| |superficial NEC S30.873
| | |insect S30.863
|thigh S71.15-
| |superficial NEC S70.37-
| | |insect S70.36-
|thorax, thoracic (wall) S21.95
| |back S21.25-
| | |with penetration into thoracic cavity
| | | S21.45-
| |breast *see* Bite, breast
| |front S21.15-
| | |with penetration into thoracic cavity
| | | S21.35-
| |superficial NEC S20.97
| | |back S20.47-
| | |front S20.37-
| | |insect S20.96
| | | |back S20.46-
| | | |front S20.36-
|throat *see* Bite, neck, throat
|thumb S61.05-
| |with
| | |damage to nail S61.15-
| |superficial NEC S60.37-
| | |insect S60.36-
|thyroid S11.15
| |superficial NEC S10.87
| | |insect S10.86
|toe(s) S91.15-
| |with
| | |damage to nail S91.25-
| |great S91.15
| | |with
| | | |damage to nail S91.25-
| |lesser S91.15-
| | |with
| | | |damage to nail S91.25-
| |superficial NEC S90.47-
| | |great S90.47-
| | |insect S90.46-
| | | |great S90.46-
|tongue S01.552
|trachea S11.025
| |superficial NEC S10.17
| | |insect S10.16
|tunica vaginalis *see* Bite, testis
|tympanum, tympanic membrane *see* Bite, ear
|umbilical region S31.155
|uvula *see* Bite, oral cavity
|vagina *see* Bite, vulva
|venomous *see* Venom
|vocal cords S11.035

Bite(s) (animal) (human) - *continued*
| |superficial NEC S10.17
| | |insect S10.16
| |vulva S31.45
| | |superficial NEC S30.874
| | | |insect S30.864
| |wrist S61.55-
| | |superficial NEC S60.87-
| | | |insect S60.86-
Biting, cheek or lip K13.1
Biventricular failure (heart) I50.82
Björck (-Thorson) syndrome (malignant
carcinoid) E34.0
Black
|death A20.9
|eye S00.1-
|hairy tongue K14.3
|heel (foot) S90.3-
Black - *continued*
|lung (disease) J60
|palm (hand) S60.22-
Blackfan-Diamond anemia or syndrome
(congenital hypoplastic anemia) D61.01
Blackhead L70.0
Blackout R55
Bladder *see* condition
Blast (air) (hydraulic) (immersion)
(underwater)
|blindness S05.8X-
|injury
| |abdomen or thorax *see* Injury, by site
| |ear (acoustic nerve trauma) *see* Injury,
| | nerve, acoustic, specified type NEC
| |syndrome NEC T70.8
Blastoma *see* Neoplasm, malignant, by site
|pulmonary *see* Neoplasm, lung, malignant
Blastomycosis, blastomycotic B40.9
|Brazilian *see* Paracoccidioidomycosis
|cutaneous B40.3
|disseminated B40.7
|European *see* Cryptococcosis
|generalized B40.7
|keloidal B48.0
|North American B40.9
|primary pulmonary B40.0
|pulmonary B40.2
| |acute B40.0
| |chronic B40.1
|skin B40.3
|South American *see* Paracoccidioidomycosis
|specified NEC B40.89
Bleb(s) R23.8
|emphysematous (lung) (solitary) J43.9
|endophthalmitis H59.43
|filtering (vitreous), after glaucoma surgery
| Z98.83
|inflamed (infected), postprocedural H59.40
| |stage 1 H59.41
| |stage 2 H59.42
| |stage 3 H59.43
|lung (ruptured) J43.9
| |congenital *see* Atelectasis
| |newborn P25.8
|subpleural (emphysematous) J43.9
Blebitis, postprocedural H59.40
|stage 1 H59.41
|stage 2 H59.42
|stage 3 H59.43
Bleeder (familial) (hereditary) *see* Hemophilia
Bleeding *see also* Hemorrhage
|anal K62.5
|anovulatory N97.0
|atonic, following delivery O72.1
|capillary I78.8
| |puerperal O72.2
|contact (postcoital) N93.0
|due to uterine subinvolution N85.3

Bleeding - *continued*
|ear *see* Otorrhagia
|excessive, associated with menopausal onset
| N92.4
|familial *see* Defect, coagulation
|following intercourse N93.0
|gastrointestinal K92.2
|hemorrhoids *see* Hemorrhoids
|intermenstrual (regular) N92.3
| |irregular N92.1
|intraoperative *see* Complication,
| intraoperative, hemorrhage
|irregular N92.6
|menopausal N92.4
|newborn, intraventricular *see* Newborn,
| affected by, hemorrhage, intraventricular
|nipple N64.59
|nose R04.0
|ovulation N92.3
|postclimacteric N95.0
|postcoital N93.0
|postmenopausal N95.0
|postoperative *see* Complication,
| postprocedural, hemorrhage
|preclimacteric N92.4
|pre-pubertal vaginal N93.1
|puberty (excessive, with onset of menstrual
| periods) N92.2
|rectum, rectal K62.5
| |newborn P54.2
|tendencies *see* Defect, coagulation
|throat R04.1
|tooth socket (post-extraction) K91.840
|umbilical stump P51.9
|uterus, uterine NEC N93.9
| |climacteric N92.4
| |dysfunctional or functional N93.8
| |menopausal N92.4
| |preclimacteric or premenopausal N92.4
| |unrelated to menstrual cycle N93.9
|vagina, vaginal (abnormal) N93.9
| |dysfunctional or functional N93.8
| |newborn P54.6
| |pre-pubertal N93.1
|vicarious N94.89
Blennorrhagia, blennorrhagic *see* Gonorrhea
Blennorrhea (acute) (chronic) *see also*
Gonorrhea
|inclusion (neonatal) (newborn) P39.1
|lower genitourinary tract (gonococcal) A54.00
|neonatorum (gonococcal ophthalmia) A54.31
Blepharelosis *see* Entropion
Blepharitis (angularis) (ciliaris) (eyelid)
(marginal) (nonulcerative) H01.009
|herpes zoster B02.39
|left H01.006
| |lower H01.005
| |upper H01.004
| |upper and lower H01.00B
| |right H01.003
| |lower H01.002
| |upper H01.001
| |upper and lower H01.00A
|squamous H01.029
| |left H01.026
| | |lower H01.025
| | |upper H01.024
| | |upper and lower H01.02B
| |right H01.023
| | |lower H01.022
| | |upper H01.021
| | |upper and lower H01.02A
|ulcerative H01.019
| |left H01.016
| | |lower H01.015
| | |upper H01.014

Blepharitis - *continued*
    |upper and lower H01.01B
  |right H01.013
    |lower H01.012
    |upper H01.011
    |upper and lower H01.01A
Blepharochalasis H02.30
 |congenital Q10.0
 |left H02.36
  |lower H02.35
  |upper H02.34
 |right H02.33
  |lower H02.32
  |upper H02.31
Blepharoclonus H02.59
Blepharoconjunctivitis H10.50-
 |angular H10.52-
 |contact H10.53-
 |ligneous H10.51-
Blepharophimosis (eyelid) H02.529
 |congenital Q10.3
 |left H02.526
  |lower H02.525
  |upper H02.524
 |right H02.523
  |lower H02.522
  |upper H02.521
Blepharoptosis H02.40-
 |congenital Q10.0
 |mechanical H02.41-
 |myogenic H02.42-
 |neurogenic H02.43-
 |paralytic H02.43-
Blepharopyorrhea, gonococcal A54.39
Blepharospasm G24.5
 |drug induced G24.01
Blighted ovum O02.0
Blind *see also* Blindness
 |bronchus (congenital) Q32.4
 |loop syndrome K90.2
  |congenital Q43.8
 |sac, fallopian tube (congenital) Q50.6
 |spot, enlarged *see* Defect, visual field,
    localized, scotoma, blind spot area
 |tract or tube, congenital NEC *see* Atresia, by
    site
Blindness (acquired) (congenital) (both eyes)
    H54.0X-
 |blast S05.8X-
 |color *see* Deficiency, color vision
 |concussion S05.8X-
 |cortical H47.619
  |left brain H47.612
  |right brain H47.611
 |day H53.11
 |due to injury (current episode) S05.9-
  |sequelae   code to injury with seventh
     character S
 |eclipse (total) *see* Retinopathy, solar
 |emotional (hysterical) F44.6
 |face H53.16
 |hysterical F44.6
 |legal (both eyes) (USA definition) H54.8
 |mind R48.8
 |night H53.60
  |abnormal dark adaptation curve H53.61
  |acquired H53.62
  |congenital H53.63
  |specified type NEC H53.69
  |vitamin A deficiency E50.5
 |one eye (other eye normal) H54.40
  |left (normal vision on right) H54.42-
   |low vision on right H54.12-
  |low vision, other eye H54.10
  |right (normal vision on left) H54.41-
   |low vision on left H54.11-
 |psychic R48.8

|river B73.01
|snow *see* Photokeratitis
|sun, solar *see* Retinopathy, solar
|transient *see* Disturbance, vision, subjective,
    loss, transient
|traumatic (current episode) S05.9-
|word (developmental) F81.0
  |acquired R48.0
  |secondary to organic lesion R48.0
Blister (nonthermal)
|abdominal wall S30.821
|alveolar process S00.522
|ankle S90.52-
|antecubital space *see* Blister, elbow
|anus S30.827
|arm (upper) S40.82-
|auditory canal *see* Blister, ear
|auricle *see* Blister, ear
|axilla *see* Blister, arm
|back, lower S30.820
|beetle dermatitis L24.89
|breast S20.12-
|brow S00.82
|calf *see* Blister, leg
|canthus *see* Blister, eyelid
|cheek S00.82
  |internal S00.522
|chest wall *see* Blister, thorax
|chin S00.82
|costal region *see* Blister, thorax
|digit(s)
  |foot *see* Blister, toe
  |hand *see* Blister, finger
|due to burn *see* Burn, by site, second degree
  |ear S00.42-
|elbow S50.32-
|epiglottis S10.12
|esophagus, cervical S10.12
|eyebrow *see* Blister, eyelid
|eyelid S00.22-
|face S00.82
|fever B00.1
|finger(s) S60.429
  |index S60.42-
  |little S60.42-
  |middle S60.42-
  |ring S60.42-
|foot (except toe(s) alone) S90.82-
  |toe *see* Blister, toe
|forearm S50.82-
  |elbow only *see* Blister, elbow
|forehead S00.82
|fracture
|omit code
|genital organ
  |female S30.826
  |male S30.825
|gum S00.522
|hand S60.52-
|head S00.92
  |ear *see* Blister, ear
  |eyelid *see* Blister, eyelid
  |lip S00.521
  |nose S00.32
  |oral cavity S00.522
  |scalp S00.02
  |specified site NEC S00.82
|heel *see* Blister, foot
|hip S70.22-
|interscapular region S20.429
|jaw S00.82
|knee S80.22-
|larynx S10.12
|leg (lower) S80.82-
  |knee *see* Blister, knee
  |upper *see* Blister, thigh
|lip S00.521
|malar region S00.82

Blister (nonthermal) - *continued*
|mammary *see* Blister, breast
|mastoid region S00.82
|mouth S00.522
|multiple, skin, nontraumatic R23.8
|nail
  |finger *see* Blister, finger
  |toe *see* Blister, toe
|nasal S00.32
|neck S10.92
  |specified site NEC S10.82
  |throat S10.12
|nose S00.32
|occipital region S00.02
|oral cavity S00.522
|orbital region *see* Blister, eyelid
|palate S00.522
|palm *see* Blister, hand
|parietal region S00.02
|pelvis S30.820
|penis S30.822
|periocular area *see* Blister, eyelid
|phalanges
  |finger *see* Blister, finger
  |toe *see* Blister, toe
|pharynx S10.12
|pinna *see* Blister, ear
|popliteal space *see* Blister, knee
|scalp S00.02
|scapular region *see* Blister, shoulder
|scrotum S30.823
|shin *see* Blister, leg
|shoulder S40.22-
|sternal region S20.329
|submaxillary region S00.82
|submental region S00.82
|subungual
  |finger(s) *see* Blister, finger
  |toe(s) *see* Blister, toe
|supraclavicular fossa S10.82
|supraorbital S00.82
|temple S00.82
|temporal region S00.82
|testis S30.823
|thermal *see* Burn, second degree, by site
|thigh S70.32-
|thorax, thoracic (wall) S20.92
  |back S20.42-
  |front S20.32-
|throat S10.12
|thumb S60.32-
|toe(s) S90.42-
  |great S90.42-
|tongue S00.522
|trachea S10.12
|tympanum, tympanic membrane *see* Blister,
  ear
|upper arm *see* Blister, arm (upper)
|uvula S00.522
|vagina S30.824
|vocal cords S10.12
|vulva S30.824
|wrist S60.82-
Bloating R14.0
Bloch-Sulzberger disease or syndrome Q82.3
Block, blocked
|alveolocapillary J84.10
|arborization (heart) I45.5
|arrhythmic I45.9
|atrioventricular (incomplete) (partial) I44.30
  |with atrioventricular dissociation I44.2
  |complete I44.2
    |congenital Q24.6
  |congenital Q24.6
  |first degree I44.0
  |second degree (types I and II) I44.1
  |specified NEC I44.39

Borderline
 |diabetes mellitus R73.03
 |hypertension R03.0
 |osteopenia M85.8-
 |pelvis, with obstruction during labor O65.1
 |personality F60.3
Borna disease A83.9
Bornholm disease B33.0
Boston exanthem A88.0
Botalli, ductus (patent) (persistent) Q25.0
Bothriocephalus latus infestation B70.0
Botulism (foodborne intoxication) A05.1
 |infant A48.51
 |non-foodborne A48.52
 |wound A48.52
Bouba *see* Yaws
Bouchard's nodes (with arthropathy) M15.2
Bouffée délirante F23
Bouillaud's disease or syndrome (rheumatic heart disease) I01.9
Bourneville's disease Q85.1
Boutonniere deformity (finger) *see* Deformity, finger, boutonniere
Bouveret (-Hoffmann) syndrome (paroxysmal tachycardia) I47.9
Bovine heart *see* Hypertrophy, cardiac
Bowel *see* condition
Bowen's
 |dermatosis (precancerous) *see* Neoplasm, skin, in situ
 |disease *see* Neoplasm, skin, in situ
 |epithelioma *see* Neoplasm, skin, in situ
 |type
  |epidermoid carcinoma-in-situ *see* Neoplasm, skin, in situ
  |intraepidermal squamous cell carcinoma *see* Neoplasm, skin, in situ
Bowing
 |femur *see also* Deformity, limb, specified type NEC, thigh
  |congenital Q68.3
 |fibula *see also* Deformity, limb, specified type NEC, lower leg
  |congenital Q68.4
 |forearm *see* Deformity, limb, specified type NEC, forearm
 |leg(s), long bones, congenital Q68.5
 |radius *see* Deformity, limb, specified type NEC, forearm
 |tibia *see also* Deformity, limb, specified type NEC, lower leg
  |congenital Q68.4
Bowleg(s) (acquired) M21.16-
 |congenital Q68.5
 |rachitic E64.3
Boyd's dysentery A03.2
Brachial *see* condition
Brachycardia R00.1
Brachycephaly Q75.0
Bradley's disease A08.19
Bradyarrhythmia, cardiac I49.8
Bradycardia (sinoatrial) (sinus) (vagal) R00.1
 |neonatal P29.12
 |reflex G90.09
 |tachycardia syndrome I49.5
Bradykinesia R25.8
Bradypnea R06.89
Bradytachycardia I49.5
Brailsford's disease or osteochondrosis *see* Osteochondrosis, juvenile, radius
Brain *see also* condition
 |death G93.82
 |syndrome *see* Syndrome, brain
Branched-Chain amino-Acid disorder E71.2

Branchial *see* condition
 |cartilage, congenital Q18.2
Branchiogenic remnant (in neck) Q18.0
Brandt's syndrome (acrodermatitis enteropathica) E83.2
Brash (water) R12
Bravais-Jacksonian epilepsy *see* Epilepsy, localization-related, symptomatic, with simple partial seizures
Braxton Hicks contractions *see* False, labor
Brazilian leishmaniasis B55.2
BRBPR K62.5
Break, retina (without detachment) H33.30-
 |with retinal detachment *see* Detachment, retina
 |horseshoe tear H33.31-
 |multiple H33.33-
 |round hole H33.32-
Breakdown
 |device, graft or implant *see also* Complications, by site and type, mechanical T85.618
  |arterial graft NEC *see* Complication, cardiovascular device, mechanical, vascular
  |breast (implant) T85.41
  |catheter NEC T85.618
   |cystostomy T83.010
   |Hopkins T83.018
   |ileostomy T83.018
   |dialysis (renal) T82.41
    |intraperitoneal T85.611
   |infusion NEC T82.514
    |cranial T85.610
    |epidural T85.610
    |intrathecal T85.610
    |spinal T85.610
    |subarachnoid T85.610
    |subdural T85.610
   |nephrostomy T83.012
   |urethral indwelling T83.011
   |urinary NEC T83.018
   |urostomy T83.018
  |electronic (electrode) (pulse generator) (stimulator)
   |bone T84.310
   |cardiac T82.119
    |electrode T82.110
    |pulse generator T82.111
    |specified type NEC T82.118
   |nervous system *see* Complication, prosthetic device, mechanical, electronic nervous system stimulator
   |urinary *see* Complication, genitourinary, device, urinary, mechanical
  |fixation, internal (orthopedic) NEC *see* Complication, fixation device, mechanical
  |gastrointestinal *see* Complications, prosthetic device, mechanical, gastrointestinal device
  |genital NEC T83.418
   |intrauterine contraceptive device T83.31
   |penile prosthesis (cylinder) (implanted) (pump) (reservoir) T83.410
   |testicular prosthesis T83.411
  |heart NEC *see* Complication, cardiovascular device, mechanical
  |intrathecal infusion pump T85.615
  |joint prosthesis *see* Complications, joint prosthesis, internal, mechanical, by site
  |nervous system, specified device NEC T85.615
  |ocular NEC *see* Complications, prosthetic device, mechanical, ocular device
  |orthopedic NEC *see* Complication, orthopedic, device, mechanical
  |specified NEC T85.618

Breakdown - *continued*
 |subcutaneous device pocket
  |nervous system prosthetic device, implant, or graft T85.890
  |other internal prosthetic device, implant, or graft T85.898
 |sutures, permanent T85.612
  |used in bone repair *see* Complications, fixation device, internal (orthopedic), mechanical
 |urinary NEC T83.118
  |graft T83.21
  |sphincter, implanted T83.111
  |stent (ileal conduit) (nephroureteral) T83.113
   |ureteral indwelling T83.112
 |vascular NEC *see* Complication, cardiovascular device, mechanical
 |ventricular intracranial shunt T85.01
 |nervous F48.8
 |perineum O90.1
 |respirator J95.850
  |specified NEC J95.859
 |ventilator J95.850
  |specified NEC J95.859
Breast *see also* condition
 |buds E30.1
  |in newborn P96.89
 |dense R92.2
 |nodule (*see also* Lump, breast) N63.0
Breath
 |foul R19.6
 |holder, child R06.89
 |holding spell R06.89
 |shortness R06.02
Breathing
 |labored *see* Hyperventilation
 |mouth R06.5
  |causing malocclusion M26.5
 |periodic R06.3
  |high altitude G47.32
Breathlessness R06.81
Breda's disease *see* Yaws
Breech presentation (mother) O32.1
 |causing obstructed labor O64.1
 |footling O32.8
  |causing obstructed labor O64.8
 |incomplete O32.8
  |causing obstructed labor O64.8
Breisky's disease N90.4
Brennemann's syndrome I88.0
Brenner
 |tumor (benign) D27.9
  |borderline malignancy D39.1-
  |malignant C56
  |proliferating D39.1-
Bretonneau's disease or angina A36.0
Breus' mole O02.0
Brevicollis Q76.49
Brickmakers' anemia B76.9 [*D63.8*]
Bridge, myocardial Q24.5
Bright red blood per rectum (BRBPR) K62.5
Bright's disease *see also* Nephritis
 |arteriosclerotic *see* Hypertension, kidney
Brill (-Zinsser) disease (recrudescent typhus) A75.1
 |flea-borne A75.2
 |louse-borne A75.1
Brill-Symmers' disease C82.90
Brion-Kayser disease *see* Fever, parathyroid
Briquet's disorder or syndrome F45.0
Brissaud's
 |infantilism or dwarfism E23.0
 |motor-verbal tic F95.2

Brittle
|bones disease Q78.0
|nails L60.3
||congenital Q84.6
Broad *see also* condition
|beta disease E78.2
|ligament laceration syndrome N83.8
Broad or floating-Betalipoproteinemia E78.2
Brock's syndrome (atelectasis due to enlarged lymph nodes) J98.19
Brocq-Duhring disease (dermatitis herpetiformis) L13.0
Brodie's abscess or disease M86.8X-
Broken
|arches *see also* Deformity, limb, flat foot
|arm (meaning upper limb) *see* Fracture, arm
|back *see* Fracture, vertebra
|bone *see* Fracture
|implant or internal device *see* Complications, by site and type, mechanical
|leg (meaning lower limb) *see* Fracture, leg
|nose S02.2
|tooth, teeth *see* Fracture, tooth
Bromhidrosis, bromidrosis L75.0
Bromidism, bromism G92.8
|due to
||correct substance properly administered *see* Table of Drugs and Chemicals, by drug, adverse effect
||overdose or wrong substance given or taken *see* Table of Drugs and Chemicals, by drug, poisoning
|chronic (dependence) F13.20
Bromidrosiphobia F40.298
Bronchi, bronchial *see* condition
Bronchiectasis (cylindrical) (diffuse) (fusiform) (localized) (saccular) J47.9
|with
||acute
|||bronchitis J47.0
|||lower respiratory infection J47.0
||exacerbation (acute) J47.1
|congenital Q33.4
|tuberculous NEC *see* Tuberculosis, pulmonary
Bronchiolectasis *see* Bronchiectasis
Bronchiolitis (acute) (infective) (subacute) J21.9
|with
||bronchospasm or obstruction J21.9
||influenza, flu or grippe *see* Influenza, with, respiratory manifestations NEC
|chemical (chronic) J68.4
||acute J68.0
|chronic (fibrosing) (obliterative) J44.9
|due to
||external agent *see* Bronchitis, acute, due to
||human metapneumovirus J21.1
||respiratory syncytial virus J21.0
||specified organism NEC J21.8
|fibrosa obliterans J44.9
|influenzal *see* Influenza, with, respiratory manifestations NEC
|obliterans J42
||with organizing pneumonia (BOOP) J84.89
|obliterative (chronic) (subacute) J44.9
||due to fumes or vapors J68.4
||due to chemicals, gases, fumes or vapors (inhalation) J68.4
|respiratory, interstitial lung disease J84.115
Bronchitis (diffuse) (fibrinous) (hypostatic) (infective) (membranous) J40
|with
||influenza, flu or grippe *see* Influenza, with, respiratory manifestations NEC
||obstruction (airway) (lung) J44.9
||tracheitis (15 years of age and above) J40
|||acute or subacute J20.9
|||chronic J42

Bronchitis - *continued*
||under 15 years of age J20.9
|acute or subacute (with bronchospasm or obstruction) J20.9
||with
|||bronchiectasis J47.0
|||chronic obstructive pulmonary disease J44.0
||chemical (due to gases, fumes or vapors) J68.0
||due to
|||fumes or vapors J68.0
|||Haemophilus influenzae J20.1
|||Mycoplasma pneumoniae J20.0
|||radiation J70.0
|||specified organism NEC J20.8
|||Streptococcus J20.2
|||virus
||||coxsackie J20.3
||||echovirus J20.7
||||parainfluenzae J20.4
||||respiratory syncytial J20.5
||||rhinovirus J20.6
||viral NEC J20.8
|allergic (acute) J45.909
||with
|||exacerbation (acute) J45.901
|||status asthmaticus J45.902
|arachidic T17.528
|aspiration (due to food and vomit) J69.0
|asthmatic J45.9
||chronic J44.9
|||with
||||acute lower respiratory infection J44.0
||||exacerbation (acute) J44.1
|capillary *see* Pneumonia, broncho
|caseous (tuberculous) A15.5
|Castellani's A69.8
|catarrhal (15 years of age and above) J40
||acute *see* Bronchitis, acute
||chronic J41.0
||under 15 years of age J20.9
|chemical (acute) (subacute) J68.0
||chronic J68.4
||due to fumes or vapors J68.0
|||chronic J68.4
|chronic J42
||with
|||airways obstruction J44.9
|||tracheitis (chronic) J42
||asthmatic (obstructive) J44.9
||catarrhal J41.0
||chemical (due to fumes or vapors) J68.4
||due to
|||chemicals, gases, fumes or vapors (inhalation) J68.4
|||radiation J70.1
|||tobacco smoking J41.0
||emphysematous J44.9
||mucopurulent J41.1
||non-obstructive J41.0
||obliterans J44.9
||obstructive J44.9
||purulent J41.1
||simple J41.0
|croupous *see* Bronchitis, acute
|due to gases, fumes or vapors (chemical) J68.0
|emphysematous (obstructive) J44.9
|exudative *see* Bronchitis, acute
|fetid J41.1
|grippal *see* Influenza, with, respiratory manifestations NEC
|in those under 15 years age *see* Bronchitis, acute
||chronic *see* Bronchitis, chronic

Bronchitis - *continued*
|influenzal *see* Influenza, with, respiratory manifestations NEC
|mixed simple and mucopurulent J41.8
|moulder's J62.8
|mucopurulent (chronic) (recurrent) J41.1
||acute or subacute J20.9
||simple (mixed) J41.8
|obliterans (chronic) J44.9
|obstructive (chronic) (diffuse) J44.9
|pituitous J41.1
|pneumococcal, acute or subacute J20.2
|pseudomembranous, acute or subacute *see* Bronchitis, acute
|purulent (chronic) (recurrent) J41.1
||acute or subacute *see* Bronchitis, acute
|putrid J41.1
|senile (chronic) J42
|simple and mucopurulent (mixed) J41.8
|smokers' J41.0
|spirochetal NEC A69.8
|subacute *see* Bronchitis, acute
|suppurative (chronic) J41.1
||acute or subacute *see* Bronchitis, acute
|tuberculous A15.5
|under 15 years of age *see* Bronchitis, acute
||chronic *see* Bronchitis, chronic
|viral NEC, acute or subacute *see also* Bronchitis, acute J20.8
Bronchoalveolitis J18.0
Bronchoaspergillosis B44.1
Bronchocele meaning goiter E04.0
Broncholithiasis J98.09
||tuberculous NEC A15.5
Bronchomalacia J98.09
|congenital Q32.2
Bronchomycosis NOS B49 [*J99*]
|candidal B37.1
Bronchopleuropneumonia *see* Pneumonia, broncho
Bronchopneumonia *see* Pneumonia, broncho
Bronchopneumonitis *see* Pneumonia, broncho
Bronchopulmonary *see* condition
Bronchopulmonitis *see* Pneumonia, broncho
Bronchorrhagia (see Hemoptysis)
Bronchorrhea J98.09
|acute J20.9
|chronic (infective) (purulent) J42
Bronchospasm (acute) J98.01
|with
||bronchiolitis, acute J21.9
||bronchitis, acute (conditions in J20) *see* Bronchitis, acute
|due to external agent *see* condition, respiratory, acute, due to
|exercise induced J45.990
Bronchospirochetosis A69.8
|Castellani A69.8
Bronchostenosis J98.09
Bronchus *see* condition
Brontophobia F40.220
Bronze baby syndrome P83.88
Brooke's tumor *see* Neoplasm, skin, benign
Brown enamel of teeth (hereditary) K00.5
Brown's sheath syndrome H50.61-
Brown-Séquard disease, paralysis or syndrome G83.81
Bruce sepsis A23.0
Brucellosis (infection) A23.9
|abortus A23.1
|canis A23.3
|dermatitis A23.9
|melitensis A23.0
|mixed A23.8
|sepsis A23.9
||melitensis A23.0
||specified NEC A23.8
|suis A23.2

Bruck-De Lange disease Q87.1
Bruck's disease *see* Deformity, limb
BRUE (brief resolved unexplained event)
   R68.13
Brugsch's syndrome Q82.8
Bruise (skin surface intact) *see also* Contusion
  |with
    |open wound *see* Wound, open
  |internal organ *see* Injury, by site
  |newborn P54.5
  |scalp, due to birth injury, newborn P12.3
  |umbilical cord O69.5
Bruit (arterial) R09.89
  |cardiac R01.1
Brush burn *see* Abrasion, by site
Bruton's X-Linked agammaglobulinemia
   D80.0
Bruxism
  |psychogenic F45.8
  |sleep related G47.63
Bubbly lung syndrome P27.0
Bubo I88.8
  |blennorrhagic (gonococcal) A54.89
  |chancroidal A57
  |climatic A55
  |due to Haemophilus ducreyi A57
  |gonococcal A54.89
  |indolent (nonspecific) I88.8
  |inguinal (nonspecific) I88.8
    |chancroidal A57
    |climatic A55
    |due to H. ducreyi A57
    |infective I88.8
  |scrofulous (tuberculous) A18.2
  |soft chancre A57
  |suppurating *see* Lymphadenitis, acute
  |syphilitic (primary) A51.0
    |congenital A50.07
  |tropical A55
  |virulent (chancroidal) A57
Bubonic plague A20.0
Bubonocele *see* Hernia, inguinal
Buccal *see* condition
Buchanan's disease or osteochondrosis M91.0
Buchem's syndrome (hyperostosis corticalis)
   M85.2
Bucket-Handle fracture or tear (semilunar
   cartilage) *see* Tear, meniscus
Budd-Chiari syndrome (hepatic vein
   thrombosis) I82.0
Budgerigar fancier's disease or lung J67.2
Buds
  |breast E30.1
    |in newborn P96.89
Buerger's disease (thromboangiitis obliterans)
   I73.1
Bulbar *see* condition
Bulbus cordis (left ventricle) (persistent)
   Q21.8
Bulimia (nervosa) F50.2
  |atypical F50.9
  |normal weight F50.9
Bulky
  |stools R19.5
  |uterus N85.2
Bulla (e) R23.8
  |lung (emphysematous) (solitary) J43.9
    |newborn P25.8
Bullet wound *see also* Wound, open
  |fracture   code as Fracture, by site
  |internal organ *see* Injury, by site
Bundle
  |branch block (complete) (false) (incomplete)
    see Block, bundle-branch
  |of His *see* condition
Bunion M21.61-
  |tailor's M21.62-

Bunionette M21.62-
Buphthalmia, buphthalmos (congenital) Q15.0
Burdwan fever B55.0
Bürger-Grütz disease or syndrome E78.3
Buried
  |penis (congenital) Q55.64
    |acquired N48.83
  |roots K08.3
Burke's syndrome K86.89
Burkitt
  |cell leukemia C91.0-
  |lymphoma (malignant) C83.7-
    |small noncleaved, diffuse C83.7-
    |spleen C83.77
    |undifferentiated C83.7-
  |tumor C83.7-
  |type
    |acute lymphoblastic leukemia C91.0-
    |undifferentiated C83.7-
Burn (electricity) (flame) (hot gas, liquid or hot
   object) (radiation) (steam) (thermal) T30.0
  |abdomen, abdominal (muscle) (wall) T21.02
    |first degree T21.12
    |second degree T21.22
    |third degree T21.32
  |above elbow T22.039
    |first degree T22.139
    |left T22.032
      |first degree T22.132
      |second degree T22.232
      |third degree T22.332
    |right T22.031
      |first degree T22.131
      |second degree T22.231
      |third degree T22.331
    |second degree T22.239
    |third degree T22.339
  |acid (caustic) (external) (internal) *see*
    Corrosion, by site
  |alimentary tract NEC T28.2
    |esophagus T28.1
    |mouth T28.0
    |pharynx T28.0
  |alkaline (caustic) (external) (internal) *see*
    Corrosion, by site
  |ankle T25.019
    |first degree T25.119
    |left T25.012
      |first degree T25.112
      |second degree T25.212
      |third degree T25.312
    |multiple with foot *see* Burn, lower, limb,
      multiple, ankle and foot
    |right T25.011
      |first degree T25.111
      |second degree T25.211
      |third degree T25.311
    |second degree T25.219
    |third degree T25.319
  |anus *see* Burn, buttock
  |arm (lower) (upper) *see* Burn, upper, limb
  |axilla T22.049
    |first degree T22.149
    |left T22.042
      |first degree T22.142
      |second degree T22.242
      |third degree T22.342
    |right T22.041
      |first degree T22.141
      |second degree T22.241
      |third degree T22.341
    |second degree T22.249
    |third degree T22.349
  |back (lower) T21.04
    |first degree T21.14
    |second degree T21.24

Burn - *continued*
    |third degree T21.34
    |upper T21.03
      |first degree T21.13
      |second degree T21.23
      |third degree T21.33
  |blisters   code as Burn, second degree, by site
  |breast(s) *see* Burn, chest wall
  |buttock(s) T21.05
    |first degree T21.15
    |second degree T21.25
    |third degree T21.35
  |calf T24.039
    |first degree T24.139
    |left T24.032
      |first degree T24.132
      |second degree T24.232
      |third degree T24.332
    |right T24.031
      |first degree T24.131
      |second degree T24.231
      |third degree T24.331
    |second degree T24.239
    |third degree T24.339
  |canthus (eye) *see* Burn, eyelid
  |caustic acid or alkaline *see* Corrosion, by site
  |cervix T28.3
  |cheek T20.06
    |first degree T20.16
    |second degree T20.26
    |third degree T20.36
  |chemical (acids) (alkalines) (caustics)
    (external) (internal) *see* Corrosion, by site
  |chest wall T21.01
    |first degree T21.11
    |second degree T21.21
    |third degree T21.31
  |chin T20.03
    |first degree T20.13
    |second degree T20.23
    |third degree T20.33
  |colon T28.2
  |conjunctiva (and cornea) *see* Burn, cornea
  |cornea (and conjunctiva) T26.1-
    |chemical *see* Corrosion, cornea
  |corrosion (external) (internal) *see* Corrosion,
    by site
  |deep necrosis of underlying tissue   code as
    Burn, third degree, by site
  |dorsum of hand T23.069
    |first degree T23.169
    |left T23.062
      |first degree T23.162
      |second degree T23.262
      |third degree T23.362
    |right T23.061
      |first degree T23.161
      |second degree T23.261
      |third degree T23.361
    |second degree T23.269
    |third degree T23.369
  |due to ingested chemical agent *see* Corrosion,
    by site
  |ear (auricle) (external) (canal) T20.01
    |first degree T20.11
    |second degree T20.21
    |third degree T20.31
  |elbow T22.029
    |first degree T22.129
    |left T22.022
      |first degree T22.122
      |second degree T22.222
      |third degree T22.322
    |right T22.021
      |first degree T22.121
      |second degree T22.221

Burn - *continued*

|third degree T22.321
|second degree T22.229
|third degree T22.329
|epidermal loss   code as Burn, second degree, by site
|erythema, erythematous   code as Burn, first degree, by site
|esophagus T28.1
|extent (percentage of body surface)
　|less than 10 percent T31.0
　|10-19 percent T31.10
　　|with 0-9 percent third degree burns T31.10
　　|with 10-19 percent third degree burns T31.11
　|20-29 percent T31.20
　　|with 0-9 percent third degree burns T31.20
　　|with 10-19 percent third degree burns T31.21
　　|with 20-29 percent third degree burns T31.22
　|30-39 percent T31.30
　　|with 0-9 percent third degree burns T31.30
　　|with 10-19 percent third degree burns T31.31
　　|with 20-29 percent third degree burns T31.32
　　|with 30-39 percent third degree burns T31.33
　|40-49 percent T31.40
　　|with 0-9 percent third degree burns T31.40
　　|with 10-19 percent third degree burns T31.41
　　|with 20-29 percent third degree burns T31.42
　　|with 30-39 percent third degree burns T31.43
　　|with 40-49 percent third degree burns T31.44
　|50-59 percent T31.50
　　|with 0-9 percent third degree burns T31.50
　　|with 10-19 percent third degree burns T31.51
　　|with 20-29 percent third degree burns T31.52
　　|with 30-39 percent third degree burns T31.53
　　|with 40-49 percent third degree burns T31.54
　　|with 50-59 percent third degree burns T31.55
　|60-69 percent T31.60
　　|with 0-9 percent third degree burns T31.60
　　|with 10-19 percent third degree burns T31.61
　　|with 20-29 percent third degree burns T31.62
　　|with 30-39 percent third degree burns T31.63
　　|with 40-49 percent third degree burns T31.64
　　|with 50-59 percent third degree burns T31.65
　　|with 60-69 percent third degree burns T31.66
　|70-79 percent T31.70
　　|with 0-9 percent third degree burns T31.70

Burn - *continued*

　　|with 10-19 percent third degree burns T31.71
　　|with 20-29 percent third degree burns T31.72
　　|with 30-39 percent third degree burns T31.73
　　|with 40-49 percent third degree burns T31.74
　　|with 50-59 percent third degree burns T31.75
　　|with 60-69 percent third degree burns T31.76
　　|with 70-79 percent third degree burns T31.77
　|80-89 percent T31.80
　　|with 0-9 percent third degree burns T31.80
　　|with 10-19 percent third degree burns T31.81
　　|with 20-29 percent third degree burns T31.82
　　|with 30-39 percent third degree burns T31.83
　　|with 40-49 percent third degree burns T31.84
　　|with 50-59 percent third degree burns T31.85
　　|with 60-69 percent third degree burns T31.86
　　|with 70-79 percent third degree burns T31.87
　　|with 80-89 percent third degree burns T31.88
　|90 percent or more T31.90
　　|with 0-9 percent third degree burns T31.90
　　|with 10-19 percent third degree burns T31.91
　　|with 20-29 percent third degree burns T31.92
　　|with 30-39 percent third degree burns T31.93
　　|with 40-49 percent third degree burns T31.94
　　|with 50-59 percent third degree burns T31.95
　　|with 60-69 percent third degree burns T31.96
　　|with 70-79 percent third degree burns T31.97
　　|with 80-89 percent third degree burns T31.98
　　|with 90 percent or more third degree burns T31.99
|extremity *see* Burn, limb
|eye(s) and adnexa T26.4-
　|with resulting rupture and destruction of eyeball T26.2-
　|conjunctival sac *see* Burn, cornea
　|cornea *see* Burn, cornea
　|lid *see* Burn, eyelid
　|periocular area *see* Burn, eyelid
　|specified site NEC T26.3-
|eyeball *see* Burn, eye　　|eyelid(s) T26.0-
　|chemical *see* Corrosion, eyelid
|face *see* Burn, head
|finger T23.029
　|first degree T23.129
　|left T23.022
　　|first degree T23.122
　　|second degree T23.222
　　|third degree T23.322
　|multiple sites (without thumb) T23.039
　　|with thumb T23.049
　　　|first degree T23.149
　　　|left T23.042

Burn - *continued*

　　|first degree T23.142
　　|second degree T23.242
　　|third degree T23.342
　|right T23.041
　　|first degree T23.141
　　|second degree T23.241
　　|third degree T23.341
　|second degree T23.249
　|third degree T23.349
|first degree T23.139
|left T23.032
　|first degree T23.132
　|second degree T23.232
　|third degree T23.332
|right T23.031
　|first degree T23.131
　|second degree T23.231
　|third degree T23.331
|second degree T23.239
　|right T23.021
　　|first degree T23.121
　　|second degree T23.221
　　|third degree T23.321
|second degree T23.229
|third degree T23.329
|flank *see* Burn, abdominal wall
|foot T25.029
　|first degree T25.129
　|left T25.022
　　|first degree T25.122
　　|second degree T25.222
　　|third degree T25.322
　|multiple with ankle *see* Burn, lower, limb, multiple, ankle and foot
　|right T25.021
　　|first degree T25.121
　　|second degree T25.221
　　|third degree T25.321
　|second degree T25.229
　|third degree T25.329
|forearm T22.019
　|first degree T22.119
　|left T22.012
　　|first degree T22.112
　　|second degree T22.212
　　|third degree T22.312
　|right T22.011
　　|first degree T22.111
　　|second degree T22.211
　　|third degree T22.311
　|second degree T22.219
　|third degree T22.319
|forehead T20.06
　|first degree T20.16
　|second degree T20.26
　|third degree T20.36
|fourth degree   code as Burn, third degree, by site
|friction *see* Burn, by site
|from swallowing caustic or corrosive substance NEC *see* Corrosion, by site
|full thickness skin loss   code as Burn, third degree, by site
|gastrointestinal tract NEC T28.2
　|from swallowing caustic or corrosive substance T28.7
|genital organs
　|external
　　|female T21.07
　　　|first degree T21.17
　　　|second degree T21.27
　　　|third degree T21.37
　　|male T21.06

Burn - *continued*
    |first degree T21.16
    |second degree T21.26
    |third degree T21.36
  |internal T28.3
  |from caustic or corrosive substance T28.8
|groin *see* Burn, abdominal wall
|hand(s) T23.009
  |back *see* Burn, dorsum of hand
  |finger *see* Burn, finger
  |first degree T23.109
  |left T23.002
    |first degree T23.102
    |second degree T23.202
    |third degree T23.302
  |multiple sites with wrist T23.099
    |first degree T23.199
    |left T23.092
      |first degree T23.192
      |second degree T23.292
      |third degree T23.392
    |right T23.091
      |first degree T23.191
      |second degree T23.291
      |third degree T23.391
    |second degree T23.299
    |third degree T23.399
  |palm *see* Burn, palm
  |right T23.001
    |first degree T23.101
    |second degree T23.201
    |third degree T23.301
  |second degree T23.209
  |third degree T23.309
  |thumb *see* Burn, thumb
|head (and face) (and neck) T20.00
  |cheek *see* Burn, cheek
  |chin *see* Burn, chin
  |ear *see* Burn, ear
  |eye(s) only *see* Burn, eye
  |first degree T20.10
  |forehead *see* Burn, forehead
  |lip *see* Burn, lip
  |multiple sites T20.09
    |first degree T20.19
    |second degree T20.29
    |third degree T20.39
  |neck *see* Burn, neck
  |nose *see* Burn, nose
  |scalp *see* Burn, scalp
  |second degree T20.20
  |third degree T20.30
|hip(s) *see* Burn, thigh
|inhalation *see* Burn, respiratory tract
  |caustic or corrosive substance (fumes) *see*
  Corrosion, respiratory tract
|internal organ(s) T28.40
  |alimentary tract T28.2
    |esophagus T28.1
  |eardrum T28.41
  |esophagus T28.1
  |from caustic or corrosive substance
  (swallowing) NEC *see* Corrosion, by site
  |genitourinary T28.3
  |mouth T28.0
  |pharynx T28.0
  |respiratory tract *see* Burn, respiratory tract
  |specified organ NEC T28.49
|interscapular region *see* Burn, back, upper
|intestine (large) (small) T28.2
|knee T24.029
  |first degree T24.129
  |left T24.022
    |first degree T24.122
    |second degree T24.222
    |third degree T24.322
  |right T24.021

Burn - *continued*
    |first degree T24.121
    |second degree T24.221
    |third degree T24.321
  |second degree T24.229
  |third degree T24.329
|labium (majus) (minus) *see* Burn, genital
  organs, external, female
|lacrimal apparatus, duct, gland or sac *see*
  Burn, eye, specified site NEC
|larynx T27.0
  |with lung T27.1
|leg(s) (lower) (upper) *see* Burn, lower, limb
|lightning *see* Burn, by site
|limb(s)
  |lower (except ankle or foot alone) *see* Burn,
  lower, limb
  |upper *see* Burn, upper limb
|lip(s) T20.02
  |first degree T20.12
  |second degree T20.22
  |third degree T20.32
|lower
  |back *see* Burn, back
  |limb T24.009
    |ankle *see* Burn, ankle
    |calf *see* Burn, calf
    |first degree T24.109
    |foot *see* Burn, foot
    |hip *see* Burn, thigh
    |knee *see* Burn, knee
    |left T24.002
      |first degree T24.102
      |second degree T24.202
      |third degree T24.302
    |multiple sites, except ankle and foot
    T24.099
      |ankle and foot T25.099
        |first degree T25.199
        |left T25.092
          |first degree T25.192
          |second degree T25.292
          |third degree T25.392
        |right T25.091
          |first degree T25.191
          |second degree T25.291
          |third degree T25.391
        |second degree T25.299
        |third degree T25.399
      |first degree T24.199
      |left T24.092
        |first degree T24.192
        |second degree T24.292
        |third degree T24.392
      |right T24.091
        |first degree T24.191
        |second degree T24.291
        |third degree T24.391
      |second degree T24.299
      |third degree T24.399
    |right T24.001
      |first degree T24.101
      |second degree T24.201
      |third degree T24.301
    |second degree T24.209
    |thigh *see* Burn, thigh
    |third degree T24.309
    |toe *see* Burn, toe
|lung (with larynx and trachea) T27.1
|mouth T28.0
|neck T20.07
  |first degree T20.17
  |second degree T20.27
  |third degree T20.37
|nose (septum) T20.04
  |first degree T20.14

Burn - *continued*
  |second degree T20.24
  |third degree T20.34
|ocular adnexa *see* Burn, eye
|orbit region *see* Burn, eyelid
|palm T23.059
  |first degree T23.159
  |left T23.052
    |first degree T23.152
    |second degree T23.252
    |third degree T23.352
  |right T23.051
    |first degree T23.151
    |second degree T23.251
    |third degree T23.351
  |second degree T23.259
  |third degree T23.359
|partial thickness - code as Burn, by site,
  second degree
|pelvis *see* Burn, trunk
|penis *see* Burn, genital organs, external, male
|perineum
  |female *see* Burn, genital organs, external,
  female
  |male *see* Burn, genital organs, external,
  male
|periocular area *see* Burn, eyelid
|pharynx T28.0
|rectum T28.2
|respiratory tract T27.3
  |larynx *see* Burn, larynx
  |specified part NEC T27.2
  |trachea *see* Burn, trachea
|sac, lacrimal *see* Burn, eye, specified site NEC
|scalp T20.05
  |first degree T20.15
  |second degree T20.25
  |third degree T20.35
|scapular region T22.069
  |first degree T22.169
  |left T22.062
    |first degree T22.162
    |second degree T22.262
    |third degree T22.362
  |right T22.061
    |first degree T22.161
    |second degree T22.261
    |third degree T22.361
  |second degree T22.269
  |third degree T22.369
|sclera *see* Burn, eye, specified site NEC
|scrotum *see* Burn, genital organs, external,
  male
|shoulder T22.059
  |first degree T22.159
  |left T22.052
    |first degree T22.152
    |second degree T22.252
    |third degree T22.352
  |right T22.051
    |first degree T22.151
    |second degree T22.251
    |third degree T22.351
  |second degree T22.259
  |third degree T22.359
|stomach T28.2
|temple *see* Burn, head
|testis *see* Burn, genital organs, external, male
|thigh T24.019
  |first degree T24.119
  |left T24.012
    |first degree T24.112
    |second degree T24.212
    |third degree T24.312
  |right T24.011

Burn - *continued*

    |first degree T24.111
    |second degree T24.211
    |third degree T24.311
  |second degree T24.219
  |third degree T24.319
|thorax (external) *see* Burn, trunk
|throat (meaning pharynx) T28.0
|thumb(s) T23.019
  |first degree T23.119
  |left T23.012
    |first degree T23.112
    |second degree T23.212
    |third degree T23.312
  |multiple sites with fingers T23.049
    |first degree T23.149
    |left T23.042
      |first degree T23.142
      |second degree T23.242
      |third degree T23.342
    |right T23.041
      |first degree T23.141
      |second degree T23.241
      |third degree T23.341
    |second degree T23.249
    |third degree T23.349
  |right T23.011
    |first degree T23.111
    |second degree T23.211
    |third degree T23.311
  |second degree T23.219
  |third degree T23.319
|toe T25.039
  |first degree T25.139
  |left T25.032
    |first degree T25.132
    |second degree T25.232
    |third degree T25.332
  |right T25.031
    |first degree T25.131
    |second degree T25.231
    |third degree T25.331
  |second degree T25.239
  |third degree T25.339
|tongue T28.0
|tonsil(s) T28.0
|trachea T27.0
  |with lung T27.1
|trunk T21.00
  |abdominal wall *see* Burn, abdominal wall
  |anus *see* Burn, buttock
  |axilla *see* Burn, upper limb
  |back *see* Burn, back
  |breast *see* Burn, chest wall
  |buttock *see* Burn, buttock
  |chest wall *see* Burn, chest wall
  |first degree T21.10
  |flank *see* Burn, abdominal wall
  |genital
    |female *see* Burn, genital organs, external,
    female
    |male *see* Burn, genital organs, external,
    male
  |groin *see* Burn, abdominal wall
  |interscapular region *see* Burn, back, upper
  |labia *see* Burn, genital organs, external,
  female
  |lower back *see* Burn, back
  |penis *see* Burn, genital organs, external,
  male
  |perineum
    |female *see* Burn, genital organs, external,
    female
    |male *see* Burn, genital organs, external,
    male
  |scapula region *see* Burn, scapular region

Burn - *continued*

  |scrotum *see* Burn, genital organs, external,
  male
  |second degree T21.20
  |specified site NEC T21.09
    |first degree T21.19
    |second degree T21.29
    |third degree T21.39
  |testes *see* Burn, genital organs, external,
  male
  |third degree T21.30
  |upper back *see* Burn, back, upper
  |vulva *see* Burn, genital organs, external,
  female
|unspecified site with extent of body surface
  involved specified
  |less than 10 percent T31.0
  |10-19 percent (0-9 percent third degree)
    T31.10
    |with 10-19 percent third degree T31.11
  |20-29 percent (0-9 percent third degree)
    T31.20
    |with
      |10-19 percent third degree T31.21
      |20-29 percent third degree T31.22
  |30-39 percent (0-9 percent third degree)
    T31.30
    |with
      |10-19 percent third degree T31.31
      |20-29 percent third degree T31.32
      |30-39 percent third degree T31.33
  |40-49 percent (0-9 percent third degree)
    T31.40
    |with
      |10-19 percent third degree T31.41
      |20-29 percent third degree T31.42
      |30-39 percent third degree T31.43
      |40-49 percent third degree T31.44
  |50-59 percent (0-9 percent third degree)
    T31.50
    |with
      |10-19 percent third degree T31.51
      |20-29 percent third degree T31.52
      |30-39 percent third degree T31.53
      |40-49 percent third degree T31.54
      |50-59 percent third degree T31.55
  |60-69 percent (0-9 percent third degree)
    T31.60
    |with
      |10-19 percent third degree T31.61
      |20-29 percent third degree T31.62
      |30-39 percent third degree T31.63
      |40-49 percent third degree T31.64
      |50-59 percent third degree T31.65
      |60-69 percent third degree T31.66
  |70-79 percent (0-9 percent third degree)
    T31.70
    |with
      |10-19 percent third degree T31.71
      |20-29 percent third degree T31.72
      |30-39 percent third degree T31.73
      |40-49 percent third degree T31.74
      |50-59 percent third degree T31.75
      |60-69 percent third degree T31.76
      |70-79 percent third degree T31.77
  |80-89 percent (0-9 percent third degree)
    T31.80
    |with
      |10-19 percent third degree T31.81
      |20-29 percent third degree T31.82
      |30-39 percent third degree T31.83
      |40-49 percent third degree T31.84
      |50-59 percent third degree T31.85
      |60-69 percent third degree T31.86
      |70-79 percent third degree T31.87
      |80-89 percent third degree T31.88

Burn - *continued*

  |90 percent or more (0-9 percent third degree)
    T31.90
    |with
      |10-19 percent third degree T31.91
      |20-29 percent third degree T31.92
      |30-39 percent third degree T31.93
      |40-49 percent third degree T31.94
      |50-59 percent third degree T31.95
      |60-69 percent third degree T31.96
      |70-79 percent third degree T31.97
      |80-89 percent third degree T31.98
      |90-99 percent third degree T31.99
|upper limb T22.00
  |above elbow *see* Burn, above elbow
  |axilla *see* Burn, axilla
  |elbow *see* Burn, elbow
  |first degree T22.10
  |forearm *see* Burn, forearm
  |hand *see* Burn, hand
  |interscapular region *see* Burn, back, upper
  |multiple sites T22.099
    |first degree T22.199
    |left T22.092
      |first degree T22.192
      |second degree T22.292
      |third degree T22.392
    |right T22.091
      |first degree T22.191
      |second degree T22.291
      |third degree T22.391
    |second degree T22.299
    |third degree T22.399
  |scapular region *see* Burn, scapular region
  |second degree T22.20
  |shoulder *see* Burn, shoulder
  |third degree T22.30
  |wrist *see* Burn, wrist
|uterus T28.3
|vagina T28.3
|vulva *see* Burn, genital organs, external,
  female
|wrist T23.079
  |first degree T23.179
  |left T23.072
    |first degree T23.172
    |second degree T23.272
    |third degree T23.372
  |multiple sites with hand T23.099
    |first degree T23.199
    |left T23.092
      |first degree T23.192
      |second degree T23.292
      |third degree T23.392
    |right T23.091
      |first degree T23.191
      |second degree T23.291
      |third degree T23.391
    |second degree T23.299
    |third degree T23.399
  |right T23.071
    |first degree T23.171
    |second degree T23.271
    |third degree T23.371
  |second degree T23.279
  |third degree T23.379
Burnett's syndrome E83.52
Burning
  |feet syndrome E53.9
  |sensation R20.8
  |tongue K14.6
Burn-Out (state) Z73.0
Burns' disease or osteochondrosis *see*
  Osteochondrosis, juvenile, ulna
Bursa *see* condition

Bursitis M71.9
|Achilles *see* Tendinitis, Achilles
|adhesive *see* Bursitis, specified NEC
|ankle *see* Enthesopathy, lower limb, ankle,
  specified type NEC
|calcaneal *see* Enthesopathy, foot, specified
  type NEC
|collateral ligament, tibial *see* Bursitis, tibial
  collateral
|due to use, overuse, pressure *see also*
  Disorder, soft tissue, due to use, specified
  type NEC
  |specified NEC *see* Disorder, soft tissue, due
    to use, specified NEC
|Duplay's M75.0
|elbow NEC M70.3-
  |olecranon M70.2-
|finger *see* Disorder, soft tissue, due to use,
  specified type NEC, hand
|foot *see* Enthesopathy, foot, specified type
  NEC
|gonococcal A54.49
|gouty *see* Gout
|hand M70.1-
|hip NEC M70.7-
  |trochanteric M70.6-
|infective NEC M71.10
  |abscess *see* Abscess, bursa
  |ankle M71.17-
  |elbow M71.12-
  |foot M71.17-
  |hand M71.14-
  |hip M71.15-
  |knee M71.16-
  |multiple sites M71.19
  |shoulder M71.11-
  |specified site NEC M71.18
  |wrist M71.13-
|ischial *see* Bursitis, hip
|knee NEC M70.5-
  |prepatellar M70.4-
|occupational NEC *see also* Disorder, soft
  tissue, due to, use
|olecranon *see* Bursitis, elbow, olecranon
|pharyngeal J39.1
|popliteal *see* Bursitis, knee
|prepatellar M70.4-
|radiohumeral M70.3-
|rheumatoid M06.20
  |ankle M06.27-
  |elbow M06.22-
  |foot joint M06.27-
  |hand joint M06.24-
  |hip M06.25-
  |knee M06.26-
  |multiple site M06.29
  |shoulder M06.21-
  |vertebra M06.28
  |wrist M06.23-
|scapulohumeral *see* Bursitis, shoulder
|semimembranous muscle (knee) *see* Bursitis,
  knee
|shoulder M75.5-
  |adhesive *see* Capsulitis, adhesive
|specified NEC M71.50
  |ankle M71.57-
  |due to use, overuse or pressure *see* Disorder,
    soft tissue, due to, use
  |elbow M71.52-
  |foot M71.57-
  |hand M71.54-
  |hip M71.55-
  |knee M71.56-
  |shoulder *see* Bursitis, shoulder
  |specified site NEC M71.58
  |tibial collateral M76.4-

Bursitis - *continued*
|wrist M71.53-
|subacromial *see* Bursitis, shoulder
|subcoracoid *see* Bursitis, shoulder
|subdeltoid *see* Bursitis, shoulder
|syphilitic A52.78
|Thornwaldt, Tornwaldt J39.2
|tibial collateral M76.4-
|toe *see* Enthesopathy, foot, specified type
  NEC
|trochanteric (area) *see* Bursitis, hip,
  trochanteric
|wrist *see* Bursitis, hand
Bursopathy M71.9
|specified type NEC M71.80
  |ankle M71.87-
  |elbow M71.82-
  |foot M71.87-
  |hand M71.84-
  |hip M71.85-
  |knee M71.86-
  |multiple sites M71.89
  |shoulder M71.81-
  |specified site NEC M71.88
  |wrist M71.83-
Burst stitches or sutures (complication of
  surgery) T81.31
|external operation wound T81.31
|internal operation wound T81.32
Buruli ulcer A31.1
Bury's disease L95.1
Buschke's
|disease   *see* Cryptococcosis by site
|scleredema *see* Sclerosis, systemic
Busse-Buschke disease   *see* Cryptococcosis by
  site
Buttock *see* condition
Button
|Biskra B55.1
|Delhi B55.1
|oriental B55.1
Buttonhole deformity (finger) *see* Deformity,
  finger, boutonniere
Bwamba fever A92.8
Byssinosis J66.0
Bywaters' syndrome T79.5

C

Cachexia R64
|cancerous R64
|cardiac *see* Disease, heart
|dehydration E86.0
|due to malnutrition R64
|exophthalmic *see* Hyperthyroidism
|heart *see* Disease, heart
|hypophyseal E23.0
|hypopituitary E23.0
|lead *see* Poisoning, lead
|malignant R64
|marsh *see* Malaria
|nervous F48.8
|old age R54
|paludal *see* Malaria
|pituitary E23.0
- pulmonary R64
|renal N28.9
|saturnine *see* Poisoning, lead
|senile R54
|Simmonds' E23.0
|splenica D73.0
|strumipriva E03.4
|tuberculous NEC *see* Tuberculosis
CADASIL (cerebral autosomal dominant
  arteriopathy with subcortical infarcts and
  leukoencephalopathy) I67.850
Café, au lait spots L81.3

Caffeine-Induced
|anxiety disorder F15.980
|sleep disorder F15.982
Caffey's syndrome Q78.8
Caisson disease T70.3
Cake kidney Q63.1
Caked breast (puerperal, postpartum) O92.79
Calabar swelling B74.3
Calcaneal spur *see* Spur, bone, calcaneal
Calcaneo-Apophysitis M92.8
Calcareous *see* condition
Calcicosis J62.8
Calciferol (vitamin D) deficiency E55.9
|with rickets E55.0
Calcification
|adrenal (capsule) (gland) E27.49
  |tuberculous E35 [*B90.8*]
|aorta I70.0
|artery (annular) *see* Arteriosclerosis
|auricle (ear) *see* Disorder, pinna, specified
  type NEC
|basal ganglia G23.8
|bladder N32.89
  |due to Schistosoma hematobium B65.0
|brain (cortex) *see* Calcification, cerebral
|bronchus J98.09
|bursa M71.40
  |ankle M71.47-
  |elbow M71.42-
  |foot M71.47-
  |hand M71.44-
  |hip M71.45-
  |knee M71.46-
  |multiple sites M71.49
  |shoulder M75.3-
  |specified site NEC M71.48
  |wrist M71.43-
|cardiac *see* Degeneration, myocardial
|cerebral (cortex) G93.89
  |artery I67.2
|cervix (uteri) N88.8
|choroid plexus G93.89
|conjunctiva *see* Concretion, conjunctiva
|corpora cavernosa (penis) N48.89
|cortex (brain) *see* Calcification, cerebral
|dental pulp (nodular) K04.2
|dentinal papilla K00.4
|fallopian tube N83.8
|falx cerebri G96.198
|gallbladder K82.8
|general E83.59
|heart *see also* Degeneration, myocardial
  |valve *see* Endocarditis
|idiopathic infantile arterial (IIAC) Q28.8
|intervertebral cartilage or disc (postinfective)
  see Disorder, disc, specified NEC
|intracranial *see* Calcification, cerebral
|joint *see* Disorder, joint, specified type NEC
|kidney N28.89
  |tuberculous N29 [*B90.1*]
|larynx (senile) J38.7
|lens *see* Cataract, specified NEC
|lung (active) (postinfectional) J98.4
  |tuberculous B90.9
|lymph gland or node (postinfectional) I89.8
  |tuberculous *see also* Tuberculosis, lymph
    gland B90.8
|mammographic R92.1
|massive (paraplegic) *see* Myositis, ossificans,
  in, quadriplegia
|medial *see* Arteriosclerosis, extremities
|meninges (cerebral) (spinal) G96.198
|metastatic E83.59
|Mönckeberg's *see* Arteriosclerosis, extremities
|muscle M61.9

Calvé's disease *see* Osteochondrosis, juvenile, spine
Calvities *see* Alopecia, androgenic
Cameroon fever *see* Malaria
Camptocormia (hysterical) F44.4
Camurati-Engelmann syndrome Q78.3
Canal *see also* condition
|atrioventricular common Q21.2
Canaliculitis (lacrimal) (acute) (subacute) H04.33-
|Actinomyces A42.89
|chronic H04.42
Canavan's disease E75.29
Canceled procedure (surgical) Z53.9
|because of
  |contraindication Z53.09
    |smoking Z53.01
  |left against medical advice (AMA) Z53.21
  |patient's decision Z53.20
    |for reasons of belief or group pressure Z53.1
    |specified reason NEC Z53.29
  |specified reason NEC Z53.8
Cancer *see also* Neoplasm, by site, malignant
|bile duct type liver C22.1
|blood *see* Leukemia
|breast *see also* Neoplasm, breast, malignant C50.91-
|hepatocellular C22.0
|lung *see also* Neoplasm, lung, malignant C34.90-
|ovarian *see also* Neoplasm ovary, malignant C56.9-
|unspecified site (primary) C80.1
Cancer (o) phobia F45.29
Cancerous *see* Neoplasm, malignant, by site
Cancrum oris A69.0
Candidiasis, candidal B37.9
|balanitis B37.42
|bronchitis B37.1
|cheilitis B37.83
|congenital P37.5
|cystitis B37.41
|disseminated B37.7
|endocarditis B37.6
|enteritis B37.82
|esophagitis B37.81
|intertrigo B37.2
|lung B37.1
|meningitis B37.5
|mouth B37.0
|nails B37.2
|neonatal P37.5
|onychia B37.2
|oral B37.0
|osteomyelitis B37.89
|otitis externa B37.84
|paronychia B37.2
|perionyxis B37.2
|pneumonia B37.1
|proctitis B37.82
|pulmonary B37.1
|pyelonephritis B37.49
|sepsis B37.7
|skin B37.2
|specified site NEC B37.89
|stomatitis B37.0
|systemic B37.7
|urethritis B37.41
|urogenital site NEC B37.49
|vagina B37.3
|vulva B37.3
|vulvovaginitis B37.3
Candidid L30.2
Candidosis *see* Candidiasis
Candiru infection or infestation B88.8

Canities (premature) L67.1
|congenital Q84.2
Canker (mouth) (sore) K12.0
|rash A38.9
Cannabinosis J66.2
Cannabis induced
|anxiety disorder F12.980
|psychotic disorder F12.959
|sleep disorder F12.988
Canton fever A75.9
Cantrell's syndrome Q87.89
Capillariasis (intestinal) B81.1
|hepatic B83.8
Capillary *see* condition
Caplan's syndrome *see* Rheumatoid, lung
Capsule *see* condition
Capsulitis (joint) *see also* Enthesopathy
|adhesive (shoulder) M75.0-
|hepatic K65.8
|labyrinthine *see* Otosclerosis, specified NEC
|thyroid E06.9
Caput
|crepitus Q75.8
|medusae I86.8
|succedaneum P12.81
Car sickness T75.3
Carapata (disease) A68.0
Carate *see* Pinta
Carbon lung J60
Carbuncle L02.93
|abdominal wall L02.231
|anus K61.0
|auditory canal, external *see* Abscess, ear, external
|auricle ear *see* Abscess, ear, external
|axilla L02.43-
|back (any part) L02.232
|breast N61.1
|buttock L02.33
|cheek (external) L02.03
|chest wall L02.233
|chin L02.03
|corpus cavernosum N48.21
|ear (any part) (external) (middle) *see* Abscess, ear, external
|external auditory canal *see* Abscess, ear, external
|eyelid *see* Abscess, eyelid
|face NEC L02.03
|femoral (region) *see* Carbuncle, lower limb
|finger *see* Carbuncle, hand
|flank L02.231
|foot L02.63-
|forehead L02.03
|genital *see* Abscess, genital
|gluteal (region) L02.33
|groin L02.234
|hand L02.53-
|head NEC L02.831
|heel *see* Carbuncle, foot
|hip *see* Carbuncle, lower limb
|kidney *see* Abscess, kidney
|knee *see* Carbuncle, lower limb
|labium (majus) (minus) N76.4
|lacrimal
  |gland *see* Dacryoadenitis
  |passages (duct) (sac) *see* Inflammation, lacrimal, passages, acute
|leg *see* Carbuncle, lower limb
|lower limb L02.43-
|malignant A22.0
|navel L02.236
|neck L02.13
|nose (external) (septum) J34.0
|orbit, orbital *see* Abscess, orbit

Carbuncle - *continued*
|palmar (space) *see* Carbuncle, hand
|partes posteriores L02.33
|pectoral region L02.233
|penis N48.21
|perineum L02.235
|pinna *see* Abscess, ear, external
|popliteal *see* Carbuncle, lower limb
|scalp L02.831
|seminal vesicle N49.0
|shoulder *see* Carbuncle, upper limb
|specified site NEC L02.838
|temple (region) L02.03
|thumb *see* Carbuncle, hand
|toe *see* Carbuncle, foot
|trunk L02.239
  |abdominal wall L02.231
  |back L02.232
  |chest wall L02.233
  |groin L02.234
  |perineum L02.235
  |umbilicus L02.236
|umbilicus L02.236
|upper limb L02.43-
|urethra N34.0
|vulva N76.4
Carbunculus *see* Carbuncle
Carcinoid (tumor) *see* Tumor, carcinoid
Carcinoidosis E34.0
Carcinoma (malignant) *see also* Neoplasm, by site, malignant
|acidophil
  |specified site *see* Neoplasm, malignant, by site
  |unspecified site C75.1
|acidophil-basophil, mixed
  |specified site *see* Neoplasm, malignant, by site
  |unspecified site C75.1
|adnexal (skin) *see* Neoplasm, skin, malignant
|adrenal cortical C74.0-
|alveolar *see* Neoplasm, lung, malignant
  |cell *see* Neoplasm, lung, malignant
|ameloblastic C41.1
  |upper jaw (bone) C41.0
|apocrine
  |breast *see* Neoplasm, breast, malignant
  |specified site NEC *see* Neoplasm, skin, malignant
  |unspecified site C44.99
|basal cell (pigmented) (*see also* Neoplasm, skin, malignant) C44.91
  |fibro-epithelial *see* Neoplasm, skin, malignant
  |morphea *see* Neoplasm, skin, malignant
  |multicentric *see* Neoplasm, skin, malignant
|basaloid
|basal-squamous cell, mixed *see* Neoplasm, skin, malignant
|basophil
  |specified site *see* Neoplasm, malignant, by site
  |unspecified site C75.1
|basophil-acidophil, mixed
  |specified site *see* Neoplasm, malignant, by site
  |unspecified site C75.1
|basosquamous *see* Neoplasm, skin, malignant
|bile duct
  |with hepatocellular, mixed C22.0
  |liver C22.1
  |specified site NEC *see* Neoplasm, malignant, by site
  |unspecified site C22.1
|branchial or branchiogenic C10.4

Carcinoma - *continued*

|bronchial or bronchogenic *see* Neoplasm, lung, malignant
|bronchiolar *see* Neoplasm, lung, malignant
|bronchioloalveolar *see* Neoplasm, lung, malignant
|C cell
    |specified site *see* Neoplasm, malignant, by site
    |unspecified site C73
|ceruminous C44.29-
|cervix uteri
    |in situ D06.9
        |endocervix D06.0
        |exocervix D06.1
        |specified site NEC D06.7
|chorionic
    |specified site *see* Neoplasm, malignant, by site
    |unspecified site
        |female C58
        |male C62.90
|chromophobe
    |specified site *see* Neoplasm, malignant, by site
    |unspecified site C75.1
|cloacogenic
    |specified site *see* Neoplasm, malignant, by site
    |unspecified site C21.2
|diffuse type
    |specified site *see* Neoplasm, malignant, by site
    |unspecified site C16.9
|duct (cell)
    |with Paget's disease *see* Neoplasm, breast, malignant
    |infiltrating
        |with lobular carcinoma (in situ)
            |specified site *see* Neoplasm, malignant, by site
            |unspecified site (female) C50.91-
                |male C50.92-
        |specified site *see* Neoplasm, malignant, by site
        |unspecified site (female) C50.91-
            |male C50.92-
|ductal
    |with lobular
        |specified site *see* Neoplasm, malignant, by site
        |unspecified site (female) C50.91-
            |male C50.92-
|ductular, infiltrating
    |specified site *see* Neoplasm, malignant, by site
    |unspecified site (female) C50.91-
        |male C50.92-
|embryonal
    |liver C22.7
|endometrioid
    |specified site *see* Neoplasm, malignant, by site
    |unspecified site
        |female C56.9
        |male C61
|eosinophil
    |specified site *see* Neoplasm, malignant, by site
    |unspecified site C75.1
|epidermoid *see also* Neoplasm, skin malignant
    |in situ, Bowen's type *see* Neoplasm, skin, in situ
|fibroepithelial, basal cell *see* Neoplasm, skin, malignant
|follicular

Carcinoma - *continued*

|with papillary (mixed) C73
|moderately differentiated C73
|pure follicle C73
|specified site *see* Neoplasm, malignant, by site
|trabecular C73
|unspecified site C73
|well differentiated C73
|generalized, with unspecified primary site C80.0
|glycogen-rich *see* Neoplasm, breast, malignant
|granulosa cell C56-
|hepatic cell C22.0
|hepatocellular C22.0
    |with bile duct, mixed C22.0
    |fibrolamellar C22.0
|hepatocholangiolitic C22.0
|Hürthle cell C73
|in
    |adenomatous
        |polyposis coli C18.9
    |pleomorphic adenoma *see* Neoplasm, salivary glands, malignant
    |situ *see* Carcinoma-in-situ
|infiltrating
    |duct
        |with lobular
            |specified site *see* Neoplasm, malignant, by site
            |unspecified site (female) C50.91-
                |male C50.92-
        |with Paget's disease *see* Neoplasm, breast, malignant
        |specified site *see* Neoplasm, malignant
        |unspecified site (female) C50.91-
            |male C50.92-
    |ductular
        |specified site *see* Neoplasm, malignant
        |unspecified site (female) C50.91-
            |male C50.92-
    |lobular
        |specified site *see* Neoplasm, malignant
        |unspecified site (female) C50.91-
            |male C50.92-
|inflammatory
    |specified site *see* Neoplasm, malignant
    |unspecified site (female) C50.91-
        |male C50.92-
|intestinal type
    |specified site *see* Neoplasm, malignant, by site
    |unspecified site C16.9
|intracystic
    |noninfiltrating *see* Neoplasm, in situ, by site
|intraductal (noninfiltrating)
    |with Paget's disease *see* Neoplasm, breast, malignant
    |breast D05.1-
    |papillary
        |with invasion
            |specified site *see* Neoplasm, malignant, by site
            |unspecified site (female) C50.91-
                |male C50.92-
        |breast D05.1-
        |specified site NEC *see* Neoplasm, in situ, by site
        |unspecified site (female) D05.1-
    |specified site NEC *see* Neoplasm, in situ, by site
    |unspecified site (female) D05.1-
|intraepidermal *see* Neoplasm, in situ
    |squamous cell, Bowen's type *see* Neoplasm, skin, in situ

Carcinoma - *continued*

|intraepithelial *see* Neoplasm, in situ, by site
    |squamous cell *see* Neoplasm, in situ, by site
|intraosseous C41.1
    |upper jaw (bone) C41.0
|islet cell
    |with exocrine, mixed
        |specified site *see* Neoplasm, malignant, by site
        |unspecified site C25.9
    |pancreas C25.4
    |specified site NEC *see* Neoplasm, malignant, by site
    |unspecified site C25.4
|juvenile, breast *see* Neoplasm, breast, malignant
|large cell
    |small cell
        |specified site *see* Neoplasm, malignant, by site
        |unspecified site C34.90
|Leydig cell (testis)
    |specified site *see* Neoplasm, malignant, by site
    |unspecified site
        |female C56.9
        |male C62.90
|lipid-rich (female) C50.91-
    |male C50.92-
|liver cell C22.0
|liver NEC C22.7
|lobular (infiltrating)
    |with intraductal
        |specified site *see* Neoplasm, malignant, by site
        |unspecified site (female) C50.91-
            |male C50.92-
    |noninfiltrating
        |breast D05.0-
        |specified site NEC *see* Neoplasm, in situ, by site
        |unspecified site D05.0-
    |specified site *see* Neoplasm, malignant, by site
    |unspecified site (female) C50.91-
        |male C50.92-
|medullary
    |with
        |amyloid stroma
            |specified site *see* Neoplasm, malignant, by site
            |unspecified site C73
        |lymphoid stroma
            |specified site *see* Neoplasm, malignant, by site
            |unspecified site (female) C50.91-
                |male C50.92-
|Merkel cell C4A.9
    |anal margin C4A.51
    |anal skin C4A.51
    |canthus C4A.1-
    |ear and external auricular canal C4A.2-
    |external auricular canal C4A.2-
    |eyelid, including canthus C4A.1-
    |face C4A.30
        |specified NEC C4A.39
    |hip C4A.7-
    |lip C4A.0
    |lower limb, including hip C4A.7-
    |neck C4A.4
    |nodal presentation C7B.1
    |nose C4A.31
    |overlapping sites C4A.8
    |perianal skin C4A.51
    |scalp C4A.4
    |secondary C7B.1

Carcinoma - *continued*
|shoulder C4A.6-
|skin of breast C4A.52
|trunk NEC C4A.59
|upper limb, including shoulder C4A.6-
|visceral metastatic C7B.1
|metastatic *see* Neoplasm, secondary, by site
|metatypical *see* Neoplasm, skin, malignant
|morphea, basal cell *see* Neoplasm, skin, malignant
|mucoid
  |cell
    |specified site *see* Neoplasm, malignant, by site
    |unspecified site C75.1
|neuroendocrine *see also* Tumor, neuroendocrine
  |high grade, any site C7A.1
  |poorly differentiated, any site C7A.1
|nonencapsulated sclerosing C73
|noninfiltrating
  |intracystic *see* Neoplasm, in situ, by site
  |intraductal
    |breast D05.1-
    |papillary
      |breast D05.1-
      |specified site NEC *see* Neoplasm, in situ, by site
      |unspecified site D05.1-
    |specified site *see* Neoplasm, in situ, by site
    |unspecified site D05.1-
  |lobular
    |breast D05.0-
    |specified site NEC *see* Neoplasm, in situ, by site
    |unspecified site (female) D05.0-
|oat cell
  |specified site *see* Neoplasm, malignant, by site
  |unspecified site C34.90
|odontogenic C41.1
  |upper jaw (bone) C41.0
|papillary
  |with follicular (mixed) C73
  |follicular variant C73
  |intraductal (noninfiltrating)
    |with invasion
      |specified site *see* Neoplasm, malignant, by site
      |unspecified site (female) C50.91-
        |male C50.92-
    |breast D05.1-
    |specified site NEC *see* Neoplasm, in situ, by site
    |unspecified site D05.1-
  |serous
    |specified site *see* Neoplasm, malignant, by site
    |surface
      |specified site *see* Neoplasm, malignant, by site
      |unspecified site C56.9
    |unspecified site C56.9
|papillocystic
  |specified site *see* Neoplasm, malignant, by site
  |unspecified site C56.9
|parafollicular cell
  |specified site *see* Neoplasm, malignant, by site
  |unspecified site C73
|pilomatrix *see* Neoplasm, skin, malignant
|pseudomucinous

Carcinoma - *continued*
  |specified site *see* Neoplasm, malignant, by site
  |unspecified site C56.9
|renal cell C64-
|Schmincke *see* Neoplasm, nasopharynx, malignant
|Schneiderian
  |specified site *see* Neoplasm, malignant, by site
  |unspecified site C30.0
|sebaceous *see* Neoplasm, skin, malignant
|secondary *see also* Neoplasm, secondary, by site
  |Merkel cell C7B.1
|secretory, breast *see* Neoplasm, breast, malignant
|serous
  |papillary
    |specified site *see* Neoplasm, malignant, by site
    |unspecified site C56.9
  |surface, papillary
    |specified site *see* Neoplasm, malignant, by site
    |unspecified site C56.9
|Sertoli cell
  |specified site *see* Neoplasm, malignant, by site
  |unspecified site C62.90
    |female C56.9
    |male C62.90
|skin appendage *see* Neoplasm, skin, malignant
|small cell
  |fusiform cell
    |specified site *see* Neoplasm, malignant, by site
    |unspecified site C34.90
  |intermediate cell
    |specified site *see* Neoplasm, malignant, by site
    |unspecified site C34.90
  |large cell
    |specified site *see* Neoplasm, malignant, by site
    |unspecified site C34.90
|solid
  |with amyloid stroma
    |specified site *see* Neoplasm, malignant, by site
    |unspecified site C73
  |microinvasive
    |specified site *see* Neoplasm, malignant, by site
    |unspecified site C53.9
|sweat gland *see* Neoplasm, skin, malignant
|theca cell C56.-
|thymic C37
|unspecified site (primary) C80.1
|water-clear cell C75.0
Carcinoma-In-Situ *see also* Neoplasm, in situ, by site
|breast NOS D05.9-
  |specified type NEC D05.8-
|epidermoid *see also* Neoplasm, in situ, by site
  |with questionable stromal invasion
    |cervix D06.9
    |specified site NEC *see* Neoplasm, in situ, by site
    |unspecified site D06.9
  |Bowen's type *see* Neoplasm, skin, in situ
|intraductal
  |breast D05.1-
  |specified site NEC *see* Neoplasm, in situ, by site
  |unspecified site D05.1-

Carcinoma-In-Situ - *continued*
|lobular
  |with
    |infiltrating duct
      |breast (female) C50.91-
        |male C50.92-
      |specified site NEC *see* Neoplasm, malignant
      |unspecified site (female) C50.91-
        |male C50.92-
  |intraductal
    |breast D05.8-
    |specified site NEC *see* Neoplasm, in situ, by site
    |unspecified site (female) D05.8-
  |breast D05.0-
  |specified site NEC *see* Neoplasm, in situ, by site
  |unspecified site D05.0-
|squamous cell *see also* Neoplasm, in situ, by site
  |with questionable stromal invasion
    |cervix D06.9
    |specified site NEC *see* Neoplasm, in situ, by site
    |unspecified site D06.9
Carcinomaphobia F45.29
Carcinomatosis C80.0
|peritonei C78.6
|unspecified site (primary) (secondary) C80.0
Carcinosarcoma *see* Neoplasm, malignant, by site
|embryonal *see* Neoplasm, malignant, by site
Cardia, cardial *see* condition
Cardiac *see also* condition
|death, sudden *see* Arrest, cardiac
|pacemaker
  |in situ Z95.0
  |management or adjustment Z45.018
|tamponade I31.4
Cardialgia *see* Pain, precordial
Cardiectasis *see* Hypertrophy, cardiac
Cardiochalasia K21.9
Cardiomalacia I51.5
Cardiomegalia glycogenica diffusa E74.02 [*I43*]
Cardiomegaly *see also* Hypertrophy, cardiac
|congenital Q24.8
|glycogen E74.02 [*I43*]
|idiopathic I51.7
Cardiomyoliposis I51.5
Cardiomyopathy (familial) (idiopathic) I42.9
|alcoholic I42.6
|amyloid E85.4 [*I43*]
  |transthyretin-related (ATTR) familial E85.4
|arteriosclerotic *see* Disease, heart, ischemic, atherosclerotic
|beriberi E51.12
|cobalt-beer I42.6
|congenital I42.4
|congestive I42.0
|constrictive NOS I42.5
|dilated I42.0
|due to
  |alcohol I42.6
  |beriberi E51.12
  |cardiac glycogenosis E74.02 [*I43*]
  |drugs I42.7
  |external agents NEC I42.7
  |Friedreich's ataxia G11.11
  |myotonia atrophica G71.11 [*I43*]
  |progressive muscular dystrophy G71.09 [*I43*]
|glycogen storage E74.02 [*I43*]
|hypertensive *see* Hypertension, heart
|hypertrophic (nonobstructive) I42.2

Cardiomyopathy - *continued*
|obstructive I42.1
||congenital Q24.8
|in
||Chagas' disease (chronic) B57.2
|||acute B57.0
||sarcoidosis D86.85
|ischemic I25.5
|metabolic E88.9 [143]
||thyrotoxic E05.90 [143]
|||with thyroid storm E05.91 [143]
|newborn I42.8
||congenital I42.4
|nutritional E63.9 [143]
||beriberi E51.12
|obscure of Africa I42.8
|peripartum O90.3
|postpartum O90.3
|restrictive NEC I42.5
|rheumatic I09.0
|secondary I42.9
|stress induced I51.81
|takotsubo I51.81
|thyrotoxic E05.90 [143]
||with thyroid storm E05.91 [143]
|toxic NEC I42.7
|transthyretin-related (ATTR) familial amyloid
|||E85.4
|tuberculous A18.84
|viral B33.24
Cardionephritis *see* Hypertension, cardiorenal
Cardionephropathy *see* Hypertension,
|||cardiorenal
Cardionephrosis *see* Hypertension, cardiorenal
Cardiopathia nigra I27.0
Cardiopathy *see also* Disease, heart I51.9
|idiopathic I42.9
|mucopolysaccharidosis E76.3 [152]
Cardiopericarditis *see* Pericarditis
Cardiophobia F45.29
Cardiorenal *see* condition
Cardiorrhexis *see* Infarct, myocardium
Cardiosclerosis *see* Disease, heart, ischemic,
|||atherosclerotic
Cardiosis *see* Disease, heart
Cardiospasm (esophagus) (reflex) (stomach)
|||K22.0
|congenital Q39.5
||with megaesophagus Q39.5
Cardiostenosis *see* Disease, heart
Cardiosymphysis I31.0
Cardiovascular *see* condition
Carditis (acute) (bacterial) (chronic) (subacute)
|||I51.89
|meningococcal A39.50
|rheumatic *see* Disease, heart, rheumatic
|rheumatoid *see* Rheumatoid, carditis
|viral B33.20
Care (of) (for) (following)
|child (routine) Z76.2
|family member (handicapped) (sick)
||creating problem for family Z63.6
||provided away from home for holiday relief
|||Z75.5
||unavailable, due to
|||absence (person rendering care) (sufferer)
||||Z74.2
|||inability (any reason) of person rendering
||||care Z74.2
|foundling Z76.1
|holiday relief Z75.5
|improper *see* Maltreatment
|lack of (at or after birth) (infant) *see*
|||Maltreatment, child, neglect
|lactating mother Z39.1
|palliative Z51.5

Care (of) (for) - *continued*
|postpartum
||immediately after delivery Z39.0
||routine follow-up Z39.2
|respite Z75.5
|unavailable, due to
||absence of person rendering care Z74.2
||inability (any reason) of person rendering
|||care Z74.2
|well-baby Z76.2
Caries
|bone NEC A18.03
|dental (dentino enamel junction) (early
|||childhood) (of dentine) (pre-eruptive)
|||(recurrent) (to the pulp) K02.9
||arrested (coronal) (root) K02.3
||chewing surface
|||limited to enamel K02.51
|||penetrating into dentin K02.52
|||penetrating into pulp K02.53
||coronal surface
|||chewing surface
||||limited to enamel K02.51
||||penetrating into dentin K02.52
||||penetrating into pulp K02.53
|||pit and fissure surface
||||limited to enamel K02.51
||||penetrating into dentin K02.52
||||penetrating into pulp K02.53
|||smooth surface
||||limited to enamel K02.61
||||penetrating into dentin K02.62
||||penetrating into pulp K02.63
||pit and fissure surface
|||limited to enamel K02.51
|||penetrating into dentin K02.52
|||penetrating into pulp K02.53
||primary, cervical origin K02.52
||root K02.7
||smooth surface
|||limited to enamel K02.61
|||penetrating into dentin K02.62
|||penetrating into pulp K02.63
|external meatus *see* Disorder, ear, external,
|||specified type NEC
|hip (tuberculous) A18.02
|initial (tooth)
||chewing surface K02.51
||pit and fissure surface K02.51
||smooth surface K02.61
|knee (tuberculous) A18.02
|labyrinth *see* subcategory H83.8
|limb NEC (tuberculous) A18.03
|mastoid process (chronic) *see* Mastoiditis,
|||chronic
||tuberculous A18.03
|middle ear *see* subcategory H74.8
|nose (tuberculous) A18.03
|orbit (tuberculous) A18.03
|ossicles, ear *see* Abnormal, ear ossicles
|petrous bone *see* Petrositis
|root (dental) (tooth) K02.7
|sacrum (tuberculous) A18.01
|spine, spinal (column) (tuberculous) A18.01
|syphilitic A52.77
||congenital (early) A50.02 [M90.80]
|tooth, teeth *see* Caries, dental
|tuberculous A18.03
|vertebra (column) (tuberculous) A18.01
Carious teeth *see* Caries, dental
Carneous mole O02.0
Carnitine insufficiency E71.40
Carotid body or sinus syndrome G90.01
Carotidynia G90.01
Carotenemia (dietary) E67.1
Carotenosis (cutis) (skin) E67.1

Carpal tunnel syndrome *see* Syndrome, carpal
|||tunnel
Carpenter's syndrome Q87.0
Carpopedal spasm *see* Tetany
Carr-Barr-Plunkett syndrome Q97.1
Carrier (suspected) of
|amebiasis Z22.1
|bacterial disease NEC Z22.39
||diphtheria Z22.2
||intestinal infectious NEC Z22.1
|||typhoid Z22.0
||meningococcal Z22.31
||sexually transmitted Z22.4
||specified NEC Z22.39
||staphylococcal (Methicillin susceptible)
|||Z22.321
|||Methicillin resistant Z22.322
||streptococcal Z22.338
|||group B Z22.330
||||complicating pregnancy or delivery
|||||O99.82-
||typhoid Z22.0
|cholera Z22.1
|diphtheria Z22.2
|gastrointestinal pathogens NEC Z22.1
|genetic Z14.8
||cystic fibrosis Z14.1
||hemophilia A (asymptomatic) Z14.01
|||symptomatic Z14.02
|gestational, pregnant Z33.1
|gonorrhea Z22.4
|HAA (hepatitis Australian-antigen) B18.8
|HB (c)(s) -AG B18.1
|hepatitis (viral) B18.9
||Australia-Antigen (HAA) B18.8
||B surface antigen (HBsAg) B18.1
|||with acute delta (super) infection B17.0
||C B18.2
||specified NEC B18.8
|human T-cell lymphotropic virus type 1
|||(HTLV 1) infection Z22.6
|infectious organism Z22.9
||specified NEC Z22.8
|meningococci Z22.31
|Salmonella typhosa Z22.0
|serum hepatitis *see* Carrier, hepatitis
|staphylococci (Methicillin susceptible)
|||Z22.321
||Methicillin resistant Z22.322
|streptococci Z22.338
||group B Z22.330
|||complicating pregnancy or delivery
||||O99.82-
|syphilis Z22.4
|typhoid Z22.0
|venereal disease NEC Z22.4
Carrion's disease A44.0
Carter's relapsing fever (Asiatic) A68.1
Cartilage *see* condition
Caruncle (inflamed)
|conjunctiva (acute) *see* Conjunctivitis, acute
|labium (majus) (minus) N90.89
|lacrimal *see* Inflammation, lacrimal, passages
|myrtiform N89.8
|urethral (benign) N36.2
Cascade stomach K31.2
Caseation lymphatic gland (tuberculous)
|||A18.2
Cassidy (-Scholte) syndrome (malignant
|||**carcinoid)** E34.0
Castellani's disease A69.8
Castration, traumatic, male S38.231
Casts in urine R82.998
Cat
|cry syndrome Q93.4
|ear Q17.3
|eye syndrome Q92.8

Cellulitis - *continued*
  |acute N73.0
  |drainage site (following operation) T81.49
  |ear (external) H60.1-
  |eosinophilic (granulomatous) L98.3
  |erysipelatous *see* Erysipelas
  |external auditory canal *see* Cellulitis, ear
  |eyelid *see* Abscess, eyelid
  |face NEC L03.211
  |finger (intrathecal) (periosteal) (subcutaneous)
      (subcuticular) L03.01-
  |foot *see* Cellulitis, lower limb
  |gangrenous *see* Gangrene
  |genital organ NEC
      |female (external) N76.4
      |male N49.9
          |multiple sites N49.8
          |specified NEC N49.8
  |gluteal (region) L03.317
  |gonococcal A54.89
  |groin L03.314
  |hand *see* Cellulitis, upper limb
  |head NEC L03.811
      |face (any part, except ear, eye and nose)
          L03.211
  |heel *see* Cellulitis, lower limb
  |hip *see* Cellulitis, lower limb
  |jaw (region) L03.211
  |knee *see* Cellulitis, lower limb
  |labium (majus) (minus) *see* Vulvitis
  |lacrimal passages *see* Inflammation, lacrimal,
      passages
  |larynx J38.7
  |leg *see* Cellulitis, lower limb
  |lip K13.0
  |lower limb L03.11-
      |toe *see* Cellulitis, toe
  |mouth (floor) K12.2
  |multiple sites, so stated L03.90
  |nasopharynx J39.1
  |navel L03.316
      |newborn P38.9
          |with mild hemorrhage P38.1
          |without hemorrhage P38.9
  |neck (region) L03.221
  |nipple (acute) (nonpuerperal) (subacute)
      N61.0
  |nose (septum) (external) J34.0
  |orbit, orbital H05.01-
  |palate (soft) K12.2
  |pectoral (region) L03.313
  |pelvis, pelvic (chronic)
      |female *see also* Disease, pelvis,
          inflammatory N73.2
          |acute N73.0
      |following ectopic or molar pregnancy O08.0
      |male K65.0
  |penis N48.22
  |perineal, perineum L03.315
  |periorbital L03.213
  |perirectal K61.1
  |peritonsillar J36
  |periurethral N34.0
  |periuterine *see also* Disease, pelvis,
      inflammatory N73.2
      |acute N73.0
  |pharynx J39.1
  |preseptal L03.213
  |rectum K61.1
  |retroperitoneal K68.9
  |round ligament
      |acute N73.0
  |scalp (any part) L03.811
  |scrotum N49.2
  |seminal vesicle N49.0
  |shoulder *see* Cellulitis, upper limb
  |specified site NEC L03.818

Cellulitis - *continued*
  |submandibular (region) (space) (triangle)
      K12.2
      |gland K11.3
  |submaxillary (region) K12.2
      |gland K11.3
  |thigh *see* Cellulitis, lower limb
  |thumb (intrathecal) (periosteal)
      (subcutaneous) (subcuticular) *see*
      Cellulitis, finger
  |toe (intrathecal) (periosteal) (subcutaneous)
      (subcuticular) L03.03-
  |tonsil J36
  |trunk L03.319
      |abdominal wall L03.311
      |back (any part) L03.312
      |buttock L03.317
      |chest wall L03.313
      |groin L03.314
      |perineal, perineum L03.315
      |umbilicus L03.316
  |tuberculous (primary) A18.4
  |umbilicus L03.316
  |upper limb L03.11-
      |axilla *see* Cellulitis, axilla
      |finger *see* Cellulitis, finger
      |thumb *see* Cellulitis, finger
  |vaccinal T88.0
  |vocal cord J38.3
  |vulva *see* Vulvitis
  |wrist *see* Cellulitis, upper limb
Cementoblastoma, benign *see* Cyst, calcifying
    odontogenic
Cementoma *see* Cyst, calcifying odontogenic
Cementoperiostitis *see* Periodontitis
Cementosis K03.4
Central auditory processing disorder H93.25
Central pain syndrome G89.0
Cephalematocele, cephal (o) hematocele
  |newborn P52.8
      |birth injury P10.8
  |traumatic *see* Hematoma, brain
Cephalematoma, cephalhematoma (calcified)
  |newborn (birth injury) P12.0
  |traumatic *see* Hematoma, brain
Cephalgia, cephalalgia *see also* Headache
      |histamine G44.009
      |intractable G44.001
      |not intractable G44.009
  |trigeminal autonomic (TAC) NEC G44.099
      |intractable G44.091
      |not intractable G44.099
Cephalic *see* condition
Cephalitis *see* Encephalitis
Cephalocele *see* Encephalocele
Cephalomenia N94.89
Cephalopelvic *see* condition
Cerclage (with cervical incompetence) in
    pregnancy *see* Incompetence, cervix, in
    pregnancy
Cerebellitis *see* Encephalitis
Cerebellum, cerebellar *see* condition
Cerebral *see* condition
Cerebritis *see* Encephalitis
Cerebro-Hepato-Renal syndrome Q87.89
Cerebromalacia *see* Softening, brain
  |sequelae of cerebrovascular disease I69.398
Cerebroside lipidosis E75.22
Cerebrospasticity (congenital) G80.1
Cerebrospinal *see* condition
Cerebrum *see* condition
Ceroid-Lipofuscinosis, neuronal E75.4
Cerumen (accumulation) (impacted) H61.2-

Cervical *see also* condition
  |auricle Q18.2
  |dysplasia in pregnancy *see* Abnormal, cervix,
      in pregnancy or childbirth
  |erosion in pregnancy *see* Abnormal, cervix, in
      pregnancy or childbirth
  |fibrosis in pregnancy *see* Abnormal, cervix, in
      pregnancy or childbirth
  |fusion syndrome Q76.1
  |rib Q76.5
  |shortening (complicating pregnancy) O26.87-
Cervicalgia M54.2
Cervicitis (acute) (chronic) (nonvenereal) (senile
    (atrophic)) (subacute) (with ulceration) N72
  |with abortion *see* Abortion, by type
      complicated by genital tract and pelvic
      infection
  |ectopic pregnancy O08.0
      |molar pregnancy O08.0
  |chlamydial A56.09
  |gonococcal A54.03
  |herpesviral A60.03
  |puerperal (postpartum) O86.11
  |syphilitic A52.76
  |trichomonal A59.09
  |tuberculous A18.16
Cervicocolpitis (emphysematosa) (*see also*
    Cervicitis) N72
Cervix *see* condition
Cesarean delivery, previous, affecting
    management of pregnancy O34.219
  |classical (vertical) scar O34.212
  |isthmocele O34.22
  |low transverse scar O34.211
  |mid-transverse T incision O34.218
  |scar
      |defect (isthmocele) O34.22
      |specified type NEC O34.218
Céstan (-Chenais) paralysis or syndrome
    G46.3
Céstan-Raymond syndrome I65.8
Cestode infestation B71.9
  |specified type NEC B71.8
Cestodiasis B71.9
Chabert's disease A22.9
Chacaleh E53.8
Chafing L30.4
Chagas' (-Mazza) disease (chronic) B57.2
  |with
      |cardiovascular involvement NEC B57.2
      |digestive system involvement B57.30
          |megacolon B57.32
          |megaesophagus B57.31
          |other specified B57.39
      |megacolon B57.32
      |megaesophagus B57.31
      |myocarditis B57.2
      |nervous system involvement B57.40
          |meningitis B57.41
          |meningoencephalitis B57.42
          |other specified B57.49
      |specified organ involvement NEC B57.5
  |acute (with) B57.1
      |cardiovascular NEC B57.0
      |myocarditis B57.0
Chagres fever B50.9
Chair ridden Z74.09
Chalasia (cardiac sphincter) K21.9
Chalazion H00.19
  |left H00.16
      |lower H00.15
      |upper H00.14
  |right H00.13
      |lower H00.12
      |upper H00.11

Chalcosis *see also* Disorder, globe, degenerative, chalcosis
|cornea *see* Deposit, cornea
|crystalline lens *see* Cataract, complicated
|retina H35.89
Chalcosis (pulmonum) J62.8
Chancre (any genital site) (hard) (hunterian) (mixed) (primary) (seronegative) (seropositive) (syphilitic) A51.0
|congenital A50.07
|conjunctiva NEC A51.2
|Ducrey's A57
|extragenital A51.2
|eyelid A51.2
|lip A51.2
|nipple A51.2
|Nisbet's A57
|of
|carate A67.0
|pinta A67.0
|yaws A66.0
|palate, soft A51.2
|phagedenic A57
|simple A57
|soft A57
|bubo A57
|palate A51.2
|urethra A51.0
|yaws A66.0
Chancroid (anus) (genital) (penis) (perineum) (rectum) (urethra) (vulva) A57
Chandler's disease (osteochondritis dissecans, hip) *see* Osteochondritis, dissecans, hip
Change(s) (in) (of) *see also* Removal
|arteriosclerotic *see* Arteriosclerosis
|bone *see also* Disorder, bone
|diabetic *see* Diabetes, bone change
|bowel habit R19.4
|cardiorenal (vascular) *see* Hypertension, cardiorenal
|cardiovascular *see* Disease, cardiovascular
|circulatory I99.9
|cognitive (mild) (organic) R41.89
|color, tooth, teeth
|during formation K00.8
|posteruptive K03.7
|contraceptive device Z30.433
|corneal membrane H18.30
|Bowman's membrane fold or rupture H18.31-
|Descemet's membrane
|fold H18.32-
|rupture H18.33-
|coronary *see* Disease, heart, ischemic
|degenerative, spine or vertebra *see* Spondylosis
|dental pulp, regressive K04.2
|dressing (nonsurgical) Z48.00
|surgical Z48.01
|heart *see* Disease, heart
|hip joint *see* Derangement, joint, hip
|hyperplastic larynx J38.7
|hypertrophic
|nasal sinus J34.89
|turbinate, nasal J34.3
|upper respiratory tract J39.8
|indwelling catheter Z46.6
|inflammatory *see also* Inflammation
|sacroiliac M46.1
|job, anxiety concerning Z56.1
|joint *see* Derangement, joint
|life *see* Menopause
|mental status R41.82
|minimal (glomerular) *see also* N00-N07 with fourth character .0 N05.0
|myocardium, myocardial *see* Degeneration, myocardial

Change(s) (in) (of) - *continued*
|of life *see* Menopause
|pacemaker Z45.018
|pulse generator Z45.010
|personality (enduring) F68.8
|due to (secondary to)
|general medical condition F07.0
|secondary (nonspecific) F60.89
|regressive, dental pulp K04.2
|renal *see* Disease, renal
|retina H35.9
|myopic (*see also* Myopia, degenerative) H44.2-
|sacroiliac joint M53.3
|senile *see also* condition R54
|sensory R20.8
|skin R23.9
|acute, due to ultraviolet radiation L56.9
|specified NEC L56.8
|chronic, due to nonionizing radiation L57.9
|specified NEC L57.8
|cyanosis R23.0
|flushing R23.2
|pallor R23.1
|petechiae R23.3
|specified change NEC R23.8
|swelling *see* Mass, localized
|texture R23.4
|trophic
|arm *see* Mononeuropathy, upper limb
|leg *see* Mononeuropathy, lower limb
|vascular I99.9
|vasomotor I73.9
|voice R49.9
|psychogenic F44.4
|specified NEC R49.8
Changing sleep-Work schedule, affecting sleep G47.26
Changuinola fever A93.1
Chapping skin T69.8
Charcot-Marie-Tooth disease, paralysis or syndrome G60.0
Charcot's
|arthropathy *see* Arthropathy, neuropathic
|cirrhosis K74.3
|disease (tabetic arthropathy) A52.16
|joint (disease) (tabetic) A52.16
|diabetic *see* Diabetes, with, arthropathy
|syringomyelic G95.0
|syndrome (intermittent claudication) I73.9
CHARGE association Q89.8
Charley-Horse (quadriceps) M62.831
|traumatic (quadriceps) S76.11-
Charlouis' disease *see* Yaws
Cheadle's disease E54
Checking (of)
|cardiac pacemaker (battery) (electrode(s)) Z45.018
|pulse generator Z45.010
|implantable subdermal contraceptive Z30.46
|intrauterine contraceptive device Z30.431
|wound Z48.0-
|due to injury   code to Injury, by site, using appropriate seventh character for subsequent encounter
Check-Up *see* Examination
Chédiak-Higashi (-Steinbrinck) syndrome (congenital gigantism of peroxidase granules) E70.330
Cheek *see* condition
Cheese itch B88.0
Cheese-Washer's lung J67.8
Cheese-Worker's lung J67.8

Cheilitis (acute) (angular) (catarrhal) (chronic) (exfoliative) (gangrenous) (glandular) (infectional) (suppurative) (ulcerative) (vesicular) K13.0
|actinic (due to sun) L56.8
|other than from sun L59.8
|candidal B37.83
Cheilodynia K13.0
Cheiloschisis *see* Cleft, lip
Cheilosis (angular) K13.0
|with pellagra E52
|due to
|vitamin B2 (riboflavin) deficiency E53.0
Cheiromegaly M79.89
Cheiropompholyx L30.1
Cheloid *see* Keloid
Chemical burn *see* Corrosion, by site
Chemodectoma *see* Paraganglioma, nonchromaffin
Chemosis, conjunctiva *see* Edema, conjunctiva
Chemotherapy (session) (for)
|cancer Z51.11
|neoplasm Z51.11
Cherubism M27.8
Chest *see* condition
Cheyne-Stokes breathing (respiration) R06.3
Chiari's
|disease or syndrome (hepatic vein thrombosis) I82.0
|malformation
|type I G93.5
|type II *see* Spina bifida
|net Q24.8
Chicago disease B40.9
Chickenpox *see* Varicella
Chiclero ulcer or sore B55.1
Chigger (infestation) B88.0
Chignon (disease) B36.8
|newborn (from vacuum extraction) (birth injury) P12.1
Chilaiditi's syndrome (subphrenic displacement, colon) Q43.3
Chilblain(s) (lupus) T69.1
Child
|custody dispute Z65.3
Childbirth *see* Delivery
Childhood
|cerebral X-linked adrenoleukodystrophy E71.520
|period of rapid growth Z00.2
Chill(s) R68.83
|with fever R50.9
|congestive in malarial regions B54
|without fever R68.83
Chilomastigiasis A07.8
Chimera 46,XX/46,XY Q99.0
Chin *see* condition
Chinese dysentery A03.9
Chionophobia F40.228
Chitral fever A93.1
Chlamydia, chlamydial A74.9
|cervicitis A56.09
|conjunctivitis A74.0
|cystitis A56.01
|endometritis A56.11
|epididymitis A56.19
|female
|pelvic inflammatory disease A56.11
|pelviperitonitis A56.11
|orchitis A56.19
|peritonitis A74.81
|pharyngitis A56.4
|proctitis A56.3
|psittaci (infection) A70
|salpingitis A56.11
|sexually-transmitted infection NEC A56.8
|specified NEC A74.89

Chlamydia - *continued*
  |urethritis A56.01
  |vulvovaginitis A56.02
Chlamydiosis *see* Chlamydia
Chloasma (skin) (idiopathic) (symptomatic)
  L81.1
  |eyelid H02.719
    |hyperthyroid E05.90 [*H02.719*]
      |with thyroid storm E05.91 [*H02.719*]
    |left H02.716
      |lower H02.715
      |upper H02.714
    |right H02.713
      |lower H02.712
      |upper H02.711
Chloroma C92.3-
Chlorosis D50.9
  |Egyptian B76.9 [*D63.8*]
  |miner's B76.9 [*D63.8*]
Chlorotic anemia D50.8
Chocolate cyst (ovary) N80.1
Choked
  |disc or disk *see* Papilledema
  |on food, phlegm, or vomitus NOS *see* Foreign
    body, by site
  |while vomiting NOS *see* Foreign body, by site
Chokes (resulting from bends) T70.3
Choking sensation R09.89
Cholangiectasis K83.8
Cholangiocarcinoma
  |with hepatocellular carcinoma, combined
    C22.0
  |liver C22.1
  |specified site NEC *see* Neoplasm, malignant,
    by site
  |unspecified site C22.1
Cholangiohepatitis K83.8
  |due to fluke infestation B66.1
Cholangiohepatoma C22.0
Cholangiolitis (acute) (chronic) (extrahepatic)
  (gangrenous) (intrahepatic) K83.09
  |paratyphoidal *see* Fever, paratyphoid
  |typhoidal A01.09
Cholangioma D13.4
  |malignant *see* Cholangiocarcinoma
Cholangitis (ascending) (primary) (recurrent)
  (sclerosing) (secondary) (stenosing)
  (suppurative) K83.09
  |with calculus, bile duct *see* Calculus, bile
    duct, with cholangitis
  |chronic nonsuppurative destructive K74.3
  |primary K83.09
    |sclerosing K83.01
  |sclerosing K83.09
Cholecystectasia K82.8
Cholecystitis K81.9
  |with
    |calculus, stones in
      |bile duct (common) (hepatic) *see*
        Calculus, bile duct, with cholecystitis
      |cystic duct *see* Calculus, gallbladder, with
        cholecystitis
      |gallbladder *see* Calculus, gallbladder, with
        cholecystitis
      |choledocholithiasis *see* Calculus, bile duct,
        with cholecystitis
      |cholelithiasis *see* Calculus, gallbladder, with
        cholecystitis
    |gangrene of gallbladder K82.A1
    |perforation of gallbladder K82.A2
  |acute (emphysematous) (gangrenous)
    (suppurative) K81.0
    |with
      |calculus, stones in
        |cystic duct *see* Calculus, gallbladder,
          with cholecystitis, acute

Cholecystitis - *continued*
      |gallbladder *see* Calculus, gallbladder,
        with cholecystitis, acute
      |choledocholithiasis *see* Calculus, bile
        duct, with cholecystitis, acute
      |cholelithiasis *see* Calculus, gallbladder,
        with cholecystitis, acute
  |chronic cholecystitis K81.2
    |with gallbladder calculus K80.12
      |with obstruction K80.13
  |chronic K81.1
    |with acute cholecystitis K81.2
      |with gallbladder calculus K80.12
        |with obstruction K80.13
  |emphysematous (acute) *see* Cholecystitis,
    acute
  |gangrenous *see* Cholecystitis, acute
  |paratyphoidal, current A01.4
  |suppurative *see* Cholecystitis, acute
  |typhoidal A01.09
Cholecystolithiasis *see* Calculus, gallbladder
Choledochitis (suppurative) K83.09
Choledocholith *see* Calculus, bile duct
Choledocholithiasis (common duct) (hepatic
  duct) *see* Calculus, bile duct
  |cystic *see* Calculus, gallbladder
  |typhoidal A01.09
Cholelithiasis (cystic duct) (gallbladder)
  (impacted) (multiple) *see* Calculus,
  gallbladder
  |bile duct (common) (hepatic) *see* Calculus,
    bile duct
  |hepatic duct *see* Calculus, bile duct
  |specified NEC K80.80
    |with obstruction K80.81
Cholemia *see also* Jaundice
  |familial (simple) (congenital) E80.4
  |Gilbert's E80.4
Choleperitoneum, choleperitonitis K65.3
Cholera (Asiatic) (epidemic) (malignant) A00.9
  |antimonial *see* Poisoning, antimony
  |classical A00.0
  |due to Vibrio cholerae 01 A00.9
    |biovar cholerae A00.0
    |biovar eltor A00.1
    |el tor A00.1
  |el tor A00.1
Cholerine *see* Cholera
Cholestasis NEC K83.1
  |with hepatocyte injury K71.0
  |due to total parenteral nutrition (TPN) K76.89
  |pure K71.0
Cholesteatoma (ear) (middle) (with reaction)
  H71.9-
  |attic H71.0-
  |external ear (canal) H60.4-
  |mastoid H71.2-
  |postmastoidectomy cavity (recurrent) *see*
    Complications, postmastoidectomy,
    recurrent cholesteatoma
  |recurrent (postmastoidectomy) *see*
    Complications, postmastoidectomy,
    recurrent cholesteatoma
  |tympanum H71.1-
Cholesteatosis, diffuse H71.3-
Cholesteremia E78.00
Cholesterin in vitreous *see* Deposit, crystalline
Cholesterol
  |deposit
    |retina H35.89
    |vitreous *see* Deposit, crystalline
  |elevated (high) E78.00
    |with elevated (high) triglycerides E78.2
    |screening for Z13.220
  |imbibition of gallbladder K82.4

Cholesterolemia (essential) (pure) E78.00
  |familial E78.01
  |hereditary E78.01
Cholesterolosis, cholesterosis (gallbladder)
  K82.4
  |cerebrotendinous E75.5
Cholocolic fistula K82.3
Choluria R82.2
Chondritis M94.8X9
  |auricle H61.03-
  |costal (Tietze's) M94.0
  |external ear H61.03-
  |patella, posttraumatic *see* Chondromalacia,
    patella
  |pinna H61.03-
  |purulent M94.8X-
  |tuberculous NEC A18.02
    |intervertebral A18.01
Chondroblastoma *see also* Neoplasm, bone,
  benign
  |malignant *see* Neoplasm, bone, malignant
Chondrocalcinosis M11.20
  |ankle M11.27-
  |elbow M11.22-
  |familial M11.10
    |ankle M11.17-
    |elbow M11.12-
    |foot joint M11.17-
    |hand joint M11.14-
    |hip M11.15-
    |knee M11.16-
    |multiple site M11.19
    |shoulder M11.11-
    |vertebrae M11.18
    |wrist M11.13-
  |foot joint M11.27-
  |hand joint M11.24-
  |hip M11.25-
  |knee M11.26-
  |multiple site M11.29
  |shoulder M11.21-
  |vertebrae M11.28
  |specified type NEC M11.20
    |ankle M11.27-
    |elbow M11.22-
    |foot joint M11.27-
    |hand joint M11.24-
    |hip M11.25-
    |knee M11.26-
    |multiple site M11.29
    |shoulder M11.21-
    |vertebrae M11.28
    |wrist M11.23-
  |wrist M11.23-
Chondrodermatitis nodularis helicis or
  anthelicis *see* Perichondritis, ear
Chondrodysplasia Q78.9
  |with hemangioma Q78.4
  |calcificans congenita Q77.3
  |fetalis Q77.4
  |metaphyseal (Jansen's) (McKusick's)
    (Schmid's) Q78.8
  |punctata Q77.3
Chondrodystrophy, chondrodystrophia
  (familial) (fetalis) (hypoplastic) Q78.9
  |calcificans congenita Q77.3
  |myotonic (congenital) G71.13
  |punctata Q77.3
Chondroectodermal dysplasia Q77.6
Chondrogenesis imperfecta Q77.4
Chondrolysis M94.35-
Chondroma *see also* Neoplasm, cartilage,
  benign
  |juxtacortical *see* Neoplasm, bone, benign
  |periosteal *see* Neoplasm, bone, benign

Chondromalacia (systemic) M94.20
| acromioclavicular joint M94.21-
| ankle M94.27-
| elbow M94.22-
| foot joint M94.27-
| glenohumeral joint M94.21-
| hand joint M94.24-
| hip M94.25-
| knee M94.26-
| | patella M22.4-
| multiple sites M94.29
| patella M22.4-
| rib M94.28
| sacroiliac joint M94.259
| shoulder M94.21-
| sternoclavicular joint M94.21-
| vertebral joint M94.28
| wrist M94.23-
Chondromatosis see also Neoplasm, cartilage, uncertain behavior
| internal Q78.4
Chondromyxosarcoma see Neoplasm, cartilage, malignant
Chondro-Osteodysplasia (Morquio-Brailsford type) E76.219
Chondro-Osteodystrophy E76.29
Chondro-Osteoma see Neoplasm, bone, benign
Chondropathia tuberosa M94.0
Chondrosarcoma see Neoplasm, cartilage, malignant
| juxtacortical see Neoplasm, bone, malignant
| mesenchymal see Neoplasm, connective tissue, malignant
| myxoid see Neoplasm, cartilage, malignant
Chordee (nonvenereal) N48.89
| congenital Q54.4
| gonococcal A54.09
Chorditis (fibrinous) (nodosa) (tuberosa) J38.2
Chordoma see Neoplasm, vertebral (column), malignant
Chorea (chronic) (gravis) (posthemiplegic) (senile) (spasmodic) G25.5
| with
| | heart involvement I02.0
| | | active or acute (conditions in I01) I02.0
| | | rheumatic I02.9
| | | | with valvular disorder I02.0
| | rheumatic heart disease (chronic) (inactive)(quiescent) code to rheumatic heart condition involved
| drug-induced G25.4
| habit F95.8
| hereditary G10
| Huntington's G10
| hysterical F44.4
| minor I02.9
| | with heart involvement I02.0
| progressive G25.5
| | hereditary G10
| rheumatic (chronic) I02.9
| | with heart involvement I02.0
| Sydenham's I02.9
| | with heart involvement see Chorea, with rheumatic heart disease
| nonrheumatic G25.5
Choreoathetosis (paroxysmal) G25.5
Chorioadenoma (destruens) D39.2
Chorioamnionitis O41.12-
Chorioangioma D26.7
Choriocarcinoma see Neoplasm, malignant, by site
| combined with
| | embryonal carcinoma see Neoplasm, malignant, by site

Choriocarcinoma - continued
| | other germ cell elements see Neoplasm, malignant, by site
| | teratoma see Neoplasm, malignant, by site
| specified site see Neoplasm, malignant, by site
| unspecified site
| | female C58
| | male C62.90
Chorioencephalitis (acute) (lymphocytic) (serous) A87.2
Chorioepithelioma see Choriocarcinoma
Choriomeningitis (acute) (lymphocytic) (serous) A87.2
Chorionepithelioma see Choriocarcinoma
Chorioretinitis see also Inflammation, chorioretinal
| disseminated see also Inflammation, chorioretinal, disseminated
| | in neurosyphilis A52.19
| Egyptian B76.9 [D63.8]
| focal see also Inflammation, chorioretinal, focal
| histoplasmic B39.9 [H32]
| in (due to)
| | histoplasmosis B39.9 [H32]
| | syphilis (secondary) A51.43
| | | late A52.71
| | toxoplasmosis (acquired) B58.01
| | | congenital (active) P37.1 [H32]
| | tuberculosis A18.53
| juxtapapillary, juxtapapillaris see Inflammation, chorioretinal, focal, juxtapapillary
| leprous A30.9 [H32]
| miner's B76.9 [D63.8]
| progressive myopia (degeneration) (see also Myopia, degenerative) H44.2-
| syphilitic (secondary) A51.43
| | congenital (early) A50.01 [H32]
| | | late A50.32
| | late A52.71
| tuberculous A18.53
Chorioretinopathy, central serous H35.71-
Choroid see condition
Choroideremia H31.21
Choroiditis see Chorioretinitis
Choroidopathy see Disorder, choroid
Choroidoretinitis see Chorioretinitis
Choroidoretinopathy, central serous see Chorioretinopathy, central serous
Christian-Weber disease M35.6
Christmas disease D67
Chromaffinoma see also Neoplasm, benign, by site
| malignant see Neoplasm, malignant, by site
Chromatopsia see Deficiency, color vision
Chromhidrosis, chromidrosis L75.1
Chromoblastomycosis see Chromomycosis
Chromoconversion R82.91
Chromomycosis B43.9
| brain abscess B43.1
| cerebral B43.1
| cutaneous B43.0
| skin B43.0
| specified NEC B43.8
| subcutaneous abscess or cyst B43.2
Chromophytosis B36.0
Chromosome see condition by chromosome involved
| D (1) see condition, chromosome 13
| E (3) see condition, chromosome 18
| G see condition, chromosome 21
Chromotrichomycosis B36.8
Chronic see condition
| fracture see Fracture, pathological

Churg-Strauss syndrome M30.1
Chyle cyst, mesentery I89.8
Chylocele (nonfilarial) I89.8
| filarial see also Infestation, filarial B74.9 [N51]
| tunica vaginalis N50.89
| | filarial see also Infestation, filarial B74.9 [N51]
Chylomicronemia (fasting) (with hyperprebetalipoproteinemia) E78.3
Chylopericardium I31.3
| acute I30.9
Chylothorax (nonfilarial) J94.0
| filarial see also Infestation, filarial B74.9 [J91.8]
Chylous see condition
Chyluria (nonfilarial) R82.0
| due to
| | bilharziasis B65.0
| | Brugia (malayi) B74.1
| | | timori B74.2
| | schistosomiasis (bilharziasis) B65.0
| | Wuchereria (bancrofti) B74.0
| filarial see Infestation, filarial
Cicatricial (deformity) see Cicatrix
Cicatrix (adherent) (contracted) (painful) (vicious) see also Scar L90.5
| adenoid (and tonsil) J35.8
| alveolar process M26.79
| anus K62.89
| auricle see Disorder, pinna, specified type NEC
| bile duct (common) (hepatic) K83.8
| bladder N32.89
| bone see Disorder, bone, specified type NEC
| brain G93.89
| cervix (postoperative) (postpartal) N88.1
| common duct K83.8
| cornea H17.9
| | tuberculous A18.59
| duodenum (bulb), obstructive K31.5
| esophagus K22.2
| eyelid see Disorder, eyelid function
| hypopharynx J39.2
| lacrimal passages see Obstruction, lacrimal
| larynx J38.7
| lung J98.4
| middle ear see subcategory H74.8
| mouth K13.79
| muscle M62.89
| | with contracture see Contraction, muscle NEC
| nasopharynx J39.2
| palate (soft) K13.79
| penis N48.89
| pharynx J39.2
| prostate N42.89
| rectum K62.89
| retina see Scar, chorioretinal
| semilunar cartilage see Derangement, meniscus
| seminal vesicle N50.89
| skin L90.5
| | infected L08.89
| | postinfective L90.5
| | tuberculous B90.8
| specified site NEC L90.5
| throat J39.2
| tongue K14.8
| tonsil (and adenoid) J35.8
| trachea J39.8
| tuberculous NEC B90.9
| urethra N36.8
| uterus N85.8
| vagina N89.8
| | postoperative N99.2
| vocal cord J38.3
| wrist, constricting (annular) L90.5

CIDP (chronic inflammatory demyelinating polyneuropathy) G61.81

CIN *see* Neoplasia, intraepithelial, cervix

CINCA (chronic infantile neurological, cutaneous and articular syndrome) M04.2

Cinchonism *see* Deafness, ototoxic
 |correct substance properly administered *see* Table of Drugs and Chemicals, by drug, adverse effect
 |overdose or wrong substance given or taken *see* Table of Drugs and Chemicals, by drug, poisoning

Circle of Willis *see* condition

Circular *see* condition

Circulating anticoagulants *see also* |Disorder, hemorrhagic D68.318
 |due to drugs *see also* |Disorder, hemorrhagic D68.32
 |following childbirth O72.3

Circulation
 |collateral, any site I99.8
 |defective (lower extremity) I99.9
  |congenital Q28.9
 |embryonic Q28.9
 |failure (peripheral) R57.9
  |newborn P29.89
 |fetal, persistent P29.38
 |heart, incomplete Q28.9

Circulatory system *see* condition

Circulus senilis (cornea) *see* Degeneration, cornea, senile

Circumcision (in absence of medical indication) (ritual) (routine) Z41.2

Circumscribed *see* condition

Circumvallate placenta O43.11-

Cirrhosis, cirrhotic (hepatic) (liver) K74.60
 |alcoholic K70.30
  |with ascites K70.31
 |atrophic *see* Cirrhosis, liver
 |Baumgarten-Cruveilhier K74.69
 |biliary (cholangiolitic) (cholangitic) (hypertrophic) (obstructive) (pericholangiolitic) K74.5
  |due to
   |Clonorchiasis B66.1
    |flukes B66.3
  |primary K74.3
  |secondary K74.4
 |cardiac (of liver) K76.1
 |Charcot's K74.3
 |cholangiolitic, cholangitic, cholestatic (primary) K74.3
 |congestive K76.1
 |Cruveilhier-Baumgarten K74.69
 |cryptogenic (liver) K74.69
 |due to
  |hepatolenticular degeneration E83.01
  |Wilson's disease E83.01
  |xanthomatosis E78.2
 |fatty K76.0
  |alcoholic K70.0
 |Hanot's (hypertrophic) K74.3
 |hepatic *see* Cirrhosis, liver
 |hypertrophic K74.3
 |Indian childhood K74.69
 |kidney *see* Sclerosis, renal
 |Laennec's K70.30
  |with ascites K70.31
  |alcoholic K70.30
   |with ascites K70.31
  |nonalcoholic K74.69
 |liver K74.60
  |alcoholic K70.30
   |with ascites K70.31
   |fatty K70.0
  |congenital P78.81

Cirrhosis - *continued*
 |syphilitic A52.74
 |lung (chronic) J84.10
 |macronodular K74.69
  |alcoholic K70.30
   |with ascites K70.31
 |micronodular K74.69
  |alcoholic K70.30
   |with ascites K70.31
 |mixed type K74.69
 |monolobular K74.3
 |nephritis *see* Sclerosis, renal
 |nutritional K74.69
  |alcoholic K70.30
   |with ascites K70.31
 |obstructive *see* Cirrhosis, biliary
 |ovarian N83.8
 |pancreas (duct) K86.89
 |pigmentary E83.110
 |portal K74.69
  |alcoholic K70.30
   |with ascites K70.31
 |postnecrotic K74.69
  |alcoholic K70.30
   |with ascites K70.31
 |pulmonary J84.10
 |renal *see* Sclerosis, renal
 |spleen D73.2
 |stasis K76.1
 |Todd's K74.3
 |unilobar K74.3
 |xanthomatous (biliary) K74.5
  |due to xanthomatosis (familial) (metabolic) (primary) E78.2

Cistern, subarachnoid R93.0

Citrullinemia E72.23

Citrullinuria E72.23

Civatte's disease or poikiloderma L57.3

Clam digger's itch B65.3

Clammy skin R23.1

Clap *see* Gonorrhea

Clarke-Hadfield syndrome (pancreatic infantilism) K86.89

Clark's paralysis G80.9

Clastothrix L67.8

Claude Bernard-Horner syndrome G90.2
 |traumatic *see* Injury, nerve, cervical sympathetic

Claude's disease or syndrome G46.3

Claudication (intermittent) I73.9
 |cerebral (artery) G45.9
 |spinal cord (arteriosclerotic) G95.19
  |syphilitic A52.09
 |venous (axillary) I87.8

Claudication venosa intermittens I87.8

Claustrophobia F40.240

Clavus (infected) L84

Clawfoot (congenital) Q66.89
 |acquired *see* Deformity, limb, clawfoot

Clawhand (acquired) *see also* Deformity, limb, clawhand
 |congenital Q68.1

Claw toe (congenital) Q66.89
 |acquired *see* Deformity, toe, specified NEC

Clay eating *see* Pica

Cleansing of artificial opening *see* Attention to, artificial, opening

Cleft (congenital) *see also* Imperfect, closure
 |alveolar process M26.79
 |branchial (persistent) Q18.2
  |cyst Q18.0
   |fistula Q18.0
   |sinus Q18.0
 |cricoid cartilage, posterior Q31.8
 |foot Q72.7
 |hand Q71.6
 |lip (unilateral) Q36.9

Cleft (congenital) - *continued*
 |with cleft palate Q37.9
  |hard Q37.1
   |with soft Q37.5
  |soft Q37.3
   |with hard Q37.5
  |bilateral Q36.0
   |with cleft palate Q37.8
    |hard Q37.0
     |with soft Q37.4
    |soft Q37.2
     |with hard Q37.4
  |median Q36.1
 |nose Q30.2
 |palate Q35.9
  |with cleft lip (unilateral) Q37.9
   |bilateral Q37.8
  |hard Q35.1
   |with
    |cleft lip (unilateral) Q37.1
     |bilateral Q37.0
    |soft Q35.5
     |with cleft lip (unilateral) Q37.5
      |bilateral Q37.4
  |medial Q35.5
  |soft Q35.3
   |with
    |cleft lip (unilateral) Q37.3
     |bilateral Q37.2
    |hard Q35.5
     |with cleft lip (unilateral) Q37.5
      |bilateral Q37.4
 |penis Q55.69
 |scrotum Q55.29
 |thyroid cartilage Q31.8
 |uvula Q35.7

Cleidocranial dysostosis Q74.0

Cleptomania F63.2

Clicking hip (newborn) R29.4

Climacteric (female) *see also* Menopause
 |arthritis (any site) NEC *see* Arthritis, specified form NEC
 |depression (single episode) F32.89
  |recurrent episode F33.8
 |melancholia (single episode) F32.89
  |recurrent episode F33.8
 |male (symptoms) (syndrome) NEC N50.89
 |paranoid state F22
 |polyarthritis NEC *see* Arthritis, specified form NEC
 |symptoms (female) N95.1

Clinical research investigation (clinical trial) (control subject) (normal comparison) (participant) Z00.6

Clitoris *see* condition

Cloaca (persistent) Q43.7

Clonorchiasis, Clonorchis infection (liver) B66.1

Clonus R25.8

Closed bite M26.29

Clostridium (C.) perfringens, as cause of disease classified elsewhere B96.7

Closure
 |congenital, nose Q30.0
 |cranial sutures, premature Q75.0
 |defective or imperfect NEC *see* Imperfect, closure
 |fistula, delayed *see* Fistula
 |foramen ovale, imperfect Q21.1
 |hymen N89.6
 |interauricular septum, defective Q21.1
 |interventricular septum, defective Q21.0
 |lacrimal duct *see also* Stenosis, lacrimal, duct
  |congenital Q10.5
 |nose (congenital) Q30.0
  |acquired M95.0

Closure - *continued*
| of artificial opening *see* Attention to, artificial, opening
| primary angle, without glaucoma damage H40.06-
| vagina N89.5
| valve *see* Endocarditis
| vulva N90.5
Clot (blood) *see also* Embolism
| artery (obstruction) (occlusion) *see* Embolism
| bladder N32.89
| brain (intradural or extradural) *see* Occlusion, artery, cerebral
| circulation I74.9
| heart *see also* Infarct, myocardium
| | not resulting in infarction I51.3
| vein *see* Thrombosis
Clouded state R40.1
| epileptic *see* Epilepsy, specified NEC
| paroxysmal *see* Epilepsy, specified NEC
Cloudy antrum, antra J32.0
Clouston's (hidrotic) ectodermal dysplasia Q82.4
Clubbed nail pachydermoperiostosis M89.40 [*L62*]
Clubbing of finger(s) (nails) R68.3
Club finger R68.3
| congenital Q68.1
Clubfoot (congenital) Q66.89
| acquired *see* Deformity, limb, clubfoot
| equinovarus Q66.0
| paralytic *see* Deformity, limb, clubfoot
Clubhand (congenital) (radial) Q71.4-
| acquired *see* Deformity, limb, clubhand
Club nail R68.3
| congenital Q84.6
Clump, kidney Q63.1
Clumsiness, clumsy child syndrome F82
Cluttering F80.81
Clutton's joints A50.51 [*M12.80*]
Coagulation, intravascular (diffuse) (disseminated) *see also* Defibrination syndrome
| complicating abortion *see* Abortion, by type, complicated by, intravascular coagulation
| following ectopic or molar pregnancy O08.1
Coagulopathy *see also* Defect, coagulation
| consumption D65
| intravascular D65
| | newborn P60
Coalition
| calcaneo-scaphoid Q66.89
| tarsal Q66.89
Coalminer's
| elbow *see* Bursitis, elbow, olecranon
| lung or pneumoconiosis J60
Coalworker's lung or pneumoconiosis J60
Coarctation
| aorta (preductal) (postductal) Q25.1
| pulmonary artery Q25.71
Coated tongue K14.3
Coats' disease (exudative retinopathy) *see* Retinopathy, exudative
Cocaine-Induced
| anxiety disorder F14.980
| bipolar and related disorder F14.94
| depressive disorder F14.94
| obsessive-compulsive and related disorder F14.988
| psychotic disorder F14.959
| sleep disorder F14.982
| sexual dysfunction F14.981
Cocainism *see* Disorder, cocaine use
Coccidioidomycosis B38.9
| cutaneous B38.3
| disseminated B38.7

Coccidioidomycosis - *continued*
| generalized B38.7
| meninges B38.4
| prostate B38.81
| pulmonary B38.2
| | acute B38.0
| | chronic B38.1
| skin B38.3
| specified NEC B38.89
Coccidioidosis *see* Coccidioidomycosis
Coccidiosis (intestinal) A07.3
Coccydynia, coccygodynia M53.3
Coccyx *see* condition
Cochin-China diarrhea K90.1
Cockayne's syndrome Q87.1
Cocked up toe *see* Deformity, toe, specified NEC
Cock's peculiar tumor L72.3
Codman's tumor *see* Neoplasm, bone, benign
Coenurosis B71.8
Coffee-Worker's lung J67.8
Cogan's syndrome H16.32-
| oculomotor apraxia H51.8
Coitus, painful (female) N94.10
| male N53.12
| psychogenic F52.6
Cold J00
| agglutinin disease or hemoglobinuria (chronic) D59.12
| bronchial *see* Bronchitis
| chest *see* Bronchitis
| common (head) J00
| effects of T69.9
| | specified effect NEC T69.8
| excessive, effects of T69.9
| | specified effect NEC T69.8
| exhaustion from T69.8
| exposure to T69.9
| | specified effect NEC T69.8
| head J00
| injury syndrome (newborn) P80.0
| on lung *see* Bronchitis
| rose J30.1
| sensitivity, auto-immune D59.12
| symptoms J00
| virus J00
| with influenza, flu, or grippe *see* Influenza, with, respiratory manifestations NEC
Cold sore B00.1
Colibacillosis A49.8
| as the cause of other disease *see also* Escherichia coli B96.20
| generalized A41.50
Colic (bilious) (infantile) (intestinal) (recurrent) (spasmodic) R10.83
| abdomen R10.83
| | psychogenic F45.8
| appendix, appendicular K38.8
| bile duct *see* Calculus, bile duct
| biliary *see* Calculus, bile duct
| common duct *see* Calculus, bile duct
| cystic duct *see* Calculus, gallbladder
| Devonshire NEC *see* Poisoning, lead
| gallbladder *see* Calculus, gallbladder
| gallstone *see* Calculus, gallbladder
| | gallbladder or cystic duct *see* Calculus, gallbladder
| hepatic (duct) *see* Calculus, bile duct
| hysterical F45.8
| kidney N23
| lead NEC *see* Poisoning, lead
| mucous K58.9
| | with diarrhea K58.0
| | psychogenic F54
| nephritic N23
| painter's NEC *see* Poisoning, lead
| pancreas K86.89

Colic - *continued*
| psychogenic F45.8
| renal N23
| saturnine NEC *see* Poisoning, lead
| ureter N23
| urethral N36.8
| | due to calculus N21.1
| uterus NEC N94.89
| | menstrual *see* Dysmenorrhea
| worm NOS B83.9
Colicystitis *see* Cystitis
Colitis (acute) (catarrhal) (chronic) (noninfective) (hemorrhagic) *see also* Enteritis K52.9
| allergic K52.29
| | with
| | | food protein-induced enterocolitis syndrome K52.21
| | | proctocolitis K52.89
| amebic (acute) *see also* Amebiasis A06.0
| | nondysenteric A06.2
| anthrax A22.2
| bacillary *see* Infection, Shigella
| balantidial A07.0
| Clostridium difficile
| | not specified as recurrent A04.72
| | recurrent A04.71
| coccidial A07.3
| collagenous K52.831
| cystica superficialis K52.89
| dietary counseling and surveillance (for) Z71.3
| dietetic *see also* Colitis, allergic K52.29
| drug-induced K52.1
| due to radiation K52.0
| eosinophilic K52.82
| food hypersensitivity *see also* Colitis, allergic K52.29
| giardial A07.1
| granulomatous *see* Enteritis, regional, large intestine
| indeterminate, so stated K52.3
| infectious *see* Enteritis, infectious
| ischemic K55.9
| | acute (subacute) *see also* Ischemia, intestine, acute K55.039
| | chronic K55.1
| | due to mesenteric artery insufficiency K55.1
| | fulminant (acute) *see also* Ischemia, intestine, acute K55.039
| left sided K51.50
| | with
| | | abscess K51.514
| | | complication K51.519
| | | | specified NEC K51.518
| | | fistula K51.513
| | | obstruction K51.512
| | | rectal bleeding K51.511
| lymphocytic K52.832
| membranous
| | psychogenic F54
| microscopic K52.839
| | specified NEC K52.838
| mucous *see* Syndrome, irritable, bowel
| | psychogenic F54
| noninfective K52.9
| | specified NEC K52.89
| polyposa *see* Polyp, colon, inflammatory
| | protozoal A07.9
| pseudomembranous
| | not specified as recurrent A04.72
| | recurrent A04.71
| pseudomucinous *see* Syndrome, irritable, bowel
| regional *see* Enteritis, regional, large intestine
| | infectious A09

Colitis - *continued*
  |segmental *see* Enteritis, regional, large intestine
  |septic *see* Enteritis, infectious
  |spastic K58.9
    |with diarrhea K58.0
    |psychogenic F54
  |staphylococcal A04.8
    |foodborne A05.0
  |subacute ischemic *see also* Ischemia, intestine, acute K55.039
  |thromboulcerative *see also* Ischemia, intestine, acute K55.039
  |toxic NEC K52.1
    |due to Clostridium difficile
      |not specified as recurrent A04.72
      |recurrent A04.71
  |transmural *see* Enteritis, regional, large intestine
  |trichomonal A07.8
  |tuberculous (ulcerative) A18.32
  |ulcerative (chronic) K51.90
    |with
      |complication K51.919
        |abscess K51.914
        |fistula K51.913
        |obstruction K51.912
        |rectal bleeding K51.911
        |specified complication NEC K51.918
    |enterocolitis *see* Enterocolitis, ulcerative
    |ileocolitis *see* Ileocolitis, ulcerative
    |mucosal proctocolitis *see* Proctocolitis, mucosal
    |proctitis *see* Proctitis, ulcerative
    |pseudopolyposis *see* Polyp, colon, inflammatory
    |psychogenic F54
    |rectosigmoiditis *see* Rectosigmoiditis, ulcerative
    |specified type NEC K51.80
      |with
        |complication K51.819
          |abscess K51.814
          |fistula K51.813
          |obstruction K51.812
          |rectal bleeding K51.811
          |specified complication NEC K51.818

Collagenosis, collagen disease (nonvascular) (vascular) M35.9
  |cardiovascular I42.8
  |reactive perforating L87.1
  |specified NEC M35.8
Collapse R55
  |adrenal E27.2
  |cardiorespiratory R57.0
  |cardiovascular R57.0
    |newborn P29.89
  |circulatory (peripheral) R57.9
    |during or after labor and delivery O75.1
    |following ectopic or molar pregnancy O08.3
    |newborn P29.89
  |during or
    |after labor and delivery O75.1
    |resulting from a procedure, not elsewhere classified T81.10
  |external ear canal *see* Stenosis, external ear canal
  |general R55
  |heart *see* Disease, heart
  |heat T67.1
  |hysterical F44.89
  |labyrinth, membranous (congenital) Q16.5
  |lung (massive) *see also* Atelectasis J98.19
    |pressure due to anesthesia (general) (local) or other sedation T88.2
      |during labor and delivery O74.1
      |in pregnancy O29.02-

Collapse - *continued*
    |postpartum, puerperal O89.09
  |myocardial *see* Disease, heart
  |nervous F48.8
  |neurocirculatory F45.8
  |nose M95.0
  |postoperative T81.10
  |pulmonary *see also* Atelectasis J98.19
    |newborn *see* Atelectasis
  |trachea J39.8
  |tracheobronchial J98.09
  |valvular *see* Endocarditis
  |vascular (peripheral) R57.9
    |during or after labor and delivery O75.1
    |following ectopic or molar pregnancy O08.3
    |newborn P29.89
  |vertebra M48.50-
    |cervical region M48.52-
    |cervicothoracic region M48.53-
    |in (due to)
      |metastasis *see* Collapse, vertebra, in, specified disease NEC
      |osteoporosis *see also* Osteoporosis M80.88
        |cervical region M80.88
        |cervicothoracic region M80.88
        |lumbar region M80.88
        |lumbosacral region M80.88
        |multiple sites M80.88
        |occipito-atlanto-axial region M80.88
        |sacrococcygeal region M80.88
        |thoracic region M80.88
        |thoracolumbar region M80.88
      |specified disease NEC M48.50-
        |cervical region M48.52-
        |cervicothoracic region M48.53-
        |lumbar region M48.56-
        |lumbosacral region M48.57-
        |occipito-atlanto-axial region M48.51-
        |sacrococcygeal region M48.58-
        |thoracic region M48.54-
        |thoracolumbar region M48.55-
    |lumbar region M48.56-
    |lumbosacral region M48.57-
    |occipito-atlanto-axial region M48.51-
    |sacrococcygeal region M48.58-
    |thoracic region M48.54-
    |thoracolumbar region M48.55-
Collateral *see also* condition
  |circulation (venous) I87.8
  |dilation, veins I87.8
Colles' fracture S52.53-
Collet (-Sicard) syndrome G52.7
Collier's asthma or lung J60
Collodion baby Q80.2
Colloid nodule (of thyroid) (cystic) E04.1
Coloboma (iris) Q13.0
  |eyelid Q10.3
  |fundus Q14.8
  |lens Q12.2
  |optic disc (congenital) Q14.2
    |acquired H47.31-
Coloenteritis *see* Enteritis
Colon *see* condition
Colonization
  |MRSA (Methicillin resistant Staphylococcus aureus) Z22.322
  |MSSA (Methicillin susceptible Staphylococcus aureus) Z22.321
  |status *see* Carrier (suspected) of
Coloptosis K63.4
Color blindness *see* Deficiency, color vision

Colostomy
  |attention to Z43.3
  |fitting or adjustment Z46.89
  |malfunctioning K94.03
  |status Z93.3
Colpitis (acute) *see* Vaginitis
Colpocele N81.5
Colpocystitis *see* Vaginitis
Colpospasm N94.2
Column, spinal, vertebral *see* condition
Coma R40.20
  |with
    |motor response (none) R40.231
      |abnormal R40.233
      |abnormal extensor posturing to pain or noxious stimuli (< 2 years of age) R40.232
      |abnormal flexure posturing to pain or noxious stimuli (0-5 years of age) R40.233
      |extension R40.232
      |extensor posturing to pain or noxious stimuli (2 5 years of age) R40.232
      |flexion withdrawal R40.234
      |flexion/decorticate posturing (< 2 years of age) R40.233
      |localizes pain (2 5 years of age) R40.235
      |normal or spontaneous movement (< 2 years of age) R40.236
      |obeys commands (2 5 years of age) R40.236
      |score of
        |1 R40.231
        |2 R40.232
        |3 R40.233
        |4 R40.234
        |5 R40.235
        |6 R40.236
    |withdraws from pain or noxious stimuli (0-5 years of age) R40.234
    |withdraws to touch (< 2 years of age) R40.235
    |opening of eyes (never) R40.211
      |in response to
        |pain R40.212
        |sound R40.213
      |score of
        |1 R40.211
        |2 R40.212
        |3 R40.213
        |4 R40.214
      |spontaneous R40.214
    |verbal response (none) R40.221
      |cooing or babbling or crying appropriately (< 2 years of age) R40.225
      |inappropriate crying or screaming (< 2 years of age) R40.223
      |confused conversation R40.224
      |inappropriate words (2 5 years of age) R40.224
      |incomprehensible words R40.222
      |oriented R40.225
      |incomprehensible sounds (2 5 years of age) R40.222
      |irritable cries (< 2 years of age) R40.224
      |moans/grunts to pain; restless (< 2 years old) R40.222
      |score of
        |1 R40.221
        |2 R40.222
        |3 R40.223
        |4 R40.224
        |5 R40.225
      |screaming (2-5 years of age) R40.223

Complication(s) - *continued*
    |breakdown T82.511
    |displacement T82.521
    |leakage T82.531
    |malposition T82.521
    |obstruction T82.591
    |perforation T82.591
    |protrusion T82.591
  |pain T82.848
  |specified type NEC T82.898
  |stenosis T82.858
  |thrombosis T82.868
|arthroplasty *see* Complications, joint
  prosthesis
|artificial
  |fertilization or insemination N98.9
    |attempted introduction (of)
      |embryo in embryo transfer N98.3
      |ovum following in vitro fertilization
        N98.2
    |hyperstimulation of ovaries N98.1
    |infection N98.0
    |specified NEC N98.8
  |heart T82.9
    |embolism T82.817
    |fibrosis T82.827
    |hemorrhage T82.837
    |infection or inflammation T82.7
    |mechanical
      |breakdown T82.512
      |displacement T82.522
      |leakage T82.532
      |malposition T82.522
      |obstruction T82.592
      |perforation T82.592
      |protrusion T82.592
    |pain T82.847
    |specified type NEC T82.897
    |stenosis T82.857
    |thrombosis T82.867
  |opening
    |cecostomy *see* Complications, colostomy
    |colostomy *see* Complications, colostomy
    |cystostomy *see* Complications,
      cystostomy
    |enterostomy *see* Complications,
      enterostomy
    |gastrostomy *see* Complications,
      gastrostomy
    |ileostomy *see* Complications, enterostomy
    |jejunostomy *see* Complications,
      enterostomy
    |nephrostomy *see* Complications, stoma,
      urinary tract
    |tracheostomy *see* Complications,
      tracheostomy
    |ureterostomy *see* Complications, stoma,
      urinary tract
    |urethrostomy *see* Complications, stoma,
      urinary tract
|balloon implant or device
  |gastrointestinal T85.9
    |embolism T85.818
    |fibrosis T85.828
    |hemorrhage T85.838
    |infection and inflammation T85.79
    |pain T85.848
    |specified type NEC T85.898
    |stenosis T85.858
    |thrombosis T85.868
  |vascular (counterpulsation) T82.9
    |embolism T82.818
    |fibrosis T82.828
    |hemorrhage T82.838
    |infection or inflammation T82.7
    |mechanical
      |breakdown T82.513

Complication(s) - *continued*
    |displacement T82.523
    |leakage T82.533
    |malposition T82.523
    |obstruction T82.593
    |perforation T82.593
    |protrusion T82.593
  |pain T82.848
  |specified type NEC T82.898
  |stenosis T82.858
  |thrombosis T82.868
|bariatric procedure
  |gastric band procedure K95.09
    |infection K95.01
  |specified procedure NEC K95.89
    |infection K95.81
|bile duct implant (prosthetic) T85.9
  |embolism T85.818
  |fibrosis T85.828
  |hemorrhage T85.838
  |infection and inflammation T85.79
  |mechanical
    |breakdown T85.510
    |displacement T85.520
    |malfunction T85.510
    |malposition T85.520
    |obstruction T85.590
    |perforation T85.590
    |protrusion T85.590
    |specified NEC T85.590
  |pain T85.848
  |specified type NEC T85.898
  |stenosis T85.858
  |thrombosis T85.868
|bladder device (auxiliary) *see* Complications,
  genitourinary, device or implant, urinary
  system
|bleeding (postoperative) *see* Complication,
  postoperative, hemorrhage
  |intraoperative *see* Complication,
    intraoperative, hemorrhage
|blood vessel graft *see* Complications, graft,
  vascular
|bone
  |device NEC T84.9
    |embolism T84.81
    |fibrosis T84.82
    |hemorrhage T84.83
    |infection or inflammation T84.7
    |mechanical
      |breakdown T84.318
      |displacement T84.328
      |malposition T84.328
      |obstruction T84.398
      |perforation T84.398
      |protrusion T84.398
    |pain T84.84
    |specified type NEC T84.89
    |stenosis T84.85
    |thrombosis T84.86
  |graft *see* Complications, graft, bone
  |growth stimulator (electrode) *see*
    Complications, electronic stimulator
    device, bone
  |marrow transplant *see* Complications,
    transplant, bone, marrow
|brain neurostimulator (electrode) *see*
  Complications, electronic stimulator
  device, brain
|breast implant (prosthetic) T85.9
  |capsular contracture T85.44
  |embolism T85.818
  |fibrosis T85.828
  |hemorrhage T85.838
  |infection and inflammation T85.79
  |mechanical

Complication(s) - *continued*
    |breakdown T85.41
    |displacement T85.42
    |leakage T85.43
    |malposition T85.42
    |obstruction T85.49
    |perforation T85.49
    |protrusion T85.49
    |specified NEC T85.49
  |pain T85.848
  |specified type NEC T85.898
  |stenosis T85.858
  |thrombosis T85.868
|bypass *see also* Complications, prosthetic
  device or implant
  |aortocoronary *see* Complications, coronary
    artery (bypass) graft
  |arterial *see also* Complications, graft,
  vascular
    |extremity *see* Complications, extremity
  artery (bypass) graft
  |cardiac *see also* Disease, heart
    |device, implant or graft T82.9
      |embolism T82.817
      |fibrosis T82.827
      |hemorrhage T82.837
      |infection or inflammation T82.7
        |valve prosthesis T82.6
      |mechanical
        |breakdown T82.519
          |specified device NEC T82.518
        |displacement T82.529
          |specified device NEC T82.528
        |leakage T82.539
          |specified device NEC T82.538
        |malposition T82.529
          |specified device NEC T82.528
        |obstruction T82.599
          |specified device NEC T82.598
        |perforation T82.599
          |specified device NEC T82.598
        |protrusion T82.599
          |specified device NEC T82.598
      |pain T82.847
      |specified type NEC T82.897
      |stenosis T82.857
      |thrombosis T82.867
|cardiovascular device, graft or implant T82.9
  |aortic graft *see* Complications, graft,
    vascular
  |arteriovenous
    |fistula, artificial *see* Complication,
      arteriovenous, fistula, surgically
      created
    |shunt *see* Complication, arteriovenous,
      shunt, surgically created
  |artificial heart *see* Complication, artificial,
    heart
  |balloon (counterpulsation) device *see*
    Complication, balloon implant, vascular
  |carotid artery graft *see* Complications, graft,
    vascular
  |coronary bypass graft *see* Complication,
    coronary artery (bypass) graft
  |dialysis catheter (vascular) *see*
    Complication, catheter, dialysis
  |electronic T82.9
    |electrode T82.9
      |embolism T82.817
      |fibrosis T82.827
      |hemorrhage T82.837
      |infection T82.7
      |mechanical
        |breakdown T82.110
        |displacement T82.120
        |leakage T82.190

Complication(s) - continued
    |obstruction T82.190
    |perforation T82.190
    |protrusion T82.190
    |specified type NEC T82.190
   |pain T82.847
   |specified NEC T82.897
   |stenosis T82.857
   |thrombosis T82.867
  |embolism T82.817
  |fibrosis T82.827
  |hemorrhage T82.837
  |infection T82.7
  |mechanical
   |breakdown T82.119
   |displacement T82.129
   |leakage T82.199
   |obstruction T82.199
   |perforation T82.199
   |protrusion T82.199
   |specified type NEC T82.199
  |pain T82.847
  |pulse generator T82.9
   |embolism T82.817
   |fibrosis T82.827
   |hemorrhage T82.837
   |infection T82.7
   |mechanical
    |breakdown T82.111
    |displacement T82.121
    |leakage T82.191
    |obstruction T82.191
    |perforation T82.191
    |protrusion T82.191
    |specified type NEC T82.191
   |pain T82.847
   |specified NEC T82.897
   |stenosis T82.857
   |thrombosis T82.867
  |specified condition NEC T82.897
  |specified device NEC T82.9
   |embolism T82.817
   |fibrosis T82.827
   |hemorrhage T82.837
   |infection T82.7
   |mechanical
    |breakdown T82.118
    |displacement T82.128
    |leakage T82.198
    |obstruction T82.198
    |perforation T82.198
    |protrusion T82.198
    |specified type NEC T82.198
   |pain T82.847
   |specified NEC T82.897
   |stenosis T82.857
   |thrombosis T82.867
  |stenosis T82.857
  |thrombosis T82.867
 |extremity artery graft *see* Complication,
    extremity artery (bypass) graft
 |femoral artery graft *see* Complication,
    extremity artery (bypass) graft
 |heart-lung transplant *see* Complication,
    transplant, heart, with lung
 |heart
  |transplant *see* Complication, transplant,
    heart
  |valve *see* Complication, prosthetic device,
    heart valve
   |graft *see* Complication, heart, valve,
    graft
 |infection or inflammation T82.7
 |umbrella device *see* Complication, umbrella
    device, vascular

Complication(s) - continued
 |vascular graft (or anastomosis) *see*
    Complication, graft, vascular
 |carotid artery (bypass) graft *see*
    Complications, graft, vascular
 |catheter (device) NEC *see also* Complications,
    prosthetic device or implant
  |cranial infusion
   |infection and inflammation T85.735
   |mechanical
    |breakdown T85.610
    |displacement T85.620
    |leakage T85.630
    |malfunction T85.690
    |malposition T85.620
    |obstruction T85.690
    |perforation T85.690
    |protrusion T85.690
    |specified NEC T85.690
  |cystostomy T83.9
   |embolism T83.81
   |fibrosis T83.82
   |hemorrhage T83.83
   |infection and inflammation T83.510
   |mechanical
    |breakdown T83.010
    |displacement T83.020
    |leakage T83.030
    |malposition T83.020
    |obstruction T83.090
    |perforation T83.090
    |protrusion T83.090
    |specified NEC T83.090
   |pain T83.84
   |specified type NEC T83.89
   |stenosis T83.85
   |thrombosis T83.86
  |dialysis (vascular) T82.9
   |embolism T82.818
   |fibrosis T82.828
   |hemorrhage T82.838
   |infection and inflammation T82.7
   |intraperitoneal *see* Complications,
    catheter, intraperitoneal
   |mechanical
    |breakdown T82.41
    |displacement T82.42
    |leakage T82.43
    |malposition T82.42
    |obstruction T82.49
    |perforation T82.49
    |protrusion T82.49
   |pain T82.848
   |specified type NEC T82.898
   |stenosis T82.858
   |thrombosis T82.868
  |epidural infusion T85.9
   |embolism T85.810
   |fibrosis T85.820
   |hemorrhage T85.830
   |infection and inflammation T85.735
   |mechanical
    |breakdown T85.610
    |displacement T85.620
    |leakage T85.630
    |malfunction T85.610
    |malposition T85.620
    |obstruction T85.690
    |perforation T85.690
    |protrusion T85.690
    |specified NEC T85.690
   |pain T85.840
   |specified type NEC T85.890
   |stenosis T85.850
   |thrombosis T85.860
  |intraperitoneal dialysis T85.9
   |embolism T85.818

Complication(s) - continued
   |fibrosis T85.828
   |hemorrhage T85.838
   |infection and inflammation T85.71
   |mechanical
    |breakdown T85.611
    |displacement T85.621
    |leakage T85.631
    |malfunction T85.611
    |malposition T85.621
    |obstruction T85.691
    |perforation T85.691
    |protrusion T85.691
    |specified NEC T85.691
   |pain T85.848
   |specified type NEC T85.898
   |stenosis T85.858
   |thrombosis T85.868
  |intrathecal infusion
   |infection and inflammation T85.735
   |mechanical
    |breakdown T85.610
    |displacement T85.620
    |leakage T85.630
    |malfunction T85.690
    |malposition T85.620
    |obstruction T85.690
    |perforation T85.690
    |protrusion T85.690
    |specified NEC T85.690
  |intravenous infusion T82.9
   |embolism T82.818
   |fibrosis T82.828
   |hemorrhage T82.838
   |infection or inflammation T82.7
   |mechanical
    |breakdown T82.514
    |displacement T82.524
    |leakage T82.534
    |malposition T82.524
    |obstruction T82.594
    |perforation T82.594
    |protrusion T82.594
   |pain T82.848
   |specified type NEC T82.898
   |stenosis T82.858
   |thrombosis T82.868
  |spinal infusion
   |infection and inflammation T85.735
   |mechanical
    |breakdown T85.610
    |displacement T85.620
    |leakage T85.630
    |malfunction T85.690
    |malposition T85.620
    |obstruction T85.690
    |perforation T85.690
    |protrusion T85.690
    |specified NEC T85.690
  |subarachnoid infusion
   |infection and inflammation T85.735
   |mechanical
    |breakdown T85.610
    |displacement T85.620
    |leakage T85.630
    |malfunction T85.690
    |malposition T85.620
    |obstruction T85.690
    |perforation T85.690
    |protrusion T85.690
    |specified NEC T85.690
  |subdural infusion T85.9
   |embolism T85.810
   |fibrosis T85.820
   |hemorrhage T85.830

Complication(s) - *continued*
- |infection and inflammation T85.735
- |mechanical
  - |breakdown T85.610
  - |displacement T85.620
  - |leakage T85.630
  - |malfunction T85.610
  - |malposition T85.620
  - |obstruction T85.690
  - |perforation T85.690
  - |protrusion T85.690
  - |specified NEC T85.690
- |pain T85.840
- |specified type NEC T85.890
- |stenosis T85.850
- |thrombosis T85.860
- |urethral T83.9
  - |displacement T83.028
  - |embolism T83.81
  - |fibrosis T83.82
  - |hemorrhage T83.83
  - |indwelling
    - |breakdown T83.011
    - |displacement T83.021
    - |infection and inflammation T83.511
    - |leakage T83.031
    - |specified complication NEC T83.091
  - |infection and inflammation T83.511
  - |leakage T83.038
  - |malposition T83.028
  - |mechanical
    - |breakdown T83.011
  - |obstruction (mechanical) T83.091
  - |pain T83.84
  - |perforation T83.091
  - |protrusion T83.091
  - |specified type NEC T83.091
  - |stenosis T83.85
  - |thrombosis T83.86
- |urinary NEC
  - |breakdown T83.018
  - |displacement T83.028
  - |infection and inflammation T83.518
  - |leakage T83.038
  - |specified complication NEC T83.098
- |cecostomy (stoma) *see* Complications, colostomy
- |cesarean delivery wound NEC O90.89
  - |disruption O90.0
  - |hematoma O90.2
  - |infection (following delivery) O86.00
- |chemotherapy (antineoplastic) NEC T88.7
- - chimeric antigen receptor (CAR-T) cell therapy T80.82
- |chin implant (prosthetic) *see* Complication, prosthetic device or implant, specified NEC
- |circulatory system I99.8
  - |intraoperative I97.88
  - |postprocedural I97.89
    - |following cardiac surgery (*see also* Infarct, myocardium, associated with revascularization procedure) I97.19-
    - |postcardiotomy syndrome I97.0
    - |hypertension I97.3
    - |lymphedema after mastectomy I97.2
    - |postcardiotomy syndrome I97.0
    - |specified NEC I97.89
- |colostomy (stoma) K94.00
  - |hemorrhage K94.01
  - |infection K94.02
  - |malfunction K94.03
  - |mechanical K94.03
  - |specified complication NEC K94.09
- |contraceptive device, intrauterine *see* Complications, intrauterine, contraceptive device

Complication(s) - *continued*
- |cord (umbilical) *see* Complications, umbilical cord
- |corneal graft *see* Complications, graft, cornea
- |coronary artery (bypass) graft T82.9
  - |atherosclerosis *see* Arteriosclerosis, coronary (artery), embolism T82.818
  - |fibrosis T82.828
  - |hemorrhage T82.838
  - |infection and inflammation T82.7
  - |mechanical
    - |breakdown T82.211
    - |displacement T82.212
    - |leakage T82.213
    - |malposition T82.212
    - |obstruction T82.218
    - |perforation T82.218
    - |protrusion T82.218
    - |specified NEC T82.218
  - |pain T82.848
  - |specified type NEC T82.898
  - |stenosis T82.858
  - |thrombosis T82.868
- |counterpulsation device (balloon), intra aortic *see* Complications, balloon implant, vascular
- |cystostomy (stoma) N99.518
  - |catheter *see* Complications, catheter, cystostomy
  - |hemorrhage N99.510
  - |infection N99.511
  - |malfunction N99.512
  - |specified type NEC N99.518
- |delivery *see also* Complications, obstetric O75.9
  - |procedure (instrumental) (manual) (surgical) O75.4
  - |specified NEC O75.89
- |dialysis (peritoneal) (renal) *see also* Complications, infusion
  - |catheter (vascular) *see* Complication, catheter, dialysis
    - |peritoneal, intraperitoneal *see* Complications, catheter, intraperitoneal
- |dorsal column (spinal) neurostimulator *see* Complications, electronic stimulator device, spinal cord
- |drug NEC T88.7
- |ear procedure *see also* Disorder, ear
  - |intraoperative H95.88
    - |hematoma *see* Complications, intraoperative, hemorrhage (hematoma) (of), ear
    - |hemorrhage *see* Complications, intraoperative, hemorrhage (hematoma) (of), ear
    - |laceration *see* Complications, intraoperative, puncture or laceration, ear
    - |specified NEC H95.88
  - |postoperative H95.89
    - |external ear canal stenosis H95.81-
    - |hematoma *see* Complications, postprocedural, hematoma (of), ear
    - |hemorrhage *see* Complications, postprocedural, hemorrhage (of), ear
    - |postmastoidectomy *see* Complications, postmastoidectomy
    - |seroma *see* Complications, postprocedural, seroma (of), mastoid process
    - |specified NEC H95.89
- |ectopic pregnancy O08.9
  - |damage to pelvic organs O08.6
  - |embolism O08.2

Complication(s) - *continued*
- |genital infection O08.0
- |hemorrhage (delayed) (excessive) O08.1
- |metabolic disorder O08.5
- |renal failure O08.4
- |shock O08.3
- |specified type NEC O08.0
- |venous complication NEC O08.7
- |electronic stimulator device
  - |bladder (urinary) *see* Complications, electronic stimulator device, urinary
  - |bone T84.9
    - |breakdown T84.310
    - |displacement T84.320
    - |embolism T84.81
    - |fibrosis T84.82
    - |hemorrhage T84.83
    - |infection or inflammation T84.7
    - |malfunction T84.310
    - |malposition T84.320
    - |mechanical NEC T84.390
    - |obstruction T84.390
    - |pain T84.84
    - |perforation T84.390
    - |protrusion T84.390
    - |specified type NEC T84.89
    - |stenosis T84.85
    - |thrombosis T84.86
  - |brain T85.9
    - |embolism T85.810
    - |fibrosis T85.820
    - |hemorrhage T85.830
    - |infection and inflammation T85.731
    - |mechanical
      - |breakdown T85.110
      - |displacement T85.120
      - |leakage T85.190
      - |malposition T85.120
      - |obstruction T85.190
      - |perforation T85.190
      - |protrusion T85.190
      - |specified NEC T85.190
    - |pain T85.840
    - |specified type NEC T85.890
    - |stenosis T85.850
    - |thrombosis T85.860
  - |cardiac (defibrillator) (pacemaker) *see* Complications, cardiovascular device or implant, electronic
  - |generator (brain) (gastric) (peripheral) (sacral) (spinal)
    - |breakdown T85.113
    - |displacement T85.123
    - |leakage T85.193
    - |malposition T85.123
    - |obstruction T85.193
    - |perforation T85.193
    - |protrusion T85.193
    - |specified type NEC T85.193
  - |muscle T84.9
    - |breakdown T84.418
    - |displacement T84.428
    - |embolism T84.81
    - |fibrosis T84.82
    - |hemorrhage T84.83
    - |infection or inflammation T84.7
    - |mechanical NEC T84.498
    - |pain T84.84
    - |specified type NEC T84.89
    - |stenosis T84.85
    - |thrombosis T84.86
  - |nervous system T85.9
    - |brain *see* Complications, electronic stimulator device, brain

Complication(s) - continued
- |cranial nerve *see* Complications, electronic stimulator device, peripheral nerve
- |embolism T85.810
- |fibrosis T85.820
- |gastric nerve *see* Complications, electronic stimulator device, peripheral nerve
- |hemorrhage T85.830
- |infection and inflammation T85.738
- |mechanical
  - |breakdown T85.118
  - |displacement T85.128
  - |leakage T85.199
  - |malposition T85.128
  - |obstruction T85.199
  - |perforation T85.199
  - |protrusion T85.199
  - |specified NEC T85.199
- |pain T85.840
- |peripheral nerve *see* Complications, electronic stimulator device, peripheral nerve
- |sacral nerve *see* Complications, electronic stimulator device, peripheral nerve
- |specified type NEC T85.890
- |spinal cord *see* Complications, electronic stimulator device, spinal cord
- |stenosis T85.850
- |thrombosis T85.860
- |vagal nerve *see* Complications, electronic stimulator device, peripheral nerve
- |peripheral nerve T85.9
  - |embolism T85.810
  - |fibrosis T85.820
  - |hemorrhage T85.830
  - |infection and inflammation T85.732
  - |mechanical
    - |breakdown T85.111
    - |displacement T85.121
    - |leakage T85.191
    - |malposition T85.121
    - |obstruction T85.191
    - |perforation T85.191
    - |protrusion T85.191
    - |specified NEC T85.191
  - |pain T85.840
  - |specified type NEC T85.890
  - |stenosis T85.850
  - |thrombosis T85.860
- |spinal cord T85.9
  - |embolism T85.810
  - |fibrosis T85.820
  - |hemorrhage T85.830
  - |infection and inflammation T85.733
  - |mechanical
    - |breakdown T85.112
    - |displacement T85.122
    - |leakage T85.192
    - |malposition T85.122
    - |obstruction T85.192
    - |perforation T85.192
    - |protrusion T85.192
    - |specified NEC T85.192
  - |pain T85.840
  - |specified type NEC T85.890
  - |stenosis T85.850
  - |thrombosis T85.860
- |urinary T83.9
  - |embolism T83.81
  - |fibrosis T83.82
  - |hemorrhage T83.83
  - |infection and inflammation T83.598
  - |mechanical
    - |breakdown T83.110
    - |displacement T83.120
    - |malposition T83.120

Complication(s) - continued
- |perforation T83.190
- |protrusion T83.190
- |specified NEC T83.190
- |pain T83.84
- |specified type NEC T83.89
- |stenosis T83.85
- |thrombosis T83.86
- |electroshock therapy T88.9
  - |specified NEC T88.8
- |endocrine E34.9
  - |postprocedural
    - |adrenal hypofunction E89.6
    - |hypoinsulinemia E89.1
    - |hypoparathyroidism E89.2
    - |hypopituitarism E89.3
    - |hypothyroidism E89.0
    - |ovarian failure E89.40
      - |asymptomatic E89.40
      - |symptomatic E89.41
    - |specified NEC E89.89
    - |testicular hypofunction E89.5
- |endodontic treatment NEC M27.59
- |enterostomy (stoma) K94.10
  - |hemorrhage K94.11
  - |infection K94.12
  - |malfunction K94.13
  - |mechanical K94.13
  - |specified complication NEC K94.19
- |episiotomy, disruption O90.1
- |esophageal anti-reflux device T85.9
  - |embolism T85.818
  - |fibrosis T85.828
  - |hemorrhage T85.838
  - |infection and inflammation T85.79
  - |mechanical
    - |breakdown T85.511
    - |displacement T85.521
    - |malfunction T85.511
    - |malposition T85.521
    - |obstruction T85.591
    - |perforation T85.591
    - |protrusion T85.591
    - |specified NEC T85.591
  - |pain T85.848
  - |specified type NEC T85.898
  - |stenosis T85.858
  - |thrombosis T85.868
- |esophagostomy K94.30
  - |hemorrhage K94.31
  - |infection K94.32
  - |malfunction K94.33
  - |mechanical K94.33
  - |specified complication NEC K94.39
- |extracorporeal circulation T80.90
- |extremity artery (bypass) graft T82.9
  - |arteriosclerosis *see* Arteriosclerosis, extremities, bypass graft
  - |embolism T82.818
  - |fibrosis T82.828
  - |hemorrhage T82.838
  - |infection and inflammation T82.7
  - |mechanical
    - |breakdown T82.318
      - |femoral artery T82.312
    - |displacement T82.328
      - |femoral artery T82.322
    - |leakage T82.338
      - |femoral artery T82.332
    - |malposition T82.328
      - |femoral artery T82.322
    - |obstruction T82.398
      - |femoral artery T82.392
    - |perforation T82.398
      - |femoral artery T82.392
    - |protrusion T82.398

Complication(s) - continued
- |femoral artery T82.392
- |pain T82.848
- |specified type NEC T82.898
- |stenosis T82.858
- |thrombosis T82.868
- |eye H57.9
  - |corneal graft *see* Complications, graft, cornea
  - |implant (prosthetic) T85.9
    - |embolism T85.818
    - |fibrosis T85.828
    - |hemorrhage T85.838
    - |infection and inflammation T85.79
    - |mechanical
      - |breakdown T85.318
      - |displacement T85.328
      - |leakage T85.398
      - |malposition T85.328
      - |obstruction T85.398
      - |perforation T85.398
      - |protrusion T85.398
      - |specified NEC T85.398
    - |pain T85.848
    - |specified type NEC T85.898
    - |stenosis T85.858
    - |thrombosis T85.868
  - |intraocular lens *see* Complications, intraocular lens
  - |orbital prosthesis *see* Complications, orbital prosthesis
- |female genital N94.9
  - |device, implant or graft NEC *see* Complications, genitourinary, device or implant, genital tract
- |femoral artery (bypass) graft *see* Complication, extremity artery (bypass) graft
- |fixation device, internal (orthopedic) T84.9
  - |infection and inflammation T84.60
    - |arm T84.61-
      - |humerus T84.61-
      - |radius T84.61-
      - |ulna T84.61-
    - |leg T84.629
      - |femur T84.62-
      - |fibula T84.62-
      - |tibia T84.62-
    - |specified site NEC T84.69
    - |spine T84.63
  - |mechanical
    - |breakdown
      - |limb T84.119
        - |carpal T84.210
        - |femur T84.11-
        - |fibula T84.11-
        - |humerus T84.11-
        - |metacarpal T84.210
        - |metatarsal T84.213
        - |phalanx
          - |foot T84.213
          - |hand T84.210
        - |radius T84.11-
        - |tarsal T84.213
        - |tibia T84.11-
        - |ulna T84.11-
      - |specified bone NEC T84.218
      - |spine T84.216
    - |displacement
      - |limb T84.129
        - |carpal T84.220
        - |femur T84.12-
        - |fibula T84.12-
        - |humerus T84.12-
        - |metacarpal T84.220

Complication(s) - *continued*
 |metatarsal T84.223
 |phalanx
  |foot T84.223
  |hand T84.220
 |radius T84.12-
 |tarsal T84.223
 |tibia T84.12-
 |ulna T84.12-
 |specified bone NEC T84.228
 |spine T84.226
 |malposition *see* Complications, fixation device, internal, mechanical, displacement
 |obstruction *see* Complications, fixation device, internal, mechanical, specified type NEC
 |perforation *see* Complications, fixation device, internal, mechanical, specified type NEC
 |protrusion *see* Complications, fixation device, internal, mechanical, specified type NEC
 |specified type NEC
  |limb T84.199
  |carpal T84.290
  |femur T84.19-
  |fibula T84.19-
  |humerus T84.19-
  |metacarpal T84.290
  |metatarsal T84.293
  |phalanx
   |foot T84.293
   |hand T84.290
  |radius T84.19-
  |tarsal T84.293
  |tibia T84.19-
  |ulna T84.19-
  |specified bone NEC T84.298
  |vertebra T84.296
 |specified type NEC T84.89
  |embolism T84.81
  |fibrosis T84.82
  |hemorrhage T84.83
  |pain T84.84
  |specified complication NEC T84.89
  |stenosis T84.85
  |thrombosis T84.86
|following
 |acute myocardial infarction NEC I23.8
 |aneurysm (false) (of cardiac wall) (of heart wall) (ruptured) I23.3
 |angina I23.7
 |atrial
  |septal defect I23.1
  |thrombosis I23.6
 |cardiac wall rupture I23.3
 |chordae tendinae rupture I23.4
 |defect
  |septal
   |atrial (heart) I23.1
   |ventricular (heart) I23.2
 |hemopericardium I23.0
 |papillary muscle rupture I23.5
 |rupture
  |cardiac wall I23.3
   |with hemopericardium I23.0
  |chordae tendineae I23.4
  |papillary muscle I23.5
 |specified NEC I23.8
 |thrombosis
  |atrium I23.6
  |auricular appendage I23.6
  |ventricle (heart) I23.6
 |ventricular
  |septal defect I23.2

Complication(s) - *continued*
  |thrombosis I23.6
 |ectopic or molar pregnancy O08.9
  |cardiac arrest O08.81
  |sepsis O08.82
  |specified type NEC O08.89
  |urinary tract infection O08.83
 |termination of pregnancy *see* Abortion
|gastrointestinal K92.9
 |bile duct prosthesis *see* Complications, bile duct implant
 |esophageal anti-reflux device *see* Complications, esophageal anti-reflux device
 |postoperative
  |colostomy *see* Complications, colostomy
  |dumping syndrome K91.1
  |enterostomy *see* Complications, enterostomy
  |gastrostomy *see* Complications, gastrostomy
  |malabsorption NEC K91.2
  |obstruction (*see also* Obstruction, intestine, postoperative) K91.30
  |postcholecystectomy syndrome K91.5
  |specified NEC K91.89
  |vomiting after GI surgery K91.0
 |prosthetic device or implant
  |bile duct prosthesis *see* Complications, bile duct implant
  |esophageal anti-reflux device *see* Complications, esophageal anti-reflux device
  |specified type NEC
   |embolism T85.818
   |fibrosis T85.828
   |hemorrhage T85.838
   |mechanical
    |breakdown T85.518
    |displacement T85.528
    |malfunction T85.518
    |malposition T85.528
    |obstruction T85.598
    |perforation T85.598
    |protrusion T85.598
    |specified NEC T85.598
   |pain T85.848
   |specified complication NEC T85.898
   |stenosis T85.858
   |thrombosis T85.868
|gastrostomy (stoma) K94.20
 |hemorrhage K94.21
 |infection K94.22
 |malfunction K94.23
 |mechanical K94.23
 |specified complication NEC K94.29
|genitourinary
 |device or implant T83.9
  |genital tract T83.9
   |infection or inflammation T83.69
   |intrauterine contraceptive device *see* Complications, intrauterine, contraceptive device
   |mechanical *see* Complications, by device, mechanical
   |mesh *see* Complications, mesh
   |penile prosthesis *see* Complications, prosthetic device, penile
   |specified type NEC T83.89
    |embolism T83.81
    |fibrosis T83.82
    |hemorrhage T83.83
    |pain T83.84
    |specified complication NEC T83.89
    |stenosis T83.85

Complication(s) - *continued*
    |thrombosis T83.86
   |vaginal mesh *see* Complications, mesh
  |urinary system T83.9
   |cystostomy catheter *see* Complication, catheter, cystostomy
   |electronic stimulator *see* Complications, electronic stimulator device, urinary
   |indwelling urethral catheter *see* Complications, catheter, urethral, indwelling
   |infection or inflammation T83.598
    |indwelling urethral catheter T83.511
   |kidney transplant *see* Complication, transplant, kidney
   |organ graft *see* Complication, graft, urinary organ
   |specified type NEC T83.89
    |embolism T83.81
    |fibrosis T83.82
    |hemorrhage T83.83
    |mechanical T83.198
     |breakdown T83.118
     |displacement T83.128
     |malfunction T83.118
     |malposition T83.128
     |obstruction T83.198
     |perforation T83.198
     |protrusion T83.198
     |specified NEC T83.198
    |sphincter, implanted T83.191
    |stent (ileal conduit) (nephroureteral) T83.193
    |ureteral indwelling T83.192
    |pain T83.84
    |specified complication NEC T83.89
    |stenosis T83.85
    |thrombosis T83.86
   |sphincter implant *see* Complications, implant, urinary sphincter
 |postprocedural
  |pelvic peritoneal adhesions N99.4
  |renal failure N99.0
  |specified NEC N99.89
  |stoma *see* Complications, stoma, urinary tract
  |urethral stricture *see* Stricture, urethra, postprocedural
  |vaginal
   |adhesions N99.2
   |vault prolapse N99.3
|graft (bypass) (patch) *see also* Complications, prosthetic device or implant
 |aorta *see* Complications, graft, vascular
 |arterial *see* Complication, graft, vascular
 |bone T86.839
  |failure T86.831
  |infection T86.832
  |mechanical T84.318
   |breakdown T84.318
   |displacement T84.328
   |protrusion T84.398
   |specified type NEC T84.398
  |rejection T86.830
  |specified type NEC T86.838
 |carotid artery *see* Complications, graft, vascular
 |cornea T86.849-
  |failure T86.841-
  |infection T86.842-
  |mechanical T85.398
   |breakdown T85.318
   |displacement T85.328
   |protrusion T85.398
   |specified type NEC T85.398
  |rejection T86.840-

Complication(s) - *continued*
　　|retroprosthetic membrane T85.398
　　|specified type NEC T86.848-
　|femoral artery (bypass) *see* Complication,
　　extremity artery (bypass) graft
　|genital organ or tract *see* Complications,
　　genitourinary, device or implant, genital
　　tract
　|muscle T84.9
　　|breakdown T84.410
　　|displacement T84.420
　　|embolism T84.81
　　|fibrosis T84.82
　　|hemorrhage T84.83
　　|infection and inflammation T84.7
　　|mechanical NEC T84.490
　　|pain T84.84
　　|specified type NEC T84.89
　　|stenosis T84.85
　　|thrombosis T84.86
　|nerve *see* Complication, prosthetic device or
　　implant, specified NEC
　|skin *see* Complications, prosthetic device or
　　implant, skin graft
　|tendon T84.9
　　|breakdown T84.410
　　|displacement T84.420
　　|embolism T84.81
　　|fibrosis T84.82
　　|hemorrhage T84.83
　　|infection and inflammation T84.7
　　|mechanical NEC T84.490
　　|pain T84.84
　　|specified type NEC T84.89
　　|stenosis T84.85
　　|thrombosis T84.86
　|urinary organ T83.9
　　|embolism T83.81
　　|fibrosis T83.82
　　|hemorrhage T83.83
　　|infection and inflammation T83.598
　　　|indwelling urethral catheter T83.511
　　|mechanical
　　　|breakdown T83.21
　　　|displacement T83.22
　　　|erosion T83.24
　　　|exposure T83.25
　　　|leakage T83.23
　　　|malposition T83.22
　　　|obstruction T83.29
　　　|perforation T83.29
　　　|protrusion T83.29
　　　|specified NEC T83.29
　　|pain T83.84
　　|specified type NEC T83.89
　　|stenosis T83.85
　　|thrombosis T83.86
　|vascular T82.9
　　|embolism T82.818
　　|femoral artery *see* Complication,
　　　extremity artery (bypass) graft
　　|fibrosis T82.828
　　|hemorrhage T82.838
　　|mechanical
　　　|breakdown T82.319
　　　　|aorta (bifurcation) T82.310
　　　　|carotid artery T82.311
　　　　|specified vessel NEC T82.318
　　　|displacement T82.329
　　　　|aorta (bifurcation) T82.320
　　　　|carotid artery T82.321
　　　　|specified vessel NEC T82.328
　　　|leakage T82.339
　　　　|aorta (bifurcation) T82.330
　　　　|carotid artery T82.331
　　　　|specified vessel NEC T82.338
　　　|malposition T82.329

Complication(s) - *continued*
　　　　|aorta (bifurcation) T82.320
　　　　|carotid artery T82.321
　　　　|specified vessel NEC T82.328
　　　|obstruction T82.399
　　　　|aorta (bifurcation) T82.390
　　　　|carotid artery T82.391
　　　　|specified vessel NEC T82.398
　　　|perforation T82.399
　　　　|aorta (bifurcation) T82.390
　　　　|carotid artery T82.391
　　　　|specified vessel NEC T82.398
　　　|protrusion T82.399
　　　　|aorta (bifurcation) T82.390
　　　　|carotid artery T82.391
　　　　|specified vessel NEC T82.398
　　|pain T82.848
　　|specified complication NEC T82.898
　　|stenosis T82.858
　　|thrombosis T82.868
　|heart I51.9
　　|assist device
　　　|infection and inflammation T82.7
　　|following acute myocardial infarction *see*
　　　Complications, following, acute
　　　myocardial infarction
　　|postoperative *see* Complications, circulatory
　　　system
　　|transplant *see* Complication, transplant,
　　　heart
　　　|and lung(s) *see* Complications, transplant,
　　　　heart, with lung
　　|valve
　　　|graft (biological) T82.9
　　　　|embolism T82.817
　　　　|fibrosis T82.827
　　　　|hemorrhage T82.837
　　　　|infection and inflammation T82.7
　　　　|mechanical T82.228
　　　　　|breakdown T82.221
　　　　　|displacement T82.222
　　　　　|leakage T82.223
　　　　　|malposition T82.222
　　　　　|obstruction T82.228
　　　　　|perforation T82.228
　　　　　|protrusion T82.228
　　　　|pain T82.847
　　　　|specified type NEC T82.897
　　　　|stenosis T82.857
　　　　|thrombosis T82.867
　　　|prosthesis T82.9
　　　　|embolism T82.817
　　　　|fibrosis T82.827
　　　　|hemorrhage T82.837
　　　　|infection or inflammation T82.6
　　　　|mechanical T82.09
　　　　　|breakdown T82.01
　　　　　|displacement T82.02
　　　　　|leakage T82.03
　　　　　|malposition T82.02
　　　　　|obstruction T82.09
　　　　　|perforation T82.09
　　　　　|protrusion T82.09
　　　　|pain T82.847
　　　　|specified type NEC T82.897
　　　　　|mechanical T82.09
　　　　|stenosis T82.857
　　　　|thrombosis T82.867
　　|hematoma
　　　|intraoperative *see* Complication,
　　　　intraoperative, hemorrhage
　　　|postprocedural *see* Complication,
　　　　postprocedural, hematoma
　　|hemodialysis *see* Complications, dialysis
　　|hemorrhage

Complication(s) - *continued*
　　　|intraoperative *see* Complication,
　　　　intraoperative, hemorrhage
　　　|postprocedural *see* Complication,
　　　　postprocedural, hemorrhage
　|IEC (immune effector cellular) therapy T80.82
　|ileostomy (stoma) *see* Complications,
　　enterostomy
　|immune effector cellular (IEC) therapy T80.82
　|immunization (procedure) *see* Complications,
　　vaccination
　|implant *see also* Complications, by site and
　　type
　　|urinary sphincter T83.9
　　　|embolism T83.81
　　　|fibrosis T83.82
　　　|hemorrhage T83.83
　　　|infection and inflammation T83.591
　　　|mechanical
　　　　|breakdown T83.111
　　　　|displacement T83.121
　　　　|leakage T83.191
　　　　|malposition T83.121
　　　　|obstruction T83.191
　　　　|perforation T83.191
　　　　|protrusion T83.191
　　　　|specified NEC T83.191
　　　|pain T83.84
　　　|specified type NEC T83.89
　　　|stenosis T83.85
　　　|thrombosis T83.86
　|infusion (procedure) T80.90
　　|air embolism T80.0
　　|blood *see* Complications, transfusion
　　|catheter *see* Complications, catheter
　　|infection T80.29
　　|pump *see* Complications, cardiovascular,
　　　device or implant
　　|sepsis T80.29
　　|serum reaction *see also* Reaction, serum
　　　T80.69
　　　|anaphylactic shock *see also* Shock,
　　　　anaphylactic T80.59
　　|specified type NEC T80.89
　|inhalation therapy NEC T81.81
　|injection (procedure) T80.90
　　|drug reaction *see* Reaction, drug
　　|infection T80.29
　　|sepsis T80.29
　　|serum (prophylactic) (therapeutic) *see*
　　　Complications, vaccination
　　|specified type NEC T80.89
　　|vaccine (any) *see* Complications,
　　　vaccination
　|inoculation (any) *see* Complications,
　　vaccination
　|insulin pump
　　|infection and inflammation T85.72
　　|mechanical
　　　|breakdown T85.614
　　　|displacement T85.624
　　　|leakage T85.633
　　　|malposition T85.624
　　　|obstruction T85.694
　　　|perforation T85.694
　　　|protrusion T85.694
　　　|specified NEC T85.694
　|intestinal pouch NEC K91.858
　|intraocular lens (prosthetic) T85.9
　　|embolism T85.818
　　|fibrosis T85.828
　　|hemorrhage T85.838
　　|infection and inflammation T85.79
　　|mechanical
　　　|breakdown T85.21

Complication(s) - *continued*
    |displacement T85.22
    |malposition T85.22
    |obstruction T85.29
    |perforation T85.29
    |protrusion T85.29
    |specified NEC T85.29
  |pain T85.848
  |specified type NEC T85.898
  |stenosis T85.858
  |thrombosis T85.868
 |intraoperative (intraprocedural)
  |cardiac arrest *see also* Infarct, myocardium, associated with revascularization procedure
    |during cardiac surgery I97.710
    |during other surgery I97.711
  |cardiac functional disturbance NEC *see also* Infarct, myocardium, associated with revascularization procedure
    |during cardiac surgery I97.790
    |during other surgery I97.791
  |hemorrhage (hematoma) (of)
    |circulatory system organ or structure
      |during cardiac bypass I97.411
      |during cardiac catheterization I97.410
      |during other circulatory system procedure I97.418
      |during other procedure I97.42
    |digestive system organ
      |during procedure on digestive system K91.61
      |during procedure on other organ K91.62
    |ear
      |during procedure on ear and mastoid process H95.21
      |during procedure on other organ H95.22
    |endocrine system organ or structure
      |during procedure on endocrine system organ or structure E36.01
      |during procedure on other organ E36.02
    |eye and adnexa
      |during ophthalmic procedure H59.11-
      |during other procedure H59.12-
    |genitourinary organ or structure
      |during procedure on genitourinary organ or structure N99.61
      |during procedure on other organ N99.62
    |mastoid process
      |during procedure on ear and mastoid process H95.21
      |during procedure on other organ H95.22
    |musculoskeletal structure
      |during musculoskeletal surgery M96.810
      |during non-orthopedic surgery M96.811
      |during orthopedic surgery M96.810
    |nervous system
      |during a nervous system procedure G97.31
      |during other procedure G97.32
    |respiratory system
      |during other procedure J95.62
      |during procedure on respiratory system organ or structure J95.61
    |skin and subcutaneous tissue
      |during a dermatologic procedure L76.01
      |during a procedure on other organ L76.02
    |spleen
      |during a procedure on other organ D78.02
      |during a procedure on the spleen D78.01
  |puncture or laceration (accidental) (unintentional) (of)

Complication(s) - *continued*
    |brain
      |during a nervous system procedure G97.48
      |during other procedure G97.49
    |circulatory system organ or structure
      |during circulatory system procedure I97.51
      |during other procedure I97.52
    |digestive system
      |during procedure on digestive system K91.71
      .|during procedure on other organ K91.72
    |ear
      |during procedure on ear and mastoid process H95.31
      |during procedure on other organ H95.32
    |endocrine system organ or structure
      |during procedure on endocrine system organ or structure E36.11
      |during procedure on other organ E36.12
    |eye and adnexa
      |during ophthalmic procedure H59.21-
      |during other procedure H59.22-
    |genitourinary organ or structure
      |during procedure on genitourinary organ or structure N99.71
      |during procedure on other organ N99.72
    |mastoid process
      |during procedure on ear and mastoid process H95.31
      |during procedure on other organ H95.32
    |musculoskeletal structure
      |during musculoskeletal surgery M96.820
      |during non-orthopedic surgery M96.821
      |during orthopedic surgery M96.820
    |nervous system
      |during a nervous system procedure G97.48
      |during other procedure G97.49
    |respiratory system
      |during other procedure J95.72
      |during procedure on respiratory system organ or structure J95.71
    |skin and subcutaneous tissue
      |during a dermatologic procedure L76.11
      |during a procedure on other organ L76.12
    |spleen
      |during a procedure on other organ D78.12
      |during a procedure on the spleen D78.11
 |specified NEC
  |circulatory system I97.88
  |digestive system K91.81
  |ear H95.88
  |endocrine system E36.8
  |eye and adnexa H59.88
  |genitourinary system N99.81
  |mastoid process H95.88
  |musculoskeletal structure M96.89
  |nervous system G97.81
  |respiratory system J95.88
  |skin and subcutaneous tissue L76.81
  |spleen D78.81
 |intraperitoneal catheter (dialysis) (infusion) *see* Complication(s), catheter, intraperitoneal dialysis
 |intrathecal infusion pump
  |infection and inflammation T85.738
  |mechanical
    |breakdown T85.615
    |displacement T85.625
    |leakage T85.635

Complication(s) (from) (of) - *continued*
    |malfunction T85.695
    |malposition T85.625
    |obstruction T85.695
    |perforation T85.695
    |protrusion T85.695
    |specified NEC T85.695
 |intrauterine
  |contraceptive device
    |embolism T83.81
    |fibrosis T83.82
    |hemorrhage T83.83
    |infection and inflammation T83.69
    |mechanical
      |breakdown T83.31
      |displacement T83.32
      |malposition T83.32
      |obstruction T83.39
      |perforation T83.39
      |protrusion T83.39
      |specified NEC T83.39
    |pain T83.84
    |specified type NEC T83.89
    |stenosis T83.85
    |thrombosis T83.86
  |procedure (fetal), to newborn P96.5
 |jejunostomy (stoma) *see* Complications, enterostomy
 |joint prosthesis, internal T84.9
  |breakage (fracture) T84.01-
  |dislocation T84.02-
  |fracture T84.01-
  |infection or inflammation T84.50
    |hip T84.5-
    |knee T84.5-
    |specified joint NEC T84.59
  |instability T84.02-
  |malposition *see* Complications, joint prosthesis, mechanical, displacement
  |mechanical
    |breakage, broken T84.01-
    |dislocation T84.02-
    |fracture T84.01-
    |instability T84.02-
    |leakage *see* Complications, joint prosthesis, mechanical, specified NEC
    |loosening T84.039
      |hip T84.03-
      |knee T84.03-
      |specified joint NEC T84.038
    |obstruction *see* Complications, joint prosthesis, mechanical, specified NEC
    |perforation *see* Complications, joint prosthesis, mechanical, specified NEC
    |periprosthetic osteolysis T84.059
      |hip T84.05-
      |knee T84.05-
      |other specified joint T84.058
    |protrusion *see* Complications, joint prosthesis, mechanical, specified NEC
    |specified complication NEC T84.099
      |hip T84.09-
      |knee T84.09-
      |other specified joint T84.098
    |subluxation T84.02-
    |wear of articular bearing surface T84.069
      |hip T84.06-
      |knee T84.06-
      |other specified joint T84.068
  |specified joint NEC T84.89
    |embolism T84.81
    |fibrosis T84.82
    |hemorrhage T84.83
    |pain T84.84
    |specified complication NEC T84.89

Complication(s) (from) (of) - *continued*

> |stenosis T84.85
> |thrombosis T84.86
>> |subluxation T84.02-
> |kidney transplant *see* Complications, transplant, kidney
> |labor O75.9
>> |specified NEC O75.89
> |liver transplant (immune or nonimmune) *see* Complications, transplant, liver
> |lumbar puncture G97.1
>> |cerebrospinal fluid leak G97.0
>> |headache or reaction G97.1
> |lung transplant *see* Complications, transplant, lung
>> |and heart *see* Complications, transplant, lung, with heart
> |male genital N50.9
>> |device, implant or graft *see* Complications, genitourinary, device or implant, genital tract
>> |postprocedural or postoperative *see* Complications, genitourinary, postprocedural
>> |specified NEC N99.89
> |mastoid (process) procedure
>> |intraoperative H95.88
>>> |hematoma *see* Complications, intraoperative, hemorrhage (hematoma) (of), mastoid process
>>> |hemorrhage *see* Complications, intraoperative, hemorrhage (hematoma) (of), mastoid process
>>> |laceration *see* Complications, intraoperative, puncture or laceration, mastoid process
>>> |specified NEC H95.88
>> |postmastoidectomy *see* Complications, postmastoidectomy
>> |postoperative H95.89
>>> |external ear canal stenosis H95.81-
>>> |hematoma *see* Complications, postprocedural, hematoma (of), mastoid process
>>> |hemorrhage *see* Complications, postprocedural, hemorrhage (of), mastoid process
>>> |postmastoidectomy *see* Complications, postmastoidectomy
>>> |seroma *see* Complications, postprocedural, seroma (of), mastoid process
>>> |specified NEC H95.89
> |mastoidectomy cavity *see* Complications, postmastoidectomy
> |mechanical *see* Complications, by site and type, mechanical
> |medical procedures *see also* Complication(s), intraoperative T88.9
> |metabolic E88.9
>> |postoperative E89.89
>>> |specified NEC E89.89
> |molar pregnancy NOS O08.9
>> |damage to pelvic organs O08.6
>> |embolism O08.2
>> |genital infection O08.0
>> |hemorrhage (delayed) (excessive) O08.1
>> |metabolic disorder O08.5
>> |renal failure O08.4
>> |shock O08.3
>> |specified type NEC O08.0
>> |venous complication NEC O08.7
> |musculoskeletal system *see also* Complication, intraoperative (intraprocedural), by site

Complication(s) (from) (of) - *continued*

> |device, implant or graft NEC *see* Complications, orthopedic, device or implant
> |internal fixation (nail) (plate) (rod) *see* Complications, fixation device, internal
> |joint prosthesis *see* Complications, joint prosthesis
> |postoperative (postprocedural) M96.89
>> |with osteoporosis *see* Osteoporosis
>> |fracture following insertion of device *see* Fracture, following insertion of orthopedic implant, joint prosthesis or bone plate
>> |joint instability after prosthesis removal M96.89
>> |lordosis M96.4
>> |postlaminectomy syndrome NEC M96.1
>>> |kyphosis M96.3
>> |pseudarthrosis M96.0
>> |specified complication NEC M96.89
> |post radiation M96.89
>> |kyphosis M96.2
>> |scoliosis M96.5
>> |specified complication NEC M96.89
> |nephrostomy (stoma) *see* Complications, stoma, urinary tract, external NEC
> |nervous system G98.8
>> |central G96.9
>> |device, implant or graft *see also* Complication, prosthetic device or implant, specified NEC
>> |electronic stimulator (electrode(s)) *see* Complications, electronic stimulator device
>> |specified NEC
>>> |infection and inflammation T85.738
>>> |mechanical T85.695
>>>> |breakdown T85.615
>>>> |displacement T85.625
>>>> |leakage T85.635
>>>> |malfunction T85.695
>>>> |malposition T85.625
>>>> |obstruction T85.695
>>>> |perforation T85.695
>>>> |protrusion T85.695
>>>> |specified NEC T85.695
>> |ventricular shunt *see* Complications, ventricular shunt
>> |electronic stimulator (electrode(s)) *see* Complications, electronic stimulator device
>> |postprocedural G97.82
>>> |intracranial hypotension G97.2
>>> |specified NEC G97.82
>>> |spinal fluid leak G97.0
> |newborn, due to intrauterine (fetal) procedure P96.5
> |nonabsorbable (permanent) sutures *see* Complication, sutures, permanent
> |obstetric O75.9
>> |procedure (instrumental) (manual) (surgical) specified NEC O75.4
>> |specified NEC O75.89
>> |surgical wound NEC O90.89
>>> |hematoma O90.2
>>> |infection O86.00
> |ocular lens implant *see* Complications, intraocular lens
> |ophthalmologic
>> |postprocedural bleb *see* Blebitis
> |orbital prosthesis T85.9
>> |embolism T85.818
>> |fibrosis T85.828
>> |hemorrhage T85.838
>> |infection and inflammation T85.79

Complication(s) (from) (of) - *continued*

> |mechanical
>> |breakdown T85.31-
>> |displacement T85.32-
>> |malposition T85.32-
>> |obstruction T85.39-
>> |perforation T85.39-
>> |protrusion T85.39-
>> |specified NEC T85.39-
> |pain T85.848
> |specified type NEC T85.898
> |stenosis T85.858
> |thrombosis T85.868
> |organ or tissue transplant (partial) (total) *see* Complications, transplant
> |orthopedic *see also* Disorder, soft tissue
>> |device or implant T84.9
>>> |bone
>>>> |device or implant *see* Complication, bone, device NEC
>>>> |graft *see* Complication, graft, bone
>>> |breakdown T84.418
>>> |displacement T84.428
>>> |electronic bone stimulator *see* Complications, electronic stimulator device, bone
>>> |embolism T84.81
>>> |fibrosis T84.82
>>> |fixation device *see* Complication, fixation device, internal
>>> |hemorrhage T84.83
>>> |infection or inflammation T84.7
>>> |joint prosthesis *see* Complication, joint prosthesis, internal
>>> |malfunction T84.418
>>> |malposition T84.428
>>> |mechanical NEC T84.498
>>> |muscle graft *see* Complications, graft, muscle
>>> |obstruction T84.498
>>> |pain T84.84
>>> |perforation T84.498
>>> |protrusion T84.498
>>> |specified complication NEC T84.89
>>> |stenosis T84.85
>>> |tendon graft *see* Complications, graft, tendon
>>> |thrombosis T84.86
>> |fracture (following insertion of device) *see* Fracture, following insertion of orthopedic implant, joint prosthesis or bone plate
>> |postprocedural M96.89
>>> |fracture *see* Fracture, following insertion of orthopedic implant, joint prosthesis or bone plate
>>> |postlaminectomy syndrome NEC M96.1
>>>> |kyphosis M96.3
>>>> |lordosis M96.4
>>> |postradiation
>>>> |kyphosis M96.2
>>>> |scoliosis M96.5
>>> |pseudarthrosis post-fusion M96.0
>>> |specified type NEC M96.89
> |pacemaker (cardiac) *see* Complications, cardiovascular device or implant, electronic
> |pancreas transplant *see* Complications, transplant, pancreas
> |penile prosthesis (implant) *see* Complications, prosthetic device, penile
> |perfusion NEC T80.90
> |perineal repair (obstetrical) NEC O90.89
>> |disruption O90.1
>> |hematoma O90.2
>> |infection (following delivery) O86.09

Complication(s) (from) (of) - *continued*

|genitourinary N99.89
|mastoid process H95.89
|metabolic E89.89
|musculoskeletal structure M96.89
|nervous system G97.82
|respiratory system J95.89
|skin and subcutaneous tissue L76.82
|spleen D78.89
|pregnancy NEC *see* Pregnancy, complicated by
|prosthetic device or implant T85.9
  |bile duct *see* Complications, bile duct implant
  |breast *see* Complications, breast implant
  |bulking agent
    |ureteral
      |erosion T83.714
      |exposure T83.724
    |urethral
      |erosion T83.713
      |exposure T83.723
  |cardiac and vascular NEC *see* Complications, cardiovascular device or implant
  |corneal transplant *see* Complications, graft, cornea
  |electronic nervous system stimulator *see* Complications, electronic stimulator device
|epidural infusion catheter *see* Complications, catheter, epidural
  |esophageal anti-reflux device *see* Complications, esophageal anti-reflux device
  |genital organ or tract *see* Complications, genitourinary, device or implant, genital tract
    |specified NEC T83.79
  |heart valve *see* Complications, heart, valve, prosthesis
  |infection or inflammation T85.79
    |intestine transplant T86.892
    |liver transplant T86.43
    |lung transplant T86.812
    |pancreas transplant T86.892
    |skin graft T86.822
  |intraocular lens *see* Complications, intraocular lens
  |intraperitoneal (dialysis) catheter *see* Complication(s), catheter, intraperitoneal dialysis
  |joint *see* Complications, joint prosthesis, internal
  |mechanical NEC T85.698
    |dialysis catheter (vascular) *see also* Complication, catheter, dialysis, mechanical
      |peritoneal *see* Complication (s), catheter, intraperitoneal dialysis
    |gastrointestinal device T85.598
    |ocular device T85.398
    |subdural (infusion) catheter T85.690
    |suture, permanent T85.692
      |that for bone repair *see* Complications, fixation device, internal (orthopedic), mechanical
    |ventricular shunt
      |breakdown T85.01
      |displacement T85.02
      |leakage T85.03
      |malposition T85.02
      |obstruction T85.09
      |perforation T85.09
      |protrusion T85.09
      |specified NEC T85.09

Complication(s) (from) (of) - *continued*

|mesh
  |erosion (to surrounding organ or tissue) T83.718
    |urethral (into pelvic floor muscles) T83.712
    |vaginal (into pelvic floor muscles) T83.711
  |exposure (into surrounding organ or tissue) T83.728
    |urethral (through urethral wall) T83.722
    |vaginal (into vagina) (through vaginal wall) T83.721
|orbital *see* Complications, orbital prosthesis
|penile T83.9
  |embolism T83.81
  |fibrosis T83.82
  |hemorrhage T83.83
  |infection and inflammation T83.61
  |mechanical
    |breakdown T83.410
    |displacement T83.420
    |leakage T83.490
    |malposition T83.420
    |obstruction T83.490
    |perforation T83.490
    |protrusion T83.490
    |specified NEC T83.490
  |pain T83.84
  |specified type NEC T83.89
  |stenosis T83.85
  |thrombosis T83.86
|prosthetic materials NEC
  |erosion (to surrounding organ or tissue) T83.718
  |exposure (into surrounding organ or tissue) T83.728
|skin graft T86.829
  |artificial skin or decellularized allodermis
    |embolism T85.818
    |fibrosis T85.828
    |hemorrhage T85.838
    |infection and inflammation T85.79
    |mechanical
      |breakdown T85.613
      |displacement T85.623
      |malfunction T85.613
      |malposition T85.623
      |obstruction T85.693
      |perforation T85.693
      |protrusion T85.693
      |specified NEC T85.693
    |pain T85.848
    |specified type NEC T85.898
    |stenosis T85.858
    |thrombosis T85.868
  |failure T86.821
  |infection T86.822
  |rejection T86.820
  |specified NEC T86.828
|sling
  |urethral (female) (male)
    |erosion T83.712
    |exposure T83.722
|specified NEC T85.9
  |embolism T85.818
  |fibrosis T85.828
  |hemorrhage T85.838
  |infection and inflammation T85.79
  |mechanical
    |breakdown T85.618
    |displacement T85.628
    |leakage T85.638
    |malfunction T85.618
    |malposition T85.628

Complication(s) (from) (of) - *continued*

    |obstruction T85.698
    |perforation T85.698
    |protrusion T85.698
    |specified NEC T85.698
  |pain T85.848
  |specified type NEC T85.898
  |stenosis T85.858
  |thrombosis T85.868
|subdural infusion catheter *see* Complications, catheter, subdural
|sutures *see* Complications, sutures
|urinary organ or tract NEC *see* Complications, genitourinary, device or implant, urinary system
|vascular *see* Complications, cardiovascular device or implant
|ventricular shunt *see* Complications, ventricular shunt (device)
|puerperium *see* Puerperal
|puncture, spinal G97.1
  |cerebrospinal fluid leak G97.0
  |headache or reaction G97.1
|pyelogram N99.89
|radiation
  |kyphosis M96.2
  |scoliosis M96.5
|reattached
  |extremity (infection) (rejection)
    |lower T87.1X-
    |upper T87.0X-
  |specified body part NEC T87.2
|reconstructed breast
  |asymmetry between native and reconstructed breast N65.1
  |deformity N65.0
  |disproportion between native and reconstructed breast N65.1
  |excess tissue N65.0
  |misshapen N65.0
|reimplant NEC *see also* Complications, prosthetic device or implant
  |limb (infection) (rejection) *see* Complications, reattached, extremity
  |organ (partial) (total) *see* Complications, transplant
  |prosthetic device NEC *see* Complications, prosthetic device
|renal N28.9
  |allograft *see* Complications, transplant, kidney
  |dialysis *see* Complications, dialysis
|respirator
  |mechanical J95.850
    |specified NEC J95.859
|respiratory system J98.9
  |device, implant or graft *see* Complication, prosthetic device or implant, specified NEC
  |lung transplant *see* Complications, prosthetic device or implant, lung transplant
  |postoperative J95.89
    |air leak J95.812
    |Mendelson's syndrome (chemical pneumonitis) J95.4
    |pneumothorax J95.811
    |pulmonary insufficiency (acute) (after nonthoracic surgery) J95.2
      |chronic J95.3
      |following thoracic surgery J95.1
    |respiratory failure (acute) J95.821
      |acute and chronic J95.822
    |specified NEC J95.89
    |subglottic stenosis J95.5

Complication(s) (from) (of) - *continued*

|tracheostomy complication *see*
   Complications, tracheostomy
|therapy T81.89
|sedation during labor and delivery O74.9
   |cardiac O74.2
   |central nervous system O74.3
   |pulmonary NEC O74.1
|shunt *see also* Complications, prosthetic
   device or implant
   |arteriovenous *see* Complications,
      arteriovenous, shunt
   |ventricular (communicating) *see*
      Complications, ventricular shunt
|skin
   |graft T86.829
      |failure T86.821
      |infection T86.822
      |rejection T86.820
      |specified type NEC T86.828
|spinal
   |anesthesia *see* Complications, anesthesia,
      spinal
   |catheter (epidural) (subdural) *see*
      Complications, catheter
   |puncture or tap G97.1
      |cerebrospinal fluid leak G97.0
      |headache or reaction G97.1
|stent
   |bile duct *see* Complications, bile duct
      prosthesis
   |ureteral indwelling
      |breakdown T83.112
      |displacement T83.122
      |leakage T83.192
      |malposition T83.122
      |obstruction T83.192
      |perforation T83.192
      |protrusion T83.192
      |specified NEC T83.192
   |urinary NEC (ileal conduit) (nephroureteral)
      T83.193
      |embolism T83.81
      |fibrosis T83.82
      |hemorrhage T83.83
      |infection and inflammation T83.593
      |mechanical
         |breakdown T83.113
         |displacement T83.123
         |leakage T83.193
         |malposition T83.123
         |obstruction T83.193
         |perforation T83.193
         |protrusion T83.193
         |specified NEC T83.193
      |pain T83.84
      |specified type NEC T83.89
      |stenosis T83.85
      |thrombosis T83.86
   |vascular
      |end stent stenosis *see* Restenosis, stent
      |in stent stenosis *see* Restenosis, stent
|stoma
   |digestive tract
      |colostomy *see* Complications, colostomy
      |enterostomy *see* Complications,
         enterostomy
      |esophagostomy *see* Complications,
         esophagostomy
      |gastrostomy *see* Complications,
         gastrostomy
   |urinary tract N99.528
      |continent N99.538
         |hemorrhage N99.530
         |herniation N99.533
         |infection N99.531

Complication(s) (from) (of) - *continued*

         |malfunction N99.532
         |specified type NEC N99.538
         |stenosis N99.534
      |cystostomy *see* Complications,
         cystostomy
      |external NOS N99.528
      |hemorrhage N99.520
      |herniation N99.523
      |incontinent N99.528
         |hemorrhage N99.520
         |herniation N99.523
         |infection N99.521
         |malfunction N99.522
         |specified type NEC N99.528
         |stenosis N99.524
      |infection N99.521
      |malfunction N99.522
      |specified type NEC N99.528
      |stenosis N99.524
|stomach banding *see* Complication(s),
   bariatric procedure
|stomach stapling *see* Complication(s),
   bariatric procedure
|surgical material, nonabsorbable *see*
   Complication, suture, permanent
|surgical procedure (on) T81.9
   |amputation stump (late) *see* Complications,
      amputation stump
   |cardiac *see* Complications, circulatory
      system
   |cholesteatoma, recurrent *see* Complications,
      postmastoidectomy, recurrent
      cholesteatoma
   |circulatory (early) *see* Complications,
      circulatory system
   |digestive system *see* Complications,
      gastrointestinal
   |dumping syndrome (postgastrectomy)
      K91.1
   |ear *see* Complications, ear
   |elephantiasis or lymphedema I97.89
      |postmastectomy I97.2
   |emphysema (surgical) T81.82
   |endocrine *see* Complications, endocrine
   |eye *see* Complications, eye
   |fistula (persistent postoperative) T81.83
   |foreign body inadvertently left in wound
      (sponge) (suture) (swab) *see* Foreign
      body, accidentally left during a procedure
   |gastrointestinal *see* Complications,
      gastrointestinal
   |genitourinary NEC N99.89 postprocedural,
      hematoma
   |hematoma
      |intraoperative *see* Complication,
         intraoperative, hemorrhage
      |postprocedural *see* Complication,
   |hemorrhage
      |intraoperative *see* Complication,
         intraoperative, hemorrhage
      |postprocedural *see* Complication,
         postprocedural, hemorrhage
   |hepatic failure K91.82
   |hyperglycemia (postpancreatectomy) E89.1
   |hypoinsulinemia (postpancreatectomy)
      E89.1
   |hypoparathyroidism
      (postparathyroidectomy) E89.2
   |hypopituitarism (posthypophysectomy)
      E89.3
   |hypothyroidism (post-thyroidectomy) E89.0
   |intestinal obstruction (*see also* Obstruction,
      intestine, postoperative) K91.30

Complication(s) (from) (of) - *continued*

|intracranial hypotension following
   ventricular shunting (ventriculostomy)
   G97.2
|lymphedema I97.89
   |postmastectomy I97.2
|malabsorption (postsurgical) NEC K91.2
   |osteoporosis *see* Osteoporosis,
      postsurgical malabsorption
|mastoidectomy cavity NEC *see*
   Complications, postmastoidectomy
|metabolic E89.89
   |specified NEC E89.89
|musculoskeletal *see* Complications,
   musculoskeletal system
|nervous system (central) (peripheral) *see*
   Complications, nervous system
|ovarian failure E89.40
   |asymptomatic E89.40
   |symptomatic E89.41
|peripheral vascular *see* Complications,
   surgical procedure, vascular
|postcardiotomy syndrome I97.0
|postcholecystectomy syndrome K91.5
|postcommissurotomy syndrome I97.0
|postgastrectomy dumping syndrome K91.1
|postlaminectomy syndrome NEC M96.1
   |kyphosis M96.3
|postmastectomy lymphedema syndrome
   I97.2
|postmastoidectomy cholesteatoma *see*
   Complications, postmastoidectomy,
   recurrent cholesteatoma
|postvagotomy syndrome K91.1
|postvalvulotomy syndrome I97.0
|pulmonary insufficiency (acute) J95.2
   |chronic J95.3
   |following thoracic surgery J95.1
|reattached body part *see* Complications,
   reattached
|respiratory *see* Complications, respiratory
   system
|shock (hypovolemic) T81.19
|spleen (postoperative) D78.89
   |intraoperative D78.81
|stitch abscess T81.41
|subglottic stenosis (postsurgical) J95.5
|testicular hypofunction E89.5
|transplant *see* Complications, organ or
   tissue transplant
|urinary NEC N99.89
|vaginal vault prolapse (posthysterectomy)
   N99.3
|vascular (peripheral)
   |artery T81.719
      |mesenteric T81.710
      |renal T81.711
      |specified NEC T81.718
   |vein T81.72
|wound infection T81.49
|suture, permanent (wire) NEC T85.9
   |with repair of bone *see* Complications,
   fixation device, internal
   |embolism T85.818
   |fibrosis T85.828
   |hemorrhage T85.838
   |infection and inflammation T85.79
   |mechanical
      |breakdown T85.612
      |displacement T85.622
      |malfunction T85.612
      |malposition T85.622
      |obstruction T85.692
      |perforation T85.692
      |protrusion T85.692
      |specified NEC T85.692

Complication(s) (from) (of) - *continued*
|pain T85.848
|specified type NEC T85.898
|stenosis T85.858
|thrombosis T85.868
|tracheostomy J95.00
|granuloma J95.09
|hemorrhage J95.01
|infection J95.02
|malfunction J95.03
|mechanical J95.03
|obstruction J95.03
|specified type NEC J95.09
|tracheo-esophageal fistula J95.04
|transfusion (blood) (lymphocytes) (plasma)
    T80.92
|air embolism T80.0
|circulatory overload E87.71
|febrile nonhemolytic transfusion reaction
    R50.84
|hemolysis T80.89
|hemochromatosis E83.111
|hemolytic reaction (antigen unspecified)
    T80.919
|incompatibility reaction (antigen
    unspecified) T80.919
|ABO T80.30
    |delayed serologic (DSTR) T80.39
    |hemolytic transfusion reaction (HTR)
        (unspecified time after transfusion)
        T80.319
        |acute (AHTR) (less than 24 hours
            after transfusion) T80.310
        |delayed (DHTR) (24 hours or more
            after transfusion) T80.311
    |specified NEC T80.39
|acute (antigen unspecified) T80.910
|delayed (antigen unspecified) T80.911
|delayed serologic (DSTR) T80.89
|Non-ABO (minor antigens (Duffy) (K)
    (Kell) (Kidd) (Lewis) (M) (N) (P) (S))
    T80.A0
    |delayed serologic (DSTR) T80.A9
    |hemolytic transfusion reaction (HTR)
        (unspecified time after transfusion)
        T80.A19
        |acute (AHTR) (less than 24 hours
            after transfusion) T80.A10
        |delayed (DHTR) (24 hours or more
            after transfusion) T80.A11
    |specified NEC T80.A9
|Rh (antigens (C) (c) (D) (E) (e)) (factor)
    T80.40
    |delayed serologic (DSTR) T80.49
    |hemolytic transfusion reaction (HTR)
        (unspecified time after transfusion)
        T80.419
        |acute (AHTR) (less than 24 hours
            after transfusion) T80.410
        |delayed (DHTR) (24 hours or more
            after transfusion) T80.411
    |specified NEC T80.49
|infection T80.29
|acute T80.22
|reaction NEC T80.89
|sepsis T80.29
|shock T80.89
|transplant T86.90
|bone T86.839
    |failure T86.831
    |infection T86.832
    |rejection T86.830
    |specified type NEC T86.838
|bone marrow T86.00
    |failure T86.02
    |infection T86.03

Complication(s) (from) (of) - *continued*
|rejection T86.01
|specified type NEC T86.09
|cornea T86.849-
    |failure T86.841-
    |infection T86.842-
    |rejection T86.840-
    |specified type NEC T86.848-
|failure T86.92
|heart T86.20
    |with lung T86.30
    |cardiac allograft vasculopathy T86.290
        |failure T86.32
        |infection T86.33
        |rejection T86.31
        |specified type NEC T86.39
    |failure T86.22
    |infection T86.23
    |rejection T86.21
    |specified type NEC T86.298
|infection T86.93
|intestine T86.859
    |failure T86.851
    |infection T86.852
    |rejection T86.850
    |specified type NEC T86.858
|kidney T86.10
    |failure T86.12
    |infection T86.13
    |rejection T86.11
    |specified type NEC T86.19
|liver T86.40
    |failure T86.42
    |infection T86.43
    |rejection T86.41
    |specified type NEC T86.49
|lung T86.819
    |with heart T86.30
        |failure T86.32
        |infection T86.33
        |rejection T86.31
        |specified type NEC T86.39
    |failure T86.811
    |infection T86.812
    |rejection T86.810
    |specified type NEC T86.818
|malignant neoplasm C80.2
|pancreas T86.899
    |failure T86.891
    |infection T86.892
    |rejection T86.890
    |specified type NEC T86.898
|peripheral blood stem cells T86.5
|post-transplant lymphoproliferative disorder
    (PTLD) D47.Z1
|rejection T86.91
|skin T86.829
    |failure T86.821
    |infection T86.822
    |rejection T86.820
    |specified type NEC T86.828
|specified
    |tissue T86.899
        |failure T86.891
        |infection T86.892
        |rejection T86.890
        |specified type NEC T86.898
    |type NEC T86.99
|stem cell (from peripheral blood) (from
    umbilical cord) T86.5
|umbilical cord stem cells T86.5
|trauma (early) T79.9
|specified NEC T79.8
|ultrasound therapy NEC T88.9
|umbilical cord NEC

Complication(s) (from) (of) - *continued*
|complicating delivery O69.9
    |specified NEC O69.89
|umbrella device, vascular T82.9
    |embolism T82.818
    |fibrosis T82.828
    |hemorrhage T82.838
    |infection or inflammation T82.7
    |mechanical
        |breakdown T82.515
        |displacement T82.525
        |leakage T82.535
        |malposition T82.525
        |obstruction T82.595
        |perforation T82.595
        |protrusion T82.595
    |pain T82.848
    |specified type NEC T82.898
    |stenosis T82.858
    |thrombosis T82.868
|urethral catheter *see* Complications, catheter,
    urethral, indwelling
|vaccination T88.1
    |anaphylaxis NEC T80.52
    |arthropathy *see* Arthropathy,
        postimmunization
    |cellulitis T88.0
    |encephalitis or encephalomyelitis G04.02
    |infection (general) (local) NEC T88.0
    |meningitis G03.8
    |myelitis G04.02
    |protein sickness T80.62
    |rash T88.1
    |reaction (allergic) T88.1
        |serum T80.62
    |sepsis T88.0
    |serum intoxication, sickness, rash, or other
        serum reaction NEC T80.62
        |anaphylactic shock T80.52
    |shock (allergic) (anaphylactic) T80.52
    |vaccinia (generalized) (localized) T88.1
|vas deferens device or implant *see*
    Complications, genitourinary, device or
    implant, genital tract
|vascular I99.9
    |device or implant T82.9
        |embolism T82.818
        |fibrosis T82.828
        |hemorrhage T82.838
        |infection or inflammation T82.7
        |mechanical
            |breakdown T82.519
                |specified device NEC T82.518
            |displacement T82.529
                |specified device NEC T82.528
            |leakage T82.539
                |specified device NEC T82.538
            |malposition T82.529
                |specified device NEC T82.528
            |obstruction T82.599
                |specified device NEC T82.598
            |perforation T82.599
                |specified device NEC T82.598
            |protrusion T82.599
                |specified device NEC T82.598
        |pain T82.848
        |specified type NEC T82.898
        |stenosis T82.858
        |thrombosis T82.868
    |dialysis catheter *see* Complication, catheter,
        dialysis
    |following infusion, therapeutic injection or
        transfusion T80.1
    |graft T82.9
        |embolism T82.818
        |fibrosis T82.828

Complication(s) (from) (of) - *continued*
|hemorrhage T82.838
|mechanical
|breakdown T82.319
|aorta (bifurcation) T82.310
|carotid artery T82.311
|specified vessel NEC T82.318
|displacement T82.329
|aorta (bifurcation) T82.320
|carotid artery T82.321
|specified vessel NEC T82.328
|leakage T82.339
|aorta (bifurcation) T82.330
|carotid artery T82.331
|specified vessel NEC T82.338
|malposition T82.329
|aorta (bifurcation) T82.320
|carotid artery T82.321
|specified vessel NEC T82.328
|obstruction T82.399
|aorta (bifurcation) T82.390
|carotid artery T82.391
|specified vessel NEC T82.398
|perforation T82.399
|aorta (bifurcation) T82.390
|carotid artery T82.391
|specified vessel NEC T82.398
|protrusion T82.399
|aorta (bifurcation) T82.390
|carotid artery T82.391
|specified vessel NEC T82.398
|pain T82.848
|specified complication NEC T82.898
|stenosis T82.858
|thrombosis T82.868
|postoperative *see* Complications,
postoperative, circulatory
|vena cava device (filter) (sieve) (umbrella) *see*
Complications, umbrella device, vascular
|ventilation therapy NEC T81.81
|ventilator
|mechanical J95.850
|specified NEC J95.859
|ventricular (communicating) shunt (device)
T85.9
|embolism T85.810
|fibrosis T85.820
|hemorrhage T85.830
|infection and inflammation T85.730
|mechanical
|breakdown T85.01
|displacement T85.02
|leakage T85.03
|malposition T85.02
|obstruction T85.09
|perforation T85.09
|protrusion T85.09
|specified NEC T85.09
|pain T85.840
|specified type NEC T85.890
|stenosis T85.850
|thrombosis T85.860
|wire suture, permanent (implanted) *see*
Complications, suture, permanent
Compressed air disease T70.3
Compression
|with injury code by Nature of injury artery
I77.1
|celiac, syndrome I77.4
|brachial plexus G54.0
|brain (stem) G93.5
|due to
| contusion (diffuse) (see also Injury,
intracranial, diffuse) S06.A0
|with herniation S06.A1
|focal (see also Injury, intracranial,
focal) S06.A0

Compression - *continued*
|with herniation S06.A1
|injury NEC (see also Injury, intracranial,
diffuse) S06.A0
|nontraumatic G93.5
|traumatic (see also Injury, intracranial,
diffuse) S06.A0
|with herniation S06.A1
|bronchus J98.09
|cauda equina G83.4
|celiac (artery) (axis) I77.4
|cerebral *see* Compression, brain
|cervical plexus G54.2
|cord
|spinal *see* Compression, spinal
|umbilical *see* Compression, umbilical cord
|cranial nerve G52.9
|eighth *see* subcategory H93.3
|eleventh G52.8
|fifth G50.8
|first G52.0
|fourth *see* Strabismus, paralytic, fourth
nerve
|ninth G52.1
|second *see* Disorder, nerve, optic
|seventh G51.8
|sixth *see* Strabismus, paralytic, sixth nerve
|tenth G52.2
|third *see* Strabismus, paralytic, third nerve
|twelfth G52.3
|diver's squeeze T70.3
|during birth (newborn) P15.9
|esophagus K22.2
|eustachian tube *see* Obstruction, eustachian
tube, cartilaginous
|facies Q67.1
|fracture
|nontraumatic NOS *see* Collapse, vertebra
|pathological *see* Fracture, pathological
|traumatic *see* Fracture, traumatic
|heart *see* Disease, heart
|intestine *see* Obstruction, intestine
|laryngeal nerve, recurrent G52.2
|with paralysis of vocal cords and larynx
J38.00
|bilateral J38.02
|unilateral J38.01
|lumbosacral plexus G54.1
|lung J98.4
|lymphatic vessel I89.0
|medulla *see* Compression, brain
|nerve *see also* Disorder, nerve G58.9
|arm NEC *see* Mononeuropathy, upper limb
|axillary G54.0
|cranial *see* Compression, cranial nerve
|leg NEC *see* Mononeuropathy, lower limb
|median (in carpal tunnel) *see* Syndrome,
carpal tunnel
|optic *see* Disorder, nerve, optic
|plantar *see* Lesion, nerve, plantar
|posterior tibial (in tarsal tunnel) *see*
Syndrome, tarsal tunnel
|root or plexus NOS (in) G54.9
|intervertebral disc disorder NEC *see*
Disorder, disc, with, radiculopathy
|with myelopathy *see* Disorder, disc,
with, myelopathy
|neoplastic disease *see also* Neoplasm
D49.9 [*G55*]
|spondylosis *see* Spondylosis, with
radiculopathy
|sciatic (acute) *see* Lesion, nerve, sciatic
|sympathetic G90.8
|traumatic *see* Injury, nerve
|ulnar *see* Lesion, nerve, ulnar

Compression - *continued*
|upper extremity NEC *see* Mononeuropathy,
upper limb
|spinal (cord) G95.20
|by displacement of intervertebral disc NEC
see also Disorder, disc, with, myelopathy
|nerve root NOS G54.9
|due to displacement of intervertebral disc
NEC *see* Disorder, disc, with,
radiculopathy
|with myelopathy *see* Disorder, disc,
with, myelopathy
|specified NEC G95.29
|spondylogenic (cervical) (lumbar,
lumbosacral) (thoracic) *see* Spondylosis,
with myelopathy NEC
|anterior *see* Syndrome, anterior, spinal
artery, compression
|traumatic *see* Injury, spinal cord, by region
|subcostal nerve (syndrome) *see*
Mononeuropathy, upper limb, specified NEC
|sympathetic nerve NEC G90.8
|syndrome T79.5
|trachea J39.8
|ulnar nerve (by scar tissue) *see* Lesion, nerve,
ulnar
|umbilical cord
|complicating delivery O69.2
|cord around neck O69.1
|prolapse O69.0
|specified NEC O69.2
|ureter N13.5
|vein I87.1
|vena cava (inferior) (superior) I87.1
Compulsion, compulsive
|gambling F63.0
|neurosis F42.8
|personality F60.5
|states F42.8
|swearing F42.8
|in Gilles de la Tourette's syndrome F95.2
|tics and spasms F95.9
Concato's disease (pericardial polyserositis)
A19.9
|nontubercular I31.1
|pleural *see* Pleurisy, with effusion
Concavity chest wall M95.4
Concealed penis Q55.64
Concern (normal) about sick person in family
Z63.6
Concrescence (teeth) K00.2
Concretio cordis I31.1
|rheumatic I09.2
Concretion *see also* Calculus
|appendicular K38.1
|canaliculus *see* Dacryolith
|clitoris N90.89
|conjunctiva H11.12-
|eyelid *see* Disorder, eyelid, specified type
NEC
|lacrimal passages *see* Dacryolith
|prepuce (male) N47.8
|salivary gland (any) K11.5
|seminal vesicle N50.89
|tonsil J35.8
Concussion (brain) (cerebral) (current)
S06.0X9
|with
|loss of consciousness of 30 minutes or less
S06.0X1
|loss of consciousness of unspecified
duration S06.0X9
|blast (air) (hydraulic) (immersion)
(underwater)
|abdomen or thorax *see* Injury, blast, by site

Concussion - *continued*
　|ear with acoustic nerve injury *see* Injury,
　　　nerve, acoustic, specified type NEC
　|cauda equina S34.3
　|conus medullaris S34.02
　|ocular S05.8X-
　|spinal (cord)
　　|cervical S14.0
　　|lumbar S34.01
　　|sacral S34.02
　　|thoracic S24.0
　|syndrome F07.81
　|without loss of consciousness S06.0X0
Condition *see also* Disease
　|post COVID-19 U09.9
Conditions arising in the perinatal period *see*
　　Newborn, affected by
Conduct disorder *see* Disorder, conduct
Condyloma A63.0
　|acuminatum A63.0
　|gonorrheal A54.09
　|latum A51.31
　|syphilitic A51.31
　　|congenital A50.07
　|venereal, syphilitic A51.31
Conflagration *see also* Burn
　|asphyxia (by inhalation of gases, fumes or
　　vapors) *see also* Table of Drugs and
　　Chemicals T59.9-
Conflict (with) *see also* Discord
　|family Z73.9
　|marital Z63.0
　　|involving divorce or estrangement Z63.5
　|parent-child Z62.820
　　|parent-adopted child Z62.821
　　|parent-biological child Z62.820
　　|parent-foster child Z62.822
　|social role NEC Z73.5
Confluent *see* condition
Confusion, confused R41.0
　|epileptic F05
　|mental state (psychogenic) F44.89
　|psychogenic F44.89
　|reactive (from emotional stress, psychological
　　trauma) F44.89
Confusional arousals G47.51
Congelation T69.9
Congenital *see also* condition
　|aortic septum Q25.49
　|intrinsic factor deficiency D51.0
　|malformation *see* Anomaly
Congestion, congestive
　|bladder N32.89
　|bowel K63.89
Congestion, congestive
　|brain G93.89
　|breast N64.59
　|bronchial J98.09
　|catarrhal J31.0
　|chest R09.89
　|chill, malarial *see* Malaria
　|circulatory NEC I99.8
　|duodenum K31.89
　|eye *see* Hyperemia, conjunctiva
　|facial, due to birth injury P15.4
　|general R68.89
　|glottis J37.0
　|heart *see* Failure, heart, congestive
　|hepatic K76.1
　|hypostatic (lung) *see* Edema, lung
　|intestine K63.89
　|kidney N28.89
　|labyrinth *see* subcategory H83.8
　|larynx J37.0
　|liver K76.1
　|lung R09.89
　　|active or acute *see* Pneumonia

Congestion, congestive - *continued*
　|malaria, malarial *see* Malaria
　|nasal R09.81
　|nose R09.81
　|orbit, orbital *see also* Exophthalmos
　　|inflammatory (chronic) *see* Inflammation,
　　　orbit
　|ovary N83.8
　|pancreas K86.89
　|pelvic, female N94.89
　|pleural J94.8
　|prostate (active) N42.1
　|pulmonary *see* Congestion, lung
　|renal N28.89
　|retina H35.81
　|seminal vesicle N50.1
　|spinal cord G95.19
　|spleen (chronic) D73.2
　|stomach K31.89
　|trachea *see* Tracheitis
　|urethra N36.8
　|uterus N85.8
　　|with subinvolution N85.3
　|venous (passive) I87.8
　|viscera R68.89
Congestive *see* Congestion
Conical
　|cervix (hypertrophic elongation) N88.4
　|cornea *see* Keratoconus
　|teeth K00.2
Conjoined twins Q89.4
Conjugal maladjustment Z63.0
　|involving divorce or estrangement Z63.5
Conjunctiva *see* condition
Conjunctivitis (staphylococcal) (streptococcal)
　　NOS H10.9
　|Acanthamoeba B60.12
　|acute H10.3-
　　|atopic H10.1-
　　|mucopurulent H10.02-
　　　|follicular H10.01-
　　|chemical *see also* Corrosion, cornea
　　　H10.21-
　　|pseudomembranous H10.22-
　　|serous except viral H10.23-
　　　|viral *see* Conjunctivitis, viral
　　|toxic H10.21-
　|adenoviral (acute) (follicular) B30.1
　|allergic (acute) *see* Conjunctivitis, acute,
　　atopic
　　|chronic H10.45
　　　|vernal H10.44
　|anaphylactic *see* Conjunctivitis, acute, atopic
　|Apollo B30.3
　|atopic (acute) *see* Conjunctivitis, acute, atopic
　|Béal's B30.2
　|blennorrhagic (gonococcal) (neonatorum)
　　A54.31
　|chemical (acute) *see also* Corrosion, cornea
　　H10.21-
　|chlamydial A74.0
　　|due to trachoma A71.1
　　|neonatal P39.1
　|chronic (nodosa) (petrificans) (phlyctenular)
　　H10.40-
　　|allergic H10.45
　　　|vernal H10.44
　　|follicular H10.43-
　　|giant papillary H10.41-
　　|simple H10.42-
　　|vernal H10.44
　|coxsackievirus 24 B30.3
　|diphtheritic A36.86
　|due to
　　|dust *see* Conjunctivitis, acute, atopic

Conjunctivitis - *continued*
　|filariasis B74.9
　|mucocutaneous leishmaniasis B55.2
　|enterovirus type 70 (hemorrhagic) B30.3
　|epidemic (viral) B30.9
　　|hemorrhagic B30.3
　|gonococcal (neonatorum) A54.31
　|granular (trachomatous) A71.1
　　|sequelae (late effect) B94.0
　|hemorrhagic (acute) (epidemic) B30.3
　|herpes zoster B02.31
　|in (due to)
　　|Acanthamoeba B60.12
　　|adenovirus (acute) (follicular) B30.1
　　|Chlamydia A74.0
　　|coxsackievirus 24 B30.3
　　|diphtheria A36.86
　　|enterovirus type 70 (hemorrhagic) B30.3
　　|filariasis B74.9
　　|gonococci A54.31
　　|herpes (simplex) virus B00.53
　　　|zoster B02.31
　　|infectious disease NEC B99
　　|meningococci A39.89
　　|mucocutaneous leishmaniasis B55.2
　　|rosacea H10.82-
　　|syphilis (late) A52.71
　　|zoster B02.31
　|inclusion A74.0
　|infantile P39.1
　　|gonococcal A54.31
　|Koch-Weeks' *see* Conjunctivitis, acute,
　　mucopurulent
　|light *see* Conjunctivitis, acute, atopic
　|ligneous *see* Blepharoconjunctivitis, ligneous
　|meningococcal A39.89
　|mucopurulent *see* Conjunctivitis, acute,
　　mucopurulent
　|neonatal P39.1
　　|gonococcal A54.31
　|Newcastle B30.8
　|of Béal B30.2
　|parasitic
　　|filariasis B74.9
　　|mucocutaneous leishmaniasis B55.2
　|Parinaud's H10.89
　|petrificans H10.89
　|rosacea H10.82-
　|specified NEC H10.89
　|swimming-pool B30.1
　|trachomatous A71.1
　　|acute A71.0
　　|sequelae (late effect) B94.0
　|traumatic NEC H10.89
　|tuberculous A18.59
　|tularemic A21.1
　|tularensis A21.1
　|viral B30.9
　　|due to
　　　|adenovirus B30.1
　　　|enterovirus B30.3
　　|specified NEC B30.8
Conjunctivochalasis H11.82-
Connective tissue *see* condition
Conn's syndrome E26.01
Conradi (-Hunermann) disease Q77.3
Consanguinity Z84.3
　|counseling Z71.89
Conscious simulation (of illness) Z76.5
Consecutive *see* condition
Consolidation lung (base) *see* Pneumonia, lobar
Constipation (atonic) (neurogenic) (simple)
　　(spastic) K59.00
　|chronic K59.09
　　|idiopathic K59.04
　|drug-induced K59.03

Constipation - *continued*
| functional K59.04
| outlet dysfunction K59.02
| psychogenic F45.8
| slow transit K59.01
| specified NEC K59.09
Constitutional *see also* condition
| substandard F60.7
Constitutionally substandard F60.7
Constriction *see also* Stricture
| auditory canal *see* Stenosis, external ear canal
| bronchial J98.09
| duodenum K31.5
| esophagus K22.2
| external
| | abdomen, abdominal (wall) S30.841
| | alveolar process S00.542
| | ankle S90.54-
| | antecubital space *see* Constriction, external, forearm
| | arm (upper) S40.84-
| | auricle *see* Constriction, external, ear
| | axilla *see* Constriction, external, arm
| | back, lower S30.840
| | breast S20.14-
| | brow S00.84
| | buttock S30.840
| | calf *see* Constriction, external, leg
| | canthus *see* Constriction, external, eyelid
| | cheek S00.84
| | | internal S00.542
| | chest wall *see* Constriction, external, thorax
| | chin S00.84
| | clitoris S30.844
| | costal region *see* Constriction, external, thorax
| | digit(s)
| | | foot *see* Constriction, external, toe
| | | hand *see* Constriction, external, finger
| | ear S00.44-
| | elbow S50.34-
| | epididymis S30.843
| | epigastric region S30.841
| | esophagus, cervical S10.14
| | eyebrow *see* Constriction, external, eyelid
| | eyelid S00.24-
| | face S00.84
| | finger(s) S60.44-
| | | index S60.44
| | | little S60.44-
| | | middle S60.44-
| | | ring S60.44-
| | flank S30.841
| | foot (except toe(s) alone) S90.84-
| | | toe *see* Constriction, external, toe
| | forearm S50.84-
| | | elbow only *see* Constriction, external, elbow
| | forehead S00.84
| | genital organs, external
| | | female S30.846
| | | male S30.845
| | groin S30.841
| | gum S00.542
| | hand S60.54-
| | head S00.94
| | | ear *see* Constriction, external, ear
| | | eyelid *see* Constriction, external, eyelid
| | | lip S00.541
| | | nose S00.34
| | | oral cavity S00.542
| | | scalp S00.04
| | | specified site NEC S00.84
| | heel *see* Constriction, external, foot
| | hip S70.24-
| | inguinal region S30.841

Constriction - *continued*
| | interscapular region S20.449
| | jaw S00.84
| | knee S80.24-
| | labium (majus) (minus) S30.844
| | larynx S10.14
| | leg (lower) S80.84-
| | | knee *see* Constriction, external, knee
| | | upper *see* Constriction, external, thigh
| | lip S00.541
| | lower back S30.840
| | lumbar region S30.840
| | malar region S00.84
| | mammary *see* Constriction, external, breast
| | mastoid region S00.84
| | mouth S00.542
| | nail
| | | finger *see* Constriction, external, finger
| | | toe *see* Constriction, external, toe
| | nasal S00.34
| | neck S10.94
| | | specified site NEC S10.84
| | | throat S10.14
| | nose S00.34
| | occipital region S00.04
| | oral cavity S00.542
| | orbital region *see* Constriction, external, eyelid
| | palate S00.542
| | palm *see* Constriction, external, hand
| | parietal region S00.04
| | pelvis S30.840
| | penis S30.842
| | perineum
| | | female S30.844
| | | male S30.840
| | periocular area *see* Constriction, external, eyelid
| | phalanges
| | | finger *see* Constriction, external, finger
| | | toe *see* Constriction, external, toe
| | pharynx S10.14
| | pinna *see* Constriction, external, ear
| | popliteal space *see* Constriction, external, knee
| | prepuce S30.842
| | pubic region S30.840
| | pudendum
| | | female S30.846
| | | male S30.845
| | sacral region S30.840
| | scalp S00.04
| | scapular region *see* Constriction, external, shoulder
| | scrotum S30.843
| | shin *see* Constriction, external, leg
| | shoulder S40.24-
| | sternal region S20.349
| | submaxillary region S00.84
| | submental region S00.84
| | subungual
| | | finger(s) *see* Constriction, external, finger
| | | toe(s) *see* Constriction, external, toe
| | supraclavicular fossa S10.84
| | supraorbital S00.84
| | temple S00.84
| | temporal region S00.84
| | testis S30.843
| | thigh S70.34-
| | thorax, thoracic (wall) S20.94
| | | back S20.44-
| | | front S20.34-
| | throat S10.14
| | thumb S60.34-
| | toe(s) (lesser) S90.44-
| | | great S90.44-
| | tongue S00.542
| | trachea S10.14

Constriction - *continued*
| | tunica vaginalis S30.843
| | uvula S00.542
| | vagina S30.844
| | vulva S30.844
| | wrist S60.84-
| gallbladder *see* Obstruction, gallbladder
| intestine *see* Obstruction, intestine
| larynx J38.6
| | congenital Q31.8
| | | specified NEC Q31.8
| | | subglottic Q31.1
| organ or site, congenital NEC *see* Atresia, by site
| prepuce (acquired) (congenital) N47.1
| pylorus (adult hypertrophic) K31.1
| | congenital or infantile Q40.0
| | newborn Q40.0
| ring dystocia (uterus) O62.4
| spastic *see also* Spasm
| | ureter N13.5
| ureter N13.5
| | with infection N13.6
| urethra *see* Stricture, urethra
| visual field (peripheral) (functional) *see* Defect, visual field
Constrictive *see* condition
Consultation
| medical *see* Counseling, medical
| religious Z71.81
| specified reason NEC Z71.89
| spiritual Z71.81
| without complaint or sickness Z71.9
| | feared complaint unfounded Z71.1
| | specified reason NEC Z71.89
Consumption *see* Tuberculosis
Contact (with) *see also* Exposure (to)
| acariasis Z20.7
| AIDS virus Z20.6
| air pollution Z77.110
| algae and algae toxins Z77.121
| algae bloom Z77.121
| anthrax Z20.810
| aromatic amines Z77.020
| aromatic (hazardous) compounds NEC Z77.028
| aromatic dyes NOS Z77.028
| arsenic Z77.010
| asbestos Z77.090
| bacterial disease NEC Z20.818
| benzene Z77.021
| blue-green algae bloom Z77.121
| body fluids (potentially hazardous) Z77.21
| brown tide Z77.121
| chemicals (chiefly nonmedicinal) (hazardous) NEC Z77.098
| cholera Z20.09
| chromium compounds Z77.018
| communicable disease Z20.9
| | bacterial NEC Z20.818
| | specified NEC Z20.89
| | viral NEC Z20.828
| | Zika virus Z20.821
| - coronavirus (disease) (novel) 2019 Z20.822
| cyanobacteria bloom Z77.121
| dyes Z77.098
| Escherichia coli (E. coli) Z20.01
| fiberglass *see* Table of Drugs and Chemicals, fiberglass
| German measles Z20.4
| gonorrhea Z20.2
| hazardous metals NEC Z77.018
| hazardous substances NEC Z77.29
| hazards in the physical environment NEC Z77.128

Contraction(s), contracture, contracted - continued
- lower leg M62.46-
- multiple sites M62.49
- neck M62.48
- pelvic region M62.45-
- shoulder region M62.41-
- specified site NEC M62.48
- thigh M62.45-
- thorax M62.48
- trunk M62.48
- upper arm M62.42-
- toe see Deformity, toe, specified NEC
- ureterovesical orifice (postinfectional) N13.5
  - with infection N13.6
- urethra see also Stricture, urethra
  - orifice N32.0
- uterus N85.8
  - abnormal NEC O62.9
  - clonic (complicating delivery) O62.4
  - dyscoordinate (complicating delivery) O62.4
  - hourglass (complicating delivery) O62.4
  - hypertonic O62.4
  - hypotonic NEC O62.2
  - inadequate
    - primary O62.0
    - secondary O62.1
  - incoordinate (complicating delivery) O62.4
  - poor O62.2
  - tetanic (complicating delivery) O62.4
- vagina (outlet) N89.5
- vesical N32.89
  - neck or urethral orifice N32.0
- visual field see Defect, visual field, generalized
- Volkmann's (ischemic) T79.6

Contusion (skin surface intact) T14.8
- abdomen, abdominal (muscle) (wall) S30.1
- adnexa, eye NEC S05.8X-
- adrenal gland S37.812
- alveolar process S00.532
- ankle S90.0-
- antecubital space see Contusion, forearm
- anus S30.3
- arm (upper) S40.02-
  - lower (with elbow) see Contusion, forearm
- auditory canal see Contusion, ear
- auricle see Contusion, ear
- axilla see Contusion, arm, upper
- back see also Contusion, thorax, back
  - lower S30.0
- bile duct S36.13
- bladder S37.22
- bone NEC T14.8
- brain (diffuse) see Injury, intracranial, diffuse
  - focal see Injury, intracranial, focal
- brainstem S06.38-
- breast S20.0-
- broad ligament S37.892
- brow S00.83
- buttock S30.0
- canthus, eye S00.1-
- cauda equina S34.3
- cerebellar, traumatic S06.37-
- cerebral S06.33-
  - left side S06.32-
  - right side S06.31-
- cheek S00.83
  - internal S00.532
- chest (wall) see Contusion, thorax
- chin S00.83
- clitoris S30.23
- colon see Injury, intestine, large, contusion
- common bile duct S36.13
- conjunctiva S05.1-

Contusion - continued
- with foreign body (in conjunctival sac) see Foreign body, conjunctival sac
- conus medullaris (spine) S34.139
- cornea see Contusion, eyeball
  - with foreign body see Foreign body, cornea
- corpus cavernosum S30.21
- cortex (brain) (cerebral) see Injury, intracranial, diffuse
  - focal see Injury, intracranial, focal
- costal region see Contusion, thorax
- cystic duct S36.13
- diaphragm S27.802
- duodenum S36.420
- ear S00.43-
- elbow S50.0-
  - with forearm see Contusion, forearm
- epididymis S30.22
- epigastric region S30.1
- epiglottis S10.0
- esophagus (thoracic) S27.812
  - cervical S10.0
- eyeball S05.1-
- eyebrow S00.1-
- eyelid (and periocular area) S00.1-
- face NEC S00.83
- fallopian tube S37.529
  - bilateral S37.522
  - unilateral S37.521
- femoral triangle S30.1
- finger(s) S60.00
  - with damage to nail (matrix) S60.10
  - index S60.02-
    - with damage to nail S60.12-
  - little S60.05-
    - with damage to nail S60.15-
  - middle S60.03-
    - with damage to nail S60.13-
  - ring S60.04-
    - with damage to nail S60.14-
  - thumb see Contusion, thumb
- flank S30.1
- foot (except toe(s) alone) S90.3-
  - toe see Contusion, toe
- forearm S50.1-
  - elbow only see Contusion, elbow
- forehead S00.83
- gallbladder S36.122
- genital organs, external
  - female S30.202
  - male S30.201
- globe (eye) see Contusion, eyeball
- groin S30.1
- gum S00.532
- hand S60.22-
  - finger(s) see Contusion, finger
  - wrist see Contusion, wrist
- head S00.93
  - ear see Contusion, ear
  - eyelid see Contusion, eyelid
  - lip S00.531
  - nose S00.33
  - oral cavity S00.532
  - scalp S00.03
  - specified part NEC S00.83
- heart see also Injury, heart S26.91
- heel see Contusion, foot
- hepatic duct S36.13
- hip S70.0-
- ileum S36.428
- iliac region S30.1
- inguinal region S30.1
- interscapular region S20.229
- intra-abdominal organ S36.92
  - colon see Injury, intestine, large, contusion
  - liver S36.112

Contusion - continued
- pancreas see Contusion, pancreas
- rectum S36.62
- small intestine see Injury, intestine, small, contusion
- specified organ NEC S36.892
- spleen see Contusion, spleen
- stomach S36.32
- iris (eye) see Contusion, eyeball
- jaw S00.83
- jejunum S36.428
- kidney S37.01-
  - major (greater than 2 cm) S37.02-
  - minor (less than 2 cm) S37.01-
- knee S80.0-
- labium (majus) (minus) S30.23
- lacrimal apparatus, gland or sac S05.8X
- larynx S10.0
- leg (lower) S80.1-
  - knee see Contusion, knee
- lens see Contusion, eyeball
- lip S00.531
- liver S36.112
- lower back S30.0
- lumbar region S30.0
- lung S27.329
  - bilateral S27.322
  - unilateral S27.321
- malar region S00.83
- mastoid region S00.83
- membrane, brain see Injury, intracranial, diffuse
  - focal see Injury, intracranial, focal
- mesentery S36.892
- mesosalpinx S37.892
- mouth S00.532
- muscle see Contusion, by site
- nail
  - finger see Contusion, finger, with damage to nail
  - toe see Contusion, toe, with damage to nail
- nasal S00.33
- neck S10.93
  - specified site NEC S10.83
  - throat S10.0
- nerve see Injury, nerve
- newborn P54.5
- nose S00.33
- occipital
  - lobe (brain) see Injury, intracranial, diffuse
    - focal see Injury, intracranial, focal
  - region (scalp) S00.03
- orbit (region) (tissues) S05.1-
- ovary S37.429
  - bilateral S37.422
  - unilateral S37.421
- palate S00.532
- pancreas S36.229
  - body S36.221
  - head S36.220
  - tail S36.222
- parietal
  - lobe (brain) see Injury, intracranial, diffuse
    - focal see Injury, intracranial, focal
  - region (scalp) S00.03
- pelvic organ S37.92
  - adrenal gland S37.812
  - bladder S37.22
  - fallopian tube see Contusion, fallopian tube
  - kidney see Contusion, kidney
  - ovary see Contusion, ovary
  - prostate S37.822
  - specified organ NEC S37.892
  - ureter S37.12
  - urethra S37.32
  - uterus S37.62

Contusion - *continued*
- pelvis S30.0
- penis S30.21
- perineum
  - female S30.23
  - male S30.0
- periocular area S00.1-
- peritoneum S36.81
- periurethral tissue *see* Contusion, urethra
- pharynx S10.0
- pinna *see* Contusion, ear
- popliteal space *see* Contusion, knee
- prepuce S30.21
- prostate S37.822
- pubic region S30.1
- pudendum
  - female S30.202
  - male S30.201
- quadriceps femoris *see* Contusion, thigh
- rectum S36.62
- retroperitoneum S36.892
- round ligament S37.892
- sacral region S30.0
- scalp S00.03
  - due to birth injury P12.3
- scapular region *see* Contusion, shoulder
- sclera *see* Contusion, eyeball
- scrotum S30.22
- seminal vesicle S37.892
- shoulder S40.01-
- skin NEC T14.8
- small intestine *see* Injury, intestine, small, contusion
- spermatic cord S30.22
- spinal cord *see* Injury, spinal cord, by region
  - cauda equina S34.3
  - conus medullaris S34.139
- spleen S36.029
  - major S36.021
  - minor S36.020
- sternal region S20.219
- stomach S36.32
- subconjunctival S05.1-
- subcutaneous NEC T14.8
- submaxillary region S00.83
- submental region S00.83
- subperiosteal NEC T14.8
- subungual
  - finger *see* Contusion, finger, with damage to nail
  - toe *see* Contusion, toe, with damage to nail
- supraclavicular fossa S10.83
- supraorbital S00.83
- suprarenal gland S37.812
- temple (region) S00.83
- temporal
  - lobe (brain) *see* Injury, intracranial, diffuse
    - focal *see* Injury, intracranial, focal
  - region S00.83
- testis S30.22
- thigh S70.1-
- thorax (wall) S20.20
  - back S20.22-
  - front S20.21-
- throat S10.0
- thumb S60.01-
  - with damage to nail S60.11-
- toe(s) (lesser) S90.12-
  - with damage to nail S90.22-
  - great S90.11-
    - with damage to nail S90.21-
- tongue S00.532
- trachea (cervical) S10.0
  - thoracic S27.52
- tunica vaginalis S30.22

Contusion - *continued*
- tympanum, tympanic membrane *see* Contusion, ear
- ureter S37.12
- urethra S37.32
- urinary organ NEC S37.892
- uterus S37.62
- uvula S00.532
- vagina S30.23
- vas deferens S37.892
- vesical S37.22
- vocal cord(s) S10.0
- vulva S30.23
- wrist S60.21-

Conus (congenital) (any type) Q14.8
- cornea *see* Keratoconus
- medullaris syndrome G95.81

Conversion hysteria, neurosis or reaction F44.9

Converter, tuberculosis (test reaction) R76.11

Conviction (legal), anxiety concerning Z65.0
- with imprisonment Z65.1

Convulsions (idiopathic) *see also* Seizure(s) R56.9
- apoplectiform (cerebral ischemia) I67.82
- dissociative F44.5
- epileptic *see* Epilepsy
- epileptiform, epileptoid *see* Seizure, epileptiform
- ether (anesthetic) *see* Table of Drugs and Chemicals, by drug
- febrile R56.00
  - with status epilepticus G40.901
  - complex R56.01
    - with status epilepticus G40.901
  - simple R56.00
- hysterical F44.5
- infantile P90
  - epilepsy *see* Epilepsy
- jacksonian *see* Epilepsy, localization-related, symptomatic, with simple partial seizures
- myoclonic G25.3
- newborn P90
- obstetrical (nephritic) (uremic) *see* Eclampsia
- paretic A52.17
- post traumatic R56.1
- psychomotor *see* Epilepsy, localization-related, symptomatic, with complex partial seizures
- recurrent R56.9
- reflex R25.8
- scarlatinal A38.8
- tetanus, tetanic *see* Tetanus
- thymic E32.8

Convulsive *see also* Convulsions

Cooley's anemia D56.1

Coolie itch B76.9

Cooper's
- disease *see* Mastopathy, cystic
- hernia *see* Hernia, abdomen, specified site NEC

Copra itch B88.0

Coprophagy F50.89

Coprophobia F40.298

Coproporphyria, hereditary E80.29

Cor
- biloculare Q20.8
- bovis, bovinum *see* Hypertrophy, cardiac
- pulmonale (chronic) I27.81
  - acute I26.09
- triatriatum, triatrium Q24.2
- triloculare Q20.8
  - biatrium Q20.4
  - biventriculare Q21.1

Corbus' disease (gangrenous balanitis) N48.1

Cord *see also* condition
- around neck
  - complicating delivery O69.81
    - with compression O69.1
- bladder G95.89
  - tabetic A52.19

Cordis ectopia Q24.8

Corditis (spermatic) N49.1

Corectopia Q13.2

Cori's disease (glycogen storage) E74.03

Cork handler's disease or lung J67.3

Corkscrew esophagus K22.4

Cork worker's disease or lung J67.3

Corn (infected) L84

Cornea *see also* condition
- donor Z52.5
- plana Q13.4

Cornelia de Lange syndrome Q87.1

Cornu cutaneum L85.8

Cornual gestation or pregnancy O00.80
- with intrauterine pregnancy O00.81

Coronary (artery) *see* condition

Coronavirus (infection)
- as cause of disease classified elsewhere B97.29
- coronavirus-19 U07.1
- COVID-19 U07.1
- SARS-associated B97.21

Corpora *see also* condition
- amylacea, prostate N42.89
- cavernosa *see* condition

Corpulence *see* Obesity

Corpus *see* condition

Corrected transposition Q20.5

Corrosion (injury) (acid) (caustic) (chemical) (lime) (external) (internal) T30.4
- abdomen, abdominal (muscle) (wall) T21.42
  - first degree T21.52
  - second degree T21.62
  - third degree T21.72
- above elbow T22.439
  - first degree T22.539
  - left T22.432
    - first degree T22.532
    - second degree T22.632
    - third degree T22.732
  - right T22.431
    - first degree T22.531
    - second degree T22.631
    - third degree T22.731
  - second degree T22.639
  - third degree T22.739
- alimentary tract NEC T28.7
- ankle T25.419
  - first degree T25.519
  - left T25.412
    - first degree T25.512
    - second degree T25.612
    - third degree T25.712
  - multiple with foot *see* Corrosion, lower, limb, multiple, ankle and foot
  - right T25.411
    - first degree T25.511
    - second degree T25.611
    - third degree T25.711
  - second degree T25.619
  - third degree T25.719
- anus *see* Corrosion, buttock
- arm(s) (meaning upper limb(s)) *see* Corrosion, upper limb
- axilla T22.449
  - first degree T22.549
  - left T22.442
    - first degree T22.542
    - second degree T22.642
    - third degree T22.742

Corrosion - *continued*

|right T22.441
|first degree T22.541
|second degree T22.641
|third degree T22.741
|second degree T22.649
|third degree T22.749
|back (lower) T21.44
|first degree T21.54
|second degree T21.64
|third degree T21.74
|upper T21.43
|first degree T21.53
|second degree T21.63
|third degree T21.73
|blisters   code as Corrosion, second degree, by site
|breast(s) *see* Corrosion, chest wall
|buttock(s) T21.45
|first degree T21.55
|second degree T21.65
|third degree T21.75
|calf T24.439
|first degree T24.539
|left T24.432
|first degree T24.532
|second degree T24.632
|third degree T24.732
|right T24.431
|first degree T24.531
|second degree T24.631
|third degree T24.731
|second degree T24.639
|third degree T24.739
|canthus (eye) *see* Corrosion, eyelid
|cervix T28.8
|cheek T20.46
|first degree T20.56
|second degree T20.66
|third degree T20.76
|chest wall T21.41
|first degree T21.51
|second degree T21.61
|third degree T21.71
|chin T20.43
|first degree T20.53
|second degree T20.63
|third degree T20.73
|colon T28.7
|conjunctiva (and cornea) *see* Corrosion, cornea
|cornea (and conjunctiva) T26.6-
|deep necrosis of underlying tissue   code as Corrosion, third degree, by site
|dorsum of hand T23.469
|first degree T23.569
|left T23.462
|first degree T23.562
|second degree T23.662
|third degree T23.762
|right T23.461
|first degree T23.561
|second degree T23.661
|third degree T23.761
|second degree T23.669
|third degree T23.769
|ear (auricle) (external) (canal) T20.41
|drum T28.91
|first degree T20.51
|second degree T20.61
|third degree T20.71
|elbow T22.429
|first degree T22.529
|left T22.422
|first degree T22.522
|second degree T22.622
|third degree T22.722

Corrosion - *continued*

|right T22.421
|first degree T22.521
|second degree T22.621
|third degree T22.721
|second degree T22.629
|third degree T22.729
|entire body *see* Corrosion, multiple body regions
|epidermal loss   code as Corrosion, second degree, by site
|epiglottis T27.4
|erythema, erythematous   code as Corrosion, first degree, by site
|esophagus T28.6
|extent (percentage of body surface)
|less than 10 percent T32.0
|10-19 percent (0-9 percent third degree) T32.10
|with 10-19 percent third degree T32.11
|20-29 percent (0-9 percent third degree) T32.20
|with
|10-19 percent third degree T32.21
|20-29 percent third degree T32.22
|30-39 percent (0-9 percent third degree) T32.30
|with
|10-19 percent third degree T32.31
|20-29 percent third degree T32.32
|30-39 percent third degree T32.33
|40-49 percent (0-9 percent third degree) T32.40
|with
|10-19 percent third degree T32.41
|20-29 percent third degree T32.42
|30-39 percent third degree T32.43
|40-49 percent third degree T32.44
|50-59 percent (0-9 percent third degree) T32.50
|with
|10-19 percent third degree T32.51
|20-29 percent third degree T32.52
|30-39 percent third degree T32.53
|40-49 percent third degree T32.54
|50-59 percent third degree T32.55
|60-69 percent (0-9 percent third degree) T32.60
|with
|10-19 percent third degree T32.61
|20-29 percent third degree T32.62
|30-39 percent third degree T32.63
|40-49 percent third degree T32.64
|50-59 percent third degree T32.65
|60-69 percent third degree T32.66
|70-79 percent (0-9 percent third degree) T32.70
|with
|10-19 percent third degree T32.71
|20-29 percent third degree T32.72
|30-39 percent third degree T32.73
|40-49 percent third degree T32.74
|50-59 percent third degree T32.75
|60-69 percent third degree T32.76
|70-79 percent third degree T32.77
|80-89 percent (0-9 percent third degree) T32.80
|with
|10-19 percent third degree T32.81
|20-29 percent third degree T32.82
|30-39 percent third degree T32.83
|40-49 percent third degree T32.84
|50-59 percent third degree T32.85
|60-69 percent third degree T32.86
|70-79 percent third degree T32.87
|80-89 percent third degree T32.88

Corrosion - *continued*

|90 percent or more (0-9 percent third degree) T32.90
|with
|10-19 percent third degree T32.91
|20-29 percent third degree T32.92
|30-39 percent third degree T32.93
|40-49 percent third degree T32.94
|50-59 percent third degree T32.95
|60-69 percent third degree T32.96
|70-79 percent third degree T32.97
|80-89 percent third degree T32.98
|90-99 percent third degree T32.99
|extremity *see* Corrosion, limb
|eye(s) and adnexa T26.9-
|with resulting rupture and destruction of eyeball T26.7-
|conjunctival sac *see* Corrosion, cornea
|cornea *see* Corrosion, cornea
|lid *see* Corrosion, eyelid
|periocular area *see* Corrosion eyelid
|specified site NEC T26.8-
|eyeball *see* Corrosion, eye
|eyelid(s) T26.5-
|face *see* Corrosion, head
|finger T23.429
|first degree T23.529
|left T23.422
|first degree T23.522
|second degree T23.622
|third degree T23.722
|multiple sites (without thumb) T23.439
|with thumb T23.449
|first degree T23.549
|left T23.442
|first degree T23.542
|second degree T23.642
|third degree T23.742
|right T23.441
|first degree T23.541
|second degree T23.641
|third degree T23.741
|second degree T23.649
|third degree T23.749
|first degree T23.539
|left T23.432
|first degree T23.532
|second degree T23.632
|third degree T23.732
|right T23.431
|first degree T23.531
|second degree T23.631
|third degree T23.731
|second degree T23.639
|third degree T23.739
|right T23.421
|first degree T23.521
|second degree T23.621
|third degree T23.721
|second degree T23.629
|third degree T23.729
|flank *see* Corrosion, abdomen
|foot T25.429
|first degree T25.529
|left T25.422
|first degree T25.522
|second degree T25.622
|third degree T25.722
|multiple with ankle *see* Corrosion, lower, limb, multiple, ankle and foot
|right T25.421
|first degree T25.521
|second degree T25.621
|third degree T25.721
|second degree T25.629

Corrosion - *continued*

|third degree T25.729
|forearm T22.419
  |first degree T22.519
  |left T22.412
   |first degree T22.512
   |second degree T22.612
   |third degree T22.712
  |right T22.411
   |first degree T22.511
   |second degree T22.611
   |third degree T22.711
  |second degree T22.619
  |third degree T22.719
|forehead T20.46
  |first degree T20.56
  |second degree T20.66
  |third degree T20.76
|fourth degree   code as Corrosion, third
  degree, by site
|full thickness skin loss   code as Corrosion,
  third degree, by site
|gastrointestinal tract NEC T28.7
|genital organs
  |external
   |female T21.47
    |first degree T21.57
    |second degree T21.67
    |third degree T21.77
   |male T21.46
    |first degree T21.56
    |second degree T21.66
    |third degree T21.76
  |internal T28.8
|groin *see* Corrosion, abdominal wall
|hand(s) T23.409
  |back *see* Corrosion, dorsum of hand
  |finger *see* Corrosion, finger
  |first degree T23.509
  |left T23.402
   |first degree T23.502
   |second degree T23.602
   |third degree T23.702
  |multiple sites with wrist T23.499
   |first degree T23.599
   |left T23.492
    |first degree T23.592
    |second degree T23.692
    |third degree T23.792
   |right T23.491
    |first degree T23.591
    |second degree T23.691
    |third degree T23.791
   |second degree T23.699
   |third degree T23.799
  |palm *see* Corrosion, palm
  |right T23.401
   |first degree T23.501
   |second degree T23.601
   |third degree T23.701
  |second degree T23.609
  |third degree T23.709
  |thumb *see* Corrosion, thumb
|head (and face) (and neck) T20.40
  |cheek *see* Corrosion, cheek
  |chin *see* Corrosion, chin
  |ear *see* Corrosion, ear
  |eye(s) only *see* Corrosion, eye
  |first degree T20.50
  |forehead *see* Corrosion, forehead
  |lip *see* Corrosion, lip
  |multiple sites T20.49
   |first degree T20.59
   |second degree T20.69
   |third degree T20.79
  |neck *see* Corrosion, neck

Corrosion - *continued*

|nose *see* Corrosion, nose
|scalp *see* Corrosion, scalp
|second degree T20.60
|third degree T20.70
|hip(s) *see* Corrosion, lower, limb
|inhalation *see* Corrosion, respiratory tract
|internal organ(s) *see also* Corrosion, by site
  T28.90
  |alimentary tract T28.7
   |esophagus T28.6
  |esophagus T28.6
  |genitourinary T28.8
  |mouth T28.5
  |pharynx T28.5
  |specified organ NEC T28.99
|interscapular region *see* Corrosion, back,
  upper
|intestine (large) (small) T28.7
|knee T24.429
  |first degree T24.529
  |left T24.422
   |first degree T24.522
   |second degree T24.622
   |third degree T24.722
  |right T24.421
   |first degree T24.521
   |second degree T24.621
   |third degree T24.721
  |second degree T24.629
  |third degree T24.729
|labium (majus) (minus) *see* Corrosion, genital
  organs, external, female
|lacrimal apparatus, duct, gland or sac *see*
  Corrosion, eye, specified site NEC
|larynx T27.4
  |with lung T27.5
|leg(s) (meaning lower limb(s)) *see* Corrosion,
  lower limb
|limb(s)
  |lower *see* Corrosion, lower, limb
  |upper *see* Corrosion, upper limb
|lip(s) T20.42
  |first degree T20.52
  |second degree T20.62
  |third degree T20.72
|lower
  |back *see* Corrosion, back
  |limb T24.409
   |ankle *see* Corrosion, ankle
   |calf *see* Corrosion, calf
   |first degree T24.509
    |foot *see* Corrosion, foot
    |knee *see* Corrosion, knee
    |left T24.402
     |first degree T24.502
     |second degree T24.602
     |third degree T24.702
    |multiple sites, except ankle and foot
     T24.499
    |ankle and foot T25.499
     |first degree T25.599
     |left T25.492
      |first degree T25.592
      |second degree T25.692
      |third degree T25.792
     |right T25.491
      |first degree T25.591
      |second degree T25.691
      |third degree T25.791
     |second degree T25.699
     |third degree T25.799
    |first degree T24.599
    |left T24.492
     |first degree T24.592
     |second degree T24.692

Corrosion - *continued*

|third degree T24.792
  |right T24.491
   |first degree T24.591
   |second degree T24.691
   |third degree T24.791
  |second degree T24.699
  |third degree T24.799
  |right T24.401
   |first degree T24.501
   |second degree T24.601
   |third degree T24.701
  |second degree T24.609
  |hip *see* Corrosion, thigh
  |thigh *see* Corrosion, thigh
  |third degree T24.709
|lung (with larynx and trachea) T27.5
|mouth T28.5
|neck T20.47
  |first degree T20.57
  |second degree T20.67
  |third degree T20.77
|nose (septum) T20.44
  |first degree T20.54
  |second degree T20.64
  |third degree T20.74
|ocular adnexa *see* Corrosion, eye
|orbit region *see* Corrosion, eyelid
|palm T23.459
  |first degree T23.559
  |left T23.452
   |first degree T23.552
   |second degree T23.652
   |third degree T23.752
  |right T23.451
   |first degree T23.551
   |second degree T23.651
   |third degree T23.751
  |second degree T23.659
  |third degree T23.759
|partial thickness   code as Corrosion,
  unspecified degree, by site
|pelvis *see* Corrosion, trunk
|penis *see* Corrosion, genital organs, external,
  male
|perineum
  |female *see* Corrosion, genital organs,
   external, female
  |male *see* Corrosion, genital organs, external,
   male
|periocular area *see* Corrosion, eyelid
|pharynx T28.5
|rectum T28.7
|respiratory tract T27.7
  |larynx *see* Corrosion, larynx
  |specified part NEC T27.6
  |trachea *see* Corrosion, larynx
|sac, lacrimal *see* Corrosion, eye, specified site
  NEC
|scalp T20.45
  |first degree T20.55
  |second degree T20.65
  |third degree T20.75
|scapular region T22.469
  |first degree T22.569
  |left T22.462
   |first degree T22.562
   |second degree T22.662
   |third degree T22.762
  |right T22.461
   |first degree T22.561
   |second degree T22.661
   |third degree T22.761
  |second degree T22.669
  |third degree T22.769
|sclera *see* Corrosion, eye, specified site NEC

Corrosion - *continued*

|scrotum *see* Corrosion, genital organs,
  external, male
|shoulder T22.459
  |first degree T22.559
  |left T22.452
    |first degree T22.552
    |second degree T22.652
    |third degree T22.752
  |right T22.451
    |first degree T22.551
    |second degree T22.651
    |third degree T22.751
  |second degree T22.659
  |third degree T22.759
|stomach T28.7
|temple *see* Corrosion, head
|testis *see* Corrosion, genital organs, external,
  male
|thigh T24.419
  |first degree T24.519
  |left T24.412
    |first degree T24.512
    |second degree T24.612
    |third degree T24.712
  |right T24.411
    |first degree T24.511
    |second degree T24.611
    |third degree T24.711
  |second degree T24.619
  |third degree T24.719
|thorax (external) *see* Corrosion, trunk
|throat (meaning pharynx) T28.5
|thumb(s) T23.419
  |first degree T23.519
  |left T23.412
    |first degree T23.512
    |second degree T23.612
    |third degree T23.712
  |multiple sites with fingers T23.449
    |first degree T23.549
    |left T23.442
      |first degree T23.542
      |second degree T23.642
      |third degree T23.742
    |right T23.441
      |first degree T23.541
      |second degree T23.641
      |third degree T23.741
    |second degree T23.649
    |third degree T23.749
  |right T23.411
    |first degree T23.511
    |second degree T23.611
    |third degree T23.711
  |second degree T23.619
  |third degree T23.719
|toe T25.439
  |first degree T25.539
  |left T25.432
    |first degree T25.532
    |second degree T25.632
    |third degree T25.732
  |right T25.431
    |first degree T25.531
    |second degree T25.631
    |third degree T25.731
  |second degree T25.639
  |third degree T25.739
|tongue T28.5
|tonsil(s) T28.5
|total body *see* Corrosion, multiple body
  regions
|trachea T27.4
  |with lung T27.5
|trunk T21.40

Corrosion - *continued*

|abdominal wall *see* Corrosion, abdominal
  wall
|anus *see* Corrosion, buttock
|axilla *see* Corrosion, upper limb
|back *see* Corrosion, back
|breast *see* Corrosion, chest wall
|buttock *see* Corrosion, buttock
|chest wall *see* Corrosion, chest wall
|first degree T21.50
|flank *see* Corrosion, abdominal wall
|genital
  |female *see* Corrosion, genital organs,
    external, female
  |male *see* Corrosion, genital organs,
    external, male
|groin *see* Corrosion, abdominal wall
|interscapular region *see* Corrosion, back,
  upper
|labia *see* Corrosion, genital organs, external,
  female
|lower back *see* Corrosion, back
|penis *see* Corrosion, genital organs,
  external, male
|perineum
  |female *see* Corrosion, genital organs,
    external, female
  |male *see* Corrosion, genital organs,
    external, male
|scapular region *see* Corrosion, upper limb
|scrotum *see* Corrosion, genital organs,
  external, male
|second degree T21.60
|shoulder *see* Corrosion, upper limb
|specified site NEC T21.49
  |first degree T21.59
  |second degree T21.69
  |third degree T21.79
|testes *see* Corrosion, genital organs,
  external, male
|third degree T21.70
|upper back *see* Corrosion, back, upper
|vagina T28.8
|vulva *see* Corrosion, genital organs,
  external, female
|unspecified site with extent of body surface
  involved specified
|less than 10 percent T32.0
|10-19 percent (0-9 percent third degree)
  T32.10
  |with 10-19 percent third degree T32.11
  |(0-9 percent third degree) T32.20
  |with
    |10-19 percent third degree T32.21
    |20-29 percent third degree T32.22
    |30-39 percent (0-9 percent third degree)
      T32.30
  |with
    |10-19 percent third degree T32.31
    |20-29 percent third degree T32.32
    |30-39 percent third degree T32.33
    |40-49 percent (0-9 percent third degree)
      T32.40
  |with
    |10-19 percent third degree T32.41
    |20-29 percent third degree T32.42
    |30-39 percent third degree T32.43
    |40-49 percent third degree T32.44
    |50-59 percent (0-9 percent third degree)
      T32.50
  |with
    |10-19 percent third degree T32.51
    |20-29 percent third degree T32.52
    |30-39 percent third degree T32.53
    |40-49 percent third degree T32.54
    |50-59 percent third degree T32.55

Corrosion - *continued*

  |60-69 percent (0-9 percent third degree)
    T32.60
  |with
    |10-19 percent third degree T32.61
    |20-29 percent third degree T32.62
    |30-39 percent third degree T32.63
    |40-49 percent third degree T32.64
    |50-59 percent third degree T32.65
    |60-69 percent third degree T32.66
    |70-79 percent (0-9 percent third degree)
      T32.70
  |with
    |10-19 percent third degree T32.71
    |20-29 percent third degree T32.72
    |30-39 percent third degree T32.73
    |40-49 percent third degree T32.74
    |50-59 percent third degree T32.75
    |60-69 percent third degree T32.76
    |70-79 percent third degree T32.77
    |80-89 percent (0-9 percent third degree)
      T32.80
  |with
    |10-19 percent third degree T32.81
    |20-29 percent third degree T32.82
    |30-39 percent third degree T32.83
    |40-49 percent third degree T32.84
    |50-59 percent third degree T32.85
    |60-69 percent third degree T32.86
    |70-79 percent third degree T32.87
    |80-89 percent third degree T32.88
    |90 percent or more (0-9 percent third
      degree) T32.90
  |with
    |10-19 percent third degree T32.91
    |20-29 percent third degree T32.92
    |30-39 percent third degree T32.93
    |40-49 percent third degree T32.94
    |50-59 percent third degree T32.95
    |60-69 percent third degree T32.96
    |70-79 percent third degree T32.97
    |80-89 percent third degree T32.98
    |90-99 percent third degree T32.99
|upper limb (axilla) (scapular region) T22.40
  |above elbow *see* Corrosion, above elbow
  |axilla *see* Corrosion, axilla
  |elbow *see* Corrosion, elbow
  |first degree T22.50
  |forearm *see* Corrosion, forearm
  |hand *see* Corrosion, hand
  |interscapular region *see* Corrosion, back,
    upper
  |multiple sites T22.499
    |first degree T22.599
    |left T22.492
      |first degree T22.592
      |second degree T22.692
      |third degree T22.792
    |right T22.491
      |first degree T22.591
      |second degree T22.691
      |third degree T22.791
    |second degree T22.699
    |third degree T22.799
  |scapular region *see* Corrosion, scapular
    region
  |second degree T22.60
  |shoulder *see* Corrosion, shoulder
  |third degree T22.70
  |wrist *see* Corrosion, hand
|uterus T28.8
|vagina T28.8
|vulva *see* Corrosion, genital organs, external,
  female
|wrist T23.479
  |first degree T23.579

Corrosion - *continued*
 |left T23.472
  |first degree T23.572
  |second degree T23.672
  |third degree T23.772
 |multiple sites with hand T23.499
  |first degree T23.599
  |left T23.492
   |first degree T23.592
   |second degree T23.692
   |third degree T23.792
  |right T23.491
   |first degree T23.591
   |second degree T23.691
   |third degree T23.791
  |second degree T23.699
  |third degree T23.799
 |right T23.471
  |first degree T23.571
  |second degree T23.671
  |third degree T23.771
 |second degree T23.679
 |third degree T23.779
Corrosive burn *see* Corrosion
Corsican fever *see* Malaria
Cortical *see* condition
Cortico-Adrenal *see* condition
Coryza (acute) J00
 |with grippe or influenza *see* Influenza, with,
  respiratory manifestations NEC
 |syphilitic
  |congenital (chronic) A50.05
Costen's syndrome or complex M26.69
Costiveness *see* Constipation
Costochondritis M94.0
Cotard's syndrome F22
Cot death R99
Cotia virus B08.8
Cotton wool spots (retinal) H35.81
Cotugno's disease *see* Sciatica
Cough (affected)(epidemic)(nervous) R05.9
 |with hemorrhage *see* Hemoptysis
 |acute R05.1
 |bronchial R05.8
  |with grippe or influenza *see* Influenza, with,
   respiratory manifestations NEC
 |functional F45.8
 |hysterical F45.8
 |laryngeal, spasmodic R05.8
 |paroxysmal, due to Bordetella pertussis
  (without pneumonia) A37.00
  |with pneumonia A37.01
 |persistent R05.3
 |psychogenic F45.8
 |refractory R05.3
 |smokers' J41.0
 |specified NEC R05.8
 |subacute R05.2
 |syncope R05.4
 |tea taster's B49
 |unexplained R05.3
Counseling (for) Z71.9
 |abuse NEC
  |perpetrator Z69.82
  |victim Z69.81
 |alcohol abuser Z71.41
  |family Z71.42
 |child abuse
  |nonparental
   |perpetrator Z69.021
   |victim Z69.020
  |parental
   |perpetrator Z69.011
   |victim Z69.010
 |consanguinity Z71.89
 |contraceptive Z30.09

Counseling - *continued*
 |dietary Z71.3
 |drug abuser Z71.51
  |family member Z71.52
 |exercise Z71.82
 |family Z71.89
 |fertility preservation (prior to cancer therapy)
  (prior to removal of gonads) Z31.62
 |for non-attending third party Z71.0
  |related to sexual behavior or orientation
   Z70.2
 |genetic
  |nonprocreative Z71.83
  |procreative NEC Z31.5
 |gestational carrier Z31.7
 |health (advice) (education) (instruction) *see*
  Counseling, medical
 |human immunodeficiency virus (HIV) Z71.7
 |impotence Z70.1
 |immunization safety Z71.85
 |insulin pump use Z46.81
 |medical (for) Z71.9
  |boarding school resident Z59.3
  |consanguinity Z71.89
  |feared complaint and no disease found
   Z71.1
  |human immunodeficiency virus (HIV)
   Z71.7
  |institutional resident Z59.3
  |on behalf of another Z71.0
   |related to sexual behavior or orientation
    Z70.2
  |person living alone Z60.2
  |specified reason NEC Z71.89
 |natural family planning
  |procreative Z31.61
  |to avoid pregnancy Z30.02
 |perpetrator (of)
  |abuse NEC Z69.82
  |child abuse
   |non-parental Z69.021
   |parental Z69.011
  |rape NEC Z69.82
  |spousal abuse Z69.12
 |procreative NEC Z31.69
  |fertility preservation (prior to cancer
   therapy) (prior to removal of gonads)
   Z31.62
  |using natural family planning Z31.61
 |promiscuity Z70.1
 |rape victim Z69.81
 |religious Z71.81
 |sex, sexual (related to) Z70.9
  |attitude(s) Z70.0
  |behavior or orientation Z70.1
  |combined concerns Z70.3
  |non-responsiveness Z70.1
  |on behalf of third party Z70.2
  |specified reason NEC Z70.8
 |specified reason NEC Z71.89
 |spiritual Z71.81
 |spousal abuse (perpetrator) Z69.12
  |victim Z69.11
 |substance abuse Z71.89
  |alcohol Z71.41
  |drug Z71.51
  |tobacco Z71.6
 |tobacco use Z71.6
 |use (of)
  |insulin pump Z46.81
 |vaccine product safety Z71.85
 |victim (of)
  |abuse Z69.81
  |child abuse
   |by parent Z69.010
   |non-parental Z69.020
  |rape NEC Z69.81

Coupled rhythm R00.8
**Couvelaire syndrome or uterus (complicating
 delivery)** O45.8X-
COVID-19 U07.1
 |condition post U09.9
 |contact (with) Z20.822
 |exposure (to) Z20.822
 |history of (personal) Z86.16
 |long (haul) U09.9
 |pneumonia J12.82
 |screening Z11.52
 |sequelae (post acute) U09.9
Cowperitis *see* Urethritis
Cowper's gland *see* condition
Cowpox B08.010
 |due to vaccination T88.1
Coxa
 |magna M91.4-
 |plana M91.2-
 |valga (acquired) *see also* Deformity, limb,
  specified type NEC, thigh
  |congenital Q65.81
  |sequelae (late effect) of rickets E64.3
 |vara (acquired) *see also* Deformity, limb,
  specified type NEC, thigh
  |congenital Q65.82
  |sequelae (late effect) of rickets E64.3
Coxalgia, coxalgic (nontuberculous) *see also*
 Pain, joint, hip
 |tuberculous A18.02
Coxitis *see* Monoarthritis, hip
Coxsackie (virus) (infection) B34.1
 |as cause of disease classified elsewhere
  B97.11
 |carditis B33.20
 |central nervous system NEC A88.8
 |endocarditis B33.21
 |enteritis A08.39
 |meningitis (aseptic) A87.0
 |myocarditis B33.22
 |pericarditis B33.23
 |pharyngitis B08.5
 |pleurodynia B33.0
 |specific disease NEC B33.8
Crabs, meaning pubic lice B85.3
Crack baby P04.41
Cracked nipple N64.0
 |associated with
  |lactation O92.13
  |pregnancy O92.11-
  |puerperium O92.12
Cracked tooth K03.81
Cradle cap L21.0
Craft neurosis F48.8
Cramp(s) R25.2
 |abdominal *see* Pain, abdominal
 |bathing T75.1
 |colic R10.83
  |psychogenic F45.8
 |due to immersion T75.1
 |fireman T67.2
 |heat T67.2
 |immersion T75.1
 |intestinal *see* Pain, abdominal
  |psychogenic F45.8
 |leg, sleep related G47.62
 |limb (lower) (upper) NEC R25.2
  |sleep related G47.62
 |linotypist's F48.8
  |organic G25.89
 |muscle (limb) (general) R25.2
  |due to immersion T75.1
  |psychogenic F45.8
 |occupational (hand) F48.8
  |organic G25.89
 |salt-depletion E87.1

Cramp(s) - continued
 |sleep related, leg G47.62
 |stoker's T67.2
 |swimmer's T75.1
 |telegrapher's F48.8
  |organic G25.89
 |typist's F48.8
  |organic G25.89
 |uterus N94.89
  |menstrual *see* Dysmenorrhea
 |writer's F48.8
  |organic G25.89
Cranial *see* condition
Craniocleidodysostosis Q74.0
Craniofenestria (skull) Q75.8
Craniolacunia (skull) Q75.8
Craniopagus Q89.4
Craniopathy, metabolic M85.2
Craniopharyngeal *see* condition
Craniopharyngioma D44.4
Craniorachischisis (totalis) Q00.1
Cranioschisis Q75.8
Craniostenosis Q75.0
Craniosynostosis Q75.0
Craniotabes (cause unknown) M83.8
 |neonatal P96.3
 |rachitic E64.3
 |syphilitic A50.56
Cranium *see* condition
Craw-Craw *see* Onchocerciasis
Creaking joint *see* Derangement, joint,
  specified type NEC
Creeping
 |eruption B76.9
 |palsy or paralysis G12.22
Crenated tongue K14.8
Creotoxism A05.9
Crepitus
 |caput Q75.8
 |joint *see* Derangement, joint, specified type
  NEC
Crescent or conus choroid, congenital Q14.3
CREST syndrome M34.1
Cretin, cretinism (congenital) (endemic)
  (nongoitrous) (sporadic) E00.9
 |pelvis
  |with disproportion (fetopelvic) O33.0
   |causing obstructed labor O65.0
 |type
  |hypothyroid E00.1
  |mixed E00.2
  |myxedematous E00.1
  |neurological E00.0
Creutzfeldt-Jakob disease or syndrome (with
  dementia) A81.00
 |familial A81.09
 |iatrogenic A81.09
 |specified NEC A81.09
 |sporadic A81.09
 |variant (vCJD) A81.01
Crib death R99
Cribriform hymen Q52.3
Cri-Du-Chat syndrome Q93.4
Crigler Najjar disease or syndrome E80.5
Crime, victim of Z65.4
Crimean hemorrhagic fever A98.0
Criminalism F60.2
Crisis
 |abdomen R10.0
 |acute reaction F43.0
 |addisonian E27.2
 |adrenal (cortical) E27.2
 |celiac K90.0
 |Dietl's N13.8
 |emotional *see also* Disorder, adjustment

Crisis - *continued*
  |acute reaction to stress F43.0
  |specific to childhood and adolescence F93.8
 |glaucomatocyclitic *see* Glaucoma, secondary,
  inflammation
 |heart *see* Failure, heart
 |nitritoid I95.2
  |correct substance properly administered *see*
   Table of Drugs and Chemicals, by drug,
   adverse effect
  |overdose or wrong substance given or taken
   see Table of Drugs and Chemicals, by
   drug, poisoning
 |oculogyric H51.8
  |psychogenic F45.8
 |Pel's (tabetic) A52.11
 |psychosexual identity F64.2
 |renal N28.0
 |sickle-cell D57.00
  |with
   |acute chest syndrome D57.01
   |cerebral vascular involvement D57.03
   |crisis (painful) D57.00
    |with complication specified NEC
     D57.09
   |splenic sequestration D57.02
   |vasoocclusive pain D57.00
 |state (acute reaction) F43.0
 |tabetic A52.11
 |thyroid *see* Thyrotoxicosis with thyroid storm
 |thyrotoxic *see* Thyrotoxicosis with thyroid
  storm
Crocq's disease (acrocyanosis) I73.89
Crohn's disease *see* Enteritis, regional
Crooked septum, nasal J34.2
Cross syndrome E70.328
Crossbite (anterior) (posterior) M26.24
Cross-Eye *see* Strabismus, convergent
  concomitant
Croup, croupous (catarrhal) (infectious)
  (inflammatory) (non diphtheritic) J05.0
 |bronchial J20.9
 |diphtheritic A36.2
 |false J38.5
 |spasmodic J38.5
  |diphtheritic A36.2
 |stridulous J38.5
  |diphtheritic A36.2
Crouzon's disease Q75.1
Crowding, tooth, teeth, fully erupted M26.31
CRST syndrome M34.1
Cruchet's disease A85.8
Cruelty in children *see also* Disorder, conduct
Crural ulcer *see* Ulcer, lower limb
Crush, crushed, crushing T14.8
 |abdomen S38.1
 |ankle S97.0-
 |arm (upper) (and shoulder) S47.
  |axilla *see* Crush, arm
 |back, lower S38.1
 |buttock S38.1
 |cheek S07.0
 |chest S28.0
 |cranium S07.1
 |ear S07.0
 |elbow S57.0-
 |extremity
  |lower
   |ankle *see* Crush, ankle
   |below knee *see* Crush, leg
   |foot *see* Crush, foot
   |hip *see* Crush, hip
   |knee *see* Crush, knee
   |thigh *see* Crush, thigh
   |toe *see* Crush, toe
  |upper

Crush - *continued*
  |below elbow S67.9-
  |elbow *see* Crush, elbow
  |finger *see* Crush, finger
  |forearm *see* Crush, forearm
  |hand *see* Crush, hand
  |thumb *see* Crush, thumb
  |upper arm *see* Crush, arm
  |wrist *see* Crush, wrist
 |face S07.0
 |finger(s) S67.1-
  |with hand (and wrist) *see* Crush, hand,
   specified site NEC
  |index S67.19-
  |little S67.19-
  |middle S67.19-
  |ring S67.19-
  |thumb *see* Crush, thumb
 |foot S97.8-
  |toe *see* Crush, toe
 |forearm S57.8-
 |genitalia, external
  |female S38.002
   |vagina S38.03
   |vulva S38.03
  |male S38.001
   |penis S38.01
   |scrotum S38.02
   |testis S38.02
 |hand (except fingers alone) S67.2-
  |with wrist S67.4-
 |head S07.9
  |specified NEC S07.8
 |heel *see* Crush, foot
 |hip S77.0-
  |with thigh S77.2-
 |internal organ (abdomen, chest, or pelvis)
  NEC T14.8
 |knee S87.0-
 |labium (majus) (minus) S38.03
 |larynx S17.0
 |leg (lower) S87.8-
  |knee *see* Crush, knee
 |lip S07.0
 |lower
  |back S38.1
  |leg *see* Crush, leg
 |neck S17.9
 |nerve *see* Injury, nerve
 |nose S07.0
 |pelvis S38.1
 |penis S38.01
 |scalp S07.8
 |scapular region *see* Crush, arm
 |scrotum S38.02
 |severe, unspecified site T14.8
 |shoulder (and upper arm) *see* Crush, arm
 |skull S07.1
 |syndrome (complication of trauma) T79.5
 |testis S38.02
 |thigh S77.1-
  |with hip S77.2-
 |throat S17.8
 |thumb S67.0-
  |with hand (and wrist) *see* Crush, hand,
   specified site NEC
 |toe(s) S97.10-
  |great S97.11-
  |lesser S97.12-
 |trachea S17.0
 |vagina S38.03
 |vulva S38.03
 |wrist S67.3-
  |with hand S67.4-
Crusta lactea L21.0
Crusts R23.4

Crutch paralysis *see* Injury, brachial plexus
Cruveilhier-Baumgarten cirrhosis, disease or **syndrome** K74.69
Cruveilhier's atrophy or disease G12.8
Crying (constant) (continuous) (excessive)
|child, adolescent, or adult R45.83
|infant (baby) (newborn) R68.11
Cryofibrinogenemia D89.2
Cryoglobulinemia (essential) (idiopathic) **(mixed) (primary) (purpura) (secondary)** **(vasculitis)** D89.1
|with lung involvement D89.1 [*J99*]
Cryptitis (anal) (rectal) K62.89
Cryptococcosis, cryptococcus (infection) **(neoformans)** B45.9
|bone B45.3
|cerebral B45.1
|cutaneous B45.2
|disseminated B45.7
|generalized B45.7
|meningitis B45.1
|meningocerebralis B45.1
|osseous B45.3
|pulmonary B45.0
|skin B45.2
|specified NEC B45.8
Cryptopapillitis (anus) K62.89
Cryptophthalmos Q11.2
|syndrome Q87.0
Cryptorchid, cryptorchism, cryptorchidism Q53.9
|bilateral Q53.20
|abdominal Q53.211
|perineal Q53.22
|unilateral Q53.10
|abdominal Q53.111
|perineal Q53.12
Cryptosporidiosis A07.2
|hepatobiliary B88.8
|respiratory B88.8
Cryptostromosis J67.6
Crystalluria R82.998
Cubitus
|congenital Q68.8
|valgus (acquired) M21.0-
|congenital Q68.8
|sequelae (late effect) of rickets E64.3
|varus (acquired) M21.1-
|congenital Q68.8
|sequelae (late effect) of rickets E64.3
Cultural deprivation or shock Z60.3
Curling esophagus K22.4
Curling's ulcer *see* Ulcer, peptic, acute
Curschmann (-Batten) (-Steinert) disease or **syndrome** G71.11
Curse, Ondine's *see* Apnea, sleep
Curvature
|organ or site, congenital NEC *see* Distortion
|penis (lateral) Q55.61
|Pott's (spinal) A18.01
|radius, idiopathic, progressive (congenital) Q74.0
|spine (acquired) (angular) (idiopathic) (incorrect) (postural) *see* Dorsopathy, deforming
|congenital Q67.5
|due to or associated with
|Charcot-Marie-Tooth disease *see also* subcategory M49.8 G60.0
|osteitis
|deformans M88.88
|fibrosa cystica *see also* subcategory M49.8 E21.0
|tuberculosis (Pott's curvature) A18.01
|sequelae (late effect) of rickets E64.3
|tuberculous A18.01

Cushingoid due to steroid therapy E24.2
|correct substance properly administered *see* Table of Drugs and Chemicals, by drug, adverse effect
|overdose or wrong substance given or taken *see* Table of Drugs and Chemicals, by drug, poisoning
Cushing's
|syndrome or disease E24.9
|drug-induced E24.2
|iatrogenic E24.2
|pituitary-dependent E24.0
|specified NEC E24.8
|ulcer *see* Ulcer, peptic, acute
Cusp, Carabelli omit code
Cut (external) *see also* Laceration
|muscle *see* Injury, muscle
Cutaneous *see also* condition
|hemorrhage R23.3
|larva migrans B76.9
Cutis *see also* condition
|hyperelastica Q82.8
|acquired L57.4
|laxa (hyperelastica) *see* Dermatolysis
|marmorata R23.8
|osteosis L94.2
|pendula *see* Dermatolysis
|rhomboidalis nuchae L57.2
|verticis gyrata Q82.8
|acquired L91.8
Cyanosis R23.0
|due to
|patent foramen botalli Q21.1
|persistent foramen ovale Q21.1
|enterogenous D74.8
|paroxysmal digital *see* Raynaud's disease
|with gangrene I73.01
|retina, retinal H35.89
Cyanotic heart disease I24.9
|congenital Q24.9
Cycle
|anovulatory N97.0
|menstrual, irregular N92.6
Cyclencephaly Q04.9
Cyclical vomiting *see also* Vomiting, cyclical G43.A0
|psychogenic F50.89
Cyclitis *see also* Iridocyclitis H20.9
|chronic *see* Iridocyclitis, chronic
|Fuchs' heterochromic H20.81-
|granulomatous *see* Iridocyclitis, chronic
|lens-induced *see* Iridocyclitis, lens-induced
|posterior H30.2-
Cycloid personality F34.0
Cyclophoria H50.54
Cyclopia, cyclops Q87.0
Cyclopism Q87.0
Cyclosporiasis A07.4
Cyclothymia F34.0
Cyclothymic personality F34.0
Cyclotropia H50.41-
Cylindroma *see also* Neoplasm, malignant, by site
|eccrine dermal *see* Neoplasm, skin, benign
|skin *see* Neoplasm, skin, benign
Cylindruria R82.998
Cynanche
|diphtheritic A36.2
|tonsillaris J36
Cynophobia F40.218
Cynorexia R63.2
Cyphosis *see* Kyphosis
Cyprus fever *see* Brucellosis
Cyst (colloid) (mucous) (simple) (retention)
|adenoid (infected) J35.8
|adrenal gland E27.8

Cyst - *continued*
|congenital Q89.1
|air, lung J98.4
|allantoic Q64.4
|alveolar process (jaw bone) M27.40
|amnion, amniotic O41.8X-
|aneurysmal M27.49
|anterior
|chamber (eye) *see* Cyst, iris
|nasopalatine K09.1
|antrum J34.1
|anus K62.89
|apical (tooth) (periodontal) K04.8
|appendix K38.8
|arachnoid, brain (acquired) G93.0
|congenital Q04.6
|arytenoid J38.7
|Baker's M71.2-
|ruptured M66.0
|tuberculous A18.02
|Bartholin's gland N75.0
|bile duct (common) (hepatic) K83.5
|bladder (multiple) (trigone) N32.89
|blue dome (breast) *see* Cyst, breast
|bone (local) NEC M85.60
|aneurysmal M85.50
|ankle M85.57-
|foot M85.57-
|forearm M85.53-
|hand M85.54-
|jaw M27.49
|lower leg M85.56-
|multiple site M85.59
|neck M85.58
|rib M85.58
|shoulder M85.51-
|skull M85.58
|specified site NEC M85.58
|thigh M85.55-
|toe M85.57-
|upper arm M85.52-
|vertebra M85.58
|solitary M85.40
|ankle M85.47-
|fibula M85.46-
|foot M85.47-
|hand M85.44-
|humerus M85.42-
|jaw M27.49
|neck M85.48
|pelvis M85.45-
|radius M85.43-
|rib M85.48
|shoulder M85.41-
|skull M85.48
|specified site NEC M85.48
|tibia M85.46-
|toe M85.47-
|ulna M85.43-
|vertebra M85.48
|specified type NEC M85.60
|ankle M85.67-
|foot M85.67-
|forearm M85.63-
|hand M85.64-
|jaw M27.40
|developmental (nonodontogenic) K09.1
|odontogenic K09.0
|latent M27.0
|lower leg M85.66-
|multiple site M85.69
|neck M85.68
|rib M85.68
|shoulder M85.61-
|skull M85.68
|specified site NEC M85.68

Cyst - *continued*

- |thigh M85.65-
- |toe M85.67-
- |upper arm M85.62-
- |vertebra M85.68
- |brain (acquired) G93.0
  - |congenital Q04.6
  - |hydatid B67.99 [*G94*]
  - |third ventricle (colloid), congenital Q04.6
- |branchial (cleft) Q18.0
- |branchiogenic Q18.0
- |breast (benign) (blue dome) (pedunculated) (solitary) N60.0-
  - |involution *see* Dysplasia, mammary, specified type NEC
  - |sebaceous *see* Dysplasia, mammary, specified type NEC
- |broad ligament (benign) N83.8
- |bronchogenic (mediastinal) (sequestration) J98.4
  - |congenital Q33.0
- |buccal K09.8
- |bulbourethral gland N36.8
- |bursa, bursal NEC M71.30
  - |with rupture *see* Rupture, synovium
  - |ankle M71.37-
  - |elbow M71.32-
  - |foot M71.37-
  - |hand M71.34-
  - |hip M71.35-
  - |multiple sites M71.39
  - |pharyngeal J39.2
  - |popliteal space *see* Cyst, Baker's
  - |shoulder M71.31-
  - |specified site NEC M71.38
  - |wrist M71.33-
- |calcifying odontogenic D16.5
  - |upper jaw (bone) (maxilla) D16.4
- |canal of Nuck (female) N94.89
  - |congenital Q52.4
- |canthus *see* Cyst, conjunctiva
- |carcinomatous *see* Neoplasm, malignant, by site
- |cauda equina G95.89
- |cavum septi pellucidi *see* Cyst, brain
- |celomic (pericardium) Q24.8
- |cerebellopontine (angle) *see* Cyst, brain
- |cerebellum *see* Cyst, brain
- |cerebral *see* Cyst, brain
- |cervical lateral Q18.0
- |cervix NEC N88.8
  - |embryonic Q51.6
  - |nabothian N88.8
- |chiasmal optic NEC *see* Disorder, optic, chiasm
- |chocolate (ovary) N80.1
- |choledochus, congenital Q44.4
- |chorion O41.8X-
- |choroid plexus G93.0
- |ciliary body *see* Cyst, iris
- |clitoris N90.7
- |colon K63.89
- |common (bile) duct K83.5
- |congenital NEC Q89.8
  - |adrenal gland Q89.1
  - |epiglottis Q31.8
  - |esophagus Q39.8
  - |fallopian tube Q50.4
  - |kidney Q61.00
    - |more than one (multiple) Q61.02
      - |specified as polycystic Q61.3
        - |adult type Q61.2
        - |infantile type NEC Q61.19
          - |collecting duct dilation Q61.11
    - |solitary Q61.01
  - |larynx Q31.8

Cyst - *continued*

- |liver Q44.6
- |lung Q33.0
- |mediastinum Q34.1
- |ovary Q50.1
- |oviduct Q50.4
- |periurethral (tissue) Q64.79
- |prepuce Q55.69
- |salivary gland (any) Q38.4
- |sublingual Q38.6
- |submaxillary gland Q38.6
- |thymus (gland) Q89.2
- |tongue Q38.3
- |ureterovesical orifice Q62.8
- |vulva Q52.79
- |conjunctiva H11.44-
- |cornea H18.89-
- |corpora quadrigemina G93.0
- |corpus
  - |albicans N83.29-
  - |luteum (hemorrhagic) (ruptured) N83.1-
- |Cowper's gland (benign) (infected) N36.8
- |cranial meninges G93.0
- |craniobuccal pouch E23.6
- |craniopharyngeal pouch E23.6
- |cystic duct K82.8
- |Cysticercus *see* Cysticercosis
- |Dandy-Walker Q03.1
  - |with spina bifida *see* Spina bifida
- |dental (root) K04.8
  - |developmental K09.0
  - |eruption K09.0
  - |primordial K09.0
- |dentigerous (mandible) (maxilla) K09.0
- |dermoid *see* Neoplasm, benign, by site
  - |with malignant transformation C56.-
  - |implantation
    - |external area or site (skin) NEC L72.0
    - |iris *see* Cyst, iris, implantation
    - |vagina N89.8
    - |vulva N90.7
  - |mouth K09.8
  - |oral soft tissue K09.8
  - |sacrococcygeal *see* Cyst, pilonidal
- |developmental K09.1
  - |odontogenic K09.0
  - |oral region (nonodontogenic) K09.1
  - |ovary, ovarian Q50.1
- |dura (cerebral) G93.0
  - |spinal G96.198
- |ear (external) Q18.1
- |echinococcal *see* Echinococcus
- |embryonic
  - |cervix uteri Q51.6
  - |fallopian tube Q50.4
  - |vagina Q52.4
- |endometrium, endometrial (uterus) N85.8
  - |ectopic *see* Endometriosis
- |enterogenous Q43.8
- |epidermal, epidermoid (inclusion) (*see also* Cyst, skin) L72.0
  - |mouth K09.8
  - |oral soft tissue K09.8
- |epididymis N50.3
- |epiglottis J38.7
- |epiphysis cerebri E34.8
- |epithelial (inclusion) L72.0
- |epoophoron Q50.5
- |eruption K09.0
- |esophagus K22.89
- |ethmoid sinus J34.1
- |external female genital organs NEC N90.7
- |eye NEC H57.89
  - |congenital Q15.8
- |eyelid (sebaceous) H02.829
  - |infected *see* Hordeolum

Cyst - *continued*

- |left H02.826
  - |lower H02.825
  - |upper H02.824
- |right H02.823
  - |lower H02.822
  - |upper H02.821
- |fallopian tube N83.8
  - |congenital Q50.4
- |fimbrial (twisted) Q50.4
- |fissural (oral region) K09.1
- |follicle (graafian) (hemorrhagic) N83.0-
  - |nabothian N88.8
- |follicular (atretic) (hemorrhagic) (ovarian) N83.0-
  - |dentigerous K09.0
  - |odontogenic K09.0
  - |skin L72.9
    - |specified NEC L72.8
- |frontal sinus J34.1
- |gallbladder K82.8
- |ganglion *see* Ganglion
- |Gartner's duct Q52.4
- |gingiva K09.0
- |gland of Moll *see* Cyst, eyelid
- |globulomaxillary K09.1
- |graafian follicle (hemorrhagic) N83.0-
- |granulosal lutein (hemorrhagic) N83.1-
- |hemangiomatous D18.00
  - |intra-abdominal D18.03
  - |intracranial D18.02
  - |skin D18.01
  - |specified site NEC D18.09
- |hemorrhagic M27.49
- |hydatid *see also* Echinococcus B67.90
  - |brain B67.99 [*G94*]
  - |liver *see also* Cyst, liver, hydatid B67.8
  - |lung NEC B67.99 [*J99*]
  - |Morgagni
    - |female Q50.5
    - |male (epididymal) Q55.4
      - |testicular Q55.29
  - |specified site NEC B67.99
- |hymen N89.8
  - |embryonic Q52.4
- |hypopharynx J39.2
- |hypophysis, hypophyseal (duct) (recurrent) E23.6
  - |cerebri E23.6
- |implantation (dermoid)
  - |external area or site (skin) NEC L72.0
  - |iris *see* Cyst, iris, implantation
  - |vagina N89.8
  - |vulva N90.7
- |incisive canal K09.1
- |inclusion (epidermal) (epithelial) (epidermoid) (squamous) L72.0
  - |not of skin   code under Cyst, by site
- |intestine (large) (small) K63.89
- |intracranial *see* Cyst, brain
- |intraligamentous *see also* Disorder, ligament
  - |knee *see* Derangement, knee
- |intrasellar E23.6
- |iris H21.309
  - |exudative H21.31-
  - |idiopathic H21.30-
  - |implantation H21.32-
  - |parasitic H21.33-
  - |pars plana (primary) H21.34-
    - |exudative H21.35-
- |jaw (bone) M27.40
  - |aneurysmal M27.49
  - |hemorrhagic M27.49
  - |traumatic M27.49
  - |developmental (odontogenic) K09.0
  - |fissural K09.1

Cyst - *continued*

|joint NEC *see* Disorder, joint, specified type
　NEC
|kidney (acquired) N28.1
　|calyceal *see* Hydronephrosis
　|congenital Q61.00
　|more than one (multiple) Q61.02
　　|specified as polycystic Q61.3
　　　|adult type (autosomal dominant) Q61.2
　　　|infantile type (autosomal recessive)
　　　　NEC Q61.19
　　　|collecting duct dilation Q61.11
　|pyelogenic *see* Hydronephrosis
　|simple N28.1
　|solitary (single) Q61.01
　　|acquired N28.1
|labium (majus) (minus) N90.7
　|sebaceous N90.7
|lacrimal *see also* Disorder, lacrimal system,
　　specified NEC
　|gland H04.13-
　|passages or sac *see* Disorder, lacrimal
　　system, specified NEC
|larynx J38.7
|lateral periodontal K09.0
|lens H27.8
　|congenital Q12.8
|lip (gland) K13.0
|liver (idiopathic) (simple) K76.89
　|congenital Q44.6
　|hydatid B67.8
　　|granulosus B67.0
　　|multilocularis B67.5
|lung J98.4
　|congenital Q33.0
　|giant bullous J43.9
|lutein N83.1-
|lymphangiomatous D18.1
|lymphoepithelial, oral soft tissue K09.8
|macula *see* Degeneration, macula, hole
|malignant *see* Neoplasm, malignant, by site
|mammary gland *see* Cyst, breast
|mandible M27.40
　|dentigerous K09.0
　|radicular K04.8
|maxilla M27.40
　|dentigerous K09.0
　|radicular K04.8
|medial, face and neck Q18.8
|median
　|anterior maxillary K09.1
　|palatal K09.1
|mediastinum, congenital Q34.1
|meibomian (gland) *see* Chalazion
　|infected *see* Hordeolum
|membrane, brain G93.0
|meninges (cerebral) G93.0
　|spinal G96.198
|meniscus, knee *see* Derangement, knee,
　　meniscus, cystic
|mesentery, mesenteric K66.8
　|chyle I89.8
|mesonephric duct
　|female Q50.5
　|male Q55.4
|milk N64.89
|Morgagni (hydatid)
　|female Q50.5
　|male (epididymal) Q55.4
　　|testicular Q55.29
|mouth K09.8
|Müllerian duct Q50.4
　|appendix testis Q55.29
　|cervix Q51.6
　|fallopian tube Q50.4
　|female Q50.4

Cyst - *continued*

|male Q55.29
　|prostatic utricle Q55.4
　|vagina (embryonal) Q52.4
|multilocular (ovary) D39.10
　|benign *see* Neoplasm, benign, by site
|myometrium N85.8
|nabothian (follicle) (ruptured) N88.8
|nasoalveolar K09.1
|nasolabial K09.1
|nasopalatine (anterior) (duct) K09.1
|nasopharynx J39.2
|neoplastic *see* Neoplasm, uncertain behavior,
　　by site
　|benign *see* Neoplasm, benign, by site
|nerve root
　|cervical G96.191
　|lumbar G96.191
　|sacral G96.191
　|thoracic G96.191
|nervous system NEC G96.89
|neuroenteric (congenital) Q06.8
|nipple *see* Cyst, breast
|nose (turbinates) J34.1
　|sinus J34.1
|odontogenic, developmental K09.0
|omentum (lesser) K66.8
　|congenital Q45.8
|ora serrata *see* Cyst, retina, ora serrata
|oral
　|region K09.9
　　|developmental (nonodontogenic) K09.1
　　|specified NEC K09.8
　|soft tissue K09.9
　　|specified NEC K09.8
|orbit H05.81-
|ovary, ovarian (twisted) N83.20-
　|adherent N83.20-
　|chocolate N80.1
　|corpus
　　|albicans N83.29-
　　|luteum (hemorrhagic) N83.1-
　|dermoid D27.9
　|developmental Q50.1
　|due to failure of involution NEC N83.20-
　|endometrial N80.1
　|follicular (graafian) (hemorrhagic) N83.0-
　|hemorrhagic N83.20-
　|in pregnancy or childbirth O34.8-
　　|with obstructed labor O65.5
　|multilocular D39.10
　|pseudomucinous D27.9
　|retention N83.29-
　|serous N83.20-
　|specified NEC N83.29-
　|theca lutein (hemorrhagic) N83.1-
　|tuberculous A18.18
|oviduct N83.8
|palate (median) (fissural) K09.1
|palatine papilla (jaw) K09.1
|pancreas, pancreatic (hemorrhagic) (true)
　　K86.2
　|congenital Q45.2
　|false K86.3
|paralabral
　|hip M24.85-
　|shoulder S43.43-
|paramesonephric duct Q50.4
　|female Q50.4
　|male Q55.29
|paranephric N28.1
|paraphysis, cerebri, congenital Q04.6
|parasitic B89
|parathyroid (gland) E21.4
|paratubal N83.8
|paraurethral duct N36.8

Cyst - *continued*

|paroophoron Q50.5
|parotid gland K11.6
|parovarian Q50.5
|pelvis, female N94.89
　|in pregnancy or childbirth O34.8-
　　|causing obstructed labor O65.5
|penis (sebaceous) N48.89
|periapical K04.8
|pericardial (congenital) Q24.8
　|acquired (secondary) I31.8
|pericoronal K09.0
|periodontal K04.8
　|lateral K09.0
|perineural G96.191
|peripelvic (lymphatic) N28.1
|peritoneum K66.8
　|chylous I89.8
|periventricular, acquired, newborn P91.1
|pharynx (wall) J39.2
|pilar L72.11
|pilonidal (infected) (rectum) L05.91
　|with abscess L05.01
　|malignant C44.59-
|pituitary (duct) (gland) E23.6
|placenta O43.19-
|pleura J94.8
|popliteal *see* Cyst, Baker's
|porencephalic Q04.6
　|acquired G93.0
|postanal (infected) *see* Cyst, pilonidal
|postmastoidectomy cavity (mucosal) *see*
　　Complications, postmastoidectomy, cyst
|preauricular Q18.1
|prepuce N47.4
　|congenital Q55.69
|primordial (jaw) K09.0
|prostate N42.83
|pseudomucinous (ovary) D27.9
|pupillary, miotic H21.27-
|radicular (residual) K04.8
|radiculodental K04.8
|ranular K11.8
|Rathke's pouch E23.6
|rectum (epithelium) (mucous) K62.89
|renal *see* Cyst, kidney
|residual (radicular) K04.8
|retention (ovary) N83.29-
　|salivary gland K11.6
|retina H33.19-
　|ora serrata H33.11-
　|parasitic H33.12-
|retroperitoneal K68.9
|sacrococcygeal (dermoid) *see* Cyst, pilonidal
|salivary gland or duct (mucous extravasation
　　or retention) K11.6
|Sampson's N80.1
|sclera H15.89
|scrotum L72.9
　|sebaceous L72.3
|sebaceous (duct) (gland) L72.3
　|breast *see* Dysplasia, mammary, specified
　　type NEC
　|eyelid *see* Cyst, eyelid
　|genital organ NEC
　　|female N94.89
　　|male N50.89
　|scrotum L72.3
|semilunar cartilage (knee) (multiple) *see*
　　Derangement, knee, meniscus, cystic
|seminal vesicle N50.89
|serous (ovary) N83.20-
|sinus (accessory) (nasal) J34.1
|Skene's gland N36.8
|skin L72.9

Cyst - *continued*

|breast *see* Dysplasia, mammary, specified
    type NEC
|epidermal, epidermoid L72.0
|epithelial L72.0
|eyelid *see* Cyst, eyelid
|genital organ NEC
  |female N90.7
  |male N50.89
|inclusion L72.0
|scrotum L72.9
|sebaceous L72.3
|sweat gland or duct L74.8
|solitary
  |bone *see* Cyst, bone, solitary
  |jaw M27.40
  |kidney N28.1
|spermatic cord N50.89
|sphenoid sinus J34.1
|spinal meninges G96.198
|spleen NEC D73.4
  |congenital Q89.09
  |hydatid *see also* Echinococcus B67.99
    [D77]
|Stafne's M27.0
|subarachnoid intrasellar R93.0
|subcutaneous, pheomycotic (chromomycotic)
  B43.2
|subdural (cerebral) G93.0
  |spinal cord G96.198
|sublingual gland K11.6
|submandibular gland K11.6
|submaxillary gland K11.6
|suburethral N36.8
|suprarenal gland E27.8
|suprasellar *see* Cyst, brain
|sweat gland or duct L74.8
|synovial *see also* Cyst, bursa
  |ruptured *see* Rupture, synovium
|Tarlov G96.191
|tarsal *see* Chalazion
|tendon (sheath) *see* Disorder, tendon,
  specified type NEC
|testis N44.2
  |tunica albuginea N44.1
|theca lutein (ovary) N83.1-
|Thornwaldt's J39.2
|thymus (gland) E32.8
|thyroglossal duct (infected) (persistent) Q89.2
|thyrolingual duct (infected) (persistent) Q89.2
|thyroid (gland) E04.1
|tongue K14.8
|tonsil J35.8
|tooth *see* Cyst, dental
|Tornwaldt's J39.2
|trichilemmal (proliferating) L72.12
|trichodermal L72.12
|tubal (fallopian) N83.8
  |inflammatory *see* Salpingitis, chronic
|tubo-ovarian N83.8
  |inflammatory N70.13
|tunica
  |albuginea testis N44.1
  |vaginalis N50.89
|turbinate (nose) J34.1
|Tyson's gland N48.89
|urachus, congenital Q64.4
|ureter N28.89
|ureterovesical orifice N28.89
|urethra, urethral (gland) N36.8
|uterine ligament N83.8
|uterus (body) (corpus) (recurrent) N85.8
  |embryonic Q51.818
  |cervix Q51.6
|vagina, vaginal (implantation) (inclusion)
  (squamous cell) (wall) N89.8

Cyst - *continued*

|embryonic Q52.4
|vallecula, vallecular (epiglottis) J38.7
|vesical (orifice) N32.89
|vitreous body H43.89
|vulva (implantation) (inclusion) N90.7
  |congenital Q52.79
  |sebaceous gland N90.7
|vulvovaginal gland N90.7
|wolffian
  |female Q50.5
  |male Q55.4

Cystadenocarcinoma *see* Neoplasm, malignant,
  by site

|bile duct C22.1
|endometrioid *see* Neoplasm, malignant, by
  site
  |specified site *see* Neoplasm, malignant, by
    site
  |unspecified site
    |female C56.9
    |male C61
|mucinous
  |papillary
    |specified site *see* Neoplasm, malignant, by
      site
    |unspecified site C56.9
  |specified site *see* Neoplasm, malignant, by
    site
  |unspecified site C56.9
|papillary
  |mucinous
    |specified site *see* Neoplasm, malignant, by
      site
    |unspecified site C56.9
  |pseudomucinous
    |specified site *see* Neoplasm, malignant, by
      site
    |unspecified site C56.9
  |serous
    |specified site *see* Neoplasm, malignant, by
      site
    |unspecified site C56.9
  |specified site *see* Neoplasm, malignant, by
    site
  |unspecified site C56.9
|pseudomucinous
  |papillary
    |specified site *see* Neoplasm, malignant, by
      site
    |unspecified site C56.9
  |specified site *see* Neoplasm, malignant, by
    site
  |unspecified site C56.9
|serous
  |papillary
    |specified site *see* Neoplasm, malignant, by
      site
    |unspecified site C56.9
  |specified site *see* Neoplasm, malignant, by
    site
  |unspecified site C56.9

Cystadenofibroma

|clear cell *see* Neoplasm, benign, by site
|endometrioid D27.9
  |borderline malignancy D39.1-
  |malignant C56.-
|mucinous
  |specified site *see* Neoplasm, benign, by site
  |unspecified site D27.9
|serous
  |specified site *see* Neoplasm, benign, by site
  |unspecified site D27.9
|specified site *see* Neoplasm, benign, by site
|unspecified site D27.9

Cystadenoma *see also* Neoplasm, benign, by
  site

|bile duct D13.4
|endometrioid *see* Neoplasm, benign, by site
  |borderline malignancy *see* Neoplasm,
    uncertain behavior, by site
  |malignant *see* Neoplasm, malignant, by site
|mucinous
  |borderline malignancy
    |ovary C56.-
    |specified site NEC *see* Neoplasm,
      uncertain behavior, by site
    |unspecified site C56.9
  |papillary
    |borderline malignancy
      |ovary C56.-
      |specified site NEC *see* Neoplasm,
        uncertain behavior, by site
      |unspecified site C56.9
    |specified site *see* Neoplasm, benign, by
      site
    |unspecified site D27.9
  |specified site *see* Neoplasm, benign, by site
  |unspecified site D27.9
|papillary
  |borderline malignancy
    |ovary C56.-
    |specified site NEC *see* Neoplasm,
      uncertain behavior, by site
    |unspecified site C56.9
  |lymphomatosum
    |specified site *see* Neoplasm, benign, by
      site
    |unspecified site D11.9
  |mucinous
    |borderline malignancy
      |ovary C56.-
      |specified site NEC *see* Neoplasm,
        uncertain behavior, by site
      |unspecified site C56.9
    |specified site *see* Neoplasm, benign, by
      site
    |unspecified site D27.9
  |pseudomucinous
    |borderline malignancy
      |ovary C56.-
      |specified site NEC *see* Neoplasm,
        uncertain behavior, by site
      |unspecified site C56.9
    |specified site *see* Neoplasm, benign, by
      site
    |unspecified site D27.9
  |serous
    |borderline malignancy
      |ovary C56.-
      |specified site NEC *see* Neoplasm,
        uncertain behavior, by site
      |unspecified site C56.9
    |specified site *see* Neoplasm, benign, by
      site
    |unspecified site D27.9
  |specified site *see* Neoplasm, benign, by site
  |unspecified site D27.9
|pseudomucinous
  |borderline malignancy
    |ovary C56.-
    |specified site NEC *see* Neoplasm,
      uncertain behavior, by site
    |unspecified site C56.9
  |papillary
    |borderline malignancy
      |ovary C56.-
      |specified site NEC *see* Neoplasm,
        uncertain behavior, by site
      |unspecified site C56.9

Cystadenoma - *continued*
  |specified site *see* Neoplasm, benign, by site
  |unspecified site D27.9
 |specified site *see* Neoplasm, benign, by site
 |unspecified site D27.9
 |serous
  |borderline malignancy
   |ovary C56.-
   |specified site NEC *see* Neoplasm, uncertain behavior, by site
   |unspecified site C56.9
  |papillary
   |borderline malignancy
    |ovary C56.-
    |specified site NEC *see* Neoplasm, uncertain behavior, by site
    |unspecified site C56.9
   |specified site *see* Neoplasm, benign, by site
   |unspecified site D27.9
  |specified site *see* Neoplasm, benign, by site
  |unspecified site D27.9
Cystathionine synthase deficiency E72.11
Cystathioninemia E72.19
Cystathioninuria E72.19
Cystic *see also* condition
 |breast (chronic) *see* Mastopathy, cystic
 |corpora lutea (hemorrhagic) N83.1-
 |duct *see* condition
 |eyeball (congenital) Q11.0
 |fibrosis *see* Fibrosis, cystic
 |kidney (congenital) Q61.9
  |adult type Q61.2
  |infantile type NEC Q61.19
   |collecting duct dilatation Q61.11
  |medullary Q61.5
 |liver, congenital Q44.6
 |lung disease J98.4
  |congenital Q33.0
 |mastitis, chronic *see* Mastopathy, cystic
 |medullary, kidney Q61.5
 |meniscus *see* Derangement, knee, meniscus, cystic
 |ovary N83.20-
Cysticercosis, cysticerciasis B69.9
 |with
  |epileptiform fits B69.0
  |myositis B69.81
 |brain B69.0
 |central nervous system B69.0
 |cerebral B69.0
 |ocular B69.1
 |specified NEC B69.89
Cysticercus cellulose infestation *see* Cysticercosis
Cystinosis (malignant) E72.04
Cystinuria E72.01
Cystitis (exudative) (hemorrhagic) (septic) (suppurative) N30.90
 |with
  |fibrosis *see* Cystitis, chronic, interstitial
  |hematuria N30.91
  |leukoplakia *see* Cystitis, chronic, interstitial
  |malakoplakia *see* Cystitis, chronic, interstitial
  |metaplasia *see* Cystitis, chronic, interstitial
  |prostatitis N41.3
 |acute N30.00
  |with hematuria N30.01
  |of trigone N30.30
   |with hematuria N30.31
 |allergic *see* Cystitis, specified type NEC
 |amebic A06.81
 |bilharzial B65.9 *[N33]*
 |blennorrhagic (gonococcal) A54.01
 |bullous *see* Cystitis, specified type NEC
 |calculous N21.0

Cystitis - *continued*
 |chlamydial A56.01
 |chronic N30.20
  |with hematuria N30.21
  |interstitial N30.10
   |with hematuria N30.11
  |of trigone N30.30
   |with hematuria N30.31
  |specified NEC N30.20
   |with hematuria N30.21
 |cystic (a) *see* Cystitis, specified type NEC
 |diphtheritic A36.85
 |echinococcal
  |granulosus B67.39
  |multilocularis B67.69
 |emphysematous *see* Cystitis, specified type NEC
 |encysted *see* Cystitis, specified type NEC
 |eosinophilic *see* Cystitis, specified type NEC
 |follicular *see* Cystitis, of trigone
 |gangrenous *see* Cystitis, specified type NEC
 |glandularis *see* Cystitis, specified type NEC
 |gonococcal A54.01
 |incrusted *see* Cystitis, specified type NEC
 |interstitial (chronic) *see* Cystitis, chronic, interstitial
 |irradiation N30.40
  |with hematuria N30.41
 |irritation *see* Cystitis, specified type NEC
 |malignant *see* Cystitis, specified type NEC
 |of trigone N30.30
  |with hematuria N30.31
 |panmural *see* Cystitis, chronic, interstitial
 |polyposa *see* Cystitis, specified type NEC
 |prostatic N41.3
 |puerperal (postpartum) O86.22
 |radiation *see* Cystitis, irradiation
 |specified type NEC N30.80
  |with hematuria N30.81
 |subacute *see* Cystitis, chronic
 |submucous *see* Cystitis, chronic, interstitial
 |syphilitic (late) A52.76
 |trichomonal A59.03
 |tuberculous A18.12
 |ulcerative *see* Cystitis, chronic, interstitial
Cystocele (-Urethrocele)
 |female N81.10
  |with prolapse of uterus *see* Prolapse, uterus
  |lateral N81.12
  |midline N81.11
  |paravaginal N81.12
 |in pregnancy or childbirth O34.8-
  |causing obstructed labor O65.5
 |male N32.89
Cystolithiasis N21.0
Cystoma *see also* Neoplasm, benign, by site
 |endometrial, ovary N80.1
 |mucinous
  |specified site *see* Neoplasm, benign, by site
  |unspecified site D27.9
 |serous
  |specified site *see* Neoplasm, benign, by site
  |unspecified site D27.9
 |simple (ovary) N83.29-
Cystoplegia N31.2
Cystoptosis N32.89
Cystopyelitis *see* Pyelonephritis
Cystorrhagia N32.89
Cystosarcoma phyllodes D48.6-
 |benign D24-
 |malignant *see* Neoplasm, breast, malignant
Cystostomy
 |attention to Z43.5
 |complication *see* Complications, cystostomy
 |status Z93.50
  |appendico-vesicostomy Z93.52
  |cutaneous Z93.51
  |specified NEC Z93.59

Cystourethritis *see* Urethritis
Cystourethrocele *see also* Cystocele
 |female N81.10
  |with uterine prolapse *see* Prolapse, uterus
  |lateral N81.12
  |midline N81.11
  |paravaginal N81.12
 |male N32.89
Cytomegalic inclusion disease
 |congenital P35.1
Cytomegalovirus infection B25.9
Cytomycosis (reticuloendothelial) B39.4
Cytopenia D75.9
 |refractory
  |with multilineage dysplasia D46.A
   |and ring sideroblasts (RCMD RS) D46.B
Czerny's disease (periodic hydrarthrosis of the knee) *see* Effusion, joint, knee

D

Daae (-Finsen) disease (epidemic pleurodynia) B33.0
Da Costa's syndrome F45.8
Dabney's grip B33.0
Dacryoadenitis, dacryadenitis H04.00-
 |acute H04.01-
 |chronic H04.02-
Dacryocystitis H04.30-
 |acute H04.32-
 |chronic H04.41-
 |neonatal P39.1
 |phlegmonous H04.31-
 |syphilitic A52.71
  |congenital (early) A50.01
 |trachomatous, active A71.1
  |sequelae (late effect) B94.0
Dacryocystoblennorrhea *see* Inflammation, lacrimal, passages, chronic
Dacryocystocele *see* Disorder, lacrimal system, changes
Dacryolith, dacryolithiasis H04.51-
Dacryoma *see* Disorder, lacrimal system, changes
Dacryopericystitis *see* Dacryocystitis
Dacryops H04.11-
Dacryostenosis *see also* Stenosis, lacrimal
 |congenital Q10.5
Dactylitis
 |bone *see* Osteomyelitis
 |sickle-cell D57.00
  |Hb C D57.219
  |Hb SS D57.00
  |specified NEC D57.819
 |skin L08.9
 |syphilitic A52.77
 |tuberculous A18.03
Dactylolysis spontanea (ainhum) L94.6
Dactylosymphysis Q70.9
 |fingers *see* Syndactylism, complex, fingers
 |toes *see* Syndactylism, complex, toes
Damage
 |arteriosclerotic *see* Arteriosclerosis
 |brain (nontraumatic) G93.9
  |anoxic, hypoxic G93.1
   |resulting from a procedure G97.82
  |child NEC G80.9
  |due to birth injury P11.2
 |cardiorenal (vascular) *see* Hypertension, cardiorenal
 |cerebral NEC *see* Damage, brain
 |coccyx, complicating delivery O71.6
 |coronary *see* Disease, heart, ischemic
 |eye, birth injury P15.3
 |liver (nontraumatic) K76.9
  |alcoholic K70.9

DEF

Damage - *continued*
| due to drugs *see* Disease, liver, toxic
| toxic *see* Disease, liver, toxic
| lung
| | dabbing (related) U07.0
| | electronic cigarette (related) U07.0
| | vaping (associated) (device) (product) (use)
| | | U07.0
| medication T88.7
| organ
| | dabbing (related) U07.0
| | electronic cigarette (related) U07.0
| | vaping (associated) (device) (product) (use)
| | | U07.0
| pelvic
| | joint or ligament, during delivery O71.6
| | organ NEC
| | | during delivery O71.5
| | | following ectopic or molar pregnancy
| | | | O08.6
| renal *see* Disease, renal
| subendocardium, subendocardial *see*
| | Degeneration, myocardial
| vascular I99.9
Dana-Putnam syndrome (subacute combined
sclerosis with pernicious anemia) *see*
Degeneration, combined
Danbolt (-Cross) syndrome (acrodermatitis
enteropathica) E83.2
Dandruff L21.0
Dandy-Walker syndrome Q03.1
| with spina bifida *see* Spina bifida
Danlos' syndrome Q79.6
Darier (-White) disease (congenital) Q82.8
| meaning erythema annulare centrifugum
| | L53.1
Darier-Roussy sarcoid D86.3
Darling's disease or histoplasmosis B39.4
Darwin's tubercle Q17.8
Dawson's (inclusion body) encephalitis A81.1
De Beurmanni (-Gougerot) disease B42.1
De la Tourette's syndrome F95.2
De Lange's syndrome Q87.1
De Morgan's spots (senile angiomas) I78.1
De Quervain's
| disease (tendon sheath) M65.4
| syndrome E34.51
| thyroiditis (subacute granulomatous
| | thyroiditis) E06.1
De Toni-Fanconi (-Debre) syndrome E72.09
| with cystinosis E72.04
Dead
| fetus, retained (mother) O36.4
| | early pregnancy O02.1
| labyrinth *see* subcategory H83.2
| ovum, retained O02.0
Deaf nonspeaking NEC H91.3
Deafmutism (acquired) (congenital) NEC
H91.3
| hysterical F44.6
| syphilitic, congenital *see also* subcategory
| | H94.8 A50.09
Deafness (acquired) (complete) (hereditary)
(partial) H91.9-
| with blue sclera and fragility of bone Q78.0
| auditory fatigue *see* Deafness, specified type
| | NEC
| aviation T70.0
| | nerve injury *see* Injury, nerve, acoustic,
| | specified type NEC
| boilermaker's *see* subcategory H83.3
| central *see* Deafness, sensorineural
| conductive H90.2
| | and sensorineural
| | | mixed H90.8
| | | | bilateral H90.6

Deafness - *continued*
| | bilateral H90.0
| | unilateral H90.1-
| | | with restricted hearing on the contralateral
| | | | side H90.A
| congenital H90.5
| | with blue sclera and fragility of bone Q78.0
| due to toxic agents *see* Deafness, ototoxic
| emotional (hysterical) F44.6
| functional (hysterical) F44.6
| high frequency H91.9-
| hysterical F44.6
| low frequency H91.9-
| mental R48.8
| mixed conductive and sensorineural H90.8
| | bilateral H90.6
| | unilateral H90.7-
| nerve *see* Deafness, sensorineural
| neural *see* Deafness, sensorineural
| noise-induced *see also* subcategory H83.3
| | nerve injury *see* Injury, nerve, acoustic,
| | specified type NEC
| nonspeaking H91.3
| ototoxic *see* subcategory H91.0
| perceptive *see* Deafness, sensorineural
| psychogenic (hysterical) F44.6
| sensorineural H90.5
| | and conductive
| | | mixed H90.8
| | | | bilateral H90.6
| | bilateral H90.3
| | unilateral H90.4-
| | | with restricted hearing on the contralateral
| | | | side H90.A
| sensory *see* Deafness, sensorineural
| specified type NEC *see* subcategory H91.8
| sudden (idiopathic) H91.2-
| syphilitic A52.15
| transient ischemic H93.01-
| | traumatic *see* Injury, nerve, acoustic,
| | specified type NEC
| word (developmental) H93.25
Death (cause unknown) (of) (unexplained)
(unspecified cause) R99
| brain G93.82
| cardiac (sudden) (with successful
| | resuscitation)   code to underlying disease
| | family history of Z82.41
| | personal history of Z86.74
| family member (assumed) Z63.4
Debility (chronic) (general) (nervous) R53.81
| congenital or neonatal NOS P96.9
| nervous R53.81
| old age R54
| senile R54
Debove's disease (splenomegaly) R16.1
Decalcification
| bone *see* Osteoporosis
| teeth K03.89
Decapsulation, kidney N28.89
Decay
| dental *see* Caries, dental
| senile R54
| tooth, teeth *see* Caries, dental
Deciduitis (acute)
| following ectopic or molar pregnancy O08.0
Decline (general) *see* Debility
| cognitive, age-associated R41.81
Decompensation
| cardiac (acute) (chronic) *see* Disease, heart
| cardiovascular *see* Disease, cardiovascular
| heart *see* Disease, heart
| hepatic *see* Failure, hepatic
| myocardial (acute) (chronic) *see* Disease,
| | heart
| respiratory J98.8

Decompression sickness T70.3
Decrease(d)
| absolute neutrophile count *see* Neutropenia
| blood
| | platelets *see* Thrombocytopenia
| | pressure R03.1
| | | due to shock following
| | | | injury T79.4
| | | | operation T81.19
| estrogen E28.39
| | postablative E89.40
| | | asymptomatic E89.40
| | | symptomatic E89.41
| fragility of erythrocytes D58.8
| function
| | lipase (pancreatic) K90.3
| | ovary in hypopituitarism E23.0
| | parenchyma of pancreas K86.89
| | pituitary (gland) (anterior) (lobe) E23.0
| | posterior (lobe) E23.0
| functional activity R68.89
| glucose R73.09
| hematocrit R71.0
| hemoglobin R71.0
| leukocytes D72.819
| | specified NEC D72.818
| libido R68.82
| lymphocytes D72.810
| platelets D69.6
| respiration, due to shock following injury
| | T79.4
| sexual desire R68.82
| tear secretion NEC *see* Syndrome, dry eye
| | tolerance
| | | fat K90.49
| | | glucose R73.09
| | | pancreatic K90.3
| | | salt and water E87.8
| vision NEC H54.7
| white blood cell count D72.819
| | specified NEC D72.818
Decubitus (ulcer) *see* Ulcer, pressure, by site
| cervix N86
Deepening acetabulum *see* Derangement, joint,
| specified type NEC, hip
Defect, defective Q89.9
| 3-beta-hydroxysteroid dehydrogenase E25.0
| 11-hydroxylase E25.0
| 21-hydroxylase E25.0
| abdominal wall, congenital Q79.59
| antibody immunodeficiency D80.9
| aorticopulmonary septum Q21.4
| atrial septal (ostium secundum type) Q21.1
| | following acute myocardial infarction
| | | (current complication) I23.1
| | ostium primum type Q21.2
| atrioventricular
| | canal Q21.2
| | septum Q21.2
| auricular septal Q21.1
| bilirubin excretion NEC E80.6
| biosynthesis, androgen (testicular) E29.1
| bulbar septum Q21.0
| catalase E80.3
| cell membrane receptor complex (CR3) D71
| circulation I99.9
| | congenital Q28.9
| | newborn Q28.9
| coagulation (factor) *see also* Deficiency,
| | factor D68.9
| | with
| | | ectopic pregnancy O08.1
| | | molar pregnancy O08.1
| | acquired D68.4

Defect, defective - *continued*
  |antepartum with hemorrhage *see*
      Hemorrhage, antepartum, with
      coagulation defect
  |due to
      |liver disease D68.4
      |vitamin K deficiency D68.4
  |hereditary NEC D68.2
  |intrapartum O67.0
  |newborn, transient P61.6
  |postpartum O99.13
      |with hemorrhage O72.3
  |specified type NEC D68.8
  |complement system D84.1
  |conduction (heart) I45.9
      |bone *see* Deafness, conductive
  |congenital, organ or site not listed *see*
      Anomaly, by site
  |coronary sinus Q21.1
  |cushion, endocardial Q21.2
  |degradation, glycoprotein E77.1
  |dental bridge, crown, fillings *see* Defect,
      dental restoration
  |dental restoration K08.50
      |specified NEC K08.59
  |dentin (hereditary) K00.5
  |Descemet's membrane, congenital Q13.89
  |developmental *see also* Anomaly
      |cauda equina Q06.3
  |diaphragm
      |with elevation, eventration or hernia *see*
          Hernia, diaphragm
      |congenital Q79.1
          |with hernia Q79.0
          |gross (with hernia) Q79.0
  |ectodermal, congenital Q82.9
  |Eisenmenger's Q21.8
  |enzyme
      |catalase E80.3
      |peroxidase E80.3
  |esophagus, congenital Q39.9
  |extensor retinaculum M62.89
  |fibrin polymerization D68.2
  |filling
      |bladder R93.41
      |kidney R93.42-
      |renal pelvis R93.41
      |stomach R93.3
      |ureter R93.41
      |urinary organs, specified NEC R93.49
  |GABA (gamma aminobutyric acid) metabolic
      E72.81
  |Gerbode Q21.0
  |glucose transport, blood-brain barrier E74.810
  |glycoprotein degradation E77.1
  |Hageman (factor) D68.2
  |hearing *see* Deafness
  |high grade F70
  |interatrial septal Q21.1
  |interauricular septal Q21.1
  |interventricular septal Q21.0
      |with dextroposition of aorta, pulmonary
          stenosis and hypertrophy of right ventricle
          Q21.3
      |in tetralogy of Fallot Q21.3
  |learning (specific) *see* Disorder, learning
  |lymphocyte function antigen 1 (LFA 1) D84.0
  |lysosomal enzyme, post-translational
      modification E77.0
  |major osseous M89.70
      |ankle M89.77-
      |carpus M89.74-
      |clavicle M89.71-
      |femur M89.75-
      |fibula M89.76-
      |fingers M89.74-

Defect, defective - *continued*
  |foot M89.77-
  |forearm M89.73-
  |hand M89.74-
  |humerus M89.72-
  |lower leg M89.76-
  |metacarpus M89.74-
  |metatarsus M89.77
  |multiple sites M89.79
  |pelvic region M89.75-
  |pelvis M89.75-
  |radius M89.73-
  |scapula M89.71-
  |shoulder region M89.71-
  |specified NEC M89.78
  |tarsus M89.77-
  |thigh M89.75-
  |tibia M89.76-
  |toes M89.77-
  |ulna M89.73-
  |mental *see* Disability, intellectual
  |modification, lysosomal enzymes, post-
      translational E77.0
  |obstructive, congenital
      |renal pelvis Q62.39
      |ureter Q62.39
          |atresia *see* Atresia, ureter
          |cecoureterocele Q62.32
          |megaureter Q62.2
          |orthotopic ureterocele Q62.31
  |osseous, major M89.70
      |ankle M89.77-
      |carpus M89.74-
      |clavicle M89.71-
      |femur M89.75-
      |fibula M89.76-
      |fingers M89.74-
      |foot M89.77-
      |forearm M89.73-
      |hand M89.74-
      |humerus M89.72-
      |lower leg M89.76-
      |metacarpus M89.74-
      |metatarsus M89.77-
      |multiple sites M89.9
      |pelvic region M89.75-
      |pelvis M89.75-
      |radius M89.73-
      |scapula M89.71-
      |shoulder region M89.71-
      |specified NEC M89.78
      |tarsus M89.77-
      |thigh M89.75-
      |tibia M89.76-
      |toes M89.77-
      |ulna M89.73-
  |osteochondral NEC *see also* Deformity M95.8
  |ostium
      |primum Q21.2
      |secundum Q21.1
  |peroxidase E80.3
  |placental blood supply *see* Insufficiency,
      placental
  |platelets, qualitative D69.1
      |constitutional D68.0
  |postural NEC, spine *see* Dorsopathy,
      deforming
  |reduction
      |limb Q73.8
          |lower Q72.9-
              |absence *see* Agenesis, leg
              |foot *see* Agenesis, foot
              |longitudinal
                  |femur Q72.4-
                  |fibula Q72.6-
                  |tibia Q72.5-

Defect, defective - *continued*
      |specified type NEC Q72.89-
      |split foot Q72.7-
  |specified type NEC Q73.8
  |upper Q71.9-
      |absence *see* Agenesis, arm
          |forearm *see* Agenesis, forearm
          |hand *see* Agenesis, hand
      |lobster-claw hand Q71.6-
      |longitudinal
          |radius Q71.4-
          |ulna Q71.5-
      |specified type NEC Q71.89-
  |renal pelvis Q63.8
      |obstructive Q62.39
  |respiratory system, congenital Q34.9
  |restoration, dental K08.50
      |specified NEC K08.59
  |retinal nerve bundle fibers H35.89
  |septal (heart) NOS Q21.9
      |acquired (atrial) (auricular) (ventricular)
          (old) I51.0
      |atrial Q21.1
          |concurrent with acute myocardial
              infarction *see* Infarct, myocardium
          |following acute myocardial infarction
              (current complication) I23.1
      |ventricular *see also* Defect, ventricular
          septal Q21.0
  |sinus venosus Q21.1
  |speech – *see* Disorder, speech
      |developmental F80.9
      |specified NEC R47.89
  |Taussig-Bing (aortic transposition and
      overriding pulmonary artery) Q20.1
  |teeth, wedge K03.1
  |vascular (local) I99.9
      |congenital Q27.9
  |ventricular septal Q21.0
      |concurrent with acute myocardial infarction
          see Infarct, myocardium
      |following acute myocardial infarction
          (current complication) I23.2
      |in tetralogy of Fallot Q21.3
  |vision NEC H54.7
  |visual field H53.40
      |bilateral
          |heteronymous H53.47
          |homonymous H53.46-
      |generalized contraction H53.48-
      |localized
          |arcuate H53.43-
          |scotoma (central area) H53.41-
              |blind spot area H53.42-
          |sector H53.43-
      |specified type NEC H53.45-
  |voice R49.9
      |specified NEC R49.8
  |wedge, tooth, teeth (abrasion) K03.1
Deferentitis N49.1
  |gonorrheal (acute) (chronic) A54.23
Defibrination (syndrome) D65
  |antepartum *see* Hemorrhage, antepartum, with
      coagulation defect, disseminated
      intravascular coagulation
  |following ectopic or molar pregnancy O08.1
  |intrapartum O67.0
  |newborn P60
  |postpartum O72.3
Deficiency, deficient
  |3-beta hydroxysteroid dehydrogenase E25.0
  |5-Alpha reductase (with male
      pseudohermaphroditism) E29.1
  |11-hydroxylase E25.0
  |21-hydroxylase E25.0

Deficiency, deficient - *continued*
- AADC (aromatic L-amino acid decarboxylase) E70.81
- abdominal muscle syndrome Q79.4
- accelerator globulin (Ac G) (blood) D68.2
- AC globulin (congenital) (hereditary) D68.2
  - acquired D68.4
- acid phosphatase E83.39
- acid sphingomyelinase (ASMD) E75.249
  - type
    - A E75.240
    - A/B E75.244
    - B E75.241
- activating factor (blood) D68.2
- adenosine deaminase (ADA) D81.3
- aldolase (hereditary) E74.19
- alpha 1-antitrypsin E88.01
- amino-acids E72.9
- anemia *see* Anemia
- aneurin E51.9
- antibody with
  - hyperimmunoglobulinemia D80.6
  - near-normal immunoglobins D80.6
- antidiuretic hormone E23.2
- anti-hemophilic
  - factor (A) D66
    - B D67
    - C D68.1
  - globulin (AHG) NEC D66
- antithrombin (antithrombin III) D68.59
- aromatic L-amino acid decarboxylase (AADC) E70.81
- ascorbic acid E54
- attention (disorder) (syndrome) F98.8
  - with hyperactivity *see* Disorder, attention-deficit hyperactivity
- autoprothrombin
  - I D68.2
  - II D67
  - C D68.2
- beta-glucuronidase E76.29
- biotin E53.8
- biotin-dependent carboxylase D81.819
- biotinidase D81.810
- brancher enzyme (amylopectinosis) E74.03
- calciferol E55.9
  - with
    - adult osteomalacia M83.8
    - rickets *see* Rickets
- calcium (dietary) E58
- calorie, severe E43
  - with marasmus E41
  - and kwashiorkor E42
- cardiac *see* Insufficiency, myocardial
- carnitine E71.40
  - due to
    - hemodialysis E71.43
    - inborn errors of metabolism E71.42
    - Valproic acid therapy E71.43
  - iatrogenic E71.43
  - muscle palmitoyltransferase E71.314
  - primary E71.41
  - secondary E71.448
- carotene E50.9
- central nervous system G96.89
- ceruloplasmin (Wilson) E83.01
- choline E53.8
- Christmas factor D67
- chromium E61.4
- chronic neurovisceral acid sphingomyelinase E75.244
- chronic visceral acid sphingomyelinase E75.241
- clotting (blood) *see also* Deficiency, coagulation factor D68.9

Deficiency, deficient - *continued*
- clotting factor NEC (hereditary) *see also* Deficiency, factor D68.2
- coagulation NOS D68.9
  - with
    - ectopic pregnancy O08.1
    - molar pregnancy O08.1
  - acquired (any) D68.4
  - antepartum hemorrhage *see* Hemorrhage, antepartum, with coagulation defect
  - clotting factor NEC *see also* Deficiency, factor D68.2
  - due to
    - hyperprothrombinemia D68.4
    - liver disease D68.4
    - vitamin K deficiency D68.4
  - newborn, transient P61.6
  - postpartum O72.3
  - specified NEC D68.8
- cognitive F09
- color vision H53.50
  - achromatopsia H53.51
  - acquired H53.52
  - deuteranomaly H53.53
  - protanomaly H53.54
  - specified type NEC H53.59
  - tritanomaly H53.55
- combined glucocorticoid and mineralocorticoid E27.49
- contact factor D68.2
- copper (nutritional) E61.0
- corticoadrenal E27.40
  - primary E27.1
- craniofacial axis Q75.0
- cyanocobalamin E53.8
- C1 esterase inhibitor (C1-INH) D84.1
- debrancher enzyme (limit dextrinosis) E74.03
- dehydrogenase
  - long chain/very long chain acyl CoA E71.310
  - medium chain acyl CoA E71.311
  - short chain acyl CoA E71.312
- diet E63.9
- dihydropyrimidine dehydrogenase (DPD) E88.89
- disaccharidase E73.9
- edema *see* Malnutrition, severe
- endocrine E34.9
- energy-supply *see* Malnutrition
- enzymes, circulating NEC E88.09
- ergosterol E55.9
  - with
    - adult osteomalacia M83.8
    - rickets *see* Rickets
- essential fatty acid (EFA) E63.0
- eye movements
  - saccadic H55.81
  - smooth pursuit H55.82
- factor *see also* Deficiency, coagulation
  - Hageman D68.2
  - I (congenital) (hereditary) D68.2
  - II (congenital) (hereditary) D68.2
  - IX (congenital) (functional) (hereditary) (with functional defect) D67
  - multiple (congenital) D68.8
    - acquired D68.4
  - V (congenital) (hereditary) D68.2
  - VII (congenital) (hereditary) D68.2
  - VIII (congenital) (functional) (hereditary) (with functional defect) D66
    - with vascular defect D68.0
  - X (congenital) (hereditary) D68.2
  - XI (congenital) (hereditary) D68.1
  - XII (congenital) (hereditary) D68.2
  - XIII (congenital) (hereditary) D68.2

Deficiency, deficient - *continued*
- femoral, proximal focal (congenital) *see* Defect, reduction, lower limb, longitudinal, femur
- fibrin-stabilizing factor (congenital) (hereditary) D68.2
  - acquired D68.4
- fibrinase D68.2
- fibrinogen (congenital) (hereditary) D68.2
  - acquired D65
- folate E53.8
- folic acid E53.8
- foreskin N47.3
- fructokinase E74.11
- fructose 1,6-diphosphatase E74.19
- fructose 1-phosphate aldolase E74.19
- galactokinase E74.29
- GABA (gamma aminobutyric acid) transaminase E72.81
- GABA-T (gamma aminobutyric acid transaminase) E72.81
- galactose 1-phosphate uridyl transferase E74.29
- gammaglobulin in blood D80.1
  - hereditary D80.0
- glass factor D68.2
- glucocorticoid E27.49
  - mineralocorticoid E27.49
- glucose 6-phosphatase E74.01
- glucose 6-phosphate dehydrogenase anemia D55.0
- glucose transporter protein type 1 E74.810
- glucuronyl transferase E80.5
- Glut1 E74.810
- glycogen synthetase E74.09
- gonadotropin (isolated) E23.0
- growth hormone (idiopathic) (isolated) E23.0
- Hageman factor D68.2
- hemoglobin D64.9
- hepatophosphorylase E74.09
- homogentisate 1,2-dioxygenase E70.29
- hormone
  - anterior pituitary (partial) NEC E23.0
    - growth E23.0
  - growth (isolated) E23.0
  - pituitary E23.0
  - testicular E29.1
- hypoxanthine (guanine)-phosphoribosyltransferase (HGPRT) (total H-PRT) E79.1
- immunity D84.9
  - cell-mediated D84.89
    - with thrombocytopenia and eczema D82.0
  - combined D81.9
  - humoral D80.9
  - IgA (secretory) D80.2
  - IgG D80.3
  - IgM D80.4
- immuno *see* Immunodeficiency
- immunoglobulin, selective
  - A (IgA) D80.2
  - G (IgG) (subclasses) D80.3
  - M (IgM) D80.4
- infantile neurovisceral acid sphingomyelinase E75.240
- inositol (B complex) E53.8
- intrinsic
  - factor (congenital) D51.0
  - sphincter N36.42
    - with urethral hypermobility N36.43
- iodine E61.8
  - congenital syndrome *see* Syndrome, iodine-deficiency, congenital
- iron E61.1
  - anemia D50.9
- kalium E87.6

Deficiency, deficient - *continued*
| kappa-light chain D80.8
| labile factor (congenital) (hereditary) D68.2
| | acquired D68.4
| lacrimal fluid (acquired) *see also* Syndrome, dry eye
| | congenital Q10.6
| | congenital E73.0
| | secondary E73.1
| lactase
| Laki-Lorand factor D68.2
| lecithin cholesterol acyltransferase E78.6
| lipocaic K86.89
| lipoprotein (familial) (high density) E78.6
| liver phosphorylase E74.09
| lysosomal alpha 1, 4 glucosidase E74.02
| magnesium E61.2
| major histocompatibility complex
| | class I D81.6
| | class II D81.7
| manganese E61.3
| menadione (vitamin K) E56.1
| | newborn P53
| mental (familial) (hereditary) *see* Disability, intellectual
| methylenetetrahydrofolate reductase (MTHFR) E72.12
| mevalonate kinase M04.1
| mineral NEC E61.8
| mineralocorticoid E27.49
| | with glucocorticoid E27.49
| molybdenum (nutritional) E61.5
| moral F60.2
| multiple nutrient elements E61.7
| multiple sulfatase (MSD) E75.26 muscle
| | carnitine (palmitoyltransferase) E71.314
| | phosphofructokinase E74.09
| myoadenylate deaminase E79.2
| myocardial *see* Insufficiency, myocardial
| myophosphorylase E74.04
| NADH diaphorase or reductase (congenital) D74.0
| NADH-methemoglobin reductase (congenital) D74.0
| natrium E87.1
| niacin (amide) (-tryptophan) E52
| nicotinamide E52
| nicotinic acid E52
| number of teeth *see* Anodontia
| nutrient element E61.9
| | multiple E61.7
| | specified NEC E61.8
| nutrition, nutritional E63.9
| | sequelae *see* Sequelae, nutritional deficiency
| | specified NEC E63.8
| of interleukin 1 receptor antagonist [DIRA] M04.8
| ornithine transcarbamylase E72.4
| ovarian E28.39
| oxygen *see* Anoxia
| pantothenic acid E53.8
| parathyroid (gland) E20.9
| perineum (female) N81.89
| phenylalanine hydroxylase E70.1
| phosphoenolpyruvate carboxykinase E74.4
| phosphofructokinase E74.19
| phosphomannomutase E74.818
| phosphomannose isomerase E74.818
| phosphomannosyl mutase E74.818
| phosphorylase kinase, liver E74.09
| pituitary hormone (isolated) E23.0
| plasma thromboplastin
| | antecedent (PTA) D68.1
| | component (PTC) D67
| plasminogen (type 1) (type 2) E88.02
| platelet NEC D69.1

Deficiency, deficient - *continued*
| | constitutional D68.0
| polyglandular E31.8
| | autoimmune E31.0
| potassium (K) E87.6
| prepuce N47.3
| proaccelerin (congenital) (hereditary) D68.2
| | acquired D68.4
| proconvertin factor (congenital) (hereditary) D68.2
| | acquired D68.4
| protein *see also* Malnutrition E46
| | anemia D53.0
| | C D68.59
| | S D68.59
| prothrombin (congenital) (hereditary) D68.2
| | acquired D68.4
| Prower factor D68.2
| pseudocholinesterase E88.09
| PTA (plasma thromboplastin antecedent) D68.1
| PTC (plasma thromboplastin component) D67
| purine nucleoside phosphorylase (PNP) D81.5
| pyracin (alpha) (beta) E53.1
| pyridoxal E53.1
| pyridoxamine E53.1
| pyridoxine (derivatives) E53.1
| pyruvate
| | carboxylase E74.4
| | dehydrogenase E74.4
| riboflavin (vitamin B2) E53.0
| salt E87.1
| secretion
| | ovary E28.39
| | salivary gland (any) K11.7
| | urine R34
| selenium (dietary) E59
| serum antitrypsin, familial E88.01
| short stature homeobox gene (SHOX)
| | with
| | dyschondrosteosis Q78.8
| | short stature (idiopathic) E34.3
| | Turner's syndrome Q96.9
| sodium (Na) E87.1
| SPCA (factor VII) D68.2
| sphincter, intrinsic N36.42
| | with urethral hypermobility N36.43
| stable factor (congenital) (hereditary) D68.2
| | acquired D68.4
| Stuart-Prower (factor X) D68.2
| succinic semialdehyde dehydrogenase E72.81
| sucrase E74.39
| sulfatase E75.26
| sulfite oxidase E72.19
| thiamin, thiaminic (chloride) E51.9
| | beriberi (dry) E51.11
| | wet E51.12
| thrombokinase D68.2
| | newborn P53
| thyroid (gland) *see* Hypothyroidism
| tocopherol E56.0
| tooth bud K00.0
| transcobalamine II (anemia) D51.2
| vanadium E61.6
| vascular I99.9
| vasopressin E23.2
| vertical ridge K06.8
| viosterol *see* Deficiency, calciferol
| vitamin (multiple) NOS E56.9
| | A E50.9
| | with
| | Bitot's spot (corneal) E50.1
| | follicular keratosis E50.8
| | keratomalacia E50.4
| | manifestations NEC E50.8
| | night blindness E50.5

Deficiency, deficient - *continued*
| | scar of cornea, xerophthalmic E50.6
| | xeroderma E50.8
| | xerophthalmia E50.7
| | xerosis
| | conjunctival E50.0
| | and Bitot's spot E50.1
| | cornea E50.2
| | and ulceration E50.3
| | sequelae E64.1
| B (complex) NOS E53.9
| | with
| | beriberi (dry) E51.11
| | wet E51.12
| | pellagra E52
| B1 NOS E51.9
| | beriberi (dry) E51.11
| | with circulatory system manifestations E51.11
| | wet E51.12
| B12 E53.8
| B2 (riboflavin) E53.0
| B6 E53.1
| C E54
| | sequelae E64.2
| D E55.9
| | with
| | adult osteomalacia M83.8
| | rickets *see* Rickets
| | 25-hydroxylase E83.32
| E E56.0
| folic acid E53.8
| G E53.0
| group B E53.9
| | specified NEC E53.8
| H (biotin) E53.8
| K E56.1
| | of newborn P53
| nicotinic E52
| P E56.8
| PP (pellagra-preventing) E52
| specified NEC E56.8
| thiamin E51.9
| | beriberi *see* Beriberi
| zinc, dietary E60

Deficit *see also* Deficiency
| attention and concentration R41.840
| | following
| | cerebral infarction I69.310
| | cerebrovascular disease I69.910
| | specified disease NEC I69.810
| | nontraumatic
| | intracerebral hemorrhage I69.110
| | specified intracranial hemorrhage NEC I69.210
| | subarachnoid hemorrhage I69.010
| | disorder *see* Attention, deficit
| cognitive
| communication R41.841
| emotional
| | following
| | cerebral infarction I69.315
| | cerebrovascular disease I69.915
| | specified disease NEC I69.815
| | nontraumatic
| | intracerebral hemorrhage I69.115
| | specified intracranial hemorrhage NEC I69.215
| | cerebral infarction I69.319
| | cerebrovascular disease I69.919
| | subarachnoid hemorrhage I69.015
| following
| | specified disease NEC I69.819
| nontraumatic
| | intracerebral hemorrhage I69.119

Deficit - *continued*
  |specified intracranial hemorrhage NEC
    I69.219
  |subarachnoid hemorrhage I69.019
|social
  |following
    |cerebral infarction I69.315
    |cerebrovascular disease I69.915
      |specified disease NEC I69.815
    |nontraumatic
      |intracerebral hemorrhage I69.115
      |specified intracranial hemorrhage
        NEC I69.215
      |subarachnoid hemorrhage I69.015
|cognitive NEC R41.89
  |following
    |cerebral infarction I69.318
    |cerebrovascular disease I69.918
      |specified disease NEC I69.818
    |nontraumatic
      |intracerebral hemorrhage I69.118
      |specified intracranial hemorrhage NEC
        I69.218
      |subarachnoid hemorrhage I69.018
|concentration R41.840
|executive function R41.844
  |following
    |cerebral infarction I69.314
    |cerebrovascular disease I69.914
      |specified disease NEC I69.814
    |nontraumatic
      |intracerebral hemorrhage I69.114
      |specified intracranial hemorrhage NEC
        I69.214
      |subarachnoid hemorrhage I69.014
|frontal lobe R41.844
  |following
    |cerebral infarction I69.314
    |cerebrovascular disease I69.914
      |specified disease NEC I69.814
    |nontraumatic
      |intracerebral hemorrhage I69.114
      |specified intracranial hemorrhage NEC
        I69.214
      |subarachnoid hemorrhage I69.014
|memory
  |following
    |cerebral infarction I69.311
    |cerebrovascular disease I69.911
      |specified disease NEC I69.811
    |nontraumatic
      |intracerebral hemorrhage I69.111
      |specified intracranial hemorrhage NEC
        I69.211
      |subarachnoid hemorrhage I69.011
|neurologic NEC R29.818
  |ischemic
    |reversible (RIND) I63.9
      |prolonged (PRIND) I63.9
|oxygen R09.02
|prolonged reversible ischemic neurologic
  (PRIND) I63.9
|psychomotor R41.843
  |following
    |cerebral infarction I69.313
    |cerebrovascular disease I69.913
      |specified disease NEC I69.813
    |nontraumatic
      |intracerebral hemorrhage I69.113
      |specified intracranial hemorrhage NEC
        I69.213
      |subarachnoid hemorrhage I69.013
|visuospatial R41.842
  |following
    |cerebral infarction I69.312
    |cerebrovascular disease I69.912

Deficit - *continued*
  |specified disease NEC I69.812
  |nontraumatic
    |intracerebral hemorrhage I69.112
    |specified intracranial hemorrhage NEC
      I69.212
    |subarachnoid hemorrhage I69.012
Deflection
|radius *see* Deformity, limb, specified type
  NEC, forearm
|septum (acquired) (nasal) (nose) J34.2
|spine *see* Curvature, spine
|turbinate (nose) J34.2
Defluvium
|capillorum *see* Alopecia
|ciliorum *see* Madarosis
|unguium L60.8
Deformity Q89.9
|abdomen, congenital Q89.9
|abdominal wall
  |acquired M95.8
  |congenital Q79.59
|acquired (unspecified site) M95.9
|adrenal gland Q89.1
|alimentary tract, congenital Q45.9
  |upper Q40.9
|ankle (joint) (acquired) *see also* Deformity,
  limb, lower leg
  |abduction *see* Contraction, joint, ankle
  |congenital Q68.8
  |contraction *see* Contraction, joint, ankle
  |specified type NEC *see* Deformity, limb,
    foot, specified NEC
|anus (acquired) K62.89
  |congenital Q43.9
|aorta (arch) (congenital) Q25.40
  |acquired I77.89
|aortic
  |arch, acquired I77.89
  |cusp or valve (congenital) Q23.8
    |acquired *see also* Endocarditis, aortic
      I35.8
|arm (acquired) (upper) *see also* Deformity,
  limb, upper arm
  |congenital Q68.8
  |forearm *see* Deformity, limb, forearm
|artery (congenital) (peripheral) NOS Q27.9
  |acquired I77.89
  |coronary (acquired) I25.9
    |congenital Q24.5
  |umbilical Q27.0
|atrial septal Q21.1
|auditory canal (external) (congenital) *see also*
  Malformation, ear, external
  |acquired *see* Disorder, ear, external,
    specified type NEC
|auricle
  |ear (congenital) *see also* Malformation, ear,
    external
    |acquired *see* Disorder, pinna, deformity
|bile duct (common) (congenital) (hepatic)
  Q44.5
|back *see* Dorsopathy, deforming
  |acquired K83.8
|biliary duct or passage (congenital) Q44.5
  |acquired K83.8
|bladder (neck) (trigone) (sphincter) (acquired)
  N32.89
  |congenital Q64.79
|bone (acquired) NOS M95.9
  |congenital Q79.9
  |turbinate M95.0
|brain (congenital) Q04.9
  |acquired G93.89
  |reduction Q04.3
|breast (acquired) N64.89

Deformity - *continued*
  |congenital Q83.9
  |reconstructed N65.0
|bronchus (congenital) Q32.4
  |acquired NEC J98.09
|bursa, congenital Q79.9
|canaliculi (lacrimalis) (acquired) *see also*
  Disorder, lacrimal system, changes
  |congenital Q10.6
|canthus, acquired *see* Disorder, eyelid,
  specified type NEC
|capillary (acquired) I78.8
|cardiovascular system, congenital Q28.9
|caruncle, lacrimal (acquired) *see also*
  Disorder, lacrimal system, changes
  |congenital Q10.6
|cascade, stomach K31.2
|cecum (congenital) Q43.9
  |acquired K63.89
|cerebral, acquired G93.89
  |congenital Q04.9
|cervix (uterus) (acquired) NEC N88.8
  |congenital Q51.9
|cheek (acquired) M95.2
  |congenital Q18.9
|chest (acquired) (wall) M95.4
  |congenital Q67.8
  |sequelae (late effect) of rickets E64.3
|chin (acquired) M95.2
  |congenital Q18.9
|choroid (congenital) Q14.3
  |acquired H31.8
  |plexus Q07.8
    |acquired G96.198
|cicatricial *see* Cicatrix
|cilia, acquired *see* Disorder, eyelid, specified
  type NEC
|clavicle (acquired) M95.8
  |congenital Q68.8
|clitoris (congenital) Q52.6
  |acquired N90.89
|clubfoot *see* Clubfoot
|coccyx (acquired) *see* subcategory M43.8
|colon (congenital) Q43.9
  |acquired K63.89
|concha (ear), congenital *see also*
  Malformation, ear, external
  |acquired *see* Disorder, pinna, deformity
|cornea (acquired) H18.70
  |congenital Q13.4
  |descemetocele *see* Descemetocele
  |ectasia *see* Ectasia, cornea
  |specified NEC H18.79-
  |staphyloma *see* Staphyloma, cornea
|coronary artery (acquired) I25.9
|cranium (acquired) *see* Deformity, skull
|cricoid cartilage (congenital) Q31.8
  |congenital Q24.5
  |acquired J38.7
|cystic duct (congenital) Q44.5
  |acquired K82.8
|Dandy-Walker Q03.1
  |with spina bifida *see* Spina bifida
|diaphragm (congenital) Q79.1
  |acquired J98.6
|digestive organ NOS Q45.9
|ductus arteriosus Q25.0
|duodenal bulb K31.89
|duodenum (congenital) Q43.9
  |acquired K31.89
|dura *see* Deformity, meninges
|ear (acquired) *see also* Disorder, pinna,
  deformity
  |congenital (external) Q17.9
    |internal Q16.5
    |middle Q16.4

Deformity - *continued*
    |ossicles Q16.3
    |ossicles Q16.3
|ectodermal (congenital) NEC Q84.9
|ejaculatory duct (congenital) Q55.4
  |acquired N50.89
|elbow (joint) (acquired) *see also* Deformity,
  limb, upper arm
  |congenital Q68.8
  |contraction *see* Contraction, joint, elbow
|endocrine gland NEC Q89.2
|epididymis (congenital) Q55.4
  |acquired N50.89
|epiglottis (congenital) Q31.8
  |acquired J38.7
|esophagus (congenital) Q39.9
  |acquired K22.89
|eustachian tube (congenital) NEC Q17.8
|eye, congenital Q15.9
|eyebrow (congenital) Q18.8
|eyelid (acquired) *see also* Disorder, eyelid,
  specified type NEC
  |congenital Q10.3
|face (acquired) M95.2
  |congenital Q18.9
|fallopian tube, acquired N83.8
|femur (acquired) *see* Deformity, limb,
  specified type NEC, thigh
|fetal
  |with fetopelvic disproportion O33.7
  |causing obstructed labor O66.3
|finger (acquired) M20.00-
  |boutonniere M20.02-
  |congenital Q68.1
  |flexion contracture *see* Contraction, joint,
    hand
  |mallet finger M20.01-
  |specified NEC M20.09-
  |swan-neck M20.03-
|flexion (joint) (acquired) *see also* Deformity,
  limb, flexion M21.20
  |congenital NOS Q74.9
    |hip Q65.89
|foot (acquired) *see also* Deformity, limb,
  lower leg
  |cavovarus (congenital) Q66.1
  |congenital NOS Q66.9
    |specified type NEC Q66.89
  |specified type NEC *see* Deformity, limb,
    foot, specified NEC
  |varus (congenital) NEC Q66.3
    |acquired *see* Deformity, varus, ankle
|forearm (acquired) *see also* Deformity, limb,
  forearm
  |congenital Q68.8
|forehead (acquired) M95.2
  |congenital Q75.8
|frontal bone (acquired) M95.2
  |congenital Q75.8
|gallbladder (congenital) Q44.1
  |acquired K82.8
|gastrointestinal tract (congenital) NOS Q45.9
  |acquired K63.89
|genitalia, genital organ(s) or system NEC
  |female (congenital) Q52.9
    |acquired N94.89
    |external Q52.70
  |male (congenital) Q55.9
    |acquired N50.89
|globe (eye) (congenital) Q15.8
  |acquired H44.89
|gum, acquired NEC K06.8
|hand (acquired) *see* Deformity, limb, hand
  |congenital Q68.1
|head (acquired) M95.2
  |congenital Q75.8

Deformity - *continued*
|heart (congenital) Q24.9
  |septum Q21.9
    |auricular Q21.1
    |ventricular Q21.0
  |valve (congenital) NEC Q24.8
    |acquired *see* Endocarditis
|heel (acquired) *see* Deformity, foot
|hepatic duct (congenital) Q44.5
  |acquired K83.8
|hip (joint) (acquired) *see also* Deformity,
  limb, thigh
  |congenital Q65.9
  |due to (previous) juvenile osteochondrosis
    see Coxa, plana
  |flexion *see* Contraction, joint, hip
|hourglass *see* Contraction, hourglass
|humerus (acquired) M21.82-
  |congenital Q74.0
|hypophyseal (congenital) Q89.2
|ileocecal (coil) (valve) (acquired) K63.89
  |congenital Q43.9
|ileum (congenital) Q43.9
  |acquired K63.89
|ilium (acquired) M95.5
  |congenital Q74.2
|integument (congenital) Q84.9
|intervertebral cartilage or disc (acquired) *see*
  Disorder, disc, specified NEC
|intestine (large) (small) (congenital) NOS
  Q43.9
  |acquired K63.89
|intrinsic minus or plus (hand) *see* Deformity,
  limb, specified type NEC, forearm
|iris (acquired) H21.89
  |congenital Q13.2
|ischium (acquired) M95.5
  |congenital Q74.2
|jaw (acquired) (congenital) M26.9
|joint (acquired) NEC M21.90
  |congenital Q68.8
  |elbow M21.92-
  |hand M21.94-
  |shoulder M21.92-
  |wrist M21.93-
  |hip M21.95-
  |knee M21.96-
|kidney(s) (calyx) (pelvis) (congenital) Q63.9
  |acquired N28.89
  |artery (congenital) Q27.2
    |acquired I77.89
|Klippel-Feil (brevicollis) Q76.1
|knee (acquired) NEC *see also* Deformity,
  limb, lower leg
  |congenital Q68.2
|labium (majus) (minus) (congenital) Q52.79
  |acquired N90.89
|lacrimal passages or duct (congenital) NEC
  Q10.6
  |acquired *see* Disorder, lacrimal system,
    changes
|larynx (muscle) (congenital) Q31.8
  |acquired J38.7
  |web (glottic) Q31.0
|leg (upper) (acquired) NEC *see also*
  Deformity, limb, thigh
  |congenital Q68.8
  |lower leg *see* Deformity, limb, lower leg
|lens (acquired) H27.8
  |congenital Q12.9
|lid (fold) (acquired) *see also* Disorder, eyelid,
  specified type NEC
  |congenital Q10.3
|ligament (acquired) *see* Disorder, ligament
  |congenital Q79.9
|limb (acquired) M21.90

Deformity - *continued*
|clawfoot M21.53-
|clawhand M21.51-
|clubfoot M21.54-
|clubhand M21.52-
|congenital, except reduction deformity
  Q74.9
|flat foot M21.4-
|flexion M21.20
  |ankle M21.27-
  |elbow M21.22-
  |finger M21.24-
  |hip M21.25-
  |knee M21.26-
  |shoulder M21.21-
  |toe M21.27-
  |wrist M21.23-
|foot
  |claw *see* Deformity, limb, clawfoot
  |club *see* Deformity, limb, clubfoot
  |drop M21.37-
  |flat *see* Deformity, limb, flat foot
  |specified NEC M21.6X-
|forearm M21.93-
|hand M21.94-
|lower leg M21.96-
|specified type NEC M21.80
  |forearm M21.83-
  |lower leg M21.86-
  |thigh M21.85-
  |upper arm M21.82-
|thigh M21.95-
|unequal length M21.70
  |short site is
    |femur M21.75-
    |fibula M21.76-
    |humerus M21.72-
    |radius M21.73-
|upper arm M21.92-
|valgus *see* Deformity, valgus
|varus *see* Deformity, varus
  |tibia M21.76-
  |ulna M21.73-
|wrist drop M21.33-
|lip (acquired) NEC K13.0
  |congenital Q38.0
|liver (congenital) Q44.7
  |acquired K76.89
|lumbosacral (congenital) (joint) (region)
  Q76.49
  |acquired *see* subcategory M43.8
  |kyphosis *see* Kyphosis, congenital
  |lordosis *see* Lordosis, congenital
|lung (congenital) Q33.9
  |acquired J98.4
|lymphatic system, congenital Q89.9
|Madelung's (radius) Q74.0
|mandible (acquired) (congenital) M26.9
|maxilla (acquired) (congenital) M26.9
|meninges or membrane (congenital) Q07.9
  |cerebral Q04.8
    |acquired G96.198
  |spinal cord (congenital) Q06.-
    |acquired G96.198
|metacarpus (acquired) *see* Deformity, limb,
  forearm
  |congenital Q74.0
|metatarsus (acquired) *see* Deformity, foot
  |congenital Q66.9
|middle ear (congenital) Q16.4
  |ossicles Q16.3
|mitral (leaflets) (valve) I05.8
  |parachute Q23.2
  |stenosis, congenital Q23.2
|mouth (acquired) K13.79
  |congenital Q38.6

Deformity - *continued*
- |multiple, congenital NEC Q89.7
- |muscle (acquired) M62.89
  - |congenital Q79.9
    - |sternocleidomastoid Q68.0
- |musculoskeletal system (acquired) M95.9
  - |congenital Q79.9
  - |specified NEC M95.8
- |nail (acquired) L60.8
  - |congenital Q84.6
- |nasal *see* Deformity, nose
- |neck (acquired) M95.3
  - |congenital Q18.9
    - |sternocleidomastoid Q68.0
- |nervous system (congenital) Q07.9
- |nipple (congenital) Q83.9
  - |acquired N64.89
- |nose (acquired) (cartilage) M95.0
  - |bone (turbinate) M95.0
  - |congenital Q30.9
    - |bent or squashed Q67.4
  - |saddle M95.0
    - |syphilitic A50.57
  - |septum (acquired) J34.2
    - |congenital Q30.8
  - |sinus (wall) (congenital) Q30.8
    - |acquired M95.0
  - |syphilitic (congenital) A50.57
    - |late A52.73
- |ocular muscle (congenital) Q10.3
  - |acquired *see* Strabismus, mechanical
- |opticociliary vessels (congenital) Q13.2
- |orbit (eye) (acquired) H05.30
  - |atrophy *see* Atrophy, orbit
  - |congenital Q10.7
  - |due to
    - |bone disease NEC H05.32-
    - |trauma or surgery H05.33-
  - |enlargement *see* Enlargement, orbit
  - |exostosis *see* Exostosis, orbit
- |organ of Corti (congenital) Q16.5
- |ovary (congenital) Q50.39
  - |acquired N83.8
- |oviduct, acquired N83.8
- |palate (congenital) Q38.5
  - |acquired M27.8
  - |cleft (congenital) *see* Cleft, palate
- |pancreas (congenital) Q45.3
  - |acquired K86.89
- |parathyroid (gland) Q89.2
- |parotid (gland) (congenital) Q38.4
  - |acquired K11.8
- |patella (acquired) *see* Disorder, patella, specified NEC
- |pelvis, pelvic (acquired) (bony) M95.5
  - |with disproportion (fetopelvic) O33.0
    - |causing obstructed labor O65.0
  - |congenital Q74.2
  - |rachitic sequelae (late effect) E64.3
- |penis (glans) (congenital) Q55.69
  - |acquired N48.89
- |pericardium (congenital) Q24.8
  - |acquired *see* Pericarditis
- |pharynx (congenital) Q38.8
  - |acquired J39.2
- |pinna, acquired *see also* Disorder, pinna, deformity
  - |congenital Q17.9
- |pituitary (congenital) Q89.2
- |posture *see* Dorsopathy, deforming
- |prepuce (congenital) Q55.69
  - |acquired N47.8
- |prostate (congenital) Q55.4
  - |acquired N42.89
- |pupil (congenital) Q13.2
  - |acquired *see* Abnormality, pupillary

Deformity - *continued*
- |pylorus (congenital) Q40.3
  - |acquired K31.89
- |rachitic (acquired), old or healed E64.3
- |radius (acquired) *see also* Deformity, limb, forearm
  - |congenital Q68.8
- |rectum (congenital) Q43.9
  - |acquired K62.89
- |reduction (extremity) (limb), congenital *see also* condition and site Q73.8
  - |brain Q04.3
  - |lower *see* Defect, reduction, lower limb
  - |upper *see* Defect, reduction, upper limb
- |renal *see* Deformity, kidney
- |respiratory system (congenital) Q34.9
- |rib (acquired) M95.4
  - |congenital Q76.6
  - |cervical Q76.5
- |rotation (joint) (acquired) *see* Deformity, limb, specified site NEC
  - |congenital Q74.9
  - |hip *see* Deformity, limb, specified type NEC, thigh
    - |congenital Q65.89
- |sacroiliac joint (congenital) Q74.2
  - |acquired *see* subcategory M43.8
- |sacrum (acquired) *see* subcategory M43.8
  - |nose M95.0
    - |syphilitic A50.57
- |saddle
  - |back *see* Lordosis
- |salivary gland or duct (congenital) Q38.4
  - |acquired K11.8
- |scapula (acquired) M95.8
  - |congenital Q68.8
- |scrotum (congenital) *see also* Malformation, testis and scrotum
  - |acquired N50.89
- |seminal vesicles (congenital) Q55.4
  - |acquired N50.89
- |septum, nasal (acquired) J34.2
- |shoulder (joint) (acquired) *see* Deformity, limb, upper arm
  - |congenital Q74.0
  - |contraction *see* Contraction, joint, shoulder
- |sigmoid (flexure) (congenital) Q43.9
  - |acquired K63.89
- |skin (congenital) Q82.9
- |skull (acquired) M95.2
  - |congenital Q75.8
    - |with
      - |anencephaly Q00.0
      - |encephalocele *see* Encephalocele
      - |hydrocephalus Q03.9
        - |with spina bifida *see* Spina bifida, by site, with hydrocephalus
      - |microcephaly Q02
- |soft parts, organs or tissues (of pelvis)
  - |in pregnancy or childbirth NEC O34.8-
    - |causing obstructed labor O65.5
- |spermatic cord (congenital) Q55.4
  - |acquired N50.89
  - |torsion *see* Torsion, spermatic cord
- |spinal *see* Dorsopathy, deforming
  - |column (acquired) *see* Dorsopathy, deforming
  - |congenital Q67.5
  - |cord (congenital) Q06.9
    - |acquired G95.89
  - |nerve root (congenital) Q07.9
- |spine (acquired) *see also* Dorsopathy, deforming
  - |congenital Q67.5
  - |rachitic E64.3

Deformity - *continued*
- |specified NEC *see* Dorsopathy, deforming, specified NEC
- |spleen
  - |acquired D73.89
  - |congenital Q89.09
- |Sprengel's (congenital) Q74.0
- |sternocleidomastoid (muscle), congenital Q68.0
- |sternum (acquired) M95.4
  - |congenital NEC Q76.7
- |stomach (congenital) Q40.3
  - |acquired K31.89
- |submandibular gland (congenital) Q38.4
- |submaxillary gland (congenital) Q38.4
  - |acquired K11.8
- |talipes *see* Talipes
- |testis (congenital) *see also* Malformation, testis and scrotum
  - |acquired N44.8
    - |torsion *see* Torsion, testis
- |thigh (acquired) *see also* Deformity, limb, thigh
  - |congenital NEC Q68.8
  - |sequelae of rickets E64.3
- |thumb (acquired) *see also* Deformity, finger
  - |congenital NEC Q68.1
- |thorax (acquired) (wall) M95.4
  - |congenital Q67.8
- |thymus (tissue) (congenital) Q89.2
- |thyroid (gland) (congenital) Q89.2
  - |cartilage Q31.8
    - |acquired J38.7
- |tibia (acquired) *see also* Deformity, limb, specified type NEC, lower leg
  - |congenital NEC Q68.8
  - |saber (syphilitic) A50.56
- |toe (acquired) M20.6-
  - |congenital Q66.9
  - |hallux rigidus M20.2-
  - |hallux valgus M20.1-
  - |hallux varus M20.3-
  - |hammer toe M20.4-
  - |specified NEC M20.5X-
- |tongue (congenital) Q38.3
  - |acquired K14.8
- |tooth, teeth K00.2
- |trachea (rings) (congenital) Q32.1
  - |acquired J39.8
- |transverse aortic arch (congenital) Q25.49
- |tricuspid (leaflets) (valve) I07.8
  - |atresia or stenosis Q22.4
  - |Ebstein's Q22.5
- |trunk (acquired) M95.8
  - |congenital Q89.9
- |ulna (acquired) *see also* Deformity, limb, forearm
  - |congenital NEC Q68.8
- |urachus, congenital Q64.4
- |ureter (opening) (congenital) Q62.8
  - |acquired N28.89
- |urethra (congenital) Q64.79
  - |acquired N36.8
- |urinary tract (congenital) Q64.9
  - |urachus Q64.4
- |uterus (congenital) Q51.9
  - |acquired N85.8
- |uvula (congenital) Q38.5
- |vagina (acquired) N89.8
  - |congenital Q52.4
- |valgus NEC M21.00
  - |ankle M21.07-
  - |elbow M21.02-
  - |hip M21.05-
  - |knee M21.06-
- |valve, valvular (congenital) (heart) Q24.8

Deformity - *continued*
|acquired *see* Endocarditis
|varus NEC M21.10
  |ankle M21.17-
  |elbow M21.12-
  |hip M21.15
  |knee M21.16-
  |tibia *see* Osteochondrosis, juvenile, tibia
|vas deferens (congenital) Q55.4
  |acquired N50.89
|vein (congenital) Q27.9
  |great Q26.9
|vertebra *see* Dorsopathy, deforming
|vertical talus (congenital) Q66.80
  |left foot Q66.82
  |right foot Q66.81
|vesicourethral orifice (acquired) N32.89
  |congenital NEC Q64.79
|vessels of optic papilla (congenital) Q14.2
|visual field (contraction) *see* Defect, visual
  field
|vitreous body, acquired H43.89
|vulva (congenital) Q52.79
  |acquired N90.89
|wrist (joint) (acquired) *see also* Deformity,
  limb, forearm
  |congenital Q68.8
  |contraction *see* Contraction, joint, wrist

Degeneration, degenerative
|adrenal (capsule) (fatty) (gland) (hyaline)
  (infectional) E27.8
|amyloid *see also* Amyloidosis E85.9
|anterior cornua, spinal cord G12.29
|anterior labral S43.49-
|aorta, aortic I70.0
  |fatty I77.89
|aortic valve (heart) *see* Endocarditis, aortic
|arteriovascular *see* Arteriosclerosis
|artery, arterial (atheromatous) (calcareous) *see*
  also Arteriosclerosis
  |cerebral, amyloid E85.4 [*I68.0*]
  |medial *see* Arteriosclerosis, extremities
|articular cartilage NEC *see* Derangement,
  joint, articular cartilage, by site
|atheromatous *see* Arteriosclerosis
|basal nuclei or ganglia G23.9
  |specified NEC G23.8
|bone NEC *see* Disorder, bone, specified type
  NEC
|brachial plexus G54.0
|brain (cortical) (progressive) G31.9
  |alcoholic G31.2
  |arteriosclerotic I67.2
  |childhood G31.9
    |specified NEC G31.89
  |cystic G31.89
    |congenital Q04.6
  |in
    |alcoholism G31.2
    |beriberi E51.2
    |cerebrovascular disease I67.9
    |congenital hydrocephalus Q03.9
      |with spina bifida *see also* Spina bifida
    |Fabry-Anderson disease E75.21
    |Gaucher's disease E75.22
    |Hunter's syndrome E76.1
    |lipidosis
      |cerebral E75.4
      |generalized E75.6
    |mucopolysaccharidosis *see*
      Mucopolysaccharidosis
    |myxedema E03.9 [*G32.89*]
    |neoplastic disease *see also* Neoplasm
      D49.6 [*G32.89*]
    |Niemann-Pick disease E75.249 [*G32.89*]
    |sphingolipidosis E75.3 [*G32.89*]
    |vitamin B12 deficiency E53.8 [*G32.89*]

Degeneration, degenerative - *continued*
|senile NEC G31.1
|breast N64.89
|Bruch's membrane *see* Degeneration, choroid
|capillaries (fatty) I78.8
  |amyloid E85.89 [*I79.8*]
|cardiac *see also* Degeneration, myocardial
  |valve, valvular *see* Endocarditis
|cardiorenal *see* Hypertension, cardiorenal
|cardiovascular *see also* Disease,
  cardiovascular
  |renal *see* Hypertension, cardiorenal
|cerebellar NOS G31.9
|cerebral *see* Degeneration, brain
|cerebrovascular I67.9
  |due to hypertension I67.4
  |alcoholic G31.2
  |primary (hereditary) (sporadic) G11.9
|cervical plexus G54.2
|cervix N88.8
  |due to radiation (intended effect) N88.8
    |adverse effect or misadventure N99.89
|chamber angle H21.21-
|changes, spine or vertebra *see* Spondylosis
|chorioretinal *see also* Degeneration, choroid
  |hereditary H31.20
|choroid (colloid) (drusen) H31.10-
  |atrophy *see* Atrophy, choroidal
  |hereditary *see* Dystrophy, choroidal,
  hereditary
|ciliary body H21.22-
|cochlear *see* subcategory H83.8
|combined (spinal cord) (subacute) E53.8
  [*G32.0*]
  |with anemia (pernicious) D51.0 [*G32.0*]
    |due to dietary vitamin B12 deficiency
      D51.3 [*G32.0*]
  |in (due to)
    |vitamin B12 deficiency E53.8 [*G32.0*]
    |anemia D51.9 [*G32.0*]
|conjunctiva H11.10
  |concretions *see* Concretion, conjunctiva
  |deposits *see* Deposit, conjunctiva
  |pigmentations *see* Pigmentation,
  conjunctiva
  |pinguecula *see* Pinguecula
  |xerosis *see* Xerosis, conjunctiva
|cornea H18.40
  |calcereous H18.43
    |band keratopathy H18.42-
  |familial, hereditary *see* Dystrophy, cornea
  |hyaline (of old scars) H18.49
  |keratomalacia *see* Keratomalacia
  |nodular H18.45-
  |peripheral H18.46-
  |senile H18.41-
  |specified type NEC H18.49
|cortical (cerebellar) (parenchymatous) G31.89
  |alcoholic G31.2
  |diffuse, due to arteriopathy I67.2
|corticobasal G31.85
|cutis L98.8
  |amyloid E85.4 [*L99*]
|dental pulp K04.2
|disc disease *see* Degeneration, intervertebral
  disc NEC
|dorsolateral (spinal cord) *see* Degeneration,
  combined
|extrapyramidal G25.9
|eye, macular *see also* Degeneration, macula
  |congenital or hereditary *see* Dystrophy,
  retina
|facet joints *see* Spondylosis
|fatty
  |liver NEC K76.0
    |alcoholic K70.0

Degeneration, degenerative - *continued*
|grey matter (brain) (Alpers') G31.81
|heart *see also* Degeneration, myocardial
  |amyloid E85.4 [*I43*]
  |atheromatous *see* Disease, heart, ischemic,
  atherosclerotic
  |ischemic *see* Disease, heart, ischemic
|hepatolenticular (Wilson's) E83.01
  |localized *see* Degeneration, by site
|infrapatellar fat pad M79.4
|intervertebral disc NOS
|hepatorenal K76.7
|hyaline (diffuse) (generalized)
  |with
    |myelopathy *see* Disorder, disc, with,
    myelopathy
    |radiculitis or radiculopathy *see* Disorder,
    disc, with, radiculopathy
  |cervical, cervicothoracic *see* Disorder, disc,
  cervical, degeneration
    |with
      |myelopathy *see* Disorder, disc, cervical,
      with myelopathy
      |neuritis, radiculitis or radiculopathy *see*
      Disorder, disc, cervical, with
      neuritis
  |lumbar region M51.36
    |with
      |myelopathy M51.06
      |neuritis, radiculitis, radiculopathy or
      sciatica M51.16
  |lumbosacral region M51.37
    |with
      |neuritis, radiculitis, radiculopathy or
      sciatica M51.17
  |sacrococcygeal region M53.3
  |thoracic region M51.34
    |with
      |myelopathy M51.04
      |neuritis, radiculitis, radiculopathy
      M51.14
  |thoracolumbar region M51.35
    |with
      |myelopathy M51.05
      |neuritis, radiculitis, radiculopathy
      M51.15
|intestine, amyloid E85.4
|iris (pigmentary) H21.23-
|ischemic *see* Ischemia
|joint disease *see* Osteoarthritis
|kidney N28.89
  |amyloid E85.4 [*N29*]
  |cystic, congenital Q61.9
  |fatty N28.89
  |polycystic Q61.3
    |adult type (autosomal dominant) Q61.2
    |infantile type (autosomal recessive) NEC
    Q61.19
      |collecting duct dilatation Q61.11
|Kuhnt-Junius *see also* Degeneration, macula
  H35.32-
|lens *see* Cataract
|lenticular (familial) (progressive) (Wilson's)
  (with cirrhosis of liver) E83.01
|liver (diffuse) NEC K76.89
  |amyloid E85.4 [*K77*]
  |cystic K76.89
    |congenital Q44.6
  |fatty NEC K76.0
    |alcoholic K70.0
  |hypertrophic K76.89
  |parenchymatous, acute or subacute K72.00
    |with coma K72.01
  |pigmentary K76.89
  |toxic (acute) K71.9
|lung J98.4

Degeneration, degenerative - *continued*
|lymph gland I89.8
  |hyaline I89.8
|macula, macular (acquired) (age-related)
  (senile) H35.30
  |angioid streaks H35.33
  |atrophic age-related H35.31-
  |congenital or hereditary *see* Dystrophy,
    retina
  |cystoid H35.35-
  |drusen H35.36-
  |dry age-related H35.31-
  |exudative H35.32-
  |hole H35.34-
  |nonexudative H35.31-
  |puckering H35.37-
  |toxic H35.38-
  |wet age-related H35.32-
|membranous labyrinth, congenital (causing
  impairment of hearing) Q16.5
|meniscus *see* Derangement, meniscus
|mitral *see* Insufficiency, mitral
|Mönckeberg's *see* Arteriosclerosis, extremities
|motor centers, senile G31.1
|multi-system G90.3
|mural *see* Degeneration, myocardial
|muscle (fatty) (fibrous) (hyaline) (progressive)
  M62.89
  |heart *see* Degeneration, myocardial
|myelin, central nervous system G37.9
|myocardial, myocardium (fatty) (hyaline)
  (senile) I51.5
  |with rheumatic fever (conditions in I00)
    I09.0
    |active, acute or subacute I01.2
      |with chorea I02.0
    |inactive or quiescent (with chorea) I09.0
  |hypertensive *see* Hypertension, heart
  |rheumatic *see* Degeneration, myocardial,
    with rheumatic fever
  |syphilitic A52.06
|nasal sinus (mucosa) J32.9
  |frontal J32.1
  |maxillary J32.0
|nerve *see* Disorder, nerve
|nervous system G31.9
  |alcoholic G31.2
  |amyloid E85.4 [*G99.8*]
  |autonomic G90.9
  |fatty G31.89
  |specified NEC G31.89
|nipple N64.89
|olivopontocerebellar (hereditary) (familial)
  G23.8
|osseous labyrinth *see* subcategory H83.8
|ovary N83.8
  |cystic N83.20-
  |microcystic N83.20-
|pallidal pigmentary (progressive) G23.0
|pancreas K86.89
  |tuberculous A18.83
|penis N48.89
|pigmentary (diffuse) (general)
  |localized *see* Degeneration, by site
  |pallidal (progressive) G23.0
|pineal gland E34.8
|pituitary (gland) E23.6
|popliteal fat pad M79.4
|posterolateral (spinal cord) *see* Degeneration,
  combined
|pulmonary valve (heart) I37.8
|pulp (tooth) K04.2
|pupillary margin H21.24-
|renal *see* Degeneration, kidney
|retina H35.9
  |hereditary (cerebroretinal) (congenital)

Degeneration, degenerative - *continued*
  (juvenile) (macula) (peripheral)
  (pigmentary) *see* Dystrophy, retina
  |Kuhnt-Junius *see also* Degeneration, macula
    H35.32-
  |macula (cystic) (exudative) (hole)
    (nonexudative) (pseudohole) (senile)
    (toxic) *see* Degeneration, macula
  |peripheral H35.40
    |lattice H35.41-
    |microcystoid H35.42-
    |paving stone H35.43-
    |secondary
      |pigmentary H35.45-
      |vitreoretinal H35.46-
    |senile reticular H35.44-
  |pigmentary (primary) *see also* Dystrophy,
    retina
  |secondary *see* Degeneration, retina,
  peripheral, secondary
  |posterior pole *see* Degeneration, macula
|saccule, congenital (causing impairment of
  hearing) Q16.5
|senile R54
  |brain G31.1
  |cardiac, heart or myocardium *see*
    Degeneration, myocardial
  |motor centers G31.1
  |vascular *see* Arteriosclerosis
|sinus (cystic) *see also* Sinusitis
  |polypoid J33.1
|skin L98.8
  |amyloid E85.4 [*L99*]
  |colloid L98.8
|spinal (cord) G31.89
  |amyloid E85.4 [*G32.89*]
  |combined (subacute) *see* Degeneration,
    combined
  |dorsolateral *see* Degeneration, combined
  |familial NEC G31.89
  |fatty G31.89
  |funicular *see* Degeneration, combined
  |posterolateral *see* Degeneration, combined
  |subacute combined *see* Degeneration,
    combined
  |tuberculous A17.81
|spleen D73.0
  |amyloid E85.4 [*D77*]
|stomach K31.89
|striatonigral G23.2
|suprarenal (capsule) (gland) E27.8
|synovial membrane (pulpy) *see* Disorder,
  synovium, specified type NEC
|tapetoretinal *see* Dystrophy, retina
|thymus (gland) E32.8
  |fatty E32.8
|thyroid (gland) E07.89
|tricuspid (heart) (valve) I07.9
|tuberculous NEC *see* Tuberculosis
|turbinate J34.89
|uterus (cystic) N85.8
|vascular (senile) *see* Arteriosclerosis
  |hypertensive *see* Hypertension
|vitreoretinal, secondary *see* Degeneration,
  retina, peripheral, secondary, vitreoretinal
|vitreous (body) H43.81-
|Wallerian *see* Disorder, nerve
|Wilson's hepatolenticular E83.01
Deglutition
|paralysis R13.0
  |hysterical F44.4
|pneumonia J69.0
Degos' disease I77.89

Dehiscence (of)
|amputation stump T87.81
|cesarean wound O90.0
|closure of
  |cornea T81.31
  |craniotomy T81.32
  |fascia (muscular) (superficial) T81.32
  |internal organ or tissue T81.32
  |laceration (external) (internal) T81.33
  |ligament T81.32
  |mucosa T81.31
  |muscle or muscle flap T81.32
  |ribs or rib cage T81.32
  |skin and subcutaneous tissue (full-thickness)
    (superficial) T81.31
  |skull T81.32
  |sternum (sternotomy) T81.32
  |tendon T81.32
  |traumatic laceration (external) (internal)
    T81.33
|episiotomy O90.1
|operation wound NEC T81.31
  |external operation wound (superficial)
    T81.31
  |internal operation wound (deep) T81.32
|perineal wound (postpartum) O90.1
|traumatic injury wound repair T81.33
|wound T81.30
  |traumatic repair T81.33
Dehydration E86.0
|newborn P74.1
Déjérine-Roussy syndrome G89.0
**Déjérine-Sottas disease or neuropathy
(hypertrophic)** G60.0
Déjérine-Thomas atrophy G23.8
Delay, delayed
|any plane in pelvis
  |complicating delivery O66.9
|birth or delivery NOS O63.9
|closure, ductus arteriosus (Botalli) P29.38
|coagulation *see* Defect, coagulation
|conduction (cardiac) (ventricular) I45.9
|delivery, second twin, triplet, etc O63.2
|development R62.50
  |global F88
  |intellectual (specific) F81.9
  |language F80.9
    |due to hearing loss F80.4
  |learning F81.9
  |pervasive F84.9
  |physiological R62.50
    |specified stage NEC R62.0
  |reading F81.0
  |sexual E30.0
  |speech F80.9
    |due to hearing loss F80.4
  |spelling F81.81
|ejaculation F52.32
|gastric emptying K30
|menarche E30.0
|menstruation (cause unknown) N91.0
|milestone R62.0
|passage of meconium (newborn) P76.0
|primary respiration P28.9
|puberty (constitutional) E30.0
|separation of umbilical cord P96.82
|sexual maturation, female E30.0
|sleep phase syndrome G47.21
|union, fracture *see* Fracture, by site
|vaccination Z28.9
Deletion(s)
|autosome Q93.9
  |identified by fluorescence in situ
    hybridization (FISH) Q93.89
  |identified by in situ hybridization (ISH)
    Q93.89

Deletion(s) - *continued*
|chromosome
|with complex rearrangements NEC Q93.7
|part of NEC Q93.59
|seen only at prometaphase Q93.89
|short arm
|4 Q93.3
|5p Q93.4
|22q11.2 Q93.81
|specified NEC Q93.89
|long arm chromosome 18 or 21 Q93.89
|with complex rearrangements NEC Q93.7
|microdeletions NEC Q93.88
Delhi boil or button B55.1
Delinquency (juvenile) (neurotic) F91.8
|group Z72.810
Delinquent immunization status Z28.3
Delirium, delirious (acute or subacute) (not alcohol-or drug-Induced) (with dementia) R41.0
|alcoholic (acute) (tremens) (withdrawal) F10.921
|with intoxication F10.921
|in
|abuse F10.121
|dependence F10.221
|due to (secondary to)
|alcohol
|intoxication F10.921
|in
|abuse F10.121
|dependence F10.221
|withdrawal F10.231
|amphetamine intoxication F15.921
|in
|abuse F15.121
|dependence F15.221
|anxiolytic
|intoxication F13.921
|in
|abuse F13.121
|dependence F13.221
|withdrawal F13.231
|cannabis intoxication (acute) F12.921
|in
|abuse F12.121
|dependence F12.221
|cocaine intoxication (acute) F14.921
|in
|abuse F14.121
|dependence F14.221
|general medical condition F05
|hallucinogen intoxication F16.921
|in
|abuse F16.121
|dependence F16.221
|hypnotic
|intoxication F13.921
|in
|abuse F13.121
|dependence F13.221
|withdrawal F13.231
|inhalant intoxication (acute) F18.921
|in
|abuse F18.121
|dependence F18.221
|multiple etiologies F05
|opioid intoxication (acute) F11.921
|in
|abuse F11.121
|dependence F11.221
|other (or unknown) substance F19.921
|phencyclidine intoxication (acute) F16.921
|in
|abuse F16.121
|dependence F16.221

Delirium, delirious - *continued*
|psychoactive substance NEC intoxication (acute) F19.921
|in
|abuse F19.121
|dependence F19.221
|sedative
|intoxication F13.921
|in
|abuse F13.121
|dependence F13.221
|withdrawal F13.231
|unknown etiology F05
|exhaustion F43.0
|hysterical F44.89
|postprocedural (postoperative) F05
|puerperal F05
|thyroid *see* Thyrotoxicosis with thyroid storm
|traumatic *see* Injury, intracranial
|tremens (alcohol-induced) F10.231
|sedative-induced F13.231
Delivery (childbirth) (labor)
|arrested active phase O62.1
|cesarean (for)
|abnormal
|pelvis (bony) (deformity) (major) NEC with disproportion (fetopelvic) O33.0
|with obstructed labor O65.0
|presentation or position O32.9
|abruptio placentae *see also* Abruptio placentae O45.9-
|acromion presentation O32.2
|atony, uterus O62.2
|breech presentation O32.1
|incomplete O32.8
|brow presentation O32.3
|cephalopelvic disproportion O33.9
|cerclage O34.3-
|chin presentation O32.3
|cicatrix of cervix O34.4-
|contracted pelvis (general)
|inlet O33.2
|outlet O33.3
|cord presentation or prolapse O69.0
|cystocele O34.8-
|deformity (acquired) (congenital)
|pelvic organs or tissues NEC O34.8-
|pelvis (bony) NEC O33.0
|disproportion NOS O33.9
|eclampsia *see* Eclampsia
|face presentation O32.3
|failed
|forceps O66.5
|induction of labor O61.9
|instrumental O61.1
|mechanical O61.1
|medical O61.0
|specified NEC O61.8
|surgical O61.1
|trial of labor NOS O66.40
|following previous cesarean delivery O66.41
|vacuum extraction O66.5
|ventouse O66.5
|fetal-maternal hemorrhage O43.01-
|hemorrhage (intrapartum) O67.9
|with coagulation defect O67.0
|specified cause NEC O67.8
|high head at term O32.4
|hydrocephalic fetus O33.6
|incarceration of uterus O34.51-
|incoordinate uterine action O62.4
|increased size, fetus O33.5
|inertia, uterus O62.2
|primary O62.0
|secondary O62.1

Delivery (childbirth) (labor) - *continued*
|isthmocele O34.22
|lateroversion, uterus O34.59-
|mal lie O32.9
|malposition
|fetus O32.9
|pelvic organs or tissues NEC O34.8-
|uterus NEC O34.59-
|malpresentation NOS O32.9
|oblique presentation O32.2
|occurring after 37 completed weeks of gestation but before 39 completed weeks gestation due to (spontaneous) onset of labor O75.82
|oversize fetus O33.5
|pelvic tumor NEC O34.8-
|placenta previa O44.0-
|complete O44.0-
|with hemorrhage O44.1-
|placental insufficiency O36.51-
|planned, occurring after 37 completed weeks of gestation but before 39 completed weeks gestation due to (spontaneous) onset of labor O75.82
|polyp, cervix O34.4-
|causing obstructed labor O65.5
|poor dilatation, cervix O62.0
|pre-eclampsia O14.94
|mild O14.04
|moderate O14.04
|severe O14.14
|with hemolysis, elevated liver enzymes and low platelet count (HELLP) O14.24
|previous
|cesarean delivery O34.219
|classical (vertical) scar O34.212
|isthmocele O34.22
|low transverse scar O34.211
|mid-transverse T incision O34.218
|scar
|defect (isthmocele) O34.22
|specified type NEC O34.218
|surgery (to)
|cervix O34.4-
|gynecological NEC O34.8-
|rectum O34.7-
|uterus O34.29
|vagina O34.6-
|prolapse
|arm or hand O32.2
|uterus O34.52-
|prolonged labor NOS O63.9
|rectocele O34.8-
|retroversion
|uterus O34.53-
|rigid
|cervix O34.4-
|pelvic floor O34.8-
|perineum O34.7-
|vagina O34.6-
|vulva O34.7-
|sacculation, pregnant uterus O34.59-
|scar(s)
|cervix O34.4-
|cesarean delivery O34.219
|classical (vertical) O34.212
|isthmocele O34.22
|low transverse O34.211
|mid-transverse T incision O34.218
|scar
|defect (isthmocele) O34.22
|specified type NEC O34.218
|transmural uterine O34.29
|uterus O34.29
|Shirodkar suture in situ O34.3-

Delivery (childbirth) (labor) - *continued*
|shoulder presentation O32.2
|stenosis or stricture, cervix O34.4-
|streptococcus group B (GBS) carrier state O99.824
|transmural uterine scar O34.29
|transverse presentation or lie O32.2
|tumor, pelvic organs or tissues NEC O34.8-
   |cervix O34.4-
|umbilical cord presentation or prolapse O69.0
|without indication O82
|completely normal case O80
|complicated O75.9
   |by
      |abnormal, abnormality (of)
         |forces of labor O62.9
            |specified type NEC O62.8
         |glucose O99.814
         |uterine contractions NOS O62.9
      |abruptio placentae *see also* Abruptio placentae O45.9-
      |abuse
         |physical O9A.32
         |psychological O9A.52
         |sexual O9A.42
      |adherent placenta O72.0
         |without hemorrhage O73.0
      |alcohol use O99.314
      |anemia (pre-existing) O99.02
      |anesthetic death O74.8
      |annular detachment of cervix O71.3
      |atony, uterus O62.2
      |attempted vacuum extraction and forceps O66.5
      |Bandl's ring O62.4
      |bariatric surgery status O99.844
      |biliary tract disorder O26.62
      |bleeding *see* Delivery, complicated by, hemorrhage
      |blood disorder NEC O99.12
      |cervical dystocia (hypotonic) O62.2
         |primary O62.0
         |secondary O62.1
      |circulatory system disorder O99.42
      |compression of cord (umbilical) NEC O69.2
      |condition NEC O99.892
      |contraction, contracted ring O62.4
      |cord (umbilical)
         |around neck
            |with compression O69.1
            |without compression O69.81
         |bruising O69.5
         |complication O69.9
            |specified NEC O69.89
         |compression NEC O69.2
         |entanglement O69.2
            |without compression O69.82
         |hematoma O69.5
         |presentation O69.0
         |prolapse O69.0
         |short O69.3
         |thrombosis (vessels) O69.5
         |vascular lesion O69.5
      |Couvelaire uterus O45.8X-
      |damage to (injury to) NEC
         |perineum O71.82
         |periurethral tissue O71.82
         |vulva O71.82
      |delay following rupture of membranes (spontaneous) *see* Pregnancy, complicated by, premature rupture of membranes
      |depressed fetal heart tones O76
      |diabetes O24.92
         |gestational O24.429

Delivery (childbirth) (labor) - *continued*
         |diet controlled O24.420
         |insulin controlled O24.424
         |oral drug controlled (antidiabetic) (hypoglycemic) O24.425
      |pre-existing O24.32
         |specified NEC O24.82
         |type 1 O24.02
         |type 2 O24.12
      |diastasis recti (abdominis) O71.89
      |dilatation
         |bladder O66.8
         |cervix incomplete, poor or slow O62.0
      |disease NEC O99.892
      |disruptio uteri *see* Delivery, complicated by, rupture, uterus
      |drug use O99.324
      |dysfunction, uterus NOS O62.9
         |hypertonic O62.4
         |hypotonic O62.2
            |primary O62.0
            |secondary O62.1
         |incoordinate O62.4
      |eclampsia O15.1
      |embolism (pulmonary) *see* Embolism, obstetric
      |endocrine, nutritional or metabolic disease NEC O99.284
      |failed
         |attempted vaginal birth after previous cesarean delivery O66.41
         |induction of labor O61.9
            |instrumental O61.1
            |mechanical O61.1
            |medical O61.0
            |specified NEC O61.8
            |surgical O61.1
         |trial of labor O66.40
      |female genital mutilation O65.5
      |fetal
         |abnormal acid-base balance O68
         |acidemia O68
         |acidosis O68
         |alkalosis O68
         |death, early O02.1
         |deformity O66.3
         |heart rate or rhythm (abnormal) (non-reassuring) O76
         |hypoxia O77.8
         |stress O77.9
            |due to drug administration O77.1
            |electrocardiographic evidence of O77.8
            |specified NEC O77.8
            |ultrasound evidence of O77.8
      |fever during labor O75.2
      |gastric banding status O99.844
      |gastric bypass status O99.844
      |gastrointestinal disease NEC O99.62
      |gestational
         |diabetes O24.429
            |diet controlled O24.420
            |insulin (and diet) controlled O24.424
            |oral drug controlled (antidiabetic) (hypoglycemic) O24.425
         |edema O12.04
            |with proteinuria O12.24
         |proteinuria O12.14
      |gonorrhea O98.22
      |hematoma O71.7
         |ischial spine O71.7
         |pelvic O71.7
         |vagina O71.7
         |vulva or perineum O71.7
      |hemorrhage (uterine) O67.9
         |associated with
            |afibrinogenemia O67.0

Delivery (childbirth) (labor) - *continued*
         |coagulation defect O67.0
         |hyperfibrinolysis O67.0
         |hypofibrinogenemia O67.0
      |due to
         |low implantation of placenta O44.5-
         |low lying placenta O44.5-
         |placenta previa O44.1-
            |marginal O44.3-
            |partial O44.3-
         |premature separation of placenta (normally implanted) *see also* Abruptio placentae O45.9-
         |retained placenta O72.0
         |uterine leiomyoma O67.8
      |placenta NEC O67.8
      |postpartum NEC (atonic) (immediate) O72.1
         |with retained or trapped placenta O72.0
         |delayed O72.2
         |secondary O72.2
         |third stage O72.0
      |hourglass contraction, uterus O62.4
      |hypertension, hypertensive (pre-existing) *see* Hypertension, complicated by, childbirth (labor)
      |hypotension O26.5-
      |incomplete dilatation (cervix) O62.0
      |incoordinate uterus contractions O62.4
      |inertia, uterus O62.2
         |during latent phase of labor O62.0
         |primary O62.0
         |secondary O62.1
      |infection (maternal) O98.92
         |carrier state NEC O99.834
         |gonorrhea O98.22
         |human immunodeficiency virus (HIV) O98.72
         |sexually transmitted NEC O98.32
         |specified NEC O98.82
         |syphilis O98.12
         |tuberculosis O98.02
         |viral hepatitis O98.42
         |viral NEC O98.52
      |injury (to mother) *see also* Delivery, complicated, by, damage to O71.9
      |nonobstetric O9A.22
         |caused by abuse *see* Delivery, complicated by, abuse
      |intrauterine fetal death, early O02.1
      |inversion, uterus O71.2
      |laceration (perineal) O70.9
         |anus (sphincter) O70.4
            |with third degree laceration *see also* Delivery, complicated, by, laceration, perineum, third degree O70.20
            |with mucosa O70.3
            |without third degree laceration O70.4
         |bladder (urinary) O71.5
         |bowel O71.5
         |cervix (uteri) O71.3
         |fourchette O70.0
         |hymen O70.0
         |labia O70.0
         |pelvic
            |floor O70.1
            |organ NEC O71.5
         |perineum, perineal O70.9
            |first degree O70.0
            |fourth degree O70.3
            |muscles O70.1
            |second degree O70.1
            |skin O70.0
            |slight O70.0

Delivery (childbirth) (labor) - *continued*

  |third degree O70.20
  |with
    |both external anal sphincter
        (EAS) and internal anal
        sphincter (IAS) torn (IIIc)
        O70.23
    |less than 50% of external anal
        sphincter (EAS) thickness torn
        (IIIa) O70.21
    |more than 50% external anal
        sphincter (EAS) thickness torn
        (IIIb) O70.22
    |IIIa O70.21
    |IIIb O70.22
    |IIIc O70.23
  |peritoneum (pelvic) O71.5
  |rectovaginal (septum) (without perineal
      laceration) O71.4
    |with perineum *see also* Delivery,
        complicated, by, laceration,
        perineum, third degree O70.20
      |with anal or rectal mucosa O70.3
  |specified NEC O71.89
  |sphincter ani *see* Delivery, complicated,
      by, laceration, anus (sphincter)
  |urethra O71.5
  |uterus O71.81
    |before labor O71.81
  |vagina, vaginal (deep) (high) (without
      perineal laceration) O71.4
    |with perineum O70.0
    |muscles, with perineum O70.1
  |vulva O70.0
  |liver disorder O26.62
  |malignancy O9A.12
  |malnutrition O25.2
  |malposition, malpresentation
    |placenta O44.0-
      |with hemorrhage O44.1-
    |uterus or cervix O65.5
    |without obstruction *see also* Delivery,
        complicated by, obstruction O32.9
      |breech O32.1
      |compound O32.6
      |face (brow) (chin) O32.3
      |footling O32.8
      |high head O32.4
      |oblique O32.2
      |specified NEC O32.8
      |transverse O32.2
      |unstable lie O32.0
  |meconium in amniotic fluid O77.0
  |mental disorder NEC O99.344
  |metrorrhexis *see* Delivery, complicated
      by, rupture, uterus
  |nervous system disorder O99.354
  |obesity (pre-existing) O99.214
  |obesity surgery status O99.844
  |obstetric trauma O71.9
    |specified NEC O71.89
  |obstructed labor
    |due to
      |breech (complete) (frank) presentation
          O64.1
        |incomplete O64.8
      |brow presentation O64.3
      |buttock presentation O64.1
      |chin presentation O64.2
      |compound presentation O64.5
      |contracted pelvis O65.1
      |deep transverse arrest O64.0
    |deformed pelvis O65.0
    |dystocia (fetal) O66.9
      |due to
        |conjoined twins O66.3

Delivery (childbirth) (labor) - *continued*

    |fetal
      |abnormality NEC O66.3
      |ascites O66.3
      |hydrops O66.3
      |meningomyelocele O66.3
      |sacral teratoma O66.3
      |tumor O66.3
    |hydrocephalic fetus O66.3
    |shoulder O66.0
  |face presentation O64.2
  |fetopelvic disproportion O65.4
  |footling presentation O64.8
  |impacted shoulders O66.0
  |incomplete rotation of fetal head
      O64.0
  |large fetus O66.2
  |locked twins O66.1
  |malposition O64.9
    |specified NEC O64.8
  |malpresentation O64.9
    |specified NEC O64.8
  |multiple fetuses NEC O66.6
  |pelvic
    |abnormality (maternal) O65.9
      |organ O65.5
      |specified NEC O65.8
    |contraction
      |inlet O65.2
      |mid-cavity O65.3
      |outlet O65.3
  |persistent (position)
    |occipitoiliac O64.0
    |occipitoposterior O64.0
    |occipitosacral O64.0
    |occipitotransverse O64.0
  |prolapsed arm O64.4
  |shoulder presentation O64.4
  |specified NEC O66.8
  |pathological retraction ring, uterus O62.4
  |penetration, pregnant uterus by instrument
      O71.1
  |perforation *see* Delivery, complicated by,
      laceration
  |placenta, placental
    |ablatio *see also* Abruptio placentae
        O45.9-
    |abnormality O43.9-
      |specified NEC O43.89-
    |abruptio *see also* Abruptio placentae
        O45.9-
    |accreta O43.21-
    |adherent (with hemorrhage) O72.0
      |without hemorrhage O73.0
    |detachment (premature) *see also*
        Abruptio placentae O45.9-
    |disorder O43.9-
      |specified NEC O43.89-
    |hemorrhage NEC O67.8
    |increta O43.22-
    |low (implantation) (lying) O44.4-
      |with hemorrhage O44.5-
    |malformation O43.10-
    |malposition O44.0-
      |without hemorrhage O44.1-
    |percreta O43.23-
    |previa (central) (complete) (lateral)
        (total) O44.0-
      |with hemorrhage O44.1-
      |marginal O44.2-
        |with hemorrhage O44.3-
      |partial O44.2-
        |with hemorrhage O44.3-
    |retained (with hemorrhage) O72.0
      |without hemorrhage O73.0
    |separation (premature) O45.9-

Delivery (childbirth) (labor) - *continued*

    |specified NEC O45.8X-
  |vicious insertion O44.1-
  |precipitate labor O62.3
  |premature rupture, membranes *see also*
      Pregnancy, complicated by, premature
      rupture of membranes O42.90
  |prolapse
    |arm or hand O32.2
    |cord (umbilical) O69.0
    |foot or leg O32.8
    |uterus O34.52-
  |prolonged labor O63.9
    |first stage O63.0
    |second stage O63.1
  |protozoal disease (maternal) O98.62
  |respiratory disease NEC O99.52
  |retained membranes or portions of
      placenta O72.2
    |without hemorrhage O73.1
  |retarded birth O63.9
  |retention of secundines (with hemorrhage)
      O72.0
    |without hemorrhage O73.0
    |partial O72.2
      |without hemorrhage O73.1
  |rupture
    |bladder (urinary) O71.5
    |cervix O71.3
    |pelvic organ NEC O71.5
    |urethra O71.5
    |uterus (during or after labor) O71.1
      |before labor O71.0-
  |separation, pubic bone (symphysis pubis)
      O71.6
  |shock O75.1
  |shoulder presentation O64.4
  |skin disorder NEC O99.72
  |spasm, cervix O62.4
  |stenosis or stricture, cervix O65.5
  |streptococcus group B (GBS) carrier state
      O99.824
  |subluxation of symphysis (pubis) O26.72
  |syphilis (maternal) O98.12
  |tear *see* Delivery, complicated by,
      laceration
  |tetanic uterus O62.4
  |trauma (obstetrical) *see also* Delivery,
      complicated, by, damage to O71.9
    |non-obstetric O9A.22
    |periurethral O71.82
    |specified NEC O71.89
  |tuberculosis (maternal) O98.02
  |tumor, pelvic organs or tissues NEC
      O65.5
  |umbilical cord around neck
    |with compression O69.1
    |without compression O69.81
  |uterine inertia O62.2
    |during latent phase of labor O62.0
    |primary O62.0
    |secondary O62.1
  |vasa previa O69.4
  |velamentous insertion of cord O43.12-
  |specified complication NEC O75.89
|delayed NOS O63.9
  |following rupture of membranes
    |artificial O75.5
  |second twin, triplet, etc. O63.2
|forceps, low following failed vacuum
    extraction O66.5
|missed (at or near term) O36.4
|normal O80
|obstructed *see* Delivery, complicated by,
    obstructed labor

Delivery (childbirth) (labor) - *continued*
|precipitate O62.3
|preterm *see also* Pregnancy, complicated by, preterm labor O60.10
|spontaneous O80
|term pregnancy NOS O80
|uncomplicated O80
|vaginal, following previous cesarean delivery O34.219
  |classical (vertical) scar O34.212
  |low transverse scar O34.211
  |mid-transverse T incision O34.218
  |scar
   |defect (isthmocele) O34.22
  |specified type NEC O34.218
Delusions (paranoid) *see* Disorder, delusional
Dementia (degenerative (primary)) (old age) (persisting) F03.90
|with
  |aggressive behavior F03.91
  |behavioral disturbance F03.91
  |combative behavior F03.91
  |Lewy bodies G31.83 *[F02.80]*
   |with behavioral disturbance G31.83 *[F02.81]*
  |Parkinsonism G31.83 *[F02.80]*
   |with behavioral disturbance G31.83 *[F02.81]*
  |Parkinson's disease G20 *[F02.80]*
   |with behavioral disturbance G20 *[F02.81]*
  |violent behavior F03.91
|alcoholic F10.97
  |with dependence F10.27
|Alzheimer's type *see* Disease, Alzheimer's
|arteriosclerotic *see* Dementia, vascular
|atypical, Alzheimer's type *see* Disease, Alzheimer's, specified NEC
|congenital *see* Disability, intellectual
|frontal (lobe) G31.09 *[F02.80]*
  |with behavioral disturbance G31.09 *[F02.81]*
|frontotemporal G31.09 *[F02.80]*
  |with behavioral disturbance G31.09 *[F02.81]*
  |specified NEC G31.09 *[F02.80]*
   |with behavioral disturbance G31.09 *[F02.81]*
|in (due to)
  |alcohol F10.97
   |with dependence F10.27
  |Alzheimer's disease *see* Disease, Alzheimer's
  |arteriosclerotic brain disease *see* Dementia, vascular
  |cerebral lipidoses E75. *[F02.80]*
   |with behavioral disturbance E75. *[F02.81]*
  |Creutzfeldt-Jakob disease *see also* Creutzfeldt-Jakob disease or syndrome (with dementia) A81.00
  |epilepsy G40. *[F02.80]*
   |with behavioral disturbance G40. *[F02.81]*
  |hepatolenticular degeneration E83.01 *[F02.80]*
   |with behavioral disturbance E83.01 *[F02.81]*
  |human immunodeficiency virus (HIV) disease B20 *[F02.80]*
   |with behavioral disturbance B20 *[F02.81]*
  |Huntington's disease or chorea G10 *[F02.80]*
   |with behavioral disturbance G10 *[F02.81]*
  |hypercalcemia E83.52 *[F02.80]*

Dementia - *continued*
   |with behavioral disturbance E83.52 *[F02.81]*
  |hypothyroidism, acquired E03.9 *[F02.80]*
   |with behavioral disturbance E03.9 *[F02.81]*
   |due to iodine deficiency E01.8 *[F02.80]*
    |with behavioral disturbance E01.8 *[F02.81]*
  |inhalants F18.97
   |with dependence F18.27
  |multiple
   |etiologies F03
   |sclerosis G35 *[F02.80]*
    |with behavioral disturbance G35 *[F02.81]*
  |neurosyphilis A52.17 *[F02.80]*
   |with behavioral disturbance A52.17 *[F02.81]*
   |juvenile A50.49 *[F02.80]*
    |with behavioral disturbance A50.49 *[F02.81]*
  |niacin deficiency E52 *[F02.80]*
   |with behavioral disturbance E52 *[F02.81]*
  |paralysis agitans G20 *[F02.80]*
   |with behavioral disturbance G20 *[F02.81]*
  |Parkinson's disease G20 *[F02.80]*
  |pellagra E52 *[F02.80]*
   |with behavioral disturbance E52 *[F02.81]*
  |Pick's G31.01 *[F02.80]*
   |with behavioral disturbance G31.01 *[F02.81]*
  |polyarteritis nodosa M30.0 *[F02.80]*
   |with behavioral disturbance M30.0 *[F02.81]*
  |psychoactive drug F19.97
   |with dependence F19.27
   |inhalants F18.97
    |with dependence F18.27
   |sedatives, hypnotics or anxiolytics F13.97
    |with dependence F13.27
  |sedatives, hypnotics or anxiolytics F13.97
   |with dependence F13.27
  |systemic lupus erythematosus M32. *[F02.80]*
   |with behavioral disturbance M32. *[F02.81]*
  |trypanosomiasis
   |African B56.9 *[F02.80]*
    |with behavioral disturbance B56.9 *[F02.81]*
  |unknown etiology F03
  |vitamin B12
   |deficiency E53.8 *[F02.80]*
   |with behavioral disturbance E53.8 *[F02.81]*
  |volatile solvents F18.97
   |with dependence F18.27
  |with behavioral disturbance G31.83 *[F02.81]*
|infantile, infantilis F84.3
|Lewy body G31.83 *[F02.80]*
  |with behavioral disturbance G31.83 *[F02.81]*
|multi-infarct *see* Dementia, vascular
|paralytica, paralytic (syphilitic) A52.17 *[F02.80]*
  |with behavioral disturbance A52.17 *[F02.81]*
  |juvenilis A50.45
|paretic A52.17
|praecox *see* Schizophrenia
|presenile F03
  |Alzheimer's type *see* Disease, Alzheimer's, early onset

Dementia - *continued*
|primary degenerative F03
|progressive, syphilitic A52.17
|senile F03
  |with acute confusional state F05
  |Alzheimer's type *see* Disease, Alzheimer's, late onset
  |depressed or paranoid type F03
|vascular (acute onset) (mixed) (multi-infarct) (subcortical) F01.50
  |with behavioral disturbance F01.51
Demineralization, bone *see* Osteoporosis
Demodex folliculorum (infestation) B88.0
Demophobia F40.248
Demoralization R45.3
Demyelination, demyelinization
|central nervous system G37.9
  |specified NEC G37.8
|corpus callosum (central) G37.1
|disseminated, acute G36.9
  |specified NEC G36.8
|global G35
|in optic neuritis G36.0
Dengue (classical) (fever) A90
|hemorrhagic A91
|sandfly A93.1
Dennie-Marfan syphilitic syndrome A50.45
Dens evaginatus, in dente or invaginatus K00.2
Dense breasts R92.2
Density
|increased, bone (disseminated) (generalized) (spotted) *see* Disorder, bone, density and structure, specified type NEC
|lung (nodular) J98.4
Dental *see also* condition
|examination Z01.20
  |with abnormal findings Z01.21
|restoration
  |aesthetically inadequate or displeasing K08.56
  |defective K08.50
   |specified NEC K08.59
  |failure of marginal integrity K08.51
  |failure of periodontal anatomical integrity K08.54
Dentia praecox K00.6
Denticles (pulp) K04.2
Dentigerous cyst K09.0
Dentin
|irregular (in pulp) K04.3
|opalescent K00.5
|secondary (in pulp) K04.3
|sensitive K03.89
Dentinogenesis imperfecta K00.5
Dentinoma *see* Cyst, calcifying odontogenic
Dentition (syndrome) K00.7
|delayed K00.6
|difficult K00.7
|precocious K00.6
|premature K00.6
|retarded K00.6
Dependence (on) (syndrome) F19.20
|with remission F19.21
|alcohol (ethyl) (methyl) (without remission) F10.20
  |in remission F10.21
  |with
   |amnestic disorder, persisting F10.26
   |anxiety disorder F10.280
   |dementia, persisting F10.27
   |intoxication F10.229
    |with delirium F10.221
    |uncomplicated F10.220
   |mood disorder F10.24

Dependence (on) (syndrome) - *continued*
 |psychotic disorder F10.259
  |with
   |delusions F10.250
   |hallucinations F10.251
 |remission F10.21
 |sexual dysfunction F10.281
 |sleep disorder F10.282
 |specified disorder NEC F10.288
 |withdrawal F10.239
  |with
   |delirium F10.231
   |perceptual disturbance F10.232
  |uncomplicated F10.230
 |counseling and surveillance Z71.41
|amobarbital *see* Dependence, drug, sedative
|amphetamine(s) (type) *see* Dependence, drug, stimulant NEC
|amytal (sodium) *see* Dependence, drug, sedative
|analgesic NEC F55.8
|anesthetic (agent) (gas) (general) (local) NEC *see* Dependence, drug, psychoactive NEC
|anxiolytic NEC *see* Dependence, drug, sedative
|barbital(s) *see* Dependence, drug, sedative
|barbiturate(s) (compounds) (drugs classifiable to T42) *see* Dependence, drug, sedative
|benzedrine *see* Dependence, drug, stimulant NEC
|bhang *see* Dependence, drug, cannabis
|bromide(s) NEC *see* Dependence, drug, sedative
|caffeine *see* Dependence, drug, stimulant NEC
|cannabis (sativa) (indica) (resin) (derivatives) (type) *see* Dependence, drug, cannabis
|chloral (betaine) (hydrate) *see* Dependence, drug, sedative
|chlordiazepoxide *see* Dependence, drug, sedative
|coca (leaf) (derivatives) *see* Dependence, drug, cocaine
|cocaine *see* Dependence, drug, cocaine
|codeine *see* Dependence, drug, opioid
|combinations of drugs F19.20
|dagga *see* Dependence, drug, cannabis
|demerol *see* Dependence, drug, opioid
|dexamphetamine *see* Dependence, drug, stimulant NEC
|dexedrine *see* Dependence, drug, stimulant NEC
|dextromethorphan *see* Dependence, drug, opioid
|dextromoramide *see* Dependence, drug, opioid
|dextro or-pseudo-ephedrine *see* Dependence, drug, stimulant NEC
|dextrorphan *see* Dependence, drug, opioid
|diazepam *see* Dependence, drug, sedative
|dilaudid *see* Dependence, drug, opioid
|D-lysergic acid diethylamide *see* Dependence, drug, hallucinogen
|drug NEC F19.20
 |with sleep disorder F19.282
 |cannabis F12.20
  |with
   |anxiety disorder F12.280
   |intoxication F12.229
    |with
     |delirium F12.221
     |perceptual disturbance F12.222
    |uncomplicated F12.220
   |other specified disorder F12.288
   |psychosis F12.259
    |delusions F12.250
    |hallucinations F12.251

Dependence (on) (syndrome) - *continued*
   |unspecified disorder F12.29
   |withdrawal F12.23
  |in remission F12.21
 |cocaine F14.20
  |with
   |anxiety disorder F14.280
   |intoxication F14.229
    |with
     |delirium F14.221
     |perceptual disturbance F14.222
    |uncomplicated F14.220
   |mood disorder F14.24
   |other specified disorder F14.288
   |psychosis F14.259
    |delusions F14.250
    |hallucinations F14.251
   |sexual dysfunction F14.281
   |sleep disorder F14.282
   |unspecified disorder F14.29
   |withdrawal F14.23
  |in remission F14.21
  |withdrawal symptoms in newborn P96.1
 |counseling and surveillance Z71.51
 |hallucinogen F16.20
  |with
   |anxiety disorder F16.280
   |flashbacks F16.283
   |intoxication F16.229
    |with delirium F16.221
    |uncomplicated F16.220
   |mood disorder F16.24
   |other specified disorder F16.288
   |perception disorder, persisting F16.283
   |psychosis F16.259
    |delusions F16.250
    |hallucinations F16.251
   |unspecified disorder F16.29
  |in remission F16.21
 |in remission F19.21
 |inhalant F18.20
  |with
   |anxiety disorder F18.280
   |dementia, persisting F18.27
   |intoxication F18.229
    |with delirium F18.221
    |uncomplicated F18.220
   |mood disorder F18.24
   |other specified disorder F18.288
   |psychosis F18.259
    |delusions F18.250
    |hallucinations F18.251
   |unspecified disorder F18.29
  |in remission F18.21
 |nicotine F17.200
  |with disorder F17.209
  |in remission F17.201
  |specified disorder NEC F17.208
  |withdrawal F17.203
  |chewing tobacco F17.220
   |with disorder F17.229
   |in remission F17.221
   |specified disorder NEC F17.228
   |withdrawal F17.223
  |cigarettes F17.210
   |with disorder F17.219
   |in remission F17.211
   |specified disorder NEC F17.218
   |withdrawal F17.213
  |specified product NEC F17.290
   |with disorder F17.299
   |remission F17.291
   |specified disorder NEC F17.298
   |withdrawal F17.293
 |opioid F11.20

Dependence (on) (syndrome) - *continued*
  |with
   |intoxication F11.229
    |with
     |delirium F11.221
     |perceptual disturbance F11.222
    |uncomplicated F11.220
   |mood disorder F11.24
   |other specified disorder F11.288
   |psychosis F11.259
    |delusions F11.250
    |hallucinations F11.251
   |sexual dysfunction F11.281
   |sleep disorder F11.282
   |unspecified disorder F11.29
   |withdrawal F11.23
  |in remission F11.21
 |psychoactive NEC F19.20
  |with
   |amnestic disorder F19.26
   |anxiety disorder F19.280
   |dementia F19.27
   |intoxication F19.229
    |with
     |delirium F19.221
     |perceptual disturbance F19.222
    |uncomplicated F19.220
   |mood disorder F19.24
   |other specified disorder F19.288
   |psychosis F19.259
    |delusions F19.250
    |hallucinations F19.251
   |sexual dysfunction F19.281
   |sleep disorder F19.282
   |unspecified disorder F19.29
   |withdrawal F19.239
    |with
     |delirium F19.231
     |perceptual disturbance F19.232
    |uncomplicated F19.230
 |sedative, hypnotic or anxiolytic F13.20
  |with
   |amnestic disorder F13.26
   |anxiety disorder F13.280
   |dementia, persisting F13.27
   |intoxication F13.229
    |with delirium F13.221
    |uncomplicated F13.220
   |mood disorder F13.24
   |other specified disorder F13.288
   |psychosis F13.259
    |delusions F13.250
    |hallucinations F13.251
   |sexual dysfunction F13.281
   |sleep disorder F13.282
   |unspecified disorder F13.29
   |withdrawal F13.239
    |with
     |delirium F13.231
     |perceptual disturbance F13.232
    |uncomplicated F13.230
  |in remission F13.21
 |stimulant NEC F15.20
  |with
   |anxiety disorder F15.280
   |intoxication F15.229
    |with
     |delirium F15.221
     |perceptual disturbance F15.222
    |uncomplicated F15.220
   |mood disorder F15.24
   |other specified disorder F15.288
   |psychosis F15.259
    |delusions F15.250
    |hallucinations F15.251

Dependence (on) (syndrome) - *continued*
    |sexual dysfunction F15.281
    |sleep disorder F15.282
    |unspecified disorder F15.29
    |withdrawal F15.23
    |in remission F15.21
  |ethyl
    |alcohol (without remission) F10.20
      |with remission F10.21
    |bromide *see* Dependence, drug, sedative
    |carbamate F19.20
    |chloride F19.20
    |morphine *see* Dependence, drug, opioid
  |ganja *see* Dependence, drug, cannabis
  |glue (airplane) (sniffing) *see* Dependence, drug, inhalant
  |glutethimide *see* Dependence, drug, sedative
  |hallucinogenics *see* Dependence, drug, hallucinogen
  |hashish *see* Dependence, drug, cannabis
  |hemp *see* Dependence, drug, cannabis
  |heroin (salt) (any) *see* Dependence, drug, opioid
  |hypnotic NEC *see* Dependence, drug, sedative
  |Indian hemp *see* Dependence, drug, cannabis
  |inhalants *see* Dependence, drug, inhalant
  |khat *see* Dependence, drug, stimulant NEC
  |laudanum *see* Dependence, drug, opioid
  |LSD (25) (derivatives) *see* Dependence, drug, hallucinogen
  |luminal *see* Dependence, drug, sedative
  |lysergic acid *see* Dependence, drug, hallucinogen
  |maconha *see* Dependence, drug, cannabis
  |marihuana *see* Dependence, drug, cannabis
  |meprobamate *see* Dependence, drug, sedative
  |mescaline *see* Dependence, drug, hallucinogen
  |methadone *see* Dependence, drug, opioid
  |methamphetamine(s) *see* Dependence, drug, stimulant NEC
  |methaqualone *see* Dependence, drug, sedative
  |methyl
    |alcohol (without remission) F10.20
      |with remission F10.21
    |bromide *see* Dependence, drug, sedative
    |morphine *see* Dependence, drug, opioid
    |phenidate *see* Dependence, drug, stimulant NEC
    |sulfonal *see* Dependence, drug, sedative
  |morphine (sulfate) (sulfite) (type) *see* Dependence, drug, opioid
  |narcotic (drug) NEC *see* Dependence, drug, opioid
  |nembutal *see* Dependence, drug, sedative
  |neraval *see* Dependence, drug, sedative
  |neravan *see* Dependence, drug, sedative
  |neurobarb *see* Dependence, drug, sedative
  |nicotine *see* Dependence, drug, nicotine
  |nitrous oxide F19.20
  |nonbarbiturate sedatives and tranquilizers with similar effect *see* Dependence, drug, sedative
  |on
    |artificial heart (fully implantable) (mechanical) Z95.812
    |aspirator Z99.0
    |care provider (because of) Z74.9
      |impaired mobility Z74.09
      |need for
        |assistance with personal care Z74.1
        |continuous supervision Z74.3
      |no other household member able to render care Z74.2
      |specified reason NEC Z74.8
    |machine Z99.89

Dependence (on) (syndrome) - *continued*
    |enabling NEC Z99.89
    |specified type NEC Z99.89
    |renal dialysis (hemodialysis) (peritoneal) Z99.2
    |respirator Z99.11
    |ventilator Z99.11
    |wheelchair Z99.3
  |opiate *see* Dependence, drug, opioid
  |opioids *see* Dependence, drug, opioid
  |opium (alkaloids) (derivatives) (tincture) *see* Dependence, drug, opioid
  |oxygen (long-term) (supplemental) Z99.81
  |paraldehyde *see* Dependence, drug, sedative
  |paregoric *see* Dependence, drug, opioid
  |PCP (phencyclidine) (or related substance) *see* Dependence, drug, hallucinogen
  |pentobarbital *see* Dependence, drug, sedative
  |pentobarbitone (sodium) *see* Dependence, drug, sedative
  |pentothal *see* Dependence, drug, sedative
  |peyote *see* Dependence, drug, hallucinogen
  |phencyclidine (PCP) (or related substance) *see* Dependence, drug, hallucinogen
  |phenmetrazine *see* Dependence, drug, stimulant NEC
  |phenobarbital *see* Dependence, drug, sedative
  |polysubstance F19.20
  |psilocybin, psilocin, psilocin, psilocyline *see* Dependence, drug, hallucinogen
  |psychostimulant NEC *see* Dependence, drug, stimulant NEC
  |secobarbital *see* Dependence, drug, sedative
  |seconal *see* Dependence, drug, sedative
  |sedative NEC *see* Dependence, drug, sedative
  |specified drug NEC *see* Dependence, drug
  |stimulant NEC *see* Dependence, drug, stimulant NEC
  |substance NEC *see* Dependence, drug
  |supplemental oxygen Z99.81
  |tobacco *see* Dependence, drug, nicotine
    |counseling and surveillance Z71.6
  |tranquilizer NEC *see* Dependence, drug, sedative
  |vitamin B6 E53.1
  |volatile solvents *see* Dependence, drug, inhalant
Dependency
  |care-provider Z74.9
  |passive F60.7
  |reactions (persistent) F60.7
Depersonalization (in neurotic state) (neurotic) (syndrome) F48.1
Depletion
  |extracellular fluid E86.9
  |plasma E86.1
  |potassium E87.6
    |nephropathy N25.89
  |salt or sodium E87.1
    |causing heat exhaustion or prostration T67.4
    |nephropathy N28.9
  |volume NOS E86.9
Deployment (current) (military) status Z56.82
  |in theater or in support of military war, peacekeeping and humanitarian operations Z56.82
  |personal history of Z91.82
    |military war, peacekeeping and humanitarian deployment (current or past conflict) Z91.82
  |returned from Z91.82
Depolarization, premature I49.40
  |atrial I49.1
  |junctional I49.2
  |specified NEC I49.49
  |ventricular I49.3

Deposit
  |bone in Boeck's sarcoid D86.89
  |calcareous, calcium *see* Calcification
  |cholesterol
    |retina H35.89
    |vitreous (body) (humor) *see* Deposit, crystalline
  |conjunctiva H11.11-
  |cornea H18.00-
    |argentous H18.02-
    |due to metabolic disorder H18.03-
    |Kayser-Fleischer ring H18.04-
    |pigmentation *see* Pigmentation, cornea
  |crystalline, vitreous (body) (humor) H43.2-
  |hemosiderin in old scars of cornea *see* Pigmentation, cornea, stromal
  |metallic in lens *see* Cataract, specified NEC
  |skin R23.8
  |tooth, teeth (betel) (black) (green) (materia alba) (orange) (tobacco) K03.6
  |urate, kidney *see* Calculus, kidney
Depraved appetite *see* Pica
Depressed
  |HDL cholesterol E78.6
Depression (acute) (mental) F32.A
  |agitated (single episode) F32.2
  |anaclitic *see* Disorder, adjustment
  |anxiety F41.8
    |persistent F34.1
  |arches *see also* Deformity, limb, flat foot
  |atypical (single episode) F32.89
    |recurrent episode F33.8
  |basal metabolic rate R94.8
  |bone marrow D75.89
  |central nervous system R09.2
  |cerebral R29.818
    |newborn P91.4
  |cerebrovascular I67.9
  |chest wall M95.4
  |climacteric (single episode) F32.89
    |recurrent episode F33.8
  |endogenous (without psychotic symptoms) F33.2
    |with psychotic symptoms F33.3
  |functional activity R68.89
  |hysterical F44.89
  |involutional (single episode) F32.89
    |recurrent episode F33.8
  |major F32.9
    |with psychotic symptoms F32.3
    |recurrent *see* Disorder, depressive, recurrent
  |manic-depressive *see* Disorder, depressive, recurrent
  |masked (single episode) F32.89
  |medullary G93.89
  |menopausal (single episode) F32.89
    |recurrent episode F33.8
  |metatarsus *see* Depression, arches
  |monopolar F33.9
  |nervous F34.1
  |neurotic F34.1
  |nose M95.0
  |postnatal (NOS) F53.0
  |postpartum (NOS) F53.0
  |post-psychotic of schizophrenia F32.89
  |post-schizophrenic F32.89
  |psychogenic (reactive) (single episode) F32.9
  |psychoneurotic F34.1
  |psychotic (single episode) F32.3
    |recurrent F33.3
  |reactive (psychogenic) (single episode) F32.9
    |psychotic (single episode) F32.3
  |recurrent *see* Disorder, depressive, recurrent
  |respiratory center G93.89
  |seasonal *see* Disorder, depressive, recurrent

Depression (acute) (mental) - *continued*
|senile F03
|severe, single episode F32.2
|situational F43.21
|skull Q67.4
|specified NEC (single episode) F32.89
|sternum M95.4
|visual field *see* Defect, visual field
|vital (recurrent) (without psychotic symptoms) F33.2
||with psychotic symptoms F33.3
||single episode F32.2
Deprivation
|cultural Z60.3
|effects NOS T73.9
||specified NEC T73.8
|emotional NEC Z65.8
||affecting infant or child *see* Maltreatment, child, psychological
|food T73.0
|protein *see* Malnutrition
|sleep Z72.820
|social Z60.4
||affecting infant or child *see* Maltreatment, child, psychological
|specified NEC T73.8
|vitamins *see* Deficiency, vitamin
|water T73.1
Derangement
|ankle (internal) *see* Derangement, joint, ankle
|cartilage (articular) NEC *see* Derangement, joint, articular cartilage, by site
||recurrent *see* Dislocation, recurrent
|cruciate ligament, anterior, current injury *see* Sprain, knee, cruciate, anterior
|elbow (internal) *see* Derangement, joint, elbow
|hip (joint) (internal) (old) *see* Derangement, joint, hip
|joint (internal) M24.9
||ankylosis *see* Ankylosis
||articular cartilage M24.10
|||ankle M24.17-
|||elbow M24.12-
|||foot M24.17-
|||hand M24.14-
|||hip M24.15-
|||knee NEC M23.9-
|||loose body *see* Loose, body
|||shoulder M24.11-
|||specified site NEC M24.19
|||wrist M24.13-
||contracture *see* Contraction, joint
||current injury *see also* Dislocation
|||knee, meniscus or cartilage *see* Tear, meniscus
||dislocation
|||pathological *see* Dislocation, pathological
|||recurrent *see* Dislocation, recurrent
||knee *see* Derangement, knee
||ligament *see* Disorder, ligament
||loose body *see* Loose, body
||recurrent *see* Dislocation, recurrent
||specified type NEC M24.80
|||ankle M24.87-
|||elbow M24.82-
|||foot joint M24.87-
|||hand joint M24.84-
|||hip M24.85-
|||shoulder M24.81-
|||specified site NEC M24.89
|||wrist M24.83-
||temporomandibular M26.69
|knee (recurrent) M23.9-
||ligament disruption, spontaneous M23.60-

Derangement - *continued*
||anterior cruciate M23.61-
||capsular M23.67-
||instability, chronic M23.5-
||lateral collateral M23.64-
||medial collateral M23.63-
||posterior cruciate M23.62-
|loose body M23.4-
|meniscus M23.30-
||cystic M23.00-
|||lateral M23.002
||||anterior horn M23.04-
||||posterior horn M23.05-
||||specified NEC M23.06-
|||medial M23.005
||||anterior horn M23.01-
||||posterior horn M23.02-
||||specified NEC M23.03-
||degenerate *see* Derangement, knee, meniscus, specified NEC
||detached *see* Derangement, knee, meniscus, specified NEC
||due to old tear or injury M23.20-
|||lateral M23.20-
||||anterior horn M23.24-
||||posterior horn M23.25-
||||specified NEC M23.26-
|||medial M23.20-
||||anterior horn M23.21-
||||posterior horn M23.22-
||||specified NEC M23.23-
||retained *see* Derangement, knee, meniscus, specified NEC
||specified NEC M23.30-
|||lateral M23.30-
||||anterior horn M23.34-
||||posterior horn M23.35-
||||specified NEC M23.36-
|||medial M23.30-
||||anterior horn M23.31-
||||posterior horn M23.32-
||||specified NEC M23.33-
||old M23.8X-
||specified NEC *see* subcategory M23.8
|low back NEC *see* Dorsopathy, specified NEC
|meniscus *see* Derangement, knee, meniscus
|mental *see* Psychosis
|patella, specified NEC *see* Disorder, patella, derangement NEC
|semilunar cartilage (knee) *see* Derangement, knee, meniscus, specified NEC
|shoulder (internal) *see* Derangement, joint, shoulder
Dercum's disease E88.2
Derealization (neurotic) F48.1
Dermal *see* condition **Dermaphytid** *see* Dermatophytosis
Dermatitis (eczematous) L30.9
|ab igne L59.0
|acarine B88.0
|actinic (due to sun) L57.8
||other than from sun L59.8 |allergic *see* Dermatitis, contact, allergic
|ambustionis, due to burn or scald *see* Burn
|amebic A06.7
|ammonia L22
|arsenical (ingested) L27.8
|artefacta L98.1
||psychogenic F54
|atopic L20.9
||psychogenic F54
||specified NEC L20.89
|autoimmune progesterone L30.8
|berlock, berloque L56.2
|blastomycotic B40.3

Dermatitis - *continued*
|blister beetle L24.89
|bullous, bullosa L13.9
||mucosynechial, atrophic L12.1
||seasonal L30.8
||specified NEC L13.8
|calorica L59.0
||due to burn or scald *see* Burn
|caterpillar L24.89
|cercarial B65.3
|combustionis L59.0
||due to burn or scald *see* Burn
|congelationis T69.1
|contact (occupational) L25.9
||allergic L23.9
|||due to
||||adhesives L23.1
||||cement L23.5
||||chemical products NEC L23.5
||||chromium L23.0
||||cosmetics L23.2
||||dander (cat) (dog) L23.81
||||drugs in contact with skin L23.3
||||dyes L23.4
||||food in contact with skin L23.6
||||hair (cat) (dog) L23.81
||||insecticide L23.5
||||metals L23.0
||||nickel L23.0
||||plants, non-food L23.7
||||plastic L23.5
||||rubber L23.5
||||specified agent NEC L23.89
||due to
|||cement L25.3
|||chemical products NEC L25.3
|||cosmetics L25.0
|||dander (cat) (dog) L23.81
|||drugs in contact with skin L25.1
|||dyes L25.2
|||food in contact with skin L25.4
|||hair (cat) (dog) L23.81
|||plants, non-food L25.5
|||specified agent NEC L25.8
||irritant L24.9
|||due to
||||body fluids L24.A0
|||||incontinence (dual) (fecal) (urinary) L24.A2
|||||saliva L24.A1
|||||specified NEC L24.A9
||||cement L24.5
||||chemical products NEC L24.5
||||cosmetics L24.3
||||detergents L24.0
||||drugs in contact with skin L24.4
||||food in contact with skin L24.6
||||oils and greases L24.1
||||plants, non-food L24.7
||||solvents L24.2
||||specified agent NEC L24.89
|||related to
||||colostomy L24.B3
||||endotracheal tube L24.A9
||||enterocutaneous fistula L24.B3
||||gastrostomy L24.B1
||||ileostomy L24.B3
||||jejunostomy L24.B1
||||saliva or spit fistula L24.B1
||||stoma or fistula L24.B0
|||||digestive L24.B1
|||||fecal or urinary L24.B3
|||||respiratory L24.B2
||||tracheostomy L24.B2
|contusiformis L52

Dermatitis - *continued*
  |desquamative L30.8
  |diabetic *see* E08-E13 with .620
  |diaper L22
  |diphtheritica A36.3
  |dry skin L85.3
  |due to
    |acetone (contact) (irritant) L24.2
    |acids (contact) (irritant) L24.5
    |adhesive(s) (allergic) (contact) (plaster)
      L23.1
      |irritant L24.5
    |alcohol (irritant) (skin contact) (substances
      in category T51) L24.2
      |taken internally L27.8
    |alkalis (contact) (irritant) L24.5
    |arsenic (ingested) L27.8
    |carbon disulfide (contact) (irritant) L24.2
    |caustics (contact) (irritant) L24.5
    |cement (contact) L25.3
    |cereal (ingested) L27.2
    |chemical(s) NEC L25.3
      |taken internally L27.8
    |chlorocompounds L24.2
    |chromium (contact) (irritant) L24.81
    |coffee (ingested) L27.2
    |cold weather L30.8
    |cosmetics (contact) L25.0
      |allergic L23.2
      |irritant L24.3
    |cyclohexanes L24.2
    |dander (cat) (dog) L23.81
    |Demodex species B88.0
    |Dermanyssus gallinae B88.0
    |detergents (contact) (irritant) L24.0
    |dichromate L24.81
    |drugs and medicaments (generalized)
      (internal use) L27.0
      |external *see* Dermatitis, due to, drugs, in
        contact with skin
      |in contact with skin L25.1
        |allergic L23.3
        |irritant L24.4
      |localized skin eruption L27.1
      |specified substance *see* Table of Drugs
        and Chemicals
    |dyes (contact) L25.2
      |allergic L23.4
      |irritant L24.89
    |epidermophytosis *see* Dermatophytosis
    |esters L24.2
    |external irritant NEC L24.9
    |fish (ingested) L27.2
    |flour (ingested) L27.2
    |food (ingested) L27.2
      |in contact with skin L25.4
    |fruit (ingested) L27.2
    |furs (allergic) (contact) L23.81
    |glues *see* Dermatitis, due to, adhesives
    |glycols L24.2
    |greases NEC (contact) (irritant) L24.1
    |hair (cat) (dog) L23.81
    |hot
      |objects and materials *see* Burn
      |weather or places L59.0
    |hydrocarbons L24.2
    |infrared rays L59.8
    |ingestion, ingested substance L27.9
      |chemical NEC L27.8
      |drugs and medicaments *see* Dermatitis,
        due to, drugs
      |food L27.2
      |specified NEC L27.8
    |insecticide in contact with skin L24.5
    |internal agent L27.9

Dermatitis - *continued*
      |drugs and medicaments (generalized) *see*
        Dermatitis, due to, drugs
        |food L27.2
      |irradiation *see* Dermatitis, due to,
        radioactive substance
      |ketones L24.2
      |lacquer tree (allergic) (contact) L23.7
      |light (sun) NEC L57.8
        |acute L56.8
        |other L59.8
      |Liponyssoides sanguineus B88.0
      |low temperature L30.8
      |meat (ingested) L27.2
      |metals, metal salts (contact) (irritant) L24.81
      |milk (ingested) L27.2
      |nickel (contact) (irritant) L24.81
      |nylon (contact) (irritant) L24.5
      |oils NEC (contact) (irritant) L24.1
      |paint solvent (contact) (irritant) L24.2
      |petroleum products (contact) (irritant)
        (substances in T52.0) L24.2
      |plants NEC (contact) L25.5
        |allergic L23.7
        |irritant L24.7
      |plasters (adhesive) (any) (allergic) (contact)
        L23.1
        |irritant L24.5
      |plastic (contact) L25.3
      |preservatives (contact) *see* Dermatitis, due
        to, chemical, in contact with skin
      |primrose (allergic) (contact) L23.7
      |primula (allergic) (contact) L23.7
      |radiation L59.8
        |nonionizing (chronic exposure) L57.8
        |sun NEC L57.8
          |acute L56.8
      |radioactive substance L58.9
        |acute L58.0
        |chronic L58.1
      |radium L58.9
        |acute L58.0
        |chronic L58.1
      |ragweed (allergic) (contact) L23.7
      |Rhus (allergic) (contact) (diversiloba)
        (radicans) (toxicodendron) (venenata)
        (verniciflua) L23.7
      |rubber (contact) L24.5
      |Senecio jacobaea (allergic) (contact) L23.7
      |solvents (contact) (irritant) (substances in
        categories T52) L24.2
      |specified agent NEC (contact) L25.8
        |allergic L23.89
        |irritant L24.89
      |sunshine NEC L57.8
        |acute L56.8
      |tetrachlorethylene (contact) (irritant) L24.2
      |toluene (contact) (irritant) L24.2
      |turpentine (contact) L24.2
      |ultraviolet rays (sun NEC) (chronic
        exposure) L57.8
        |acute L56.8
      |vaccine or vaccination L27.0
        |specified substance *see* Table of Drugs
        and Chemicals
      |varicose veins *see* Varix, leg, with,
        inflammation
      |X-rays L58.9
        |acute L58.0
        |chronic L58.1
  |dyshidrotic L30.1
  |dysmenorrheica N94.6
  |escharotica *see* Burn
  |exfoliative, exfoliativa (generalized) L26
    |neonatorum L00

Dermatitis - *continued*
  |eyelid *(see also* Dermatosis, eyelid) H01.9
  specified NEC H01.8
    |allergic H01.119
      |left H01.116
        |lower H01.115
        |upper H01.114
      |right H01.113
        |lower H01.112
        |upper H01.111
    |contact *see* Dermatitis, eyelid, allergic
    |due to
      |Demodex species B88.0
      |herpes (zoster) B02.39
        |simplex B00.59
    |eczematous H01.139
      |left H01.136
        |lower H01.135
        |upper H01.134
      |right H01.133
        |lower H01.132
        |upper H01.131
  |facta, factitia, factitial L98.1
    |psychogenic F54
  |flexural NEC L20.82
  |friction L30.4
  |fungus B36.9
    |specified type NEC B36.8
  |gangrenosa, gangrenous infantum L08.0
  |harvest mite B88.0
  |heat L59.0
  |herpesviral, vesicular (ear) (lip) B00.1
  |herpetiformis (bullous) (erythematous)
    (pustular) (vesicular) L13.0
    |juvenile L12.2
    |senile L12.0
  |hiemalis L30.8
  |hypostatic, hypostatica *see* Varix, leg, with,
    inflammation
  |infectious eczematoid L30.3
  |infective L30.3
  |irritant *see* Dermatitis, contact, irritant
  |Jacquet's (diaper dermatitis) L22
  |Leptus B88.0
  |lichenified NEC L28.0
  |medicamentosa (generalized) (internal use)
    see Dermatitis, due to drugs
  |mite B88.0
  |multiformis L13.0
    |juvenile L12.2
  |napkin L22
  |neurotica L13.0
  |nummular L30.0
  |papillaris capillitii L73.0
  |pellagrous E52
  |perioral L71.0
  |photocontact L56.2
  |polymorpha dolorosa L13.0
  |pruriginosa L13.0
  |pruritic NEC L30.8
  |psychogenic F54
  |purulent L08.0
  |pustular
    |contagious B08.02
    |subcorneal L13.1
  |pyococcal L08.0
  |pyogenica L08.0
  |repens L40.2
  |Ritter's (exfoliativa) L00
  |Schamberg's L81.7
  |schistosome B65.3
  |seasonal bullous L30.8
  |seborrheic L21.9
    |infantile L21.1
    |specified NEC L21.8

Dermatitis - *continued*
|sensitization NOS L23.9
|septic L08.0
|solare L57.8
|specified NEC L30.8
|stasis I87.2
 |with
  |varicose ulcer *see* Varix, leg, with ulcer, with inflammation
  |varicose veins *see* Varix, leg, with, inflammation
 |due to postthrombotic syndrome *see* Syndrome, postthrombotic
|suppurative L08.0
|traumatic NEC L30.4
|trophoneurotica L13.0
|ultraviolet (sun) (chronic exposure) L57.8
 |acute L56.8
|varicose *see* Varix, leg, with, inflammation
|vegetans L10.1
|verrucosa B43.0
|vesicular, herpesviral B00.1
Dermatoarthritis, lipoid E78.81
Dermatochalasis, eyelid H02.839
|left H02.836
 |lower H02.835
 |upper H02.834
|right H02.833
 |lower H02.832
 |upper H02.831
Dermatofibroma (lenticulare) *see* Neoplasm, skin, benign
|protuberans *see* Neoplasm, skin, uncertain behavior
Dermatofibrosarcoma (pigmented) (protuberans) *see* Neoplasm, skin, malignant
Dermatographia L50.3
Dermatolysis (exfoliativa) (congenital) Q82.8
|acquired L57.4
|eyelids *see* Blepharochalasis
|palpebrarum *see* Blepharochalasis
|senile L57.4
Dermatomegaly NEC Q82.8
Dermatomucosomyositis M33.10
|with
 |myopathy M33.12
 |respiratory involvement M33.11
 |specified organ involvement NEC M33.19
Dermatomycosis B36.9
|furfuracea B36.0
|specified type NEC B36.8
Dermatomyositis (acute) (chronic) *see also* Dermatopolymyositis
|adult (*see also* Dermatomyositis, specified NEC) M33.10
|in (due to) neoplastic disease *see also* Neoplasm D49.9 *[M36.0]*
|juvenile M33.00
 |with
  |myopathy M33.02
  |respiratory involvement M33.01
  |specified organ involvement NEC M33.09
 |without myopathy M33.03
|specified NEC M33.10
 |with
  |myopathy M33.12
  |respiratory involvement M33.11
  |specified organ involvement NEC M33.19
 |without myopathy M33.13
Dermatoneuritis of children *see* Poisoning, mercury
Dermatophilosis A48.8
Dermatophytid L30.2
Dermatophytid *see* Dermatophytosis

Dermatophytosis (epidermophyton) (infection) (Microsporum) (tinea) (Trichophyton) B35.9
|beard B35.0
|body B35.4
|capitis B35.0
|corporis B35.4
|deep-seated B35.8
|disseminated B35.8
|foot B35.3
|granulomatous B35.8
|groin B35.6
|hand B35.2
|nail B35.1
|perianal (area) B35.6
|scalp B35.0
|specified NEC B35.8
Dermatopolymyositis M33.90
|with
 |myopathy M33.92
 |respiratory involvement M33.91
 |specified organ involvement NEC M33.99
|in neoplastic disease *see also* Neoplasm D49.9 *[M36.0]*
|juvenile M33.00
 |with
  |myopathy M33.02
  |respiratory involvement M33.01
  |specified organ involvement NEC M33.09
|specified NEC M33.10
 |myopathy M33.12
 |respiratory involvement M33.11
 |specified organ involvement NEC M33.19
|without myopathy M33.93
Dermatopolyneuritis *see* Poisoning, mercury
Dermatorrhexis Q79.6
|acquired L57.4
Dermatosclerosis *see also* Scleroderma
|localized L94.0
Dermatosis L98.9
|Andrews' L08.89
|Bowen's *see* Neoplasm, skin, in situ
|bullous L13.9
 |specified NEC L13.8
|exfoliativa L26
|eyelid (noninfectious) (see also Dermatitis, eyelid) H01.9
 |discoid lupus erythematosus *see* Lupus, erythematosus, eyelid
 |xeroderma *see* Xeroderma, acquired, eyelid
|factitial L98.1
|febrile neutrophilic L98.2
|gonococcal A54.89
|herpetiformis L13.0
 |juvenile L12.2
|linear IgA L13.8
|menstrual NEC L98.8
|neutrophilic, febrile L98.2
|occupational *see* Dermatitis, contact
|papulosa nigra L82.1
|pigmentary L81.9
 |progressive L81.7
 |Schamberg's L81.7
|psychogenic F54
|purpuric, pigmented L81.7
|pustular, subcorneal L13.1
|transient acantholytic L11.1
Dermographia, dermographism L50.3
Dermoid (cyst) *see also* Neoplasm, benign, by site
|with malignant transformation C56-
|due to radiation (nonionizing) L57.8

Dermopathy
|infiltrative with thyrotoxicosis *see* Thyrotoxicosis
|nephrogenic fibrosing L90.8
Dermophytosis *see* Dermatophytosis
Descemetocele H18.73-
Descemet's membrane *see* condition
Descending *see* condition
Descensus uteri *see* Prolapse, uterus
Desert
|rheumatism B38.0
|sore *see* Ulcer, skin
Desertion (newborn) *see* Maltreatment
Desmoid (extra-Abdominal) (tumor) *see* Neoplasm, connective tissue, uncertain behavior
|abdominal D48.1
Despondency F32.A
Desquamation, skin R23.4
Destruction, destructive *see also* Damage
|articular facet *see also* Derangement, joint, specified type NEC
 |knee M23.8X-
 |vertebra *see* Spondylosis
|bone *see also* Disorder, bone, specified type NEC
 |syphilitic A52.77
|joint *see also* Derangement, joint, specified type NEC
 |sacroiliac M53.3
|rectal sphincter K62.89
|septum (nasal) J34.89
|tuberculous NEC *see* Tuberculosis
|tympanum, tympanic membrane (nontraumatic) *see* Disorder, tympanic membrane, specified NEC
|vertebral disc *see* Degeneration, intervertebral disc
Destructiveness *see also* Disorder, conduct
|adjustment reaction *see* Disorder, adjustment
Desultory labor O62.2
Detachment
|cartilage *see* Sprain
|cervix, annular N88.8
 |complicating delivery O71.3
|choroid (old) (postinfectional) (simple) (spontaneous) H31.40-
 |hemorrhagic H31.41-
 |serous H31.42-
|ligament *see* Sprain
|meniscus (knee) *see also* Derangement, knee, meniscus, specified NEC
 |current injury *see* Tear, meniscus
 |due to old tear or injury *see* Derangement, knee, meniscus, due to old tear
|retina (without retinal break) (serous) H33.2-
 |with retinal:
  |break H33.00-
   |giant H33.03-
   |multiple H33.02-
   |single H33.01-
   |dialysis H33.04-
 |pigment epithelium *see* Degeneration, retina, separation of layers, pigment epithelium detachment
 |rhegmatogenous *see* Detachment, retina, with retinal, break
 |specified NEC H33.8
 |total H33.05-
 |traction H33.4-
|vitreous (body) H43.81
Detergent asthma J69.8
Deterioration
|epileptic F06.8
|general physical R53.81

Deterioration - *continued*
  |heart, cardiac *see* Degeneration, myocardial
  |mental *see* Psychosis
  |myocardial, myocardium *see* Degeneration, myocardial
  |senile (simple) R54
Deuteranomaly (anomalous trichromat) H53.53
Deuteranopia (complete) (incomplete) H53.53
Development
  |abnormal, bone Q79.9
  |arrested R62.50
    |bone *see* Arrest, development or growth, bone
    |child R62.50
    |due to malnutrition E45
  |defective, congenital *see also* Anomaly, by site
    |cauda equina Q06.3
    |left ventricle Q24.8
      |in hypoplastic left heart syndrome Q23.4
    |valve Q24.8
      |pulmonary Q22.3
  |delayed *see also* Delay, development R62.50
    |arithmetical skills F81.2
    |language (skills) (expressive) F80.1
    |learning skill F81.9
    |mixed skills F88
    |motor coordination F82
    |reading F81.0
    |specified learning skill NEC F81.89
    |speech F80.9
    |spelling F81.81
    |written expression F81.81
  |imperfect, congenital *see also* Anomaly, by site
    |heart Q24.9
    |lungs Q33.6
  |incomplete
    |bronchial tree Q32.4
    |organ or site not listed *see* Hypoplasia, by site
    |respiratory system Q34.9
  |sexual, precocious NEC E30.1
  |tardy, mental *see also* Disability, intellectual F79
Developmental *see* condition
  |testing, infant or child *see* Examination, child
Devergie's disease (pityriasis rubra pilaris) L44.0
Deviation (in)
  |conjugate palsy (eye) (spastic) H51.0
  |esophagus (acquired) K22.89
  |eye, skew H51.8
  |midline (jaw) (teeth) (dental arch) M26.29
    |specified site NEC *see* Malposition
  |nasal septum J34.2
    |congenital Q67.4
  |opening and closing of the mandible M26.53
  |organ or site, congenital NEC *see* Malposition, congenital
  |septum (nasal) (acquired) J34.2
    |congenital Q67.4
  |sexual F65.9
    |bestiality F65.89
    |erotomania F52.8
    |exhibitionism F65.2
    |fetishism, fetishistic F65.0
      |transvestism F65.1
    |frotteurism F65.81
    |masochism F65.51
    |multiple F65.89
    |necrophilia F65.89
    |nymphomania F52.8
    |pederosis F65.4

Deviation - *continued*
    |pedophilia F65.4
    |sadism, sadomasochism F65.52
    |satyriasis F52.8
    |specified type NEC F65.89
    |transvestism F64.1
    |voyeurism F65.3
  |teeth, midline M26.29
  |trachea J39.8
  |ureter, congenital Q62.61
Device
  |cerebral ventricle (communicating) in situ Z98.2
  |contraceptive *see* Contraceptive, device
  |drainage, cerebrospinal fluid, in situ Z98.2
Devic's disease G36.0
Devil's
  |grip B33.0
  |pinches (purpura simplex) D69.2
Devitalized tooth K04.99
Devonshire colic *see* Poisoning, lead
Dextrinosis, limit (debrancher enzyme deficiency) E74.03
Dextrocardia (true) Q24.0
  |with
    |complete transposition of viscera Q89.3
    |situs inversus Q89.3
Dextroposition, aorta Q20.3
  |in tetralogy of Fallot Q21.3
Dextrotransposition, aorta Q20.3
d-Glycericacidemia E72.59
Dhat syndrome F48.8
Dhobi itch B35.6
Di George's syndrome D82.1
Di Guglielmo's disease C94.0-
Diabetes, diabetic (mellitus) (sugar) E11.9
  |with
    |amyotrophy E11.44
    |arthropathy NEC E11.618
    |autonomic (poly) neuropathy E11.43
    |cataract E11.36
    |Charcot's joints E11.610
    |chronic kidney disease E11.22
    |circulatory complication NEC E11.59
    |coma due to
      |hyperosmolarity E11.01
      |hypoglycemia E11.641
      |ketoacidosis E11.11
    |complication E11.8
      |specified NEC E11.69
    |dermatitis E11.620
    |foot ulcer E11.621
    |gangrene E11.52
    |gastroparalysis E11.43
    |gastroparesis E11.43
    |glomerulonephrosis, intracapillary E11.21
    |glomerulosclerosis, intercapillary E11.21
    |hyperglycemia E11.65
    |hyperosmolarity E11.00
      |with coma E11.01
    |hypoglycemia E11.649
      |with coma E11.641
    |ketoacidosis E11.10
      |with coma E11.11
    |kidney complications NEC E11.29
    |Kimmelstiel-Wilson disease E11.21
    |loss of protective sensation (LOPS) *see* Diabetes, by type, with neuropathy
    |mononeuropathy E11.41
    |myasthenia E11.44
    |necrobiosis lipoidica E11.620
    |nephropathy E11.21
    |neuralgia E11.42
    |neurologic complication NEC E11.49
    |neuropathic arthropathy E11.610

Diabetes, diabetic - *continued*
    |neuropathy E11.40
    |ophthalmic complication NEC E11.39
    |oral complication NEC E11.638
    |osteomyelitis E11.69
    |periodontal disease E11.630
    |peripheral angiopathy E11.51
      |with gangrene E11.52
    |polyneuropathy E11.42
    |renal complication NEC E11.29
    |renal tubular degeneration E11.29
    |retinopathy E11.319
      |with macular edema E11.311
        |resolved following treatment E11.37
      |nonproliferative E11.329
        |with macular edema E11.321
        |mild E11.329
          |with macular edema E11.321
        |moderate E11.339
          |with macular edema E11.331
        |severe E11.349
          |with macular edema E11.341
      |proliferative E11.359
        |with
          |combined traction retinal detachment and rhegmatogenous retinal detachment E11.354
          |macular edema E11.351
          |stable proliferative diabetic retinopathy E11.355
          |traction retinal detachment involving the macula E11.352
          |traction retinal detachment not involving the macula E11.353
    |skin complication NEC E11.628
    |skin ulcer NEC E11.622
  |brittle *see* Diabetes, type 1
  |bronzed E83.110
  |complicating pregnancy *see* Pregnancy, complicated by, diabetes
  |dietary counseling and surveillance Z71.3
  |due to
    |autoimmune process *see* Diabetes, type 1
    |immune mediated pancreatic islet beta-cell destruction *see* Diabetes, type 1
  |due to drug or chemical E09.9
    |with
      |amyotrophy E09.44
      |arthropathy NEC E09.618
      |autonomic (poly) neuropathy E09.43
      |cataract E09.36
      |Charcot's joints E09.610
      |chronic kidney disease E09.22
      |circulatory complication NEC E09.59
      |complication E09.8
        |specified NEC E09.69
      |dermatitis E09.620
      |foot ulcer E09.621
      |gangrene E09.52
      |gastroparalysis E09.43
      |gastroparesis E09.43
      |glomerulonephrosis, intracapillary E09.21
      |glomerulosclerosis, intercapillary E09.21
      |hyperglycemia E09.65
      |hyperosmolarity E09.00
        |with coma E09.01
      |hypoglycemia E09.649
        |with coma E09.641
      |ketoacidosis E09.10
        |with coma E09.11
      |kidney complications NEC E09.29
      |Kimmelstiel-Wilson disease E09.21
      |mononeuropathy E09.41
      |myasthenia E09.44
      |necrobiosis lipoidica E09.620

Diabetes, diabetic - *continued*
  |nephropathy E09.21
  |neuralgia E09.42
  |neurologic complication NEC E09.49
  |neuropathic arthropathy E09.610
  |neuropathy E09.40
  |ophthalmic complication NEC E09.39
  |oral complication NEC E09.638
  |periodontal disease E09.630
  |peripheral angiopathy E09.51
    |with gangrene E09.52
  |polyneuropathy E09.42
  |renal complication NEC E09.29
  |renal tubular degeneration E09.29
  |retinopathy E09.319
    |with macular edema E09.311
    |resolved following treatment E09.37
    |nonproliferative E09.329
      |with macular edema E09.321
      |mild E09.329
        |with macular edema E09.321
      |moderate E09.339
        |with macular edema E09.331
      |severe E09.349
        |with macular edema E09.341
    |proliferative E09.359
      |with
        |combined traction retinal
          detachment and rhegmatogenous
          retinal detachment E09.354
        |macular edema E09.351
        |stable proliferative diabetic
          retinopathy E09.355
        |traction retinal detachment
          involving the macula E09.352
        |traction retinal detachment not
          involving the macula E09.353
  |skin complication NEC E09.628
  |skin ulcer NEC E09.622
|due to underlying condition E08.9
  |with
    |amyotrophy E08.44
    |arthropathy NEC E08.618
    |autonomic (poly) neuropathy E08.43
    |cataract E08.36
    |Charcot's joints E08.610
    |chronic kidney disease E08.22
    |circulatory complication NEC E08.59
    |complication E08.8
      |specified NEC E08.69
    |dermatitis E08.620
    |foot ulcer E08.621
    |gangrene E08.52
    |gastroparalysis E08.43
    |gastroparesis E08.43
    |glomerulonephrosis, intracapillary E08.21
    |glomerulosclerosis, intercapillary E08.21
    |hyperglycemia E08.65
    |hyperosmolarity E08.00
      |with coma E08.01
    |hypoglycemia E08.649
      |with coma E08.641
    |ketoacidosis E08.10
      |with coma E08.11
    |kidney complications NEC E08.29
    |Kimmelstiel-Wilson disease E08.21
    |mononeuropathy E08.41
    |myasthenia E08.44
    |necrobiosis lipoidica E08.620
    |nephropathy E08.21
    |neuralgia E08.42
    |neurologic complication NEC E08.49
    |neuropathic arthropathy E08.610
    |neuropathy E08.40
    |ophthalmic complication NEC E08.39

    |oral complication NEC E08.638
    |periodontal disease E08.630
    |peripheral angiopathy E08.51
      |with gangrene E08.52
    |polyneuropathy E08.42
    |renal complication NEC E08.29
    |renal tubular degeneration E08.29
    |retinopathy E08.319
      |with macular edema E08.311
      |resolved following treatment E08.37
      |nonproliferative E08.329
        |with macular edema E08.321
        |mild E08.329
          |with macular edema E08.321
        |moderate E08.339
          |with macular edema E08.331
        |severe E08.349
          |with macular edema E08.341
    |proliferative E08.359
      |with
        |combined traction retinal
          detachment and rhegmatogenous
          retinal detachment E08.354
        |macular edema E08.351
        |stable proliferative diabetic
          retinopathy E08.355
        |traction retinal detachment
          involving the macula E08.352
        |traction retinal detachment not
          involving the macula E08.353
    |skin complication NEC E08.628
    |skin ulcer NEC E08.622
|gestational (in pregnancy) O24.419
  |affecting newborn P70.0
  |diet controlled O24.410
  |in childbirth O24.429
    |diet controlled O24.420
    |insulin (and diet) controlled O24.424
    |oral drug controlled (antidiabetic)
      (hypoglycemic) O24.425
  |insulin (and diet) controlled O24.414
  |oral drug controlled (antidiabetic)
    (hypoglycemic) O24.415
  |puerperal O24.439
    |diet controlled O24.430
    |insulin (and diet) controlled O24.434
    |oral drug controlled (antidiabetic)
      (hypoglycemic) O24.435
|hepatogenous E13.9
|idiopathic *see* Diabetes, type 1
|inadequately controlled   code to Diabetes, by
  type, with hyperglycemia
|insipidus E23.2
  |nephrogenic N25.1
  |pituitary E23.2
  |vasopressin resistant N25.1
|insulin dependent   code to type of diabetes
|juvenile-onset *see* Diabetes, type 1
|ketosis-prone *see* Diabetes, type 1
|latent R73.03
|neonatal (transient) P70.2
|non-insulin dependent   code to type of
  diabetes
|out of control   code to Diabetes, by type, with
  hyperglycemia
|phosphate E83.39
|poorly controlled   code to Diabetes, by type,
  with hyperglycemia
|postpancreatectomy *see* Diabetes, specified
  type NEC
|postprocedural *see* Diabetes, specified type
  NEC
|secondary diabetes mellitus NEC *see*
  Diabetes, specified type NEC

|specified type NEC E13.9
  |with
    |amyotrophy E13.44
    |arthropathy NEC E13.618
    |autonomic (poly) neuropathy E13.43
    |cataract E13.36
    |Charcot's joints E13.610
    |chronic kidney disease E13.22
    |circulatory complication NEC E13.59
    |complication E13.8
      |specified NEC E13.69
    |dermatitis E13.620
    |foot ulcer E13.621
    |gangrene E13.52
    |gastroparalysis E13.43
    |gastroparesis E13.43
    |glomerulonephrosis, intracapillary E13.21
    |glomerulosclerosis, intercapillary E13.21
    |hyperglycemia E13.65
    |hyperosmolarity E13.00
      |with coma E13.01
    |hypoglycemia E13.649
      |with coma E13.641
    |ketoacidosis E13.10
      |with coma E13.11
    |kidney complications NEC E13.29
    |Kimmelstiel-Wilson disease E13.21
    |mononeuropathy E13.41
    |myasthenia E13.44
    |necrobiosis lipoidica E13.620
    |nephropathy E13.21
    |neuralgia E13.42
    |neurologic complication NEC E13.49
    |neuropathic arthropathy E13.610
    |neuropathy E13.40
    |ophthalmic complication NEC E13.39
    |oral complication NEC E13.638
    |periodontal disease E13.630
    |peripheral angiopathy E13.51
      |with gangrene E13.52
    |polyneuropathy E13.42
    |renal complication NEC E13.29
    |renal tubular degeneration E13.29
    |retinopathy E13.319
      |with macular edema E13.311
      |resolved following treatment E13.37
      |nonproliferative E13.329
        |with macular edema E13.321
        |mild E13.329
          |with macular edema E13.321
        |moderate E13.339
          |with macular edema E13.331
        |severe E13.349
          |with macular edema E13.341
    |proliferative E13.359
      |with
        |combined traction retinal
          detachment and
          rhegmatogenous retinal
          detachment E13.354
        |macular edema E13.351
        |stable proliferative diabetic
          retinopathy E13.355
        |traction retinal detachment
          involving the macula E13.352
        |traction retinal detachment not
          involving the macula E13.353
    |skin complication NEC E13.628
    |skin ulcer NEC E13.622
|steroid-induced *see* Diabetes, due to, drug or
  chemical
|type 1 E10.9
  |with
    |amyotrophy E10.44

Diabetes, diabetic - *continued*
- arthropathy NEC E10.618
- autonomic (poly) neuropathy E10.43
- cataract E10.36
- Charcot's joints E10.610
- chronic kidney disease E10.22
- circulatory complication NEC E10.59
- coma due to
  - hyperosmolarity E11.01
  - hypoglycemia E11.641
  - ketoacidosis
- complication E10.8
  - specified NEC E10.69
- dermatitis E10.620
- foot ulcer E10.621
- gangrene E10.52
- gastroparalysis E10.43
- gastroparesis E10.43
- glomerulonephrosis, intracapillary E10.21
- glomerulosclerosis, intercapillary E10.21
- hyperglycemia E10.65
- hypoglycemia E10.649
  - with coma E10.641
- ketoacidosis E10.10
  - with coma E10.11
- kidney complications NEC E10.29
- Kimmelstiel-Wilson disease E10.21
- mononeuropathy E10.41
- myasthenia E10.44
- necrobiosis lipoidica E10.620
- nephropathy E10.21
- neuralgia E10.42
- neurologic complication NEC E10.49
- neuropathic arthropathy E10.610
- neuropathy E10.40
- ophthalmic complication NEC E10.39
- oral complication NEC E10.638
- osteomyelitis E10.69
- periodontal disease E10.630
- peripheral angiopathy E10.51
  - with gangrene E10.52
- polyneuropathy E10.42
- renal complication NEC E10.29
- renal tubular degeneration E10.29
- retinopathy E10.319
  - with macular edema E10.311
  - resolved following treatment E10.37
  - nonproliferative E10.329
    - with macular edema E10.321
    - mild E10.329
      - with macular edema E10.321
    - moderate E10.339
      - with macular edema E10.331
    - severe E10.349
      - with macular edema E10.341
  - proliferative E10.359
    - with
      - combined traction retinal detachment and rhegmatogenous retinal detachment E10.354
      - macular edema E10.351
      - stable proliferative diabetic retinopathy E10.355
      - traction retinal detachment involving the macula E10.352
      - traction retinal detachment not involving the macula E10.353
- skin complication NEC E10.628
- skin ulcer NEC E10.622
- type 2 E11.9
  - with
    - amyotrophy E11.44
    - arthropathy NEC E11.618
    - autonomic (poly) neuropathy E11.43

Diabetes, diabetic - *continued*
- cataract E11.36
- Charcot's joints E11.610
- chronic kidney disease E11.22
- circulatory complication NEC E11.59
- complication E11.8
  - specified NEC E11.69
- dermatitis E11.620
- foot ulcer E11.621
- gangrene E11.52
- gastroparalysis E11.43
- gastroparesis E11.43
- glomerulonephrosis, intracapillary E11.21
- glomerulosclerosis, intercapillary E11.21
- hyperglycemia E11.65
- hyperosmolarity E11.00
  - with coma E11.01
- hypoglycemia E11.649
  - with coma E11.641
- ketoacidosis E11.10
  - with coma E11.11
- kidney complications NEC E11.29
- Kimmelstiel-Wilson disease E11.21
- mononeuropathy E11.41
- myasthenia E11.44
- necrobiosis lipoidica E11.620
- nephropathy E11.21
- neuralgia E11.42
- neurologic complication NEC E11.49
- neuropathic arthropathy E11.610
- neuropathy E11.40
- ophthalmic complication NEC E11.39
- oral complication NEC E11.638
- osteomyelitis E11.69
- periodontal disease E11.630
- peripheral angiopathy E11.51
  - with gangrene E11.52
- polyneuropathy E11.42
- renal complication NEC E11.29
- renal tubular degeneration E11.29
- retinopathy E11.319
  - with macular edema E11.311
  - resolved following treatment E11.37
  - nonproliferative E11.329
    - with macular edema E11.321
    - mild E11.329
      - with macular edema E11.321
    - moderate E11.339
      - with macular edema E11.331
    - severe E11.349
      - with macular edema E11.341
  - proliferative E11.359
    - with
      - combined traction retinal detachment and rhegmatogenous retinal detachment E11.354
      - macular edema E11.351
      - stable proliferative diabetic retinopathy E11.355
      - traction retinal detachment involving the macula E11.352
      - traction retinal detachment not involving the macula E11.353
- skin complication NEC E11.628
- skin ulcer NEC E11.622
- uncontrolled
  - meaning
    - hyperglycemia *see* Diabetes, by type, with, hyperglycemia
    - hypoglycemia *see* Diabetes, by type, with, hypoglycemia

Diacyclothrombopathia D69.1
Diagnosis deferred R69

Dialysis (intermittent) (treatment)
- noncompliance (with) Z91.15
- renal (hemodialysis) (peritoneal), status Z99.2
- retina, retinal *see* Detachment, retina, with retinal, dialysis

Diamond-Blackfan anemia (congenital hypoplastic) D61.01
Diamond-Gardener syndrome (autoerythrocyte sensitization) D69.2
Diaper rash L22
Diaphoresis (excessive) R61
Diaphragm *see* condition
Diaphragmalgia R07.1
Diaphragmatitis, diaphragmitis J98.6
Diaphysial aclasis Q78.6
Diaphysitis *see* Osteomyelitis, specified type NEC
Diarrhea, diarrheal (disease) (infantile) (inflammatory) R19.7
- achlorhydric K31.83
- allergic K52.29
  - due to
    - colitis *see* Colitis, allergic
    - enteritis *see* Enteritis, allergic
- amebic *see also* Amebiasis A06.0
  - with abscess *see* Abscess, amebic
  - acute A06.0
  - chronic A06.1
  - nondysenteric A06.2
- bacillary *see* Dysentery, bacillary
- balantidial A07.0
- cachectic NEC K52.89
- Chilomastix A07.8
- choleriformis A00.1
- chronic (noninfectious) K52.9
- coccidial A07.3
- Cochin-China K90.1
  - strongyloidiasis B78.0
- Dientamoeba A07.8
- dietetic *see also* Diarrhea, allergic K52.29
- drug-induced K52.1
- due to
  - bacteria A04.9
    - specified NEC A04.8
  - Campylobacter A04.5
  - Capillaria philippinensis B81.1
  - Clostridium difficile
    - not specified as recurrent A04.72
    - recurrent A04.71
  - Clostridium perfringens (C) (F) A04.8
  - Cryptosporidium A07.2
  - drugs K52.1
  - Escherichia coli A04.4
    - enteroaggregative A04.4
    - enterohemorrhagic A04.3
    - enteroinvasive A04.2
    - enteropathogenic A04.0
    - enterotoxigenic A04.1
    - specified NEC A04.4
  - food hypersensitivity *see also* Diarrhea, allergic K52.29
  - Necator americanus B76.1
  - S. japonicum B65.2
  - specified organism NEC A08.8
    - bacterial A04.8
    - viral A08.39
  - Staphylococcus A04.8
  - Trichuris trichiura B79
  - virus *see* Enteritis, viral
  - Yersinia enterocolitica A04.6
- dysenteric A09
- endemic A09
- epidemic A09
- flagellate A07.9
- Flexner's (ulcerative) A03.1

Diarrhea, diarrheal - *continued*
  |functional K59.1
    |following gastrointestinal surgery K91.89
    |psychogenic F45.8
  |Giardia lamblia A07.1
  |giardial A07.1
  |hill K90.1
  |infectious A09
  |malarial *see* Malaria
  |mite B88.0
  |mycotic NEC B49
  |neonatal (noninfectious) P78.3
  |nervous F45.8
  |neurogenic K59.1
  |noninfectious K52.9
  |postgastrectomy K91.1
  |postvagotomy K91.1
  |protozoal A07.9
    |specified NEC A07.8
  |psychogenic F45.8
  |specified
    |bacterium NEC A04.8
    |virus NEC A08.39
  |strongyloidiasis B78.0
  |toxic K52.1
  |trichomonal A07.8
  |tropical K90.1
  |tuberculous A18.32
  |viral *see* Enteritis, viral
Diastasis
  |cranial bones M84.88
    |congenital NEC Q75.8
  |joint (traumatic) *see* Dislocation
  |muscle M62.00
    |ankle M62.07-
    |congenital Q79.8
    |foot M62.07-
    |forearm M62.03-
    |hand M62.04-
    |lower leg M62.06-
    |pelvic region M62.05-
    |shoulder region M62.01-
    |specified site NEC M62.08
    |thigh M62.05-
    |upper arm M62.02-
  |recti (abdomen)
    |complicating delivery O71.89
    |congenital Q79.59
Diastema, tooth, teeth, fully erupted M26.32
Diastematomyelia Q06.2
Diataxia, cerebral G80.4
Diathesis
  |allergic *see* History, allergy bleeding
    (familial) D69.9
  |cystine (familial) E72.00
  |gouty *see* Gout
  |hemorrhagic (familial) D69.9
    |newborn NEC P53
  |spasmophilic R29.0
Diaz's disease or osteochondrosis (juvenile)
    (talus) *see* Osteochondrosis, juvenile, tarsus
Dibothriocephalus, dibothriocephaliasis
    (latus) (infection) (infestation) B70.0
  |larval B70.1
Dicephalus, dicephaly Q89.4
Dichotomy, teeth K00.2
Dichromat, dichromatopsia (congenital) *see*
    Deficiency, color vision
Dichuchwa A65
Dicroceliasis B66.2
Didelphia, didelphys *see* Double uterus
Didymitis N45.1
  |with orchitis N45.3
Dietary
  |inadequacy or deficiency E63.9
  |surveillance and counseling Z71.3

Dietl's crisis N13.8
Dieulafoy lesion (hemorrhagic)
  |duodenum K31.82
  |esophagus K22.89
  |intestine (colon) K63.81
  |stomach K31.82
Difficult, difficulty (in)
  |acculturation Z60.3
  |feeding R63.30
    |newborn P92.9
      |breast P92.5
      |specified NEC P92.8
    |nonorganic (infant or child) F98.29
  |intubation, in anesthesia T88.4
  |mechanical, gastroduodenal stoma K91.89
    |causing obstruction (*see also* Obstruction,
    intestine, postoperative) K91.30
  |micturition
    |need to immediately re-void R39.191
    |position dependent R39.192
    |specified NEC R39.198
  |reading (developmental) F81.0
    |secondary to emotional disorders F93.9
  |spelling (specific) F81.81
    |with reading disorder F81.89
    |due to inadequate teaching Z55.8
  |swallowing *see* Dysphagia
  |walking R26.2
  |work
    |conditions NEC Z56.5
    |schedule Z56.3
Diffuse *see* condition
Digeorge's syndrome (thymic hypoplasia)
    D82.1
Digestive *see* condition
Dihydropyrimidine dehydrogenase disease
    (DPD) E88.89
Diktyoma *see* Neoplasm, malignant, by site
Dilaceration, tooth K00.4
Dilatation
  |anus K59.89
    |venule *see* Hemorrhoids
  |aorta (focal) (general) *see* Ectasia, aorta
    |with aneurysm *see* Aneurysm, aorta
    |congenital Q25.44
  |artery *see* Aneurysm
  |bladder (sphincter) N32.89
    |congenital Q64.79
  |blood vessel I99.8
  |bronchial J47.9
    |with
      |exacerbation (acute) J47.1
      |lower respiratory infection J47.0
  |calyx N28.89
- - due to obstruction - see Hydronephrosis
  |capillaries I78.8
  |cardiac (acute) (chronic) *see also*
    Hypertrophy, cardiac
    |congenital Q24.8
      |valve NEC Q24.8
        |pulmonary Q22.3
    |valve *see* Endocarditis
  |cavum septi pellucidi Q06.8
  |cervix (uteri) *see also* Incompetency, cervix
    |incomplete, poor, slow complicating
    delivery O62.0
  |colon K59.39
    |congenital Q43.1
    |psychogenic F45.8
    |toxic K59.31
  |common duct (acquired) K83.8
    |congenital Q44.5
  |cystic duct (acquired) K82.8
    |congenital Q44.5
  |duct, mammary *see* Ectasia, mammary duct

Dilatation - *continued*
  |duodenum K59.89
  |esophagus K22.89
    |congenital Q39.5
    |due to achalasia K22.0
  |eustachian tube, congenital Q17.8
  |gallbladder K82.8
  |gastric *see* Dilatation, stomach
  |heart (acute) (chronic) *see also* Hypertrophy,
    cardiac
    |congenital Q24.8
    |valve *see* Endocarditis
  |ileum K59.89
    |psychogenic F45.8
  |jejunum K59.89
    |psychogenic F45.8
  |kidney (calyx) (collecting structures) (cystic)
    (parenchyma) (pelvis) (idiopathic) N28.89
    |due to obstruction - see Hydronephrosis
  |lacrimal passages or duct *see* Disorder,
    lacrimal system, changes
  |lymphatic vessel I89.0
  |mammary duct *see* Ectasia, mammary duct
  |Meckel's diverticulum (congenital) Q43.0
    |malignant *see* Table of Neoplasms, small
    intestine, malignant
  |myocardium (acute) (chronic) *see*
    Hypertrophy, cardiac
  |organ or site, congenital NEC *see* Distortion
  |pancreatic duct K86.89
  |pericardium *see* Pericarditis
  |pharynx J39.2
  |prostate N42.89
  |pulmonary
    |artery (idiopathic) I28.8
    |valve, congenital Q22.3
  |pupil H57.04
  |rectum K59.39
  |saccule, congenital Q16.5
  |salivary gland (duct) K11.8
  |sphincter ani K62.89
  |stomach K31.89
    |acute K31.0
    |psychogenic F45.8
  |submaxillary duct K11.8
  |trachea, congenital Q32.1
  |ureter (idiopathic) N28.82
    |congenital Q62.2
    |due to obstruction N13.4
  |urethra (acquired) N36.8
  |vasomotor I73.9
  |vein I86.8
  |ventricular, ventricle (acute) (chronic) *see also*
    Hypertrophy, cardiac
    |cerebral, congenital Q04.8
  |venule NEC I86.8
  |vesical orifice N32.89
Dilated, dilation *see* Dilatation
Diminished, diminution
  |hearing (acuity) *see* Deafness
  |sense or sensation (cold) (heat) (tactile)
    (vibratory) R20.8
  |vision NEC H54.7
  |vital capacity R94.2
Diminuta taenia B71.0
Dimitri-Sturge-Weber disease Q85.8
Dimple
  |congenital sacral Q82.6
  |parasacral Q82.6
  |pilonidal or postanal *see* Cyst, pilonidal
Dioctophyma renalis (infection) (infestation)
    B83.8
Dipetalonemiasis B74.4
Diphallus Q55.69

Diphtheria, diphtheritic (gangrenous) (hemorrhagic) A36.9
|carrier (suspected) Z22.2
|cutaneous A36.3
|faucial A36.0
|infection of wound A36.3
|laryngeal A36.2
|myocarditis A36.81
|nasal, anterior A36.89
|nasopharyngeal A36.1
|neurological complication A36.89
|pharyngeal A36.0
|specified site NEC A36.89
|tonsillar A36.0
Diphyllobothriasis (intestine) B70.0
|larval B70.1
Diplacusis H93.22-
Diplegia (upper limbs) G83.0
|congenital (cerebral) G80.8
|facial G51.0
|lower limbs G82.20
|spastic G80.1
Diplococcus, diplococcal see condition
Diplopia H53.2
Dipsomania F10.20
|with
|psychosis see Psychosis, alcoholic
|remission F10.21
Dipylidiasis B71.1
DIRA (deficiency of interleukin 1 receptor antagonist) M04.8
Direction, teeth, abnormal, fully erupted M26.30
Dirofilariasis B74.8
Dirt-Eating child F98.3
Disability, disabilities
|heart see Disease, heart
|intellectual F79
|with
|autistic features F84.9
|pathogenic CHAMP1 (genetic) (variant) F78.A9
|pathogenic HNRNPH2 (genetic) (variant) F78.A9
|pathogenic SATB2 (genetic) (variant) F78.A9
|pathogenic SETBP1 (genetic) (variant) F78.A9
|pathogenic STXBP1 (genetic) (variant) F78.A9
|pathogenic SYNGAP1 (genetic) (variant) F78.A1
|pathogenic HNRNPH2 (genetic) (variant) F78.A9
|pathogenic SATB2 (genetic) (variant) F78.A9
|pathogenic SETBP1 (genetic) (variant) F78.A9
|pathogenic STXBP1 (genetic) (variant) F78.A9
|pathogenic SYNGAP1 (genetic) (variant) F78.A1
|autosomal dominant F78.A9
|autosomal recessive F78.A9
|genetic related F78.A9
|with
|pathogenic CHAMP1 (variant) F78.A9
|pathogenic HNRNPH2 (variant) F78.A9
|pathogenic SATB2 (variant) F78.A9
|pathogenic SETBP1 (variant) F78.A9
|pathogenic STXBP1 (variant) F78.A9
|pathogenic SYNGAP1 (variant) F78.A1

Disability, disabilities - continued
|specified NEC F78.A9
|SYNGAP1-related F78.A1
|in
|autosomal dominant mental retardation F78.A9
|autosomal recessive mental retardation F78.A9
|SATB2-associated syndrome F78.A9
|SETBP1 disorder F78.A9
|STXBP1 encephalopathy with epilepsy (see also Encephalopathy; and see also Epilepsy) F78.A9
|X-linked mental retardation (syndromic) (Bain type) F78.A9
|mild (I.Q.50-69) F70
|moderate (I.Q.35 49) F71
|profound (I.Q. under 20) F73
|severe (I.Q.20-34) F72
|specified level NEC F78
|SYNGAP1-related F78.A1
|X-linked (syndromic) (Bain type) F78.A9
|knowledge acquisition F81.9
|learning F81.9
|limiting activities Z73.6
|spelling, specific F81.81
Disappearance of family member Z63.4
Disarticulation see Amputation
|meaning traumatic amputation see Amputation, traumatic
Discharge (from)
|abnormal finding in see Abnormal, specimen
|breast (female) (male) N64.52
|diencephalic autonomic idiopathic see Epilepsy, specified NEC
|ear see also Otorrhea
|blood see Otorrhagia
|excessive urine R35.89
|nipple N64.52
|penile R36.9
|postnasal R09.82
|prison, anxiety concerning Z65.2
|urethral R36.9
|without blood R36.0
|hematospermia R36.1
|vaginal N89.8
Discitis, diskitis M46.40
|cervical region M46.42
|cervicothoracic region M46.43
|lumbar region M46.46
|lumbosacral region M46.47
|multiple sites M46.49
|occipito-atlanto-axial region M46.41
|pyogenic see Infection, intervertebral disc, pyogenic
|sacrococcygeal region M46.48
|thoracic region M46.44
|thoracolumbar region M46.45
Discoid
|meniscus (congenital) Q68.6
|semilunar cartilage (congenital) see Derangement, knee, meniscus, specified NEC
Discoloration
|nails L60.8
|teeth (posteruptive) K03.7
|during formation K00.8
Discomfort
|chest R07.89
|visual H53.14-
Discontinuity, ossicles, ear H74.2-

Discord (with)
|boss Z56.4
|classmates Z55.4
|counselor Z64.4
|employer Z56.4
|family Z63.8
|fellow employees Z56.4
|in-laws Z63.1
|landlord Z59.2
|lodgers Z59.2
|neighbors Z59.2
|probation officer Z64.4
|social worker Z64.4
|teachers Z55.4
|workmates Z56.4
Discordant connection
|atrioventricular (congenital) Q20.5
|ventriculoarterial Q20.3
Discrepancy
|centric occlusion maximum intercuspation M26.55
|leg length (acquired) see Deformity, limb, unequal length
|congenital see Defect, reduction, lower limb
|uterine size date O26.84-
Discrimination
|ethnic Z60.5
|political Z60.5
|racial Z60.5
|religious Z60.5
|sex Z60.5
Disease, diseased see also Syndrome
|absorbent system I87.8
|acid-peptic K30
|Acosta's T70.29
|Adams-Stokes (-Morgagni) (syncope with heart block) I45.9
|Addison's anemia (pernicious) D51.0
|adenoids (and tonsils) J35.9
|adrenal (capsule) (cortex) (gland) (medullary) E27.9
|hyperfunction E27.0
|specified NEC E27.8
|ainhum L94.6
|airway
|obstructive, chronic J44.9
|due to
|cotton dust J66.0
|specific organic dusts NEC J66.8
|reactive see Asthma
|akamushi (scrub typhus) A75.3
|Albers-Schonberg (marble bones) Q78.2
|Albert's see Tendinitis, Achilles
|alimentary canal K63.9
|alligator-skin Q80.9
|acquired L85.0
|alpha heavy chain C88.3
|alpine T70.29
|altitude T70.20
|alveolar ridge
|edentulous K06.9
|specified NEC K06.8
|alveoli, teeth K08.9
|Alzheimer's G30.9 [F02.80]
|with behavioral disturbance G30.9 [F02.81]
|early onset G30.0 [F02.80]
|with behavioral disturbance G30.0 [F02.81]
|late onset G30.1 [F02.80]
|with behavioral disturbance G30.1 [F02.81]
|specified NEC G30.8 [F02.80]
|with behavioral disturbance G30.8 [F02.81]
|amyloid see Amyloidosis

Disease, diseased - *continued*
- |Andersen's (glycogenosis IV) E74.09
- |Andes T70.29
- |Andrews' (bacterid) L08.89
- |angiospastic I73.9
  - |cerebral G45.9
  - |vein I87.8
- |anterior
  - |chamber H21.9
  - |horn cell G12.29
- |antiglomerular basement membrane (antiGBM) antibody M31.0
  - |tubulo-interstitial nephritis N12
- |antral *see* Sinusitis, maxillary
- |anus K62.9
  - |specified NEC K62.89
- |aorta (nonsyphilitic) I77.9
  - |syphilitic NEC A52.02
- |aortic (heart) (valve) I35.9
  - |rheumatic I06.9
- |Apollo B30.3
- |aponeuroses *see* Enthesopathy
- |appendix K38.9
  - |specified NEC K38.8
- |aqueous (chamber) H21.9
- |Arnold-Chiari *see* Arnold-Chiari disease
- |arterial I77.9
  - |occlusive *see* Occlusion, by site
    - |due to stricture or stenosis I77.1
- |arteriocardiorenal *see* Hypertension, cardiorenal
- |arteriolar (generalized) (obliterative) I77.9
- |arteriorenal *see* Hypertension, kidney
- |arteriosclerotic *see also* Arteriosclerosis
  - |cardiovascular *see* Disease, heart, ischemic, atherosclerotic
  - |coronary (artery) *see* Disease, heart, ischemic, atherosclerotic
  - |heart *see* Disease, heart, ischemic, atherosclerotic
- |artery I77.9
  - |cerebral I67.9
  - |coronary I25.10
    - |with angina pectoris *see* Arteriosclerosis, coronary (artery),
- |arthropod-borne NOS (viral) A94
  - |specified type NEC A93.8
- |atticoantral, chronic H66.20
  - |left H66.22
    - |with right H66.23
  - |right H66.21
    - |with left H66.23
- |auditory canal *see* Disorder, ear, external
- |auricle, ear NEC *see* Disorder, pinna
- |Australian X A83.4
- |autoimmune (systemic) NOS M35.9
  - |hemolytic D59.1
    - |cold type (primary) (secondary) (symptomatic) D59.12
    - |drug-induced D59.0
    - |mixed type (primary) (secondary) (symptomatic) D59.13
    - |warm type (primary) (secondary) (symptomatic) D59.11
  - |thyroid E06.3
- |autoinflammatory M04.9
  - |NOD2-associated M04.8
  - |specified type NEC M04.8
- |aviator's *see* Effect, adverse, high altitude
- |Ayerza's (pulmonary artery sclerosis with pulmonary hypertension) I27.0
- |Babington's (familial hemorrhagic telangiectasia) I78.0
- |bacterial A49.9
  - |specified NEC A48.8

Disease, diseased - *continued*
- |zoonotic A28.9
  - |specified type NEC A28.8
- |Baelz's (cheilitis glandularis apostematosa) K13.0
- |bagasse J67.1
- |balloon *see* Effect, adverse, high altitude
- |Bang's (brucella abortus) A23.1
- |Bannister's T78.3
- |barometer makers' *see* Poisoning, mercury
- |Barraquer (-Simons') (progressive lipodystrophy) E88.1
- |Barrett's *see* Barrett's, esophagus
- |Bartholin's gland N75.9
- |basal ganglia G25.9
  - |degenerative G23.9
    - |specified NEC G23.8
  - |specified NEC G25.89
- |Basedow's (exophthalmic goiter) *see* Hyperthyroidism, with, goiter (diffuse)
- |Bateman's B08.1
- |Batten-Steinert G71.11
- |Battey A31.0
- |Beard's (neurasthenia) F48.8
- |Becker
  - |idiopathic mural endomyocardial I42.3
  - |myotonia congenita G71.12
- |Begbie's (exophthalmic goiter) *see* Hyperthyroidism, with, goiter (diffuse)
- |behavioral, organic F07.9
- |Beigel's (white piedra) B36.2
- |Benson's *see* Deposit, crystalline
- |Bernard-Soulier (thrombopathy) D69.1
- |Bernhardt (-Roth) *see* Mononeuropathy, lower limb, meralgia paresthetica
- |Biermer's (pernicious anemia) D51.0
- |bile duct (common) (hepatic) K83.9
  - |with calculus, stones *see* Calculus, bile duct
  - |specified NEC K83.8
- |biliary (tract) K83.9
  - |specified NEC K83.8
- |Billroth's *see* Spina bifida
- |bird fancier's J67.2
- |black lung J60
- |bladder N32.9
  - |in (due to)
    - |schistosomiasis (bilharziasis) B65.0 *[N33]*
  - |specified NEC N32.89
- |bleeder's D66
- |blood D75.9
  - |forming organs D75.9
  - |vessel I99.9
- |Bloodgood's *see* Mastopathy, cystic
- |Blount M92.51-
- |Bodechtel-Guttmann (subacute sclerosing panencephalitis) A81.1
- |bone *see also* Disorder, bone
  - |aluminum M83.4
  - |fibrocystic NEC
    - |jaw M27.49
- |bone-marrow D75.9
- |Borna A83.9
- |Bornholm (epidemic pleurodynia) B33.0
- |Bouchard's (myopathic dilatation of the stomach) K31.0
- |Bouillaud's (rheumatic heart disease) I01.9
- |Bourneville (-Brissaud) (tuberous sclerosis) Q85.1
- |Bouveret (-Hoffmann) (paroxysmal tachycardia) I47.9
- |bowel K63.9
  - |functional K59.9
    - |psychogenic F45.8
- |brain G93.9
  - |arterial, artery I67.9

Disease, diseased - *continued*
- |arteriosclerotic I67.2
- |congenital Q04.9
- |degenerative *see* Degeneration, brain
- |inflammatory *see* Encephalitis
- |organic G93.9
  - |arteriosclerotic I67.2
- |parasitic NEC B71.9 *[G94]*
- |senile NEC G31.1
- |specified NEC G93.89
- |breast *see also* Disorder, breast N64.9
  - |cystic (chronic) *see* Mastopathy, cystic
  - |fibrocystic *see* Mastopathy, cystic
  - |Paget's
    - |female, unspecified side C50.91-
    - |male, unspecified side C50.92-
  - |specified NEC N64.89
- |Breda's *see* Yaws
- |Bretonneau's (diphtheritic malignant angina) A36.0
- |Bright's *see* Nephritis
  - |arteriosclerotic *see* Hypertension, kidney
- |Brill's (recrudescent typhus) A75.1
- |Brill-Zinsser (recrudescent typhus) A75.1
- |Brion-Kayser *see* Fever, paratyphoid
- |broad
  - |beta E78.2
  - |ligament (noninflammatory) N83.9
    - |inflammatory *see* Disease, pelvis, inflammatory
    - |specified NEC N83.8
- |Brocq-Duhring (dermatitis herpetiformis) L13.0
- |Brocq's
  - |meaning
    - |dermatitis herpetiformis L13.0
    - |prurigo L28.2
- |bronchopulmonary J98.4
- |bronchus NEC J98.09
- |bronze Addison's E27.1
  - |tuberculous A18.7
- |budgerigar fancier's J67.2
- |bullous L13.9
  - |chronic of childhood L12.2
  - |specified NEC L13.8
- |Buerger's (thromboangiitis obliterans) I73.1
- |Bürger-Grütz (essential familial hyperlipemia) E78.3
- |bursa *see* Bursopathy
- |caisson T70.3
- |California *see* Coccidioidomycosis
- |capillaries I78.9
  - |specified NEC I78.8
- |Carapata A68.0
- |cardiac *see* Disease, heart
- |cardiopulmonary, chronic I27.9
- |cardiorenal (hepatic) (hypertensive) (vascular) *see* Hypertension, cardiorenal
- |cardiovascular (atherosclerotic) I25.10
  - |with angina pectoris *see* Arteriosclerosis, coronary (artery),
  - |congenital Q28.9
  - |newborn P29.9
    - |specified NEC P29.89
  - |hypertensive *see* Hypertension, heart
  - |renal (hypertensive) *see* Hypertension, cardiorenal
  - |syphilitic (asymptomatic) A52.00
- |cartilage *see* Disorder, cartilage
- |Castellani's A69.8
- |Castleman (unicentric) (multicentric) D47.Z2
  - |HHV 8-associated *see also* Herpesvirus, human, 8 D47.Z2
- |cat-scratch A28.1
- |Cavare's (familial periodic paralysis) G72.3

Disease, diseased - *continued*
|cecum K63.9
|celiac (adult) (infantile) (with steatorrhea) K90.0
|cellular tissue L98.9
|central core G71.29
|cerebellar, cerebellum *see* Disease, brain
|cerebral *see also* Disease, brain
| |degenerative *see* Degeneration, brain
|cerebrospinal G96.9
|cerebrovascular I67.9
| |acute I67.89
| | |embolic I63.4-
| | |thrombotic I63.3-
| |arteriosclerotic I67.2
| |hereditary NEC I67.858
| |specified NEC I67.89
|cervix (uteri) (noninflammatory) N88.9
| |inflammatory *see* Cervicitis
| |specified NEC N88.8
|Chabert's A22.9
|Chandler's (osteochondritis dissecans, hip) *see* Osteochondritis, dissecans, hip
|Charlouis *see* Yaws
|Chédiak-Steinbrinck (-Higashi) (congenital gigantism of peroxidase granules) E70.330
|chest J98.9
|Chiari's (hepatic vein thrombosis) I82.0
|Chicago B40.9
|Chignon B36.8
|chigo, chigoe B88.1
|childhood granulomatous D71
|Chinese liver fluke B66.1
|chlamydial A74.9
| |specified NEC A74.89
|cholecystic K82.9
|choroid H31.9
| |specified NEC H31.8
|Christmas D67
|chronic bullous of childhood L12.2
|chylomicron retention E78.3
|ciliary body H21.9
| |specified NEC H21.89
|circulatory (system) NEC I99.8
| |newborn P29.9
| |syphilitic A52.00
| | |congenital A50.54
|coagulation factor deficiency (congenital) *see* Defect, coagulation
|coccidioidal *see* Coccidioidomycosis
|cold
| |agglutinin or hemoglobinuria D59.12
| | |paroxysmal D59.6
| |hemagglutinin (chronic) D59.12
|collagen NOS (nonvascular) (vascular) M35.9
| |specified NEC M35.8
|colon K63.9
| |functional K59.9
| | |congenital Q43.2
| |ischemic *see also* Ischemia, intestine, acute K55.039
|colonic inflammatory bowel, unclassified (IBDU) K52.3
|combined system *see* Degeneration, combined
|compressed air T70.3
|Concato's (pericardial polyserositis) A19.9
| |nontubercular I31.1
| |pleural *see* Pleurisy, with effusion
|conjunctiva H11.9
| |chlamydial A74.0
| |specified NEC H11.89
| |viral B30.9
| | |specified NEC B30.8
|connective tissue, systemic (diffuse) M35.9
| |in (due to)

Disease, diseased - *continued*
| |hypogammaglobulinemia D80.1 *[M36.8]*
| |ochronosis E70.29 *[M36.8]*
| |specified NEC M35.8
|Conor and Bruch's (boutonneuse fever) A77.1
|Cooper's *see* Mastopathy, cystic
|Cori's (glycogenosis III) E74.03
|cork handler's or cork worker's J67.3
|cornea H18.9
| |specified NEC H18.89-
|coronary (artery) *see* Disease, heart, ischemic, atherosclerotic
| |congenital Q24.5
| |ostial, syphilitic (aortic) (mitral) (pulmonary) A52.03
|corpus cavernosum N48.9
| |specified NEC N48.89
|Cotugno's *see* Sciatica
|COVID-19 U07.1
|coxsackie (virus) NEC B34.1
|cranial nerve NOS G52.9
|Creutzfeldt-Jakob *see* Creutzfeldt-Jakob disease or syndrome
|Crocq's (acrocyanosis) I73.89
|Crohn's *see* Enteritis, regional
|Curschmann G71.11
|cystic
| |breast (chronic) *see* Mastopathy, cystic
| |kidney, congenital Q61.9
| |liver, congenital Q44.6
| |lung J98.4
| | |congenital Q33.0
|cytomegalic inclusion (generalized) B25.9
| |with pneumonia B25.0
| |congenital P35.1
|cytomegaloviral B25.9
| |specified NEC B25.8
|Czerny's (periodic hydrarthrosis of the knee) *see* Effusion, joint, knee
|Daae (-Finsen) (epidemic pleurodynia) B33.0
|Darling's *see* Histoplasmosis capsulati
|Debove's (splenomegaly) R16.1
|deer fly *see* Tularemia
|Degos' I77.89
|demyelinating, demyelinizating (nervous system) G37.9
| |multiple sclerosis G35
| |specified NEC G37.8
|dense deposit *see also* N00-N07 with fourth character .6 N05.6
|deposition, hydroxyapatite *see* Disease, hydroxyapatite deposition
|de Quervain's (tendon sheath) M65.4
| |thyroid (subacute granulomatous thyroiditis) E06.1
|Devergie's (pityriasis rubra pilaris) L44.0
|Devic's G36.0
|diaphorase deficiency D74.0
|diaphragm J98.6
|diarrheal, infectious NEC A09
|digestive system K92.9
| |specified NEC K92.89
|disc, degenerative *see* Degeneration, intervertebral disc
|discogenic *see also* Displacement, intervertebral disc NEC
| |with myelopathy *see* Disorder, disc, with, myelopathy
|diverticular *see* Diverticula
|Dubois (thymus) A50.59 *[E35]*
|Duchenne-Griesinger G71.01
|Duchenne's
| |muscular dystrophy G71.01
| |pseudohypertrophy, muscles G71.01
|ductless glands E34.9

Disease, diseased - *continued*
|Duhring's (dermatitis herpetiformis) L13.0
|duodenum K31.9
| |specified NEC K31.89
|Dupré's (meningism) R29.1
|Dupuytren's (muscle contracture) M72.0
|Durand-Nicholas-Favre (climatic bubo) A55
|Duroziez's (congenital mitral stenosis) Q23.2
|ear *see* Disorder, ear
|Eberth's *see* Fever, typhoid
|Ebola (virus) A98.4
|Ebstein's heart Q22.5
|Echinococcus *see* Echinococcus
|echovirus NEC B34.1
|Eddowes' (brittle bones and blue sclera) Q78.0
|edentulous (alveolar) ridge K06.9
| |specified NEC K06.8
|Edsall's T67.2
|Eichstedt's (pityriasis versicolor) B36.0
|Eisenmenger's (irreversible) I27.83
|Ellis-Van Creveld (chondroectodermal dysplasia) Q77.6
|end stage renal (ESRD) N18.6
| |due to hypertension I12.0
|endocrine glands or system NEC E34.9
|endomyocardial (eosinophilic) I42.3
|English (rickets) E55.0
|enteroviral, enterovirus NEC B34.1
| |central nervous system NEC A88.8
|epidemic B99.9
| |specified NEC B99.8
|epididymis N50.9
|Erb (-Landouzy) G71.02
|Erdheim-Chester (ECD) E88.89
|esophagus K22.9
| |functional K22.4
| |psychogenic F45.8
| |specified NEC K22.89
|Eulenburg's (congenital paramyotonia) G71.19
|eustachian tube *see* Disorder, eustachian tube
|external
| |auditory canal *see* Disorder, ear, external
| |ear *see* Disorder, ear, external
|extrapyramidal G25.9
| |specified NEC G25.89
|eye H57.9
| |anterior chamber H21.9
| |inflammatory NEC H57.89
| |muscle (external) *see* Strabismus
| |specified NEC H57.89
| |syphilitic *see* Oculopathy, syphilitic
|eyeball H44.9
| |specified NEC H44.89
|eyelid *see* Disorder, eyelid
| |specified NEC *see* Disorder, eyelid, specified type NEC
|eyeworm of Africa B74.3
|facial nerve (seventh) G51.9
| |newborn (birth injury) P11.3
|Fahr (of brain) G23.8
|Fahr Volhard (of kidney) I12.-
|fallopian tube (noninflammatory) N83.9
| |inflammatory *see* Salpingo-oophoritis
| |specified NEC N83.8
|familial periodic paralysis G72.3
|Fanconi's (congenital pancytopenia) D61.09
|fascia NEC *see also* Disorder, muscle
| |inflammatory *see* Myositis
| |specified NEC M62.89
|Fauchard's (periodontitis) *see* Periodontitis
|Favre-Durand-Nicolas (climatic bubo) A55
|Fede's K14.0
|Feer's *see* Poisoning, mercury

Disease, diseased - *continued*

|female pelvic inflammatory *see also* Disease, pelvic, inflammatory N73.9
  |syphilitic (secondary) A51.42
  |tuberculous A18.17
|Fernels' (aortic aneurysm) I71.9
|fibrocaseous of lung *see* Tuberculosis, pulmonary
|fibrocystic *see* Fibrocystic disease
|Fiedler's (leptospiral jaundice) A27.0
|fifth B08.3
|file-cutter's *see* Poisoning, lead
|fish-skin Q80.9
  |acquired L85.0
|Flajani (-Basedow) (exophthalmic goiter) *see* Hyperthyroidism, with, goiter (diffuse)
|flax-dresser's J66.1
|fluke *see* Infestation, fluke |foot and mouth B08.8
|foot process N04.9
|Forbes' (glycogenosis III) E74.03
|Fordyce-Fox (apocrine miliaria) L75.2
|Fordyce's (ectopic sebaceous glands) (mouth) Q38.6
|Forestier's (rhizomelic pseudopolyarthritis) M35.3
  |meaning ankylosing hyperostosis *see* Hyperostosis, ankylosing
|Fothergill's
  |neuralgia *see* Neuralgia, trigeminal
  |scarlatina anginosa A38.9
|Fournier (gangrene) N49.3
  |female N76.89
|fourth B08.8
|Fox (-Fordyce) (apocrine miliaria) L75.2
|Francis' *see* Tularemia
|Franklin C88.2
|Frei's (climatic bubo) A55
|Friedreich's
  |combined systemic or ataxia G11.11
  |myoclonia G25.3
|frontal sinus *see* Sinusitis, frontal
|fungus NEC B49
|Gaisböck's (polycythemia hypertonica) D75.1
|gallbladder K82.9
  |calculus *see* Calculus, gallbladder
  |cholecystitis *see* Cholecystitis
  |cholesterolosis K82.4
  |fistula *see* Fistula, gallbladder
  |hydrops K82.1
  |obstruction *see* Obstruction, gallbladder
  |perforation K82.2
  |specified NEC K82.8
|gamma heavy chain C88.2
|Gamna's (siderotic splenomegaly) D73.2
|Gamstorp's (adynamia episodica hereditaria) G72.3
|Gandy-Nanta (siderotic splenomegaly) D73.2
|ganister J62.8
|gastric *see* Disease, stomach
|gastroesophageal reflux (GERD) K21.9
  |with esophagitis (without bleeding) K21.00
    |with bleeding K21.01
|gastrointestinal (tract) K92.9
  |amyloid E85.4
  |functional K59.9
    |psychogenic F45.8
  |specified NEC K92.89
|Gee (-Herter) (-Heubner) (-Thaysen) (nontropical sprue) K90.0
|genital organs
  |female N94.9
  |male N50.9
|Gerhardt's (erythromelalgia) I73.81
|Gibert's (pityriasis rosea) L42

Disease, diseased - *continued*

|Gierke's (glycogenosis I) E74.01
|Gilles de la Tourette's (motor-verbal tic) F95.2
|gingiva K06.9
  |plaque induced K05.00
  |specified NEC K06.8
|gland (lymph) I89.9
|Glanzmann's (hereditary hemorrhagic thrombasthenia) D69.1
|glass-blower's (cataract) *see* Cataract, specified NEC
  |salivary gland hypertrophy K11.1
|Glisson's *see* Rickets
|globe H44.9
  |specified NEC H44.89
|glomerular *see also* Glomerulonephritis
  |with edema *see* Nephrosis
  |acute *see* Nephritis, acute
  |chronic *see* Nephritis, chronic
  |minimal change N05.0
  |rapidly progressive N01.9
|glycogen storage E74.00
  |Andersen's E74.09
  |Cori's E74.03
  |Forbes' E74.03
  |generalized E74.00
  |glucose 6-phosphatase deficiency E74.01
  |heart E74.02 [143]
  |hepatorenal E74.09
  |Hers' E74.09
  |liver and kidney E74.09
  |McArdle's E74.04
  |muscle phosphofructokinase E74.09
  |myocardium E74.02 [143]
  |Pompe's E74.02
  |Tauri's E74.09
  |type 0 E74.09
  |type I E74.01
  |type II E74.02
  |type III E74.03
  |type IV E74.09
  |type V E74.04
  |type VI-XI E74.09
  |Von Gierke's E74.01
|Goldstein's (familial hemorrhagic telangiectasia) I78.0
|gonococcal NOS A54.9
|graft-versus-host (GVH) D89.813
  |acute D89.810
  |acute on chronic D89.812
  |chronic D89.811
|grain handler's J67.8
|granulomatous (childhood) (chronic) D71
|Graves' (exophthalmic goiter) *see* Hyperthyroidism, with, goiter (diffuse)
|Griesinger's *see* Ancylostomiasis
|Grisel's M43.6
|Gruby's (tinea tonsurans) B35.0
|Guillain-Barré G61.0
|Guinon's (motor-verbal tic) F95.2
|gum K06.9
|gynecological N94.9
|H (Hartnup's) E72.02
|Haff *see* Poisoning, mercury
|Hageman (congenital factor XII deficiency) D68.2
|hair (color) (shaft) L67.9
  |follicles L73.9
    |specified NEC L73.8
|Hamman's (spontaneous mediastinal emphysema) J98.2
|hand, foot and mouth B08.4
|Hansen's *see* Leprosy
|Hantavirus, with pulmonary manifestations B33.4

Disease, diseased - *continued*

|with renal manifestations A98.5
|Harada's H30.81-
|Hartnup (pellagra-cerebellar ataxia-renal aminoaciduria) E72.02
|Hart's (pellagra-cerebellar ataxia-renal aminoaciduria) E72.02
|Hashimoto's (struma lymphomatosa) E06.3
|Hb *see* Disease, hemoglobin
|heart (organic) I51.9
  |with
    |pulmonary edema (acute) *see also* Failure, ventricular, left I50.1
    |rheumatic fever (conditions in I00)
      |active I01.9
        |with chorea I02.0
        |specified NEC I01.8
      |inactive or quiescent (with chorea) I09.9
        |specified NEC I09.89
|amyloid E85.4 [143]
|aortic (valve) I35.9
|arteriosclerotic or sclerotic (senile) *see* Disease, heart, ischemic, atherosclerotic
|artery, arterial *see* Disease, heart, ischemic, atherosclerotic
|beer drinkers' I42.6
|beriberi (wet) E51.12
|black I27.0
|congenital Q24.9
  |cyanotic Q24.9
  |specified NEC Q24.8
|coronary *see* Disease, heart, ischemic
|cryptogenic I51.9
|fibroid *see* Myocarditis
|functional I51.89
  |psychogenic F45.8
|glycogen storage E74.02 [143]
|gonococcal A54.83
|hypertensive *see* Hypertension, heart
|hyperthyroid *see also* Hyperthyroidism E05.90 [143]
  |with thyroid storm E05.91 [143]
|ischemic (chronic or with a stated duration of over 4 weeks) I25.9
  |atherosclerotic (of) I25.10
    |with angina pectoris *see* Arteriosclerosis, coronary (artery)
    |coronary artery bypass graft *see* Arteriosclerosis, coronary (artery),
  |cardiomyopathy I25.5
  |diagnosed on ECG or other special investigation, but currently presenting no symptoms I25.6
  |silent I25.6
  |specified form NEC I25.89
|kyphoscoliotic I27.1
|meningococcal A39.50
  |endocarditis A39.51
  |myocarditis A39.52
  |pericarditis A39.53
|mitral I05.9
  |specified NEC I05.8
|muscular *see* Degeneration, myocardial
|psychogenic (functional) F45.8
|pulmonary (chronic) I27.9
  |in schistosomiasis B65.9 [152]
  |specified NEC I27.89
|rheumatic (chronic) (inactive) (old) (quiescent) (with chorea) I09.9
  |active or acute I01.9
    |with chorea (acute) (rheumatic) (Sydenham's) I02.0
  |specified NEC I09.89
|senile *see* Myocarditis
|syphilitic A52.06

Disease, diseased - *continued*
- |aortic A52.03
  - |aneurysm A52.01
  - |congenital A50.54 *[152]*
- |thyrotoxic *see also* Thyrotoxicosis E05.90 *[143]*
  - |with thyroid storm E05.91 *[143]*
- |valve, valvular (obstructive) (regurgitant) *see also* Endocarditis
  - |congenital NEC Q24.8
    - |pulmonary Q22.3
- |vascular *see* Disease, cardiovascular
- |heavy chain NEC C88.2
  - |alpha C88.3
  - |gamma C88.2
  - |mu C88.2
- |Hebra's
  - |pityriasis
    - |maculata et circinata L42
    - |rubra pilaris L44.0
  - |prurigo L28.2
- |hematopoietic organs D75.9
- |hemoglobin or Hb
  - |abnormal (mixed) NEC D58.2
    - |with thalassemia D56.9
  - |AS genotype D57.3
  - |Bart's D56.0
  - |C (Hb-C) D58.2
    - |with other abnormal hemoglobin NEC D58.2
    - |elliptocytosis D58.1
    - |Hb-S D57.2-
    - |sickle-cell D57.2-
    - |thalassemia D56.8
  - |Constant Spring D58.2
  - |D (Hb-D) D58.2
  - |E (Hb-E) D58.2
  - |E-beta thalassemia D56.5
  - |elliptocytosis D58.1
  - |H (Hb-H) (thalassemia) D56.0
    - |with other abnormal hemoglobin NEC D56.9
    - |Constant Spring D56.0
  - |I thalassemia D56.9
  - |M D74.0
  - |S or SS D57.1
    - |with
      - |acute chest syndrome D57.01
      - |cerebral vascular involvement D57.03
      - |crisis (painful) D57.00
        - |with complication specified NEC D57.09
      - |splenic sequestration D57.02
      - |vasoocclusive pain D57.00
    - |beta plus D57.44
      - |with
        - |acute chest syndrome D57.451
        - |cerebral vascular involvement D57.453
        - |crisis D57.459
          - |with specified complication NEC D57.458
        - |splenic sequestration D57.452
        - |vasoocclusive pain D57.459
      - |without crisis D57.44
    - |beta zero D57.42
      - |with
        - |acute chest syndrome D57.431
        - |cerebral vascular involvement D57.433
        - |crisis D57.439
          - |with specified complication NEC D57.438
        - |splenic sequestration D57.432
        - |vasoocclusive pain D57.439

Disease, diseased - *continued*
- |without crisis D57.42
- |SC D57.2-
- |SD D57.8-
- |SE D57.8-
- |spherocytosis D58.0
- |unstable, hemolytic D58.2
- |hemolytic (newborn) P55.9
  - |autoimmune D59.10
    - |cold type (primary) (secondary) (symptomatic) D59.12
    - |mixed type (primary) (secondary) (symptomatic) D59.13
    - |warm type (primary) (secondary) (symptomatic) D59.11
  - |drug-induced D59.0
  - |due to or with
    - |incompatibility
      - |ABO (blood group) P55.1
      - |blood (group) (Duffy) (K) (Kell) (Kidd) (Lewis) (M) (S) NEC P55.8
      - |Rh (blood group) (factor) P55.0
    - |Rh negative mother P55.0
  - |specified type NEC P55.8
  - |unstable hemoglobin D58.2
- |hemorrhagic D69.9
  - |newborn P53
- |Henoch (-Schönlein) (purpura nervosa) D69.0
- |hepatic *see* Disease, liver
- |hepatobiliary K83.9
  - |toxic K71.9
- |hepatolenticular E83.01
- |heredodegenerative NEC
  - |spinal cord G95.89
- |herpesviral, disseminated B00.7
- |Hers' (glycogenosis VI) E74.09
- |Herter (-Gee) (-Heubner) (nontropical sprue) K90.0
- |Heubner-Herter (nontropical sprue) K90.0
- |high fetal gene or hemoglobin thalassemia D56.9
- |Hildebrand's *see* Typhus
- |hip (joint) M25.9
  - |congenital Q65.89
  - |suppurative M00.9
  - |tuberculous A18.02
- |His (-Werner) (trench fever) A79.0
- |Hodgson's I71.2
  - |ruptured I71.1
- |Holla *see* Spherocytosis
- |hookworm B76.9
  - |specified NEC B76.8
- |host-versus-graft D89.813
  - |acute D89.810
  - |acute on chronic D89.812
  - |chronic D89.811
- |human immunodeficiency virus (HIV) B20
- |Huntington's G10
  - |with dementia G10 *[F02.80]*
- |Hutchinson's (cheiropompholyx) *see* Hutchinson's disease
- |hyaline (diffuse) (generalized)
  - |membrane (lung) (newborn) P22.0
  - |adult J80
- |hydatid *see* Echinococcus
- |hydroxyapatite deposition M11.00
  - |ankle M11.07-
  - |elbow M11.02-
  - |foot joint M11.07-
  - |hand joint M11.04-
  - |hip M11.05-
  - |knee M11.06-
  - |multiple site M11.09
  - |shoulder M11.01-
  - |vertebra M11.08

Disease, diseased - *continued*
- |wrist M11.03-
- |hyperkinetic *see* Hyperkinesia
- |hypertensive *see* Hypertension
- |hypophysis E23.7
- |Iceland G93.3
- |I-cell E77.0
- |immune D89.9
- |immunoproliferative (malignant) C88.9
  - |small intestinal C88.3
  - |specified NEC C88.8
- |inclusion B25.9
  - |salivary gland B25.9
- |infectious, infective B99.9
  - |congenital P37.9
    - |specified NEC P37.8
    - |viral P35.9
      - |specified type NEC P35.8
  - |specified NEC B99.8
- |inflammatory
  - |penis N48.29
    - |abscess N48.21
    - |cellulitis N48.22
  - |prepuce N47.7
    - |balanoposthitis N47.6
  - |tubo-ovarian *see* Salpingo-oophoritis
- |intervertebral disc *see also* Disorder, disc
  - |with myelopathy *see* Disorder, disc, with, myelopathy
  - |cervical, cervicothoracic *see* Disorder, disc, cervical
    - |with
      - |myelopathy *see* Disorder, disc, cervical, with myelopathy
      - |neuritis, radiculitis or radiculopathy *see* Disorder, disc, cervical, with neuritis
      - |specified NEC *see* Disorder, disc, cervical, specified type NEC
  - |lumbar (with)
    - |myelopathy M51.06
    - |neuritis, radiculitis, radiculopathy or sciatica M51.16
    - |specified NEC M51.86
  - |lumbosacral (with)
    - |neuritis, radiculitis, radiculopathy or sciatica M51.17
    - |specified NEC M51.87
  - |specified NEC *see* Disorder, disc, specified NEC
  - |thoracic (with)
    - |myelopathy M51.04
    - |neuritis, radiculitis or radiculopathy M51.14
    - |specified NEC M51.84
  - |thoracolumbar (with)
    - |myelopathy M51.05
    - |neuritis, radiculitis or radiculopathy M51.15
    - |specified NEC M51.85
- |intestine K63.9
  - |functional K59.9
    - |psychogenic F45.8
    - |specified NEC K59.89
  - |organic K63.9
  - |protozoal A07.9
  - |specified NEC K63.89
- |iris H21.9
  - |specified NEC H21.89
- |iron metabolism or storage E83.10
- |island (scrub typhus) A75.3
- |Itai-Itai *see* Poisoning, cadmium
- |Jakob-Creutzfeldt *see* Creutzfeldt-Jakob disease or syndrome
- |jaw M27.9
  - |fibrocystic M27.49

Disease, diseased - *continued*
  |specified NEC M27.8
|jigger B88.1
|joint *see also* Disorder, joint
  |Charcot's *see* Arthropathy, neuropathic
    (Charcot)
  |degenerative *see* Osteoarthritis
    |multiple M15.9
    |spine *see* Spondylosis
  facet joint (see also Spondylosis) M47.819
  |hypertrophic *see* Osteoarthritis
  |sacroiliac M53.3
  |specified NEC *see* Disorder, joint, specified
    type NEC
  |spine NEC *see* Dorsopathy
  |suppurative *see* Arthritis, pyogenic or
    pyemic
|Jourdain's (acute gingivitis) K05.00
  |nonplaque induced K05.01
  |plaque induced K05.00
|Kaschin-Beck (endemic polyarthritis) M12.10
  |ankle M12.17-
  |elbow M12.12-
  |foot joint M12.17-
  |hand joint M12.14-
  |hip M12.15-
  |knee M12.16-
  |multiple site M12.19
  |shoulder M12.11-
  |vertebra M12.18
  |wrist M12.13-
|Katayama B65.2
|Kedani (scrub typhus) A75.3
|Keshan E59
|kidney (functional) (pelvis) N28.9
  |chronic N18.9
    |hypertensive *see* Hypertension, kidney
    |stage 1 N18.1
    |stage 2(mild) N18.2
    |stage 3(moderate) N18.30
    |stage 3a N18.31
    |stage 3b N18.32
    |stage 4(severe) N18.4
    |stage 5 N18.5
  |complicating pregnancy *see* Pregnancy,
    complicated by, renal disease
  |cystic (congenital) Q61.9
  |diabetic *see* E08-E13 with .22
  |fibrocystic (congenital) Q61.8
  |hypertensive *see* Hypertension, kidney
  |in (due to)
    |schistosomiasis (bilharziasis) B65.9 *[N29]*
  |multicystic Q61.4
  |polycystic Q61.3
    |adult type Q61.2
    |childhood type NEC Q61.19
      |collecting duct dilatation Q61.11
  |Kimmelstiel (-Wilson) (intercapillary
    polycystic (congenital) glomerulosclerosis)
    see E08-E13 with .21
|Kimura D21.9
  |specified site (*see* Neoplasm, connective
    tissue benign)
|Kinnier Wilson's (hepatolenticular
  degeneration) E83.01
|kissing *see* Mononucleosis, infectious
|Klebs' *see also* Glomerulonephritis N05.
|Klippel-Feil (brevicollis) Q76.1
|Köhler-Pellegrini-Stieda (calcification, knee
  joint) *see* Bursitis, tibial collateral
|Kok Q89.8
|Koenig's (osteochondritis dissecans) *see*
  Osteochondritis, dissecans
|Korsakoff's (nonalcoholic) F04
  |alcoholic F10.96

Disease, diseased - *continued*
    |with dependence F10.26
|Kostmann's (infantile genetic agranulocytosis)
  D70.0
|kuru A81.81
|Kyasanur Forest A98.2
|labyrinth, ear *see* Disorder, ear, inner
|lacrimal system *see* Disorder, lacrimal system
|Lafora's *see* Epilepsy, generalized, idiopathic
|Lancereaux-Mathieu (leptospiral jaundice)
  A27.0
|Landry's G61.0
|Larrey-Weil (leptospiral jaundice) A27.0
|larynx J38.7
|legionnaires' A48.1
  |nonpneumonic A48.2
|Lenegre's I44.2
|lens H27.9
  |specified NEC H27.8
|Lev's (acquired complete heart block) I44.2
|Lewy body (dementia) G31.83 *[F02.80]*
  |with behavioral disturbance G31.83
    [F02.81]
|Lichtheim's (subacute combined sclerosis with
  pernicious anemia) D51.0
|Lightwood's (renal tubular acidosis) N25.89
|Lignac's (cystinosis) E72.04
|lip K13.0
|lipid-storage E75.6
  |specified NEC E75.5
|Lipschütz's N76.6
|liver (chronic) (organic) K76.9
  |alcoholic (chronic) K70.9
    |acute *see* Disease, liver, alcoholic,
      hepatitis
    |cirrhosis K70.30
      |with ascites K70.31
    |failure K70.40
      |with coma K70.41
    |fatty liver K70.0
    |fibrosis K70.2
    |hepatitis K70.10
      |with ascites K70.11
    |sclerosis K70.2
  |cystic, congenital Q44.6
  |drug-induced (idiosyncratic) (toxic)
    (predictable) (unpredictable) *see* Disease,
    liver, toxic
  |end stage K72.10
    |due to hepatitis *see* Hepatitis
  with coma K72.11
  |fatty, nonalcoholic (NAFLD) K76.0
    |alcoholic K70.0
  |fibrocystic (congenital) Q44.6
  |fluke
    |Chinese B66.1
    |oriental B66.1
    |sheep B66.3
  |gestational alloimmune (GALD) P78.84
  |glycogen storage E74.09 *[K77]*
  |in (due to)
    |schistosomiasis (bilharziasis) B65.9 *[K77]*
  |inflammatory K75.9
    |alcoholic K70.1
    |specified NEC K75.89
  |polycystic (congenital) Q44.6
  |toxic K71.9
    |with
      |cholestasis K71.0
      |cirrhosis (liver) K71.7
      |fibrosis (liver) K71.7
      |focal nodular hyperplasia K71.8
      |hepatic granuloma K71.8
      |hepatic necrosis K71.10
        |with coma K71.11

Disease, diseased - *continued*
    |hepatitis NEC K71.6
    |acute K71.2
    |chronic
      |active K71.50
        |with ascites K71.51
      |lobular K71.4
      |persistent K71.3
    |lupoid K71.50
      |with ascites K71.51
    |peliosis hepatis K71.8
    |veno-occlusive disease (VOD) of liver
      K71.8
  |veno-occlusive K76.5
|Lobo's (keloid blastomycosis) B48.0
|Lobstein's (brittle bones and blue sclera)
  Q78.0
|Ludwig's (submaxillary cellulitis) K12.2
|lumbosacral region M53.87
|lung J98.4
  |black J60
  |congenital Q33.9
  |cystic J98.4
    |congenital Q33.0
  |dabbing (related) U07.0
  |electronic cigarette (related) U07.0
  |fibroid (chronic) *see* Fibrosis, lung
  |fluke B66.4
    |oriental B66.4
  |in
    |amyloidosis E85.4 *[J99]*
    |sarcoidosis D86.0
    |Sjögren's syndrome M35.02
    |systemic
      |lupus erythematosus M32.13
      |sclerosis M34.81
  |interstitial J84.9
    |of childhood, specified NEC J84.848
    |respiratory bronchiolitis J84.115
    |specified NEC J84.89
    |with progressive fibrotic phenotype, in
      diseases classified elsewhere J84.170
  |obstructive (chronic) J44.9
    |with
      |acute
        |bronchitis J44.0
        |exacerbation NEC J44.1
        |lower respiratory infection J44.0
      |alveolitis, allergic J67.9
      |asthma J44.9
      |bronchiectasis J47.9
        |with
          |exacerbation (acute) J47.1
          |lower respiratory infection J47.0
      |bronchitis J44.9
        |with
          |exacerbation (acute) J44.1
          |lower respiratory infection J44.0
      |emphysema J43.9
      |hypersensitivity pneumonitis J67.9
    |vaping (associated) (device) (product) (use)
      U07.0
    |decompensated J44.1
      |with
        |exacerbation (acute) J44.1
  |polycystic J98.4
    |congenital Q33.0
  |rheumatoid (diffuse) (interstitial) *see*
    Rheumatoid, lung
|Lutembacher's (atrial septal defect with mitral
  stenosis) Q21.1
|Lyme A69.20
|lymphatic (gland) (system) (channel) (vessel)
  I89.9
|lymphoproliferative D47.9

Disease, diseased - *continued*
| |specified NEC D47.Z9
| | |T-gamma D47.Z9
| | |X-linked D82.3
| |Magitot's M27.2
| |malarial *see* Malaria
| |malignant *see also* Neoplasm, malignant, by
| site
| |Manson's B65.1
| |maple bark J67.6
| |maple-syrup-urine E71.0
| |Marburg (virus) A98.3
| |Marion's (bladder neck obstruction) N32.0
| |Marsh's (exophthalmic goiter) *see*
| Hyperthyroidism, with, goiter (diffuse)
| |mastoid (process) *see* Disorder, ear, middle
| |Mathieu's (leptospiral jaundice) A27.0
| |Maxcy's A75.2
| |McArdle (-Schmid-Pearson) (glycogenosis V)
| E74.04
| |mediastinum J98.59
| |medullary center (idiopathic) (respiratory)
| G93.89
| |Meige's (chronic hereditary edema) Q82.0
| |meningococcal *see* Infection, meningococcal
| |mental F99
| | |organic F09
| |mesenchymal M35.9
| |mesenteric embolic *see also* Ischemia,
| intestine, acute K55.039
| |metabolic, metabolism E88.9
| | |bilirubin E80.7
| |metal-polisher's J62.8
| |metastatic *see also* Neoplasm, secondary, by
| site C79.9
| |microvascular   code to condition
| |microvillus
| | |atrophy Q43.8
| | |inclusion (MVD) Q43.8
| |middle ear *see* Disorder, ear, middle
| |Mikulicz' (dryness of mouth, absent or
| decreased lacrimation) K11.8
| |Milroy's (chronic hereditary edema) Q82.0
| |Minamata *see* Poisoning, mercury
| |minicore G71.29
| |Minor's G95.19
| |Minot's (hemorrhagic disease, newborn) P53
| |Minot-Von Willebrand-Jurgens
| (angiohemophilia) D68.0
| |Mitchell's (erythromelalgia) I73.81
| |mitral (valve) I05.9
| | |nonrheumatic I34.9
| |mixed connective tissue M35.1
| |moldy hay J67.0
| |Monge's T70.29
| |Morgagni-Adams-Stokes (syncope with heart
| block) I45.9
| |Morgagni's (syndrome) (hyperostosis frontalis
| interna) M85.2
| |Morton's (with metatarsalgia) *see* Lesion,
| nerve, plantar
| |Morvan's G60.8
| |motor neuron (bulbar) (mixed type) (spinal)
| G12.20
| | |amyotrophic lateral sclerosis G12.21
| | |familial G12.24
| | |progressive bulbar palsy G12.22
| | |specified NEC G12.29
| |moyamoya I67.5
| |mu heavy chain disease C88.2
| |multicore G71.29
| |multiminicore G71.29
| |muscle *see also* Disorder, muscle
| | |inflammatory *see* Myositis
| | |ocular (external) *see* Strabismus

Disease, diseased - *continued*
| |musculoskeletal system, soft tissue *see also*
| Disorder, soft tissue
| | |specified NEC *see* Disorder, soft tissue,
| specified type NEC
| |mushroom workers' J67.5
| |mycotic B49
| |myelodysplastic, not classified C94.6
| |myeloproliferative, (see also Syndrome,
| myelodysplasia) C94.6
| | |chronic D47.1
| |myocardium, myocardial *see also*
| Degeneration, myocardial I51.5
| | |primary (idiopathic) I42.9
| |myoneural G70.9
| |Naegeli's D69.1
| |nails L60.9
| | |specified NEC L60.8
| |Nairobi (sheep virus) A93.8
| |nasal J34.9
| |nemaline body G71.21
| |nerve *see* Disorder, nerve
| |nervous system G98.8
| | |autonomic G90.9
| | |central G96.9
| | | |specified NEC G96.89
| | |congenital Q07.9
| | |parasympathetic G90.9
| | |specified NEC G98.8
| | |sympathetic G90.9
| | |vegetative G90.9
| |neuromuscular system G70.9
| |Newcastle B30.8
| |Nicolas (-Durand)-Favre (climatic bubo) A55
| |nipple N64.9
| | |Paget's C50.01-
| | | |female C50.01-
| | | |male C50.02-
| |Nishimoto (-Takeuchi) I67.5
| |nonarthropod-borne NOS (viral) B34.9
| | |enterovirus NEC B34.1
| |nonautoimmune hemolytic D59.4
| | |drug-induced D59.2
| |Nonne-Milroy-Meige (chronic hereditary
| edema) Q82.0
| |nose J34.9
| |nucleus pulposus *see* Disorder, disc
| |nutritional E63.9
| |oast-house-urine E72.19
| | |ocular
| | | |herpesviral B00.50
| | | |zoster B02.30
| |obliterative vascular I77.1
| |Ohara's *see* Tularemia
| |Opitz's (congestive splenomegaly) D73.2
| |Oppenheim-Urbach (necrobiosis lipoidica
| diabeticorum) *see* E08-E13 with .620
| |optic nerve NEC *see* Disorder, nerve, optic
| |orbit *see* Disorder, orbit
| |organ
| | |dabbing (related) U07.0
| | |electronic cigarette (related) U07.0
| | |vaping (associated) (device) (product) (use)
| | U07.0
| |Oriental liver fluke B66.1
| |Oriental lung fluke B66.4
| |Ormond's N13.5
| |Oropouche virus A93.0
| |Osler-Rendu (familial hemorrhagic
| telangiectasia) I78.0
| |osteofibrocystic E21.0
| |Otto's M24.7
| |outer ear *see* Disorder, ear, external
| |ovary (noninflammatory) N83.9
| | |cystic N83.20-

Disease, diseased - *continued*
| |inflammatory *see* Salpingo-oophoritis
| | |polycystic E28.2
| | |specified NEC N83.8
| |Owren's (congenital) *see* Defect, coagulation
| |pancreas K86.9
| | |cystic K86.2
| | |fibrocystic E84.9
| | |specified NEC K86.89
| |panvalvular I08.9
| | |specified NEC I08.8
| |parametrium (noninflammatory) N83.9
| |parasitic B89
| | |cerebral NEC B71.9 *[G94]*
| | |intestinal NOS B82.9
| | |mouth B37.0
| | |skin NOS B88.9
| | |specified type *see* Infestation
| | |tongue B37.0
| |parathyroid (gland) E21.5
| | |specified NEC E21.4
| |Parkinson's G20
| |parodontal K05.6
| |Parrot's (syphilitic osteochondritis) A50.02
| |Parry's (exophthalmic goiter) *see*
| Hyperthyroidism, with, goiter (diffuse)
| |Parson's (exophthalmic goiter) *see*
| Hyperthyroidism, with, goiter (diffuse)
| |Paxton's (white piedra) B36.2
| |pearl-worker's *see* Osteomyelitis, specified
| type NEC
| |Pellegrini-Stieda (calcification, knee joint) *see*
| Bursitis, tibial collateral
| |pelvis, pelvic
| | |female NOS N94.9
| | | |specified NEC N94.89
| | |gonococcal (acute) (chronic) A54.24
| | |inflammatory (female) N73.9
| | | |acute N73.0
| | | |chlamydial A56.11
| | | |chronic N73.1
| | | |specified NEC N73.8
| | | |syphilitic (secondary) A51.42
| | | | |late A52.76
| | | |tuberculous A18.17
| | |organ, female N94.9
| | |peritoneum, female NEC N94.89
| |penis N48.9
| | |inflammatory N48.29
| | | |abscess N48.21
| | | |cellulitis N48.22
| | |specified NEC N48.89
| |periapical tissues NOS K04.90
| |periodontal K05.6
| | |specified NEC K05.5
| |periosteum *see* Disorder, bone, specified type
| NEC
| |peripheral
| | |arterial I73.9
| | |autonomic nervous system G90.9
| | |nerves *see* Polyneuropathy
| | |vascular NOS I73.9
| |peritoneum K66.9
| | |pelvic, female NEC N94.89
| | |specified NEC K66.8
| |persistent mucosal (middle ear) H66.20
| | |left H66.22
| | | |with right H66.23
| | |right H66.21
| | | |with left H66.23
| |Petit's *see* Hernia, abdomen, specified site
| NEC
| |pharynx J39.2
| | |specified NEC J39.2
| |Phocas' *see* Mastopathy, cystic

Disease, diseased - *continued*
|photochromogenic (acid-fast bacilli) (pulmonary) A31.0
|nonpulmonary A31.9
|Pick's G31.01 *[F02.80]*
  |with behavioral disturbance G31.01 *[F02.81]*
  |brain G31.01 *[F02.80]*
    |with behavioral disturbance G31.01 *[F02.81]*
  |of pericardium (pericardial pseudocirrhosis of liver) I31.1
|pigeon fancier's J67.2
|pineal gland E34.8
|pink *see* Poisoning, mercury
|Pinkus' (lichen nitidus) L44.1
|pinworm B80
|Piry virus A93.8
|pituitary (gland) E23.7
|pituitary-snuff-taker's J67.8
|pleura (cavity) J94.9
  |specified NEC J94.8
|pneumatic drill (hammer) T75.21
|Pollitzer's (hidradenitis suppurativa) L73.2
|polycystic
  |kidney or renal Q61.3
    |adult type Q61.2
    |childhood type NEC Q61.19
      |collecting duct dilatation Q61.11
  |liver or hepatic Q44.6
  |lung or pulmonary J98.4
    |congenital Q33.0
  |ovary, ovaries E28.2
  |spleen Q89.09
|polyethylene T84.05-
|Pompe's (glycogenosis II) E74.02
|Posadas-Wernicke B38.9
|Potain's (pulmonary edema) *see* Edema, lung
|prepuce N47.8
  |inflammatory N47.7
    |balanoposthitis N47.6
|Pringle's (tuberous sclerosis) Q85.1
|prion, central nervous system A81.9
  |specified NEC A81.89
|prostate N42.9
  |specified NEC N42.89
|protozoal B64
  |acanthamebiasis *see* Acanthamebiasis
  |African trypanosomiasis *see* African trypanosomiasis
  |babesiosis B60.00
  |Chagas disease *see* Chagas disease
  |intestine, intestinal A07.9
  |leishmaniasis *see* Leishmaniasis
  |malaria *see* Malaria
  |naegleriasis B60.2
  |pneumocystosis B59
  |specified organism NEC B60.8
  |toxoplasmosis *see* Toxoplasmosis
|pseudo-Hurler's E77.0
|psychiatric F99
|psychotic *see* Psychosis
|Puente's (simple glandular cheilitis) K13.0
|puerperal *see also* Puerperal O90.89
|pulmonary *see also* Disease, lung
  |artery I28.9
  |chronic obstructive J44.9
    |with
      |acute bronchitis J44.0
      |exacerbation (acute) J44.1
      |lower respiratory infection (acute) J44.0
    |decompensated J44.1
      |with
        |exacerbation (acute) J44.1
  |heart I27.9

Disease, diseased - *continued*
  |specified NEC I27.89
|hypertensive (vascular) (*see also* Hypertension, pulmonary) I27.20
  |primary (idiopathic) I27.0
|valve I37.9
  |rheumatic I09.89
|pulp (dental) NOS K04.90
|pulseless M31.4
|Putnam's (subacute combined sclerosis with pernicious anemia) D51.0
|Pyle (-Cohn) (metaphyseal dysplasia) Q78.5
|ragpicker's or ragsorter's A22.1
|Raynaud's *see* Raynaud's disease |reactive airway *see* Asthma
|Reclus' (cystic) *see* Mastopathy, cystic
|rectum K62.9
  |specified NEC K62.89
|Refsum's (heredopathia atactica polyneuritiformis) G60.1
|renal (functional) (pelvis) *see also* Disease, kidney N28.9
  |with
    |edema *see* Nephrosis
    |glomerular lesion *see* Glomerulonephritis
      |with edema *see* Nephrosis
    |interstitial nephritis N12
  |acute N28.9
  |chronic *see also* Disease, kidney, chronic N18.9
  |cystic, congenital Q61.9
  |diabetic *see* E08-E13 with .22
  |end-stage (failure) N18.6
    |due to hypertension I12.0
  |fibrocystic (congenital) Q61.8
  |hypertensive *see* Hypertension, kidney
  |lupus M32.14
  |phosphate-losing (tubular) N25.0
  |polycystic (congenital) Q61.3
    |adult type Q61.2
    |childhood type NEC Q61.19
      |collecting duct dilatation Q61.11
  |rapidly progressive N01.9
  |subacute N01.9
|Rendu-Osler-Weber (familial hemorrhagic telangiectasia) I78.0
|renovascular (arteriosclerotic) *see* Hypertension, kidney
|respiratory (tract) J98.9
  |acute or subacute NOS J06.9
    |due to
      |chemicals, gases, fumes or vapors (inhalation) J68.3
      |external agent J70.9
        |specified NEC J70.8
      |radiation J70.0
      |smoke inhalation J70.5
    |noninfectious J39.8
  |chronic NOS J98.9
    |due to
      |chemicals, gases, fumes or vapors J68.4
      |external agent J70.9
        |specified NEC J70.8
      |radiation J70.1
  |newborn P27.9
    |specified NEC P27.8
  |due to
    |chemicals, gases, fumes or vapors J68.9
      |acute or subacute NEC J68.3
      |chronic J68.4
    |external agent J70.9
      |specified NEC J70.8
  |newborn P28.9
    |specified type NEC P28.89
  |upper J39.9

Disease, diseased - *continued*
  |acute or subacute J06.9
  |noninfectious NEC J39.8
  |specified NEC J39.8
  |streptococcal J06.9
|retina, retinal H35.9
  |Batten's or Batten-Mayou E75.4 *[H36]*
  |specified NEC H35.89
|rheumatoid *see* Arthritis, rheumatoid
|rickettsial NOS A79.9
  |specified type NEC A79.89
|Riga (-Fede) (cachectic aphthae) K14.0
|Riggs' (compound periodontitis) *see* Periodontitis
|Ritter's L00
|Rivalta's (cervicofacial actinomycosis) A42.2
|Robles' (onchocerciasis) B73.01
|rod body G71.21
|Roger's (congenital interventricular septal defect) Q21.0
|Rosenthal's (factor XI deficiency) D68.1
|Rossbach's (hyperchlorhydria) K30
|Ross River B33.1
|Rotes Quérol *see* Hyperostosis, ankylosing
|Roth (-Bernhardt) *see* Mononeuropathy, lower limb, meralgia paresthetica
|Runeberg's (progressive pernicious anemia) D51.0
|sacroiliac NEC M53.3
|salivary gland or duct K11.9
  |inclusion B25.9
  |specified NEC K11.8
  |virus B25.9
|sandworm B76.9
|Schimmelbusch's *see* Mastopathy, cystic
|Schmorl's *see* Schmorl's disease or nodes
|Schönlein (-Henoch) (purpura rheumatica) D69.0
|Schottmüller's *see* Fever, paratyphoid
|Schultz's (agranulocytosis) *see* Agranulocytosis
|Schwalbe-Ziehen-Oppenheim G24.1
|Schwartz-Jampel G71.13
|sclera H15.9
  |specified NEC H15.89
|scrofulous (tuberculous) A18.2
|scrotum N50.9
|sebaceous glands L73.9
|semilunar cartilage, cystic *see also* Derangement, knee, meniscus, cystic
|seminal vesicle N50.9
|serum NEC *see also* Reaction, serum T80.69
|sexually transmitted A64
  |anogenital
    |herpesviral infection *see* Herpes, anogenital
    |warts A63.0
  |chancroid A57
  |chlamydial infection *see* Chlamydia
  |gonorrhea *see* Gonorrhea
  |granuloma inguinale A58
  |specified organism NEC A63.8
  |syphilis *see* Syphilis
  |trichomoniasis *see* Trichomoniasis
|Sézary C84.1-
|shimamushi (scrub typhus) A75.3
|shipyard B30.0
|sickle-cell D57.1
  |with
    |acute chest syndrome D57.01
    |cerebral vascular involvement D57.03
    |crisis (painful) D57.00
      |with complication specified NEC D57.09
    |splenic sequestration D57.02

Disease, diseased - *continued*

|vasoocclusive pain D57.00
|elliptocytosis D57.8-
|Hb-C D57.20
|with
|acute chest syndrome D57.211
|cerebral vascular involvement D57.213
|crisis D57.219
|with specified complication NEC D57.218
|splenic sequestration D57.212
|vasoocclusive pain D57.219
|Hb-SD D57.80
|with
|acute chest syndrome D57.811
|cerebral vascular involvement D57.813
|crisis D57.819
|with complication specified NEC D57.818
|splenic sequestration D57.812
|vasoocclusive pain D57.819
|without crisis D57.80
|Hb-SE D57.80
|with
|acute chest syndrome D57.811
|cerebral vascular involvement D57.813
|crisis D57.819
|with complication specified NEC D57.818
|splenic sequestration D57.812
|vasoocclusive pain D57.819
|without crisis D57.80
|specified NEC D57.80
|with
|acute chest syndrome D57.811
|cerebral vascular involvement D57.813
|crisis D57.819
|with complication specified NEC D57.818
|splenic sequestration D57.812
|vasoocclusive pain D57.819
|without crisis D57.80
|spherocytosis D57.80
|with
|acute chest syndrome D57.811
|cerebral vascular involvement D57.813
|crisis D57.819
|with complication specified NEC D57.818
|splenic sequestration D57.812
|vasoocclusive pain D57.819
|without crisis D57.80
|thalassemia D57.40
|with
|acute chest syndrome D57.411
|cerebral vascular involvement D57.413
|crisis (painful) D57.419
|with specified complication NEC D57.418
|splenic sequestration D57.412
|vasoocclusive pain D57.419
|beta plus D57.44
|with
|acute chest syndrome D57.451
|cerebral vascular involvement D57.453
|crisis D57.459
|with specified complication NEC D57.458
|splenic sequestration D57.452
|vasoocclusive pain D57.459

Disease, diseased - *continued*

|without crisis D57.44
|beta zero D57.42
|with
|acute chest syndrome D57.431
|cerebral vascular involvement D57.433
|crisis D57.439
|with specified complication NEC D57.438
|splenic sequestration D57.432
|vasoocclusive pain D57.439
|without crisis D57.42
|Silo-Filler's J68.8
|bronchitis J68.0
|pneumonitis J68.0
|pulmonary edema J68.1
|simian B B00.4
|Simons' (progressive lipodystrophy) E88.1
|sin nombre virus B33.4
|sinus *see* Sinusitis
|Sirkari's B55.0
|sixth B08.20
|due to human herpesvirus 6 B08.21
|due to human herpesvirus 7 B08.22
|skin L98.9
|due to metabolic disorder NEC E88.9 [*L99*]
|specified NEC L98.8
|slim (HIV) B20
|small vessel I73.9
|Sneddon-Wilkinson (subcorneal pustular dermatosis) L13.1
|South African creeping B88.0
|spinal (cord) G95.9
|congenital Q06.9
|specified NEC G95.89
|spine *see also* Spondylopathy
|joint *see* Dorsopathy
|tuberculous A18.01
|spinocerebellar (hereditary) G11.9
|specified NEC G11.8
|spleen D73.9
|amyloid E85.4 [*D77*]
|organic D73.9
|polycystic Q89.09
|postinfectional D73.89
|sponge-diver's *see* Toxicity, venom, marine animal, sea anemone
|Startle Q89.8
|Steinert's G71.11
|Sticker's (erythema infectiosum) B08.3
|Stieda's (calcification, knee joint) *see* Bursitis, tibial collateral
|Stokes' (exophthalmic goiter) *see* Hyperthyroidism, with, goiter (diffuse)
|Stokes-Adams (syncope with heart block) I45.9
|stomach K31.9
|functional, psychogenic F45.8
|specified NEC K31.89
|stonemason's J62.8
|storage
|glycogen *see* Disease, glycogen storage
|mucopolysaccharide *see* Mucopolysaccharidosis
|striatopallidal system NEC G25.89
|Stuart-Prower (congenital factor X deficiency) D68.2
|Stuart's (congenital factor X deficiency) D68.2
|subcutaneous tissue *see* Disease, skin
|supporting structures of teeth K08.9
|specified NEC K08.89
|suprarenal (capsule) (gland) E27.9
|hyperfunction E27.0
|specified NEC E27.8
|sweat glands L74.9

Disease, diseased - *continued*

|specified NEC L74.8
|Sweeley-Klionsky E75.21
|Swift (-Feer) *see* Poisoning, mercury
|swimming-pool granuloma A31.1
|Sylvest's (epidemic pleurodynia) B33.0
|sympathetic nervous system G90.9
|synovium *see* Disorder, synovium
|syphilitic *see* Syphilis
|systemic tissue mast cell C96.20
|tanapox (virus) B08.71
|Tangier E78.6
|Tarral-Besnier (pityriasis rubra pilaris) L44.0
|Tauri's E74.09
|tear duct *see* Disorder, lacrimal system
|tendon, tendinous *see also* Disorder, tendon
|nodular *see* Trigger finger
|terminal vessel I73.9
|testis N50.9
|thalassemia Hb-S *see* Disease, sickle-cell, thalassemia
|Thaysen-Gee (nontropical sprue) K90.0
|Thomsen G71.12
|throat J39.2
|septic J02.0
|thromboembolic *see* Embolism
|thymus (gland) E32.9
|specified NEC E32.8
|thyroid (gland) E07.9
|heart *see also* Hyperthyroidism E05.90 [*I43*]
|with thyroid storm E05.91 [*I43*]
|specified NEC E07.89
|Tietze's M94.0
|tongue K14.9
|specified NEC K14.8
|tonsils, tonsillar (and adenoids) J35.9
|tooth, teeth K08.9
|hard tissues K03.9
|specified NEC K03.89
|pulp NEC K04.99
|specified NEC K08.89
|Tourette's F95.2
|trachea NEC J39.8
|tricuspid I07.9
|nonrheumatic I36.9
|triglyceride-storage E75.5
|trophoblastic *see* Mole, hydatidiform
|tsutsugamushi A75.3
|tube (fallopian) (noninflammatory) N83.9
|inflammatory *see* Salpingitis
|specified NEC N83.8
|tuberculous NEC *see* Tuberculosis
|tubo-ovarian (noninflammatory) N83.9
|inflammatory *see* Salpingo-oophoritis
|specified NEC N83.8
|tubotympanic, chronic *see* Otitis, media, suppurative, chronic, tubotympanic
|tubulo-interstitial N15.9
|specified NEC N15.8
|tympanum *see* Disorder, tympanic membrane
|Uhl's Q24.8
|Underwood's (sclerema neonatorum) P83.0
|Unverricht (-Lundborg) *see* Epilepsy, generalized, idiopathic
|Urbach-Oppenheim (necrobiosis lipoidica diabeticorum) *see* E08-E13 with .620
|ureter N28.9
|in (due to)
|schistosomiasis (bilharziasis) B65.0 [*N29*]
|urethra N36.9
|specified NEC N36.8
|urinary (tract) N39.9
|bladder N32.9
|specified NEC N32.89

Disease, diseased - continued

|specified NEC N39.8
|uterus (noninflammatory) N85.9
  |infective see Endometritis
  |inflammatory see Endometritis
  |specified NEC N85.8
|uveal tract (anterior) H21.9
  |posterior H31.9
|vagabond's B85.1
|vagina, vaginal (noninflammatory) N89.9
  |inflammatory NEC N76.89
  |specified NEC N89.8
|valve, valvular I38
  |multiple I08.9
    |specified NEC I08.8
|van Creveld-Von Gierke (glycogenosis I)
  E74.01
|vas deferens N50.9
|vascular I99.9
  |arteriosclerotic see Arteriosclerosis
  |ciliary body NEC see Disorder, iris,
  vascular
  |hypertensive see Hypertension
  |iris NEC see Disorder, iris, vascular
  |obliterative I77.1
    |peripheral I73.9
  |occlusive I99.8
  |peripheral (occlusive) I73.9
    |in diabetes mellitus see E08-E13 with .51
|vasomotor I73.9
|vasospastic I73.9
|vein I87.9
|venereal see also Disease, sexually
  transmitted A64
  |chlamydial NEC A56.8
    |anus A56.3
    |genitourinary NOS A56.2
    |pharynx A56.4
    |rectum A56.3
  |fifth A55
  |sixth A55
  |specified nature or type NEC A63.8
|vertebra, vertebral see also Spondylopathy
  |disc see Disorder, disc
|vibration see Vibration, adverse effects
|viral, virus see also Disease, by type of virus
  B34.9
  |arbovirus NOS A94
  |arthropod-borne NOS A94
  |congenital P35.9
    |specified NEC P35.8
  |Hanta (with renal manifestations) (Dobrava)
    (Puumala) (Seoul) A98.5
    |with pulmonary manifestations (Andes)
      (Bayou) (Bermejo) (Black Creek
      Canal) (Choclo) (Juquitiba) (Laguna
      negra)(Lechiguanas) (New York)
      (Oran) (Sin nombre) B33.4
  |Hantaan (Korean hemorrhagic fever) A98.5
  |human immunodeficiency (HIV) B20
  |Kunjin A83.4
  |nonarthropod-borne NOS B34.9
  |Powassan A84.81
  |Rocio (encephalitis) A83.6
  |Sin nombre (Hantavirus) (cardio)-
    pulmonary syndrome) B33.4
  |Tahyna B33.8
  |vesicular stomatitis A93.8
|vitreous H43.9
  |specified NEC H43.89
|vocal cord J38.3
|Volkmann's, acquired T79.6
|von Eulenburg's (congenital paramyotonia)
  G71.19
|von Gierke's (glycogenosis I) E74.01

Disease, diseased - continued

|von Graefe's see Strabismus, paralytic,
  ophthalmoplegia, progressive
|von Willebrand (-Jurgens) (angiohemophilia)
  D68.0
|Vrolik's (osteogenesis imperfecta) Q78.0
|vulva (noninflammatory) N90.9
  |inflammatory NEC N76.89
  |specified NEC N90.89
|Wallgren's (obstruction of splenic vein with
  collateral circulation) I87.8
|Wassilieff's (leptospiral jaundice) A27.0
|wasting NEC R64
  |due to malnutrition E43
with marasmus E41
|Waterhouse-Friderichsen A39.1
|Wegner's (syphilitic osteochondritis) A50.02
|Weil's (leptospiral jaundice of lung) A27.0
|Weir Mitchell's (erythromelalgia) I73.81
|Werdnig-Hoffmann G12.0
|Wermer's E31.21
|Werner-His (trench fever) A79.0
|Werner-Schultz (neutropenic splenomegaly)
  D73.81
|Wernicke-Posadas B38.9
|whipworm B79
|white blood cells D72.9
  |specified NEC D72.89
|white matter R90.82
|white-spot, meaning lichen sclerosus et
  atrophicus L90.0
  |penis N48.0
  |vulva N90.4
|Wilkie's K55.1
|Wilkinson-Sneddon (subcorneal pustular
  dermatosis) L13.1
|Willis' see Diabetes
|Wilson's (hepatolenticular degeneration)
  E83.01
|woolsorter's A22.1
|yaba monkey tumor B08.72
|yaba pox (virus) B08.72
|Zika virus A92.5
  |congenital P35.4
|zoonotic, bacterial A28.9
  |specified type NEC A28.8

Disfigurement (due to scar) L90.5
Disgerminoma see Dysgerminoma
DISH (diffuse idiopathic skeletal hyperostosis)
  see Hyperostosis, ankylosing
Disinsertion, retina see Detachment, retina
Dislocatable hip, congenital Q65.6
Dislocation (articular)
|with fracture see Fracture
|acromioclavicular (joint) S43.10-
  |with displacement
    |100% 200% S43.12-
    |more than 200% S43.13-
  |inferior S43.14-
  |posterior S43.15-
|ankle S93.0-
|astragalus see Dislocation, ankle
|atlantoaxial S13.121
|atlantooccipital S13.111
|atloido-occipital S13.111
|breast bone S23.29
|capsule, joint   code by site under Dislocation
|carpal (bone) see Dislocation, wrist
|carpometacarpal (joint) NEC S63.05-
  |thumb S63.04-
|cartilage (joint)   code by site under
  Dislocation
|cervical spine (vertebra) see Dislocation,
  vertebra, cervical
|chronic see Dislocation, recurrent

Dislocation (articular) - continued

|clavicle see Dislocation, acromioclavicular
  joint
|coccyx S33.2
|congenital NEC Q68.8
|coracoid see Dislocation, shoulder
|costal cartilage S23.29
|costochondral S23.29
|cricoarytenoid articulation S13.29
|cricothyroid articulation S13.29
|dorsal vertebra see Dislocation, vertebra,
  thoracic
|ear ossicle see Discontinuity, ossicles, ear
|elbow S53.10-
  |congenital Q68.8
  |pathological see Dislocation, pathological
    NEC, elbow
  |radial head alone see Dislocation, radial
    head
  |recurrent see Dislocation, recurrent, elbow
  |traumatic S53.10-
    |anterior S53.11-
    |lateral S53.14-
    |medial S53.13-
    |posterior S53.12-
    |specified type NEC S53.19-
|eye, nontraumatic see Luxation, globe
|eyeball, nontraumatic see Luxation, globe
|femur
  |distal end see Dislocation, knee
  |proximal end see Dislocation, hip
|fibula
  |distal end see Dislocation, ankle
  |proximal end see Dislocation, knee
|finger S63.25-
  |index S63.25-
  |interphalangeal S63.27-
    |distal S63.29-
      |index S63.29-
      |little S63.29-
      |middle S63.29-
      |ring S63.29-
    |index S63.27-
    |little S63.27-
    |middle S63.27-
    |proximal S63.28-
      |index S63.28-
      |little S63.28-
      |middle S63.28-
      |ring S63.28-
    |ring S63.27-
  |little S63.25-
  |metacarpophalangeal S63.26-
    |index S63.26-
    |little S63.26-
    |middle S63.26-
    |ring S63.26-
  |middle S63.25-
  |recurrent see Dislocation, recurrent, finger
  |ring S63.25-
  |thumb see Dislocation, thumb
|foot S93.30-
  |recurrent see Dislocation, recurrent, foot
  |specified site NEC S93.33-
  |tarsal joint S93.31-
  |tarsometatarsal joint S93.32-
  |toe see Dislocation, toe
|fracture see Fracture
|glenohumeral (joint) see Dislocation, shoulder
|glenoid see Dislocation, shoulder
|habitual see Dislocation, recurrent
|hip S73.00-
  |anterior S73.03-
    |obturator S73.02-
  |central S73.04-

Dislocation (articular) - *continued*
  |great S93.10-
    |interphalangeal joint S93.11-
    |metatarsophalangeal joint S93.12-
  |interphalangeal joint S93.119
  |lesser S93.106
    |interphalangeal joint S93.11-
    |metatarsophalangeal joint S93.12-
  |metatarsophalangeal joint S93.12-
  |tooth S03.2
  |trachea S23.29
  |ulna
    |distal end S63.07-
    |proximal end *see* Dislocation, elbow
  |ulnohumeral (joint) *see* Dislocation, elbow
  |vertebra (articular process) (body) (traumatic)
    |cervical S13.101
      |atlantoaxial joint S13.121
      |atlantooccipital joint S13.111
      |atloido-occipital joint S13.111
      |joint between
        |C0 and C1 S13.111
        |C1 and C2 S13.121
        |C2 and C3 S13.131
        |C3 and C4 S13.141
        |C4 and C5 S13.151
        |C5 and C6 S13.161
        |C6 and C7 S13.171
        |C7 and T1 S13.181
      |occipitoatloid joint S13.111
    |congenital Q76.49
    |lumbar S33.101
      |joint between
        |L1 and L2 S33.111
        |L2 and L3 S33.121
        |L3 and L4 S33.131
        |L4 and L5 S33.141
    |nontraumatic *see* Displacement,
      intervertebral disc
    |partial *see* Subluxation, by site
    |recurrent NEC *see* subcategory M43.5
    |thoracic S23.101
      |joint between
        |T1 and T2 S23.111
        |T2 and T3 S23.121
        |T3 and T4 S23.123
        |T4 and T5 S23.131
        |T5 and T6 S23.133
        |T6 and T7 S23.141
        |T7 and T8 S23.143
        |T8 and T9 S23.151
        |T9 and T10 S23.153
        |T10 and T11 S23.161
        |T11 and T12 S23.163
        |T12 and L1 S23.171
  |wrist (carpal bone) S63.006
    |carpometacarpal joint *see* Dislocation,
      carpometacarpal (joint)
    |distal radioulnar joint *see* Dislocation,
      radioulnar (joint), distal
    |metacarpal bone, proximal *see* Dislocation,
      metacarpal (bone), proximal end
    |midcarpal *see* Dislocation, midcarpal (joint)
    |radiocarpal joint *see* Dislocation,
      radiocarpal (joint)
    |recurrent *see* Dislocation, recurrent, wrist
    |specified site NEC S63.09-
    |ulna *see* Dislocation, ulna, distal end
  |xiphoid cartilage S23.29
Disorder (of) *see also* Disease
  |acantholytic L11.9
    |specified NEC L11.8
  |acute
    |psychotic *see* Psychosis, acute
    |stress F43.0

Disorder (of) - *continued*
  |adjustment (grief) F43.20
    |with
      |anxiety F43.22
        |with depressed mood F43.23
      |conduct disturbance F43.24
        |with emotional disturbance F43.25
      |depressed mood F43.21
        |with anxiety F43.23
      |other specified symptom F43.29
  |adrenal (capsule) (gland) (medullary) E27.9
    |specified NEC E27.8
  |adrenogenital E25.9
    |drug-induced E25.8
    |iatrogenic E25.8
    |idiopathic E25.8
  |adult personality (and behavior) F69
    |specified NEC F68.8
  |affective (mood) *see* Disorder, mood
  |aggressive, unsocialized F91.1
  |alcohol-related F10.99
    |with
      |amnestic disorder, persisting F10.96
      |anxiety disorder F10.980
      |dementia, persisting F10.97
      |intoxication F10.929
        |with delirium F10.921
        |uncomplicated F10.920
      |mood disorder F10.94
      |other specified F10.988
      |psychotic disorder F10.959
        |with
          |delusions F10.950
          |hallucinations F10.951
      |sexual dysfunction F10.981
      |sleep disorder F10.982
  |alcohol use
    |mild F10.10
      |in remission (early) (sustained) F10.11
      |with
        |alcohol-induced
          |anxiety disorder F10.180
          |bipolar and related disorder F10.14
          |depressive disorder F10.14
          |psychotic disorder F10.159
          |sexual dysfunction F10.181
          |sleep disorder F10.182
        |alcohol intoxication F10.129
          |delirium F10.121
    |moderate or severe F10.20
      |in remission (early) (sustained) F10.21
      |with
        |alcohol-induced
          |anxiety disorder F10.280
          |bipolar and related disorder F10.24
          |depressive disorder F10.24
          |major neurocognitive disorder,
            amnestic-confabulatory type
            F10.26
          |major neurocognitive disorder, non-
            amnestic-confabulatory type
            F10.27
          |mild neurocognitive disorder F10.288
          |psychotic disorder F10.259
          |sexual dysfunction F10.281
          |sleep disorder F10.282
        |alcohol intoxication F10.229
          |delirium F10.221
  |allergic *see* Allergy
  |alveolar NEC J84.09
  |amino-acid
    |cystathioninuria E72.19
    |cystinosis E72.04
    |cystinuria E72.01
    |glycinuria E72.09

Disorder (of) - *continued*
  |homocystinuria E72.11
  |metabolism *see* Disturbance, metabolism,
    amino-acid
    |specified NEC E72.89
  |neonatal, transitory P74.8
  |renal transport NEC E72.09
  |transport NEC E72.09
  |amnesic, amnestic
    |alcohol-induced F10.96
      |with dependence F10.26
    |due to (secondary to) general medical
      condition F04
    |psychoactive NEC-induced F19.96
      |with
        |abuse F19.16
        |dependence F19.26
    |sedative, hypnotic or anxiolytic-induced
      F13.96
      |with dependence F13.26
  |amphetamine-type substance use
    |mild F15.10
      |in remission (early) (sustained) F15.11
    |moderate F15.20
      |in remission (early) (sustained) F15.21
    |severe F15.20
      |in remission (early) (sustained) F15.21
  |amphetamine (or other stimulant) use
    |mild
      |with
        |amphetamine (or other stimulant) -
          induced
          |anxiety disorder F15.180
          |bipolar and related disorder F15.14
          |depressive disorder F15.14
          |obsessive-compulsive and related
            disorder F15.188
          |psychotic disorder F15.159
          |sexual dysfunction F15.181
        |amphetamine, cocaine, or other
          stimulant intoxication
          |with perceptual disturbances F15.122
          |without perceptual disturbances
            F15.129
        |intoxication delirium F15.121
    |moderate or severe
      |with
        |amphetamine (or other stimulant) -
          induced
          |anxiety disorder F15.280
          |obsessive-compulsive and related
            disorder F15.288
          |sexual dysfunction F15.281
          |bipolar and related disorder F15.24
          |depressive disorder F15.24
          |psychotic disorder F15.259
        |amphetamine, cocaine, or other
          stimulant intoxication
          |with perceptual disturbances F15.222
          |without perceptual disturbances
            F15.229
        |intoxication delirium F15.221
  |anaerobic glycolysis with anemia D55.29
  |anxiety F41.9
    |due to (secondary to)
      |alcohol F10.980
      |amphetamine F15.980
        |in
          |abuse F15.180
          |dependence F15.280
      |anxiolytic F13.980
        |in
          |abuse F13.180
          |dependence F13.280

Disorder (of) - continued
   |caffeine F15.980
     |in
       |abuse F15.180
       |dependence F15.280
   |cannabis F12.980
     |in
       |abuse F12.180
       |dependence F12.280
   |cocaine F14.980
     |in
       |abuse F14.180
       |dependence F14.180
   |general medical condition F06.4
   |hallucinogen F16.980
     |in
       |abuse F16.180
       |dependence F16.280
   |hypnotic F13.980
     |in
       |abuse F13.180
       |dependence F13.280
   |inhalant F18.980
     |in
       |abuse F18.180
       |dependence F18.280
   |phencyclidine F16.980
     |in
       |abuse F16.180
       |dependence F16.280
   |psychoactive substance NEC F19.980
     |in
       |abuse F19.180
       |dependence F19.280
   |sedative F13.980
     |in
       |abuse F13.180
       |dependence F13.280
   |volatile solvents F18.980
     |in
       |abuse F18.180
       |dependence F18.280
   |generalized F41.1
   |illness F45.21
   |mixed
     |with depression (mild) F41.8
     |specified NEC F41.3
   |organic F06.4
   |phobic F40.9
     |of childhood F40.8
   |specified NEC F41.8
  |aortic valve *see* Endocarditis, aortic
  |aromatic amino-acid metabolism E70.9
    |specified NEC E70.89
  |arteriole NEC I77.89
  |artery NEC I77.89
  |articulation *see* Disorder, joint
  |attachment (childhood)
   |disinhibited F94.2
   |reactive F94.1
  |attention-deficit hyperactivity (adolescent) (adult) (child) F90.9
   |combined
    |presentation F90.2
    |type F90.2
   |hyperactive
    |impulsive presentation F90.1
    |type F90.1
   |inattentive
    |presentation F90.0
    |type F90.0
   |specified type NEC F90.8
  |attention-deficit without hyperactivity (adolescent) (adult) (child) F98.8

Disorder (of) - continued
  |auditory processing (central) H93.25
  |autistic F84.0
  |autism spectrum F84.0
  |autoimmune D89.89
  |autonomic nervous system G90.9
   |specified NEC G90.8
  |avoidant
   |child or adolescent F40.10
   |restrictive food intake F50.82
  |balance
   |acid-base E87.8
    |mixed E87.4
   |electrolyte E87.8
   |fluid NEC E87.8
  |behavioral (disruptive) *see* Disorder, conduct
  |beta-amino-acid metabolism E72.89
  |bile acid and cholesterol metabolism E78.70
   |Barth syndrome E78.71
   |other specified E78.79
   |Smith-Lemli-Opitz syndrome E78.72
  |bilirubin excretion E80.6
  |binge eating F50.81
  |binocular
   |movement H51.9
    |convergence
     |excess H51.12
     |insufficiency H51.11
    |internuclear ophthalmoplegia *see* Ophthalmoplegia, internuclear
    |palsy of conjugate gaze H51.0
    |specified type NEC H51.8
   |vision NEC *see* Disorder, vision, binocular
  |bipolar (I) (type 1) F31.9
   |and related due to a known physiological condition
    |with
     |manic features F06.33
     |manic or hypomanic-like episodes F06.33
     |mixed features F06.34
   |current (or most recent) episode
    |depressed F31.9
     |with psychotic features F31.5
     |without psychotic features F31.30
      |mild F31.31
      |moderate F31.32
      |severe (without psychotic features) F31.4
      |with psychotic features F31.5
    |hypomanic F31.0
    |manic F31.9
     |with psychotic features F31.2
     |without psychotic features F31.10
      |mild F31.11
      |moderate F31.12
      |severe (without psychotic features) F31.13
      |with psychotic features F31.2
    |mixed F31.60
     |mild F31.61
     |moderate F31.62
     |severe (without psychotic features) F31.63
     |with psychotic features F31.64
    |severe depression (without psychotic features) F31.4
     |with psychotic features F31.5
   |in remission (currently) F31.70
    |in full remission
     |most recent episode
      |depressed F31.76
      |hypomanic F31.72
      |manic F31.74
      |mixed F31.78

Disorder (of) - continued
   |in partial remission
    |most recent episode
     |depressed F31.75
     |hypomanic F31.71
     |manic F31.73
     |mixed F31.77
   |specified NEC F31.89
  |II (type 2) F31.81
  |organic F06.30
  |single manic episode F30.9
   |mild F30.11
   |moderate F30.12
   |severe (without psychotic symptoms) F30.13
    |with psychotic symptoms F30.2
  |bladder N32.9
   |functional NEC N31.9
   |in schistosomiasis B65.0 *[N33]*
   |specified NEC N32.89
  |bleeding D68.9
  |blood D75.9
   |in congenital early syphilis A50.09 *[D77]*
  |body dysmorphic F45.22
  |bone M89.9
   |continuity M84.9
    |specified type NEC M84.80
     |ankle M84.87-
     |fibula M84.86-
     |foot M84.87-
     |hand M84.84-
     |humerus M84.82-
     |neck M84.88
     |pelvis M84.859
     |radius M84.83-
     |rib M84.88
     |shoulder M84.81-
     |skull M84.88
     |thigh M84.85-
     |tibia M84.86-
     |ulna M84.83-
     |vertebra M84.88
   |density and structure M85.9
    |cyst *see also* Cyst, bone, specified type NEC
    |aneurysmal *see* Cyst, bone, aneurysmal
    |solitary *see* Cyst, bone, solitary
    |diffuse idiopathic skeletal hyperostosis *see* Hyperostosis, ankylosing
    |fibrous dysplasia (monostotic) *see* Dysplasia, fibrous, bone
    |fluorosis *see* Fluorosis, skeletal
    |hyperostosis of skull M85.2
    |osteitis condensans *see* Osteitis, condensans
    |specified type NEC M85.8-
     |ankle M85.87-
     |foot M85.87-
     |forearm M85.83-
     |hand M85.84-
     |lower leg M85.86-
     |multiple sites M85.89
     |neck M85.88
     |rib M85.88
     |shoulder M85.81-
     |skull M85.88
     |thigh M85.85-
     |upper arm M85.82-
     |vertebra M85.88
   |development and growth NEC M89.20
    |carpus M89.24-
    |clavicle M89.21-
    |femur M89.25-
    |fibula M89.26-
    |finger M89.24-

Disorder (of) - *continued*

|humerus M89.22-
|ilium M89.259
|ischium M89.259
|metacarpus M89.24-
|metatarsus M89.27-
|multiple sites M89.29
|neck M89.28
|radius M89.23-
|rib M89.28
|scapula M89.21-
|skull M89.28
|tarsus M89.27-
|tibia M89.26-
|toe M89.27-
|ulna M89.23-
|vertebra M89.28
|specified type NEC M89.8X
|brachial plexus G54.0
|branched-chain amino-acid metabolism E71.2
|specified NEC E71.19
|breast N64.9
|agalactia *see* Agalactia
|associated with
|lactation O92.70
|specified NEC O92.79
|pregnancy O92.20
|specified NEC O92.29
|puerperium O92.20
|specified NEC O92.29
|cracked nipple *see* Cracked nipple
|galactorrhea *see* Galactorrhea
|hypogalactia O92.4
|lactation disorder NEC O92.79
|mastitis *see* Mastitis
|nipple infection *see* Infection, nipple
|retracted nipple *see* Retraction, nipple
|specified type NEC N64.89
|Briquet's F45.0
|bullous, in diseases classified elsewhere L14
|caffeine use
|mild
|with
|caffeine-induced
|anxiety disorder F15.180
|sleep disorder F15.182
|moderate or severe
|with
|caffeine-induced
|anxiety disorder F15.280
|sleep disorder F15.282
|cannabis use
|mild F12.10
|in remission (early) (sustained) F12.11
|with
|cannabis-induced
|anxiety disorder F12.180
|psychotic disorder F12.159
|sleep disorder F12.188
|cannabis intoxication delirium F12.121
|with perceptual disturbances F12.122
|without perceptual disturbances
F12.129
|moderate or severe F12.20
|in remission (early) (sustained) F12.21
|with
|cannabis-induced
|anxiety disorder F12.280
|psychotic disorder F12.259
|sleep disorder F12.288
|cannabis intoxication
|with perceptual disturbances F12.222
|without perceptual disturbances
F12.229
|delirium F12.221

Disorder (of) - *continued*

|carbohydrate
|absorption, intestinal NEC E74.39
|metabolism (congenital) E74.9
|specified NEC E74.89
|cardiac, functional I51.89
|carnitine metabolism E71.40
|cartilage M94.9
|articular NEC *see* Derangement, joint,
articular cartilage
|chondrocalcinosis *see* Chondrocalcinosis
|specified type NEC M94.8X-
|articular *see* Derangement, joint, articular
cartilage
|multiple sites M94.8X0
|catatonia (due to known physiological
condition) (with another mental disorder)
F06.1
|catatonic
|due to (secondary to) known physiological
condition F06.1
|organic F06.1
|central auditory processing H93.25
|cervical
|region NEC M53.82
|root (nerve) NEC G54.2
|character NOS F60.9
|childhood disintegrative NEC F84.3
|cholesterol and bile acid metabolism E78.70
|Barth syndrome E78.71
|other specified E78.79
|Smith-Lemli-Opitz syndrome E78.72
|choroid H31.9
|atrophy *see* Atrophy, choroid
|degeneration *see* Degeneration, choroid
|detachment *see* Detachment, choroid
|dystrophy *see* Dystrophy, choroid
|hemorrhage *see* Hemorrhage, choroid
|rupture *see* Rupture, choroid
|scar *see* Scar, chorioretinal
|solar retinopathy *see* Retinopathy, solar
|specified type NEC H31.8
|ciliary body *see* Disorder, iris
|degeneration *see* Degeneration, ciliary body
|coagulation (factor) *see also* Defect,
coagulation D68.9
|newborn, transient P61.6
|cocaine use
|mild F14.10
|in remission (early) (sustained) F14.11
|with
|amphetamine, cocaine, or other
stimulant intoxication
|with perceptual disturbances F14.122
|without perceptual disturbances
F14.129
|cocaine-induced
|anxiety disorder F14.180
|bipolar and related disorder F14.14
|depressive disorder F14.14
|obsessive-compulsive and related
disorder F14.188
|psychotic disorder F14.159
|sexual dysfunction F14.181
|sleep disorder F14.182
|cocaine intoxication delirium F14.121
|moderate or severe F14.20
|in remission (early) (sustained) F14.21
|with
|amphetamine, cocaine, or other
stimulant intoxication
|with perceptual disturbances F14.222
|without perceptual disturbances
F14.229
|cocaine-induced

Disorder (of) - *continued*

|anxiety disorder F14.280
|bipolar and related disorder F14.24
|depressive disorder F14.24
|obsessive-compulsive and related
disorder F14.288
|psychotic disorder F14.259
|sexual dysfunction F14.281
|sleep disorder F14.282
|cocaine intoxication delirium F14.221
|coccyx NEC M53.3
|cognitive F09
|due to (secondary to) general medical
condition F09
|persisting R41.89
|due to
|alcohol F10.97
|with dependence F10.27
|anxiolytics F13.97
|with dependence F13.27
|hypnotics F13.97
|with dependence F13.27
|sedatives F13.97
|with dependence F13.27
|specified substance NEC F19.97
|with
|abuse F19.17
|dependence F19.27
|communication F80.9
|social pragmatic F80.82
|conduct (childhood) F91.9
|adjustment reaction *see* Disorder,
adjustment
|adolescent onset type F91.2
|childhood onset type F91.1
|compulsive F63.9
|confined to family context F91.0
|depressive F91.8
|group type F91.2
|hyperkinetic *see* Disorder, attention-deficit
hyperactivity
|oppositional defiance F91.3
|socialized F91.2
|solitary aggressive type F91.1
|specified NEC F91.8
|unsocialized (aggressive) F91.1
|conduction, heart I45.9
|congenital glycosylation (CDG) E74.89
|conjunctiva H11.9
|infection *see* Conjunctivitis
|connective tissue, localized L94.9
|specified NEC L94.8
|conversion (functional neurological symptom
disorder)
|with
|abnormal movement F44.4
|anesthesia or sensory loss F44.6
|attacks or seizures F44.5
|mixed symptoms F44.7
|special sensory symptoms F44.6
|speech symptoms F44.4
|swallowing symptoms F44.4
|weakness or paralysis F44.4
|convulsive (secondary) *see* Convulsions
|cornea H18.9
|deformity *see* Deformity, cornea
|degeneration *see* Degeneration, cornea
|deposits *see* Deposit, cornea
|due to contact lens H18.82-
|specified as edema *see* Edema, cornea
|edema *see* Edema, cornea
|keratitis *see* Keratitis
|keratoconjunctivitis *see* Keratoconjunctivitis
|membrane change *see* Change, corneal
membrane

Disorder (of) - *continued*
- |neovascularization *see* Neovascularization, cornea
- |scar *see* Opacity, cornea
- |specified type NEC H18.89-
- |ulcer *see* Ulcer, cornea
- |corpus cavernosum N48.9
- |cranial nerve *see* Disorder, nerve, cranial
- |Cyclin-Dependent Kinase-Like 5 Deficiency (CDKL5) G40.42
- |cyclothymic F34.0
- |defiant oppositional F91.3
- |delusional (persistent) (systematized) F22
  - |induced F24
- |depersonalization F48.1
- |depressive F32.A
  - |due to known physiological condition
    - |with
      - |depressive features F06.31
      - |major depressive-like episode F06.32
      - |mixed features F06.34
  - |major F32.9
    - |with psychotic symptoms F32.3
    - |in remission (full) F32.5
      - |partial F32.4
    - |recurrent F33.9
      - |with psychotic features F33.3
    - |single episode F32.9
      - |mild F32.0
      - |moderate F32.1
      - |severe (without psychotic symptoms) F32.2
        - |with psychotic symptoms F32.3
  - |organic F06.31
  - |persistent F34.1
  - |recurrent F33.9
    - |current episode
      - |mild F33.0
      - |moderate F33.1
      - |severe (without psychotic symptoms) F33.2
        - |with psychotic symptoms F33.3
    - |in remission F33.40
      - |full F33.42
      - |partial F33.41
    - |specified NEC F33.8
  - |single episode *see* Episode, depressive
  - |specified NEC F32.89
- |developmental F89
  - |arithmetical skills F81.2
  - |coordination (motor) F82
  - |expressive writing F81.81
  - |language F80.9
    - |expressive F80.1
    - |mixed receptive and expressive F80.2
    - |receptive type F80.2
    - |specified NEC F80.89
  - |learning F81.9
    - |arithmetical F81.2
    - |reading F81.0
  - |mixed F88
  - |motor coordination or function F82
  - |pervasive F84.9
    - |specified NEC F84.8
  - |phonological F80.0
  - |reading F81.0
  - |scholastic skills *see also* Disorder, learning
    - |mixed F81.89
  - |specified NEC F88
  - |speech F80.9
    - |articulation F80.0
    - |specified NEC F80.89
  - |written expression F81.81
- |diaphragm J98.6
- |digestive (system) K92.9

Disorder (of) - *continued*
- |newborn P78.9
  - |specified NEC P78.89
- |postprocedural *see* Complication, gastrointestinal
- |psychogenic F45.8
- |disc (intervertebral) M51.9
  - |with
    - |myelopathy
      - |cervical region M50.00
      - |cervicothoracic region M50.03
      - |high cervical region M50.01
      - |lumbar region M51.06
      - |mid-cervical region M50.020
      - |sacrococcygeal region M53.3
      - |thoracic region M51.04
      - |thoracolumbar region M51.05
    - |radiculopathy
      - |cervical region M50.10
      - |cervicothoracic region M50.13
      - |high cervical region M50.11
      - |lumbar region M51.16
      - |lumbosacral region M51.17
      - |mid-cervical region M50.120
      - |sacrococcygeal region M53.3
      - |thoracic region M51.14
      - |thoracolumbar region M51.15
  - |cervical M50.90
    - |with
      - |myelopathy M50.00
        - |C2-C3 M50.01
        - |C3-C4 M50.01
        - |C4-C5 M50.021
        - |C5-C6 M50.022
        - |C6-C7 M50.023
        - |C7-T1 M50.03
      - |cervicothoracic region M50.03
      - |high cervical region M50.01
      - |mid-cervical region M50.020
      - |neuritis, radiculitis or radiculopathy M50.10
        - |C2-C3 M50.11
        - |C3-C4 M50.11
        - |C4-C5 M50.121
        - |C5-C6 M50.122
        - |C6-C7 M50.123
        - |C7-T1 M50.13
      - |cervicothoracic region M50.13
      - |high cervical region M50.11
      - |mid-cervical region M50.120
    - |C2-C3 M50.91
    - |C3-C4 M50.91
    - |C4-C5 M50.921
    - |C5-C6 M50.922
    - |C6-C7 M50.923
    - |C7-T1 M50.93
    - |cervicothoracic region M50.93
    - |degeneration M50.30
      - |C2-C3 M50.31
      - |C3-C4 M50.31
      - |C4-C5 M50.321
      - |C5-C6 M50.322
      - |C6-C7 M50.323
      - |C7-T1 M50.33
      - |cervicothoracic region M50.33
      - |high cervical region M50.31
      - |mid-cervical region M50.320
    - |displacement M50.20
      - |C2-C3 M50.21
      - |C3-C4 M50.21
      - |C4-C5 M50.221
      - |C5-C6 M50.222
      - |C6-C7 M50.223
      - |C7-T1 M50.23
      - |cervicothoracic region M50.23

Disorder (of) - *continued*
- |high cervical region M50.21
- |mid-cervical region M50.220
- |high cervical region M50.91
- |mid-cervical region M50.920
- |NEC M50.80
  - |C2-C3 M50.81
  - |C3-C4 M50.81
  - |C4-C5 M50.821
  - |C5-C6 M50.822
  - |C6-C7 M50.823
  - |C7-T1 M50.83
  - |cervicothoracic region M50.83
  - |high cervical region M50.81
  - |mid-cervical region M50.820
- |specified NEC
  - |lumbar region M51.86
  - |lumbosacral region M51.87
  - |sacrococcygeal region M53.3
  - |thoracic region M51.84
  - |thoracolumbar region M51.85
- |disinhibited attachment (childhood) F94.2
- |disintegrative, childhood NEC F84.3
- |disruptive F91.9
  - |mood dysregulation F34.81
  - |specified NEC F91.8
- |disruptive behavior *see* Disorder, conduct
- |dissocial personality F60.2
- |dissociative F44.9
  - |affecting
    - |motor function F44.4
      - |and sensation F44.7
    - |sensation F44.6
      - |and motor function F44.7
  - |brief reactive F43.0
  - |due to (secondary to) general medical condition F06.8
  - |mixed F44.7
  - |organic F06.8
  - |other specified NEC F44.89
- |double heterozygous sickling *see* Disease, sickle-cell
- |dream anxiety F51.5
- |drug induced hemorrhagic D68.32
- |drug related F19.99
  - |abuse *see* Abuse, drug
  - |dependence *see* Dependence, drug
- |dysmorphic body F45.22
- |dysthymic F34.1
- |ear H93.9-
  - |bleeding *see* Otorrhagia
  - |deafness *see* Deafness
  - |degenerative H93.09-
  - |discharge *see* Otorrhea
  - |external H61.9-
    - |auditory canal stenosis *see* Stenosis, external ear canal
    - |exostosis *see* Exostosis, external ear canal
    - |impacted cerumen *see* Impaction, cerumen
    - |otitis *see* Otitis, externa
    - |perichondritis *see* Perichondritis, ear
    - |pinna *see* Disorder, pinna
    - |specified type NEC H61.89-
      - |in diseases classified elsewhere H62.8X-
  - |inner H83.9-
    - |vestibular dysfunction *see* Disorder, vestibular function
  - |middle H74.9-
    - |adhesive H74.1-
    - |ossicle *see* Abnormal, ear ossicles
    - |polyp *see* Polyp, ear (middle)
    - |specified NEC, in diseases classified elsewhere H75.8-

Disorder (of) - *continued*

|postprocedural *see* Complications, ear, procedure
|specified NEC, in diseases classified elsewhere H94.8-
|eating (adult) (psychogenic) F50.9
  |anorexia *see* Anorexia
  |binge F50.81
  |bulimia F50.2
  |child F98.29
    |pica F98.3
    |rumination disorder F98.21
  |pica F50.89
    |childhood F98.3
|electrolyte (balance) NEC E87.8
  |with
    |abortion *see* Abortion by type complicated by specified condition NEC
    |ectopic pregnancy O08.5
    |molar pregnancy O08.5
  |acidosis (metabolic) (respiratory) E87.2
  |alkalosis (metabolic) (respiratory) E87.3
|elimination, transepidermal L87.9
  |specified NEC L87.8
|emotional (persistent) F34.9
  |of childhood F93.9
    |specified NEC F93.8
|endocrine E34.9
  |postprocedural E89.89
    |specified NEC E89.89
|erectile (male) (organic) *see also* Dysfunction, sexual, male, erectile N52.9
  |nonorganic F52.21
|erythematous *see* Erythema
|esophagus K22.9
  |functional K22.4
  |psychogenic F45.8
|eustachian tube H69.9-
  |infection *see* Salpingitis, eustachian
  |obstruction *see* Obstruction, eustachian tube
  |patulous *see* Patulous, eustachian tube
  |specified NEC H69.8-
|exhibitionistic F65.2
|extrapyramidal G25.9
  |in diseases classified elsewhere *see* category G26
  |specified type NEC G25.89
|eye H57.9
  |postprocedural *see* Complication, postprocedural, eye
|eyelid H02.9
  |cyst *see* Cyst, eyelid
  |degenerative H02.70
    |chloasma *see* Chloasma, eyelid
    |madarosis *see* Madarosis
    |specified type NEC H02.79
    |vitiligo *see* Vitiligo, eyelid
    |xanthelasma *see* Xanthelasma
  |dermatochalasis *see* Dermatochalasis
  |edema *see* Edema, eyelid
  |elephantiasis *see* Elephantiasis, eyelid
  |foreign body, retained *see* Foreign body, retained, eyelid
  |function H02.59
    |abnormal innervation syndrome *see* Syndrome, abnormal innervation
    |blepharochalasis *see* Blepharochalasis
    |blepharoclonus *see* Blepharoclonus
    |blepharophimosis *see* Blepharophimosis
    |blepharoptosis *see* Blepharoptosis
    |lagophthalmos *see* Lagophthalmos
    |lid retraction *see* Retraction, lid
  |hypertrichosis *see* Hypertrichosis, eyelid
  |specified type NEC H02.89
  |vascular H02.879

Disorder (of) - *continued*

    |left H02.876
      |lower H02.875
      |upper H02.874
    |right H02.873
      |lower H02.872
      |upper H02.871
|factitious F68.10
  |by proxy F68.A
  |imposed on another F68.A
  |imposed on self F68.10
    |with predominantly
      |psychological symptoms F68.11
        |with physical symptoms F68.13
      |physical symptoms F68.12
        |with psychological symptoms F68.13
|factor, coagulation *see* Defect, coagulation
|fatty acid
  |metabolism E71.30
    |specified NEC E71.39
  |oxidation
    |LCAD E71.310
    |MCAD E71.311
    |SCAD E71.312
    |specified deficiency NEC E71.318
|feeding (infant or child) *see also* Disorder, eating R63.30
    |pediatric
acute R63.31
chronic R63.32
  |or eating disorder F50.9
  |specified NEC F50.9
|feigned (with obvious motivation) Z76.5
  |without obvious motivation *see* Disorder, factitious
|female
  |hypoactive sexual desire F52.0
  |orgasmic F52.31
  |sexual interest/arousal F52.22
|fetishistic F65.0
|fibroblastic M72.9
  |specified NEC M72.8
|fluency
  |adult onset F98.5
  |childhood onset F80.81
  |following
    |cerebral infarction I69.323
    |cerebrovascular disease I69.923
      |specified disease NEC I69.823
    |intracerebral hemorrhage I69.123
    |nontraumatic intracranial hemorrhage NEC I69.223
    |subarachnoid hemorrhage I69.023
  |in conditions classified elsewhere R47.82
|fluid balance E87.8
|follicular (skin) L73.9
  |specified NEC L73.8
|frotteuristic F65.81
|fructose metabolism E74.10
  |essential fructosuria E74.11
  |fructokinase deficiency E74.11
  |fructose 1, 6-diphosphatase deficiency E74.19
  |hereditary fructose intolerance E74.12
  |other specified E74.19
|functional polymorphonuclear neutrophils D71
|gallbladder, biliary tract and pancreas in diseases classified elsewhere K87
|gambling F63.0
|gamma aminobutyric acid (GABA) metabolism E72.81
|gamma-glutamyl cycle E72.89
|gastric (functional) K31.9
  |motility K30

Disorder (of) - *continued*

  |psychogenic F45.8
  |secretion K30
|gastrointestinal (functional) NOS K92.9
  |newborn P78.9
  |psychogenic F45.8
|gender-identity or -role F64.9
  |childhood F64.2
  |effect on relationship F66
  |of adolescence or adulthood F64.0
    |nontranssexual F64.8
  |specified NEC F64.8
  |uncertainty F66
|genito-pelvic pain penetration F52.6
|genitourinary system
  |female N94.9
  |male N50.9
  |psychogenic F45.8
|globe H44.9
  |degenerated condition H44.50
    |absolute glaucoma H44.51-
    |atrophy H44.52-
    |leucocoria H44.53-
  |degenerative H44.30
    |chalcosis H44.31-
    |myopia (*see also* Myopia, degenerative) H44.2-
    |siderosis H44.32-
    |specified type NEC H44.39-
  |endophthalmitis *see* Endophthalmitis
  |foreign body, retained *see* Foreign body, intraocular, old, retained
  |hemophthalmos *see* Hemophthalmos
  |hypotony H44.40
    |due to
      |ocular fistula H44.42-
      |specified disorder NEC H44.43-
    |flat anterior chamber H44.41-
    |primary H44.44-
  |luxation *see* Luxation, globe
  |specified type NEC H44.89
|glomerular (in) N05.9
  |amyloidosis E85.4 *[N08]*
  |cryoglobulinemia D89.1 *[N08]*
  |disseminated intravascular coagulation D65 *[N08]*
  |Fabry's disease E75.21 *[N08]*
  |familial lecithin cholesterol acyltransferase deficiency E78.6 *[N08]*
  |Goodpasture's syndrome M31.0
  |hemolytic-uremic syndrome D59.3
  |Henoch (-Schönlein) purpura D69.0 *[N08]*
  |malariae malaria B52.0
  |microscopic polyangiitis M31.7 *[N08]*
  |multiple myeloma C90.0 *[N08]*
  |mumps B26.83
  |schistosomiasis B65.9 *[N08]*
  |sepsis NEC A41. *[N08]*
    |streptococcal A40. *[N08]*
  |sickle-cell disorders D57. *[N08]*
  |strongyloidiasis B78.9 *[N08]*
  |subacute bacterial endocarditis I33.0 *[N08]*
  |syphilis A52.75
  |systemic lupus erythematosus M32.14
  |thrombotic thrombocytopenic purpura M31.19 *[N08]*
  |Waldenström macroglobulinemia C88.0 *[N08]*
  |Wegener's granulomatosis M31.31
|gluconeogenesis E74.4
|glucosaminoglycan metabolism *see* Disorder, metabolism, glucosaminoglycan
|glucose transport E74.819
  |specified NEC E74.818
|glycine metabolism E72.50

Disorder (of) - *continued*
- d-glycericacidemia E72.59
- hyperhydroxyprolinemia E72.59
- hyperoxaluria R82.992
  - primary E72.53
- hyperprolinemia E72.59
- non-ketotic hyperglycinemia E72.51
- oxalosis E72.53
- oxaluria E72.53
- sarcosinemia E72.59
- trimethylaminuria E72.52
- glycoprotein metabolism E77.9
  - specified NEC E77.8
- habit (and impulse) F63.9
  - involving sexual behavior NEC F65.9
  - specified NEC F63.89
- hallucinogen use
  - mild F16.10
    - in remission (early) (sustained) F16.11
    - with
      - hallucinogen-induced
        - anxiety disorder F16.180
        - bipolar and related disorder F16.14
        - depressive disorder F16.14
        - psychotic disorder F16.159
      - hallucinogen intoxication delirium F16.121
      - other hallucinogen intoxication F16.129
  - moderate or severe F16.20
    - in remission (early) (sustained) F16.21
    - with
      - hallucinogen-induced
        - anxiety disorder F16.280
        - bipolar and related disorder F16.24
        - depressive disorder F16.24
        - psychotic disorder F16.259
      - hallucinogen intoxication delirium F16.221
      - other hallucinogen intoxication F16.229
- heart action I49.9
- hematological D75.9
  - newborn (transient) P61.9
  - specified NEC P61.8
- hematopoietic organs D75.9
- hemorrhagic NEC D69.9
  - drug-induced D68.32
  - due to
    - extrinsic circulating anticoagulants D68.32
    - increase in
      - anti-IIa D68.32
      - anti-Xa D68.32
    - intrinsic
      - circulating anticoagulants D68.318
      - increase in
        - antithrombin D68.318
        - anti-VIIIa D68.318
        - anti-IXa D68.318
        - anti-XIa D68.318
  - following childbirth O72.3
- hemostasis *see* Defect, coagulation
- histidine metabolism E70.40
  - histidinemia E70.41
  - other specified E70.49
- hoarding F42.3
- hyperkinetic *see* Disorder, attention-deficit hyperactivity
- hyperleucine-isoleucinemia E71.19
- hypervalinemia E71.19
- hypoactive sexual desire F52.0
- hypochondriacal F45.20
  - body dysmorphic F45.22
  - neurosis F45.21
  - other specified F45.29
- identity

Disorder (of) - *continued*
- dissociative F44.81
- of childhood F93.8
- illness anxiety F45.21
- immune mechanism (immunity) D89.9
  - specified type NEC D89.89
- impaired renal tubular function N25.9
  - specified NEC N25.89
- impulse (control) F63.9
- inflammatory
  - pelvic, in diseases classified elsewhere *see* category N74
  - penis N48.29
    - abscess N48.21
    - cellulitis N48.22
- inhalant use
  - mild F18.10
    - in remission (early) (sustained) F18.11
    - with
      - inhalant-induced
        - anxiety disorder F18.180
        - depressive disorder F18.14
        - major neurocognitive disorder F18.17
        - mild neurocognitive disorder F18.188
        - psychotic disorder F18.159
      - inhalant intoxication F18.129
      - inhalant intoxication delirium F18.121
  - moderate or severe F18.20
    - in remission (early) (sustained) F18.21
    - with
      - inhalant-induced
        - anxiety disorder F18.280
        - depressive disorder F18.24
        - major neurocognitive disorder F18.27
        - mild neurocognitive disorder F18.288
        - psychotic disorder F18.259
      - inhalant intoxication F18.229
      - inhalant intoxication delirium F18.221
- integument, newborn P83.9
  - specified NEC P83.88
- intermittent explosive F63.81
- internal secretion pancreas *see* Increased, secretion, pancreas, endocrine
- intestine, intestinal
  - carbohydrate absorption NEC E74.39
    - postoperative K91.2
  - functional NEC K59.9
    - postoperative K91.89
  - psychogenic F45.8
  - vascular K55.9
    - chronic K55.1
    - specified NEC K55.8
- intraoperative (intraprocedural) *see* Complications, intraoperative
- involuntary emotional expression (IEED) F48.2
- iris H21.9
  - adhesions *see* Adhesions, iris
  - atrophy *see* Atrophy, iris
  - chamber angle recession *see* Recession, chamber angle
  - cyst *see* Cyst, iris
  - degeneration *see* Degeneration, iris
  - in diseases classified elsewhere H22
  - iridodialysis *see* Iridodialysis
  - iridoschisis *see* Iridoschisis
  - miotic pupillary cyst *see* Cyst, pupillary
  - pupillary
    - abnormality *see* Abnormality, pupillary
    - membrane *see* Membrane, pupillary
  - specified type NEC H21.89
  - vascular NEC H21.1X-
- iron metabolism E83.10
  - specified NEC E83.19
- isovaleric acidemia E71.110

Disorder (of) - *continued*
- jaw, developmental M27.0
  - temporomandibular *see also* Anomaly, dentofacial, temporomandibular joint M26.60-
- joint M25.9
  - derangement *see* Derangement, joint
  - effusion *see* Effusion, joint
  - fistula *see* Fistula, joint
  - hemarthrosis *see* Hemarthrosis
  - instability *see* Instability, joint
  - osteophyte *see* Osteophyte
  - pain *see* Pain, joint
  - psychogenic F45.8
  - specified type NEC M25.80
    - ankle M25.87-
    - elbow M25.82-
    - foot joint M25.87-
    - hand joint M25.84-
    - hip M25.85-
    - knee M25.86-
    - shoulder M25.81-
    - wrist M25.83-
  - stiffness *see* Stiffness, joint
- ketone metabolism E71.32
- kidney N28.9
  - functional (tubular) N25.9
  - in
    - schistosomiasis B65.9 *[N29]*
  - tubular function N25.9
    - specified NEC N25.89
- lacrimal system H04.9
  - changes H04.69
    - fistula *see* Fistula, lacrimal
  - gland H04.19
    - atrophy *see* Atrophy, lacrimal gland
    - cyst *see* Cyst, lacrimal, gland
    - dacryops *see* Dacryops
    - dislocation *see* Dislocation, lacrimal gland
    - dry eye syndrome *see* Syndrome, dry eye
    - infection *see* Dacryoadenitis
  - granuloma *see* Granuloma, lacrimal
  - inflammation *see* Inflammation, lacrimal
  - obstruction *see* Obstruction, lacrimal
  - specified NEC H04.89
- lactation NEC O92.79
- language (developmental) F80.9
  - expressive F80.1
  - mixed receptive and expressive F80.2
  - receptive F80.2
- late luteal phase dysphoric N94.89
- learning (specific) F81.9
  - acalculia R48.8
  - alexia R48.0
  - mathematics F81.2
  - reading F81.0
  - specified
    - with impairment in
      - mathematics F81.2
      - reading F81.0
      - written expression F81.81
  - specified NEC F81.89
  - spelling F81.81
  - written expression F81.81
- lens H27.9
  - aphakia *see* Aphakia
  - cataract *see* Cataract
  - dislocation *see* Dislocation, lens
  - specified type NEC H27.8
- ligament M24.20
  - ankle M24.27-
  - attachment, spine *see* Enthesopathy, spinal
  - elbow M24.22-
  - foot joint M24.27-
  - hand joint M24.24-

Disorder (of) - *continued*
|hip M24.25-
|knee *see* Derangement, knee, specified NEC
|shoulder M24.21-
|specified site NEC M24.29
|vertebra M24.28
|wrist M24.23-
|ligamentous attachments *see also*
   Enthesopathy
|spine *see* Enthesopathy, spinal
|lipid
|metabolism, congenital E78.9
|storage E75.6
|specified NEC E75.5
|lipoprotein
|deficiency (familial) E78.6
|metabolism E78.9
|specified NEC E78.89
|liver K76.9
|malarial B54 [*K77*]
|low back *see also* Dorsopathy, specified NEC
|lumbosacral
|plexus G54.1
|root (nerve) NEC G54.4
|lung, interstitial, drug-induced J70.4
|acute J70.2
|chronic J70.3
|dabbing (related) U07.0
|e-cigarette (related) U07.0
|electronic cigarette (related) U07.0
|vaping (associated) (device) (product)
   (related) (use) U07.0
|lymphoproliferative, post-transplant (PTLD)
   D47.Z1
|lysine and hydroxylysine metabolism E72.3
|major neurocognitive *see* Dementia, in (due
   to)
|male
|erectile (organic) *see also* Dysfunction,
   sexual, male, erectile N52.9
|nonorganic F52.21
|hypoactive sexual desire F52.0
|orgasmic F52.32
|manic F30.9
|organic F06.33
|mast cell activation *see* Activation, mast cell
|mastoid *see also* Disorder, ear, middle
|postprocedural *see* Complications, ear,
   procedure
|meninges, specified type NEC G96.198
|meniscus *see* Derangement, knee, meniscus
|menopausal N95.9
|specified NEC N95.8
|menstrual N92.6
|psychogenic F45.8
|specified NEC N92.5
|mental (or behavioral) (nonpsychotic) F99
|due to (secondary to)
|amphetamine
|due to drug abuse *see* Abuse, drug,
   stimulant
|due to drug dependence *see*
   Dependence, drug, stimulant
|brain disease, damage and dysfunction
   F09
|caffeine use
|due to drug abuse *see* Abuse, drug,
   stimulant
|due to drug dependence *see*
   Dependence, drug, stimulant
|cannabis use
|due to drug abuse *see* Abuse, drug,
   cannabis
|due to drug dependence *see*
   Dependence, drug, cannabis

Disorder (of) - *continued*
|general medical condition F09
|sedative or hypnotic use
|due to drug abuse *see* Abuse, drug,
   sedative
|due to drug dependence *see*
   Dependence, drug, sedative
|tobacco (nicotine) use *see* Dependence,
   drug, nicotine
|following organic brain damage F07.9
|frontal lobe syndrome F07.0
|personality change F07.0
|postconcussional syndrome F07.81
|specified NEC F07.89
|infancy, childhood or adolescence F98.9
|neurotic *see* Neurosis
|organic or symptomatic F09
|presenile, psychotic F03
|problem NEC
|psychoneurotic *see* Neurosis
|psychotic *see* Psychosis
|puerperal F53.0
|senile, psychotic NEC F03
|metabolic, amino acid, transitory, newborn
   P74.8
|metabolism NOS E88.9
|amino-acid E72.9
|aromatic E70.9
|albinism *see* Albinism
|histidine E70.40
|histidinemia E70.41
|other specified E70.49
|hyperphenylalaninemia E70.1
|classical phenylketonuria E70.0
|other specified E70.89
|tryptophan E70.5
|tyrosine E70.20
|hypertyrosinemia E70.21
|other specified E70.29
|branched chain E71.2
|3-methylglutaconic aciduria E71.111
|hyperleucine-isoleucinemia E71.19
|hypervalinemia E71.19
|isovaleric acidemia E71.110
|maple syrup urine disease E71.0
|methylmalonic acidemia E71.120
|organic aciduria NEC E71.118
|other specified E71.19
|propionate NEC E71.128
|propionic acidemia E71.121
|glycine E72.50
|d-glycericacidemia E72.59
|hyperhydroxyprolinemia E72.59
|hyperoxaluria R82.992
|primary E72.53
|hyperprolinemia E72.59
|non-ketotic hyperglycinemia E72.51
|other specified E72.59
|sarcosinemia E72.59
|trimethylaminuria E72.52
|hydroxylysine E72.3
|lysine E72.3
|ornithine E72.4
|other specified E72.89
|beta-amino acid E72.89
|gamma-glutamyl cycle E72.89
|straight-chain E72.89
|sulfur-bearing E72.10
|homocystinuria E72.11
|methylenetetrahydrofolate reductase
   deficiency E72.12
|other specified E72.19
|bile acid and cholesterol metabolism E78.70
|bilirubin E80.7
|specified NEC E80.6

Disorder (of) - *continued*
|calcium E83.50
|hypercalcemia E83.52
|hypocalcemia E83.51
|other specified E83.59
|carbohydrate E74.9
|specified NEC E74.89
|cholesterol and bile acid metabolism E78.70
|congenital E88.9
|copper E83.00
|Wilson's disease E83.01
|specified type NEC E83.09
|cystinuria E72.01
|fructose E74.10
|galactose E74.20
|glucosaminoglycan E76.9
|mucopolysaccharidosis *see*
   Mucopolysaccharidosis
|specified NEC E76.8
|glutamine E72.89
|glycine E72.50
|glycogen storage (hepatorenal) E74.09
|glycoprotein E77.9
|specified NEC E77.8
|glycosaminoglycan E76.9
|specified NEC E76.8
|in labor and delivery O75.89
|iron E83.10
|isoleucine E71.19
|leucine E71.19
|lipoid E78.9
|lipoprotein E78.9
|specified NEC E78.89
|magnesium E83.40
|hypermagnesemia E83.41
|hypomagnesemia E83.42
|other specified E83.49
|mineral E83.9
|specified NEC E83.89
|mitochondrial E88.40
|MELAS syndrome E88.41
|MERRF syndrome (myoclonic epilepsy
   associated with ragged-red fibers)
   E88.42
|other specified E88.49
|ornithine E72.4
|phosphatases E83.30
|phosphorus E83.30
|acid phosphatase deficiency E83.39
|hypophosphatasia E83.39
|hypophosphatemia E83.39
|familial E83.31
|other specified E83.39
|pseudovitamin D deficiency E83.32
|plasma protein NEC E88.09
|porphyrin *see* Porphyria
|postprocedural E89.89
|specified NEC E89.89
|purine E79.9
|specified NEC E79.8
|pyrimidine E79.9
|specified NEC E79.8
|pyruvate E74.4
|serine E72.89
|sodium E87.8
|specified NEC E88.89
|threonine E72.89
|valine E71.19
|zinc E83.2
|methylmalonic acidemia E71.120
|micturition NEC *see also* Difficulty,
   micturition R39.198
|feeling of incomplete emptying R39.14
|hesitancy R39.11
|poor stream R39.12

Disorder (of) - _continued_
  |psychogenic F45.8
  |split stream R39.13
  |straining R39.16
  |urgency R39.15
  |mild neurocognitive G31.84
  |mitochondrial metabolism E88.40
  |mitral (valve) _see_ Endocarditis, mitral
  |mixed
    |anxiety and depressive F41.8
    |of scholastic skills (developmental) F81.89
    |receptive expressive language F80.2
  |mood F39
    |bipolar _see_ Disorder, bipolar
    |depressive _see_ Disorder, depressive
    |due to (secondary to)
      |alcohol F10.94
      |amphetamine F15.94
        |in
          |abuse F15.14
          |dependence F15.24
      |anxiolytic F13.94
        |in
          |abuse F13.14
          |dependence F13.24
      |cocaine F14.94
        |in
          |abuse F14.14
          |dependence F14.24
      |general medical condition F06.30
      |hallucinogen F16.94
        |in
          |abuse F16.14
          |dependence F16.24
      |hypnotic F13.94
        |in
          |abuse F13.14
          |dependence F13.24
      |inhalant F18.94
        |in
          |abuse F18.14
          |dependence F18.24
      |opioid F11.94
        |in
          |abuse F11.14
          |dependence F11.24
      |phencyclidine (PCP) F16.94
        |in
          |abuse F16.14
          |dependence F16.24
      |physiological condition F06.30
        |with
          |depressive features F06.31
          |major depressive-like episode F06.32
          |manic features F06.33
          |mixed features F06.34
      |psychoactive substance NEC F19.94
        |in
          |abuse F19.14
          |dependence F19.24
      |sedative F13.94
        |in
          |abuse F13.14
          |dependence F13.24
      |volatile solvents F18.94
        |in
          |abuse F18.14
          |dependence F18.24
  |manic episode F30.9
    |with psychotic symptoms F30.2
    |in remission (full) F30.4
      |partial F30.3
    |specified type NEC F30.8
    |without psychotic symptoms F30.10
      |mild F30.11

Disorder (of) - _continued_
      |moderate F30.12
      |severe F30.13
    |organic F06.30
      |right hemisphere F07.89
    |persistent F34.9
      |cyclothymia F34.0
      |dysthymia F34.1
      |specified type NEC F34.89
    |recurrent F39
    |right hemisphere organic F07.89
  |movement G25.9
    |drug-induced G25.70
      |akathisia G25.71
      |specified NEC G25.79
    |hysterical F44.4
    |in diseases classified elsewhere _see_ category G26
    |periodic limb G47.61
      |sleep related G47.61
    |specified NEC G25.89
    |sleep related NEC G47.69
    |stereotyped F98.4
    |treatment-induced G25.9
  |multiple personality F44.81
  |muscle M62.9
    |attachment, spine _see_ Enthesopathy, spinal
    |in trichinellosis _see_ Trichinellosis, with muscle disorder
    |psychogenic F45.8
    |specified type NEC M62.89
    |tone, newborn P94.9
      |specified NEC P94.8
  |muscular
    |attachments _see also_ Enthesopathy
      |spine _see_ Enthesopathy, spinal
    |urethra N36.44
  |musculoskeletal system, soft tissue _see_ Disorder, soft tissue
    |postprocedural M96.89
    |psychogenic F45.8
  |myoneural G70.9
    |due to lead G70.1
    |specified NEC G70.89
    |toxic G70.1
  |myotonic NEC G71.19
  |nail, in diseases classified elsewhere L62
  |neck region NEC _see_ Dorsopathy, specified NEC
  |neonatal onset multisystemic inflammatory (NOMID) M04.2
  |nerve G58.9
    |abducent NEC _see_ Strabismus, paralytic, sixth nerve
    |accessory G52.8
    |acoustic _see_ subcategory H93.3
    |auditory _see_ subcategory H93.3
    |auriculotemporal G50.8
    |axillary G54.0
    |cerebral _see_ Disorder, nerve, cranial
    |cranial G52.9
      |eighth _see_ subcategory H93.3
      |eleventh G52.8
      |fifth G50.9
      |first G52.0
      |fourth NEC _see_ Strabismus, paralytic, fourth nerve
      |multiple G52.7
      |ninth G52.1
      |second NEC _see_ Disorder, nerve, optic
      |seventh NEC G51.8
      |sixth NEC _see_ Strabismus, paralytic, sixth nerve
      |specified NEC G52.8
      |tenth G52.2

Disorder (of) - _continued_
      |third NEC _see_ Strabismus, paralytic, third nerve
      |twelfth G52.3
    |entrapment _see_ Neuropathy, entrapment
    |facial G51.9
      |specified NEC G51.8
    |femoral _see_ Lesion, nerve, femoral
    |glossopharyngeal NEC G52.1
    |hypoglossal G52.3
    |intercostal G58.0
    |lateral
      |cutaneous of thigh _see_ Mononeuropathy, lower limb, meralgia paresthetica
      |popliteal _see_ Lesion, nerve, popliteal
    |lower limb _see_ Mononeuropathy, lower limb
    |medial popliteal _see_ Lesion, nerve, popliteal, medial
    |median NEC _see_ Lesion, nerve, median
    |multiple G58.7
    |oculomotor NEC _see_ Strabismus, paralytic, third nerve
    |olfactory G52.0
    |optic NEC H47.09-
      |hemorrhage into sheath _see_ Hemorrhage, optic nerve
      |ischemic H47.01-
    |peroneal _see_ Lesion, nerve, popliteal
    |phrenic G58.8
    |plantar _see_ Lesion, nerve, plantar
    |pneumogastric G52.2
    |posterior tibial _see_ Syndrome, tarsal tunnel
    |radial _see_ Lesion, nerve, radial
    |recurrent laryngeal G52.2
    |root G54.9
      |cervical G54.2
      |lumbosacral G54.1
      |specified NEC G54.8
      |thoracic G54.3
    |sciatic NEC _see_ Lesion, nerve, sciatic
    |specified NEC G58.8
      |lower limb _see_ Mononeuropathy, lower limb, specified NEC
      |upper limb _see_ Mononeuropathy, upper limb, specified NEC
    |sympathetic G90.9
    |tibial _see_ Lesion, nerve, popliteal, medial
    |trigeminal G50.9
      |specified NEC G50.8
    |trochlear NEC _see_ Strabismus, paralytic, fourth nerve
    |ulnar _see_ Lesion, nerve, ulnar
    |upper limb _see_ Mononeuropathy, upper limb
    |vagus G52.2
  |nervous system G98.8
    |autonomic (peripheral) G90.9
      |specified NEC G90.8
    |central G96.9
      |specified NEC G96.89
    |parasympathetic G90.9
    |specified NEC G98.8
    |sympathetic G90.9
    |vegetative G90.9
  |neurocognitive R41.9
    |major
      |with
        |aggressive behavior F01.51
        |combative behavior F01.51
        |violent behavior F01.51
      |due to vascular disease, with behavioral disturbance F01.51
      |in (due to) (other diseases classified elsewhere) _see also_ Dementia, in (due to) F02.80
        |with

Disorder (of) - *continued*
> |aggressive behavior F02.81
> |combative behavior F02.81
> |violent behavior F02.81
> |without behavioral disturbance F01.50
> |mild G31.84
|neurodevelopmental F89
> |specified NEC F88
|neurohypophysis NEC E23.3
|neurological NEC R29.818
|neuromuscular G70.9
> |hereditary NEC G71.9
> |specified NEC G70.89
> |toxic G70.1
|neurotic F48.9
> |specified NEC F48.8
|neutrophil, polymorphonuclear D71
|nicotine use *see* Dependence, drug, nicotine
|nightmare F51.5
|non-rapid eye movement sleep arousal
> |sleep terror type F51.4
> |sleepwalking type F51.3
|nose J34.9
> |specified NEC J34.89
|obsessive-compulsive F42.9
> |and related disorder due to a known physiological condition F06.8
|odontogenesis NOS K00.9
|opioid use
> |with
>> |opioid-induced psychotic disorder F11.959
>>> |with
>>>> |delusions F11.950
>>>> |hallucinations F11.951
> |due to drug abuse *see* Abuse, drug, opioid
> |due to drug dependence *see* Dependence, drug, opioid
> |mild F11.10
>> |in remission (early) (sustained) F11.11
>> |with
>>> |opioid-induced
>>>> |anxiety disorder F11.188
>>>> |depressive disorder F11.14
>>>> |sexual dysfunction F11.181
>>> |opioid intoxication
>>>> |with perceptual disturbances F11.122
>>>> |delirium F11.121
>>>> |without perceptual disturbances F11.129
> |moderate or severe F11.20
>> |in remission (early) (sustained) F11.21
>> |with
>>> |opioid-induced
>>>> |anxiety disorder F11.288
>>>> |anxiety disorder F11.988
>>>> |depressive disorder F11.24
>>>> |depressive disorder F11.94
>>>> |sexual dysfunction F11.281
>>>> |sexual dysfunction F11.981
>>> |opioid intoxication
>>>> |with perceptual disturbances F11.222
>>>> |delirium F11.221
>>>> |without perceptual disturbances F11.229
|oppositional defiant F91.3
|optic
> |chiasm H47.49
>> |due to
>>> |inflammatory disorder H47.41
>>> |neoplasm H47.42
>>> |vascular disorder H47.43
> |disc H47.39-
>> |coloboma *see* Coloboma, optic disc
>> |drusen *see* Drusen, optic disc

Disorder (of) - *continued*
> |pseudopapilledema *see* Pseudopapilledema
> |radiations *see* Disorder, visual, pathway
> |tracts *see* Disorder, visual, pathway |orbit H05.9
> |cyst *see* Cyst, orbit
> |deformity *see* Deformity, orbit
> |edema *see* Edema, orbit
> |enophthalmos *see* Enophthalmos
> |exophthalmos *see* Exophthalmos
> |hemorrhage *see* Hemorrhage, orbit
> |inflammation *see* Inflammation, orbit
> |myopathy *see* Myopathy, extraocular muscles
> |retained foreign body *see* Foreign body, orbit, old
> |specified type NEC H05.89
|organic
> |anxiety F06.4
> |catatonic F06.1
> |delusional F06.2
> |dissociative F06.8
> |emotionally labile (asthenic) F06.8
> |mood (affective) F06.30
> |schizophrenia-like F06.2
|orgasmic (female) F52.31
> |male F52.32
|ornithine metabolism E72.4
|overanxious F41.1
> |of childhood F93.8
|pain
> |with related psychological factors F45.42
> |exclusively related to psychological factors F45.41
> |genito-pelvic penetration disorder F52.6
|pancreatic internal secretion E16.9
> |specified NEC E16.8
|panic F41.0
> |with agoraphobia F40.01
|papulosquamous L44.9
> |in diseases classified elsewhere L45
> |specified NEC L44.8
|paraphilic F65.9
> |specified NEC F65.89
|paranoid F22
> |induced F24
> |shared F24
|parathyroid (gland) E21.5
> |specified NEC E21.4
|parietoalveolar NEC J84.09
|paroxysmal, mixed R56.9
|patella M22.9-
> |chondromalacia *see* Chondromalacia, patella
> |derangement NEC M22.3X-
> |recurrent
>> |dislocation *see* Dislocation, patella, recurrent
>> |subluxation *see* Dislocation, patella, recurrent, incomplete
> |specified NEC M22.8X-
|patellofemoral M22.2X
|pedophilic F65.4
|pentose phosphate pathway with anemia D55.1
|perception, due to hallucinogens F16.983
> |in
>> |abuse F16.183
>> |dependence F16.283
|peripheral nervous system NEC G64
|peroxisomal E71.50
> |biogenesis
>> |neonatal adrenoleukodystrophy E71.511
>> |specified disorder NEC E71.518

Disorder (of) - *continued*
> |Zellweger syndrome E71.510
> |rhizomelic chondrodysplasia punctata E71.540
> |specified form NEC E71.548
>> |group 1 E71.518
>> |group 2 E71.53
>> |group 3 E71.542
> |X-linked adrenoleukodystrophy E71.529
>> |adolescent E71.521
>> |adrenomyeloneuropathy E71.522
>> |childhood E71.520
>> |specified form NEC E71.528
> |Zellweger-like syndrome E71.541
|persistent
> |(somatoform) pain F45.41
> |affective (mood) F34.9
|personality *see also* Personality F60.9
> |affective F34.0
> |aggressive F60.3
> |amoral F60.2
> |anankastic F60.5
> |antisocial F60.2
> |anxious F60.6
> |asocial F60.2
> |asthenic F60.7
> |avoidant F60.6
> |borderline F60.3
> |change (secondary) due to general medical condition F07.0
> |compulsive F60.5
> |cyclothymic F34.0
> |dependent (passive) F60.7
> |depressive F34.1
> |dissocial F60.2
> |emotional instability F60.3
> |expansive paranoid F60.0
> |explosive F60.3
> |following organic brain damage F07.9
> |histrionic F60.4
> |hyperthymic F34.0
> |hypothymic F34.1
> |hysterical F60.4
> |immature F60.89
> |inadequate F60.7
> |labile F60.3
> |mixed (nonspecific) F60.89
> |moral deficiency F60.2
> |narcissistic F60.81
> |negativistic F60.89
> |obsessional F60.5
> |obsessive (-compulsive) F60.5
> |organic F07.9
> |overconscientious F60.5
> |paranoid F60.0
> |passive (-dependent) F60.7
> |passive-aggressive F60.89
> |pathological NEC F60.9
> |pseudosocial F60.2
> |psychopathic F60.2
> |schizoid F60.1
> |schizotypal F21
> |self-defeating F60.7
> |specified NEC F60.89
> |type A F60.5
> |unstable (emotional) F60.3
|pervasive, developmental F84.9
|phencyclidine use
> |mild F16.10
>> |in remission (early) (sustained) F16.11
>> |with
>>> |phencyclidine-induced
>>>> |anxiety disorder F16.180
>>>> |bipolar and related disorder F16.14
>>>> |depressive disorder F16.14

Disorder (of) - continued

|psychotic disorder F16.159
|phencyclidine intoxication F16.129
|phencyclidine intoxication delirium F16.121
|moderate or severe F16.20
|in remission (early) (sustained) F16.21
|with
|phencyclidine-induced
|anxiety disorder F16.280
|bipolar and related disorder F16.24
|depressive disorder F16.24
|psychotic disorder F16.259
|phencyclidine intoxication F16.229
|phencyclidine intoxication delirium F16.221
|phobic anxiety, childhood F40.8
|phosphate-losing tubular N25.0
|pigmentation L81.9
|choroid, congenital Q14.3
|diminished melanin formation L81.6
|iron L81.8
|specified NEC L81.8
|pinna (noninfective) H61.10-
|deformity, acquired H61.11-
|hematoma H61.12-
|perichondritis see Perichondritis, ear
|specified type NEC H61.19-
|pituitary gland E23.7
|iatrogenic (postprocedural) E89.3
|specified NEC E23.6
|platelets D69.1
|plexus G54.9
|specified NEC G54.8
|polymorphonuclear neutrophils D71
|porphyrin metabolism see Porphyria
|postconcussional F07.81
|posthallucinogen perception F16.983
|in
|abuse F16.183
|dependence F16.283
|postmenopausal N95.9
|specified NEC N95.8
|postprocedural (postoperative) see Complications, postprocedural
|post-transplant lymphoproliferative D47.Z1
|post-traumatic stress (PTSD) F43.10
|acute F43.11
|chronic F43.12
|premenstrual dysphoric (PMDD) F32.81
|prepuce N47.8
|propionic acidemia E71.121
|prostate N42.9
|specified NEC N42.89
|psychogenic NOS see also condition F45.9
|anxiety F41.8
|appetite F50.9
|asthenic F48.8
|cardiovascular (system) F45.8
|compulsive F42.8
|cutaneous F54
|depressive F32.9
|digestive (system) F45.8
|dysmenorrheic F45.8
|dyspneic F45.8
|endocrine (system) F54
|eye NEC F45.8
|feeding see Disorder, eating
|functional NEC F45.8
|gastric F45.8
|gastrointestinal (system) F45.8
|genitourinary (system) F45.8
|heart (function) (rhythm) F45.8
|hyperventilatory F45.8

Disorder (of) - continued

|hypochondriacal see Disorder, hypochondriacal
|intestinal F45.8
|joint F45.8
|learning F81.9
|limb F45.8
|lymphatic (system) F45.8
|menstrual F45.8
|micturition F45.8
|monoplegic NEC F44.4
|motor F44.4
|muscle F45.8
|musculoskeletal F45.8
|neurocirculatory F45.8
|obsessive F42.8
|occupational F48.8
|organ or part of body NEC F45.8
|paralytic NEC F44.4
|phobic F40.9
|physical NEC F45.8
|rectal F45.8
|respiratory (system) F45.8
|rheumatic F45.8
|sexual (function) F52.9
|skin (allergic) (eczematous) F54
|sleep F51.9
|specified part of body NEC F45.8
|stomach F45.8
|psychological F99
|associated with
|disease classified elsewhere F54
|sexual
|development F66
|relationship F66
|uncertainty about gender identity F64.9
|psychomotor NEC F44.4
|hysterical F44.4
|psychoneurotic see also Neurosis
|mixed NEC F48.8
|psychophysiologic see Disorder, somatoform
|psychosexual F65.9
|development F66
|identity of childhood F64.2
|psychosomatic NOS see Disorder, somatoform
|multiple F45.0
|undifferentiated F45.1
|psychotic see Psychosis
|transient (acute) F23
|puberty E30.9
|specified NEC E30.8
|pulmonary (valve) see Endocarditis, pulmonary
|purine metabolism E79.9
|pyrimidine metabolism E79.9
|pyruvate metabolism E74.4
|reactive attachment (childhood) F94.1
|reading R48.0
|developmental (specific) F81.0
|receptive language F80.2
|receptor, hormonal, peripheral see also Syndrome, androgen insensitivity E34.50
|recurrent brief depressive F33.8
|reflex R29.2
|refraction H52.7
|aniseikonia H52.32
|anisometropia H52.31
|astigmatism see Astigmatism
|hypermetropia see Hypermetropia
|myopia see Myopia
|presbyopia H52.4
|specified NEC H52.6
|relationship F68.8
|due to sexual orientation F66

Disorder (of) - continued

|REM sleep behavior G47.52
|renal function, impaired (tubular) N25.9
|resonance R49.9
|specified NEC R49.8
|respiratory function, impaired see also Failure, respiration
|postprocedural see Complication, postoperative, respiratory system
|psychogenic F45.8
|retina H35.9
|angioid streaks H35.33
|changes in vascular appearance H35.01-
|degeneration see Degeneration, retina
|dystrophy (hereditary) see Dystrophy, retina
|edema H35.81
|hemorrhage see Hemorrhage, retina
|ischemia H35.82
|macular degeneration see Degeneration, macula
|microaneurysms H35.04-
|microvascular abnormality NEC H35.09
|neovascularization see Neovascularization, retina
|retinopathy see Retinopathy
|separation of layers H35.70
|central serous chorioretinopathy H35.71-
|pigment epithelium detachment (serous) H35.72-
|hemorrhagic H35.73-
|specified type NEC H35.89
|telangiectasis see Telangiectasis, retina
|vasculitis see Vasculitis, retina
|retroperitoneal K68.9
|right hemisphere organic affective F07.89
|rumination (infant or child) F98.21
|sacrum, sacrococcygeal NEC M53.3
|schizoaffective F25.9
|bipolar type F25.0
|depressive type F25.1
|manic type F25.0
|mixed type F25.0
|specified NEC F25.8
|schizoid of childhood F84.5
|schizophrenia spectrum and other psychotic disorder F29
|specified NEC F28
|schizophreniform F20.81
|brief F23
|schizotypal (personality) F21
|secretion, thyrocalcitonin E07.0
|sedative, hypnotic, or anxiolytic use
|mild F13.10
|in remission (early) (sustained) F13.11
|with
|sedative, hypnotic, or anxiolytic-induced
|anxiety disorder F13.180
|bipolar and related disorder F13.14
|depressive disorder F13.14
|psychotic disorder F13.159
|sexual dysfunction F13.181
|sedative, hypnotic, or anxiolytic intoxication F13.129
|sedative, hypnotic, or anxiolytic intoxication delirium F13.121
|moderate or severe F13.20
|in remission (early) (sustained) F13.21
|with
|sedative, hypnotic, or anxiolytic-induced
|anxiety disorder F13.280
|bipolar and related disorder F13.24
|depressive disorder F13.24
|major neurocognitive disorder F13.27

Disorder (of) - *continued*
|spine *see also* Dorsopathy
  |ligamentous or muscular attachments,
      peripheral *see* Enthesopathy, spinal
  |specified NEC *see* Dorsopathy, specified
      NEC
|stereotyped, habit or movement F98.4
|stimulant use (other) (unspecified)
  |mild F15.10
    |in remission (early) (sustained) F15.11
  |moderate or severe F15.20
    |in remission (early) (sustained) F15.21
|stomach (functional) *see* Disorder, gastric
|stress F43.9
  |acute F43.0
  |post-traumatic F43.10
    |acute F43.11
    |chronic F43.12
|substance use (other) (unknown)
  |mild F19.10
    |with substance-induced
      |anxiety disorder F19.180
      |bipolar and related disorder F19.14
      |depressive disorder F19.14
      |major neurocognitive disorder F19.17
      |mild neurocognitive disorder F19.188
      |obsessive-compulsive and related
          disorder F19.188
      |sexual dysfunction F19.181
      |substance intoxication F19.129
      |substance intoxication delirium F19.121
  |moderate or severe F19.20
    |in remission (early) (sustained) F19.21
    |with substance-induced
      |anxiety disorder F19.280
      |bipolar and related disorder F19.24
      |depressive disorder F19.24
      |major neurocognitive disorder F19.27
      |mild neurocognitive disorder F19.288
      |obsessive-compulsive and related
          disorder F19.288
      |sexual dysfunction F19.281
      |substance intoxication F19.229
      |substance intoxication delirium F19.221
|sulfur-bearing amino-acid metabolism E72.10
|sweat gland (eccrine) L74.9
  |apocrine L75.9
    |specified NEC L75.8
  |specified NEC L74.8
|synovium M67.90
  |acromioclavicular M67.91-
  |ankle M67.97-
  |elbow M67.92-
  |foot M67.97-
  |forearm M67.93-
  |hand M67.94-
  |hip M67.95-
  |knee M67.96-
  |multiple sites M67.99
  |rupture *see* Rupture, synovium
  |shoulder M67.91-
  |specified type NEC M67.80
    |acromioclavicular M67.81-
    |ankle M67.87-
    |elbow M67.82-
    |foot M67.87-
    |hand M67.84-
    |hip M67.85-
    |knee M67.86-
    |multiple sites M67.89
    |wrist M67.83-
  |synovitis *see* Synovitis
  |upper arm M67.92-
  |wrist M67.93-
|temperature regulation, newborn P81.9

Disorder (of) - *continued*
  |specified NEC P81.8
|temporomandibular joint M26.60-
|tendon M67.90
  |acromioclavicular M67.91-
  |ankle M67.97-
  |contracture *see* Contracture, tendon
  |elbow M67.92-
  |foot M67.97-
  |forearm M67.93-
  |hand M67.94-
  |hip M67.95-
  |knee M67.96-
  |multiple sites M67.99
  |rupture *see* Rupture, tendon
  |shoulder M67.91-
  |specified type NEC M67.80
    |acromioclavicular M67.81-
    |ankle M67.87-
    |elbow M67.82-
    |foot M67.87-
    |hand M67.84-
    |hip M67.85-
    |knee M67.86-
    |multiple sites M67.89
    |trunk M67.88
    |wrist M67.83-
  |synovitis *see* Synovitis
  |tendinitis *see* Tendinitis
  |tenosynovitis *see* Tenosynovitis
  |trunk M67.98
  |upper arm M67.92-
  |wrist M67.93-
|thoracic root (nerve) NEC G54.3
|thyrocalcitonin hypersecretion E07.0
|thyroid (gland) E07.9
  |function NEC, neonatal, transitory P72.2
  |iodine-deficiency related E01.8
  |specified NEC E07.89
|tic *see* Tic
|tobacco use
  |chewing tobacco (mild) (moderate) (severe)
    |in remission (early) (sustained) F17.221
  |cigarettes (mild) (moderate) (severe)
    |in remission (early) (sustained) F17.211
  |mild Z72.00
    |in remission (early) (sustained) F17.201
  |moderate F17.200
    |in remission (early) (sustained) F17.201
  |severe F17.200
    |in remission (early) (sustained) F17.201
  |specified product NEC (mild) (moderate)
      (severe)
    |in remission (early) (sustained) F17.291
|tooth K08.9
  |development K00.9
|transvestic F65.1
|voyeuristic F65.3
    |specified NEC K00.8
  |eruption K00.6
|Tourette's F95.2
|trance and possession F44.89
|trauma and stressor-related F43.9
  |other specified F43.8
|tricuspid (valve) *see* Endocarditis, tricuspid
|tryptophan metabolism E70.5
|tubular, phosphate-losing N25.0
|tubulo-interstitial (in)
  |brucellosis A23.9 *[N16]*
  |cystinosis E72.04
  |diphtheria A36.84
  |glycogen storage disease E74.00 *[N16]*
  |leukemia NEC C95.9 *[N16]*
  |lymphoma NEC C85.9 *[N16]*
  |mixed cryoglobulinemia D89.1 *[N16]*

Disorder (of) - *continued*
  |multiple myeloma C90.0 *[N16]*
  |Salmonella infection A02.25
  |sarcoidosis D86.84
  |sepsis A41.9 *[N16]*
    |streptococcal A40.9 *[N16]*
  |systemic lupus erythematosus M32.15
  |toxoplasmosis B58.83
  |transplant rejection T86.91 *[N16]*
  |Wilson's disease E83.01 *[N16]*
|tubulo-renal function, impaired N25.9
  |specified NEC N25.89
|tympanic membrane H73.9-
  |atrophy *see* Atrophy, tympanic membrane
  |infection *see* Myringitis
  |perforation *see* Perforation, tympanum
  |specified NEC H73.89-
|unsocialized aggressive F91.1
|urea cycle metabolism E72.20
  |argininemia E72.21
  |argininosuccinic aciduria E72.22
  |citrullinemia E72.23
  |ornithine transcarbamylase deficiency E72.4
  |other specified E72.29
|ureter (in) N28.9
  |schistosomiasis B65.0 *[N29]*
  |tuberculosis A18.11
|urethra N36.9
  |specified NEC N36.8
|urinary system N39.9
  |specified NEC N39.8
|valve, heart
  |aortic *see* Endocarditis, aortic
  |mitral *see* Endocarditis, mitral
  |pulmonary *see* Endocarditis, pulmonary
  |rheumatic
    |aortic *see* Endocarditis, aortic, rheumatic
    |mitral *see* Endocarditis, mitral
    |pulmonary *see* Endocarditis, pulmonary,
        rheumatic
    |tricuspid *see* Endocarditis, tricuspid
  |tricuspid *see* Endocarditis, tricuspid
|vestibular function H81.9-
  |specified NEC *see* subcategory H81.8
  |in diseases classified elsewhere H82.-
|vertigo *see* Vertigo
|vision, binocular H53.30
  |abnormal retinal correspondence H53.31
  |diplopia H53.2
  |fusion with defective stereopsis H53.32
  |simultaneous perception H53.33
  |suppression H53.34
|visual
  |cortex
    |blindness H47.619
      |left brain H47.612
      |right brain H47.611
    |due to
      |inflammatory disorder H47.629
        |left brain H47.622
        |right brain H47.621
      |neoplasm H47.639
        |left brain H47.632
        |right brain H47.631
      |vascular disorder H47.649
        |left brain H47.642
        |right brain H47.641
  |pathway H47.9
    |due to
      |inflammatory disorder H47.51-
      |neoplasm H47.52-
      |vascular disorder H47.53-
    |optic chiasm *see* Disorder, optic, chiasm
|vitreous body H43.9
  |crystalline deposits *see* Deposit, crystalline

Disorder (of) - *continued*

|degeneration *see* Degeneration, vitreous
|hemorrhage *see* Hemorrhage, vitreous
|opacities *see* Opacity, vitreous
|prolapse *see* Prolapse, vitreous
|specified type NEC H43.89
|voice R49.9
|specified type NEC R49.8
|volatile solvent use
|due to drug abuse *see* Abuse, drug, inhalant
|due to drug dependence *see* Dependence, drug, inhalant
|white blood cells D72.9
|specified NEC D72.89
|withdrawing, child or adolescent F40.10

Disorientation R41.0

Displacement, displaced

|acquired traumatic of bone, cartilage, joint, tendon NEC *see* Dislocation
|adrenal gland (congenital) Q89.1
|appendix, retrocecal (congenital) Q43.8
|auricle (congenital) Q17.4
|bladder (acquired) N32.89
|congenital Q64.19
|brachial plexus (congenital) Q07.8
|brain stem, caudal (congenital) Q04.8
|canaliculus (lacrimalis), congenital Q10.6
|cardia through esophageal hiatus (congenital) Q40.1
|cerebellum, caudal (congenital) Q04.8
|cervix *see* Malposition, uterus
|colon (congenital) Q43.3
|device, implant or graft *see also* Complications, by site and type, mechanical T85.628
|arterial graft NEC *see* Complication, cardiovascular device, mechanical, vascular
|breast (implant) T85.42
|catheter NEC T85.628
|dialysis (renal) T82.42
|intraperitoneal T85.621
|infusion NEC T82.524
|spinal (epidural) (subdural) T85.620
|urinary
|cystostomy T83.020
|Hopkins T83.028
|ileostomy T83.028
|indwelling T83.021
|nephrostomy T83.022
|specified NEC T83.028
|urostomy T83.028
|electronic (electrode) (pulse generator) (stimulator) *see* Complication, electronic stimulator
|fixation, internal (orthopedic) NEC *see* Complication, fixation device, mechanical
|gastrointestinal *see* Complications, prosthetic device, mechanical, gastrointestinal device
|genital NEC T83.428
|intrauterine contraceptive device (string) T83.32
|penile prosthesis (cylinder) (implanted) (pump) (reservoir) T83.420
|testicular prosthesis T83.421
|heart NEC *see* Complication, cardiovascular device, mechanical
|joint prosthesis *see* Complications, joint prosthesis, mechanical
|ocular *see* Complications, prosthetic device, mechanical, ocular device
|orthopedic NEC *see* Complication, orthopedic, device or graft, mechanical
|specified NEC T85.628

Displacement, displaced - *continued*

|urinary NEC T83.128
|graft T83.22
|sphincter, implanted T83.121
|stent (ileal conduit) (nephroureteral) T83.123
|ureteral indwelling T83.122
|vascular NEC *see* Complication, cardiovascular device, mechanical
|ventricular intracranial shunt T85.02
|electronic stimulator
|bone T84.320
|cardiac *see* Complications, cardiac device, electronic
|nervous system *see* Complication, prosthetic device, mechanical, electronic nervous system stimulator
|urinary *see* Complications, electronic stimulator, urinary
|esophageal mucosa into cardia of stomach, congenital Q39.8
|esophagus (acquired) K22.89
|congenital Q39.8
|eyeball (acquired) (lateral) (old) *see* Displacement, globe
|congenital Q15.8
|current *see* Avulsion, eye
|fallopian tube (acquired) N83.4-
|congenital Q50.6
|opening (congenital) Q50.6
|gallbladder (congenital) Q44.1
|gastric mucosa (congenital) Q40.2
|globe (acquired) (old) (lateral) H05.21-
|current *see* Avulsion, eye
|heart (congenital) Q24.8
|acquired I51.89
|hymen (upward) (congenital) Q52.4
|intervertebral disc NEC
|with myelopathy *see* Disorder, disc, with, myelopathy
|cervical, cervicothoracic (with) M50.20
|myelopathy *see* Disorder, disc, cervical, with myelopathy
|neuritis, radiculitis or radiculopathy *see* Disorder, disc, cervical, with neuritis
|due to trauma *see* Dislocation, vertebra
|lumbar region M51.26
|with
|myelopathy M51.06
|neuritis, radiculitis, radiculopathy or sciatica M51.16
|lumbosacral region M51.27
|with
|neuritis, radiculitis, radiculopathy or sciatica M51.17
|sacrococcygeal region M53.3
|thoracic region M51.24
|with
|myelopathy M51.04
|neuritis, radiculitis, radiculopathy M51.14
|thoracolumbar region M51.25
|with
|myelopathy M51.05
|neuritis, radiculitis, radiculopathy M51.15
|intrauterine device (string) T83.32
|kidney (acquired) N28.83
|congenital Q63.2
|lachrymal, lacrimal apparatus or duct (congenital) Q10.6
|lens, congenital Q12.1
|macula (congenital) Q14.1
|Meckel's diverticulum Q43.0

Displacement, displaced - *continued*

|malignant *see* Table of Neoplasms, small intestine, malignant
|nail (congenital) Q84.6
|acquired L60.8
|opening of Wharton's duct in mouth Q38.4
|organ or site, congenital NEC *see* Malposition, congenital
|ovary (acquired) N83.4-
|congenital Q50.39
|free in peritoneal cavity (congenital) Q50.39
|into hernial sac N83.4-
|oviduct (acquired) N83.4-
|congenital Q50.6
|parathyroid (gland) E21.4
|parotid gland (congenital) Q38.4
|punctum lacrimale (congenital) Q10.6
|sacro-iliac (joint) (congenital) Q74.2
|current injury S33.2
|old *see* subcategory M53.2
|salivary gland (any) (congenital) Q38.4
|spleen (congenital) Q89.09
|stomach, congenital Q40.2
|sublingual duct Q38.4
|tongue (downward) (congenital) Q38.3
|tooth, teeth, fully erupted M26.30
|horizontal M26.33
|vertical M26.34
|trachea (congenital) Q32.1
|ureter or ureteric opening or orifice (congenital) Q62.62
|uterine opening of oviducts or fallopian tubes Q50.6
|uterus, uterine *see* Malposition, uterus
|ventricular septum Q21.0
|with rudimentary ventricle Q20.4

Disproportion

|between native and reconstructed breast N65.1
|fiber-type G71.20
|congenital G71.29

Disruptio uteri *see* Rupture, uterus

Disruption (of)

|ciliary body NEC H21.89
|closure of
|cornea T81.31
|craniotomy T81.32
|fascia (muscular) (superficial) T81.32
|internal organ or tissue T81.32
|laceration (external) (internal) T81.33
|ligament T81.32
|mucosa T81.31
|muscle or muscle flap T81.32
|ribs or rib cage T81.32
|skin and subcutaneous tissue (full-thickness) (superficial) T81.31
|skull T81.32
|sternum (sternotomy) T81.32
|tendon T81.32
|traumatic laceration (external) (internal) T81.33
|family Z63.8
|due to
|absence of family member due to military deployment Z63.31
|absence of family member NEC Z63.32
|alcoholism and drug addiction in family Z63.72
|bereavement Z63.4
|death (assumed) or disappearance of family member Z63.4
|divorce or separation Z63.5
|drug addiction in family Z63.72
|return of family member from military deployment (current or past conflict) Z63.71

Disruption (of) - *continued*
  |stressful life events NEC Z63.79
  |iris NEC H21.89
  |ligament(s) *see also* Sprain
    |knee
      |current injury *see* Dislocation, knee
      |old (chronic) *see* Derangement, knee, ligament, instability, chronic
      |spontaneous NEC *see* Derangement, knee, disruption ligament
  |ossicular chain *see* Discontinuity, ossicles, ear
  |pelvic ring (stable) S32.810
    |unstable S32.811
  |wound T81.30
    |episiotomy O90.1
    |operation T81.31
      |cesarean O90.0
      |external operation wound (superficial) T81.31
      |internal operation wound (deep) T81.32
    |perineal (obstetric) O90.1
    |traumatic injury repair T81.33
    |traumatic injury wound repair T81.33

Dissatisfaction with
  |employment Z56.9
  |school environment Z55.4

Dissecting *see* condition

Dissection
  |aorta I71.00
    |abdominal I71.02
    |thoracic I71.01
    |thoracoabdominal I71.03
  |artery I77.70
    |basilar (trunk) I77.75
    |carotid I77.71
    |cerebral (nonruptured) I67.0
      |ruptured *see* Hemorrhage, intracranial, subarachnoid
    |coronary I25.42
    |extremity
      |lower I77.77
      |upper I77.76
    |iliac I77.72
    |precerebral
      |congenital (nonruptured) Q28.1
      |specified site NEC I77.75
    |renal I77.73
    |specified NEC I77.79
    |vertebral I77.74
  |precerebral artery, congential (nonruptured) Q28.1
  |Heartland A93.8
  |traumatic *see* Wound, open, by site
  |vascular I99.8
  |wound *see* Wound, open

Disseminated *see* condition

Dissociation
  |auriculoventricular or atrioventricular (AV) (any degree) (isorhythmic) I45.89
    |with heart block I44.2
  |interference I45.89

Dissociative reaction, state F44.9

Dissolution, vertebra *see* Osteoporosis

Distension, distention
  |abdomen R14.0
  |bladder N32.89
  |cecum K63.89
  |colon K63.89
  |gallbladder K82.8
  |intestine K63.89
  |kidney N28.89
  |liver K76.89
  |seminal vesicle N50.89
  |stomach K31.89
    |acute K31.0

Distension, distention - *continued*
  |psychogenic F45.8
  |ureter *see* Dilatation, ureter
  |uterus N85.8

Distoma hepaticum infestation B66.3

Distomiasis B66.9
  |bile passages B66.3
  |hemic B65.9
  |hepatic B66.3
    |due to Clonorchis sinensis B66.1
  |intestinal B66.5
  |liver B66.3
    |due to Clonorchis sinensis B66.1
  |lung B66.4
  |pulmonary B66.4

Distomolar (fourth molar) K00.1

Disto-Occlusion (Division I) (Division II) M26.212

Distortion(s) (congenital)
  |adrenal (gland) Q89.1
  |arm NEC Q68.8
  |bile duct or passage Q44.5
  |bladder Q64.79
  |brain Q04.9
  |cervix (uteri) Q51.9
  |chest (wall) Q67.8
    |bones Q76.8
  |clavicle Q74.0
  |clitoris Q52.6
  |coccyx Q76.49
  |common duct Q44.5
  |coronary Q24.5
  |cystic duct Q44.5
  |ear (auricle) (external) Q17.3
    |inner Q16.5
    |middle Q16.4
      |ossicles Q16.3
  |endocrine NEC Q89.2
  |eustachian tube Q17.8
  |eye (adnexa) Q15.8
  |face bone(s) NEC Q75.8
  |fallopian tube Q50.6
  |femur NEC Q68.8
  |fibula NEC Q68.8
  |finger(s) Q68.1
  |foot Q66.9
  |genitalia, genital organ(s)
    |female Q52.8
      |external Q52.79
      |internal NEC Q52.8
  |gyri Q04.8
  |hand bone(s) Q68.1
  |heart (auricle) (ventricle) Q24.8
    |valve (cusp) Q24.8
  |hepatic duct Q44.5
  |humerus NEC Q68.8
  |hymen Q52.4
  |intrafamilial communications Z63.8
  |jaw NEC M26.89
  |labium (majus) (minus) Q52.79
  |leg NEC Q68.8
  |lens Q12.8
  |liver Q44.7
  |lumbar spine Q76.49
    |with disproportion O33.8
      |causing obstructed labor O65.0
  |lumbosacral (joint) (region) Q76.49
    |kyphosis *see* Kyphosis, congenital
    |lordosis *see* Lordosis, congenital
  |nerve Q07.8
  |nose Q30.8
  |organ
    |of Corti Q16.5
    |or site not listed *see* Anomaly, by site
  |ossicles, ear Q16.3

Distortion(s) (congenital) - *continued*
  |oviduct Q50.6
  |pancreas Q45.3
  |parathyroid (gland) Q89.2
  |pituitary (gland) Q89.2
  |radius NEC Q68.8
  |sacroiliac joint Q74.2
  |sacrum Q76.49
  |scapula Q74.0
  |shoulder girdle Q74.0
  |skull bone(s) NEC Q75.8
    |with
      |anencephalus Q00.0
      |encephalocele *see* Encephalocele
      |hydrocephalus Q03.9
        |with spina bifida *see* Spina bifida, with hydrocephalus
      |microcephaly Q02
  |spinal cord Q06.8
  |spine Q76.49
    |kyphosis *see* Kyphosis, congenital
    |lordosis *see* Lordosis, congenital
  |spleen Q89.09
  |sternum NEC Q76.7
  |thorax (wall) Q67.8
    |bony Q76.8
  |thymus (gland) Q89.2
  |thyroid (gland) Q89.2
  |tibia NEC Q68.8
  |toe(s) Q66.9
  |tongue Q38.3
  |trachea (cartilage) Q32.1
  |ulna NEC Q68.8
  |ureter Q62.8
  |urethra Q64.79
    |causing obstruction Q64.39
  |uterus Q51.9
  †vagina Q52.4
  |vertebra Q76.49
    |kyphosis *see* Kyphosis, congenital
    |lordosis *see* Lordosis, congenital
  |visual *see also* Disturbance, vision
    |shape and size H53.15
  |vulva Q52.79
  |wrist (bones) (joint) Q68.8

Distress
  |abdomen *see* Pain, abdominal
  |acute respiratory R06.03
    |syndrome (adult) (child) J80
  |epigastric R10.13
  |fetal P84
    |complicating pregnancy *see* Stress, fetal
  |gastrointestinal (functional) K30
    |psychogenic F45.8
  |intestinal (functional) NOS K59.9
    |psychogenic F45.8
  |maternal, during labor and delivery O75.0
  |relationship, with spouse or intimate partner Z63.0
  |respiratory (adult) (child) R06.03
    |newborn P22.9
      |specified NEC P22.8
    |orthopnea R06.01
    |psychogenic F45.8
    |shortness of breath R06.02
    |specified type NEC R06.09

Distribution vessel, atypical Q27.9
  |coronary artery Q24.5
  |precerebral Q28.1

Districhiasis L68.8

Disturbance(s) *see also* Disease
  |absorption K90.9
    |calcium E58
    |carbohydrate K90.49
    |fat K90.49

Disturbance(s) - _continued_
 |pancreatic K90.3
 |protein K90.49
 |starch K90.49
 |vitamin _see_ Deficiency, vitamin
|acid-base equilibrium E87.8
 |mixed E87.4
|activity and attention (with hyperkinesis) _see_
  Disorder, attention-deficit hyperactivity
|amino acid transport E72.00
|assimilation, food K90.9
|auditory nerve, except deafness _see_
  subcategory H93.3
|behavior _see_ Disorder, conduct
|blood clotting (mechanism) _see also_ Defect,
  coagulation D68.9
|cerebral
 |nerve _see_ Disorder, nerve, cranial
 |status, newborn P91.9
  |specified NEC P91.88
|circulatory I99.9
|conduct _see also_ Disorder, conduct F91.9
 |adjustment reaction _see_ Disorder,
   adjustment
 |compulsive F63.9
 |disruptive F91.9
 |hyperkinetic _see_ Disorder, attention-deficit
   hyperactivity
 |socialized F91.2
 |specified NEC F91.8
 |unsocialized F91.1
|coordination R27.8
|cranial nerve _see_ Disorder, nerve, cranial
|deep sensibility _see_ Disturbance, sensation
|digestive K30
 |psychogenic F45.8
|electrolyte _see also_ Imbalance, electrolyte
 |newborn, transitory P74.49
  |hyperammonemia P74.6
  |hyperchloremia P74.421
  |hyperchloremic metabolic acidosis
    P74.421
  |hypochloremia P74.422
  |potassium balance
   |hyperkalemia P74.31
   |hypokalemia P74.32
  |sodium balance
   |hypernatremia P74.21
   |hyponatremia P74.22
  |specified type NEC P74.49
|emotions specific to childhood and
  adolescence F93.9
 |with
  |anxiety and fearfulness NEC F93.8
  |elective mutism F94.0
  |oppositional disorder F91.3
  |sensitivity (withdrawal) F40.10
  |shyness F40.10
  |social withdrawal F40.10
 |involving relationship problems F93.8
 |mixed F93.8
 |specified NEC F93.8
|endocrine (gland) E34.9
 |neonatal, transitory P72.9
  |specified NEC P72.8
|equilibrium R42
|fructose metabolism E74.10
|gait _see_ Gait
 |hysterical F44.4
 |psychogenic F44.4
|gastrointestinal (functional) K30
 |psychogenic F45.8
|habit, child F98.9
|hearing, except deafness and tinnitus _see_
  Abnormal, auditory perception

Disturbance(s) - _continued_
|heart, functional (conditions in I44-I50)
 |due to presence of (cardiac) prosthesis
   I97.19-
 |postoperative I97.89
  |cardiac surgery (_see also_ Infarct,
    myocardium, associated with
    revascularization procedure) I97.19-
|hormones E34.9
|innervation uterus (parasympathetic)
  (sympathetic) N85.8
|keratinization NEC
 |gingiva K05.10
  |nonplaque induced K05.11
  |plaque induced K05.10
 |lip K13.0
 |oral (mucosa) (soft tissue) K13.29
 |tongue K13.29
|learning (specific) _see_ Disorder, learning
|memory _see_ Amnesia
 |mild, following organic brain damage F06.8
|mental F99
 |associated with diseases classified
   elsewhere F54
|metabolism E88.9
 |with
  |abortion _see_ Abortion, by type with other
  specified complication
   |ectopic pregnancy O08.5
   |molar pregnancy O08.5
 |amino-acid E72.9
  |aromatic E70.9
  |branched-chain E71.2
  |straight-chain E72.89
  |sulfur-bearing E72.10
 |ammonia E72.20
 |arginine E72.21
 |argininosuccinic acid E72.22
 |carbohydrate E74.9
 |cholesterol E78.9
 |citrulline E72.23
 |cystathionine E72.19
 |general E88.9
 |glutamine E72.89
 |histidine E70.40
 |homocystine E72.19
 |hydroxylysine E72.3
 |in labor or delivery O75.89
 |iron E83.10
 |lipoid E78.9
 |lysine E72.3
 |methionine E72.19
 |neonatal, transitory P74.9
  |calcium and magnesium P71.9
   |specified type NEC P71.8
  |carbohydrate metabolism P70.9
   |specified type NEC P70.8
  |specified NEC P74.8
 |ornithine E72.4
 |phosphate E83.39
 |sodium NEC E87.8
 |threonine E72.89
 |tryptophan E70.5
 |tyrosine E70.20
 |urea cycle E72.20
|motor R29.2
|nervous, functional R45.0
|neuromuscular mechanism (eye), due to
  syphilis A52.15
|nutritional E63.9
 |nail L60.3
|ocular motion H51.9
 |psychogenic F45.8
|oculogyric H51.8
 |psychogenic F45.8

Disturbance(s) - _continued_
|oculomotor H51.9
 |psychogenic F45.8
|olfactory nerve R43.1
|optic nerve NEC _see_ Disorder, nerve, optic
|oral epithelium, including tongue NEC
  K13.29
|perceptual due to
 |alcohol withdrawal F10.232
 |amphetamine intoxication F15.922
  |in
   |abuse F15.122
   |dependence F15.222
 |anxiolytic withdrawal F13.232
 |cannabis intoxication (acute) F12.922
  |in
   |abuse F12.122
   |dependence F12.222
 |cocaine intoxication (acute) F14.922
  |in
   |abuse F14.122
   |dependence F14.222
 |hypnotic withdrawal F13.232
 |opioid intoxication (acute) F11.922
  |in
   |abuse F11.122
   |dependence F11.222
 |phencyclidine intoxication (acute) F16.122
 |sedative withdrawal F13.232
|personality (pattern) (trait) _see also_ Disorder,
  personality F60.9
 |following organic brain damage F07.9
|polyglandular E31.9
 |specified NEC E31.8
|potassium balance, newborn
 |hyperkalemia P74.31
 |hypokalemia P74.32
|psychogenic F45.9
|psychomotor F44.4
|psychophysical visual H53.16
|pupillary _see_ Anomaly, pupil, function
|reflex R29.2
|rhythm, heart I49.9
|salivary secretion K11.7
|sensation (cold) (heat) (localization) (tactile
  discrimination) (texture) (vibratory) NEC
  R20.9
 |hysterical F44.6
 |skin R20.9
  |anesthesia R20.0
  |hyperesthesia R20.3
  |hypoesthesia R20.1
  |paresthesia R20.2
  |specified type NEC R20.8
 |smell R43.9
  |and taste (mixed) R43.8
  |anosmia R43.0
  |parosmia R43.1
  |specified NEC R43.8
 |taste R43.9
  |and smell (mixed) R43.8
  |parageusia R43.2
  |specified NEC R43.8
|sensory _see_ Disturbance, sensation
|situational (transient) _see also_ Disorder,
  adjustment
 |acute F43.0
|sleep G47.9
 |nonorganic origin F51.9
|smell _see_ Disturbance, sensation, smell
|sociopathic F60.2
|sodium balance, newborn
 |hypernatremia P74.21
 |hyponatremia P74.22
|speech R47.9

Disturbance(s) - *continued*
- developmental F80.9
- specified NEC R47.89
- stomach (functional) K31.9
- sympathetic (nerve) G90.9
- taste *see* Disturbance, sensation, taste
- temperature
  - regulation, newborn P81.9
    - specified NEC P81.8
  - sense R20.8
    - hysterical F44.6
- tooth
  - eruption K00.6
  - formation K00.4
  - structure, hereditary NEC K00.5
- touch *see* Disturbance, sensation
- vascular I99.9
  - arteriosclerotic *see* Arteriosclerosis
- vasomotor I73.9
- vasospastic I73.9
- vision, visual H53.9
  - following
    - cerebral infarction I69.398
    - cerebrovascular disease I69.998
      - specified NEC I69.898
    - intracerebral hemorrhage I69.198
    - nontraumatic intracranial hemorrhage NEC I69.298
    - specified disease NEC I69.898
    - subarachnoid hemorrhage I69.098
  - psychophysical H53.16
  - specified NEC H53.8
  - subjective H53.10
    - day blindness H53.11
    - discomfort H53.14-
    - distortions of shape and size H53.15
    - loss
      - sudden H53.13-
      - transient H53.12-
    - specified type NEC H53.19
- voice R49.9
  - psychogenic F44.4
  - specified NEC R49.8
Diuresis R35.89
Diver's palsy, paralysis or squeeze T70.3
Diverticulitis (acute) K57.92
- bladder *see* Cystitis
- ileum *see* Diverticulitis, intestine, small
- intestine K57.92
  - with
    - abscess, perforation K57.80
      - with bleeding K57.81
    - bleeding K57.93
  - congenital Q43.8
  - large K57.32
    - with
      - abscess, perforation K57.20
        - with bleeding K57.21
      - bleeding K57.33
      - small intestine K57.52
        - with
          - abscess, perforation K57.40
            - with bleeding K57.41
          - bleeding K57.53
  - small K57.12
    - with
      - abscess, perforation K57.00
        - with bleeding K57.01
      - bleeding K57.13
      - large intestine K57.52
        - with
          - abscess, perforation K57.40
            - with bleeding K57.41
          - bleeding K57.53

Diverticulosis K57.90
- with bleeding K57.91
- large intestine K57.30
  - with
    - bleeding K57.31
    - small intestine K57.50
      - with bleeding K57.51
- small intestine K57.10
  - with
    - bleeding K57.11
    - large intestine K57.50
      - with bleeding K57.51
Diverticulum, diverticula (multiple) K57.90
- appendix (noninflammatory) K38.2
- bladder (sphincter) N32.3
  - congenital Q64.6
- bronchus (congenital) Q32.4
  - acquired J98.09
- calyx, calyceal (kidney) N28.89
- cardia (stomach) K31.4
- cecum *see* Diverticulosis, intestine, large
  - congenital Q43.8
- colon *see* Diverticulosis, intestine, large
  - congenital Q43.8
- duodenum *see* Diverticulosis, intestine, small
  - congenital Q43.8
- epiphrenic (esophagus) K22.5
- esophagus (congenital) Q39.6
  - acquired (epiphrenic) (pulsion) (traction) K22.5
- eustachian tube *see* Disorder, eustachian tube, specified NEC
- fallopian tube N83.8
- gastric K31.4
- heart (congenital) Q24.8
- ileum *see* Diverticulosis, intestine, small
- jejunum *see* Diverticulosis, intestine, small
- kidney (pelvis) (calyces) N28.89
  - with calculus *see* Calculus, kidney
- Meckel's (displaced) (hypertrophic) Q43.0
  - malignant *see* Table of Neoplasms, small intestine, malignant
- midthoracic K22.5
- organ or site, congenital NEC *see* Distortion
- pericardium (congenital) (cyst) Q24.8
  - acquired I31.8
- pharyngoesophageal (congenital) Q39.6
  - acquired K22.5
- pharynx (congenital) Q38.7
- rectosigmoid *see* Diverticulosis, intestine, large
  - congenital Q43.8
- rectum *see* Diverticulosis, intestine, large
- Rokitansky's K22.5
- seminal vesicle N50.89
- sigmoid *see* Diverticulosis, intestine, large
  - congenital Q43.8
- stomach (acquired) K31.4
  - congenital Q40.2
- trachea (acquired) J39.8
- ureter (acquired) N28.89
  - congenital Q62.8
- ureterovesical orifice N28.89
- urethra (acquired) N36.1
  - congenital Q64.79
- ventricle, left (congenital) Q24.8
- vesical N32.3
  - congenital Q64.6
- Zenker's (esophagus) K22.5
Division
- cervix uteri (acquired) N88.8
- glans penis Q55.69
- labia minora (congenital) Q52.79
- ligament (partial or complete) (current) *see also* Sprain

Division - *continued*
- with open wound *see* Wound, open
- muscle (partial or complete) (current) *see also* Injury, muscle
  - with open wound *see* Wound, open
- nerve (traumatic) *see* Injury, nerve
- spinal cord *see* Injury, spinal cord, by region
- vein I87.8
Divorce, causing family disruption Z63.5
Dix-Hallpike neurolabyrinthitis *see* Neuronitis, vestibular
Dizziness R42
- hysterical F44.89
- psychogenic F45.8
DMAC (disseminated mycobacterium avium intracellulare complex) A31.2
DNR (do not resuscitate) Z66
Doan-Wiseman syndrome (primary splenic neutropenia) *see* Agranulocytosis
Doehle-Heller aortitis A52.02
Dog bite *see* Bite
Dohle body panmyelopathic syndrome D72.0
Dolichocephaly Q67.2
Dolichocolon Q43.8
Dolichostenomelia *see* Syndrome, Marfan's
Donohue's syndrome E34.8
Donor (organ or tissue) Z52.9
- blood (whole) Z52.000
  - autologous Z52.010
  - specified component (lymphocytes) (platelets) NEC Z52.008
    - autologous Z52.018
    - specified donor NEC Z52.098
  - specified donor NEC Z52.090
  - stem cells Z52.001
    - autologous Z52.011
    - specified donor NEC Z52.091
- bone Z52.20
  - autologous Z52.21
  - marrow Z52.3
  - specified type NEC Z52.29
- cornea Z52.5
- egg (Oocyte) Z52.819
  - age 35 and over Z52.812
    - anonymous recipient Z52.812
    - designated recipient Z52.813
  - under age 35 Z52.810
    - anonymous recipient Z52.810
    - designated recipient Z52.811
- kidney Z52.4
- liver Z52.6
- lung Z52.89
- lymphocyte *see* Donor, blood, specified components NEC
- Oocyte *see* Donor, egg
- platelets Z52.008
- potential, examination of Z00.5
- semen Z52.89
- skin Z52.10
  - autologous Z52.11
  - specified type NEC Z52.19
- specified organ or tissue NEC Z52.89
- sperm Z52.89
Donovanosis A58
Dorsalgia M54.9
- psychogenic F45.41
- specified NEC M54.89
Dorsopathy M53.9
- deforming M43.9
  - specified NEC *see* subcategory M43.8
- specified NEC M53.80
  - cervical region M53.82
  - cervicothoracic region M53.83
  - lumbar region M53.86
  - lumbosacral region M53.87

Dorsopathy - *continued*
    |occipito-atlanto-axial region M53.81
    |sacrococcygeal region M53.88
    |thoracic region M53.84
    |thoracolumbar region M53.85

Double
    |albumin E88.09
    |aortic arch Q25.45
    |auditory canal Q17.8
    |auricle (heart) Q20.8
    |bladder Q64.79
    |cervix Q51.820
      |with doubling of uterus (and vagina) Q51.10
        |with obstruction Q51.11
    |inlet ventricle Q20.4
    |kidney with double pelvis (renal) Q63.0
    |meatus urinarius Q64.75
    |monster Q89.4
    |outlet
      |left ventricle Q20.2
      |right ventricle Q20.1
    |pelvis (renal) with double ureter Q62.5
    |tongue Q38.3
    |ureter (one or both sides) Q62.5
      |with double pelvis (renal) Q62.5
    |urethra Q64.74
    |urinary meatus Q64.75
    |uterus Q51.28
      |complete Q51.21
      |partial Q51.22
      |specified NEC Q51.28
      |with
        |doubling of cervix (and vagina) Q51.10
          |with obstruction Q51.11
      |in pregnancy or childbirth O34.59-
        |causing obstructed labor O65.5
    |vagina Q52.10
      |with doubling of uterus (and cervix) Q51.10
        |with obstruction Q51.11
    |vision H53.2
    |vulva Q52.79

Doubled up Z59.01
Douglas' pouch, cul-De-Sac *see* condition
Down syndrome Q90.9
    |meiotic nondisjunction Q90.0
    |mitotic nondisjunction Q90.1
    |mosaicism Q90.1
    |translocation Q90.2
DPD (dihydropyrimidine dehydrogenase deficiency) E88.89
Dracontiasis B72
Dracunculiasis, dracunculosis B72
Dream state, hysterical F44.89
Dreschlera (hawaiiensis) (infection) B43.8
Drepanocytic anemia *see* Disease, sickle-cell
Dresbach's syndrome (elliptocytosis) D58.1
Dressler's syndrome I24.1
Drift, ulnar *see* Deformity, limb, specified type NEC, forearm
Drinking (alcohol)
    |excessive, to excess NEC (without dependence) F10.10
      |habitual (continual) (without remission) F10.20
        |with remission F10.21
Drip, postnasal (chronic) R09.82
    |due to
      |allergic rhinitis *see* Rhinitis, allergic
      |common cold J00
      |gastroesophageal reflux *see* Reflux, gastroesophageal
      |nasopharyngitis *see* Nasopharyngitis
      |other know condition   code to condition
      |sinusitis *see* Sinusitis

Droop
    |facial R29.810
      |cerebrovascular disease I69.992
        |cerebral infarction I69.392
        |intracerebral hemorrhage I69.192
        |nontraumatic intracranial hemorrhage NEC I69.292
        |specified disease NEC I69.892
        |subarachnoid hemorrhage I69.092
Drop (in)
    |attack NEC R55
    |finger *see* Deformity, finger
    |foot *see* Deformity, limb, foot, drop
    |hematocrit (precipitous) R71.0
    |hemoglobin R71.0
    |toe *see* Deformity, toe, specified NEC
    |wrist *see* Deformity, limb, wrist drop
Dropped heart beats I45.9
Dropsy, dropsical *see also* Hydrops
    |abdomen R18.8
    |brain *see* Hydrocephalus
    |cardiac, heart *see* Failure, heart, congestive
    |gangrenous *see* Gangrene
    |heart *see* Failure, heart, congestive
    |kidney *see* Nephrosis
    |lung *see* Edema, lung
    |newborn due to isoimmunization P56.0
    |pericardium *see* Pericarditis
Drowned, drowning (near) T75.1
Drowsiness R40.0
Drug
    |abuse counseling and surveillance Z71.51
    |addiction *see* Dependence
    |dependence *see* Dependence
    |habit *see* Dependence
    |harmful use *see* Abuse, drug
    |induced fever R50.2
    |overdose *see* Table of Drugs and Chemicals, by drug, poisoning
    |poisoning *see* Table of Drugs and Chemicals, by drug, poisoning
    |resistant organism infection *see also* Resistant, organism, to, drug Z16.30
    |therapy
      |long term (current) (prophylactic) *see* Therapy, drug long-term (current) (prophylactic)
      |short term
    |omit code
    |wrong substance given or taken in error *see* Table of Drugs and Chemicals, by drug, poisoning
Drunkenness (without dependence) F10.129
    |acute in alcoholism F10.229
    |chronic (without remission) F10.20
      |with remission F10.21
    |pathological (without dependence) F10.129
      |with dependence F10.229
    |sleep F51.9
Drusen
    |macula (degenerative) (retina) *see* Degeneration, macula, drusen
    |optic disc H47.32-
Dry, dryness *see also* condition
    |larynx J38.7
    |mouth R68.2
      |due to dehydration E86.0
    |nose J34.89
    |socket (teeth) M27.3
    |throat J39.2
DSAP L56.5
Duane's syndrome H50.81-
Dubin-Johnson disease or syndrome E80.6

Dubois' disease (thymus gland) A50.59 [*E35*]
Dubowitz' syndrome Q87.1
Duchenne-Aran muscular atrophy G12.21
Duchenne-Griesinger disease G71.01
Duchenne's
    |disease or syndrome
      |motor neuron disease G12.22
      |muscular dystrophy G71.01
    |locomotor ataxia (syphilitic) A52.11
    |paralysis
      |birth injury P14.0
      |due to or associated with
        |motor neuron disease G12.22
        |muscular dystrophy G71.01
Ducrey's chancre A57
Duct, ductus *see* condition
Duhring's disease (dermatitis herpetiformis) L13.0
Dullness, cardiac (decreased) (increased) R01.2
Dumb ague *see* Malaria
Dumbness *see* Aphasia
Dumdum fever B55.0
Dumping syndrome (postgastrectomy) K91.1
Duodenitis (nonspecific) (peptic) K29.80
    |with bleeding K29.81
Duodenocholangitis *see* Cholangitis
Duodenum, duodenal *see* condition
Duplay's bursitis or periarthritis M75.0
Duplication, duplex *see also* Accessory
    |alimentary tract Q45.8
    |anus Q43.4
    |appendix (and cecum) Q43.4
    |biliary duct (any) Q44.5
    |bladder Q64.79
    |cecum (and appendix) Q43.4
    |cervix Q51.820
    |chromosome NEC
      |with complex rearrangements NEC Q92.5
      |seen only at prometaphase Q92.8
    |cystic duct Q44.5
    |digestive organs Q45.8
    |esophagus Q39.8
    |frontonasal process Q75.8
    |intestine (large) (small) Q43.4
    |kidney Q63.0
    |liver Q44.7
    |pancreas Q45.3
    |penis Q55.69
    |respiratory organs NEC Q34.8
    |salivary duct Q38.4
    |spinal cord (incomplete) Q06.2
    |stomach Q40.2
Dupré's disease (meningism) R29.1
Dupuytren's contraction or disease M72.0
Durand Nicolas-Favre disease A55
Durotomy (inadvertent) (incidental) G97.41
Duroziez's disease (congenital mitral stenosis) Q23.2
Dutton's relapsing fever (West African) A68.1
Dwarfism E34.3
    |achondroplastic Q77.4
    |congenital E34.3
    |constitutional E34.3
    |hypochondroplastic Q77.4
    |hypophyseal E23.0
    |infantile E34.3
    |Laron-Type E34.3
    |Lorain (-Lévi) type E23.0
    |metatropic Q77.8
    |nephrotic-glycosuric (with hypophosphatemic rickets) E72.09
    |nutritional E45
    |pancreatic K86.89
    |pituitary E23.0
    |renal N25.0
    |thanatophoric Q77.1

Dyke-Young anemia (secondary)
(symptomatic) D59.19
Dysacusis *see* Abnormal, auditory perception
Dysadrenocortism E27.9
|hyperfunction E27.0
Dysarthria R47.1
|following
|cerebral infarction I69.322
|cerebrovascular disease I69.922
|specified disease NEC I69.822
|intracerebral hemorrhage I69.122
|nontraumatic intracranial hemorrhage NEC
I69.222
|subarachnoid hemorrhage I69.022
Dysautonomia (familial) G90.1
Dysbarism T70.3
Dysbasia R26.2
|angiosclerotica intermittens I73.9
|hysterical F44.4
|lordotica (progressiva) G24.1
|nonorganic origin F44.4
|psychogenic F44.4
Dysbetalipoproteinemia (familial) E78.2
Dyscalculia R48.8
|developmental F81.2
Dyschezia K59.00
Dyschondroplasia (with hemangiomata) Q78.4
Dyschromia (skin) L81.9
Dyscollagenosis M35.9
Dyscranio-Pygo-Phalangy Q87.0
Dyscrasia
|blood (with) D75.9
|antepartum hemorrhage *see* Hemorrhage,
antepartum, with coagulation defect
|newborn P61.9
|specified type NEC P61.8
|intrapartum hemorrhage O67.0
|puerperal, postpartum O72.3
|polyglandular, pluriglandular E31.9
Dysendocrinism E34.9
Dysentery, dysenteric (catarrhal) (diarrhea)
(epidemic) (hemorrhagic) (infectious)
(sporadic) (tropical) A09
|abscess, liver A06.4
|amebic *see also* Amebiasis A06.0
|with abscess *see* Abscess, amebic
|acute A06.0
|chronic A06.1
|arthritis *see also* category M01 A09
|bacillary *see also* category M01 A03.9
|bacillary A03.9
|arthritis *see also* category M01 A03.9
|Boyd A03.2
|Flexner A03.1
|Schmitz (-Stutzer) A03.0
|Shiga (-Kruse) A03.0
|Shigella A03.9
|boydii A03.2
|dysenteriae A03.0
|flexneri A03.1
|group A A03.0
|group B A03.1
|group C A03.2
|group D A03.3
|sonnei A03.3
|specified type NEC A03.8
|Sonne A03.3
|specified type NEC A03.8
|balantidial A07.0
|Balantidium coli A07.0
|Boyd's A03.2
|candidal B37.82
|Chilomastix A07.8
|Chinese A03.9
|coccidial A07.3

Dysentery, dysenteric - *continued*
|Dientamoeba (fragilis) A07.8
|Embadomonas A07.8
|Entamoeba, entamebic *see* Dysentery, amebic
|Flexner-Boyd A03.2
|Flexner's A03.1
|Giardia lamblia A07.1
|Hiss-Russell A03.1
|Lamblia A07.1
|leishmanial B55.0
|malarial *see* Malaria
|metazoal B82.0
|monilial B37.82
|protozoal A07.9
|Salmonella A02.0
|schistosomal B65.1
|Schmitz (-Stutzer) A03.0
|Shiga (-Kruse) A03.0
|Shigella NOS *see* Dysentery, bacillary
|Sonne A03.3
|strongyloidiasis B78.0
|trichomonal A07.8
|viral *see also* Enteritis, viral A08.4
Dysequilibrium R42
Dysesthesia R20.8
|hysterical F44.6
Dysfibrinogenemia (congenital) D68.2
Dysfunction
|adrenal E27.9
|hyperfunction E27.0
|autonomic
|due to alcohol G31.2
|somatoform F45.8
|bladder N31.9
|neurogenic NOS *see* Dysfunction, bladder,
neuromuscular
|neuromuscular NOS N31.9
|atonic (motor) (sensory) N31.2
|autonomous N31.2
|flaccid N31.2
|nonreflex N31.2
|reflex N31.1
|specified NEC N31.8
|uninhibited N31.0
|bleeding, uterus N93.8
|cerebral G93.89
|colon K59.9
|psychogenic F45.8
|colostomy K94.03
|cystic duct K82.8
|cystostomy (stoma) *see* Complications,
cystostomy
|ejaculatory N53.19
|anejaculatory orgasm N53.13
|painful N53.12
|premature F52.4
|retarded N53.11
|endocrine NOS E34.9
|endometrium N85.8
|enterostomy K94.13
|erectile *see* Dysfunction, sexual, male, erectile
|feeding, pediatric
|acute R63.31
|chronic R63.32
|gallbladder K82.8
|gastrostomy (stoma) K94.23
|gland, glandular NOS E34.9
|meibomian, of eyelid *see* Dysfunction,
meibomian gland
|heart I51.89
|hemoglobin D75.89
|hepatic K76.89
|hypophysis E23.7
|hypothalamic NEC E23.3

Dysfunction - *continued*
|ileostomy (stoma) K94.13
|jejunostomy (stoma) K94.13
|kidney *see* Disease, renal
|labyrinthine *see* subcategory H83.2
|left ventricular, following sudden emotional
stress I51.81
|liver K76.89
|male *see* Dysfunction, sexual, male
|meibomian gland, of eyelid H02.889
|left H02.886
|lower H02.885
|upper H02.884
|upper and lower eyelids H02.88B
|right H02.883
|lower H02.882
|upper H02.881
|upper and lower eyelids H02.88A
|orgasmic (female) F52.31
|male F52.32
|ovary E28.9
|specified NEC E28.8
|papillary muscle I51.89
|parathyroid E21.4
|physiological NEC R68.89
|psychogenic F59
|pineal gland E34.8
|pituitary (gland) E23.3
|platelets D69.1
|polyglandular E31.9
|specified NEC E31.8
|psychophysiologic F59
|psychosexual F52.9
|with
|dyspareunia F52.6
|premature ejaculation F52.4
|vaginismus F52.5
|pylorus K31.9
|rectum K59.9
|psychogenic F45.8
|reflex (sympathetic) *see* Syndrome, pain,
complex regional I
|segmental *see* Dysfunction, somatic
|senile R54
|sexual (due to) R37
|alcohol F10.981
|amphetamine F15.981
|in
|abuse F15.181
|dependence F15.281
|anxiolytic F13.981
|in
|abuse F13.181
|dependence F13.281
|cocaine F14.981
|in
|abuse F14.181
|dependence F14.281
|excessive sexual drive F52.8
|failure of genital response (male) F52.21
|female F52.22
|female N94.9
|aversion F52.1
|dyspareunia N94.10
|psychogenic F52.6
|frigidity F52.22
|nymphomania F52.8
|orgasmic F52.31
|psychogenic F52.9
|aversion F52.1
|dyspareunia F52.6
|frigidity F52.22
|nymphomania F52.8
|orgasmic F52.31
|vaginismus F52.5

Dysfunction - *continued*
|vaginismus N94.2
|psychogenic F52.5
|hypnotic F13.981
|in
|abuse F13.181
|dependence F13.281
|inhibited orgasm (female) F52.31
|male F52.32
|lack
|of sexual enjoyment F52.1
|or loss of sexual desire F52.0
|male N53.9
|anejaculatory orgasm N53.13
|ejaculatory N53.19
|painful N53.12
|premature F52.4
|retarded N53.11
|erectile N52.9
|drug induced N52.2
|due to
|disease classified elsewhere N52.1
|drug N52.2
|postoperative (postprocedural) N52.39
|following
|cryotherapy N52.37
|interstitial seed therapy N52.36
|prostate ablative therapy N52.37
|prostatectomy N52.34
|radical N52.31
|radiation therapy N52.35
|radical cystectomy N52.32
|ultrasound ablative therapy N52.37
|urethral surgery N52.33
|psychogenic F52.21
|specified cause NEC N52.8
|vasculogenic
|arterial insufficiency N52.01
|with corporo-venous occlusive N52.03
|corporo-venous occlusive N52.02
|with arterial insufficiency N52.03
|impotence *see* Dysfunction, sexual, male, erectile
|psychogenic F52.9
|aversion F52.1
|erectile F52.21
|orgasmic F52.32
|premature ejaculation F52.4
|satyriasis F52.8
|specified type NEC F52.8
|specified type NEC N53.8
|nonorganic F52.9
|specified NEC F52.8
|opioid F11.981
|in
|abuse F11.181
|dependence F11.281
|orgasmic dysfunction (female) F52.31
|male F52.32
|premature ejaculation F52.4
|psychoactive substances NEC F19.981
|in
|abuse F19.181
|dependence F19.281
|psychogenic F52.9
|sedative F13.981
|in
|abuse F13.181
|dependence F13.281
|sexual aversion F52.1
|vaginismus (nonorganic) (psychogenic) F52.5
|sinoatrial node I49.5
|somatic M99.09

Dysfunction - *continued*
|abdomen M99.09
|acromioclavicular M99.07
|cervical region M99.01
|cervicothoracic M99.01
|costochondral M99.08
|costovertebral M99.08
|head region M99.00
|hip M99.05
|lower extremity M99.06
|lumbar region M99.03
|lumbosacral M99.03
|occipitocervical M99.00
|pelvic region M99.05
|pubic M99.05
|rib cage M99.08
|sacral region M99.04
|sacrococcygeal M99.04
|sacroiliac M99.04
|specified NEC M99.09
|sternochondral M99.08
|sternoclavicular M99.07
|thoracic region M99.02
|thoracolumbar M99.02
|upper extremity M99.07
|somatoform autonomic F45.8
|stomach K31.89
|psychogenic F45.8
|suprarenal E27.9
|hyperfunction E27.0
|symbolic R48.9
|specified type NEC R48.8
|temporomandibular (joint) M26.69
|joint-pain syndrome M26.62-
|testicular (endocrine) E29.9
|specified NEC E29.8
|thymus E32.9
|thyroid E07.9
|ureterostomy (stoma) *see* Complications, stoma, urinary tract
|uterus, complicating delivery O62.9
|hypertonic O62.4
|hypotonic O62.2
|primary O62.0
|secondary O62.1
|ventricular I51.9
|with congestive heart failure (*see also* Failure, heart) I50.9
|left, reversible, following sudden emotional stress I51.81
Dysgenesis
|gonadal (due to chromosomal anomaly) Q96.9
|pure Q99.1
|renal Q60.5
|bilateral Q60.4
|unilateral Q60.3
|reticular D72.0
|tidal platelet D69.3
Dysgerminoma
|specified site *see* Neoplasm, malignant, by site
|unspecified site
|female C56.9
|male C62.90
Dysgeusia R43.2
Dysgraphia R27.8
Dyshidrosis, dysidrosis L30.1
Dyskaryotic cervical smear R87.619
Dyskeratosis L85.8
|cervix *see* Dysplasia, cervix
|congenital Q82.8
|uterus NEC N85.8
Dyskinesia G24.9
|biliary (cystic duct or gallbladder) K82.8
|drug induced
|orofacial G24.01

Dyskinesia - *continued*
|esophagus K22.4
|hysterical F44.4
|intestinal K59.89
|nonorganic origin F44.4
|orofacial (idiopathic) G24.4
|drug induced G24.01
|psychogenic F44.4
|subacute, drug induced G24.01
|tardive G24.01
|neuroleptic induced G24.01
|trachea J39.8
|tracheobronchial J98.09
Dyslalia (developmental) F80.0
Dyslexia R48.0
|developmental F81.0
Dyslipidemia E78.5
|depressed HDL cholesterol E78.6
|elevated fasting triglycerides E78.1
Dysmaturity *see also* Light for dates
|pulmonary (newborn) (Wilson-Mikity) P27.0
Dysmenorrhea (essential) (exfoliative) N94.6
|congestive (syndrome) N94.6
|primary N94.4
|psychogenic F45.8
|secondary N94.5
Dysmetabolic syndrome X E88.81
Dysmetria R27.8
Dysmorphism (due to)
|alcohol Q86.0
|exogenous cause NEC Q86.8
|hydantoin Q86.1
|warfarin Q86.2
Dysmorphophobia (nondelusional) F45.22
|delusional F22
Dysnomia R47.01
Dysorexia R63.0
|psychogenic F50.89
Dysostosis
|cleidocranial, cleidocranialis Q74.0
|craniofacial Q75.1
|Fairbank's (idiopathic familial generalized osteophytosis) Q78.9
|mandibulofacial (incomplete) Q75.4
|multiplex E76.01
|oculomandibular Q75.5
Dyspareunia (female) N94.10
|deep N94.12
|male N53.12
|nonorganic F52.6
|psychogenic F52.6
|secondary N94.19
|specified NEC N94.19
|superficial (introital) N94.11
Dyspepsia R10.13
|atonic K30
|functional (allergic) (congenital) (gastrointestinal) (occupational) (reflex) K30
|intestinal K59.89
|nervous F45.8
|neurotic F45.8
|psychogenic F45.8
Dysphagia R13.10
|cervical R13.19
|following
|cerebral infarction I69.391
|cerebrovascular disease I69.991
|specified NEC I69.891
|intracerebral hemorrhage I69.191
|nontraumatic intracranial hemorrhage NEC I69.291
|specified disease NEC I69.891
|subarachnoid hemorrhage I69.091
|functional (hysterical) F45.8

Dystrophy, dystrophia - *continued*
|Duchenne's type G71.01
|due to malnutrition E45
|Erb's G71.02
|Fuchs' H18.51-
|Gower's muscular G71.01
|hair L67.8
|infantile neuraxonal G31.89
|Landouzy-Déjérine G71.02
|Leyden-Mobius G71.09
|muscular G71.00
  |autosomal recessive, childhood type,
    muscular dystrophy resembling Duchenne
    or Becker G71.01
  |benign (Becker type) G71.01
    |scapuloperoneal with early contractures
      [Emery-Dreifuss] G71.09
  |congenital (hereditary) (progressive) (with
    specific morphological abnormalities of
    the muscle fiber) G71.09
    |myotonic G71.11
  |distal G71.09
  |Duchenne type G71.01
  |Emery-Dreifuss G71.09
  |Erb type G71.02
  |facioscapulohumeral G71.02
  |Gower's G71.01
  |hereditary (progressive) G71.09
  |Landouzy-Déjérine type G71.02
  |limb-girdle G71.09
  |myotonic G71.11
  |progressive (hereditary) G71.09
    |Charcot-Marie (-Tooth) type G60.0
  |pseudohypertrophic (infantile) G71.01
  |scapulohumeral G71.02
  |scapuloperoneal G71.09
  |severe (Duchenne type) G71.01
  |specified type NEC G71.09
|myocardium, myocardial *see* Degeneration,
  myocardial
|myotonic, myotonica G71.11
|nail L60.3
  |congenital Q84.6
|nutritional E45
|ocular G71.09
|oculocerebrorenal E72.03
|oculopharyngeal G71.09
|ovarian N83.8
|polyglandular E31.8
|reflex (neuromuscular) (sympathetic) *see*
  Syndrome, pain, complex regional I
|retinal (hereditary) H35.50
  |in
    |lipid storage disorders E75.6 [*H36*]
    |systemic lipidoses E75.6 [*H36*]
  |involving
    |pigment epithelium H35.54
    |sensory area H35.53
  |pigmentary H35.52
  |vitreoretinal H35.51
|Salzmann's nodular *see* Degeneration, cornea,
  nodular
|scapuloperoneal G71.09
|skin NEC L98.8
|sympathetic (reflex) *see* Syndrome, pain,
  complex regional I
  |cervical G90.2
|tapetoretinal H35.54
|thoracic, asphyxiating Q77.2
|unguium L60.3
  |congenital Q84.6
|vitreoretinal H35.51
|vulva N90.4
|yellow (liver) *see* Failure, hepatic

Dysuria R30.0
|psychogenic F45.8

E

Eales' disease H35.06-
Ear *see also* condition
|piercing Z41.3
|tropical NEC B36.9 [*H62.40*]
  in
    |aspergillosis B44.89
    |candidiasis B37.84
    |moniliasis B37.84
|wax (impacted) H61.20
  |left H61.22
    |with right H61.23
  |right H61.21
    |with left H61.23
Earache *see* subcategory H92.0
Early satiety R68.81
Eaton-Lambert syndrome *see* Syndrome,
  Lambert-Eaton
Eberth's disease (typhoid fever) A01.00
Ebola virus disease A98.4
Ebstein's anomaly or syndrome (heart) Q22.5
Eccentro-Osteochondrodysplasia E76.29
Ecchondroma *see* Neoplasm, bone, benign
Ecchondrosis D48.0
Ecchymosis R58
|conjunctiva *see* Hemorrhage, conjunctiva
|eye (traumatic) *see* Contusion, eyeball
|eyelid (traumatic) *see* Contusion, eyelid
|newborn P54.5
|spontaneous R23.3
|traumatic *see* Contusion
Echinococciasis *see* Echinococcus
Echinococcus (infection) B67.90
|granulosus B67.4
  |bone B67.2
  |liver B67.0
  |lung B67.1
  |multiple sites B67.32
  |specified site NEC B67.39
  |thyroid B67.31
|liver NOS B67.8
  |granulosus B67.0
  |multilocularis B67.5
|lung NEC B67.99
  |granulosus B67.1
  |multilocularis B67.69
|multilocularis B67.7
  |liver B67.5
  |multiple sites B67.61
  |specified site NEC B67.69
|specified site NEC B67.99
  |granulosus B67.39
  |multilocularis B67.69
|thyroid NEC B67.99
  |granulosus B67.31
  |multilocularis B67.69 [*E35*]
Echinorhynchiasis B83.8
Echinostomiasis B66.8
Echolalia R48.8
Echovirus, as cause of disease classified
  elsewhere B97.12
Eclampsia, eclamptic (coma) (convulsions)
  (delirium) (with hypertension) NEC O15.9
|complicating
  |labor and delivery O15.1
  |postpartum O15.2
  |pregnancy O15.0-
  |puerperium O15.2
Economic circumstances affecting care Z59.9
Economo's disease A85.8

Ectasia, ectasis
|annuloaortic I35.8
|aorta I77.819
  |with aneurysm *see* Aneurysm, aorta
  |abdominal I77.811
  |thoracic I77.810
  |thoracoabdominal I77.812
|breast *see* Ectasia, mammary duct
|capillary I78.8
|cornea H18.71-
|gastric antral vascular (GAVE) K31.819
  |with hemorrhage K31.811
  |without hemorrhage K31.819
|mammary duct N60.4-
|salivary gland (duct) K11.8
|sclera *see* Sclerectasia
Ecthyma L08.0
|contagiosum B08.02
|gangrenosum L08.0
|infectiosum B08.02
Ectocardia Q24.8
Ectodermal dysplasia (anhidrotic) Q82.4
Ectodermosis erosiva pluriorificialis L51.1
Ectopic, ectopia (congenital)
|abdominal viscera Q45.8
  |due to defect in anterior abdominal wall
    Q79.59
|ACTH syndrome E24.3
|adrenal gland Q89.1
|anus Q43.5
|atrial beats I49.1
|beats I49.49
  |atrial I49.1
  |ventricular I49.3
|bladder Q64.10
|bone and cartilage in lung Q33.5
|brain Q04.8
|breast tissue Q83.8
|cardiac Q24.8
|cerebral Q04.8
|cordis Q24.8
|endometrium *see* Endometriosis
|gastric mucosa Q40.2
|gestation *see* Pregnancy, by site
|heart Q24.8
|hormone secretion NEC E34.2
|kidney (crossed) (pelvis) Q63.2
|lens, lentis Q12.1
|mole *see* Pregnancy, by site
|organ or site NEC *see* Malposition, congenital
|pancreas Q45.3
|pregnancy *see* Pregnancy, ectopic
|pupil *see* Abnormality, pupillary
|renal Q63.2
|sebaceous glands of mouth Q38.6
|spleen Q89.09
|testis Q53.00
  |bilateral Q53.02
  |unilateral Q53.01
|thyroid Q89.2
|tissue in lung Q33.5
|ureter Q62.63
|ventricular beats I49.3
|vesicae Q64.10
Ectromelia Q73.8
|lower limb *see* Defect, reduction, limb, lower,
  specified type NEC
|upper limb *see* Defect, reduction, limb, upper,
  specified type NEC
Ectropion H02.109
|cervix N86
  |with cervicitis N72
|congenital Q10.1
|eyelid H02.109
  |cicatricial H02.119

Ectropion - *continued*
|left H02.116
||lower H02.115
||upper H02.114
|right H02.113
||lower H02.112
||upper H02.111
|congenital Q10.1
|left H02.106
||lower H02.105
||upper H02.104
|mechanical H02.129
||left H02.126
|||lower H02.125
|||upper H02.124
||right H02.123
|||lower H02.122
|||upper H02.121
|right H02.103
||lower H02.102
||upper H02.101
|paralytic H02.159
||left H02.156
|||lower H02.155
|||upper H02.154
||right H02.153
|||lower H02.152
|||upper H02.151
|senile H02.139
||left H02.136
|||lower H02.135
|||upper H02.134
||right H02.133
|||lower H02.132
|||upper H02.131
|spastic H02.149
||left H02.146
|||lower H02.145
|||upper H02.144
||right H02.143
|||lower H02.142
|||upper H02.141
|iris H21.89
|lip (acquired) K13.0
||congenital Q38.0
|urethra N36.8
|uvea H21.89
Eczema (acute) (chronic) (erythematous) (fissum) (rubrum) (squamous) *see also* Dermatitis L30.9
|contact *see* Dermatitis, contact
|dyshidrotic L30.1
|external ear *see* Otitis, externa, acute, eczematoid
|flexural L20.82
|herpeticum B00.0
|hypertrophicum L28.0
|hypostatic *see* Varix, leg, with, inflammation
|impetiginous L01.1
|infantile (due to any substance) L20.83
||intertriginous L21.1
||seborrheic L21.1
|intertriginous NEC L30.4
||infantile L21.1
|intrinsic (allergic) L20.84
|lichenified NEC L28.0
|marginatum (hebrae) B35.6
|pustular L30.3
|stasis I87.2
||with varicose veins *see* Varix, leg, with, inflammation
|vaccination, vaccinatum T88.1
|varicose *see* Varix, leg, with, inflammation
Eczematid L30.2
Eddowes (-Spurway) syndrome Q78.0

Edema, edematous (infectious) (pitting) (toxic) R60.9
|with nephritis *see* Nephrosis
|allergic T78.3
|amputation stump (surgical) (sequelae (late effect)) T87.89
|angioneurotic (allergic) (any site) (with urticaria) T78.3
||hereditary D84.1
|angiospastic I73.9
|Berlin's (traumatic) S05.8X-
|brain (cytotoxic) (vasogenic) G93.6
||due to birth injury P11.0
||newborn (anoxia or hypoxia) P52.4
|||birth injury P11.0
||traumatic *see* Injury, intracranial, cerebral edema
|cardiac *see* Failure, heart, congestive
|cardiovascular *see* Failure, heart, congestive
|cerebral *see* Edema, brain
|cerebrospinal *see* Edema, brain
|cervix (uteri) (acute) N88.8
||puerperal, postpartum O90.89
|chronic hereditary Q82.0
|circumscribed, acute T78.3
||hereditary D84.1
|conjunctiva H11.42-
|cornea H18.2-
||idiopathic H18.22-
||secondary H18.23-
|||due to contact lens H18.21-
|due to
||lymphatic obstruction I89.0
||salt retention E87.0
|epiglottis *see* Edema, glottis
|essential, acute T78.3
||hereditary D84.1
|extremities, lower *see* Edema, legs
|eyelid NEC H02.849
||left H02.846
|||lower H02.845
|||upper H02.844
||right H02.843
|||lower H02.842
|||upper H02.841
|familial, hereditary Q82.0
|famine *see* Malnutrition, severe
|generalized R60.1
|glottis, glottic, glottidis (obstructive) (passive) J38.4
||allergic T78.3
|||hereditary D84.1
|heart *see* Failure, heart, congestive
|heat T67.7
|hereditary Q82.0
|inanition *see* Malnutrition, severe
|intracranial G93.6
|iris H21.89
|joint *see* Effusion, joint
|larynx *see* Edema, glottis
|legs R60.0
||due to venous obstruction I87.1
||hereditary Q82.0
|localized R60.0
||due to venous obstruction I87.1
|lower limbs *see* Edema, legs
|lung J81.1
||with heart condition or failure *see* Failure, ventricular, left
||acute J81.0
||chemical (acute) J68.1
|||chronic J68.1
||chronic J81.1
|||due to

Edema, edematous - *continued*
||chemicals, gases, fumes or vapors (inhalation) J68.1
||external agent J70.9
|||specified NEC J70.8
||radiation J70.1
|due to
||chemicals, fumes or vapors (inhalation) J68.1
||external agent J70.9
|||specified NEC J70.8
||high altitude T70.29
||near drowning T75.1
||radiation J70.0
|meaning failure, left ventricle I50.1
|lymphatic I89.0
||due to mastectomy I97.2
|macula H35.81
||cystoid, following cataract surgery *see* Complications, postprocedural, following cataract surgery
||diabetic *see* Diabetes, by type, with, retinopathy, with macular edema
|malignant *see* Gangrene, gas
|Milroy's Q82.0
|nasopharynx J39.2
|newborn P83.30
||hydrops fetalis *see* Hydrops, fetalis
||specified NEC P83.39
|nutritional *see also* Malnutrition, severe
||with dyspigmentation, skin and hair E40
|optic disc or nerve *see* Papilledema
|orbit H05.22-
|pancreas K86.89
|papilla, optic *see* Papilledema
|penis N48.89
|periodic T78.3
||hereditary D84.1
|pharynx J39.2
|pulmonary *see* Edema, lung
|Quincke's T78.3
||hereditary D84.1
|renal *see* Nephrosis
|retina H35.81
||diabetic *see* Diabetes, by type, with, retinopathy, with macular edema
|salt E87.0
|scrotum N50.89
|seminal vesicle N50.89
|spermatic cord N50.89
|spinal (cord) (vascular) (nontraumatic) G95.19
|starvation *see* Malnutrition, severe
|stasis *see* Hypertension, venous, (chronic)
|subglottic *see* Edema, glottis
|supraglottic *see* Edema, glottis
|testis N44.8
|tunica vaginalis N50.89
|vas deferens N50.89
|vulva (acute) N90.89
Edentulism *see* Absence, teeth, acquired
Edsall's disease T67.2
Educational handicap Z55.9
|less than a high school diploma Z55.5
|no general equivalence degree (GED) Z55.5
|specified NEC Z55.8
Edward's syndrome *see* Trisomy, 18
Effect, adverse
|abnormal gravitational (G) forces or states T75.81
|abuse *see* Maltreatment
|air pressure T70.9
||specified NEC T70.8
|altitude (high) *see* Effect, adverse, high altitude
|anesthesia *see also* Anesthesia T88.59

Effect, adverse - *continued*
|in labor and delivery O74.9
|local, toxic
|in labor and delivery O74.4
|in pregnancy NEC O29.3-
|postpartum, puerperal O89.3
|postpartum, puerperal O89.9
|specified NEC T88.59
|in labor and delivery O74.8
|postpartum, puerperal O89.8
|spinal and epidural T88.59
|headache T88.59
|in labor and delivery O74.5
|postpartum, puerperal O89.4
|specified NEC
|in labor and delivery O74.6
|postpartum, puerperal O89.5
|antitoxin *see* Complications, vaccination
|atmospheric pressure T70.9
|due to explosion T70.8
|high T70.3
|low *see* Effect, adverse, high altitude
|specified effect NEC T70.8
|biological, correct substance properly
    administered *see* Effect, adverse, drug
|blood (derivatives) (serum) (transfusion) *see*
    Complications, transfusion
|chemical substance *see* Table of Drugs and
    Chemicals
|cold (temperature) (weather) T69.9
|chilblains T69.1
|frostbite *see* Frostbite
|specified effect NEC T69.8
|drugs and medicaments T88.7
|specified drug *see* Table of Drugs and
    Chemicals, by drug, adverse effect
|specified effect   code to condition
|electric current, electricity (shock) T75.4
|burn *see* Burn
|exertion (excessive) T73.3
|exposure *see* Exposure
|external cause NEC T75.89
|foodstuffs T78.1
|allergic reaction *see* Allergy, food
|causing anaphylaxis *see* Shock,
    anaphylactic, due to food
|noxious *see* Poisoning, food, noxious
|gases, fumes, or vapors T59.9-
|specified agent *see* Table of Drugs and
    Chemicals
|glue (airplane) sniffing
|due to drug abuse *see* Abuse, drug, inhalant
|due to drug dependence *see* Dependence,
    drug, inhalant
|heat *see* Heat
|high altitude NEC T70.29
|anoxia T70.29
|on
|ears T70.0
|sinuses T70.1
|polycythemia D75.1
|high pressure fluids T70.4
|hot weather *see* Heat
|hunger T73.0
|immersion, foot *see* Immersion
|immunization *see* Complications, vaccination
|immunological agents *see* Complications,
    vaccination
|infrared (radiation) (rays) NOS T66
|dermatitis or eczema L59.8
|infusion *see* Complications, infusion
|lack of care of infants *see* Maltreatment, child
|lightning *see* Lightning
|medical care T88.9
|specified NEC T88.8

Effect, adverse - *continued*
|medicinal substance, correct, properly
    administered *see* Effect, adverse, drug
|motion T75.3
|noise, on inner ear *see* subcategory H83.3
|overheated places *see* Heat
|psychosocial, of work environment Z56.5
|radiation (diagnostic) (infrared) (natural
    source) (therapeutic) (ultraviolet) (X-ray)
    NOS T66
|dermatitis or eczema *see* Dermatitis, due to,
    radiation
|fibrosis of lung J70.1
|pneumonitis J70.0
|pulmonary manifestations
|acute J70.0
|chronic J70.1
|skin L59.9
|radioactive substance NOS
|dermatitis or eczema *see* Radiodermatitis
|reduced temperature T69.9
|immersion foot or hand *see* Immersion
|specified effect NEC T69.8
|serum NEC *see also* Reaction, serum T80.69
|specified NEC T78.8
|external cause NEC T75.89
|strangulation *see* Asphyxia, traumatic
|submersion T75.1
|thirst T73.1
|toxic *see* Toxicity
|transfusion *see* Complications, transfusion
|ultraviolet (radiation) (rays) NOS T66
|burn *see* Burn
|dermatitis or eczema *see* Dermatitis, due to,
    ultraviolet rays
|acute L56.8
|vaccine (any) *see* Complications, vaccination
|vibration *see* Vibration, adverse effects
|water pressure NEC T70.9
|specified NEC T70.8
|weightlessness T75.82
|whole blood *see* Complications, transfusion
|work environment Z56.5
Effect(s) (of) (from) *see* Effect, adverse NEC
Effects, late *see* Sequelae
Effluvium
|anagen L65.1
|telogen L65.0
Effort syndrome (psychogenic) F45.8
Effusion
|amniotic fluid *see* Pregnancy, complicated by,
    premature rupture of membranes
|brain (serous) G93.6
|bronchial *see* Bronchitis
|cerebral G93.6
|cerebrospinal *see also* Meningitis
|vessel G93.6
|chest *see* Effusion, pleura
|chylous, chyliform (pleura) J94.0
|intracranial G93.6
|joint M25.40
|ankle M25.47-
|elbow M25.42-
|foot joint M25.47-
|hand joint M25.44-
|hip M25.45-
|knee M25.46-
|shoulder M25.41-
|specified joint NEC M25.48
|wrist M25.43-
|malignant pleural J91.0
|meninges *see* Meningitis
|pericardium, pericardial (noninflammatory)
    I31.3
|acute *see* Pericarditis, acute
|peritoneal (chronic) R18.8

Effusion - *continued*
|pleura, pleurisy, pleuritic, pleuropericardial
    J90
|chylous, chyliform J94.0
|due to systemic lupus erythematosus
    M32.13
|in conditions classified elsewhere J91.8
|influenzal *see* Influenza, with, respiratory
    manifestations NEC
|malignant J91.0
|newborn P28.89
|tuberculous NEC A15.6
|primary (progressive) A15.7
|spinal *see* Meningitis
|thorax, thoracic *see* Effusion, pleura
Egg shell nails L60.3
|congenital Q84.6
**EGPA (eosinophilic granulomatosis with
  polyangiitis)** M30.1
Egyptian splenomegaly B65.1
Ehrlichiosis A77.40
|due to
|E. chafeensis A77.41
|E. ewingii A77.49
|E. muris euclairensis A77.49
|E. sennetsu A79.81
|specified organism NEC A77.49
Ehlers-Danlos syndrome Q79.6
Eichstedt's disease B36.0
Eisenmenger's
|complex or syndrome I27.83
|defect Q21.8
Ejaculation
|delayed F52.32
|painful N53.12
|premature F52.4
|retarded N53.11
|retrograde N53.14
|semen, painful N53.12
|psychogenic F52.6
Ekbom's syndrome (restless legs) G25.81
**Ekman's syndrome (brittle bones and blue
  sclera)** Q78.0
Elastic skin Q82.8
|acquired L57.4
Elastofibroma *see* Neoplasm, connective tissue,
  benign
Elastoma (juvenile) Q82.8
|Miescher's L87.2
Elastomyofibrosis I42.4
Elastosis
|actinic, solar L57.8
|atrophicans (senile) L57.4
|perforans serpiginosa L87.2
|senilis L57.4
Elbow *see* condition
**Electric current, electricity, effects
  (concussion) (fatal) (nonfatal) (shock)**
  T75.4
|burn *see* Burn
Electric feet syndrome E53.8
Electrocution T75.4
|from electroshock gun (taser) T75.4
Electrolyte imbalance E87.8
|with
|abortion *see* Abortion by type, complicated
    by, electrolyte imbalance
|ectopic pregnancy O08.5
|molar pregnancy O08.5
Elephantiasis (nonfilarial) I89.0
|arabicum *see* Infestation, filarial
|bancroftian B74.0
|congenital (any site) (hereditary) Q82.0
|due to
|Brugia (malayi) B74.1
|timori B74.2

Elephantiasis - *continued*
- |mastectomy I97.2
- |Wuchereria (bancrofti) B74.0
- |eyelid H02.859
  - |left H02.856
    - |lower H02.855
    - |upper H02.854
  - |right H02.853
    - |lower H02.852
    - |upper H02.851
- |filarial, filariensis *see* Infestation, filarial
- |glandular I89.0
- |graecorum A30.9
- |lymphangiectatic I89.0
- |lymphatic vessel I89.0
  - |due to mastectomy I97.2
- |scrotum (nonfilarial) I89.0
- |streptococcal I89.0
- |surgical I97.89
- |postmastectomy I97.2
- |telangiectodes I89.0
- |vulva (nonfilarial) N90.89

Elevated, elevation
- |alanine transaminase (ALT) R74.01
- |ALT (alanine transaminase) R74.01
- |antibody titer R76.0
- |aspartate transaminase (AST) R74.01
- |AST (aspartate transaminase) R74.01
- |basal metabolic rate R94.8
- |blood pressure *see also* Hypertension
  - |reading (incidental) (isolated) (nonspecific), no diagnosis of hypertension R03.0
- |blood sugar R73.9
- |body temperature (of unknown origin) R50.9
- |C-reactive protein (CRP) R79.82
- |cancer antigen 125 [CA 125] R97.1
- |carcinoembryonic antigen [CEA] R97.0
- |cholesterol E78.00
  - |with high triglycerides E78.2
- |conjugate, eye H51.0
- |diaphragm, congenital Q79.1
- |erythrocyte sedimentation rate R70.0
- |fasting glucose R73.01
- |fasting triglycerides E78.1
- |finding on laboratory examination *see* Findings, abnormal, inconclusive, without diagnosis, by type of exam
- |GFR (glomerular filtration rate) *see* Findings, abnormal, inconclusive, without diagnosis, by type of exam
- |glucose tolerance (oral) R73.02
- |immunoglobulin level R76.8
- |indoleacetic acid R82.5
- |lactic acid dehydrogenase (LDH) level R74.02
- |leukocytes D72.829
- |lipoprotein a (Lp(a)) level E78.41
- |liver function
  - |study R94.5
  - |test R79.89
    - |alkaline phosphatase R74.8
    - |aminotransferase R74.01
    - |bilirubin R17
    - |hepatic enzyme R74.8
    - |lactate dehydrogenase R74.02
- |Lp(a) (lipoprotein(a)) E78.41
- |lymphocytes D72.820
- |prostate specific antigen [PSA] R97.20
- |Rh titer *see* Complication(s), transfusion, incompatibility reaction, Rh (factor)
- |scapula, congenital Q74.0
- |sedimentation rate R70.0
- |SGOT R74.01
- |SGPT R74.01
- |transaminase level R74.01
- |triglycerides E78.1

Elevated, elevation- *continued*
- |with high cholesterol E78.2
- |troponin R77.8
- |tumor associated antigens [TAA] NEC R97.8
- |tumor specific antigens [TSA] NEC R97.8
- |urine level of
  - |catecholamine R82.5
  - |indoleacetic acid R82.5
  - |17-ketosteroids R82.5
  - |steroids R82.5
  - |vanillylmandelic acid (VMA) R82.5
- |venous pressure I87.8
- |white blood cell count D72.829
  - |specified NEC D72.828
Elliptocytosis (congenital) (hereditary) D58.1
- |Hb C (disease) D58.1
- |hemoglobin disease D58.1
- |sickle-cell (disease) D57.8-
  - |trait D57.3
Ellison-Zollinger syndrome E16.4
Ellis-Van Creveld syndrome (chondroectodermal dysplasia) Q77.6
Elongated, elongation (congenital) *see also* Distortion
- |bone Q79.9
- |cervix (uteri) Q51.828
  - |acquired N88.4
  - |hypertrophic N88.4
- |colon Q43.8
- |common bile duct Q44.5
- |cystic duct Q44.5
- |frenulum, penis Q55.69
- |labia minora (acquired) N90.69
- |ligamentum patellae Q74.1
- |petiolus (epiglottidis) Q31.8
- |tooth, teeth K00.2
- |uvula Q38.6
Eltor cholera A00.1
Emaciation R64
- - due to malnutrition E43
Embadomoniasis A07.8
Embedded tooth, teeth K01.0
- |root only K08.3
Embolic *see* condition
Embolism (multiple) (paradoxical) I74.9
- |air (any site) (traumatic) T79.0
  - |following
    - |abortion *see* Abortion by type complicated by embolism
    - |ectopic pregnancy O08.2
    - |infusion, therapeutic injection or transfusion T80.0
    - |molar pregnancy O08.2
    - |procedure NEC
      - |artery T81.719
        - |mesenteric T81.710
        - |renal T81.711
        - |specified NEC T81.718
      - |vein T81.72
  - |in pregnancy, childbirth or puerperium *see* Embolism, obstetric
- |amniotic fluid (pulmonary) *see also* Embolism, obstetric
  - |following
    - |abortion *see* Abortion by type complicated by embolism
    - |ectopic pregnancy O08.2
    - |molar pregnancy O08.2
- |aorta, aortic I74.10
  - |abdominal I74.09
    - |saddle I74.01
  - |bifurcation I74.09
  - |saddle I74.01
  - |thoracic I74.11

Embolism - *continued*
- |artery I74.9
  - |auditory, internal I65.8
  - |basilar *see* Occlusion, artery, basilar
  - |carotid (common) (internal) *see* Occlusion, artery, carotid
  - |cerebellar (anterior inferior) (posterior inferior) (superior) I66.3
  - |cerebral *see* Occlusion, artery, cerebral
  - |choroidal (anterior) I65.8
  - |communicating posterior I65.8
  - |coronary *see also* Infarct, myocardium
    - |not resulting in infarction I24.0
  - |extremity I74.4
    - |lower I74.3
    - |upper I74.2
  - |hypophyseal I65.8
  - |iliac I74.5
  - |limb I74.4
    - |lower I74.3
    - |upper I74.2
  - |mesenteric (with gangrene) *see also* Ischemia, intestine, acute K55.059
  - |ophthalmic *see* Occlusion, artery, retina
  - |peripheral I74.4
  - |pontine I65.8
  - |precerebral *see* Occlusion, artery, precerebral
  - |pulmonary *see* Embolism, pulmonary
  - |renal N28.0
  - |retinal *see* Occlusion, artery, retina
  - |septic I76
  - |specified NEC I74.8
  - |vertebral *see* Occlusion, artery, vertebral
- |basilar (artery) I65.1
- |blood clot
  - |following
    - |abortion *see* Abortion by type complicated by embolism
    - |ectopic or molar pregnancy O08.2
  - |in pregnancy, childbirth or puerperium *see* Embolism, obstetric
- |brain *see also* Occlusion, artery, cerebral
  - |following
    - |abortion *see* Abortion by type complicated by embolism
    - |ectopic or molar pregnancy O08.2
  - |puerperal, postpartum, childbirth *see* Embolism, obstetric
- |capillary I78.8
- |cardiac *see also* Infarct, myocardium
  - |not resulting in infarction I51.3
- |carotid (artery) (common) (internal) *see* Occlusion, artery, carotid
- |cavernous sinus (venous) *see* Embolism, intracranial venous sinus
- |cerebral *see* Occlusion, artery, cerebral
- |cholesterol *see* Atheroembolism
- |coronary (artery or vein) (systemic) *see* Occlusion, coronary
- |due to device, implant or graft *see also* Complications, by site and type, specified NEC
  - |arterial graft NEC T82.818
  - |breast (implant) T85.818
  - |catheter NEC T85.818
    - |dialysis (renal) T82.818
      - |intraperitoneal T85.818
    - |infusion NEC T82.818
      - |spinal (epidural) (subdural) T85.810
    - |urinary (indwelling) T83.81
  - |electronic (electrode) (pulse generator) (stimulator)
    - |bone T84.81
    - |cardiac T82.817

Embolism - *continued*

|nervous system (brain) (peripheral nerve)
(spinal) T85.810
|urinary T83.81
|fixation, internal (orthopedic) NEC T84.81
|gastrointestinal (bile duct) (esophagus)
T85.818
|genital NEC T83.81
|heart (graft) (valve) T82.817
|joint prosthesis T84.81
|ocular (corneal graft) (orbital implant)
T85.818
|orthopedic (bone graft) NEC T86.838
|specified NEC T85.818
|urinary (graft) NEC T83.81
|vascular NEC T82.818
|ventricular intracranial shunt T85.810
|extremities
|lower *see* Embolism, vein, lower extremity
|arterial I74.3
|upper I74.2
|eye H34.9
|fat (cerebral) (pulmonary) (systemic) T79.1
|following
|abortion *see* Abortion by type complicated
by embolism
|ectopic or molar pregnancy O08.2
|complicating delivery *see* Embolism,
obstetric
|following
|abortion *see* Abortion by type complicated
by embolism
|ectopic or molar pregnancy O08.2
|infusion, therapeutic injection or transfusion
|air T80.0
|heart (fatty) *see also* Infarct, myocardium
|not resulting in infarction I51.3
|hepatic (vein) I82.0
|in pregnancy, childbirth or puerperium *see*
Embolism, obstetric
|intestine (artery) (vein) (with gangrene) *see*
also Ischemia, intestine, acute K55.039
|intracranial *see also* Occlusion, artery,
cerebral
|venous sinus (any) G08
|nonpyogenic I67.6
|intraspinal venous sinuses or veins G08
|nonpyogenic G95.19
|kidney (artery) N28.0
|lateral sinus (venous) *see* Embolism,
intracranial, venous sinus
|leg *see* Embolism, vein, lower extremity
|arterial I74.3
|longitudinal sinus (venous) *see* Embolism,
intracranial, venous sinus
|lung (massive) *see* Embolism, pulmonary
|meninges I66.8
|mesenteric (artery) (vein) (with gangrene) *see*
also Ischemia, intestine, acute K55.059
|obstetric (in) (pulmonary)
|childbirth O88.22
|air O88.02
|amniotic fluid O88.12
|blood clot O88.22
|fat O88.82
|pyemic O88.32
|septic O88.32
|specified type NEC O88.82
|pregnancy O88.21-
|air O88.01-
|amniotic fluid O88.11-
|blood clot O88.21-
|fat O88.81-
|pyemic O88.31-
|septic O88.31-

Embolism - *continued*

|specified type NEC O88.81-
|puerperal O88.23
|air O88.03
|amniotic fluid O88.13
|blood clot O88.23
|fat O88.83
|pyemic O88.33
|septic O88.33
|specified type NEC O88.83
|ophthalmic *see* Occlusion, artery, retina
|penis N48.81
|peripheral artery NOS I74.4
|pituitary E23.6
|popliteal (artery) I74.3
|portal (vein) I81
|postoperative, postprocedural
|artery T81.719
|mesenteric T81.710
|renal T81.711
|specified NEC T81.718
|vein T81.72
|precerebral artery *see* Occlusion, artery,
precerebral
|puerperal *see* Embolism, obstetric
|pulmonary (acute) (artery) (vein) I26.99
|with acute cor pulmonale I26.09
|chronic I27.82
|following
|abortion *see* Abortion by type complicated
by embolism
|ectopic or molar pregnancy O08.2
|healed or old Z86.711
|in pregnancy, childbirth or puerperium *see*
Embolism, obstetric
|personal history of Z86.711
|saddle I26.92
|with acute cor pulmonale I26.02
|septic I26.90
|with acute cor pulmonale I26.01
|pyemic (multiple) I76
|following
|abortion *see* Abortion by type complicated
by embolism
|ectopic or molar pregnancy O08.2
|Hemophilus influenzae A41.3
|pneumococcal A40.3
|with pneumonia J13
|puerperal, postpartum, childbirth (any
organism) *see* Embolism, obstetric
|specified organism NEC A41.89
|staphylococcal A41.2
|streptococcal A40.9
|renal (artery) N28.0
|vein I82.3
|retina, retinal *see* Occlusion, artery, retina
|saddle
|abdominal aorta I74.01
|pulmonary artery I26.92
|with acute cor pulmonale I26.02
|septic (arterial) I76
|complicating abortion *see* Abortion, by type,
complicated by, embolism
|sinus *see* Embolism, intracranial, venous sinus
|soap complicating abortion *see* Abortion, by
type, complicated by, embolism
|spinal cord G95.19
|pyogenic origin G06.1
|spleen, splenic (artery) I74.8
|upper extremity I74.2
|vein (acute) I82.90
|antecubital I82.61-
|chronic I82.71-
|axillary I82.A1-
|chronic I82.A2-

Embolism - *continued*

|basilic I82.61-
|chronic I82.71-
|brachial I82.62-
|chronic I82.72-
|brachiocephalic (innominate) I82.290
|chronic I82.291
|cephalic I82.61-
|chronic I82.71-
|chronic I82.91
|deep (DVT) I82.40-
|calf I82.4Z-
|chronic I82.5Z-
|lower leg I82.4Z-
|chronic I82.5Z-
|thigh I82.4Y-
|chronic I82.5Y-
|upper leg I82.4Y
|chronic I82.5Y-
|femoral I82.41-
|chronic I82.51-
|iliac (iliofemoral) I82.42-
|chronic I82.52-
|innominate I82.290
|chronic I82.291
|internal jugular I82.C1-
|chronic I82.C2-
|lower extremity
|deep I82.40-
|chronic I82.50-
|specified NEC I82.49-
|chronic NEC I82.59-
|distal
|deep I82.4Z-
|proximal
|deep I82.4Y-
|chronic I82.5Y-
|superficial I82.81-
|popliteal I82.43-
|chronic I82.53-
|radial I82.62-
|chronic I82.72-
|renal I82.3
|saphenous (greater) (lesser) I82.81-
|specified NEC I82.890
|chronic NEC I82.891
|subclavian I82.B1-
|chronic I82.B2-
|thoracic NEC I82.290
|chronic I82.291
|tibial I82.44-
|chronic I82.54-
|ulnar I82.62-
|chronic I82.72-
|upper extremity I82.60-
|chronic I82.70-
|deep I82.62-
|chronic I82.72-
|superficial I82.61-
|chronic I82.71-
|vena cava
|inferior (acute) I82.220
|chronic I82.221
|superior (acute) I82.210
|chronic I82.211
|venous sinus G08
|vessels of brain *see* Occlusion, artery, cerebral
Embolus *see* Embolism
Embryoma *see also* Neoplasm, uncertain
behavior, by site
|benign *see* Neoplasm, benign, by site
|kidney C64.-
|liver C22.0
|malignant *see also* Neoplasm, malignant, by
site

Embryoma - *continued*
|kidney C64.-
|liver C22.0
|testis C62.9-
|descended (scrotal) C62.1-
|undescended C62.0-
|testis C62.9-
|descended (scrotal) C62.1-
|undescended C62.0-
Embryonic
|circulation Q28.9
|heart Q28.9
|vas deferens Q55.4
Embryopathia NOS Q89.9
Embryotoxon Q13.4
Emesis *see* Vomiting
Emotional lability R45.86
Emotionality, pathological F60.3
Emotogenic disease *see* Disorder, psychogenic
Emphysema (atrophic) (bullous) (chronic) (interlobular) (lung) (obstructive) (pulmonary) (senile) (vesicular) J43.9
|cellular tissue (traumatic) T79.7
|surgical T81.82
|centrilobular J43.2
|compensatory J98.3
|congenital (interstitial) P25.0
|conjunctiva H11.89
|connective tissue (traumatic) T79.7
|surgical T81.82
|due to chemicals, gases, fumes or vapors J68.4
|eyelid(s) *see* Disorder, eyelid, specified type NEC
|surgical T81.82
|traumatic T79.7
|interstitial J98.2
|congenital P25.0
|perinatal period P25.0
|laminated tissue T79.7
|surgical T81.82
|mediastinal J98.2
|newborn P25.2
|orbit, orbital *see* Disorder, orbit, specified type NEC
|panacinar J43.1
|panlobular J43.1
|specified NEC J43.8
|subcutaneous (traumatic) T79.7
|nontraumatic J98.2
|postprocedural T81.82
|surgical T81.82
|surgical T81.82
|thymus (gland) (congenital) E32.8
|traumatic (subcutaneous) T79.7
|unilateral J43.0
Empty nest syndrome Z60.0
Empyema (acute) (chest) (double) (pleura) (supradiaphragmatic) (thorax) J86.9
|with fistula J86.0
|accessory sinus (chronic) *see* Sinusitis
|antrum (chronic) *see* Sinusitis, maxillary
|brain (any part) *see* Abscess, brain
|ethmoidal (chronic) (sinus) *see* Sinusitis, ethmoidal
|extradural *see* Abscess, extradural
|frontal (chronic) (sinus) *see* Sinusitis, frontal
|gallbladder K81.0
|mastoid (process) (acute) *see* Mastoiditis, acute
|maxilla, maxillary M27.2
|sinus (chronic) *see* Sinusitis, maxillary
|nasal sinus (chronic) *see* Sinusitis
|sinus (accessory) (chronic) (nasal) *see* Sinusitis

Empyema - *continued*
|sphenoidal (sinus) (chronic) *see* Sinusitis, sphenoidal
|subarachnoid *see* Abscess, extradural
|subdural *see* Abscess, subdural
|tuberculous A15.6
|ureter *see* Ureteritis
|ventricular *see* Abscess, brain
En coup de sabre lesion L94.1
Enamel pearls K00.2
Enameloma K00.2
Enanthema, viral B09
Encephalitis (chronic) (hemorrhagic) (idiopathic) (nonepidemic) (spurious) (subacute) G04.90
|acute *see also* Encephalitis, viral A86
|disseminated G04.00
|infectious G04.01
|noninfectious G04.81
|postimmunization (postvaccination) G04.02
|postinfectious G04.01
|inclusion body A85.8
|necrotizing hemorrhagic G04.30
|postimmunization G04.32
|postinfectious G04.31
|specified NEC G04.39
|arboviral, arbovirus NEC A85.2
|arthropod-borne NEC (viral) A85.2
|Australian A83.4
|California (virus) A83.5
|Central European (tick-borne) A84.1
|Czechoslovakian A84.1
|Dawson's (inclusion body) A81.1
|diffuse sclerosing A81.1
|disseminated, acute G04.00
|due to
|cat scratch disease A28.1
|human immunodeficiency virus (HIV) disease B20 [*G05.3*]
|malaria *see* Malaria
|rickettsiosis *see* Rickettsiosis
|smallpox inoculation G04.02
|typhus *see* Typhus
|Eastern equine A83.2
|endemic (viral) A86
|epidemic NEC (viral) A86
|equine (acute) (infectious) (viral) A83.9
|Eastern A83.2
|Venezuelan A92.2
|Western A83.1
|Far Eastern (tick-borne) A84.0
|following vaccination or other immunization procedure G04.02
|herpes zoster B02.0
|herpesviral B00.4
|due to herpesvirus 6 B10.01
|due to herpesvirus 7 B10.09
|specified NEC B10.09
|Ilhéus (virus) A83.8
|inclusion body A81.1
|in (due to)
|actinomycosis A42.82
|adenovirus A85.1
|African trypanosomiasis B56.9 [*G05.3*]
|Chagas' disease (chronic) B57.42
|cytomegalovirus B25.8
|enterovirus A85.0
|herpes (simplex) virus B00.4
|due to herpesvirus 6 B10.01
|due to herpesvirus 7 B10.09
|specified NEC B10.09
|infectious disease NEC B99 [*G05.3*]
|influenza *see* Influenza, with, encephalopathy

Encephalitis - *continued*
|listeriosis A32.12
|measles B05.0
|mumps B26.2
|naegleriasis B60.2
|parasitic disease NEC B89 [*G05.3*]
|poliovirus A80.9 [*G05.3*]
|rubella B06.01
|syphilis
|congenital A50.42
|late A52.14
|systemic lupus erythematosus M32.19
|toxoplasmosis (acquired) B58.2
|congenital P37.1
|tuberculosis A17.82
|zoster B02.0
|infectious (acute) (virus) NEC A86
|Japanese (B type) A83.0
|La Crosse A83.5
|lead *see* Poisoning, lead
|lethargica (acute) (infectious) A85.8
|louping ill A84.89
|lupus erythematosus, systemic M32.19
|lymphatica A87.2
|Mengo A85.8
|meningococcal A39.81
|Murray Valley A83.4
|otitic NEC H66.40 [*G05.3*]
|parasitic NOS B71.9
|periaxial G37.0
|periaxialis (concentrica) (diffuse) G37.5
|post chickenpox B01.11
|postexanthematous NEC B09
|postimmunization G04.02
|postinfectious NEC G04.01
|postmeasles B05.0
|postvaccinal G04.02
|post varicella B01.11
|postviral NEC A86
|Powassan A84.81
|Rasmussen G04.81
|Rio Bravo A85.8
|Russian
|autumnal A83.0
|spring-summer (taiga) A84.0
|saturnine *see* Poisoning, lead
|specified NEC G04.81
|St. Louis A83.3
|subacute sclerosing A81.1
|summer A83.0
|suppurative G04.81
|tick-borne A84.9
|Torula, torular (cryptococcal) B45.1
|toxic NEC G92.8
|trichinosis B75 [*G05.3*]
|type
|B A83.0
|C A83.3
|van Bogaert's A81.1
|Venezuelan equine A92.2
|Vienna A85.8
|viral, virus A86
|arthropod-borne NEC A85.2
|mosquito-borne A83.9
|Australian X disease A83.4
|California virus A83.5
|Eastern equine A83.2
|Japanese (B type) A83.0
|Murray Valley A83.4
|specified NEC A83.8
|St. Louis A83.3
|type B A83.0
|type C A83.3
|Western equine A83.1
|tick-borne A84.9

Encephalitis - *continued*
    |biundulant A84.1
    |central European A84.1
    |Czechoslovakian A84.1
    |diphasic meningoencephalitis A84.1
    |Far Eastern A84.0
    |Russian spring-summer (taiga) A84.0
    |specified NEC A84.89
  |specified type NEC A85.8
  |tick-borne, specified NEC A84.89
  |Western equine A83.1
Encephalocele Q01.9
  |frontal Q01.0
  |nasofrontal Q01.1
  |occipital Q01.2
  |specified NEC Q01.8
Encephalocystocele *see* Encephalocele
Encephaloduroarteriomyosynangiosis
  (EDAMS) I67.5
Encephalomalacia (brain) (cerebellar)
  (cerebral) *see* Softening, brain
Encephalomeningitis *see* Meningoencephalitis
Encephalomeningocele *see* Encephalocele
Encephalomeningomyelitis *see*
  Meningoencephalitis
Encephalomyelitis *see also* Encephalitis G04.90
  |acute disseminated G04.00
    |infectious G04.01
    |noninfectious G04.81
    |postimmunization G04.02
    |postinfectious G04.01
  |acute necrotizing hemorrhagic G04.30
    |postimmunization G04.32
    |postinfectious G04.31
    |specified NEC G04.39
  |benign myalgic G93.3
  |equine A83.9
    |Eastern A83.2
    |Venezuelan A92.2
    |Western A83.1
  |in diseases classified elsewhere G05.3
  |myalgic, benign G93.3
  |post chickenpox B01.11
  |postinfectious NEC G04.01
  |postmeasles B05.0
  |postvaccinal G04.02
  |post varicella B01.11
  |rubella B06.01
  |specified NEC G04.81
  |Venezuelan equine A92.2
Encephalomyelocele *see* Encephalocele
Encephalomyelomeningitis *see*
  Meningoencephalitis
Encephalomyelopathy G96.9
Encephalomyeloradiculitis (acute) G61.0
Encephalomyeloradiculoneuritis (acute)
  (Guillain-Barré) G61.0
Encephalomyeloradiculopathy G96.9
Encephalopathia hyperbilirubinemic,
  newborn P57.9
  |due to isoimmunization (conditions in P55)
    P57.0
Encephalopathy (acute) G93.40
  |acute necrotizing hemorrhagic G04.30
    |postimmunization G04.32
    |postinfectious G04.31
    |specified NEC G04.39
  |alcoholic G31.2
  |anoxic *see* Damage, brain, anoxic
  |arteriosclerotic I67.2
  |centrolobar progressive (Schilder) G37.0
  |congenital Q07.9
  |degenerative, in specified disease NEC
    G32.89
  |demyelinating callosal G37.1

Encephalopathy - *continued*
  |due to
    |drugs Table of Drugs and Chemicals G92.8
  |hepatic *see* Failure, hepatic
  |hyperbilirubinemic, newborn P57.9
    |due to isoimmunization (conditions in P55)
      P57.0
  |hypertensive I67.4
  |hypoglycemic E16.2
  |hypoxic *see* Damage, brain, anoxic
  |hypoxic ischemic P91.60
    |mild P91.61
    |moderate P91.62
    |severe P91.63
  |in (due to) (with)
    |birth injury P11.1
    |hyperinsulinism E16.1 *[G94]*
    |influenza *see* Influenza, with,
      encephalopathy
    |lack of vitamin *see also* Deficiency, vitamin
      E56.9 *[G32.89]*
    |neoplastic disease (*see also* Neoplasm)
      D49.9 *[G13.1]*
    |serum *see also* Reaction, serum T80.69
    |syphilis A52.17
    |trauma (postconcussional) F07.81
      |current injury *see* Injury, intracranial
    |vaccination G04.02
  |lead *see* Poisoning, lead
  |metabolic G93.41
    |drug induced G92.8
    |toxic G92.8
  |myoclonic, early, symptomatic *see* Epilepsy,
    generalized, specified NEC
  |necrotizing, subacute (Leigh) G31.82
  |neonatal P91.819
    |in diseases classified elsewhere P91.811
  |pellagrous E52 *[G32.89]*
  |portosystemic *see* Failure, hepatic
  |postcontusional F07.81
    |current injury *see* Injury, intracranial,
      diffuse
  |posthypoglycemic (coma) E16.1 *[G94]*
  |postradiation G93.89
  |saturnine *see* Poisoning, lead
  |septic G93.41
  |specified NEC G93.49
  |spongiform, subacute (viral) A81.09
  |toxic G92.8
    |metabolic G92.8
  |traumatic (postconcussional) F07.81
    |current injury *see* Injury, intracranial
  |vitamin B deficiency NEC E53.9 *[G32.89]*
  | vitamin B1 E51.2
  |Wernicke's E51.2
Encephalorrhagia *see* Hemorrhage, intracranial,
  intracerebral
Encephalosis, posttraumatic F07.81
Enchondroma *see also* Neoplasm, bone, benign
Enchondromatosis (cartilaginous) (multiple)
  Q78.4
Encopresis R15.9
  |functional F98.1
  |nonorganic origin F98.1
  |psychogenic F98.1
Encounter (with health service) (for) Z76.89
  |adjustment and management (of)
    |breast implant Z45.81
    |implanted device NEC Z45.89
    |myringotomy device (stent) (tube) Z45.82
  |administrative purpose only Z02.9
    |examination for
      |adoption Z02.82
      |armed forces Z02.3
      |disability determination Z02.71

Encounter (with health service) - *continued*
    |driving license Z02.4
    |employment Z02.1
    |insurance Z02.6
    |medical certificate NEC Z02.79
    |paternity testing Z02.81
    |residential institution admission Z02.2
    |school admission Z02.0
    |sports Z02.5
    |specified reason NEC Z02.89
  |aftercare *see* Aftercare
  |antenatal screening Z36.9
    |cervical length Z36.86
    |chromosomal anomalies Z36.0
    |congenital cardiac abnormalities Z36.83
    |elevated maternal serum alphafetoprotein
      level Z36.1
    |fetal growth retardation Z36.4
    |fetal lung maturity Z36.84
    |fetal macrosomia Z36.88
    |hydrops fetalis Z36.81
    |intrauterine growth restriction (IUGR)/
      small-for-dates Z36.4
    |isoimmunization Z36.5
    |large-for-dates Z36.88
    |malformations Z36.3
    |non-visualized anatomy on a previous scan
      Z36.2
    |nuchal translucency Z36.82
    |raised alphafetoprotein level Z36.1
    |risk of pre-term labor Z36.86
    |specified type NEC Z36.89
    |specified follow-up NEC Z36.2
    |specified genetic defects NEC Z36.8A
    |Streptococcus B Z36.85
    |suspected anomaly Z36.3
    |uncertain dates Z36.87
  |assisted reproductive fertility procedure cycle
    Z31.83
  |blood typing Z01.83
    |Rh typing Z01.83
  |breast augmentation or reduction Z41.1
  |breast implant exchange (different material)
    (different size) Z45.81
  |breast reconstruction following mastectomy
    Z42.1
  |check-up *see* Examination
  |chemotherapy for neoplasm Z51.11
  |colonoscopy, screening Z12.11
  |counseling *see* Counseling
  |delivery, full-term, uncomplicated O80
    |cesarean, without indication O82
  |desensitization to allergens Z51.6
  |ear piercing Z41.3
  |examination *see* Examination
  |expectant parent(s) (adoptive) pre-birth
    pediatrician visit Z76.81
  |fertility preservation procedure (prior to
    cancer therapy) (prior to removal of
    gonads) Z31.84
  |fitting (of) *see* Fitting (and adjustment) (of)
  |genetic
    |counseling
      |nonprocreative Z71.83
      |procreative Z31.5
    |testing *see* Test, genetic
  |hearing conservation and treatment Z01.12
  |immunotherapy for neoplasm Z51.12
  |in vitro fertilization cycle Z31.83
  |instruction (in)
    |childbirth Z32.2
    |child care (postpartal) (prenatal) Z32.3
    |natural family planning
      |procreative Z31.61
      |to avoid pregnancy Z30.02

Encounter (with health service) - *continued*
 |insulin pump titration Z46.81
 |joint prosthesis insertion following prior
  explantation of joint prosthesis (staged
  procedure)
  |hip Z47.32
  |knee Z47.33
  |shoulder Z47.31
 |laboratory (as part of a general medical
  examination) Z00.00
  |with abnormal findings Z00.01
 |mental health services (for)
  |abuse NEC
   |perpetrator Z69.82
   |victim Z69.81
  |child abuse
   |nonparental
  |child neglect
   |nonparental
    |perpetrator Z69.021
    |victim Z69.020
   |parental
    |perpetrator Z69.011
    |victim Z69.010
  |child psychological abuse
   |nonparental
    |perpetrator Z69.021
    |victim Z69.020
   |parental
    |perpetrator Z69.011
    |victim Z69.010
  |child sexual abuse
   |nonparental
    |perpetrator Z69.021
    |victim Z69.020
   |parental
    |perpetrator Z69.011
    |victim Z69.010
  |non-spousal adult abuse (perpetrator)
   (victim) Z69.81
  |spousal or partner
   |abuse
    |perpetrator Z69.12
    |victim Z69.11
   |neglect
    |perpetrator Z69.12
    |victim Z69.11
   |psychological abuse
    |perpetrator Z69.12
    |victim Z69.11
   |violence
    |perpetrator (physical) (sexual) Z69.12
    |victim (physical) Z69.11
    |sexual Z69.81
 |placental sample (taken vaginally) (*see also*
  Encounter, antenatal screening) Z36.9
   |perpetrator Z69.021
   |victim Z69.020
  |parental
   |perpetrator Z69.011
   |victim Z69.010
 |observation (for) (ruled out)
  |exposure to (suspected)
   |anthrax Z03.810
   |biological agent NEC Z03.818
 |pediatrician visit, by expectant parent(s)
  (adoptive) Z76.81
 |plastic and reconstructive surgery following
  medical procedure or healed injury NEC
  Z42.8
 |pregnancy
  |supervision of *see* Pregnancy, supervision of
  |test Z32.00
   |result negative Z32.02
   |result positive Z32.01

Encounter (with health service) - *continued*
 |procreative management and counseling for
  gestational carrier Z31.7
 |prophylactic measures Z29.9
  |antivenin Z29.12
  |fluoride administration Z29.3
  |immunotherapy for respiratory syncytial
   virus (RSV) Z29.11
  |rabies immune globin Z29.14
  |Rho (D) immune globulin Z29.13
  |specified NEC Z29.8
 |radiation therapy (antineoplastic) Z51.0
 |radiological (as part of a general medical
  examination) Z00.00
  |with abnormal findings Z00.01
 |reconstructive surgery following medical
  procedure or healed injury NEC Z42.8
 |removal (of) *see also* Removal
  |artificial
   |arm Z44.00-
    |complete Z44.01-
    |partial Z44.02-
   |eye Z44.2-
   |leg Z44.10-
    |complete Z44.11-
    |partial Z44.12-
  |breast implant Z45.81
   |tissue expander (without synchronous
    insertion of permanent implant) Z45.81
  |device Z46.9
   |specified NEC Z46.89
  |external
   |fixation device   code to fracture with
 seventh character D
   |prosthesis, prosthetic device Z44.9
    |breast Z44.3-
    |specified NEC Z44.8
  |implanted device NEC Z45.89
  |insulin pump Z46.81
  |internal fixation device Z47.2
  |myringotomy device (stent) (tube) Z45.82
  |nervous system device NEC Z46.2
   |brain neuropacemaker Z46.2
   |visual substitution device Z46.2
    |implanted Z45.31
  |non-vascular catheter Z46.82
  |orthodontic device Z46.4
  |stent
   |ureteral Z46.6
  |urinary device Z46.6
 |repeat cervical smear to confirm findings of
  recent normal smear following initial
  abnormal smear Z01.42
 |respirator [ventilator] use during power failure
  Z99.12
 |Rh typing Z01.83
 |screening *see* Screening
 |specified NEC Z76.89
 |sterilization Z30.2
 |suspected condition, ruled out
  |amniotic cavity and membrane Z03.71
  |cervical shortening Z03.75
  |fetal anomaly Z03.73
  |fetal growth Z03.74
  |maternal and fetal conditions NEC Z03.79
  |oligohydramnios Z03.71
  |placental problem Z03.72
  |polyhydramnios Z03.71
 |suspected exposure (to), ruled out
  |anthrax Z03.810
  |biological agents NEC Z03.818
 |termination of pregnancy, elective Z33.2
 |testing *see* Test
 |therapeutic drug level monitoring Z51.81
 |titration, insulin pump Z46.81

Encounter (with health service) - *continued*
 |to determine fetal viability of pregnancy
  O36.80
 |training
  |insulin pump Z46.81
 |X-ray of chest (as part of a general medical
  examination) Z00.00
  |with abnormal findings Z00.01
Encystment *see* Cyst
Endarteritis (bacterial, subacute) (infective)
 I77.6
 |brain I67.7
 |cerebral or cerebrospinal I67.7
 |deformans *see* Arteriosclerosis
 |embolic *see* Embolism
 |obliterans *see also* Arteriosclerosis
  |pulmonary I28.8
 |pulmonary I28.8
 |retina *see* Vasculitis, retina
 |senile *see* Arteriosclerosis
 |syphilitic A52.09
  |brain or cerebral A52.04
  |congenital A50.54 *[179.8]*
 |tuberculous A18.89
Endemic *see* condition
Endocarditis (chronic) (marantic)
 (nonbacterial) (thrombotic) (valvular) I38
 |with rheumatic fever (conditions in I00)
  |active *see* Endocarditis, acute, rheumatic
  |inactive or quiescent (with chorea) I09.1
 |acute or subacute I33.9
  |infective I33.0
  |rheumatic (aortic) (mitral) (pulmonary)
   (tricuspid) I01.1
   |with chorea (acute) (rheumatic)
    (Sydenham's) I02.0
 |aortic (heart) (nonrheumatic) (valve) I35.8
  |with
   |mitral disease I08.0
    |with tricuspid (valve) disease I08.3
   |active or acute I01.1
    |with chorea (acute) (rheumatic)
     (Sydenham's) I02.0
   |rheumatic fever (conditions in I00)
    |active *see* Endocarditis, acute,
     rheumatic
    |inactive or quiescent (with chorea) I06.9
   |tricuspid (valve) disease I08.2
    |with mitral (valve) disease I08.3
 |acute or subacute I33.9
 |arteriosclerotic I35.8
 |rheumatic I06.9
  |with mitral disease I08.0
   |with tricuspid (valve) disease I08.3
   |active or acute I01.1
    |with chorea (acute) (rheumatic)
     (Sydenham's) I02.0
  |active or acute I01.1
   |with chorea (acute) (rheumatic)
    (Sydenham's) I02.0
  |specified NEC I06.8
 |specified cause NEC I35.8
 |syphilitic A52.03
 |arteriosclerotic I38
 |atypical verrucous (Libman-Sacks) M32.11
 |bacterial (acute) (any valve) (subacute) I33.0
 |candidal B37.6
 |congenital Q24.8
 |constrictive I33.0
 |Coxiella burnetii A78 *[139]*
 |Coxsackie B33.21
 |due to
  |prosthetic cardiac valve T82.6
  |Q fever A78 *[139]*
  |Serratia marcescens I33.0

Endocarditis - *continued*
  |typhoid (fever) A01.02
  |gonococcal A54.83
  |infectious or infective (acute) (any valve)
    (subacute) I33.0
  |lenta (acute) (any valve) (subacute) I33.0
  |Libman-Sacks M32.11
  |listerial A32.82
  |Löffler's I42.3
  |malignant (acute) (any valve) (subacute) I33.0
  |meningococcal A39.51
  |mitral (chronic) (double) (fibroid) (heart)
    (inactive) (valve) (with chorea) I05.9
    |with
      |aortic (valve) disease I08.0
        |with tricuspid (valve) disease I08.3
        |active or acute I01.1
          |with chorea (acute) (rheumatic)
            (Sydenham's) I02.0
      |rheumatic fever (conditions in I00)
        |active *see* Endocarditis, acute,
          rheumatic
        |inactive or quiescent (with chorea) I05.9
      |tricuspid (valve) disease I08.1
        |with aortic (valve) disease I08.3
    |active or acute I01.1
      |with chorea (acute) (rheumatic)
        (Sydenham's) I02.0
      |bacterial I33.0
    |arteriosclerotic I34.8
    |nonrheumatic I34.8
      |acute or subacute I33.9
    |specified NEC I05.8
  |monilial B37.6
  |multiple valves I08.9
    |specified disorders I08.8
  |mycotic (acute) (any valve) (subacute) I33.0
  |pneumococcal (acute) (any valve) (subacute)
    I33.0
  |pulmonary (chronic) (heart) (valve) I37.8
    |with rheumatic fever (conditions in I00)
      |active *see* Endocarditis, acute, rheumatic
      |inactive or quiescent (with chorea) I09.89
        |with aortic, mitral or tricuspid disease
          I08.8
    |acute or subacute I33.9
      |rheumatic I01.1
        |with chorea (acute) (rheumatic)
          (Sydenham's) I02.0
    |arteriosclerotic I37.8
    |congenital Q22.2
    |rheumatic (chronic) (inactive) (with chorea)
      I09.89
      |active or acute I01.1
        |with chorea (acute) (rheumatic)
          (Sydenham's) I02.0
    |syphilitic A52.03
  |purulent (acute) (any valve) (subacute) I33.0
  |Q fever A78 [*I39*]
  |rheumatic (chronic) (inactive) (with chorea)
    I09.1
    |active or acute (aortic) (mitral) (pulmonary)
      (tricuspid) I01.1
      |with chorea (acute) (rheumatic)
        (Sydenham's) I02.0
  |rheumatoid *see* Rheumatoid, carditis
  |septic (acute) (any valve) (subacute) I33.0
  |streptococcal (acute) (any valve) (subacute)
    I33.0
  |subacute *see* Endocarditis, acute
  |suppurative (acute) (any valve) (subacute)
    I33.0
  |syphilitic A52.03
  |toxic I33.9

Endocarditis - *continued*
  |tricuspid (chronic) (heart) (inactive)
    (rheumatic) (valve) (with chorea) I07.9
    |with
      |aortic (valve) disease I08.2
        |mitral (valve) disease I08.3
      |mitral (valve) disease I08.1
        |aortic (valve) disease I08.3
      |rheumatic fever (conditions in I00)
        |active *see* Endocarditis, acute,
          rheumatic
        |inactive or quiescent (with chorea) I07.8
    |active or acute I01.1
      |with chorea (acute) (rheumatic)
        (Sydenham's) I02.0
    |arteriosclerotic I36.8
    |nonrheumatic I36.8
      |acute or subacute I33.9
    |specified cause, except rheumatic I36.8
  |tuberculous *see* Tuberculosis, endocarditis
  |typhoid A01.02
  |ulcerative (acute) (any valve) (subacute) I33.0
  |vegetative (acute) (any valve) (subacute) I33.0
  |verrucous (atypical) (nonbacterial)
    (nonrheumatic) M32.11
Endocardium, endocardial *see also* condition
  |cushion defect Q21.2
Endocervicitis *see also* Cervicitis
  |due to intrauterine (contraceptive) device
    T83.69
  |hyperplastic N72
Endocrine *see* condition
Endocrinopathy, pluriglandular E31.9
Endodontic
  |overfill M27.52
  |underfill M27.53
Endodontitis K04.01
  |irreversible K04.02
  |reversible K04.01
Endomastoiditis *see* Mastoiditis
Endometrioma N80.9
Endometriosis N80.9
  |appendix N80.5
  |bladder N80.8
  |bowel N80.5
  |broad ligament N80.3
  |cervix N80.0
  |colon N80.5
  |cul-de-sac (Douglas') N80.3
  |exocervix N80.0
  |fallopian tube N80.2
  |female genital organ NEC N80.8
  |gallbladder N80.8
  |in scar of skin N80.6
  |internal N80.0
  |intestine N80.5
  |lung N80.8
  |myometrium N80.0
  |ovary N80.1
  |parametrium N80.3
  |pelvic peritoneum N80.3
  |peritoneal (pelvic) N80.3
  |rectovaginal septum N80.4
  |rectum N80.5
  |round ligament N80.3
  |skin (scar) N80.6
  |specified site NEC N80.8
  |stromal D39.0
  |thorax N80.8
  |umbilicus N80.8
  |uterus (internal) N80.0
  |vagina N80.4
  |vulva N80.8

Endometritis (decidual) (nonspecific)
  (purulent) (senile) (atrophic) (suppurative)
  N71.9
  |with ectopic pregnancy O08.0
  |acute N71.0
  |blenorrhagic (gonococcal) (acute) (chronic)
    A54.24
  |cervix, cervical (with erosion or ectropion) *see*
    also Cervicitis
    |hyperplastic N72
  |chlamydial A56.11
  |chronic N71.1
  |following
    |abortion *see* Abortion by type complicated
      by genital infection
    |ectopic or molar pregnancy O08.0
  |gonococcal, gonorrheal (acute) (chronic)
    A54.24
  |hyperplastic *see also* Hyperplasia, endometrial
    N85.00-
    |cervix N72
  |puerperal, postpartum, childbirth O86.12
  |subacute N71.0
  |tuberculous A18.17
Endometrium *see* condition
Endomyocardiopathy, South African I42.3
Endomyocarditis *see* Endocarditis
Endomyofibrosis I42.3
Endomyometritis *see* Endometritis
Endopericarditis *see* Endocarditis
Endoperineuritis *see* Disorder, nerve
Endophlebitis *see* Phlebitis
Endophthalmia *see* Endophthalmitis, purulent
Endophthalmitis (acute) (infective)
  (metastatic) (subacute) H44.009
  |bleb associated H59.4 *see also* Bleb, inflamed
    (infected), postprocedural
  |gonorrheal A54.39
  |in (due to)
    |cysticercosis B69.1
    |onchocerciasis B73.01
    |toxocariasis B83.0
  |panuveitis *see* Panuveitis
  |parasitic H44.12-
  |purulent H44.00-
    |panophthalmitis *see* Panophthalmitis
    |vitreous abscess H44.02-
  |specified NEC H44.19
  |sympathetic *see* Uveitis, sympathetic
Endosalpingoma D28.2
Endosalpingiosis N94.89
Endosteitis *see* Osteomyelitis
Endothelioma, bone *see* Neoplasm, bone,
  malignant
Endotheliosis (hemorrhagic infectional) D69.8
Endotoxemia   code to condition
Endotrachelitis *see* Cervicitis
Engelmann (-Camurati) syndrome Q78.3
English disease *see* Rickets
Engman's disease L30.3
Engorgement
  |breast N64.59
    |newborn P83.4
    |puerperal, postpartum O92.79
  |lung (passive) *see* Edema, lung
  |pulmonary (passive) *see* Edema, lung
  |stomach K31.89
  |venous, retina *see* Occlusion, retina, vein,
    engorgement
Enlargement, enlarged *see also* Hypertrophy
  |adenoids J35.2
    |with tonsils J35.3
  |alveolar ridge K08.89
    |congenital *see* Anomaly, alveolar
  |apertures of diaphragm (congenital) Q79.1

Enlargement - *continued*
|gingival K06.1
|heart, cardiac *see* Hypertrophy, cardiac
|labium majus, childhood asymmetric (CALME) N90.61
|lacrimal gland, chronic H04.03-
|liver *see* Hypertrophy, liver
|lymph gland or node R59.9
| |generalized R59.1
| |localized R59.0
|orbit H05.34-
|organ or site, congenital NEC *see* Anomaly, by site
|parathyroid (gland) E21.0
|pituitary fossa R93.0
|prostate N40.0
| |with lower urinary tract symptoms (LUTS) N40.1
| |without lower urinary tract symptoms (LUTS) N40.0
|sella turcica R93.0
|spleen *see* Splenomegaly
|thymus (gland) (congenital) E32.0
|thyroid (gland) *see* Goiter
|tongue K14.8
|tonsils J35.1
| |with adenoids J35.3
|uterus N85.2
|vestibular aqueduct Q16.5
Enophthalmos H05.40-
|due to
| |orbital tissue atrophy H05.41-
| |trauma or surgery H05.42-
Enostosis M27.8
Entamebic, entamebiasis *see* Amebiasis
Entanglement
|umbilical cord(s) O69.82
| |with compression O69.2
| |around neck (with compression) O69.81
| |with compression O69.1
| |without compression O69.82
| |without compression O69.81
| |of twins in monoamniotic sac O69.2
Enteralgia *see* Pain, abdominal
Enteric *see* condition
Enteritis (acute) (diarrheal) (hemorrhagic) (noninfective) K52.9
|adenovirus A08.2
|aertrycke infection A02.0
|allergic K52.29
| |with
| |eosinophilic gastritis or gastroenteritis K52.81
| |food protein-induced enterocolitis syndrome K52.21
| |food protein-induced enteropathy K52.22
| |FPIES K52.21
|amebic (acute) A06.0
| |with abscess *see* Abscess, amebic
| |chronic A06.1
| |with abscess *see* Abscess, amebic
| |nondysenteric A06.2
| |nondysenteric A06.2
|astrovirus A08.32
|bacillary NOS A03.9
|bacterial A04.9
| |specified NEC A04.8
|calicivirus A08.31
|candidal B37.82
|Chilomastix A07.8
|choleriformis A00.1
|chronic (noninfectious) K52.9
| |ulcerative *see* Colitis, ulcerative

Enteritis - *continued*
|cicatrizing (chronic) *see* Enteritis, regional, small intestine
|Clostridium
| |botulinum (food poisoning) A05.1
| |difficile
| |not specified as recurrent A04.72
| |recurrent A04.71
|coccidial A07.3
|coxsackie virus A08.39
|dietetic *see also* Enteritis, allergic K52.29
|drug-induced K52.1
|due to
| |astrovirus A08.32
| |calicivirus A08.31
| |coxsackie virus A08.39
| |drugs K52.1
| |echovirus A08.39
| |enterovirus NEC A08.39
| |food hypersensitivity *see also* Enteritis, allergic K52.29
| |infectious organism (bacterial) (viral) *see* Enteritis, infectious
| |torovirus A08.39
| |Yersinia enterocolitica A04.6
|echovirus A08.39
|eltor A00.1
|enterovirus NEC A08.39
|eosinophilic K52.81
|epidemic (infectious) A09
|fulminant *see also* Ischemia, intestine, acute K55.019
|gangrenous *see* Enteritis, infectious
|giardial A07.1
|infectious NOS A09
| |due to
| |adenovirus A08.2
| |Aerobacter aerogenes A04.8
| |Arizona (bacillus) A02.0
| |bacteria NOS A04.9
| |specified NEC A04.8
| |Campylobacter A04.5
| |Clostridium difficile
| |not specified as recurrent A04.72
| |recurrent A04.71
| |Clostridium perfringens A04.8
| |Enterobacter aerogenes A04.8
| |enterovirus A08.39
| |Escherichia coli A04.4
| |enteroaggregative A04.4
| |enterohemorrhagic A04.3
| |enteroinvasive A04.2
| |enteropathogenic A04.0
| |enterotoxigenic A04.1
| |specified NEC A04.4
| |specified
| |bacteria NEC A04.8
| |virus NEC A08.39
| |Staphylococcus A04.8
| |virus NEC A08.4
| |specified type NEC A08.39
| |Yersinia enterocolitica A04.6
| |specified organism NEC A08.8
|influenzal *see* Influenza, with, digestive manifestations
|ischemic K55.9
| |acute *see also* Ischemia, intestine, acute K55.019
| |chronic K55.1
|microsporidial A07.8
|mucomembranous, myxomembranous *see* Syndrome, irritable bowel
|mucous *see* Syndrome, irritable bowel
|necroticans A05.2

Enteritis - *continued*
|necrotizing of newborn *see* Enterocolitis, necrotizing, in newborn
|neurogenic *see* Syndrome, irritable bowel
|newborn necrotizing *see* Enterocolitis, necrotizing, in newborn
|noninfectious K52.9
|norovirus A08.11
|parasitic NEC B82.9
|paratyphoid (fever) *see* Fever, paratyphoid
|protozoal A07.9
| |specified NEC A07.8
|radiation K52.0
|regional (of) K50.90
| |with
| |complication K50.919
| |abscess K50.914
| |fistula K50.913
| |intestinal obstruction K50.912
| |rectal bleeding K50.911
| |specified complication NEC K50.918
| |colon *see* Enteritis, regional, large intestine
| |duodenum *see* Enteritis, regional, small intestine
| |ileum *see* Enteritis, regional, small intestine
| |jejunum *see* Enteritis, regional, small intestine
| |large bowel *see* Enteritis, regional, large intestine
| |large intestine (colon) (rectum) K50.10
| |with
| |complication K50.119
| |abscess K50.114
| |fistula K50.113
| |intestinal obstruction K50.112
| |rectal bleeding K50.111
| |small intestine (duodenum) (ileum) (jejunum) involvement K50.80
| |with
| |complication K50.819
| |abscess K50.814
| |fistula K50.813
| |intestinal obstruction K50.812
| |rectal bleeding K50.811
| |specified complication NEC K50.818
| |specified complication NEC K50.118
| |rectum *see* Enteritis, regional, large intestine
| |small intestine (duodenum) (ileum) (jejunum) K50.00
| |with
| |complication K50.019
| |abscess K50.014
| |fistula K50.013
| |intestinal obstruction K50.012
| |large intestine (colon) (rectum) involvement K50.80
| |with
| |complication K50.819
| |abscess K50.814
| |fistula K50.813
| |intestinal obstruction K50.812
| |rectal bleeding K50.811
| |specified complication NEC K50.818
| |rectal bleeding K50.011
| |specified complication NEC K50.018
|Rotaviral A08.0
|Salmonella, salmonellosis (arizonae) (cholerae-suis) (enteritidis) (typhimurium) A02.0
|segmental *see* Enteritis, regional
|septic A09
|Shigella *see* Infection, Shigella
|small round structured NEC A08.19

Enteritis - *continued*
|spasmodic, spastic *see* Syndrome, irritable
  bowel
|staphylococcal A04.8
  |due to food A05.0
|torovirus A08.39
|toxic NEC K52.1
  |due to Clostridium difficile
    |not specified as recurrent A04.72
    |recurrent A04.71
|trichomonal A07.8
|tuberculous A18.32
|typhosa A01.00
|ulcerative (chronic) *see* Colitis, ulcerative
|viral A08.4
  |adenovirus A08.2
  |enterovirus A08.39
  |Rotavirus A08.0
  |small round structured NEC A08.19
  |specified NEC A08.39
  |virus specified NEC A08.39
Enterobiasis B80
Enterobius vermicularis (infection)
  (infestation) B80
Enterocele *see also* Hernia, abdomen
|pelvic, pelvis (acquired) (congenital) N81.5
|vagina, vaginal (acquired) (congenital) NEC
  N81.5
Enterocolitis *see also* Enteritis K52.9
|due to Clostridium difficile
  |not specified as recurrent A04.72
  |recurrent A04.71
|fulminant ischemic *see also* Ischemia,
  intestine, acute K55.059
|granulomatous *see* Enteritis, regional
|hemorrhagic (acute) *see also* Ischemia,
  intestine, acute K55.059
  |chronic K55.1
|infectious NEC A09
|ischemic K55.9
|necrotizing K55.30
  |with
    |perforation K55.33
    |pneumatosis K55.32
      |and perforation K55.33
  |due to Clostridium difficile
    |not specified as recurrent A04.72
    |recurrent A04.71
  |in non-newborn K55.30
    |stage 1 (without pneumatosis, without
      perforation) K55.31
    |stage 2 (with pneumatosis, without
      perforation) K55.32
    |stage 3 (with pneumatosis, with
      perforation) K55.33
  |in newborn P77.9
    |stage 1 (without pneumatosis, without
      perforation) P77.1
    |stage 2 (with pneumatosis, without
      perforation) P77.2
    |stage 3 (with pneumatosis, with
      perforation) P77.3
  |without pneumatosis or perforation K55.31
|noninfectious K52.9
  |newborn *see* Enterocolitis, necrotizing, in
    newborn
|pseudomembranous (newborn)
  |not specified as recurrent A04.72
  |recurrent A04.71
|radiation K52.0
  |newborn *see* Enterocolitis, necrotizing, in
    newborn
|ulcerative (chronic) *see* Pancolitis, ulcerative
  (chronic)
Enterogastritis *see* Enteritis

Enteropathy K63.9
|celiac-gluten-sensitive K90.0
  |non-celiac K90.41
|food protein-induced enterocolitis (FPIES)
  K52.22
|hemorrhagic, terminal *see also* Ischemia,
  intestine, acute K55.059
|protein-losing K90.49
Enteroperitonitis *see* Peritonitis
Enteroptosis K63.4
Enterorrhagia K92.2
Enterospasm *see also* Syndrome, irritable,
  bowel
|psychogenic F45.8
Enterostenosis (see also Obstruction, intestine,
  specified NEC) K56.699
Enterostomy
|complication *see* Complication, enterostomy
|status Z93.4
Enterovirus, as cause of disease classified
  elsewhere B97.10
|coxsackievirus B97.11
|echovirus B97.12
|other specified B97.19
Enthesopathy (peripheral) M77.9
|Achilles tendinitis *see* Tendinitis, Achilles
|ankle and tarsus M77.9
  |specified type NEC *see* Enthesopathy, foot,
    specified type NEC
|anterior tibial syndrome M76.81-
|calcaneal spur *see* Spur, bone, calcaneal
|elbow region M77.8
  |lateral epicondylitis *see* Epicondylitis,
    lateral
  |medial epicondylitis *see* Epicondylitis,
    medial
|foot NEC M77.8
  |metatarsalgia *see* Metatarsalgia
  |specified type NEC M77.5-
|forearm M77.8
|gluteal tendinitis *see* Tendinitis, gluteal
|hand M77.8
|hip *see* Enthesopathy, lower limb, specified
  type NEC
|iliac crest spur *see* Spur, bone, iliac crest
|iliotibial band syndrome *see* Syndrome,
  iliotibial band
|knee *see* Enthesopathy, lower limb, lower leg,
  specified type NEC
|lateral epicondylitis *see* Epicondylitis, lateral
|lower limb (excluding foot) M76.9
  |Achilles tendinitis *see* Tendinitis, Achilles
  |anterior tibial syndrome M76.81-
  |gluteal tendinitis *see* Tendinitis, gluteal
  |iliac crest spur *see* Spur, bone, iliac crest
  |iliotibial band syndrome *see* Syndrome,
    iliotibial band
  |patellar tendinitis *see* Tendinitis, patellar
  |pelvic region *see* Enthesopathy, lower limb,
    specified type NEC
  |peroneal tendinitis *see* Tendinitis, peroneal
  |posterior tibial syndrome M76.82-
  |psoas tendinitis *see* Tendinitis, psoas
  |shoulder M77.8
  |specified type NEC M76.89-
  |tibial collateral bursitis *see* Bursitis, tibial
    collateral
|medial epicondylitis *see* Epicondylitis, medial
|metatarsalgia *see* Metatarsalgia
|multiple sites M77.8
|patellar tendinitis *see* Tendinitis, patellar
|pelvis M77.8
|periarthritis of wrist *see* Periarthritis, wrist
|peroneal tendinitis *see* Tendinitis, peroneal
|posterior tibial syndrome M76.82-

Enthesopathy - *continued*
|psoas tendinitis *see* Tendinitis, psoas
|shoulder region *see* Lesion, shoulder
|specified type NEC M77.8
|spinal M46.00
  |cervical region M46.02
  |cervicothoracic region M46.03
  |lumbar region M46.06
  |lumbosacral region M46.07
  |multiple sites M46.09
  |occipito-atlanto-axial region M46.01
  |sacrococcygeal region M46.08
  |thoracic region M46.04
  |thoracolumbar region M46.05
|tibial collateral bursitis *see* Bursitis, tibial
  collateral
|upper arm M77.8
|wrist and carpus NEC M77.8
  |calcaneal spur *see* Spur, bone, calcaneal
  |periarthritis of wrist *see* Periarthritis, wrist
Entomophobia F40.218
Entomophthoromycosis B46.8
Entrance, air into vein *see* Embolism, air
Entrapment, nerve *see* Neuropathy, entrapment
Entropion (eyelid) (paralytic) H02.009
|cicatricial H02.019
  |left H02.016
    |lower H02.015
    |upper H02.014
  |right H02.013
    |lower H02.012
    |upper H02.011
|congenital Q10.2
|left H02.006
  |lower H02.005
  |upper H02.004
|mechanical H02.029
  |left H02.026
    |lower H02.025
    |upper H02.024
  |right H02.023
    |lower H02.022
    |upper H02.021
|right H02.003
  |lower H02.002
  |upper H02.001
|senile H02.039
  |left H02.036
    |lower H02.035
    |upper H02.034
  |right H02.033
    |lower H02.032
    |upper H02.031
|spastic H02.049
  |left H02.046
    |lower H02.045
    |upper H02.044
  |right H02.043
    |lower H02.042
    |upper H02.041
Enucleated eye (traumatic, current) S05.7-
Enuresis R32
|functional F98.0
|habit disturbance F98.0
|nocturnal N39.44
  |psychogenic F98.0
|nonorganic origin F98.0
|psychogenic F98.0
Eosinopenia *see* Agranulocytosis
Eosinophilia (allergic)(idiopathic) (secondary)
  D72.1
|with
  |angiolymphoid hyperplasia (ALHE) D18.01
|familial D72.19
|hereditary D72.19

Eosinophilia - *continued*
|in disease classified elsewhere D72.18
|infiltrative *see* Eosinophilia, pulmonary
|Löffler's J82.89
|peritoneal *see* Peritonitis, eosinophilic
|pulmonary NEC J82.89
  |acute J82.82
  |asthmatic J82.83
  |chronic J82.81
|specified NEC D72.19
|tropical (pulmonary) J82.89
Eosinophilia-Myalgia syndrome M35.8
Ependymitis (acute) (cerebral) (chronic) (granular) *see* Encephalomyelitis
Ependymoblastoma
|specified site *see* Neoplasm, malignant, by site
|unspecified site C71.9
Ependymoma (epithelial) (malignant)
|anaplastic
  |specified site *see* Neoplasm, malignant, by site
  |unspecified site C71.9
|benign
  |specified site *see* Neoplasm, benign, by site
  |unspecified site D33.2
|myxopapillary D43.2
  |specified site *see* Neoplasm, uncertain behavior, by site
  |unspecified site D43.2
|papillary D43.2
  |specified site *see* Neoplasm, uncertain behavior, by site
  |unspecified site D43.2
|specified site *see* Neoplasm, malignant, by site
|unspecified site C71.9
Ependymopathy G93.89
Ephelis, ephelides L81.2
Epiblepharon (congenital) Q10.3
Epicanthus, epicanthic fold (eyelid) (congenital) Q10.3
Epicondylitis (elbow)
|lateral M77.1-
|medial M77.0-
Epicystitis *see* Cystitis
Epidemic *see* condition
Epidermidalization, cervix *see* Dysplasia, cervix
Epidermis, epidermal *see* condition
Epidermodysplasia verruciformis B07.8
Epidermolysis
|bullosa (congenital) Q81.9
  |acquired L12.30
    |drug-induced L12.31
    |specified cause NEC L12.35
  |dystrophica Q81.2
  |letalis Q81.1
  |simplex Q81.0
  |specified NEC Q81.8
|necroticans combustiformis L51.2
  |due to drug *see* Table of Drugs and Chemicals, by drug
Epidermophytid *see* Dermatophytosis
Epidermophytosis (infected) *see* Dermatophytosis
Epididymis *see* condition
Epididymitis (acute) (nonvenereal) (recurrent) (residual) N45.1
|with orchitis N45.3
|blennorrhagic (gonococcal) A54.23
|caseous (tuberculous) A18.15
|chlamydial A56.19
|filarial *see also* Infestation, filarial B74.9 *[N51]*
|gonococcal A54.23
|syphilitic A52.76
|tuberculous A18.15

Epididymo-Orchitis *see also* Epididymitis N45.3
Epidural *see* condition
Epigastrium, epigastric *see* condition
Epigastrocele *see* Hernia, ventral
Epiglottis *see* condition
Epiglottitis, epiglottiditis (acute) J05.10
|with obstruction J05.11
|chronic J37.0
Epignathus Q89.4
Epilepsia partialis continua *see also* Kozhevnikov's epilepsy G40.1-
Epilepsy, epileptic, epilepsia (attack) (cerebral) (convulsion) (fit) (seizure) G40.909
|Note: the following terms are to be considered equivalent to intractable: pharmacoresistent (pharmacologically resistant), treatment resistant, refractory (medically) and poorly controlled
|with
  |complex partial seizures *see* Epilepsy, localization-related, symptomatic, with complex partial seizures
  |grand mal seizures on awakening *see* Epilepsy, generalized, specified NEC
  |myoclonic absences *see* Epilepsy, generalized, specified NEC
  |myoclonic-astatic seizures *see* Epilepsy, generalized, specified NEC
  |simple partial seizures *see* Epilepsy, localization-related, symptomatic, with simple partial seizures
|akinetic *see* Epilepsy, generalized, specified NEC
|benign childhood with centrotemporal EEG spikes *see* Epilepsy, localization-related, idiopathic
|benign myoclonic in infancy G40.80-
|Bravais-Jacksonian *see* Epilepsy, localization-related, symptomatic, with simple partial seizures
|childhood
  |with occipital EEG paroxysms *see* Epilepsy, localization-related, idiopathic
  |absence G40.A09
    |intractable G40.A19
      |with status epilepticus G40.A11
      |without status epilepticus G40.A19
    |not intractable G40.A09
      |with status epilepticus G40.A01
      |without status epilepticus G40.A09
|climacteric *see* Epilepsy, specified NEC
|cysticercosis B69.0
|deterioration (mental) F06.8
|due to syphilis A52.19
|focal *see* Epilepsy, localization-related, symptomatic, with simple partial seizures
|generalized
  |idiopathic G40.309
    |intractable G40.319
      |with status epilepticus G40.311
      |without status epilepticus G40.319
    |not intractable G40.309
      |with status epilepticus G40.301
      |without status epilepticus G40.309
  |specified NEC G40.409
    |intractable G40.419
      |with status epilepticus G40.411
      |without status epilepticus G40.419
    |not intractable G40.409
      |with status epilepticus G40.401
      |without status epilepticus G40.409

Epilepsy, epileptic, epilepsia - *continued*
|impulsive petit mal *see* Epilepsy, juvenile myoclonic
|intractable G40.919
  |with status epilepticus G40.911
  |without status epilepticus G40.919
|juvenile absence G40.A09
  |intractable G40.A19
    |with status epilepticus G40.A11
    |without status epilepticus G40.A19
  |not intractable G40.A09
    |with status epilepticus G40.A01
    |without status epilepticus G40.A09
|juvenile myoclonic G40.B09
  |intractable G40.B19
    |with status epilepticus G40.B11
    |without status epilepticus G40.B19
  |not intractable G40.B09
    |with status epilepticus G40.B01
    |without status epilepticus G40.B09
|localization-related (focal) (partial)
  |idiopathic G40.009
    |with seizures of localized onset G40.009
      |intractable G40.019
        |with status epilepticus G40.011
        |without status epilepticus G40.019
      |not intractable G40.009
        |with status epilepticus G40.001
        |without status epilepticus G40.009
  |symptomatic
    |with complex partial seizures G40.209
      |intractable G40.219
        |with status epilepticus G40.211
        |without status epilepticus G40.219
      |not intractable G40.209
        |with status epilepticus G40.201
        |without status epilepticus G40.209
    |with simple partial seizures G40.109
      |intractable G40.119
        |with status epilepticus G40.111
        |without status epilepticus G40.119
      |not intractable G40.109
        |with status epilepticus G40.101
        |without status epilepticus G40.109
|myoclonus, myoclonic *see also* Epilepsy, generalized, specified NEC
|progressive *see* Epilepsy, generalized, idiopathic
|severe, in infancy (SMEI) G40.83-
|not intractable G40.909
  |with status epilepticus G40.901
  |without status epilepticus G40.909
|on awakening *see* Epilepsy, generalized, specified NEC
|parasitic NOS B71.9 *[G94]*
|partialis continua *see also* Kozhevnikov's epilepsy G40.1-
|peripheral *see* Epilepsy, specified NEC
|polymorphic, in infancy (PMEI) G40.83-
|procursiva *see* Epilepsy, localization-related, symptomatic, with simple partial seizures
|progressive (familial) myoclonic *see* Epilepsy, generalized, idiopathic
|reflex *see* Epilepsy, specified NEC
|related to
  |alcohol G40.509
    |not intractable G40.509
      |with status epilepticus G40.501
      |without status epilepticus G40.509
  |drugs G40.509
    |not intractable G40.509
      |with status epilepticus G40.501
      |without status epilepticus G40.509
  |external causes G40.509
    |not intractable G40.509

Epilepsy, epileptic, epilepsia - *continued*
  |with status epilepticus G40.501
  |without status epilepticus G40.509
 |hormonal changes G40.509
  |not intractable G40.509
   |with status epilepticus G40.501
   |without status epilepticus G40.509
 |sleep deprivation G40.509
  |not intractable G40.509
   |with status epilepticus G40.501
   |without status epilepticus G40.509
 |stress G40.509
  |not intractable G40.509
   |with status epilepticus G40.501
   |without status epilepticus G40.509
 |somatomotor *see* Epilepsy, localization-
  related, symptomatic, with simple partial
  seizures
 |somatosensory *see* Epilepsy, localization-
  related, symptomatic, with simple partial
  seizures
 |spasms G40.822
  |intractable G40.824
   |with status epilepticus G40.823
   |without status epilepticus G40.824
  |not intractable G40.822
   |with status epilepticus G40.821
   |without status epilepticus G40.822
 |specified NEC G40.802
  |intractable G40.804
   |with status epilepticus G40.803
   |without status epilepticus G40.804
  |not intractable G40.802
   |with status epilepticus G40.801
   |without status epilepticus G40.802
 |syndromes
  |generalized
   |idiopathic G40.309
    |intractable G40.319
     |with status epilepticus G40.311
     |without status epilepticus G40.319
    |not intractable G40.309
     |with status epilepticus G40.301
     |without status epilepticus G40.309
   |specified NEC G40.409
    |intractable G40.419
     |with status epilepticus G40.411
     |without status epilepticus G40.419
    |not intractable G40.409
     |with status epilepticus G40.401
     |without status epilepticus G40.409
  |localization-related (focal) (partial)
   |idiopathic G40.009
    |with seizures of localized onset
     G40.009
    |intractable G40.019
     |with status epilepticus G40.011
     |without status epilepticus G40.019
    |not intractable G40.009
     |with status epilepticus G40.001
     |without status epilepticus G40.009
   |symptomatic
    |with complex partial seizures G40.209
     |intractable G40.219
      |with status epilepticus G40.211
      |without status epilepticus G40.219
     |not intractable G40.209
      |with status epilepticus G40.201
      |without status epilepticus G40.209
    |with simple partial seizures G40.109
     |intractable G40.119
      |with status epilepticus G40.111
      |without status epilepticus G40.119
     |not intractable G40.109
      |with status epilepticus G40.101
      |without status epilepticus G40.109
 |specified NEC G40.802
  |intractable G40.804

Epilepsy, epileptic, epilepsia - *continued*
  |with status epilepticus G40.803
  |without status epilepticus G40.804
  |not intractable G40.802
   |with status epilepticus G40.801
   |without status epilepticus G40.802
 |tonic (-clonic) *see* Epilepsy, generalized,
  specified NEC
 |twilight F05
 |uncinate (gyrus) *see* Epilepsy, localization-
  related, symptomatic, with complex partial
  seizures
 |Unverricht (-Lundborg) (familial myoclonic)
  see Epilepsy, generalized, idiopathic
 |visceral *see* Epilepsy, specified NEC
 |visual *see* Epilepsy, specified NEC
Epiloia Q85.1
Epimenorrhea N92.0
Epipharyngitis *see* Nasopharyngitis
Epiphora H04.20-
 |due to
  |excess lacrimation H04.21-
  |insufficient drainage H04.22-
Epiphyseal arrest *see* Arrest, epiphyseal
Epiphyseolysis, epiphysiolysis *see*
 Osteochondropathy
Epiphysitis *see also* Osteochondropathy
 |juvenile M92.9
 |syphilitic (congenital) A50.02
Epiplocele *see* Hernia, abdomen
Epiploitis *see* Peritonitis
Epiplosarcomphalocele *see* Hernia, umbilicus
Episcleritis (suppurative) H15.10-
 |in (due to)
  |syphilis A52.71
  |tuberculosis A18.51
 |nodular H15.12-
 |periodica fugax H15.11-
  |angioneurotic *see* Edema, angioneurotic
 |syphilitic (late) A52.71
 |tuberculous A18.51
Episode
 |affective, mixed F39
 |depersonalization (in neurotic state) F48.1
 |depressive F32.A
  |major F32.9
   |mild F32.0
   |moderate F32.1
   |severe (without psychotic symptoms)
    F32.2
    |with psychotic symptoms F32.3
  |recurrent F33.9
   |brief F33.8
  |specified NEC F32.89
 |hypomanic F30.8
 |manic F30.9
  |with
   |psychotic symptoms F30.2
   |remission (full) F30.4
    |partial F30.3
  |other specified F30.8
  |recurrent F31.89
  |without psychotic symptoms F30.10
   |mild F30.11
   |moderate F30.12
   |severe (without psychotic symptoms)
    F30.13
    |with psychotic symptoms F30.2
 |psychotic F23
  |organic F06.8
 |schizophrenic (acute) NEC, brief F23
Epispadias (female) (male) Q64.0
Episplenitis D73.89
Epistaxis (multiple) R04.0
 |hereditary I78.0
 |vicarious menstruation N94.89

Epithelioma (malignant) *see also* Neoplasm,
 malignant, by site
 |adenoides cysticum *see* Neoplasm, skin,
  benign
 |basal cell *see* Neoplasm, skin, malignant
 |benign *see* Neoplasm, benign, by site
 |Bowen's *see* Neoplasm, skin, in situ
 |calcifying, of Malherbe *see* Neoplasm, skin,
  benign
 |external site *see* Neoplasm, skin, malignant
 |intraepidermal, Jadassohn *see* Neoplasm, skin,
  benign
 |squamous cell *see* Neoplasm, malignant, by
  site
Epitheliomatosis pigmented Q82.1
Epitheliopathy, multifocal placoid pigment
 H30.14-
Epithelium, epithelial *see* condition
Epituberculosis (with atelectasis) (allergic)
 A15.7
Eponychia Q84.6
Epstein's
 |nephrosis or syndrome *see* Nephrosis
 |pearl K09.8
Epulis (gingiva) (fibrous) (giant cell) K06.8
Equinia A24.0
Equinovarus (congenital) (talipes) Q66.0
 |acquired *see* Deformity, limb, clubfoot
Equivalent
 |convulsive (abdominal) *see* Epilepsy,
  specified NEC
 |epileptic (psychic) *see* Epilepsy, localization-
  related, symptomatic, with complex partial
  seizures
Erb (-Duchenne) paralysis (birth injury)
 (newborn) P14.0
Erb-Goldflam disease or syndrome G70.00
 |with exacerbation (acute) G70.01
 |in crisis G70.01
Erb's
 |disease G71.02
 |palsy, paralysis (brachial) (birth) (newborn)
  P14.0
  |spinal (spastic) syphilitic A52.17
 |pseudohypertrophic muscular dystrophy
  G71.02
Erdheim's syndrome (acromegalic
 macrospondylitis) E22.0
Erection, painful (persistent) *see* Priapism
Ergosterol deficiency (vitamin D) E55.9
 |with
  |adult osteomalacia M83.8
  |rickets *see* Rickets
Ergotism *see also* Poisoning, food, noxious,
 plant
 |from ergot used as drug (migraine therapy) *see*
  Table of Drugs and Chemicals
Erosio interdigitalis blastomycetica B37.2
Erosion
 |artery I77.2
  |without rupture I77.89
 |bone *see* Disorder, bone, density and structure,
  specified NEC
 |bronchus J98.09
 |cartilage (joint) *see* Disorder, cartilage,
  specified type NEC
 |cervix (uteri) (acquired) (chronic) (congenital)
  N86
  |with cervicitis N72
 |cornea (nontraumatic) *see* Ulcer, cornea
  |recurrent H18.83
  |traumatic *see* Abrasion, cornea
 |dental (idiopathic) (occupational) (due to diet,
  drugs or vomiting) K03.2
 |duodenum, postpyloric *see* Ulcer, duodenum
 |esophagus K22.10

Erosion - *continued*
 |with bleeding K22.11
 |gastric *see* Ulcer, stomach
 |gastrojejunal *see* Ulcer, gastrojejunal
 |implanted mesh *see* Complications, prosthetic
  device or implant, mesh
 |intestine K63.3
 |lymphatic vessel I89.8
 |pylorus, pyloric (ulcer) *see* Ulcer, stomach
 |spine, aneurysmal A52.09
 |stomach *see* Ulcer, stomach
 |subcutaneous device pocket
  |nervous system prosthetic device, implant,
   or graft T85.890
  |other internal prosthetic device, implant, or
   graft T85.898
 |teeth (idiopathic) (occupational) (due to diet,
  drugs or vomiting) K03.2
 |urethra N36.8
 |uterus N85.8
Erotomania F52.8
Error
 |metabolism, inborn *see* Disorder, metabolism
 |refractive *see* Disorder, refraction
Eructation R14.2
 |nervous or psychogenic F45.8
Eruption
 |creeping B76.9
 |drug (generalized) (taken internally) L27.0
  |fixed L27.1
  |in contact with skin *see* Dermatitis, due to
   drugs
  |localized L27.1
 |Hutchinson, summer L56.4
 |Kaposi's varicelliform B00.0
 |napkin L22
 |polymorphous light (sun) L56.4
 |recalcitrant pustular L13.8
 |ringed R23.8
 |skin (nonspecific) R21
  |creeping (meaning hookworm) B76.9
  |due to inoculation/vaccination (generalized)
   see also Dermatitis, due to, vaccine L27.0
   |localized L27.1
  |erysipeloid A26.0
  |feigned L98.1
  |Kaposi's varicelliform B00.0
  |lichenoid L28.0
  |meaning dermatitis *see* Dermatitis
  |toxic NEC L53.0
 |tooth, teeth, abnormal (incomplete) (late)
  (premature) (sequence) K00.6
 |vesicular R23.8
Erysipelas (gangrenous) (infantile) (newborn)
 (phlegmonous) (suppurative) A46
 |external ear A46 [*H62.40*]
 |puerperal, postpartum O86.89
Erysipeloid A26.9
 |cutaneous (Rosenbach's) A26.0
 |disseminated A26.8
 |sepsis A26.7
 |specified NEC A26.8
Erythema, erythematous (infectional)
 (inflammation) L53.9
 |ab igne L59.0
 |annulare (centrifugum) (rheumaticum) L53.1
 |arthriticum epidemicum A25.1
 |brucellum *see* Brucellosis
 |chronic figurate NEC L53.3
 |chronicum migrans (Borrelia burgdorferi)
  A69.20
 |diaper L22
 |due to
  |chemical NEC L53.0
   |in contact with skin L24.5
  |drug (internal use) *see* Dermatitis, due to,
   drugs
 |elevatum diutinum L95.1

Erythema, erythematous - *continued*
 |endemic E52
 |epidemic, arthritic A25.1
 |figuratum perstans L53.3
 |gluteal L22
 |heat code by site under Burn, first degree
 |ichthyosiforme congenitum bullous Q80.3
 |in diseases classified elsewhere L54
 |induratum (nontuberculous) L52
  |tuberculous A18.4
 |infectiosum B08.3
 |intertrigo L30.4
 |iris L51.9
 |marginatum L53.2
  |in (due to) acute rheumatic fever I00
 |medicamentosum *see* Dermatitis, due to, drugs
 |migrans A26.0
  |chronicum A69.20
  |tongue K14.1
 |multiforme (major) (minor) L51.9
  |bullous, bullosum L51.1
  |conjunctiva L51.1
  |nonbullous L51.0
  |pemphigoides L12.0
  |specified NEC L51.8
 |napkin L22
 |neonatorum P83.88
  |toxic P83.1
 |nodosum L52
  |tuberculous A18.4
 |palmar L53.8
 |pernio T69.1
 |rash, newborn P83.88
 |scarlatiniform (recurrent) (exfoliative) L53.8
 |solare L55.0
 |specified NEC L53.8
 |toxic, toxicum NEC L53.0
  |newborn P83.1
 |tuberculous (primary) A18.4
Erythematous, erythematosus *see* condition
Erythermalgia (primary) I73.81
Erythralgia I73.81
Erythrasma L08.1
Erythredema (polyneuropathy) *see* Poisoning,
 mercury
Erythremia (acute) C94.0-
 |chronic D45
 |secondary D75.1
Erythroblastopenia *see also* Aplasia, red cell
 D60.9
 |congenital D61.01
Erythroblastophthisis D61.09
Erythroblastosis (fetalis) (newborn) P55.9
 |due to
  |ABO (antibodies) (incompatibility)
   (isoimmunization) P55.1
  |Rh (antibodies) (incompatibility)
   (isoimmunization) P55.0
Erythrocyanosis (crurum) I73.89
Erythrocythemia *see* Erythremia
Erythrocytosis (megalosplenic) (secondary)
 D75.1
 |familial D75.0
 |oval, hereditary *see* Elliptocytosis
 |secondary D75.1
 |stress D75.1
Erythroderma (secondary) *see also* Erythema
 L53.9
 |bullous ichthyosiform, congenital Q80.3
 |desquamativum L21.1
 |ichthyosiform, congenital (bullous) Q80.3
 |neonatorum P83.88
 |psoriaticum L40.8
Erythrodysesthesia, palmar plantar (PPE)
 L27.1
Erythrogenesis imperfecta D61.09

Erythroleukemia C94.0-
Erythromelalgia I73.81
Erythrophagocytosis D75.89
Erythrophobia F40.298
Erythroplakia, oral epithelium, and tongue
 K13.29
Erythroplasia (Queyrat) D07.4
 |specified site *see* Neoplasm, skin, in situ
 |unspecified site D07.4
Escherichia coli (E. coli), as cause of disease
 classified elsewhere B96.20
 |non-O157 Shiga toxin-producing (with known
  O group) B96.22
 |non-Shiga toxin-producing B96.29
 |O157 with confirmation of Shiga toxin when
  H antigen is unknown, or is not H7 B96.21
 |O157:H (nonmotile) with confirmation of
  Shiga toxin B96.21
 |Shiga toxin-producing (with unspecified O
  group) (STEC) B96.23
 |O157 B96.21
 |O157:H7 with or without confirmation of
  Shiga toxin-production B96.21
  |specified NEC B96.22
 |specified NEC B96.29
Esophagismus K22.4
Esophagitis (acute) (alkaline) (chemical)
 (chronic) (infectional) (necrotic) (peptic)
 (postoperative)(without bleeding) K20.90
 |with bleeding K20.91
 |candidal B37.81
 |due to gastrointestinal reflux disease (without
  bleeding) K21.00
  |with bleeding K21.01
 |eosinophilic K20.0
 |reflux K21.00
 |specified NEC K20.80
  |with bleeding K20.81
 |tuberculous A18.83
 |ulcerative K22.10
  |with bleeding K22.11
Esophagocele K22.5
Esophagomalacia K22.89
Esophagospasm K22.4
Esophagostenosis K22.2
Esophagostomiasis B81.8
Esophagotracheal *see* condition
Esophagus *see* condition
Esophoria H50.51
 |convergence, excess H51.12
 |divergence, insufficiency H51.8
Esotropia *see* Strabismus, convergent
 concomitant
Espundia B55.2
Essential *see* condition
Esthesioneuroblastoma C30.0
Esthesioneurocytoma C30.0
Esthesioneuroepithelioma C30.0
Esthiomene A55
Estivo-Autumnal malaria (fever) B50.9
Estrangement (marital) Z63.5
 |parent-child NEC Z62.890
Estriasis *see* Myiasis
Ethanolism *see* Alcoholism
Etherism *see* Dependence, drug, inhalant
Ethmoid, ethmoidal *see* condition
Ethmoiditis (chronic) (nonpurulent)
 (purulent) *see also* Sinusitis, ethmoidal
 |influenzal *see* Influenza, with, respiratory
  manifestations NEC
 |Woakes' J33.1
Ethylism *see* Alcoholism
Eulenburg's disease (congenital
 paramyotonia) G71.19
Eumycetoma B47.0
Eunuchoidism E29.1
 |hypogonadotropic E23.0

European blastomycosis *see* Cryptococcosis
Eustachian *see* condition
Evaluation (for) (of)
|development state
  |adolescent Z00.3
  |period of
    |delayed growth in childhood Z00.70
      |with abnormal findings Z00.71
    |rapid growth in childhood Z00.2
  |puberty Z00.3
|growth and developmental state (period of
    rapid growth) Z00.2
  |delayed growth Z00.70
    |with abnormal findings Z00.71
|mental health (status) Z00.8
  |requested by authority Z04.6
|period of
  |delayed growth in childhood Z00.70
    |with abnormal findings Z00.71
  |rapid growth in childhood Z00.2
|suspected condition *see* Observation
Evans syndrome D69.41
Event
|apparent life threatening in newborn and
    infant (ALTE) R68.13
|brief resolved unexplained event (BRUE)
    R68.13
Eventration *see also* Hernia, ventral
|colon into chest *see* Hernia, diaphragm
|diaphragm (congenital) Q79.1
Eversion
|bladder N32.89
|cervix (uteri) N86
  |with cervicitis N72
|foot NEC *see also* Deformity, valgus, ankle
  |congenital Q66.6
|punctum lacrimale (postinfectional) (senile)
    H04.52-
|ureter (meatus) N28.89
|urethra (meatus) N36.8
|uterus N81.4
Evidence
|cytologic
  |of malignancy on anal smear R85.614
  |of malignancy on cervical smear R87.614
  |of malignancy on vaginal smear R87.624
Evisceration
|birth injury P15.8
|traumatic NEC
  |eye *see* Enucleated eye
Evulsion *see* Avulsion
Ewing's sarcoma or tumor *see* Neoplasm,
  bone, malignant
Examination (for) (following) (general) (of)
(routine) Z00.00
|with abnormal findings Z00.01
|abuse, physical (alleged), ruled out
  |adult Z04.71
  |child Z04.72
|adolescent (development state) Z00.3
|alleged rape or sexual assault (victim), ruled
    out
  |adult Z04.41
  |child Z04.42
|allergy Z01.82
|annual (adult) (periodic) (physical) Z00.00
  |with abnormal findings Z00.01
  |gynecological Z01.419
    |with abnormal findings Z01.411
|antibody response Z01.84
|blood *see* Examination, laboratory |blood
    pressure Z01.30
  |with abnormal findings Z01.31
|cancer staging *see* Neoplasm, malignant, by
    site
|cervical Papanicolaou smear Z12.4

Examination - *continued*
|as part of routine gynecological examination
    Z01.419
  |with abnormal findings Z01.411
|child (over 28 days old) Z00.129
  |with abnormal findings Z00.121
  |under 28 days old *see* Newborn,
    examination
|clinical research control or normal comparison
    (control) (participant) Z00.6
|contraceptive (drug) maintenance (routine)
    Z30.8
  |device (intrauterine) Z30.431
|dental Z01.20
  |with abnormal findings Z01.21
|developmental *see* Examination, child
  |donor (potential) Z00.5
|ear Z01.10
  |with abnormal findings NEC Z01.118
|eye Z01.00
  |with abnormal findings Z01.01
|following
  |accident NEC Z04.3
    |transport Z04.1
    |work Z04.2
  |assault, alleged, ruled out
    |adult Z04.71
    |child Z04.72
  |motor vehicle accident Z04.1
  |treatment (for) Z09
    |combined NEC Z09
      |fracture Z09
      |malignant neoplasm Z08
    |malignant neoplasm Z08
    |mental disorder Z09
    |specified condition NEC Z09
|follow-up (routine) (following) Z09
  |chemotherapy NEC Z09
    |malignant neoplasm Z08
  |fracture Z09
  |malignant neoplasm Z08
  |postpartum Z39.2
  |psychotherapy Z09
  |radiotherapy NEC Z09
    |malignant neoplasm Z08
  |surgery NEC Z09
    |malignant neoplasm Z08
|forced sexual exploitation Z04.81
|forced labor exploitation Z04.82
|gynecological Z01.419
  |with abnormal findings Z01.411
  |for contraceptive maintenance Z30.8
|health *see* Examination, medical
|hearing Z01.10
  |infant or child (over 28 days old) Z00.129
    |with abnormal findings Z00.121
  |with abnormal findings NEC Z01.118
    |following failed hearing screening Z01.110
|immunity status testing Z01.84
|laboratory (as part of a general medical
    examination) Z00.00
  |with abnormal findings Z00.01
  |preprocedural Z01.812
|lactating mother Z39.1
|medical (adult) (for) (of) Z00.00
  |with abnormal findings Z00.01
  |administrative purpose only Z02.9
    |specified NEC Z02.89
  |admission to
    |armed forces Z02.3
    |old age home Z02.2
    |prison Z02.89
    |residential institution Z02.2
    |school Z02.0

Examination - *continued*
  |following illness or medical treatment
    Z02.0
  |summer camp Z02.89
|adoption Z02.82
|blood alcohol or drug level Z02.83
|camp (summer) Z02.89
|clinical research, normal subject (control)
    (participant) Z00.6
|control subject in clinical research (normal
    comparison) (participant) Z00.6
|donor (potential) Z00.5
|driving license Z02.4
|general (adult) Z00.00
  |with abnormal findings Z00.01
|immigration Z02.89
|insurance purposes Z02.6
|marriage Z02.89
|medicolegal reasons NEC Z04.89
|naturalization Z02.89
|participation in sport Z02.5
|paternity testing Z02.81
|population survey Z00.8
|pre-employment Z02.1
|pre-operative *see* Examination, pre-
    procedural
|pre-procedural
  |cardiovascular Z01.810
  |respiratory Z01.811
  |specified NEC Z01.818
|preschool children
  |for admission to school Z02.0
|prisoners
  |for entrance into prison Z02.89
|recruitment for armed forces Z02.3
|specified NEC Z00.8
|sport competition Z02.5
|medicolegal reason NEC Z04.89
  |following
    |forced sexual exploitation Z04.81
    |forced labor exploitation Z04.82
|newborn *see* Newborn, examination
|pelvic (annual) (periodic) Z01.419
  |with abnormal findings Z01.411
|period of rapid growth in childhood Z00.2
|periodic (adult) (annual) (routine) Z00.00
  |with abnormal findings Z00.01
|physical (adult) *see also* Examination, medical
    Z00.00
  |sports Z02.5
|postpartum
  |immediately after delivery Z39.0
  |routine follow-up Z39.2
|prenatal (normal pregnancy) *see also*
    Pregnancy, normal Z34.9-
|pre-chemotherapy (antineoplastic) Z01.818
|pre-procedural (pre-operative)
  |cardiovascular Z01.810
  |laboratory Z01.812
  |respiratory Z01.811
  |specified NEC Z01.818
|prior to chemotherapy (antineoplastic)
    Z01.818
|psychiatric NEC Z00.8
  |follow-up not needing further care Z09
  |requested by authority Z04.6
|radiological (as part of a general medical
    examination) Z00.00
  |with abnormal findings Z00.01
|repeat cervical smear to confirm findings of
    recent normal smear following initial
    abnormal smear Z01.42
|skin (hypersensitivity) Z01.82
|special *see also* Examination, by type Z01.89
  |specified type NEC Z01.89

Examination - *continued*
| specified type or reason NEC Z04.89
| teeth Z01.20
| | with abnormal findings Z01.21
| urine *see* Examination, laboratory
| vision Z01.00
| | with abnormal findings Z01.01
| vision Z01.00
| | infant or child (over 28 days old) Z00.129
| | | with abnormal findings Z00.121
Exanthem, exanthema *see also* Rash
| with enteroviral vesicular stomatitis B08.4
| Boston A88.0
| epidemic with meningitis A88.0 [*G02*]
| subitum B08.20
| | due to human herpesvirus 6 B08.21
| | due to human herpesvirus 7 B08.22
| viral, virus B09
| | specified type NEC B08.8
Excess, excessive, excessively
| alcohol level in blood R78.0
| androgen (ovarian) E28.1
| attrition, tooth, teeth K03.0
| carotene, carotin (dietary) E67.1
| cold, effects of T69.9
| | specified effect NEC T69.8
| convergence H51.12
| crying
| | in child, adolescent, or adult R45.83
| | in infant R68.11
| development, breast N62
| divergence H51.8
| drinking (alcohol) NEC (without dependence)
| | F10.10
| | habitual (continual) (without remission)
| | | F10.20
| eating R63.2
| estrogen E28.0
| fat *see also* Obesity
| | in heart *see* Degeneration, myocardial
| | localized E65
| foreskin N47.8
| gas R14.0
| glucagon E16.3
| heat *see* Heat
| intermaxillary vertical dimension of fully
| | erupted teeth M26.37
| interocclusal distance of fully erupted teeth
| | M26.37
| kalium E87.5
| large
| | colon K59.39
| | | congenital Q43.8
| | infant P08.0
| | organ or site, congenital NEC *see* Anomaly,
| | | by site
| long
| | organ or site, congenital NEC *see* Anomaly,
| | | by site
| menstruation (with regular cycle) N92.0
| | with irregular cycle N92.1
| napping Z72.821
| natrium E87.0
| number of teeth K00.1
| nutrient (dietary) NEC R63.2
| potassium (K) E87.5
| salivation K11.7
| secretion *see also* Hypersecretion
| | milk O92.6
| | sputum R09.3
| | sweat R61
| sexual drive F52.8
| short
| | organ or site, congenital NEC *see* Anomaly,
| | | by site
| | umbilical cord in labor or delivery O69.3
| skin L98.7

Excess, excessive, excessively - *continued*
| | and subcutaneous tissue L98.7
| | eyelid (acquired) *see* Blepharochalasis
| | | congenital Q10.3
| sodium (Na) E87.0
| spacing of fully erupted teeth M26.32
| sputum R09.3
| sweating R61
| thirst R63.1
| | due to deprivation of water T73.1
| tuberosity of jaw M26.07
| vitamin
| | A (dietary) E67.0
| | | administered as drug (prolonged intake)
| | | | *see* Table of Drugs and Chemicals,
| | | | vitamins, adverse effect
| | | overdose or wrong substance given or
| | | | taken *see* Table of Drugs and
| | | | Chemicals, vitamins, poisoning
| | D (dietary) E67.3
| | | administered as drug (prolonged intake)
| | | | *see* Table of Drugs and Chemicals,
| | | | vitamins, adverse effect
| | | overdose or wrong substance given or
| | | | taken *see* Table of Drugs and
| | | | Chemicals, vitamins, poisoning
| weight
| | gain R63.5
| | loss R63.4
Excitability, abnormal, under minor stress
(personality disorder) F60.3
Excitation
| anomalous atrioventricular I45.6
| psychogenic F30.8
| reactive (from emotional stress, psychological
| | trauma) F30.8
Excitement
| hypomanic F30.8
| manic F30.9
| mental, reactive (from emotional stress,
| | psychological trauma) F30.8
| state, reactive (from emotional stress,
| | psychological trauma) F30.8
Excoriation (traumatic) *see also* Abrasion
| neurotic L98.1
| skin picking disorder F42.4
Exfoliation
| due to erythematous conditions according to
| | extent of body surface involved L49.0
| | 10-19 percent of body surface L49.1
| | 20-29 percent of body surface L49.2
| | 30-39 percent of body surface L49.3
| | 40-49 percent of body surface L49.4
| | 50-59 percent of body surface L49.5
| | 60-69 percent of body surface L49.6
| | 70-79 percent of body surface L49.7
| | 80-89 percent of body surface L49.8
| | 90-99 percent of body surface L49.9
| | less than 10 percent of body surface L49.0
| teeth, due to systemic causes K08.0
Exfoliative *see* condition
Exhaustion, exhaustive (physical NEC) R53.83
| battle F43.0
| cardiac *see* Failure, heart
| delirium F43.0
| due to
| | cold T69.8
| | excessive exertion T73.3
| | exposure T73.2
| | neurasthenia F48.8
| heart *see* Failure, heart
| heat *see also* Heat, exhaustion T67.5
| | due to
| | | salt depletion T67.4
| | | water depletion T67.3
| maternal, complicating delivery O75.81

Exhaustion - *continued*
| mental F48.8
| myocardium, myocardial *see* Failure, heart
| nervous F48.8
| old age R54
| psychogenic F48.8
| psychosis F43.0
| senile R54
| vital NEC Z73.0
Exhibitionism F65.2
Exocervicitis *see* Cervicitis
Exomphalos Q79.2
| meaning hernia *see* Hernia, umbilicus
Exophoria H50.52
| convergence, insufficiency H51.11
| divergence, excess H51.8
Exophthalmos H05.2-
| congenital Q15.8
| constant NEC H05.24-
| displacement, globe *see* Displacement, globe
| due to thyrotoxicosis (hyperthyroidism) *see*
| | Hyperthyroidism, with, goiter (diffuse)
| dysthyroid *see* Hyperthyroidism, with, goiter
| | (diffuse)
| goiter *see* Hyperthyroidism, with, goiter
| | (diffuse)
| intermittent NEC H05.25-
| malignant *see* Hyperthyroidism, with, goiter
| | (diffuse)
| orbital
| | edema *see* Edema, orbit
| | hemorrhage *see* Hemorrhage, orbit
| | pulsating NEC H05.26-
| thyrotoxic, thyrotropic *see* Hyperthyroidism,
| | with, goiter (diffuse)
Exostosis *see also* Disorder, bone
| cartilaginous *see* Neoplasm, bone, benign
| congenital (multiple) Q78.6
| external ear canal H61.81-
| gonococcal A54.49
| jaw (bone) M27.8
| multiple, congenital Q78.6
| orbit H05.35-
| osteocartilaginous *see* Neoplasm, bone,
| | benign
| syphilitic A52.77
Exotropia *see* Strabismus, divergent
concomitant
Explanation of
| investigation finding Z71.2
| medication Z71.89
Exploitation
| labor
| | confirmed
| | | adult forced T74.61
| | | child forced T74.62
| | suspected
| | | adult forced T76.61
| | | child forced T76.62
| sexual
| | confirmed
| | | adult forced T74.51
| | | child T74.52
| | suspected
| | | adult forced T76.51
| | | child T76.52
Exposure (to) *see also* Contact, with T75.89
| acariasis Z20.7
| AIDS virus Z20.6
| air pollution Z77.110
| algae and algae toxins Z77.121
| algae bloom Z77.121
| anthrax Z20.810
| aromatic amines Z77.020

Exposure (to) - *continued*
|aromatic (hazardous) compounds NEC
    Z77.028
|aromatic dyes NOS Z77.028
|arsenic Z77.010
|asbestos Z77.090
|bacterial disease NEC Z20.818
|benzene Z77.021
|blue-green algae bloom Z77.121
|body fluids (potentially hazardous) Z77.21
|brown tide Z77.121
|chemicals (chiefly nonmedicinal) (hazardous)
    NEC Z77.098
|cholera Z20.09
|chromium compounds Z77.018
|cold, effects of T69.9
    |specified effect NEC T69.8
|communicable disease Z20.9
    |bacterial NEC Z20.818
    |specified NEC Z20.89
    |viral NEC Z20.828
    |Zika virus Z20.821
|coronavirus (disease) (novel) 2019 Z20.822
|cyanobacteria bloom Z77.121
|disaster Z65.5
|discrimination Z60.5
|dyes Z77.098
|effects of T73.9
|environmental tobacco smoke (acute)
    (chronic) Z77.22
|Escherichia coli (E. coli) Z20.01
|exhaustion due to T73.2
|fiberglass *see* Table of Drugs and Chemicals,
    fiberglass
|German measles Z20.4
|gonorrhea Z20.2
|hazardous metals NEC Z77.018
|hazardous substances NEC Z77.29
|hazards in the physical environment NEC
    Z77.128
|hazards to health NEC Z77.9
|human immunodeficiency virus (HIV) Z20.6
|human T-lymphotropic virus type 1 (HTLV-
    1) Z20.89
|implanted
    |mesh *see* Complications, prosthetic device
        or implant, mesh
    |prosthetic materials NEC *see*
        Complications, prosthetic materials NEC
|infestation (parasitic) NEC Z20.7
|intestinal infectious disease NEC Z20.09
    |Escherichia coli (E. coli) Z20.01
|lead Z77.011
|meningococcus Z20.811
|mold (toxic) Z77.120
|nickel dust Z77.018
|noise Z77.122
|occupational
    |air contaminants NEC Z57.39
    |dust Z57.2
    |environmental tobacco smoke Z57.31
    |extreme temperature Z57.6
    |noise Z57.0
    |radiation Z57.1
    |risk factors Z57.9
        |specified NEC Z57.8
    |toxic agents (gases) (liquids) (solids)
        (vapors) in agriculture Z57.4
    |toxic agents (gases) (liquids) (solids)
        (vapors) in industry NEC Z57.5
    |vibration Z57.7
|parasitic disease NEC Z20.7
|pediculosis Z20.7
|persecution Z60.5
|pfiesteria piscicida Z77.121

Exposure (to) - *continued*
|poliomyelitis Z20.89
|polycyclic aromatic hydrocarbons Z77.028
|pollution
    |air Z77.110
    |environmental NEC Z77.118
    |soil Z77.112
    |water Z77.111
|prenatal (drugs) (toxic chemicals) *see*
    Newborn, affected by, noxious substances
        transmitted via placenta or breast milk
|rabies Z20.3
|radiation, naturally occurring NEC Z77.123
|radon Z77.123
|red tide (Florida) Z77.121
|rubella Z20.4
|second hand tobacco smoke (acute) (chronic)
    Z77.22
    |in the perinatal period P96.81
|sexually-transmitted disease Z20.2
|smallpox (laboratory) Z20.89
|syphilis Z20.2
|terrorism Z65.4
|torture Z65.4
|tuberculosis Z20.1
|uranium Z77.012
|varicella Z20.820
|venereal disease Z20.2
|viral disease NEC Z20.828
|war Z65.5
|water pollution Z77.111
|Zika virus Z20.821
Exsanguination *see* Hemorrhage
Exstrophy
|abdominal contents Q45.8
|bladder Q64.10
    |cloacal Q64.12
    |specified type NEC Q64.19
    |supravesical fissure Q64.11
Extensive *see* condition
Extra *see also* Accessory
|marker chromosomes (normal individual)
    Q92.61
    |in abnormal individual Q92.62
|rib Q76.6
    |cervical Q76.5
Extrasystoles (supraventricular) I49.49
|atrial I49.1
|auricular I49.1
|junctional I49.2
|ventricular I49.3
Extrauterine gestation or pregnancy *see*
    Pregnancy, by site
Extravasation
|blood R58
|chyle into mesentery I89.8
|pelvicalyceal N13.8
|pyelosinus N13.8
|urine (from ureter) R39.0
|vesicant agent
    |antineoplastic chemotherapy T80.810
    |other agent NEC T80.818
Extremity *see* condition, limb
Extrophy *see* Exstrophy
Extroversion
|bladder Q64.19
|uterus N81.4
    |complicating delivery O71.2
    |postpartal (old) N81.4
Extruded tooth (teeth) M26.34
Extrusion
|breast implant (prosthetic) T85.42
|eye implant (globe) (ball) T85.328
|intervertebral disc *see* Displacement,
    intervertebral disc

Extrusion - *continued*
|ocular lens implant (prosthetic) *see*
    Complications, intraocular lens
|vitreous *see* Prolapse, vitreous
Exudate
|pleural *see* Effusion, pleura
|retina H35.89
|wound fluids L24.A9
Exudative *see* condition
Eye, eyeball, eyelid *see* condition
Eyestrain *see* Disturbance, vision, subjective
Eyeworm disease of Africa B74.3

F

Faber's syndrome (achlorhydric anemia)
    D50.9
Fabry (-Anderson) disease E75.21
Facet syndrome M47.89-
Faciocephalalgia, autonomic *see also*
    Neuropathy, peripheral, autonomic G90.09
Factor(s)
|psychic, associated with diseases classified
    elsewhere F54
|psychological
    |affecting physical conditions F54
    |or behavioral
        |affecting general medical condition F54
        |associated with disorders or diseases
            classified elsewhere F54
Fahr disease (of brain) G23.8
Fahr Volhard disease (of kidney) I12.
Failure, failed
|abortion *see* Abortion, attempted
|aortic (valve) I35.8
    |rheumatic I06.8
|attempted abortion *see* Abortion, attempted
|biventricular I50.82
    |due to left heart failure I50.814
|bone marrow *see* Anemia, aplastic
|cardiac *see* Failure, heart
|cardiorenal (chronic) (*see also* Failure, renal,
    and Failure, heart) I50.9
    |hypertensive I13.2
|cardiorespiratory *see also* Failure, heart R09.2
|cardiovascular (chronic) *see* Failure, heart
|cerebrovascular I67.9
|cervical dilatation in labor O62.0
|circulation, circulatory (peripheral) R57.9
    |newborn P29.89
|compensation *see* Disease, heart
|compliance with medical treatment or regimen
    see Noncompliance
|congestive *see* Failure, heart, congestive
|dental implant (endosseous) M27.69
    |due to
        |failure of dental prosthesis M27.63
        |lack of attached gingiva M27.62
        |occlusal trauma (poor prosthetic design)
            M27.62
        |parafunctional habits M27.62
        |periodontal infection (peri-implantitis)
            M27.62
        |poor oral hygiene M27.62
    |osseointegration M27.61
        |due to
            |complications of systemic disease
                M27.61
            |poor bone quality M27.61
        |iatrogenic M27.61
    |post-osseointegration
        |biological M27.62
        |due to complications of systemic disease
            M27.62

Failure, failed - *continued*

|iatrogenic M27.62
|mechanical M27.63
|pre-integration M27.61
|pre-osseointegration M27.61
|specified NEC M27.69
|descent of head (at term) of pregnancy (mother) O32.4
|endosseous dental implant *see* Failure, dental implant
|engagement of head (term of pregnancy) (mother) O32.4
|erection (penile) *see also* Dysfunction, sexual, male, erectile N52.9
|nonorganic F52.21
|examination(s), anxiety concerning Z55.2
|expansion terminal respiratory units (newborn) (primary) P28.0
|forceps NOS (with subsequent cesarean delivery) O66.5
|gain weight (child over 28 days old) R62.51
|adult R62.7
|newborn P92.6
|genital response (male) F52.21
|female F52.22
|heart (acute) (senile) (sudden) I50.9
|with
|acute pulmonary edema *see* Failure, ventricular, left
|decompensation I50.9
|with
|normal ejection fraction I50.33
|preserved ejection fraction I50.33
|reduced ejection fraction I50.23
|with diastolic dysfunction I50.43
|combined systolic and diastolic I50.43
|diastolic I50.33
|right I50.813
|systolic I50.23
|dilatation *see* Disease, heart
|normal ejection fraction *see* Failure, heart, diastolic
|preserved ejection fraction *see* Failure, heart, diastolic
|reduced ejection fraction *see* Failure, heart, systolic
|arteriosclerotic I70.90
|biventricular I50.82
|due to left heart failure I50.814
|combined left-right sided I50.82
|due to left heart failure I50.814
|compensated (*see also* Failure, heart, by type as diastolic or systolic, chronic) I50.9
|complicating
|anesthesia (general) (local) or other sedation
|in labor and delivery O74.2
|in pregnancy O29.12-
|postpartum, puerperal O89.1
|delivery (cesarean) (instrumental) O75.4
|congestive I50.9
|with rheumatic fever (conditions in I00)
|active I01.8
|inactive or quiescent (with chorea) I09.81
|newborn P29.0
|rheumatic (chronic) (inactive) (with chorea) I09.81
|active or acute I01.8
|with chorea I02.0
|decompensated (*see also* Failure, heart, by type as diastolic or systolic, acute and chronic) I50.9
|degenerative *see* Degeneration, myocardial

Failure, failed - *continued*

|diastolic (congestive) (left ventricular) I50.30
|acute (congestive) I50.31
|and (on) chronic (congestive) I50.33
|chronic (congestive) I50.32
|and (on) acute (congestive) I50.33
|combined with systolic (congestive) I50.40
|acute (congestive) I50.41
|and (on) chronic (congestive) I50.43
|chronic (congestive) I50.42
|and (on) acute (congestive) I50.43
|due to presence of cardiac prosthesis I97.13-
|end stage (*see also* Failure, heart, by type as diastolic or systolic, chronic) I50.84
|following cardiac surgery I97.13-
|high output NOS I50.83
|hypertensive *see* Hypertension, heart
|left (ventricular) *see also* Failure, ventricular, left
|combined diastolic and systolic *see* Failure, heart, diastolic, combined with systolic
|diastolic *see* Failure, heart, diastolic
|systolic *see* Failure, heart, systolic
|low output (syndrome) NOS I50.9
|newborn P29.0
|organic *see* Disease, heart
|peripartum O90.3
|postprocedural I97.13-
|rheumatic (chronic) (inactive) I09.9
|right (isolated) (ventricular) I50.810
|acute I50.811
|and (on) chronic I50.813
|chronic I50.812
|and acute I50.813
|secondary to left heart failure I50.814
|specified NEC I50.89
|Note: heart failure stages A, B, C, and D are based on the American College of Cardiology and American Heart Association stages of heart failure, which complement and should not be confused with the New York Heart Association Classification of Heart Failure, into Class I, Class II, Class III, and Class IV
|stage A Z91.89
|stage B (*see also* Failure, heart, by type as diastolic or systolic) I50.9
|stage C (*see also* Failure, heart, by type as diastolic or systolic) I50.9
|stage D (*see also* Failure, heart, by type as diastolic or systolic, chronic) I50.84
|systolic (congestive) (left ventricular) I50.20
|acute (congestive) I50.21
|and (on) chronic (congestive) I50.23
|chronic (congestive) I50.22
|and (on) acute (congestive) I50.23
|combined with diastolic (congestive) I50.40
|acute (congestive) I50.41
|and (on) chronic (congestive) I50.43
|chronic (congestive) I50.42
|and (on) acute (congestive) I50.43
|thyrotoxic (*see also* Thyrotoxicosis) E05.90 [I43]
|with
|high output (*see also* Thyrotoxicosis) I50.83
|thyroid storm E05.91 [I43]
|high output (*see also* Thyrotoxicosis) I50.83
|valvular *see* Endocarditis
|hepatic K72.90

Failure, failed - *continued*

|with coma K72.91
|acute or subacute K72.00
|with coma K72.01
|due to drugs K71.10
|with coma K71.11
|alcoholic (acute) (chronic) (subacute) K70.40
|with coma K70.41
|chronic K72.10
|with coma K72.11
|due to drugs (acute) (subacute) (chronic) K71.10
|with coma K71.11
|due to drugs (acute) (subacute) (chronic) K71.10
|with coma K71.11
|postprocedural K91.82
|hepatorenal K76.7
|induction (of labor) O61.9
|abortion *see* Abortion, attempted
|by
|oxytocic drugs O61.0
|prostaglandins O61.0
|instrumental O61.1
|mechanical O61.1
|medical O61.0
|specified NEC O61.8
|surgical O61.1
|intubation during anesthesia T88.4
|in pregnancy O29.6-
|labor and delivery O74.7
|postpartum, puerperal O89.6
|involution, thymus (gland) E32.0
|kidney *see also* Disease, kidney, chronic N19
|acute *see also* Failure, renal, acute N17.9-
|diabetic *see* E08-E13 with .22
|lactation (complete) O92.3
|partial O92.4
|Leydig's cell, adult E29.1
|liver *see* Failure, hepatic
|menstruation at puberty N91.0
|mitral I05.8
|myocardial, myocardium *see also* Failure, heart I50.9
|chronic *see also* Failure, heart, congestive I50.9
|congestive *see also* Failure, heart, congestive I50.9
|newborn screening - see Abnormal, neonatal screening
|neonatal congenital heart disease P09.5
|orgasm (female) (psychogenic) F52.31
|male F52.32
|ovarian (primary) E28.39
|iatrogenic E89.40
|asymptomatic E89.40
|symptomatic E89.41
|postprocedural (postablative) (postirradiation) (postsurgical) E89.40
|asymptomatic E89.40
|symptomatic E89.41
|ovulation causing infertility N97.0
|polyglandular, autoimmune E31.0
|prosthetic joint implant *see* Complications, joint prosthesis, mechanical, breakdown, by site
|renal N19
|with
|tubular necrosis (acute) N17.0
|acute N17.9
|with
|cortical necrosis N17.1
|medullary necrosis N17.2
|tubular necrosis N17.0

Failure, failed - *continued*
  |specified NEC N17.8
  |chronic N18.9
    |hypertensive *see* Hypertension, kidney
  |congenital P96.0
  |end stage (chronic) N18.6
    |due to hypertension I12.0
  |following
    |abortion *see* Abortion by type complicated
      by specified condition NEC
    |crushing T79.5
    |ectopic or molar pregnancy O08.4
    |labor and delivery (acute) O90.4
  |hypertensive *see* Hypertension, kidney
  |postprocedural N99.0
  |respiration, respiratory J96.90
    |with
      |hypercapnia J96.92
      |hypercarbia J96.02
      |hypoxia J96.91
    |acute J96.00
      |with
        |hypercapnia J96.02
        |hypercarbia J96.02
        |hypoxia J96.01
      |center G93.89
    |acute and (on) chronic J96.20
      |with
        |hypercapnia J96.22
        |hypercarbia J96.22
        |hypoxia J96.21
    |chronic J96.10
      |with
        |hypercapnia J96.12
        |hypercarbia J96.12
        |hypoxia J96.11
    |newborn P28.5
    |postprocedural (acute) J95.821
      |acute and chronic J95.822
  |rotation
    |cecum Q43.3
    |colon Q43.3
    |intestine Q43.3
    |kidney Q63.2
  |sedation (conscious) (moderate) during
    procedure T88.52
    |history of Z92.83
  |segmentation *see also* Fusion
    |fingers *see* Syndactylism, complex, fingers
    |vertebra Q76.49
      |with scoliosis Q76.3
  |seminiferous tubule, adult E29.1
  |senile (general) R54
  |sexual arousal (male) F52.21
    |female F52.22
  |testicular endocrine function E29.1
  |to thrive (child over 28 days old) R62.51
    |adult R62.7
    |newborn P92.6
  |transplant T86.92
    |bone T86.831
      |marrow T86.02
    |cornea T86.841-
    |heart T86.22
      |with lung(s) T86.32
    |intestine T86.851
    |kidney T86.12
    |liver T86.42
    |lung(s) T86.811
      |with heart T86.32
    |pancreas T86.891
    |skin (allograft) (autograft) T86.821
    |specified organ or tissue NEC T86.891
    |stem cell (peripheral blood) (umbilical cord)
      T86.5

Failure, failed - *continued*
  |trial of labor (with subsequent cesarean
    delivery) O66.40
    |following previous cesarean delivery
      O66.41
  |tubal ligation N99.89
  |urinary *see* Disease, kidney, chronic
  |vacuum extraction NOS (with subsequent
    cesarean delivery) O66.5
  |vasectomy N99.89
  |ventouse NOS (with subsequent cesarean
    delivery) O66.5
  |ventricular *see also* Failure, heart I50.9
    |left (*see also* Failure, heart, left) I50.1
      |with rheumatic fever (conditions in I00)
        |active I01.8
          |with chorea I02.0
        |inactive or quiescent (with chorea)
          I09.81
      |rheumatic (chronic) (inactive) (with
        chorea) I09.81
        |active or acute I01.8
          |with chorea I02.0
    |right *see* Failure, heart, right
  |vital centers, newborn P91.88
Fainting (fit) R55
Fallen arches *see* Deformity, limb, flat foot
Falling, falls (repeated) R29.6
  |any organ or part *see* Prolapse
Fallopian
  |insufflation Z31.41
  |tube *see* condition
Fallot's
  |pentalogy Q21.8
  |tetrad or tetralogy Q21.3
  |triad or trilogy Q22.3
False *see also* condition
  |croup J38.5
  |joint *see* Nonunion, fracture
  |labor (pains) O47.9
    |at or after 37 completed weeks of gestation
      O47.1
    |before 37 completed weeks of gestation
      O47.0-
  |passage, urethra (prostatic) N36.5
  |pregnancy F45.8
Family, familial *see also* condition
  |disruption Z63.8
    |involving divorce or separation Z63.5
  |Li-Fraumeni (syndrome) Z15.01
  |planning advice Z30.09
  |problem Z63.9
    |specified NEC Z63.8
  |retinoblastoma C69.2-
Famine (effects of) T73.0
  |edema *see* Malnutrition, severe
Fanconi (-De Toni)(-Debre) syndrome E72.09
  |with cystinosis E72.04
Fanconi's anemia (congenital pancytopenia)
  D61.09
Farber's disease or syndrome E75.29
Farcy A24.0
Farmer's
  |lung J67.0
  |skin L57.8
Farsightedness *see* Hypermetropia
Fascia *see* condition
Fasciculation R25.3
Fasciitis M72.9
  |diffuse (eosinophilic) M35.4
  |infective M72.8
    |necrotizing M72.6
  |necrotizing M72.6
  |nodular M72.4
  |perirenal (with ureteral obstruction) N13.5

Fasciitis - *continued*
  |with infection N13.6
  |plantar M72.2
  |specified NEC M72.8
  |traumatic (old) M72.8
    |current code by site under Sprain
Fascioliasis B66.3
Fasciolopsis, fasciolopsiasis (intestinal) B66.5
Fascioscapulohumeral myopathy G71.02
Fast pulse R00.0
Fat
  |embolism *see* Embolism, fat
  |excessive *see also* Obesity
    |in heart *see* Degeneration, myocardial
  |in stool R19.5
  |localized (pad) E65
    |heart *see* Degeneration, myocardial
    |knee M79.4
    |retropatellar M79.4
  |necrosis
    |breast N64.1
    |mesentery K65.4
    |omentum K65.4
  |pad E65
    |knee M79.4
Fatigue R53.83
  |auditory deafness *see* Deafness
  |chronic R53.82
  |combat F43.0
  |general R53.83
    |psychogenic F48.8
  |heat (transient) T67.6
  |muscle M62.89
  |myocardium *see* Failure, heart
  |neoplasm-related R53.0
  |nervous, neurosis F48.8
  |operational F48.8
  |psychogenic (general) F48.8
  |senile R54
  |voice R49.8
Fatness *see* Obesity
Fatty *see also* condition
  |apron E65
  |degeneration *see* Degeneration, fatty
  |heart (enlarged) *see* Degeneration, myocardial
  |liver NEC K76.0
    |alcoholic K70.0
    |nonalcoholic K76.0
  |necrosis *see* Degeneration, fatty
Fauces *see* condition
Fauchard's disease (periodontitis) *see*
  Periodontitis
Faucitis J02.9
Favism (anemia) D55.0
Favus *see* Dermatophytosis
Fazio-Londe disease or syndrome G12.1
Fear complex or reaction F40.9
Fear of *see* Phobia
Feared complaint unfounded Z71.1
Febris, febrile *see also* Fever
  |flava *see also* Fever, yellow A95.9
  |melitensis A23.0
  |pestis *see* Plague
  |recurrens *see* Fever, relapsing
  |rubra A38.9
Fecal
  |incontinence R15.9
  |smearing R15.1
  |soiling R15.1
  |urgency R15.2
Fecalith (impaction) K56.41
  |appendix K38.1
  |congenital P76.8
Fede's disease K14.0
**Feeble rapid pulse due to shock following
  injury** T79.4
Feeble-Minded F70

Feeding
| difficulties R63.30
| problem (elderly) (infant) R63.39
|| newborn P92.9
||| specified NEC P92.8
|| nonorganic (adult) *see* Disorder, eating
Feeling (of)
| foreign body in throat R09.89
Feer's disease *see* Poisoning, mercury
Feet *see* condition
Feigned illness Z76.5
Feil-Klippel syndrome (brevicollis) Q76.1
Feinmesser's (hidrotic) ectodermal dysplasia
| Q82.4
Felinophobia F40.218
Felon *see also* Cellulitis, digit
| with lymphangitis *see* Lymphangitis, acute,
| digit
Felty's syndrome M05.00
| ankle M05.07-
| elbow M05.02-
| foot joint M05.07-
| hand joint M05.04-
| hip M05.05-
| knee M05.06-
| multiple site M05.09
| shoulder M05.01-
| vertebra *see* Spondylitis, ankylosing
| wrist M05.03-
Female genital cutting status *see* Female
| genital mutilation status (FGM)
Female genital mutilation status (FGM)
| N90.810
| specified NEC N90.818
| type I (clitorectomy status) N90.811
| type II (clitorectomy with excision of labia
| minora status) N90.812
| type III (infibulation status) N90.813
| type IV N90.818
Femur, femoral *see* condition
Fenestration, fenestrated *see also* Imperfect,
| closure
| aortico-pulmonary Q21.4
| cusps, heart valve NEC Q24.8
|| pulmonary Q22.3
| pulmonic cusps Q22.3
Fernell's disease (aortic aneurysm) I71.9
Fertile eunuch syndrome E23.0
Fetid
| breath R19.6
| sweat L75.0
Fetishism F65.0
| transvestic F65.1
Fetus, fetal *see also* condition
| alcohol syndrome (dysmorphic) Q86.0
| compressus O31.0-
| hydantoin syndrome Q86.1
| lung tissue P28.0
| papyraceous O31.0-
Fever (inanition) (of unknown origin)
| **(persistent) (with chills) (with rigor)** R50.9
| abortus A23.1
| Aden (dengue) A90
| African tick bite A77.8
| African tick-borne A68.1
| American
|| mountain (tick) A93.2
|| spotted A77.0
| aphthous B08.8
| arbovirus, arboviral A94
|| hemorrhagic A94
|| specified NEC A93.8
| Argentinian hemorrhagic A96.0

Fever - *continued*
| Assam B55.0
| Australian Q A78
| Bangkok hemorrhagic A91
| Barmah forest A92.8
| Bartonella A44.0
| bilious, hemoglobinuric B50.8
| blackwater B50.8
| blister B00.1
| Bolivian hemorrhagic A96.1
| Bonvale dam T73.3
| boutonneuse A77.1
| brain *see* Encephalitis
| Brazilian purpuric A48.4
| breakbone A90
| Bullis A77.0
| Bunyamwera A92.8
| Burdwan B55.0
| Bwamba A92.8
| Cameroon *see* Malaria
| Canton A75.9
| catarrhal (acute) J00
|| chronic J31.0
| cat-scratch A28.1
| Central Asian hemorrhagic A98.0
| cerebral *see* Encephalitis
| cerebrospinal meningococcal A39.0
| Chagres B50.9
| Chandipura A92.8
| Changuinola A93.1
| Charcot's (biliary) (hepatic) (intermittent) *see*
|| Calculus, bile duct
| Chikungunya (viral) (hemorrhagic) A92.0
| Chitral A93.1
| Colombo *see* Fever, paratyphoid
| Colorado tick (virus) A93.2
| congestive (remittent) *see* Malaria
| Congo virus A98.0
| continued malarial B50.9
| Corsican *see* Malaria
| Crimean-Congo hemorrhagic A98.0
| Cyprus *see* Brucellosis
| dandy A90
| deer fly *see* Tularemia
| dengue (virus) A90
|| hemorrhagic A91
|| sandfly A93.1
| desert B38.0
| drug induced R50.2
| due to
|| conditions classified elsewhere R50.81
|| heat T67.0
| enteric A01.00
| enteroviral exanthematous (Boston exanthem)
|| A88.0
| ephemeral (of unknown origin) R50.9
| epidemic hemorrhagic A98.5
| erysipelatous *see* Erysipelas
| estivo-autumnal (malarial) B50.9
| famine A75.0
| five day A79.0
| following delivery O86.4
| Fort Bragg A27.89
| gastroenteric A01.00
| gastromalarial *see* Malaria
| Gibraltar *see* Brucellosis
| glandular *see* Mononucleosis, infectious
| Guama (viral) A92.8
| Haverhill A25.1
| hay (allergic) J30.1
|| with asthma (bronchial) J45.909
||| with
|||| exacerbation (acute) J45.901
|||| status asthmaticus J45.902
| due to

Fever - *continued*
| allergen other than pollen J30.89
| pollen, any plant or tree J30.1
| heat (effects) T67.0
| hematuric, bilious B50.8
| hemoglobinuric (malarial) (bilious) B50.8
| hemorrhagic (arthropod-borne) NOS A94
|| with renal syndrome A98.5
|| arenaviral A96.9
||| specified NEC A96.8
|| Argentinian A96.0
|| Bangkok A91
|| Bolivian A96.1
|| Central Asian A98.0
|| Chikungunya A92.0
|| Crimean-Congo A98.0
|| dengue (virus) A91
|| epidemic A98.5
|| Junin (virus) A96.0
|| Korean A98.5
|| Kyasanur forest A98.2
|| Machupo (virus) A96.1
|| mite-borne A93.8
|| mosquito-borne A92.8
|| Omsk A98.1
|| Philippine A91
|| Russian A98.5
|| Singapore A91
|| Southeast Asia A91
|| Thailand A91
|| tick-borne NEC A93.8
|| viral A99
||| specified NEC A98.8
| hepatic *see* Cholecystitis
| herpetic *see* Herpes
| icterohemorrhagic A27.0
| Indiana A93.8
| infective B99.9
|| specified NEC B99.8
| intermittent (bilious) *see also* Malaria
|| of unknown origin R50.9
|| pernicious B50.9
| iodide R50.2
| Japanese river A75.3
| jungle *see also* Malaria
|| yellow A95.0
| Junin (virus) hemorrhagic A96.0
| Katayama B65.2
| kedani A75.3
| Kenya (tick) A77.1
| Kew Garden A79.1
| Korean hemorrhagic A98.5
| Lassa A96.2
| Lone Star A77.0
| Machupo (virus) hemorrhagic A96.1
| malaria, malarial *see* Malaria
| Malta A23.9
| Marseilles A77.1
| marsh *see* Malaria
| Mayaro (viral) A92.8
| Mediterranean *see also* Brucellosis A23.9
|| familial M04.1
|| tick A77.1
| meningeal *see* Meningitis
| Meuse A79.0
| Mexican A75.2
| mianeh A68.1
| miasmatic *see* Malaria
| mosquito-borne (viral) A92.9
|| hemorrhagic A92.8
| mountain *see also* Brucellosis
|| meaning Rocky Mountain spotted fever
||| A77.0
|| tick (American) (Colorado) (viral) A93.2
| Mucambo (viral) A92.8

Fever - *continued*
|mud A27.9
|Neapolitan *see* Brucellosis
|neutropenic D70.9
|newborn P81.9
  |environmental P81.0
|Nine-mile A78
|non-exanthematous tick A93.2
|North Asian tick-borne A77.2
|Omsk hemorrhagic A98.1
|O'nyong-Nyong (viral) A92.1
|Oropouche (viral) A93.0
|Oroya A44.0
|pacific coast tick A77.8
|paludal *see* Malaria
|Panama (malarial) B50.9
|Pappataci A93.1
|paratyphoid A01.4
  |A A01.1
  |B A01.2
  |C A01.3
|parrot A70
|periodic (Mediterranean) M04.1
|persistent (of unknown origin) R50.9
|petechial A39.0
|pharyngoconjunctival B30.2
|Philippine hemorrhagic A91
|phlebotomus A93.1
|Piry (virus) A93.8
|Pixuna (viral) A92.8
|Plasmodium ovale B53.0
|polioviral (nonparalytic) A80.4
|Pontiac A48.2
|postimmunization R50.83
|postoperative R50.82
  |due to infection T81.40
|posttransfusion R50.84
|postvaccination R50.83
|presenting with conditions classified
    elsewhere R50.81
|pretibial A27.89
|puerperal O86.4
|Q A78
|quadrilateral A78
|quartan (malaria) B52.9
|Queensland (coastal) (tick) A77.3
|quintan A79.0
|rabbit *see* Tularemia
|rat-bite A25.9
  |due to
    |Spirillum A25.0
    |Streptobacillus moniliformis A25.1
|recurrent *see* Fever, relapsing
|relapsing (Borrelia) A68.9
  |Carter's (Asiatic) A68.1
  |Dutton's (West African) A68.1
  |Koch's A68.9
  |louse-borne A68.0
  |Novy's
    |louse-borne A68.0
    |tick-borne A68.1
  |Obermeyer's (European) A68.0
  |tick-borne A68.1
|remittent (bilious) (congestive) (gastric) *see*
    Malaria
|rheumatic (active) (acute) (chronic) (subacute)
    I00
  |with central nervous system involvement
      I02.9
  |active with heart involvement *see* category
      I01
  |inactive or quiescent with
    |cardiac hypertrophy I09.89
    |carditis I09.9

Fever - *continued*
  |endocarditis I09.1
    |aortic (valve) I06.9
      |with mitral (valve) disease I08.0
    |mitral (valve) I05.9
      |with aortic (valve) disease I08.0
    |pulmonary (valve) I09.89
    |tricuspid (valve) I07.8
  |heart disease NEC I09.89
  |heart failure (congestive) (conditions in
      category I50.) I09.81
  |left ventricular failure (conditions in
      I50.1-I50.4-) I09.81
  |myocarditis, myocardial degeneration
      (conditions in I51.4) I09.0
  |pancarditis I09.9
  |pericarditis I09.2
|Rift Valley (viral) A92.4
|Rocky Mountain spotted A77.0
|rose J30.1
|Ross River B33.1
|Russian hemorrhagic A98.5
|San Joaquin (Valley) B38.0
|sandfly A93.1
|Sao Paulo A77.0
|scarlet A38.9
|seven day (leptospirosis) (autumnal)
    (Japanese) A27.89
  |dengue A90
|shin-bone A79.0
|Singapore hemorrhagic A91
|solar A90
|Songo A98.5
|sore B00.1
|South African tick-bite A68.1
|Southeast Asia hemorrhagic A91
|spinal *see* Meningitis
|spirillary A25.0
|splenic *see* Anthrax
|spotted A77.9
  |American A77.0
  |Brazilian A77.0
  |cerebrospinal meningitis A39.0
  |Colombian A77.0
  |due to Rickettsia
    |africae (African tick bite fever) A77.8
    |australis A77.3
    |conorii A77.1
    |parkeri A77.8
    |rickettsii A77.0
    |sibirica A77.2
    |specified type NEC A77.8
  |Ehrlichiosis A77.40
    |due to
      |E. chafeensis A77.41
      |specified organism NEC A77.49
  |Rocky Mountain A77.0
|steroid R50.2
|streptobacillary A25.1
|subtertian B50.9
|Sumatran mite A75.3
|sun A90
|swamp A27.9
|swine A02.8
|sylvatic, yellow A95.0
|Tahyna B33.8
|tertian *see* Malaria, tertian
|Thailand hemorrhagic A91
|thermic T67.0
|three-day A93.1
|tick
  |American mountain A93.2
  |Colorado A93.2
  |Kemerovo A93.8
  |Mediterranean A77.1

Fever - *continued*
  |mountain A93.2
  |nonexanthematous A93.2
  |Quaranfil A93.8
|tick-bite NEC A93.8
|tick-borne (hemorrhagic) NEC A93.8
|trench A79.0
|tsutsugamushi A75.3
|typhogastric A01.00
|typhoid (abortive) (hemorrhagic)
    (intermittent) (malignant) A01.00
  |complicated by
    |arthritis A01.04
    |heart involvement A01.02
    |meningitis A01.01
    |osteomyelitis A01.05
    |pneumonia A01.03
    |specified NEC A01.09
|typhomalarial *see* Malaria
|typhus *see* Typhus (fever)
|undulant *see* Brucellosis
|unknown origin R50.9
|uveoparotid D86.89
|valley B38.0
|Venezuelan equine A92.2
|vesicular stomatitis A93.8
|viral hemorrhagic *see* Fever, hemorrhagic, by
    type of virus
|Volhynian A79.0
|Wesselsbron (viral) A92.8
|West
  |African B50.8
  |Nile (viral) A92.30
    |with
      |complications NEC A92.39
      |cranial nerve disorders A92.32
      |encephalitis A92.31
      |encephalomyelitis A92.31
      |neurologic manifestation NEC A92.32
      |optic neuritis A92.32
      |polyradiculitis A92.32
|Whitmore's *see* Melioidosis
|Wolhynian A79.0
|worm B83.9
|yellow A95.9
  |jungle A95.0
  |sylvatic A95.0
  |urban A95.1
|Zika virus A92.5
Fibrillation
|atrial or auricular (established) I48.91
  |chronic I48.2
  |paroxysmal I48.0
  |permanent I48.2
  |persistent I48.1
|cardiac I49.8
|heart I49.8
|muscular M62.89
|ventricular I49.01
Fibrin
|ball or bodies, pleural (sac) J94.1
|chamber, anterior (eye) (gelatinous exudate)
    see Iridocyclitis, acute
Fibrinogenolysis *see* Fibrinolysis
Fibrinogenopenia D68.8
|acquired D65
|congenital D68.2
Fibrinolysis (hemorrhagic) (acquired) D65
|antepartum hemorrhage *see* Hemorrhage,
    antepartum, with coagulation defect
|following
  |abortion *see* Abortion by type complicated
      by hemorrhage
  |ectopic or molar pregnancy O08.1
|intrapartum O67.0
|newborn, transient P60
|postpartum O72.3

Fibrinopenia (hereditary) D68.2
|acquired D68.4
Fibrinopurulent *see* condition
Fibrinous *see* condition
Fibroadenoma
|cellular intracanalicular D24-
|giant D24-
|intracanalicular
||cellular D24-
||giant D24-
||specified site *see* Neoplasm, benign, by site
||unspecified site D24-
|juvenile D24-
|pericanalicular
||specified site *see* Neoplasm, benign, by site
||unspecified site D24-
|phyllodes D24-
|prostate D29.1
|specified site NEC *see* Neoplasm, benign, by
||site
|unspecified site D24-
Fibroadenosis, breast (chronic) (cystic)
|(diffuse) (periodic) (segmental) N60.2-
Fibroangioma *see also* Neoplasm, benign, by
|site
|juvenile
||specified site *see* Neoplasm, benign, by site
||unspecified site D10.6
Fibrochondrosarcoma *see* Neoplasm, cartilage,
|malignant
Fibrocystic
|disease *see also* Fibrosis, cystic
||breast *see* Mastopathy, cystic
||jaw M27.49
||kidney (congenital) Q61.8
||liver Q44.6
||pancreas E84.9
|kidney (congenital) Q61.8
Fibrodysplasia ossificans progressiva *see*
|Myositis, ossificans, progressiva
Fibroelastosis (cordis) (endocardial)
|(endomyocardial) I42.4
Fibroid (tumor) *see also* Neoplasm, connective
|tissue, benign
|disease, lung (chronic) *see* Fibrosis, lung
|heart (disease) *see* Myocarditis
|in pregnancy or childbirth O34.1-
||causing obstructed labor O65.5
|induration, lung (chronic) *see* Fibrosis, lung
|lung *see* Fibrosis, lung
|pneumonia (chronic) *see* Fibrosis, lung
|uterus (*see also* Leiomyoma, uterus) D25.9
Fibrolipoma *see* Lipoma
Fibroliposarcoma *see* Neoplasm, connective
|tissue, malignant
Fibroma *see also* Neoplasm, connective tissue,
|benign
|ameloblastic *see* Cyst, calcifying odontogenic
|bone (nonossifying) *see* Disorder, bone,
||specified type NEC
||ossifying *see* Neoplasm, bone, benign
|cementifying *see* Neoplasm, bone, benign
|chondromyxoid *see* Neoplasm, bone, benign
|desmoplastic *see* Neoplasm, connective tissue,
||uncertain behavior
|durum *see* Neoplasm, connective tissue,
||benign
|fascial *see* Neoplasm, connective tissue,
||benign
|invasive *see* Neoplasm, connective tissue,
||uncertain behavior
|molle *see* Lipoma
|myxoid *see* Neoplasm, connective tissue,
||benign
|nasopharynx, nasopharyngeal (juvenile) D10.6

Fibroma - *continued*
|nonosteogenic (nonossifying) *see* Dysplasia,
||fibrous
|odontogenic (central) *see* Cyst, calcifying
||odontogenic
|ossifying *see* Neoplasm, bone, benign
|periosteal *see* Neoplasm, bone, benign
|soft *see* Lipoma
Fibromatosis M72.9
|abdominal *see* Neoplasm, connective tissue,
||uncertain behavior
|aggressive *see* Neoplasm, connective tissue,
||uncertain behavior
|congenital generalized *see* Neoplasm,
||connective tissue, uncertain behavior
|Dupuytren's M72.0
|gingival K06.1
|palmar (fascial) M72.0
|plantar (fascial) M72.2
|pseudosarcomatous (proliferative)
||(subcutaneous) M72.4
|retroperitoneal D48.3
|specified NEC M72.8
Fibromyalgia M79.7
Fibromyoma *see also* Neoplasm, connective
|tissue, benign
|uterus (corpus) *see also* Leiomyoma, uterus
||in pregnancy or childbirth *see* Fibroid, in
|||pregnancy or childbirth
||causing obstructed labor O65.5
Fibromyositis M79.7
Fibromyxolipoma D17.9
Fibromyxoma *see* Neoplasm, connective tissue,
|benign
Fibromyxosarcoma *see* Neoplasm, connective
|tissue, malignant
Fibro-Odontoma, ameloblastic *see* Cyst,
|calcifying odontogenic
Fibro-Osteoma *see* Neoplasm, bone, benign
Fibroplasia, retrolental H35.17-
Fibropurulent *see* condition
Fibrosarcoma *see also* Neoplasm, connective
|tissue, malignant
|ameloblastic C41.1
||upper jaw (bone) C41.0
|congenital *see* Neoplasm, connective tissue,
||malignant
|fascial *see* Neoplasm, connective tissue,
||malignant
|infantile *see* Neoplasm, connective tissue,
||malignant
|odontogenic C41.1
||upper jaw (bone) C41.0
|periosteal *see* Neoplasm, bone, malignant
Fibrosclerosis
|breast N60.3-
|multifocal M35.5
|penis (corpora cavernosa) N48.6
Fibrosis, fibrotic
|adrenal (gland) E27.8
|amnion O41.8X-
|anal papillae K62.89
|arteriocapillary *see* Arteriosclerosis
|bladder N32.89
||interstitial *see* Cystitis, chronic, interstitial
||localized submucosal *see* Cystitis, chronic,
|||interstitial
||panmural *see* Cystitis, chronic, interstitial
|breast *see* Fibrosclerosis, breast
|capillary *see also* Arteriosclerosis I70.90
||lung (chronic) *see* Fibrosis, lung
|cardiac *see* Myocarditis
|cervix N88.8
|chorion O41.8X-
|corpus cavernosum (sclerosing) N48.6

Fibrosis, fibrotic - *continued*
|cystic (of pancreas) E84.9
||with
|||distal intestinal obstruction syndrome
||||E84.19
|||fecal impaction E84.19
|||intestinal manifestations NEC E84.19
|||pulmonary manifestations E84.0
|||specified manifestations NEC E84.8
|due to device, implant or graft *see also*
||Complications, by site and type, specified
||NEC T85.828
|arterial graft NEC T82.828
|breast (implant) T85.828
|catheter NEC T85.828
||dialysis (renal) T82.828
|||intraperitoneal T85.828
||infusion NEC T82.828
|||spinal (epidural) (subdural) T85.820
||urinary (indwelling) T83.82
|electronic (electrode) (pulse generator)
||(stimulator)
||bone T84.82
||cardiac T82.827
||nervous system (brain) (peripheral nerve)
|||(spinal) T85.820
||urinary T83.82
|fixation, internal (orthopedic) NEC T84.82
|gastrointestinal (bile duct) (esophagus)
||T85.828
|genital NEC T83.82
|heart NEC T82.827
|joint prosthesis T84.82
|ocular (corneal graft) (orbital implant) NEC
||T85.828
|orthopedic NEC T84.82
|specified NEC T85.828
|urinary NEC T83.82
|vascular NEC T82.828
|ventricular intracranial shunt T85.820
|ejaculatory duct N50.89
|endocardium *see* Endocarditis
|endomyocardial (tropical) I42.3
|epididymis N50.89
|eye muscle *see* Strabismus, mechanical
|heart *see* Myocarditis
|hepatic *see* Fibrosis, liver
|hepatolienal (portal hypertension) K76.6
|hepatosplenic (portal hypertension) K76.6
|infrapatellar fat pad M79.4
|intrascrotal N50.89
|kidney N26.9
|liver K74.00
||with sclerosis K74.2
||advanced K74.02
||alcoholic K70.2
||early K74.01
||stage
|||F1 or F2 K74.01
|||F3 K74.02
|lung (atrophic) (chronic) (confluent) (massive)
||(perialveolar) (peribronchial) J84.10
||with
|||anthracosilicosis J60
|||anthracosis J60
|||asbestosis J61
|||bagassosis J67.1
|||bauxite J63.1
|||berylliosis J63.2
|||byssinosis J66.0
|||calcicosis J62.8
|||chalicosis J62.8
|||dust reticulation J64
|||farmer's lung J67.0
|||ganister disease J62.8

Fibrosis, fibrotic - *continued*
    |graphite J63.3
    |pneumoconiosis NOS J64
    |siderosis J63.4
    |silicosis J62.8
    |capillary J84.10
    |congenital P27.8
    |diffuse (idiopathic) J84.10
      |chemicals, gases, fumes or vapors
        (inhalation) J68.4
      |interstitial J84.10
        |acute J84.114
      |talc J62.0
    |following radiation J70.1
    |idiopathic J84.112
    |postinflammatory J84.10
    |silicotic J62.8
    |tuberculous *see* Tuberculosis, pulmonary
    lymphatic gland I89.8
    |median bar *see* Hyperplasia, prostate
    |mediastinum (idiopathic) J98.59
    |meninges G96.198
    |myocardium, myocardial *see* Myocarditis
    |ovary N83.8
    |oviduct N83.8
    |pancreas K86.89
    |penis NEC N48.6
    |pericardium I31.0
    |perineum, in pregnancy or childbirth O34.7-
      |causing obstructed labor O65.5
    |pleura J94.1
    |popliteal fat pad M79.4
    |prostate (chronic) *see* Hyperplasia, prostate
    |pulmonary *see also* Fibrosis, lung J84.10
      |congenital P27.8
      |idiopathic J84.112
    |rectal sphincter K62.89
    |retroperitoneal, idiopathic (with ureteral
      obstruction) N13.5
      |with infection N13.6
    |sclerosing mesenteric (idiopathic) K65.4
    |scrotum N50.89
    |seminal vesicle N50.89
    |senile R54
    |skin L90.5
    |spermatic cord N50.89
    |spleen D73.89
      |in schistosomiasis (bilharziasis) B65.9
        [D77]
    |subepidermal nodular *see* Neoplasm, skin,
      benign
    |submucous (oral) (tongue) K13.5
    |testis N44.8
      |chronic, due to syphilis A52.76
    |thymus (gland) E32.8
    |tongue, submucous K13.5
    |tunica vaginalis N50.89
    |uterus (non-neoplastic) N85.8
    |vagina N89.8
    |valve, heart *see* Endocarditis
    |vas deferens N50.89
    |vein I87.8
Fibrositis (periarticular) M79.7
    |nodular, chronic (Jaccoud's) (rheumatoid) *see*
      Arthropathy, postrheumatic, chronic
Fibrothorax J94.1
Fibrotic *see* Fibrosis
Fibrous *see* condition
Fibroxanthoma *see also* Neoplasm, connective
    tissue, benign
    |atypical *see* Neoplasm, connective tissue,
      uncertain behavior
    |malignant *see* Neoplasm, connective tissue,
      malignant

Fibroxanthosarcoma *see* Neoplasm, connective
    tissue, malignant
Fiedler's
    |disease (icterohemorrhagic leptospirosis)
      A27.0
    |myocarditis (acute) I40.1
Fifth disease B08.3
    |venereal A55
Filaria, filarial, filariasis *see* Infestation, filarial
Filatov's disease *see* Mononucleosis, infectious
File-Cutter's disease *see* Poisoning, lead
Filling defect
    |biliary tract R93.2
    |bladder R93.41
    |duodenum R93.3
    |gallbladder R93.2
    |gastrointestinal tract R93.3
    |intestine R93.3
    |kidney R93.42-
    |stomach R93.3
    |ureter R93.41
    |urinary organs, specified NEC R93.49
Fimbrial cyst Q50.4
Financial problem affecting care NOS Z59.9
    |bankruptcy Z59.89
    |foreclosure on loan Z59.89
    home loan Z59.81-
Findings, abnormal, inconclusive, without
    diagnosis *see also* Abnormal
    |17-ketosteroids, elevated R82.5
    |acetonuria R82.4
    |alcohol in blood R78.0
    |anisocytosis R71.8
    |antenatal screening of mother O28.9
      |biochemical O28.1
      |chromosomal O28.5
      |cytological O28.2
      |genetic O28.5
      |hematological O28.0
      |radiological O28.4
      |specified NEC O28.8
      |ultrasonic O28.3
    |antibody titer, elevated R76.0
    |anticardiolipin antibody R76.0
    |antiphosphatidylglycerol antibody R76.0
    |antiphosphatidylinositol antibody R76.0
    |antiphosphatidylserine antibody R76.0
    |antiphospholipid antibody R76.0
    |bacteriuria R82.71
    |bicarbonate E87.8
    |bile in urine R82.2
    |blood sugar R73.09
      |high R73.9
      |low (transient) E16.2
    |body fluid or substance, specified NEC R88.8
    |casts, urine R82.998
    |catecholamines R82.5
    |cells, urine R82.998
    |chloride E87.8
    |cholesterol E78.9
      |high E78.00
        |with high triglycerides E78.2
    |chyluria R82.0
    |cloudy
      |dialysis effluent R88.0
      |urine R82.90
    |creatinine clearance R94.4
    |crystals, urine R82.998
    |culture
      |blood R78.81
      |positive *see* Positive, culture
    |echocardiogram R93.1
    |electrolyte level, urinary R82.99
    |function study NEC R94.8
      |bladder R94.8

Findings - *continued*
    |endocrine NEC R94.7
      |thyroid R94.6
    |kidney R94.4
    |liver R94.5
    |pancreas R94.8
    |placenta R94.8
    |pulmonary R94.2
    |spleen R94.8
    |gallbladder, nonvisualization R93.2
    |glucose (tolerance test) (non-fasting) R73.09
    |glycosuria R81
    |heart
      |shadow R93.1
      |sounds R01.2
    |hematinuria R82.3
    |hematocrit drop (precipitous) R71.0
    |hemoglobinuria R82.3
    |human papillomavirus (HPV) DNA test
      positive
      |cervix
        |high risk R87.810
        |low risk R87.820
      |vagina
        |high risk R87.811
        |low risk R87.821
    |in blood (of substance not normally found in
      blood) R78.9
      |addictive drug NEC R78.4
      |alcohol (excessive level) R78.0
      |cocaine R78.2
      |hallucinogen R78.3
      |heavy metals (abnormal level) R78.79
      |lead R78.71
      |lithium (abnormal level) R78.89
      |opiate drug R78.1
      |psychotropic drug R78.5
      |specified substance NEC R78.89
      |steroid agent R78.6
    |indoleacetic acid, elevated R82.5
    |ketonuria R82.4
    |lactic acid dehydrogenase (LDH) R74.02
    |liver function test (see also Elevated, liver
      function, test) R79.89
    |mammogram NEC R92.8
      |calcification (calculus) R92.1
      |inconclusive result (due to dense breasts)
        R92.2
      |microcalcification R92.0
    |mediastinal shift R93.89
    |melanin, urine R82.998
    |myoglobinuria R82.1
    |neonatal screening - see Abnormal, neonatal
      screening
  - newborn screens, state mandated - see
      Abnormal, neonatal
    |nonvisualization of gallbladder R93.2
    |odor of urine NOS R82.90
    |Papanicolaou cervix R87.619
      |non-atypical endometrial cells R87.618
    |pneumoencephalogram R93.0
    |poikilocytosis R71.8
    |potassium (deficiency) E87.6
      |excess E87.5
    |PPD R76.11
    |radiologic (X-ray) R93.89
      |abdomen R93.5
      |biliary tract R93.2
      |breast R92.8
      |gastrointestinal tract R93.3
      |genitourinary organs R93.89
      |head R93.0
      |inconclusive due to excess body fat of
        patient R93.9
      |intrathoracic organs NEC R93.1
      |placenta R93.89

Findings - *continued*

|retroperitoneum R93.5
|skin R93.89
|skull R93.0
|subcutaneous tissue R93.89
|testis R93.81-
|red blood cell (count) (morphology) (sickling)
(volume) R71.8
|scan NEC R94.8
|bladder R94.8
|bone R94.8
|kidney R94.4
|liver R93.2
|lung R94.2
|pancreas R94.8
|placental R94.8
|spleen R94.8
|thyroid R94.6
|sedimentation rate, elevated R70.0
|SGOT R74.01
|SGPT R74.01
|sodium (deficiency) E87.1
|excess E87.0
|specified body fluid NEC R88.8
|stress test R94.39
|thyroid (function) (metabolic rate) (scan)
(uptake) R94.6
|transaminase (level) R74.01
|triglycerides E78.9
|high E78.1
|with high cholesterol E78.2
|tuberculin skin test (without active
tuberculosis) R76.11
|urine R82.90
|acetone R82.4
|bacteria R82.71
|bile R82.2
|casts or cells R82.998
|chyle R82.0
|culture positive R82.79
|glucose R81
|hemoglobin R82.3
|ketone R82.4
|sugar R81
|vanillylmandelic acid (VMA), elevated R82.5
|vectorcardiogram (VCG) R94.39
|ventriculogram R93.0
|white blood cell (count) (differential)
(morphology) D72.9
|xerography R92.8
Finger *see* condition
Fire, Saint Anthony's *see* Erysipelas
Fire-Setting
|pathological (compulsive) F63.1
Fish hook stomach K31.89
Fishmeal-Worker's lung J67.8
Fissure, fissured
|anus, anal K60.2
|acute K60.0
|chronic K60.1
|congenital Q43.8
|ear, lobule, congenital Q17.8
|epiglottis (congenital) Q31.8
|larynx J38.7
|congenital Q31.8
|lip K13.0
|congenital *see* Cleft, lip
|nipple N64.0
|associated with
|lactation O92.13
|pregnancy O92.11-
|puerperium O92.12
|nose Q30.2
|palate (congenital) *see* Cleft, palate
|skin R23.4

Fissure, fissured - *continued*

|spine (congenital) *see also* Spina bifida
|with hydrocephalus *see* Spina bifida, by site,
with hydrocephalus
|tongue (acquired) K14.5
|congenital Q38.3
Fistula (cutaneous) L98.8
|abdomen (wall) K63.2
|bladder N32.2
|intestine NEC K63.2
|ureter N28.89
|uterus N82.5
|abdominorectal K63.2
|abdominosigmoidal K63.2
|abdominothoracic J86.0
|abdominouterine N82.5
|congenital Q51.7
|abdominovesical N32.2
|accessory sinuses *see* Sinusitis
|actinomycotic *see* Actinomycosis
|alveolar antrum *see* Sinusitis, maxillary
|alveolar process K04.6
|anorectal K60.5
|antrobuccal *see* Sinusitis, maxillary
|antrum *see* Sinusitis, maxillary
|anus, anal (recurrent) (infectional) K60.3
|congenital Q43.6
|with absence, atresia and stenosis Q42.2
|tuberculous A18.32
|aorta-duodenal I77.2
|appendix, appendicular K38.3
|arteriovenous (acquired) (nonruptured) I77.0
|brain I67.1
|congenital Q28.2
|ruptured I60.8
|ruptured I60.8
|cerebral *see* Fistula, arteriovenous, brain
|congenital (peripheral) *see also*
Malformation, arteriovenous
|brain Q28.2
|ruptured I60.8
|coronary Q24.5
|pulmonary Q25.72
|coronary I25.41
|congenital Q24.5
|pulmonary I28.0
|congenital Q25.72
|surgically created (for dialysis) Z99.2
|complication *see* Complication,
arteriovenous, fistula, surgically created
|traumatic *see* Injury, blood vessel
|artery I77.2
|aural (mastoid) *see* Mastoiditis, chronic
|auricle *see also* Disorder, pinna, specified type
NEC
|congenital Q18.1
|Bartholin's gland N82.8
|bile duct (common) (hepatic) K83.3
|with calculus, stones (*see also* Calculus,
bile duct) K83.3
|biliary (tract) *see* Fistula, bile duct
|bladder (sphincter) NEC *see also* Fistula,
vesico N32.2
|into seminal vesicle N32.2
|bone *see also* Disorder, bone, specified type
NEC
|with osteomyelitis, chronic *see*
Osteomyelitis, chronic, with draining
sinus
|brain G93.89
|arteriovenous (acquired) I67.1
|congenital Q28.2
|branchial (cleft) Q18.0
|branchiogenous Q18.0
|breast N61.0

Fistula (cutaneous) - *continued*

|puerperal, postpartum or gestational, due to
mastitis (purulent) *see* Mastitis, obstetric,
purulent
|bronchial J86.0
|bronchocutaneous, bronchomediastinal,
bronchopleural, bronchopleuromediastinal
(infective) J86.0
|tuberculous NEC A15.5
|bronchoesophageal J86.0
|congenital Q39.2
|with atresia of esophagus Q39.1
|bronchovisceral J86.0
|buccal cavity (infective) K12.2
|cecosigmoidal K63.2
|cecum K63.2
|cerebrospinal (fluid) G96.08
|cervical, lateral Q18.1
|cervicoaural Q18.1
|cervicosigmoidal N82.4
|cervicovesical N82.1
|cervix N82.8
|chest (wall) J86.0
|cholecystenteric *see* Fistula, gallbladder
|cholecystocolic *see* Fistula, gallbladder
|cholecystocolonic *see* Fistula, gallbladder
|cholecystoduodenal *see* Fistula, gallbladder
|cholecystogastric *see* Fistula, gallbladder
|cholecystointestinal *see* Fistula, gallbladder
|choledochoduodenal *see* Fistula, bile duct
|cholocolic K82.3
|coccyx *see* Sinus, pilonidal
|colon K63.2
|colostomy K94.09
|common duct *see* Fistula, bile duct
|congenital, site not listed *see* Anomaly, by site
|coronary, arteriovenous I25.41
|congenital Q24.5
|costal region J86.0
|cul-de-sac, Douglas' N82.8
|cystic duct *see also* Fistula, gallbladder
|congenital Q44.5
|dental K04.6
|diaphragm J86.0
|duodenum K31.6
|ear (external) (canal) *see* Disorder, ear,
external, specified type NEC
|enterocolic K63.2
|enterocutaneous K63.2
|enterouterine N82.4
|congenital Q51.7
|enterovaginal N82.4
|congenital Q52.2
|large intestine N82.3
|small intestine N82.2
|enterovesical N32.1
|epididymis N50.89
|tuberculous A18.15
|esophagobronchial J86.0
|congenital Q39.2
|with atresia of esophagus Q39.1
|esophagocutaneous K22.89
|esophagopleural-cutaneous J86.0
|esophagotracheal J86.0
|congenital Q39.2
|with atresia of esophagus Q39.1
|esophagus K22.89
|congenital Q39.2
|with atresia of esophagus Q39.1
|ethmoid *see* Sinusitis, ethmoidal
|eyeball (cornea) (sclera) *see* Disorder, globe,
hypotony
|eyelid H01.8
|fallopian tube, external N82.5
|fecal K63.2

Fistula (cutaneous) - *continued*
|congenital Q43.6
|from periapical abscess K04.6
|frontal sinus *see* Sinusitis, frontal
|gallbladder K82.3
　|with calculus, cholelithiasis, stones *see*
　　Calculus, gallbladder
|gastric K31.6
|gastrocolic K31.6
　|congenital Q40.2
　|tuberculous A18.32
|gastroenterocolic K31.6
|gastroesophageal K31.6
|gastrojejunal K31.6
|gastrojejunocolic K31.6
|genital tract (female) N82.9
　|specified NEC N82.8
　|to intestine NEC N82.4
　|to skin N82.5
|hepatic artery-portal vein, congenital Q26.6
|hepatopleural J86.0
|hepatopulmonary J86.0
|ileorectal or ileosigmoidal K63.2
|ileovaginal N82.2
|ileovesical N32.1
|ileum K63.2
|in ano K60.3
　|tuberculous A18.32
|inner ear (labyrinth) *see* subcategory H83.1
|intestine NEC K63.2
|intestinocolonic (abdominal) K63.2
|intestinoureteral N28.89
|intestinouterine N82.4
|intestinovaginal N82.4
　|large intestine N82.3
　|small intestine N82.2
|intestinovesical N32.1
|ischiorectal (fossa) K61.39
|jejunum K63.2
|joint M25.10
　|ankle M25.17-
　|elbow M25.12-
　|foot joint M25.17-
　|hand joint M25.14-
　|hip M25.15-
　|knee M25.16-
　|shoulder M25.11-
　|specified joint NEC M25.18
　|tuberculous *see* Tuberculosis, joint
　|vertebrae M25.18
　|wrist M25.13-
|kidney N28.89
|labium (majus) (minus) N82.8
|labyrinth *see* subcategory H83.1
|lacrimal (gland) (sac) H04.61-
|lacrimonasal duct *see* Fistula, lacrimal
|laryngotracheal, congenital Q34.8
|larynx J38.7
|lip K13.0
　|congenital Q38.0
|lumbar, tuberculous A18.01
|lung J86.0
|lymphatic I89.8
|mammary (gland) N61.0
|mastoid (process) (region) *see* Mastoiditis,
　chronic
|maxillary J32.0
|medial, face and neck Q18.8
|mediastinal J86.0
|mediastinobronchial J86.0
|mediastinocutaneous J86.0
|middle ear *see* subcategory H74.8
|mouth K12.2
|nasal J34.89
　|sinus *see* Sinusitis

Fistula (cutaneous) - *continued*
|nasopharynx J39.2
|nipple N64.0
|nose J34.89
|oral (cutaneous) K12.2
　|maxillary J32.0
　|nasal (with cleft palate) *see* Cleft, palate
|orbit, orbital *see* Disorder, orbit, specified type
　NEC
|oroantral J32.0
|oviduct, external N82.5
|palate (hard) M27.8
|pancreatic K86.89
|pancreaticoduodenal K86.89
|parotid (gland) K11.4
　|region K12.2
|penis N48.89
|perianal K60.3
|pericardium (pleura) (sac) *see* Pericarditis
|pericecal K63.2
|perineorectal K60.4
|perineosigmoidal K63.2
|perineum, perineal (with urethral
　involvement) NEC N36.0
　|tuberculous A18.13
　|ureter N28.89
|perirectal K60.4
　|tuberculous A18.32
|peritoneum K65.9
|pharyngoesophageal J39.2
|pharynx J39.2
　|branchial cleft (congenital) Q18.0
|pilonidal (infected) (rectum) *see* Sinus,
　pilonidal
|pleura, pleural, pleurocutaneous,
　pleuroperitoneal J86.0
　|tuberculous NEC A15.6
|pleuropericardial I31.8
|portal vein-hepatic artery, congenital Q26.6
|postauricular H70.81-
|postoperative, persistent T81.83
　|specified site *see* Fistula, by site
|preauricular (congenital) Q18.1
|prostate N42.89
|pulmonary J86.0
　|arteriovenous I28.0
　　|congenital Q25.72
　|tuberculous *see* Tuberculosis, pulmonary
|pulmonoperitoneal J86.0
|rectolabial N82.4
|rectosigmoid (intercommunicating) K63.2
|rectoureteral N28.89
|rectourethral N36.0
　|congenital Q64.73
|rectouterine N82.4
　|congenital Q51.7
|rectovaginal N82.3
　|congenital Q52.2
　|tuberculous A18.18
|rectovesical N32.1
　|congenital Q64.79
|rectovesicovaginal N82.3
|rectovulval N82.4
　|congenital Q52.79
|rectum (to skin) K60.4
　|congenital Q43.6
　　|with absence, atresia and stenosis Q42.0
　|tuberculous A18.32
|renal N28.89
|retroauricular *see* Fistula, postauricular
|salivary duct or gland (any) K11.4
　|congenital Q38.4
|scrotum (urinary) N50.89
　|tuberculous A18.15
|semicircular canals *see* subcategory H83.1

Fistula (cutaneous) - *continued*
|sigmoid K63.2
　|to bladder N32.1
|sinus *see* Sinusitis
|skin L98.8
　|to genital tract (female) N82.5
|splenocolic D73.89
|stercoral K63.2
|stomach K31.6
|sublingual gland K11.4
|submandibular gland K11.4
|submaxillary (gland) K11.4
　|region K12.2
|thoracic J86.0
　|duct I89.8
|thoracoabdominal J86.0
|thoracogastric J86.0
|thoracointestinal J86.0
|thorax J86.0
|thyroglossal duct Q89.2
|thyroid E07.89
|trachea, congenital (external) (internal) Q32.1
|tracheoesophageal J86.0
　|congenital Q39.2
　　|with atresia of esophagus Q39.1
　|following tracheostomy J95.04
|traumatic arteriovenous *see* Injury, blood
　vessel, by site
|tuberculous　code by site under Tuberculosis
|typhoid A01.09
|umbilicourinary Q64.8
|urachus, congenital Q64.4
|ureter (persistent) N28.89
|ureteroabdominal N28.89
|ureterorectal N28.89
|ureterosigmoido-abdominal N28.89
|ureterovaginal N82.1
|ureterovesical N32.2
|urethra N36.0
　|congenital Q64.79
　|tuberculous A18.13
|urethroperineal N36.0
|urethroperineovesical N32.2
|urethrorectal N36.0
　|congenital Q64.73
|urethroscrotal N50.89
|urethrovaginal N82.1
|urethrovesical N32.2
|urinary (tract) (persistent) (recurrent) N36.0
|uteroabdominal N82.5
　|congenital Q51.7
|uteroenteric, uterointestinal N82.4
　|congenital Q51.7
|uterorectal N82.4
　|congenital Q51.7
|uteroureteric N82.1
|uterourethral Q51.7
|uterovaginal N82.8
|uterovesical N82.1
　|congenital Q51.7
|uterus N82.8
|vagina (postpartal) (wall) N82.8
|vaginocutaneous (postpartal) N82.5
|vaginointestinal NEC N82.4
　|large intestine N82.3
　|small intestine N82.2
|vaginoperineal N82.5
|vasocutaneous, congenital Q55.7
|vesical NEC N32.2
|vesicoabdominal N32.2
|vesicocervicovaginal N82.1
|vesicocolic N32.1
|vesicocutaneous N32.2
|vesicoenteric N32.1
|vesicointestinal N32.1
|vesicometrorectal N82.4

Fistula (cutaneous) - *continued*
|vesicoperineal N32.2
|vesicorectal N32.1
  |congenital Q64.79
|vesicosigmoidal N32.1
|vesicosigmoidovaginal N82.3
|vesicoureteral N32.2
|vesicourethrovaginal N82.1
|vesicourethral N32.2
|vesicourethrorectal N32.1
|vesicouterine N82.1
  |congenital Q51.7
|vesicovaginal N82.0
|vulvorectal N82.4
  |congenital Q52.79
Fit R56.9
|epileptic *see* Epilepsy
|fainting R55
|hysterical F44.5
|newborn P90
Fitting (and adjustment) (of)
|artificial
  |arm *see* Admission, adjustment, artificial,
    arm
  |breast Z44.3
  |eye Z44.2
  |leg *see* Admission, adjustment, artificial, leg
|automatic implantable cardiac defibrillator
    (with synchronous cardiac pacemaker)
    Z45.02
|brain neuropacemaker Z46.2
  |implanted Z45.42
|cardiac defibrillator *see* Fitting (and
    adjustment) (of), automatic implantable
    cardiac defibrillator
|catheter, non-vascular Z46.82
|colostomy belt Z46.89
|contact lenses Z46.0
|CRT-D (resynchronization therapy
    defibrillator) Z45.02
|CRT-P (cardiac resynchronization therapy
    pacemaker) Z45.018
  |pulse generator Z45.010
|cystostomy device Z46.6
|defibrillator, cardiac *see* Fitting (and
    adjustment) (of), automatic implantable
    cardiac defibrillator
|dentures Z46.3
|device NOS Z46.9
  |abdominal Z46.89
  |gastrointestinal NEC Z46.59
  |implanted NEC Z45.89
  |nervous system Z46.2
    |implanted *see* Admission, adjustment,
        device, implanted, nervous system
  |orthodontic Z46.4
  |orthoptic Z46.0
  |orthotic Z46.89
  |prosthetic (external) Z44.9
    |breast Z44.3
    |dental Z46.3
    |eye Z44.2
    |specified NEC Z44.8
  |specified NEC Z46.89
  |substitution
    |auditory Z46.2
      |implanted *see* Admission, adjustment,
          device, implanted, hearing device
    |nervous system Z46.2
      |implanted *see* Admission, adjustment,
          device, implanted, nervous system
    |visual Z46.2
      |implanted Z45.31
  |urinary Z46.6
|gastric lap band Z46.51

Fitting (and adjustment) (of) - *continued*
|gastrointestinal appliance NEC Z46.59
|glasses (reading) Z46.0
|hearing aid Z46.1
|ileostomy device Z46.89
|insulin pump Z46.81
|intestinal appliance NEC Z46.89
|myringotomy device (stent) (tube) Z45.82
|neuropacemaker Z46.2
  |implanted Z45.42
|non-vascular catheter Z46.82
|orthodontic device Z46.4
|orthopedic device (brace) (cast) (corset)
    (shoes) Z46.89
|pacemaker (cardiac) (cardiac
    resynchronization therapy (CRT-P))
    Z45.018
  |nervous system (brain) (peripheral nerve)
      (spinal cord) Z46.2
    |implanted Z45.42
  |pulse generator Z45.010
|portacath (port-a-cath) Z45.2
|prosthesis (external) Z44.9
  |arm *see* Admission, adjustment, artificial,
    arm
  |breast Z44.3
  |dental Z46.3
  |eye Z44.2
  |leg *see* Admission, adjustment, artificial, leg
  |specified NEC Z44.8
|spectacles Z46.0
|wheelchair Z46.89
Fitzhugh-Curtis syndrome
|due to
  |Chlamydia trachomatis A74.81
  |Neisseria gonorrhorea (gonococcal
      peritonitis) A54.85
**Fitz's syndrome (acute hemorrhagic
pancreatitis)** *see also* Pancreatitis, acute
K85.80
Fixation
|joint *see* Ankylosis
|larynx J38.7
|stapes *see* Ankylosis, ear ossicles
  |deafness *see* Deafness, conductive
|uterus (acquired) *see* Malposition, uterus
|vocal cord J38.3
Flabby ridge K06.8
Flaccid *see also* condition
|palate, congenital Q38.5
Flail
|chest S22.5
  |newborn (birth injury) P13.8
|joint (paralytic) M25.20
  |ankle M25.27-
  |elbow M25.22-
  |foot joint M25.27-
  |hand joint M25.24-
  |hip M25.25-
  |knee M25.26-
  |shoulder M25.21-
  |specified joint NEC M25.28
  |wrist M25.23-
Flajani's disease *see* Hyperthyroidism, with,
goiter (diffuse)
Flap, liver K71.3
Flashbacks (residual to hallucinogen use)
F16.283
Flat
|chamber (eye) *see* Disorder, globe, hypotony,
    flat anterior chamber
|chest, congenital Q67.8
|foot (acquired) (fixed type) (painful)
    (postural) *see also* Deformity, limb, flat
    foot

Flat - *continued*
|congenital (rigid) (spastic (everted)) Q66.5-
  |rachitic sequelae (late effect) E64.3
|organ or site, congenital NEC *see* Anomaly,
    by site
|pelvis M95.5
  |with disproportion (fetopelvic) O33.0
    |causing obstructed labor O65.0
  |congenital Q74.2
Flatau-Schilder disease G37.0
Flatback syndrome M40.30
|lumbar region M40.36
|lumbosacral region M40.37
|thoracolumbar region M40.35
Flattening
|head, femur M89.8X5
|hip *see* Coxa, plana
|lip (congenital) Q18.8
|nose (congenital) Q67.4
  |acquired M95.0
Flatulence R14.3
|psychogenic F45.8
Flatus R14.3
|vaginalis N89.8
Flax-Dresser's disease J66.1
Flea bite *see* Injury, bite, by site, superficial,
insect
Flecks, glaucomatous (subcapsular) *see*
Cataract, complicated
Fleischer (-Kayser) ring (cornea) H18.04-
Fleshy mole O02.0
Flexibilitas cerea *see* Catalepsy
Flexion
|amputation stump (surgical) T87.89
|cervix *see* Malposition, uterus
|contracture, joint *see* Contraction, joint
|deformity, joint *see also* Deformity, limb,
    flexion M21.20
  |hip, congenital Q65.89
|uterus *see also* Malposition, uterus
  |lateral *see* Lateroversion, uterus
Flexner-Boyd dysentery A03.2
Flexner's dysentery A03.1
Flexure *see* Flexion
Flint murmur (aortic insufficiency) I35.1
Floater, vitreous *see* Opacity, vitreous
Floating
|cartilage (joint) *see also* Loose, body, joint
  |knee *see* Derangement, knee, loose body
|gallbladder, congenital Q44.1
|kidney N28.89
  |congenital Q63.8
|spleen D73.89
Flooding N92.0
Floor *see* condition
Floppy
|baby syndrome (nonspecific) P94.2
|iris syndrome (intraoperative) (IFIS) H21.81
|nonrheumatic mitral valve syndrome I34.1
Flu *see also* Influenza
|avian *see also* Influenza, due to, identified
    novel influenza A virus J09.X2
|bird *see also* Influenza, due to, identified
    novel influenza A virus J09.X2
|intestinal NEC A08.4
|swine (viruses that normally cause infections
    in pigs) *see also* Influenza, due to,
    identified novel influenza A virus J09.X2
Fluctuating blood pressure I99.8
Fluid
|abdomen R18.8
|chest J94.8
|heart *see* Failure, heart, congestive
|joint *see* Effusion, joint
|loss (acute) E86.9

Fluid - *continued*
|lung *see* Edema, lung
|overload E87.70
  |specified NEC E87.79
|peritoneal cavity R18.8
|pleural cavity J94.8
|retention R60.9
Flukes NEC *see also* Infestation, fluke
|blood NEC *see* Schistosomiasis
|liver B66.3
Fluor (vaginalis) N89.8
|trichomonal or due to Trichomonas (vaginalis)
  A59.00
Fluorosis
|dental K00.3
|skeletal M85.10
  |ankle M85.17-
  |foot M85.17-
  |forearm M85.13-
  |hand M85.14-
  |lower leg M85.16-
  |multiple site M85.19
  |neck M85.18
  |rib M85.18
  |shoulder M85.11-
  |skull M85.18
  |specified site NEC M85.18
  |thigh M85.15-
  |toe M85.17-
  |upper arm M85.12-
  |vertebra M85.18
Flush syndrome E34.0
Flushing R23.2
|menopausal N95.1
Flutter
|atrial or auricular I48.92
  |atypical I48.4
  |type I I48.3
  |type II I48.4
  |typical I48.3
|heart I49.8
  |atrial or auricular I48.92
    |atypical I48.4
    |type I I48.3
    |type II I48.4
    |typical I48.3
  |ventricular I49.02
|ventricular I49.02
**FNHTR (febrile nonhemolytic transfusion
  reaction)** R50.84
Fochier's abscess   code by site under Abscess
Focus, Assmann's *see* Tuberculosis, pulmonary
Fogo selvagem L10.3
Foix-Alajouanine syndrome G95.19
Fold, folds (anomalous) *see also* Anomaly, by
  site
|Descemet's membrane *see* Change, corneal
  membrane, Descemet's, fold
|epicanthic Q10.3
|heart Q24.8
Folie à deux F24
Follicle
|cervix (nabothian) (ruptured) N88.8
|graafian, ruptured, with hemorrhage N83.0-
|nabothian N88.8
Follicular *see* condition
Folliculitis (superficial) L73.9
|abscedens et suffodiens L66.3
|cyst N83.0-
|decalvans L66.2
|deep *see* Furuncle, by site
|gonococcal (acute) (chronic) A54.01
|keloid, keloidalis L73.0
|pustular L01.02
|ulerythematosa reticulata L66.4

Folliculome lipidique
|specified site *see* Neoplasm, benign, by site
|unspecified site
  |female D27.9
  |male D29.20
Følling's disease E70.0
Follow-Up *see* Examination, follow-up
**Fong's syndrome (hereditary osteo-
  Onychodysplasia)** Q87.2
Food
|allergy L27.2
|asphyxia (from aspiration or inhalation) *see*
  Foreign body, by site
|choked on *see* Foreign body, by site
|deprivation T73.0
  |specified kind of food NEC E63.8
|intoxication *see* Poisoning, food
|insecurity Z59.41
|lack of T73.0
|poisoning *see* Poisoning, food
|rejection NEC *see* Disorder, eating
|strangulation or suffocation *see* Foreign body,
  by site
|toxemia *see* Poisoning, food
Foot *see* condition
**Foramen ovale (nonclosure) (patent)
  (persistent)** Q21.1
Forbes' glycogen storage disease E74.03
Fordyce-Fox disease L75.2
Fordyce's disease (mouth) Q38.6
Forearm *see* condition
Foreclosure on loan Z59.89
Foreign body
  with
  |laceration *see* Laceration, by site, with
    foreign body
  |puncture wound *see* Puncture, by site, with
    foreign body
|accidentally left following a procedure
  T81.509
|aspiration T81.506
  |resulting in
    |adhesions T81.516
    |obstruction T81.526
    |perforation T81.536
    |specified complication NEC T81.596
|cardiac catheterization T81.505
  |resulting in
    |acute reaction T81.60
      |aseptic peritonitis T81.61
      |specified NEC T81.69
    |adhesions T81.515
    |obstruction T81.525
    |perforation T81.535
    |specified complication NEC T81.595
|causing
  |acute reaction T81.60
    |aseptic peritonitis T81.61
    |specified complication NEC T81.69
  |adhesions T81.519
  |aseptic peritonitis T81.61
  |obstruction T81.529
  |perforation T81.539
  |specified complication NEC T81.599
|endoscopy T81.504
  |resulting in
    |adhesions T81.514
    |obstruction T81.524
    |perforation T81.534
    |specified complication NEC T81.594
|immunization T81.503
  |resulting in
    |adhesions T81.513
    |obstruction T81.523
    |perforation T81.533

Foreign body - *continued*
    |specified complication NEC T81.593
|infusion T81.501
  |resulting in
    |adhesions T81.511
    |obstruction T81.521
    |perforation T81.531
    |specified complication NEC T81.591
|injection T81.503
  |resulting in
    |adhesions T81.513
    |obstruction T81.523
    |perforation T81.533
    |specified complication NEC T81.593
|kidney dialysis T81.502
  |resulting in
    |adhesions T81.512
    |obstruction T81.522
    |perforation T81.532
    |specified complication NEC T81.592
|packing removal T81.507
  |resulting in
    |acute reaction T81.60
      |aseptic peritonitis T81.61
      |specified NEC T81.69
    |adhesions T81.517
    |obstruction T81.527
    |perforation T81.537
    |specified complication NEC T81.597
|puncture T81.506
  |resulting in
    |adhesions T81.516
    |obstruction T81.526
    |perforation T81.536
    |specified complication NEC T81.596
|specified procedure NEC T81.508
  |resulting in
    |acute reaction T81.60
      |aseptic peritonitis T81.61
      |specified NEC T81.69
    |adhesions T81.518
    |obstruction T81.528
    |perforation T81.538
    |specified complication NEC T81.598
|surgical operation T81.500
  |resulting in
    |acute reaction T81.60
      |aseptic peritonitis T81.61
      |specified NEC T81.69
    |adhesions T81.510
    |obstruction T81.520
    |perforation T81.530
    |specified complication NEC T81.590
|transfusion T81.501
  |resulting in
    |adhesions T81.511
    |obstruction T81.521
    |perforation T81.531
    |specified complication NEC T81.591
|alimentary tract T18.9
  |anus T18.5
  |colon T18.4
  |esophagus *see* Foreign body, esophagus
  |mouth T18.0
  |multiple sites T18.8
  |rectosigmoid (junction) T18.5
  |rectum T18.5
  |small intestine T18.3
  |specified site NEC T18.8
  |stomach T18.2
|anterior chamber (eye) S05.5-
|auditory canal *see* Foreign body, entering
  through orifice, ear
|bronchus T17.508
  |causing

Foreign body - *continued*
   |asphyxiation T17.500
     |food (bone) (seed) T17.520
     |gastric contents (vomitus) T17.510
     |specified type NEC T17.590
   |injury NEC T17.508
     |food (bone) (seed) T17.528
     |gastric contents (vomitus) T17.518
     |specified type NEC T17.598
  |canthus *see* Foreign body, conjunctival sac
  |ciliary body (eye) S05.5-
  |conjunctival sac T15.1-
  |cornea T15.0-
  |entering through orifice
   |accessory sinus T17.0
   |alimentary canal T18.9
    |multiple parts T18.8
    |specified part NEC T18.8
   |alveolar process T18.0
   |antrum (Highmore's) T17.0
   |anus T18.5
   |appendix T18.4
   |auditory canal *see* Foreign body, entering
     through orifice, ear
   |auricle *see* Foreign body, entering through
     orifice, ear
   |bladder T19.1
   |bronchioles *see* Foreign body, respiratory
     tract, specified site NEC
   |bronchus (main) *see* Foreign body, bronchus
   |buccal cavity T18.0
   |canthus (inner) *see* Foreign body,
     conjunctival sac
   |cecum T18.4
   |cervix (canal) (uteri) T19.3
   |colon T18.4
   |conjunctival sac *see* Foreign body,
     conjunctival sac
   |cornea *see* Foreign body, cornea
   |digestive organ or tract NOS T18.9
    |multiple parts T18.8
    |specified part NEC T18.8
   |duodenum T18.3
   |ear (external) T16.-
   |esophagus *see* Foreign body, esophagus
   |eye (external) NOS T15.9-
    |conjunctival sac *see* Foreign body,
     conjunctival sac
    |cornea *see* Foreign body, cornea
    |specified part NEC T15.8-
   |eyeball *see also* Foreign body, entering
     through orifice, eye, specified part NEC
    |with penetrating wound *see* Puncture,
     eyeball
   |eyelid *see also* Foreign body, conjunctival
     sac
    |with
     |laceration *see* Laceration, eyelid, with
      foreign body
     |puncture *see* Puncture, eyelid, with
      foreign body
     |superficial injury *see* Foreign body,
      superficial, eyelid
   |gastrointestinal tract T18.9
    |multiple parts T18.8
    |specified part NEC T18.8
   |genitourinary tract T19.9
    |multiple parts T19.8
    |specified part NEC T19.8
   |globe *see* Foreign body, entering through
     orifice, eyeball
   |gum T18.0
   |Highmore's antrum T17.0
   |hypopharynx *see* Foreign body, pharynx
   |ileum T18.3

Foreign body - *continued*
   |intestine (small) T18.3
    |large T18.4
   |lacrimal apparatus (punctum) *see* Foreign
     body, entering through orifice, eye,
     specified part NEC
   |large intestine T18.4
   |larynx *see* Foreign body, larynx
   |lung *see* Foreign body, respiratory tract,
     specified site NEC
   |maxillary sinus T17.0
   |mouth T18.0
   |nasal sinus T17.0
   |nasopharynx *see* Foreign body, pharynx
   |nose (passage) T17.1
   |nostril T17.1
   |oral cavity T18.0
   |palate T18.0
   |penis T19.4
   |pharynx *see* Foreign body, pharynx
   |piriform sinus *see* Foreign body, pharynx
   |rectosigmoid (junction) T18.5
   |rectum T18.5
   |respiratory tract *see* Foreign body,
     respiratory tract
   |sinus (accessory) (frontal) (maxillary)
     (nasal) T17.0
    |piriform *see* Foreign body, pharynx
   |small intestine T18.3
   |stomach T18.2
   |suffocation by *see* Foreign body, by site
   |tear ducts or glands *see* Foreign body,
     entering through orifice, eye, specified
     part NEC
   |throat *see* Foreign body, pharynx
   |tongue T18.0
   |tonsil, tonsillar (fossa) *see* Foreign body,
     pharynx
   |trachea *see* Foreign body, trachea
   |ureter T19.8
   |urethra T19.0
   |uterus (any part) T19.3
   |vagina T19.2
   |vulva T19.2
  |esophagus T18.108
   |causing
    |injury NEC T18.108
     |food (bone) (seed) T18.128
     |gastric contents (vomitus) T18.118
     |specified type NEC T18.198
    |tracheal compression T18.100
     |food (bone) (seed) T18.120
     |gastric contents (vomitus) T18.110
     |specified type NEC T18.190
  |feeling of, in throat R09.89
  |fragment *see* Retained, foreign body
    fragments (type of)
  |genitourinary tract T19.9
   |bladder T19.1
   |multiple parts T19.8
   |penis T19.4
   |specified site NEC T19.8
   |urethra T19.0
   |uterus T19.3
    |IUD Z97.5
   |vagina T19.2
    |contraceptive device Z97.5
   |vulva T19.2
  |granuloma (old) (soft tissue) *see also*
    Granuloma, foreign body
   |skin L92.3
  |in
   |laceration *see* Laceration, by site, with
     foreign body

Foreign body - *continued*
   |puncture wound *see* Puncture, by site, with
     foreign body
   |soft tissue (residual) M79.5
  |inadvertently left in operation wound *see*
    Foreign body, accidentally left during a
    procedure
  |ingestion, ingested NOS T18.9
  |inhalation or inspiration *see* Foreign body, by
    site
  |internal organ, not entering through a natural
    orifice   code as specific injury with
    foreign body
  |intraocular S05.5-
   |old, retained (nonmagnetic) H44.70-
    |anterior chamber H44.71-
    |ciliary body H44.72-
    |iris H44.72-
    |lens H44.73-
    |magnetic H44.60-
     |anterior chamber H44.61-
     |ciliary body H44.62-
     |iris H44.62-
     |lens H44.63-
     |posterior wall H44.64-
     |specified site NEC H44.69-
     |vitreous body H44.65-
    |posterior wall H44.74-
    |specified site NEC H44.79-
    |vitreous body H44.75-
  |iris *see* Foreign body, intraocular
  |lacrimal punctum *see* Foreign body, entering
    through orifice, eye, specified part NEC
  |larynx T17.308
   |causing
    |asphyxiation T17.300
     |food (bone) (seed) T17.320
     |gastric contents (vomitus) T17.310
     |specified type NEC T17.390
    |injury NEC T17.308
     |food (bone) (seed) T17.328
     |gastric contents (vomitus) T17.318
     |specified type NEC T17.398
  |lens *see* Foreign body, intraocular
  |ocular muscle S05.4-
   |old, retained *see* Foreign body, orbit, old
  |old or residual
   |soft tissue (residual) M79.5
  |operation wound, left accidentally *see* Foreign
    body, accidentally left during a procedure
  |orbit S05.4-
   |old, retained H05.5-
  |pharynx T17.208
   |causing
    |asphyxiation T17.200
     |food (bone) (seed) T17.220
     |gastric contents (vomitus) T17.210
     |specified type NEC T17.290
    |injury NEC T17.208
     |food (bone) (seed) T17.228
     |gastric contents (vomitus) T17.218
     |specified type NEC T17.298
  |respiratory tract T17.908
   |bronchioles *see* Foreign body, respiratory
     tract, specified site NEC
   |bronchus *see* Foreign body, bronchus
   |causing
    |asphyxiation T17.900
     |food (bone) (seed) T17.920
     |gastric contents (vomitus) T17.910
     |specified type NEC T17.990
    |injury NEC T17.908
     |food (bone) (seed) T17.928
     |gastric contents (vomitus) T17.918
     |specified type NEC T17.998

Foreign body - *continued*

|larynx *see* Foreign body, larynx
|lung *see* Foreign body, respiratory tract,
   specified site NEC
|multiple parts *see* Foreign body, respiratory
   tract, specified site NEC
|nasal sinus T17.0
|nasopharynx *see* Foreign body, pharynx
|nose T17.1
|nostril T17.1
|pharynx *see* Foreign body, pharynx
|specified site NEC T17.808
   |causing
      |asphyxiation T17.800
         |food (bone) (seed) T17.820
         |gastric contents (vomitus) T17.810
         |specified type NEC T17.890
      |injury NEC T17.808
         |food (bone) (seed) T17.828
         |gastric contents (vomitus) T17.818
         |specified type NEC T17.898
|throat *see* Foreign body, pharynx
|trachea *see* Foreign body, trachea
|retained (old) (nonmagnetic) (in)
   |anterior chamber (eye) *see* Foreign body,
      intraocular, old, retained, anterior
      chamber
      |magnetic *see* Foreign body, intraocular,
         old, retained, magnetic, anterior
         chamber
   |ciliary body *see* Foreign body, intraocular,
      old, retained, ciliary body
      |magnetic *see* Foreign body, intraocular,
         old, retained, magnetic, ciliary body
   |eyelid H02.819
      |left H02.816
         |lower H02.815
         |upper H02.814
      |right H02.813
         |lower H02.812
         |upper H02.811
   |fragments *see* Retained, foreign body
      fragments (type of)
   |globe *see* Foreign body, intraocular, old,
      retained
      |magnetic *see* Foreign body, intraocular,
         old, retained, magnetic
   |intraocular *see* Foreign body, intraocular,
      old, retained
      |magnetic *see* Foreign body, intraocular,
         old, retained, magnetic
   |iris *see* Foreign body, intraocular, old,
      retained, iris
      |magnetic *see* Foreign body, intraocular,
         old, retained, magnetic, iris
   |lens *see* Foreign body, intraocular, old,
      retained, lens
      |magnetic *see* Foreign body, intraocular,
         old, retained, magnetic, lens
   |muscle *see* Foreign body, retained, soft
      tissue
   |orbit *see* Foreign body, orbit, old
   |posterior wall of globe *see* Foreign body,
      intraocular, old, retained, posterior wall
      |magnetic *see* Foreign body, intraocular,
         old, retained, magnetic, posterior wall
   |retrobulbar *see* Foreign body, orbit, old,
      retrobulbar
   |soft tissue M79.5
   |vitreous *see* Foreign body, intraocular, old,
      retained, vitreous body
      |magnetic *see* Foreign body, intraocular,
         old, retained, magnetic, vitreous body
|retina S05.5-
|superficial, without open wound

Foreign body - *continued*

|abdomen, abdominal (wall) S30.851
|alveolar process S00.552
|ankle S90.55-
|antecubital space *see* Foreign body,
   superficial, forearm
|anus S30.857
|arm (upper) S40.85-
|auditory canal *see* Foreign body, superficial,
   ear
|auricle *see* Foreign body, superficial, ear
|axilla *see* Foreign body, superficial, arm
|back, lower S30.850
|breast S20.15-
|brow S00.85
|buttock S30.850
|calf *see* Foreign body, superficial, leg
|canthus *see* Foreign body, superficial, eyelid
|cheek S00.85
   |internal S00.552
|chest wall *see* Foreign body, superficial,
   thorax
|chin S00.85
|clitoris S30.854
|costal region *see* Foreign body, superficial,
   thorax
|digit(s)
   |hand *see* Foreign body, superficial, finger
   |foot *see* Foreign body, superficial, toe
|ear S00.45-
|elbow S50.35-
|epididymis S30.853
|epigastric region S30.851
|epiglottis S10.15
|esophagus, cervical S10.15
|eyebrow *see* Foreign body, superficial,
   eyelid
|eyelid S00.25-
|face S00.85
|finger(s) S60.459
   |index S60.45-
   |little S60.45-
   |middle S60.45-
   |ring S60.45-
|flank S30.851
|foot (except toe(s) alone) S90.85-
   |toe *see* Foreign body, superficial, toe
|forearm S50.85-
   |elbow only *see* Foreign body, superficial,
      elbow
|forehead S00.85
|genital organs, external
   |female S30.856
   |male S30.855
|groin S30.851
|gum S00.552
|hand S60.55-
|head S00.95
   |ear *see* Foreign body, superficial, ear
   |eyelid *see* Foreign body, superficial,
      eyelid
   |lip S00.551
   |nose S00.35
   |oral cavity S00.552
   |scalp S00.05
   |specified site NEC S00.85
|heel *see* Foreign body, superficial, foot
|hip S70.25-
|inguinal region S30.851
|interscapular region S20.459
|jaw S00.85
|knee S80.25-
|labium (majus) (minus) S30.854
|larynx S10.15
|leg (lower) S80.85-

Foreign body - *continued*

|knee *see* Foreign body, superficial, knee
   |upper *see* Foreign body, superficial, thigh
|lip S00.551
|lower back S30.850
|lumbar region S30.850
|malar region S00.85
|mammary *see* Foreign body, superficial,
   breast
|mastoid region S00.85
|mouth S00.552
|nail
   |finger *see* Foreign body, superficial,
      finger
   |toe *see* Foreign body, superficial, toe
|nape S10.85
|nasal S00.35
|neck S10.95
   |specified site NEC S10.85
   |throat S10.15
|nose S00.35
|occipital region S00.05
|oral cavity S00.552
|orbital region *see* Foreign body, superficial,
   eyelid
|palate S00.552
|palm *see* Foreign body, superficial, hand
|parietal region S00.05
|pelvis S30.850
|penis S30.852
|perineum
   |female S30.854
   |male S30.850
|periocular area *see* Foreign body,
   superficial, eyelid
|phalanges
   |finger *see* Foreign body, superficial,
      finger
   |toe *see* Foreign body, superficial, toe
|pharynx S10.15
|pinna *see* Foreign body, superficial, ear
|popliteal space *see* Foreign body,
   superficial, knee
|prepuce S30.852
|pubic region S30.850
|pudendum
   |female S30.856
   |male S30.855
|sacral region S30.850
|scalp S00.05
|scapular region *see* Foreign body,
   superficial, shoulder
|scrotum S30.853
|shin *see* Foreign body, superficial, leg
|shoulder S40.25-
|sternal region S20.359
|submaxillary region S00.85
|submental region S00.85
|subungual
   |finger(s) *see* Foreign body, superficial,
      finger
   |toe(s) *see* Foreign body, superficial, toe
|supraclavicular fossa S10.85
|supraorbital S00.85
|temple S00.85
|temporal region S00.85
|testis S30.853
|thigh S70.35-
|thorax, thoracic (wall) S20.95
   |back S20.45-
   |front S20.35-
|throat S10.15
|thumb S60.35-
|toe(s) (lesser) S90.456
   |great S90.45-

Foreign body - *continued*
|tongue S00.552
|trachea S10.15
|tunica vaginalis S30.853
|tympanum, tympanic membrane *see* Foreign body, superficial, ear
|uvula S00.552
|vagina S30.854
|vocal cords S10.15
|vulva S30.854
|wrist S60.85-
|swallowed T18.9
|trachea T17.408
|causing
|asphyxiation T17.400
|food (bone) (seed) T17.420
|gastric contents (vomitus) T17.410
|specified type NEC T17.490
|injury NEC T17.408
|food (bone) (seed) T17.428
|gastric contents (vomitus) T17.418
|specified type NEC T17.498
|type of fragment *see* Retained, foreign body fragments (type of)
|vitreous (humor) S05.5-
Forestier's disease (rhizomelic pseudopolyarthritis) M35.3
|meaning ankylosing hyperostosis *see* Hyperostosis, ankylosing
Formation
|hyalin in cornea *see* Degeneration, cornea
|sequestrum in bone (due to infection) *see* Osteomyelitis, chronic
|valve
|colon, congenital Q43.8
|ureter (congenital) Q62.39
Formication R20.2
Fort Bragg fever A27.89
Fossa *see also* condition
|pyriform *see* condition
Foster-Kennedy syndrome H47.14-
Fothergill's
|disease (trigeminal neuralgia) *see also* Neuralgia, trigeminal
|scarlatina anginosa A38.9
Foul breath R19.6
Foundling Z76.1
Fournier disease or gangrene N49.3
|female N76.89
Fourth
|cranial nerve *see* condition
|molar K00.1
Foville's (peduncular) disease or syndrome G46.3
Fox (-Fordyce) disease (apocrine miliaria) L75.2
FPIES (food protein-Induced enteropathy syndrome) K52.21
Fracture, burst *see* Fracture, traumatic, by site
Fracture, chronic *see* Fracture, pathological, by site
Fracture, nontraumatic, NEC
|atypical
|femur M84.750-
|complete
|oblique M84.759
|left side M84.758
|right side M84.757
|transverse M84.756
|left side M84.755
|right side M84.754
|incomplete M84.753
|left side M84.752
|right side M84.751

Fracture, pathological (pathologic) *see also* Fracture, traumatic M84.40
|ankle M84.47-
|carpus M84.44-
|clavicle M84.41-
|compression (not due to trauma) *see also* Collapse, vertebra M48.50-
|dental implant M27.63
|dental restorative material K08.539
|with loss of material K08.531
|without loss of material K08.530
|due to
|neoplastic disease NEC *see also* Neoplasm M84.50
|ankle M84.57
|carpus M84.54-
|clavicle M84.51-
|femur M84.55-
|fibula M84.56-
|finger M84.54-
|hip M84.559
|humerus M84.52-
|ilium M84.550
|ischium M84.550
|metacarpus M84.54-
|metatarsus M84.57-
|neck M84.58
|pelvis M84.550
|radius M84.53-
|rib M84.58
|scapula M84.51-
|skull M84.58
|specified site NEC M84.58
|tarsus M84.57-
|tibia M84.56-
|toe M84.57-
|ulna M84.53-
|vertebra M84.58
|osteoporosis M80.00
|disuse *see* Osteoporosis, specified type NEC, with pathological fracture
|drug-induced *see* Osteoporosis, drug induced, with pathological fracture
|idiopathic *see* Osteoporosis, specified type NEC, with pathological fracture
|postmenopausal *see* Osteoporosis, postmenopausal, with pathological fracture
|postoophorectomy *see* Osteoporosis, postoophorectomy, with pathological fracture
|postsurgical malabsorption *see* Osteoporosis, specified type NEC, with pathological fracture
|specified cause NEC *see* Osteoporosis, specified type NEC, with pathological fracture
|specified disease NEC M84.60
|ankle M84.67-
|carpus M84.64-
|clavicle M84.61-
|femur M84.65-
|fibula M84.66-
|finger M84.64-
|hip M84.65-
|humerus M84.62-
|ilium M84.650
|ischium M84.650
|metacarpus M84.64-
|metatarsus M84.67-
|neck M84.68
|radius M84.63-
|rib M84.68
|scapula M84.61-
|skull M84.68

Fracture, pathological - *continued*
|tarsus M84.67-
|tibia M84.66-
|toe M84.67-
|ulna M84.63-
|vertebra M84.68
|femur M84.45-
|fibula M84.46-
|finger M84.44-
|hip M84.459
|humerus M84.42-
|ilium M84.454
|ischium M84.454
|joint prosthesis *see* Complications, joint prosthesis, mechanical, breakdown, by site
|periprosthetic *see* Fracture, pathological, periprosthetic
|metacarpus M84.44-
|metatarsus M84.47-
|neck M84.48
|pelvis M84.454
|periprosthetic M97.9
|ankle M97.2-
|elbow M97.4-
|finger M97.8
|hip M97.0-
|knee M97.1-
|other specified joint M97.8
|shoulder M97.3-
|spinal joint M97.8
|toe joint M97.8
|wrist joint M97.8
|radius M84.43-
|restorative material (dental) K08.539
|with loss of material K08.531
|without loss of material K08.530
|rib M84.48
|scapula M84.41-
|skull M84.48
|tarsus M84.47-
|tibia M84.46-
|toe M84.47-
|ulna M84.43-
|vertebra M84.48
Fracture, traumatic (abduction) (adduction) (separation) *see also* Fracture, pathological T14.8
|acetabulum S32.40-
|column
|anterior (displaced) (iliopubic) S32.43-
|nondisplaced S32.436
|posterior (displaced) (ilioischial) S32.443
|nondisplaced S32.44-
|dome (displaced) S32.48-
|nondisplaced S32.48
|specified NEC S32.49-
|transverse (displaced) S32.45-
|with associated posterior wall fracture (displaced) S32.46-
|nondisplaced S32.46-
|nondisplaced S32.45-
|wall
|anterior (displaced) S32.41-
|nondisplaced S32.41-
|medial (displaced) S32.47-
|nondisplaced S32.47-
|posterior (displaced) S32.42-
|with associated transverse fracture (displaced) S32.46-
|nondisplaced S32.46-
|nondisplaced S32.42-
|acromion *see* Fracture, scapula, acromial process
|ankle S82.899
|bimalleolar (displaced) S82.84-

Fracture, traumatic - *continued*

|nondisplaced S82.84-
|lateral malleolus only (displaced) S82.6-
|nondisplaced S82.6-
|medial malleolus (displaced) S82.5-
|associated with Maisonneuve's fracture
see Fracture, Maisonneuve's
|nondisplaced S82.5-
|talus *see* Fracture, tarsal, talus
|trimalleolar (displaced) S82.85-
|nondisplaced S82.85-
|arm (upper) *see also* Fracture, humerus, shaft
|humerus *see* Fracture, humerus
|radius *see* Fracture, radius
|ulna *see* Fracture, ulna
|astragalus *see* Fracture, tarsal, talus
|atlas *see* Fracture, neck, cervical vertebra, first
|axis *see* Fracture, neck, cervical vertebra, second
|back *see* Fracture, vertebra
|Barton's *see* Barton's fracture
|base of skull *see* Fracture, skull, base
|basicervical (basal) (femoral) S72.0
|Bennett's *see* Bennett's fracture
|bimalleolar *see* Fracture, ankle, bimalleolar
|blow-out S02.3-
|bone NEC T14.8
|birth injury P13.9
|following insertion of orthopedic implant, joint prosthesis or bone plate *see* Fracture, following insertion of orthopedic implant, joint prosthesis or bone plate
|in (due to) neoplastic disease NEC *see* Fracture, pathological, due to, neoplastic disease
|pathological (cause unknown) *see* Fracture, pathological
|breast bone *see* Fracture, sternum
|bucket handle (semilunar cartilage) *see* Tear, meniscus
|burst *see* Fracture, traumatic, by site
|calcaneus *see* Fracture, tarsal, calcaneus
|carpal bone(s) S62.10-
|capitate (displaced) S62.13-
|nondisplaced S62.13-
|cuneiform *see* Fracture, carpal bone, triquetrum
|hamate (body) (displaced) S62.143
|hook process (displaced) S62.15-
|nondisplaced S62.15-
|nondisplaced S62.14-
|larger multangular *see* Fracture, carpal bones, trapezium
|lunate (displaced) S62.12-
|nondisplaced S62.12-
|navicular S62.00-
|distal pole (displaced) S62.01-
|nondisplaced S62.01-
|middle third (displaced) S62.02-
|nondisplaced S62.02-
|proximal third (displaced) S62.03-
|nondisplaced S62.03-
|volar tuberosity *see* Fracture, carpal bones, navicular, distal pole
|os magnum *see* Fracture, carpal bones, capitate
|pisiform (displaced) S62.16-
|nondisplaced S62.16-
|semilunar *see* Fracture, carpal bones, lunate
|smaller multangular *see* Fracture, carpal bones, trapezoid
|trapezium (displaced) S62.17-
|nondisplaced S62.17-
|trapezoid (displaced) S62.18-
|nondisplaced S62.18-

Fracture, traumatic - *continued*

|triquetrum (displaced) S62.11-
|nondisplaced S62.11-
|unciform *see* Fracture, carpal bones, hamate
|buckle   *see* Fracture, by site, torus
|cervical *see* Fracture, vertebra, cervical
|clavicle S42.00-
|acromial end (displaced) S42.03-
|nondisplaced S42.03-
|birth injury P13.4
|lateral end *see* Fracture, clavicle, acromial end
|shaft (displaced) S42.02-
|nondisplaced S42.02-
|sternal end (anterior) (displaced) S42.01-
|nondisplaced S42.01-
|posterior S42.01-
|coccyx S32.2
|collapsed *see* Collapse, vertebra
|collar bone *see* Fracture, clavicle
|Colles' *see* Colles' fracture
|coronoid process *see* Fracture, ulna, upper end, coronoid process
|corpus cavernosum penis S39.840
|costochondral cartilage S23.41
|costochondral, costosternal junction *see* Fracture, rib
|cranium *see* Fracture, skull
|cricoid cartilage S12.8
|cuboid (ankle) *see* Fracture, tarsal, cuboid
|cuneiform
|foot *see* Fracture, tarsal, cuneiform
|wrist *see* Fracture, carpal, triquetrum
|delayed union *see* Delay, union, fracture
|dental restorative material K08.539
|with loss of material K08.531
|without loss of material K08.530
|due to
|birth injury *see* Birth, injury, fracture
|osteoporosis *see* Osteoporosis, with fracture
|Dupuytren's *see* Fracture, ankle, lateral malleolus
|elbow S42.40-
|ethmoid (bone) (sinus) *see* Fracture, skull, base
|face bone S02.92
|fatigue *see also* Fracture, stress
|vertebra M48.40
|cervical region M48.42
|cervicothoracic region M48.43
|lumbar region M48.46
|lumbosacral region M48.47
|occipito-atlanto-axial region M48.41
|sacrococcygeal region M48.48
|thoracic region M48.44
|thoracolumbar region M48.45
|femur, femoral S72.9-
|basicervical (basal) S72.0
|birth injury P13.2
|capital epiphyseal S79.01-
|condyles, epicondyles *see* Fracture, femur, lower end
|distal end *see* Fracture, femur, lower end
|epiphysis
|head *see* Fracture, femur, upper end, epiphysis
|lower *see* Fracture, femur, lower end, epiphysis
|upper *see* Fracture, femur, upper end, epiphysis
|following insertion of implant, prosthesis or plate M96.66-
|head *see* Fracture, femur, upper end, head
|intertrochanteric *see* Fracture, femur, trochanteric

Fracture, traumatic - *continued*

|intratrochanteric *see* Fracture, femur, trochanteric
|lower end S72.40-
|condyle (displaced) S72.41-
|lateral (displaced) S72.42-
|nondisplaced S72.42-
|medial (displaced) S72.43-
|nondisplaced S72.43-
|nondisplaced S72.41-
|epiphysis (displaced) S72.44-
|nondisplaced S72.44-
|physeal S79.10-
|Salter-Harris
|Type I S79.11-
|Type II S79.12-
|Type III S79.13-
|Type IV S79.14-
|specified NEC S79.19-
|specified NEC S72.49-
|supracondylar (displaced) S72.45-
|with intracondylar extension (displaced) S72.46-
|nondisplaced S72.46-
|nondisplaced S72.45-
|torus S72.47-
|metaphyseal   *see* Fracture, traumatic, by site, shaft
|neck *see* Fracture, femur, upper end, neck
|pertrochanteric *see* Fracture, femur, trochanteric
|shaft (lower third) (middle third) (upper third) S72.30-
|comminuted (displaced) S72.35-
|nondisplaced S72.35-
|oblique (displaced) S72.33-
|nondisplaced S72.33-
|segmental (displaced) S72.36-
|nondisplaced S72.36-
|specified NEC S72.39-
|spiral (displaced) S72.34-
|nondisplaced S72.34-
|transverse (displaced) S72.32-
|nondisplaced S72.32-
|specified site NEC *see* subcategory S72.8
|subcapital (displaced) S72.01-
|subtrochanteric (region) (section) (displaced) S72.2-
|nondisplaced S72.2-
|transcervical *see* Fracture, femur, upper end, neck
|transtrochanteric *see* Fracture, femur, trochanteric
|trochanteric S72.10-
|apophyseal (displaced) S72.13-
|nondisplaced S72.13-
|greater trochanter (displaced) S72.11-
|nondisplaced S72.11-
|intertrochanteric (displaced) S72.14-
|nondisplaced S72.14-
|lesser trochanter (displaced) S72.12-
|nondisplaced S72.12-
|upper end S72.00-
|apophyseal (displaced) S72.13-
|nondisplaced S72.13-
|cervicotrochanteric *see* Fracture, femur, upper end, neck, base
|epiphysis (displaced) S72.02-
|nondisplaced S72.02-
|head S72.05-
|articular (displaced) S72.06-
|nondisplaced S72.06-
|specified NEC S72.09-
|intertrochanteric (displaced) S72.14-
|nondisplaced S72.14-

Fracture, traumatic - *continued*
|intracapsular S72.01-
|midcervical (displaced) S72.03-
|nondisplaced S72.03-
|neck S72.00-
|base (displaced) S72.04-
|nondisplaced S72.04-
|specified NEC S72.09-
|pertrochanteric *see* Fracture, femur, upper
end, trochanteric
|physeal S79.00-
|Salter-Harris type I S79.01-
|specified NEC S79.09-
|subcapital (displaced) S72.01-
|subtrochanteric (displaced) S72.2-
|nondisplaced S72.2-
|transcervical *see* Fracture, femur, upper
end, midcervical
|trochanteric S72.10-
|greater (displaced) S72.11-
|nondisplaced S72.11-
|lesser (displaced) S72.12-
|nondisplaced S72.12-
|fibula (shaft) (styloid) S82.40-
|comminuted (displaced) S82.45-
|nondisplaced S82.45-
|following insertion of implant, prosthesis or
plate M96.67-
|involving ankle or malleolus *see* Fracture,
fibula, lateral malleolus
|lateral malleolus (displaced) S82.6-
|nondisplaced S82.6-
|lower end
|physeal S89.30-
|Salter-Harris
|Type I S89.31-
|Type II S89.32-
|specified NEC S89.39-
|specified NEC S82.83-
|torus S82.82-
|oblique (displaced) S82.43-
|nondisplaced S82.43-
|segmental (displaced) S82.46-
|nondisplaced S82.46-
|specified NEC S82.49-
|spiral (displaced) S82.44-
|nondisplaced S82.44-
|transverse (displaced) S82.42-
|nondisplaced S82.42-
|upper end
|physeal S89.20-
|Salter-Harris
|Type I S89.21-
|Type II S89.22-
|specified NEC S89.29-
|specified NEC S82.83-
|torus S82.81-
|finger (except thumb) S62.60-
|distal phalanx (displaced) S62.63-
|nondisplaced S62.66-
|index S62.60-
|distal phalanx (displaced) S62.63-
|nondisplaced S62.66-
|middle phalanx (displaced) S62.62-
|nondisplaced S62.65-
|proximal phalanx (displaced) S62.61-
|nondisplaced S62.64
|little S62.60-
|distal phalanx (displaced) S62.63-
|nondisplaced S62.66-
|middle phalanx (displaced) S62.62-
|nondisplaced S62.65-
|proximal phalanx (displaced) S62.61-
|nondisplaced S62.64-
|middle phalanx (displaced) S62.62-

Fracture, traumatic - *continued*
|nondisplaced S62.65-
|middle S62.60-
|distal phalanx (displaced) S62.63-
|nondisplaced S62.66-
|middle phalanx (displaced) S62.62-
|nondisplaced S62.65-
|proximal phalanx (displaced) S62.61-
|nondisplaced S62.64-
|proximal phalanx (displaced) S62.61-
|nondisplaced S62.64-
|ring S62.60-
|distal phalanx (displaced) S62.63-
|nondisplaced S62.66-
|middle phalanx (displaced) S62.62-
|nondisplaced S62.65-
|proximal phalanx (displaced) S62.61-
|nondisplaced S62.64-
|thumb *see* Fracture, thumb
|following insertion (intraoperative)
(postoperative) of orthopedic implant, joint
prosthesis or bone plate M96.69
|femur M96.66-
|fibula M96.67-
|humerus M96.62-
|pelvis M96.65
|radius M96.63-
|specified bone NEC M96.69
|tibia M96.67-
|ulna M96.63-
|foot S92.90-
|astragalus *see* Fracture, tarsal, talus
|calcaneus *see* Fracture, tarsal, calcaneus
|cuboid *see* Fracture, tarsal, cuboid
|cuneiform *see* Fracture, tarsal, cuneiform
|metatarsal *see* Fracture, metatarsal
|navicular *see* Fracture, tarsal, navicular
|sesamoid S92.81-
|specified NEC S92.81-
|talus *see* Fracture, tarsal, talus
|tarsal *see* Fracture, tarsal
|toe *see* Fracture, toe
|forearm S52.9-
|radius *see* Fracture, radius
|ulna *see* Fracture, ulna
|fossa (anterior) (middle) (posterior) S02.19
|frontal (bone) (skull) S02.0
|sinus S02.19
|glenoid (cavity) (scapula) *see* Fracture,
scapula, glenoid cavity
|greenstick *see* Fracture, by site
|hallux *see* Fracture, toe, great
|hand S62.9-
|carpal *see* Fracture, carpal bone
|finger (except thumb) *see* Fracture, finger
|metacarpal *see* Fracture, metacarpal
|navicular (scaphoid) (hand) *see* Fracture,
carpal bone, navicular
|thumb *see* Fracture, thumb
|healed or old
|with complications   code by Nature of the
complication
|heel bone *see* Fracture, tarsal, calcaneus
|Hill-Sachs S42.29-
|hip *see* Fracture, femur, neck
|humerus S42.30-
|anatomical neck *see* Fracture, humerus,
upper end
|articular process *see* Fracture, humerus,
lower end
|capitellum *see* Fracture, humerus, lower
end, condyle, lateral
|distal end *see* Fracture, humerus, lower end
|epiphysis

Fracture, traumatic - *continued*
|lower *see* Fracture, humerus, lower end,
physeal
|upper *see* Fracture, humerus, upper end,
physeal
|external condyle *see* Fracture, humerus,
lower end, condyle, lateral
|following insertion of implant, prosthesis or
plate M96.62-
|great tuberosity *see* Fracture, humerus,
upper end, greater tuberosity
|intercondylar *see* Fracture, humerus, lower
end
|internal epicondyle *see* Fracture, humerus,
lower end, epicondyle, medial
|lesser tuberosity *see* Fracture, humerus,
upper end, lesser tuberosity
|lower end S42.40-
|condyle
|lateral (displaced) S42.45-
|nondisplaced S42.45-
|medial (displaced) S42.46-
|nondisplaced S42.46-
|epicondyle
|lateral (displaced) S42.43-
|nondisplaced S42.43-
|medial (displaced) S42.44-
|incarcerated S42.44-
|nondisplaced S42.44-
|physeal S49.10-
|Salter-Harris
|Type I S49.11-
|Type II S49.12-
|Type III S49.13-
|Type IV S49.14-
|specified NEC S49.19-
|specified NEC (displaced) S42.49-
|nondisplaced S42.49-
|supracondylar (simple) (displaced)
S42.41-
|with intercondylar fracture *see* Fracture,
humerus, lower end
|comminuted (displaced) S42.42-
|nondisplaced S42.42-
|nondisplaced S42.41-
|torus S42.48-
|transcondylar (displaced) S42.47-
|nondisplaced S42.47-
|proximal end *see* Fracture, humerus, upper
end
|shaft S42.30-
|comminuted (displaced) S42.35-
|nondisplaced S42.35-
|greenstick S42.31-
|oblique (displaced) S42.33-
|nondisplaced S42.33-
|segmental (displaced) S42.36-
|nondisplaced S42.36-
|specified NEC S42.39-
|spiral (displaced) S42.34-
|nondisplaced S42.34-
|transverse (displaced) S42.32-
|nondisplaced S42.32-
|supracondylar *see* Fracture, humerus, lower
end
|surgical neck *see* Fracture, humerus, upper
end, surgical neck
|trochlea *see* Fracture, humerus, lower end,
condyle, medial
|tuberosity *see* Fracture, humerus, upper end
|upper end S42.20-
|anatomical neck *see* Fracture, humerus,
upper end, specified NEC
|articular head *see* Fracture, humerus,
upper end, specified NEC

Fracture, traumatic - *continued*
- |epiphysis *see* Fracture, humerus, upper end, physeal
- |greater tuberosity (displaced) S42.25-
  - |nondisplaced S42.25-
- |lesser tuberosity (displaced) S42.26-
  - |nondisplaced S42.26-
- |physeal S49.00-
  - |Salter-Harris
    - |Type I S49.01-
    - |Type II S49.02-
    - |Type III S49.03-
    - |Type IV S49.04-
  - |specified NEC S49.09-
- |specified NEC (displaced) S42.29-
  - |nondisplaced S42.29-
- |surgical neck (displaced) S42.21-
  - |four-part S42.24-
  - |nondisplaced S42.21-
  - |three-part S42.23-
  - |two-part (displaced) S42.22-
    - |nondisplaced S42.22-
- |torus S42.27-
- |transepiphyseal *see* Fracture, humerus, upper end, physeal
- |hyoid bone S12.8
- |ilium S32.30-
  - |with disruption of pelvic ring *see* Disruption, pelvic ring
  - |avulsion (displaced) S32.31-
    - |nondisplaced S32.31-
  - |specified NEC S32.39-
- |impaction, impacted   code as Fracture, by site
- |innominate bone *see* Fracture, ilium
- |instep *see* Fracture, foot
- |ischium S32.60-
  - |with disruption of pelvic ring *see* Disruption, pelvic ring
  - |avulsion (displaced) S32.61-
    - |nondisplaced S32.61-
  - |specified NEC S32.69-
- |jaw (bone) (lower) *see* Fracture, mandible
  - |upper *see* Fracture, maxilla
- |joint prosthesis *see* Complications, joint prosthesis, mechanical, breakdown, by site
  - |periprosthetic *see* Fracture, traumatic, periprosthetic
- |knee cap *see* Fracture, patella
- |larynx S12.8
- |late effects *see* Sequelae, fracture
- |leg (lower) S82.9-
  - |ankle *see* Fracture, ankle
  - |femur *see* Fracture, femur
  - |fibula *see* Fracture, fibula
  - |malleolus *see* Fracture, ankle
  - |patella *see* Fracture, patella
  - |specified site NEC S82.89-
  - |tibia *see* Fracture, tibia
- |lumbar spine *see* Fracture, vertebra, lumbar
- |lumbosacral spine S32.9
- |Maisonneuve's (displaced) S82.86-
  - |nondisplaced S82.86-
- |malar bone *see also* Fracture, maxilla S02.400
  - |left side S02.40B
  - |right side S02.40A
- |malleolus *see* Fracture, ankle
- |malunion *see* Fracture, by site
- |mandible (lower jaw (bone)) S02.609
  - |alveolus S02.67-
  - |angle (of jaw) S02.65-
  - |body, unspecified S02.600
    - |left side S02.602
    - |right side S02.601
  - |condylar process S02.61-

Fracture, traumatic - *continued*
- |coronoid process S02.63-
- |ramus, unspecified S02.64-
- |specified site NEC S02.69-
- |subcondylar process S02.62-
- |symphysis S02.66
- |manubrium (sterni) S22.21
  - |dissociation from sternum S22.23
- |march *see* Fracture, traumatic, stress, by site
- |maxilla, maxillary (bone) (sinus) (superior) (upper jaw) S02.401
  - |alveolus S02.42
  - |inferior *see* Fracture, mandible
  - |LeFort I S02.411
  - |LeFort II S02.412
  - |LeFort III S02.413
  - |left side S02.40D
  - |right side S02.40C
- |metacarpal S62.309
  - |base (displaced) S62.319
    - |nondisplaced S62.349
  - |fifth S62.30-
    - |base (displaced) S62.31-
      - |nondisplaced S62.34-
    - |neck (displaced) S62.33-
      - |nondisplaced S62.36-
    - |shaft (displaced) S62.32-
      - |nondisplaced S62.35-
    - |specified NEC S62.398
  - |first S62.20-
    - |base NEC (displaced) S62.23-
      - |nondisplaced S62.23-
    - |Bennett's *see* Bennett's fracture
    - |neck (displaced) S62.25-
      - |nondisplaced S62.25-
    - |shaft (displaced) S62.24-
      - |nondisplaced S62.24-
    - |specified NEC S62.29-
  - |fourth S62.30-
    - |base (displaced) S62.31-
      - |nondisplaced S62.34-
    - |neck (displaced) S62.33-
      - |nondisplaced S62.36-
    - |shaft (displaced) S62.32-
      - |nondisplaced S62.35-
    - |specified NEC S62.39-
  - |neck (displaced) S62.33-
    - |nondisplaced S62.36-
  - |Rolando's *see* Rolando's fracture
  - |second S62.30-
    - |base (displaced) S62.31-
      - |nondisplaced S62.34-
    - |neck (displaced) S62.33-
      - |nondisplaced S62.36-
    - |shaft (displaced) S62.32-
      - |nondisplaced S62.35-
    - |specified NEC S62.39-
  - |shaft (displaced) S62.32-
    - |nondisplaced S62.35-
  - |third S62.30-
    - |base (displaced) S62.31-
      - |nondisplaced S62.34-
    - |neck (displaced) S62.33-
      - |nondisplaced S62.36-
    - |shaft (displaced) S62.32-
      - |nondisplaced S62.35-
    - |specified NEC S62.39-
  - |specified NEC S62.399
- |metastatic *see* Fracture, pathological, due to, neoplastic disease *see also* Neoplasm
- |metatarsal bone S92.30-
  - |fifth (displaced) S92.35-
    - |nondisplaced S92.35-
  - |first (displaced) S92.31-
    - |nondisplaced S92.31-

Fracture, traumatic - *continued*
- |fourth (displaced) S92.34-
  - |nondisplaced S92.34-
- |physeal S99.10-
  - |Salter-Harris
    - |Type I S99.11-
    - |Type II S99.12-
    - |Type III S99.13-
    - |Type IV S99.14-
  - |specified NEC S99.19-
- |second (displaced) S92.32-
  - |nondisplaced S92.32-
- |third (displaced) S92.33-
  - |nondisplaced S92.33-
- |Monteggia's *see* Monteggia's fracture
- |multiple
  - |hand (and wrist) NEC *see* Fracture, by site
  - |ribs *see* Fracture, rib, multiple
- |nasal (bone(s)) S02.2
- |navicular (scaphoid) (foot) *see also* Fracture, tarsal, navicular
  - |hand *see* Fracture, carpal, navicular
- |neck S12.9
  - |cervical vertebra S12.9
    - |fifth (displaced) S12.400
      - |nondisplaced S12.401
      - |specified type NEC (displaced) S12.490
        - |nondisplaced S12.491
    - |first (displaced) S12.000
      - |burst (stable) S12.01
        - |unstable S12.02
      - |lateral mass (displaced) S12.040
        - |nondisplaced S12.041
      - |nondisplaced S12.001
      - |posterior arch (displaced) S12.030
        - |nondisplaced S12.031
      - |specified type NEC (displaced) S12.090
        - |nondisplaced S12.091
    - |fourth (displaced) S12.300
      - |nondisplaced S12.301
      - |specified type NEC (displaced) S12.390
        - |nondisplaced S12.391
    - |second (displaced) S12.100
      - |nondisplaced S12.101
      - |dens (anterior) (displaced) (type II) S12.110
        - |nondisplaced S12.112
        - |posterior S12.111
      - |specified type NEC (displaced) S12.120
        - |nondisplaced S12.121
      - |specified type NEC (displaced) S12.190
        - |nondisplaced S12.191
    - |seventh (displaced) S12.600
      - |nondisplaced S12.601
      - |specified type NEC (displaced) S12.690
        - |nondisplaced S12.691
    - |sixth (displaced) S12.500
      - |nondisplaced S12.501
      - |specified type NEC (displaced) S12.590
        - |nondisplaced S12.591
    - |third (displaced) S12.200
      - |nondisplaced S12.201
      - |specified type NEC (displaced) S12.290
        - |nondisplaced S12.291
  - |hyoid bone S12.8
  - |larynx S12.8
  - |specified site NEC S12.8
  - |thyroid cartilage S12.8
  - |trachea S12.8
- |neoplastic NEC *see* Fracture, pathological, due to, neoplastic disease
- |neural arch *see* Fracture, vertebra
- |newborn *see* Birth, injury, fracture
- |nontraumatic *see* Fracture, pathological

Fracture, traumatic - *continued*
- nonunion *see* Nonunion, fracture
- nose, nasal (bone) (septum) S02.2
- occiput *see* Fracture, skull, base, occiput
- odontoid process *see* Fracture, neck, cervical vertebra, second
- olecranon (process) (ulna) *see* Fracture, ulna, upper end, olecranon process
- orbit, orbital (bone) (region) S02.8-
  - floor (blow-out) S02.3-
  - roof S02.19
- os
  - calcis *see* Fracture, tarsal, calcaneus
  - magnum *see* Fracture, carpal, capitate
  - pubis *see* Fracture, pubis
- palate S02.8-
- parietal bone (skull) S02.0
- patella S82.00-
  - comminuted (displaced) S82.04-
    - nondisplaced S82.04-
  - longitudinal (displaced) S82.02-
    - nondisplaced S82.02-
  - osteochondral (displaced) S82.01-
    - nondisplaced S82.01-
  - specified NEC S82.09-
  - transverse (displaced) S82.03-
    - nondisplaced S82.03-
- pedicle (of vertebral arch) *see* Fracture, vertebra
- pelvis, pelvic (bone) S32.9
  - acetabulum *see* Fracture, acetabulum
  - circle *see* Disruption, pelvic ring
  - following insertion of implant, prosthesis or plate M96.65
  - ilium *see* Fracture, ilium
  - ischium *see* Fracture, ischium
  - multiple
    - with disruption of pelvic ring (circle) *see* Disruption, pelvic ring
    - without disruption of pelvic ring (circle) S32.82
  - pubis *see* Fracture, pubis
  - specified site NEC S32.89
  - sacrum *see* Fracture, sacrum
- periprosthetic, around internal prosthetic joint M97.9
  - ankle M97.2-
  - elbow M97.4-
  - finger M97.8
  - hip M97.0-
  - knee M97.1-
  - shoulder M97.3-
  - specified joint NEC M97.8
  - spine M97.8
  - toe M97.8
  - wrist M97.8
- phalanx
  - foot *see* Fracture, toe
  - hand *see* Fracture, finger
- pisiform *see* Fracture, carpal, pisiform
- pond *see* Fracture, skull
- prosthetic device, internal *see* Complications, prosthetic device, by site, mechanical
- pubis S32.50-
  - with disruption of pelvic ring *see* Disruption, pelvic ring
  - specified site NEC S32.59-
  - superior rim S32.51-
- radius S52.9-
  - distal end *see* Fracture, radius, lower end
  - following insertion of implant, prosthesis or plate M96.63-
  - head *see* Fracture, radius, upper end, head
  - lower end S52.50-
    - Barton's *see* Barton's fracture

Fracture, traumatic - *continued*
  - Colles' *see* Colles' fracture
  - extraarticular NEC S52.55-
  - intraarticular NEC S52.57-
  - physeal S59.20-
    - Salter-Harris
      - Type I S59.21-
      - Type II S59.22-
      - Type III S59.23-
      - Type IV S59.24-
    - specified NEC S59.29-
  - Smith's *see* Smith's fracture
  - specified NEC S52.59-
  - styloid process (displaced) S52.51-
    - nondisplaced S52.51-
  - torus S52.52-
  - neck *see* Fracture, radius, upper end
  - proximal end *see* Fracture, radius, upper end
  - shaft S52.30-
    - bent bone S52.38-
    - comminuted (displaced) S52.35-
      - nondisplaced S52.35-
    - Galeazzi's *see* Galeazzi's fracture
    - greenstick S52.31-
    - oblique (displaced) S52.33-
      - nondisplaced S52.33-
    - segmental (displaced) S52.36-
      - nondisplaced S52.36-
    - specified NEC S52.39-
    - spiral (displaced) S52.34-
      - nondisplaced S52.34-
    - transverse (displaced) S52.32-
      - nondisplaced S52.32-
  - upper end S52.10-
    - head (displaced) S52.12-
      - nondisplaced S52.12-
    - neck (displaced) S52.13-
      - nondisplaced S52.13-
    - specified NEC S52.18-
    - physeal S59.10-
      - Salter-Harris
        - Type I S59.11-
        - Type II S59.12-
        - Type III S59.13-
        - Type IV S59.14-
      - specified NEC S59.19-
    - torus S52.11-
- ramus
  - inferior or superior, pubis *see* Fracture, pubis
  - mandible *see* Fracture, mandible
- restorative material (dental) K08.539
  - with loss of material K08.531
  - without loss of material K08.530
- rib S22.3-
  - with flail chest *see* Flail, chest
  - multiple S22.4-
    - with flail chest *see* Flail, chest
- root, tooth *see* Fracture, tooth
- sacrum S32.10
  - specified NEC S32.19
  - Type
    - 1 S32.14
    - 2 S32.15
    - 3 S32.16
    - 4 S32.17
  - Zone
    - I S32.119
      - displaced (minimally) S32.111
        - severely S32.112
      - nondisplaced S32.110
    - II S32.129
      - displaced (minimally) S32.121
        - severely S32.122
      - nondisplaced S32.120

Fracture, traumatic - *continued*
    - III S32.139
      - displaced (minimally) S32.131
        - severely S32.132
      - nondisplaced S32.130
- scaphoid (hand) *see also* Fracture, carpal, navicular
  - foot *see* Fracture, tarsal, navicular
- scapula S42.10-
  - acromial process (displaced) S42.12-
    - nondisplaced S42.12-
  - body (displaced) S42.11-
    - nondisplaced S42.11-
  - coracoid process (displaced) S42.13-
    - nondisplaced S42.13-
  - glenoid cavity (displaced) S42.14-
    - nondisplaced S42.14-
  - neck (displaced) S42.15-
    - nondisplaced S42.15-
  - specified NEC S42.19-
- semilunar bone, wrist *see* Fracture, carpal, lunate
- sequelae *see* Sequelae, fracture
- sesamoid bone
  - foot S92.81-
  - hand *see* Fracture, carpal
  - other *see* Fracture, traumatic, by site
- shepherd's *see* Fracture, tarsal, talus
- shoulder (girdle) S42.9-
  - blade *see* Fracture, scapula
- sinus (ethmoid) (frontal) S02.19
- skull S02.91
  - base S02.10-
    - occiput S02.119
      - condyle S02.113
        - type I S02.110
          - left side S02.11B
          - right side S02.11A
        - type II S02.111
          - left side S02.11D
          - right side S02.11C
        - type III S02.112
          - left side S02.11F
          - right side S02.11E
      - specified NEC S02.118
        - left side S02.11H
        - right side S02.11G
    - specified NEC S02.19
  - birth injury P13.0
  - frontal bone S02.0
  - parietal bone S02.0
  - specified site NEC S02.8-
  - temporal bone S02.19
  - vault S02.0
- Smith's *see* Smith's fracture
- sphenoid (bone) (sinus) S02.19
- spine *see* Fracture, vertebra
- spinous process *see* Fracture, vertebra
- spontaneous (cause unknown) *see* Fracture, pathological
- stave (of thumb) *see* Fracture, metacarpal, first
- sternum S22.20
  - with flail chest *see* Flail, chest
  - body S22.22
  - manubrium S22.21
  - xiphoid (process) S22.24
- stress M84.30
  - ankle M84.37-
  - carpus M84.34-
  - clavicle M84.31-
  - femoral neck M84.359
  - femur M84.35-
  - fibula M84.36-
  - finger M84.34-
  - hip M84.359

Fracture, traumatic - *continued*

| humerus M84.32-
| ilium M84.350
| ischium M84.350
| metacarpus M84.34-
| metatarsus M84.37-
| neck *see* Fracture, fatigue, vertebra
| pelvis M84.350
| radius M84.33-
| rib M84.38
| scapula M84.31-
| skull M84.38
| tarsus M84.37-
| tibia M84.36-
| toe M84.37-
| ulna M84.33-
| vertebra *see* Fracture, fatigue, vertebra
| supracondylar, elbow *see* Fracture, humerus,
    lower end, supracondylar
| symphysis pubis *see* Fracture, pubis
| talus (ankle bone) *see* Fracture, tarsal, talus
| tarsal bone(s) S92.20-
  | astragalus *see* Fracture, tarsal, talus
  | calcaneus S92.00-
    | anterior process (displaced) S92.02-
     | nondisplaced S92.02-
    | body (displaced) S92.01-
     | nondisplaced S92.01-
    | extraarticular NEC (displaced) S92.05-
     | nondisplaced S92.05-
    | intraarticular (displaced) S92.06-
     | nondisplaced S92.06
    | physeal S99.00-
     | Salter-Harris
      | Type I S99.01-
      | Type II S99.02-
      | Type III S99.03-
      | Type IV S99.04-
     | specified NEC S99.09-
    | tuberosity (displaced) S92.04-
     | avulsion (displaced) S92.03-
      | nondisplaced S92.03-
     | nondisplaced S92.04-
  | cuboid (displaced) S92.21-
    | nondisplaced S92.21-
  | cuneiform
    | intermediate (displaced) S92.23-
     | nondisplaced S92.23-
    | lateral (displaced) S92.22-
     | nondisplaced S92.22-
    | medial (displaced) S92.24-
     | nondisplaced S92.24-
  | navicular (displaced) S92.25-
    | nondisplaced S92.25-
  | scaphoid *see* Fracture, tarsal, navicular
  | talus S92.10-
    | avulsion (displaced) S92.15-
     | nondisplaced S92.15-
    | body (displaced) S92.12-
     | nondisplaced S92.12-
    | dome (displaced) S92.14-
     | nondisplaced S92.14-
    | head (displaced) S92.12-
     | nondisplaced S92.12-
    | lateral process (displaced) S92.14-
     | nondisplaced S92.14-
    | neck (displaced) S92.11-
     | nondisplaced S92.11-
    | posterior process (displaced) S92.13-
     | nondisplaced S92.13-
    | specified NEC S92.19-
| temporal bone (styloid) S02.19
| thorax (bony) S22.9
  | with flail chest *see* Flail, chest
  | rib S22.3-

Fracture, traumatic - *continued*

| multiple S22.4-
  | with flail chest *see* Flail, chest
| sternum S22.20
  | body S22.22
  | manubrium S22.21
  | xiphoid process S22.24
| vertebra (displaced) S22.009
  | burst (stable) S22.001
    | unstable S22.002
  | eighth S22.069
    | burst (stable) S22.061
     | unstable S22.062
    | specified type NEC S22.068
    | wedge compression S22.060
  | eleventh S22.089
    | burst (stable) S22.081
     | unstable S22.082
    | specified type NEC S22.088
    | wedge compression S22.080
  | fifth S22.059
    | burst (stable) S22.051
     | unstable S22.052
    | specified type NEC S22.058
    | wedge compression S22.050
  | first S22.019
    | burst (stable) S22.011
     | unstable S22.012
    | specified type NEC S22.018
    | wedge compression S22.010
  | fourth S22.049
    | burst (stable) S22.041
     | unstable S22.042
    | specified type NEC S22.048
    | wedge compression S22.040
  | ninth S22.079
    | burst (stable) S22.071
     | unstable S22.072
    | specified type NEC S22.078
    | wedge compression S22.070
  | nondisplaced S22.001
  | second S22.029
    | burst (stable) S22.021
     | unstable S22.022
    | specified type NEC S22.028
    | wedge compression S22.020
  | seventh S22.069
    | burst (stable) S22.061
     | unstable S22.062
    | specified type NEC S22.068
    | wedge compression S22.060
  | sixth S22.059
    | burst (stable) S22.051
     | unstable S22.052
    | specified type NEC S22.058
    | wedge compression S22.050
  | specified type NEC S22.008
  | tenth S22.079
    | burst (stable) S22.071
     | unstable S22.072
    | specified type NEC S22.078
    | wedge compression S22.070
  | third S22.039
    | burst (stable) S22.031
     | unstable S22.032
    | specified type NEC S22.038
    | wedge compression S22.030
  | twelfth S22.089
    | burst (stable) S22.081
     | unstable S22.082
    | specified type NEC S22.088
    | wedge compression S22.080
  | wedge compression S22.000
| thumb S62.50-
  | distal phalanx (displaced) S62.52-

Fracture, traumatic - *continued*

  | nondisplaced S62.52-
  | proximal phalanx (displaced) S62.51-
    | nondisplaced S62.51-
| thyroid cartilage S12.8
| tibia (shaft) S82.20-
  | comminuted (displaced) S82.25-
    | nondisplaced S82.25-
  | condyles *see* Fracture, tibia, upper end
  | distal end *see* Fracture, tibia, lower end
  | epiphysis
    | lower *see* Fracture, tibia, lower end
    | upper *see* Fracture, tibia, upper end
  | following insertion of implant, prosthesis or
    plate M96.67-
  | head (involving knee joint) *see* Fracture,
    tibia, upper end
  | intercondyloid eminence *see* Fracture, tibia,
    upper end
  | involving ankle or malleolus *see* Fracture,
    ankle, medial malleolus
  | lower end S82.30-
    | physeal S89.10-
     | Salter-Harris
      | Type I S89.11-
      | Type II S89.12-
      | Type III S89.13-
      | Type IV S89.14-
     | specified NEC S89.19-
    | pilon (displaced) S82.87-
     | nondisplaced S82.87-
    | specified NEC S82.39-
    | torus S82.31-
  | malleolus *see* Fracture, ankle, medial
    malleolus
  | oblique (displaced) S82.23-
    | nondisplaced S82.23-
  | pilon *see* Fracture, tibia, lower end, pilon
  | proximal end *see* Fracture, tibia, upper end
  | segmental (displaced) S82.26-
    | nondisplaced S82.26-
  | specified NEC S82.29-
  | spine *see* Fracture, tibia, upper end, spine
  | spiral (displaced) S82.24-
    | nondisplaced S82.24-
  | transverse (displaced) S82.22-
    | nondisplaced S82.22-
  | tuberosity *see* Fracture, tibia, upper end,
    tuberosity
  | upper end S82.10-
    | bicondylar (displaced) S82.14-
     | nondisplaced S82.14-
    | lateral condyle (displaced) S82.12-
     | nondisplaced S82.12-
    | medial condyle (displaced) S82.13-
     | nondisplaced S82.13-
    | physeal S89.00-
     | Salter-Harris
      | Type I S89.01-
      | Type II S89.02-
      | Type III S89.03-
      | Type IV S89.04-
     | specified NEC S89.09-
    | plateau *see* Fracture, tibia, upper end,
     bicondylar
    | spine (displaced) S82.11-
     | nondisplaced S82.11-
    | torus S82.16-
    | specified NEC S82.19-
    | tuberosity (displaced) S82.15-
     | nondisplaced S82.15-
| toe S92.91-
  | great (displaced) S92.40-
    | distal phalanx (displaced) S92.42-
     | nondisplaced S92.42-

Fracture, traumatic - *continued*
  |nondisplaced S92.40-
  |proximal phalanx (displaced) S92.41-
    |nondisplaced S92.41-
  |specified NEC S92.49-
 |lesser (displaced) S92.50-
  |distal phalanx (displaced) S92.53-
    |nondisplaced S92.53-
  |medial phalanx (displaced) S92.52-
    |nondisplaced S92.52-
  |nondisplaced S92.50-
  |proximal phalanx (displaced) S92.51-
    |nondisplaced S92.51-
  |specified NEC S92.59-
 |physeal
  |phalanx S99.20-
    |Salter-Harris
      |Type I S99.21-
      |Type II S99.22-
      |Type III S99.23-
      |Type IV S99.24-
    |specified NEC S99.29-
 |tooth (root) S02.5
 |trachea (cartilage) S12.8
 |transverse process *see* Fracture, vertebra
 |trapezium or trapezoid bone *see* Fracture,
   carpal
 |trimalleolar *see* Fracture, ankle, trimalleolar
 |triquetrum (cuneiform of carpus) *see* Fracture,
   carpal, triquetrum
 |trochanter *see* Fracture, femur, trochanteric
 |tuberosity (external) *see* Fracture, traumatic,
   by site
 |ulna (shaft) S52.20-
  |bent bone S52.28-
  |coronoid process *see* Fracture, ulna, upper
    end, coronoid process
  |distal end *see* Fracture, ulna, lower end
  |following insertion of implant, prosthesis or
    plate M96.63-
  |head S52.60-
  |lower end S52.60-
    |physeal S59.00-
      |Salter-Harris
        |Type I S59.01-
        |Type II S59.02-
        |Type III S59.03-
        |Type IV S59.04-
      |specified NEC S59.09-
    |specified NEC S52.69-
    |styloid process (displaced) S52.61-
      |nondisplaced S52.61-
    |torus S52.62-
  |proximal end *see* Fracture, ulna, upper end
  |shaft S52.20-
    |comminuted (displaced) S52.25-
      |nondisplaced S52.25-
    |greenstick S52.21-
    |Monteggia's *see* Monteggia's fracture
    |oblique (displaced) S52.23-
      |nondisplaced S52.23-
    |segmental (displaced) S52.26-
      |nondisplaced S52.26-
    |specified NEC S52.29-
    |spiral (displaced) S52.24-
      |nondisplaced S52.24-
    |transverse (displaced) S52.22-
      |nondisplaced S52.22-
  |upper end S52.00-
    |coronoid process (displaced) S52.04-
      |nondisplaced S52.04-
    |olecranon process (displaced) S52.02-
      |with intraarticular extension S52.03-
      |nondisplaced S52.02-
        |with intraarticular extension S52.03-

Fracture, traumatic - *continued*
  |specified NEC S52.09-
  |torus S52.01-
 |unciform *see* Fracture, carpal, hamate
 |vault of skull S02.0
 |vertebra, vertebral (arch) (body) (column)
   (neural arch) (pedicle) (spinous process)
   (transverse process)
  |atlas *see* Fracture, neck, cervical vertebra,
    first
  |axis *see* Fracture, neck, cervical vertebra,
    second
  |cervical (teardrop) S12.9
    |axis *see* Fracture, neck, cervical vertebra,
      second
    |first (atlas) *see* Fracture, neck, cervical
      vertebra, first
    |second (axis) *see* Fracture, neck, cervical
      vertebra, second
  |chronic M84.48
  |coccyx S32.2
  |dorsal *see* Fracture, thorax, vertebra
  |lumbar S32.009
    |burst (stable) S32.001
      |unstable S32.002
    |fifth S32.059
      |burst (stable) S32.051
        |unstable S32.052
      |specified type NEC S32.058
      |wedge compression S32.050
    |first S32.019
      |burst (stable) S32.011
        |unstable S32.012
      |specified type NEC S32.018
      |wedge compression S32.010
    |fourth S32.049
      |burst (stable) S32.041
        |unstable S32.042
      |specified type NEC S32.048
      |wedge compression S32.040
    |second S32.029
      |burst (stable) S32.021
        |unstable S32.022
      |specified type NEC S32.028
      |wedge compression S32.020
    |specified type NEC S32.008
    |third S32.039
      |burst (stable) S32.031
        |unstable S32.032
      |specified type NEC S32.038
      |wedge compression S32.030
    |wedge compression S32.000
  |metastatic *see* Collapse, vertebra, in,
    specified disease NEC *see also* Neoplasm
  |newborn (birth injury) P11.5
  |sacrum S32.10
    |specified NEC S32.19
    |Type
      |1 S32.14
      |2 S32.15
      |3 S32.16
      |4 S32.17
    |Zone
      |I S32.119
        |displaced (minimally) S32.111
          |severely S32.112
        |nondisplaced S32.110
      |II S32.129
        |displaced (minimally) S32.121
          |severely S32.122
        |nondisplaced S32.120
      |III S32.139
        |displaced (minimally) S32.131
          |severely S32.132
        |nondisplaced S32.130
  |thoracic *see* Fracture, thorax, vertebra
 |vertex S02.0

Fracture, traumatic - *continued*
  |vomer (bone) S02.2
  |wrist S62.10-
    |carpal *see* Fracture, carpal bone
    |navicular (scaphoid) (hand) *see* Fracture,
      carpal, navicular
  |xiphisternum, xiphoid (process) S22.24
  |zygoma S02.402
    |left side S02.40F
    |right side S02.40E
Fragile, fragility
  |autosomal site Q95.5
  |bone, congenital (with blue sclera) Q78.0
  |capillary (hereditary) D69.8
  |hair L67.8
  |nails L60.3
  |non-sex chromosome site Q95.5
  |X chromosome Q99.2
Fragilitas
  |crinium L67.8
  |ossium (with blue sclerae) (hereditary) Q78.0
  |unguium L60.3
  |congenital Q84.6
Fragments, cataract (lens), following cataract
  surgery H59.02-
  |retained foreign body *see* Retained, foreign
    body fragments (type of)
Frailty (frail) R54
  |mental R41.81
Frambesia, frambesial (tropica) *see also* Yaws
  |initial lesion or ulcer A66.0
  |primary A66.0
Frambeside
  |gummatous A66.4
  |of early yaws A66.2
Frambesioma A66.1
Franceschetti-Klein (-Wildervanck) disease or
  syndrome Q75.4
Francis' disease *see* Tularemia
Franklin disease C88.2
Frank's essential thrombocytopenia D69.3
Fraser's syndrome Q87.0
Freckle(s) L81.2
  |malignant melanoma in *see* Melanoma
  |melanotic (Hutchinson's) *see* Melanoma, in
    situ
  |retinal D49.81
Frederickson's hyperlipoproteinemia, type
  |I and V E78.3
  |IIA E78.00
  |IIB and III E78.2
  |IV E78.1
Freeman Sheldon syndrome Q87.0
Freezing *see also* Effect, adverse, cold T69.9
Freiberg's disease (infraction of metatarsal
  head or osteochondrosis) *see*
  Osteochondrosis, juvenile, metatarsus
Frei's disease A55
Fremitus, friction, cardiac R01.2
Frenum, frenulum
  |external os Q51.828
  |tongue (shortening) (congenital) Q38.1
Frequency micturition (nocturnal) R35.0
  |psychogenic F45.8
Frey's syndrome
  |auriculotemporal G50.8
  |hyperhidrosis L74.52
Friction
  |burn *see* Burn, by site
  |fremitus, cardiac R01.2
  |precordial R01.2
  |sounds, chest R09.89
Friderichsen-Waterhouse syndrome or
  disease A39.1

Friedländer's B (bacillus) NEC *see also*
  condition A49.8
Friedreich's
  |ataxia G11.11
  |combined systemic disease G11.11
  |facial hemihypertrophy Q67.4
  |sclerosis (cerebellum) (spinal cord) G11.11
Frigidity F52.22
Fröhlich's syndrome E23.6
Frontal *see also* condition
  |lobe syndrome F07.0
Frostbite (superficial) T33.90
  |with
    |partial thickness skin loss *see* Frostbite
      (superficial), by site
    |tissue necrosis T34.90
  |abdominal wall T33.3
    |with tissue necrosis T34.3
  |ankle T33.81-
Frostbite (superficial) - *continued*
  |with tissue necrosis T34.81-
  |arm T33.4-
    |with tissue necrosis T34.4-
    |finger(s) *see* Frostbite, finger
    |hand *see* Frostbite, hand
    |wrist *see* Frostbite, wrist
  |ear T33.01-
    |with tissue necrosis T34.01-
  |face T33.09
    |with tissue necrosis T34.09
  |finger T33.53-
    |with tissue necrosis T34.53-
  |foot T33.82-
    |with tissue necrosis T34.82-
  |hand T33.52-
    |with tissue necrosis T34.52-
  |head T33.09
    |with tissue necrosis T34.09
    |ear *see* Frostbite, ear
    |nose *see* Frostbite, nose
  |hip (and thigh) T33.6-
    |with tissue necrosis T34.6-
  |knee T33.7-
    |with tissue necrosis T34.7-
  |leg T33.9-
    |with tissue necrosis T34.9-
    |ankle *see* Frostbite, ankle
    |foot *see* Frostbite, foot
    |knee *see* Frostbite, knee
    |lower T33.7-
      |with tissue necrosis T34.7-
    |thigh *see* Frostbite, hip
    |toe *see* Frostbite, toe
  |limb
    |lower T33.99
      |with tissue necrosis T34.99
    |upper *see* Frostbite, arm
  |neck T33.1
    |with tissue necrosis T34.1
  |nose T33.02
    |with tissue necrosis T34.02
  |pelvis T33.3
    |with tissue necrosis T34.3
  |specified site NEC T33.99
    |with tissue necrosis T34.99
  |thigh *see* Frostbite, hip
  |thorax T33.2
    |with tissue necrosis T34.2
  |toes T33.83-
    |with tissue necrosis T34.83-
  |trunk T33.99
    |with tissue necrosis T34.99
  |wrist T33.51-
    |with tissue necrosis T34.51-
Frotteurism F65.81

Frozen *see also* Effect, adverse, cold T69.9
  |pelvis (female) N94.89
    |male K66.8
  |shoulder *see* Capsulitis, adhesive
Fructokinase deficiency E74.11
Fructose 1,6 diphosphatase deficiency E74.19
Fructosemia (benign) (essential) E74.12
Fructosuria (benign) (essential) E74.11
Fuchs'
  |black spot (myopic) (*see also* Myopia,
    degenerative) H44.2-
  |dystrophy (corneal endothelium) H18.51-
  |heterochromic cyclitis *see* Cyclitis, Fuchs'
    heterochromic
Fucosidosis E77.1
Fugue R68.89
  |dissociative F44.1
  |hysterical (dissociative) F44.1
  |postictal in epilepsy *see* Epilepsy
  |reaction to exceptional stress (transient) F43.0
Fulminant, fulminating *see* condition
Functional *see also* condition
  |bleeding (uterus) N93.8
Functioning, intellectual, borderline R41.83
Fundus *see* condition
Fungemia NOS B49
Fungus, fungous
  |cerebral G93.89
  |disease NOS B49
  |infection *see* Infection, fungus
Funiculitis (acute) (chronic) (endemic) N49.1
  |gonococcal (acute) (chronic) A54.23
  |tuberculous A18.15
Funnel
  |breast (acquired) M95.4
    |congenital Q67.6
    |sequelae (late effect) of rickets E64.3
  |chest (acquired) M95.4
    |congenital Q67.6
    |sequelae (late effect) of rickets E64.3
  |pelvis (acquired) M95.5
    |with disproportion (fetopelvic) O33.3
      |causing obstructed labor O65.3
    |congenital Q74.2
FUO (fever of unknown origin) R50.9
Furfur L21.0
  |microsporon B36.0
Furrier's lung J67.8
Furrowed K14.5
  |nail(s) (transverse) L60.4
    |congenital Q84.6
  |tongue K14.5
    |congenital Q38.3
Furuncle L02.92
  |abdominal wall L02.221
  |ankle *see* Furuncle, lower limb
  |anus K61.0
  |antecubital space *see* Furuncle, upper limb
  |arm *see* Furuncle, upper limb
  |auditory canal, external *see* Abscess, ear,
    external
  |auricle (ear) *see* Abscess, ear, external
  |axilla (region) L02.42-
  |back (any part) L02.222
  |breast N61.1
  |buttock L02.32
  |cheek (external) L02.02
  |chest wall L02.223
  |chin L02.02
  |corpus cavernosum N48.21
  |ear, external *see* Abscess, ear, external
  |external auditory canal *see* Abscess, ear,
    external
  |eyelid *see* Abscess, eyelid
  |face L02.02
  |femoral (region) *see* Furuncle, lower limb

Furuncle - *continued*
  |finger *see* Furuncle, hand
  |flank L02.221
  |foot L02.62-
  |forehead L02.02
  |gluteal (region) L02.32
  |groin L02.224
  |hand L02.52-
  |head L02.821
    |face L02.02
  |hip *see* Furuncle, lower limb
  |kidney *see* Abscess, kidney
  |knee *see* Furuncle, lower limb
  |labium (majus) (minus) N76.4
  |lacrimal
    |gland *see* Dacryoadenitis
    |passages (duct) (sac) *see* Inflammation,
    lacrimal, passages, acute
  |leg (any part) *see* Furuncle, lower limb
  |lower limb L02.42-
  |malignant A22.0
  |mouth K12.2
  |navel L02.226
  |neck L02.12
  |nose J34.0
  |orbit, orbital *see* Abscess, orbit
  |palmar (space) *see* Furuncle, hand
  |partes posteriores L02.32
  |pectoral region L02.223
  |penis N48.21
  |perineum L02.225
  |pinna *see* Abscess, ear, external
  |popliteal *see* Furuncle, lower limb
  |prepatellar *see* Furuncle, lower limb
  |scalp L02.821
  |seminal vesicle N49.0
  |shoulder *see* Furuncle, upper limb
  |specified site NEC L02.828
  |submandibular K12.2
  |temple (region) L02.02
  |thumb *see* Furuncle, hand
  |toe *see* Furuncle, foot
  |trunk L02.229
    |abdominal wall L02.221
    |back L02.222
    |chest wall L02.223
    |groin L02.224
    |perineum L02.225
    |umbilicus L02.226
  |umbilicus L02.226
  |upper limb L02.42-
  |vulva N76.4
Furunculosis *see* Furuncle
Fused *see* Fusion, fused
Fusion, fused (congenital)
  |astragaloscaphoid Q74.2
  |atria Q21.1
  |auditory canal Q16.1
  |auricles, heart Q21.1
  |binocular with defective stereopsis H53.32
  |bone Q79.8
  |cervical spine M43.22
  |choanal Q30.0
  |commissure, mitral valve Q23.2
  |cusps, heart valve NEC Q24.8
    |mitral Q23.2
    |pulmonary Q22.1
    |tricuspid Q22.4
  |ear ossicles Q16.3
  |fingers Q70.0-
  |hymen Q52.3
  |joint (acquired) *see also* Ankylosis
    |congenital Q74.8
  |kidneys (incomplete) Q63.1
  |labium (majus) (minus) Q52.5

Fusion, fused - *continued*
|larynx and trachea Q34.8
|limb, congenital Q74.8
||lower Q74.2
||upper Q74.0
|lobes, lung Q33.8
|lumbosacral (acquired) M43.27
||arthrodesis status Z98.1
||congenital Q76.49
||postprocedural status Z98.1
|nares, nose, nasal, nostril(s) Q30.0
|organ or site not listed *see* Anomaly, by site
|ossicles Q79.9
||auditory Q16.3
|pulmonic cusps Q22.1
|ribs Q76.6
|sacroiliac (joint) (acquired) M43.28
||arthrodesis status Z98.1
||congenital Q74.2
||postprocedural status Z98.1
|spine (acquired) NEC M43.20
||arthrodesis status Z98.1
||cervical region M43.22
||cervicothoracic region M43.23
||congenital Q76.49
||lumbar M43.26
||lumbosacral region M43.27
||occipito-atlanto-axial region M43.21
||postoperative status Z98.1
||sacrococcygeal region M43.28
||thoracic region M43.24
||thoracolumbar region M43.25
|sublingual duct with submaxillary duct at
   opening in mouth Q38.4
|testes Q55.1
|toes Q70.2-
|tooth, teeth K00.2
|trachea and esophagus Q39.8
|twins Q89.4
|vagina Q52.4
|ventricles, heart Q21.0
|vertebra (arch) *see* Fusion, spine
|vulva Q52.5
Fusospirillosis (mouth) (tongue) (tonsil) A69.1
Fussy baby R68.12

G

Gain in weight (abnormal) (excessive) *see also*
   Weight, gain
Gaisböck's disease (polycythemia
   hypertonica) D75.1
Gait abnormality R26.9
|ataxic R26.0
|falling R29.6
|hysterical (ataxic) (staggering) F44.4
|paralytic R26.1
|spastic R26.1
|specified type NEC R26.89
|staggering R26.0
|unsteadiness R26.81
|walking difficulty NEC R26.2
Galactocele (breast) N64.89
|puerperal, postpartum O92.79
Galactokinase deficiency E74.29
Galactophoritis N61.0
|gestational, puerperal, postpartum O91.2-
Galactorrhea O92.6
|not associated with childbirth N64.3
Galactosemia (classic) (congenital) E74.21
Galactosuria E74.29
Galacturia R82.0
|schistosomiasis (bilharziasis) B65.0

GALD (gestational alloimmune liver disease)
   P78.84
Galeazzi's fracture S52.37-
Galen's vein *see* condition
Galeophobia F40.218
Gall duct *see* condition
Gallbladder *see also* condition
|acute K81.0
Gallop rhythm R00.8
Gallstone (colic) (cystic duct) (gallbladder)
   (impacted) (multiple) *see also* Calculus,
   gallbladder
|with
||cholecystitis *see* Calculus, gallbladder, with
    cholecystitis
||bile duct (common) (hepatic) *see* Calculus,
    bile duct
|causing intestinal obstruction K56.3
|specified NEC K80.80
||with obstruction K80.81
Gambling Z72.6
|pathological (compulsive) F63.0
Gammopathy (of undetermined significance
   [MGUS]) D47.2
|associated with lymphoplasmacytic dyscrasia
   D47.2
|monoclonal D47.2
|polyclonal D89.0
Gamna's disease (siderotic splenomegaly)
   D73.1
Gamophobia F40.298
Gampsodactylia (congenital) Q66.7
Gamstorp's disease (adynamia episodica
   hereditaria) G72.3
Gandy Nanta disease (siderotic splenomegaly)
   D73.1
Gang
|membership offenses Z72.810
Gangliocytoma D36.10
Ganglioglioma *see* Neoplasm, uncertain
   behavior, by site
Ganglion (compound) (diffuse) (joint) (tendon
   (sheath)) M67.40
|ankle M67.47-
|foot M67.47-
|forearm M67.43-
|hand M67.44-
|lower leg M67.46-
|multiple sites M67.49
|of yaws (early) (late) A66.6
|pelvic region M67.45-
|periosteal *see* Periostitis
|shoulder region M67.41-
|specified site NEC M67.48
|thigh region M67.45-
|tuberculous A18.09
|upper arm M67.42-
|wrist M67.43-
Ganglioneuroblastoma *see* Neoplasm, nerve,
   malignant
Ganglioneuroma D36.10
|malignant *see* Neoplasm, nerve, malignant
Ganglioneuromatosis D36.10
Ganglionitis
|fifth nerve *see* Neuralgia, trigeminal
|gasserian (postherpetic) (postzoster) B02.21
|geniculate G51.1
||newborn (birth injury) P11.3
||postherpetic, postzoster B02.21
|herpes zoster B02.21
|postherpetic geniculate B02.21
Gangliosidosis E75.10
|GM1 E75.19
|GM2 E75.00
||other specified E75.09

Gangliosidosis - *continued*
|Sandhoff disease E75.01
|Tay-Sachs disease E75.02
|GM3 E75.19
|mucolipidosis IV E75.11
Gangosa A66.5
Gangrene, gangrenous (connective tissue)
   (dropsical) (dry) (moist) (skin) (ulcer) *see*
   also Necrosis I96
|with diabetes (mellitus) *see* Diabetes, with,
   gangrene
|abdomen (wall) I96
|alveolar M27.3
|appendix K35.80
||with
|||peritonitis, localized (*see also*
     Appendicitis) K35.31
|arteriosclerotic (general) (senile) *see*
   Arteriosclerosis, extremities, with,
   gangrene
|auricle I96
|Bacillus welchii A48.0
|bladder (infectious) *see* Cystitis, specified
   type NEC
|bowel, cecum, or colon *see* Gangrene,
   intestine
|Clostridium perfringens or welchii A48.0
|cornea H18.89-
|corpora cavernosa N48.29
||noninfective N48.89
|cutaneous, spreading I96
|decubital *see* Ulcer, pressure, by site
|diabetic (any site) *see* Diabetes, with,
   gangrene
|epidemic *see* Poisoning, food, noxious, plant
|epididymis (infectional) N45.1
|erysipelas *see* Erysipelas
|emphysematous *see* Gangrene, gas
|extremity (lower) (upper) I96
|Fournier N49.3
||female N76.89
|fusospirochetal A69.0
|gallbladder *see* Cholecystitis, acute
|gas (bacillus) A48.0
||following
|||abortion *see* Abortion by type complicated
     by infection
|||ectopic or molar pregnancy O08.0
|glossitis K14.0
|hernia *see* Hernia, by site, with gangrene
|intestine, intestinal (hemorrhagic) (massive)
   see also Infarct, intestine K55.069
|with
|||mesenteric embolism *see also* Infarct,
     intestine K55.069
|||obstruction *see* Obstruction, intestine
|laryngitis J04.0
|limb (lower) (upper) I96
|lung J85.0
||spirochetal A69.8
|lymphangitis I89.1
|Meleney's (synergistic) *see* Ulcer, skin
|mesentery *see also* Infarct, intestine K55.069
||with
|||embolism *see also* Infarct, intestine
     K55.069
|||intestinal obstruction *see* Obstruction,
     intestine
|mouth A69.0
|ovary *see* Oophoritis
|pancreas *see* Pancreatitis, acute
|penis N48.29
||noninfective N48.89

Gangrene, gangrenous - *continued*
|perineum I96
|pharynx *see also* Pharyngitis
  |Vincent's A69.1
|presenile I73.1
|progressive synergistic *see* Ulcer, skin
|pulmonary J85.0
|pulpal (dental) K04.1
|quinsy J36
|Raynaud's (symmetric gangrene) I73.01
|retropharyngeal J39.2
|scrotum N49.3
  |noninfective N50.89
|senile (atherosclerotic) *see* Arteriosclerosis,
  extremities, with, gangrene
|spermatic cord N49.1
  |noninfective N50.89
|spine I96
|spirochetal NEC A69.8
|spreading cutaneous I96
|stomatitis A69.0
|symmetrical I73.01
|testis (infectional) N45.2
  |noninfective N44.8
|throat *see also* Pharyngitis
  |diphtheritic A36.0
  |Vincent's A69.1
|thyroid (gland) E07.89
|tooth (pulp) K04.1
|tuberculous NEC *see* Tuberculosis
|tunica vaginalis N49.1
  |noninfective N50.89
|umbilicus I96
|uterus *see* Endometritis
|uvulitis K12.2
|vas deferens N49.1
  |noninfective N50.89
|vulva N76.89
Ganister disease J62.8
Ganser's syndrome (hysterical) F44.89
Gardner-Diamond syndrome
  (autoerythrocyte sensitization) D69.2
Gargoylism E76.01
Garré's disease, osteitis (sclerosing),
  osteomyelitis *see* Osteomyelitis, specified
  type NEC
Garrod's pad, knuckle M72.1
Gartner's duct
  |cyst Q52.4
  |persistent Q50.6
Gas R14.3
  |asphyxiation, inhalation, poisoning,
    suffocation NEC *see* Table of Drugs and
    Chemicals
  |excessive R14.0
  |gangrene A48.0
    |following
      |abortion *see* Abortion by type complicated
        by infection
      |ectopic or molar pregnancy O08.0
  |on stomach R14.0
  |pains R14.1
Gastralgia *see also* Pain, abdominal
Gastrectasis K31.0
  |psychogenic F45.8
Gastric *see* condition
Gastrinoma
  |malignant
    |pancreas C25.4
    |specified site NEC *see* Neoplasm,
      malignant, by site
    |unspecified site C25.4

Gastrinoma - *continued*
  |specified site *see* Neoplasm, uncertain
    behavior
  |unspecified site D37.9
Gastritis (simple) K29.70
  |with bleeding K29.71
  |acute (erosive) K29.00
    |with bleeding K29.01
  |alcoholic K29.20
    |with bleeding K29.21
  |allergic K29.60
    |with bleeding K29.61
  |atrophic (chronic) K29.40
    |with bleeding K29.41
  |chronic (antral) (fundal) K29.50
    |with bleeding K29.51
    |atrophic K29.40
      |with bleeding K29.41
    |superficial K29.30
      |with bleeding K29.31
  |dietary counseling and surveillance Z71.3
  |due to diet deficiency E63.9
  |eosinophilic K52.81
  |giant hypertrophic K29.60
    |with bleeding K29.61
  |granulomatous K29.60
    |with bleeding K29.61
  |hypertrophic (mucosa) K29.60
    |with bleeding K29.61
  |nervous F54
  |spastic K29.60
    |with bleeding K29.61
  |specified NEC K29.60
    |with bleeding K29.61
  |superficial chronic K29.30
    |with bleeding K29.31
  |tuberculous A18.83
  |viral NEC A08.4
Gastrocarcinoma *see* Neoplasm, malignant,
  stomach
Gastrocolic *see* condition
Gastrodisciasis, gastrodiscoidiasis B66.8
Gastroduodenitis K29.90
  |with bleeding K29.91
  |virus, viral A08.4
    |specified type NEC A08.39
Gastrodynia *see* Pain, abdominal
Gastroenteritis (acute) (chronic)
  (noninfectious) *see also* Enteritis K52.9
  |allergic K52.29
    |with
      |eosinophilic gastritis or gastroenteritis
        K52.81
      |food protein-induced enterocolitis
        syndrome K52.21
      |food protein-induced enteropathy K52.22
  |dietetic *see also* Gastroenteritis, allergic
    K52.29
  |drug-induced K52.1
  |due to
    |Cryptosporidium A07.2
    |drugs K52.1
    |food poisoning *see* Intoxication, foodborne
    |radiation K52.0
  |eosinophilic K52.81
  |epidemic (infectious) A09
  |food hypersensitivity *see also* Gastroenteritis,
    allergic K52.29
  |infectious *see* Enteritis, infectious
  |influenzal *see* Influenza, with gastroenteritis
  |noninfectious K52.9
    |specified NEC K52.89
  |Rotaviral A08.0
  |Salmonella A02.0
  |toxic K52.1

Gastroenteritis - *continued*
  |viral NEC A08.4
    |acute infectious A08.39
      |type Norwalk A08.11
    |infantile (acute) A08.39
    |Norwalk agent A08.11
    |Rotaviral A08.0
    |severe of infants A08.39
    |specified type NEC A08.39
Gastroenteropathy *see also* Gastroenteritis
  K52.9
  |acute, due to Norwalk agent A08.11
  |acute, due to Norovirus A08.11
  |infectious A09
Gastroenteroptosis K63.4
Gastroesophageal laceration hemorrhage
  syndrome K22.6
Gastrointestinal *see* condition
Gastrojejunal *see* condition
Gastrojejunitis *see also* Enteritis K52.9
Gastrojejunocolic *see* condition
Gastroliths K31.89
Gastromalacia K31.89
Gastroparalysis K31.84
  |diabetic *see* Diabetes, gastroparalysis
Gastroparesis K31.84
  |diabetic *see* Diabetes, by type, with
    gastroparesis
Gastropathy K31.9
  |congestive portal (see also, Hypertension,
    portal) K31.89
  |erythematous K29.70
  |exudative K90.89
  |portal hypertensive (see also, Hypertension,
    portal) K31.89
Gastroptosis K31.89
Gastrorrhagia K92.2
  |psychogenic F45.8
Gastroschisis (congenital) Q79.3
Gastrospasm (neurogenic) (reflex) K31.89
  |neurotic F45.8
  |psychogenic F45.8
Gastrostaxis *see* Gastritis, with bleeding
Gastrostenosis K31.89
Gastrostomy
  |attention to Z43.1
  |status Z93.1
Gastrosuccorrhea (continuous) (intermittent)
  K31.89
  |neurotic F45.8
  |psychogenic F45.8
Gatophobia F40.218
Gaucher's disease or splenomegaly (adult)
  (infantile) E75.22
Gee (-Herter)(-Thaysen) disease (nontropical
  sprue) K90.0
Gélineau's syndrome G47.419
  |with cataplexy G47.411
Gemination, tooth, teeth K00.2
Gemistocytoma
  |specified site *see* Neoplasm, malignant, by site
  |unspecified site C71.9
General, generalized *see* condition
Genetic
  |carrier (status)
    |cystic fibrosis Z14.1
    |hemophilia A (asymptomatic) Z14.01
      |symptomatic Z14.02
    |specified NEC Z14.8
  |susceptibility to disease NEC Z15.89
    |malignant neoplasm Z15.09
      |breast Z15.01
      |endometrium Z15.04
      |ovary Z15.02
      |prostate Z15.03
      |specified NEC Z15.09
    |multiple endocrine neoplasia Z15.81

Genital *see* condition
Genito-Anorectal syndrome A55
Genitourinary system *see* condition
Genu
| congenital Q74.1
| extrorsum (acquired) *see also* Deformity,
    varus, knee
| | congenital Q74.1
| | sequelae (late effect) of rickets E64.3
| introrsum (acquired) *see also* Deformity,
    valgus, knee
| | congenital Q74.1
| | sequelae (late effect) of rickets E64.3
| rachitic (old) E64.3
| recurvatum (acquired) *see also* Deformity,
    limb, specified type NEC, lower leg
| | congenital Q68.2
| | sequelae (late effect) of rickets E64.3
| valgum (acquired) (knock-knee) M21.06-
| | congenital Q74.1
| | sequelae (late effect) of rickets E64.3
| varum (acquired) (bowleg) M21.16-
| | congenital Q74.1
| | sequelae (late effect) of rickets E64.3
Geographic tongue K14.1
Geophagia *see* Pica Geotrichosis B48.3
| stomatitis B48.3
Gephyrophobia F40.242
Gerbode defect Q21.0
GERD (gastroesophageal reflux disease)
    K21.9
Gerhardt's
| disease (erythromelalgia) I73.81
| syndrome (vocal cord paralysis) J38.00
| | bilateral J38.02
| | unilateral J38.01
German measles *see also* Rubella
| exposure to Z20.4
Germinoblastoma (diffuse) C85.9-
| follicular C82.9-
Germinoma *see* Neoplasm, malignant, by site
Gerontoxon *see* Degeneration, cornea, senile
Gerstmann-Sträussler-Scheinker syndrome
    (GSS) A81.82
Gerstmann's syndrome R48.8
| developmental F81.2
Gestation (period) *see also* Pregnancy
| ectopic *see* Pregnancy, by site
| multiple O30.9-
| | greater than quadruplets *see* Pregnancy,
      multiple (gestation), specified NEC
| | specified NEC *see* Pregnancy, multiple
      (gestation), specified NEC
Gestational
| mammary abscess O91.11-
| purulent mastitis O91.11-
| subareolar abscess O91.11-
Ghon tubercle, primary infection A15.7
Ghost
| teeth K00.4
| vessels (cornea) H16.41
Ghoul hand A66.3
Gianotti-Crosti disease L44.4
Giant
| cell
| | epulis K06.8
| | peripheral granuloma K06.8
| esophagus, congenital Q39.5
| kidney, congenital Q63.3
| urticaria T78.3
| | hereditary D84.1
Giardiasis A07.1
Gibert's disease or pityriasis L42
Giddiness R42
| hysterical F44.89
| psychogenic F45.8
Gierke's disease (glycogenosis I) E74.01

Gigantism (cerebral) (hypophyseal)
    (pituitary) E22.0
| constitutional E34.4
Gilbert's disease or syndrome E80.4
Gilchrist's disease B40.9
Gilford-Hutchinson disease E34.8
Gilles de la Tourette's disease or syndrome
    (motor-Verbal tic) F95.2
Gingivitis K05.10
| acute (catarrhal) K05.00
| | necrotizing A69.1
| | nonplaque induced K05.01
| | plaque induced K05.00
| chronic (desquamative) (hyperplastic) (simple
    marginal) (pregnancy associated)
    (ulcerative) K05.10
| | nonplaque induced K05.11
| | plaque induced K05.10
| expulsiva *see* Periodontitis
| necrotizing ulcerative (acute) A69.1
| pellagrous E52
| | acute necrotizing A69.1
| Vincent's A69.1
Gingivoglossitis K14.0
Gingivopericementitis *see* Periodontitis
Gingivosis *see* Gingivitis, chronic
Gingivostomatitis K05.10
| herpesviral B00.2
| necrotizing ulcerative (acute) A69.1
Gland, glandular *see* condition
Glanders A24.0
Glanzmann (Naegeli) disease or
    thrombasthenia D69.1
Glasgow coma scale
| total score
| | 3-8 R40.243
| | 9-12 R40.242
| | 13-15 R40.241
Glass-Blower's disease (cataract) *see* Cataract,
    specified NEC
Glaucoma H40.9
| with
| | increased episcleral venous pressure
      H40.81-
| | pseudoexfoliation of lens *see* Glaucoma,
      open angle, primary, capsular
| absolute H44.51-
| angle-closure (primary) H40.20-
| | acute (attack) (crisis) H40.21-
| | chronic H40.22-
| | intermittent H40.23-
| | residual stage H40.24-
| borderline H40.00-
| capsular (with pseudoexfoliation of lens) *see*
    Glaucoma, open angle, primary, capsular
| childhood Q15.0
| closed angle *see* Glaucoma, angle-closure
| congenital Q15.0
| corticosteroid-induced *see* Glaucoma,
    secondary, drugs
| hypersecretion H40.82-
| in (due to)
| | amyloidosis E85.4 [*H42*]
| | aniridia Q13.1 [*H42*]
| | concussion of globe *see* Glaucoma,
      secondary, trauma
| | dislocation of lens *see* Glaucoma, secondary
| | disorder of lens NEC *see* Glaucoma,
      secondary
| | drugs *see* Glaucoma, secondary, drugs
| | endocrine disease NOS E34.9 [*H42*]
| | eye
| | | inflammation *see* Glaucoma, secondary,
       inflammation
| | | trauma *see* Glaucoma, secondary, trauma

Glaucoma- *continued*
| | hypermature cataract *see* Glaucoma,
      secondary
| | iridocyclitis *see* Glaucoma, secondary,
      inflammation
| | lens disorder *see* Glaucoma, secondary,
| | Lowe's syndrome E72.03 [*H42*]
| | metabolic disease NOS E88.9 [*H42*]
| | ocular disorders NEC *see* Glaucoma,
      secondary
| | onchocerciasis B73.02
| | pupillary block *see* Glaucoma, secondary
| | retinal vein occlusion *see* Glaucoma,
      secondary
| | Rieger's anomaly Q13.81 [*H42*]
| | rubeosis of iris *see* Glaucoma, secondary
| | tumor of globe *see* Glaucoma, secondary
| infantile Q15.0
| low tension *see* Glaucoma, open angle,
    primary, low-tension
| malignant H40.83-
| narrow angle *see* Glaucoma, angle-closure
| newborn Q15.0
| noncongestive (chronic) *see* Glaucoma, open
    angle
| nonobstructive *see* Glaucoma, open angle
| obstructive *see also* Glaucoma, angle-closure
| | due to lens changes *see* Glaucoma,
      secondary
| open angle H40.10-
| | primary H40.11-
| | | capsular (with pseudoexfoliation of lens)
       H40.14-
| | | low-tension H40.12
| | | pigmentary H40.13-
| | | residual stage H40.15-
| phacolytic *see* Glaucoma, secondary
| pigmentary *see* Glaucoma, open angle,
    primary, pigmentary
| postinfectious *see* Glaucoma, secondary,
    inflammation
| secondary (to) H40.5-
| | drugs H40.6-
| | inflammation H40.4-
| | trauma H40.3-
| simple (chronic) H40.11-
| simplex H40.11-
| specified type NEC H40.89
| suspect H40.00-
| syphilitic A52.71
| traumatic *see also* Glaucoma, secondary,
    trauma
| | newborn (birth injury) P15.3
| tuberculous A18.59
Glaucomatous flecks (subcapsular) *see*
    Cataract, complicated
Glazed tongue K14.4
Gleet (gonococcal) A54.01
Glénard's disease K63.4
Glioblastoma (multiforme)
| with sarcomatous component
| | specified site *see* Neoplasm, malignant, by
      site
| | unspecified site C71.9
| giant cell
| | specified site *see* Neoplasm, malignant, by
      site
| | unspecified site C71.9
| specified site *see* Neoplasm, malignant, by site
| unspecified site C71.9
Glioma (malignant)
| astrocytic
| | specified site *see* Neoplasm, malignant, by
      site
| | unspecified site C71.9

Glioma - *continued*
| mixed
| | specified site *see* Neoplasm, malignant, by
| | | site
| | unspecified site C71.9
| nose Q30.8
| specified site NEC *see* Neoplasm, malignant,
| | by site
| subependymal D43.2
| | specified site *see* Neoplasm, uncertain
| | | behavior, by site
| | unspecified site D43.2
| unspecified site C71.9
Gliomatosis cerebri C71.0
Glioneuroma *see* Neoplasm, uncertain behavior,
| by site
Gliosarcoma
| specified site *see* Neoplasm, malignant, by site
| unspecified site C71.9
Gliosis (cerebral) G93.89
| spinal G95.89
Glisson's disease *see* Rickets
Globinuria R82.3
Globus (hystericus) F45.8
Glomangioma D18.00
| intra-abdominal D18.03
| intracranial D18.02
| skin D18.01
| specified site NEC D18.09
Glomangiomyoma D18.00
| intra-abdominal D18.03
| intracranial D18.02
| skin D18.01
| specified site NEC D18.09
Glomangiosarcoma *see* Neoplasm, connective
| tissue, malignant
Glomerular
| disease in syphilis A52.75
| nephritis *see* Glomerulonephritis
Glomerulitis *see* Glomerulonephritis
Glomerulonephritis *see also* Nephritis N05.9
| with
| | C3
| | | glomerulonephritis N05.A
| | | glomerulopathy N05.A
| | | | with dense deposit disease N05.6
| | edema *see* Nephrosis
| | minimal change N05.0
| | minor glomerular abnormality N05.0
| acute N00.9
| chronic N03.9
| crescentic (diffuse) NEC *see also* N00-N07
| | with fourth character .7 N05.7
| dense deposit *see also* N00-N07 with fourth
| | character .6 N05.6
| diffuse
| | crescentic *see also* N00-N07 with fourth
| | | character .7 N05.7
| | endocapillary proliferative *see also* N00-
| | | N07 with fourth character .4 N05.4
| | membranous *see also* N00-N07 with fourth
| | | character .2 N05.2
| | mesangial proliferative *see also* N00-N07
| | | with fourth character .3 N05.3
| | mesangiocapillary *see also* N00-N07 with
| | | fourth character .5 N05.5
| | sclerosing N18.9
| endocapillary proliferative (diffuse) NEC *see*
| | *also* N00-N07 with fourth character .4
| | N05.4
| extracapillary NEC *see also* N00-N07 with
| | fourth character .7 N05.7
| focal (and segmental) *see also* N00-N07 with
| | fourth character .1 N05.1

Glomerulonephritis - *continued*
| hypocomplementemic *see* Glomerulonephritis,
| | membranoproliferative
| IgA *see* Nephropathy, IgA
| immune complex (circulating) NEC N05.8
| in (due to)
| | amyloidosis E85.4 *[N08]*
| | bilharziasis B65.9 *[N08]*
| | cryoglobulinemia D89.1 *[N08]*
| | defibrination syndrome D65 *[N08]*
| | diabetes mellitus *see* Diabetes,
| | | glomerulosclerosis
| | disseminated intravascular coagulation D65
| | | *[N08]*
| | Fabry (-Anderson) disease E75.21 *[N08]*
| | Goodpasture's syndrome M31.0
| | hemolytic-uremic syndrome D59.3
| | Henoch (-Schönlein) purpura D69.0 *[N08]*
| | lecithin cholesterol acyltransferase
| | | deficiency E78.6 *[N08]*
| | microscopic polyangiitis M31.7 *[N08]*
| | multiple myeloma C90.0 *[N08]*
| | Plasmodium malariae B52.0
| | schistosomiasis B65.9 *[N08]*
| | sepsis A41.9 *[N08]*
| | | streptococcal A40 *[N08]*
| | sickle-cell disorders D57. *[N08]*
| | strongyloidiasis B78.9 *[N08]*
| | subacute bacterial endocarditis I33.0 *[N08]*
| | syphilis (late) congenital A50.59 *[N08]*
| | systemic lupus erythematosus M32.14
| | thrombotic thrombocytopenic purpura
| | | M31.19 *[N08]*
| | typhoid fever A01.09
| | Waldenström macroglobulinemia C88.0
| | . *[N08]*
| | Wegener's granulomatosis M31.31
| latent or quiescent N03.9
| lobular, lobulonodular *see*
| | Glomerulonephritis,
| | membranoproliferative
| membranoproliferative (diffuse)(type 1 or 3)
| | *see also* N00-N07 with fourth character .5
| | N05.5
| | dense deposit (type 2) NEC *see also* N00-
| | | N07 with fourth character .6 N05.6
| membranous (diffuse) NEC *see also* N00-N07
| | with fourth character .2 N05.2
| mesangial
| | IgA/IgG *see* Nephropathy, IgA
| | proliferative (diffuse) NEC *see also* N00-
| | | N07 with fourth character .3 N05.3
| mesangiocapillary (diffuse) NEC *see also*
| | N00-N07 with fourth character .5 N05.5
| necrotic, necrotizing NEC *see also* N00-N07
| | with fourth character .8 N05.8
| nodular *see* Glomerulonephritis,
| | membranoproliferative
| poststreptococcal NEC N05.9
| | acute N00.9
| | chronic N03.9
| | rapidly progressive N01.9
| proliferative NEC *see also* N00-N07 with
| | fourth character .8 N05.8
| | diffuse (lupus) M32.14
| rapidly progressive N01.9
| sclerosing, diffuse N18.9
| specified pathology NEC *see also* N00-N07
| | with fourth character .8 N05.8
| subacute N01.9
Glomerulopathy *see* Glomerulonephritis
Glomerulosclerosis *see also* Sclerosis, renal
| intercapillary (nodular) (with diabetes) *see*
| | Diabetes, glomerulosclerosis
| intracapillary *see* Diabetes, glomerulosclerosis

Glossagra K14.6
Glossalgia K14.6
Glossitis (chronic superficial) (gangrenous)
| **(Moeller's)** K14.0
| areata exfoliativa K14.1
| atrophic K14.4
| benign migratory K14.1
| cortical superficial, sclerotic K14.0
| Hunter's D51.0
| interstitial, sclerous K14.0
| median rhomboid K14.2
| pellagrous E52
| superficial, chronic K14.0
Glossocele K14.8
Glossodynia K14.6
| exfoliativa K14.4
Glossoncus K14.8
Glossopathy K14.9
Glossophytia K14.3
Glossoplegia K14.8
Glossoptosis K14.8
Glossopyrosis K14.6
Glossotrichia K14.3
Glossy skin L90.8
Glottis *see* condition
Glottitis *see also* Laryngitis J04.0
Glucagonoma
| pancreas
| | benign D13.7
| | malignant C25.4
| | uncertain behavior D37.8
| specified site NEC
| | benign *see* Neoplasm, benign, by site
| | malignant *see* Neoplasm, malignant, by site
| | uncertain behavior *see* Neoplasm, uncertain
| | | behavior, by site
| unspecified site
| | benign D13.7
| | malignant C25.4
| | uncertain behavior D37.8
Glucoglycinuria E72.51
Glucose-Galactose malabsorption E74.39
Glue
| ear *see* Otitis, media, nonsuppurative, chronic,
| | mucoid
| sniffing (airplane) *see* Abuse, drug, inhalant
| | dependence *see* Dependence, drug, inhalant
GLUT1 deficiency syndrome 1, infantile onset
| E74.810
GLUT1 deficiency syndrome 2, childhood
| **onset** E74.810
Glutaric aciduria E72.3
Glycinemia E72.51
Glycinuria (renal) (with ketosis) E72.09
Glycogen
| infiltration *see* Disease, glycogen storage
| storage disease *see* Disease, glycogen storage
Glycogenosis (diffuse) (generalized) *see also*
| Disease, glycogen storage
| cardiac E74.02 *[I43]*
| diabetic, secondary *see* Diabetes,
| | glycogenosis, secondary
| pulmonary interstitial J84.842
Glycopenia E16.2
Glycosuria R81
| renal (familial) E74.818
Gnathostoma spinigerum (infection)
| **(infestation), gnathostomiasis (wandering**
| **swelling)** B83.1
Goiter (plunging) (substernal) E04.9
| with
| | hyperthyroidism (recurrent) *see*
| | | Hyperthyroidism, with, goiter

Goiter - *continued*
  |thyrotoxicosis *see* Hyperthyroidism, with, goiter
  |adenomatous *see* Goiter, nodular
  |cancerous C73
  |congenital (nontoxic) E03.0
    |diffuse E03.0
    |parenchymatous E03.0
    |transitory, with normal functioning P72.0
  |cystic E04.2
    |due to iodine-deficiency E01.1
  |due to
    |enzyme defect in synthesis of thyroid hormone E07.1
    |iodine-deficiency (endemic) E01.2
  |dyshormonogenetic (familial) E07.1
  |endemic (iodine-deficiency) E01.2
    |diffuse E01.0
    |multinodular E01.1
  |exophthalmic *see* Hyperthyroidism, with, goiter
  |iodine-deficiency (endemic) E01.2
    |diffuse E01.0
    |multinodular E01.1
    |nodular E01.1
  |lingual Q89.2
  |lymphadenoid E06.3
  |malignant C73
  |multinodular (cystic) (nontoxic) E04.2
    |toxic or with hyperthyroidism E05.20
      |with thyroid storm E05.21
  |neonatal NEC P72.0
  |nodular (nontoxic) (due to) E04.9
    |with
      |hyperthyroidism E05.20
        |with thyroid storm E05.21
      |thyrotoxicosis E05.20
        |with thyroid storm E05.21
    |endemic E01.1
    |iodine-deficiency E01.1
    |sporadic E04.9
    |toxic E05.20
      |with thyroid storm E05.21
  |nontoxic E04.9
    |diffuse (colloid) E04.0
    |multinodular E04.2
    |simple E04.0
    |specified NEC E04.8
    |uninodular E04.1
  |simple E04.0
  |toxic *see* Hyperthyroidism, with, goiter
  |uninodular (nontoxic) E04.1
    |toxic or with hyperthyroidism E05.10
      |with thyroid storm E05.11
Goiter-Deafness syndrome E07.1
Goldberg syndrome Q89.8
Goldberg-Maxwell syndrome E34.51
Goldblatt's hypertension or kidney I70.1
Goldenhar (-Gorlin) syndrome Q87.0
Goldflam-Erb disease or syndrome G70.00
  |with exacerbation (acute) G70.01
  |in crisis G70.01
Goldscheider's disease Q81.8
Goldstein's disease (familial hemorrhagic telangiectasia) I78.0
Golfer's elbow *see* Epicondylitis, medial
Gonadoblastoma
  |specified site *see* Neoplasm, uncertain behavior, by site
  |unspecified site
    |female D39.10
    |male D40.10
Gonecystitis *see* Vesiculitis
Gongylonemiasis B83.8

Goniosynechiae *see* Adhesions, iris, goniosynechiae
Gonococcemia A54.86
Gonococcus, gonococcal (disease) (infection) *see also* condition A54.9
  |anus A54.6
  |bursa, bursitis A54.49
  |conjunctiva, conjunctivitis (neonatorum) A54.31
  |endocardium A54.83
  |eye A54.30
    |conjunctivitis A54.31
    |iridocyclitis A54.32
    |keratitis A54.33
    |newborn A54.31
    |other specified A54.39
  |fallopian tubes (acute) (chronic) A54.24
  |genitourinary (organ) (system) (tract) (acute)
    |lower A54.00
      |with abscess (accessory gland) (periurethral) A54.1
    |upper *see also* condition A54.29
  |heart A54.83
  |iridocyclitis A54.32
  |joint A54.42
  |lymphatic (gland) (node) A54.89
  |meninges, meningitis A54.81
  |musculoskeletal A54.40
    |arthritis A54.42
    |osteomyelitis A54.43
    |other specified A54.49
    |spondylopathy A54.41
  |pelviperitonitis A54.24
  |pelvis (acute) (chronic) A54.24
  |pharynx A54.5
  |proctitis A54.6
  |pyosalpinx (acute) (chronic) A54.24
  |rectum A54.6
  |skin A54.89
  |specified site NEC A54.89
  |tendon sheath A54.49
  |throat A54.5
  |urethra (acute) (chronic) A54.01
    |with abscess (accessory gland) (periurethral) A54.1
  |vulva (acute) (chronic) A54.02
Gonocytoma
  |specified site *see* Neoplasm, uncertain behavior, by site
  |unspecified site
    |female D39.10
    |male D40.10
Gonorrhea (acute) (chronic) A54.9
  |Bartholin's gland (acute) (chronic) (purulent) A54.02
    |with abscess (accessory gland) (periurethral) A54.1
  |bladder A54.01
  |cervix A54.03
  |conjunctiva, conjunctivitis (neonatorum) A54.31
  |contact Z20.2
  |Cowper's gland (with abscess) A54.1
  |exposure to Z20.2
  |fallopian tube (acute) (chronic) A54.24
  |kidney (acute) (chronic) A54.21
  |lower genitourinary tract A54.00
    |with abscess (accessory gland) (periurethral) A54.1
  |ovary (acute) (chronic) A54.24
  |pelvis (acute) (chronic) A54.24
    |female pelvic inflammatory disease A54.24
  |penis A54.09
  |prostate (acute) (chronic) A54.22
  |seminal vesicle (acute) (chronic) A54.23

Gonorrhea - *continued*
  |specified site not listed *see also* Gonococcus A54.89
  |spermatic cord (acute) (chronic) A54.23
  |urethra A54.01
    |with abscess (accessory gland) (periurethral) A54.1
  |vagina A54.02
  |vas deferens (acute) (chronic) A54.23
  |vulva A54.02
Goodall's disease A08.19
Goodpasture's syndrome M31.0
Gopalan's syndrome (burning feet) E53.0
Gorlin-Chaudry-Moss syndrome Q87.0
Gottron's papules L94.4
Gougerot's syndrome (trisymptomatic) L81.7
Gougerot-Blum syndrome (pigmented purpuric lichenoid dermatitis) L81.7
Gougerot-Carteaud disease or syndrome (confluent reticulate papillomatosis) L83
Gouley's syndrome (constrictive pericarditis) I31.1
Goundou A66.6
Gout, gouty (acute) (attack) (flare) *see also* Gout, chronic M10.9
  |drug-induced M10.20
    |ankle M10.27-
    |elbow M10.22-
    |foot joint M10.27-
    |hand joint M10.24-
    |hip M10.25-
    |knee M10.26-
    |multiple site M10.29
    |shoulder M10.21-
    |vertebrae M10.28
    |wrist M10.23-
  |idiopathic M10.00
    |ankle M10.07-
    |elbow M10.02-
    |foot joint M10.07-
    |hand joint M10.04-
    |hip M10.05-
    |knee M10.06-
    |multiple site M10.09
    |shoulder M10.01-
    |vertebrae M10.08
    |wrist M10.03-
  |in (due to) renal impairment M10.30
    |ankle M10.37-
    |elbow M10.32-
    |foot joint M10.37-
    |hand joint M10.34-
    |hip M10.35-
    |knee M10.36-
    |multiple site M10.39
    |shoulder M10.31-
    |vertebrae M10.38
    |wrist M10.33-
  |lead-induced M10.10
    |ankle M10.17-
    |elbow M10.12-
    |foot joint M10.17-
    |hand joint M10.14-
    |hip M10.15-
    |knee M10.16-
    |multiple site M10.19
    |shoulder M10.11-
    |vertebrae M10.18
    |wrist M10.13-
  |primary *see* Gout, idiopathic
  |saturnine *see* Gout, lead-induced
  |secondary NEC M10.40
    |ankle M10.47-
    |elbow M10.42-
    |foot joint M10.47-

Gout, gouty (acute) - *continued*
|hand joint M10.44-
|hip M10.45-
|knee M10.46-
|multiple site M10.49
|shoulder M10.41-
|vertebrae M10.48
|wrist M10.43-
|syphilitic *see also* subcategory M14.8
  A52.77
|tophi *see* Gout, chronic
Gout, chronic *see also* Gout, gouty M1A.9
|drug-induced M1A.20
  |ankle M1A.27-
  |elbow M1A.22-
  |foot joint M1A.27-
  |hand joint M1A.24-
  |hip M1A.25-
  |knee M1A.26-
  |multiple site M1A.29-
  |shoulder M1A.21-
  |vertebrae M1A.28
  |wrist M1A.23-
|idiopathic M1A.00
  |ankle M1A.07-
  |elbow M1A.02-
  |foot joint M1A.07-
  |hand joint M1A.04-
  |hip M1A.05-
  |knee M1A.06-
  |multiple site M1A.09
  |shoulder M1A.01-
  |vertebrae M1A.08
  |wrist M1A.03-
|in (due to) renal impairment M1A.30
  |ankle M1A.37-
  |elbow M1A.32-
  |foot joint M1A.37-
  |hand joint M1A.34-
  |hip M1A.35-
  |knee M1A.36-
  |multiple site M1A.39
  |shoulder M1A.31-
  |vertebrae M1A.38
  |wrist M1A.33-
|lead-induced M1A.10
  |ankle M1A.17-
  |elbow M1A.12-
  |foot joint M1A.17-
  |hand joint M1A.14-
  |hip M1A.15-
  |knee M1A.16-
  |multiple site M1A.19
  |shoulder M1A.11-
  |vertebrae M1A.18
  |wrist M1A.13-
|primary *see* Gout, chronic, idiopathic
|saturnine *see* Gout, chronic, lead-induced
|secondary NEC M1A.40
  |ankle M1A.47-
  |elbow M1A.42-
  |foot joint M1A.47-
  |hand joint M1A.44-
  |hip M1A.45-
  |knee M1A.46-
  |multiple site M1A.49
  |shoulder M1A.41-
  |vertebrae M1A.48
  |wrist M1A.43-
|syphilitic *see also* subcategory M14.8
  A52.77
|tophi M1A.9
Gower's
|muscular dystrophy G71.01
|syndrome (vasovagal attack) R55

Gradenigo's syndrome *see* Otitis, media,
  suppurative, acute
Graefe's disease *see* Strabismus, paralytic,
  ophthalmoplegia, progressive
Graft-Versus-Host disease D89.813
|acute D89.810
|acute on chronic D89.812
|chronic D89.811
Grain handler's disease or lung J67.8
Grain mite (itch) B88.0
Grand mal *see* Epilepsy, generalized, specified
  NEC
Grand multipara status only (not pregnant)
  Z64.1
|pregnant *see* Pregnancy, complicated by,
  grand multiparity
Granite worker's lung J62.8
Granular *see also* condition
|inflammation, pharynx J31.2
|kidney (contracting) *see* Sclerosis, renal
|liver K74.69
Granulation tissue (abnormal) (excessive)
  L92.9
|postmastoidectomy cavity *see* Complications,
  postmastoidectomy, granulation
Granulocytopenia (primary) (malignant) *see*
  Agranulocytosis
Granuloma L92.9
|abdomen K66.8
  |from residual foreign body L92.3
  |pyogenicum L98.0
|actinic L57.5
|annulare (perforating) L92.0
|apical K04.5
|aural *see* Otitis, externa, specified NEC
|beryllium (skin) L92.3
|bone
  |eosinophilic C96.6
  |from residual foreign body *see*
    Osteomyelitis, specified type NEC
  |lung C96.6
|brain (any site) G06.0
  |schistosomiasis B65.9 [*G07*]
|canaliculus lacrimalis *see* Granuloma, lacrimal
|candidal (cutaneous) B37.2
|cerebral (any site) G06.0
|coccidioidal (primary) (progressive) B38.7
  |lung B38.1
  |meninges B38.4
|colon K63.89
|conjunctiva H11.22-
|dental K04.5
|ear, middle *see* Cholesteatoma
|eosinophilic C96.6
  |bone C96.6
  |lung C96.6
  |oral mucosa K13.4
  |skin L92.2
|eyelid H01.8
|facial (e) L92.2
|foreign body (in soft tissue) NEC M60.20
  |ankle M60.27-
  |foot M60.27-
  |forearm M60.23-
  |hand M60.24-
  |in operation wound *see* Foreign body,
    accidentally left during a procedure
  |lower leg M60.26-
  |pelvic region M60.25-
  |shoulder region M60.21-
  |skin L92.3
  |specified site NEC M60.28
  |subcutaneous tissue L92.3
  |thigh M60.25-
  |upper arm M60.22-

Granuloma - *continued*
|gangraenescens M31.2
|genito-inguinale A58
|giant cell (central) (reparative) (jaw) M27.1
  |gingiva (peripheral) K06.8
|gland (lymph) I88.8
|hepatic NEC K75.3
  |in (due to)
    |berylliosis J63.2 [*K77*]
    |sarcoidosis D86.89
|Hodgkin C81.9
|ileum K63.89
|infectious B99.9
  |specified NEC B99.8
|inguinale (Donovan) (venereal) A58
|intestine NEC K63.89
|intracranial (any site) G06.0
|intraspinal (any part) G06.1
|iridocyclitis *see* Iridocyclitis, chronic
|jaw (bone) (central) M27.1
  |reparative giant cell M27.1
|kidney *see also* Infection, kidney N15.8
|lacrimal H04.81-
|larynx J38.7
|lethal midline (faciale(e)) M31.2
|liver NEC *see* Granuloma, hepatic
|lung (infectious) *see also* Fibrosis, lung
  |coccidioidal B38.1
  |eosinophilic C96.6
|Majocchi's B35.8
|malignant (facial(e)) M31.2
|mandible (central) M27.1
|midline (lethal) M31.2
|monilial (cutaneous) B37.2
|nasal sinus *see* Sinusitis
|operation wound T81.89
  |foreign body *see* Foreign body, accidentally
    left during a procedure
  |stitch T81.89
  |talc *see* Foreign body, accidentally left
    during a procedure
|oral mucosa K13.4
|orbit, orbital H05.11-
|paracoccidioidal B41.8
|penis, venereal A58
|periapical K04.5
|peritoneum K66.8
  |due to ova of helminths NOS *see also*
    Helminthiasis B83.9 [*K67*]
|postmastoidectomy cavity *see* Complications,
  postmastoidectomy, recurrent
  cholesteatoma
|prostate N42.89
|pudendi (ulcerating) A58
|pulp, internal (tooth) K03.3
|pyogenic, pyogenicum (of) (skin) L98.0
  |gingiva K06.8
  |maxillary alveolar ridge K04.5
  |oral mucosa K13.4
|rectum K62.89
|reticulohistiocytic D76.3
|rubrum nasi L74.8
|Schistosoma *see* Schistosomiasis
|septic (skin) L98.0
|silica (skin) L92.3
|sinus (accessory) (infective) (nasal) *see*
  Sinusitis
|skin L92.9
  |from residual foreign body L92.3
  |pyogenicum L98.0
|spine
  |syphilitic (epidural) A52.19
  |tuberculous A18.01
|stitch (postoperative) T81.89
|suppurative (skin) L98.0

Granuloma - *continued*
|swimming pool A31.1
|talc *see also* Granuloma, foreign body
  |in operation wound *see* Foreign body,
    accidentally left during a procedure
|telangiectaticum (skin) L98.0
|tracheostomy J95.09
|trichophyticum B35.8
|tropicum A66.4
|umbilical P83.81
|umbilicus P83.81
|urethra N36.8
|uveitis *see* Iridocyclitis, chronic
|vagina A58
|venereum A58
|vocal cord J38.3
Granulomatosis L92.9
|with polyangiitis M31.3
|eosinophilic, with polyangiitis [EGPA] M30.1
|lymphoid C83.8-
|miliary (listerial) A32.89
|necrotizing, respiratory M31.30
|progressive septic D71
|specified NEC L92.8
|Wegener's M31.30
  |with renal involvement M31.31
Granulomatous tissue (abnormal) (excessive) L92.9
Granulosis rubra nasi L74.8
Graphite fibrosis (of lung) J63.3
Graphospasm F48.8
|organic G25.89
Grating scapula M89.8X1
Gravel (urinary) *see* Calculus, urinary
Graves' disease *see* Hyperthyroidism, with, goiter
Gravis *see* condition
Grawitz tumor C64.-
Gray syndrome (newborn) P93.0
Grayness, hair (premature) L67.1
|congenital Q84.2
Green sickness D50.8
Greenfield's disease
|meaning
  |concentric sclerosis (encephalitis periaxialis concentrica) G37.5
  |metachromatic leukodystrophy E75.25
Greenstick fracture   code as Fracture, by site
Grey syndrome (newborn) P93.0
Grief F43.21
|prolonged F43.29
|reaction *see also* Disorder, adjustment F43.20
Griesinger's disease B76.9
Grinder's lung or pneumoconiosis J62.8
Grinding, teeth
|psychogenic F45.8
|sleep related G47.63
Grip
|Dabney's B33.0
|devil's B33.0
Grippe, grippal *see also* Influenza
|Balkan A78
|summer, of Italy A93.1
Grisel's disease M43.6
Groin *see* condition
Grooved tongue K14.5
Ground itch B76.9
Grover's disease or syndrome L11.1
Growing pains, children R29.898
Growth (fungoid) (neoplastic) (new) *see also* Neoplasm
|adenoid (vegetative) J35.8
|benign *see* Neoplasm, benign, by site
|malignant *see* Neoplasm, malignant, by site
|rapid, childhood Z00.2
|secondary *see* Neoplasm, secondary, by site

Gruby's disease B35.0
Gubler-Millard paralysis or syndrome G46.3
Guerin-Stern syndrome Q74.3
Guidance, insufficient anterior (occlusal) M26.54
Guillain-Barré disease or syndrome G61.0
|sequelae G65.0
Guinea worms (infection) (infestation) B72
Guinon's disease (motor-Verbal tic) F95.2
Gull's disease E03.4
Gum *see* condition
Gumboil K04.7
|with sinus K04.6
Gumma (syphilitic) A52.79
|artery A52.09
  |cerebral A52.04
|bone A52.77
  |of yaws (late) A66.6
|brain A52.19
|cauda equina A52.19
|central nervous system A52.3
|ciliary body A52.71
|congenital A50.59
|eyelid A52.71
|heart A52.06
|intracranial A52.19
|iris A52.71
|kidney A52.75
|larynx A52.73
|leptomeninges A52.19
|liver A52.74
|meninges A52.19
|myocardium A52.06
|nasopharynx A52.73
|neurosyphilitic A52.3
|nose A52.73
|orbit A52.71
|palate (soft) A52.79
|penis A52.76
|pericardium A52.06
|pharynx A52.73
|pituitary A52.79
|scrofulous (tuberculous) A18.4
|skin A52.79
|specified site NEC A52.79
|spinal cord A52.19
|tongue A52.79
|tonsil A52.73
|trachea A52.73
|tuberculous A18.4
|ulcerative due to yaws A66.4
|ureter A52.75
|yaws A66.4
  |bone A66.6
Gunn's syndrome Q07.8
Gunshot wound *see also* Puncture, open
|fracture   code as Fracture, by site
|internal organs *see* Injury, by site
Gynandrism Q56.0
Gynandroblastoma
|specified site *see* Neoplasm, uncertain behavior, by site
|unspecified site
  |female D39.10
  |male D40.10
Gynecological examination (periodic) (routine) Z01.419
|with abnormal findings Z01.411
Gynecomastia N62
Gynephobia F40.291
Gyrate scalp Q82.8

H

H (Hartnup's) disease E72.02
Haas' disease or osteochondrosis (juvenile) (head of humerus) *see* Osteochondrosis, juvenile, humerus
Habit, habituation
|bad sleep Z72.821
|chorea F95.8
|disturbance, child F98.9
|drug *see* Dependence, drug
|irregular sleep Z72.821
|laxative F55.2
|spasm *see* Tic
|tic *see* Tic
Haemophilus (H.) influenzae, as cause of disease classified elsewhere B96.3
Haff disease *see* Poisoning, mercury
Hageman's factor defect, deficiency or disease D68.2
Haglund's disease or osteochondrosis (juvenile) (os tibiale externum) *see* Osteochondrosis, juvenile, tarsus
Hailey-Hailey disease Q82.8
Hair *see also* condition
|plucking F63.3
  |in stereotyped movement disorder F98.4
|tourniquet syndrome *see also* Constriction, external, by site
  |finger S60.44-
  |penis S30.842
  |thumb S60.34-
  |toe S90.44-
Hairball in stomach T18.2
Hair-Pulling, pathological (compulsive) F63.3
Hairy black tongue K14.3
Half vertebra Q76.49
Halitosis R19.6
Hallerman-Streiff syndrome Q87.0
Hallervorden-Spatz disease G23.0
Hallopeau's acrodermatitis or disease L40.2
Hallucination R44.3
|auditory R44.0
|gustatory R44.2
|olfactory R44.2
|specified NEC R44.2
|tactile R44.2
|visual R44.1
Hallucinosis (chronic) F28
|alcoholic (acute) F10.951
  |in
    |abuse F10.151
    |dependence F10.251
|drug-induced F19.951
  |cannabis F12.951
  |cocaine F14.951
  |hallucinogen F16.151
  |in
    |abuse F19.151
      |cannabis F12.151
    |cocaine F14.151
      |hallucinogen F16.151
      |inhalant F18.151
      |opioid F11.151
      |sedative, anxiolytic or hypnotic F13.151
      |stimulant NEC F15.151
    |dependence F19.251
      |cannabis F12.251
      |hallucinogen F16.251
      |inhalant F18.251
      |cocaine F14.251
      |opioid F11.251
      |sedative, anxiolytic or hypnotic F13.251
      |stimulant NEC F15.251
  |inhalant F18.951
  |opioid F11.951
  |sedative, anxiolytic or hypnotic F13.951
  |stimulant NEC F15.951
|organic F06.0

Hallux
|deformity (acquired) NEC M20.5X
|limitus M20.5X-
|malleus (acquired) NEC M20.3-
|rigidus M20.2-
  |congenital Q74.2
  |sequelae (late effect) of rickets E64.3
|valgus (acquired) M20.1-
  |congenital Q66.6
|varus (acquired) M20.3-
  |congenital Q66.3
Halo, visual H53.19
Hamartoma, hamartoblastoma Q85.9
|epithelial (gingival), odontogenic, central or
  peripheral *see* Cyst, calcifying odontogenic
Hamartoses Q85.9
Hamman-Rich syndrome J84.114
Hammer toe (acquired) NEC *see also*
  Deformity, toe, hammer toe
|congenital Q66.89
|sequelae (late effect) of rickets E64.3
Hand *see* condition
Hand-Foot syndrome L27.1
Handicap, handicapped
|educational Z55.9
  |specified NEC Z55.8
Hand-Schüller-Christian disease or syndrome
  C96.5
Hanging (asphyxia) (strangulation)
  (suffocation) *see* Asphyxia, traumatic, due to
  mechanical threat
Hangnail *see also* Cellulitis, digit
|with lymphangitis *see* Lymphangitis, acute,
  digit
Hangover (alcohol) F10.129
Hanhart's syndrome Q87.0
Hanot-Chauffard (-Troisier) syndrome E83.19
Hanot's cirrhosis or disease K74.3
Hansen's disease *see* Leprosy
Hantaan virus disease (Korean hemorrhagic
  fever) A98.5
Hantavirus disease (with renal
  manifestations) (Dobrava) (Puumala)
  (Seoul) A98.5
|with pulmonary manifestations (Andes)
  (Bayou) (Bermejo) (Black Creek Canal)
  (Choclo) (Juquitiba) (Laguna negra)
  (Lechiguanas) (New York) (Oran) (Sin
  nombre) B33.4
Happy puppet syndrome Q93.51
Harada's disease or syndrome H30.81-
Hardening
|artery *see* Arteriosclerosis
|brain G93.89
Harelip (complete) (incomplete) *see* Cleft, lip
Harlequin (newborn) Q80.4
Harley's disease D59.6
Harmful use (of)
|alcohol F10.10
|anxiolytics *see* Abuse, drug, sedative
|cannabinoids *see* Abuse, drug, cannabis
|cocaine *see* Abuse, drug, cocaine
|drug *see* Abuse, drug
|hallucinogens *see* Abuse, drug, hallucinogen
|hypnotics *see* Abuse, drug, sedative
|opioids *see* Abuse, drug, opioid
|PCP (phencyclidine) *see* Abuse, drug,
  hallucinogen
|sedatives *see* Abuse, drug, sedative
|stimulants NEC *see* Abuse, drug, stimulant
Harris' lines *see* Arrest, epiphyseal
Hartnup's disease E72.02
Harvester's lung J67.0
Harvesting ovum for in vitro fertilization
  Z31.83

Hashimoto's disease or thyroiditis E06.3
Hashitoxicosis (transient) E06.3
Hassal-Henle bodies or warts (cornea) H18.49
Haut mal *see* Epilepsy, generalized, specified
  NEC
Haverhill fever A25.1
Hay fever *see also* Fever, hay J30.1
Hayem-Widal syndrome D59.8
Haygarth's nodes M15.8
Haymaker's lung J67.0
Hb (abnormal)
|Bart's disease D56.0
|disease *see* Disease, hemoglobin
|trait *see* Trait
Head *see* condition
Headache R51.9
|with
  |orthostatic component NEC R51.0
  |positional component NEC R51.0
|allergic NEC G44.89
|associated with sexual activity G44.82
- cervicogenic G44.86
|chronic daily R51.9
|cluster G44.009
  |chronic G44.029
    |intractable G44.021
    |not intractable G44.029
  |episodic G44.019
    |intractable G44.011
    |not intractable G44.019
  |intractable G44.001
  |not intractable G44.009
|cough (primary) G44.83
|daily chronic R51.9
|drug-induced NEC G44.40
  |intractable G44.41
  |not intractable G44.40
|exertional (primary) G44.84
|histamine G44.009
  |intractable G44.001
  |not intractable G44.009
|hypnic G44.81
|lumbar puncture G97.1
|medication overuse G44.40
  |intractable G44.41
  |not intractable G44.40
|menstrual *see* Migraine, menstrual
|migraine (type) *see also* Migraine G43.909
|nasal septum R51.9
|neuralgiform, short lasting unilateral, with
  conjunctival injection and tearing
  (SUNCT) G44.059
  |intractable G44.051
  |not intractable G44.059
|new daily persistent (NDPH) G44.52
|orgasmic G44.82
|periodic syndromes in adults and children
  G43.C0
  |with refractory migraine G43.C1
  |intractable G43.C1
  |not intractable G43.C0
  |without refractory migraine G43.C0
|postspinal puncture G97.1
|post-traumatic G44.309
  |acute G44.319
    |intractable G44.311
    |not intractable G44.319
  |chronic G44.329
    |intractable G44.321
    |not intractable G44.329
  |intractable G44.301
  |not intractable G44.309
|pre-menstrual *see* Migraine, menstrual
|preorgasmic G44.82
|primary

Headache - *continued*
|cough G44.83
|exertional G44.84
|stabbing G44.85
|thunderclap G44.53
|rebound G44.40
  |intractable G44.41
  |not intractable G44.40
|short lasting unilateral neuralgiform, with
  conjunctival injection and tearing
  (SUNCT) G44.059
  |intractable G44.051
  |not intractable G44.059
* |specified syndrome NEC G44.89
|spinal and epidural anesthesia
|induced T88.59
  |in labor and delivery O74.5
  |in pregnancy O29.4-
  |postpartum, puerperal O89.4
|spinal fluid loss (from puncture) G97.1
|stabbing (primary) G44.85
|tension (-type) G44.209
  |chronic G44.229
    |intractable G44.221
    |not intractable G44.229
  |episodic G44.219
    |intractable G44.211
    |not intractable G44.219
  |intractable G44.201
  |not intractable G44.209
|thunderclap (primary) G44.53
|vascular NEC G44.1
Healthy
|infant
  |accompanying sick mother Z76.3
  |receiving care Z76.2
|person accompanying sick person Z76.3
Hearing examination Z01.10
|with abnormal findings NEC Z01.118
|following failed hearing screening Z01.110
|for hearing conservation and treatment Z01.12
|infant or child (over 28 days old) Z00.129
  |with abnormal findings Z00.121
Heart *see* condition
Heart beat
|abnormality R00.9
  |specified NEC R00.8
|awareness R00.2
|rapid R00.0
|slow R00.1
Heartburn R12
|psychogenic F45.8
Heartland virus disease A93.8
Heat (effects) T67.9
|apoplexy T67.0
|burn *see also* Burn L55.9
|collapse T67.1
|cramps T67.2
|dermatitis or eczema L59.0
|edema T67.7
|erythema   code by site under Burn, first
  degree
|excessive T67.9
  |specified effect NEC T67.8
|exhaustion T67.5
  |anhydrotic T67.3
  |due to
    |salt (and water) depletion T67.4
    |water depletion T67.3
      |with salt depletion T67.4
|fatigue (transient) T67.6
|fever T67.0
|hyperpyrexia T67.0
|prickly L74.0
|prostration *see* Heat, exhaustion
|pyrexia T67.0

Heat (effects) - *continued*
- rash L74.0
- specified effect NEC T67.8
- stroke T67.0
- sunburn *see* Sunburn
- syncope T67.1

Heavy-For-Dates NEC (infant) (4000g to 4499g) P08.1
- exceptionally (4500g or more) P08.0

Hebephrenia, hebephrenic (schizophrenia) F20.1

Heberden's disease or nodes (with arthropathy) M15.1

Hebra's
- pityriasis L26
- prurigo L28.2

Heel *see* condition Heerfordt's disease D86.89

Hegglin's anomaly or syndrome D72.0

Heilmeyer-Schoner disease D45

Heine-Medin disease A80.9

Heinz body anemia, congenital D58.2

Heliophobia F40.228

Heller's disease or syndrome F84.3

HELLP syndrome (hemolysis, elevated liver enzymes and low platelet count) O14.2-
- complicating
  - childbirth O14.24
  - puerperium O14.25

Helminthiasis *see also* Infestation, helminth
- Ancylostoma B76.0
- intestinal B82.0
  - mixed types (types classifiable to more than one of the titles B65.0-B81.3 and B81.8) B81.4
  - specified type NEC B81.8
- mixed types (intestinal) (types classifiable to more than one of the titles B65.0-B81.3 and B81.8) B81.4
- Necator (americanus) B76.1
- specified type NEC B83.8

Heloma L84

Hemangioblastoma *see* Neoplasm, connective tissue, uncertain behavior
- malignant *see* Neoplasm, connective tissue, malignant

Hemangioendothelioma *see also* Neoplasm, uncertain behavior, by site
- benign D18.00
  - intra-abdominal D18.03
  - intracranial D18.02
  - skin D18.01
  - specified site NEC D18.09
- bone (diffuse) *see* Neoplasm, bone, malignant
- epithelioid *see also* Neoplasm, uncertain behavior, by site
  - malignant *see* Neoplasm, malignant, by site
- malignant *see* Neoplasm, connective tissue, malignant

Hemangiofibroma *see* Neoplasm, benign, by site

Hemangiolipoma *see* Lipoma

Hemangioma D18.00
- arteriovenous D18.00
  - intra-abdominal D18.03
  - intracranial D18.02
  - skin D18.01
  - specified site NEC D18.09
- capillary D18.00
  - intra-abdominal D18.03
  - intracranial D18.02
  - skin D18.01
  - specified site NEC D18.09
- cavernous D18.00
  - intra-abdominal D18.03
  - intracranial D18.02
  - skin D18.01

Hemangioma - *continued*
- specified site NEC D18.09
- epithelioid D18.00
  - intra-abdominal D18.03
  - intracranial D18.02
  - skin D18.01
  - specified site NEC D18.09
- histiocytoid D18.00
  - intra-abdominal D18.03
  - intracranial D18.02
  - skin D18.01
  - specified site NEC D18.09
- infantile D18.00
  - intra-abdominal D18.03
  - intracranial D18.02
  - skin D18.01
  - specified site NEC D18.09
- intra-abdominal D18.03
- intracranial D18.02
- intramuscular D18.00
  - intra-abdominal D18.03
  - intracranial D18.02
  - skin D18.01
  - specified site NEC D18.09
- intrathoracic structures D18.09
- juvenile D18.00
- malignant *see* Neoplasm, connective tissue, malignant
- plexiform D18.00
  - intra-abdominal D18.03
  - intracranial D18.02
  - skin D18.01
  - specified site NEC D18.09
- racemose D18.00
  - intra-abdominal D18.03
  - intracranial D18.02
  - skin D18.01
  - specified site NEC D18.09
- sclerosing *see* Neoplasm, skin, benign
- simplex D18.00
  - intra-abdominal D18.03
  - intracranial D18.02
  - skin D18.01
  - specified site NEC D18.09
- skin D18.01
- specified site NEC D18.09
- venous D18.00
  - intra-abdominal D18.03
  - intracranial D18.02
  - skin D18.01
  - specified site NEC D18.09
- verrucous keratotic D18.00
  - intra-abdominal D18.03
  - intracranial D18.02
  - skin D18.01
  - specified site NEC D18.09

Hemangiomatosis (systemic) I78.8
- involving single site *see* Hemangioma

Hemangiopericytoma *see also* Neoplasm, connective tissue, uncertain behavior
- benign *see* Neoplasm, connective tissue, benign
- malignant *see* Neoplasm, connective tissue, malignant

Hemangiosarcoma *see* Neoplasm, connective tissue, malignant

Hemarthrosis (nontraumatic) M25.00
- ankle M25.07-
- elbow M25.02-
- foot joint M25.07-
- hand joint M25.04-
- hip M25.05-
- in hemophilic arthropathy *see* Arthropathy, hemophilic
- knee M25.06-

Hemarthrosis - *continued*
- shoulder M25.01-
- specified joint NEC M25.08
- traumatic *see* Sprain, by site
- vertebrae M25.08
- wrist M25.03-

Hematemesis K92.0
- with ulcer   code by site under Ulcer, with hemorrhage K27.4
- newborn, neonatal P54.0
  - due to swallowed maternal blood P78.2

Hematidrosis L74.8

Hematinuria *see also* Hemoglobinuria
- malarial B50.8

Hematobilia K83.8

Hematocele
- female NEC N94.89
  - with ectopic pregnancy O00.90
    - with intrauterine pregnancy O00.91
  - ovary N83.8
- male N50.1

Hematochezia *see also* Melena K92.1

Hematochyluria *see also* Infestation, filarial
- schistosomiasis (bilharziasis) B65.0

Hematocolpos (with hematometra or hematosalpinx) N89.7

Hematocornea *see* Pigmentation, cornea, stromal

Hematogenous *see* condition

Hematoma (traumatic) (skin surface intact) *see also* Contusion
- with
  - injury of internal organs *see* Injury, by site
  - open wound *see* Wound, open
- amputation stump (surgical) (late) T87.89
- aorta, dissecting I71.00
  - abdominal I71.02
  - thoracic I71.01
  - thoracoabdominal I71.03
- aortic intramural *see* Dissection, aorta
- arterial (complicating trauma) *see* Injury, blood vessel, by site
- auricle *see* Contusion, ear
  - nontraumatic *see* Disorder, pinna, hematoma
- birth injury NEC P15.8
- brain (traumatic)
  - with
    - cerebral laceration or contusion (diffuse) *see* Injury, intracranial, diffuse
    - focal *see* Injury, intracranial, focal cerebellar, traumatic S06.37-
  - newborn NEC P52.4
    - birth injury P10.1
  - intracerebral, traumatic *see* Injury, intracranial, intracerebral hemorrhage
  - nontraumatic *see* Hemorrhage, intracranial
  - subarachnoid, arachnoid, traumatic *see* Injury, intracranial, subarachnoid hemorrhage
  - subdural, traumatic *see* Injury, intracranial, subdural hemorrhage
- breast (nontraumatic) N64.89
- broad ligament (nontraumatic) N83.7
  - traumatic S37.892
- cerebellar, traumatic S06.37-
- cerebral *see* Hematoma, brain
- cerebrum S06.36-
  - left S06.35-
  - right S06.34-
- cesarean delivery wound O90.2
- complicating delivery (perineal) (pelvic) (vagina) (vulva) O71.7
- corpus cavernosum (nontraumatic) N48.89

Hematoma - *continued*
|epididymis (nontraumatic) N50.1
|epidural (traumatic) *see* Injury, intracranial,
   epidural hemorrhage
 |spinal *see* Injury, spinal cord, by region
|episiotomy O90.2
|face, birth injury P15.4
|genital organ NEC (nontraumatic)
 |female (nonobstetric) N94.89
  |traumatic S30.202
 |male N50.1
  |traumatic S30.201
|internal organs *see* Injury, by site
|intracerebral, traumatic *see* Injury,
   intracranial, intracerebral hemorrhage
|intraoperative *see* Complications,
   intraoperative, hemorrhage
|labia (nontraumatic) (nonobstetric) N90.89
|liver (subcapsular) (nontraumatic) K76.89
 |birth injury P15.0
|mediastinum *see* Injury, intrathoracic
|mesosalpinx (nontraumatic) N83.7
  |traumatic S37.898
|muscle   code by site under Contusion
|nontraumatic
 |muscle M79.81
 |soft tissue M79.81
|obstetrical surgical wound O90.2
|orbit, orbital (nontraumatic) *see also*
   Hemorrhage, orbit
 |traumatic *see* Contusion, orbit
|pelvis (female) (nontraumatic) (nonobstetric)
   N94.89
 |obstetric O71.7
 |traumatic *see* Injury, by site
|penis (nontraumatic) N48.89
 |birth injury P15.5
|perianal (nontraumatic) K64.5
|perineal S30.23
 |complicating delivery O71.7
|perirenal *see* Injury, kidney
|pinna *see* Contusion, ear
 |nontraumatic *see* Disorder, pinna,
   hematoma
|placenta O43.89-
|postoperative (postprocedural) *see*
   Complication, postprocedural, hematoma
|retroperitoneal (nontraumatic) K66.1
 |traumatic S36.892
|scrotum, superficial S30.22
 |birth injury P15.5
|seminal vesicle (nontraumatic) N50.1
 |traumatic S37.892
|spermatic cord (traumatic) S37.892
 |nontraumatic N50.1
|spinal (cord) (meninges) *see also* Injury,
   spinal cord, by region
 |newborn (birth injury) P11.5
|spleen D73.5
 |intraoperative *see* Complications,
   intraoperative, hemorrhage, spleen
 |postprocedural (postoperative) *see*
   Complications, postprocedural,
   hemorrhage, spleen
|sternocleidomastoid, birth injury P15.2
|sternomastoid, birth injury P15.2
|subarachnoid (traumatic) *see* Injury,
   intracranial, subarachnoid hemorrhage
 |newborn (nontraumatic) P52.5
  |due to birth injury P10.3
 |nontraumatic *see* Hemorrhage, intracranial,
   subarachnoid
|subdural (traumatic) *see* Injury, intracranial,
   subdural hemorrhage
 |newborn (localized) P52.8

Hematoma - *continued*
 |birth injury P10.0
|nontraumatic *see* Hemorrhage, intracranial,
   subdural
|superficial, newborn P54.5
|testis (nontraumatic) N50.1
 |birth injury P15.5
|tunica vaginalis (nontraumatic) N50.1
|umbilical cord, complicating delivery O69.5
|uterine ligament (broad) (nontraumatic) N83.7
 |traumatic S37.892
|vagina (ruptured) (nontraumatic) N89.8
 |complicating delivery O71.7
|vas deferens (nontraumatic) N50.1
 |traumatic S37.892
|vitreous *see* Hemorrhage, vitreous
|vulva (nontraumatic) (nonobstetric) N90.89
 |complicating delivery O71.7
 |newborn (birth injury) P15.5
Hematometra N85.7
|with hematocolpos N89.7
Hematomyelia (central) G95.19
|newborn (birth injury) P11.5
|traumatic T14.8
Hematomyelitis G04.90
Hematoperitoneum *see* Hemoperitoneum
Hematophobia F40.230
Hematopneumothorax (see Hemothorax)
Hematopoiesis, cyclic D70.4
Hematoporphyria *see* Porphyria
Hematorachis, hematorrhachis G95.19
|newborn (birth injury) P11.5
Hematosalpinx N83.6
|with
 |hematocolpos N89.7
 |hematometra N85.7
  |with hematocolpos N89.7
|infectional *see* Salpingitis
Hematospermia R36.1
Hematothorax (see Hemothorax)
Hematuria R31.9
|due to sulphonamide, sulfonamide *see* Table
   of Drugs and Chemicals, by drug
|benign (familial) (of childhood) *see also*
   Hematuria, idiopathic
 |essential microscopic R31.1
|endemic *see also* Schistosomiasis B65.0
|gross R31.0
|idiopathic N02.9
 |with glomerular lesion
  |C3
   |glomerulonephritis N02.A
   |glomerulopathy N02.A
    |with dense deposit disease N02.6
  |crescentic (diffuse) glomerulonephritis
   N02.7
  |dense deposit disease N02.6
  |endocapillary proliferative
   glomerulonephritis N02.4
  |focal and segmental hyalinosis or sclerosis
   N02.1
  |membranoproliferative (diffuse) N02.5
  |membranous (diffuse) N02.2
  |mesangial proliferative (diffuse) N02.3
  |mesangiocapillary (diffuse) N02.5
  |minor abnormality N02.0
  |proliferative NEC N02.8
  |specified pathology NEC N02.8
|intermittent *see* Hematuria, idiopathic
|malarial B50.8
|microscopic NEC (with symptoms) R31.29
 |asymptomatic R31.21
 |benign essential R31.1
|paroxysmal *see also* Hematuria, idiopathic
 |nocturnal D59.5

Hematuria - *continued*
|persistent *see* Hematuria, idiopathic
|recurrent *see* Hematuria, idiopathic
|tropical *see also* Schistosomiasis B65.0
|tuberculous A18.13
Hemeralopia (day blindness) H53.11
|vitamin A deficiency E50.5
Hemi-Akinesia R41.4
Hemianalgesia R20.0
Hemianencephaly Q00.0
Hemianesthesia R20.0
Hemianopia, hemianopsia (heteronymous)
  H53.47
|homonymous H53.46-
|syphilitic A52.71
Hemiathetosis R25.8
Hemiatrophy R68.89
|cerebellar G31.9
|face, facial, progressive (Romberg) G51.8
|tongue K14.8
Hemiballism (us) G25.5
Hemicardia Q24.8
Hemicephalus, hemicephaly Q00.0
Hemichorea G25.5
Hemicolitis, left *see* Colitis, left sided
Hemicrania
|congenital malformation Q00.0
|continua G44.51
|meaning migraine *see also* Migraine G43.909
|paroxysmal G44.039
 |chronic G44.049
  |intractable G44.041
  |not intractable G44.049
 |episodic G44.039
  |intractable G44.031
  |not intractable G44.039
 |intractable G44.031
 |not intractable G44.039
Hemidystrophy *see* Hemiatrophy
Hemiectromelia Q73.8
Hemihypalgesia R20.8
Hemihypesthesia R20.1
Hemi-Inattention R41.4
Hemimelia Q73.8
|lower limb *see* Defect, reduction, lower limb,
   specified type NEC
|upper limb *see* Defect, reduction, upper limb,
   specified type NEC
Hemiparalysis *see* Hemiplegia
Hemiparesis *see* Hemiplegia
Hemiparesthesia R20.2
Hemiparkinsonism G20
Hemiplegia G81.9-
|alternans facialis G83.89
|ascending NEC G81.90
 |spinal G95.89
|congenital (cerebral) G80.8
 |spastic G80.2
|embolic (current episode) I63.4-
|flaccid G81.0-
|following
 |cerebrovascular disease I69.959
  |cerebral infarction I69.35-
  |intracerebral hemorrhage I69.15-
  |nontraumatic intracranial hemorrhage
   NEC I69.25-
  |specified disease NEC I69.85-
  |stroke NOS I69.35-
  |subarachnoid hemorrhage I69.05-
|hysterical F44.4
|newborn NEC P91.88
 |birth injury P11.9
|spastic G81.1-
 |congenital G80.2
|thrombotic (current episode) I63.3-

Hemisection, spinal cord *see* Injury, spinal
   cord, by region
Hemispasm (facial) R25.2
Hemisporosis B48.8
Hemitremor R25.1
Hemivertebra Q76.49
  |failure of segmentation with scoliosis Q76.3
  |fusion with scoliosis Q76.3
Hemochromatosis E83.119
  |with refractory anemia D46.1
  |due to repeated red blood cell transfusion
    E83.111
  |hereditary (primary) E83.110
  |neonatal P78.84
  |primary E83.110
  |specified NEC E83.118
Hemoglobin *see also* condition
  |abnormal (disease) *see* Disease, hemoglobin
  |AS genotype D57.3
  |Constant Spring D58.2
  |E-beta thalassemia D56.5
  |fetal, hereditary persistence (HPFH) D56.4
  |H Constant Spring D56.0
  |low NOS D64.9
  |S (Hb S), heterozygous D57.3
Hemoglobinemia D59.9
  |due to blood transfusion T80.89
  |paroxysmal D59.6
    |nocturnal D59.5
Hemoglobinopathy (mixed) D58.2
  |with thalassemia D56.8
  |sickle-cell D57.1
    |with thalassemia D57.40
      |with
        |acute chest syndrome D57.411
        |cerebral vascular involvement D57.413
        |crisis (painful) D57.419
          |with specified complication NEC
            D57.418
        |splenic sequestration D57.412
        |vasoocclusive pain D57.419
    |without crisis D57.40
Hemoglobinuria R82.3
  |with anemia, hemolytic, acquired (chronic)
    NEC D59.6
  |cold (paroxysmal) (with Raynaud's syndrome)
    D59.6
    |agglutinin D59.12
  |due to exertion or hemolysis NEC D59.6
  |intermittent D59.6
  |malarial B50.8
  |march D59.6
  |nocturnal (paroxysmal) D59.5
  |paroxysmal (cold) D59.6
    |nocturnal D59.5
Hemolymphangioma D18.1
Hemolysis
  |intravascular
    |with
      |abortion *see* Abortion, by type,
        complicated by, hemorrhage
      |ectopic or molar pregnancy O08.1
      |hemorrhage
        |antepartum *see* Hemorrhage,
          antepartum, with coagulation defect
        |intrapartum *see also* Hemorrhage,
          complicating, delivery O67.0
    |postpartum O72.3
  |neonatal (excessive) P58.9
    |specified NEC P58.8
Hemolytic *see* condition
Hemopericardium I31.2
  |following acute myocardial infarction (current
    complication) I23.0
  |newborn P54.8
  |traumatic *see* Injury, heart, with
    hemopericardium

Hemoperitoneum K66.1
  |infectional K65.9
  |traumatic S36.899
    |with open wound *see* Wound, open, with
      penetration into peritoneal cavity
Hemophilia (classical) (familial) (hereditary)
  D66
  |A D66
  |B D67
  |C D68.1
  |acquired D68.311
  |autoimmune D68.311
  |calcipriva *see also* Defect, coagulation D68.4
  |nonfamilial *see also* Defect, coagulation D68.4
  |secondary D68.311
  |vascular D68.0
Hemophthalmos H44.81-
Hemopneumothorax *see also* Hemothorax
  |traumatic S27.2
Hemoptysis R04.2
  |newborn P26.9
  |tuberculous *see* Tuberculosis, pulmonary
Hemorrhage, hemorrhagic (concealed) R58
  |abdomen R58
  |accidental antepartum *see* Hemorrhage,
    antepartum
  |acute idiopathic pulmonary, in infants R04.81
  |adenoid J35.8
  |adrenal (capsule) (gland) E27.49
    |medulla E27.8
    |newborn P54.4
  |after delivery *see* Hemorrhage, postpartum
  |alveolar
    |lung, newborn P26.8
    |process K08.89
  |alveolus K08.89
  |amputation stump (surgical) T87.89
  |anemia (chronic) D50.0
    |acute D62
  |antepartum (with) O46.90
    |with coagulation defect O46.00-
      |afibrinogenemia O46.01-
      |disseminated intravascular coagulation
        O46.02-
      |hypofibrinogenemia O46.01-
      |specified defect NEC O46.09-
    |before 20 weeks gestation O20.9
      |specified type NEC O20.8
      |threatened abortion O20.0
    |due to
      |abruptio placenta *see also* Abruptio
        placentae O45.9-
      |leiomyoma, uterus *see* Hemorrhage,
        antepartum, specified cause NEC
      |placenta previa O44.1-
    |specified cause NEC *see* subcategory
      O46.8X-
  |anus (sphincter) K62.5
  |apoplexy (stroke) *see* Hemorrhage,
    intracranial, intracerebral
  |arachnoid *see* Hemorrhage, intracranial,
    subarachnoid
  |artery R58
    |brain *see* Hemorrhage, intracranial,
      intracerebral
  |basilar (ganglion) I61.0
  |bladder N32.89
  |bowel K92.2
    |newborn P54.3
  |brain (miliary) (nontraumatic) *see*
    Hemorrhage, intracranial, intracerebral
    |due to
      |birth injury P10.1
      |syphilis A52.05

Hemorrhage, hemorrhagic - *continued*
  |epidural or extradural (traumatic) *see* Injury,
    intracranial, epidural hemorrhage
  |newborn P52.4
    |birth injury P10.1
  |subarachnoid *see* Hemorrhage, intracranial,
    subarachnoid
  |subdural *see* Hemorrhage, intracranial,
    subdural
  |brainstem (nontraumatic) I61.3
    |traumatic S06.38-
  |breast N64.59
  |bronchial tube *see* Hemorrhage, lung
  |bronchopulmonary *see* Hemorrhage, lung
  |bronchus *see* Hemorrhage, lung
  |bulbar I61.5
  |capillary I78.8
    |primary D69.8
  |cecum K92.2
  |cerebellar, cerebellum (nontraumatic) I61.4
    |newborn P52.6
    |traumatic S06.37-
  |cerebral, cerebrum *see also* Hemorrhage,
    intracranial, intracerebral
    |newborn (anoxic) P52.4
      |birth injury P10.1
    |lobe I61.1
  |cerebromeningeal I61.8
  |cerebrospinal *see* Hemorrhage, intracranial,
    intracerebral
  |cervix (uteri) (stump) NEC N88.8
  |chamber, anterior (eye) *see* Hyphema
  |childbirth *see* Hemorrhage, complicating,
    delivery
  |choroid H31.30-
    |expulsive H31.31-
  |ciliary body *see* Hyphema
  |cochlea *see* subcategory H83.8
  |colon K92.2
  |complicating
    |abortion *see* Abortion, by type, complicated
      by, hemorrhage
    |delivery O67.9
      |associated with coagulation defect
        (afibrinogenemia) (DIC)
        (hyperfibrinolysis) O67.0
      |specified cause NEC O67.8
    |surgical procedure *see* Hemorrhage,
      intraoperative
  |conjunctiva H11.3-
    |newborn P54.8
  |cord, newborn (stump) P51.9
  |corpus luteum (ruptured) cyst N83.1-
  |cortical (brain) I61.1
  |cranial *see* Hemorrhage, intracranial
  |cutaneous R23.3
    |due to autosensitivity, erythrocyte D69.2
    |newborn P54.5
  |delayed
    |following ectopic or molar pregnancy O08.1
    |postpartum O72.2
  |diathesis (familial) D69.9
  |disease D69.9
    |newborn P53
    |specified type NEC D69.8
  |due to or associated with
    |afibrinogenemia or other coagulation defect
      (conditions in categories D65-D69)
      |antepartum *see* Hemorrhage, antepartum,
        with coagulation defect
      |intrapartum O67.0
  |dental implant M27.61
  |device, implant or graft *see also*
    Complications, by site and type, specified
    NEC T85.838

Hemorrhage, hemorrhagic - *continued*
- |arterial graft NEC T82.838
- |breast T85.838
- |catheter NEC T85.838
  - |dialysis (renal) T82.838
    - |intraperitoneal T85.838
  - |infusion NEC T82.838
    - |spinal (epidural) (subdural) T85.830
  - |urinary (indwelling) T83.83
- |electronic (electrode) (pulse generator) (stimulator)
  - |bone T84.83
  - |cardiac T82.837
  - |nervous system (brain) (peripheral nerve) (spinal) T85.830
  - |urinary T83.83
- |fixation, internal (orthopedic) NEC T84.83
- |gastrointestinal (bile duct) (esophagus) T85.838
- |genital NEC T83.83
- |heart NEC T82.837
- |joint prosthesis T84.83
- |ocular (corneal graft) (orbital implant) NEC T85.838
- |orthopedic NEC T84.83
  - |bone graft T86.838
- |specified NEC T85.838
- |urinary NEC T83.83
- |vascular NEC T82.838
- |ventricular intracranial shunt T85.830
- |duodenum, duodenal K92.2
  - |ulcer *see* Ulcer, duodenum, with hemorrhage
- |dura mater *see* Hemorrhage, intracranial, subdural
- |endotracheal *see* Hemorrhage, lung
- |epicranial subaponeurotic (massive), birth injury P12.2
- |epidural (traumatic) *see also* Injury, intracranial, epidural hemorrhage
  - |nontraumatic I62.1
- |esophagus K22.89
  - |varix I85.01
    - |secondary I85.11
- |excessive, following ectopic gestation (subsequent episode) O08.1
- |extradural (traumatic) *see* Injury, intracranial, epidural hemorrhage
  - |birth injury P10.8
  - |newborn (anoxic) (nontraumatic) P52.8
  - |nontraumatic I62.1
- |eye NEC H57.89
  - |fundus *see* Hemorrhage, retina
  - |lid *see* Disorder, eyelid, specified type NEC
- |fallopian tube N83.6
- |fibrinogenolysis *see* Fibrinolysis
- |fibrinolytic (acquired) *see* Fibrinolysis
- |from
  - |ear (nontraumatic) *see* Otorrhagia
  - |tracheostomy stoma J95.01
- |fundus, eye *see* Hemorrhage, retina
- |funis *see* Hemorrhage, umbilicus, cord
- |gastric *see* Hemorrhage, stomach
- |gastroenteric K92.2
  - |newborn P54.3
- |gastrointestinal (tract) K92.2
  - |newborn P54.3
- |genital organ, male N50.1
- |genitourinary (tract) NOS R31.9
- |gingiva K06.8
- |globe (eye) *see* Hemophthalmos
- |graafian follicle cyst (ruptured) N83.0-
- |gum K06.8
- |heart I51.89

Hemorrhage, hemorrhagic - *continued*
- |hypopharyngeal (throat) R04.1
- |intermenstrual (regular) N92.3
  - |irregular N92.1
- |internal (organs) NEC R58
  - |capsule I61.0
  - |ear *see* subcategory H83.8
  - |newborn P54.8
- |intestine K92.2
  - |newborn P54.3
- |intra-abdominal R58
- |intra-alveolar (lung), newborn P26.8
- |intracerebral (nontraumatic) *see* Hemorrhage, intracranial, intracerebral
- |intracranial (nontraumatic) I62.9
  - |birth injury P10.9
  - |epidural, nontraumatic I62.1
  - |extradural, nontraumatic I62.1
  - |newborn P52.9
    - |specified NEC P52.8
  - |intracerebral (nontraumatic) (in) I61.9
    - |brain stem I61.3
    - |cerebellum I61.4
    - |newborn P52.4
      - |birth injury P10.1
    - |hemisphere I61.2
      - |cortical (superficial) I61.1
      - |subcortical (deep) I61.0
    - |intraoperative
      - |during a nervous system procedure G97.31
      - |during other procedure G97.32
    - |intraventricular I61.5
    - |multiple localized I61.6
    - |postprocedural
      - |following a nervous system procedure G97.51
      - |following other procedure G97.52
    - |specified NEC I61.8
    - |superficial I61.1
    - |traumatic (diffuse) *see* Injury, intracranial, diffuse
      - |focal *see* Injury, intracranial, focal
  - |subarachnoid (nontraumatic) (from) I60.9
    - |newborn P52.5
      - |birth injury P10.3
    - |intracranial (cerebral) artery I60.7
      - |anterior communicating I60.2
      - |basilar I60.4
      - |carotid siphon and bifurcation I60.0-
      - |communicating I60.7
        - |anterior I60.2
        - |posterior I60.3-
      - |middle cerebral I60.1-
      - |posterior communicating I60.3-
      - |specified artery NEC I60.6
      - |vertebral I60.5-
    - |specified NEC I60.8
    - |traumatic S06.6X-
  - |subdural (nontraumatic) I62.00
    - |acute I62.01
    - |birth injury P10.0
    - |chronic I62.03
    - |newborn (anoxic) (hypoxic) P52.8
      - |birth injury P10.0
    - |spinal G95.19
    - |subacute I62.02
    - |traumatic *see* Injury, intracranial, subdural hemorrhage
  - |traumatic *see* Injury, intracranial, focal brain injury
- |intramedullary NEC G95.19
- |intraocular *see* Hemophthalmos

Hemorrhage, hemorrhagic - *continued*
- |intraoperative, intraprocedural *see* Complication, hemorrhage (hematoma), intraoperative (intraprocedural), by site
- |intrapartum *see* Hemorrhage, complicating, delivery
- |intrapelvic
  - |female N94.89
  - |male K66.1
- |intraperitoneal K66.1
- |intrapontine I61.3
- |intraprocedural *see* Complication, hemorrhage (hematoma), intraoperative (intraprocedural), by site
- |intrauterine N85.7
  - |complicating delivery *see also* Hemorrhage, complicating, delivery O67.9
  - |postpartum *see* Hemorrhage, postpartum
- |intraventricular I61.5
  - |newborn (nontraumatic) *see also* Newborn, affected by, hemorrhage P52.3
    - |due to birth injury P10.2
    - |grade
      - |1 P52.0
      - |2 P52.1
      - |3 P52.21
      - |4 P52.22
- |intravesical N32.89
- |iris (postinfectional) (postinflammatory) (toxic) *see* Hyphema
- |joint (nontraumatic) *see* Hemarthrosis
- |kidney N28.89
- |knee (joint) (nontraumatic) *see* Hemarthrosis, knee
- |labyrinth *see* subcategory H83.8
- |lenticular striate artery I61.0
- |ligature, vessel *see* Hemorrhage, postoperative
- |liver K76.89
- |lung R04.89
  - |newborn P26.9
    - |massive P26.1
    - |specified NEC P26.8
  - |tuberculous *see* Tuberculosis, pulmonary
- |massive umbilical, newborn P51.0
- |mediastinum *see* Hemorrhage, lung
- |medulla I61.3
- |membrane (brain) I60.8
  - |spinal cord *see* Hemorrhage, spinal cord
- |meninges, meningeal (brain) (middle) I60.8
  - |spinal cord *see* Hemorrhage, spinal cord
- |mesentery K66.1
- |metritis *see* Endometritis
- |mouth K13.79
- |mucous membrane NEC R58
  - |newborn P54.8
- |muscle M62.89
- |nail (subungual) L60.8
- |nasal turbinate R04.0
  - |newborn P54.8
- |navel, newborn P51.9
- |newborn P54.9
  - |specified NEC P54.8
- |nipple N64.59
- |nose R04.0
  - |newborn P54.8
- |omentum K66.1
- |optic nerve (sheath) H47.02-
- |orbit, orbital H05.23-
- |ovary NEC N83.8
- |oviduct N83.6
- |pancreas K86.89
- |parathyroid (gland) (spontaneous) E21.4
- |parturition *see* Hemorrhage, complicating, delivery
- |penis N48.89

Hemorrhage, hemorrhagic - *continued*
- pericardium, pericarditis I31.2
- peritoneum, peritoneal K66.1
- peritonsillar tissue J35.8
  - due to infection J36
- petechial R23.3
  - due to autosensitivity, erythrocyte D69.2
- pituitary (gland) E23.6
- pleura *see* Hemorrhage, lung
- polioencephalitis, superior E51.2
- polymyositis *see* Polymyositis
- pons, pontine I61.3
- posterior fossa (nontraumatic) I61.8
  - newborn P52.6
- postmenopausal N95.0
- postnasal R04.0
- postoperative *see* Complications, postprocedural, hemorrhage, by site
- postpartum NEC (following delivery of placenta) O72.1
  - delayed or secondary O72.2
  - retained placenta O72.0
  - third stage O72.0
- pregnancy *see* Hemorrhage, antepartum
- preretinal *see* Hemorrhage, retina
- prostate N42.1
- puerperal *see* Hemorrhage, postpartum
  - delayed or secondary O72.2
- pulmonary R04.89
  - newborn P26.9
    - massive P26.1
    - specified NEC P26.8
  - tuberculous *see* Tuberculosis, pulmonary
- purpura (primary) D69.3
- rectum (sphincter) K62.5
  - newborn P54.2
- recurring, following initial hemorrhage at time of injury T79.2
- renal N28.89
- respiratory passage or tract R04.9
  - specified NEC R04.89
- retina, retinal (vessels) H35.6-
  - diabetic *see* Diabetes, retinal, hemorrhage
- retroperitoneal R58
- scalp R58
- scrotum N50.1
- secondary (nontraumatic) R58
  - following initial hemorrhage at time of injury T79.2
- seminal vesicle N50.1
- skin R23.3
  - newborn P54.5
- slipped umbilical ligature P51.8
- spermatic cord N50.1
- spinal (cord) G95.19
  - newborn (birth injury) P11.5
- spleen D73.5
  - intraoperative *see* Complications, intraoperative, hemorrhage, spleen
  - postprocedural *see* Complications, postprocedural, hemorrhage, spleen
- stomach K92.2
  - newborn P54.3
  - ulcer *see* Ulcer, stomach, with hemorrhage
- subarachnoid (nontraumatic) *see* Hemorrhage, intracranial, subarachnoid
- subconjunctival *see also* Hemorrhage, conjunctiva
  - birth injury P15.3
- subcortical (brain) I61.0
- subcutaneous R23.3
- subdiaphragmatic R58
- subdural (acute) (nontraumatic) *see* Hemorrhage, intracranial, subdural
- subependymal

Hemorrhage, hemorrhagic - *continued*
- newborn P52.0
  - with intraventricular extension P52.1
    - and intracerebral extension P52.22
- subgaleal P12.2
- subhyaloid *see* Hemorrhage, retina
- subperiosteal *see* Disorder, bone, specified type NEC
- subretinal *see* Hemorrhage, retina
- subtentorial *see* Hemorrhage, intracranial, subdural
- subungual L60.8
- suprarenal (capsule) (gland) E27.49
  - newborn P54.4
- tentorium (traumatic) NEC *see* Hemorrhage, brain
  - newborn (birth injury) P10.4
- testis N50.1
- third stage (postpartum) O72.0
- thorax *see* Hemorrhage, lung
- throat R04.1
- thymus (gland) E32.8
- thyroid (cyst) (gland) E07.89
- tongue K14.8
- tonsil J35.8
- trachea *see* Hemorrhage, lung
- tracheobronchial R04.89
  - newborn P26.0
- traumatic code to specific injury
  - cerebellar *see* Hemorrhage, brain
  - intracranial *see* Hemorrhage, brain
  - recurring or secondary (following initial hemorrhage at time of injury) T79.2
- tuberculous NEC *see also* Tuberculosis, pulmonary A15.0
- tunica vaginalis N50.1
- ulcer code by site under Ulcer, with hemorrhage K27.4
- umbilicus, umbilical
  - cord
    - after birth, newborn P51.9
    - complicating delivery O69.5
  - newborn P51.9
    - massive P51.0
    - slipped ligature P51.8
  - stump P51.9
- urethra (idiopathic) N36.8
- uterus, uterine (abnormal) N93.9
  - climacteric N92.4
  - complicating delivery *see* Hemorrhage, complicating, delivery
  - dysfunctional or functional N93.8
  - intermenstrual (regular) N92.3
    - irregular N92.1
  - postmenopausal N95.0
  - postpartum *see* Hemorrhage, postpartum
  - preclimacteric or premenopausal N92.4
  - prepubertal N93.8
  - pubertal N92.2
- vagina (abnormal) N93.9
  - newborn P54.6
- vas deferens N50.1
- vasa previa O69.4
- ventricular I61.5
- vesical N32.89
- viscera NEC R58
  - newborn P54.8
- vitreous (humor) (intraocular) H43.1-
- vulva N90.89

Hemorrhoids (bleeding) (without mention of degree) K64.9
- 1st degree (grade/stage I) (without prolapse outside of anal canal) K64.0
- 2nd degree (grade/stage II) (that prolapse with straining but retract spontaneously) K64.1

Hemorrhoids - *continued*
- 3rd degree (grade/stage III) (that prolapse with straining and require manual replacement back inside anal canal) K64.2
- 4th degree (grade/stage IV) (with prolapsed tissue that cannot be manually replaced) K64.3
- complicating
  - pregnancy O22.4
  - puerperium O87.2
- external K64.4
  - with
    - thrombosis K64.5
- internal (without mention of degree) K64.8
- prolapsed K64.8
- skin tags
  - anus K64.4
  - residual K64.4
- specified NEC K64.8
- strangulated *see also* Hemorrhoids, by degree K64.8
- thrombosed *see also* Hemorrhoids, by degree K64.5
- ulcerated *see also* Hemorrhoids, by degree K64.8
Hemosalpinx N83.6
- with
  - hematocolpos N89.7
  - hematometra N85.7
    - with hematocolpos N89.7
Hemosiderosis (dietary) E83.19
- pulmonary, idiopathic E83.1 *[J84.03]*
- transfusion T80.89
Hemothorax (bacterial) (nontuberculous) J94.2
- newborn P54.8
- traumatic S27.1
  - with pneumothorax S27.2
- tuberculous NEC A15.6
Henoch (-Schönlein) disease or syndrome (purpura) D69.0
Henpue, henpuye A66.6
Hepar lobatum (syphilitic) A52.74
Hepatalgia K76.89
Hepatitis K75.9
- acute B17.9
  - with coma K72.01
  - with hepatic failure *see* Failure, hepatic
  - alcoholic *see* Hepatitis, alcoholic
  - infectious B17.9
  - non-viral K72.0
  - viral B17.9
- alcoholic (acute) (chronic) K70.10
  - with ascites K70.11
- amebic *see* Abscess, liver, amebic
- anicteric, (viral) *see* Hepatitis, viral
- antigen-associated (HAA) *see* Hepatitis, B
- Australia-antigen (positive) *see* Hepatitis, B
- autoimmune K75.4
- B B19.10
  - with hepatic coma B19.11
  - acute B16.9
    - with
      - delta-agent (coinfection) (without hepatic coma) B16.1
        - with hepatic coma B16.0
      - hepatic coma (without delta-agent coinfection) B16.2
  - chronic B18.1
    - with delta-agent B18.0
- bacterial NEC K75.89
- C (viral) B19.20
  - with hepatic coma B19.21
  - acute B17.10
    - with hepatic coma B17.11

Hepatitis - *continued*
 |chronic B18.2
 |catarrhal (acute) B15.9
  |with hepatic coma B15.0
 |cholangiolitic K75.89
 |cholestatic K75.89
 |chronic K73.9
  |active NEC K73.2
  |lobular NEC K73.1
  |persistent NEC K73.0
  |specified NEC K73.8
 |cytomegaloviral B25.1
 |due to ethanol (acute) (chronic) *see* Hepatitis, alcoholic
 |epidemic B15.9
  |with hepatic coma B15.0
 |fulminant NEC (viral) *see* Hepatitis, viral
 |neonatal giant cell P59.29
 |granulomatous NEC K75.3
 |herpesviral B00.81
 |history of
  |B Z86.19
  |C Z86.19
 |homologous serum *see* Hepatitis, viral, type B
 |in (due to)
  |mumps B26.81
  |toxoplasmosis (acquired) B58.1
   |congenital (active) P37.1 [*K77*]
 |infectious, infective B15.9
  |acute (subacute) B17.9
  |chronic B18.9
 |inoculation *see* Hepatitis, viral, type B
 |interstitial (chronic) K74.69
 |ischemia, ischemic K72.00
 |lupoid NEC K75.4
 |malignant NEC (with hepatic failure) K72.90
  |with coma K72.91
 |neonatal (idiopathic) (toxic) P59.29
 |newborn P59.29
 |postimmunization *see* Hepatitis, viral, type B
 |post-transfusion *see* Hepatitis, viral, type B
 |reactive, nonspecific K75.2
 |serum *see* Hepatitis, viral, type B
 |shock K72.00
 |specified type NEC
  |with hepatic failure *see* Failure, hepatic
 |syphilitic (late) A52.74
  |congenital (early) A50.08 [*K77*]
   |late A50.59 [*K77*]
  |secondary A51.45
 |toxic *see also* Disease, liver, toxic K71.6
 |tuberculous A18.83
 |viral, virus B19.9
  |with hepatic coma B19.0
  |acute B17.9
  |chronic B18.9
   |specified NEC B18.8
   |type
    |B B18.1
     |with delta-agent B18.0
    |C B18.2
  |congenital P35.3
  |coxsackie B33.8 [*K77*]
  |cytomegalic inclusion B25.1
  |in remission, any type   code to Hepatitis, chronic, by type
  |non-A, non-B B17.8
  |specified type NEC (with or without coma) B17.8
  |type
   |A B15.9
    |with hepatic coma B15.0
   |B B19.10
    |with hepatic coma B19.11
    |acute B16.9

Hepatitis - *continued*
  |with
   |delta-agent (coinfection) (without hepatic coma) B16.1
    |with hepatic coma B16.0
   |hepatic coma (without delta-agent coinfection) B16.2
  |chronic B18.1
   |with delta-agent B18.0
  |C B19.20
   |with hepatic coma B19.21
   |acute B17.10
    |with hepatic coma B17.11
   |chronic B18.2
  |E B17.2
  |non-A, non-B B17.8
Hepatization lung (acute) *see* Pneumonia, lobar
Hepatoblastoma C22.2
Hepatocarcinoma C22.0
Hepatocholangiocarcinoma C22.0
Hepatocholangioma, benign D13.4
Hepatocholangitis K75.89
Hepatolenticular degeneration E83.01
Hepatoma (malignant) C22.0
 |benign D13.4
 |embryonal C22.0
Hepatomegaly *see also* Hypertrophy, liver
 |with splenomegaly R16.2
 |congenital Q44.7
 |in mononucleosis
  |gammaherpesviral B27.09
  |infectious specified NEC B27.89
Hepatoptosis K76.89
Hepatorenal syndrome following labor and delivery O90.4
Hepatosis K76.89
Hepatosplenomegaly R16.2
 |hyperlipemic (Bürger-Grütz type) E78.3 [*K77*]
Hereditary *see* condition
Hereditary alpha tryptasemia (syndrome) D89.44
Heredodegeneration, macular *see* Dystrophy, retina
Heredopathia atactica polyneuritiformis G60.1
Heredosyphilis *see* Syphilis, congenital
Herlitz' syndrome Q81.1
Hermansky-Pudlak syndrome E70.331
Hermaphrodite, hermaphroditism (true) Q56.0
 |46,XX with streak gonads Q99.1
 |46,XX/46,XY Q99.0
 |46,XY with streak gonads Q99.1
 |chimera 46,XX/46,XY Q99.0
Hernia, hernial (acquired) (recurrent) K46.9
 |with
  |gangrene *see* Hernia, by site, with, gangrene
  |incarceration *see* Hernia, by site, with, obstruction
  |irreducible *see* Hernia, by site, with, obstruction
  |obstruction *see* Hernia, by site, with, obstruction
  |strangulation *see* Hernia, by site, with, obstruction
 |abdomen, abdominal K46.9
  |with
   |gangrene (and obstruction) K46.1
   |obstruction K46.0
  |femoral *see* Hernia, femoral
  |incisional *see* Hernia, incisional
  |inguinal *see* Hernia, inguinal
  |specified site NEC K45.8
   |with

Hernia, hernial - *continued*
   |gangrene (and obstruction) K45.1
   |obstruction K45.0
  |umbilical *see* Hernia, umbilical
  |wall *see* Hernia, ventral
 |appendix *see* Hernia, abdomen
 |bladder (mucosa) (sphincter)
  |congenital (female) (male) Q79.51
  |female *see* Cystocele
  |male N32.89
 |brain, congenital *see* Encephalocele
 |cartilage, vertebra *see* Displacement, intervertebral disc
 |cerebral, congenital *see also* Encephalocele
  |endaural Q01.8
 |ciliary body (traumatic) S05.2-
 |colon *see* Hernia, abdomen
 |Cooper's *see* Hernia, abdomen, specified site NEC
 |crural *see* Hernia, femoral
 |diaphragm, diaphragmatic K44.9
  |with
   |gangrene (and obstruction) K44.1
   |obstruction K44.0
  |congenital Q79.0
 |direct (inguinal) *see* Hernia, inguinal
 |diverticulum, intestine *see* Hernia, abdomen
 |double (inguinal) *see* Hernia, inguinal, bilateral
 |due to adhesions (with obstruction) K56.50
 |epigastric *see also* Hernia, ventral K43.9
 |esophageal hiatus *see* Hernia, hiatal
 |external (inguinal) *see* Hernia, inguinal
 |fallopian tube N83.4-
 |fascia M62.89
 |femoral K41.90
  |with
   |gangrene (and obstruction) K41.40
    |not specified as recurrent K41.40
    |recurrent K41.41
   |obstruction K41.30
    |not specified as recurrent K41.30
    |recurrent K41.31
  |bilateral K41.20
   |with
    |gangrene (and obstruction) K41.10
     |not specified as recurrent K41.10
     |recurrent K41.11
    |obstruction K41.00
     |not specified as recurrent K41.00
     |recurrent K41.01
   |not specified as recurrent K41.20
   |recurrent K41.21
  |unilateral K41.90
   |with
    |gangrene (and obstruction) K41.40
     |not specified as recurrent K41.40
     |recurrent K41.41
    |obstruction K41.30
     |not specified as recurrent K41.30
     |recurrent K41.31
   |not specified as recurrent K41.90
   |recurrent K41.91
  |not specified as recurrent K41.90
  |recurrent K41.91
 |foramen magnum G93.5
  |congenital Q01.8
 |funicular (umbilical) *see also* Hernia, umbilicus
  |spermatic (cord) *see* Hernia, inguinal
 |gastrointestinal tract *see* Hernia, abdomen
 |Hesselbach's *see* Hernia, femoral, specified site NEC
 |hiatal (esophageal) (sliding) K44.9
  |with

Hernia, hernial - *continued*
> |gangrene (and obstruction) K44.1
> |obstruction K44.0
> |congenital Q40.1
> |hypogastric *see* Hernia, ventral
> |incarcerated *see also* Hernia, by site, with obstruction
>> |with gangrene *see* Hernia, by site, with gangrene
> |incisional K43.2
>> |with
>>> |gangrene (and obstruction) K43.1
>>> |obstruction K43.0
> |indirect (inguinal) *see* Hernia, inguinal
> |inguinal (direct) (external) (funicular) (indirect) (internal) (oblique) (scrotal) (sliding) K40.90
>> |with
>>> |gangrene (and obstruction) K40.40
>>>> |not specified as recurrent K40.40
>>>> |recurrent K40.41
>>> |obstruction K40.30
>>>> |not specified as recurrent K40.30
>>>> |recurrent K40.31
>> |not specified as recurrent K40.90
>> |recurrent K40.91
>> |bilateral K40.20
>>> |with
>>>> |gangrene (and obstruction) K40.10
>>>>> |not specified as recurrent K40.10
>>>>> |recurrent K40.11
>>>> |obstruction K40.00
>>>>> |not specified as recurrent K40.00
>>>>> |recurrent K40.01
>>> |not specified as recurrent K40.20
>>> |recurrent K40.21
>> |unilateral K40.90
>>> |with
>>>> |gangrene (and obstruction) K40.40
>>>>> |not specified as recurrent K40.40
>>>>> |recurrent K40.41
>>>> |obstruction K40.30
>>>>> |not specified as recurrent K40.30
>>>>> |recurrent K40.31
>>> |not specified as recurrent K40.90
>>> |recurrent K40.91
> |internal *see also* Hernia, abdomen
>> |inguinal *see* Hernia, inguinal
> |interstitial *see* Hernia, abdomen
> |intervertebral cartilage or disc *see* Displacement, intervertebral disc
> |intestine, intestinal *see* Hernia, by site
> |intra-abdominal *see* Hernia, abdomen
> |iris (traumatic) S05.2-
> |irreducible *see also* Hernia, by site, with obstruction
>> |with gangrene *see* Hernia, by site, with gangrene
> |ischiatic *see* Hernia, abdomen, specified site NEC
> |ischiorectal *see* Hernia, abdomen, specified site NEC
> |lens (traumatic) S05.2-
> |linea (alba) (semilunaris) *see* Hernia, ventral
> |Littre's *see* Hernia, abdomen
> |lumbar *see* Hernia, abdomen, specified site NEC
> |lung (subcutaneous) J98.4
> |mediastinum J98.59
> |mesenteric (internal) *see* Hernia, abdomen
> |midline *see* Hernia, ventral
> |muscle (sheath) M62.89
> |nucleus pulposus *see* Displacement, intervertebral disc
> |oblique (inguinal) *see* Hernia, inguinal

Hernia, hernial - *continued*
> |obstructive *see also* Hernia, by site, with obstruction
>> |with gangrene *see* Hernia, by site, with gangrene
> |obturator *see* Hernia, abdomen, specified site NEC
> |omental *see* Hernia, abdomen
> |ovary N83.4-
> |oviduct N83.4-
> |paraesophageal *see also* Hernia, diaphragm
>> |congenital Q40.1
> |parastomal K43.5
>> |with
>>> |gangrene (and obstruction) K43.4
>>> |obstruction K43.3
> |paraumbilical *see* Hernia, umbilicus
> |perineal *see* Hernia, abdomen, specified site NEC
> |Petit's *see* Hernia, abdomen, specified site NEC
> |postoperative *see* Hernia, incisional
> |pregnant uterus *see* Abnormal, uterus in pregnancy or childbirth
> |prevesical N32.89
> |properitoneal *see* Hernia, abdomen, specified site NEC
> |pudendal *see* Hernia, abdomen, specified site NEC
> |rectovaginal N81.6
> |retroperitoneal *see* Hernia, abdomen, specified site NEC
> |Richter's *see* Hernia, abdomen, with obstruction
> |Rieux's, Riex's *see* Hernia, abdomen, specified site NEC
> |sac condition (adhesion) (dropsy) (inflammation) (laceration) (suppuration) code by site under Hernia
> |sciatic *see* Hernia, abdomen, specified site NEC
> |scrotum, scrotal *see* Hernia, inguinal
> |sliding (inguinal) *see also* Hernia, inguinal
>> |hiatus *see* Hernia, hiatal
> |spigelian *see* Hernia, ventral
> |spinal *see* Spina bifida
> |strangulated *see also* Hernia, by site, with obstruction
>> |with gangrene *see* Hernia, by site, with gangrene
> |subxiphoid *see* Hernia, ventral
> |supra-umbilicus *see* Hernia, ventral
> |tendon *see* Disorder, tendon, specified type NEC
> |Treitz's (fossa) *see* Hernia, abdomen, specified site NEC
> |tunica vaginalis Q55.29
> |umbilicus, umbilical K42.9
>> |with
>>> |gangrene (and obstruction) K42.1
>>> |obstruction K42.0
> |ureter N28.89
> |urethra, congenital Q64.79
> |urinary meatus, congenital Q64.79
> |uterus N81.4
>> |pregnant *see* Abnormal, uterus in pregnancy or childbirth
> |vaginal (anterior) (wall) *see* Cystocele
> |Velpeau's *see* Hernia, femoral
> |ventral K43.9
>> |with
>>> |gangrene (and obstruction) K43.7
>>> |obstruction K43.6
>> |recurrent *see* Hernia, incisional
>> |incisional K43.2

Hernia, hernial - *continued*
> |with
>> |gangrene (and obstruction) K43.1
>> |obstruction K43.0
> |specified NEC K43.9
>> |with
>>> |gangrene (and obstruction) K43.7
>>> |obstruction K43.6
> |vesical
>> |congenital (female) (male) Q79.51
>> |female *see* Cystocele
>> |male N32.89
> |vitreous (into wound) S05.2-
>> |into anterior chamber *see* Prolapse, vitreous
Herniation *see also* Hernia
> |brain (stem) G93.5
>> |nontraumatic G93.5
>> |traumatic S06.A1
>>> |cerebellar S06.A1
>>> |subfalcine (cingulate) S06.A1
>>> |tonsillar S06.A1
>>> |transtentorial (central) (upward cerebellar) S06.A1
>>> |uncal S06.A1
> |cerebral G93.5
>> |nontraumatic G93.5
>> |traumatic S06.A1
> |mediastinum J98.59
> |nucleus pulposus *see* Displacement, intervertebral disc
Herpangina B08.5
Herpes, herpesvirus, herpetic B00.9
> |anogenital A60.9
>> |perianal skin A60.1
>> |rectum A60.1
>> |urogenital tract A60.00
>>> |cervix A60.03
>>> |male genital organ NEC A60.02
>>> |penis A60.01
>>> |specified site NEC A60.09
>>> |vagina A60.04
>>> |vulva A60.04
> |blepharitis (zoster) B02.39
>> |simplex B00.59
> |circinatus B35.4
>> |bullosus L12.0
> |conjunctivitis (simplex) B00.53
>> |zoster B02.31
> |cornea B02.33
> |encephalitis B00.4
>> |due to herpesvirus 6 B10.01
>> |due to herpesvirus 7 B10.09
>> |specified NEC B10.09
> |eye (zoster) B02.30
>> |simplex B00.50
> |eyelid (zoster) B02.39
>> |simplex B00.59
> |facialis B00.1
> |febrilis B00.1
> |geniculate ganglionitis B02.21
> |genital, genitalis A60.00
>> |female A60.09
>> |male A60.02
> |gestational, gestationis O26.4-
> |gingivostomatitis B00.2
> |human B00.9
>> |1 *see* Herpes, simplex
>> |2 *see* Herpes, simplex
>> |3 *see* Varicella
>> |4 *see* Mononucleosis, Epstein-Barr (virus)
>> |5 *see* Disease, cytomegalic inclusion (generalized)
>> |6
>>> |encephalitis B10.01

Herpes, herpesvirus, herpetic - *continued*
|specified NEC B10.81
|7
|encephalitis B10.09
|specified NEC B10.82
|8 B10.89
|infection NEC B10.89
|Kaposi's sarcoma associated B10.89
|iridocyclitis (simplex) B00.51
|zoster B02.32
|iris (vesicular erythema multiforme) L51.9
|iritis (simplex) B00.51
|Kaposi's sarcoma associated B10.89
|keratitis (simplex) (dendritic) (disciform)
(interstitial) B00.52
|zoster (interstitial) B02.33
|keratoconjunctivitis (simplex) B00.52
|zoster B02.33
|labialis B00.1
|lip B00.1
|meningitis (simplex) B00.3
|zoster B02.1
|ophthalmicus (zoster) NEC B02.30
|simplex B00.50
|penis A60.01
|perianal skin A60.1
|pharyngitis, pharyngotonsillitis B00.2
|rectum A60.1
|scrotum A60.02
|sepsis B00.7
|simplex B00.9
|complicated NEC B00.89
|congenital P35.2
|conjunctivitis B00.53
|external ear B00.1
|eyelid B00.59
|hepatitis B00.81
|keratitis (interstitial) B00.52
|myelitis B00.82
|specified complication NEC B00.89
|visceral B00.89
|stomatitis B00.2
|tonsurans B35.0
|visceral B00.89
|vulva A60.04
|whitlow B00.89
|zoster *see also* condition B02.9
|auricularis B02.21
|complicated NEC B02.8
|conjunctivitis B02.31
|disseminated B02.7
|encephalitis B02.0
|eye (lid) B02.39
|geniculate ganglionitis B02.21
|keratitis (interstitial) B02.33
|meningitis B02.1
|myelitis B02.24
|neuritis, neuralgia B02.29
|ophthalmicus NEC B02.30
|oticus B02.21
|polyneuropathy B02.23
|specified complication NEC B02.8
|trigeminal neuralgia B02.22
Herpesvirus (human) *see* Herpes
Herpetophobia F40.218
Herrick's anemia *see* Disease, sickle-cell
Hers' disease E74.09
Herter-Gee syndrome K90.0
Herxheimer's reaction R68.89
Hesitancy
|of micturition R39.11
|urinary R39.11
Hesselbach's hernia *see* Hernia, femoral,
specified site NEC

Heterochromia (congenital) Q13.2
|cataract *see* Cataract, complicated
|cyclitis (Fuchs) *see* Cyclitis, Fuchs'
heterochromic
|hair L67.1
|iritis *see* Cyclitis, Fuchs' heterochromic
|retained metallic foreign body (nonmagnetic)
see Foreign body, intraocular, old, retained
|magnetic *see* Foreign body, intraocular, old,
retained, magnetic
|uveitis *see* Cyclitis, Fuchs' heterochromic
Heterophoria *see* Strabismus, heterophoria
Heterophyes, heterophyiasis (small intestine)
B66.8
Heterotopia, heterotopic *see also* Malposition,
congenital
|cerebralis Q04.8
Heterotropia *see* Strabismus
Heubner-Herter disease K90.0
Hexadactylism Q69.9
**HGSIL (cytology finding) (high grade
squamous intraepithelial lesion on cytologic
smear) (Pap smear finding)**
|anus R85.613
|cervix R87.613
|biopsy (histology) finding *see* Neoplasia,
intraepithelial, cervix, grade II or grade
III
|vagina R87.623
|biopsy (histology) finding *see* Neoplasia,
intraepithelial, vagina, grade II or grade
III
Hibernoma *see* Lipoma
Hiccup, hiccough R06.6
|epidemic B33.0
|psychogenic F45.8
Hidden penis (congenital) Q55.64
|acquired N48.83
Hidradenitis (axillaris) (suppurative) L73.2
Hidradenoma (nodular) *see also* Neoplasm,
skin, benign
|clear cell *see* Neoplasm, skin, benign
|papillary *see* Neoplasm, skin, benign
Hidrocystoma *see* Neoplasm, skin, benign
High
|altitude effects T70.20
|anoxia T70.29
|on
|ears T70.0
|sinuses T70.1
|polycythemia D75.1
|arch
|foot Q66.7
|palate, congenital Q38.5
|arterial tension *see* Hypertension
|basal metabolic rate R94.8
|blood pressure *see also* Hypertension
|borderline R03.0
|reading (incidental) (isolated) (nonspecific),
without diagnosis of hypertension R03.0
|cholesterol E78.00
|with high triglycerides E78.2
|diaphragm (congenital) Q79.1
|expressed emotional level within family Z63.8
|head at term O32.4
|palate, congenital Q38.5
|risk
|infant NEC Z76.2
|sexual behavior (heterosexual) Z72.51
|bisexual Z72.53
|homosexual Z72.52
|scrotal testis, testes
|bilateral Q53.23
|unilateral Q53.13
|temperature (of unknown origin) R50.9

High - *continued*
|thoracic rib Q76.6
|triglycerides E78.1
|with high cholesterol E78.2
Hildebrand's disease A75.0
Hilum *see* condition
Hip *see* condition
Hippel's disease Q85.8
Hippophobia F40.218
Hippus H57.09
Hirschsprung's disease or megacolon Q43.1
Hirsutism, hirsuties L68.0
Hirudiniasis
|external B88.3
|internal B83.4
Hiss-Russell dysentery A03.1
Histidinemia, histidinuria E70.41
Histiocytoma *see also* Neoplasm, skin, benign
|fibrous *see also* Neoplasm, skin, benign
|atypical *see* Neoplasm, connective tissue,
uncertain behavior
|malignant *see* Neoplasm, connective tissue,
malignant
Histiocytosis D76.3
|acute differentiated progressive C96.0
|Langerhans' cell NEC C96.6
|multifocal X
|multisystemic (disseminated) C96.0
|unisystemic C96.5
|pulmonary, adult (adult PLCH) J84.82
|unifocal (X) C96.6
|lipid, lipoid D76.3
|essential E75.29
|malignant C96.A
|mononuclear phagocytes NEC D76.1
|Langerhans' cells C96.6
|non-Langerhans cell D76.3
|polyostotic sclerosing D76.3
|sinus, with massive lymphadenopathy D76.3
|syndrome NEC D76.3
|X NEC C96.6
|acute (progressive) C96.0
|chronic C96.6
|multifocal C96.5
|multisystemic C96.0
|unifocal C96.6
Histoplasmosis B39.9
|with pneumonia NEC B39.2
|African B39.5
|American *see* Histoplasmosis, capsulati
|capsulati B39.4
|disseminated B39.3
|generalized B39.3
|pulmonary B39.2
|acute B39.0
|chronic B39.1
|Darling's B39.4
|duboisii B39.5
|lung NEC B39.2
History
|family (of) *see also* History, personal (of)
|alcohol abuse Z81.1
|allergy NEC Z84.89
|anemia Z83.2
|arthritis Z82.61
|asthma Z82.5
|blindness Z82.1
|cardiac death (sudden) Z82.41
|carrier of genetic disease Z84.81
|chromosomal anomaly Z82.79
|chronic
|disabling disease NEC Z82.8
|lower respiratory disease Z82.5
|colonic polyps Z83.71

History - *continued*

   |congenital malformations and deformations Z82.79
    |polycystic kidney Z82.71
  |consanguinity Z84.3
  |deafness Z82.2
  |diabetes mellitus Z83.3
  |disability NEC Z82.8
  |disease or disorder (of)
   |allergic NEC Z84.89
   |behavioral NEC Z81.8
   |blood and blood-forming organs Z83.2
   |cardiovascular NEC Z82.49
   |chronic disabling NEC Z82.8
   |digestive Z83.79
   |ear NEC Z83.52
   |elevated lipoprotein(a) (Lp(a)) Z83.430
   |endocrine NEC Z83.49
   |eye NEC Z83.518
    |glaucoma Z83.511
   |familial hypercholesterolemia Z83.42
   |genitourinary NEC Z84.2
   |glaucoma Z83.511
   |hematological Z83.2
   |immune mechanism Z83.2
   |infectious NEC Z83.1
   |ischemic heart Z82.49
   |kidney Z84.1
   |lipoprotein metabolism Z83.438
   |mental NEC Z81.8
   |metabolic Z83.49
   |musculoskeletal NEC Z82.69
   |neurological NEC Z82.0
   |nutritional Z83.49
   |parasitic NEC Z83.1
   |psychiatric NEC Z81.8
   |respiratory NEC Z83.6
   |skin and subcutaneous tissue NEC Z84.0
   |specified NEC Z84.89
  |drug abuse NEC Z81.3
  |elevated lipoprotein(a) (Lp(a)) Z83.430
   epilepsy Z82.0
  |familial hypercholesterolemia Z83.42
  |genetic disease carrier Z84.81
  |glaucoma Z83.511
  |hearing loss Z82.2
  |human immunodeficiency virus (HIV) infection Z83.0
  |Huntington's chorea Z82.0
  |hyperlipidemia, familial combined Z83.438
  |intellectual disability Z81.0
  |leukemia Z80.6
  |lipidemia NEC Z83.438
  |malignant neoplasm (of) NOS Z80.9
   |bladder Z80.52
   |breast Z80.3
   |bronchus Z80.1
   |digestive organ Z80.0
   |gastrointestinal tract Z80.0
   |genital organ Z80.49
    |ovary Z80.41
    |prostate Z80.42
    |specified organ NEC Z80.49
    |testis Z80.43
   |hematopoietic NEC Z80.7
   |intrathoracic organ NEC Z80.2
   |kidney Z80.51
   |lung Z80.1
   |lymphatic NEC Z80.7
   |ovary Z80.41
   |prostate Z80.42
   |respiratory organ NEC Z80.2
   |specified site NEC Z80.8
   |testis Z80.43
   |trachea Z80.1

History - *continued*

   |urinary organ or tract Z80.59
    |bladder Z80.52
    |kidney Z80.51
  |mental
   |disorder NEC Z81.8
  |multiple endocrine neoplasia (MEN) syndrome Z83.41
  |osteoporosis Z82.62
  |polycystic kidney Z82.71
  |polyps (colon) Z83.71
  |psychiatric disorder Z81.8
  |psychoactive substance abuse NEC Z81.3
  |respiratory condition NEC Z83.6
   |asthma and other lower respiratory conditions Z82.5
  |self-harmful behavior Z81.8
  |SIDS (sudden infant death syndrome) Z84.82
  |skin condition Z84.0
  |specified condition NEC Z84.89
  |stroke (cerebrovascular) Z82.3
  |substance abuse NEC Z81.4
   |alcohol Z81.1
   |drug NEC Z81.3
   |psychoactive NEC Z81.3
   |tobacco Z81.2
  |sudden
   |cardiac death Z82.41
   |infant death syndrome (SIDS) Z84.82
  |tobacco abuse Z81.2
  |violence, violent behavior Z81.8
  |visual loss Z82.1
 |personal (of) *see also* History, family (of)
  |abuse
   |childhood Z62.819
    |forced labor or sexual exploitation in childhood Z62
    |physical Z62.810
    |psychological Z62.811
    |sexual Z62.810
   |adult Z91.419
    |forced labor or sexual exploitation Z91.42
    |physical and sexual Z91.410
    |psychological Z91.411
  |alcohol dependence F10.21
  |allergy (to) Z88.9
   |analgesic agent NEC Z88.6
   |anesthetic Z88.4
   |antibiotic agent NEC Z88.1
   |anti-infective agent NEC Z88.3
   |contrast media Z91.041
   |drugs, medicaments and biological substances Z88.9
    |specified NEC Z88.8
   |food Z91.018
    |additives Z91.02
    |beef Z91.014
    |eggs Z91.012
    |milk products Z91.011
    |lamb Z91.014
    |mammalian meats Z91.014
    |peanuts Z91.010
    |pork Z91.014
    |red meats Z91.014
    |seafood Z91.013
    |specified food NEC Z91.018
   |insect Z91.038
    |bee Z91.030
   |latex Z91.040
   |medicinal agents Z88.9
    |specified NEC Z88.8
   |narcotic agent NEC Z88.5
   |nonmedicinal agents Z91.048

History - *continued*

   |penicillin Z88.0
   |serum Z88.7
   |specified NEC Z91.09
   |sulfonamides Z88.2
   |vaccine Z88.7
  |anaphylactic shock Z87.892
  |anaphylaxis Z87.892
  |behavioral disorders Z86.59
  |benign carcinoid tumor Z86.012
  |benign neoplasm Z86.018
   |carcinoid Z86.012
   |brain Z86.011
   |colonic polyps Z86.010
  |brain injury (traumatic) Z87.820
  |breast implant removal Z98.86
  |calculi, renal Z87.442
  |cancer *see* History, personal (of), malignant neoplasm (of)
  |cardiac arrest (death), successfully resuscitated Z86.74
  |CAR-T (Chimeric Antigen Receptor T-cell) therapy Z92.850
  |cellular therapy Z92.859
   |specified NEC Z92.858
  |cerebral infarction without residual deficit Z86.73
  |cervical dysplasia Z87.410
  |chemotherapy for neoplastic condition Z92.21
  |childhood abuse *see* History, personal (of), abuse
  |Chimeric Antigen Receptor T-cell (CAR-T) therapy Z92.850
  |cleft lip (corrected) Z87.730
  |cleft palate (corrected) Z87.730
  |collapsed vertebra (healed) Z87.311
   |due to osteoporosis Z87.310
  |combat and operational stress reaction Z86.51
  |congenital malformation (corrected) Z87.798
   |circulatory system (corrected) Z87.74
   |digestive system (corrected) NEC Z87.738
   |ear (corrected) Z87.721
   |eye (corrected) Z87.720
   |face and neck (corrected) Z87.790
   |genitourinary system (corrected) NEC Z87.718
   |heart (corrected) Z87.74
   |integument (corrected) Z87.76
   |limb(s) (corrected) Z87.76
   |musculoskeletal system (corrected) Z87.76
   |neck (corrected) Z87.790
   |nervous system (corrected) NEC Z87.728
   |respiratory system (corrected) Z87.75
   |sense organs (corrected) NEC Z87.728
   |specified NEC Z87.798
  |contraception Z92.0
  |coronavirus (disease) (novel) 2019 Z86.16
  |COVID-19 Z86.16
  |deployment (military) Z91.82
  |diabetic foot ulcer Z86.31
  |disease or disorder (of) Z87.898
   |blood and blood-forming organs Z86.2
   |circulatory system Z86.79
    |specified condition NEC Z86.79
   |connective tissue NEC Z87.39
   |digestive system Z87.19
    |colonic polyp Z86.010
    |peptic ulcer disease Z87.11
    |specified condition NEC Z87.19
   |ear Z86.69

History - *continued*

    |endocrine Z86.39
      |diabetic foot ulcer Z86.31
      |gestational diabetes Z86.32
      |specified type NEC Z86.39
    |eye Z86.69
    |genital (track) system NEC
      |female Z87.42
      |male Z87.438
    |hematological Z86.2
    |Hodgkin Z85.71
    |immune mechanism Z86.2
    |infectious Z86.19
      |malaria Z86.13
      |Methicillin resistant Staphylococcus
        aureus (MRSA) Z86.14
      |poliomyelitis Z86.12
      |specified NEC Z86.19
      |tuberculosis Z86.11
    |mental NEC Z86.59
    |metabolic Z86.39
      |diabetic foot ulcer Z86.31
      |gestational diabetes Z86.32
      |specified type NEC Z86.39
    |musculoskeletal NEC Z87.39
    |nervous system Z86.69
    |nutritional Z86.39
    |parasitic Z86.19
    |respiratory system NEC Z87.09
    |sense organs Z86.69
    |skin Z87.2
    |specified site or type NEC Z87.898
    |subcutaneous tissue Z87.2
    |trophoblastic Z87.59
    |urinary system NEC Z87.448
  |drug dependence *see* Dependence, drug, by
    type, in remission
- - |drug therapy
    |antineoplastic chemotherapy Z92.21
    |estrogen Z92.23
    |immunosuppression Z92.25
    |inhaled steroids Z92.240
    |monoclonal drug Z92.22
    |specified NEC Z92.29
    |steroid Z92.241
    |systemic steroids Z92.241
  |dysplasia
    |cervical (mild) (moderate) Z87.410
      |severe (grade III) Z86.001
    |prostatic Z87.430
    |vaginal (mild) (moderate) Z87.411
      |severe (grade III) Z86.008
    |vulvar (mild) (moderate) Z87.412
      |severe (grade III) Z86.008
  |embolism (venous) Z86.718
    |pulmonary Z86.711
  |encephalitis Z86.61
  |estrogen therapy Z92.23
  |extracorporeal membrane oxygenation
    (ECMO) Z92.81
  |failed moderate sedation Z92.83
  |failed conscious sedation Z92.83
  |fall, falling Z91.81
  |forced labor or sexual exploitation Z91.42
    |in childhood Z62.813
  |fracture (healed)
    |fatigue Z87.312
    |fragility Z87.310
    |osteoporosis Z87.310
    |pathological NEC Z87.311
    |stress Z87.312
    |traumatic Z87.81
gene therapy Z92.86
  |gestational diabetes Z86.32
  |hepatitis

History - *continued*

  |B Z86.19
  |C Z86.19
|Hodgkin disease Z85.71
|hyperthermia, malignant Z88.4
|hypospadias (corrected) Z87.710
|hysterectomy Z90.710
|immunosuppression therapy Z92.25
|in situ neoplasm
  |breast Z86.000
  |cervix uteri Z86.001
  |specified NEC Z86.008
|infection NEC Z86.19
  |central nervous system Z86.61
  |Methicillin resistant Staphylococcus
    aureus (MRSA) Z86.14
  |urinary (recurrent) (tract) Z87.440
|injury NEC Z87.828
|in utero procedure during pregnancy
  Z98.870
|in utero procedure while a fetus Z98.871
|irradiation Z92.3
|kidney stones Z87.442
|leukemia Z85.6
|lymphoma (non-hodgkin) Z85.72
|malignant melanoma (skin) Z85.820
|malignant neoplasm (of) Z85.9
  |accessory sinuses Z85.22
  |anus NEC Z85.048
    |carcinoid Z85.040
  |bladder Z85.51
  |bone Z85.830
  |brain Z85.841
  |breast Z85.3
  |bronchus NEC Z85.118
    |carcinoid Z85.110
  |carcinoid *see* History, personal (of),
    malignant neoplasm, by site, carcinoid
  |cervix Z85.41
  |colon NEC Z85.038
    |carcinoid Z85.030
  |digestive organ Z85.00
    |specified NEC Z85.09
  |endocrine gland NEC Z85.858
  |epididymis Z85.48
  |esophagus Z85.01
  |eye Z85.840
  |gastrointestinal tract *see* History,
    malignant neoplasm, digestive organ
  |genital organ
    |female Z85.40
      |specified NEC Z85.44
    |male Z85.45
      |specified NEC Z85.49
  |hematopoietic NEC Z85.79
  |intrathoracic organ Z85.20
  |kidney NEC Z85.528
    |carcinoid Z85.520
  |large intestine NEC Z85.038
    |carcinoid Z85.030
  |larynx Z85.21
  |liver Z85.05
  |lung NEC Z85.118
    |carcinoid Z85.110
  |mediastinum Z85.29
  |Merkel cell Z85.821
  |middle ear Z85.22
  |nasal cavities Z85.22
  |nervous system NEC Z85.848
  |oral cavity Z85.819
    |specified site NEC Z85.818
  |ovary Z85.43
  |pancreas Z85.07
  |pharynx Z85.819
    |specified site NEC Z85.818

History - *continued*

  |pelvis Z85.53
  |pleura Z85.29
  |prostate Z85.46
  |rectosigmoid junction NEC Z85.048
    |carcinoid Z85.040
  |rectum NEC Z85.048
    |carcinoid Z85.040
  |respiratory organ Z85.20
  |sinuses, accessory Z85.22
  |skin NEC Z85.828
    |melanoma Z85.820
    |Merkel cell Z85.821
  |small intestine NEC Z85.068
    |carcinoid Z85.060
  |soft tissue Z85.831
  |specified site NEC Z85.89
  |stomach NEC Z85.028
    |carcinoid Z85.020
  |testis Z85.47
  |thymus NEC Z85.238
    |carcinoid Z85.230
  |thyroid Z85.850
  |tongue Z85.810
  |trachea Z85.12
  |ureter Z85.54
  |urinary organ or tract Z85.50
    |specified NEC Z85.59
  |uterus Z85.42
|maltreatment Z91.89
|medical treatment NEC Z92.89
|melanoma (malignant) (skin) Z85.820
|meningitis Z86.61
|mental disorder Z86.59
|Merkel cell carcinoma (skin) Z85.821
|Methicillin resistant Staphylococcus aureus
  (MRSA) Z86.14
|military deployment Z91.82
|military war, peacekeeping and
  humanitarian deployment (current or past
  conflict) Z91.82
|myocardial infarction (old) I25.2
|neglect (in)
  |adult Z91.412
  |childhood Z62.812
|neoplasm
  |benign Z86.018
    |brain Z86.011
    |colon polyp Z86.010
  |in situ
    |breast Z86.000
    |cervix uteri Z86.001
    |specified NEC Z86.008
  |malignant *see* History of, malignant
    neoplasm
  |uncertain behavior Z86.03
|nephrotic syndrome Z87.441
|nicotine dependence Z87.891
|noncompliance with medical treatment or
  regimen *see* Noncompliance
|nutritional deficiency Z86.39
|obstetric complications Z87.59
  |childbirth Z87.59
  |pregnancy Z87.59
  |pre-term labor Z87.51
  |puerperium Z87.59
|osteoporosis fractures Z87.31
|parasuicide (attempt) Z91.51
|physical trauma NEC Z87.828
  |self-harm or suicide attempt Z91.51
|poisoning NEC Z91.89
  |self-harm or suicide attempt Z91.51
|poor personal hygiene Z91.89
|pneumonia (recurrent) Z87.01
|preterm labor Z87.51

History - *continued*
|prolonged reversible ischemic neurologic deficit (PRIND) Z86.73
|procedure during pregnancy Z98.870
|procedure while a fetus Z98.871
|prostatic dysplasia Z87.430
|psychological
  |abuse
    |adult Z91.411
    |child Z62.811
  |trauma, specified NEC Z91.49
|radiation therapy Z92.3
|removal
  |implant
    |breast Z98.86
|renal calculi Z87.442
|respiratory condition NEC Z87.09
|retained foreign body fully removed Z87.821
|risk factors NEC Z91.89
|SARS-CoV-2 infection Z86.16
|self-harm Z91.51
  |nonsuicidal Z91.52
  |suicidal Z91.51
|self-inflicted injury without suicidal intent Z91.52
|self-injury
  |nonsuicidal Z91.52
|self-mutilation Z91.52
|self-poisoning attempt Z91.51
|sex reassignment Z87.890
|sleep-wake cycle problem Z72.821
|specified NEC Z87.898
|steroid therapy (systemic) Z92.241
  |inhaled Z92.240
|stroke without residual deficits Z86.73
|substance abuse NEC F10-F19
|sudden cardiac arrest Z86.74
|sudden cardiac death successfully resuscitated Z86.74
|suicide attempt Z91.51
|suicidal behavior Z91.51
|surgery NEC Z98.890
  |with uterine scar Z98.891
  |sex reassignment Z87.890
  |transplant *see* Transplant
|thrombophlebitis Z86.72
|thrombosis (venous) Z86.718
  |pulmonary Z86.711
|tobacco dependence Z87.891
|transient ischemic attack (TIA) without residual deficits Z86.73
|trauma (physical) NEC Z87.828
  |psychological NEC Z91.49
  |self-harm Z91.5
|traumatic brain injury Z87.820
|unhealthy sleep-wake cycle Z72.821
|unintended awareness under general anesthesia Z92.84
|urinary calculi Z87.442
|urinary (recurrent) (tract) infection(s) Z87.440
|uterine scar from previous surgery Z98.891
|vaginal dysplasia Z87.411
|venous thrombosis or embolism Z86.718
  |pulmonary Z86.711
|vulvar dysplasia Z87.412
His-Werner disease A79.0
HIV *see also* Human, immunodeficiency virus B20
|laboratory evidence (nonconclusive) R75
|positive, seropositive Z21
|nonconclusive test (in infants) R75
Hives (bold) *see* Urticaria
Hoarseness R49.0

Hobo Z59.00
Hodgkin disease *see* Lymphoma, Hodgkin
Hodgson's disease I71.2
|ruptured I71.1
Hoffa-Kastert disease E88.89
Hoffa's disease E88.89
Hoffmann-Bouveret syndrome I47.9
Hoffmann's syndrome E03.9 *[G73.7]*
Hole (round)
|macula H35.34-
|retina (without detachment) *see* Break, retina, round hole
  |with detachment *see* Detachment, retina, with retinal, break
Holiday relief care Z75.5
Hollenhorst's plaque *see* Occlusion, artery, retina
Hollow foot (congenital) Q66.7
|acquired *see* Deformity, limb, foot, specified NEC
Holoprosencephaly Q04.2
Holt-Oram syndrome Q87.2
Homelessness Z59.00
- sheltered Z59.01
- unsheltered Z59.02
Homesickness *see* Disorder, adjustment
Homocysteinemia R79.83
Homocystinemia, homocystinuria E72.11
Homogentisate 1,2-Dioxygenase deficiency E70.29
Homologous serum hepatitis (prophylactic) (therapeutic) *see* Hepatitis, viral, type B
Honeycomb lung J98.4
|congenital Q33.0
Hooded
|clitoris Q52.6
|penis Q55.69
Hookworm (anemia) (disease) (infection) (infestation) B76.9
|specified NEC B76.8
Hordeolum (eyelid) (externum) (recurrent) H00.019
|internum H00.029
  |left H00.026
    |lower H00.025
    |upper H00.024
  |right H00.023
    |lower H00.022
    |upper H00.021
|left H00.016
  |lower H00.015
  |upper H00.014
|right H00.013
  |lower H00.012
  |upper H00.011
Horn
|cutaneous L85.8
|nail L60.2
  |congenital Q84.6
Horner (-Claude Bernard) syndrome G90.2
|traumatic *see* Injury, nerve, cervical sympathetic
Horseshoe kidney (congenital) Q63.1
Horton's headache or neuralgia G44.099
|intractable G44.091
|not intractable G44.099
Hospital hopper syndrome *see* Disorder, factitious
Hospitalism in children *see* Disorder, adjustment
Hostility R45.5
|towards child Z62.3
Hot flashes
|menopausal N95.1

Hourglass (contracture) *see also* Contraction, hourglass
|stomach K31.89
  |congenital Q40.2
  |stricture K31.2
Household, housing circumstance affecting care Z59.9
|specified NEC Z59.89
Housemaid's knee *see* Bursitis, prepatellar
HSCT-TMA (hematopoietic stem cell transplantation-associated thrombotic microangiopathy) M31.11
Hudson (-Stähli) line (cornea) *see* Pigmentation, cornea, anterior
Human
|bite (open wound) *see also* Bite
  |intact skin surface *see* Bite, superficial
|herpesvirus *see* Herpes
|immunodeficiency virus (HIV) disease (infection) B20
  |asymptomatic status Z21
  |contact Z20.6
  |counseling Z71.7
  |dementia B20 *[F02.80]*
    |with behavioral disturbance B20 *[F02.81]*
  |exposure to Z20.6
  |laboratory evidence R75
  |type 2 (HIV 2) as cause of disease classified elsewhere B97.35
|papillomavirus (HPV)
  |DNA test positive
    |high risk
      |cervix R87.810
      |vagina R87.811
    |low risk
      |cervix R87.820
      |vagina R87.821
  |screening for Z11.51
|T-cell lymphotropic virus
  |type 1(HTLV-I) infection B33.3
    |as cause of disease classified elsewhere B97.33
  |carrier Z22.6
  |type 2 (HTLV-II) as cause of disease classified elsewhere B97.34
Humidifier lung or pneumonitis J67.7
Humiliation (experience) in childhood Z62.898
Humpback (acquired) *see* Kyphosis
Hunchback (acquired) *see* Kyphosis
Hunger T73.0
|air, psychogenic F45.8
Hungry bone syndrome E83.81
Hunner's ulcer *see* Cystitis, chronic, interstitial
Hunter's
|glossitis D51.0
|syndrome E76.1
Huntington's disease or chorea G10
|with dementia G10 *[F02.80]*
  |with behavioral disturbance G10 *[F02.81]*
Hunt's
|disease or syndrome (herpetic geniculate ganglionitis) B02.21
  |dyssynergia cerebellaris myoclonica G11.19
|neuralgia B02.21
Hurler (-Scheie) disease or syndrome E76.02
Hurst's disease G36.1
Hürthle cell
|adenocarcinoma C73
|adenoma D34
|carcinoma C73
|tumor D34
Hutchinson-Boeck disease or syndrome *see* Sarcoidosis

Hutchinson-Gilford disease or syndrome
E34.8
Hutchinson's
|disease, meaning
||angioma serpiginosum L81.7
||pompholyx (cheiropompholyx) L30.1
||prurigo estivalis L56.4
||summer eruption or summer prurigo L56.4
|melanotic freckle *see* Melanoma, in situ
||malignant melanoma in *see* Melanoma
|teeth or incisors (congenital syphilis) A50.52
|triad (congenital syphilis) A50.53
Hyalin plaque, sclera, senile H15.89
Hyaline membrane (disease) (lung)
(pulmonary) (newborn) P22.0
Hyalinosis
|cutis (et mucosae) E78.89
|focal and segmental (glomerular) *see also*
|N00-N07 with fourth character .1N05.1
Hyalitis, hyalosis, asteroid *see also* Deposit,
crystalline
|syphilitic (late) A52.71
Hydatid
|cyst or tumor *see* Echinococcus
|mole *see* Hydatidiform mole
|Morgagni
||female Q50.5
||male (epididymal) Q55.4
|||testicular Q55.29
Hydatidiform mole (benign) (complicating
pregnancy) (delivered) (undelivered) O01.9
|classical O01.0
|complete O01.0
|incomplete O01.1
|invasive D39.2
|malignant D39.2
|partial O01.1
Hydatidosis *see* Echinococcus
Hydradenitis (axillaris) (suppurative) L73.2
Hydradenoma *see* Hidradenoma
Hydramnios O40.-
Hydrancephaly, hydranencephaly Q04.3
|with spina bifida *see* Spina bifida, with
hydrocephalus
Hydrargyrism NEC *see* Poisoning, mercury
Hydrarthrosis *see also* Effusion, joint
|gonococcal A54.42
|intermittent M12.40
||ankle M12.47-
||elbow M12.42-
||foot joint M12.47-
||hand joint M12.44-
||hip M12.45-
||knee M12.46-
||multiple site M12.49
||shoulder M12.41-
||specified joint NEC M12.48
||wrist M12.43-
|of yaws (early) (late) *see also* subcategory
M14.8   A66.6
|syphilitic (late) A52.77
||congenital A50.55 [M12.80]
Hydremia D64.89
Hydrencephalocele (congenital) *see*
Encephalocele
Hydrencephalomeningocele (congenital) *see*
Encephalocele
Hydroa R23.8
|aestivale L56.4
|vacciniforme L56.4
Hydroadenitis (axillaris) (suppurative) L73.2
Hydrocalycosis *see* Hydronephrosis
Hydrocele (spermatic cord) (testis) (tunica
vaginalis) N43.3
|canal of Nuck N94.89

Hydrocele - *continued*
|communicating N43.2
||congenital P83.5
|congenital P83.5
|encysted N43.0
|female NEC N94.89
|infected N43.1
|newborn P83.5
|round ligament N94.89
|specified NEC N43.2
|spinalis *see* Spina bifida
|vulva N90.89
Hydrocephalus (acquired) (external)
(internal) (malignant) (recurrent) G91.9
|aqueduct Sylvius stricture Q03.0
|causing disproportion O33.6
||with obstructed labor O66.3
|communicating G91.0
|congenital (external) (internal) Q03.9
||with spina bifida Q05.4
|||cervical Q05.0
|||dorsal Q05.1
|||lumbar Q05.2
|||lumbosacral Q05.2
|||sacral Q05.3
|||thoracic Q05.1
|||thoracolumbar Q05.1
||specified NEC Q03.8
|due to toxoplasmosis (congenital) P37.1
|foramen Magendie block (acquired) G91.1
||congenital *see also* Hydrocephalus,
congenital Q03.1
|in (due to)
||infectious disease NEC B89 [*G91.4*]
||neoplastic disease NEC (*see also*
Neoplasm) G91.4
||parasitic disease B89 [*G91.4*]
|newborn Q03.9
||with spina bifida *see* Spina bifida, with
hydrocephalus
|noncommunicating G91.1
|normal pressure G91.2
||secondary G91.0
|obstructive G91.1
|otitic G93.2
|post-traumatic NEC G91.3
|secondary G91.4
||post-traumatic G91.3
|specified NEC G91.8
|syphilitic, congenital A50.49
Hydrocolpos (congenital) N89.8
Hydrocystoma *see* Neoplasm, skin, benign
Hydroencephalocele (congenital) *see*
Encephalocele
Hydroencephalomeningocele (congenital) *see*
Encephalocele
Hydrohematopneumothorax *see* Hemothorax
Hydromeningitis *see* Meningitis
Hydromeningocele (spinal) *see also* Spina
bifida
|cranial *see* Encephalocele
Hydrometra N85.8
Hydrometrocolpos N89.8
Hydromicrocephaly Q02
Hydromphalus (since birth) Q45.8
Hydromyelia Q06.4
Hydromyelocele *see* Spina bifida
Hydronephrosis (atrophic) (early)
(functionless) (intermittent) (primary)
(secondary) NEC N13.30
|with
||infection N13.6
||obstruction (by) (of)
|||renal calculus N13.2
||||with infection N13.6

Hydronephrosis - *continued*
|ureteral NEC N13.1
||with infection N13.6
||calculus N13.2
|||with infection N13.6
|ureteropelvic junction (congenital)
Q62.11
||acquired N13.0
|||with infection N13.6
|ureteral stricture NEC N13.1
||with infection N13.6
|congenital Q62.0
|due to acquired occlusion of ureteropelvic
junction N13.0
|specified type NEC N13.39
|tuberculous A18.11
Hydropericarditis *see* Pericarditis
Hydropericardium *see* Pericarditis
Hydroperitoneum R18.8
Hydrophobia *see* Rabies
Hydrophthalmos Q15.0
Hydropneumohemothorax *see* Hemothorax
Hydropneumopericarditis *see* Pericarditis
Hydropneumopericardium *see* Pericarditis
Hydropneumothorax J94.8
|traumatic *see* Injury, intrathoracic, lung
|tuberculous NEC A15.6
Hydrops R60.9
|abdominis R18.8
|articulorum intermittens *see* Hydrarthrosis,
intermittent
|cardiac *see* Failure, heart, congestive
|causing obstructed labor (mother) O66.3
|endolymphatic H81.0-
|fetal *see* Pregnancy, complicated by, hydrops,
fetalis
|fetalis P83.2
||due to
|||ABO isoimmunization P56.0
|||alpha thalassemia D56.0
|||hemolytic disease P56.90
||||specified NEC P56.99
|||isoimmunization (ABO) (Rh) P56.0
|||other specified nonhemolytic disease NEC
P83.2
|||Rh incompatibility P56.0
||during pregnancy *see* Pregnancy,
complicated by, hydrops, fetalis
|gallbladder K82.1
|joint *see* Effusion, joint
|labyrinth H81.0-
|newborn (idiopathic) P83.2
||due to
|||ABO isoimmunization P56.0
|||alpha thalassemia D56.0
|||hemolytic disease P56.90
||||specified NEC P56.99
|||isoimmunization (ABO) (Rh) P56.0
|||Rh incompatibility P56.0
|nutritional *see* Malnutrition, severe
|pericardium *see* Pericarditis
|pleura *see* Hydrothorax
|spermatic cord *see* Hydrocele
Hydropyonephrosis N13.6
Hydrorachis Q06.4
Hydrorrhea (nasal) J34.89
|pregnancy *see* Rupture, membranes,
premature
Hydrosadenitis (axillaris) (suppurative) L73.2
Hydrosalpinx (fallopian tube) (follicularis)
N70.11
Hydrothorax (double) (pleura) J94.8
|chylous (nonfilarial) I89.8
||filarial *see also* Infestation, filarial B74.9
[*J91.8*]
|traumatic *see* Injury, intrathoracic
|tuberculous NEC (non primary) A15.6

Hydroureter *see also* Hydronephrosis N13.4
|with infection N13.6
|congenital Q62.39
Hydroureteronephrosis *see* Hydronephrosis
Hydrourethra N36.8
Hydroxykynureninuria E70.89
Hydroxylysinemia E72.3
Hydroxyprolinemia E72.59
Hygiene, sleep
|abuse Z72.821
|inadequate Z72.821
|poor Z72.821
Hygroma (congenital) (cystic) D18.1
|praepatellare, prepatellar *see* Bursitis,
prepatellar
Hymen *see* condition
Hymenolepis, hymenolepiasis (diminuta)
(infection) (infestation) (nana) B71.0
Hypalgesia R20.8
Hyperacidity (gastric) K31.89
|psychogenic F45.8
Hyperactive, hyperactivity F90.9
|basal cell, uterine cervix *see* Dysplasia, cervix
|bowel sounds R19.12
|cervix epithelial (basal) *see* Dysplasia, cervix
|child F90.9
|attention deficit *see* Disorder, attention-
deficit hyperactivity
|detrusor muscle N32.81
|gastrointestinal K31.89
|psychogenic F45.8
|nasal mucous membrane J34.3
|stomach K31.89
|thyroid (gland) *see* Hyperthyroidism
Hyperacusis H93.23-
Hyperadrenalism E27.5
Hyperadrenocorticism E24.9
|congenital E25.0
|iatrogenic E24.2
|correct substance properly administered *see*
Table of Drugs and Chemicals, by drug,
adverse effect
|overdose or wrong substance given or taken
see Table of Drugs and Chemicals, by
drug, poisoning
|not associated with Cushing's syndrome E27.0
|pituitary-dependent E24.0
Hyperaldosteronism E26.9
|familial (type I) E26.02
|glucocorticoid-remediable E26.02
|primary (due to (bilateral) adrenal
hyperplasia) E26.09
|primary NEC E26.09
|secondary E26.1
|specified NEC E26.89
Hyperalgesia R20.8
Hyperalimentation R63.2
|carotene, carotin E67.1
|specified NEC E67.8
|vitamin
|A E67.0
|D E67.3
Hyperaminoaciduria arginine E72.21
|cystine E72.01
|lysine E72.3
|ornithine E72.4
Hyperammonemia (congenital) E72.20
Hyperazotemia *see* Uremia
Hyperbetalipoproteinemia (familial) E78.00
|with prebetalipoproteinemia E78.2
Hyperbicarbonatemia P74.41
Hyperbilirubinemia
|constitutional E80.6
|familial conjugated E80.6
|neonatal (transient) *see* Jaundice, newborn
Hypercalcemia, hypocalciuric, familial E83.52
Hypercalciuria, idiopathic R82.994

Hypercapnia R06.89
|newborn P84
Hypercarotenemia (dietary) E67.1
Hypercementosis K03.4
Hyperchloremia E87.8
Hyperchlorhydria K31.89
|neurotic F45.8
|psychogenic F45.8
Hypercholesterinemia *see*
Hypercholesterolemia
Hypercholesterolemia (essential) (primary)
(pure) E78.00
|with hyperglyceridemia, endogenous E78.2
|dietary counseling and surveillance Z71.3
|familial E78.01
|hereditary E78.01
Hyperchylia gastrica, psychogenic F45.8
Hyperchylomicronemia (familial) (primary)
E78.3
|with hyperbetalipoproteinemia E78.3
Hypercoagulable (state) D68.59
|activated protein C resistance D68.51
|antithrombin (III) deficiency D68.59
|factor V Leiden mutation D68.51
|primary NEC D68.59
|protein C deficiency D68.59
|protein S deficiency D68.59
|prothrombin gene mutation D68.52
|secondary D68.69
|specified NEC D68.69
Hypercoagulation (state) D68.59
Hypercorticalism, pituitary-Dependent E24.0
Hypercorticosolism *see* Cushing's, syndrome
Hypercorticosteronism E24.2
|correct substance properly administered *see*
Table of Drugs and Chemicals, by drug,
adverse effect
|overdose or wrong substance given or taken
see Table of Drugs and Chemicals, by
drug, poisoning
Hypercortisonism E24.2
|correct substance properly administered *see*
Table of Drugs and Chemicals, by drug,
adverse effect
|overdose or wrong substance given or taken
see Table of Drugs and Chemicals, by
drug, poisoning
Hyperekplexia Q89.8
Hyperelectrolytemia E87.8
Hyperemesis R11.10
|with nausea R11.2
|gravidarum (mild) O21.0
|with
|carbohydrate depletion O21.1
|dehydration O21.1
|electrolyte imbalance O21.1
|metabolic disturbance O21.1
|severe (with metabolic disturbance) O21.1
|projectile R11.12
|psychogenic F45.8
Hyperemia (acute) (passive) R68.89
|anal mucosa K62.89
|bladder N32.89
|cerebral I67.89
|conjunctiva H11.43-
|ear internal, acute *see* subcategory H83.0
|enteric K59.89
|eye *see* Hyperemia, conjunctiva
|eyelid (active) (passive) *see* Disorder, eyelid,
specified type NEC
|intestine K59.89
|iris *see* Disorder, iris, vascular
|kidney N28.89
|labyrinth *see* subcategory H83.0
|liver (active) K76.89

Hyperemia - *continued*
|lung (passive) *see* Edema, lung
|pulmonary (passive) *see* Edema, lung
|renal N28.89
|retina H35.89
|stomach K31.89
Hyperesthesia (body surface) R20.3
|larynx (reflex) J38.7
|hysterical F44.89
|pharynx (reflex) J39.2
|hysterical F44.89
Hyperestrogenism (drug-Induced)
(iatrogenic) E28.0
Hyperexplexia Q89.8
Hyperfibrinolysis *see* Fibrinolysis
Hyperfructosemia E74.19
Hyperfunction
|adrenal cortex, not associated with Cushing's
syndrome E27.0
|medulla E27.5
|adrenomedullary E27.5
|virilism E25.9
|congenital E25.0
|ovarian E28.8
|pancreas K86.89
|parathyroid (gland) E21.3
|pituitary (gland) (anterior) E22.9
|specified NEC E22.8
|polyglandular E31.1
|testicular E29.0
Hypergammaglobulinemia D89.2
|polyclonal D89.0
|Waldenström D89.0
Hypergastrinemia E16.4
Hyperglobulinemia R77.1
Hyperglycemia, hyperglycemic (transient)
R73.9
|coma *see* Diabetes, by type, with coma
|postpancreatectomy E89.1
Hyperglyceridemia (endogenous) (essential)
(familial) (hereditary) (pure) E78.1
|mixed E78.3
Hyperglycinemia (non-Ketotic) E72.51
Hypergonadism
|ovarian E28.8
|testicular (primary) (infantile) E29.0
Hyperheparinemia D68.32
Hyperhidrosis, hyperidrosis R61
|focal
|primary L74.519
|axilla L74.510
|face L74.511
|palms L74.512
|soles L74.513
|secondary L74.52
|generalized R61
|localized
|primary L74.519
|axilla L74.510
|face L74.511
|palms L74.512
|soles L74.513
|secondary L74.52
|psychogenic F45.8
|secondary R61
|focal L74.52
Hyperhistidinemia E70.41
Hyperhomocysteinemia E72.11
Hyperhydroxyprolinemia E72.59
Hyperinsulinism (functional) E16.1
|with
|coma (hypoglycemic) E15
|encephalopathy E16.1 [*G94*]
|ectopic E16.1
|therapeutic misadventure (from administration
of insulin) *see* subcategory T38.3

Hyperkalemia E87.5
Hyperkeratosis *see also* Keratosis L85.9
 |cervix N88.0
 |due to yaws (early) (late) (palmar or plantar) A66.3
 |follicularis Q82.8
   |penetrans (in cutem) L87.0
 |palmoplantaris climacterica L85.1
 |pinta A67.1
 |senile (with pruritus) L57.0
 |universalis congenita Q80.8
 |vocal cord J38.3
 |vulva N90.4
Hyperkinesia, hyperkinetic (disease) (reaction) (syndrome) (childhood) (adolescence) *see also* Disorder, attention-deficit hyperactivity
 |heart I51.89
Hyperleucine-Isoleucinemia E71.19
Hyperlipemia, hyperlipidemia E78.5
 |combined E78.2
   |familial E78.49
 |group
   |A E78.00
   |B E78.1
   |C E78.2
   |D E78.3
 |mixed E78.2
 |specified NEC E78.49
Hyperlipidosis E75.6
 |hereditary NEC E75.5
Hyperlipoproteinemia E78.5
 |Fredrickson's type
   |I E78.3
   |IIa E78.00
   |IIb E78.2
   |III E78.2
   |IV E78.1
   |V E78.3
 |low-density-lipoprotein-type (LDL) E78.00
 |very-low-density-lipoprotein-type (VLDL) E78.1
Hyperlucent lung, unilateral J43.0
Hyperlysinemia E72.3
Hypermagnesemia E83.41
 |neonatal P71.8
Hypermenorrhea N92.0
Hypermethioninemia E72.19
Hypermetropia (congenital) H52.0-
Hypermobility, hypermotility
 |cecum *see* Syndrome, irritable bowel
 |coccyx *see* subcategory M53.2
 |colon *see* Syndrome, irritable bowel
   |psychogenic F45.8
 |ileum K58.9
 |intestine *see also* Syndrome, irritable bowel K58.9
   |psychogenic F45.8
 |meniscus (knee) *see* Derangement, knee, meniscus
 |scapula *see* Instability, joint, shoulder
 |stomach K31.89
   |psychogenic F45.8
 |syndrome M35.7
 |urethra N36.41
   |with intrinsic sphincter deficiency N36.43
Hypernasality R49.21
Hypernatremia E87.0
Hypernephroma C64.
Hyperopia *see* Hypermetropia
Hyperorexia nervosa F50.2
Hyperornithinemia E72.4
Hyperosmia R43.1
Hyperosmolality E87.0

Hyperostosis (monomelic) *see also* Disorder, bone, density and structure, specified NEC
 |ankylosing (spine) M48.10
   |cervical region M48.12
   |cervicothoracic region M48.13
   |lumbar region M48.16
   |lumbosacral region M48.17
   |multiple sites M48.19
   |occipito-atlanto-axial region M48.11
   |sacrococcygeal region M48.18
   |thoracic region M48.14
   |thoracolumbar region M48.15
 |cortical (skull) M85.2
   |infantile M89.8X-
 |frontal, internal of skull M85.2
 |interna frontalis M85.2
 |skeletal, diffuse idiopathic *see* Hyperostosis, ankylosing
 |skull M85.2
   |congenital Q75.8
 |vertebral, ankylosing *see* Hyperostosis, ankylosing
Hyperovarism E28.8
Hyperoxaluria (primary) R82.992
 |primary E72.53
Hyperparathyroidism E21.3
 |primary E21.0
 |secondary (renal) N25.81
   |non-renal E21.1
 |specified NEC E21.2
 |tertiary E21.2
Hyperpathia R20.8
Hyperperistalsis R19.2
 |psychogenic F45.8
Hyperpermeability, capillary I78.8
Hyperphagia R63.2
Hyperphenylalaninemia NEC E70.1
Hyperphoria (alternating) H50.53
Hyperphosphatemia E83.39
Hyperpiesis, hyperpiesia *see* Hypertension
Hyperpigmentation *see also* Pigmentation
 |melanin NEC L81.4
 |postinflammatory L81.0
Hyperpinealism E34.8
Hyperpituitarism E22.9
Hyperplasia, hyperplastic
 |adenoids J35.2
 |adrenal (capsule) (cortex) (gland) E27.8
   |with
     |sexual precocity (male) E25.9
       |congenital E25.0
     |virilism, adrenal E25.9
       |congenital E25.0
     |virilization (female) E25.9
       |congenital E25.0
   |congenital E25.0
   |salt-losing E25.0
 |adrenomedullary E27.5
 |angiolymphoid, eosinophilia (ALHE) D18.01
 |appendix (lymphoid) K38.0
 |artery, fibromuscular I77.3
 |bone *see also* Hypertrophy, bone
   |marrow D75.89
 |breast *see also* Hypertrophy, breast
   |ductal (atypical) N60.9-
 |C-cell, thyroid E07.0
 |cementation (tooth) (teeth) K03.4
 |cervical gland R59.0
 |cervix (uteri) (basal cell) (endometrium) (polypoid) *see also* Dysplasia, cervix
   |congenital Q51.828
 |clitoris, congenital Q52.6
 |denture K06.2
 |endocervicitis N72

Hyperplasia, hyperplastic - *continued*
 |endometrium, endometrial (adenomatous) (benign) (cystic) (glandular) (glandular-cystic) (polypoid) N85.00
   |with atypia N85.02
   |cervix *see* Dysplasia, cervix
   |complex (without atypia) N85.01
   |simple (without atypia) N85.01
 |epithelial L85.9
   |focal, oral, including tongue K13.29
   |nipple N62
   |skin L85.9
   |tongue K13.29
   |vaginal wall N89.3
 |erythroid D75.89
 |fibromuscular of artery (carotid) (renal) I77.3
 |genital
   |female NEC N94.89
   |male N50.89
 |gingiva K06.1
 |glandularis cystica uteri (interstitialis) *see also* Hyperplasia, endometrial N85.00-
 |gum K06.1
 |hymen, congenital Q52.4
 |irritative, edentulous (alveolar) K06.2
 |jaw M26.09
   |alveolar M26.79
   |lower M26.03
     |alveolar M26.72
   |upper M26.01
     |alveolar M26.71
 |kidney (congenital) Q63.3
 |labia N90.69
   |epithelial N90.3
 |liver (congenital) Q44.7
   |nodular, focal K76.89
 |lymph gland or node R59.9
 |mandible, mandibular M26.03
   |alveolar M26.72
   |unilateral condylar M27.8
 |maxilla, maxillary M26.01
   |alveolar M26.71
 |myometrium, myometrial N85.2
 |neuroendocrine cell, of infancy J84.841
 |nose
   |lymphoid J34.89
   |polypoid J33.9
 |oral mucosa (irritative) K13.6
 |organ or site, congenital NEC *see* Anomaly, by site
 |ovary N83.8
 |palate, papillary (irritative) K13.6
 |pancreatic islet cells E16.9
   |alpha E16.8
     |with excess
       |gastrin E16.4
       |glucagon E16.3
   |beta E16.1
 |parathyroid (gland) E21.0
 |pharynx (lymphoid) J39.2
 |prostate (adenofibromatous) (nodular) N40.0
   |with lower urinary tract symptoms (LUTS) N40.1
   |without lower urinary tract symptoms (LUTS) N40.0
 |renal artery I77.89
 |reticulo-endothelial (cell) D75.89
 |salivary gland (any) K11.1
 |Schimmelbusch's *see* Mastopathy, cystic
 |suprarenal capsule (gland) E27.8
 |thymus (gland) (persistent) E32.0
 |thyroid (gland) *see* Goiter
 |tonsils (faucial) (infective) (lingual) (lymphoid) J35.1
   |with adenoids J35.3

Hyperplasia, hyperplastic - *continued*
  |unilateral condylar M27.8
  |uterus, uterine N85.2
    |endometrium (glandular) *see also*
      Hyperplasia, endometrial N85.00-
  |vulva N90.69
    |epithelial N90.3
Hyperpnea *see* Hyperventilation
Hyperpotassemia E87.5
Hyperprebetalipoproteinemia (familial) E78.1
Hyperprolactinemia E22.1
Hyperprolinemia (type I) (type II) E72.59
Hyperproteinemia E88.09
Hyperprothrombinemia, causing coagulation
    factor deficiency D68.4
Hyperpyrexia R50.9
  |heat (effects) T67.0
  |malignant, due to anesthetic T88.3
  |rheumatic *see* Fever, rheumatic
  |unknown origin R50.9
Hyper-Reflexia R29.2
Hypersalivation K11.7
Hypersecretion
  |ACTH (not associated with Cushing's
    syndrome) E27.0
    |pituitary E24.0
  |adrenaline E27.5
  |adrenomedullary E27.5
  |androgen (testicular) E29.0
    |ovarian (drug-induced) (iatrogenic) E28.1
  |calcitonin E07.0
  |catecholamine E27.5
  |corticoadrenal E24.9
  |cortisol E24.9
  |epinephrine E27.5
  |estrogen E28.0
  |gastric K31.89
    |psychogenic F45.8
  |gastrin E16.4
  |glucagon E16.3
  |hormone(s)
    |ACTH (not associated with Cushing's
      syndrome) E27.0
      |pituitary E24.0
    |antidiuretic E22.2
    |growth E22.0
    |intestinal NEC E34.1
    |ovarian androgen E28.1
    |pituitary E22.9
    |testicular E29.0
    |thyroid stimulating E05.80
      |with thyroid storm E05.81
  |insulin *see* Hyperinsulinism
  |lacrimal glands *see* Epiphora
  |medulloadrenal E27.5
  |milk O92.6
  |ovarian androgens E28.1
  |salivary gland (any) K11.7
  |thyrocalcitonin E07.0
  |upper respiratory J39.8
Hypersegmentation, leukocytic, hereditary
  D72.0
Hypersensitive, hypersensitiveness,
  hypersensitivity *see also* Allergy
  |carotid sinus G90.01
  |colon *see* Irritable, colon
  |drug T88.7
  |gastrointestinal K52.29
    |immediate K52.29
    |psychogenic F45.8
  |labyrinth *see* subcategory H83.2
  |pain R20.8
  |pneumonitis *see* Pneumonitis, allergic
  |reaction T78.40
    |upper respiratory tract NEC J39.3

Hypersomnia (organic) G47.10
  |due to
    |alcohol
      |abuse F10.182
      |dependence F10.282
      |use F10.982
    |amphetamines
      |abuse F15.182
      |dependence F15.282
      |use F15.982
    |caffeine
      |abuse F15.182
      |dependence F15.282
      |use F15.982
    |cocaine
      |abuse F14.182
      |dependence F14.282
      |use F14.982
    |drug NEC
      |abuse F19.182
      |dependence F19.282
      |use F19.982
    |medical condition G47.14
    |mental disorder F51.13
    |opioid
      |abuse F11.182
      |dependence F11.282
      |use F11.982
    |psychoactive substance NEC
      |abuse F19.182
      |dependence F19.282
      |use F19.982
    |sedative, hypnotic, or anxiolytic
      |abuse F13.182
      |dependence F13.282
      |use F13.982
    |stimulant NEC
      |abuse F15.182
      |dependence F15.282
      |use F15.982
  |idiopathic G47.11
    |with long sleep time G47.11
    |without long sleep time G47.12
  |menstrual related G47.13
  |nonorganic origin F51.11
    |specified NEC F51.19
  |not due to a substance or known physiological
    condition F51.11
    |specified NEC F51.19
  |primary F51.11
  |recurrent G47.13
  |specified NEC G47.19
Hypersplenia, hypersplenism D73.1
Hyperstimulation, ovaries (associated with
  induced ovulation) N98.1
Hypersusceptibility *see* Allergy
Hypertelorism (ocular) (orbital) Q75.2
Hypertension, hypertensive (accelerated)
  (benign) (essential) (idiopathic)
  (malignant) (systemic) I10
  |with
    |heart failure (congestive) I11.0
    |heart involvement (conditions in I50.- or
      I51.4-I51.7, I51.89, I51.9, due to
      hypertension) *see* Hypertension, Heart
    |kidney involvement *see* Hypertension,
      kidney
  |benign, intracranial G93.2
  |borderline R03.0
  |cardiorenal (disease) I13.10
    |with heart failure I13.0
      |with stage 1 through stage 4 chronic
        kidney disease I13.0
      |with stage 5 or end stage renal disease
        I13.2

Hypertension, hypertensive - *continued*
  |without heart failure I13.10
    |with stage 1 through stage 4 chronic
      kidney disease I13.10
    |with stage 5 or end stage renal disease
      I13.11
  |cardiovascular
    |disease (arteriosclerotic) (sclerotic) *see*
      Hypertension, heart
    |renal (disease) *see* Hypertension,
      cardiorenal
  |chronic venous *see* Hypertension, venous
    (chronic)
  |complicating
    |childbirth (labor) O16.4
      |pre-existing O10.92
        |with
          |heart disease O10.12
            |with renal disease O10.32
          |pre-eclampsia O11.4
          |renal disease O10.22
            |with heart disease O10.32
        |essential O10.02
      |secondary O10.42
    |pregnancy O16.-
      |with edema *see also* Pre-eclampsia O14.9-
      |gestational (pregnancy induced) (without
        proteinuria) O13.-
        |with proteinuria O14.9-
          |mild pre-eclampsia O14.0-
          |moderate pre-eclampsia O14.0-
          |severe pre-eclampsia O14.1-
            |with hemolysis, elevated liver
              enzymes and low platelet count
              (HELLP) O14.2-
      |pre-existing O10.91-
        |with
          |heart disease O10.11-
            |with renal disease O10.31-
          |pre-eclampsia *see* category O11
          |renal disease O10.21-
            |with heart disease O10.31-
        |essential O10.01-
        |secondary O10.41-
    |transient O13.-
    |puerperium, pre-existing O16.5
      |pre-existing
        |with
          |heart disease O10.13
            |with renal disease O10.33
          |pre-eclampsia O11.5
          |renal disease O10.23
            |with heart disease O10.33
        |essential O10.03
    |pregnancy-induced O13.9
    |secondary O10.43
  |crisis I16.9
  |due to
    |endocrine disorders I15.2
    |pheochromocytoma I15.2
    |renal disorders NEC I15.1
      |arterial I15.0
    |renovascular disorders I15.0
    |specified disease NEC I15.8
  |emergency I16.1
  |encephalopathy I67.4
  |gestational (without significant proteinuria)
    (pregnancy-induced) (transient) O13.-
    |with significant proteinuria *see* Pre-
      eclampsia
    |complicating
      |delivery O13.4
      |puerperium O13.5
  |Goldblatt's I70.1

Hypertension, hypertensive - *continued*
|heart (disease) (conditions in I51.4-I51.9 due to hypertension) I11.9
| |with
| | |heart failure (congestive) I11.0
| | |kidney disease (chronic) *see* Hypertension, cardiorenal
|intracranial benign G93.2
|kidney I12.9
| |with
| | |heart disease *see* Hypertension, cardiorenal
| | |stage 5 chronic kidney disease (CKD) or end stage renal disease (ESRD) I12.0
| | |stage 1 through stage 4 chronic kidney disease I12.9
|lesser circulation I27.0
|maternal O16.-
|newborn P29.2
| |pulmonary (persistent) P29.30
|ocular H40.05-
|pancreatic duct   code to underlying condition
| |with chronic pancreatitis K86.1
|portal (due to chronic liver disease) (idiopathic) K76.6
| |gastropathy K31.89
| |in (due to) schistosomiasis (bilharziasis) B65.9 [*K77*]
|postoperative I97.3
|psychogenic F45.8
|pulmonary I27.20
| |with
| | |cor pulmonale (chronic) I27.29
| | | |acute I26.09
| | |right heart ventricular strain/failure I27.29
| | | |acute I26.09
| | |right to left shunt related to congenital heart disease I27.83
| | |unclear multifactorial mechanisms I27.29
| |arterial (associated) (drug-induced) (toxin-induced) I27.21
| |chronic thromboembolic I27.24
| |due to
| | |hematologic disorders I27.29
- - - kyphoscoliotic heart disease I27.1
| | |left heart disease I27.22
| | |lung diseases and hypoxia I27.23
| | |metabolic disorders I27.29
| | |specified systemic disorders NEC I27.29
| |group 1 (associated) (drug-induced) (toxin-induced) I27.21
| |group 2 I27.22
| |group 3 I27.23
| |group 4 I27.24
| |group 5 I27.29
| |of newborn (persistent) P29.30
| |primary (idiopathic) I27.0
| |secondary
| | |arterial I27.21
| | |specified NEC I27.29
|renal *see* Hypertension, kidney
|renovascular I15.0
|secondary NEC I15.9
| |due to
| | |endocrine disorders I15.2
| | |pheochromocytoma I15.2
| | |renal disorders NEC I15.1
| | | |arterial I15.0
| | |renovascular disorders I15.0
| |specified NEC I15.8
|transient R03.0
| |of pregnancy O13.-
|urgency I16.0
|venous (chronic)
| |due to

Hypertension, hypertensive - *continued*
| |deep vein thrombosis *see* Syndrome, postthrombotic
|idiopathic I87.309
| |with
| | |inflammation I87.32-
| | | |with ulcer I87.33-
| | |specified complication NEC I87.39-
| | |ulcer I87.31-
| | | |with inflammation I87.33-
| |asymptomatic I87.30-
Hypertensive urgency *see* Hypertension
Hyperthecosis ovary E28.8
Hyperthermia (of unknown origin) *see also* Hyperpyrexia
|malignant, due to anesthesia T88.3
|newborn P81.9
| |environmental P81.0
Hyperthyroid (recurrent) *see* Hyperthyroidism
Hyperthyroidism (latent) (pre-Adult) (recurrent) E05.90
|with
| |goiter (diffuse) E05.00
| | |with thyroid storm E05.01
| | |nodular (multinodular) E05.20
| | | |with thyroid storm E05.21
| | | |uninodular E05.10
| | | | |with thyroid storm E05.11
| |storm E05.91
|due to ectopic thyroid tissue E05.30
| |with thyroid storm E05.31
|neonatal, transitory P72.1
|specified NEC E05.80
| |with thyroid storm E05.81
Hypertony, hypertonia, hypertonicity
|bladder N31.8
|congenital P94.1
|stomach K31.89
| |psychogenic F45.8
|uterus, uterine (contractions) (complicating delivery) O62.4
Hypertrichosis L68.9
|congenital Q84.2
|eyelid H02.869
| |left H02.866
| | |lower H02.865
| | |upper H02.864
| |right H02.863
| | |lower H02.862
| | |upper H02.861
|lanuginosa Q84.2
| |acquired L68.1
|localized L68.2
|specified NEC L68.8
Hypertriglyceridemia, essential E78.1
Hypertrophy, hypertrophic
|adenofibromatous, prostate *see* Enlargement, enlarged, prostate
|adenoids (infective) J35.2
| |with tonsils J35.3
|adrenal cortex E27.8
|alveolar process or ridge *see* Anomaly, alveolar
|anal papillae K62.89
|artery I77.89
| |congenital NEC Q27.8
| | |digestive system Q27.8
| | |lower limb Q27.8
| | |specified site NEC Q27.8
| | |upper limb Q27.8
|auricular *see* Hypertrophy, cardiac
| |Bartholin's gland N75.8
|bile duct (common) (hepatic) K83.8
|bladder (sphincter) (trigone) N32.89
|bone M89.30

Hypertrophy, hypertrophic - *continued*
|carpus M89.34-
|clavicle M89.31-
|femur M89.35-
|fibula M89.36-
|finger M89.34-
|humerus M89.32-
|ilium M89.359
|ischium M89.359
|metacarpus M89.34-
|metatarsus M89.37-
|multiple sites M89.39
|neck M89.38
|radius M89.33-
|rib M89.38
|scapula M89.31-
|skull M89.38
|tarsus M89.37-
|tibia M89.36-
|toe M89.37-
|ulna M89.33-
|vertebra M89.38
|brain G93.89
|breast N62
| |cystic *see* Mastopathy, cystic
| |newborn P83.4
| |pubertal, massive N62
| |puerperal, postpartum *see* Disorder, breast, specified type NEC
| |senile (parenchymatous) N62
|cardiac (chronic) (idiopathic) I51.7
| |with rheumatic fever (conditions in I00)
| | |active I01.8
| | |inactive or quiescent (with chorea) I09.89
| |congenital NEC Q24.8
| |fatty *see* Degeneration, myocardial
| |hypertensive *see* Hypertension, heart
| |rheumatic (with chorea) I09.89
| | |active or acute I01.8
| | | |with chorea I02.0
| |valve *see* Endocarditis
|cartilage *see* Disorder, cartilage, specified type NEC
|cecum *see* Megacolon
|cervix (uteri) N88.8
| |congenital Q51.828
| |elongation N88.4
|clitoris (cirrhotic) N90.89
| |congenital Q52.6
|colon *see also* Megacolon
| |congenital Q43.2
|conjunctiva, lymphoid H11.89
|corpora cavernosa N48.89
|cystic duct K82.8
|duodenum K31.89
|endometrium (glandular) *see also* Hyperplasia, endometrial N85.00-
| |cervix N88.8
|epididymis N50.89
|esophageal hiatus (congenital) Q79.1
| |with hernia *see* Hernia, hiatal
|eyelid *see* Disorder, eyelid, specified type NEC
|facet joint (see also Spondylosis) M47.819
|fat pad E65
| |knee (infrapatellar) (popliteal) (prepatellar) (retropatellar) M79.4
|foot (congenital) Q74.2
|frenulum, frenum (tongue) K14.8
| |lip K13.0
|gallbladder K82.8
|gastric mucosa K29.60
| |with bleeding K29.61
|gland, glandular R59.9
| |generalized R59.1

Hypertrophy, hypertrophic - *continued*
|localized R59.0
|gum (mucous membrane) K06.1
|heart (idiopathic) *see also* Hypertrophy, cardiac
|valve *see also* Endocarditis I38
|hemifacial Q67.4
|hepatic *see* Hypertrophy, liver
|hiatus (esophageal) Q79.1
|hilus gland R59.0
|hymen, congenital Q52.4
|ileum K63.89
|intestine NEC K63.89
|jejunum K63.89
|kidney (compensatory) N28.81
|congenital Q63.3
|labium (majus) (minus) N90.60
|ligament *see* Disorder, ligament
|lingual tonsil (infective) J35.1
|with adenoids J35.3
|lip K13.0
|congenital Q18.6
|liver R16.0
|acute K76.89
|congenital Q44.7
|cirrhotic *see* Cirrhosis, liver
|fatty *see* Fatty, liver
|lymph, lymphatic gland R59.9
|generalized R59.1
|localized R59.0
|tuberculous *see* Tuberculosis, lymph gland
|mammary gland *see* Hypertrophy, breast
|Meckel's diverticulum (congenital) Q43.0
|malignant *see* Table of Neoplasms, small intestine, malignant
|median bar *see* Hyperplasia, prostate
|meibomian gland *see* Chalazion
|meniscus, knee, congenital Q74.1
|metatarsal head *see* Hypertrophy, bone, metatarsus
|metatarsus *see* Hypertrophy, bone, metatarsus
|mucous membrane
|alveolar ridge K06.2
|gum K06.1
|nose (turbinate) J34.3
|muscle M62.89
|muscular coat, artery I77.89
|myocardium *see also* Hypertrophy, cardiac
|idiopathic I42.2
|myometrium N85.2
|nail L60.2
|congenital Q84.5
|nasal J34.89
|alae J34.89
|bone J34.89
|cartilage J34.89
|mucous membrane (septum) J34.3
|sinus J34.89
|turbinate J34.3
|nasopharynx, lymphoid (infectional) (tissue) (wall) J35.2
|nipple N62
|organ or site, congenital NEC *see* Anomaly, by site
|ovary N83.8
|palate (hard) M27.8
|soft K13.79
|pancreas, congenital Q45.3
|parathyroid (gland) E21.0
|parotid gland K11.1
|penis N48.89
|pharyngeal tonsil J35.2
|pharynx J39.2
|lymphoid (infectional) (tissue) (wall) J35.2
|pituitary (anterior) (fossa) (gland) E23.6

Hypertrophy, hypertrophic - *continued*
|prepuce (congenital) N47.8
|female N90.89
|prostate *see* Enlargement, enlarged, prostate
|congenital Q55.4
|pseudomuscular G71.09
|pylorus (adult) (muscle) (sphincter) K31.1
|congenital or infantile Q40.0
|rectal, rectum (sphincter) K62.89
|rhinitis (turbinate) J31.0
|salivary gland (any) K11.1
|congenital Q38.4
|scaphoid (tarsal) *see* Hypertrophy, bone, tarsus
|scar L91.0
|scrotum N50.89
|seminal vesicle N50.89
|sigmoid *see* Megacolon
|skin L91.9
|specified NEC L91.8
|spermatic cord N50.89
|spleen *see* Splenomegaly
|spondylitis *see* Spondylosis
|stomach K31.89
|sublingual gland K11.1
|submandibular gland K11.1
|suprarenal cortex (gland) E27.8
|synovial NEC M67.20
|acromioclavicular M67.21-
|ankle M67.27-
|elbow M67.22-
|foot M67.27-
|hand M67.24-
|hip M67.25-
|knee M67.26-
|multiple sites M67.29
|specified site NEC M67.28
|wrist M67.23-
|tendon *see* Disorder, tendon, specified type NEC
|testis N44.8
|congenital Q55.29
|thymic, thymus (gland) (congenital) E32.0
|thyroid (gland) *see* Goiter
|toe (congenital) Q74.2
|acquired *see also* Deformity, toe, specified NEC
|tongue K14.8
|congenital Q38.2
|papillae (foliate) K14.3
|tonsils (faucial) (infective) (lingual) (lymphoid) J35.1
|with adenoids J35.3
|tunica vaginalis N50.89
|ureter N28.89
|urethra N36.8
|uterus N85.2
|neck (with elongation) N88.4
|puerperal O90.89
|uvula K13.79
|vagina N89.8
|vas deferens N50.89
|vein I87.8
|ventricle, ventricular (heart) *see also* Hypertrophy, cardiac
|congenital Q24.8
|in tetralogy of Fallot Q21.3
|verumontanum N36.8
|vocal cord J38.3
|vulva N90.60
|stasis (nonfilarial) N90.69
Hypertropia H50.2-
Hypertyrosinemia E70.21
Hyperuricemia (asymptomatic) E79.0
Hyperuricosuria R82.993

Hypervalinemia E71.19
Hyperventilation (tetany) R06.4
|hysterical F45.8
|psychogenic F45.8
|syndrome F45.8
Hypervitaminosis (dietary) NEC E67.8
|A E67.0
|administered as drug (prolonged intake) *see* Table of Drugs and Chemicals, vitamins, adverse effect
|overdose or wrong substance given or taken *see* Table of Drugs and Chemicals, vitamins, poisoning
|B6 E67.2
|D E67.3
|administered as drug (prolonged intake) *see* Table of Drugs and Chemicals, vitamins, adverse effect
|overdose or wrong substance given or taken *see* Table of Drugs and Chemicals, vitamins, poisoning
|K E67.8
|administered as drug (prolonged intake) *see* Table of Drugs and Chemicals, vitamins, adverse effect
|overdose or wrong substance given or taken *see* Table of Drugs and Chemicals, vitamins, poisoning
Hypervolemia E87.70
|specified NEC E87.79
Hypesthesia R20.1
|cornea *see* Anesthesia, cornea
Hyphema H21.0-
|traumatic S05.1-
Hypoacidity, gastric K31.89
|psychogenic F45.8
Hypoadrenalism, hypoadrenia E27.40
|primary E27.1
|tuberculous A18.7
Hypoadrenocorticism E27.40
|pituitary E23.0
|primary E27.1
Hypoalbuminemia E88.09
Hypoaldosteronism E27.40
Hypoalphalipoproteinemia E78.6
Hypobarism T70.29
Hypobaropathy T70.29
Hypobetalipoproteinemia (familial) E78.6
Hypocalcemia E83.51
|dietary E58
|neonatal P71.1
|due to cow's milk P71.0
|phosphate-loading (newborn) P71.1
Hypochloremia E87.8
Hypochlorhydria K31.89
|neurotic F45.8
|psychogenic F45.8
Hypochondria, hypochondriac, hypochondriasis (reaction) F45.21
|sleep F51.03
Hypochondrogenesis Q77.0
Hypochondroplasia Q77.4
Hypochromasia, blood cells D50.8
Hyperuricoscuria R82.993
Hypodontia *see* Anodontia
Hypoeosinophilia D72.89
Hypoesthesia R20.1
Hypofibrinogenemia D68.8
|acquired D65
|congenital (hereditary) D68.2
Hypofunction
|adrenocortical E27.40
|drug-induced E27.3
|postprocedural E89.6
|primary E27.1
|adrenomedullary, postprocedural E89.6
|cerebral R29.818

Hypofunction - *continued*
| corticoadrenal NEC E27.40
| intestinal K59.89
| labyrinth *see* subcategory H83.2
| ovary E28.39
| pituitary (gland) (anterior) E23.0
| testicular E29.1
| | postprocedural (postsurgical)
| | | (postirradiation) (iatrogenic) E89.5
Hypogalactia O92.4
Hypogammaglobulinemia *see also*
    Agammaglobulinemia D80.1
| hereditary D80.0
| nonfamilial D80.1
| transient, of infancy D80.7
Hypogenitalism (congenital) *see*
    Hypogonadism
Hypoglossia Q38.3
Hypoglycemia (spontaneous) E16.2
| coma E15
 diabetic *see* Diabetes, by type, with
   hypoglycemia, with coma
| diabetic *see* Diabetes, hypoglycemia
| dietary counseling and surveillance Z71.3
| drug-induced E16.0
| | with coma (nondiabetic) E15
| due to insulin E16.0
| | with coma (nondiabetic) E15
| | therapeutic misadventure *see* subcategory
| | | T38.3
| functional, nonhyperinsulinemic E16.1
| iatrogenic E16.0
| | with coma (nondiabetic) E15
| in infant of diabetic mother P70.1
| | gestational diabetes P70.0
| infantile E16.1
| leucine-induced E71.19
| neonatal (transitory) P70.4
| | iatrogenic P70.3
| reactive (not drug-induced) E16.1
| transitory neonatal P70.4
Hypogonadism
| female E28.39
| hypogonadotropic E23.0
| male E29.1
| ovarian (primary) E28.39
| pituitary E23.0
| testicular (primary) E29.1
Hypohidrosis, hypoidrosis L74.4
Hypoinsulinemia, postprocedural E89.1
Hypokalemia E87.6
Hypoleukocytosis *see* Agranulocytosis
Hypolipoproteinemia (alpha) (beta) E78.6
Hypomagnesemia E83.42
| neonatal P71.2
Hypomania, hypomanic reaction F30.8
Hypomenorrhea *see* Oligomenorrhea
Hypometabolism R63.8
Hypomotility
| gastrointestinal (tract) K31.89
| | psychogenic F45.8
| intestine K59.89
| | psychogenic F45.8
| stomach K31.89
| | psychogenic F45.8
Hyponasality R49.22
Hyponatremia E87.1
Hypo-Osmolality E87.1
Hypo-Ovarianism, hypo-Ovarism E28.39
Hypoparathyroidism E20.9
| familial E20.8
| idiopathic E20.0
| neonatal, transitory P71.4
| postprocedural E89.2
| specified NEC E20.8

Hypoperfusion (in)
| newborn P96.89
Hypopharyngitis *see* Laryngopharyngitis
Hypophoria H50.53
Hypophosphatemia, hypophosphatasia
    (acquired) (congenital) (renal) E83.39
| familial E83.31
Hypophyseal, hypophysis *see also* condition
| dwarfism E23.0
| gigantism E22.0
Hypoplasminogenemia E88.02
Hypopiesis *see* Hypotension
Hypopinealism E34.8
Hypopituitarism (juvenile) E23.0
| drug-induced E23.1
| due to
| | hypophysectomy E89.3
| | radiotherapy E89.3
| iatrogenic NEC E23.1
| postirradiation E89.3
| postpartum O99.285
| postprocedural E89.3
Hypoplasia, hypoplastic
| adrenal (gland), congenital Q89.1
| alimentary tract, congenital Q45.8
| | upper Q40.8
| anus, anal (canal) Q42.3
| | with fistula Q42.2
| aorta, aortic Q25.42
| | ascending, in hypoplastic left heart
| | | syndrome Q23.4
| | valve Q23.1
| | | in hypoplastic left heart syndrome Q23.4
| areola, congenital Q83.8
| arm (congenital) *see* Defect, reduction, upper
| | limb
| artery (peripheral) Q27.8
| | brain (congenital) Q28.3
| | coronary Q24.5
| | digestive system Q27.8
| | lower limb Q27.8
| | pulmonary Q25.79
| | | functional, unilateral J43.0
| | retinal (congenital) Q14.1
| | specified site NEC Q27.8
| | umbilical Q27.0
| | upper limb Q27.8
| auditory canal Q17.8
| | causing impairment of hearing Q16.9
| biliary duct or passage Q44.5
| bone NOS Q79.9
| | face Q75.8
| | marrow D61.9
| | | megakaryocytic D69.49
| | skull *see* Hypoplasia, skull
| brain Q02
| | gyri Q04.3
| | part of Q04.3
| breast (areola) N64.82
| bronchus Q32.4
| cardiac Q24.8
| carpus *see* Defect, reduction, upper limb,
| | specified type NEC
| cartilage hair Q78.8
| cecum Q42.8
| cementum K00.4
| cephalic Q02
| cerebellum Q04.3
| cervix (uteri), congenital Q51.821
| clavicle (congenital) Q74.0
| coccyx Q76.49
| colon Q42.9
| | specified NEC Q42.8
| corpus callosum Q04.0

Hypoplasia, hypoplastic - *continued*
| cricoid cartilage Q31.2
| digestive organ(s) or tract NEC Q45.8
| | upper (congenital) Q40.8
| ear (auricle) (lobe) Q17.2
| | middle Q16.4
| enamel of teeth (neonatal) (postnatal)
| | (prenatal) K00.4
| endocrine (gland) NEC Q89.2
| endometrium N85.8
| epididymis (congenital) Q55.4
| epiglottis Q31.2
| erythroid, congenital D61.01
| esophagus (congenital) Q39.8
| eustachian tube Q17.8
| eye Q11.2
| eyelid (congenital) Q10.3
| face Q18.8
| | bone(s) Q75.8
| femur (congenital) *see* Defect, reduction,
| | lower limb, specified type NEC
| fibula (congenital) *see* Defect, reduction,
| | lower limb, specified type NEC
| finger (congenital) *see* Defect, reduction,
| | upper limb, specified type NEC
| focal dermal Q82.8
| foot *see* Defect, reduction, lower limb,
| | specified type NEC
| gallbladder Q44.0
| genitalia, genital organ(s)
| | female, congenital Q52.8
| | | external Q52.79
| | | internal NEC Q52.8
| | in adiposogenital dystrophy E23.6
| glottis Q31.2
| hair Q84.2
| hand (congenital) *see* Defect, reduction, upper
| | limb, specified type NEC
| heart Q24.8
| humerus (congenital) *see* Defect, reduction,
| | upper limb, specified type NEC
| intestine (small) Q41.9
| | large Q42.9
| | | specified NEC Q42.8
| jaw M26.09
| | alveolar M26.79
| | lower M26.04
| | | alveolar M26.74
| | upper M26.02
| | | alveolar M26.73
| kidney(s) Q60.5
| | bilateral Q60.4
| | unilateral Q60.3
| labium (majus) (minus), congenital Q52.79
| larynx Q31.2
| left heart syndrome Q23.4
| leg (congenital) *see* Defect, reduction, lower
| | limb
| limb Q73.8
| | lower (congenital) *see* Defect, reduction,
| | | lower limb
| | upper (congenital) *see* Defect, reduction,
| | | upper limb
| liver Q44.7
| lung (lobe) (not associated with short
| | gestation) Q33.6
| | associated with immaturity, low birth
| | | weight, prematurity, or short gestation
| | | P28.0
| mammary (areola), congenital Q83.8
| mandible, mandibular M26.04
| | alveolar M26.74
| | unilateral condylar M27.8
| maxillary M26.02
| | alveolar M26.73

Hypoplasia, hypoplastic - *continued*
|medullary D61.9
|megakaryocytic D69.49
|metacarpus *see* Defect, reduction, upper limb,
    specified type NEC
|metatarsus *see* Defect, reduction, lower limb,
    specified type NEC
|muscle Q79.8
|nail(s) Q84.6
|nose, nasal Q30.1
|optic nerve H47.03-
|osseous meatus (ear) Q17.8
|ovary, congenital Q50.39
|pancreas Q45.0
|parathyroid (gland) Q89.2
|parotid gland Q38.4
|patella Q74.1
|pelvis, pelvic girdle Q74.2
|penis (congenital) Q55.62
|peripheral vascular system Q27.8
    |digestive system Q27.8
    |lower limb Q27.8
    |specified site NEC Q27.8
    |upper limb Q27.8
|pituitary (gland) (congenital) Q89.2
|pulmonary (not associated with short
    gestation) Q33.6
    |artery, functional J43.0
    |associated with short gestation P28.0
|radioulnar *see* Defect, reduction, upper limb,
    specified type NEC
|radius *see* Defect, reduction, upper limb
|rectum Q42.1
    |with fistula Q42.0
|respiratory system NEC Q34.8
|rib Q76.6
|right heart syndrome Q22.6
|sacrum Q76.49
|scapula Q74.0
|scrotum Q55.1
|shoulder girdle Q74.0
|skin Q82.8
|skull (bone) Q75.8
    |with
        |anencephaly Q00.0
        |encephalocele *see* Encephalocele
        |hydrocephalus Q03.9
            |with spina bifida *see* Spina bifida, by
                site, with hydrocephalus
        |microcephaly Q02
|spinal (cord) (ventral horn cell) Q06.1
|spine Q76.49
|sternum Q76.7
|tarsus *see* Defect, reduction, lower limb,
    specified type NEC
|testis Q55.1
|thymic, with immunodeficiency D82.1
|thymus (gland) Q89.2
    |with immunodeficiency D82.1
|thyroid (gland) E03.1
    |cartilage Q31.2
|tibiofibular (congenital) *see* Defect, reduction,
    lower limb, specified type NEC
|toe *see* Defect, reduction, lower limb,
    specified type NEC
|tongue Q38.3
|Turner's K00.4
|ulna (congenital) *see* Defect, reduction, upper
    limb
|umbilical artery Q27.0
|unilateral condylar M27.8
|ureter Q62.8
|uterus, congenital Q51.811
|vagina Q52.4
|vascular NEC peripheral Q27.8

Hypoplasia, hypoplastic - *continued*
|brain Q28.3
|digestive system Q27.8
|lower limb Q27.8
|specified site NEC Q27.8
|upper limb Q27.8
|vein(s) (peripheral) Q27.8
    |brain Q28.3
    |digestive system Q27.8
    |great Q26.8
    |lower limb Q27.8
    |specified site NEC Q27.8
    |upper limb Q27.8
|vena cava (inferior) (superior) Q26.8
|vertebra Q76.49
|vulva, congenital Q52.79
|zonule (ciliary) Q12.8
Hypopnea, obstructive sleep apnea G47.33
Hypopotassemia E87.6
Hypoproconvertinemia, congenital
    (hereditary) D68.2
Hypoproteinemia E77.8
Hypoprothrombinemia (congenital)
    (hereditary) (idiopathic) D68.2
|acquired D68.4
|newborn, transient P61.6
Hypoptyalism K11.7
Hypopyon (eye) (anterior chamber) *see*
    Iridocyclitis, acute, hypopyon
Hypopyrexia R68.0
Hyporeflexia R29.2
Hyposecretion
|ACTH E23.0
|antidiuretic hormone E23.2
|ovary E28.39
|salivary gland (any) K11.7
|vasopressin E23.2
Hyposegmentation, leukocytic, hereditary
    D72.0
Hyposiderinemia D50.9
Hypospadias Q54.9
|balanic Q54.0
|coronal Q54.0
|glandular Q54.0
|penile Q54.1
|penoscrotal Q54.2
|perineal Q54.3
|specified NEC Q54.8
Hypospermatogenesis *see* Oligospermia
Hyposplenism D73.0
Hypostasis pulmonary, passive *see* Edema,
    lung
Hypostatic *see* condition
Hyposthenuria N28.89
Hypotension (arterial) (constitutional) I95.9
|chronic I95.89
|due to (of) hemodialysis I95.3
|drug-induced I95.2
|iatrogenic I95.89
|idiopathic (permanent) I95.0
|intracranial G96.810
    |following
        |lumbar cerebrospinal fluid shunting
            G97.83
        |specified procedure NEC G97.84
        |ventricular shunting (ventriculostomy)
            G97.2
    |specified NEC G96.819
    |spontaneous G96.811
|intra-dialytic I95.3
|maternal, syndrome (following labor and
    delivery) O26.5-
|neurogenic, orthostatic G90.3
|orthostatic (chronic) I95.1
    |due to drugs I95.2
    |neurogenic G90.3

Hypotension - *continued*
|postoperative I95.81
|postural I95.1
|specified NEC I95.89
Hypothermia (accidental) T68
|due to anesthesia, anesthetic T88.51
|low environmental temperature T68
|neonatal P80.9
    |environmental (mild) NEC P80.8
    |mild P80.8
    |severe (chronic) (cold injury syndrome)
        P80.0
    |specified NEC P80.8
|not associated with low environmental
    temperature R68.0
Hypothyroidism (acquired) E03.9
|autoimmune *see* Thyroiditis, autoimmune
|congenital (without goiter) E03.1
    |with goiter (diffuse) E03.0
|due to
    |exogenous substance NEC E03.2
    |iodine-deficiency, acquired E01.8
        |subclinical E02
    |irradiation therapy E89.0
    |medicament NEC E03.2
    |P-aminosalicylic acid (PAS) E03.2
    |phenylbutazone E03.2
    |resorcinol E03.2
    |sulfonamide E03.2
    |surgery E89.0
    |thiourea group drugs E03.2
|iatrogenic NEC E03.2
|iodine-deficiency (acquired) E01.8
    |congenital *see* Syndrome, iodine
    |deficiency, congenital
    |subclinical E02
|neonatal, transitory P72.2
|postinfectious E03.3
|postirradiation E89.0
|postprocedural E89.0
|postsurgical E89.0
|specified NEC E03.8
|subclinical, iodine-deficiency related E02
Hypotonia, hypotonicity, hypotony
|bladder N31.2
|congenital (benign) P94.2
|eye *see* Disorder, globe, hypotony
Hypotrichosis *see* Alopecia
Hypotropia H50.2-
Hypoventilation R06.89
|congenital central alveolar G47.35
|sleep related
    |idiopathic nonobstructive alveolar G47.34
    |in conditions classified elsewhere G47.36
Hypovitaminosis *see* Deficiency, vitamin
Hypovolemia E86.1
|surgical shock T81.19
|traumatic (shock) T79.4
Hypoxemia R09.02
|newborn P84
|sleep related, in conditions classified
    elsewhere G47.36
Hypoxia *see also* Anoxia R09.02
|cerebral, during a procedure NEC G97.81
    |postprocedural NEC G97.82
|intrauterine P84
|myocardial *see* Insufficiency, coronary
|newborn P84
|sleep-related G47.34
Hypsarhythmia *see* Epilepsy, generalized,
    specified NEC
Hysteralgia, pregnant uterus O26.89-

Hysteria, hysterical (conversion) (dissociative state) F44.9
|anxiety F41.8
|convulsions F44.5
|psychosis, acute F44.9
Hysteroepilepsy F44.5

I

IBDU (colonic inflammatory bowel disease unclassified) K52.3
ICANS (immune effector cell-associated neurotoxicity syndrome) - *see* Syndrome, immune effector cell- associated neurotoxicity
Ichthyoparasitism due to Vandellia cirrhosa B88.8
Ichthyosis (congenital) Q80.9
|acquired L85.0
|fetalis Q80.4
|hystrix Q80.8
|lamellar Q80.2
|lingual K13.29
|palmaris and plantaris Q82.8
|simplex Q80.0
|vera Q80.8
|vulgaris Q80.0
|X-linked Q80.1
Ichthyotoxism *see* Poisoning, fish
|bacterial *see* Intoxication, foodborne
Icteroanemia, hemolytic (acquired) D59.9
|congenital *see* Spherocytosis
Icterus *see also* Jaundice
|conjunctiva R17
|newborn P59.9
|gravis, newborn P55.0
|hematogenous (acquired) D59.9
|hemolytic (acquired) D59.9
|congenital *see* Spherocytosis
|hemorrhagic (acute) (leptospiral) (spirochetal) A27.0
|newborn P53
|infectious B15.9
|with hepatic coma B15.0
|leptospiral A27.0
|spirochetal A27.0
|neonatorum *see* Jaundice, newborn
|spirochetal A27.0
Ictus solaris, solis T67.0
Ideation
|homicidal R45.850
|suicidal R45.851
Identity disorder (child) F64.9
|gender role F64.2
|psychosexual F64.2
Id reaction (due to bacteria) L30.2
Idioglossia F80.0
Idiopathic *see* condition
Idiot, idiocy (congenital) F73
|amaurotic (Bielschowsky(-Jansky)) (family) (infantile (late)) (juvenile (late)) (Vogt-Spielmeyer) E75.4
|microcephalic Q02
IgE asthma J45.909
IIAC (idiopathic infantile arterial calcification) Q28.8
Ileitis (chronic) (noninfectious) *see also* Enteritis K52.9
|backwash *see* Pancolitis, ulcerative (chronic)
|infectious A09
|regional (ulcerative) *see* Enteritis, regional, small intestine
|segmental *see* Enteritis, regional
|terminal (ulcerative) *see* Enteritis, regional, small intestine

Ileocolitis *see also* Enteritis K52.9
|regional *see* Enteritis, regional
|infectious A09
|ulcerative K51.0-
Ileostomy
|attention to Z43.2
|malfunctioning K94.13
|status Z93.2
|with complication *see* Complications, enterostomy
Ileotyphus *see* Typhoid
Ileum *see* condition
Ileus (bowel) (colon) (inhibitory) (intestine) K56.7
|adynamic K56.0
|due to gallstone (in intestine) K56.3
|duodenal (chronic) K31.5
|gallstone K56.3
|mechanical NEC (*see also* Obstruction, intestine, specified NEC) K56.699
|meconium P76.0
|in cystic fibrosis E84.11
|meaning meconium plug (without cystic fibrosis) P76.0
|myxedema K59.89
|neurogenic K56.0
|Hirschsprung's disease or megacolon Q43.1
|newborn
|due to meconium P76.0
|in cystic fibrosis E84.11
|meaning meconium plug (without cystic fibrosis) P76.0
|transitory P76.1
|obstructive (*see also* Obstruction, intestine, specified NEC) K56.699
|postoperative K91.89
|paralytic K56.0
Iliac *see* condition
Iliotibial band syndrome M76.3-
Illiteracy Z55.0
Illness *see also* Disease R69
|manic-depressive *see* Disorder, bipolar
Imbalance R26.89
|autonomic G90.8
|constituents of food intake E63.1
|electrolyte E87.8
|with
|abortion *see* Abortion by type, complicated by, electrolyte imbalance
|molar pregnancy O08.5
|due to hyperemesis gravidarum O21.1
|following ectopic or molar pregnancy O08.5
|neonatal, transitory NEC P74.49
|potassium
|hyperkalemia P74.31
|hypokalemia P74.32
|sodium
|hypernatremia P74.21
|hyponatremia P74.22
|endocrine E34.9
|eye muscle NOS H50.9
|hormone E34.9
|hysterical F44.4
|labyrinth *see* subcategory H83.2
|posture R29.3
|protein-energy *see* Malnutrition
|sympathetic G90.8
Imbecile, imbecility (I.Q.35 49) F71
Imbedding, intrauterine device T83.39
Imbibition, cholesterol (gallbladder) K82.4
Imbrication, teeth,, fully erupted M26.30
Imerslund (-Grasbeck) syndrome D51.1
Immature *see also* Immaturity
|birth (less than 37 completed weeks) *see* Preterm, newborn

Immature - *continued*
|extremely (less than 28 completed weeks) *see* Immaturity, extreme
|personality F60.89
Immaturity (less than 37 completed weeks) *see also* Preterm, newborn
|extreme of newborn (less than 28 completed weeks of gestation) (less than 196 completed days of gestation) (unspecified weeks of gestation) P07.20
|gestational age
|23 completed weeks (23 weeks, 0 days through 23 weeks, 6 days) P07.22
|24 completed weeks (24 weeks, 0 days through 24 weeks, 6 days) P07.23
|25 completed weeks (25 weeks, 0 days through 25 weeks, 6 days) P07.24
|26 completed weeks (26 weeks, 0 days through 26 weeks, 6 days) P07.25
|27 completed weeks (27 weeks, 0 days through 27 weeks, 6 days) P07.26
|less than 23 completed weeks P07.21
|fetus or infant light-for-dates *see* Light-for-dates
|lung, newborn P28.0
|organ or site NEC *see* Hypoplasia
|pulmonary, newborn P28.0
|reaction F60.89
|sexual (female) (male), after puberty E30.0
Immersion T75.1
|hand T69.01-
|foot T69.02-
Immobile, immobility
|complete, due to severe physical disability or frailty R53.2
|intestine K59.89
|syndrome (paraplegic) M62.3
Immune reconstitution (inflammatory) syndrome [IRIS] D89.3
Immunization *see also* Vaccination
|ABO *see* Incompatibility, ABO
|in newborn P55.1
|appropriate for age
|child (over 28 days old) Z00.129
|with abnormal findings Z00.121
|complication *see* Complications, vaccination
|encounter for Z23
|not done (not carried out) Z28.9
|because (of)
|acute illness of patient Z28.01
|allergy to vaccine (or component) Z28.04
|caregiver refusal Z28.82
|chronic illness of patient Z28.02
|contraindication NEC Z28.09
|delay in delivery of vaccine Z28.83
|group pressure Z28.1
|guardian refusal Z28.82
|immune compromised state of patient Z28.03
|lack of availability of vaccine Z28.83
|manufacturer delay of vaccine Z28.83
|parent refusal Z28.82
|patient's belief Z28.1
|patient had disease being vaccinated against Z28.81
|patient refusal Z28.21
|religious beliefs of patient Z28.1
|specified reason NEC Z28.89
|of patient Z28.29
|unavailability of vaccine Z28.83
|unspecified patient reason Z28.20
|Rh factor
|affecting management of pregnancy NEC O36.09-
|anti-D antibody O36.01-
|from transfusion *see* Complication(s), transfusion, incompatibility reaction, Rh (factor)

Immunocompromised NOS D84.9
Immunocytoma C83.0-
Immunodeficiency D84.9
  |with
    |adenosine-deaminase deficiency D81.3
    |antibody defects D80.9
      |specified type NEC D80.8
    |hyperimmunoglobulinemia D80.6
    |increased immunoglobulin M (IgM) D80.5
    |major defect D82.9
      |specified type NEC D82.8
    |partial albinism D82.8
    |short-limbed stature D82.2
    |thrombocytopenia and eczema D82.0
  |antibody with
    |hyperimmunoglobulinemia D80.6
    |near-normal immunoglobulins D80.6
  |autosomal recessive, Swiss type D80.0
  |combined D81.9
    |biotin-dependent carboxylase D81.819
      |biotinidase D81.810
      |holocarboxylase synthetase D81.818
      |specified type NEC D81.818
    |severe (SCID) D81.9
      |with
        |low or normal B-cell numbers D81.2
        |low T |and B-cell numbers D81.1
        |reticular dysgenesis D81.0
    |specified type NEC D81.89
  |common variable D83.9
    |with
      |abnormalities of B-cell numbers and
        function D83.0
      |autoantibodies to B |or T-cells D83.2
      |immunoregulatory T-cell disorders D83.1
    |specified type NEC D83.8
  |due to
    |conditions classified elsewhere D84.81
    |drugs D84.821
    |external causes D84.822
    |medication (current or past) D84.821
  |following hereditary defective response to
    Epstein-Barr virus (EBV) D82.3
  |selective, immunoglobulin
    |A (IgA) D80.2
    |G (IgG) (subclasses) D80.3
    |M (IgM) D80.4
  |severe combined (SCID) D81.9
  |specified type NEC D84.89
  |X-linked, with increased IgM D80.5
Immunodeficient NOS D84.9
Immunosuppressed NOS D84.9
Immunotherapy (encounter for)
  |antineoplastic Z51.12
Impaction, impacted
  |bowel, colon, rectum see also Impaction, fecal
    K56.49
    |by gallstone K56.3
  |calculus see Calculus
  |cerumen (ear) (external) H61.2-
  |cuspid see Impaction, tooth
  |dental (same or adjacent tooth) K01.1
  |fecal, feces K56.41
  |fracture see Fracture, by site
  |gallbladder see Calculus, gallbladder
  |gallstone(s) see Calculus, gallbladder
    |bile duct (common) (hepatic) see Calculus,
      bile duct
    |cystic duct see Calculus, gallbladder
    |in intestine, with obstruction (any part)
      K56.3
  |intestine (calculous) NEC see also Impaction,
    fecal K56.49
    |gallstone, with ileus K56.3
  |intrauterine device (IUD) T83.39

Impaction, impacted - *continued*
  |molar see Impaction, tooth
  |shoulder, causing obstructed labor O66.0
  |tooth, teeth K01.1
  |turbinate J34.89
Impaired, impairment (function)
  |auditory discrimination see Abnormal,
    auditory perception
  |cognitive, mild, so stated G31.84
  |dual sensory Z73.82
  |fasting glucose R73.01
  |glucose tolerance (oral) R73.02
  |hearing see Deafness
  |heart see Disease, heart
  |kidney N28.9
    |disorder resulting from N25.9
      |specified NEC N25.89
  |liver K72.90
    |with coma K72.91
  |mastication K08.89
  |mild cognitive, so stated G31.84
  |mobility
    |ear ossicles see Ankylosis, ear ossicles
    |requiring care provider Z74.09
  |myocardium, myocardial see Insufficiency,
    myocardial
  |rectal sphincter R19.8
  |renal (acute) (chronic) N28.9
    |disorder resulting from N25.9
      |specified NEC N25.89
  |vision NEC H54.7
    |both eyes H54.3
Impediment, speech (*see also* Disorder,
    speech) R47.9
  |psychogenic (childhood) F98.8
  |slurring R47.81
  |specified NEC R47.89
Impending
  |coronary syndrome I20.0
  |delirium tremens F10.239
  |myocardial infarction I20.0
Imperception auditory (acquired) see also
    Deafness
  |congenital H93.25
Imperfect
  |aeration, lung (newborn) NEC see Atelectasis
  |closure (congenital)
    |alimentary tract NEC Q45.8
      |lower Q43.8
      |upper Q40.8
    |atrioventricular ostium Q21.2
    |atrium (secundum) Q21.1
    |branchial cleft NOS Q18.2
      |cyst Q18.0
      |fistula Q18.0
      |sinus Q18.0
    |choroid Q14.3
    |cricoid cartilage Q31.8
    |cusps, heart valve NEC Q24.8
      |pulmonary Q22.3
    |ductus
      |arteriosus Q25.0
      |Botalli Q25.0
    |ear drum (causing impairment of hearing)
      Q16.4
    |esophagus with communication to bronchus
      or trachea Q39.1
    |eyelid Q10.3
    |foramen
      |botalli Q21.1
      |ovale Q21.1
    |genitalia, genital organ(s) or system
      |female Q52.8
        |external Q52.79
        |internal NEC Q52.8
      |male Q55.8
    |glottis Q31.8

Imperfect - *continued*
    |interatrial ostium or septum Q21.1
    |interauricular ostium or septum Q21.1
    |interventricular ostium or septum Q21.0
    |larynx Q31.8
    |lip see Cleft, lip
    |nasal septum Q30.3
    |nose Q30.2
    |omphalomesenteric duct Q43.0
    |optic nerve entry Q14.2
    |organ or site not listed see Anomaly, by site
    |ostium
      |interatrial Q21.1
      |interauricular Q21.1
      |interventricular Q21.0
    |palate see Cleft, palate
    |preauricular sinus Q18.1
    |retina Q14.1
    |roof of orbit Q75.8
    |sclera Q13.5
    |septum
      |aorticopulmonary Q21.4
      |atrial (secundum) Q21.1
      |between aorta and pulmonary artery
        Q21.4
      |heart Q21.9
      |interatrial (secundum) Q21.1
      |interauricular (secundum) Q21.1
      |interventricular Q21.0
        |in tetralogy of Fallot Q21.3
      |nasal Q30.3
      |ventricular Q21.0
        |with pulmonary stenosis or atresia,
          dextroposition of aorta, and
          hypertrophy of right ventricle Q21.3
        |in tetralogy of Fallot Q21.3
    |skull Q75.0
      |with
        |anencephaly Q00.0
        |encephalocele see Encephalocele
        |hydrocephalus Q03.9
          |with spina bifida see Spina bifida, by
            site, with hydrocephalus
        |microcephaly Q02
    |spine (with meningocele) see Spina bifida
    |trachea Q32.1
    |tympanic membrane (causing impairment of
      hearing) Q16.4
    |uterus Q51.818
    |vitelline duct Q43.0
  |erection see Dysfunction, sexual, male,
    erectile
  |fusion see Imperfect, closure
  |inflation, lung (newborn) see Atelectasis
  |posture R29.3
  |rotation, intestine Q43.3
  |septum, ventricular Q21.0
Imperfectly descended testis see Cryptorchid
Imperforate (congenital) see also Atresia
  |anus Q42.3
    |with fistula Q42.2
  |cervix (uteri) Q51.828
  |esophagus Q39.0
    |with tracheoesophageal fistula Q39.1
  |hymen Q52.3
  |jejunum Q41.1
  |pharynx Q38.8
  |rectum Q42.1
    |with fistula Q42.0
  |urethra Q64.39
  |vagina Q52.4
Impervious (congenital) see also Atresia
  |anus Q42.3
    |with fistula Q42.2
  |bile duct Q44.2
  |esophagus Q39.0

Impervious (congenital) - *continued*
 |with tracheoesophageal fistula Q39.1
 |intestine (small) Q41.9
  |large Q42.9
   |specified NEC Q42.8
 |rectum Q42.1
  |with fistula Q42.0
 |ureter *see* Atresia, ureter
 |urethra Q64.39
Impetiginization of dermatoses L01.1
Impetigo (any organism) (any site) (circinate)
 (contagiosa) (simplex) (vulgaris) L01.00
 |Bockhart's L01.02
 |bullous, bullosa L01.03
 |external ear L01.00 [*H62.40*]
 |follicularis L01.02
 |furfuracea L30.5
 |herpetiformis L40.1
  |nonobstetrical L40.1
 |neonatorum L01.03
 |nonbullous L01.01
 |specified type NEC L01.09
 |ulcerative L01.09
Impingement (on teeth)
 |soft tissue
  |anterior M26.81
  |posterior M26.82
Implant, endometrial N80.9
Implantation
 |anomalous *see* Anomaly, by site
  |ureter Q62.63
 |cyst
  |external area or site (skin) NEC L72.0
  |iris *see* Cyst, iris, implantation
  |vagina N89.8
  |vulva N90.7
 |dermoid (cyst) *see* Implantation, cyst
Impotence (sexual) N52.9
 |counseling Z70.1
 |organic origin *see also* Dysfunction, sexual,
  male, erectile N52.9
 |psychogenic F52.21
Impression, basilar Q75.8
Imprisonment, anxiety concerning Z65.1
Improper care (child) (newborn) *see*
 Maltreatment
Improperly tied umbilical cord (causing
 hemorrhage) P51.8
Impulsiveness (impulsive) R45.87
Inability to swallow *see* Aphagia
Inaccessible, inaccessibility
 |health care NEC Z75.3
  |due to
   |waiting period Z75.2
    |for admission to facility elsewhere
     Z75.1
 |other helping agencies Z75.4
Inactive *see* condition
Inadequate, inadequacy
 |aesthetics of dental restoration K08.56
 |biologic, constitutional, functional, or social
  F60.7
 |development
  |child R62.50
  |genitalia
   |after puberty NEC E30.0
   |congenital
    |female Q52.8
     |external Q52.79
     |internal Q52.8
    |male Q55.8
 |lungs Q33.6
  |associated with short gestation P28.0
 |organ or site not listed *see* Anomaly, by site
 |diet (causing nutritional deficiency) E63.9

Inadequate, inadequacy - *continued*
 |drinking-water supply Z58.6
 |eating habits Z72.4
 |environment, household Z59.1
 |family support Z63.8
 |food (supply) NEC Z59.48
  |hunger effects T73.0
 |functional F60.7
 |household care, due to
  |family member
   |handicapped or ill Z74.2
   |on vacation Z75.5
   |temporarily away from home Z74.2
  |technical defects in home Z59.1
  |temporary absence from home of person
   rendering care Z74.2
 |housing (heating) (space) Z59.1
 |income (financial) Z59.6
 |intrafamilial communication Z63.8
 |material resources Z59.9
 |mental *see* Disability, intellectual
 |parental supervision or control of child Z62.0
 |personality F60.7
 |pulmonary
  |function R06.89
   |newborn P28.5
  |ventilation, newborn P28.5
 |sample of cytologic smear
  |anus R85.615
  |cervix R87.615
  |vagina R87.625
 |social F60.7
  |insurance Z59.7
  |skills NEC Z73.4
 |supervision of child by parent Z62.0
 |teaching affecting education Z55.8
 |welfare support Z59.7
Inanition R64
 |with edema *see* Malnutrition, severe
 |due to
  |deprivation of food T73.0
  |malnutrition *see* Malnutrition
 |fever R50.9
Inappropriate
 |change in quantitative human chorionic
  gonadotropin (hCG) in early pregnancy
  O02.81
 |diet or eating habits Z72.4
 |level of quantitative human chorionic
  gonadotropin (hCG) for gestational age in
  early pregnancy O02.81
 |secretion
  |antidiuretic hormone (ADH) (excessive)
   E22.2
   |deficiency E23.2
  |pituitary (posterior) E22.2
Inattention at or after birth *see* Neglect
Incarceration, incarcerated
 |enterocele K46.0
  |gangrenous K46.1
 |epiplocele K46.0
  |gangrenous K46.1
 |exomphalos K42.0
  |gangrenous K42.1
 |hernia *see also* Hernia, by site, with
  obstruction
  |with gangrene *see* Hernia, by site, with
   gangrene
 |iris, in wound *see* Injury, eye, laceration, with
  prolapse
 |lens, in wound *see* Injury, eye, laceration, with
  prolapse
 |omphalocele K42.0
 |prison, anxiety concerning Z65.1
 |rupture *see* Hernia, by site
 |sarcoepiplocele K46.0
  |gangrenous K46.1
 |sarcoepiplomphalocele K42.0

Incarceration - *continued*
 |with gangrene K42.1
 |uterus N85.8
  |gravid O34.51-
   |causing obstructed labor O65.5
Incised wound
 |external *see* Laceration
 |internal organs *see* Injury, by site
Incision, incisional
 |hernia K43.2
  |with
   |gangrene (and obstruction) K43.1
   |obstruction K43.0
 |surgical, complication *see* Complications,
  surgical procedure
 |traumatic
  |external *see* Laceration
  |internal organs *see* Injury, by site
Inclusion
 |azurophilic leukocytic D72.0
 |blennorrhea (neonatal) (newborn) P39.1
 |gallbladder in liver (congenital) Q44.1
Incompatibility
 |ABO
  |affecting management of pregnancy
   O36.11-
   |anti-A sensitization O36.11-
   |anti-B sensitization O36.19-
   |specified NEC O36.19-
  |infusion or transfusion reaction *see*
   Complication(s), transfusion, incompatibility
   reaction, ABO
  |newborn P55.1
 |blood (group) (Duffy) (K) (Kell) (Kidd)
  (Lewis) (M) (S) NEC
  |affecting management of pregnancy
   O36.11-
   |anti-A sensitization O36.11-
   |anti-B sensitization O36.19
  |infusion or transfusion reaction T80.89
  |newborn P55.8
 |divorce or estrangement Z63.5
 |Rh (blood group) (factor) Z31.82
  |affecting management of pregnancy NEC
   O36.09-
   |anti-D antibody O36.01-
  |infusion or transfusion reaction *see*
   Complication(s), transfusion, incompatibility
   reaction, Rh (factor)
  |newborn P55.0
 |rhesus *see* Incompatibility, Rh
Incompetency, incompetent, incompetence
 |annular
  |aortic (valve) *see* Insufficiency, aortic
  |mitral (valve) I34.0
  |pulmonary valve (heart) I37.1
 |aortic (valve) *see* Insufficiency, aortic
 |cardiac valve *see* Endocarditis
 |cervix, cervical (os) N88.3
  |in pregnancy O34.3-
 |chronotropic I45.89
  |with
   |autonomic dysfunction G90.8
   |ischemic heart disease I25.89
   |left ventricular dysfunction I51.89
   |sinus node dysfunction I49.8
 |esophagogastric (junction) (sphincter) K22.0
 |mitral (valve) *see* Insufficiency, mitral
 |pelvic fundus N81.89
 |pubocervical tissue N81.82
 |pulmonary valve (heart) I37.1
  |congenital Q22.3
 |rectovaginal tissue N81.83
 |tricuspid (annular) (valve) *see* Insufficiency,
  tricuspid
 |valvular *see* Endocarditis
  |congenital Q24.8
 |vein, venous (saphenous) (varicose) *see* Varix,
  leg

Incomplete *see also* condition
  |bladder, emptying R33.9
  |defecation R15.0
  |expansion lungs (newborn) NEC *see*
    Atelectasis
  |rotation, intestine Q43.3
Inconclusive
  |diagnostic imaging due to excess body fat of
    patient R93.9
  |findings on diagnostic imaging of breast NEC
    R92.8
  |mammogram (due to dense breasts) R92.2
Incontinence R32
  |anal sphincter R15.9
  |coital N39.491
  |feces R15.9
    |nonorganic origin F98.1
  |insensible (urinary) N39.42
  |overflow N39.490
  |postural (urinary) N39.492
  |psychogenic F45.8
  |rectal R15.9
  |reflex N39.498
  |stress (female) (male) N39.3
    |and urge N39.46
  |urethral sphincter R32
  |urge N39.41
    |and stress (female) (male) N39.46
  |urine (urinary) R32
    |continuous N39.45
    |due to cognitive impairment, or severe
    physical disability or immobility R39.81
    |functional R39.81
    |insensible N39.42
    |mixed (stress and urge) N39.46
    |nocturnal N39.44
    |nonorganic origin F98.0
    |overflow N39.490
    |post dribbling N39.43
    |postural N39.492
    |reflex N39.498
    |specified NEC N39.498
    |stress (female) (male) N39.3
      |and urge N39.46
    |total N39.498
    |unaware N39.42
    |urge N39.41
      |and stress (female) (male) N39.46
Incontinentia pigmenti Q82.3
Incoordinate, incoordination
  |esophageal-pharyngeal (newborn) *see*
    Dysphagia
  |muscular R27.8
  |uterus (action) (contractions) (complicating
    delivery) O62.4
Increase, increased
  |abnormal, in development R63.8
  |androgens (ovarian) E28.1
  |anticoagulants (antithrombin) (anti-VIIIa)
    (anti-IXa) (anti-Xa) (anti-XIa) *see*
    Circulating anticoagulants
  |cold sense R20.8
  |estrogen E28.0
  |function
    |adrenal
      |cortex *see* Cushing's, syndrome
      |medulla E27.5
    |pituitary (gland) (anterior) (lobe) E22.9
      |posterior E22.2
  |heat sense R20.8
  |intracranial pressure (benign) G93.2
  |permeability, capillaries I78.8
  |pressure, intracranial G93.2
  |secretion
    |gastrin E16.4

Increase, increased - *continued*
    |glucagon E16.3
  |pancreas, endocrine E16.9
    |growth hormone-releasing hormone E16.8
    |pancreatic polypeptide E16.8
    |somatostatin E16.8
    |vasoactive-intestinal polypeptide E16.8
  |sphericity, lens Q12.4
  |splenic activity D73.1
  |venous pressure I87.8
  |portal K76.6
Increta placenta O43.22-
Incrustation, cornea, foreign body (lead)(zinc)
  see Foreign body, cornea
Incyclophoria H50.54
Incyclotropia *see* Cyclotropia Indeterminate
  sex Q56.4
India rubber skin Q82.8
Indigestion (acid) (bilious) (functional) K30
  |catarrhal K31.89
  |due to decomposed food NOS A05.9
  |nervous F45.8
  |psychogenic F45.8
Indirect *see* condition
Induration penis plastica N48.6
Induration, indurated
  |brain G93.89
  |breast (fibrous) N64.51
    |puerperal, postpartum O92.29
  |broad ligament N83.8
  |chancre
    |anus A51.1
    |congenital A50.07
    |extragenital NEC A51.2
  |corpora cavernosa (penis) (plastic) N48.6
  |liver (chronic) K76.89
  |lung (black) (chronic) (fibroid) *see also*
    Fibrosis, lung J84.10
    |essential brown J84.03
  |penile (plastic) N48.6
  |phlebitic *see* Phlebitis
  |skin R23.4
Inebriety (without dependence) *see* Alcohol,
  intoxication
Inefficiency, kidney N28.9
Inelasticity, skin R23.4
Inequality, leg (length) (acquired) *see also*
  Deformity, limb, unequal length
  |congenital *see* Defect, reduction, lower limb
  |lower leg *see* Deformity, limb, unequal length
Inertia
  |bladder (neurogenic) N31.2
  |stomach K31.89
    |psychogenic F45.8
  |uterus, uterine during labor O62.2
    |during latent phase of labor O62.0
    |primary O62.0
    |secondary O62.1
  |vesical (neurogenic) N31.2
Infancy, infantile, infantilism *see also*
  condition
  |celiac K90.0
  |genitalia, genitals (after puberty) E30.0
  |Herter's (nontropical sprue) K90.0
  |intestinal K90.0
  |Lorain E23.0
  |pancreatic K86.89
  |pelvis M95.5
    |with disproportion (fetopelvic) O33.1
      |causing obstructed labor O65.1
  |pituitary E23.0
  |renal N25.0
  |uterus *see* Infantile, genitalia

Infant(s) *see also* Infancy
  |excessive crying R68.11
  |irritable child R68.12
  |lack of care *see* Neglect
  |liveborn (singleton) Z38.2
    |born in hospital Z38.00
      |by cesarean Z38.01
    |born outside hospital Z38.1
    |multiple NEC Z38.8
      |born in hospital Z38.68
        |by cesarean Z38.69
      |born outside hospital Z38.7
    |quadruplet Z38.8
      |born in hospital Z38.63
        |by cesarean Z38.64
      |born outside hospital Z38.7
    |quintuplet Z38.8
      |born in hospital Z38.65
        |by cesarean Z38.66
      |born outside hospital Z38.7
    |triplet Z38.8
      |born in hospital Z38.61
        |by cesarean Z38.62
      |born outside hospital Z38.7
    |twin Z38.5
      |born in hospital Z38.30
        |by cesarean Z38.31
      |born outside hospital Z38.4
  |of diabetic mother (syndrome of) P70.1
    |gestational diabetes P70.0
Infantile *see also* condition
  |genitalia, genitals E30.0
  |os, uterine E30.0
  |penis E30.0
  |testis E29.1
  |uterus E30.0
Infantilism *see* Infancy
Infarct, infarction
  |adrenal (capsule) (gland) E27.49
  |appendices epiploicae *see also* Infarct,
    intestine K55.069
  |bowel *see also* Infarct, intestine K55.069
  |brain (stem) *see* Infarct, cerebral
  |breast N64.89
  |brewer's (kidney) N28.0
  |cardiac *see* Infarct, myocardium
  |cerebellar *see* Infarct, cerebral
  |cerebral *see also* Occlusion, artery cerebral or
    precerebral, with infarction I63.9-
    |aborted I63.9
    |cortical I63.9
    |due to
      |cerebral venous thrombosis, nonpyogenic
        I63.6
      |embolism
        |cerebral arteries I63.4-
        |precerebral arteries I63.1-
      |occlusion NEC
        |cerebral arteries I63.5-
        |precerebral arteries I63.2-
        |small artery I63.81
      |stenosis NEC
        |cerebral arteries I63.5-
        |precerebral arteries I63.2-
        |small artery I63.81
      |thrombosis
        |cerebral artery I63.3-
        |precerebral artery I63.0-
    |intraoperative
      |during cardiac surgery I97.810
      |during other surgery I97.811
    |neonatal P91.82-
    |perinatal (arterial ischemic) P91.82-
    |postprocedural
      |following cardiac surgery I97.820

Infarct, infarction - *continued*
    |following other surgery I97.821
  |specified NEC I63.89
|colon (acute) (agnogenic) (embolic)
  (hemorrhagic) (nonocclusive)
  (nonthrombotic) (occlusive) (segmental)
  (thrombotic)(with gangrene) *see also*
  Infarct, intestine K55.049
|coronary artery *see* Infarct, myocardium
|embolic *see* Embolism
|fallopian tube N83.8
|gallbladder K82.8
|heart *see* Infarct, myocardium
|hepatic K76.3
|hypophysis (anterior lobe) E23.6
|impending (myocardium) I20.0
|intestine (acute) (agnogenic) (embolic)
  (hemorrhagic) (nonocclusive)
  (nonthrombotic) (occlusive) (thrombotic)
  (with
|gangrene) K55.069
  |diffuse K55.062
  |focal K55.061
  |large K55.049
    |diffuse K55.042
    |focal K55.041
  |small K55.029
    |diffuse K55.022
    |focal K55.021
|kidney N28.0
|lacunar I63.81
|liver K76.3
|lung (embolic) (thrombotic) *see* Embolism,
  pulmonary
|lymph node I89.8
|mesentery, mesenteric (embolic) (thrombotic)
  (with gangrene) *see also* Infarct, intestine
  K55.069
|muscle (ischemic) M62.20
  |ankle M62.27-
  |foot M62.27-
  |forearm M62.23-
  |hand M62.24-
  |lower leg M62.26-
  |pelvic region M62.25-
  |shoulder region M62.21-
  |specified site NEC M62.28
  |thigh M62.25-
  |upper arm M62.22-
|myocardium, myocardial (acute) (with stated
  duration of 4weeks or less) I21.9
  |associated with revascularization procedure
    I21.A9
  |diagnosed on ECG, but presenting no
    symptoms I25.2
  |due to
    |demand ischemia I21.A1
    |ischemic imbalance I21.A1
  |healed or old I25.2
  |intraoperative *see also* Infarct, myocardium,
    associated with revascularization
    procedure
    |during cardiac surgery I97.790
    |during other surgery I97.791
  |non-Q wave I21.4
  |non-ST elevation (NSTEMI) I21.4
    |subsequent I22.2
  |nontransmural I21.4
  |past (diagnosed on ECG or other
    investigation, but currently presenting no
    symptoms) I25.2
  |postprocedural *see also* Infarct,
    myocardium, associated with
    revascularization procedure

Infarct, infarction - *continued*
  |following cardiac surgery (*see also*
    Infarct, myocardium, type 4 or type 5)
    I97.190
  |following other surgery I97.191
|Q wave (*see also* , Infarct, myocardium, by
  site) I21.3
|secondary to
  |demand ischemia I21.A1
  |ischemic imbalance I21.A1
|ST elevation (STEMI) I21.3
  |anterior (anteroapical) (anterolateral)
    (anteroseptal) (Q wave) (wall) I21.09
    |subsequent I22.0
  |inferior (diaphragmatic) (inferolateral)
    (inferoposterior) (wall) NEC I21.19
    |subsequent I22.1
  |inferoposterior transmural (Q wave)
    I21.11
  |involving
    |coronary artery of anterior wall NEC
      I21.09
    |coronary artery of inferior wall NEC
      I21.19
    |diagonal coronary artery I21.02
    |left anterior descending coronary artery
      I21.02
    |left circumflex coronary artery I21.21
    |left main coronary artery I21.01
    |oblique marginal coronary artery I21.21
    |right coronary artery I21.11
  |lateral (apical-lateral) (basal-lateral)
    (high) I21.29
    |subsequent I22.8
  |posterior (posterobasal) (posterolateral)
    (posteroseptal) (true) I21.29
    |subsequent I22.8
  |septal I21.29
    |subsequent I22.8
  |specified NEC I21.29
    |subsequent I22.8
  |subsequent I22.9
|subsequent (recurrent) (reinfarction) I22.9
  |anterior (anteroapical) (anterolateral)
    (anteroseptal) (wall) I22.0
  |diaphragmatic (wall) I22.1
  |inferior (diaphragmatic) (inferolateral)
    (inferoposterior) (wall) I22.1
  |lateral (apical-lateral) (basal-lateral)
    (high) I22.8
  |non-ST elevation (NSTEMI) I22.2
  |posterior (posterobasal) (posterolateral)
    (posteroseptal) (true) I22.8
  |septal I22.8
  |specified NEC I22.8
  |ST elevation I22.9
    |anterior (anteroapical) (anterolateral)
      (anteroseptal) (wall) I22.0
    |inferior (diaphragmatic) (inferolateral)
      (inferoposterior) (wall) I22.1
    |specified NEC I22.8
  |subendocardial I22.2
  |transmural I21.3
    |anterior (anteroapical) (anterolateral)
      (anteroseptal) (wall) I22.0
    |diaphragmatic (wall) I22.1
    |inferior (diaphragmatic) (inferolateral)
      (inferoposterior) (wall) I22.1
    |lateral (apical-lateral) (basal-lateral)
      (high) I22.8
    |posterior (posterobasal) (posterolateral)
      (posteroseptal) (true) I22.8
    |specified NEC I22.8

Infarct, infarction - *continued*
  |type 1 (*see also* Infarction, myocardial,
    subsequent, by site, or by ST elevation
    or non-ST elevation) I22.9
  |type 2 I21.A1
  |type 3 I21.A9
  |type 4 I21.A9
  |type 5 I21.A9
  |syphilitic A52.06
  |transmural I21.9
    |anterior (anteroapical) (anterolateral)
      (anteroseptal) (Q wave) (wall) NEC
      I21.09
    |inferior (diaphragmatic) (inferolateral)
      (inferoposterior) (Q wave) (wall) NEC
      I21.19
    |inferoposterior (Q wave) I21.11
    |lateral (apical-lateral) (basal-lateral)
      (high) NEC I21.29
    |posterior (posterobasal) (posterolateral)
      (posteroseptal) (true) NEC I21.29
    |septal NEC I21.29
    |specified NEC I21.29
  |type 1 (*see also* Infarction, myocardial, by
    site, or by ST elevation or non-ST
    elevation) I21.9
  |type 2 I21.A1
  |type 3 I21.A9
  |type 4 (a) (b) (c) I21.A9
  |type 5 I21.A9
|nontransmural I21.4
|omentum *see also* Infarct, intestine K55.069
|ovary N83.8
|pancreas K86.89
|papillary muscle *see* Infarct, myocardium
|parathyroid gland E21.4
|pituitary (gland) E23.6
|placenta O43.81-
|prostate N42.89
|pulmonary (artery) (vein) (hemorrhagic) *see*
  Embolism, pulmonary
|renal (embolic) (thrombotic) N28.0
|retina, retinal (artery) *see* Occlusion, artery,
  retina
|spinal (cord) (acute) (embolic) (nonembolic)
  G95.11
|spleen D73.5
  |embolic or thrombotic I74.8
|subendocardial (acute) (nontransmural) I21.4
|suprarenal (capsule) (gland) E27.49
|testis N50.1
|thrombotic *see also* Thrombosis
  |artery, arterial *see* Embolism
|thyroid (gland) E07.89
|ventricle (heart) *see* Infarct, myocardium
Infecting *see* condition
Infection, infected, infective (opportunistic)
  B99.9
  |with
    |drug resistant organism *see* Resistance (to),
    drug *see also* specific organism
    |lymphangitis *see* Lymphangitis
    |organ dysfunction (acute) R65.20
      |with septic shock R65.21
  |abscess (skin) code by site under Abscess
  |Absidia *see* Mucormycosis
  |Acanthamoeba *see* Acanthamebiasis
  |Acanthocheilonema (perstans) (streptocerca)
    B74.4
  |accessory sinus (chronic) *see* Sinusitis
  |achorion *see* Dermatophytosis
  |Acremonium falciforme B47.0
  |acromioclavicular M00.9
  |Actinobacillus (actinomycetem-comitans)
    A28.8
    |mallei A24.0

Infection, infected, infective - *continued*

|muris A25.1
|Actinomadura B47.1
|Actinomyces (israelii) *see also* Actinomycosis
A42.9
|Actinomycetales *see* Actinomycosis
|actinomycotic NOS *see* Actinomycosis
|adenoid (and tonsil) J03.90
|chronic J35.02
|adenovirus NEC
|as cause of disease classified elsewhere
B97.0
|unspecified nature or site B34.0
|aerogenes capsulatus A48.0
|aertrycke *see* Infection, salmonella
|alimentary canal NOS *see* Enteritis, infectious
|Allescheria boydii B48.2
|Alternaria B48.8
|alveolus, alveolar (process) K04.7
|Ameba, amebic (histolytica) *see* Amebiasis
|amniotic fluid, sac or cavity O41.10-
|chorioamnionitis O41.12-
|placentitis O41.14-
|amputation stump (surgical) *see* Complication,
amputation stump, infection
|Ancylostoma (duodenalis) B76.0
|Anisakiasis, Anisakis larvae B81.0
|anthrax *see* Anthrax
|antrum (chronic) *see* Sinusitis, maxillary
|anus, anal (papillae) (sphincter) K62.89
|arbovirus (arbor virus) A94
|specified type NEC A93.8
|artificial insemination N98.0
|Ascaris lumbricoides *see* Ascariasis
|Ascomycetes B47.0
|Aspergillus (flavus) (fumigatus) (terreus) *see*
Aspergillosis
|atypical
|acid-fast (bacilli) *see* Mycobacterium,
atypical
|mycobacteria *see* Mycobacterium, atypical
|virus A81.9
|specified type NEC A81.89
|auditory meatus (external) *see* Otitis, externa,
infective
|auricle (ear) *see* Otitis, externa, infective
|axillary gland (lymph) L04.2
|Bacillus A49.9
|abortus A23.1
|anthracis *see* Anthrax
|Ducrey's (any location) A57
|Flexner's A03.1
|Friedländer's NEC A49.8
|gas (gangrene) A48.0
|mallei A24.0
|melitensis A23.0
|paratyphoid, paratyphosus A01.4
|A A01.1
|B A01.2
|C A01.3
|Shiga (-Kruse) A03.0
|suipestifer *see* Infection, salmonella
|swimming pool A31.1
|typhosa A01.00
|welchii *see* Gangrene, gas
|bacterial NOS A49.9
|as cause of disease classified elsewhere
B96.89
|Clostridium perfringens [C. perfringens]
B96.7
|Bacteroides fragilis [B. fragilis] B96.6
|Enterobacter sakazakii B96.89
|Enterococcus B95.2
|Escherichia coli [E. coli] *see also*
Escherichia coli B96.20

Infection, infected, infective - *continued*

|Helicobacter pylori [H. pylori] B96.81
|Hemophilus influenzae [H. influenzae]
B96.3
|Klebsiella pneumoniae [K. pneumoniae]
B96.1
|Mycoplasma pneumoniae [M.
pneumoniae] B96.0
|Proteus (mirabilis) (morganii) B96.4
|Pseudomonas (aeruginosa) (mallei)
(pseudomallei) B96.5
|Staphylococcus B95.8
|aureus (methicillin susceptible) (MSSA)
B95.61
|methicillin resistant (MRSA) B95.62
|specified NEC B95.7
|Streptococcus B95.5
|group A B95.0
|group B B95.1
|pneumoniae B95.3
|specified NEC B95.4
|Vibrio vulnificus B96.82
|specified NEC A48.8
|Bacterium
|paratyphosum A01.4
|A A01.1
|B A01.2
|C A01.3
|typhosum A01.00
|Bacteroides NEC A49.8
|fragilis, as cause of disease classified
elsewhere B96.6
|Balantidium coli A07.0
|Bartholin's gland N75.8
|Basidiobolus B46.8
|bile duct (common) (hepatic) *see* Cholangitis
|bladder *see* Cystitis
|Blastomyces, blastomycotic *see also*
Blastomycosis
|brasiliensis *see* Paracoccidioidomycosis
|dermatitidis *see* Blastomycosis
|European *see* Cryptococcosis
|Loboi B48.0
|North American B40.9
|South American *see*
Paracoccidioidomycosis
|bleb, postprocedure *see* Blebitis
|bone *see* Osteomyelitis
|Bordetella *see* Whooping cough
|Borrelia bergdorfi A69.20
|brain *see also* Encephalitis G04.90
|membranes *see* Meningitis
|septic G06.0
|meninges *see* Meningitis, bacterial
|branchial cyst Q18.0
|breast *see* Mastitis
|bronchus *see* Bronchitis
|Brucella A23.9
|abortus A23.1
|canis A23.3
|melitensis A23.0
|mixed A23.8
|specified NEC A23.8
|suis A23.2
|Brugia (malayi) B74.1
|timori B74.2
|bursa *see* Bursitis, infective
|buttocks (skin) L08.9
|Campylobacter, intestinal A04.5
|as cause of disease classified elsewhere
B96.81
|Candida (albicans) (tropicalis) *see* Candidiasis
|candiru B88.8
|Capillaria (intestinal) B81.1
|hepatica B83.8

Infection, infected, infective - *continued*

|philippinensis B81.1
|cartilage *see* Disorder, cartilage, specified type
NEC
|catheter-related bloodstream (CRBSI)
T80.211
|cat liver fluke B66.0
|cellulitis code by site under Cellulitis
|central line-associated T80.219
|bloodstream (CLABSI) T80.211
|specified NEC T80.218
|Cephalosporium falciforme B47.0
|cerebrospinal *see* Meningitis
|cervical gland (lymph) L04.0
|cervix *see* Cervicitis
|cesarean delivery wound (puerperal) O86.00
|cestodes *see* Infestation, cestodes
|chest J22
|Chilomastix (intestinal) A07.8
|Chlamydia, chlamydial A74.9
|anus A56.3
|genitourinary tract A56.2
|lower A56.00
|specified NEC A56.19
|lymphogranuloma A55
|pharynx A56.4
|psittaci A70
|rectum A56.3
|sexually transmitted NEC A56.8
|cholera *see* Cholera
|Cladosporium
|bantianum (brain abscess) B43.1
|carrionii B43.0
|castellanii B36.1
|trichoides (brain abscess) B43.1
|werneckii B36.1
|Clonorchis (sinensis) (liver) B66.1
|Clostridium NEC
|bifermentans A48.0
|botulinum (food poisoning) A05.1
|infant A48.51
|wound A48.52
|difficile
|as cause of disease classified elsewhere
B96.89
|foodborne (disease)
|not specified as recurrent A04.72
|recurrent A04.71
|gas gangrene A48.0
|necrotizing enterocolitis
|not specified as recurrent A04.72
|recurrent A04.71
|sepsis A41.4
|gas-forming NEC A48.0
|histolyticum A48.0
|novyi, causing gas gangrene A48.0
|oedematiens A48.0
|perfringens
|as cause of disease classified elsewhere
B96.7
|due to food A05.2
|foodborne (disease) A05.2
|gas gangrene A48.0
|sepsis A41.4
|septicum, causing gas gangrene A48.0
|sordellii, causing gas gangrene A48.0
|welchii
|as cause of disease classified elsewhere
B96.7
|foodborne (disease) A05.2
|gas gangrene A48.0
|necrotizing enteritis A05.2
|sepsis A41.4
|Coccidioides (immitis) *see*
Coccidioidomycosis

Infection, infected, infective - *continued*
- |colon *see* Enteritis, infectious
- |colostomy K94.02
- |common duct *see* Cholangitis
- |congenital P39.9
  - |Candida (albicans) P37.5
  - |cytomegalovirus P35.1
  - |hepatitis, viral P35.3
  - |herpes simplex P35.2
  - |infectious or parasitic disease P37.9
    - |specified NEC P37.8
  - |listeriosis (disseminated) P37.2
  - |malaria NEC P37.4
    - |falciparum P37.3
  - |Plasmodium falciparum P37.3
  - |poliomyelitis P35.8
  - |rubella P35.0
  - |skin P39.4
  - |toxoplasmosis (acute) (subacute) (chronic) P37.1
  - |tuberculosis P37.0
  - |urinary (tract) P39.3
  - |vaccinia P35.8
  - |virus P35.9
    - |specified type NEC P35.8
- |Conidiobolus B46.8
- |coronavirus-2019 U07.1
- |coronavirus NEC B34.2
  - |as cause of disease classified elsewhere B97.29
  - |severe acute respiratory syndrome (SARS associated) B97.21
- |corpus luteum *see* Salpingo-oophoritis
- |Corynebacterium diphtheriae *see* Diphtheria
- |cotia virus B08.8
- |COVID-19 U07.1
- |Coxiella burnetii A78
- |coxsackie *see* Coxsackie
- |Cryptococcus neoformans *see* Cryptococcosis
- |Cryptosporidium A07.2
- |Cunninghamella *see* Mucormycosis
- |cyst *see* Cyst
- |cystic duct *see also* Cholecystitis K81.9
- |Cysticercus cellulosae *see* Cysticercosis
- |cytomegalovirus, cytomegaloviral B25.9
  - |congenital P35.1
  - |maternal, maternal care for (suspected) damage to fetus O35.3
  - |mononucleosis B27.10
    - |with
      - |complication NEC B27.19
      - |meningitis B27.12
      - |polyneuropathy B27.11
- |delta-agent (acute), in hepatitis B carrier B17.0
- |dental (pulpal origin) K04.7
- |Deuteromycetes B47.0
- |Dicrocoelium dendriticum B66.2
- |Dipetalonema (perstans) (streptocerca) B74.4
- |diphtherial *see* Diphtheria
- |Diphyllobothrium (adult) (latum) (pacificum) B70.0
  - |larval B70.1
- |Diplogonoporus (grandis) B71.8
- |Dipylidium caninum B67.4
- |Dirofilaria B74.8
- |Dracunculus medinensis B72
- |Drechslera (hawaiiensis) B43.8
- |Ducrey Haemophilus (any location) A57
- |due to or resulting from
  - |artificial insemination N98.0
  - |Babesia
    - |divergens (-like) strain B60.03
    - |duncani (-type) species B60.02
    - |microti B60.01

Infection, infected, infective - *continued*
- |species
  - |specified NEC B60.09
- |central venous catheter T80.219
  - |bloodstream T80.211
  - |exit or insertion site T80.212
  - |localized T80.212
  - |port or reservoir T80.212
  - |specified NEC T80.218
  - |tunnel T80.212
- |device, implant or graft *see also* Complications, by site and type, infection or inflammation T85.79
  - |arterial graft NEC T82.7
  - |breast (implant) T85.79
  - |catheter NEC T85.79
    - |dialysis (renal) T82.7
      - |central line T80.211
      - |intraperitoneal T85.71
      - |Hopkins T83.518
      - |ileostomy T83.518
      - |nephrostomy T83.512
      - |specified NEC T83.518
      - |urethral indwelling T83.511
      - |urostomy T83.518
  - |electronic (electrode) (pulse generator) (stimulator)
    - |bone T84.7
    - |cardiac T82.7
    - |nervous system T85.738
      - |brain T85.731
      - |cranial nerve T85.732
      - |gastric nerve T85.732
      - |generator pocket T85.734
      - |neurostimulator generator T85.734
      - |peripheral nerve T85.732
      - |sacral nerve T85.732
      - |spinal cord T85.733
      - |vagal nerve T85.732
    - |urinary T83.590
  - |fixation, internal (orthopedic) NEC *see* Complication, fixation device, infection
  - |gastrointestinal (bile duct) (esophagus) T85.79
    - |neurostimulator electrode (lead) T85.732
  - |genital NEC T83.69
  - |heart NEC T82.7
    - |valve (prosthesis) T82.6
    - |graft T82.7
  - |joint prosthesis *see* Complication, joint prosthesis, infection
  - |ocular (corneal graft) (orbital implant) NEC T85.79
  - |orthopedic NEC T84.7
  - |penile (cylinder) (pump) (reservoir) T83.61
  - |protozoa of the order Piroplasmida NEC B60.09
  - |specified NEC T85.79
  - |testicular T83.62
  - |urinary NEC T83.598
    - |ileal conduit stent T83.593
    - |implanted neurostimulation T83.590
    - |implanted sphincter T83.591
    - |indwelling ureteral stent T83.592
    - |nephroureteral stent T83.593
    - |specified stent NEC T83.593
  - |vascular NEC T82.7
  - |ventricular intracranial (communicating) shunt T85.730
- |Hickman catheter T80.219
  - |bloodstream T80.211
  - |localized T80.212

Infection, infected, infective - *continued*
- |specified NEC T80.218
- |immunization or vaccination T88.0
- |infusion, injection or transfusion NEC T80.29
  - |acute T80.22
- |injury NEC   code by site under Wound, open
- |peripherally inserted central catheter (PICC) T80.219
  - |bloodstream T80.211
  - |localized T80.212
  - |specified NEC T80.218
- |portacath (port-a-cath) T80.219
  - |bloodstream T80.211
  - |localized T80.212
  - |specified NEC T80.218
- |pulmonary artery catheter *see* Infection, due to or resulting from, central venous catheter
- |surgery T81.40
- |Swan Ganz catheter *see* Infection, due to or resulting from, central venous catheter
- |triple lumen catheter T80.219
  - |bloodstream T80.211
  - |localized T80.212
  - |specified NEC T80.218
- |umbilical venous catheter T80.219
  - |bloodstream T80.211
  - |localized T80.212
  - |specified NEC T80.218
- |during labor NEC O75.3
- |ear (middle) *see also* Otitis media
  - |external *see* Otitis, externa, infective
  - |inner *see* subcategory H83.0
- |Eberthella typhosa A01.00
- |Echinococcus *see* Echinococcus
- |echovirus
  - |as cause of disease classified elsewhere B97.12
  - |unspecified nature or site B34.1
- |endocardium I33.0
- |endocervix *see* Cervicitis
- |Entamoeba *see* Amebiasis
- |enteric *see* Enteritis, infectious
- |Enterobacter sakazakii B96.89
- |Enterobius vermicularis B80
- |enterostomy K94.12
- |enterovirus B34.1
  - |as cause of disease classified elsewhere B97.10
  - |coxsackievirus B97.11
  - |echovirus B97.12
  - |specified NEC B97.19
- |Entomophthora B46.8
- |Epidermophyton *see* Dermatophytosis
- |epididymis *see* Epididymitis
- |episiotomy (puerperal) O86.09
- |Erysipelothrix (insidiosa) (rhusiopathiae) *see* Erysipeloid
- |erythema infectiosum B08.3
- |Escherichia (E.) coli NEC A49.8
  - |as cause of disease classified elsewhere *see also* Escherichia coli B96.20
  - |congenital P39.8
    - |sepsis P36.4
  - |generalized A41.51
  - |intestinal *see* Enteritis, infectious, due to, Escherichia coli
- |ethmoidal (chronic) (sinus) *see* Sinusitis, ethmoidal
- |eustachian tube (ear) *see* Salpingitis, eustachian
- |external auditory canal (meatus) NEC *see* Otitis, externa, infective

Infection, infected, infective - *continued*
|eye (purulent) *see* Endophthalmitis, purulent
|eyelid *see* Inflammation, eyelid
|fallopian tube *see* Salpingo-oophoritis
|Fasciola (gigantica) (hepatica) (indica) B66.3
|Fasciolopsis (buski) B66.5
|filarial *see* Infestation, filarial
|finger (skin) L08.9
  |nail L03.01-
    |fungus B35.1
|fish tapeworm B70.0
  |larval B70.1
|flagellate, intestinal A07.9
|fluke *see* Infestation, fluke
|focal
  |teeth (pulpal origin) K04.7
  |tonsils J35.01
|Fonsecaea (compactum) (pedrosoi) B43.0
|food *see* Intoxication, foodborne
|foot (skin) L08.9
  |dermatophytic fungus B35.3
|Francisella tularensis *see* Tularemia
|frontal (sinus) (chronic) *see* Sinusitis, frontal
|fungus NOS B49
  |beard B35.0
  |dermatophytic *see* Dermatophytosis
  |foot B35.3
  |groin B35.6
  |hand B35.2
  |nail B35.1
  |pathogenic to compromised host only B48.8
  |perianal (area) B35.6
  |scalp B35.0
  |skin B36.9
    |foot B35.3
    |hand B35.2
    |toenails B35.1
|Fusarium B48.8
|gallbladder *see* Cholecystitis
|gas bacillus *see* Gangrene, gas
|gastrointestinal *see* Enteritis, infectious
|generalized NEC *see* Sepsis
|generator pocket, implanted electronic
  neurostimulator T85.734
|genital organ or tract
  |female *see* Disease, pelvis, inflammatory
  |male N49.9
    |multiple sites N49.8
    |specified NEC N49.8
|Ghon tubercle, primary A15.7
|Giardia lamblia A07.1
|gingiva (chronic) K05.10
  |acute K05.00
    |nonplaque induced K05.01
    |plaque induced K05.00
  |nonplaque induced K05.11
  |plaque induced K05.10
|glanders A24.0
|glenosporosis B48.0
|Gnathostoma (spinigerum) B83.1
|Gongylonema B83.8
|gonococcal *see* Gonococcus
|gram-negative bacilli NOS A49.9
|guinea worm B72
|gum (chronic) K05.10
  |acute K05.00
    |nonplaque induced K05.01
    |plaque induced K05.00
  |nonplaque induced K05.11
  |plaque induced K05.10
|Haemophilus *see* Infection, Hemophilus
|heart *see* Carditis
|Helicobacter pylori A04.8
  |as cause of disease classified elsewhere
    B96.81

Infection, infected, infective - *continued*
|helminths B83.9
  |intestinal B82.0
    |mixed (types classifiable to more than one
      of the titles B65.0-B81.3 and B81.8)
      B81.4
    |specified type NEC B81.8
  |specified type NEC B83.8
|Hemophilus
  |aegyptius, systemic A48.4
  |Ducrey (any location) A57
  |influenzae NEC A49.2
    |as cause of disease classified elsewhere
      B96.3
  |generalized A41.3
|herpes (simplex) *see also* Herpes
  |congenital P35.2
  |disseminated B00.7
  |zoster B02.9
|herpesvirus, herpesviral *see* Herpes
|hip (joint) NEC M00.9
  |due to internal joint prosthesis
    |left T84.52
    |right T84.51
  |skin NEC L08.9
|Heterophyes (heterophyes) B66.8
|Histoplasma *see* Histoplasmosis
  |American B39.4
  |capsulatum B39.4
|hookworm B76.9
|human
  |papilloma virus A63.0
  |T-cell lymphotropic virus type 1(HTLV 1)
    B33.3
|hydrocele N43.0
|Hymenolepis B71.0
|hypopharynx *see* Pharyngitis
|inguinal (lymph) glands L04.1
  |due to soft chancre A57
|intervertebral disc, pyogenic M46.30
  |cervical region M46.32
  |cervicothoracic region M46.33
  |lumbar region M46.36
  |lumbosacral region M46.37
  |multiple sites M46.39
  |occipito-atlanto-axial region M46.31
  |sacrococcygeal region M46.38
  |thoracic region M46.34
  |thoracolumbar region M46.35
|intestine, intestinal *see* Enteritis, infectious
  |specified NEC A08.8
|intra-amniotic affecting newborn NEC P39.2
|intrauterine inflammation O41.12-
|Isospora belli or hominis A07.3
|Japanese B encephalitis A83.0
|jaw (bone) (lower) (upper) M27.2
|joint NEC M00.9
  |due to internal joint prosthesis T84.50
|kidney (cortex) (hematogenous) N15.9
  |with calculus N20.0
    |with hydronephrosis N13.6
  |following ectopic gestation O08.83
  |pelvis and ureter (cystic) N28.85
  |puerperal (postpartum) O86.21
  |specified NEC N15.8
|Klebsiella (K.) pneumoniae NEC A49.8
  |as cause of disease classified elsewhere
    B96.1
|knee (joint) NEC M00.9
  |joint M00.9
  |due to internal joint prosthesis
    |left T84.54
    |right T84.53
  |skin L08.9
|Koch's *see* Tuberculosis

Infection, infected, infective - *continued*
|labia (majora) (minora) (acute) *see* Vulvitis
|lacrimal
  |gland *see* Dacryoadenitis
  |passages (duct) (sac) *see* Inflammation,
    lacrimal, passages
|lancet fluke B66.2
|larynx NEC J38.7
|leg (skin) NOS L08.9
|Legionella pneumophila A48.1
  |nonpneumonic A48.2
|Leishmania *see also* Leishmaniasis
  |aethiopica B55.1
  |braziliensis B55.2
  |chagasi B55.0
  |donovani B55.0
  |infantum B55.0
  |major B55.1
  |mexicana B55.1
  |tropica B55.1
|lentivirus, as cause of disease classified
  elsewhere B97.31
|Leptosphaeria senegalensis B47.0
|Leptospira interrogans A27.9
  |autumnalis A27.89
  |canicola A27.89
  |hebdomadis A27.89
  |icterohaemorrhagiae A27.0
  |pomona A27.89
  |specified type NEC A27.89
|leptospirochetal NEC *see* Leptospirosis
|Listeria monocytogenes *see also* Listeriosis
  |congenital P37.2
|Loa Loa B74.3
  |with conjunctival infestation B74.3
  |eyelid B74.3
|Loboa loboi B48.0
|local, skin (staphylococcal) (streptococcal)
  L08.9
  |abscess - code by site under Abscess
  |cellulitis - code by site under Cellulitis
  |specified NEC L08.89
  |ulcer *see* Ulcer, skin
|Loefflerella mallei A24.0
|lung *see also* Pneumonia J18.9
  |atypical Mycobacterium A31.0
  |spirochetal A69.8
  |tuberculous *see* Tuberculosis, pulmonary
  |virus *see* Pneumonia, viral
|lymph gland *see also* Lymphadenitis, acute
  |mesenteric I88.0
|lymphoid tissue, base of tongue or posterior
  pharynx, NEC (chronic) J35.03
|Madurella (grisea) (mycetomii) B47.0
|major
  |following ectopic or molar pregnancy O08.0
  |puerperal, postpartum, childbirth O85
|Malassezia furfur B36.0
|Malleomyces
  |mallei A24.0
  |pseudomallei (whitmori) *see* Melioidosis
|mammary gland N61.0
|Mansonella (ozzardi) (perstans) (streptocerca)
  B74.4
|mastoid *see* Mastoiditis
|maxilla, maxillary M27.2
  |sinus (chronic) *see* Sinusitis, maxillary
|mediastinum J98.51
|Medina (worm) B72
|meibomian cyst or gland *see* Hordeolum
|meninges *see* Meningitis, bacterial
|meningococcal *see also* condition A39.9
  |adrenals A39.1
  |brain A39.81
  |cerebrospinal A39.0

Infection, infected, infective - *continued*
- conjunctiva A39.89
- endocardium A39.51
- heart A39.50
  - endocardium A39.51
  - myocardium A39.52
  - pericardium A39.53
- joint A39.83
- meninges A39.0
- meningococcemia A39.4
  - acute A39.2
  - chronic A39.3
- myocardium A39.52
- pericardium A39.53
- retrobulbar neuritis A39.82
- specified site NEC A39.89
- mesenteric lymph nodes or glands NEC I88.0
- Metagonimus B66.8
- metatarsophalangeal M00.9
- methicillin
  - resistant Staphylococcus aureus (MRSA) A49.02
  - susceptible Staphylococcus aureus (MSSA) A49.01
- Microsporum, microsporic *see* Dermatophytosis
- mixed flora (bacterial) NEC A49.8
- Monilia *see* Candidiasis
- Monosporium apiospermum B48.2
- mouth, parasitic B37.0
- Mucor *see* Mucormycosis
- muscle NEC *see* Myositis, infective
- mycelium NOS B49
- mycetoma B47.9
  - actinomycotic NEC B47.1
  - mycotic NEC B47.0
- Mycobacterium, mycobacterial *see* Mycobacterium
- Mycoplasma NEC A49.3
  - pneumoniae, as cause of disease classified elsewhere B96.0
- mycotic NOS B49
  - pathogenic to compromised host only B48.8
  - skin NOS B36.9
- myocardium NEC I40.0
- nail (chronic)
  - with lymphangitis *see* Lymphangitis, acute, digit
  - finger L03.01-
    - fungus B35.1
  - ingrowing L60.0
  - toe L03.03-
    - fungus B35.1
- nasal sinus (chronic) *see* Sinusitis
- nasopharynx *see* Nasopharyngitis
- navel L08.82
- Necator americanus B76.1
- Neisseria *see* Gonococcus
- Neotestudina rosati B47.0
- newborn P39.9
  - intra-amniotic NEC P39.2
  - skin P39.4
  - specified type NEC P39.8
- nipple N61.0
  - associated with
    - lactation O91.03
    - pregnancy O91.01-
    - puerperium O91.02
- Nocardia *see* Nocardiosis
- obstetrical surgical wound (puerperal) O86.00
  - incisional site
    - deep O86.02
    - superficial O86.01
  - organ and space site O86.03
  - surgical site specified NEC O86.09

Infection, infected, infective - *continued*
- Oesophagostomum (apiostomum) B81.8
- Oestrus ovis *see* Myiasis
- Oidium albicans B37.9
- Onchocerca (volvulus) *see* Onchocerciasis
- oncovirus, as cause of disease classified elsewhere B97.32
- operation wound T81.49
- Opisthorchis (felineus) (viverrini) B66.0
- orbit, orbital *see* Inflammation, orbit
- orthopoxvirus NEC B08.09
- ovary *see* Salpingo-oophoritis
- Oxyuris vermicularis B80
- pancreas (acute) *see* Pancreatitis, acute
  - abscess *see* Pancreatitis, acute
  - specified NEC *see also* Pancreatitis, acute K85.80
- papillomavirus, as cause of disease classified elsewhere B97.7
- papovavirus NEC B34.4
- Paracoccidioides brasiliensis *see* Paracoccidioidomycosis
- Paragonimus (westermani) B66.4
- parainfluenza virus B34.8
- parameningococcus NOS A39.9
- parapoxvirus B08.60
  - specified NEC B08.69
- parasitic B89
- Parastrongylus
  - cantonensis B83.2
  - costaricensis B81.3
- paratyphoid A01.4
  - Type A A01.1
  - Type B A01.2
  - Type C A01.3
- paraurethral ducts N34.2
- parotid gland *see* Sialoadenitis
- parvovirus NEC B34.3
  - as cause of disease classified elsewhere B97.6
- Pasteurella NEC A28.0
  - multocida A28.0
  - pestis *see* Plague
  - pseudotuberculosis A28.0
  - septica (cat bite) (dog bite) A28.0
  - tularensis *see* Tularemia
- pelvic, female *see* Disease, pelvis, inflammatory
- Penicillium (marneffei) B48.4
- penis (glans) (retention) NEC N48.29
- periapical K04.5
- peridental, periodontal K05.20
  - generalized *see* Periodontitis, aggressive, generalized
  - localized *see* Periodontitis, aggressive, localized
- perinatal period P39.9
  - specified type NEC P39.8
- perineal repair (puerperal) O86.09
- periorbital *see* Inflammation, orbit
- perirectal K62.89
- perirenal *see* Infection, kidney
- peritoneal *see* Peritonitis
- periureteral N28.89
- Petriellidium boydii B48.2
- pharynx *see also* Pharyngitis
  - coxsackievirus B08.5
  - posterior, lymphoid (chronic) J35.03
- Phialophora
  - gougerotii (subcutaneous abscess or cyst) B43.2
  - jeanselmei (subcutaneous abscess or cyst) B43.2
  - verrucosa (skin) B43.0
- Piedraia hortae B36.3

Infection, infected, infective - *continued*
- pinta A67.9
  - intermediate A67.1
  - late A67.2
  - mixed A67.3
  - primary A67.0
- pinworm B80
- Pityrosporum furfur B36.0
- Pleuro-pneumonia-like Organism (PPLO) NEC A49.3
  - as cause of disease classified elsewhere B96.0
- pneumococcus, pneumococcal NEC A49.1
  - as cause of disease classified elsewhere B95.3
  - generalized (purulent) A40.3
    - with pneumonia J13
- Pneumocystis carinii (pneumonia) B59
- Pneumocystis jiroveci (pneumonia) B59
- port or reservoir T80.212
- postoperative T81.4
- postoperative wound T81.49
  - surgical site
    - deep incisional T81.42
    - organ and space T81.43
    - specified NEC T81.49
    - superficial incisional T81.41
- postprocedural T81.40
- postvaccinal T88.0
- prepuce NEC N47.7
  - with penile inflammation N47.6
- prion *see* Disease, prion, central nervous system
- prostate (capsule) *see* Prostatitis
- Proteus (mirabilis) (morganii) (vulgaris) NEC A49.8
  - as cause of disease classified elsewhere B96.4
- protozoal NEC B64
  - intestinal A07.9
    - specified NEC A07.8
  - specified NEC B60.8
- Pseudoallescheria boydii B48.2
- Pseudomonas NEC A49.8
  - as cause of disease classified elsewhere B96.5
  - mallei A24.0
  - pneumonia J15.1
  - pseudomallei *see* Melioidosis
- puerperal O86.4
  - genitourinary tract NEC O86.89
  - major or generalized O85
  - minor O86.4
  - specified NEC O86.89
- pulmonary *see* Infection, lung
- purulent *see* Abscess
- Pyrenochaeta romeroi B47.0
- Q fever A78
- rectum (sphincter) K62.89
- renal *see also* Infection, kidney
  - pelvis and ureter (cystic) N28.85
- reovirus, as cause of disease classified elsewhere B97.5
- respiratory (tract) NEC J98.8
  - acute J22
  - chronic J98.8
  - influenzal (upper) (acute) *see* Influenza, with, respiratory manifestations NEC
  - lower (acute) J22
    - chronic *see* Bronchitis, chronic
  - rhinovirus J00
  - syncytial virus, as cause of disease classified elsewhere B97.4
  - upper (acute) NOS J06.9
    - chronic J39.8

Infection, infected, infective - *continued*

|streptococcal J06.9
|viral NOS J06.9
|resulting from
|presence of internal prosthesis, implant,
graft *see* Complications, by site and type,
infection
|retortamoniasis A07.8
|retroperitoneal NEC K68.9
|retrovirus B33.3
|as cause of disease classified elsewhere
B97.30
|human
|immunodeficiency, type 2 (HIV 2)
B97.35
|T-cell lymphotropic
|type I (HTLV-I) B97.33
|type II (HTLV-II) B97.34
|lentivirus B97.31
|oncovirus B97.32
|specified NEC B97.39
|Rhinosporidium (seeberi) B48.1
|rhinovirus
|as cause of disease classified elsewhere
B97.89
|unspecified nature or site B34.8
|Rhizopus *see* Mucormycosis
|rickettsial NOS A79.9
|roundworm (large) NEC B82.0
|Ascariasis *see also* Ascariasis B77.9
|rubella *see* Rubella
|Saccharomyces *see* Candidiasis
|salivary duct or gland (any) *see* Sialoadenitis
|Salmonella (aertrycke) (arizonae) (gallinarum)
(cholerae-suis) (enteritidis) (suipestifer)
(typhimurium) A02.9
|with
(gastro) enteritis A02.0
|sepsis A02.1
|specified manifestation NEC A02.8
|due to food (poisoning) A02.9
|hirschfeldii A01.3
|localized A02.20
|arthritis A02.23
|meningitis A02.21
|osteomyelitis A02.24
|pneumonia A02.22
|pyelonephritis A02.25
|specified NEC A02.29
|paratyphi A01.4
|A A01.1
|B A01.2
|C A01.3
|schottmuelleri A01.2
|typhi, typhosa *see* Typhoid
|Sarcocystis A07.8
|scabies B86
|Schistosoma *see* Infestation, Schistosoma
|scrotum (acute) NEC N49.2
|seminal vesicle *see* Vesiculitis
|septic
|localized, skin *see* Abscess
|sheep liver fluke B66.3
|Shigella A03.9
|boydii A03.2
|dysenteriae A03.0
|flexneri A03.1
|group
|A A03.0
|B A03.1
|C A03.2
|D A03.3
|Schmitz (-Stutzer) A03.0
|schmitzii A03.0
|shigae A03.0
|sonnei A03.3
|specified NEC A03.8
|shoulder (joint) NEC M00.9

Infection, infected, infective - *continued*

|due to internal joint prosthesis T84.59
|skin NEC L08.9
|sinus (accessory) (chronic) (nasal) *see also*
Sinusitis
|pilonidal *see* Sinus, pilonidal
|skin NEC L08.89
|Skene's duct or gland *see* Urethritis
|skin (local) (staphylococcal) (streptococcal)
L08.9
|abscess   code by site under Abscess
|cellulitis   code by site under Cellulitis
|due to fungus B36.9
|specified type NEC B36.8
|mycotic B36.9
|specified type NEC B36.8
|newborn P39.4
|ulcer *see* Ulcer, skin
|slow virus A81.9
|specified NEC A81.89
|Sparganum (mansoni) (proliferum) (baxteri)
B70.1
|specific *see also* Syphilis
|to perinatal period *see* Infection, congenital
|specified NEC B99.8
|spermatic cord NEC N49.1
|sphenoidal (sinus) *see* Sinusitis, sphenoidal
|spinal cord NOS *see also* Myelitis G04.91
|abscess G06.1
|meninges *see* Meningitis
|streptococcal G04.89
|Spirillum A25.0
|spirochetal NOS A69.9
|lung A69.8
|specified NEC A69.8
|Spirometra larvae B70.1
|spleen D73.89
|Sporotrichum, Sporothrix (schenckii) *see*
Sporotrichosis
|staphylococcal, unspecified site
|aureus (methicillin susceptible) (MSSA)
A49.01
|methicillin resistant (MRSA) A49.02
|as cause of disease classified elsewhere
B95.8
|aureus (methicillin susceptible) (MSSA)
B95.61
|methicillin resistant (MRSA) B95.62
|specified NEC B95.7
|food poisoning A05.0
|generalized (purulent) A41.2
|pneumonia *see* Pneumonia, staphylococcal
|Stellantchasmus falcatus B66.8
|streptobacillus moniliformis A25.1
|streptococcal NEC A49.1
|as cause of disease classified elsewhere
B95.5
|B genitourinary complicating
|childbirth O98.82
|pregnancy O98.81-
|puerperium O98.83
|congenital
|sepsis P36.10
|group B P36.0
|specified NEC P36.19
|generalized (purulent) A40.9
|Streptomyces B47.1
|Strongyloides (stercoralis) *see*
Strongyloidiasis
|stump (amputation) (surgical) *see*
Complication, amputation stump, infection
|subcutaneous tissue, local L08.9
|suipestifer *see* Infection, salmonella
|swimming pool bacillus A31.1
|Taenia *see* Infestation, Taenia
|Taeniarhynchus saginatus B68.1

Infection, infected, infective - *continued*

|tapeworm *see* Infestation, tapeworm
|tendon (sheath) *see* Tenosynovitis, infective
NEC
|Ternidens diminutus B81.8
|testis *see* Orchitis
|threadworm B80
|throat *see* Pharyngitis
|thyroglossal duct K14.8
|toe (skin) L08.9
|cellulitis L03.03-
|fungus B35.1
|nail L03.03-
|fungus B35.1
|tongue NEC K14.0
|parasitic B37.0
|tonsil (and adenoid) (faucial) (lingual)
(pharyngeal) *see* Tonsillitis
|tooth, teeth K04.7
|periapical K04.7
|peridental, periodontal K05.20
|generalized *see* Periodontitis, aggressive,
generalized
|localized *see* Periodontitis, aggressive,
localized
|pulp K04.01
|irreversible K04.02
|reversible K04.01
|socket M27.3
|TORCH *see* Infection, congenital
|without active infection P00.2
|Torula histolytica *see* Cryptococcosis
|Toxocara (canis) (cati) (felis) B83.0
|Toxoplasma gondii *see* Toxoplasma
|trachea, chronic J42
|trematode NEC *see* Infestation, fluke
|trench fever A79.0
|Treponema pallidum *see* Syphilis
|Trichinella (spiralis) B75
|Trichomonas A59.9
|cervix A59.09
|intestine A07.8
|prostate A59.02
|specified site NEC A59.8
|urethra A59.03
|urogenitalis A59.00
|vagina A59.01
|vulva A59.01
|Trichophyton, trichophytic *see*
Dermatophytosis
|Trichosporon (beigelii) cutaneum B36.2
|Trichostrongylus B81.2
|Trichuris (trichiura) B79
|Trombicula (irritans) B88.0
|Trypanosoma
|brucei
|gambiense B56.0
|rhodesiense B56.1
|cruzi *see* Chagas' disease
|tubal *see* Salpingo-oophoritis
|tuberculous NEC *see* Tuberculosis
|tubo-ovarian *see* Salpingo-oophoritis
|tunnel T80.212
|tunica vaginalis N49.1
|tympanic membrane NEC *see* Myringitis
|typhoid (abortive) (ambulant) (bacillus) *see*
Typhoid
|typhus A75.9
|flea-borne A75.2
|mite-borne A75.3
|recrudescent A75.1
|tick-borne A77.9
|African A77.1
|North Asian A77.2
|umbilicus L08.82

Infection, infected, infective - *continued*
|ureter N28.86
|urethra *see* Urethritis
|urinary (tract) N39.0
  |bladder *see* Cystitis
  |complicating
    |pregnancy O23.4-
      |specified type NEC O23.3-
  |kidney *see* Infection, kidney
  |newborn P39.3
  |puerperal (postpartum) O86.20
  |tuberculous A18.13
  |urethra *see* Urethritis
|uterus, uterine *see* Endometritis
|vaccination T88.0
|vaccinia not from vaccination B08.011
|vagina (acute) *see* Vaginitis
|varicella B01.9
|varicose veins *see* Varix
|vas deferens NEC N49.1
|vesical *see* Cystitis
|Vibrio
  |cholerae A00.0
    |El Tor A00.1
  |parahaemolyticus (food poisoning) A05.3
  |vulnificus
    |as cause of disease classified elsewhere
      B96.82
    |foodborne intoxication A05.5
|Vincent's (gum) (mouth) (tonsil) A69.1
|virus, viral NOS B34.9
  |adenovirus
    |as cause of disease classified elsewhere
      B97.0
    |unspecified nature or site B34.0
  |arborvirus, arbovirus arthropod-borne A94
  |as cause of disease classified elsewhere
    B97.89
    |adenovirus B97.0
    |coronavirus B97.29
      |SARS-associated B97.21
    |coxsackievirus B97.11
    |echovirus B97.12
    |enterovirus B97.10
      |coxsackievirus B97.11
      |echovirus B97.12
      |specified NEC B97.19
    |human
      |immunodeficiency, type 2 (HIV 2)
        B97.35
      |T-cell lymphotropic,
        |type I (HTLV-I) B97.33
        |type II (HTLV-II) B97.34
      |metapneumovirus B97.81
    |papillomavirus B97.7
    |parvovirus B97.6
    |reovirus B97.5
    |respiratory syncytial B97.4
    |retrovirus B97.30
      |human
        |immunodeficiency, type 2 (HIV 2)
          B97.35
        |T-cell lymphotropic,
          |type I (HTLV-I) B97.33
          |type II (HTLV-II) B97.34
      |lentivirus B97.31
      |oncovirus B97.32
      |specified NEC B97.39
    |specified NEC B97.89
  |central nervous system A89
  |atypical A81.9
    |specified NEC A81.89
  |enterovirus NEC A88.8
    |meningitis A87.0
  |slow virus A81.9

Infection, infected, infective - *continued*
    |specified NEC A81.89
    |specified NEC A88.8
|chest J98.8
|cotia B08.8
|COVID-19 U07.1
|coxsackie *see also* Infection, coxsackie
  B34.1
  |as cause of disease classified elsewhere
    B97.11
|ECHO
  |as cause of disease classified elsewhere
    B97.12
  |unspecified nature or site B34.1
|encephalitis, tick-borne A84.9
|enterovirus, as cause of disease classified
  elsewhere B97.10
  |coxsackievirus B97.11
  |echovirus B97.12
  |specified NEC B97.19
|exanthem NOS B09
|human papilloma as cause of disease
  classified elsewhere B97.7
|human metapneumovirus as cause of disease
  classified elsewhere B97.81
|intestine *see* Enteritis, viral
|respiratory syncytial
  |as cause of disease classified elsewhere
    B97.4
  |bronchopneumonia J12.1
  |common cold syndrome J00
  |nasopharyngitis (acute) J00
|rhinovirus
  |as cause of disease classified elsewhere
    B97.89
  |unspecified nature or site B34.8
|slow A81.9
  |specified NEC A81.89
|specified type NEC B33.8
  |as cause of disease classified elsewhere
    B97.89
  |unspecified nature or site B34.8
|unspecified nature or site B34.9
|West Nile *see* Virus, West Nile
|vulva (acute) *see* Vulvitis
|West Nile *see* Virus, West Nile
|whipworm B79
|worms B83.9
  |specified type NEC B83.8
|Wuchereria (bancrofti) B74.0
  |malayi B74.1
|yatapoxvirus B08.70
  |specified NEC B08.79
|yeast *see also* Candidiasis B37.9
|yellow fever *see* Fever, yellow
|Yersinia
  |enterocolitica (intestinal) A04.6
  |pestis *see* Plague
  |pseudotuberculosis A28.2
|Zeis' gland *see* Hordeolum
|Zika virus A92.5
  |congenital P35.4
|zoonotic bacterial NOS A28.9
|Zofia senagalensis B47.0
Infective, infectious *see* condition
Infertility
|female N97.9
  |age-related N97.8
  |associated with
    |anovulation N97.0
    |cervical (mucus) disease or anomaly
      N88.3
    |congenital anomaly
      |cervix N88.3
      |fallopian tube N97.1
      |uterus N97.2

Infertility - *continued*
      |vagina N97.8
    |dysmucorrhea N88.3
    |fallopian tube disease or anomaly N97.1
    |pituitary-hypothalamic origin E23.0
    |specified origin NEC N97.8
    |Stein-Leventhal syndrome E28.2
    |uterine disease or anomaly N97.2
    |vaginal disease or anomaly N97.8
  |due to
    |cervical anomaly N88.3
    |fallopian tube anomaly N97.1
    |ovarian failure E28.39
    |Stein-Leventhal syndrome E28.2
    |uterine anomaly N97.2
    |vaginal anomaly N97.8
  |nonimplantation N97.2
  |origin
    |cervical N88.3
    |tubal (block) (occlusion) (stenosis) N97.1
    |uterine N97.2
    |vaginal N97.8
|male N46.9
  |azoospermia N46.01
    |extratesticular cause N46.029
      |drug therapy N46.021
      |efferent duct obstruction N46.023
      |infection N46.022
      |radiation N46.024
      |specified cause NEC N46.029
      |systemic disease N46.025
  |oligospermia N46.11
    |extratesticular cause N46.129
      |drug therapy N46.121
      |efferent duct obstruction N46.123
      |infection N46.122
      |radiation N46.124
      |specified cause NEC N46.129
      |systemic disease N46.125
  |specified type NEC N46.8
Infestation B88.9
|Acanthocheilonema (perstans) (streptocerca)
  B74.4
|Acariasis B88.0
  |demodex folliculorum B88.0
  |sarcoptes scabiei B86
  |trombiculae B88.0
|Agamofilaria streptocerca B74.4
|Ancylostoma, ankylostoma (braziliense)
  (caninum) (ceylanicum) (duodenale) B76.0
  |americanum B76.1
  |new world B76.1
|Anisakis larvae, anisakiasis B81.0
|arthropod NEC B88.2
|Ascaris lumbricoides *see* Ascariasis
|Balantidium coli A07.0
|beef tapeworm B68.1
|Bothriocephalus (latus) B70.0
  |larval B70.1
|broad tapeworm B70.0
  |larval B70.1
|Brugia (malayi) B74.1
  |timori B74.2
|candiru B88.8
|Capillaria
  |hepatica B83.8
  |philippinensis B81.1
|cat liver fluke B66.0
|cestodes B71.9
  |diphyllobothrium *see* Infestation,
    diphyllobothrium
  |dipylidiasis B71.1
  |hymenolepiasis B71.0
  |specified type NEC B71.8
|chigger B88.0

Infestation - *continued*

|chigo, chigoe B88.1
|Clonorchis (sinensis) (liver) B66.1
|coccidial A07.3
|crab-lice B85.3
|Cysticercus cellulosae *see* Cysticercosis
|Demodex (folliculorum) B88.0
|Dermanyssus gallinae B88.0
|Dermatobia (hominis) *see* Myiasis
|Dibothriocephalus (latus) B70.0
  |larval B70.1
|Dicrocoelium dendriticum B66.2
|Diphyllobothrium (adult) (latum) (intestinal) (pacificum) B70.0
  |larval B70.1
|Diplogonoporus (grandis) B71.8
|Dipylidium caninum B67.4
|Distoma hepaticum B66.3
|dog tapeworm B67.4
|Dracunculus medinensis B72
|dragon worm B72
|dwarf tapeworm B71.0
|Echinococcus *see* Echinococcus
|Echinostomum ilocanum B66.8
|Entamoeba (histolytica) *see* Infection, Ameba
|Enterobius vermicularis B80
|eyelid
  |in (due to)
    |leishmaniasis B55.1
    |loiasis B74.3
    |onchocerciasis B73.09
    |phthiriasis B85.3
  |parasitic NOS B89
|eyeworm B74.3
|Fasciola (gigantica) (hepatica) (indica) B66.3
|Fasciolopsis (buski) (intestine) B66.5
|filarial B74.9
  |bancroftian B74.0
  |conjunctiva B74.9
  |due to
    |Acanthocheilonema (perstans) (streptocerca) B74.4
    |Brugia (malayi) B74.1
      |timori B74.2
    |Dracunculus medinensis B72
    |guinea worm B72
    |Loa Loa B74.3
    |Mansonella (ozzardi) (perstans) (streptocerca) B74.4
    |Onchocerca volvulus B73.00
      |eye B73.00
      |eyelid B73.09
    |Wuchereria (bancrofti) B74.0
  |Malayan B74.1
  |ozzardi B74.4
  |specified type NEC B74.8
|fish tapeworm B70.0
  |larval B70.1
|fluke B66.9
  |blood NOS *see* Schistosomiasis
  |cat liver B66.0
  |intestinal B66.5
  |liver (sheep) B66.3
    |cat B66.0
    |Chinese B66.1
    |due to clonorchiasis B66.1
    |oriental B66.1
  |lancet B66.2
  |lung (oriental) B66.4
  |sheep liver B66.3
  |specified type NEC B66.8
|fly larvae *see* Myiasis
|Gasterophilus (intestinalis) *see* Myiasis
|Gastrodiscoides hominis B66.8

Infestation - *continued*

|Giardia lamblia A07.1
|Gnathostoma (spinigerum) B83.1
|Gongylonema B83.8
|guinea worm B72
|helminth B83.9
  |angiostrongyliasis B83.2
    |intestinal B81.3
  |gnathostomiasis B83.1
  |hirudiniasis, internal B83.4
  |intestinal B82.0
    |angiostrongyliasis B81.3
    |anisakiasis B81.0
    |ascariasis *see* Ascariasis
    |capillariasis B81.1
    |cysticercosis *see* Cysticercosis
    |diphyllobothriasis *see* Infestation, diphyllobothriasis
    |dracunculiasis B72
    |echinococcus *see* Echinococcosis
    |enterobiasis B80
    |filariasis *see* Infestation, filarial
    |fluke *see* Infestation, fluke
    |hookworm *see* Infestation, hookworm
    |mixed (types classifiable to more than one of the titles B65.0-B81.3 and B81.8) B81.4
    |onchocerciasis *see* Onchocerciasis
    |schistosomiasis *see* Infestation, Schistosoma
    |specified
      |cestode NEC *see* Infestation, cestode
      |type NEC B81.8
    |strongyloidiasis *see* Strongyloidiasis
    |taenia *see* Infestation, taenia
    |trichinellosis B75
    |trichostrongyliasis B81.2
    |trichuriasis B79
  |specified type NEC B83.8
  |syngamiasis B83.3
  |visceral larva migrans B83.0
|Heterophyes (heterophyes) B66.8
|hookworm B76.9
  |ancylostomiasis B76.0
  |necatoriasis B76.1
  |specified type NEC B76.8
|Hymenolepis (diminuta) (nana) B71.0
|intestinal NEC B82.9
|leeches (aquatic) (land) *see* Hirudiniasis
|Leishmania *see* Leishmaniasis
|lice, louse *see* Infestation, Pediculus
|Linguatula B88.8
|Liponyssoides sanguineus B88.0
|Loa Loa B74.3
  |conjunctival B74.3
  |eyelid B74.3
|louse *see* Infestation, Pediculus
|maggots *see* Myiasis
|Mansonella (ozzardi) (perstans) (streptocerca) B74.4
|Medina (worm) B72
|Metagonimus (yokogawai) B66.8
|microfilaria streptocerca *see* Onchocerciasis
  |eye B73.00
  |eyelid B73.09
|mites B88.9
  |scabic B86
|Monilia (albicans) *see* Candidiasis
|mouth B37.0
|Necator americanus B76.1
|nematode NEC (intestinal) B82.0
  |Ancylostoma B76.0
  |conjunctiva NEC B83.9
  |Enterobius vermicularis B80
  |Gnathostoma spinigerum B83.1

Infestation - *continued*

|physaloptera B80
|specified NEC B81.8
|trichostrongylus B81.2
|trichuris (trichuria) B79
|Oesophagostomum (apiostomum) B81.8
|Oestrus ovis *see also* Myiasis B87.9
|Onchocerca (volvulus) *see* Onchocerciasis
|Opisthorchis (felineus) (viverrini) B66.0
|orbit, parasitic NOS B89
|Oxyuris vermicularis B80
|Paragonimus (westermani) B66.4
|parasite, parasitic B89
  |eyelid B89
  |intestinal NOS B82.9
  |mouth B37.0
  |skin B88.9
  |tongue B37.0
|Parastrongylus
  |cantonensis B83.2
  |costaricensis B81.3
|Pediculus B85.2
  |body B85.1
  |capitis (humanus) (any site) B85.0
  |corporis (humanus) (any site) B85.1
  |head B85.0
  |mixed (classifiable to more than one of the titles B85.0-B85.3) B85.4
  |pubis (any site) B85.3
|Pentastoma B88.8
|Phthirus (pubis) (any site) B85.3
  |with any infestation classifiable to B85.0-B85.2 B85.4
|pinworm B80
|pork tapeworm (adult) B68.0
|protozoal NEC B64
  |intestinal A07.9
    |specified NEC A07.8
  |specified NEC B60.8
|pubic, louse B85.3
|rat tapeworm B71.0
|red bug B88.0
|roundworm (large) NEC B82.0
  |Ascariasis *see also* Ascariasis B77.9
|sandflea B88.1
|Sarcoptes scabiei B86
|scabies B86
|Schistosoma B65.9
  |bovis B65.8
  |cercariae B65.3
  |haematobium B65.0
  |intercalatum B65.8
  |japonicum B65.2
  |mansoni B65.1
  |mattheei B65.8
  |mekongi B65.8
  |specified type NEC B65.8
  |spindale B65.8
|screw worms *see* Myiasis
|skin NOS B88.9
|Sparganum (mansoni) (proliferum) (baxteri) B70.1
  |larval B70.1
|specified type NEC B88.8
|Spirometra larvae B70.1
|Stellantchasmus falcatus B66.8
|Strongyloides stercoralis *see* Strongyloidiasis
|Taenia B68.9
  |diminuta B71.0
  |echinococcus *see* Echinococcus
  |mediocanellata B68.1
  |nana B71.0
  |saginata B68.1
  |solium (intestinal form) B68.0
    |larval form *see* Cysticercosis

Infestation - *continued*
|Taeniarhynchus saginatus B68.1
|tapeworm B71.9
  |beef B68.1
  |broad B70.0
    |larval B70.1
  |dog B67.4
  |dwarf B71.0
  |fish B70.0
    |larval B70.1
  |pork B68.0
  |rat B71.0
|Ternidens diminutus B81.8
|Tetranychus molestissimus B88.0
|threadworm B80
|tongue B37.0
|Toxocara (canis) (cati) (felis) B83.0
|trematode(s) NEC *see* Infestation, fluke
|Trichinella (spiralis) B75
|Trichocephalus B79
|Trichomonas *see* Trichomoniasis
|Trichostrongylus B81.2
|Trichuris (trichiura) B79
|Trombicula (irritans) B88.0
|Tunga penetrans B88.1
|Uncinaria americana B76.1
|Vandellia cirrhosa B88.8
|whipworm B79
|worms B83.9
  |intestinal B82.0
|Wuchereria (bancrofti) B74.0
Infiltrate, infiltration
|amyloid (generalized) (localized) *see*
  Amyloidosis
|calcareous NEC R89.7
  |localized *see* Degeneration, by site
|calcium salt R89.7
|cardiac
  |fatty *see* Degeneration, myocardial
  |glycogenic E74.02 [*143*]
|corneal *see* Edema, cornea
|eyelid *see* Inflammation, eyelid
|glycogen, glycogenic *see* Disease, glycogen
  storage
|heart, cardiac
  |fatty *see* Degeneration, myocardial
  |glycogenic E74.02 [*143*]
|inflammatory in vitreous H43.89
|kidney N28.89
|leukemic *see* Leukemia
|liver K76.89
  |fatty *see* Fatty, liver NEC
  |glycogen *see also* Disease, glycogen storage
    E74.03 [*K77*]
|lung R91.8
  |eosinophilic   *see* Eosinophilia, pulmonary
  |lymphatic *see also* Leukemia, lymphatic
    C91.9-
  |gland I88.9
|muscle, fatty M62.89
|myocardium, myocardial
  |fatty *see* Degeneration, myocardial
  |glycogenic E74.02 [*143*]
|on chest x-ray R91.8
|pulmonary R91.8
  |with eosinophilia – *see* Eosinophilia,
    pulmonary
|skin (lymphocytic) L98.6
|thymus (gland) (fatty) E32.8
|urine R39.0
|vesicant agent
  |antineoplastic chemotherapy T80.810
  |other agent NEC T80.818
|vitreous body H43.89

Infirmity R68.89
|senile R54
Inflammation, inflamed, inflammatory (with exudation)
|abducent (nerve) *see* Strabismus, paralytic,
  sixth nerve
|accessory sinus (chronic) *see* Sinusitis
|adrenal (gland) E27.8
|alveoli, teeth M27.3
  |scorbutic E54
|anal canal, anus K62.89
|antrum (chronic) *see* Sinusitis, maxillary
|appendix *see* Appendicitis
|arachnoid *see* Meningitis
|areola N61.0
  |puerperal, postpartum or gestational *see*
  |Infection, nipple
|areolar tissue NOS L08.9
|artery *see* Arteritis
|auditory meatus (external) *see* Otitis, externa
|Bartholin's gland N75.8
|bile duct (common) (hepatic) or passage *see*
  Cholangitis
|bladder *see* Cystitis
|bone *see* Osteomyelitis
|brain *see also* Encephalitis
  |membrane *see* Meningitis
|breast N61.0
  |puerperal, postpartum, gestational *see*
  Mastitis, obstetric
|broad ligament *see* Disease, pelvis,
  inflammatory
|bronchi *see* Bronchitis
|catarrhal J00
|cecum *see* Appendicitis
|cerebral *see also* Encephalitis
  |membrane *see* Meningitis
|cerebrospinal
  |meningococcal A39.0
|cervix (uteri) *see* Cervicitis
|chest J98.8
|chorioretinal H30.9-
  |cyclitis *see* Cyclitis
  |disseminated H30.10-
    |generalized H30.13-
    |peripheral H30.12-
    |posterior pole H30.11-
  |epitheliopathy *see* Epitheliopathy
  |focal H30.00-
    |juxtapapillary H30.01-
    |macular H30.04-
    |paramacular *see* Inflammation,
  chorioretinal, focal, macular
    |peripheral H30.03-
    |posterior pole H30.02-
  |specified type NEC H30.89-
|choroid *see* Inflammation, chorioretinal
|chronic, postmastoidectomy cavity *see*
  Complications, postmastoidectomy,
  inflammation
|colon *see* Enteritis
|connective tissue (diffuse) NEC *see* Disorder,
  soft tissue, specified type NEC
|cornea *see* Keratitis
|corpora cavernosa N48.29
|cranial nerve *see* Disorder, nerve, cranial
|Douglas' cul-de-sac or pouch (chronic) N73.0
|due to device, implant or graft *see also*
  Complications, by site and type, infection
  or inflammation
  |arterial graft T82.7
  |breast (implant) T85.79
  |catheter T85.79
    |dialysis (renal) T82.7
      |intraperitoneal T85.71

Inflammation - *continued*
|infusion T82.7
  |cranial T85.735
  |intrathecal T85.735
  |spinal (epidural) (subdural) T85.735
  |subarachnoid T85.735
  |urinary T83.518
    |cystostomy T83.510
    |Hopkins T83.518
    |ileostomy T83.518
    |nephrostomy T83.512
    |specified NEC T83.518
    |urethral indwelling T83.511
    |urostomy T83.518
|electronic (electrode) (pulse generator)
  (stimulator)
  |bone T84.7
  |cardiac T82.7
  |nervous system T85.738
    |brain T85.731
    |cranial nerve T85.732
    |gastric nerve T85.732
    |neurostimulator generator T85.734
    |peripheral nerve T85.732
    |sacral nerve T85.732
    |spinal cord T85.733
    |vagal nerve T85.732
  |urinary T83.590
|fixation, internal (orthopedic) NEC *see*
  Complication, fixation device, infection
|gastrointestinal (bile duct) (esophagus)
  T85.79
|neurostimulator electrode (lead) T85.732
|genital NEC T83.69
|heart NEC T82.7
  |valve (prosthesis) T82.6
    |graft T82.7
|joint prosthesis *see* Complication, joint
  prosthesis, infection
|ocular (corneal graft) (orbital implant) NEC
  T85.79
|orthopedic NEC T84.7
|penile (cylinder) (pump) (reservoir) T83.61
|specified NEC T85.79
|testicular T83.62
|urinary NEC T83.598
  |ileal conduit stent T83.593
  |implanted neurostimulation T83.590
  |implanted sphincter T83.591
  |indwelling ureteral stent T83.592
  |nephroureteral stent T83.593
  |specified stent NEC T83.593
|vascular NEC T82.7
|ventricular intracranial (communicating)
  shunt T85.730
|duodenum K29.80
  |with bleeding K29.81
|dura mater *see* Meningitis
|ear (middle) *see also* Otitis, media
  |external *see* Otitis, externa
  |inner *see* subcategory H83.0
|epididymis *see* Epididymitis
|esophagus – *see* Esophagitis
|ethmoidal (sinus) (chronic) *see* Sinusitis,
  ethmoidal
|eustachian tube (catarrhal) *see* Salpingitis,
  eustachian
|eyelid H01.9
  |abscess *see* Abscess, eyelid
  |blepharitis *see* Blepharitis
  |chalazion *see* Chalazion
  |dermatosis (noninfectious) *see* Dermatosis,
    eyelid
  |hordeolum *see* Hordeolum
  |specified NEC H01.8

Inflammation - continued

| fallopian tube *see* Salpingo-oophoritis
| fascia *see* Myositis
| follicular, pharynx J31.2
| frontal (sinus) (chronic) *see* Sinusitis, frontal
| gallbladder *see* Cholecystitis
| gastric *see* Gastritis
| gastrointestinal *see* Enteritis
| genital organ (internal) (diffuse)
　| female *see* Disease, pelvis, inflammatory
　| male N49.9
　　| multiple sites N49.8
　　| specified NEC N49.8
| gland (lymph) *see* Lymphadenitis
| glottis *see* Laryngitis
| granular, pharynx J31.2
| gum K05.10
　| nonplaque induced K05.11
　| plaque induced K05.10
| heart *see* Carditis
| hepatic duct *see* Cholangitis
| ileoanal (internal) pouch K91.850
| ileum *see also* Enteritis
　| regional or terminal *see* Enteritis, regional
| intestine (any part) *see* Enteritis
| intestinal pouch K91.850
| jaw (acute) (bone) (chronic) (lower) (suppurative) (upper) M27.2
| joint NEC *see* Arthritis
　| sacroiliac M46.1
| kidney *see* Nephritis
| knee (joint) M13.169
　| tuberculous A18.02
| labium (majus) (minus) *see* Vulvitis
| lacrimal
　| gland *see* Dacryoadenitis
　| passages (duct) (sac) *see also* Dacryocystitis
　　| canaliculitis *see* Canaliculitis, lacrimal
| larynx *see* Laryngitis
| leg NOS L08.9
| lip K13.0
| liver (capsule) *see also* Hepatitis
　| chronic K73.9
　| suppurative K75.0
| lung (acute) *see also* Pneumonia
　| chronic J98.4
| lymph gland or node *see* Lymphadenitis
| lymphatic vessel *see* Lymphangitis
| maxilla, maxillary M27.2
　| sinus (chronic) *see* Sinusitis, maxillary
| membranes of brain or spinal cord *see* Meningitis
| meninges *see* Meningitis
| mouth K12.1
| muscle *see* Myositis
| myocardium *see* Myocarditis
| nasal sinus (chronic) *see* Sinusitis
| nasopharynx *see* Nasopharyngitis
| navel L08.82
| nerve NEC *see* Neuritis
| nipple N61.0
　| puerperal, postpartum or gestational *see* Infection, nipple
| nose *see* Rhinitis
| oculomotor (nerve) *see* Strabismus, paralytic, third nerve
| optic nerve *see* Neuritis, optic
| orbit (chronic) H05.10
　| acute H05.00
　　| abscess *see* Abscess, orbit
　　| cellulitis *see* Cellulitis, orbit
　　| osteomyelitis *see* Osteomyelitis, orbit
　　| periostitis *see* Periostitis, orbital
　　| tenonitis *see* Tenonitis, eye

Inflammation - continued

　| granuloma *see* Granuloma, orbit
　| myositis *see* Myositis, orbital
| ovary *see* Salpingo-oophoritis
| oviduct *see* Salpingo-oophoritis
| pancreas (acute) *see* Pancreatitis
| parametrium N73.0
| parotid region L08.9
| pelvis, female *see* Disease, pelvis, inflammatory
| penis (corpora cavernosa) N48.29
| perianal K62.89
| pericardium *see* Pericarditis
| perineum (female) (male) L08.9
| perirectal K62.89
| peritoneum *see* Peritonitis
| periuterine *see* Disease, pelvis, inflammatory
| perivesical *see* Cystitis
| petrous bone (acute) (chronic) *see* Petrositis
| pharynx (acute) *see* Pharyngitis
| pia mater *see* Meningitis
| pleura *see* Pleurisy
| polyp, colon *see also* Polyp, colon, inflammatory K51.40
| prostate *see also* Prostatitis
　| specified type NEC N41.8
| rectosigmoid *see* Rectosigmoiditis
| rectum *see also* Proctitis K62.89
| respiratory, upper *see also* Infection, respiratory, upper J06.9
　| acute, due to radiation J70.0
　| chronic, due to external agent *see* condition, respiratory, chronic, due to
　| due to
　　| chemicals, gases, fumes or vapors (inhalation) J68.2
　　| radiation J70.1
| retina *see* Chorioretinitis
| retrocecal *see* Appendicitis
| retroperitoneal *see* Peritonitis
| salivary duct or gland (any) (suppurative) *see* Sialoadenitis
| scorbutic, alveoli, teeth E54
| scrotum N49.2
| seminal vesicle *see* Vesiculitis
| sigmoid *see* Enteritis
| sinus *see* Sinusitis
| Skene's duct or gland *see* Urethritis
| skin L08.9
| spermatic cord N49.1
| sphenoidal (sinus) *see* Sinusitis, sphenoidal
| spinal
　| cord *see* Encephalitis
　| membrane *see* Meningitis
　| nerve *see* Disorder, nerve
| spine *see* Spondylopathy, inflammatory
| spleen (capsule) D73.89
| stomach *see* Gastritis
| subcutaneous tissue L08.9
| suprarenal (gland) E27.8
| synovial *see* Tenosynovitis
| tendon (sheath) NEC *see* Tenosynovitis
| testis *see* Orchitis
| throat (acute) *see* Pharyngitis
| thymus (gland) E32.8
| thyroid (gland) *see* Thyroiditis
| tongue K14.0
| tonsil *see* Tonsillitis
| trachea *see* Tracheitis
| trochlear (nerve) *see* Strabismus, paralytic, fourth nerve
| tubal *see* Salpingo-oophoritis
| tuberculous NEC *see* Tuberculosis
| tubo-ovarian *see* Salpingo-oophoritis

Inflammation - continued

| tunica vaginalis N49.1
| tympanic membrane *see* Tympanitis
| umbilicus, umbilical L08.82
| uterine ligament *see* Disease, pelvis, inflammatory
| uterus (catarrhal) *see* Endometritis
| uveal tract (anterior) NOS *see also* Iridocyclitis
　| posterior *see* Chorioretinitis
| vagina *see* Vaginitis
| vas deferens N49.1
| vein *see also* Phlebitis
　| intracranial or intraspinal (septic) G08
　| thrombotic I80.9
　　| leg *see* Phlebitis, leg
　　| lower extremity *see* Phlebitis, leg
| vocal cord J38.3
| vulva *see* Vulvitis
| Wharton's duct (suppurative) *see* Sialoadenitis

Inflation, lung, imperfect (newborn) *see* Atelectasis

Influenza (bronchial) (epidemic) (respiratory (upper)) (unidentified influenza virus) J11.1

| with
　| digestive manifestations J11.2
　| encephalopathy J11.81
　| enteritis J11.2
　| gastroenteritis J11.2
　| gastrointestinal manifestations J11.2
　| laryngitis J11.1
　| myocarditis J11.82
　| otitis media J11.83
　| pharyngitis J11.1
　| pneumonia J11.00
　　| specified type J11.08
　| respiratory manifestations NEC J11.1
　| specified manifestation NEC J11.89
| A (non-novel) J10-
| A/H5N1 *see also* Influenza, due to, identified novel influenza A virus J09.X2
| avian *see also* Influenza, due to, identified novel influenza A virus J09.X2
| B J10
| bird *see also* Influenza, due to, identified novel influenza A virus J09.X2
| C J10-
| novel (2009) H1N1 influenza *see also* Influenza, due to, identified influenza virus NEC J10.1
| novel influenza A/H1N1 *see also* Influenza, due to, identified influenza virus NEC J10.1
| due to
　| avian *see also* Influenza, due to, identified novel influenza A virus J09.X2
　| identified influenza virus NEC J10.1
　　| with
　　　| digestive manifestations J10.2
　　　| encephalopathy J10.81
　　　| enteritis J10.2
　　　| gastroenteritis J10.2
　　　| gastrointestinal manifestations J10.2
　　　| laryngitis J10.1
　　　| myocarditis J10.82
　　　| otitis media J10.83
　　　| pharyngitis J10.1
　　　| pneumonia (unspecified type) J10.00
　　　　| with same identified influenza virus J10.01
　　　　| specified type NEC J10.08
　　　| respiratory manifestations NEC J10.1
　　　| specified manifestation NEC J10.89

Influenza - *continued*
  |identified novel influenza A virus J09.X2
  |with
    |digestive manifestations J09.X3
    |encephalopathy J09.X9
    |enteritis J09.X3
    |gastroenteritis J09.X3
    |gastrointestinal manifestations J09.X3
    |laryngitis J09.X2
    |myocarditis J09.X9
    |otitis media J09.X9
    |pharyngitis J09.X2
    |pneumonia J09.X1
    |respiratory manifestations NEC J09.X2
    |specified manifestation NEC J09.X9
    |upper respiratory symptoms J09.X2
  |of other animal origin, not bird or swine *see also* Influenza, due to, identified novel influenza A virus J09.X2
  |swine (viruses that normally cause infections in pigs) *see also* Influenza, due to, identified novel influenza A virus J09.X2
Influenza-Like disease *see* Influenza
Influenzal *see* Influenza
Infraction, Freiberg's (metatarsal head) *see* Osteochondrosis, juvenile, metatarsus
Infraeruption of tooth (teeth) M26.34
Infusion complication, misadventure, or reaction *see* Complications, infusion
Ingestion
  |chemical *see* Table of Drugs and Chemicals, by substance, poisoning
  |drug or medicament
    |correct substance properly administered *see* Table of Drugs and Chemicals, by drug, adverse effect
    |overdose or wrong substance given or taken *see* Table of Drugs and Chemicals, by drug, poisoning
  |foreign body *see* Foreign body, alimentary tract
  |tularemia A21.3
Ingrowing
  |hair (beard) L73.1
  |nail (finger) (toe) L60.0
Inguinal *see also* condition
  |testicle Q53.9
    |bilateral Q53.212
    |unilateral Q53.112
Inhalant-Induced
  |anxiety disorder F18.980
  |depressive disorder F18.94
  |major neurocognitive disorder F18.97
  |mild neurocognitive disorder F18.988
  |psychotic disorder F18.959
Inhalation
  |anthrax A22.1
  |flame T27.3
  |food or foreign body *see* Foreign body, by site
  |gases, fumes, or vapors T59.9-
    |specified agent NEC *see* Table of Drugs and Chemicals, by substance T59.89-
  |liquid or vomitus *see* Asphyxia
  |meconium (newborn) P24.00
    |with
      |pneumonia (pneumonitis) P24.01
      |with respiratory symptoms P24.01
  |mucus *see* Asphyxia, mucus
  |oil or gasoline (causing suffocation) *see* Foreign body, by site
  |smoke T59.81
    |with respiratory conditions J70.5
      |due to chemicals, gases, fumes and vapors J68.9

Inhalation - *continued*
  |steam (see also Burn, respiratory tract) T59.9-
  |stomach contents or secretions *see* Foreign body, by site
    |due to anesthesia (general) (local) or other sedation T88.59
      |in labor and delivery O74.0
      |in pregnancy O29.01-
      |postpartum, puerperal O89.01
Inhibition, orgasm
  |female F52.31
  |male F52.32
Inhibitor, systemic lupus erythematosus (presence of) D68.62
Iniencephalus, iniencephaly Q00.2
Injection, traumatic jet (air) (industrial) (water) (paint or dye) T70.4
Injury *see also* specified injury type T14.90
  |abdomen, abdominal S39.91
    |blood vessel *see* Injury, blood vessel, abdomen
    |cavity *see* Injury, intra-abdominal
    |contusion S30.1
    |internal *see* Injury, intra-abdominal
    |intra-abdominal organ *see* Injury, intra-abdominal
    |nerve *see* Injury, nerve, abdomen
    |open *see* Wound, open, abdomen
    |specified NEC S39.81
    |superficial *see* Injury, superficial, abdomen
  |Achilles tendon S86.00-
    |laceration S86.02-
    |specified type NEC S86.09-
    |strain S86.01-
  |acoustic, resulting in deafness *see* Injury, nerve, acoustic
  |adrenal (gland) S37.819
    |contusion S37.812
    |laceration S37.813
    |specified type NEC S37.818
  |alveolar (process) S09.93
  |ankle S99.91-
    |contusion *see* Contusion, ankle
    |dislocation *see* Dislocation, ankle
    |fracture *see* Fracture, ankle
    |nerve *see* Injury, nerve, ankle
    |open *see* Wound, open, ankle
    |specified type NEC S99.81-
    |sprain *see* Sprain, ankle
    |superficial *see* Injury, superficial, ankle
  |anterior chamber, eye *see* Injury, eye, specified site NEC
  |anus *see* Injury, abdomen
  |aorta (thoracic) S25.00
    |abdominal S35.00
      |laceration (minor) (superficial) S35.01
        |major S35.02
      |specified type NEC S35.09
    |laceration (minor) (superficial) S25.01
      |major S25.02
    |specified type NEC S25.09
  |arm (upper) S49.9-
    |blood vessel *see* Injury, blood vessel, arm
    |contusion *see* Contusion, arm, upper
    |fracture *see* Fracture, humerus
    |lower *see* Injury, forearm
    |muscle *see* Injury, muscle, shoulder
    |nerve *see* Injury, nerve, arm
    |open *see* Wound, open, arm
    |specified type NEC S49.8-
    |superficial *see* Injury, superficial, arm
  |artery (complicating trauma) *see also* Injury, blood vessel, by site

Injury - *continued*
  |cerebral or meningeal *see* Injury, intracranial
  |auditory canal (external) (meatus) S09.91
  |auricle, auris, ear S09.91
  |axilla *see* Injury, shoulder
  |back *see* Injury, back, lower
  |bile duct S36.13
  |birth *see also* Birth, injury P15.9
  |bladder (sphincter) S37.20
    |at delivery O71.5
    |contusion S37.22
    |laceration S37.23
    |obstetrical trauma O71.5
    |specified type NEC S37.29
  |blast (air) (hydraulic) (immersion) (underwater) NEC T14.8
    |acoustic nerve trauma *see* Injury, nerve, acoustic
    |bladder *see* Injury, bladder
    |brain *see* Concussion
    |colon *see* Injury, intestine, large, blast injury
    |ear (primary) S09.31-
      |secondary S09.39-
    |generalized T70.8
    |lung *see* Injury, intrathoracic, lung, blast injury
    |multiple body organs T70.8
    |peritoneum S36.81
    |rectum S36.61
    |retroperitoneum S36.898
    |small intestine S36.419
      |duodenum S36.410
      |specified site NEC S36.418
    |specified
      |intra-abdominal organ NEC S36.898
      |pelvic organ NEC S37.899
  |blood vessel NEC T14.8
    |abdomen S35.9-
      |aorta *see* Injury, aorta, abdominal
      |celiac artery *see* Injury, blood vessel, celiac artery
      |iliac vessel *see* Injury, blood vessel, iliac
      |laceration S35.91
      |mesenteric vessel *see* Injury, mesenteric
      |portal vein *see* Injury, blood vessel, portal vein
      |renal vessel *see* Injury, blood vessel, renal
      |specified vessel NEC S35.8X-
      |splenic vessel *see* Injury, blood vessel, splenic
      |vena cava *see* Injury, vena cava, inferior
    |ankle *see* Injury, blood vessel, foot
    |aorta (abdominal) (thoracic) *see* Injury, aorta
    |arm (upper) NEC S45.90-
      |forearm *see* Injury, blood vessel, forearm
      |laceration S45.91-
      |specified
        |site NEC S45.80-
          |laceration S45.81-
          |specified type NEC S45.89-
        |type NEC S45.99-
      |superficial vein S45.30-
        |laceration S45.31-
        |specified type NEC S45.39-
    |axillary
      |artery S45.00-
        |laceration S45.01-
        |specified type NEC S45.09-
      |vein S45.20-
        |laceration S45.21-

Injury - *continued*

|specified type NEC S45.29-
|azygos vein *see* Injury, blood vessel, thoracic, specified site NEC
|brachial
|artery S45.10-
|laceration S45.11-
|specified type NEC S45.19-
|vein S45.20-
|laceration S45.219
|specified type NEC S45.29-
|carotid artery (common) (external) (internal, extracranial) S15.00-
|internal, intracranial S06.8-
|laceration (minor) (superficial) S15.01-
|major S15.02-
|specified type NEC S15.09-
|celiac artery S35.219
|branch S35.299
|laceration (minor) (superficial) S35.291
|major S35.292
|specified NEC S35.298
|laceration (minor) (superficial) S35.211
|major S35.212
|specified type NEC S35.218
|cerebral *see* Injury, intracranial
|deep plantar *see* Injury, blood vessel, plantar artery
|digital (hand) *see* Injury, blood vessel, finger
|dorsal
|artery (foot) S95.00-
|laceration S95.01-
|specified type NEC S95.09-
|vein (foot) S95.20-
|laceration S95.21-
|specified type NEC S95.29-
|due to accidental laceration during procedure *see* Laceration, accidental complicating surgery
|extremity *see* Injury, blood vessel, limb
|femoral
|artery (common) (superficial) S75.00-
|laceration (minor) (superficial) S75.01-
|major S75.02-
|specified type NEC S75.09-
|vein (hip level) (thigh level) S75.10-
|laceration (minor) (superficial) S75.11-
|major S75.12-
|specified type NEC S75.19-
|finger S65.50-
|index S65.50-
|laceration S65.51-
|specified type NEC S65.59-
|laceration S65.51-
|little S65.50-
|laceration S65.51-
|specified type NEC S65.59-
|middle S65.50-
|laceration S65.51-
|specified type NEC S65.59-
|specified type NEC S65.59-
|thumb *see* Injury, blood vessel, thumb
|foot S95.90-
|dorsal
|artery *see* Injury, blood vessel, dorsal, artery
|vein *see* Injury, blood vessel, dorsal, vein
|laceration S95.91-
|plantar artery *see* Injury, blood vessel, plantar artery
|specified
|site NEC S95.80-

Injury - *continued*

|laceration S95.81-
|specified type NEC S95.89-
|specified type NEC S95.99-
|forearm S55.90-
|laceration S55.91-
|radial artery *see* Injury, blood vessel, radial artery
|specified
|site NEC S55.80-
|laceration S55.81-
|specified type NEC S55.89-
|type NEC S55.99-
|ulnar artery *see* Injury, blood vessel, ulnar artery
|vein S55.20-
|laceration S55.21-
|specified type NEC S55.29-
|gastric
|artery *see* Injury, mesenteric, artery, branch
|vein *see* Injury, blood vessel, abdomen
|gastroduodenal artery *see* Injury, mesenteric, artery, branch
|greater saphenous vein (lower leg level) S85.30-
|hip (and thigh) level S75.20-
|laceration (minor) (superficial) S75.21-
|major S75.22-
|specified type NEC S75.29-
|laceration S85.31-
|specified type NEC S85.39-
|hand (level) S65.90-
|finger *see* Injury, blood vessel, finger
|laceration S65.91-
|palmar arch *see* Injury, blood vessel, palmar arch
|radial artery *see* Injury, blood vessel, radial artery, hand
|specified
|site NEC S65.80-
|laceration S65.81-
|specified type NEC S65.89-
|type NEC S65.99-
|thumb *see* Injury, blood vessel, thumb
|ulnar artery *see* Injury, blood vessel, ulnar artery, hand
|head S09.0
|intracranial *see* Injury, intracranial
|multiple S09.0
|hepatic
|artery *see* Injury, mesenteric, artery
|vein *see* Injury, vena cava, inferior
|hip S75.90-
|femoral artery *see* Injury, blood vessel, femoral, artery
|femoral vein *see* Injury, blood vessel, femoral, vein
|greater saphenous vein *see* Injury, blood vessel, greater saphenous, hip level
|laceration S75.91-
|specified
|site NEC S75.80-
|laceration S75.81-
|specified type NEC S75.89-
|type NEC S75.99-
|hypogastric (artery) (vein) *see* Injury, blood vessel, iliac
|iliac S35.5-
|artery S35.51-
|specified vessel NEC S35.5-
|uterine vessel *see* Injury, blood vessel, uterine
|vein S35.51-

Injury - *continued*

|innominate *see* Injury, blood vessel, thoracic, innominate
|intercostal (artery) (vein) *see* Injury, blood vessel, thoracic, intercostal
|jugular vein (external) S15.20-
|internal S15.30-
|laceration (minor) (superficial) S15.31-
|major S15.32-
|specified type NEC S15.39-
|laceration (minor) (superficial) S15.21-
|major S15.22-
|specified type NEC S15.29-
|leg (level) (lower) S85.90-
|greater saphenous *see* Injury, blood vessel, greater saphenous
|laceration S85.91-
|lesser saphenous *see* Injury, blood vessel, lesser saphenous
|peroneal artery *see* Injury, blood vessel, peroneal artery
|popliteal
|artery *see* Injury, blood vessel, popliteal, artery
|vein *see* Injury, blood vessel, popliteal, vein
|specified
|site NEC S85.80-
|laceration S85.81-
|specified type NEC S85.89-
|type NEC S85.99-
|thigh *see* Injury, blood vessel, hip
|tibial artery *see* Injury, blood vessel, tibial artery
|lesser saphenous vein (lower leg level) S85.40-
|laceration S85.41-
|specified type NEC S85.49-
|limb
|lower *see* Injury, blood vessel, leg
|upper *see* Injury, blood vessel, arm
|lower back *see* Injury, blood vessel, abdomen
|specified NEC *see* Injury, blood vessel, abdomen, specified, site NEC
|mammary (artery) (vein) *see* Injury, blood vessel, thoracic, specified site NEC
|mesenteric (inferior) (superior)
|artery *see* Injury, mesenteric, artery
|vein *see* Injury, mesenteric, vein
|neck S15.9
|specified site NEC S15.8
|ovarian (artery) (vein) *see* subcategory S35.8
|palmar arch (superficial) S65.20-
|deep S65.30-
|laceration S65.31-
|specified type NEC S65.39-
|laceration S65.21-
|specified type NEC S65.29-
|pelvis *see* Injury, blood vessel, abdomen
|specified NEC *see* Injury, blood vessel, abdomen, specified, site NEC
|peroneal artery S85.20-
|laceration S85.21-
|specified type NEC S85.29-
|plantar artery (deep) (foot) S95.10-
|laceration S95.11-
|specified type NEC S95.19-
|popliteal
|artery S85.00-
|laceration S85.01-
|specified type NEC S85.09-
|vein S85.50-
|laceration S85.51-

Injury - *continued*

|specified type NEC S85.59-
|portal vein S35.319
  |laceration S35.311
  |specified type NEC S35.318
|precerebral *see* Injury, blood vessel, neck
|pulmonary (artery) (vein) *see* Injury, blood
  vessel, thoracic, pulmonary
|radial artery (forearm level) S55.10-
  |hand and wrist (level) S65.10-
    |laceration S65.11-
    |specified type NEC S65.19-
  |laceration S55.11-
  |specified type NEC S55.19-
|renal
  |artery S35.40-
    |laceration S35.41-
    |specified NEC S35.49-
  |vein S35.40-
    |laceration S35.41-
    |specified NEC S35.49-
|saphenous vein (greater) (lower leg level)
  see Injury, blood vessel, greater
  saphenous
  |hip and thigh level *see* Injury, blood
    vessel, greater saphenous, hip level
  |lesser *see* Injury, blood vessel, lesser
    saphenous
|shoulder
  |specified NEC *see* Injury, blood vessel,
    arm, specified site NEC
  |superficial vein *see* Injury, blood vessel,
    arm, superficial vein
|specified NEC T14.8
|splenic
  |artery *see* Injury, blood vessel, celiac
    artery, branch
  |vein S35.329
    |laceration S35.321
    |specified NEC S35.328
|subclavian *see* Injury, blood vessel,
  thoracic, innominate
|thigh *see* Injury, blood vessel, hip
|thoracic S25.90
  |aorta S25.00
    |laceration (minor) (superficial) S25.01
      |major S25.02
    |specified type NEC S25.09
  |azygos vein *see* Injury, blood vessel,
    thoracic, specified, site NEC
  |innominate
    |artery S25.10-
      |laceration (minor) (superficial)
        S25.11-
        |major S25.12-
      |specified type NEC S25.19-
    |vein S25.30-
      |laceration (minor) (superficial)
        S25.31-
        |major S25.32
      |specified type NEC S25.39-
  |intercostal S25.50-
    |laceration S25.51-
    |specified type NEC S25.59-
  |laceration S25.91
  |mammary vessel *see* Injury, blood vessel,
    thoracic, specified, site NEC
  |pulmonary S25.40-
    |laceration (minor) (superficial) S25.41-
      |major S25.42-
    |specified type NEC S25.49-
  |specified
    |site NEC S25.80-
      |laceration S25.81-
      |specified type NEC S25.89-
  |type NEC S25.99

Injury - *continued*

|subclavian *see* Injury, blood vessel,
  thoracic, innominate
|vena cava (superior) S25.20
  |laceration (minor) (superficial) S25.21
    |major S25.22
  |specified type NEC S25.29
|thumb S65.40-
  |laceration S65.41-
  |specified type NEC S65.49-
|tibial artery S85.10-
  |anterior S85.13-
    |laceration S85.14-
    |specified injury NEC S85.15-
  |laceration S85.11-
  |posterior S85.16-
    |laceration S85.17-
    |specified injury NEC S85.18-
  |specified injury NEC S85.12-
|ulnar artery (forearm level) S55.00-
  |hand and wrist (level) S65.00-
    |laceration S65.01-
    |specified type NEC S65.09-
  |laceration S55.01-
  |specified type NEC S55.09-
|upper arm (level) *see* Injury, blood vessel,
  arm
  |superficial vein *see* Injury, blood vessel,
    arm, superficial vein
|uterine S35.5-
  |artery S35.53-
  |vein S35.53-
|vena cava *see* Injury, vena cava
|vertebral artery S15.10-
  |laceration (minor) (superficial) S15.11-
    |major S15.12-
  |specified type NEC S15.19-
|wrist (level) *see* Injury, blood vessel, hand
|brachial plexus S14.3
  |newborn P14.3
|brain (traumatic) S06.9-
  |diffuse (axonal) S06.2X-
  |focal S06.30-
|brainstem S06.38-
|breast NOS S29.9
|broad ligament *see* Injury, pelvic organ,
  specified site NEC
|bronchus, bronchi *see* Injury, intrathoracic,
  bronchus
|brow S09.90
|buttock S39.92
|canthus, eye S05.90
|cardiac plexus *see* Injury, nerve, thorax,
  sympathetic
|cauda equina S34.3
|cavernous sinus *see* Injury, intracranial
|cecum *see* Injury, colon
|celiac ganglion or plexus *see* Injury, nerve,
  lumbosacral, sympathetic
|cerebellum *see* Injury, intracranial
|cerebral *see* Injury, intracranial
|cervix (uteri) *see* Injury, uterus
|cheek (wall) S09.93
|chest *see* Injury, thorax
|childbirth (newborn) *see also* Birth, injury
  |maternal NEC O71.9
|chin S09.93
|choroid (eye) *see* Injury, eye, specified site
  NEC
|clitoris S39.94
|coccyx *see also* Injury, back, lower
  |complicating delivery O71.6
|colon *see* Injury, intestine, large
|common bile duct *see* Injury, liver

Injury - *continued*

|conjunctiva (superficial) *see* Injury, eye,
  conjunctiva
|conus medullaris *see* Injury, spinal, sacral
|cord
  |spermatic (pelvic region) S37.898
    |scrotal region S39.848
  |spinal *see* Injury, spinal cord, by region
|cornea *see* Injury, eye, specified site NEC
  |abrasion *see* Injury, eye, cornea, abrasion
|cortex (cerebral) *see also* Injury, intracranial
  |visual *see* Injury, nerve, optic
|costal region NEC S29.9
|costochondral NEC S29.9
|cranial
  |cavity *see* Injury, intracranial
  |nerve *see* Injury, nerve, cranial
|crushing *see* Crush
|cutaneous sensory nerve
|cystic duct *see* Injury, liver
|deep tissue *see* Contusion, by site
  |meaning pressure ulcer *see* Ulcer, pressure,
    L89 with final character .6 |delivery
    (newborn) P15.9
  |maternal NEC O71.9
|Descemet's membrane *see* Injury, eyeball,
  penetrating
|diaphragm *see* Injury, intrathoracic,
  diaphragm
|duodenum *see* Injury, intestine, small,
  duodenum
|ear (auricle) (external) (canal) S09.91
  |abrasion *see* Abrasion, ear
  |bite *see* Bite, ear
  |blister *see* Blister, ear
  |bruise *see* Contusion, ear
  |contusion *see* Contusion, ear
  |external constriction *see* Constriction,
    external, ear
  |hematoma *see* Hematoma, ear
  |inner *see* Injury, ear, middle
  |laceration *see* Laceration, ear
  |middle S09.30-
    |blast *see* Injury, blast, ear
    |specified NEC S09.39-
  |puncture *see* Puncture, ear
  |superficial *see* Injury, superficial, ear
|eighth cranial nerve (acoustic or auditory) *see*
  Injury, nerve, acoustic
|elbow S59.90-
  |contusion *see* Contusion, elbow
  |dislocation *see* Dislocation, elbow
  |fracture *see* Fracture, ulna, upper end
  |open *see* Wound, open, elbow
  |specified NEC S59.80-
  |sprain *see* Sprain, elbow
  |superficial *see* Injury, superficial, elbow
|eleventh cranial nerve (accessory) *see* Injury,
  nerve, accessory
|epididymis S39.94
|epigastric region S39.91
|epiglottis NEC S19.89
|esophageal plexus *see* Injury, nerve, thorax,
  sympathetic
|esophagus (thoracic part) *see also* Injury,
  intrathoracic, esophagus
  |cervical NEC S19.85
|eustachian tube S09.30-
|eye S05.9-
  |avulsion S05.7-
  |ball *see* Injury, eyeball
  |conjunctiva S05.0-
  |cornea
    |abrasion S05.0-
  |laceration S05.3-

Injury - *continued*

|with prolapse S05.2-
|lacrimal apparatus S05.8X-
|orbit penetration S05.4-
|specified site NEC S05.8X
|eyeball S05.8X-
|contusion S05.1-
|penetrating S05.6-
|with
|foreign body S05.5-
|prolapse or loss of intraocular tissue S05.2-
|without prolapse or loss of intraocular tissue S05.3-
|specified type NEC S05.8-
|eyebrow S09.93
|eyelid S09.93
|abrasion *see* Abrasion, eyelid
|contusion *see* Contusion, eyelid
|open *see* Wound, open, eyelid
|face S09.93
|fallopian tube S37.509
|bilateral S37.502
|blast injury S37.512
|contusion S37.522
|laceration S37.532
|specified type NEC S37.592
|blast injury (primary) S37.519
|bilateral S37.512
|secondary *see* Injury, fallopian tube, specified type NEC
|unilateral S37.511
|contusion S37.529
|bilateral S37.522
|unilateral S37.521
|laceration S37.539
|bilateral S37.532
|unilateral S37.531
|specified type NEC S37.599
|bilateral S37.592
|unilateral S37.591
|unilateral S37.501
|blast injury S37.511
|contusion S37.521
|laceration S37.531
|specified type NEC S37.591
|fascia *see* Injury, muscle
|fifth cranial nerve (trigeminal) *see* Injury, nerve, trigeminal
|finger (nail) S69.9-
|blood vessel *see* Injury, blood vessel, finger
|contusion *see* Contusion, finger
|dislocation *see* Dislocation, finger
|fracture *see* Fracture, finger
|muscle *see* Injury, muscle, finger
|nerve *see* Injury, nerve, digital, finger
|open *see* Wound, open, finger
|specified NEC S69.8-
|sprain *see* Sprain, finger
|superficial *see* Injury, superficial, finger
|first cranial nerve (olfactory) *see* Injury, nerve, olfactory
|flank *see* Injury, abdomen
|foot S99.92-
|blood vessel *see* Injury, blood vessel, foot
|contusion *see* Contusion, foot
|dislocation *see* Dislocation, foot
|fracture *see* Fracture, foot
|muscle *see* Injury, muscle, foot
|open *see* Wound, open, foot
|specified type NEC S99.82-
|sprain *see* Sprain, foot
|superficial *see* Injury, superficial, foot
|forceps NOS P15.9
|forearm S59.91-

Injury - *continued*

|blood vessel *see* Injury, blood vessel, forearm
|contusion *see* Contusion, forearm
|fracture *see* Fracture, forearm
|muscle *see* Injury, muscle, forearm
|nerve *see* Injury, nerve, forearm
|open *see* Wound, open, forearm
|specified NEC S59.81-
|superficial *see* Injury, superficial, forearm
|forehead S09.90
|fourth cranial nerve (trochlear) *see* Injury, nerve, trochlear
|gallbladder S36.129
|contusion S36.122
|laceration S36.123
|specified NEC S36.128
|ganglion
|celiac, coeliac *see* Injury, nerve, lumbosacral, sympathetic
|gasserian *see* Injury, nerve, trigeminal
|stellate *see* Injury, nerve, thorax, sympathetic
|thoracic sympathetic *see* Injury, nerve, thorax, sympathetic
|gasserian ganglion *see* Injury, nerve, trigeminal
|gastric artery *see* Injury, blood vessel, celiac artery, branch
|gastroduodenal artery *see* Injury, blood vessel, celiac artery, branch
|gastrointestinal tract *see* Injury, intra-abdominal
|with open wound into abdominal cavity *see* Wound, open, with penetration into peritoneal cavity
|colon *see* Injury, intestine, large
|rectum *see* Injury, intestine, large, rectum
|with open wound into abdominal cavity S36.61
|specified site NEC *see* Injury, intra-abdominal, specified, site NEC
|stomach *see* Injury, stomach
|small intestine *see* Injury, intestine, small
|genital organ(s)
|external S39.94
|specified NEC S39.848
|internal S37.90
|fallopian tube *see* Injury, fallopian tube
|ovary *see* Injury, ovary
|prostate *see* Injury, prostate
|seminal vesicle *see* Injury, pelvis, organ, specified site NEC
|uterus *see* Injury, uterus
|vas deferens *see* Injury, pelvis, organ, specified site NEC
|obstetrical trauma O71.9
|gland
|lacrimal laceration *see* Injury, eye, specified site NEC
|salivary S09.93
|thyroid NEC S19.84
|globe (eye) S05.90
|specified NEC S05.8X-
|groin *see* Injury, abdomen
|gum S09.90
|hand S69.9-
|blood vessel *see* Injury, blood vessel, hand
|contusion *see* Contusion, hand
|fracture *see* Fracture, hand
|muscle *see* Injury, muscle, hand
|nerve *see* Injury, nerve, hand
|open *see* Wound, open, hand
|specified NEC S69.8-
|sprain *see* Sprain, hand

Injury - *continued*

|superficial *see* Injury, superficial, hand
|head S09.90
|with loss of consciousness S06.9-
|specified NEC S09.8
|heart (traumatic) S26.90
|with hemopericardium S26.00
|contusion S26.01
|laceration (mild) S26.020
|moderate S26.021
|major S26.022
|specified type NEC S26.09
|contusion S26.91
|laceration S26.92
|non-traumatic (acute) (chronic) (non-ischemic) I5A
|specified type NEC S26.99
|without hemopericardium S26.10
|contusion S26.11
|laceration S26.12
|specified type NEC S26.19
|heel *see* Injury, foot
|hepatic
|artery *see* Injury, blood vessel, celiac artery, branch
|duct *see* Injury, liver
|vein *see* Injury, vena cava, inferior
|hip S79.91-
|blood vessel *see* Injury, blood vessel, hip
|contusion *see* Contusion, hip
|dislocation *see* Dislocation, hip
|fracture *see* Fracture, femur, neck
|muscle *see* Injury, muscle, hip
|nerve *see* Injury, nerve, hip
|open *see* Wound, open, hip
|sprain *see* Sprain, hip
|superficial *see* Injury, superficial, hip
|specified NEC S79.81-
|hymen S39.94
|hypogastric
|blood vessel *see* Injury, blood vessel, iliac
|plexus *see* Injury, nerve, lumbosacral, sympathetic
|ileum *see* Injury, intestine, small
|iliac region S39.91
|instrumental (during surgery) *see* Laceration, accidental complicating surgery
|birth injury *see* Birth, injury
|nonsurgical *see* Injury, by site
|obstetrical O71.9
|bladder O71.5
|cervix O71.3
|high vaginal O71.4
|perineal NOS O70.9
|urethra O71.5
|uterus O71.5
|with rupture or perforation O71.1
|internal T14.8
|aorta *see* Injury, aorta
|bladder (sphincter) *see* Injury, bladder
|with
|ectopic or molar pregnancy O08.6
|following ectopic or molar pregnancy O08.6
|obstetrical trauma O71.5
|bronchus, bronchi *see* Injury, intrathoracic, bronchus
|cecum *see* Injury, intestine, large
|cervix (uteri) *see also* Injury, uterus
|with ectopic or molar pregnancy O08.6
|following ectopic or molar pregnancy O08.6
|obstetrical trauma O71.3
|chest *see* Injury, intrathoracic

Injury - *continued*

|gastrointestinal tract *see* Injury, intra-
   abdominal
|heart *see* Injury, heart
|intestine NEC *see* Injury, intestine
|intrauterine *see* Injury, uterus
|mesentery *see* Injury, intra-abdominal,
   specified, site NEC
|pelvis, pelvic (organ) S37.90
   |following ectopic or molar pregnancy
      (subsequent episode) O08.6
   |obstetrical trauma NEC O71.5
     |rupture or perforation O71.1
   |specified NEC S39.83
|rectum *see* Injury, intestine, large, rectum
|stomach *see* Injury, stomach
|ureter *see* Injury, ureter
|urethra (sphincter) following ectopic or
|molar pregnancy O08.6
|uterus *see* Injury, uterus
|interscapular area *see* Injury, thorax
|intestine
   |large S36.509
     |ascending (right) S36.500
       |blast injury (primary) S36.510
         |secondary S36.590
       |contusion S36.520
       |laceration S36.530
       |specified type NEC S36.590
     |blast injury (primary) S36.519
       |ascending (right) S36.510
       |descending (left) S36.512
       |rectum S36.61
       |sigmoid S36.513
       |specified site NEC S36.518
       |transverse S36.511
     |contusion S36.529
       |ascending (right) S36.520
       |descending (left) S36.522
       |rectum S36.62
       |sigmoid S36.523
       |specified site NEC S36.528
       |transverse S36.521
     |descending (left) S36.502
       |blast injury (primary) S36.512
         |secondary S36.592
       |contusion S36.522
       |laceration S36.532
       |specified type NEC S36.592
     |laceration S36.539
       |ascending (right) S36.530
       |descending (left) S36.532
       |rectum S36.63
       |sigmoid S36.533
       |specified site NEC S36.538
       |transverse S36.531
     |rectum S36.60
       |blast injury (primary) S36.61
         |secondary S36.69
       |contusion S36.62
       |laceration S36.63
       |specified type NEC S36.69
     |sigmoid S36.503
       |blast injury (primary) S36.513
         |secondary S36.593
       |contusion S36.523
       |laceration S36.533
       |specified type NEC S36.593
     |specified
       |site NEC S36.508
         |blast injury (primary) S36.518
           |secondary S36.598
         |contusion S36.528
         |laceration S36.538
         |specified type NEC S36.598

Injury - *continued*

        |type NEC S36.599
          |ascending (right) S36.590
          |descending (left) S36.592
          |rectum S36.69
          |sigmoid S36.593
          |specified site NEC S36.598
          |transverse S36.591
     |transverse S36.501
       |blast injury (primary) S36.511
         |secondary S36.591
       |contusion S36.521
       |laceration S36.531
       |specified type NEC S36.591
   |small S36.409
     |blast injury (primary) S36.419
       |duodenum S36.410
       |secondary S36.499
         |duodenum S36.490
         |specified site NEC S36.498
       |specified site NEC S36.418
     |contusion S36.429
       |duodenum S36.420
       |specified site NEC S36.428
     |duodenum S36.400
       |blast injury (primary) S36.410
         |secondary S36.490
       |contusion S36.420
       |laceration S36.430
       |specified NEC S36.490
     |laceration S36.439
       |duodenum S36.430
       |specified site NEC S36.438
     |specified
       |type NEC S36.499
         |duodenum S36.490
         |specified site NEC S36.498
       |site NEC S36.408
|intra-abdominal S36.90
   |adrenal gland *see* Injury, adrenal gland
   |bladder *see* Injury, bladder
   |colon *see* Injury, intestine, large
   |contusion S36.92
   |fallopian tube *see* Injury, fallopian tube
   |gallbladder *see* Injury, gallbladder
   |intestine *see* Injury, intestine
   |laceration S36.93
   |liver *see* Injury, liver
   |kidney *see* Injury, kidney
   |ovary *see* Injury, ovary
   |pancreas *see* Injury, pancreas
   |pelvic NOS S37.90
   |peritoneum *see* Injury, intra-abdominal,
     specified, site NEC
   |prostate *see* Injury, prostate
   |rectum *see* Injury, intestine, large, rectum
   |retroperitoneum *see* Injury, intra-abdominal,
     specified, site NEC
   |seminal vesicle *see* Injury, pelvis, organ,
     specified site NEC
   |small intestine *see* Injury, intestine, small
   |specified
     |site NEC S36.899
       |contusion S36.892
       |laceration S36.893
       |specified type NEC S36.898
     |type NEC S36.99
   |pelvic S37.90
     |specified
       |site NEC S37.899
         |specified type NEC S37.898
       |type NEC S37.99
   |spleen *see* Injury, spleen
   |stomach *see* Injury, stomach
   |ureter *see* Injury, ureter

Injury - *continued*

   |urethra *see* Injury, urethra
   |uterus *see* Injury, uterus
   |vas deferens *see* Injury, pelvis, organ,
     specified site NEC
|intracranial (traumatic) (see also, if applicable,
   Compression, brain, traumatic) S06.9-
   |cerebellar hemorrhage, traumatic *see* Injury,
     intracranial, focal
   |cerebral edema, traumatic S06.1X-
     |diffuse S06.1X-
     |focal S06.1X-
   |diffuse (axonal) S06.2X-
   |epidural hemorrhage (traumatic) S06.4X-
   |focal brain injury S06.30-
     |contusion *see* Contusion, cerebral
     |laceration *see* Laceration, cerebral
   |intracerebral hemorrhage, traumatic S06.36-
     |left side S06.35-
     |right side S06.34-
   |subarachnoid hemorrhage, traumatic
     S06.6X-
   |subdural hemorrhage, traumatic S06.5X-
|intraocular *see* Injury, eyeball, penetrating
|intrathoracic S27.9
   |bronchus S27.409
     |bilateral S27.402
     |blast injury (primary) S27.419
       |bilateral S27.412
       |secondary *see* Injury, intrathoracic,
         bronchus, specified type NEC
       |unilateral S27.411
     |contusion S27.429
       |bilateral S27.422
       |unilateral S27.421
     |laceration S27.439
       |bilateral S27.432
       |unilateral S27.431
     |specified type NEC S27.499
       |bilateral S27.492
       |unilateral S27.491
     |unilateral S27.401
   |diaphragm S27.809
     |contusion S27.802
     |laceration S27.803
     |specified type NEC S27.808
   |esophagus (thoracic) S27.819
     |contusion S27.812
     |laceration S27.813
     |specified type NEC S27.818
   |heart *see* Injury, heart
   |hemopneumothorax S27.2
   |hemothorax S27.1
   |lung S27.309
     |aspiration J69.0
     |bilateral S27.302
     |blast injury (primary) S27.319
       |bilateral S27.312
       |secondary *see* Injury, intrathoracic,
         lung, specified type NEC
       |unilateral S27.311
     |contusion S27.329
       |bilateral S27.322
       |unilateral S27.321
     |laceration S27.339
       |bilateral S27.332
       |unilateral S27.331
     |specified type NEC S27.399
       |bilateral S27.392
       |unilateral S27.391
     |unilateral S27.301
   |pleura S27.60
     |laceration S27.63
     |specified type NEC S27.69
   |pneumothorax S27.0

Injury - *continued*

|specified organ NEC S27.899
|contusion S27.892
|laceration S27.893
|specified type NEC S27.898
|thoracic duct *see* Injury, intrathoracic, specified organ NEC
|thymus gland *see* Injury, intrathoracic, specified organ NEC
|trachea, thoracic S27.50
|blast (primary) S27.51
|contusion S27.52
|laceration S27.53
|specified type NEC S27.59
|iris *see* Injury, eye, specified site NEC
|penetrating *see* Injury, eyeball, penetrating
|jaw S09.93
|jejunum *see* Injury, intestine, small
|joint NOS T14.8
|old or residual *see* Disorder, joint, specified type NEC
|kidney S37.00-
|acute (nontraumatic) N17.9
|contusion *see* Contusion, kidney
|laceration *see* Laceration, kidney
|specified NEC S37.09-
|knee S89.9-
|contusion *see* Contusion, knee
|dislocation *see* Dislocation, knee
|meniscus (lateral) (medial) *see* Sprain, knee, specified site NEC
|old injury or tear *see* Derangement, knee, meniscus, due to old injury
|open *see* Wound, open, knee
|specified NEC S89.8-
|sprain *see* Sprain, knee
|superficial *see* Injury, superficial, knee
|labium (majus) (minus) S39.94
|labyrinth, ear S09.30-
|lacrimal apparatus, duct, gland, or sac *see* Injury, eye, specified site NEC
|larynx NEC S19.81
|leg (lower) S89.9-
|blood vessel *see* Injury, blood vessel, leg
|contusion *see* Contusion, leg
|fracture *see* Fracture, leg
|muscle *see* Injury, muscle, leg
|nerve *see* Injury, nerve, leg
|open *see* Wound, open, leg
|specified NEC S89.8-
|superficial *see* Injury, superficial, leg
|lens, eye *see* Injury, eye, specified site NEC
|penetrating *see* Injury, eyeball, penetrating
|limb NEC T14.8
|lip S09.93
|liver S36.119
|contusion S36.112
|laceration S36.113
|major (stellate) S36.116
|minor S36.114
|moderate S36.115
|specified NEC S36.118
|lower back S39.92
|specified NEC S39.82
|lumbar, lumbosacral (region) S39.92
|plexus *see* Injury, lumbosacral plexus
|lumbosacral plexus S34.4
|lung *see also* Injury, intrathoracic, lung
|aspiration J69.0
|dabbing (related) U07.0
|electronic cigarette (related) U07.0
|EVALI   [e-cigarette, or vaping, product use associated] U07.0
|transfusion-related (TRALI) J95.84

Injury - *continued*

|vaping (associated) (device) (product) (use) U07.0
|lymphatic thoracic duct *see* Injury, intrathoracic, specified organ NEC
|malar region S09.93
|mastoid region S09.90
|maxilla S09.93
|mediastinum *see* Injury, intrathoracic, specified organ NEC
|membrane, brain *see* Injury, intracranial
|meningeal artery *see* Injury, intracranial, subdural hemorrhage
|meninges (cerebral) *see* Injury, intracranial
|mesenteric
|artery
|branch S35.299
|laceration (minor) (superficial) S35.291
|major S35.292
|specified NEC S35.298
|inferior S35.239
|laceration (minor) (superficial) S35.231
|major S35.232
|specified NEC S35.238
|superior S35.229
|laceration (minor) (superficial) S35.221
|major S35.222
|specified NEC S35.228
|plexus (inferior) (superior) *see* Injury, nerve, lumbosacral, sympathetic
|vein
|inferior S35.349
|laceration S35.341
|specified NEC S35.348
|superior S35.339
|laceration S35.331
|specified NEC S35.338
|mesentery *see* Injury, intra-abdominal, specified site NEC
|mesosalpinx *see* Injury, pelvic organ, specified site NEC
|middle ear S09.30-
|midthoracic region NOS S29.9
|mouth S09.93
|multiple NOS T07
|muscle (and fascia) (and tendon)
|abdomen S39.001
|laceration S39.021
|specified type NEC S39.091
|strain S39.011
|abductor
|thumb, forearm level *see* Injury, muscle, thumb, abductor
|adductor
|thigh S76.20-
|laceration S76.22-
|specified type NEC S76.29-
|strain S76.21-
|ankle *see* Injury, muscle, foot
|anterior muscle group, at leg level (lower) S86.20-
|laceration S86.22-
|specified type NEC S86.29-
|strain S86.21-
|arm (upper) *see* Injury, muscle, shoulder
|biceps (parts NEC) S46.20-
|laceration S46.22-
|long head S46.10-
|laceration S46.12-
|strain S46.11-
|specified type NEC S46.19-
|specified type NEC S46.29-
|strain S46.21-
|extensor

Injury - *continued*

|finger(s) (other than thumb) *see* Injury, muscle, finger by site, extensor
|forearm level, specified NEC *see* Injury, muscle, forearm, extensor
|thumb *see* Injury, muscle, thumb, extensor
|toe (large) (ankle level) (foot level) *see* Injury, muscle, toe, extensor
|finger
|extensor (forearm level) S56.40-
|hand level S66.309
|laceration S66.329
|specified type NEC S66.399
|strain S66.319
|laceration S56.429
|specified type NEC S56.499
|strain S56.419
|flexor (forearm level) S56.10-
|hand level S66.109
|laceration S66.129
|specified type NEC S66.199
|strain S66.119
|laceration S56.129
|specified type NEC S56.199
|strain S56.119
|intrinsic S66.509
|laceration S66.529
|specified type NEC S66.599
|strain S66.519
|index
|extensor (forearm level)
|hand level S66.308
|laceration S66.32-
|specified type NEC S66.39-
|strain S66.31-
|specified type NEC S56.492-
|flexor (forearm level)
|hand level S66.108
|laceration S66.12-
|specified type NEC S66.19-
|strain S66.11-
|specified type NEC S56.19-
|strain S56.11-
|intrinsic S66.50-
|laceration S66.52-
|specified type NEC S66.59-
|strain S66.51-
|little
|extensor (forearm level)
|hand level S66.30-
|laceration S66.32-
|specified type NEC S66.39-
|strain S66.31-
|laceration S56.42-
|specified type NEC S56.49-
|strain S56.41-
|flexor (forearm level)
|hand level S66.10-
|laceration S66.12-
|specified type NEC S66.19-
|strain S66.11-
|laceration S56.12-
|specified type NEC S56.19-
|strain S56.11-
|intrinsic S66.50-
|laceration S66.52-
|specified type NEC S66.59-
|strain S66.51-
|middle
|extensor (forearm level)
|hand level S66.30-
|laceration S66.32-
|specified type NEC S66.39-
|strain S66.31-
|laceration S56.42-

Injury - *continued*
- |specified type NEC S56.49-
- |strain S56.41-
- |flexor (forearm level)
  - |hand level S66.10-
    - |laceration S66.12-
    - |specified type NEC S66.19-
    - |strain S66.11-
  - |laceration S56.12-
  - |specified type NEC S56.19-
  - |strain S56.11-
  - |intrinsic S66.50-
    - |laceration S66.52-
    - |specified type NEC S66.59-
    - |strain S66.51-
- |ring
  - |extensor (forearm level)
    - |hand level S66.30-
      - |laceration S66.32-
      - |specified type NEC S66.39-
      - |strain S66.31-
    - |laceration S56.42-
    - |specified type NEC S56.49-
    - |strain S56.41-
  - |flexor (forearm level)
    - |hand level S66.10-
      - |laceration S66.12-
      - |specified type NEC S66.19-
      - |strain S66.11-
    - |laceration S56.12-
    - |specified type NEC S56.19-
    - |strain S56.11-
    - |intrinsic S66.50-
      - |laceration S66.52-
      - |specified type NEC S66.59-
      - |strain S66.51-
- |flexor
  - |finger(s) (other than thumb) *see* Injury, muscle, finger
  - |forearm level, specified NEC *see* Injury, muscle, forearm, flexor
  - |thumb *see* Injury, muscle, thumb, flexor
  - |toe (long) (ankle level) (foot level) *see* Injury, muscle, toe, flexor
- |foot S96.90-
  - |intrinsic S96.20-
    - |laceration S96.22-
    - |specified type NEC S96.29-
    - |strain S96.21-
  - |laceration S96.92-
  - |long extensor, toe *see* Injury, muscle, toe, extensor
  - |long flexor, toe *see* Injury, muscle, toe, flexor
  - |specified
    - |site NEC S96.80-
      - |laceration S96.82-
      - |specified type NEC S96.89-
      - |strain S96.81-
    - |type NEC S96.99-
  - |strain S96.91-
- |forearm (level) S56.90-
  - |extensor S56.50-
    - |laceration S56.52-
    - |specified type NEC S56.59-
    - |strain S56.51-
  - |flexor S56.20-
    - |laceration S56.22-
    - |specified type NEC S56.29-
    - |strain S56.21-
  - |laceration S56.92-
  - |specified S56.99-
    - |site NEC S56.80-
      - |laceration S56.82-
      - |strain S56.81-

Injury - *continued*
- |type NEC S56.89-
- |strain S56.91-
- |hand (level) S66.90-
  - |laceration S66.92-
  - |specified
    - |site NEC S66.80-
      - |laceration S66.82-
      - |specified type NEC S66.89-
      - |strain S66.81-
    - |type NEC S66.99-
  - |strain S66.91-
- |head S09.10-
  - |laceration S09.12
  - |specified type NEC S09.19
  - |strain S09.11
- |hip NEC S76.00-
  - |laceration S76.02-
  - |specified type NEC S76.09-
  - |strain S76.01-
- |intrinsic
  - |ankle and foot level *see* Injury, muscle, foot, intrinsic
  - |finger (other than thumb) *see* Injury, muscle, finger by site, intrinsic
  - |foot (level) *see* Injury, muscle, foot, intrinsic
  - |thumb *see* Injury, muscle, thumb, intrinsic
- |leg (level) (lower) S86.90-
  - |Achilles tendon *see* Injury, Achilles tendon
  - |anterior muscle group *see* Injury, muscle, anterior muscle group
  - |laceration S86.92-
  - |peroneal muscle group *see* Injury, muscle, peroneal muscle group
  - |posterior muscle group *see* Injury, muscle, posterior muscle group, leg level
  - |specified
    - |site NEC S86.80-
      - |laceration S86.82-
      - |specified type NEC S86.89-
      - |strain S86.81-
    - |type NEC S86.99-
  - |strain S86.91-
- |long
  - |extensor toe, at ankle and foot level *see* Injury, muscle, toe, extensor
  - |flexor, toe, at ankle and foot level *see* Injury, muscle, toe, flexor
  - |head, biceps *see* Injury, muscle, biceps, long head
- |lower back S39.002
  - |laceration S39.022
  - |specified type NEC S39.092
  - |strain S39.012
- |neck (level) S16.9
  - |laceration S16.2
  - |specified type NEC S16.8
  - |strain S16.1
- |pelvis S39.003
  - |laceration S39.023
  - |specified type NEC S39.093
  - |strain S39.013
- |peroneal muscle group, at leg level (lower) S86.30-
  - |laceration S86.32-
  - |specified type NEC S86.39-
  - |strain S86.31-
- |posterior muscle (group)
  - |leg level (lower) S86.10-
    - |laceration S86.12-
    - |specified type NEC S86.19-
    - |strain S86.11-
  - |thigh level S76.30-

Injury - *continued*
- |laceration S76.32-
- |specified type NEC S76.39-
- |strain S76.31-
- |quadriceps (thigh) S76.10-
  - |laceration S76.12-
  - |specified type NEC S76.19-
  - |strain S76.11-
- |shoulder S46.90-
  - |laceration S46.92-
  - |rotator cuff *see* Injury, rotator cuff
  - |specified site NEC S46.80-
    - |laceration S46.82-
    - |strain S46.81-
    - |specified type NEC S46.89-
  - |strain S46.91-
  - |specified type NEC S46.99-
- |thigh NEC (level) S76.90-
  - |adductor *see* Injury, muscle, adductor, thigh
  - |laceration S76.92-
  - |posterior muscle (group) *see* Injury, muscle, posterior muscle, thigh level
  - |quadriceps *see* Injury, muscle, quadriceps
  - |specified
    - |site NEC S76.80-
      - |laceration S76.82-
      - |specified type NEC S76.89-
      - |strain S76.81-
    - |type NEC S76.99-
  - |strain S76.91-
- |thorax (level) S29.009
  - |back wall S29.002
  - |front wall S29.001
  - |laceration S29.029
    - |back wall S29.022
    - |front wall S29.021
  - |specified type NEC S29.099
    - |back wall S29.092
    - |front wall S29.091
  - |strain S29.019
    - |back wall S29.012
    - |front wall S29.011
- |thumb
  - |abductor (forearm level) S56.30-
    - |laceration S56.32-
    - |specified type NEC S56.39-
    - |strain S56.31-
  - |extensor (forearm level) S56.30-
    - |hand level S66.20-
      - |laceration S66.22-
      - |specified type NEC S66.29-
      - |strain S66.21-
    - |laceration S56.32-
    - |specified type NEC S56.39-
    - |strain S56.31-
  - |flexor (forearm level) S56.00-
    - |hand level S66.00-
      - |laceration S66.02-
      - |specified type NEC S66.09-
      - |strain S66.01-
    - |laceration S56.02-
    - |specified type NEC S56.09-
    - |strain S56.01-
    - |wrist level *see* Injury, muscle, thumb, flexor, hand level
  - |intrinsic S66.40-
    - |laceration S66.42-
    - |specified type NEC S66.49-
    - |strain S66.41-
- |toe *see also* Injury, muscle, foot
  - |extensor, long S96.10-
    - |laceration S96.12-
    - |specified type NEC S96.19-
    - |strain S96.11-

Injury - *continued*

|flexor, long S96.00-
||laceration S96.02-
|||specified type NEC S96.09-
|||strain S96.01-
|triceps S46.30-
||laceration S46.32-
||specified type NEC S46.39-
||strain S46.31-
|wrist (and hand) level *see* Injury, muscle, hand
|musculocutaneous nerve *see* Injury, nerve, musculocutaneous
|myocardial (acute) (chronic) (non-ischemic) (non-traumatic) I5A
||traumatic - see Injury, heart
|myocardium *see also* Injury, heart
||non-traumatic - see Injury, myocardial
|nape *see* Injury, neck
|nasal (septum) (sinus) S09.92
|nasopharynx S09.92
|neck S19.9
||specified NEC S19.80
|||specified site NEC S19.89
|nerve NEC T14.8
||abdomen S34.9
|||peripheral S34.6
|||specified site NEC S34.8
||abducens S04.4-
|||contusion S04.4-
|||laceration S04.4-
|||specified type NEC S04.4-
||abducent *see* Injury, nerve, abducens
||accessory S04.7-
|||contusion S04.7-
|||laceration S04.7-
|||specified type NEC S04.7-
||acoustic S04.6-
|||contusion S04.6-
|||laceration S04.6-
|||specified type NEC S04.6-
||ankle S94.9-
|||cutaneous sensory S94.3-
|||specified site NEC *see* subcategory S94.8
||anterior crural, femoral *see* Injury, nerve, femoral
||arm (upper) S44.9-
|||axillary *see* Injury, nerve, axillary
|||cutaneous *see* Injury, nerve, cutaneous, arm
|||median *see* Injury, nerve, median, upper arm
|||musculocutaneous *see* Injury, nerve, musculocutaneous
|||radial *see* Injury, nerve, radial, upper arm
|||specified site NEC *see* subcategory S44.8
|||ulnar *see* Injury, nerve, ulnar, arm
||auditory *see* Injury, nerve, acoustic
||axillary S44.3-
||brachial plexus *see* Injury, brachial plexus
||cervical sympathetic S14.5
||cranial S04.9
|||contusion S04.9
|||eighth (acoustic or auditory) *see* Injury, nerve, acoustic
|||eleventh (accessory) *see* Injury, nerve, accessory
|||fifth (trigeminal) *see* Injury, nerve, trigeminal
|||first (olfactory) *see* Injury, nerve, olfactory
|||fourth (trochlear) *see* Injury, nerve, trochlear
|||laceration S04.9

Injury - *continued*

|||ninth (glossopharyngeal) *see* Injury, nerve, glossopharyngeal
|||second (optic) *see* Injury, nerve, optic
|||seventh (facial) *see* Injury, nerve, facial
|||sixth (abducent) *see* Injury, nerve, abducens
|||specified
||||nerve NEC S04.89-
|||||contusion S04.89-
|||||laceration S04.89-
|||||specified type NEC S04.89-
||||type NEC S04.9
|||tenth (pneumogastric or vagus) *see* Injury, nerve, vagus
|||third (oculomotor) *see* Injury, nerve, oculomotor
|||twelfth (hypoglossal) *see* Injury, nerve, hypoglossal
||cutaneous sensory
|||ankle (level) S94.3-
|||arm (upper) (level) S44.5-
|||foot (level) *see* Injury, nerve, cutaneous sensory, ankle
|||forearm (level) S54.3-
|||hip (level) S74.2-
|||leg (lower level) S84.2-
|||shoulder (level) *see* Injury, nerve, cutaneous sensory, arm
|||thigh (level) *see* Injury, nerve, cutaneous sensory, hip
||deep peroneal *see* Injury, nerve, peroneal, foot
||digital
|||finger S64.4-
||||index S64.49-
||||little S64.49-
||||middle S64.49-
||||ring S64.49-
|||thumb S64.3-
|||toe *see* Injury, nerve, ankle, specified site NEC
||eighth cranial (acoustic or auditory) *see* Injury, nerve, acoustic
||eleventh cranial (accessory) *see* Injury, nerve, accessory
||facial S04.5-
|||contusion S04.5-
|||laceration S04.5-
|||newborn P11.3
|||specified type NEC S04.5-
||femoral (hip level) (thigh level) S74.1-
||fifth cranial (trigeminal) *see* Injury, nerve, trigeminal
||finger (digital) *see* Injury, nerve, digital, finger
||first cranial (olfactory) *see* Injury, nerve, olfactory
||foot S94.9-
|||cutaneous sensory S94.3-
|||deep peroneal S94.2-
|||lateral plantar S94.0-
|||medial plantar S94.1-
|||specified site NEC *see* subcategory S94.8
||forearm (level) S54.9-
|||cutaneous sensory *see* Injury, nerve, cutaneous sensory, forearm
|||median *see* Injury, nerve, median
|||radial *see.*Injury, nerve, radial
|||specified site NEC *see* subcategory S54.8
|||ulnar *see* Injury, nerve, ulnar
||fourth cranial (trochlear) *see* Injury, nerve, trochlear
||glossopharyngeal S04.89-

Injury - *continued*

|||specified type NEC S04.89-
||hand S64.9-
|||median *see* Injury, nerve, median, hand
|||radial *see* Injury, nerve, radial, hand
|||specified NEC *see* subcategory S64.8
|||ulnar *see* Injury, nerve, ulnar, hand
||hip (level) S74.9-
|||cutaneous sensory *see* Injury, nerve, cutaneous sensory, hip
|||femoral *see* Injury, nerve, femoral
|||sciatic *see* Injury, nerve, sciatic
|||specified site NEC *see* subcategory S74.8
||hypoglossal S04.89-
|||specified type NEC S04.89-
||lateral plantar S94.0-
||leg (lower) S84.9-
|||cutaneous sensory *see* Injury, nerve, cutaneous sensory, leg
|||peroneal *see* Injury, nerve, peroneal
|||specified site NEC *see* subcategory S84.8
|||tibial *see* Injury, nerve, tibial
|||upper *see* Injury, nerve, thigh
||lower
|||back *see* Injury, nerve, abdomen, specified site NEC
|||peripheral *see* Injury, nerve, abdomen, peripheral
|||limb *see* Injury, nerve, leg
||lumbar spinal
|||peripheral S34.6
|||root S34.21
||| sympathetic S34.5
||lumbar plexus *see* Injury, nerve, lumbosacral, sympathetic
||lumbosacral
|||plexus *see* Injury, nerve, lumbosacral, sympathetic
|||sympathetic S34.5
||medial plantar S94.1-
||median (forearm level) S54.1-
|||hand (level) S64.1-
|||upper arm (level) S44.1-
|||wrist (level) *see* Injury, nerve, median, hand
||musculocutaneous S44.4-
||musculospiral (upper arm level) *see* Injury, nerve, radial, upper arm
||neck S14.9
|||peripheral S14.4
|||specified site NEC S14.8
|||sympathetic S14.5
||ninth cranial (glossopharyngeal) *see* Injury, nerve, glossopharyngeal
||oculomotor S04.1-
|||contusion S04.1-
|||laceration S04.1-
|||specified type NEC S04.1-
||olfactory S04.81-
|||specified type NEC S04.81-
||optic S04.01-
|||contusion S04.01-
|||laceration S04.01-
|||specified type NEC S04.01-
||pelvic girdle *see* Injury, nerve, hip
||pelvis *see* Injury, nerve, abdomen, specified site NEC
|||peripheral *see* Injury, nerve, abdomen, peripheral
||peripheral NEC T14.8
|||abdomen *see* Injury, nerve, abdomen, peripheral
|||lower back *see* Injury, nerve, abdomen, peripheral
|||neck *see* Injury, nerve, neck, peripheral

Injury - *continued*

|pelvis *see* Injury, nerve, abdomen, peripheral
|specified NEC T14.8
|peroneal (lower leg level) S84.1-
  |foot S94.2-
|plexus
  |brachial *see* Injury, brachial plexus
  |celiac, coeliac *see* Injury, nerve, lumbosacral, sympathetic
  |mesenteric, inferior *see* Injury, nerve, lumbosacral, sympathetic
  |sacral *see* Injury, lumbosacral plexus
  |spinal
    |brachial *see* Injury, brachial plexus
    |lumbosacral *see* Injury, lumbosacral plexus
|pneumogastric *see* Injury, nerve, vagus
|radial (forearm level) S54.2-
  |hand (level) S64.2-
  |upper arm (level) S44.2-
  |wrist (level) *see* Injury, nerve, radial, hand
|root *see* Injury, nerve, spinal, root
|sacral plexus *see* Injury, lumbosacral plexus
|sacral spinal
  |peripheral S34.6
  |root S34.22
  |sympathetic S34.5
|sciatic (hip level) (thigh level) S74.0-
|second cranial (optic) *see* Injury, nerve, optic
|self-inflicted, without suicidal intent R45.88
|seventh cranial (facial) *see* Injury, nerve, facial
|shoulder *see* Injury, nerve, arm
|sixth cranial (abducent) *see* Injury, nerve, abducens
|spinal
  |plexus *see* Injury, nerve, plexus, spinal
  |root
    |cervical S14.2
    |dorsal S24.2
    |lumbar S34.21
    |sacral S34.22
    |thoracic *see* Injury, nerve, spinal, root, dorsal
|splanchnic *see* Injury, nerve, lumbosacral, sympathetic
|sympathetic NEC *see* Injury, nerve, lumbosacral, sympathetic
  |cervical *see* Injury, nerve, cervical sympathetic
|tenth cranial (pneumogastric or vagus) *see* Injury, nerve, vagus
|thigh (level) *see* Injury, nerve, hip
  |cutaneous sensory *see* Injury, nerve, cutaneous sensory, hip
  |femoral *see* Injury, nerve, femoral
  |sciatic *see* Injury, nerve, sciatic
  |specified NEC *see* Injury, nerve, hip
|third cranial (oculomotor) *see* Injury, nerve, oculomotor
|thorax S24.9
  |peripheral S24.3
  |specified site NEC S24.8
  |sympathetic S24.4
|thumb, digital *see* Injury, nerve, digital, thumb
|tibial (lower leg level) (posterior) S84.0-
|toe *see* Injury, nerve, ankle
|trigeminal S04.3-
  |contusion S04.3-
  |laceration S04.3-
  |specified type NEC S04.3-
|trochlear S04.2-

Injury - *continued*

  |contusion S04.2-
  |laceration S04.2-
  |specified type NEC S04.2-
|twelfth cranial (hypoglossal) *see* Injury, nerve, hypoglossal
|ulnar (forearm level) S54.0-
  |arm (upper) (level) S44.0-
  |hand (level) S64.0-
  |wrist (level) *see* Injury, nerve, ulnar, hand
|vagus S04.89-
  |specified type NEC S04.89-
  |wrist (level) *see* Injury, nerve, hand
|ninth cranial nerve (glossopharyngeal) *see* Injury, nerve, glossopharyngeal
|nose (septum) S09.92
|obstetrical O71.9
  |specified NEC O71.89
|occipital (region) (scalp) S09.90
  |lobe *see* Injury, intracranial
|optic chiasm S04.02
|optic radiation S04.03-
|optic tract and pathways S04.03-
|orbit, orbital (region) *see* Injury, eye
  |penetrating (with foreign body) *see* Injury, eye, orbit, penetrating
  |specified NEC *see* Injury, eye, specified site NEC
|ovary, ovarian S37.409
  |bilateral S37.402
    |contusion S37.422
    |laceration S37.432
    |specified type NEC S37.492
  |blood vessel *see* Injury, blood vessel, ovarian
  |contusion S37.429
    |bilateral S37.422
    |unilateral S37.421
  |laceration S37.439
    |bilateral S37.432
    |unilateral S37.431
  |specified type NEC S37.499
    |bilateral S37.492
    |unilateral S37.491
  |unilateral S37.401
    |contusion S37.421
    |laceration S37.431
    |specified type NEC S37.491
|palate (hard) (soft) S09.93
|pancreas S36.209
  |body S36.201
    |contusion S36.221
    |laceration S36.231
      |major S36.261
      |minor S36.241
      |moderate S36.251
    |specified type NEC S36.291
  |contusion S36.229
  |head S36.200
    |contusion S36.220
    |laceration S36.230
      |major S36.260
      |minor S36.240
      |moderate S36.250
    |specified type NEC S36.290
  |laceration S36.239
    |major S36.269
    |minor S36.249
    |moderate S36.259
  |specified type NEC S36.299
  |tail S36.202
    |contusion S36.222
    |laceration S36.232
      |major S36.262
      |minor S36.242

Injury - *continued*

    |moderate S36.252
  |specified type NEC S36.292
|parietal (region) (scalp) S09.90
  |lobe *see* Injury, intracranial
|patellar ligament (tendon) S76.10-
  |laceration S76.12-
  |specified NEC S76.19-
  |strain S76.11-
|pelvis, pelvic (floor) S39.93
  |complicating delivery O70.1
  |joint or ligament, complicating delivery O71.6
  |organ S37.90
    |with ectopic or molar pregnancy O08.6
    |complication of abortion *see* Abortion
    |contusion S37.92
    |following ectopic or molar pregnancy O08.6
    |laceration S37.93
    |obstetrical trauma NEC O71.5
    |specified
      |site NEC S37.899
        |contusion S37.892
        |laceration S37.893
        |specified type NEC S37.898
      |type NEC S37.99
  |specified NEC S39.83
|penis S39.94
|perineum S39.94
|peritoneum S36.81
  |laceration S36.893
|periurethral tissue *see* Injury, urethra
  |complicating delivery O71.82
|phalanges
  |foot *see* Injury, foot
  |hand *see* Injury, hand
|pharynx NEC S19.85
|pleura *see* Injury, intrathoracic, pleura
|plexus
  |brachial *see* Injury, brachial plexus
  |cardiac *see* Injury, nerve, thorax, sympathetic
  |celiac, coeliac *see* Injury, nerve, lumbosacral, sympathetic
  |esophageal *see* Injury, nerve, thorax, sympathetic
  |hypogastric *see* Injury, nerve, lumbosacral, sympathetic
  |lumbar, lumbosacral *see* Injury, lumbosacral plexus
  |mesenteric *see* Injury, nerve, lumbosacral, sympathetic
  |pulmonary *see* Injury, nerve, thorax, sympathetic
|postcardiac surgery (syndrome) I97.0
|prepuce S39.94
|prostate S37.829
  |contusion S37.822
  |laceration S37.823
  |specified type NEC S37.828
|pubic region S39.94
|pudendum S39.94
|pulmonary plexus *see* Injury, nerve, thorax, sympathetic
|rectovaginal septum NEC S39.83
|rectum *see* Injury, intestine, large, rectum
|retina *see* Injury, eye, specified site NEC
  |penetrating *see* Injury, eyeball, penetrating
|retroperitoneal *see* Injury, intra-abdominal, specified site NEC
|rotator cuff (muscle(s)) (tendon(s)) S46.00-
  |laceration S46.02-
  |specified type NEC S46.09
  |strain S46.01-

Injury - *continued*

|round ligament *see* Injury, pelvic organ,
  specified site NEC
|sacral plexus *see* Injury, lumbosacral plexus
|salivary duct or gland S09.93
|scalp S09.90
  |newborn (birth injury) P12.9
    |due to monitoring (electrode) (sampling
    incision) P12.4
      |specified NEC P12.89
        |caput succedaneum P12.81
|scapular region *see* Injury, shoulder
|sclera *see* Injury, eye, specified site NEC
  |penetrating *see* Injury, eyeball, penetrating
|scrotum S39.94
|second cranial nerve (optic) *see* Injury, nerve,
  optic
|seminal vesicle *see* Injury, pelvic organ,
  specified site NEC
|seventh cranial nerve (facial) *see* Injury,
  nerve, facial
|shoulder S49.9-
  |blood vessel *see* Injury, blood vessel, arm
  |contusion *see* Contusion, shoulder
  |dislocation *see* Dislocation, shoulder
  |fracture *see* Fracture, shoulder
  |muscle *see* Injury, muscle, shoulder
  |nerve *see* Injury, nerve, shoulder
  |open *see* Wound, open, shoulder
  |specified type NEC S49.8-
  |sprain *see* Sprain, shoulder girdle
  |superficial *see* Injury, superficial, shoulder
|sinus
  |cavernous *see* Injury, intracranial
  |nasal S09.92
|sixth cranial nerve (abducent) *see* Injury,
  nerve, abducens
|skeleton, birth injury P13.9
  |specified part NEC P13.8
|skin NEC T14.8
  |surface intact *see* Injury, superficial
|skull NEC S09.90
|specified NEC T14.8
|spermatic cord (pelvic region) S37.898
  |scrotal region S39.848
|spinal (cord)
  |cervical (neck) S14.109
    |anterior cord syndrome S14.139
      |C1 level S14.131
      |C2 level S14.132
      |C3 level S14.133
      |C4 level S14.134
      |C5 level S14.135
      |C6 level S14.136
      |C7 level S14.137
      |C8 level S14.138
    |Brown-Séquard syndrome S14.149
      |C1 level S14.141
      |C2 level S14.142
      |C3 level S14.143
      |C4 level S14.144
      |C5 level S14.145
      |C6 level S14.146
      |C7 level S14.147
      |C8 level S14.148
    |C1 level S14.101
    |C2 level S14.102
    |C3 level S14.103
    |C4 level S14.104
    |C5 level S14.105
    |C6 level S14.106
    |C7 level S14.107
    |C8 level S14.108
    |central cord syndrome S14.129

Injury - *continued*

      |C1 level S14.121
      |C2 level S14.122
      |C3 level S14.123
      |C4 level S14.124
      |C5 level S14.125
      |C6 level S14.126
      |C7 level S14.127
      |C8 level S14.128
    |complete lesion S14.119
      |C1 level S14.111
      |C2 level S14.112
      |C3 level S14.113
      |C4 level S14.114
      |C5 level S14.115
      |C6 level S14.116
      |C7 level S14.117
      |C8 level S14.118
    |concussion S14.0
    |edema S14.0
    |incomplete lesion specified NEC S14.159
      |C1 level S14.151
      |C2 level S14.152
      |C3 level S14.153
      |C4 level S14.154
      |C5 level S14.155
      |C6 level S14.156
      |C7 level S14.157
      |C8 level S14.158
    |posterior cord syndrome S14.159
      |C1 level S14.151
      |C2 level S14.152
      |C3 level S14.153
      |C4 level S14.154
      |C5 level S14.155
      |C6 level S14.156
      |C7 level S14.157
      |C8 level S14.158
  |dorsal *see* Injury, spinal, thoracic
  |lumbar S34.109
    |complete lesion S34.119
      |L1 level S34.111
      |L2 level S34.112
      |L3 level S34.113
      |L4 level S34.114
      |L5 level S34.115
    |concussion S34.01
    |edema S34.01
    |incomplete lesion S34.129
      |L1 level S34.121
      |L2 level S34.122
      |L3 level S34.123
      |L4 level S34.124
      |L5 level S34.125
    |L1 level S34.101
    |L2 level S34.102
    |L3 level S34.103
    |L4 level S34.104
    |L5 level S34.105
  |nerve root NEC
    |cervical *see* Injury, nerve, spinal, root,
    cervical
    |dorsal *see* Injury, nerve, spinal, root,
    dorsal
    |lumbar S34.21
    |sacral S34.22
    |thoracic *see* Injury, nerve, spinal, root,
    dorsal
  |plexus
    |brachial *see* Injury, brachial plexus
    |lumbosacral *see* Injury, lumbosacral
    plexus
  |sacral S34.139
    |complete lesion S34.131
    |incomplete lesion S34.132

Injury - *continued*

  |thoracic S24.109
    |anterior cord syndrome S24.139
      |T1 level S24.131
      |T2-T6 level S24.132
      |T7-T10 level S24.133
      |T11-T12 level S24.134
    |Brown-Séquard syndrome S24.149
      |T1 level S24.141
      |T2-T6 level S24.142
      |T7-T10 level S24.143
      |T11-T12 level S24.144
    |complete lesion S24.119
      |T1 level S24.111
      |T2-T6 level S24.112
      |T7-T10 level S24.113
      |T11-T12 level S24.114
    |concussion S24.0
    |edema S24.0
    |incomplete lesion specified NEC S24.159
      |T1 level S24.151
      |T2-T6 level S24.152
      |T7-T10 level S24.153
      |T11-T12 level S24.154
    |posterior cord syndrome S24.159
      |T1 level S24.151
      |T2-T6 level S24.152
      |T7-T10 level S24.153
      |T11-T12 level S24.154
    |T1 level S24.101
    |T2-T6 level S24.102
    |T7-T10 level S24.103
    |T11-T12 level S24.104
|splanchnic nerve *see* Injury, nerve,
  lumbosacral, sympathetic
|spleen S36.00
  |contusion S36.029
    |major S36.021
    |minor S36.020
  |laceration S36.039
    |major (massive) (stellate) S36.032
    |moderate S36.031
    |superficial (capsular) (minor) S36.030
  |specified type NEC S36.09
|splenic artery *see* Injury, blood vessel, celiac
  artery, branch
|stellate ganglion *see* Injury, nerve, thorax,
  sympathetic
|sternal region S29.9
|stomach S36.30
  |contusion S36.32
  |laceration S36.33
  |specified type NEC S36.39
|subconjunctival *see* Injury, eye, conjunctiva
|subcutaneous NEC T14.8
|submaxillary region S09.93
|submental region S09.93
|subungual
  |fingers *see* Injury, hand
  |toes *see* Injury, foot
|superficial NEC T14.8
  |abdomen, abdominal (wall) S30.92
    |abrasion S30.811
    |bite S30.871
      |insect S30.861
    |contusion S30.1
    |external constriction S30.841
    |foreign body S30.851
  |abrasion *see* Abrasion, by site
  |adnexa, eye NEC *see* Injury, eye, specified
  site NEC
  |alveolar process *see* Injury, superficial, oral
  cavity
  |ankle S90.91-
    |abrasion *see* Abrasion, ankle

Injury - *continued*

|blister *see* Blister, ankle
|bite *see* Bite, ankle
|contusion *see* Contusion, ankle
|external constriction *see* Constriction, external, ankle
|foreign body *see* Foreign body, superficial, ankle
|anus S30.98
|arm (upper) S40.92-
|abrasion *see* Abrasion, arm
|bite *see* Bite, superficial, arm
|blister *see* Blister, arm (upper)
|contusion *see* Contusion, arm
|external constriction *see* Constriction, external, arm
|foreign body *see* Foreign body, superficial, arm
|auditory canal (external) (meatus) *see* Injury, superficial, ear
|auricle *see* Injury, superficial, ear
|axilla *see* Injury, superficial, arm
|back *see also* Injury, superficial, thorax, back
|lower S30.91
|abrasion S30.810
|contusion S30.0
|external constriction S30.840
|superficial
|bite NEC S30.870
|insect S30.860
|foreign body S30.850
|bite NEC *see* Bite, superficial NEC, by site
|blister *see* Blister, by site
|breast S20.10-
|abrasion *see* Abrasion, breast
|bite *see* Bite, superficial, breast
|contusion *see* Contusion, breast
|external constriction *see* Constriction, external, breast
|foreign body *see* Foreign body, superficial, breast
|brow *see* Injury, superficial, head, specified NEC
|buttock S30.91
|calf *see* Injury, superficial, leg
|canthus, eye *see* Injury, superficial, periocular area
|cheek (external) *see* Injury, superficial, head, specified NEC
|internal *see* Injury, superficial, oral cavity
|chest wall *see* Injury, superficial, thorax
|chin *see* Injury, superficial, head NEC
|clitoris S30.95
|conjunctiva *see* Injury, eye, conjunctiva
|with foreign body (in conjunctival sac) *see* Foreign body, conjunctival sac
|contusion *see* Contusion, by site
|costal region *see* Injury, superficial, thorax
|digit(s)
|hand *see* Injury, superficial, finger
|ear (auricle) (canal) (external) S00.40-
|abrasion *see* Abrasion, ear
|bite *see* Bite, superficial, ear
|contusion *see* Contusion, ear
|external constriction *see* Constriction, external, ear
|foreign body *see* Foreign body, superficial, ear
|elbow S50.90-
|abrasion *see* Abrasion, elbow
|bite *see* Bite, superficial, elbow
|blister *see* Blister, elbow
|contusion *see* Contusion, elbow

|external constriction *see* Constriction, external, elbow
|foreign body *see* Foreign body, superficial, elbow
|epididymis S30.94
|epigastric region S30.92
|epiglottis *see* Injury, superficial, throat
|esophagus
|cervical *see* Injury, superficial, throat
|external constriction *see* Constriction, external, by site
|extremity NEC T14.8
|eyeball NEC *see* Injury, eye, specified site NEC
|eyebrow *see* Injury, superficial, periocular area
|eyelid S00.20-
|abrasion *see* Abrasion, eyelid
|bite *see* Bite, superficial, eyelid
|contusion *see* Contusion, eyelid
|external constriction *see* Constriction, external, eyelid
|foreign body *see* Foreign body, superficial, eyelid
|face NEC *see* Injury, superficial, head, specified NEC
|finger(s) S60.949
|abrasion *see* Abrasion, finger
|bite *see* Bite, superficial, finger
|blister *see* Blister, finger
|contusion *see* Contusion, finger
|external constriction *see* Constriction, external, finger
|foreign body *see* Foreign body, superficial, finger
|insect bite *see* Bite, by site, superficial, insect
|index S60.94-
|little S60.94-
|middle S60.94-
|ring S60.94-
|flank S30.92
|foot S90.92-
|abrasion *see* Abrasion, foot
|bite *see* Bite, foot
|blister *see* Blister, foot
|contusion *see* Contusion, foot
|external constriction *see* Constriction, external, foot
|foreign body *see* Foreign body, superficial, foot
|forearm S50.91-
|abrasion *see* Abrasion, forearm
|bite *see* Bite, forearm, superficial
|blister *see* Blister, forearm
|contusion *see* Contusion, forearm
|elbow only *see* Injury, superficial, elbow
|external constriction *see* Constriction, external, forearm
|foreign body *see* Foreign body, superficial, forearm
|forehead *see* Injury, superficial, head NEC
|foreign body *see* Foreign body, superficial
|genital organs, external
|female S30.97
|male S30.96
|globe (eye) *see* Injury, eye, specified site NEC
|groin S30.92
|gum *see* Injury, superficial, oral cavity
|hand S60.92-
|abrasion *see* Abrasion, hand
|bite *see* Bite, superficial, hand

|contusion *see* Contusion, hand
|external constriction *see* Constriction, external, hand
|foreign body *see* Foreign body, superficial, hand
|head S00.90
|ear *see* Injury, superficial, ear
|eyelid *see* Injury, superficial, eyelid
|nose S00.30
|oral cavity S00.502
|scalp S00.00
|specified site NEC S00.80
|heel *see* Injury, superficial, foot
|hip S70.91-
|abrasion *see* Abrasion, hip
|bite *see* Bite, superficial, hip
|blister *see* Blister, hip
|contusion *see* Contusion, hip
|external constriction *see* Constriction, external, hip
|foreign body *see* Foreign body, superficial, hip
|iliac region *see* Injury, superficial, abdomen
|inguinal region *see* Injury, superficial, abdomen
|insect bite *see* Bite, by site, superficial, insect
|interscapular region *see* Injury, superficial, thorax, back
|jaw *see* Injury, superficial, head, specified NEC
|knee S80.91-
|abrasion *see* Abrasion, knee
|bite *see* Bite, superficial, knee
|blister *see* Blister, knee
|contusion *see* Contusion, knee
|external constriction *see* Constriction, external, knee
|foreign body *see* Foreign body, superficial, knee
|labium (majus) (minus) S30.95
|lacrimal (apparatus) (gland) (sac) *see* Injury, eye, specified site NEC
|larynx *see* Injury, superficial, throat
|leg (lower) S80.92-
|abrasion *see* Abrasion, leg
|bite *see* Bite, superficial, leg
|contusion *see* Contusion, leg
|external constriction *see* Constriction, external, leg
|foreign body *see* Foreign body, superficial, leg
|knee *see* Injury, superficial, knee
|limb NEC T14.8
|lip S00.501
|lower back S30.91
|lumbar region S30.91
|malar region *see* Injury, superficial, head, specified NEC
|mammary *see* Injury, superficial, breast
|mastoid region *see* Injury, superficial, head, specified NEC
|mouth *see* Injury, superficial, oral cavity
|muscle NEC T14.8
|nail NEC T14.8
|finger *see* Injury, superficial, finger
|toe *see* Injury, superficial, toe
|nasal (septum) *see* Injury, superficial, nose
|neck S10.90
|specified site NEC S10.80
|nose (septum) S00.30
|occipital region *see* Injury, superficial, scalp
|oral cavity S00.502

Injury - *continued*
- orbital region *see* Injury, superficial, periocular area
- palate *see* Injury, superficial, oral cavity
- palm *see* Injury, superficial, hand
- parietal region *see* Injury, superficial, scalp
- pelvis S30.91
  - girdle *see* Injury, superficial, hip
- penis S30.93
- perineum
  - female S30.95
  - male S30.91
- periocular area S00.20-
  - abrasion *see* Abrasion, eyelid
  - bite *see* Bite, superficial, eyelid
  - contusion *see* Contusion, eyelid
  - external constriction *see* Constriction, external, eyelid
  - foreign body *see* Foreign body, superficial, eyelid
- phalanges
  - finger *see* Injury, superficial, finger
  - toe *see* Injury, superficial, toe
- pharynx *see* Injury, superficial, throat
- pinna *see* Injury, superficial, ear
- popliteal space *see* Injury, superficial, knee
- prepuce S30.93
- pubic region S30.91
- pudendum
  - female S30.97
  - male S30.96
- sacral region S30.91
- scalp S00.00
- scapular region *see* Injury, superficial, shoulder
- sclera *see* Injury, eye, specified site NEC
- scrotum S30.94
- shin *see* Injury, superficial, leg
- shoulder S40.91-
  - abrasion *see* Abrasion, shoulder
  - bite *see* Bite, superficial, shoulder
  - blister *see* Blister, shoulder
  - contusion *see* Contusion, shoulder
  - external constriction *see* Constriction, external, shoulder
  - foreign body *see* Foreign body, superficial, shoulder
- skin NEC T14.8
- sternal region *see* Injury, superficial, thorax, front
- subconjunctival *see* Injury, eye, specified site NEC
- subcutaneous NEC T14.8
- submaxillary region *see* Injury, superficial, head, specified NEC
- submental region *see* Injury, superficial, head, specified NEC
- subungual
  - finger(s) *see* Injury, superficial, finger
  - toe(s) *see* Injury, superficial, toe
- supraclavicular fossa *see* Injury, superficial, neck
- supraorbital *see* Injury, superficial, head, specified NEC
- temple *see* Injury, superficial, head, specified NEC
- temporal region *see* Injury, superficial, head, specified NEC
- testis S30.94
- thigh S70.92-
  - abrasion *see* Abrasion, thigh
  - bite *see* Bite, superficial, thigh
  - blister *see* Blister, thigh
  - contusion *see* Contusion, thigh

Injury - *continued*
- external constriction *see* Constriction, external, thigh
- foreign body *see* Foreign body, superficial, thigh
- thorax, thoracic (wall) S20.90
  - abrasion *see* Abrasion, thorax
  - back S20.40-
  - bite *see* Bite, thorax, superficial
  - blister *see* Blister, thorax
  - contusion *see* Contusion, thorax
  - external constriction *see* Constriction, external, thorax
  - foreign body *see* Foreign body, superficial, thorax
  - front S20.30-
- throat S10.10
  - abrasion S10.11
  - bite S10.17
    - insect S10.16
  - blister S10.12
  - contusion S10.0
  - external constriction S10.14
  - foreign body S10.15
- thumb S60.93-
  - abrasion *see* Abrasion, thumb
  - bite *see* Bite, superficial, thumb
  - blister *see* Blister, thumb
  - contusion *see* Contusion, thumb
  - external constriction *see* Constriction, external, thumb
  - foreign body *see* Foreign body, superficial, thumb
  - insect bite *see* Bite, by site, superficial, insect
  - specified type NEC S60.39-
- toe(s) S90.93-
  - abrasion *see* Abrasion, toe
  - bite *see* Bite, toe
  - blister *see* Blister, toe
  - contusion *see* Contusion, toe
  - external constriction *see* Constriction, external, toe
  - foreign body *see* Foreign body, superficial, toe
  - great S90.93-
- tongue *see* Injury, superficial, oral cavity
- tooth, teeth *see* Injury, superficial, oral cavity
- trachea S10.10
- tunica vaginalis S30.94
- tympanum, tympanic membrane *see* Injury, superficial, ear
- uvula *see* Injury, superficial, oral cavity
- vagina S30.95
- vocal cords *see* Injury, superficial, throat
- vulva S30.95
- wrist S60.91-
- supraclavicular region *see* Injury, neck
- supraorbital S09.93
- suprarenal gland (multiple) *see* Injury, adrenal
- surgical complication (external or internal site) *see* Laceration, accidental complicating surgery
- temple S09.90
- temporal region S09.90
- tendon *see also* Injury, muscle, by site
  - abdomen *see* Injury, muscle, abdomen
  - Achilles *see* Injury, Achilles tendon
  - lower back *see* Injury, muscle, lower back
  - pelvic organs *see* Injury, muscle, pelvis
- tenth cranial nerve (pneumogastric or vagus) *see* Injury, nerve, vagus
- testis S39.94

Injury - *continued*
- thigh S79.92-
  - blood vessel *see* Injury, blood vessel, hip
  - contusion *see* Contusion, thigh
  - fracture *see* Fracture, femur
  - muscle *see* Injury, muscle, thigh
  - nerve *see* Injury, nerve, thigh
  - open *see* Wound, open, thigh
  - specified NEC S79.82-
  - superficial *see* Injury, superficial, thigh
- third cranial nerve (oculomotor) *see* Injury, nerve, oculomotor
- thorax, thoracic S29.9
  - blood vessel *see* Injury, blood vessel, thorax
  - cavity *see* Injury, intrathoracic
  - dislocation *see* Dislocation, thorax
  - external (wall) S29.9
    - contusion *see* Contusion, thorax
    - nerve *see* Injury, nerve, thorax
    - open *see* Wound, open, thorax
    - specified NEC S29.8
    - sprain *see* Sprain, thorax
    - superficial *see* Injury, superficial, thorax
  - fracture *see* Fracture, thorax
  - internal *see* Injury, intrathoracic
  - intrathoracic organ *see* Injury, intrathoracic
  - sympathetic ganglion *see* Injury, nerve, thorax, sympathetic
- throat *see also* Injury, neck S19.9
- thumb S69.9-
  - blood vessel *see* Injury, blood vessel, thumb
  - contusion *see* Contusion, thumb
  - dislocation *see* Dislocation, thumb
  - fracture *see* Fracture, thumb
  - muscle *see* Injury, muscle, thumb
  - nerve *see* Injury, nerve, digital, thumb
  - open *see* Wound, open, thumb
  - specified NEC S69.8
  - sprain *see* Sprain, thumb
  - superficial *see* Injury, superficial, thumb
- thymus (gland) *see* Injury, intrathoracic, specified organ NEC
- thyroid (gland) NEC S19.84
- toe S99.92-
  - contusion *see* Contusion, toe
  - dislocation *see* Dislocation, toe
  - fracture *see* Fracture, toe
  - muscle *see* Injury, muscle, toe
  - open *see* Wound, open, toe
  - specified type NEC S99.82-
  - sprain *see* Sprain, toe
  - superficial *see* Injury, superficial, toe
- tongue S09.93
- tonsil S09.93
- tooth S09.93
- trachea (cervical) NEC S19.82
  - thoracic *see* Injury, intrathoracic, trachea, thoracic
- transfusion-related acute lung (TRALI) J95.84
- tunica vaginalis S39.94
- twelfth cranial nerve (hypoglossal) *see* Injury, nerve, hypoglossal
- ureter S37.10
  - contusion S37.12
  - laceration S37.13
  - specified type NEC S37.19
- urethra (sphincter) S37.30
  - at delivery O71.5
  - contusion S37.32
  - laceration S37.33
  - specified type NEC S37.39
- urinary organ S37.90
  - contusion S37.92
  - laceration S37.93
  - specified

Injury - *continued*
- site NEC S37.899
  - contusion S37.892
  - laceration S37.893
  - specified type NEC S37.898
  - type NEC S37.99
- uterus, uterine S37.60
  - with ectopic or molar pregnancy O08.6
  - blood vessel *see* Injury, blood vessel, iliac
  - contusion S37.62
  - laceration S37.63
    - cervix at delivery O71.3
  - rupture associated with obstetrics *see* Rupture, uterus
  - specified type NEC S37.69
- uvula S09.93
- vagina S39.93
  - abrasion S30.814
  - bite S31.45
    - insect S30.864
    - superficial NEC S30.874
  - contusion S30.23
  - crush S38.03
  - during delivery *see* Laceration, vagina, during delivery
  - external constriction S30.844
  - insect bite S30.864
  - laceration S31.41
    - with foreign body S31.42
  - open wound S31.40
  - puncture S31.43
    - with foreign body S31.44
  - superficial S30.95
    - foreign body S30.854
- vas deferens *see* Injury, pelvic organ, specified site NEC
- vascular NEC T14.8
- vein *see* Injury, blood vessel
- vena cava (superior) S25.20
  - inferior S35.10
    - laceration (minor) (superficial) S35.11
      - major S35.12
    - specified type NEC S35.19
  - laceration (minor) (superficial) S25.21
    - major S25.22
  - specified type NEC S25.29
- vesical (sphincter) *see* Injury, bladder
- visual cortex S04.04-
- vitreous (humor) S05.90
  - specified NEC S05.8X   vocal cord NEC S19.83
- vulva S39.94
  - abrasion S30.814
  - bite S31.45
    - insect S30.864
    - superficial NEC S30.874
  - contusion S30.23
  - crush S38.03
  - during delivery *see* Laceration, perineum, female, during delivery
  - external constriction S30.844
  - insect bite S30.864
  - laceration S31.41
    - with foreign body S31.42
  - open wound S31.40
  - puncture S31.43
    - with foreign body S31.44
  - superficial S30.95
    - foreign body S30.854
- whiplash (cervical spine) S13.4
- wrist S69.9-
  - blood vessel *see* Injury, blood vessel, hand
  - contusion *see* Contusion, wrist
  - dislocation *see* Dislocation, wrist
  - fracture *see* Fracture, wrist

Injury - *continued*
- muscle *see* Injury, muscle, hand
- nerve *see* Injury, nerve, hand
- open *see* Wound, open, wrist
- specified NEC S69.8-
- sprain *see* Sprain, wrist
- superficial *see* Injury, superficial, wrist

Inoculation *see also* Vaccination
- complication or reaction *see* Complications, vaccination

Insanity, insane *see also* Psychosis
- adolescent *see* Schizophrenia
- confusional F28
  - acute or subacute F05
- delusional F22
- senile F03

Insect
- bite *see* Bite, by site, superficial, insect
- venomous, poisoning NEC (by) *see* Venom, arthropod

Insecurity, food Z59.41

Insensitivity
- adrenocorticotropin hormone (ACTH) E27.49
- androgen E34.50
  - complete E34.51
  - partial E34.52

Insertion
- cord (umbilical) lateral or velamentous O43.12-
- intrauterine contraceptive device (encounter for) *see* Intrauterine contraceptive device

Insolation (sunstroke) T67.0

Insomnia (organic) G47.00
- adjustment F51.02
- adjustment disorder F51.02
- behavioral, of childhood Z73.819
  - combined type Z73.812
  - limit setting type Z73.811
  - sleep-onset association type Z73.810
- childhood Z73.819
- chronic F51.04
  - somatized tension F51.04
- conditioned F51.04
- due to
  - alcohol
    - abuse F10.182
    - dependence F10.282
    - use F10.982
  - amphetamines
    - abuse F15.182
    - dependence F15.282
    - use F15.982
  - anxiety disorder F51.05
  - caffeine
    - abuse F15.182
    - dependence F15.282
    - use F15.982
  - cocaine
    - abuse F14.182
    - dependence F14.282
    - use F14.982
  - depression F51.05
  - drug NEC
    - abuse F19.182
    - dependence F19.282
    - use F19.982
  - medical condition G47.01
  - mental disorder NEC F51.05
  - opioid
    - abuse F11.182
    - dependence F11.282
    - use F11.982
  - psychoactive substance NEC
    - abuse F19.182
    - dependence F19.282

Insomnia (organic) - *continued*
  - use F19.982
  - sedative, hypnotic, or anxiolytic
    - abuse F13.182
    - dependence F13.282
    - use F13.982
  - stimulant NEC
    - abuse F15.182
    - dependence F15.282
    - use F15.982
- fatal familial (FFI) A81.83
- idiopathic F51.01
- learned F51.3
- nonorganic origin F51.01
- not due to a substance or known physiological condition F51.01
  - specified NEC F51.09
- paradoxical F51.03
- primary F51.01
- psychiatric F51.05
- psychophysiologic F51.04
- related to psychopathology F51.05
- short-term F51.02
- specified NEC G47.09
- stress-related F51.02
- transient F51.02
- without objective findings F51.02

Inspiration
- food or foreign body *see* Foreign body, by site
- mucus *see* Asphyxia, mucus

Inspissated bile syndrome (newborn) P59.1

Instability
- emotional (excessive) F60.3
- joint (post-traumatic) M25.30
  - ankle M25.37-
  - due to old ligament injury *see* Disorder, ligament
  - elbow M25.32-
  - flail *see* Flail, joint
  - foot M25.37-
  - hand M25.34-
  - hip M25.35-
- housing
- - housed Z59.819
- - - with risk of homelessness Z59.811
- - - homelessness in past 12 months Z59.812
  - knee M25.36-
  - lumbosacral *see* subcategory M53.2
  - prosthesis *see* Complications, joint prosthesis, mechanical, displacement, by site
  - sacroiliac *see* subcategory M53.2
  - secondary to
    - old ligament injury *see* Disorder, ligament
    - removal of joint prosthesis M96.89
  - shoulder (region) M25.31-
  - specified site NEC M25.39
  - spine *see* subcategory M53.2
  - wrist M25.33-
- knee (chronic) M23.5-
- lumbosacral *see* subcategory M53.2
- nervous F48.8
- personality (emotional) F60.3
- spine *see* Instability, joint, spine
- vasomotor R55

Institutional syndrome (childhood) F94.2

Institutionalization, affecting child Z62.22
- disinhibited attachment F94.2

Insufficiency, insufficient
- accommodation, old age H52.4
- adrenal (gland) E27.40
  - primary E27.1
- adrenocortical E27.40
  - drug-induced E27.3
  - iatrogenic E27.3

Insufficiency - *continued*
  |primary E27.1
  |anatomic crown height K08.89
  |anterior (occlusal) guidance M26.54
  |anus K62.89
  |aortic (valve) I35.1
    |with
      |mitral (valve) disease I08.0
        |with tricuspid (valve) disease I08.3
      |stenosis I35.2
      |tricuspid (valve) disease I08.2
        |with mitral (valve) disease I08.3
    |congenital Q23.1
    |rheumatic I06.1
      |with
        |mitral (valve) disease I08.0
          |with tricuspid (valve) disease I08.3
        |stenosis I06.2
          |with mitral (valve) disease I08.0
            |with tricuspid (valve) disease I08.3
        |tricuspid (valve) disease I08.2
          |with mitral (valve) disease I08.3
    |specified cause NEC I35.1
    |syphilitic A52.03
  |arterial I77.1
    |basilar G45.0
    |carotid (hemispheric) G45.1
    |cerebral I67.81
    |coronary (acute or subacute) I24.8
    |mesenteric K55.1
    |peripheral I73.9
    |precerebral (multiple) (bilateral) G45.2
    |vertebral G45.0
  |arteriovenous I99.8
  |biliary K83.8
  |cardiac *see also* Insufficiency, myocardial
    |due to presence of (cardiac) prosthesis
      I97.11-
    |postprocedural I97.11-
  |cardiorenal, hypertensive I13.2
  |cardiovascular *see* Disease, cardiovascular
  |cerebrovascular (acute) I67.81
    |with transient focal neurological signs and
      symptoms G45.8
  |circulatory NEC I99.8
    |newborn P29.89
  |clinical crown length K08.89
  |convergence H51.11
  |coronary (acute or subacute) I24.8
    |chronic or with a stated duration of over 4
      weeks I25.89
  |corticoadrenal E27.40
    |primary E27.1
  |dietary E63.9
  |divergence H51.8
  |food T73.0
  |gastroesophageal K22.89
  |gonadal
    |ovary E28.39
    |testis E29.1
  |heart *see also* Insufficiency, myocardial
    |newborn P29.0
    |valve *see* Endocarditis
  |hepatic *see* Failure, hepatic
  |idiopathic autonomic G90.09
  |interocclusal distance of fully erupted teeth
    (ridge) M26.36
  |kidney N28.9
    |acute N28.9
    |chronic N18.9
  |lacrimal (secretion) H04.12-
    |passages *see* Stenosis, lacrimal
  |liver *see* Failure, hepatic

Insufficiency - *continued*
  |lung *see* Insufficiency, pulmonary
  |mental (congenital) *see* Disability, intellectual
  |mesenteric K55.1
  |mitral (valve) I34.0
    |with
      |aortic valve disease I08.0
        |with tricuspid (valve) disease I08.3
      |obstruction or stenosis I05.2
        |with aortic valve disease I08.0
      |tricuspid (valve) disease I08.1
        |with aortic (valve) disease I08.3
    |congenital Q23.3
    |rheumatic I05.1
      |with
        |aortic valve disease I08.0
          |with tricuspid (valve) disease I08.3
        |obstruction or stenosis I05.2
          |with aortic valve disease I08.0
            |with tricuspid (valve) disease I08.3
        |tricuspid (valve) disease I08.1
          |with aortic (valve) disease I08.3
      |active or acute I01.1
        |with chorea, rheumatic (Sydenham's)
          I02.0
    |specified cause, except rheumatic I34.0
  |muscle *see also* Disease, muscle
    |heart *see* Insufficiency, myocardial
    |ocular NEC H50.9
  |myocardial, myocardium (with
    arteriosclerosis) (*see also* Failure, heart)
    I50.9
    |with
      |rheumatic fever (conditions in I00) I09.0
        |active, acute or subacute I01.2
          |with chorea I02.0
        |inactive or quiescent (with chorea) I09.0
    |congenital Q24.8
    |hypertensive *see* Hypertension, heart
    |newborn P29.0
    |rheumatic I09.0
      |active, acute, or subacute I01.2
    |syphilitic A52.06
  |nourishment T73.0
  |pancreatic K86.89
    |exocrine K86.81
  |parathyroid (gland) E20.9
  |peripheral vascular (arterial) I73.9
  |pituitary E23.0
  |placental (mother) O36.51-
  |platelets D69.6
  |prenatal care affecting management of
    pregnancy O09.3-
  |progressive pluriglandular E31.0
  |pulmonary J98.4
    |acute, following surgery (nonthoracic) J95.2
      |thoracic J95.1
    |chronic, following surgery J95.3
    |following
      |shock J98.4
      |trauma J98.4
    |newborn P28.5
    |valve I37.1
      |with stenosis I37.2
      |congenital Q22.2
      |rheumatic I09.89
        |with aortic, mitral or tricuspid (valve)
        disease I08.8
  |pyloric K31.89
  |renal (acute) N28.9
    |chronic N18.9
  |respiratory R06.89
    |newborn P28.5
  |rotation *see* Malrotation

Insufficiency - *continued*
  |sleep syndrome F51.12
  |social insurance Z59.7
  |suprarenal E27.40
    |primary E27.1
  |tarso-orbital fascia, congenital Q10.3
  |testis E29.1
  |thyroid (gland) (acquired) E03.9
    |congenital E03.1
  |tricuspid (valve) (rheumatic) I07.1
    |with
      |aortic (valve) disease I08.2
        |with mitral (valve) disease I08.3
      |mitral (valve) disease I08.1
        |with aortic (valve) disease I08.3
      |obstruction or stenosis I07.2
        |with aortic (valve) disease I08.2
          |with mitral (valve) disease I08.3
    |congenital Q22.8
    |nonrheumatic I36.1
      |with stenosis I36.2
  |urethral sphincter R32
  |valve, valvular (heart) I38
    |aortic *see* Insufficiency, aortic (valve)
    |mitral *see* Insufficiency, mitral (valve)
    |pulmonary *see* Insufficiency, pulmonary,
      valve
    |tricuspid *see* Insufficiency, tricuspid (valve)
      |congenital Q24.8
  |vascular I99.8
    |intestine K55.9
      |acute *see also* Ischemia, intestine, acute
        K55.059
    |mesenteric K55.1
    |peripheral I73.9
    |renal *see* Hypertension, kidney
  |velopharyngeal
    |acquired K13.79
    |congenital Q38.8
  |venous (chronic) (peripheral) I87.2
  |ventricular *see* Insufficiency, myocardial
  |welfare support Z59.7
Insufflation, fallopian Z31.41
Insular *see* condition **Insulinoma**
  |pancreas
    |benign D13.7
    |malignant C25.4
    |uncertain behavior D37.8
  |specified site
    |benign *see* Neoplasm, by site, benign
    |malignant *see* Neoplasm, by site, malignant
    |uncertain behavior *see* Neoplasm, by site,
      uncertain behavior
  |unspecified site
    |benign D13.7
    |malignant C25.4
    |uncertain behavior D37.8
Insuloma *see* Insulinoma
Interference
  |balancing side M26.56
  |non-working side M26.56
Intermenstrual *see* condition
Intermittent *see* condition
Internal *see* condition
Interrogation
  |cardiac defibrillator (automatic) (implantable)
    Z45.02
  |cardiac pacemaker Z45.018
  |cardiac (event) (loop) recorder Z45.09
  |infusion pump (implanted) (intrathecal) Z45.1
  |neurostimulator Z46.2

Interruption
|aortic arch Q25.21
|bundle of His I44.30
|phase-shift, sleep cycle *see* Disorder, sleep,
 circadian rhythm
|sleep phase-shift, or 24 hour sleep-wake cycle
 see Disorder, sleep, circadian rhythm
Interstitial *see* condition
Intertrigo L30.4
|labialis K13.0
Intervertebral disc *see* condition
Intestine, intestinal *see* condition
Intolerance
|carbohydrate K90.49
|disaccharide, hereditary E73.0
|fat NEC K90.49
 |pancreatic K90.3
|food K90.49
 |dietary counseling and surveillance Z71.3
|fructose E74.10
 |hereditary E74.12
|glucose (-galactose) E74.39
|gluten K90.41
|lactose E73.9
 |specified NEC E73.8
|lysine E72.3
|milk NEC K90.49
 |lactose E73.9
|protein K90.49
|starch NEC K90.49
|sucrose (-isomaltose) E74.31
Intoxicated NEC (without dependence) *see*
 Alcohol, intoxication
Intoxication
|acid E87.2
|alcoholic (acute) (without dependence) *see*
 Alcohol, intoxication
|alimentary canal K52.1
|amphetamine (without dependence) *see*
 Abuse, drug, stimulant, with intoxication
 |with dependence *see* Dependence, drug,
 stimulant, with intoxication
|anxiolytic (acute) (without dependence) *see*
 Abuse, drug, sedative, with intoxication
 |with dependence *see* Dependence, drug,
 sedative, with intoxication
|caffeine F15.929
 |with dependence *see* Dependence, drug,
 stimulant, with intoxication
|cannabinoids (acute) (without dependence)
 see Use, cannabis, with intoxication
 |with
 |abuse *see* Abuse, drug, cannabis, with
 intoxication
 |dependence *see* Dependence, drug,
 cannabis, with intoxication
|chemical *see* Table of Drugs and Chemicals
 |via placenta or breast milk *see*
 |Absorption, chemical, through placenta
|cocaine (acute) (without dependence) *see*
 Abuse, drug, cocaine, with intoxication
 |with dependence *see* Dependence, drug,
 cocaine, with intoxication
|drug
 |acute (without dependence) *see* Abuse,
 drug, by type with intoxication
 |with dependence *see* Dependence, drug,
 by type with intoxication
 |addictive
 |via placenta or breast milk *see*
 Absorption, drug, addictive, through
 placenta
 |newborn P93.8
 |gray baby syndrome P93.0

Intoxication - *continued*
|overdose or wrong substance given or taken
 see Table of Drugs and Chemicals, by
 drug, poisoning
|enteric K52.1
|foodborne A05.9
 |bacterial A05.9
 |classical (Clostridium botulinum) A05.1
 |due to
 |Bacillus cereus A05.4
 |bacterium A05.9
 |specified NEC A05.8
 |Clostridium
 |botulinum A05.1
 |perfringens A05.2
 |welchii A05.2
 |Salmonella A02.9
 |with
 |(gastro) enteritis A02.0
 |localized infection(s) A02.20
 |arthritis A02.23
 |meningitis A02.21
 |osteomyelitis A02.24
 |pneumonia A02.22
 |pyelonephritis A02.25
 |specified NEC A02.29
 |sepsis A02.1
 |specified manifestation NEC A02.8
 |Staphylococcus A05.0
 |Vibrio
 |parahaemolyticus A05.3
 |vulnificus A05.5
 |enterotoxin, staphylococcal A05.0
 |noxious *see* Poisoning, food, noxious
|gastrointestinal K52.1
|hallucinogenic (without dependence) *see*
 Abuse, drug, hallucinogen, with
 intoxication
 |with dependence *see* Dependence, drug,
 hallucinogen, with intoxication
|hypnotic (acute) (without dependence) *see*
 Abuse, drug, sedative, with intoxication
 |with dependence *see* Dependence, drug,
 sedative, with intoxication
|inhalant (acute) (without dependence) *see*
 Abuse, drug, inhalant, with intoxication
 |with dependence *see* Dependence, drug,
 inhalant, with intoxication
|meaning
 |inebriation *see* category F10
 |poisoning *see* Table of Drugs and
 Chemicals
|methyl alcohol (acute) (without dependence)
 see Alcohol, intoxication
|opioid (acute) (without dependence) *see*
 Abuse, drug, opioid, with intoxication
 |with dependence *see* Dependence, drug,
 opioid, with intoxication
|pathologic NEC (without dependence) *see*
 Alcohol, intoxication
|phencyclidine (without dependence) *see*
 Abuse, drug, hallucinogen, with
 intoxication
 |with dependence *see* Dependence, drug,
 hallucinogen, with intoxication
|potassium (K) E87.5
|psychoactive substance NEC (without
 dependence) *see* Abuse, drug, psychoactive
 NEC, with intoxication
 |with dependence *see* Dependence, drug,
 psychoactive NEC, with intoxication
|sedative (acute) (without dependence) *see*
 Abuse, drug, sedative, with intoxication
 |with dependence *see* Dependence, drug,
 sedative, with intoxication
|serum *see also* Reaction, serum T80.69

Intoxication - *continued*
|uremic *see* Uremia
|volatile solvents (acute) (without dependence)
 see Abuse, drug, inhalant, with intoxication
 |with dependence *see* Dependence, drug,
 inhalant, with intoxication
|water E87.79
Intraabdominal testis, testes
|bilateral Q53.211
|unilateral Q53.111
Intracranial *see* condition
Intrahepatic gallbladder Q44.1
Intraligamentous *see* condition
Intrathoracic *see also* condition
|kidney Q63.2
Intrauterine contraceptive device
|checking Z30.431
|insertion Z30.430
 |immediately following removal Z30.433
|in situ Z97.5
|management Z30.431
|reinsertion Z30.433
|removal Z30.432
|replacement Z30.433
|retention in pregnancy O26.3
Intraventricular *see* condition
Intrinsic deformity *see* Deformity
Intubation, difficult or failed T88.4
Intumescence, lens (eye) (cataract) *see*
 Cataract
Intussusception (bowel) (colon) (enteric)
 (ileocecal) (ileocolic) (intestine) (rectum)
 K56.1
|appendix K38.8
|congenital Q43.8
|ureter (with obstruction) N13.5
Invagination (bowel, colon, intestine or
 rectum) K56.1
Inversion
|albumin-globulin (A-G) ratio E88.09
|bladder N32.89
|cecum *see* Intussusception
|cervix N88.8
|chromosome in normal individual Q95.1
|circadian rhythm *see* Disorder, sleep,
 circadian rhythm
|nipple N64.59
 |congenital Q83.8
 |gestational *see* Retraction, nipple
 |puerperal, postpartum *see* Retraction, nipple
|nyctohemeral rhythm *see* Disorder, sleep,
 circadian rhythm
|optic papilla Q14.2
|organ or site, congenital NEC *see* Anomaly,
 by site
|sleep rhythm *see* Disorder, sleep, circadian
 rhythm
|testis (congenital) Q55.29
|uterus (chronic) (postinfectional) (postpartal,
 old) N85.5
 |postpartum O71.2
|vagina (posthysterectomy) N99.3
|ventricular Q20.5
Investigation *see also* Examination Z04.9
|clinical research subject (control) (normal
 comparison) (participant) Z00.6
Involuntary movement, abnormal R25.9
Involution, involutional *see also* condition
|breast, cystic *see* Dysplasia, mammary,
 specified type NEC
|depression (single episode) F32.89
 |recurrent episode F33.9
|melancholia (single episode) F32.89
 |recurrent episode F33.8
|ovary, senile *see* Atrophy, ovary
|thymus failure E32.8

I.Q.
|under 20 F73
|20-34 F72
|35 49 F71
|50-69 F70
IRDS (type I) P22.0
|type II P22.1
Irideremia Q13.1
Iridis rubeosis *see* Disorder, iris, vascular
Iridochoroiditis (panuveitis) *see* Panuveitis
Iridocyclitis H20.9
|acute H20.0-
||hypopyon H20.05-
||primary H20.01-
||recurrent H20.02-
||secondary (noninfectious) H20.04-
|||infectious H20.03-
|chronic H20.1-
|due to allergy *see* Iridocyclitis, acute, secondary
|endogenous *see* Iridocyclitis, acute, primary
|Fuchs' *see* Cyclitis, Fuchs' heterochromic
|gonococcal A54.32
|granulomatous *see* Iridocyclitis, chronic
|herpes, herpetic (simplex) B00.51
||zoster B02.32
|hypopyon *see* Iridocyclitis, acute, hypopyon
|in (due to)
||ankylosing spondylitis M45.9
||gonococcal infection A54.32
||herpes (simplex) virus B00.51
|||zoster B02.32
||infectious disease NOS B99
||parasitic disease NOS B89 [H22]
||sarcoidosis D86.83
||syphilis A51.43
||tuberculosis A18.54
||zoster B02.32
|lens-induced H20.2-
|nongranulomatous *see* Iridocyclitis, acute
|recurrent *see* Iridocyclitis, acute, recurrent
|rheumatic *see* Iridocyclitis, chronic
|subacute *see* Iridocyclitis, acute
|sympathetic *see* Uveitis, sympathetic
|syphilitic (secondary) A51.43
|tuberculous (chronic) A18.54
|Vogt-Koyanagi H20.82-
Iridocyclochoroiditis (panuveitis) *see* Panuveitis
Iridodialysis H21.53-
Iridodonesis H21.89
Iridoplegia (complete) (partial) (reflex) H57.09
Iridoschisis H21.25-
Iris *see also* condition
|bombé *see* Membrane, pupillary
Iritis *see also* Iridocyclitis
|chronic *see* Iridocyclitis, chronic
|diabetic *see* E08-E13 with .39
|due to
||herpes simplex B00.51
||leprosy A30.9 [H22]
|gonococcal A54.32
|gouty *see also* Gout, by type M10.9 [H22]
|granulomatous *see* Iridocyclitis, chronic
|lens induced *see* Iridocyclitis, lens-induced
|papulosa (syphilitic) A52.71
|rheumatic *see* Iridocyclitis, chronic
|syphilitic (secondary) A51.43
||congenital (early) A50.01
||late A52.71
|tuberculous A18.54
Iron *see* condition
Iron-Miner's lung J63.4
Irradiated enamel (tooth, teeth) K03.89

Irradiation effects, adverse T66
Irreducible, irreducibility *see* condition
Irregular, irregularity
|action, heart I49.9
|alveolar process K08.89
|bleeding N92.6
|breathing R06.89
|contour of cornea (acquired) *see* Deformity, cornea
||congenital Q13.4
|contour, reconstructed breast N65.0
|dentin (in pulp) K04.3
|eye movements H55.89
||deficient
|||saccadic H55.81
|||smooth H55.82
||nystagmus *see* Nystagmus
|labor O62.2
|menstruation (cause unknown) N92.6
|periods N92.6
|prostate N42.9
|pupil *see* Abnormality, pupillary
|reconstructed breast N65.0
|respiratory R06.89
|septum (nasal) J34.2
|shape, organ or site, congenital NEC *see* Distortion
|sleep-wake pattern (rhythm) G47.23
Irritable, irritability R45.4
|bladder N32.89
|bowel (syndrome) K58.9
||with
|||constipation K58.1
|||diarrhea K58.0
||mixed K58.2
||psychogenic F45.8
||specified NEC K58.8
|bronchial *see* Bronchitis
|cerebral, in newborn P91.3
|colon *see also* Irritable, bowel K58.9
||with diarrhea K58.0
||psychogenic F45.8
|duodenum K59.89
|heart (psychogenic) F45.8
|hip *see* Derangement, joint, specified type NEC, hip
|ileum K59.89
|infant R68.12
|jejunum K59.89
|rectum K59.89
|stomach K31.89
||psychogenic F45.8
|sympathetic G90.8
|urethra N36.8
Irritation
|anus K62.89
|axillary nerve G54.0
|bladder N32.89
|brachial plexus G54.0
|bronchial *see* Bronchitis
|cervical plexus G54.2
|cervix *see* Cervicitis
|choroid, sympathetic *see* Endophthalmitis
|cranial nerve *see* Disorder, nerve, cranial
|gastric K31.89
||psychogenic F45.8
|globe, sympathetic *see* Uveitis, sympathetic
|labyrinth *see* subcategory H83.2
|lumbosacral plexus G54.1
|meninges (traumatic) *see* Injury, intracranial
||nontraumatic *see* Meningismus
|nerve *see* Disorder, nerve
|nervous R45.0
|penis N48.89
|perineum NEC L29.3

Irritation - *continued*
|peripheral autonomic nervous system G90.8
|peritoneum *see* Peritonitis
|pharynx J39.2
|plantar nerve *see* Lesion, nerve, plantar
|spinal (cord) (traumatic) *see also* Injury, spinal cord, by region
||nerve G58.9
|||root NEC *see* Radiculopathy
||nontraumatic *see* Myelopathy
|stomach K31.89
||psychogenic F45.8
|sympathetic nerve NEC G90.8
|ulnar nerve *see* Lesion, nerve, ulnar
|vagina N89.8
Ischemia, ischemic I99.8
|brain *see* Ischemia, cerebral
|bowel (transient)
||acute *see also* Ischemia, intestine, acute K55.059
||chronic K55.1
||due to mesenteric artery insufficiency K55.1
|cardiac (*see* Disease, heart, ischemic)
|cardiomyopathy I25.5
|cerebral (chronic) (generalized) I67.82
||arteriosclerotic I67.2
||intermittent G45.9
||newborn P91.0
||recurrent focal G45.8
||transient G45.9
|colon chronic (due to mesenteric artery insufficiency) K55.1
|coronary *see* Disease, heart, ischemic
|demand (coronary) *see also* Angina I24.8
||with myocardial infarction I21.A1
||resulting in myocardial infarction I21.A1
|heart (chronic or with a stated duration of over 4weeks) I25.9
||acute or with a stated duration of 4 weeks or less I24.9
||subacute I24.9
|infarction, muscle *see* Infarct, muscle
|intestine (large) (small) (transient) K55.9
||acute K55.059
|||diffuse K55.052
|||focal K55.051
|||large K55.039
||||diffuse K55.032
||||focal K55.031
|||small K55.019
||||diffuse K55.012
||||focal K55.011
||chronic K55.1
||due to mesenteric artery insufficiency K55.1
|kidney N28.0
|limb, critical   *see* Arteriosclerosis, with critical limb ischemia
|limb-threatening, chronic *see* Arteriosclerosis, with critical limb ischemia
|mesenteric, acute *see also* Ischemia, intestine, acute K55.059
|muscle, traumatic T79.6
|myocardium, myocardial (chronic or with a stated duration of over 4 weeks) I25.9
||acute, without myocardial infarction I51.3
||silent (asymptomatic) I25.6
||transient of newborn P29.4
|renal N28.0
|retina, retinal *see* Occlusion, artery, retina
|small bowel
||acute K55.019
|||diffuse K55.012
|||focal K55.011
||chronic K55.1

Ischemia, ischemic - *continued*
   |due to mesenteric artery insufficiency K55.1
  |spinal cord G95.11
  |subendocardial *see* Insufficiency, coronary
  |supply (coronary) *see also* Angina I25.9
   |due to vasospasm I20.1
Ischial spine *see* condition
Ischialgia *see* Sciatica
Ischiopagus Q89.4
Ischium, ischial *see* condition
Ischuria R34
Iselin's disease or osteochondrosis *see*
  Osteochondrosis, juvenile, metatarsus
Islands of
  |parotid tissue in
   |lymph nodes Q38.6
   |neck structures Q38.6
  |submaxillary glands in
   |fascia Q38.6
   |lymph nodes Q38.6
   |neck muscles Q38.6
Islet cell tumor, pancreas D13.7
Isoimmunization NEC *see also* Incompatibility
  |affecting management of pregnancy (ABO)
   (with hydrops fetalis) O36.11-
   |anti-A sensitization O36.11-
   |anti-B sensitization O36.19-
   |anti-C sensitization O36.09-
   |anti-C sensitization O36.09-
   |anti-E sensitization O36.09-
   |anti-E sensitization O36.09-
   |Rh NEC O36.09-
    |anti-D antibody O36.01-
   |specified NEC O36.19-
  |newborn P55.9
   |with
    |hydrops fetalis P56.0
    |kernicterus P57.0
   |ABO (blood groups) P55.1
   |Rhesus (Rh) factor P55.0
   |specified type NEC P55.8
Isolation, isolated
  |dwelling Z59.89
  |family Z63.79
  |social Z60.4
Isoleucinosis E71.19
Isomerism atrial appendages (with asplenia or polysplenia) Q20.6
Isosporiasis, isosporosis A07.3
Isovaleric acidemia E71.110
Issue of
  |medical certificate Z02.79
   |for disability determination Z02.71
  |repeat prescription (appliance) (glasses)
   (medicinal substance, medicament,
   medicine) Z76.0
   |contraception *see* Contraception
Itch, itching *see also* Pruritus
  |baker's L23.6
  |barber's B35.0
  |bricklayer's L24.5
  |cheese B88.0
  |clam digger's B65.3
  |coolie B76.9
  |copra B88.0
  |dew B76.9
  |dhobi B35.6
  |filarial *see* Infestation, filarial
  |grain B88.0
  |grocer's B88.0
  |ground B76.9
  |harvest B88.0
  |jock B35.6
  |Malabar B35.5
   |beard B35.0

Itch, itching - *continued*
  |foot B35.3
   |scalp B35.0
  |meaning scabies B86
  |Norwegian B86
  |perianal L29.0
  |poultry men's B88.0
  |sarcoptic B86
  |scabies B86
  |scrub B88.0
  |straw B88.0
  |swimmer's B65.3
  |water B76.9
  |winter L29.8
Ivemark's syndrome (asplenia with congenital heart disease) Q89.01
Ivory bones Q78.2
Ixodiasis NEC B88.8

J

Jaccoud's syndrome *see* Arthropathy,
  postrheumatic, chronic
Jackson's
  |membrane Q43.3
  |paralysis or syndrome G83.89
  |veil Q43.3
Jacquet's dermatitis (diaper dermatitis) L22
Jadassohn-Pellizari's disease or anetoderma L90.2
Jadassohn's
  |blue nevus *see* Nevus
  |intraepidermal epithelioma *see* Neoplasm,
  skin, benign
Jaffe-Lichtenstein (-Uehlinger) syndrome *see*
  Dysplasia, fibrous, bone NEC
Jakob-Creutzfeldt disease or syndrome *see*
  Creutzfeldt-Jakob disease or syndrome
Jaksch-Luzet disease D64.89
Jamaican
  |neuropathy G92.8
  |paraplegic tropical ataxic-spastic syndrome
  G92.8
Janet's disease F48.8
Janiceps Q89.4
Jansky-Bielschowsky amaurotic idiocy E75.4
Japanese
  |B-type encephalitis A83.0
  |river fever A75.3
Jaundice (yellow) R17
  |acholuric (familial) (splenomegalic) *see also*
   Spherocytosis
   |acquired D59.8
  |breast-milk (inhibitor) P59.3
  |catarrhal (acute) B15.9
   |with hepatic coma B15.0
  |cholestatic (benign) R17
  |due to or associated with
   |delayed conjugation P59.8
    |associated with (due to) preterm delivery
    P59.0
   |preterm delivery P59.0
  |epidemic (catarrhal) B15.9
   |with hepatic coma B15.0
   |leptospiral A27.0
   |spirochetal A27.0
  |familial nonhemolytic (congenital) (Gilbert)
   E80.4
   |Crigler-Najjar E80.5
  |febrile (acute) B15.9
   |with hepatic coma B15.0
   |leptospiral A27.0
   |spirochetal A27.0
  |hematogenous D59.9

Jaundice (yellow) - *continued*
  |hemolytic (acquired) D59.9
   |congenital *see* Spherocytosis
  |hemorrhagic (acute) (leptospiral) (spirochetal)
   A27.0
  |infectious (acute) (subacute) B15.9
   |with hepatic coma B15.0
   |leptospiral A27.0
   |spirochetal A27.0
  |leptospiral (hemorrhagic) A27.0
  |malignant (without coma) K72.90
   |with coma K72.91
  |newborn P59.9
   |due to or associated with
    |ABO
     |antibodies P55.1
     |incompatibility, maternal/fetal P55.1
     |isoimmunization P55.1
    |absence or deficiency of enzyme system
    for bilirubin conjugation (congenital)
    P59.8
    |bleeding P58.1
    |breast milk inhibitors to conjugation
    P59.3
     |associated with preterm delivery P59.0
    |bruising P58.0
    |Crigler-Najjar syndrome E80.5
    |delayed conjugation P59.8
     |associated with preterm delivery P59.0
    |drugs or toxins
     |given to newborn P58.42
     |transmitted from mother P58.41
    |excessive hemolysis P58.9
     |due to
      |bleeding P58.1
      |bruising P58.0
      |drugs or toxins
       |given to newborn P58.42
       |transmitted from mother P58.41
      |infection P58.2
      |polycythemia P58.3
      |swallowed maternal blood P58.5
     |specified type NEC P58.8
   |galactosemia E74.21
   |Gilbert syndrome E80.4
   |hemolytic disease P55.9
    |ABO isoimmunization P55.1
    |Rh isoimmunization P55.0
    |specified NEC P55.8
   |hepatocellular damage P59.20
    |specified NEC P59.29
   |hereditary hemolytic anemia P58.8
   |hypothyroidism, congenital E03.1
   |incompatibility, maternal/fetal NOS P55.9
   |infection P58.2
   |inspissated bile syndrome P59.1
   |isoimmunization NOS P55.9
   |mucoviscidosis E84.9
   |polycythemia P58.3
   |preterm delivery P59.0
   |Rh
    |antibodies P55.0
    |incompatibility, maternal/fetal P55.0
    |isoimmunization P55.0
   |specified cause NEC P59.8
   |swallowed maternal blood P58.5
   |spherocytosis (congenital) D58.0
  |neonatal *see* Jaundice, newborn
  |nonhemolytic congenital familial (Gilbert)
   E80.4
  |nuclear, newborn *see also* Kernicterus of
   newborn P57.9
  |obstructive *see also* Obstruction, bile duct
   K83.1

Jaundice (yellow) - *continued*
  |post-immunization *see* Hepatitis, viral, type, B
  |post-transfusion *see* Hepatitis, viral, type, B
  |regurgitation *see also* Obstruction, bile duct
     K83.1
  |serum (homologous) (prophylactic)
     (therapeutic) *see* Hepatitis, viral, type, B
  |spirochetal (hemorrhagic) A27.0
  |symptomatic R17
     |newborn P59.9
Jaw *see* condition
Jaw-Winking phenomenon or syndrome
  Q07.8
Jealousy
  |alcoholic F10.988
  |childhood F93.8
  |sibling F93.8
Jejunitis *see* Enteritis
Jejunostomy status Z93.4
Jejunum, jejunal *see* condition
Jensen's disease *see* Inflammation,
  chorioretinal, focal, juxtapapillary
Jerks, myoclonic G25.3
Jervell-Lange Nielsen syndrome I45.81
Jeune's disease Q77.2
Jigger disease B88.1
Job's syndrome (chronic granulomatous
  disease) D71
Joint *see also* condition
  |mice *see* Loose, body, joint
     |knee M23.4-
Jordan's anomaly or syndrome D72.0
Joseph-Diamond-Blackfan anemia (congenital
  hypoplastic) D61.01
Jungle yellow fever A95.0
Jüngling's disease *see* Sarcoidosis
Juvenile *see* condition

K

Kahler's disease C90.0-
Kakke E51.11
Kala-Azar B55.0
Kallmann's syndrome E23.0
Kanner's syndrome (autism) *see* Psychosis,
  childhood
Kaposi's
  |dermatosis (xeroderma pigmentosum) Q82.1
  |lichen ruber L44.0
     |acuminatus L44.0
  |sarcoma
     |colon C46.4
     |connective tissue C46.1
     |gastrointestinal organ C46.4
     |lung C46.5-
     |lymph node (multiple) C46.3
     |palate (hard) (soft) C46.2
     |rectum C46.4
     |skin (multiple sites) C46.0
     |specified site NEC C46.7
     |stomach C46.4
     |unspecified site C46.9
  |varicelliform eruption B00.0
     |vaccinia T88.1
Kartagener's syndrome or triad (sinusitis,
  bronchiectasis, situs inversus) Q89.3
Karyotype
  |with abnormality except iso (Xq) Q96.2
  |45,X Q96.0
  |46,X
     |iso (Xq) Q96.1
  |46,XX Q98.3
     |with streak gonads Q50.32
     |hermaphrodite (true) Q99.1
     |male Q98.3
  |46,XY

Karyotype - *continued*
     |with streak gonads Q56.1
     |female Q97.3
     |hermaphrodite (true) Q99.1
  |47,XXX Q97.0
  |47,XXY Q98.0
  |47,XYY Q98.5
Kaschin-Beck disease *see* Disease, Kaschin-
  Beck
Katayama's disease or fever B65.2
Kawasaki's syndrome M30.3
Kayser-Fleischer ring (cornea)
  (pseudosclerosis) H18.04-
Kaznelson's syndrome (congenital hypoplastic
  anemia) D61.01
Kearns-Sayre syndrome H49.81-
Kedani fever A75.3
Kelis L91.0
Kelly (-Patterson) syndrome (sideropenic
  dysphagia) D50.1
Keloid, cheloid L91.0
  |acne L73.0
  |Addison's L94.0
  |cornea *see* Opacity, cornea
  |Hawkin's L91.0
  |scar L91.0
Keloma L91.0
Kenya fever A77.1
Keratectasia *see also* Ectasia, cornea
  |congenital Q13.4
Keratinization of alveolar ridge mucosa
  excessive K13.23
  |minimal K13.22
Keratinized residual ridge mucosa   excessive
  K13.23
  |minimal K13.22
Keratitis (nodular) (nonulcerative) (simple)
  (zonular) H16.9
  |with ulceration (central) (marginal)
     (perforated) (ring) *see* Ulcer, cornea
  |actinic *see* Photokeratitis
  |arborescens (herpes simplex) B00.52
  |areolar H16.11-
  |bullosa H16.8
  |deep H16.309
     |specified type NEC H16.399
  |dendritic (a) (herpes simplex) B00.52
  |disciform (is) (herpes simplex) B00.52
     |varicella B01.81
  |filamentary H16.12-
  |gonococcal (congenital or prenatal) A54.33
  |herpes, herpetic (simplex) B00.52
     |zoster B02.33
  |in (due to)
     |acanthamebiasis B60.13
     |adenovirus B30.0
     |exanthema *see also* Exanthem B09
     |herpes (simplex) virus B00.52
     |measles B05.81
     |syphilis A50.31
     |tuberculosis A18.52
     |zoster B02.33
  |interstitial (nonsyphilitic) H16.30-
     |diffuse H16.32-
     |herpes, herpetic (simplex) B00.52
        |zoster B02.33
     |sclerosing H16.33-
     |specified type NEC H16.39
     |syphilitic (congenital) (late) A50.31
     |tuberculous A18.52
  |macular H16.11-
  |nummular H16.11-
  |oyster shuckers' H16.8
  |parenchymatous *see* Keratitis, interstitial

Keratitis - *continued*
  |petrificans H16.8
  |postmeasles B05.81
  |punctata
     |leprosa A30.9 [*H16.14*]
     |syphilitic (profunda) A50.31
  |punctate H16.14-
  |purulent H16.8
  |rosacea L71.8
  |sclerosing H16.33-
  |specified type NEC H16.8
  |stellate H16.11-
  |striate H16.11-
  |superficial H16.10-
     |with conjunctivitis *see* Keratoconjunctivitis
     |due to light *see* Photokeratitis
  |suppurative H16.8
  |syphilitic (congenital) (prenatal) A50.31
  |trachomatous A71.1
     |sequelae B94.0
  |tuberculous A18.52
  |vesicular H16.8
  |xerotic *see also* Keratomalacia H16.8
     |vitamin A deficiency E50.4
Keratoacanthoma L85.8
Keratocele *see* Descemetocele
Keratoconjunctivitis H16.20-
  |Acanthamoeba B60.13
  |adenoviral B30.0
  |epidemic B30.0
  |exposure H16.21-
  |herpes, herpetic (simplex) B00.52
     |zoster B02.33
  |in exanthema *see also* Exanthem B09
  |infectious B30.0
  |lagophthalmic *see* Keratoconjunctivitis,
     specified type NEC
  |neurotrophic H16.23-
  |phlyctenular H16.25-
  |postmeasles B05.81
  |shipyard B30.0
  |sicca (Sjogren's) M35.0-
     |not Sjogren's H16.22-
  |specified type NEC H16.29-
  |tuberculous (phlyctenular) A18.52
  |vernal H16.26-
Keratoconus H18.60-
  |congenital Q13.4
  |stable H18.61-
  |unstable H18.62-
Keratocyst (dental) (odontogenic) *see* Cyst,
  calcifying odontogenic
Keratoderma, keratodermia (congenital)
  (palmaris et plantaris) (symmetrical) Q82.8
  |acquired L85.1
     |in diseases classified elsewhere L86
  |climactericum L85.1
  |gonococcal A54.89
  |gonorrheal A54.89
  |punctata L85.2
  |Reiter's *see* Reiter's disease
Keratodermatocele *see* Descemetocele
Keratoglobus H18.79
  |congenital Q15.8
     |with glaucoma Q15.0
Keratohemia *see* Pigmentation, cornea, stromal
Keratoiritis *see also* Iridocyclitis
  |syphilitic A50.39
  |tuberculous A18.54
Keratoma L57.0
  |palmaris and plantaris hereditarium Q82.8
  |senile L57.0
Keratomalacia H18.44-
  |vitamin A deficiency E50.4

Keratomegaly Q13.4
Keratomycosis B49
|nigrans, nigricans (palmaris) B36.1
Keratopathy H18.9
|band H18.42-
|bullous H18.1-
|bullous (aphakic), following cataract surgery
H59.01-
Keratoscleritis, tuberculous A18.52
Keratosis L57.0
|actinic L57.0
|arsenical L85.8
|congenital, specified NEC Q80.8
|female genital NEC N94.89
|follicularis Q82.8
|acquired L11.0
|congenita Q82.8
|et parafollicularis in cutem penetrans L87.0
|spinulosa (decalvans) Q82.8
|vitamin A deficiency E50.8
|gonococcal A54.89
|male genital (external) N50.89
|nigricans L83
|obturans, external ear (canal) see
Cholesteatoma, external ear
|palmaris et plantaris (inherited) (symmetrical)
Q82.8
|acquired L85.1
|penile N48.89
|pharynx J39.2
|pilaris, acquired L85.8
|punctata (palmaris et plantaris) L85.2
|scrotal N50.89
|seborrheic L82.1
|inflamed L82.0
|senile L57.0
|solar L57.0
|tonsillaris J35.8
|vagina N89.4
|vegetans Q82.8
|vitamin A deficiency E50.8
|vocal cord J38.3
Kerato-Uveitis see Iridocyclitis
Keraunoparalysis T75.09
Kerion (celsi) B35.0
Kernicterus of newborn (not due to
isoimmunization) P57.9
|due to isoimmunization (conditions in P55.0-
P55.9) P57.0
|specified type NEC P57.8
Keshan disease E59
Ketoacidosis E87.2
|diabetic see Diabetes, by type, with
ketoacidosis
Ketonuria R82.4
Ketosis NEC E88.89
|diabetic see Diabetes, by type, with
ketoacidosis
Kew Garden fever A79.1
Kidney see condition
Kienböck's disease see also Osteochondrosis,
juvenile, hand, carpal lunate
|adult M93.1
Kimmelstiel (-Wilson) disease see Diabetes,
Kimmelstiel (-Wilson) disease
Kimura disease D21.9
|specified site (see Neoplasm, connective
tissue benign)
Kink, kinking
|artery I77.1
|hair (acquired) L67.8
|ileum or intestine see Obstruction, intestine
|Lane's see Obstruction, intestine
|organ or site, congenital NEC see Anomaly,
by site

Kink, kinking - continued
|ureter (pelvic junction) N13.5
|with
|hydronephrosis N13.1
|with infection N13.6
|pyelonephritis (chronic) N11.1
|congenital Q62.39
|vein(s) I87.8
|caval I87.1
|peripheral I87.1
Kinnier Wilson's disease (hepatolenticular
degeneration) E83.01
Kissing spine M48.20
|cervical region M48.22
|cervicothoracic region M48.23
|lumbar region M48.26
|lumbosacral region M48.27
|occipito-atlanto-axial region M48.21
|thoracic region M48.24
|thoracolumbar region M48.25
Klatskin's tumor C24.0
Klauder's disease A26.8
Klebs' disease see also Glomerulonephritis
N05.-
Klebsiella (K.) pneumoniae, as cause of
disease classified elsewhere B96.1
Klein (e) -Levin syndrome G47.13
Kleptomania F63.2
Klinefelter's syndrome Q98.4
|karyotype 47,XXY Q98.0
|male with more than two X chromosomes
Q98.1
Klippel-Feil deficiency, disease, or syndrome
(brevicollis) Q76.1
Klippel's disease I67.2
Klippel-Trenaunay (-Weber) syndrome Q87.2
Klumpke (-Déjérine) palsy, paralysis (birth)
(newborn) P14.1
Knee see condition
Knock knee (acquired) M21.06-
|congenital Q74.1
Knot(s)
|intestinal, syndrome (volvulus) K56.2
|surfer S89.8-
|umbilical cord (true) O69.2
Knotting (of)
|hair L67.8
|intestine K56.2
Knuckle pad (Garrod's) M72.1
Koch's
|infection see Tuberculosis
|relapsing fever A68.9
Koch-Weeks' conjunctivitis see Conjunctivitis,
acute, mucopurulent
Köebner's syndrome Q81.8
Köenig's disease (osteochondritis dissecans)
see Osteochondritis, dissecans
Köhler-Pellegrini-Steida disease or syndrome
(calcification, knee joint) see Bursitis, tibial
collateral
Köhler's disease
|patellar see Osteochondrosis, juvenile, patella
|tarsal navicular see Osteochondrosis, juvenile,
tarsus
Koilonychia L60.3
|congenital Q84.6
Kojevnikov's, epilepsy see Kozhevnikov's
epilepsy
Koplik's spots B05.9
Kopp's asthma E32.8
Korsakoff's (Wernicke) disease, psychosis or
syndrome (alcoholic) F10.96
|with dependence F10.26
|drug-induced

Korsakoff's - continued
|due to drug abuse see Abuse, drug, by type,
with amnestic disorder
|due to drug dependence see Dependence,
drug, by type, with amnestic disorder
|nonalcoholic F04
Korsakov's disease, psychosis or syndrome see
Korsakoff's disease
Korsakow's disease, psychosis or syndrome
see Korsakoff's disease
Kostmann's disease or syndrome (infantile
genetic agranulocytosis) see Agranulocytosis
Kozhevnikov's epilepsy G40.109
|intractable G40.119
|with status epilepticus G40.111
|without status epilepticus G40.119
|not intractable G40.109
|with status epilepticus G40.101
|without status epilepticus G40.109
Krabbe's
|disease E75.23
|syndrome, congenital muscle hypoplasia
Q79.8
Kraepelin-Morel disease see Schizophrenia
Kraft-Weber-Dimitri disease Q85.8
Kraurosis
|ani K62.89
|penis N48.0
|vagina N89.8
|vulva N90.4
Kreotoxism A05.9
Krukenberg's
|spindle see Pigmentation, cornea, posterior
|tumor C79.6-
Kufs' disease E75.4
Kugelberg-Welander disease G12.1
Kuhnt-Junius degeneration see also
Degeneration, macula H35.32-
Kümmell's disease or spondylitis see
Spondylopathy, traumatic
Kupffer cell sarcoma C22.3
Kuru A81.81
Kussmaul's
|disease M30.0
|respiration E87.2
|in diabetic acidosis see Diabetes, by type,
with ketoacidosis
Kwashiorkor E40
|marasmic, marasmus type E42
Kyasanur Forest disease A98.2
Kyphoscoliosis, kyphoscoliotic (acquired) see
also Scoliosis M41.9
|congenital Q67.5
|heart (disease) I27.1
|sequelae of rickets E64.3
|tuberculous A18.01
Kyphosis, kyphotic (acquired) M40.209
|cervical region M40.202
|cervicothoracic region M40.203
|congenital Q76.419
|cervical region Q76.412
|cervicothoracic region Q76.413
|occipito-atlanto-axial region Q76.411
|thoracic region Q76.414
|thoracolumbar region Q76.415
|Morquio-Brailsford type (spinal) see also
subcategory M49.8 E76.219
|postlaminectomy M96.3
|postradiation therapy M96.2
|postural (adolescent) M40.00
|cervicothoracic region M40.03
|thoracic region M40.04
|thoracolumbar region M40.05
|secondary NEC M40.10
|cervical region M40.12

Kyphosis, kyphotic - continued
    |cervicothoracic region M40.13
    |thoracic region M40.14
    |thoracolumbar region M40.15
 |sequelae of rickets E64.3
 |specified type NEC M40.299
    |cervical region M40.292
    |cervicothoracic region M40.293
    |thoracic region M40.294
    |thoracolumbar region M40.295
 |syphilitic, congenital A50.56
 |thoracic region M40.204
 |thoracolumbar region M40.205
 |tuberculous A18.01
Kyrle disease L87.0

L

Labia, labium see condition
Labile
 |blood pressure R09.89
 |vasomotor system I73.9
Labioglossal paralysis G12.29
Labium leporinum see Cleft, lip
Labor see Delivery
Labored breathing see Hyperventilation
Labyrinthitis (circumscribed) (destructive)
  (diffuse) (inner ear) (latent) (purulent)
  (suppurative) see also subcategory H83.0
 |syphilitic A52.79
Laceration
 |with abortion see Abortion, by type,
   complicated by laceration of pelvic organs
 |abdomen, abdominal
   |wall S31.119
    |with
     |foreign body S31.129
     |penetration into peritoneal cavity
      S31.619
      |with foreign body S31.629
   |epigastric region S31.112
    |with
     |foreign body S31.122
     |penetration into peritoneal cavity
      S31.612
      |with foreign body S31.622
   |left
    |lower quadrant S31.114
     |with
      |foreign body S31.124
      |penetration into peritoneal cavity
       S31.614
       |with foreign body S31.624
    |upper quadrant S31.111
     |with
      |foreign body S31.121
      |penetration into peritoneal cavity
       S31.611
       |with foreign body S31.621
   |periumbilic region S31.115
    |with
     |foreign body S31.125
     |penetration into peritoneal cavity
      S31.615
      |with foreign body S31.625
   |right
    |lower quadrant S31.113
     |with
      |foreign body S31.123
      |penetration into peritoneal cavity
       S31.613
       |with foreign body S31.623
    |upper quadrant S31.110
     |with

Laceration - continued
      |foreign body S31.120
      |penetration into peritoneal cavity
       S31.610
       |with foreign body S31.620
 |accidental, complicating surgery see
   Complications, surgical, accidental
   puncture or laceration
 |Achilles tendon S86.02-
 |adrenal gland S37.813
 |alveolar (process) see Laceration, oral cavity
 |ankle S91.01-
   |with
    |foreign body S91.02-
 |antecubital space see Laceration, elbow
 |anus (sphincter) S31.831
   |with
    |ectopic or molar pregnancy O08.6
    |foreign body S31.832
   |complicating delivery see Delivery,
    complicated, by, laceration, anus
    (sphincter)
   |following ectopic or molar pregnancy O08.6
   |nontraumatic, nonpuerperal see Fissure,
    anus
 |arm (upper) S41.11-
   |with foreign body S41.12-
   |lower see Laceration, forearm
 |auditory canal (external) (meatus) see
   Laceration, ear
 |auricle, ear see Laceration, ear
 |axilla see Laceration, arm
 |back see also Laceration, thorax, back
   |lower S31.010
    |with
     |foreign body S31.020
      |with penetration into retroperitoneal
       space S31.021
     |penetration into retroperitoneal space
      S31.011
 |bile duct S36.13
 |bladder S37.23
   |with ectopic or molar pregnancy O08.6
   |following ectopic or molar pregnancy O08.6
   |obstetrical trauma O71.5
 |blood vessel see Injury, blood vessel
 |bowel see also Laceration, intestine
   |with ectopic or molar pregnancy O08.6
   |complicating abortion see Abortion, by type,
    complicated by, specified condition NEC
   |following ectopic or molar pregnancy O08.6
   |obstetrical trauma O71.5
 |brain (any part) (cortex) (diffuse) (membrane)
   see also Injury, intracranial, diffuse
   |during birth P10.8
    |with hemorrhage P10.1
   |focal see Injury, intracranial, focal brain
    injury
 |brainstem S06.38-
 |breast S21.01-
   |with foreign body S21.02-
 |broad ligament S37.893
   |with ectopic or molar pregnancy O08.6
   |following ectopic or molar pregnancy O08.6
   |laceration syndrome N83.8
   |obstetrical trauma O71.6
   |syndrome (laceration) N83.8
 |buttock S31.801
   |with foreign body S31.802
   |left S31.821
    |with foreign body S31.822
   |right S31.811
    |with foreign body S31.812
 |calf see Laceration, leg
 |canaliculus lacrimalis see Laceration, eyelid

Laceration - continued
 |canthus, eye see Laceration, eyelid
 |capsule, joint see Sprain
 |causing eversion of cervix uteri (old) N86
 |central (perineal), complicating delivery
   O70.9
 |cerebellum, traumatic S06.37-
 |cerebral S06.33-
   |left side S06.32-
   |during birth P10.8
    |with hemorrhage P10.1
   |right side S06.31-
 |cervix (uteri)
   |with ectopic or molar pregnancy O08.6
   |following ectopic or molar pregnancy O08.6
   |nonpuerperal, nontraumatic N88.1
   |obstetrical trauma (current) O71.3
   |old (postpartal) N88.1
   |traumatic S37.63
 |cheek (external) S01.41-
   |with foreign body S01.42-
   |internal see Laceration, oral cavity
 |chest wall see Laceration, thorax
 |chin see Laceration, head, specified site NEC
 |chordae tendinae NEC I51.1
   |concurrent with acute myocardial infarction
    see Infarct, myocardium
   |following acute myocardial infarction
    (current complication) I23.4
 |clitoris see Laceration, vulva
 |colon see Laceration, intestine, large, colon
 |common bile duct S36.13
 |cortex (cerebral) see Injury, intracranial,
   diffuse
 |costal region see Laceration, thorax
 |cystic duct S36.13
 |diaphragm S27.803
 |digit(s)
   |hand see Laceration, finger
   |foot see Laceration, toe
 |duodenum S36.430
 |ear (canal) (external) S01.31-
   |with foreign body S01.32-
   |drum S09.2-
 |elbow S51.01-
   |with
    |foreign body S51.02-
 |epididymis see Laceration, testis
 |epigastric region see Laceration, abdomen,
   wall, epigastric region
 |esophagus K22.89
   |traumatic
    |cervical S11.21
     |with foreign body S11.22
    |thoracic S27.813
 |eye (ball) S05.3-
   |with prolapse or loss of intraocular tissue
    S05.2-
   |penetrating S05.6-
 |eyebrow see Laceration, eyelid
 |eyelid S01.11-
   |with foreign body S01.12-
 |face NEC see Laceration, head, specified site
   NEC
 |fallopian tube S37.539
   |bilateral S37.532
   |unilateral S37.531
 |finger(s) S61.219
   |with
    |damage to nail S61.319
     |with
      |foreign body S61.329
    |foreign body S61.229
   |index S61.218
    |with

Laceration - *continued*
|damage to nail S61.318
　|with
　　|foreign body S61.328
　|foreign body S61.228
|left S61.211
　|with
　　|damage to nail S61.311
　　　|with
　　　　|foreign body S61.321
　　|foreign body S61.221
|right S61.210
　|with
　　|damage to nail S61.310
　　　|with
　　　　|foreign body S61.320
　　|foreign body S61.220
|little S61.218
　|with
　　|damage to nail S61.318
　　　|with
　　　　|foreign body S61.328
　　|foreign body S61.228
|left S61.217
　|with
　　|damage to nail S61.317
　　　|with
　　　　|foreign body S61.327
　　|foreign body S61.227
|right S61.216
　|with
　　|damage to nail S61.316
　　　|with
　　　　|foreign body S61.326
　　|foreign body S61.226
|middle S61.218
　|with
　　|damage to nail S61.318
　　　|with
　　　　|foreign body S61.328
　　|foreign body S61.228
|left S61.213
　|with
　　|damage to nail S61.313
　　　|with
　　　　|foreign body S61.323
　　|foreign body S61.223
|right S61.212
　|with
　　|damage to nail S61.312
　　　|with
　　　　|foreign body S61.322
　　|foreign body S61.222
|ring S61.218
　|with
　　|damage to nail S61.318
　　　|with
　　　　|foreign body S61.328
　　|foreign body S61.228
|left S61.215
　|with
　　|damage to nail S61.315
　　　|with
　　　　|foreign body S61.325
　　|foreign body S61.225
|right S61.214
　|with
　　|damage to nail S61.314
　　　|with
　　　　|foreign body S61.324
　　|foreign body S61.224
|flank S31.119
　|with foreign body S31.129
|foot (except toe(s) alone) S91.319
　|with foreign body S91.329

Laceration - *continued*
|left S91.312
　|with foreign body S91.322
|right S91.311
　|with foreign body S91.321
|toe *see* Laceration, toe
|forearm S51.819
　|with
　　|foreign body S51.829
　|elbow only *see* Laceration, elbow
　|left S51.812
　　|with
　　　|foreign body S51.822
　|right S51.811
　　|with
　　　|foreign body S51.821
|forehead S01.81
　|with foreign body S01.82
|fourchette O70.0
　|with ectopic or molar pregnancy O08.6
　|complicating delivery O70.0
　|following ectopic or molar pregnancy O08.6
|gallbladder S36.123
|genital organs, external
　|female S31.512
　　|with foreign body S31.522
　　|vagina *see* Laceration, vagina
　　|vulva *see* Laceration, vulva
　|male S31.511
　　|with foreign body S31.521
　　|penis *see* Laceration, penis
　　|scrotum *see* Laceration, scrotum
　　|testis *see* Laceration, testis
|groin *see* Laceration, abdomen, wall
|gum *see* Laceration, oral cavity
|hand S61.419
　|with
　　|foreign body S61.429
　|finger *see* Laceration, finger
　|left S61.412
　　|with
　　　|foreign body S61.422
　|right S61.411
　　|with
　　　|foreign body S61.421
　|thumb *see* Laceration, thumb
|head S01.91
　|with foreign body S01.92
　|cheek *see* Laceration, cheek
　|ear *see* Laceration, ear
　|eyelid *see* Laceration, eyelid
　|lip *see* Laceration, lip
　|nose *see* Laceration, nose
　|oral cavity *see* Laceration, oral cavity
　|scalp S01.01
　　|with foreign body S01.02
　|specified site NEC S01.81
　　|with foreign body S01.82
　|temporomandibular area *see* Laceration, cheek
|heart *see* Injury, heart, laceration
|heel *see* Laceration, foot
|hepatic duct S36.13
|hip S71.019
　|with foreign body S71.029
　|left S71.012
　　|with foreign body S71.022
　|right S71.011
　　|with foreign body S71.021
|hymen *see* Laceration, vagina
|hypochondrium *see* Laceration, abdomen, wall
|hypogastric region *see* Laceration, abdomen, wall

Laceration - *continued*
|ileum S36.438
|inguinal region *see* Laceration, abdomen, wall
|instep *see* Laceration, foot
|internal organ *see* Injury, by site
|interscapular region *see* Laceration, thorax, back
|intestine
　|large
　　|colon S36.539
　　　|ascending S36.530
　　　|descending S36.532
　　　|sigmoid S36.533
　　　|specified site NEC S36.538
　　|rectum S36.63
　　　|transverse S36.531
　|small S36.439
　　|duodenum S36.430
　　|specified site NEC S36.438
|intra-abdominal organ S36.93
　|intestine *see* Laceration, intestine
　|liver *see* Laceration, liver
　|pancreas *see* Laceration, pancreas
　|peritoneum S36.81
　|specified site NEC S36.893
　|spleen *see* Laceration, spleen
　|stomach *see* Laceration, stomach
|intracranial NEC *see also* Injury, intracranial, diffuse
　|birth injury P10.9
|jaw *see* Laceration, head, specified site NEC
|jejunum S36.438
|joint capsule *see* Sprain, by site
|kidney S37.03-
　|major (greater than 3 cm) (massive) (stellate) S37.06-
　|minor (less than 1 cm) S37.04-
　|moderate (1 to 3 cm) S37.05-
　　|multiple S37.06-
|knee S81.01-
　|with foreign body S81.02-
|labium (majus) (minus) *see* Laceration, vulva
|lacrimal duct *see* Laceration, eyelid
|large intestine *see* Laceration, intestine, large
|larynx S11.011
　|with foreign body S11.012
|leg (lower) S81.819
　|with foreign body S81.829
　|foot *see* Laceration, foot
　|knee *see* Laceration, knee
　|left S81.812
　　|with foreign body S81.822
　|right S81.811
　　|with foreign body S81.821
　|upper *see* Laceration, thigh
|ligament *see* Sprain
|lip S01.511
　|with foreign body S01.521
|liver S36.113
　|major (stellate) S36.116
　|minor S36.114
　|moderate S36.115
|loin *see* Laceration, abdomen, wall
|lower back *see* Laceration, back, lower
|lumbar region *see* Laceration, back, lower
|lung S27.339
　|bilateral S27.332
　|unilateral S27.331
|malar region *see* Laceration, head, specified site NEC
|mammary *see* Laceration, breast
|mastoid region *see* Laceration, head, specified site NEC
|meninges *see* Injury, intracranial, diffuse

Laceration - *continued*

|meniscus *see* Tear, meniscus
|mesentery S36.893
|mesosalpinx S37.893
|mouth *see* Laceration, oral cavity
|muscle *see* Injury, muscle, by site, laceration
|nail
  |finger *see* Laceration, finger, with damage
    to nail
  |toe *see* Laceration, toe, with damage to nail
|nasal (septum) (sinus) *see* Laceration, nose
|nasopharynx *see* Laceration, head, specified
  site NEC
|neck S11.91
  |with foreign body S11.92
  |involving
    |cervical esophagus S11.21
      |with foreign body S11.22
    |larynx *see* Laceration, larynx
    |pharynx *see* Laceration, pharynx
    |thyroid gland *see* Laceration, thyroid
      gland
    |trachea *see* Laceration, trachea
  |specified site NEC S11.81
    |with foreign body S11.82
|nerve *see* Injury, nerve
|nose (septum) (sinus) S01.21
  |with foreign body S01.22
|ocular NOS S05.3-
  |adnexa NOS S01.11-
|oral cavity S01.512
  |with foreign body S01.522
|orbit (eye) *see* Wound, open, ocular, orbit
|ovary S37.439
  |bilateral S37.432
  |unilateral S37.431
|palate *see* Laceration, oral cavity
|palm *see* Laceration, hand
|pancreas S36.239
  |body S36.231
    |major S36.261
    |minor S36.241
    |moderate S36.251
  |head S36.230
    |major S36.260
    |minor S36.240
    |moderate S36.250
  |major S36.269
  |minor S36.249
  |moderate S36.259
  |tail S36.232
    |major S36.262
    |minor S36.242
    |moderate S36.252
|pelvic S31.010
  |with
    |foreign body S31.020
      |penetration into retroperitoneal cavity
        S31.021
    |penetration into retroperitoneal cavity
      S31.011
  |floor *see also* Laceration, back, lower
    |with ectopic or molar pregnancy O08.6
    |complicating delivery O70.1
    |following ectopic or molar pregnancy
      O08.6
    |old (postpartal) N81.89
  |organ S37.93
    |with ectopic or molar pregnancy O08.6
    |adrenal gland S37.813
    |bladder S37.23
    |fallopian tube *see* Laceration, fallopian
      tube
    |following ectopic or molar pregnancy
      O08.6

Laceration - *continued*

  |kidney *see* Laceration, kidney
  |obstetrical trauma O71.5
  |ovary *see* Laceration, ovary
  |prostate S37.823
  |specified site NEC S37.893
  |ureter S37.13
  |urethra S37.33
  |uterus S37.63
|penis S31.21
  |with foreign body S31.22
|perineum
  |female S31.41
    |with
      |ectopic or molar pregnancy O08.6
      |foreign body S31.42
    |during delivery O70.9
      |first degree O70.0
      |fourth degree O70.3
      |second degree O70.1
      |third degree *see also* Delivery,
        complicated, by, laceration,
        perineum, third degree O70.20
    |old (postpartal) N81.89
    |postpartal N81.89
    |secondary (postpartal) O90.1
  |male S31.119
    |with foreign body S31.129
|periocular area (with or without lacrimal
  passages) *see* Laceration, eyelid
|peritoneum S36.893
|periumbilic region *see* Laceration, abdomen,
  wall, periumbilic
|periurethral tissue *see* Laceration, urethra
|phalanges
  |finger *see* Laceration, finger
  |toe *see* Laceration, toe
|pharynx S11.21
  |with foreign body S11.22
|pinna *see* Laceration, ear
|popliteal space *see* Laceration, knee
|prepuce *see* Laceration, penis
|prostate S37.823
|pubic region S31.119
  |with foreign body S31.129
|pudendum *see* Laceration, genital organs,
  external
|rectovaginal septum *see* Laceration, vagina
|rectum S36.63
|retroperitoneum S36.893
|round ligament S37.893
|sacral region *see* Laceration, back, lower
|sacroiliac region *see* Laceration, back, lower
|salivary gland *see* Laceration, oral cavity
|scalp S01.01
  |with foreign body S01.02
|scapular region *see* Laceration, shoulder
|scrotum S31.31
  |with foreign body S31.32
|seminal vesicle S37.893
|shin *see* Laceration, leg
|shoulder S41.019
  |with foreign body S41.029
  |left S41.012
    |with foreign body S41.022
  |right S41.011
    |with foreign body S41.021
|small intestine *see* Laceration, intestine, small
|spermatic cord *see* Laceration, testis
|spinal cord (meninges) *see also* Injury, spinal
  cord, by region

Laceration - *continued*

  |due to injury at birth P11.5
  |newborn (birth injury) P11.5
|spleen S36.039
  |major (massive) (stellate) S36.032
  |moderate S36.031
  |superficial (minor) S36.030
|sternal region *see* Laceration, thorax, front
|stomach S36.33
|submaxillary region *see* Laceration, head,
  specified site NEC
|submental region *see* Laceration, head,
  specified site NEC
|subungual
  |finger(s) *see* Laceration, finger, with
    damage to nail
  |toe(s) *see* Laceration, toe, with damage to
    nail
|suprarenal gland *see* Laceration, adrenal gland
|temple, temporal region *see* Laceration, head,
  specified site NEC
|temporomandibular area *see* Laceration, cheek
|tendon *see* Injury, muscle, by site, laceration
  |Achilles S86.02-
|tentorium cerebelli *see* Injury, intracranial,
  diffuse
|testis S31.31
  |with foreign body S31.32
|thigh S71.11-
  |with foreign body S71.12-
|thorax, thoracic (wall) S21.91
  |with foreign body S21.92
    |back S21.22-
      |with penetration into thoracic cavity
        S21.42-
    |front S21.12-
      |with penetration into thoracic cavity
        S21.32-
  |back S21.21-
    |with
      |foreign body S21.22-
        |with penetration into thoracic cavity
          S21.42-
      |penetration into thoracic cavity S21.41-
  |breast *see* Laceration, breast
  |front S21.11-
    |with
      |foreign body S21.12-
        |with penetration into thoracic cavity
          S21.32-
      |penetration into thoracic cavity S21.31-
|thumb S61.019
  |with
    |damage to nail S61.119
      |with
        |foreign body S61.129
    |foreign body S61.029
  |left S61.012
    |with
      |damage to nail S61.112
        |with
          |foreign body S61.122
      |foreign body S61.022
  |right S61.011
    |with
      |damage to nail S61.111
        |with
          |foreign body S61.121
      |foreign body S61.021
|thyroid gland S11.11
  |with foreign body S11.12
|toe(s) S91.119

Laceration - *continued*
| with
| | damage to nail S91.219
| | | with
| | | | foreign body S91.229
| | | foreign body S91.129
| | great S91.113
| | | with
| | | | damage to nail S91.213
| | | | | with
| | | | | | foreign body S91.223
| | | | | foreign body S91.123
| | | | left S91.112
| | | | | with
| | | | | | damage to nail S91.212
| | | | | | | with
| | | | | | | | foreign body S91.222
| | | | | | foreign body S91.122
| | | | right S91.111
| | | | | with
| | | | | | damage to nail S91.211
| | | | | | | with
| | | | | | | | foreign body S91.221
| | | | | | foreign body S91.121
| | lesser S91.116
| | | with
| | | | damage to nail S91.216
| | | | | with
| | | | | | foreign body S91.226
| | | | foreign body S91.126
| | | left S91.115
| | | | with
| | | | | damage to nail S91.215
| | | | | | with
| | | | | | | foreign body S91.225
| | | | | foreign body S91.125
| | | right S91.114
| | | | with
| | | | | damage to nail S91.214
| | | | | | with
| | | | | | | foreign body S91.224
| | | | | foreign body S91.124
| tongue *see* Laceration, oral cavity trachea
| | S11.021
| | with foreign body S11.022
| tunica vaginalis *see* Laceration, testis
| tympanum, tympanic membrane *see*
| | Laceration, ear, drum
| umbilical region S31.115
| | with foreign body S31.125
| ureter S37.13
| urethra S37.33
| | with or following ectopic or molar
| | | pregnancy O08.6
| | obstetrical trauma O71.5
| urinary organ NEC S37.893
| uterus S37.63
| | with ectopic or molar pregnancy O08.6
| | following ectopic or molar pregnancy O08.6
| | nonpuerperal, nontraumatic N85.8
| | obstetrical trauma NEC O71.81
| | old (postpartal) N85.8
| uvula *see* Laceration, oral cavity
| vagina S31.41
| | with
| | | ectopic or molar pregnancy O08.6
| | | foreign body S31.42
| | during delivery O71.4
| | | with perineal laceration *see* Laceration,
| | perineum, female, during delivery
| | following ectopic or molar pregnancy O08.6
| | nonpuerperal, nontraumatic N89.8

Laceration - *continued*
| old (postpartal) N89.8
| vas deferens S37.893
| vesical *see* Laceration, bladder
| vocal cords S11.031
| | with foreign body S11.032
| vulva S31.41
| | with
| | | ectopic or molar pregnancy O08.6
| | | foreign body S31.42
| | complicating delivery O70.0
| | following ectopic or molar pregnancy O08.6
| | nonpuerperal, nontraumatic N90.89
| | old (postpartal) N90.89
| wrist S61.519
| | with
| | | foreign body S61.529
| | left S61.512
| | | with
| | | | foreign body S61.522
| | right S61.511
| | | with
| | | | foreign body S61.521

Lack of
| achievement in school Z55.3
| adequate
| | food Z59.48
| | intermaxillary vertical dimension of fully
| | | erupted teeth M26.36
| | sleep Z72.820
| appetite (*see* Anorexia) R63.0
| awareness R41.9
| care
| | in home Z74.2
| | of infant (at or after birth) T76.02
| | | confirmed T74.02
| cognitive functions R41.9
| coordination R27.9
| | ataxia R27.0
| | specified type NEC R27.8
| development (physiological) R62.50
| | failure to thrive (child over 28 days old)
| | | R62.51
| | adult R62.7
| | newborn P92.6
| | short stature R62.52
| | specified type NEC R62.59
| energy R53.83
| financial resources Z59.6
| food Z59.48
| growth R62.52
| heating Z59.1
| housing (permanent) (temporary) Z59.00
| | adequate Z59.1
| learning experiences in childhood Z62.898
| leisure time (affecting life-style) Z73.2
| material resources Z59.9
| memory *see also* Amnesia
| | mild, following organic brain damage F06.8
| ovulation N97.0
| parental supervision or control of child Z62.0
| person able to render necessary care Z74.2
| physical exercise Z72.3
| play experience in childhood Z62.898
| posterior occlusal support M26.57
| relaxation (affecting life-style) Z73.2
| safe drinking water Z58.6
| sexual
| | desire F52.0
| | enjoyment F52.1
| shelter Z59.02
| sleep (adequate) Z72.820
| supervision of child by parent Z62.0
| support, posterior occlusal M26.57
| water T73.1
| | safe drinking Z58.6

Lacrimal *see* condition
Lacrimation, abnormal *see* Epiphora
Lacrimonasal duct *see* condition
Lactation, lactating (breast) (puerperal,
postpartum)
| associated
| | cracked nipple O92.13
| | retracted nipple O92.03
| defective O92.4
Lactation
| disorder NEC O92.79
| excessive O92.6
| failed (complete) O92.3
| | partial O92.4
| mastitis NEC *see* Mastitis, obstetric
| mother (care and/or examination) Z39.1
| nonpuerperal N64.3
Lacticemia, excessive E87.2
Lacunar skull Q75.8
Laennec's cirrhosis K70.30
| with ascites K70.31
| nonalcoholic K74.69
Lafora's disease *see* Epilepsy, generalized,
idiopathic
Lag, lid (nervous) *see* Retraction, lid
Lagophthalmos (eyelid) (nervous) H02.209
| bilateral, upper and lower eyelids H02.20C
| cicatricial H02.219
| | bilateral, upper and lower eyelids H02.21C
| | left H02.216
| | | lower H02.215
| | | upper H02.214
| | | upper and lower eyelids H02.21B
| | right H02.213
| | | lower H02.212
| | | upper H02.211
| | | upper and lower eyelids H02.21A
| keratoconjunctivitis *see* Keratoconjunctivitis
| left H02.206
| | lower H02.205
| | upper H02.204
| | upper and lower eyelids H02.20B
| mechanical H02.229
| | bilateral, upper and lower eyelids H02.22C
| | left H02.226
| | | lower H02.225
| | | upper H02.224
| | | upper and lower eyelids H02.22B
| | right H02.223
| | | lower H02.222
| | | upper H02.221
| | | upper and lower eyelids H02.22B
| paralytic H02.239
| | bilateral, upper and lower eyelids H02.23C
| | left H02.236
| | | lower H02.235
| | | upper H02.234
| | | upper and lower eyelids H02.23B
| | right H02.233
| | | lower H02.232
| | | upper H02.231
| | | upper and lower eyelids H02.23A
| right H02.203
| | lower H02.202
| | upper H02.201
| | upper and lower eyelids H02.20A
Laki-Lorand factor deficiency *see* Defect,
coagulation, specified type NEC
Lalling F80.0
Lambert-Eaton syndrome *see* Syndrome,
Lambert-Eaton
Lambliasis, lambliosis A07.1
Landau-Kleffner syndrome *see* Epilepsy,
specified NEC

Landouzy-Déjérine dystrophy or
facioscapulohumeral atrophy G71.02
Landouzy's disease (icterohemorrhagic
leptospirosis) A27.0
Landry-Guillain-Barré, syndrome or
paralysis G61.0
Landry's disease or paralysis G61.0
Lane's
|band Q43.3
|kink *see* Obstruction, intestine
|syndrome K90.2
Langdon Down syndrome *see* Trisomy, 21
Lapsed immunization schedule status Z28.3
Large
|baby (regardless of gestational age) (4000g to
    4499g) P08.1
|ear, congenital Q17.1
|physiological cup Q14.2
|stature R68.89
Large-For-Dates NEC (infant) (4000g to
4499g) P08.1
|affecting management of pregnancy O36.6-
|exceptionally (4500g or more) P08.0
Larsen-Johansson disease or osteochondrosis
see Osteochondrosis, juvenile, patella
Larsen's syndrome (flattened facies and
multiple congenital dislocations) Q74.8
Larva migrans
|cutaneous B76.9
    |Ancylostoma B76.0
|visceral B83.0
Laryngeal *see* condition
Laryngismus (stridulus) J38.5
|congenital P28.89
|diphtheritic A36.2
Laryngitis (acute) (edematous) (fibrinous)
(infective) (infiltrative) (malignant)
(membranous) (phlegmonous)
(pneumococcal) (pseudomembranous)
(septic) (subglottic) (suppurative)
(ulcerative) J04.0
|with
    |influenza, flu, or grippe *see* Influenza, with,
        laryngitis
    |tracheitis (acute) *see* Laryngotracheitis
|atrophic J37.0
|catarrhal J37.0
|chronic J37.0
    |with tracheitis (chronic) J37.1
|diphtheritic A36.2
|due to external agent *see* Inflammation,
    respiratory, upper, due to
|Hemophilus influenzae J04.0
|H. influenzae J04.0
|hypertrophic J37.0
|influenzal *see* Influenza, with, respiratory
    manifestations NEC
|obstructive J05.0
|sicca J37.0
|spasmodic J05.0
    |acute J04.0
|streptococcal J04.0
|stridulous J05.0
|syphilitic (late) A52.73
    |congenital A50.59 [*J99*]
        |early A50.03 [*J99*]
|tuberculous A15.5
|Vincent's A69.1
Laryngocele (congenital) (ventricular) Q31.3
Laryngofissure J38.7
|congenital Q31.8
Laryngomalacia (congenital) Q31.5
Laryngopharyngitis (acute) J06.0
|chronic J37.0
|due to external agent *see* Inflammation,
    respiratory, upper, due to
Laryngoplegia J38.00
|bilateral J38.02
|unilateral J38.01

Laryngoptosis J38.7
Laryngospasm J38.5
Laryngostenosis J38.6
Laryngotracheitis (acute) (Infectional)
(infective) (viral) J04.2
|atrophic J37.1
|catarrhal J37.1
|chronic J37.1
|diphtheritic A36.2
|due to external agent *see* Inflammation,
    respiratory, upper, due to
|Hemophilus influenzae J04.2
|hypertrophic J37.1
|influenzal *see* Influenza, with, respiratory
    manifestations NEC
|pachydermic J38.7
|sicca J37.1
|spasmodic J38.5
    |acute J05.0
|streptococcal J04.2
|stridulous J38.5
|syphilitic (late) A52.73
    |congenital A50.59 [*J99*]
        |early A50.03 [*J99*]
|tuberculous A15.5
|Vincent's A69.1
Laryngotracheobronchitis *see* Bronchitis
Larynx, laryngeal *see* condition
Lassa fever A96.2
Lassitude *see* Weakness
Late
|talker R62.0
|walker R62.0
Late effect(s) *see* Sequelae
Latent *see* condition
Laterocession *see* Lateroversion
Lateroflexion *see* Lateroversion
Lateroversion
|cervix *see* Lateroversion, uterus
|uterus, uterine (cervix) (postinfectional)
    (postpartal, old) N85.4
    |congenital Q51.818
    |in pregnancy or childbirth O34.59-
Lathyrism *see* Poisoning, food, noxious, plant
Launois' syndrome (pituitary gigantism)
E22.0
Launois-Bensaude adenolipomatosis E88.89
Laurence-Moon (-Bardet) -Biedl syndrome
Q87.89
Lax, laxity *see also* Relaxation
|ligament (ous) *see also* Disorder, ligament
    |familial M35.7
    |knee *see* Derangement, knee
|skin (acquired) L57.4
    |congenital Q82.8
Laxative habit F55.2
Lazy leukocyte syndrome D70.8
Lead miner's lung J63.6
Leak, leakage
|air NEC J93.82
    |postprocedural J95.812
|amniotic fluid *see* Rupture, membranes,
    premature
|blood (microscopic), fetal, into maternal
    circulation affecting management of
    pregnancy *see* Pregnancy, complicated by
|cerebrospinal fluid G96.00
    |cranial
        |postoperative G96.08
        |specified NEC G96.08
        |spontaneous G96.01
        |traumatic G96.08
    |spinal
        |postoperative G96.09
        |post-traumatic G96.09
        |specified NEC G96.09

Leak, leakage - *continued*
    |spontaneous G96.02
    |spontaneous
        |from
            |skull base G96.01
            |spine G96.02
    |from spinal (lumbar) puncture G97.0
|CSF *see* Leak, cerebrospinal fluid
|device, implant or graft *see also*
    Complications, by site and type,
    mechanical
    |arterial graft NEC *see* Complication,
        cardiovascular device, mechanical,
        vascular
    |breast (implant) T85.43
    |catheter NEC T85.638
        |urinary T83.038
            |cystostomy T83.030
            |Hopkins T83.038
            |ileostomy T83.038
            |indwelling T83.031
            |nephrostomy T83.032
            |specified NEC T83.038
            |urostomy T83.038
    |dialysis (renal) T82.43
        |intraperitoneal T85.631
    |infusion NEC T82.534
        |spinal (epidural) (subdural) T85.630
    |gastrointestinal *see* Complications,
        prosthetic device, mechanical,
        gastrointestinal device
    |genital NEC T83.498
        |penile prosthesis (cylinder) (implanted)
            (pump) (reservoir) T83.490
        |testicular prosthesis T83.491
    |heart NEC *see* Complication, cardiovascular
        device, mechanical
    |joint prosthesis *see* Complications, joint
        prosthesis, mechanical, specified NEC, by
        site
    |ocular NEC *see* Complications, prosthetic
        device, mechanical, ocular device
    |orthopedic NEC *see* Complication,
        orthopedic, device, mechanical
    |persistent air J93.82
    |specified NEC T85.638
    |urinary NEC *see also* Complication,
        genitourinary, device, urinary, mechanical
        |graft T83.23
    |vascular NEC *see* Complication,
        cardiovascular device, mechanical
    |ventricular intracranial shunt T85.03
|urine *see* Incontinence
Leaky heart *see* Endocarditis
Learning defect (specific) F81.9
Leather bottle stomach C16.9
Leber's
|congenital amaurosis H35.50
|optic atrophy (hereditary) H47.22
Lederer's anemia D59.19
Leeches (external) *see* Hirudiniasis
Leg *see* condition
Legg (-Calvé) -Perthes disease, syndrome or
osteochondrosis M91.1-
Legionellosis A48.1
|nonpneumonic A48.2
Legionnaires'
|disease A48.1
    |nonpneumonic A48.2
|pneumonia A48.1
Leigh's disease G31.82
Leiner's disease L21.1
Leiofibromyoma *see* Leiomyoma
Leiomyoblastoma *see* Neoplasm, connective
tissue, benign

Leiomyofibroma *see also* Neoplasm, connective
 tissue, benign
 |uterus (cervix) (corpus) D25.9
Leiomyoma *see also* Neoplasm, connective
 tissue, benign
 |bizarre *see* Neoplasm, connective tissue,
  benign
 |cellular *see* Neoplasm, connective tissue,
  benign
 |epithelioid *see* Neoplasm, connective tissue,
  benign
 |uterus (cervix) (corpus) D25.9
  |intramural D25.1
  |submucous D25.0
  |subserosal D25.2
 |vascular *see* Neoplasm, connective tissue,
  benign
Leiomyoma, leiomyomatosis (intravascular)
 see Neoplasm, connective tissue, uncertain
 behavior
Leiomyosarcoma *see also* Neoplasm,
 connective tissue, malignant
 |epithelioid *see* Neoplasm, connective tissue,
  malignant
 |myxoid *see* Neoplasm, connective tissue,
  malignant
Leishmaniasis B55.9
 |American (mucocutaneous) B55.2
  |cutaneous B55.1
 |Asian Desert B55.1
 |Brazilian B55.2
 |cutaneous (any type) B55.1
 |dermal *see also* Leishmaniasis, cutaneous
  |post-Kala-Azar B55.0
 |eyelid B55.1
 |infantile B55.0
 |Mediterranean B55.0
 |mucocutaneous (American) (New World)
  B55.2
 |naso-oral B55.2
 |nasopharyngeal B55.2
 |old world B55.1
 |tegumentaria diffusa B55.1
 |visceral B55.0
Leishmanoid, dermal *see also* Leishmaniasis,
 cutaneous
 |post-Kala-Azar B55.0
Lenegre's disease I44.2
Lengthening, leg *see* Deformity, limb, unequal
 length
Lennert's lymphoma *see* Lymphoma, Lennert's
Lennox-Gastaut syndrome G40.812
 |intractable G40.814
  |with status epilepticus G40.813
  |without status epilepticus G40.814
 |not intractable G40.812
  |with status epilepticus G40.811
  |without status epilepticus G40.812
Lens *see* condition
Lenticonus (anterior) (posterior) (congenital)
 Q12.8
Lenticular degeneration, progressive E83.01
Lentiglobus (posterior) (congenital) Q12.8
Lentigo (congenital) L81.4
 |maligna *see also* Melanoma, in situ
  |melanoma *see* Melanoma
Lentivirus, as cause of disease classified
 elsewhere B97.31
Leontiasis
 |ossium M85.2
 |syphilitic (late) A52.78
  |congenital A50.59
Lepothrix A48.8
Lepra *see* Leprosy
Leprechaunism E34.8

Leprosy A30.-
 |with muscle disorder A30.9 *[M63.80]*
  |ankle A30.9 *[M63.87]*
  |foot A30.9 *[M63.87]*
  |forearm A30.9 *[M63.83]*
  |hand A30.9 *[M63.84]*
  |lower leg A30.9 *[M63.86]*
  |multiple sites A30.9 *[M63.89]*
  |pelvic region A30.9 *[M63.85]*
  |shoulder region A30.9 *[M63.81]*
  |specified site NEC A30.9 *[M63.88]*
  |thigh A30.9 *[M63.85]*
  |upper arm A30.9 *[M63.82]*
 |anesthetic A30.9
 |BB A30.3
 |BL A30.4
 |borderline (infiltrated) (neuritic) A30.3
  |lepromatous A30.4
  |tuberculoid A30.2
 |BT A30.2
 |dimorphous (infiltrated) (neuritic) A30.3
 |I A30.0
 |indeterminate (macular) (neuritic) A30.0
 |lepromatous (diffuse) (infiltrated) (macular)
  (neuritic) (nodular) A30.5
 |LL A30.5
 |macular (early) (neuritic) (simple) A30.9
 |maculoanesthetic A30.9
 |mixed A30.3
 |neural A30.9
 |nodular A30.5
 |primary neuritic A30.3
 |specified type NEC A30.8
 |TT A30.1
 |tuberculoid (major) (minor) A30.1
Leptocytosis, hereditary D56.9
Leptomeningitis (chronic) (circumscribed)
 (hemorrhagic) (nonsuppurative) *see*
 Meningitis
Leptomeningopathy G96.198
Leptospiral *see* condition
Leptospirochetal *see* condition **Leptospirosis**
 A27.9
 |canicola A27.89
 |due to Leptospira interrogans serovar
  icterohaemorrhagiae A27.0
 |icterohemorrhagica A27.0
 |pomona A27.89
 |Weil's disease A27.0
Leptus dermatitis B88.0
Leriche's syndrome (aortic bifurcation
 occlusion) I74.09
Leri's pleonosteosis Q78.8
Leri-Weill syndrome Q77.8
Lermoyez' syndrome *see* Vertigo, peripheral
 NEC
Lesch Nyhan syndrome E79.1
Leser-Trélat disease L82.1
 |inflamed L82.0
Lesion(s) (nontraumatic)
 |abducens nerve *see* Strabismus, paralytic,
  sixth nerve
 |alveolar process K08.9
 |angiocentric immunoproliferative D47.Z9
 |anorectal K62.9
 |aortic (valve) I35.9
 |auditory nerve *see* subcategory H93.3
 |basal ganglion G25.9
 |bile duct *see* Disease, bile duct
 |biomechanical M99.9
  |specified type NEC M99.89
   |abdomen M99.89
   |acromioclavicular M99.87
   |cervical region M99.81
   |cervicothoracic M99.81

Lesion(s) (nontraumatic) - *continued*
 |costochondral M99.88
 |costovertebral M99.88
 |head region M99.80
 |hip M99.85
 |lower extremity M99.86
 |lumbar region M99.83
 |lumbosacral M99.83
 |occipitocervical M99.80
 |pelvic region M99.85
 |pubic M99.85
 |rib cage M99.88
 |sacral region M99.84
 |sacrococcygeal M99.84
 |sacroiliac M99.84
 |specified NEC M99.89
 |sternochondral M99.88
 |sternoclavicular M99.87
 |thoracic region M99.82
 |thoracolumbar M99.82
 |upper extremity M99.87
|bladder N32.9
|bone *see* Disorder, bone
|brachial plexus G54.0
|brain G93.9
 |congenital Q04.9
 |vascular I67.9
  |degenerative I67.9
  |hypertensive I67.4
|buccal cavity K13.79
|calcified *see* Calcification
|canthus *see* Disorder, eyelid
|carate *see* Pinta, lesions
|cardia K31.9
|cardiac *see also* Disease, heart I51.9
 |congenital Q24.9
 |valvular *see* Endocarditis
|cauda equina G83.4
|cecum K63.9
|cerebral *see* Lesion, brain
|cerebrovascular I67.9
 |degenerative I67.9
 |hypertensive I67.4
|cervical (nerve) root NEC G54.2
|chiasmal *see* Disorder, optic, chiasm
|chorda tympani G51.8
|coin, lung R91.1
|colon K63.9
|combined periodontic
 endodontic K05.5
|congenital *see* Anomaly, by site
|conjunctiva H11.9
|conus medullaris *see* Injury, conus medullaris
|coronary artery *see* Ischemia, heart
|cranial nerve G52.9
 |eighth *see* Disorder, ear
 |eleventh G52.9
 |fifth G50.9
 |first G52.0
 |fourth *see* Strabismus, paralytic, fourth
  nerve
 |seventh G51.9
 |sixth *see* Strabismus, paralytic, sixth nerve
 |tenth G52.2
 |twelfth G52.3
|cystic *see* Cyst
|degenerative *see* Degeneration
|duodenum K31.9
|edentulous (alveolar) ridge, associated with
 trauma, due to traumatic occlusion K06.2
|en coup de sabre L94.1
|eyelid *see* Disorder, eyelid
|gasserian ganglion G50.8
|gastric K31.9
|gastroduodenal K31.9

Lesion(s) (nontraumatic) - *continued*
- gastrointestinal K63.9
- gingiva, associated with trauma K06.2
- glomerular
  - focal and segmental *see also* N00-N07 with fourth character .1 N05.1
  - minimal change *see also* N00-N07 with fourth character .0 N05.0
- heart (organic) *see* Disease, heart
- hyperchromic, due to pinta (carate) A67.1
- hyperkeratotic *see* Hyperkeratosis
- hypothalamic E23.7
- ileocecal K63.9
- ileum K63.9
- iliohypogastric nerve G57.8-
- inflammatory *see* Inflammation
- intestine K63.9
- intracerebral *see* Lesion, brain
- intrachiasmal (optic) *see* Disorder, optic, chiasm
- intracranial, space-occupying R90.0
- joint *see* Disorder, joint
  - sacroiliac (old) M53.3
- keratotic *see* Keratosis
- kidney *see* Disease, renal
- laryngeal nerve (recurrent) G52.2
- lip K13.0
- liver K76.9
- lumbosacral
  - plexus G54.1
  - root (nerve) NEC G54.4
- lung (coin) R91.1
- maxillary sinus J32.0
- mitral I05.9
- Morel-Lavallée *see* Hematoma, by site
- motor cortex NEC G93.89
- mouth K13.79
- nerve G58.9
  - femoral G57.2-
  - median G56.1-
    - carpal tunnel syndrome *see* Syndrome, carpal tunnel
  - plantar G57.6-
  - popliteal (lateral) G57.3-
    - medial G57.4-
  - radial G56.3-
  - sciatic G57.0-
  - spinal *see* Injury, nerve, spinal
  - ulnar G56.2-
- nervous system, congenital Q07.9
- nonallopathic *see* Lesion, biomechanical
- nose (internal) J34.89
- obstructive *see* Obstruction
- obturator nerve G57.8-
- oral mucosa K13.70
- organ or site NEC *see* Disease, by site
- osteolytic *see* Osteolysis
- peptic K27.9
- periodontal, due to traumatic occlusion K05.5
- pharynx J39.2
- pigment, pigmented (skin) L81.9
- pinta *see* Pinta, lesions
- polypoid *see* Polyp
- prechiasmal (optic) *see* Disorder, optic, chiasm
- primary *see also* Syphilis, primary A51.0
  - carate A67.0
  - pinta A67.0
  - yaws A66.0
- pulmonary J98.4
  - valve I37.9
- pylorus K31.9
- rectosigmoid K63.9
- retina, retinal H35.9
- sacroiliac (joint) (old) M53.3

Lesion(s) (nontraumatic) - *continued*
- salivary gland K11.9
  - benign lymphoepithelial K11.8
- saphenous nerve G57.8-
- sciatic nerve G57.0-
- secondary *see* Syphilis, secondary
- shoulder (region) M75.9-
  - specified NEC M75.8-
- sigmoid K63.9
- sinus (accessory) (nasal) J34.89
- skin L98.9
  - suppurative L08.0
- SLAP S43.43-
- spinal cord G95.9
  - congenital Q06.9
- spleen D73.89
- stomach K31.9
- superior glenoid labrum S43.43-
- syphilitic *see* Syphilis
- tertiary *see* Syphilis, tertiary
- thoracic root (nerve) NEC G54.3
- tonsillar fossa J35.9
- tooth, teeth K08.9
  - white spot
    - chewing surface K02.51
    - pit and fissure surface K02.51
    - smooth surface K02.61
- traumatic *see* specific type of injury by site
- tricuspid (valve) I07.9
  - nonrheumatic I36.9
- trigeminal nerve G50.9
- ulcerated or ulcerative *see* Ulcer, skin
- uterus N85.9
- vagina N89.8
- vagus nerve G52.2
- valvular *see* Endocarditis
- vascular I99.9
  - affecting central nervous system I67.9
  - following trauma NEC T14.8
  - umbilical cord, complicating delivery O69.5
- vulva N90.89
- warty *see* Verruca
- white spot (tooth)
  - chewing surface K02.51
  - pit and fissure surface K02.51
  - smooth surface K02.61

Less than a high school diploma Z55.5
Lethargic *see* condition
Lethargy R53.83
Letterer-Siwe's disease C96.0
Leukemia, leukemic C95.9-
- acute basophilic C94.8-
- acute bilineal C95.0-
- acute erythroid C94.0-
- acute lymphoblastic C91.0-
- acute megakaryoblastic C94.2-
- acute megakaryocytic C94.2-
- acute mixed lineage C95.0-
- acute monoblastic (monoblastic/monocytic) C93.0-
- acute monocytic (monoblastic/monocytic) C93.0-
- acute myeloblastic (minimal differentiation) (with maturation) C92.0-
- acute myeloid, NOS C92.0-
  - with
    - 11q23-abnormality C92.6-
    - dysplasia of remaining hematopoesis and/or myelodysplastic disease in its history C92.A-
    - multilineage dysplasia C92.A-
    - variation of MLL-gene C92.6-
  - M6 (a)(b) C94.0-
  - M7 C94.2-
- acute myelomonocytic C92.5-
- acute promyelocytic C92.4-

Leukemia, leukemic - *continued*
- adult T-cell (HTLV 1-associated) (acute variant) (chronic variant) (lymphomatoid variant) (smouldering variant) C91.5-
- aggressive NK-cell C94.8-
- AML (1/ETO) (M0) (M1) (M2) (without a FAB classification) C92.0-
- AML M3 C92.4-
- AML M4 (EO with inv(16) or t(16;16)) C92.5-
- AML M5 C93.0-
- AML M5a C93.0-
- AML M5b C93.0-
- AML Me with t (15;17) and variants C92.4-
- atypical chronic myeloid, BCR/ABL-negative C92.2-
- biphenotypic acute C95.0-
- blast cell C95.0-
- Burkitt-type, mature B-cell C91.A-
- chronic eosinophilic (*see also* Syndrome, hypereosinophilic, myeloid) C94.8-
- chronic lymphocytic, of B-cell type C91.1-
- chronic monocytic C93.1-
- chronic myelogenous (Philadelphia chromosome (Ph1) positive) (t(9;22)) (q34;q11) (with crisis of blast cells) C92.1-
- chronic myeloid, BCR/ABL-Positive C92.1-
  - atypical, BCR/ABL-negative C92.2-
- chronic myelomonocytic C93.1-
- chronic neutrophilic D47.1
- CMML (1) (2) (with eosinophilia) C93.1-
- granulocytic *see also* Category C92 C92.9-
- hairy cell C91.4-
- juvenile myelomonocytic C93.3-
- lymphoid C91.9-
  - specified NEC C91.Z
- mast cell C94.3-
- mature B-cell, Burkitt-type C91.A
- monocytic (subacute) C93.9-
  - specified NEC C93.Z-
- myelogenous *see also* Category C92 C92.9-
- myeloid C92.9-
  - specified NEC C92.Z
- plasma cell C90.1-
- plasmacytic C90.1-
- prolymphocytic
  - of B-cell type C91.3-
  - of T-cell type C91.6-
- specified NEC C94.8-
- stem cell, of unclear lineage C95.0-
- subacute lymphocytic C91.9-
- T-cell large granular lymphocytic C91.Z
- unspecified cell type C95.9-
  - acute C95.0-
  - chronic C95.1-

Leukemoid reaction *see also* Reaction, leukemoid D72.823-
Leukoaraiosis (hypertensive) I67.81
Leukoariosis *see* Leukoaraiosis
Leukocoria *see* Disorder, globe, degenerated condition, leucocoria
Leukocytopenia D72.819
Leukocytosis D72.829
- eosinophilic D72.19
Leukoderma, leukodermia NEC L81.5
- syphilitic A51.39
  - late A52.79
Leukodystrophy E75.29
Leukoedema, oral epithelium K13.29
Leukoencephalitis G04.81
- acute (subacute) hemorrhagic G36.1
  - postimmunization or postvaccinal G04.02
- postinfectious G04.01
- subacute sclerosing A81.1
- van Bogaert's (sclerosing) A81.1

Leukoencephalopathy *see also* Encephalopathy G93.49
| Binswanger's I67.3
| heroin vapor G92.8
| metachromatic E75.25
| multifocal (progressive) A81.2
| postimmunization and postvaccinal G04.02
| progressive multifocal A81.2
| reversible, posterior G93.6
| van Bogaert's (sclerosing) A81.1
| vascular, progressive I67.3
Leukoerythroblastosis D75.9
Leukokeratosis *see also* Leukoplakia
| mouth K13.21
| nicotina palati K13.24
| oral mucosa K13.21
| tongue K13.21
| vocal cord J38.3
Leukokraurosis vulva (e) N90.4
Leukoma (cornea) *see also* Opacity, cornea
| adherent H17.0-
| interfering with central vision *see* Opacity, cornea, central
Leukomalacia, cerebral, newborn P91.2
| periventricular P91.2
Leukomelanopathy, hereditary D72.0
Leukonychia (punctata) (striata) L60.8
| congenital Q84.4
Leukopathia unguium L60.8
| congenital Q84.4
Leukopenia D72.819
| basophilic D72.818
| chemotherapy (cancer) induced D70.1
| congenital D70.0
| cyclic D70.0
| drug induced NEC D70.2
|| due to cytoreductive cancer chemotherapy D70.1
| eosinophilic D72.818
| familial D70.0
| infantile genetic D70.0
| malignant D70.9
| periodic D70.0
| transitory neonatal P61.5
Leukopenic *see* condition
Leukoplakia
| anus K62.89
| bladder (postinfectional) N32.89
| buccal K13.21
| cervix (uteri) N88.0
| esophagus K22.89
| gingiva K13.21
| hairy (oral mucosa) (tongue) K13.3
| kidney (pelvis) N28.89
| larynx J38.7
| lip K13.21
| mouth K13.21
| oral epithelium, including tongue (mucosa) K13.21
| palate K13.21
| pelvis (kidney) N28.89
| penis (infectional) N48.0
| rectum K62.89
| syphilitic (late) A52.79
| tongue K13.21
| ureter (postinfectional) N28.89
| urethra (postinfectional) N36.8
| uterus N85.8
| vagina N89.4
| vocal cord J38.3
| vulva N90.4
Leukorrhea N89.8
| due to Trichomonas (vaginalis) A59.00
| trichomonal A59.00
Leukosarcoma C85.9-

Levocardia (isolated) Q24.1
| with situs inversus Q89.3
Levotransposition Q20.5
Lev's disease or syndrome (acquired complete heart block) I44.2
Levulosuria *see* Fructosuria
Levurid L30.2
Lewy body (ies) (dementia) (disease) G31.83
Leyden-Moebius dystrophy G71.09
Leydig cell
| carcinoma
|| specified site *see* Neoplasm, malignant, by site
|| unspecified site
||| female C56.9
||| male C62.9-
| tumor
|| benign
||| specified site *see* Neoplasm, benign, by site
||| unspecified site
|||| female D27.-
|||| male D29.2-
|| malignant
||| specified site *see* Neoplasm, malignant, by site
||| unspecified site
|||| female C56.-
|||| male C62.9-
|| specified site *see* Neoplasm, uncertain behavior, by site
|| unspecified site
||| female D39.1-
||| male D40.1-
Leydig-Sertoli cell tumor
| specified site *see* Neoplasm, benign, by site
| unspecified site
|| female D27.-
|| male D29.2-
LGSIL (Low grade squamous intraepithelial lesion on cytologic smear of)
| anus R85.612
| cervix R87.612
| vagina R87.622
Liar, pathologic F60.2
Libido
| decreased R68.82
Libman-Sacks disease M32.11
Lice (infestation) B85.2
| body (Pediculus corporis) B85.1
| crab B85.3
| head (Pediculus capitis) B85.0
| mixed (classifiable to more than one of the titles B85.0-B85.3) B85.4
| pubic (Phthirus pubis) B85.3
Lichen L28.0
| albus L90.0
|| penis N48.0
|| vulva N90.4
| amyloidosis E85.4 [L99]
| atrophicus L90.0
|| penis N48.0
|| vulva N90.4
| congenital Q82.8
| myxedematosus L98.5
| nitidus L44.1
| pilaris Q82.8
|| acquired L85.8
| planopilaris L66.1
| planus (chronicus) L43.9
|| annularis L43.8
|| bullous L43.1

Lichen . *- continued*
| follicular L66.1
| hypertrophic L43.0
| moniliformis L44.3
| of Wilson L43.9
| specified NEC L43.8
| subacute (active) L43.3
| tropicus L43.3
| ruber
|| acuminatus L44.0
|| moniliformis L44.3
|| planus L43.9
| sclerosus (et atrophicus) L90.0
|| penis N48.0
|| vulva N90.4
| scrofulosus (primary) (tuberculous) A18.4
| simplex (chronicus) (circumscriptus) L28.0
| striatus L44.2
| urticatus L28.2
Lichenification L28.0
Lichenoides tuberculosis (primary) A18.4
Lichtheim's disease or syndrome *see* Degeneration, combined
Lien migrans D73.89
Ligament *see* condition
Light
| for gestational age *see* Light for dates
| headedness R42
Light-For-Dates (infant) P05.00
| with weight of
|| 499 grams or less P05.01
|| 500-749 grams P05.02
|| 750-999 grams P05.03
|| 1000-1249 grams P05.04
|| 1250-1499 grams P05.05
|| 1500-1749 grams P05.06
|| 1750-1999 grams P05.07
|| 2000-2499 grams P05.08
|| 2500 grams and over P05.09
| specified NEC P05.09
| and small-for-dates *see* Small for dates
| affecting management of pregnancy O36.59-
Lightning (effects) (stroke) (struck by) T75.00
| burn *see* Burn
| foot E53.8
| shock T75.01
| specified effect NEC T75.09
Lightwood-Albright syndrome N25.89
Lightwood's disease or syndrome (renal tubular acidosis) N25.89
Lignac (-De Toni) (-Fanconi) (-Debre) disease or syndrome E72.09
| with cystinosis E72.04
Ligneous thyroiditis E06.5
Likoff's syndrome I20.8
Limb *see* condition
Limbic epilepsy personality syndrome F07.0
Limitation, limited
| activities due to disability Z73.6
| cardiac reserve *see* Disease, heart
| eye muscle duction, traumatic *see* Strabismus, mechanical
| mandibular range of motion M26.52
Lindau (-Von Hippel) disease Q85.8
Line(s)
| Beau's L60.4
| Harris' *see* Arrest, epiphyseal
| Hudson's (cornea) *see* Pigmentation, cornea, anterior
| Stähli's (cornea) *see* Pigmentation, cornea, anterior
Linea corneae senilis *see* Change, cornea, senile

Lingua
|geographica K14.1
|nigra (villosa) K14.3
|plicata K14.5
|tylosis K13.29
Lingual *see* condition
Linguatulosis B88.8
Linitis (gastric) plastica C16.9
Lip *see* condition
Lipedema *see* Edema
Lipemia *see also* Hyperlipidemia
|retina, retinalis E78.3
Lipidosis E75.6
|cerebral (infantile) (juvenile) (late) E75.4
|cerebroretinal E75.4
|cerebroside E75.22
|cholesterol (cerebral) E75.5
|glycolipid E75.21
|hepatosplenomegalic E78.3
|sphingomyelin *see* Niemann-Pick disease or
  syndrome
|sulfatide E75.29
Lipoadenoma *see* Neoplasm, benign, by site
Lipoblastoma *see* Lipoma
Lipoblastomatosis *see* Lipoma
Lipochondrodystrophy E76.01
Lipodermatosclerosis *see* Varix, leg, with,
  inflammation
|ulcerated *see* Varix, leg, with, ulcer, with
  inflammation by site
Lipochrome histiocytosis (familial) D71
Lipodystrophia progressiva E88.1
Lipodystrophy (progressive) E88.1
|insulin E88.1
|intestinal K90.81
|mesenteric K65.4
Lipofibroma *see* Lipoma
Lipofuscinosis, neuronal (with ceroidosis)
  E75.4
Lipogranuloma, sclerosing L92.8
Lipogranulomatosis E78.89
Lipoid *see also* condition
|histiocytosis D76.3
  |essential E75.29
|nephrosis N04.9
|proteinosis of Urbach E78.89
Lipoidemia *see* Hyperlipidemia
Lipoidosis *see* Lipidosis
Lipoma D17.9
|fetal D17.9
|fat cell D17.9
|infiltrating D17.9
|intramuscular D17.9
|pleomorphic D17.9
|site classification
  |arms (skin) (subcutaneous) D17.2-
  |connective tissue D17.30
    |intra-abdominal D17.5
    |intrathoracic D17.4
    |peritoneum D17.79
    |retroperitoneum D17.79
    |specified site NEC D17.39
    |spermatic cord D17.6
  |face (skin) (subcutaneous) D17.0
  |genitourinary organ NEC D17.72
  |head (skin) (subcutaneous) D17.0
  |intra-abdominal D17.5
  |intrathoracic D17.4
  |kidney D17.71
  |legs (skin) (subcutaneous) D17.2-
  |neck (skin) (subcutaneous) D17.0
  |peritoneum D17.79
  |retroperitoneum D17.79
  |skin D17.30
    |specified site NEC D17.39

Lipoma - *continued*
|specified site NEC D17.79
|spermatic cord D17.6
|subcutaneous D17.30
  |specified site NEC D17.39
|trunk (skin) (subcutaneous) D17.1
|unspecified D17.9
|spindle cell D17.9
Lipomatosis E88.2
|dolorosa (Dercum) E88.2
|fetal *see* Lipoma
|Launois-Bensaude E88.89
Lipomyoma *see* Lipoma
Lipomyxoma *see* Lipoma
Lipomyxosarcoma *see* Neoplasm, connective
  tissue, malignant
Lipoprotein metabolism disorder E78.9
Lipoproteinemia E78.5
|broad-beta E78.2
|floating-beta E78.2
|hyper-pre-beta E78.1
Liposarcoma *see also* Neoplasm, connective
  tissue, malignant
|dedifferentiated *see* Neoplasm, connective
  tissue, malignant
|differentiated type *see* Neoplasm, connective
  tissue, malignant
|embryonal *see* Neoplasm, connective tissue,
  malignant
|mixed type *see* Neoplasm, connective tissue,
  malignant
|myxoid *see* Neoplasm, connective tissue,
  malignant
|pleomorphic *see* Neoplasm, connective tissue,
  malignant
|round cell *see* Neoplasm, connective tissue,
  malignant
|well differentiated type *see* Neoplasm,
  connective tissue, malignant
Liposynovitis prepatellaris E88.89
Lipping, cervix N86
Lipschütz disease or ulcer N76.6
Lipuria R82.90
|schistosomiasis (bilharziasis) B65.0
Lisping F80.0
Lissauer's paralysis A52.17
Lissencephalia, lissencephaly Q04.3
Listeriosis, listerellosis A32.9
|congenital (disseminated) P37.2
|cutaneous A32.0
|neonatal, newborn (disseminated) P37.2
|oculoglandular A32.81
|specified NEC A32.89
Lithemia E79.0
Lithiasis *see* Calculus
Lithosis J62.8
Lithuria R82.998
Litigation, anxiety concerning Z65.3
Little leaguer's elbow *see* Epicondylitis, medial
Little's disease G80.9
Littre's
|gland *see* condition
|hernia *see* Hernia, abdomen
Littritis *see* Urethritis
Livedo (annularis) (racemosa) (reticularis)
  R23.1
Living in a shelter (motel) (scattered site
  housing) (temporary or transitional living
  situation) Z59.01
Liver *see* condition
Living alone (problems with) Z60.2
|with handicapped person Z74.2
Lloyd's syndrome *see* Adenomatosis, endocrine
Loa Loa, loaiasis, loiasis B74.3
Lobar *see* condition

Lobomycosis B48.0
Lobo's disease B48.0
Lobotomy syndrome F07.0
Lobstein (-Ekman) disease or syndrome Q78.0
Lobster-Claw hand Q71.6-
Lobulation (congenital) *see also* Anomaly, by
  site
|kidney, Q63.1
|liver, abnormal Q44.7
|spleen Q89.09
Lobule, lobular *see* condition
Local, localized *see* condition
Locked-In state G83.5
Locked twins causing obstructed labor O66.1
Locking
|joint *see* Derangement, joint, specified type
  NEC
  |knee *see* Derangement, knee
Lockjaw *see* Tetanus
Löffler's
|endocarditis I42.3
|eosinophilia J82.89
|pneumonia J82.89
|syndrome (eosinophilic pneumonitis) J82.89
Loiasis (with conjunctival infestation) (eyelid)
  B74.3
Lone Star fever A77.0
Long
|COVID (-19) (see also COVID-19) U09.9
|labor O63.9
  |first stage O63.0
  |second stage O63.1
|QT syndrome I45.81
Long-Term (current) (prophylactic) drug
  therapy (use of)
|agents affecting estrogen receptors and
  estrogen levels NEC Z79.818
|anastrozole (Arimidex) Z79.811
|antibiotics Z79.2
  |short-term use |omit code
|anticoagulants Z79.01
|anti-inflammatory, non-steroidal (NSAID)
  Z79.1
|antiplatelet Z79.02
|antithrombotics Z79.02
|aromatase inhibitors Z79.811
|aspirin Z79.82
|birth control pill or patch Z79.3
|bisphosphonates Z79.83
|contraceptive, oral Z79.3
|drug, specified NEC Z79.899
|estrogen receptor downregulators Z79.818
|Evista Z79.810
|exemestane (Aromasin) Z79.811
|Fareston Z79.810
|fulvestrant (Faslodex) Z79.818
|gonadotropin-releasing hormone (GnRH)
  agonist Z79.818
|goserelin acetate (Zoladex) Z79.818
|hormone replacement Z79.890
|insulin Z79.4
|letrozole (Femara) Z79.811
|leuprolide acetate (leuprorelin) (Lupron)
  Z79.818
|megestrol acetate (Megace) Z79.818
|methadone for pain management Z79.891
|Nolvadex Z79.810
|non-insulin antidiabetic drug, injectable
  Z79.899
|non-steroidal anti-inflammatories (NSAID)
  Z79.1
|opiate analgesic Z79.891
|oral
  |antidiabetic Z79.84
  |contraceptive Z79.3
  |hypoglycemic Z79.84
|raloxifene (Evista) Z79.810

Long-Term (current) (prophylactic) drug therapy
|selective estrogen receptor modulators (SERMs) Z79.810
|steroids
|inhaled Z79.51
|systemic Z79.52
|tamoxifen (Nolvadex) Z79.810
|toremifene (Fareston) Z79.810
Longitudinal stripes or grooves, nails L60.8
|congenital Q84.6
Loop
|intestine *see* Volvulus
|vascular on papilla (optic) Q14.2
Loose *see also* condition
|body
|joint M24.00
|ankle M24.07-
|elbow M24.02-
|hand M24.04-
|hip M24.05-
|knee M23.4-
|shoulder (region) M24.01-
|specified site NEC M24.08
|vertebra M24.08
|toe M24.07-
|wrist M24.03-
|knee M23.4-
|sheath, tendon *see* Disorder, tendon, specified type NEC
|cartilage *see* Loose, body, joint
|skin and subcutaneous tissue (following bariatric surgery weight loss) (following dietary weight loss) L98.7
|tooth, teeth K08.89
Loosening
|aseptic
|joint prosthesis *see* Complications, joint prosthesis, mechanical, loosening, by site
|epiphysis *see* Osteochondropathy
|mechanical
|joint prosthesis *see* Complications, joint prosthesis, mechanical, loosening, by site
Looser-Milkman (-Debray) syndrome M83.8
Lop ear (deformity) Q17.3
Lorain (-Lévi) short stature syndrome E23.0
Lordosis M40.50
|acquired *see* Lordosis, specified type NEC
|congenital Q76.429
|lumbar region Q76.426
|lumbosacral region Q76.427
|sacral region Q76.428
|sacrococcygeal region Q76.428
|thoracolumbar region Q76.425
|lumbar region M40.56
|lumbosacral region M40.57
|postsurgical M96.4
|postural *see* Lordosis, specified type NEC
|rachitic (late effect) (sequelae) E64.3
|sequelae of rickets E64.3
|specified type NEC M40.40
|lumbar region M40.46
|lumbosacral region M40.47
|thoracolumbar region M40.45
|thoracolumbar region M40.55
|tuberculous A18.01
Loss (of)
|appetite (*see* Anorexia) R63.0
|hysterical F50.89
|nonorganic origin F50.89
|psychogenic F50.89
|blood *see* Hemorrhage
|bone *see* Loss, substance of, bone
|control, sphincter, rectum R15.9
|nonorganic origin F98.1
|consciousness, transient R55

Loss (of) - *continued*
|traumatic *see* Injury, intracranial
|elasticity, skin R23.4
|family (member) in childhood Z62.898
|fluid (acute) E86.9
|function of labyrinth *see* subcategory H83.2
|hair, nonscarring *see* Alopecia
|hearing *see also* Deafness
|central NOS H90.5
|conductive H90.2
|bilateral H90.0
|unilateral
|with
|restricted hearing on the contralateral side H90.A1-
|unrestricted hearing on the contralateral side H90.1-
|mixed conductive and sensorineural hearing loss H90.8
|bilateral H90.6
|unilateral
|with
|restricted hearing on the contralateral side H90.A3-
|unrestricted hearing on the contralateral side H90.7-
|neural NOS H90.5
|perceptive NOS H90.5
|sensorineural NOS H90.5
|bilateral H90.3
|unilateral
|with
|restricted hearing on the contralateral side H90.A2-
|unrestricted hearing on the contralateral side H90.4-
|sensory NOS H90.5
|height R29.890
|limb or member, traumatic, current *see* Amputation, traumatic
|love relationship in childhood Z62.898
|memory *see also* Amnesia
|mild, following organic brain damage F06.8
|mind *see* Psychosis
|occlusal vertical dimension of fully erupted teeth M26.37
|organ or part *see* Absence, by site, acquired
|ossicles, ear (partial) H74.32-
|parent in childhood Z63.4
|pregnancy, recurrent N96
|care in current pregnancy O26.2-
|without current pregnancy N96
|recurrent pregnancy *see* Loss, pregnancy, recurrent
|self-esteem, in childhood Z62.898
|sense of
|smell *see* Disturbance, sensation, smell
|taste *see* Disturbance, sensation, taste
|touch R20.8
|sensory R44.9
|dissociative F44.6
|sexual desire F52.0
|sight (acquired) (complete) (congenital) *see* Blindness
|substance of
|bone *see* Disorder, bone, density and structure, specified NEC
|horizontal alveolar K06.3
|cartilage *see* Disorder, cartilage, specified type NEC
|auricle (ear) *see* Disorder, pinna, specified type NEC
|vitreous (humor) H15.89
|tooth, teeth *see* Absence, teeth, acquired
|vision, visual H54.7

Loss (of) - *continued*
|both eyes H54.3
|one eye H54.60
|left (normal vision on right) H54.62
|right (normal vision on left) H54.61
|specified as blindness *see* Blindness
|subjective
|sudden H53.13-
|transient H53.12-
|vitreous *see* Prolapse, vitreous
|voice *see* Aphonia
|weight (abnormal) (cause unknown) R63.4
Louis-Bar syndrome (ataxia-Telangiectasia) G11.3
Louping ill (encephalitis) A84.89
Louse, lousiness *see* Lice
Low
|achiever, school Z55.3
|back syndrome M54.50
|basal metabolic rate R94.8
|birthweight (2499 grams or less) P07.10
|with weight of
|1000-1249 grams P07.14
|1250-1499 grams P07.15
|1500-1749 grams P07.16
|1750-1999 grams P07.17
|2000-2499 grams P07.18
|extreme (999 grams or less) P07.00
|with weight of
|499 grams or less P07.01
|500-749 grams P07.02
|750-999 grams P07.03
|for gestational age *see* Light for dates
|blood pressure *see also* Hypotension
|reading (incidental) (isolated) (nonspecific) R03.1
|cardiac reserve *see* Disease, heart
|function *see also* Hypofunction
|kidney N28.9
|hematocrit D64.9
|hemoglobin D64.9
|income Z59.6
|level of literacy Z55.0
|lying
|kidney N28.89
|organ or site, congenital *see* Malposition, congenital
|output syndrome (cardiac) *see* Failure, heart
|platelets (blood) *see* Thrombocytopenia
|reserve, kidney N28.89
|salt syndrome E87.1
|self esteem R45.81
|set ears Q17.4
|vision H54.2X-
|one eye (other eye normal) H54.50
|left (normal vision on right) H54.52A-
|other eye blind *see* Blindness
|right (normal vision on left) H54.511-
Low-Density-Lipoprotein-Type (LDL) hyperlipoproteinemia E78.00
Lowe's syndrome E72.03
Lown-Ganong-Levine syndrome I45.6
LSD reaction (acute) (without dependence) F16.90
|with dependence F16.20
L-Shaped kidney Q63.8
Ludwig's angina or disease K12.2
Lues (venerea), luetic *see* Syphilis
Luetscher's syndrome (dehydration) E86.0
Lumbago, lumbalgia M54.50
|with sciatica M54.4-
|due to intervertebral disc disorder M51.17
|due to displacement, intervertebral disc M51.27
|with sciatica M51.17

Lumbar *see* condition
Lumbarization, vertebra, congenital Q76.49
Lumbermen's itch B88.0
Lump *see also* Mass
  |breast N63.0
    |axillary tail
      |left N63.32
      |right N63.31
    |left
      |lower inner quadrant N63.24
      |lower outer quadrant N63.23
      |unspecified quadrant N63.20
      |upper inner quadrant N63.22
      |upper outer quadrant N63.21
    |right
      |lower inner quadrant N63.14
      |lower outer quadrant N63.13
      |unspecified quadrant N63.10
      |upper inner quadrant N63.12
      |upper outer quadrant N63.11
    |subareolar
      |left N63.42
      |right N63.41
Lunacy *see* Psychosis
Lung *see* condition
Lupoid (miliary) of Boeck D86.3
Lupus
  |anticoagulant D68.62
    |with
      |hemorrhagic disorder D68.312
      |hypercoagulable state D68.62
    |finding without diagnosis R76.0
  |discoid (local) L93.0
  |erythematosus (discoid) (local) L93.0
    |disseminated *see* Lupus, erythematosus,
      systemic
    |eyelid H01.129
      |left H01.126
        |lower H01.125
        |upper H01.124
      |right H01.123
        |lower H01.122
        |upper H01.121
  |profundus L93.2
  |specified NEC L93.2
  |subacute cutaneous L93.1
  |systemic M32.9
    |with organ or system involvement M32.10
      |endocarditis M32.11
      |lung M32.13
      |pericarditis M32.12
      |renal (glomerular) M32.14
        |tubulo-interstitial M32.15
      |specified organ or system NEC M32.19
    |drug-induced M32.0
    |inhibitor (presence of) D68.62
      |with
        |hemorrhagic disorder D68.312
        |hypercoagulable state D68.62
      |finding without diagnosis R76.0
    |specified NEC M32.8
  |exedens A18.4
  |hydralazine M32.0
    |correct substance properly administered *see*
      Table of Drugs and Chemicals, by drug,
      adverse effect
    |overdose or wrong substance given or taken
      see Table of Drugs and Chemicals, by
      drug, poisoning
  |nephritis (chronic) M32.14
  |nontuberculous, not disseminated L93.0
  |panniculitis L93.2
  |pernio (Besnier) D86.3
  |systemic *see* Lupus, erythematosus, systemic
  |tuberculous A18.4

Lupus - *continued*
  |eyelid A18.4
  |vulgaris A18.4
    |eyelid A18.4
Luteinoma D27.-
**Lutembacher's disease or syndrome (atrial
  septal defect with mitral stenosis)** Q21.1
Luteoma D27.-
Lutz (-Splendore-De Almeida) disease *see*
  Paracoccidioidomycosis
Luxation *see also* Dislocation
  |eyeball (nontraumatic) *see* Luxation, globe
    |birth injury P15.3
  |globe, nontraumatic H44.82-
  |lacrimal gland *see* Dislocation, lacrimal gland
  |lens (old) (partial) (spontaneous)
    |congenital Q12.1
    |syphilitic A50.39
Lycanthropy F22
Lyell's syndrome L51.2
  |due to drug L51.2
    |correct substance properly administered *see*
      Table of Drugs and Chemicals, by drug,
      adverse effect
    |overdose or wrong substance given or taken
      see Table of Drugs and Chemicals, by
      drug, poisoning
Lyme disease A69.20
Lymph
  |gland or node *see* condition
  |scrotum *see* Infestation, filarial
Lymphadenitis I88.9
  |with ectopic or molar pregnancy O08.0
  |acute L04.9
    |axilla L04.2
    |face L04.0
    |head L04.0
    |hip L04.3
    |limb
      |lower L04.3
      |upper L04.2
    |neck L04.0
    |shoulder L04.2
    |specified site NEC L04.8
    |trunk L04.1
  |anthracosis (occupational) J60
  |any site, except mesenteric I88.9
    |chronic I88.1
    |subacute I88.1
  |breast
    |gestational *see* Mastitis, obstetric
    |puerperal, postpartum (nonpurulent) O91.22
  |chancroidal (congenital) A57
  |chronic I88.1
    |mesenteric I88.0
  |due to
    |Brugia (malayi) B74.1
      |timori B74.2
    |chlamydial lymphogranuloma A55
    |diphtheria (toxin) A36.89
    |lymphogranuloma venereum A55
    |Wuchereria bancrofti B74.0
  |following ectopic or molar pregnancy O08.0
  |gonorrheal A54.89
  |infective *see* Lymphadenitis, acute
  |mesenteric (acute) (chronic) (nonspecific)
    (subacute) I88.0
    |due to Salmonella typhi A01.09
    |tuberculous A18.39
  |mycobacterial A31.8
  |purulent *see* Lymphadenitis, acute
  |pyogenic *see* Lymphadenitis, acute
  |regional, nonbacterial I88.8
  |septic *see* Lymphadenitis, acute

Lymphadenitis - *continued*
  |subacute, unspecified site I88.1
  |suppurative *see* Lymphadenitis, acute
  |syphilitic (early) (secondary) A51.49
    |late A52.79
  |tuberculous *see* Tuberculosis, lymph gland
  |venereal (chlamydial) A55
Lymphadenoid goiter E06.3
Lymphadenopathy (generalized) R59.1
  |angioimmunoblastic, with dysproteinemia
    (AILD) C86.5
  |due to toxoplasmosis (acquired) B58.89
    |congenital (acute) (subacute) (chronic)
      P37.1
  |localized R59.0
  |syphilitic (early) (secondary) A51.49
Lymphadenosis R59.1
Lymphangiectasis I89.0
  |conjunctiva H11.89
  |postinfectional I89.0
  |scrotum I89.0
Lymphangiectatic elephantiasis, nonfilarial
  I89.0
Lymphangioendothelioma D18.1
  |malignant *see* Neoplasm, connective tissue,
    malignant
Lymphangioleiomyomatosis J84.81
Lymphangioma D18.1
  |capillary D18.1
  |cavernous D18.1
  |cystic D18.1
  |malignant *see* Neoplasm, connective tissue,
    malignant
Lymphangiomyoma D18.1
Lymphangiomyomatosis J84.81
Lymphangiosarcoma *see* Neoplasm, connective
  tissue, malignant
Lymphangitis I89.1
  |with
    |abscess - code by site under Abscess
    |cellulitis - code by site under Cellulitis
    |ectopic or molar pregnancy O08.0
  |acute L03.91
    |abdominal wall L03.321
    |ankle *see* Lymphangitis, acute, lower limb
    |arm *see* Lymphangitis, acute, upper limb
    |auricle (ear) *see* Lymphangitis, acute, ear
    |axilla L03.12-
    |back (any part) L03.322
    |buttock L03.327
    |cervical (meaning neck) L03.222
    |cheek (external) L03.212
    |chest wall L03.323
    |digit
      |finger *see* Lymphangitis, acute, finger
      |toe *see* Lymphangitis, acute, toe
    |ear (external) H60.1-
    |external auditory canal *see* Lymphangitis,
      acute, ear
    |eyelid *see* Abscess, eyelid
    |face NEC L03.212
    |finger (intrathecal) (periosteal)
      (subcutaneous) (subcuticular) L03.02-
    |foot *see* Lymphangitis, acute, lower limb
    |gluteal (region) L03.327
    |groin L03.324
    |hand *see* Lymphangitis, acute, upper limb
    |head NEC L03.891
      |face (any part, except ear, eye and nose)
        L03.212
    |heel *see* Lymphangitis, acute, lower limb
    |hip *see* Lymphangitis, acute, lower limb
    |jaw (region) L03.212
    |knee *see* Lymphangitis, acute, lower limb
    |leg *see* Lymphangitis, acute, lower limb
    |lower limb L03.12-

Lymphangitis - *continued*
　　|toe *see* Lymphangitis, acute, toe
　|navel L03.326
　|neck (region) L03.222
　|orbit, orbital *see* Cellulitis, orbit
　|pectoral (region) L03.323
　|perineal, perineum L03.325
　|scalp (any part) L03.891
　|shoulder *see* Lymphangitis, acute, upper
　　　limb
　|specified site NEC L03.898
　|thigh *see* Lymphangitis, acute, lower limb
　|thumb (intrathecal) (periosteal)
　　　(subcutaneous) (subcuticular) *see*
　　　Lymphangitis, acute, finger
　|toe (intrathecal) (periosteal) (subcutaneous)
　　　(subcuticular) L03.04-
　|trunk L03.329
　　|abdominal wall L03.321
　　|back (any part) L03.322
　　|buttock L03.327
　　|chest wall L03.323
　　|groin L03.324
　　|perineal, perineum L03.325
　　|umbilicus L03.326
　|umbilicus L03.326
　|upper limb L03.12-
　　|axilla *see* Lymphangitis, acute, axilla
　　|finger *see* Lymphangitis, acute, finger
　　|thumb *see* Lymphangitis, acute, finger
　|wrist *see* Lymphangitis, acute, upper limb
　|breast
　　|gestational *see* Mastitis, obstetric
　|chancroidal A57
　|chronic (any site) I89.1
　|due to
　　|Brugia (malayi) B74.1
　　　|timori B74.2
　　|Wuchereria bancrofti B74.0
　|following ectopic or molar pregnancy O08.89
　|penis
　　|acute N48.29
　　|gonococcal (acute) (chronic) A54.09
　|puerperal, postpartum, childbirth O86.89
　|strumous, tuberculous A18.2
　|subacute (any site) I89.1
　|tuberculous *see* Tuberculosis, lymph gland
Lymphatic (vessel) *see* condition
Lymphatism E32.8
Lymphectasia I89.0
Lymphedema (acquired) *see also* Elephantiasis
　|congenital Q82.0
　|hereditary (chronic) (idiopathic) Q82.0
　|postmastectomy I97.2
　|praecox I89.0
　|secondary I89.0
　|surgical NEC I97.89
　　|postmastectomy (syndrome) I97.2
Lymphoblastic *see* condition
Lymphoblastoma (diffuse) *see* Lymphoma,
　　lymphoblastic (diffuse)
　|giant follicular *see* Lymphoma, lymphoblastic
　　　(diffuse)
　|macrofollicular *see* Lymphoma, lymphoblastic
　　　(diffuse)
Lymphocele I89.8
Lymphocytic
　|chorioencephalitis (acute) (serous) A87.2
　|choriomeningitis (acute) (serous) A87.2
　|meningoencephalitis A87.2
Lymphocytoma, benign cutis L98.8
Lymphocytopenia D72.810
Lymphocytosis (symptomatic) D72.820
　|infectious (acute) B33.8

Lymphoepithelioma *see* Neoplasm, malignant,
　　by site
Lymphogranuloma (malignant) *see also*
　　Lymphoma, Hodgkin
　|chlamydial A55
　|inguinale A55
　|venereum (any site) (chlamydial) (with
　　　stricture of rectum) A55
Lymphogranulomatosis (malignant) *see also*
　　Lymphoma, Hodgkin
　|benign (Boeck's sarcoid) (Schaumann's)
　　　D86.1
**Lymphohistiocytosis, hemophagocytic
　　(familial)** D76.1
Lymphoid *see* condition
Lymphoma (of) (malignant) C85.90
　|adult T-cell (HTLV 1-associated) (acute
　　　variant) (chronic variant) (lymphomatoid
　　　variant) (smouldering variant) C91.5-
　|anaplastic large cell
　　|ALK-negative C84.7-
　　|ALK-positive C84.6-
　　|breast implant associated (BIA-ALCL)
　　　　C84.7A
　　|CD30-positive C84.6-
　　|primary cutaneous C86.6
　|angioimmunoblastic T-cell C86.5
　|BALT C88.4
　|B-cell C85.1-
　|B-precursor C83.5-
　|blastic NK-cell C86.4
　|blastic plasmacytoid dendritic cell neoplasm
　　　(BPDCN) C86.4
　|bronchial-associated lymphoid tissue [BALT-
　　　lymphoma] C88.4
　|Burkitt (atypical) C83.7-
　|Burkitt-like C83.7-
　|centrocytic C83.1-
　|cutaneous follicle center C82.6-
　|cutaneous T-cell C84.A-
　|diffuse follicle center C82.5-
　|diffuse large cell C83.3-
　　|anaplastic C83.3-
　　|B-cell C83.3-
　　|CD30-positive C83.3-
　　|centroblastic C83.3-
　　|immunoblastic C83.3-
　　|plasmablastic C83.3-
　　|subtype not specified C83.3-
　　|T-cell rich C83.3-
　|enteropathy-type (associated) (intestinal) T-
　　　cell C86.2
　|extranodal NK/T-cell, nasal type C86.0
　|extranodal marginal zone B-cell lymphoma of
　　　mucosa-associated lymphoid tissue [MALT-
　　　lymphoma] C88.4
　|follicular C82.9-
　　|grade
　　　|I C82.0-
　　　|II C82.1-
　　　|III C82.2-
　　　|IIIa C82.3-
　　　|IIIb C82.4-
　　|specified NEC C82.8-
　|hepatosplenic T-cell (alpha-beta) (gamma-
　　　delta) C86.1
　|histiocytic C85.9-
　　|true C96.A
　|Hodgkin C81.9
　　|lymphocyte-rich (classical) C81.4-
　　|lymphocyte depleted (classical) C81.3-
　　|mixed cellularity (classical) C81.2-
　　|nodular sclerosis (classical) C81.1-
　　|specified NEC (classical) C81.7-
　　|lymphocyte-rich classical C81.4-

Lymphoma - *continued*
　|lymphocyte depleted classical C81.3-
　|mixed cellularity classical C81.2-
　|nodular
　　|lymphocyte predominant C81.0-
　　|sclerosis (classical) C81.1-
　|intravascular large B-cell C83.8-
　|Lennert's C84.4-
　|lymphoblastic B-cell C83.5-
　|lymphoblastic (diffuse) C83.5-
　|lymphoblastic T-cell C83.5-
　|lymphoepithelioid C84.4-
　|lymphoplasmacytic C83.0-
　　|with IgM-production C88.0
　|MALT C88.4
　|mantle cell C83.1-
　|mature T-cell NEC C84.4-
　|mature T/NK-cell C84.9-
　　|specified NEC C84.Z-
　|mediastinal (thymic) large B-Cell C85.2-
　|Mediterranean C88.3
　|mucosa-associated lymphoid tissue [MALT-
　　　lymphoma] C88.4
　|NK/T cell C84.9-
　|nodal marginal zone C83.0-
　|non-follicular (diffuse) C83.9-
　　|specified NEC C83.8-
　|non-hodgkin *see also* Lymphoma, by type
　　　C85.9-
　　|specified NEC C85.8-
　|non-leukemic variant of B-cLL C83.0-
　|peripheral T-cell, not classified C84.4-
　|primary cutaneous
　　|anaplastic large cell C86.6
　　|CD30-positive large T-cell C86.6
　|primary effusion B-cell C83.8-
　|SALT C88.4
　|skin-associated lymphoid tissue [SALT-
　　　lymphoma] C88.4
　|small cell B-cell C83.0-
　|splenic marginal zone C83.0-
　|subcutaneous panniculitis-like T-cell C86.3
　|T-precursor C83.5-
　|true histiocytic C96.A
Lymphomatosis *see* Lymphoma
Lymphopathia venereum, veneris A55
Lymphopenia D72.810
Lymphoplasmacytic leukemia *see* Leukemia,
　　chronic lymphocytic, B-cell type
Lymphoproliferation, X-Linked disease D82.3
Lymphoreticulosis, benign (of inoculation)
　　A28.1
Lymphorrhea I89.8
Lymphosarcoma (diffuse) *see also* Lymphoma
　　C85.9-
Lymphostasis I89.8
Lypemania *see* Melancholia
**Lysine and hydroxylysine metabolism
　　disorder** E72.3
Lyssa *see* Rabies

M

Macacus ear Q17.3
Maceration, wet feet, tropical (syndrome)
　　T69.02-
MacLeod's syndrome J43.0
Macrocephalia, macrocephaly Q75.3
Macrocheilia, macrochilia (congenital) Q18.6
Macrocolon *see also* Megacolon Q43.1
Macrocornea Q15.8
　|with glaucoma Q15.0
Macrocytic *see* condition Macrocytosis D75.89
Macrocytosis *see* condition Macrocytosis D75.89
**Macrodactylia, macrodactylism (fingers)
　　(thumbs)** Q74.0
　|toes Q74.2
Macrodontia K00.2

ONMJ

Macrogenia M26.05
Macrogenitosomia (adrenal) (male) (praecox)
  E25.9
  |congenital E25.0
Macroglobulinemia (idiopathic) (primary)
  C88.0
  |monoclonal (essential) D47.2
  |Waldenström C88.0
Macroglossia (congenital) Q38.2
  |acquired K14.8
Macrognathia, macrognathism (congenital)
  (mandibular) (maxillary) M26.09
Macrogyria (congenital) Q04.8
Macrohydrocephalus see Hydrocephalus
Macromastia see Hypertrophy, breast
Macrophthalmos Q11.3
  |in congenital glaucoma Q15.0
Macropsia H53.15
Macrosigmoid K59.39
  |congenital Q43.2
Macrospondylitis , acromegalic E22.0
Macrostomia (congenital) Q18.4
Macrotia (external ear) (congenital) Q17.1
Macula
  |cornea, corneal see Opacity, cornea
  |degeneration (atrophic) (exudative) (senile)
    see also Degeneration, macula
    |hereditary see Dystrophy, retina
Maculae ceruleae B85.1
Maculopathy, toxic see Degeneration, macula,
  toxic
Madarosis (eyelid) H02.729
  |left H02.726
    |lower H02.725
    |upper H02.724
  |right H02.723
    |lower H02.722
    |upper H02.721
Madelung's
  |deformity (radius) Q74.0
  |disease
    |radial deformity Q74.0
    |symmetrical lipomas, neck E88.89
Madness see Psychosis
Madura
  |foot B47.9
    |actinomycotic B47.1
    |mycotic B47.0
Maduromycosis B47.0
Maffucci's syndrome Q78.4
Magnesium metabolism disorder see Disorder,
  metabolism, magnesium
Main en griffe (acquired) see also Deformity,
  limb, clawhand
  |congenital Q74.0
Maintenance (encounter for)
  |antineoplastic chemotherapy Z51.11
  |antineoplastic radiation therapy Z51.0
  |methadone F11.20
Majocchi's
  |disease L81.7
  |granuloma B35.8
Major see condition
Malabar itch (any site) B35.5
Malabsorption K90.9
  |calcium K90.89
  |carbohydrate K90.49
  |disaccharide E73.9
  |fat K90.49
  |galactose E74.20
  |glucose (-galactose) E74.39
  |intestinal K90.9
    |specified NEC K90.89
  |isomaltose E74.31
  |lactose E73.9

Malabsorption - continued
  |methionine E72.19
  |monosaccharide E74.39
  |postgastrectomy K91.2
  |postsurgical K91.2
  |protein K90.49
  |starch K90.49
  |sucrose E74.39
  |syndrome K90.9
    |postsurgical K91.2
Malacia, bone (adult) M83.9
  |juvenile see Rickets
Malacoplakia
  |bladder N32.89
  |pelvis (kidney) N28.89
  |ureter N28.89
  |urethra N36.8
Malacosteon, juvenile see Rickets
Maladaptation see Maladjustment
Maladie de Roger Q21.0
Maladjustment
  |conjugal Z63.0
    |involving divorce or estrangement Z63.5
  |educational Z55.4
  |family Z63.9
  |marital Z63.0
    |involving divorce or estrangement Z63.5
  |occupational NEC Z56.89
  |simple, adult see Disorder, adjustment
  |situational see Disorder, adjustment
  |social Z60.9
    |due to
      |acculturation difficulty Z60.3
      |discrimination and persecution
        (perceived) Z60.5
      |exclusion and isolation Z60.4
      |life-cycle (phase of life) transition Z60.0
      |rejection Z60.4
      |specified reason NEC Z60.8
Malaise R53.81
Malakoplakia see Malacoplakia
Malaria, malarial (fever) B54
  |with
    |blackwater fever B50.8
      |hemoglobinuric (bilious) B50.8
    |hemoglobinuria B50.8
  |accidentally induced (therapeutically) code by
    type under Malaria algid B50.9
  |cerebral B50.0 *[G94]*
  |clinically diagnosed (without parasitological
    confirmation) B54
  |congenital NEC P37.4
    |falciparum P37.3
  |congestion, congestive B54
  |continued (fever) B50.9
  |estivo-autumnal B50.9
  |falciparum B50.9
    |with complications NEC B50.8
      |cerebral B50.0 *[G94]*
    |severe B50.8
  |hemorrhagic B54
  |malariae B52.9
    |with
      |complications NEC B52.8
      |glomerular disorder B52.0
  |malignant (tertian) see Malaria, falciparum
  |mixed infections   code to first listed type in
    B50-B53
  |ovale B53.0
  |parasitologically confirmed NEC B53.8
  |pernicious, acute see Malaria, falciparum
  |Plasmodium (P.)
    |falciparum NEC see Malaria, falciparum
    |malariae NEC B52.9
      |with Plasmodium
        |falciparum (and or vivax) see Malaria,
        falciparum

Malaria, malarial - continued
    |vivax see also Malaria, vivax
      and falciparum see Malaria,
      falciparum
  |ovale B53.0
    |with Plasmodium malariae see also
      Malaria, malariae
    |and vivax see also Malaria, vivax
      |and falciparum see Malaria,
      falciparum
  |simian B53.1
    |with Plasmodium malariae see also
      Malaria, malariae
    |and vivax see also Malaria, vivax
      |and falciparum see Malaria,
      falciparum
  |vivax NEC B51.9
    |with Plasmodium falciparum see Malaria,
      falciparum
  |quartan see Malaria, malariae
  |quotidian see Malaria, falciparum
  |recurrent B54
  |remittent B54
  |specified type NEC (parasitologically
    confirmed) B53.8
  |spleen B54
  |subtertian (fever) see Malaria, falciparum
  |tertian (benign) see also Malaria, vivax
    |malignant B50.9
  |tropical B50.9
  |typhoid B54
  |vivax B51.9
    |with
      |complications NEC B51.8
      |ruptured spleen B51.0
Malassimilation K90.9
Malassez's disease (cystic) N50.89
Mal de los pintos see Pinta
Mal de mer T75.3
Maldescent, testis Q53.9
  |bilateral Q53.20
    |abdominal Q53.211
    |perineal Q53.22
  |unilateral Q53.10
    |abdominal Q53.111
    |perineal Q53.12
Maldevelopment see also Anomaly
  |brain Q07.9
  |colon Q43.9
  |hip Q74.2
    |congenital dislocation Q65.2
      |bilateral Q65.1
      |unilateral Q65.0-
  |mastoid process Q75.8
  |middle ear Q16.4
    |except ossicles Q16.4
    |ossicles Q16.3
  |ossicles Q16.3
  |spine Q76.49
  |toe Q74.2
Male type pelvis Q74.2
  |with disproportion (fetopelvic) O33.3
    |causing obstructed labor O65.3
Malformation (congenital) see also Anomaly
  |adrenal gland Q89.1
  |affecting multiple systems with skeletal
    changes NEC Q87.5
  |alimentary tract Q45.9
    |specified type NEC Q45.8
    |upper Q40.9
      |specified type NEC Q40.8
  |aorta Q25.40
    |absence Q25.41
    |aneurysm, congenital Q25.43
    |aplasia Q25.41
    |atresia Q25.29

Malformation - *continued*
> |aortic arch Q25.21
> |coarctation (preductal) (postductal) Q25.1
> |dilatation, congenital Q25.44
> |hypoplasia Q25.42
> |patent ductus arteriosus Q25.0
> |specified type NEC Q25.49
> |stenosis Q25.1
> |supravalvular Q25.3
> |aortic valve Q23.9
> |specified NEC Q23.8
> |arteriovenous, aneurysmatic (congenital) Q27.30
> |brain Q28.2
> |cerebral Q28.2
> |peripheral Q27.30
> |digestive system Q27.33
> |lower limb Q27.32
> |other specified site Q27.39
> |renal vessel Q27.34
> |upper limb Q27.31
> |precerebral vessels (nonruptured) Q28.0
> |auricle
> |ear (congenital) Q17.3
> |acquired H61.119
> |left H61.112
> |with right H61.113
> |right H61.111
> |with left H61.113
> |bile duct Q44.5
> |bladder Q64.79
> |aplasia Q64.5
> |diverticulum Q64.6
> |exstrophy *see* Exstrophy, bladder
> |neck obstruction Q64.31
> |bone Q79.9
> |face Q75.9
> |specified type NEC Q75.8
> |skull Q75.9
> |specified type NEC Q75.8
> |brain (multiple) Q04.9
> |arteriovenous Q28.2
> |specified type NEC Q04.8
> |branchial cleft Q18.2
> |breast Q83.9
> |specified type NEC Q83.8
> |broad ligament Q50.6
> |bronchus Q32.4
> |bursa Q79.9
> |cardiac
> |chambers Q20.9
> |specified type NEC Q20.8
> |septum Q21.9
> |specified type NEC Q21.8
> |cerebral Q04.9
> |vessels Q28.3
> |cervix uteri Q51.9
> |specified type NEC Q51.828
> |Chiari
> |Type I G93.5
> |Type II Q07.01
> |choroid (congenital) Q14.3
> |plexus Q07.8
> |circulatory system Q28.9
> |cochlea Q16.5
> |cornea Q13.4
> |coronary vessels Q24.5
> |corpus callosum (congenital) Q04.0
> |diaphragm Q79.1
> |digestive system NEC, specified type NEC Q45.8
> |dura Q07.9
> |brain Q04.9
> |spinal Q06.9
> |ear Q17.9

Malformation - *continued*
> |causing impairment of hearing Q16.9
> |external Q17.9
> |accessory auricle Q17.0
> |causing impairment of hearing Q16.9
> |absence of
> |auditory canal Q16.1
> |auricle Q16.0
> |macrotia Q17.1
> |microtia Q17.2
> |misplacement Q17.4
> |misshapen NEC Q17.3
> |prominence Q17.5
> |specified type NEC Q17.8
> |inner Q16.5
> |middle Q16.4
> |absence of eustachian tube Q16.2
> |ossicles (fusion) Q16.3
> |ossicles Q16.3
> |specified type NEC Q17.8
> |epididymis Q55.4
> |esophagus Q39.9
> |specified type NEC Q39.8
> |eye Q15.9
> |lid Q10.3
> |specified NEC Q15.8
> |fallopian tube Q50.6
> |genital organ *see* Anomaly, genitalia
> |great
> |artery Q25.9
> |aorta *see* Malformation, aorta
> |pulmonary artery *see* Malformation, pulmonary, artery
> |specified type NEC Q25.8
> |vein Q26.9
> |anomalous
> |portal venous connection Q26.5
> |pulmonary venous connection Q26.4
> |partial Q26.3
> |total Q26.2
> |persistent left superior vena cava Q26.1
> |portal vein-hepatic artery fistula Q26.6
> |specified type NEC Q26.8
> |vena cava stenosis, congenital Q26.0
> |gum Q38.6
> |hair Q84.2
> |heart Q24.9
> |specified type NEC Q24.8
> |integument Q84.9
> |specified type NEC Q84.8
> |internal ear Q16.5
> |intestine Q43.9
> |specified type NEC Q43.8
> |iris Q13.2
> |joint Q74.9
> |ankle Q74.2
> |lumbosacral Q76.49
> |sacroiliac Q74.2
> |specified type NEC Q74.8
> |kidney Q63.9
> |accessory Q63.0
> |giant Q63.3
> |horseshoe Q63.1
> |hydronephrosis Q62.0
> |malposition Q63.2
> |specified type NEC Q63.8
> |lacrimal apparatus Q10.6
> |lip Q38.0
> |lingual Q38.3
> |liver Q44.7
> |lung Q33.9
> |meninges or membrane (congenital) Q07.9
> |cerebral Q04.8
> |spinal (cord) Q06.9
> |middle ear Q16.4

Malformation - *continued*
> |ossicles Q16.3
> |mitral valve Q23.9
> |specified NEC Q23.8
> |Mondini's (congenital) (malformation, cochlea) Q16.5
> |mouth (congenital) Q38.6
> |multiple types NEC Q89.7
> |musculoskeletal system Q79.9
> |myocardium Q24.8
> |nail Q84.6
> |nervous system (central) Q07.9
> |nose Q30.9
> |specified type NEC Q30.8
> |optic disc Q14.2
> |orbit Q10.7
> |ovary Q50.39
> |palate Q38.5
> |parathyroid gland Q89.2
> |pelvic organs or tissues NEC
> |in pregnancy or childbirth O34.8-
> |causing obstructed labor O65.5
> |penis Q55.69
> |aplasia Q55.5
> |curvature (lateral) Q55.61
> |hypoplasia Q55.62
> |pericardium Q24.8
> |peripheral vascular system Q27.9
> |specified type NEC Q27.8
> |pharynx Q38.8
> |precerebral vessels Q28.1
> |prostate Q55.4
> |pulmonary
> |arteriovenous Q25.72
> |artery Q25.9
> |atresia Q25.5
> |specified type NEC Q25.79
> |stenosis Q25.6
> |valve Q22.3
> |renal artery Q27.2
> |respiratory system Q34.9
> |retina Q14.1
> |scrotum *see* Malformation, testis and scrotum
> |seminal vesicles Q55.4
> |sense organs NEC Q07.9
> |skin Q82.9
> |specified NEC Q89.8
> |spinal
> |cord Q06.9
> |nerve root Q07.8
> |spine Q76.49
> |kyphosis *see* Kyphosis, congenital
> |lordosis *see* Lordosis, congenital
> |spleen Q89.09
> |stomach Q40.3
> |specified type NEC Q40.2
> |teeth, tooth K00.9
> |tendon Q79.9
> |testis and scrotum Q55.20
> |aplasia Q55.0
> |hypoplasia Q55.1
> |polyorchism Q55.21
> |retractile testis Q55.22
> |scrotal transposition Q55.23
> |specified NEC Q55.29
> |throat Q38.8
> |thorax, bony Q76.9
> |thyroid gland Q89.2
> |tongue (congenital) Q38.3
> |hypertrophy Q38.2
> |tie Q38.1
> |trachea Q32.1
> |tricuspid valve Q22.9
> |specified type NEC Q22.8

Malformation - *continued*

|umbilical cord NEC (complicating delivery) O69.89
|umbilicus Q89.9
|ureter Q62.8
  |agenesis Q62.4
  |duplication Q62.5
  |malposition *see* Malposition, congenital, ureter
  |obstructive defect *see* Defect, obstructive, ureter
  |vesico-uretero-renal reflux Q62.7
|urethra Q64.79
  |aplasia Q64.5
  |duplication Q64.74
  |posterior valves Q64.2
  |prolapse Q64.71
  |stricture Q64.32
|urinary system Q64.9
|uterus Q51.9
  |specified type NEC Q51.818
|vagina Q52.4
|vascular system, peripheral Q27.9
|vas deferens Q55.4
  |atresia Q55.3
|venous *see* Anomaly, vein(s)
|vulva Q52.70

Malfunction *see also* Dysfunction

|cardiac electronic device T82.119
  |electrode T82.110
  |pulse generator T82.111
  |specified type NEC T82.118
|catheter device NEC T85.618
  |cystostomy T83.010
  |dialysis (renal) (vascular) T82.41
    |intraperitoneal T85.611
  |infusion NEC T82.514
    |cranial T85.610
    |epidural T85.610
    |intrathecal T85.610
    |spinal T85.610
    |subarachnoid T85.610
    |subdural T85.610
  |urinary *see also* Breakdown, device, catheter T83.018
|colostomy K94.03
  |valve K94.03
|cystostomy (stoma) N99.512
  |catheter T83.010
|enteric stoma K94.13
|enterostomy K94.13
|esophagostomy K94.33
|gastroenteric K31.89
|gastrostomy K94.23
|ileostomy K94.13
  |valve K94.13
|intrathecal infusion pump T85.615
|jejunostomy K94.13
|nervous system device, implant or graft, specified NEC T85.615
|pacemaker *see* Malfunction, cardiac electronic device
|prosthetic device, internal *see* Complications, prosthetic device, by site, mechanical
|tracheostomy J95.03
|urinary device NEC *see* Complication, genitourinary, device, urinary, mechanical
|valve
  |colostomy K94.03
  |heart T82.09
  |ileostomy K94.13
|vascular graft or shunt NEC *see* Complication, cardiovascular device, mechanical, vascular
|ventricular (communicating shunt) T85.01

Malherbe's tumor *see* Neoplasm, skin, benign
Malibu disease L98.8
Malignancy *see also* Neoplasm, malignant, by site
|unspecified site (primary) C80.1
Malignant *see* condition
Malingerer, malingering Z76.5
Mallet finger (acquired) *see* Deformity, finger, mallet finger
|congenital Q74.0
|sequelae of rickets E64.3
Malleus A24.0
Mallory's bodies R89.7
Mallory-Weiss syndrome K22.6
Malnutrition E46
|degree
  |first E44.1
  |mild (protein) E44.1
  |moderate (protein) E44.0
  |second E44.0
  |severe (protein-energy) E43
    |intermediate form E42
      |with
        |kwashiorkor (and marasmus) E42
        |marasmus E41
  |third E43
|following gastrointestinal surgery K91.2
|intrauterine
  |light-for-dates *see* Light for dates
  |small-for-dates *see* Small for dates
|lack of care, or neglect (child) (infant) T76.02
  |confirmed T74.02
|malignant E40
|protein E46
  |calorie E46
    |mild E44.1
    |moderate E44.0
    |severe E43
      |intermediate form E42
        |with
          |kwashiorkor (and marasmus) E42
          |marasmus E41
  |energy E46
    |mild E44.1
    |moderate E44.0
    |severe E43
      |intermediate form E42
        |with
          |kwashiorkor (and marasmus) E42
          |marasmus E41
|severe (protein-energy) E43
  |with
    |kwashiorkor (and marasmus) E42
    |marasmus E41
Malocclusion (teeth) M26.4
|Angle's M26.219
  |class I M26.211
  |class II M26.212
  |class III M26.213
|due to
  |abnormal swallowing M26.59
  |mouth breathing M26.59
  |tongue, lip or finger habits M26.59
|temporomandibular (joint) M26.69
Malposition
|cervix *see* Malposition, uterus
|congenital
  |adrenal (gland) Q89.1
  |alimentary tract Q45.8
    |lower Q43.8
    |upper Q40.8
  |aorta Q25.49
  |appendix Q43.8

Malposition - *continued*

  |arterial trunk Q20.0
  |artery (peripheral) Q27.8
    |coronary Q24.5
    |digestive system Q27.8
    |lower limb Q27.8
    |pulmonary Q25.79
    |specified site NEC Q27.8
    |upper limb Q27.8
  |auditory canal Q17.8
    |causing impairment of hearing Q16.9
  |auricle (ear) Q17.4
    |causing impairment of hearing Q16.9
    |cervical Q18.2
  |biliary duct or passage Q44.5
  |bladder (mucosa) *see* Exstrophy, bladder
  |brachial plexus Q07.8
  |brain tissue Q04.8
  |breast Q83.8
  |bronchus Q32.4
  |cecum Q43.8
  |clavicle Q74.0
  |colon Q43.8
  |digestive organ or tract NEC Q45.8
    |lower Q43.8
    |upper Q40.8
  |ear (auricle) (external) Q17.4
    |ossicles Q16.3
  |endocrine (gland) NEC Q89.2
  |epiglottis Q31.8
  |eustachian tube Q17.8
  |eye Q15.8
  |facial features Q18.8
  |fallopian tube Q50.6
  |finger(s) Q68.1
    |supernumerary Q69.0
  |foot Q66.9
  |gallbladder Q44.1
  |gastrointestinal tract Q45.8
  |genitalia, genital organ(s) or tract
    |female Q52.8
      |external Q52.79
      |internal NEC Q52.8
    |male Q55.8
  |glottis Q31.8
  |hand Q68.1
  |heart Q24.8
    |dextrocardia Q24.0
      |with complete transposition of viscera Q89.3
  |hepatic duct Q44.5
  |hip (joint) Q65.89
  |intestine (large) (small) Q43.8
    |with anomalous adhesions, fixation or malrotation Q43.3
  |joint NEC Q68.8
  |kidney Q63.2
  |larynx Q31.8
  |limb Q68.8
    |lower Q68.8
    |upper Q68.8
  |liver Q44.7
  |lung (lobe) Q33.8
  |nail(s) Q84.6
  |nerve Q07.8
  |nervous system NEC Q07.8
  |nose, nasal (septum) Q30.8
  |organ or site not listed *see* Anomaly, by site
  |ovary Q50.39
  |pancreas Q45.3
  |parathyroid (gland) Q89.2
  |patella Q74.1
  |peripheral vascular system Q27.8
  |pituitary (gland) Q89.2
  |respiratory organ or system NEC Q34.8

Malposition - *continued*
  |rib (cage) Q76.6
    |supernumerary in cervical region Q76.5
  |scapula Q74.0
  |shoulder Q74.0
  |spinal cord Q06.8
  |spleen Q89.09
  |sternum NEC Q76.7
  |stomach Q40.2
  |symphysis pubis Q74.2
  |thymus (gland) Q89.2
  |thyroid (gland) (tissue) Q89.2
    |cartilage Q31.8
  |toe(s) Q66.9
    |supernumerary Q69.2
  |tongue Q38.3
  |trachea Q32.1
  |ureter Q62.60
    |deviation Q62.61
    |displacement Q62.62
    |ectopia Q62.63
    |specified type NEC Q62.69
  |uterus Q51.818
  |vein(s) (peripheral) Q27.8
    |great Q26.8
  |vena cava (inferior) (superior) Q26.8
  |device, implant or graft *see also*
    Complications, by site and type,
    mechanical T85.628
  |arterial graft NEC *see* Complication,
    cardiovascular device, mechanical,
    vascular
  |breast (implant) T85.42
  |catheter NEC T85.628
    |cystostomy T83.020
    |dialysis (renal) T82.42
      |intraperitoneal T85.621
    |infusion NEC T82.524
      |spinal (epidural) (subdural) T85.620
    |urinary *see also* Displacement, device,
      catheter, urinary T83.028
  |electronic (electrode) (pulse generator)
    (stimulator)
    |bone T84.320
    |cardiac T82.129
      |electrode T82.120
      |pulse generator T82.121
      |specified type NEC T82.128
    |nervous system *see* Complication,
      prosthetic device, mechanical,
      electronic nervous system stimulator
    |urinary *see* Complication, genitourinary,
      device, urinary, mechanical
  |fixation, internal (orthopedic) NEC *see*
    Complication, fixation device, mechanical
  |gastrointestinal *see* Complications,
    prosthetic device, mechanical,
    gastrointestinal device
  |genital NEC T83.428
    |intrauterine contraceptive device (string)
      T83.32
    |penile prosthesis (cylinder) (implanted)
      (pump) (reservoir) T83.420
    |testicular prosthesis T83.421
  |heart NEC *see* Complication, cardiovascular
    device, mechanical
  |joint prosthesis *see* Complication, joint
    prosthesis, mechanical
  |ocular NEC *see* Complications, prosthetic
    device, mechanical, ocular device
  |orthopedic NEC *see* Complication,
    orthopedic, device, mechanical
  |specified NEC T85.628
  |urinary NEC *see also* Complication,
    genitourinary, device, urinary, mechanical
    |graft T83.22

Malposition - *continued*
  |vascular NEC *see* Complication,
    cardiovascular device, mechanical
  |ventricular intracranial shunt T85.02
  |fetus *see* Pregnancy, complicated by
    (management affected by), presentation,
    fetal
  |gallbladder K82.8
  |gastrointestinal tract, congenital Q45.8
  |heart, congenital NEC Q24.8
  |joint prosthesis *see* Complications, joint
    prosthesis, mechanical, displacement, by
    site
  |stomach K31.89
    |congenital Q40.2
  |tooth, teeth, fully erupted M26.30
  |uterus (acute) (acquired) (adherent)
    (asymptomatic) (postinfectional)
    (postpartal, old) N85.4
    |anteflexion or anteversion N85.4
      |congenital Q51.818
    |flexion N85.4
      |lateral *see* Lateroversion, uterus
    |inversion N85.5
    |lateral (flexion) (version) *see* Lateroversion,
      uterus
    |in pregnancy or childbirth *see* subcategory
      O34.5
    |retroflexion or retroversion *see*
      Retroversion, uterus
Malposture R29.3
Malrotation
  |cecum Q43.3
  |colon Q43.3
  |intestine Q43.3
  |kidney Q63.2
Maltreatment
  |adult
    |abandonment
      |confirmed T74.01
      |suspected T76.01
    |bullying
      |confirmed T74.31
      |suspected T76.31
    |confirmed T74.91
    |history of Z91.419
    |intimidation (through social media)
      |confirmed T74.31
      |suspected T76.31
    |neglect
      |confirmed T74.01
      |suspected T76.01
    |physical abuse
      |confirmed T74.11
      |suspected T76.11
    |psychological abuse
      |confirmed T74.31
      |suspected T76.31
      |history of Z91.411
    |sexual abuse
      |confirmed T74.21
      |suspected T76.21
    |suspected T76.91
  |child
    |abandonment
      |confirmed T74.02
      |suspected T76.02
    |bullying
      |confirmed T74.32
      |suspected T76.32
    |confirmed T74.92
    |history of *see* History, personal (of), abuse
    |intimidation (through social media)
      |confirmed T74.32
      |suspected T76.32
    |neglect

Maltreatment - *continued*
    |confirmed T74.02
    |history of *see* History, personal (of), abuse
    |suspected T76.02
  |physical abuse
    |confirmed T74.12
    |history of *see* History, personal (of), abuse
    |suspected T76.12
  |psychological abuse
    |confirmed T74.32
    |history of *see* History, personal (of), abuse
    |suspected T76.32
  |sexual abuse
    |confirmed T74.22
    |history of *see* History, personal (of), abuse
    |suspected T76.22
  |suspected T76.92
  |personal history of Z91.89
Malta fever *see* Brucellosis
Maltworker's lung J67.4
Malunion, fracture *see* Fracture, by site
Mammillitis N61.0
  |puerperal, postpartum O91.02
Mammitis *see* Mastitis
Mammogram (examination) Z12.39
  |routine Z12.31
Mammoplasia N62
Management (of)
  |bone conduction hearing device (implanted)
    Z45.320
  |cardiac pacemaker NEC Z45.018
  |cerebrospinal fluid drainage device Z45.41
  |cochlear device (implanted) Z45.321
  |contraceptive Z30.9
    |specified NEC Z30.8
  |implanted device Z45.9
    |specified NEC Z45.89
  |infusion pump Z45.1
  |procreative Z31.9
    |male factor infertility in female Z31.81
    |specified NEC Z31.89
  |prosthesis (external) *see also* Fitting Z44.9
    |implanted Z45.9
      |specified NEC Z45.89
  |renal dialysis catheter Z49.01
  |vascular access device Z45.2
Mangled *see* specified injury by site
Mania (monopolar) *see also* Disorder, mood,
    manic episode
  |with psychotic symptoms F30.2
  |without psychotic symptoms F30.10
    |mild F30.11
    |moderate F30.12
    |severe F30.13
  |Bell's F30.8
  |chronic (recurrent) F31.89
  |hysterical F44.89
  |puerperal F30.8
  |recurrent F31.89
Manic depression F31.9
Manic-Depressive insanity, psychosis, or
    syndrome *see* Disorder, bipolar
Mannosidosis E77.1
Mansonelliasis, mansonellosis B74.4
Manson's
  |disease B65.1
  |schistosomiasis B65.1
Manual *see* condition
Maple-Bark-Stripper's lung (disease) J67.6
Maple-Syrup-Urine disease E71.0
Marable's syndrome (celiac artery
    compression) I77.4
Marasmus E41
  |due to malnutrition E41
  |intestinal E41
  |nutritional E41
  |senile R54
  |tuberculous NEC *see* Tuberculosis

Marble
 |bones Q78.2
 |skin R23.8
Marburg virus disease A98.3
March
 |fracture *see* Fracture, traumatic, stress, by site
 |hemoglobinuria D59.6
Marchesani (-Weill) syndrome Q87.0
Marchiafava (-Bignami) syndrome or disease
  G37.1
Marchiafava-Micheli syndrome D59.5
Marcus Gunn's syndrome Q07.8
Marfan's syndrome *see* Syndrome, Marfan's
Marie-Bamberger disease *see*
  Osteoarthropathy, hypertrophic, specified
  NEC
Marie-Charcot-Tooth neuropathic muscular
  atrophy G60.0
Marie's
 |cerebellar ataxia (late-onset) G11.2
 |disease or syndrome (acromegaly) E22.0
Marie-Strumpell arthritis, disease or
  spondylitis *see* Spondylitis, ankylosing
Marion's disease (bladder neck obstruction)
  N32.0
Marital conflict Z63.0
Mark
 |port wine Q82.5
 |raspberry Q82.5
 |strawberry Q82.5
 |stretch L90.6
 |tattoo L81.8
Marker heterochromatin *see* Extra, marker
  chromosomes
Maroteaux-Lamy syndrome (mild) (severe)
  E76.29
Marrow (bone)
 |arrest D61.9
 |poor function D75.89
Marseilles fever A77.1
Marsh fever *see* Malaria
Marshall's (hidrotic) ectodermal dysplasia
  Q82.4
Marsh's disease (exophthalmic goiter) E05.00
 |with storm E05.01
Masculinization (female) with adrenal
  hyperplasia E25.9
 |congenital E25.0
Masculinovoblastoma D27.-
Masochism (sexual) F65.51
Mason's lung J62.8
Mass
 |abdominal R19.00
  |epigastric R19.06
  |generalized R19.07
  |left lower quadrant R19.04
  |left upper quadrant R19.02
  |periumbilic R19.05
  |right lower quadrant R19.03
  |right upper quadrant R19.01
  |specified site NEC R19.09
 |breast (*see also* Lump, breast) N63.0
 |chest R22.2
 |cystic *see* Cyst
 |ear H93.8-
 |head R22.0
 |intra-abdominal (diffuse) (generalized) *see*
   Mass, abdominal
 |kidney N28.89
 |liver R16.0
 |localized (skin) R22.9
  |chest R22.2
  |head R22.0
  |limb
   |lower R22.4-
   |upper R22.3-

Mass - *continued*
  |neck R22.1
  |trunk R22.2
 |lung R91.8
 |malignant *see* Neoplasm, malignant, by site
 |neck R22.1
 |pelvic (diffuse) (generalized) *see* Mass,
   abdominal
 |specified organ NEC *see* Disease, by site
 |splenic R16.1
 |substernal thyroid *see* Goiter
 |superficial (localized) R22.9
 |umbilical (diffuse) (generalized) R19.09
Massive *see* condition
Mast cell
 |disease, systemic tissue D47.02
 |leukemia C94.3-
 |neoplasm
  |malignant C96.20
   |specified type NEC C96.29
  |of uncertain behavior NEC D47.09
 |sarcoma C96.22
 |tumor D47.09
Mastalgia N64.4
Masters-Allen syndrome N83.8
Mastitis (acute) (diffuse) (nonpuerperal)
  (subacute) N61.0
 |with abscess N61.1
 |chronic (cystic) *see* Mastopathy, cystic
 |cystic (Schimmelbusch's type) *see*
   Mastopathy, cystic
 |granulomatous N61.2-
 |fibrocystic *see* Mastopathy, cystic
 |infective N61.0
  |newborn P39.0
 |interstitial, gestational or puerperal *see*
   Mastitis, obstetric
 |neonatal (noninfective) P83.4
  |infective P39.0
 |obstetric (interstitial) (nonpurulent)
   |associated with
    |lactation O91.23
    |pregnancy O91.21-
    |puerperium O91.22
   |purulent
    |associated with
     |lactation O91.13
     |pregnancy O91.11-
     |puerperium O91.12
 |periductal *see* Ectasia, mammary duct
 |phlegmonous *see* Mastopathy, cystic
 |plasma cell *see* Ectasia, mammary duct
 |without abscess N61.0
Mastocytoma (extracutaneous) D47.09
 |malignant C96.2
 |solitary D47.01
Mastocytosis D47.09
 |aggressive systemic C96.21
 |cutaneous (diffuse) (maculopapular) D47.01
  |congenital Q82.2
  |of neonatal onset Q82.2
  |of newborn onset Q82.2
 |indolent systemic D47.02
 |isolated bone marrow D47.02
 |malignant C96.29
 |systemic (indolent) (smoldering)
  |with an associated hematological non-mast
    cell lineage disease (SM-AHNMD)
    D47.02
Mastodynia N64.4
Mastoid *see* condition
Mastoidalgia *see* subcategory H92.0
Mastoiditis (coalescent) (hemorrhagic)
  (suppurative) H70.9-
 |acute, subacute H70.00-
  |complicated NEC H70.09-

Mastoiditis - *continued*
  |subperiosteal H70.01-
 |chronic (necrotic) (recurrent) H70.1-
 |in (due to)
   |infectious disease NEC B99 [*H75.0*]
   |parasitic disease NEC B89 [*H75.0*]
   |tuberculosis A18.03
 |petrositis *see* Petrositis
 |postauricular fistula *see* Fistula, postauricular
 |specified NEC H70.89-
 |tuberculous A18.03
Mastopathy, mastopathia N64.9
 |chronica cystica *see* Mastopathy, cystic
 |cystic (chronic) (diffuse) N60.1-
  |with epithelial proliferation N60.3-
 |diffuse cystic *see* Mastopathy, cystic
 |estrogenic, oestrogenica N64.89
 |ovarian origin N64.89
Mastoplasia, mastoplastia N62
Masturbation (excessive) F98.8
Maternal care (for) *see* Pregnancy (complicated
  by) (management affected by)
Matheiu's disease (leptospiral jaundice) A27.0
Mauclaire's disease or osteochondrosis *see*
  Osteochondrosis, juvenile, hand, metacarpal
Maxcy's disease A75.2
Maxilla, maxillary *see* condition
May (-Hegglin) anomaly or syndrome D72.0
McArdle (-Schmid)(-Pearson) disease
  (glycogen storage) E74.04
McCune-Albright syndrome Q78.1
McQuarrie's syndrome (idiopathic familial
  hypoglycemia) E16.2
Meadow's syndrome Q86.1
Measles (black) (hemorrhagic) (suppressed)
  B05.9
 |with
  |complications NEC B05.89
  |encephalitis B05.0
  |intestinal complications B05.4
  |keratitis (keratoconjunctivitis) B05.81
  |meningitis B05.1
  |otitis media B05.3
  |pneumonia B05.2
 |French *see* Rubella
 |German *see* Rubella
 |Liberty *see* Rubella
Meatitis, urethral *see* Urethritis
Meatus, meatal *see* condition
Meat-Wrappers' asthma J68.9
Meckel-Gruber syndrome Q61.9
Meckel's diverticulitis, diverticulum
  (displaced) (hypertrophic) Q43.0
 |malignant *see* Table of Neoplasms, small
   intestine, malignant
Meconium
 |ileus, newborn P76.0
  |in cystic fibrosis E84.11
  |meaning meconium plug (without cystic
    fibrosis) P76.0
 |obstruction, newborn P76.0
  |due to fecaliths P76.0
  |in mucoviscidosis E84.11
 |peritonitis P78.0
 |plug syndrome (newborn) NEC P76.0
Median *see also* condition
 |arcuate ligament syndrome I77.4
 |bar (prostate) (vesical orifice) *see*
   Hyperplasia, prostate
 |rhomboid glossitis K14.2
Mediastinal shift R93.89
Mediastinitis (acute) (chronic) J98.51
 |syphilitic A52.73
 |tuberculous A15.8

Mediastinopericarditis *see also* Pericarditis
|acute I30.9
|adhesive I31.0
|chronic I31.8
  |rheumatic I09.2
Mediastinum, mediastinal *see* condition
Medicine poisoning *see* Table of Drugs and
  Chemicals, by drug, poisoning
Mediterranean
|fever *see* Brucellosis
  |familial M04.1
  |tick A77.1
|kala-Azar B55.0
|leishmaniasis B55.0
|tick fever A77.1
Medulla *see* condition
Medullary cystic kidney Q61.5
Medullated fibers
|optic (nerve) Q14.8
|retina Q14.1
Medulloblastoma
|desmoplastic C71.6
|specified site *see* Neoplasm, malignant, by site
|unspecified site C71.6
Medulloepithelioma *see also* Neoplasm,
  malignant, by site
|teratoid *see* Neoplasm, malignant, by site
Medullomyoblastoma
|specified site *see* Neoplasm, malignant, by site
|unspecified site C71.6
Meekeren-Ehlers-Danlos syndrome Q79.6
Megacolon (acquired) (functional) (not
  Hirschsprung's disease) (in) K59.39
|Chagas' disease B57.32
|congenital, congenitum (aganglionic) Q43.1
|Hirschsprung's (disease) Q43.1
|toxic NEC K59.31
  |due to Clostridium difficile
    |not specified as recurrent A04.72
    |recurrent A04.71
Megaesophagus (functional) K22.0
|congenital Q39.5
|in (due to) Chagas' disease B57.31
Megalencephaly Q04.5
Megalerythema (epidemic) B08.3
Megaloappendix Q43.8
Megalocephalous, megalocephaly NEC Q75.3
Megalocornea Q15.8
|with glaucoma Q15.0
Megalocytic anemia D53.1
Megalodactylia (fingers) (thumbs)
  (congenital) Q74.0
|toes Q74.2
Megaloduodenum Q43.8
Megaloesophagus (functional) K22.0
|congenital Q39.5
Megalogastria (acquired) K31.89
|congenital Q40.2
Megalophthalmos Q11.3
Megalopsia H53.15
Megalosplenia *see* Splenomegaly
Megaloureter N28.82
|congenital Q62.2
Megarectum K62.89
Megasigmoid K59.39
|congenital Q43.2
Megaureter N28.82
|congenital Q62.2
Megavitamin-B6
syndrome E67.2
Megrim *see* Migraine
Meibomian
|cyst, infected *see* Hordeolum
|gland *see* condition
|sty, stye *see* Hordeolum
Meibomitis *see* Hordeolum

Meige-Milroy disease (chronic hereditary
  edema) Q82.0
Meige's syndrome Q82.0
Melalgia, nutritional E53.8
Melancholia F32.A
|climacteric (single episode) F32.89
  |recurrent episode F33.8
|hypochondriac F45.29
|intermittent (single episode) F32.89
  |recurrent episode F33.8
|involutional (single episode) F32.89
  |recurrent episode F33.8
|menopausal (single episode) F32.89
  |recurrent episode F33.8
|puerperal F32.89
|reactive (emotional stress or trauma) F32.3
|recurrent F33.9
|senile F03
|stuporous (single episode) F32.89
  |recurrent episode F33.8
Melanemia R79.89
Melanoameloblastoma *see* Neoplasm, bone,
  benign
Melanoblastoma *see* Melanoma
Melanocarcinoma *see* Melanoma
Melanocytoma, eyeball D31.9-
Melanocytosis, neurocutaneous Q82.8
Melanoderma, melanodermia L81.4
Melanodontia, infantile K03.89
Melanodontoclasia K03.89
Melanoepithelioma *see* Melanoma (malignant)
  C43.9
Melanoma (malignant) C43.9
|acral lentiginous, malignant *see* Melanoma,
  skin, by site
|amelanotic *see* Melanoma, skin, by site
|balloon cell *see* Melanoma, skin, by site
|benign *see* Nevus
|desmoplastic, malignant *see* Melanoma, skin,
  by site
|epithelioid cell *see* Melanoma, skin, by site
  |with spindle cell, mixed *see* Melanoma,
    skin, by site
|in
  |giant pigmented nevus *see* Melanoma, skin,
    by site
  |Hutchinson's melanotic freckle *see*
    Melanoma, skin, by site
  |junctional nevus *see* Melanoma, skin, by
    site
  |precancerous melanosis *see* Melanoma,
    skin, by site
|in situ D03.9
  |abdominal wall D03.59
  |ala nasi D03.39
  |ankle D03.7-
  |anus, anal (margin) (skin) D03.51
  |arm D03.6-
  |auditory canal D03.2-
  |auricle (ear) D03.2-
  |auricular canal (external) D03.2-
  |axilla, axillary fold D03.59
  |back D03.59
  |breast D03.52
  |brow D03.39
  |buttock D03.59
  |canthus (eye) D03.1-
  |cheek (external) D03.39
  |chest wall D03.59
  |chin D03.39
  |choroid D03.8
  |conjunctiva D03.8
  |ear (external) D03.2-
  |external meatus (ear) D03.2-
  |eye D03.8
  |eyebrow D03.39
  |eyelid (lower) (upper) D03.1-
  |face D03.30

Melanoma (malignant) - *continued*
  |specified NEC D03.39
|female genital organ (external) NEC D03.8
|finger D03.6-
|flank D03.59
|foot D03.7-
|forearm D03.6-
|forehead D03.39
|foreskin D03.8
|gluteal region D03.59
|groin D03.59
|hand D03.6-
|heel D03.7-
|helix D03.2-
|hip D03.7-
|interscapular region D03.59
|iris D03.8
|jaw D03.39
|knee D03.7-
|labium (majus) (minus) D03.8
|lacrimal gland D03.8
|leg D03.7-
|lip (lower) (upper) D03.0
|lower limb NEC D03.7-
|male genital organ (external) NEC D03.8
|nail D03.9
  |finger D03.6-
  |toe D03.7-
|neck D03.4
|nose (external) D03.39
|orbit D03.8
|penis D03.8
|perianal skin D03.51
|perineum D03.51
|pinna D03.2-
|popliteal fossa or space D03.7-
|prepuce D03.8
|pudendum D03.8
|retina D03.8
|retrobulbar D03.8
|scalp D03.4
|scrotum D03.8
|shoulder D03.6
|specified site NEC D03.8
|submammary fold D03.52
|temple D03.39
|thigh D03.7-
|toe D03.7-
|trunk NEC D03.59
|umbilicus D03.59
|upper limb NEC D03.6-
|vulva D03.8
|juvenile *see* Nevus
|malignant, of soft parts except skin *see*
  Neoplasm, connective tissue, malignant
|metastatic
  |breast C79.81
  |genital organ C79.82
  |specified site NEC C79.89
|neurotropic, malignant *see* Melanoma, skin,
  by site
|nodular *see* Melanoma, skin, by site
|regressing, malignant *see* Melanoma, skin, by
  site
|skin C43.9
  |abdominal wall C43.59
  |ala nasi C43.31
  |ankle C43.7-
  |anus, anal (skin) C43.51
  |arm C43.6-
  |auditory canal (external) C43.2-
  |auricle (ear) C43.2-
  |auricular canal (external) C43.2-
  |axilla, axillary fold C43.59
  |back C43.59
  |breast (female) (male) C43.52

Melanoma (malignant) - *continued*
| brow C43.39
| buttock C43.59
| canthus (eye) C43.1-
| cheek (external) C43.39
| chest wall C43.59
| chin C43.39
| ear (external) C43.2-
| elbow C43.6-
| external meatus (ear) C43.2-
| eyebrow C43.39
| eyelid (lower) (upper) C43.1-
| face C43.30
| | specified NEC C43.39
| female genital organ (external) NEC C51.9
| finger C43.6-
| flank C43.59
| foot C43.7-
| forearm C43.6-
| forehead C43.39
| foreskin C60.0
| glabella C43.39
| gluteal region C43.59
| groin C43.59
| hand C43.6-
| heel C43.7-
| helix C43.2-
| hip C43.7-
| interscapular region C43.59
| jaw (external) C43.39
| knee C43.7-
| labium C51.9
| | majus C51.0
| | minus C51.1
| leg C43.7-
| lip (lower) (upper) C43.0
| lower limb NEC C43.7-
| male genital organ (external) NEC C63.9
| nail
| | finger C43.6-
| | toe C43.7-
| nasolabial groove C43.39
| nates C43.59
| neck C43.4
| nose (external) C43.31
| overlapping site C43.8
| palpebra C43.1-
| penis C60.9
| perianal skin C43.51
| perineum C43.51
| pinna C43.2-
| popliteal fossa or space C43.7-
| prepuce C60.0
| pudendum C51.9
| scalp C43.4
| scrotum C63.2
| shoulder C43.6-
| skin NEC C43.9
| submammary fold C43.52
| temple C43.39
| thigh C43.7-
| toe C43.7-
| trunk NEC C43.59
| umbilicus C43.59
| upper limb NEC C43.6-
| vulva C51.9
| | overlapping sites C51.8
| spindle cell
| | with epithelioid, mixed *see* Melanoma, skin, by site
| | type A C69.4-
| | type B C69.4-
| superficial spreading *see* Melanoma, skin, by site
Melanosarcoma *see also* Melanoma
| epithelioid cell *see* Melanoma

Melanosis L81.4
| addisonian E27.1
| | tuberculous A18.7
| adrenal E27.1
| colon K63.89
| conjunctiva *see* Pigmentation, conjunctiva
| | congenital Q13.89
| cornea (presenile) (senile) *see also* Pigmentation, cornea
| | congenital Q13.4
| eye NEC H57.89
| | congenital Q15.8
| lenticularis progressiva Q82.1
| liver K76.89
| precancerous *see also* Melanoma, in situ
| | malignant melanoma in *see* Melanoma
| Riehl's L81.4
| sclera H15.89
| | congenital Q13.89
| suprarenal E27.1
| tar L81.4
| toxic L81.4
Melanuria R82.998
MELAS syndrome E88.41
Melasma L81.1
| adrenal (gland) E27.1
| suprarenal (gland) E27.1
Melena K92.1
| with ulcer   code by site under Ulcer, with hemorrhage K27.4
| due to swallowed maternal blood P78.2
| newborn, neonatal P54.1
| | due to swallowed maternal blood P78.2
Meleney's
| gangrene (cutaneous) *see* Ulcer, skin
| ulcer (chronic undermining) *see* Ulcer, skin
Melioidosis A24.9
| acute A24.1
| chronic A24.2
| fulminating A24.1
| pneumonia A24.1
| pulmonary (chronic) A24.2
| | acute A24.1
| | subacute A24.2
| sepsis A24.1
| specified NEC A24.3
| subacute A24.2
Melitensis, febris A23.0
Melkersson (-Rosenthal) syndrome G51.2
Mellitus, diabetes *see* Diabetes
Melorheostosis (bone) *see* Disorder, bone, density and structure, specified NEC
Meloschisis Q18.4
Melotia Q17.4
Membrana
| capsularis lentis posterior Q13.89
| epipapillaris Q14.2
Membranacea placenta O43.19-
Membranaceous uterus N85.8
Membrane(s), membranous *see also* condition
| cyclitic *see* Membrane, pupillary
| folds, congenital *see* Web | Jackson's Q43.3
| over face of newborn P28.9
| premature rupture *see* Rupture, membranes, premature
| pupillary H21.4-
| | persistent Q13.89
| retained (with hemorrhage) (complicating delivery) O72.2
| | without hemorrhage O73.1
| secondary cataract *see* Cataract, secondary
| unruptured (causing asphyxia) *see* Asphyxia, newborn
| vitreous *see* Opacity, vitreous, membranes and strands

Membranitis *see* Chorioamnionitis
Memory disturbance, lack or loss *see also* Amnesia
| mild, following organic brain damage F06.8
Menadione deficiency E56.1
Menarche
| delayed E30.0
| precocious E30.1
Mendacity, pathologic F60.2
Mendelson's syndrome (due to anesthesia) J95.4
| in labor and delivery O74.0
| in pregnancy O29.01-
| obstetric O74.0
| postpartum, puerperal O89.01
Ménétrier's disease or syndrome K29.60
| with bleeding K29.61
Ménière's disease, syndrome or vertigo H81.0-
Meninges, meningeal *see* condition
Meningioma *see also* Neoplasm, meninges, benign
| angioblastic *see* Neoplasm, meninges, benign
| angiomatous *see* Neoplasm, meninges, benign
| atypical   *see* Neoplasm, meninges, uncertain behavior
| endotheliomatous *see* Neoplasm, meninges, benign
| fibroblastic *see* Neoplasm, meninges, benign
| fibrous *see* Neoplasm, meninges, benign
| hemangioblastic *see* Neoplasm, meninges, benign
| hemangiopericytic *see* Neoplasm, meninges, benign
| malignant *see* Neoplasm, meninges, malignant
| meningothelial *see* Neoplasm, meninges, benign
| meningotheliomatous *see* Neoplasm, meninges, benign
| mixed *see* Neoplasm, meninges, benign
| multiple *see* Neoplasm, meninges, uncertain behavior
| papillary *see* Neoplasm, meninges, uncertain behavior
| psammomatous *see* Neoplasm, meninges, benign
| syncytial *see* Neoplasm, meninges, benign
| transitional *see* Neoplasm, meninges, benign
Meningiomatosis (diffuse) *see* Neoplasm, meninges, uncertain behavior
Meningism *see* Meningismus
Meningismus (infectional) (pneumococcal) R29.1
| due to serum or vaccine R29.1
| influenzal *see* Influenza, with, manifestations NEC
Meningitis (basal) (basic) (brain) (cerebral) (cervical) (congestive) (diffuse) (hemorrhagic) (infantile) (membranous) (metastatic) (nonspecific) (pontine) (progressive) (simple) (spinal) (subacute) (sympathetic) (toxic) G03.9
| abacterial G03.0
| actinomycotic A42.81
| adenoviral A87.1
| arbovirus A87.8
| aseptic (acute) G03.0
| bacterial G00.9
| | Escherichia coli (E. coli) G00.8
| | Friedländer (bacillus) G00.8
| | gram-negative G00.9
| | H. influenzae G00.0
| | Klebsiella G00.8
| | pneumococcal G00.1
| | specified organism NEC G00.8
| | staphylococcal G00.3

Meningitis - *continued*
 |streptococcal (acute) G00.2
 |benign recurrent (Mollaret) G03.2
 |candidal B37.5
 |caseous (tuberculous) A17.0
 |cerebrospinal A39.0
 |chronic NEC G03.1
 |clear cerebrospinal fluid NEC G03.0
 |coxsackievirus A87.0
 |cryptococcal B45.1
 |diplococcal (gram positive) A39.0
 |echovirus A87.0
 |enteroviral A87.0
 |eosinophilic B83.2
 |epidemic NEC A39.0
 |Escherichia coli (E. coli) G00.8
 |fibrinopurulent G00.9
   |specified organism NEC G00.8
 |Friedländer (bacillus) G00.8
 |gonococcal A54.81
 |gram-negative cocci G00.9
 |gram-positive cocci G00.9
 |Haemophilus (influenzae) G00.0
 |H. influenzae G00.0
 |in (due to)
   |adenovirus A87.1
   |African trypanosomiasis B56.9 [G02]
   |anthrax A22.8
   |bacterial disease NEC A48.8 [G01]
   |Chagas' disease (chronic) B57.41
   |chickenpox B01.0
   |coccidioidomycosis B38.4
   |Diplococcus pneumoniae G00.1
   |enterovirus A87.0
   |herpes (simplex) virus B00.3
     |zoster B02.1
   |infectious mononucleosis B27.92
   |leptospirosis A27.81
   |Listeria monocytogenes A32.11
   |Lyme disease A69.21
   |measles B05.1
   |mumps (virus) B26.1
   |neurosyphilis (late) A52.13
   |parasitic disease NEC B89 [G02]
   |poliovirus A80.9 [G02]
   |preventive immunization, inoculation or
     vaccination G03.8
   |rubella B06.02
   |Salmonella infection A02.21
   |specified cause NEC G03.8
   |Streptococcal pneumoniae G00.1
   |typhoid fever A01.01
   |varicella B01.0
   |viral disease NEC A87.8
   |whooping cough A37.90
   |zoster B02.1
 |infectious G00.9
 |influenzal (H. influenzae) G00.0
 |Klebsiella G00.8
 |leptospiral (aseptic) A27.81
 |lymphocytic (acute) (benign) (serous) A87.2
 |meningococcal A39.0
 |Mima polymorpha G00.8
 |Mollaret (benign recurrent) G03.2
 |monilial B37.5
 |mycotic NEC B49 [G02]
 |Neisseria A39.0
 |nonbacterial G03.0
 |nonpyogenic NEC G03.0
 |ossificans G96.198
 |pneumococcal streptococcus pneumoniae
   G00.1
 |poliovirus A80.9 [G02]
 |postmeasles B05.1
 |purulent G00.9

Meningitis - *continued*
 |specified organism NEC G00.8
 |pyogenic G00.9
   |specified organism NEC G00.8
 |Salmonella (arizonae) (Cholerae-Suis)
   (enteritidis) (typhimurium) A02.21
 |septic G00.9
   |specified organism NEC G00.8
 |serosa circumscripta NEC G03.0
 |serous NEC G93.2
 |specified organism NEC G00.8
 |sporotrichosis B42.81
 |staphylococcal G00.3
 |sterile G03.0
 |Streptococcal (acute) G00.2
   |pneumoniae G00.1
 |suppurative G00.9
   |specified organism NEC G00.8
 |syphilitic (late) (tertiary) A52.13
   |acute A51.41
   |congenital A50.41
   |secondary A51.41
 |Torula histolytica (cryptococcal) B45.1
 |traumatic (complication of injury) T79.8
 |tuberculous A17.0
 |typhoid A01.01
 |viral NEC A87.9
 |Yersinia pestis A20.3
Meningocele (spinal) *see also* Spina bifida
 |with hydrocephalus *see* Spina bifida, by site,
   with hydrocephalus
 |acquired (traumatic) G96.198
 |cerebral *see* Encephalocele
Meningocerebritis *see* Meningoencephalitis
Meningococcemia A39.4
 |acute A39.2
 |chronic A39.3
Meningococcus, meningococcal *see also*
   condition A39.9
 |adrenalitis, hemorrhagic A39.1
 |carrier (suspected) of Z22.31
 |meningitis (cerebrospinal) A39.0
Meningoencephalitis *see also* Encephalitis
   G04.90
 |acute NEC *see also* Encephalitis, viral A86
 |bacterial NEC G04.2
 |California A83.5
 |diphasic A84.1
 |eosinophilic B83.2
 |epidemic A39.81
 |herpesviral, herpetic B00.4
   |due to herpesvirus 6 B10.01
   |due to herpesvirus 7 B10.09
   |specified NEC B10.09
 |in (due to)
   |blastomycosis NEC B40.81
   |diseases classified elsewhere G05.3
   |free-living amebae B60.2
   |Hemophilus influenzae (H .influenzae)
     G00.0
   |herpes B00.4
     |due to herpesvirus 6 B10.01
     |due to herpesvirus 7 B10.09
     |specified NEC B10.09
   |H. influenzae G00.0
   |Lyme disease A69.22
   |mercury *see* subcategory T56.1
   |mumps B26.2
   |Naegleria (amebae) (organisms) (fowleri)
     B60.2
   |Parastrongylus cantonensis B83.2
   |toxoplasmosis (acquired) B58.2
     |congenital P37.1
 |infectious (acute) (viral) A86
 |influenzal (H. influenzae) G00.0

Meningoencephalitis - *continued*
 |Listeria monocytogenes A32.12
 |lymphocytic (serous) A87.2
 |mumps B26.2
 |parasitic NEC B89 [G05.3]
 |pneumococcal G04.2
 |primary amebic B60.2
 |specific (syphilitic) A52.14
 |specified organism NEC G04.81
 |staphylococcal G04.2
 |streptococcal G04.2
 |syphilitic A52.14
 |toxic NEC G92.8
   |due to mercury *see* subcategory T56.1
 |tuberculous A17.82
 |virus NEC A86
Meningoencephalocele *see also* Encephalocele
 |syphilitic A52.19
   |congenital A50.49
Meningoencephalomyelitis *see also*
   Meningoencephalitis
 |acute NEC (viral) A86
   |disseminated G04.00
     |postimmunization or postvaccination
       G04.02
     |postinfectious G04.01
 |due to
   |actinomycosis A42.82
   |Torula B45.1
   |Toxoplasma or toxoplasmosis (acquired)
     B58.2
     |congenital P37.1
 |postimmunization or postvaccination G04.02
Meningoencephalomyelopathy G96.9
Meningoencephalopathy G96.9
Meningomyelitis *see also* Meningoencephalitis
 |bacterial NEC G04.2
 |blastomycotic NEC B40.81
 |cryptococcal B45.1
 |in diseases classified elsewhere G05.4
 |meningococcal A39.81
 |syphilitic A52.14
 |tuberculous A17.82
Meningomyelocele *see also* Spina bifida
 |syphilitic A52.19
Meningomyeloneuritis *see* Meningoencephalitis
Meningoradiculitis *see* Meningitis
Meningovascular *see* condition
Menkes' disease or syndrome E83.09
 |meaning maple-syrup-urine disease E71.0
Menometrorrhagia N92.1
**Menopause, menopausal (asymptomatic)
   (state)** Z78.0
 |arthritis (any site) NEC *see* Arthritis, specified
   form NEC
 |bleeding N92.4
 |depression (single episode) F32.89
   |agitated (single episode) F32.2
     |recurrent episode F33.9
   |psychotic (single episode) F32.89
     |recurrent episode F33.9
   |recurrent episode F33.8
 |melancholia (single episode) F32.89
   |recurrent episode F33.8
 |paranoid state F22
 |premature E28.319
   |asymptomatic E28.319
     |postirradiation E89.40
     |postsurgical E89.40
   |symptomatic E28.310
     |postirradiation E89.41
     |postsurgical E89.41
 |psychosis NEC F28
 |symptomatic N95.1
 |toxic polyarthritis NEC *see* Arthritis, specified
   form NEC

Menorrhagia (primary) N92.0
  |climacteric N92.4
    |menopausal N92.4
  |menopausal N92.4
  |postclimacteric N95.0
  |postmenopausal N95.0
  |preclimacteric or premenopausal N92.4
  |pubertal (menses retained) N92.2
Menostaxis N92.0
Menses, retention N94.89
Menstrual *see* Menstruation
  |absent *see* Amenorrhea
  |anovulatory N97.0
  |cycle, irregular N92.6
  |disorder N93.9
    |psychogenic F45.8
  |during pregnancy O20.8
  |excessive (with regular cycle) N92.0
    |with irregular cycle N92.1
    |at puberty N92.2
  |frequent N92.0
  |infrequent *see* Oligomenorrhea
  |irregular N92.6
    |specified NEC N92.5
  |latent N92.5
  |membranous N92.5
  |painful *see also* Dysmenorrhea N94.6
    |primary N94.4
    |psychogenic F45.8
    |secondary N94.5
  |passage of clots N92.0
  |precocious E30.1
  |protracted N92.5
  |rare *see* Oligomenorrhea
  |retained N94.89
  |retrograde N92.5
  |scanty *see* Oligomenorrhea
  |suppression N94.89
  |vicarious (nasal) N94.89
Mental *see also* condition
  |deficiency *see* Disability, intellectual
  |deterioration *see* Psychosis
  |disorder *see* Disorder, mental
  |exhaustion F48.8
  |insufficiency (congenital) *see* Disability,
    intellectual
  |observation without need for further medical
    care Z03.89
  |retardation *see* Disability, intellectual
  |subnormality *see* Disability, intellectual
  |upset *see* Disorder, mental
Meralgia paresthetica G57.1-
Mercurial *see* condition
Mercurialism *see* subcategory T56.1
MERRF syndrome (myoclonic epilepsy
  associated with ragged-Red fiber) E88.42
Merkel cell tumor *see* Carcinoma, Merkel cell
Merocele *see* Hernia, femoral
Meromelia
  |lower limb *see* Defect, reduction, lower limb
    |intercalary
      |femur *see* Defect, reduction, lower limb,
        specified type NEC
        |tibiofibular (complete) (incomplete) *see*
          Defect, reduction, lower limb
  |upper limb *see* Defect, reduction, upper limb
    |intercalary, humeral, radioulnar *see*
      Agenesis, arm, with hand present
Merzbacher-Pelizaeus disease E75.29
Mesaortitis *see* Aortitis
Mesarteritis *see* Arteritis
Mesencephalitis *see* Encephalitis

Mesenchymoma *see also* Neoplasm, connective
  tissue, uncertain behavior
  |benign *see* Neoplasm, connective tissue,
    benign
  |malignant *see* Neoplasm, connective tissue,
    malignant
Mesenteritis
  |retractile K65.4
  |sclerosing K65.4
Mesentery, mesenteric *see* condition
Mesiodens, mesiodentes K00.1
Mesio-Occlusion M26.213
Mesocolon *see* condition
Mesonephroma (malignant) *see* Neoplasm,
  malignant, by site
  |benign *see* Neoplasm, benign, by site
Mesophlebitis *see* Phlebitis
Mesostromal dysgenesia Q13.89
Mesothelioma (malignant) C45.9
  |benign
    |mesentery D19.1
    |mesocolon D19.1
    |omentum D19.1
    |peritoneum D19.1
    |pleura D19.0
    |specified site NEC D19.7
    |unspecified site D19.9
  |biphasic C45.9
    |benign
      |mesentery D19.1
      |mesocolon D19.1
      |omentum D19.1
      |peritoneum D19.1
      |pleura D19.0
      |specified site NEC D19.7
      |unspecified site D19.9
  |cystic D48.4
  |epithelioid C45.9
    |benign
      |mesentery D19.1
      |mesocolon D19.1
      |omentum D19.1
      |peritoneum D19.1
      |pleura D19.0
      |specified site NEC D19.7
      |unspecified site D19.9
  |fibrous C45.9
    |benign
      |mesentery D19.1
      |mesocolon D19.1
      |omentum D19.1
      |peritoneum D19.1
      |pleura D19.0
      |specified site NEC D19.7
      |unspecified site D19.9
  |site classification
    |liver C45.7
    |lung C45.7
    |mediastinum C45.7
    |mesentery C45.1
    |mesocolon C45.1
    |omentum C45.1
    |pericardium C45.2
    |peritoneum C45.1
    |pleura C45.0
      |parietal C45.0
    |retroperitoneum C45.7
    |specified site NEC C45.7
    |unspecified C45.9
Metabolic syndrome E88.81
Metagonimiasis B66.8
Metagonimus infestation (intestine) B66.8
Metal
  |pigmentation L81.8
  |polisher's disease J62.8
Metamorphopsia H53.15

Metaplasia
  |apocrine (breast) *see* Dysplasia, mammary,
    specified type NEC
  |cervix (squamous) *see* Dysplasia, cervix
  |endometrium (squamous) (uterus) N85.8
  |esophagus K22.7-
  |gastric intestinal K31.A0
    |with dysplasia K31.A29
      |high grade K31.A22
      |low grade K31.A21
    |indefinite for dysplasia K31.A0
    |without dysplasia K31.A19
      |involving
        |antrum K31.A11
        |body (corpus) K31.A12
        |cardia K31.A14
        |fundus K31.A13
        |multiple sites K31.A15
  |kidney (pelvis) (squamous) N28.89
  |myelogenous D73.1
  |myeloid (agnogenic) (megakaryocytic) D73.1
  |spleen D73.1
  |squamous cell, bladder N32.89
Metastasis, metastatic
  |abscess *see* Abscess
  |calcification E83.59
  |cancer
    |from specified site *see* Neoplasm,
      malignant, by site
    |to specified site *see* Neoplasm, secondary,
      by site
  |deposits (in) *see* Neoplasm, secondary, by site
  |disease *see also* Neoplasm, secondary, by site
    C79.9
  |spread (to) *see* Neoplasm, secondary, by site
Metastrongyliasis B83.8
Metatarsalgia M77.4-
  |anterior G57.6-
  |Morton's G57.6-
Metatarsus, metatarsal *see also* condition
  |adductus, congenital Q66.22
  |valgus (abductus), congenital Q66.6
  |varus (congenital) Q66.22
    |primus Q66.21
Methadone use *see* Use, opioid
Methemoglobinemia D74.9
  |acquired (with sulfhemoglobinemia) D74.8
  |congenital D74.0
  |enzymatic (congenital) D74.0
  |Hb M disease D74.0
  |hereditary D74.0
  |toxic D74.8
Methemoglobinuria *see* Hemoglobinuria
Methioninemia E72.19
Methylmalonic acidemia E71.120
Metritis (catarrhal) (hemorrhagic) (septic)
  (suppurative) *see also* Endometritis
  |cervical *see* Cervicitis
Metropathia hemorrhagica N93.8
Metroperitonitis *see* Peritonitis, pelvic, female
Metrorrhagia N92.1
  |climacteric N92.4
  |menopausal N92.4
  |postpartum NEC (atonic) (following delivery
    of placenta) O72.1
    |delayed or secondary O72.2
  |preclimacteric or premenopausal N92.4
  |psychogenic F45.8
Metrorrhexis *see* Rupture, uterus
Metrosalpingitis N70.91
Metrostaxis N93.8
Metrovaginitis *see* Endometritis
Meyer-Schwickerath and Weyers syndrome
  Q87.0

Meynert's amentia (nonalcoholic) F04
  |alcoholic F10.96
    |with dependence F10.26
Mibelli's disease (porokeratosis) Q82.8
Mice, joint see Loose, body, joint
  |knee M23.4-
Micrencephalon, micrencephaly Q02
Microalbuminuria R80.9
Microaneurysm, retinal see also Disorder,
  retina, microaneurysms
  |diabetic see E08-E13 with .31
Microangiopathy (peripheral) I73.9
  |thrombotic M31.10
    |hematopoietic stem cell transplantation-
  associated [HSCT-TMA] M31.10
Microcalcifications, breast R92.0
Microcephalus, microcephalic, microcephaly
  Q02
  |due to toxoplasmosis (congenital) P37.1
Microcheilia Q18.7
Microcolon (congenital) Q43.8
Microcornea (congenital) Q13.4
Microcytic see condition **Microdeletions NEC**
  Q93.88
Microdontia K00.2
Microdrepanocytosis D57.40
  |with
    |acute chest syndrome D57.411
    |cerebral vascular involvement D57.413
    |crisis (painful) D57.419
      |with specified complication NEC
      D57.418
    |splenic sequestration D57.412
    |vasoocclusive pain D57.419
Microembolism
  |atherothrombotic see Atheroembolism
  |retinal see Occlusion, artery, retina
Microencephalon Q02
Microfilaria streptocerca infestation see
  Onchocerciasis
Microgastria (congenital) Q40.2
Microgenia M26.06
Microgenitalia, congenital
  |female Q52.8
  |male Q55.8
Microglioma see Lymphoma, non-hodgkin,
  specified NEC
Microglossia (congenital) Q38.3
Micrognathia, micrognathism (congenital)
  (mandibular) (maxillary) M26.09
Microgyria (congenital) Q04.3
Microinfarct of heart see Insufficiency,
  coronary
Microlentia (congenital) Q12.8
Microlithiasis, alveolar, pulmonary J84.02
Micromastia N64.82
Micromyelia (congenital) Q06.8
Micropenis Q55.62
Microphakia (congenital) Q12.8
Microphthalmos, microphthalmia
  (congenital) Q11.2
  |due to toxoplasmosis P37.1
Micropsia H53.15
Microscopic polyangiitis (polyarteritis) M31.7
Microsporidiosis B60.8
  |intestinal A07.8
Microsporon furfur infestation B36.0
Microsporosis see also Dermatophytosis
  |nigra B36.1
Microstomia (congenital) Q18.5
Microtia (congenital) (external ear) Q17.2
Microtropia H50.40
Microvillus inclusion disease (MVD) (MVID)
  Q43.8
Micturition

Micturition - continued
  |disorder NEC see also Difficulty, micturition
  R39.198
    |psychogenic F45.8
  |frequency R35.0
    |psychogenic F45.8
  |hesitancy R39.11
  |incomplete emptying R39.14
  |nocturnal R35.1
  |painful R30.9
    |dysuria R30.0
    |psychogenic F45.8
    |tenesmus R30.1
  |poor stream R39.12
  |position dependent R39.192
  |split stream R39.13
  |straining R39.16
  |urgency R39.15
Mid plane see condition
Middle
  |ear see condition
  |lobe (right) syndrome J98.19
Miescher's elastoma L87.2
Mietens' syndrome Q87.2
Migraine (idiopathic) G43.909
  |with refractory migraine G43.919
    |with status migrainosus G43.911
    |without status migrainosus G43.919
  |with aura (acute-onset) (prolonged) (typical)
  (without headache) G43.109
    |with refractory migraine G43.119
      |with status migrainosus G43.111
      |without status migrainosus G43.119
    |intractable G43.119
      |with status migrainosus G43.111
      |without status migrainosus G43.119
    |not intractable G43.109
      |with status migrainosus G43.101
      |without status migrainosus G43.109
    |persistent G43.509
      |with cerebral infarction G43.609
        |with refractory migraine G43.619
          |with status migrainosus G43.611
          |without status migrainosus G43.619
        |intractable G43.619
          |with status migrainosus G43.611
          |without status migrainosus G43.619
        |not intractable G43.609
          |with status migrainosus G43.601
          |without status migrainosus G43.609
        |without refractory migraine G43.609
          |with status migrainosus G43.601
          |without status migrainosus G43.609
      |without cerebral infarction G43.509
        |with refractory migraine G43.519
          |with status migrainosus G43.511
          |without status migrainosus G43.519
        |intractable G43.519
          |with status migrainosus G43.511
          |without status migrainosus G43.519
        |not intractable G43.509
          |with status migrainosus G43.501
          |without status migrainosus G43.509
        |without refractory migraine G43.509
          |with status migrainosus G43.501
          |without status migrainosus G43.509
    |without mention of refractory migraine
    G43.109
      |with status migrainosus G43.101
      |without status migrainosus G43.109
  |abdominal G43.D0
    |with refractory migraine G43.D1
    |intractable G43.D1
    |not intractable G43.D0
    |without refractory migraine G43.D0

Migraine - continued
  |basilar see Migraine, with aura
  |classical see Migraine, with aura
  |common see Migraine, without aura
  |complicated G43.109
  |equivalents see Migraine, with aura
  |familiar see Migraine, hemiplegic
  |hemiplegic G43.409
    |with refractory migraine G43.419
      |with status migrainosus G43.411
      |without status migrainosus G43.419
    |intractable G43.419
      |with status migrainosus G43.411
      |without status migrainosus G43.419
    |not intractable G43.409
      |with status migrainosus G43.401
      |without status migrainosus G43.409
    |without refractory migraine G43.409
      |with status migrainosus G43.401
      |without status migrainosus G43.409
  |intractable G43.919
    |with status migrainosus G43.911
    |without status migrainosus G43.919
  |menstrual G43.829
    |with refractory migraine G43.839
      |with status migrainosus G43.831
      |without status migrainosus G43.839
    |intractable G43.839
      |with status migrainosus G43.831
      |without status migrainosus G43.839
    |not intractable G43.829
      |with status migrainosus G43.821
      |without status migrainosus G43.829
    |without refractory migraine G43.829
      |with status migrainosus G43.821
      |without status migrainosus G43.829
  |menstrually related see Migraine, menstrual
  |not intractable G43.909
    |with status migrainosus G43.901
    |without status migrainosus G43.919
  |ophthalmoplegic G43.B0
    |with refractory migraine G43.B1
    |intractable G43.B1
    |not intractable G43.B0
    |without refractory migraine G43.B0
  |persistent aura (with, without) cerebral
  infarction see Migraine, with aura, persistent
  |preceded or accompanied by transient focal
  neurological phenomena see Migraine, with
  aura
  |pre-menstrual see Migraine, menstrual
  |pure menstrual see Migraine, menstrual
  |retinal see Migraine, with aura
  |specified NEC G43.809
    |intractable G43.819
      |with status migrainosus G43.811
      |without status migrainosus G43.819
    |not intractable G43.809
      |with status migrainosus G43.801
      |without status migrainosus G43.809
  |sporadic see Migraine, hemiplegic
  |transformed see Migraine, without aura,
  chronic
  |triggered seizures see Migraine, with aura
  |without aura G43.009
    |with refractory migraine G43.019
      |with status migrainosus G43.011
      |without status migrainosus G43.019
    |chronic G43.709
      |with refractory migraine G43.719
        |with status migrainosus G43.711
        |without status migrainosus G43.719
      |intractable
        |with status migrainosus G43.711
        |without status migrainosus G43.719

Migraine - *continued*
|not intractable
||with status migrainosus G43.701
||without status migrainosus G43.709
|without refractory migraine G43.709
||with status migrainosus G43.701
||without status migrainosus G43.709
|intractable
||with status migrainosus G43.011
||without status migrainosus G43.019
|not intractable
||with status migrainosus G43.001
||without status migrainosus G43.009
|without mention of refractory migraine
|| G43.009
||with status migrainosus G43.001
||without status migrainosus G43.009
|without refractory migraineG43.909
||with status migrainosus G43.901
||without status migrainosus G43.919
Migrant, social Z59.00
Migration, anxiety concerning Z60.3
Migratory, migrating *see also* condition
|person Z59.00
|testis Q55.29
Mikity-Wilson disease or syndrome P27.0
Mikulicz' disease or syndrome K11.8
Miliaria L74.3
|alba L74.1
|apocrine L75.2
|crystallina L74.1
|profunda L74.2
|rubra L74.0
|tropicalis L74.2
Miliary *see* condition
Milium L72.0
|colloid L57.8
Milk
|crust L21.0
|excessive secretion O92.6
|poisoning *see* Poisoning, food, noxious
|retention O92.79
|sickness *see* Poisoning, food, noxious
|spots I31.0
Milk-Alkali disease or syndrome E83.52
Milk-Leg (deep vessels) (nonpuerperal) *see*
Embolism, vein, lower extremity
|complicating pregnancy O22.3-
|puerperal, postpartum, childbirth O87.1
Milkman's disease or syndrome M83.8
Milky urine *see* Chyluria
Millard-Gubler (-Foville) paralysis or
syndrome G46.3
Millar's asthma J38.5
Miller Fisher syndrome G61.0
Mills' disease *see* Hemiplegia
Millstone maker's pneumoconiosis J62.8
Milroy's disease (chronic hereditary edema)
Q82.0
Minamata disease T56.1
Miners' asthma or lung J60
Minkowski-Chauffard syndrome *see*
Spherocytosis
Minor *see* condition
Minor's disease (hematomyelia) G95.19
Minot's disease (hemorrhagic disease),
newborn P53
Minot-Von Willebrand-Jurgens disease or
syndrome (angiohemophilia) D68.0
Minus (and plus) hand (intrinsic) *see*
Deformity, limb, specified type NEC, forearm
Miosis (pupil) H57.03
Mirizzi's syndrome (hepatic duct stenosis)
K83.1
Mirror writing F81.0

Misadventure (of) (prophylactic)
(therapeutic) *see also* Complications T88.9
|administration of insulin (by accident) *see*
subcategory T38.3
|infusion *see* Complications, infusion
|local applications (of fomentations, plasters,
etc.) T88.9
||burn or scald *see* Burn
||specified NEC T88.8
|medical care (early) (late) T88.9
||adverse effect of drugs or chemicals *see*
Table of Drugs and Chemicals
|medical care (early) (late)
||burn or scald *see* Burn
||specified NEC T88.8
|specified NEC T88.8
|surgical procedure (early) (late) *see*
Complications, surgical procedure
|transfusion *see* Complications, transfusion
|vaccination or other immunological procedure
see Complications, vaccination
Miscarriage O03.9
Misdirection, aqueous H40.83-
Misperception, sleep state F51.02
Misplaced, misplacement
|ear Q17.4
|kidney (acquired) N28.89
||congenital Q63.2
|organ or site, congenital NEC *see*
Malposition, congenital
Missed
|abortion O02.1
|delivery O36.4
Missing *see also* Absence
|string of intrauterine contraceptive device
T83.32
Misuse of drugs F19.99
Mitchell's disease (erythromelalgia) I73.81
Mite(s) (infestation) B88.9
|diarrhea B88.0
|grain (itch) B88.0
|hair follicle (itch) B88.0
|in sputum B88.0
Mitral *see* condition **Mittelschmerz** N94.0
Mixed *see* condition
MMN (multifocal motor neuropathy) G61.82
MNGIE (Mitochondrial Neurogastrointestinal
Encephalopathy) syndrome E88.49
Mobile, mobility
|cecum Q43.3
|excessive *see* Hypermobility
|gallbladder, congenital Q44.1
|kidney N28.89
|organ or site, congenital NEC *see*
Malposition, congenital
Mobitz heart block (atrioventricular) I44.1
Moebius, Möbius
|disease (ophthalmoplegic migraine) *see*
Migraine, ophthalmoplegic
|syndrome Q87.0
||congenital oculofacial paralysis (with other
anomalies) Q87.0
||ophthalmoplegic migraine *see* Migraine,
ophthalmoplegic
Moeller's glossitis K14.0
Mohr's syndrome (Types I and II) Q87.0
Mola destruens D39.2
Molar pregnancy O02.0
Molarization of premolars K00.2
Molding, head (during birth) omit code
Mole (pigmented) *see also* Nevus
|blood O02.0
|Breus' O02.0
|cancerous *see* Melanoma
|carneous O02.0

Mole (pigmented) - *continued*
|destructive D39.2
|fleshy O02.0
|hydatid, hydatidiform (benign) (complicating
pregnancy) (delivered) (undelivered) O01.9
||classical O01.0
||complete O01.0
||incomplete O01.1
||invasive D39.2
||malignant D39.2
||partial O01.1
|intrauterine O02.0
|invasive (hydatidiform) D39.2
|malignant
||meaning
|||malignant hydatidiform mole D39.2
|||melanoma *see* Melanoma
|nonhydatidiform O02.0
|nonpigmented *see* Nevus
|pregnancy NEC O02.0
|skin *see* Nevus
|tubal O00.10-
||with intrauterine pregnancy O00.11-
|vesicular *see* Mole, hydatidiform
Molimen, molimina (menstrual) N94.3
Molluscum contagiosum (epitheliale) B08.1
Mönckeberg's arteriosclerosis, disease, or
sclerosis *see* Arteriosclerosis, extremities
Mondini's malformation (cochlea) Q16.5
Mondor's disease I80.8
Monge's disease T70.29
Monilethrix (congenital) Q84.1
Moniliasis *see also* Candidiasis B37.9
|neonatal P37.5
Monitoring (encounter for)
|therapeutic drug level Z51.81
Monkey malaria B53.1
Monkeypox B04
Monoarthritis M13.10
|ankle M13.17-
|elbow M13.12-
|foot joint M13.17-
|hand joint M13.14-
|hip M13.15-
|knee M13.16-
|shoulder M13.11-
|wrist M13.13-
Monoblastic *see* condition
Monochromat (ism), monochromatopsia
(acquired) (congenital) H53.51
Monocytic *see* condition
Monocytopenia D72.818
Monocytopenia D72.818
Monocytosis (symptomatic) D72.821
Monomania *see* Psychosis
Mononeuritis G58.9
|cranial nerve *see* Disorder, nerve, cranial
|femoral nerve G57.2-
|lateral
||cutaneous nerve of thigh G57.1-
||popliteal nerve G57.3-
|lower limb G57.9-
||specified nerve NEC G57.8-
|medial popliteal nerve G57.4-
|median nerve G56.1-
|multiplex G58.7
|plantar nerve G57.6-
|posterior tibial nerve G57.5-
|radial nerve G56.3-
|sciatic nerve G57.0-
|specified NEC G58.8
|tibial nerve G57.4-
|ulnar nerve G56.2-
|upper limb G56.9-
||specified nerve NEC G56.8-
|vestibular *see* subcategory H93.3

Mononeuropathy G58.9
|carpal tunnel syndrome *see* Syndrome, carpal
tunnel
|diabetic NEC *see* E08-E13 with .41
|femoral nerve *see* Lesion, nerve, femoral
|ilioinguinal nerve G57.8-
|in diseases classified elsewhere *see* category
G59
|intercostal G58.0
|lower limb G57.9-
|causalgia *see* Causalgia, lower limb
|femoral nerve *see* Lesion, nerve, femoral
|meralgia paresthetica G57.1-
|plantar nerve *see* Lesion, nerve, plantar
|popliteal nerve *see* Lesion, nerve, popliteal
|sciatic nerve *see* Lesion, nerve, sciatic
|specified NEC G57.8-
|tarsal tunnel syndrome *see* Syndrome, tarsal
tunnel
|median nerve *see* Lesion, nerve, median
|multiplex G58.7
|obturator nerve G57.8-
|popliteal nerve *see* Lesion, nerve, popliteal
|radial nerve *see* Lesion, nerve, radial
|saphenous nerve G57.8-
|specified NEC G58.8
|tarsal tunnel syndrome *see* Syndrome, tarsal
tunnel
|tuberculous A17.83
|ulnar nerve *see* Lesion, nerve, ulnar
|upper limb G56.9-
|carpal tunnel syndrome *see* Syndrome,
carpal tunnel
|causalgia *see* Causalgia
|median nerve *see* Lesion, nerve, median
|radial nerve *see* Lesion, nerve, radial
|specified site NEC G56.8-
|ulnar nerve *see* Lesion, nerve, ulnar
Mononucleosis, infectious B27.90
|with
|complication NEC B27.99
|meningitis B27.92
|polyneuropathy B27.91
|cytomegaloviral B27.10
|with
|complication NEC B27.19
|meningitis B27.12
|polyneuropathy B27.11
|Epstein-Barr (virus) B27.00
|with
|complication NEC B27.09
|meningitis B27.02
|polyneuropathy B27.01
|gammaherpesviral B27.00
|with
|complication NEC B27.09
|meningitis B27.02
|polyneuropathy B27.01
|specified NEC B27.80
|with
|complication NEC B27.89
|meningitis B27.82
|polyneuropathy B27.81
Monoplegia G83.3-
|congenital (cerebral) G80.8
|spastic G80.1
|embolic (current episode) I63.4-
|following
|cerebrovascular disease
|cerebral infarction
|lower limb I69.34-
|upper limb I69.33-
|intracerebral hemorrhage
|lower limb I69.14-
|upper limb I69.13-

Monoplegia - *continued*
|lower limb I69.94-
|nontraumatic intracranial hemorrhage
NEC
|lower limb I69.24-
|upper limb I69.23-
|specified disease NEC
|lower limb I69.84-
|upper limb I69.83-
|stroke NOS
|lower limb I69.34-
|upper limb I69.33-
|subarachnoid hemorrhage
|lower limb I69.04-
|upper limb I69.03-
|upper limb I69.93-
|hysterical (transient) F44.4
|lower limb G83.1-
|psychogenic (conversion reaction) F44.4
|thrombotic (current episode) I63.3-
|transient R29.818
|upper limb G83.2-
Monorchism, monorchidism Q55.0
Monosomy *see also* Deletion, chromosome
Q93.9
|specified NEC Q93.89
|whole chromosome
|meiotic nondisjunction Q93.0
|mitotic nondisjunction Q93.1
|mosaicism Q93.1
|X Q96.9
Monster, monstrosity (single) Q89.7
|acephalic Q00.0
|twin Q89.4
Monteggia's fracture (-Dislocation) S52.27-
Mooren's ulcer (cornea) *see* Ulcer, cornea,
Mooren's
Moore's syndrome *see* Epilepsy, specified NEC
Mooser Neill reaction A75.2
Mooser's bodies A75.2
Morbidity not stated or unknown R69
Morbilli *see* Measles
Morbus *see also* Disease
|angelicus, anglorum E55.0
|Beigel B36.2
|caducus *see* Epilepsy
|celiacus K90.0
|comitialis *see* Epilepsy
|cordis *see also* Disease, heart I51.9
|valvulorum *see* Endocarditis
|coxae senilis M16.9
|tuberculous A18.02
|hemorrhagicus neonatorum P53
|maculosus neonatorum P54.5
Morel (-Stewart)(-Morgagni) syndrome M85.2
Morel-Kraepelin disease *see* Schizophrenia
Morel-Moore syndrome M85.2
Morgagni's
|cyst, organ, hydatid, or appendage
|female Q50.5
|male (epididymal) Q55.4
|testicular Q55.29
|syndrome M85.2
Morgagni-Stokes-Adams syndrome I45.9
Morgagni-Stewart-Morel syndrome M85.2
Morgagni-Turner (-Albright) syndrome Q96.9
Moria F07.0
Moron (I.Q.50-69) F70
Morphea L94.0
Morphinism (without remission) F11.20
|with remission F11.21
Morphinomania (without remission) F11.20
|with remission F11.21
Morquio (-Ullrich)(-Brailsford) disease or
syndrome *see* Mucopolysaccharidosis

Mortification (dry) (moist) *see* Gangrene
Morton's metatarsalgia (neuralgia)(neuroma)
(syndrome) G57.6-
Morvan's disease or syndrome G60.8
Mosaicism, mosaic (autosomal)
(chromosomal)
|45,X/other cell lines NEC with abnormal sex
chromosome Q96.4
|45,X/46,XX Q96.3
|sex chromosome
|female Q97.8
|lines with various numbers of X
chromosomes Q97.2
|male Q98.7
|XY Q96.3
Moschowitz' disease M31.19
Mother yaw A66.0
Motion sickness (from travel, any vehicle)
(from roundabouts or swings) T75.3
Mottled, mottling, teeth (enamel) (endemic)
(nonendemic) K00.3
Mounier-Kuhn syndrome Q32.4
|with bronchiectasis J47.9
|exacerbation (acute) J47.1
|lower respiratory infection J47.0
|acquired J98.09
|with bronchiectasis J47.9
|with
|exacerbation (acute) J47.1
|lower respiratory infection J47.0
Mountain
|sickness T70.29
|with polycythemia , acquired (acute) D75.1
|tick fever A93.2
Mouse, joint *see* Loose, body, joint
|knee M23.4-
Mouth *see* condition **Movable**
|coccyx *see* subcategory M53.2
|kidney N28.89
|congenital Q63.8
|spleen D73.89
Movements, dystonic R25.8
Moyamoya disease I67.5
MRSA (Methicillin resistant Staphylococcus
aureus)
|infection A49.02
|as the cause of diseases classified elsewhere
B95.62
|sepsis A41.02
MSD (multiple sulfatase deficiency) E75.26
MSSA (Methicillin susceptible Staphylococcus
aureus)
|infection A49.01
|as the cause of diseases classified elsewhere
B95.61
|sepsis A41.01
Mucha-Habermann disease L41.0
Mucinosis (cutaneous) (focal) (papular)
(reticular erythematous) (skin) L98.5
|oral K13.79
Mucocele
|appendix K38.8
|buccal cavity K13.79
|gallbladder K82.1
|lacrimal sac, chronic H04.43-
|nasal sinus J34.1
|nose J34.1
|salivary gland (any) K11.6
|sinus (accessory) (nasal) J34.1
|turbinate (bone) (middle) (nasal) J34.1
|uterus N85.8
Mucolipidosis
|I E77.1
|II, III E77.0
|IV E75.11

Mucopolysaccharidosis E76.3
  |beta-gluduronidase deficiency E76.29
  |cardiopathy E76.3 *[I52]*
  |Hunter's syndrome E76.1
  |Hurler's syndrome E76.01
  |Hurler-Scheie syndrome E76.02
  |Maroteaux-Lamy syndrome E76.29
  |Morquio syndrome E76.219
    |A E76.210
    |B E76.211
    |classic E76.210
  |Sanfilippo syndrome E76.22
  |Scheie's syndrome E76.03
  |specified NEC E76.29
  |type
    |I
      |Hurler's syndrome E76.01
      |Hurler-Scheie syndrome E76.02
      |Scheie's syndrome E76.03
    |II E76.1
    |III E76.22
    |IV E76.219
    |IVA E76.210
    |IVB E76.211
    |VI E76.29
    |VII E76.29
Mucormycosis B46.5
  |cutaneous B46.3
  |disseminated B46.4
  |gastrointestinal B46.2
  |generalized B46.4
  |pulmonary B46.0
  |rhinocerebral B46.1
  |skin B46.3
  |subcutaneous B46.3
Mucositis (ulcerative) K12.30
  |due to drugs NEC K12.32
  |gastrointestinal K92.81
  |mouth (oral) (oropharyngeal) K12.30
    |due to antineoplastic therapy K12.31
    |due to drugs NEC K12.32
    |due to radiation K12.33
    |specified NEC K12.39
    |viral K12.39
  |nasal J34.81
  |oral cavity *see* Mucositis, mouth
  |oral soft tissues *see* Mucositis, mouth
  |vagina and vulva N76.81
Mucositis necroticans agranulocytica *see*
  Agranulocytosis
Mucous *see also* condition
  |patches (syphilitic) A51.39
    |congenital A50.07
Mucoviscidosis E84.9
  |with meconium obstruction E84.11
Mucus
  |asphyxia or suffocation *see* Asphyxia, mucus
  |in stool R19.5
  |plug *see* Asphyxia, mucus
Muguet B37.0
Mulberry molars (congenital syphilis) A50.52
Müllerian mixed tumor
  |specified site *see* Neoplasm, malignant, by site
  |unspecified site C54.9
Multicystic kidney (development) Q61.4
Multiparity (grand) Z64.1
  |affecting management of pregnancy, labor and
    delivery (supervision only) O09.4-
  |requiring contraceptive management *see*
    Contraception
Multipartita placenta O43.19-
**Multisystem inflammatory syndrome (in
  adult) (in children)** M35.81
Multiple, multiplex *see also* condition
  |digits (congenital) Q69.9
  |endocrine neoplasia *see* Neoplasia, endocrine,
    multiple (MEN)
  |personality F44.81

Mumps B26.9
  |arthritis B26.85
  |complication NEC B26.89
  |encephalitis B26.2
  |hepatitis B26.81
  |meningitis (aseptic) B26.1
  |meningoencephalitis B26.2
  |myocarditis B26.82
  |oophoritis B26.89
  |orchitis B26.0
  |pancreatitis B26.3
  |polyneuropathy B26.84
Mumu *see also* Infestation, filarial B74.9 *[N51]*
Münchhausen's syndrome *see* Disorder,
  factitious
Münchmeyer's syndrome *see* Myositis,
  ossificans, progressiva
Mural *see* condition
Murmur (cardiac) (heart) (organic) R01.1
  |abdominal R19.15
  |aortic (valve) *see* Endocarditis, aortic
  |benign R01.0
  |diastolic *see* Endocarditis
  |Flint I35.1
  |functional R01.0
  |Graham Steell I37.1
  |innocent R01.0
  |mitral (valve) *see* Insufficiency, mitral
  |nonorganic R01.0
  |presystolic, mitral *see* Insufficiency, mitral
  |pulmonic (valve) I37.8
  |systolic R01.1
  |tricuspid (valve) I07.9
  |valvular *see* Endocarditis
Murri's disease (intermittent hemoglobinuria)
  D59.6
Muscle, muscular *see also* condition
  |carnitine (palmitoyltransferase) deficiency
    E71.314
Musculoneuralgia *see* Neuralgia
**Mushroom-Workers' (pickers') disease or
  lung** J67.5
Mushrooming hip *see* Derangement, joint,
  specified NEC, hip
Mutation(s)
  |factor V Leiden D68.51
  |surfactant, of lung J84.83
  |prothrombin gene D68.52
Mutism *see also* Aphasia
  |deaf (acquired) (congenital) NEC H91.3
  |elective (adjustment reaction) (childhood)
    F94.0
  |hysterical F44.4
  |selective (childhood) F94.0
MVD (microvillus inclusion disease) Q43.8
MVID (microvillus inclusion disease) Q43.8
Myalgia M79.10
  |auxiliary muscles, head and neck M79.12
  |epidemic (cervical) B33.0
  |mastication muscle M79.11
  |site specified NEC M79.18
  |traumatic NEC T14.8
Myasthenia G70.9
  |congenital G70.2
  |cordis *see* Failure, heart
  |developmental G70.2
  |gravis G70.00
    |with exacerbation (acute) G70.01
    |in crisis G70.01
    |neonatal, transient P94.0
    |pseudoparalytica G70.00
      |with exacerbation (acute) G70.01
      |in crisis G70.01
  |stomach, psychogenic F45.8
  |syndrome

Myasthenia - *continued*
  |in
    |diabetes mellitus *see* E08-E13 with .44
    |neoplastic disease *see also* Neoplasm
      D49.9 *[G73.3]*
    |pernicious anemia D51.0 *[G73.3]*
    |thyrotoxicosis E05.90 *[G73.3]*
      |with thyroid storm E05.91 *[G73.3]*
Myasthenic M62.81
Mycelium infection B49
Mycetismus *see* Poisoning, food, noxious,
  mushroom
Mycetoma B47.9
  |actinomycotic B47.1
  |bone (mycotic) B47.9 *[M90.80]*
  |eumycotic B47.0
  |foot B47.9
    |actinomycotic B47.1
    |mycotic B47.0
  |madurae NEC B47.9
    |mycotic B47.0
  |maduromycotic B47.0
  |mycotic B47.0
  |nocardial B47.1
Mycobacteriosis *see* Mycobacterium
Mycobacterium, mycobacterial (infection)
  A31.9
  |anonymous A31.9
  |atypical A31.9
    |cutaneous A31.1
    |pulmonary A31.0
      |tuberculous *see* Tuberculosis, pulmonary
    |specified site NEC A31.8
  |avium (intracellulare complex) A31.0
  |balnei A31.1
  |Battey A31.0
  |chelonei A31.8
  |cutaneous A31.1
  |extrapulmonary systemic A31.8
  |fortuitum A31.8
  |intracellulare (Battey bacillus) A31.0
  |kansasii (yellow bacillus) A31.0
  |kakaferifu A31.8
  |kasongo A31.8
  |leprae *see also* Leprosy A30.9
  |luciflavum A31.1
  |marinum (M. balnei) A31.1
  |nonspecific *see* Mycobacterium, atypical
  |pulmonary (atypical) A31.0
    |tuberculous *see* Tuberculosis, pulmonary
  |scrofulaceum A31.8
  |simiae A31.8
  |systemic, extrapulmonary A31.8
  |szulgai A31.8
  |terrae A31.8
  |triviale A31.8
  |tuberculosis (human, bovine) *see* Tuberculosis
  |ulcerans A31.1
  |xenopi A31.8
**Mycoplasma (M.) pneumoniae, as cause of
  disease classified elsewhere** B96.0
Mycosis, mycotic B49
  |cutaneous NEC B36.9
  |ear B36.9
    |in
      |aspergillosis B44.89
      |candidiasis B37.84
      |moniliasis B37.84
  |fungoides (extranodal) (solid organ) C84.0-
  |mouth B37.0
  |nails B35.1
  |opportunistic B48.8
  |skin NEC B36.9
  |specified NEC B48.8
  |stomatitis B37.0
  |vagina, vaginitis (candidal) B37.3

Mydriasis (pupil) H57.04
Myelatelia Q06.1
Myelinolysis, pontine, central G37.2
Myelitis (acute) (ascending) (childhood)
    (chronic) (descending) (diffuse)
    (disseminated) (idiopathic) (pressure)
    (progressive) (spinal cord) (subacute) *see*
    also Encephalitis G04.91
  |flaccid G04.82
  |herpes simplex B00.82
  |herpes zoster B02.24
  |in diseases classified elsewhere G05.4
  |necrotizing, subacute G37.4
  |optic neuritis in G36.0
  |post chickenpox B01.12
  |postherpetic B02.24
  |postimmunization G04.02
  |postinfectious NEC G04.89
  |postvaccinal G04.02
  |specified NEC G04.89
  |syphilitic (transverse) A52.14
  |toxic G92.9
  |transverse (in demyelinating diseases of
    central nervous system) G37.3
  |tuberculous A17.82
  |varicella B01.12
Myeloblastic *see* condition
Myeloblastoma
  |granular cell *see also* Neoplasm, connective
    tissue
    |malignant *see* Neoplasm, connective tissue,
      malignant
    |tongue D10.1
Myelocele *see* Spina bifida
Myelocystocele *see* Spina bifida
Myelocytic *see* condition
Myelodysplasia D46.9
  |specified NEC D46.Z
  |spinal cord (congenital) Q06.1
Myelodysplastic syndrome (see also Syndrome,
  myelodysplastic**)** D46.9
  |with
    |5q deletion D46.C
    |isolated del (5q) chromosomal abnormality
      D46.C
  |specified NEC D46.Z
Myeloencephalitis *see* Encephalitis
Myelofibrosis D75.81
  |with myeloid metaplasia D47.4
  |acute C94.4-
  |idiopathic (chronic) D47.4
  |primary D47.1
  |secondary D75.81
    |in myeloproliferative disease D47.4
Myelogenous *see* condition
Myeloid *see* condition
Myelokathexis D70.9
Myeloleukodystrophy E75.29
Myelolipoma *see* Lipoma
Myeloma (multiple) C90.0-
  |monostotic C90.3
    |plasma cell C90.0-
  |plasma cell C90.0-
  |solitary *see also* Plasmacytoma, solitary
    C90.3-
Myelomalacia G95.89
Myelomatosis C90.0-
Myelomeningitis *see* Meningoencephalitis
Myelomeningocele (spinal cord) *see* Spina
  bifida
Myelo-Osteo-Musculodysplasia hereditaria
  Q79.8
Myelopathic
  |anemia D64.89
  |muscle atrophy *see* Atrophy, muscle, spinal
  |pain syndrome G89.0

Myelopathy (spinal cord) G95.9
  |drug-induced G95.89
  |in (due to)
    |degeneration or displacement, intervertebral
      disc NEC *see* Disorder, disc, with,
      myelopathy
    |infection *see* Encephalitis
    |intervertebral disc disorder *see also*
      Disorder, disc, with, myelopathy
    |mercury *see* subcategory T56.1
    |neoplastic disease *see also* Neoplasm D49.9
      [*G99.2*]
    pernicious anemia D51.0 [*G99.2*]
    |spondylosis *see* Spondylosis, with
      myelopathy NEC
  |necrotic (subacute) (vascular) G95.19
  |radiation-induced G95.89
  |spondylogenic NEC *see* Spondylosis, with
    myelopathy NEC
  |toxic G95.89
  |transverse, acute G37.3
  |vascular G95.19
  |vitamin B12 E53.8 [*G32.0*]
Myelophthisis D61.82
Myeloradiculitis G04.91
Myeloradiculodysplasia (spinal) Q06.1
Myelosarcoma C92.3-
Myelosclerosis D75.89
  |with myeloid metaplasia D47.4
  |disseminated, of nervous system G35
  |megakaryocytic D47.4
    |with myeloid metaplasia D47.4
Myelosis
  |acute C92.0-
  |aleukemic C92.9-
  |chronic D47.1
  |erythremic (acute) C94.0-
  |megakaryocytic C94.2-
  |nonleukemic D72.828
  |subacute C92.9-
Myiasis (cavernous) B87.9
  |aural B87.4
  |creeping B87.0
  |cutaneous B87.0
  |dermal B87.0
  |ear (external) (middle) B87.4
  |eye B87.2
  |genitourinary B87.81
  |intestinal B87.82
  |laryngeal B87.3
  |nasopharyngeal B87.3
  |ocular B87.2
  |orbit B87.2
  |skin B87.0
  |specified site NEC B87.89
  |traumatic B87.1
  |wound B87.1
Myoadenoma, prostate *see* Hyperplasia,
  prostate
Myoblastoma
  |granular cell *see also* Neoplasm, connective
    tissue, benign
    |malignant *see* Neoplasm, connective tissue,
      malignant
  |tongue D10.1
Myocardial *see* condition
Myocardiopathy (congestive) (constrictive)
  (familial) (hypertrophic nonobstructive)
  (idiopathic) (infiltrative) (obstructive)
  (primary) (restrictive) (sporadic) *see also*
  Cardiomyopathy I42.9
  |alcoholic I42.6
  |cobalt-beer I42.6
  |glycogen storage E74.02 [*143*]
  |hypertrophic obstructive I42.1
  |in (due to)

Myocardiopathy - *continued*
  |beriberi E51.12
  |cardiac glycogenosis E74.02 [*143*]
  |Friedreich's ataxia G11.11 [*143*]
  |myotonia atrophica G71.11 [*143*]
  |progressive muscular dystrophy G71.09
    [*143*]
  |obscure (African) I42.8
  |secondary I42.9
  |thyrotoxic E05.90 [*143*]
    |with storm E05.91 [*143*]
  |toxic NEC I42.7
Myocarditis (with arteriosclerosis) (chronic)
  (fibroid) (interstitial) (old) (progressive)
  (senile) I51.4
  |with
    |rheumatic fever (conditions in I00) I09.0
      |active *see* Myocarditis, acute, rheumatic
      |inactive or quiescent (with chorea) I09.0
  |active I40.9
    |rheumatic I01.2
      |with chorea (acute) (rheumatic)
        (Sydenham's) I02.0
  |acute or subacute (interstitial) I40.9
    |due to
      |streptococcus (beta-hemolytic) I01.2
    |idiopathic I40.1
    |rheumatic I01.2
      |with chorea (acute) (rheumatic)
        (Sydenham's) I02.0
    |specified NEC I40.8
  |aseptic of newborn B33.22
  |bacterial (acute) I40.0
  |Coxsackie (virus) B33.22
  |diphtheritic A36.81
  |eosinophilic I40.1
  |epidemic of newborn (Coxsackie) B33.22
  |Fiedler's (acute) (isolated) I40.1
  |giant cell (acute) (subacute) I40.1
  |gonococcal A54.83
  |granulomatous (idiopathic) (isolated)
    (nonspecific) I40.1
  |hypertensive *see* Hypertension, heart
  |idiopathic (granulomatous) I40.1
  |in (due to)
    |diphtheria A36.81
    |epidemic louse-borne typhus A75.0 [*141*]
    |Lyme disease A69.29
    |sarcoidosis D86.85
    |scarlet fever A38.1
    |toxoplasmosis (acquired) B58.81
    |typhoid A01.02
    |typhus NEC A75.9 [*141*]
  |infective I40.0
  |influenzal *see* Influenza, with, myocarditis
  |isolated (acute) I40.1
  |meningococcal A39.52
  |mumps B26.82
  |nonrheumatic, active I40.9
  |parenchymatous I40.9
  |pneumococcal I40.0
  |rheumatic (chronic) (inactive) (with chorea)
    I09.0
    |active or acute I01.2
      |with chorea (acute) (rheumatic)
        (Sydenham's) I02.0
  |rheumatoid *see* Rheumatoid, carditis
  |septic I40.0
  |staphylococcal I40.0
  |suppurative I40.0
  |syphilitic (chronic) A52.06
  |toxic I40.8
    |rheumatic *see* Myocarditis, acute, rheumatic
  |tuberculous A18.84
  |typhoid A01.02
  |valvular *see* Endocarditis
  |virus, viral I40.0
    |of newborn (Coxsackie) B33.22

Myocardium, myocardial *see* condition
Myocardosis *see* Cardiomyopathy
Myoclonus, myoclonic, myoclonia (familial) (essential) (multifocal) (simplex) G25.3
|drug-induced G25.3
|epilepsy *see also* Epilepsy, generalized, specified NEC G40.4-
||familial (progressive) G25.3
|epileptica G40.409
||with status epilepticus G40.401
|facial G51.3-
|familial progressive G25.3
|Friedreich's G25.3
|jerks G25.3
|massive G25.3
|palatal G25.3
|pharyngeal G25.3
Myocytolysis I51.5
Myodiastasis *see* Diastasis, muscle
Myoendocarditis *see* Endocarditis
Myoepithelioma *see* Neoplasm, benign, by site
Myofasciitis (acute) *see* Myositis
Myofibroma *see also* Neoplasm, connective tissue, benign
|uterus (cervix) (corpus) *see* Leiomyoma
Myofibromatosis D48.1
|infantile Q89.8
Myofibrosis M62.89
|heart *see* Myocarditis
|scapulohumeral *see* Lesion, shoulder, specified NEC
Myofibrositis M79.7
|scapulohumeral *see* Lesion, shoulder, specified NEC
Myoglobulinuria, myoglobinuria (primary) R82.1
Myokymia, facial G51.4
Myolipoma *see* Lipoma
Myoma *see also* Neoplasm, connective tissue, benign
|malignant *see* Neoplasm, connective tissue, malignant
|prostate D29.1
|uterus (cervix) (corpus) *see* Leiomyoma
Myomalacia M62.89
Myometritis *see* Endometritis
Myometrium *see* condition
Myonecrosis, clostridial A48.0
Myopathy G72.9
|acute
||necrotizing G72.81
||quadriplegic G72.81
|alcoholic G72.1
|benign congenital G71.20
|central core G71.29
|centronuclear G71.228
||autosomal (dominant) (recessive) G71.228
||other specified NEC G71.228
|congenital (benign) G71.20
|critical illness G72.81
|distal G71.09
|drug-induced G72.0
|endocrine NEC E34.9 [*G73.7*]
|extraocular muscles H05.82-
|facioscapulohumeral G71.02
|hereditary G71.9
||specified NEC G71.8
|hyaline body G71.29
|immune NEC G72.49
|in (due to)
||Addison's disease E27.1 [*G73.7*]
||alcohol G72.1
||amyloidosis E85.0 [*G73.7*]
||cretinism E00.9 [*G73.7*]

Myopathy - *continued*
||Cushing's syndrome E24.9 [*G73.7*]
||drugs G72.0
||endocrine disease NEC E34.9 [*G73.7*]
||giant cell arteritis M31.6 [*G73.7*]
||glycogen storage disease E74.00 [*G73.7*]
||hyperadrenocorticism E24.9 [*G73.7*]
||hyperparathyroidism NEC E21.3 [*G73.7*]
||hypoparathyroidism E20.9 [*G73.7*]
||hypopituitarism E23.0 [*G73.7*]
||hypothyroidism E03.9 [*G73.7*]
||infectious disease NEC B99 [*G73.7*]
||lipid storage disease E75.6 [*G73.7*]
||metabolic disease NEC E88.9 [*G73.7*]
||myxedema E03.9 [*G73.7*]
||parasitic disease NEC B89 [*G73.7*]
||polyarteritis nodosa M30.0 [*G73.7*]
||rheumatoid arthritis *see* Rheumatoid, myopathy
||sarcoidosis D86.87
||scleroderma M34.82
||sicca syndrome M35.03
||Sjögren's syndrome M35.03
||systemic lupus erythematosus M32.19
||thyrotoxicosis (hyperthyroidism) E05.90 [*G73.7*]
|||with thyroid storm E05.91 [*G73.7*]
||toxic agent NEC G72.2
|inflammatory NEC G72.49
|intensive care (ICU) G72.81
|limb-girdle G71.09
|mitochondrial NEC G71.3
|mytonic, proximal (PROMM) G71.11
|myosin storage G71.29
|myotubular (centronuclear) G71.220
||X-linked G71.220
|nemaline G71.21
|ocular G71.09
|oculopharyngeal G71.09
|of critical illness G72.81
|primary G71.9
||specified NEC G71.8
|progressive NEC G72.89
|proximal myotonic (PROMM) G71.11
|rod (body) G71.21
|scapulohumeral G71.02
|specified NEC G72.89
|toxic G72.2
Myopericarditis *see also* Pericarditis
|chronic rheumatic I09.2
Myopia (axial) (congenital) H52.1-
|degenerative (malignant) H44.20-
||with
|||choroidal neovascularization H44.2A-
|||foveoschisis H44.2D-
|||macular hole H44.2B-
|||retinal detachment H44.2C-
|||specified maculopathy NEC H44.2E-
||bilateral H44.23
||left eye H44.22
||right eye H44.21
|malignant (*see also* Myopia, degenerative) H44.2-
|pernicious (*see also* Myopia, degenerative) H44.2-
|progressive high (degenerative) (*see also* Myopia, degenerative) H44.2-
Myosarcoma *see* Neoplasm, connective tissue, malignant
Myosis (pupil) H57.03
|stromal (endolymphatic) D39.0
Myositis M60.9
|clostridial A48.0
|due to posture *see* Myositis, specified type NEC

Myositis - *continued*
|epidemic B33.0
|fibrosa or fibrous (chronic), Volkmann's T79.6
|foreign body granuloma *see* Granuloma, foreign body
|in (due to)
||bilharziasis B65.9 [*M63.8*]
||cysticercosis B69.81
||leprosy A30.9 [*M63.8*]
||mycosis B49 [*M63.8*]
||sarcoidosis D86.87
||schistosomiasis B65.9 [*M63.8*]
||syphilis
|||late A52.78
|||secondary A51.49
||toxoplasmosis (acquired) B58.82
||trichinellosis B75 [*M63.8*]
||tuberculosis A18.09
|inclusion body [IBM] G72.41
|infective M60.009
||arm M60.002
|||left M60.001
|||right M60.000
||leg M60.005
|||left M60.004
|||right M60.003
||lower limb M60.005
|||ankle M60.07-
|||foot M60.07-
|||lower leg M60.06-
|||thigh M60.05-
|||toe M60.07-
||multiple sites M60.09
||specified site NEC M60.08
||upper limb M60.002
|||finger M60.04-
|||forearm M60.03-
|||hand M60.04-
|||shoulder region M60.01-
|||upper arm M60.02-
|interstitial M60.10
||ankle M60.17-
||foot M60.17-
||forearm M60.13-
||hand M60.14-
||lower leg M60.16-
||multiple sites M60.19
||shoulder region M60.11-
||specified site NEC M60.18
||thigh M60.15-
||upper arm M60.12-
|mycotic B49 [*M63.8*]
|orbital, chronic H05.12-
|ossificans or ossifying (circumscripta) *see also* Ossification, muscle, specified NEC
||in (due to)
|||burns M61.30
||||ankle M61.37-
||||foot M61.37-
||||forearm M61.33-
||||hand M61.34-
||||lower leg M61.36-
||||multiple sites M61.39
||||pelvic region M61.35-
||||shoulder region M61.31-
||||specified site NEC M61.38
||||thigh M61.35-
||||upper arm M61.32-
||quadriplegia or paraplegia M61.20
||||ankle M61.27-
||||foot M61.27-
||||forearm M61.23-
||||hand M61.24-
||||lower leg M61.26-

Myositis - *continued*
    |multiple sites M61.29
    |pelvic region M61.25-
    |shoulder region M61.21-
    |specified site NEC M61.28
    |thigh M61.25-
    |upper arm M61.22-
  |progressiva M61.10
    |ankle M61.17-
    |finger M61.14-
    |foot M61.17-
    |forearm M61.13-
    |hand M61.14-
    |lower leg M61.16-
    |multiple sites M61.19
    |pelvic region M61.15-
    |shoulder region M61.11-
    |specified site NEC M61.18
    |thigh M61.15-
    |toe M61.17-
    |upper arm M61.12-
  |traumatica M61.00
    |ankle M61.07-
    |foot M61.07-
    |forearm M61.03-
    |hand M61.04-
    |lower leg M61.06-
    |multiple sites M61.09
    |pelvic region M61.05-
    |shoulder region M61.01-
    |specified site NEC M61.08
    |thigh M61.05-
    |upper arm M61.02-
  |purulent *see* Myositis, infective
  |specified type NEC M60.80
    |ankle M60.87-
    |foot M60.87-
    |forearm M60.83-
    |hand M60.84-
    |lower leg M60.86-
    |multiple sites M60.89
    |pelvic region M60.85-
    |shoulder region M60.81-
    |specified site NEC M60.88
    |thigh M60.85-
    |upper arm M60.82-
  |suppurative *see* Myositis, infective
  |traumatic (old) *see* Myositis, specified type NEC
Myospasia impulsiva F95.2
Myotonia (acquisita) (intermittens) M62.89
  |atrophica G71.11
  |chondrodystrophic G71.13
  |congenita (acetazolamide responsive) (dominant) (recessive) G71.12
  |drug-induced G71.14
  |dystrophica G71.11
  |fluctuans G71.19
  |levior G71.12
  |permanens G71.19
  |symptomatic G71.19
Myotonic pupil *see* Anomaly, pupil, function, tonic pupil
Myriapodiasis B88.2
Myringitis H73.2-
  |with otitis media *see* Otitis, media
  |acute H73.00-
    |bullous H73.01-
    |specified NEC H73.09-
  |bullous *see* Myringitis, acute, bullous
  |chronic H73.1-
Mysophobia F40.228
Mytilotoxism *see* Poisoning, fish
Myxadenitis labialis K13.0

Myxedema (adult) (idiocy) (infantile) (juvenile) *see also* Hypothyroidism E03.9
  |circumscribed E05.90
    |with storm E05.91
  |coma E03.5
  |congenital E00.1
  |cutis L98.5
  |localized (pretibial) E05.90
    |with storm E05.91
  |papular L98.5
Myxochondrosarcoma *see* Neoplasm, cartilage, malignant
Myxofibroma *see* Neoplasm, connective tissue, benign
  |odontogenic *see* Cyst, calcifying odontogenic
Myxofibrosarcoma *see* Neoplasm, connective tissue, malignant
Myxolipoma D17.9
Myxoliposarcoma *see* Neoplasm, connective tissue, malignant
Myxoma *see also* Neoplasm, connective tissue, benign
  |nerve sheath *see* Neoplasm, nerve, benign
  |odontogenic *see* Cyst, calcifying odontogenic
Myxosarcoma *see* Neoplasm, connective tissue, malignant

N

Naegeli's
  |disease Q82.8
  |leukemia, monocytic C93.1-
Naegleriasis (with meningoencephalitis) B60.2
Naffziger's syndrome G54.0
Naga sore *see* Ulcer, skin
Nägele's pelvis M95.5
  |with disproportion (fetopelvic) O33.0
    |causing obstructed labor O65.0
Nail *see also* condition
  |biting F98.8
  |patella syndrome Q87.2
Nanism, nanosomia *see* Dwarfism
Nanophyetiasis B66.8
Nanukayami A27.89
Napkin rash L22
Narcolepsy G47.419
  |with cataplexy G47.411
  |in conditions classified elsewhere G47.429
    |with cataplexy G47.421
Narcosis R06.89
Narcotism *see* Dependence
NARP (Neuropathy, Ataxia and Retinitis pigmentosa) syndrome E88.49
Narrow
  |anterior chamber angle H40.03-
  |gingival width (of periodontal soft tissue) K05.5
  |pelvis *see* Contraction, pelvis
Narrowing *see also* Stenosis
  |artery I77.1
    |auditory, internal I65.8
    |basilar *see* Occlusion, artery, basilar
    |carotid *see* Occlusion, artery, carotid
    |cerebellar *see* Occlusion, artery, cerebellar
    |cerebral *see* Occlusion artery, cerebral
    |choroidal *see* Occlusion, artery, cerebral, specified NEC
    |communicating posterior *see* Occlusion, artery, cerebral, specified NEC
    |coronary *see also* Disease, heart, ischemic, atherosclerotic
      |congenital Q24.5
        |syphilitic A50.54 [*152*]
    |due to syphilis NEC A52.06

Narrowing - *continued*
  |hypophyseal *see* Occlusion, artery, cerebral, specified NEC
  |pontine *see* Occlusion, artery, cerebral, specified NEC
  |precerebral *see* Occlusion, artery, precerebral
  |vertebral *see* Occlusion, artery, vertebral
  |auditory canal (external) *see* Stenosis, external ear canal
  |eustachian tube *see* Obstruction, eustachian tube
  |eyelid *see* Disorder, eyelid function
  |larynx J38.6
  |mesenteric artery *see also* Ischemia, intestine, acute K55.059
  |palate M26.89
  |palpebral fissure *see* Disorder, eyelid function
  |ureter N13.5
    |with infection N13.6
  |urethra *see* Stricture, urethra
Narrowness, abnormal, eyelid Q10.3
Nasal *see* condition
Nasolachrymal, nasolacrimal *see* condition
Nasopharyngeal *see also* condition
  |pituitary gland Q89.2
  |torticollis M43.6
Nasopharyngitis (acute) (infective) (streptococcal) (subacute) J00
  |chronic (suppurative) (ulcerative) J31.1
Nasopharynx, nasopharyngeal *see* condition
Natal tooth, teeth K00.6
Nausea (without vomiting) R11.0
  |with vomiting R11.2
  |gravidarum *see* Hyperemesis, gravidarum
  |marina T75.3
  |navalis T75.3
Navel *see* condition
Neapolitan fever *see* Brucellosis
Near drowning T75.1
Nearsightedness *see* Myopia
Near-Syncope R55
Nebula, cornea *see* Opacity, cornea
Necator americanus infestation B76.1
Necatoriasis B76.1
Neck *see* condition **Necrobiosis** R68.89
  |lipoidica NEC L92.1
    |with diabetes *see* E08-E13 with .620
Necrolysis, toxic epidermal L51.2
  |due to drug
    |correct substance properly administered *see* Table of Drugs and Chemicals, by drug, adverse effect
    |overdose or wrong substance given or taken *see* Table of Drugs and Chemicals, by drug, poisoning
Necrophilia F65.89
Necrosis, necrotic (ischemic) *see also* Gangrene
  |adrenal (capsule) (gland) E27.49
  |amputation stump (surgical) (late) T87.50
    |arm T87.5-
    |leg T87.5-
  |antrum J32.0
  |aorta (hyaline) *see also* Aneurysm, aorta
    |cystic medial *see* Dissection, aorta
  |artery I77.5
  |bladder (aseptic) (sphincter) N32.89
  |bone *see also* Osteonecrosis M87.9
    |aseptic or avascular *see* Osteonecrosis
      |idiopathic M87.00
    |ethmoid J32.2
    |jaw M27.2
    |tuberculous *see* Tuberculosis, bone
  |brain I67.89
  |breast (aseptic) (fat) (segmental) N64.1

Necrosis, necrotic - *continued*
 |bronchus J98.09
 |central nervous system NEC I67.89
 |cerebellar I67.89
 |cerebral I67.89
 |colon *see also* Infarct, intestine K55.049
 |cornea H18.89-
 |cortical (acute) (renal) N17.1
 |cystic medial (aorta) *see* Dissection, aorta
 |dental pulp K04.1
 |esophagus K22.89
 |ethmoid (bone) J32.2
 |eyelid *see* Disorder, eyelid, degenerative
 |fat, fatty (generalized) *see also* Disorder, soft
  tissue, specified type NEC
   |abdominal wall K65.4
   |breast (aseptic) (segmental) N64.1
   |localized *see* Degeneration, by site, fatty
   |mesentery K65.4
   |omentum K65.4
   |pancreas K86.89
   |peritoneum K65.4
   |skin (subcutaneous), newborn P83.0
   |subcutaneous, due to birth injury P15.6
 |gallbladder *see* Cholecystitis, acute
 |heart *see* Infarct, myocardium
 |hip, aseptic or avascular *see* Osteonecrosis, by
  type, femur
 |intestine (acute) (hemorrhagic) (massive) *see
  also* Infarct, intestine K55.069
 |jaw M27.2
 |kidney (bilateral) N28.0
   |acute N17.9
   |cortical (acute) (bilateral) N17.1
    |with ectopic or molar pregnancy O08.4
   |medullary (bilateral) (in acute renal failure)
    (papillary) N17.2
   |papillary (bilateral) (in acute renal failure)
    N17.2
   |tubular N17.0
    |with ectopic or molar pregnancy O08.4
    |complicating
     |abortion *see* Abortion, by type,
      complicated by, tubular necrosis
     |ectopic or molar pregnancy O08.4
     |pregnancy *see* Pregnancy, complicated
      by, diseases of, specified type or
      system NEC
    |following ectopic or molar pregnancy
     O08.4
    |traumatic T79.5
 |larynx J38.7
 |liver (with hepatic failure) (cell) *see* Failure,
  hepatic
   |hemorrhagic, central K76.2
 |lung J85.0
 |lymphatic gland *see* Lymphadenitis, acute
 |mammary gland (fat) (segmental) N64.1
 |mastoid (chronic) *see* Mastoiditis, chronic
 |medullary (acute) (renal) N17.2
 |mesentery *see also* Infarct, intestine K55.069
   |fat K65.4
 |mitral valve *see* Insufficiency, mitral
 |myocardium, myocardial *see* Infarct,
  myocardium
 |nose J34.0
 |omentum (with mesenteric infarction) *see also*
  Infarct, intestine K55.069
   |fat K65.4
 |orbit, orbital *see* Osteomyelitis, orbit
 |ossicles, ear *see* Abnormal, ear ossicles
 |ovary N70.92
 |pancreas (aseptic) (duct) (fat) K86.89
   |acute (infective) *see* Pancreatitis, acute
   |infective *see* Pancreatitis, acute

Necrosis, necrotic - *continued*
 |papillary (acute) (renal) N17.2
 |perineum N90.89
 |peritoneum (with mesenteric infarction) *see
  also* Infarct, intestine K55.069
   |fat K65.4
 |pharynx J02.9
   |in granulocytopenia *see* Neutropenia
   |Vincent's A69.1
 |phosphorus *see* subcategory T54.2
 |pituitary (gland) E23.0
   |postpartum O99.285
   |Sheehan O99.285
 |pressure *see* Ulcer, pressure, by site
 |pulmonary J85.0
 |pulp (dental) K04.1
 |radiation *see* Necrosis, by site
 |radium *see* Necrosis, by site
 |renal *see* Necrosis, kidney
 |sclera H15.89
 |scrotum N50.89
 |skin or subcutaneous tissue NEC I96
 |spine, spinal (column) *see also* Osteonecrosis,
  by type, vertebra
   |cord G95.19
 |spleen D73.5
 |stomach K31.89
 |stomatitis (ulcerative) A69.0
 |subcutaneous fat, newborn P83.88
 |subendocardial (acute) I21.4
   |chronic I25.89
 |suprarenal (capsule) (gland) E27.49
 |testis N50.89
 |thymus (gland) E32.8
 |tonsil J35.8
 |trachea J39.8
 |tuberculous NEC *see* Tuberculosis
 |tubular (acute) (anoxic) (renal) (toxic) N17.0
   |postprocedural N99.0
 |vagina N89.8
 |vertebra *see also* Osteonecrosis, by type,
  vertebra
   |tuberculous A18.01
 |vulva N90.89
 |X-ray *see* Necrosis, by site
Necrospermia *see* Infertility, male
Need (for)
 |care provider because of (of)
   |assistance with personal care Z74.1
   |continuous supervision required Z74.3
   |impaired mobility Z74.09
   |no other household member able to render
    care Z74.2
   |specified reason NEC Z74.8
 |immunization *see* Vaccination
 |vaccination *see* Vaccination
Neglect
 |adult
   |confirmed T74.01
   |history of Z91.412
   |suspected T76.01
 |child (childhood)
   |confirmed T74.02
   |history of Z62.812
   |suspected T76.02
 |emotional, in childhood Z62.898
 |hemispatial R41.4
 |left-sided R41.4
 |sensory R41.4
 |visuospatial R41.4
Neisserian infection NEC *see* Gonococcus
Nélaton's syndrome G60.8
Nelson's syndrome E24.1
Nematodiasis (intestinal) B82.0
 |Ancylostoma B76.0

Neonatal *see also* Newborn
 |acne L70.4
 |bradycardia P29.12
 |tachycardia P29.11
 |screening, abnormal findings on - *see*
  Abnormal, neonatal screening
 |tooth, teeth K00.6
Neonatorum *see* condition
Neoplasia
 |endocrine, multiple (MEN) E31.20
   |type I E31.21
   |type IIA E31.22
   |type IIB E31.23
 |intraepithelial (histologically confirmed)
   |anal (AIN) (histologically confirmed)
    K62.82
    |grade I K62.82
    |grade II K62.82
    |severe D01.3
   |cervical glandular (histologically confirmed)
    D06.9
   |cervix (uteri) (CIN) (histologically
    confirmed) N87.9
    |glandular D06.9
    |grade I N87.0
    |grade II N87.1
    |grade III (severe dysplasia) *see also*
     Carcinoma, cervix uteri, in situ D06.9
   |prostate (histologically confirmed) (PIN)
    N42.31
    |grade I N42.31
    |grade II N42.31
    |grade III (severe dysplasia) D07.5
   |vagina (histologically confirmed) (VAIN)
    N89.3
    |grade I N89.0
    |grade II N89.1
    |grade III (severe dysplasia) D07.2
   |vulva (histologically confirmed) (VIN)
    N90.3
    |grade I N90.0
    |grade II N90.1
    |grade III (severe dysplasia) D07.1
Neoplasm, neoplastic *see also* Table of
 Neoplasms
 |malignant mast cell C96.20
   |specified type NEC C96.29
 |mast cell, of uncertain behavior NEC D47.09
 |lipomatous, benign *see* Lipoma
Neovascularization
 |ciliary body *see* Disorder, iris, vascular
 |cornea H16.40-
   |deep H16.44-
   |ghost vessels *see* Ghost, vessels
   |localized H16.43-
   |pannus *see* Pannus
 |iris *see* Disorder, iris, vascular
 |retina H35.05-
Nephralgia N23
**Nephritis, nephritic (albuminuric) (azotemic)
 (congenital) (disseminated) (epithelial)
 (familial) (focal) (granulomatous)
 (hemorrhagic) (infantile) (nonsuppurative,
 excretory) (uremic)** N05.9
 |with
   |C3
    |glomerulonephritis N05.A
    |glomerulopathy N05.A
     |with dense deposit disease N05.6
   |dense deposit disease N05.6
   |diffuse
    |crescentic glomerulonephritis N05.7
    |endocapillary proliferative
     glomerulonephritis N05.4
    |membranous glomerulonephritis N05.2

Nephritis, nephritic - *continued*
  |mesangial proliferative glomerulonephritis N05.3
    |mesangiocapillary glomerulonephritis N05.5
  |edema *see* Nephrosis
  |focal and segmental glomerular lesions N05.1
  |foot process disease N04.9
  |glomerular lesion
    |diffuse sclerosing N05.8
    |hypocomplementemic *see* Nephritis, membranoproliferative
    |IgA *see* Nephropathy, IgA
    |lobular, lobulonodular *see* Nephritis, membranoproliferative
    |nodular *see* Nephritis, membranoproliferative
  |lesion of
    |glomerulonephritis, proliferative N05.8
    |renal necrosis N05.9
  |minor glomerular abnormality N05.0
  |specified morphological changes NEC N05.8
  |acute N00.9
    |with
      |C3
        |glomerulonephritis N00.A
        |glomerulopathy N00.A
          |with dense deposit disease N00.6
      |dense deposit disease N00.6
      |diffuse
        |crescentic glomerulonephritis N00.7
        |endocapillary proliferative glomerulonephritis N00.4
        |membranous glomerulonephritis N00.2
        |mesangial proliferative glomerulonephritis N00.3
        |mesangiocapillary glomerulonephritis N00.5
      |focal and segmental glomerular lesions N00.1
      |minor glomerular abnormality N00.0
      |specified morphological changes NEC N00.8
  |amyloid E85.4 *[N08]*
  |antiglomerular basement membrane (anti-GBM) antibody NEC
    |in Goodpasture's syndrome M31.0
  |antitubular basement membrane (tubulo-interstitial) NEC N12
    |toxic *see* Nephropathy, toxic
  |arteriolar *see* Hypertension, kidney
  |arteriosclerotic *see* Hypertension, kidney
  |ascending *see* Nephritis, tubulo-interstitial
  |atrophic N03.9
  |Balkan (endemic) N15.0
  |calculous, calculus *see* Calculus, kidney
  |cardiac *see* Hypertension, kidney
  |cardiovascular *see* Hypertension, kidney
  |chronic N03.9
    |with
      |C3
        |glomerulonephritis N03.A
        |glomerulopathy N03.A
          |with dense deposit disease N03.6
      |dense deposit disease N03.6
      |diffuse
        |crescentic glomerulonephritis N03.7
        |endocapillary proliferative glomerulonephritis N03.4
        |membranous glomerulonephritis N03.2
        |mesangial proliferative glomerulonephritis N03.3

Nephritis, nephritic - *continued*
        |mesangiocapillary glomerulonephritis N03.5
      |focal and segmental glomerular lesions N03.1
      |minor glomerular abnormality N03.0
      |specified morphological changes NEC N03.8
    |arteriosclerotic *see* Hypertension, kidney
  |cirrhotic N26.9
  |complicating pregnancy O26.83
  |croupous N00.9
  |degenerative *see* Nephrosis
  |diffuse sclerosing N05.8
  |due to
    |diabetes mellitus *see* E08-E13 with .21
    |subacute bacterial endocarditis I33.0
    |systemic lupus erythematosus (chronic) M32.14
    |typhoid fever A01.09
  |gonococcal (acute) (chronic) A54.21
  |hypocomplementemic *see* Nephritis, membranoproliferative
  |IgA *see* Nephropathy, IgA
  |immune complex (circulating) NEC N05.8
  |infective *see* Nephritis, tubulo-interstitial
  |interstitial *see* Nephritis, tubulo-interstitial
  |lead N14.3
  |membranoproliferative (diffuse) (type 1 or 3) *see also* N00-N07 with fourth character .5 N05.5
    |type 2 *see also* N00-N07 with fourth character .6 N05.6
  |minimal change N05.0
  |necrotic, necrotizing NEC *see also* N00-N07 with fourth character .8 N05.8
  |nephrotic *see* Nephrosis
  |nodular *see* Nephritis, membranoproliferative
  |polycystic Q61.3
    |adult type Q61.2
    |autosomal
      |dominant Q61.2
      |recessive NEC Q61.19
    |childhood type NEC Q61.19
    |infantile type NEC Q61.19
  |poststreptococcal N05.9
    |acute N00.9
    |chronic N03.9
    |rapidly progressive N01.9
  |proliferative NEC *see also* N00-N07 with fourth character .8 N05.8
  |purulent *see* Nephritis, tubulo-interstitial
  |rapidly progressive N01.9
    |with
      |C3
        |glomerulonephritis N01.A
        |glomerulopathy N01.A
          |with dense deposit disease N01.6
      |dense deposit disease N01.6
      |diffuse
        |crescentic glomerulonephritis N01.7
        |endocapillary proliferative glomerulonephritis N01.4
        |membranous glomerulonephritis N01.2
        |mesangial proliferative glomerulonephritis N01.3
        |mesangiocapillary glomerulonephritis N01.5
      |focal and segmental glomerular lesions N01.1
      |minor glomerular abnormality N01.0
      |specified morphological changes NEC N01.8
  |salt losing or wasting NEC N28.89
  |saturnine N14.3
  |sclerosing, diffuse N05.8

Nephritis, nephritic - *continued*
  |septic *see* Nephritis, tubulo-interstitial
  |specified pathology NEC *see also* N00-N07 with fourth character .8 N05.8
  |subacute N01.9
  |suppurative *see* Nephritis, tubulo-interstitial
  |syphilitic (late) A52.75
    |congenital A50.59 *[N08]*
    |early (secondary) A51.44
  |toxic *see* Nephropathy, toxic
  |tubal, tubular *see* Nephritis, tubulo-interstitial
  |tuberculous A18.11
  |tubulo-interstitial (in) N12
    |acute (infectious) N10
    |chronic (infectious) N11.9
      |nonobstructive N11.8
        |reflux-associated N11.0
      |obstructive N11.1
      |specified NEC N11.8
    |due to
      |brucellosis A23.9 *[N16]*
      |cryoglobulinemia D89.1 *[N16]*
      |glycogen storage disease E74.00 *[N16]*
      |*Sjögren's* syndrome M35.04
  |vascular *see* Hypertension, kidney
  |war N00.9
Nephroblastoma (epithelial) (mesenchymal) C64-
Nephrocalcinosis E83.59 *[N29]*
Nephrocystitis, pustular *see* Nephritis, tubulo-interstitial
Nephrolithiasis (congenital) (pelvis) (recurrent) *see also* Calculus, kidney
Nephroma C64-
  |mesoblastic D41.0-
Nephronephritis *see* Nephrosis
Nephronophthisis Q61.5
Nephropathia epidemica A98.5
Nephropathy *see also* Nephritis N28.9
  |with
    |edema *see* Nephrosis
    |glomerular lesion *see* Glomerulonephritis
  |amyloid, hereditary E85.0
  |analgesic N14.0
    |with medullary necrosis, acute N17.2
  |Balkan (endemic) N15.0
  |chemical *see* Nephropathy, toxic
  |diabetic *see* E08-E13 with .21
  |drug-induced N14.2
    |specified NEC N14.1
  |focal and segmental hyalinosis or sclerosis N02.1
  |heavy metal-induced N14.3
  |hereditary NEC N07.9
    |with
      |C3
        |glomerulonephritis N07.A
        |glomerulopathy N07.A
          |with dense deposit disease N07.6
      |dense deposit disease N07.6
      |diffuse
        |crescentic glomerulonephritis N07.7
        |endocapillary proliferative glomerulonephritis N07.4
        |membranous glomerulonephritis N07.2
        |mesangial proliferative glomerulonephritis N07.3
        |mesangiocapillary glomerulonephritis N07.5
      |focal and segmental glomerular lesions N07.1
      |minor glomerular abnormality N07.0
      |specified morphological changes NEC N07.8
  |hypercalcemic N25.89
  |hypertensive *see* Hypertension, kidney

Neuritis (rheumatoid) - *continued*
|olfactory nerve G52.0
|optic (nerve) (hereditary) (sympathetic) H46.9
  |with demyelination G36.0
  |in myelitis G36.0
  |nutritional H46.2
  |papillitis *see* Papillitis, optic
  |retrobulbar H46.1-
  |specified type NEC H46.8
  |toxic H46.3
|peripheral (nerve) G62.9
  |multiple *see* Polyneuropathy
  |single *see* Mononeuritis
|pneumogastric (nerve) G52.2
|postherpetic, postzoster B02.29
|progressive hypertrophic interstitial G60.0
|retrobulbar *see also* Neuritis, optic,
    retrobulbar
  |in (due to)
    |late syphilis A52.15
    |meningococcal infection A39.82
  |meningococcal A39.82
  |syphilitic A52.15
|sciatic (nerve) *see also* Sciatica
  |due to displacement of intervertebral disc
    see Disorder, disc, with, radiculopathy
|serum *see also* Reaction, serum T80.69
|shoulder-girdle G54.5
|specified nerve NEC G58.8
|spinal (nerve) root *see* Radiculopathy
|syphilitic A52.15
|thenar (median) G56.1-
|thoracic M54.14
|toxic NEC G62.2
|trochlear (nerve) *see* Strabismus, paralytic,
    fourth nerve
|vagus (nerve) G52.2
Neuroastrocytoma *see* Neoplasm, uncertain
    behavior, by site
Neuroavitaminosis E56.9 [*G99.8*]
Neuroblastoma olfactory C30.0
|specified site *see* Neoplasm, malignant, by site
|unspecified site C74.90
Neurochorioretinitis *see* Chorioretinitis
Neurocirculatory asthenia F45.8
Neurocysticercosis B69.0
Neurocytoma *see* Neoplasm, benign, by site
Neurodermatitis (circumscribed)
    (circumscripta) (local) L28.0
|atopic L20.81
|diffuse (Brocq) L20.81
|disseminated L20.81
Neuroencephalomyelopathy, optic G36.0
Neuroepithelioma *see also* Neoplasm,
    malignant, by site
|olfactory C30.0
Neurofibroma *see also* Neoplasm, nerve,
    benign
|melanotic *see* Neoplasm, nerve, benign
|multiple *see* Neurofibromatosis
|plexiform *see* Neoplasm, nerve, benign
Neurofibromatosis (multiple) (nonmalignant)
    Q85.00
|acoustic Q85.02
|malignant *see* Neoplasm, nerve, malignant
|specified NEC Q85.09
|type 1 (von Recklinghausen) Q85.01
|type 2 Q85.02
Neurofibrosarcoma *see* Neoplasm, nerve,
    malignant
Neurogenic *see also* condition
|bladder *see also* Dysfunction, bladder,
    neuromuscular N31.9
  |cauda equina syndrome G83.4
|bowel NEC K59.2
|heart F45.8

Neuroglioma *see* Neoplasm, uncertain behavior,
    by site
Neurolabyrinthitis (of Dix and Hallpike) *see*
    Neuronitis, vestibular
Neurolathyrism *see* Poisoning, food, noxious,
    plant
Neuroleprosy A30.9
Neuroma *see also* Neoplasm, nerve, benign
|acoustic (nerve) D33.3
|amputation (stump) (traumatic) (surgical
    complication) (late) T87.3-
  |arm T87.3-
  |leg T87.3-
|digital (toe) G57.6-
|interdigital G58.8
  |lower limb (toe) G57.8-
  |upper limb G56.8-
|intermetatarsal G57.8-
|Morton's G57.6-
|nonneoplastic
  |arm G56.9-
  |leg G57.9-
  |lower extremity G57.9-
  |upper extremity G56.9-
|optic (nerve) D33.3
|plantar G57.6-
|plexiform *see* Neoplasm, nerve, benign
|surgical (nonneoplastic)
  |arm G56.9-
  |leg G57.9-
  |lower extremity G57.9-
  |upper extremity G56.9-
Neuromyalgia *see* Neuralgia
Neuromyasthenia (epidemic) (postinfectious)
    G93.3
Neuromyelitis G36.9
|ascending G61.0
|optica G36.0
Neuromyopathy G70.9
|paraneoplastic D49.9 [*G13.0*]
Neuromyotonia (Isaacs) G71.19
Neuronevus *see* Nevus
Neuronitis G58.9
|ascending (acute) G57.2-
|vestibular H81.2-
Neuroparalytic *see* condition
Neuropathy, neuropathic G62.9
|acute motor G62.81
|alcoholic G62.1
  |with psychosis *see* Psychosis, alcoholic
|arm G56.9-
|autonomic, peripheral *see* Neuropathy,
    peripheral, autonomic
|axillary G56.9-
|bladder N31.9
  |atonic (motor) (sensory) N31.2
  |autonomous N31.2
  |flaccid N31.2
  |nonreflex N31.2
  |reflex N31.1
  |uninhibited N31.0
|brachial plexus G54.0
|cervical plexus G54.2
|chronic
  |progressive segmentally demyelinating
    G62.89
  |relapsing demyelinating G62.89
|Déjérine-Sottas G60.0
|diabetic *see* E08-E13 with .40
  |mononeuropathy *see* E08-E13 with .41
  |polyneuropathy *see* E08-E13 with .42
|entrapment G58.9
  |iliohypogastric nerve G57.8-
  |ilioinguinal nerve G57.8-
  |lateral cutaneous nerve of thigh G57.1-

Neuropathy, neuropathic - *continued*
  |median nerve G56.0-
  |obturator nerve G57.8-
  |peroneal nerve G57.3-
  |posterior tibial nerve G57.5-
  |saphenous nerve G57.8-
  |ulnar nerve G56.2-
|facial nerve G51.9
|hereditary G60.9
  |motor and sensory (types I-IV) G60.0
  |sensory G60.8
  |specified NEC G60.8
|hypertrophic G60.0
  |Charcot-Marie-Tooth G60.0
  |Déjérine-Sottas G60.0
  |interstitial progressive G60.0
  |of infancy G60.0
  |Refsum G60.1
|idiopathic G60.9
  |progressive G60.3
  |specified NEC G60.8
|in association with hereditary ataxia G60.2
|intercostal G58.0
|ischemic *see* Disorder, nerve
|Jamaica (ginger) G62.2
|leg NEC G57.9-
|lower extremity G57.9-
|lumbar plexus G54.1
|median nerve G56.1-
|motor and sensory *see also* Polyneuropathy
  |hereditary (types I-IV) G60.0
|multifocal motor (MMN) G61.82
|multiple (acute) (chronic) *see* Polyneuropathy
|optic (nerve) *see also* Neuritis, optic
  |ischemic H47.01-
|paraneoplastic (sensorial) (Denny Brown)
    D49.9 [*G13.0*]
|peripheral (nerve) *see also* Polyneuropathy
    G62.9
  |autonomic G90.9
    |idiopathic G90.09
    |in (due to)
      |amyloidosis E85.4 [*G99.0*]
      |diabetes mellitus *see* E08-E13 with .43
      |endocrine disease NEC E34.9 [*G99.0*]
      |gout M10.00 [*G99.0*]
      |hyperthyroidism E05.90 [*G99.0*]
        |with thyroid storm E05.91 [*G99.0*]
      |metabolic disease NEC E88.9 [*G99.0*]
  |idiopathic G60.9
    |progressive G60.3
  |in (due to)
    |antitetanus serum G62.0
    |arsenic G62.2
    |drugs NEC G62.0
    |lead G62.2
    |organophosphate compounds G62.2
    |toxic agent NEC G62.2
|plantar nerves G57.6-
|progressive
  |hypertrophic interstitial G60.0
  |inflammatory G62.81
|radicular NEC *see* Radiculopathy
|sacral plexus G54.1
|sciatic G57.0-
|serum G61.1
|toxic NEC G62.2
|trigeminal sensory G50.8
|ulnar nerve G56.2-
|uremic N18.9 [*G63*]
|vitamin B12 E53.8 [*G63*]
  |with anemia (pernicious) D51.0 [*G63*]
  |due to dietary deficiency D51.3 [*G63*]
Neurophthisis *see also* Disorder, nerve
|peripheral, diabetic *see* E08-E13 with .42

Neuroretinitis *see* Chorioretinitis
Neuroretinopathy, hereditary optic H47.22
Neurosarcoma *see* Neoplasm, nerve, malignant
Neurosclerosis *see* Disorder, nerve
Neurosis, neurotic F48.9
  |anankastic F42.8
  |anxiety (state) F41.1
    |panic type F41.0
  |asthenic F48.8
  |bladder F45.8
  |cardiac (reflex) F45.8
  |cardiovascular F45.8
  |character F60.9
  |colon F45.8
  |compensation F68.10
  |compulsive, compulsion F42.8
  |conversion F44.9
  |craft F48.8
  |cutaneous F45.8
  |depersonalization F48.1
  |depressive (reaction) (type) F34.1
  |environmental F48.8
  |excoriation L98.1
  |fatigue F48.8
  |functional *see* Disorder, somatoform
  |gastric F45.8
  |gastrointestinal F45.8
  |heart F45.8
  |hypochondriacal F45.21
  |hysterical F44.9
  |incoordination F45.8
    |larynx F45.8
    |vocal cord F45.8
  |intestine F45.8
  |larynx (sensory) F45.8
    |hysterical F44.4
  |mixed NEC F48.8
  |musculoskeletal F45.8
  |obsessional F42.8
  |obsessive-compulsive F42.8
  |occupational F48.8
  |ocular NEC F45.8
  |organ *see* Disorder, somatoform
  |pharynx F45.8
  |phobic F40.9
  |posttraumatic (situational) F43.10
    |acute F43.11
    |chronic F43.12
  |psychasthenic (type) F48.8
  |railroad F48.8
  |rectum F45.8
  |respiratory F45.8
  |rumination F45.8
  |sexual F65.9
  |situational F48.8
  |social F40.10
    |generalized F40.11
  |specified type NEC F48.8
  |state F48.9
    |with depersonalization episode F48.1
  |stomach F45.8
  |traumatic F43.10
    |acute F43.11
    |chronic F43.12
  |vasomotor F45.8
  |visceral F45.8
  |war F48.8
Neurospongioblastosis diffusa Q85.1
Neurosyphilis (arrested) (early) (gumma)
  (late) (latent) (recurrent) (relapse) A52.3
  |with ataxia (cerebellar) (locomotor) (spastic)
    (spinal) A52.19
  |aneurysm (cerebral) A52.05
  |arachnoid (adhesive) A52.13
  |arteritis (any artery) (cerebral) A52.04
  |asymptomatic A52.2

Neurosyphilis - *continued*
  |congenital A50.40
  |dura (mater) A52.13
  |general paresis A52.17
  |hemorrhagic A52.05
  |juvenile (asymptomatic) (meningeal) A50.40
  |leptomeninges (aseptic) A52.13
  |meningeal, meninges (adhesive) A52.13
  |meningitis A52.13
  |meningovascular (diffuse) A52.13
  |optic atrophy A52.15
  |parenchymatous (degenerative) A52.19
  |paresis, paretic A52.17
    |juvenile A50.45
  |remission in (sustained) A52.3
  |serological (without symptoms) A52.2
  |specified nature or site NEC A52.19
  |tabes, tabetic (dorsalis) A52.11
    |juvenile A50.45
  |taboparesis A52.17
    |juvenile A50.45
  |thrombosis (cerebral) A52.05
  |vascular (cerebral) NEC A52.05
Neurothekeoma *see* Neoplasm, nerve, benign
Neurotic *see* Neurosis
Neurotoxemia *see* Toxemia
Neutroclusion M26.211
Neutropenia, neutropenic (chronic) (genetic)
  (idiopathic) (immune) (infantile)
  (malignant) (pernicious) (splenic) D70.9
  |congenital (primary) D70.0
  |cyclic D70.4
  |cytoreductive cancer chemotherapy sequela
    D70.1
  |drug-induced D70.2
    |due to cytoreductive cancer chemotherapy
      D70.1
  |due to infection D70.3
  |fever D70.9
  |neonatal, transitory (isoimmune) (maternal
    transfer) P61.5
  |periodic D70.4
  |secondary (cyclic) (periodic) (splenic) D70.4
    |drug-induced D70.2
      |due to cytoreductive cancer chemotherapy
        D70.1
  |toxic D70.8
Neutrophilia, hereditary giant D72.0
Nevocarcinoma *see* Melanoma
Nevus D22.9
  |achromic *see* Neoplasm, skin, benign
  |amelanotic *see* Neoplasm, skin, benign
  |angiomatousD18.00
    |intra-abdominal D18.03
    |intracranial D18.02
    |skin D18.01
    |specified site NEC D18.09
  |araneus I78.1
  |balloon cell *see* Neoplasm, skin, benign
  |bathing trunk D48.5
  |blue *see* Neoplasm, skin, benign
    |cellular *see* Neoplasm, skin, benign
    |giant *see* Neoplasm, skin, benign
    |Jadassohn's *see* Neoplasm, skin, benign
    |malignant *see* Melanoma
  |capillary D18.00
    |intra-abdominal D18.03
    |intracranial D18.02
    |skin D18.01
    |specified site NEC D18.09
  |cavernous D18.00
    |intra-abdominal D18.03
    |intracranial D18.02
    |skin D18.01
    |specified site NEC D18.09
  |cellular *see* Neoplasm, skin, benign

Nevus - *continued*
  |blue *see* Neoplasm, skin, benign
  |choroid D31.3-
  |comedonicus Q82.5
  |conjunctiva D31.0-
  |dermal *see* Neoplasm, skin, benign
    |with epidermal nevus *see* Neoplasm, skin,
      benign
  |dysplastic *see* Neoplasm, skin, benign
  |eye D31.9-
  |flammeus Q82.5
  |hemangiomatous D18.00
    |intra-abdominal D18.03
    |intracranial D18.02
    |skin D18.01
    |specified site NEC D18.09
  |iris D31.4-
  |lacrimal gland D31.5-
  |lymphatic D18.1
  |magnocellular
    |specified site *see* Neoplasm, benign, by site
    |unspecified site D31.40
  |malignant *see* Melanoma
  |meaning hemangioma D18.00
    |intra-abdominal D18.03
    |intracranial D18.02
    |skin D18.01
    |specified site NEC D18.09
  |mouth (mucosa) D10.30
    |specified site NEC D10.39
    |white sponge Q38.6
  |multiplex Q85.1
  |non-neoplastic I78.1
  |oral mucosa D10.30
    |specified site NEC D10.39
    |white sponge Q38.6
  |orbit D31.6-
  |pigmented
    |giant *see also* Neoplasm, skin, uncertain
      behavior D48.5
      |malignant melanoma in *see* Melanoma
  |portwine Q82.5
  |retina D31.2-
  |retrobulbar D31.6-
  |sanguineous Q82.5
  |senile I78.1
  |skin D22.9
    |abdominal wall D22.5
    |ala nasi D22.39
    |ankle D22.7-
    |anus, anal D22.5
    |arm D22.6-
    |auditory canal (external) D22.2-
    |auricle (ear) D22.2-
    |auricular canal (external) D22.2-
    |axilla, axillary fold D22.5
    |back D22.5
    |breast D22.5
    |brow D22.39
    |buttock D22.5
    |canthus (eye) D22.1-
    |cheek (external) D22.39
    |chest wall D22.5
    |chin D22.39
    |ear (external) D22.2-
    |external meatus (ear) D22.2-
    |eyebrow D22.39
    |eyelid (lower) (upper) D22.1-
    |face D22.30
      |specified NEC D22.39
    |female genital organ (external) NEC D28.0
    |finger D22.6-
    |flank D22.5
    |foot D22.7-
    |forearm D22.6-

Nevus - *continued*
|forehead D22.39
|foreskin D29.0
|genital organ (external) NEC
||female D28.0
||male D29.9
|gluteal region D22.5
|groin D22.5
|hand D22.6-
|heel D22.7-
|helix D22.2-
|hip D22.7-
|interscapular region D22.5
|jaw D22.39
|knee D22.7-
|labium (majus) (minus) D28.0
|leg D22.7-
|lip (lower) (upper) D22.0
|lower limb D22.7-
|male genital organ (external) D29.9
|nail D22.9
||finger D22.6-
||toe D22.7-
|nasolabial groove D22.39
|nates D22.5
|neck D22.4
|nose (external) D22.39
|palpebra D22.1-
|penis D29.0
|perianal skin D22.5
|perineum D22.5
|pinna D22.2-
|popliteal fossa or space D22.7-
|prepuce D29.0
|pudendum D28.0
|scalp D22.4
|scrotum D29.4
|shoulder D22.6-
|submammary fold D22.5
|temple D22.39
|thigh D22.7-
|toe D22.7-
|trunk NEC D22.5
|umbilicus D22.5
|upper limb D22.6-
|vulva D28.0
|specified site NEC *see* Neoplasm, by site,
|| benign
|spider I78.1
|stellar I78.1
|strawberry Q82.5
|Sutton's benign D22.9
|unius lateris Q82.5
|Unna's Q82.5
|vascular Q82.5
|verrucous Q82.5

Newborn (infant) (liveborn) (singleton) Z38.2
|acne L70.4
|abstinence syndrome P96.1
|affected by
||abnormalities of membranes P02.9
|||specified NEC P02.8
||abruptio placenta P02.1
||amino-acid metabolic disorder, transitory
||| P74.8
||amniocentesis (while in utero) P00.6
||amnionitis P02.78
||apparent life threatening event (ALTE)
||| R68.13
||bleeding (into)
|||cerebral cortex P52.22
|||germinal matrix P52.0
|||ventricles P52.1
||breech delivery P03.0
||cardiac arrest P29.81

Newborn - *continued*
|cardiomyopathy I42.8
||congenital I42.4
|cerebral ischemia P91.0
|Cesarean delivery P03.4
|chemotherapy agents P04.11
|chorioamnionitis P02.78
|cocaine (crack) P04.41
|complications of labor and delivery P03.9
||specified NEC P03.89
|compression of umbilical cord NEC P02.5
|contracted pelvis P03.1
|delivery P03.9
||Cesarean P03.4
||forceps P03.2
||vacuum extractor P03.3
|drugs of Addiction P04.40
||cocaine P04.41
||hallucinogens P04.42
||specified drug NEC P04.49
|environmental chemicals P04.6
|entanglement (knot) in umbilical cord P02.5
|fetal (intrauterine)
||growth retardation P05.9
||inflammatory response syndrome (FIRS)
||| P02.70
||malnutrition not light or small for
||| gestational age P05.2
|FIRS (fetal inflammatory response
|| syndrome) P02.70
|forceps delivery P03.2
|heart rate abnormalities
||bradycardia P29.12
||intrauterine P03.819
|||before onset of labor P03.810
|||during labor P03.811
||tachycardia P29.11
|hemorrhage (antepartum) P02.1
||cerebellar (nontraumatic) P52.6
||intracerebral (nontraumatic) P52.4
||intracranial (nontraumatic) P52.9
|||specified NEC P52.8
||intraventricular (nontraumatic) P52.3
|||grade 1 P52.0
|||grade 2 P52.1
|||grade 3 P52.21
|||grade 4 P52.22
||posterior fossa (nontraumatic) P52.6
||subarachnoid (nontraumatic) P52.5
||subependymal P52.0
|||with intracerebral extension P52.22
|||with intraventricular extension P52.1
||||with enlargement of ventricles P52.21
|||without intraventricular extension P52.0
|hypoxic ischemic encephalopathy [HIE]
|| P91.60
||mild P91.61
||moderate P91.62
||severe P91.63
|induction of labor P03.89
|intestinal perforation P78.0
|intrauterine (fetal) blood loss P50.9
||due to (from)
|||cut end of co-twin cord P50.5
|||hemorrhage into
||||co-twin P50.3
||||maternal circulation P50.4
|||placenta P50.2
|||ruptured cord blood P50.1
|||vasa previa P50.0
||specified NEC P50.8
|intrauterine (fetal) hemorrhage P50.9
|intrauterine (in utero) procedure P96.5
|malpresentation (malposition) NEC P03.1
|maternal (complication of) (use of)
||group B streptococcus (GBS) colonization
||| (positive) P00.82

Newborn - *continued*
|alcohol P04.3
|amphetamines P04.16
|analgesia (maternal) P04.0
|anesthesia (maternal) P04.0
|anticonvulsants P04.13
|antidepressants P04.15
|antineoplastic chemotherapy P04.11
|anxiolytics P04.1A
|blood loss P02.1
|cannabis P04.81
|circulatory disease P00.3
|condition P00.9
||specified NEC P00.89
|cytotoxic drugs P04.12
|delivery P03.9
||Cesarean P03.4
||forceps P03.2
||vacuum extractor P03.3
|diabetes mellitus (pre-existing) P70.1
|disorder P00.9
||specified NEC P00.89
|drugs (addictive) (illegal) NEC P04.49
|ectopic pregnancy P01.4
|gestational diabetes P70.0
|hemorrhage P02.1
|hypertensive disorder P00.0
|incompetent cervix P01.0
|infectious disease P00.2
|injury P00.5
|labor and delivery P03.9
|malpresentation before labor P01.7
|maternal death P01.6
|medical procedure P00.7
|medication P04.19
||specified type NEC P04.18
||tranquilizers administered for procedures
||| during pregnancy or labor and delivery
||| P04.0
|multiple pregnancy P01.5
|nutritional disorder P00.4
|oligohydramnios P01.2
|opiates P04.14
||administered for procedures during
||| pregnancy or labor and delivery
||| P04.0
|parasitic disease P00.2
|periodontal disease P00.81
|placenta previa P02.0
|polyhydramnios P01.3
|precipitate delivery P03.5
|pregnancy P01.9
||specified P01.8
|premature rupture of membranes P01.1
|renal disease P00.1
|respiratory disease P00.3
|sedative-hypnotics P04.17
|surgical procedure P00.6
|tranquilizers administered for procedures
|| during pregnancy or labor and delivery
|| P04.0
|urinary tract disease P00.1
|uterine contraction (abnormal) P03.6
|meconium peritonitis P78.0
|medication (legal) (maternal use)
|| (prescribed) P04.19
|membrane abnormalities P02.9
||specified NEC P02.8
|membranitis P02.78
|methamphetamine(s) P04.49
|mixed metabolic and respiratory acidosis
|| P84
|neonatal abstinence syndrome P96.1
|noxious substances transmitted via placenta
|| or breast milk P04.9

Newborn - *continued*
- |cannabis P04.81
- |specified NEC P04.89
- |nutritional supplements P04.5
- |placenta previa P02.0
- |placental
  - |abnormality (functional) (morphological)
    - P02.20
    - |specified NEC P02.29
  - |dysfunction P02.29
  - |infarction P02.29
  - |insufficiency P02.29
  - |separation NEC P02.1
  - |transfusion syndromes P02.3
- |placentitis P02.78
- |precipitate delivery P03.5
- |prolapsed cord P02.4
- |respiratory arrest P28.81
- |slow intrauterine growth P05.9
- |tobacco P04.2
- |twin to twin transplacental transfusion P02.3
- |umbilical cord (tightly) around neck P02.5
- |umbilical cord condition P02.60
  - |short cord P02.69
  - |specified NEC P02.69
- |uterine contractions (abnormal) P03.6
- |vasa previa P02.69
  - |from intrauterine blood loss P50.0
- |apnea P28.4
  - |primary P28.3
  - |obstructive P28.4
  - |sleep (central) (obstructive) (primary) P28.3
- |born in hospital Z38.00
  - |by cesarean Z38.01
- |born outside hospital Z38.1
- |breast buds P96.89
- |breast engorgement P83.4
- |check-up *see* Newborn, examination
- |convulsion P90
- |dehydration P74.1
- |examination
  - |8 to 28 days old Z00.111
  - |under 8 days old Z00.110
- |fever P81.9
  - |environmentally-induced P81.0
- |hyperbilirubinemia P59.9
  - |of prematurity P59.0
- |hypernatremia P74.21
- |hyponatremia P74.22
- |infection P39.9
  - |candidal P37.5
  - |specified NEC P39.8
  - |urinary tract P39.3
- |jaundice P59.9
  - |due to
    - |breast milk inhibitor P59.3
    - |hepatocellular damage P59.20
      - |specified NEC P59.29
    - |preterm delivery P59.0
  - |of prematurity P59.0
  - |specified NEC P59.8
- |late metabolic acidosis P74.0
- |mastitis P39.0
  - |infective P39.0
  - |noninfective P83.4
- |multiple born NEC Z38.8
  - |born in hospital Z38.68
    - |by cesarean Z38.69
  - |born outside hospital Z38.7
- |omphalitis P38.9
  - |with mild hemorrhage P38.1
  - |without hemorrhage P38.9
- |post-term P08.21
- |prolonged gestation (over 42 completed
  - weeks) P08.22

Newborn - *continued*
- |quadruplet Z38.8
  - |born in hospital Z38.63
    - |by cesarean Z38.64
  - |born outside hospital Z38.7
- |quintuplet Z38.8
  - |born in hospital Z38.65
    - |by cesarean Z38.66
  - |born outside hospital Z38.7
- |seizure P90
- |sepsis (congenital) P36.9
  - |due to
    - |anaerobes NEC P36.5
    - |Escherichia coli P36.4
    - |Staphylococcus P36.30
      - |aureus P36.2
      - |specified NEC P36.39
    - |Streptococcus P36.10
      - |group B P36.0
      - |specified NEC P36.19
  - |specified NEC P36.8
- |triplet Z38.8
  - |born in hospital Z38.61
    - |by cesarean Z38.62
  - |born outside hospital Z38.7
- |twin Z38.5
  - |born in hospital Z38.30
    - |by cesarean Z38.31
  - |born outside hospital Z38.4
- |vomiting P92.09
  - |bilious P92.01
- |weight check Z00.111
Newcastle conjunctivitis or disease B30.8
Nezelof's syndrome (pure alymphocytosis)
  D81.4
Niacin (amide) deficiency E52
Nicolas (-Durand) -Favre disease A55
Nicotine *see* Tobacco
Nicotinic acid deficiency E52
Niemann-Pick disease or syndrome E75.249
- |specified NEC E75.248
- |type
  - |A E75.240
  - |A/B E75.244
  - |B E75.241
  - |C E75.242
  - |D E75.243
Night
- |blindness *see* Blindness, night
- |sweats R61
- |terrors (child) F51.4
Nightmares (REM sleep type) F51.5
NIHSS (National Institutes of Health Stroke
  Scale) score R29.7-
Nipple *see* condition
Nisbet's chancre A57
Nishimoto (-Takeuchi) disease I67.5
Nitritoid crisis or reaction *see* Crisis, nitritoid
Nitrosohemoglobinemia D74.8
Njovera A65
No general equivalence degree (GED) Z55.5
Nocardiosis, nocardiasis A43.9
- |cutaneous A43.1
- |lung A43.0
- |pneumonia A43.0
- |pulmonary A43.0
- |specified site NEC A43.8
Nocturia R35.1
- |psychogenic F45.8
Nocturnal *see* condition
Nodal rhythm I49.8
Node(s) *see also* Nodule
- |Bouchard's (with arthropathy) M15.2
- |Haygarth's M15.8
- |Heberden's (with arthropathy) M15.1

Node(s) - *continued*
- |larynx J38.7
- |lymph *see* condition
- |milker's B08.03
- |Osler's I33.0
- |Schmorl's *see* Schmorl's disease
- |singer's J38.2
- |teacher's J38.2
- |tuberculous *see* Tuberculosis, lymph gland
- |vocal cord J38.2
Nodule(s), nodular
- |actinomycotic *see* Actinomycosis
- |breast NEC (*see also* Lump, breast) N63.0
- |colloid (cystic), thyroid E04.1
- |cutaneous *see* Swelling, localized
- |endometrial (stromal) D26.1
- |Haygarth's M15.8
- |inflammatory *see* Inflammation
- |juxta-articular
  - |syphilitic A52.77
  - |yaws A66.7
- |larynx J38.7
- |lung, solitary (subsegmental branch of the
  - bronchial tree) R91.1
  - |multiple R91.8
- |milker's B08.03
- |prostate N40.2
  - |with lower urinary tract symptoms (LUTS)
    - N40.3
  - |without lower urinary tract symptoms
    - (LUTS) N40.2
- |pulmonary, solitary (subsegmental branch of
  - the bronchial tree) R91.1
- |retrocardiac R09.89
- |rheumatoid M06.30
  - |ankle M06.37-
  - |elbow M06.32-
  - |foot joint M06.37-
  - |hand joint M06.34-
  - |hip M06.35-
  - |knee M06.36-
  - |multiple site M06.39
  - |shoulder M06.31-
  - |vertebra M06.38
  - |wrist M06.33-
- |scrotum (inflammatory) N49.2
- |singer's J38.2
- |solitary, lung (subsegmental branch of the
  - bronchial tree) R91.1
  - |multiple R91.8
- |subcutaneous *see* Swelling, localized
- |teacher's J38.2
- |thyroid (cold) (gland) (nontoxic) E04.1
  - |with thyrotoxicosis E05.20
    - |with thyroid storm E05.21
  - |toxic or with hyperthyroidism E05.20
    - |with thyroid storm E05.21
- |vocal cord J38.2
Noma (gangrenous) (hospital) (infective)
  A69.0
- |auricle I96
- |mouth A69.0
- |pudendi N76.89
- |vulvae N76.89
Nomad, nomadism Z59.00
NOMID (neonatal onset multisystemic
  inflammatory disorder) M04.2
Nonadherence to medical treatment Z91.19
Nonautoimmune hemolytic anemia D59.4
- |drug-induced D59.2
Nonclosure *see also* Imperfect, closure
- |ductus arteriosus (Botallo's) Q25.0
- |foramen
  - |botalli Q21.1
  - |ovale Q21.1

Noncompliance Z91.19
|with
  |dietary regimen Z91.11
  |dialysis Z91.15
  |medical treatment Z91.19
  |medication regimen NEC Z91.14
    |underdosing *see also* Table of Drugs and
        Chemicals, categories T36-T50, with
        final character 6 Z91.14
    |intentional NEC Z91.128
      |due to financial hardship of patient
          Z91.120
    |unintentional NEC Z91.138
      |due to patient's age related debility
          Z91.130
  |renal dialysis Z91.15
Nondescent (congenital) *see also* Malposition,
    congenital
|cecum Q43.3
|colon Q43.3
|testicle Q53.9
  |bilateral Q53.20
    |abdominal Q53.211
    |perineal Q53.22
  |unilateral Q53.10
    |abdominal Q53.111
    |perineal Q53.12
Nondevelopment
|brain Q02
  |part of Q04.3
|heart Q24.8
|organ or site, congenital NEC *see* Hypoplasia
Nonengagement
|head NEC O32.4
  |in labor, causing obstructed labor O64.8
Nonexanthematous tick fever A93.2
Nonexpansion, lung (newborn) P28.0
Nonfunctioning
|cystic duct *see also* Disease, gallbladder
    K82.8
|gallbladder *see also* Disease, gallbladder
    K82.8
|kidney N28.9
|labyrinth *see* subcategory H83.2
Non-Hodgkin lymphoma NEC *see* Lymphoma,
    non-hodgkin
Nonimplantation, ovum N97.2
Noninsufflation, fallopian tube N97.1
Non-Ketotic hyperglycinemia E72.51
Nonne-Milroy syndrome Q82.0
Nonovulation N97.0
Non-Palpable testicle(s)
|bilateral R39.84
|unilateral R39.83
Nonpatent fallopian tube N97.1
Nonpneumatization, lung NEC P28.0
Nonrotation *see* Malrotation
Nonsecretion, urine *see* Anuria
Nonunion
|fracture *see* Fracture, by site
|joint, following fusion or arthrodesis M96.0
|organ or site, congenital NEC *see* Imperfect,
    closure
|symphysis pubis, congenital Q74.2
Nonvisualization, gallbladder R93.2
Nonvital, nonvitalized tooth K04.99
Non-Working side interference M26.56
Noonan's syndrome Q87.1
**Normocytic anemia (infectional) due to blood
    loss (chronic)** D50.0
|acute D62
Norrie's disease (congenital) Q15.8
North American blastomycosis B40.9
Norwegian itch B86
Nose, nasal *see* condition

Nosebleed R04.0
Nose-Picking F98.8
Nosomania F45.21
Nosophobia F45.22
Nostalgia F43.20
Notch of iris Q13.2
Notching nose, congenital (tip) Q30.2
Nothnagel's
|syndrome *see* Strabismus, paralytic, third
    nerve
|vasomotor acroparesthesia I73.89
Novy's relapsing fever A68.9
|louse-borne A68.0
|tick-borne A68.1
Noxious
|foodstuffs, poisoning by *see* Poisoning, food,
    noxious, plant
|substances transmitted through placenta or
    breast milk P04.9
Nucleus pulposus *see* condition
Numbness R20.0
Nuns' knee *see* Bursitis, prepatellar
Nursemaid's elbow S53.03-
Nutcracker esophagus K22.4
Nutmeg liver K76.1
Nutrient element deficiency E61.9
|specified NEC E61.8
Nutrition deficient or insufficient *see also*
    Malnutrition E46
|due to
  |insufficient food T73.0
  |lack of
    |care (child) T76.02
      |adult T76.01
    |food T73.0
Nutritional stunting E45
Nyctalopia (night blindness) *see* Blindness,
    night
Nycturia R35.1
|psychogenic F45.8
Nymphomania F52.8
Nystagmus H55.00
|benign paroxysmal *see* Vertigo, benign
    paroxysmal
|central positional H81.4-
|congenital H55.01
|dissociated H55.04
|latent H55.02
|miners' H55.09
|positional
  |benign paroxysmal H81.4-
  |central H81.4-
|specified form NEC H55.09
|visual deprivation H55.03

O

Obermeyer's relapsing fever (European)
    A68.0
Obesity E66.9
|with alveolar hypoventilation E66.2
|adrenal E27.8
|complicating
  |childbirth O99.214
  |pregnancy O99.21-
  |puerperium O99.215
|constitutional E66.8
|dietary counseling and surveillance Z71.3
|drug-induced E66.1
|due to
  |drug E66.1
  |excess calories E66.09
    |morbid E66.01
    |severe E66.01
|endocrine E66.8
|endogenous E66.8

Obesity *- continued*
|exogenous E66.09
|familial E66.8
|glandular E66.8
|hypothyroid *see* Hypothyroidism
|hypoventilation syndrome (OHS) E66.2
|morbid E66.01
  |with
    |alveolar hypoventilation E66.2
    |obesity hypoventilation syndrome (OHS)
        E66.2
  |due to excess calories E66.01
|nutritional E66.09
|pituitary E23.6
|severe E66.01
|specified type NEC E66.8
Oblique *see* condition
Obliteration
|appendix (lumen) K38.8
|artery I77.1
|bile duct (noncalculous) K83.1
|common duct (noncalculous) K83.1
|cystic duct *see* Obstruction, gallbladder
|disease, arteriolar I77.1
|endometrium N85.8
|eye, anterior chamber *see* Disorder, globe,
    hypotony
|fallopian tube N97.1
|lymphatic vessel I89.0
  |due to mastectomy I97.2
|organ or site, congenital NEC *see* Atresia, by
    site
|ureter N13.5
  |with infection N13.6
|urethra *see* Stricture, urethra
|vein I87.8
|vestibule (oral) K08.89
**Observation (following) (for) (without need
    for further medical care)** Z04.9
|accident NEC Z04.3
  |at work Z04.2
  |transport Z04.1
|adverse effect of drug Z03.6
|alleged rape or sexual assault (victim), ruled
    out
  |adult Z04.41
  |child Z04.42
|criminal assault Z04.89
|development state
  |adolescent Z00.3
  |period of rapid growth in childhood Z00.2
  |puberty Z00.3
|disease, specified NEC Z03.89
|following work accident Z04.2
|forced sexual exploitation Z04.81
|forced labor exploitation Z04.82
|growth and development state *see*
    Observation, development state
|injuries (accidental) NEC *see also*
    Observation, accident
|newborn (for)
  |suspected condition, related to exposure
      from the mother or birth process *see*
      Newborn, affected by, maternal
  |ruled out Z05.9
    |cardiac Z05.0
    |connective tissue Z05.73
    |gastrointestinal Z05.5
    |genetic Z05.41
    |genitourinary Z05.6
    |immunologic Z05.43
    |infectious Z05.1
    |metabolic Z05.42
    |musculoskeletal Z05.72
    |neurological Z05.2

Observation - *continued*
|respiratory Z05.3
|skin and subcutaneous tissue Z05.71
|specified condition NEC Z05.8
|postpartum
|immediately after delivery Z39.0
|routine follow-up Z39.2
|pregnancy (normal) (without complication)
  Z34.9-
|high risk O09.9-
|suicide attempt, alleged NEC Z03.89
|self-poisoning Z03.6
|suspected, ruled out *see also* Suspected
  condition, ruled out
|abuse, physical
  |adult Z04.71
  |child Z04.72
|accident at work Z04.2
|adult battering victim Z04.71
|child battering victim Z04.72
|condition NEC Z03.89
  |newborn *see also* Observation, newborn
    (for), suspected condition, ruled out
    Z05.9
|drug poisoning or adverse effect Z03.6
|exposure (to)
  |anthrax Z03.810
  |biological agent NEC Z03.818
|foreign body
  |aspirated (inhaled) Z03.822
  |ingested Z03.821
  |inserted (injected), in (eye) (orifice) (skin)
    Z03.823
|inflicted injury NEC Z04.89
|suicide attempt, alleged Z03.89
  |self-poisoning Z03.6
|toxic effects from ingested substance (drug)
  (poison) Z03.6
|toxic effects from ingested substance (drug)
  (poison) Z03.6

Obsession, obsessional state F42.8
|mixed thoughts and acts F42.2

Obsessive-Compulsive neurosis or reaction
F42.8

Obstetric embolism, septic *see* Embolism,
obstetric, septic

Obstetrical trauma (complicating delivery)
O71.9
|with or following ectopic or molar pregnancy
  O08.6
|specified type NEC O71.89

Obstipation *see* Constipation

Obstruction, obstructed, obstructive
|airway J98.8
|with
  |allergic alveolitis J67.9
  |asthma J45.909
    |with
      |exacerbation (acute) J45.901
      |status asthmaticus J45.902
  |bronchiectasis J47.9
    |with
      |exacerbation (acute) J47.1
      |lower respiratory infection J47.0
  |bronchitis (chronic) J44.9
  |emphysema J43.9
|chronic J44.9
  |with
    |allergic alveolitis *see* Pneumonitis,
      hypersensitivity
    |bronchiectasis J47.9
      |with
        |exacerbation (acute) J47.1
        |lower respiratory infection J47.0
|due to

Obstruction - *continued*
|foreign body *see* Foreign body, by site,
causing asphyxia
  |inhalation of fumes or vapors J68.9
  |laryngospasm J38.5
|ampulla of Vater K83.1
|aortic (heart) (valve) *see* Stenosis, aortic
|aortoiliac I74.09
|aqueduct of Sylvius G91.1
|congenital Q03.0
  |with spina bifida *see* Spina bifida, by site,
    with hydrocephalus
|Arnold-Chiari *see* Arnold-Chiari disease
|artery (*see also* Atherosclerosis, artery) I70.9
  |stent *see* Restenosis, stent
  |basilar (complete) (partial) *see* Occlusion,
    artery, basilar
  |carotid (complete) (partial) *see* Occlusion,
    artery, carotid
  |cerebellar *see* Occlusion, artery, cerebellar
  |cerebral (anterior) (middle) (posterior) *see*
    Occlusion, artery, cerebral
  |precerebral *see* Occlusion, artery,
    precerebral
  |renal N28.0
  |retinal NEC *see* Occlusion, artery, retina
  |vertebral (complete) (partial) *see* Occlusion,
    artery, vertebral
|band (intestinal) (*see also* Obstruction,
  intestine, specified NEC) K56.699
|bile duct or passage (common) (hepatic)
  (noncalculous) K83.1
  |with calculus K80.51
  |congenital (causing jaundice) Q44.3
|biliary (duct) (tract) K83.1
  |gallbladder K82.0
|bladder-neck (acquired) N32.0
  |congenital Q64.31
  |due to hyperplasia (hypertrophy) of prostate
    see Hyperplasia, prostate
|bowel *see* Obstruction, intestine
|bronchus J98.09
|canal, ear *see* Stenosis, external ear canal
|cardia K22.2
|caval veins (inferior) (superior) I87.1
|cecum *see* Obstruction, intestine
|circulatory I99.8
|colon *see* Obstruction, intestine
|common duct (noncalculous) K83.1
|coronary (artery) *see* Occlusion, coronary
|cystic duct *see also* Obstruction, gallbladder
  |with calculus K80.21
|device, implant or graft *see also*
  Complications, by site and type,
  mechanical T85.698
  |arterial graft NEC *see* Complication,
    cardiovascular device, mechanical,
    vascular
  |catheter NEC T85.628
    |cystostomy T83.090
    |dialysis (renal) T82.49
      |intraperitoneal T85.691
    |Hopkins T83.098
    |ileostomy T83.098
    |infusion NEC T82.594
      |spinal (epidural) (subdural) T85.690
    |nephrostomy T83.092
    |urethral indwelling T83.091
    |urinary T83.098
    |urostomy T83.098
  |due to infection T85.79
  |gastrointestinal *see* Complications,
    prosthetic device, mechanical,
    gastrointestinal device
  |genital NEC T83.498

Obstruction - *continued*
|intrauterine contraceptive device T83.39
|penile prosthesis (cylinder) (implanted)
  (pump) (reservoir) T83.490
|testicular prosthesis T83.491
|heart NEC *see* Complication, cardiovascular
  device, mechanical
|joint prosthesis *see* Complications, joint
  prosthesis, mechanical, specified NEC, by
  site
|orthopedic NEC *see* Complication,
  orthopedic, device, mechanical
|specified NEC T85.628
|urinary NEC *see* Complication,
  genitourinary, device, urinary, mechanical
  |graft T83.29
|vascular NEC *see* Complication,
  cardiovascular device, mechanical
|ventricular intracranial shunt T85.09
|due to foreign body accidentally left in
  operative wound T81.529
|duodenum K31.5
|ejaculatory duct N50.89
|esophagus K22.2
|eustachian tube (complete) (partial) H68.10-
  |cartilaginous (extrinsic) H68.13-
  |intrinsic H68.12-
  |osseous H68.11-
|fallopian tube (bilateral) N97.1
|fecal K56.41
  |with hernia *see* Hernia, by site, with
    obstruction
|foramen of Monro (congenital) Q03.8
  |with spina bifida *see* Spina bifida, by site,
    with hydrocephalus
|foreign body *see* Foreign body
|gallbladder K82.0
  |with calculus, stones K80.21
  |congenital Q44.1
|gastric outlet K31.1
|gastrointestinal *see* Obstruction, intestine
|hepatic K76.89
  |duct (noncalculous) K83.1
|hepatobiliary K83.1
|ileum *see* Obstruction, intestine
|iliofemoral (artery) I74.5
|intestine K56.609
  |complete K56.601
  |incomplete K56.600
  |partial K56.600
  |with
    |adhesions (intestinal) (peritoneal) K56.50
      |complete K56.52
      |incomplete K56.51
      |partial K56.51
  |adynamic K56.0
  |by gallstone K56.3
  |congenital (small) Q41.9
    |large Q42.9
    |specified part NEC Q42.8
  |neurogenic K56.0
    |Hirschsprung's disease or megacolon
      Q43.1
  |newborn P76.9
    |due to
      |fecaliths P76.8
      |inspissated milk P76.2
      |meconium (plug) P76.0
        |in mucoviscidosis E84.11
    |specified NEC P76.8
  |postoperative K91.30
    |complete K91.32
    |incomplete K91.31
    |partial K91.31
  |reflex K56.0

Obstruction - *continued*
- specified NEC K56.699
  - complete K56.691
  - incomplete K56.690
  - partial K56.690
- volvulus K56.2
- intracardiac ball valve prosthesis T82.09
- jejunum *see* Obstruction, intestine
- joint prosthesis *see* Complications, joint prosthesis, mechanical, specified NEC, by site
- kidney (calices) (see also Hydronephrosis) N28.89
- labor *see* Delivery
- lacrimal (passages) (duct)
  - by
    - dacryolith *see* Dacryolith
    - stenosis *see* Stenosis, lacrimal
  - congenital Q10.5
  - neonatal H04.53-
- lacrimonasal duct *see* Obstruction, lacrimal
- lacteal, with steatorrhea K90.2
- laryngitis *see* Laryngitis
- larynx NEC J38.6
  - congenital Q31.8
- lung J98.4
  - disease, chronic J44.9
- lymphatic I89.0
- meconium (plug)
  - newborn P76.0
    - due to fecaliths P76.0
    - in mucoviscidosis E84.11
- mitral *see* Stenosis, mitral
- nasal J34.89
- nasolacrimal duct *see also* Obstruction, lacrimal
  - congenital Q10.5
- nasopharynx J39.2
- nose J34.89
- organ or site, congenital NEC *see* Atresia, by site
- pancreatic duct K86.89
- parotid duct or gland K11.8
- pelviureteral junction N13.5
  - with hydronephrosis N13.0
  - congenital Q62.39
- pharynx J39.2
- portal (circulation) (vein) I81
- prostate *see also* Hyperplasia, prostate
  - valve (urinary) N32.0
- pulmonary valve (heart) I37.0
- pyelonephritis (chronic) N11.1
- pylorus
  - adult K31.1
  - congenital or infantile Q40.0
- rectosigmoid *see* Obstruction, intestine
- rectum K62.4
- renal (see also Hydronephrosis) N28.89
  - outflow N13.8
  - pelvis, congenital Q62.39
- respiratory J98.8
  - chronic J44.9
- retinal (vessels) H34.9
- salivary duct (any) K11.8
  - with calculus K11.5
- sigmoid *see* Obstruction, intestine
- sinus (accessory) (nasal) J34.89
- Stensen's duct K11.8
- stomach NEC K31.89
  - acute K31.0
  - congenital Q40.2
  - due to pylorospasm K31.3
- submandibular duct K11.8
- submaxillary gland K11.8
  - with calculus K11.5
- thoracic duct I89.0

Obstruction - *continued*
- thrombotic *see* Thrombosis
- trachea J39.8
- tracheostomy airway J95.03
- tricuspid (valve) *see* Stenosis, tricuspid
- upper respiratory, congenital Q34.8
- ureter (functional) (pelvic junction) NEC N13.5
  - with
    - hydronephrosis N13.1
      - with infection N13.6
    - pyelonephritis (chronic) N11.1
  - congenital Q62.39
  - due to calculus *see* Calculus, ureter
- urethra NEC N36.8
  - congenital Q64.39
- urinary (moderate) N13.9
  - due to hyperplasia (hypertrophy) of prostate *see* Hyperplasia, prostate
  - organ or tract (lower) N13.9
  - prostatic valve N32.0
  - specified NEC N13.8
- uropathy N13.9
- uterus N85.8
- vagina N89.5
- valvular *see* Endocarditis
- vein, venous I87.1
  - caval (inferior) (superior) I87.1
  - thrombotic *see* Thrombosis
- vena cava (inferior) (superior) I87.1
- vesical NEC N32.0
- vesicourethral orifice N32.0
  - congenital Q64.31
- vessel NEC I99.8
  - stent *see* Restenosis, stent

Obturator *see* condition
Occlusal wear, teeth K03.0
Occlusio pupillae *see* Membrane, pupillary
Occlusion, occluded
- anus K62.4
  - congenital Q42.3
    - with fistula Q42.2
- aortoiliac (chronic) I74.09
- aqueduct of Sylvius G91.1
  - congenital Q03.0
    - with spina bifida *see* Spina bifida, by site, with hydrocephalus
- artery (*see also* Atherosclerosis, artery) I70.9
  - auditory, internal I65.8
  - basilar I65.1
    - with
      - infarction I63.22
        - due to
          - embolism I63.12
          - thrombosis I63.02
  - brain or cerebral I66.9
    - with infarction (due to) I63.5-
      - embolism I63.4-
      - thrombosis I63.3-
  - carotid I65.2-
    - with
      - infarction I63.23-
        - due to
          - embolism I63.13-
          - thrombosis I63.03-
  - cerebellar (anterior inferior) (posterior inferior) (superior) I66.3
    - with infarction I63.54-
      - due to
        - embolism I63.44-
        - thrombosis I63.34-
  - cerebral I66.9
    - with infarction I63.50
      - due to
        - embolism I63.40

Occlusion, occluded - *continued*
- specified NEC I63.49
  - thrombosis I63.30
    - specified NEC I63.39
- anterior I66.1-
  - with infarction I63.52-
    - due to
      - embolism I63.42-
      - thrombosis I63.32-
- middle I66.0-
  - with infarction I63.51-
    - due to
      - embolism I63.41-
      - thrombosis I63.31-
- posterior I66.2-
  - with infarction I63.53-
    - due to
      - embolism I63.43-
      - thrombosis I63.33-
- specified NEC I66.8
  - with infarction I63.59
    - due to
      - embolism I63.4-
      - thrombosis I63.3-
- choroidal (anterior) *see* Occlusion, artery, precerebral, specified NEC
- communicating posterior *see* Occlusion, artery, precerebral, specified NEC
- complete
  - coronary I25.82
  - extremities I70.92
- coronary (acute) (thrombotic) (without myocardial infarction) I24.0
  - with myocardial infarction *see* Infarction, myocardium
  - chronic total I25.82
  - complete I25.82
  - healed or old I25.2
  - total (chronic) I25.82
- hypophyseal *see* Occlusion, artery, precerebral, specified NEC
- iliac I74.5
- lower extremities due to stenosis or stricture I77.1
- mesenteric (embolic) (thrombotic) *see also* Infarct, intestine K55.069
- perforating *see* Occlusion, artery, cerebral, specified NEC
- peripheral I77.9
  - thrombotic or embolic I74.4
- pontine *see* Occlusion, artery, precerebral, specified NEC
- precerebral I65.9
  - with infarction I63.20
    - specified NEC I63.29
    - due to
      - embolism I63.10
        - specified NEC I63.19
      - thrombosis I63.00
        - specified NEC I63.09
  - basilar *see* Occlusion, artery, basilar
  - carotid *see* Occlusion, artery, carotid
  - puerperal O88.23
  - specified NEC I65.8
    - with infarction I63.29
      - due to
        - embolism I63.19
        - thrombosis I63.09
  - vertebral *see* Occlusion, artery, vertebral
- renal N28.0
- retinal
  - central H34.1-
  - partial H34.21-
  - branch H34.23-
  - transient H34.0-

Occlusion, occluded - *continued*
|spinal *see* Occlusion, artery, precerebral, vertebral
|total (chronic)
||coronary I25.82
||extremities I70.92
|vertebral I65.0-
||with
|||infarction I63.21-
||||due to
|||||embolism I63.11-
|||||thrombosis I63.01-
|basilar artery *see* Occlusion, artery, basilar
|bile duct (common) (hepatic) (noncalculous) K83.1
|bowel *see* Obstruction, intestine
|carotid (artery) (common) (internal) *see* Occlusion, artery, carotid
|centric (of teeth) M26.59
||maximum intercuspation discrepancy M26.55
|cerebellar (artery) *see* Occlusion, artery, cerebellar
|cerebral (artery) *see* Occlusion, artery, cerebral
|cerebrovascular *see also* Occlusion, artery, cerebral
||with infarction I63.5-
|cervical canal *see* Stricture, cervix
|cervix (uteri) *see* Stricture, cervix
|choanal Q30.0
|choroidal (artery) *see* Occlusion, artery, precerebral, specified NEC
|colon *see* Obstruction, intestine
|communicating posterior artery *see* Occlusion, artery, precerebral, specified NEC
|coronary (artery) (vein) (thrombotic) *see also* Infarct, myocardium
||chronic total I25.82
||healed or old I25.2
||not resulting in infarction I24.0
||total (chronic) I25.82
|cystic duct *see* Obstruction, gallbladder
|embolic *see* Embolism
|fallopian tube N97.1
||congenital Q50.6
|gallbladder *see also* Obstruction, gallbladder
||congenital (causing jaundice) Q44.1
|gingiva, traumatic K06.2
|hymen N89.6
||congenital Q52.3
|hypophyseal (artery) *see* Occlusion, artery, precerebral, specified NEC
|iliac artery I74.5
|intestine *see* Obstruction, intestine
|lacrimal passages *see* Obstruction, lacrimal
|lung J98.4
|lymph or lymphatic channel I89.0
|mammary duct N64.89
|mesenteric artery (embolic) (thrombotic) *see also* Infarct, intestine K55.069
|nose J34.89
||congenital Q30.0
|organ or site, congenital NEC *see* Atresia, by site
|oviduct N97.1
||congenital Q50.6
|peripheral arteries
||due to stricture or stenosis I77.1
||upper extremity I74.2
|pontine (artery) *see* Occlusion, artery, precerebral, specified NEC
|posterior lingual, of mandibular teeth M26.29
|precerebral artery *see* Occlusion, artery, precerebral

Occlusion, occluded - *continued*
|punctum lacrimale *see* Obstruction, lacrimal
|pupil *see* Membrane, pupillary
|pylorus, adult *see also* Stricture, pylorus K31.1
|renal artery N28.0
|retina, retinal
||artery *see* Occlusion, artery, retinal
||vein (central) H34.81-
|||engorgement H34.82-
|||tributary H34.83-
||vessels H34.9
|spinal artery *see* Occlusion, artery, precerebral, vertebral
|teeth (mandibular) (posterior lingual) M26.29
|thoracic duct I89.0
|thrombotic *see* Thrombosis, artery
|traumatic
||edentulous (alveolar) ridge K06.2
||gingiva K06.2
||periodontal K05.5
|tubal N97.1
|ureter (complete) (partial) N13.5
||congenital Q62.10
|ureteropelvic junction N13.5
||congenital Q62.11
|ureterovesical orifice N13.5
||congenital Q62.12
|urethra *see* Stricture, urethra
|uterus N85.8
|vagina N89.5
|vascular NEC I99.8
|vein *see* Thrombosis
||retinal *see* Occlusion, retinal, vein
|vena cava (inferior) (superior) *see* Embolism, vena cava
|ventricle (brain) NEC G91.1
|vertebral (artery) *see* Occlusion, artery, vertebral
|vessel (blood) I99.8
|vulva N90.5
Occult
|blood in feces (stools) R19.5
Occupational
|problems NEC Z56.89
Ochlophobia *see* Agoraphobia
Ochronosis (endogenous) E70.29
Ocular muscle *see* condition
Oculogyric crisis or disturbance H51.8
|psychogenic F45.8
Oculomotor syndrome H51.9
Oculopathy
|syphilitic NEC A52.71
||congenital
|||early A50.01
|||late A50.30
||early (secondary) A51.43
||late A52.71
Oddi's sphincter spasm K83.4
Odontalgia K08.89
Odontoameloblastoma *see* Cyst, calcifying odontogenic
Odontoclasia K03.89
Odontodysplasia, regional K00.4
Odontogenesis imperfecta K00.5
Odontoma (ameloblastic) (complex) (compound) (fibroameloblastic) *see* Cyst, calcifying odontogenic
Odontomyelitis (closed) (open) K04.01
|irreversible K04.02
|reversible K04.01
Odontorrhagia K08.89
Odontosarcoma, ameloblastic C41.1
|upper jaw (bone) C41.0
Oestriasis *see* Myiasis

Oguchi's disease H53.63
Ohara's disease *see* Tularemia
OHS (obesity hypoventilation syndrome) E66.2
Oidiomycosis *see* Candidiasis
Oidium albicans infection *see* Candidiasis
Old age (without mention of debility) R54
|dementia F03
Old (previous) myocardial infarction I25.2
Olfactory *see* condition
Oligemia *see* Anemia
Oligoastrocytoma
|specified site *see* Neoplasm, malignant, by site
|unspecified site C71.9
Oligocythemia D64.9
Oligodendroblastoma
|specified site *see* Neoplasm, malignant
|unspecified site C71.9
Oligodendroglioma
|anaplastic type
||specified site *see* Neoplasm, malignant, by site
||unspecified site C71.9
|specified site *see* Neoplasm, malignant, by site
|unspecified site C71.9
Oligodontia *see* Anodontia
Oligoencephalon Q02
Oligohidrosis L74.4
Oligohydramnios O41.0-
Oligohidrosis L74.4
Oligomenorrhea N91.5
|primary N91.3
|secondary N91.4
Oligophrenia *see also* Disability, intellectual
|phenylpyruvic E70.0
Oligospermia N46.11
|due to
||drug therapy N46.121
||efferent duct obstruction N46.123
||infection N46.122
||radiation N46.124
||specified cause NEC N46.129
||systemic disease N46.125
Oligotrichia *see* Alopecia
Oliguria R34
|with, complicating or following ectopic or molar pregnancy O08.4
|postprocedural N99.0
Ollier's disease Q78.4
Omentitis *see* Peritonitis
Omenotocele *see* Hernia, abdomen, specified site NEC
Omentum, omental *see* condition
Omphalitis (congenital) (newborn) P38.9
|with mild hemorrhage P38.1
|without hemorrhage P38.9
|not of newborn L08.82
|tetanus A33
Omphalocele Q79.2
Omphalomesenteric duct, persistent Q43.0
Omphalorrhagia, newborn P51.9
Omsk hemorrhagic fever A98.1
Onanism (excessive) F98.8
Onchocerciasis, onchocercosis B73.1
|with
||eye disease B73.00
|||endophthalmitis B73.01
|||eyelid B73.09
|||glaucoma B73.02
|||specified NEC B73.09
|eye NEC B73.00
|eyelid B73.09
Oncocytoma *see* Neoplasm, benign, by site
Oncovirus, as cause of disease classified elsewhere B97.32
Ondine's curse *see* Apnea, sleep

Oneirophrenia F23
Onychauxis L60.2
  |congenital Q84.5
Onychia *see also* Cellulitis, digit
  |with lymphangitis *see* Lymphangitis, acute,
    digit
  |candidal B37.2
  |dermatophytic B35.1
Onychitis *see also* Cellulitis, digit
  |with lymphangitis *see* Lymphangitis, acute,
    digit
Onychocryptosis L60.0
Onychodystrophy L60.3
  |congenital Q84.6
Onychogryphosis, onychogryposis L60.2
Onycholysis L60.1
Onychomadesis L60.8
Onychomalacia L60.3
Onychomycosis (finger) (toe) B35.1
Onycho-Osteodysplasia Q87.2
Onychophagia F98.8
Onychophosis L60.8
Onychoptosis L60.8
Onychorrhexis L60.3
  |congenital Q84.6
Onychoschizia L60.3
Onyxis (finger) (toe) L60.0
Onyxitis *see also* Cellulitis, digit
  |with lymphangitis *see* Lymphangitis, acute,
    digit
Oophoritis (cystic) (infectional) (interstitial)
  N70.92
  |with salpingitis N70.93
  |acute N70.02
    |with salpingitis N70.03
  |chronic N70.12
    |with salpingitis N70.13
  |complicating abortion *see* Abortion, by type,
    complicated by, oophoritis
Oophorocele N83.4-
Opacity, opacities   cornea H17.-
  |central H17.1-
  |congenital Q13.3
  |degenerative *see* Degeneration, cornea
  |hereditary *see* Dystrophy, cornea
  |inflammatory *see* Keratitis
  |minor H17.81-
  |peripheral H17.82-
  |sequelae of trachoma (healed) B94.0
  |specified NEC H17.89
  |enamel (teeth) (fluoride) (nonfluoride) K00.3
  |lens *see* Cataract
  |snowball *see* Deposit, crystalline
  |vitreous (humor) NEC H43.39-
    |congenital Q14.0
    |membranes and strands H43.31-
Opalescent dentin (hereditary) K00.5
Open, opening
  |abnormal, organ or site, congenital *see*
    Imperfect, closure
  |angle with
    |borderline
      |findings
        |high risk H40.02-
        |low risk H40.01-
      |intraocular pressure H40.00-
    |cupping of discs H40.01-
    |glaucoma (primary) *see* Glaucoma, open
      angle
  |bite
    |anterior M26.220
    |posterior M26.221
  |false *see* Imperfect, closure
  |margin on tooth restoration K08.51
  |restoration margins of tooth K08.51
  |wound *see* Wound, open
Operational fatigue F48.8
Operative *see* condition

Operculitis *see* Periodontitis
Operculum *see* Break, retina
Ophiasis L63.2
Ophthalmia *see also* Conjunctivitis H10.9
  |actinic rays *see* Photokeratitis
  |allergic (acute) *see* Conjunctivitis, acute,
    atopic
  |blennorrhagic (gonococcal) (neonatorum)
    A54.31
  |diphtheritic A36.86
  |Egyptian A71.1
  |electrica *see* Photokeratitis
  |gonococcal (neonatorum) A54.31
  |metastatic *see* Endophthalmitis, purulent
  |migraine *see* Migraine, ophthalmoplegic
  |neonatorum, newborn P39.1
    |gonococcal A54.31
  |nodosa H16.24-
  |purulent *see* Conjunctivitis, acute,
    mucopurulent
  |spring *see* Conjunctivitis, acute, atopic
  |sympathetic *see* Uveitis, sympathetic
Ophthalmitis *see* Ophthalmia
Ophthalmocele (congenital) Q15.8
Ophthalmoneuromyelitis G36.0
Ophthalmoplegia *see also* Strabismus, paralytic
  |anterior internuclear *see* Ophthalmoplegia,
    internuclear
  |ataxia-areflexia G61.0
  |diabetic *see* E08-E13 with .39
  |exophthalmic E05.00
    |with thyroid storm E05.01
  |external H49.88-
    |progressive H49.4-
      |with pigmentary retinopathy *see* Kearns-
        Sayre syndrome
    |total H49.3-
  |internal (complete) (total) H52.51-
  |internuclear H51.2-
  |migraine *see* Migraine, ophthalmoplegic
  |Parinaud's H49.88-
  |progressive external *see* Ophthalmoplegia,
    external, progressive
  |supranuclear, progressive G23.1
  |total (external) *see* Ophthalmoplegia, external,
    total
Opioid(s)
  |abuse *see* Abuse, drug, opioids
  |dependence *see* Dependence, drug, opioids
  |induced, without use disorder
    |anxiety disorder F11.988
    |delirium F11.921
    |depressive disorder F11.94
    |sexual dysfunction F11.981
    |sleep disorder F11.982
Opisthognathism M26.09
Opisthorchiasis (felineus) (viverrini) B66.0
Opitz' disease D73.2
Opiumism *see* Dependence, drug, opioid
Oppenheim's disease G70.2
Oppenheim-Urbach disease (necrobiosis
  lipoidica diabeticorum) *see* E08-E13 with
  .620
Optic nerve *see* condition
Orbit *see* condition
Orchioblastoma C62.9-
Orchitis (gangrenous) (nonspecific) (septic)
  (suppurative) N45.2
  |blennorrhagic (gonococcal) (acute) (chronic)
    A54.23
  |chlamydial A56.19
  |filarial *see also* Infestation, filarial B74.9
    [N51]

Orchitis - *continued*
  |filarial *see also* Infestation, filarial B74.9
    [N51]
  |gonococcal (acute) (chronic) A54.23
  |mumps B26.0
  |syphilitic A52.76
  |tuberculous A18.15
ORF (virus disease) B08.02
Organic *see also* condition
  |brain syndrome F09
  |heart *see* Disease, heart
  |mental disorder F09
  |psychosis F09
Orgasm
  |anejaculatory N53.13
Oriental
  |bilharziasis B65.2
  |schistosomiasis B65.2
Orifice *see* condition
Origin of both great vessels from right
  ventricle Q20.1
Ormond's disease (with ureteral obstruction)
  N13.5
  |with infection N13.6
Ornithine metabolism disorder E72.4
Ornithinemia (Type I) (Type II) E72.4
Ornithosis A70
Orotaciduria, oroticaciduria (congenital)
  (hereditary) (pyrimidine deficiency) E79.8
  |anemia D53.0
Orthodontics
  |adjustment Z46.4
  |fitting Z46.4
Orthopnea R06.01
Orthopoxvirus B08.09
  |specified NEC B08.09
Os, uterus *see* condition
Osgood-Schlatter disease or osteochondrosis
  M92.52-
Osler (-Weber) -Rendu disease I78.0
Osler's nodes I33.0
Osmidrosis L75.0
Osseous *see* condition
Ossification
  |artery *see* Arteriosclerosis
  |auricle (ear) *see* Disorder, pinna, specified
    type NEC
  |bronchial J98.09
  |cardiac *see* Degeneration, myocardial
  |cartilage (senile) *see* Disorder, cartilage,
    specified type NEC
  |coronary (artery) *see* Disease, heart, ischemic,
    atherosclerotic
  |diaphragm J98.6
  |ear, middle *see* Otosclerosis
  |falx cerebri G96.198
  |fontanel, premature Q75.0
  |heart *see also* Degeneration, myocardial
    |valve *see* Endocarditis
  |larynx J38.7
  |ligament *see* Disorder, tendon, specified type
    NEC
    |posterior longitudinal *see* Spondylopathy,
      specified NEC
  |meninges (cerebral) (spinal) G96.198
  |multiple, eccentric centers *see* Disorder, bone,
    development or growth
  |muscle *see also* Calcification, muscle
    |due to burns *see* Myositis, ossificans, in,
      burns
    |paralytic *see* Myositis, ossificans, in,
      quadriplegia
    |progressive *see* Myositis, ossificans,
      progressiva
    |specified NEC M61.50

Osteochondroarthrosis deformans endemica
  see Disease, Kaschin-Beck
Osteochondritis *see also* Osteochondropathy,
  by site
  |Brailsford's *see* Osteochondrosis, juvenile,
    radius
  |dissecans M93.20
    |ankle M93.27-
    |elbow M93.22-
    |foot M93.27-
    |hand M93.24-
    |hip M93.25-
    |knee M93.26-
    |multiple sites M93.29
    |shoulder joint M93.21-
    |specified site NEC M93.28
    |wrist M93.23-
  |juvenile M92.9
    |patellar *see* Osteochondrosis, juvenile,
      patella
  |syphilitic (congenital) (early) A50.02
      [M90.80]
    |ankle A50.02 *[M90.87]*
    |elbow A50.02 *[M90.82]*
    |foot A50.02 *[M90.87]*
    |forearm A50.02 *[M90.83]*
    |hand A50.02 *[M90.84]*
    |hip A50.02 *[M90.85]*
    |knee A50.02 *[M90.86]*
    |multiple sites A50.02 *[M90.89]*
    |shoulder joint A50.02 *[M90.81]*
    |specified site NEC A50.02 *[M90.88]*
Osteochondrodysplasia Q78.9
  |with defects of growth of tubular bones and
    spine Q77.9
  |specified NEC Q77.8
  |specified NEC Q78.8
Osteochondrodystrophy E78.9
Osteochondrolysis *see* Osteochondritis,
  dissecans
Osteochondroma *see* Neoplasm, bone, benign
Osteochondromatosis D48.0
  |syndrome Q78.4
Osteochondromyxosarcoma *see* Neoplasm,
  bone, malignant
Osteochondropathy M93.90
  |ankle M93.97-
  |elbow M93.92-
  |foot M93.97-
  |hand M93.94-
  |hip M93.95-
  |Kienböck's disease of adults M93.1
  |knee M93.96-
  |multiple joints M93.99
  |osteochondritis dissecans *see* Osteochondritis,
    dissecans
  |osteochondrosis *see* Osteochondrosis
  |shoulder region M93.91-
  |slipped upper femoral epiphysis *see* Slipped,
    epiphysis, upper femoral
  |specified joint NEC M93.98
  |specified type NEC M93.80
    |ankle M93.87-
    |elbow M93.82-
    |foot M93.87-
    |hand M93.84-
    |hip M93.85-
    |knee M93.86-
    |multiple joints M93.89
    |shoulder region M93.81-
    |specified joint NEC M93.88
    |wrist M93.83-
  |syphilitic, congenital
    |early A50.02 *[M90.80]*

Osteochondropathy - *continued*
  |late A50.56 *[M90.80]*
  |wrist M93.93-
Osteochondrosarcoma *see* Neoplasm, bone,
  malignant
Osteochondrosis *see also* Osteochondropathy,
  by site
  |acetabulum (juvenile) M91.0
  |adult *see* Osteochondropathy, specified type
    NEC, by site
  |astragalus (juvenile) *see* Osteochondrosis,
    juvenile, tarsus
  |Blount M92.51-
  |Buchanan's M91.0
  |Burns' *see* Osteochondrosis, juvenile, ulna
  |calcaneus (juvenile) *see* Osteochondrosis,
    juvenile, tarsus
  |capitular epiphysis (femur) (juvenile) *see*
    Legg-Calvé-Perthes disease
  |carpal (juvenile) (lunate) (scaphoid) *see*
    Osteochondrosis, juvenile, hand, carpal
    lunate
    |adult M93.1
  |coxae juvenilis *see* Legg-Calvé-Perthes
    disease
  |deformans juvenilis, coxae *see* Legg-Calvé-
    Perthes disease
  |Diaz's *see* Osteochondrosis, juvenile, tarsus
  |dissecans (knee) (shoulder) *see*
    Osteochondritis, dissecans
  |femoral capital epiphysis (juvenile) *see* Legg-
    Calvé-Perthes disease
  |femur (head), juvenile *see* Legg-Calvé-Perthes
    disease
  |fibula (juvenile) *see* Osteochondrosis,
    juvenile, fibula
  |foot NEC (juvenile) M92.8
  |Freiberg's *see* Osteochondrosis, juvenile,
    metatarsus
  |Haas' (juvenile) *see* Osteochondrosis, juvenile,
    humerus
  |Haglund's *see* Osteochondrosis, juvenile,
    tarsus
  |hip (juvenile) *see* Legg-Calvé-Perthes disease
  |humerus (capitulum) (head) (juvenile) *see*
    Osteochondrosis, juvenile, humerus
  |ilium, iliac crest (juvenile) M91.0
  |ischiopubic synchondrosis M91.0
  |Iselin's *see* Osteochondrosis, juvenile,
    metatarsus
  |juvenile, juvenilis M92.9
    |after congenital dislocation of hip reduction
      see Osteochondrosis, juvenile, hip,
      specified NEC
    |arm *see* Osteochondrosis, juvenile, upper
      limb NEC
    |capitular epiphysis (femur) *see* Legg-Calvé-
      Perthes disease
    |clavicle, sternal epiphysis *see*
      Osteochondrosis, juvenile, upper limb
      NEC
    |coxae *see* Legg-Calvé-Perthes disease
    |deformans M92.9
    |fibula M92.50-
    |foot NEC M92.8
    |hand M92.20-
      |carpal lunate M92.21-
      |metacarpal head M92.22-
      |specified site NEC M92.29-
    |head of femur *see* Legg-Calvé-Perthes
      disease
    |hip and pelvis M91.9-
      |coxa plana *see* Coxa, plana
      |femoral head *see* Legg-Calvé-Perthes
        disease

Osteochondrosis - *continued*
  |pelvis M91.0
  |pseudocoxalgia *see* Pseudocoxalgia
  |specified NEC M91.8-
  |humerus M92.0-
  |limb
    |lower NEC M92.8
    |upper NEC *see* Osteochondrosis, juvenile,
      upper limb NEC
  |medial cuneiform bone *see*
    Osteochondrosis, juvenile, tarsus
  |metatarsus M92.7-
  |patella M92.4-
  |radius M92.1-
  |specified
    |site NEC M92.8
      |type NEC M92.8
      |tibia and fibula M92.59-
  |spine M42.00
    |cervical region M42.02
    |cervicothoracic region M42.03
    |lumbar region M42.06
    |lumbosacral region M42.07
    |multiple sites M42.09
    |occipito-atlanto-axial region M42.01
    |sacrococcygeal region M42.08
    |thoracic region M42.04
    |thoracolumbar region M42.05
  |tarsus M92.6-
  |tibia M92.50-
    |proximal M92.51-
    |tubercle M92.52-
  |ulna M92.1-
  |upper limb NEC M92.3-
  |vertebra (body) (epiphyseal plates) (Calvé's)
    (Scheuermann's) *see* Osteochondrosis,
    juvenile, spine
  |Kienböck's *see* Osteochondrosis, juvenile,
    hand, carpal lunate
    |adult M93.1
  |Köhler's
    |patellar *see* Osteochondrosis, juvenile,
      patella
    |tarsal navicular *see* Osteochondrosis,
      juvenile, tarsus
  |Legg-Perthes (-Calvé)(-Waldenström) *see*
    Legg-Calvé-Perthes disease
  |limb
    |lower NEC (juvenile) M92.8
      |tibia and fibula M92.59-
    |upper NEC (juvenile) *see* Osteochondrosis,
      juvenile, upper limb NEC
  |lunate bone (carpal) (juvenile) *see also*
    Osteochondrosis, juvenile, hand, carpal
    lunate
    |adult M93.1
  |Mauclaire's *see* Osteochondrosis, juvenile,
    hand, metacarpal
  |metacarpal (head) (juvenile) *see*
    Osteochondrosis, juvenile, hand,
    metacarpal
  |metatarsus (fifth) (head) (juvenile) (second)
    see Osteochondrosis, juvenile, metatarsus
  |navicular (juvenile) *see* Osteochondrosis,
    juvenile, tarsus
  |os
    |calcis (juvenile) *see* Osteochondrosis,
      juvenile, tarsus
    |tibiale externum (juvenile) *see*
      Osteochondrosis, juvenile, tarsus
  |Osgood-Schlatter M92.52-
  |Panner's *see* Osteochondrosis, juvenile,
    humerus

Osteochondrosis - *continued*
|patellar center (juvenile) (primary)
   (secondary) *see* Osteochondrosis, juvenile,
   patella
|pelvis (juvenile) M91.0
|Pierson's M91.0
|radius (head) (juvenile) *see* Osteochondrosis,
   juvenile, radius
|Scheuermann's *see* Osteochondrosis, juvenile,
   spine
|Sever's *see* Osteochondrosis, juvenile, tarsus
|Sinding-Larsen *see* Osteochondrosis, juvenile,
   patella
|spine M42.9
   |adult M42.10
      |cervical region M42.12
      |cervicothoracic region M42.13
      |lumbar region M42.16
      |lumbosacral region M42.17
      |multiple sites M42.19
      |occipito-atlanto-axial region M42.11
      |sacrococcygeal region M42.18
      |thoracic region M42.14
      |thoracolumbar region M42.15
   |juvenile *see* Osteochondrosis, juvenile,
      spine
|symphysis pubis (juvenile) M91.0
|syphilitic (congenital) A50.02
|talus (juvenile) *see* Osteochondrosis, juvenile,
   tarsus
|tarsus (navicular) (juvenile) *see*
   Osteochondrosis, juvenile, tarsus
|tibia (proximal) (tubercle) (juvenile) *see*
   Osteochondrosis, juvenile, tibia
|tuberculous *see* Tuberculosis, bone
|ulna (lower) (juvenile) *see* Osteochondrosis,
   juvenile, ulna
|van Neck's M91.0
|vertebral *see* Osteochondrosis, spine
Osteoclastoma D48.0
|malignant *see* Neoplasm, bone, malignant
Osteodynia *see* Disorder, bone, specified type
   NEC
Osteodystrophy Q78.9
|azotemic N25.0
|congenital Q78.9
|parathyroid, secondary E21.1
|renal N25.0
Osteofibroma *see* Neoplasm, bone, benign
Osteofibrosarcoma *see* Neoplasm, bone,
   malignant
Osteogenesis imperfecta Q78.0
Osteogenic *see* condition
Osteolysis M89.50
|carpus M89.54-
|clavicle M89.51-
|femur M89.55-
|fibula M89.56-
|finger M89.54-
|humerus M89.52-
|ilium M89.559
|ischium M89.559
|joint prosthesis (periprosthetic) *see*
   Complications, joint prosthesis, mechanical,
   periprosthetic, osteolysis, by site
|metacarpus M89.54-
|metatarsus M89.57-
|multiple sites M89.59
|neck M89.58
|periprosthetic *see* Complications, joint
   prosthesis, mechanical, periprosthetic,
   osteolysis, by site
|radius M89.53-
|rib M89.58
|scapula M89.51-

Osteolysis - *continued*
|skull M89.58
|tarsus M89.57-
|tibia M89.56-
|toe M89.57-
|ulna M89.53-
|vertebra M89.58
Osteoma *see also* Neoplasm, bone, benign
|osteoid *see also* Neoplasm, bone, benign
   |giant *see* Neoplasm, bone, benign
Osteomalacia M83.9
|adult M83.9
   |drug-induced NEC M83.5
   |due to
      |malabsorption (postsurgical) M83.2
      |malnutrition M83.3
   |specified NEC M83.8
|aluminium-induced M83.4
|infantile *see* Rickets
|juvenile *see* Rickets
|oncogenic E83.89
|pelvis M83.8
|puerperal M83.0
|senile M83.1
|vitamin-D-resistant in adults E83.31 *[M90.8]*
   |carpus E83.31 *[M90.84]*
   |clavicle E83.31 *[M90.81]*
   |femur E83.31 *[M90.85]*
   |fibula E83.31 *[M90.86]*
   |finger E83.31 *[M90.84]*
   |humerus E83.31 *[M90.82]*
   |ilium E83.31 *[M90.859]*
   |ischium E83.31 *[M90.859]*
   |metacarpus E83.31 *[M90.84]*
   |metatarsus E83.31 *[M90.87]*
   |multiple sites E83.31 *[M90.89]*
   |neck E83.31 *[M90.88]*
   |radius E83.31 *[M90.83]*
   |rib E83.31 *[M90.88]*
   |scapula E83.31 *[M90.819]*
   |skull E83.31 *[M90.88]*
   |tarsus E83.31 *[M90.879]*
   |tibia E83.31 *[M90.869]*
   |toe E83.31 *[M90.879]*
   |ulna E83.31 *[M90.839]*
   |vertebra E83.31 *[M90.88]*
Osteomyelitis (general) (infective) (localized)
   (neonatal) (purulent) (septic)
   (staphylococcal) (streptococcal)
   (suppurative) (with periostitis) M86.9
|acute M86.10
   |carpus M86.14-
   |clavicle M86.11-
   |femur M86.15-
   |fibula M86.16-
   |finger M86.14-
   |hematogenous M86.00
      |carpus M86.04-
      |clavicle M86.01-
      |femur M86.05-
      |fibula M86.06-
      |finger M86.04-
      |humerus M86.02-
      |ilium M86.08
      |ischium M86.08
      |mandible M27.2
      |metacarpus M86.04-
      |metatarsus M86.07-
      |multiple sites M86.09
      |neck M86.08
      |orbit H05.02-
      |petrous bone *see* Petrositis
      |radius M86.03-
      |rib M86.08
      |scapula M86.01-

Osteomyelitis - *continued*
|skull M86.08
|tarsus M86.07-
|tibia M86.06-
|toe M86.07-
|ulna M86.03-
|vertebra *see* Osteomyelitis, vertebra
|humerus M86.12-
|ilium M86.159
|ischium M86.159
|mandible M27.2
|metacarpus M86.14-
|metatarsus M86.17-
|multiple sites M86.19
|neck M86.18
|orbit H05.02-
|petrous bone *see* Petrositis
|radius M86.13-
|rib M86.18
|scapula M86.11-
|skull M86.18
|tarsus M86.17-
|tibia M86.16-
|toe M86.17-
|ulna M86.13-
|vertebra *see* Osteomyelitis, vertebra
|chronic (or old) M86.60
   |with draining sinus M86.40
      |carpus M86.44-
      |clavicle M86.41-
      |femur M86.45-
      |fibula M86.46-
      |finger M86.44-
      |humerus M86.42-
      |ilium M86.459
      |ischium M86.459
      |mandible M27.2
      |metacarpus M86.44-
      |metatarsus M86.47-
      |multiple sites M86.49
      |neck M86.48
      |orbit H05.02-
      |petrous bone *see* Petrositis
      |radius M86.43-
      |rib M86.48
      |scapula M86.41-
      |skull M86.48
      |tarsus M86.47-
      |tibia M86.46-
      |toe M86.47-
      |ulna M86.43-
      |vertebra *see* Osteomyelitis, vertebra
   |carpus M86.64-
   |clavicle M86.61-
   |femur M86.65-
   |fibula M86.66-
   |finger M86.64-
   |hematogenous NEC M86.50
      |carpus M86.54-
      |clavicle M86.51-
      |femur M86.55-
      |fibula M86.56-
      |finger M86.54-
      |humerus M86.52-
      |ilium M86.559
      |ischium M86.559
      |mandible M27.2
      |metacarpus M86.54-
      |metatarsus M86.57-
      |multifocal M86.30
         |carpus M86.34-
         |clavicle M86.31-
         |femur M86.35-
         |fibula M86.36-
         |finger M86.34-

Osteomyelitis - *continued*
- |humerus M86.32-
- |ilium M86.359
- |ischium M86.359
- |metacarpus M86.34-
- |metatarsus M86.37-
- |multiple sites M86.39
- |neck M86.38
- |radius M86.33-
- |rib M86.38
  - |scapula M86.31-
  - |skull M86.38
  - |tarsus M86.37-
  - |tibia M86.36-
  - |toe M86.37-
  - |ulna M86.33-
  - |vertebra *see* Osteomyelitis, vertebra
- |multiple sites M86.59
- |neck M86.58
- |orbit H05.02-
- |petrous bone *see* Petrositis
- |radius M86.53-
- |rib M86.58
- |scapula M86.51-
- |skull M86.58
- |tarsus M86.57-
- |tibia M86.56-
- |toe M86.57-
- |ulna M86.53-
- |vertebra *see* Osteomyelitis, vertebra
- |humerus M86.62-
- |ilium M86.659
- |ischium M86.659
- |mandible M27.2
- |metacarpus M86.64-
- |metatarsus M86.67-
- |multifocal *see* Osteomyelitis, chronic, hematogenous, multifocal
- |multiple sites M86.69
- |neck M86.68
- |orbit H05.02-
- |petrous bone *see* Petrositis
- |radius M86.63-
- |rib M86.68
- |scapula M86.61-
- |skull M86.68
- |tarsus M86.67-
- |tibia M86.66-
- |toe M86.67-
- |ulna M86.63-
- |vertebra *see* Osteomyelitis, vertebra
- |echinococcal B67.2
- |Garr's *see* Osteomyelitis, specified type NEC
- |in diabetes mellitus *see* E08-E13 with .69
- |jaw (acute) (chronic) (lower) (neonatal) (suppurative) (upper) M27.2
- |nonsuppurating *see* Osteomyelitis, specified type NEC
- |orbit H05.02-
- |petrous bone *see* Petrositis
- |Salmonella (arizonae) (cholerae-Suis) (enteritidis) (typhimurium) A02.24
- |sclerosing, nonsuppurative *see* Osteomyelitis, specified type NEC
- |specified type NEC *see also* subcategory M86.8X-
  - |mandible M27.2
  - |orbit H05.02-
  - |petrous bone *see* Petrositis
  - |vertebra *see* Osteomyelitis, vertebra
- |subacute M86.20
  - |carpus M86.24-
  - |clavicle M86.21-
  - |femur M86.25-
  - |fibula M86.26-

Osteomyelitis - *continued*
- |finger M86.24-
- |humerus M86.22-
- |mandible M27.2
- |metacarpus M86.24-
- |metatarsus M86.27-
- |multiple sites M86.29
- |neck M86.28
- |orbit H05.02-
- |petrous bone *see* Petrositis
- |radius M86.23-
- |rib M86.28
- |scapula M86.21-
- |skull M86.28
- |tarsus M86.27-
- |tibia M86.26-
- |toe M86.27-
- |ulna M86.23-
- |vertebra *see* Osteomyelitis, vertebra
- |syphilitic A52.77
  - |congenital (early) A50.02 *[M90.80]*
- |tuberculous *see* Tuberculosis, bone
- |typhoid A01.05
- |vertebra M46.20
  - |cervical region M46.22
  - |cervicothoracic region M46.23
  - |lumbar region M46.26
  - |lumbosacral region M46.27
  - |occipito-atlanto-axial region M46.21
  - |sacrococcygeal region M46.28
  - |thoracic region M46.24
  - |thoracolumbar region M46.25

Osteomyelofibrosis D47.4

Osteomyelosclerosis D75.89

Osteonecrosis M87.9
- |due to
  - |drugs *see* Osteonecrosis, secondary, due to, drugs
  - |trauma *see* Osteonecrosis, secondary, due to, trauma
- |idiopathic aseptic M87.00
  - |ankle M87.07-
  - |carpus M87.03-
  - |clavicle M87.01-
  - |femur M87.05-
  - |fibula M87.06-
  - |finger M87.04-
  - |humerus M87.02-
  - |ilium M87.050
  - |ischium M87.050
  - |metacarpus M87.04-
  - |metatarsus M87.07-
  - |multiple sites M87.09
  - |neck M87.08
  - |pelvis M87.050
  - |radius M87.03-
  - |rib M87.08
  - |scapula M87.01-
  - |skull M87.08
  - |tarsus M87.07-
  - |tibia M87.06-
  - |toe M87.07-
  - |ulna M87.03-
  - |vertebra M87.08
- |secondary NEC M87.30
  - |carpus M87.33-
  - |clavicle M87.31-
  - |due to
    - |drugs M87.10
      - |carpus M87.13-
      - |clavicle M87.11-
      - |femur M87.15-
      - |fibula M87.16-
      - |finger M87.14-
      - |humerus M87.12-

Osteonecrosis - *continued*
- |ilium M87.159
- |ischium M87.159
- |jaw M87.180
- |metacarpus M87.14-
- |metatarsus M87.17-
- |multiple sites M87.19
- |neck M87.18
- |radius M87.13-
- |rib M87.18
- |scapula M87.11-
- |skull M87.18
- |tarsus M87.17-
- |tibia M87.16-
- |toe M87.17-
- |ulna M87.13-
- |vertebra M87.18
- |hemoglobinopathy NEC D58.2 *[M90.50]*
  - |carpus D58.2 *[M90.54]*
  - |clavicle D58.2 *[M90.51]*
  - |femur D58.2 *[M90.55]*
  - |fibula D58.2 *[M90.56]*
  - |finger D58.2 *[M90.54]*
  - |humerus D58.2 *[M90.52]*
  - |ilium D58.2 *[M90.55]*
  - |ischium D58.2 *[M90.55]*
  - |metacarpus D58.2 *[M90.54]*
  - |metatarsus D58.2 *[M90.57]*
  - |multiple sites D58.2 *[M90.58]*
  - |neck D58.2 *[M90.58]*
  - |radius D58.2 *[M90.53]*
  - |rib D58.2 *[M90.58]*
  - |scapula D58.2 *[M90.51]*
  - |skull D58.2 *[M90.58]*
  - |tarsus D58.2 *[M90.57]*
  - |tibia D58.2 *[M90.56]*
  - |toe D58.2 *[M90.57]*
  - |ulna D58.2 *[M90.53]*
  - |vertebra D58.2 *[M90.58]*
- |trauma (previous) M87.20
  - |carpus M87.23-
  - |clavicle M87.21-
  - |femur M87.25-
  - |fibula M87.26-
  - |finger M87.24-
  - |humerus M87.22-
  - |ilium M87.25-
  - |ischium M87.25-
  - |metacarpus M87.24-
  - |metatarsus M87.27-
  - |multiple sites M87.29
  - |neck M87.28
  - |radius M87.23-
  - |rib M87.28
  - |scapula M87.21-
  - |skull M87.28
  - |tarsus M87.27-
  - |tibia M87.26-
  - |toe M87.27-
  - |ulna M87.23-
  - |vertebra M87.28
- |femur M87.35-
- |fibula M87.36-
- |finger M87.34-
- |humerus M87.32-
- |ilium M87.350
- |in
  - |caisson disease T70.3 *[M90.50]*
    - |carpus T70.3 *[M90.54]*
    - |clavicle T70.3 *[M90.51]*
    - |femur T70.3 *[M90.55]*
    - |fibula T70.3 *[M90.56]*
    - |finger T70.3 *[M90.54]*
    - |humerus T70.3 *[M90.52]*
    - |ilium T70.3 *[M90.55]*

Osteonecrosis - *continued*
|ischium T70.3 *[M90.55]*
|metacarpus T70.3 *[M90.54]*
|metatarsus T70.3 *[M90.57]*
|multiple sites T70.3 *[M90.59]*
|neck T70.3 *[M90.58]*
|radius T70.3 *[M90.53]*
|rib T70.3 *[M90.58]*
|scapula T70.3 *[M90.51]*
|skull T70.3 *[M90.58]*
|tarsus T70.3 *[M90.57]*
|tibia T70.3 *[M90.56]*
|toe T70.3 *[M90.57]*
|ulna T70.3 *[M90.53]*
|vertebra T70.3 *[M90.58]*
|ischium M87.350
|metacarpus M87.34-
|metatarsus M87.37-
|multiple site M87.39
|neck M87.38
|radius M87.33-
|rib M87.38
|scapula M87.319
|skull M87.38
|tarsus M87.379
|tibia M87.366
|toe M87.379
|ulna M87.33-
|vertebra M87.38
|specified type NEC M87.80
|carpus M87.83-
|clavicle M87.81-
|femur M87.85-
|fibula M87.86-
|finger M87.84-
|humerus M87.82-
|ilium M87.85-
|ischium M87.85-
|metacarpus M87.84-
|metatarsus M87.87-
|multiple sites M87.89
|neck M87.88
|radius M87.83-
|rib M87.88
|scapula M87.81-
|skull M87.88
|tarsus M87.87-
|tibia M87.86-
|toe M87.87-
|ulna M87.83-
|vertebra M87.88
Osteo-Onycho-Arthro-Dysplasia Q87.2
Osteo-Onychodysplasia, hereditary Q87.2
Osteopathia condensans disseminata Q78.8
Osteopathy *see also* Osteomyelitis, Osteonecrosis, Osteoporosis
|after poliomyelitis M89.60
|carpus M89.64-
|clavicle M89.61-
|femur M89.65-
|fibula M89.66-
|finger M89.64-
|humerus M89.62-
|ilium M89.659
|ischium M89.659
|metacarpus M89.64-
|metatarsus M89.67-
|multiple sites M89.69
|neck M89.68
|radius M89.63-
|rib M89.68
|scapula M89.61-
|skull M89.68
|tarsus M89.67-
|tibia M89.66-

Osteopathy - *continued*
|toe M89.67-
|ulna M89.63-
|vertebra M89.68
|in (due to)
|renal osteodystrophy N25.0
|specified diseases classified elsewhere *see* subcategory M90.8
Osteopenia M85.8-
|borderline M85.8-
Osteoperiostitis *see* Osteomyelitis, specified type NEC
Osteopetrosis (familial) Q78.2
Osteophyte M25.70
|ankle M25.77-
|elbow M25.72-
|foot joint M25.77-
|hand joint M25.74-
|hip M25.75-
|knee M25.76-
|shoulder M25.71-
|spine M25.78
|vertebrae M25.78
|wrist M25.73-
Osteopoikilosis Q78.8
Osteoporosis (female) (male) M81.0
|with current pathological fracture M80.00
|age-related M81.0
|with current pathologic fracture M80.00
|carpus M80.04-
|clavicle M80.01-
|fibula M80.06-
|finger M80.04-
|humerus M80.02-
|ilium M80.05-
|ischium M80.05-
|metacarpus M80.04-
|metatarsus M80.07-
|pelvis M80.05-
|radius M80.03-
|scapula M80.01-
|site specified NEC M80.0A
|tarsus M80.07-
|tibia M80.06-
|toe M80.07-
|ulna M80.03-
|vertebra M80.08
|disuse M81.8
|with current pathological fracture M80.80
|carpus M80.84-
|clavicle M80.81-
|fibula M80.86-
|finger M80.84-
|humerus M80.82-
|ilium M80.85-
|ischium M80.85-
|metacarpus M80.84-
|metatarsus M80.87-
|pelvis M80.85-
|radius M80.83-
|scapula M80.81-
|site specified NEC M80.8A
|tarsus M80.87-
|tibia M80.86-
|toe M80.87-
|ulna M80.83-
|vertebra M80.88
|drug-induced *see* Osteoporosis, specified type NEC
|idiopathic *see* Osteoporosis, specified type NEC
|involutional *see* Osteoporosis, age-related
|Lequesne M81.6
|localized M81.6
|postmenopausal M81.0

Osteoporosis - *continued*
|with pathological fracture M80.00
|carpus M80.04-
|clavicle M80.01-
|fibula M80.06-
|finger M80.04-
|humerus M80.02-
|ilium M80.05-
|ischium M80.05-
|metacarpus M80.04-
|metatarsus M80.07-
|pelvis M80.05-
|radius M80.03-
|scapula M80.01-
|site specified NEC M80.0A
|tarsus M80.07-
|tibia M80.06-
|toe M80.07-
|ulna M80.03-
|vertebra M80.08
|postoophorectomy *see* Osteoporosis, specified type NEC
|postsurgical malabsorption *see* Osteoporosis, specified type NEC
|post-traumatic *see* Osteoporosis, specified type NEC
|senile *see* Osteoporosis, age-related
|specified type NEC M81.8
|with pathological fracture M80.80
|carpus M80.84-
|clavicle M80.81-
|fibula M80.86-
|finger M80.84-
|humerus M80.82-
|ilium M80.85-
|ischium M80.85-
|metacarpus M80.84-
|metatarsus M80.87-
|pelvis M80.85-
|radius M80.83-
|scapula M80.81-
|site specified NEC M80.8A
|tarsus M80.87-
|tibia M80.86-
|toe M80.87-
|ulna M80.83-
|vertebra M80.88
Osteopsathyrosis (idiopathica) Q78.0
Osteoradionecrosis, jaw (acute) (chronic) (lower) (suppurative) (upper) M27.2
Osteosarcoma (any form) *see* Neoplasm, bone, malignant
Osteosclerosis Q78.2
|acquired M85.8-
|congenita Q77.4
|fragilitas (generalisata) Q78.2
|myelofibrosis D75.81
Osteosclerotic anemia D64.89
Osteosis
|cutis L94.2
|renal fibrocystic N25.0
Österreicher-Turner syndrome Q87.2
Ostium
|atrioventriculare commune Q21.2
|primum (arteriosum) (defect) (persistent) Q21.2
|secundum (arteriosum) (defect) (patent) (persistent) Q21.1
Ostrum-Furst syndrome Q75.8
Otalgia *see* subcategory H92.0
Otitis (acute) H66.90
|with effusion *see also* Otitis, media, nonsuppurative
|purulent *see* Otitis, media, suppurative
|adhesive *see* subcategory H74.1

Otitis (acute) - *continued*
|chronic *see also* Otitis, media, chronic
  |with effusion *see also* Otitis, media,
    nonsuppurative, chronic
|externa H60.9-
  |abscess *see* Abscess, ear, external
  |acute (noninfective) H60.50-
    |actinic H60.51-
    |chemical H60.52-
    |contact H60.53-
    |eczematoid H60.54-
    |infective *see* Otitis, externa, infective
    |reactive H60.55-
    |specified NEC H60.59-
  |cellulitis *see* Cellulitis, ear
  |chronic H60.6-
  |diffuse *see* Otitis, externa, infective, diffuse
  |hemorrhagic *see* Otitis, externa, infective,
    hemorrhagic
  |in (due to)
    |aspergillosis B44.89
    |candidiasis B37.84
    |erysipelas A46 [*H62.40*]
    |herpes (simplex) virus infection B00.1
      |zoster B02.8
    |impetigo L01.00 [*H62.40*]
    |infectious disease NEC B99 [*H62.4*]
    |mycosis NEC B36.9 [*H62.40*]
    |parasitic disease NEC B89 [*H62.40*]
    |viral disease NEC B34.9 [*H62.40*]
    |zoster B02.8
  |infective NEC H60.39-
    |abscess *see* Abscess, ear, external
    |cellulitis *see* Cellulitis, ear
    |diffuse H60.31-
    |hemorrhagic H60.32-
    |swimmer's ear *see* Swimmer's, ear
  |malignant H60.2-
  |mycotic NEC B36.9 [*H62.40*]
    |in
      |aspergillosis B44.89
      |candidiasis B37.84
      |moniliasis B37.84
  |necrotizing *see* Otitis, externa, malignant
  |Pseudomonas aeruginosa *see* Otitis, externa,
    malignant
  |reactive *see* Otitis, externa, acute, reactive
  |specified NEC *see* subcategory H60.8
  |tropical NEC B36.9 [*H62.40*]
    |in
      |aspergillosis B44.89
      |candidiasis B37.84
      |moniliasis B37.84
|insidiosa *see* Otosclerosis
|interna *see* subcategory H83.0
|media (hemorrhagic) (staphylococcal)
  (streptococcal) H66.9-
  |with effusion (nonpurulent) *see* Otitis,
    media, nonsuppurative
  |acute, subacute H66.90
    |allergic *see* Otitis, media, nonsuppurative,
      acute, allergic
    |exudative *see* Otitis, media, suppurative,
      acute
    |mucoid *see* Otitis, media, nonsuppurative,
      acute
    |necrotizing *see also* Otitis, media,
      suppurative, acute
    |in
      |measles B05.3
      |scarlet fever A38.0
    |nonsuppurative NEC *see* Otitis, media,
      nonsuppurative, acute
    |purulent *see* Otitis, media, suppurative,
      acute

Otitis (acute) - *continued*
    |sanguinous *see* Otitis, media,
      nonsuppurative, acute
    |secretory *see* Otitis, media,
      nonsuppurative, acute, serous
    |seromucinous *see* Otitis, media,
      nonsuppurative, acute
    |serous *see* Otitis, media, nonsuppurative,
      acute, serous
    |suppurative *see* Otitis, media, suppurative,
      acute
  |allergic *see* Otitis, media, nonsuppurative
  |catarrhal *see* Otitis, media, nonsuppurative
  |chronic H66.90
    |with effusion (nonpurulent) *see* Otitis,
      media, nonsuppurative, chronic
    |allergic *see* Otitis, media, nonsuppurative,
      chronic, allergic
    |benign suppurative *see* Otitis, media,
      suppurative, chronic, tubotympanic
    |catarrhal *see* Otitis, media,
      nonsuppurative, chronic, serous
    |exudative *see* Otitis, media,
      nonsuppurative, chronic
    |mucinous *see* Otitis, media,
      nonsuppurative, chronic, mucoid
    |mucoid *see* Otitis, media, nonsuppurative,
      chronic, mucoid
    |nonsuppurative NEC *see* Otitis, media,
      nonsuppurative, chronic
    |purulent *see* Otitis, media, suppurative,
      chronic
    |secretory *see* Otitis, media,
      nonsuppurative, chronic, mucoid
    |seromucinous *see* Otitis, media,
      nonsuppurative, chronic
    |serous *see* Otitis, media, nonsuppurative,
      chronic, serous
    |suppurative *see* Otitis, media, suppurative,
      chronic
    |transudative *see* Otitis, media,
      nonsuppurative, chronic, mucoid
  |exudative *see* Otitis, media, suppurative
  |in (due to) (with)
    |influenza *see* Influenza, with, otitis media
    |measles B05.3
    |scarlet fever A38.0
    |tuberculosis A18.6
    |viral disease NEC B34. [*H67.*]
  |mucoid *see* Otitis, media, nonsuppurative
  |nonsuppurative H65.9-
    |acute or subacute NEC H65.19-
      |allergic H65.11-
        |recurrent H65.11-
      |recurrent H65.19-
      |secretory *see* Otitis, media,
        nonsuppurative, serous
      |serous H65.0-
        |recurrent H65.0-
    |chronic H65.49-
      |allergic H65.41-
      |mucoid H65.3-
      |serous H65.2-
    |postmeasles B05.3
  |purulent *see* Otitis, media, suppurative
  |secretory *see* Otitis, media, nonsuppurative
  |seromucinous *see* Otitis, media,
    nonsuppurative
  |serous *see* Otitis, media, nonsuppurative
  |suppurative H66.4-
    |acute H66.00-
      |with rupture of ear drum H66.01-
      |recurrent H66.00-
        |with rupture of ear drum H66.01-
    |chronic *see also* subcategory H66.3

Otitis (acute) - *continued*
    |atticoantral H66.2-
    |benign *see* Otitis, media, suppurative,
    chronic, tubotympanic
    |tubotympanic H66.1-
  |transudative *see* Otitis, media,
    nonsuppurative
  |tuberculous A18.6
Otocephaly Q18.2
Otolith syndrome *see* subcategory H81.8
Otomycosis (diffuse) NEC B36.9 [*H62.40*]
|in
  |aspergillosis B44.89
  |candidiasis B37.84
  |moniliasis B37.84
Otoporosis *see* Otosclerosis
Otorrhagia (nontraumatic) H92.2-
|traumatic   code by Type of injury
Otorrhea H92.1-
|cerebrospinal (fluid) G96.01
  |postoperative G96.08
  |specified NEC G96.08
  |spontaneous G96.01
  |traumatic G96.08
Otosclerosis (general) H80.9-
|cochlear (endosteal) H80.2-
|involving
  |otic capsule *see* Otosclerosis, cochlear
  |oval window
    |nonobliterative H80.0-
    |obliterative H80.1-
  |round window *see* Otosclerosis, cochlear
|nonobliterative *see* Otosclerosis, involving,
  oval window, nonobliterative
|obliterative *see* Otosclerosis, involving, oval
  window, obliterative
|specified NEC H80.8-
Otospongiosis *see* Otosclerosis
Otto's disease or pelvis M24.7
Outcome of delivery Z37.9
|multiple births Z37.9
  |all liveborn Z37.50
    |quadruplets Z37.52
    |quintuplets Z37.53
    |sextuplets Z37.54
    |specified number NEC Z37.59
    |triplets Z37.51
  |all stillborn Z37.7
  |some liveborn Z37.60
    |quadruplets Z37.62
    |quintuplets Z37.63
    |sextuplets Z37.64
    |specified number NEC Z37.69
    |triplets Z37.61
|single NEC Z37.9
  |liveborn Z37.0
  |stillborn Z37.1
|twins NEC Z37.9
  |both liveborn Z37.2
  |both stillborn Z37.4
  |one liveborn, one stillborn Z37.3
Outlet *see* condition
Ovalocytosis (congenital) (hereditary) *see*
  Elliptocytosis
Ovarian *see* Condition
Ovariocele N83.4-
Ovaritis (cystic) *see* Oophoritis
Ovary, ovarian *see also* condition
|resistant syndrome E28.39
|vein syndrome N13.8
Overactive *see also* Hyperfunction
|adrenal cortex NEC E27.0
|bladder N32.81
|hypothalamus E23.3
|thyroid *see* Hyperthyroidism

Overactivity R46.3
|child *see* Disorder, attention-deficit
  hyperactivity
Overbite (deep) (excessive) (horizontal)
  (vertical) M26.29
Overbreathing *see* Hyperventilation
Overconscientious personality F60.5
Overdevelopment *see* Hypertrophy
Overdistension *see* Distension
Overdose, overdosage (drug) *see* Table of
  Drugs and Chemicals, by drug, poisoning
Overeating R63.2
|nonorganic origin F50.89
|psychogenic F50.89
Overexertion (effects) (exhaustion) T73.3
Overexposure (effects) T73.9
|exhaustion T73.2
Overfeeding *see* Overeating
|newborn P92.4
Overfill, endodontic M27.52
Overgrowth, bone *see* Hypertrophy, bone
Overhanging of dental restorative material
  (unrepairable) K08.52
Overheated (places) (effects) *see* Heat
Overjet (excessive horizontal) M26.23
Overlaid, overlying (suffocation) *see* Asphyxia,
  traumatic, due to mechanical threat
Overlap, excessive horizontal (teeth) M26.23
Overlapping toe (acquired) *see also* Deformity,
  toe, specified NEC
|congenital (fifth toe) Q66.89
Overload
|circulatory, due to transfusion (blood) (blood
  components) (TACO) E87.71
|fluid E87.70
  |due to transfusion (blood) (blood
    components) E87.71
  |specified NEC E87.79
|iron, due to repeated red blood cell
  transfusions E83.111
|potassium (K) E87.5
|sodium (Na) E87.0
Overnutrition *see* Hyperalimentation
Overproduction *see also* Hypersecretion
|ACTH E27.0
|catecholamine E27.5
|growth hormone E22.0
Overprotection, child by parent Z62.1
Overriding
|aorta Q25.49
|finger (acquired) *see* Deformity, finger
  |congenital Q68.1
|toe (acquired) *see also* Deformity, toe,
  specified NEC
  |congenital Q66.89
Overstrained R53.83
|heart *see* Hypertrophy, cardiac
Overuse, muscle NEC M70.8-
Overweight E66.3
Overworked R53.83
Oviduct *see* condition
Ovotestis Q56.0
Ovulation (cycle)
|failure or lack of N97.0
|pain N94.0
Ovum *see* condition
Owren's disease or syndrome
  (parahemophilia) D68.2
Ox heart *see* Hypertrophy, cardiac
Oxalosis E72.53
Oxaluria E72.53
Oxycephaly, oxycephalic Q75.0
|syphilitic, congenital A50.02
Oxyuriasis B80
Oxyuris vermicularis (infestation) B80

Ozena J31.0

P

Pachyderma, pachydermia L85.9
|larynx (verrucosa) J38.7
Pachydermatocele (congenital) Q82.8
Pachydermoperiostosis *see also*
  Osteoarthropathy, hypertrophic, specified type
  NEC
|clubbed nail M89.40 [*L62*]
Pachygyria Q04.3
Pachymeningitis (adhesive) (basal) (brain)
  (cervical) (chronic)(circumscribed)
  (external) (fibrous) (hemorrhagic)
  (hypertrophic) (internal) (purulent)
  (spinal) (suppurative) *see* Meningitis
Pachyonychia (congenital) Q84.5
Pacinian tumor *see* Neoplasm, skin, benign
Pad, knuckle or Garrod's M72.1
Paget-Schroetter syndrome I82.890
Paget's disease
|with infiltrating duct carcinoma *see*
  Neoplasm, breast, malignant
|bone M88.9
  |carpus M88.84-
  |clavicle M88.81-
  |femur M88.85-
  |fibula M88.86-
  |finger M88.84-
  |humerus M88.82-
  |ilium M88.85-
  |in neoplastic disease *see* Osteitis,
    deformans, in neoplastic disease
  |ischium M88.85-
  |metacarpus M88.84-
  |metatarsus M88.87-
  |multiple sites M88.89
  |neck M88.88
  |radius M88.83-
  |rib M88.88
  |scapula M88.81-
  |skull M88.0
  |tarsus M88.87-
  |tibia M88.86-
  |toe M88.87-
  |ulna M88.83-
  |vertebra M88.88
|breast (female) C50.01-
  |male C50.02-
|extramammary *see also* Neoplasm, skin,
  malignant
  |anus C21.0
    |margin C44.590
    |skin C44.590
|intraductal carcinoma *see* Neoplasm, breast,
  malignant
|malignant *see* Neoplasm, skin, malignant
  |breast (female) C50.01-
    |male C50.02-
  |unspecified site (female) C50.01-
    |male C50.02-
|mammary *see* Paget's disease, breast
|nipple *see* Paget's disease, breast
|osteitis deformans *see* Paget's disease, bone
Pain(s) *see also* Painful R52
|abdominal R10.9
  |colic R10.83
  |generalized R10.84
    |with acute abdomen R10.0
  |lower R10.30
    |left quadrant R10.32
    |pelvic or perineal R10.2
    |periumbilical R10.33

Pain(s) - *continued*
|right quadrant R10.31
|rebound *see* Tenderness, abdominal,
  rebound
|severe with abdominal rigidity R10.0
|tenderness *see* Tenderness, abdominal
|upper R10.10
  |epigastric R10.13
  |left quadrant R10.12
  |right quadrant R10.11
|acute R52
|due to trauma G89.11
|neoplasm related G89.3
|postprocedural NEC G89.18
|post-thoracotomy G89.12
|specified by site   code to Pain, by site
|adnexa (uteri) R10.2
|anginoid *see* Pain, precordial
|anus K62.89
|arm *see* Pain, limb, upper
|axillary (axilla) M79.62-
|back (postural) M54.9
|bladder R39.89
  |associated with micturition *see* Micturition,
    painful
  |chronic R39.82
|bone *see* Disorder, bone, specified type NEC
|breast N64.4
|broad ligament R10.2
|cancer associated (acute) (chronic) G89.3
|cecum *see* Pain, abdominal
|cervicobrachial M53.1
|chest (central) R07.9
  |anterior wall R07.89
  |atypical R07.89
  |ischemic I20.9
  |musculoskeletal R07.89
  |non-cardiac R07.89
  |on breathing R07.1
  |pleurodynia R07.81
  |precordial R07.2
  |wall (anterior) R07.89
|chronic G89.29
  |associated with significant psychosocial
    dysfunction G89.4
  |due to trauma G89.21
  |neoplasm related G89.3
  |postoperative NEC G89.28
  |postprocedural NEC G89.28
  |post-thoracotomy G89.22
  |specified NEC G89.29
|coccyx M53.3
|colon *see* Pain, abdominal
|coronary *see* Angina
|costochondral R07.1
|diaphragm R07.1
|due to cancer G89.3
|due to device, implant or graft *see also*
  Complications, by site and type, specified
  NEC T85.848
  |arterial graft NEC T82.848
  |breast (implant) T85.848
  |catheter NEC T85.848
    |dialysis (renal) T82.848
      |intraperitoneal T85.848
    |infusion NEC T82.848
      |spinal (epidural) (subdural) T85.840
    |urinary (indwelling) T83.84
  |electronic (electrode) (pulse generator)
    (stimulator)
    |bone T84.84
    |cardiac T82.847
    |nervous system (brain) (peripheral nerve)
      (spinal) T85.840
    |urinary T83.84

Pain(s) - *continued*
   |fixation, internal (orthopedic) NEC T84.84
   |gastrointestinal (bile duct) (esophagus)
     T85.848
   |genital NEC T83.84
   |heart NEC T82.847
   |infusion NEC T85.848
   |joint prosthesis T84.84
   |ocular (corneal graft) (orbital implant) NEC
     T85.848
   |orthopedic NEC T84.84
   |specified NEC T85.848
   |urinary NEC T83.84
   |vascular NEC T82.848
   |ventricular intracranial shunt T85.840
  |due to malignancy (primary) (secondary)
    G89.3
  |ear *see* subcategory H92.0
  |epigastric, epigastrium R10.13
  |eye *see* Pain, ocular
  |face, facial R519
   |atypical G50.1
  |female genital organs NEC N94.89
  |finger *see* Pain, limb, upper
  |flank *see* Pain, abdominal
  |foot *see* Pain, limb, lower
  |gallbladder K82.9
  |gas (intestinal) R14.1
  |gastric *see* Pain, abdominal
  |generalized NOS R52
  |genital organ
   |female N94.89
   |male N50.89
  |groin *see* Pain, abdominal, lower
  |hand *see* Pain, limb, upper
  |head *see* Headache
  |heart *see* Pain, precordial
  |infra-orbital *see* Neuralgia, trigeminal
  |intercostal R07.82
  |intermenstrual N94.0
  |jaw R68.84
  |joint M25.50
   |ankle M25.57-
   |elbow M25.52-
   |finger M25.54-
   |foot M25.57-
   |hand M25.54-
   |hip M25.55-
   |knee M25.56-
   |shoulder M25.51-
   |specified site NEC M25.59
   |toe M25.57-
   |wrist M25.53-
  |kidney N23
  |laryngeal R07.0
  |leg *see* Pain, limb, lower
  |limb M79.609
   |lower M79.60-
    |foot M79.67-
    |lower leg M79.66-
    |thigh M79.65-
    |toe M79.67-
   |upper M79.60-
    |axilla M79.62-
    |finger M79.64-
    |forearm M79.63-
    |hand M79.64-
    |upper arm M79.62-
  |loin M54.50
  |low back M54.50
   |specified NEC M54.59
   |vertebral end plate M54.51
   |vertebrogenic M54.51
  |lumbar region M54.50
   |vertebral end plate M54.51

Pain(s) - *continued*
   |vertebrogenic M54.51
  |mandibular R68.84
  |mastoid *see* subcategory H92.0
  |maxilla R68.84
  |menstrual *see also* Dysmenorrhea N94.6
  |metacarpophalangeal (joint) *see* Pain, joint,
    hand
  |metatarsophalangeal (joint) *see* Pain, joint,
    foot
  |mouth K13.79
  |muscle *see* Myalgia
  |musculoskeletal *see also* Pain, by site M79.18
  |myofascial M79.18
  |nasal J34.89
  |nasopharynx J39.2
  |neck NEC M54.2
  |nerve NEC *see* Neuralgia
  |neuromuscular *see* Neuralgia
  |nose J34.89
  |ocular H57.1-
  |ophthalmic *see* Pain, ocular
  |orbital region *see* Pain, ocular
  |ovary N94.89
  |over heart *see* Pain, precordial
  |ovulation N94.0
  |pelvic (female) R10.2
  |penis N48.89
  |pericardial *see* Pain, precordial
  |perineal, perineum R10.2
  |pharynx J39.2
  |pleura, pleural, pleuritic R07.81
  |postoperative NOS G89.18
  |postprocedural NOS G89.18
  |post-thoracotomy G89.12
  |precordial (region) R07.2
  |premenstrual N94.3
  |psychogenic (persistent) (any site) F45.41
  |radicular (spinal) *see* Radiculopathy
  |rectum K62.89
  |respiration R07.1
  |retrosternal R07.2
  |rheumatoid, muscular *see* Myalgia rib R07.81
  |root (spinal) *see* Radiculopathy
  |round ligament (stretch) R10.2
  |sacroiliac M53.3
  |sciatic *see* Sciatica
  |scrotum N50.82
  |seminal vesicle N50.89
  |shoulder M25.51-
  |spermatic cord N50.89
  |spinal root *see* Radiculopathy
  |spine M54.9
   |cervical M54.2
   |low back M54.50
    |with sciatica M54.4-
   |thoracic M54.6
  |stomach *see* Pain, abdominal
  |substernal R07.2
  |temporomandibular (joint) M26.62-
  |testis N50.81-
  |thoracic spine M54.6
   |with radicular and visceral pain M54.14
  |throat R07.0
  |tibia *see* Pain, limb, lower
  |toe *see* Pain, limb, lower
  |tongue K14.6
  |tooth K08.89
  |trigeminal *see* Neuralgia, trigeminal
  |tumor associated G89.3
  |ureter N23
  |urinary (organ) (system) N23
  |uterus NEC N94.89
  |vagina R10.2
  |vertebral end plate - see Pain, vertebrogenic

Pain(s) - *continued*
  |vertebrogenic M54.89
   |low back M54.51
   |lumbar M54.51
   |syndrome M54.89
  |vesical R39.89
   |associated with micturition *see* Micturition,
    painful
  |vulva R10.2
Painful *see also* Pain
  |coitus
   |female N94.10
   |male N53.12
   |psychogenic F52.6
  |ejaculation (semen) N53.12
   |psychogenic F52.6
  |erection *see* Priapism
  |feet syndrome E53.8
  |joint replacement (hip) (knee) T84.84
  |menstruation *see* Dysmenorrhea
   |psychogenic F45.8
  |micturition *see* Micturition, painful
  |respiration R07.1
  |scar NEC L90.5
  |wire sutures T81.89
Painter's colic *see* subcategory T56.0
Palate *see* condition
Palatoplegia K13.79
Palatoschisis *see* Cleft, palate
Palilalia R48.8
Palliative care Z51.5
Pallor R23.1
  |optic disc, temporal *see* Atrophy, optic
Palmar *see also* condition
  |fascia *see* condition
Palpable
  |cecum K63.89
  |kidney N28.89
  |ovary N83.8
  |prostate N42.9
  |spleen *see* Splenomegaly
Palpitations (heart) R00.2
  |psychogenic F45.8
Palsy *see also* Paralysis G83.9
  |atrophic diffuse (progressive) G12.22
  |Bell's *see also* Palsy, facial
   |newborn P11.3
  |brachial plexus NEC G54.0
   |newborn (birth injury) P14.3
  |brain *see* Palsy, cerebral
  |bulbar (progressive) (chronic) G12.22
   |of childhood (Fazio-Londe) G12.1
   |pseudo NEC G12.29
   |supranuclear (progressive) G23.1
  |cerebral (congenital) G80.9
   |ataxic G80.4
   |athetoid G80.3
   |choreoathetoid G80.3
   |diplegic G80.8
    |spastic G80.1
   |dyskinetic G80.3
    |athetoid G80.3
    |choreoathetoid G80.3
    |dystonic G80.3
   |dystonic G80.3
   |hemiplegic G80.8
    |spastic G80.2
   |mixed G80.8
   |monoplegic G80.8
    |spastic G80.1
   |paraplegic G80.8
    |spastic G80.1
   |quadriplegic G80.8
    |spastic G80.0
   |spastic G80.1

PQR

Palsy - *continued*
 |diplegic G80.1
 |hemiplegic G80.2
 |monoplegic G80.1
 |quadriplegic G80.0
 |specified NEC G80.1
 |tetraplegic G80.0
 |specified NEC G80.8
 |syphilitic A52.12
 |congenital A50.49
 |tetraplegic G80.8
 |spastic G80.0
 |cranial nerve *see also* Disorder, nerve, cranial
 |multiple G52.7
 |in
 |infectious disease B99 [*G53*]
 |neoplastic disease *see also* Neoplasm
 D49.9 [*G53*]
 |parasitic disease B89 [*G53*]
 |sarcoidosis D86.82
 |creeping G12.22
 |diver's T70.3
 |Erb's P14.0
 |facial G51.0
 |newborn (birth injury) P11.3
 |glossopharyngeal G52.1
 |Klumpke (-Déjérine) P14.1
 |lead *see* subcategory T56.0
 |median nerve (tardy) G56.1-
 |nerve G58.9
 |specified NEC G58.8
 |peroneal nerve (acute) (tardy) G57.3-
 |progressive supranuclear G23.1
 |pseudobulbar NEC G12.29
 |radial nerve (acute) G56.3-
 |seventh nerve *see also* Palsy, facial
 |newborn P11.3
 |shaking *see* Parkinsonism
 |spastic (cerebral) (spinal) G80.1
 |ulnar nerve (tardy) G56.2-
 |wasting G12.29
Paludism *see* Malaria
Panangiitis M30.0
Panaris, panaritium *see also* Cellulitis, digit
 |with lymphangitis *see* Lymphangitis, acute,
 digit
Panarteritis nodosa M30.0
 |brain or cerebral I67.7
Pancake heart R93.1
 |with cor pulmonale (chronic) I27.81
Pancarditis (acute) (chronic) I51.89
 |rheumatic I09.89
 |active or acute I01.8
Pancoast's syndrome or tumor C34.1-
Pancolitis, ulcerative (chronic) K51.00
 |with
 |complication K51.019
 |abscess K51.014
 |fistula K51.013
 |obstruction K51.012
 |rectal bleeding K51.011
 |specified complication NEC K51.018
Pancreas, pancreatic *see* condition
Pancreatitis (annular) (apoplectic)
 (calcareous) (edematous) (hemorrhagic)
 (malignant) (subacute)(suppurative) K85.90
 |with necrosis (uninfected) K85.91
 |infected K85.92
 |acute (without necrosis or infection) K85.90
 |with necrosis (uninfected) K85.91
 |infected K85.92
 |alcohol induced (without necrosis or
 infection) K85.20
 |with necrosis (uninfected) K85.21
 |infected K85.22

Pancreatitis - *continued*
 |biliary (without necrosis or infection)
 K85.10
 |with necrosis (uninfected) K85.11
 |infected K85.12
 |drug induced (without necrosis or infection)
 K85.30
 |with necrosis (uninfected) K85.31
 |infected K85.32
 |gallstone (without necrosis or infection)
 K85.10
 |with necrosis (uninfected) K85.11
 |infected K85.12
 |idiopathic (without necrosis or infection)
 K85.00
 |with necrosis (uninfected) K85.01
 |infected K85.02
 |specified NEC (without necrosis or
 infection) K85.80
 |with necrosis (uninfected) K85.81
 |infected K85.82
 |chronic (infectious) K86.1
 |alcohol-induced K86.0
 |recurrent K86.1
 |relapsing K86.1
 |cystic (chronic) K86.1
 |cytomegaloviral B25.2
 |fibrous (chronic) K86.1
 |gangrenous *see* Pancreatitis, acute
 |gallstone (without necrosis or infection)
 K85.10
 |with necrosis (uninfected) K85.11
 |infected K85.12
 |interstitial (chronic) K86.1
 |acute *see also* Pancreatitis, acute K85.80
 |mumps B26.3
 |recurrent
 |acute - see Pancreatitis, acute by type
 |chronic K86.1
 |relapsing, chronic K86.1
 |syphilitic A52.74
Pancreatoblastoma *see* Neoplasm, pancreas,
 malignant
Pancreolithiasis K86.89
Pancytolysis D75.89
Pancytopenia (acquired) D61.818
 |with
 |malformations D61.09
 |myelodysplastic syndrome *see* Syndrome,
 myelodysplastic
 |antineoplastic chemotherapy induced D61.810
 |congenital D61.09
 |drug-induced NEC D61.811
PANDAS (pediatric autoimmune
 neuropsychiatric disorders associated with
 streptococcal infections syndrome) D89.89
Panencephalitis, subacute, sclerosing A81.1
Panhematopenia D61.9
 |congenital D61.09
 |constitutional D61.09
 |splenic, primary D73.1
Panhemocytopenia D61.9
 |congenital D61.09
 |constitutional D61.09
Panhypogonadism E29.1
Panhypopituitarism E23.0
 |prepubertal E23.0
Panic (attack) (state) F41.0
 |reaction to exceptional stress (transient) F43.0
Panmyelopathy, familial, constitutional
 D61.09
Panmyelophthisis D61.82
 |congenital D61.09
Panmyelosis (acute) (with myelofibrosis)
 C94.4-

Panner's disease *see* Osteochondrosis, juvenile,
 humerus
Panneuritis endemica E51.11
Panniculitis (nodular) (nonsuppurative)
 M79.3
 |back M54.00
 |cervical region M54.02
 |cervicothoracic region M54.03
 |lumbar region M54.06
 |lumbosacral region M54.07
 |multiple sites M54.09
 |occipito-atlanto-axial region M54.01
 |sacrococcygeal region M54.08
 |thoracic region M54.04
 |thoracolumbar region M54.05
 |lupus L93.2
 |mesenteric K65.4
 |neck M54.02
 |cervicothoracic region M54.03
 |occipito-atlanto-axial region M54.01
 |relapsing M35.6
Panniculus adiposus (abdominal) E65
Pannus (allergic) (cornea) (degenerativus)
 (keratic) H16.42-
 |abdominal (symptomatic) E65
 |trachomatosus, trachomatous (active) A71.1
Panophthalmitis H44.01-
Pansinusitis (chronic) (hyperplastic)
 (nonpurulent) (purulent) J32.4
 |acute J01.40
 |recurrent J01.41
 |tuberculous A15.8
Panuveitis (sympathetic) H44.11-
Panvalvular disease I08.9
 |specified NEC I08.8
PAPA (pyogenic arthritis, pyoderma
 gangrenosum, and acne syndrome) M04.8
Papanicolaou smear, cervix Z12.4
 |as part of routine gynecological examination
 Z01.419
 |with abnormal findings Z01.411
 |for suspected neoplasm Z12.4
 |nonspecific abnormal finding R87.619
 |routine Z01.419
 |with abnormal findings Z01.411
Papilledema (choked disc) H47.10
 |associated with
 |decreased ocular pressure H47.12
 |increased intracranial pressure H47.11
 |retinal disorder H47.13
 |Foster-Kennedy syndrome H47.14-
Papillitis H46.00
 |anus K62.89
 |chronic lingual K14.4
 |necrotizing, kidney N17.2
 |optic H46.0-
 |rectum K62.89
 |renal, necrotizing N17.2
 |tongue K14.0
Papilloma *see also* Neoplasm, benign, by site
 |acuminatum (female) (male) (anogenital)
 A63.0
 |basal cell L82.1
 |inflamed L82.0
 |benign pinta (primary) A67.0
 |bladder (urinary) (transitional cell) D41.4
 |choroid plexus (lateral ventricle) (third
 ventricle) D33.0
 |anaplastic C71.5
 |fourth ventricle D33.1
 |malignant C71.5
 |renal pelvis (transitional cell) D41.1-
 |benign D30.1-
 |Schneiderian
 |specified site *see* Neoplasm, benign, by site

Papilloma - *continued*
  |unspecified site D14.0
 |serous surface
  |borderline malignancy
   |specified site *see* Neoplasm, uncertain
    behavior, by site
    |unspecified site D39.10
  |specified site *see* Neoplasm, benign, by site
  |unspecified site D27.9
 |transitional (cell)
  |bladder (urinary) D41.4
  |inverted type *see* Neoplasm, uncertain
   behavior, by site
  |renal pelvis D41.1-
  |ureter D41.2-
 |ureter (transitional cell) D41.2-
  |benign D30.2-
 |urothelial *see* Neoplasm, uncertain behavior,
  by site
 |villous *see* Neoplasm, uncertain behavior, by
  site
  |adenocarcinoma in *see* Neoplasm,
   malignant, by site
   |in situ *see* Neoplasm, in situ
 |yaws, plantar or palmar A66.1
Papillomata, multiple, of yaws A66.1
Papillomatosis *see also* Neoplasm, benign, by
  site
 |confluent and reticulated L83
 |cystic, breast *see* Mastopathy, cystic
 |ductal, breast *see* Mastopathy, cystic
 |intraductal (diffuse) *see* Neoplasm, benign, by
  site
 |subareolar duct D24-
Papillomavirus, as cause of disease classified
  elsewhere B97.7
Papillon-Léage and Psaume syndrome Q87.0
Papule(s) R23.8
 |carate (primary) A67.0
 |fibrous, of nose D22.39
 |Gottron's L94.4
 |pinta (primary) A67.0
Papulosis
 |lymphomatoid C86.6
 |malignant I77.89
Papyraceous fetus O31.0-
Para-Albuminemia E88.09
Paracephalus Q89.7
Parachute mitral valve Q23.2
Paracoccidioidomycosis B41.9
 |disseminated B41.7
 |generalized B41.7
 |mucocutaneous-lymphangitic B41.8
 |pulmonary B41.0
 |specified NEC B41.8
 |visceral B41.8
Paradentosis K05.4
Paraffinoma T88.8
Paraganglioma D44.7
 |adrenal D35.0-
  |malignant C74.1-
 |aortic body D44.7
  |malignant C75.5
 |carotid body D44.6
  |malignant C75.4
 |chromaffin *see also* Neoplasm, benign, by site
  |malignant *see* Neoplasm, malignant, by site
 |extra-adrenal D44.7
  |malignant C75.5
   |specified site *see* Neoplasm, malignant, by
    site
   |unspecified site C75.5
  |specified site *see* Neoplasm, uncertain
   behavior, by site
  |unspecified site D44.7

Paraganglioma - *continued*
 |gangliocytic D13.2
  |specified site *see* Neoplasm, benign, by site
  |unspecified site D13.2
 |glomus jugulare D44.7
  |malignant C75.5
 |jugular D44.7
 |malignant C75.5
  |specified site *see* Neoplasm, malignant, by
   site
  |unspecified site C75.5
 |nonchromaffin D44.7
  |malignant C75.5
   |specified site *see* Neoplasm, malignant, by
    site
   |unspecified site C75.5
  |specified site *see* Neoplasm, uncertain
   behavior, by site
  |unspecified site D44.7
 |parasympathetic D44.7
  |specified site *see* Neoplasm, uncertain
   behavior, by site
  |unspecified site D44.7
 |specified site *see* Neoplasm, uncertain
  behavior, by site
 |sympathetic D44.7
  |specified site *see* Neoplasm, uncertain
   behavior, by site
  |unspecified site D44.7
 |unspecified site D44.7
Parageusia R43.2
 |psychogenic F45.8
Paragonimiasis B66.4
Paragranuloma, Hodgkin *see* Lymphoma,
  Hodgkin, specified NEC
Parahemophilia *see also* Defect, coagulation
  D68.2
Parakeratosis R23.4
 |variegata L41.0
Paralysis, paralytic (complete) (incomplete)
  G83.9
 |with
  |syphilis A52.17
 |abducens, abducent (nerve) *see* Strabismus,
  paralytic, sixth nerve
 |abductor, lower extremity G57.9-
 |accessory nerve G52.8
 |accommodation *see also* Paresis, of
  accommodation
  |hysterical F44.89
 |acoustic nerve (except Deafness) *see*
  subcategory H93.3
 |agitans *see also* Parkinsonism G20
  |arteriosclerotic G21.4
 |alternating (oculomotor) G83.89
 |amyotrophic G12.21
 |ankle G57.9-
 |anus (sphincter) K62.89
 |arm *see* Monoplegia, upper limb
 |ascending (spinal), acute G61.0
 |association G12.29
 |asthenic bulbar G70.00
  |with exacerbation (acute) G70.01
  |in crisis G70.01
 |ataxic (hereditary) G11.9
  |general (syphilitic) A52.17
 |atrophic G58.9
  |infantile, acute *see* Poliomyelitis, paralytic
  |progressive G12.22
  |spinal (acute) *see* Poliomyelitis, paralytic
 |axillary G54.0
 |Babinski-Nageotte's G83.89
 |Bell's G51.0
  |newborn P11.3
 |Benedikt's G46.3

Paralysis, paralytic - *continued*
 |birth injury P14.9
  |spinal cord P11.5
 |bladder (neurogenic) (sphincter) N31.2
 |bowel, colon or intestine K56.0
 |brachial plexus G54.0
  |birth injury P14.3
  |newborn (birth injury) P14.3
 |brain G83.9
  |diplegia G83.0
  |triplegia G83.89
 |bronchial J98.09
 |Brown-Séquard G83.81
 |bulbar (chronic) (progressive) G12.22
  |infantile *see* Poliomyelitis, paralytic
  |poliomyelitic *see* Poliomyelitis, paralytic
  |pseudo G12.29
 |bulbospinal G70.00
  |with exacerbation (acute) G70.01
  |in crisis G70.01
 |cardiac *see also* Failure, heart I50.9
 |cerebrocerebellar, diplegic G80.1
 |cervical
  |plexus G54.2
  |sympathetic G90.09
 |Céstan-Chenais G46.3
 |Charcot-Marie-Tooth type G60.0
 |Clark's G80.9
 |colon K56.0
 |compressed air T70.3
 |compression
  |arm G56.9-
  |leg G57.9-
  |lower extremity G57.9-
  |upper extremity G56.9-
 |congenital (cerebral) *see* Palsy, cerebral
 |conjugate movement (gaze) (of eye) H51.0
  |cortical (nuclear) (supranuclear) H51.0
 |cordis *see* Failure, heart
 |cranial or cerebral nerve G52.9
 |creeping G12.22
 |crossed leg G83.89
 |crutch *see* Injury, brachial plexus
 |deglutition R13.0
  |hysterical F44.4
 |dementia A52.17
 |descending (spinal) NEC G12.29
 |diaphragm (flaccid) J98.6
  |due to accidental dissection of phrenic nerve
   during procedure *see* Puncture, accidental
   complicating surgery
 |digestive organs NEC K59.89
 |diplegic *see* Diplegia
 |divergence (nuclear) H51.8
 |diver's T70.3
 |Duchenne's
  |birth injury P14.0
  |due to or associated with
   |motor neuron disease G12.22
   |muscular dystrophy G71.01
 |due to intracranial or spinal birth injury *see*
  Palsy, cerebral
 |embolic (current episode) I63.4-
 |Erb (-Duchenne) (birth) (newborn) P14.0
 |Erb's syphilitic spastic spinal A52.17
 |esophagus K22.89
 |eye muscle (extrinsic) H49.9
  |intrinsic *see also* Paresis, of accommodation
 |facial (nerve) G51.0
  |birth injury P11.3
  |congenital P11.3
  |following operation NEC *see* Puncture,
   accidental complicating surgery
  |newborn (birth injury) P11.3
 |familial (recurrent) (periodic) G72.3

Paralysis, paralytic - *continued*
  |spastic G11.4
  |fauces J39.2
  |finger G56.9-
  |gait R26.1
  |gastric nerve (nondiabetic) G52.2
  |gaze, conjugate H51.0
  |general (progressive) (syphilitic) A52.17
    |juvenile A50.45
  |glottis J38.00
    |bilateral J38.02
    |unilateral J38.01
  |gluteal G54.1
  |Gubler (-Millard) G46.3
  |hand *see* Monoplegia, upper limb
  |heart *see* Arrest, cardiac
  |hemiplegic *see* Hemiplegia
  |hyperkalemic periodic (familial) G72.3
  |hypoglossal (nerve) G52.3
  |hypokalemic periodic G72.3
  |hysterical F44.4
  |ileus K56.0
  |infantile *see also* Poliomyelitis, paralytic
      A80.30
    |bulbar *see* Poliomyelitis, paralytic
    |cerebral *see* Palsy, cerebral
    |spastic *see* Palsy, cerebral, spastic
  |infective *see* Poliomyelitis, paralytic
  |inferior nuclear G83.9
  |internuclear *see* Ophthalmoplegia,
      internuclear
  |intestine K56.0
  |iris H57.09
    |due to diphtheria (toxin) A36.89
  |ischemic, Volkmann's (complicating trauma)
      T79.6
  |Jackson's G83.89
  |jake *see* Poisoning, food, noxious, plant
  |Jamaica ginger (jake) G62.2
  |juvenile general A50.45
  |Klumpke (-Déjérine) (birth) (newborn) P14.1
  |labioglossal (laryngeal) (pharyngeal) G12.29
  |Landry's G61.0
  |laryngeal nerve (recurrent) (superior)
      (unilateral) J38.00
    |bilateral J38.02
    |unilateral J38.01
  |larynx J38.00
    |bilateral J38.02
    |due to diphtheria (toxin) A36.2
    |unilateral J38.01
  |lateral G12.23
  |lead *see* subcategory T56.0
  |left side *see* Hemiplegia
  |leg G83.1-
    |both *see* Paraplegia
    |crossed G83.89
    |hysterical F44.4
    |psychogenic F44.4
    |transient or transitory R29.818
      |traumatic NEC *see* Injury, nerve, leg
  |levator palpebrae superioris *see*
      Blepharoptosis, paralytic
  |limb *see* Monoplegia
  |lip K13.0
  |Lissauer's A52.17
  |lower limb *see* Monoplegia, lower limb
    |both *see* Paraplegia
  |lung J98.4
  |median nerve G56.1-
  |medullary (tegmental) G83.89
  |mesencephalic NEC G83.89
    |tegmental G83.89
  |middle alternating G83.89
  |Millard-Gubler-Foville G46.3

Paralysis, paralytic - *continued*
  |monoplegic *see* Monoplegia
  |motor G83.9
  |muscle, muscular NEC G72.89
    |due to nerve lesion G58.9
    |eye (extrinsic) H49.9
      |intrinsic *see* Paresis, of accommodation
      |oblique *see* Strabismus, paralytic, fourth
          nerve
    |iris sphincter H21.9
    |ischemic (Volkmann's) (complicating
        trauma) T79.6
    |progressive G12.21
    |pseudohypertrophic G71.09
  |musculocutaneous nerve G56.9-
  |musculospiral G56.9-
  |nerve *see also* Disorder, nerve
    |abducent *see* Strabismus, paralytic, sixth
        nerve
    |accessory G52.8
    |auditory (except Deafness) *see* subcategory
        H93.3
    |birth injury P14.9
    |cranial or cerebral G52.9
    |facial G51.0
      |birth injury P11.3
      |congenital P11.3
      |newborn (birth injury) P11.3
    |fourth or trochlear *see* Strabismus, paralytic,
        fourth nerve
    |newborn (birth injury) P14.9
    |oculomotor *see* Strabismus, paralytic, third
        nerve
    |phrenic (birth injury) P14.2
    |radial G56.3-
    |seventh or facial G51.0
      |newborn (birth injury) P11.3
    |sixth or abducent *see* Strabismus, paralytic,
        sixth nerve
    |syphilitic A52.15
    |third or oculomotor *see* Strabismus,
        paralytic, third nerve
    |trigeminal G50.9
    |trochlear *see* Strabismus, paralytic, fourth
        nerve
    |ulnar G56.2-
  |normokalemic periodic G72.3
  |ocular H49.9
    |alternating G83.89
  |oculofacial, congenital (Moebius) Q87.0
  |oculomotor (external bilateral) (nerve) *see*
      Strabismus, paralytic, third nerve
  |palate (soft) K13.79
  |paratrigeminal G50.9
  |periodic (familial) (hyperkalemic)
      (hypokalemic) (myotonic) (normokalemic)
      (potassium sensitive) (secondary) G72.3
  |peripheral autonomic nervous system *see*
      Neuropathy, peripheral, autonomic
  |peroneal (nerve) G57.3-
  |pharynx J39.2
  |phrenic nerve G56.8-
  |plantar nerve(s) G57.6-
  |pneumogastric nerve G52.2
  |poliomyelitis (current) *see* Poliomyelitis,
      paralytic
  |popliteal nerve G57.3-
  |postepileptic transitory G83.84
  |progressive (atrophic) (bulbar) (spinal)
      G12.22
    |general A52.17
    |infantile acute *see* Poliomyelitis, paralytic
    |supranuclear G23.1
  |pseudobulbar G12.29
  |pseudohypertrophic (muscle) G71.0

Paralysis, paralytic - *continued*
  |psychogenic F44.4
  |quadriceps G57.9-
  |quadriplegic *see* Tetraplegia
  |radial nerve G56.3-
  |rectus muscle (eye) H49.9
  |recurrent isolated sleep G47.53
  |respiratory (muscle) (system) (tract) R06.81
    |center NEC G93.89
    |congenital P28.89
    |newborn P28.89
  |right side *see* Hemiplegia
  |saturnine *see* subcategory T56.0
  |sciatic nerve G57.0-
  |senile G83.9
  |shaking *see* Parkinsonism
  |shoulder G56.9-
  |sleep, recurrent isolated G47.53
  |spastic G83.9
    |cerebral *see* Palsy, cerebral, spastic
    |congenital (cerebral) *see* Palsy, cerebral,
        spastic
    |familial G11.4
    |hereditary G11.4
    |quadriplegic G80.0
    |syphilitic (spinal) A52.17
  |sphincter, bladder *see* Paralysis, bladder
  |spinal (cord) G83.9
    |accessory nerve G52.8
    |acute *see* Poliomyelitis, paralytic
    |ascending acute G61.0
    |atrophic (acute) *see also* Poliomyelitis,
        paralytic
      |spastic, syphilitic A52.17
    |congenital NEC *see* Palsy, cerebral
    |infantile *see* Poliomyelitis, paralytic
    |hereditary G95.89
    |progressive G12.21
    |sequelae NEC G83.89
  |sternomastoid G52.8
  |stomach K31.84
    |diabetic *see* Diabetes, by type, with
        gastroparesis
    |nerve G52.2
      |diabetic *see* Diabetes, by type, with
          gastroparesis
  |stroke *see* Infarct, brain
  |subcapsularis G56.8-
  |supranuclear (progressive) G23.1
  |sympathetic G90.8
    |cervical G90.09
    |nervous system *see* Neuropathy, peripheral,
        autonomic
  |syndrome G83.9
    |specified NEC G83.89
  |syphilitic spastic spinal (Erb's) A52.17
  |thigh G57.9-
  |throat J39.2
    |diphtheritic A36.0
    |muscle J39.2
  |thrombotic (current episode) I63.3-
  |thumb G56.9-
  |tick *see* Toxicity, venom, arthropod, specified
      NEC
  |Todd's (postepileptic transitory paralysis)
      G83.84
  |toe G57.6-
  |tongue K14.8
  |transient R29.5
    |arm or leg NEC R29.818
    |traumatic NEC *see* Injury, nerve
  |trapezius G52.8
  |traumatic, transient NEC *see* Injury, nerve
  |trembling *see* Parkinsonism
  |triceps brachii G56.9-

Paralysis, paralytic - *continued*
|trigeminal nerve G50.9
|trochlear (nerve) *see* Strabismus, paralytic, fourth nerve
|ulnar nerve G56.2-
|upper limb *see* Monoplegia, upper limb
|uremic N18.9 [*G99.8*]
|uveoparotitic D86.89
|uvula K13.79
|postdiphtheritic A36.0
|vagus nerve G52.2
|vasomotor NEC G90.8
|velum palati K13.79
|vesical *see* Paralysis, bladder
|vestibular nerve (except Vertigo) *see* subcategory H93.3
|vocal cords J38.00
|bilateral J38.02
|unilateral J38.01
|Volkmann's (complicating trauma) T79.6
|wasting G12.29
|Weber's G46.3
|wrist G56.9-
Paramedial urethrovesical orifice Q64.79
Paramenia N92.6
Parametritis *see also* Disease, pelvis, inflammatory N73.2
|acute N73.0
|complicating abortion *see* Abortion, by type, complicated by, parametritis
Parametrium, parametric *see* condition
Paramnesia *see* Amnesia
Paramolar K00.1
Paramyloidosis E85.89
Paramyoclonus multiplex G25.3
Paramyotonia (congenita) G71.19
Parangi *see* Yaws
Paranoia (querulans) F22
|senile F03
Paranoid
|dementia (senile) F03
|praecox *see* Schizophrenia
|personality F60.0
|psychosis (climacteric) (involutional) (menopausal) F22
|psychogenic (acute) F23
|senile F03
|reaction (acute) F23
|chronic F22
|schizophrenia F20.0
|state (climacteric) (involutional) (menopausal) (simple) F22
|senile F03
|tendencies F60.0
|traits F60.0
|trends F60.0
|type, psychopathic personality F60.0
Paraparesis *see* Paraplegia
Paraphasia R47.02
Paraphilia F65.9
Paraphimosis (congenital) N47.2
|chancroidal A57
Paraphrenia, paraphrenic (late) F22
|schizophrenia F20.0
Paraplegia (lower) G82.20
|ataxic *see* Degeneration, combined, spinal cord
|complete G82.21
|congenital (cerebral) G80.8
|spastic G80.1
|familial spastic G11.4
|functional (hysterical) F44.4
|hereditary, spastic G11.4
|hysterical F44.4
|incomplete G82.22

Paraplegia - *continued*
|Pott's A18.01
|psychogenic F44.4
|spastic
|Erb's spinal, syphilitic A52.17
|hereditary G11.4
|tropical G04.1
|syphilitic (spastic) A52.17
|traumatic
|current injury   code to injury with seventh character A
|sequela of previous injury   code to injury with seventh character S
|tropical spastic G04.1
Parapoxvirus B08.60
|specified NEC B08.69
Paraproteinemia D89.2
|benign (familial) D89.2
|monoclonal D47.2
|secondary to malignant disease D47.2
Parapsoriasis L41.9
|en plaques L41.4
|guttata L41.1
|large plaque L41.4
|retiform, retiformis L41.5
|small plaque L41.3
|specified NEC L41.8
|varioliformis (acuta) L41.0
Parasitic *see also* condition
|disease NEC B89
|stomatitis B37.0
|sycosis (beard) (scalp) B35.0
|twin Q89.4
Parasitism B89
|intestinal B82.9
|skin B88.9
|specified *see* Infestation
Parasitophobia F40.218
Parasomnia G47.50
|due to
|alcohol
|abuse F10.182
|dependence F10.282
|use F10.982
|amphetamines
|abuse F15.182
|dependence F15.282
|use F15.982
|caffeine
|abuse F15.182
|dependence F15.282
|use F15.982
|cocaine
|abuse F14.182
|dependence F14.282
|use F14.982
|drug NEC
|abuse F19.182
|dependence F19.282
|use F19.982
|opioid
|abuse F11.182
|dependence F11.282
|use F11.982
|psychoactive substance NEC
|abuse F19.182
|dependence F19.282
|use F19.982
|sedative, hypnotic, or anxiolytic
|abuse F13.182
|dependence F13.282
|use F13.982
|stimulant NEC
|abuse F15.182
|dependence F15.282

Parasomnia - *continued*
|use F15.982
|in conditions classified elsewhere G47.54
|nonorganic origin F51.8
|organic G47.50
|specified NEC G47.59
Paraspadias Q54.9
Paraspasmus facialis G51.8
Parasuicide (attempt)
|history of (personal) Z91.51
|in family Z81.8
Parathyroid gland *see* condition
Parathyroid tetany E20.9
Paratrachoma A74.0
Paratyphlitis *see* Appendicitis
Paratyphoid (fever) *see* Fever, paratyphoid
Paratyphus *see* Fever, paratyphoid
Paraurethral duct Q64.79
|nonorganic origin F51.5
Paraurethritis *see also* Urethritis
|gonococcal (acute) (chronic) (with abscess) A54.1
Paravaccinia NEC B08.04
Paravaginitis *see* Vaginitis
Parencephalitis *see also* Encephalitis
|sequelae G09
Parent-Child conflict *see* Conflict, parent-child
|estrangement NEC Z62.890
Paresis *see also* Paralysis
|accommodation *see* Paresis, of accommodation
|Bernhardt's G57.1-
|bladder (sphincter) *see also* Paralysis, bladder
|tabetic A52.17
|bowel, colon or intestine K56.0
|extrinsic muscle, eye H49.9
|general (progressive) (syphilitic) A52.17
|juvenile A50.45
|heart *see* Failure, heart
|insane (syphilitic) A52.17
|juvenile (general) A50.45
|of accommodation H52.52-
|peripheral progressive (idiopathic) G60.3
|pseudohypertrophic G71.09
|senile G83.9
|syphilitic (general) A52.17
|congenital A50.45
|vesical NEC N31.2
Paresthesia (see also Disturbance, sensation, skin) R20.2
|Bernhardt G57.1-
Paretic *see* condition
Parinaud's
|conjunctivitis H10.89
|oculoglandular syndrome H10.89
|ophthalmoplegia H49.88-
Parkinsonism (idiopathic) (primary) G20
|with neurogenic orthostatic hypotension (symptomatic) G90.3
|arteriosclerotic G21.4
|dementia G31.83 [*F02.80*]
|with behavioral disturbance G31.83 [*F02.81*]
|due to
|drugs NEC G21.19
|neuroleptic G21.11
|medication-induced NEC G21.19
|neuroleptic induced G21.11
|postencephalitic G21.3
|secondary G21.9
|due to
|arteriosclerosis G21.4
|drugs NEC G21.19
|neuroleptic G21.11
|encephalitis G21.3
|external agents NEC G21.2
|syphilis A52.19
|specified NEC G21.8

Parkinsonism - *continued*
|syphilitic A52.19
|treatment-induced NEC G21.19
|vascular G21.4
Parkinson's disease, syndrome or tremor *see* Parkinsonism
Parodontitis *see* Periodontitis
Parodontosis K05.4
Paronychia *see also* Cellulitis, digit
|with lymphangitis *see* Lymphangitis, acute, digit
|candidal (chronic) B37.2
|tuberculous (primary) A18.4
Parorexia (psychogenic) F50.89
Parosmia R43.1
|psychogenic F45.8
Parotid gland *see* condition
Parotitis, parotiditis (allergic)(nonspecific toxic) (purulent) (septic) (suppurative) *see also* Sialoadenitis
|epidemic *see* Mumps
|infectious *see* Mumps
|postoperative K91.89
|surgical K91.89
Parrot fever A70
Parrot's disease (early congenital syphilitic pseudoparalysis) A50.02
Parry-Romberg syndrome G51.8
Parry's disease or syndrome E05.00
|with thyroid storm E05.01
Pars planitis *see* Cyclitis
Parsonage (-Aldren) -Turner syndrome G54.5
Parson's disease (exophthalmic goiter) E05.00
|with thyroid storm E05.01
Particolored infant Q82.8
Parturition *see* Delivery **Parulis** K04.7
|with sinus K04.6
Parvovirus, as cause of disease classified elsewhere B97.6
Pasini and Pierini's atrophoderma L90.3
Passage
|false, urethra N36.5
|meconium (newborn) during delivery P03.82
|of sounds or bougies *see* Attention to, artificial, opening
Passive *see* condition
|smoking Z77.22
Past due on rent or mortgage Z59.81-
Pasteurella septica A28.0
Pasteurellosis *see* Infection, Pasteurella
PAT (paroxysmal atrial tachycardia) I47.1
Patau's syndrome *see* Trisomy, 13
Patches
|mucous (syphilitic) A51.39
|congenital A50.07
|smokers' (mouth) K13.24
Patellar *see* condition
Patent *see also* Imperfect, closure
|canal of Nuck Q52.4
|cervix N88.3
|ductus arteriosus or Botallo's Q25.0
|foramen
|botalli Q21.1
|ovale Q21.1
|interauricular septum Q21.1
|interventricular septum Q21.0
|omphalomesenteric duct Q43.0
|os (uteri) *see* Patent, cervix
|ostium secundum Q21.1
|urachus Q64.4
|vitelline duct Q43.0
Paterson (-Brown)(-Kelly) syndrome or web D50.1

Pathologic, pathological *see also* condition
|asphyxia R09.01
|fire-setting F63.1
|gambling F63.0
|ovum O02.0
|resorption, tooth K03.3
|stealing F63.2
Pathology (of) *see* Disease
|periradicular, associated with previous endodontic treatment NEC M27.59
Pattern, sleep-Wake, irregular G47.23
Patulous *see also* Imperfect, closure (congenital)
|alimentary tract Q45.8
|lower Q43.8
|upper Q40.8
|eustachian tube H69.0-
Pause, sinoatrial I49.5
Paxton's disease B36.2
Pearl(s)
|enamel K00.2
|Epstein's K09.8
Pearl-Worker's disease *see* Osteomyelitis, specified type NEC
Pectenosis K62.4
Pectoral *see* condition
Pectus
|carinatum (congenital) Q67.7
|acquired M95.4
|rachitic sequelae (late effect) E64.3
|excavatum (congenital) Q67.6
|acquired M95.4
|rachitic sequelae (late effect) E64.3
|recurvatum (congenital) Q67.6
Pedatrophia E41
Pederosis F65.4
Pediculosis (infestation) B85.2
|capitis (head-louse) (any site) B85.0
|corporis (body-louse) (any site) B85.1
|eyelid B85.0
|mixed (classifiable to more than one of the titles B85.0-B85.3) B85.4
|pubis (pubic louse) (any site) B85.3
|vestimenti B85.1
|vulvae B85.3
Pediculus (infestation) *see* Pediculosis
Pedophilia F65.4
Peg-Shaped teeth K00.2
Pelade *see* Alopecia, areata
Pelger-Huët anomaly or syndrome D72.0
Peliosis (rheumatica) D69.0
|hepatis K76.4
|with toxic liver disease K71.8
Pelizaeus-Merzbacher disease E75.29
Pellagra (alcoholic) (with polyneuropathy) E52
Pellagra-Cerebellar-Ataxia-Renal aminoaciduria syndrome E72.02
Pellegrini (-Stieda) disease or syndrome *see* Bursitis, tibial collateral
Pellizzi's syndrome E34.8
Pel's crisis A52.11
Pelvic *see also* condition
|examination (periodic) (routine) Z01.419
|with abnormal findings Z01.411
|kidney, congenital Q63.2
Pelviolithiasis *see* Calculus, kidney
Pelviperitonitis *see also* Peritonitis, pelvic
|gonococcal A54.24
|puerperal O85
Pelvis *see* condition or type
Pemphigoid L12.9
|benign, mucous membrane L12.1
|bullous L12.0
|cicatricial L12.1
|juvenile L12.2
|ocular L12.1
|specified NEC L12.8

Pemphigus L10.9
|benign familial (chronic) Q82.8
|Brazilian L10.3
|circinatus L13.0
|conjunctiva L12.1
|drug-induced L10.5
|erythematosus L10.4
|foliaceous L10.2
|gangrenous *see* Gangrene
|neonatorum L01.03
|ocular L12.1
|paraneoplastic L10.81
|specified NEC L10.89
|syphilitic (congenital) A50.06
|vegetans L10.1
|vulgaris L10.0
|wildfire L10.3
Pendred's syndrome E07.1
Pendulous
|abdomen, in pregnancy *see* Pregnancy, complicated by, abnormal, pelvic organs or tissues NEC
|breast N64.89
Penetrating wound *see also* Puncture
|with internal injury *see* Injury, by site
|eyeball *see* Puncture, eyeball
|orbit (with or without foreign body) *see* Puncture, orbit
|uterus by instrument with or following ectopic or molar pregnancy O08.6
Penicillosis B48.4
Penis *see* condition
Penitis N48.29
Pentalogy of Fallot Q21.8
Pentasomy X syndrome Q97.1
Pentosuria (essential) E74.89
Percreta placenta O43.23-
Peregrinating patient *see* Disorder, factitious
Perforation, perforated (nontraumatic) (of)
|accidental during procedure (blood vessel) (nerve) (organ) *see* Complication, accidental puncture or laceration
|antrum *see* Sinusitis, maxillary
|appendix K35.32
|with localized peritonitis K35.32
|atrial septum, multiple Q21.1
|attic, ear *see* Perforation, tympanum, attic
|bile duct (common) (hepatic) K83.2
|cystic K82.2
|bladder (urinary)
|with or following ectopic or molar pregnancy O08.6
|obstetrical trauma O71.5
|traumatic S37.29
|at delivery O71.5
|bowel K63.1
|with or following ectopic or molar pregnancy O08.6
|newborn P78.0
|obstetrical trauma O71.5
|traumatic *see* Laceration, intestine
|broad ligament N83.8
|with or following ectopic or molar pregnancy O08.6
|obstetrical trauma O71.6
|by
|device, implant or graft *see also* Complications, by site and type, mechanical T85.628
|arterial graft NEC *see* Complication, cardiovascular device, mechanical, vascular
|breast (implant) T85.49
|catheter NEC T85.698
|cystostomy T83.090
|dialysis (renal) T82.49

Perforation, perforated - *continued*
    |intraperitoneal T85.691
    |infusion NEC T82.594
        |spinal (epidural) (subdural) T85.690
    |urinary *see also* Complications,
        catheter, urinary T83.098
    |electronic (electrode) (pulse generator)
        (stimulator)
        |bone T84.390
        |cardiac T82.199
            |electrode T82.190
            |pulse generator T82.191
            |specified type NEC T82.198
        |nervous system *see* Complication,
            prosthetic device, mechanical,
            electronic nervous system stimulator
        |urinary *see* Complication, genitourinary,
            device, urinary, mechanical
    |fixation, internal (orthopedic) NEC *see*
        Complication, fixation device,
        mechanical
    |gastrointestinal *see* Complications,
        prosthetic device, mechanical,
        gastrointestinal device
    |genital NEC T83.498
        |intrauterine contraceptive device T83.39
        |penile prosthesis T83.490
    |heart NEC *see* Complication,
        cardiovascular device, mechanical
    |joint prosthesis *see* Complications, joint
        prosthesis, mechanical, specified NEC,
        by site
    |ocular NEC *see* Complications, prosthetic
        device, mechanical, ocular device
    |orthopedic NEC *see* Complication,
        orthopedic, device, mechanical
    |specified NEC T85.628
    |urinary NEC *see also* Complication,
        genitourinary, device, urinary,
        mechanical
        |graft T83.29
    |vascular NEC *see* Complication,
        cardiovascular device, mechanical
    |ventricular intracranial shunt T85.09
    |foreign body left accidentally in operative
        wound T81.539
    |instrument (any) during a procedure,
        accidental *see* Puncture, accidental
        complicating surgery
    |cecum K35.2
    |cecum K35.32
        |with localized peritonitis K35.32
    |cervix (uteri) N88.8
        |with or following ectopic or molar
            pregnancy O08.6
        |obstetrical trauma O71.3
    |colon K63.1
        |newborn P78.0
        |obstetrical trauma O71.5
        |traumatic *see* Laceration, intestine, large
    |common duct (bile) K83.2
    |cornea (due to ulceration) *see* Ulcer, cornea,
        perforated
    |cystic duct K82.2
    |diverticulum (intestine) K57.80
        |with bleeding K57.81
        |large intestine K57.20
            |with
                |bleeding K57.21
                |small intestine K57.40
                    |with bleeding K57.41
        |small intestine K57.00
            |with
                |bleeding K57.01
                |large intestine K57.40

Perforation, perforated - *continued*
                    |with bleeding K57.41
    |ear drum *see* Perforation, tympanum
    |esophagus K22.3
    |ethmoidal sinus *see* Sinusitis, ethmoidal
    |frontal sinus *see* Sinusitis, frontal
    |gallbladder K82.2
    |heart valve *see* Endocarditis
    |ileum K63.1
        |newborn P78.0
        |obstetrical trauma O71.5
        |traumatic *see* Laceration, intestine, small
    |instrumental, surgical (accidental) (blood
        vessel) (nerve) (organ) *see* Puncture,
        accidental complicating surgery intestine
        NEC K63.1
        |with ectopic or molar pregnancy O08.6
        |newborn P78.0
        |obstetrical trauma O71.5
        |traumatic *see* Laceration, intestine
        |ulcerative NEC K63.1
            |newborn P78.0
    |jejunum, jejunal K63.1
        |obstetrical trauma O71.5
        |traumatic *see* Laceration, intestine, small
        |ulcer *see* Ulcer, gastrojejunal, with
            perforation
    |joint prosthesis *see* Complications, joint
        prosthesis, mechanical, specified NEC, by
        site
    |mastoid (antrum) (cell) *see* Disorder, mastoid,
        specified NEC
    |maxillary sinus *see* Sinusitis, maxillary
    |membrana tympani *see* Perforation,
        tympanum
    |nasal
        |septum J34.89
            |congenital Q30.3
            |syphilitic A52.73
        |sinus J34.89
            |congenital Q30.8
            |due to sinusitis *see* Sinusitis
    |palate *see also* Cleft, palate Q35.9
        |syphilitic A52.79
    |palatine vault *see also* Cleft, palate, hard
        Q35.1
        |syphilitic A52.79
        |congenital A50.59
    |pars flaccida (ear drum) *see* Perforation,
        tympanum, attic
    |pelvic
        |floor S31.030
            |with
                |ectopic or molar pregnancy O08.6
                |penetration into retroperitoneal space
                    S31.031
                |retained foreign body S31.040
                    |with penetration into retroperitoneal
                        space S31.041
            |following ectopic or molar pregnancy
                O08.6
            |obstetrical trauma O70.1
        |organ S37.99
            |adrenal gland S37.818
            |bladder *see* Perforation, bladder
            |fallopian tube S37.599
                |bilateral S37.592
                |unilateral S37.591
            |kidney S37.09-
            |obstetrical trauma O71.5
            |ovary S37.499
                |bilateral S37.492
                |unilateral S37.491
            |prostate S37.828
            |specified organ NEC S37.898

Perforation, perforated - *continued*
    |ureter *see* Perforation, ureter
    |urethra *see* Perforation, urethra
    |uterus *see* Perforation, uterus
    |perineum *see* Laceration, perineum
    |pharynx J39.2
    |rectum K63.1
        |newborn P78.0
        |obstetrical trauma O71.5
        |traumatic S36.63
    |root canal space due to endodontic treatment
        M27.51
    |sigmoid K63.1
        |newborn P78.0
        |obstetrical trauma O71.5
        |traumatic S36.533
    |sinus (accessory) (chronic) (nasal) J34.89
    |sphenoidal sinus *see* Sinusitis, sphenoidal
    |surgical (accidental) (by instrument) (blood
        vessel) (nerve) (organ) *see* Puncture,
        accidental complicating surgery
    |traumatic
        |external *see* Puncture
        |eye *see* Puncture, eyeball
        |internal organ *see* Injury, by site
    |tympanum, tympanic (membrane) (persistent
        post-traumatic) (postinflammatory) H72.9-
        |attic H72.1-
            |multiple *see* Perforation, tympanum,
                multiple
            |total *see* Perforation, tympanum, total
        |central H72.0-
            |multiple *see* Perforation, tympanum,
                multiple
            |total *see* Perforation, tympanum, total
        |marginal NEC *see* subcategory H72.2
        |multiple H72.81-
        |pars flaccida *see* Perforation, tympanum,
            attic
        |total H72.82-
        |traumatic, current episode S09.2-
    |typhoid, gastrointestinal *see* Typhoid
    |ulcer *see* Ulcer, by site, with perforation
    |ureter N28.89
        |traumatic S37.19
    |urethra N36.8
        |with ectopic or molar pregnancy O08.6
        |following ectopic or molar pregnancy O08.6
        |obstetrical trauma O71.5
        |traumatic S37.39
            |at delivery O71.5
    |uterus
        |with ectopic or molar pregnancy O08.6
        |by intrauterine contraceptive device T83.39
        |following ectopic or molar pregnancy O08.6
        |obstetrical trauma O71.1
        |traumatic S37.69
            |obstetric O71.1
    |uvula K13.79
        |syphilitic A52.79
    |vagina
        |obstetrical trauma O71.4
        |other trauma *see* Puncture, vagina
Periadenitis mucosa necrotica recurrens
    K12.0
Periappendicitis (acute) *see* Appendicitis
Periarteritis nodosa (disseminated)
    (infectious) (necrotizing) M30.0
Periarthritis (joint) *see also* Enthesopathy
    |Duplay's M75.0-
    |gonococcal A54.42
    |humeroscapularis *see* Capsulitis, adhesive
    |scapulohumeral *see* Capsulitis, adhesive
    |shoulder *see* Capsulitis, adhesive
    |wrist M77.2-

Periarthrosis (angioneural) *see* Enthesopathy
Pericapsulitis, adhesive (shoulder) *see*
  Capsulitis, adhesive
Pericarditis (with decompensation) (with
  effusion) I31.9
  |with rheumatic fever (conditions in I00)
    |active *see* Pericarditis, rheumatic
    |inactive or quiescent I09.2
  |acute (hemorrhagic) (nonrheumatic) (Sicca)
    I30.9
    |with chorea (acute) (rheumatic)
      (Sydenham's) I02.0
    |benign I30.8
    |nonspecific I30.0
    |rheumatic I01.0
      |with chorea (acute) (Sydenham's) I02.0
  |adhesive or adherent (chronic) (external)
    (internal) I31.0
    |acute *see* Pericarditis, acute
    |rheumatic I09.2
  |bacterial (acute) (subacute) (with serous or
    seropurulent effusion) I30.1
  |calcareous I31.1
  |cholesterol (chronic) I31.8
    |acute I30.9
  |chronic (nonrheumatic) I31.9
    |rheumatic I09.2
  |constrictive (chronic) I31.1
  |coxsackie B33.23
  |fibrinocaseous (tuberculous) A18.84
  |fibrinopurulent I30.1
  |fibrinous I30.8
  |fibrous I31.0
  |gonococcal A54.83
  |idiopathic I30.0
  |in systemic lupus erythematosus M32.12
  |infective I30.1
  |meningococcal A39.53
  |neoplastic (chronic) I31.8
    |acute I30.9
  |obliterans, obliterating I31.0
  |plastic I31.0
  |pneumococcal I30.1
  |postinfarction I24.1
  |purulent I30.1
  |rheumatic (active) (acute) (with effusion)
    (with pneumonia) I01.0
    |with chorea (acute) (rheumatic)
      (Sydenham's) I02.0
    |chronic or inactive (with chorea) I09.2
  |rheumatoid *see* Rheumatoid, carditis
  |septic I30.1
  |serofibrinous I30.8
  |staphylococcal I30.1
  |streptococcal I30.1
  |suppurative I30.1
  |syphilitic A52.06
  |tuberculous A18.84
  |uremic N18.9 *[132]*
  |viral I30.1
Pericardium, pericardial *see* condition
Pericellulitis *see* Cellulitis
Pericementitis (chronic) (suppurative) *see also*
  Periodontitis
  |acute K05.20
    |generalized *see* Periodontitis, aggressive,
      generalized
    |localized *see* Periodontitis, aggressive,
      localized
Perichondritis
  |auricle *see* Perichondritis, ear
  |bronchus J98.09
  |ear (external) H61.00-
    |acute H61.01
    |chronic H61.02-
  |external auditory canal *see* Perichondritis, ear

Perichondritis - *continued*
  |larynx J38.7
    |syphilitic A52.73
    |typhoid A01.09
  |nose J34.89
  |pinna *see* Perichondritis, ear
  |trachea J39.8
Periclasia K05.4
Pericoronitis *see* Periodontitis
Pericystitis N30.90
  |with hematuria N30.91
Peridiverticulitis (intestine) K57.92
  |cecum *see* Diverticulitis, intestine, large
  |colon *see* Diverticulitis, intestine, large
  |duodenum *see* Diverticulitis, intestine, small
  |intestine *see* Diverticulitis, intestine
  |jejunum *see* Diverticulitis, intestine, small
  |rectosigmoid *see* Diverticulitis, intestine, large
  |rectum *see* Diverticulitis, intestine, large
  |sigmoid *see* Diverticulitis, intestine, large
Periendocarditis *see* Endocarditis
Periepididymitis N45.1
Perifolliculitis L01.02
  |abscedens, caput, scalp L66.3
  |capitis, abscedens (et suffodiens) L66.3
  |superficial pustular L01.02
Perihepatitis K65.8
Perilabyrinthitis (acute) *see* subcategory H83.0
Perimeningitis *see* Meningitis
Perimetritis *see* Endometritis
Perimetrosalpingitis *see* Salpingo-oophoritis
Perineocele N81.81
Perinephric, perinephritic *see* condition
Perinephritis *see also* Infection, kidney
  |purulent *see* Abscess, kidney
Perineum, perineal *see* condition
Perineuritis NEC *see* Neuralgia **Periodic** *see*
  condition
Periodontitis (chronic) (complex) (compound)
  (local) (simplex) K05.30
  |acute K05.20
    |generalized K05.229
      |moderate K05.222
      |severe K05.223
      |slight K05.221
    |localized K05.219
      |moderate K05.212
      |severe K05.213
      |slight K05.211
  |apical K04.5
    |acute (pulpal origin) K04.4
  |generalized K05.329
    |moderate K05.322
    |severe K05.323
    |slight K05.321
  |localized K05.319
    |moderate K05.312
    |severe K05.313
    |slight K05.311
Periodontoclasia K05.4
Periodontosis (juvenile) K05.4
Periods *see also* Menstruation
  |heavy N92.0
  |irregular N92.6
  |shortened intervals (irregular) N92.1
Perionychia *see also* Cellulitis, digit
  |with lymphangitis *see* Lymphangitis, acute,
    digit
Perioophoritis *see* Salpingo-oophoritis
Periorchitis N45.2
Periosteum, periosteal *see* condition
Periostitis (albuminosa) (circumscribed)
  (diffuse) (infective) (monomelic) *see also*
  Osteomyelitis
  |alveolar M27.3
  |alveolodental M27.3

Periostitis - *continued*
  |dental M27.3
  |gonorrheal A54.43
  |jaw (lower) (upper) M27.2
  |orbit H05.03-
  |syphilitic A52.77
    |congenital (early) A50.02 *[M90.80]*
    |secondary A51.46
  |tuberculous *see* Tuberculosis, bone
  |yaws (hypertrophic) (early) (late) A66.6
    [M90.80]
Periostosis (hyperplastic) *see also* Disorder,
  bone, specified type NEC
  |with osteomyelitis *see* Osteomyelitis,
    specified type NEC
Peripartum
  |cardiomyopathy O90.3
Periphlebitis *see* Phlebitis
Periproctitis K62.89
Periprostatitis *see* Prostatitis
Perirectal *see* condition
Perirenal *see* condition
Perisalpingitis *see* Salpingo-oophoritis
Perisplenitis (infectional) D73.89
Peristalsis, visible or reversed R19.2
Peritendinitis *see* Enthesopathy
Peritoneum, peritoneal *see* condition
Peritonitis (adhesive) (bacterial) (fibrinous)
  (hemorrhagic) (idiopathic) (localized)
  (perforative) (primary) (with adhesions)
  (with effusion) K65.9
  |with or following
    |abscess K65.1
    |appendicitis
      |with perforation or rupture K35.32
      |generalized (*see also* Appendicitis)
        K35.20
      |localized (*see also* Appendicitis) K35.30
    |diverticular disease (intestine) K57.80
      |with bleeding K57.81
      |large intestine K57.20
        |with
          |bleeding K57.21
          |small intestine K57.40
            |with bleeding K57.41
      |small intestine K57.00
        |with
          |bleeding K57.01
          |large intestine K57.40
            |with bleeding K57.41
    |ectopic or molar pregnancy O08.0
  |acute (generalized) K65.0
  |aseptic T81.61
  |bile, biliary K65.3
  |chemical T81.61
  |chlamydial A74.81
  |complicating abortion *see* Abortion, by type,
    complicated by, pelvic peritonitis
  |congenital P78.1
  |chronic proliferative K65.8
  |diaphragmatic K65.0
  |diffuse K65.0
  |diphtheritic A36.89
  |disseminated K65.0
  |due to
    |bile K65.3
    |foreign
      |body or object accidentally left during a
        procedure (instrument) (sponge)
        (swab) T81.599
      |substance accidentally left during a
        procedure (chemical) (powder) (talc)
        T81.61
    |talc T81.61
    |urine K65.8

Peritonitis - *continued*
|eosinophilic K65.8
    |acute K65.0
|fibrocaseous (tuberculous) A18.31
|fibropurulent K65.0
|following ectopic or molar pregnancy O08.0
|general (ized) K65.0
|gonococcal A54.85
|meconium (newborn) P78.0
|neonatal P78.1
    |meconium P78.0
|pancreatic K65.0
|paroxysmal, familial E85.0
    |benign E85.0
|pelvic
    |female N73.5
        |acute N73.3
        |chronic N73.4
            |with adhesions N73.6
    |male K65.0
|periodic, familial E85.0
|proliferative, chronic K65.8
|puerperal, postpartum, childbirth O85
|purulent K65.0
|septic K65.0
|specified NEC K65.8
|spontaneous bacterial K65.2
|subdiaphragmatic K65.0
|subphrenic K65.0
|suppurative K65.0
|syphilitic A52.74
    |congenital (early) A50.08 *[K67]*
|talc T81.61
|tuberculous A18.31
|urine K65.8
Peritonsillar *see* condition
Peritonsillitis J36
Perityphlitis K37
Periureteritis N28.89
Periurethral *see* condition
Periurethritis (gangrenous) *see* Urethritis
Periuterine *see* condition
Perivaginitis *see* Vaginitis
Perivasculitis, retinal H35.06-
Perivasitis (chronic) N49.1
Perivesiculitis (seminal) *see* Vesiculitis
Perlèche NEC K13.0
|due to
    |candidiasis B37.83
    |moniliasis B37.83
    |riboflavin deficiency E53.0
    |vitamin B2 (riboflavin) deficiency E53.0
Pernicious *see* condition
Pernio, perniosis T69.1
Perpetrator (of abuse) *see* Index to External
    Causes of Injury, Perpetrator
Persecution
|delusion F22
|social Z60.5
Perseveration (tonic) R48.8
Persistence, persistent (congenital)
|anal membrane Q42.3
    |with fistula Q42.2
|arteria stapedia Q16.3
|atrioventricular canal Q21.2
|branchial cleft NOS Q18.2
    |cyst Q18.0
    |fistula Q18.0
    |sinus Q18.0
|bulbus cordis in left ventricle Q21.8
|canal of Cloquet Q14.0
|capsule (opaque) Q12.8
|cilioretinal artery or vein Q14.8
|cloaca Q43.7
|communication *see* Fistula, congenital

Persistence, persistent - *continued*
|convolutions
    |aortic arch Q25.46
    |fallopian tube Q50.6
    |oviduct Q50.6
    |uterine tube Q50.6
|double aortic arch Q25.45
|ductus arteriosus (Botalli) Q25.0
|fetal
    |circulation P29.38
    |form of cervix (uteri) Q51.828
    |hemoglobin, hereditary (HPFH) D56.4
|foramen
    |Botalli Q21.1
    |ovale Q21.1
|Gartner's duct Q52.4
|hemoglobin, fetal (hereditary) (HPFH) D56.4
|hyaloid
    |artery (generally incomplete) Q14.0
    |system Q14.8
|hymen, in pregnancy or childbirth *see*
    Pregnancy, complicated by, abnormal,
    vulva
|lanugo Q84.2
|left
    |posterior cardinal vein Q26.8
    |root with right arch of aorta Q25.49
    |superior vena cava Q26.1
|Meckel's diverticulum Q43.0
    |malignant *see* Table of Neoplasms, small
        intestine, malignant
|mucosal disease (middle ear) *see* Otitis,
    media, suppurative, chronic, tubotympanic
|nail(s), anomalous Q84.6
|omphalomesenteric duct Q43.0
|organ or site not listed *see* Anomaly, by site
|ostium
    |atrioventriculare commune Q21.2
    |primum Q21.2
    |secundum Q21.1
|ovarian rests in fallopian tube Q50.6
|pancreatic tissue in intestinal tract Q43.8
|primary (deciduous)
    |teeth K00.6
    |vitreous hyperplasia Q14.0
|pupillary membrane Q13.89
|right aortic arch Q25.47
|rhesus (Rh) titer *see* Complication(s),
    transfusion, incompatibility reaction, Rh
    (factor)
|sinus
    |urogenitalis
        |female Q52.8
        |male Q55.8
    |venosus with imperfect incorporation in
        right auricle Q26.8
|thymus (gland) (hyperplasia) E32.0
|thyroglossal duct Q89.2
|thyrolingual duct Q89.2
|truncus arteriosus or communis Q20.0
|tunica vasculosa lentis Q12.2
|umbilical sinus Q64.4
|urachus Q64.4
|vitelline duct Q43.0
Person (with)
|admitted for clinical research, as a control
    subject (normal comparison) (participant)
    Z00.6
|awaiting admission to adequate facility
    elsewhere Z75.1
|concern (normal) about sick person in family
    Z63.6
|consulting on behalf of another Z71.0

Person (with) - *continued*
|feigning illness Z76.5
|living (in)
    |alone Z60.2
    |boarding school Z59.3
    |residential institution Z59.3
    |without
        |adequate housing (heating) (space) Z59.1
        |housing (permanent) (temporary) Z59.00
        |person able to render necessary care Z74.2
        |shelter Z59.02
|on waiting list Z75.1
|sick or handicapped in family Z63.6
Personality (disorder) F60.9
|accentuation of traits (type A pattern) Z73.1
|affective F34.0
|aggressive F60.3
|amoral F60.2
|anancastic, anankastic F60.5
|antisocial F60.2
|anxious F60.6
|asocial F60.2
|asthenic F60.7
|avoidant F60.6
|borderline F60.3
|change due to organic condition (enduring)
    F07.0
|compulsive F60.5
|cycloid F34.0
|cyclothymic F34.0
|dependent F60.7
|depressive F34.1
|dissocial F60.2
|dual F44.81
|eccentric F60.89
|emotionally unstable F60.3
|expansive paranoid F60.0
|explosive F60.3
|fanatic F60.0
|haltlose type F60.89
|histrionic F60.4
|hyperthymic F34.0
|hypothymic F34.1
|hysterical F60.4
|immature F60.89
|inadequate F60.7
|labile (emotional) F60.3
|mixed (nonspecific) F60.89
|morally defective F60.2
|multiple F44.81
|narcissistic F60.81
|obsessional F60.5
|obsessive (-compulsive) F60.5
|organic F07.0
|overconscientious F60.5
|paranoid F60.0
|passive (-dependent) F60.7
|passive-aggressive F60.89
|pathologic F60.9
|pattern defect or disturbance F60.9
|pseudopsychopathic (organic) F07.0
|pseudoretarded (organic) F07.0
|psychoinfantile F60.4
|psychoneurotic NEC F60.89
|psychopathic F60.2
|querulant F60.0
|sadistic F60.89
|schizoid F60.1
|self-defeating F60.7
|sensitive paranoid F60.0
|sociopathic (amoral) (antisocial) (asocial)
    (dissocial) F60.2
|specified NEC F60.89
|type A Z73.1
|unstable (emotional) F60.3

Perthes' disease *see* Legg-Calvé-Perthes disease
Pertussis *see also* Whooping cough A37.90
Perversion, perverted
　|appetite F50.89
　　|psychogenic F50.89
　|function
　　|pituitary gland E23.2
　　　|posterior lobe E22.2
　|sense of smell and taste R43.8
　　|psychogenic F45.8
　|sexual *see* Deviation, sexual
Pervious, congenital *see also* Imperfect, closure
　|ductus arteriosus Q25.0
Pes (congenital) *see also* Talipes
　|acquired *see also* Deformity, limb, foot,
　　specified NEC
　　|planus *see* Deformity, limb, flat foot
　|adductus Q66.89
　|cavus Q66.7
　|deformity NEC, acquired *see* Deformity, limb,
　　foot, specified NEC
　|planus (acquired) (any degree) *see also*
　　Deformity, limb, flat foot
　　|rachitic sequelae (late effect) E64.3
　|valgus Q66.6
Pest, pestis *see* Plague
Petechia, petechiae R23.3
　|newborn P54.5
Petechial typhus A75.9
Peter's anomaly Q13.4
Petit mal seizure *see* Epilepsy, generalized,
　specified NEC
Petit's hernia *see* Hernia, abdomen, specified
　site NEC
Petriellidiosis B48.2
Petrositis H70.20-
　|acute H70.21-
　|chronic H70.22-
Peutz-Jeghers disease or syndrome Q85.8
Peyronie's disease N48.6
PFAPA (periodic fever, aphthous stomatitis,
　pharyngitis, and adenopathy syndrome)
　M04.8
Pfeiffer's disease *see* Mononucleosis, infectious
Phagedena (dry) (moist) (sloughing) *see also*
　Gangrene
　|geometric L88
　|penis N48.29
　|tropical *see* Ulcer, skin
　|vulva N76.6
Phagedenic *see* condition
Phakoma H35.89
Phakomatosis *see also* specific eponymous
　syndromes Q85.9
　|Bourneville's Q85.1
　|specified NEC Q85.8
Phantom limb syndrome (without pain) G54.7
　|with pain G54.6
Pharyngeal pouch syndrome D82.1
Pharyngitis (acute) (catarrhal)(gangrenous)
　(infective) (malignant) (membranous)
　(phlegmonous) (pseudomembranous)
　(simple) (subacute) (suppurative)
　(ulcerative) (viral) J02.9
　|with influenza, flu, or grippe *see* Influenza,
　　with, pharyngitis
　|aphthous B08.5
　|atrophic J31.2
　|chlamydial A56.4
　|chronic (atrophic) (granular) (hypertrophic)
　　J31.2
　|coxsackievirus B08.5
　|diphtheritic A36.0
　|enteroviral vesicular B08.5
　|follicular (chronic) J31.2

Pharyngitis – *continued*
　|fusospirochetal A69.1
　|gonococcal A54.5
　|granular (chronic) J31.2
　|herpesviral B00.2
　|hypertrophic J31.2
　|infectional, chronic J31.2
　|influenzal *see* Influenza, with, respiratory
　　manifestations NEC
　|lymphonodular, acute (enteroviral) B08.8
　|pneumococcal J02.8
　|purulent J02.9
　|putrid J02.9
　|septic J02.0
　|sicca J31.2
　|specified organism NEC J02.8
　|staphylococcal J02.8
　|streptococcal J02.0
　|syphilitic, congenital (early) A50.03
　|tuberculous A15.8
　|vesicular, enteroviral B08.5
　|viral NEC J02.8
Pharyngoconjunctivitis, viral B30.2
Pharyngolaryngitis (acute) J06.0
　|chronic J37.0
Pharyngoplegia J39.2
Pharyngotonsillitis, herpesviral B00.2
Pharyngotracheitis, chronic J42
Pharynx, pharyngeal *see* condition
Phencyclidine-Induced
　|anxiety disorder F16.980
　|bipolar and related disorder F16.94
　|depressive disorder F16.94
　|psychotic disorder F16.959
Phenomenon
　|Arthus' *see* Arthus' phenomenon
　|jaw-winking Q07.8
　|lupus erythematosus (LE) cell M32.9
　|Raynaud's (secondary) I73.00
　　|with gangrene I73.01
　|vasomotor R55
　|vasospastic I73.9
　|vasovagal R55
　|Wenckebach's I44.1
Phenylketonuria E70.1
　|classical E70.0
　|maternal E70.1
Pheochromoblastoma
　|specified site *see* Neoplasm, malignant, by site
　|unspecified site C74.10
Pheochromocytoma malignant
　　|specified site *see* Neoplasm, malignant, by
　　　site
　　|unspecified site C74.10
　|specified site *see* Neoplasm, benign, by site
　|unspecified site D35.00
Phaeohyphomycosis *see* Chromomycosis
Pheomycosis *see* Chromomycosis
Phimosis (congenital) (due to infection) N47.1
　|chancroidal A57
Phlebectasia *see also* Varix
　|congenital Q27.4
Phlebitis (infective) (pyemic) (septic)
　(suppurative) I80.9
　|antepartum *see* Thrombophlebitis, antepartum
　|blue *see* Phlebitis, leg, deep
　|breast, superficial I80.8
　|cavernous (venous) sinus *see* Phlebitis,
　　intracranial (venous) sinus
　|cerebral (venous) sinus *see* Phlebitis,
　　intracranial (venous) sinus
　|chest wall, superficial I80.8
　|cranial (venous) sinus *see* Phlebitis,
　　intracranial (venous) sinus
　|deep (vessels) *see* Phlebitis, leg, deep

Phlebitis – *continued*
　|due to implanted device *see* Complications, by
　　site and type, specified NEC
　|during or resulting from a procedure T81.72
　|femoral vein (superficial) I80.1-
　|femoropopliteal vein I80.0-
　|gestational *see* Phlebopathy, gestational
　|hepatic veins I80.8
　|iliofemoral *see* Phlebitis, femoral vein
　|intracranial (venous) sinus (any) G08
　　|nonpyogenic I67.6
　|intraspinal venous sinuses and veins G08
　　|nonpyogenic G95.19
　|lateral (venous) sinus *see* Phlebitis,
　　intracranial (venous) sinus
　|leg I80.3
　　|antepartum *see* Thrombophlebitis,
　　　antepartum
　　|deep (vessels) NEC I80.20-
　　　|iliac I80.21-
　　　|popliteal vein I80.22-
　　　|specified vessel NEC I80.29-
　　　|tibial vein I80.23-
　　|femoral vein (superficial) I80.1-
　　|superficial (vessels) I80.0-
　|longitudinal sinus *see* Phlebitis, intracranial
　　(venous) sinus
　|lower limb *see* Phlebitis, leg
　|migrans, migrating (superficial) I82.1
　|pelvic
　　|with ectopic or molar pregnancy O08.0
　　|following ectopic or molar pregnancy O08.0
　　|puerperal, postpartum O87.1
　|popliteal vein *see* Phlebitis, leg, deep,
　　popliteal
　|portal (vein) K75.1
　|postoperative T81.72
　|pregnancy *see* Thrombophlebitis, antepartum
　|puerperal, postpartum, childbirth O87.0
　　|deep O87.1
　　|pelvic O87.1
　　|superficial O87.0
　|retina *see* Vasculitis, retina
　|saphenous (accessory) (great) (long) (small)
　　see Phlebitis, leg, superficial
　|sinus (meninges) *see* Phlebitis, intracranial
　　(venous) sinus
　|specified site NEC I80.8
　|syphilitic A52.09
　|tibial vein *see* Phlebitis, leg, deep, tibial
　|ulcerative I80.9
　　|leg *see* Phlebitis, leg
　|umbilicus I80.8
　|uterus (septic) *see* Endometritis
　|varicose (leg) (lower limb) *see* Varix, leg,
　　with, inflammation
Phlebofibrosis I87.8
Phleboliths I87.8
Phlebopathy,
　|gestational O22.9-
　|puerperal O87.9
Phlebosclerosis I87.8
Phlebothrombosis *see also* Thrombosis
　|antepartum *see* Thrombophlebitis, antepartum
　|pregnancy *see* Thrombophlebitis, antepartum
　|puerperal *see* Thrombophlebitis, puerperal
Phlebotomus fever A93.1
Phlegmasia
　|alba dolens O87.1
　　|nonpuerperal *see* Phlebitis, femoral vein
　|cerulea dolens *see* Phlebitis, leg, deep
Phlegmon *see* Abscess
Phlegmonous *see* condition

Phlyctenulosis (allergic) (keratoconjunctivitis) (nontuberculous) *see also* Keratoconjunctivitis
|cornea *see* Keratoconjunctivitis
|tuberculous A18.52
Phobia, phobic F40.9
|animal F40.218
||spiders F40.210
|examination F40.298
|reaction F40.9
|simple F40.298
|social F40.10
||generalized F40.11
|specific (isolated) F40.298
||animal F40.218
|||spiders F40.210
||blood F40.230
||injection F40.231
||injury F40.233
||men F40.290
||natural environment F40.228
|||thunderstorms F40.220
||situational F40.248
|||bridges F40.242
|||closed in spaces F40.240
|||flying F40.243
|||heights F40.241
||specified focus NEC F40.298
||transfusion F40.231
||women F40.291
|specified NEC F40.8
||medical care NEC F40.232
|state F40.9
Phocas' disease *see* Mastopathy, cystic
Phocomelia Q73.1
|lower limb *see* Agenesis, leg, with foot present
|upper limb *see* Agenesis, arm, with hand present
Phoria H50.50
Phosphate-Losing tubular disorder N25.0
Phosphatemia E83.39
Phosphaturia E83.39
Photodermatitis (sun) L56.8
|chronic L57.8
|due to drug L56.8
|light other than sun L59.8
Photokeratitis H16.13-
Photophobia H53.14-
Photophthalmia *see* Photokeratitis
Photopsia H53.19
Photoretinitis *see* Retinopathy, solar
Photosensitivity, photosensitization (sun) skin L56.8
|light other than sun L59.8
Phrenitis *see* Encephalitis
Phrynoderma (vitamin A deficiency) E50.8
Phthiriasis (pubis) B85.3
|with any infestation classifiable to B85.0-B85.2, B85.4
Phthirus infestation *see* Phthiriasis
Phthisis *see also* Tuberculosis
|bulbi (infectional) *see* Disorder, globe, degenerated condition, atrophy
|eyeball (due to infection) *see* Disorder, globe, degenerated condition, atrophy
Phycomycosis *see* Zygomycosis
Physalopteriasis B81.8
Physical restraint status Z78.1
Phytobezoar T18.9
|intestine T18.3
|stomach T18.2
Pian *see* Yaws
Pianoma A66.1

Pica F50.89
|in adults F50.89
|infant or child F98.3
Picking, nose F98.8
Pick Niemann disease *see* Niemann-Pick disease or syndrome
Pick's
|cerebral atrophy G31.01 *[F02.80]*
||with behavioral disturbance G31.01 *[F02.81]*
|disease or syndrome (brain) G31.01 *[F02.80]*
||with behavioral disturbance G31.01 *[F02.81]*
||brain G31.01 *[F02.80]*
|||with behavioral disturbance G31.01 *[F02.81]*
||pericardium (pericardial pseudocirrhosis of liver) I31.1
|syndrome
||brain G31.01 *[F02.80]*
|||with behavioral disturbance G31.01 *[F02.81]*
||of heart (pericardial pseudocirrhosis of liver) I31.1
Pickwickian syndrome E66.2
Piebaldism E70.39
Piedra (beard) (scalp) B36.8
|black B36.3
|white B36.2
Pierre Robin deformity or syndrome Q87.0
Pierson's disease or osteochondrosis M91.0
Pig-Bel A05.2
Pigeon
|breast or chest (acquired) M95.4
||congenital Q67.7
||rachitic sequelae (late effect) E64.3
|breeder's disease or lung J67.2
|fancier's disease or lung J67.2
|toe *see* Deformity, toe, specified NEC
Pigmentation (abnormal) (anomaly) L81.9
|conjunctiva H11.13-
|cornea (anterior) H18.01-
||posterior H18.05-
||stromal H18.06-
|diminished melanin formation NEC L81.6
|iron L81.8
|lids, congenital Q82.8
|limbus corneae *see* Pigmentation, cornea
|metals L81.8
|optic papilla, congenital Q14.2
|retina, congenital (grouped) (nevoid) Q14.1
|scrotum, congenital Q82.8
|tattoo L81.8
Piles *see also* Hemorrhoids K64.9
Pili
|annulati or torti (congenital) Q84.1
|incarnati L73.1
Pill roller hand (intrinsic) *see* Parkinsonism
Pilomatrixoma *see* Neoplasm, skin, benign
|malignant *see* Neoplasm, skin, malignant
Pilonidal *see* condition
Pimple R23.8
PIN *see* Neoplasia, intraepithelial, prostate
Pinched nerve *see* Neuropathy, entrapment
Pindborg tumor *see* Cyst, calcifying odontogenic
Pineal body or gland *see* condition
Pinealoblastoma C75.3
Pinealoma D44.5
|malignant C75.3
Pineoblastoma C75.3
Pineocytoma D44.5
Pinguecula H11.15-
Pingueculitis H10.81-

Pinhole meatus *see also* Stricture, urethra N35.919
Pink
|disease *see* subcategory T56.1
|eye *see* Conjunctivitis, acute, mucopurulent
Pinkus' disease (lichen nitidus) L44.1
Pinpoint
|meatus *see* Stricture, urethra
|os (uteri) *see* Stricture, cervix
Pins and needles R20.2
Pinta A67.9
|cardiovascular lesions A67.2
|chancre (primary) A67.0
|erythematous plaques A67.1
|hyperchromic lesions A67.1
|hyperkeratosis A67.1
|lesions A67.9
||cardiovascular A67.2
||hyperchromic A67.1
||intermediate A67.1
||late A67.2
||mixed A67.3
||primary A67.0
||skin (achromic) (cicatricial) (dyschromic) A67.2
|||hyperchromic A67.1
|||mixed (achromic and hyperchromic) A67.3
|papule (primary) A67.0
|skin lesions (achromic) (cicatricial) (dyschromic) A67.2
||hyperchromic A67.1
||mixed (achromic and hyperchromic) A67.3
|vitiligo A67.2
Pintids A67.1
Pinworm (disease) (infection) (infestation) B80
Piroplasmosis (see also Babesiosis) B60.0
|specified NEC B60.09
Pistol wound *see* Gunshot wound
Pitchers' elbow *see* Derangement, joint, specified type NEC, elbow
Pithecoid pelvis Q74.2
|with disproportion (fetopelvic) O33.0
||causing obstructed labor O65.0
Pithiatism F48.8
Pitted *see* Pitting
Pitting *see also* Edema R60.9
|lip R60.0
|nail L60.8
|teeth K00.4
Pituitary gland *see* condition
Pituitary-Snuff-Taker's disease J67.8
Pityriasis (capitis) L21.0
|alba L30.5
|circinata (et maculata) L42
|furfuracea L21.0
|Hebra's L26
|lichenoides L41.0
||chronica L41.1
||et varioliformis (acuta) L41.0
|maculata (et circinata) L30.5
|nigra B36.1
|pilaris, Hebra's L44.0
|rosea L42
|rotunda L44.8
|rubra (Hebra) pilaris L44.0
|simplex L30.5
|specified type NEC L30.5
|streptogenes L30.5
|versicolor (scrotal) B36.0
Placenta, placental *see* Pregnancy, complicated by (care of) (management affected by), specified condition
Placentitis O41.14-

Plagiocephaly Q67.3
Plague A20.9
 |abortive A20.8
 |ambulatory A20.8
 |asymptomatic A20.8
 |bubonic A20.0
 |cellulocutaneous A20.1
 |cutaneobubonic A20.1
 |lymphatic gland A20.0
 |meningitis A20.3
 |pharyngeal A20.8
 |pneumonic (primary) (secondary) A20.2
 |pulmonary, pulmonic A20.2
 |septicemic A20.7
 |tonsillar A20.8
  |septicemic A20.7
Planning, family
 |contraception Z30.9
 |procreation Z31.69
Plaque(s)
 |artery, arterial see Arteriosclerosis
 |calcareous see Calcification
 |coronary, lipid rich I25.83
 |epicardial I31.8
 |erythematous, of pinta A67.1
 |Hollenhorst's see Occlusion, artery, retina
 |lipid rich, coronary I25.83
 |pleural (without asbestos) J92.9
  |with asbestos J92.0
 |tongue K13.29
Plasmacytoma C90.3-
 |extramedullary C90.2-
 |medullary C90.0-
 |solitary C90.3-
Plasmacytopenia D72.818
Plasmacytosis D72.822
Plaster ulcer see Ulcer, pressure, by site
Plateau iris syndrome (post-Iridectomy)
  (postprocedural) (without glaucoma)
  H21.82
 |with glaucoma H40.22-
Platybasia Q75.8
Platyonychia (congenital) Q84.6
 |acquired L60.8
Platypelloid pelvis M95.5
 |with disproportion (fetopelvic) O33.0
  |causing obstructed labor O65.0
 |congenital Q74.2
Platyspondylisis Q76.49
Plaut (-Vincent) disease see also Vincent's
  A69.1
Plethora R23.2
 |newborn P61.1
Pleura, pleural see condition
Pleuralgia R07.81
Pleurisy (acute) (adhesive) (chronic) (costal)
  (diaphragmatic) (double) (dry) (fibrinous)
  (fibrous) (interlobar) (latent) (plastic)
  (primary) (residual) (sicca) (sterile)
  (subacute) (unresolved) R09.1
 |with
  |adherent pleura J86.0
  |effusion J90
   |chylous, chyliform J94.0
   |tuberculous (non primary) A15.6
    |primary (progressive) A15.7
  |tuberculosis see Pleurisy, tuberculous (non
     primary)
 |encysted see Pleurisy, with effusion
 |exudative see Pleurisy, with effusion
 |fibrinopurulent, fibropurulent see Pyothorax
  |hemorrhagic see Hemothorax
 |pneumococcal J90
 |purulent see Pyothorax
 |septic see Pyothorax
 |serofibrinous see Pleurisy, with effusion

Pleurisy - continued
 |seropurulent see Pyothorax
 |serous see Pleurisy, with effusion
 |staphylococcal J86.9
 |streptococcal J90
 |suppurative see Pyothorax
 |traumatic (post) (current) see Injury,
    intrathoracic, pleura
 |tuberculous (with effusion) (non primary)
    A15.6
  |primary (progressive) A15.7
Pleuritis sicca see Pleurisy
Pleurobronchopneumonia see Pneumonia,
  broncho-
Pleurodynia R07.81
 |epidemic B33.0
 |viral B33.0
Pleuropericarditis see also Pericarditis
 |acute I30.9
Pleuropneumonia (acute) (bilateral) (double)
  (septic) see also Pneumonia J18.8
 |chronic see Fibrosis, lung
Pleuro-Pneumonia-Like-Organism (PPLO),
  as cause of disease classified elsewhere
  B96.0
Pleurorrhea see Pleurisy, with effusion
Plexitis, brachial G54.0
Plica
 |polonica B85.0
 |syndrome, knee M67.5-
 |tonsil J35.8
Plicated tongue K14.5
Plug
 |bronchus NEC J98.09
 |meconium (newborn) NEC syndrome P76.0
 |mucus see Asphyxia, mucus
Plumbism see subcategory T56.0
Plummer's disease E05.20
 |with thyroid storm E05.21
Plummer-Vinson syndrome D50.1
Pluricarential syndrome of infancy E40
Plus (and minus) hand (intrinsic) see
  Deformity, limb, specified type NEC, forearm
PMEI (polymorphic epilepsy in infancy)
  G40.83-
Pneumathemia see Air, embolism
Pneumatic hammer (drill) syndrome T75.21
Pneumatocele (lung) J98.4
 |intracranial G93.89
 |tension J44.9
Pneumatosis
 |cystoides intestinalis K63.89
 |intestinalis K63.89
 |peritonei K66.8
Pneumaturia R39.89
Pneumoblastoma see Neoplasm, lung,
  malignant
Pneumocephalus G93.89
Pneumococcemia A40.3
Pneumococcus, pneumococcal see condition
Pneumoconiosis (due to) (inhalation of) J64
 |with tuberculosis (any type in A15) J65
 |aluminum J63.0
 |asbestos J61
 |bagasse, bagassosis J67.1
 |bauxite J63.1
 |beryllium J63.2
 |coal miners' (simple) J60
 |Coalworker's' (simple) J60
 |collier's J60
 |cotton dust J66.0
 |diatomite (diatomaceous earth) J62.8
 |dust
  |inorganic NEC J63.6
  |lime J62.8

Pneumoconiosis – continued
 |marble J62.8
 |organic NEC J66.8
 |fumes or vapors (from silo) J68.9
 |graphite J63.3
 |grinder's J62.8
 |kaolin J62.8
 |mica J62.8
 |millstone maker's J62.8
 |mineral fibers NEC J61
 |miner's J60
 |moldy hay J67.0
 |potter's J62.8
 |rheumatoid see Rheumatoid, lung
 |sandblaster's J62.8
 |silica, silicate NEC J62.8
  |with carbon J60
 |stonemason's J62.8
 |talc (dust) J62.0
Pneumocystis carinii pneumonia B59
Pneumocystis jiroveci (pneumonia) B59
Pneumocystosis (with pneumonia) B59
Pneumohemopericardium I31.2
Pneumohemothorax J94.2
 |traumatic S27.2
Pneumohydropericardium see Pericarditis
Pneumohydrothorax see Hydrothorax
Pneumomediastinum J98.2
 |congenital or perinatal P25.2
Pneumomycosis B49 [J99]
Pneumonia (acute) (double) (migratory)
  (purulent) (septic) (unresolved) J18.9
 |2019 (novel) coronavirus J12.82
 |with
  |lung abscess J85.1
   |due to specified organism see Pneumonia,
     in (due to)
  |influenza see Influenza, with, pneumonia
 |adenoviral J12.0
 |adynamic J18.2
 |alba A50.04
 |allergic (see also Pneumonitis,
    hypersensitivity) J82.89
 |alveolar see Pneumonia, lobar
 |anaerobes J15.8
 |anthrax A22.1
 |apex, apical see Pneumonia, lobar
 |Ascaris B77.81
 |aspiration J69.0
  |due to
   |aspiration of microorganisms
    |bacterial J15.9
    |viral J12.9
   |food (regurgitated) J69.0
   |gastric secretions J69.0
   |milk (regurgitated) J69.0
   |oils, essences J69.1
   |solids, liquids NEC J69.8
   |vomitus J69.0
  |newborn P24.81
   |amniotic fluid (clear) P24.11
   |blood P24.21
   |liquor (amnii) P24.11
   |meconium P24.01
   |milk P24.31
   |mucus P24.11
   |food (regurgitated) P24.31
   |specified NEC P24.81
   |stomach contents P24.31
  |postprocedural J95.4
 |atypical NEC J18.9
 |bacillus J15.9
  |specified NEC J15.8
 |bacterial J15.9
  |specified NEC J15.8

Pneumonia - *continued*
|Bacteroides (fragilis) (oralis) (melaninogenicus) J15.8
|basal, basic, basilar *see* Pneumonia, by type
|bronchiolitis obliterans organized (BOOP) J84.89
|broncho, bronchial (confluent) (croupous) (diffuse) (disseminated) (hemorrhagic) (involving lobes) (lobar) (terminal) J18.0
||allergic (*see also* Pneumonitis, hypersensitivity) J82.89
||aspiration *see* Pneumonia, aspiration
||bacterial J15.9
|||specified NEC J15.8
||chronic *see* Fibrosis, lung
||diplococcal J13
||Eaton's agent J15.7
||Escherichia coli (E. coli) J15.5
||Friedländer's bacillus J15.0
||Hemophilus influenzae J14
||hypostatic J18.2
||inhalation *see also* Pneumonia, aspiration
|||due to fumes or vapors (chemical) J68.0
|||of oils or essences J69.1
||Klebsiella (pneumoniae) J15.0
||lipid, lipoid J69.1
|||endogenous J84.89
||Mycoplasma (pneumoniae) J15.7
||pleuro-pneumonia-like-organisms (PPLO) J15.7
||pneumococcal J13
||Proteus J15.6
||Pseudomonas J15.1
||Serratia marcescens J15.6
||specified organism NEC J16.8
||staphylococcal *see* Pneumonia, staphylococcal
||streptococcal NEC J15.4
|||group B J15.3
|||pneumoniae J13
||viral, virus *see* Pneumonia, viral
|Butyrivibrio (fibriosolvens) J15.8
|Candida B37.1
|caseous *see* Tuberculosis, pulmonary
|catarrhal *see* Pneumonia, broncho
|chlamydial J16.0
||congenital P23.1
|cholesterol J84.89
|cirrhotic (chronic) *see* Fibrosis, lung
|Clostridium (haemolyticum) (novyi) J15.8
|confluent *see* Pneumonia, broncho
|congenital (infective) P23.9
||due to
|||bacterium NEC P23.6
|||Chlamydia P23.1
|||Escherichia coli P23.4
|||Haemophilus influenzae P23.6
|||infective organism NEC P23.8
|||Klebsiella pneumoniae P23.6
|||Mycoplasma P23.6
|||Pseudomonas P23.5
|||Staphylococcus P23.2
|||Streptococcus (except group B) P23.6
||||group B P23.3
|||viral agent P23.0
||specified NEC P23.8
|coronavirus (novel) (disease) 2019 J12.82
|croupous *see* Pneumonia, lobar
|cryptogenic organizing J84.116
|cytomegalic inclusion B25.0
|cytomegaloviral B25.0
|deglutition *see* Pneumonia, aspiration
|desquamative interstitial J84.117
|diffuse *see* Pneumonia, broncho

Pneumonia - *continued*
|diplococcal, diplococcus (broncho) (lobar) J13
|disseminated (focal) *see* Pneumonia, broncho
|Eaton's agent J15.7
|embolic, embolism *see* Embolism, pulmonary
|Enterobacter J15.6
|eosinophilic J82.81
||acute J82.82
||chronic J82.81
|Escherichia coli (E. coli) J15.5
|Eubacterium J15.8
|fibrinous *see* Pneumonia, lobar
|fibroid, fibrous (chronic) *see* Fibrosis, lung
|Friedländer's bacillus J15.0
|Fusobacterium (nucleatum) J15.8
|gangrenous J85.0
|giant cell (measles) B05.2
|gonococcal A54.84
|gram-negative bacteria NEC J15.6
||anaerobic J15.8
|Hemophilus influenzae (broncho) (lobar) J14
|human metapneumovirus J12.3
|hypostatic (broncho) (lobar) J18.2
|in (due to)
||actinomycosis A42.0
||adenovirus J12.0
||anthrax A22.1
||ascariasis B77.81
||aspergillosis B44.9
||Bacillus anthracis A22.1
||Bacterium anitratum J15.6
||candidiasis B37.1
||chickenpox B01.2
||Chlamydia J16.0
|||neonatal P23.1
||coccidioidomycosis B38.2
|||acute B38.0
|||chronic B38.1
||cytomegalovirus disease B25.0
||Diplococcus (pneumoniae) J13
||Eaton's agent J15.7
||Enterobacter J15.6
||Escherichia coli (E. coli) J15.5
||Friedländer's bacillus J15.0
||fumes and vapors (chemical) (inhalation) J68.0
||gonorrhea A54.84
||Hemophilus influenzae (H. influenzae) J14
||Herellea J15.6
||histoplasmosis B39.2
|||acute B39.0
|||chronic B39.1
||human metapneumovirus J12.3
||Klebsiella (pneumoniae) J15.0
||measles B05.2
||Mycoplasma (pneumoniae) J15.7
||nocardiosis, nocardiasis A43.0
||ornithosis A70
||parainfluenza virus J12.2
||pleuro-pneumonia-like-organism (PPLO) J15.7
||pneumococcus J13
||pneumocystosis (Pneumocystis carinii) (Pneumocystis jiroveci) B59
||Proteus J15.6
||Pseudomonas NEC J15.1
|||pseudomallei A24.1
||psittacosis A70
||Q fever A78
||respiratory syncytial virus J12.1
||rheumatic fever I00 [*J17*]
||rubella B06.81
||Salmonella (infection) A02.22
|||typhi A01.03

Pneumonia - *continued*
||schistosomiasis B65.9 [*J17*]
||Serratia marcescens J15.6
||specified
|||bacterium NEC J15.8
|||organism NEC J16.8
||spirochetal NEC A69.8
||Staphylococcus J15.20
|||aureus (methicillin susceptible) (MSSA) J15.211
||||methicillin resistant (MRSA) J15.212
|||specified NEC J15.29
||Streptococcus J15.4
|||group B J15.3
|||pneumoniae J13
|||specified NEC J15.4
||toxoplasmosis B58.3
||tularemia A21.2
||typhoid (fever) A01.03
||varicella B01.2
||virus *see* Pneumonia, viral
||whooping cough A37.91
|||due to
||||Bordetella parapertussis A37.11
||||Bordetella pertussis A37.01
|||specified NEC A37.81
||Yersinia pestis A20.2
|inhalation of food or vomit *see* Pneumonia, aspiration
|interstitial J84.9
||chronic J84.111
||desquamative J84.117
||due to
|||collagen vascular disease J84.178
|||known underlying cause J84.178
||idiopathic NOS J84.111
||in disease classified elsewhere J84.178
||lymphocytic (due to collagen vascular disease) (in diseases classified elsewhere) J84.178
||lymphoid J84.2
||non-specific J84.89
|||due to
||||collagen vascular disease J84.178
||||known underlying cause J84.178
|||idiopathic J84.113
|||in diseases classified elsewhere J84.178
||plasma cell B59
||pseudomonas J15.1
||usual J84.112
|||due to collagen vascular disease J84.178
|||idiopathic J84.112
|||in diseases classified elsewhere J84.178
|Klebsiella (pneumoniae) J15.0
|lipid, lipoid (exogenous) J69.1
||endogenous J84.89
|lobar (disseminated) (double) (interstitial) J18.1
||bacterial J15.9
|||specified NEC J15.8
||chronic *see* Fibrosis, lung
||Escherichia coli (E. coli) J15.5
||Friedländer's bacillus J15.0
||Hemophilus influenzae J14
||hypostatic J18.2
||Klebsiella (pneumoniae) J15.0
||pneumococcal J13
||Proteus J15.6
||Pseudomonas J15.1
||specified organism NEC J16.8
||staphylococcal *see* Pneumonia, staphylococcal
||streptococcal NEC J15.4
||Streptococcus pneumoniae J13
||viral, virus *see* Pneumonia, viral

Pneumonia - *continued*
  |lobular *see* Pneumonia, broncho
  |Löffler's J82.89
  |lymphoid interstitial J84.2
  |massive *see* Pneumonia, lobar
  |meconium P24.01
  |MRSA (Methicillin resistant Staphylococcus
    aureus) J15.212
  |MSSA (methicillin susceptible
    Staphylococcus aureus) J15.211
  |multilobar *see* Pneumonia, by type
  |Mycoplasma (pneumoniae) J15.7
  |necrotic J85.0
  |neonatal P23.9
    |aspiration *see* Aspiration, by substance, with
      pneumonia
  |nitrogen dioxide J68.0
  |organizing J84.89
    |due to
      |collagen vascular disease J84.178
      |known underlying cause J84.178
    |in diseases classified elsewhere J84.178
  |orthostatic J18.2
  |parainfluenza virus J12.2
  |parenchymatous *see* Fibrosis, lung
  |passive J18.2
  |patchy *see* Pneumonia, broncho
  |Peptococcus J15.8
  |Peptostreptococcus J15.8
  |plasma cell (of infants) B59
  |pleurolobar *see* Pneumonia, lobar
  |pleuro-pneumonia-like organism (PPLO)
    J15.7
  |pneumococcal (broncho) (lobar) J13
  |Pneumocystis (carinii) (jiroveci) B59
  |postinfectional NEC B99 [*J17*]
  |postmeasles B05.2
  |Proteus J15.6
  |Pseudomonas J15.1
  |psittacosis A70
  |radiation J70.0
  |respiratory syncytial virus J12.1
  |resulting from a procedure J95.89
  |rheumatic I00 [*J17*]
  |Salmonella (arizonae) (cholerae-Suis)
    (enteritidis) (typhimurium) A02.22
    |typhi A01.03
    |typhoid fever A01.03
  |SARS-associated coronavirus J12.81
  |segmented, segmental *see* Pneumonia,
    broncho
  |Serratia marcescens J15.6
  |specified NEC J18.8
    |bacterium NEC J15.8
    |organism NEC J16.8
    |virus NEC J12.89
  |spirochetal NEC A69.8
  |staphylococcal (broncho) (lobar) J15.20
    |aureus (methicillin susceptible) (MSSA)
      J15.211
      |methicillin resistant (MRSA) J15.212
    |specified NEC J15.29
  |static, stasis J18.2
  |streptococcal NEC (broncho) (lobar) J15.4
    |group
      |A J15.4
      |B J15.3
      |specified NEC J15.4
  |Streptococcus pneumoniae J13
  |syphilitic, congenital (early) A50.04
  |traumatic (complication) (early) (secondary)
    T79.8
  |tuberculous (any) *see* Tuberculosis,
    pulmonary
  |tularemic A21.2

Pneumonia - *continued*
  |varicella B01.2
  |Veillonella J15.8
  |ventilator associated J95.851
  |viral, virus (broncho) (interstitial) (lobar)
    J12.9
    |adenoviral J12.0
    |congenital P23.0
    |human metapneumovirus J12.3
    |parainfluenza J12.2
    |respiratory syncytial J12.1
    |SARS-associated coronavirus J12.81
    |specified NEC J12.89
  |white (congenital) A50.04
Pneumonic *see* condition
Pneumonitis (acute) (primary) *see also*
    Pneumonia
  |air-conditioner J67.7
  |allergic (due to) J67.9
    |organic dust NEC J67.8
    |red cedar dust J67.8
    |sequoiosis J67.8
    |wood dust J67.8
  |aspiration J69.0
    |due to
      |anesthesia J95.4
        |during
          |labor and delivery O74.0
          |pregnancy O29.01-
          |puerperium O89.01
      |fumes or gases J68.0
    |obstetric O74.0
  |chemical (due to gases, fumes or vapors)
    (inhalation) J68.0
    |due to anesthesia J95.4
  |cholesterol J84.89
  |chronic *see* Fibrosis, lung
  |congenital rubella P35.0
  |due to
    |beryllium J68.0
    |cadmium J68.0
    |crack (cocaine) J68.0
    |detergent J69.8
    |fluorocarbon-polymer J68.0
    |food, vomit (aspiration) J69.0
    |fumes or vapors J68.0
    |gases, fumes or vapors (inhalation) J68.0
    |inhalation
      |blood J69.8
      |essences J69.1
      |food (regurgitated), milk, vomit J69.0
      |oils, essences J69.1
      |saliva J69.0
      |solids, liquids NEC J69.8
    |manganese J68.0
    |nitrogen dioxide J68.0
    |oils, essences J69.1
    |solids, liquids NEC J69.8
    |toxoplasmosis (acquired) B58.3
      |congenital P37.1
    |vanadium J68.0
    |ventilator J95.851
  |eosinophilic J82.81
    |acute J82.82
    |chronic J82.81
  |hypersensitivity J67.9
    |air conditioner lung J67.7
    |bagassosis J67.1
    |bird fancier's lung J67.2
    |farmer's lung J67.0
    |Maltworker's lung J67.4
    |maple bark-stripper's lung J67.6
    |mushroom worker's lung J67.5
    |specified organic dust NEC J67.8

Pneumonitis (acute) (primary) - *continued*
    |suberosis J67.3
  |interstitial (chronic) J84.89
    |acute J84.114
    |lymphoid J84.2
    |non-specific J84.89
      |idiopathic J84.113
  |lymphoid, interstitial J84.2
  |meconium P24.01
  |postanesthetic J95.4
    |correct substance properly administered *see*
      Table of Drugs and Chemicals, by drug,
      adverse effect
    |in labor and delivery O74.0
    |in pregnancy O29.01-
    |obstetric O74.0
    |overdose or wrong substance given or taken
      (by accident) *see* Table of Drugs and
      Chemicals, by drug, poisoning
    |postpartum, puerperal O89.01
  |postoperative J95.4
    |obstetric O74.0
  |radiation J70.0
  |rubella, congenital P35.0
  |ventilation (air-conditioning) J67.7
  |ventilator associated J95.851
  |wood-dust J67.8
Pneumonoconiosis *see* Pneumoconiosis
Pneumoparotid K11.8
Pneumopathy NEC J98.4
  |alveolar J84.09
  |due to organic dust NEC J66.8
  |parietoalveolar J84.09
Pneumopericarditis *see also* Pericarditis
  |acute I30.9
Pneumopericardium *see also* Pericarditis
  |congenital P25.3
  |newborn P25.3
  |traumatic (post) *see* Injury, heart
Pneumophagia (psychogenic) F45.8
Pneumopleurisy, pneumopleuritis *see also*
    Pneumonia J18.8
Pneumopyopericardium I30.1
Pneumopyothorax *see* Pyopneumothorax
  |with fistula J86.0
Pneumorrhagia *see also* Hemorrhage, lung
  |tuberculous *see* Tuberculosis, pulmonary
Pneumothorax NOS J93.9
  |acute J93.83
  |chronic J93.81
  |congenital P25.1
  |perinatal period P25.1
  |postprocedural J95.811
  |specified NEC J93.83
  |spontaneous NOS J93.83
    |newborn P25.1
    |primary J93.11
    |secondary J93.12
    |tension J93.0
  |tense valvular, infectional J93.0
  |tension (spontaneous) J93.0
  |traumatic S27.0
    |with hemothorax S27.2
  |tuberculous *see* Tuberculosis, pulmonary
Podagra *see also* Gout M10.9
Podencephalus Q01.9
Poikilocytosis R71.8
Poikiloderma L81.6
  |Civatte's L57.3
  |congenital Q82.8
  |vasculare atrophicans L94.5
Poikilodermatomyositis M33.10
  |with
    |myopathy M33.12
    |respiratory involvement M33.11
    |specified organ involvement NEC M33.19

Pointed ear (congenital) Q17.3
Poison ivy, oak, sumac or other plant dermatitis (allergic) (contact) L23.7
Poisoning (acute) *see also* Table of Drugs and Chemicals
|algae and toxins T65.82-
|Bacillus B (aertrycke) (cholerae (suis)) (paratyphosus) (suipestifer) A02.9
|botulinus A05.1
|bacterial toxins A05.9
|berries, noxious *see* Poisoning, food, noxious, berries
|botulism A05.1
|ciguatera fish T61.0-
|Clostridium botulinum A05.1
|death-cap (Amanita phalloides) (Amanita verna) *see* Poisoning, food, noxious, mushrooms
|drug *see* Table of Drugs and Chemicals, by drug, poisoning
|epidemic, fish (noxious) *see* Poisoning, seafood
|bacterial A05.9
|fava bean D55.0
|fish (noxious) T61.9-
|bacterial *see* Intoxication, foodborne, by agent
|ciguatera fish *see* Poisoning, ciguatera fish
|scombroid fish *see* Poisoning, scombroid fish
|specified type NEC T61.77-
|food (acute) (diseased) (infected) (noxious) NEC T62.9-
|bacterial *see* Intoxication, foodborne, by agent
|due to
|Bacillus (aertrycke) (choleraesuis) (paratyphosus) (suipestifer) A02.9
|botulinus A05.1
|Clostridium (perfringens) (Welchii) A05.2
|salmonella (aertrycke) (gallinarum) (choleraesuis) (enteritidis) (paratyphi) (suipestifer) A02.9
|with
|gastroenteritis A02.0
|sepsis A02.1
|staphylococcus A05.0
|Vibrio
|parahaemolyticus A05.3
|vulnificus A05.5
|noxious or naturally toxic T62.9-
|berries *see* subcategory T62.1-
|fish *see* Poisoning, seafood
|mushrooms *see* subcategory T62.0X-
|plants NEC *see* subcategory T62.2X-
|seafood *see* Poisoning, seafood
|specified NEC *see* subcategory T62.8X
|ichthyotoxism *see* Poisoning, seafood
|kreotoxism, food A05.9
|latex T65.81-
|lead T56.0-
|mushroom *see* Poisoning, food, noxious, mushroom
|mussels *see also* Poisoning, shellfish
|bacterial *see* Intoxication, foodborne, by agent
|nicotine (tobacco) T65.2-
|noxious foodstuffs *see* Poisoning, food, noxious
|plants, noxious *see* Poisoning, food, noxious, plants NEC
|ptomaine *see* Poisoning, food
|radiation J70.0
|Salmonella (arizonae) (cholerae-suis) (enteritidis) (typhimurium) A02.9
|scombroid fish T61.1-
|seafood (noxious) T61.9-

Poisoning (acute) - *continued*
|bacterial *see* Intoxication, foodborne, by agent
|fish *see* Poisoning, fish
|shellfish *see* Poisoning, shellfish
|specified NEC *see* subcategory T61.8X-
|shellfish (amnesic) (azaspiracid) (diarrheic) (neurotoxic) (noxious) (paralytic) T61.78-
|bacterial *see* Intoxication, foodborne, by agent
|ciguatera mollusk *see* Poisoning, ciguatera fish
|specified substance NEC T65.891
|Staphylococcus, food A05.0
|tobacco (nicotine) T65.2-
|water E87.79
Poker spine *see* Spondylitis, ankylosing
Poland syndrome Q79.8
Polioencephalitis (acute) (bulbar) A80.9
|inferior G12.22
|influenzal *see* Influenza, with, encephalopathy
|superior hemorrhagic (acute) (Wernicke's) E51.2
|Wernicke's E51.2
Polioencephalomyelitis (acute) (anterior) A80.9
|with beriberi E51.2
Polioencephalopathy, superior hemorrhagic E51.2
|with
|beriberi E51.11
|pellagra E52
Poliomeningoencephalitis *see* Meningoencephalitis
Poliomyelitis (acute) (anterior) (epidemic) A80.9
|with paralysis (bulbar) *see* Poliomyelitis, paralytic
|abortive A80.4
|ascending (progressive) *see* Poliomyelitis, paralytic
|bulbar (paralytic) *see* Poliomyelitis, paralytic
|congenital P35.8
|nonepidemic A80.9
|nonparalytic A80.4
|paralytic A80.30
|specified NEC A80.39
|vaccine-associated A80.0
|wild virus
|imported A80.1
|indigenous A80.2
|spinal, acute A80.9
Poliosis (eyebrow) (eyelashes) L67.1
|circumscripta, acquired L67.1
Pollakiuria R35.0
|psychogenic F45.8
Pollinosis J30.1
Pollitzer's disease L73.2
Polyadenitis *see also* Lymphadenitis
|malignant A20.0
Polyalgia M79.89
Polyangiitis M30.0
|microscopic M31.7
|overlap syndrome M30.8
Polyarteritis
|microscopic M31.7
|nodosa M30.0
|with lung involvement M30.1
|juvenile M30.2
|related condition NEC M30.8
Polyarthralgia *see* Pain, joint
Polyarthritis, polyarthropathy *see also* Arthritis M13.0

Polyarthritis - *continued*
|due to or associated with other specified conditions *see* Arthritis
|epidemic (Australian) (with exanthema) B33.1
|infective *see* Arthritis, pyogenic or pyemic
|inflammatory M06.4
|juvenile (chronic) (seronegative) M08.3
|migratory *see* Fever, rheumatic
|rheumatic, acute *see* Fever, rheumatic
Polyarthrosis M15.9
|post-traumatic M15.3
|primary M15.0
|specified NEC M15.8
Polycarential syndrome of infancy E40
Polychondritis (atrophic) (chronic) *see also* Disorder, cartilage, specified type NEC
|relapsing M94.1
Polycoria Q13.2
Polycystic (disease)
|degeneration, kidney Q61.3
|autosomal dominant (adult type) Q61.2
|autosomal recessive (infantile type) NEC Q61.19
|kidney Q61.3
|autosomal
|dominant Q61.2
|recessive NEC Q61.19
|autosomal dominant (adult type) Q61.2
|autosomal recessive (childhood type) NEC Q61.19
|infantile type NEC Q61.19
|liver Q44.6
|lung J98.4
|congenital Q33.0
|ovary, ovaries E28.2
|spleen Q89.09
Polycythemia (secondary) D75.1
|acquired D75.1
|benign (familial) D75.0
|due to
|donor twin P61.1
|erythropoietin D75.1
|fall in plasma volume D75.1
|high altitude D75.1
|maternal-fetal transfusion P61.1
|stress D75.1
|emotional D75.1
|erythropoietin D75.1
|familial (benign) D75.0
|Gaisböck's (hypertonica) D75.1
|high altitude D75.1
|hypertonica D75.1
|hypoxemic D75.1
|neonatorum P61.1
|nephrogenous D75.1
|relative D75.1
|secondary D75.1
|spurious D75.1
|stress D75.1
|vera D45
Polycytosis cryptogenica D75.1
Polydactylism, polydactyly Q69.9
|toes Q69.2
Polydipsia R63.1
Polydystrophy, pseudo-Hurler E77.0
Polyembryoma *see* Neoplasm, malignant, by site
Polyglandular
|deficiency E31.0
|dyscrasia E31.9
|dysfunction E31.9
|syndrome E31.8
Polyhydramnios O40.-
Polymastia Q83.1

Polymenorrhea N92.0
Polymyalgia M35.3
 |arteritica, giant cell M31.5
 |rheumatica M35.3
  |with giant cell arteritis M31.5
Polymyositis (acute) (chronic) (hemorrhagic)
  M33.20
 |with
  |myopathy M33.22
  |respiratory involvement M33.21
  |skin involvement *see* Dermatopolymyositis
  |specified organ involvement NEC M33.29
 |ossificans (generalisata) (progressiva) *see*
  Myositis, ossificans, progressiva
Polyneuritis, polyneuritic *see also*
  Polyneuropathy
 |acute (post) infective G61.0
 |alcoholic G62.1
 |cranialis G52.7
 |demyelinating, chronic inflammatory (CIDP)
  G61.81
 |diabetic *see* Diabetes, polyneuropathy
 |diphtheritic A36.83
 |due to lack of vitamin NEC E56.9 [*G63*]
 |endemic E51.11
 |erythredema *see* subcategory T56.1
 |febrile, acute G61.0
 |hereditary ataxic G60.1
 |idiopathic, acute G61.0
 |infective (acute) G61.0
 |inflammatory, chronic demyelinating (CIDP)
  G61.81
 |nutritional E63.9 [*G63*]
 |postinfective (acute) G61.0
 |specified NEC G62.89
Polyneuropathy (peripheral) G62.9
 |alcoholic G62.1
 |amyloid (Portuguese) E85.1 [*G63*]
  |transthyretin-related (ATTR) familial E85.1
 |arsenical G62.2
 |critical illness G62.81
 |demyelinating, chronic inflammatory (CIDP)
  G61.81
 |diabetic *see* Diabetes, polyneuropathy
 |drug-induced G62.0
 |hereditary G60.9
  |specified NEC G60.8
 |idiopathic G60.9
  |progressive G60.3
 |in (due to)
  |alcohol G62.1
   |sequelae G65.2
  |amyloidosis, familial (Portuguese) E85.1
   [*G63*]
  |antitetanus serum G61.1
  |arsenic G62.2
   |sequelae G65.2
  |avitaminosis NEC E56.9 [*G63*]
  |beriberi E51.11
  |collagen vascular disease NEC M35.9
   [*G63*]
  |deficiency (of)
   |B (-complex) vitamins E53.9 [*G63*]
   |vitamin B6 E53.1 [*G63*]
  |diabetes *see* Diabetes, polyneuropathy
  |diphtheria A36.83
  |drug or medicament G62.0
   |correct substance properly administered
    see Table of Drugs and Chemicals, by
    drug, adverse effect
   |overdose or wrong substance given or
    taken *see* Table of Drugs and
    Chemicals, by drug, poisoning
  |endocrine disease NEC E34.9 [*G63*]

Polyneuropathy - *continued*
  |herpes zoster B02.23
  |hypoglycemia E16.2 [*G63*]
  |infectious
   |disease NEC B99 [*G63*]
   |mononucleosis B27.91
  |lack of vitamin NEC E56.9 [*G63*]
  |lead G62.2
   |sequelae G65.2
  |leprosy A30.9 [*G63*]
  |Lyme disease A69.22
  |metabolic disease NEC E88.9 [*G63*]
  |microscopic polyangiitis M31.7 [*G63*]
  |mumps B26.84
  |neoplastic disease *see also* Neoplasm D49.9
   [*G63*]
  |nutritional deficiency NEC E63.9 [*G63*]
  |organophosphate compounds G62.2
   |sequelae G65.2
  |parasitic disease NEC B89 [*G63*]
  |pellagra E52 [*G63*]
  |polyarteritis nodosa M30.0
  |porphyria E80.20 [*G63*]
  |radiation G62.82
  |rheumatoid arthritis *see* Rheumatoid,
   polyneuropathy
  |sarcoidosis D86.89
  |serum G61.1
  |syphilis (late) A52.15
   |congenital A50.43
  |systemic
   |connective tissue disorder M35.9 [*G63*]
   |lupus erythematosus M32.19
  |toxic agent NEC G62.2
   |sequelae G65.2
  |transthyretin-related (ATTR) familial
   amyloid E85.1
  |triorthocresyl phosphate G62.2
   |sequelae G65.2
  |tuberculosis A17.89
  |uremia N18.9 [*G63*]
  |vitamin B12 deficiency E53.8 [G63]
   |with anemia (pernicious) D51.0 [G63]
    |due to dietary deficiency D51.3 [G63]
  |zoster B02.23
 |inflammatory G61.9
  |chronic demyelinating (CIDP) G61.81
  |sequelae G65.1
  |specified NEC G61.89
 |lead G62.2
  |sequelae G65.2
 |nutritional NEC E63.9 [*G63*]
 |postherpetic (zoster) B02.23
 |progressive G60.3
 |radiation-induced G62.82
 |sensory (hereditary) (idiopathic) G60.8
 |specified NEC G62.89
 |syphilitic (late) A52.15
  |congenital A50.43
Polyopia H53.8
Polyorchism, polyorchidism Q55.21
Polyosteoarthritis *see also* Osteoarthritis,
  generalized M15.9-
 |post-traumatic M15.3
 |specified NEC M15.8
Polyostotic fibrous dysplasia Q78.1
Polyotia Q17.0
Polyp, polypus
  accessory sinus J33.8
 |adenocarcinoma in *see* Neoplasm, malignant,
  by site
 |adenocarcinoma in situ in *see* Neoplasm, in
  situ, by site
 |adenoid tissue J33.0

Polyp, polypus - *continued*
 |adenomatous *see also* Neoplasm, benign, by
  site
  |adenocarcinoma in *see* Neoplasm,
   malignant, by site
  |adenocarcinoma in situ in *see* Neoplasm, in
   situ, by site
  |carcinoma in *see* Neoplasm, malignant, by
   site
  |carcinoma in situ in *see* Neoplasm, in situ,
   by site
  |multiple *see* Neoplasm, benign
   |adenocarcinoma in *see* Neoplasm,
    malignant, by site
   |adenocarcinoma in situ in *see* Neoplasm,
   in situ, by site
 |antrum J33.8
 |anus, anal (canal) K62.0
 |Bartholin's gland N84.3
 |bladder D41.4
 |carcinoma in *see* Neoplasm, malignant, by site
 |carcinoma in situ in *see* Neoplasm, in situ, by
  site
 |cecum D12.0
 |cervix (uteri) N84.1
  |in pregnancy or childbirth *see* Pregnancy,
   complicated by, abnormal, cervix
  |mucous N84.1
  |nonneoplastic N84.1
 |choanal J33.0
 |cholesterol K82.4
 |clitoris N84.3
 |colon K63.5
  |adenomatous D12.6
  |sigmoid D12.5
  |transverse D12.3
 |ascending K63.5
 |cecum K63.5
 |descending K63.5
 |inflammatory K51.40
  |with
   |abscess K51.414
   |complication K51.419
    |specified NEC K51.418
   |fistula K51.413
   |intestinal obstruction K51.412
   |rectal bleeding K51.411
  |sigmoid D63.5
  |transverse D63.5
 |corpus uteri N84.0
 |dental K04.01
  |irreversible K04.02
  |reversible K04.01
 |duodenum K31.7
 |ear (middle) H74.4-
 |endometrium N84.0
 |esophageal K22.81
 |esophagogastric junction K22.82
 |ethmoidal (sinus) J33.8
 |fallopian tube N84.8
 |female genital tract N84.9
  |specified NEC N84.8
 |frontal (sinus) J33.8
 |gallbladder K82.4
 |gingiva, gum K06.8
 |labia, labium (majus) (minus) N84.3
 |larynx (mucous) J38.1
  |adenomatous D14.1
 |malignant *see* Neoplasm, malignant, by site
 |maxillary (sinus) J33.8
 |middle ear *see* Polyp, ear (middle)
 |myometrium N84.0
 |nares
  |anterior J33.9
  |posterior J33.0

Polyp, polypus - continued
  |nasal (mucous) J33.9
    |cavity J33.0
    |septum J33.0
  |nasopharyngeal J33.0
  |nose (mucous) J33.9
  |oviduct N84.8
  |pharynx J39.2
  |placenta O90.89
  |prostate see Enlargement, enlarged, prostate
  |pudenda, pudendum N84.3
  |pulpal (dental) K04.01
    |irreversible K04.02
    |reversible K04.01
  |rectum (nonadenomatous) K62.1
    |adenomatous see Polyp, adenomatous
  |septum (nasal) J33.0
  |sinus (accessory) (ethmoidal) (frontal)
    (maxillary) (sphenoidal) J33.8
  |sphenoidal (sinus) J33.8
  |stomach K31.7
    |adenomatous D13.1
  |tube, fallopian N84.8
  |turbinate, mucous membrane J33.8
  |umbilical, newborn P83.6
  |ureter N28.89
  |urethra N36.2
  |uterus (body) (corpus) (mucous) N84.0
    |cervix N84.1
    |in pregnancy or childbirth see Pregnancy,
      complicated by, tumor, uterus
  |vagina N84.2
  |vocal cord (mucous) J38.1
  |vulva N84.3
Polyphagia R63.2
Polyploidy Q92.7
Polypoid see condition
Polyposis see also Polyp
  |coli (adenomatous) D12.6
    |adenocarcinoma in C18.9
    |adenocarcinoma in situ in see Neoplasm, in
      situ, by site
    |carcinoma in C18.9
  |colon (adenomatous) D12.6
  |familial D12.6
    |adenocarcinoma in situ in see Neoplasm, in
      situ, by site
  |intestinal (adenomatous) D12.6
  |malignant lymphomatous C83.1-
  |multiple, adenomatous see also Neoplasm,
    benign D36.9
Polyradiculitis see Polyneuropathy
Polyradiculoneuropathy (acute)
  (postinfective) (segmentally demyelinating)
  G61.0
Polyserositis
  |due to pericarditis I31.1
  |pericardial I31.1
  |periodic, familial E85.0
  |tuberculous A19.9
    |acute A19.1
    |chronic A19.8
Polysplenia syndrome Q89.09
Polysyndactyly see also Syndactylism,
  syndactyly Q70.4
Polytrichia L68.3
Polyunguia Q84.6
Polyuria R35.89
  |nocturnal R35.81
  |psychogenic F45.8
- specified NEC R35.89
Pompe's disease (glycogen storage) E74.02
Pompholyx L30.1
Poncet's disease (tuberculous rheumatism)
  A18.09
Pond fracture see Fracture, skull
Ponos B55.0

Pons, pontine see condition **Poor**
  |aesthetic of existing restoration of tooth
    K08.56
  |contractions, labor O62.2
  |gingival margin to tooth restoration K08.51
  |personal hygiene R46.0
  |prenatal care, affecting management of
    pregnancy see Pregnancy, complicated by,
    insufficient, prenatal care
  |sucking reflex (newborn) R29.2
  |urinary stream R39.12
  |vision NEC H54.7
Poradenitis, nostras inguinalis or venerea A55
Porencephaly (congenital) (developmental)
  (true) Q04.6
  |acquired G93.0
  |nondevelopmental G93.0
  |traumatic (post) F07.89
Porocephaliasis B88.8
Porokeratosis Q82.8
Poroma, eccrine see Neoplasm, skin, benign
Porphyria (South African) E80.20
  |acquired E80.20
  |acute intermittent (hepatic) (Swedish) E80.21
  |cutanea tarda (hereditary) (symptomatic)
    E80.1
  |due to drugs E80.20
    |correct substance properly administered see
      Table of Drugs and Chemicals, by drug,
      adverse effect
    |overdose or wrong substance given or taken
      see Table of Drugs and Chemicals, by
      drug, poisoning
  |erythropoietic (congenital) (hereditary) E80.0
  |hepatocutaneous type E80.1
  |secondary E80.20
  |toxic NEC E80.20
  |variegata E80.20
Porphyrinuria see Porphyria
Porphyruria see Porphyria
Portal see condition
Port wine nevus, mark, or stain Q82.5
Posadas-Wernicke disease B38.9
Positive
  |culture (nonspecific)
    |blood R78.81
    |bronchial washings R84.5
    |cerebrospinal fluid R83.5
    |cervix uteri R87.5
    |nasal secretions R84.5
    |nipple discharge R89.5
    |nose R84.5
      |staphylococcus (Methicillin susceptible)
        Z22.321
      |Methicillin resistant Z22.322
    |peritoneal fluid R85.5
    |pleural fluid R84.5
    |prostatic secretions R86.5
    |saliva R85.5
    |seminal fluid R86.5
    |sputum R84.5
    |synovial fluid R89.5
    |throat scrapings R84.5
    |urine R82.79
    |vagina R87.5
    |vulva R87.5
    |wound secretions R89.5
  |PPD (skin test) R76.11
  |serology for syphilis A53.0
    |false R76.8
    |with signs or symptoms   code as Syphilis,
      by site and stage
  |skin test, tuberculin (without active
    tuberculosis) R76.11

Positive - continued
  |test, human immunodeficiency virus (HIV)
    R75
  |VDRL A53.0
    |with signs or symptoms   code by site and
      stage under Syphilis A53.9
  |Wassermann reaction A53.0
Post COVID-19 condition, unspecified U09.9
Postcardiotomy syndrome I97.0
Postcaval ureter Q62.62
Postcholecystectomy syndrome K91.5
Postclimacteric bleeding N95.0
Postcommissurotomy syndrome I97.0
Postconcussional syndrome F07.81
Postcontusional syndrome F07.81
Postcricoid region see condition
Post-Dates (40-42 weeks) (pregnancy)
  (mother) O48.0
  |more than 42 weeks gestation O48.1
Postencephalitic syndrome F07.89
Posterior see condition
Posterolateral sclerosis (spinal cord) see
  Degeneration, combined
Postexanthematous see condition
Postfebrile see condition
Postgastrectomy dumping syndrome K91.1
Posthemiplegic chorea see Monoplegia
Posthemorrhagic anemia (chronic) D50.0
  |acute D62
  |newborn P61.3
Postherpetic neuralgia (zoster) B02.29
  |trigeminal B02.22
Posthitis N47.7
Postimmunization complication or reaction
  see Complications, vaccination
Postinfectious see condition
Postlaminectomy syndrome NEC M96.1
Postleukotomy syndrome F07.0
Postmastectomy lymphedema (syndrome)
  I97.2
Postmaturity, postmature (over 42 weeks)
  |maternal (over 42weeks gestation) O48.1
  |newborn P08.22
Postmeasles complication NEC see also
  condition B05.89
Postmenopausal
  |endometrium (atrophic) N95.8
    |suppurative see also Endometritis N71.9
  |osteoporosis see Osteoporosis,
    postmenopausal
Postnasal drip R09.82
  |due to
    |allergic rhinitis see Rhinitis, allergic
    |common cold J00
    |gastroesophageal reflux see Reflux,
      gastroesophageal
    |nasopharyngitis see Nasopharyngitis
    |other know condition   code to condition
    |sinusitis see Sinusitis
Postnatal see condition
Postoperative (postprocedural) see
  Complication, postoperative
  |pneumothorax, therapeutic Z98.3
  |state NEC Z98.890
Postpancreatectomy hyperglycemia E89.1
Postpartum see Puerperal
Postphlebitic syndrome see Syndrome,
  postthrombotic
Postpoliomyelitic see also condition
  |osteopathy see Osteopathy, after poliomyelitis
Postpolio (myelitic) syndrome G14
Postprocedural see also Postoperative
  |hypoinsulinemia E89.1
Postschizophrenic depression F32.89

Postsurgery status *see also* Status (post)
  |pneumothorax, therapeutic Z98.3
Post-Term (40-42 weeks) (pregnancy)
  (mother) O48.0
  |infant P08.21
  |more than 42 weeks gestation (mother) O48.1
Post-Traumatic brain syndrome,
  nonpsychotic F07.81
Post-Typhoid abscess A01.09
Postures, hysterical F44.2
Postvaccinal reaction or complication *see*
  Complications, vaccination
Postvalvulotomy syndrome I97.0
Potain's
  |disease (pulmonary edema) *see* Edema, lung
  |syndrome (gastrectasis with dyspepsia) K31.0
Potter's
  |asthma J62.8
  |facies Q60.6
  |lung J62.8
  |syndrome (with renal agenesis) Q60.6
Pott's
  |curvature (spinal) A18.01
  |disease or paraplegia A18.01
  |spinal curvature A18.01
  |tumor, puffy *see* Osteomyelitis, specified type
    NEC
Pouch
  |bronchus Q32.4
  |Douglas' *see* condition
  |esophagus, esophageal, congenital Q39.6
    |acquired K22.5
  |gastric K31.4
  |Hartmann's K82.8
  |pharynx, pharyngeal (congenital) Q38.7
Pouchitis K91.850
Poultry men's itch B88.0
Poverty NEC Z59.6
  |extreme Z59.5
Poxvirus NEC B08.8
Prader-Willi syndrome Q87.1
Preauricular appendage or tag Q17.0
Prebetalipoproteinemia (acquired) (essential)
  (familial) (hereditary) (primary)
  (secondary) E78.1
  |with chylomicronemia E78.3
Precipitate labor or delivery O62.3
Preclimacteric bleeding (menorrhagia) N92.4
Precocious
  |adrenarche E30.1
  |menarche E30.1
  |menstruation E30.1
  |pubarche E30.1
  |puberty E30.1
    |central E22.8
  |sexual development NEC E30.1
  |thelarche E30.8
Precocity, sexual (constitutional)
  (cryptogenic) (female) (idiopathic) (male)
  E30.1
  |with adrenal hyperplasia E25.9
  |congenital E25.0
Precordial pain R07.2
Predeciduous teeth K00.2
Prediabetes, prediabetic R73.03
  |complicating
    |pregnancy *see* Pregnancy, complicated by,
      diseases of, specified type or system NEC
    |puerperium O99.893
Predislocation status of hip at birth Q65.6
Pre-Eclampsia O14.9-
  |with pre-existing hypertension *see*
    Hypertension, complicating pregnancy,
    pre-existing, with, pre-eclampsia
  |complicating

Pre-Eclampsia *- continued*
    |childbirth O14.94
    |puerperium O14.95
  |mild O14.0-
    |complicating
      |childbirth O14.04
      |puerperium O14.05
  |moderate O14.0-
    |complicating
      |childbirth O14.04
      |puerperium O14.05
  |severe O14.1-
    |with hemolysis, elevated liver enzymes and
    low platelet count (HELLP) O14.2-
      |complicating
        |childbirth O14.24
        |puerperium O14.25
    |complicating
      |childbirth O14.14
      |puerperium O14.15
Pre-Eruptive color change, teeth, tooth K00.8
Pre-Excitation atrioventricular conduction
  I45.6
Preglaucoma H40.00-
Pregnancy (single) (uterine) *see also* Delivery
  and Puerperal
  |Note: The Tabular must be reviewed for
    assignment of the appropriate character
    indicating the trimester of the pregnancy
  |Note: The Tabular must be reviewed for
    assignment of appropriate seventh
    character for multiple gestation codes in
    Chapter 15
  |abdominal (ectopic) O00.00
    |with intrauterine pregnancy O00.01
    |with viable fetus O36.7-
  |ampullar O00.10-
    |with intrauterine pregnancy O00.11-
  |biochemical O02.81
  |broad ligament O00.80
    |with intrauterine pregnancy O00.81
  |cervical O00.80
    |with intrauterine pregnancy O00.81
  |chemical O02.81
  |complicated NOS O26.9-
  |complicated by (care of) (management
    affected by)
    |abnormal, abnormality
      |cervix O34.4-
        |causing obstructed labor O65.5
      |cord (umbilical) O69.9
      |fetal heart rate or rhythm O36.83-
      |findings on antenatal screening of mother
        O28.9
        |biochemical O28.1
        |cytological O28.2
        |chromosomal O28.5
        |genetic O28.5
        |hematological O28.0
        |radiological O28.4
        |specified NEC O28.8
        |ultrasonic O28.3
      |glucose (tolerance) NEC O99.810
      |pelvic organs O34.9-
        |specified NEC O34.8-
          |causing obstructed labor O65.5
      |pelvis (bony) (major) NEC O33.0
      |perineum O34.7-
      |position
        |placenta O44.0-
          |with hemorrhage O44.1-
        |uterus O34.59-
      |uterus O34.59-
        |causing obstructed labor O65.5
        |congenital O34.0-

Pregnancy *- continued*
    |vagina O34.6-
      |causing obstructed labor O65.5
    |vulva O34.7-
      |causing obstructed labor O65.5
  |abruptio placentae *see* Abruptio placentae
  |abscess or cellulitis
    |bladder O23.1-
    |breast O91.11-
    |genital organ or tract O23.9-
  |abuse
    |physical O9A.31-
    |psychological O9A.51-
    |sexual O9A.41-
  |adverse effect anesthesia O29.9-
    |aspiration pneumonitis O29.01-
    |cardiac arrest O29.11-
    |cardiac complication NEC O29.19-
    |cardiac failure O29.12-
    |central nervous system complication NEC
      O29.29-
    |cerebral anoxia O29.21-
    |failed or difficult intubation O29.6-
    |inhalation of stomach contents or
      secretions NOS O29.01-
    |local, toxic reaction O29.3X
    |Mendelson's syndrome O29.01-
    |pressure collapse of lung O29.02-
    |pulmonary complications NEC O29.09-
    |specified NEC O29.8X-
    |spinal and epidural type NEC O29.5X
      |induced headache O29.4-
  |albuminuria *see also* Proteinuria, gestational
    O12.1-
  |alcohol use O99.31-
  |amnionitis O41.12
  |anaphylactoid syndrome of pregnancy
    O88.01-
  |anemia (conditions in D50-D64) (pre-
    existing) O99.01-
    |complicating the puerperium O99.03
  |antepartum hemorrhage O46.9-
    |with coagulation defect *see* Hemorrhage,
      antepartum, with coagulation defect
    |specified NEC O46.8X-
  |appendicitis O99.61-
  |atrophy (yellow) (acute) liver (subacute)
    O26.61-
  |bariatric surgery status O99.84-
  |bicornis or bicornuate uterus O34.0-
  |biliary tract problems O26.61-
  |breech presentation O32.1
  |cardiovascular diseases (conditions in I00-
    I09, I20-I52, I70-I99) O99.41-
  |cerebrovascular disorders (conditions in
    I60-I69) O99.41-
  |cervical shortening O26.87-
  |cervicitis O23.51-
  |cesarean scar defect (isthmocele) O34.22
  |chloasma (gravidarum) O26.89-
  |cholestasis (intrahepatic) O26.61-
  |cholecystitis O99.61-
  |chorioamnionitis O41.12-
  |circulatory system disorder (conditions in
    I00-I09, I20-I99, O99.41)
  |compound presentation O32.6
  |conjoined twins O30.02-
  |connective system disorders (conditions in
    M00-M99) O99.891
  |contracted pelvis (general) O33.1
    |inlet O33.2
    |outlet O33.3
  |convulsions (eclamptic) (uremic) *see also*
    Eclampsia O15.9-
  |cracked nipple O92.11-

Pregnancy - *continued*
|cystitis O23.1-
|cystocele O34.8-
|death of fetus (near term) O36.4
  |early pregnancy O02.1
  |of one fetus or more in multiple gestation
    O31.2-
|deciduitis O41.14-
|decreased fetal movement O36.81-
|dental problems O99.61-
|diabetes (mellitus) O24.91-
  |gestational (pregnancy induced) *see*
    Diabetes, gestational
  |pre-existing O24.31-
    |specified NEC O24.81-
    |type 1 O24.01-
    |type 2 O24.11-
|digestive system disorders (conditions in
    K00-K93) O99.61-
|diseases of *see* Pregnancy, complicated by,
    specified body system disease
  |biliary tract O26.61-
  |blood NEC (conditions in D65-D77)
    O99.11-
  |liver O26.61-
  |specified NEC O99.891
|disorders of *see* Pregnancy, complicated by,
    specified body system disorder
  |amniotic fluid and membranes O41.9-
    |specified NEC O41.8X-
  |biliary tract O26.61-
  |ear and mastoid process (conditions in
    H60-H95) O99.891
  |eye and adnexa (conditions in H00-H59)
    O99.891
  |liver O26.61-
  |skin (conditions in L00-L99) O99.71-
  |specified NEC O99.891
|displacement, uterus NEC O34.59-
  |causing obstructed labor O65.5
|disproportion (due to) O33.9
  |fetal (ascites) (hydrops)
      (meningomyelocele) (sacral teratoma)
      (tumor) deformities NEC O33.7
  |generally contracted pelvis O33.1
  |hydrocephalic fetus O33.6
  |inlet contraction of pelvis O33.2
  |mixed maternal and fetal origin O33.4
  |specified NEC O33.8
|double uterus O34.0-
  |causing obstructed labor O65.5
|drug use (conditions in F11-F19) O99.32-
|eclampsia, eclamptic (coma) (convulsions)
    (delirium) (nephritis) (uremia) *see also*
    Eclampsia O15.-
|ectopic pregnancy *see* Pregnancy, ectopic
|edema O12.0-
  |with
    |gestational hypertension, mild *see also*
      Pre-eclampsia O14.0-
    |proteinuria O12.2-
|effusion, amniotic fluid *see* Pregnancy,
    complicated by, premature rupture of
    membranes
|elderly
  |multigravida O09.52-
  |primigravida O09.51-
|embolism *see also* Embolism, obstetric,
    pregnancy O88.-
|endocrine diseases NEC O99.28-
|endometritis O86.12
|excessive weight gain O26.0-
|exhaustion O26.81-
  |during labor and delivery O75.81
|face presentation O32.3

Pregnancy - *continued*
|failed induction of labor O61.9
  |instrumental O61.1
  |mechanical O61.1
  |medical O61.0
  |specified NEC O61.8
  |surgical O61.1
|failed or difficult intubation for anesthesia
    O29.6-
|false labor (pains) O47.9
  |at or after 37 completed weeks of
    pregnancy O47.1
  |before 37 completed weeks of pregnancy
    O47.0-
|fatigue O26.81-
  |during labor and delivery O75.81
|fatty metamorphosis of liver O26.61-
|female genital mutilation O34.8 *[N90.81]*
|fetal (maternal care for)
  |abnormality or damage O35.9
    |acid-base balance O68
    |specified type NEC O35.8
  |acidemia O68
  |acidosis O68
  |alkalosis O68
  |anemia and thrombocytopenia O36.82-
  |anencephaly O35.0
  |chromosomal abnormality (conditions in
    Q90-Q99) O35.1
  |conjoined twins O30.02-
  |damage from
    |amniocentesis O35.7
    |biopsy procedures O35.7
    |drug addiction O35.5
    |hematological investigation O35.7
    |intrauterine contraceptive device O35.7
    |maternal
      |alcohol addiction O35.4
      |cytomegalovirus infection O35.3
      |disease NEC O35.8
      |drug addiction O35.5
      |listeriosis O35.8
      |rubella O35.3
      |toxoplasmosis O35.8
      |viral infection O35.3
    |medical procedure NEC O35.7
    |radiation O35.6
  |death (near term) O36.4
    |early pregnancy O02.1
  |decreased movement O36.81-
  |disproportion due to deformity (fetal)
    O33.7
  |excessive growth (large for dates) O36.6-
  |growth retardation O36.59-
    |light for dates O36.59-
    |small for dates O36.59-
  |heart rate irregularity (bradycardia)
    (decelerations) (tachycardia) O76
  |hereditary disease O35.2
  |hydrocephalus O35.0
  |intrauterine death O36.4
  |poor growth O36.59-
    |light for dates O36.59-
    |small for dates O36.59-
  |problem O36.9-
    |specified NEC O36.89-
  |reduction (elective) O31.3-
  |selective termination O31.3-
  |spina bifida O35.0
  |thrombocytopenia O36.82-
|fibroid (tumor) (uterus) O34.1-
|fissure of nipple O92.11-
|gallstones O99.61-
|gastric banding status O99.84-
|gastric bypass status O99.84-

Pregnancy - *continued*
|genital herpes (asymptomatic) (history of)
    (inactive) O98.3-
|genital tract infection O23.9-
|glomerular diseases (conditions in N00-
    N07) O26.83-
  |with hypertension, pre-existing *see*
    Hypertension, complicating,
    pregnancy, pre-existing, with, renal
    disease
|gonorrhea O98.21-
|grand multiparity O09.4
|habitual aborter *see* Pregnancy, complicated
    by, recurrent pregnancy loss
|HELLP syndrome (hemolysis, elevated liver
    enzymes and low platelet count) O14.2-
|hemorrhage
  |antepartum *see* Hemorrhage, antepartum
  |before 20 completed weeks gestation
    O20.9
    |specified NEC O20.8
  |due to premature separation, placenta *see
    also* Abruptio placentae O45.9-
  |early O20.9
    |specified NEC O20.8
  |threatened abortion O20.0
|hemorrhoids O22.4-
|hepatitis (viral) O98.41-
|herniation of uterus O34.59-
|high
  |head at term O32.4
  |risk *see* Supervision (of) (for), high-risk
|history of in utero procedure during
    previous pregnancy O09.82-
|HIV O98.71-
|human immunodeficiency virus (HIV)
    disease O98.71-
|hydatidiform mole *see also* Mole,
    hydatidiform O01.9-
|hydramnios O40.-
|hydrocephalic fetus (disproportion) O33.6
|hydrops
  |amnii O40.-
  |fetalis O36.2-
    |associated with isoimmunization *see
      also* Pregnancy, complicated by,
      isoimmunization O36.11-
|hydrorrhea O42.90
|hyperemesis (gravidarum) (mild) *see also*
    Hyperemesis, gravidarum O21.0-
|hypertension *see* Hypertension,
complicating pregnancy
|hypertensive
  |heart and renal disease, pre-existing *see*
    Hypertension, complicating,
    pregnancy, pre-existing, with, heart
    disease, with renal disease
  |heart disease, pre-existing *see*
    Hypertension, complicating,
    pregnancy, pre-existing, with, heart
    disease
  |renal disease, pre-existing *see*
    Hypertension, complicating,
    pregnancy, pre-existing, with, renal
    disease
|hypotension O26.5-
|immune disorders NEC (conditions in D80-
    D89) O99.11-
|incarceration, uterus O34.51-
|incompetent cervix O34.3-
|inconclusive fetal viability O36.80
|infection(s) O98.91-
  |amniotic fluid or sac O41.10-
  |bladder O23.1-
  |carrier state NEC O99.830

Pregnancy - *continued*
- |streptococcus B O99.820
- |genital organ or tract O23.9-
  - |specified NEC O23.59-
- |genitourinary tract O23.9-
- |gonorrhea O98.21-
- |hepatitis (viral) O98.41-
- |HIV O98.71-
- |human immunodeficiency virus (HIV) O98.71-
- |intrauterine O41.12
- |kidney O23.0-
- |nipple O91.01-
- |parasitic disease O98.91-
  - |specified NEC O98.81-
- |protozoal disease O98.61-
- |sexually transmitted NEC O98.31-
- |specified type NEC O98.81-
- |syphilis O98.11-
- |tuberculosis O98.01-
- |urethra O23.2-
- |urinary (tract) O23.4-
  - |specified NEC O23.3-
- |viral disease O98.51-
- - - inflammation
- - - - intrauterine O41.12
- |injury or poisoning (conditions in S00-T88) O9A.21-
  - |due to abuse
    - |physical O9A.31-
    - |psychological O9A.51-
    - |sexual O9A.41-
- |insufficient
  - |prenatal care O09.3-
  - |weight gain O26.1-
- |insulin resistance O26.89
- |intrauterine fetal death (near term) O36.4
  - |early pregnancy O02.1
  - |multiple gestation (one fetus or more) O31.2-
- |isoimmunization O36.11-
  - |anti-A sensitization O36.11-
  - |anti-B sensitization O36.19-
  - |Rh O36.09-
    - |anti-D antibody O36.01-
  - |specified NEC O36.19-
- |laceration of uterus NEC O71.81
- |malformation
  - |placenta, placental (vessel) O43.10-
    - |specified NEC O43.19-
  - |uterus (congenital) O34.0-
- |malnutrition (conditions in E40-E46) O25.1-
- |maternal hypotension syndrome O26.5-
- |mental disorders (conditions in F01-F09, F20-F52 and F54-F99) O99.34
  - |alcohol use O99.31-
  - |drug use O99.32-
  - |smoking O99.33-
- |mentum presentation O32.3
- |metabolic disorders O99.28-
- |missed
  - |abortion O02.1
  - |delivery O36.4
- |multiple gestations O30.9-
  - |conjoined twins O30.02-
  - |specified number of multiples NEC *see* Pregnancy, multiple (gestation), specified NEC
  - |quadruplet *see* Pregnancy, quadruplet
  - |specified complication NEC O31.8X-
  - |triplet *see* Pregnancy, triplet
  - |twin *see* Pregnancy, twin
- |musculoskeletal condition (conditions is M00-M99) O99.891
- |necrosis, liver (conditions in K72) O26.61-
- |neoplasm

Pregnancy - *continued*
- |benign
  - |cervix O34.4-
  - |corpus uteri O34.1-
  - |uterus O34.1-
- |malignant O9A.11-
- |nephropathy NEC O26.83-
- |nervous system condition (conditions in G00-G99) O99.35-
- |nutritional diseases NEC O99.28-
- |obesity (pre-existing) O99.21-
- |obesity surgery status O99.84-
- |oblique lie or presentation O32.2
- |older mother *see* Pregnancy, complicated by, elderly
- |oligohydramnios O41.0-
  - |with premature rupture of membranes *see also* Pregnancy, complicated by, premature rupture of membranes O42.-
- |onset (spontaneous) of labor after 37 completed weeks of gestation but before 39 completed weeks gestation, with delivery by (planned) cesarean section O75.82
- |oophoritis O23.52-
- |overdose, drug *see also* Table of Drugs and Chemicals, by drug, poisoning O9A.21-
- |oversize fetus O33.5
- |papyraceous fetus O31.0-
- |pelvic inflammatory disease O99.891
- |periodontal disease O99.61-
- |peripheral neuritis O26.82-
- |peritoneal (pelvic) adhesions O99.891
- |phlebitis O22.9-
- |phlebopathy O22.9-
- |phlebothrombosis (superficial) O22.2-
  - |deep O22.3-
- |placenta accreta O43.21-
- |placenta increta O43.22-
- |placenta percreta O43.23-
- |placenta previa O44.0-
  - |complete O44.0-
    - |with hemorrhage O44.1-
  - |marginal O44.2-
    - |with hemorrhage O44.3-
  - |partial O44.2-
    - |with hemorrhage O44.3-
- |placental disorder O43.9-
  - |specified NEC O43.89-
- |placental dysfunction O43.89-
- |placental infarction O43.81-
- |placental insufficiency O36.51-
- |placental transfusion syndromes
  - |fetomaternal O43.01-
  - |fetus to fetus O43.02-
  - |maternofetal O43.01-
- |placentitis O41.14-
- |pneumonia O99.51-
- |poisoning *see also* Table of Drugs and Chemicals O9A.21-
- |polyhydramnios O40-
- |polymorphic eruption of pregnancy O26.86
- |poor obstetric history NEC O09.29-
- |postmaturity (post-term) (40 to 42 weeks) O48.0
  - |more than 42 completed weeks gestation (prolonged) O48.1
- |pre-eclampsia O14.9-
  - |mild O14.0-
  - |moderate O14.0-
  - |severe O14.1-
    - |with hemolysis, elevated liver enzymes and low platelet count (HELLP) O14.2-

Pregnancy - *continued*
- |premature labor *see* Pregnancy, complicated by, preterm labor
- |premature rupture of membranes O42.90
  - |full-term, unspecified as to length of time between rupture and onset of labor O42.92
  - |with onset of labor
    - |within 24 hours O42.00
      - |at or after 37 weeks gestation, onset of labor within 24 hours of rupture O42.02
      - |pre-term (before 37 completed weeks of gestation) O42.01
    - |after 24 hours O42.10
      - |at or after 37 weeks gestation, onset of labor more than 24 hours following rupture O42.12
      - |pre-term (before 37 completed weeks of gestation) O42.11-
    - |at or after 37 weeks gestation, unspecified as to length of time between rupture and onset of labor O42.92
  - |pre-term (before 37 completed weeks of gestation) O42.91-
- |premature separation of placenta *see also* Abruptio placentae O45.9-
- |presentation, fetal *see* Delivery, complicated by, malposition
- |preterm delivery O60.10
- |preterm labor
  - |with delivery O60.10
    - |preterm O60.10
    - |term O60.20
  - |second trimester
    - |with term delivery O60.22
    - |without delivery O60.02
    - |with preterm delivery
      - |second trimester O60.12
      - |third trimester O60.13
  - |third trimester
    - |with term delivery O60.23
    - |without delivery O60.03
    - |with third trimester preterm delivery O60.14
  - |without delivery O60.00
    - |second trimester O60.02
    - |third trimester O60.03
- |previous history of *see* Pregnancy, supervision of, high-risk
- |prolapse, uterus O34.52-
- |proteinuria (gestational) *see also* Proteinuria, gestational O12.1-
  - |with edema O12.2-
- |pruritic urticarial papules and plaques of pregnancy (PUPPP) O26.86
- |pruritus (neurogenic) O26.89-
- |psychosis or psychoneurosis (puerperal) F53.1
- |ptyalism O26.89-
- |PUPPP (pruritic urticarial papules and plaques of pregnancy) O26.86
- |pyelitis O23.0-
- |recurrent pregnancy loss O26.2-
- |renal disease or failure NEC O26.83-
  - |with secondary hypertension, pre-existing *see* Hypertension, complicating, pregnancy, pre-existing, secondary
  - |hypertensive, pre-existing *see* Hypertension, complicating, pregnancy, pre-existing, with, renal disease
- |respiratory condition (conditions in J00-J99) O99.51-
- |retained, retention

Pregnancy - *continued*

|dead ovum O02.0
|intrauterine contraceptive device O26.3-
|retroversion, uterus O34.53-
|Rh immunization, incompatibility or sensitization NEC O36.09-
|anti-D antibody O36.01-
|rupture
|amnion (premature) *see also* Pregnancy, complicated by, premature rupture of membranes O42-
|membranes (premature) *see also* Pregnancy, complicated by, premature rupture of membranes O42-
|uterus (during labor) O71.1
|before onset of labor O71.0-
|salivation (excessive) O26.89-
|salpingitis O23.52-
|salpingo-oophoritis O23.52-
|sepsis (conditions in A40, A41) O98.81-
|size date discrepancy (uterine) O26.84-
|skin condition (conditions in L00-L99) O99.71-
|smoking (tobacco) O99.33-
|social problem O09.7-
|specified condition NEC O26.89-
|spotting O26.85-
|streptococcus group B (GBS) carrier state O99.820
|subluxation of symphysis (pubis) O26.71-
|syphilis (conditions in A50-A53) O98.11-
|threatened
|abortion O20.0
|labor O47.9
|at or after 37 completed weeks of gestation O47.1
|before 37 completed weeks of gestation O47.0-
|thrombophlebitis (superficial) O22.2-
|thrombosis O22.9-
|cerebral venous O22.5-
|cerebrovenous sinus O22.5-
|deep O22.3-
|tobacco use disorder (smoking) O99.33-
|torsion of uterus O34.59-
|toxemia O14.9-
|transverse lie or presentation O32.2
|tuberculosis (conditions in A15-A19) O98.01-
|tumor (benign)
|cervix O34.4-
|malignant O9A.11-
|uterus O34.1-
|unstable lie O32.0
|upper respiratory infection O99.51-
|urethritis O23.2-
|uterine size date discrepancy O26.84-
|vaginitis or vulvitis O23.59-
|varicose veins (lower extremities) O22.0-
|genitals O22.1-
|legs O22.0-
|perineal O22.1-
|vaginal or vulval O22.1-
|venereal disease NEC (conditions in A63.8) O98.31-
|venous disorders O22.9-
|specified NEC O22.8X-
|viral diseases (conditions in A80-B09, B25-B34) O98.51-
|very young mother *see* Pregnancy, complicated by, young mother
|vomiting O21.9
|due to diseases classified elsewhere O21.8
|hyperemesis gravidarum (mild) *see also* Hyperemesis, gravidarum O21.0-

Pregnancy - *continued*

|late (occurring after 20 weeks of gestation) O21.2
|young mother
|multigravida O09.62-
|primigravida O09.61-
|concealed O09.3-
|continuing following
|elective fetal reduction of one or more fetus O31.3-
|intrauterine death of one or more fetus O31.2-
|spontaneous abortion of one or more fetus O31.1-
|cornual O00.80
|with intrauterine pregnancy O00.81
|ectopic (ruptured) O00.90
|with intrauterine pregnancy O00.91
|abdominal O00.00
|with
|intrauterine pregnancy O00.01
|viable fetus O36.7-
|cervical O00.80
|with intrauterine pregnancy O00.81
|complicated (by) O08.9
|afibrinogenemia O08.1
|cardiac arrest O08.81
|chemical damage of pelvic organ(s) O08.6
|circulatory collapse O08.3
|defibrination syndrome O08.1
|electrolyte imbalance O08.5
|embolism (amniotic fluid) (blood clot) (pulmonary) (septic) O08.2
|endometritis O08.0
|genital tract and pelvic infection O08.0
|hemorrhage (delayed) (excessive) O08.1
|infection
|genital tract or pelvic O08.0
|kidney O08.83
|urinary tract O08.83
|intravascular coagulation O08.1
|laceration of pelvic organ(s) O08.6
|metabolic disorder O08.5
|oliguria O08.4
|oophoritis O08.0
|parametritis O08.0
|pelvic peritonitis O08.0
|perforation of pelvic organ(s) O08.6
|renal failure or shutdown O08.4
|salpingitis or salpingo-oophoritis O08.0
|sepsis O08.82
|shock O08.83
|septic O08.82
|specified condition NEC O08.89
|tubular necrosis (renal) O08.4
|uremia O08.4
|urinary infection O08.83
|venous complication NEC O08.7
|embolism O08.2
|cornual O00.80
|with intrauterine pregnancy O00.81
|intraligamentous O00.80
|with intrauterine pregnancy O00.81
|mural O00.80
|with intrauterine pregnancy O00.81
|ovarian O00.20-
|with intrauterine pregnancy O00.21-
|specified site NEC O00.80
|with intrauterine pregnancy O00.81
|tubal (ruptured) O00.10-
|with intrauterine pregnancy O00.11-
|examination (normal) Z34.9-
|high-risk *see* Pregnancy, supervision of, high-risk
|first Z34.0-

Pregnancy - *continued*

|specified Z34.8-
|extrauterine *see* Pregnancy, ectopic
|fallopian O00.10-
|with intrauterine pregnancy O00.11-
|false F45.8
|gestational carrier Z33.3
|heptachorionic, hepta-amniotic (septuplets) O30.83-
|hexachorionic, hexa-amniotic (sextuplets) O30.83-
|hidden O09.3-
|high-risk *see* Pregnancy, supervision of, high-risk
|incidental finding Z33.1
|interstitial O00.80
|with intrauterine pregnancy O00.81
|intraligamentous O00.80
|with intrauterine pregnancy O00.81
|intramural O00.80
|with intrauterine pregnancy O00.81
|intraperitoneal O00.00
|with intrauterine pregnancy O00.01
|isthmian O00.10-
|with intrauterine pregnancy O00.11-
|mesometric (mural) O00.80
|with intrauterine pregnancy O00.81
|molar NEC O02.0
|complicated (by) O08.9
|afibrinogenemia O08.1
|cardiac arrest O08.81
|chemical damage of pelvic organ(s) O08.6
|circulatory collapse O08.3
|defibrination syndrome O08.1
|electrolyte imbalance O08.5
|embolism (amniotic fluid) (blood clot) (pulmonary) (septic) O08.2
|endometritis O08.0
|genital tract and pelvic infection O08.0
|hemorrhage (delayed) (excessive) O08.1
|infection
|genital tract or pelvic O08.0
|kidney O08.83
|urinary tract O08.83
|intravascular coagulation O08.1
|laceration of pelvic organ(s) O08.6
|metabolic disorder O08.5
|oliguria O08.4
|oophoritis O08.0
|parametritis O08.0
|pelvic peritonitis O08.0
|perforation of pelvic organ(s) O08.6
|renal failure or shutdown O08.4
|salpingitis or salpingo-oophoritis O08.0
|sepsis O08.82
|shock O08.3
|septic O08.82
|specified condition NEC O08.89
|tubular necrosis (renal) O08.4
|uremia O08.4
|urinary infection O08.83
|venous complication NEC O08.7
|embolism O08.2
|hydatidiform *see also* Mole, hydatidiform O01.9-
|multiple (gestation) O30.9-
|greater than quadruplets *see* Pregnancy, multiple (gestation), specified NEC
|specified NEC O30.80-
|number of chorions and amnions are both equal to the number of fetuses O30.83-
|with
|two or more monoamniotic fetuses O30.82-

Pregnancy - *continued*

- two or more monochorionic fetuses O30.81-
- two or more monoamniotic fetuses O30.82-
- two or more monochorionic fetuses O30.81-
- unable to determine number of placenta and number of amniotic sacs O30.89-
- unspecified number of placenta and unspecified number of amniotic sacs O30.80-
- mural O00.80
  - with intrauterine pregnancy O00.81
- normal (supervision of) Z34.9-
  - high-risk *see* Pregnancy, supervision of, high-risk
  - first Z34.0-
  - specified Z34.8-
- ovarian O00.20-
  - with intrauterine pregnancy O00.21-
- pentachorionic, penta-amniotic (quintuplets) O30.83-
- postmature (40 to 42 weeks) O48.0
  - more than 42 weeks gestation O48.1
- post-term (40 to 42 weeks) O48.0
- prenatal care only Z34.9-
  - high-risk *see* Pregnancy, supervision of, high-risk
  - first Z34.0-
  - specified Z34.8-
- prolonged (more than 42 weeks gestation) O48.1
- quadruplet O30.20-
  - quadrachorionic/quadra-amniotic O30.23-
  - with
    - two or more monoamniotic fetuses O30.22-
    - two or more monochorionic fetuses O30.21-
  - two or more monoamniotic fetuses O30.22-
  - two or more monochorionic fetuses O30.21-
  - unable to determine number of placenta and number of amniotic sacs O30.29-
  - unspecified number of placenta and unspecified number of amniotic sacs O30.20-
- quintuplet *see* Pregnancy, multiple (gestation), specified NEC
- sextuplet *see* Pregnancy, multiple (gestation), specified NEC
- supervision of
  - concealed pregnancy O09.3-
  - elderly mother
    - multigravida O09.52-
    - primigravida O09.51-
  - hidden pregnancy O09.3-
  - high-risk O09.9-
    - due to (history of)
      - ectopic pregnancy O09.1-
      - elderly *see* Pregnancy, supervision, elderly mother
      - grand multiparity O09.4
      - infertility O09.0-
      - insufficient prenatal care O09.3-
      - in utero procedure during previous pregnancy O09.82-
      - in vitro fertilization O09.81-
      - molar pregnancy O09.A-
      - multiple previous pregnancies O09.4-
      - older mother *see* Pregnancy, supervision of, elderly mother
      - poor reproductive or obstetric history NEC O09.29-
      - pre-term labor O09.21-

Pregnancy - *continued*

- previous
  - neonatal death O09.29-
  - social problems O09.7-
  - specified NEC O09.89-
  - very young mother *see* Pregnancy, supervision, young mother
- resulting from in vitro fertilization O09.81-
- normal Z34.9-
  - first Z34.0-
  - specified NEC Z34.8-
- young mother
  - multigravida O09.62-
  - primigravida O09.61-
- triplet O30.10-
  - trichorionic/triamniotic O30.13-
  - with
    - two or more monoamniotic fetuses O30.12-
    - two or more monochorionic fetuses O30.11-
  - two or more monoamniotic fetuses O30.12-
  - two or more monochorionic fetuses O30.11-
  - unable to determine number of placenta and number of amniotic sacs O30.19-
  - unspecified number of placenta and unspecified number of amniotic sacs O30.10-
- tubal (with abortion) (with rupture) O00.10-
  - with intrauterine pregnancy O00.11-
- twin O30.00-
  - conjoined O30.02-
  - dichorionic/diamniotic (two placenta, two amniotic sacs) O30.04-
  - monochorionic/diamniotic (one placenta, two amniotic sacs) O30.03-
  - monochorionic/monoamniotic (one placenta, one amniotic sac) O30.01-
  - unable to determine number of placenta and number of amniotic sacs O30.09-
  - unspecified number of placenta and unspecified number of amniotic sacs O30.00-
- unwanted Z64.0
- weeks of gestation
  - 8 weeks Z3A.08
  - 9 weeks Z3A.09
  - 10 weeks Z3A.10
  - 11 weeks Z3A.11
  - 12 weeks Z3A.12
  - 13 weeks Z3A.13
  - 14 weeks Z3A.14
  - 15 weeks Z3A.15
  - 16 weeks Z3A.16
  - 17 weeks Z3A.17
  - 18 weeks Z3A.18
  - 19 weeks Z3A.19
  - 20 weeks Z3A.20
  - 21 weeks Z3A.21
  - 22 weeks Z3A.22
  - 23 weeks Z3A.23
  - 24 weeks Z3A.24
  - 25 weeks Z3A.25
  - 26 weeks Z3A.26
  - 27 weeks Z3A.27
  - 28 weeks Z3A.28
  - 29 weeks Z3A.29
  - 30 weeks Z3A.30
  - 31 weeks Z3A.31
  - 32 weeks Z3A.32
  - 33 weeks Z3A.33
  - 34 weeks Z3A.34
  - 35 weeks Z3A.35

Pregnancy - *continued*

- 36 weeks Z3A.36
- 37 weeks Z3A.37
- 38 weeks Z3A.38
- 39 weeks Z3A.39
- 40 weeks Z3A.40
- 41 weeks Z3A.41
- 42 weeks Z3A.42
- greater than 42 weeks Z3A.49
- less than 8 weeks Z3A.01
- not specified Z3A.00

Preiser's disease *see* Osteonecrosis, secondary, due to, trauma, metacarpus

Pre-Kwashiorkor *see* Malnutrition, severe

Preleukemia (syndrome) D46.9

Preluxation, hip, congenital Q65.6

Premature *see also* condition
- adrenarche E27.0
- aging E34.8
- beats I49.40
  - atrial I49.1
  - auricular I49.1
  - supraventricular I49.1
- birth NEC *see* Preterm, newborn
- closure, foramen ovale Q21.8
- contraction
  - atrial I49.1
  - atrioventricular I49.2
  - auricular I49.1
  - auriculoventricular I49.49
  - heart (extrasystole) I49.49
  - junctional I49.2
  - ventricular I49.3
- delivery *see also* Pregnancy, complicated by, preterm labor O60.10
- ejaculation F52.4
- infant NEC *see* Preterm, newborn
  - light-for-dates *see* Light for dates
- labor *see* Pregnancy, complicated by, preterm labor
- lungs P28.0
- menopause E28.319
  - asymptomatic E28.319
  - symptomatic E28.310
- newborn
  - extreme (less than 28 completed weeks) *see* Immaturity, extreme
  - less than 37 completed weeks *see* Preterm, newborn
- puberty E30.1
- rupture membranes or amnion *see* Pregnancy, complicated by, premature rupture of membranes
- senility E34.8
- thelarche E30.8
- ventricular systole I49.3

Prematurity NEC (less than 37 completed weeks) *see* Preterm, newborn
- extreme (less than 28 completed weeks) *see* Immaturity, extreme

Premenstrual
- dysphoric disorder (PMDD) F32.81
- tension (syndrome) N94.3

Premolarization, cuspids K00.2

Prenatal
- care, normal pregnancy *see* Pregnancy, normal
- screening of mother (*see also* Encounter, antenatal screening) Z36.9
- teeth K00.6

Preparatory care for subsequent treatment NEC
- for dialysis Z49.01
  - peritoneal Z49.02

Prepartum *see* condition

Preponderance, left or right ventricular I51.7

Prepuce *see* condition
PRES (posterior reversible encephalopathy syndrome) I67.83
Presbycardia R54
Presbycusis, presbyacusia H91.1-
Presbyesophagus K22.89
Presbyophrenia F03
Presbyopia H52.4
Prescription of contraceptives (initial) Z30.019
|barrier Z30.018
|diaphragm Z30.018
|emergency (postcoital) Z30.012
|implantable subdermal Z30.017
|injectable Z30.013
|intrauterine contraceptive device Z30.014
|pills Z30.011
|postcoital (emergency) Z30.012
|repeat Z30.40
    |barrier Z30.49
    |diaphragm Z30.49
    |implantable subdermal Z30.46
    |injectable Z30.42
    |pills Z30.41
    |specified type NEC Z30.49
    |transdermal patch hormonal Z30.45
    |vaginal ring hormonal Z30.44
|specified type NEC Z30.018
    |transdermal patch hormonal Z30.016
    |vaginal ring hormonal Z30.015
Presence (of)
|ankle-joint implant (functional) (prosthesis) Z96.66-
|aortocoronary (bypass) graft Z95.1
|arterial-venous shunt (dialysis) Z99.2
|artificial
    |eye (globe) Z97.0
    |heart (fully implantable) (mechanical) Z95.812
        |valve Z95.2
    |larynx Z96.3
    |lens (intraocular) Z96.1
    |limb (complete) (partial) Z97.1-
        |arm Z97.1-
            |bilateral Z97.15
        |leg Z97.1-
            |bilateral Z97.16
|audiological implant (functional) Z96.29
|bladder implant (functional) Z96.0
|bone
    |conduction hearing device Z96.29
    |implant (functional) NEC Z96.7
    |joint (prosthesis) *see* Presence, joint implant
|cardiac
    |defibrillator (functional) (with synchronous cardiac pacemaker) Z95.810
    |implant or graft Z95.9
        |specified type NEC Z95.818
    |pacemaker Z95.0
    |resynchronization therapy
        |defibrillator Z95.810
        |pacemaker Z95.0
|cerebrospinal fluid drainage device Z98.2
|cochlear implant (functional) Z96.21
|contact lens (es) Z97.3
|coronary artery graft or prosthesis Z95.5
|CRT-D (cardiac resynchronization therapy defibrillator) Z95.810
|CRT-P (cardiac resynchronization therapy pacemaker) Z95.0
|cardioverter-defibrillator (ICD) Z95.810
|CSF shunt Z98.2
|dental prosthesis device Z97.2
|dentures Z97.2
|device (external) NEC Z97.8

Presence (of) - *continued*
|cardiac NEC Z95.818
|heart assist Z95.811
|implanted (functional) Z96.9
    |specified NEC Z96.89
|prosthetic Z97.8
|ear implant Z96.20
    |cochlear implant Z96.21
    |myringotomy tube Z96.22
    |specified type NEC Z96.29
|elbow-joint implant (functional) (prosthesis) Z96.62-
|endocrine implant (functional) NEC Z96.49
|eustachian tube stent or device (functional) Z96.29
|external hearing-aid or device Z97.4
|finger-joint implant (functional) (prosthetic) Z96.69-
|functional implant Z96.9
    |specified NEC Z96.89
|graft
    |cardiac NEC Z95.818
    |vascular NEC Z95.828
|hearing-aid or device (external) Z97.4
    |implant (bone) (cochlear) (functional) Z96.21
|heart assist device Z95.811
|heart valve implant (functional) Z95.2
    |prosthetic Z95.2
    |specified type NEC Z95.4
    |xenogenic Z95.3
|hip-joint implant (functional) (prosthesis) Z96.64-
|ICD (cardioverter-defibrillator) Z95.810
|implanted device (artificial) (functional) (prosthetic) Z96.9
    |automatic cardiac defibrillator (with synchronous cardiac pacemaker) Z95.810
    |cardiac pacemaker Z95.0
    |cochlear Z96.21
    |dental Z96.5
    |heart Z95.812
    |heart valve Z95.2
        |prosthetic Z95.2
        |specified NEC Z95.4
        |xenogenic Z95.3
    |insulin pump Z96.41
    |intraocular lens Z96.1
    |joint Z96.60
        |ankle Z96.66-
        |elbow Z96.62-
        |finger Z96.69-
        |hip Z96.64-
        |knee Z96.65-
        |shoulder Z96.61-
        |specified NEC Z96.698
        |wrist Z96.63-
    |larynx Z96.3
    |myringotomy tube Z96.22
    |otological Z96.20
        |cochlear Z96.21
        |eustachian stent Z96.29
        |myringotomy Z96.22
        |specified NEC Z96.29
        |stapes Z96.29
    |skin Z96.81
    |skull plate Z96.7
    |specified NEC Z96.89
    |urogenital Z96.0
|insulin pump (functional) Z96.41
|intestinal bypass or anastomosis Z98.0
|intraocular lens (functional) Z96.1
|intrauterine contraceptive device (IUD) Z97.5
|intravascular implant (functional) (prosthetic) NEC Z95.9

Presence (of) - *continued*
|coronary artery Z95.5
|defibrillator (with synchronous cardiac pacemaker) Z95.810
|peripheral vessel (with angioplasty) Z95.820
|joint implant (prosthetic) (any) Z96.60
    |ankle *see* Presence, ankle joint implant
    |elbow *see* Presence, elbow joint implant
    |finger *see* Presence, finger joint implant
    |hip *see* Presence, hip joint implant
    |knee *see* Presence, knee joint implant
    |shoulder *see* Presence, shoulder joint implant
    |specified joint NEC Z96.698
    |wrist *see* Presence, wrist joint implant
|knee-joint implant (functional) (prosthesis) Z96.65-
|laryngeal implant (functional) Z96.3
|mandibular implant (dental) Z96.5
|myringotomy tube(s) Z96.22
|orthopedic-joint implant (prosthetic) (any) *see* Presence, joint implant
|otological implant (functional) Z96.29
|shoulder-joint implant (functional) (prosthesis) Z96.61-
|skull-plate implant Z96.7
|spectacles Z97.3
|stapes implant (functional) Z96.29
|systemic lupus erythematosus [SLE] inhibitor D68.62
|tendon implant (functional) (graft) Z96.7
|tooth root(s) implant Z96.5
|ureteral stent Z96.0
|urethral stent Z96.0
|urogenital implant (functional) Z96.0
|vascular implant or device Z95.9
    |access port device Z95.828
    |specified type NEC Z95.828
|wrist-joint implant (functional) (prosthesis) Z96.63-
Presenile *see also* condition
|dementia F03
|premature aging E34.8
Presentation, fetal *see* Delivery , complicated by, malposition
Prespondylolisthesis (congenital) Q76.2
Pressure
|area, skin *see* Ulcer, pressure, by site
|brachial plexus G54.0
|brain G93.5
    |injury at birth NEC P11.1
|cerebral *see* Pressure, brain
|chest R07.89
|cone, tentorial G93.5
|hyposystolic *see also* Hypotension
    |incidental reading, without diagnosis of hypotension R03.1
|increased
    |intracranial benign G93.2
        |injury at birth P11.0
    |intraocular H40.05-
|lumbosacral plexus G54.1
|mediastinum J98.59
|necrosis (chronic) *see* Ulcer, pressure, by site
|parental, inappropriate (excessive) Z62.6
|sore (chronic) *see* Ulcer, pressure, by site
|spinal cord G95.20
|ulcer (chronic) *see* Ulcer, pressure, by site
|venous, increased I87.8
Pre-Syncope R55
Preterm
|delivery *see also* Pregnancy, complicated by, preterm labor O60.10
|labor *see* Pregnancy, complicated by, preterm labor
|newborn (infant) P07.30
    |gestational age

Preterm - *continued*

|28 completed weeks (28 weeks, 0 days through 28 weeks, 6 days) P07.31
|29 completed weeks (29 weeks, 0 days through 29 weeks, 6 days) P07.32
|30 completed weeks (30 weeks, 0 days through 30 weeks, 6 days) P07.33
|31 completed weeks (31 weeks, 0 days through 31 weeks, 6 days) P07.34
|32 completed weeks (32 weeks, 0 days through 32 weeks, 6 days) P07.35
|33 completed weeks (33 weeks, 0 days through 33 weeks, 6 days) P07.36
|34 completed weeks (34 weeks, 0 days through 34 weeks, 6 days) P07.37
|35 completed weeks (35 weeks, 0 days through 35 weeks, 6 days) P07.38
|36 completed weeks (36 weeks, 0 days through 36 weeks, 6 days) P07.39

Previa

|placenta (total) (without hemorrhage) O44.0-
|with hemorrhage O44.1-
|complete O44.0-
|with hemorrhage O44.1-
|low *see also* Delivery, complicated, by, placenta, low O44.4-
|with hemorrhage O44.5-
|marginal O44.2-
|with hemorrhage O44.3-
|partial O44.2-
|with hemorrhage O44.3-
|vasa O69.4

Priapism N48.30

|due to
|disease classified elsewhere N48.32
|drug N48.33
|specified cause NEC N48.39
|trauma N48.31

Prickling sensation (skin) R20.2

Prickly heat L74.0

Primary *see* condition **Primigravida**

|elderly, affecting management of pregnancy, labor and delivery (supervision only) *see* Pregnancy, complicated by, elderly, primigravida
|older, affecting management of pregnancy, labor and delivery (supervision only) *see* Pregnancy, complicated by elderly, primigravida
|very young, affecting management of pregnancy, labor and delivery (supervision only) *see* Pregnancy, complicated by, young mother, primigravida

Primipara

|elderly, affecting management of pregnancy, labor and delivery (supervision only) *see* Pregnancy, complicated by, elderly, primigravida
|older, affecting management of pregnancy, labor and delivery (supervision only) *see* Pregnancy, complicated by, elderly, primigravida
|very young, affecting management of pregnancy, labor and delivery (supervision only) *see* Pregnancy, complicated by, young mother, primigravida

Primus varus (bilateral) Q66.2

PRIND (Prolonged reversible ischemic neurologic deficit) I63.9

Pringle's disease (tuberous sclerosis) Q85.1

Prinzmetal angina I20.1

Prizefighter ear *see* Cauliflower ear

Problem (with) (related to)

|academic Z55.8
|acculturation Z60.3
|adjustment (to)

Problem (with) (related to) - *continued*

|change of job Z56.1
|life-cycle transition Z60.0
|pension Z60.0
|retirement Z60.0
|adopted child Z62.821
|alcoholism in family Z63.72
|atypical parenting situation Z62.9
|bankruptcy Z59.89
|behavioral (adult) F69
|drug seeking Z76.5
|birth of sibling affecting child Z62.898
|care (of)
|provider dependency Z74.9
|specified NEC Z74.8
|sick or handicapped person in family or household Z63.6
|child
|abuse (affecting the child) *see* Maltreatment, child
|custody or support proceedings Z65.3
|in welfare custody Z62.21
|in care of non-parental family member Z62.21
|in foster care Z62.21
|living in orphanage or group home Z62.22
|child-rearing Z62.9
|specified NEC Z62.898
|communication (developmental) F80.9
|conflict or discord (with)
|boss Z56.4
|classmates Z55.4
|counselor Z64.4
|employer Z56.4
|family Z63.9
|specified NEC Z63.8
|probation officer Z64.4
|social worker Z64.4
|teachers Z55.4
|workmates Z56.4
|conviction in legal proceedings Z65.0
|with imprisonment Z65.1
|counselor Z64.4
|creditors Z59.89
|digestive K92.9
|drug addict in family Z63.72
|ear *see* Disorder, ear
|economic Z59.9
|affecting care Z59.9
|specified NEC Z59.8
|education Z55.9
|specified NEC Z55.89
|employment Z56.9
|change of job Z56.1
|discord Z56.4
|environment Z56.5
|sexual harassment Z56.81
|specified NEC Z56.89
|stress NEC Z56.6
|stressful schedule Z56.3
|threat of job loss Z56.2
|unemployment Z56.0
|enuresis, child F98.0
|eye H57.9
|failed examinations (school) Z55.2
|falling Z91.81
|family *see also* Disruption, family Z63.9-
|specified NEC Z63.8
|feeding (elderly) (infant) R63.39
|newborn P92.9
|breast P92.5
|overfeeding P92.4
|slow P92.2
|specified NEC P92.8
|underfeeding P92.3

Problem (with) (related to) - *continued*

|nonorganic F50.89
|finance Z59.9
|specified NEC Z59.89
|foreclosure on loan Z59.89
|foster child Z62.822
|frightening experience(s) in childhood Z62.898
|genital NEC
|female N94.9
|male N50.9
|health care Z75.9
|specified NEC Z75.8
|hearing *see* Deafness
|homelessness Z59.00
|housing Z59.9
|inadequate Z59.1
|isolated Z59.89
|specified NEC Z59.89
|identity (of childhood) F93.8
|illegitimate pregnancy (unwanted) Z64.0
|illiteracy Z55.0
|impaired mobility Z74.09
|imprisonment or incarceration Z65.1
|inadequate teaching affecting education Z55.8
|inappropriate (excessive) parental pressure Z62.6
|influencing health status NEC Z78.9
|in-law Z63.1
|institutionalization, affecting child Z62.22
|intrafamilial communication Z63.8
|jealousy, child F93.8
|landlord Z59.2
|language (developmental) F80.9
|learning (developmental) F81.9
|legal Z65.3
|conviction without imprisonment Z65.0
|imprisonment Z65.1
|release from prison Z65.2
|life-management Z73.9
|specified NEC Z73.89
|life-style Z72.9
|gambling Z72.6
|high-risk sexual behavior (heterosexual) Z72.51
|bisexual Z72.53
|homosexual Z72.52
|inappropriate eating habits Z72.4
|self-damaging behavior NEC Z72.89
|specified NEC Z72.89
|tobacco use Z72.0
|literacy Z55.9
|low level Z55.0
|specified NEC Z55.8
|living alone Z60.2
|lodgers Z59.2
|loss of love relationship in childhood Z62.898
|marital Z63.0
|involving
|divorce Z63.5
|estrangement Z63.5
|gender identity F66
|mastication K08.89
|medical
|care, within family Z63.6
|facilities Z75.9
|specified NEC Z75.8
|mental F48.9
|multiparity Z64.1
|negative life events in childhood Z62.9
|altered pattern of family relationships Z62.898
|frightening experience Z62.898
|loss of
|love relationship Z62.898

Problem (with) (related to) - *continued*
|self-esteem Z62.898
|physical abuse (alleged) *see* Maltreatment, child
|removal from home Z62.29
|specified event NEC Z62.898
|neighbor Z59.2
|neurological NEC R29.818
|new step-parent affecting child Z62.898
|none (feared complaint unfounded) Z71.1
|occupational NEC Z56.89
|parent-child *see* Conflict, parent-child
|personal hygiene Z91.89
|personality F69
|phase-of-life transition, adjustment Z60.0
|presence of sick or disabled person in family or household Z63.79
|needing care Z63.6
|primary support group (family) Z63.9
|specified NEC Z63.8
|probation officer Z64.4
|psychiatric F99
|psychosexual (development) F66
|psychosocial Z65.9
|religious or spiritual Z65.8
|specified NEC Z65.8
|relationship Z63.9
|childhood F93.8
|release from prison Z65.2
|religious or spiritual Z65.8
|removal from home affecting child Z62.29
|seeking and accepting known hazardous and harmful
|behavioral or psychological interventions Z65.8
|chemical, nutritional or physical interventions Z65.8
|sexual function (nonorganic) F52.9
|sight H54.7
|sleep disorder, child F51.9
|smell *see* Disturbance, sensation, smell
|social
|environment Z60.9
|specified NEC Z60.8
|exclusion and rejection Z60.4
|worker Z64.4
|speech R47.9
|developmental F80.9
|specified NEC R47.89
|swallowing *see* Dysphagia
|taste *see* Disturbance, sensation, taste
|tic, child F95.0
|underachievement in school Z55.3
|unemployment Z56.0
|threatened Z56.2
|unwanted pregnancy Z64.0
|upbringing Z62.9
|specified NEC Z62.898
|urinary N39.9
|voice production R47.89
|work schedule (stressful) Z56.3
Procedure (surgical)
|converted
|arthroscopic to open Z53.33
|laparoscopic to open Z53.31
|specified procedure NEC to open Z53.39
|thoracoscopic to open Z53.32
|for purpose other than remedying health state Z41.9
|specified NEC Z41.8
|not done Z53.9
|because of
|administrative reasons Z53.8
|contraindication Z53.09
|smoking Z53.01

Procedure (surgical) - *continued*
|patient's decision Z53.20
|for reasons of belief or group pressure Z53.1
|left against medical advice (AMA) Z53.29
|left without being seen Z53.21
|specified reason NEC Z53.29
|specified reason NEC Z53.8
Procidentia (uteri) N81.3
Proctalgia K62.89
|fugax K59.4
|spasmodic K59.4
Proctitis K62.89
|amebic (acute) A06.0
|chlamydial A56.3
|gonococcal A54.6
|granulomatous *see* Enteritis, regional, large intestine
|herpetic A60.1
|radiation K62.7
|tuberculous A18.32
|ulcerative (chronic) K51.20
|with
|complication K51.219
|abscess K51.214
|fistula K51.213
|obstruction K51.212
|rectal bleeding K51.211
|specified NEC K51.218
Proctocele
|female (without uterine prolapse) N81.6
|with uterine prolapse N81.2
|complete N81.3
|male K62.3
Proctocolitis
|allergic K52.29
|food-induced eosinophilic K52.29
|food protein-induced K52.29
|milk protein-induced K52.29
|mucosal *see* Rectosigmoiditis, ulcerative
Proctoptosis K62.3
Proctorrhagia K62.5
Proctosigmoiditis K63.89
|ulcerative (chronic) *see* Rectosigmoiditis, ulcerative
Proctospasm K59.4
|psychogenic F45.8
Profichet's disease *see* Disorder, soft tissue, specified type NEC
Progeria E34.8
Prognathism (mandibular) (maxillary) M26.19
Progonoma (melanotic) *see* Neoplasm, benign, by site
Progressive *see* condition
Prolactinoma
|specified site *see* Neoplasm, benign, by site
|unspecified site D35.2
Prolapse, prolapsed
|anus, anal (canal) (sphincter) K62.2
|arm or hand O32.2
|causing obstructed labor O64.4
|bladder (mucosa) (sphincter) (acquired)
|congenital Q79.4
|female *see* Cystocele
|male N32.89
|breast implant (prosthetic) T85.49
|cecostomy K94.09
|cecum K63.4
|cervix, cervical (hypertrophied) N81.2
|anterior lip, obstructing labor O65.5
|congenital Q51.828
|postpartal, old N81.2
|stump N81.85

Prolapse, prolapsed - *continued*
|ciliary body (traumatic) *see* Laceration, eye(ball), with prolapse or loss of interocular tissue
|colon (pedunculated) K63.4
|colostomy K94.09
|disc (intervertebral) *see* Displacement, intervertebral disc |eye implant (orbital) T85.398
|lens (ocular) *see* Complications, intraocular lens
|fallopian tube N83.4-
|gastric (mucosa) K31.89
|genital, female N81.9
|specified NEC N81.89
|globe, nontraumatic *see* Luxation, globe
|ileostomy bud K94.19
|intervertebral disc *see* Displacement, intervertebral disc
|intestine (small) K63.4
|iris (traumatic) *see* Laceration, eye(ball), with prolapse or loss of interocular tissue
|nontraumatic H21.89
|kidney N28.83
|congenital Q63.2
|laryngeal muscles or ventricle J38.7
|liver K76.89
|meatus urinarius N36.8
|mitral (valve) I34.1
|ocular lens implant *see* Complications, intraocular lens
|organ or site, congenital NEC *see* Malposition, congenital
|ovary N83.4-
|pelvic floor, female N81.89
|perineum, female N81.89
|rectum (mucosa) (sphincter) K62.3
|due to trichuris trichuria B79
|spleen D73.89
|stomach K31.89
|umbilical cord
|complicating delivery O69.0
|urachus, congenital Q64.4
|ureter N28.89
|with obstruction N13.5
|with infection N13.6
|ureterovesical orifice N28.89
|urethra (acquired) (infected) (mucosa) N36.8
|congenital Q64.71
|urinary meatus N36.8
|congenital Q64.72
|uterovaginal N81.4
|complete N81.3
|incomplete N81.2
|uterus (with prolapse of vagina) N81.4
|complete N81.3
|congenital Q51.818
|first degree N81.2
|in pregnancy or childbirth *see* Pregnancy, complicated by, abnormal, uterus
|incomplete N81.2
|postpartal (old) N81.4
|second degree N81.2
|third degree N81.3
|uveal (traumatic) *see* Laceration, eye(ball), with prolapse or loss of interocular tissue
|vagina (anterior) (wall) *see* Cystocele
|with prolapse of uterus N81.4
|complete N81.3
|incomplete N81.2
|posterior wall N81.6
|posthysterectomy N99.3
|vitreous (humor) H43.0-

Prolapse, prolapsed - *continued*
　|in wound *see* Laceration, eye(ball), with
　　　prolapse or loss of interocular tissue
　|womb *see* Prolapse, uterus
Prolapsus, female N81.9
　|specified NEC N81.89
Proliferation(s)
　|prostate, atypical small acinar N42.32
　|primary cutaneous CD30-positive large T-cell
　　　C86.6
Proliferative *see* condition
Prolonged, prolongation (of)
　|bleeding (time) (idiopathic) R79.1
　|coagulation (time) R79.1
　|gestation (over 42 completed weeks)
　　|mother O48.1
　　|newborn P08.22
　|interval I44.0
　|labor O63.9
　　|first stage O63.0
　　|second stage O63.1
　|partial thromboplastin time (PTT) R79.1
　|pregnancy (more than 42 weeks gestation)
　　　O48.1
　|prothrombin time R79.1
　|QT interval I45.81
　|uterine contractions in labor O62.4
Prominence, prominent
　|auricle (congenital) (ear) Q17.5
　|ischial spine or sacral promontory with
　　　disproportion (fetopelvic) O33.0
　　|causing obstructed labor O65.0
　|nose (congenital) acquired M95.0
Promiscuity *see* High, risk, sexual behavior
Pronation
　|ankle *see* Deformity, limb, foot, specified
　　　NEC
　|foot *see also* Deformity, limb, foot, specified
　　　NEC
　　|congenital Q74.2
Prophylactic
　|administration of
　　|antibiotics, long-term Z79.2
　　　|short-term use　omit code
　　|drug *see also* Long-term (current) drug
　　　therapy (use of) Z79.899-
　|medication Z79.899
　|organ removal (for neoplasia management)
　　　Z40.00
　　|breast Z40.01
　　|fallopian tube(s) Z40.03
　　　|with ovary(s) Z40.02
　　|ovary(s) Z40.02
　　|specified site NEC Z40.09
　|surgery Z40.9
　　|for risk factors related to malignant
　　　neoplasm *see* Prophylactic, organ removal
　　|specified NEC Z40.8
　|vaccination Z23
Propionic acidemia E71.121
Proptosis (ocular) *see also* Exophthalmos
　|thyroid *see* Hyperthyroidism, with goiter
Prosecution, anxiety concerning Z65.3
Prosopagnosia R48.3
Prostadynia N42.81
Prostate, prostatic *see* condition
Prostatism *see* Hyperplasia, prostate
Prostatitis (congestive) (suppurative) (with
　cystitis) N41.9
　|acute N41.0
　|cavitary N41.8
　|chronic N41.1
　|diverticular N41.8

Prostatitis - *continued*
　|due to Trichomonas (vaginalis) A59.02
　|fibrous N41.1
　|gonococcal (acute) (chronic) A54.22
　|granulomatous N41.4
　|hypertrophic N41.1
　|subacute N41.1
　|trichomonal A59.02
　|tuberculous A18.14
Prostatocystitis N41.3
Prostatorrhea N42.89
Prostatosis N42.82
Prostration R53.83
　|heat *see also* Heat, exhaustion
　　|anhydrotic T67.3
　　|due to
　　　|salt (and water) depletion T67.4
　　　|water depletion T67.3
　|nervous F48.8
　|senile R54
Protanomaly (anomalous trichromat) H53.54
Protanopia (complete) (incomplete) H53.54
Protection (against) (from) *see* Prophylactic
Protein
　|deficiency NEC *see* Malnutrition
　|malnutrition *see* Malnutrition
　|sickness *see also* Reaction, serum T80.69
Proteinemia R77.9
Proteinosis
　|alveolar (pulmonary) J84.01
　|lipid or lipoid (of Urbach) E78.89
Proteinuria R80.9
　|Bence Jones R80.3
　|complicating pregnancy *see* Proteinuria,
　　　gestational
　|gestational
　　|complicating
　　　|childbirth O12.14
　　　|pregnancy O12.1-
　　　　|with edema O12.2-
　　|puerperium O12.15
　|idiopathic R80.0
　|isolated R80.0
　　|with glomerular lesion N06.9
　　　|C3
　　　　|glomerulonephritis N06.A
　　　　|glomerulopathy N06.A
　　　　　|with dense deposit disease N06.6
　　　|dense deposit disease N06.6
　　　|diffuse
　　　　|crescentic glomerulonephritis N06.7
　　　　|endocapillary proliferative
　　　　　glomerulonephritis N06.4
　　　　|mesangiocapillary glomerulonephritis
　　　　　N06.5
　　　|focal and segmental hyalinosis or sclerosis
　　　　　N06.1
　　　|membranous (diffuse) N06.2
　　　|mesangial proliferative (diffuse) N06.3
　　　|minimal change N06.0
　　　|specified pathology NEC N06.8
　|orthostatic R80.2
　　|with glomerular lesion *see* Proteinuria,
　　　isolated, with glomerular lesion
　|persistent R80.1
　　|with glomerular lesion *see* Proteinuria,
　　　isolated, with glomerular lesion
　|postural R80.2
　　|with glomerular lesion *see* Proteinuria,
　　　isolated, with glomerular lesion
　|pre-eclamptic *see* Pre-eclampsia
　|puerperal O12.15
　|specified type NEC R80.8
Proteolysis, pathologic D65

Proteus (mirabilis) (morganii), as cause of
　disease classified elsewhere B96.4
Prothrombin gene mutation D68.52
Protoporphyria, erythropoietic E80.0
Protozoal *see also* condition
　|disease B64
　　|specified NEC B60.8
Protrusion, protrusio　acetabuli M24.7
　|acetabulum (into pelvis) M24.7
　|device, implant or graft *see also*
　　　Complications, by site and type,
　　　mechanical T85.698
　　|arterial graft NEC *see* Complication,
　　　cardiovascular device, mechanical,
　　　vascular
　　|breast (implant) T85.49
　　|catheter NEC T85.698
　　　|cystostomy T83.090
　　　|dialysis (renal) T82.49
　　　　|intraperitoneal T85.691
　　　|infusion NEC T82.594
　　　　|spinal (epidural) (subdural) T85.690
　　　|urinary *see also* Complications, catheter,
　　　　urinary T83.098
　　|electronic (electrode) (pulse generator)
　　　(stimulator)
　　　|bone T84.390
　　　|nervous system *see* Complication,
　　　　prosthetic device, mechanical,
　　　　electronic nervous system stimulator
　　|fixation, internal (orthopedic) NEC *see*
　　　Complication, fixation device, mechanical
　　|gastrointestinal *see* Complications,
　　　prosthetic device, mechanical,
　　　gastrointestinal device
　　|genital NEC T83.498
　　　|intrauterine contraceptive device T83.39
　　　|penile prosthesis (cylinder) (implanted)
　　　　(pump) (reservoir) T83.490
　　　|testicular prosthesis T83.491
　　|heart NEC *see* Complication, cardiovascular
　　　device, mechanical
　　|joint prosthesis *see* Complications, joint
　　　prosthesis, mechanical, specified NEC, by
　　　site
　　|ocular NEC *see* Complications, prosthetic
　　　device, mechanical, ocular device
　　|orthopedic NEC *see* Complication,
　　　orthopedic, device, mechanical
　　|specified NEC T85.628
　　|urinary NEC *see also* Complication,
　　　genitourinary, device, urinary, mechanical
　　　|graft T83.29
　　|vascular NEC *see* Complication,
　　　cardiovascular device, mechanical
　　|ventricular intracranial shunt T85.09
　|intervertebral disc *see* Displacement,
　　　intervertebral disc
　|joint prosthesis *see* Complications, joint
　　　prosthesis, mechanical, specified NEC, by
　　　site
　|nucleus pulposus *see* Displacement,
　　　intervertebral disc
Prune belly (syndrome) Q79.4
Prurigo (ferox) (gravis) (Hebrae) (Hebra's)
　(mitis) (simplex) L28.2
　|Besnier's L20.0
　|estivalis L56.4
　|nodularis L28.1
　|psychogenic F45.8
Pruritus, pruritic (essential) L29.9
　|ani, anus L29.0
　　|psychogenic F45.8
　|anogenital L29.3
　　|psychogenic F45.8

Pruritus, pruritic (essential) - continued
|due to onchocerca volvulus B73.1
|gravidarum *see* Pregnancy, complicated by, specified pregnancy-related condition NEC
|hiemalis L29.8
|neurogenic (any site) F45.8
|perianal L29.0
|psychogenic (any site) F45.8
|scroti, scrotum L29.1
  |psychogenic F45.8
|senile, senilis L29.8
|specified NEC L29.8
  |psychogenic F45.8
|Trichomonas A59.9
|vulva, vulvae L29.2
  |psychogenic F45.8
Pseudarthrosis, pseudoarthrosis (bone) *see* Nonunion, fracture
|clavicle, congenital Q74.0
|joint, following fusion or arthrodesis M96.0
Pseudoaneurysm *see* Aneurysm
Pseudoangioma I81
Pseudoangina (pectoris) *see* Angina
Pseudoarteriosus Q28.8
Pseudoarthrosis *see* Pseudarthrosis
Pseudobulbar affect (PBA) F48.2
Pseudochromhidrosis L67.8
Pseudocirrhosis, liver, pericardial I31.1
Pseudocowpox B08.03
Pseudocoxalgia M91.3-
Pseudocroup J38.5
Pseudo-Cushing's syndrome, alcohol-Induced E24.4
Pseudocyesis F45.8
Pseudocyst
|lung J98.4
|pancreas K86.3
|retina *see* Cyst, retina
Pseudoelephantiasis neuroarthritica Q82.0
Pseudoexfoliation, capsule (lens) *see* Cataract, specified NEC
Pseudofolliculitis barbae L73.1
Pseudoglioma H44.89
Pseudohemophilia (Bernuth's) (hereditary) (type B) D68.0
|Type A D69.8
|vascular D69.8
Pseudohermaphroditism Q56.3
|adrenal E25.2
|female Q56.2
  |with adrenocortical disorder E25.8
  |without adrenocortical disorder Q56.2
  |adrenal (congenital) E25.0
  |unspecified E25.9
|male Q56.1
  |with
    |adrenocortical disorder E25.8
    |androgen resistance E34.51
    |cleft scrotum Q56.1
    |feminizing testis E34.51
    |5-alpha-reductase deficiency E29.1
  |without gonadal disorder Q56.1
  |adrenal E25.8
  |unspecified E25.9
Pseudo-Hurler's polydystrophy E77.0
Pseudohydrocephalus G93.2
Pseudohypertrophic muscular dystrophy (Erb's) G71.02
Pseudohypertrophy, muscle G71.02
Pseudohypoparathyroidism E20.1
Pseudoinsomnia F51.03
Pseudoleukemia, infantile D64.89
Pseudomembranous *see* condition
Pseudomenses (newborn) P54.6

Pseudomenstruation (newborn) P54.6
Pseudomeningocele (cerebral) (infective) (post-Traumatic) G96.198
|postprocedural (spinal) G97.82
Pseudomonas
|aeruginosa, as cause of disease classified elsewhere B96.5
|mallei infection A24.0
  |as cause of disease classified elsewhere B96.5
|pseudomallei, as cause of disease classified elsewhere B96.5
Pseudomyotonia G71.19
Pseudomyxoma peritonei C78.6
Pseudoneuritis, optic (nerve) (disc) (papilla), congenital Q14.2
Pseudo-Obstruction intestine (acute) (chronic) (idiopathic) (intermittent secondary) (primary) K59.89
|colonic K59.81
Pseudopapilledema H47.33-
|congenital Q14.2
Pseudoparalysis
|arm or leg R29.818
|atonic, congenital P94.2
Pseudopelade L66.0
Pseudophakia Z96.1
Pseudopolyarthritis, rhizomelic M35.3
Pseudopolycythemia D75.1
Pseudopseudohypoparathyroidism E20.1
Pseudopterygium H11.81-
Pseudoptosis (eyelid) *see* Blepharochalasis
Pseudopuberty, precocious
|female heterosexual E25.8
|male isosexual E25.8
Pseudorickets (renal) N25.0
Pseudorubella B08.20
Pseudosclerema, newborn P83.88
Pseudosclerosis (brain)
|of Westphal (Strümpell) E83.01
|Jakob's *see* Creutzfeldt-Jakob disease or syndrome
|spastic *see* Creutzfeldt-Jakob disease or syndrome
Pseudotetanus *see* Convulsions
Pseudotetany R29.0
|hysterical F44.5
Pseudotruncus arteriosus Q25.49
Pseudotuberculosis A28.2
|enterocolitis A04.8
|pasteurella (infection) A28.0
Pseudotumor G93.2
|cerebri G93.2
|orbital H05.11-
Pseudoxanthoma elasticum Q82.8
Psilosis (sprue) (tropical) K90.1
|nontropical K90.0
Psittacosis A70
Psoitis M60.88
Psoriasis L40.9
|arthropathic L40.50
  |arthritis mutilans L40.52
  |distal interphalangeal L40.51
  |juvenile L40.54
  |other specified L40.59
  |spondylitis L40.53
|buccal K13.29
|flexural L40.8
|guttate L40.4
|mouth K13.29
|nummular L40.0
|plaque L40.0
|psychogenic F54
|pustular (generalized) L40.1
  |palmaris et plantaris L40.3
|specified NEC L40.8
|vulgaris L40.0

Psychasthenia F48.8
Psychiatric disorder or problem F99
Psychogenic *see also* condition
|factors associated with physical conditions F54
Psychological and behavioral factors affecting medical condition F59
Psychoneurosis, psychoneurotic *see also* Neurosis
|anxiety (state) F41.1
|depersonalization F48.1
|hypochondriacal F45.21
|hysteria F44.9
|neurasthenic F48.8
|personality NEC F60.89
Psychopathy, psychopathic
|affectionless F94.2
|autistic F84.5
|constitution, post-traumatic F07.81
|personality *see* Disorder, personality
|sexual *see* Deviation, sexual
|state F60.2
Psychosexual identity disorder of childhood F64.2
Psychosis, psychotic F29
|acute (transient) F23
  |hysterical F44.9
|affective *see* Disorder, mood
|alcoholic F10.959
  |with
    |abuse F10.159
    |anxiety disorder F10.980
      |with
        |abuse F10.180
        |dependence F10.280
    |delirium tremens F10.231
    |delusions F10.950
      |with
        |abuse F10.150
        |dependence F10.250
    |dementia F10.97
      |with dependence F10.27
    |dependence F10.259
    |hallucinosis F10.951
      |with
        |abuse F10.151
        |dependence F10.251
    |mood disorder F10.94
      |with
        |abuse F10.14
        |dependence F10.24
    |paranoia F10.950
      |with
        |abuse F10.150
        |dependence F10.250
    |persisting amnesia F10.96
      |with dependence F10.26
  |amnestic confabulatory F10.96
    |with dependence F10.26
  |delirium tremens F10.231
  |Korsakoff's, Korsakov's, Korsakow's F10.26
  |paranoid type F10.950
    |with
      |abuse F10.150
      |dependence F10.250
|anergastic *see* Psychosis, organic
|arteriosclerotic (simple type) (uncomplicated) F01.50
  |with behavioral disturbance F01.51
|childhood F84.0
  |atypical F84.8
|climacteric *see* Psychosis, involutional
|confusional F29
  |acute or subacute F05
  |reactive F23

Psychosis, psychotic - *continued*
- cycloid F23
- depressive *see* Disorder, depressive
- disintegrative (childhood) F84.3
- drug-induced *see* F11-F19 with .x59
  - paranoid and hallucinatory states *see* F11-F19 with .x50 or .x51
- due to or associated with
  - addiction, drug *see* F11-F19 with .x59
  - dependence
    - alcohol F10.259
    - drug *see* F11-F19 with .x59
  - epilepsy F06.8
  - Huntington's chorea F06.8
  - ischemia, cerebrovascular (generalized) F06.8
  - multiple sclerosis F06.8
  - physical disease F06.8
  - presenile dementia F03
  - senile dementia F03
  - vascular disease (arteriosclerotic) (cerebral) F01.50
    - with behavioral disturbance F01.51
- epileptic F06.8
- episode F23
  - due to or associated with physical condition F06.8
- exhaustive F43.0
- hallucinatory, chronic F28
- hypomanic F30.8
- hysterical (acute) F44.9
- induced F24
- infantile F84.0
  - atypical F84.8
- infective (acute) (subacute) F05
- involutional F28
  - depressive *see* Disorder, depressive
  - melancholic *see* Disorder, depressive
  - paranoid (state) F22
- Korsakoff's, Korsakov's, Korsakow's (nonalcoholic) F04
  - alcoholic F10.96
    - in dependence F10.26
  - induced by other psychoactive substance *see* categories F11-F19 with .x5x
- mania, manic (single episode) F30.2
  - recurrent type F31.89
- manic-depressive *see* Disorder, bipolar
- menopausal *see* Psychosis, involutional
- mixed schizophrenic and affective F25.8
- multi-infarct (cerebrovascular) F01.50
  - with behavioral disturbance F01.51
- nonorganic F29
  - specified NEC F28
- organic F09
  - due to or associated with
    - arteriosclerosis (cerebral) *see* Psychosis, arteriosclerotic
    - cerebrovascular disease, arteriosclerotic *see* Psychosis, arteriosclerotic
    - childbirth *see* Psychosis, puerperal
    - Creutzfeldt-Jakob disease or syndrome *see* Creutzfeldt-Jakob disease or syndrome
    - dependence, alcohol F10.259
    - disease
      - alcoholic liver F10.259
      - brain, arteriosclerotic *see* Psychosis, arteriosclerotic
      - cerebrovascular F01.50
        - with behavioral disturbance F01.51
      - Creutzfeldt-Jakob *see* Creutzfeldt-Jakob disease or syndrome
      - endocrine or metabolic F06.8
        - acute or subacute F05

Psychosis, psychotic - *continued*
- liver, alcoholic F10.259
- epilepsy transient (acute) F05
- infection
  - brain (intracranial) F06.8
    - acute or subacute F05
- intoxication
  - alcoholic (acute) F10.259
  - drug F11-F19 with .x59
- ischemia, cerebrovascular (generalize *see* Psychosis, arteriosclerotic
- puerperium *see* Psychosis, puerperal
- trauma, brain (birth) (from electric current) (surgical) F06.8
  - acute or subacute F05
- infective F06.8
  - acute or subacute F05
- post-traumatic F06.8
  - acute or subacute F05
- paranoiac F22
- paranoid (climacteric) (involutional) (menopausal) F22
  - psychogenic (acute) F23
  - schizophrenic F20.0
  - senile F03
- postpartum (NOS) F53.1
- presbyophrenic (type) F03
- presenile F03
- psychogenic (paranoid) F23
  - depressive F32.3
- puerperal (NOS) F53.1
  - specified type *see* Psychosis, by type
- reactive (brief) (transient) (emotional stress) (psychological trauma) F23
  - depressive F32.3
    - recurrent F33.3
  - excitative type F30.8
- schizoaffective F25.9
  - depressive type F25.1
  - manic type F25.0
- schizophrenia, schizophrenic *see* Schizophrenia
- schizophrenia-like, in epilepsy F06.2
- schizophreniform F20.81
  - affective type F25.9
  - brief F23
  - confusional type F23
  - mixed type F25.0
- senile NEC F03
  - depressed or paranoid type F03
  - simple deterioration F03
  - specified type code to condition
- shared F24
- situational (reactive) F23
- symbiotic (childhood) F84.3
- symptomatic F09

Psychosomatic *see* Disorder, psychosomatic
Psychosyndrome, organic F07.9
Psychotic episode due to or associated with physical condition F06.8
Pterygium (eye) H11.00-
- amyloid H11.01-
- central H11.02-
- colli Q18.3
- double H11.03-
- peripheral
  - progressive H11.05-
  - stationary H11.04-
- recurrent H11.06-

Ptilosis (eyelid) *see* Madarosis
Ptomaine (poisoning) *see* Poisoning, food
Ptosis *see also* Blepharoptosis
- adiposa (false) *see* Blepharoptosis
- breast N64.81
- brow H57.81-
- cecum K63.4

Ptosis - *continued*
- colon K63.4
- congenital (eyelid) Q10.0
  - specified site NEC *see* Anomaly, by site
- eyebrow H57.81-
- eyelid *see* Blepharoptosis
  - congenital Q10.0
- gastric K31.89
- intestine K63.4
- kidney N28.83
- liver K76.89
- renal N28.83
- splanchnic K63.4
- spleen D73.89
- stomach K31.89
- viscera K63.4

PTP D69.51
Ptyalism (periodic) K11.7
- hysterical F45.8
- pregnancy *see* Pregnancy, complicated by, specified pregnancy-related condition NEC
- psychogenic F45.8

Ptyalolithiasis K11.5
Pubarche, precocious E30.1
Pubertas praecox E30.1
Puberty (development state) Z00.3
- bleeding (excessive) N92.2
- delayed E30.0
- precocious (constitutional) (cryptogenic) (idiopathic) E30.1
  - central E22.8
  - due to
    - ovarian hyperfunction E28.1
      - estrogen E28.0
    - testicular hyperfunction E29.0
- premature E30.1
  - due to
    - adrenal cortical hyperfunction E25.8
    - pineal tumor E34.8
    - pituitary (anterior) hyperfunction E22.8

Puckering, macula *see* Degeneration, macula, puckering
Pudenda, pudendum *see* condition
Puente's disease (simple glandular cheilitis) K13.0
Puerperal, puerperium (complicated by, complications)
- abnormal glucose (tolerance test) O99.815
- abscess
  - areola O91.02
    - associated with lactation O91.03
  - Bartholin's gland O86.19
  - breast O91.12
    - associated with lactation O91.13
  - cervix (uteri) O86.11
  - genital organ NEC O86.19
  - kidney O86.21
  - mammary O91.12
    - associated with lactation O91.13
  - nipple O91.02
    - associated with lactation O91.03
  - peritoneum O85
  - subareolar O91.12
    - associated with lactation O91.13
  - urinary tract *see* Puerperal, infection, urinary
  - uterus O86.12
  - vagina (wall) O86.13
  - vaginorectal O86.13
  - vulvovaginal gland O86.13
- adnexitis O86.19
- afibrinogenemia, or other coagulation defect O72.3
- albuminuria (acute) (subacute) *see* Proteinuria, gestational

Puerperal, puerperium - *continued*
|alcohol use O99.315
|anemia O90.81
||pre-existing (pre-pregnancy) O99.03
|anesthetic death O89.8
|apoplexy O99.43
|bariatric surgery status O99.845
|blood disorder NEC O99.13
|blood dyscrasia O72.3
|cardiomyopathy O90.3
|cerebrovascular disorder (conditions in I60-
  I69) O99.43
|cervicitis O86.11
|circulatory system disorder O99.43
|coagulopathy (any) O99.13
||with hemorrhage O72.3
|complications O90.9
||specified NEC O90.89
|convulsions *see* Eclampsia
|cystitis O86.22
|cystopyelitis O86.29
|delirium NEC F05
|diabetes O24.93
||gestational *see* Puerperal, gestational
  diabetes
||pre-existing O24.33
|||specified NEC O24.83
|||type 1 O24.03
|||type 2 O24.13
|digestive system disorder O99.63
|disease O90.9
||breast NEC O92.29
||cerebrovascular (acute) O99.43
||nonobstetric NEC O99.893
||tubo-ovarian O86.19
||Valsuani's O99.03
|disorder O90.9
||biliary tract O26.63
||lactation O92.70
||liver O26.63
||nonobstetric NEC O99.893
|disruption
||cesarean wound O90.0
||episiotomy wound O90.1
||perineal laceration wound O90.1
|drug use O99.325
|eclampsia (with pre-existing hypertension)
  O15.2
|embolism (pulmonary) (blood clot) *see*
  Embolism, obstetric, puerperal
|endocrine, nutritional or metabolic disease
  NEC O99.285
|endophlebitis *see* Puerperal, phlebitis
|endotrachelitis O86.11
|failure
||lactation (complete) O92.3
|||partial O92.4
||renal, acute O90.4
|fever (of unknown origin) O86.4
||septic O85
|fissure, nipple O92.12
||associated with lactation O92.13
|fistula
||breast (due to mastitis) O91.12
|||associated with lactation O91.13
||nipple O91.02
|||associated with lactation O91.03
|galactophoritis O91.22
||associated with lactation O91.23
|galactorrhea O92.6
|gastric banding status O99.845
|gastric bypass status O99.845
|gastrointestinal disease NEC O99.63
|gestational
||diabetes O24.439

Puerperal, puerperium - *continued*
||diet controlled O24.430
||insulin (and diet) controlled O24.434
||oral drug controlled (antidiabetic)
    (hypoglycemic) O24.435
|edema O12.05
||with proteinuria O12.25
||proteinuria O12.15
|gonorrhea O98.23
|hematoma, subdural O99.43
|hemiplegia, cerebral O99.355
||due to cerebrovascular disorder O99.43
|hemorrhage O72.1
||brain O99.43
||bulbar O99.43
||cerebellar O99.43
||cerebral O99.43
||cortical O99.43
||delayed or secondary O72.2
||extradural O99.43
||internal capsule O99.43
||intracranial O99.43
||intrapontine O99.43
||meningeal O99.43
||pontine O99.43
||retained placenta O72.0
||subarachnoid O99.43
||subcortical O99.43
||subdural O99.43
||third stage O72.0
||uterine, delayed O72.2
||ventricular O99.43
|hemorrhoids O87.2
|hepatorenal syndrome O90.4
|hypertension *see* Hypertension, complicating,
  puerperium
|hypertrophy, breast O92.29
|induration breast (fibrous) O92.29
|infection O86.4
||cervix O86.11
||generalized O85
||genital tract NEC O86.19
|||obstetric surgical wound O86.09
||kidney (bacillus coli) O86.21
||maternal O98.93
|||carrier state NEC O99.835
|||gonorrhea O98.23
|||human immunodeficiency virus (HIV)
      O98.73
|||protozoal O98.63
|||sexually transmitted NEC O98.33
|||specified NEC O98.83
|||streptococcus group B (GBS) carrier state
      O99.825
|||syphilis O98.13
|||tuberculosis O98.03
|||viral hepatitis O98.43
|||viral NEC O98.53
||nipple O91.02
|||associated with lactation O91.03
||peritoneum O85
||renal O86.21
||specified NEC O86.89
||urinary (asymptomatic) (tract) NEC O86.20
|||bladder O86.22
|||kidney O86.21
|||specified site NEC O86.29
|||urethra O86.22
||vagina O86.13
||vein *see* Puerperal, phlebitis
|ischemia, cerebral O99.43
|lymphangitis O86.89
||breast O91.22
|||associated with lactation O91.23
|malignancy O9A.13

Puerperal, puerperium - *continued*
|malnutrition O25.3
|mammillitis O91.02
||associated with lactation O91.03
|mammitis O91.22
||associated with lactation O91.23
|mania F30.8
|mastitis O91.22
||associated with lactation O91.23
||purulent O91.12
|||associated with lactation O91.13
|melancholia *see* Disorder, depressive
|mental disorder NEC O99.345
|metroperitonitis O85
|metrorrhagia *see* Hemorrhage, postpartum
|metrosalpingitis O86.19
|metrovaginitis O86.13
|milk leg O87.1
|monoplegia, cerebral O99.43
|mood disturbance O90.6
|necrosis, liver (acute) (subacute) (conditions
  in subcategory K72.0) O26.63
||with renal failure O90.4
|nervous system disorder O99.355
|neuritis O90.89
|obesity (pre-existing prior to pregnancy)
  O99.215
|obesity surgery status O99.845
|occlusion, precerebral artery O99.43
|paralysis
||bladder (sphincter) O90.89
||cerebral O99.43
|paralytic stroke O99.43
|parametritis O85
|paravaginitis O86.13
|pelviperitonitis O85
|perimetritis O86.12
|perimetrosalpingitis O86.19
|perinephritis O86.21
|periphlebitis *see* Puerperal phlebitis
|peritoneal infection O85
|peritonitis (pelvic) O85
|perivaginitis O86.13
|phlebitis O87.0
||deep O87.1
||pelvic O87.1
||superficial O87.0
|phlebothrombosis, deep O87.1
|phlegmasia alba dolens O87.1
|placental polyp O90.89
|pneumonia, embolic *see* Embolism, obstetric,
  puerperal
|pre-eclampsia *see* Pre-eclampsia
|psychosis (NOS) F53.1
|pyelitis O86.21
|pyelocystitis O86.29
|pyelonephritis O86.21
|pyelonephrosis O86.21
|pyemia O85
|pyocystitis O86.29
|pyohemia O85
|pyometra O86.12
|pyonephritis O86.21
|pyosalpingitis O86.19
|pyrexia (of unknown origin) O86.4
|renal
||disease NEC O90.89
||failure O90.4
|respiratory disease NEC O99.53
|retention
||decidua *see* Retention, decidua
||placenta O72.0
||secundines *see* Retention, secundines
|retracted nipple O92.02
|salpingo-ovaritis O86.19

Puerperal, puerperium - continued

|salpingoperitonitis O85
|secondary perineal tear O90.1
|sepsis (pelvic) O85
|sepsis O85
|septic thrombophlebitis O86.81
|skin disorder NEC O99.73
|specified condition NEC O99.893
|stroke O99.43
|subinvolution (uterus) O90.89
|subluxation of symphysis (pubis) O26.73
|suppuration *see* Puerperal, abscess
|tetanus A34
|thelitis O91.02
  |associated with lactation O91.03
|thrombocytopenia O72.3
|thrombophlebitis (superficial) O87.0
  |deep O87.1
  |pelvic O87.1
  |septic O86.81
|thrombosis (venous) *see* Thrombosis, puerperal
|thyroiditis O90.5
|toxemia (eclamptic) (pre-eclamptic) (with convulsions) O15.2
|trauma, non-obstetric O9A.23
  |caused by abuse (physical) (suspected) O9A.33
    |confirmed O9A.33
    |psychological (suspected) O9A.53
      |confirmed O9A.53
    |sexual (suspected) O9A.43
      |confirmed O9A.43
|uremia (due to renal failure) O90.4
|urethritis O86.22
|vaginitis O86.13
|varicose veins (legs) O87.4
  |vulva or perineum O87.8
|venous O87.9
|vulvitis O86.19
|vulvovaginitis O86.13
|white leg O87.1

Puerperium *see* Puerperal
Pulmolithiasis J98.4
Pulmonary *see* condition
Pulpitis (acute) (anachoretic) (chronic) (hyperplastic) (putrescent) (suppurative) (ulcerative) K04.01
|irreversible K04.02
|reversible K04.01
Pulpless tooth K04.99
Pulse
|alternating R00.8
|bigeminal R00.8
|fast R00.0
|feeble, rapid due to shock following injury T79.4
|rapid R00.0
|weak R09.89
Pulsus alternans or trigeminus R00.8
Punch drunk F07.81
Punctum lacrimale occlusion *see* Obstruction, lacrimal
Puncture
|abdomen, abdominal
  |wall S31.139
    |with
      |foreign body S31.149
      |penetration into peritoneal cavity S31.639
        |with foreign body S31.649
    |epigastric region S31.132
      |with
        |foreign body S31.142

Puncture - continued

        |penetration into peritoneal cavity S31.632
          |with foreign body S31.642
  |left
    |lower quadrant S31.134
      |with
        |foreign body S31.144
        |penetration into peritoneal cavity S31.634
          |with foreign body S31.644
    |upper quadrant S31.131
      |with
        |foreign body S31.141
        |penetration into peritoneal cavity S31.631
          |with foreign body S31.641
  |periumbilic region S31.135
    |with
      |foreign body S31.145
      |penetration into peritoneal cavity S31.635
        |with foreign body S31.645
  |right
    |lower quadrant S31.133
      |with
        |foreign body S31.143
        |penetration into peritoneal cavity S31.633
          |with foreign body S31.643
    |upper quadrant S31.130
      |with
        |foreign body S31.140
        |penetration into peritoneal cavity S31.630
          |with foreign body S31.640
|accidental, complicating surgery *see* Complication, accidental puncture or laceration
|alveolar (process) *see* Puncture, oral cavity
|ankle S91.039
  |with
    |foreign body S91.049
  |left S91.032
    |with
      |foreign body S91.042
  |right S91.031
    |with
      |foreign body S91.041
|anus S31.833
  |with foreign body S31.834
|arm (upper) S41.139
  |with foreign body S41.149
  |left S41.132
    |with foreign body S41.142
  |lower *see* Puncture, forearm
  |right S41.131
    |with foreign body S41.141
|auditory canal (external) (meatus) *see* Puncture, ear
|auricle, ear *see* Puncture, ear
|axilla *see* Puncture, arm
|back *see also* Puncture, thorax, back
  |lower S31.030
    |with
      |foreign body S31.040
        |with penetration into retroperitoneal space S31.041
      |penetration into retroperitoneal space S31.031
|bladder (traumatic) S37.29
  |nontraumatic N32.89
|breast S21.039
  |with foreign body S21.049

Puncture - continued

    |left S21.032
      |with foreign body S21.042
    |right S21.031
      |with foreign body S21.041
  |buttock S31.803
    |with foreign body S31.804
    |left S31.823
      |with foreign body S31.824
    |right S31.813
      |with foreign body S31.814
  |by
    |device, implant or graft *see* Complications, by site and type, mechanical
    |foreign body left accidentally in operative wound T81.539
    |instrument (any) during a procedure, accidental *see* Puncture, accidental complicating surgery
  |calf *see* Puncture, leg
  |canaliculus lacrimalis *see* Puncture, eyelid
  |canthus, eye *see* Puncture, eyelid
  |cervical esophagus S11.23
    |with foreign body S11.24
  |cheek (external) S01.439
    |with foreign body S01.449
    |left S01.432
      |with foreign body S01.442
    |right S01.431
      |with foreign body S01.441
    |internal *see* Puncture, oral cavity
  |chest wall *see* Puncture, thorax
  |chin *see* Puncture, head, specified site NEC
  |clitoris *see* Puncture, vulva
  |costal region *see* Puncture, thorax
  |digit(s)
    |hand *see* Puncture, finger
    |foot *see* Puncture, toe
  |ear (canal) (external) S01.339
    |with foreign body S01.349
    |left S01.332
      |with foreign body S01.342
    |right S01.331
      |with foreign body S01.341
    |drum S09.2-
  |elbow S51.039
    |with
      |foreign body S51.049
    |left S51.032
      |with
        |foreign body S51.042
    |right S51.031
      |with
        |foreign body S51.041
  |epididymis *see* Puncture, testis
  |epigastric region *see* Puncture, abdomen, wall, epigastric
  |epiglottis S11.83
    |with foreign body S11.84
  |esophagus
    |cervical S11.23
      |with foreign body S11.24
    |thoracic S27.818
  |eyeball S05.6-
    |with foreign body S05.5-
  |eyebrow *see* Puncture, eyelid
  |eyelid S01.13-
    |with foreign body S01.14-
    |left S01.132
      |with foreign body S01.142
    |right S01.131
      |with foreign body S01.141
  |face NEC *see* Puncture, head, specified site NEC
  |finger(s) S61.239

Purpura - *continued*
| symptomatica D69.0
| telangiectasia annularis L81.7
| thrombocytopenic D69.49
  | congenital D69.42
  | hemorrhagic D69.3
  | hereditary D69.42
  | idiopathic D69.3
  | immune D69.3
  | neonatal, transitory P61.0
  | thrombotic M31.19
| thrombohemolytic *see* Fibrinolysis
| thrombolytic *see* Fibrinolysis
| thrombopenic D69.49
| thrombotic, thrombocytopenic M31.19
| toxic D69.0
| vascular D69.0
| visceral symptoms D69.0
Purpuric spots R23.3
Purulent *see* condition
Pus
| in
  | stool R19.5
  | urine N39.0
| tube (rupture) *see* Salpingo-oophoritis
Pustular rash L08.0
Pustule (nonmalignant) L08.9
| malignant A22.0
Pustulosis palmaris et plantaris L40.3
Putnam (-Dana) disease or syndrome *see*
  Degeneration, combined
Putrescent pulp (dental) K04.1
Pyarthritis, pyarthrosis *see* Arthritis, pyogenic
  or pyemic
| tuberculous *see* Tuberculosis, joint
Pyelectasis *see* Hydronephrosis
Pyelitis (congenital) (uremic) *see also*
  Pyelonephritis
| with
  | calculus *see* category N20
    | with hydronephrosis N13.2
  | contracted kidney N11.9
| acute N10
| chronic N11.9
  | with calculus *see* category N20
    | with hydronephrosis N13.2
| cystica N28.84
| puerperal (postpartum) O86.21
| tuberculous A18.11
Pyelocystitis *see* Pyelonephritis
Pyelonephritis *see also* Nephritis, tubulo-
  interstitial
| with
  | calculus *see* category N20
    | with hydronephrosis N13.2
  | contracted kidney N11.9
| acute N10
| calculous *see* category N20
  | with hydronephrosis N13.2
| chronic N11.9
  | with calculus *see* category N20
    | with hydronephrosis N13.2
  | associated with ureteral obstruction or
    stricture N11.1
  | nonobstructive N11.8
    | with reflux (vesicoureteral) N11.0
  | obstructive N11.1
  | specified NEC N11.8
| in (due to)
  | brucellosis A23.9 *[N16]*
  | cryoglobulinemia (mixed) D89.1 *[N16]*
  | cystinosis E72.04
  | diphtheria A36.84
  | glycogen storage disease E74.09 *[N16]*
  | leukemia NEC C95.9 *[N16]*

Pyelonephritis - *continued*
  | lymphoma NEC C85.90 *[N16]*
  | multiple myeloma C90.0 *[N16]*
  | obstruction N11.1
  | Salmonella infection A02.25
  | sarcoidosis D86.84
  | sepsis A41.9 *[N16]*
  | Sjögren's disease M35.04
  | toxoplasmosis B58.83
  | transplant rejection T86.91 *[N16]*
  | Wilson's disease E83.01 *[N16]*
| nonobstructive N12
  | with reflux (vesicoureteral) N11.0
  | chronic N11.8
| syphilitic A52.75
Pyelonephrosis (obstructive) N11.1
| chronic N11.9
Pyelophlebitis I80.8
Pyeloureteritis cystica N28.85
Pyemia, pyemic (fever) (infection) (purulent)
  see also Sepsis
| joint *see* Arthritis, pyogenic or pyemic
| liver K75.1
| pneumococcal A40.3
| portal K75.1
| postvaccinal T88.0
| puerperal, postpartum, childbirth O85
| specified organism NEC A41.89
| tuberculous *see* Tuberculosis, miliary
Pygopagus Q89.4
Pyknoepilepsy (idiopathic) *see* Pyknolepsy
Pyknolepsy G40.A09
| intractable G40.A19
  | with status epilepticus G40.A11
  | without status epilepticus G40.A19
| not intractable G40.A09
  | with status epilepticus G40.A01
  | without status epilepticus G40.A09
Pylephlebitis K75.1
Pyle's syndrome Q78.5
Pylethrombophlebitis K75.1
Pylethrombosis K75.1
Pyloritis K29.90
| with bleeding K29.91
Pylorospasm (reflex) NEC K31.3
| congenital or infantile Q40.0
| newborn Q40.0
| neurotic F45.8
| psychogenic F45.8
Pylorus, pyloric *see* condition
Pyoarthrosis *see* Arthritis, pyogenic or pyemic
Pyocele
| mastoid *see* Mastoiditis, acute
| sinus (accessory) *see* Sinusitis
| turbinate (bone) J32.9
| urethra *see also* Urethritis N34.0
Pyocolpos *see* Vaginitis
Pyocystitis N30.80
| with hematuria N30.81
Pyoderma, pyodermia L08.0
| gangrenosum L88
| newborn P39.4
| phagedenic L88
| vegetans L08.81
Pyodermatitis L08.0
| vegetans L08.81
Pyogenic *see* condition
Pyohydronephrosis N13.6
Pyometra, pyometrium, pyometritis *see*
  Endometritis
Pyomyositis (tropical) *see* Myositis, infective
Pyonephritis N12
Pyonephrosis N13.6
| tuberculous A18.11

Pyo-Oophoritis *see* Salpingo-oophoritis
Pyo-Ovarium *see* Salpingo-oophoritis
Pyopericarditis, pyopericardium I30.1
Pyophlebitis *see* Phlebitis
Pyopneumopericardium I30.1
Pyopneumothorax (infective) J86.9
| with fistula J86.0
| tuberculous NEC A15.6
Pyosalpinx, pyosalpingitis *see also* Salpingo-
  oophoritis
Pyothorax J86.9
| with fistula J86.0
| tuberculous NEC A15.6
Pyoureter N28.89
| tuberculous A18.11
Pyramidopallidonigral syndrome G20
Pyrexia (of unknown origin) R50.9
| atmospheric T67.0
| during labor NEC O75.2
| heat T67.0
| newborn P81.9
  | environmentally-induced P81.0
| persistent R50.9
| puerperal O86.4
Pyroglobulinemia NEC E88.09
Pyromania F63.1
Pyrosis R12
Pyuria (bacterial) N39.0

Q

Q fever A78
| with pneumonia A78
Quadricuspid aortic valve Q23.8
Quadrilateral fever A78
Quadriparesis *see* Quadriplegia
| meaning muscle weakness M62.81
Quadriplegia G82.50
| complete
  | C1-C4 level G82.51
  | C5-C7 level G82.53
| congenital (cerebral) (spinal) G80.8
  | spastic G80.0
| embolic (current episode) I63.4-
| functional R53.2
| incomplete
  | C1-C4 level G82.52
  | C5-C7 level G82.54
| thrombotic (current episode) I63.3-
| traumatic code to injury with seventh
  character S
  | current episode *see* Injury, spinal (cord),
    cervical
Quadruplet, pregnancy *see* Pregnancy,
  quadruplet
Quarrelsomeness F60.3
Queensland fever A77.3
Quervain's disease M65.4
| thyroid E06.1
Queyrat's erythroplasia D07.4
| penis D07.4
| specified site *see* Neoplasm, skin, in situ
| unspecified site D07.4
Quincke's disease or edema T78.3
| hereditary D84.1
Quinsy (gangrenous) J36
Quintan fever A79.0
Quintuplet, pregnancy *see* Pregnancy,
  quintuplet

R

Rabbit fever *see* Tularemia
Rabies A82.9
| contact Z20.3
| exposure to Z20.3

Rabies - continued
|inoculation reaction see Complications, vaccination
|sylvatic A82.0
|urban A82.1
Rachischisis see Spina bifida
Rachitic see also condition
|deformities of spine (late effect) (sequelae) E64.3
|pelvis (late effect) (sequelae) E64.3
|with disproportion (fetopelvic) O33.0
|causing obstructed labor O65.0
Rachitis, rachitism (acute) (tarda) see also Rickets
|renalis N25.0
|sequelae E64.3
Radial nerve see condition
Radiation
|burn see Burn
|effects NOS T66
|sickness NOS T66
|therapy, encounter for Z51.0
Radiculitis (pressure) (vertebrogenic) see Radiculopathy
Radiculomyelitis see also Encephalitis
|toxic, due to
|Clostridium tetani A35
|Corynebacterium diphtheriae A36.82
Radiculopathy M54.10
|cervical region M54.12
|cervicothoracic region M54.13
|due to
|disc disorder
|C3 M50.11
|C4 M50.11
|C5 M50.121
|C6 M50.122
|C7 M50.123
|C8 M50.13
|displacement of intervertebral disc see Disorder, disc, with, radiculopathy
|leg M54.1-
|lumbar region M54.16
|lumbosacral region M54.17
|occipito-atlanto-axial region M54.11
|postherpetic B02.29
|sacrococcygeal region M54.18
|syphilitic A52.11
|thoracic region (with visceral pain) M54.14
|thoracolumbar region M54.15
Radiodermal burns (acute, chronic, or occupational) see Burn
Radiodermatitis L58.9
|acute L58.0
|chronic L58.1
Radiotherapy session Z51.0
RAEB (refractory anemia with excess blasts) D46.2-
Rage, meaning rabies see Rabies
Ragpicker's disease A22.1
Ragsorter's disease A22.1
Raillietiniasis B71.8
Railroad neurosis F48.8
Railway spine F48.8
Raised see also Elevated
|antibody titer R76.0
Rake teeth, tooth M26.39
Rales R09.89
Ramifying renal pelvis Q63.8
Ramsay-Hunt disease or syndrome see also Hunt's disease B02.21
|meaning dyssynergia cerebellaris myoclonica G11.19
Ranula K11.6
|congenital Q38.4

Rape
|adult
|confirmed T74.21
|suspected T76.21
|alleged, observation or examination, ruled out
|adult Z04.41
|child Z04.42
|child
|confirmed T74.22
|suspected T76.22
Rapid
|feeble pulse, due to shock, following injury T79.4
|heart (beat) R00.0
|psychogenic F45.8
|second stage (delivery) O62.3
|time-zone change syndrome G47.25
Rarefaction, bone see Disorder, bone, density and structure, specified NEC
Rash (toxic) R21
|canker A38.9
|diaper L22
|drug (internal use) L27.0
|contact see also Dermatitis, due to, drugs, external L25.1
|following immunization T88.1
|food see Dermatitis, due to, food
|heat L74.0
|napkin (psoriasiform) L22
|nettle see Urticaria
|pustular L08.0
|rose R21
|epidemic B06.9
|scarlet A38.9
|serum see also Reaction, serum T80.69
|wandering tongue K14.1
Rasmussen aneurysm see Tuberculosis, pulmonary
Rasmussen encephalitis G04.81
Rat-Bite fever A25.9
|due to Streptobacillus moniliformis A25.1
|spirochetal (morsus muris) A25.0
Rathke's pouch tumor D44.3
Raymond (-Cestan) syndrome I65.8
Raynaud's disease, phenomenon or syndrome (secondary) I73.00
|with gangrene (symmetric) I73.01
RDS (newborn) (type I) P22.0
|type II P22.1
Reaction see also Disorder
|adaptation see Disorder, adjustment
|adjustment (anxiety) (conduct disorder) (depressiveness) (distress) see Disorder, adjustment
|with
|mutism, elective (child) (adolescent) F94.0
|adverse
|food (any) (ingested) NEC T78.1
|anaphylactic see Shock, anaphylactic, due to food
|affective see Disorder, mood
|allergic see Allergy
|anaphylactic see Shock, anaphylactic
|anaphylactoid see Shock, anaphylactic
|anesthesia see Anesthesia, complication
|antitoxin (prophylactic) (therapeutic) see Complications, vaccination
|anxiety F41.1
|Arthus see Arthus' phenomenon
|asthenic F48.8
|combat and operational stress F43.0
|compulsive F42.8
|conversion F44.9
|crisis, acute F43.0

Reaction - continued
|deoxyribonuclease (DNA) (DNase) hypersensitivity D69.2
|depressive (single episode) F32.9
|affective (single episode) F31.4
|recurrent episode F33.9
|neurotic F34.1
|psychoneurotic F34.1
|psychotic F32.3
|recurrent see Disorder, depressive, recurrent
|dissociative F44.9
|drug NEC T88.7
|addictive see Dependence, drug
|transmitted via placenta or breast milk see Absorption, drug, addictive, through placenta
|allergic see Allergy, drug
|lichenoid L43.2
|newborn P93.8
|gray baby syndrome P93.0
|overdose or poisoning (by accident) see Table of Drugs and Chemicals, by drug, poisoning
|photoallergic L56.1
|phototoxic L56.0
|withdrawal see Dependence, by drug, with, withdrawal
|infant of dependent mother P96.1
|newborn P96.1
|wrong substance given or taken (by accident) see Table of Drugs and Chemicals, by drug, poisoning
|fear F40.9
|child (abnormal) F93.8
|febrile nonhemolytic transfusion (FNHTR) R50.84
|fluid loss, cerebrospinal G97.1
|foreign
|body NEC see Granuloma, foreign body
|in operative wound (inadvertently left) see Foreign body, accidentally left during a procedure
|substance accidentally left during a procedure (chemical) (powder) (talc) T81.60
|aseptic peritonitis T81.61
|body or object (instrument) (sponge) (swab) see Foreign body, accidentally left during a procedure
|specified reaction NEC T81.69
|grief see Disorder, adjustment
|Herxheimer's R68.89
|hyperkinetic see Hyperkinesia
|hypochondriacal F45.20
|hypoglycemic, due to insulin E16.0
|with coma (diabetic) see Diabetes, coma
|nondiabetic E15
|therapeutic misadventure see subcategory T38.3
|hypomanic F30.8
|hysterical F44.9
|immunization see Complications, vaccination
|incompatibility
|ABO blood group (infusion) (transfusion) see Complication(s), transfusion, incompatibility reaction, ABO
|delayed serologic T80.39
|minor blood group (Duffy) (E) (K) (Kell) (Kidd) (Lewis) (M) (N) (P) (S) T80.89
|Rh (factor) (infusion) (transfusion) see Complication(s), transfusion, incompatibility reaction, Rh (factor)
|inflammatory see Infection
|infusion see Complications, infusion
|inoculation (immune serum) see Complications, vaccination

Reaction - *continued*
|insulin T38.3-
|involutional psychotic *see* Disorder, depressive
|leukemoid D72.823
  |basophilic D72.823
  |lymphocytic D72.823
  |monocytic D72.823
  |myelocytic D72.823
  |neutrophilic D72.823
|LSD (acute)
  |due to drug abuse *see* Abuse, drug, hallucinogen
  |due to drug dependence *see* Dependence, drug, hallucinogen
|lumbar puncture G97.1
|manic-depressive *see* Disorder, bipolar
|neurasthenic F48.8
|neurogenic *see* Neurosis
|neurotic F48.9
|neurotic-depressive F34.1
|nitritoid *see* Crisis, nitritoid
|nonspecific
  |to
    |cell mediated immunity measurement of gamma interferon antigen response without active tuberculosis R76.12
    |QuantiFERON-TB test (QFT) without active tuberculosis R76.12
    |tuberculin test *see also* Reaction, tuberculin skin test R76.11
|obsessive-compulsive F42.8
|organic, acute or subacute *see* Delirium
|paranoid (acute) F23
  |chronic F22
  |senile F03
|passive dependency F60.7
|phobic F40.9
|post-traumatic stress, uncomplicated Z73.3
|psychogenic F99
|psychoneurotic *see also* Neurosis
  |compulsive F42.8
  |depersonalization F48.1
  |depressive F34.1
  |hypochondriacal F45.20
  |neurasthenic F48.8
  |obsessive F42.8
|psychophysiologic *see* Disorder, somatoform
|psychosomatic *see* Disorder, somatoform
|psychotic *see* Psychosis
|scarlet fever toxin *see* Complications, vaccination
|schizophrenic F23
  |acute (brief) (undifferentiated) F23
  |latent F21
  |undifferentiated (acute) (brief) F23
|serological for syphilis *see* Serology for syphilis
|serum T80.69
  |anaphylactic (immediate) *see also* Shock, anaphylactic T80.59
  |specified reaction NEC
    |due to
      |administration of blood and blood products T80.61
        |immunization T80.62
        |serum specified NEC T80.69
        |vaccination T80.62
|situational *see* Disorder, adjustment
|somatization *see* Disorder, somatoform
|spinal puncture G97.1
  |dural G97.1
|stress (severe) F43.9

Reaction - *continued*
|acute (agitation) ("daze") (disorientation) (disturbance of consciousness) (flight reaction) (fugue) F43.0
  |specified NEC F43.8
|surgical procedure *see* Complications, surgical procedure
|tetanus antitoxin *see* Complications, vaccination
|toxic, to local anesthesia T88.59
  |in labor and delivery O74.4
  |in pregnancy O29.3X-
  |postpartum, puerperal O89.3
|toxin-antitoxin *see* Complications, vaccination
|transfusion (blood) (bone marrow) (lymphocytes) (allergic) *see* Complications, transfusion
|tuberculin skin test, abnormal R76.11
|vaccination (any) *see* Complications, vaccination
|withdrawing, child or adolescent F93.8
Reactive airway disease *see* Asthma
Reactive depression *see* Reaction, depressive
Rearrangement
|chromosomal
  |balanced (in) Q95.9
    |abnormal individual (autosomal) Q95.2
      |non-sex (autosomal) chromosomes Q95.2
    |sex/non-sex chromosomes Q95.3
  |specified NEC Q95.8
Recalcitrant patient *see* Noncompliance
Recanalization, thrombus *see* Thrombosis
Recession, receding
|chamber angle (eye) H21.55-
|chin M26.09
|gingival (postinfective) (postoperative)
  |generalized K06.020
    |minimal K06.021
    |moderate K06.022
    |severe K06.023
  |localized K06.010
    |minimal K06.011
    |moderate K06.012
    |severe K06.013
Recklinghausen disease Q85.01
|bones E21.0
Reclus' disease (cystic) *see* Mastopathy, cystic
Recrudescent typhus (fever) A75.1
Recruitment, auditory H93.21-
Rectalgia K62.89
Rectitis K62.89
Rectocele
|female (without uterine prolapse) N81.6
  |with uterine prolapse N81.4
    |incomplete N81.2
|in pregnancy *see* Pregnancy, complicated by, abnormal, pelvic organs or tissues NEC
|male K62.3
Rectosigmoid junction *see* condition
Rectosigmoiditis K63.89
|ulcerative (chronic) K51.30
  |with
    |complication K51.319
      |abscess K51.314
      |fistula K51.313
      |obstruction K51.312
      |rectal bleeding K51.311
      |specified NEC K51.318
Rectourethral *see* condition
Rectovaginal *see* condition
Rectovesical *see* condition
Rectum, rectal *see* condition

Recurrent *see* condition
|pregnancy loss *see* Loss (of), pregnancy, recurrent
Red bugs B88.0
Red-Cedar lung or pneumonitis J67.8
Red tide *see also* Table of Drugs and Chemicals T65.82-
Reduced
|mobility Z74.09
|ventilatory or vital capacity R94.2
Redundant, redundancy
|anus (congenital) Q43.8
|clitoris N90.89
|colon (congenital) Q43.8
|foreskin (congenital) N47.8
|intestine (congenital) Q43.8
|labia N90.69
|organ or site, congenital NEC *see* Accessory
|panniculus (abdominal) E65
|prepuce (congenital) N47.8
|pylorus K31.89
|rectum (congenital) Q43.8
|scrotum N50.89
|sigmoid (congenital) Q43.8
|skin L98.7
  |and subcutaneous tissue L98.7
  |of face L57.4
    |eyelids *see* Blepharochalasis
|stomach K31.89
Reduplication *see* Duplication
Reflex R29.2
|hyperactive gag J39.2
|pupillary, abnormal *see* Anomaly, pupil, function
|vasoconstriction I73.9
|vasovagal R55
Reflux K21.9
|acid K21.9
|esophageal K21.9
  |with esophagitis K21.0
  |newborn P78.83
|gastroesophageal K21.9
  |with esophagitis (without bleeding) K21.00
    |with bleeding K21.01
|mitral *see* Insufficiency, mitral
|ureteral *see* Reflux, vesicoureteral
|vesicoureteral (with scarring) N13.70
  |with
    |nephropathy N13.729
      |with hydroureter N13.739
        |bilateral N13.732
        |unilateral N13.731
      |bilateral N13.722
      |unilateral N13.721
    |without hydroureter N13.729
      |bilateral N13.722
      |unilateral N13.721
    |pyelonephritis (chronic) N11.0
  |congenital Q62.7
  |without nephropathy N13.71
Reforming, artificial openings *see* Attention to, artificial, opening
Refractive error *see* Disorder, refraction
Refsum's disease or syndrome G60.1
Refusal of
|food, psychogenic F50.89
|treatment (because of) Z53.20
  |left against medical advice (AMA) Z53.29
  |left without being seen Z53.21
  |patient's decision NEC Z53.29
  |reasons of belief or group pressure Z53.1
Regional *see* condition
Regurgitation R11.10
|aortic (valve) *see* Insufficiency, aortic
|food *see also* Vomiting
  |with reswallowing *see* Rumination
  |newborn P92.1

Regurgitation - *continued*
|gastric contents *see* Vomiting
|heart *see* Endocarditis
|mitral (valve) *see* Insufficiency, mitral
| |congenital Q23.3
|myocardial *see* Endocarditis
|pulmonary (valve) (heart) I37.1
| |congenital Q22.2
| |syphilitic A52.03
|tricuspid *see* Insufficiency, tricuspid
|valve, valvular *see* Endocarditis
| |congenital Q24.8
|vesicoureteral *see* Reflux, vesicoureteral
Reifenstein syndrome E34.52
Reinsertion
|implantable subdermal contraceptive Z30.46
|intrauterine contraceptive device Z30.433
Reiter's disease, syndrome, or urethritis
   M02.30
|ankle M02.37-
|elbow M02.32-
|foot joint M02.37-
|hand joint M02.34-
|hip M02.35-
|knee M02.36-
|multiple site M02.39
|shoulder M02.31-
|vertebra M02.38
|wrist M02.33-
Reichmann's disease or syndrome K31.89
Rejection
|food, psychogenic F50.89
|transplant T86.91
| |bone T86.830
| | |marrow T86.01
| |cornea T86.840-
| |heart T86.21
| | |with lung(s) T86.31
| |intestine T86.850
| |kidney T86.11
| |liver T86.41
| |lung(s) T86.810
| | |with heart T86.31
| |organ (immune or nonimmune cause)
| | T86.91
| |pancreas T86.890
| |skin (allograft) (autograft) T86.820
| |specified NEC T86.890
| |stem cell (peripheral blood) (umbilical cord)
| | T86.5
Relapsing fever A68.9
|Carter's (Asiatic) A68.1
|Dutton's (West African) A68.1
|Koch's A68.9
|louse-borne (epidemic) A68.0
|Novy's (American) A68.1
|Obermeyer's (European) A68.0
|Spirillum A68.9
|tick-borne (endemic) A68.1
Relationship
|occlusal
| |open anterior M26.220
| |open posterior M26.221
Relaxation
|anus (sphincter) K62.89
| |psychogenic F45.8
|arch (foot) *see also* Deformity, limb, flat foot
|back ligaments *see* Instability, joint, spine
|bladder (sphincter) N31.2
|cardioesophageal K21.9
|cervix *see* Incompetency, cervix
|diaphragm J98.6
|joint (capsule) (ligament) (paralytic) *see* Flail,
| joint
| |congenital NEC Q74.8
|lumbosacral (joint) *see* subcategory M53.2

Relaxation - *continued*
|pelvic floor N81.89
|perineum N81.89
|posture R29.3
|rectum (sphincter) K62.89
|sacroiliac (joint) *see* subcategory M53.2
|scrotum N50.89
|urethra (sphincter) N36.44
|vesical N31.2
Release from prison, anxiety concerning Z65.2
Remains
|canal of Cloquet Q14.0
|capsule (opaque) Q14.8
Remittent fever (malarial) B54
Remnant
|canal of Cloquet Q14.0
|capsule (opaque) Q14.8
|cervix, cervical stump (acquired)
| (postoperative) N88.8
|cystic duct, postcholecystectomy K91.5
|fingernail L60.8
| |congenital Q84.6
|meniscus, knee *see* Derangement, knee,
| meniscus, specified NEC
|thyroglossal duct Q89.2
|tonsil J35.8
| |infected (chronic) J35.01
|urachus Q64.4
Removal (from) (of)
|artificial
| |arm Z44.00-
| | |complete Z44.01-
| | |partial Z44.02-
| |eye Z44.2-
| |leg Z44.10-
| | |complete Z44.11-
| | |partial Z44.12-
|breast implant Z45.81
|cardiac pulse generator (battery) (end-of-life)
| Z45.010
|catheter (urinary) (indwelling) Z46.6
| |from artificial opening *see* Attention to,
| | artificial, opening
| |non-vascular Z46.82
| |vascular NEC Z45.2
|drains Z48.03
|device Z46.9
| |contraceptive Z30.432
| | |implantable subdermal Z30.46
| |implanted NEC Z45.89
| |specified NEC Z46.89
|dressing (nonsurgical) Z48.00
| |surgical Z48.01
|external
| |fixation device   code to fracture with
| | seventh character D
| |prosthesis, prosthetic device Z44.9
| | |breast Z44.3-
| | |specified NEC Z44.8
|home in childhood (to foster home or
| institution) Z62.29
|ileostomy Z43.2
|insulin pump Z46.81
|myringotomy device (stent) (tube) Z45.82
|nervous system device NEC Z46.2
| |brain neuropacemaker Z46.2
| |visual substitution device Z46.2
| | |implanted Z45.31
|non-vascular catheter Z46.82
|orthodontic device Z46.4
|organ, prophylactic (for neoplasia
| management) *see* Prophylactic, organ
| removal
|staples Z48.02
|stent

Removal (from) (of) - *continued*
|ureteral Z46.6
|suture Z48.02
|urinary device Z46.6
|vascular access device or catheter Z45.2
Ren
|arcuatus Q63.1
|mobile, mobilis N28.89
| |congenital Q63.8
|unguliformis Q63.1
Renal *see* condition
Rendu-Osler-Weber disease or syndrome
   I78.0
Reninoma D41.0-
Renon-Delille syndrome E23.3
Reovirus, as cause of disease classified
   elsewhere B97.5
Repeated falls NEC R29.6
Replaced chromosome by dicentric ring Q93.2
Replacement by artificial or mechanical
   device or prosthesis of
|bladder Z96.0
|blood vessel NEC Z95.828
|bone NEC Z96.7
|cochlea Z96.21
|coronary artery Z95.5
|eustachian tube Z96.29
|eye globe Z97.0
|heart Z95.812
| |valve Z95.2
| | |prosthetic Z95.2
| | |specified NEC Z95.4
| | |xenogenic Z95.3
|intestine Z96.89
|joint Z96.60
| |hip *see* Presence, hip joint implant
| |knee *see* Presence, knee joint implant
| |specified site NEC Z96.698
|larynx Z96.3
|lens Z96.1
|limb(s) *see* Presence, artificial, limb
|mandible NEC (for tooth root implant(s))
| Z96.5
|organ NEC Z96.89
|peripheral vessel NEC Z95.828
|stapes Z96.29
|teeth Z97.2
|tendon Z96.7
|tissue NEC Z96.89
|tooth root(s) Z96.5
|vessel NEC Z95.828
| |coronary (artery) Z95.5
Request for expert evidence Z04.89
Reserve, decreased or low
|cardiac *see* Disease, heart
|kidney N28.89
Residing
- in place not meant for human habitation
(abandoned building) (car) (park) (sidewalk)
Z59.02
- on the street Z59.02
Residual *see also* condition
|ovary syndrome N99.83
|state, schizophrenic F20.5
|urine R39.198
Resistance, resistant (to)
|activated protein C D68.51
|complicating pregnancy O26.89
|insulin E88.81
|organism(s)
| |to
| | |drug Z16.30
| | | |aminoglycosides Z16.29
| | | |amoxicillin Z16.11
| | | |ampicillin Z16.11

Resistance, resistant (to) - *continued*
  |antibiotic(s) Z16.20
    |multiple Z16.24
    |specified NEC Z16.29
  |antifungal Z16.32
  |antimicrobial (single) Z16.30
    |multiple Z16.35
    |specified NEC Z16.39
  |antimycobacterial (single) Z16.341
    |multiple Z16.342
  |antiparasitic Z16.31
  |antiviral Z16.33
  |beta lactam antibiotics Z16.10
    |specified NEC Z16.19
  |cephalosporins Z16.19
  |extended beta lactamase (ESBL) Z16.12
  |fluoroquinolones Z16.23
  |macrolides Z16.29
  |methicillin *see* MRSA
  |multiple drugs (MDRO)
    |antibiotics Z16.24
    |antimicrobial Z16.35
    |antimycobacterials Z16.342
  |penicillins Z16.11
  |quinine (and related compounds)
  Z16.31
    |quinolones Z16.23
    |sulfonamides Z16.29
    |tetracyclines Z16.29
  |tuberculostatics (single) Z16.341
    |multiple Z16.342
  |vancomycin Z16.21
    |related antibiotics Z16.22
  |thyroid hormone E07.89
Resorption
  |dental (roots) K03.3
    |alveoli M26.79
  |teeth (external) (internal) (pathological)
  (roots) K03.3
Respiration
  |Cheyne-Stokes R06.3
  |decreased due to shock, following injury
  T79.4
  |disorder of, psychogenic F45.8
  |insufficient, or poor R06.89
    |newborn P28.5
  |painful R07.1
  |sighing, psychogenic F45.8
Respiratory *see also* condition
  |distress syndrome (newborn) (type I) P22.0
    |type II P22.1
  |syncytial virus, as cause of disease classified
  elsewhere B97.4
Respite care Z75.5
Response (drug)
  |photoallergic L56.1
  |phototoxic L56.0
Restenosis
  |stent
    |vascular
      |end stent
        |adjacent to stent *see* Arteriosclerosis
        |within the stent
          |coronary T82.855
          |peripheral T82.856
      |in stent
        |coronary vessel T82.855
        |peripheral vessel T82.856
Restless legs (syndrome) G25.81
Restlessness R45.1
Restriction of housing space Z59.1

Restoration (of)
  |dental
    |aesthetically inadequate or displeasing
    K08.56
    |defective K08.50
      |specified NEC K08.59
    |failure of marginal integrity K08.51
    |failure of periodontal anatomical integrity
    K08.54
  |organ continuity from previous sterilization
  (tuboplasty) (vasoplasty) Z31.0
    |aftercare Z31.42
  |tooth (existing)
    |contours biologically incompatible with oral
    health K08.54
    |open margins K08.51
    |overhanging K08.52
    |poor aesthetic K08.56
    |poor gingival margins K08.51
    |unsatisfactory, of tooth K08.50
      |specified NEC K08.59
Restorative material (dental)
  |allergy to K08.55
  |fractured K08.539
    |with loss of material K08.531
    |without loss of material K08.530
  |unrepairable overhanging of K08.52
Rests, ovarian, in fallopian tube Q50.6
Restzustand (schizophrenic) F20.5
Retained *see also* Retention
  |cholelithiasis following cholecystectomy
  K91.86
  |foreign body fragments (type of) Z18.9
    |acrylics Z18.2
    |animal quill(s) or spines Z18.31
    |cement Z18.83
    |concrete Z18.83
    |crystalline Z18.83
    |depleted isotope Z18.09
    |depleted uranium Z18.01
    |diethylhexyl phthalates Z18.2
    |glass Z18.81
    |isocyanate Z18.2
    |magnetic metal Z18.11
    |metal Z18.10
    |nonmagnetic metal Z18.12
    |nontherapeutic radioactive Z18.09
    |organic NEC Z18.39
    |plastic Z18.2
    |quill(s) (animal) Z18.31
    |radioactive (nontherapeutic) NEC Z18.09
    |specified NEC Z18.89
    |spine(s) (animal) Z18.31
    |stone Z18.83
    |tooth (teeth) Z18.32
    |wood Z18.33
  |fragments (type of) Z18.9
    |acrylics Z18.2
    |animal quill(s) or spines Z18.31
    |cement Z18.83
    |concrete Z18.83
    |crystalline Z18.83
    |depleted isotope Z18.09
    |depleted uranium Z18.01
    |diethylhexyl phthalates Z18.2
    |glass Z18.81
    |isocyanate Z18.2
    |magnetic metal Z18.11
    |metal Z18.10
    |nonmagnetic metal Z18.12
    |nontherapeutic radioactive Z18.09
    |organic NEC Z18.39
    |plastic Z18.2

Retained - *continued*
    |quill(s) (animal) Z18.31
    |radioactive (nontherapeutic) NEC Z18.09
    |specified NEC Z18.89
    |spine(s) (animal) Z18.31
    |stone Z18.83
    |tooth (teeth) Z18.32
    |wood Z18.33
  |gallstones, following cholecystectomy K91.86
Retardation
  |development, developmental, specific *see*
  Disorder, developmental
  |endochondral bone growth *see* Disorder, bone,
  development or growth
  |growth R62.50
    |due to malnutrition E45
  |mental *see* Disability, intellectual
  |motor function, specific F82
  |physical (child) R62.52
    |due to malnutrition E45
  |reading (specific) F81.0
  |spelling (specific) (without reading disorder)
  F81.81
Retching *see* Vomiting
Retention *see also* Retained
  |bladder *see* Retention, urine
  |carbon dioxide E87.2
  |cholelithiasis following cholecystectomy
  K91.86
  |cyst *see* Cyst
  |dead
    |fetus (at or near term) (mother) O36.4
      |early fetal death O02.1
    |ovum O02.0
  |decidua (fragments) (following delivery) (with
  hemorrhage) O72.2
    |without hemorrhage O73.1
  |deciduous tooth K00.6
  |dental root K08.3
  |fecal *see* Constipation
  |fetus
    |dead O36.4
      |early O02.1
  |fluid R60.9
  |foreign body *see also* Foreign body, retained
    |current trauma   code as Foreign body, by
    site or type
  |gallstones, following cholecystectomy K91.86
  |gastric K31.89
  |intrauterine contraceptive device, in
  pregnancy *see* Pregnancy, complicated by,
  retention, intrauterine device
  |membranes (complicating delivery) (with
  hemorrhage) O72.2
    |with abortion *see* Abortion, by type
    |without hemorrhage O73.1
  |meniscus *see* Derangement, meniscus
  |menses N94.89
  |milk (puerperal, postpartum) O92.79
  |nitrogen, extrarenal R39.2
  |ovary syndrome N99.83
  |placenta (total) (with hemorrhage) O72.0
    |without hemorrhage O73.0
    |portions or fragments (with hemorrhage)
    O72.2
    |without hemorrhage O73.1
  |products of conception
    |early pregnancy (dead fetus) O02.1
    |following
      |delivery (with hemorrhage) O72.2
        |without hemorrhage O73.1
  |secundines (following delivery) (with
  hemorrhage) O72.0
    |without hemorrhage O73.0

Retention - *continued*
- |complicating puerperium (delayed hemorrhage) O72.2
- |partial O72.2
  - |without hemorrhage O73.1
- |smegma, clitoris N90.89
- |urine R33.9
  - |due to hyperplasia (hypertrophy) of prostate *see* Hyperplasia, prostate
  - |drug-induced R33.0
  - |organic R33.8
    - |drug-induced R33.0
  - |psychogenic F45.8
  - |specified NEC R33.8
- |water (in tissues) *see* Edema

Reticular erythematous mucinosis L98.5
Reticulation, dust *see* Pneumoconiosis
Reticulocytosis R70.1
Reticuloendotheliosis
- |acute infantile C96.0
- |leukemic C91.4-
- |nonlipid C96.0

Reticulohistiocytoma (giant-Cell) D76.3
Reticuloid, actinic L57.1
Reticulosis (skin)
- |acute of infancy C96.0
- |hemophagocytic, familial D76.1
- |histiocytic medullary C96.A
- |lipomelanotic I89.8
- |malignant (midline) C86.0
- |polymorphic C86.0
- |Sézary *see* Sézary disease

Retina, retinal *see also* condition
- |dark area D49.81

Retinitis *see also* Inflammation, chorioretinal
- |albuminurica N18.9 *[H32]*
- |diabetic *see* Diabetes, retinitis
- |disciformis *see* Degeneration, macula
- |focal *see* Inflammation, chorioretinal, focal
- |gravidarum *see* Pregnancy, complicated by, specified pregnancy-related condition NEC
- |juxtapapillaris *see* Inflammation, chorioretinal, focal, juxtapapillary
- |luetic *see* Retinitis, syphilitic
- |pigmentosa H35.52
- |proliferans *see* Disorder, globe, degenerative, specified type NEC
- |proliferating *see* Disorder, globe, degenerative, specified type NEC
- |renal N18.9 *[H32]*
- |syphilitic (early) (secondary) A51.43
  - |central, recurrent A52.71
  - |congenital (early) A50.01 *[H32]*
  - |late A52.71
- |tuberculous A18.53

Retinoblastoma C69.2-
- |differentiated C69.2-
- |undifferentiated C69.2-

Retinochoroiditis *see also* Inflammation, chorioretinal
- |disseminated *see* Inflammation, chorioretinal, disseminated
  - |syphilitic A52.71
- |focal *see* Inflammation, chorioretinal
- |juxtapapillaris *see* Inflammation, chorioretinal, focal, juxtapapillary

Retinopathy (background) H35.00
- |arteriosclerotic I70.8 *[H35.0]*
- |atherosclerotic I70.8 *[H35.0]*
- |central serous *see* Chorioretinopathy, central serous
- |Coats H35.02-

Retinopathy (background) - *continued*
- |diabetic *see* Diabetes, retinopathy
- |exudative H35.02-
- |hypertensive H35.03-
- |in (due to)
  - |diabetes *see* Diabetes, retinopathy
  - |sickle-cell disorders D57. *[H36]*
- |of prematurity H35.10-
  - |stage 0 H35.11-
  - |stage 1 H35.12-
  - |stage 2 H35.13-
  - |stage 3 H35.14-
  - |stage 4 H35.15-
  - |stage 5 H35.16-
- |pigmentary, congenital *see* Dystrophy, retina
- |proliferative NEC H35.2-
  - |diabetic *see* Diabetes, retinopathy, proliferative
  - |sickle-cell D57. *[H36]*
- |solar H31.02-

Retinoschisis H33.10-
- |congenital Q14.1
- |specified type NEC H33.19-

Retortamoniasis A07.8
Retractile testis Q55.22
Retraction
- |cervix *see* Retroversion, uterus
- |drum (membrane) *see* Disorder, tympanic membrane, specified NEC
- |finger *see* Deformity, finger
- |lid H02.539
  - |left H02.536
    - |lower H02.535
    - |upper H02.534
  - |right H02.533
    - |lower H02.532
    - |upper H02.531
- |lung J98.4
- |mediastinum J98.59
- |nipple N64.53
  - |associated with
    - |lactation O92.03
    - |pregnancy O92.01-
    - |puerperium O92.02
  - |congenital Q83.8
- |palmar fascia M72.0
- |pleura *see* Pleurisy
- |ring, uterus (Bandl's) (pathological) O62.4
- |sternum (congenital) Q76.7
  - |acquired M95.4
- |uterus *see* Retroversion, uterus
- |valve (heart) *see* Endocarditis

Retrobulbar *see* condition
Retrocecal *see* condition
Retrocession *see* Retroversion
Retrodisplacement *see* Retroversion
Retroflection, retroflexion *see* Retroversion
Retrognathia, retrognathism (mandibular) (maxillary) M26.19
Retrograde menstruation N92.5
Retroperineal *see* condition
Retroperitoneal *see* condition
Retroperitonitis K68.9
Retropharyngeal *see* condition
Retroplacental *see* condition
Retroposition *see* Retroversion
Retroprosthetic membrane T85.398
Retrosternal thyroid (congenital) Q89.2
Retroversion, retroverted
- |cervix *see* Retroversion, uterus
- |female NEC *see* Retroversion, uterus
- |iris H21.89
- |testis (congenital) Q55.29

Retroversion, retroverted - *continued*
- |uterus (acquired) (acute) (any degree) (asymptomatic) (cervix) (postinfectional) (postpartal, old) N85.4
  - |congenital Q51.818
  - |in pregnancy O34.53-

Retrovirus, as cause of disease classified elsewhere B97.30
- |human
  - |immunodeficiency, type 2 (HIV 2) B97.35
  - |T-cell lymphotropic
    - |type I (HTLV-I) B97.33
    - |type II (HTLV-II) B97.34
- |lentivirus B97.31
- |oncovirus B97.32
- |specified NEC B97.39

Retrusion, premaxilla (developmental) M26.09
Rett's disease or syndrome F84.2
Reverse peristalsis R19.2
Reye's syndrome G93.7
Rh (factor)
- |hemolytic disease (newborn) P55.0
- |incompatibility, immunization or sensitization
  - |affecting management of pregnancy NEC O36.09-
    - |anti-D antibody O36.01-
  - |newborn P55.0
  - |transfusion reaction *see* Complication(s), transfusion, incompatibility reaction, Rh (factor)
- |negative mother affecting newborn P55.0
- |titer elevated *see* Complication(s), transfusion, incompatibility reaction, Rh (factor)
- |transfusion reaction *see* Complication(s), transfusion, incompatibility reaction, Rh (factor)

Rhabdomyolysis (idiopathic) NEC M62.82
- |traumatic T79.6

Rhabdomyoma *see also* Neoplasm, connective tissue, benign
- |adult *see* Neoplasm, connective tissue, benign
- |fetal *see* Neoplasm, connective tissue, benign
- |glycogenic *see* Neoplasm, connective tissue, benign

Rhabdomyosarcoma (any type) *see* Neoplasm, connective tissue, malignant
Rhabdosarcoma *see* Rhabdomyosarcoma
Rhesus (factor) incompatibility *see* Rh, incompatibility
Rheumatic (acute) (subacute) (chronic)
- |adherent pericardium I09.2
- |coronary arteritis I01.9
- |degeneration, myocardium I09.0
- |fever (acute) *see* Fever, rheumatic
- |heart *see* Disease, heart, rheumatic
- |myocardial degeneration *see* Degeneration, myocardium
- |myocarditis (chronic) (inactive) (with chorea) I09.0
  - |active or acute I01.2
    - |with chorea (acute) (rheumatic) (Sydenham's) I02.0
- |pancarditis, acute I01.8
  - |with chorea (acute) (rheumatic) Sydenham's I02.0
- |pericarditis (active) (acute) (with effusion) (with pneumonia) I01.0
  - |with chorea (acute) (rheumatic) (Sydenham's) I02.0
  - |chronic or inactive I09.2
- |pneumonia I00 *[J17]*
- |torticollis M43.6
- |typhoid fever A01.09

Rheumatism (articular) (neuralgic) (nonarticular) M79.0
|gout *see* Arthritis, rheumatoid
|intercostal, meaning Tietze's disease M94.0
|palindromic (any site) M12.30
  |ankle M12.37-
  |elbow M12.32-
  |foot joint M12.37-
  |hand joint M12.34-
  |hip M12.35-
  |knee M12.36-
  |multiple site M12.39
  |shoulder M12.31-
  |specified joint NEC M12.38
  |vertebrae M12.38
  |wrist M12.33-
|sciatic M54.4-
Rheumatoid *see also* condition
|arthritis *see also* Arthritis, rheumatoid
  |with involvement of organs NEC M05.60
    |ankle M05.67-
    |elbow M05.62-
    |foot joint M05.67-
    |hand joint M05.64-
    |hip M05.65-
    |knee M05.66-
    |multiple site M05.69
    |shoulder M05.61-
    |vertebra *see* Spondylitis, ankylosing
    |wrist M05.63-
  |seronegative *see* Arthritis, rheumatoid, seronegative
  |seropositive *see* Arthritis, rheumatoid, seropositive
|carditis M05.30
  |ankle M05.37-
  |elbow M05.32-
  |foot joint M05.37-
  |hand joint M05.34-
  |hip M05.35-
  |knee M05.36-
  |multiple site M05.39
  |shoulder M05.31-
  |vertebra *see* Spondylitis, ankylosing
  |wrist M05.33-
|endocarditis *see* Rheumatoid, carditis
|lung (disease) M05.10
  |ankle M05.17-
  |elbow M05.12-
  |foot joint M05.17-
  |hand joint M05.14-
  |hip M05.15-
  |knee M05.16-
  |multiple site M05.19
  |shoulder M05.11-
  |vertebra *see* Spondylitis, ankylosing
  |wrist M05.13-
|myocarditis *see* Rheumatoid, carditis
|myopathy M05.40
  |ankle M05.47-
  |elbow M05.42-
  |foot joint M05.47-
  |hand joint M05.44-
  |hip M05.45-
  |knee M05.46-
  |multiple site M05.49
  |shoulder M05.41-
  |vertebra *see* Spondylitis, ankylosing
  |wrist M05.43-
|pericarditis *see* Rheumatoid, carditis
|polyarthritis *see* Arthritis, rheumatoid
|polyneuropathy M05.50
  |ankle M05.57-
  |elbow M05.52-
  |foot joint M05.57-

Rheumatoid - *continued*
|hand joint M05.54-
|hip M05.55-
|knee M05.56-
|multiple site M05.59
|shoulder M05.51-
|vertebra *see* Spondylitis, ankylosing
|wrist M05.53-
|vasculitis M05.20
  |ankle M05.27-
  |elbow M05.22-
  |foot joint M05.27-
  |hand joint M05.24-
  |hip M05.25-
  |knee M05.26-
  |multiple site M05.29
  |shoulder M05.21-
  |vertebra *see* Spondylitis, ankylosing
  |wrist M05.23-
Rhinitis (atrophic) (catarrhal) (chronic) (croupous) (fibrinous) (granulomatous) (hyperplastic) (hypertrophic) (membranous) (obstructive) (purulent) (suppurative) (ulcerative) J31.0
|with
  |sore throat *see* Nasopharyngitis
|acute J00
|allergic J30.9
  |with asthma J45.909
    |with
      |exacerbation (acute) J45.901
      |status asthmaticus J45.902
  |due to
    |food J30.5
    |pollen J30.1
  |nonseasonal J30.89
  |perennial J30.89
  |seasonal NEC J30.2
  |specified NEC J30.89
|infective J00
|pneumococcal J00
|syphilitic A52.73
  |congenital A50.05 [*J99*]
|tuberculous A15.8
|vasomotor J30.0
Rhinoantritis (chronic) *see* Sinusitis, maxillary
Rhinodacryolith *see* Dacryolith
Rhinolith (nasal sinus) J34.89
Rhinomegaly J34.89
Rhinopharyngitis (acute) (subacute) *see also* Nasopharyngitis
|chronic J31.1
|destructive ulcerating A66.5
|mutilans A66.5
Rhinophyma L71.1
Rhinorrhea J34.89
|cerebrospinal (fluid) G96.01
  |postoperative G96.08
  |specified NEC G96.08
  |spontaneous G96.01
  |traumatic G96.08
|paroxysmal *see* Rhinitis, allergic
|spasmodic *see* Rhinitis, allergic
Rhinosalpingitis *see* Salpingitis, eustachian
Rhinoscleroma A48.8
Rhinosporidiosis B48.1
Rhinovirus infection NEC B34.8
Rhizomelic chondrodysplasia punctata E71.540
Rhythm
|atrioventricular nodal I49.8
|disorder I49.9
  |coronary sinus I49.8
  |ectopic I49.8
  |nodal I49.8

Rhythm - *continued*
|escape I49.9
|heart, abnormal I49.9
|idioventricular I44.2
|nodal I49.8
|sleep, inversion G47.2-
  |nonorganic origin *see* Disorder, sleep, circadian rhythm, psychogenic
Rhytidosis facialis L98.8
Rib *see also* condition
|cervical Q76.5
Riboflavin deficiency E53.0
Rice bodies *see also* Loose, body, joint
|knee M23.4-
Richter syndrome *see* Leukemia, chronic lymphocytic, B-cell type
Richter's hernia *see* Hernia, abdomen, with obstruction
Ricinism *see* Poisoning, food, noxious, plant
Rickets (active) (acute) (adolescent) (chest wall) (congenital) (current) (infantile) (intestinal) E55.0
|adult *see* Osteomalacia
|celiac K90.0
|hypophosphatemic with nephrotic-glycosuric dwarfism E72.09
|inactive E64.3
|kidney N25.0
|renal N25.0
|sequelae, any E64.3
|vitamin-D-resistant E83.31 [*M90.80*]
Rickettsial disease A79.9
|specified type NEC A79.89
Rickettsialpox (Rickettsia akari) A79.1
Rickettsiosis A79.9
|due to
  |Ehrlichia sennetsu A79.81
  |Neorickettsia sennetsu A79.81
  |Rickettsia akari (rickettsialpox) A79.1
|specified type NEC A79.89
|tick-borne A77.9
|vesicular A79.1
Rider's bone *see* Ossification, muscle, specified NEC
Ridge, alveolus *see also* condition
|flabby K06.8
Ridged ear, congenital Q17.3
Riedel's
|lobe, liver Q44.7
|struma, thyroiditis or disease E06.5
Rieger's anomaly or syndrome Q13.81
Riehl's melanosis L81.4
Rietti-Grippe-Micheli anemia D56.9
Rieux's hernia *see* Hernia, abdomen, specified site NEC
Riga (-Feed) disease K14.0
Riggs' disease *see* Periodontitis
Right aortic arch Q25.47
Right middle lobe syndrome J98.11
Rigid, rigidity *see also* condition
|abdominal R19.30
  |with severe abdominal pain R10.0
  |epigastric R19.36
  |generalized R19.37
  |left lower quadrant R19.34
  |left upper quadrant R19.32
  |periumbilic R19.35
  |right lower quadrant R19.33
  |right upper quadrant R19.31
|articular, multiple, congenital Q68.8
|cervix (uteri) in pregnancy *see* Pregnancy, complicated by, abnormal, cervix
|hymen (acquired) (congenital) N89.6
|nuchal R29.1

Rigid, rigidity - *continued*
|pelvic floor in pregnancy *see* Pregnancy,
  complicated by, abnormal, pelvic organs or
  tissues NEC
|perineum or vulva in pregnancy *see*
  Pregnancy, complicated by, abnormal, vulva
|spine *see* Dorsopathy, specified NEC
|vagina in pregnancy *see* Pregnancy,
  complicated by, abnormal, vagina
Rigors R68.89
|with fever R50.9
Riley-Day syndrome G90.1
RIND (reversible ischemic neurologic deficit)
  I63.9
Ring(s)
|aorta (vascular) Q25.45
|Bandl's O62.4
|contraction, complicating delivery O62.4
|esophageal, lower (muscular) K22.2
|Fleischer's (cornea) H18.04-
|hymenal, tight (acquired) (congenital) N89.6
|Kayser-Fleischer (cornea) H18.04-
|retraction, uterus, pathological O62.4
|Schatzki's (esophagus) (lower) K22.2
  |congenital Q39.3
|Soemmerring's *see* Cataract, secondary
|vascular (congenital) Q25.8
  |aorta Q25.45
Ringed hair (congenital) Q84.1
Ringworm B35.9
|beard B35.0
|black dot B35.0
|body B35.4
|Burmese B35.5
|corporeal B35.4
|foot B35.3
|groin B35.6
|hand B35.2
|honeycomb B35.0
|nails B35.1
|perianal (area) B35.6
|scalp B35.0
|specified NEC B35.8
|Tokelau B35.5
Rise, venous pressure I87.8
Rising, PSA following treatment for
  malignant neoplasm of prostate R97.21
Risk
|for
  |dental caries Z91.849
    |high Z91.843
    |low Z91.841
    |moderate Z91.842
  |homelessness, imminent Z59.811
|suicidal
  |meaning personal history of attempted
    suicide Z91.51
  |meaning suicidal ideation *see* Ideation,
    suicidal
Ritter's disease L00
Rivalry, sibling Z62.891
Rivalta's disease A42.2
River blindness B73.01
Robert's pelvis Q74.2
|with disproportion (fetopelvic) O33.0
  |causing obstructed labor O65.0
Robin (-Pierre) syndrome Q87.0
Robinow-Silvermann-Smith syndrome Q87.1
Robinson's (hidrotic) ectodermal dysplasia or
  syndrome Q82.4
Robles' disease B73.01
Rocky Mountain (spotted) fever A77.0
Roetheln *see* Rubella
Roger's disease Q21.0

Rokitansky-Aschoff sinuses (gallbladder)
  K82.8
Rolando's fracture (displaced) S62.22-
|nondisplaced S62.22-
Romano-Ward (prolonged QT interval)
  syndrome I45.81
Romberg's disease or syndrome G51.8
Roof, mouth *see* condition **Rosacea** L71.9
|acne L71.9
|keratitis L71.8
|specified NEC L71.8
Rosary, rachitic E55.0
Rose
|cold J30.1
|fever J30.1
|rash R21
  |epidemic B06.9
Rosenbach's erysipeloid A26.0
Rosenthal's disease or syndrome D68.1
Roseola B09
|infantum B08.20
  |due to human herpesvirus 6 B08.21
  |due to human herpesvirus 7 B08.22
Rossbach's disease K31.89
|psychogenic F45.8
Ross River disease or fever B33.1
Rostan's asthma (cardiac) *see* Failure,
  ventricular, left
Rotation
|anomalous, incomplete or insufficient,
  intestine Q43.3
|cecum (congenital) Q43.3
|colon (congenital) Q43.3
|spine, incomplete or insufficient *see*
  Dorsopathy, deforming, specified NEC
|tooth, teeth, fully erupted M26.35
|vertebra, incomplete or insufficient *see*
  Dorsopathy, deforming, specified NEC
Rotes Quérol disease or syndrome *see*
  Hyperostosis, ankylosing
Roth (-Bernhardt) disease or syndrome *see*
  Meralgia paraesthetica
Rothmund (-Thomson) syndrome Q82.8
Rotor's disease or syndrome E80.6
Round
|back (with wedging of vertebrae) *see*
  Kyphosis
  |sequelae (late effect) of rickets E64.3
|worms (large) (infestation) NEC B82.0
  |Ascariasis *see also* Ascariasis B77.9
Roussy-Lévy syndrome G60.0
Rubella (German measles) B06.9
|complication NEC B06.09
  |neurological B06.00
|congenital P35.0
|contact Z20.4
|exposure to Z20.4
|maternal
  |manifest rubella in infant P35.0
  |care for (suspected) damage to fetus O35.3
  |suspected damage to fetus affecting
    management of pregnancy O35.3
|specified complications NEC B06.89
Rubeola (meaning measles) *see* Measles
|meaning rubella *see* Rubella
Rubeosis, iris *see* Disorder, iris, vascular
Rubinstein-Taybi syndrome Q87.2
Rudimentary (congenital) *see also* Agenesis
|arm *see* Defect, reduction, upper limb
|bone Q79.9
|cervix uteri Q51.828
|eye Q11.2
|lobule of ear Q17.3

Rudimentary (congenital) - *continued*
|patella Q74.1
|respiratory organs in thoracopagus Q89.4
|tracheal bronchus Q32.4
|uterus Q51.818
  |in male Q56.1
|vagina Q52.0
Ruled out condition *see* Observation, suspected
Rumination R11.10
|with nausea R11.2
|disorder of infancy F98.21
|neurotic F42.8
|newborn P92.1
|obsessional F42.8
|psychogenic F42.8
Runeberg's disease D51.0
Runny nose R09.89
Rupia (syphilitic) A51.39
|congenital A50.06
|tertiary A52.79
Rupture, ruptured
|abscess (spontaneous) code by site under
  Abscess
|aneurysm *see* Aneurysm
|anus (sphincter) *see* Laceration, anus
|aorta, aortic I71.8
  |abdominal I71.3
  |arch I71.1
  |ascending I71.1
  |descending I71.8
    |abdominal I71.3
    |thoracic I71.1
  |syphilitic A52.01
  |thoracoabdominal I71.5
  |thorax, thoracic I71.1
  |transverse I71.1
  |traumatic *see* Injury, aorta, laceration, major
  |valve or cusp *see also* Endocarditis, aortic
    I35.8
|appendix (with peritonitis) (*see also*
  Appendicitis) K35.32
  |with localized peritonitis (*see also*
    Appendicitis) K35.32
|arteriovenous fistula, brain I60.8
|artery I77.2
  |brain *see* Hemorrhage, intracranial,
    intracerebral
  |coronary *see* Infarct, myocardium
  |heart *see* Infarct, myocardium
  |pulmonary I28.8
  |traumatic (complication) *see* Injury, blood
    vessel
|bile duct (common) (hepatic) K83.2
  |cystic K82.2
|bladder (sphincter) (nontraumatic)
    (spontaneous) N32.89
  |following ectopic or molar pregnancy O08.6
  |obstetrical trauma O71.5
  |traumatic S37.29
|blood vessel *see also* Hemorrhage
  |brain *see* Hemorrhage, intracranial,
    intracerebral
  |heart *see* Infarct, myocardium
  |traumatic (complication) *see* Injury, blood
    vessel, laceration, major, by site
|bone *see* Fracture
|bowel (nontraumatic) K63.1
|brain
  |aneurysm (congenital) *see also* Hemorrhage,
    intracranial, subarachnoid
    |syphilitic A52.05
  |hemorrhagic *see* Hemorrhage, intracranial,
    intracerebral
|capillaries I78.8
|cardiac (auricle) (ventricle) (wall) I23.3

Rupture, ruptured - *continued*
 |with hemopericardium I23.0
 |infectional I40.9
 |traumatic *see* Injury, heart
|cartilage (articular) (current) *see also* Sprain
 |knee S83.3-
 |semilunar *see* Tear, meniscus
|cecum (with peritonitis) K65.0
 |with peritoneal abscess K35.33
 |traumatic S36.598
|celiac artery, traumatic *see* Injury, blood
  vessel, celiac artery, laceration, major
|cerebral aneurysm (congenital) (*see*
  Hemorrhage, intracranial, subarachnoid)
|cervix (uteri)
 |with ectopic or molar pregnancy O08.6
 |following ectopic or molar pregnancy O08.6
 |obstetrical trauma O71.3
 |traumatic S37.69
|chordae tendineae NEC I51.1
 |concurrent with acute myocardial infarction
   see Infarct, myocardium
 |following acute myocardial infarction
   (current complication) I23.4
|choroid (direct) (indirect) (traumatic) H31.32-
|circle of Willis I60.6
|colon (nontraumatic) K63.1
 |traumatic *see* Injury, intestine, large
|cornea (traumatic) *see* Injury, eye, laceration
|coronary (artery) (thrombotic) *see* Infarct,
  myocardium
|corpus luteum (infected) (ovary) N83.1-
|cyst *see* Cyst
|cystic duct K82.2
|Descemet's membrane *see* Change, corneal
  membrane, Descemet's, rupture
 |traumatic *see* Injury, eye, laceration
|diaphragm, traumatic *see* Injury, intrathoracic,
  diaphragm
|disc *see* Rupture, intervertebral disc
|diverticulum (intestine) K57.80
 |with bleeding K57.81
 |bladder N32.3
 |large intestine K57.20
  |with
   |bleeding K57.21
   |small intestine K57.40
    |with bleeding K57.41
 |small intestine K57.00
  |with
   |bleeding K57.01
   |large intestine K57.40
    |with bleeding K57.41
|duodenal stump K31.89
|ear drum (nontraumatic) *see also* Perforation,
  tympanum
 |traumatic S09.2-
  |due to blast injury *see* Injury, blast, ear
|esophagus K22.3
|eye (without prolapse or loss of intraocular
  tissue) *see* Injury, eye, laceration
|fallopian tube NEC (nonobstetric)
   (nontraumatic) N83.8
 |due to pregnancy O00.10-
  |with intrauterine pregnancy O00.11-
|fontanel P13.1
|gallbladder K82.2
 |traumatic S36.128
|gastric *see also* Rupture, stomach
 |vessel K92.2
|globe (eye) (traumatic) *see* Injury, eye,
  laceration
|graafian follicle (hematoma) N83.0-
|heart *see* Rupture, cardiac
|hymen (nontraumatic) (nonintentional) N89.8

Rupture, ruptured - *continued*
 |internal organ, traumatic *see* Injury, by site
|intervertebral disc *see* Displacement,
  intervertebral disc
 |traumatic *see* Rupture, traumatic,
   intervertebral disc
|intestine NEC (nontraumatic) K63.1
 |traumatic *see* Injury, intestine
|iris *see also* Abnormality, pupillary
 |traumatic *see* Injury, eye, laceration
|joint capsule, traumatic *see* Sprain
|kidney (traumatic) S37.06-
 |birth injury P15.8
 |nontraumatic N28.89
|lacrimal duct (traumatic) *see* Injury, eye,
  specified site NEC
|lens (cataract) (traumatic) *see* Cataract,
  traumatic
|ligament, traumatic *see* Rupture, traumatic,
  ligament, by site
|liver S36.116
 |birth injury P15.0
|lymphatic vessel I89.8
|marginal sinus (placental) (with hemorrhage)
  see Hemorrhage, antepartum, specified cause
  NEC
|membrana tympani (nontraumatic) *see*
  Perforation, tympanum
|membranes (spontaneous)
 |artificial
  |delayed delivery following O75.5
 |delayed delivery following *see* Pregnancy,
   complicated by, premature rupture of
   membranes
|meningeal artery I60.8
|meniscus (knee) *see also* Tear, meniscus
 |old *see* Derangement, meniscus
 |site other than knee   code as Sprain
|mesenteric artery, traumatic *see* Injury,
  mesenteric, artery, laceration, major
|mesentery (nontraumatic) K66.8
 |traumatic *see* Injury, intra-abdominal,
   specified, site NEC
|mitral (valve) I34.8
|muscle (traumatic) *see also* Strain
 |diastasis *see* Diastasis, muscle
 |nontraumatic M62.10
  |ankle M62.17-
  |foot M62.17-
  |forearm M62.13-
  |hand M62.14-
  |lower leg M62.16-
  |pelvic region M62.15-
  |shoulder region M62.11-
  |specified site NEC M62.18
  |thigh M62.15-
  |upper arm M62.12-
 |traumatic *see* Strain, by site
|musculotendinous junction NEC,
  nontraumatic *see* Rupture, tendon,
  spontaneous
|mycotic aneurysm causing cerebral
  hemorrhage *see* Hemorrhage, intracranial,
  subarachnoid
|myocardium, myocardial *see* Rupture, cardiac
 |traumatic *see* Injury, heart
|nontraumatic, meaning hernia *see* Hernia
|obstructed *see* Hernia, by site, obstructed
|operation wound *see* Disruption, wound,
  operation
|ovary, ovarian N83.8
 |corpus luteum cyst N83.1-
 |follicle (graafian) N83.0-
|oviduct (nonobstetric) (nontraumatic) N83.8
 |due to pregnancy O00.10-

Rupture, ruptured - *continued*
 |with intrauterine pregnancy O00.11-
|pancreas (nontraumatic) K86.89
 |traumatic S36.299
|papillary muscle NEC I51.2
 |following acute myocardial infarction
   (current complication) I23.5
|pelvic
 |floor, complicating delivery O70.1
 |organ NEC, obstetrical trauma O71.5
|perineum (nonobstetric) (nontraumatic)
   N90.89
 |complicating delivery *see* Delivery,
   complicated, by, laceration, anus (sphincter)
|postoperative wound *see* Disruption, wound,
  operation
|prostate (traumatic) S37.828
|pulmonary
 |artery I28.8
 |valve (heart) I37.8
 |vein I28.8
 |vessel I28.8
|pus tube *see* Salpingitis
|pyosalpinx *see* Salpingitis
|rectum (nontraumatic) K63.1
 |traumatic S36.69
|retina, retinal (traumatic) (without
  detachment) *see also* Break, retina
 |with detachment *see* Detachment, retina,
   with retinal, break
|rotator cuff (nontraumatic) M75.10-
 |complete M75.12-
 |incomplete M75.11-
|sclera *see* Injury, eye, laceration
|sigmoid (nontraumatic) K63.1
 |traumatic S36.593
|spinal cord *see also* Injury, spinal cord, by
  region
 |due to injury at birth P11.5
 |newborn (birth injury) P11.5
|spleen (traumatic) S36.09
 |birth injury P15.1
 |congenital (birth injury) P15.1
 |due to P. vivax malaria B51.0
 |nontraumatic D73.5
 |spontaneous D73.5
|splenic vein R58
 |traumatic *see* Injury, blood vessel, splenic
   vein
|stomach (nontraumatic) (spontaneous) K31.89
 |traumatic S36.39
|supraspinatus (complete) (incomplete)
  (nontraumatic) *see* Tear, rotator cuff
|symphysis pubis
 |obstetric O71.6
 |traumatic S33.4
|synovium (cyst) M66.10
 |ankle M66.17-
 |elbow M66.12-
 |finger M66.14-
 |foot M66.17-
 |forearm M66.13-
 |hand M66.14-
 |pelvic region M66.15-
 |shoulder region M66.11-
 |specified site NEC M66.18
 |thigh M66.15-
 |toe M66.17-
 |upper arm M66.12-
 |wrist M66.13-
|tendon (traumatic) *see* Strain
 |nontraumatic (spontaneous) M66.9
  |ankle M66.87-
  |extensor M66.20
   |ankle M66.27-

Rupture, ruptured - *continued*
|foot M66.27-
|forearm M66.23-
|hand M66.24-
|lower leg M66.26-
|multiple sites M66.29
|pelvic region M66.25-
|shoulder region M66.21-
|specified site NEC M66.28
|thigh M66.25-
|upper arm M66.22-
|flexor M66.30
|ankle M66.37-
|foot M66.37-
|forearm M66.33-
|hand M66.34-
|lower leg M66.36-
|multiple sites M66.39
|pelvic region M66.35-
|shoulder region M66.31-
|specified site NEC M66.38
|thigh M66.35-
|upper arm M66.32-
|foot M66.87-
|forearm M66.83-
|hand M66.84-
|lower leg M66.86-
|multiple sites M66.89
|pelvic region M66.85-
|shoulder region M66.81-
|specified
|site NEC M66.88
|tendon M66.80
|thigh M66.85-
|upper arm M66.82-
|thoracic duct I89.8
|tonsil J35.8
|traumatic
|aorta *see* Injury, aorta, laceration, major
|diaphragm *see* Injury, intrathoracic, diaphragm
|external site *see* Wound, open, by site
|eye *see* Injury, eye, laceration
|internal organ *see* Injury, by site
|intervertebral disc
|cervical S13.0
|lumbar S33.0
|thoracic S23.0
|kidney S37.06-
|ligament *see also* Sprain
|ankle *see* Sprain, ankle
|carpus *see* Rupture, traumatic, ligament, wrist
|collateral (hand) *see* Rupture, traumatic, ligament, finger, collateral
|finger (metacarpophalangeal) (interphalangeal) S63.40-
|collateral S63.41-
|index S63.41-
|little S63.41-
|middle S63.41-
|ring S63.41-
|index S63.40-
|little S63.40-
|middle S63.40-
|palmar S63.42-
|index S63.42-
|little S63.42-
|middle S63.42-
|ring S63.42-
|ring S63.40-
|specified site NEC S63.499
|index S63.49-
|little S63.49-
|middle S63.49-

Rupture, ruptured - *continued*
|ring S63.49-
|volar plate S63.43-
|index S63.43-
|little S63.43-
|middle S63.43-
|ring S63.43-
|foot *see* Sprain, foot
|radial collateral S53.2-
|radiocarpal *see* Rupture, traumatic, ligament, wrist, radiocarpal
|ulnar collateral S53.3-
|ulnocarpal *see* Rupture, traumatic, ligament, wrist, ulnocarpal
|wrist S63.30-
|collateral S63.31-
|radiocarpal S63.32-
|specified site NEC S63.39-
|ulnocarpal (palmar) S63.33-
|liver S36.116
|membrana tympani *see* Rupture, ear drum, traumatic
|muscle or tendon *see* Strain
|myocardium *see* Injury, heart
|pancreas S36.299
|rectum S36.69
|sigmoid S36.593
|spleen S36.09
|stomach S36.39
|symphysis pubis S33.4
|tympanum, tympanic (membrane) *see* Rupture, ear drum, traumatic
|ureter S37.19
|uterus S37.69
|vagina *see* Injury, vagina
|vena cava *see* Injury, vena cava, laceration, major
|tricuspid (heart) (valve) I07.8
|tube, tubal (nonobstetric) (nontraumatic) N83.8
|abscess *see* Salpingitis
|due to pregnancy O00.10-
|with intrauterine pregnancy O00.11-
|tympanum, tympanic (membrane) (nontraumatic) *see also* Perforation, tympanic membrane H72.9-
|traumatic *see* Rupture, ear drum, traumatic
|umbilical cord, complicating delivery O69.89
|ureter (traumatic) S37.19
|nontraumatic N28.89
|urethra (nontraumatic) N36.8
|with ectopic or molar pregnancy O08.6
|following ectopic or molar pregnancy O08.6
|obstetrical trauma O71.5
|traumatic S37.39
|uterosacral ligament (nonobstetric) (nontraumatic) N83.8
|uterus (traumatic) S37.69
|before labor O71.0-
|during or after labor O71.1
|nonpuerperal, nontraumatic N85.8
|pregnant (during labor) O71.1
|before labor O71.0-
|vagina *see* Injury, vagina
|valve, valvular (heart) *see* Endocarditis
|varicose vein *see* Varix
|varix *see* Varix
|vena cava R58
|traumatic *see* Injury, vena cava, laceration, major
|vesical (urinary) N32.89
|vessel (blood) R58
|pulmonary I28.8
|traumatic *see* Injury, blood vessel
|viscus R19.8
|vulva complicating delivery O70.0

Russell-Silver syndrome Q87.1
Russian spring-Summer type encephalitis A84.0
Rust's disease (tuberculous cervical spondylitis) A18.01
Ruvalcaba-Myhre-Smith syndrome E71.440
Rytand-Lipsitch syndrome I44.2

S

Saber, sabre shin or tibia (syphilitic) A50.56 [M90.8]
Sac lacrimal *see* condition
Saccharomyces infection B37.9
Saccharopinuria E72.3
Saccular *see* condition **Sacculation**
|aorta (nonsyphilitic) *see* Aneurysm, aorta
|bladder N32.3
|intralaryngeal (congenital) (ventricular) Q31.3
|larynx (congenital) (ventricular) Q31.3
|organ or site, congenital *see* Distortion
|pregnant uterus *see* Pregnancy, complicated by, abnormal, uterus
|ureter N28.89
|urethra N36.1
|vesical N32.3
Sachs' amaurotic familial idiocy or disease E75.02
Sachs-Tay disease E75.02
Sacks-Libman disease M32.11
Sacralgia M53.3
Sacralization Q76.49
Sacrodynia M53.3
Sacroiliac joint *see* condition
Sacroiliitis NEC M46.1
Sacrum *see* condition
Saddle
|back *see* Lordosis
|embolus
|abdominal aorta I74.01
|pulmonary artery I26.92
|with acute cor pulmonale I26.02
|injury   code to condition
|nose M95.0
|due to syphilis A50.57
Sadism (sexual) F65.52
Sadness, postpartal O90.6
Sadomasochism F65.50
Saemisch's ulcer (cornea) *see* Ulcer, cornea, central
Sagging
|skin and subcutaneous tissue (following bariatric surgery weight loss) (following dietary weight loss) L98.7
Sahib disease B55.0
Sailors' skin L57.8
Saint
|Anthony's fire *see* Erysipelas
|triad *see* Hernia, diaphragm
|Vitus' dance *see* Chorea, Sydenham's
Salaam
|attack(s) *see* Epilepsy, spasms
|tic R25.8
Salicylism
|abuse F55.8
|overdose or wrong substance given *see* Table of Drugs and Chemicals, by drug, poisoning
Salivary duct or gland *see* condition
Salivation, excessive K11.7
Salmonella *see* Infection, Salmonella
Salmonellosis A02.0

Salpingitis (catarrhal) (fallopian tube)
  (nodular) (pseudofollicular) (purulent)
  (septic) N70.91
  |with oophoritis N70.93
  |acute N70.01
    |with oophoritis N70.03
  |chlamydial A56.11
  |chronic N70.11
    |with oophoritis N70.13
  |complicating abortion *see* Abortion, by type,
    complicated by, salpingitis
  |ear *see* Salpingitis, eustachian
  |eustachian (tube) H68.00-
    |acute H68.01-
    |chronic H68.02-
  |follicularis N70.11
    |with oophoritis N70.13
  |gonococcal (acute) (chronic) A54.24
  |interstitial, chronic N70.11
    |with oophoritis N70.13
  |isthmica nodosa N70.11
    |with oophoritis N70.13
  |specific (gonococcal) (acute) (chronic) A54.24
  |tuberculous (acute) (chronic) A18.17
  |venereal (gonococcal) (acute) (chronic)
    A54.24
Salpingocele N83.4-
Salpingo-Oophoritis (catarrhal) (purulent)
  (ruptured) (septic) (suppurative) N70.93
  |acute N70.03
    |with ectopic or molar pregnancy O08.0
    |following ectopic or molar pregnancy O08.0
    |gonococcal A54.24
  |chronic N70.13
  |following ectopic or molar pregnancy O08.0
  |gonococcal (acute) (chronic) A54.24
  |puerperal O86.19
  |specific (gonococcal) (acute) (chronic) A54.24
  |subacute N70.03
  |tuberculous (acute) (chronic) A18.17
  |venereal (gonococcal) (acute) (chronic)
    A54.24
Salpingo-Ovaritis *see* Salpingo-oophoritis
Salpingoperitonitis *see* Salpingo-oophoritis
Salzmann's nodular dystrophy *see*
  Degeneration, cornea, nodular
Sampson's cyst or tumor N80.1
San Joaquin (Valley) fever B38.0
Sandblaster's asthma, lung or pneumoconiosis
  J62.8
Sander's disease (paranoia) F22
Sandfly fever A93.1
Sandhoff's disease E75.01
Sanfilippo (Type B) (Type C) (Type D)
  syndrome E76.22
Sanger-Brown ataxia G11.2
Sao Paulo fever or typhus A77.0
Saponification, mesenteric K65.8
Sarcocele (benign)
  |syphilitic A52.76
    |congenital A50.59
Sarcocystosis A07.8
Sarcoepiplocele *see* Hernia
Sarcoepiplomphalocele Q79.2
Sarcoid *see also* Sarcoidosis
  |arthropathy D86.86
  |Boeck's D86.9
  |Darier-Roussy D86.3
  |iridocyclitis D86.83
  |meningitis D86.81
  |myocarditis D86.85
  |myositis D86.87
  |pyelonephritis D86.84
  |Spiegler-Fendt L08.89

Sarcoidosis D86.9
  |with
    |cranial nerve palsies D86.82
    |hepatic granuloma D86.89
    |polyarthritis D86.86
    |tubulo-interstitial nephropathy D86.84
  |combined sites NEC D86.89
  |lung D86.0
    |and lymph nodes D86.2
  |lymph nodes D86.1
    |and lung D86.2
  |meninges D86.81
  |skin D86.3
  |specified type NEC D86.89
Sarcoma (of) *see also* Neoplasm, connective
  tissue, malignant
  |alveolar soft part *see* Neoplasm, connective
    tissue, malignant
  |ameloblastic C41.1
    |upper jaw (bone) C41.0
  |botryoid *see* Neoplasm, connective tissue,
    malignant
  |botryoides *see* Neoplasm, connective tissue,
    malignant
  |cerebellar C71.6
    |circumscribed (arachnoidal) C71.6
  |circumscribed (arachnoidal) cerebellar C71.6
  |clear cell *see also* Neoplasm, connective
    tissue, malignant
    |kidney C64.-
  |dendritic cells (accessory cells) C96.4
  |embryonal *see* Neoplasm, connective tissue,
    malignant
  |endometrial (stromal) C54.1
    |isthmus C54.0
  |epithelioid (cell) *see* Neoplasm, connective
    tissue, malignant
  |Ewing's *see* Neoplasm, bone, malignant
  |follicular dendritic cell C96.4
  |germinoblastic (diffuse) *see* Lymphoma,
    diffuse large cell
    |follicular *see* Lymphoma, follicular,
      specified NEC
  |giant cell (except of bone) *see also* Neoplasm,
    connective tissue, malignant
    |bone *see* Neoplasm, bone, malignant
  |glomoid *see* Neoplasm, connective tissue,
    malignant
  |granulocytic C92.3-
  |hemangioendothelial *see* Neoplasm,
    connective tissue, malignant
  |hemorrhagic, multiple *see* Sarcoma, Kaposi's
  |histiocytic C96.A
  |Hodgkin *see* Lymphoma, Hodgkin
  |immunoblastic (diffuse) *see* Lymphoma,
    diffuse large cell
  |interdigitating dendritic cell C96.4
  |Kaposi's
    |colon C46.4
    |connective tissue C46.1
    |gastrointestinal organ C46.4
    |lung C46.5-
    |lymph node(s) C46.3
    |palate (hard) (soft) C46.2
    |rectum C46.4
    |skin C46.0
    |specified site NEC C46.7
    |stomach C46.4
    |unspecified site C46.9
  |Kupffer cell C22.3
  |Langerhans cell C96.4
  |leptomeningeal *see* Neoplasm, meninges,
    malignant
  |liver NEC C22.4

Sarcoma (of) - *continued*
  |lymphangioendothelial *see* Neoplasm,
    connective tissue, malignant
  |lymphoblastic *see* Lymphoma, lymphoblastic
    (diffuse)
  |lymphocytic *see* Lymphoma, small cell B-cell
  |mast cell C96.22
  |melanotic *see* Melanoma
  |meningeal *see* Neoplasm, meninges,
    malignant
  |meningothelial *see* Neoplasm, meninges,
    malignant
  |mesenchymal *see also* Neoplasm, connective
    tissue, malignant
    |mixed *see* Neoplasm, connective tissue,
      malignant
  |mesothelial *see* Mesothelioma
  |monstrocellular
    |specified site *see* Neoplasm, malignant, by
      site
    |unspecified site C71.9
  |myeloid C92.3-
  |neurogenic *see* Neoplasm, nerve, malignant
  |odontogenic C41.1
    |upper jaw (bone) C41.0
  |osteoblastic *see* Neoplasm, bone, malignant
  |osteogenic *see also* Neoplasm, bone,
    malignant
    |juxtacortical *see* Neoplasm, bone, malignant
    |periosteal *see* Neoplasm, bone, malignant
  |periosteal *see also* Neoplasm, bone, malignant
    |osteogenic *see* Neoplasm, bone, malignant
  |pleomorphic cell *see* Neoplasm, connective
    tissue, malignant
  |reticulum cell (diffuse) *see* Lymphoma,
    diffuse large cell
    |nodular *see* Lymphoma, follicular
    |pleomorphic cell type *see* Lymphoma,
      diffuse large cell
  |rhabdoid *see* Neoplasm, malignant, by site
  |round cell *see* Neoplasm, connective tissue,
    malignant
  |small cell *see* Neoplasm, connective tissue,
    malignant
  |soft tissue *see* Neoplasm, connective tissue,
    malignant
  |spindle cell *see* Neoplasm, connective tissue,
    malignant
  |stromal (endometrial) C54.1
    |isthmus C54.0
  |synovial *see also* Neoplasm, connective tissue,
    malignant
    |biphasic *see* Neoplasm, connective tissue,
      malignant
    |epithelioid cell *see* Neoplasm, connective
      tissue, malignant
    |spindle cell *see* Neoplasm, connective
      tissue, malignant
Sarcomatosis
  |meningeal *see* Neoplasm, meninges,
    malignant
  |specified site NEC *see* Neoplasm, connective
    tissue, malignant
  |unspecified site C80.1
Sarcopenia (age-Related) M62.84
Sarcosinemia E72.59
Sarcosporidiosis (intestinal) A07.8
SARS-CoV-2 - see also COVID-19
- sequelae (post acute) U09.9
Satiety, early R68.81
Saturnine *see* condition
Saturnism
  |overdose or wrong substance given or taken
    see Table of Drugs and Chemicals, by
    drug, poisoning

STUV

Satyriasis F52.8
Sauriasis *see* Ichthyosis
SBE (subacute bacterial endocarditis) I33.0
Scabs R23.4
Scabies (any site) B86
Scaglietti-Dagnini syndrome E22.0
Scald *see* Burn
Scalenus anticus (anterior) syndrome G54.0
Scales R23.4
Scaling, skin R23.4
Scalp *see* condition
Scapegoating affecting child Z62.3
Scaphocephaly Q75.0
Scapulalgia M89.8X1
Scapulohumeral myopathy G71.02
Scar, scarring *see also* Cicatrix L90.5
|adherent L90.5
|atrophic L90.5
|cervix
||in pregnancy or childbirth *see* Pregnancy,
||complicated by, abnormal cervix
|cheloid L91.0
|chorioretinal H31.00-
||posterior pole macula H31.01-
||postsurgical H59.81-
||solar retinopathy H31.02-
||specified type NEC H31.09-
|choroid *see* Scar, chorioretinal
|conjunctiva H11.24-
|defect (isthmocele) O34.22
|cornea H17.9
||xerophthalmic *see also* Opacity, cornea
|||vitamin A deficiency E50.6
|duodenum, obstructive K31.5
|hypertrophic L91.0
|keloid L91.0
|labia N90.89
|lung (base) J98.4
|macula *see* Scar, chorioretinal, posterior pole
|muscle M62.89
|myocardium, myocardial I25.2
|painful L90.5
|posterior pole (eye) *see* Scar, chorioretinal,
||posterior pole
|retina *see* Scar, chorioretinal
|trachea J39.8
|transmural uterine, in pregnancy O34.29
|uterus N85.8
||in pregnancy O34.29
|vagina N89.8
||postoperative N99.2
|vulva N90.89
Scarabiasis B88.2
Scarlatina (anginosa) (maligna) A38.9
|myocarditis (acute) A38.1
|, |old *see* Myocarditis
|otitis media A38.0
|ulcerosa A38.8
Scarlet fever (albuminuria) (angina) A38.9
**Schamberg's disease (progressive pigmentary
dermatosis)** L81.7
Schatzki's ring (acquired) (esophagus) (lower)
K22.2
|congenital Q39.3
Schaufenster krankheit I20.8
Schaumann's
|benign lymphogranulomatosis D86.1
|disease or syndrome *see* Sarcoidosis
Scheie's syndrome E76.03
Schenck's disease B42.1
Scheuermann's disease or osteochondrosis *see*
Osteochondrosis, juvenile, spine
Schilder (-Flatau) disease G37.0
Schilling-Type monocytic leukemia C93.0-

**Schimmelbusch's disease, cystic mastitis, or
hyperplasia** *see* Mastopathy, cystic
Schistosoma infestation *see* Infestation,
Schistosoma
Schistosomiasis B65.9
|with muscle disorder B65.9 *[M63.80]*
||ankle B65.9 *[M63.87]*
||foot B65.9 *[M63.87]*
||forearm B65.9 *[M63.83]*
||hand B65.9 *[M63.84]*
||lower leg B65.9 *[M63.86]*
||multiple sites B65.9 *[M63.89]*
||pelvic region B65.9 *[M63.85]*
||shoulder region B65.9 *[M63.81]*
||specified site NEC B65.9 *[M63.88]*
||thigh B65.9 *[M63.85]*
||upper arm B65.9 *[M63.82]*
|Asiatic B65.2
|bladder B65.0
|chestermani B65.8
|colon B65.1
|cutaneous B65.3
|due to
||S. haematobium B65.0
||S. japonicum B65.2
||S. mansoni B65.1
||S. mattheii B65.8
|Eastern B65.2
|genitourinary tract B65.0
|intestinal B65.1
|lung NEC B65.9 *[J99]*
||pneumonia B65.9 *[J17]*
|Manson's (intestinal) B65.1
|oriental B65.2
|pulmonary NEC B65.9 *[J99]*
||pneumonia B65.9
|Schistosoma
||haematobium B65.0
||japonicum B65.2
||mansoni B65.1
|specified type NEC B65.8
|urinary B65.0
|vesical B65.0
Schizencephaly Q04.6
Schizoaffective psychosis F25.9
Schizodontia K00.2
Schizoid personality F60.1
Schizophrenia, schizophrenic F20.9
|acute (brief) (undifferentiated) F23
|atypical (form) F20.3
|borderline F21
|catalepsy F20.2
|catatonic (type) (excited) (withdrawn) F20.2
|cenesthopathic, cenesthesiopathic F20.89
|childhood type F84.5
|chronic undifferentiated F20.9
|cyclic F25.0
|disorganized (type) F20.1
|flexibilitas cerea F20.2
|hebephrenic (type) F20.1
|incipient F21
|latent F21
|negative type F20.5
|paranoid (type) F20.0
|paraphrenic F20.0
|post-psychotic depression F32.89
|prepsychotic F21
|prodromal F21
|pseudoneurotic F21
|pseudopsychopathic F21
|reaction F23
|residual (state) (type) F20.5
|restzustand F20.5
|schizoaffective (type) *see* Psychosis,
||schizoaffective
|simple (type) F20.89
|simplex F20.89

Schizophrenia, schizophrenic - *continued*
|specified type NEC F20.89
|spectrum and other psychotic disorder F29
||specified NEC F28
|stupor F20.2
|syndrome of childhood F84.5
|undifferentiated (type) F20.3
||chronic F20.5
Schizothymia (persistent) F60.1
Schlatter-Osgood disease or osteochondrosis
M92.52-
Schlatter's tibia *see* Osteochondrosis, juvenile,
tibia
**Schmidt's syndrome (polyglandular,
autoimmune)** E31.0
Schmincke's carcinoma or tumor *see*
Neoplasm, nasopharynx, malignant
Schmitz (-Stutzer) dysentery A03.0
Schmorl's disease or nodes   lumbar region
M51.46
|lumbosacral region M51.47
|sacrococcygeal region M53.3
|thoracic region M51.44
|thoracolumbar region M51.45
Schneiderian
|papilloma *see* Neoplasm, nasopharynx, benign
||specified site *see* Neoplasm, benign, by site
||unspecified site D14.0
|specified site *see* Neoplasm, malignant, by site
||unspecified site C30.0
Scholte's syndrome (malignant carcinoid)
E34.0
**Scholz (-Bielchowsky-Henneberg) disease or
syndrome** E75.25
**Schönlein (-Henoch) disease or purpura
(primary) (rheumatic)** D69.0
Schottmuller's disease A01.4
**Schroeder's syndrome (endocrine
hypertensive)** E27.0
Schüller-Christian disease or syndrome C96.5
Schultze's type acroparesthesia, simple I73.89
Schultz's disease or syndrome *see*
Agranulocytosis
Schwalbe-Ziehen-Oppenheim disease G24.1
Schwannoma *see also* Neoplasm, nerve, benign
|malignant *see also* Neoplasm, nerve,
||malignant
|||with rhabdomyoblastic differentiation *see*
|||Neoplasm, nerve, malignant
|melanocytic *see* Neoplasm, nerve, benign
|pigmented *see* Neoplasm, nerve, benign
Schwannomatosis Q85.03
Schwartz (-Jampel) syndrome G71.13
Schwartz-Bartter syndrome E22.2
Schweniger-Buzzi anetoderma L90.1
Sciatic *see* condition
Sciatica (infective) M54.3
|with lumbago M54.4-
||due to intervertebral disc disorder *see*
||Disorder, disc, with, radiculopathy
|due to displacement of intervertebral disc
||(with lumbago) *see* Disorder, disc, with,
||radiculopathy
|wallet M54.3-
Scimitar syndrome Q26.8
Sclera *see* condition
Sclerectasia H15.84-
Scleredema
|adultorum *see* Sclerosis, systemic
|Buschke's *see* Sclerosis, systemic
|newborn P83.0
**Sclerema (adiposum) (edematosum)
(neonatorum) (newborn)** P83.0
|adultorum *see* Sclerosis, systemic
Scleriasis *see* Scleroderma

Scleritis H15.00-
|with corneal involvement H15.04-
|anterior H15.01-
|brawny H15.02-
|in (due to) zoster B02.34
|posterior H15.03-
|specified type NEC H15.09-
|syphilitic A52.71
|tuberculous (nodular) A18.51
Sclerochoroiditis H31.8
Scleroconjunctivitis see Scleritis
Sclerocystic ovary syndrome E28.2
Sclerodactyly, sclerodactylia L94.3
Scleroderma, sclerodermia (acrosclerotic)
(diffuse) (generalized) (progressive)
(pulmonary) see also Sclerosis, systemic
M34.9-
|circumscribed L94.0
|linear L94.1
|localized L94.0
|newborn P83.88
|systemic M34.9
Sclerokeratitis H16.8
|tuberculous A18.52
Scleroma nasi A48.8
Scleromalacia (perforans) H15.05-
Scleromyxedema L98.5
Sclérose en plaques G35
Sclerosis, sclerotic
|adrenal (gland) E27.8
|Alzheimer's see Disease, Alzheimer's
|amyotrophic (lateral) G12.21
|aorta, aortic I70.0
  |valve see Endocarditis, aortic
|artery, arterial, arteriolar, arteriovascular see
  Arteriosclerosis
|ascending multiple G35
|brain (generalized) (lobular) G37.9
  |artery, arterial I67.2
  |diffuse G37.0
  |disseminated G35
  |insular G35
  |Krabbe's E75.23
  |miliary G35
  |multiple G35
  |presenile (Alzheimer's) see Disease,
    Alzheimer's, early onset
  |senile (arteriosclerotic) I67.2
  |stem, multiple G35
  |tuberous Q85.1
|bulbar, multiple G35
|bundle of His I44.39
|cardiac see Disease, heart, ischemic,
  atherosclerotic
|cardiorenal see Hypertension, cardiorenal
|cardiovascular see also Disease,
  cardiovascular
  |renal see Hypertension, cardiorenal
|cerebellar see Sclerosis, brain
|cerebral see Sclerosis, brain
|cerebrospinal (disseminated) (multiple) G35
|cerebrovascular I67.2
|choroid see Degeneration, choroid
|combined (spinal cord) see also Degeneration,
  combined
  |multiple G35
|concentric (Balo) G37.5
|cornea see Opacity, cornea
|coronary (artery) I25.10
  |with angina pectoris see Arteriosclerosis,
    coronary (artery)
|corpus cavernosum
  |female N90.89
  |male N48.6

Sclerosis, sclerotic - *continued*
|diffuse (brain) (spinal cord) G37.0
|disseminated G35
|dorsal G35
|dorsolateral (spinal cord) see Degeneration,
  combined
|endometrium N85.5
|extrapyramidal G25.9
|eye, nuclear (senile) see Cataract, senile,
  nuclear
|focal and segmental (glomerular) see also
  N00-N07 with fourth character .1 N05.1
|Friedreich's (spinal cord) G11.11
|funicular (spermatic cord) N50.89
|general (vascular) see Arteriosclerosis
|gland (lymphatic) I89.8
|hepatic K74.1
  |alcoholic K70.2
|hereditary
  |cerebellar G11.9
  |spinal (Friedreich's ataxia) G11.11
|hippocampal G93.81
|insular G35
|kidney see Sclerosis, renal
|larynx J38.7
|lateral (amyotrophic) (descending) (spinal)
  G12.21
  |primary G12.23
|lens, senile nuclear see Cataract, senile,
  nuclear
|liver K74.1
  |with fibrosis K74.2
    |alcoholic K70.2
  |alcoholic K70.2
  |cardiac K76.1
|lung see Fibrosis, lung
|mastoid see Mastoiditis, chronic
|mesial temporal G93.81
|mitral I05.8
|Mönckeberg's (medial) see Arteriosclerosis,
  extremities
|multiple (brain stem) (cerebral) (generalized)
  (spinal cord) G35
|myocardium, myocardial see Disease, heart,
  ischemic, atherosclerotic
|nuclear (senile), eye see Cataract, senile,
  nuclear
|ovary N83.8
|pancreas K86.89
|penis N48.6
|peripheral arteries see Arteriosclerosis,
  extremities
|plaques G35
|pluriglandular E31.8
|polyglandular E31.8
|posterolateral (spinal cord) see Degeneration,
  combined
|presenile (Alzheimer's) see Disease,
  Alzheimer's, early onset
|primary, lateral G12.23
|progressive, systemic M34.0
|pulmonary see Fibrosis, lung
  |artery I27.0
  |valve (heart) see Endocarditis, pulmonary
|renal N26.9
  |with
    |cystine storage disease E72.09
    |hypertensive heart disease (conditions in
      I11) see Hypertension, cardiorenal
  |arteriolar (hyaline) (hyperplastic) see
    Hypertension, kidney
|retina (senile) (vascular) H35.00
|senile (vascular) see Arteriosclerosis
|spinal (cord) (progressive) G95.89
  |ascending G61.0
  |combined see also Degeneration, combined

Sclerosis, sclerotic - *continued*
  |multiple G35
    |syphilitic A52.11
  |disseminated G35
  |dorsolateral see Degeneration, combined
  |hereditary (Friedreich's) (mixed form)
    G11.11
  |lateral (amyotrophic) G12.23
  |multiple G35
  |posterior (syphilitic) A52.11
|stomach K31.89
|subendocardial, congenital I42.4
|systemic M34.9
  |with
    |lung involvement M34.81
    |myopathy M34.82
    |polyneuropathy M34.83
  |drug-induced M34.2
  |due to chemicals NEC M34.2
  |progressive M34.0
  |specified NEC M34.89
|temporal (mesial) G93.81
|tricuspid (heart) (valve) I07.8
|tuberous (brain) Q85.1
|tympanic membrane see Disorder, tympanic
  membrane, specified NEC
|valve, valvular (heart) see Endocarditis
|vascular see Arteriosclerosis
|vein I87.8
Scoliosis (acquired) (postural) M41.9
|adolescent (idiopathic) see Scoliosis,
  idiopathic, adolescent
|congenital Q67.5
  |due to bony malformation Q76.3
  |failure of segmentation (hemivertebra)
    Q76.3
  |hemivertebra fusion Q76.3
  |postural Q67.5
|degenerative M41.8-
|idiopathic M41.20
  |adolescent M41.129
    |cervical region M41.122
    |cervicothoracic region M41.123
    |lumbar region M41.126
    |lumbosacral region M41.127
    |thoracic region M41.124
    |thoracolumbar region M41.125
  |cervical region M41.22
  |cervicothoracic region M41.23
  |infantile M41.00
    |cervical region M41.02
    |cervicothoracic region M41.03
    |lumbar region M41.06
    |lumbosacral region M41.07
    |sacrococcygeal region M41.08
    |thoracic region M41.04
    |thoracolumbar region M41.05
  |juvenile M41.119
    |cervical region M41.112
    |cervicothoracic region M41.113
    |lumbar region M41.116
    |lumbosacral region M41.117
    |thoracic region M41.114
    |thoracolumbar region M41.115
  |lumbar region M41.26
  |lumbosacral region M41.27
  |thoracic region M41.24
  |thoracolumbar region M41.25
|infantile see Scoliosis, idiopathic, infantile
|neuromuscular M41.40
  |cervical region M41.42
  |cervicothoracic region M41.43
  |lumbar region M41.46
  |lumbosacral region M41.47
  |occipito-atlanto-axial region M41.41

Scoliosis (acquired) - *continued*
    |thoracic region M41.44
    |thoracolumbar region M41.45
  |paralytic *see* Scoliosis, neuromuscular
  |postradiation therapy M96.5
  |rachitic (late effect or sequelae) E64.3
      [M49.80]
    |cervical region E64.3 *[M49.82]*
    |cervicothoracic region E64.3 *[M49.83]*
    |lumbar region E64.3 *[M49.86]*
    |lumbosacral region E64.3 *[M49.87]*
    |multiple sites E64.3 *[M49.89]*
    |occipito-atlanto-axial region E64.3
        [M49.81]
    |sacrococcygeal region E64.3 *[M49.88]*
    |thoracic region E64.3 *[M49.84]*
    |thoracolumbar region E64.3 *[M49.85]*
  |sciatic M54.4-
  |secondary (to) NEC M41.50
    |cerebral palsy, Friedreich's ataxia,
        poliomyelitis, neuromuscular disorders
        see Scoliosis, neuromuscular
    |cervical region M41.52
    |cervicothoracic region M41.53
    |lumbar region M41.56
    |lumbosacral region M41.57
    |thoracic region M41.54
    |thoracolumbar region M41.55
  |specified form NEC M41.80
    |cervical region M41.82
    |cervicothoracic region M41.83
    |lumbar region M41.86
    |lumbosacral region M41.87
    |thoracic region M41.84
    |thoracolumbar region M41.85
  |thoracogenic M41.30
    |thoracic region M41.34
    |thoracolumbar region M41.35
  |tuberculous A18.01
Scoliotic pelvis
  |with disproportion (fetopelvic) O33.0
    |causing obstructed labor O65.0
Scorbutus, scorbutic *see also* Scurvy
  |anemia D53.2
**Score, NIHSS (National Institutes of Health
    Stroke Scale)** R29.7-
Scotoma (arcuate) (Bjerrum) (central) (ring)
    see also Defect, visual field, localized,
    scotoma
  |scintillating H53.19
Scratch *see* Abrasion
Scratchy throat R09.89
Screening (for) Z13.9
  |alcoholism Z13.39
  |anemia Z13.0
  |anomaly, congenital Z13.89
  |antenatal, of mother (*see also* Encounter,
    antenatal screening) Z36.9
  |arterial hypertension Z13.6
  |arthropod-borne viral disease NEC Z11.59
  |autism Z13.41
  |bacteriuria, asymptomatic Z13.89
  |behavioral disorder Z13.30
    |specified NEC Z13.39
  |brain injury, traumatic Z13.850
  |bronchitis, chronic Z13.83
  |brucellosis Z11.2
  |cardiovascular disorder Z13.6
  |cataract Z13.5
  |chlamydial diseases Z11.8
  |cholera Z11.0
  |chromosomal abnormalities (nonprocreative)
    NEC Z13.79
  |colonoscopy Z12.11
  |congenital
    |dislocation of hip Z13.89

Screening (for) - *continued*
  |eye disorder Z13.5
    |malformation or deformation Z13.89
  |contamination NEC Z13.88
  |cystic fibrosis Z13.228
  |dengue fever Z11.59
  |dental disorder Z13.84
  |depression (adult) (adolescent) (child) Z13.31
    |maternal Z13.32
    |perinatal Z13.32
  |developmental
    |delays Z13.40
      |global (milestones) Z13.42
      |specified NEC Z13.49
    |handicap Z13.42
    |in early childhood Z13.42
  |diabetes mellitus Z13.1
  |diphtheria Z11.2
  |disability, intellectual Z13.39
  |disease or disorder Z13.9
    |bacterial NEC Z11.2
      |intestinal infectious Z11.0
      |respiratory tuberculosis Z11.1
    |behavioral Z13.30
      |specified NEC Z13.39
    |blood or blood-forming organ Z13.0
    |cardiovascular Z13.6
    |Chagas' Z11.6
    |chlamydial Z11.8
    |coronavirus (novel) 2019 Z11.52
    |dental Z13.89
    |developmental delays Z13.40
      |global (milestones) Z13.42
      |specified NEC Z13.49
    |digestive tract NEC Z13.818
      |lower GI Z13.811
      |upper GI Z13.810
    |ear Z13.5
    |endocrine Z13.29
    |eye Z13.5
    |genitourinary Z13.89
    |heart Z13.6
    |human immunodeficiency virus (HIV)
        infection Z11.4
    |immunity Z13.0
    |infection
      |intestinal Z11.0
        |specified NEC Z11.6
    |infectious Z11.9
    |mental health and behavioral Z13.30
      |specified NEC Z13.39
    |metabolic Z13.228
    |neurological Z13.89
    |nutritional Z13.21
      |metabolic Z13.228
        |lipoid disorders Z13.220
    |protozoal Z11.6
      |intestinal Z11.0
    |respiratory Z13.83
    |rheumatic Z13.828
    |rickettsial Z11.8
    |sexually-transmitted NEC Z11.3
      |human immunodeficiency virus (HIV)
        Z11.4
    |sickle-cell (trait) Z13.0
    |skin Z13.89
    |specified NEC Z13.89
    |spirochetal Z11.8
    |thyroid Z13.29
    |vascular Z13.6
    |venereal Z11.3
    |viral NEC Z11.59
      |human immunodeficiency virus (HIV)
        Z11.4
      |intestinal Z11.0

Screening (for) - *continued*
  |elevated titer Z13.89
  |emphysema Z13.83
  |encephalitis, viral (mosquito or tick-borne)
    Z11.59
  |exposure to contaminants (toxic) Z13.88
  |fever
    |dengue Z11.59
    |hemorrhagic Z11.59
    |yellow Z11.59
  |filariasis Z11.6
  |galactosemia Z13.228
  |gastrointestinal condition Z13.818
  |genetic (nonprocreative)
  |for procreative management *see* Testing,
      genetic, for procreative management
    |disease carrier status (nonprocreative)
      Z13.71
    |specified NEC (nonprocreative) Z13.79
  |genitourinary condition Z13.89
  |glaucoma Z13.5
  |gonorrhea Z11.3
  |gout Z13.89
  |helminthiasis (intestinal) Z11.6
  |hematopoietic malignancy Z12.89
  |hemoglobinopathies NEC Z13.0
  |hemorrhagic fever Z11.59
  |Hodgkin disease Z12.89
  |human immunodeficiency virus (HIV) Z11.4
  |human papillomavirus Z11.51
  |hypertension Z13.6
  |immunity disorders Z13.0
  |infant or child (over 28 days old) Z00.129
    |with abnormal findings Z00.121
  |infection
    |mycotic Z11.8
    |parasitic Z11.8
  |ingestion of radioactive substance Z13.88
  |intellectual disability Z13.39
  |intestinal
    |helminthiasis Z11.6
    |infectious disease Z11.0
  |leishmaniasis Z11.6
  |leprosy Z11.2
  |leptospirosis Z11.8
  |leukemia Z12.89
  |lymphoma Z12.89
  |malaria Z11.6
  |malnutrition Z13.29
    |metabolic Z13.228
    |nutritional Z13.21
  |measles Z11.59
  |mental health disorder Z13.30
    |specified NEC Z13.39
  |metabolic errors, inborn Z13.228
  |multiphasic Z13.89
  |musculoskeletal disorder Z13.828
    |osteoporosis Z13.820
  |mycoses Z11.8
  |myocardial infarction (acute) Z13.6
  |neoplasm (malignant) (of) Z12.9
    |bladder Z12.6
    |blood Z12.89
    |breast Z12.39
      |routine mammogram Z12.31
    |cervix Z12.4
    |colon Z12.11
    |genitourinary organs NEC Z12.79
      |bladder Z12.6
      |cervix Z12.4
      |ovary Z12.73
      |prostate Z12.5
      |testis Z12.71
      |vagina Z12.72
    |hematopoietic system Z12.89

Screening (for) - *continued*
|intestinal tract Z12.10
  |colon Z12.11
  |rectum Z12.12
  |small intestine Z12.13
|lung Z12.2
|lymph (glands) Z12.89
|nervous system Z12.82
|oral cavity Z12.81
|prostate Z12.5
|rectum Z12.12
|respiratory organs Z12.2
|skin Z12.83
|small intestine Z12.13
|specified site NEC Z12.89
|stomach Z12.0
|nephropathy Z13.89
|nervous system disorders NEC Z13.858
|neurological condition Z13.89
|osteoporosis Z13.820
|parasitic infestation Z11.9
  |specified NEC Z11.8
|phenylketonuria Z13.228
|plague Z11.2
|poisoning (chemical) (heavy metal) Z13.88
|poliomyelitis Z11.59
|postnatal, chromosomal abnormalities Z13.89
|prenatal, of mother (*see also* Encounter, antenatal screening) Z36.9
|protozoal disease Z11.6
  |intestinal Z11.0
|pulmonary tuberculosis Z11.1
|radiation exposure Z13.88
|respiratory condition Z13.83
|respiratory tuberculosis Z11.1
|rheumatoid arthritis Z13.828
|rubella Z11.59
|schistosomiasis Z11.6
|sexually-transmitted disease NEC Z11.3
  |human immunodeficiency virus (HIV) Z11.4
|sickle-cell disease or trait Z13.0
|skin condition Z13.89
|sleeping sickness Z11.6
|special Z13.9
  |specified NEC Z13.89
|syphilis Z11.3
|tetanus Z11.2
|trachoma Z11.8
|traumatic brain injury Z13.850
|trypanosomiasis Z11.6
|tuberculosis, respiratory Z11.1
|venereal disease Z11.3
|viral encephalitis (mosquito or tick-Borne) Z11.59
|whooping cough Z11.2
|worms, intestinal Z11.6
|yaws Z11.8
|yellow fever Z11.59
Scrofula, scrofulosis (tuberculosis of cervical lymph glands) A18.2
Scrofulide (primary) (tuberculous) A18.4
Scrofuloderma, scrofulodermia (any site) (primary) A18.4
Scrofulosus lichen (primary) (tuberculous) A18.4
Scrofulous *see* condition
Scrotal tongue K14.5
Scrotum *see* condition
Scurvy, scorbutic E54
|anemia D53.2
|gum E54
|infantile E54
|rickets E55.0 *[M90.80]*
Sealpox B08.62

Seasickness T75.3
Seatworm (infection) (infestation) B80
Sebaceous *see also* condition
|cyst *see* Cyst, sebaceous
Seborrhea, seborrheic L21.9
|capillitii R23.8
|capitis L21.0
|dermatitis L21.9
  |infantile L21.1
|eczema L21.9
  |infantile L21.1
|sicca L21.0
Seckel's syndrome Q87.1
Seclusion, pupil *see* Membrane, pupillary
Second hand tobacco smoke exposure (acute) (chronic) Z77.22
|in the perinatal period P96.81
Secondary
|dentin (in pulp) K04.3
|neoplasm, secondaries *see* Table of Neoplasms, secondary
Secretion
|antidiuretic hormone, inappropriate E22.2
|catecholamine, by pheochromocytoma E27.5
|hormone
  |antidiuretic, inappropriate (syndrome) E22.2
  |by
    |carcinoid tumor E34.0
    |pheochromocytoma E27.5
  |ectopic NEC E34.2
|urinary
  |excessive R35.89
  |suppression R34
Section
|nerve, traumatic *see* Injury, nerve
Sedative, hypnotic, or anxiolytic-Induced
|anxiety disorder F13.980
|bipolar and related disorder F13.94
|delirium F13.921
|depressive disorder F13.94
|major neurocognitive disorder F13.97
|mild neurocognitive disorder F13.988
|psychotic disorder F13.959
|sexual dysfunction F13.981
|sleep disorder F13.982
Segmentation, incomplete (congenital) *see also* Fusion
|bone NEC Q78.8
|lumbosacral (joint) (vertebra) Q76.49
Seitelberger's syndrome (infantile neuraxonal dystrophy) G31.89
Seizure(s) *see also* Convulsions R56.9
|akinetic *see* Epilepsy, generalized, specified NEC
|atonic *see* Epilepsy, generalized, specified NEC
|autonomic (hysterical) F44.5
|convulsive *see* Convulsions
|cortical (focal) (motor) *see* Epilepsy, localization-related, symptomatic, with simple partial seizures
|disorder *see also* Epilepsy G40.909
|due to stroke *see* Sequelae (of), disease, cerebrovascular, by type, specified NEC
|epileptic *see* Epilepsy
|febrile (simple) R56.00
  |with status epilepticus G40.901
  |complex (atypical) (complicated) R56.01
    |with status epilepticus G40.901
|grand mal G40.409
  |intractable G40.419
    |with status epilepticus G40.411
    |without status epilepticus G40.419
  |not intractable G40.409
    |with status epilepticus G40.401

Seizure(s) - *continued*
|without status epilepticus G40.409
|heart *see* Disease, heart
|hysterical F44.5
|intractable G40.919
  |with status epilepticus G40.911
|Jacksonian (focal) (motor type) (sensory type) *see* Epilepsy, localization-related, symptomatic, with simple partial seizures
|newborn P90
|nonspecific epileptic
  |atonic *see* Epilepsy, generalized, specified NEC
  |clonic *see* Epilepsy, generalized, specified NEC
  |myoclonic *see* Epilepsy, generalized, specified NEC
  |tonic *see* Epilepsy, generalized, specified NEC
  |tonic-clonic *see* Epilepsy, generalized, specified NEC
|partial, developing into secondarily generalized seizures
  |complex *see* Epilepsy, localization-related, symptomatic, with complex partial seizures
  |simple *see* Epilepsy, localization-related, symptomatic, with simple partial seizures
|petit mal G40.A
  |intractable G40.A1
    |with status epilepticus G40.A11
    |without status epilepticus G40.A19
  |not intractable G40.A0-
    |with status epilepticus G40.A01
    |without status epilepticus G40.A09
|post traumatic R56.1
|recurrent G40.909
|specified NEC G40.89
|uncinate *see* Epilepsy, localization-related, symptomatic, with complex partial seizures
Selenium deficiency, dietary E59
Self-Damaging behavior (life-Style) Z72.89
Self-Harm (attempted)
|history (personal)
  |in family Z81.8
  |nonsuicidal Z91.52
  |suicidal Z91.51
|nonsuicidal R45.88
Self-injury, nonsuicidal R45.88
|personal history Z91.52
Self-Mutilation (attempted)
|history (personal)
  |in family Z81.8
  |nonsuicidal Z91.52
  |suicidal Z91.51
|nonsuicidal R45.88
Self-Poisoning
|history (personal) Z91.51
  |in family Z81.8
|observation following (alleged) attempt Z03.6
Semicoma R40.1
Seminal vesiculitis N49.0
Seminoma C62.9-
|specified site *see* Neoplasm, malignant, by site
Senear-Usher disease or syndrome L10.4
Senectus R54
Senescence (without mention of psychosis) R54
Senile, senility *see also* condition R41.81
|with
  |acute confusional state F05
  |mental changes NOS F03
  |psychosis NEC *see* Psychosis, senile
|asthenia R54

Senile, senility - *continued*
|cervix (atrophic) N88.8
|debility R54
|endometrium (atrophic) N85.8
|fallopian tube (atrophic) *see* Atrophy, fallopian tube
|heart (failure) R54
|ovary (atrophic) *see* Atrophy, ovary
|premature E34.8
|vagina, vaginitis (atrophic) N95.2
|wart L82.1
Sensation
|burning (skin) R20.8
||tongue K14.6
|loss of R20.8
|prickling (skin) R20.2
|tingling (skin) R20.2
Sense loss
|smell *see* Disturbance, sensation, smell
|taste *see* Disturbance, sensation, taste
|touch R20.8
Sensibility disturbance (cortical) (deep) (vibratory) R20.9
Sensitive, sensitivity *see also* Allergy
|carotid sinus G90.01
|child (excessive) F93.8
|cold, autoimmune D59.12
|dentin K03.89
|gluten (non-celiac) K90.41
|latex Z91.040
|methemoglobin D74.8
|tuberculin, without clinical or radiological symptoms R76.11
|visual
||glare H53.71
||impaired contrast H53.72
Sensitiver Beziehungswahn F22
Sensitization, auto-Erythrocytic D69.2
Separation
|anxiety, abnormal (of childhood) F93.0
|apophysis, traumatic   code as Fracture, by site
|choroid *see* Detachment, choroid
|epiphysis, epiphyseal
||nontraumatic *see also* Osteochondropathy, specified type NEC
|||upper femoral *see* Slipped, epiphysis, upper femoral
||traumatic   code as Fracture, by site
|fracture *see* Fracture
|infundibulum cardiac from right ventricle by a partition Q24.3
|joint (traumatic) (current)   code by site under Dislocation
|pubic bone, obstetrical trauma O71.6
|retina, retinal *see* Detachment, retina
|symphysis pubis, obstetrical trauma O71.6
|tracheal ring, incomplete, congenital Q32.1
Sepsis (generalized) (unspecified organism) A41.9
|with
||organ dysfunction (acute) (multiple) R65.20
|||with septic shock R65.21
|actinomycotic A42.7
|adrenal hemorrhage syndrome (meningococcal) A39.1
|anaerobic A41.4
|Bacillus anthracis A22.7
|Brucella *see also* Brucellosis A23.9
|candidal B37.7
|cryptogenic A41.9
|due to device, implant or graft T85.79
||arterial graft NEC T82.7
||breast (implant) T85.79
||catheter NEC T85.79
|||dialysis (renal) T82.7

Sepsis - *continued*
||intraperitoneal T85.71
||infusion NEC T82.7
|||spinal (cranial) (epidural) (intrathecal) (spinal) (subarachnoid) (subdural) T85.735
||urethral indwelling T83.511
||urinary T83.518
|ectopic or molar pregnancy O08.82
|electronic (electrode) (pulse generator) (stimulator)
||bone T84.7
||cardiac T82.7
||nervous system T85.738
|||brain T85.731
|||neurostimulator generator T85.734
|||peripheral nerve T85.732
|||spinal cord T85.733
||urinary T83.590
|fixation, internal (orthopedic) *see* Complication, fixation device, infection
|gastrointestinal (bile duct) (esophagus) T85.79
||neurostimulator electrode (lead) T85.732
|genital T83.69
|heart NEC T82.7
||valve (prosthesis) T82.6
|||graft T82.7
|joint prosthesis *see* Complication, joint prosthesis, infection
|ocular (corneal graft) (orbital implant) T85.79
|orthopedic NEC T84.7
||fixation device, internal *see* Complication, fixation device, infection
|specified NEC T85.79
|vascular T82.7
|ventricular intracranial (communicating) shunt T85.730
|during labor O75.3
|Enterococcus A41.81
|Erysipelothrix (rhusiopathiae) (erysipeloid) A26.7
|Escherichia coli (E. coli) A41.5
|extraintestinal yersiniosis A28.2
|following
||abortion (subsequent episode) O08.0
|||current episode *see* Abortion
||ectopic or molar pregnancy O08.82
||immunization T88.0
||infusion, therapeutic injection or transfusion NEC T80.29
||obstetrical procedure O86.04
|gangrenous A41.9
|gonococcal A54.86
|Gram negative (organism) A41.5
||anaerobic A41.4
|Haemophilus influenzae A41.3
|herpesviral B00.7
|intra-abdominal K65.1
|intraocular *see* Endophthalmitis, purulent
|Listeria monocytogenes A32.7
|localized   code to specific localized infection
||in operation wound T81.49
||skin *see* Abscess
|malleus A24.0
|melioidosis A24.1
|meningeal *see* Meningitis
|meningococcal A39.4
||acute A39.2
||chronic A39.3
|MSSA (Methicillin susceptible Staphylococcus aureus) A41.01
|newborn P36.9
||due to

Sepsis - *continued*
|||anaerobes NEC P36.5
|||Escherichia coli P36.4
|||Staphylococcus P36.30
||||aureus P36.2
||||specified NEC P36.39
|||Streptococcus P36.10
||||group B P36.0
||||specified NEC P36.19
|||specified NEC P36.8
|Pasteurella multocida A28.0
|pelvic, puerperal, postpartum, childbirth O85
|postprocedural T81.44
|pneumococcal A40.3
|puerperal, postpartum, childbirth (pelvic) O85
|Salmonella (arizonae) (cholerae-suis) (enteritidis) (typhimurium) A02.1
|severe R65.20
||with septic shock R65.21
|skin, localized *see* Abscess
|Shigella *see also* Dysentery, bacillary A03.9
|specified organism NEC A41.89
|Staphylococcus, staphylococcal A41.2
||aureus (methicillin susceptible) (MSSA) A41.01
||methicillin resistant (MRSA) A41.02
||coagulase-negative A41.1
||specified NEC A41.1
|Streptococcus, streptococcal A40.9
||agalactiae A40.1
||group
|||A A40.0
|||B A40.1
|||D A41.81
||neonatal P36.10
|||group B P36.0
|||specified NEC P36.19
||pneumoniae A40.3
||pyogenes A40.0
||specified NEC A40.8
|tracheostomy stoma J95.02
|tularemic A21.7
|umbilical, umbilical cord (newborn) *see* Sepsis, newborn
|Yersinia pestis A20.7
Septate *see* Septum
Septic *see* condition
|arm *see* Cellulitis, upper limb
||with lymphangitis *see* Lymphangitis, acute, upper limb
|embolus *see* Embolism
|finger *see* Cellulitis, digit
||with lymphangitis *see* Lymphangitis, acute, digit
|foot *see* Cellulitis, lower limb
||with lymphangitis *see* Lymphangitis, acute, lower limb
|gallbladder (acute) K81.0
|hand *see* Cellulitis, upper limb
||with lymphangitis *see* Lymphangitis, acute, upper limb
|joint *see* Arthritis, pyogenic or pyemic
|leg *see* Cellulitis, lower limb
||with lymphangitis *see* Lymphangitis, acute, lower limb
|nail *see also* Cellulitis, digit
||with lymphangitis *see* Lymphangitis, acute, digit
|sore *see also* Abscess
||throat J02.0
|||streptococcal J02.0
|spleen (acute) D73.89
|teeth, tooth (pulpal origin) K04.4
|throat *see* Pharyngitis

Septic - *continued*
|thrombus *see* Thrombosis
|toe *see* Cellulitis, digit
|with lymphangitis *see* Lymphangitis, acute, digit
|tonsils, chronic J35.01
|with adenoiditis J35.03
|uterus *see* Endometritis
Septicemia A41.9
|meaning sepsis *see* Sepsis
Septum, septate (congenital) *see also* Anomaly, by site
|anal Q42.3
|with fistula Q42.2
|aqueduct of Sylvius Q03.0
|with spina bifida *see* Spina bifida, by site, with hydrocephalus
|uterus Q51.28
|complete Q51.21
|partial Q51.22
|specified NEC Q51.28
|vagina Q52.10
|in pregnancy *see* Pregnancy, complicated by, abnormal vagina
|causing obstructed labor O65.5
|longitudinal Q52.129
|microperforate
|left side Q52.124
|right side Q52.123
|nonobstruction Q52.120
|obstructing Q52.129
|left side Q52.122
|right side Q52.121
|transverse Q52.11
Sequelae (of) *see also* condition
|abscess, intracranial or intraspinal (conditions in G06) G09
|amputation   code to injury with seventh character S
|burn and corrosion   code to injury with seventh character S
|calcium deficiency E64.8
|cerebrovascular disease *see* Sequelae, disease, cerebrovascular
|childbirth O94
|contusion   code to injury with seventh character S
|corrosion *see* Sequelae, burn and corrosion
|COVID-19 (post acute) U09.9
|crushing injury   code to injury with seventh character S
|disease
|cerebrovascular I69.90
|alteration of sensation I69.998
|aphasia I69.920
|apraxia I69.990
|ataxia I69.993
|cognitive deficits I69.91
|disturbance of vision I69.998
|dysarthria I69.922
|dysphagia I69.991
|dysphasia I69.921
|facial droop I69.992
|facial weakness I69.992
|fluency disorder I69.923
|hemiplegia I69.95-
|hemorrhage
|intracerebral *see* Sequelae, hemorrhage, intracerebral
|intracranial, nontraumatic NEC *see* Sequelae, hemorrhage, intracranial, nontraumatic

Sequelae (of) - *continued*
|subarachnoid *see* Sequelae, hemorrhage, subarachnoid
|language deficit I69.928
|monoplegia
|lower limb I69.94-
|upper limb I69.93-
|paralytic syndrome I69.96-
|specified effect NEC I69.998
|specified type NEC I69.80
|alteration of sensation I69.898
|aphasia I69.820
|apraxia I69.890
|ataxia I69.893
|cognitive deficits I69.81
|disturbance of vision I69.898
|dysarthria I69.822
|dysphagia I69.891
|dysphasia I69.821
|facial droop I69.892
|facial weakness I69.892
|fluency disorder I69.823
|hemiplegia I69.85-
|language deficit I69.828
|monoplegia
|lower limb I69.84-
|upper limb I69.83-
|paralytic syndrome I69.86-
|specified effect NEC I69.898
|speech deficit I69.928
|speech deficit I69.828
|stroke NOS *see* Sequelae, stroke NOS
|dislocation   code to injury with seventh character S
|encephalitis or encephalomyelitis (conditions in G04) G09
|in infectious disease NEC B94.8
|viral B94.1
|external cause - code to injury with seventh character S
|foreign body entering natural orifice - code to injury with seventh character S
|fracture - code to injury with seventh character S
|frostbite - code to injury with seventh character S
|Hansen's disease B92
|hemorrhage
|intracerebral I69.10
|alteration of sensation I69.198
|aphasia I69.120
|apraxia I69.190
|ataxia I69.193
|cognitive deficits I69.11
|disturbance of vision I69.198
|dysarthria I69.122
|dysphagia I69.191
|dysphasia I69.121
|facial droop I69.192
|facial weakness I69.192
|fluency disorder I69.123
|hemiplegia I69.15-
|language deficit NEC I69.128
|monoplegia
|lower limb I69.14-
|upper limb I69.13-
|paralytic syndrome I69.16-
|specified effect NEC I69.198
|speech deficit NEC I69.128
|intracranial, nontraumatic NEC I69.20
|alteration of sensation I69.298
|aphasia I69.220
|apraxia I69.290
|ataxia I69.293
|cognitive deficits I69.21

Sequelae (of) - *continued*
|disturbance of vision I69.298
|dysarthria I69.222
|dysphagia I69.291
|dysphasia I69.221
|facial droop I69.292
|facial weakness I69.292
|fluency disorder I69.223
|hemiplegia I69.25-
|language deficit NEC I69.228
|monoplegia
|lower limb I69.24-
|upper limb I69.23-
|paralytic syndrome I69.26-
|specified effect NEC I69.298
|speech deficit NEC I69.228
|subarachnoid I69.00
|alteration of sensation I69.098
|aphasia I69.020
|apraxia I69.090
|ataxia I69.093
|cognitive deficits *see* subcategory I69.01-
|disturbance of vision I69.098
|dysarthria I69.022
|dysphagia I69.091
|dysphasia I69.021
|facial droop I69.092
|facial weakness I69.092
|fluency disorder I69.023
|hemiplegia I69.05-
|language deficit NEC I69.028
|monoplegia
|lower limb I69.04-
|upper limb I69.03-
|paralytic syndrome I69.06-
|specified effect NEC I69.098
|speech deficit NEC I69.028
|hepatitis, viral B94.2
|hyperalimentation E68
|infarction
|cerebral I69.30
|alteration of sensation I69,398
|aphasia I69.320
|apraxia I69.390
|ataxia I69.393
|cognitive deficits I69.31
|disturbance of vision I69.398
|dysarthria I69.322
|dysphagia I69.391
|dysphasia I69.321
|facial droop I69.392
|facial weakness I69.392
|fluency disorder I69.323
|hemiplegia I69.35-
|language deficit NEC I69.328
|monoplegia
|lower limb I69.34-
|upper limb I69.33-
|paralytic syndrome I69.36-
|specified effect NEC I69.398
|speech deficit NEC I69.328
|infection, pyogenic, intracranial or intraspinal G09
|infectious disease B94.9
|specified NEC B94.8
|injury   code to injury with seventh character S
|leprosy B92
|meningitis
|bacterial (conditions in G00) G09
|other or unspecified cause (conditions in G03) G09
|muscle (and tendon) injury   code to injury with seventh character S
|myelitis *see* Sequelae, encephalitis

Sequelae (of) - continued
|niacin deficiency E64.8
|nutritional deficiency E64.9
  |specified NEC E64.8
|obstetrical condition O94
|parasitic disease B94.9
|phlebitis or thrombophlebitis of intracranial or
  intraspinal venous sinuses and veins
  (conditions in G08) G09
|poisoning - code to poisoning with seventh
  character S
  |nonmedicinal substance *see* Sequelae, toxic
    effect, nonmedicinal substance
|poliomyelitis (acute) B91
|pregnancy O94
|protein-energy malnutrition E64.0
|puerperium O94
|rickets E64.3
|SARS-CoV-2 (post acute) U09.9
|selenium deficiency E64.8
|sprain and strain - code to injury with seventh
  character S
|stroke NOS I69.30
  |alteration in sensation I69.398
  |aphasia I69.320
  |apraxia I69.390
  |ataxia I69.393
  |cognitive deficits I69.31
  |disturbance of vision I69.398
  |dysarthria I69.322
  |dysphagia I69.391
  |dysphasia I69.321
  |facial droop I69.392
  |facial weakness I69.392
  |hemiplegia I69.35-
  |language deficit NEC I69.328
  |monoplegia
    |lower limb I69.34-
    |upper limb I69.33-
  |paralytic syndrome I69.36-
  |specified effect NEC I69.398
  |speech deficit NEC I69.328
|tendon and muscle injury   code to injury with
  seventh character S
|thiamine deficiency E64.8
|trachoma B94.0
|tuberculosis B90.9
  |bones and joints B90.2
  |central nervous system B90.0
  |genitourinary B90.1
  |pulmonary (respiratory) B90.9
  |specified organs NEC B90.8
|viral
  |encephalitis B94.1
  |hepatitis B94.2
|vitamin deficiency NEC E64.8
  |A E64.1
  |B E64.8
  |C E64.2
|wound, open - code to injury with seventh
  character S
Sequestration *see also* Sequestrum
|disc *see* Displacement, intervertebral disk
|lung, congenital Q33.2
Sequestrum
|bone *see* Osteomyelitis, chronic
|dental M27.2
|jaw bone M27.2
|orbit *see* Osteomyelitis, orbit
|sinus (accessory) (nasal) *see* Sinusitis
Sequoiosis lung or pneumonitis J67.8
Serology for syphilis
|doubtful
  |with signs or symptoms   code by site and
    stage under Syphilis

Serology for syphilis - continued
  |follow-up of latent syphilis *see* Syphilis,
    latent
|negative, with signs or symptoms - code by
  site and stage under Syphilis
|positive A53.0
  |with signs or symptoms - code by site and
    stage under Syphilis
|reactivated A53.0
Seroma *see also* Hematoma
|postprocedural *see* Complication,
  postprocedural, seroma
|traumatic, secondary and recurrent T79.2
Seropurulent *see* condition
Serositis, multiple K65.8
|pericardial I31.1
|peritoneal K65.8
Serous *see* condition
Sertoli cell
|adenoma
  |specified site *see* Neoplasm, benign, by site
  |unspecified site
    |female D27.9
    |male D29.20
|carcinoma
  |specified site *see* Neoplasm, malignant, by
    site
  |unspecified site (male) C62.9-
    |female C56.9
|tumor
  |with lipid storage
    |specified site *see* Neoplasm, benign, by
      site
    |unspecified site
      |female D27.9
      |male D29.20
  |specified site *see* Neoplasm, benign, by site
  |unspecified site
    |female D27.9
    |male D29.20
Sertoli-Leydig cell tumor *see* Neoplasm,
  benign, by site
|specified site *see* Neoplasm, benign, by site
|unspecified site
  |female D27.9
  |male D29.20
Serum
|allergy, allergic reaction *see also* Reaction,
  serum T80.69
  |shock *see also* Shock, anaphylactic T80.59
|arthritis *see also* Reaction, serum T80.69
|complication or reaction NEC *see also*
  Reaction, serum T80.69
|disease NEC *see also* Reaction, serum T80.69
|hepatitis *see also* Hepatitis, viral, type B
  |carrier (suspected) of B18.1
|intoxication *see also* Reaction, serum T80.69
|neuritis *see also* Reaction, serum T80.69
|neuropathy G61.1
|poisoning NEC *see also* Reaction, serum
  T80.69
|rash NEC *see also* Reaction, serum T80.69
|reaction NEC *see also* Reaction, serum
  T80.69
|sickness NEC *see also* Reaction, serum
  T80.69
|urticaria *see also* Reaction, serum T80.69
Sesamoiditis M25.8-
Sever's disease or osteochondrosis *see*
  Osteochondrosis, juvenile, tarsus
Severe sepsis R65.20
|with septic shock R65.21
Sex
|chromosome mosaics Q97.8
  |lines with various numbers of X
    chromosomes Q97.2
|education Z70.8
|reassignment surgery status Z87.890

Sextuplet pregnancy *see* Pregnancy, sextuplet
Sexual
|function, disorder of (psychogenic) F52.9
|immaturity (female) (male) E30.0
|impotence (psychogenic) organic origin NEC
  see Dysfunction, sexual, male
|precocity (constitutional)
  (cryptogenic)(female) (idiopathic) (male)
  E30.1
Sexuality, pathologic *see* Deviation, sexual
Sézary disease C84.1-
Shadow, lung R91.8
Shaking palsy or paralysis *see* Parkinsonism
Shallowness, acetabulum *see* Derangement,
  joint, specified type NEC, hip
Shaver's disease J63.1
Sheath (tendon) *see* condition
Sheathing, retinal vessels H35.01-
Shedding
|nail L60.8
|premature, primary (deciduous) teeth K00.6
Sheehan's disease or syndrome E23.0
Shelf, rectal K62.89
Shell teeth K00.5
Shellshock (current) F43.0
|lasting state *see* Disorder, post-traumatic
  stress
Shield kidney Q63.1
Shift
|auditory threshold (temporary) H93.24-
|mediastinal R93.89
Shifting sleep-Work schedule (affecting sleep)
  G47.26
Shiga (-Kruse) dysentery A03.0
Shiga's bacillus A03.0
Shigella (dysentery) *see* Dysentery, bacillary
Shigellosis A03.9
|Group A A03.0
|Group B A03.1
|Group C A03.2
|Group D A03.3
Shin splints S86.89
Shingles *see* Herpes, zoster
Shipyard disease or eye B30.0
Shirodkar suture, in pregnancy *see* Pregnancy,
  complicated by, incompetent cervix
Shock R57.9
|with ectopic or molar pregnancy O08.3
|adrenal (cortical) (Addisonian) E27.2
|adverse food reaction (anaphylactic) *see*
  Shock, anaphylactic, due to food
|allergic *see* Shock, anaphylactic
|anaphylactic T78.2
  |chemical *see* Table of Drugs and Chemicals
  |due to drug or medicinal substance
    |correct substance properly administered
      T88.6
    |overdose or wrong substance given or
      taken (by accident) *see* Table of Drugs
      and Chemicals, by drug, poisoning
  |due to food (nonpoisonous) T78.00
    |additives T78.06
    |dairy products T78.07
    |eggs T78.08
    |fish T78.03
      |shellfish T78.02
    |fruit T78.04
    |milk T78.07
    |nuts T78.05
      |multiple types T78.05
      |peanuts T78.01
    |peanuts T78.01
    |seeds T78.05
    |specified type NEC T78.09
    |vegetable T78.04

Shock - *continued*
|following sting(s) *see* Venom
|immunization T80.52
|serum T80.59
||blood and blood products T80.51
||immunization T80.52
||specified NEC T80.59
||vaccination T80.52
|anaphylactoid *see* Shock, anaphylactic
|anesthetic
||correct substance properly administered
|||T88.2
||overdose or wrong substance given or taken
|||*see* Table of Drugs and Chemicals, by
|||drug, poisoning
||specified anesthetic *see* Table of Drugs
|||and Chemicals, by drug, poisoning
|cardiogenic R57.0
|chemical substance *see* Table of Drugs and
||Chemicals
|complicating ectopic or molar pregnancy
||O08.3
|culture *see* Disorder, adjustment
|drug
||due to correct substance properly
|||administered T88.6
||overdose or wrong substance given or taken
|||(by accident) *see* Table of Drugs and
|||Chemicals, by drug, poisoning
|during or after labor and delivery O75.1
|electric T75.4
||(taser) T75.4
|endotoxic R65.21
||postprocedural (resulting from a procedure,
|||not elsewhere classified) T81.12
|following
||ectopic or molar pregnancy O08.3
||injury (immediate) (delayed) T79.4
||labor and delivery O75.1
|food (anaphylactic) *see* Shock, anaphylactic,
||due to food
|from electroshock gun (taser) T75.4
|gram-negative R65.21
||postprocedural (resulting from a procedure,
|||not elsewhere classified) T81.12
|hematologic R57.8
|hemorrhagic R57.8
||surgery (intraoperative) (postoperative)
|||T81.19
||trauma T79.4
|hypovolemic R57.1
||surgical T81.19
||traumatic T79.4
|insulin E15
||therapeutic misadventure *see* subcategory
|||T38.3
|kidney N17.0
||traumatic (following crushing) T79.5
|liver K72.00
|lightning T75.01
|lung J80
|obstetric O75.1
||with ectopic or molar pregnancy O08.3
||following ectopic or molar pregnancy O08.3
|pleural (surgical) T81.19
||due to trauma T79.4
|postprocedural (postoperative) T81.10
||with ectopic or molar pregnancy O08.3
||cardiogenic T81.11
||endotoxic T81.12
||following ectopic or molar pregnancy O08.3
||gram-negative T81.12
||hypovolemic T81.19
||septic T81.12
||specified type NEC T81.19

Shock - *continued*
|psychic F43.0
|septic (due to severe sepsis) R65.21
|specified NEC R57.8
|surgical T81.10
|taser gun (taser) T75.4
|therapeutic misadventure NEC T81.10
|thyroxin
||overdose or wrong substance given or taken
|||*see* Table of Drugs and Chemicals, by
|||drug, poisoning
|toxic, syndrome A48.3
|transfusion *see* Complications, transfusion
|traumatic (immediate) (delayed) T79.4
Shoemaker's chest M95.4
Short, shortening, shortness
|arm (acquired) *see also* Deformity, limb,
||unequal length
||congenital Q71.81-
||forearm *see* Deformity, limb, unequal length
|bowel syndrome K91.2
|breath R06.02
|cervical (complicating pregnancy) O26.87-
||non-gravid uterus N88.3
|common bile duct, congenital Q44.5
|cord (umbilical), complicating delivery O69.3
|cystic duct, congenital Q44.5
|esophagus (congenital) Q39.8
|femur (acquired) *see* Deformity, limb, unequal
||length
||congenital *see* Defect, reduction, lower
|||limb, longitudinal, femur
|frenum, frenulum, linguae (congenital) Q38.1
|hip (acquired) *see also* Deformity, limb,
||unequal length
||congenital Q65.89
|leg (acquired) *see also* Deformity, limb,
||unequal length
||congenital Q72.81-
||lower leg *see also* Deformity, limb, unequal
|||length
|limbed stature, with immunodeficiency D82.2
|lower limb (acquired) *see also* Deformity,
||limb, unequal length
||congenital Q72.81-
|organ or site, congenital NEC *see* Distortion
|palate, congenital Q38.5
|radius (acquired) *see also* Deformity, limb,
||unequal length
||congenital *see* Defect, reduction, upper
|||limb, longitudinal, radius
|rib syndrome Q77.2
|stature (child) (hereditary) (idiopathic) NEC
||R62.52
||constitutional E34.3
||due to endocrine disorder E34.3
||Laron-type E34.3
|tendon *see also* Contraction, tendon
||with contracture of joint *see* Contraction,
|||joint
||Achilles (acquired) M67.0-
|||congenital Q66.89
||congenital Q79.8
|thigh (acquired) *see also* Deformity, limb,
||unequal length, femur
||congenital *see* Defect, reduction, lower
|||limb, longitudinal, femur
|tibialis anterior (tendon) *see* Contraction,
||tendon
|umbilical cord
||complicating delivery O69.3
|upper limb, congenital *see* Defect, reduction,
||upper limb, specified type NEC
|urethra N36.8
|uvula, congenital Q38.5
|vagina (congenital) Q52.4

Shortsightedness *see* Myopia
Shoshin (acute fulminating beriberi) E51.11
Shoulder *see* condition
Shovel-Shaped incisors K00.2
Shower, thromboembolic *see* Embolism
Shunt
|arterial-venous (dialysis) Z99.2
|arteriovenous, pulmonary (acquired) I28.0
||congenital Q25.72
|cerebral ventricle (communicating) in situ
||Z98.2
|surgical, prosthetic, with complications *see*
||Complications, cardiovascular, device or
||implant
Shutdown, renal N28.9
Shy-Drager syndrome G90.3
Sialadenitis, sialadenosis (any gland) (chronic)
(periodic) (suppurative) *see* Sialoadenitis
Sialectasia K11.8
Sialidosis E77.1
Sialitis, silitis (any gland) (chronic)
(suppurative) *see* Sialoadenitis
Sialoadenitis (any gland) (periodic)
(suppurative) K11.20
|acute K11.21
||recurrent K11.22
|chronic K11.23
Sialadenopathy K11.9
Sialoangitis *see* Sialoadenitis
Sialodochitis (fibrinosa) *see* Sialoadenitis
Sialodocholithiasis K11.5
Sialolithiasis K11.5
Sialometaplasia, necrotizing K11.8
Sialorrhea *see also* Ptyalism
|periodic *see* Sialoadenitis
Sialosis K11.7
Siamese twin Q89.4
Sibling rivalry Z62.891
Sicard's syndrome G52.7
Sicca syndrome - see Syndrome, Sjögren
Sick R69
|or handicapped person in family Z63.79
||needing care at home Z63.6
|sinus (syndrome) I49.5
Sick-Euthyroid syndrome E07.81
Sickle-Cell
|anemia *see* Disease, sickle-cell
|beta plus *see* Disease, sickle-cell, thalassemia,
||beta plus
|beta zero *see* Disease, sickle-cell, thalassemia,
||beta zero
|trait D57.3
Sicklemia *see also* Disease, sickle-cell
|trait D57.3
Sickness
|air (travel) T75.3
|airplane T75.3
|alpine T70.29
|altitude T70.20
|Andes T70.29
|aviator's T70.29
|balloon T70.29
|car T75.3
|compressed air T70.3
|decompression T70.3
|green D50.8
|milk *see* Poisoning, food, noxious
|motion T75.3
|mountain T70.29
||acute D75.1
|protein *see also* Reaction, serum T80.69
|radiation T66
|roundabout (motion) T75.3
|sea T75.3
|serum NEC *see also* Reaction, serum T80.69

Sickness - *continued*
| sleeping (African) B56.9
| | by Trypanosoma B56.9
| | | brucei
| | | | gambiense B56.0
| | | | rhodesiense B56.1
| | East African B56.1
| | Gambian B56.0
| | Rhodesian B56.1
| | West African B56.0
| swing (motion) T75.3
| train (railway) (travel) T75.3
| travel (any vehicle) T75.3
Sideropenia *see* Anemia, iron deficiency
Siderosilicosis J62.8
Siderosis (lung) J63.4
| brain G93.89
| eye (globe) *see* Disorder, globe, degenerative,
| | siderosis
Siemens' syndrome (ectodermal dysplasia)
| Q82.8
Sighing R06.89
| psychogenic F45.8
Sigmoid *see also* condition
| flexure *see* condition
| kidney Q63.1
Sigmoiditis *see also* Enteritis K52.9
| infectious A09
| noninfectious K52.9
Silfversköld's syndrome Q78.9
Silicosiderosis J62.8
Silicosis, silicotic (simple) (complicated) J62.8
| with tuberculosis J65
Silicotuberculosis J65
Silo-Fillers' disease J68.8
| bronchitis J68.0
| pneumonitis J68.0
| pulmonary edema J68.1
Silver's syndrome Q87.1
Simian malaria B53.1
Simmonds' cachexia or disease E23.0
Simons' disease or syndrome (progressive
| **lipodystrophy)** E88.1
Simple, simplex *see* condition
Simulation, conscious (of illness) Z76.5
Simultanagnosia (asimultagnosia) R48.3
Sin Nombre virus disease (Hantavirus)
| **(cardio)-Pulmonary syndrome)** B33.4
Sinding-Larsen disease or osteochondrosis *see*
| Osteochondrosis, juvenile, patella
Singapore hemorrhagic fever A91
Singer's node or nodule J38.2
Single
| atrium Q21.2
| coronary artery Q24.5
| umbilical artery Q27.0
| ventricle Q20.4
Singultus R06.6
| epidemicus B33.0
Sinus *see also* Fistula
| abdominal K63.89
| arrest I45.5
| arrhythmia I49.8
| bradycardia R00.1
| branchial cleft (internal) (external) Q18.0
| coccygeal *see* Sinus, pilonidal
| dental K04.6
| dermal (congenital) Q06.8
| | with abscess Q06.8
| | coccygeal, pilonidal *see* Sinus, coccygeal
| infected, skin NEC L08.89
| marginal, ruptured or bleeding *see*
| | Hemorrhage, antepartum, specified cause
| | NEC
| medial, face and neck Q18.8
| pause I45.5
| pericranii Q01.9

| pilonidal (infected) (rectum) L05.92**S**
| | with abscess L05.02
| preauricular Q18.1
| rectovaginal N82.3
| Rokitansky-Aschoff (gallbladder) K82.8
| sacrococcygeal (dermoid) (infected) *see* Sinus,
| | pilonidal
| tachycardia R00.0
| | paroxysmal I47.1
| tarsi syndrome M25.57-
| testis N50.89
| tract (postinfective) *see* Fistula
| urachus Q64.4
Sinusitis (accessory) (chronic) (hyperplastic)
| **(nasal) (nonpurulent) (purulent)** J32.9
| acute J01.90
| | ethmoidal J01.20
| | | recurrent J01.21
| | frontal J01.10
| | | recurrent J01.11
| | involving more than one sinus, other than
| | | pansinusitis J01.80
| | | recurrent J01.81
| | maxillary J01.00
| | | recurrent J01.01
| | pansinusitis J01.40
| | | recurrent J01.41
| | recurrent J01.91
| | specified NEC J01.80
| | | recurrent J01.81
| | sphenoidal J01.30
| | | recurrent J01.31
| allergic *see* Rhinitis, allergic
| due to high altitude T70.1
| ethmoidal J32.2
| | acute J01.20
| | | recurrent J01.21
| frontal J32.1
| | acute J01.10
| | | recurrent J01.11
| influenzal *see* Influenza, with, respiratory
| | manifestations NEC
| involving more than one sinus but not
| | pansinusitis J32.8
| | acute J01.80
| | | recurrent J01.81
| maxillary J32.0
| | acute J01.00
| | | recurrent J01.01
| sphenoidal J32.3
| | acute J01.30
| | | recurrent J01.31
| tuberculous, any sinus A15.8
Sinusitis-Bronchiectasis-Situs inversus
| **(syndrome) (triad)** Q89.3
Sipple's syndrome E31.22
Sirenomelia (syndrome) Q87.2
Siriasis T67.0
Sirkari's disease B55.0
Siti A65
Situation, psychiatric F99
Situational
| disturbance (transient) *see* Disorder,
| | adjustment
| | acute F43.0
| maladjustment *see* Disorder, adjustment
| reaction *see* Disorder, adjustment
| | acute F43.0
Situs inversus or transversus (abdominalis)
| **(thoracis)** Q89.3
Sixth disease B08.20
| due to human herpesvirus 6 B08.21
| due to human herpesvirus 7 B08.22
Sjögren-Larsson syndrome Q87.1

Sjögren's syndrome or disease *see* - see
| Syndrome, Sjögren
Skeletal *see* condition
Skene's gland *see* condition
Skenitis *see* Urethritis
Skerljevo A65
Skevas-Zerfus disease *see* Toxicity, venom,
| marine animal, sea anemone
Skin *see also* condition
| clammy R23.1
| donor *see* Donor, skin
| dry L85.3
| hidebound M35.9
Slate-Dressers' or slate-Miners' lung J62.8
Sleep
| apnea *see* Apnea, sleep
| deprivation Z72.820
| disorder or disturbance G47.9
| | child F51.9
| | nonorganic origin F51.9
| | specified NEC G47.8
| disturbance G47.9
| | nonorganic origin F51.9
| drunkenness F51.9
| rhythm inversion G47.2-
| terrors F51.4
| walking F51.3
| | hysterical F44.89
Sleep hygiene
| abuse Z72.821
| inadequate Z72.821
| poor Z72.821
Sleeping sickness *see* Sickness, sleeping
Sleeplessness *see* Insomnia
| menopausal N95.1
Sleep-Wake schedule disorder G47.20
Slim disease (in HIV infection) B20
Slipped, slipping
| epiphysis (traumatic) *see also*
| | Osteochondropathy, specified type NEC
| | capital femoral (traumatic)
| | | acute (on chronic) S79.01-
| | current traumatic - code as Fracture, by site
| | upper femoral (nontraumatic) M93.00-
| | | acute M93.01-
| | | | on chronic M93.03-
| | | chronic M93.02-
| intervertebral disc *see* Displacement,
| | intervertebral disc
| ligature, umbilical P51.8
| patella *see* Disorder, patella, derangement
| | NEC
| rib M89.8X8
| sacroiliac joint *see* subcategory M53.2
| tendon *see* Disorder, tendon
| ulnar nerve, nontraumatic *see* Lesion, nerve,
| | ulnar
| vertebra NEC *see* Spondylolisthesis
Slocumb's syndrome E27.0
Sloughing (multiple) (phagedena) (skin) *see*
| *also* Gangrene
| abscess *see* Abscess
| appendix K38.8
| fascia *see* Disorder, soft tissue, specified type
| | NEC
| scrotum N50.89
| tendon *see* Disorder, tendon
| transplanted organ *see* Rejection, transplant
| ulcer *see* Ulcer, skin
Slow
| feeding, newborn P92.2
| flow syndrome, coronary I20.8
| heart (beat) R00.1
Slowing, urinary stream R39.198

Sluder's neuralgia (syndrome) G44.89
Slurred, slurring speech R47.81
Small (ness)
|for gestational age *see* Small for dates
|introitus, vagina N89.6
|kidney (unknown cause) N27.9
||bilateral N27.1
||unilateral N27.0
|ovary (congenital) Q50.39
|pelvis
||with disproportion (fetopelvic) O33.1
|||causing obstructed labor O65.1
|uterus N85.8
|white kidney N03.9
Small-And-Light-For-Dates *see* Small for dates
Small-For-Dates (infant) P05.10
|with weight of
||499 grams or less P05.11
||500-749 grams P05.12
||750-999 grams P05.13
||1000-1249 grams P05.14
||1250-1499 grams P05.15
||1500-1749 grams P05.16
||1750-1999 grams P05.17
||2000-2499 grams P05.18
||2500 grams and over P05.19
|specified NEC P05.19
SMEI (severe myoclonic epilepsy in infancy)
  G40.83-
Smallpox B03
Smearing, fecal R15.1
Smith-Lemli-Opitz syndrome E78.72
Smith's fracture S52.54-
Smoker *see* Dependence, drug, nicotine
Smoker's
|bronchitis J41.0
|cough J41.0
|palate K13.24
|throat J31.2
|tongue K13.24
Smoking
|passive Z77.22
Smothering spells R06.81
Snaggle teeth, tooth M26.39
Snapping
|finger *see* Trigger finger
|hip *see* Derangement, joint, specified type
  NEC, hip
||involving the iliotibial band M76.3-
|knee *see* Derangement, knee
||involving the iliotibial band M76.3-
Sneddon-Wilkinson disease or syndrome (sub-
  Corneal pustular dermatosis) L13.1
Sneezing (intractable) R06.7
Sniffing
|cocaine
||abuse *see* Abuse, drug, cocaine
||dependence *see* Dependence, drug, cocaine
|gasoline
||abuse *see* Abuse, drug, inhalant
||dependence *see* Dependence, drug, inhalant
|glue (airplane)
||abuse *see* Abuse, drug, inhalant
||drug dependence *see* Dependence, drug,
  inhalant
Sniffles
|newborn P28.89
Snoring R06.83
Snow blindness *see* Photokeratitis
Snuffles (non-Syphilitic) R06.5
|newborn P28.89
|syphilitic (infant) A50.05 [*J99*]

Social
|exclusion Z60.4
||due to discrimination or persecution
  (perceived) Z60.5
|migrant Z59.00
||acculturation difficulty Z60.3
|rejection Z60.4
||due to discrimination or persecution Z60.5
|role conflict NEC Z73.5
|skills inadequacy NEC Z73.4
|transplantation Z60.3
Sodoku A25.0
Soemmerring's ring *see* Cataract, secondary
Soft *see also* condition
|nails L60.3
Softening
|bone *see* Osteomalacia
|brain (necrotic) (progressive) G93.89
||congenital Q04.8
||embolic I63.4-
||hemorrhagic *see* Hemorrhage, intracranial,
  intracerebral
||occlusive I63.5-
||thrombotic I63.3-
|cartilage M94.2-
||patella M22.4-
|cerebellar *see* Softening, brain
|cerebral *see* Softening, brain
|cerebrospinal *see* Softening, brain
|myocardial, heart *see* Degeneration,
  myocardial
|spinal cord G95.89
|stomach K31.89
Soldier's
|heart F45.8
|patches I31.0
Solitary
|cyst, kidney N28.1
|kidney, congenital Q60.0
Solvent abuse *see* Abuse, drug, inhalant
|dependence *see* Dependence, drug, inhalant
Somatization reaction, somatic reaction *see*
  Disorder, somatoform
Somnambulism F51.3
|hysterical F44.89
Somnolence R40.0
|nonorganic origin F51.11
Sonne dysentery A03.3
Soor B37.0
Sore
|bed *see* Ulcer, pressure, by site
|chiclero B55.1
|Delhi B55.1
|desert *see* Ulcer, skin
|eye H57.1-
|Lahore B55.1
|mouth K13.79
||canker K12.0
|muscle M79.10
|Naga *see* Ulcer, skin
|of skin *see* Ulcer, skin
|oriental B55.1
|pressure *see* Ulcer, pressure, by site
|skin L98.9
|soft A57
|throat (acute) *see also* Pharyngitis
||with influenza, flu, or grippe *see* Influenza,
  with, respiratory manifestations NEC
||chronic J31.2
||coxsackie (virus) B08.5
||diphtheritic A36.0
||herpesviral B00.2
||influenzal *see* Influenza, with, respiratory
  manifestations NEC
||septic J02.0
||streptococcal (ulcerative) J02.0

Sore - *continued*
|viral NEC J02.8
||coxsackie B08.5
|tropical *see* Ulcer, skin
|veldt *see* Ulcer, skin
Soto's syndrome (cerebral gigantism) Q87.3
South African cardiomyopathy syndrome
  I42.8
Southeast Asian hemorrhagic fever A91
Spacing
|abnormal, tooth, teeth, fully erupted M26.30
|excessive, tooth, fully erupted M26.32
Spade-Like hand (congenital) Q68.1
Spading nail L60.8
|congenital Q84.6
Spanish collar N47.1
Sparganosis B70.1
Spasm(s), spastic, spasticity *see also* condition
  R25.2
|accommodation *see* Spasm, of
  accommodation
|ampulla of Vater K83.4
|anus, ani (sphincter) (reflex) K59.4
||psychogenic F45.8
|artery I73.9
||cerebral G45.9
|Bell's G51.3-
|bladder (sphincter, external or internal)
  N32.89
||psychogenic F45.8
|bronchus, bronchiole J98.01
|cardia K22.0
|cardiac I20.1
|carpopedal *see* Tetany
|cerebral (arteries) (vascular) G45.9
|cervix, complicating delivery O62.4
|ciliary body (of accommodation) *see* Spasm,
  of accommodation
|colon *see also* Irritable, bowel K58.9
||with diarrhea K58.0
||psychogenic F45.8
|common duct K83.8
|compulsive *see* Tic
|conjugate H51.8
|coronary (artery) I20.1
|diaphragm (reflex) R06.6
||epidemic B33.0
||psychogenic F45.8
|duodenum K59.89
|epidemic diaphragmatic (transient) B33.0
|esophagus (diffuse) K22.4
||psychogenic F45.8
|facial G51.3-
|fallopian tube N83.8
|gastrointestinal (tract) K31.89
||psychogenic F45.8
|glottis J38.5
||hysterical F44.4
||psychogenic F45.8
|||conversion reaction F44.4
||reflex through recurrent laryngeal nerve
  J38.5
|habit *see* Tic
|heart I20.1
|hemifacial (clonic) G51.3-
|hourglass *see* Contraction, hourglass
|hysterical F44.4
|infantile *see* Epilepsy, spasms
|inferior oblique, eye H51.8
|intestinal *see also* Syndrome, irritable bowel
  K58.9
||psychogenic F45.8
|larynx, laryngeal J38.5
||hysterical F44.4
||psychogenic F45.8

Spasm(s), spastic, spasticity - continued
|conversion reaction F44.4
|levator palpebrae superioris see Disorder, eyelid function
|muscle NEC M62.838
||back M62.830
|nerve, trigeminal G51.0
|nervous F45.8
|nodding F98.4
|occupational F48.8
|oculogyric H51.8
||psychogenic F45.8
|of accommodation H52.53-
|ophthalmic artery see Occlusion, artery, retina
|perineal, female N94.89
|peroneo-extensor see also Deformity, limb, flat foot
|pharynx (reflex) J39.2
||hysterical F45.8
||psychogenic F45.8
|psychogenic F45.8
|pylorus NEC K31.3
||adult hypertrophic K31.89
||congenital or infantile Q40.0
||psychogenic F45.8
|rectum (sphincter) K59.4
||psychogenic F45.8
|retinal (artery) see Occlusion, artery, retina
|sigmoid see also Syndrome, irritable bowel K58.9
||psychogenic F45.8
|sphincter of Oddi K83.4
|stomach K31.89
||neurotic F45.8
|throat J39.2
||hysterical F45.8
||psychogenic F45.8
|tic F95.9
||chronic F95.1
||transient of childhood F95.0
|tongue K14.8
|torsion (progressive) G24.1
|trigeminal nerve see Neuralgia, trigeminal
|ureter N13.5
|urethra (sphincter) N35.919
|uterus N85.8
||complicating labor O62.4
|vagina N94.2
||psychogenic F52.5
|vascular I73.9
|vasomotor I73.9
|vein NEC I87.8
|viscera see Pain, abdominal
Spasmodic see condition
Spasmophilia see Tetany
Spasmus nutans F98.4
Spastic, spasticity see also Spasm
|child (cerebral) (congenital) (paralysis) G80.1
Speaker's throat R49.8
Specific, specified see condition
Speech
|defect, disorder, disturbance, impediment see Disorder, speech R47.9
||psychogenic, in childhood and adolescence F98.8
||slurring R47.81
||specified NEC R47.89
Spencer's disease A08.19
Spens' syndrome (syncope with heart block) I45.9
Sperm counts (fertility testing) Z31.41
|postvasectomy Z30.8
||reversal Z31.42
Spermatic cord see condition

Spermatocele N43.40
|congenital Q55.4
|multiple N43.42
|single N43.41
Spermatocystitis N49.0
Spermatocytoma C62.9-
|specified site see Neoplasm, malignant, by site
Spermatorrhea N50.89
Sphacelus see Gangrene
Sphenoidal see condition
Sphenoiditis (chronic) see Sinusitis, sphenoidal
Sphenopalatine ganglion neuralgia G90.09
Sphericity, increased, lens (congenital) Q12.4
Spherocytosis (congenital) (familial) (hereditary) D58.0
|hemoglobin disease D58.0
|sickle-cell (disease) D57.8-
Spherophakia Q12.4
Sphincter see condition
Sphincteritis, sphincter of Oddi see Cholangitis
Sphingolipidosis E75.3
|specified NEC E75.29
Sphingomyelinosis E75.3
Spicule tooth K00.2
Spider
|bite see Toxicity, venom, spider
||nonvenomous see Bite, by site, superficial, insect
|fingers see Syndrome, Marfan's
|nevus I78.1
|toes see Syndrome, Marfan's
|vascular I78.1
Spiegler-Fendt
|benign lymphocytoma L98.8
|sarcoid L08.89
Spielmeyer-Vogt disease E75.4
Spina bifida (aperta) Q05.9
|with hydrocephalus NEC Q05.4
|cervical Q05.5
||with hydrocephalus Q05.0
|dorsal Q05.6
||with hydrocephalus Q05.1
|lumbar Q05.7
||with hydrocephalus Q05.2
|lumbosacral Q05.7
||with hydrocephalus Q05.2
|occulta Q76.0
|sacral Q05.8
||with hydrocephalus Q05.3
|thoracic Q05.6
||with hydrocephalus Q05.1
|thoracolumbar Q05.6
||with hydrocephalus Q05.1
Spindle, Krukenberg's see Pigmentation, cornea, posterior
Spine, spinal see condition
Spiradenoma (eccrine) see Neoplasm, skin, benign
Spirillosis A25.0
Spirillum
|minus A25.0
|obermeieri infection A68.0
Spirochetal see condition
Spirochetosis A69.9
|arthritic, arthritica A69.9
|bronchopulmonary A69.8
|icterohemorrhagic A27.0
|lung A69.8
Spirometrosis B70.1
Spitting blood see Hemoptysis
Splanchnoptosis K63.4
Spleen, splenic see condition
Splenectasis see Splenomegaly

Splenitis (interstitial) (malignant) (nonspecific) D73.89
|malarial see also Malaria B54 [D77]
|tuberculous A18.85
Splenocele D73.89
Splenomegaly, splenomegalia (Bengal) (cryptogenic) (idiopathic) (tropical) R16.1
|with hepatomegaly R16.2
|cirrhotic D73.2
|congenital Q89.09
|congestive, chronic D73.2
|Egyptian B65.1
|Gaucher's E75.22
|malarial see also Malaria B54 [D77]
|neutropenic D73.81
|Niemann-Pick see Niemann-Pick disease or syndrome
|siderotic D73.2
|syphilitic A52.79
||congenital (early) A50.08 [D77]
Splenopathy D73.9
Splenoptosis D73.89
Splenosis D73.89
Splinter see Foreign body, superficial, by site
Split, splitting
|foot Q72.7-
|hand Q71.6
|heart sounds R01.2
|lip, congenital see Cleft, lip
|nails L60.3
|urinary stream R39.13
Spondylarthrosis see Spondylosis
Spondylitis (chronic) see also Spondylopathy, inflammatory
|ankylopoietica see Spondylitis, ankylosing
|ankylosing (chronic) M45.9
||with lung involvement M45.9 [J99]
||cervical region M45.2
||cervicothoracic region M45.3
||juvenile M08.1
||lumbar region M45.6
||lumbosacral region M45.7
||multiple sites M45.0
||occipito-atlanto-axial region M45.1
||sacrococcygeal region M45.8
||thoracic region M45.4
||thoracolumbar region M45.5
|atrophic (ligamentous) see Spondylitis, ankylosing
|deformans (chronic) see Spondylosis
|gonococcal A54.41
|gouty see also Gout, by type, vertebrae M10.08
|in (due to)
||brucellosis A23.9 [M49.80]
|||cervical region A23.9 [M49.82]
|||cervicothoracic region A23.9 [M49.83]
|||lumbar region A23.9 [M49.86]
|||lumbosacral region A23.9 [M49.87]
|||multiple sites A23.9 [M49.89]
|||occipito-atlanto-axial region A23.9 [M49.81]
|||sacrococcygeal region A23.9 [M49.88]
|||thoracic region A23.9 [M49.84]
|||thoracolumbar region A23.9 [M49.85]
||enterobacteria see also subcategory M49.8 A04.9
||tuberculosis A18.01
|infectious NEC see Spondylopathy, infective
|juvenile ankylosing (chronic) M08.1
|Kümmell's see Spondylopathy, traumatic
|Marie-Strümpell see Spondylitis, ankylosing
|muscularis see Spondylopathy, specified NEC
|psoriatic L40.53
|rheumatoid see Spondylitis, ankylosing

Spondylitis - *continued*
|rhizomelica *see* Spondylitis, ankylosing
|sacroiliac NEC M46.1
|senescent, senile *see* Spondylosis
|traumatic (chronic) or post-traumatic *see*
    Spondylopathy, traumatic
|tuberculous A18.01
|typhosa A01.05
Spondyloarthritis
|axial *see also* Spondlyitis, ankylosing
    |non-radiographic M45.A0
        |cervical M46.A2
        |cervicothoracic M46.A3
        |lumbar M46.A6
        |lumbosacral M46.A7
        |multiple sites M45.AB
        |occipito-atlanto-axial region M46.A1
        |sacral and sacrococcygeal M45.A8
        |thoracic M45.A4
        |thoracolumbar M45.A5
Spondylolisthesis (acquired) (degenerative)
    M43.10
|with disproportion (fetopelvic) O33.0
    |causing obstructed labor O65.0
|cervical region M43.12
|cervicothoracic region M43.13
|congenital Q76.2
|lumbar region M43.16
|lumbosacral region M43.17
|multiple sites M43.19
|occipito-atlanto-axial region M43.11
|sacrococcygeal region M43.18
|thoracic region M43.14
|thoracolumbar region M43.15
|traumatic (old) M43.10
    |acute
        |fifth cervical (displaced) S12.430
            |nondisplaced S12.431
            |specified type NEC (displaced) S12.450
                |nondisplaced S12.451
            |type III S12.44
        |fourth cervical (displaced) S12.330
            |nondisplaced S12.331
            |specified type NEC (displaced) S12.350
                |nondisplaced S12.351
            |type III S12.34
        |second cervical (displaced) S12.130
            |nondisplaced S12.131
            |specified type NEC (displaced) S12.150
                |nondisplaced S12.151
            |type III S12.14
        |seventh cervical (displaced) S12.630
            |nondisplaced S12.631
            |specified type NEC (displaced) S12.650
                |nondisplaced S12.651
            |type III S12.64
        |sixth cervical (displaced) S12.530
            |nondisplaced S12.531
            |specified type NEC (displaced) S12.550
                |nondisplaced S12.551
            |type III S12.54
        |third cervical (displaced) S12.230
            |nondisplaced S12.231
            |specified type NEC (displaced) S12.250
                |nondisplaced S12.251
            |type III S12.24
Spondylolysis (acquired) M43.00
|cervical region M43.02
|cervicothoracic region M43.03
|congenital Q76.2
|lumbar region M43.06
|lumbosacral region M43.07
    |with disproportion (fetopelvic) O33.0
        |causing obstructed labor O65.8
|multiple sites M43.09
|occipito-atlanto-axial region M43.01

Spondylolysis (acquired) - *continued*
|sacrococcygeal region M43.08
|thoracic region M43.04
|thoracolumbar region M43.05
Spondylopathy M48.9
|infective NEC M46.50
    |cervical region M46.52
    |cervicothoracic region M46.53
    |lumbar region M46.56
    |lumbosacral region M46.57
    |multiple sites M46.59
    |occipito-atlanto-axial region M46.51
    |sacrococcygeal region M46.58
    |thoracic region M46.54
    |thoracolumbar region M46.55
|inflammatory M46.90
    |cervical region M46.92
    |cervicothoracic region M46.93
    |lumbar region M46.96
    |lumbosacral region M46.97
    |multiple sites M46.99
    |occipito-atlanto-axial region M46.91
    |sacrococcygeal region M46.98
|specified type NEC M46.80
    |cervical region M46.82
    |cervicothoracic region M46.83
    |lumbar region M46.86
    |lumbosacral region M46.87
    |multiple sites M46.89
    |occipito-atlanto-axial region M46.81
    |sacrococcygeal region M46.88
    |thoracic region M46.84
    |thoracolumbar region M46.85
|thoracic region M46.94
|thoracolumbar region M46.95
|neuropathic, in
    |syringomyelia and syringobulbia G95.0
    |tabes dorsalis A52.11
|specified NEC *see* subcategory M48.8
|traumatic M48.30
    |cervical region M48.32
    |cervicothoracic region M48.33
    |lumbar region M48.36
    |lumbosacral region M48.37
    |occipito-atlanto-axial region M48.31
    |sacrococcygeal region M48.38
    |thoracic region M48.34
    |thoracolumbar region M48.35
Spondylosis M47.9
|with
    |disproportion (fetopelvic) O33.0
        |causing obstructed labor O65.0
    |myelopathy NEC M47.10
        |cervical region M47.12
        |cervicothoracic region M47.13
        |lumbar region M47.16
        |occipito-atlanto-axial region M47.11
        |thoracic region M47.14
        |thoracolumbar region M47.15
    |radiculopathy M47.20
        |cervical region M47.22
        |cervicothoracic region M47.23
        |lumbar region M47.26
        |lumbosacral region M47.27
        |occipito-atlanto-axial region M47.21
        |sacrococcygeal region M47.28
        |thoracic region M47.24
        |thoracolumbar region M47.25
|specified NEC M47.899
    |cervical region M47.892
    |cervicothoracic region M47.893
    |facet joint (see also Spondylosis) M47.819
    |lumbar region M47.896
    |lumbosacral region M47.897
    |occipito-atlanto-axial region M47.891
    |sacrococcygeal region M47.898
    |thoracic region M47.894

Spondylosis - *continued*
    |thoracolumbar region M47.895
    |traumatic *see* Spondylopathy, traumatic
    |without myelopathy or radiculopathy M47.819
        |cervical region M47.812
        |cervicothoracic region M47.813
        |lumbar region M47.816
        |lumbosacral region M47.817
        |occipito-atlanto-axial region M47.811
        |sacrococcygeal region M47.818
        |thoracic region M47.814
        |thoracolumbar region M47.815
Sponge
|inadvertently left in operation wound *see*
    Foreign body, accidentally left during a
    procedure
|kidney (medullary) Q61.5
Sponge-Diver's disease *see* Toxicity, venom,
    marine animal, sea anemone
Spongioblastoma (any type) *see* Neoplasm,
    malignant, by site
|specified site *see* Neoplasm, malignant, by site
|unspecified site C71.9
Spongioneuroblastoma *see* Neoplasm,
    malignant, by site
Spontaneous *see also* condition
|fracture (cause unknown) *see* Fracture,
    pathological **S**
Spoon nail L60.3
|congenital Q84.6
Sporadic *see* condition
Sporothrix schenckii infection *see*
    Sporotrichosis
Sporotrichosis B42.9
|arthritis B42.82
|disseminated B42.7
|generalized B42.7
|lymphocutaneous (fixed) (progressive) B42.1
|pulmonary B42.0
|specified NEC B42.89
Spots, spotting (in) (of)
|Bitot's *see also* Pigmentation, conjunctiva
    |in the young child E50.1
    |vitamin A deficiency E50.1
|café, au lait L81.3
|Cayenne pepper I78.1
|cotton wool, retina *see* Occlusion, artery,
    retina
|de Morgan's (senile angiomas) I78.1
|Fuchs' black (myopic) (*see also* Myopia,
    degenerative) H44.2-
|intermenstrual (regular) N92.0
    |irregular N92.1
|Koplik's B05.9
|liver L81.4
|pregnancy O26.85-
|purpuric R23.3
|ruby I78.1
Spotted fever *see* Fever, spotted A77.9
Sprain (joint) (ligament)
|acromioclavicular joint or ligament S43.5-
|ankle S93.40-
    |calcaneofibular ligament S93.41-
    |deltoid ligament S93.42-
    |internal collateral ligament *see* Sprain,
        ankle, specified ligament NEC
    |specified ligament NEC S93.49-
    |talofibular ligament *see* Sprain, ankle,
        specified ligament NEC
    |tibiofibular ligament S93.43-
|anterior longitudinal, cervical S13.4
|atlas, atlanto-axial, atlanto-occipital S13.4
|breast bone *see* Sprain, sternum
|calcaneofibular *see* Sprain, ankle

Sprain - *continued*

|carpal *see* Sprain, wrist
|carpometacarpal *see* Sprain, hand, specified
  site NEC
|cartilage
  |costal S23.41
  |semilunar (knee) *see* Sprain, knee, specified
    site NEC
    |with current tear *see* Tear, meniscus
  |thyroid region S13.5
  |xiphoid *see* Sprain, sternum
|cervical, cervicodorsal, cervicothoracic S13.4
|chondrosternal S23.421
|coracoclavicular S43.8-
|coracohumeral S43.41-
|coronary, knee *see* Sprain, knee, specified site
  NEC
|costal cartilage S23.41
|cricoarytenoid articulation or ligament S13.5
|cricothyroid articulation S13.5
|cruciate, knee *see* Sprain, knee, cruciate
|deltoid, ankle *see* Sprain, ankle
|dorsal (spine) S23.3
|elbow S53.40-
  |radial collateral ligament S53.43-
  |radiohumeral S53.41-
  |rupture
    |radial collateral ligament *see* Rupture,
      traumatic, ligament, radial collateral
    |ulnar collateral ligament *see* Rupture,
      traumatic, ligament, ulnar collateral
  |specified type NEC S53.49-
  |ulnar collateral ligament S53.44-
  |ulnohumeral S53.42-
|femur, head *see* Sprain, hip
|fibular collateral, knee *see* Sprain, knee,
  collateral
|fibulocalcaneal *see* Sprain, ankle
|finger(s) S63.61-
  |index S63.61-
  |interphalangeal (joint) S63.63-
    |index S63.63-
    |little S63.63
    |middle S63.63
    |ring S63.63-
  |little S63.61-
  |middle S63.61-
  |ring S63.61-
  |metacarpophalangeal (joint) S63.65-
  |specified site NEC S63.69-
    |index S63.69-
    |little S63.69-
    |middle S63.69-
    |ring S63.69-
|foot S93.60-
  |specified ligament NEC S93.69-
  |tarsal ligament S93.61-
  |tarsometatarsal ligament S93.62-
  |toe *see* Sprain, toe
|hand S63.9-
  |finger *see* Sprain, finger
  |specified site NEC subcategory S63.8
  |thumb *see* Sprain, thumb
|head S03.9
|hip S73.10-
  |iliofemoral ligament S73.11-
  |ischiocapsular (ligament) S73.12-
  |specified NEC S73.19-
|iliofemoral *see* Sprain, hip
|innominate
  |acetabulum *see* Sprain, hip
  |sacral junction S33.6
|internal
  |collateral, ankle *see* Sprain, ankle

Sprain - *continued*

  |semilunar cartilage *see* Sprain, knee,
    specified site NEC
|interphalangeal
  |finger *see* Sprain, finger, interphalangeal
    (joint)
  |toe *see* Sprain, toe, interphalangeal joint
|ischiocapsular *see* Sprain, hip
|ischiofemoral *see* Sprain, hip
|jaw (articular disc) (cartilage) (meniscus)
  S03.4-
  |old M26.69
|knee S83.9-
  |collateral ligament S83.40-
    |lateral (fibular) S83.42-
    |medial (tibial) S83.41-
  |cruciate ligament S83.50-
    |anterior S83.51-
    |posterior S83.52-
  |lateral (fibular) collateral ligament S83.42-
  |medial (tibial) collateral ligament S83.41-
  |patellar ligament S76.11-
  |specified site NEC S83.8X-
  |superior tibiofibular joint (ligament) S83.6-
|lateral collateral, knee *see* Sprain, knee,
  collateral
|lumbar (spine) S33.5
|lumbosacral S33.9
|mandible (articular disc) S03.4-
  |old M26.69
|medial collateral, knee *see* Sprain, knee,
  collateral
|meniscus
  |jaw S03.4-
    |old M26.69
  |knee *see* Sprain, knee, specified site NEC
    |with current tear *see* Tear, meniscus
      |old *see* Derangement, knee, meniscus,
        due to old tear
  |mandible S03.4-
    |old M26.69
|metacarpal (distal) (proximal) *see* Sprain,
  hand, specified site NEC
|metacarpophalangeal *see* Sprain, finger,
  metacarpophalangeal (joint)
|metatarsophalangeal *see* Sprain, toe,
  metatarsophalangeal joint
|midcarpal *see* Sprain, hand, specified site
  NEC
|midtarsal *see* Sprain, foot, specified site NEC
|neck S13.9
  |anterior longitudinal cervical ligament S13.4
  |atlanto-axial joint S13.4
  |atlanto-occipital joint S13.4
  |cervical spine S13.4
  |cricoarytenoid ligament S13.5
  |cricothyroid ligament S13.5
  |specified site NEC S13.8
  |thyroid region (cartilage) S13.5
|nose S03.8
|orbicular, hip *see* Sprain, hip
|patella *see* Sprain, knee, specified site NEC
|patellar ligament S76.11-
|pelvis NEC S33.8
|phalanx
  |finger *see* Sprain, finger
  |toe *see* Sprain, toe
|pubofemoral *see* Sprain, hip
|radiocarpal *see* Sprain, wrist
|radiohumeral *see* Sprain, elbow
|radius, collateral *see* Rupture, traumatic,
  ligament, radial collateral
|rib (cage) S23.41
|rotator cuff (capsule) S43.42-
|sacroiliac (region)

Sprain - *continued*

  |chronic or old *see* subcategory M53.2
  |joint S33.6
|scaphoid (hand) *see* Sprain, hand, specified
  site NEC
|scapula (r) *see* Sprain, shoulder girdle,
  specified site NEC
|semilunar cartilage (knee) *see* Sprain, knee,
  specified site NEC
  |with current tear *see* Tear, meniscus
    |old *see* Derangement, knee, meniscus, due
      to old tear
|shoulder joint S43.40-
  |acromioclavicular joint (ligament) *see*
    Sprain, acromioclavicular joint
  |blade *see* Sprain, shoulder, girdle, specified
    site NEC
  |coracoclavicular joint (ligament) *see* Sprain,
    coracoclavicular joint
  |coracohumeral ligament *see* Sprain,
    coracohumeral joint
  |girdle S43.9-
    |specified site NEC S43.8-
  |rotator cuff *see* Sprain, rotator cuff
  |specified site NEC S43.49-
  |sternoclavicular joint (ligament) *see* Sprain,
    sternoclavicular joint
|spine
  |cervical S13.4
  |lumbar S33.5
  |thoracic S23.3
|sternoclavicular joint S43.6-
|sternum S23.429
  |chondrosternal joint S23.421
  |specified site NEC S23.428
  |sternoclavicular (joint) (ligament) S23.420
|symphysis
  |jaw S03.4-
    |old M26.69
  |mandibular S03.4-
    |old M26.69
|talofibular *see* Sprain, ankle
|tarsal *see* Sprain, foot, specified site NEC
|tarsometatarsal *see* Sprain, foot, specified site
  NEC
|temporomandibular S03.4-
  |old M26.69
|thorax S23.9
  |ribs S23.41
  |specified site NEC S23.8
  |spine S23.3
  |sternum *see* Sprain, sternum
|thumb S63.60-
  |interphalangeal (joint) S63.62-
  |metacarpophalangeal (joint) S63.64-
  |specified site NEC S63.68-
|thyroid cartilage or region S13.5
|tibia (proximal end) *see* Sprain, knee,
  specified site NEC
|tibial collateral, knee *see* Sprain, knee,
  collateral
|tibiofibular
  |distal *see* Sprain, ankle
  |superior *see* Sprain, knee, specified site
    NEC
|toe(s) S93.50-
  |great S93.50-
  |interphalangeal joint S93.51-
    |great S93.51-
    |lesser S93.51-
  |lesser S93.50-
  |metatarsophalangeal joint S93.52-
    |great S93.52-
    |lesser S93.52-

Sprain - *continued*
| ulna, collateral *see* Rupture, traumatic,
   ligament, ulnar collateral
| ulnohumeral *see* Sprain, elbow
| wrist S63.50-
   | carpal S63.51-
   | radiocarpal S63.52-
   | specified site NEC S63.59-
| xiphoid cartilage *see* Sprain, sternum
Sprengel's deformity (congenital) Q74.0
Sprue (tropical) K90.1
| celiac K90.0
| idiopathic K90.49
| meaning thrush B37.0
| nontropical K90.0
Spur, bone *see also* Enthesopathy
| calcaneal M77.3-
| iliac crest M76.2-
| nose (septum) J34.89
Spurway's syndrome Q78.0
Sputum
| abnormal (amount) (color) (odor) (purulent)
   R09.3
| blood-stained R04.2
| excessive (cause unknown) R09.3
Squamous *see also* condition
| epithelium in
   | cervical canal (congenital) Q51.828
   | uterine mucosa (congenital) Q51.818
Squashed nose M95.0
| congenital Q67.4
Squeeze, diver's T70.3
Squint *see also* Strabismus
| accommodative *see* Strabismus, convergent
   concomitant
**SSADHD (succinic semialdehyde
   dehydrogenase deficiency)** E72.81
St. Hubert's disease A82.9
Stab *see also* Laceration
| internal organs *see* Injury, by site
Stafne's cyst or cavity M27.0
Staggering gait R26.0
| hysterical F44.4
Staghorn calculus *see* Calculus, kidney
Stähli's line (cornea) (pigment) *see*
   Pigmentation, cornea, anterior
Stain, staining
| meconium (newborn) P96.83
| port wine Q82.5
| tooth, teeth (hard tissues) (extrinsic) K03.6
   | due to
      | accretions K03.6
      | deposits (betel) (black) (green) (materia
   alba) (orange) (soft) (tobacco) K03.6
      | metals (copper) (silver) K03.7
      | nicotine K03.6
      | pulpal bleeding K03.7
      | tobacco K03.6
   | intrinsic K00.8
Stammering *see also* Disorder, fluency F80.81
Standstill
| auricular I45.5
| cardiac *see* Arrest, cardiac
| sinoatrial I45.5
| ventricular *see* Arrest, cardiac
Stannosis J63.5
Stanton's disease *see* Melioidosis
**Staphylitis (acute) (catarrhal) (chronic)
   (gangrenous) (membranous) (suppurative)
   (ulcerative)** K12.2
Staphylococcal scalded skin syndrome L00
Staphylococcemia A41.2

Staphylococcus, staphylococcal *see also*
   condition
| as cause of disease classified elsewhere B95.8
   | aureus (methicillin susceptible) (MSSA)
      B95.61
      | methicillin resistant (MRSA) B95.62
| specified NEC, as cause of disease classified
   elsewhere B95.7
Staphyloma (sclera)
| cornea H18.72-
| equatorial H15.81-
| localized (anterior) H15.82-
| posticum H15.83-
| ring H15.85-
Stargardt's disease *see* Dystrophy, retina
Starvation (inanition) (due to lack of food)
   T73.0
| edema *see* Malnutrition, severe
Stasis
| bile (noncalculous) K83.1
| bronchus J98.09
   | with infection *see* Bronchitis
| cardiac *see* Failure, heart, congestive
| cecum K59.89
| colon K59.89
| dermatitis I87.2
   | with
      | varicose ulcer *see* Varix, leg, with ulcer,
         with inflammation
      | varicose veins *see* Varix, leg, with,
         inflammation
   | due to postthrombotic syndrome *see*
      Syndrome, postthrombotic
| duodenal K31.5
| eczema *see* Varix, leg, with, inflammation
| edema *see* Hypertension, venous (chronic),
   idiopathic
| foot T69.0-
| ileocecal coil K59.89
| ileum K59.89
| intestinal K59.8
| jejunum K59.89
| kidney N19
| liver (cirrhotic) K76.1
| lymphatic I89.8
| pneumonia J18.2
| pulmonary *see* Edema, lung
| rectal K59.89
| renal N19
   | tubular N17.0
| ulcer *see* Varix, leg, with, ulcer
   | without varicose veins I87.2
| urine *see* Retention, urine
| venous I87.8
State (of)
| affective and paranoid, mixed, organic
   psychotic F06.8
| agitated R45.1
   | acute reaction to stress F43.0
| anxiety (neurotic) F41.1
| apprehension F41.1
| burn-out Z73.0
| climacteric, female Z78.0
   | symptomatic N95.1
| compulsive F42.8
   | mixed with obsessional thoughts F42.2
| confusional (psychogenic) F44.89
   | acute *see also* Delirium
      | with
         | arteriosclerotic dementia F01.50
            | with behavioral disturbance F01.51
         | senility or dementia F05
      | alcoholic F10.231
   | epileptic F05

State (of) - *continued*
| reactive (from emotional stress,
   psychological trauma) F44.89
| subacute *see* Delirium
| convulsive *see* Convulsions
| crisis F43.0
| depressive F32.A
   | neurotic F34.1
| dissociative F44.9
| emotional shock (stress) R45.7
| hypercoagulation *see* Hypercoagulable
| locked-in G83.5
| menopausal Z78.0
   | symptomatic N95.1
| neurotic F48.9
   | with depersonalization F48.1
| obsessional F42.8
| oneiroid (schizophrenia-like) F23
| organic
   | hallucinatory (nonalcoholic) F06.0
   | paranoid (-hallucinatory) F06.2
| panic F41.0
| paranoid F22
   | climacteric F22
   | involutional F22
   | menopausal F22
   | organic F06.2
   | senile F03
   | simple F22
| persistent vegetative R40.3
| phobic F40.9
| postleukotomy F07.0
| pregnant
   | gestational carrier Z33.3
   | incidental Z33.1
| psychogenic, twilight F44.89
| psychopathic (constitutional) F60.2
| psychotic, organic *see also* Psychosis, organic
   | mixed paranoid and affective F06.8
   | senile or presenile F03
   | transient NEC F06.8
      | with
         | hallucinations F06.0
         | depression F06.31
| residual schizophrenic F20.5
| restlessness R45.1
| stress (emotional) R45.7
| tension (mental) F48.9
   | specified NEC F48.8
| transient organic psychotic NEC F06.8
   | depressive type F06.31
   | hallucinatory type F06.0
| twilight
   | epileptic F05
   | psychogenic F44.89
| vegetative, persistent R40.3
| vital exhaustion Z73.0
| withdrawal, *see* Withdrawal, state
Status (post) *see also* Presence (of)
| absence, epileptic *see* Epilepsy, by type, with
   status epilepticus
| administration of tPA (rtPA) in a different
   facility within the last 24 hours prior to
   admission to current facility Z92.82
| adrenalectomy (unilateral) (bilateral) E89.6
| anastomosis Z98.0
| angioplasty (peripheral) Z98.62
   | with implant Z95.820
   | coronary artery Z98.61
      | with implant Z95.5
| anginosus I20.9
| aortocoronary bypass Z95.1
| arthrodesis Z98.1
| artificial opening (of) Z93.9
   | gastrointestinal tract Z93.4

Status (post) - *continued*
|specified NEC Z93.8
|urinary tract Z93.6
|vagina Z93.8
|asthmaticus *see* Asthma, by type, with status asthmaticus
|awaiting organ transplant Z76.82
|bariatric surgery Z98.84
|bed confinement Z74.01
|bleb, filtering (vitreous), after glaucoma surgery Z98.83
|breast implant Z98.82
  |removal Z98.86
|cataract extraction Z98.4-
|cholecystectomy Z90.49
|clitorectomy N90.811
  |with excision of labia minora N90.812
|colectomy (complete) (partial) Z90.49
|colonization *see* Carrier (suspected) of
|colostomy Z93.3
|convulsivus idiopathicus *see* Epilepsy, by type, with status epilepticus
|coronary artery angioplasty *see* Status, angioplasty, coronary artery
|coronary artery bypass graft Z95.1
|cystectomy (urinary bladder) Z90.6
|cystostomy Z93.50
  |appendico-vesicostomy Z93.52
  |cutaneous Z93.51
  |specified NEC Z93.59
|delinquent immunization Z28.3
|dental Z98.818
  |crown Z98.811
  |fillings Z98.811
  |restoration Z98.811
  |sealant Z98.810
  |specified NEC Z98.818
|deployment (current) (military) Z56.82
|dialysis (hemodialysis) (peritoneal) Z99.2
|do not resuscitate (DNR) Z66
|donor *see* Donor
|embedded fragments *see* Retained, foreign body fragments (type of)
|embedded splinter *see* Retained, foreign body fragments (type of)
|enterostomy Z93.4
|epileptic, epilepticus *see also* Epilepsy, by type, with status epilepticus G40.901
|estrogen receptor
  |negative Z17.1
  |positive Z17.0
|female genital cutting *see* Female genital mutilation status
|female genital mutilation *see* Female genital mutilation status
|filtering (vitreous) bleb after glaucoma surgery Z98.83
|gastrectomy (complete) (partial) Z90.3
|gastric banding Z98.84
|gastric bypass for obesity Z98.84
|gastrostomy Z93.1
|human immunodeficiency virus (HIV) infection, asymptomatic Z21
|hysterectomy (complete) (total) Z90.710
  |partial (with remaining cervical stump) Z90.711
|ileostomy Z93.2
|implant
  |breast Z98.82
|infibulation N90.813
|intestinal bypass Z98.0
|jejunostomy Z93.4
|laryngectomy Z90.02
|lapsed immunization schedule Z28.3
|lymphaticus E32.8

Status (post) - *continued*
|malignancy
  |castrate resistant prostate Z19.2
  |hormone resistant Z19.2
  |hormone sensitive Z19.1
|marmoratus G80.3
|mastectomy (unilateral) (bilateral) Z90.1-
|military deployment status (current) Z56.82
  |in theater or in support of military war, peacekeeping and humanitarian operations Z56.82
|nephrectomy (unilateral) (bilateral) Z90.5
|nephrostomy Z93.6
|obesity surgery Z98.84
|oophorectomy
  |bilateral Z90.722
  |unilateral Z90.721
|organ replacement
  |by artificial or mechanical device or prosthesis of
    artery Z95.828
    bladder Z96.0
    blood vessel Z95.828
    breast Z97.8
    eye globe Z97.0
    heart Z95.812
      |valve Z95.2
    intestine Z97.8
    joint Z96.60
      |hip *see* Presence, hip joint implant
      |knee *see* Presence, knee joint implant
      |specified site NEC Z96.698
    kidney Z97.8
    larynx Z96.3
    lens Z96.1
    limbs *see* Presence, artificial, limb
    liver Z97.8
    lung Z97.8
    pancreas Z97.8
  |by organ transplant (heterologous)(homologous) *see* Transplant pacemaker
    brain Z96.89
    cardiac Z95.0
    specified NEC Z96.89
|pancreatectomy Z90.410
  |complete Z90.410
  |partial Z90.411
  |total Z90.410
|physical restraint Z78.1
|pneumonectomy (complete) (partial) Z90.2
|pneumothorax, therapeutic Z98.3
|postcommotio cerebri F07.81
|postoperative (postprocedural) NEC Z98.890
  |breast implant Z98.82
  |dental Z98.818
    |crown Z98.811
    |fillings Z98.811
    |restoration Z98.811
    |sealant Z98.810
    |specified NEC Z98.818
  |uterine scar Z98.891
  |pneumothorax, therapeutic Z98.3
|postpartum (routine follow-up) Z39.2
  |care immediately after delivery Z39.0
|postsurgical (postprocedural) NEC Z98.890
  |pneumothorax, therapeutic Z98.3
|pregnancy, incidental Z33.1
|prosthesis coronary angioplasty Z95.5
|pseudophakia Z96.1
|renal dialysis (hemodialysis) (peritoneal) Z99.2
|retained foreign body *see* Retained, foreign body fragments (type of)

Status (post) - *continued*
|reversed jejunal transposition (for bypass) Z98.0
|salpingo-oophorectomy
  |bilateral Z90.722
  |unilateral Z90.721
|sex reassignment surgery status Z87.890
|shunt
  |arteriovenous (for dialysis) Z99.2
  |cerebrospinal fluid Z98.2
  |ventricular (communicating) (for drainage) Z98.2
|splenectomy Z90.81
|thymicolymphaticus E32.8
|thymicus E32.8
|thymolymphaticus E32.8
|thyroidectomy (hypothyroidism) E89.0
|tooth (teeth) extraction *see also* Absence, teeth, acquired K08.409
|tPA (rtPA) administration in a different facility within the last 24 hours prior to admission to current facility Z92.82
|tracheostomy Z93.0
|transplant *see* Transplant
  |organ removed Z98.85
|tubal ligation Z98.51
|underimmunization Z28.3
|ureterostomy Z93.6
|urethrostomy Z93.6
|vagina, artificial Z93.8
|vasectomy Z98.52
|wheelchair confinement Z99.3
Stealing
|child problem F91.8
  |in company with others Z72.810
|pathological (compulsive) F63.2
Steam burn *see* Burn
Steatocystoma multiplex L72.2
Steatohepatitis (nonalcoholic) (NASH) K75.81
Steatoma L72.3
|eyelid (cystic) *see* Dermatosis, eyelid
|infected *see* Hordeolum
Steatorrhea (chronic) K90.9
|with lacteal obstruction K90.2
|idiopathic (adult) (infantile) K90.9
|pancreatic K90.3
|primary K90.0
|tropical K90.1
Steatosis E88.89
|heart *see* Degeneration, myocardial
|kidney N28.89
|liver NEC K76.0
Steele-Richardson-Olszewski disease or syndrome G23.1
Steinbrocker's syndrome G90.8
Steinert's disease G71.11
Stein-Leventhal syndrome E28.2
Stein's syndrome E28.2
STEMI *see also* Infarct, myocardium, ST elevation I21.3
Stenocardia I20.8
Stenocephaly Q75.8
Stenosis, stenotic (cicatricial) *see also* Stricture
|ampulla of Vater K83.1
|anus, anal (canal) (sphincter) K62.4
  |and rectum K62.4
  |congenital Q42.3
    |with fistula Q42.2
|aorta (ascending) (supraventricular) (congenital) Q25.1
  |arteriosclerotic I70.0
  |calcified I70.0
  |supravalvular Q25.3
|aortic (valve) I35.0
  |with insufficiency I35.2

Stenosis, stenotic - *continued*
|congenital Q23.0
|rheumatic I06.0
||with
|||incompetency, insufficiency or
||||regurgitation I06.2
|||||with mitral (valve) disease I08.0
||||||with tricuspid (valve) disease I08.3
||||mitral (valve) disease I08.0
|||||with tricuspid (valve) disease I08.3
||||tricuspid (valve) disease I08.2
|||||with mitral (valve) disease I08.3
||specified cause NEC I35.0
||syphilitic A52.03
|aqueduct of Sylvius (congenital) Q03.0
||with spina bifida *see* Spina bifida, by site,
|||with hydrocephalus
||acquired G91.1
|artery NEC *see also* Arteriosclerosis I77.1
||celiac I77.4
||cerebral *see* Occlusion, artery, cerebral
||extremities *see* Arteriosclerosis, extremities
||precerebral *see* Occlusion, artery,
|||precerebral
||pulmonary (congenital) Q25.6
|||acquired I28.8
||renal I70.1
||stent
|||coronary T82.855
|||peripheral T82.856
|bile duct (common) (hepatic) K83.1
||congenital Q44.3
|bladder-neck (acquired) N32.0
||congenital Q64.31
|brain G93.89
|bronchus J98.09
||congenital Q32.3
||syphilitic A52.72
|cardia (stomach) K22.2
||congenital Q39.3
|cardiovascular *see* Disease, cardiovascular
|caudal M48.08
|cervix, cervical (canal) N88.2
||congenital Q51.828
||in pregnancy or childbirth *see* Pregnancy,
|||complicated by, abnormal cervix
|colon *see also* Obstruction, intestine
||congenital Q42.9
|||specified NEC Q42.8
|colostomy K94.03
|common (bile) duct K83.1
||congenital Q44.3
|coronary (artery) *see* Disease, heart, ischemic,
||atherosclerotic
|cystic duct *see* Obstruction, gallbladder
|due to presence of device, implant or graft *see*
||*also* Complications, by site and type,
||*specified NEC T85.858
|arterial graft NEC T82.858
|breast (implant) T85.858
|catheter T85.858
||dialysis (renal) T82.858
|||intraperitoneal T85.858
||infusion NEC T82.858
|||spinal (epidural) (subdural) T85.850
||urinary (indwelling) T83.85
|fixation, internal (orthopedic) NEC T84.85
|gastrointestinal (bile duct) (esophagus)
||T85.858
|genital NEC T83.85
|heart NEC T82.857
|joint prosthesis T84.85
|ocular (corneal graft) (orbital implant) NEC
||T85.858
|orthopedic NEC T84.85

Stenosis, stenotic - *continued*
|specified NEC T85.858
|urinary NEC T83.85
|vascular NEC T82.858
|ventricular intracranial shunt T85.850
|duodenum K31.5
||congenital Q41.0
|ejaculatory duct NEC N50.89
|endocervical os *see* Stenosis, cervix
|enterostomy K94.13
|esophagus K22.2
||congenital Q39.3
||syphilitic A52.79
|||congenital A50.59 *[K23]*
|eustachian tube *see* Obstruction, eustachian
||tube
|external ear canal (acquired) H61.30-
||congenital Q16.1
||due to
|||inflammation H61.32-
|||trauma H61.31-
||postprocedural H95.81-
||specified cause NEC H61.39-
|gallbladder *see* Obstruction, gallbladder
|glottis J38.6
|heart valve (see also Endocarditis) I38
||aortic - see Stenosis, aortic
- - congenital Q24.8
||mitral - see Stenosis, mitral
||pulmonary - see Stenosis, pulmonary, valve
||tricuspid - see Stenosis, tricuspid Q22.4
|hepatic duct K83.1
|hymen N89.6
|hypertrophic subaortic (idiopathic) I42.1
|ileum (*see also* Obstruction, intestine,
||specified NEC) K56.699
||congenital Q41.2
|infundibulum cardia Q24.3
|intervertebral foramina *see also* Lesion,
||biomechanical, specified NEC
||connective tissue M99.79
|||abdomen M99.79
|||cervical region M99.71
|||cervicothoracic M99.71
|||head region M99.70
|||lumbar region M99.73
|||lumbosacral M99.73
|||occipitocervical M99.70
|||sacral region M99.74
|||sacrococcygeal M99.74
|||sacroiliac M99.74
|||specified NEC M99.79
|||thoracic region M99.72
|||thoracolumbar M99.72
||disc M99.79
|||abdomen M99.79
|||cervical region M99.71
|||cervicothoracic M99.71
|||head region M99.70
|||lower extremity M99.76
|||lumbar region M99.73
|||lumbosacral M99.73
|||occipitocervical M99.70
|||pelvic M99.75
|||rib cage M99.78
|||sacral region M99.74
|||sacrococcygeal M99.74
|||sacroiliac M99.74
|||specified NEC M99.79
|||thoracic region M99.72
|||thoracolumbar M99.72
|||upper extremity M99.77
||osseous M99.69
|||abdomen M99.69
|||cervical region M99.61

Stenosis, stenotic - *continued*
|||cervicothoracic M99.61
|||head region M99.60
|||lower extremity M99.66
|||lumbar region M99.63
|||lumbosacral M99.63
|||occipitocervical M99.60
|||pelvic M99.65
|||rib cage M99.68
|||sacral region M99.64
|||sacrococcygeal M99.64
|||sacroiliac M99.64
|||specified NEC M99.69
|||thoracic region M99.62
|||thoracolumbar M99.62
|||upper extremity M99.67
||subluxation *see* Stenosis, intervertebral
|||foramina, osseous
|intestine *see also* Obstruction, intestine
||congenital (small) Q41.9
|||large Q42.9
||||specified NEC Q42.8
|||specified NEC Q41.8
|jejunum (*see also* Obstruction, intestine,
||specified NEC) K56.699
||congenital Q41.1
|lacrimal (passage)
||canaliculi H04.54-
||congenital Q10.5
||duct H04.55-
||punctum H04.56-
|sac H04.57-
|lacrimonasal duct *see* Stenosis, lacrimal, duct
||congenital Q10.5
|larynx J38.6
||congenital NEC Q31.8
|||subglottic Q31.1
||syphilitic A52.73
|||congenital A50.59 *[J99]*
|mitral (chronic) (inactive) (valve) I05.0
||with
|||aortic valve disease I08.0
|||incompetency, insufficiency or
||||regurgitation I05.2
||active or acute I01.1
|||with rheumatic or Sydenham's chorea
||||I02.0
||congenital Q23.2
||specified cause, except rheumatic I34.2
||syphilitic A52.03
|myocardium, myocardial *see also*
||Degeneration, myocardial
||hypertrophic subaortic (idiopathic) I42.1
|nares (anterior) (posterior) J34.89
||congenital Q30.0
|nasal duct *see also* Stenosis, lacrimal, duct
||congenital Q10.5
|nasolacrimal duct *see also* Stenosis, lacrimal,
||duct
||congenital Q10.5
|neural canal *see also* Lesion, biomechanical,
||specified NEC
||connective tissue M99.49
|||abdomen M99.49
|||cervical region M99.41
|||cervicothoracic M99.41
|||head region M99.40
|||lower extremity M99.46
|||lumbar region M99.43
|||lumbosacral M99.43
|||occipitocervical M99.40
|||pelvic M99.45
|||rib cage M99.48
|||sacral region M99.44
|||sacrococcygeal M99.44

Stenosis, stenotic - *continued*
- |sacroiliac M99.44
- |specified NEC M99.49
- |thoracic region M99.42
- |thoracolumbar M99.42
- |upper extremity M99.47
- |intervertebral disc M99.59
  - |abdomen M99.59
  - |cervical region M99.51
  - |cervicothoracic M99.51
  - |head region M99.50
  - |lower extremity M99.56
  - |lumbar region M99.53
  - |lumbosacral M99.53
  - |occipitocervical M99.50
  - |pelvic M99.55
  - |rib cage M99.58
  - |sacral region M99.54
  - |sacrococcygeal M99.54
  - |sacroiliac M99.54
  - |specified NEC M99.59
  - |thoracic region M99.52
  - |thoracolumbar M99.52
  - |upper extremity M99.57
- |osseous M99.39
  - |abdomen M99.39
  - |cervical region M99.31
  - |cervicothoracic M99.31
  - |head region M99.30
  - |lower extremity M99.36
  - |lumbar region M99.33
  - |lumbosacral M99.33
  - |pelvic M99.35
  - |rib cage M99.38
  - |occipitocervical M99.30
  - |sacral region M99.34
  - |sacrococcygeal M99.34
  - |sacroiliac M99.34
  - |specified NEC M99.39
  - |thoracic region M99.32
  - |thoracolumbar M99.32
  - |upper extremity M99.37
- |subluxation M99.29
  - |cervical region M99.21
  - |cervicothoracic M99.21
  - |head region M99.20
  - |lower extremity M99.26
  - |lumbar region M99.23
  - |lumbosacral M99.23
  - |occipitocervical M99.20
  - |pelvic M99.25
  - |rib cage M99.28
  - |sacral region M99.24
  - |sacrococcygeal M99.24
  - |sacroiliac M99.24
  - |specified NEC M99.29
  - |thoracic region M99.22
  - |thoracolumbar M99.22
  - |upper extremity M99.27
- |organ or site, congenital NEC *see* Atresia, by site
- |papilla of Vater K83.1
- |pulmonary (artery) (congenital) Q25.6
  - |with ventricular septal defect, transposition of aorta, and hypertrophy of right ventricle Q21.3
  - |acquired I28.8
  - |in tetralogy of Fallot Q21.3
  - |infundibular Q24.3
  - |subvalvular Q24.3
  - |supravalvular Q25.6
  - |valve I37.0
    - |with insufficiency I37.2
    - |congenital Q22.1
    - |rheumatic I09.89

Stenosis, stenotic - *continued*
- |with aortic, mitral or tricuspid (valve) disease I08.8
- |vein, acquired I28.8
- |vessel NEC I28.8
- |pulmonic (congenital) Q22.1
  - |infundibular Q24.3
  - |subvalvular Q24.3
- |pylorus (hypertrophic) (acquired) K31.1
  - |adult K31.1
  - |congenital Q40.0
  - |infantile Q40.0
- |rectum (sphincter) *see* Stricture, rectum
- |renal artery I70.1
  - |congenital Q27.1
- |salivary duct (any) K11.8
- |sphincter of Oddi K83.1
- |spinal M48.00
  - |cervical region M48.02
  - |cervicothoracic region M48.03
  - |lumbar region M48.06
  - |lumbar region (NOS) (without neurogenic claudication) M48.061
    - |with neurogenic claudication M48.062
  - |occipito-atlanto-axial region M48.01
  - |sacrococcygeal region M48.08
  - |thoracic region M48.04
  - |thoracolumbar region M48.05
- |stent
  - |vascular
    - |end stent
      - |adjacent to stent *see* Arteriosclerosis
      - |within the stent
        - |coronary T82.855
        - |peripheral T82.856
    - |in stent
      - |coronary vessel T82.855
      - |peripheral vessel T82.856
- |stomach, hourglass K31.2
- |subaortic (congenital) Q24.4
  - |hypertrophic (idiopathic) I42.1
- |subglottic J38.6
  - |congenital Q31.1
  - |postprocedural J95.5
- |trachea J39.8
  - |congenital Q32.1
  - |syphilitic A52.73
  - |tuberculous NEC A15.5
- |tracheostomy J95.03
- |tricuspid (valve) I07.0
  - |with
    - |aortic (valve) disease I08.2
    - |incompetency, insufficiency or regurgitation I07.2
      - |with aortic (valve) disease I08.2
        - |with mitral (valve) disease I08.3
      - |mitral (valve) disease I08.1
        - |with aortic (valve) disease I08.3
  - |congenital Q22.4
  - |nonrheumatic I36.0
    - |with insufficiency I36.2
- |tubal N97.1
- |ureter *see* Atresia, ureter
- |ureteropelvic junction, congenital Q62.11
- |ureterovesical orifice, congenital Q62.12
- |urethra (valve) *see also* Stricture, urethra
  - |congenital Q64.32
- |urinary meatus, congenital Q64.33
- |vagina N89.5
  - |congenital Q52.4
  - |in pregnancy *see* Pregnancy, complicated by, abnormal vagina
    - |causing obstructed labor O65.5
- |valve (cardiac) (heart) *see also* Endocarditis I38

Stenosis, stenotic - *continued*
- |congenital Q24.8
  - |aortic Q23.0
  - |mitral Q23.2
  - |pulmonary Q22.1
  - |tricuspid Q22.4
- |vena cava (inferior) (superior) I87.1
  - |congenital Q26.0
- |vesicourethral orifice Q64.31
- |vulva N90.5
Stent jail T82.897
Stercolith (impaction) K56.41
- |appendix K38.1
Stercoraceous, stercoral ulcer K63.3
- |anus or rectum K62.6
Stereotypies NEC F98.4
Sterility *see* Infertility
Sterilization *see* Encounter (for), sterilization
Sternalgia *see* Angina
Sternopagus Q89.4
Sternum bifidum Q76.7
Steroid
- |effects (adverse) (adrenocortical) (iatrogenic)
  - |cushingoid E24.2
    - |correct substance properly administered *see* Table of Drugs and Chemicals, by drug, adverse effect
    - |overdose or wrong substance given or taken *see* Table of Drugs and Chemicals, by drug, poisoning
  - |diabetes *see* category E09
    - |correct substance properly administered *see* Table of Drugs and Chemicals, by drug, adverse effect
    - |overdose or wrong substance given or taken *see* Table of Drugs and Chemicals, by drug, poisoning
  - |fever R50.2
  - |insufficiency E27.3
  - |correct substance properly administered *see* Table of Drugs and Chemicals, by drug, adverse effect
    - |overdose or wrong substance given or taken *see* Table of Drugs and Chemicals, by drug, poisoning
- |responder H40.04-
Stevens-Johnson disease or syndrome L51.1
- |toxic epidermal necrolysis overlap L51.3
Stewart-Morel syndrome M85.2
Sticker's disease B08.3
Sticky eye *see* Conjunctivitis, acute, mucopurulent
Stieda's disease *see* Bursitis, tibial collateral
Stiff neck *see* Torticollis
Stiff-Man syndrome G25.82
Stiffness, joint NEC M25.60-
- |ankle M25.67-
- |ankylosis *see* Ankylosis, joint
- |contracture *see* Contraction, joint
- |elbow M25.62-
- |foot M25.67-
- |hand M25.64-
- |hip M25.65-
- |knee M25.66-
- |shoulder M25.61-
- |specified site NEC M25.69
- |wrist M25.63-
Stigmata congenital syphilis A50.59
Stillbirth P95
Still-Felty syndrome *see* Felty's syndrome
Still's disease or syndrome (juvenile) M08.20
- |adult-onset M06.1
- |ankle M08.27-
- |elbow M08.22-
- |foot joint M08.27-
- |hand joint M08.24-
- |hip M08.25-

Still's disease - *continued*
| knee M08.26-
| multiple site M08.29
| shoulder M08.21-
| specified site NEC M08.2A
| vertebra M08.28
| wrist M08.23-
Stimulation, ovary E28.1
Sting (venomous) (with allergic or anaphylactic shock) *see* Table of Drugs and Chemicals, by animal or substance, poisoning
Stippled epiphyses Q78.8
Stitch
| abscess T81.41
| burst (in operation wound) *see* Disruption, wound, operation
Stokes-Adams disease or syndrome I45.9
Stokes' disease E05.00
| with thyroid storm E05.01
Stokvis (-Talma) disease D74.8
Stoma malfunction
| colostomy K94.03
| enterostomy K94.13
| gastrostomy K94.23
| ileostomy K94.13
| tracheostomy J95.03
Stomach *see* condition
Stomatitis (denture) (ulcerative) K12.1
| angular K13.0
| | due to dietary or vitamin deficiency E53.0
| aphthous K12.0
| bovine B08.61
| candidal B37.0
| catarrhal K12.1
| diphtheritic A36.89
| due to
| | dietary deficiency E53.0
| | thrush B37.0
| | vitamin deficiency
| | | B group NEC E53.9
| | | B2 (riboflavin) E53.0
| epidemic B08.8
| epizootic B08.8
| follicular K12.1
| gangrenous A69.0
| Geotrichum B48.3
| herpesviral, herpetic B00.2
| herpetiformis K12.0
| malignant K12.1
| membranous acute K12.1
| monilial B37.0
| mycotic B37.0
| necrotizing ulcerative A69.0
| parasitic B37.0
| septic K12.1
| spirochetal A69.1
| suppurative (acute) K12.2
| ulceromembranous A69.1
| vesicular K12.1
| | with exanthem (enteroviral) B08.4
| | virus disease A93.8
| Vincent's A69.1
Stomatocytosis D58.8
Stomatomycosis B37.0
Stomatorrhagia K13.79
Stone(s) *see also* Calculus
| bladder (diverticulum) N21.0
| cystine E72.09
| heart syndrome I50.1
| kidney N20.0
| prostate N42.0
| pulpal (dental) K04.2
| renal N20.0
| salivary gland or duct (any) K11.5

Stone(s) - *continued*
| urethra (impacted) N21.1
| urinary (duct) (impacted) (passage) N20.9
| | bladder (diverticulum) N21.0
| | lower tract N21.9
| | specified NEC N21.8
| xanthine E79.8 *[N22]*
Stonecutter's lung J62.8
Stonemason's asthma, disease, lung or pneumoconiosis J62.8
Stoppage
| heart *see* Arrest, cardiac
| urine *see* Retention, urine **Storm, thyroid** *see* Thyrotoxicosis
Strabismus (congenital) (nonparalytic) H50.9
| concomitant H50.40
| | convergent *see* Strabismus, convergent concomitant
| | divergent *see* Strabismus, divergent concomitant
| convergent concomitant H50.00
| | accommodative component H50.43
| | alternating H50.05
| | | with
| | | | A pattern H50.06
| | | | specified nonconcomitances NEC H50.08
| | | | V pattern H50.07
| | monocular H50.01-
| | | with
| | | | A pattern H50.02-
| | | | specified nonconcomitances NEC H50.04-
| | | | V pattern H50.03-
| | | intermittent H50.31-
| | | | alternating H50.32
| cyclotropia H50.41
| divergent concomitant H50.10
| | alternating H50.15
| | | with
| | | | A pattern H50.16
| | | | specified noncomitances NEC H50.18
| | | | V pattern H50.17
| | monocular H50.11-
| | | with
| | | | A pattern H50.12-
| | | | specified noncomitances NEC H50.14-
| | | | V pattern H50.13-
| | | intermittent H50.33
| | | | alternating H50.34
| Duane's syndrome H50.81-
| due to adhesions, scars H50.69
| heterophoria H50.50
| | alternating H50.55
| | cyclophoria H50.54
| | esophoria H50.51
| | exophoria H50.52
| | vertical H50.53
| heterotropia H50.40
| | intermittent H50.30
| hypertropia H50.2-
| hypotropia *see* Hypertropia
| latent H50.50
| mechanical H50.60
| | Brown's sheath syndrome H50.61-
| | specified type NEC H50.69
| monofixation syndrome H50.42
| paralytic H49.9
| | abducens nerve H49.2-
| | fourth nerve H49.1-
| | Kearns-Sayre syndrome H49.81-
| | ophthalmoplegia (external)
| | | progressive H49.4-
| | | | with pigmentary retinopathy H49.81-
| | total H49.3-

Strabismus - *continued*
| sixth nerve H49.2-
| specified type NEC H49.88-
| third nerve H49.0-
| trochlear nerve H49.1-
| specified type NEC H50.89
| vertical H50.2-
Strain
| back S39.012
| cervical S16.1
| eye NEC *see* Disturbance, vision, subjective
| heart *see* Disease, heart
| low back S39.012
| mental NOS Z73.3
| | work-related Z56.6
| muscle (tendon) *see* Injury, muscle, by site, strain
| neck S16.1
| postural *see also* Disorder, soft tissue, due to use
| physical NOS Z73.3
| | work-related Z56.6
| psychological NEC Z73.3
| tendon *see* Injury, muscle, by site, strain
Straining, on urination R39.16
Strand, vitreous *see* Opacity, vitreous, membranes and strands
Strangulation, strangulated *see also* Asphyxia, traumatic
| appendix K38.8
| bladder-neck N32.0
| bowel or colon K56.2
| food or foreign body *see* Foreign body, by site
| hemorrhoids *see* Hemorrhoids, with complication
| hernia *see also* Hernia, by site, with obstruction
| | with gangrene *see* Hernia, by site, with gangrene
| intestine (large) (small) K56.2
| | with hernia *see also* Hernia, by site, with obstruction
| | | with gangrene *see* Hernia, by site, with gangrene
| mesentery K56.2
| mucus *see* Asphyxia, mucus
| omentum K56.2
| organ or site, congenital NEC *see* Atresia, by site
| ovary *see* Torsion, ovary
| penis N48.89
| | foreign body T19.4
| rupture *see* Hernia, by site, with obstruction
| stomach due to hernia *see also* Hernia, by site, with obstruction
| | with gangrene *see* Hernia, by site, with gangrene
| vesicourethral orifice N32.0
Strangury R30.0
Straw itch B88.0
Strawberry
| gallbladder K82.4
| mark Q82.5
| tongue (red) (white) K14.3
Streak(s)
| macula, angioid H35.33
| ovarian Q50.32
Strephosymbolia F81.0
| secondary to organic lesion R48.8
Streptobacillary fever A25.1
Streptobacillosis A25.1
Streptobacillus moniliformis A25.1

Stricture - *continued*
|gastrostomy K94.23
|ileostomy K94.13
|tracheostomy J95.03
|stomach K31.89
|congenital Q40.2
|hourglass K31.2
|subaortic Q24.4
|hypertrophic (acquired) (idiopathic) I42.1
|subglottic J38.6
|syphilitic NEC A52.79
|trachea J39.8
|congenital Q32.1
|syphilitic A52.73
|tuberculous NEC A15.5
|tracheostomy J95.03
|tricuspid (valve) *see* Stenosis, tricuspid
|tunica vaginalis N50.89
|ureter (postoperative) N13.5
|with
|hydronephrosis N13.1
|with infection N13.6
|pyelonephritis (chronic) N11.1
|congenital *see* Atresia, ureter
|tuberculous A18.11
|ureteropelvic junction (congenital) Q62.11
|acquired, with hydronephrosis N13.0
|ureterovesical orifice N13.5
|with infection N13.6
|urethra (organic) (spasmodic) (*see also*
Stricture, urethra, male) N35.919
|associated with schistosomiasis B65.0
[N37]
|congenital Q64.39
|valvular (posterior) Q64.2
|due to
|infection *see* Stricture, urethra,
postinfective
|female N35.92
|male N35.919
|anterior urethra N35.914
|bulbous urethra N35.912
|meatal N35.911
|membranous urethra N35.913
|overlapping sites N35.916
|trauma *see* Stricture, urethra, post-
traumatic
|gonococcal, gonorrheal A54.01
|infective NEC *see* Stricture, urethra,
postinfective
|late effect (sequelae) of injury *see* Stricture,
urethra, post-traumatic
|postcatheterization *see* Stricture, urethra,
postprocedural
|postinfective NEC
|female N35.12
|male N35.119
|anterior urethra N35.114
|bulbous urethra N35.112
|meatal N35.111
|membranous urethra N35.113
|overlapping sites N35.116
|postobstetric N35.021
|postoperative *see* Stricture, urethra,
postprocedural
|postprocedural
|female N99.12
|male N99.114
|anterior bulbous urethra N99.113
|bulbous urethra N99.111
|fossa navicularis N99.115
|meatal N99.110
|membranous urethra N99.112
|overlapping sites N99.116
|post-traumatic

Stricture - *continued*
|female N35.028
|due to childbirth N35.021
|male N35.014
|anterior urethra N35.013
|bulbous urethra N35.011
|meatal N35.010
|membranous urethra N35.012
|overlapping sites N35.016
|sequela (late effect) of
|childbirth N35.021
|injury *see* Stricture, urethra, post-
traumatic
|specified cause NEC N35.8
|female N35.82
|male N35.819
|anterior urethra N35.814
|bulbous urethra N35.812
|meatal N35.811
|membranous urethra N35.813
|overlapping sites N35.816
|syphilitic A52.76
|traumatic *see* Stricture, urethra, post-
traumatic
|valvular (posterior), congenital Q64.2
|urinary meatus *see* Stricture, urethra
|uterus, uterine (synechiae) N85.6
|os (external) (internal) *see* Stricture, cervix
|vagina (outlet) *see* Stenosis, vagina
|valve (cardiac) (heart) *see also* Endocarditis
|congenital
|aortic Q23.0
|mitral Q23.2
|pulmonary Q22.1
|tricuspid Q22.4
|vas deferens N50.89
|congenital Q55.4
|vein I87.1
|vena cava (inferior) (superior) NEC I87.1
|congenital Q26.0
|vesicourethral orifice N32.0
|congenital Q64.31
|vulva (acquired) N90.5
Stridor R06.1
|congenital (larynx) P28.89
Stridulous *see* condition
Stroke (apoplectic) (brain) (embolic)
(ischemic) (paralytic) (thrombotic) I63.9
|cerebral, perinatal P91.82-
|epileptic *see* Epilepsy
|heat T67.0
|in evolution I63.9
|intraoperative
|during cardiac surgery I97.810
|during other surgery I97.811
|ischemic, perinatal arterial P91.82-
|lightning *see* Lightning
|meaning
|cerebral hemorrhage   code to Hemorrhage,
intracranial
|cerebral infarction   code to Infarction,
cerebral
|cryptogenic (*see also* infarction, cerebral)
I63.9
|neonatal P91.82-
|postprocedural
|following cardiac surgery I97.820
|following other surgery I97.821
|unspecified (NOS) I63.9
Stromatosis, endometrial D39.0
Strongyloidiasis, strongyloidosis B78.9
|cutaneous B78.1
|disseminated B78.7
|intestinal B78.0
Strophulus pruriginosus L28.2

Struck by lightning *see* Lightning
Struma *see also* Goiter
|Hashimoto E06.3
|lymphomatosa E06.3
|nodosa (simplex) E04.9
|endemic E01.2
|multinodular E01.1
|multinodular E04.2
|iodine-deficiency related E01.1
|toxic or with hyperthyroidism E05.20
|with thyroid storm E05.21
|multinodular E05.20
|with thyroid storm E05.21
|uninodular E05.10
|with thyroid storm E05.11
|toxicosa E05.20
|with thyroid storm E05.21
|multinodular E05.20
|with thyroid storm E05.21
|uninodular E05.10
|with thyroid storm E05.11
|uninodular E04.1
|ovarii D27.-
|Riedel's E06.5
Strumipriva cachexia E03.4
Strümpell-Marie spine *see* Spondylitis,
ankylosing
Strümpell-Westphal pseudosclerosis E83.01
Stuart deficiency disease (factor X) D68.2
Stuart-Prower factor deficiency (factor X)
D68.2
Student's elbow *see* Bursitis, elbow, olecranon
Stump *see* Amputation
Stunting, nutritional E45
Stupor (catatonic) R40.1
|depressive (single episode) F32.89
|recurrent episode F33.8
|dissociative F44.2
|manic F30.2
|manic-depressive F31.89
|psychogenic (anergic) F44.2
|reaction to exceptional stress (transient) F43.0
Sturge (-Weber) (-Dimitri) (-Kalischer)
disease or syndrome Q85.8
Stuttering F80.81
|adult onset F98.5
|childhood onset F80.81
|following cerebrovascular disease *see*
Disorder, fluency. following cerebro-
vascular disease in conditions classified
elsewhere R47.82
Sty, stye (external) (internal) (meibomian)
(zeisian) *see* Hordeolum
Subacidity, gastric K31.89
|psychogenic F45.8
Subacute *see* condition
Subarachnoid *see* condition
Subcortical *see* condition
Subcostal syndrome, nerve compression *see*
Mononeuropathy, upper limb, specified site
NEC
Subcutaneous, subcuticular *see* condition
Sundowning F05
Subdural *see* condition
Subendocardium *see* condition
Subependymoma
|specified site *see* Neoplasm, uncertain
behavior, by site
|unspecified site D43.2
Suberosis J67.3
Subglossitis *see* Glossitis **S**
Subhemophilia D66
Subinvolution
|breast (postlactational) (postpuerperal) N64.89
|puerperal O90.89
|uterus (chronic) (nonpuerperal) N85.3
|puerperal O90.89

Sublingual *see* condition
Sublinguitis *see* Sialoadenitis
Subluxatable hip Q65.6
Subluxation *see also* Dislocation
|acromioclavicular S43.11-
|ankle S93.0-
|atlantoaxial, recurrent M43.4
|with myelopathy M43.3
|carpometacarpal (joint) NEC S63.05-
|thumb S63.04-
|complex, vertebral *see* Complex, subluxation
|congenital *see also* Malposition, congenital
|hip *see* Dislocation, hip, congenital, partial
|joint (excluding hip)
|lower limb Q68.8
|shoulder Q68.8
|upper limb Q68.8
|elbow (traumatic) S53.10-
|anterior S53.11-
|lateral S53.14-
|medial S53.13-
|posterior S53.12-
|specified type NEC S53.19-
|finger S63.20-
|index S63.20-
|interphalangeal S63.22-
|distal S63.24-
|index S63.24-
|little S63.24-
|middle S63.24-
|ring S63.24-
|index S63.22-
|little S63.22-
|middle S63.22-
|proximal S63.23-
|index S63.23-
|little S63.23-
|middle S63.23-
|ring S63.23-
|ring S63.22-
|little S63.20-
|metacarpophalangeal S63.21-
|index S63.21-
|little S63.21-
|middle S63.21-
|ring S63.21-
|middle S63.20-
|ring S63.20-
|foot S93.30-
|specified site NEC S93.33-
|tarsal joint S93.31-
|tarsometatarsal joint S93.32-
|toe *see* Subluxation, toe
|hip S73.00-
|anterior S73.03-
|obturator S73.02-
|central S73.04-
|posterior S73.01-
|interphalangeal (joint)
|finger S63.22-
|distal joint S63.24-
|index S63.24-
|little S63.24-
|middle S63.24-
|ring S63.24-
|index S63.22-
|little S63.22-
|middle S63.22-
|proximal joint S63.23-
|index S63.23-
|little S63.23-
|middle S63.23-
|ring S63.23-
|ring S63.22-
|thumb S63.12-

Subluxation - *continued*
|toe S93.13-
|great S93.13-
|lesser S93.13-
|joint prosthesis *see* Complications, joint
prosthesis, mechanical, displacement, by site
|knee S83.10-
|cap *see* Subluxation, patella
|patella *see* Subluxation, patella
|proximal tibia
|anteriorly S83.11-
|laterally S83.14-
|medially S83.13-
|posteriorly S83.12-
|specified type NEC S83.19-
|lens *see* Dislocation, lens, partial
|ligament, traumatic *see* Sprain, by site
|metacarpal (bone)
|proximal end S63.06-
|metacarpophalangeal (joint)
|finger S63.21-
|index S63.21-
|little S63.21-
|middle S63.21-
|ring S63.21-
|thumb S63.11-
|metatarsophalangeal joint S93.14-
|great toe S93.14-
|lesser toe S93.14-
|midcarpal (joint) S63.03-
|patella S83.00-
|lateral S83.01-
|recurrent (nontraumatic) *see* Dislocation,
patella, recurrent, incomplete
|specified type NEC S83.09-
|pathological *see* Dislocation, pathological
|radial head S53.00-
|anterior S53.01-
|nursemaid's elbow S53.03-
|posterior S53.02-
|specified type NEC S53.09-
|radiocarpal (joint) S63.02-
|radioulnar (joint)
|distal S63.01-
|proximal *see* Subluxation, elbow
|shoulder
|congenital Q68.8
|girdle S43.30-
|scapula S43.31-
|specified site NEC S43.39-
|traumatic S43.00-
|anterior S43.01-
|inferior S43.03-
|posterior S43.02-
|specified type NEC S43.08-
|sternoclavicular (joint) S43.20-
|anterior S43.21-
|posterior S43.22-
|symphysis (pubis)
|thumb S63.103
|interphalangeal joint *see* Subluxation,
interphalangeal (joint), thumb
|metacarpophalangeal joint *see* Subluxation,
metacarpophalangeal (joint), thumb
|toe(s) S93.10-
|great S93.10-
|interphalangeal joint S93.13-
|metatarsophalangeal joint S93.14-
|interphalangeal joint S93.13-
|lesser S93.10-
|interphalangeal joint S93.13-
|metatarsophalangeal joint S93.14-
|metatarsophalangeal joint S93.149
|ulnohumeral joint *see* Subluxation, elbow
|vertebral

Subluxation - *continued*
|recurrent NEC *see* subcategory M43.5
|traumatic
|cervical S13.100
|atlantoaxial joint S13.120
|atlantooccipital joint S13.110
|atloido-occipital joint S13.110
|joint between
|C0 and C1 S13.110
|C1 and C2 S13.120
|C2 and C3 S13.130
|C3 and C4 S13.140
|C4 and C5 S13.150
|C5and C6 S13.160
|C6and C7 S13.170
|C7and T1 S13.180
|occipitoatloid joint S13.110
|lumbar S33.100
|joint between
|L1and L2 S33.110
|L2and L3 S33.120
|L3 and L4 S33.130
|L4and L5 S33.140
|thoracic S23.100
|joint between
|T1and T2 S23.110
|T2and T3 S23.120
|T3 and T4 S23.122
|T4 and T5 S23.130
|T5 and T6 S23.132
|T6 and T7 S23.140
|T7 and T8 S23.142
|T8 and T9 S23.150
|T9 and T10 S23.152
|T10 and T11 S23.160
|T11 and T12 S23.162
|T12 and L1 S23.170
|ulna
|distal end S63.07-
|proximal end *see* Subluxation, elbow
|wrist (carpal bone) S63.00-
|carpometacarpal joint *see* Subluxation,
carpometacarpal (joint)
|distal radioulnar joint *see* Subluxation,
radioulnar (joint), distal
|metacarpal bone, proximal *see* Subluxation,
metacarpal (bone), proximal end
|midcarpal *see* Subluxation, midcarpal (joint)
|radiocarpal joint *see* Subluxation,
radiocarpal (joint)
|recurrent *see* Dislocation, recurrent, wrist
|specified site NEC S63.09-
|ulna *see* Subluxation, ulna, distal end
Submaxillary *see* condition
Submersion (fatal) (nonfatal) T75.1
Submucous *see* condition
Subnormal, subnormality
|accommodation (old age) H52.4
|mental *see* Disability, intellectual
|temperature (accidental) T68
Subphrenic *see* condition
Subscapular nerve *see* condition
Subseptus uterus Q51.28
Subsiding appendicitis K36
Substance (other psychoactive) -Induced
|anxiety disorder F19.980
|bipolar and related disorder F19.94
|delirium F19.921
|depressive disorder F19.94
|major neurocognitive disorder F19.97
|mild neurocognitive disorder F19.988
|obsessive-compulsive and related disorder
F19.988
|psychotic disorder F19.959
|sexual dysfunction F19.981
|sleep disorder F19.982

Substernal thyroid E04.9
|congenital Q89.2
Substitution disorder F44.9
Subtentorial *see* condition
Subthyroidism (acquired) *see also*
  Hypothyroidism
|congenital E03.1
Succenturiate placenta O43.19-
Sucking thumb, child (excessive) F98.8
Sudamen, sudamina L74.1
Sudanese kala-Azar B55.0
Sudden
|heart failure *see* Failure, heart
|hearing loss *see* Deafness, sudden
Sudeck's atrophy, disease, or syndrome *see*
  Algoneurodystrophy
Suffocation *see* Asphyxia, traumatic
Sugar
|blood
  |high (transient) R73.9
  |low (transient) E16.2
|in urine R81
Suicide, suicidal (attempted) T14.91
|by poisoning *see* Table of Drugs and
  Chemicals
|history of (personal) Z91.51
  |in family Z81.8
|ideation *see* Ideation, suicidal
|risk
  |meaning personal history of attempted
    suicide Z91.51
  |meaning suicidal ideation *see* Ideation,
    suicidal
|tendencies
  |meaning personal history of attempted
    suicide Z91.51
  |meaning suicidal ideation *see* Ideation,
    suicidal
|trauma *see* nature of injury by site
Suipestifer infection *see* Infection, salmonella
**Sulfhemoglobinemia, sulphemoglobinemia
  (acquired) (with methemoglobinemia)**
  D74.8
Sumatran mite fever A75.3
Summer *see* condition
Sunburn L55.9
|due to
  |tanning bed (acute) L56.8
    |chronic L57.8
  |ultraviolet radiation (acute) L56.8
    |chronic L57.8
|first degree L55.0
|second degree L55.1
|third degree L55.2
**SUNCT (short lasting unilateral neuralgiform
  headache with conjunctival injection and
  tearing)** G44.059
|intractable G44.051
|not intractable G44.059
Sunken acetabulum *see* Derangement, joint,
  specified type NEC, hip
Sunstroke T67.0
Superfecundation *see* Pregnancy, multiple
Superfetation *see* Pregnancy, multiple
Superinvolution (uterus) N85.8
Supernumerary (congenital)
|aortic cusps Q23.8
|auditory ossicles Q16.3
|bone Q79.8
|breast Q83.1
|carpal bones Q74.0
|cusps, heart valve NEC Q24.8
  |aortic Q23.8
  |mitral Q23.2
  |pulmonary Q22.3

Supernumerary (congenital)
|digit(s) Q69.9
|ear (lobule) Q17.0
|fallopian tube Q50.6
|finger Q69.0
|hymen Q52.4
|kidney Q63.0
|lacrimonasal duct Q10.6
|lobule (ear) Q17.0
|mitral cusps Q23.2
|muscle Q79.8
|nipple(s) Q83.3
|organ or site not listed *see* Accessory
|ossicles, auditory Q16.3
|ovary Q50.31
|oviduct Q50.6
|pulmonary, pulmonic cusps Q22.3
|rib Q76.6
  |cervical or first (syndrome) Q76.5
|roots (of teeth) K00.2
|spleen Q89.09
|tarsal bones Q74.2
|teeth K00.1
|testis Q55.29
|thumb Q69.1
|toe Q69.2
|uterus Q51.28
|vagina Q52.1
|vertebra Q76.49
Supervision (of)
|contraceptive *see* Prescription, contraceptives
|dietary (for) Z71.3
  |allergy (food) Z71.3
  |colitis Z71.3
  |diabetes mellitus Z71.3
  |food allergy or intolerance Z71.3
  |gastritis Z71.3
  |hypercholesterolemia Z71.3
  |hypoglycemia Z71.3
  |intolerance (food) Z71.3
  |obesity Z71.3
  |specified NEC Z71.3
|healthy infant or child Z76.2
  |foundling Z76.1
|high-risk pregnancy *see* Pregnancy,
  complicated by, high, risk
|lactation Z39.1
|pregnancy *see* Pregnancy, supervision of
Supplemental teeth K00.1
Suppression
|binocular vision H53.34
|lactation O92.5
|menstruation N94.89
|ovarian secretion E28.39
|renal N28.9
|urine, urinary secretion R34
Suppuration, suppurative *see also* condition
|accessory sinus (chronic) *see* Sinusitis
|adrenal gland
|antrum (chronic) *see* Sinusitis, maxillary
|bladder *see* Cystitis
|brain G06.0
  |sequelae G09
|breast N61.1
  |puerperal, postpartum or gestational *see*
    Mastitis, obstetric, purulent
|dental periosteum M27.3
|ear (middle) *see also* Otitis, media
  |external NEC *see* Otitis, externa, infective
  |internal *see* subcategory H83.0
|ethmoidal (chronic) (sinus) *see* Sinusitis,
  ethmoidal
|fallopian tube *see* Salpingo-oophoritis
|frontal (chronic) (sinus) *see* Sinusitis, frontal
|gallbladder (acute) K81.0

Suppuration, suppurative - *continued*
|gum K05.20
  |generalized *see* Periodontitis, aggressive,
    generalized
  |localized *see* Periodontitis, aggressive,
    localized
|intracranial G06.0
|joint *see* Arthritis, pyogenic or pyemic
|labyrinthine *see* subcategory H83.0
|lung *see* Abscess, lung
|mammary gland N61.1
  |puerperal, postpartum O91.12
    |associated with lactation O91.13
|maxilla, maxillary M27.2
  |sinus (chronic) *see* Sinusitis, maxillary
|muscle *see* Myositis, infective
|nasal sinus (chronic) *see* Sinusitis
|pancreas, acute *see also* Pancreatitis, acute
  K85.80
|parotid gland *see* Sialoadenitis
|pelvis, pelvic
  |female *see* Disease, pelvis, inflammatory
  |male K65.0
|pericranial *see* Osteomyelitis
|salivary duct or gland (any) *see* Sialoadenitis
|sinus (accessory) (chronic) (nasal) *see*
  Sinusitis
|sphenoidal sinus (chronic) *see* Sinusitis,
  sphenoidal
|thymus (gland) E32.1
|thyroid (gland) E06.0
|tonsil *see* Tonsillitis
|uterus *see* Endometritis
Supraeruption of tooth (teeth) M26.34
Supraglottitis J04.30
|with obstruction J04.31
Suprarenal (gland) *see* condition
Suprascapular nerve *see* condition
Suprasellar *see* condition
Surfer's knots or nodules S89.8-
Surgical
|emphysema T81.82
|procedures, complication or misadventure *see*
  Complications, surgical procedures
|shock T81.10
Surveillance (of) (for) *see also* Observation
|alcohol abuse Z71.41
|contraceptive *see* Prescription, contraceptives
|dietary Z71.3
|drug abuse Z71.51
Susceptibility to disease, genetic Z15.89
|malignant neoplasm Z15.09
  |breast Z15.01
  |endometrium Z15.04
  |ovary Z15.02
  |prostate Z15.03
  |specified NEC Z15.09
|multiple endocrine neoplasia Z15.81
Suspected condition, ruled out *see also*
  Observation, suspected
|amniotic cavity and membrane Z03.71
|cervical shortening Z03.75
|fetal anomaly Z03.73
|fetal growth Z03.74
|maternal and fetal conditions NEC Z03.79
|newborn *see also* Observation, newborn,
  suspected condition ruled out Z05.9
|oligohydramnios Z03.71
|placental problem Z03.72
|polyhydramnios Z03.71
Suspended uterus
|in pregnancy or childbirth *see* Pregnancy,
  complicated by, abnormal uterus
Sutton's nevus D22.9

Suture
|burst (in operation wound) T81.31
||external operation wound T81.31
||internal operation wound T81.32
|inadvertently left in operation wound *see*
    Foreign body, accidentally left during a
    procedure
|removal Z48.02
Swab inadvertently left in operation wound
    see Foreign body, accidentally left during a
    procedure
Swallowed, swallowing
|difficulty *see* Dysphagia
|foreign body *see* Foreign body, alimentary
    tract
Swan-neck deformity (finger) *see* Deformity,
    finger, swan-neck
Swearing, compulsive F42.8
|in Gilles de la Tourette's syndrome F95.2
Sweat, sweats
|fetid L75.0
|night R61
Sweating, excessive R61
Sweeley-Klionsky disease E75.21
Sweet's disease or dermatosis L98.2
Swelling (of) R60.9
|abdomen, abdominal (not referable to any
    particular organ) *see* Mass, abdominal
|ankle *see* Effusion, joint, ankle
|arm M79.89
||forearm M79.89
|breast (*see also* Lump, breast) N63.0
|Calabar B74.3
|cervical gland R59.0
|chest, localized R22.2
|ear H93.8-
|extremity (lower) (upper) *see* Disorder, soft
    tissue, specified type NEC
|finger M79.89
|foot M79.89
|glands R59.9
||generalized R59.1
||localized R59.0
|hand M79.89
|head (localized) R22.0
|inflammatory *see* Inflammation
|intra-abdominal *see* Mass, abdominal
|joint *see* Effusion, joint
|leg M79.89
||lower M79.89
|limb *see* Disorder, soft tissue, specified type
    NEC
|localized (skin) R22.9
||chest R22.2
||head R22.0
||limb
|||lower *see* Mass, localized, limb, lower
|||upper *see* Mass, localized, limb, upper
||neck R22.1
||trunk R22.2
|neck (localized) R22.1
|pelvic *see* Mass, abdominal
|scrotum N50.89
|splenic *see* Splenomegaly
|testis N50.89
|toe M79.89
|umbilical R19.09
|wandering, due to Gnathostoma (spinigerum)
    B83.1
|white *see* Tuberculosis, arthritis
Swift (-Feer) disease
|overdose or wrong substance given or taken
    see Table of Drugs and Chemicals, by drug,
    poisoning

Swimmer's
|cramp T75.1
|ear H60.33-
|itch B65.3
Swimming in the head R42
Swollen *see* Swelling
Swyer syndrome Q99.1
Sycosis L73.8
|barbae (not parasitic) L73.8
|contagiosa (mycotic) B35.0
|lupoides L73.8
|mycotic B35.0
|parasitic B35.0
|vulgaris L73.8
Sydenham's chorea *see* Chorea, Sydenham's
Sylvatic yellow fever A95.0
Sylvest's disease B33.0
Symblepharon H11.23-
|congenital Q10.3
Symond's syndrome G93.2
Sympathetic *see* condition
Sympatheticotonia G90.8
Sympathicoblastoma
|specified site *see* Neoplasm, malignant, by site
|unspecified site C74.90
Sympathogonioma *see* Sympathicoblastoma
Symphalangy (fingers) (toes) Q70.9
Symptoms NEC R68.89
|breast NEC N64.59
|cold J00
|development NEC R63.8
|factitious, self-induced *see* Disorder, factitious
|genital organs, female R10.2
|involving
||abdomen NEC R19.8
||appearance NEC R46.89
||awareness R41.9
|||altered mental status R41.82
|||amnesia *see* Amnesia
|||borderline intellectual functioning R41.83
|||coma *see* Coma
|||disorientation R41.0
|||neurologic neglect syndrome R41.4
|||senile cognitive decline R41.81
|||specified symptom NEC R41.89
||behavior NEC R46.89
||cardiovascular system NEC R09.89
||chest NEC R09.89
||circulatory system NEC R09.89
||cognitive functions R41.9
|||altered mental status R41.82
|||amnesia *see* Amnesia
|||borderline intellectual functioning R41.83
|||coma *see* Coma
|||disorientation R41.0
|||neurologic neglect syndrome R41.4
|||senile cognitive decline R41.81
|||specified symptom NEC R41.89
||development NEC R62.50
||digestive system NEC R19.8
||emotional state NEC R45.89
|||emotional lability R45.86
||food and fluid intake R63.8
||general perceptions and sensations R44.9
|||specified NEC R44.8
||musculoskeletal system R29.91
|||specified NEC R29.898
||nervous system R29.90
|||specified NEC R29.818
||pelvis NEC R19.8
||respiratory system NEC R09.89
||skin and integument NEC R23.9
||urinary system R39.9
|menopausal N95.1
|metabolism NEC R63.8

Symptoms - *continued*
|neurotic F48.8
|of infancy R68.19
|pelvis NEC, female R10.2
|skin and integument NEC R23.9
|subcutaneous tissue NEC R23.9
|viral cold J00
Sympus Q74.2
Syncephalus Q89.4
Synchondrosis
|abnormal (congenital) Q78.8
|ischiopubic M91.0
Synchysis (scintillans) (senile) (vitreous body)
    H43.89
Syncope (near) (pre) R55
|anginosa I20.8
|bradycardia R00.1
|cardiac R55
|carotid sinus G90.01
|due to spinal (lumbar) puncture G97.1
|heart R55
|heat T67.1
|laryngeal R05.4
|psychogenic F48.8
|tussive R05.8
|vasoconstriction R55
|vasodepressor R55
|vasomotor R55
|vasovagal R55
Syndactylism, syndactyly Q70.9
|complex (with synostosis)
||fingers Q70.0-
||toes Q70.2-
|simple (without synostosis)
||fingers Q70.1-
||toes Q70.3-
Syndrome *see also* Disease
|5q minus NOS D46.C
|48,XXXX Q97.1
|49,XXXXX Q97.1
|abdominal
||acute R10.0
||muscle deficiency Q79.4
|abnormal innervation H02.519
||left H02.516
|||lower H02.515
|||upper H02.514
||right H02.513
|||lower H02.512
|||upper H02.511
|abstinence, neonatal P96.1
|acid pulmonary aspiration, obstetric O74.0
|acquired immunodeficiency *see* Human,
    immunodeficiency virus (HIV) disease
|acute abdominal R10.0
|acute respiratory distress (adult) (child) J80
||idiopathic J84.114
|Adair-Dighton Q78.0
|Adams-Stokes (-Morgagni) I45.9
|adiposogenital E23.6
|adrenal
||hemorrhage (meningococcal) A39.1
||meningococcic A39.1
|adrenocortical *see* Cushing's, syndrome
|adrenogenital E25.9
||congenital, associated with enzyme
    deficiency E25.0
|afferent loop NEC K91.89
|Alagille's Q44.7
|alcohol withdrawal (without convulsions) *see*
    Dependence, alcohol, with, withdrawal
|Alder's D72.0
|Aldrich (-Wiskott) D82.0
|alien hand R41.4
|Alport Q87.81

Syndrome - *continued*
   |compartment (deep) (posterior) (traumatic)
      T79.A0
      |abdomen T79.A3
      |lower extremity (hip, buttock, thigh, leg,
         foot, toes) T79.A2
      |nontraumatic
         |abdomen M79.A3
         |lower extremity (hip, buttock, thigh, leg,
            foot, toes) M79.A2-
         |specified site NEC M79.A9
         |upper extremity (shoulder, arm, forearm,
            wrist, hand, fingers) M79.A1-
      |postprocedural *see* Syndrome, compartment,
         nontraumatic
      |specified site NEC T79.A9
      |upper extremity (shoulder, arm, forearm,
         wrist, hand, fingers) T79.A1
   |complex regional pain *see* Syndrome, pain,
      complex regional
   |compression T79.5
      |anterior spinal *see* Syndrome, anterior,
         spinal artery, compression
      |cauda equina G83.4
      |celiac artery I77.4
      |vertebral artery M47.029
         |occipito-atlanto-axial region M47.021
         |cervical region M47.022
   |concussion F07.81
   |congenital
      |affecting multiple systems NEC Q87.89
      |central alveolar hypoventilation G47.35
      |facial diplegia Q87.0
      |muscular hypertrophy-cerebral Q87.89
      |oculo-auriculovertebral Q87.0
      |oculofacial diplegia (Moebius) Q87.0
      |rubella (manifest) P35.0
   |congestion-fibrosis (pelvic), female N94.89
   |congestive dysmenorrhea N94.6
   |Conn's E26.01
   |connective tissue M35.9
      |overlap NEC M35.1
   |conus medullaris G95.81
   |cord
      |anterior G83.82
      |posterior G83.83
   |coronary
      |acute NEC I24.9
      |insufficiency or intermediate I20.0
      |slow flow I20.8
   |Costen's (complex) M26.69
   |costochondral junction M94.0
   |costoclavicular G54.0
   |costovertebral E22.0
   |Cowden Q85.8
   |craniovertebral M53.0
   |Creutzfeldt-Jakob *see* Creutzfeldt-Jakob
      disease or syndrome
   |cri-du-Chat Q93.4
   |crib death R99
   |cricopharyngeal *see* Dysphagia
   |croup J05.0
   |CRPS I *see* Syndrome, pain, complex regional
      I
   |crush T79.5
   |cubital tunnel *see* Lesion, nerve, ulnar
   |Curschmann (-Batten) (-Steinert) G71.11
   |Cushing's E24.9
      |alcohol-induced E24.4
      |due to
         |alcohol
         |drugs E24.2
         |ectopic ACTH E24.3
         |overproduction of pituitary ACTH E24.0
      |drug-induced E24.2

Syndrome - *continued*
      |overdose or wrong substance given or taken
         see Table of Drugs and Chemicals, by
         drug, poisoning
      |pituitary-dependent E24.0
      |specified type NEC E24.8
   |Cryopyrin-associated periodic M04.2
   |cryptophthalmos Q87.0
   |cystic duct stump K91.5
   |cytokine release D89.839
      |grade 1 D89.831
      |grade 2 D89.832
      |grade 3 D89.833
      |grade 4 D89.834
      |grade 5 D89.835
   |Dana-Putnam D51.0
   |Danbolt (-Cross) (acrodermatitis
      enteropathica) E83.2
   |Dandy-Walker Q03.1
      |with spina bifida Q07.01
   |Danlos' Q79.6
   |defibrination *see also* Fibrinolysis
      |with
         |antepartum hemorrhage *see* Hemorrhage,
            antepartum, with coagulation defect
         |intrapartum hemorrhage *see* Hemorrhage,
            complicating, delivery
      |newborn P60
      |postpartum O72.3
   |Degos' I77.89
   |Déjérine-Roussy G89.0
   |delayed sleep phase G47.21
   |demyelinating G37.9
   |dependence *see* F10-F19 with fourth character
      .2
   |depersonalization (-derealization) F48.1
   |De Quervain E34.51
   |de Toni-Fanconi (-Debre) E72.09
      |with cystinosis E72.04
   |de Vivo syndrome E74.810
   |diabetes mellitus-hypertension-nephrosis *see*
      Diabetes, nephrosis
   |diabetes mellitus in newborn infant P70.2
   |diabetes-nephrosis *see* Diabetes, nephrosis
   |diabetic amyotrophy *see* Diabetes,
      amyotrophy
   |dialysis associated steal T82.898-
   |Diamond-Blackfan D61.01
   |Diamond-Gardener D69.2
   |DIC (diffuse or disseminated intravascular
      coagulopathy) D65
   |di George's D82.1
   |Dighton's Q78.0
   |disequilibrium E87.8
   |Döhle body-panmyelopathic D72.0
   |dorsolateral medullary G46.4
   |double athetosis G80.3
   |Down *see also* Down syndrome Q90.9
   |Dravet (intractable) G40.834
      |with status epilepticus G40.833
      |without status epilepticus G40.834
   |Dresbach's (elliptocytosis) D58.1
   |DRESS (drug rash with eosinophilia and
      systemic symptoms) D72.12
   |Dressler's (postmyocardial infarction) I24.1
      |postcardiotomy I97.0
   |drug rash with eosinophilia and systemic
      symptoms (DRESS) D72.12
   |drug withdrawal, infant of dependent mother
      P96.1
   |dry eye H04.12-
   |due to abnormality
      |chromosomal Q99.9
         |sex
            |female phenotype Q97.9

Syndrome - *continued*
      |male phenotype Q98.9
      |specified NEC Q99.8
   |dumping (postgastrectomy) K91.1
      |nonsurgical K31.89
   |Dupré's (meningism) R29.1
   |dysmetabolic X E88.81
   |dyspraxia, developmental F82
   |Eagle-Barrett Q79.4
   |Eaton-Lambert *see* Syndrome, Lambert-Eaton
   |Ebstein's Q22.5
   |ectopic ACTH E24.3
   |eczema-thrombocytopenia D82.0
   |Eddowes' Q78.0
   |effort (psychogenic) F45.8
   |Eisenmenger's I27.83
   |Ehlers-Danlos Q79.6
   |Ekman's Q78.0
   |electric feet E53.8
   |Ellis-Van Creveld Q77.6
   |empty nest Z60.0
   |endocrine-hypertensive E27.0
   |entrapment *see* Neuropathy, entrapment
   |eosinophilia-myalgia M35.8
   |epileptic *see also* Epilepsy, by type
      |absence G40.A09
         |intractable G40.A19
            |with status epilepticus G40.A11
            |without status epilepticus G40.A19
         |not intractable G40.A09
            |with status epilepticus G40.A01
            |without status epilepticus G40.A09
   |Erdheim-Chester (ECD) E88.89
   |Erdheim's E22.0
   |erythrocyte fragmentation D59.4
   |Evans D69.41
   |exhaustion F48.8
   |extrapyramidal G25.9
      |specified NEC G25.89
   |eye retraction *see* Strabismus
   |eyelid-malar-mandible Q87.0
   |Faber's D50.9
   |facet M47.89-
   |facet joint (see also Spondylosis) M47.819
   |facial pain, paroxysmal G50.0
   |Fallot's Q21.3
   |familial cold autoinflammatory M04.2
   |familial eczema-thrombocytopenia (Wiskott-
      Aldrich) D82.0
   |Fanconi (-De Toni) (-Debre) E72.09
      |with cystinosis E72.04
   |Fanconi's (anemia) (congenital pancytopenia)
      D61.09
   |fatigue
      |chronic R53.82
      |psychogenic F48.8
   |faulty bowel habit K59.39
   |Feil-Klippel (brevicollis) Q76.1
   |Felty's *see* Felty's syndrome
   |fertile eunuch E23.0
   |fetal
      |alcohol (dysmorphic) Q86.0
      |hydantoin Q86.1
   |Fiedler's I40.1
   |first arch Q87.0
   |fish odor E72.89
   |Fisher's G61.0
   |Fitzhugh-Curtis
      |due to
         |Chlamydia trachomatis A74.81
         |Neisseria gonorrhorea (gonococcal
            peritonitis) A54.85
   |Fitz's *see also* Pancreatitis, acute K85.80
   |Flajani (-Basedow) E05.00
      |with thyroid storm E05.01

Syndrome - *continued*

|flatback *see* Flatback syndrome
|floppy
  |baby P94.2
  |iris (intraoperative) (IFIS) H21.81
  |mitral valve I34.1
|flush E34.0
|Foix-Alajouanine G95.19
|Fong's Q87.2
|food protein-induced enterocolitis (FPIES)
  K52.21
|foramen magnum G93.5
|Foster-Kennedy H47.14-
|Foville's (peduncular) G46.3
|fragile X Q99.2
|Franceschetti Q75.4
|Frey's
  |auriculotemporal G50.8
  |hyperhidrosis L74.52
|Friderichsen-Waterhouse A39.1
|Froin's G95.89
|frontal lobe F07.0
|Fukuhara E88.49
|functional
  |bowel K59.9
  |prepubertal castrate E29.1
|Gaisböck's D75.1
|ganglion (basal ganglia brain) G25.9
  |geniculi G51.1
|Gardner-Diamond D69.2
|gastroesophageal
  |junction K22.0
  |laceration-hemorrhage K22.6
|gastrojejunal loop obstruction K91.89
|Gee-Herter-Heubner K90.0
|Gelineau's G47.419
  |with cataplexy G47.411
|genito-anorectal A55
|Gerstmann-Sträussler-Scheinker (GSS)
  A81.82
|Gianotti-Crosti L44.4
|giant platelet (Bernard-Soulier) D69.1
|Gilles de la Tourette's F95.2
|Gleich's D72.118
|goiter-Deafness E07.1
|Goldberg Q89.8
|Goldberg-Maxwell E34.51
|Good's D83.8
|Gopalan' (burning feet) E53.8
|Gorlin's Q87.89
|Gougerot-Blum L81.7
|Gouley's I31.1
|Gower's R55
|gray or grey (newborn) P93.0
  |platelet D69.1
|Gubler-Millard G46.3
|Guillain-Barré (-Strohl) G61.0
|gustatory sweating G50.8
|Hadfield-Clarke K86.89
|hair tourniquet *see* Constriction, external, by
  site
|Hamman's J98.19
|hand-foot L27.1
|hand-shoulder G90.8
|hantavirus (cardio)-pulmonary (HPS) (HCPS)
  B33.4
|happy puppet Q93.51
|Harada's H30.81-
|Hayem-Faber D50.9
|headache NEC G44.89
  |complicated NEC G44.59
|Heberden's I20.8
|Hedinger's E34.0
|Hegglin's D72.0

Syndrome - *continued*

|HELLP (hemolysis, elevated liver enzymes
  and low platelet count) O14.2-
  |complicating
    |childbirth O14.24
    |puerperium O14.25
|hemolytic-uremic D59.3
|hemophagocytic, infection-associated D76.2
|Henoch-Schönlein D69.0
|hepatic flexure K59.89
|hepatopulmonary K76.81
|hepatorenal K76.7
  |following delivery O90.4
  |postoperative or postprocedural K91.83
  |postpartum, puerperal O90.4
|hepatourologic K76.7
|hereditary alpha tryptasemia D89.44
|Herter (-Gee) (nontropical sprue) K90.0
|Heubner-Herter K90.0
|Heyd's K76.7
|Hilger's G90.09
|histamine-like (fish poisoning) *see* Poisoning,
  fish
|histiocytic D76.3
|histiocytosis NEC D76.3
|HIV infection, acute B20
|Hoffmann-Werdnig G12.0
|Hollander-Simons E88.1
|Hoppe-Goldflam G70.00
  |with exacerbation (acute) G70.01
  |in crisis G70.01
|Horner's G90.2
|hungry bone E83.81
|hunterian glossitis D51.0
|Hutchinson's triad A50.53
|hyperabduction G54.0
|hyperammonemia-hyperornithinemia-
  homocitrullinemia E72.4
|hypereosinophilic (HES) D72.119
  |idiopathic (IHES) D72.110
  |lymphocytic variant (LHES) D72.111
  |myeloid D72.118
  |specified NEC D72.118
|hyperimmunoglobulin D M04.1
|hyperimmunoglobulin E (IgE) D82.4
|hyperkalemic E87.5
|hyperkinetic *see* Hyperkinesia
|hypermobility M35.7
|hypernatremia E87.0
|hyperosmolarity E87.0
|hyperperfusion G97.82
|hypersplenic D73.1
|hypertransfusion, newborn P61.1
|hyperventilation F45.8
|hyperviscosity (of serum)
  |polycythemic D75.1
  |sclerothymic D58.8
|hypoglycemic (familial) (neonatal) E16.2
|hypokalemic E87.6
|hyponatremic E87.1
|hypoventilation, obesity (OHS) E66.2
|ICF (intravascular coagulation-fibrinolysis)
  D65
|idiopathic
  |cardiorespiratory distress, newborn P22.0
  |nephrotic (infantile) N04.9
|iliotibial band M76.3-
|immobility, immobilization (paraplegic)
  M62.3
|immune effector cell-associated neurotoxicity
  (ICANS) G92.00
  |grade
    |1 G92.01
    |2 G92.02
    |3 G92.03

Syndrome - *continued*

    |4 G92.04
    |5 G92.05
  |unspecified G92.00
|immune reconstitution D89.3
|immune reconstitution inflammatory [IRIS]
  D89.3
|immunity deficiency, combined D81.9
|immunodeficiency
  |acquired *see* Human, immunodeficiency
    virus (HIV) disease
  |combined D81.9
|impending coronary I20.0
|impingement, shoulder M75.4-
|inappropriate secretion of antidiuretic
  hormone E22.2
|infant
  |of diabetic mother P70.1
  |gestational diabetes P70.0
|infantilism (pituitary) E23.0
|inferior vena cava I87.1
|inspissated bile (newborn) P59.1
|institutional (childhood) F94.2
|insufficient sleep F51.12
|intermediate coronary (artery) I20.0
|interspinous ligament *see* Spondylopathy,
  specified NEC
|intestinal
  |carcinoid E34.0
  |knot K56.2
|intravascular coagulation-fibrinolysis (ICF)
  D65
|iodine-Deficiency, congenital E00.9
  |type
    |mixed E00.2
    |myxedematous E00.1
    |neurological E00.0
|IRDS (idiopathic respiratory distress,
  newborn) P22.0
|irritable
  |bowel K58.9
    |with
      |constipation K58.1
      |diarrhea K58.0
    |mixed K58.2
    |psychogenic F45.8
    |specified NEC K58.8
  |heart (psychogenic) F45.8
  |weakness F48.8
|ischemic
  |bowel (transient) K55.9
    |chronic K55.1
    |due to mesenteric artery insufficiency
      K55.1
  |steal T82.898
|IVC (intravascular coagulopathy) D65
|Ivemark's Q89.01
|Jaccoud's *see* Arthropathy, postrheumatic,
  chronic
|Jackson's G83.89
|Jakob-Creutzfeldt *see* Creutzfeldt-Jakob
  disease or syndrome
|jaw-winking Q07.8
|Jervell-Lange-Nielsen I45.81
|jet lag G47.25
|Job's D71
|Joseph-Diamond-Blackfan D61.01
|jugular foramen G52.7
|Kabuki Q89.8
|Kanner's (autism) F84.0
|Kartagener's Q89.3
|Kelly's D50.1
|Kimmelstiel-Wilson *see* Diabetes, specified
  type, with Kimmelstiel-Wilson disease
|Klein (e) -Levine G47.13

Syndrome - *continued*
|Klippel-Feil (brevicollis) Q76.1
|Köhler-Pellegrini-Steida *see* Bursitis, tibial collateral
|Koenig's K59.89
|Korsakoff (-Wernicke) (nonalcoholic) F04
|alcoholic F10.26
|Kostmann's D70.0
|Krabbe's congenital muscle hypoplasia Q79.8
|labyrinthine *see* subcategory H83.2
|lacunar NEC G46.7
|Lambert-Eaton G70.80
|in
|neoplastic disease G73.1
|specified disease NEC G70.81
|Landau-Kleffner *see* Epilepsy, specified NEC
|Larsen's Q74.8
|lateral
|cutaneous nerve of thigh G57.1-
|medullary G46.4
|Launois' E22.0
|lazy
|leukocyte D70.8
|posture M62.3
|Lemiere I80.8
|Lennox-Gastaut G40.812
|intractable G40.814
|with status epilepticus G40.813
|without status epilepticus G40.814
|not intractable G40.812
|with status epilepticus G40.811
|without status epilepticus G40.812
|lenticular, progressive E83.01
|Leopold-Levi's E05.90
|Lev's I44.2
|Li-Fraumeni Z15.01
|Lichtheim's D51.0
|Lightwood's N25.89
|Lignac (de Toni) (-Fanconi) (-Debre) E72.09
|with cystinosis E72.04
|Likoff's I20.8
|limbic epilepsy personality F07.0
|liver-kidney K76.7
|lobotomy F07.0
|Loffler's J82.89
|long arm 18 or 21 deletion Q93.89
|long QT I45.81
|Louis-Barré G11.3
|low
|atmospheric pressure T70.29
|back M54.50
|output (cardiac) I50.9
|lower radicular, newborn (birth injury) P14.8
|Luetscher's (dehydration) E86.0
|Lupus anticoagulant D68.62
|Lutembacher's Q21.1
|macrophage activation D76.1
|due to infection D76.2
|magnesium-Deficiency R29.0
|Majeed M04.8
|Mal de Debarquement R42
|malabsorption K90.9
|postsurgical K91.2
|malformation, congenital, due to
|alcohol Q86.0
|exogenous cause NEC Q86.8
|hydantoin Q86.1
|warfarin Q86.2
|malignant
|carcinoid E34.0
|neuroleptic G21.0
|Mallory-Weiss K22.6
|mandibulofacial dysostosis Q75.4
|manic-Depressive *see* Disorder, bipolar
|maple-syrup-urine E71.0

Syndrome - *continued*
|Marable's I77.4
|Marfan's Q87.40
|with
|cardiovascular manifestations Q87.418
|aortic dilation Q87.410
|ocular manifestations Q87.42
|skeletal manifestations Q87.43
|Marie's (acromegaly) E22.0
|mast cell activation *see* Activation, mast cell
|maternal hypotension *see* Syndrome, hypotension, maternal
|May (-Hegglin) D72.0
|McArdle (-Schmidt) (-Pearson) E74.04
|McQuarrie's E16.2
|meconium plug (newborn) P76.0
|median arcuate ligament I77.4
|Meekeren-Ehlers-Danlos Q79.6
|megavitamin-B6 E67.2
|Meige G24.4
|MELAS E88.41
|Mendelson's O74.0
|MERRF (myoclonic epilepsy associated with ragged-red fibers) E88.42
|mesenteric
|artery (superior) K55.1
|vascular insufficiency K55.1
|metabolic E88.81
|metastatic carcinoid E34.0
|micrognathia-glossoptosis Q87.0
|midbrain NEC G93.89
|middle lobe (lung) J98.19
|middle radicular G54.0
|migraine *see also* Migraine G43.909-
|Mikulicz' K11.8
|milk-alkali E83.52
|Millard-Gubler G46.3
|Miller-Dieker Q93.88
|Miller-Fisher G61.0
|Minkowski-Chauffard D58.0
|Mirizzi's K83.1
|MNGIE (Mitochondrial Neurogastrointestinal Encephalopathy) E88.49
|Möbius, ophthalmoplegic migraine *see* Migraine, ophthalmoplegic
|monofixation H50.42
|Morel-More M85.2
|Morel-Morgagni M85.2
|Morgagni (-Morel) (-Stewart) M85.2
|Morgagni-Adams-Stokes I45.9
|Muckle-Wells M04.2
|mucocutaneous lymph node (acute febrile) (MCLS) M30.3
|multiple endocrine neoplasia (MEN) *see* Neoplasia, endocrine, multiple (MEN)
|multiple operations *see* Disorder, factitious
|Mounier-Kuhn Q32.4
|with bronchiectasis J47.9
|with
|exacerbation (acute) J47.1
|lower respiratory infection J47.0
|acquired J98.09
|with bronchiectasis J47.9
|with
|exacerbation (acute) J47.1
|lower respiratory infection J47.0
|myasthenic G70.9
|in
|diabetes mellitus *see* Diabetes, amyotrophy
|endocrine disease NEC E34.9 *[G73.3]*
|neoplastic disease *see also* Neoplasm D49.9 *[G73.3]*
|thyrotoxicosis (hyperthyroidism) E05.90 *[G73.3]*

Syndrome - *continued*
|with thyroid storm E05.91 *[G73.3]*
|myelodysplastic D46.9
|with
|5q deletion D46.C
|isolated del (5q) chromosomal abnormality D46.C
|multilineage dysplasia D46.A
|with ringed sideroblasts D46.B
|lesions, low grade D46.20
|myeloid hypereosinophilic D72.118
|specified NEC D46.Z
|myelopathic pain G89.0
|myeloproliferative (chronic) D47.1
|myofascial pain M79.18
|Naffziger's G54.0
|nail patella Q87.2
|NARP (Neuropathy, Ataxia and Retinitis pigmentosa) E88.49
|neonatal abstinence P96.1
|nephritic *see also* Nephritis
|with edema *see* Nephrosis
|acute N00.9
|chronic N03.9
|rapidly progressive N01.9
|nephrotic (congenital) *see also* Nephrosis N04.9
|with
|C3
|glomerulonephritis N04.A
|glomerulopathy N04.A
|with dense deposit disease N04.6
|dense deposit disease N04.6
|diffuse
|crescentic glomerulonephritis N04.7
|endocapillary proliferative glomerulonephritis N04.4
|membranous glomerulonephritis N04.2
|mesangial proliferative glomerulonephritis N04.3
|mesangiocapillary glomerulonephritis N04.5
|focal and segmental glomerular lesions N04.1
|minor glomerular abnormality N04.0
|specified morphological changes NEC N04.8
|diabetic *see* Diabetes, nephrosis
|neurologic neglect R41.4
|Nezelof's D81.4
|Nonne-Milroy-Meige Q82.0
|Nothnagel's vasomotor acroparesthesia I73.89
|obesity hypoventilation (OHS) E66.2
|oculomotor H51.9
|Ogilvie K59.81
|ophthalmoplegia-cerebellar ataxia *see* Strabismus, paralytic, third nerve
|oral allergy T78.1
|oral-facial-Digital Q87.0
|organic
|affective F06.30
|amnesic (not alcohol or drug-induced) F04
|brain F09
|depressive F06.31
|hallucinosis F06.0
|personality F07.0
|Ormond's N13.5
|oro-facial-digital Q87.0
|os trigonum Q68.8
|Osler-Weber-Rendu I78.0
|osteoporosis-osteomalacia M83.8
|Osterreicher-Turner Q87.2
|otolith *see* subcategory H81.8
|oto-palatal-Digital Q87.0
|outlet (thoracic) G54.0

Syndrome - *continued*

|scimitar Q26.8
|sclerocystic ovary E28.2
|Seitelberger's G31.89
|septicemic adrenal hemorrhage A39.1
|seroconversion, retroviral (acute) Z21
|serous meningitis G93.2
|severe acute respiratory (SARS) J12.81
|shaken infant T74.4
|shock (traumatic) T79.4
  |kidney N17.0
    |following crush injury T79.5
  |toxic A48.3
|shock-lung J80
|Shone's   code to specific anomalies
|short
  |bowel K91.2
  |rib Q77.2
|shoulder-hand *see* Algoneurodystrophy
|Shwachman's D70.4
|sicca - *see* Syndrome, Sjögren
|sick
  |cell E87.1
  |sinus I49.5
|sick-euthyroid E07.81
|sideropenic D50.1
|Siemens' ectodermal dysplasia Q82.4
|Silfversköld's Q78.9
|Simons' E88.1
|sinus tarsi M25.57-
|sinusitis-bronchiectasis-situs inversus Q89.3
|Sipple's E31.22
|sirenomelia Q87.2
|Sjögren M35.00
  |with
    |central nervous system involvement
      M35.07
    |dental involvement M35.0C
    |gastrointestinal involvement M35.08
    |glomerular disease M35.0A
    |inflammatory arthritis M35.05
    |keratoconjunctivitis M35.01
    |lung involvement M35.02
    |myopathy M35.03
    |peripheral nervous system involvement
      M35.06
    |renal tubular acidosis M35.04
    |specified organ involvement, NEC
      M35.09
    |tubulo-interstitial nephropathy M35.04
    |vasculitis M35.0B
|Slocumb's E27.0
|slow flow, coronary I20.8
|Sluder's G44.89
|Smith-Magenis Q93.88
|Sneddon-Wilkinson L13.1
|Soto's Q87.3
|South African cardiomyopathy I42.8
|spasmodic
  |upward movement, eyes H51.8
  |winking F95.8
|Spen's I45.9
|splenic
  |agenesis Q89.01
  |flexure K59.89
  |neutropenia D73.81
|Spurway's Q78.0
|staphylococcal scalded skin L00
|steal
  |arteriovenous T82.898-
  |ischemic T82.898-
  |subclavian G45.8
|Stein-Leventhal E28.2

Syndrome - *continued*

|Stein's E28.2
|Stevens-Johnson syndrome L51.1
  |toxic epidermal necrolysis overlap L51.3
|Stewart-Morel M85.2
|Stickler Q89.8
|stiff baby Q89.8
|stiff man G25.82
|Still-Felty *see* Felty's syndrome
|Stokes (-Adams) I45.9
|stone heart I50.1
|straight back, congenital Q76.49
|subclavian steal G45.8
|subcoracoid-pectoralis minor G54.0
|subcostal nerve compression I77.89
|subphrenic interposition Q43.3
|superior
  |cerebellar artery I63.89
  |mesenteric artery K55.1
  |semi-circular canal dehiscence H83.8X-
  |vena cava I87.1
|supine hypotensive (maternal) *see* Syndrome,
  hypotension, maternal
|suprarenal cortical E27.0
|supraspinatus *see also* Tear, rotator cuff
  M75.10-
|Susac G93.49
|swallowed blood P78.2
|sweat retention L74.0
|Swyer Q99.1
|Symond's G93.2
|sympathetic
  |cervical paralysis G90.2
  |pelvic, female N94.89
|systemic inflammatory response (SIRS), of
  non-infectious origin (without organ
  dysfunction) R65.10
  |with acute organ dysfunction R65.11
|tachycardia-bradycardia I49.5
|takotsubo I51.81
|TAR (thrombocytopenia with absent radius)
  Q87.2
|tarsal tunnel G57.5-
|teething K00.7
|tegmental G93.89
|telangiectasic-pigmentation-cataract Q82.8
|temporal pyramidal apex *see* Otitis, media,
  suppurative, acute
|temporomandibular joint-pain-Dysfunction
  M26.62-
|Terry's (*see also* Myopia, degenerative)
  H44.2-
|testicular feminization *see also* Syndrome,
  androgen insensitivity E34.51
|thalamic pain (hyperesthetic) G89.0
|thoracic outlet (compression) G54.0
|Thorson-Björck E34.0
|thrombocytopenia with absent radius (TAR)
  Q87.2
|thyroid-adrenocortical insufficiency E31.0
|tibial
  |anterior M76.81-
  |posterior M76.82-
|Tietze's M94.0
|time-zone (rapid) G47.25
|Toni-Fanconi E72.09
  |with cystinosis E72.04
|Touraine's Q79.8
|tourniquet *see* Constriction, external, by site
|toxic shock A48.3
|transient left ventricular apical ballooning
  I51.81
|traumatic vasospastic T75.22
|Treacher Collins Q75.4
|triple X, female Q97.0

Syndrome - *continued*

|trisomy Q92.9
  |13 Q91.7
    |meiotic nondisjunction Q91.4
    |mitotic nondisjunction Q91.5
    |mosaicism Q91.5
    |translocation Q91.6
  |18 Q91.3
    |meiotic nondisjunction Q91.0
    |mitotic nondisjunction Q91.1
    |mosaicism Q91.1
    |translocation Q91.2
  |20 (q)(p) Q92.8
  |21 Q90.9
    |meiotic nondisjunction Q90.0
    |mitotic nondisjunction Q90.1
    |mosaicism Q90.1
    |translocation Q90.2
  |22 Q92.8
|tropical wet feet T69.0-
|Trousseau's I82.1
|tumor lysis (following antineoplastic
  chemotherapy) (spontaneous) NEC E88.3
|tumor necrosis factor receptor associated
  periodic (TRAPS) M04.1
|Twiddler's (due to)
  |automatic implantable defibrillator T82.198
  |cardiac pacemaker T82.198
|Unverricht (-Lundborg) *see* Epilepsy,
  generalized, idiopathic
|upward gaze H51.8
|uremia, chronic *see also* Disease, kidney,
  chronic N18.9
|urethral N34.3
|urethro-oculo-articular *see* Reiter's disease
|urohepatic K76.7
|vago-hypoglossal G52.7
|vascular NEC in cerebrovascular disease
  G46.8
|vasoconstriction, reversible cerebrovascular
  I67.841
|vasomotor I73.9
|vasospastic (traumatic) T75.22
|vasovagal R55
|van Buchem's M85.2
|van der Hoeve's Q78.0
|VATER Q87.2
|velo-cardio-facial Q93.81
|vena cava (inferior) (superior) (obstruction)
  I87.1
|vertebral
  |artery G45.0
    |compression *see* Syndrome, anterior,
      spinal artery, compression
  |steal G45.0
|vertebro-basilar artery G45.0
|vertebrogenic (pain) (*see also* Pain,
  vertebrogenic) M54.89
|vertiginous *see* Disorder, vestibular function
|Vinson-Plummer D50.1
|virus B34.9
|visceral larva migrans B83.0
|visual disorientation H53.8
|vitamin B6 deficiency E53.1
|vitreal corneal H59.01-
|vitreous (touch) H59.01-
|Vogt-Koyanagi H20.82-
|Volkmann's T79.6
|von Schroetter's I82.890
|von Willebrand (-Jürgen) D68.0
|Waldenström-Kjellberg D50.1
|Wallenberg's G46.3
|water retention E87.79
|Waterhouse (-Friderichsen) A39.1
|Weber-Gubler G46.3

Syndrome - *continued*
 |Weber-Leyden G46.3
 |Weber's G46.3
 |Wegener's M31.30
   |with
     |kidney involvement M31.31
     |lung involvement M31.30
       |with kidney involvement M31.31
 |Weingarten's (tropical eosinophilia) J82.89
 |Weiss-Baker G90.09
 |Werdnig-Hoffman G12.0
 |Wermer's E31.21
 |Werner's E34.8
 |Wernicke-Korsakoff (nonalcoholic) F04
   |alcoholic F10.26
 |West's *see* Epilepsy, spasms
 |Westphal-Strümpell E83.01
 |wet
   |feet (maceration) (tropical) T69.0-
   |lung, newborn P22.1
 |whiplash S13.4
 |whistling face Q87.0
 |Wilkie's K55.1
 |Wilkinson-Sneddon L13.1
 |Willebrand (-Jurgens) D68.0
 |Williams Q93.82
 |Wilson's (hepatolenticular degeneration)
   E83.01
 |Wiskott-Aldrich D82.0
 |withdrawal *see* Withdrawal, state
   |drug
     |infant of dependent mother P96.1
     |therapeutic use, newborn P96.2
 |Woakes' (ethmoiditis) J33.1
 |Wright's (hyperabduction) G54.0
 |X I20.9
 |XXXX Q97.1
 |XXXXX Q97.1
 |XXXXY Q98.1
 |XXY Q98.0
 |Yao M04.8
 |yellow nail L60.5
 |Zahorsky's B08.5
 |Zellweger syndrome E71.510
 |Zellweger-like syndrome E71.541
Synechia (anterior) (iris) (posterior) (pupil)
   see also Adhesions, iris
 |intra-uterine (traumatic) N85.6
Synesthesia R20.8
Syngamiasis, syngamosis B83.3
Synodontia K00.2
Synorchidism, synorchism Q55.1
Synostosis (congenital) Q78.8
 |astragalo-scaphoid Q74.2
 |radioulnar Q74.0
Synovial sarcoma *see* Neoplasm, connective
   tissue, malignant
Synovioma (malignant) *see also* Neoplasm,
   connective tissue, malignant
 |benign *see* Neoplasm, connective tissue,
   benign
Synoviosarcoma *see* Neoplasm, connective
   tissue, malignant
Synovitis *see also* Tenosynovitis M65.9
 |crepitant
   |hand M70.0-
   |wrist M70.03-
 |gonococcal A54.49
 |gouty *see* Gout
 |in (due to)
   |crystals M65.8-
   |gonorrhea A54.49
   |syphilis (late) A52.78
   |use, overuse, pressure *see* Disorder, soft
     tissue, due to use

Synovitis - *continued*
 |infective NEC *see* Tenosynovitis, infective
   NEC
 |specified NEC *see* Tenosynovitis, specified
   type NEC
 |syphilitic A52.78
   |congenital (early) A50.02
 |toxic *see* Synovitis, transient
 |transient M67.3-
   |ankle M67.37-
   |elbow M67.32-
   |foot joint M67.37-
   |hand joint M67.34-
   |hip M67.35-
   |knee M67.36-
   |multiple site M67.39
   |pelvic region M67.35-
   |shoulder M67.31-
   |specified joint NEC M67.38
   |wrist M67.33-
 |traumatic, current *see* Sprain
 |tuberculous *see* Tuberculosis, synovitis
 |villonodular (pigmented) M12.2-
   |ankle M12.27-
   |elbow M12.22-
   |foot joint M12.27-
   |hand joint M12.24-
   |hip M12.25-
   |knee M12.26-
   |multiple site M12.29
   |pelvic region M12.25-
   |shoulder M12.21-
   |specified joint NEC M12.28
   |vertebrae M12.28
   |wrist M12.23-
Syphilid A51.39
 |congenital A50.06
 |newborn A50.06
 |tubercular (late) A52.79
Syphilis, syphilitic (acquired) A53.9
 |abdomen (late) A52.79
 |acoustic nerve A52.15
 |adenopathy (secondary) A51.49
 |adrenal (gland) (with cortical hypofunction)
   A52.79
 |age under 2 years NOS *see also* Syphilis,
   congenital, early
   |acquired A51.9
 |alopecia (secondary) A51.32
 |anemia (late) A52.79 [D63.8]
 |aneurysm (aorta) (ruptured) A52.01
   |central nervous system A52.05
   |congenital A50.54 [I79.0]
 |anus (late) A52.74
   |primary A51.1
   |secondary A51.39
 |aorta (arch) (abdominal) (thoracic) A52.02
   |aneurysm A52.01
 |aortic (insufficiency) (regurgitation) (stenosis)
   A52.03
   |aneurysm A52.01
 |arachnoid (adhesive) (cerebral) (spinal)
   A52.13
 |asymptomatic *see* Syphilis, latent
 |ataxia (locomotor) A52.11
 |atrophoderma maculatum A51.39
 |auricular fibrillation A52.06
 |bladder (late) A52.76
 |bone A52.77
   |secondary A51.46
 |brain A52.17
 |breast (late) A52.79
 |bronchus (late) A52.72
 |bubo (primary) A51.0
 |bulbar palsy A52.19

Syphilis, syphilitic - *continued*
 |bursa (late) A52.78
 |cardiac decompensation A52.06
 |cardiovascular A52.00
 |central nervous system (late) (recurrent)
   (relapse) (tertiary) A52.3
   |with
     |ataxia A52.11
     |general paralysis A52.17
       |juvenile A50.45
     |paresis (general) A52.17
       |juvenile A50.45
     |tabes (dorsalis) A52.11
       |juvenile A50.45
     |taboparesis A52.17
       |juvenile A50.45
   |aneurysm A52.05
   |congenital A50.40
     |juvenile A50.40
   |remission in (sustained) A52.3
   |serology doubtful, negative, or positive
     A52.3
   |specified nature or site NEC A52.19
   |vascular A52.05
 |cerebral A52.17
   |meningovascular A52.13
   |nerves (multiple palsies) A52.15
   |sclerosis A52.17
   |thrombosis A52.05
 |cerebrospinal (tabetic type) A52.12
 |cerebrovascular A52.05
 |cervix (late) A52.76
 |chancre (multiple) A51.0
   |extragenital A51.2
   |Rollet's A51.0
 |Charcot's joint A52.16
 |chorioretinitis A51.43
   |congenital A50.01
   |late A52.71
   |prenatal A50.01
 |choroiditis *see* Syphilitic chorioretinitis
 |choroidoretinitis *see* Syphilitic chorioretinitis
 |ciliary body (secondary) A51.43
   |late A52.71
 |colon (late) A52.74
 |combined spinal sclerosis A52.11
 |condyloma (latum) A51.31
 |congenital A50.9
   |with
     |paresis (general) A50.45
     |tabes (dorsalis) A50.45
     |taboparesis A50.45
   |chorioretinitis, choroiditis A50.01 [H32]
   |early, or less than 2 years after birth NEC
     A50.2
   |with manifestations *see* Syphilis,
   congenital, early, symptomatic
     |latent (without manifestations) A50.1
       |negative spinal fluid test A50.1
       |serology positive A50.1
     |symptomatic A50.09
       |cutaneous A50.06
       |mucocutaneous A50.07
       |oculopathy A50.01
       |osteochondropathy A50.02
       |pharyngitis A50.03
       |pneumonia A50.04
       |rhinitis A50.05
       |visceral A50.08
   |interstitial keratitis A50.31
   |juvenile neurosyphilis A50.45
   |late, or 2 years or more after birth NEC
     A50.7
     |chorioretinitis, choroiditis A50.32
     |interstitial keratitis A50.31

Syphilis, syphilitic - *continued*
- │juvenile neurosyphilis A50.45
- │latent (without manifestations) A50.6
  - │negative spinal fluid test A50.6
  - │serology positive A50.6
- │symptomatic or with manifestations NEC A50.59
  - │arthropathy A50.55
  - │cardiovascular A50.54
  - │Clutton's joints A50.51
  - │Hutchinson's teeth A50.52
  - │Hutchinson's triad A50.53
  - │osteochondropathy A50.56
  - │saddle nose A50.57
- │conjugal A53.9
  - │tabes A52.11
- │conjunctiva (late) A52.71
- │contact Z20.2
- │cord bladder A52.19
- │cornea, late A52.71
- │coronary (artery) (sclerosis) A52.06
- │coryza, congenital A50.05
- │cranial nerve A52.15
  - │multiple palsies A52.15
- │cutaneous *see* Syphilis, skin
- │dacryocystitis (late) A52.71
- │degeneration, spinal cord A52.12
- │dementia paralytica A52.17
  - │juvenilis A50.45
- │destruction of bone A52.77
- │dilatation, aorta A52.01
- │due to blood transfusion A53.9
- │dura mater A52.13
- │ear A52.79
  - │inner A52.79
    - │nerve (eighth) A52.15
    - │neurorecurrence A52.15
- │early A51.9
  - │cardiovascular A52.00
  - │central nervous system A52.3
  - │latent (without manifestations) (less than 2 years after infection) A51.5
    - │negative spinal fluid test A51.5
    - │serological relapse after treatment A51.5
    - │serology positive A51.5
  - │relapse (treated, untreated) A51.9
  - │skin A51.39
  - │symptomatic A51.9
    - │extragenital chancre A51.2
    - │primary, except extragenital chancre A51.0
    - │secondary *see also* Syphilis, secondary A51.39
      - │relapse (treated, untreated) A51.49
    - │ulcer A51.39
- │eighth nerve (neuritis) A52.15
- │endemic A65
- │endocarditis A52.03
  - │aortic A52.03
  - │pulmonary A52.03
- │epididymis (late) A52.76
- │epiglottis (late) A52.73
- │epiphysitis (congenital) (early) A50.02
- │episcleritis (late) A52.71
- │esophagus A52.79
- │eustachian tube A52.73
- │exposure to Z20.2
- │eye A52.71
- │eyelid (late) (with gumma) A52.71
- │fallopian tube (late) A52.76
- │fracture A52.77
- │gallbladder (late) A52.74
- │gastric (polyposis) (late) A52.74
- │general A53.9
  - │paralysis A52.17

Syphilis, syphilitic - *continued*
- │juvenile A50.45
- │genital (primary) A51.0
- │glaucoma A52.71
- │gumma NEC A52.79
  - │cardiovascular system A52.00
  - │central nervous system A52.3
  - │congenital A50.59
- │heart (block) (decompensation) (disease) (failure) A52.06 [*152*]
  - │valve NEC A52.03
- │hemianesthesia A52.19
- │hemianopsia A52.71
- │hemiparesis A52.17
- │hemiplegia A52.17
- │hepatic artery A52.09
- │hepatis A52.74
- │hepatomegaly, congenital A50.08
- │hereditaria tarda *see* Syphilis, congenital, late
- │hereditary *see* Syphilis, congenital
- │Hutchinson's teeth A50.52
- │hyalitis A52.71
- │inactive *see* Syphilis, latent
- │infantum *see* Syphilis, congenital
- │inherited *see* Syphilis, congenital
- │internal ear A52.79
- │intestine (late) A52.74
- │iris, iritis (secondary) A51.43
  - │late A52.71
- │joint (late) A52.77
- │keratitis (congenital) (interstitial) (late) A50.31
- │kidney (late) A52.75
- │lacrimal passages (late) A52.71
- │larynx (late) A52.73
- │late A52.9
  - │cardiovascular A52.00
  - │central nervous system A52.3
  - │kidney A52.75
  - │latent or 2 years or more after infection (without manifestations) A52.8
    - │negative spinal fluid test A52.8
    - │serology positive A52.8
  - │paresis A52.17
  - │specified site NEC A52.79
  - │symptomatic or with manifestations A52.79
  - │tabes A52.11
- │latent A53.0
  - │with signs or symptoms   code by site and stage under Syphilis
  - │central nervous system A52.2
  - │date of infection unspecified A53.0
  - │early, or less than 2 years after infection A51.5
  - │follow-up of latent syphilis A53.0
    - │date of infection unspecified A53.0
    - │late, or 2 years or more after infection A52.8
  - │late, or 2 years or more after infection A52.8
  - │positive serology (only finding) A53.0
    - │date of infection unspecified A53.0
    - │early, or less than 2 years after infection A51.5
    - │late, or 2 years or more after infection A52.8
- │lens (late) A52.71
- │leukoderma A51.39
  - │late A52.79
- │lienitis A52.79
- │lip A51.39
  - │chancre (primary) A51.2
  - │late A52.79
- │Lissauer's paralysis A52.17
- │liver A52.74
- │locomotor ataxia A52.11

Syphilis, syphilitic - *continued*
- │lung A52.72
- │lymph gland (early) (secondary) A51.49
  - │late A52.79
- │lymphadenitis (secondary) A51.49
- │macular atrophy of skin A51.39
  - │striated A52.79
- │mediastinum (late) A52.73
- │meninges (adhesive) (brain) (spinal cord) A52.13
- │meningitis A52.13
  - │acute (secondary) A51.41
  - │congenital A50.41
- │meningoencephalitis A52.14
- │meningovascular A52.13
  - │congenital A50.41
- │mesarteritis A52.09
  - │brain A52.04
- │middle ear A52.77
- │mitral stenosis A52.03
- │monoplegia A52.17
- │mouth (secondary) A51.39
  - │late A52.79
- │mucocutaneous (secondary) A51.39
  - │late A52.79
- │mucous
  - │membrane (secondary) A51.39
    - │late A52.79
  - │patches A51.39
    - │congenital A50.07
- │mulberry molars A50.52
- │muscle A52.78
- │myocardium A52.06
- │nasal sinus (late) A52.73
- │neonatorum *see* Syphilis, congenital
- │nephrotic syndrome (secondary) A51.44
- │nerve palsy (any cranial nerve) A52.15
  - │multiple A52.15
- │nervous system, central A52.3
- │neuritis A52.15
  - │acoustic A52.15
- │neurorecidive of retina A52.19
- │neuroretinitis A52.19
- │newborn *see* Syphilis, congenital
- │nodular superficial (late) A52.79
- │nonvenereal A65
- │nose (late) A52.73
  - │saddle back deformity A50.57
- │occlusive arterial disease A52.09
- │oculopathy A52.71
- │ophthalmic (late) A52.71
- │optic nerve (atrophy) (neuritis) (papilla) A52.15
- │orbit (late) A52.71
- │organic A53.9
- │osseous (late) A52.77
- │osteochondritis (congenital) (early) A50.02 [*M90.80*]
- │osteoporosis A52.77
- │ovary (late) A52.76
- │oviduct (late) A52.76
- │palate (late) A52.79
- │pancreas (late) A52.74
- │paralysis A52.17
  - │general A52.17
    - │juvenile A50.45
- │paresis (general) A52.17
  - │juvenile A50.45
- │paresthesia A52.19
- │Parkinson's disease or syndrome A52.19
- │paroxysmal tachycardia A52.06
- │pemphigus (congenital) A50.06
- │penis (chancre) A51.0
  - │late A52.76
- │pericardium A52.06

Syphilis, syphilitic - *continued*
| perichondritis, larynx (late) A52.73
| periosteum (late) A52.77
| | congenital (early) A50.02 *[M90.80]*
| | early (secondary) A51.46
| peripheral nerve A52.79
| petrous bone (late) A52.77
| pharynx (late) A52.73
| | secondary A51.39
| pituitary (gland) A52.79
| pleura (late) A52.73
| pneumonia, white A50.04
| pontine lesion A52.17
| portal vein A52.09
| primary A51.0
| | anal A51.1
| | and secondary *see* Syphilis, secondary
| | central nervous system A52.3
| | extragenital chancre NEC A51.2
| | fingers A51.2
| | genital A51.0
| | lip A51.2
| | specified site NEC A51.2
| | tonsils A51.2
| prostate (late) A52.76
| ptosis (eyelid) A52.71
| pulmonary (late) A52.72
| | artery A52.09
| pyelonephritis (late) A52.75
| recently acquired, symptomatic A51.9
| rectum (late) A52.74
| respiratory tract (late) A52.73
| retina, late A52.71
| retrobulbar neuritis A52.15
| salpingitis A52.76
| sclera (late) A52.71
| sclerosis
| | cerebral A52.17
| | coronary A52.06
| | multiple A52.11
| scotoma (central) A52.71
| scrotum (late) A52.76
| secondary (and primary) A51.49
| | adenopathy A51.49
| | anus A51.39
| | bone A51.46
| | chorioretinitis, choroiditis A51.43
| | hepatitis A51.45
| | liver A51.45
| | lymphadenitis A51.49
| | meningitis (acute) A51.41
| | mouth A51.39
| | mucous membranes A51.39
| | periosteum, periostitis A51.46
| | pharynx A51.39
| | relapse (treated, untreated) A51.49
| | skin A51.39
| | specified form NEC A51.49
| | tonsil A51.39
| | ulcer A51.39
| | viscera NEC A51.49
| | vulva A51.39
| seminal vesicle (late) A52.76
| seronegative with signs or symptoms   code
| | by site and stage under Syphilis
| seropositive
| | with signs or symptoms   code by site and
| | | stage under Syphilis
| | follow-up of latent syphilis *see* Syphilis,
| | | latent
| | only finding *see* Syphilis, latent
| seventh nerve (paralysis) A52.15
| sinus, sinusitis (late) A52.73
| skeletal system A52.77

Syphilis, syphilitic - *continued*
| skin (with ulceration) (early) (secondary)
| | A51.39
| | late or tertiary A52.79
| small intestine A52.74
| spastic spinal paralysis A52.17
| spermatic cord (late) A52.76
| spinal (cord) A52.12
| spleen A52.79
| splenomegaly A52.79
| spondylitis A52.77
| staphyloma A52.71
| stigmata (congenital) A50.59
| stomach A52.74
| synovium A52.78
| tabes dorsalis (late) A52.11
| | juvenile A50.45
| tabetic type A52.11
| | juvenile A50.45
| taboparesis A52.17
| | juvenile A50.45
| tachycardia A52.06
| tendon (late) A52.78
| tertiary A52.9
| | with symptoms NEC A52.79
| | cardiovascular A52.00
| | central nervous system A52.3
| | multiple NEC A52.79
| | specified site NEC A52.79
| testis A52.76
| thorax A52.73
| throat A52.73
| thymus (gland) (late) A52.79
| thyroid (late) A52.79
| tongue (late) A52.79
| tonsil (lingual) (late) A52.73
| | primary A51.2
| | secondary A51.39
| trachea (late) A52.73
| tunica vaginalis (late) A52.76
| ulcer (any site) (early) (secondary) A51.39
| | late A52.79
| | perforating A52.79
| | | foot A52.11
| urethra (late) A52.76
| urogenital (late) A52.76
| uterus (late) A52.76
| uveal tract (secondary) A51.43
| | late A52.71
| uveitis (secondary) A51.43
| | late A52.71
| uvula (late) (perforated) A52.79
| vagina A51.0
| | late A52.76
| valvulitis NEC A52.03
| vascular A52.00
| | brain (cerebral) A52.05
| ventriculi A52.74
| vesicae urinariae (late) A52.76
| viscera (abdominal) (late) A52.74
| | secondary A51.49
| vitreous (opacities) (late) A52.71
| | hemorrhage A52.71
| vulva A51.0
| | late A52.76
| | secondary A51.39
Syphiloma A52.79
| cardiovascular system A52.00
| central nervous system A52.3
| circulatory system A52.00
| congenital A50.59
Syphilophobia F45.29
Syringadenoma *see also* Neoplasm, skin,
| benign
| papillary *see* Neoplasm, skin, benign

Syringobulbia G95.0
Syringocystadenoma *see* Neoplasm, skin,
| benign
| papillary *see* Neoplasm, skin, benign
Syringoma *see also* Neoplasm, skin, benign
| chondroid *see* Neoplasm, skin, benign
Syringomyelia G95.0
Syringomyelitis *see* Encephalitis
Syringomyelocele *see* Spina bifida
Syringopontia G95.0
System, systemic *see also* condition
| disease, combined *see* Degeneration,
| | combined
| inflammatory response syndrome (SIRS) of
| | non-infectious origin (without organ
| | dysfunction) R65.10
| | with acute organ dysfunction R65.11
| lupus erythematosus M32.9
| | inhibitor present D68.62

T

Tabacism, tabacosis, tabagism *see also*
| Poisoning, tobacco
| meaning dependence (without remission)
| | F17.200
| | with
| | | disorder F17.299
| | | | in remission F17.211
| | | | specified disorder NEC F17.298
| | | withdrawal F17.203
Tabardillo A75.9
| flea-borne A75.2
| louse-borne A75.0
Tabes, tabetic A52.10
| with
| | central nervous system syphilis A52.10
| | Charcot's joint A52.16
| | cord bladder A52.19
| | crisis, viscera (any) A52.19
| | paralysis, general A52.17
| | paresis (general) A52.17
| | perforating ulcer (foot) A52.19
| arthropathy (Charcot) A52.16
| bladder A52.19
| bone A52.11
| cerebrospinal A52.12
| congenital A50.45
| conjugal A52.10
| dorsalis A52.11
| | juvenile A50.49
| juvenile A50.49
| latent A52.19
| mesenterica A18.39
| paralysis, insane, general A52.17
| spasmodic A52.17
| syphilis (cerebrospinal) A52.12
Taboparalysis A52.17
Taboparesis (remission) A52.17
| juvenile A50.45
TAC (trigeminal autonomic cephalgia) NEC
| G44.099
| intractable G44.091
| not intractable G44.099
Tache noir S60.22-
Tachyalimentation K91.2
Tachyarrhythmia, tachyrhythmia *see*
| Tachycardia
Tachycardia R00.0
| atrial (paroxysmal) I47.1
| auricular I47.1
| AV nodal re-entry (re-entrant) I47.1
| junctional (paroxysmal) I47.1
| newborn P29.11

Tachycardia - *continued*
|nodal (paroxysmal) I47.1
|non-paroxysmal AV nodal I45.89
|paroxysmal (sustained) (nonsustained) I47.9
   |with sinus bradycardia I49.5
   |atrial (PAT) I47.1
   |atrioventricular (AV) (re-entrant) I47.1
      |psychogenic F54
   |junctional I47.1
      |ectopic I47.1
   |nodal I47.1
   |psychogenic (atrial) (supraventricular)
      (ventricular) F54
   |supraventricular (sustained) I47.1
      |psychogenic F54
   |ventricular I47.2
      |psychogenic F54
|psychogenic F45.8
|sick sinus I49.5
|sinoauricular NOS R00.0
   |paroxysmal I47.1
|sinus [sinusal] NOS R00.0
   |paroxysmal I47.1
|supraventricular I47.1
|ventricular (paroxysmal) (sustained) I47.2
   |psychogenic F54
Tachygastria K31.89
Tachypnea R06.82
|hysterical F45.8
|newborn (idiopathic) (transitory) P22.1
|psychogenic F45.8
|transitory, of newborn P22.1
Taenia (infection) (infestation) B68.9
|diminuta B71.0
|echinococcal infestation B67.90
|mediocanellata B68.1
|nana B71.0
|saginata B68.1
|solium (intestinal form) B68.0
|larval form *see* Cysticercosis
Taeniasis (intestine) *see* Taenia
TACO (transfusion associated circulatory
   overload) E87.71
Tag (hypertrophied skin) (infected) L91.8
|adenoid J35.8
|anus K64.4
|hemorrhoidal K64.4
|hymen N89.8
|perineal N90.89
|preauricular Q17.0
|sentinel K64.4
|skin L91.8
   |accessory (congenital) Q82.8
   |anus K64.4
   |congenital Q82.8
   |preauricular Q17.0
|tonsil J35.8
|urethra, urethral N36.8
|vulva N90.89
Tahyna fever B33.8
Takahara's disease E80.3
Takayasu's disease or syndrome M31.4
Talaromycosis B48.4
Talcosis (pulmonary) J62.0
Talipes (congenital) Q66.89
|acquired, planus *see* Deformity, limb, flat foot
|asymmetric Q66.89
|calcaneovalgus Q66.4
|calcaneovarus Q66.1
|calcaneus Q66.89
|cavus Q66.7
|equinovalgus Q66.6
|equinovarus Q66.0
|equinus Q66.89
|percavus Q66.7
|planovalgus Q66.6

Talipes - *continued*
|planus (acquired) (any degree) *see also*
   Deformity, limb, flat foot
   |congenital Q66.5-
   |due to rickets (sequelae) E64.3
|valgus Q66.6
|varus Q66.3
Tall stature, constitutional E34.4
Talma's disease M62.89
Talon noir S90.3-
|hand S60.22-
|heel S90.3-
|toe S90.1-
Tamponade, heart I31.4
Tanapox (virus disease) B08.71
Tangier disease E78.6
Tantrum, child problem F91.8
Tapeworm (infection) (infestation) *see*
   Infestation, tapeworm
Tapia's syndrome G52.7
TAR (thrombocytopenia with absent radius)
   syndrome Q87.2
Tarral-Besnier disease L44.0
Tarsal tunnel syndrome *see* Syndrome, tarsal
   tunnel
Tarsalgia *see* Pain, limb, lower
Tarsitis (eyelid) H01.8
|syphilitic A52.71
|tuberculous A18.4
Tartar (teeth) (dental calculus) K03.6
Tattoo (mark) L81.8
Tauri's disease E74.09
Taurodontism K00.2
Taussig-Bing syndrome Q20.1
Taybi's syndrome Q87.2
Tay-Sachs amaurotic familial idiocy or
   disease E75.02
TBI (traumatic brain injury) S06.9
Teacher's node or nodule J38.2
Tear, torn (traumatic) *see also* Laceration
|with abortion *see* Abortion
|annular fibrosis M51.35
|anus, anal (sphincter) S31.831
   |complicating delivery
      |with third degree perineal laceration *see*
         also Delivery, complicated, by,
         laceration, perineum, third degree
         O70.20
         |with mucosa O70.3
      |without third degree perineal laceration
         O70.4
   |nontraumatic (healed) (old) K62.81
|articular cartilage, old *see* Derangement, joint,
   articular cartilage, by site
|bladder
   |with ectopic or molar pregnancy O08.6
   |following ectopic or molar pregnancy O08.6
   |obstetrical O71.5
   |traumatic *see* Injury, bladder
|bowel
   |with ectopic or molar pregnancy O08.6
   |following ectopic or molar pregnancy O08.6
   |obstetrical trauma O71.5
|broad ligament
   |with ectopic or molar pregnancy O08.6
   |following ectopic or molar pregnancy O08.6
   |obstetrical trauma O71.6
|bucket handle (knee) (meniscus) *see* Tear,
   meniscus
|capsule, joint *see* Sprain
|cartilage *see also* Sprain
   |articular, old *see* Derangement, joint,
      articular cartilage, by site
|cervix
   |with ectopic or molar pregnancy O08.6

Tear, torn - *continued*
|following ectopic or molar pregnancy O08.6
|obstetrical trauma (current) O71.3
|old N88.1
|traumatic *see* Injury, uterus
|dural G97.41
|nontraumatic G96.11
|internal organ *see* Injury, by site
|knee cartilage
   |articular (current) S83.3-
   |old *see* Derangement, knee, meniscus, due
      to old tear
|ligament *see* Sprain
|meniscus (knee) (current injury) S83.209
   |bucket-handle S83.20-
   |lateral
      |bucket-handle S83.25-
      |complex S83.27-
      |peripheral S83.26-
      |specified type NEC S83.28-
   |medial
      |bucket-handle S83.21-
      |complex S83.23-
      |peripheral S83.22-
      |specified type NEC S83.24-
   |old *see* Derangement, knee, meniscus, due
      to old tear
   |site other than knee   code as Sprain
   |specified type NEC S83.20-
|muscle *see* Strain
|pelvic
   |floor, complicating delivery O70.1
   |organ NEC, obstetrical trauma O71.5
      |with ectopic or molar pregnancy O08.6
      |following ectopic or molar pregnancy
         O08.6
|perineal, secondary O90.1
|periurethral tissue, obstetrical trauma O71.82
   |with ectopic or molar pregnancy O08.6
   |following ectopic or molar pregnancy O08.6
|rectovaginal septum *see* Laceration, vagina
|retina, retinal (without detachment)
      (horseshoe) *see also* Break, retina,
      horseshoe
   |with detachment *see* Detachment, retina,
      with retinal, break
|rotator cuff (nontraumatic) M75.10-
   |complete M75.12-
   |incomplete M75.11-
   |traumatic S46.01-
      |capsule S43.42-
|semilunar cartilage, knee *see* Tear, meniscus
|supraspinatus (complete) (incomplete)
   (nontraumatic) *see also* Tear, rotator cuff
   M75.10-
|tendon *see* Strain
|tentorial, at birth P10.4
|umbilical cord
   |complicating delivery O69.89
|urethra
   |with ectopic or molar pregnancy O08.6
   |following ectopic or molar pregnancy O08.6
   |obstetrical trauma O71.5
|uterus *see* Injury, uterus
|vagina *see* Laceration, vagina
|vessel, from catheter *see* Puncture, accidental
   complicating surgery
|vulva, complicating delivery O70.0
Tear-Stone *see* Dacryolith
Teeth *see also* condition
|grinding
   |psychogenic F45.8
   |sleep related G47.63
Teething (syndrome) K00.7

Telangiectasia, telangiectasis (verrucous)
I78.1
|ataxic (cerebellar) (Louis-Bar) G11.3
|familial I78.0
|hemorrhagic, hereditary (congenital) (senile)
I78.0
|hereditary, hemorrhagic (congenital) (senile)
I78.0
|juxtafoveal H35.07-
|macular H35.07-
|macularis eruptiva perstans D47.01
|parafoveal H35.07-
|retinal (idiopathic) (juxtafoveal) (macular)
(parafoveal) H35.07-
|spider I78.1
Telephone scatologia F65.89
Telescoped bowel or intestine K56.1
|congenital Q43.8
Temperature
|body, high (of unknown origin) R50.9
|cold, trauma from T69.9
|newborn P80.0
|specified effect NEC T69.8
Temple *see* condition
Temporal *see* condition
Temporomandibular joint pain-Dysfunction
syndrome M26.62-
Temporosphenoidal *see* condition
Tendency
|bleeding *see* Defect, coagulation
|suicide
|meaning personal history of attempted
suicide Z91.51
|meaning suicidal ideation *see* Ideation,
suicidal
|to fall R29.6
Tenderness, abdominal R10.819
|epigastric R10.816
|generalized R10.817
|left lower quadrant R10.814
|left upper quadrant R10.812
|periumbilic R10.815
|right lower quadrant R10.813
|right upper quadrant R10.811
|rebound R10.829
|epigastric R10.826
|generalized R10.827
|left lower quadrant R10.824
|left upper quadrant R10.822
|periumbilic R10.825
|right lower quadrant R10.823
|right upper quadrant R10.821
Tendinitis, tendonitis *see also* Enthesopathy
|Achilles M76.6-
|adhesive *see* Tenosynovitis, specified type
NEC
|shoulder *see* Capsulitis, adhesive
|bicipital M75.2-
|calcific M65.2-
|ankle M65.27-
|foot M65.27-
|forearm M65.23-
|hand M65.24-
|lower leg M65.26-
|multiple sites M65.29
|pelvic region M65.25-
|shoulder M75.3-
|specified site NEC M65.28
|thigh M65.25-
|upper arm M65.22-
|due to use, overuse, pressure *see also*
Disorder, soft tissue, due to use
|specified NEC *see* Disorder, soft tissue, due
to use, specified NEC
|gluteal M76.0-
|patellar M76.5-

Tendinitis, tendonitis - *continued*
|peroneal M76.7-
|psoas M76.1-
|tibial (posterior) M76.82-
|anterior M76.81-
|trochanteric *see* Bursitis, hip, trochanteric
Tendon *see* condition
Tendosynovitis *see* Tenosynovitis
Tenesmus (rectal) R19.8
|vesical R30.1
Tennis elbow *see* Epicondylitis, lateral
Tenonitis *see also* Tenosynovitis
|eye (capsule) H05.04-
Tenontosynovitis *see* Tenosynovitis
Tenontothecitis *see* Tenosynovitis
Tenophyte *see* Disorder, synovium, specified
type NEC
Tenosynovitis *see also* Synovitis M65.9
|adhesive *see* Tenosynovitis, specified type
NEC
|shoulder *see* Capsulitis, adhesive
|bicipital (calcifying) *see* Tendinitis, bicipital
|gonococcal A54.49
|in (due to)
|crystals M65.8-
|gonorrhea A54.49
|syphilis (late) A52.78
|use, overuse, pressure *see also* Disorder,
soft tissue, due to use
|specified NEC *see* Disorder, soft tissue,
due to use, specified NEC
|infective NEC M65.1-
|ankle M65.17-
|foot M65.17-
|forearm M65.13-
|hand M65.14-
|lower leg M65.16-
|multiple sites M65.19
|pelvic region M65.15-
|shoulder region M65.11-
|specified site NEC M65.18
|thigh M65.15-
|upper arm M65.12-
|radial styloid M65.4
|shoulder region M65.81-
|adhesive *see* Capsulitis, adhesive
|specified type NEC M65.88
|ankle M65.87-
|foot M65.87-
|forearm M65.83-
|hand M65.84-
|lower leg M65.86-
|multiple sites M65.89
|pelvic region M65.85-
|shoulder region M65.81-
|specified site NEC M65.88
|thigh M65.85-
|upper arm M65.82-
|tuberculous *see* Tuberculosis, tenosynovitis
Tenovaginitis *see* Tenosynovitis
Tension
|arterial, high *see also* Hypertension
|without diagnosis of hypertension R03.0
|headache G44.209
|intractable G44.201
|not intractable G44.209
|nervous R45.0
|pneumothorax J93.0
|premenstrual N94.3
|state (mental) F48.9
Tentorium *see* condition
Teratencephalus Q89.8
Teratism Q89.7

Teratoblastoma (malignant) *see* Neoplasm,
malignant, by site
Teratocarcinoma *see also* Neoplasm,
malignant, by site
|liver C22.7
Teratoma (solid) *see also* Neoplasm, uncertain
behavior, by site
|with embryonal carcinoma, mixed *see*
Neoplasm, malignant, by site
|with malignant transformation *see* Neoplasm,
malignant, by site
|adult (cystic) *see* Neoplasm, benign, by site
|benign *see* Neoplasm, benign, by site
|combined with choriocarcinoma *see*
Neoplasm, malignant, by site
|cystic (adult) *see* Neoplasm, benign, by site
|differentiated *see* Neoplasm, benign, by site
|embryonal *see also* Neoplasm, malignant, by
site
|liver C22.7
|immature *see* Neoplasm, malignant, by site
|liver C22.7
|adult, benign, cystic, differentiated type or
mature D13.4
|malignant *see also* Neoplasm, malignant, by
site
|anaplastic *see* Neoplasm, malignant, by site
|intermediate *see* Neoplasm, malignant, by
site
|specified site *see* Neoplasm, malignant, by
site
|unspecified site C62.90
|undifferentiated *see* Neoplasm, malignant,
by site
|mature *see* Neoplasm, uncertain behavior, by
site
|malignant *see* Neoplasm, by site, malignant,
by site
|ovary D27.-
|embryonal, immature or malignant C56-
|solid *see* Neoplasm, uncertain behavior, by
site
|testis C62.9-
|adult, benign, cystic, differentiated type or
mature D29.2-
|scrotal C62.1-
|undescended C62.0-
Termination
|anomalous *see also* Malposition, congenital
|right pulmonary vein Q26.3
|pregnancy, elective Z33.2
Ternidens diminutus infestation B81.8
Ternidensiasis B81.8
Terror(s) night (child) F51.4
Terrorism, victim of Z65.4
Terry's syndrome (see also Myopia,
degenerative) H44.2-
Tertiary *see* condition
Test, tests, testing (for)
|adequacy (for dialysis)
|hemodialysis Z49.31
|peritoneal Z49.32
|blood pressure Z01.30
|abnormal reading *see* Blood, pressure
|blood-alcohol Z04.83
|positive *see* Findings, abnormal, in blood
|blood-Drug Z04.83
|positive *see* Findings, abnormal, in blood
|blood typing Z01.83
|Rh typing Z01.83
|cardiac pulse generator (battery) Z45.010
|fertility Z31.41
|genetic
|disease carrier status for procreative
management

Test, tests, testing - *continued*

|female Z31.430
|male Z31.440
|male partner of patient with recurrent
  pregnancy loss Z31.441
|procreative management NEC
  |female Z31.438
  |male Z31.448
|hearing Z01.10
|infant or child (over 28 days old) Z00.129
  |with abnormal findings Z00.121
|with abnormal findings NEC Z01.118
|HIV (human immunodeficiency virus)
  |nonconclusive (in infants) R75
  |positive Z21
  |seropositive Z21
|immunity status Z01.84
|intelligence NEC Z01.89
|laboratory (as part of a general medical
  examination) Z00.00
  |with abnormal finding Z00.01
  |for medicolegal reason NEC Z04.89
|male partner of patient with recurrent
  pregnancy loss Z31.441
|Mantoux (for tuberculosis) Z11.1
  |abnormal result R76.11
|pregnancy, positive first pregnancy *see*
  Pregnancy, normal, first
|procreative Z31.49
  |fertility Z31.41
|skin, diagnostic
  |allergy Z01.82
    |special screening examination *see*
      Screening, by name of disease
    |Mantoux Z11.1
    |tuberculin Z11.1
|specified NEC Z01.89
|tuberculin Z11.1
  |abnormal result R76.11
|vision Z01.00
  |infant or child (over 28 days old) Z00.129
    |with abnormal findings Z00.121
  |with abnormal findings Z01.01
|Wassermann Z11.3
  |positive *see* Serology for syphilis, positive
Testicle, testicular, testis *see also* condition
|feminization syndrome *see also* Syndrome,
  androgen insensitivity E34.51
|migrans Q55.29
Tetanus, tetanic (cephalic) (convulsions) A35
|with
  |abortion A34
  |ectopic or molar pregnancy O08.0
|following ectopic or molar pregnancy O08.0
|inoculation reaction (due to serum) *see*
  Complications, vaccination
|neonatorum A33
|obstetrical A34
|puerperal, postpartum, childbirth A34
Tetany (due to) R29.0
|alkalosis E87.3
|associated with rickets E55.0
|convulsions R29.0
  |hysterical F44.5
|functional (hysterical) F44.5
|hyperkinetic R29.0
  |hysterical F44.5
  |hyperpnea R06.4
  |hysterical F44.5
  |psychogenic F45.8
|hyperventilation *see also* Hyperventilation
  R06.4
  |hysterical F44.5
|neonatal (without calcium or magnesium
  deficiency) P71.3

Tetany - *continued*
|parathyroid (gland) E20.9
|parathyroprival E89.2
|post-(para) thyroidectomy E89.2
|postoperative E89.2
|pseudotetany R29.0
|psychogenic (conversion reaction) F44.5
Tetralogy of Fallot Q21.3
Tetraplegia (chronic) *see also* Quadriplegia
  G82.50
Thailand hemorrhagic fever A91
Thalassanemia *see* Thalassemia
Thalassemia (anemia) (disease) D56.9
|with other hemoglobinopathy D56.8
|alpha (major) (severe) (triple gene defect)
  D56.0
  |minor D56.3
  |silent carrier D56.3
  |trait D56.3
|beta (severe) D56.1
  |homozygous D56.1
  |major D56.1
  |minor D56.3
  |trait D56.3
|delta-beta (homozygous) D56.2
  |minor D56.3
  |trait D56.3
|dominant D56.8
|hemoglobin
  |C D56.8
  |E-beta D56.5
|intermedia D56.1
|major D56.1
|minor D56.3
|mixed D56.8
|sickle-cell *see* Disease, sickle-cell,
  thalassemia
|specified type NEC D56.8
|trait D56.3
|variants D56.8
Thanatophoric dwarfism or short stature
  Q77.1
Thaysen-Gee disease (nontropical sprue)
  K90.0
Thaysen's disease K90.0
Thecoma D27-
|luteinized D27-
|malignant C56-
Thelarche, premature E30.8
Thelaziasis B83.8
Thelitis N61.0
|puerperal, postpartum or gestational *see*
  Infection, nipple
Therapeutic *see* condition
Therapy
|drug, long-term (current) (prophylactic)
  |agents affecting estrogen receptors and
    estrogen levels NEC Z79.818
  |anastrozole (Arimidex) Z79.811
  |antibiotics Z79.2
    |short-term use |omit code
  |anticoagulants Z79.01
  |anti-inflammatory Z79.1
  |antiplatelet Z79.02
  |antithrombotics Z79.02
  |aromatase inhibitors Z79.811
  |aspirin Z79.82
  |birth control pill or patch Z79.3
  |bisphosphonates Z79.83
  |contraceptive, oral Z79.3
  |drug, specified NEC Z79.899
  |estrogen receptor downregulators Z79.818
  |Evista Z79.810
  |exemestane (Aromasin) Z79.811
  |Fareston Z79.810

Therapy - *continued*
|fulvestrant (Faslodex) Z79.818
|gonadotropin-releasing hormone (GnRH)
  agonist Z79.818
|goserelin acetate (Zoladex) Z79.818
|hormone replacement Z79.890
|insulin Z79.4
|letrozole (Femara) Z79.811
|leuprolide acetate (leuprorelin) (Lupron)
  Z79.818
|megestrol acetate (Megace) Z79.818
|methadone
  |for pain management Z79.891
  |maintenance therapy F11.20
|Nolvadex Z79.810
|opiate analgesic Z79.891
|oral contraceptive Z79.3
|raloxifene (Evista) Z79.810
|selective estrogen receptor modulators
  (SERMs) Z79.810
|short term
|omit code
|steroids
  |inhaled Z79.51
  |systemic Z79.52
|tamoxifen (Nolvadex) Z79.810
|toremifene (Fareston) Z79.810
Thermic *see* condition
Thermography (abnormal) *see also* Abnormal,
  diagnostic imaging R93.89
|breast R92.8
Thermoplegia T67.0
Thesaurismosis, glycogen *see* Disease,
  glycogen storage
Thiamin deficiency E51.9
|specified NEC E51.8
Thiaminic deficiency with beriberi E51.11
Thibierge-Weissenbach syndrome *see*
  Sclerosis, systemic
Thickening
|bone *see* Hypertrophy, bone
|breast N64.59
|endometrium R93.89
|epidermal L85.9
  |specified NEC L85.8
|hymen N89.6
|larynx J38.7
|nail L60.2
  |congenital Q84.5
|periosteal *see* Hypertrophy, bone
|pleura J92.9
  |with asbestos J92.0
|skin R23.4
|subepiglottic J38.7
|tongue K14.8
|valve, heart *see* Endocarditis
Thigh *see* condition
Thinning vertebra *see* Spondylopathy,
  specified NEC
Thirst, excessive R63.1
|due to deprivation of water T73.1
Thomsen disease G71.12
Thoracic *see also* condition
|kidney Q63.2
|outlet syndrome G54.0
Thoracogastroschisis (congenital) Q79.8
Thoracopagus Q89.4
Thorax *see* condition
Thorn's syndrome N28.89
Thorson-Björck syndrome E34.0
Threadworm (infection) (infestation) B80
Threatened
|abortion O20.0
  |with subsequent abortion O03.9
|job loss, anxiety concerning Z56.2
|labor (without delivery) O47.9

Threatened - *continued*
- at or after 37 completed weeks of gestation O47.1
- before 37 completed weeks of gestation O47.0-
- loss of job, anxiety concerning Z56.2
- miscarriage O20.0
- unemployment, anxiety concerning Z56.2

Three-Day fever A93.1

Threshers' lung J67.0

Thrix annulata (congenital) Q84.1

Throat *see* condition

Thrombasthenia (Glanzmann) (hemorrhagic) (hereditary) D69.1

Thromboangiitis I73.1
- obliterans (general) I73.1
  - cerebral I67.89
  - vessels
    - brain I67.89
    - spinal cord I67.89

Thromboarteritis *see* Arteritis

Thromboasthenia (Glanzmann) (hemorrhagic) (hereditary) D69.1

Thrombocytasthenia (Glanzmann) D69.1

Thrombocythemia (hemorrhagic) (see also Thrombocytosis) D75.839
- essential D47.3
- idiopathic D47.3
- primary D47.3

Thrombocytopathy (dystrophic) (granulopenic) D69.1

Thrombocytopenia, thrombocytopenic D69.6
- with absent radius (TAR) Q87.2
- congenital D69.42
- dilutional D69.59
- due to
  - drugs D69.59
  - extracorporeal circulation of blood D69.59
  - (massive) blood transfusion D69.59
  - platelet alloimmunization D69.59
- essential D69.3
- heparin induced (HIT) D75.82
- hereditary D69.42
- idiopathic D69.3
- neonatal, transitory P61.0
  - due to
    - exchange transfusion P61.0
    - idiopathic maternal thrombocytopenia P61.0
    - isoimmunization P61.0
- primary NEC D69.49
  - idiopathic D69.3
- puerperal, postpartum O72.3
- secondary D69.59
- transient neonatal P61.0

Thrombocytosis D75.839
- essential D47.3
- idiopathic D47.3
- primary D47.3
- reactive D75.838
- secondary D75.838
- specified NEC D75.838

Thromboembolism *see* Embolism

Thrombopathy (Bernard-Soulier) D69.1
- constitutional D68.0
- Willebrand-Jurgens D68.0

Thrombopenia *see* Thrombocytopenia

Thrombophilia D68.59
- primary NEC D68.59
- secondary NEC D68.69
- specified NEC D68.69

Thrombophlebitis I80.9
- antepartum O22.2-
  - deep O22.3-
  - superficial O22.2-

Thrombophlebitis - *continued*
- cavernous (venous) sinus G08
  - complicating pregnancy O22.5-
  - nonpyogenic I67.6
- cerebral (sinus) (vein) G08
  - nonpyogenic I67.6
  - sequelae G09
- due to implanted device *see* Complications, by site and type, specified NEC
- during or resulting from a procedure NEC T81.72
- femoral vein (superficial) I80.1-
- femoropopliteal vein I80.0-
- hepatic (vein) I80.8
- idiopathic, recurrent I82.1
- iliofemoral I80.1-
- intracranial venous sinus (any) G08
  - nonpyogenic I67.6
  - sequelae G09
- intraspinal venous sinuses and veins G08
  - nonpyogenic G95.19
- lateral (venous) sinus G08
  - nonpyogenic I67.6
- leg I80.3
  - superficial I80.0-
- longitudinal (venous) sinus G08
  - nonpyogenic I67.6
- lower extremity I80.299
- migrans, migrating I82.1
- pelvic
  - with ectopic or molar pregnancy O08.0
  - following ectopic or molar pregnancy O08.0
  - puerperal O87.1
- popliteal vein *see* Phlebitis, leg, deep, popliteal
- portal (vein) K75.1
- postoperative T81.72
- pregnancy *see* Thrombophlebitis, antepartum
- puerperal, postpartum, childbirth O87.0
  - deep O87.1
  - pelvic O87.1
  - septic O86.81
  - superficial O87.0
- saphenous (greater) (lesser) I80.0-
- sinus (intracranial) G08
  - nonpyogenic I67.6
- specified site NEC I80.8
- tibial vein I80.23-

Thrombosis, thrombotic (bland) (multiple) (progressive) (silent) (vessel) I82.90
- anal K64.5
- antepartum *see* Thrombophlebitis, antepartum
- aorta, aortic I74.10
  - abdominal I74.09
    - saddle I74.01
  - bifurcation I74.09
  - saddle I74.01
  - specified site NEC I74.19
  - terminal I74.09
  - thoracic I74.11
  - valve *see* Endocarditis, aortic
- apoplexy I63.3-
- artery, arteries (postinfectional) I74.9
  - auditory, internal *see* Occlusion, artery, precerebral, specified NEC
  - basilar *see* Occlusion, artery, basilar
  - carotid (common) (internal) *see* Occlusion, artery, carotid
  - cerebellar (anterior inferior) (posterior inferior) (superior) *see* Occlusion, artery, cerebellar
  - cerebral *see* Occlusion, artery, cerebral
  - choroidal (anterior) *see* Occlusion, artery, precerebral, specified NEC

Thrombosis, thrombotic - *continued*
- communicating, posterior *see* Occlusion, artery, precerebral, specified NEC
- coronary *see also* Infarct, myocardium
  - not resulting in infarction I24.0
- hepatic I74.8
- hypophyseal *see* Occlusion, artery, precerebral, specified NEC
- iliac I74.5
- limb I74.4
  - lower I74.3
  - upper I74.2
- meningeal, anterior or posterior *see* Occlusion, artery, cerebral, specified NEC
- mesenteric (with gangrene) *see also* Infarct, intestine K55.069
- ophthalmic *see* Occlusion, artery, retina
- pontine *see* Occlusion, artery, precerebral, specified NEC
- precerebral *see* Occlusion, artery, precerebral
- pulmonary (iatrogenic) *see* Embolism, pulmonary
- renal N28.0
- retinal *see* Occlusion, artery, retina
- spinal, anterior or posterior G95.11
- traumatic NEC T14.8
- vertebral *see* Occlusion, artery, vertebral
- atrium, auricular *see also* Infarct, myocardium
  - following acute myocardial infarction (current complication) I23.6
  - not resulting in infarction I51.3
  - old I51.3
- basilar (artery) *see* Occlusion, artery, basilar
- brain (artery) (stem) *see also* Occlusion, artery, cerebral
  - due to syphilis A52.05
  - puerperal O99.43
  - sinus *see* Thrombosis, intracranial venous sinus
- capillary I78.8
- cardiac *see also* Infarct, myocardium
  - not resulting in infarction I51.3
  - old I51.3
  - valve *see* Endocarditis
- carotid (artery) (common) (internal) *see* Occlusion, artery, carotid
- cavernous (venous) sinus *see* Thrombosis, intracranial venous sinus
- cerebellar artery (anterior inferior) (posterior inferior) (superior) I66.3
- cerebral (artery) *see* Occlusion, artery, cerebral
- cerebrovenous sinus *see also* Thrombosis, intracranial venous sinus
  - puerperium O87.3
- chronic I82.91
- coronary (artery) (vein) *see also* Infarct, myocardium
  - not resulting in infarction I24.0
- corpus cavernosum N48.89
- cortical I66.9
- deep *see* Embolism, vein, lower extremity
- due to device, implant or graft *see also* Complications, by site and type, specified NEC T85.868
  - arterial graft NEC T82.868
  - breast (implant) T85.868
  - catheter NEC T85.868
    - dialysis (renal) T82.868
      - intraperitoneal T85.868
    - infusion NEC T82.868
      - spinal (epidural) (subdural) T85.860
    - urinary (indwelling) T83.86

Thrombosis, thrombotic - *continued*
|electronic (electrode) (pulse generator)
(stimulator)
|bone T84.86
|cardiac T82.867
|nervous system (brain) (peripheral nerve)
(spinal) T85.860
|urinary T83.86
|fixation, internal (orthopedic) NEC T84.86
|gastrointestinal (bile duct) (esophagus)
T85.868
|genital NEC T83.86
|heart T82.867
|joint prosthesis T84.86
|ocular (corneal graft) (orbital implant) NEC
T85.868
|orthopedic NEC T84.86
|specified NEC T85.868
|urinary NEC T83.86
|vascular NEC T82.868
|ventricular intracranial shunt T85.860
|during the puerperium *see* Thrombosis,
puerperal
|endocardial *see also* Infarct, myocardium
|not resulting in infarction I51.3
|eye *see* Occlusion, retina
|genital organ
|female NEC N94.89
|pregnancy *see* Thrombophlebitis,
antepartum
|male N50.1
|gestational *see* Phlebopathy, gestational
|heart (chamber) *see also* Infarct, myocardium
|not resulting in infarction I51.3
|old I51.3
|hepatic (vein) I82.0
|artery I74.8
|history (of) Z86.718
|intestine (with gangrene) *see also* Infarct,
intestine K55.069
|intracardiac NEC (apical) (atrial) (auricular)
(ventricular) (old) I51.3
|intracranial (arterial) I66.9
|venous sinus (any) G08
|nonpyogenic origin I67.6
|puerperium O87.3
|intramural *see also* Infarct, myocardium
|not resulting in infarction I51.3
|old I51.3
|intraspinal venous sinuses and veins G08
|nonpyogenic G95.19
|kidney (artery) N28.0
|lateral (venous) sinus *see* Thrombosis,
intracranial venous sinus
|leg *see* Thrombosis, vein, lower extremity
|arterial I74.3
|liver (venous) I82.0
|artery I74.8
|portal vein I81
|longitudinal (venous) sinus *see* Thrombosis,
intracranial venous sinus
|lower limb *see* Thrombosis, vein, lower
extremity
|lung (iatrogenic) (postoperative) *see*
Embolism, pulmonary
|meninges (brain) (arterial) I66.8
|mesenteric (artery) (with gangrene) *see also*
Infarct, intestine K55.069
|vein (inferior) (superior) K55.0-
|mitral I34.8
|mural *see also* Infarct, myocardium
|due to syphilis A52.06
|not resulting in infarction I51.3
|old I51.3

Thrombosis, thrombotic - *continued*
|omentum (with gangrene) *see also* Infarct,
intestine K55.069
|ophthalmic *see* Occlusion, retina
|pampiniform plexus (male) N50.1
|parietal *see also* Infarct, myocardium
|not resulting in infarction I24.0
|penis, superficial vein N48.81
|perianal venous K64.5
|peripheral arteries I74.4
|upper I74.2
|personal history (of) Z86.718
|portal I81
|due to syphilis A52.09
|precerebral artery *see* Occlusion, artery,
precerebral
|puerperal, postpartum O87.0
|brain (artery) O99.43
|venous (sinus) O87.3
|cardiac O99.43
|cerebral (artery) O99.43
|venous (sinus) O87.3
|superficial O87.0
|pulmonary (artery) (iatrogenic)
(postoperative) (vein) *see* Embolism,
pulmonary
|renal (artery) N28.0
|vein I82.3
|resulting from presence of device, implant or
graft *see* Complications, by site and type,
specified NEC
|retina, retinal *see* Occlusion, retina
|scrotum N50.1
|seminal vesicle N50.1
|sigmoid (venous) sinus *see* Thrombosis,
intracranial venous sinus
|sinus, intracranial (any) *see* Thrombosis,
intracranial venous sinus
|specified site NEC I82.890
|chronic I82.891
|spermatic cord N50.1
|spinal cord (arterial) G95.11
|due to syphilis A52.09
|pyogenic origin G06.1
|spleen, splenic D73.5
|artery I74.8
|testis N50.1
|tumor *see* Neoplasm, unspecified behavior, by
site
|traumatic NEC T14.8
|tricuspid I07.8
|tunica vaginalis N50.1
|umbilical cord (vessels), complicating
delivery O69.5
|vas deferens N50.1
|vein (acute) I82.90
|antecubital I82.61-
|chronic I82.71-
|axillary I82.A1-
|chronic I82.A2-
|basilic I82.61-
|chronic I82.71-
|brachial I82.62-
|chronic I82.72-
|brachiocephalic (innominate) I82.290
|chronic I82.291
|cerebral, nonpyogenic I67.6
|cephalic I82.61-
|chronic I82.71-
|chronic I82.91
|deep (DVT) I82.40-
|calf I82.4Z-
|chronic I82.5Z-
|lower leg I82.4Z-
|chronic I82.5Z-

Thrombosis, thrombotic - *continued*
|thigh I82.4Y-
|chronic I82.5Y-
|upper leg I82.4Y-
|chronic I82.5Y-
|femoral I82.41-
|chronic I82.51-
|iliac (iliofemoral) I82.42-
|chronic I82.52-
|innominate I82.290
|chronic I82.291
|internal jugular I82.C1-
|chronic I82.C2-
|lower extremity
|deep I82.40-
|chronic I82.50-
|specified NEC I82.49-
|chronic NEC I82.59-
|distal
|deep I82.4Z-
|proximal
|deep I82.4Y-
|chronic I82.5Y-
|superficial I82.81-
|perianal K64.5
|popliteal I82.43-
|chronic I82.53-
|radial I82.62-
|chronic I82.72-
|renal I82.3
|saphenous (greater) (lesser) I82.81-
|specified NEC I82.890
|chronic NEC I82.891
|subclavian I82.B1-
|chronic I82.B2-
|thoracic NEC I82.290
|chronic I82.291
|tibial I82.44-
|chronic I82.54-
|ulnar I82.62-
|chronic I82.72-
|upper extremity I82.60-
|chronic I82.70-
|deep I82.62-
|chronic I82.72-
|superficial I82.61-
|chronic I82.71-
|vena cava
|inferior I82.220
|chronic I82.221
|superior I82.210
|chronic I82.211
|venous, perianal K64.5
|ventricle *see also* Infarct, myocardium
|following acute myocardial infarction
(current complication) I23.6
|not resulting in infarction I24.0
|old I51.3
Thrombus *see* Thrombosis
Thrush *see also* Candidiasis
|oral B37.0
|newborn P37.5
|vaginal B37.3
Thumb *see also* condition
|sucking (child problem) F98.8
Thymitis E32.8
Thymoma *see also* Neoplasm, thymus, by type
|malignant C37
|metaplastic C37
|microscopic D15.0
|sclerosing C37
|type A C37
|type AB C37
|type B1 C37
|type B2 C37
|type B3 C37

Thymus, thymic (gland) *see* condition
Thyrocele *see* Goiter
Thyroglossal *see also* condition
　|cyst Q89.2
　|duct, persistent Q89.2
Thyroid (gland) (body) *see also* condition
　|hormone resistance E07.89
　|lingual Q89.2
　|nodule (cystic) (nontoxic) (single) E04.1
Thyroiditis E06.9
　|acute (nonsuppurative) (pyogenic)
　　(suppurative) E06.0
　|autoimmune E06.3
　|chronic (nonspecific) (sclerosing) E06.5
　　|with thyrotoxicosis, transient E06.2
　　|fibrous E06.5
　　|lymphadenoid E06.3
　　|lymphocytic E06.3
　　|lymphoid E06.3
　|de Quervain's E06.1
　|drug-induced E06.4
　|fibrous (chronic) E06.5
　|giant-cell (follicular) E06.1
　|granulomatous (de Quervain) (subacute)
　　E06.1
　|Hashimoto's (struma lymphomatosa) E06.3
　|iatrogenic E06.4
　|ligneous E06.5
　|lymphocytic (chronic) E06.3
　|lymphoid E06.3
　|lymphomatous E06.3
　|nonsuppurative E06.1
　|postpartum, puerperal O90.5
　|pseudotuberculous E06.1
　|pyogenic E06.0
　|radiation E06.4
　|Riedel's E06.5
　|subacute (granulomatous) E06.1
　|suppurative E06.0
　|tuberculous A18.81
　|viral E06.1
　|woody E06.5
Thyrolingual duct, persistent Q89.2
Thyromegaly E01.0
Thyrotoxic
　|crisis *see* Thyrotoxicosis
　|heart disease or failure *see also*
　　Thyrotoxicosis E05.90 [*I43*]
　　with thyroid storm E05.91 [*I43*]
　|storm *see* Thyrotoxicosis
Thyrotoxicosis (recurrent) E05.90
　|with
　　|goiter (diffuse) E05.00
　　　|with thyroid storm E05.01
　　　|adenomatous uninodular E05.10
　　　　|with thyroid storm E05.11
　　　|multinodular E05.20
　　　　|with thyroid storm E05.21
　　　|nodular E05.20
　　　　|with thyroid storm E05.21
　　　|uninodular E05.10
　　　　|with thyroid storm E05.11
　　|infiltrative
　　　|dermopathy E05.00
　　　　|with thyroid storm E05.01
　　　|ophthalmopathy E05.00
　　　　|with thyroid storm E05.01
　　|single thyroid nodule E05.10
　　　|with thyroid storm E05.11
　　|thyroid storm E05.91
　|due to
　　|ectopic thyroid nodule or tissue E05.30
　　　|with thyroid storm E05.31
　　|ingestion of (excessive) thyroid material
　　　E05.40

Thyrotoxicosis - *continued*
　　|with thyroid storm E05.41
　　|overproduction of thyroid-stimulating
　　　hormone E05.80
　　　|with thyroid storm E05.81
　　|specified cause NEC E05.80
　　　|with thyroid storm E05.81
　|factitia E05.40
　　|with thyroid storm E05.41
　|heart (*see also* Failure, heart, high-output)
　　E05.90 [*I43*]
　　|with thyroid storm (*see also* Failure, heart,
　　　high-output) E05.91 [*I43*]
　　|failure (*see also* Failure, heart, high-
　　　output) E05.90 [*I43*]
　|neonatal (transient) P72.1
　|transient with chronic thyroiditis E06.2
Tibia vara M92.51-
Tic (disorder) F95.9
　|breathing F95.8
　|child problem F95.0
　|compulsive F95.1
　|de la Tourette F95.2
　|degenerative (generalized) (localized) G25.69
　　|facial G25.69
　|disorder
　　|chronic
　　　|motor F95.1
　　　|vocal F95.1
　　|combined vocal and multiple motor F95.2
　　|transient F95.0
　|douloureux G50.0
　　|atypical G50.1
　　|postherpetic, postzoster B02.22
　|drug-induced G25.61
　|eyelid F95.8
　|habit F95.9
　　|chronic F95.1
　　|transient of childhood F95.0
　|lid, transient of childhood F95.0
　|motor-verbal F95.2
　|occupational F48.8
　|orbicularis F95.8
　　|transient of childhood F95.0
　|organic origin G25.69
　|postchoreic G25.69
　|provisional F95.0
　|psychogenic, compulsive F95.1
　|salaam R25.8
　|spasm (motor or vocal) F95.9
　　|chronic F95.1
　　|transient of childhood F95.0
　|specified NEC F95.8
Tick-Borne *see* condition
Tietze's disease or syndrome M94.0
Tight, tightness
　|anus K62.89
　|chest R07.89
　|fascia (lata) M62.89
　|foreskin (congenital) N47.1
　|hymen, hymenal ring N89.6
　|introitus (acquired) (congenital) N89.6
　|rectal sphincter K62.89
　|tendon *see* Short, tendon
　|urethral sphincter N35.919
Tilting vertebra *see* Dorsopathy, deforming,
　specified NEC
Timidity, child F93.8
Tin-Miner's lung J63.5
Tinea (intersecta) (tarsi) B35.9
　|amiantacea L44.8
　|asbestina B35.0
　|barbae B35.0
　|beard B35.0
　|black dot B35.0

Tinea - *continued*
　|blanca B36.2
　|capitis B35.0
　|corporis B35.4
　|cruris B35.6
　|flava B36.0
　|foot B35.3
　|furfuracea B36.0
　|imbricata (Tokelau) B35.5
　|kerion B35.0
　|manuum B35.2
　|microsporic *see* Dermatophytosis
　|nigra B36.1
　|nodosa *see* Piedra
　|pedis B35.3
　|scalp B35.0
　|specified NEC B35.8
　|sycosis B35.0
　|tonsurans B35.0
　|trichophytic *see* Dermatophytosis
　|unguium B35.1
　|versicolor B36.0
Tingling sensation (skin) R20.2
Tinnitus NOS H93.1-
　|audible H93.1-
　|aurium H93.1-
　|pulsatile H93.A-
　|subjective H93.1-
Tipped tooth (teeth) M26.33
Tipping
　|pelvis M95.5
　　|with disproportion (fetopelvic) O33.0
　　　|causing obstructed labor O65.0
　|tooth (teeth), fully erupted M26.33
Tiredness R53.83
Tissue *see* condition
Tobacco (nicotine)
　|abuse *see* Tobacco, use
　|dependence *see* Dependence, drug, nicotine
　|harmful use Z72.0
　|heart *see* Tobacco, toxic effect
　|maternal use, affecting newborn P04.2
　|toxic effect *see* Table of Drugs and
　　Chemicals, by substance, poisoning
　　|chewing tobacco *see* Table of Drugs and
　　　Chemicals, by substance, poisoning
　　|cigarettes *see* Table of Drugs and
　　　Chemicals, by substance, poisoning
　|use Z72.0
　　|complicating
　　　|childbirth O99.334
　　　|pregnancy O99.33-
　　　|puerperium O99.335
　　|counseling and surveillance Z71.6
　　|history Z87.891
　|withdrawal state *see also* Dependence, drug,
　　nicotine F17.203
Tocopherol deficiency E56.0
Todd's
　|cirrhosis K74.3
　|paralysis (postepileptic) (transitory) G83.84
Toe *see* condition
Toilet, artificial opening *see* Attention to,
　artificial, opening
Tokelau (ringworm) B35.5
Tollwut *see* Rabies
Tommaselli's disease R31.9
　|correct substance properly administered *see*
　　Table of Drugs and Chemicals, by drug,
　　adverse effect
　|overdose or wrong substance given or taken
　　see Table of Drugs and Chemicals, by
　　drug, poisoning
Tongue *see also* condition
　|tie Q38.1

Tonic pupil *see* Anomaly, pupil, function, tonic
pupil
Toni-Fanconi syndrome (cystinosis) E72.09
|with cystinosis E72.04
Tonsil *see* condition
Tonsillitis (acute) (catarrhal) (croupous)
(follicular) (gangrenous) (infective)
(lacunar) (lingual) (malignant)
(membranous) (parenchymatous)
(phlegmonous) (pseudomembranous)
(purulent) (septic) (subacute) (suppurative)
(toxic) (ulcerative) (vesicular) (viral) J03.90
|chronic J35.01
|with adenoiditis J35.03
|diphtheritic A36.0
|hypertrophic J35.01
|with adenoiditis J35.03
|recurrent J03.91
|specified organism NEC J03.80
|recurrent J03.81
|staphylococcal J03.80
|recurrent J03.81
|streptococcal J03.00
|recurrent J03.01
|tuberculous A15.8
|Vincent's A69.1
Tooth, teeth *see* condition
Toothache K08.89
Topagnosis R20.8
Tophi *see* Gout, chronic
TORCH infection *see* Infection, congenital
|without active infection P00.2
Torn *see* Tear
Tornwaldt's cyst or disease J39.2
Torsion
|accessory tube *see* Torsion, fallopian tube
|adnexa (female) *see* Torsion, fallopian tube
|aorta, acquired I77.1
|appendix epididymis N44.04
|appendix testis N44.03
|bile duct (common) (hepatic) K83.8
|congenital Q44.5
|bowel, colon or intestine K56.2
|cervix *see* Malposition, uterus
|cystic duct K82.8
|dystonia *see* Dystonia, torsion
|epididymis (appendix) N44.04
|fallopian tube N83.52-
|with ovary N83.53
|gallbladder K82.8
|congenital Q44.1
|hydatid of Morgagni
|female N83.52-
|male N44.03
|kidney (pedicle) (leading to infarction) N28.0
|Meckel's diverticulum (congenital) Q43.0
|malignant *see* Table of Neoplasms, small
intestine, malignant
|mesentery K56.2
|omentum K56.2
|organ or site, congenital NEC *see* Anomaly,
by site
|ovary (pedicle) N83.51-
|with fallopian tube N83.53
|congenital Q50.2
|oviduct *see* Torsion, fallopian tube
|penis (acquired) N48.82
|congenital Q55.63
|spasm *see* Dystonia, torsion
|spermatic cord N44.02
|extravaginal N44.01
|intravaginal N44.02
|spleen D73.5
|testis, testicle N44.00
|appendix N44.03

Torsion - *continued*
|tibia *see* Deformity, limb, specified type NEC,
lower leg
|uterus *see* Malposition, uterus
Torticollis (intermittent) (spastic) M43.6
|congenital (sternomastoid) Q68.0
|due to birth injury P15.8
|hysterical F44.4
|ocular R29.891
|psychogenic F45.8
|conversion reaction F44.4
|rheumatic M43.6
|rheumatoid M06.88
|spasmodic G24.3
|traumatic, current S13.4
Tortipelvis G24.1
Tortuous
|aortic arch Q25.46
|artery I77.1
|organ or site, congenital NEC *see* Distortion
|retinal vessel, congenital Q14.1
|ureter N13.8
|urethra N36.8
|vein *see* Varix
Torture, victim of Z65.4
Torula, torular (histolytica) (infection) *see*
Cryptococcosis
Torulosis *see* Cryptococcosis
Torus (mandibularis) (palatinus) M27.0
|fracture *see* Fracture, by site, torus
Touraine's syndrome Q79.8
Tourette's syndrome F95.2
Tourniquet syndrome *see* Constriction,
external, by site
Tower skull Q75.0
|with exophthalmos Q87.0
Toxemia R68.89
|bacterial *see* Sepsis
|burn *see* Burn
|eclamptic (with pre-existing hypertension) *see*
Eclampsia
|erysipelatous *see* Erysipelas
|fatigue R68.89
|food *see* Poisoning, food
|gastrointestinal K52.1
|intestinal K52.1
|kidney *see* Uremia
|malarial *see* Malaria
|myocardial *see* Myocarditis, toxic
|of pregnancy *see* Pre-eclampsia
|pre-eclamptic *see* Pre-eclampsia
|small intestine K52.1
|staphylococcal, due to food A05.0
|stasis R68.89
|uremic *see* Uremia
|urinary *see* Uremia
Toxemica cerebropathia psychica
(nonalcoholic) F04
|alcoholic *see* Alcohol, amnestic disorder
Toxic (poisoning) *see also* condition T65.91
|effect *see* Table of Drugs and Chemicals, by
substance, poisoning
|shock syndrome A48.3
|thyroid (gland) *see* Thyrotoxicosis
Toxicemia *see* Toxemia
Toxicity *see* Table of Drugs and Chemicals, by
substance, poisoning
|fava bean D55.0
|food, noxious *see* Poisoning, food
|from drug or nonmedicinal substance *see*
Table of Drugs and Chemicals, by drug
Toxicosis *see also* Toxemia
|capillary, hemorrhagic D69.0
Toxinfection, gastrointestinal K52.1
Toxocariasis B83.0

Toxoplasma, toxoplasmosis (acquired) B58.9
|with
|hepatitis B58.1
|meningoencephalitis B58.2
|ocular involvement B58.00
|other organ involvement B58.89
|pneumonia, pneumonitis B58.3
|congenital (acute) (subacute) (chronic) P37.1
|maternal, manifest toxoplasmosis in infant
(acute) (subacute) (chronic) P37.1
tPA (rtPA) administration in a different
facility within the last 24 hours prior to
admission to current facility Z92.82
Trabeculation, bladder N32.89
Trachea *see* condition
Tracheitis (catarrhal) (infantile)
(membranous) (plastic) (septal)
(suppurative) (viral) J04.10
|with
|bronchitis (15 years of age and above) J40
|acute or subacute *see* Bronchitis, acute
|chronic J42
|tuberculous NEC A15.5
|under 15 years of age J20.9
|laryngitis (acute) J04.2
|chronic J37.1
|tuberculous NEC A15.5
|acute J04.10
|with obstruction J04.11
|chronic J42
|with
|bronchitis (chronic) J42
|laryngitis (chronic) J37.1
|diphtheritic (membranous) A36.89
|due to external agent *see* Inflammation,
respiratory, upper, due to
|syphilitic A52.73
|tuberculous A15.5
Trachelitis (nonvenereal) *see* Cervicitis
Tracheobronchial *see* condition
Tracheobronchitis (15 years of age and above)
see also Bronchitis
|due to
|Bordetella bronchiseptica A37.80
|with pneumonia A37.81
|Francisella tularensis A21.8
Tracheobronchomegaly Q32.4
|with bronchiectasis J47.9
|with
|exacerbation (acute) J47.1
|lower respiratory infection J47.0
|acquired J98.09
|with bronchiectasis J47.9
|with
|exacerbation (acute) J47.1
|lower respiratory infection J47.0
Tracheobronchopneumonitis *see* Pneumonia,
broncho-
Tracheocele (external) (internal) J39.8
|congenital Q32.1
Tracheomalacia J39.8
|congenital Q32.0
Tracheopharyngitis (acute) J06.9
|chronic J42
|due to external agent *see* Inflammation,
respiratory, upper, due to
Tracheostenosis J39.8
Tracheostomy
|complication *see* Complication, tracheostomy
|status Z93.0
|attention to Z43.0
|malfunctioning J95.03
Trachoma, trachomatous A71.9
|active (stage) A71.1
|contraction of conjunctiva A71.1
|dubium A71.0
|initial (stage) A71.0
|healed or sequelae B94.0

Trachoma - *continued*
|pannus A71.1
|Türck's J37.0
Traction, vitreomacular H43.82-
Train sickness T75.3
Trait(s)
|Hb-S D57.3
|hemoglobin
|abnormal NEC D58.2
|with thalassemia D56.3
|C *see* Disease, hemoglobin C
|S (Hb-S) D57.3
|Lepore D56.3
|personality, accentuated Z73.1
|sickle-cell D57.3
|with elliptocytosis or spherocytosis D57.3
|type A personality Z73.1
Tramp Z59.00
Trance R41.89
|hysterical F44.89
Transection
|abdomen (partial) S38.3
|aorta (incomplete) *see also* Injury, aorta
|complete *see* Injury, aorta, laceration, major
|carotid artery (incomplete) *see also* Injury,
blood vessel, carotid, laceration
|complete *see* Injury, blood vessel, carotid,
laceration, major
|celiac artery (incomplete) S35.211
|branch (incomplete) S35.291
|complete S35.292
|complete S35.212
|innominate
|artery (incomplete) *see also* Injury, blood
vessel, thoracic, innominate, artery,
laceration
|complete *see* Injury, blood vessel,
thoracic, innominate, artery, laceration,
major
|vein (incomplete) *see also* Injury, blood
vessel, thoracic, innominate, vein, laceration
|complete *see* Injury, blood vessel,
thoracic, innominate, vein, laceration, major
|jugular vein (external) (incomplete) *see also*
Injury, blood vessel, jugular vein,
laceration
|complete *see* Injury, blood vessel, jugular
vein, laceration, major
|internal (incomplete) *see also* Injury, blood
vessel, jugular vein, internal, laceration
|complete *see* Injury, blood vessel, jugular
vein, internal, laceration, major
|mesenteric artery (incomplete) *see also* Injury,
mesenteric, artery, laceration
|complete *see* Injury, mesenteric artery,
laceration, major
|pulmonary vessel (incomplete) *see also*
Injury, blood vessel, thoracic, pulmonary,
laceration
|complete *see* Injury, blood vessel, thoracic,
pulmonary, laceration, major
|subclavian *see* Transection, innominate
|vena cava (incomplete) *see also* Injury, vena
cava
|complete *see* Injury, vena cava, laceration,
major
|vertebral artery (incomplete) *see also* Injury,
blood vessel, vertebral, laceration
|complete *see* Injury, blood vessel, vertebral,
laceration, major
Transaminasemia R74.01
Transfusion
|associated (red blood cell) hemochromatosis
E83.111
|blood

Transfusion - *continued*
|ABO incompatible *see* Complication(s),
transfusion, incompatibility reaction,
ABO
|minor blood group (Duffy) (E) (K) (Kell)
(Kidd) (Lewis) (M) (N) (P) (S) T80.89
|reaction or complication *see* Complications,
transfusion
|fetomaternal (mother) *see* Pregnancy,
complicated by, placenta, transfusion
syndrome
|maternofetal (mother) *see* Pregnancy,
complicated by, placenta, transfusion
syndrome
|placental (syndrome) (mother) *see* Pregnancy,
complicated by, placenta, transfusion
syndrome
|reaction (adverse) *see* Complications,
transfusion
|related acute lung injury (TRALI) J95.84
|twin-to-twin *see* Pregnancy, complicated by,
placenta, transfusion syndrome, fetus to
fetus
Transient (meaning homeless) *see also*
condition Z59.00
Translocation
|balanced autosomal Q95.9
|in normal individual Q95.0
|chromosomes NEC Q99.8
|balanced and insertion in normal individual
Q95.0
|Down syndrome Q90.2
|trisomy
|13 Q91.6
|18 Q91.2
|21 Q90.2
Translucency, iris *see* Degeneration, iris
**Transmission of chemical substances through
the placenta *see*** Absorption, chemical,
through placenta
Transparency, lung, unilateral J43.0
Transplant (ed) (status) Z94.9
|awaiting organ Z76.82
|bone Z94.6
|marrow Z94.81
|candidate Z76.82
|complication *see* Complication, transplant
|cornea Z94.7
|heart Z94.1
|and lung(s) Z94.3
|valve Z95.2
|prosthetic Z95.2
|specified NEC Z95.4
|xenogenic Z95.3
|intestine Z94.82
|kidney Z94.0
|liver Z94.4
|lung(s) Z94.2
|and heart Z94.3
|organ (failure) (infection) (rejection) Z94.9
|removal status Z98.85
|pancreas Z94.83
|skin Z94.5
|social Z60.3
|specified organ or tissue NEC Z94.89
|stem cells Z94.84
|tissue Z94.9
Transplants, ovarian, endometrial N80.1
Transposed *see* Transposition
Transposition (congenital) *see also*
Malposition, congenital
|abdominal viscera Q89.3
|aorta (dextra) Q20.3
|appendix Q43.8

Transposition - *continued*
|colon Q43.8
|corrected Q20.5
|great vessels (complete) (partial) Q20.3
|heart Q24.0
|with complete transposition of viscera
Q89.3
|intestine (large) (small) Q43.8
|reversed jejunal (for bypass) (status) Z98.0
|scrotum Q55.23
|stomach Q40.2
|with general transposition of viscera Q89.3
|tooth, teeth, fully erupted M26.30
|vessels, great (complete) (partial) Q20.3
|viscera (abdominal) (thoracic) Q89.3
Transsexualism F64.0
Transverse *see also* condition
|arrest (deep), in labor O64.0
|lie (mother) O32.2
|causing obstructed labor O64.8
Transvestism, transvestitism (dual-Role)
F64.1
|fetishistic F65.1
Trapped placenta (with hemorrhage) O72.0
|without hemorrhage O73.0
**TRAPS (tumor necrosis factor receptor
associated periodic syndrome)** M04.1
Trauma, traumatism *see also* Injury
|acoustic *see* subcategory H83.3
|birth *see* Birth, injury
|complicating ectopic or molar pregnancy
O08.6
|during delivery O71.9
|following ectopic or molar pregnancy O08.6
|obstetric O71.9
|specified NEC O71.89
|occlusal
|primary K08.81
|secondary K08.82
Traumatic *see also* condition
|brain injury S06.9
Treacher Collins syndrome Q75.4
Treitz's hernia *see* Hernia, abdomen, specified
site NEC
Trematode infestation *see* Infestation, fluke
Trematodiasis *see* Infestation, fluke
Trembling paralysis *see* Parkinsonism
Tremor(s) R25.1
|drug induced G25.1
|essential (benign) G25.0
|familial G25.0
|hereditary G25.0
|hysterical F44.4
|intention G25.2
|medication induced postural G25.1
|mercurial *see* subcategory T56.1
|Parkinson's *see* Parkinsonism
|psychogenic (conversion reaction) F44.4
|senilis R54
|specified type NEC G25.2
Trench
|fever A79.0
|foot *see* Immersion, foot
|mouth A69.1
Treponema pallidum infection *see* Syphilis
Treponematosis
|due to
|T. pallidum *see* Syphilis
|T. pertenue *see* Yaws
Triad
|Hutchinson's (congenital syphilis) A50.53
|Kartagener's Q89.3
|Saint's *see* Hernia, diaphragm

Trichiasis (eyelid) H02.059
 |with entropion *see* Entropion
 |left H02.056
  |lower H02.055
  |upper H02.054
 |right H02.053
  |lower H02.052
  |upper H02.051
Trichinella spiralis (infection) (infestation) B75
Trichinellosis, trichiniasis, trichinelliasis, trichinosis B75
 |with muscle disorder B75 *[M63.80]*
  |ankle B75 *[M63.87]*
  |foot B75 *[M63.87]*
  |forearm B75 *[M63.83]*
  |hand B75 *[M63.84]*
  |lower leg B75 *[M63.86]*
  |multiple sites B75 *[M63.89]*
  |pelvic region B75 *[M63.85]*
  |shoulder region B75 *[M63.81]*
  |specified site NEC B75 *[M63.88]*
  |thigh B75 *[M63.85]*
  |upper arm B75 *[M63.82]*
Trichobezoar T18.9
 |intestine T18.3
 |stomach T18.2
Trichocephaliasis, trichocephalosis B79
Trichocephalus infestation B79
Trichoclasis L67.8
Trichoepithelioma *see also* Neoplasm, skin, benign
 |malignant *see* Neoplasm, skin, malignant
Trichofolliculoma *see* Neoplasm, skin, benign
Tricholemmoma *see* Neoplasm, skin, benign
Trichomoniasis A59.9
 |bladder A59.03
 |cervix A59.09
 |intestinal A07.8
 |prostate A59.02
 |seminal vesicles A59.09
 |specified site NEC A59.8
 |urethra A59.03
 |urogenitalis A59.00
 |vagina A59.01
 |vulva A59.01
Trichomycosis
 |axillaris A48.8
 |nodosa, nodularis B36.8
Trichonodosis L67.8
Trichophytid, trichophyton infection *see* Dermatophytosis
Trichophytobezoar T18.9
 |intestine T18.3
 |stomach T18.2
Trichophytosis *see* Dermatophytosis
Trichoptilosis L67.8
Trichorrhexis (nodosa) (invaginata) L67.0
Trichosis axillaris A48.8
Trichosporosis nodosa B36.2
Trichostasis spinulosa (congenital) Q84.1
Trichostrongyliasis, trichostrongylosis (small intestine) B81.2
Trichostrongylus infection B81.2
Trichotillomania F63.3
Trichromat, trichromatopsia, anomalous (congenital) H53.55
Trichuriasis B79
Trichuris trichiura (infection) (infestation) (any site) B79
Tricuspid (valve) *see* condition
Trifid *see also* Accessory
 |kidney (pelvis) Q63.8
 |tongue Q38.3
Trigeminal neuralgia *see* Neuralgia, trigeminal

Trigeminy R00.8
Trigger finger (acquired) M65.30
 |congenital Q74.0
 |index finger M65.32-
 |little finger M65.35-
 |middle finger M65.33-
 |ring finger M65.34-
 |thumb M65.31-
Trigonitis (bladder) (chronic) (pseudomembranous) N30.30
 |with hematuria N30.31
Trigonocephaly Q75.0
Trilocular heart *see* Cor triloculare
Trimethylaminuria E72.52
Tripartite placenta O43.19-
Triphalangeal thumb Q74.0
Triple *see also* Accessory
 |kidneys Q63.0
 |uteri Q51.818
 |X, female Q97.0
Triple I O41.12-
Triplegia G83.89
 |congenital G80.8
Triplet (newborn) *see also* Newborn, triplet
 |complicating pregnancy *see* Pregnancy, triplet
Triplication *see* Accessory
Triploidy Q92.7
Trismus R25.2
 |neonatorum A33
 |newborn A33
Trisomy (syndrome) Q92.9
 |autosomes Q92.9
 |chromosome specified NEC Q92.8
  |partial Q92.2
   |due to unbalanced translocation Q92.5
  |whole (nonsex chromosome)
   |meiotic nondisjunction Q92.0
   |mitotic nondisjunction Q92.1
   |mosaicism Q92.1
  |specified NEC Q92.8
 |due to
  |dicentrics *see* Extra, marker chromosomes
  |extra rings *see* Extra, marker chromosomes
  |isochromosomes *see* Extra, marker chromosomes
 |specified NEC Q92.8
 |whole chromosome Q92.9
  |meiotic nondisjunction Q92.0
  |mitotic nondisjunction Q92.1
  |mosaicism Q92.1
  |partial Q92.9
  |specified NEC Q92.8
 |13 (partial) Q91.7
  |meiotic nondisjunction Q91.4
  |mitotic nondisjunction Q91.5
  |mosaicism Q91.5
  |translocation Q91.6
 |18 (partial) Q91.3
  |meiotic nondisjunction Q91.0
  |mitotic nondisjunction Q91.1
  |mosaicism Q91.1
  |translocation Q91.2
 |20 Q92.8
 |21 (partial) Q90.9
  |meiotic nondisjunction Q90.0
  |mitotic nondisjunction Q90.1
  |mosaicism Q90.1
  |translocation Q90.2
 |22 Q92.8
Tritanomaly, tritanopia H53.55
Trombiculosis, trombiculiasis, trombidiosis B88.0
Trophedema (congenital) (hereditary) Q82.0
Trophoblastic disease *see also* Mole, hydatidiform O01.9

Tropholymphedema Q82.0
Trophoneurosis NEC G96.89
 |disseminated M34.9
Tropical *see* condition
Trouble *see also* Disease
 |heart *see* Disease, heart
 |kidney *see* Disease, renal
 |nervous R45.0
 |sinus *see* Sinusitis
Trousseau's syndrome (thrombophlebitis migrans) I82.1
Truancy, childhood
 |from school Z72.810
Truncus
 |arteriosus (persistent) Q20.0
 |communis Q20.0
Trunk *see* condition
Trypanosomiasis
 |African B56.9
  |by Trypanosoma brucei
   |gambiense B56.0
   |rhodesiense B56.1
 |American *see* Chagas' disease
 |Brazilian *see* Chagas' disease
 |by Trypanosoma
  |brucei gambiense B56.0
  |brucei rhodesiense B56.1
  |cruzi *see* Chagas' disease
 |gambiensis, Gambian B56.0
 |rhodesiensis, Rhodesian B56.1
 |South American *see* Chagas' disease
 |where
  |African trypanosomiasis is prevalent B56.9
  |Chagas' disease is prevalent B57.2
Tryptasemia, hereditary alpha D89.44
T-Shaped incisors K00.2
Tsutsugamushi (disease) (fever) A75.3
Tube, tubal, tubular *see* condition
Tubercle *see also* Tuberculosis
 |brain, solitary A17.81
 |Darwin's Q17.8
 |Ghon, primary infection A15.7
Tuberculid, tuberculide (indurating, subcutaneous) (lichenoid) (miliary) (papulonecrotic) (primary) (skin) A18.4
Tuberculoma *see also* Tuberculosis
 |brain A17.81
 |meninges (cerebral) (spinal) A17.1
 |spinal cord A17.81
Tuberculosis, tubercular, tuberculous (calcification) (calcified) (caseous) (chromogenic acid-Fast bacilli) (degeneration) (fibrocaseous) (fistula) (interstitial) (isolated circumscribed lesions) (necrosis) (parenchymatous) (ulcerative) A15.9
 |with pneumoconiosis (any condition in J60-J64) J65
 |abdomen (lymph gland) A18.39
 |abscess (respiratory) A15.9
  |bone A18.03
   |hip A18.02
   |knee A18.02
   |sacrum A18.01
   |specified site NEC A18.03
   |spinal A18.01
   |vertebra A18.01
  |brain A17.81
  |breast A18.89
  |Cowper's gland A18.15
  |dura (mater) (cerebral) (spinal) A17.81
  |epidural (cerebral) (spinal) A17.81
  |female pelvis A18.17
  |frontal sinus A15.8

Tuberculosis - *continued*
- |genital organs NEC A18.10
- |genitourinary A18.10
- |gland (lymphatic) *see* Tuberculosis, lymph gland
- |hip A18.02
- |intestine A18.32
- |ischiorectal A18.32
- |joint NEC A18.02
  - |hip A18.02
  - |knee A18.02
  - |specified NEC A18.02
  - |vertebral A18.01
- |kidney A18.11
- |knee A18.02
- |latent R76.11
- |lumbar (spine) A18.01
- |lung *see* Tuberculosis, pulmonary
- |meninges (cerebral) (spinal) A17.0
- |muscle A18.09
- |perianal (fistula) A18.32
- |perinephritic A18.11
- |perirectal A18.32
- |rectum A18.32
- |retropharyngeal A15.8
- |sacrum A18.01
- |scrofulous A18.2
- |scrotum A18.15
- |skin (primary) A18.4
- |spinal cord A17.81
- |spine or vertebra (column) A18.01
- |subdiaphragmatic A18.31
- |testis A18.15
- |urinary A18.13
- |uterus A18.17
- |accessory sinus *see* Tuberculosis, sinus
- |Addison's disease A18.7
- |adenitis *see* Tuberculosis, lymph gland
- |adenoids A15.8
- |adenopathy *see* Tuberculosis, lymph gland
- |adherent pericardium A18.84
- |adnexa (uteri) A18.17
- |adrenal (capsule) (gland) A18.7
- |alimentary canal A18.32
- |anemia A18.89
- |ankle (joint) (bone) A18.02
- |anus A18.32
- |apex, apical *see* Tuberculosis, pulmonary
- |appendicitis, appendix A18.32
- |arachnoid A17.0
- |artery, arteritis A18.89
  - |cerebral A18.89
- |arthritis (chronic) (synovial) A18.02
  - |spine or vertebra (column) A18.01
- |articular *see* Tuberculosis, joint
- |ascites A18.31
- |asthma *see* Tuberculosis, pulmonary
- |axilla, axillary (gland) A18.2
- |bladder A18.12
- |bone A18.03
  - |hip A18.02
  - |knee A18.02
  - |limb NEC A18.03
  - |sacrum A18.01
  - |spine or vertebral column A18.01
- |bowel (miliary) A18.32
- |brain A17.81
- |breast A18.89
- |broad ligament A18.17
- |bronchi, bronchial, bronchus A15.5
  - |ectasia, ectasis (bronchiectasis) *see* Tuberculosis, pulmonary
  - |fistula A15.5
    - |primary (progressive) A15.7
  - |gland or node A15.4

Tuberculosis - *continued*
- |primary (progressive) A15.7
- |lymph gland or node A15.4
  - |primary (progressive) A15.7
- |bronchiectasis *see* Tuberculosis, pulmonary
- |bronchitis A15.5
- |bronchopleural A15.6
- |bronchopneumonia, bronchopneumonic *see* Tuberculosis, pulmonary
- |bronchorrhagia A15.5
- |bronchotracheal A15.5
- |bronze disease A18.7
- |buccal cavity A18.83
- |bulbourethral gland A18.15
- |bursa A18.09
- |cachexia A15.9
- |cardiomyopathy A18.84
- |caries *see* Tuberculosis, bone
- |cartilage A18.02
  - |intervertebral A18.01
- |catarrhal *see* Tuberculosis, respiratory
- |cecum A18.32
- |cellulitis (primary) A18.4
- |cerebellum A17.81
- |cerebral, cerebrum A17.81
- |cerebrospinal A17.81
  - |meninges A17.0
- |cervical (lymph gland or node) A18.2
- |cervicitis, cervix (uteri) A18.16
- |chest *see* Tuberculosis, respiratory
- |chorioretinitis A18.53
- |choroid, choroiditis A18.53
- |ciliary body A18.54
- |colitis A18.32
- |collier's J65
- |colliquativa (primary) A18.4
- |colon A18.32
- |complex, primary A15.7
- |congenital P37.0
- |conjunctiva A18.59
- |connective tissue (systemic) A18.89
- |contact Z20.1
- |cornea (ulcer) A18.52
- |Cowper's gland A18.15
- |coxae A18.02
- |coxalgia A18.02
- |cul-de-sac of Douglas A18.17
- |curvature, spine A18.01
- |cutis (colliquativa) (primary) A18.4
- |cyst, ovary A18.18
- |cystitis A18.12
- |dactylitis A18.03
- |diarrhea A18.32
- |diffuse *see* Tuberculosis, miliary
- |digestive tract A18.32
- |disseminated *see* Tuberculosis, miliary
- |duodenum A18.32
- |dura (mater) (cerebral) (spinal) A17.0
  - |abscess (cerebral) (spinal) A17.81
- |dysentery A18.32
- |ear (inner) (middle) A18.6
  - |bone A18.03
  - |external (primary) A18.4
  - |skin (primary) A18.4
- |elbow A18.02
- |emphysema *see* Tuberculosis, pulmonary
- |empyema A15.6
- |encephalitis A17.82
- |endarteritis A18.89
- |endocarditis A18.84
  - |aortic A18.84
  - |mitral A18.84
  - |pulmonary A18.84
  - |tricuspid A18.84
- |endocrine glands NEC A18.82

Tuberculosis - *continued*
- |endometrium A18.17
- |enteric, enterica, enteritis A18.32
- |enterocolitis A18.32
- |epididymis, epididymitis A18.15
- |epidural abscess (cerebral) (spinal) A17.81
- |epiglottis A15.5
- |episcleritis A18.51
- |erythema (induratum) (nodosum) (primary) A18.4
- |esophagus A18.83
- |eustachian tube A18.6
- |exposure (to) Z20.1
- |exudative *see* Tuberculosis, pulmonary
- |eye A18.50
- |eyelid (primary) (lupus) A18.4
- |fallopian tube (acute) (chronic) A18.17
- |fascia A18.09
- |fauces A15.8
- |female pelvic inflammatory disease A18.17
- |finger A18.03
- |first infection A15.7
- |gallbladder A18.83
- |ganglion A18.09
- |gastritis A18.83
- |gastrocolic fistula A18.32
- |gastroenteritis A18.32
- |gastrointestinal tract A18.32
- |general, generalized *see* Tuberculosis, miliary
- |genital organs A18.10
- |genitourinary A18.10
- |genu A18.02
- |glandula suprarenalis A18.7
- |glandular, general A18.2
- |glottis A15.5
- |grinder's J65
- |gum A18.83
- |hand A18.03
- |heart A18.84
- |hematogenous *see* Tuberculosis, miliary
- |hemoptysis *see* Tuberculosis, pulmonary
- |hemorrhage NEC *see* Tuberculosis, pulmonary
- |hemothorax A15.6
- |hepatitis A18.83
- |hilar lymph nodes A15.4
  - |primary (progressive) A15.7
- |hip (joint) (disease) (bone) A18.02
- |hydropneumothorax A15.6
- |hydrothorax A15.6
- |hypoadrenalism A18.7
- |hypopharynx A15.8
- |ileocecal (hyperplastic) A18.32
- |ileocolitis A18.32
- |ileum A18.32
- |iliac spine (superior) A18.03
- |immunological findings only A15.7
- |indurativa (primary) A18.4
- |infantile A15.7
- |infection A15.9
  - |without clinical manifestations A15.7
- |infraclavicular gland A18.2
- |inguinal gland A18.2
- |inguinalis A18.2
- |intestine (any part) A18.32
- |iridocyclitis A18.54
- |iris, iritis A18.54
- |ischiorectal A18.32
- |jaw A18.03
- |jejunum A18.32
- |joint A18.02
  - |vertebral A18.01
- |keratitis (interstitial) A18.52
- |keratoconjunctivitis A18.52
- |kidney A18.11

Tuberculosis - *continued*

|knee (joint) A18.02
|kyphosis, kyphoscoliosis A18.01
|laryngitis A15.5
|larynx A15.5
|latent R76.11
|leptomeninges, leptomeningitis (cerebral)
    (spinal) A17.0
|lichenoides (primary) A18.4
|linguae A18.83
|lip A18.83
|liver A18.83
|lordosis A18.01
|lung *see* Tuberculosis, pulmonary
|lupus vulgaris A18.4
|lymph gland or node (peripheral) A18.2
    |abdomen A18.39
    |bronchial A15.4
        |primary (progressive) A15.7
    |cervical A18.2
    |hilar A15.4
        |primary (progressive) A15.7
    |intrathoracic A15.4
        |primary (progressive) A15.7
    |mediastinal A15.4
        |primary (progressive) A15.7
    |mesenteric A18.39
    |retroperitoneal A18.39
    |tracheobronchial A15.4
        |primary (progressive) A15.7
|lymphadenitis *see* Tuberculosis, lymph gland
|lymphangitis *see* Tuberculosis, lymph gland
|lymphatic (gland) (vessel) *see* Tuberculosis,
    lymph gland
|mammary gland A18.89
|marasmus A15.9
|mastoiditis A18.03
|mediastinal lymph gland or node A15.4
    |primary (progressive) A15.7
|mediastinitis A15.8
    |primary (progressive) A15.7
|mediastinum A15.8
    |primary (progressive) A15.7
|medulla A17.81
|melanosis, Addisonian A18.7
|meninges, meningitis (basilar) (cerebral)
    (cerebrospinal) (spinal) A17.0
|meningoencephalitis A17.82
|mesentery, mesenteric (gland or node) A18.39
|miliary A19.9
    |acute A19.2
        |multiple sites A19.1
        |single specified site A19.0
    |chronic A19.8
    |specified NEC A19.8
|millstone makers' J65
|miner's J65
|molder's J65
|mouth A18.83
|multiple A19.9
    |acute A19.1
    |chronic A19.8
|muscle A18.09
|myelitis A17.82
|myocardium, myocarditis A18.84
|nasal (passage) (sinus) A15.8
|nasopharynx A15.8
|neck gland A18.2
|nephritis A18.11
|nerve (mononeuropathy) A17.83
|nervous system A17.9
|nose (septum) A15.8
|ocular A18.50
|omentum A18.31
|oophoritis (acute) (chronic) A18.17

Tuberculosis - *continued*

|optic (nerve trunk) (papilla) A18.59
|orbit A18.59
|orchitis A18.15
|organ, specified NEC A18.89
|osseous *see* Tuberculosis, bone
|osteitis *see* Tuberculosis, bone
|osteomyelitis *see* Tuberculosis, bone
|otitis media A18.6
|ovary, ovaritis (acute) (chronic) A18.17
|oviduct (acute) (chronic) A18.17
|pachymeningitis A17.0
|palate (soft) A18.83
|pancreas A18.83
|papulonecrotic (a) (primary) A18.4
|parathyroid glands A18.82
|paronychia (primary) A18.4
|parotid gland or region A18.83
|pelvis (bony) A18.03
|penis A18.15
|peribronchitis A15.5
|pericardium, pericarditis A18.84
|perichondritis, larynx A15.5
|periostitis *see* Tuberculosis, bone
|perirectal fistula A18.32
|peritoneum NEC A18.31
|peritonitis A18.31
|pharynx, pharyngitis A15.8
|phlyctenulosis (keratoconjunctivitis) A18.52
|phthisis NEC *see* Tuberculosis, pulmonary
|pituitary gland A18.82
|pleura, pleural, pleurisy, pleuritis (fibrinous)
    (obliterative) (purulent) (simple plastic)
    (with effusion) A15.6
    |primary (progressive) A15.7
|pneumonia, pneumonic *see* Tuberculosis,
    pulmonary
|pneumothorax (spontaneous) (tense valvular)
    see Tuberculosis, pulmonary
|polyneuropathy A17.89
|polyserositis A19.9
    |acute A19.1
    |chronic A19.8
|potter's J65
|prepuce A18.15
|primary (complex) A15.7
|proctitis A18.32
|prostate, prostatitis A18.14
|pulmonalis *see* Tuberculosis, pulmonary
|pulmonary (cavitated) (fibrotic) (infiltrative)
    (nodular) A15.0
    |childhood type or first infection A15.7
    |primary (complex) A15.7
|pyelitis A18.11
|pyelonephritis A18.11
|pyemia *see* Tuberculosis, miliary
|pyonephrosis A18.11
|pyopneumothorax A15.6
|pyothorax A15.6
|rectum (fistula) (with abscess) A18.32
|reinfection stage *see* Tuberculosis, pulmonary
|renal A18.11
|renis A18.11
|respiratory A15.9
    |primary A15.7
    |specified site NEC A15.8
|retina, retinitis A18.53
|retroperitoneal (lymph gland or node) A18.39
|rheumatism NEC A18.09
|rhinitis A15.8
|sacroiliac (joint) A18.01
|sacrum A18.01
|salivary gland A18.83
|salpingitis (acute) (chronic) A18.17
|sandblaster's J65

Tuberculosis - *continued*

|sclera A18.51
|scoliosis A18.01
|scrofulous A18.2
|scrotum A18.15
|seminal tract or vesicle A18.15
|senile A15.9
|septic *see* Tuberculosis, miliary
|shoulder (joint) A18.02
    |blade A18.03
|sigmoid A18.32
|sinus (any nasal) A15.8
    |bone A18.03
    |epididymis A18.15
|skeletal NEC A18.03
|skin (any site) (primary) A18.4
|soft palate A18.83
|spermatic cord A18.15
|spine, spinal (column) A18.01
    |cord A17.81
    |medulla A17.81
    |membrane A17.0
    |meninges A17.0
|spleen, splenitis A18.85
|spondylitis A18.01
|sternoclavicular joint A18.02
|stomach A18.83
|stonemason's J65
|subcutaneous tissue (cellular) (primary) A18.4
|subcutis (primary) A18.4
|subdeltoid bursa A18.83
|submaxillary (region) A18.83
|supraclavicular gland A18.2
|suprarenal (capsule) (gland) A18.7
|swelling, joint (*see also* category M01) *see*
    also Tuberculosis, joint A18.02
|symphysis pubis A18.02
|synovitis A18.09
    |articular A18.02
    |spine or vertebra A18.01
|systemic *see* Tuberculosis, miliary
|tarsitis A18.4
|tendon (sheath) *see* Tuberculosis,
    tenosynovitis
|tenosynovitis A18.09
    |spine or vertebra A18.01
|testis A18.15
|throat A15.8
|thymus gland A18.82
|thyroid gland A18.81
|tongue A18.83
|tonsil, tonsillitis A15.8
|trachea, tracheal A15.5
    |lymph gland or node A15.4
        |primary (progressive) A15.7
|tracheobronchial A15.5
    |lymph gland or node A15.4
        |primary (progressive) A15.7
|tubal (acute) (chronic) A18.17
|tunica vaginalis A18.15
|ulcer (skin) (primary) A18.4
    |bowel or intestine A18.32
    |specified NEC code under Tuberculosis, by
        site
|unspecified site A15.9
|ureter A18.11
|urethra, urethral (gland) A18.13
|urinary organ or tract A18.13
|uterus A18.17
|uveal tract A18.54
|uvula A18.83
|vagina A18.18
|vas deferens A18.15
|verruca, verrucosa (cutis) (primary) A18.4
|vertebra (column) A18.01

Tuberculosis - *continued*
|vesiculitis A18.15
|vulva A18.18
|wrist (joint) A18.02
Tuberculum
|Carabelli *see* Note at K00.2
|occlusal *see* Note at K00.2
|paramolare K00.2
Tuberosity, entire maxillary M26.07
Tuberous sclerosis (brain) Q85.1
Tubo-Ovarian *see* condition
Tuboplasty, after previous sterilization Z31.0
|aftercare Z31.42
Tubotympanitis, catarrhal (chronic) *see* Otitis,
media, nonsuppurative, chronic, serous
Tularemia A21.9
|with
|conjunctivitis A21.1
|pneumonia A21.2
|abdominal A21.3
|bronchopneumonic A21.2
|conjunctivitis A21.1
|cryptogenic A21.3
|enteric A21.3
|gastrointestinal A21.3
|generalized A21.7
|ingestion A21.3
|intestinal A21.3
|oculoglandular A21.1
|ophthalmic A21.1
|pneumonia (any), pneumonic A21.2
|pulmonary A21.2
|sepsis A21.7
|specified NEC A21.8
|typhoidal A21.7
|ulceroglandular A21.0
Tularensis conjunctivitis A21.1
Tumefaction *see also* Swelling
|liver *see* Hypertrophy, liver
Tumor *see also* Neoplasm, unspecified
behavior, by site
|acinar cell *see* Neoplasm, uncertain behavior,
by site
|acinic cell *see* Neoplasm, uncertain behavior,
by site
|adenocarcinoid *see* Neoplasm, malignant, by
site
|adenomatoid *see also* Neoplasm, benign, by
site
|odontogenic *see* Cyst, calcifying
odontogenic
|adnexal (skin) *see* Neoplasm, skin, benign, by
site
|adrenal
|cortical (benign) D35.0-
|malignant C74.0-
|rest *see* Neoplasm, benign, by site
|alpha-cell
|malignant
|pancreas C25.4
|specified site NEC *see* Neoplasm,
malignant, by site
|unspecified site C25.4
|pancreas D13.7
|specified site NEC *see* Neoplasm, benign,
by site
|unspecified site D13.7
|aneurysmal *see* Aneurysm
|aortic body D44.7
|malignant C75.5
|Askin's *see* Neoplasm, connective tissue,
malignant
|basal cell *see also* Neoplasm, skin, uncertain
behavior D48.5
|Bednar *see* Neoplasm, skin, malignant

Tumor - *continued*
|benign (unclassified) *see* Neoplasm, benign,
by site
|beta-cell
|malignant
|pancreas C25.4
|specified site NEC *see* Neoplasm,
malignant, by site
|unspecified site C25.4
|pancreas D13.7
|specified site NEC *see* Neoplasm, benign,
by site
|unspecified site D13.7
|Brenner D27.9
|borderline malignancy D39.1-
|malignant C56-
|proliferating D39.1-
|bronchial alveolar, intravascular D38.1
|Brooke's *see* Neoplasm, skin, benign
|brown fat *see* Lipoma
|Burkitt *see* Lymphoma, Burkitt
|calcifying epithelial odontogenic *see* Cyst,
calcifying odontogenic
|carcinoid D3A.00
|benign D3A.00
|appendix D3A.020
|ascending colon D3A.022
|bronchus (lung) D3A.090
|cecum D3A.021
|colon D3A.029
|descending colon D3A.024
|duodenum D3A.010
|foregut NOS D3A.094
|hindgut NOS D3A.096
|ileum D3A.012
|jejunum D3A.011
|kidney D3A.093
|large intestine D3A.029
|lung (bronchus) D3A.090
|midgut NOS D3A.095
|rectum D3A.026
|sigmoid colon D3A.025
|small intestine D3A.019
|specified NEC D3A.098
|stomach D3A.092
|thymus D3A.091
|transverse colon D3A.023
|malignant C7A.00
|appendix C7A.020
|ascending colon C7A.022
|bronchus (lung) C7A.090
|cecum C7A.021
|colon C7A.029
|descending colon C7A.024
|duodenum C7A.010
|foregut NOS C7A.094
|hindgut NOS C7A.096
|ileum C7A.012
|jejunum C7A.011
|kidney C7A.093
|large intestine C7A.029
|lung (bronchus) C7A.090
|midgut NOS C7A.095
|rectum C7A.026
|sigmoid colon C7A.025
|small intestine C7A.019
|specified NEC C7A.098
|stomach C7A.092
|thymus C7A.091
|transverse colon C7A.023
|mesentery metastasis C7B.04
|secondary C7B.00
|bone C7B.03
|distant lymph nodes C7B.01
|liver C7B.02

Tumor - *continued*
|peritoneum C7B.04
|specified NEC C7B.09
|carotid body D44.6
|malignant C75.4
|cells *see also* Neoplasm, unspecified behavior,
by site
|benign *see* Neoplasm, benign, by site
|malignant *see* Neoplasm, malignant, by site
|uncertain whether benign or malignant *see*
Neoplasm, uncertain behavior, by site
|cervix, in pregnancy or childbirth *see*
Pregnancy, complicated by, tumor, cervix
|chondromatous giant cell *see* Neoplasm, bone,
benign
|chromaffin *see also* Neoplasm, benign, by site
|malignant *see* Neoplasm, malignant, by site
|Cock's peculiar L72.3
|Codman's *see* Neoplasm, bone, benign
|dentigerous, mixed *see* Cyst, calcifying
odontogenic
|dermoid *see* Neoplasm, benign, by site
|with malignant transformation C56-
|desmoid (extra-abdominal) *see also*
Neoplasm, connective tissue, uncertain
behavior
|abdominal *see* Neoplasm, connective tissue,
uncertain behavior
|embolus *see* Neoplasm, secondary, by site
|embryonal (mixed) *see also* Neoplasm,
uncertain behavior, by site
|liver C22.7
|endodermal sinus
|specified site *see* Neoplasm, malignant, by
site
|unspecified site
|female C56.-
|male C62.90
|epithelial
|benign *see* Neoplasm, benign, by site
|malignant *see* Neoplasm, malignant, by site
|Ewing's *see* Neoplasm, bone, malignant, by
site
|fatty *see* Lipoma
|fibroid *see* Leiomyoma
|G cell
|malignant
|pancreas C25.4
|specified site NEC *see* Neoplasm,
malignant, by site
|unspecified site C25.4
|specified site *see* Neoplasm, uncertain
behavior, by site
|unspecified site D37.8
|germ cell *see also* Neoplasm, malignant, by
site
|mixed *see* Neoplasm, malignant, by site
|ghost cell, odontogenic *see* Cyst, calcifying
odontogenic
|giant cell *see also* Neoplasm, uncertain
behavior, by site
|bone D48.0
|malignant *see* Neoplasm, bone, malignant
|chondromatous *see* Neoplasm, bone, benign
|malignant *see* Neoplasm, malignant, by site
|soft parts *see* Neoplasm, connective tissue,
uncertain behavior
|malignant *see* Neoplasm, connective
tissue, malignant
|glomus D18.00
|intra-abdominal D18.03
|intracranial D18.02
|jugulare D44.7
|malignant C75.5
|skin D18.01

Tumor - *continued*

|specified site NEC D18.09
|gonadal stromal *see* Neoplasm, uncertain behavior, by site
|granular cell *see also* Neoplasm, connective tissue, benign
|malignant *see* Neoplasm, connective tissue, malignant
|granulosa cell D39.1-
|juvenile D39.1-
|malignant C56-
|granulosa cell-theca cell D39.1-
|malignant C56-
|Grawitz's C64-
|hemorrhoidal *see* Hemorrhoids
|hilar cell D27-
|hilus cell D27-
|Hürthle cell (benign) D34
|malignant C73
|hydatid *see* Echinococcus
|hypernephroid *see also* Neoplasm, uncertain behavior, by site
|interstitial cell *see also* Neoplasm, uncertain behavior, by site
|benign *see* Neoplasm, benign, by site
|malignant *see* Neoplasm, malignant, by site
|intravascular bronchial alveolar D38.1
|islet cell *see* Neoplasm, benign, by site
|malignant *see* Neoplasm, malignant, by site
|pancreas C25.4
|specified site NEC *see* Neoplasm, malignant, by site
|unspecified site C25.4
|pancreas D13.7
|specified site NEC *see* Neoplasm, benign, by site
|unspecified site D13.7
|juxtaglomerular D41.0-
|Klatskin's C24.0
|Krukenberg's C79.6-
|Leydig cell *see* Neoplasm, uncertain behavior, by site
|benign *see* Neoplasm, benign, by site
|specified site *see* Neoplasm, benign, by site
|unspecified site
|female D27.9
|male D29.20
|malignant *see* Neoplasm, malignant, by site
|specified site *see* Neoplasm, malignant, by site
|unspecified site
|female C56.9
|male C62.90
|specified site *see* Neoplasm, uncertain behavior, by site
|unspecified site
|female D39.10
|male D40.10
|lipid cell, ovary D27-
|lipoid cell, ovary D27-
|malignant *see also* Neoplasm, malignant, by site C80.1
|fusiform cell (type) C80.1
|giant cell (type) C80.1
|localized, plasma cell *see* Plasmacytoma, solitary
|mixed NEC C80.1
|small cell (type) C80.1
|spindle cell (type) C80.1
|unclassified C80.1
|mast cell D47.09
|melanotic, neuroectodermal *see* Neoplasm, benign, by site
|Merkel cell *see* Carcinoma, Merkel cell

Tumor - *continued*

|mesenchymal
|malignant *see* Neoplasm, connective tissue, malignant
|mixed *see* Neoplasm, connective tissue, uncertain behavior
|mesodermal, mixed *see also* Neoplasm, malignant, by site
|liver C22.4
|mesonephric *see also* Neoplasm, uncertain behavior, by site
|malignant *see* Neoplasm, malignant, by site
|metastatic
|from specified site *see* Neoplasm, malignant, by site
|of specified site *see* Neoplasm, malignant, by site
|to specified site *see* Neoplasm, secondary, by site
|mixed NEC *see also* Neoplasm, benign, by site
|malignant *see* Neoplasm, malignant, by site
|mucinous of low malignant potential
|specified site *see* Neoplasm, malignant, by site
|unspecified site C56.9
|mucocarcinoid
|specified site *see* Neoplasm, malignant, by site
|unspecified site C18.1
|mucoepidermoid *see* Neoplasm, uncertain behavior, by site
|Müllerian, mixed
|specified site *see* Neoplasm, malignant, by site
|unspecified site C54.9
|myoepithelial *see* Neoplasm, benign, by site
|neuroectodermal (peripheral) *see* Neoplasm, malignant, by site
|primitive
|specified site *see* Neoplasm, malignant, by site
|unspecified site C71.9
|neuroendocrine D3A.8
|malignant poorly differentiated C7A.1
|secondary NEC C7B.8
|specified NEC C7A.8
|neurogenic olfactory C30.0
|nonencapsulated sclerosing C73
|odontogenic (adenomatoid) (benign) (calcifying epithelial) (keratocystic) (squamous) *see* Cyst, calcifying odontogenic
|malignant C41.1
|upper jaw (bone) C41.0
|ovarian stromal D39.1-
|ovary, in pregnancy *see* Pregnancy, complicated by
|pacinian *see* Neoplasm, skin, benign
|Pancoast's *see* Pancoast's syndrome
|papillary *see also* Papilloma
|cystic D37.9
|mucinous of low malignant potential C56-
|specified site *see* Neoplasm, malignant, by site
|unspecified site C56.9
|serous of low malignant potential
|specified site *see* Neoplasm, malignant, by site
|unspecified site C56.9
|pelvic, in pregnancy or childbirth *see* Pregnancy, complicated by
|phantom F45.8
|phyllodes D48.6-
|benign D24-
|malignant *see* Neoplasm, breast, malignant

Tumor - *continued*

|Pindborg *see* Cyst, calcifying odontogenic
|placental site trophoblastic D39.2
|plasma cell (malignant) (localized) *see* Plasmacytoma, solitary
|polyvesicular vitelline
|specified site *see* Neoplasm, malignant, by site
|unspecified site
|female C56.9
|male C62.90
|Pott's puffy *see* Osteomyelitis, specified NEC
|Rathke's pouch D44.3
|retinal anlage *see* Neoplasm, benign, by site
|salivary gland type, mixed *see* Neoplasm, salivary gland, benign
|malignant *see* Neoplasm, salivary gland, malignant
|Sampson's N80.1
|Schmincke's *see* Neoplasm, nasopharynx, malignant
|sclerosing stromal D27-
|sebaceous *see* Cyst, sebaceous
|secondary *see* Neoplasm, secondary, by site
|carcinoid C7B.00
|bone C7B.03
|distant lymph nodes C7B.01
|liver C7B.02
|peritoneum C7B.04
|specified NEC C7B.09
|neuroendocrine NEC C7B.8
|serous of low malignant potential
|specified site *see* Neoplasm, malignant, by site
|unspecified site C56.9
|Sertoli cell *see* Neoplasm, benign, by site
|with lipid storage
|specified site *see* Neoplasm, benign, by site
|unspecified site
|female D27.9
|male D29.20
|specified site *see* Neoplasm, benign, by site
|unspecified site
|female D27.9
|male D29.20
|Sertoli-Leydig cell *see* Neoplasm, benign, by site
|specified site *see* Neoplasm, benign, by site
|unspecified site
|female D27.9
|male D29.20
|sex cord (-Stromal) *see* Neoplasm, uncertain behavior, by site
|with annular tubules D39.1-
|skin appendage *see* Neoplasm, skin, benign
|smooth muscle *see* Neoplasm, connective tissue, uncertain behavior
|soft tissue
|benign *see* Neoplasm, connective tissue, benign
|malignant *see* Neoplasm, connective tissue, malignant
|sternomastoid (congenital) Q68.0
|stromal
|endometrial D39.0
|gastric D48.1
|benign D21.4
|malignant C16.9
|uncertain behavior D48.1
|gastrointestinal C49.A-
|benign D21.4
|esophagus C49.A1
|malignant C49.A0
|colon C49.A4

Tumor - *continued*
|duodenum C49.A3
|esophagus C49.A1
|ileum C49.A3
|jejunum C49.A3
|Meckel diverticulum C49.A3
|large intestine C49.A4
|omentum C49.A9
|peritoneum C49.A9
|rectum C49.A5
|small intestine C49.A3
|specified site NEC C49.A9
|stomach C49.A2
|large intestine C49.A4
|rectum C49.A5
|small intestine C49.A3
|specified site NEC C49.A9
|stomach C49.A2
|uncertain behavior D48.1
|intestine
|benign D21.4
|malignant
|large C49.A4
|small C49.A3
|uncertain behavior D48.1
|ovarian D39.1-
|stomach C49.A2
|benign D21.4
|malignant C49.A2
|uncertain behavior D48.1
|testicular D40.10
|sweat gland *see also* Neoplasm, skin,
uncertain behavior
|benign *see* Neoplasm, skin, benign
|malignant *see* Neoplasm, skin, malignant
|syphilitic, brain A52.17
|testicular stromal D40.1-
|theca cell D27.-
|theca cell-granulosa cell D39.1-
|Triton, malignant *see* Neoplasm, nerve,
malignant
|trophoblastic, placental site D39.2
|turban D23.4
|uterus (body), in pregnancy or childbirth *see*
Pregnancy, complicated by, tumor, uterus
|vagina, in pregnancy or childbirth *see*
Pregnancy, complicated by
|varicose *see* Varix
|von Recklinghausen's *see* Neurofibromatosis
|vulva or perineum, in pregnancy or childbirth
see Pregnancy, complicated by
|causing obstructed labor O65.5
|Warthin's *see* Neoplasm, salivary gland,
benign
|Wilms' C64-
|yolk sac *see* Neoplasm, malignant, by site
|specified site *see* Neoplasm, malignant, by
site
|unspecified site
|female C56.9
|male C62.90
**Tumor lysis syndrome (following
antineoplastic chemotherapy)
(spontaneous) NEC** E88.3
Tumorlet *see* Neoplasm, uncertain behavior, by
site
Tungiasis B88.1
Tunica vasculosa lentis Q12.2
Turban tumor D23.4
Türck's trachoma J37.0
Turner-Kieser syndrome Q87.2
Turner-Like syndrome Q87.1
Turner's
|hypoplasia (tooth) K00.4
|syndrome Q96.9
|specified NEC Q96.8
|tooth K00.4

Turner-Ullrich syndrome Q96.9
Tussis convulsiva *see* Whooping cough
Twiddler's syndrome (due to)
|automatic implantable defibrillator T82.198
|cardiac pacemaker T82.198
Twilight state
|epileptic F05
|psychogenic F44.89
Twin (newborn) *see also* Newborn, twin
|conjoined Q89.4
|pregnancy *see* Pregnancy, twin
Twinning, teeth K00.2
Twist, twisted
|bowel, colon or intestine K56.2
|hair (congenital) Q84.1
|mesentery K56.2
|omentum K56.2
|organ or site, congenital NEC *see* Anomaly,
by site
|ovarian pedicle *see* Torsion, ovary
Twitching R25.3
Tylosis (acquired) L84
|buccalis K13.29
|linguae K13.29
|palmaris et plantaris (congenital) (inherited)
Q82.8
|acquired L85.1
Tympanism R14.0
Tympanites (abdominal) (intestinal) R14.0
Tympanitis *see* Myringitis
Tympanosclerosis *see* subcategory H74.0
Tympanum *see* condition
Tympany
|abdomen R14.0
|chest R09.89
Type A behavior pattern Z73.1
Typhlitis *see* Appendicitis
Typhoenteritis *see* Typhoid
**Typhoid (abortive) (ambulant) (any site)
(clinical) (fever) (hemorrhagic) (infection)
(intermittent) (malignant) (rheumatic)
(Widal negative)** A01.00
|with pneumonia A01.03
|abdominal A01.09
|arthritis A01.04
|carrier (suspected) of Z22.0
|cholecystitis (current) A01.09
|endocarditis A01.02
|heart involvement A01.02
|inoculation reaction *see* Complications,
vaccination
|meningitis A01.01
|mesenteric lymph nodes A01.09
|myocarditis A01.02
|osteomyelitis A01.05
|perichondritis, larynx A01.09
|pneumonia A01.03
|spine A01.05
|specified NEC A01.09
|ulcer (perforating) A01.09
Typhomalaria (fever) *see* Malaria
Typhomania A01.00
Typhoperitonitis A01.09
Typhus (fever) A75.9
|abdominal, abdominalis *see* Typhoid
|African tick A77.1
|amarillic A95.9
|brain A75.9 [G94]
|cerebral A75.9 [G94]
|classical A75.0
|due to Rickettsia
|prowazekii A75.0
|recrudescent A75.1
|tsutsugamushi A75.3
|typhi A75.2

Typhus - *continued*
|endemic (flea-borne) A75.2
|epidemic (louse-borne) A75.0
|exanthematic NEC A75.0
|exanthematicus SAI A75.0
|brillii SAI A75.1
|mexicanus SAI A75.2
|typhus murinus A75.2
|flea-borne A75.2
|India tick A77.1
|Kenya (tick) A77.1
|louse-borne A75.0
|Mexican A75.2
|mite-borne A75.3
|murine A75.2
|North Asian tick-borne A77.2
|Orientia Tsutsugamushi (scrub typhus) A75.3
|petechial A75.9
|Queensland tick A77.3
|rat A75.2
|recrudescent A75.1
|recurrens *see* Fever, relapsing
|Sao Paulo A77.0
|scrub (China) (India) (Malaysia) (New
Guinea) A75.3
|shop (of Malaysia) A75.2
|Siberian tick A77.2
|tick-borne A77.9
|tropical (mite-borne) A75.3
Tyrosinemia E70.21
|newborn, transitory P74.5
Tyrosinosis E70.21
Tyrosinuria E70.29

U

Uhl's anomaly or disease Q24.8
**Ulcer, ulcerated, ulcerating, ulceration,
ulcerative**
|alveolar process M27.3
|amebic (intestine) A06.1
|skin A06.7
|anastomotic *see* Ulcer, gastrojejunal
|anorectal K62.6
|antral *see* Ulcer, stomach
|anus (sphincter) (solitary) K62.6
|aorta *see* Aneurysm
|aphthous (oral) (recurrent) K12.0
|genital organ(s)
|female N76.6
|male N50.89
|artery I77.2
|atrophic *see* Ulcer, skin
|decubitus *see* Ulcer, pressure, by site
|back L98.429
|with
|bone involvement without evidence of
necrosis L98.426
|bone necrosis L98.424
|exposed fat layer L98.422
|muscle involvement without evidence of
necrosis L98.425
|muscle necrosis L98.423
|skin breakdown only L98.421
|specified severity NEC L98.428
|Barrett's (esophagus) K22.10
|with bleeding K22.11
|bile duct (common) (hepatic) K83.8
|bladder (solitary) (sphincter) NEC N32.89
|bilharzial B65.9 [N33]
|in schistosomiasis (bilharzial) B65.9 [N33]
|submucosal *see* Cystitis, interstitial
|tuberculous A18.12
|bleeding K27.4

Ulcer - *continued*

- |bone *see* Osteomyelitis, specified type NEC
- |bowel *see* Ulcer, intestine
- |breast N61.1
- |bronchus J98.09
- |buccal (cavity) (traumatic) K12.1
- |Buruli A31.1
- |buttock L98.419
  - |with
    - |bone involvement without evidence of
      - necrosis L98.416
    - |bone necrosis L98.414
    - |exposed fat layer L98.412
    - |muscle involvement without evidence of
      - necrosis L98.415
    - |muscle necrosis L98.413
    - |skin breakdown only L98.411
    - |specified severity NEC L98.418
- |cancerous *see* Neoplasm, malignant, by site
- |cardia K22.10
  - |with bleeding K22.11
- |cardioesophageal (peptic) K22.10
  - |with bleeding K22.11
- |cecum *see* Ulcer, intestine
- |cervix (uteri) (decubitus) (trophic) N86
  - |with cervicitis N72
- |chancroidal A57
- |chiclero B55.1
- |chronic (cause unknown) *see* Ulcer, skin
- |Cochin-China B55.1
- |colon *see* Ulcer, intestine
- |conjunctiva H10.89
- |cornea H16.00-
  - |with hypopyon H16.03-
  - |central H16.01-
  - |dendritic (herpes simplex) B00.52
  - |marginal H16.04-
  - |Mooren's H16.05-
  - |mycotic H16.06-
  - |perforated H16.07-
  - |ring H16.02-
  - |tuberculous (phlyctenular) A18.52
- |corpus cavernosum (chronic) N48.5
- |crural *see* Ulcer, lower limb
- |Curling's *see* Ulcer, peptic, acute
- |Cushing's *see* Ulcer, peptic, acute
- |cystic duct K82.8
- |cystitis (interstitial) *see* Cystitis, interstitial
- |decubitus *see* Ulcer, pressure, by site
- |dendritic, cornea (herpes simplex) B00.52
- |diabetes, diabetic *see* Diabetes, ulcer
- |Dieulafoy's K25.0
- |due to
  - |infection NEC *see* Ulcer, skin
  - |radiation NEC L59.8
  - |trophic disturbance (any region) *see* Ulcer, skin
  - |X-ray L58.1
- |duodenum, duodenal (eroded) (peptic) K26.9
  - |with
    - |hemorrhage K26.4
      - |and perforation K26.6
    - |perforation K26.5
  - |acute K26.3
    - |with
      - |hemorrhage K26.0
        - |and perforation K26.2
      - |perforation K26.1
  - |chronic K26.7
    - |with
      - |hemorrhage K26.4
        - |and perforation K26.6
      - |perforation K26.5
- |dysenteric A09
- |elusive *see* Cystitis, interstitial

Ulcer - *continued*

- |endocarditis (acute) (chronic) (subacute) I28.8
- |epiglottis J38.7
- |esophagus (peptic) K22.10
  - |with bleeding K22.11
  - |due to
    - |aspirin K22.10
      - |with bleeding K22.11
    - |gastrointestinal reflux disease (without
      - bleeding) K21.00
      - |with bleeding K21.01
    - |ingestion of chemical or medicament
      - K22.10
      - |with bleeding K22.11
  - |fungal K22.10
    - |with bleeding K22.11
  - |infective K22.10
    - |with bleeding K22.11
  - |varicose *see* Varix, esophagus
- |eyelid (region) H01.8
- |fauces J39.2
- |Fenwick (-Hunner) (solitary) *see* Cystitis,
  - interstitial
- |fistulous *see* Ulcer, skin
- |foot (indolent) (trophic) *see* Ulcer, lower limb
- |frambesial, initial A66.0
- |frenum (tongue) K14.0
- |gallbladder or duct K82.8
- |gangrenous *see* Gangrene
- |gastric *see* Ulcer, stomach
- |gastrocolic *see* Ulcer, gastrojejunal
- |gastroduodenal *see* Ulcer, peptic
- |gastroesophageal *see* Ulcer, stomach
- |gastrointestinal *see* Ulcer, gastrojejunal
- |gastrojejunal (peptic) K28.9
  - |with
    - |hemorrhage K28.4
      - |and perforation K28.6
    - |perforation K28.5
  - |acute K28.3
    - |with
      - |hemorrhage K28.0
        - |and perforation K28.2
      - |perforation K28.1
  - |chronic K28.7
    - |with
      - |hemorrhage K28.4
        - |and perforation K28.6
      - |perforation K28.5
- |gastrojejunocolic *see* Ulcer, gastrojejunal
- |gingiva K06.8
- |gingivitis K05.10
  - |nonplaque induced K05.11
  - |plaque induced K05.10
- |glottis J38.7
- |granuloma of pudenda A58
- |gum K06.8
- |gumma, due to yaws A66.4
- |heel *see* Ulcer, lower limb
- |hemorrhoid *see also* Hemorrhoids, by degree
  - K64.8
- |Hunner's *see* Cystitis, interstitial
- |hypopharynx J39.2
- |hypopyon (chronic) (subacute) *see* Ulcer,
  - cornea, with hypopyon
- |hypostaticum *see* Ulcer, varicose
- |ileum *see* Ulcer, intestine
- |intestine, intestinal K63.3
  - |with perforation K63.1
  - |amebic A06.1
  - |duodenal *see* Ulcer, duodenum
  - |granulocytopenic (with hemorrhage) *see*
    - Neutropenia
  - |marginal *see* Ulcer, gastrojejunal
  - |perforating K63.1

Ulcer - *continued*

- |newborn P78.0
- |primary, small intestine K63.3
- |rectum K62.6
- |stercoraceous, stercoral K63.3
- |tuberculous A18.32
- |typhoid (fever) *see* Typhoid
- |varicose I86.8
- |jejunum, jejunal *see* Ulcer, gastrojejunal
- |keratitis *see* Ulcer, cornea
- |knee *see* Ulcer, lower limb
- |labium (majus) (minus) N76.6
- |laryngitis *see* Laryngitis
- |larynx (aphthous) (contact) J38.7
  - |diphtheritic A36.2
- |leg *see* Ulcer, lower limb
- |lip K13.0
- |Lipschütz's N76.6
- |lower limb (atrophic) (chronic) (neurogenic)
  - (perforating) (pyogenic) (trophic) (tropical)
  - L97.909
  - |with
    - |bone involvement without evidence of
      - necrosis L97.906
    - |bone necrosis L97.904
    - |exposed fat layer L97.902
    - |muscle involvement without evidence of
      - necrosis L97.905
    - |muscle necrosis L97.903
    - |skin breakdown only L97.901
    - |specified severity NEC L97.908
    - |with
      - |bone involvement without evidence of
        - necrosis L97.306
      - |bone necrosis L97.304
      - |exposed fat layer L97.302
      - |muscle involvement without evidence
        - of necrosis L97.305
      - |muscle necrosis L97.303
      - |skin breakdown only L97.301
      - |specified severity NEC L97.308
  - |left L97.329
    - |with
      - |bone involvement without evidence of
        - necrosis L97.326
      - |bone necrosis L97.324
      - |exposed fat layer L97.322
      - |muscle involvement without evidence
        - of necrosis L97.325
      - |specified severity NEC L97.328
      - |muscle necrosis L97.323
      - |skin breakdown only L97.321
  - |right L97.319
    - |with
      - |bone involvement without evidence of
        - necrosis L97.316
      - |bone necrosis L97.314
      - |exposed fat layer L97.312
      - |muscle involvement without evidence
        - of necrosis L97.315
      - |muscle necrosis L97.313
      - |skin breakdown only L97.311
      - |specified severity NEC L97.318
- |calf L97.209
  - |with
    - |bone involvement without evidence of
      - necrosis L97.206
    - |bone necrosis L97.204
    - |exposed fat layer L97.202
    - |muscle involvement without evidence
      - of necrosis L97.205
    - |muscle necrosis L97.203
    - |skin breakdown only L97.201
    - |specified severity NEC L97.208
  - |left L97.229

Ulcer - *continued*
|with
|bone involvement without evidence of
necrosis L97.226
|bone necrosis L97.224
|exposed fat layer L97.222
|muscle involvement without evidence
of necrosis L97.225
|muscle necrosis L97.223
|skin breakdown only L97.221
|specified severity NEC L97.228
|right L97.219
|with
|bone involvement without evidence of
necrosis L97.216
|bone necrosis L97.214
|exposed fat layer L97.212
|muscle involvement without evidence
of necrosis L97.215
|muscle necrosis L97.213
|skin breakdown only L97.211
|specified severity NEC L97.218
|decubitus *see* Ulcer, pressure, by site
|foot specified NEC L97.509
|with
|bone involvement without evidence of
necrosis L97.506
|bone necrosis L97.504
|exposed fat layer L97.502
|muscle involvement without evidence
of necrosis L97.505
|muscle necrosis L97.503
|skin breakdown only L97.501
|specified severity NEC L97.508
|left L97.529
|with
|bone involvement without evidence of
necrosis L97.526
|bone necrosis L97.524
|exposed fat layer L97.522
|muscle involvement without evidence
of necrosis L97.525
|muscle necrosis L97.523
|skin breakdown only L97.521
|specified severity NEC L97.528
|right L97.519
|with
|bone involvement without evidence of
necrosis L97.516
|bone necrosis L97.514
|exposed fat layer L97.512
|muscle involvement without evidence
of necrosis L97.515
|muscle necrosis L97.513
|skin breakdown only L97.511
|specified severity NEC L97.518
|heel L97.409
|with
|bone involvement without evidence of
necrosis L97.406
|bone necrosis L97.404
|exposed fat layer L97.402
|muscle involvement without evidence
of necrosis L97.405
|muscle necrosis L97.403
|skin breakdown only L97.401
|specified severity NEC L97.408
|left L97.429
|with
|bone involvement without evidence of
necrosis L97.426
|bone necrosis L97.424
|exposed fat layer L97.422
|muscle involvement without evidence
of necrosis L97.425

Ulcer - *continued*
|muscle necrosis L97.423
|skin breakdown only L97.421
|specified severity NEC L97.428
|right L97.419
|with
|bone involvement without evidence of
necrosis L97.416
|bone necrosis L97.414
|exposed fat layer L97.412
|muscle involvement without evidence
of necrosis L97.415
|muscle necrosis L97.413
|skin breakdown only L97.411
|specified severity NEC L97.418
|left L97.929
|with
|bone necrosis L97.924
|exposed fat layer L97.922
|bone involvement without evidence of
necrosis L97.926
|muscle involvement without evidence
of necrosis L97.925
|muscle necrosis L97.923
|skin breakdown only L97.921
|specified severity NEC L97.928
|lower leg NOS L97.909
|with
|bone necrosis L97.904
|exposed fat layer L97.902
|bone involvement without evidence of
necrosis L97.906
|muscle involvement without evidence
of necrosis L97.905
|muscle necrosis L97.903
|skin breakdown only L97.901
|specified severity NEC L97.908
|left L97.929
|with
|bone involvement without evidence of
necrosis L97.926
|bone necrosis L97.924
|exposed fat layer L97.922
|muscle involvement without evidence
of necrosis L97.925
|muscle necrosis L97.923
|skin breakdown only L97.921
|specified severity NEC L97.928
|right L97.919
|with
|bone involvement without evidence of
necrosis L97.916
|bone necrosis L97.914
|exposed fat layer L97.912
|muscle involvement without evidence
of necrosis L97.915
|muscle necrosis L97.913
|skin breakdown only L97.911
|specified severity NEC L97.918
|specified site NEC L97.809
|with
|bone involvement without evidence of
necrosis L97.806
|bone necrosis L97.804
|exposed fat layer L97.802
|muscle involvement without evidence
of necrosis L97.805
|muscle necrosis L97.803
|skin breakdown only L97.801
|specified severity NEC L97.808
|left L97.829
|with
|bone involvement without evidence
of necrosis L97.826
|bone necrosis L97.824

Ulcer - *continued*
|exposed fat layer L97.822
|muscle involvement without
evidence of necrosis L97.825
|muscle necrosis L97.823
|skin breakdown only L97.821
|specified severity NEC L97.828
|right L97.819
|with
|bone involvement without evidence
of necrosis L97.816
|bone necrosis L97.814
|exposed fat layer L97.812
|muscle involvement without
evidence of necrosis L97.815
|muscle necrosis L97.813
|skin breakdown only L97.811
|specified severity NEC L97.818
|midfoot L97.409
|with
|bone involvement without evidence of
necrosis L97.406
|bone necrosis L97.404
|exposed fat layer L97.402
|muscle involvement without evidence
of necrosis L97.405
|muscle necrosis L97.403
|skin breakdown only L97.401
|specified severity NEC L97.408
|left L97.429
|with
|bone involvement without evidence of
necrosis L97.426
|bone necrosis L97.424
|exposed fat layer L97.422
|muscle involvement without evidence
of necrosis L97.425
|muscle necrosis L97.423
|skin breakdown only L97.421
|specified severity NEC L97.428
|right L97.419
|with
|bone involvement without evidence of
necrosis L97.416
|bone necrosis L97.414
|exposed fat layer L97.412
|muscle involvement without evidence
of necrosis L97.415
|muscle necrosis L97.413
|skin breakdown only L97.411
|specified severity NEC L97.418
|right L97.919
|with
|bone involvement without evidence of
necrosis L97.916
|bone necrosis L97.914
|exposed fat layer L97.912
|muscle involvement without evidence
of necrosis L97.915
|muscle necrosis L97.913
|skin breakdown only L97.911
|specified severity NEC L97.918
|thigh L97.109
|with
|bone involvement without evidence of
necrosis L97.106
|muscle involvement without evidence
of necrosis L97.105
|bone necrosis L97.104
|exposed fat layer L97.102
|specified severity NEC L97.108
|muscle necrosis L97.103
|skin breakdown only L97.101
|left L97.129
|with

Ulcer - *continued*

|bone involvement without evidence of
  necrosis L97.126
|bone necrosis L97.124
|exposed fat layer L97.122
|muscle involvement without evidence
  of necrosis L97.125
|muscle necrosis L97.123
|skin breakdown only L97.121
|specified severity NEC L97.128
|right L97.119
|with
|bone involvement without evidence of
  necrosis L97.116
|bone necrosis L97.114
|exposed fat layer L97.112
|muscle involvement without evidence
  of necrosis L97.115
|muscle necrosis L97.113
|skin breakdown only L97.111
|specified severity NEC L97.118
|toe L97.509
|with
|bone involvement without evidence of
  necrosis L97.506
|bone necrosis L97.504
|exposed fat layer L97.502
|muscle involvement without evidence
  of necrosis L97.505
|muscle necrosis L97.503
|skin breakdown only L97.501
|specified severity NEC L97.508
|left L97.529
|with
|bone involvement without evidence of
  necrosis L97.526
|bone necrosis L97.524
|exposed fat layer L97.522
|muscle involvement without evidence
  of necrosis L97.525
|muscle necrosis L97.523
|skin breakdown only L97.521
|specified severity NEC L97.528
|right L97.519
|with
|bone involvement without evidence of
  necrosis L97.516
|bone necrosis L97.514
|exposed fat layer L97.512
|muscle involvement without evidence
  of necrosis L97.515
|muscle necrosis L97.513
|skin breakdown only L97.511
|specified severity NEC L97.518
|leprous A30.1
|syphilitic A52.19
|varicose *see* Varix, leg, with, ulcer
|luetic *see* Ulcer, syphilitic
|lung J98.4
|tuberculous *see* Tuberculosis, pulmonary
|malignant *see* Neoplasm, malignant, by site
|marginal NEC *see* Ulcer, gastrojejunal
|meatus (urinarius) N34.2
|Meckel's diverticulum Q43.0
|malignant *see* Table of Neoplasms, small
  intestine, malignant
|Meleney's (chronic undermining) *see* Ulcer,
  skin
|Mooren's (cornea) *see* Ulcer, cornea, Mooren's
|mycobacterial (skin) A31.1
|nasopharynx J39.2
|neck, uterus N86
|neurogenic NEC *see* Ulcer, skin
|nose, nasal (passage) (infective) (septum)
  J34.0

Ulcer - *continued*

|skin *see* Ulcer, skin
|spirochetal A69.8
|varicose (bleeding) I86.8
|oral mucosa (traumatic) K12.1
|palate (soft) K12.1
|penis (chronic) N48.5
|peptic (site unspecified) K27.9
|with
|hemorrhage K27.4
|and perforation K27.6
|perforation K27.5
|acute K27.3
|with
|hemorrhage K27.0
|and perforation K27.2
|perforation K27.1
|chronic K27.7
|with
|hemorrhage K27.4
|and perforation K27.6
|perforation K27.5
|esophagus K22.10
|with bleeding K22.11
|newborn P78.82
|perforating K27.5
|skin *see* Ulcer, skin
|peritonsillar J35.8
|phagedenic (tropical) *see* Ulcer, skin
|pharynx J39.2
|phlebitis *see* Phlebitis
|plaster *see* Ulcer, pressure, by site
|popliteal space *see* Ulcer, lower limb
|postpyloric *see* Ulcer, duodenum
|prepuce N47.7
|prepyloric *see* Ulcer, stomach
|pressure (pressure area) L89.9-
|ankle L89.5-
|back L89.1-
|buttock L89.3-
|coccyx L89.15-
|contiguous site of back, buttock, hip L89.4-
|elbow L89.0-
|face L89.81-
|head L89.81-
|heel L89.6-
|hip L89.2-
|sacral region (tailbone) L89.15-
|specified site NEC L89.89-
|stage 1 (healing) (pre-ulcer skin changes
  limited to persistent focal edema)
|ankle L89.5-
|back L89.1-
|buttock L89.3-
|coccyx L89.15-
|contiguous site of back, buttock, hip
  L89.4-
|elbow L89.0-
|face L89.81-
|head L89.81-
|heel L89.6-
|hip L89.2-
|sacral region (tailbone) L89.15-
|specified site NEC L89.89-
|stage 2 (healing) (abrasion, blister, partial
  thickness skin loss involving epidermis
  and/or dermis)
|ankle L89.5-
|back L89.1-
|buttock L89.3-
|coccyx L89.15-
|contiguous site of back, buttock, hip
  L89.4-
|elbow L89.0-
|face L89.81-

Ulcer - *continued*

|head L89.81-
|heel L89.6-
|hip L89.2-
|sacral region (tailbone) L89.15-
|specified site NEC L89.89-
|stage 3 (healing) (full thickness skin loss
  involving damage or necrosis of
  subcutaneous tissue)
|ankle L89.5-
|back L89.1-
|buttock L89.3-
|coccyx L89.15-
|contiguous site of back, buttock, hip
  L89.4-
|elbow L89.0-
|face L89.81-
|head L89.81-
|heel L89.6-
|hip L89.2-
|sacral region (tailbone) L89.15-
|specified site NEC L89.89-
|stage 4 (healing) (necrosis of soft tissues
  through to underlying muscle, tendon, or
  bone)
|ankle L89.5-
|back L89.1-
|buttock L89.3-
|coccyx L89.15-
|contiguous site of back, buttock, hip
  L89.4-
|elbow L89.0-
|face L89.81-
|head L89.81-
|heel L89.6-
|hip L89.2-
|sacral region (tailbone) L89.15-
|specified site NEC L89.89-
|unspecified stage
|ankle L89.5-
|back L89.1-
|buttock L89.3-
|coccyx L89.15-
|contiguous site of back, buttock, hip
  L89.4-
|elbow L89.0-
|face L89.81-
|head L89.81-
|heel L89.6-
|hip L89.2-
|sacral region (tailbone) L89.15-
|specified site NEC L89.89-
|unstageable
|ankle L89.5-
|back L89.1-
|buttock L89.3-
|coccyx L89.15-
|contiguous site of back, buttock, hip
  L89.4-
|elbow L89.0-
|face L89.81-
|head L89.81-
|heel L89.6-
|hip L89.2-
|sacral region (tailbone) L89.15-
|specified site NEC L89.89-
|primary of intestine K63.3
|with perforation K63.1
|prostate N41.9
|pyloric *see* Ulcer, stomach
|rectosigmoid K63.3
|with perforation K63.1
|rectum (sphincter) (solitary) K62.6
|stercoraceous, stercoral K62.6
|retina *see* Inflammation, chorioretinal

Ulcer - *continued*
|rodent *see also* Neoplasm, skin, malignant
|sclera *see* Scleritis
|scrofulous (tuberculous) A18.2
|scrotum N50.89
  |tuberculous A18.15
  |varicose I86.1
|seminal vesicle N50.89
|sigmoid *see* Ulcer, intestine
|skin (atrophic) (chronic) (neurogenic) (non-
  healing) (perforating) (pyogenic) (trophic)
  (tropical) L98.499
  |with gangrene *see* Gangrene
  |amebic A06.7
  |back *see* Ulcer, back
  |buttock *see* Ulcer, buttock
  |decubitus *see* Ulcer, pressure
  |lower limb *see* Ulcer, lower limb
  |mycobacterial A31.1
  |specified site NEC L98.499
    |with
      |bone involvement without evidence of
        necrosis L98.496
      |bone necrosis L98.494
      |exposed fat layer L98.492
      |muscle involvement without evidence
        of necrosis L98.495
      |muscle necrosis L98.493
      |skin breakdown only L98.491
      |specified severity NEC L98.498
  |tuberculous (primary) A18.4
  |varicose *see* Ulcer, varicose
|sloughing *see* Ulcer, skin
|solitary, anus or rectum (sphincter) K62.6
|sore throat J02.9
  |streptococcal J02.0
|spermatic cord N50.89
|spine (tuberculous) A18.01
|stasis (venous) *see* Varix, leg, with, ulcer
  |without varicose veins I87.2
|stercoraceous, stercoral K63.3
  |with perforation K63.1
  |anus or rectum K62.6
|stoma, stomal *see* Ulcer, gastrojejunal
|stomach (eroded) (peptic) (round) K25.9
  |with
    |hemorrhage K25.4
      |and perforation K25.6
    |perforation K25.5
  |acute K25.3
    |with
      |hemorrhage K25.0
        |and perforation K25.2
      |perforation K25.1
  |chronic K25.7
    |with
      |hemorrhage K25.4
        |and perforation K25.6
      |perforation K25.5
|stomal *see* Ulcer, gastrojejunal
|stomatitis K12.1
|stress *see* Ulcer, peptic
|strumous (tuberculous) A18.2
|submucosal, bladder *see* Cystitis, interstitial
|syphilitic (any site) (early) (secondary)
  A51.39
  |late A52.79
  |perforating A52.79
    |foot A52.11
|testis N50.89
|thigh *see* Ulcer, lower limb
|throat J39.2
  |diphtheritic A36.0
|toe *see* Ulcer, lower limb
|tongue (traumatic) K14.0

Ulcer - *continued*
|tonsil J35.8
  |diphtheritic A36.0
|trachea J39.8
|trophic *see* Ulcer, skin
|tropical *see* Ulcer, skin
|tuberculous *see* Tuberculosis, ulcer
|tunica vaginalis N50.89
|turbinate J34.89
|typhoid (perforating) *see* Typhoid
|unspecified site *see* Ulcer, skin
|urethra (meatus) *see* Urethritis
|uterus N85.8
  |cervix N86
    |with cervicitis N72
  |neck N86
    |with cervicitis N72
  |vagina N76.5
    |in Behçet's disease M35.2 *[N77.0]*
  |pessary N89.8
|valve, heart I33.0
|varicose (lower limb, any part) *see also* Varix,
  leg, with, ulcer
  |broad ligament I86.2
  |esophagus *see* Varix, esophagus
  |inflamed or infected *see* Varix, leg, with
    ulcer, with inflammation
  |nasal septum I86.8
  |perineum I86.3
  |scrotum I86.1
  |specified site NEC I86.8
  |sublingual I86.0
  |vulva I86.3
|vas deferens N50.89
|vulva (acute) (infectional) N76.6
  |in (due to)
    |Behçet's disease M35.2 *[N77.0]*
    |herpesviral (herpes simplex) infection
      A60.04
    |tuberculosis A18.18
  |vulvobuccal, recurring N76.6
|X-ray L58.1
|yaws A66.4
Ulcerosa scarlatina A38.8
Ulcus *see also* Ulcer
|cutis tuberculosum A18.4
|duodeni *see* Ulcer, duodenum
|durum (syphilitic) A51.0
  |extragenital A51.2
|gastrojejunale *see* Ulcer, gastrojejunal
|hypostaticum *see* Ulcer, varicose
|molle (cutis) (skin) A57
|serpens corneae *see* Ulcer, cornea, central
|ventriculi *see* Ulcer, stomach
Ulegyria Q04.8
Ulerythema
|ophryogenes, congenital Q84.2
|sycosiforme L73.8
Ullrich (-Bonnevie)(-Turner) syndrome *see*
  also Turner's syndrome Q87.1
Ullrich-Feichtiger syndrome Q87.0
Ulnar *see* condition
Ulorrhagia, ulorrhea K06.8
Umbilicus, umbilical *see* condition
Unacceptable
|contours of tooth K08.54
|morphology of tooth K08.54
Unavailability (of)
|bed at medical facility Z75.1
|health service-related agencies Z75.4
|medical facilities (at) Z75.3
  |due to
    |investigation by social service agency
      Z75.2
    |lack of services at home Z75.0

Unavailability - *continued*
    |remoteness from facility Z75.3
    |waiting list Z75.1
  |home Z75.0
  |outpatient clinic Z75.3
|schooling Z55.1
|social service agencies Z75.4
Uncinaria americana infestation B76.1
Uncinariasis B76.9
Uncongenial work Z56.5
Unconscious (ness) *see* Coma
Under observation *see* Observation
Underachievement in school Z55.3
Underdevelopment *see also* Undeveloped
|nose Q30.1
|sexual E30.0
Underdosing *see also* Table of Drugs and
  Chemicals, categories T36-T50, with final
  character 6 Z91.14
|intentional NEC Z91.128
  |due to financial hardship of patient Z91.120
|unintentional NEC Z91.138
  |due to patient's age related debility Z91.130
Underfeeding, newborn P92.3
Underfill, endodontic M27.53
Underimmunization status Z28.3
Undernourishment *see* Malnutrition
Undernutrition *see* Malnutrition
Underweight R63.6
|for gestational age *see* Light for dates
Underwood's disease P83.0
Undescended *see also* Malposition, congenital
|cecum Q43.3
|colon Q43.3
|testicle *see* Cryptorchid
Undeveloped, undevelopment *see also*
  Hypoplasia
|brain (congenital) Q02
|cerebral (congenital) Q02
|heart Q24.8
|lung Q33.6
|testis E29.1
|uterus E30.0
Undiagnosed (disease) R69
Undulant fever *see* Brucellosis
Unemployment, anxiety concerning Z56.0
|threatened Z56.2
Unequal length (acquired) (limb) *see also*
  Deformity, limb, unequal length
|leg *see also* Deformity, limb, unequal length
  |congenital Q72.9-
Unextracted dental root K08.3
Unguis incarnatus L60.0
Unhappiness R45.2
Unicornate uterus Q51.4
|in pregnancy or childbirth O34.00
Unilateral *see also* condition
|development, breast N64.89
|organ or site, congenital NEC *see* Agenesis,
  by site
Unilocular heart Q20.8
Union, abnormal *see also* Fusion
|larynx and trachea Q34.8
Universal mesentery Q43.3
Unrepairable overhanging of dental
  restorative materials K08.52
Unsatisfactory
|restoration of tooth K08.50
  |specified NEC K08.59
|sample of cytologic smear
  |anus R85.615
  |cervix R87.615
  |vagina R87.625
|surroundings Z59.1
|work Z56.5

Unsoundness of mind *see* Psychosis
Unstable
|back NEC *see* Instability, joint, spine
|hip (congenital) Q65.6
| |acquired *see* Derangement, joint, specified
| | type NEC, hip
|joint *see* Instability, joint
| |secondary to removal of joint prosthesis
| | M96.89
|lie (mother) O32.0
|lumbosacral joint (congenital)
| |acquired *see* subcategory M53.2
|sacroiliac *see* subcategory M53.2
|spine NEC *see* Instability, joint, spine
Unsteadiness on feet R26.81
Untruthfulness, child problem F91.8
Unwanted
|multiple moves in the last 12 months Z59.81-
|pregnancy Z64.0
Unverricht (-Lundborg) disease or epilepsy
| *see* Epilepsy, generalized, idiopathic
Upbringing, institutional Z62.22
|away from parents NEC Z62.29
|in care of non-parental family member Z62.21
|in foster care Z62.21
|in orphanage or group home Z62.22
|in welfare custody Z62.21
Upper respiratory *see* condition
Upset
|gastric K30
|gastrointestinal K30
| |psychogenic F45.8
|intestinal (large) (small) K59.9
| |psychogenic F45.8
|menstruation N93.9
|mental F48.9
|stomach K30
| |psychogenic F45.8
Urachus *see also* condition
|patent or persistent Q64.4
Urbach-Oppenheim disease (necrobiosis
| **lipoidica diabeticorum)** *see* E08-E13 with
| .620
Urbach's lipoid proteinosis E78.89
Urbach-Wiethe disease E78.89
Urban yellow fever A95.1
Urea
|blood, high *see* Uremia
|cycle metabolism disorder *see* Disorder, urea
| cycle metabolism
Uremia, uremic N19
|with
| |ectopic or molar pregnancy O08.4
| |polyneuropathy N18.9 [*G63*]
|chronic NOS (*see also* Disease, kidney,
| chronic) N18.9
| |due to hypertension *see* Hypertensive,
| | kidney
| |ectopic or molar pregnancy O08.4
|congenital P96.0
|extrarenal R39.2
|following ectopic or molar pregnancy O08.4
|newborn P96.0
|prerenal R39.2
Ureter, ureteral *see* condition
Ureteralgia N23
Ureterectasis *see* Hydroureter
Ureteritis N28.89
|cystica N28.86
|due to calculus N20.1
| |with calculus, kidney N20.2
| | |with hydronephrosis N13.2
|gonococcal (acute) (chronic) A54.21
|nonspecific N28.89

Ureterocele N28.89
|congenital (orthotopic) Q62.31
|ectopic Q62.32
Ureterolith, ureterolithiasis *see* Calculus,
| ureter
Ureterostomy
|attention to Z43.6
|status Z93.6
Urethra, urethral *see* condition
Urethralgia R39.89
Urethritis (anterior) (posterior) N34.2
|calculous N21.1
|candidal B37.41
|chlamydial A56.01
|diplococcal (gonococcal) A54.01
| |with abscess (accessory gland) (periurethral)
| | A54.1
|gonococcal A54.01
| |with abscess (accessory gland) (periurethral)
| | A54.1
|nongonococcal N34.1
| |Reiter's *see* Reiter's disease
|nonspecific N34.1
|nonvenereal N34.1
|postmenopausal N34.2
|puerperal O86.22
|Reiter's *see* Reiter's disease
|specified NEC N34.2
|trichomonal or due to Trichomonas (vaginalis)
| A59.03
Urethrocele N81.0
|with
| |cystocele *see* Cystocele
| |prolapse of uterus *see* Prolapse, uterus
Urethrolithiasis (with colic or infection) N21.1
Urethrorectal *see* condition
Urethrorrhagia N36.8
Urethrorrhea R36.9
Urethrostomy
|attention to Z43.6
|status Z93.6
Urethrotrigonitis *see* Trigonitis
Urethrovaginal *see* condition
Urgency
|fecal R15.2
|hypertensive *see* Hypertension
|urinary R39.15
Urhidrosis, uridrosis L74.8
Uric acid in blood (increased) E79.0
Uricacidemia (asymptomatic) E79.0
Uricemia (asymptomatic) E79.0
Uricosuria R82.998
Urinary *see* condition
Urination
|frequent R35.0
|painful R30.9
Urine
|blood in *see* Hematuria
|discharge, excessive R35.89
|enuresis, nonorganic origin F98.0
|extravasation R39.0
|frequency R35.0
|incontinence R32
| |nonorganic origin F98.0
|intermittent stream R39.198
|pus in N39.0
|retention or stasis R33.9
| |organic R33.8
| | |drug-induced R33.0
| |psychogenic F45.8
|secretion
| |deficient R34
| |excessive R35.89
| |frequency R35.0
|stream
| |intermittent R39.198

Urine
|slowing R39.198
|splitting R39.13
|weak R39.12
Urinemia *see* Uremia
Urinoma, urethra N36.8
Uroarthritis, infectious (Reiter's) *see* Reiter's
| disease
Urodialysis R34
Urolithiasis *see* Calculus, urinary
Uronephrosis *see* Hydronephrosis
Uropathy N39.9
|obstructive N13.9
| |specified NEC N13.8
|reflux N13.9
| |specified NEC N13.8
|vesicoureteral reflux-associated *see* Reflux,
| vesicoureteral
Urosepsis   code to condition
Urticaria L50.9
|with angioneurotic edema T78.3
| |hereditary D84.1
|allergic L50.0
|cholinergic L50.5
|chronic L50.8
|cold, familial L50.2
|contact L50.6
|dermatographic L50.3
|due to
| |cold or heat L50.2
| |drugs L50.0
| |food L50.0
| |inhalants L50.0
| |plants L50.6
| |serum *see also* Reaction, serum T80.69
|factitial L50.3
|familial cold M04.2
|giant T78.3
| |hereditary D84.1
|gigantea T78.3
|idiopathic L50.1
|larynx T78.3
| |hereditary D84.1
|neonatorum P83.88
|nonallergic L50.1
|papulosa (Hebra) L28.2
|pigmentosa D47.01
| |congenital Q82.2
| |of neonatal onset Q82.2
| |of newborn onset Q82.2
|recurrent periodic L50.8
|serum *see also* Reaction, serum T80.69
|solar L56.3
|specified type NEC L50.8
|thermal (cold) (heat) L50.2
|vibratory L50.4
|xanthelasmoidea *see* Urticaria pigmentosa
Use (of)
|alcohol Z72.89
| |with
| | |intoxication F10.929
| | |sleep disorder F10.982
| | |withdrawal F10.939
| | | |with
| | | | |perceptual disturbance F10.932
| | | | |delirium F10.931
| | | | |uncomplicated F10.930
| |harmful *see* Abuse, alcohol
|amphetamines *see* Use, stimulant NEC
|caffeine *see* Use, stimulant NEC
|cannabis F12.90
| |with
| | |anxiety disorder F12.980
| | |intoxication F12.929
| | | |with

Use (of) - continued
   |delirium F12.921
      |perceptual disturbance F12.922
   |uncomplicated F12.920
   |withdrawal F12.93
      |other specified disorder F12.988
      |psychosis F12.959
         |delusions F12.950
         |hallucinations F12.951
      |unspecified disorder F12.99
|cocaine F14.90
   |with
      |anxiety disorder F14.980
      |intoxication F14.929
         |with
            |delirium F14.921
            |perceptual disturbance F14.922
         |uncomplicated F14.920
      |other specified disorder F14.988
      |psychosis F14.959
         |delusions F14.950
         |hallucinations F14.951
      |sexual dysfunction F14.981
      |sleep disorder F14.982
      |unspecified disorder F14.99
   |withdrawal F14.93
   |harmful see Abuse, drug, cocaine
|drug(s) NEC F19.90
   |with sleep disorder F19.982
   |harmful see Abuse, drug, by type
|hallucinogen NEC F16.90
   |with
      |anxiety disorder F16.980
      |intoxication F16.929
         |with
            |delirium F16.921
         |uncomplicated F16.920
      |mood disorder F16.94
      |other specified disorder F16.988
      |perception disorder (flashbacks) F16.983
      |psychosis F16.959
         |delusions F16.950
         |hallucinations F16.951
      |unspecified disorder F16.99
   |harmful see Abuse, drug, hallucinogen NEC
|inhalants F18.90
   |with
      |anxiety disorder F18.980
      |intoxication F18.929
         |with delirium F18.921
         |uncomplicated F18.920
      |mood disorder F18.94
      |other specified disorder F18.988
      |persisting dementia F18.97
      |psychosis F18.959
         |delusions F18.950
         |hallucinations F18.951
      |unspecified disorder F18.99
   |harmful see Abuse, drug, inhalant
|methadone see Use, opioid
|nonprescribed drugs F19.90
   |harmful see Abuse, non-psychoactive
      substance
|opioid F11.90
   |with
      |disorder F11.99
         |mood F11.94
         |sleep F11.982
         |specified type NEC F11.988
      |intoxication F11.929
         |with
            |delirium F11.921
            |perceptual disturbance F11.922
         |uncomplicated F11.920
      |withdrawal F11.93

Use (of) - continued
   |harmful see Abuse, drug, opioid
|patent medicines F19.90
   |harmful see Abuse, non-psychoactive
      substance
|psychoactive drug NEC F19.90
   |with
      |anxiety disorder F19.980
      |intoxication F19.929
         |with
            |delirium F19.921
            |perceptual disturbance F19.922
         |uncomplicated F19.920
      |mood disorder F19.94
      |other specified disorder F19.988
      |persisting
         |amnestic disorder F19.96
         |dementia F19.97
      |psychosis F19.959
         |delusions F19.950
         |hallucinations F19.951
      |sexual dysfunction F19.981
      |sleep disorder F19.982
      |unspecified disorder F19.99
      |withdrawal F19.939
         |with
            |delirium F19.931
            |perceptual disturbance F19.932
         |uncomplicated F19.930
   |harmful see Abuse, drug NEC, psychoactive
      NEC
|sedative, hypnotic, or anxiolytic F13.90
   |with
      |anxiety disorder F13.980
      |intoxication F13.929
         |with
            |delirium F13.921
         |uncomplicated F13.920
      |other specified disorder F13.988
      |persisting
         |amnestic disorder F13.96
         |dementia F13.97
      |psychosis F13.959
         |delusions F13.950
         |hallucinations F13.951
      |sexual dysfunction F13.981
      |sleep disorder F13.982
      |unspecified disorder F13.99
   |harmful see Abuse, drug, sedative, hypnotic,
      or anxiolytic
|stimulant NEC F15.90
   |with
      |anxiety disorder F15.980
      |intoxication F15.929
         |with
            |delirium F15.921
            |perceptual disturbance F15.922
         |uncomplicated F15.920
      |mood disorder F15.94
      |other specified disorder F15.988
      |psychosis F15.959
         |delusions F15.950
         |hallucinations F15.951
      |sexual dysfunction F15.981
      |sleep disorder F15.982
      |unspecified disorder F15.99
      |withdrawal F15.93
   |harmful see Abuse, drug, stimulant NEC
|tobacco Z72.0
   |with dependence see Dependence, drug,
      nicotine
|volatile solvents see also Use, inhalant F18.90
   |harmful see Abuse, drug, inhalant

Usher-Senear disease or syndrome L10.4
Uta B55.1
Uteromegaly N85.2
Uterovaginal see condition
Uterovesical see condition
Uveal see condition
Uveitis (anterior) see also Iridocyclitis
   |acute see Iridocyclitis, acute
   |chronic see Iridocyclitis, chronic
   |due to toxoplasmosis (acquired) B58.09
      |congenital P37.1
   |granulomatous see Iridocyclitis, chronic
   |heterochromic see Cyclitis, Fuchs'
      heterochromic
   |lens-induced see Iridocyclitis, lens-induced
   |posterior see Chorioretinitis
   |sympathetic H44.13-
   |syphilitic (secondary) A51.43
      |congenital (early) A50.01
      |late A52.71
   |tuberculous A18.54
Uveoencephalitis see Inflammation,
   chorioretinal
Uveokeratitis see Iridocyclitis
Uveoparotitis D86.89
Uvula see condition
**Uvulitis (acute) (catarrhal) (chronic)
   (membranous) (suppurative) (ulcerative)**
   K12.2

V

Vaccination (prophylactic)
   |complication or reaction see Complications,
      vaccination
   |delayed Z28.9
   |encounter for Z23
   |not done see Immunization, not done, because
      (of)
Vaccinia (generalized) (localized) T88.1
   |congenital P35.8
   |without vaccination B08.011
Vacuum, in sinus (accessory) (nasal) J34.89
Vagabond, vagabondage Z59.00
Vagabond's disease B85.1
Vagina, vaginal see condition
Vaginalitis (tunica) (testis) N49.1
Vaginismus (reflex) N94.2
   |functional F52.5
   |nonorganic F52.5
   |psychogenic F52.5
   |secondary N94.2
**Vaginitis (acute) (circumscribed) (diffuse)
   (emphysematous) (nonvenereal)
   (ulcerative)** N76.0
   |with ectopic or molar pregnancy O08.0
   |amebic A06.82
   |atrophic, postmenopausal N95.2
   |bacterial N76.0
   |blennorrhagic (gonococcal) A54.02
   |candidal B37.3
   |chlamydial A56.02
   |chronic N76.1
   |due to Trichomonas (vaginalis) A59.01
   |following ectopic or molar pregnancy O08.0
   |gonococcal A54.02
      |with abscess (accessory gland) (periurethral)
         A54.1
   |granuloma A58
   |in (due to)
      |candidiasis B37.3
      |herpesviral (herpes simplex) infection
         A60.04
      |pinworm infection B80 [N77.1]

Vaginitis - *continued*
| monilial B37.3
| mycotic (candidal) B37.3
| postmenopausal atrophic N95.2
| puerperal (postpartum) O86.13
| senile (atrophic) N95.2
| subacute or chronic N76.1
| syphilitic (early) A51.0
| | late A52.76
| trichomonal A59.01
| tuberculous A18.18
Vaginosis *see* Vaginitis
Vagotonia G52.2
Vagrancy Z59.00
VAIN *see* Neoplasia, intraepithelial, vagina
Vallecula *see* condition
Valley fever B38.0
Valsuani's disease *see* Anemia, obstetric
Valve, valvular (formation) *see also* condition
| cerebral ventricle (communicating) in situ Z98.2
| cervix, internal os Q51.828
| congenital NEC *see* Atresia, by site
| ureter (pelvic junction) (vesical orifice) Q62.39
| urethra (congenital) (posterior) Q64.2
Valvulitis (chronic) *see* Endocarditis
Valvulopathy *see* Endocarditis
Van Bogaert's leukoencephalopathy (sclerosing) (subacute) A81.1
Van Bogaert-Scherer-Epstein disease or syndrome E75.5
Van Buchem's syndrome M85.2
Van Creveld-Von Gierke disease E74.01
Van der Hoeve (-De Kleyn) syndrome Q78.0
Van der Woude's syndrome Q38.0
Van Neck's disease or osteochondrosis M91.0
Vanishing lung J44.9
Vapor asphyxia or suffocation T59.9
| specified agent *see* Table of Drugs and Chemicals
Variance, lethal ball, prosthetic heart valve T82.09
Variants, thalassemic D56.8
Variations in hair color L67.1
Varicella B01.9
| with
| | complications NEC B01.89
| | encephalitis B01.11
| | encephalomyelitis B01.11
| | meningitis B01.0
| | myelitis B01.12
| | pneumonia B01.2
| congenital P35.8
Varices *see* Varix
Varicocele (scrotum) (thrombosed) I86.1
| ovary I86.2
| perineum I86.3
| spermatic cord (ulcerated) I86.1
Varicose
| aneurysm (ruptured) I77.0
| dermatitis *see* Varix, leg, with, inflammation
| eczema *see* Varix, leg, with, inflammation
| phlebitis *see* Varix, with, inflammation
| tumor *see* Varix
| ulcer (lower limb, any part) *see also* Varix, leg, with, ulcer
| | anus *see also* Hemorrhoids K64.8
| | esophagus *see* Varix, esophagus
| | inflamed or infected *see* Varix, leg, with ulcer, with inflammation
| | nasal septum I86.8
| | perineum I86.3
| | scrotum I86.1
| | specified site NEC I86.8
| vein *see* Varix
| vessel *see* Varix, leg

Varicosis, varicosities, varicosity *see* Varix
Variola (major) (minor) B03
Varioloid B03
Varix (lower limb) (ruptured) I83.90
| with
| | edema I83.899
| | inflammation I83.10
| | | with ulcer (venous) I83.209
| | pain I83.819
| | specified complication NEC I83.899
| | stasis dermatitis I83.10
| | | with ulcer (venous) I83.209
| | swelling I83.899
| | ulcer I83.0-
| | | with inflammation I83.2-
| aneurysmal I77.0
| asymptomatic I83.9-
| bladder I86.2
| broad ligament I86.2
| complicating
| | childbirth (lower extremity) O87.4
| | | anus or rectum O87.2
| | | genital (vagina, vulva or perineum) O87.8
| | pregnancy (lower extremity) O22.0-
| | | anus or rectum O22.4-
| | | genital (vagina, vulva or perineum) O22.1-
| | puerperium (lower extremity) O87.4
| | | anus or rectum O87.2
| | | genital (vagina, vulva, perineum) O87.8
| congenital (any site) Q27.8
| esophagus (idiopathic) (primary) (ulcerated) I85.00
| | bleeding I85.01
| | congenital Q27.8
| | in (due to)
| | | alcoholic liver disease I85.10
| | | | bleeding I85.11
| | | cirrhosis of liver I85.10
| | | | bleeding I85.11
| | | portal hypertension I85.10
| | | | bleeding I85.11
| | | schistosomiasis I85.10
| | | | bleeding I85.11
| | | toxic liver disease I85.10
| | | | bleeding I85.11
| | secondary I85.10
| | | bleeding I85.11
| gastric I86.4
| inflamed or infected I83.10
| | ulcerated I83.209
| labia (majora) I86.3
| leg (asymptomatic) I83.9-
| | with
| | | edema I83.899
| | | inflammation I83.10
| | | | with ulcer *see* Varix, leg, with, ulcer, with inflammation by site
| | | pain I83.819
| | | specified complication NEC I83.899
| | | swelling I83.899
| | | ulcer I83.009
| | | | with inflammation I83.209
| | | | ankle I83.003
| | | | | with inflammation I83.203
| | | | calf I83.002
| | | | | with inflammation I83.202
| | | | foot NEC I83.005
| | | | | with inflammation I83.205
| | | | heel I83.004
| | | | | with inflammation I83.204
| | | | lower leg NEC I83.008
| | | | | with inflammation I83.208
| | | | midfoot I83.004
| | | | | with inflammation I83.204
| | | | thigh I83.001

Varix - *continued*
| | with inflammation I83.201
| bilateral (asymptomatic) I83.93
| | with
| | | edema I83.893
| | | pain I83.813
| | | specified complication NEC I83.893
| | | swelling I83.893
| | | ulcer I83.0-
| | | | with inflammation I83.209
| left (asymptomatic) I83.92
| | with
| | | edema I83.892
| | | pain I83.812
| | | specified complication NEC I83.892
| | | swelling I83.892
| | | inflammation I83.12
| | | | with ulcer *see* Varix, leg, with, ulcer, with inflammation by site
| | | ulcer I83.029
| | | | with inflammation I83.229
| | | | ankle I83.023
| | | | | with inflammation I83.223
| | | | calf I83.022
| | | | | with inflammation I83.222
| | | | foot NEC I83.025
| | | | | with inflammation I83.225
| | | | heel I83.024
| | | | | with inflammation I83.224
| | | | lower leg NEC I83.028
| | | | | with inflammation I83.228
| | | | midfoot I83.024
| | | | | with inflammation I83.224
| | | | thigh I83.021
| | | | | with inflammation I83.221
| right (asymptomatic) I83.91
| | with
| | | edema I83.891
| | | pain I83.811
| | | specified complication NEC I83.891
| | | swelling I83.891
| | | inflammation I83.11
| | | | with ulcer *see* Varix, leg, with, ulcer, with inflammation by site
| | | ulcer I83.019
| | | | with inflammation I83.219
| | | | ankle I83.013
| | | | | with inflammation I83.213
| | | | calf I83.012
| | | | | with inflammation I83.212
| | | | foot NEC I83.015
| | | | | with inflammation I83.215
| | | | heel I83.014
| | | | | with inflammation I83.214
| | | | lower leg NEC I83.018
| | | | | with inflammation I83.218
| | | | midfoot I83.014
| | | | | with inflammation I83.214
| | | | thigh I83.011
| | | | | with inflammation I83.211
| nasal septum I86.8
| orbit I86.8
| | congenital Q27.8
| ovary I86.2
| papillary I78.1
| pelvis I86.2
| perineum I86.3
| pharynx I86.8
| placenta O43.89-
| renal papilla I86.8
| retina H35.09
| scrotum (ulcerated) I86.1
| sigmoid colon I86.8
| specified site NEC I86.8
| spinal (cord) (vessels) I86.8

Varix - *continued*
 |spleen, splenic (vein) (with phlebolith) I86.8
 |stomach I86.4
 |sublingual I86.0
 |ulcerated I83.009
  |inflamed or infected I83.209
 |uterine ligament I86.2
 |vagina I86.8
 |vocal cord I86.8
 |vulva I86.3
Vas deferens *see* condition
Vas deferentitis N49.1
Vasa previa O69.4
 |hemorrhage from, affecting newborn P50.0
Vascular *see also* condition
 |loop on optic papilla Q14.2
 |spasm I73.9
 |spider I78.1
Vascularization, cornea *see*
  Neovascularization, cornea
Vasculitis I77.6
 |allergic D69.0
 |cryoglobulinemic D89.1
 |disseminated I77.6
 |hypocomplementemic M31.8
 |kidney I77.89
 |leukocytoclastic M31.0
 |livedoid L95.0
 |nodular L95.8
 |retina H35.06-
 |rheumatic *see* Fever, rheumatic
 |rheumatoid *see* Rheumatoid, vasculitis
 |skin (limited to) L95.9
  |specified NEC L95.8
 |systemic M31.8
Vasculopathy, necrotizing M31.9
 |cardiac allograft T86.290
 |specified NEC M31.8
Vasitis (nodosa) N49.1
 |tuberculous A18.15
Vasodilation I73.9
Vasomotor *see* condition
Vasoplasty, after previous sterilization Z31.0
 |aftercare Z31.42
Vasospasm (vasoconstriction) I73.9
 |cerebral (cerebrovascular) (artery) I67.848
  |reversible I67.841
 |coronary I20.1
 |nerve
  |arm *see* Mononeuropathy, upper limb
  |brachial plexus G54.0
  |cervical plexus G54.2
  |leg *see* Mononeuropathy, lower limb
 |peripheral NOS I73.9
 |retina (artery) *see* Occlusion, artery, retina
Vasospastic *see* condition
Vasovagal attack (paroxysmal) R55
 |psychogenic F45.8
VATER syndrome Q87.2
Vater's ampulla *see* condition
Vegetation, vegetative
 |adenoid (nasal fossa) J35.8
 |endocarditis (acute) (any valve) (subacute)
  I33.0
 |heart (mycotic) (valve) I33.0
Veil
 |Jackson's Q43.3
Vein, venous *see* condition
Veldt sore *see* Ulcer, skin
Velpeau's hernia *see* Hernia, femoral
Venereal
 |bubo A55
 |disease A64
 |granuloma inguinale A58
 |lymphogranuloma (Durand-Nicolas-Favre)
  A55

Venofibrosis I87.8
Venom, venomous *see* Table of Drugs and
  Chemicals, by animal or substance,
  poisoning
Venous *see* condition
Ventilator lung, newborn P27.8
Ventral *see* condition
Ventricle, ventricular *see also* condition
 |escape I49.3
 |inversion Q20.5
Ventriculitis (cerebral) *see also* Encephalitis
  G04.90
Ventriculostomy status Z98.2
Vernet's syndrome G52.7
Verneuil's disease (syphilitic bursitis) A52.78
Verruca (due to HPV) (filiformis) (simplex)
  (viral) (vulgaris) B07.9
 |acuminata A63.0
 |necrogenica (primary) (tuberculosa) A18.4
 |plana B07.8
 |plantaris B07.0
 |seborrheica L82.1
  |inflamed L82.0
 |senile (seborrheic) L82.1
  |inflamed L82.0
 |tuberculosa (primary) A18.4
 |venereal A63.0
Verrucosities *see* Verruca
Verruga peruana, peruviana A44.1
Version
 |cervix *see* Malposition, uterus
 |uterus (postinfectional) (postpartal, old) *see*
  Malposition, uterus
Vertebra, vertebral *see* condition
Vertical talus (congenital) Q66.80
 |left foot Q66.82
 |right foot Q66.81
Vertigo R42
 |auditory *see* Vertigo, aural
 |aural H81.31-
 |benign paroxysmal (positional) H81.1-
 |central (origin) H81.4-
 |cerebral H81.4-
 |Dix and Hallpike (epidemic) *see* Neuronitis,
  vestibular
 |due to infrasound T75.23
 |epidemic A88.1
  |Dix and Hallpike *see* Neuronitis, vestibular
  |Pedersen's *see* Neuronitis, vestibular
  |vestibular neuronitis *see* Neuronitis,
   vestibular
 |hysterical F44.89
 |infrasound T75.23
 |labyrinthine *see* subcategory H81.0
 |laryngeal R05.4
 |malignant positional H81.4-
 |Ménière's *see* subcategory H81.0
 |menopausal N95.1
 |otogenic *see* Vertigo, aural
 |paroxysmal positional, benign *see* Vertigo,
  benign paroxysmal
 |Pedersen's (epidemic) *see* Neuronitis,
  vestibular
 |peripheral NEC H81.39-
 |positional
  |benign paroxysmal *see* Vertigo, benign
   paroxysmal
  |malignant H81.4-
Very-Low-Density-Lipoprotein-Type (VLDL)
  hyperlipoproteinemia E78.1
Vesania *see* Psychosis
Vesical *see* condition
Vesicle
 |cutaneous R23.8
 |seminal *see* condition
 |skin R23.8

Vesicocolic *see* condition
Vesicoperineal *see* condition
Vesicorectal *see* condition
Vesicourethrorectal *see* condition
Vesicovaginal *see* condition
Vesicular *see* condition
Vesiculitis (seminal) N49.0
 |amebic A06.82
 |gonorrheal (acute) (chronic) A54.23
 |trichomonal A59.09
 |tuberculous A18.15
Vestibulitis (ear) *see also* subcategory H83.0
 |nose (external) J34.89
 |vulvar N94.810
Vestibulopathy , acute peripheral (recurrent)
  see Neuronitis, vestibular
Vestige, vestigial *see also* Persistence
 |branchial Q18.0
 |structures in vitreous Q14.0
Vibration
 |adverse effects T75.20
  |pneumatic hammer syndrome T75.21
  |specified effect NEC T75.29
  |vasospastic syndrome T75.22
  |vertigo from infrasound T75.23
 |exposure (occupational) Z57.7
 |vertigo T75.23
Vibriosis A28.9
Victim (of)
 |crime Z65.4
 |disaster Z65.5
 |terrorism Z65.4
 |torture Z65.4
 |war Z65.5
Vidal's disease L28.0
Villaret's syndrome G52.7
Villous *see* condition
VIN *see* Neoplasia, intraepithelial, vulva
Vincent's infection (angina) (gingivitis) A69.1
 |stomatitis NEC A69.1
Vinson-Plummer syndrome D50.1
Violence, physical R45.6
Viosterol deficiency *see* Deficiency, calciferol
Vipoma *see* Neoplasm, malignant, by site
Viremia B34.9
Virilism (adrenal) E25.9
 |congenital E25.0
Virilization (female) (suprarenal) E25.9
 |congenital E25.0
 |isosexual E28.2
Virulent bubo A57
Virus, viral *see also* condition
 |as cause of disease classified elsewhere
  B97.89
   |respiratory syncytial virus (RSV) - *see*
    Virus, respiratory syncytial (RSV)
 |cytomegalovirus B25.9
 |human immunodeficiency (HIV) *see* Human,
  immunodeficiency virus (HIV) disease
 |infection *see* Infection, virus
 |specified NEC B34.8
 |swine influenza (viruses that normally cause
  infections in pigs) *see also* Influenza, due to,
  identified novel influenza A virus J09.X2
 |West Nile (fever) A92.30
  |with
   |complications NEC A92.39
   |cranial nerve disorders A92.32
   |encephalitis A92.31
   |encephalomyelitis A92.31
   |neurologic manifestation NEC A92.32
   |optic neuritis A92.32
   |polyradiculitis A92.32
Viscera, visceral *see* condition

Visceroptosis K63.4
Visible peristalsis R19.2
Vision, visual
|binocular, suppression H53.34
|blurred, blurring H53.8
  |hysterical F44.6
|defect, defective NEC H54.7
|disorientation (syndrome) H53.8
|disturbance H53.9
  |hysterical F44.6
|double H53.2
|examination Z01.00
  |with abnormal findings Z01.01
|field, limitation (defect) *see* Defect, visual
  field
|hallucinations R44.1
|halos H53.19
|loss *see* Loss, vision
  |sudden *see* Disturbance, vision, subjective,
  loss, sudden
|low (both eyes) *see* Low, vision
|perception, simultaneous without fusion
  H53.33
Vitality, lack or want of R53.83
|newborn P96.89
Vitamin deficiency *see* Deficiency, vitamin
Vitelline duct, persistent Q43.0
Vitiligo L80
|eyelid H02.739
  |left H02.736
    |lower H02.735
    |upper H02.734
  |right H02.733
    |lower H02.732
    |upper H02.731
|pinta A67.2
|vulva N90.89
Vitreal corneal syndrome H59.01-
Vitreoretinopathy, proliferative *see also*
  Retinopathy, proliferative
|with retinal detachment *see* Detachment,
  retina, traction
Vitreous *see also* condition
|touch syndrome *see* Complication,
  postprocedural, following cataract surgery
Vocal cord *see* condition
Vogt-Koyanagi syndrome H20.82-
Vogt's disease or syndrome G80.3
Vogt-Spielmeyer amaurotic idiocy or disease
  E75.4
Voice
|change R49.9
  |specified NEC R49.8
|loss *see* Aphonia
Volhynian fever A79.0
Volkmann's ischemic contracture or paralysis
  (complicating trauma) T79.6
Volvulus (bowel) (colon) (intestine) K56.2
|with perforation K56.2
|congenital Q43.8
|duodenum K31.5
|fallopian tube *see* Torsion, fallopian tube
|oviduct *see* Torsion, fallopian tube
|stomach (due to absence of gastrocolic
  ligament) K31.89
Vomiting R11.10
|with nausea R11.2
|asphyxia *see* Foreign body, by site, causing
  asphyxia, gastric contents
|bilious (cause unknown) R11.14
  |in newborn P92.01
  |following gastro-intestinal surgery K91.0
|blood *see* Hematemesis
|causing asphyxia, choking, or suffocation *see*
  Foreign body, by site

Vomiting - *continued*
|cyclical G43.A0
  |with refractory migraine G43.A1
  |intractable G43.A1
  |not intractable G43.A0
  |psychogenic F50.89
  |without refractory migraine G43.A0
|fecal mater R11.13
|following gastrointestinal surgery K91.0
  |psychogenic F50.89
|functional K31.89
|hysterical F50.89
|nervous F50.89
|neurotic F50.89
|newborn NEC P92.09
  |bilious P92.01
|periodic R11.10
  |psychogenic F50.89
|projectile R11.12
|psychogenic F50.89
|uremic *see* Uremia
|without nausea R11.11
Vomito negro *see* Fever, yellow
Von Bezold's abscess *see* Mastoiditis, acute
Von Economo-Cruchet disease A85.8
Von Eulenburg's disease G71.19
Von Gierke's disease E74.01
Von Hippel (-Lindau) disease or syndrome
  Q85.8
Von Jaksch's anemia or disease D64.89
Von Recklinghausen
|disease (neurofibromatosis) Q85.01
  |bones E21.0
Von Schroetter's syndrome I82.890
Von Willebrand (-Jurgens)(-Minot) disease or
  syndrome D68.0
Von Zumbusch's disease L40.1
Voyeurism F65.3
Vrolik's disease Q78.0
Vulva *see* condition
Vulvismus N94.2
Vulvitis (acute) (allergic) (atrophic)
  (hypertrophic) (intertriginous) (senile)
  N76.2
|with ectopic or molar pregnancy O08.0
|adhesive, congenital Q52.79
|blennorrhagic (gonococcal) A54.02
|candidal B37.3
|chlamydial A56.02
|due to Haemophilus ducreyi A57
|following ectopic or molar pregnancy O08.0
|gonococcal A54.02
  |with abscess (accessory gland) (periurethral)
  A54.1
|herpesviral A60.04
|leukoplakic N90.4
|monilial B37.3
|puerperal (postpartum) O86.19
|subacute or chronic N76.3
|syphilitic (early) A51.0
  |late A52.76
|trichomonal A59.01
|tuberculous A18.18
Vulvodynia N94.819
|specified NEC N94.818
Vulvorectal *see* condition
Vulvovaginitis (acute) *see* Vaginitis

W

Waiting list, person on Z75.1
|for organ transplant Z76.82
|undergoing social agency investigation Z75.2
Waldenström-Kjellberg syndrome D50.1

Waldenström
|hypergammaglobulinemia D89.0
|syndrome or macroglobulinemia C88.0
Walking
|difficulty R26.2
  |psychogenic F44.4
|sleep F51.3
  |hysterical F44.89
Wall, abdominal *see* condition
Wallenberg's disease or syndrome G46.3
Wallgren's disease I87.8
Wandering
|gallbladder, congenital Q44.1
|in diseases classified elsewhere Z91.83
|kidney, congenital Q63.8
|organ or site, congenital NEC *see*
  Malposition, congenital, by site
|pacemaker (heart) I49.8
|spleen D73.89
War neurosis F48.8
Wart (due to HPV) (filiform) (infectious)
  (viral) B07.9
|anogenital region (venereal) A63.0
|common B07.8
|external genital organs (venereal) A63.0
|flat B07.8
|Hassal-Henle's (of cornea) H18.49
|Peruvian A44.1
|plantar B07.0
|prosector (tuberculous) A18.4
|seborrheic L82.1
  |inflamed L82.0
|senile (seborrheic) L82.1
  |inflamed L82.0
|tuberculous A18.4
|venereal A63.0
Warthin's tumor *see* Neoplasm, salivary gland,
  benign
Wassilieff's disease A27.0
Wasting
|disease R64
  |due to malnutrition E43
    |with marasmus E41
  |extreme (due to malnutrition) E43
    |with marasmus E41
|muscle NEC *see* Atrophy, muscle
Water
|clefts (senile cataract) *see* Cataract, senile,
  incipient
|deprivation of T73.1
|intoxication E87.79
|itch B76.9
|lack of T73.1
  |safe drinking Z58.6
|loading E87.70
|on
  |brain *see* Hydrocephalus
  |chest J94.8
|poisoning E87.79
Waterbrash R12
Waterhouse (-Friderichsen) syndrome or
  disease (meningococcal) A39.1
Water-Losing nephritis N25.89
Watermelon stomach K31.819
|with hemorrhage K31.811
|without hemorrhage K31.819
Watsoniasis B66.8
Wax in ear *see* Impaction, cerumen
Weak, weakening, weakness (generalized)
  R53.1
|arches (acquired) *see also* Deformity, limb,
  flat foot
|bladder (sphincter) R32
|facial R29.810
  |following

Weak, weakening - *continued*
|cerebrovascular disease I69.992
|cerebral infarction I69.392
|intracerebral hemorrhage I69.192
|nontraumatic intracranial hemorrhage
NEC I69.292
|specified disease NEC I69.892
|stroke I69.392
|subarachnoid hemorrhage I69.092
|foot (double) *see* Weak, arches
|heart, cardiac *see* Failure, heart
|mind F70
|muscle M62.81
|myocardium *see* Failure, heart
|newborn P96.89
|pelvic fundus N81.89
|pubocervical tissue N81.82
|senile R54
|rectovaginal tissue N81.83
|urinary stream R39.12
|valvular *see* Endocarditis
Wear, worn (with normal or routine use)
|articular bearing surface of internal joint
prosthesis *see* Complications, joint
prosthesis, mechanical, wear of articular
bearing surfaces, by site
|device, implant or graft *see* Complications, by
site, mechanical complication
|tooth, teeth (approximal) (hard tissues)
(interproximal) (occlusal) K03.0
Weather, weathered
|effects of
|cold T69.9
|specified effect NEC T69.8
|hot *see* Heat
|skin L57.8
Weaver's syndrome Q87.3
Web, webbed (congenital)
|duodenal Q43.8
|esophagus Q39.4
|fingers Q70.1-
|larynx (glottic) (subglottic) Q31.0
|neck (pterygium colli) Q18.3
|Paterson-Kelly D50.1
|popliteal syndrome Q87.89
|toes Q70.3-
Weber-Christian disease M35.6
**Weber-Cockayne syndrome (epidermolysis
bullosa)** Q81.8
Weber-Gubler syndrome G46.3
Weber-Leyden syndrome G46.3
Weber-Osler syndrome I78.0
Weber's paralysis or syndrome G46.3
Wedge-Shaped or wedging vertebra *see*
Collapse, vertebra NEC
Wegener's granulomatosis or syndrome
M31.30
|with
|kidney involvement M31.31
|lung involvement M31.30
|with kidney involvement M31.31
Wegner's disease A50.02
Weight
|1000-2499 grams at birth (low) *see* Low,
birthweight
|999 grams or less at birth (extremely low) *see*
Low, birthweight, extreme
|and length below 10th percentile for
gestational age P05.1-
|below but length above 10th percentile for
gestational age P05.0-
|gain (abnormal) (excessive) R63.5
|in pregnancy *see* Pregnancy, complicated
by, excessive weight gain
|low *see* Pregnancy, complicated by,
insufficient, weight gain
|loss (abnormal) (cause unknown) R63.4

Weightlessness (effect of) T75.82
Weil (l) -Marchesani syndrome Q87.1
Weil's disease A27.0
Weingarten's syndrome J82.89
Weir Mitchell's disease I73.81
Weiss-Baker syndrome G90.09
Wells' disease L98.3
Wen *see* Cyst, sebaceous
Wenckebach's block or phenomenon I44.1
**Werdnig-Hoffmann syndrome (muscular
atrophy)** G12.0
Werlhof's disease D69.3
Wermer's disease or syndrome E31.21
Werner-His disease A79.0
Werner's disease or syndrome E34.8
**Wernicke-Korsakoff's syndrome or psychosis
(alcoholic)** F10.96
|with dependence F10.26
|drug-induced
|due to drug abuse *see* Abuse, drug, by type,
with amnestic disorder
|due to drug dependence *see* Dependence,
drug, by type, with amnestic disorder
|nonalcoholic F04
Wernicke-Posadas disease B38.9
Wernicke's
|developmental aphasia F80.2
|disease or syndrome E51.2
|encephalopathy E51.2
|polioencephalitis, superior E51.2
West African fever B50.8
Westphal-Strumpell syndrome E83.01
West's syndrome *see* Epilepsy, spasms
Wet
|feet, tropical (maceration) (syndrome) *see*
Immersion, foot
|lung (syndrome), newborn P22.1
Wharton's duct *see* condition
Wheal *see* Urticaria
Wheezing R06.2
Whiplash injury S13.4
Whipple's disease *see also* subcategory M14.8 -
K90.81
Whipworm (disease) (infection) (infestation)
B79
Whistling face Q87.0
White *see also* condition
|kidney, small N03.9
|leg, puerperal, postpartum, childbirth O87.1
|mouth B37.0
|patches of mouth K13.29
|spot lesions, teeth
|chewing surface K02.51
|pit and fissure surface K02.51
|smooth surface K02.61
Whitehead L70.0
Whitlow *see also* Cellulitis, digit
|with lymphangitis *see* Lymphangitis, acute,
digit
|herpesviral B00.89
Whitmore's disease or fever *see* Melioidosis
Whooping cough A37.90
|with pneumonia A37.91
|due to Bordetella
|bronchiseptica A37.81
|parapertussis A37.11
|pertussis A37.01
|specified organism NEC A37.81
|due to
|Bordetella
|bronchiseptica A37.80
|with pneumonia A37.81
|parapertussis A37.10
|with pneumonia A37.11
|pertussis A37.00
|with pneumonia A37.01
|specified NEC A37.80
|with pneumonia A37.81

Wichman's asthma J38.5
Wide cranial sutures, newborn P96.3
Widening aorta *see* Ectasia, aorta
|with aneurysm *see* Aneurysm, aorta
Wilkie's disease or syndrome K55.1
Wilkinson-Sneddon disease or syndrome
L13.1
Willebrand (-Jurgens) thrombopathy D68.0
Williams syndrome Q93.82
Willige-Hunt disease or syndrome G23.1
Wilms' tumor C64-
Wilson-Mikity syndrome P27.0
Wilson's
|disease or syndrome E83.01
|hepatolenticular degeneration E83.01
|lichen ruber L43.9
Window *see also* Imperfect, closure
|aorticopulmonary Q21.4
Winter *see* condition
Wiskott-Aldrich syndrome D82.0
Withdrawal state *see also* Dependence, drug by
type, with withdrawal
|alcohol
|with perceptual disturbances F10.232
|without perceptual disturbances F10.239
|caffeine F15.93
|cannabis F12.23
|newborn
|correct therapeutic substance properly
administered P96.2
|infant of dependent mother P96.1
|therapeutic substance, neonatal P96.2
Witts' anemia D50.8
Witzelsucht F07.0
Woakes' ethmoiditis or syndrome J33.1
Wolff-Hirschorn syndrome Q93.3
Wolff-Parkinson-White syndrome I45.6
Wolhynian fever A79.0
Wolman's disease E75.5
Wood lung or pneumonitis J67.8
Woolly, wooly hair (congenital) (nevus) Q84.1
Woolsorter's disease A22.1
Word
|blindness (congenital) (developmental) F81.0
|deafness (congenital) (developmental) H93.25
Worm(s) (infection) (infestation) *see also*
Infestation, helminth
|guinea B72
|in intestine NEC B82.0
Worm-Eaten soles A66.3
Worn out *see* Exhaustion
|cardiac
|defibrillator (with synchronous cardiac
pacemaker) Z45.02
|pacemaker
|battery Z45.010
|lead Z45.018
|device, implant or graft *see* Complications, by
site, mechanical
Worried well Z71.1
Worries R45.82
Wound check Z48.0-
|due to injury code to Injury, by site, using
appropriate seventh character for
subsequent encounter
Wound, open T14.8-
|abdomen, abdominal
|wall S31.109
|with penetration into peritoneal cavity
S31.609
|bite *see* Bite, abdomen, wall
|epigastric region S31.102
|with penetration into peritoneal cavity
S31.602

WXYZ

Wound, open - *continued*
- |bite *see* Bite, abdomen, wall, epigastric region
- |laceration *see* Laceration, abdomen, wall, epigastric region
- |puncture *see* Puncture, abdomen, wall, epigastric region
- |laceration *see* Laceration, abdomen, wall
- |left
  - |lower quadrant S31.104
    - |with penetration into peritoneal cavity S31.604
    - |bite *see* Bite, abdomen, wall, left, lower quadrant
    - |laceration *see* Laceration, abdomen, wall, left, lower quadrant
    - |puncture *see* Puncture, abdomen, wall, left, lower quadrant
  - |upper quadrant S31.101
    - |with penetration into peritoneal cavity S31.601
    - |bite *see* Bite, abdomen, wall, left, upper quadrant
    - |laceration *see* Laceration, abdomen, wall, left, upper quadrant
    - |puncture *see* Puncture, abdomen, wall, left, upper quadrant
  - |periumbilic region S31.105
    - |with penetration into peritoneal cavity S31.605
    - |bite *see* Bite, abdomen, wall, periumbilic region
    - |laceration *see* Laceration, abdomen, wall, periumbilic region
    - |puncture *see* Puncture, abdomen, wall, periumbilic region
- |puncture *see* Puncture, abdomen, wall
- |right
  - |lower quadrant S31.103
    - |with penetration into peritoneal cavity S31.603
    - |bite *see* Bite, abdomen, wall, right, lower quadrant
    - |laceration *see* Laceration, abdomen, wall, right, lower quadrant
    - |puncture *see* Puncture, abdomen, wall, right, lower quadrant
  - |upper quadrant S31.100
    - |with penetration into peritoneal cavity S31.600
    - |bite *see* Bite, abdomen, wall, right, upper quadrant
    - |laceration *see* Laceration, abdomen, wall, right, upper quadrant
    - |puncture *see* Puncture, abdomen, wall, right, upper quadrant
- |alveolar (process) *see* Wound, open, oral cavity
- |ankle S91.00-
  - |bite *see* Bite, ankle
  - |laceration *see* Laceration, ankle
  - |puncture *see* Puncture, ankle
- |antecubital space *see* Wound, open, elbow
- |anterior chamber, eye *see* Wound, open, ocular
- |anus S31.839
  - |bite S31.835
  - |laceration *see* Laceration, anus
  - |puncture *see* Puncture, anus
- |arm (upper) S41.10-
  - |with amputation *see* Amputation, traumatic, arm
  - |bite *see* Bite, arm
  - |forearm *see* Wound, open, forearm
  - |laceration *see* Laceration, arm

Wound, open - *continued*
- |puncture *see* Puncture, arm
- |auditory canal (external) (meatus) *see* Wound, open, ear
- |auricle, ear *see* Wound, open, ear
- |axilla *see* Wound, open, arm
- |back *see also* Wound, open, thorax, back
  - |lower S31.000
    - |with penetration into retroperitoneal space S31.001
    - |bite *see* Bite, back, lower
    - |laceration *see* Laceration, back, lower
    - |puncture *see* Puncture, back, lower
- |bite *see* Bite
- |blood vessel *see* Injury, blood vessel
- |breast S21.00-
  - |with amputation *see* Amputation, traumatic, breast
  - |bite *see* Bite, breast
  - |laceration *see* Laceration, breast
  - |puncture *see* Puncture, breast
- |buttock S31.809
  - |bite *see* Bite, buttock
  - |laceration *see* Laceration, buttock
  - |left S31.829
  - |puncture *see* Puncture, buttock
  - |right S31.819
- |calf *see* Wound, open, leg
- |canaliculus lacrimalis *see* Wound, open, eyelid
- |canthus, eye *see* Wound, open, eyelid
- |cervical esophagus S11.20
  - |bite S11.25
  - |laceration *see* Laceration, esophagus, traumatic, cervical
  - |puncture *see* Puncture, cervical esophagus
- |cheek (external) S01.40-
  - |bite *see* Bite, cheek
  - |laceration *see* Laceration, cheek
  - |puncture *see* Puncture, cheek
  - |internal *see* Wound, open, oral cavity
  - |chest wall *see* Wound, open, thorax
- |chin *see* Wound, open, head, specified site NEC
- |choroid *see* Wound, open, ocular
- |ciliary body (eye) *see* Wound, open, ocular
- |clitoris S31.40
  - |with amputation *see* Amputation, traumatic, clitoris
  - |bite S31.45
  - |laceration *see* Laceration, vulva
  - |puncture *see* Puncture, vulva
- |conjunctiva *see* Wound, open, ocular
- |cornea *see* Wound, open, ocular
- |costal region *see* Wound, open, thorax
- |Descemet's membrane *see* Wound, open, ocular
- |digit(s)
  - |foot *see* Wound, open, toe
  - |hand *see* Wound, open, finger
- |ear (canal) (external) S01.30-
  - |with amputation *see* Amputation, traumatic, ear
  - |bite *see* Bite, ear
  - |laceration *see* Laceration, ear
  - |puncture *see* Puncture, ear
  - |drum S09.2-
- |elbow S51.00-
  - |bite *see* Bite, elbow
  - |laceration *see* Laceration, elbow
  - |puncture *see* Puncture, elbow
- |epididymis *see* Wound, open, testis
- |epigastric region S31.102
  - |with penetration into peritoneal cavity S31.602

Wound, open - *continued*
- |bite *see* Bite, abdomen, wall, epigastric region
- |laceration *see* Laceration, abdomen, wall, epigastric region
- |puncture *see* Puncture, abdomen, wall, epigastric region
- |epiglottis *see* Wound, open, neck, specified site NEC
- |esophagus (thoracic) S27.819
  - |cervical *see* Wound, open, cervical esophagus
  - |laceration S27.813
  - |specified type NEC S27.818
- |eye *see* Wound, open, ocular
- |eyeball *see* Wound, open, ocular
- |eyebrow *see* Wound, open, eyelid
- |eyelid S01.10-
  - |bite *see* Bite, eyelid
  - |laceration *see* Laceration, eyelid
  - |puncture *see* Puncture, eyelid
- |face NEC *see* Wound, open, head, specified site NEC
- |finger(s) S61.209
  - |with
    - |amputation *see* Amputation, traumatic, finger
    - |damage to nail S61.309
  - |bite *see* Bite, finger
  - |index S61.208
    - |with
      - |damage to nail S61.308
    - |left S61.201
      - |with
        - |damage to nail S61.301
    - |right S61.200
      - |with
        - |damage to nail S61.300
  - |laceration *see* Laceration, finger
  - |little S61.208
    - |with
      - |damage to nail S61.308
    - |left S61.207
      - |with damage to nail S61.307
    - |right S61.206
      - |with damage to nail S61.306
  - |middle S61.208
    - |with
      - |damage to nail S61.308
    - |left S61.203
      - |with damage to nail S61.303
    - |right S61.202
      - |with damage to nail S61.302
  - |puncture *see* Puncture, finger
  - |ring S61.208
    - |with
      - |damage to nail S61.308
    - |left S61.205
      - |with damage to nail S61.305
    - |right S61.204
      - |with damage to nail S61.304
- |flank *see* Wound, open, abdomen, wall
- |foot (except toe(s) alone) S91.30-
  - |with amputation *see* Amputation, traumatic, foot
  - |bite *see* Bite, foot
  - |laceration *see* Laceration, foot
  - |puncture *see* Puncture, foot
  - |toe *see* Wound, open, toe
- |forearm S51.80-
  - |with
    - |amputation *see* Amputation, traumatic, forearm
  - |bite *see* Bite, forearm
  - |elbow only *see* Wound, open, elbow

Wound, open - *continued*

|laceration *see* Laceration, forearm
|puncture *see* Puncture, forearm
|forehead *see* Wound, open, head, specified
site NEC
|genital organs, external
|with amputation *see* Amputation, traumatic,
genital organs
|bite *see* Bite, genital organ
|female S31.502
|vagina S31.40
|vulva S31.40
|laceration *see* Laceration, genital organ
|male S31.501
|penis S31.20
|scrotum S31.30
|testes S31.30
|puncture *see* Puncture, genital organ
|globe (eye) *see* Wound, open, ocular
|groin *see* Wound, open, abdomen, wall
|gum *see* Wound, open, oral cavity
|hand S61.40-
|with
|amputation *see* Amputation, traumatic,
hand
|bite *see* Bite, hand
|finger(s) *see* Wound, open, finger
|laceration *see* Laceration, hand
|puncture *see* Puncture, hand
|thumb *see* Wound, open, thumb
|head S01.90
|bite *see* Bite, head
|cheek *see* Wound, open, cheek
|ear *see* Wound, open, ear
|eyelid *see* Wound, open, eyelid
|laceration *see* Laceration, head
|lip *see* Wound, open, lip
|nose S01.20
|oral cavity *see* Wound, open, oral cavity
|puncture *see* Puncture, head
|scalp *see* Wound, open, scalp
|specified site NEC S01.80
|temporomandibular area *see* Wound, open,
cheek
|heel *see* Wound, open, foot
|hip S71.00-
|with amputation *see* Amputation, traumatic,
hip
|bite *see* Bite, hip
|laceration *see* Laceration, hip
|puncture *see* Puncture, hip
|hymen S31.40
|bite *see* Bite, vulva
|laceration *see* Laceration, vagina
|puncture *see* Puncture, vagina
|hypochondrium S31.109
|bite *see* Bite, hypochondrium
|laceration *see* Laceration, hypochondrium
|puncture *see* Puncture, hypochondrium
|hypogastric region S31.109
|bite *see* Bite, hypogastric region
|laceration *see* Laceration, hypogastric
region
|puncture *see* Puncture, hypogastric region
|iliac (region) *see* Wound, open, inguinal
region
|inguinal region S31.109
|bite *see* Bite, abdomen, wall, lower quadrant
|laceration *see* Laceration, inguinal region
|puncture *see* Puncture, inguinal region
|instep *see* Wound, open, foot
|interscapular region *see* Wound, open, thorax,
back
|intraocular *see* Wound, open, ocular
|iris *see* Wound, open, ocular

Wound, open - *continued*

|jaw *see* Wound, open, head, specified site
NEC
|knee S81.00-
|bite *see* Bite, knee
|laceration *see* Laceration, knee
|puncture *see* Puncture, knee
|labium (majus) (minus) *see* Wound, open,
vulva
|laceration *see* Laceration, by site
|lacrimal duct *see* Wound, open, eyelid
|larynx S11.019
|bite *see* Bite, larynx
|laceration *see* Laceration, larynx
|puncture *see* Puncture, larynx
|left
|lower quadrant S31.104
|with penetration into peritoneal cavity
S31.604
|bite *see* Bite, abdomen, wall, left, lower
quadrant
|laceration *see* Laceration, abdomen, wall,
left, lower quadrant
|puncture *see* Puncture, abdomen, wall,
left, lower quadrant
|upper quadrant S31.101
|with penetration into peritoneal cavity
S31.601
|bite *see* Bite, abdomen, wall, left, upper
quadrant
|laceration *see* Laceration, abdomen, wall,
left, upper quadrant
|puncture *see* Puncture, abdomen, wall,
left, upper quadrant
|leg (lower) S81.80-
|with amputation *see* Amputation, traumatic,
leg
|ankle *see* Wound, open, ankle
|bite *see* Bite, leg
|foot *see* Wound, open, foot
|knee *see* Wound, open, knee
|laceration *see* Laceration, leg
|puncture *see* Puncture, leg
|toe *see* Wound, open, toe
|upper *see* Wound, open, thigh
|lip S01.501
|bite *see* Bite, lip
|laceration *see* Laceration, lip
|puncture *see* Puncture, lip
|loin S31.109
|bite *see* Bite, abdomen, wall
|laceration *see* Laceration, loin
|puncture *see* Puncture, loin
|lower back *see* Wound, open, back, lower
|lumbar region *see* Wound, open, back, lower
|malar region *see* Wound, open, head, specified
site NEC
|mammary *see* Wound, open, breast
|mastoid region *see* Wound, open, head,
specified site NEC
|mouth *see* Wound, open, oral cavity
|nail
|finger *see* Wound, open, finger, with
damage to nail
|toe *see* Wound, open, toe, with damage to
nail
|nape (neck) *see* Wound, open, neck
|nasal (septum) (sinus) *see* Wound, open, nose
|nasopharynx *see* Wound, open, head,
specified site NEC
|neck S11.90
|bite *see* Bite, neck
|involving
|cervical esophagus S11.20
|larynx *see* Wound, open, larynx

Wound, open - *continued*

|pharynx S11.20
|thyroid S11.10
|trachea (cervical) S11.029
|bite *see* Bite, trachea
|laceration S11.021
|with foreign body S11.022
|puncture S11.023
|with foreign body S11.024
|laceration *see* Laceration, neck
|puncture *see* Puncture, neck
|specified site NEC S11.80
|specified type NEC S11.89
|nose (septum) (sinus) S01.20
|with amputation *see* Amputation, traumatic,
nose
|bite *see* Bite, nose
|laceration *see* Laceration, nose
|puncture *see* Puncture, nose
|ocular S05.90
|avulsion (traumatic enucleation) S05.7-
|eyeball S05.6-
|with foreign body S05.5-
|eyelid *see* Wound, open, eyelid
|laceration and rupture S05.3-
|with prolapse or loss of intraocular tissue
S05.2-
|orbit (penetrating) (with or without foreign
body) S05.4-
|periocular area *see* Wound, open, eyelid
|specified NEC S05.8X
|oral cavity S01.502
|bite S01.552
|laceration *see* Laceration, oral cavity
|puncture *see* Puncture, oral cavity
|orbit *see* Wound, open, ocular, orbit
|palate *see* Wound, open, oral cavity
|palm *see* Wound, open, hand
|pelvis, pelvic *see also* Wound, open, back,
lower
|girdle *see* Wound, open, hip
|penetrating *see* Puncture, by site
|penis S31.20
|with amputation *see* Amputation, traumatic,
penis
|bite S31.25
|laceration *see* Laceration, penis
|puncture *see* Puncture, penis
|perineum
|bite *see* Bite, perineum
|female S31.502
|laceration *see* Laceration, perineum
|male S31.501
|puncture *see* Puncture, perineum
|periocular area (with or without lacrimal
passages) *see* Wound, open, eyelid
|periumbilic region S31.105
|with penetration into peritoneal cavity
S31.605
|bite *see* Bite, abdomen, wall, periumbilic
region
|laceration *see* Laceration, abdomen, wall,
periumbilic region
|puncture *see* Puncture, abdomen, wall,
periumbilic region
|phalanges
|finger *see* Wound, open, finger
|toe *see* Wound, open, toe
|pharynx S11.20
|pinna *see* Wound, open, ear
|popliteal space *see* Wound, open, knee
|prepuce *see* Wound, open, penis
|pubic region *see* Wound, open, back, lower
|pudendum *see* Wound, open, genital organs,
external

Wound, open - *continued*
|puncture wound *see* Puncture
|rectovaginal septum *see* Wound, open, vagina
|right
  |lower quadrant S31.103
    |with penetration into peritoneal cavity
      S31.603
    |bite *see* Bite, abdomen, wall, right, lower
      quadrant
    |laceration *see* Laceration, abdomen, wall,
      right, lower quadrant
    |puncture *see* Puncture, abdomen, wall,
      right, lower quadrant
  |upper quadrant S31.100
    |with penetration into peritoneal cavity
      S31.600
    |bite *see* Bite, abdomen, wall, right, upper
      quadrant
    |laceration *see* Laceration, abdomen, wall,
      right, upper quadrant
    |puncture *see* Puncture, abdomen, wall,
      right, upper quadrant
|sacral region *see* Wound, open, back, lower
|sacroiliac region *see* Wound, open, back,
  lower
|salivary gland *see* Wound, open, oral cavity
|scalp S01.00
  |bite S01.05
  |laceration *see* Laceration, scalp
  |puncture *see* Puncture, scalp
|scalpel, newborn (birth injury) P15.8
|scapular region *see* Wound, open, shoulder
|sclera *see* Wound, open, ocular
|scrotum S31.30
  |with amputation *see* Amputation, traumatic,
    scrotum
  |bite S31.35
  |laceration *see* Laceration, scrotum
  |puncture *see* Puncture, scrotum
|shin *see* Wound, open, leg
|shoulder S41.00-
  |with amputation *see* Amputation, traumatic,
    arm
  |bite *see* Bite, shoulder
  |laceration *see* Laceration, shoulder
  |puncture *see* Puncture, shoulder
|skin NOS T14.8
|spermatic cord *see* Wound, open, testis
|sternal region *see* Wound, open, thorax, front
  wall
|submaxillary region *see* Wound, open, head,
  specified site NEC
|submental region *see* Wound, open, head,
  specified site NEC
|subungual
  |finger(s) *see* Wound, open, finger
  |toe(s) *see* Wound, open, toe
|supraclavicular region *see* Wound, open, neck,
  specified site NEC
|temple, temporal region *see* Wound, open,
  head, specified site NEC
|temporomandibular area *see* Wound, open,
  cheek
|testis S31.30
  |with amputation *see* Amputation, traumatic,
    testes
  |bite S31.35
  |laceration *see* Laceration, testis
  |puncture *see* Puncture, testis
|thigh S71.10-
  |with amputation *see* Amputation, traumatic,
    hip
  |bite *see* Bite, thigh
  |laceration *see* Laceration, thigh
  |puncture *see* Puncture, thigh

Wound, open - *continued*
|thorax, thoracic (wall) S21.90
  |back S21.20-
    |with penetration S21.40
  |bite *see* Bite, thorax
  |breast *see* Wound, open, breast
  |front S21.10-
    |with penetration S21.30
  |laceration *see* Laceration, thorax
  |puncture *see* Puncture, thorax
|throat *see* Wound, open, neck
|thumb S61.009
  |with
    |amputation *see* Amputation, traumatic,
      thumb
    |damage to nail S61.109
  |bite *see* Bite, thumb
  |laceration *see* Laceration, thumb
  |left S61.002
    |with
      |damage to nail S61.102
  |puncture *see* Puncture, thumb
  |right S61.001
    |with
      |damage to nail S61.101
|thyroid (gland) *see* Wound, open, neck,
  thyroid
|toe(s) S91.109
  |with
    |amputation *see* Amputation, traumatic, toe
    |damage to nail S91.209
  |bite *see* Bite, toe
  |great S91.103
    |with
      |damage to nail S91.203
    |left S91.102
      |with
        |damage to nail S91.202
    |right S91.101
      |with
        |damage to nail S91.201
  |laceration *see* Laceration, toe
  |lesser S91.106
    |with
      |damage to nail S91.206
    |left S91.105
      |with
        |damage to nail S91.205
    |right S91.104
      |with
        |damage to nail S91.204
  |puncture *see* Puncture, toe
|tongue *see* Wound, open, oral cavity
|trachea (cervical region) *see* Wound, open,
  neck, trachea
|tunica vaginalis *see* Wound, open, testis
|tympanum, tympanic membrane S09.2-
  |laceration *see* Laceration, ear, drum
  |puncture *see* Puncture, tympanum
|umbilical region *see* Wound, open, abdomen,
  wall, periumbilic region
|uvula *see* Wound, open, oral cavity
|vagina S31.40
  |bite S31.45
  |laceration *see* Laceration, vagina
  |puncture *see* Puncture, vagina
|vocal cord S11.039
  |bite *see* Bite, vocal cord
  |laceration S11.031
    |with foreign body S11.032
  |puncture S11.033
    |with foreign body S11.034
|vitreous (humor) *see* Wound, open, ocular
|vulva S31.40

Wound, open - *continued*
  |with amputation *see* Amputation, traumatic,
    vulva
  |bite S31.45
  |laceration *see* Laceration, vulva
  |puncture *see* Puncture, vulva
|wrist S61.50-
  |bite *see* Bite, wrist
  |laceration *see* Laceration, wrist
  |puncture *see* Puncture, wrist
Wound, superficial *see* Injury *see also* specified
  injury type
Wright's syndrome G54.0
Wrist *see* condition
Wrong drug (by accident) (given in error) *see*
  Table of Drugs and Chemicals, by drug,
  poisoning
Wry neck *see* Torticollis
Wuchereria (bancrofti) infestation B74.0
Wuchereriasis B74.0
Wuchernde Struma Langhans C73

X

Xanthelasma (eyelid) (palpebrarum) H02.60
  |left H02.66
    |lower H02.65
    |upper H02.64
  |right H02.63
    |lower H02.62
    |upper H02.61
Xanthelasmatosis (essential) E78.2
Xanthinuria, hereditary E79.8
Xanthoastrocytoma
  |specified site *see* Neoplasm, malignant, by site
  |unspecified site C71.9
Xanthofibroma *see* Neoplasm, connective
  tissue, benign
Xanthogranuloma D76.3
Xanthoma(s), xanthomatosis (primary)
  (familial) (hereditary) E75.5
  |with
    |hyperlipoproteinemia
      |Type I E78.3
      |Type III E78.2
      |Type IV E78.1
      |Type V E78.3
  |bone (generalisata) C96.5
  |cerebrotendinous E75.5
  |cutaneotendinous E75.5
  |disseminatum (skin) E78.2
  |eruptive E78.2
  |hypercholesterinemic E78.00
  |hypercholesterolemic E78.00
  |hyperlipidemic E78.5
  |joint E75.5
  |multiple (skin) E78.2
  |tendon (sheath) E75.5
  |tubo-eruptive E78.2
  |tuberosum E78.2
  |tuberous E78.2
  |verrucous, oral mucosa K13.4
Xanthosis R23.8
Xenophobia F40.10
Xeroderma *see also* Ichthyosis
  |acquired L85.0
  |eyelid H01.149
    |left H01.146
      |lower H01.145
      |upper H01.144
    |right H01.143
      |lower H01.142
      |upper H01.141
  |pigmentosum Q82.1
  |vitamin A deficiency E50.8
Xerophthalmia (vitamin A deficiency) E50.7
  |unrelated to vitamin A deficiency *see*
    Keratoconjunctivitis

Xerosis
|conjunctiva H11.14-
  |with Bitot's spots *see also* Pigmentation,
    conjunctiva
    |vitamin A deficiency E50.1
  |vitamin A deficiency E50.0
|cornea H18.89-
  |with ulceration *see* Ulcer, cornea
    |vitamin A deficiency E50.3
  |vitamin A deficiency E50.2
|cutis (dry skin) L85.3
|skin L85.3
Xerostomia K11.7
Xiphopagus Q89.4
XO syndrome Q96.9
X-Ray (of)
|abnormal findings *see* Abnormal, diagnostic
  imaging
|breast (mammogram) (routine) Z12.31
|chest
  |routine (as part of a general medical
    examination) Z00.00
    |with abnormal findings Z00.01
  |routine (as part of a general medical
    examination) Z00.00
    |with abnormal findings Z00.01
XXXXY syndrome Q98.1
XXY syndrome Q98.0

Y

Yaba pox (virus disease) B08.72
Yatapoxvirus B08.70
|specified NEC B08.79
Yawning R06.89
|psychogenic F45.8
Yaws A66.9
|bone lesions A66.6
|butter A66.1
|chancre A66.0
|cutaneous, less than five years after infection
  A66.2
|early (cutaneous) (macular) (maculopapular)
  (micropapular) (papular) A66.2
  |frambeside A66.2
  |skin lesions NEC A66.2
|eyelid A66.2
|ganglion A66.6
|gangosis, gangosa A66.5
|gumma, gummata A66.4
  |bone A66.6
|gummatous
  |frambeside A66.4
  |osteitis A66.6
  |periostitis A66.6
|hydrarthrosis *see also* subcategory M14.8
  A66.6
|hyperkeratosis (early) (late) A66.3
|initial lesions A66.0
|joint lesions *see also* subcategory M14.8 -
  A66.6
|juxta-articular nodules A66.7
|late nodular (ulcerated) A66.4
|latent (without clinical manifestations) (with
  positive serology) A66.8
|mother A66.0
|mucosal A66.7
|multiple papillomata A66.1
|nodular, late (ulcerated) A66.4
|osteitis A66.6
|papilloma, plantar or palmar A66.1
|periostitis (hypertrophic) A66.6
|specified NEC A66.7
|ulcers A66.4
|wet crab A66.1

Yeast infection *see also* Candidiasis B37.9
Yellow
|atrophy (liver) *see* Failure, hepatic
|fever *see* Fever, yellow
|jack *see* Fever, yellow
|jaundice *see* Jaundice
|nail syndrome L60.5
Yersiniosis *see also* Infection, Yersinia
|extraintestinal A28.2
|intestinal A04.6

Z

Zahorsky's syndrome (herpangina) B08.5
Zellweger's syndrome Q87.89
Zenker's diverticulum (esophagus) K22.5
Ziehen-Oppenheim disease G24.1
Zieve's syndrome K70.0
Zika NOS A92.5
|congenital P35.4
Zinc
|deficiency, dietary E60
|metabolism disorder E83.2
Zollinger-Ellison syndrome E16.4
Zona *see* Herpes, zoster
Zoophobia F40.218
Zoster (herpes) *see* Herpes, zoster
Zygomycosis B46.9
|specified NEC B46.8
Zymotic *see* condition

Neoplasm Table

The list below gives the code numbers for neoplasms by anatomical site. For each site there are six possible code numbers according to whether the neoplasm in question is malignant, benign, in situ, of uncertain behavior, or of unspecified nature. The description of the neoplasm will often indicate which of the six columns is appropriate; e.g., malignant melanoma of skin, benign fibroadenoma of breast, carcinoma in situ of cervix uteri.

Where such descriptors are not present, the remainder of the Index should be consulted where guidance is given to the appropriate column for each morphological (histological) variety listed; e.g., Mesonephroma -see Neoplasm, malignant; Embryoma -see also Neoplasm, uncertain behavior; Disease, Bowen's -see Neoplasm, skin, in situ. However, the guidance in the Index can be overridden if one of the descriptors mentioned above is present; e.g., malignant adenoma of colon is coded to C18.9 and not to D12.6 as the adjective 'malignant' overrides the Index entry 'Adenoma - see also Neoplasm, benign.'

Codes listed with a dash (-) following the code have a required additional character for laterality. The Tabular List must be reviewed for the complete code.

	Malignant Primary	Malignant Secondary	CA in Situ	Benign	Uncertain Behavior	Unspecified Behavior
Neoplasm, neoplastic	C80.1	C79.9	D09.9	D36.9	D48.9	D49.9
- abdomen, abdominal	C76.2	C79.8-	D09.8	D36.7	D48.7	D49.89
- - cavity	C76.2	C79.8-	D09.8	D36.7	D48.7	D49.89
- - organ	C76.2	C79.8-	D09.8	D36.7	D48.7	D49.89
- - viscera	C76.2	C79.8-	D09.8	D36.7	D48.7	D49.89
- - wall—*see also Neoplasm, abdomen, wall, skin*	C44.509	C79.2-	D04.5	D23.5	D48.5	D49.2
- - - connective tissue	C49.4	C79.8-	-	D21.4	D48.1	D49.2
- - - skin	C44.509					
- - - - basal cell carcinoma	C44.519	-	-	-	-	-
- - - - specified type NEC	C44.599	-	-	-	-	-
- - - - squamous cell carcinoma	C44.529	-	-	-	-	-
- abdominopelvic	C76.8	C79.8-		D36.7	D48.7	D49.89
- accessory sinus—*see Neoplasm, sinus*						
- acoustic nerve	C72.4-	C79.49	-	D33.3	D43.3	D49.7
- adenoid (pharynx) (tissue)	C11.1	C79.89	D00.08	D10.6	D37.05	D49.0
- adipose tissue—*see also Neoplasm, connective tissue*	C49.4	C79.89	-	D21.9	D48.1	D49.2
- adnexa (uterine)	C57.4	C79.89	D07.39	D28.7	D39.8	D49.59
- adrenal	C74.9-	C79.7-	D09.3	D35.0-	D44.1-	D49.7
- - capsule	C74.9-	C79.7-	D09.3	D35.0-	D44.1-	D49.7
- - cortex	C74.0-	C79.7-	D09.3	D35.0-	D44.1-	D49.7
- - gland	C74.9-	C79.7-	D09.3	D35.0-	D44.1-	D49.7
- - medulla	C74.1-	C79.7-	D09.3	D35.0-	D44.1-	D49.7
- ala nasi (external)—*see also Neoplasm, skin, nose*	C44.301	C79.2	D04.39	D23.39	D48.5	D49.2
- alimentary canal or tract NEC	C26.9	C78.80	D01.9	D13.9	D37.9	D49.0
- alveolar	C03.9	C79.89	D00.03	D10.39	D37.09	D49.0
- - mucosa	C03.9	C79.89	D00.03	D10.39	D37.09	D49.0
- - - lower	C03.1	C79.89	D00.03	D10.39	D37.09	D49.0
- - - upper	C03.0	C79.89	D00.03	D10.39	D37.09	D49.0
- - ridge or process	C41.1	C79.51	-	D16.5-	D48.0	D49.2
- - - carcinoma	C03.9	C79.8-	-	-	-	-
- - - - lower	C03.1	C79.8-	-	-	-	-
- - - - upper	C03.0	C79.8-	-	-	-	-
- - - lower	C41.1	C79.51	-	D16.5-	D48.0	D49.2
- - - mucosa	C03.9	C79.89	D00.03	D10.39	D37.09	D49.0
- - - - lower	C03.1	C79.89	D00.03	D10.39	D37.09	D49.0
- - - - upper	C03.0	C79.89	D00.03	D10.39	D37.09	D49.0
- - - upper	C41.0	C79.51	-	D16.4-	D48.0	D49.2
- - sulcus	C06.1	C79.89	D00.02	D10.39	D37.09	D49.0
- alveolus	C03.9	C79.89	D00.03	D10.39	D37.09	D49.0
- - lower	C03.1	C79.89	D00.03	D10.39	D37.09	D49.0
- - upper	C03.0	C79.89	D00.03	D10.39	D37.09	D49.0
- ampulla of Vater	C24.1	C78.89	D01.5	D13.5	D37.6	D49.0
- ankle NEC	C76.5-	C79.89	D04.7-	D36.7	D48.7	D49.89
- anorectum, anorectal (junction)	C21.8	C78.5	D01.3	D12.9	D37.8	D49.0
- antecubital fossa or space	C76.4-	C79.89	D04.6-	D36.7	D48.7	D49.89
- antrum (Highmore) (maxillary)	C31.0	C78.39	D02.3	D14.0	D38.5	D49.1
- - pyloric	C16.3	C78.89	D00.2	D13.1	D37.1	D49.0
- - tympanicum	C30.1	C78.39	D02.3	D14.0	D38.5	D49.1
- anus, anal	C21.0	C78.5	D01.3	D12.9	D37.8	D49.0
- - canal	C21.1	C78.5	D01.3	D12.9	D37.8	D49.0
- - cloacogenic zone	C21.2	C78.5	D01.3	D12.9	D37.8	D49.0
- - margin—*see also Neoplasm, anus, skin*	C44.500	C79.2	D04.5	D23.5	D48.5	D49.2

	Malignant Primary	Malignant Secondary	CA in Situ	Benign	Uncertain Behavior	Unspecified Behavior
- - overlapping lesion with rectosigmoid junction or rectum	C21.8	-	-	-	-	-
- - skin	C44.500	C79.2	D04.5	D23.5	D48.5	D49.2
- - - basal cell carcinoma	C44.510	-	-	-	-	-
- - - specified type NEC	C44.590	-	-	-	-	-
- - - squamous cell carcinoma	C44.520	-	-	-	-	-
- - sphincter	C21.1	C78.5	D01.3	D12.9	D37.8	D49.0
- aorta (thoracic)	C49.3	C79.89	-	D21.3	D48.1	D49.2
- - abdominal	C49.4	C79.89	-	D21.4	D48.1	D49.2
- aortic body	C75.5	C79.89	-	D35.6	D44.7	D49.7
- aponeurosis	C49.9	C79.89	-	D21.9	D48.1	D49.2
- - palmar	C49.1-	C79.89	-	D21.1-	D48.1	D49.2
- - plantar	C49.2-	C79.89	-	D21.2-	D48.1	D49.2
- appendix	C18.1	C78.5	D01.0	D12.1	D37.3	D49.0
- arachnoid	C70.9	C79.49	-	D32.9	D42.9	D49.7
- - cerebral	C70.0	C79.32	-	D32.0	D42.0	D49.7
- - spinal	C70.1	C79.49	-	D32.1	D42.1	D49.7
- areola	C50.0-	C79.81	D05.-	D24.-	D48.6-	D49.3
- arm NEC	C76.4-	C79.89	D04.6-	D36.7	D48.7	D49.89
- artery—*see Neoplasm, connective tissue*						
- aryepiglottic fold	C13.1	C79.89	D00.08	D10.7	D37.05	D49.0
- - hypopharyngeal aspect	C13.1	C79.89	D00.08	D10.7	D37.05	D49.0
- - laryngeal aspect	C32.1	C78.39	D02.0	D14.1	D38.0	D49.1
- - marginal zone	C13.1	C79.89	D00.08	D10.7	D37.05	D49.0
- arytenoid (cartilage)	C32.3	C78.39	D02.0	D14.1	D38.0	D49.1
- - fold—*see Neoplasm, aryepiglottic*						
- associated with transplanted organ	C80.2	-	-	-	-	-
- atlas	C41.2	C79.51	-	D16.6	D48.0	D49.2
- atrium, cardiac	C38.0	C79.89	-	D15.1	D48.7	D49.89
- auditory						
- - canal (external) (skin)	C44.20-	C79.2	D04.2-	D23.2-	D48.5	D49.2
- - - internal	C30.1	C78.39	D02.3	D14.0	D38.5	D49.1
- - nerve	C72.4-	C79.49	-	D33.3	D43.3	D49.7
- - tube	C30.1	C78.39	D02.3	D14.0	D38.5	D49.1
- - - opening	C11.2	C79.89	D00.08	D10.6	D37.05	D49.0
- auricle, ear—*see also Neoplasm, skin, ear*	C44.20-	C79.2	D04.2-	D23.2-	D48.5	D49.2
- auricular canal (external)—*see also Neoplasm, skin, ear*	C44.20-	C79.2	D04.2-	D23.2-	D48.5	D49.2
- - internal	C30.1	C78.39	D02.3	D14.0	D38.5	D49.2
- autonomic nerve or nervous system NEC (see Neoplasm, nerve, peripheral)						
- axilla, axillary	C76.1	C79.89	D09.8	D36.7	D48.7	D49.89
- - fold—*see also Neoplasm, skin, trunk*	C44.509	C79.2	D04.5	D23.5	D48.5	D49.2
- back NEC	C76.8	C79.89	D04.5	D36.7	D48.7	D49.89
- Bartholin's gland	C51.0	C79.82	D07.1	D28.0	D39.8	D49.59
- basal ganglia	C71.0	C79.31	-	D33.0	D43.0	D49.6
- basis pedunculi	C71.7	C79.31	-	D33.1	D43.1	D49.6
- bile or biliary (tract)	C24.9	C78.89	D01.5	D13.5	D37.6	D49.0
- - canaliculi (biliferi) (intrahepatic)	C22.1	C78.7	D01.5	D13.4	D37.6	D49.0
- - canals, interlobular	C22.1	C78.89	D01.5	D13.4	D37.6	D49.0
- - duct or passage (common) (cystic) (extrahepatic)	C24.0	C78.89	D01.5	D13.5	D37.6	D49.0
- - - interlobular	C22.1	C78.89	D01.5	D13.4	D37.6	D49.0
- - - intrahepatic	C22.1	C78.7	D01.5	D13.4	D37.6	D49.0
- - - - and extrahepatic	C24.8	C78.89	D01.5	D13.5	D37.6	D49.0
- bladder (urinary)	C67.9	C79.11	D09.0	D30.3	D41.4	D49.4
- - dome	C67.1	C79.11	D09.0	D30.3	D41.4	D49.4
- - neck	C67.5	C79.11	D09.0	D30.3	D41.4	D49.4
- - orifice	C67.9	C79.11	D09.0	D30.3	D41.4	D49.4
- - - ureteric	C67.6	C79.11	D09.0	D30.3	D41.4	D49.4
- - - urethral	C67.5	C79.11	D09.0	D30.3	D41.4	D49.4
- - overlapping lesion	C67.8	-	-	-	-	-
- - sphincter	C67.8	C79.11	D09.0	D30.3	D41.4	D49.4
- - trigone	C67.0	C79.11	D09.0	D30.3	D41.4	D49.4
- - urachus	C67.7	C79.11	D09.0	D30.3	D41.4	D49.4
- - wall	C67.9	C79.11	D09.0	D30.3	D41.4	D49.4
- - - anterior	C67.3	C79.11	D09.0	D30.3	D41.4	D49.4
- - - lateral	C67.2	C79.11	D09.0	D30.3	D41.4	D49.4
- - - posterior	C67.4	C79.11	D09.0	D30.3	D41.4	D49.4
- blood vessel—*see Neoplasm, connective tissue*						
- bone (periosteum)	C41.9	C79.51	-	D16.9-	D48.0	D49.2
- - acetabulum	C41.4	C79.51	-	D16.8-	D48.0	D49.2

	Malignant Primary	Malignant Secondary	CA in Situ	Benign	Uncertain Behavior	Unspecified Behavior
- - ankle	C40.3-	C79.51	-	D16.3-	-	-
- - arm NEC	C40.0-	C79.51	-	D16.0-	-	-
- - astragalus	C40.3-	C79.51	-	D16.3-	-	-
- - atlas	C41.2	C79.51	-	D16.6-	D48.0	D49.2
- - axis	C41.2	C79.51	-	D16.6-	D48.0	D49.2
- - back NEC	C41.2	C79.51	-	D16.6-	D48.0	D49.2
- - calcaneus	C40.3-	C79.51	-	D16.3-	-	-
- - calvarium	C41.0	C79.51	-	D16.4-	D48.0	D49.2
- - carpus (any)	C40.1-	C79.51	-	D16.1-	-	-
- - cartilage NEC	C41.9	C79.51	-	D16.9-	D48.0	D49.2
- - clavicle	C41.3	C79.51	-	D16.7-	D48.0	D49.2
- - clivus	C41.0	C79.51	-	D16.4-	D48.0	D49.2
- - coccygeal vertebra	C41.4	C79.51	-	D16.8-	D48.0	D49.2
- - coccyx	C41.4	C79.51	-	D16.8-	D48.0	D49.2
- - costal cartilage	C41.3	C79.51	-	D16.7-	D48.0	D49.2
- - costovertebral joint	C41.3	C79.51	-	D16.7-	D48.0	D49.2
- - cranial	C41.0	C79.51	-	D16.4-	D48.0	D49.2
- - cuboid	C40.3-	C79.51	-	D16.3-	-	-
- - cuneiform	C41.9	C79.51	-	D16.9-	D48.0	D49.2
- - elbow	C40.0-	C79.51	-	D16.0-	-	-
- - ethmoid (labyrinth)	C41.0	C79.51	-	D16.4-	D48.0	D49.2
- - face	C41.0	C79.51	-	D16.4-	D48.0	D49.2
- - femur (any part)	C40.2-	C79.51	-	D16.2-	-	-
- - fibula (any part)	C40.2-	C79.51	-	D16.2-	-	-
- - finger (any)	C40.1-	C79.51	-	D16.1-	-	-
- - foot	C40.3-	C79.51	-	D16.3-	-	-
- - forearm	C40.0-	C79.51	-	D16.0-	-	-
- - frontal	C41.0	C79.51	-	D16.4-	D48.0	D49.2
- - hand	C40.1-	C79.51	-	D16.1-	-	-
- - heel	C40.3-	C79.51	-	D16.3-	-	-
- - hip	C41.4	C79.51	-	D16.8-	D48.0	D49.2
- - humerus (any part)	C40.0-	C79.51	-	D16.0-	-	-
- - hyoid	C41.0	C79.51	-	D16.4-	D48.0	D49.2
- - ilium	C41.4	C79.51	-	D16.8-	D48.0	D49.2
- - innominate	C41.4	C79.51	-	D16.8-	D48.0	D49.2
- - intervertebral cartilage or disc	C41.2	C79.51	-	D16.6-	D48.0	D49.2
- - ischium	C41.4	C79.51	-	D16.8-	D48.0	D49.2
- - jaw (lower)	C41.1	C79.51	-	D16.5-	D48.0	D49.2
- - knee	C40.2-	C79.51	-	D16.2-	-	-
- - leg NEC	C40.2-	C79.51	-	D16.2-	-	-
- - limb NEC	C40.9-	C79.51	-	D16.9-	-	-
- - - lower (long bones)	C40.2-	C79.51	-	D16.2-	-	-
- - - - short bones	C40.3-	C79.51	-	D16.3-	-	-
- - - upper (long bones)	C40.0-	C79.51	-	D16.0-	-	-
- - - - short bones	C40.1-	C79.51	-	D16.1-	-	-
- - malar	C41.0	C79.51	-	D16.4-	D48.0	D49.2
- - mandible	C41.1	C79.51	-	D16.5-	D48.0	D49.2
- - marrow NEC (any bone)	C96.9	C79.52	-	-	D47.9	D49.89
- - mastoid	C41.0	C79.51	-	D16.4-	D48.0	D49.2
- - maxilla, maxillary (superior)	C41.0	C79.51	-	D16.4-	D48.0	D49.2
- - - inferior	C41.1	C79.51	-	D16.5-	D48.0	D49.2
- - metacarpus (any)	C40.1-	C79.51	-	D16.1-	-	-
- - metatarsus (any)	C40.3-	C79.51	-	D16.3-	-	-
- - overlapping sites	C40.8-	-	-	-	-	-
- - navicular						
- - - ankle	C40.3-	C79.51	-	-	-	-
- - - hand	C40.1-	C79.51	-	-	-	-
- - nose, nasal	C41.0	C79.51	-	D16.4-	D48.0	D49.2
- - occipital	C41.0	C79.51	-	D16.4-	D48.0	D49.2
- - orbit	C41.0	C79.51	-	D16.4-	D48.0	D49.2
- - parietal	C41.0	C79.51	-	D16.4-	D48.0	D49.2
- - patella	C40.2-	C79.51	-	-	-	-
- - pelvic	C41.4	C79.51	-	D16.8	D48.0	D49.2
- - phalanges						
- - - foot	C40.3-	C79.51	-	-	-	-
- - - hand	C40.1-	C79.51	-	-	-	-
- - pubic	C41.4	C79.51	-	D16.8	D48.0	D49.2
- - radius (any part)	C40.0-	C79.51	-	D16.0-	-	-
- - rib	C41.3	C79.51	-	D16.7	D48.0	D49.2
- - sacral vertebra	C41.4	C79.51	-	D16.8	D48.0	D49.2
- - sacrum	C41.4	C79.51	-	D16.8	D48.0	D49.2

	Malignant Primary	Malignant Secondary	CA in Situ	Benign	Uncertain Behavior	Unspecified Behavior
- - scaphoid					-	-
- - - of ankle	C40.3-	C79.51	-	-	-	-
- - - of hand	C40.1-	C79.51	-	-	-	-
- - scapula (any part)	C40.0-	C79.51	-	D16.0-	-	-
- - sella turcica	C41.0	C79.51	-	D16.4-	D48.0	D49.2
- - shoulder	C40.0-	C79.51	-	D16.0-	-	-
- - skull	C41.0	C79.51	-	D16.4-	D48.0	D49.2
- - sphenoid	C41.0	C79.51	-	D16.4-	D48.0	D49.2
- - spine, spinal (column)	C41.2	C79.51	-	D16.6	D48.0	D49.2
- - - coccyx	C41.4	C79.51	-	D16.8	D48.0	D49.2
- - - sacrum	C41.4	C79.51	-	D16.8	D48.0	D49.2
- - sternum	C41.3	C79.51	-	D16.7	D48.0	D49.2
- - tarsus (any)	C40.3-	C79.51	-	-	-	-
- - temporal	C41.0	C79.51	-	D16.4-	D48.0	D49.2
- - thumb	C40.1-	C79.51	-	-	-	-
- - tibia (any part)	C40.2-	C79.51	-	-	-	-
- - toe (any)	C40.3-	C79.51	-	-	-	-
- - trapezium	C40.1-	C79.51	-	-	-	-
- - trapezoid	C40.1-	C79.51	-	-	-	-
- - turbinate	C41.0	C79.51	-	D16.4-	D48.0	D49.2
- - ulna (any part)	C40.0-	C79.51	-	D16.0-	-	-
- - unciform	C40.1-	C79.51	-	-	-	-
- - vertebra (column)	C41.2	C79.51	-	D16.6	D48.0	D49.2
- - - coccyx	C41.4	C79.51	-	D16.8	D48.0	D49.2
- - - sacrum	C41.4	C79.51	-	D16.8	D48.0	D49.2
- - vomer	C41.0	C79.51	-	D16.4-	D48.0	D49.2
- - wrist	C40.1-	C79.51		-	-	-
- - xiphoid process	C41.3	C79.51	-	D16.7	D48.0	D49.2
- - zygomatic	C41.0	C79.51	-	D16.4-	D48.0	D49.2
- book-leaf (mouth)	C06.89	C79.89	D00.00	D10.39	D37.09	D49.0
- bowel—*see* Neoplasm, intestine						
- brachial plexus	C47.1-	C79.89	-	D36.12	D48.2	D49.2
- brain NEC	C71.9	C79.31	-	D33.2	D43.2	D49.6
- - basal ganglia	C71.0	C79.31	-	D33.0	D43.0	D49.6
- - cerebellopontine angle	C71.6	C79.31	-	D33.1	D43.1	D49.6
- - cerebellum NOS	C71.6	C79.31	-	D33.1	D43.1	D49.6
- - cerebrum	C71.0	C79.31	-	D33.0	D43.0	D49.6
- - choroid plexus	C71.7	C79.31	-	D33.1	D43.1	D49.6
- - corpus callosum	C71.8	C79.31	-	D33.2	D43.2	D49.6
- - corpus striatum	C71.0	C79.31	-	D33.0	D43.0	D49.6
- - cortex (cerebral)	C71.0	C79.31	-	D33.0	D43.0	D49.6
- - frontal lobe	C71.1	C79.31	-	D33.0	D43.0	D49.6
- - globus pallidus	C71.0	C79.31	-	D33.0	D43.0	D49.6
- - hippocampus	C71.2	C79.31	-	D33.0	D43.0	D49.6
- - hypothalamus	C71.0	C79.31	-	D33.0	D43.0	D49.6
- - internal capsule	C71.0	C79.31	-	D33.0	D43.0	D49.6
- - medulla oblongata	C71.7	C79.31	-	D33.1	D43.1	D49.6
- - meninges	C70.0	C79.32	-	D32.0	D42.0	D49.7
- - midbrain	C71.7	C79.31	-	D33.1	D43.1	D49.6
- - occipital lobe	C71.4	C79.31	-	D33.0	D43.0	D49.6
- - overlapping lesion	C71.8	C79.31	-	-	-	-
- - parietal lobe	C71.3	C79.31	-	D33.0	D43.0	D49.6
- - peduncle	C71.7	C79.31	-	D33.1	D43.1	D49.6
- - pons	C71.7	C79.31	-	D33.1	D43.1	D49.6
- - stem	C71.7	C79.31	-	D33.1	D43.1	D49.6
- - tapetum	C71.8	C79.31	-	D33.2	D43.2	D49.6
- - temporal lobe	C71.2	C79.31	-	D33.0	D43.0	D49.6
- - thalamus	C71.0	C79.31	-	D33.0	D43.0	D49.6
- - uncus	C71.2	C79.31	-	D33.0	D43.0	D49.6
- - ventricle (floor)	C71.5	C79.31	-	D33.0	D43.0	D49.6
- - - fourth	C71.7	C79.31	-	D33.1	D43.1	D49.6
- branchial (cleft) (cyst) (vestiges)	C10.4	C79.89	D00.08	D10.5	D37.05	D49.0
- breast (connective tissue) (glandular tissue) (soft parts)	C50.9-	C79.81	D05.-	D24.-	D48.6-	D49.3
- - areola	C50.0-	C79.81	D05.-	D24.-	D48.6-	D49.3
- - axillary tail	C50.6-	C79.81	D05.-	D24.-	D48.6-	D49.3
- - central portion	C50.1-	C79.81	D05.-	D24.-	D48.6-	D49.3
- - inner	C50.8-	C79.81	D05.-	D24.-	D48.6-	D49.3
- - lower	C50.8-	C79.81	D05.-	D24.-	D48.6-	D49.3
- - lower-inner quadrant	C50.3-	C79.81	D05.-	D24.-	D48.6-	D49.3
- - lower-outer quadrant	C50.5-	C79.81	D05.-	D24.-	D48.6-	D49.3

	Malignant Primary	Malignant Secondary	CA in Situ	Benign	Uncertain Behavior	Unspecified Behavior
- - mastectomy site (skin)—*see also Neoplasm, breast, skin*	C44.501	C79.2	-	-	-	-
- - - specified as breast tissue	C50.8-	C79.81	-	-	-	-
- - midline	C50.8-	C79.81	D05.-	D24.-	D48.6-	D49.3
- - nipple	C50.0-	C79.81	D05.-	D24.-	D48.6-	D49.3
- - outer	C50.8-	C79.81	D05.-	D24.-	D48.6-	D49.3
- - overlapping lesion	C50.8-	-	-	-	-	-
- - skin	C44.501	C79.2	D04.5	D23.5	D48.5	D49.2
- - - basal cell carcinoma	C44.511	-	-	-	-	-
- - - specified type NEC	C44.591	-	-	-	-	-
- - - squamous cell carcinoma	C44.521	-	-	-	-	-
- - tail (axillary)	C50.6-	C79.81	D05.-	D24.-	D48.6-	D49.3
- - upper	C50.8-	C79.81	D05.-	D24.-	D48.6-	D49.3
- - upper-inner quadrant	C50.2-	C79.81	D05.-	D24.-	D48.6-	D49.3
- - upper-outer quadrant	C50.4-	C79.81	D05.-	D24.-	D48.6-	D49.3
- broad ligament	C57.1	C79.82	D07.39	D28.2	D39.8	D49.59
- bronchogenic, bronchogenic (lung)	C34.9-	C78.0-	D02.2-	D14.3-	D38.1	D49.1
- bronchiole	C34.9-	C78.0-	D02.2-	D14.3-	D38.1	D49.1
- bronchus	C34.9-	C78.0-	D02.2-	D14.3-	D38.1	D49.1
- - carina	C34.0-	C78.0-	D02.2-	D14.3-	D38.1	D49.1
- - lower lobe of lung	C34.3-	C78.0-	D02.2-	D14.3-	D38.1	D49.1
- - main	C34.0-	C78.0-	D02.2-	D14.3-	D38.1	D49.1
- - middle lobe of lung	C34.2	C78.0-	D02.21	D14.31	D38.1	D49.1
- - overlapping lesion	C34.8-	-	-	-	-	-
- - upper lobe of lung	C34.1-	C78.0-	D02.2-	D14.3-	D38.1	D49.1
- brow	C44.309	C79.2	D04.39	D23.39	D48.5	D49.2
- - basal cell carcinoma	C44.319	-	-	-	-	-
- - specified type NEC	C44.399	-	-	-	-	-
- - squamous cell carcinoma	C44.329	-	-	-	-	-
- buccal (cavity)	C06.9	C79.89	D00.00	D10.39	D37.09	D49.0
- - commissure	C06.0	C79.89	D00.02	D10.39	D37.09	D49.0
- - groove (lower) (upper)	C06.1	C79.89	D00.02	D10.39	D37.09	D49.0
- - mucosa	C06.0	C79.89	D00.02	D10.39	D37.09	D49.0
- - sulcus (lower) (upper)	C06.1	C79.89	D00.02	D10.39	D37.09	D49.0
- bulbourethral gland	C68.0	C79.19	D09.19	D30.4	D41.3	D49.59
- bursa—*see Neoplasm, connective tissue*						
- buttock NEC	C76.3	C79.89	D04.5	D36.7	D48.7	D49.89
- calf	C76.5-	C79.89	D04.7-	D36.7	D48.7	D49.89
- calvarium	C41.0	C79.51	-	D16.4-	D48.0	D49.2
- calyx, renal	C65.-	C79.0-	D09.19	D30.1-	D41.1-	D49.59
- canal						
- - anal	C21.1	C78.5	D01.3	D12.9	D37.8	D49.0
- - auditory (external)—*see also Neoplasm, skin, ear*	C44.20-	C79.2	D04.2-	D23.2-	D48.5	D49.2
- - auricular (external)—*see also Neoplasm, skin, ear*	C44.20-	C79.2	D04.2-	D23.2-	D48.5	D49.2
- canaliculi, biliary (biliferi) (intrahepatic)	C22.1	C78.7	D01.5	D13.4	D37.6	D49.0
- canthus (eye) (inner) (outer)	C44.10-	C79.2	D04.1-	D23.1-	D48.5	D49.2
- - basal cell carcinoma	C44.11-	-	-	-	-	-
- - sebaceous cyst	C44.13-	-	-	-	-	-
- - specified type NEC	C44.19-	-	-	-	-	-
- - squamous cell carcinoma	C44.12-	-	-	-	-	-
- capillary—*see Neoplasm, connective tissue*						
- caput coli	C18.0	C78.5	D01.0	D12.0	D37.4	D49.0
- carcinoid—*see Tumor, carcinoid*						
- cardia (gastric)	C16.0	C78.89	D00.2	D13.1	D37.1	D49.0
- cardiac orifice (stomach)	C16.0	C78.89	D00.2	D13.1	D37.1	D49.0
- cardio-esophageal junction	C16.0	C78.89	D00.2	D13.1	D37.1	D49.0
- cardio-esophagus	C16.0	C78.89	D00.2	D13.1	D37.1	D49.0
- carina (bronchus)	C34.0-	C78.0-	D02.2-	D14.3-	D38.1	D49.1
- carotid (artery)	C49.0	C79.89	-	D21.0	D48.1	D49.2
- - body	C75.4	C79.89	-	D35.5	D44.6	D49.7
- carpus (any bone)	C40.1-	C79.51	-	D16.1-	-	-
- cartilage (articular) (joint)NEC—*see also Neoplasm, bone*	C41.9	C79.51	-	D16.9-	D48.0	D49.2
- - arytenoid	C32.3	C78.39	D02.0	D14.1	D38.0	D49.1
- - auricular	C49.0	C79.89	-	D21.0	D48.1	D49.2
- - bronchi	C34.0-	C78.39	-	D14.3-	D38.1	D49.1
- - costal	C41.3	C79.51	-	D16.7	D48.0	D49.2
- - cricoid	C32.3	C78.39	D02.0	D14.1	D38.0	D49.1
- - cuneiform	C32.3	C78.39	D02.0	D14.1	D38.0	D49.1
- - ear (external)	C49.0	C79.89	-	D21.0	D48.1	D49.2
- - ensiform	C41.3	C79.51	-	D16.7	D48.0	D49.2

	Malignant Primary	Malignant Secondary	CA in Situ	Benign	Uncertain Behavior	Unspecified Behavior
- - epiglottis	C32.1	C78.39	D02.0	D14.1	D38.0	D49.1
- - - anterior surface	C10.1	C79.89	D00.08	D10.5	D37.05	D49.0
- - eyelid	C49.0	C79.89	-	D21.0	D48.1	D49.2
- - intervertebral	C41.2	C79.51	-	D16.6	D48.0	D49.2
- - larynx, laryngeal	C32.3	C78.39	D02.0	D14.1	D38.0	D49.1
- - nose, nasal	C30.0	C78.39	D02.3	D14.0	D38.5	D49.1
- - pinna	C49.0	C79.89	-	D21.0	D48.1	D49.2
- - rib	C41.3	C79.51	-	D16.7	D48.0	D49.2
- - semilunar (knee)	C40.2-	C79.51	-	D16.2-	D48.0	D49.2
- - thyroid	C32.3	C78.39	D02.0	D14.1	D38.0	D49.1
- - trachea	C33	C78.39	D02.1	D14.2	D38.1	D49.1
- cauda equina	C72.1	C79.49	-	D33.4	D43.4	D49.7
- cavity						
- - buccal	C06.9	C79.89	D00.00	D10.30	D37.09	D49.0
- - nasal	C30.0	C78.39	D02.3	D14.0	D38.5	D49.1
- - oral	C06.9	C79.89	D00.00	D10.30	D37.09	D49.0
- - peritoneal	C48.2	C78.6	-	D20.1	D48.4	D49.0
- - tympanic	C30.1	C78.39	D02.3	D14.0	D38.5	D49.1
- cecum	C18.0	C78.5	D01.0	D12.0	D37.4	D49.0
- central nervous system	C72.9	C79.40	-	-	-	-
- cerebellopontine (angle)	C71.6	C79.31	-	D33.1	D43.1	D49.6
- cerebellum, cerebellar	C71.6	C79.31	-	D33.1	D43.1	D49.6
- cerebrum, cerebra (cortex) (hemisphere) (white matter)	C71.0	C79.31	-	D33.0	D43.0	D49.6
- - meninges	C70.0	C79.32	-	D32.0	D42.0	D49.7
- - peduncle	C71.7	C79.31	-	D33.1	D43.1	D49.6
- - ventricle	C71.5	C79.31	-	D33.0	D43.0	D49.6
- - - fourth	C71.7	C79.31	-	D33.1	D43.1	D49.6
- cervical region	C76.0	C79.89	D09.8	D36.7	D48.7	D49.89
- cervix (cervical) (uteri) (uterus)	C53.9	C79.82	D06.9	D26.0	D39.0	D49.59
- - canal	C53.0	C79.82	D06.0	D26.0	D39.0	D49.59
- - endocervix (canal) (gland)	C53.0	C79.82	D06.0	D26.0	D39.0	D49.59
- - exocervix	C53.1	C79.82	D06.1	D26.0	D39.0	D49.59
- - external os	C53.1	C79.82	D06.1	D26.0	D39.0	D49.59
- - internal os	C53.0	C79.82	D06.0	D26.0	D39.0	D49.59
- - nabothian gland	C53.0	C79.82	D06.0	D26.0	D39.0	D49.59
- - overlapping lesion	C53.8	-	-	-	-	-
- - squamocolumnar junction	C53.8	C79.82	D06.7	D26.0	D39.0	D49.59
- - stump	C53.8	C79.82	D06.7	D26.0	D39.0	D49.59
- cheek	C76.0	C79.89	D09.8	D36.7	D48.7	D49.89
- - external	C44.309	C79.2	D04.39	D23.39	D48.5	D49.2
- - - basal cell carcinoma	C44.319	-	-	-	-	-
- - - specified type NEC	C44.399	-	-	-	-	-
- - - squamous cell carcinoma	C44.329	-	-	-	-	-
- - inner aspect	C06.0	C79.89	D00.02	D10.39	D37.09	D49.0
- - internal	C06.0	C79.89	D00.02	D10.39	D37.09	D49.0
- - mucosa	C06.0	C79.89	D00.02	D10.39	D37.09	D49.0
- chest (wall)NEC	C76.1	C79.89	D09.8	D36.7	D48.7	D49.89
- chiasma opticum	C72.3-	C79.49	-	D33.3	D43.3	D49.7
- chin	C44.309	C79.2	D04.39	D23.39	D48.5	D49.2
- - basal cell carcinoma	C44.319	-	-	-	-	-
- - specified type NEC	C44.399	-	-	-	-	-
- - squamous cell carcinoma	C44.329	-	-	-	-	-
-choana	C11.3	C79.89	D00.08	D10.6	D37.05	D49.0
- cholangiole	C22.1	C78.89	D01.5	D13.4	D37.6	D49.0
- choledochal duct	C24.0	C78.89	D01.5	D13.5	D37.6	D49.0
- choroid	C69.3-	C79.49	D09.2-	D31.3-	D48.7	D49.81
- - plexus	C71.5	C79.31	-	D33.0	D43.0	D49.6
- ciliary body	C69.4-	C79.49	D09.2-	D31.4-	D48.7	D49.89
- clavicle	C41.3	C79.51	-	D16.7	D48.0	D49.2
- clitoris	C51.2	C79.82	D07.1	D28.0	D39.8	D49.59
- clivus	C41.0	C79.51	-	D16.4-	D48.0	D49.2
- cloacogenic zone	C21.2	C78.5	D01.3	D12.9	D37.8	D49.0
- coccygeal						
- - body or glomus	C49.5	C79.89	-	D21.5	D48.1	D49.2
- - vertebra	C41.4	C79.51	-	D16.8	D48.0	D49.2
- coccyx	C41.4	C79.51	-	D16.8	D48.0	D49.2
- colon—see also Neoplasm, intestine, large	C18.9	C78.5	-	-	-	-
- - with rectum	C19	C78.5	D01.1	D12.7	D37.5	D49.0
- column, spinal—see Neoplasm, spine						
- columnella—see also Neoplasm, skin, face	C44.390	C79.2	D04.39	D23.39	D48.5	D49.2

	Malignant Primary	Malignant Secondary	CA in Situ	Benign	Uncertain Behavior	Unspecified Behavior
- commissure						
- - labial, lip	C00.6	C79.89	D00.01	D10.39	D37.01	D49.0
- - laryngeal	C32.0	C78.39	D02.0	D14.1	D38.0	D49.1
- common (bile)duct	C24.0	C78.89	D01.5	D13.5	D37.6	D49.0
- concha—*see also Neoplasm, skin, ear*	C44.20-	C79.2	D04.2-	D23.2-	D48.5	D49.2
- - nose	C30.0	C78.39	D02.3	D14.0	D38.5	D49.1
- conjunctiva	C69.0-	C79.49	D09.2-	D31.0-	D48.7	D49.89
- connective tissue NEC	C49.9	C79.89	-	D21.9	D48.1	D49.2

Note: For neoplasms of connective tissue (blood vessel, bursa, fascia, ligament, muscle, peripheral nerves, sympathetic and parasympathetic nerves and ganglia, synovia, tendon, etc.) or of morphological types that indicate connective tissue, code according to the list under "Neoplasm, connective tissue". For sites that do not appear in this list, code to neoplasm of that site; e.g., fibrosarcoma, pancreas (C25.9)

Note: Morphological types that indicate connective tissue appear in their proper place in the alphabetic index with the instruction "see Neoplasm, connective tissue ...."

	Malignant Primary	Malignant Secondary	CA in Situ	Benign	Uncertain Behavior	Unspecified Behavior
- - abdomen	C49.4	C79.89	-	D21.4	D48.1	D49.2
- - abdominal wall	C49.4	C79.89	-	D21.4	D48.1	D49.2
- - ankle	C49.2-	C79.89	-	D21.2-	D48.1	D49.2
- - antecubital fossa or space	C49.1-	C79.89	-	D21.1-	D48.1	D49.2
- - arm	C49.1-	C79.89	-	D21.1-	D48.1	D49.2
- - auricle (ear)	C49.0	C79.89	-	D21.0	D48.1	D49.2
- - axilla	C49.3	C79.89	-	D21.3	D48.1	D49.2
- - back	C49.6	C79.89	-	D21.6	D48.1	D49.2
- - breast—*see Neoplasm, breast*						
- - buttock	C49.5	C79.89	-	D21.5	D48.1	D49.2
- - calf	C49.2-	C79.89	-	D21.2-	D48.1	D49.2
- - cervical region	C49.0	C79.89	-	D21.0	D48.1	D49.2
- - cheek	C49.0	C79.89	-	D21.0	D48.1	D49.2
- - chest (wall)	C49.3	C79.89	-	D21.3	D48.1	D49.2
- - chin	C49.0	C79.89	-	D21.0	D48.1	D49.2
- - diaphragm	C49.3	C79.89	-	D21.3	D48.1	D49.2
- - ear (external)	C49.0	C79.89	-	D21.0	D48.1	D49.2
- - elbow	C49.1-	C79.89	-	D21.1-	D48.1	D49.2
- - extra rectal	C49.5	C79.89	-	D21.5	D48.1	D49.2
- - extremity	C49.9	C79.89	-	D21.9	D48.1	D49.2
- - - lower	C49.2-	C79.89	-	D21.2-	D48.1	D49.2
- - - upper	C49.1-	C79.89	-	D21.1-	D48.1	D49.2
- - eyelid	C49.0	C79.89	-	D21.0	D48.1	D49.2
- - face	C49.0	C79.89	-	D21.0	D48.1	D49.2
- - finger	C49.1-	C79.89	-	D21.1-	D48.1	D49.2
- - flank	C49.6	C79.89	-	D21.6	D48.1	D49.2
- - foot	C49.2-	C79.89	-	D21.2-	D48.1	D49.2
- - forearm	C49.1-	C79.89	-	D21.1-	D48.1	D49.2
- - forehead	C49.0	C79.89	-	D21.0	D48.1	D49.2
- - gastric	C49.4	C79.89	-	D21.4	D48.1	D49.2
- - gastrointestinal	C49.4	C79.89	-	D21.4	D48.1	D49.2
- - gluteal region	C49.5	C79.89	-	D21.5	D48.1	D49.2
- - great vessels NEC	C49.3	C79.89	-	D21.3	D48.1	D49.2
- - groin	C49.5	C79.89	-	D21.5	D48.1	D49.2
- - hand	C49.1-	C79.89	-	D21.1-	D48.1	D49.2
- - head	C49.0	C79.89	-	D21.0	D48.1	D49.2
- - heel	C49.2-	C79.89	-	D21.2-	D48.1	D49.2
- - hip	C49.2-	C79.89	-	D21.2-	D48.1	D49.2
- - hypochondrium	C49.4	C79.89	-	D21.4	D48.1	D49.2
- - iliopsoas muscle	C49.5	C79.89	-	D21.5	D48.1	D49.2
- - infraclavicular region	C49.3	C79.89	-	D21.3	D48.1	D49.2
- - inguinal (canal) (region)	C49.5	C79.89	-	D21.5	D48.1	D49.2
- - intestinal	C49.4	C79.89	-	D21.4	D48.1	D49.2
- - intrathoracic	C49.3	C79.89	-	D21.3	D48.1	D49.2
- - ischiorectal fossa	C49.5	C79.89	-	D21.5	D48.1	D49.2
- - jaw	C03.9	C79.89	D00.03	D10.39	D48.1	D49.0
- - knee	C49.2-	C79.89	-	D21.2-	D48.1	D49.2
- - leg	C49.2-	C79.89	-	D21.2-	D48.1	D49.2
- - limb NEC	C49.9	C79.89	-	D21.9	D48.1	D49.2
- - - lower	C49.2-	C79.89	-	D21.2-	D48.1	D49.2
- - - upper	C49.1-	C79.89	-	D21.1-	D48.1	D49.2
- - nates	C49.5	C79.89	-	D21.5	D48.1	D49.2
- - neck	C49.0	C79.89	-	D21.0	D48.1	D49.2
- - orbit	C69.6-	C79.49	D09.2-	D31.6-	D48.1	D49.89
- - overlapping lesion	C49.8	-	-	-	-	-
- - pararectal	C49.5	C79.89	-	D21.5	D48.1	D49.2
- - para-urethral	C49.5	C79.89	-	D21.5	D48.1	D49.2
- - paravaginal	C49.5	C79.89	-	D21.5	D48.1	D49.2
- - pelvis (floor)	C49.5	C79.89	-	D21.5	D48.1	D49.2

	Malignant Primary	Malignant Secondary	CA in Situ	Benign	Uncertain Behavior	Unspecified Behavior
- - pelvo-abdominal	C49.8	C79.89	-	D21.6	D48.1	D49.2
- - perineum	C49.5	C79.89	-	D21.5	D48.1	D49.2
- - perirectal (tissue)	C49.5	C79.89	-	D21.5	D48.1	D49.2
- - periurethral (tissue)	C49.5	C79.89	-	D21.5	D48.1	D49.2
- - popliteal fossa or space	C49.2-	C79.89	-	D21.2-	D48.1	D49.2
- - presacral	C49.5	C79.89	-	D21.5	D48.1	D49.2
- - psoas muscle	C49.4	C79.89	-	D21.4	D48.1	D49.2
- - pterygoid fossa	C49.0	C79.89	-	D21.0	D48.1	D49.2
- - rectovaginal septum or wall	C49.5	C79.89	-	D21.5	D48.1	D49.2
- - rectovesical	C49.5	C79.89	-	D21.5	D48.1	D49.2
- - retroperitoneum	C48.0	C78.6	-	D20.0	D48.3	D49.0
- - sacrococcygeal region	C49.5	C79.89	-	D21.5	D48.1	D49.2
- - scalp	C49.0	C79.89	-	D21.0	D48.1	D49.2
- - scapular region	C49.3	C79.89	-	D21.3	D48.1	D49.2
- - shoulder	C49.1-	C79.89	-	D21.1-	D48.1	D49.2
- - skin (dermis)NEC—*see also Neoplasm, skin, by site*	C44.90	C79.2	D04.9	D23.9	D48.5	D49.2
- - stomach	C49.4	C79.89	-	D21.4	D48.1	D49.2
- - submental	C49.0	C79.89	-	D21.0	D48.1	D49.2
- - supraclavicular region	C49.0	C79.89	-	D21.0	D48.1	D49.2
- - temple	C49.0	C79.89	-	D21.0	D48.1	D49.2
- - temporal region	C49.0	C79.89	-	D21.0	D48.1	D49.2
- - thigh	C49.2-	C79.89	-	D21.2-	D48.1	D49.2
- - thoracic (duct) (wall)	C49.3	C79.89	-	D21.3	D48.1	D49.2
- - thorax	C49.3	C79.89	-	D21.3	D48.1	D49.2
- - thumb	C49.1-	C79.89	-	D21.1-	D48.1	D49.2
- - toe	C49.2-	C79.89	-	D21.2-	D48.1	D49.2
- - trunk	C49.6	C79.89	-	D21.6	D48.1	D49.2
- - umbilicus	C49.4	C79.89	-	D21.4	D48.1	D49.2
- - vesicorectal	C49.5	C79.89	-	D21.5	D48.1	D49.2
- - wrist	C49.1-	C79.89	-	D21.1-	D48.1	D49.2
- conus medullaris	C72.0	C79.49	-	D33.4	D43.4	D49.7
- cord (true) (vocal)	C32.0	C78.39	D02.0	D14.1	D38.0	D49.1
- - false	C32.1	C78.39	D02.0	D14.1	D38.0	D49.1
- - spermatic	C63.1-	C79.82	D07.69	D29.8	D40.8	D49.59
- - spinal (cervical) (lumbar) (thoracic)	C72.0	C79.49	-	D33.4	D43.4	D49.7
- cornea (limbus)	C69.1-	C79.49	D09.2-	D31.1-	D48.7	D49.89
- corpus						
- - albicans	C56.-	C79.6-	D07.39	D27.-	D39.1-	D49.59
- - callosum, brain	C71.0	C79.31	-	D33.2	D43.2	D49.6
- - cavernosum	C60.2	C79.82	D07.4	D29.0	D40.8	D49.59
- - gastric	C16.2	C78.89	D00.2	D13.1	D37.1	D49.0
- - overlapping sites	C54.8	-	-	-	-	-
- - penis	C60.2	C79.82	D07.4	D29.0	D40.8	D49.59
- - striatum, cerebrum	C71.0	C79.31	-	D33.0	D43.0	D49.6
- - uteri	C54.9	C79.82	D07.0	D26.1	D39.0	D49.59
- - - isthmus	C54.0	C79.82	D07.0	D26.1	D39.0	D49.59
- cortex						
- - adrenal	C74.0-	C79.7-	D09.3	D35.0-	D44.1-	D49.7
- - cerebral	C71.0	C79.31	-	D33.0	D43.0	D49.6
- costal cartilage	C41.3	C79.51	-	D16.7	D48.0	D49.2
- costovertebral joint	C41.3	C79.51	-	D16.7	D48.0	D49.2
- Cowper's gland	C68.0	C79.19	D09.19	D30.4	D41.3	D49.59
- cranial (fossa, any)	C71.9	C79.31	-	D33.2	D43.2	D49.6
- - meninges	C70.0	C79.32	-	D32.0	D42.0	D49.7
- - nerve	C72.50	C79.49	-	D33.3	D43.3	D49.7
- - - specified NEC	C72.59	C79.49	-	D33.3	D43.3	D49.7
- craniobuccal pouch	C75.2	C79.89	D09.3	D35.2	D44.3	D49.7
- craniopharyngeal (duct) (pouch)	C75.2	C79.89	D09.3	D35.3	D44.4	D49.7
- cricoid	C13.0	C79.89	D00.08	D10.7	D37.05	D49.0
- - cartilage	C32.3	C79.89	D02.0	D14.1	D38.0	D49.1
- cricopharynx	C13.0	C79.89	D00.08	D10.7	D37.05	D49.0
- crypt of Morgagni	C21.8	C78.5	D01.3	D12.9	D37.8	D49.0
- crystalline lens	C69.4-	C79.49	D09.2-	D31.4-	D48.7	D49.89
- cul-de-sac (Douglas')	C48.1	C78.6	-	D20.1	D48.4	D49.0
- cuneiform cartilage	C32.3	C78.39	D02.0	D14.1	D38.0	D49.1
- cutaneous—*see Neoplasm, skin*						
- cutis—*see Neoplasm, skin*						
- cystic (bile) duct (common)	C24.0	C78.89	D01.5	D13.5	D37.6	D49.0
- dermis—*see Neoplasm, skin*						
- diaphragm	C49.3	C79.89	-	D21.3	D48.1	D49.2

	Malignant Primary	Malignant Secondary	CA in Situ	Benign	Uncertain Behavior	Unspecified Behavior
- digestive organs, system, tube, or tract NEC	C26.9	C78.89	D01.9	D13.9	D37.9	D49.0
- disc, intervertebral	C41.2	C79.51	-	D16.6	D48.0	D49.2
- disease, generalized	C80.0	-	-	-	-	-
- disseminated	C80.0	-	-	-	-	-
- Douglas' cul-de-sac or pouch	C48.1	C78.6	-	D20.1	D48.4	D49.0
- duodenojejunal junction	C17.8	C78.4	D01.49	D13.39	D37.2	D49.0
- duodenum	C17.0	C78.4	D01.49	D13.2	D37.2	D49.0
- dura (cranial) (mater)	C70.9	C79.49	-	D32.9	D42.9	D49.7
- - cerebral	C70.0	C79.32	-	D32.0	D42.0	D49.7
- - spinal	C70.1	C79.49	-	D32.1	D42.1	D49.7
- ear (external)—see also Neoplasm, skin, ear	C44.20-	C79.2	D04.2-	D23.2-	D48.5	D49.2
- - auricle or auris—see also Neoplasm, skin, ear	C44.20-	C79.2	D04.2-	D23.2-	D48.5	D49.2
- - canal, external—see also Neoplasm, skin, ear	C44.20-	C79.2	D04.2-	D23.2-	D48.5	D49.2
- - cartilage	C49.0	C79.89	-	D21.0	D48.1	D49.2
- - external meatus—see also Neoplasm, skin, ear	C44.20-	C79.2	D04.2-	D23.2-	D48.5	D49.2
- - inner	C30.1	C78.39	D02.3	D14.0	D38.5	D49.1
- - lobule—see also Neoplasm, skin, ear	C44.20-	C79.2	D04.2-	D23.2-	D48.5	D49.2
- - middle	C30.1	C78.39	D02.3	D14.0	D38.5	D49.1
- - overlapping lesion with accessory sinuses	C31.8	-	-	-	-	-
- - skin	C44.20-	C79.2	D04.2-	D23.2-	D48.5	D49.2
- - - basal cell carcinoma	C44.21-	-	-	-	-	-
- - - specified type NEC	C44.29-	-	-	-	-	-
- - - squamous cell carcinoma	C44.22-	-	-	-	-	-
- earlobe	C44.20-	C79.2	D04.2-	D23.2-	D48.5	D49.2
- - basal cell carcinoma	C44.21-	-	-	-	-	-
- - specified type NEC	C44.29-	-	-	-	-	-
- - squamous cell carcinoma	C44.22-	-	-	-	-	-
- ejaculatory duct	C63.7	C79.82	D07.69	D29.8	D40.8	D49.59
- elbow NEC	C76.4-	C79.89	D04.6-	D36.7	D48.7	D49.89
- endocardium	C38.0	C79.89	-	D15.1	D48.7	D49.89
- endocervix (canal) (gland)	C53.0	C79.82	D06.0	D26.0	D39.0	D49.59
- endocrine gland NEC	C75.9	C79.89	D09.3	D35.9	D44.9	D49.7
- - pluriglandular	C75.8	C79.89	D09.3	D35.7	D44.9	D49.7
- endometrium (gland) (stroma)	C54.1	C79.82	D07.0	D26.1	D39.0	D49.59
- ensiform cartilage	C41.3	C79.51	-	D16.7	D48.0	D49.2
- enteric—see Neoplasm, intestine						
- ependyma (brain)	C71.5	C79.31	-	D33.0	D43.0	D49.6
- - fourth ventricle	C71.7	C79.31	-	D33.1	D43.1	D49.6
- epicardium	C38.0	C79.89	-	D15.1	D48.7	D49.89
- epididymis	C63.0-	C79.82	D07.69	D29.3-	D40.8	D49.59
- epidural	C72.9	C79.49	-	D33.9	D43.9	D49.7
- epiglottis	C32.1	C78.39	D02.0	D14.1	D38.0	D49.1
- - anterior aspect or surface	C10.1	C79.89	D00.08	D10.5	D37.05	D49.0
- - cartilage	C32.3	C78.39	D02.0	D14.1	D38.0	D49.1
- - free border (margin)	C10.1	C79.89	D00.08	D10.5	D37.05	D49.0
- - junctional region	C10.8	C79.89	D00.08	D10.5	D37.05	D49.0
- - posterior (laryngeal)surface	C32.1	C78.39	D02.0	D14.1	D38.0	D49.1
- - suprahyoid portion	C32.1	C78.39	D02.0	D14.1	D38.0	D49.1
- esophagogastric junction	C16.0	C78.89	D00.2	D13.1	D37.1	D49.0
- esophagus	C15.9	C78.89	D00.1	D13.0	D37.8	D49.0
- - abdominal	C15.5	C78.89	D00.1	D13.0	D37.8	D49.0
- - cervical	C15.3	C78.89	D00.1	D13.0	D37.8	D49.0
- - distal (third)	C15.5	C78.89	D00.1	D13.0	D37.8	D49.0
- - lower (third)	C15.5	C78.89	D00.1	D13.0	D37.8	D49.0
- - middle (third)	C15.4	C78.89	D00.1	D13.0	D37.8	D49.0
- - overlapping lesion	C15.8	-	-	-	-	-
- - proximal (third)	C15.3	C78.89	D00.1	D13.0	D37.8	D49.0
- - thoracic	C15.4	C78.89	D00.1	D13.0	D37.8	D49.0
- - upper (third)	C15.3	C78.89	D00.1	D13.0	D37.8	D49.0
- ethmoid (sinus)	C31.1	C78.39	D02.3	D14.0	D38.5	D49.1
- - bone or labyrinth	C41.0	C79.51	-	D16.4-	D48.0	D49.2
- eustachian tube	C30.1	C78.39	D02.3	D14.0	D38.5	D49.1
- exocervix	C53.1	C79.82	D06.1	D26.0	D39.0	D49.59
- external						
- - meatus (ear)—see also Neoplasm, skin, ear	C44.20-	C79.2	D04.2-	D23.2-	D48.5	D49.2
- - os, cervix uteri	C53.1	C79.82	D06.1	D26.0	D39.0	D49.59
- extradural	C72.9	C79.49	-	D33.9	D43.9	D49.7
- extrahepatic (bile)duct	C24.0	C78.89	D01.5	D13.5	D37.6	D49.0
- - overlapping lesion with gallbladder	C24.8	-	-	-	-	-
- extraocular muscle	C69.6-	C79.49	D09.2-	D31.6-	D48.7	D49.89
- extra rectal	C76.3	C79.89	D09.8	D36.7	D48.7	D49.89

	Malignant Primary	Malignant Secondary	CA in Situ	Benign	Uncertain Behavior	Unspecified Behavior
- extremity	C76.8	C79.89	D04.8	D36.7	D48.7	D49.89
- - lower	C76.5-	C79.89	D04.7-	D36.7	D48.7	D49.89
- - upper	C76.4-	C79.89	D04.6-	D36.7	D48.7	D49.89
- eye NEC	C69.9-	C79.49	D09.2	D31.9	D48.7	D49.89
- - overlapping sites	C69.8	-	-	-	-	-
- eyeball	C69.9-	C79.49	D09.2-	D31.9-	D48.7	D49.89
- eyebrow	C44.309	C79.2	D04.39	D23.39	D48.5	D49.2
- - basal cell carcinoma	C44.319	-	-	-	-	-
- - specified type NEC	C44.399	-	-	-	-	-
- - squamous cell carcinoma	C44.329	-	-	-	-	-
- eyelid (lower) (skin) (upper)	C44.10-	-	-	-	-	-
- - basal cell carcinoma	C44.11-	-	-	-	-	-
- - sebaceous cell	C44.13-	-	-	-	-	-
- - specified type NEC	C44.19-	-	-	-	-	-
- - squamous cell carcinoma	C44.12-	-	-	-	-	-
- - cartilage	C49.0	C79.89	-	D21.0	D48.1	D49.2
- face NEC	C76.0	C79.89	D04.39	D36.7	D48.7	D49.89
- fallopian tube (accessory)	C57.0-	C79.82	D07.39	D28.2	D39.8	D49.59
- falx (cerebella) (cerebri)	C70.0	C79.32	-	D32.0	D42.0	D49.7
- fascia—see also Neoplasm, connective tissue						
- - palmar	C49.1-	C79.89	-	D21.1-	D48.1	D49.2
- - plantar	C49.2-	C79.89	-	D21.2-	D48.1	D49.2
- fatty tissue—see Neoplasm, connective tissue						
- fauces, faucial NEC	C10.9	C79.89	D00.08	D10.5	D37.05	D49.0
- - pillars	C09.1	C79.89	D00.08	D10.5	D37.05	D49.0
- - tonsil	C09.9	C79.89	D00.08	D10.4	D37.05	D49.0
- femur (any part)	C40.2-	-	-	D16.2-	-	-
- fetal membrane	C58	C79.82	D07.0	D26.7	D39.2	D49.59
- fibrous tissue—see Neoplasm, connective tissue						
- fibula (any part)	C40.2-	C79.51	-	D16.2-	-	-
- filum terminale	C72.0	C79.49	-	D33.4	D43.4	D49.7
- finger NEC	C76.4-	C79.89	D04.6-	D36.7	D48.7	D49.89
- flank NEC	C76.8	C79.89	D04.5	D36.7	D48.7	D49.89
- follicle, nabothian	C53.0	C79.82	D06.0	D26.0	D39.0	D49.59
- foot NEC	C76.5-	C79.89	D04.7-	D36.7	D48.7	D49.89
- forearm NEC	C76.4-	C79.89	D04.6-	D36.7	D48.7	D49.89
- forehead (skin)	C44.309	C79.2	D04.39	D23.39	D48.5	D49.2
- - basal cell carcinoma	C44.319	-	-	-	-	-
- - specified type NEC	C44.399	-	-	-	-	-
- - squamous cell carcinoma	C44.329	-	-	-	-	-
- foreskin	C60.0	C79.82	D07.4	D29.0	D40.8	D49.59
- fornix						
- - pharyngeal	C11.3	C79.89	D00.08	D10.6	D37.05	D49.0
- - vagina	C52	C79.82	D07.2	D28.1	D39.8	D49.59
- fossa (of)						
- - anterior (cranial)	C71.9	C79.31	-	D33.2	D43.2	D49.6
- - cranial	C71.9	C79.31	-	D33.2	D43.2	D49.6
- - ischiorectal	C76.3	C79.89	D09.8	D36.7	D48.7	D49.89
- - middle (cranial)	C71.9	C79.31	-	D33.2	D43.2	D49.6
- - piriform	C12	C79.89	D00.08	D10.7	D37.05	D49.0
- - pituitary	C75.1	C79.89	D09.3	D35.2	D44.3	D49.7
- - posterior (cranial)	C71.9	C79.31	-	D33.2	D43.2	D49.6
- - pterygoid	C49.0	C79.89	-	D21.0	D48.1	D49.2
- - pyriform	C12	C79.89	D00.08	D10.7	D37.05	D49.0
- - Rosenmüller	C11.2	C79.89	D00.08	D10.6	D37.05	D49.0
- - tonsillar	C09.0	C79.89	D00.08	D10.5	D37.05	D49.0
- fourchette	C51.9	C79.82	D07.1	D28.0	D39.8	D49.59
- frenulum						
- - labii—see Neoplasm, lip, internal						
- - linguae	C02.2	C79.89	D00.07	D10.1	D37.02	D49.0
- frontal						
- - bone	C41.0	C79.51	-	D16.4-	D48.0	D49.2
- - lobe, brain	C71.1	C79.31	-	D33.0	D43.0	D49.6
- - pole	C71.1	C79.31	-	D33.0	D43.0	D49.6
- - sinus	C31.2	C78.39	D02.3	D14.0	D38.5	D49.1
- fundus						
- - stomach	C16.1	C78.89	D00.2	D13.1	D37.1	D49.0
- - uterus	C54.3	C79.82	D07.0	D26.1	D39.0	D49.59
- gall duct (extrahepatic)	C24.0	C78.89	D01.5	D13.5	D37.6	D49.0
- - intrahepatic	C22.1	C78.7	D01.5	D13.4	D37.6	D49.0
- gallbladder	C23	C78.89	D01.5	D13.5	D37.6	D49.0

	Malignant Primary	Malignant Secondary	CA in Situ	Benign	Uncertain Behavior	Unspecified Behavior
- - overlapping lesion with extrahepatic bile ducts	C24.8	-	-	-	-	-
- ganglia—*see also Neoplasm, nerve, peripheral*	C47.9	C79.89	-	D36.10	D48.2	D49.2
- - basal	C71.0	C79.31	-	D33.0	D43.0	D49.6
- - cranial nerve	C72.50	C79.49	-	D33.3	D43.3	D49.7
- Gartner's duct	C52	C79.82	D07.2	D28.1	D39.8	D49.59
- gastric—*see Neoplasm, stomach*						
- gastrocolic	C26.9	C78.89	D01.9	D13.9	D37.9	D49.0
- gastroesophageal junction	C16.0	C78.89	D00.2	D13.1	D37.1	D49.0
- gastrointestinal (tract)NEC	C26.9	C78.89	D01.9	D13.9	D37.9	D49.0
- generalized	C80.0	-	-	-	-	-
- genital organ or tract						
- - female NEC	C57.9	C79.82	D07.30	D28.9	D39.9	D49.59
- - - overlapping lesion	C57.8	-	-	-	-	-
- - - specified site NEC	C57.7	C79.82	D07.39	D28.7	D39.8	D49.59
- - male NEC	C63.9	C79.82	D07.60	D29.9	D40.9	D49.59
- - - overlapping lesion	C63.8	-	-	-	-	-
- - - specified site NEC	C63.7	C79.82	D07.69	D29.8	D40.8	D49.59
- genitourinary tract						
- - female	C57.9	C79.82	D07.30	D28.9	D39.9	D49.59
- - male	C63.9	C79.82	D07.60	D29.9	D40.9	D49.59
- gingiva (alveolar) (marginal)	C03.9	C79.89	D00.03	D10.39	D37.09	D49.0
- - lower	C03.1	C79.89	D00.03	D10.39	D37.09	D49.0
- - mandibular	C03.1	C79.89	D00.03	D10.39	D37.09	D49.0
- - maxillary	C03.0	C79.89	D00.03	D10.39	D37.09	D49.0
- - upper	C03.0	C79.89	D00.03	D10.39	D37.09	D49.0
- gland, glandular (lymphatic) (system)—*see also Neoplasm, lymph gland*						
- - endocrine NEC	C75.9	C79.89	D09.3	D35.9	D44.9	D49.7
- - salivary—*see Neoplasm, salivary gland*						
- glans penis	C60.1	C79.82	D07.4	D29.0	D40.8	D49.59
- globus pallidus	C71.0	C79.31	-	D33.0	D43.0	D49.6
- glomus						
- - coccygeal	C49.5	C79.89	-	D21.5	D48.1	D49.2
- - jugularis	C75.5	C79.89	-	D35.6	D44.7	D49.7
- glosso-epiglottic fold (s)	C10.1	C79.89	D00.08	D10.5	D37.05	D49.0
- glossopalatine fold	C09.1	C79.89	D00.08	D10.5	D37.05	D49.0
- glossopharyngeal sulcus	C09.0	C79.89	D00.08	D10.5	D37.05	D49.0
- glottis	C32.0	C78.39	D02.0	D14.1	D38.0	D49.1
- gluteal region	C76.3	C79.89	D04.5	D36.7	D48.7	D49.89
- great vessels NEC	C49.3	C79.89	-	D21.3	D48.1	D49.2
- groin NEC	C76.3	C79.89	D04.5	D36.7	D48.7	D49.89
- gum	C03.9	C79.89	D00.03	D10.39	D37.09	D49.0
- - lower	C03.1	C79.89	D00.03	D10.39	D37.09	D49.0
- - upper	C03.0	C79.89	D00.03	D10.39	D37.09	D49.0
- hand NEC	C76.4-	C79.89	D04.6-	D36.7	D48.7	D49.89
- head NEC	C76.0	C79.89	D04.4	D36.7	D48.7	D49.89
- heart	C38.0	C79.89	-	D15.1	D48.7	D49.89
- heel NEC	C76.5-	C79.89	D04.7-	D36.7	D48.7	D49.89
- helix—*see also Neoplasm, skin, ear*	C44.20-	C79.2	D04.2-	D23.2-	D48.5	D49.2
- hematopoietic, hemopoietic tissue NEC	C96.9	-	-	-	-	-
- - specified NEC	C96.Z	-	-	-	-	-
- hemisphere, cerebral	C71.0	C79.31	-	D33.0	D43.0	D49.6
- hemorrhoidal zone	C21.1	C78.5	D01.3	D12.9	D37.8	D49.0
- hepatic—*see also Index to disease, by histology*	C22.9	C78.7	D01.5	D13.4	D37.6	D49.0
- - duct (bile)	C24.0	C78.89	D01.5	D13.5	D37.6	D49.0
- - flexure (colon)	C18.3	C78.5	D01.0	D12.3	D37.4	D49.0
- - primary	C22.8	C78.7	D01.5	D13.4	D37.6	D49.0
- hepatobiliary	C24.9	C78.89	D01.5	D13.5	D37.6	D49.0
- hepatoblastoma	C22.2	C78.7	D01.5	D13.4	D37.6	D49.0
- hepatoma	C22.0	C78.7	D01.5	D13.4	D37.6	D49.0
- hilus of lung	C34.0-	C78.0-	D02.2-	D14.3-	D38.1	D49.1
- hip NEC	C76.5-	C79.89	D04.7-	D36.7	D48.7	D49.89
- hippocampus, brain	C71.2	C79.31	-	D33.0	D43.0	D49.6
- humerus (any part)	C40.0-	C79.51	-	D16.0-		
- hymen	C52	C79.82	D07.2	D28.1	D39.8	D49.59
- hypopharynx, hypopharyngeal NEC	C13.9	C79.89	D00.08	D10.7	D37.05	D49.0
- - overlapping lesion	C13.8	-	-	-	-	-
- - postcricoid region	C13.0	C79.89	D00.08	D10.7	D37.05	D49.0
- - posterior wall	C13.2	C79.89	D00.08	D10.7	D37.05	D49.0
- - pyriform fossa (sinus)	C12	C79.89	D00.08	D10.7	D37.05	D49.0
- hypophysis	C75.1	C79.89	D09.3	D35.2	D44.3	D49.7

	Malignant Primary	Malignant Secondary	CA in Situ	Benign	Uncertain Behavior	Unspecified Behavior
- hypothalamus	C71.0	C79.31	-	D33.0	D43.0	D49.6
- ileocecum, ileocecal (coil) (junction) (valve)	C18.0	C78.5	D01.0	D12.0	D37.4	D49.0
- ileum	C17.2	C78.4	D01.49	D13.39	D37.2	D49.0
- ilium	C41.4	C79.51	-	D16.8	D48.0	D49.2
- immunoproliferative NEC	C88.9	-	-	-	-	-
- infraclavicular (region)	C76.1	C79.89	D04.5	D36.7	D48.7	D49.89
- inguinal (region)	C76.3	C79.89	D04.5	D36.7	D48.7	D49.89
- insula	C71.0	C79.31	-	D33.0	D43.0	D49.6
- insular tissue (pancreas)	C25.4	C78.89	D01.7	D13.7	D37.8	D49.0
- - brain	C71.0	C79.31	-	D33.0	D43.0	D49.6
- interarytenoid fold	C13.1	C79.89	D00.08	D10.7	D37.05	D49.0
- - hypopharyngeal aspect	C13.1	C79.89	D00.08	D10.7	D37.05	D49.0
- - laryngeal aspect	C32.1	C79.89	D02.0	D14.1	D38.0	D49.1
- - marginal zone	C13.1	C79.89	D00.08	D10.7	D37.05	D49.0
- interdental papillae	C03.9	C79.89	D00.03	D10.39	D37.09	D49.0
- - lower	C03.1	C79.89	D00.03	D10.39	D37.09	D49.0
- - upper	C03.0	C79.89	D00.03	D10.39	D37.09	D49.0
- internal						
- - capsule	C71.0	C79.31	-	D33.0	D43.0	D49.6
- - os (cervix)	C53.0	C79.82	D06.0	D26.0	D39.0	D49.59
- intervertebral cartilage or disc	C41.2	C79.51	-	D16.6	D48.0	D49.2
- intestine, intestinal	C26.0	C78.80	D01.40	D13.9	D37.8	D49.0
- - large	C18.9	C78.5	D01.0	D12.6	D37.4	D49.0
- - - appendix	C18.1	C78.5	D01.0	D12.1	D37.3	D49.0
- - - caput coli	C18.0	C78.5	D01.0	D12.0	D37.4	D49.0
- - - cecum	C18.0	C78.5	D01.0	D12.0	D37.4	D49.0
- - - colon	C18.9	C78.5	D01.0	D12.6	D37.4	D49.0
- - - - and rectum	C19	C78.5	D01.1	D12.7	D37.5	D49.0
- - - - ascending	C18.2	C78.5	D01.0	D12.2	D37.4	D49.0
- - - - caput	C18.0	C78.5	D01.0	D12.0	D37.4	D49.0
- - - - descending	C18.6	C78.5	D01.0	D12.4	D37.4	D49.0
- - - - distal	C18.6	C78.5	D01.0	D12.4	D37.4	D49.0
- - - - left	C18.6	C78.5	D01.0	D12.4	D37.4	D49.0
- - - - overlapping lesion	C18.8	-	-	-	-	-
- - - - pelvic	C18.7	C78.5	D01.0	D12.5	D37.4	D49.0
- - - - right	C18.2	C78.5	D01.0	D12.2	D37.4	D49.0
- - - - sigmoid (flexure)	C18.7	C78.5	D01.0	D12.5	D37.4	D49.0
- - - - transverse	C18.4	C78.5	D01.0	D12.3	D37.4	D49.0
- - - hepatic flexure	C18.3	C78.5	D01.0	D12.3	D37.4	D49.0
- - - ileocecum, ileocecal (coil) (valve)	C18.0	C78.5	D01.0	D12.0	D37.4	D49.0
- - - overlapping lesion	C18.8	-	-	-	-	-
- - - sigmoid flexure (lower) (upper)	C18.7	C78.5	D01.0	D12.5	D37.4	D49.0
- - - splenic flexure	C18.5	C78.5	D01.0	D12.3	D37.4	D49.0
- - small	C17.9	C78.4	D01.40	D13.30	D37.2	D49.0
- - - duodenum	C17.0	C78.4	D01.49	D13.2	D37.2	D49.0
- - - ileum	C17.2	C78.4	D01.49	D13.39	D37.2	D49.0
- - - jejunum	C17.1	C78.4	D01.49	D13.39	D37.2	D49.0
- - - overlapping lesion	C17.8	-	-	-	-	-
- - tract NEC	C26.0	C78.89	D01.40	D13.9	D37.8	D49.0
- intra-abdominal	C76.2	C79.89	D09.8	D36.7	D48.7	D49.89
- intracranial NEC	C71.9	C79.31	-	D33.2	D43.2	D49.6
- intrahepatic (bile)duct	C22.1	C78.7	D01.5	D13.4	D37.6	D49.0
- intraocular	C69.9-	C79.49	D09.2-	D31.9-	D48.7	D49.89
- intraorbital	C69.6-	C79.49	D09.2-	D31.6-	D48.7	D49.89
- intrasellar	C75.1	C79.89	D09.3	D35.2	D44.3	D49.7
- intrathoracic (cavity) (organs)	C76.1	C79.89	D09.8	D15.9	D48.7	D49.89
- - specified NEC	C76.1	C79.89	D09.8	D15.7	-	-
- iris	C69.4-	C79.49	D09.2-	D31.4-	D48.7	D49.89
- ischiorectal (fossa)	C76.3	C79.89	D09.8	D36.7	D48.7	D49.89
- ischium	C41.4	C79.51	-	D16.8	D48.0	D49.2
- island of Reil	C71.0	C79.31	-	D33.0	D43.0	D49.6
- islands or islets of Langerhans	C25.4	C78.89	D01.7	D13.7	D37.8	D49.0
- isthmus uteri	C54.0	C79.82	D07.0	D26.1	D39.0	D49.59
- jaw	C76.0	C79.89	D09.8	D36.7	D48.7	D49.89
- - bone	C41.1	C79.51	-	D16.5-	D48.0	D49.2
- - - lower	C41.1	C79.51	-	D16.5-	-	-
- - - upper	C41.0	C79.51	-	D16.4-	-	-
- - carcinoma (any type) (lower) (upper)	C76.0	C79.89	-	-	-	-
- - skin—*see also Neoplasm, skin, face*	C44.309	C79.2	D04.39	D23.39	D48.5	D49.2
- - soft tissues	C03.9	C79.89	D00.03	D10.39	D37.09	D49.0
- - - lower	C03.1	C79.89	D00.03	D10.39	D37.09	D49.0

	Malignant Primary	Malignant Secondary	CA in Situ	Benign	Uncertain Behavior	Unspecified Behavior
- - - upper	C03.0	C79.89	D00.03	D10.39	D37.09	D49.0
- jejunum	C17.1	C78.4	D01.49	D13.39	D37.2	D49.0
- joint NEC—*see also Neoplasm, bone*	C41.9	C79.51	-	D16.9-	D48.0	D49.2
- - acromioclavicular	C40.0-	C79.51	-	D16.0-	-	-
- - bursa or synovial membrane—*see Neoplasm, connective tissue*						
- - costovertebral	C41.3	C79.51	-	D16.7	D48.0	D49.2
- - sternocostal	C41.3	C79.51	-	D16.7	D48.0	D49.2
- - temporomandibular	C41.1	C79.51	-	D16.5-	D48.0	D49.2
- junction						
- - anorectal	C21.8	C78.5	D01.3	D12.9	D37.8	D49.0
- - cardioesophageal	C16.0	C78.89	D00.2	D13.1	D37.1	D49.0
- - esophagogastric	C16.0	C78.89	D00.2	D13.1	D37.1	D49.0
- - gastroesophageal	C16.0	C78.89	D00.2	D13.1	D37.1	D49.0
- - hard and soft palate	C05.9	C79.89	D00.00	D10.39	D37.09	D49.0
- - ileocecal	C18.0	C78.5	D01.0	D12.0	D37.4	D49.0
- - pelvirectal	C19	C78.5	D01.1	D12.7	D37.5	D49.0
- - pelviureteric	C65.-	C79.0-	D09.19	D30.1-	D41.1-	D49.59
- - rectosigmoid	C19	C78.5	D01.1	D12.7	D37.5	D49.0
- - squamocolumnar, of cervix	C53.8	C79.82	D06.7	D26.0	D39.0	D49.59
- Kaposi's sarcoma—*see Kaposi's, sarcoma*						
- kidney (parenchymal)	C64.-	C79.0-	D09.19	D30.0-	D41.0-	D49.51
- - calyx	C65.-	C79.0-	D09.19	D30.1-	D41.1-	D49.51
- - hilus	C65.-	C79.0-	D09.19	D30.1-	D41.1-	D49.51
- - pelvis	C65.-	C79.0-	D09.19	D30.1-	D41.1-	D49.51
- knee NEC	C76.5-	C79.89	D04.7-	D36.7	D48.7	D49.89
- labia (skin)	C51.9	C79.82	D07.1	D28.0	D39.8	D49.59
- - majora	C51.0	C79.82	D07.1	D28.0	D39.8	D49.59
- - minora	C51.1	C79.82	D07.1	D28.0	D39.8	D49.59
- labial—*see also Neoplasm, lip*	C00.9	C79.89	D00.01	D10.0	D37.01	D49.0
- - sulcus (lower) (upper)	C06.1	C79.89	D00.02	D10.39	D37.09	D49.0
- labium (skin)	C51.9	C79.82	D07.1	D28.0	D39.8	D49.59
- - majus	C51.0	C79.82	D07.1	D28.0	D39.8	D49.59
- - minus	C51.1	C79.82	D07.1	D28.0	D39.8	D49.59
- lacrimal						
- - canaliculi	C69.5-	C79.49	D09.2-	D31.5-	D48.7	D49.89
- - duct (nasal)	C69.5-	C79.49	D09.2-	D31.5-	D48.7	D49.89
- - gland	C69.5-	C79.49	D09.2-	D31.5-	D48.7	D49.89
- - punctum	C69.5-	C79.49	D09.2-	D31.5-	D48.7	D49.89
- - sac	C69.5-	C79.49	D09.2-	D31.5-	D48.7	D49.89
- Langerhans, islands or islets	C25.4	C78.89	D01.7	D13.7	D37.8	D49.0
- laryngopharynx	C13.9	C79.89	D00.08	D10.7	D37.05	D49.0
- larynx, laryngeal NEC	C32.9	C78.39	D02.0	D14.1	D38.0	D49.1
- - aryepiglottic fold	C32.1	C78.39	D02.0	D14.1	D38.0	D49.1
- - cartilage (arytenoid) (cricoid) (cuneiform) (thyroid)	C32.3	C78.39	D02.0	D14.1	D38.0	D49.1
- - commissure (anterior) (posterior)	C32.0	C78.39	D02.0	D14.1	D38.0	D49.1
- - extrinsic NEC	C32.1	C78.39	D02.0	D14.1	D38.0	D49.1
- - - meaning hypopharynx	C13.9	C79.89	D00.08	D10.7	D37.05	D49.0
- - interarytenoid fold	C32.1	C78.39	D02.0	D14.1	D38.0	D49.1
- - intrinsic	C32.0	C78.39	D02.0	D14.1	D38.0	D49.1
- - overlapping lesion	C32.8	-	-	-	-	-
- - ventricular band	C32.1	C78.39	D02.0	D14.1	D38.0	D49.1
- leg NEC	C76.5-	C79.89	D04.7-	D36.7	D48.7	D49.89
- lens, crystalline	C69.4-	C79.49	D09.2-	D31.4-	D48.7	D49.89
- lid (lower) (upper)	C44.10-	C79.2	D04.1-	D23.1-	D48.5	D49.2
- - basal cell carcinoma	C44.11-	-	-	-	-	-
- - sebaceous cell	C44.13-	-	-	-	-	-
- - specified type NEC	C44.19-	-	-	-	-	-
- - squamous cell carcinoma	C44.12-	-	-	-	-	-
- ligament—*see also Neoplasm, connective tissue*						
- - broad	C57.1	C79.82	D07.39	D28.2	D39.8	D49.59
- - Mackenrodt's	C57.7	C79.82	D07.39	D28.7	D39.8	D49.59
- - non-uterine—*see Neoplasm, connective tissue*						
- - round	C57.2	C79.82	-	D28.2	D39.8	D49.59
- - sacro-uterine	C57.3	C79.82	-	D28.2	D39.8	D49.59
- - uterine	C57.3	C79.82	-	D28.2	D39.8	D49.59
- - utero-ovarian	C57.7	C79.82	D07.39	D28.2	D39.8	D49.59
- - uterosacral	C57.3	C79.82	-	D28.2	D39.8	D49.59
- limb	C76.8	C79.89	D04.8	D36.7	D48.7	D49.89
- - lower	C76.5-	C79.89	D04.7-	D36.7	D48.7	D49.89
- - upper	C76.4-	C79.89	D04.6-	D36.7	D48.7	D49.89

	Malignant Primary	Malignant Secondary	CA in Situ	Benign	Uncertain Behavior	Unspecified Behavior
- limbus of cornea	C69.1-	C79.49	D09.2-	D31.1-	D48.7	D49.89
- lingual NEC—*see also Neoplasm, tongue*	C02.9	C79.89	D00.07	D10.1	D37.02	D49.0
- lingula, lung	C34.1-	C78.0-	D02.2-	D14.3-	D38.1	D49.1
- lip	C00.9	C79.89	D00.01	D10.0	D37.01	D49.0
- - buccal aspect—*see Neoplasm, lip, internal*						
- - commissure	C00.6	C79.89	D00.01	D10.0	D37.01	D49.0
- - external	C00.2	C79.89	D00.01	D10.0	D37.01	D49.0
- - - lower	C00.1	C79.89	D00.01	D10.0	D37.01	D49.0
- - - upper	C00.0	C79.89	D00.01	D10.0	D37.01	D49.0
- - frenulum—*see Neoplasm, lip, internal*						
- - inner aspect—*see Neoplasm, lip, internal*						
- - internal	C00.5	C79.89	D00.01	D10.0	D37.01	D49.0
- - - lower	C00.4	C79.89	D00.01	D10.0	D37.01	D49.0
- - - upper	C00.3	C79.89	D00.01	D10.0	D37.01	D49.0
- - lipstick area	C00.2	C79.89	D00.01	D10.0	D37.01	D49.0
- - - lower	C00.1	C79.89	D00.01	D10.0	D37.01	D49.0
- - - upper	C00.0	C79.89	D00.01	D10.0	D37.01	D49.0
- - lower	C00.1	C79.89	D00.01	D10.0	D37.01	D49.0
- - - internal	C00.4	C79.89	D00.01	D10.0	D37.01	D49.0
- - mucosa—*see Neoplasm, lip, internal*						
- - oral aspect—*see Neoplasm, lip, internal*						
- - overlapping lesion	C00.8	-	-	-	-	-
- - - with oral cavity or pharynx	C14.8	-	-	-	-	-
- - skin (commissure) (lower) (upper)	C44.00	C79.2	D04.0	D23.0	D48.5	D49.2
- - - basal cell carcinoma	C44.01	-	-	-	-	-
- - - specified type NEC	C44.09	-	-	-	-	-
- - - squamous cell carcinoma	C44.02	-	-	-	-	-
- - upper	C00.0	C79.89	D00.01	D10.0	D37.01	D49.0
- - - internal	C00.3	C79.89	D00.01	D10.0	D37.01	D49.0
- - vermilion border	C00.2	C79.89	D00.01	D10.0	D37.01	D49.0
- - - lower	C00.1	C79.89	D00.01	D10.0	D37.01	D49.0
- - - upper	C00.0	C79.89	D00.01	D10.0	D37.01	D49.0
- lipomatous—*see Lipoma, by site*						
- liver—*see also Index to disease, by histology*	C22.9	C78.7	D01.5	D13.4	D37.6	D49.0
- - primary	C22.8	C78.7	D01.5	D13.4	D37.6	D49.0
- lumbosacral plexus	C47.5	C79.89	-	D36.16	D48.2	D49.2
- lung	C34.9-	C78.0-	D02.2-	D14.3-	D38.1	D49.1
- - azygos lobe	C34.1-	C78.0-	D02.2-	D14.3-	D38.1	D49.1
- - carina	C34.0-	C78.0-	D02.2-	D14.3-	D38.1	D49.1
- - hilus	C34.0-	C78.0-	D02.2-	D14.3-	D38.1	D49.1
- - lingula	C34.1-	C78.0-	D02.2-	D14.3-	D38.1	D49.1
- - lobe NEC	C34.9-	C78.0-	D02.2-	D14.3-	D38.1	D49.1
- - lower lobe	C34.3-	C78.0-	D02.2-	D14.3-	D38.1	D49.1
- - main bronchus	C34.0-	C78.0-	D02.2-	D14.3-	D38.1	D49.1
- - mesothelioma—*see Mesothelioma*						
- - middle lobe	C34.2	C78.0-	D02.21	D14.31	D38.1	D49.1
- - overlapping lesion	C34.8-	-	-	-	-	-
- - upper lobe	C34.1-	C78.0-	D02.2-	D14.3-	D38.1	D49.1
- lymph, lymphatic channel NEC	C49.9	C79.89	-	D21.9	D48.1	D49.2
- - gland (secondary)	-	C77.9	-	D36.0	D48.7	D49.89
- - - abdominal	-	C77.2	-	D36.0	D48.7	D49.89
- - - aortic	-	C77.2	-	D36.0	D48.7	D49.89
- - - arm	-	C77.3	-	D36.0	D48.7	D49.89
- - - auricular (anterior) (posterior)	-	C77.0	-	D36.0	D48.7	D49.89
- - - axilla, axillary	-	C77.3	-	D36.0	D48.7	D49.89
- - - brachial	-	C77.3	-	D36.0	D48.7	D49.89
- - - bronchial	-	C77.1	-	D36.0	D48.7	D49.89
- - - bronchopulmonary	-	C77.1	-	D36.0	D48.7	D49.89
- - - celiac	-	C77.2	-	D36.0	D48.7	D49.89
- - - cervical	-	C77.0	-	D36.0	D48.7	D49.89
- - - cervicofacial	-	C77.0	-	D36.0	D48.7	D49.89
- - - Cloquet	-	C77.4	-	D36.0	D48.7	D49.89
- - - colic	-	C77.2	-	D36.0	D48.7	D49.89
- - - common duct	-	C77.2	-	D36.0	D48.7	D49.89
- - - cubital	-	C77.3	-	D36.0	D48.7	D49.89
- - - diaphragmatic	-	C77.1	-	D36.0	D48.7	D49.89
- - - epigastric, inferior	-	C77.1	-	D36.0	D48.7	D49.89
- - - epitrochlear	-	C77.3	-	D36.0	D48.7	D49.89
- - - esophageal	-	C77.1	-	D36.0	D48.7	D49.89
- - - face	-	C77.0	-	D36.0	D48.7	D49.89
- - - femoral	-	C77.4	-	D36.0	D48.7	D49.89

	Malignant Primary	Malignant Secondary	CA in Situ	Benign	Uncertain Behavior	Unspecified Behavior
- - - gastric	-	C77.2	-	D36.0	D48.7	D49.89
- - - groin	-	C77.4	-	D36.0	D48.7	D49.89
- - - head	-	C77.0	-	D36.0	D48.7	D49.89
- - - hepatic	-	C77.2	-	D36.0	D48.7	D49.89
- - - hilar (pulmonary)	-	C77.1	-	D36.0	D48.7	D49.89
- - - - splenic	-	C77.2	-	D36.0	D48.7	D49.89
- - - hypogastric	-	C77.5	-	D36.0	D48.7	D49.89
- - - ileocolic	-	C77.2	-	D36.0	D48.7	D49.89
- - - iliac	-	C77.5	-	D36.0	D48.7	D49.89
- - - infraclavicular	-	C77.3	-	D36.0	D48.7	D49.89
- - - inguina, inguinal	-	C77.4	-	D36.0	D48.7	D49.89
- - - innominate	-	C77.1	-	D36.0	D48.7	D49.89
- - - intercostal	-	C77.1	-	D36.0	D48.7	D49.89
- - - intestinal	-	C77.2	-	D36.0	D48.7	D49.89
- - - intraabdominal	-	C77.2	-	D36.0	D48.7	D49.89
- - - intrapelvic	-	C77.5	-	D36.0	D48.7	D49.89
- - - intrathoracic	-	C77.1	-	D36.0	D48.7	D49.89
- - - jugular	-	C77.0	-	D36.0	D48.7	D49.89
- - - leg	-	C77.4	-	D36.0	D48.7	D49.89
- - - limb						
- - - - lower	-	C77.4	-	D36.0	D48.7	D49.89
- - - - upper	-	C77.3	-	D36.0	D48.7	D49.89
- - - lower limb	-	C77.4	-	D36.0	D48.7	D49.89
- - - lumbar	-	C77.2	-	D36.0	D48.7	D49.89
- - - mandibular	-	C77.0	-	D36.0	D48.7	D49.89
- - - mediastinal	-	C77.1	-	D36.0	D48.7	D49.89
- - - mesenteric (inferior) (superior)	-	C77.2	-	D36.0	D48.7	D49.89
- - - midcolic	-	C77.2	-	D36.0	D48.7	D49.89
- - - multiple sites in categories C77.0 - C77.5	-	C77.8	-	D36.0	D48.7	D49.89
- - - neck	-	C77.0	-	D36.0	D48.7	D49.89
- - - obturator	-	C77.5	-	D36.0	D48.7	D49.89
- - - occipital	-	C77.0	-	D36.0	D48.7	D49.89
- - - pancreatic	-	C77.2	-	D36.0	D48.7	D49.89
- - - para-aortic	-	C77.2	-	D36.0	D48.7	D49.89
- - - paracervical	-	C77.5	-	D36.0	D48.7	D49.89
- - - parametrial	-	C77.5	-	D36.0	D48.7	D49.89
- - - parasternal	-	C77.1	-	D36.0	D48.7	D49.89
- - - parotid	-	C77.0	-	D36.0	D48.7	D49.89
- - - pectoral	-	C77.3	-	D36.0	D48.7	D49.89
- - - pelvic	-	C77.5	-	D36.0	D48.7	D49.89
- - - peri-aortic	-	C77.2	-	D36.0	D48.7	D49.89
- - - peripancreatic	-	C77.2	-	D36.0	D48.7	D49.89
- - - popliteal	-	C77.4	-	D36.0	D48.7	D49.89
- - - porta hepatis	-	C77.2	-	D36.0	D48.7	D49.89
- - - portal	-	C77.2	-	D36.0	D48.7	D49.89
- - - preauricular	-	C77.0	-	D36.0	D48.7	D49.89
- - - prelaryngeal	-	C77.0	-	D36.0	D48.7	D49.89
- - - presymphyseal	-	C77.5	-	D36.0	D48.7	D49.89
- - - pretracheal	-	C77.0	-	D36.0	D48.7	D49.89
- - - primary (any site) NEC	C96.9	-	-	-	-	-
- - - pulmonary (hiler)	-	C77.1	-	D36.0	D48.7	D49.89
- - - pyloric	-	C77.2	-	D36.0	D48.7	D49.89
- - - retroperitoneal	-	C77.2	-	D36.0	D48.7	D49.89
- - - retropharyngeal	-	C77.0	-	D36.0	D48.7	D49.89
- - - Rosenmüller's	-	C77.4	-	D36.0	D48.7	D49.89
- - - sacral	-	C77.5	-	D36.0	D48.7	D49.89
- - - scalene	-	C77.0	-	D36.0	D48.7	D49.89
- - - site NEC	-	C77.9	-	D36.0	D48.7	D49.89
- - - splenic (hilar)	-	C77.2	-	D36.0	D48.7	D49.89
- - - subclavicular	-	C77.3	-	D36.0	D48.7	D49.89
- - - subinguinal	-	C77.4	-	D36.0	D48.7	D49.89
- - - sublingual	-	C77.0	-	D36.0	D48.7	D49.89
- - - submandibular	-	C77.0	-	D36.0	D48.7	D49.89
- - - submaxillary	-	C77.0	-	D36.0	D48.7	D49.89
- - - submental	-	C77.0	-	D36.0	D48.7	D49.89
- - - subscapular	-	C77.3	-	D36.0	D48.7	D49.89
- - - supraclavicular	-	C77.0	-	D36.0	D48.7	D49.89
- - - thoracic	-	C77.1	-	D36.0	D48.7	D49.89
- - - tibial	-	C77.4	-	D36.0	D48.7	D49.89
- - - tracheal	-	C77.1	-	D36.0	D48.7	D49.89
- - - tracheobronchial	-	C77.1	-	D36.0	D48.7	D49.89

	Malignant Primary	Malignant Secondary	CA in Situ	Benign	Uncertain Behavior	Unspecified Behavior
- - - upper limb	-	C77.3	-	D36.0	D48.7	D49.89
- - - Virchow's	-	C77.0	-	D36.0	D48.7	D49.89
- - node—*see also Neoplasm, lymph gland*						
- - - primary NEC	C96.9	-	-	-	-	-
- - vessel—*see also Neoplasm, connective tissue*	C49.9	C79.89	-	D21.9	D48.1	D49.2
- Mackenrodt's ligament	C57.7	C79.82	D07.39	D28.7	D39.8	D49.59
- malar	C41.0	C79.51	-	D16.4-	D48.0	D49.2
- - region—*see Neoplasm, cheek*						
- mammary gland—*see Neoplasm, breast*						
- mandible	C41.1	C79.51	-	D16.5-	D48.0	D49.2
- - alveolar						
- - - mucosa (carcinoma)	C03.1	C79.89	D00.03	D10.39	D37.09	D49.0
- - - ridge or process	C41.1	C79.51	-	D16.5-	D48.0	D49.2
- marrow (bone)NEC	C96.9	C79.52	-	-	D47.9	D49.89
- mastectomy site (skin)—*see also Neoplasm, breast, skin*	C44.501	C79.2	-	-	-	-
- - specified as breast tissue	C50.8-	C79.81	-	-	-	-
- mastoid (air cells) (antrum) (cavity)	C30.1	C78.39	D02.3	D14.0	D38.5	D49.1
- - bone or process	C41.0	C79.51	-	D16.4-	D48.0	D49.2
- maxilla, maxillary (superior)	C41.0	C79.51	-	D16.4-	D48.0	D49.2
- - alveolar						
- - - mucosa	C03.0	C79.89	D00.03	D10.39	D37.09	D49.0
- - - ridge or process (carcinoma)	C41.0	C79.51	-	D16.4-	D48.0	D49.2
- - antrum	C31.0	C78.39	D02.3	D14.0	D38.5	D49.1
- - carcinoma	C03.0	C79.51	-	-	-	-
- - inferior—*see Neoplasm, mandible*						
- - sinus	C31.0	C78.39	D02.3	D14.0	D38.5	D49.1
- meatus external (ear)—*see also Neoplasm, skin, ear*	C44.20-	C79.2	D04.2-	D23.2-	D48.5	D49.2
- Meckel diverticulum, malignant	C17.3	C78.4	D01.49	D13.39	D37.2	D49.0
- mediastinum, mediastinal	C38.3	C78.1	-	D15.2	D38.3	D49.89
- - anterior	C38.1	C78.1	-	D15.2	D38.3	D49.89
- - posterior	C38.2	C78.1	-	D15.2	D38.3	D49.89
- medulla						
- - adrenal	C74.1-	C79.7-	D09.3	D35.0-	D44.1-	D49.7
- - oblongata	C71.7	C79.31	-	D33.1	D43.1	D49.6
- meibomian gland	C44.10-	C79.2	D04.1-	D23.1-	D48.5	D49.2
- - basal cell carcinoma	C44.11-	-	-	-	-	-
- - sebaceous cell	C44.13-	-	-	-	-	-
- - specified type NEC	C44.19-	-	-	-	-	-
- - squamous cell carcinoma	C44.12-	-	-	-	-	-
- melanoma—*see Melanoma*						
- meninges	C70.9	C79.49	-	D32.9	D42.9	D49.7
- - brain	C70.0	C79.32	-	D32.0	D42.0	D49.7
- - cerebral	C70.0	C79.32	-	D32.0	D42.0	D49.7
- - cranial	C70.0	C79.32	-	D32.0	D42.0	D49.7
- - intracranial	C70.0	C79.32	-	D32.0	D42.0	D49.7
- - spinal (cord)	C70.1	C79.49	-	D32.1	D42.1	D49.7
- meniscus, knee joint (lateral) (medial)	C40.2-	C79.51	-	D16.2-	D48.0	D49.2
- Merkel cell—*see Carcinoma, Merkel cell*						
- mesentery, mesenteric	C48.1	C78.6	-	D20.1	D48.4	D49.0
- mesoappendix	C48.1	C78.6	-	D20.1	D48.4	D49.0
- mesocolon	C48.1	C78.6	-	D20.1	D48.4	D49.0
- mesopharynx—*see Neoplasm, oropharynx*						
- mesosalpinx	C57.1	C79.82	D07.39	D28.2	D39.8	D49.59
- mesothelial tissue—*see Mesothelioma*						
- mesothelioma—*see Mesothelioma*						
- mesovarium	C57.1	C79.82	D07.39	D28.2	D39.8	D49.59
- metacarpus (any bone)	C40.1-	C79.51	-	D16.1-	-	-
- metastatic NEC—*see also Neoplasm, by site, secondary*	-	C79.9	-	-	-	-
- metatarsus (any bone)	C40.3-	C79.51	-	D16.3-	-	-
- midbrain	C71.7	C79.31	-	D33.1	D43.1	D49.6
- milk duct—*see Neoplasm, breast*						
- mons						
- - pubis	C51.9	C79.82	D07.1	D28.0	D39.8	D49.59
- - veneris	C51.9	C79.82	D07.1	D28.0	D39.8	D49.59
- motor tract	C72.9	C79.49	-	D33.9	D43.9	D49.7
- - brain	C71.9	C79.31	-	D33.2	D43.2	D49.6
- - cauda equina	C72.1	C79.49	-	D33.4	D43.4	D49.7
- - spinal	C72.0	C79.49	-	D33.4	D43.4	D49.7
- mouth	C06.9	C79.89	D00.00	D10.30	D37.09	D49.0

	Malignant Primary	Malignant Secondary	CA in Situ	Benign	Uncertain Behavior	Unspecified Behavior
- - book-leaf	C06.89	C79.89	-	-	-	-
- - floor	C04.9	C79.89	D00.06	D10.2	D37.09	D49.0
- - - anterior portion	C04.0	C79.89	D00.06	D10.2	D37.09	D49.0
- - - lateral portion	C04.1	C79.89	D00.06	D10.2	D37.09	D49.0
- - - overlapping lesion	C04.8	-	-	-	-	-
- - overlapping NEC	C06.80	-	-	-	-	-
- - roof	C05.9	C79.89	D00.00	D10.39	D37.09	D49.0
- - specified part NEC	C06.89	C79.89	D00.00	D10.39	D37.09	D49.0
- - vestibule	C06.1	C79.89	D00.00	D10.39	D37.09	D49.0
- mucosa						
- - alveolar (ridge or process)	C03.9	C79.89	D00.03	D10.39	D37.09	D49.0
- - - lower	C03.1	C79.89	D00.03	D10.39	D37.09	D49.0
- - - upper	C03.0	C79.89	D00.03	D10.39	D37.09	D49.0
- - buccal	C06.0	C79.89	D00.02	D10.39	D37.09	D49.0
- - cheek	C06.0	C79.89	D00.02	D10.39	D37.09	D49.0
- - lip—see Neoplasm, lip, internal						
- - nasal	C30.0	C78.39	D02.3	D14.0	D38.5	D49.1
- - oral	C06.0	C79.89	D00.02	D10.39	D37.09	D49.0
- Mullerian duct						
- - female	C57.7	C79.82	D07.39	D28.7	D39.8	D49.59
- - male	C63.7	C79.82	D07.69	D29.8	D40.8	D49.59
- muscle—see also Neoplasm, connective tissue						
- - extraocular	C69.6-	C79.49	D09.2-	D31.6-	D48.7	D49.89
- myocardium	C38.0	C79.89	-	D15.1	D48.7	D49.89
- myometrium	C54.2	C79.82	D07.0	D26.1	D39.0	D49.59
- myopericardium	C38.0	C79.89	-	D15.1	D48.7	D49.89
- nabothian gland (follicle)	C53.0	C79.82	D06.0	D26.0	D39.0	D49.59
- nail—see also Neoplasm, skin, limb	C44.90	C79.2	D04.9	D23.9	D48.5	D49.2
- - finger—see also Neoplasm, skin, limb, upper	C44.60-	C79.2	D04.6-	D23.6-	D48.5	D49.2
- - toe—see also Neoplasm, skin, limb, lower	C44.70-	C79.2	D04.7-	D23.7-	D48.5	D49.2
- nares, naris (anterior) (posterior)	C30.0	C78.39	D02.3	D14.0	D38.5	D49.1
- nasal—see Neoplasm, nose						
- nasolabial groove—see also Neoplasm, skin, face	C44.309	C79.2	D04.39	D23.39	D48.5	D49.2
- nasolacrimal duct	C69.5-	C79.49	D09.2-	D31.5-	D48.7	D49.89
- nasopharynx, nasopharyngeal	C11.9	C79.89	D00.08	D10.6	D37.05	D49.0
- - floor	C11.3	C79.89	D00.08	D10.6	D37.05	D49.0
- - overlapping lesion	C11.8	-	-	-	-	-
- - roof	C11.0	C79.89	D00.08	D10.6	D37.05	D49.0
- - wall	C11.9	C79.89	D00.08	D10.6	D37.05	D49.0
- - - anterior	C11.3	C79.89	D00.08	D10.6	D37.05	D49.0
- - - lateral	C11.2	C79.89	D00.08	D10.6	D37.05	D49.0
- - - posterior	C11.1	C79.89	D00.08	D10.6	D37.05	D49.0
- - - superior	C11.0	C79.89	D00.08	D10.6	D37.05	D49.0
- nates—see also Neoplasm, skin, trunk	C44.509	C79.2	D04.5	D23.5	D48.5	D49.2
- neck NEC	C76.0	C79.89	D09.8	D36.7	D48.7	D49.89
- - skin	C44.40	-	-	-	-	-
- - - basal cell carcinoma	C44.41	-	-	-	-	-
- - - specified type NEC	C44.49	-	-	-	-	-
- - - squamous cell carcinoma	C44.42	-	-	-	-	-
- nerve (ganglion)	C47.9	C79.89	-	D36.10	D48.2	D49.2
- - abducens	C72.59	C79.49	-	D33.3	D43.3	D49.7
- - accessory (spinal)	C72.59	C79.49	-	D33.3	D43.3	D49.7
- - acoustic	C72.4-	C79.49	-	D33.3	D43.3	D49.7
- - auditory	C72.4-	C79.49	-	D33.3	D43.3	D49.7
- - autonomic NEC—see also Neoplasm, nerve, peripheral	C47.9	C79.89	-	D36.10	D48.2	D49.2
- - brachial	C47.1-	C79.89	-	D36.12	D48.2	D49.2
- - cranial	C72.50	C79.49	-	D33.3	D43.3	D49.7
- - - specified NEC	C72.59	C79.49	-	D33.3	D43.3	D49.7
- - facial	C72.59	C79.49	-	D33.3	D43.3	D49.7
- - femoral	C47.2-	C79.89	-	D36.13	D48.2	D49.2
- - ganglion NEC—see also Neoplasm, nerve, peripheral	C47.9	C79.89	-	D36.10	D48.2	D49.2
- - glossopharyngeal	C72.59	C79.49	-	D33.3	D43.3	D49.7
- - hypoglossal	C72.59	C79.49	-	D33.3	D43.3	D49.7
- - intercostal	C47.3	C79.89	-	D36.14	D48.2	D49.2
- - lumbar	C47.6	C79.89	-	D36.17	D48.2	D49.2
- - median	C47.1-	C79.89	-	D36.12	D48.2	D49.2
- - obturator	C47.2-	C79.89	-	D36.13	D48.2	D49.2
- - oculomotor	C72.59	C79.49	-	D33.3	D43.3	D49.7
- - olfactory	C47.2-	C79.49	-	D33.3	D43.3	D49.7

	Malignant Primary	Malignant Secondary	CA in Situ	Benign	Uncertain Behavior	Unspecified Behavior
- - optic	C72.3-	C79.49	-	D33.3	D43.3	D49.7
- - parasympathetic NEC	C47.9	C79.89	-	D36.10	D48.2	D49.2
- - peripheral NEC	C47.9	C79.89	-	D36.10	D48.2	D49.2
- - - abdomen	C47.4	C79.89	-	D36.15	D48.2	D49.2
- - - abdominal wall	C47.4	C79.89	-	D36.15	D48.2	D49.2
- - - ankle	C47.2-	C79.89	-	D36.13	D48.2	D49.2
- - - antecubital fossa or space	C47.1-	C79.89	-	D36.12	D48.2	D49.2
- - - arm	C47.1-	C79.89	-	D36.12	D48.2	D49.2
- - - auricle (ear)	C47.0	C79.89	-	D36.11	D48.2	D49.2
- - - axilla	C47.3	C79.89	-	D36.12	D48.2	D49.2
- - - back	C47.6	C79.89	-	D36.17	D48.2	D49.2
- - - buttock	C47.5	C79.89	-	D36.16	D48.2	D49.2
- - - calf	C47.2-	C79.89	-	D36.13	D48.2	D49.2
- - - cervical region	C47.0	C79.89	-	D36.11	D48.2	D49.2
- - - cheek	C47.0	C79.89	-	D36.11	D48.2	D49.2
- - - chest (wall)	C47.3	C79.89	-	D36.14	D48.2	D49.2
- - - chin	C47.0	C79.89	-	D36.11	D48.2	D49.2
- - - ear (external)	C47.0	C79.89	-	D36.11	D48.2	D49.2
- - - elbow	C47.1-	C79.89	-	D36.12	D48.2	D49.2
- - - extra rectal	C47.5	C79.89	-	D36.16	D48.2	D49.2
- - - extremity	C47.9	C79.89	-	D36.10	D48.2	D49.2
- - - - lower	C47.2-	C79.89	-	D36.13	D48.2	D49.2
- - - - upper	C47.1-	C79.89	-	D36.12	D48.2	D49.2
- - - eyelid	C47.0	C79.89	-	D36.11	D48.2	D49.2
- - - face	C47.0	C79.89	-	D36.11	D48.2	D49.2
- - - finger	C47.1-	C79.89	-	D36.12	D48.2	D49.2
- - - flank	C47.6	C79.89	-	D36.17	D48.2	D49.2
- - - foot	C47.2-	C79.89	-	D36.13	D48.2	D49.2
- - - forearm	C47.1-	C79.89	-	D36.12	D48.2	D49.2
- - - forehead	C47.0	C79.89	-	D36.11	D48.2	D49.2
- - - gluteal region	C47.5	C79.89	-	D36.16	D48.2	D49.2
- - - groin	C47.5	C79.89	-	D36.16	D48.2	D49.2
- - - hand	C47.1-	C79.89	-	D36.12	D48.2	D49.2
- - - head	C47.0	C79.89	-	D36.11	D48.2	D49.2
- - - heel	C47.2-	C79.89	-	D36.13	D48.2	D49.2
- - - hip	C47.2-	C79.89	-	D36.13	D48.2	D49.2
- - - infraclavicular region	C47.3	C79.89	-	D36.14	D48.2	D49.2
- - - inguinal (canal) (region)	C47.5	C79.89	-	D36.16	D48.2	D49.2
- - - intrathoracic	C47.3	C79.89	-	D36.14	D48.2	D49.2
- - - ischiorectal fossa	C47.5	C79.89	-	D36.16	D48.2	D49.2
- - - knee	C47.2-	C79.89	-	D36.13	D48.2	D49.2
- - - leg	C47.2-	C79.89	-	D36.13	D48.2	D49.2
- - - limb NEC	C47.9	C79.89	-	D36.10	D48.2	D49.2
- - - - lower	C47.2-	C79.89	-	D36.13	D48.2	D49.2
- - - - upper	C47.1-	C79.89	-	D36.12	D48.2	D49.2
- - - nates	C47.5	C79.89	-	D36.16	D48.2	D49.2
- - - neck	C47.0	C79.89	-	D36.11	D48.2	D49.2
- - - orbit	C69.6-	C79.49	-	D31.6-	D48.7	D49.2
- - - pararectal	C47.5	C79.89	-	D36.16	D48.2	D49.2
- - - paraurethral	C47.5	C79.89	-	D36.16	D48.2	D49.2
- - - paravaginal	C47.5	C79.89	-	D36.16	D48.2	D49.2
- - - pelvis (floor)	C47.5	C79.89	-	D36.16	D48.2	D49.2
- - - pelvoabdominal	C47.8	C79.89	-	D36.17	D48.2	D49.2
- - - perineum	C47.5	C79.89	-	D36.16	D48.2	D49.2
- - - perirectal (tissue)	C47.5	C79.89	-	D36.16	D48.2	D49.2
- - - periurethral (tissue)	C47.5	C79.89	-	D36.16	D48.2	D49.2
- - - popliteal fossa or space	C47.2-	C79.89	-	D36.13	D48.2	D49.2
- - - presacral	C47.5	C79.89	-	D36.16	D48.2	D49.2
- - - pterygoid fossa	C47.0	C79.89	-	D36.11	D48.2	D49.2
- - - rectovaginal septum or wall	C47.5	C79.89	-	D36.16	D48.2	D49.2
- - - rectovesical	C47.5	C79.89	-	D36.16	D48.2	D49.2
- - - sacrococcygeal region	C47.5	C79.89	-	D36.16	D48.2	D49.2
- - - scalp	C47.0	C79.89	-	D36.11	D48.2	D49.2
- - - scapular region	C47.3	C79.89	-	D36.14	D48.2	D49.2
- - - shoulder	C47.1-	C79.89	-	D36.12	D48.2	D49.2
- - - submental	C47.0	C79.89	-	D36.11	D48.2	D49.2
- - - supraclavicular region	C47.0	C79.89	-	D36.11	D48.2	D49.2
- - - temple	C47.0	C79.89	-	D36.11	D48.2	D49.2
- - - temporal region	C47.0	C79.89	-	D36.11	D48.2	D49.2
- - - thigh	C47.2-	C79.89	-	D36.13	D48.2	D49.2
- - - thoracic (duct) (wall)	C47.3	C79.89	-	D36.14	D48.2	D49.2

	Malignant Primary	Malignant Secondary	CA in Situ	Benign	Uncertain Behavior	Unspecified Behavior
- - - thorax	C47.3	C79.89	-	D36.14	D48.2	D49.2
- - - thumb	C47.1-	C79.89	-	D36.12	D48.2	D49.2
- - - toe	C47.2-	C79.89	-	D36.13	D48.2	D49.2
- - - trunk	C47.6	C79.89	-	D36.17	D48.2	D49.2
- - - umbilicus	C47.4	C79.89	-	D36.15	D48.2	D49.2
- - - vesicorectal	C47.5	C79.89	-	D36.16	D48.2	D49.2
- - - wrist	C47.1-	C79.89	-	D36.12	D48.2	D49.2
- - radial	C47.1-	C79.89	-	D36.12	D48.2	D49.2
- - sacral	C47.5	C79.89	-	D36.16	D48.2	D49.2
- - sciatic	C47.2-	C79.89	-	D36.13	D48.2	D49.2
- - spinal NEC	C47.9	C79.89	-	D36.10	D48.2	D49.2
- - - accessory	C72.59	C79.49	-	D33.3	D43.3	D49.7
- - sympathetic NEC—see also Neoplasm, nerve, peripheral	C47.9	C79.89	-	D36.10	D48.2	D49.2
- - trigeminal	C72.59	C79.49	-	D33.3	D43.3	D49.7
- - trochlear	C72.59	C79.49	-	D33.3	D43.3	D49.7
- - ulnar	C47.1-	C79.89	-	D36.12	D48.2	D49.2
- - vagus	C72.59	C79.49	-	D33.3	D43.3	D49.7
- nervous system (central)	C72.9	C79.40	-	D33.9	D43.9	D49.7
- - autonomic—see Neoplasm, nerve, peripheral						
- - parasympathetic—see Neoplasm, nerve, peripheral						
- - specified site NEC	-	C79.49	-	D33.7	D43.8	-
- - sympathetic—see Neoplasm, nerve, peripheral						
- nevus—see Nevus						
- nipple	C50.0-	C79.81	D05.-	D24.-	-	-
- nose, nasal	C76.0	C79.89	D09.8	D36.7	D48.7	D49.89
- - ala (external) (nasi)—see also Neoplasm, nose, skin	C44.301	C79.2	D04.39	D23.39	D48.5	D49.2
- - bone	C41.0	C79.51	-	D16.4-	D48.0	D49.2
- - cartilage	C30.0	C78.39	D02.3	D14.0	D38.5	D49.1
- - cavity	C30.0	C78.39	D02.3	D14.0	D38.5	D49.1
- -choana	C11.3	C79.89	D00.08	D10.6	D37.05	D49.0
- - external (skin)—see also Neoplasm, nose, skin	C44.301	C79.2	D04.39	D23.39	D48.5	D49.2
- - fossa	C30.0	C78.39	D02.3	D14.0	D38.5	D49.1
- - internal	C30.0	C78.39	D02.3	D14.0	D38.5	D49.1
- - mucosa	C30.0	C78.39	D02.3	D14.0	D38.5	D49.1
- - septum	C30.0	C78.39	D02.3	D14.0	D38.5	D49.1
- - - posterior margin	C11.3	C79.89	D00.08	D10.6	D37.05	D49.0
- - sinus—see Neoplasm, sinus						
- - skin	C44.301	C79.2	D04.39	D23.39	D48.5	D49.2
- - - basal cell carcinoma	C44.311	-	-	-	-	-
- - - specified type NEC	C44.391	-	-	-	-	-
- - - squamous cell carcinoma	C44.321	-	-	-	-	-
- - turbinate (mucosa)	C30.0	C78.39	D02.3	D14.0	D38.5	D49.1
- - - bone	C41.0	C79.51	-	D16.4-	D48.0	D49.2
- - vestibule	C30.0	C78.39	D02.3	D14.0	D38.5	D49.1
- nostril	C30.0	C78.39	D02.3	D14.0	D38.5	D49.1
- nucleus pulposus	C41.2	C79.51	-	D16.6	D48.0	D49.2
- occipital						
- - bone	C41.0	C79.51	-	D16.4-	D48.0	D49.2
- - lobe or pole, brain	C71.4	C79.31	-	D33.0	D43.0	D49.6
- odontogenic—see Neoplasm, jaw bone						
- olfactory nerve or bulb	C72.2-	C79.49	-	D33.3	D43.3	D49.7
- olive (brain)	C71.7	C79.31	-	D33.1	D43.1	D49.6
- omentum	C48.1	C78.6	-	D20.1	D48.4	D49.0
- operculum (brain)	C71.0	C79.31	-	D33.0	D43.0	D49.6
- optic nerve, chiasm, or tract	C72.3-	C79.49	-	D33.3	D43.3	D49.7
- oral (cavity)	C06.9	C79.89	D00.00	D10.30	D37.09	D49.0
- - ill-defined	C14.8	C79.89	D00.00	D10.30	D37.09	D49.0
- - mucosa	C06.0	C79.89	D00.02	D10.39	D37.09	D49.0
- orbit	C69.6-	C79.49	D09.2-	D31.6-	D48.7	D49.89
- - autonomic nerve	C69.6-	C79.49	-	D31.6-	D48.7	D49.2
- - bone	C41.0	C79.51	-	D16.4-	D48.0	D49.2
- - eye	C69.6-	C79.49	D09.2-	D31.6-	D48.7	D49.89
- - peripheral nerves	C69.6-	C79.49	-	D31.6-	D48.7	D49.2
- - soft parts	C69.6-	C79.49	D09.2-	D31.6-	D48.7	D49.89
- organ of Zuckerkandl	C75.5	C79.89	-	D35.6	D44.7	D49.7
- oropharynx	C10.9	C79.89	D00.08	D10.5	D37.05	D49.0
- - branchial cleft (vestige)	C10.4	C79.89	D00.08	D10.5	D37.05	D49.0
- - junctional region	C10.8	C79.89	D00.08	D10.5	D37.05	D49.0
- - lateral wall	C10.2	C79.89	D00.08	D10.5	D37.05	D49.0

	Malignant Primary	Malignant Secondary	CA in Situ	Benign	Uncertain Behavior	Unspecified Behavior
- - overlapping lesion	C10.8	-	-	-	-	-
- - pillars or fauces	C09.1	C79.89	D00.08	D10.5	D37.05	D49.0
- - posterior wall	C10.3	C79.89	D00.08	D10.5	D37.05	D49.0
- - vallecula	C10.0	C79.89	D00.08	D10.5	D37.05	D49.0
- os						
- - external	C53.1	C79.82	D06.1	D26.0	D39.0	D49.59
- - internal	C53.0	C79.82	D06.0	D26.0	D39.0	D49.59
- ovary	C56.-	C79.6-	D07.39	D27.-	D39.1-	D49.59
- oviduct	C57.0-	C79.82	D07.39	D28.2	D39.8	D49.59
- palate	C05.9	C79.89	D00.00	D10.39	D37.09	D49.0
- - hard	C05.0	C79.89	D00.05	D10.39	D37.09	D49.0
- - junction of hard and soft palate	C05.9	C79.89	D00.00	D10.39	D37.09	D49.0
- - overlapping lesions	C05.8	-	-	-	-	-
- - soft	C05.1	C79.89	D00.04	D10.39	D37.09	D49.0
- - - nasopharyngeal surface	C11.3	C79.89	D00.08	D10.6	D37.05	D49.0
- - - posterior surface	C11.3	C79.89	D00.08	D10.6	D37.05	D49.0
- - - superior surface	C11.3	C79.89	D00.08	D10.6	D37.05	D49.0
- palatoglossal arch	C09.1	C79.89	D00.00	D10.5	D37.09	D49.0
- palatopharyngeal arch	C09.1	C79.89	D00.00	D10.5	D37.09	D49.0
- pallium	C71.0	C79.31		D33.0	D43.0	D49.6
- palpebra	C44.10-	C79.2	D04.1-	D23.1-	D48.5	D49.2
- - basal cell carcinoma	C44.11-	-	-	-	-	-
- - sebaceous cell	C44.13-	-	-	-	-	-
- - specified type NEC	C44.19-	-	-	-	-	-
- - squamous cell carcinoma	C44.12-	-	-	-	-	-
- pancreas	C25.9	C78.89	D01.7	D13.6	D37.8	D49.0
- - body	C25.1	C78.89	D01.7	D13.6	D37.8	D49.0
- - duct (of Santorini) (of Wirsung)	C25.3	C78.89	D01.7	D13.6	D37.8	D49.0
- - ectopic tissue	C25.7	C78.89	-	D13.6	D37.8	D49.0
- - head	C25.0	C78.89	D01.7	D13.6	D37.8	D49.0
- - islet cells	C25.4	C78.89	D01.7	D13.7	D37.8	D49.0
- - neck	C25.7	C78.89	D01.7	D13.6	D37.8	D49.0
- - overlapping lesion	C25.8	-	-	-	-	-
- - tail	C25.2	C78.89	D01.7	D13.6	D37.8	D49.0
- para-aortic body	C75.5	C79.89	-	D35.6	D44.7	D49.7
- paraganglion NEC	C75.5	C79.89	-	D35.6	D44.7	D49.7
- parametrium	C57.3	C79.82	-	D28.2	D39.8	D49.59
- paranephric	C48.0	C78.6		D20.0	D48.3	D49.0
- pararectal	C76.3	C79.89	-	D36.7	D48.7	D49.89
- parasagittal (region)	C76.0	C79.89	D09.8	D36.7	D48.7	D49.89
- parasellar	C72.9	C79.49	-	D33.9	D43.8	D49.7
- parathyroid (gland)	C75.0	C79.89	D09.3	D35.1	D44.2	D49.7
- paraurethral	C76.3	C79.89	-	D36.7	D48.7	D49.89
- - gland	C68.1	C79.19	D09.19	D30.8	D41.8	D49.59
- paravaginal	C76.3	C79.89	-	D36.7	D48.7	D49.89
- parenchyma, kidney	C64.-	C79.0-	D09.19	D30.0-	D41.0-	D49.59
- parietal						
- - bone	C41.0	C79.51	-	D16.4-	D48.0	D49.2
- - lobe, brain	C71.3	C79.31	-	D33.0	D43.0	D49.6
- paroophoron	C57.1	C79.82	D07.39	D28.2	D39.8	D49.59
- parotid (duct) (gland)	C07	C79.89	D00.00	D11.0	D37.030	D49.0
- parovarium	C57.1	C79.82	D07.39	D28.2	D39.8	D49.59
- patella	C40.20	C79.51	-	-	-	-
- peduncle, cerebral	C71.7	C79.31	-	D33.1	D43.1	D49.6
- pelvirectal junction	C19	C78.5	D01.1	D12.7	D37.5	D49.0
- pelvis, pelvic	C76.3	C79.89	D09.8	D36.7	D48.7	D49.89
- - bone	C41.4	C79.51	-	D16.8	D48.0	D49.2
- - floor	C76.3	C79.89	D09.8	D36.7	D48.7	D49.89
- - renal	C65.-	C79.0-	D09.19	D30.1-	D41.1-	D49.59
- - viscera	C76.3	C79.89	D09.8	D36.7	D48.7	D49.89
- - wall	C76.3	C79.89	D09.8	D36.7	D48.7	D49.89
- pelvo-abdominal	C76.8	C79.89	D09.8	D36.7	D48.7	D49.89
- penis	C60.9	C79.82	D07.4	D29.0	D40.8	D49.59
- - body	C60.2	C79.82	D07.4	D29.0	D40.8	D49.59
- - corpus (cavernosum)	C60.2	C79.82	D07.4	D29.0	D40.8	D49.59
- - glans	C60.1	C79.82	D07.4	D29.0	D40.8	D49.59
- - overlapping sites	C60.8	-	-	-	-	-
- - skin NEC	C60.9	C79.82	D07.4	D29.0	D40.8	D49.59
- periadrenal (tissue)	C48.0	C78.6	-	D20.0	D48.3	D49.0
- perianal (skin)—*see also Neoplasm, anus, skin*	C44.500	C79.2	D04.5	D23.5	D48.5	D49.2
- pericardium	C38.0	C79.89	-	D15.1	D48.7	D49.89

	Malignant Primary	Malignant Secondary	CA in Situ	Benign	Uncertain Behavior	Unspecified Behavior
- perinephric	C48.0	C78.6	-	D20.0	D48.3	D49.0
- perineum	C76.3	C79.89	D09.8	D36.7	D48.7	D49.89
- periodontal tissue NEC	C03.9	C79.89	D00.03	D10.39	D37.09	D49.0
- periosteum—*see Neoplasm, bone*						
- peripancreatic	C48.0	C78.6	-	D20.0	D48.3	D49.0
- peripheral nerve NEC	C47.9	C79.89	-	D36.10	D48.2	D49.2
- perirectal (tissue)	C76.3	C79.89	-	D36.7	D48.7	D49.89
- perirenal (tissue)	C48.0	C78.6	-	D20.0	D48.3	D49.0
- peritoneum, peritoneal (cavity)	C48.2	C78.6	-	D20.1	D48.4	D49.0
- - benign mesothelial tissue—*see Mesothelioma, benign*						
- - overlapping lesion	C48.8	-	-	-	-	-
- - - with digestive organs	C26.9	-	-	-	-	-
- - parietal	C48.1	C78.6	-	D20.1	D48.4	D49.0
- - pelvic	C48.1	C78.6	-	D20.1	D48.4	D49.0
- - specified part NEC	C48.1	C78.6	-	D20.1	D48.4	D49.0
- peritonsillar (tissue)	C76.0	C79.89	D09.8	D36.7	D48.7	D49.89
- periurethral tissue	C76.3	C79.89	-	D36.7	D48.7	D49.89
- phalanges						
- - foot	C40.3-	C79.51	-	D16.3-	-	-
- - hand	C40.1-	C79.51	-	D16.1-	-	-
- pharynx, pharyngeal	C14.0	C79.89	D00.08	D10.9	D37.05	D49.0
- - bursa	C11.1	C79.89	D00.08	D10.6	D37.05	D49.0
- - fornix	C11.3	C79.89	D00.08	D10.6	D37.05	D49.0
- - recess	C11.2	C79.89	D00.08	D10.6	D37.05	D49.0
- - region	C14.0	C79.89	D00.08	D10.9	D37.05	D49.0
- - tonsil	C11.1	C79.89	D00.08	D10.6	D37.05	D49.0
- - wall (lateral) (posterior)	C14.0	C79.89	D00.08	D10.9	D37.05	D49.0
- pia mater	C70.9	C79.40	-	D32.9	D42.9	D49.7
- - cerebral	C70.0	C79.32	-	D32.0	D42.0	D49.7
- - cranial	C70.0	C79.32	-	D32.0	D42.0	D49.7
- - spinal	C70.1	C79.49	-	D32.1	D42.1	D49.7
- pillars of fauces	C09.1	C79.89	D00.08	D10.5	D37.05	D49.0
- pineal (body) (gland)	C75.3	C79.89	D09.3	D35.4	D44.5	D49.7
- pinna (ear) NEC—*see also Neoplasm, skin, ear*	C44.20-	C79.2	D04.2-	D23.2-	D48.5	D49.2
- piriform fossa or sinus	C12	C79.89	D00.08	D10.7	D37.05	D49.0
- pituitary (body) (fossa) (gland) (lobe)	C75.1	C79.89	D09.3	D35.2	D44.3	D49.7
- placenta	C58	C79.82	D07.0	D26.7	D39.2	D49.59
- pleura, pleural (cavity)	C38.4	C78.2	-	D19.0	D38.2	D49.1
- - overlapping lesion with heart or mediastinum	C38.8	-	-	-	-	-
- - parietal	C38.4	C78.2	-	D19.0	D38.2	D49.1
- - visceral	C38.4	C78.2	-	D19.0	D38.2	D49.1
- plexus						
- - brachial	C47.1-	C79.89	-	D36.12	D48.2	D49.2
- - cervical	C47.0	C79.89	-	D36.11	D48.2	D49.2
- - choroid	C71.5	C79.31	-	D33.0	D43.0	D49.6
- - lumbosacral	C47.5	C79.89	-	D36.16	D48.2	D49.2
- - sacral	C47.5	C79.89	-	D36.16	D48.2	D49.2
- pluriendocrine	C75.8	C79.89	D09.3	D35.7	D44.9	D49.7
- pole						
- - frontal	C71.1	C79.31	-	D33.0	D43.0	D49.6
- - occipital	C71.4	C79.31	-	D33.0	D43.0	D49.6
- pons (varolii)	C71.7	C79.31	-	D33.1	D43.1	D49.6
- popliteal fossa or space	C76.5-	C79.89	D04.7-	D36.7	D48.7	D49.89
- postcricoid (region)	C13.0	C79.89	D00.08	D10.7	D37.05	D49.0
- posterior fossa (cranial)	C71.9	C79.31	-	D33.2	D43.2	D49.6
- postnasal space	C11.9	C79.89	D00.08	D10.6	D37.05	D49.0
- prepuce	C60.0	C79.82	D07.4	D29.0	D40.8	D49.59
- prepylorus	C16.4	C78.89	D00.2	D13.1	D37.1	D49.0
- presacral (region)	C76.3	C79.89	-	D36.7	D48.7	D49.89
- prostate (gland)	C61	C79.82	D07.5	D29.1	D40.0	D49.59
- - utricle	C68.0	C79.19	D09.19	D30.4	D41.3	D49.59
- pterygoid fossa	C49.0	C79.89	-	D21.0	D48.1	D49.2
- pubic bone	C41.4	C79.51	-	D16.8	D48.0	D49.2
- pudenda, pudendum (female)	C51.9	C79.82	D07.1	D28.0	D39.8	D49.59
- pulmonary—*see also Neoplasm, lung*	C34.9-	C78.0-	D02.2-	D14.3-	D38.1	D49.1
- putamen	C71.0	C79.31	-	D33.0	D43.0	D49.6
- pyloric						
- - antrum	C16.3	C78.89	D00.2	D13.1	D37.1	D49.0
- - canal	C16.4	C78.89	D00.2	D13.1	D37.1	D49.0
- pylorus	C16.4	C78.89	D00.2	D13.1	D37.1	D49.0

	Malignant Primary	Malignant Secondary	CA in Situ	Benign	Uncertain Behavior	Unspecified Behavior
- pyramid (brain)	C71.7	C79.31	-	D33.1	D43.1	D49.6
- pyriform fossa or sinus	C12	C79.89	D00.08	D10.7	D37.05	D49.0
- radius (any part)	C40.0-	C79.51	-	D16.0-	-	-
- Rathke's pouch	C75.1	C79.89	D09.3	D35.2	D44.3	D49.7
- rectosigmoid (junction)	C19	C78.5	D01.1	D12.7	D37.5	D49.0
- - overlapping lesion with anus or rectum	C21.8	-	-	-	-	-
- rectouterine pouch	C48.1	C78.6	-	D20.1	D48.4	D49.0
- rectovaginal septum or wall	C76.3	C79.89	D09.8	D36.7	D48.7	D49.89
- rectovesical septum	C76.3	C79.89	D09.8	D36.7	D48.7	D49.89
- rectum (ampulla)	C20	C78.5	D01.2	D12.8	D37.5	D49.0
- - and colon	C19	C78.5	D01.1	D12.7	D37.5	D49.0
- - overlapping lesion with anus or rectosigmoid junction	C21.8	-	-	-	-	-
- renal	C64.-	C79.0-	D09.19	D30.0-	D41.0-	D49.51
- - calyx	C65.-	C79.0-	D09.19	D30.1-	D41.1-	D49.51
- - hilus	C65.-	C79.0-	D09.19	D30.1-	D41.1-	D49.51
- - parenchyma	C64.-	C79.0-	D09.19	D30.0-	D41.0-	D49.51
- - pelvis	C65.-	C79.0-	D09.19	D30.1-	D41.1-	D49.51
- respiratory						
- - organs or system NEC	C39.9	C78.30	D02.4	D14.4	D38.6	D49.1
- - tract NEC	C39.9	C78.30	D02.4	D14.4	D38.5	D49.1
- - - upper	C39.0	C78.30	D02.4	D14.4	D38.5	D49.1
- retina	C69.2-	C79.49	D09.2-	D31.2-	D48.7	D49.81
- retrobulbar	C69.6-	C79.49	-	D31.6-	D48.7	D49.89
- retrocecal	C48.0	C78.6	-	D20.0	D48.3	D49.0
- retromolar (area) (triangle) (trigone)	C06.2	C79.89	D00.00	D10.39	D37.09	D49.0
- retro-orbital	C76.0	C79.89	D09.8	D36.7	D48.7	D49.89
- retroperitoneal (space) (tissue)	C48.0	C78.6	-	D20.0	D48.3	D49.0
- retroperitoneum	C48.0	C78.6	-	D20.0	D48.3	D49.0
- retropharyngeal	C14.0	C79.89	D00.08	D10.9	D37.05	D49.0
- retrovesical (septum)	C76.3	C79.89	D09.8	D36.7	D48.7	D49.89
- rhinencephalon	C71.0	C79.31	-	D33.0	D43.0	D49.6
- rib	C41.3	C79.51	-	D16.7	D48.0	D49.2
- Rosenmüller's fossa	C11.2	C79.89	D00.08	D10.6	D37.05	D49.0
- round ligament	C57.2	C79.82	-	D28.2	D39.8	D49.59
- sacrococcyx, sacrococcygeal	C41.4	C79.51	-	D16.8	D48.0	D49.2
- - region	C76.3	C79.89	D09.8	D36.7	D48.7	D49.89
- sacrouterine ligament	C57.3	C79.82	-	D28.2	D39.8	D49.59
- sacrum, sacral (vertebra)	C41.4	C79.51	-	D16.8	D48.0	D49.2
- salivary gland or duct (major)	C08.9	C79.89	D00.00	D11.9	D37.039	D49.0
- - minor NEC	C06.9	C79.89	D00.00	D10.39	D37.04	D49.0
- - overlapping lesion	C08.9	-	-	-	-	-
- - parotid	C07	C79.89	D00.00	D11.0	D37.030	D49.0
- - pluriglandular	C08.9	C79.89	D00.00	D11.9	D37.039	D49.0
- - sublingual	C08.1	C79.89	D00.00	D11.7	D37.031	D49.0
- - submandibular	C08.0	C79.89	D00.00	D11.7	D37.032	D49.0
- - submaxillary	C08.0	C79.89	D00.00	D11.7	D37.032	D49.0
- salpinx (uterine)	C57.0-	C79.82	D07.39	D28.2	D39.8	D49.59
- Santorini's duct	C25.3	C78.89	D01.7	D13.6	D37.8	D49.0
- scalp	C44.40	C79.2	D04.4	D23.4	D48.5	D49.2
- - basal cell carcinoma	C44.41	-	-	-	-	-
- - specified type NEC	C44.49	-	-	-	-	-
- - squamous cell carcinoma	C44.42	-	-	-	-	-
- scapula (any part)	C40.0-	C79.51	-	D16.0-	-	-
- scapular region	C76.1	C79.89	D09.8	D36.7	D48.7	D49.89
- scar NEC—see also Neoplasm, skin, by site	C44.90	C79.2	D04.9	D23.9	D48.5	D49.2
- sciatic nerve	C47.2-	C79.89	-	D36.13	D48.2	D49.2
- sclera	C69.4-	C79.49	D09.2-	D31.4-	D48.7	D49.89
- scrotum (skin)	C63.2	C79.82	D07.61	D29.4	D40.8	D49.59
- sebaceous gland—see Neoplasm, skin						
- sella turcica	C75.1	C79.89	D09.3	D35.2	D44.3	D49.7
- - bone	C41.0	C79.51	-	D16.4-	D48.0	D49.2
- semilunar cartilage (knee)	C40.2-	C79.51	-	D16.2-	D48.0	D49.2
- seminal vesicle	C63.7	C79.82	D07.69	D29.8	D40.8	D49.59
- septum						
- - nasal	C30.0	C78.39	D02.3	D14.0	D38.5	D49.1
- - - posterior margin	C11.3	C79.89	D00.08	D10.6	D37.05	D49.0
- - rectovaginal	C76.3	C79.89	D09.8	D36.7	D48.7	D49.89
- - rectovesical	C76.3	C79.89	D09.8	D36.7	D48.7	D49.89
- - urethrovaginal	C57.9	C79.82	D07.30	D28.9	D39.9	D49.59
- - vesicovaginal	C57.9	C79.82	D07.30	D28.9	D39.9	D49.59

	Malignant Primary	Malignant Secondary	CA in Situ	Benign	Uncertain Behavior	Unspecified Behavior
- shoulder NEC	C76.4-	C79.89	D04.6-	D36.7	D48.7	D49.89
- sigmoid flexure (lower) (upper)	C18.7	C78.5	D01.0	D12.5	D37.4	D49.0
- sinus (accessory)	C31.9	C78.39	D02.3	D14.0	D38.5	D49.1
- - bone (any)	C41.0	C79.51	-	D16.4-	D48.0	D49.2
- - ethmoidal	C31.1	C78.39	D02.3	D14.0	D38.5	D49.1
- - frontal	C31.2	C78.39	D02.3	D14.0	D38.5	D49.1
- - maxillary	C31.0	C78.39	D02.3	D14.0	D38.5	D49.1
- - nasal, paranasal NEC	C31.9	C78.39	D02.3	D14.0	D38.5	D49.1
- - overlapping lesion	C31.8	-	-	-	-	-
- - pyriform	C12	C79.89	D00.08	D10.7	D37.05	D49.0
- - sphenoid	C31.3	C78.39	D02.3	D14.0	D38.5	D49.1
- skeleton, skeletal NEC	C41.9	C79.51	-	D16.9-	D48.0	D49.2
- Skene's gland	C68.1	C79.19	D09.19	D30.8	D41.8	D49.59
- skin NOS	C44.90	C79.2	D04.9	D23.9	D48.5	D49.2
- - abdominal wall	C44.509	C79.2	D04.5	D23.5	D48.5	D49.2
- - - basal cell carcinoma	C44.519	-	-	-	-	-
- - - specified type NEC	C44.599	-	-	-	-	-
- - - squamous cell carcinoma	C44.529	-	-	-	-	-
- - ala nasi—*see also Neoplasm, nose, skin*	C44.301	C79.2	D04.39	D23.39	D48.5	D49.2
- - ankle—*see also Neoplasm, skin, limb, lower*	C44.70-	C79.2	D04.7-	D23.7-	D48.5	D49.2
- - antecubital space—*see also Neoplasm, skin, limb, upper*	C44.60-	C79.2	D04.6-	D23.6-	D48.5	D49.2
- - anus	C44.500	C79.2	D04.5	D23.5	D48.5	D49.2
- - - basal cell carcinoma	C44.510	-	-	-	-	-
- - - specified type NEC	C44.590	-	-	-	-	-
- - - squamous cell carcinoma	C44.520	-	-	-	-	-
- - arm—*see also Neoplasm, skin, limb, upper*	C44.60-	C79.2	D04.6-	D23.6-	D48.5	D49.2
- - auditory canal (external)—*see also Neoplasm, skin, ear*	C44.20-	C79.2	D04.2-	D23.2-	D48.5	D49.2
- - auricle (ear)—*see also Neoplasm, skin, ear*	C44.20-	C79.2	D04.2-	D23.2-	D48.5	D49.2
- - auricular canal (external)—*see also Neoplasm, skin, ear*	C44.20-	C79.2	D04.2-	D23.2-	D48.5	D49.2
- - axilla, axillary fold—*see also Neoplasm, skin, trunk*	C44.509	C79.2	D04.5	D23.5	D48.5	D49.2
- - back—*see also Neoplasm, skin, trunk*	C44.509	C79.2	D04.5	D23.5	D48.5	D49.2
- - basal cell carcinoma	C44.91					
- - breast	C44.501	C79.2	D04.5	D23.5	D48.5	D49.2
- - - basal cell carcinoma	C44.511	-	-	-	-	-
- - - specified type NEC	C44.591	-	-	-	-	-
- - - squamous cell carcinoma	C44.521	-	-	-	-	-
- - brow—*see also Neoplasm, skin, face*	C44.309	C79.2	D04.39	D23.39	D48.5	D49.2
- - buttock—*see also Neoplasm, skin, trunk*	C44.509	C79.2	D04.5	D23.5	D48.5	D49.2
- - calf—*see also Neoplasm, skin, limb, lower*	C44.70-	C79.2	D04.7-	D23.7-	D48.5	D49.2
- - canthus (eye) (inner) (outer)	C44.10-	C79.2	D04.1-	D23.1-	D48.5	D49.2
- - - basal cell carcinoma	C44.11-	-	-	-	-	-
- - - sebaceous cell	C44.13-	-	-	-	-	-
- - - specified type NEC	C44.19-	-	-	-	-	-
- - - squamous cell carcinoma	C44.12-	-	-	-	-	-
- - cervical region—*see also Neoplasm, skin, neck*	C44.40	C79.2	D04.4	D23.4	D48.5	D49.2
- - cheek (external)—*see also Neoplasm, skin, face*	C44.309	C79.2	D04.39	D23.39	D48.5	D49.2
- - chest (wall)—*see also Neoplasm, skin, trunk*	C44.509	C79.2	D04.5	D23.5	D48.5	D49.2
- - chin—*see also Neoplasm, skin, face*	C44.309	C79.2	D04.39	D23.39	D48.5	D49.2
- - clavicular area—*see also Neoplasm, skin, trunk*	C44.509	C79.2	D04.5	D23.5	D48.5	D49.2
- - clitoris	C51.2	C79.82	D07.1	D28.0	D39.8	D49.59
- - columnella—*see also Neoplasm, skin, face*	C44.309	C79.2	D04.39	D23.39	D48.5	D49.2
- - concha—*see also Neoplasm, skin, ear*	C44.20-	C79.2	D04.2-	D23.2-	D48.5	D49.2
- - ear (external)	C44.20-	C79.2	D04.2-	D23.2-	D48.5	D49.2
- - - basal cell carcinoma	C44.21-	-	-	-	-	-
- - - specified type NEC	C44.29-	-	-	-	-	-
- - - squamous cell carcinoma	C44.22-	-	-	-	-	-
- - elbow—*see also Neoplasm, skin, limb, upper*	C44.60-	C79.2	D04.6-	D23.6-	D48.5	D49.2
- - eyebrow—*see also Neoplasm, skin, face*	C44.309	C79.2	D04.39	D23.39	D48.5	D49.2
- - eyelid	C44.10-	C79.2	D04.1-	D23.1-	D48.5	D49.2
- - - basal cell carcinoma	C44.11-	-	-	-	-	-
- - - sebaceous cell	C44.13-	-	-	-	-	-
- - - specified type NEC	C44.19-	-	-	-	-	-
- - - squamous cell carcinoma	C44.12-	-	-	-	-	-
- - face NOS	C44.300	C79.2	D04.30	D23.30	D48.5	D49.2
- - - basal cell carcinoma	C44.310	-	-	-	-	-
- - - specified type NEC	C44.390	-	-	-	-	-
- - - squamous cell carcinoma	C44.320	-	-	-	-	-

	Malignant Primary	Malignant Secondary	CA in Situ	Benign	Uncertain Behavior	Unspecified Behavior
- - female genital organs (external)	C51.9	C79.82	D07.1	D28.0	D39.8	D49.59
- - - clitoris	C51.2	C79.82	D07.1	D28.0	D39.8	D49.59
- - - labium NEC	C51.9	C79.82	D07.1	D28.0	D39.8	D49.59
- - - - majus	C51.0	C79.82	D07.1	D28.0	D39.8	D49.59
- - - - minus	C51.1	C79.82	D07.1	D28.0	D39.8	D49.59
- - - pudendum	C51.9	C79.82	D07.1	D28.0	D39.8	D49.59
- - - vulva	C51.9	C79.82	D07.1	D28.0	D39.8	D49.59
- - finger—*see also Neoplasm, skin, limb, upper*	C44.60-	C79.2	D04.6-	D23.6-	D48.5	D49.2
- - flank—*see also Neoplasm, skin, trunk*	C44.509	C79.2	D04.5	D23.5	D48.5	D49.2
- - foot—*see also Neoplasm, skin, limb, lower*	C44.70-	C79.2	D04.7-	D23.7-	D48.5	D49.2
- - forearm—*see also Neoplasm, skin, limb, upper*	C44.60-	C79.2	D04.6-	D23.6-	D48.5	D49.2
- - forehead—*see also Neoplasm, skin, face*	C44.309	C79.2	D04.39	D23.39	D48.5	D49.2
- - glabella—*see also Neoplasm, skin, face*	C44.309	C79.2	D04.39	D23.39	D48.5	D49.2
- - gluteal region—*see also Neoplasm, skin, trunk*	C44.509	C79.2	D04.5	D23.5	D48.5	D49.2
- - groin—*see also Neoplasm, skin, trunk*	C44.509	C79.2	D04.5	D23.5	D48.5	D49.2
- - hand—*see also Neoplasm, skin, limb, upper*	C44.60-	C79.2	D04.6-	D23.6-	D48.5	D49.2
- - head NEC—*see also Neoplasm, skin, scalp*	C44.40	C79.2	D04.4	D23.4	D48.5	D49.2
- - heel—*see also Neoplasm, skin, limb, lower*	C44.70-	C79.2	D04.7-	D23.7-	D48.5	D49.2
- - helix—*see also Neoplasm, skin, ear*	C44.20-	C79.2	D04.2-	D23.2-	D48.5	D49.2
- - hip—*see also Neoplasm, skin, limb, lower*	C44.70-	C79.2	D04.7-	D23.7-	D48.5	D49.2
- - infraclavicular region—*see also Neoplasm, skin, trunk*	C44.509	C79.2	D04.5	D23.5	D48.5	D49.2
- - inguinal region—*see also Neoplasm, skin, trunk*	C44.509	C79.2	D04.5	D23.5	D48.5	D49.2
- - jaw—*see also Neoplasm, skin, face*	C44.309	C79.2	D04.39	D23.39	D48.5	D49.2
- - Kaposi's sarcoma—*see Kaposi's, sarcoma, skin*						
- - knee—*see also Neoplasm, skin, limb, lower*	C44.70-	C79.2	D04.7-	D23.7-	D48.5	D49.2
- - labia						
- - - majora	C51.0	C79.82	D07.1	D28.0	D39.8	D49.59
- - - minora	C51.1	C79.82	D07.1	D28.0	D39.8	D49.59
- - leg—*see also Neoplasm, skin, limb, lower*	C44.70-	C79.2	D04.7-	D23.7-	D48.5	D49.2
- - lid (lower) (upper)	C44.10-	C79.2	D04.1-	D23.1-	D48.5	D49.2
- - - basal cell carcinoma	C44.11-	-	-	-	-	-
- - - sebaceous cell	C44.13-	-	-	-	-	-
- - - specified type NEC	C44.19-	-	-	-	-	-
- - - squamous cell carcinoma	C44.12-	-	-	-	-	-
- - limb NEC	C44.90	C79.2	D04.9	D23.9	D48.5	D49.2
- - - basal cell carcinoma	C44.91					
- - - lower	C44.70-	C79.2	D04.7-	D23.7-	D48.5	D49.2
- - - - basal cell carcinoma	C44.71-	-	-	-	-	-
- - - - specified type NEC	C44.79-	-	-	-	-	-
- - - - squamous cell carcinoma	C44.72-	-	-	-	-	-
- - - upper	C44.60-	C79.2	D04.6-	D23.6-	D48.5	D49.2
- - - - basal cell carcinoma	C44.61-	-	-	-	-	-
- - - - specified type NEC	C44.69-	-	-	-	-	-
- - - - squamous cell carcinoma	C44.62-	-	-	-	-	-
- - lip (lower) (upper)	C44.00	C79.2	D04.0	D23.0	D48.5	D49.2
- - - basal cell carcinoma	C44.01	-	-	-	-	-
- - - specified type NEC	C44.09	-	-	-	-	-
- - - squamous cell carcinoma	C44.02	-	-	-	-	-
- - male genital organs	C63.9	C79.82	D07.60	D29.9	D40.8	D49.59
- - - penis	C60.9	C79.82	D07.4	D29.0	D40.8	D49.59
- - - prepuce	C60.0	C79.82	D07.4	D29.0	D40.8	D49.59
- - - scrotum	C63.2	C79.82	D07.61	D29.4	D40.8	D49.59
- - mastectomy site (skin)—*see also Neoplasm, skin, breast*	C44.501	C79.2	-	-	-	-
- - - specified as breast tissue	C50.8-	C79.81	-	-	-	-
- - meatus, acoustic (external)—*see also Neoplasm, skin, ear*	C44.20-	C79.2	D04.2-	D23.2-	D48.5	D49.2
- - melanotic—*see Melanoma*						
- - Merkel cell—*see Carcinoma, Merkel cell*						
- - nates—*see also Neoplasm, skin, trunk*	C44.509	C79.2	D04.5	D23.5	D48.5	D49.2
- - neck	C44.40	C79.2	D04.4	D23.4	D48.5	D49.2
- - - basal cell carcinoma	C44.41	-	-	-	-	-
- - - specified type NEC	C44.49	-	-	-	-	-
- - - squamous cell carcinoma	C44.42	-	-	-	-	-
- - nevus—*see Nevus, skin*						
- - nose (external)—*see also Neoplasm, nose, skin*	C44.301	C79.2	D04.39	D23.39	D48.5	D49.2
- - overlapping lesion	C44.80	-	-	-	-	-
- - - basal cell carcinoma	C44.81	-	-	-	-	-
- - - specified type NEC	C44.89	-	-	-	-	-
- - - squamous cell carcinoma	C44.82	-	-	-	-	-

	Malignant Primary	Malignant Secondary	CA in Situ	Benign	Uncertain Behavior	Unspecified Behavior
- - palm—*see also Neoplasm, skin, limb, upper*	C44.60-	C79.2	D04.6-	D23.6-	D48.5	D49.2
- - palpebra	C44.10-	C79.2	D04.1-	D23.1-	D48.5	D49.2
- - - basal cell carcinoma	C44.11-	-	-	-	-	-
- - - sebaceous cell	C44.13-	-	-	-	-	-
- - - specified type NEC	C44.19-	-	-	-	-	-
- - - squamous cell carcinoma	C44.12-	-	-	-	-	-
- - penis NEC	C60.9	C79.82	D07.4	D29.0	D40.8	D49.59
- - perianal—*see also Neoplasm, skin, anus*	C44.500	C79.2	D04.5	D23.5	D48.5	D49.2
- - perineum—*see also Neoplasm, skin, anus*	C44.500	C79.2	D04.5	D23.5	D48.5	D49.2
- - pinna—*see also Neoplasm, skin, ear*	C44.20-	C79.2	D04.2-	D23.2-	D48.5	D49.2
- - plantar—*see also Neoplasm, skin, limb, lower*	C44.70-	C79.2	D04.7-	D23.7-	D48.5	D49.2
- - popliteal fossa or space—*see also Neoplasm, skin, limb, lower*	C44.70-	C79.2	D04.7-	D23.7-	D48.5	D49.2
- - prepuce	C60.0	C79.82	D07.4	D29.0	D40.8	D49.59
- - pubes—*see also Neoplasm, skin, trunk*	C44.509	C79.2	D04.5	D23.5	D48.5	D49.2
- - sacrococcygeal region—*see also Neoplasm, skin, trunk*	C44.509	C79.2	D04.5	D23.5	D48.5	D49.2
- - scalp	C44.40	C79.2	D04.4	D23.4	D48.5	D49.2
- - - basal cell carcinoma	C44.41	-	-	-	-	-
- - - specified type NEC	C44.49	-	-	-	-	-
- - - squamous cell carcinoma	C44.42	-	-	-	-	-
- - scapular region—*see also Neoplasm, skin, trunk*	C44.509	C79.2	D04.5	D23.5	D48.5	D49.2
- - scrotum	C63.2	C79.82	D07.61	D29.4	D40.8	D49.59
- - shoulder—*see also Neoplasm, skin, limb, upper*	C44.60-	C79.2	D04.6-	D23.6-	D48.5	D49.2
- - sole (foot)—*see also Neoplasm, skin, limb, lower*	C44.70-	C79.2	D04.7-	D23.7-	D48.5	D49.2
- - specified sites NEC	C44.80	C79.2	D04.8	D23.9	D48.5	D49.2
- - - basal cell carcinoma	C44.81	-	-	-	-	-
- - - specified type NEC	C44.89	-	-	-	-	-
- - - squamous cell carcinoma	C44.82	-	-	-	-	-
- - specified type NEC	C44.99	-	-	-	-	-
- - squamous cell carcinoma	C44.92	-	-	-	-	-
- - submammary fold—*see also Neoplasm, skin, trunk*	C44.509	C79.2	D04.5	D23.5	D48.5	D49.2
- - supraclavicular region—*see also Neoplasm, skin, neck*	C44.40	C79.2	D04.4	D23.4	D48.5	D49.2
- - temple—*see also Neoplasm, skin, face*	C44.309	C79.2	D04.39	D23.39	D48.5	D49.2
- - thigh—*see also Neoplasm, skin, limb, lower*	C44.70-	C79.2	D04.7-	D23.7-	D48.5	D49.2
- - thoracic wall—*see also Neoplasm, skin, trunk*	C44.509	C79.2	D04.5	D23.5	D48.5	D49.2
- - thumb—*see also Neoplasm, skin, limb, upper*	C44.60-	C79.2	D04.6-	D23.6-	D48.5	D49.2
- - toe—*see also Neoplasm, skin, limb, lower*	C44.70-	C79.2	D04.7-	D23.7-	D48.5	D49.2
- - tragus—*see also Neoplasm, skin, ear*	C44.20-	C79.2	D04.2-	D23.2-	D48.5	D49.2
- - trunk	C44.509	C79.2	D04.5	D23.5	D48.5	D49.2
- - - basal cell carcinoma	C44.519	-	-	-	-	-
- - - specified type NEC	C44.599	-	-	-	-	-
- - - squamous cell carcinoma	C44.529	-	-	-	-	-
- - umbilicus—*see also Neoplasm, skin, trunk*	C44.509	C79.2	D04.5	D23.5	D48.5	D49.2
- - vulva	C51.9	C79.82	D07.1	D28.0	D39.8	D49.59
- - - overlapping lesion	C51.8	-	-	-		
- - wrist—*see also Neoplasm, skin, limb, upper*	C44.60-	C79.2	D04.6-	D23.6-	D48.5	D49.2
- skull	C41.0	C79.51	-	D16.4-	D48.0	D49.2
- soft parts or tissues—*see Neoplasm, connective tissue*						
- specified site NEC	C76.8	C79.89	D09.8	D36.7	D48.7	D49.89
- spermatic cord	C63.1-	C79.82	D07.69	D29.8	D40.8	D49.59
- sphenoid	C31.3	C78.39	D02.3	D14.0	D38.5	D49.1
- - bone	C41.0	C79.51	-	D16.4-	D48.0	D49.2
- - sinus	C31.3	C78.39	D02.3	D14.0	D38.5	D49.1
- sphincter						
- - anal	C21.1	C78.5	D01.3	D12.9	D37.8	D49.0
- - of Oddi	C24.0	C78.89	D01.5	D13.5	D37.6	D49.0
- spine, spinal (column)	C41.2	C79.51	-	D16.6	D48.0	D49.2
- - bulb	C71.7	C79.31	-	D33.1	D43.1	D49.6
- - coccyx	C41.4	C79.51	-	D16.8	D48.0	D49.2
- - cord (cervical) (lumbar) (sacral) (thoracic)	C72.0	C79.49	-	D33.4	D43.4	D49.7
- - dura mater	C70.1	C79.49	-	D32.1	D42.1	D49.7
- - lumbosacral	C41.2	C79.51	-	D16.6	D48.0	D49.2
- - marrow NEC	C96.9	C79.52	-	-	D47.9	D49.89
- - membrane	C70.1	C79.49	-	D32.1	D42.1	D49.7
- - meninges	C70.1	C79.49	-	D32.1	D42.1	D49.7
- - nerve (root)	C47.9	C79.89	-	D36.10	D48.2	D49.2
- - pia mater	C70.1	C79.49	-	D32.1	D42.1	D49.7
- - root	C47.9	C79.89	-	D36.10	D48.2	D49.2
- - sacrum	C41.4	C79.51	-	D16.8	D48.0	D49.2

	Malignant Primary	Malignant Secondary	CA in Situ	Benign	Uncertain Behavior	Unspecified Behavior
- spleen, splenic NEC	C26.1	C78.89	D01.7	D13.9	D37.8	D49.0
- - flexure (colon)	C18.5	C78.5	D01.0	D12.3	D37.4	D49.0
- stem, brain	C71.7	C79.31	-	D33.1	D43.1	D49.6
- Stensen's duct	C07	C79.89	D00.00	D11.0	D37.030	D49.0
- sternum	C41.3	C79.51	-	D16.7	D48.0	D49.2
- stomach	C16.9	C78.89	D00.2	D13.1	D37.1	D49.0
- - antrum (pyloric)	C16.3	C78.89	D00.2	D13.1	D37.1	D49.0
- - body	C16.2	C78.89	D00.2	D13.1	D37.1	D49.0
- - cardia	C16.0	C78.89	D00.2	D13.1	D37.1	D49.0
- - cardiac orifice	C16.0	C78.89	D00.2	D13.1	D37.1	D49.0
- - corpus	C16.2	C78.89	D00.2	D13.1	D37.1	D49.0
- - fundus	C16.1	C78.89	D00.2	D13.1	D37.1	D49.0
- - greater curvature NEC	C16.6	C78.89	D00.2	D13.1	D37.1	D49.0
- - lesser curvature NEC	C16.5	C78.89	D00.2	D13.1	D37.1	D49.0
- - overlapping lesion	C16.8	-	-	-	-	-
- - prepylorus	C16.4	C78.89	D00.2	D13.1	D37.1	D49.0
- - pylorus	C16.4	C78.89	D00.2	D13.1	D37.1	D49.0
- - wall NEC	C16.9	C78.89	D00.2	D13.1	D37.1	D49.0
- - - anterior NEC	C16.8	C78.89	D00.2	D13.1	D37.1	D49.0
- - - posterior NEC	C16.8	C78.89	D00.2	D13.1	D37.1	D49.0
- stroma, endometrial	C54.1	C79.82	D07.0	D26.1	D39.0	D49.59
- stump, cervical	C53.8	C79.82	D06.7	D26.0	D39.0	D49.59
- subcutaneous (nodule) (tissue)NEC—*see Neoplasm, connective tissue*						
- subdural	C70.9	C79.32	-	D32.9	D42.9	D49.7
- subglottis, subglottic	C32.2	C78.39	D02.0	D14.1	D38.0	D49.1
- sublingual	C04.9	C79.89	D00.06	D10.2	D37.09	D49.0
- - gland or duct	C08.1	C79.89	D00.00	D11.7	D37.031	D49.0
- submandibular gland	C08.0	C79.89	D00.00	D11.7	D37.032	D49.0
- submaxillary gland or duct	C08.0	C79.89	D00.00	D11.7	D37.032	D49.0
- submental	C76.0	C79.89	D09.8	D36.7	D48.7	D49.89
- subpleural	C34.9-	C78.0-	D02.2-	D14.3-	D38.1	D49.1
- substernal	C38.1	C78.1	-	D15.2	D38.3	D49.89
- sudoriferous, sudoriparous gland, site unspecified	C44.90	C79.2	D04.9	D23.9	D48.5	D49.2
- - specified site—*see Neoplasm, skin*						
- supraclavicular region	C76.0	C79.89	D09.8	D36.7	D48.7	D49.89
- supraglottis	C32.1	C78.39	D02.0	D14.1	D38.0	D49.1
- suprarenal	C74.9-	C79.7-	D09.3	D35.0-	D44.1-	D49.7
- - capsule	C74.9-	C79.7-	D09.3	D35.0-	D44.1-	D49.7
- - cortex	C74.0-	C79.7-	D09.3	D35.0-	D44.1-	D49.7
- - gland	C74.9-	C79.7-	D09.3	D35.0-	D44.1-	D49.7
- - medulla	C74.1-	C79.7-	D09.3	D35.0-	D44.1-	D49.7
- suprasellar (region)	C71.9	C79.31	-	D33.2	D43.2	D49.6
- supratentorial (brain)NEC	C71.0	C79.31	-	D33.0	D43.0	D49.6
- sweat gland (apocrine) (eccrine), site unspecified	C44.90	C79.2	D04.9	D23.9	D48.5	D49.2
- - specified site—*see Neoplasm, skin*						
- sympathetic nerve or nervous system NEC	C47.9	C79.89		D36.10	D48.2	D49.2
- symphysis pubis	C41.4	C79.51		D16.8	D48.0	D49.2
- synovial membrane—*see Neoplasm, connective tissue*						
- tapetum, brain	C71.8	C79.31	-	D33.2	D43.2	D49.6
- tarsus (any bone)	C40.3-	C79.51	-	D16.3-	-	-
- temple (skin)—*see also Neoplasm, skin, face*	C44.309	C79.2	D04.39	D23.39	D48.5	D49.2
- temporal						
- - bone	C41.0	C79.51		D16.4-	D48.0	D49.2
- - lobe or pole	C71.2	C79.31	-	D33.0	D43.0	D49.6
- - region	C76.0	C79.89	D09.8	D36.7	D48.7	D49.89
- - - skin—*see also Neoplasm, skin, face*	C44.309	C79.2	D04.39	D23.39	D48.5	D49.2
- tendon (sheath)—*see Neoplasm, connective tissue*						
- tentorium (cerebelli)	C70.0	C79.32	-	D32.0	D42.0	D49.7
- testis, testes	C62.9-	C79.82	D07.69	D29.2-	D40.1-	D49.59
- - descended	C62.1-	C79.82	D07.69	D29.2-	D40.1-	D49.59
- - ectopic	C62.0-	C79.82	D07.69	D29.2-	D40.1-	D49.59
- - retained	C62.0-	C79.82	D07.69	D29.2-	D40.1-	D49.59
- - scrotal	C62.1-	C79.82	D07.69	D29.2-	D40.1-	D49.59
- - undescended	C62.0-	C79.82	D07.69	D29.2-	D40.1-	D49.59
- - unspecified whether descended or undescended	C62.9-	C79.82	D07.69	D29.2-	D40.1-	D49.59
- thalamus	C71.0	C79.31	-	D33.0	D43.0	D49.6
- thigh NEC	C76.5-	C79.89	D04.7-	D36.7	D48.7	D49.89
- thorax, thoracic (cavity) (organs NEC)	C76.1	C79.89	D09.8	D36.7	D48.7	D49.89
- - duct	C49.3	C79.89	-	D21.3	D48.1	D49.2

	Malignant Primary	Malignant Secondary	CA in Situ	Benign	Uncertain Behavior	Unspecified Behavior
- - wall NEC	C76.1	C79.89	D09.8	D36.7	D48.7	D49.89
- throat	C14.0	C79.89	D00.08	D10.9	D37.05	D49.0
- thumb NEC	C76.4-	C79.89	D04.6-	D36.7	D48.7	D49.89
- thymus (gland)	C37	C79.89	D09.3	D15.0	D38.4	D49.89
- thyroglossal duct	C73	C79.89	D09.3	D34	D44.0	D49.7
- thyroid (gland)	C73	C79.89	D09.3	D34	D44.0	D49.7
- - cartilage	C32.3	C78.39	D02.0	D14.1	D38.0	D49.1
- tibia (any part)	C40.2-	C79.51	-	D16.2-	-	-
- toe NEC	C76.5-	C79.89	D04.7-	D36.7	D48.7	D49.89
- tongue	C02.9	C79.89	D00.07	D10.1	D37.02	D49.0
- - anterior (two-thirds)NEC	C02.3	C79.89	D00.07	D10.1	D37.02	D49.0
- - - dorsal surface	C02.0	C79.89	D00.07	D10.1	D37.02	D49.0
- - - ventral surface	C02.2	C79.89	D00.07	D10.1	D37.02	D49.0
- - base (dorsal surface)	C01	C79.89	D00.07	D10.1	D37.02	D49.0
- - border (lateral)	C02.1	C79.89	D00.07	D10.1	D37.02	D49.0
- - dorsal surface NEC	C02.0	C79.89	D00.07	D10.1	D37.02	D49.0
- - fixed part NEC	C01	C79.89	D00.07	D10.1	D37.02	D49.0
- - foramen cecum	C02.0	C79.89	D00.07	D10.1	D37.02	D49.0
- - frenulum linguae	C02.2	C79.89	D00.07	D10.1	D37.02	D49.0
- - junctional zone	C02.8	C79.89	D00.07	D10.1	D37.02	D49.0
- - margin (lateral)	C02.1	C79.89	D00.07	D10.1	D37.02	D49.0
- - midline NEC	C02.0	C79.89	D00.07	D10.1	D37.02	D49.0
- - mobile part NEC	C02.3	C79.89	D00.07	D10.1	D37.02	D49.0
- - overlapping lesion	C02.8	-	-	-	-	-
- - posterior (third)	C01	C79.89	D00.07	D10.1	D37.02	D49.0
- - root	C01	C79.89	D00.07	D10.1	D37.02	D49.0
- - surface (dorsal)	C02.0	C79.89	D00.07	D10.1	D37.02	D49.0
- - - base	C01	C79.89	D00.07	D10.1	D37.02	D49.0
- - - ventral	C02.2	C79.89	D00.07	D10.1	D37.02	D49.0
- - tip	C02.1	C79.89	D00.07	D10.1	D37.02	D49.0
- - tonsil	C02.4	C79.89	D00.07	D10.1	D37.02	D49.0
- tonsil	C09.9	C79.89	D00.08	D10.4	D37.05	D49.0
- - fauces, faucial	C09.9	C79.89	D00.08	D10.4	D37.05	D49.0
- - lingual	C02.4	C79.89	D00.07	D10.1	D37.02	D49.0
- - overlapping sites	C09.8	-	-	-	-	-
- - palatine	C09.9	C79.89	D00.08	D10.4	D37.05	D49.0
- - pharyngeal	C11.1	C79.89	D00.08	D10.6	D37.05	D49.0
- - pillar (anterior) (posterior)	C09.1	C79.89	D00.08	D10.5	D37.05	D49.0
- - tonsillar fossa	C09.0	C79.89	D00.08	D10.5	D37.05	D49.0
- tooth socket NEC	C03.9	C79.89	D00.03	D10.39	D37.09	D49.0
- trachea (cartilage) (mucosa)	C33	C78.39	D02.1	D14.2	D38.1	D49.1
- - overlapping lesion with bronchus or lung	C34.8-	-	-	-	-	-
- tracheobronchial	C34.8-	C78.39	D02.1	D14.2	D38.1	D49.1
- - overlapping lesion with lung	C34.8-	-	-	-	-	-
- tragus—*see also Neoplasm, skin, ear*	C44.20-	C79.2	D04.2-	D23.2-	D48.5	D49.2
- trunk NEC	C76.8	C79.89	D04.5	D36.7	D48.7	D49.89
- tubo-ovarian	C57.8	C79.82	D07.39	D28.7	D39.8	D49.59
- tunica vaginalis	C63.7	C79.82	D07.69	D29.8	D40.8	D49.59
- turbinate (bone)	C41.0	C79.51	-	D16.4-	D48.0	D49.2
- - nasal	C30.0	C78.39	D02.3	D14.0	D38.5	D49.1
- tympanic cavity	C30.1	C78.39	D02.3	D14.0	D38.5	D49.1
- ulna (any part)	C40.0-	C79.51	-	D16.0-	-	-
- umbilicus, umbilical—*see also Neoplasm, skin, trunk*	C44.509	C79.2	D04.5	D23.5	D48.5	D49.2
- uncus, brain	C71.2	C79.31	-	D33.0	D43.0	D49.6
- unknown site or unspecified	C80.1	C79.9	D09.9	D36.9	D48.9	D49.9
- urachus	C67.7	C79.11	D09.0	D30.3	D41.4	D49.4
- ureter, ureteral	C66.-	C79.19	D09.19	D30.2-	D41.2-	D49.59
- - orifice (bladder)	C67.6	C79.11	D09.0	D30.3	D41.4	D49.4
- ureter-bladder (junction)	C67.6	C79.11	D09.0	D30.3	D41.4	D49.4
- urethra, urethral (gland)	C68.0	C79.19	D09.19	D30.4	D41.3	D49.59
- - orifice, internal	C67.5	C79.11	D09.0	D30.3	D41.4	D49.4
- urethrovaginal (septum)	C57.9	C79.82	D07.30	D28.9	D39.8	D49.59
- urinary organ or system	C68.9	C79.10	D09.10	D30.9	D41.9	D49.59
- - bladder—*see Neoplasm, bladder*						
- - overlapping lesion	C68.8	-	-	-	-	-
- - specified sites NEC	C68.8	C79.19	D09.19	D30.8	D41.8	D49.59
- utero-ovarian	C57.8	C79.82	D07.39	D28.7	D39.8	D49.59
- - ligament	C57.1	C79.82	D07.39	D28.2	D39.8	D49.59
- uterosacral ligament	C57.3	C79.82	-	D28.2	D39.8	D49.59
- uterus, uteri, uterine	C55	C79.82	D07.0	D26.9	D39.0	D49.59

	Malignant Primary	Malignant Secondary	CA in Situ	Benign	Uncertain Behavior	Unspecified Behavior
- - adnexa NEC	C57.4	C79.82	D07.39	D28.7	D39.8	D49.59
- - body	C54.9	C79.82	D07.0	D26.1	D39.0	D49.59
- - cervix	C53.9	C79.82	D06.9	D26.0	D39.0	D49.59
- - cornu	C54.9	C79.82	D07.0	D26.1	D39.0	D49.59
- - corpus	C54.9	C79.82	D07.0	D26.1	D39.0	D49.59
- - endocervix (canal) (gland)	C53.0	C79.82	D06.0	D26.0	D39.0	D49.59
- - endometrium	C54.1	C79.82	D07.0	D26.1	D39.0	D49.59
- - exocervix	C53.1	C79.82	D06.1	D26.0	D39.0	D49.59
- - external os	C53.1	C79.82	D06.1	D26.0	D39.0	D49.59
- - fundus	C54.3	C79.82	D07.0	D26.1	D39.0	D49.59
- - internal os	C53.0	C79.82	D06.0	D26.0	D39.0	D49.59
- - isthmus	C54.0	C79.82	D07.0	D26.1	D39.0	D49.59
- - ligament	C57.3	C79.82	-	D28.2	D39.8	D49.59
- - - broad	C57.1	C79.82	D07.39	D28.2	D39.8	D49.59
- - - round	C57.2	C79.82	-	D28.2	D39.8	D49.59
- - lower segment	C54.0	C79.82	D07.0	D26.1	D39.0	D49.59
- - myometrium	C54.2	C79.82	D07.0	D26.1	D39.0	D49.59
- - overlapping sites	C54.8	-	-	-	-	-
- - squamocolumnar junction	C53.8	C79.82	D06.7	D26.0	D39.0	D49.59
- - tube	C57.0-	C79.82	D07.39	D28.2	D39.8	D49.59
- utricle, prostatic	C68.0	C79.19	D09.19	D30.4	D41.3	D49.59
- uveal tract	C69.4-	C79.49	D09.2-	D31.4-	D48.7	D49.89
- uvula	C05.2	C79.89	D00.04	D10.39	D37.09	D49.0
- vagina, vaginal (fornix) (vault) (wall)	C52	C79.82	D07.2	D28.1	D39.8	D49.59
- vaginovesical	C57.9	C79.82	D07.30	D28.9	D39.9	D49.59
- - septum	C57.9	C79.82	D07.30	D28.9	D39.9	D49.59
- vallecula (epiglottis)	C10.0	C79.89	D00.08	D10.5	D37.05	D49.0
- vas deferens	C63.1-	C79.82	D07.69	D29.8	D40.8	D49.59
- vascular—*see Neoplasm, connective tissue*						
- Vater's ampulla	C24.1	C78.89	D01.5	D13.5	D37.6	D49.0
- vein, venous—*see Neoplasm, connective tissue*						
- vena cava (abdominal) (inferior)	C49.4	C79.89	-	D21.4	D48.1	D49.2
- - superior	C49.3	C79.89	-	D21.3	D48.1	D49.2
- ventricle (cerebral) (floor) (lateral) (third)	C71.5	C79.31	-	D33.0	D43.0	D49.6
- - cardiac (left) (right)	C38.0	C79.89	-	D15.1	D48.7	D49.89
- - fourth	C71.7	C79.31	-	D33.1	D43.1	D49.6
- ventricular band of larynx	C32.1	C78.39	D02.0	D14.1	D38.0	D49.1
- ventriculus—*see Neoplasm, stomach*						
- vermillion border—*see Neoplasm, lip*						
- vermis, cerebellum	C71.6	C79.31	-	D33.1	D43.1	D49.6
- vertebra (column)	C41.2	C79.51	-	D16.6	D48.0	D49.2
- - coccyx	C41.4	C79.51	-	D16.8-	D48.0	D49.2
- - marrow NEC	C96.9	C79.52	-	-	D47.9	D49.89
- - sacrum	C41.4	C79.51	-	D16.8-	D48.0	D49.2
- vesical—*see Neoplasm, bladder*						
- vesicle, seminal	C63.7	C79.82	D07.69	D29.8	D40.8	D49.59
- vesicocervical tissue	C57.9	C79.82	D07.30	D28.9	D39.9	D49.59
- vesicorectal	C76.3	C79.82	D09.8	D36.7	D48.7	D49.89
- vesicovaginal	C57.9	C79.82	D07.30	D28.9	D39.9	D49.59
- - septum	C57.9	C79.82	D07.30	D28.9	D39.8	D49.59
- vessel (blood)—*see Neoplasm, connective tissue*						
- vestibular gland, greater	C51.0	C79.82	D07.1	D28.0	D39.8	D49.59
- vestibule						
- - mouth	C06.1	C79.89	D00.00	D10.39	D37.09	D49.0
- - nose	C30.0	C78.39	D02.3	D14.0	D38.5	D49.1
- Virchow's gland	C77.0	C77.0	-	D36.0	D48.7	D49.89
- viscera NEC	C76.8	C79.89	D09.8	D36.7	D48.7	D49.89
- vocal cords (true)	C32.0	C78.39	D02.0	D14.1	D38.0	D49.1
- - false	C32.1	C78.39	D02.0	D14.1	D38.0	D49.1
- vomer	C41.0	C79.51	-	D16.4-	D48.0	D49.2
- vulva	C51.9	C79.82	D07.1	D28.0	D39.8	D49.59
- vulvovaginal gland	C51.0	C79.82	D07.1	D28.0	D39.8	D49.59
- Waldeyer's ring	C14.2	C79.89	D00.08	D10.9	D37.05	D49.0
- Wharton's duct	C08.0	C79.89	D00.00	D11.7	D37.032	D49.0
- white matter (central) (cerebral)	C71.0	C79.31	-	D33.0	D43.0	D49.6
- windpipe	C33	C78.39	D02.1	D14.2	D38.1	D49.1
- Wirsung's duct	C25.3	C78.89	D01.7	D13.6	D37.8	D49.0
- wolffian (body) (duct)						
- - female	C57.7	C79.82	D07.39	D28.7	D39.8	D49.59
- - male	C63.7	C79.82	D07.69	D29.8	D40.8	D49.59
- womb—*see Neoplasm, uterus*						

	Malignant Primary	Malignant Secondary	CA in Situ	Benign	Uncertain Behavior	Unspecified Behavior
- wrist NEC	C76.4-	C79.89	D04.6-	D36.7	D48.7	D49.89
- xiphoid process	C41.3	C79.51	-	D16.7	D48.0	D49.2
- Zuckerkandl organ	C75.5	C79.89	-	D35.6	D44.7	D49.7

Table Of Drugs And Chemicals

Substance	Poisoning, Accidental (unintentional)	Poisoning, Intentional Self-harm	Poisoning, Assault	Poisoning, Undetermined	Adverse effect	Underdosing
1-propanol	T51.3X1	T51.3X2	T51.3X3	T51.3X4	--	--
2-propanol	T51.2X1	T51.2X2	T51.2X3	T51.2X4	--	--
2,4-D (dichlorophen-oxyacetic acid)	T60.3X1	T60.3X2	T60.3X3	T60.3X4	--	--
2,4-toluene diisocyanate	T65.0X1	T65.0X2	T65.0X3	T65.0X4	--	--
2,4,5-T (trichloro-phenoxyacetic acid)	T60.1X1	T60.1X2	T60.1X3	T60.1X4	--	--
14-hydroxydihydro-morphinone	T40.2X1	T40.2X2	T40.2X3	T40.2X4	T40.2X5	T40.2X6
3,4- methylenedioxymethamphetamine	T43.641	T43.642	T43.643	T43.644	--	--
ABOB	T37.5X1	T37.5X2	T37.5X3	T37.5X4	T37.5X5	T37.5X6
Abrine	T62.2X1	T62.2X2	T62.2X3	T62.2X4	--	--
Abrus (seed)	T62.2X1	T62.2X2	T62.2X3	T62.2X4	--	--
Absinthe	T51.0X1	T51.0X2	T51.0X3	T51.0X4	--	--
- beverage	T51.0X1	T51.0X2	T51.0X3	T51.0X4	--	--
Acaricide	T60.8X1	T60.8X2	T60.8X3	T60.8X4	--	--
Acebutolol	T44.7X1	T44.7X2	T44.7X3	T44.7X4	T44.7X5	T44.7X6
Acecarbromal	T42.6X1	T42.6X2	T42.6X3	T42.6X4	T42.6X5	T42.6X6
Aceclidine	T44.1X1	T44.1X2	T44.1X3	T44.1X4	T44.1X5	T44.1X6
Acedapsone	T37.0X1	T37.0X2	T37.0X3	T37.0X4	T37.0X5	T37.0X6
Acefylline piperazine	T48.6X1	T48.6X2	T48.6X3	T48.6X4	T48.6X5	T48.6X6
Acemorphan	T40.2X1	T40.2X2	T40.2X3	T40.2X4	T40.2X5	T40.2X6
Acenocoumarin	T45.511	T45.512	T45.513	T45.514	T45.515	T45.516
Acenocoumarol	T45.511	T45.512	T45.513	T45.514	T45.515	T45.516
Acepifylline	T48.6X1	T48.6X2	T48.6X3	T48.6X4	T48.6X5	T48.6X6
Acepromazine	T43.3X1	T43.3X2	T43.3X3	T43.3X4	T43.3X5	T43.3X6
Acesulfamethoxypyridazine	T37.0X1	T37.0X2	T37.0X3	T37.0X4	T37.0X5	T37.0X6
Acetal	T52.8X1	T52.8X2	T52.8X3	T52.8X4	--	--
Acetaldehyde (vapor)	T52.8X1	T52.8X2	T52.8X3	T52.8X4	--	--
- liquid	T65.891	T65.892	T65.893	T65.894	--	--
P-Acetamidophenol	T39.1X1	T39.1X2	T39.1X3	T39.1X4	T39.1X5	T39.1X6
Acetaminophen	T39.1X1	T39.1X2	T39.1X3	T39.1X4	T39.1X5	T39.1X6
Acetaminosalol	T39.1X1	T39.1X2	T39.1X3	T39.1X4	T39.1X5	T39.1X6
Acetanilide	T39.1X1	T39.1X2	T39.1X3	T39.1X4	T39.1X5	T39.1X6
Acetarsol	T37.3X1	T37.3X2	T37.3X3	T37.3X4	T37.3X5	T37.3X6
Acetazolamide	T50.2X1	T50.2X2	T50.2X3	T50.2X4	T50.2X5	T50.2X6
Acetiamine	T45.2X1	T45.2X2	T45.2X3	T45.2X4	T45.2X5	T45.2X6
Acetic						
- acid	T54.2X1	T54.2X2	T54.2X3	T54.2X4	--	--
- - with sodium acetate (ointment)	T49.3X1	T49.3X2	T49.3X3	T49.3X4	T49.3X5	T49.3X6
- - ester (solvent) (vapor)	T52.8X1	T52.8X2	T52.8X3	T52.8X4	--	--
- - irrigating solution	T50.3X1	T50.3X2	T50.3X3	T50.3X4	T50.3X5	T50.3X6
- - medicinal (lotion)	T49.2X1	T49.2X2	T49.2X3	T49.2X4	T49.2X5	T49.2X6
- anhydride	T65.891	T65.892	T65.893	T65.894	--	--
- ether (vapor)	T52.8X1	T52.8X2	T52.8X3	T52.8X4	--	--
Acetohexamide	T38.3X1	T38.3X2	T38.3X3	T38.3X4	T38.3X5	T38.3X6
Acetohydroxamic acid	T50.991	T50.992	T50.993	T50.994	T50.995	T50.996
Acetomenaphthone	T45.7X1	T45.7X2	T45.7X3	T45.7X4	T45.7X5	T45.7X6
Acetomorphine	T40.1X1	T40.1X2	T40.1X3	T40.1X4	T40.1X5	--
Acetone (oils)	T52.4X1	T52.4X2	T52.4X3	T52.4X4	--	--
- chlorinated	T52.4X1	T52.4X2	T52.4X3	T52.4X4	--	--
- vapor	T52.4X1	T52.4X2	T52.4X3	T52.4X4	--	--
Acetonitrile	T52.8X1	T52.8X2	T52.8X3	T52.8X4	--	--
Acetophenazine	T43.3X1	T43.3X2	T43.3X3	T43.3X4	T43.3X5	T43.3X6
Acetophenetidin	T39.1X1	T39.1X2	T39.1X3	T39.1X4	T39.1X5	T39.1X6
Acetophenone	T52.4X1	T52.4X2	T52.4X3	T52.4X4	--	--
Acetorphine	T40.2X1	T40.2X2	T40.2X3	T40.2X4	--	--
Acetosulfone (sodium)	T37.1X1	T37.1X2	T37.1X3	T37.1X4	T37.1X5	T37.1X6
Acetrizoate (sodium)	T50.8X1	T50.8X2	T50.8X3	T50.8X4	T50.8X5	T50.8X6

Substance	Poisoning, Accidental (unintentional)	Poisoning, Intentional Self-harm	Poisoning, Assault	Poisoning, Undetermined	Adverse effect	Underdosing
Acetrizoic acid	T50.8X1	T50.8X2	T50.8X3	T50.8X4	T50.8X5	T50.8X6
Acetyl						
- bromide	T53.6X1	T53.6X2	T53.6X3	T53.6X4	--	--
- chloride	T53.6X1	T53.6X2	T53.6X3	T53.6X4	--	--
Acetylcarbromal	T42.6X1	T42.6X2	T42.6X3	T42.6X4	T42.6X5	T42.6X6
Acetylcholine						
- chloride	T44.1X1	T44.1X2	T44.1X3	T44.1X4	T44.1X5	T44.1X6
- derivative	T44.1X1	T44.1X2	T44.1X3	T44.1X4	T44.1X5	T44.1X6
Acetylcysteine	T48.4X1	T48.4X2	T48.4X3	T48.4X4	T48.4X5	T48.4X6
Acetyldigitoxin	T46.0X1	T46.0X2	T46.0X3	T46.0X4	T46.0X5	T46.0X6
Acetyldigoxin	T46.0X1	T46.0X2	T46.0X3	T46.0X4	T46.0X5	T46.0X6
Acetyldihydrocodeine	T40.2X1	T40.2X2	T40.2X3	T40.2X4	--	--
Acetyldihydrocodeinone	T40.2X1	T40.2X2	T40.2X3	T40.2X4	--	--
Acetylene (gas)	T59.891	T59.892	T59.893	T59.894	--	--
- dichloride	T53.6X1	T53.6X2	T53.6X3	T53.6X4	--	--
- incomplete combustion of	T58.11	T58.12	T58.13	T58.14	--	--
- industrial	T59.891	T59.892	T59.893	T59.894	--	--
- tetrachloride	T53.6X1	T53.6X2	T53.6X3	T53.6X4	--	--
- - vapor	T53.6X1	T53.6X2	T53.6X3	T53.6X4	--	--
Acetylpheneturide	T42.6X1	T42.6X2	T42.6X3	T42.6X4	T42.6X5	T42.6X6
Acetylphenylhydrazine	T39.8X1	T39.8X2	T39.8X3	T39.8X4	T39.8X5	T39.8X6
Acetylsalicylic acid (salts)	T39.011	T39.012	T39.013	T39.014	T39.015	T39.016
- enteric coated	T39.011	T39.012	T39.013	T39.014	T39.015	T39.016
Acetylsulfamethoxypyridazine	T37.0X1	T37.0X2	T37.0X3	T37.0X4	T37.0X5	T37.0X6
Achromycin	T36.4X1	T36.4X2	T36.4X3	T36.4X4	T36.4X5	T36.4X6
- ophthalmic preparation	T49.5X1	T49.5X2	T49.5X3	T49.5X4	T49.5X5	T49.5X6
- topical NEC	T49.0X1	T49.0X2	T49.0X3	T49.0X4	T49.0X5	T49.0X6
Aciclovir	T37.5X1	T37.5X2	T37.5X3	T37.5X4	T37.5X5	T37.5X6
Acid (corrosive) NEC	T54.2X1	T54.2X2	T54.2X3	T54.2X4	--	--
Acidifying agent NEC	T50.901	T50.902	T50.903	T50.904	T50.905	T50.906
Acipimox	T46.6X1	T46.6X2	T46.6X3	T46.6X4	T46.6X5	T46.6X6
Acitretin	T50.991	T50.992	T50.993	T50.994	T50.995	T50.996
Aclarubicin	T45.1X1	T45.1X2	T45.1X3	T45.1X4	T45.1X5	T45.1X6
Aclatonium napadisilate	T48.1X1	T48.1X2	T48.1X3	T48.1X4	T48.1X5	T48.1X6
Aconite (wild)	T46.991	T46.992	T46.993	T46.994	T46.995	T46.996
Aconitine	T46.991	T46.992	T46.993	T46.994	T46.995	T46.996
Aconitum ferox	T46.991	T46.992	T46.993	T46.994	T46.995	T46.996
Acridine	T65.6X1	T65.6X2	T65.6X3	T65.6X4	--	--
- vapor	T59.891	T59.892	T59.893	T59.894	--	--
Acriflavine	T37.91	T37.92	T37.93	T37.94	T37.95	T37.96
Acriflavinium chloride	T49.0X1	T49.0X2	T49.0X3	T49.0X4	T49.0X5	T49.0X6
Acrinol	T49.0X1	T49.0X2	T49.0X3	T49.0X4	T49.0X5	T49.0X6
Acrisorcin	T49.0X1	T49.0X2	T49.0X3	T49.0X4	T49.0X5	T49.0X6
Acrivastine	T45.0X1	T45.0X2	T45.0X3	T45.0X4	T45.0X5	T45.0X6
Acrolein (gas)	T59.891	T59.892	T59.893	T59.894	--	--
- liquid	T54.1X1	T54.1X2	T54.1X3	T54.1X4	--	--
Acrylamide	T65.891	T65.892	T65.893	T65.894	--	--
Acrylic resin	T49.3X1	T49.3X2	T49.3X3	T49.3X4	T49.3X5	T49.3X6
Acrylonitrile	T65.891	T65.892	T65.893	T65.894	--	--
Actaea spicata	T62.2X1	T62.2X2	T62.2X3	T62.2X4	--	--
- berry	T62.1X1	T62.1X2	T62.1X3	T62.1X4	--	--
Acterol	T37.3X1	T37.3X2	T37.3X3	T37.3X4	T37.3X5	T37.3X6
ACTH	T38.811	T38.812	T38.813	T38.814	T38.815	T38.816
Actinomycin C	T45.1X1	T45.1X2	T45.1X3	T45.1X4	T45.1X5	T45.1X6
Actinomycin D	T45.1X1	T45.1X2	T45.1X3	T45.1X4	T45.1X5	T45.1X6
Activated charcoal—see also Charcoal, medicinal	T47.6X1	T47.6X2	T47.6X3	T47.6X4	T47.6X5	T47.6X6
Acyclovir	T37.5X1	T37.5X2	T37.5X3	T37.5X4	T37.5X5	T37.5X6
Adenine	T45.2X1	T45.2X2	T45.2X3	T45.2X4	T45.2X5	T45.2X6

Substance	Poisoning, Accidental (unintentional)	Poisoning, Intentional Self-harm	Poisoning, Assault	Poisoning, Undetermined	Adverse effect	Underdosing
- arabinoside	T37.5X1	T37.5X2	T37.5X3	T37.5X4	T37.5X5	T37.5X6
Adenosine (phosphate)	T46.2X1	T46.2X2	T46.2X3	T46.2X4	T46.2X5	T46.2X6
ADH	T38.891	T38.892	T38.893	T38.894	T38.895	T38.896
Adhesive NEC	T65.891	T65.892	T65.893	T65.894	--	--
Adicillin	T36.0X1	T36.0X2	T36.0X3	T36.0X4	T36.0X5	T36.0X6
Adiphenine	T44.3X1	T44.3X2	T44.3X3	T44.3X4	T44.3X5	T44.3X6
Adipiodone	T50.8X1	T50.8X2	T50.8X3	T50.8X4	T50.8X5	T50.8X6
Adjunct, pharmaceutical	T50.901	T50.902	T50.903	T50.904	T50.905	T50.906
Adrenal (extract, cortex or medulla) (gluco-orticoids)(hormones)(mineralocorticoids)	T38.0X1	T38.0X2	T38.0X3	T38.0X4	T38.0X5	T38.0X6
- ENT agent	T49.6X1	T49.6X2	T49.6X3	T49.6X4	T49.6X5	T49.6X6
- ophthalmic preparation	T49.5X1	T49.5X2	T49.5X3	T49.5X4	T49.5X5	T49.5X6
- topical NEC	T49.0X1	T49.0X2	T49.0X3	T49.0X4	T49.0X5	T49.0X6
Adrenaline	T44.5X1	T44.5X2	T44.5X3	T44.5X4	T44.5X5	T44.5X6
Adrenalin—see Adrenaline						
Adrenergic NEC	T44.901	T44.902	T44.903	T44.904	T44.905	T44.906
- blocking agent NEC	T44.8X1	T44.8X2	T44.8X3	T44.8X4	T44.8X5	T44.8X6
- - beta, heart	T44.7X1	T44.7X2	T44.7X3	T44.7X4	T44.7X5	T44.7X6
- specified NEC	T44.991	T44.992	T44.993	T44.994	T44.995	T44.996
Adrenochrome						
- (mono) semicarbazone	T46.991	T46.992	T46.993	T46.994	T46.995	T46.996
- derivative	T46.991	T46.992	T46.993	T46.994	T46.995	T46.996
Adrenocorticotrophic hormone	T38.811	T38.812	T38.813	T38.814	T38.815	T38.816
Adrenocorticotrophin	T38.811	T38.812	T38.813	T38.814	T38.815	T38.816
Adriamycin	T45.1X1	T45.1X2	T45.1X3	T45.1X4	T45.1X5	T45.1X6
Aerosol spray NEC	T65.91	T65.92	T65.93	T65.94	--	--
Aerosporin	T36.8X1	T36.8X2	T36.8X3	T36.8X4	T36.8X5	T36.8X6
- ENT agent	T49.6X1	T49.6X2	T49.6X3	T49.6X4	T49.6X5	T49.6X6
- ophthalmic preparation	T49.5X1	T49.5X2	T49.5X3	T49.5X4	T49.5X5	T49.5X6
- topical NEC	T49.0X1	T49.0X2	T49.0X3	T49.0X4	T49.0X5	T49.0X6
Aethusa cynapium	T62.2X1	T62.2X2	T62.2X3	T62.2X4	--	--
Afghanistan black	T40.711	T40.712	T40.713	T40.714	T40.715	T40.716
Aflatoxin	T64.01	T64.02	T64.03	T64.04	--	--
Afloqualone	T42.8X1	T42.8X2	T42.8X3	T42.8X4	T42.8X5	T42.8X6
African boxwood	T62.2X1	T62.2X2	T62.2X3	T62.2X4	--	--
Agar	T47.4X1	T47.4X2	T47.4X3	T47.4X4	T47.4X5	T47.4X6
Agonist						
- predominantly						
- - alpha-adrenoreceptor	T44.4X1	T44.4X2	T44.4X3	T44.4X4	T44.4X5	T44.4X6
- - beta-adrenoreceptor	T44.5X1	T44.5X2	T44.5X3	T44.5X4	T44.5X5	T44.5X6
Agricultural agent NEC	T65.91	T65.92	T65.93	T65.94	--	--
Agrypnal	T42.3X1	T42.3X2	T42.3X3	T42.3X4	T42.3X5	T42.3X6
AHLG	T50.Z11	T50.Z12	T50.Z13	T50.Z14	T50.Z15	T50.Z16
Air contaminant (s) , source/type NOS	T65.91	T65.92	T65.93	T65.94	--	--
Ajmaline	T46.2X1	T46.2X2	T46.2X3	T46.2X4	T46.2X5	T46.2X6
Akee	T62.1X1	T62.1X2	T62.1X3	T62.1X4	--	--
Akrinol	T49.0X1	T49.0X2	T49.0X3	T49.0X4	T49.0X5	T49.0X6
Akritoin	T37.8X1	T37.8X2	T37.8X3	T37.8X4	T37.8X5	T37.8X6
Alacepril	T46.4X1	T46.4X2	T46.4X3	T46.4X4	T46.4X5	T46.4X6
Alantolactone	T37.4X1	T37.4X2	T37.4X3	T37.4X4	T37.4X5	T37.4X6
Albamycin	T36.8X1	T36.8X2	T36.8X3	T36.8X4	T36.8X5	T36.8X6
Albendazole	T37.4X1	T37.4X2	T37.4X3	T37.4X4	T37.4X5	T37.4X6
Albumin						
- bovine	T45.8X1	T45.8X2	T45.8X3	T45.8X4	T45.8X5	T45.8X6
- human serum	T45.8X1	T45.8X2	T45.8X3	T45.8X4	T45.8X5	T45.8X6
- - salt-poor	T45.8X1	T45.8X2	T45.8X3	T45.8X4	T45.8X5	T45.8X6
- normal human serum	T45.8X1	T45.8X2	T45.8X3	T45.8X4	T45.8X5	T45.8X6
Albuterol	T48.6X1	T48.6X2	T48.6X3	T48.6X4	T48.6X5	T48.6X6
Albutoin	T42.0X1	T42.0X2	T42.0X3	T42.0X4	T42.0X5	T42.0X6

Substance	Poisoning, Accidental (unintentional)	Poisoning, Intentional Self-harm	Poisoning, Assault	Poisoning, Undetermined	Adverse effect	Underdosing
Alclometasone	T49.0X1	T49.0X2	T49.0X3	T49.0X4	T49.0X5	T49.0X6
Alcohol	T51.91	T51.92	T51.93	T51.94	--	--
- absolute	T51.0X1	T51.0X2	T51.0X3	T51.0X4	--	--
- - beverage	T51.0X1	T51.0X2	T51.0X3	T51.0X4	--	--
- allyl	T51.8X1	T51.8X2	T51.8X3	T51.8X4	--	--
- amyl	T51.3X1	T51.3X2	T51.3X3	T51.3X4	--	--
- antifreeze	T51.1X1	T51.1X2	T51.1X3	T51.1X4	--	--
- beverage	T51.0X1	T51.0X2	T51.0X3	T51.0X4	--	--
- butyl	T51.3X1	T51.3X2	T51.3X3	T51.3X4	--	--
- dehydrated	T51.0X1	T51.0X2	T51.0X3	T51.0X4	--	--
- - beverage	T51.0X1	T51.0X2	T51.0X3	T51.0X4	--	--
- denatured	T51.0X1	T51.0X2	T51.0X3	T51.0X4	--	--
- deterrent NEC	T50.6X1	T50.6X2	T50.6X3	T50.6X4	T50.6X5	T50.6X6
- diagnostic (gastric function)	T50.8X1	T50.8X2	T50.8X3	T50.8X4	T50.8X5	T50.8X6
- ethyl	T51.0X1	T51.0X2	T51.0X3	T51.0X4	--	--
- - beverage	T51.0X1	T51.0X2	T51.0X3	T51.0X4	--	--
- grain	T51.0X1	T51.0X2	T51.0X3	T51.0X4	--	--
- - beverage	T51.0X1	T51.0X2	T51.0X3	T51.0X4	--	--
- industrial	T51.0X1	T51.0X2	T51.0X3	T51.0X4	--	--
- isopropyl	T51.2X1	T51.2X2	T51.2X3	T51.2X4	--	--
- methyl	T51.1X1	T51.1X2	T51.1X3	T51.1X4	--	--
- preparation for consumption	T51.0X1	T51.0X2	T51.0X3	T51.0X4	--	--
- propyl	T51.3X1	T51.3X2	T51.3X3	T51.3X4	--	--
- - secondary	T51.2X1	T51.2X2	T51.2X3	T51.2X4	--	--
- radiator	T51.1X1	T51.1X2	T51.1X3	T51.1X4	--	--
- rubbing	T51.2X1	T51.2X2	T51.2X3	T51.2X4	--	--
- specified type NEC	T51.8X1	T51.8X2	T51.8X3	T51.8X4	--	--
- surgical	T51.0X1	T51.0X2	T51.0X3	T51.0X4	--	--
- vapor (from any type of Alcohol)	T59.891	T59.892	T59.893	T59.894	--	--
- wood	T51.1X1	T51.1X2	T51.1X3	T51.1X4	--	--
Alcuronium (chloride)	T48.1X1	T48.1X2	T48.1X3	T48.1X4	T48.1X5	T48.1X6
Aldactone	T50.0X1	T50.0X2	T50.0X3	T50.0X4	T50.0X5	T50.0X6
Aldesulfone sodium	T37.1X1	T37.1X2	T37.1X3	T37.1X4	T37.1X5	T37.1X6
Aldicarb	T60.0X1	T60.0X2	T60.0X3	T60.0X4	--	--
Aldomet	T46.5X1	T46.5X2	T46.5X3	T46.5X4	T46.5X5	T46.5X6
Aldosterone	T50.0X1	T50.0X2	T50.0X3	T50.0X4	T50.0X5	T50.0X6
Aldrin (dust)	T60.1X1	T60.1X2	T60.1X3	T60.1X4	--	--
Aleve—see Naproxen						
Alexitol sodium	T47.1X1	T47.1X2	T47.1X3	T47.1X4	T47.1X5	T47.1X6
Alfacalcidol	T45.2X1	T45.2X2	T45.2X3	T45.2X4	T45.2X5	T45.2X6
Alfadolone	T41.1X1	T41.1X2	T41.1X3	T41.1X4	T41.1X5	T41.1X6
Alfaxalone	T41.1X1	T41.1X2	T41.1X3	T41.1X4	T41.1X5	T41.1X6
Alfentanil	T40.411	T40.412	T40.413	T40.414	T40.415	T40.416
Alfuzosin (hydrochloride)	T44.8X1	T44.8X2	T44.8X3	T44.8X4	T44.8X5	T44.8X6
Algae (harmful) (toxin)	T65.821	T65.822	T65.823	T65.824	--	--
Algeldrate	T47.1X1	T47.1X2	T47.1X3	T47.1X4	T47.1X5	T47.1X6
Algin	T47.8X1	T47.8X2	T47.8X3	T47.8X4	T47.8X5	T47.8X6
Alglucerase	T45.3X1	T45.3X2	T45.3X3	T45.3X4	T45.3X5	T45.3X6
Alidase	T45.3X1	T45.3X2	T45.3X3	T45.3X4	T45.3X5	T45.3X6
Alimemazine	T43.3X1	T43.3X2	T43.3X3	T43.3X4	T43.3X5	T43.3X6
Aliphatic thiocyanates	T65.0X1	T65.0X2	T65.0X3	T65.0X4	--	--
Alizapride	T45.0X1	T45.0X2	T45.0X3	T45.0X4	T45.0X5	T45.0X6
Alkali (caustic)	T54.3X1	T54.3X2	T54.3X3	T54.3X4	--	--
Alkaline antiseptic solution (aromatic)	T49.6X1	T49.6X2	T49.6X3	T49.6X4	T49.6X5	T49.6X6
Alkalinizing agents (medicinal)	T50.901	T50.902	T50.903	T50.904	T50.905	T50.906
Alkalizing agent NEC	T50.901	T50.902	T50.903	T50.904	T50.905	T50.906
Alka-seltzer	T39.011	T39.012	T39.013	T39.014	T39.015	T39.016
Alkavervir	T46.5X1	T46.5X2	T46.5X3	T46.5X4	T46.5X5	T46.5X6
Alkonium (bromide)	T49.0X1	T49.0X2	T49.0X3	T49.0X4	T49.0X5	T49.0X6

Substance	Poisoning, Accidental (unintentional)	Poisoning, Intentional Self-harm	Poisoning, Assault	Poisoning, Undetermined	Adverse effect	Underdosing
Alkylating drug NEC	T45.1X1	T45.1X2	T45.1X3	T45.1X4	T45.1X5	T45.1X6
- antimyeloproliferative	T45.1X1	T45.1X2	T45.1X3	T45.1X4	T45.1X5	T45.1X6
- lymphatic	T45.1X1	T45.1X2	T45.1X3	T45.1X4	T45.1X5	T45.1X6
Alkylisocyanate	T65.0X1	T65.0X2	T65.0X3	T65.0X4	--	--
Allantoin	T49.4X1	T49.4X2	T49.4X3	T49.4X4	T49.4X5	T49.4X6
Allegron	T43.011	T43.012	T43.013	T43.014	T43.015	T43.016
Allethrin	T49.0X1	T49.0X2	T49.0X3	T49.0X4	T49.0X5	T49.0X6
Allobarbital	T42.3X1	T42.3X2	T42.3X3	T42.3X4	T42.3X5	T42.3X6
Allopurinol	T50.4X1	T50.4X2	T50.4X3	T50.4X4	T50.4X5	T50.4X6
Allyl						
- Alcohol	T51.8X1	T51.8X2	T51.8X3	T51.8X4	--	--
- disulfide	T46.6X1	T46.6X2	T46.6X3	T46.6X4	T46.6X5	T46.6X6
Allylestrenol	T38.5X1	T38.5X2	T38.5X3	T38.5X4	T38.5X5	T38.5X6
Allylisopropylacetylurea	T42.6X1	T42.6X2	T42.6X3	T42.6X4	T42.6X5	T42.6X6
Allylisopropylmalonylurea	T42.3X1	T42.3X2	T42.3X3	T42.3X4	T42.3X5	T42.3X6
Allylthiourea	T49.3X1	T49.3X2	T49.3X3	T49.3X4	T49.3X5	T49.3X6
Allyltribromide	T42.6X1	T42.6X2	T42.6X3	T42.6X4	T42.6X5	T42.6X6
Allypropymal	T42.3X1	T42.3X2	T42.3X3	T42.3X4	T42.3X5	T42.3X6
Almagate	T47.1X1	T47.1X2	T47.1X3	T47.1X4	T47.1X5	T47.1X6
Almasilate	T47.1X1	T47.1X2	T47.1X3	T47.1X4	T47.1X5	T47.1X6
Almitrine	T50.7X1	T50.7X2	T50.7X3	T50.7X4	T50.7X5	T50.7X6
Aloes	T47.2X1	T47.2X2	T47.2X3	T47.2X4	T47.2X5	T47.2X6
Aloglutamol	T47.1X1	T47.1X2	T47.1X3	T47.1X4	T47.1X5	T47.1X6
Aloin	T47.2X1	T47.2X2	T47.2X3	T47.2X4	T47.2X5	T47.2X6
Aloxidone	T42.2X1	T42.2X2	T42.2X3	T42.2X4	T42.2X5	
Alpha						
- acetyldigoxin	T46.0X1	T46.0X2	T46.0X3	T46.0X4	T46.0X5	T46.0X6
- adrenergic blocking drug	T44.6X1	T44.6X2	T44.6X3	T44.6X4	T44.6X5	T44.6X6
- amylase	T45.3X1	T45.3X2	T45.3X3	T45.3X4	T45.3X5	T45.3X6
- tocoferol (acetate)	T45.2X1	T45.2X2	T45.2X3	T45.2X4	T45.2X5	T45.2X6
- tocopherol	T45.2X1	T45.2X2	T45.2X3	T45.2X4	T45.2X5	T45.2X6
Alphadolone	T41.1X1	T41.1X2	T41.1X3	T41.1X4	T41.1X5	T41.1X6
Alphaprodine	T40.491	T40.492	T40.493	T40.494	T40.495	T40.496
Alphaxalone	T41.1X1	T41.1X2	T41.1X3	T41.1X4	T41.1X5	T41.1X6
Alprazolam	T42.4X1	T42.4X2	T42.4X3	T42.4X4	T42.4X5	T42.4X6
Alprenolol	T44.7X1	T44.7X2	T44.7X3	T44.7X4	T44.7X5	T44.7X6
Alprostadil	T46.7X1	T46.7X2	T46.7X3	T46.7X4	T46.7X5	T46.7X6
Alsactide	T38.811	T38.812	T38.813	T38.814	T38.815	T38.816
Alseroxylon	T46.5X1	T46.5X2	T46.5X3	T46.5X4	T46.5X5	T46.5X6
Alteplase	T45.611	T45.612	T45.613	T45.614	T45.615	T45.616
Altizide	T50.2X1	T50.2X2	T50.2X3	T50.2X4	T50.2X5	T50.2X6
Altretamine	T45.1X1	T45.1X2	T45.1X3	T45.1X4	T45.1X5	T45.1X6
Alum (medicinal)	T49.4X1	T49.4X2	T49.4X3	T49.4X4	T49.4X5	T49.4X6
- nonmedicinal (ammonium) (potassium)	T56.891	T56.892	T56.893	T56.894	--	--
Aluminium, aluminum						
- acetate	T49.2X1	T49.2X2	T49.2X3	T49.2X4	T49.2X5	T49.2X6
- - solution	T49.0X1	T49.0X2	T49.0X3	T49.0X4	T49.0X5	T49.0X6
- aspirin	T39.011	T39.012	T39.013	T39.014	T39.015	T39.016
- bis (acetylsalicylate)	T39.011	T39.012	T39.013	T39.014	T39.015	T39.016
- carbonate (gel, basic)	T47.1X1	T47.1X2	T47.1X3	T47.1X4	T47.1X5	T47.1X6
- chlorhydroxide-complex	T47.1X1	T47.1X2	T47.1X3	T47.1X4	T47.1X5	T47.1X6
- chloride	T49.2X1	T49.2X2	T49.2X3	T49.2X4	T49.2X5	T49.2X6
- clofibrate	T46.6X1	T46.6X2	T46.6X3	T46.6X4	T46.6X5	T46.6X6
- diacetate	T49.2X1	T49.2X2	T49.2X3	T49.2X4	T49.2X5	T49.2X6
- glycinate	T47.1X1	T47.1X2	T47.1X3	T47.1X4	T47.1X5	T47.1X6
- hydroxide (gel)	T47.1X1	T47.1X2	T47.1X3	T47.1X4	T47.1X5	T47.1X6
- hydroxide-magnesium carb. gel	T47.1X1	T47.1X2	T47.1X3	T47.1X4	T47.1X5	T47.1X6
- magnesium silicate	T47.1X1	T47.1X2	T47.1X3	T47.1X4	T47.1X5	T47.1X6

Substance	Poisoning, Accidental (unintentional)	Poisoning, Intentional Self-harm	Poisoning, Assault	Poisoning, Undetermined	Adverse effect	Underdosing
- nicotinate	T46.7X1	T46.7X2	T46.7X3	T46.7X4	T46.7X5	T46.7X6
- ointment (surgical) (topical)	T49.3X1	T49.3X2	T49.3X3	T49.3X4	T49.3X5	T49.3X6
- phosphate	T47.1X1	T47.1X2	T47.1X3	T47.1X4	T47.1X5	T47.1X6
- salicylate	T39.091	T39.092	T39.093	T39.094	T39.095	T39.096
- silicate	T47.1X1	T47.1X2	T47.1X3	T47.1X4	T47.1X5	T47.1X6
- sodium silicate	T47.1X1	T47.1X2	T47.1X3	T47.1X4	T47.1X5	T47.1X6
- subacetate	T49.2X1	T49.2X2	T49.2X3	T49.2X4	T49.2X5	T49.2X6
- sulfate	T49.0X1	T49.0X2	T49.0X3	T49.0X4	T49.0X5	T49.0X6
- tannate	T47.6X1	T47.6X2	T47.6X3	T47.6X4	T47.6X5	T47.6X6
- topical NEC	T49.3X1	T49.3X2	T49.3X3	T49.3X4	T49.3X5	T49.3X6
Alurate	T42.3X1	T42.3X2	T42.3X3	T42.3X4	T42.3X5	T42.3X6
Alverine	T44.3X1	T44.3X2	T44.3X3	T44.3X4	T44.3X5	T44.3X6
Alvodine	T40.2X1	T40.2X2	T40.2X3	T40.2X4	T40.2X5	T40.2X6
Amanita phalloides	T62.0X1	T62.0X2	T62.0X3	T62.0X4	--	--
Amanitine	T62.0X1	T62.0X2	T62.0X3	T62.0X4	--	--
Amantadine	T42.8X1	T42.8X2	T42.8X3	T42.8X4	T42.8X5	T42.8X6
Ambazone	T49.6X1	T49.6X2	T49.6X3	T49.6X4	T49.6X5	T49.6X6
Ambenonium (chloride)	T44.0X1	T44.0X2	T44.0X3	T44.0X4	T44.0X5	T44.0X6
Ambroxol	T48.4X1	T48.4X2	T48.4X3	T48.4X4	T48.4X5	T48.4X6
Ambuphylline	T48.6X1	T48.6X2	T48.6X3	T48.6X4	T48.6X5	T48.6X6
Ambutonium bromide	T44.3X1	T44.3X2	T44.3X3	T44.3X4	T44.3X5	T44.3X6
Amcinonide	T49.0X1	T49.0X2	T49.0X3	T49.0X4	T49.0X5	T49.0X6
Amdinocillin	T36.0X1	T36.0X2	T36.0X3	T36.0X4	T36.0X5	T36.0X6
Ametazole	T50.8X1	T50.8X2	T50.8X3	T50.8X4	T50.8X5	T50.8X6
Amethocaine	T41.3X1	T41.3X2	T41.3X3	T41.3X4	T41.3X5	T41.3X6
- regional	T41.3X1	T41.3X2	T41.3X3	T41.3X4	T41.3X5	T41.3X6
- spinal	T41.3X1	T41.3X2	T41.3X3	T41.3X4	T41.3X5	T41.3X6
Amethopterin	T45.1X1	T45.1X2	T45.1X3	T45.1X4	T45.1X5	T45.1X6
Amezinium metilsulfate	T44.991	T44.992	T44.993	T44.994	T44.995	T44.996
Amfebutamone	T43.291	T43.292	T43.293	T43.294	T43.295	T43.296
Amfepramone	T50.5X1	T50.5X2	T50.5X3	T50.5X4	T50.5X5	T50.5X6
Amfetamine	T43.621	T43.622	T43.623	T43.624	T43.625	T43.626
Amfetaminil	T43.621	T43.622	T43.623	T43.624	T43.625	T43.626
Amfomycin	T36.8X1	T36.8X2	T36.8X3	T36.8X4	T36.8X5	T36.8X6
Amidefrine mesilate	T48.5X1	T48.5X2	T48.5X3	T48.5X4	T48.5X5	T48.5X6
Amidone	T40.3X1	T40.3X2	T40.3X3	T40.3X4	T40.3X5	T40.3X6
Amidopyrine	T39.2X1	T39.2X2	T39.2X3	T39.2X4	T39.2X5	T39.2X6
Amidotrizoate	T50.8X1	T50.8X2	T50.8X3	T50.8X4	T50.8X5	T50.8X6
Amiflamine	T43.1X1	T43.1X2	T43.1X3	T43.1X4	T43.1X5	T43.1X6
Amikacin	T36.5X1	T36.5X2	T36.5X3	T36.5X4	T36.5X5	T36.5X6
Amikhelline	T46.3X1	T46.3X2	T46.3X3	T46.3X4	T46.3X5	T46.3X6
Amiloride	T50.2X1	T50.2X2	T50.2X3	T50.2X4	T50.2X5	T50.2X6
Aminacrine	T49.0X1	T49.0X2	T49.0X3	T49.0X4	T49.0X5	T49.0X6
Amineptine	T43.011	T43.012	T43.013	T43.014	T43.015	T43.016
Aminitrozole	T37.3X1	T37.3X2	T37.3X3	T37.3X4	T37.3X5	T37.3X6
Amino acids	T50.3X1	T50.3X2	T50.3X3	T50.3X4	T50.3X5	T50.3X6
Aminoacetic acid (derivatives)	T50.3X1	T50.3X2	T50.3X3	T50.3X4	T50.3X5	T50.3X6
Aminoacridine	T49.0X1	T49.0X2	T49.0X3	T49.0X4	T49.0X5	T49.0X6
Aminobenzoic acid (-p)	T49.3X1	T49.3X2	T49.3X3	T49.3X4	T49.3X5	T49.3X6
4-Aminobutyric acid	T43.8X1	T43.8X2	T43.8X3	T43.8X4	T43.8X5	T43.8X6
Aminocaproic acid	T45.621	T45.622	T45.623	T45.624	T45.625	T45.626
Aminoethylisothiourium	T45.8X1	T45.8X2	T45.8X3	T45.8X4	T45.8X5	T45.8X6
Aminofenazone	T39.2X1	T39.2X2	T39.2X3	T39.2X4	T39.2X5	T39.2X6
Aminoglutethimide	T45.1X1	T45.1X2	T45.1X3	T45.1X4	T45.1X5	T45.1X6
Aminohippuric acid	T50.8X1	T50.8X2	T50.8X3	T50.8X4	T50.8X5	T50.8X6
Aminomethylbenzoic acid	T45.691	T45.692	T45.693	T45.694	T45.695	T45.696
Aminometradine	T50.2X1	T50.2X2	T50.2X3	T50.2X4	T50.2X5	T50.2X6
Aminopentamide	T44.3X1	T44.3X2	T44.3X3	T44.3X4	T44.3X5	T44.3X6
Aminophenazone	T39.2X1	T39.2X2	T39.2X3	T39.2X4	T39.2X5	T39.2X6

Substance	Poisoning, Accidental (unintentional)	Poisoning, Intentional Self-harm	Poisoning, Assault	Poisoning, Undetermined	Adverse effect	Underdosing
Aminophenol	T54.0X1	T54.0X2	T54.0X3	T54.0X4	--	--
4-Aminophenol derivatives	T39.1X1	T39.1X2	T39.1X3	T39.1X4	T39.1X5	T39.1X6
Aminophenylpyridone	T43.591	T43.592	T43.593	T43.594	T43.595	T43.596
Aminophylline	T48.6X1	T48.6X2	T48.6X3	T48.6X4	T48.6X5	T48.6X6
Aminopterin sodium	T45.1X1	T45.1X2	T45.1X3	T45.1X4	T45.1X5	T45.1X6
Aminopyrine	T39.2X1	T39.2X2	T39.2X3	T39.2X4	T39.2X5	T39.2X6
8-Aminoquinoline drugs	T37.2X1	T37.2X2	T37.2X3	T37.2X4	T37.2X5	T37.2X6
Aminorex	T50.5X1	T50.5X2	T50.5X3	T50.5X4	T50.5X5	T50.5X6
Aminosalicylic acid	T37.1X1	T37.1X2	T37.1X3	T37.1X4	T37.1X5	T37.1X6
Aminosalylum	T37.1X1	T37.1X2	T37.1X3	T37.1X4	T37.1X5	T37.1X6
Amiodarone	T46.2X1	T46.2X2	T46.2X3	T46.2X4	T46.2X5	T46.2X6
Amiphenazole	T50.7X1	T50.7X2	T50.7X3	T50.7X4	T50.7X5	T50.7X6
Amiquinsin	T46.5X1	T46.5X2	T46.5X3	T46.5X4	T46.5X5	T46.5X6
Amisometradine	T50.2X1	T50.2X2	T50.2X3	T50.2X4	T50.2X5	T50.2X6
Amisulpride	T43.591	T43.592	T43.593	T43.594	T43.595	T43.596
Amitriptyline	T43.011	T43.012	T43.013	T43.014	T43.015	T43.016
Amitriptylinoxide	T43.011	T43.012	T43.013	T43.014	T43.015	T43.016
Amlexanox	T48.6X1	T48.6X2	T48.6X3	T48.6X4	T48.6X5	T48.6X6
Ammonia (fumes) (gas) (vapor)	T59.891	T59.892	T59.893	T59.894	--	--
- aromatic spirit	T48.991	T48.992	T48.993	T48.994	T48.995	T48.996
- liquid (household)	T54.3X1	T54.3X2	T54.3X3	T54.3X4	--	--
Ammoniated mercury	T49.0X1	T49.0X2	T49.0X3	T49.0X4	T49.0X5	T49.0X6
Ammonium						
- acid tartrate	T49.5X1	T49.5X2	T49.5X3	T49.5X4	T49.5X5	T49.5X6
- bromide	T42.6X1	T42.6X2	T42.6X3	T42.6X4	T42.6X5	T42.6X6
- carbonate	T54.3X1	T54.3X2	T54.3X3	T54.3X4	--	--
- chloride	T50.991	T50.992	T50.993	T50.994	T50.995	T50.996
- - expectorant	T48.4X1	T48.4X2	T48.4X3	T48.4X4	T48.4X5	T48.4X6
- compounds (household) NEC	T54.3X1	T54.3X2	T54.3X3	T54.3X4	--	--
- - fumes (any usage)	T59.891	T59.892	T59.893	T59.894	--	--
- - industrial	T54.3X1	T54.3X2	T54.3X3	T54.3X4	--	--
- ichthyosulronate	T49.4X1	T49.4X2	T49.4X3	T49.4X4	T49.4X5	T49.4X6
- mandelate	T37.91	T37.92	T37.93	T37.94	T37.95	T37.96
- sulfamate	T60.3X1	T60.3X2	T60.3X3	T60.3X4	--	--
- sulfonate resin	T47.8X1	T47.8X2	T47.8X3	T47.8X4	T47.8X5	T47.8X6
Amobarbital (sodium)	T42.3X1	T42.3X2	T42.3X3	T42.3X4	T42.3X5	T42.3X6
Amodiaquine	T37.2X1	T37.2X2	T37.2X3	T37.2X4	T37.2X5	T37.2X6
Amopyroquin (e)	T37.2X1	T37.2X2	T37.2X3	T37.2X4	T37.2X5	T37.2X6
Amoxapine	T43.011	T43.012	T43.013	T43.014	T43.015	T43.016
Amoxicillin	T36.0X1	T36.0X2	T36.0X3	T36.0X4	T36.0X5	T36.0X6
Amperozide	T43.591	T43.592	T43.593	T43.594	T43.595	T43.596
Amphenidone	T43.591	T43.592	T43.593	T43.594	T43.595	T43.596
Amphetamine NEC	T43.621	T43.622	T43.623	T43.624	T43.625	T43.626
Amphomycin	T36.8X1	T36.8X2	T36.8X3	T36.8X4	T36.8X5	T36.8X6
Amphotalide	T37.4X1	T37.4X2	T37.4X3	T37.4X4	T37.4X5	T37.4X6
Amphotericin B	T36.7X1	T36.7X2	T36.7X3	T36.7X4	T36.7X5	T36.7X6
- topical	T49.0X1	T49.0X2	T49.0X3	T49.0X4	T49.0X5	T49.0X6
Ampicillin	T36.0X1	T36.0X2	T36.0X3	T36.0X4	T36.0X5	T36.0X6
Amprotropine	T44.3X1	T44.3X2	T44.3X3	T44.3X4	T44.3X5	T44.3X6
Amsacrine	T45.1X1	T45.1X2	T45.1X3	T45.1X4	T45.1X5	T45.1X6
Amygdaline	T62.2X1	T62.2X2	T62.2X3	T62.2X4	--	--
Amyl						
- acetate	T52.8X1	T52.8X2	T52.8X3	T52.8X4	--	--
- - vapor	T59.891	T59.892	T59.893	T59.894	--	--
- alcohol	T51.3X1	T51.3X2	T51.3X3	T51.3X4	--	--
- chloride	T53.6X1	T53.6X2	T53.6X3	T53.6X4	--	--
- formate	T52.8X1	T52.8X2	T52.8X3	T52.8X4	--	--
- nitrite	T46.3X1	T46.3X2	T46.3X3	T46.3X4	T46.3X5	T46.3X6

Substance	Poisoning, Accidental (unintentional)	Poisoning, Intentional Self-harm	Poisoning, Assault	Poisoning, Undetermined	Adverse effect	Underdosing
- propionate	T65.891	T65.892	T65.893	T65.894	--	--
Amylase	T47.5X1	T47.5X2	T47.5X3	T47.5X4	T47.5X5	T47.5X6
Amyleine, regional	T41.3X1	T41.3X2	T41.3X3	T41.3X4	T41.3X5	T41.3X6
Amylene						
- dichloride	T53.6X1	T53.6X2	T53.6X3	T53.6X4	--	--
- hydrate	T51.3X1	T51.3X2	T51.3X3	T51.3X4	--	--
Amylmetacresol	T49.6X1	T49.6X2	T49.6X3	T49.6X4	T49.6X5	T49.6X6
Amylobarbitone	T42.3X1	T42.3X2	T42.3X3	T42.3X4	T42.3X5	T42.3X6
Amylocaine, regional	T41.3X1	T41.3X2	T41.3X3	T41.3X4	T41.3X5	T41.3X6
- infiltration (subcutaneous)	T41.3X1	T41.3X2	T41.3X3	T41.3X4	T41.3X5	T41.3X6
- nerve block (peripheral) (plexus)	T41.3X1	T41.3X2	T41.3X3	T41.3X4	T41.3X5	T41.3X6
- spinal	T41.3X1	T41.3X2	T41.3X3	T41.3X4	T41.3X5	T41.3X6
- topical (surface)	T41.3X1	T41.3X2	T41.3X3	T41.3X4	T41.3X5	T41.3X6
Amylopectin	T47.6X1	T47.6X2	T47.6X3	T47.6X4	T47.6X5	T47.6X6
Amytal (sodium)	T42.3X1	T42.3X2	T42.3X3	T42.3X4	T42.3X5	T42.3X6
Anabolic steroid	T38.7X1	T38.7X2	T38.7X3	T38.7X4	T38.7X5	T38.7X6
Analeptic NEC	T50.7X1	T50.7X2	T50.7X3	T50.7X4	T50.7X5	T50.7X6
Analgesic	T39.91	T39.92	T39.93	T39.94	T39.95	T39.96
- anti-inflammatory NEC	T39.91	T39.92	T39.93	T39.94	T39.95	T39.96
- - propionic acid derivative	T39.311	T39.312	T39.313	T39.314	T39.315	T39.316
- antirheumatic NEC	T39.4X1	T39.4X2	T39.4X3	T39.4X4	T39.4X5	T39.4X6
- aromatic NEC	T39.1X1	T39.1X2	T39.1X3	T39.1X4	T39.1X5	T39.1X6
- narcotic NEC	T40.601	T40.602	T40.603	T40.604	T40.605	T40.606
- - combination	T40.601	T40.602	T40.603	T40.604	T40.605	T40.606
- - obstetric	T40.601	T40.602	T40.603	T40.604	T40.605	T40.606
- non-narcotic NEC	T39.91	T39.92	T39.93	T39.94	T39.95	T39.96
- - combination	T39.91	T39.92	T39.93	T39.94	T39.95	T39.96
- pyrazole	T39.2X1	T39.2X2	T39.2X3	T39.2X4	T39.2X5	T39.2X6
- specified NEC	T39.8X1	T39.8X2	T39.8X3	T39.8X4	T39.8X5	T39.8X6
Analgin	T39.2X1	T39.2X2	T39.2X3	T39.2X4	T39.2X5	T39.2X6
Anamirta cocculus	T62.1X1	T62.1X2	T62.1X3	T62.1X4	--	--
Ancillin	T36.0X1	T36.0X2	T36.0X3	T36.0X4	T36.0X5	T36.0X6
Ancrod	T45.691	T45.692	T45.693	T45.694	T45.695	T45.696
Androgen	T38.7X1	T38.7X2	T38.7X3	T38.7X4	T38.7X5	T38.7X6
Androgen-estrogen mixture	T38.7X1	T38.7X2	T38.7X3	T38.7X4	T38.7X5	T38.7X6
Androstalone	T38.7X1	T38.7X2	T38.7X3	T38.7X4	T38.7X5	T38.7X6
Androstanolone	T38.7X1	T38.7X2	T38.7X3	T38.7X4	T38.7X5	T38.7X6
Androsterone	T38.7X1	T38.7X2	T38.7X3	T38.7X4	T38.7X5	T38.7X6
Anemone pulsatilla	T62.2X1	T62.2X2	T62.2X3	T62.2X4	--	--
Anesthesia						
- caudal	T41.3X1	T41.3X2	T41.3X3	T41.3X4	T41.3X5	T41.3X6
- endotracheal	T41.0X1	T41.0X2	T41.0X3	T41.0X4	T41.0X5	T41.0X6
- epidural	T41.3X1	T41.3X2	T41.3X3	T41.3X4	T41.3X5	T41.3X6
- inhalation	T41.0X1	T41.0X2	T41.0X3	T41.0X4	T41.0X5	T41.0X6
- local	T41.3X1	T41.3X2	T41.3X3	T41.3X4	T41.3X5	T41.3X6
- mucosal	T41.3X1	T41.3X2	T41.3X3	T41.3X4	T41.3X5	T41.3X6
- muscle relaxation	T48.1X1	T48.1X2	T48.1X3	T48.1X4	T48.1X5	T48.1X6
- nerve blocking	T41.3X1	T41.3X2	T41.3X3	T41.3X4	T41.3X5	T41.3X6
- plexus blocking	T41.3X1	T41.3X2	T41.3X3	T41.3X4	T41.3X5	T41.3X6
- potentiated	T41.201	T41.202	T41.203	T41.204	T41.205	T41.206
- rectal	T41.201	T41.202	T41.203	T41.204	T41.205	T41.206
- - general	T41.201	T41.202	T41.203	T41.204	T41.205	T41.206
- - local	T41.3X1	T41.3X2	T41.3X3	T41.3X4	T41.3X5	T41.3X6
- regional	T41.3X1	T41.3X2	T41.3X3	T41.3X4	T41.3X5	T41.3X6
- surface	T41.3X1	T41.3X2	T41.3X3	T41.3X4	T41.3X5	T41.3X6
Anesthetic NEC—see also Anesthesia	T41.41	T41.42	T41.43	T41.44	T41.45	T41.46
- with muscle relaxant	T41.201	T41.202	T41.203	T41.204	T41.205	T41.206
- - general	T41.201	T41.202	T41.203	T41.204	T41.205	T41.206
- - local	T41.3X1	T41.3X2	T41.3X3	T41.3X4	T41.3X5	T41.3X6

Substance	Poisoning, Accidental (unintentional)	Poisoning, Intentional Self-harm	Poisoning, Assault	Poisoning, Undetermined	Adverse effect	Underdosing
- gaseous NEC	T41.0X1	T41.0X2	T41.0X3	T41.0X4	T41.0X5	T41.0X6
- general NEC	T41.201	T41.202	T41.203	T41.204	T41.205	T41.206
- halogenated hydrocarbon derivatives NEC	T41.0X1	T41.0X2	T41.0X3	T41.0X4	T41.0X5	T41.0X6
- infiltration NEC	T41.3X1	T41.3X2	T41.3X3	T41.3X4	T41.3X5	T41.3X6
- intravenous NEC	T41.1X1	T41.1X2	T41.1X3	T41.1X4	T41.1X5	T41.1X6
- local NEC	T41.3X1	T41.3X2	T41.3X3	T41.3X4	T41.3X5	T41.3X6
- rectal	T41.201	T41.202	T41.203	T41.204	T41.205	T41.206
- - general	T41.201	T41.202	T41.203	T41.204	T41.205	T41.206
- - local	T41.3X1	T41.3X2	T41.3X3	T41.3X4	T41.3X5	T41.3X6
- regional NEC	T41.3X1	T41.3X2	T41.3X3	T41.3X4	T41.3X5	T41.3X6
- spinal NEC	T41.3X1	T41.3X2	T41.3X3	T41.3X4	T41.3X5	T41.3X6
- thiobarbiturate	T41.1X1	T41.1X2	T41.1X3	T41.1X4	T41.1X5	T41.1X6
- topical	T41.3X1	T41.3X2	T41.3X3	T41.3X4	T41.3X5	T41.3X6
Aneurine	T45.2X1	T45.2X2	T45.2X3	T45.2X4	T45.2X5	T45.2X6
Angio-Conray	T50.8X1	T50.8X2	T50.8X3	T50.8X4	T50.8X5	T50.8X6
Angiotensin	T44.5X1	T44.5X2	T44.5X3	T44.5X4	T44.5X5	T44.5X6
Angiotensinamide	T44.991	T44.992	T44.993	T44.994	T44.995	T44.996
Anhydrohydroxy-progesterone	T38.5X1	T38.5X2	T38.5X3	T38.5X4	T38.5X5	T38.5X6
Anhydron	T50.2X1	T50.2X2	T50.2X3	T50.2X4	T50.2X5	T50.2X6
Anileridine	T40.491	T40.492	T40.493	T40.494	T40.495	T40.496
Aniline (dye) (liquid)	T65.3X1	T65.3X2	T65.3X3	T65.3X4	--	--
- analgesic	T39.1X1	T39.1X2	T39.1X3	T39.1X4	T39.1X5	T39.1X6
- derivatives, therapeutic NEC	T39.1X1	T39.1X2	T39.1X3	T39.1X4	T39.1X5	T39.1X6
- vapor	T65.3X1	T65.3X2	T65.3X3	T65.3X4	--	--
Aniscoropine	T44.3X1	T44.3X2	T44.3X3	T44.3X4	T44.3X5	T44.3X6
Anise oil	T47.5X1	T47.5X2	T47.5X3	T47.5X4	T47.5X5	T47.5X6
Anisidine	T65.3X1	T65.3X2	T65.3X3	T65.3X4	--	--
Anisindione	T45.511	T45.512	T45.513	T45.514	T45.515	T45.516
Anisotropine methyl-bromide	T44.3X1	T44.3X2	T44.3X3	T44.3X4	T44.3X5	T44.3X6
Anistreplase	T45.611	T45.612	T45.613	T45.614	T45.615	T45.616
Anorexiant (central)	T50.5X1	T50.5X2	T50.5X3	T50.5X4	T50.5X5	T50.5X6
Anorexic agents	T50.5X1	T50.5X2	T50.5X3	T50.5X4	T50.5X5	T50.5X6
Ansamycin	T36.6X1	T36.6X2	T36.6X3	T36.6X4	T36.6X5	T36.6X6
Ant (bite) (sting)	T63.421	T63.422	T63.423	T63.424	--	--
Ant poison—see Insecticide						
Antabuse	T50.6X1	T50.6X2	T50.6X3	T50.6X4	T50.6X5	T50.6X6
Antacid NEC	T47.1X1	T47.1X2	T47.1X3	T47.1X4	T47.1X5	T47.1X6
Antagonist						
- Aldosterone	T50.0X1	T50.0X2	T50.0X3	T50.0X4	T50.0X5	T50.0X6
- alpha-adrenoreceptor	T44.6X1	T44.6X2	T44.6X3	T44.6X4	T44.6X5	T44.6X6
- anticoagulant	T45.7X1	T45.7X2	T45.7X3	T45.7X4	T45.7X5	T45.7X6
- beta-adrenoreceptor	T44.7X1	T44.7X2	T44.7X3	T44.7X4	T44.7X5	T44.7X6
- extrapyramidal NEC	T44.3X1	T44.3X2	T44.3X3	T44.3X4	T44.3X5	T44.3X6
- folic acid	T45.1X1	T45.1X2	T45.1X3	T45.1X4	T45.1X5	T45.1X6
- H2 receptor	T47.0X1	T47.0X2	T47.0X3	T47.0X4	T47.0X5	T47.0X6
- heavy metal	T45.8X1	T45.8X2	T45.8X3	T45.8X4	T45.8X5	T45.8X6
- narcotic analgesic	T50.7X1	T50.7X2	T50.7X3	T50.7X4	T50.7X5	T50.7X6
- opiate	T50.7X1	T50.7X2	T50.7X3	T50.7X4	T50.7X5	T50.7X6
- pyrimidine	T45.1X1	T45.1X2	T45.1X3	T45.1X4	T45.1X5	T45.1X6
- serotonin	T46.5X1	T46.5X2	T46.5X3	T46.5X4	T46.5X5	T46.5X6
Antazolin (e)	T45.0X1	T45.0X2	T45.0X3	T45.0X4	T45.0X5	T45.0X6
Anterior pituitary hormone NEC	T38.811	T38.812	T38.813	T38.814	T38.815	T38.816
Anthelmintic NEC	T37.4X1	T37.4X2	T37.4X3	T37.4X4	T37.4X5	T37.4X6
Anthiolimine	T37.4X1	T37.4X2	T37.4X3	T37.4X4	T37.4X5	T37.4X6
Anthralin	T49.4X1	T49.4X2	T49.4X3	T49.4X4	T49.4X5	T49.4X6
Anthramycin	T45.1X1	T45.1X2	T45.1X3	T45.1X4	T45.1X5	T45.1X6
Antiadrenergic NEC	T44.8X1	T44.8X2	T44.8X3	T44.8X4	T44.8X5	T44.8X6
Antiallergic NEC	T45.0X1	T45.0X2	T45.0X3	T45.0X4	T45.0X5	T45.0X6

Substance	Poisoning, Accidental (unintentional)	Poisoning, Intentional Self-harm	Poisoning, Assault	Poisoning, Undetermined	Adverse effect	Underdosing
Anti-anemic (drug) (preparation)	T45.8X1	T45.8X2	T45.8X3	T45.8X4	T45.8X5	T45.8X6
Antiandrogen NEC	T38.6X1	T38.6X2	T38.6X3	T38.6X4	T38.6X5	T38.6X6
Antianxiety drug NEC	T43.501	T43.502	T43.503	T43.504	T43.505	T43.506
Antiaris toxicaria	T65.891	T65.892	T65.893	T65.894	--	--
Antiarteriosclerotic drug	T46.6X1	T46.6X2	T46.6X3	T46.6X4	T46.6X5	T46.6X6
Antiasthmatic drug NEC	T48.6X1	T48.6X2	T48.6X3	T48.6X4	T48.6X5	T48.6X6
Antibiotic NEC	T36.91	T36.92	T36.93	T36.94	T36.95	T36.96
- aminoglycoside	T36.5X1	T36.5X2	T36.5X3	T36.5X4	T36.5X5	T36.5X6
- anticancer	T45.1X1	T45.1X2	T45.1X3	T45.1X4	T45.1X5	T45.1X6
- antifungal	T36.7X1	T36.7X2	T36.7X3	T36.7X4	T36.7X5	T36.7X6
- antimycobacterial	T36.5X1	T36.5X2	T36.5X3	T36.5X4	T36.5X5	T36.5X6
- antineoplastic	T45.1X1	T45.1X2	T45.1X3	T45.1X4	T45.1X5	T45.1X6
- cephalosporin (group)	T36.1X1	T36.1X2	T36.1X3	T36.1X4	T36.1X5	T36.1X6
- chloramphenicol (group)	T36.2X1	T36.2X2	T36.2X3	T36.2X4	T36.2X5	T36.2X6
- ENT	T49.6X1	T49.6X2	T49.6X3	T49.6X4	T49.6X5	T49.6X6
- eye	T49.5X1	T49.5X2	T49.5X3	T49.5X4	T49.5X5	T49.5X6
- fungicidal (local)	T49.0X1	T49.0X2	T49.0X3	T49.0X4	T49.0X5	T49.0X6
- intestinal	T36.8X1	T36.8X2	T36.8X3	T36.8X4	T36.8X5	T36.8X6
- b-lactam NEC	T36.1X1	T36.1X2	T36.1X3	T36.1X4	T36.1X5	T36.1X6
- local	T49.0X1	T49.0X2	T49.0X3	T49.0X4	T49.0X5	T49.0X6
- macrolides	T36.3X1	T36.3X2	T36.3X3	T36.3X4	T36.3X5	T36.3X6
- polypeptide	T36.8X1	T36.8X2	T36.8X3	T36.8X4	T36.8X5	T36.8X6
- specified NEC	T36.8X1	T36.8X2	T36.8X3	T36.8X4	T36.8X5	T36.8X6
- tetracycline (group)	T36.4X1	T36.4X2	T36.4X3	T36.4X4	T36.4X5	T36.4X6
- throat	T49.6X1	T49.6X2	T49.6X3	T49.6X4	T49.6X5	T49.6X6
Anticancer agents NEC	T45.1X1	T45.1X2	T45.1X3	T45.1X4	T45.1X5	T45.1X6
Anticholesterolemic drug NEC	T46.6X1	T46.6X2	T46.6X3	T46.6X4	T46.6X5	T46.6X6
Anticholinergic NEC	T44.3X1	T44.3X2	T44.3X3	T44.3X4	T44.3X5	T44.3X6
Anticholinesterase	T44.0X1	T44.0X2	T44.0X3	T44.0X4	T44.0X5	T44.0X6
- organophosphorus	T44.0X1	T44.0X2	T44.0X3	T44.0X4	T44.0X5	T44.0X6
- - insecticide	T60.0X1	T60.0X2	T60.0X3	T60.0X4	--	--
- - nerve gas	T59.891	T59.892	T59.893	T59.894	--	--
- reversible	T44.0X1	T44.0X2	T44.0X3	T44.0X4	T44.0X5	T44.0X6
- - ophthalmological	T49.5X1	T49.5X2	T49.5X3	T49.5X4	T49.5X5	T49.5X6
Anticoagulant NEC	T45.511	T45.512	T45.513	T45.514	T45.515	T45.516
- Antagonist	T45.7X1	T45.7X2	T45.7X3	T45.7X4	T45.7X5	T45.7X6
Anti-common-cold drug NEC	T48.5X1	T48.5X2	T48.5X3	T48.5X4	T48.5X5	T48.5X6
Anticonvulsant	T42.71	T42.72	T42.73	T42.74	T42.75	T42.76
- barbiturate	T42.3X1	T42.3X2	T42.3X3	T42.3X4	T42.3X5	T42.3X6
- combination (with barbiturate)	T42.3X1	T42.3X2	T42.3X3	T42.3X4	T42.3X5	T42.3X6
- hydantoin	T42.0X1	T42.0X2	T42.0X3	T42.0X4	T42.0X5	T42.0X6
- hypnotic NEC	T42.6X1	T42.6X2	T42.6X3	T42.6X4	T42.6X5	T42.6X6
- oxazolidinedione	T42.2X1	T42.2X2	T42.2X3	T42.2X4	T42.2X5	T42.2X6
- pyrimidinedione	T42.6X1	T42.6X2	T42.6X3	T42.6X4	T42.6X5	T42.6X6
- specified NEC	T42.6X1	T42.6X2	T42.6X3	T42.6X4	T42.6X5	T42.6X6
- succinimide	T42.2X1	T42.2X2	T42.2X3	T42.2X4	T42.2X5	T42.2X6
Anti-D immunoglobulin (human)	T50.Z11	T50.Z12	T50.Z13	T50.Z14	T50.Z15	T50.Z16
Antidepressant	T43.201	T43.202	T43.203	T43.204	T43.205	T43.206
- monoamine oxidase inhibitor	T43.1X1	T43.1X2	T43.1X3	T43.1X4	T43.1X5	T43.1X6
- selective serotonin norepinephrine reuptake inhibitor	T43.211	T43.212	T43.213	T43.214	T43.215	T43.216
- selective serotonin reuptake inhibitor	T43.221	T43.222	T43.223	T43.224	T43.225	T43.226
- specified NEC	T43.291	T43.292	T43.293	T43.294	T43.295	T43.296
- tetracyclic	T43.021	T43.022	T43.023	T43.024	T43.025	T43.026
- triazolopyridine	T43.211	T43.212	T43.213	T43.214	T43.215	T43.216
- tricyclic	T43.011	T43.012	T43.013	T43.014	T43.015	T43.016
Antidiabetic NEC	T38.3X1	T38.3X2	T38.3X3	T38.3X4	T38.3X5	T38.3X6
- biguanide	T38.3X1	T38.3X2	T38.3X3	T38.3X4	T38.3X5	T38.3X6
- - and sulfonyl combined	T38.3X1	T38.3X2	T38.3X3	T38.3X4	T38.3X5	T38.3X6

Substance	Poisoning, Accidental (unintentional)	Poisoning, Intentional Self-harm	Poisoning, Assault	Poisoning, Undetermined	Adverse effect	Underdosing
- combined	T38.3X1	T38.3X2	T38.3X3	T38.3X4	T38.3X5	T38.3X6
- sulfonylurea	T38.3X1	T38.3X2	T38.3X3	T38.3X4	T38.3X5	T38.3X6
Antidiarrheal drug NEC	T47.6X1	T47.6X2	T47.6X3	T47.6X4	T47.6X5	T47.6X6
- absorbent	T47.6X1	T47.6X2	T47.6X3	T47.6X4	T47.6X5	T47.6X6
Antidiphtheria serum	T50.Z11	T50.Z12	T50.Z13	T50.Z14	T50.Z15	T50.Z16
Antidiuretic hormone	T38.891	T38.892	T38.893	T38.894	T38.895	T38.896
Antidote NEC	T50.6X1	T50.6X2	T50.6X3	T50.6X4	T50.6X5	T50.6X6
- heavy metal	T45.8X1	T45.8X2	T45.8X3	T45.8X4	T45.8X5	T45.8X6
Antidysrhythmic NEC	T46.2X1	T46.2X2	T46.2X3	T46.2X4	T46.2X5	T46.2X6
Antiemetic drug	T45.0X1	T45.0X2	T45.0X3	T45.0X4	T45.0X5	T45.0X6
Antiepilepsy agent	T42.71	T42.72	T42.73	T42.74	T42.75	T42.76
- combination	T42.5X1	T42.5X2	T42.5X3	T42.5X4	T42.5X5	T42.5X6
- mixed	T42.5X1	T42.5X2	T42.5X3	T42.5X4	T42.5X5	T42.5X6
- specified, NEC	T42.6X1	T42.6X2	T42.6X3	T42.6X4	T42.6X5	T42.6X6
Antiestrogen NEC	T38.6X1	T38.6X2	T38.6X3	T38.6X4	T38.6X5	T38.6X6
Antifertility pill	T38.4X1	T38.4X2	T38.4X3	T38.4X4	T38.4X5	T38.4X6
Antifibrinolytic drug	T45.621	T45.622	T45.623	T45.624	T45.625	T45.626
Antifilarial drug	T37.4X1	T37.4X2	T37.4X3	T37.4X4	T37.4X5	T37.4X6
Antiflatulent	T47.5X1	T47.5X2	T47.5X3	T47.5X4	T47.5X5	T47.5X6
Antifreeze	T65.91	T65.92	T65.93	T65.94	--	--
- alcohol	T51.1X1	T51.1X2	T51.1X3	T51.1X4	--	--
- ethylene glycol	T51.8X1	T51.8X2	T51.8X3	T51.8X4	--	--
Antifungal						
- antibiotic (systemic)	T36.7X1	T36.7X2	T36.7X3	T36.7X4	T36.7X5	T36.7X6
- anti-infective NEC	T37.91	T37.92	T37.93	T37.94	T37.95	T37.96
- disinfectant, local	T49.0X1	T49.0X2	T49.0X3	T49.0X4	T49.0X5	T49.0X6
- nonmedicinal (spray)	T60.3X1	T60.3X2	T60.3X3	T60.3X4	--	--
- topical	T49.0X1	T49.0X2	T49.0X3	T49.0X4	T49.0X5	T49.0X6
Anti-gastric-secretion drug NEC	T47.1X1	T47.1X2	T47.1X3	T47.1X4	T47.1X5	T47.1X6
Antigonadotrophin NEC	T38.6X1	T38.6X2	T38.6X3	T38.6X4	T38.6X5	T38.6X6
Antihallucinogen	T43.501	T43.502	T43.503	T43.504	T43.505	T43.506
Antihelmintics	T37.4X1	T37.4X2	T37.4X3	T37.4X4	T37.4X5	T37.4X6
Antihemophilic						
- factor	T45.8X1	T45.8X2	T45.8X3	T45.8X4	T45.8X5	T45.8X6
- fraction	T45.8X1	T45.8X2	T45.8X3	T45.8X4	T45.8X5	T45.8X6
- globulin concentrate	T45.7X1	T45.7X2	T45.7X3	T45.7X4	T45.7X5	T45.7X6
- human plasma	T45.8X1	T45.8X2	T45.8X3	T45.8X4	T45.8X5	T45.8X6
- plasma, dried	T45.7X1	T45.7X2	T45.7X3	T45.7X4	T45.7X5	T45.7X6
Antihemorrhoidal preparation	T49.2X1	T49.2X2	T49.2X3	T49.2X4	T49.2X5	T49.2X6
Antiheparin drug	T45.7X1	T45.7X2	T45.7X3	T45.7X4	T45.7X5	T45.7X6
Antihistamine	T45.0X1	T45.0X2	T45.0X3	T45.0X4	T45.0X5	T45.0X6
Antihookworm drug	T37.4X1	T37.4X2	T37.4X3	T37.4X4	T37.4X5	T37.4X6
Anti-human lymphocytic globulin	T50.Z11	T50.Z12	T50.Z13	T50.Z14	T50.Z15	T50.Z16
Antihyperlipidemic drug	T46.6X1	T46.6X2	T46.6X3	T46.6X4	T46.6X5	T46.6X6
Antihypertensive drug NEC	T46.5X1	T46.5X2	T46.5X3	T46.5X4	T46.5X5	T46.5X6
Anti-infective NEC	T37.91	T37.92	T37.93	T37.94	T37.95	T37.96
- anthelmintic	T37.4X1	T37.4X2	T37.4X3	T37.4X4	T37.4X5	T37.4X6
- antibiotics	T36.91	T36.92	T36.93	T36.94	T36.95	T36.96
- - specified NEC	T36.8X1	T36.8X2	T36.8X3	T36.8X4	T36.8X5	T36.8X6
- antimalarial	T37.2X1	T37.2X2	T37.2X3	T37.2X4	T37.2X5	T37.2X6
- antimycobacterial NEC	T37.1X1	T37.1X2	T37.1X3	T37.1X4	T37.1X5	T37.1X6
- - antibiotics	T36.5X1	T36.5X2	T36.5X3	T36.5X4	T36.5X5	T36.5X6
- antiprotozoal NEC	T37.3X1	T37.3X2	T37.3X3	T37.3X4	T37.3X5	T37.3X6
- - blood	T37.2X1	T37.2X2	T37.2X3	T37.2X4	T37.2X5	T37.2X6
- antiviral	T37.5X1	T37.5X2	T37.5X3	T37.5X4	T37.5X5	T37.5X6
- arsenical	T37.8X1	T37.8X2	T37.8X3	T37.8X4	T37.8X5	T37.8X6
- bismuth, local	T49.0X1	T49.0X2	T49.0X3	T49.0X4	T49.0X5	T49.0X6
- ENT	T49.6X1	T49.6X2	T49.6X3	T49.6X4	T49.6X5	T49.6X6

Substance	Poisoning, Accidental (unintentional)	Poisoning, Intentional Self-harm	Poisoning, Assault	Poisoning, Undetermined	Adverse effect	Underdosing
- eye NEC	T49.5X1	T49.5X2	T49.5X3	T49.5X4	T49.5X5	T49.5X6
- heavy metals NEC	T37.8X1	T37.8X2	T37.8X3	T37.8X4	T37.8X5	T37.8X6
- local NEC	T49.0X1	T49.0X2	T49.0X3	T49.0X4	T49.0X5	T49.0X6
- - specified NEC	T49.0X1	T49.0X2	T49.0X3	T49.0X4	T49.0X5	T49.0X6
- mixed	T37.91	T37.92	T37.93	T37.94	T37.95	T37.96
- ophthalmic preparation	T49.5X1	T49.5X2	T49.5X3	T49.5X4	T49.5X5	T49.5X6
- topical NEC	T49.0X1	T49.0X2	T49.0X3	T49.0X4	T49.0X5	T49.0X6
Anti-inflammatory drug NEC	T39.391	T39.392	T39.393	T39.394	T39.395	T39.396
- local	T49.0X1	T49.0X2	T49.0X3	T49.0X4	T49.0X5	T49.0X6
- nonsteroidal NEC	T39.391	T39.392	T39.393	T39.394	T39.395	T39.396
- - propionic acid derivative	T39.311	T39.312	T39.313	T39.314	T39.315	T39.316
- specified NEC	T39.391	T39.392	T39.393	T39.394	T39.395	T39.396
Antikaluretic	T50.3X1	T50.3X2	T50.3X3	T50.3X4	T50.3X5	T50.3X6
Antiknock (tetraethyl lead)	T56.0X1	T56.0X2	T56.0X3	T56.0X4	--	--
Antilipemic drug NEC	T46.6X1	T46.6X2	T46.6X3	T46.6X4	T46.6X5	T46.6X6
Antimalarial	T37.2X1	T37.2X2	T37.2X3	T37.2X4	T37.2X5	T37.2X6
- prophylactic NEC	T37.2X1	T37.2X2	T37.2X3	T37.2X4	T37.2X5	T37.2X6
- pyrimidine derivative	T37.2X1	T37.2X2	T37.2X3	T37.2X4	T37.2X5	T37.2X6
Antimetabolite	T45.1X1	T45.1X2	T45.1X3	T45.1X4	T45.1X5	T45.1X6
Antimitotic agent	T45.1X1	T45.1X2	T45.1X3	T45.1X4	T45.1X5	T45.1X6
Antimony (compounds) (vapor) NEC	T56.891	T56.892	T56.893	T56.894	--	--
- anti-infectives	T37.8X1	T37.8X2	T37.8X3	T37.8X4	T37.8X5	T37.8X6
- dimercaptosuccinate	T37.3X1	T37.3X2	T37.3X3	T37.3X4	T37.3X5	T37.3X6
- hydride	T56.891	T56.892	T56.893	T56.894	--	--
- pesticide (vapor)	T60.8X1	T60.8X2	T60.8X3	T60.8X4	--	--
- potassium (sodium) tartrate	T37.8X1	T37.8X2	T37.8X3	T37.8X4	T37.8X5	T37.8X6
- sodium dimercaptosuccinate	T37.3X1	T37.3X2	T37.3X3	T37.3X4	T37.3X5	T37.3X6
- tartrated	T37.8X1	T37.8X2	T37.8X3	T37.8X4	T37.8X5	T37.8X6
Antimuscarinic NEC	T44.3X1	T44.3X2	T44.3X3	T44.3X4	T44.3X5	T44.3X6
Antimycobacterial drug NEC	T37.1X1	T37.1X2	T37.1X3	T37.1X4	T37.1X5	T37.1X6
- antibiotics	T36.5X1	T36.5X2	T36.5X3	T36.5X4	T36.5X5	T36.5X6
- combination	T37.1X1	T37.1X2	T37.1X3	T37.1X4	T37.1X5	T37.1X6
Antinausea drug	T45.0X1	T45.0X2	T45.0X3	T45.0X4	T45.0X5	T45.0X6
Antinematode drug	T37.4X1	T37.4X2	T37.4X3	T37.4X4	T37.4X5	T37.4X6
Antineoplastic NEC	T45.1X1	T45.1X2	T45.1X3	T45.1X4	T45.1X5	T45.1X6
- alkaloidal	T45.1X1	T45.1X2	T45.1X3	T45.1X4	T45.1X5	T45.1X6
- antibiotics	T45.1X1	T45.1X2	T45.1X3	T45.1X4	T45.1X5	T45.1X6
- combination	T45.1X1	T45.1X2	T45.1X3	T45.1X4	T45.1X5	T45.1X6
- - estrogen	T38.5X1	T38.5X2	T38.5X3	T38.5X4	T38.5X5	T38.5X6
- steroid	T38.7X1	T38.7X2	T38.7X3	T38.7X4	T38.7X5	T38.7X6
Antiparasitic drug (systemic)	T37.91	T37.92	T37.93	T37.94	T37.95	T37.96
- local	T49.0X1	T49.0X2	T49.0X3	T49.0X4	T49.0X5	T49.0X6
- specified NEC	T37.8X1	T37.8X2	T37.8X3	T37.8X4	T37.8X5	T37.8X6
Antiparkinsonism drug NEC	T42.8X1	T42.8X2	T42.8X3	T42.8X4	T42.8X5	T42.8X6
Antiperspirant NEC	T49.2X1	T49.2X2	T49.2X3	T49.2X4	T49.2X5	T49.2X6
Antiphlogistic NEC	T39.4X1	T39.4X2	T39.4X3	T39.4X4	T39.4X5	T39.4X6
Antiplatyhelmintic drug	T37.4X1	T37.4X2	T37.4X3	T37.4X4	T37.4X5	T37.4X6
Antiprotozoal drug NEC	T37.3X1	T37.3X2	T37.3X3	T37.3X4	T37.3X5	T37.3X6
- blood	T37.2X1	T37.2X2	T37.2X3	T37.2X4	T37.2X5	T37.2X6
- local	T49.0X1	T49.0X2	T49.0X3	T49.0X4	T49.0X5	T49.0X6
Antipruritic drug NEC	T49.1X1	T49.1X2	T49.1X3	T49.1X4	T49.1X5	T49.1X6
Antipsychotic drug	T43.501	T43.502	T43.503	T43.504	T43.505	T43.506
- specified NEC	T43.591	T43.592	T43.593	T43.594	T43.595	T43.596
Antipyretic	T39.91	T39.92	T39.93	T39.94	T39.95	T39.96
- specified NEC	T39.8X1	T39.8X2	T39.8X3	T39.8X4	T39.8X5	T39.8X6
Antipyrine	T39.2X1	T39.2X2	T39.2X3	T39.2X4	T39.2X5	T39.2X6
Antirabies hyperimmune serum	T50.Z11	T50.Z12	T50.Z13	T50.Z14	T50.Z15	T50.Z16
Antirheumatic NEC	T39.4X1	T39.4X2	T39.4X3	T39.4X4	T39.4X5	T39.4X6
Antirigidity drug NEC	T42.8X1	T42.8X2	T42.8X3	T42.8X4	T42.8X5	T42.8X6

Substance	Poisoning, Accidental (unintentional)	Poisoning, Intentional Self-harm	Poisoning, Assault	Poisoning, Undetermined	Adverse effect	Underdosing
Antischistosomal drug	T37.4X1	T37.4X2	T37.4X3	T37.4X4	T37.4X5	T37.4X6
Antiscorpion sera	T50.Z11	T50.Z12	T50.Z13	T50.Z14	T50.Z15	T50.Z16
Antiseborrheics	T49.4X1	T49.4X2	T49.4X3	T49.4X4	T49.4X5	T49.4X6
Antiseptics (external) (medicinal)	T49.0X1	T49.0X2	T49.0X3	T49.0X4	T49.0X5	T49.0X6
Antistine	T45.0X1	T45.0X2	T45.0X3	T45.0X4	T45.0X5	T45.0X6
Antitapeworm drug	T37.4X1	T37.4X2	T37.4X3	T37.4X4	T37.4X5	T37.4X6
Antitetanus immunoglobulin	T50.Z11	T50.Z12	T50.Z13	T50.Z14	T50.Z15	T50.Z16
Antithrombotic	T45.521	T45.522	T45.523	T45.524	T45.525	T45.526
Antithyroid drug NEC	T38.2X1	T38.2X2	T38.2X3	T38.2X4	T38.2X5	T38.2X6
Antitoxin	T50.Z11	T50.Z12	T50.Z13	T50.Z14	T50.Z15	T50.Z16
- diphtheria	T50.Z11	T50.Z12	T50.Z13	T50.Z14	T50.Z15	T50.Z16
- gas gangrene	T50.Z11	T50.Z12	T50.Z13	T50.Z14	T50.Z15	T50.Z16
- tetanus	T50.Z11	T50.Z12	T50.Z13	T50.Z14	T50.Z15	T50.Z16
Antitrichomonal drug	T37.3X1	T37.3X2	T37.3X3	T37.3X4	T37.3X5	T37.3X6
Antituberculars	T37.1X1	T37.1X2	T37.1X3	T37.1X4	T37.1X5	T37.1X6
- antibiotics	T36.5X1	T36.5X2	T36.5X3	T36.5X4	T36.5X5	T36.5X6
Antitussive NEC	T48.3X1	T48.3X2	T48.3X3	T48.3X4	T48.3X5	T48.3X6
- codeine mixture	T40.2X1	T40.2X2	T40.2X3	T40.2X4	T40.2X5	T40.2X6
- opiate	T40.2X1	T40.2X2	T40.2X3	T40.2X4	T40.2X5	T40.2X6
Antivaricose drug	T46.8X1	T46.8X2	T46.8X3	T46.8X4	T46.8X5	T46.8X6
Antivenin, antivenom (sera)	T50.Z11	T50.Z12	T50.Z13	T50.Z14	T50.Z15	T50.Z16
- crotaline	T50.Z11	T50.Z12	T50.Z13	T50.Z14	T50.Z15	T50.Z16
- spider bite	T50.Z11	T50.Z12	T50.Z13	T50.Z14	T50.Z15	T50.Z16
Antivertigo drug	T45.0X1	T45.0X2	T45.0X3	T45.0X4	T45.0X5	T45.0X6
Antiviral drug NEC	T37.5X1	T37.5X2	T37.5X3	T37.5X4	T37.5X5	T37.5X6
- eye	T49.5X1	T49.5X2	T49.5X3	T49.5X4	T49.5X5	T49.5X6
Antiwhipworm drug	T37.4X1	T37.4X2	T37.4X3	T37.4X4	T37.4X5	T37.4X6
Antrol—see also by specific chemical substance	T60.91	T60.92	T60.93	T60.94	--	--
- fungicide	T60.91	T60.92	T60.93	T60.94	--	--
ANTU (alpha naphthylthiourea)	T60.4X1	T60.4X2	T60.4X3	T60.4X4	--	--
Apalcillin	T36.0X1	T36.0X2	T36.0X3	T36.0X4	T36.0X5	T36.0X6
APC	T48.5X1	T48.5X2	T48.5X3	T48.5X4	T48.5X5	T48.5X6
Aplonidine	T44.4X1	T44.4X2	T44.4X3	T44.4X4	T44.4X5	T44.4X6
Apomorphine	T47.7X1	T47.7X2	T47.7X3	T47.7X4	T47.7X5	T47.7X6
Appetite depressants, central	T50.5X1	T50.5X2	T50.5X3	T50.5X4	T50.5X5	T50.5X6
Apraclonidine (hydrochloride)	T44.4X1	T44.4X2	T44.4X3	T44.4X4	T44.4X5	T44.4X6
Apresoline	T46.5X1	T46.5X2	T46.5X3	T46.5X4	T46.5X5	T46.5X6
Aprindine	T46.2X1	T46.2X2	T46.2X3	T46.2X4	T46.2X5	T46.2X6
Aprobarbital	T42.3X1	T42.3X2	T42.3X3	T42.3X4	T42.3X5	T42.3X6
Apronalide	T42.6X1	T42.6X2	T42.6X3	T42.6X4	T42.6X5	T42.6X6
Aprotinin	T45.621	T45.622	T45.623	T45.624	T45.625	T45.626
Aptocaine	T41.3X1	T41.3X2	T41.3X3	T41.3X4	T41.3X5	T41.3X6
Aqua fortis	T54.2X1	T54.2X2	T54.2X3	T54.2X4	--	--
Ara-A	T37.5X1	T37.5X2	T37.5X3	T37.5X4	T37.5X5	T37.5X6
Ara-C	T45.1X1	T45.1X2	T45.1X3	T45.1X4	T45.1X5	T45.1X6
Arachis oil	T49.3X1	T49.3X2	T49.3X3	T49.3X4	T49.3X5	T49.3X6
- cathartic	T47.4X1	T47.4X2	T47.4X3	T47.4X4	T47.4X5	T47.4X6
Aralen	T37.2X1	T37.2X2	T37.2X3	T37.2X4	T37.2X5	T37.2X6
Arecoline	T44.1X1	T44.1X2	T44.1X3	T44.1X4	T44.1X5	T44.1X6
Arginine	T50.991	T50.992	T50.993	T50.994	T50.995	T50.996
- glutamate	T50.991	T50.992	T50.993	T50.994	T50.995	T50.996
Argyrol	T49.0X1	T49.0X2	T49.0X3	T49.0X4	T49.0X5	T49.0X6
- ENT agent	T49.6X1	T49.6X2	T49.6X3	T49.6X4	T49.6X5	T49.6X6
- ophthalmic preparation	T49.5X1	T49.5X2	T49.5X3	T49.5X4	T49.5X5	T49.5X6
Aristocort	T38.0X1	T38.0X2	T38.0X3	T38.0X4	T38.0X5	T38.0X6
- ENT agent	T49.6X1	T49.6X2	T49.6X3	T49.6X4	T49.6X5	T49.6X6
- ophthalmic preparation	T49.5X1	T49.5X2	T49.5X3	T49.5X4	T49.5X5	T49.5X6
- topical NEC	T49.0X1	T49.0X2	T49.0X3	T49.0X4	T49.0X5	T49.0X6

Substance	Poisoning, Accidental (unintentional)	Poisoning, Intentional Self-harm	Poisoning, Assault	Poisoning, Undetermined	Adverse effect	Underdosing
Aromatics, corrosive	T54.1X1	T54.1X2	T54.1X3	T54.1X4	--	--
- disinfectants	T54.1X1	T54.1X2	T54.1X3	T54.1X4	--	--
Arsenate of lead	T57.0X1	T57.0X2	T57.0X3	T57.0X4	--	--
- herbicide	T57.0X1	T57.0X2	T57.0X3	T57.0X4	--	--
Arsenic, arsenicals (compounds) (dust) (vapor) NEC	T57.0X1	T57.0X2	T57.0X3	T57.0X4	--	--
- anti-infectives	T37.8X1	T37.8X2	T37.8X3	T37.8X4	T37.8X5	T37.8X6
- pesticide (dust) (fumes)	T57.0X1	T57.0X2	T57.0X3	T57.0X4	--	--
Arsine (gas)	T57.0X1	T57.0X2	T57.0X3	T57.0X4	--	--
Arsphenamine (silver)	T37.8X1	T37.8X2	T37.8X3	T37.8X4	T37.8X5	T37.8X6
Arsthinol	T37.3X1	T37.3X2	T37.3X3	T37.3X4	T37.3X5	T37.3X6
Artane	T44.3X1	T44.3X2	T44.3X3	T44.3X4	T44.3X5	T44.3X6
Arthropod (venomous) NEC	T63.481	T63.482	T63.483	T63.484	--	--
Articaine	T41.3X1	T41.3X2	T41.3X3	T41.3X4	T41.3X5	T41.3X6
Asbestos	T57.8X1	T57.8X2	T57.8X3	T57.8X4	--	--
Ascaridole	T37.4X1	T37.4X2	T37.4X3	T37.4X4	T37.4X5	T37.4X6
Ascorbic acid	T45.2X1	T45.2X2	T45.2X3	T45.2X4	T45.2X5	T45.2X6
Asiaticoside	T49.0X1	T49.0X2	T49.0X3	T49.0X4	T49.0X5	T49.0X6
Asparaginase	T45.1X1	T45.1X2	T45.1X3	T45.1X4	T45.1X5	T45.1X6
Aspidium (oleoresin)	T37.4X1	T37.4X2	T37.4X3	T37.4X4	T37.4X5	T37.4X6
Aspirin (aluminum) (soluble)	T39.011	T39.012	T39.013	T39.014	T39.015	T39.016
Aspoxicillin	T36.0X1	T36.0X2	T36.0X3	T36.0X4	T36.0X5	T36.0X6
Astemizole	T45.0X1	T45.0X2	T45.0X3	T45.0X4	T45.0X5	T45.0X6
Astringent (local)	T49.2X1	T49.2X2	T49.2X3	T49.2X4	T49.2X5	T49.2X6
- specified NEC	T49.2X1	T49.2X2	T49.2X3	T49.2X4	T49.2X5	T49.2X6
Astromicin	T36.5X1	T36.5X2	T36.5X3	T36.5X4	T36.5X5	T36.5X6
Ataractic drug NEC	T43.501	T43.502	T43.503	T43.504	T43.505	T43.506
Atenolol	T44.7X1	T44.7X2	T44.7X3	T44.7X4	T44.7X5	T44.7X6
Atonia drug, intestinal	T47.4X1	T47.4X2	T47.4X3	T47.4X4	T47.4X5	T47.4X6
Atophan	T50.4X1	T50.4X2	T50.4X3	T50.4X4	T50.4X5	T50.4X6
Atracurium besilate	T48.1X1	T48.1X2	T48.1X3	T48.1X4	T48.1X5	T48.1X6
Atropine	T44.3X1	T44.3X2	T44.3X3	T44.3X4	T44.3X5	T44.3X6
- derivative	T44.3X1	T44.3X2	T44.3X3	T44.3X4	T44.3X5	T44.3X6
- methonitrate	T44.3X1	T44.3X2	T44.3X3	T44.3X4	T44.3X5	T44.3X6
Attapulgite	T47.6X1	T47.6X2	T47.6X3	T47.6X4	T47.6X5	T47.6X6
Auramine	T65.891	T65.892	T65.893	T65.894	--	--
- dye	T65.6X1	T65.6X2	T65.6X3	T65.6X4	--	--
- fungicide	T60.3X1	T60.3X2	T60.3X3	T60.3X4	--	--
Auranofin	T39.4X1	T39.4X2	T39.4X3	T39.4X4	T39.4X5	T39.4X6
Aurantiin	T46.991	T46.992	T46.993	T46.994	T46.995	T46.996
Aureomycin	T36.4X1	T36.4X2	T36.4X3	T36.4X4	T36.4X5	T36.4X6
- ophthalmic preparation	T49.5X1	T49.5X2	T49.5X3	T49.5X4	T49.5X5	T49.5X6
- topical NEC	T49.0X1	T49.0X2	T49.0X3	T49.0X4	T49.0X5	T49.0X6
Aurothioglucose	T39.4X1	T39.4X2	T39.4X3	T39.4X4	T39.4X5	T39.4X6
Aurothioglycanide	T39.4X1	T39.4X2	T39.4X3	T39.4X4	T39.4X5	T39.4X6
Aurothiomalate sodium	T39.4X1	T39.4X2	T39.4X3	T39.4X4	T39.4X5	T39.4X6
Aurotioprol	T39.4X1	T39.4X2	T39.4X3	T39.4X4	T39.4X5	T39.4X6
Automobile fuel	T52.0X1	T52.0X2	T52.0X3	T52.0X4	--	--
Autonomic nervous system agent NEC	T44.901	T44.902	T44.903	T44.904	T44.905	T44.906
Avlosulfon	T37.1X1	T37.1X2	T37.1X3	T37.1X4	T37.1X5	T37.1X6
Avomine	T42.6X1	T42.6X2	T42.6X3	T42.6X4	T42.6X5	T42.6X6
Axerophthol	T45.2X1	T45.2X2	T45.2X3	T45.2X4	T45.2X5	T45.2X6
Azacitidine	T45.1X1	T45.1X2	T45.1X3	T45.1X4	T45.1X5	T45.1X6
Azacyclonol	T43.591	T43.592	T43.593	T43.594	T43.595	T43.596
Azadirachta	T60.2X1	T60.2X2	T60.2X3	T60.2X4	--	--
Azanidazole	T37.3X1	T37.3X2	T37.3X3	T37.3X4	T37.3X5	T37.3X6
Azapetine	T46.7X1	T46.7X2	T46.7X3	T46.7X4	T46.7X5	T46.7X6
Azapropazone	T39.2X1	T39.2X2	T39.2X3	T39.2X4	T39.2X5	T39.2X6
Azaribine	T45.1X1	T45.1X2	T45.1X3	T45.1X4	T45.1X5	T45.1X6

Substance	Poisoning, Accidental (unintentional)	Poisoning, Intentional Self-harm	Poisoning, Assault	Poisoning, Undetermined	Adverse effect	Underdosing
Azaserine	T45.1X1	T45.1X2	T45.1X3	T45.1X4	T45.1X5	T45.1X6
Azatadine	T45.0X1	T45.0X2	T45.0X3	T45.0X4	T45.0X5	T45.0X6
Azatepa	T45.1X1	T45.1X2	T45.1X3	T45.1X4	T45.1X5	T45.1X6
Azathioprine	T45.1X1	T45.1X2	T45.1X3	T45.1X4	T45.1X5	T45.1X6
Azelaic acid	T49.0X1	T49.0X2	T49.0X3	T49.0X4	T49.0X5	T49.0X6
Azelastine	T45.0X1	T45.0X2	T45.0X3	T45.0X4	T45.0X5	T45.0X6
Azidocillin	T36.0X1	T36.0X2	T36.0X3	T36.0X4	T36.0X5	T36.0X6
Azidothymidine	T37.5X1	T37.5X2	T37.5X3	T37.5X4	T37.5X5	T37.5X6
Azinphos (ethyl) (methyl)	T60.0X1	T60.0X2	T60.0X3	T60.0X4	--	--
Aziridine (chelating)	T54.1X1	T54.1X2	T54.1X3	T54.1X4	--	--
Azithromycin	T36.3X1	T36.3X2	T36.3X3	T36.3X4	T36.3X5	T36.3X6
Azlocillin	T36.0X1	T36.0X2	T36.0X3	T36.0X4	T36.0X5	T36.0X6
Azobenzene smoke	T65.3X1	T65.3X2	T65.3X3	T65.3X4	--	--
- acaricide	T60.8X1	T60.8X2	T60.8X3	T60.8X4	--	--
Azosulfamide	T37.0X1	T37.0X2	T37.0X3	T37.0X4	T37.0X5	T37.0X6
AZT	T37.5X1	T37.5X2	T37.5X3	T37.5X4	T37.5X5	T37.5X6
Aztreonam	T36.1X1	T36.1X2	T36.1X3	T36.1X4	T36.1X5	T36.1X6
Azulfidine	T37.0X1	T37.0X2	T37.0X3	T37.0X4	T37.0X5	T37.0X6
Azuresin	T50.8X1	T50.8X2	T50.8X3	T50.8X4	T50.8X5	T50.8X6
Bacampicillin	T36.0X1	T36.0X2	T36.0X3	T36.0X4	T36.0X5	T36.0X6
Bacillus						
- lactobacillus	T47.8X1	T47.8X2	T47.8X3	T47.8X4	T47.8X5	T47.8X6
- subtilis	T47.6X1	T47.6X2	T47.6X3	T47.6X4	T47.6X5	T47.6X6
Bacimycin	T49.0X1	T49.0X2	T49.0X3	T49.0X4	T49.0X5	T49.0X6
- ophthalmic preparation	T49.5X1	T49.5X2	T49.5X3	T49.5X4	T49.5X5	T49.5X6
Bacitracin zinc	T49.0X1	T49.0X2	T49.0X3	T49.0X4	T49.0X5	T49.0X6
- with neomycin	T49.0X1	T49.0X2	T49.0X3	T49.0X4	T49.0X5	T49.0X6
- ENT agent	T49.6X1	T49.6X2	T49.6X3	T49.6X4	T49.6X5	T49.6X6
- ophthalmic preparation	T49.5X1	T49.5X2	T49.5X3	T49.5X4	T49.5X5	T49.5X6
- topical NEC	T49.0X1	T49.0X2	T49.0X3	T49.0X4	T49.0X5	T49.0X6
Baclofen	T42.8X1	T42.8X2	T42.8X3	T42.8X4	T42.8X5	T42.8X6
Baking soda	T50.991	T50.992	T50.993	T50.994	T50.995	T50.996
BAL	T45.8X1	T45.8X2	T45.8X3	T45.8X4	T45.8X5	T45.8X6
Bambuterol	T48.6X1	T48.6X2	T48.6X3	T48.6X4	T48.6X5	T48.6X6
Bamethan (sulfate)	T46.7X1	T46.7X2	T46.7X3	T46.7X4	T46.7X5	T46.7X6
Bamifylline	T48.6X1	T48.6X2	T48.6X3	T48.6X4	T48.6X5	T48.6X6
Bamipine	T45.0X1	T45.0X2	T45.0X3	T45.0X4	T45.0X5	T45.0X6
Baneberry—see Actaea spicata						
Banewort—see Belladonna						
Barbenyl	T42.3X1	T42.3X2	T42.3X3	T42.3X4	T42.3X5	T42.3X6
Barbexaclone	T42.6X1	T42.6X2	T42.6X3	T42.6X4	T42.6X5	T42.6X6
Barbital	T42.3X1	T42.3X2	T42.3X3	T42.3X4	T42.3X5	T42.3X6
- sodium	T42.3X1	T42.3X2	T42.3X3	T42.3X4	T42.3X5	T42.3X6
Barbitone	T42.3X1	T42.3X2	T42.3X3	T42.3X4	T42.3X5	T42.3X6
Barbiturate NEC	T42.3X1	T42.3X2	T42.3X3	T42.3X4	T42.3X5	T42.3X6
- with tranquilizer	T42.3X1	T42.3X2	T42.3X3	T42.3X4	T42.3X5	T42.3X6
- anesthetic (intravenous)	T41.1X1	T41.1X2	T41.1X3	T41.1X4	T41.1X5	T41.1X6
Barium (carbonate) (chloride) (sulfite)	T57.8X1	T57.8X2	T57.8X3	T57.8X4	--	--
- diagnostic agent	T50.8X1	T50.8X2	T50.8X3	T50.8X4	T50.8X5	T50.8X6
- pesticide	T60.4X1	T60.4X2	T60.4X3	T60.4X4	--	--
- rodenticide	T60.4X1	T60.4X2	T60.4X3	T60.4X4	--	--
- sulfate (medicinal)	T50.8X1	T50.8X2	T50.8X3	T50.8X4	T50.8X5	T50.8X6
Barrier cream	T49.3X1	T49.3X2	T49.3X3	T49.3X4	T49.3X5	T49.3X6
Basic fuchsin	T49.0X1	T49.0X2	T49.0X3	T49.0X4	T49.0X5	T49.0X6
Battery acid or fluid	T54.2X1	T54.2X2	T54.2X3	T54.2X4	--	--
Bay rum	T51.8X1	T51.8X2	T51.8X3	T51.8X4	--	--
BCG (vaccine)	T50.A91	T50.A92	T50.A93	T50.A94	T50.A95	T50.A96
BCNU	T45.1X1	T45.1X2	T45.1X3	T45.1X4	T45.1X5	T45.1X6

Substance	Poisoning, Accidental (unintentional)	Poisoning, Intentional Self-harm	Poisoning, Assault	Poisoning, Undetermined	Adverse effect	Underdosing
Bearsfoot	T62.2X1	T62.2X2	T62.2X3	T62.2X4	--	--
Beclamide	T42.6X1	T42.6X2	T42.6X3	T42.6X4	T42.6X5	T42.6X6
Beclomethasone	T44.5X1	T44.5X2	T44.5X3	T44.5X4	T44.5X5	T44.5X6
Bee (sting) (venom)	T63.441	T63.442	T63.443	T63.444	--	--
Befunolol	T49.5X1	T49.5X2	T49.5X3	T49.5X4	T49.5X5	T49.5X6
Bekanamycin	T36.5X1	T36.5X2	T36.5X3	T36.5X4	T36.5X5	T36.5X6
Belladonna—see also Nightshade						
- alkaloids	T44.3X1	T44.3X2	T44.3X3	T44.3X4	T44.3X5	T44.3X6
- extract	T44.3X1	T44.3X2	T44.3X3	T44.3X4	T44.3X5	T44.3X6
- herb	T44.3X1	T44.3X2	T44.3X3	T44.3X4	T44.3X5	T44.3X6
Bemegride	T50.7X1	T50.7X2	T50.7X3	T50.7X4	T50.7X5	T50.7X6
Benactyzine	T44.3X1	T44.3X2	T44.3X3	T44.3X4	T44.3X5	T44.3X6
Benadryl	T45.0X1	T45.0X2	T45.0X3	T45.0X4	T45.0X5	T45.0X6
Benaprizine	T44.3X1	T44.3X2	T44.3X3	T44.3X4	T44.3X5	T44.3X6
Benazepril	T46.4X1	T46.4X2	T46.4X3	T46.4X4	T46.4X5	T46.4X6
Bencyclane	T46.7X1	T46.7X2	T46.7X3	T46.7X4	T46.7X5	T46.7X6
Bendazol	T46.3X1	T46.3X2	T46.3X3	T46.3X4	T46.3X5	T46.3X6
Bendrofluazide	T50.2X1	T50.2X2	T50.2X3	T50.2X4	T50.2X5	T50.2X6
Bendroflumethiazide	T50.2X1	T50.2X2	T50.2X3	T50.2X4	T50.2X5	T50.2X6
Benemid	T50.4X1	T50.4X2	T50.4X3	T50.4X4	T50.4X5	T50.4X6
Benethamine penicillin	T36.0X1	T36.0X2	T36.0X3	T36.0X4	T36.0X5	T36.0X6
Benexate	T47.1X1	T47.1X2	T47.1X3	T47.1X4	T47.1X5	T47.1X6
Benfluorex	T46.6X1	T46.6X2	T46.6X3	T46.6X4	T46.6X5	T46.6X6
Benfotiamine	T45.2X1	T45.2X2	T45.2X3	T45.2X4	T45.2X5	T45.2X6
Benisone	T49.0X1	T49.0X2	T49.0X3	T49.0X4	T49.0X5	T49.0X6
Benomyl	T60.0X1	T60.0X2	T60.0X3	T60.0X4	--	--
Benoquin	T49.8X1	T49.8X2	T49.8X3	T49.8X4	T49.8X5	T49.8X6
Benoxinate	T41.3X1	T41.3X2	T41.3X3	T41.3X4	T41.3X5	T41.3X6
Benperidol	T43.4X1	T43.4X2	T43.4X3	T43.4X4	T43.4X5	T43.4X6
Benproperine	T48.3X1	T48.3X2	T48.3X3	T48.3X4	T48.3X5	T48.3X6
Benserazide	T42.8X1	T42.8X2	T42.8X3	T42.8X4	T42.8X5	T42.8X6
Bentazepam	T42.4X1	T42.4X2	T42.4X3	T42.4X4	T42.4X5	T42.4X6
Bentiromide	T50.8X1	T50.8X2	T50.8X3	T50.8X4	T50.8X5	T50.8X6
Bentonite	T49.3X1	T49.3X2	T49.3X3	T49.3X4	T49.3X5	T49.3X6
Benzalbutyramide	T46.6X1	T46.6X2	T46.6X3	T46.6X4	T46.6X5	T46.6X6
Benzalkonium (chloride)	T49.0X1	T49.0X2	T49.0X3	T49.0X4	T49.0X5	T49.0X6
- ophthalmic preparation	T49.5X1	T49.5X2	T49.5X3	T49.5X4	T49.5X5	T49.5X6
Benzamidosalicylate (calcium)	T37.1X1	T37.1X2	T37.1X3	T37.1X4	T37.1X5	T37.1X6
Benzamine	T41.3X1	T41.3X2	T41.3X3	T41.3X4	T41.3X5	T41.3X6
- lactate	T49.1X1	T49.1X2	T49.1X3	T49.1X4	T49.1X5	T49.1X6
Benzamphetamine	T50.5X1	T50.5X2	T50.5X3	T50.5X4	T50.5X5	T50.5X6
Benzapril hydrochloride	T46.5X1	T46.5X2	T46.5X3	T46.5X4	T46.5X5	T46.5X6
Benzathine benzylpenicillin	T36.0X1	T36.0X2	T36.0X3	T36.0X4	T36.0X5	T36.0X6
Benzathine penicillin	T36.0X1	T36.0X2	T36.0X3	T36.0X4	T36.0X5	T36.0X6
Benzatropine	T42.8X1	T42.8X2	T42.8X3	T42.8X4	T42.8X5	T42.8X6
Benzbromarone	T50.4X1	T50.4X2	T50.4X3	T50.4X4	T50.4X5	T50.4X6
Benzcarbimine	T45.1X1	T45.1X2	T45.1X3	T45.1X4	T45.1X5	T45.1X6
Benzedrex	T44.991	T44.992	T44.993	T44.994	T44.995	T44.996
Benzedrine (amphetamine)	T43.621	T43.622	T43.623	T43.624	T43.625	T43.626
Benzenamine	T65.3X1	T65.3X2	T65.3X3	T65.3X4	--	--
Benzene	T52.1X1	T52.1X2	T52.1X3	T52.1X4	--	--
- homologues (acetyl) (dimethyl) (methyl) (solvent)	T52.2X1	T52.2X2	T52.2X3	T52.2X4	--	--
Benzethonium (chloride)	T49.0X1	T49.0X2	T49.0X3	T49.0X4	T49.0X5	T49.0X6
Benzfetamine	T50.5X1	T50.5X2	T50.5X3	T50.5X4	T50.5X5	T50.5X6
Benzhexol	T44.3X1	T44.3X2	T44.3X3	T44.3X4	T44.3X5	T44.3X6
Benzhydramine (chloride)	T45.0X1	T45.0X2	T45.0X3	T45.0X4	T45.0X5	T45.0X6
Benzidine	T65.891	T65.892	T65.893	T65.894	--	--
Benzilonium bromide	T44.3X1	T44.3X2	T44.3X3	T44.3X4	T44.3X5	T44.3X6

Substance	Poisoning, Accidental (unintentional)	Poisoning, Intentional Self-harm	Poisoning, Assault	Poisoning, Undetermined	Adverse effect	Underdosing
Benzimidazole	T60.3X1	T60.3X2	T60.3X3	T60.3X4	--	--
Benzin (e) —see Ligroin						
Benziodarone	T46.3X1	T46.3X2	T46.3X3	T46.3X4	T46.3X5	T46.3X6
Benznidazole	T37.3X1	T37.3X2	T37.3X3	T37.3X4	T37.3X5	T37.3X6
Benzocaine	T41.3X1	T41.3X2	T41.3X3	T41.3X4	T41.3X5	T41.3X6
Benzodiapin	T42.4X1	T42.4X2	T42.4X3	T42.4X4	T42.4X5	T42.4X6
Benzodiazepine NEC	T42.4X1	T42.4X2	T42.4X3	T42.4X4	T42.4X5	T42.4X6
Benzoic acid	T49.0X1	T49.0X2	T49.0X3	T49.0X4	T49.0X5	T49.0X6
- with salicylic acid	T49.0X1	T49.0X2	T49.0X3	T49.0X4	T49.0X5	T49.0X6
Benzoin (tincture)	T48.5X1	T48.5X2	T48.5X3	T48.5X4	T48.5X5	T48.5X6
Benzol (benzene)	T52.1X1	T52.1X2	T52.1X3	T52.1X4	--	--
- vapor	T52.0X1	T52.0X2	T52.0X3	T52.0X4	--	--
Benzomorphan	T40.2X1	T40.2X2	T40.2X3	T40.2X4	T40.2X5	T40.2X6
Benzonatate	T48.3X1	T48.3X2	T48.3X3	T48.3X4	T48.3X5	T48.3X6
Benzophenones	T49.3X1	T49.3X2	T49.3X3	T49.3X4	T49.3X5	T49.3X6
Benzopyrone	T46.991	T46.992	T46.993	T46.994	T46.995	T46.996
Benzothiadiazides	T50.2X1	T50.2X2	T50.2X3	T50.2X4	T50.2X5	T50.2X6
Benzoxonium chloride	T49.0X1	T49.0X2	T49.0X3	T49.0X4	T49.0X5	T49.0X6
Benzoyl peroxide	T49.0X1	T49.0X2	T49.0X3	T49.0X4	T49.0X5	T49.0X6
Benzoylpas calcium	T37.1X1	T37.1X2	T37.1X3	T37.1X4	T37.1X5	T37.1X6
Benzperidin	T43.591	T43.592	T43.593	T43.594	T43.595	T43.596
Benzperidol	T43.591	T43.592	T43.593	T43.594	T43.595	T43.596
Benzphetamine	T50.5X1	T50.5X2	T50.5X3	T50.5X4	T50.5X5	T50.5X6
Benzpyrinium bromide	T44.1X1	T44.1X2	T44.1X3	T44.1X4	T44.1X5	T44.1X6
Benzquinamide	T45.0X1	T45.0X2	T45.0X3	T45.0X4	T45.0X5	T45.0X6
Benzthiazide	T50.2X1	T50.2X2	T50.2X3	T50.2X4	T50.2X5	T50.2X6
Benztropine						
- anticholinergic	T44.3X1	T44.3X2	T44.3X3	T44.3X4	T44.3X5	T44.3X6
- antiparkinson	T42.8X1	T42.8X2	T42.8X3	T42.8X4	T42.8X5	T42.8X6
Benzydamine	T49.0X1	T49.0X2	T49.0X3	T49.0X4	T49.0X5	T49.0X6
Benzyl						
- acetate	T52.8X1	T52.8X2	T52.8X3	T52.8X4	--	--
- alcohol	T49.0X1	T49.0X2	T49.0X3	T49.0X4	T49.0X5	T49.0X6
- benzoate	T49.0X1	T49.0X2	T49.0X3	T49.0X4	T49.0X5	T49.0X6
- Benzoic acid	T49.0X1	T49.0X2	T49.0X3	T49.0X4	T49.0X5	T49.0X6
- morphine	T40.2X1	T40.2X2	T40.2X3	T40.2X4	--	--
- nicotinate	T46.6X1	T46.6X2	T46.6X3	T46.6X4	T46.6X5	T46.6X6
- penicillin	T36.0X1	T36.0X2	T36.0X3	T36.0X4	T36.0X5	T36.0X6
Benzylhydrochlorthia-zide	T50.2X1	T50.2X2	T50.2X3	T50.2X4	T50.2X5	T50.2X6
Benzylpenicillin	T36.0X1	T36.0X2	T36.0X3	T36.0X4	T36.0X5	T36.0X6
Benzylthiouracil	T38.2X1	T38.2X2	T38.2X3	T38.2X4	T38.2X5	T38.2X6
Bephenium hydroxy-naphthoate	T37.4X1	T37.4X2	T37.4X3	T37.4X4	T37.4X5	T37.4X6
Bepridil	T46.1X1	T46.1X2	T46.1X3	T46.1X4	T46.1X5	T46.1X6
Bergamot oil	T65.891	T65.892	T65.893	T65.894	--	--
Bergapten	T50.991	T50.992	T50.993	T50.994	T50.995	T50.996
Berries, poisonous	T62.1X1	T62.1X2	T62.1X3	T62.1X4	--	--
Beryllium (compounds)	T56.7X1	T56.7X2	T56.7X3	T56.7X4	--	--
b-acetyldigoxin	T46.0X1	T46.0X2	T46.0X3	T46.0X4	T46.0X5	T46.0X6
beta adrenergic blocking agent, heart	T44.7X1	T44.7X2	T44.7X3	T44.7X4	T44.7X5	T44.7X6
b-benzalbutyramide	T46.6X1	T46.6X2	T46.6X3	T46.6X4	T46.6X5	T46.6X6
Betacarotene	T45.2X1	T45.2X2	T45.2X3	T45.2X4	T45.2X5	T45.2X6
b-eucaine	T49.1X1	T49.1X2	T49.1X3	T49.1X4	T49.1X5	T49.1X6
Beta-Chlor	T42.6X1	T42.6X2	T42.6X3	T42.6X4	T42.6X5	T42.6X6
b-galactosidase	T47.5X1	T47.5X2	T47.5X3	T47.5X4	T47.5X5	T47.5X6
Betahistine	T46.7X1	T46.7X2	T46.7X3	T46.7X4	T46.7X5	T46.7X6
Betaine	T47.5X1	T47.5X2	T47.5X3	T47.5X4	T47.5X5	T47.5X6
Betamethasone	T49.0X1	T49.0X2	T49.0X3	T49.0X4	T49.0X5	T49.0X6
- topical	T49.0X1	T49.0X2	T49.0X3	T49.0X4	T49.0X5	T49.0X6

Substance	Poisoning, Accidental (unintentional)	Poisoning, Intentional Self-harm	Poisoning, Assault	Poisoning, Undetermined	Adverse effect	Underdosing
Betamicin	T36.8X1	T36.8X2	T36.8X3	T36.8X4	T36.8X5	T36.8X6
Betanidine	T46.5X1	T46.5X2	T46.5X3	T46.5X4	T46.5X5	T46.5X6
b-sitosterol (s)	T46.6X1	T46.6X2	T46.6X3	T46.6X4	T46.6X5	T46.6X6
Betaxolol	T44.7X1	T44.7X2	T44.7X3	T44.7X4	T44.7X5	T44.7X6
Betazole	T50.8X1	T50.8X2	T50.8X3	T50.8X4	T50.8X5	T50.8X6
Bethanechol	T44.1X1	T44.1X2	T44.1X3	T44.1X4	T44.1X5	T44.1X6
- chloride	T44.1X1	T44.1X2	T44.1X3	T44.1X4	T44.1X5	T44.1X6
Bethanidine	T46.5X1	T46.5X2	T46.5X3	T46.5X4	T46.5X5	T46.5X6
Betoxycaine	T41.3X1	T41.3X2	T41.3X3	T41.3X4	T41.3X5	T41.3X6
Betula oil	T49.3X1	T49.3X2	T49.3X3	T49.3X4	T49.3X5	T49.3X6
Bevantolol	T44.7X1	T44.7X2	T44.7X3	T44.7X4	T44.7X5	T44.7X6
Bevonium metilsulfate	T44.3X1	T44.3X2	T44.3X3	T44.3X4	T44.3X5	T44.3X6
Bezafibrate	T46.6X1	T46.6X2	T46.6X3	T46.6X4	T46.6X5	T46.6X6
Bezitramide	T40.491	T40.492	T40.493	T40.494	T40.495	T40.496
BHA	T50.991	T50.992	T50.993	T50.994	T50.995	T50.996
Bhang	T40.711	T40.712	T40.713	T40.714	T40.715	T40.716
BHC (medicinal)	T49.0X1	T49.0X2	T49.0X3	T49.0X4	T49.0X5	T49.0X6
- nonmedicinal (vapor)	T53.6X1	T53.6X2	T53.6X3	T53.6X4	--	--
Bialamicol	T37.3X1	T37.3X2	T37.3X3	T37.3X4	T37.3X5	T37.3X6
Bibenzonium bromide	T48.3X1	T48.3X2	T48.3X3	T48.3X4	T48.3X5	T48.3X6
Bibrocathol	T49.5X1	T49.5X2	T49.5X3	T49.5X4	T49.5X5	T49.5X6
Bichloride of mercury—see Mercury, chloride						
Bichromates (calcium) (potassium) (sodium) (crystals)	T57.8X1	T57.8X2	T57.8X3	T57.8X4	--	--
- fumes	T56.2X1	T56.2X2	T56.2X3	T56.2X4	--	--
Biclotymol	T49.6X1	T49.6X2	T49.6X3	T49.6X4	T49.6X5	T49.6X6
Bicucculine	T50.7X1	T50.7X2	T50.7X3	T50.7X4	T50.7X5	T50.7X6
Bifemelane	T43.291	T43.292	T43.293	T43.294	T43.295	T43.296
Biguanide derivatives, oral	T38.3X1	T38.3X2	T38.3X3	T38.3X4	T38.3X5	T38.3X6
Bile salts	T47.5X1	T47.5X2	T47.5X3	T47.5X4	T47.5X5	T47.5X6
Biligrafin	T50.8X1	T50.8X2	T50.8X3	T50.8X4	T50.8X5	T50.8X6
Bilopaque	T50.8X1	T50.8X2	T50.8X3	T50.8X4	T50.8X5	T50.8X6
Binifibrate	T46.6X1	T46.6X2	T46.6X3	T46.6X4	T46.6X5	T46.6X6
Binitrobenzol	T65.3X1	T65.3X2	T65.3X3	T65.3X4	--	--
Bioflavonoid (s)	T46.991	T46.992	T46.993	T46.994	T46.995	T46.996
Biological substance NEC	T50.901	T50.902	T50.903	T50.904	T50.905	T50.906
Biotin	T45.2X1	T45.2X2	T45.2X3	T45.2X4	T45.2X5	T45.2X6
Biperiden	T44.3X1	T44.3X2	T44.3X3	T44.3X4	T44.3X5	T44.3X6
Bisacodyl	T47.2X1	T47.2X2	T47.2X3	T47.2X4	T47.2X5	T47.2X6
Bisbentiamine	T45.2X1	T45.2X2	T45.2X3	T45.2X4	T45.2X5	T45.2X6
Bisbutiamine	T45.2X1	T45.2X2	T45.2X3	T45.2X4	T45.2X5	T45.2X6
Bisdequalinium (salts) (diacetate)	T49.6X1	T49.6X2	T49.6X3	T49.6X4	T49.6X5	T49.6X6
Bishydroxycoumarin	T45.511	T45.512	T45.513	T45.514	T45.515	T45.516
Bismarsen	T37.8X1	T37.8X2	T37.8X3	T37.8X4	T37.8X5	T37.8X6
Bismuth salts	T47.6X1	T47.6X2	T47.6X3	T47.6X4	T47.6X5	T47.6X6
- aluminate	T47.1X1	T47.1X2	T47.1X3	T47.1X4	T47.1X5	T47.1X6
- anti-infectives	T37.8X1	T37.8X2	T37.8X3	T37.8X4	T37.8X5	T37.8X6
- formic iodide	T49.0X1	T49.0X2	T49.0X3	T49.0X4	T49.0X5	T49.0X6
- glycolylarsenate	T49.0X1	T49.0X2	T49.0X3	T49.0X4	T49.0X5	T49.0X6
- nonmedicinal (compounds) NEC	T65.91	T65.92	T65.93	T65.94	--	--
- subcarbonate	T47.6X1	T47.6X2	T47.6X3	T47.6X4	T47.6X5	T47.6X6
- subsalicylate	T37.8X1	T37.8X2	T37.8X3	T37.8X4	T37.8X5	T37.8X6
- sulfarsphenamine	T37.8X1	T37.8X2	T37.8X3	T37.8X4	T37.8X5	T37.8X6
Bisoprolol	T44.7X1	T44.7X2	T44.7X3	T44.7X4	T44.7X5	T44.7X6
Bisoxatin	T47.2X1	T47.2X2	T47.2X3	T47.2X4	T47.2X5	T47.2X6
Bisulepin (hydrochloride)	T45.0X1	T45.0X2	T45.0X3	T45.0X4	T45.0X5	T45.0X6
Bithionol	T37.8X1	T37.8X2	T37.8X3	T37.8X4	T37.8X5	T37.8X6
- anthelminthic	T37.4X1	T37.4X2	T37.4X3	T37.4X4	T37.4X5	T37.4X6
Bitolterol	T48.6X1	T48.6X2	T48.6X3	T48.6X4	T48.6X5	T48.6X6

Substance	Poisoning, Accidental (unintentional)	Poisoning, Intentional Self-harm	Poisoning, Assault	Poisoning, Undetermined	Adverse effect	Underdosing
Bitoscanate	T37.4X1	T37.4X2	T37.4X3	T37.4X4	T37.4X5	T37.4X6
Bitter almond oil	T62.8X1	T62.8X2	T62.8X3	T62.8X4	--	--
Bittersweet	T62.2X1	T62.2X2	T62.2X3	T62.2X4	--	--
Black						
- flag	T60.91	T60.92	T60.93	T60.94	--	--
- henbane	T62.2X1	T62.2X2	T62.2X3	T62.2X4	--	--
- leaf.(40)	T60.91	T60.92	T60.93	T60.94	--	--
- widow spider (bite)	T63.311	T63.312	T63.313	T63.314	--	--
- - antivenin	T50.Z11	T50.Z12	T50.Z13	T50.Z14	T50.Z15	T50.Z16
Blast furnace gas (carbon monoxide from)	T58.8X1	T58.8X2	T58.8X3	T58.8X4	--	--
Bleach	T54.91	T54.92	T54.93	T54.94	--	--
Bleaching agent (medicinal)	T49.4X1	T49.4X2	T49.4X3	T49.4X4	T49.4X5	T49.4X6
Bleomycin	T45.1X1	T45.1X2	T45.1X3	T45.1X4	T45.1X5	T45.1X6
Blockain	T41.3X1	T41.3X2	T41.3X3	T41.3X4	T41.3X5	T41.3X6
- infiltration (subcutaneous)	T41.3X1	T41.3X2	T41.3X3	T41.3X4	T41.3X5	T41.3X6
- nerve block (peripheral) (plexus)	T41.3X1	T41.3X2	T41.3X3	T41.3X4	T41.3X5	T41.3X6
- topical (surface)	T41.3X1	T41.3X2	T41.3X3	T41.3X4	T41.3X5	T41.3X6
Blockers, calcium channel	T46.1X1	T46.1X2	T46.1X3	T46.1X4	T46.1X5	T46.1X6
Blood (derivatives) (natural) (plasma) (whole)	T45.8X1	T45.8X2	T45.8X3	T45.8X4	T45.8X5	T45.8X6
- dried	T45.8X1	T45.8X2	T45.8X3	T45.8X4	T45.8X5	T45.8X6
- drug affecting NEC	T45.91	T45.92	T45.93	T45.94	T45.95	T45.96
- expander NEC	T45.8X1	T45.8X2	T45.8X3	T45.8X4	T45.8X5	T45.8X6
- fraction NEC	T45.8X1	T45.8X2	T45.8X3	T45.8X4	T45.8X5	T45.8X6
- substitute (macromolecular)	T45.8X1	T45.8X2	T45.8X3	T45.8X4	T45.8X5	T45.8X6
Blue velvet	T40.2X1	T40.2X2	T40.2X3	T40.2X4	--	--
Bone meal	T62.8X1	T62.8X2	T62.8X3	T62.8X4	--	--
Bonine	T45.0X1	T45.0X2	T45.0X3	T45.0X4	T45.0X5	T45.0X6
Bopindolol	T44.7X1	T44.7X2	T44.7X3	T44.7X4	T44.7X5	T44.7X6
Boracic acid	T49.0X1	T49.0X2	T49.0X3	T49.0X4	T49.0X5	T49.0X6
- ENT agent	T49.6X1	T49.6X2	T49.6X3	T49.6X4	T49.6X5	T49.6X6
- ophthalmic preparation	T49.5X1	T49.5X2	T49.5X3	T49.5X4	T49.5X5	T49.5X6
Borane complex	T57.8X1	T57.8X2	T57.8X3	T57.8X4	--	--
Borate (s)	T57.8X1	T57.8X2	T57.8X3	T57.8X4	--	--
- buffer	T50.991	T50.992	T50.993	T50.994	T50.995	T50.996
- cleanser	T54.91	T54.92	T54.93	T54.94	--	--
- sodium	T57.8X1	T57.8X2	T57.8X3	T57.8X4	--	--
Borax (cleanser)	T54.91	T54.92	T54.93	T54.94	--	--
Bordeaux mixture	T60.3X1	T60.3X2	T60.3X3	T60.3X4	--	--
Boric acid	T49.0X1	T49.0X2	T49.0X3	T49.0X4	T49.0X5	T49.0X6
- ENT agent	T49.6X1	T49.6X2	T49.6X3	T49.6X4	T49.6X5	T49.6X6
- ophthalmic preparation	T49.5X1	T49.5X2	T49.5X3	T49.5X4	T49.5X5	T49.5X6
Bornaprine	T44.3X1	T44.3X2	T44.3X3	T44.3X4	T44.3X5	T44.3X6
Boron	T57.8X1	T57.8X2	T57.8X3	T57.8X4	--	--
- hydride NEC	T57.8X1	T57.8X2	T57.8X3	T57.8X4	--	--
- - fumes or gas	T57.8X1	T57.8X2	T57.8X3	T57.8X4	--	--
- trifluoride	T59.891	T59.892	T59.893	T59.894	--	--
Botox	T48.291	T48.292	T48.293	T48.294	T48.295	T48.296
Botulinus anti-toxin (type A, B)	T50.Z11	T50.Z12	T50.Z13	T50.Z14	T50.Z15	T50.Z16
Brake fluid vapor	T59.891	T59.892	T59.893	T59.894	--	--
Brallobarbital	T42.3X1	T42.3X2	T42.3X3	T42.3X4	T42.3X5	T42.3X6
Bran (wheat)	T47.4X1	T47.4X2	T47.4X3	T47.4X4	T47.4X5	T47.4X6
Brass (fumes)	T56.891	T56.892	T56.893	T56.894	--	--
Brasso	T52.0X1	T52.0X2	T52.0X3	T52.0X4	--	--
Bretylium tosilate	T46.2X1	T46.2X2	T46.2X3	T46.2X4	T46.2X5	T46.2X6
Brevital (sodium)	T41.1X1	T41.1X2	T41.1X3	T41.1X4	T41.1X5	T41.1X6
Brinase	T45.3X1	T45.3X2	T45.3X3	T45.3X4	T45.3X5	T45.3X6
British antilewisite	T45.8X1	T45.8X2	T45.8X3	T45.8X4	T45.8X5	T45.8X6
Brodifacoum	T60.4X1	T60.4X2	T60.4X3	T60.4X4	--	--

Substance	Poisoning, Accidental (unintentional)	Poisoning, Intentional Self-harm	Poisoning, Assault	Poisoning, Undetermined	Adverse effect	Underdosing
Bromal (hydrate)	T42.6X1	T42.6X2	T42.6X3	T42.6X4	T42.6X5	T42.6X6
Bromazepam	T42.4X1	T42.4X2	T42.4X3	T42.4X4	T42.4X5	T42.4X6
Bromazine	T45.0X1	T45.0X2	T45.0X3	T45.0X4	T45.0X5	T45.0X6
Brombenzylcyanide	T59.3X1	T59.3X2	T59.3X3	T59.3X4	--	--
Bromelains	T45.3X1	T45.3X2	T45.3X3	T45.3X4	T45.3X5	T45.3X6
Bromethalin	T60.4X1	T60.4X2	T60.4X3	T60.4X4	--	--
Bromhexine	T48.4X1	T48.4X2	T48.4X3	T48.4X4	T48.4X5	T48.4X6
Bromide salts	T42.6X1	T42.6X2	T42.6X3	T42.6X4	T42.6X5	T42.6X6
Bromindione	T45.511	T45.512	T45.513	T45.514	T45.515	T45.516
Bromine						
- compounds (medicinal)	T42.6X1	T42.6X2	T42.6X3	T42.6X4	T42.6X5	T42.6X6
- sedative	T42.6X1	T42.6X2	T42.6X3	T42.6X4	T42.6X5	T42.6X6
- vapor	T59.891	T59.892	T59.893	T59.894	--	--
Bromisoval	T42.6X1	T42.6X2	T42.6X3	T42.6X4	T42.6X5	T42.6X6
Bromisovalum	T42.6X1	T42.6X2	T42.6X3	T42.6X4	T42.6X5	T42.6X6
Bromobenzylcyanide	T59.3X1	T59.3X2	T59.3X3	T59.3X4	--	--
Bromochlorosalicylani-lide	T49.0X1	T49.0X2	T49.0X3	T49.0X4	T49.0X5	T49.0X6
Bromocriptine	T42.8X1	T42.8X2	T42.8X3	T42.8X4	T42.8X5	T42.8X6
Bromodiphenhydramine	T45.0X1	T45.0X2	T45.0X3	T45.0X4	T45.0X5	T45.0X6
Bromoform	T42.6X1	T42.6X2	T42.6X3	T42.6X4	T42.6X5	T42.6X6
Bromophenol blue reagent	T50.991	T50.992	T50.993	T50.994	T50.995	T50.996
Bromopride	T47.8X1	T47.8X2	T47.8X3	T47.8X4	T47.8X5	T47.8X6
Bromosalicylchloranitide	T49.0X1	T49.0X2	T49.0X3	T49.0X4	T49.0X5	T49.0X6
Bromosalicylhydroxamic acid	T37.1X1	T37.1X2	T37.1X3	T37.1X4	T37.1X5	T37.1X6
Bromo-seltzer	T39.1X1	T39.1X2	T39.1X3	T39.1X4	T39.1X5	T39.1X6
Bromoxynil	T60.3X1	T60.3X2	T60.3X3	T60.3X4	--	--
Bromperidol	T43.4X1	T43.4X2	T43.4X3	T43.4X4	T43.4X5	T43.4X6
Brompheniramine	T45.0X1	T45.0X2	T45.0X3	T45.0X4	T45.0X5	T45.0X6
Bromsulfophthalein	T50.8X1	T50.8X2	T50.8X3	T50.8X4	T50.8X5	T50.8X6
Bromural	T42.6X1	T42.6X2	T42.6X3	T42.6X4	T42.6X5	T42.6X6
Bromvaletone	T42.6X1	T42.6X2	T42.6X3	T42.6X4	T42.6X5	T42.6X6
Bronchodilator NEC	T48.6X1	T48.6X2	T48.6X3	T48.6X4	T48.6X5	T48.6X6
Brotizolam	T42.4X1	T42.4X2	T42.4X3	T42.4X4	T42.4X5	T42.4X6
Brovincamine	T46.7X1	T46.7X2	T46.7X3	T46.7X4	T46.7X5	T46.7X6
Brown recluse spider (bite) (venom)	T63.331	T63.332	T63.333	T63.334	--	--
Brown spider (bite) (venom)	T63.391	T63.392	T63.393	T63.394	--	--
Broxaterol	T48.6X1	T48.6X2	T48.6X3	T48.6X4	T48.6X5	T48.6X6
Broxuridine	T45.1X1	T45.1X2	T45.1X3	T45.1X4	T45.1X5	T45.1X6
Broxyquinoline	T37.8X1	T37.8X2	T37.8X3	T37.8X4	T37.8X5	T37.8X6
Bruceine	T48.291	T48.292	T48.293	T48.294	T48.295	T48.296
Brucia	T62.2X1	T62.2X2	T62.2X3	T62.2X4	--	--
Brucine	T65.1X1	T65.1X2	T65.1X3	T65.1X4	--	--
Brunswick green—see Copper						
Bruten—see Ibuprofen						
Bryonia	T47.2X1	T47.2X2	T47.2X3	T47.2X4	T47.2X5	T47.2X6
Buclizine	T45.0X1	T45.0X2	T45.0X3	T45.0X4	T45.0X5	T45.0X6
Buclosamide	T49.0X1	T49.0X2	T49.0X3	T49.0X4	T49.0X5	T49.0X6
Budesonide	T44.5X1	T44.5X2	T44.5X3	T44.5X4	T44.5X5	T44.5X6
Budralazine	T46.5X1	T46.5X2	T46.5X3	T46.5X4	T46.5X5	T46.5X6
Bufferin	T39.011	T39.012	T39.013	T39.014	T39.015	T39.016
Buflomedil	T46.7X1	T46.7X2	T46.7X3	T46.7X4	T46.7X5	T46.7X6
Buformin	T38.3X1	T38.3X2	T38.3X3	T38.3X4	T38.3X5	T38.3X6
Bufotenine	T40.991	T40.992	T40.993	T40.994	--	--
Bufrolin	T48.6X1	T48.6X2	T48.6X3	T48.6X4	T48.6X5	T48.6X6
Bufylline	T48.6X1	T48.6X2	T48.6X3	T48.6X4	T48.6X5	T48.6X6
Bulk filler	T50.5X1	T50.5X2	T50.5X3	T50.5X4	T50.5X5	T50.5X6
- cathartic	T47.4X1	T47.4X2	T47.4X3	T47.4X4	T47.4X5	T47.4X6
Bumetanide	T50.1X1	T50.1X2	T50.1X3	T50.1X4	T50.1X5	T50.1X6
Bunaftine	T46.2X1	T46.2X2	T46.2X3	T46.2X4	T46.2X5	T46.2X6

Substance	Poisoning, Accidental (unintentional)	Poisoning, Intentional Self-harm	Poisoning, Assault	Poisoning, Undetermined	Adverse effect	Underdosing
Bunamiodyl	T50.8X1	T50.8X2	T50.8X3	T50.8X4	T50.8X5	T50.8X6
Bunazosin	T44.6X1	T44.6X2	T44.6X3	T44.6X4	T44.6X5	T44.6X6
Bunitrolol	T44.7X1	T44.7X2	T44.7X3	T44.7X4	T44.7X5	T44.7X6
Buphenine	T46.7X1	T46.7X2	T46.7X3	T46.7X4	T46.7X5	T46.7X6
Bupivacaine	T41.3X1	T41.3X2	T41.3X3	T41.3X4	T41.3X5	T41.3X6
- infiltration (subcutaneous)	T41.3X1	T41.3X2	T41.3X3	T41.3X4	T41.3X5	T41.3X6
- nerve block (peripheral) (plexus)	T41.3X1	T41.3X2	T41.3X3	T41.3X4	T41.3X5	T41.3X6
- spinal	T41.3X1	T41.3X2	T41.3X3	T41.3X4	T41.3X5	T41.3X6
Bupranolol	T44.7X1	T44.7X2	T44.7X3	T44.7X4	T44.7X5	T44.7X6
Buprenorphine	T40.491	T40.492	T40.493	T40.494	T40.495	T40.496
Bupropion	T43.291	T43.292	T43.293	T43.294	T43.295	T43.296
Burimamide	T47.1X1	T47.1X2	T47.1X3	T47.1X4	T47.1X5	T47.1X6
Buserelin	T38.891	T38.892	T38.893	T38.894	T38.895	T38.896
Buspirone	T43.591	T43.592	T43.593	T43.594	T43.595	T43.596
Busulfan, busulphan	T45.1X1	T45.1X2	T45.1X3	T45.1X4	T45.1X5	T45.1X6
Butabarbital (sodium)	T42.3X1	T42.3X2	T42.3X3	T42.3X4	T42.3X5	T42.3X6
Butabarbitone	T42.3X1	T42.3X2	T42.3X3	T42.3X4	T42.3X5	T42.3X6
Butabarpal	T42.3X1	T42.3X2	T42.3X3	T42.3X4	T42.3X5	T42.3X6
Butacaine	T41.3X1	T41.3X2	T41.3X3	T41.3X4	T41.3X5	T41.3X6
Butalamine	T46.7X1	T46.7X2	T46.7X3	T46.7X4	T46.7X5	T46.7X6
Butalbital	T42.3X1	T42.3X2	T42.3X3	T42.3X4	T42.3X5	T42.3X6
Butallylonal	T42.3X1	T42.3X2	T42.3X3	T42.3X4	T42.3X5	T42.3X6
Butamben	T41.3X1	T41.3X2	T41.3X3	T41.3X4	T41.3X5	T41.3X6
Butamirate	T48.3X1	T48.3X2	T48.3X3	T48.3X4	T48.3X5	T48.3X6
Butane (distributed in mobile container)	T59.891	T59.892	T59.893	T59.894	--	--
- distributed through pipes	T59.891	T59.892	T59.893	T59.894	--	--
- incomplete combustion	T58.11	T58.12	T58.13	T58.14	--	--
Butanilicaine	T41.3X1	T41.3X2	T41.3X3	T41.3X4	T41.3X5	T41.3X6
Butanol	T51.3X1	T51.3X2	T51.3X3	T51.3X4	--	--
Butanone, 2-butanone	T52.4X1	T52.4X2	T52.4X3	T52.4X4	--	--
Butantrone	T49.4X1	T49.4X2	T49.4X3	T49.4X4	T49.4X5	T49.4X6
Butaperazine	T43.3X1	T43.3X2	T43.3X3	T43.3X4	T43.3X5	T43.3X6
Butazolidin	T39.2X1	T39.2X2	T39.2X3	T39.2X4	T39.2X5	T39.2X6
Butetamate	T48.6X1	T48.6X2	T48.6X3	T48.6X4	T48.6X5	T48.6X6
Butethal	T42.3X1	T42.3X2	T42.3X3	T42.3X4	T42.3X5	T42.3X6
Butethamate	T44.3X1	T44.3X2	T44.3X3	T44.3X4	T44.3X5	T44.3X6
Buthalitone (sodium)	T41.1X1	T41.1X2	T41.1X3	T41.1X4	T41.1X5	T41.1X6
Butisol (sodium)	T42.3X1	T42.3X2	T42.3X3	T42.3X4	T42.3X5	T42.3X6
Butizide	T50.2X1	T50.2X2	T50.2X3	T50.2X4	T50.2X5	T50.2X6
Butobarbital	T42.3X1	T42.3X2	T42.3X3	T42.3X4	T42.3X5	T42.3X6
- sodium	T42.3X1	T42.3X2	T42.3X3	T42.3X4	T42.3X5	T42.3X6
Butobarbitone	T42.3X1	T42.3X2	T42.3X3	T42.3X4	T42.3X5	T42.3X6
Butoconazole (nitrate)	T49.0X1	T49.0X2	T49.0X3	T49.0X4	T49.0X5	T49.0X6
Butorphanol	T40.491	T40.492	T40.493	T40.494	T40.495	T40.496
Butriptyline	T43.011	T43.012	T43.013	T43.014	T43.015	T43.016
Butropium bromide	T44.3X1	T44.3X2	T44.3X3	T44.3X4	T44.3X5	T44.3X6
Butter of antimony—see Antimony						
Buttercups	T62.2X1	T62.2X2	T62.2X3	T62.2X4	--	--
Butyl						
- acetate (secondary)	T52.8X1	T52.8X2	T52.8X3	T52.8X4	--	--
- alcohol	T51.3X1	T51.3X2	T51.3X3	T51.3X4	--	--
- aminobenzoate	T41.3X1	T41.3X2	T41.3X3	T41.3X4	T41.3X5	T41.3X6
- butyrate	T52.8X1	T52.8X2	T52.8X3	T52.8X4	--	--
- carbinol	T51.3X1	T51.3X2	T51.3X3	T51.3X4	--	--
- carbitol	T52.3X1	T52.3X2	T52.3X3	T52.3X4	--	--
- cellosolve	T52.3X1	T52.3X2	T52.3X3	T52.3X4	--	--
- chloral (hydrate)	T42.6X1	T42.6X2	T42.6X3	T42.6X4	T42.6X5	T42.6X6
- formate	T52.8X1	T52.8X2	T52.8X3	T52.8X4	--	--

Substance	Poisoning, Accidental (unintentional)	Poisoning, Intentional Self-harm	Poisoning, Assault	Poisoning, Undetermined	Adverse effect	Underdosing
- lactate	T52.8X1	T52.8X2	T52.8X3	T52.8X4	--	--
- propionate	T52.8X1	T52.8X2	T52.8X3	T52.8X4	--	--
- scopolamine bromide	T44.3X1	T44.3X2	T44.3X3	T44.3X4	T44.3X5	T44.3X6
- thiobarbital sodium	T41.1X1	T41.1X2	T41.1X3	T41.1X4	T41.1X5	T41.1X6
Butylated hydroxy-anisole	T50.991	T50.992	T50.993	T50.994	T50.995	T50.996
Butylchloral hydrate	T42.6X1	T42.6X2	T42.6X3	T42.6X4	T42.6X5	T42.6X6
Butyltoluene	T52.2X1	T52.2X2	T52.2X3	T52.2X4	--	--
Butyn	T41.3X1	T41.3X2	T41.3X3	T41.3X4	T41.3X5	T41.3X6
Butyrophenone (-based tranquilizers)	T43.4X1	T43.4X2	T43.4X3	T43.4X4	T43.4X5	T43.4X6
Cabergoline	T42.8X1	T42.8X2	T42.8X3	T42.8X4	T42.8X5	T42.8X6
Cacodyl, cacodylic acid	T57.0X1	T57.0X2	T57.0X3	T57.0X4	--	--
Cactinomycin	T45.1X1	T45.1X2	T45.1X3	T45.1X4	T45.1X5	T45.1X6
Cade oil	T49.4X1	T49.4X2	T49.4X3	T49.4X4	T49.4X5	T49.4X6
Cadexomer iodine	T49.0X1	T49.0X2	T49.0X3	T49.0X4	T49.0X5	T49.0X6
Cadmium (chloride) (fumes) (oxide)	T56.3X1	T56.3X2	T56.3X3	T56.3X4	--	--
- sulfide (medicinal) NEC	T49.4X1	T49.4X2	T49.4X3	T49.4X4	T49.4X5	T49.4X6
Cadralazine	T46.5X1	T46.5X2	T46.5X3	T46.5X4	T46.5X5	T46.5X6
Caffeine	T43.611	T43.612	T43.613	T43.614	T43.615	T43.616
Calabar bean	T62.2X1	T62.2X2	T62.2X3	T62.2X4	--	--
Caladium seguinum	T62.2X1	T62.2X2	T62.2X3	T62.2X4	--	--
Calamine (lotion)	T49.3X1	T49.3X2	T49.3X3	T49.3X4	T49.3X5	T49.3X6
Calcifediol	T45.2X1	T45.2X2	T45.2X3	T45.2X4	T45.2X5	T45.2X6
Calciferol	T45.2X1	T45.2X2	T45.2X3	T45.2X4	T45.2X5	T45.2X6
Calcitonin	T50.991	T50.992	T50.993	T50.994	T50.995	T50.996
Calcitriol	T45.2X1	T45.2X2	T45.2X3	T45.2X4	T45.2X5	T45.2X6
Calcium	T50.3X1	T50.3X2	T50.3X3	T50.3X4	T50.3X5	T50.3X6
- actylsalicylate	T39.011	T39.012	T39.013	T39.014	T39.015	T39.016
- benzamidosalicylate	T37.1X1	T37.1X2	T37.1X3	T37.1X4	T37.1X5	T37.1X6
- bromide	T42.6X1	T42.6X2	T42.6X3	T42.6X4	T42.6X5	T42.6X6
- bromolactobionate	T42.6X1	T42.6X2	T42.6X3	T42.6X4	T42.6X5	T42.6X6
- carbaspirin	T39.011	T39.012	T39.013	T39.014	T39.015	T39.016
- carbimide	T50.6X1	T50.6X2	T50.6X3	T50.6X4	T50.6X5	T50.6X6
- carbonate	T47.1X1	T47.1X2	T47.1X3	T47.1X4	T47.1X5	T47.1X6
- chloride	T50.991	T50.992	T50.993	T50.994	T50.995	T50.996
- - anhydrous	T50.991	T50.992	T50.993	T50.994	T50.995	T50.996
- cyanide	T57.8X1	T57.8X2	T57.8X3	T57.8X4	--	--
- dioctyl sulfosuccinate	T47.4X1	T47.4X2	T47.4X3	T47.4X4	T47.4X5	T47.4X6
- disodium edathamil	T45.8X1	T45.8X2	T45.8X3	T45.8X4	T45.8X5	T45.8X6
- disodium edetate	T45.8X1	T45.8X2	T45.8X3	T45.8X4	T45.8X5	T45.8X6
- dobesilate	T46.991	T46.992	T46.993	T46.994	T46.995	T46.996
- EDTA	T45.8X1	T45.8X2	T45.8X3	T45.8X4	T45.8X5	T45.8X6
- ferrous citrate	T45.4X1	T45.4X2	T45.4X3	T45.4X4	T45.4X5	T45.4X6
- folinate	T45.8X1	T45.8X2	T45.8X3	T45.8X4	T45.8X5	T45.8X6
- glubionate	T50.3X1	T50.3X2	T50.3X3	T50.3X4	T50.3X5	T50.3X6
- gluconate	T50.3X1	T50.3X2	T50.3X3	T50.3X4	T50.3X5	T50.3X6
- gluconogalactogluc-onate	T50.3X1	T50.3X2	T50.3X3	T50.3X4	T50.3X5	T50.3X6
- hydrate, hydroxide	T54.3X1	T54.3X2	T54.3X3	T54.3X4	--	--
- hypochlorite	T54.3X1	T54.3X2	T54.3X3	T54.3X4	--	--
- iodide	T48.4X1	T48.4X2	T48.4X3	T48.4X4	T48.4X5	T48.4X6
- ipodate	T50.8X1	T50.8X2	T50.8X3	T50.8X4	T50.8X5	T50.8X6
- lactate	T50.3X1	T50.3X2	T50.3X3	T50.3X4	T50.3X5	T50.3X6
- leucovorin	T45.8X1	T45.8X2	T45.8X3	T45.8X4	T45.8X5	T45.8X6
- mandelate	T37.91	T37.92	T37.93	T37.94	T37.95	T37.96
- oxide	T54.3X1	T54.3X2	T54.3X3	T54.3X4	--	--
- pantothenate	T45.2X1	T45.2X2	T45.2X3	T45.2X4	T45.2X5	T45.2X6
- phosphate	T50.3X1	T50.3X2	T50.3X3	T50.3X4	T50.3X5	T50.3X6
- salicylate	T39.091	T39.092	T39.093	T39.094	T39.095	T39.096
- salts	T50.3X1	T50.3X2	T50.3X3	T50.3X4	T50.3X5	T50.3X6
Calculus-dissolving drug	T50.991	T50.992	T50.993	T50.994	T50.995	T50.996

Substance	Poisoning, Accidental (unintentional)	Poisoning, Intentional Self-harm	Poisoning, Assault	Poisoning, Undetermined	Adverse effect	Underdosing
Calomel	T49.0X1	T49.0X2	T49.0X3	T49.0X4	T49.0X5	T49.0X6
Caloric agent	T50.3X1	T50.3X2	T50.3X3	T50.3X4	T50.3X5	T50.3X6
Calusterone	T38.7X1	T38.7X2	T38.7X3	T38.7X4	T38.7X5	T38.7X6
Camazepam	T42.4X1	T42.4X2	T42.4X3	T42.4X4	T42.4X5	T42.4X6
Camomile	T49.0X1	T49.0X2	T49.0X3	T49.0X4	T49.0X5	T49.0X6
Camoquin	T37.2X1	T37.2X2	T37.2X3	T37.2X4	T37.2X5	T37.2X6
Camphor						
- insecticide	T60.2X1	T60.2X2	T60.2X3	T60.2X4	--	--
- medicinal	T49.8X1	T49.8X2	T49.8X3	T49.8X4	T49.8X5	T49.8X6
Camylofin	T44.3X1	T44.3X2	T44.3X3	T44.3X4	T44.3X5	T44.3X6
Cancer chemotherapy drug regimen	T45.1X1	T45.1X2	T45.1X3	T45.1X4	T45.1X5	T45.1X6
Candeptin	T49.0X1	T49.0X2	T49.0X3	T49.0X4	T49.0X5	T49.0X6
Candicidin	T49.0X1	T49.0X2	T49.0X3	T49.0X4	T49.0X5	T49.0X6
Cannabinoids, synthetic	T40.721	T40.722	T40.723	T40.724	T40.725	T40.726
Cannabinol	T40.711	T40.712	T40.713	T40.714	T40.715	T40.716
Cannabis (derivatives)	T40.711	T40.712	T40.713	T40.714	T40.715	T40.716
Canned heat	T51.1X1	T51.1X2	T51.1X3	T51.1X4	--	--
Canrenoic acid	T50.0X1	T50.0X2	T50.0X3	T50.0X4	T50.0X5	T50.0X6
Canrenone	T50.0X1	T50.0X2	T50.0X3	T50.0X4	T50.0X5	T50.0X6
Cantharides, cantharidin, cantharis	T49.8X1	T49.8X2	T49.8X3	T49.8X4	T49.8X5	T49.8X6
Canthaxanthin	T50.991	T50.992	T50.993	T50.994	T50.995	T50.996
Capillary-active drug NEC	T46.901	T46.902	T46.903	T46.904	T46.905	T46.906
Capreomycin	T36.8X1	T36.8X2	T36.8X3	T36.8X4	T36.8X5	T36.8X6
Capsicum	T49.4X1	T49.4X2	T49.4X3	T49.4X4	T49.4X5	T49.4X6
Captafol	T60.3X1	T60.3X2	T60.3X3	T60.3X4	--	--
Captan	T60.3X1	T60.3X2	T60.3X3	T60.3X4	--	--
Captodiame, captodiamine	T43.591	T43.592	T43.593	T43.594	T43.595	T43.596
Captopril	T46.4X1	T46.4X2	T46.4X3	T46.4X4	T46.4X5	T46.4X6
Caramiphen	T44.3X1	T44.3X2	T44.3X3	T44.3X4	T44.3X5	T44.3X6
Carazolol	T44.7X1	T44.7X2	T44.7X3	T44.7X4	T44.7X5	T44.7X6
Carbachol	T44.1X1	T44.1X2	T44.1X3	T44.1X4	T44.1X5	T44.1X6
Carbacrylamine (resin)	T50.3X1	T50.3X2	T50.3X3	T50.3X4	T50.3X5	T50.3X6
Carbamate (insecticide)	T60.0X1	T60.0X2	T60.0X3	T60.0X4	--	--
Carbamate (sedative)	T42.6X1	T42.6X2	T42.6X3	T42.6X4	T42.6X5	T42.6X6
- herbicide	T60.0X1	T60.0X2	T60.0X3	T60.0X4	--	--
- insecticide	T60.0X1	T60.0X2	T60.0X3	T60.0X4	--	--
Carbamazepine	T42.1X1	T42.1X2	T42.1X3	T42.1X4	T42.1X5	T42.1X6
Carbamide	T47.3X1	T47.3X2	T47.3X3	T47.3X4	T47.3X5	T47.3X6
- peroxide	T49.0X1	T49.0X2	T49.0X3	T49.0X4	T49.0X5	T49.0X6
- topical	T49.8X1	T49.8X2	T49.8X3	T49.8X4	T49.8X5	T49.8X6
Carbamylcholine chloride	T44.1X1	T44.1X2	T44.1X3	T44.1X4	T44.1X5	T44.1X6
Carbaril	T60.0X1	T60.0X2	T60.0X3	T60.0X4	--	--
Carbarsone	T37.3X1	T37.3X2	T37.3X3	T37.3X4	T37.3X5	T37.3X6
Carbaryl	T60.0X1	T60.0X2	T60.0X3	T60.0X4	--	--
Carbaspirin	T39.011	T39.012	T39.013	T39.014	T39.015	T39.016
Carbazochrome (salicylate) (sodium sulfonate)	T49.4X1	T49.4X2	T49.4X3	T49.4X4	T49.4X5	T49.4X6
Carbenicillin	T36.0X1	T36.0X2	T36.0X3	T36.0X4	T36.0X5	T36.0X6
Carbenoxolone	T47.1X1	T47.1X2	T47.1X3	T47.1X4	T47.1X5	T47.1X6
Carbetapentane	T48.3X1	T48.3X2	T48.3X3	T48.3X4	T48.3X5	T48.3X6
Carbethyl salicylate	T39.091	T39.092	T39.093	T39.094	T39.095	T39.096
Carbidopa (with levodopa)	T42.8X1	T42.8X2	T42.8X3	T42.8X4	T42.8X5	T42.8X6
Carbimazole	T38.2X1	T38.2X2	T38.2X3	T38.2X4	T38.2X5	T38.2X6
Carbinol	T51.1X1	T51.1X2	T51.1X3	T51.1X4	--	--
Carbinoxamine	T45.0X1	T45.0X2	T45.0X3	T45.0X4	T45.0X5	T45.0X6
Carbiphene	T39.8X1	T39.8X2	T39.8X3	T39.8X4	T39.8X5	T39.8X6
Carbitol	T52.3X1	T52.3X2	T52.3X3	T52.3X4	--	--
Carbo medicinalis	T47.6X1	T47.6X2	T47.6X3	T47.6X4	T47.6X5	T47.6X6

Substance	Poisoning, Accidental (unintentional)	Poisoning, Intentional Self-harm	Poisoning, Assault	Poisoning, Undetermined	Adverse effect	Underdosing
Carbocaine	T41.3X1	T41.3X2	T41.3X3	T41.3X4	T41.3X5	T41.3X6
- infiltration (subcutaneous)	T41.3X1	T41.3X2	T41.3X3	T41.3X4	T41.3X5	T41.3X6
- nerve block (peripheral) (plexus)	T41.3X1	T41.3X2	T41.3X3	T41.3X4	T41.3X5	T41.3X6
- topical (surface)	T41.3X1	T41.3X2	T41.3X3	T41.3X4	T41.3X5	T41.3X6
Carbocisteine	T48.4X1	T48.4X2	T48.4X3	T48.4X4	T48.4X5	T48.4X6
Carbocromen	T46.3X1	T46.3X2	T46.3X3	T46.3X4	T46.3X5	T46.3X6
Carbol fuchsin	T49.0X1	T49.0X2	T49.0X3	T49.0X4	T49.0X5	T49.0X6
Carbolic acid—see also Phenol	T54.0X1	T54.0X2	T54.0X3	T54.0X4	--	--
Carbolonium (bromide)	T48.1X1	T48.1X2	T48,1X3	T48.1X4	T48.1X5	T48.1X6
Carbomycin	T36.8X1	T36.8X2	T36.8X3	T36.8X4	T36.8X5	T36.8X6
- bisulfide (liquid)	T65.4X1	T65.4X2	T65.4X3	T65.4X4	--	--
- - vapor	T65.4X1	T65.4X2	T65.4X3	T65.4X4	--	--
- dioxide (gas)	T59.7X1	T59.7X2	T59.7X3	T59.7X4	--	--
- - medicinal	T41.5X1	T41.5X2	T41.5X3	T41.5X4	T41.5X5	T41.5X6
- - nonmedicinal	T59.7X1	T59.7X2	T59.7X3	T59.7X4	--	--
- - snow	T49.4X1	T49.4X2	T49.4X3	T49.4X4	T49.4X5	T49.4X6
- disulfide (liquid)	T65.4X1	T65.4X2	T65.4X3	T65.4X4	--	--
- - vapor	T65.4X1	T65.4X2	T65.4X3	T65.4X4	--	--
- monoxide (from incomplete combustion)	T58.91	T58.92	T58.93	T58.94	--	--
- - blast furnace gas	T58.8X1	T58.8X2	T58.8X3	T58.8X4	--	--
- - butane (distributed in mobile container)	T58.11	T58.12	T58.13	T58.14	--	--
- - - distributed through pipes	T58.11	T58.12	T58.13	T58.14	--	--
- - charcoal fumes	T58.2X1	T58.2X2	T58.2X3	T58.2X4	--	--
- - coal	T58.2X1	T58.2X2	T58.2X3	T58.2X4	--	--
- - coke (in domestic stoves, fireplaces)	T58.2X1	T58.2X2	T58.2X3	T58.2X4	--	--
- - gas (piped)	T58.11	T58.12	T58.13	T58.14	--	--
- - solid (in domestic stoves, fireplaces)	T58.2X1	T58.2X2	T58.2X3	T58.2X4	--	--
- - exhaust gas (motor) not in transit	T58.01	T58.02	T58.03	T58.04	--	--
- - - combustion engine, any not in watercraft	T58.01	T58.02	T58.03	T58.04	--	--
- - - farm tractor, not in transit	T58.01	T58.02	T58.03	T58.04	--	--
- - - gas engine	T58.01	T58.02	T58.03	T58.04	--	--
- - - motor pump	T58.01	T58.02	T58.03	T58.04	--	--
- - - motor vehicle, not in transit	T58.01	T58.02	T58.03	T58.04	--	--
- - fuel (in domestic use)	T58.2X1	T58.2X2	T58.2X3	T58.2X4	--	--
- - - gas (piped)	T58.11	T58.12	T58.13	T58.14	--	--
- - - - in mobile container	T58.11	T58.12	T58.13	T58.14	--	--
- - - piped (natural)	T58.11	T58.12	T58.13	T58.14	--	--
- - - utility	T58.11	T58.12	T58.13	T58.14	--	--
- - - - in mobile container	T58.11	T58.12	T58.13	T58.14	--	--
- - illuminating gas	T58.11	T58.12	T58.13	T58.14	--	--
- - industrial fuels or gases, any	T58.8X1	T58.8X2	T58.8X3	T58.8X4	--	--
- - kerosene (in domestic stoves, fireplaces)	T58.2X1	T58.2X2	T58.2X3	T58.2X4	--	--
- - kiln gas or vapor	T58.8X1	T58.8X2	T58.8X3	T58.8X4	--	--
- - motor exhaust gas, not in transit	T58.01	T58.02	T58.03	T58.04	--	--
- - piped gas (manufactured) (natural)	T58.11	T58.12	T58.13	T58.14	--	--
- - producer gas	T58.8X1	T58.8X2	T58.8X3	T58.8X4	--	--
- - propane (distributed in mobile container)	T58.11	T58.12	T58.13	T58.14	--	--
- - - distributed through pipes	T58.11	T58.12	T58.13	T58.14	--	--
- - specified source NEC	T58.8X1	T58.8X2	T58.8X3	T58.8X4	--	--
- - stove gas	T58.11	T58.12	T58.13	T58.14	--	--
- - - piped	T58.11	T58.12	T58.13	T58.14	--	--
- - utility gas	T58.11	T58.12	T58.13	T58.14	--	--
- - - piped	T58.11	T58.12	T58.13	T58.14	--	--
- - water gas	T58.11	T58.12	T58.13	T58.14	--	--
- - wood (in domestic stoves, fireplaces)	T58.2X1	T58.2X2	T58.2X3	T58.2X4	--	--
- tetrachloride (vapor) NEC	T53.0X1	T53.0X2	T53.0X3	T53.0X4	--	--
- - liquid (cleansing agent) NEC	T53.0X1	T53.0X2	T53.0X3	T53.0X4	--	--
- - solvent	T53.0X1	T53.0X2	T53.0X3	T53.0X4	--	--
Carbonic acid gas	T59.7X1	T59.7X2	T59.7X3	T59.7X4	--	--

Substance	Poisoning, Accidental (unintentional)	Poisoning, Intentional Self-harm	Poisoning, Assault	Poisoning, Undetermined	Adverse effect	Underdosing
- anhydrase inhibitor NEC	T50.2X1	T50.2X2	T50.2X3	T50.2X4	T50.2X5	T50.2X6
Carbophenothion	T60.0X1	T60.0X2	T60.0X3	T60.0X4	--	--
Carboplatin	T45.1X1	T45.1X2	T45.1X3	T45.1X4	T45.1X5	T45.1X6
Carboprost	T48.0X1	T48.0X2	T48.0X3	T48.0X4	T48.0X5	T48.0X6
Carboquone	T45.1X1	T45.1X2	T45.1X3	T45.1X4	T45.1X5	T45.1X6
Carbowax	T49.3X1	T49.3X2	T49.3X3	T49.3X4	T49.3X5	T49.3X6
Carboxymethyl-cellulose	T47.4X1	T47.4X2	T47.4X3	T47.4X4	T47.4X5	T47.4X6
S-Carboxymethyl-cysteine	T48.4X1	T48.4X2	T48.4X3	T48.4X4	T48.4X5	T48.4X6
Carbrital	T42.3X1	T42.3X2	T42.3X3	T42.3X4	T42.3X5	T42.3X6
Carbromal	T42.6X1	T42.6X2	T42.6X3	T42.6X4	T42.6X5	T42.6X6
Carbutamide	T38.3X1	T38.3X2	T38.3X3	T38.3X4	T38.3X5	T38.3X6
Carbuterol	T48.6X1	T48.6X2	T48.6X3	T48.6X4	T48.6X5	T48.6X6
Cardiac						
- depressants	T46.2X1	T46.2X2	T46.2X3	T46.2X4	T46.2X5	T46.2X6
- rhythm regulator	T46.2X1	T46.2X2	T46.2X3	T46.2X4	T46.2X5	T46.2X6
- - specified NEC	T46.2X1	T46.2X2	T46.2X3	T46.2X4	T46.2X5	T46.2X6
Cardiografin	T50.8X1	T50.8X2	T50.8X3	T50.8X4	T50.8X5	T50.8X6
Cardio-green	T50.8X1	T50.8X2	T50.8X3	T50.8X4	T50.8X5	T50.8X6
Cardiotonic (glycoside) NEC	T46.0X1	T46.0X2	T46.0X3	T46.0X4	T46.0X5	T46.0X6
Cardiovascular drug NEC	T46.901	T46.902	T46.903	T46.904	T46.905	T46.906
Cardrase	T50.2X1	T50.2X2	T50.2X3	T50.2X4	T50.2X5	T50.2X6
Carfecillin	T36.0X1	T36.0X2	T36.0X3	T36.0X4	T36.0X5	T36.0X6
Carfenazine	T43.3X1	T43.3X2	T43.3X3	T43.3X4	T43.3X5	T43.3X6
Carfusin	T49.0X1	T49.0X2	T49.0X3	T49.0X4	T49.0X5	T49.0X6
Carindacillin	T36.0X1	T36.0X2	T36.0X3	T36.0X4	T36.0X5	T36.0X6
Carisoprodol	T42.8X1	T42.8X2	T42.8X3	T42.8X4	T42.8X5	T42.8X6
Carmellose	T47.4X1	T47.4X2	T47.4X3	T47.4X4	T47.4X5	T47.4X6
Carminative	T47.5X1	T47.5X2	T47.5X3	T47.5X4	T47.5X5	T47.5X6
Carmofur	T45.1X1	T45.1X2	T45.1X3	T45.1X4	T45.1X5	T45.1X6
Carmustine	T45.1X1	T45.1X2	T45.1X3	T45.1X4	T45.1X5	T45.1X6
Carotene	T45.2X1	T45.2X2	T45.2X3	T45.2X4	T45.2X5	T45.2X6
Carphenazine	T43.3X1	T43.3X2	T43.3X3	T43.3X4	T43.3X5	T43.3X6
Carpipramine	T42.4X1	T42.4X2	T42.4X3	T42.4X4	T42.4X5	T42.4X6
Carprofen	T39.311	T39.312	T39.313	T39.314	T39.315	T39.316
Carpronium chloride	T44.3X1	T44.3X2	T44.3X3	T44.3X4	T44.3X5	T44.3X6
Carrageenan	T47.8X1	T47.8X2	T47.8X3	T47.8X4	T47.8X5	T47.8X6
Carteolol	T44.7X1	T44.7X2	T44.7X3	T44.7X4	T44.7X5	T44.7X6
Carter's Little Pills	T47.2X1	T47.2X2	T47.2X3	T47.2X4	T47.2X5	T47.2X6
Cascara (sagrada)	T47.2X1	T47.2X2	T47.2X3	T47.2X4	T47.2X5	T47.2X6
Cassava	T62.2X1	T62.2X2	T62.2X3	T62.2X4	--	--
Castellani's paint	T49.0X1	T49.0X2	T49.0X3	T49.0X4	T49.0X5	T49.0X6
Castor						
- bean	T62.2X1	T62.2X2	T62.2X3	T62.2X4	--	--
- oil	T47.2X1	T47.2X2	T47.2X3	T47.2X4	T47.2X5	T47.2X6
Catalase	T45.3X1	T45.3X2	T45.3X3	T45.3X4	T45.3X5	T45.3X6
Caterpillar (sting)	T63.431	T63.432	T63.433	T63.434	--	--
Catha (edulis) (tea)	T43.691	T43.692	T43.693	T43.694	--	--
Cathartic NEC	T47.4X1	T47.4X2	T47.4X3	T47.4X4	T47.4X5	T47.4X6
- anthacene derivative	T47.2X1	T47.2X2	T47.2X3	T47.2X4	T47.2X5	T47.2X6
- bulk	T47.4X1	T47.4X2	T47.4X3	T47.4X4	T47.4X5	T47.4X6
- contact	T47.2X1	T47.2X2	T47.2X3	T47.2X4	T47.2X5	T47.2X6
- emollient NEC	T47.4X1	T47.4X2	T47.4X3	T47.4X4	T47.4X5	T47.4X6
- irritant NEC	T47.2X1	T47.2X2	T47.2X3	T47.2X4	T47.2X5	T47.2X6
- mucilage	T47.4X1	T47.4X2	T47.4X3	T47.4X4	T47.4X5	T47.4X6
- saline	T47.3X1	T47.3X2	T47.3X3	T47.3X4	T47.3X5	T47.3X6
- vegetable	T47.2X1	T47.2X2	T47.2X3	T47.2X4	T47.2X5	T47.2X6
Cathine	T50.5X1	T50.5X2	T50.5X3	T50.5X4	T50.5X5	T50.5X6
Cathomycin	T36.8X1	T36.8X2	T36.8X3	T36.8X4	T36.8X5	T36.8X6

Substance	Poisoning, Accidental (unintentional)	Poisoning, Intentional Self-harm	Poisoning, Assault	Poisoning, Undetermined	Adverse effect	Underdosing
Cation exchange resin	T50.3X1	T50.3X2	T50.3X3	T50.3X4	T50.3X5	T50.3X6
Caustic (s) NEC	T54.91	T54.92	T54.93	T54.94	--	--
- alkali	T54.3X1	T54.3X2	T54.3X3	T54.3X4	--	--
- hydroxide	T54.3X1	T54.3X2	T54.3X3	T54.3X4	--	--
- potash	T54.3X1	T54.3X2	T54.3X3	T54.3X4	--	--
- soda	T54.3X1	T54.3X2	T54.3X3	T54.3X4	--	--
- specified NEC	T54.91	T54.92	T54.93	T54.94	--	--
Ceepryn	T49.0X1	T49.0X2	T49.0X3	T49.0X4	T49.0X5	T49.0X6
- ENT agent	T49.6X1	T49.6X2	T49.6X3	T49.6X4	T49.6X5	T49.6X6
- lozenges	T49.6X1	T49.6X2	T49.6X3	T49.6X4	T49.6X5	T49.6X6
Cefacetrile	T36.1X1	T36.1X2	T36.1X3	T36.1X4	T36.1X5	T36.1X6
Cefaclor	T36.1X1	T36.1X2	T36.1X3	T36.1X4	T36.1X5	T36.1X6
Cefadroxil	T36.1X1	T36.1X2	T36.1X3	T36.1X4	T36.1X5	T36.1X6
Cefalexin	T36.1X1	T36.1X2	T36.1X3	T36.1X4	T36.1X5	T36.1X6
Cefaloglycin	T36.1X1	T36.1X2	T36.1X3	T36.1X4	T36.1X5	T36.1X6
Cefaloridine	T36.1X1	T36.1X2	T36.1X3	T36.1X4	T36.1X5	T36.1X6
Cefalosporins	T36.1X1	T36.1X2	T36.1X3	T36.1X4	T36.1X5	T36.1X6
Cefalotin	T36.1X1	T36.1X2	T36.1X3	T36.1X4	T36.1X5	T36.1X6
Cefamandole	T36.1X1	T36.1X2	T36.1X3	T36.1X4	T36.1X5	T36.1X6
Cefamycin antibiotic	T36.1X1	T36.1X2	T36.1X3	T36.1X4	T36.1X5	T36.1X6
Cefapirin	T36.1X1	T36.1X2	T36.1X3	T36.1X4	T36.1X5	T36.1X6
Cefatrizine	T36.1X1	T36.1X2	T36.1X3	T36.1X4	T36.1X5	T36.1X6
Cefazedone	T36.1X1	T36.1X2	T36.1X3	T36.1X4	T36.1X5	T36.1X6
Cefazolin	T36.1X1	T36.1X2	T36.1X3	T36.1X4	T36.1X5	T36.1X6
Cefbuperazone	T36.1X1	T36.1X2	T36.1X3	T36.1X4	T36.1X5	T36.1X6
Cefetamet	T36.1X1	T36.1X2	T36.1X3	T36.1X4	T36.1X5	T36.1X6
Cefixime	T36.1X1	T36.1X2	T36.1X3	T36.1X4	T36.1X5	T36.1X6
Cefmenoxime	T36.1X1	T36.1X2	T36.1X3	T36.1X4	T36.1X5	T36.1X6
Cefmetazole	T36.1X1	T36.1X2	T36.1X3	T36.1X4	T36.1X5	T36.1X6
Cefminox	T36.1X1	T36.1X2	T36.1X3	T36.1X4	T36.1X5	T36.1X6
Cefonicid	T36.1X1	T36.1X2	T36.1X3	T36.1X4	T36.1X5	T36.1X6
Cefoperazone	T36.1X1	T36.1X2	T36.1X3	T36.1X4	T36.1X5	T36.1X6
Ceforanide	T36.1X1	T36.1X2	T36.1X3	T36.1X4	T36.1X5	T36.1X6
Cefotaxime	T36.1X1	T36.1X2	T36.1X3	T36.1X4	T36.1X5	T36.1X6
Cefotetan	T36.1X1	T36.1X2	T36.1X3	T36.1X4	T36.1X5	T36.1X6
Cefotiam	T36.1X1	T36.1X2	T36.1X3	T36.1X4	T36.1X5	T36.1X6
Cefoxitin	T36.1X1	T36.1X2	T36.1X3	T36.1X4	T36.1X5	T36.1X6
Cefpimizole	T36.1X1	T36.1X2	T36.1X3	T36.1X4	T36.1X5	T36.1X6
Cefpiramide	T36.1X1	T36.1X2	T36.1X3	T36.1X4	T36.1X5	T36.1X6
Cefradine	T36.1X1	T36.1X2	T36.1X3	T36.1X4	T36.1X5	T36.1X6
Cefroxadine	T36.1X1	T36.1X2	T36.1X3	T36.1X4	T36.1X5	T36.1X6
Cefsulodin	T36.1X1	T36.1X2	T36.1X3	T36.1X4	T36.1X5	T36.1X6
Ceftazidime	T36.1X1	T36.1X2	T36.1X3	T36.1X4	T36.1X5	T36.1X6
Cefteram	T36.1X1	T36.1X2	T36.1X3	T36.1X4	T36.1X5	T36.1X6
Ceftezole	T36.1X1	T36.1X2	T36.1X3	T36.1X4	T36.1X5	T36.1X6
Ceftizoxime	T36.1X1	T36.1X2	T36.1X3	T36.1X4	T36.1X5	T36.1X6
Ceftriaxone	T36.1X1	T36.1X2	T36.1X3	T36.1X4	T36.1X5	T36.1X6
Cefuroxime	T36.1X1	T36.1X2	T36.1X3	T36.1X4	T36.1X5	T36.1X6
Cefuzonam	T36.1X1	T36.1X2	T36.1X3	T36.1X4	T36.1X5	T36.1X6
Celestone	T38.0X1	T38.0X2	T38.0X3	T38.0X4	T38.0X5	T38.0X6
- topical	T49.0X1	T49.0X2	T49.0X3	T49.0X4	T49.0X5	T49.0X6
Celiprolol	T44.7X1	T44.7X2	T44.7X3	T44.7X4	T44.7X5	T44.7X6
Cell stimulants and proliferants	T49.8X1	T49.8X2	T49.8X3	T49.8X4	T49.8X5	T49.8X6
Cellosolve	T52.91	T52.92	T52.93	T52.94	--	--
Cellulose						
- cathartic	T47.4X1	T47.4X2	T47.4X3	T47.4X4	T47.4X5	T47.4X6
- hydroxyethyl	T47.4X1	T47.4X2	T47.4X3	T47.4X4	T47.4X5	T47.4X6
- nitrates (topical)	T49.3X1	T49.3X2	T49.3X3	T49.3X4	T49.3X5	T49.3X6
- oxidized	T49.4X1	T49.4X2	T49.4X3	T49.4X4	T49.4X5	T49.4X6

Substance	Poisoning, Accidental (unintentional)	Poisoning, Intentional Self-harm	Poisoning, Assault	Poisoning, Undetermined	Adverse effect	Underdosing
Centipede (bite)	T63.411	T63.412	T63.413	T63.414	--	--
Central nervous system						
- depressants	T42.71	T42.72	T42.73	T42.74	T42.75	T42.76
- - anesthetic (general) NEC	T41.201	T41.202	T41.203	T41.204	T41.205	T41.206
- - - gases NEC	T41.0X1	T41.0X2	T41.0X3	T41.0X4	T41.0X5	T41.0X6
- - - intravenous	T41.1X1	T41.1X2	T41.1X3	T41.1X4	T41.1X5	T41.1X6
- - barbiturates	T42.3X1	T42.3X2	T42.3X3	T42.3X4	T42.3X5	T42.3X6
- - benzodiazepines	T42.4X1	T42.4X2	T42.4X3	T42.4X4	T42.4X5	T42.4X6
- - bromides	T42.6X1	T42.6X2	T42.6X3	T42.6X4	T42.6X5	T42.6X6
- - cannabis sativa	T40.711	T40.712	T40.713	T40.714	T40.715	T40.716
- - chloral hydrate	T42.6X1	T42.6X2	T42.6X3	T42.6X4	T42.6X5	T42.6X6
- - ethanol	T51.0X1	T51.0X2	T51.0X3	T51.0X4	--	--
- - hallucinogenics	T40.901	T40.902	T40.903	T40.904	T40.905	T40.906
- - hypnotics	T42.71	T42.72	T42.73	T42.74	T42.75	T42.76
- - - specified NEC	T42.6X1	T42.6X2	T42.6X3	T42.6X4	T42.6X5	T42.6X6
- - muscle relaxants	T42.8X1	T42.8X2	T42.8X3	T42.8X4	T42.8X5	T42.8X6
- - paraldehyde	T42.6X1	T42.6X2	T42.6X3	T42.6X4	T42.6X5	T42.6X6
- - sedatives; sedative-hypnotics	T42.71	T42.72	T42.73	T42.74	T42.75	T42.76
- - - mixed NEC	T42.6X1	T42.6X2	T42.6X3	T42.6X4	T42.6X5	T42.6X6
- - - specified NEC	T42.6X1	T42.6X2	T42.6X3	T42.6X4	T42.6X5	T42.6X6
- muscle-tone depressants	T42.8X1	T42.8X2	T42.8X3	T42.8X4	T42.8X5	T42.8X6
- stimulants	T43.601	T43.602	T43.603	T43.604	T43.605	T43.606
- - amphetamines	T43.621	T43.622	T43.623	T43.624	T43.625	T43.626
- - analeptics	T50.7X1	T50.7X2	T50.7X3	T50.7X4	T50.7X5	T50.7X6
- - antidepressants	T43.201	T43.202	T43.203	T43.204	T43.205	T43.206
- - opiate antagonists	T50.7X1	T50.7X2	T50.7X3	T50.7X4	T50.7X5	T50.7X6
- - specified NEC	T43.691	T43.692	T43.693	T43.694	T43.695	T43.696
Cephalexin	T36.1X1	T36.1X2	T36.1X3	T36.1X4	T36.1X5	T36.1X6
Cephaloglycin	T36.1X1	T36.1X2	T36.1X3	T36.1X4	T36.1X5	T36.1X6
Cephaloridine	T36.1X1	T36.1X2	T36.1X3	T36.1X4	T36.1X5	T36.1X6
Cephalosporins	T36.1X1	T36.1X2	T36.1X3	T36.1X4	T36.1X5	T36.1X6
- N (adicillin)	T36.0X1	T36.0X2	T36.0X3	T36.0X4	T36.0X5	T36.0X6
Cephalothin	T36.1X1	T36.1X2	T36.1X3	T36.1X4	T36.1X5	T36.1X6
Cephalotin	T36.1X1	T36.1X2	T36.1X3	T36.1X4	T36.1X5	T36.1X6
Cephradine	T36.1X1	T36.1X2	T36.1X3	T36.1X4	T36.1X5	T36.1X6
Cerbera (odallam)	T62.2X1	T62.2X2	T62.2X3	T62.2X4	--	--
Cerberin	T46.0X1	T46.0X2	T46.0X3	T46.0X4	T46.0X5	T46.0X6
Cerebral stimulants	T43.601	T43.602	T43.603	T43.604	T43.605	T43.606
- psychotherapeutic	T43.601	T43.602	T43.603	T43.604	T43.605	T43.606
- specified NEC	T43.691	T43.692	T43.693	T43.694	T43.695	T43.696
Cerium oxalate	T45.0X1	T45.0X2	T45.0X3	T45.0X4	T45.0X5	T45.0X6
Cerous oxalate	T45.0X1	T45.0X2	T45.0X3	T45.0X4	T45.0X5	T45.0X6
Ceruletide	T50.8X1	T50.8X2	T50.8X3	T50.8X4	T50.8X5	T50.8X6
Cetalkonium (chloride)	T49.0X1	T49.0X2	T49.0X3	T49.0X4	T49.0X5	T49.0X6
Cethexonium chloride	T49.0X1	T49.0X2	T49.0X3	T49.0X4	T49.0X5	T49.0X6
Cetiedil	T46.7X1	T46.7X2	T46.7X3	T46.7X4	T46.7X5	T46.7X6
Cetirizine	T45.0X1	T45.0X2	T45.0X3	T45.0X4	T45.0X5	T45.0X6
Cetomacrogol	T50.991	T50.992	T50.993	T50.994	T50.995	T50.996
Cetotiamine	T45.2X1	T45.2X2	T45.2X3	T45.2X4	T45.2X5	T45.2X6
Cetoxime	T45.0X1	T45.0X2	T45.0X3	T45.0X4	T45.0X5	T45.0X6
Cetraxate	T47.1X1	T47.1X2	T47.1X3	T47.1X4	T47.1X5	T47.1X6
Cetrimide	T49.0X1	T49.0X2	T49.0X3	T49.0X4	T49.0X5	T49.0X6
Cetrimonium (bromide)	T49.0X1	T49.0X2	T49.0X3	T49.0X4	T49.0X5	T49.0X6
Cetylpyridinium chloride	T49.0X1	T49.0X2	T49.0X3	T49.0X4	T49.0X5	T49.0X6
- ENT agent	T49.6X1	T49.6X2	T49.6X3	T49.6X4	T49.6X5	T49.6X6
- lozenges	T49.6X1	T49.6X2	T49.6X3	T49.6X4	T49.6X5	T49.6X6
Cevadilla—see Sabadilla						
Cevitamic acid	T45.2X1	T45.2X2	T45.2X3	T45.2X4	T45.2X5	T45.2X6

Substance	Poisoning, Accidental (unintentional)	Poisoning, Intentional Self-harm	Poisoning, Assault	Poisoning, Undetermined	Adverse effect	Underdosing
Chalk, precipitated	T47.1X1	T47.1X2	T47.1X3	T47.1X4	T47.1X5	T47.1X6
Chamomile	T49.0X1	T49.0X2	T49.0X3	T49.0X4	T49.0X5	T49.0X6
Ch'an su	T46.0X1	T46.0X2	T46.0X3	T46.0X4	T46.0X5	T46.0X6
Charcoal	T47.6X1	T47.6X2	T47.6X3	T47.6X4	T47.6X5	T47.6X6
- activated—see also Charcoal, medicinal	T47.6X1	T47.6X2	T47.6X3	T47.6X4	T47.6X5	T47.6X6
- fumes (Carbon monoxide)	T58.2X1	T58.2X2	T58.2X3	T58.2X4	--	--
- - industrial	T58.8X1	T58.8X2	T58.8X3	T58.8X4	--	--
- medicinal (activated)	T47.6X1	T47.6X2	T47.6X3	T47.6X4	T47.6X5	T47.6X6
- - antidiarrheal	T47.6X1	T47.6X2	T47.6X3	T47.6X4	T47.6X5	T47.6X6
- - poison control	T47.8X1	T47.8X2	T47.8X3	T47.8X4	T47.8X5	T47.8X6
- - specified use other than for diarrhea	T47.8X1	T47.8X2	T47.8X3	T47.8X4	T47.8X5	T47.8X6
- - topical	T49.8X1	T49.8X2	T49.8X3	T49.8X4	T49.8X5	T49.8X6
Chaulmosulfone	T37.1X1	T37.1X2	T37.1X3	T37.1X4	T37.1X5	T37.1X6
Chelating agent NEC	T50.6X1	T50.6X2	T50.6X3	T50.6X4	T50.6X5	T50.6X6
Chelidonium majus	T62.2X1	T62.2X2	T62.2X3	T62.2X4	--	--
Chemical substance NEC	T65.91	T65.92	T65.93	T65.94	--	--
Chenodeoxycholic acid	T47.5X1	T47.5X2	T47.5X3	T47.5X4	T47.5X5	T47.5X6
Chenodiol	T47.5X1	T47.5X2	T47.5X3	T47.5X4	T47.5X5	T47.5X6
Chenopodium	T37.4X1	T37.4X2	T37.4X3	T37.4X4	T37.4X5	T37.4X6
Cherry laurel	T62.2X1	T62.2X2	T62.2X3	T62.2X4	--	--
Chinidin (e)	T46.2X1	T46.2X2	T46.2X3	T46.2X4	T46.2X5	T46.2X6
Chiniofon	T37.8X1	T37.8X2	T37.8X3	T37.8X4	T37.8X5	T37.8X6
Chlophedianol	T48.3X1	T48.3X2	T48.3X3	T48.3X4	T48.3X5	T48.3X6
Chloral	T42.6X1	T42.6X2	T42.6X3	T42.6X4	T42.6X5	T42.6X6
- derivative	T42.6X1	T42.6X2	T42.6X3	T42.6X4	T42.6X5	T42.6X6
- hydrate	T42.6X1	T42.6X2	T42.6X3	T42.6X4	T42.6X5	T42.6X6
Chloralamide	T42.6X1	T42.6X2	T42.6X3	T42.6X4	T42.6X5	T42.6X6
Chloralodol	T42.6X1	T42.6X2	T42.6X3	T42.6X4	T42.6X5	T42.6X6
Chloralose	T60.4X1	T60.4X2	T60.4X3	T60.4X4	--	--
Chlorambucil	T45.1X1	T45.1X2	T45.1X3	T45.1X4	T45.1X5	T45.1X6
Chloramine	T57.8X1	T57.8X2	T57.8X3	T57.8X4	--	--
- T	T49.0X1	T49.0X2	T49.0X3	T49.0X4	T49.0X5	T49.0X6
- topical	T49.0X1	T49.0X2	T49.0X3	T49.0X4	T49.0X5	T49.0X6
Chloramphenicol	T36.2X1	T36.2X2	T36.2X3	T36.2X4	T36.2X5	T36.2X6
- ENT agent	T49.6X1	T49.6X2	T49.6X3	T49.6X4	T49.6X5	T49.6X6
- ophthalmic preparation	T49.5X1	T49.5X2	T49.5X3	T49.5X4	T49.5X5	T49.5X6
- topical NEC	T49.0X1	T49.0X2	T49.0X3	T49.0X4	T49.0X5	T49.0X6
Chlorate (potassium) (sodium) NEC	T60.3X1	T60.3X2	T60.3X3	T60.3X4	--	--
- herbicide	T60.3X1	T60.3X2	T60.3X3	T60.3X4	--	--
Chlorazanil	T50.2X1	T50.2X2	T50.2X3	T50.2X4	T50.2X5	T50.2X6
Chlorbenzene, chlorbenzol	T53.7X1	T53.7X2	T53.7X3	T53.7X4	--	--
Chlorbenzoxamine	T44.3X1	T44.3X2	T44.3X3	T44.3X4	T44.3X5	T44.3X6
Chlorbutol	T42.6X1	T42.6X2	T42.6X3	T42.6X4	T42.6X5	T42.6X6
Chlorcyclizine	T45.0X1	T45.0X2	T45.0X3	T45.0X4	T45.0X5	T45.0X6
Chlordan (e) (dust)	T60.1X1	T60.1X2	T60.1X3	T60.1X4	--	--
Chlordantoin	T49.0X1	T49.0X2	T49.0X3	T49.0X4	T49.0X5	T49.0X6
Chlordiazepoxide	T42.4X1	T42.4X2	T42.4X3	T42.4X4	T42.4X5	T42.4X6
Chlordiethyl benzamide	T49.3X1	T49.3X2	T49.3X3	T49.3X4	T49.3X5	T49.3X6
Chloresium	T49.8X1	T49.8X2	T49.8X3	T49.8X4	T49.8X5	T49.8X6
Chlorethiazol	T42.6X1	T42.6X2	T42.6X3	T42.6X4	T42.6X5	T42.6X6
Chlorethyl—see Ethyl chloride						
Chloretone	T42.6X1	T42.6X2	T42.6X3	T42.6X4	T42.6X5	T42.6X6
Chlorex	T53.6X1	T53.6X2	T53.6X3	T53.6X4	--	--
- insecticide	T60.1X1	T60.1X2	T60.1X3	T60.1X4	--	--
Chlorfenvinphos	T60.0X1	T60.0X2	T60.0X3	T60.0X4	--	--
Chlorhexadol	T42.6X1	T42.6X2	T42.6X3	T42.6X4	T42.6X5	T42.6X6
Chlorhexamide	T45.1X1	T45.1X2	T45.1X3	T45.1X4	T45.1X5	T45.1X6
Chlorhexidine	T49.0X1	T49.0X2	T49.0X3	T49.0X4	T49.0X5	T49.0X6
Chlorhydroxyquinolin	T49.0X1	T49.0X2	T49.0X3	T49.0X4	T49.0X5	T49.0X6

Substance	Poisoning, Accidental (unintentional)	Poisoning, Intentional Self-harm	Poisoning, Assault	Poisoning, Undetermined	Adverse effect	Underdosing
Chloride of lime (bleach)	T54.3X1	T54.3X2	T54.3X3	T54.3X4	--	--
Chlorimipramine	T43.011	T43.012	T43.013	T43.014	T43.015	T43.016
Chlorinated						
- camphene	T53.6X1	T53.6X2	T53.6X3	T53.6X4	--	--
- diphenyl	T53.7X1	T53.7X2	T53.7X3	T53.7X4	--	--
- hydrocarbons NEC	T53.91	T53.92	T53.93	T53.94	--	--
- - solvents	T53.91	T53.92	T53.93	T53.94	--	--
- lime (bleach)	T54.3X1	T54.3X2	T54.3X3	T54.3X4	--	--
- - and boric acid solution	T49.0X1	T49.0X2	T49.0X3	T49.0X4	T49.0X5	T49.0X6
- naphthalene (insecticide)	T60.1X1	T60.1X2	T60.1X3	T60.1X4	--	--
- - industrial (non-pesticide)	T53.7X1	T53.7X2	T53.7X3	T53.7X4	--	--
- pesticide NEC	T60.8X1	T60.8X2	T60.8X3	T60.8X4	--	--
- soda—see also sodium hypochlorite						
- - solution	T49.0X1	T49.0X2	T49.0X3	T49.0X4	T49.0X5	T49.0X6
Chlorine (fumes) (gas)	T59.4X1	T59.4X2	T59.4X3	T59.4X4	--	--
- bleach	T54.3X1	T54.3X2	T54.3X3	T54.3X4	--	
- compound gas NEC	T59.4X1	T59.4X2	T59.4X3	T59.4X4	--	--
- disinfectant	T59.4X1	T59.4X2	T59.4X3	T59.4X4	--	--
- releasing agents NEC	T59.4X1	T59.4X2	T59.4X3	T59.4X4	--	--
Chlorisondamine chloride	T46.991	T46.992	T46.993	T46.994	T46.995	T46.996
Chlormadinone	T38.5X1	T38.5X2	T38.5X3	T38.5X4	T38.5X5	T38.5X6
Chlormephos	T60.0X1	T60.0X2	T60.0X3	T60.0X4	--	--
Chlormerodrin	T50.2X1	T50.2X2	T50.2X3	T50.2X4	T50.2X5	T50.2X6
Chlormethiazole	T42.6X1	T42.6X2	T42.6X3	T42.6X4	T42.6X5	T42.6X6
Chlormethine	T45.1X1	T45.1X2	T45.1X3	T45.1X4	T45.1X5	T45.1X6
Chlormethylenecycline	T36.4X1	T36.4X2	T36.4X3	T36.4X4	T36.4X5	T36.4X6
Chlormezanone	T42.6X1	T42.6X2	T42.6X3	T42.6X4	T42.6X5	T42.6X6
Chloroacetic acid	T60.3X1	T60.3X2	T60.3X3	T60.3X4	--	--
Chloroacetone	T59.3X1	T59.3X2	T59.3X3	T59.3X4	--	--
Chloroacetophenone	T59.3X1	T59.3X2	T59.3X3	T59.3X4	--	--
Chloroaniline	T53.7X1	T53.7X2	T53.7X3	T53.7X4	--	--
Chlorobenzene, chlorobenzol	T53.7X1	T53.7X2	T53.7X3	T53.7X4	--	--
Chlorobromomethane (fire extinguisher)	T53.6X1	T53.6X2	T53.6X3	T53.6X4	--	--
Chlorobutanol	T49.0X1	T49.0X2	T49.0X3	T49.0X4	T49.0X5	T49.0X6
Chlorocresol	T49.0X1	T49.0X2	T49.0X3	T49.0X4	T49.0X5	T49.0X6
Chlorodehydro-methyltestosterone	T38.7X1	T38.7X2	T38.7X3	T38.7X4	T38.7X5	T38.7X6
Chlorodinitrobenzene	T53.7X1	T53.7X2	T53.7X3	T53.7X4	--	--
- dust or vapor	T53.7X1	T53.7X2	T53.7X3	T53.7X4	--	--
Chlorodiphenyl	T53.7X1	T53.7X2	T53.7X3	T53.7X4	--	--
Chloroethane—see Ethyl chloride						
Chloroethylene	T53.6X1	T53.6X2	T53.6X3	T53.6X4	--	--
Chlorofluorocarbons	T53.5X1	T53.5X2	T53.5X3	T53.5X4	--	--
Chloroform (fumes) (vapor)	T53.1X1	T53.1X2	T53.1X3	T53.1X4	--	--
- anesthetic	T41.0X1	T41.0X2	T41.0X3	T41.0X4	T41.0X5	T41.0X6
- solvent	T53.1X1	T53.1X2	T53.1X3	T53.1X4	--	--
- water, concentrated	T41.0X1	T41.0X2	T41.0X3	T41.0X4	T41.0X5	T41.0X6
Chloroguanide	T37.2X1	T37.2X2	T37.2X3	T37.2X4	T37.2X5	T37.2X6
Chloromycetin	T36.2X1	T36.2X2	T36.2X3	T36.2X4	T36.2X5	T36.2X6
- ENT agent	T49.6X1	T49.6X2	T49.6X3	T49.6X4	T49.6X5	T49.6X6
- ophthalmic preparation	T49.5X1	T49.5X2	T49.5X3	T49.5X4	T49.5X5	T49.5X6
- otic solution	T49.6X1	T49.6X2	T49.6X3	T49.6X4	T49.6X5	T49.6X6
- topical NEC	T49.0X1	T49.0X2	T49.0X3	T49.0X4	T49.0X5	T49.0X6
Chloronitrobenzene	T53.7X1	T53.7X2	T53.7X3	T53.7X4	--	--
- dust or vapor	T53.7X1	T53.7X2	T53.7X3	T53.7X4	--	--
Chlorophacinone	T60.4X1	T60.4X2	T60.4X3	T60.4X4	--	--
Chlorophenol	T53.7X1	T53.7X2	T53.7X3	T53.7X4	--	--
Chlorophenothane	T60.1X1	T60.1X2	T60.1X3	T60.1X4	--	--
Chlorophyll	T50.991	T50.992	T50.993	T50.994	T50.995	T50.996

Substance	Poisoning, Accidental (unintentional)	Poisoning, Intentional Self-harm	Poisoning, Assault	Poisoning, Undetermined	Adverse effect	Underdosing
Chloropicrin (fumes)	T53.6X1	T53.6X2	T53.6X3	T53.6X4	--	--
- fumigant	T60.8X1	T60.8X2	T60.8X3	T60.8X4	--	--
- fungicide	T60.3X1	T60.3X2	T60.3X3	T60.3X4	--	--
- pesticide	T60.8X1	T60.8X2	T60.8X3	T60.8X4	--	--
Chloroprocaine	T41.3X1	T41.3X2	T41.3X3	T41.3X4	T41.3X5	T41.3X6
- infiltration (subcutaneous)	T41.3X1	T41.3X2	T41.3X3	T41.3X4	T41.3X5	T41.3X6
- nerve block (peripheral) (plexus)	T41.3X1	T41.3X2	T41.3X3	T41.3X4	T41.3X5	T41.3X6
- spinal	T41.3X1	T41.3X2	T41.3X3	T41.3X4	T41.3X5	T41.3X6
Chloroptic	T49.5X1	T49.5X2	T49.5X3	T49.5X4	T49.5X5	T49.5X6
Chloropurine	T45.1X1	T45.1X2	T45.1X3	T45.1X4	T45.1X5	T45.1X6
Chloropyramine	T45.0X1	T45.0X2	T45.0X3	T45.0X4	T45.0X5	T45.0X6
Chloropyrifos	T60.0X1	T60.0X2	T60.0X3	T60.0X4	--	--
Chloropyrilene	T45.0X1	T45.0X2	T45.0X3	T45.0X4	T45.0X5	T45.0X6
Chloroquine	T37.2X1	T37.2X2	T37.2X3	T37.2X4	T37.2X5	T37.2X6
Chlorothalonil	T60.3X1	T60.3X2	T60.3X3	T60.3X4	--	--
Chlorothen	T45.0X1	T45.0X2	T45.0X3	T45.0X4	T45.0X5	T45.0X6
Chlorothiazide	T50.2X1	T50.2X2	T50.2X3	T50.2X4	T50.2X5	T50.2X6
Chlorothymol	T49.4X1	T49.4X2	T49.4X3	T49.4X4	T49.4X5	T49.4X6
Chlorotrianisene	T38.5X1	T38.5X2	T38.5X3	T38.5X4	T38.5X5	T38.5X6
Chlorovinyldichloro-arsine, not in war	T57.0X1	T57.0X2	T57.0X3	T57.0X4	--	--
Chloroxine	T49.4X1	T49.4X2	T49.4X3	T49.4X4	T49.4X5	T49.4X6
Chloroxylenol	T49.0X1	T49.0X2	T49.0X3	T49.0X4	T49.0X5	T49.0X6
Chlorphenamine	T45.0X1	T45.0X2	T45.0X3	T45.0X4	T45.0X5	T45.0X6
Chlorphenesin	T42.8X1	T42.8X2	T42.8X3	T42.8X4	T42.8X5	T42.8X6
- topical (antifungal)	T49.0X1	T49.0X2	T49.0X3	T49.0X4	T49.0X5	T49.0X6
Chlorpheniramine	T45.0X1	T45.0X2	T45.0X3	T45.0X4	T45.0X5	T45.0X6
Chlorphenoxamine	T45.0X1	T45.0X2	T45.0X3	T45.0X4	T45.0X5	T45.0X6
Chlorphentermine	T50.5X1	T50.5X2	T50.5X3	T50.5X4	T50.5X5	T50.5X6
Chlorprocaine—see Chloroprocaine						
Chlorproguanil	T37.2X1	T37.2X2	T37.2X3	T37.2X4	T37.2X5	T37.2X6
Chlorpromazine	T43.3X1	T43.3X2	T43.3X3	T43.3X4	T43.3X5	T43.3X6
Chlorpropamide	T38.3X1	T38.3X2	T38.3X3	T38.3X4	T38.3X5	T38.3X6
Chlorprothixene	T43.4X1	T43.4X2	T43.4X3	T43.4X4	T43.4X5	T43.4X6
Chlorquinaldol	T49.0X1	T49.0X2	T49.0X3	T49.0X4	T49.0X5	T49.0X6
Chlorquinol	T49.0X1	T49.0X2	T49.0X3	T49.0X4	T49.0X5	T49.0X6
Chlortalidone	T50.2X1	T50.2X2	T50.2X3	T50.2X4	T50.2X5	T50.2X6
Chlortetracycline	T36.4X1	T36.4X2	T36.4X3	T36.4X4	T36.4X5	T36.4X6
Chlorthalidone	T50.2X1	T50.2X2	T50.2X3	T50.2X4	T50.2X5	T50.2X6
Chlorthiophos	T60.0X1	T60.0X2	T60.0X3	T60.0X4	--	--
Chlortrianisene	T38.5X1	T38.5X2	T38.5X3	T38.5X4	T38.5X5	T38.5X6
Chlor-Trimeton	T45.0X1	T45.0X2	T45.0X3	T45.0X4	T45.0X5	T45.0X6
Chlorthion	T60.0X1	T60.0X2	T60.0X3	T60.0X4	--	--
Chlorzoxazone	T42.8X1	T42.8X2	T42.8X3	T42.8X4	T42.8X5	T42.8X6
Choke damp	T59.7X1	T59.7X2	T59.7X3	T59.7X4	--	--
Cholagogues	T47.5X1	T47.5X2	T47.5X3	T47.5X4	T47.5X5	T47.5X6
Cholebrine	T50.8X1	T50.8X2	T50.8X3	T50.8X4	T50.8X5	T50.8X6
Cholecalciferol	T45.2X1	T45.2X2	T45.2X3	T45.2X4	T45.2X5	T45.2X6
Cholecystokinin	T50.8X1	T50.8X2	T50.8X3	T50.8X4	T50.8X5	T50.8X6
Cholera vaccine	T50.A91	T50.A92	T50.A93	T50.A94	T50.A95	T50.A96
Choleretic	T47.5X1	T47.5X2	T47.5X3	T47.5X4	T47.5X5	T47.5X6
Cholesterol-lowering agents	T46.6X1	T46.6X2	T46.6X3	T46.6X4	T46.6X5	T46.6X6
Cholestyramine (resin)	T46.6X1	T46.6X2	T46.6X3	T46.6X4	T46.6X5	T46.6X6
Cholic acid	T47.5X1	T47.5X2	T47.5X3	T47.5X4	T47.5X5	T47.5X6
Choline	T48.6X1	T48.6X2	T48.6X3	T48.6X4	T48.6X5	T48.6X6
- chloride	T50.991	T50.992	T50.993	T50.994	T50.995	T50.996
- dihydrogen citrate	T50.991	T50.992	T50.993	T50.994	T50.995	T50.996
- salicylate	T39.091	T39.092	T39.093	T39.094	T39.095	T39.096
- theophyllinate	T48.6X1	T48.6X2	T48.6X3	T48.6X4	T48.6X5	T48.6X6
Cholinergic (drug) NEC	T44.1X1	T44.1X2	T44.1X3	T44.1X4	T44.1X5	T44.1X6

Substance	Poisoning, Accidental (unintentional)	Poisoning, Intentional Self-harm	Poisoning, Assault	Poisoning, Undetermined	Adverse effect	Underdosing
- muscle tone enhancer	T44.1X1	T44.1X2	T44.1X3	T44.1X4	T44.1X5	T44.1X6
- organophosphorus	T44.0X1	T44.0X2	T44.0X3	T44.0X4	T44.0X5	T44.0X6
- - insecticide	T60.0X1	T60.0X2	T60.0X3	T60.0X4	--	--
- - nerve gas	T59.891	T59.892	T59.893	T59.894	--	--
- trimethyl ammonium propanediol	T44.1X1	T44.1X2	T44.1X3	T44.1X4	T44.1X5	T44.1X6
Cholinesterase reactivator	T50.6X1	T50.6X2	T50.6X3	T50.6X4	T50.6X5	T50.6X6
Cholografin	T50.8X1	T50.8X2	T50.8X3	T50.8X4	T50.8X5	T50.8X6
Chorionic gonadotropin	T38.891	T38.892	T38.893	T38.894	T38.895	T38.896
Chromate	T56.2X1	T56.2X2	T56.2X3	T56.2X4	--	--
- dust or mist	T56.2X1	T56.2X2	T56.2X3	T56.2X4	--	--
- lead—see also lead	T56.0X1	T56.0X2	T56.0X3	T56.0X4	--	--
- - paint	T56.0X1	T56.0X2	T56.0X3	T56.0X4	--	--
Chromic						
- acid	T56.2X1	T56.2X2	T56.2X3	T56.2X4	--	--
- - dust or mist	T56.2X1	T56.2X2	T56.2X3	T56.2X4	--	--
- phosphate 32P	T45.1X1	T45.1X2	T45.1X3	T45.1X4	T45.1X5	T45.1X6
Chromium	T56.2X1	T56.2X2	T56.2X3	T56.2X4	--	--
- compounds—see Chromate						
- sesquioxide	T50.8X1	T50.8X2	T50.8X3	T50.8X4	T50.8X5	T50.8X6
Chromomycin A3	T45.1X1	T45.1X2	T45.1X3	T45.1X4	T45.1X5	T45.1X6
Chromonar	T46.3X1	T46.3X2	T46.3X3	T46.3X4	T46.3X5	T46.3X6
Chromyl chloride	T56.2X1	T56.2X2	T56.2X3	T56.2X4	--	--
Chrysarobin	T49.4X1	T49.4X2	T49.4X3	T49.4X4	T49.4X5	T49.4X6
Chrysazin	T47.2X1	T47.2X2	T47.2X3	T47.2X4	T47.2X5	T47.2X6
Chymar	T45.3X1	T45.3X2	T45.3X3	T45.3X4	T45.3X5	T45.3X6
- ophthalmic preparation	T49.5X1	T49.5X2	T49.5X3	T49.5X4	T49.5X5	T49.5X6
Chymopapain	T45.3X1	T45.3X2	T45.3X3	T45.3X4	T45.3X5	T45.3X6
Chymotrypsin	T45.3X1	T45.3X2	T45.3X3	T45.3X4	T45.3X5	T45.3X6
- ophthalmic preparation	T49.5X1	T49.5X2	T49.5X3	T49.5X4	T49.5X5	T49.5X6
Cianidanol	T50.991	T50.992	T50.993	T50.994	T50.995	T50.996
Cianopramine	T43.011	T43.012	T43.013	T43.014	T43.015	T43.016
Cibenzoline	T46.2X1	T46.2X2	T46.2X3	T46.2X4	T46.2X5	T46.2X6
Ciclacillin	T36.0X1	T36.0X2	T36.0X3	T36.0X4	T36.0X5	T36.0X6
Ciclobarbital—see Hexobarbital						
Ciclonicate	T46.7X1	T46.7X2	T46.7X3	T46.7X4	T46.7X5	T46.7X6
Ciclopirox (olamine)	T49.0X1	T49.0X2	T49.0X3	T49.0X4	T49.0X5	T49.0X6
Ciclosporin	T45.1X1	T45.1X2	T45.1X3	T45.1X4	T45.1X5	T45.1X6
Cicuta maculata or virosa	T62.2X1	T62.2X2	T62.2X3	T62.2X4	--	--
Cicutoxin	T62.2X1	T62.2X2	T62.2X3	T62.2X4	--	--
Cigarette lighter fluid	T52.0X1	T52.0X2	T52.0X3	T52.0X4	--	--
Cigarettes (tobacco)	T65.221	T65.222	T65.223	T65.224	--	--
Ciguatoxin	T61.01	T61.02	T61.03	T61.04	--	--
Cilazapril	T46.4X1	T46.4X2	T46.4X3	T46.4X4	T46.4X5	T46.4X6
Cimetidine	T47.0X1	T47.0X2	T47.0X3	T47.0X4	T47.0X5	T47.0X6
Cimetropium bromide	T44.3X1	T44.3X2	T44.3X3	T44.3X4	T44.3X5	T44.3X6
Cinchocaine	T41.3X1	T41.3X2	T41.3X3	T41.3X4	T41.3X5	T41.3X6
- topical (surface)	T41.3X1	T41.3X2	T41.3X3	T41.3X4	T41.3X5	T41.3X6
Cinchona	T37.2X1	T37.2X2	T37.2X3	T37.2X4	T37.2X5	T37.2X6
Cinchonine alkaloids	T37.2X1	T37.2X2	T37.2X3	T37.2X4	T37.2X5	T37.2X6
Cinchophen	T50.4X1	T50.4X2	T50.4X3	T50.4X4	T50.4X5	T50.4X6
Cinepazide	T46.7X1	T46.7X2	T46.7X3	T46.7X4	T46.7X5	T46.7X6
Cinnamedrine	T48.5X1	T48.5X2	T48.5X3	T48.5X4	T48.5X5	T48.5X6
Cinnarizine	T45.0X1	T45.0X2	T45.0X3	T45.0X4	T45.0X5	T45.0X6
Cinoxacin	T37.8X1	T37.8X2	T37.8X3	T37.8X4	T37.8X5	T37.8X6
Ciprofibrate	T46.6X1	T46.6X2	T46.6X3	T46.6X4	T46.6X5	T46.6X6
Ciprofloxacin	T36.8X1	T36.8X2	T36.8X3	T36.8X4	T36.8X5	T36.8X6
Cisapride	T47.8X1	T47.8X2	T47.8X3	T47.8X4	T47.8X5	T47.8X6
Cisplatin	T45.1X1	T45.1X2	T45.1X3	T45.1X4	T45.1X5	T45.1X6

Substance	Poisoning, Accidental (unintentional)	Poisoning, Intentional Self-harm	Poisoning, Assault	Poisoning, Undetermined	Adverse effect	Underdosing
Citalopram	T43.221	T43.222	T43.223	T43.224	T43.225	T43.226
Citanest	T41.3X1	T41.3X2	T41.3X3	T41.3X4	T41.3X5	T41.3X6
- infiltration (subcutaneous)	T41.3X1	T41.3X2	T41.3X3	T41.3X4	T41.3X5	T41.3X6
- nerve block (peripheral) (plexus)	T41.3X1	T41.3X2	T41.3X3	T41.3X4	T41.3X5	T41.3X6
Citric acid	T47.5X1	T47.5X2	T47.5X3	T47.5X4	T47.5X5	T47.5X6
Citrovorum (factor)	T45.8X1	T45.8X2	T45.8X3	T45.8X4	T45.8X5	T45.8X6
Claviceps purpurea	T62.2X1	T62.2X2	T62.2X3	T62.2X4	--	--
Clavulanic acid	T36.1X1	T36.1X2	T36.1X3	T36.1X4	T36.1X5	T36.1X6
Cleaner, cleansing agent, type not specified	T65.891	T65.892	T65.893	T65.894	--	--
- of paint or varnish	T52.91	T52.92	T52.93	T52.94	--	--
- specified type NEC	T65.891	T65.892	T65.893	T65.894	--	--
Clebopride	T47.8X1	T47.8X2	T47.8X3	T47.8X4	T47.8X5	T47.8X6
Clefamide	T37.3X1	T37.3X2	T37.3X3	T37.3X4	T37.3X5	T37.3X6
Clemastine	T45.0X1	T45.0X2	T45.0X3	T45.0X4	T45.0X5	T45.0X6
Clematis vitalba	T62.2X1	T62.2X2	T62.2X3	T62.2X4	--	--
Clemizole	T45.0X1	T45.0X2	T45.0X3	T45.0X4	T45.0X5	T45.0X6
- penicillin	T36.0X1	T36.0X2	T36.0X3	T36.0X4	T36.0X5	T36.0X6
Clenbuterol	T48.6X1	T48.6X2	T48.6X3	T48.6X4	T48.6X5	T48.6X6
Clidinium bromide	T44.3X1	T44.3X2	T44.3X3	T44.3X4	T44.3X5	T44.3X6
Clindamycin	T36.8X1	T36.8X2	T36.8X3	T36.8X4	T36.8X5	T36.8X6
Clinofibrate	T46.6X1	T46.6X2	T46.6X3	T46.6X4	T46.6X5	T46.6X6
Clioquinol	T37.8X1	T37.8X2	T37.8X3	T37.8X4	T37.8X5	T37.8X6
Cliradon	T40.2X1	T40.2X2	T40.2X3	T40.2X4	--	--
Clobazam	T42.4X1	T42.4X2	T42.4X3	T42.4X4	T42.4X5	T42.4X6
Clobenzorex	T50.5X1	T50.5X2	T50.5X3	T50.5X4	T50.5X5	T50.5X6
Clobetasol	T49.0X1	T49.0X2	T49.0X3	T49.0X4	T49.0X5	T49.0X6
Clobetasone	T49.0X1	T49.0X2	T49.0X3	T49.0X4	T49.0X5	T49.0X6
Clobutinol	T48.3X1	T48.3X2	T48.3X3	T48.3X4	T48.3X5	T48.3X6
Clocortolone	T38.0X1	T38.0X2	T38.0X3	T38.0X4	T38.0X5	T38.0X6
Clodantoin	T49.0X1	T49.0X2	T49.0X3	T49.0X4	T49.0X5	T49.0X6
Clodronic acid	T50.991	T50.992	T50.993	T50.994	T50.995	T50.996
Clofazimine	T37.1X1	T37.1X2	T37.1X3	T37.1X4	T37.1X5	T37.1X6
Clofedanol	T48.3X1	T48.3X2	T48.3X3	T48.3X4	T48.3X5	T48.3X6
Clofenamide	T50.2X1	T50.2X2	T50.2X3	T50.2X4	T50.2X5	T50.2X6
Clofenotane	T49.0X1	T49.0X2	T49.0X3	T49.0X4	T49.0X5	T49.0X6
Clofezone	T39.2X1	T39.2X2	T39.2X3	T39.2X4	T39.2X5	T39.2X6
Clofibrate	T46.6X1	T46.6X2	T46.6X3	T46.6X4	T46.6X5	T46.6X6
Clofibride	T46.6X1	T46.6X2	T46.6X3	T46.6X4	T46.6X5	T46.6X6
Cloforex	T50.5X1	T50.5X2	T50.5X3	T50.5X4	T50.5X5	T50.5X6
Clomethiazole	T42.6X1	T42.6X2	T42.6X3	T42.6X4	T42.6X5	T42.6X6
Clometocillin	T36.0X1	T36.0X2	T36.0X3	T36.0X4	T36.0X5	T36.0X6
Clomifene	T38.5X1	T38.5X2	T38.5X3	T38.5X4	T38.5X5	T38.5X6
Clomiphene	T38.5X1	T38.5X2	T38.5X3	T38.5X4	T38.5X5	T38.5X6
Clomipramine	T43.011	T43.012	T43.013	T43.014	T43.015	T43.016
Clomocycline	T36.4X1	T36.4X2	T36.4X3	T36.4X4	T36.4X5	T36.4X6
Clonazepam	T42.4X1	T42.4X2	T42.4X3	T42.4X4	T42.4X5	T42.4X6
Clonidine	T46.5X1	T46.5X2	T46.5X3	T46.5X4	T46.5X5	T46.5X6
Clonixin	T39.8X1	T39.8X2	T39.8X3	T39.8X4	T39.8X5	T39.8X6
Clopamide	T50.2X1	T50.2X2	T50.2X3	T50.2X4	T50.2X5	T50.2X6
Clopenthixol	T43.4X1	T43.4X2	T43.4X3	T43.4X4	T43.4X5	T43.4X6
Cloperastine	T48.3X1	T48.3X2	T48.3X3	T48.3X4	T48.3X5	T48.3X6
Clophedianol	T48.3X1	T48.3X2	T48.3X3	T48.3X4	T48.3X5	T48.3X6
Cloponone	T36.2X1	T36.2X2	T36.2X3	T36.2X4	T36.2X5	T36.2X6
Cloprednol	T38.0X1	T38.0X2	T38.0X3	T38.0X4	T38.0X5	T38.0X6
Cloral betaine	T42.6X1	T42.6X2	T42.6X3	T42.6X4	T42.6X5	T42.6X6
Cloramfenicol	T36.2X1	T36.2X2	T36.2X3	T36.2X4	T36.2X5	T36.2X6
Clorazepate (dipotassium)	T42.4X1	T42.4X2	T42.4X3	T42.4X4	T42.4X5	T42.4X6
Clorexolone	T50.2X1	T50.2X2	T50.2X3	T50.2X4	T50.2X5	T50.2X6
Clorfenamine	T45.0X1	T45.0X2	T45.0X3	T45.0X4	T45.0X5	T45.0X6

Substance	Poisoning, Accidental (unintentional)	Poisoning, Intentional Self-harm	Poisoning, Assault	Poisoning, Undetermined	Adverse effect	Underdosing
Clorgiline	T43.1X1	T43.1X2	T43.1X3	T43.1X4	T43.1X5	T43.1X6
Clorotepine	T44.3X1	T44.3X2	T44.3X3	T44.3X4	T44.3X5	T44.3X6
Clorox (bleach)	T54.91	T54.92	T54.93	T54.94	--	--
Clorprenaline	T48.6X1	T48.6X2	T48.6X3	T48.6X4	T48.6X5	T48.6X6
Clortermine	T50.5X1	T50.5X2	T50.5X3	T50.5X4	T50.5X5	T50.5X6
Clotiapine	T43.591	T43.592	T43.593	T43.594	T43.595	T43.596
Clotiazepam	T42.4X1	T42.4X2	T42.4X3	T42.4X4	T42.4X5	T42.4X6
Clotibric acid	T46.6X1	T46.6X2	T46.6X3	T46.6X4	T46.6X5	T46.6X6
Clotrimazole	T49.0X1	T49.0X2	T49.0X3	T49.0X4	T49.0X5	T49.0X6
Cloxacillin	T36.0X1	T36.0X2	T36.0X3	T36.0X4	T36.0X5	T36.0X6
Cloxazolam	T42.4X1	T42.4X2	T42.4X3	T42.4X4	T42.4X5	T42.4X6
Cloxiquine	T49.0X1	T49.0X2	T49.0X3	T49.0X4	T49.0X5	T49.0X6
Clozapine	T42.4X1	T42.4X2	T42.4X3	T42.4X4	T42.4X5	T42.4X6
Coagulant NEC	T45.7X1	T45.7X2	T45.7X3	T45.7X4	T45.7X5	T45.7X6
Coal (carbon monoxide from) —see also Carbon, monoxide, coal	T58.2X1	T58.2X2	T58.2X3	T58.2X4	--	--
- oil—see Kerosene						
- tar	T49.1X1	T49.1X2	T49.1X3	T49.1X4	T49.1X5	T49.1X6
- - fumes	T59.891	T59.892	T59.893	T59.894	--	--
- - medicinal (ointment)	T49.4X1	T49.4X2	T49.4X3	T49.4X4	T49.4X5	T49.4X6
- - - analgesics NEC	T39.2X1	T39.2X2	T39.2X3	T39.2X4	T39.2X5	T39.2X6
- - naphtha (solvent)	T52.0X1	T52.0X2	T52.0X3	T52.0X4	--	--
Cobalamine	T45.2X1	T45.2X2	T45.2X3	T45.2X4	T45.2X5	T45.2X6
Cobalt (nonmedicinal) (fumes) (industrial)	T56.891	T56.892	T56.893	T56.894	--	--
- medicinal (trace) (chloride)	T45.8X1	T45.8X2	T45.8X3	T45.8X4	T45.8X5	T45.8X6
Cobra (venom)	T63.041	T63.042	T63.043	T63.044	--	--
Coca (leaf)	T40.5X1	T40.5X2	T40.5X3	T40.5X4	T40.5X5	T40.5X6
Cocaine	T40.5X1	T40.5X2	T40.5X3	T40.5X4	T40.5X5	T40.5X6
- topical anesthetic	T41.3X1	T41.3X2	T41.3X3	T41.3X4	T41.3X5	T41.3X6
Cocarboxylase	T45.3X1	T45.3X2	T45.3X3	T45.3X4	T45.3X5	T45.3X6
Coccidioidin	T50.8X1	T50.8X2	T50.8X3	T50.8X4	T50.8X5	T50.8X6
Cocculus indicus	T62.1X1	T62.1X2	T62.1X3	T62.1X4	--	--
Cochineal	T65.6X1	T65.6X2	T65.6X3	T65.6X4	--	--
- medicinal products	T50.991	T50.992	T50.993	T50.994	T50.995	T50.996
Codeine	T40.2X1	T40.2X2	T40.2X3	T40.2X4	T40.2X5	T40.2X6
Cod-liver oil	T45.2X1	T45.2X2	T45.2X3	T45.2X4	T45.2X5	T45.2X6
Coenzyme A	T50.991	T50.992	T50.993	T50.994	T50.995	T50.996
Coffee	T62.8X1	T62.8X2	T62.8X3	T62.8X4	--	--
Cogalactoiso-merase	T50.991	T50.992	T50.993	T50.994	T50.995	T50.996
Cogentin	T44.3X1	T44.3X2	T44.3X3	T44.3X4	T44.3X5	T44.3X6
Coke fumes or gas (carbon monoxide)	T58.2X1	T58.2X2	T58.2X3	T58.2X4	--	--
- industrial use	T58.8X1	T58.8X2	T58.8X3	T58.8X4	--	--
Colace	T47.4X1	T47.4X2	T47.4X3	T47.4X4	T47.4X5	T47.4X6
Colaspase	T45.1X1	T45.1X2	T45.1X3	T45.1X4	T45.1X5	T45.1X6
Colchicine	T50.4X1	T50.4X2	T50.4X3	T50.4X4	T50.4X5	T50.4X6
Colchicum	T62.2X1	T62.2X2	T62.2X3	T62.2X4	--	--
Cold cream	T49.3X1	T49.3X2	T49.3X3	T49.3X4	T49.3X5	T49.3X6
Colecalciferol	T45.2X1	T45.2X2	T45.2X3	T45.2X4	T45.2X5	T45.2X6
Colestipol	T46.6X1	T46.6X2	T46.6X3	T46.6X4	T46.6X5	T46.6X6
Colestyramine	T46.6X1	T46.6X2	T46.6X3	T46.6X4	T46.6X5	T46.6X6
Colimycin	T36.8X1	T36.8X2	T36.8X3	T36.8X4	T36.8X5	T36.8X6
Colistimethate	T36.8X1	T36.8X2	T36.8X3	T36.8X4	T36.8X5	T36.8X6
Colistin	T36.8X1	T36.8X2	T36.8X3	T36.8X4	T36.8X5	T36.8X6
- sulfate (eye preparation)	T49.5X1	T49.5X2	T49.5X3	T49.5X4	T49.5X5	T49.5X6
Collagen	T50.991	T50.992	T50.993	T50.994	T50.995	T50.996
Collagenase	T49.4X1	T49.4X2	T49.4X3	T49.4X4	T49.4X5	T49.4X6
Collodion	T49.3X1	T49.3X2	T49.3X3	T49.3X4	T49.3X5	T49.3X6
Colocynth	T47.2X1	T47.2X2	T47.2X3	T47.2X4	T47.2X5	T47.2X6
Colophony adhesive	T49.3X1	T49.3X2	T49.3X3	T49.3X4	T49.3X5	T49.3X6

Substance	Poisoning, Accidental (unintentional)	Poisoning, Intentional Self-harm	Poisoning, Assault	Poisoning, Undetermined	Adverse effect	Underdosing
Colorant—see also Dye	T50.991	T50.992	T50.993	T50.994	T50.995	T50.996
Coloring matter—see Dye (s)						
Combustion gas (after combustion) —see Carbon, monoxide						
- prior to combustion	T59.891	T59.892	T59.893	T59.894	--	--
Compazine	T43.3X1	T43.3X2	T43.3X3	T43.3X4	T43.3X5	T43.3X6
Compound						
- 42 (warfarin)	T60.4X1	T60.4X2	T60.4X3	T60.4X4	--	--
- 269 (endrin)	T60.1X1	T60.1X2	T60.1X3	T60.1X4	--	--
- 497 (dieldrin)	T60.1X1	T60.1X2	T60.1X3	T60.1X4	--	--
- 1080 (sodium fluoroacetate)	T60.4X1	T60.4X2	T60.4X3	T60.4X4	--	--
- 3422 (parathion)	T60.0X1	T60.0X2	T60.0X3	T60.0X4	--	--
- 3911 (phorate)	T60.0X1	T60.0X2	T60.0X3	T60.0X4	--	--
- 3956 (toxaphene)	T60.1X1	T60.1X2	T60.1X3	T60.1X4	--	--
- 4049 (malathion)	T60.0X1	T60.0X2	T60.0X3	T60.0X4	--	--
- 4069 (malathion)	T60.0X1	T60.0X2	T60.0X3	T60.0X4	--	--
- 4124 (dicapthon)	T60.0X1	T60.0X2	T60.0X3	T60.0X4	--	--
- E (cortisone)	T38.0X1	T38.0X2	T38.0X3	T38.0X4	T38.0X5	T38.0X6
- F (hydrocortisone)	T38.0X1	T38.0X2	T38.0X3	T38.0X4	T38.0X5	T38.0X6
Congener, anabolic	T38.7X1	T38.7X2	T38.7X3	T38.7X4	T38.7X5	T38.7X6
Congo red	T50.8X1	T50.8X2	T50.8X3	T50.8X4	T50.8X5	T50.8X6
Coniine, conine	T62.2X1	T62.2X2	T62.2X3	T62.2X4	--	--
Conium (maculatum)	T62.2X1	T62.2X2	T62.2X3	T62.2X4	--	--
Conjugated estrogenic substances	T38.5X1	T38.5X2	T38.5X3	T38.5X4	T38.5X5	T38.5X6
Contac	T48.5X1	T48.5X2	T48.5X3	T48.5X4	T48.5X5	T48.5X6
Contact lens solution	T49.5X1	T49.5X2	T49.5X3	T49.5X4	T49.5X5	T49.5X6
Contraceptive (oral)	T38.4X1	T38.4X2	T38.4X3	T38.4X4	T38.4X5	T38.4X6
- vaginal	T49.8X1	T49.8X2	T49.8X3	T49.8X4	T49.8X5	T49.8X6
Contrast medium, radiography	T50.8X1	T50.8X2	T50.8X3	T50.8X4	T50.8X5	T50.8X6
Convallaria glycosides	T46.0X1	T46.0X2	T46.0X3	T46.0X4	T46.0X5	T46.0X6
Convallaria majalis	T62.2X1	T62.2X2	T62.2X3	T62.2X4	--	--
- berry	T62.1X1	T62.1X2	T62.1X3	T62.1X4	--	--
Copper (dust) (fumes) (nonmedicinal) NEC	T56.4X1	T56.4X2	T56.4X3	T56.4X4	--	--
- arsenate, arsenite	T57.0X1	T57.0X2	T57.0X3	T57.0X4	--	--
- - insecticide	T60.2X1	T60.2X2	T60.2X3	T60.2X4	--	--
- emetic	T47.7X1	T47.7X2	T47.7X3	T47.7X4	T47.7X5	T47.7X6
- fungicide	T60.3X1	T60.3X2	T60.3X3	T60.3X4	--	--
- gluconate	T49.0X1	T49.0X2	T49.0X3	T49.0X4	T49.0X5	T49.0X6
- insecticide	T60.2X1	T60.2X2	T60.2X3	T60.2X4	--	--
- medicinal (trace)	T45.8X1	T45.8X2	T45.8X3	T45.8X4	T45.8X5	T45.8X6
- oleate	T49.0X1	T49.0X2	T49.0X3	T49.0X4	T49.0X5	T49.0X6
- sulfate	T56.4X1	T56.4X2	T56.4X3	T56.4X4	--	--
- - cupric	T56.4X1	T56.4X2	T56.4X3	T56.4X4	--	--
- - - fungicide	T60.3X1	T60.3X2	T60.3X3	T60.3X4	--	--
- - - medicinal						
- - - - ear	T49.6X1	T49.6X2	T49.6X3	T49.6X4	T49.6X5	T49.6X6
- - - - emetic	T47.7X1	T47.7X2	T47.7X3	T47.7X4	T47.7X5	T47.7X6
- - - - eye	T49.5X1	T49.5X2	T49.5X3	T49.5X4	T49.5X5	T49.5X6
- - cuprous	T56.4X1	T56.4X2	T56.4X3	T56.4X4	--	--
- - fungicide	T60.3X1	T60.3X2	T60.3X3	T60.3X4	--	--
- - medicinal						
- - - ear	T49.6X1	T49.6X2	T49.6X3	T49.6X4	T49.6X5	T49.6X6
- - - emetic	T47.7X1	T47.7X2	T47.7X3	T47.7X4	T47.7X5	T47.7X6
- - - eye	T49.5X1	T49.5X2	T49.5X3	T49.5X4	T49.5X5	T49.5X6
Copperhead snake (bite) (venom)	T63.061	T63.062	T63.063	T63.064	--	--
Coral (sting)	T63.691	T63.692	T63.693	T63.694	--	--
- snake (bite) (venom)	T63.021	T63.022	T63.023	T63.024	--	--
Corbadrine	T49.6X1	T49.6X2	T49.6X3	T49.6X4	T49.6X5	T49.6X6
Cordite	T65.891	T65.892	T65.893	T65.894	--	--

Substance	Poisoning, Accidental (unintentional)	Poisoning, Intentional Self-harm	Poisoning, Assault	Poisoning, Undetermined	Adverse effect	Underdosing
- vapor	T59.891	T59.892	T59.893	T59.894	--	--
Cordran	T49.0X1	T49.0X2	T49.0X3	T49.0X4	T49.0X5	T49.0X6
Corn cures	T49.4X1	T49.4X2	T49.4X3	T49.4X4	T49.4X5	T49.4X6
Corn starch	T49.3X1	T49.3X2	T49.3X3	T49.3X4	T49.3X5	T49.3X6
Cornhusker's lotion	T49.3X1	T49.3X2	T49.3X3	T49.3X4	T49.3X5	T49.3X6
Coronary vasodilator NEC	T46.3X1	T46.3X2	T46.3X3	T46.3X4	T46.3X5	T46.3X6
Corrosive NEC	T54.91	T54.92	T54.93	T54.94	--	--
- acid NEC	T54.2X1	T54.2X2	T54.2X3	T54.2X4	--	--
- aromatics	T54.1X1	T54.1X2	T54.1X3	T54.1X4	--	--
- - disinfectant	T54.1X1	T54.1X2	T54.1X3	T54.1X4	--	--
- fumes NEC	T54.91	T54.92	T54.93	T54.94	--	--
- specified NEC	T54.91	T54.92	T54.93	T54.94	--	--
- sublimate	T56.1X1	T56.1X2	T56.1X3	T56.1X4	--	--
Cortate	T38.0X1	T38.0X2	T38.0X3	T38.0X4	T38.0X5	T38.0X6
Cort-Dome	T38.0X1	T38.0X2	T38.0X3	T38.0X4	T38.0X5	T38.0X6
- ENT agent	T49.6X1	T49.6X2	T49.6X3	T49.6X4	T49.6X5	T49.6X6
- ophthalmic preparation	T49.5X1	T49.5X2	T49.5X3	T49.5X4	T49.5X5	T49.5X6
- topical NEC	T49.0X1	T49.0X2	T49.0X3	T49.0X4	T49.0X5	T49.0X6
Cortef	T38.0X1	T38.0X2	T38.0X3	T38.0X4	T38.0X5	T38.0X6
- ENT agent	T49.6X1	T49.6X2	T49.6X3	T49.6X4	T49.6X5	T49.6X6
- ophthalmic preparation	T49.5X1	T49.5X2	T49.5X3	T49.5X4	T49.5X5	T49.5X6
- topical NEC	T49.0X1	T49.0X2	T49.0X3	T49.0X4	T49.0X5	T49.0X6
Corticosteroid	T38.0X1	T38.0X2	T38.0X3	T38.0X4	T38.0X5	T38.0X6
- ENT agent	T49.6X1	T49.6X2	T49.6X3	T49.6X4	T49.6X5	T49.6X6
- mineral	T50.0X1	T50.0X2	T50.0X3	T50.0X4	T50.0X5	T50.0X6
- ophthalmic	T49.5X1	T49.5X2	T49.5X3	T49.5X4	T49.5X5	T49.5X6
- topical NEC	T49.0X1	T49.0X2	T49.0X3	T49.0X4	T49.0X5	T49.0X6
Corticotropin	T38.811	T38.812	T38.813	T38.814	T38.815	T38.816
Cortisol	T49.0X1	T49.0X2	T49.0X3	T49.0X4	T49.0X5	T49.0X6
- ENT agent	T49.6X1	T49.6X2	T49.6X3	T49.6X4	T49.6X5	T49.6X6
- ophthalmic preparation	T49.5X1	T49.5X2	T49.5X3	T49.5X4	T49.5X5	T49.5X6
- topical NEC	T49.0X1	T49.0X2	T49.0X3	T49.0X4	T49.0X5	T49.0X6
Cortisone (acetate)	T38.0X1	T38.0X2	T38.0X3	T38.0X4	T38.0X5	T38.0X6
- ENT agent	T49.6X1	T49.6X2	T49.6X3	T49.6X4	T49.6X5	T49.6X6
- ophthalmic preparation	T49.5X1	T49.5X2	T49.5X3	T49.5X4	T49.5X5	T49.5X6
- topical NEC	T49.0X1	T49.0X2	T49.0X3	T49.0X4	T49.0X5	T49.0X6
Cortivazol	T38.0X1	T38.0X2	T38.0X3	T38.0X4	T38.0X5	T38.0X6
Cortogen	T38.0X1	T38.0X2	T38.0X3	T38.0X4	T38.0X5	T38.0X6
- ENT agent	T49.6X1	T49.6X2	T49.6X3	T49.6X4	T49.6X5	T49.6X6
- ophthalmic preparation	T49.5X1	T49.5X2	T49.5X3	T49.5X4	T49.5X5	T49.5X6
Cortone	T38.0X1	T38.0X2	T38.0X3	T38.0X4	T38.0X5	T38.0X6
- ENT agent	T49.6X1	T49.6X2	T49.6X3	T49.6X4	T49.6X5	T49.6X6
- ophthalmic preparation	T49.5X1	T49.5X2	T49.5X3	T49.5X4	T49.5X5	T49.5X6
Cortril	T38.0X1	T38.0X2	T38.0X3	T38.0X4	T38.0X5	T38.0X6
- ENT agent	T49.6X1	T49.6X2	T49.6X3	T49.6X4	T49.6X5	T49.6X6
- ophthalmic preparation	T49.5X1	T49.5X2	T49.5X3	T49.5X4	T49.5X5	T49.5X6
- topical NEC	T49.0X1	T49.0X2	T49.0X3	T49.0X4	T49.0X5	T49.0X6
Corynebacterium parvum	T45.1X1	T45.1X2	T45.1X3	T45.1X4	T45.1X5	T45.1X6
Cosmetic preparation	T49.8X1	T49.8X2	T49.8X3	T49.8X4	T49.8X5	T49.8X6
Cosmetics	T49.8X1	T49.8X2	T49.8X3	T49.8X4	T49.8X5	T49.8X6
Cosyntropin	T38.811	T38.812	T38.813	T38.814	T38.815	T38.816
Cotarnine	T45.7X1	T45.7X2	T45.7X3	T45.7X4	T45.7X5	T45.7X6
Co-trimoxazole	T36.8X1	T36.8X2	T36.8X3	T36.8X4	T36.8X5	T36.8X6
Cottonseed oil	T49.3X1	T49.3X2	T49.3X3	T49.3X4	T49.3X5	T49.3X6
Cough mixture (syrup)	T48.4X1	T48.4X2	T48.4X3	T48.4X4	T48.4X5	T48.4X6
- containing opiates	T40.2X1	T40.2X2	T40.2X3	T40.2X4	T40.2X5	T40.2X6
- expectorants	T48.4X1	T48.4X2	T48.4X3	T48.4X4	T48.4X5	T48.4X6
Coumadin	T45.511	T45.512	T45.513	T45.514	T45.515	T45.516

Substance	Poisoning, Accidental (unintentional)	Poisoning, Intentional Self-harm	Poisoning, Assault	Poisoning, Undetermined	Adverse effect	Underdosing
- rodenticide	T60.4X1	T60.4X2	T60.4X3	T60.4X4	--	--
Coumaphos	T60.0X1	T60.0X2	T60.0X3	T60.0X4	--	--
Coumarin	T45.511	T45.512	T45.513	T45.514	T45.515	T45.516
Coumetarol	T45.511	T45.512	T45.513	T45.514	T45.515	T45.516
Cowbane	T62.2X1	T62.2X2	T62.2X3	T62.2X4	--	--
Cozyme	T45.2X1	T45.2X2	T45.2X3	T45.2X4	T45.2X5	T45.2X6
Crack	T40.5X1	T40.5X2	T40.5X3	T40.5X4	--	--
Crataegus extract	T46.0X1	T46.0X2	T46.0X3	T46.0X4	T46.0X5	T46.0X6
Creolin	T54.1X1	T54.1X2	T54.1X3	T54.1X4	--	--
- disinfectant	T54.1X1	T54.1X2	T54.1X3	T54.1X4	--	--
Creosol (compound)	T49.0X1	T49.0X2	T49.0X3	T49.0X4	T49.0X5	T49.0X6
Creosote (coal tar) (beechwood)	T49.0X1	T49.0X2	T49.0X3	T49.0X4	T49.0X5	T49.0X6
- medicinal (expectorant)	T48.4X1	T48.4X2	T48.4X3	T48.4X4	T48.4X5	T48.4X6
- syrup	T48.4X1	T48.4X2	T48.4X3	T48.4X4	T48.4X5	T48.4X6
Cresol (s)	T49.0X1	T49.0X2	T49.0X3	T49.0X4	T49.0X5	T49.0X6
- and soap solution	T49.0X1	T49.0X2	T49.0X3	T49.0X4	T49.0X5	T49.0X6
Cresyl acetate	T49.0X1	T49.0X2	T49.0X3	T49.0X4	T49.0X5	T49.0X6
Cresylic acid	T49.0X1	T49.0X2	T49.0X3	T49.0X4	T49.0X5	T49.0X6
Crimidine	T60.4X1	T60.4X2	T60.4X3	T60.4X4	--	--
Croconazole	T37.8X1	T37.8X2	T37.8X3	T37.8X4	T37.8X5	T37.8X6
Cromoglicic acid	T48.6X1	T48.6X2	T48.6X3	T48.6X4	T48.6X5	T48.6X6
Cromolyn	T48.6X1	T48.6X2	T48.6X3	T48.6X4	T48.6X5	T48.6X6
Cromonar	T46.3X1	T46.3X2	T46.3X3	T46.3X4	T46.3X5	T46.3X6
Cropropamide	T39.8X1	T39.8X2	T39.8X3	T39.8X4	T39.8X5	T39.8X6
- with crotethamide	T50.7X1	T50.7X2	T50.7X3	T50.7X4	T50.7X5	T50.7X6
Crotamiton	T49.0X1	T49.0X2	T49.0X3	T49.0X4	T49.0X5	T49.0X6
Crotethamide	T39.8X1	T39.8X2	T39.8X3	T39.8X4	T39.8X5	T39.8X6
- with cropropamide	T50.7X1	T50.7X2	T50.7X3	T50.7X4	T50.7X5	T50.7X6
Croton (oil)	T47.2X1	T47.2X2	T47.2X3	T47.2X4	T47.2X5	T47.2X6
- chloral	T42.6X1	T42.6X2	T42.6X3	T42.6X4	T42.6X5	T42.6X6
Crude oil	T52.0X1	T52.0X2	T52.0X3	T52.0X4	--	--
Cryogenine	T39.8X1	T39.8X2	T39.8X3	T39.8X4	T39.8X5	T39.8X6
Cryolite (vapor)	T60.1X1	T60.1X2	T60.1X3	T60.1X4	--	--
- insecticide	T60.1X1	T60.1X2	T60.1X3	T60.1X4	--	--
Cryptenamine (tannates)	T46.5X1	T46.5X2	T46.5X3	T46.5X4	T46.5X5	T46.5X6
Crystal violet	T49.0X1	T49.0X2	T49.0X3	T49.0X4	T49.0X5	T49.0X6
Cuckoopint	T62.2X1	T62.2X2	T62.2X3	T62.2X4	--	--
Cumetharol	T45.511	T45.512	T45.513	T45.514	T45.515	T45.516
Cupric						
- acetate	T60.3X1	T60.3X2	T60.3X3	T60.3X4	--	--
- acetoarsenite	T57.0X1	T57.0X2	T57.0X3	T57.0X4	--	--
- arsenate	T57.0X1	T57.0X2	T57.0X3	T57.0X4	--	--
- gluconate	T49.0X1	T49.0X2	T49.0X3	T49.0X4	T49.0X5	T49.0X6
- oleate	T49.0X1	T49.0X2	T49.0X3	T49.0X4	T49.0X5	T49.0X6
- sulfate	T56.4X1	T56.4X2	T56.4X3	T56.4X4	--	--
Cuprous sulfate—see also Copper sulfate	T56.4X1	T56.4X2	T56.4X3	T56.4X4	--	--
Curare, curarine	T48.1X1	T48.1X2	T48.1X3	T48.1X4	T48.1X5	T48.1X6
Cyamemazine	T43.3X1	T43.3X2	T43.3X3	T43.3X4	T43.3X5	T43.3X6
Cyamopsis tetragono-loba	T46.6X1	T46.6X2	T46.6X3	T46.6X4	T46.6X5	T46.6X6
Cyanacetyl hydrazide	T37.1X1	T37.1X2	T37.1X3	T37.1X4	T37.1X5	T37.1X6
Cyanic acid (gas)	T59.891	T59.892	T59.893	T59.894	--	--
Cyanide (s) (compounds) (potassium) (sodium) NEC	T65.0X1	T65.0X2	T65.0X3	T65.0X4	--	--
- dust or gas (inhalation) NEC	T57.3X1	T57.3X2	T57.3X3	T57.3X4	--	--
- fumigant	T65.0X1	T65.0X2	T65.0X3	T65.0X4	--	--
- hydrogen	T57.3X1	T57.3X2	T57.3X3	T57.3X4	--	--
- mercuric—see Mercury						
- pesticide (dust) (fumes)	T65.0X1	T65.0X2	T65.0X3	T65.0X4	--	--
Cyanoacrylate adhesive	T49.3X1	T49.3X2	T49.3X3	T49.3X4	T49.3X5	T49.3X6

Substance	Poisoning, Accidental (unintentional)	Poisoning, Intentional Self-harm	Poisoning, Assault	Poisoning, Undetermined	Adverse effect	Underdosing
Cyanocobalamin	T45.8X1	T45.8X2	T45.8X3	T45.8X4	T45.8X5	T45.8X6
Cyanogen (chloride) (gas) NEC	T59.891	T59.892	T59.893	T59.894	--	--
Cyclacillin	T36.0X1	T36.0X2	T36.0X3	T36.0X4	T36.0X5	T36.0X6
Cyclaine	T41.3X1	T41.3X2	T41.3X3	T41.3X4	T41.3X5	T41.3X6
Cyclamate	T50.991	T50.992	T50.993	T50.994	T50.995	T50.996
Cyclamen europaeum	T62.2X1	T62.2X2	T62.2X3	T62.2X4	--	--
Cyclandelate	T46.7X1	T46.7X2	T46.7X3	T46.7X4	T46.7X5	T46.7X6
Cyclazocine	T50.7X1	T50.7X2	T50.7X3	T50.7X4	T50.7X5	T50.7X6
Cyclizine	T45.0X1	T45.0X2	T45.0X3	T45.0X4	T45.0X5	T45.0X6
Cyclobarbital	T42.3X1	T42.3X2	T42.3X3	T42.3X4	T42.3X5	T42.3X6
Cyclobarbitone	T42.3X1	T42.3X2	T42.3X3	T42.3X4	T42.3X5	T42.3X6
Cyclobenzaprine	T48.1X1	T48.1X2	T48.1X3	T48.1X4	T48.1X5	T48.1X6
Cyclodrine	T44.3X1	T44.3X2	T44.3X3	T44.3X4	T44.3X5	T44.3X6
Cycloguanil embonate	T37.2X1	T37.2X2	T37.2X3	T37.2X4	T37.2X5	T37.2X6
Cyclohexane	T52.8X1	T52.8X2	T52.8X3	T52.8X4	--	--
Cyclohexanol	T51.8X1	T51.8X2	T51.8X3	T51.8X4	--	--
Cyclohexanone	T52.4X1	T52.4X2	T52.4X3	T52.4X4	--	--
Cycloheximide	T60.3X1	T60.3X2	T60.3X3	T60.3X4	--	--
Cyclohexyl acetate	T52.8X1	T52.8X2	T52.8X3	T52.8X4	--	--
Cycloleucin	T45.1X1	T45.1X2	T45.1X3	T45.1X4	T45.1X5	T45.1X6
Cyclomethycaine	T41.3X1	T41.3X2	T41.3X3	T41.3X4	T41.3X5	T41.3X6
Cyclopentamine	T44.4X1	T44.4X2	T44.4X3	T44.4X4	T44.4X5	T44.4X6
Cyclopenthiazide	T50.2X1	T50.2X2	T50.2X3	T50.2X4	T50.2X5	T50.2X6
Cyclopentolate	T44.3X1	T44.3X2	T44.3X3	T44.3X4	T44.3X5	T44.3X6
Cyclophosphamide	T45.1X1	T45.1X2	T45.1X3	T45.1X4	T45.1X5	T45.1X6
Cycloplegic drug	T49.5X1	T49.5X2	T49.5X3	T49.5X4	T49.5X5	T49.5X6
Cyclopropane	T41.291	T41.292	T41.293	T41.294	T41.295	T41.296
Cyclopyrabital	T39.8X1	T39.8X2	T39.8X3	T39.8X4	T39.8X5	T39.8X6
Cycloserine	T37.1X1	T37.1X2	T37.1X3	T37.1X4	T37.1X5	T37.1X6
Cyclosporin	T45.1X1	T45.1X2	T45.1X3	T45.1X4	T45.1X5	T45.1X6
Cyclothiazide	T50.2X1	T50.2X2	T50.2X3	T50.2X4	T50.2X5	T50.2X6
Cycrimine	T44.3X1	T44.3X2	T44.3X3	T44.3X4	T44.3X5	T44.3X6
Cyhalothrin	T60.1X1	T60.1X2	T60.1X3	T60.1X4	--	--
Cymarin	T46.0X1	T46.0X2	T46.0X3	T46.0X4	T46.0X5	T46.0X6
Cypermethrin	T60.1X1	T60.1X2	T60.1X3	T60.1X4	--	--
Cyphenothrin	T60.2X1	T60.2X2	T60.2X3	T60.2X4	--	--
Cyproheptadine	T45.0X1	T45.0X2	T45.0X3	T45.0X4	T45.0X5	T45.0X6
Cyproterone	T38.6X1	T38.6X2	T38.6X3	T38.6X4	T38.6X5	T38.6X6
Cysteamine	T50.6X1	T50.6X2	T50.6X3	T50.6X4	T50.6X5	T50.6X6
Cytarabine	T45.1X1	T45.1X2	T45.1X3	T45.1X4	T45.1X5	T45.1X6
Cytisus						
- laburnum	T62.2X1	T62.2X2	T62.2X3	T62.2X4	--	--
- scoparius	T62.2X1	T62.2X2	T62.2X3	T62.2X4	--	--
Cytochrome C	T47.5X1	T47.5X2	T47.5X3	T47.5X4	T47.5X5	T47.5X6
Cytomel	T38.1X1	T38.1X2	T38.1X3	T38.1X4	T38.1X5	T38.1X6
Cytosine arabinoside	T45.1X1	T45.1X2	T45.1X3	T45.1X4	T45.1X5	T45.1X6
Cytoxan	T45.1X1	T45.1X2	T45.1X3	T45.1X4	T45.1X5	T45.1X6
Cytozyme	T45.7X1	T45.7X2	T45.7X3	T45.7X4	T45.7X5	T45.7X6
2,4-D	T60.3X1	T60.3X2	T60.3X3	T60.3X4	--	--
Dacarbazine	T45.1X1	T45.1X2	T45.1X3	T45.1X4	T45.1X5	T45.1X6
Dactinomycin	T45.1X1	T45.1X2	T45.1X3	T45.1X4	T45.1X5	T45.1X6
DADPS	T37.1X1	T37.1X2	T37.1X3	T37.1X4	T37.1X5	T37.1X6
Dakin's solution	T49.0X1	T49.0X2	T49.0X3	T49.0X4	T49.0X5	T49.0X6
Dalapon (sodium)	T60.3X1	T60.3X2	T60.3X3	T60.3X4	--	--
Dalmane	T42.4X1	T42.4X2	T42.4X3	T42.4X4	T42.4X5	T42.4X6
Danazol	T38.6X1	T38.6X2	T38.6X3	T38.6X4	T38.6X5	T38.6X6
Danilone	T45.511	T45.512	T45.513	T45.514	T45.515	T45.516
Danthron	T47.2X1	T47.2X2	T47.2X3	T47.2X4	T47.2X5	T47.2X6

Substance	Poisoning, Accidental (unintentional)	Poisoning, Intentional Self-harm	Poisoning, Assault	Poisoning, Undetermined	Adverse effect	Underdosing
Dantrolene	T42.8X1	T42.8X2	T42.8X3	T42.8X4	T42.8X5	T42.8X6
Dantron	T47.2X1	T47.2X2	T47.2X3	T47.2X4	T47.2X5	T47.2X6
Daphne (gnidium) (mezereum)	T62.2X1	T62.2X2	T62.2X3	T62.2X4	--	--
- berry	T62.1X1	T62.1X2	T62.1X3	T62.1X4	--	--
Dapsone	T37.1X1	T37.1X2	T37.1X3	T37.1X4	T37.1X5	T37.1X6
Daraprim	T37.2X1	T37.2X2	T37.2X3	T37.2X4	T37.2X5	T37.2X6
Darnel	T62.2X1	T62.2X2	T62.2X3	T62.2X4	--	--
Darvon	T39.8X1	T39.8X2	T39.8X3	T39.8X4	T39.8X5	T39.8X6
Daunomycin	T45.1X1	T45.1X2	T45.1X3	T45.1X4	T45.1X5	T45.1X6
Daunorubicin	T45.1X1	T45.1X2	T45.1X3	T45.1X4	T45.1X5	T45.1X6
DBI	T38.3X1	T38.3X2	T38.3X3	T38.3X4	T38.3X5	T38.3X6
D-Con	T60.91	T60.92	T60.93	T60.94	--	--
- insecticide	T60.2X1	T60.2X2	T60.2X3	T60.2X4	--	--
- rodenticide	T60.4X1	T60.4X2	T60.4X3	T60.4X4	--	--
DDAVP	T38.891	T38.892	T38.893	T38.894	T38.895	T38.896
DDE (bis (chlorophenyl) -dichloroethylene)	T60.2X1	T60.2X2	T60.2X3	T60.2X4	--	--
DDS	T37.1X1	T37.1X2	T37.1X3	T37.1X4	T37.1X5	T37.1X6
DDT (dust)	T60.1X1	T60.1X2	T60.1X3	T60.1X4	--	--
Deadly nightshade—see also Belladonna	T62.2X1	T62.2X2	T62.2X3	T62.2X4	--	--
- berry	T62.1X1	T62.1X2	T62.1X3	T62.1X4	--	--
Deamino-D-arginine vasopressin	T38.891	T38.892	T38.893	T38.894	T38.895	T38.896
Deanol (aceglumate)	T50.991	T50.992	T50.993	T50.994	T50.995	T50.996
Debrisoquine	T46.5X1	T46.5X2	T46.5X3	T46.5X4	T46.5X5	T46.5X6
Decaborane	T57.8X1	T57.8X2	T57.8X3	T57.8X4	--	--
- fumes	T59.891	T59.892	T59.893	T59.894	--	--
Decadron	T38.0X1	T38.0X2	T38.0X3	T38.0X4	T38.0X5	T38.0X6
- ENT agent	T49.6X1	T49.6X2	T49.6X3	T49.6X4	T49.6X5	T49.6X6
- ophthalmic preparation	T49.5X1	T49.5X2	T49.5X3	T49.5X4	T49.5X5	T49.5X6
- topical NEC	T49.0X1	T49.0X2	T49.0X3	T49.0X4	T49.0X5	T49.0X6
Decahydronaphthalene	T52.8X1	T52.8X2	T52.8X3	T52.8X4	--	--
Decalin	T52.8X1	T52.8X2	T52.8X3	T52.8X4	--	--
Decamethonium (bromide)	T48.1X1	T48.1X2	T48.1X3	T48.1X4	T48.1X5	T48.1X6
Decholin	T47.5X1	T47.5X2	T47.5X3	T47.5X4	T47.5X5	T47.5X6
Declomycin	T36.4X1	T36.4X2	T36.4X3	T36.4X4	T36.4X5	T36.4X6
Decongestant, nasal (mucosa)	T48.5X1	T48.5X2	T48.5X3	T48.5X4	T48.5X5	T48.5X6
- combination	T48.5X1	T48.5X2	T48.5X3	T48.5X4	T48.5X5	T48.5X6
Deet	T60.8X1	T60.8X2	T60.8X3	T60.8X4	--	--
Deferoxamine	T45.8X1	T45.8X2	T45.8X3	T45.8X4	T45.8X5	T45.8X6
Deflazacort	T38.0X1	T38.0X2	T38.0X3	T38.0X4	T38.0X5	T38.0X6
Deglycyrrhizinized extract of licorice	T48.4X1	T48.4X2	T48.4X3	T48.4X4	T48.4X5	T48.4X6
Dehydrocholic acid	T47.5X1	T47.5X2	T47.5X3	T47.5X4	T47.5X5	T47.5X6
Dehydroemetine	T37.3X1	T37.3X2	T37.3X3	T37.3X4	T37.3X5	T37.3X6
Dekalin	T52.8X1	T52.8X2	T52.8X3	T52.8X4	--	--
Delalutin	T38.5X1	T38.5X2	T38.5X3	T38.5X4	T38.5X5	T38.5X6
Delorazepam	T42.4X1	T42.4X2	T42.4X3	T42.4X4	T42.4X5	T42.4X6
Delphinium	T62.2X1	T62.2X2	T62.2X3	T62.2X4	--	--
Deltamethrin	T60.1X1	T60.1X2	T60.1X3	T60.1X4	--	--
Deltasone	T38.0X1	T38.0X2	T38.0X3	T38.0X4	T38.0X5	T38.0X6
Deltra	T38.0X1	T38.0X2	T38.0X3	T38.0X4	T38.0X5	T38.0X6
Delvinal	T42.3X1	T42.3X2	T42.3X3	T42.3X4	T42.3X5	T42.3X6
Demecarium (bromide)	T49.5X1	T49.5X2	T49.5X3	T49.5X4	T49.5X5	T49.5X6
Demeclocycline	T36.4X1	T36.4X2	T36.4X3	T36.4X4	T36.4X5	T36.4X6
Demecolcine	T45.1X1	T45.1X2	T45.1X3	T45.1X4	T45.1X5	T45.1X6
Demegestone	T38.5X1	T38.5X2	T38.5X3	T38.5X4	T38.5X5	T38.5X6
Demelanizing agents	T49.8X1	T49.8X2	T49.8X3	T49.8X4	T49.8X5	T49.8X6
Demephion -O and -S	T60.0X1	T60.0X2	T60.0X3	T60.0X4	--	--
Demerol	T40.2X1	T40.2X2	T40.2X3	T40.2X4	T40.2X5	T40.2X6
Demethylchlortetracycline	T36.4X1	T36.4X2	T36.4X3	T36.4X4	T36.4X5	T36.4X6
Demethyltetracycline	T36.4X1	T36.4X2	T36.4X3	T36.4X4	T36.4X5	T36.4X6

Substance	Poisoning, Accidental (unintentional)	Poisoning, Intentional Self-harm	Poisoning, Assault	Poisoning, Undetermined	Adverse effect	Underdosing
Demeton -O and -S	T60.0X1	T60.0X2	T60.0X3	T60.0X4	--	--
Demulcent (external)	T49.3X1	T49.3X2	T49.3X3	T49.3X4	T49.3X5	T49.3X6
- specified NEC	T49.3X1	T49.3X2	T49.3X3	T49.3X4	T49.3X5	T49.3X6
Demulen	T38.4X1	T38.4X2	T38.4X3	T38.4X4	T38.4X5	T38.4X6
Denatured alcohol	T51.0X1	T51.0X2	T51.0X3	T51.0X4	--	--
Dendrid	T49.5X1	T49.5X2	T49.5X3	T49.5X4	T49.5X5	T49.5X6
Dental drug, topical application NEC	T49.7X1	T49.7X2	T49.7X3	T49.7X4	T49.7X5	T49.7X6
Dentifrice	T49.7X1	T49.7X2	T49.7X3	T49.7X4	T49.7X5	T49.7X6
Deodorant spray (feminine hygiene)	T49.8X1	T49.8X2	T49.8X3	T49.8X4	T49.8X5	T49.8X6
Deoxycortone	T50.0X1	T50.0X2	T50.0X3	T50.0X4	T50.0X5	T50.0X6
2-Deoxy-5-fluorouridine	T45.1X1	T45.1X2	T45.1X3	T45.1X4	T45.1X5	T45.1X6
5-Deoxy-5-fluorouridine	T45.1X1	T45.1X2	T45.1X3	T45.1X4	T45.1X5	T45.1X6
Deoxyribonuclease (pancreatic)	T45.3X1	T45.3X2	T45.3X3	T45.3X4	T45.3X5	T45.3X6
Depilatory	T49.4X1	T49.4X2	T49.4X3	T49.4X4	T49.4X5	T49.4X6
Deprenalin	T42.8X1	T42.8X2	T42.8X3	T42.8X4	T42.8X5	T42.8X6
Deprenyl	T42.8X1	T42.8X2	T42.8X3	T42.8X4	T42.8X5	T42.8X6
Depressant, appetite	T50.5X1	T50.5X2	T50.5X3	T50.5X4	T50.5X5	T50.5X6
Depressant						
- appetite (central)	T50.5X1	T50.5X2	T50.5X3	T50.5X4	T50.5X5	T50.5X6
- cardiac	T46.2X1	T46.2X2	T46.2X3	T46.2X4	T46.2X5	T46.2X6
central nervous system (anesthetic) —see also Central nervous system, depressants	T42.71	T42.72	T42.73	T42.74	T42.75	T42.76
- - general anesthetic	T41.201	T41.202	T41.203	T41.204	T41.205	T41.206
- - muscle tone	T42.8X1	T42.8X2	T42.8X3	T42.8X4	T42.8X5	T42.8X6
- muscle tone, central	T42.8X1	T42.8X2	T42.8X3	T42.8X4	T42.8X5	T42.8X6
- psychotherapeutic	T43.501	T43.502	T43.503	T43.504	T43.505	T43.506
Deptropine	T45.0X1	T45.0X2	T45.0X3	T45.0X4	T45.0X5	T45.0X6
Dequalinium (chloride)	T49.0X1	T49.0X2	T49.0X3	T49.0X4	T49.0X5	T49.0X6
Derris root	T60.2X1	T60.2X2	T60.2X3	T60.2X4	--	--
Deserpidine	T46.5X1	T46.5X2	T46.5X3	T46.5X4	T46.5X5	T46.5X6
Desferrioxamine	T45.8X1	T45.8X2	T45.8X3	T45.8X4	T45.8X5	T45.8X6
Desipramine	T43.011	T43.012	T43.013	T43.014	T43.015	T43.016
Deslanoside	T46.0X1	T46.0X2	T46.0X3	T46.0X4	T46.0X5	T46.0X6
Desloughing agent	T49.4X1	T49.4X2	T49.4X3	T49.4X4	T49.4X5	T49.4X6
Desmethylimipramine	T43.011	T43.012	T43.013	T43.014	T43.015	T43.016
Desmopressin	T38.891	T38.892	T38.893	T38.894	T38.895	T38.896
Desocodeine	T40.2X1	T40.2X2	T40.2X3	T40.2X4	T40.2X5	T40.2X6
Desogestrel	T38.5X1	T38.5X2	T38.5X3	T38.5X4	T38.5X5	T38.5X6
Desomorphine	T40.2X1	T40.2X2	T40.2X3	T40.2X4	--	--
Desonide	T49.0X1	T49.0X2	T49.0X3	T49.0X4	T49.0X5	T49.0X6
Desoximetasone	T49.0X1	T49.0X2	T49.0X3	T49.0X4	T49.0X5	T49.0X6
Desoxycorticosteroid	T50.0X1	T50.0X2	T50.0X3	T50.0X4	T50.0X5	T50.0X6
Desoxycortone	T50.0X1	T50.0X2	T50.0X3	T50.0X4	T50.0X5	T50.0X6
Desoxyephedrine	T43.621	T43.622	T43.623	T43.624	T43.625	T43.626
Detaxtran	T46.6X1	T46.6X2	T46.6X3	T46.6X4	T46.6X5	T46.6X6
Detergent	T49.2X1	T49.2X2	T49.2X3	T49.2X4	T49.2X5	T49.2X6
- external medication	T49.2X1	T49.2X2	T49.2X3	T49.2X4	T49.2X5	T49.2X6
- local	T49.2X1	T49.2X2	T49.2X3	T49.2X4	T49.2X5	T49.2X6
- medicinal	T49.2X1	T49.2X2	T49.2X3	T49.2X4	T49.2X5	T49.2X6
- nonmedicinal	T55.1X1	T55.1X2	T55.1X3	T55.1X4	--	--
- specified NEC	T55.1X1	T55.1X2	T55.1X3	T55.1X4	--	--
Deterrent, alcohol	T50.6X1	T50.6X2	T50.6X3	T50.6X4	T50.6X5	T50.6X6
Detoxifying agent	T50.6X1	T50.6X2	T50.6X3	T50.6X4	T50.6X5	T50.6X6
Detrothyronine	T38.1X1	T38.1X2	T38.1X3	T38.1X4	T38.1X5	T38.1X6
Dettol (external medication)	T49.0X1	T49.0X2	T49.0X3	T49.0X4	T49.0X5	T49.0X6
Dexamethasone	T38.0X1	T38.0X2	T38.0X3	T38.0X4	T38.0X5	T38.0X6
- ENT agent	T49.6X1	T49.6X2	T49.6X3	T49.6X4	T49.6X5	T49.6X6
- ophthalmic preparation	T49.5X1	T49.5X2	T49.5X3	T49.5X4	T49.5X5	T49.5X6

Substance	Poisoning, Accidental (unintentional)	Poisoning, Intentional Self-harm	Poisoning, Assault	Poisoning, Undetermined	Adverse effect	Underdosing
- topical NEC	T49.0X1	T49.0X2	T49.0X3	T49.0X4	T49.0X5	T49.0X6
Dexamfetamine	T43.621	T43.622	T43.623	T43.624	T43.625	T43.626
Dexamphetamine	T43.621	T43.622	T43.623	T43.624	T43.625	T43.626
Dexbrompheniramine	T45.0X1	T45.0X2	T45.0X3	T45.0X4	T45.0X5	T45.0X6
Dexchlorpheniramine	T45.0X1	T45.0X2	T45.0X3	T45.0X4	T45.0X5	T45.0X6
Dexedrine	T43.621	T43.622	T43.623	T43.624	T43.625	T43.626
Dexetimide	T44.3X1	T44.3X2	T44.3X3	T44.3X4	T44.3X5	T44.3X6
Dexfenfluramine	T50.5X1	T50.5X2	T50.5X3	T50.5X4	T50.5X5	T50.5X6
Dexpanthenol	T45.2X1	T45.2X2	T45.2X3	T45.2X4	T45.2X5	T45.2X6
Dextran (40) (70) (150)	T45.8X1	T45.8X2	T45.8X3	T45.8X4	T45.8X5	T45.8X6
Dextriferron	T45.4X1	T45.4X2	T45.4X3	T45.4X4	T45.4X5	T45.4X6
Dextro calcium pantothenate	T45.2X1	T45.2X2	T45.2X3	T45.2X4	T45.2X5	T45.2X6
Dextro pantothenyl alcohol	T45.2X1	T45.2X2	T45.2X3	T45.2X4	T45.2X5	T45.2X6
Dextroamphetamine	T43.621	T43.622	T43.623	T43.624	T43.625	T43.626
Dextromethorphan	T48.3X1	T48.3X2	T48.3X3	T48.3X4	T48.3X5	T48.3X6
Dextromoramide	T40.491	T40.492	T40.493	T40.494	--	--
- topical	T49.8X1	T49.8X2	T49.8X3	T49.8X4	T49.8X5	T49.8X6
Dextropropoxyphene	T40.491	T40.492	T40.493	T40.494	T40.495	T40.496
Dextrorphan	T40.2X1	T40.2X2	T40.2X3	T40.2X4	T40.2X5	T40.2X6
Dextrose	T50.3X1	T50.3X2	T50.3X3	T50.3X4	T50.3X5	T50.3X6
- concentrated solution, intravenous	T46.8X1	T46.8X2	T46.8X3	T46.8X4	T46.8X5	T46.8X6
Dextrothyroxin	T38.1X1	T38.1X2	T38.1X3	T38.1X4	T38.1X5	T38.1X6
Dextrothyroxine sodium	T38.1X1	T38.1X2	T38.1X3	T38.1X4	T38.1X5	T38.1X6
DFP	T44.0X1	T44.0X2	T44.0X3	T44.0X4	T44.0X5	T44.0X6
DHE	T37.3X1	T37.3X2	T37.3X3	T37.3X4	T37.3X5	T37.3X6
- 45	T46.5X1	T46.5X2	T46.5X3	T46.5X4	T46.5X5	T46.5X6
Diabinese	T38.3X1	T38.3X2	T38.3X3	T38.3X4	T38.3X5	T38.3X6
Diacetone alcohol	T52.4X1	T52.4X2	T52.4X3	T52.4X4	--	--
Diacetyl monoxime	T50.991	T50.992	T50.993	T50.994	--	--
Diacetylmorphine	T40.1X1	T40.1X2	T40.1X3	T40.1X4	T40.1X5	--
Diachylon plaster	T49.4X1	T49.4X2	T49.4X3	T49.4X4	T49.4X5	T49.4X6
Diaethylstilboestrolum	T38.5X1	T38.5X2	T38.5X3	T38.5X4	T38.5X5	T38.5X6
Diagnostic agent NEC	T50.8X1	T50.8X2	T50.8X3	T50.8X4	T50.8X5	T50.8X6
Dial (soap)	T49.2X1	T49.2X2	T49.2X3	T49.2X4	T49.2X5	T49.2X6
- sedative	T42.3X1	T42.3X2	T42.3X3	T42.3X4	T42.3X5	T42.3X6
Dialkyl carbonate	T52.91	T52.92	T52.93	T52.94	--	--
Diallylbarbituric acid	T42.3X1	T42.3X2	T42.3X3	T42.3X4	T42.3X5	T42.3X6
Diallymal	T42.3X1	T42.3X2	T42.3X3	T42.3X4	T42.3X5	T42.3X6
Dialysis solution (intraperitoneal)	T50.3X1	T50.3X2	T50.3X3	T50.3X4	T50.3X5	T50.3X6
Diaminodiphenylsulfone	T37.1X1	T37.1X2	T37.1X3	T37.1X4	T37.1X5	T37.1X6
Diamorphine	T40.1X1	T40.1X2	T40.1X3	T40.1X4	T40.1X5	--
Diamox	T50.2X1	T50.2X2	T50.2X3	T50.2X4	T50.2X5	T50.2X6
Diamthazole	T49.0X1	T49.0X2	T49.0X3	T49.0X4	T49.0X5	T49.0X6
Dianthone	T47.2X1	T47.2X2	T47.2X3	T47.2X4	T47.2X5	T47.2X6
Diaphenylsulfone	T37.0X1	T37.0X2	T37.0X3	T37.0X4	T37.0X5	T37.0X6
Diasone (sodium)	T37.1X1	T37.1X2	T37.1X3	T37.1X4	T37.1X5	T37.1X6
Diastase	T47.5X1	T47.5X2	T47.5X3	T47.5X4	T47.5X5	T47.5X6
Diatrizoate	T50.8X1	T50.8X2	T50.8X3	T50.8X4	T50.8X5	T50.8X6
Diazepam	T42.4X1	T42.4X2	T42.4X3	T42.4X4	T42.4X5	T42.4X6
Diazinon	T60.0X1	T60.0X2	T60.0X3	T60.0X4	--	--
Diazomethane (gas)	T59.891	T59.892	T59.893	T59.894	--	--
Diazoxide	T46.5X1	T46.5X2	T46.5X3	T46.5X4	T46.5X5	T46.5X6
Dibekacin	T36.5X1	T36.5X2	T36.5X3	T36.5X4	T36.5X5	T36.5X6
Dibenamine	T44.6X1	T44.6X2	T44.6X3	T44.6X4	T44.6X5	T44.6X6
Dibenzepin	T43.011	T43.012	T43.013	T43.014	T43.015	T43.016
Dibenzheptropine	T45.0X1	T45.0X2	T45.0X3	T45.0X4	T45.0X5	T45.0X6
Dibenzyline	T44.6X1	T44.6X2	T44.6X3	T44.6X4	T44.6X5	T44.6X6
Diborane (gas)	T59.891	T59.892	T59.893	T59.894	--	--
Dibromochloropropane	T60.8X1	T60.8X2	T60.8X3	T60.8X4	--	--

Substance	Poisoning, Accidental (unintentional)	Poisoning, Intentional Self-harm	Poisoning, Assault	Poisoning, Undetermined	Adverse effect	Underdosing
Dibromodulcitol	T45.1X1	T45.1X2	T45.1X3	T45.1X4	T45.1X5	T45.1X6
Dibromoethane	T53.6X1	T53.6X2	T53.6X3	T53.6X4	--	--
Dibromomannitol	T45.1X1	T45.1X2	T45.1X3	T45.1X4	T45.1X5	T45.1X6
Dibromopropamidine isethionate	T49.0X1	T49.0X2	T49.0X3	T49.0X4	T49.0X5	T49.0X6
Dibrompropamidine	T49.0X1	T49.0X2	T49.0X3	T49.0X4	T49.0X5	T49.0X6
Dibucaine	T41.3X1	T41.3X2	T41.3X3	T41.3X4	T41.3X5	T41.3X6
- topical (surface)	T41.3X1	T41.3X2	T41.3X3	T41.3X4	T41.3X5	T41.3X6
Dibunate sodium	T48.3X1	T48.3X2	T48.3X3	T48.3X4	T48.3X5	T48.3X6
Dibutoline sulfate	T44.3X1	T44.3X2	T44.3X3	T44.3X4	T44.3X5	T44.3X6
Dicamba	T60.3X1	T60.3X2	T60.3X3	T60.3X4	--	--
Dicapthon	T60.0X1	T60.0X2	T60.0X3	T60.0X4	--	--
Dichlobenil	T60.3X1	T60.3X2	T60.3X3	T60.3X4	--	--
Dichlone	T60.3X1	T60.3X2	T60.3X3	T60.3X4	--	--
Dichloralphenozone	T42.6X1	T42.6X2	T42.6X3	T42.6X4	T42.6X5	T42.6X6
Dichlorbenzidine	T65.3X1	T65.3X2	T65.3X3	T65.3X4	--	--
Dichlorhydrin	T52.8X1	T52.8X2	T52.8X3	T52.8X4	--	--
Dichlorhydroxyquinoline	T37.8X1	T37.8X2	T37.8X3	T37.8X4	T37.8X5	T37.8X6
Dichlorobenzene	T53.7X1	T53.7X2	T53.7X3	T53.7X4	--	--
Dichlorobenzyl alcohol	T49.6X1	T49.6X2	T49.6X3	T49.6X4	T49.6X5	T49.6X6
Dichlorodifluoromethane	T53.5X1	T53.5X2	T53.5X3	T53.5X4	--	--
Dichloroethane	T52.8X1	T52.8X2	T52.8X3	T52.8X4	--	--
Sym-Dichloroethyl ether	T53.6X1	T53.6X2	T53.6X3	T53.6X4	--	--
Dichloroethyl sulfide, not in war	T59.891	T59.892	T59.893	T59.894	--	--
Dichloroethylene	T53.6X1	T53.6X2	T53.6X3	T53.6X4	--	--
Dichloroformoxine, not in war	T59.891	T59.892	T59.893	T59.894	--	--
Dichlorohydrin, alpha-dichlorohydrin	T52.8X1	T52.8X2	T52.8X3	T52.8X4	--	--
Dichloromethane (solvent)	T53.4X1	T53.4X2	T53.4X3	T53.4X4	--	--
- vapor	T53.4X1	T53.4X2	T53.4X3	T53.4X4	--	--
Dichloronaphthoquinone	T60.3X1	T60.3X2	T60.3X3	T60.3X4	--	--
Dichlorophen	T37.4X1	T37.4X2	T37.4X3	T37.4X4	T37.4X5	T37.4X6
2,4-Dichlorophenoxyacetic acid	T60.3X1	T60.3X2	T60.3X3	T60.3X4	--	--
Dichloropropene	T60.3X1	T60.3X2	T60.3X3	T60.3X4	--	--
Dichloropropionic acid	T60.3X1	T60.3X2	T60.3X3	T60.3X4	--	--
Dichlorphenamide	T50.2X1	T50.2X2	T50.2X3	T50.2X4	T50.2X5	T50.2X6
Dichlorvos	T60.0X1	T60.0X2	T60.0X3	T60.0X4	--	--
Diclofenac	T39.391	T39.392	T39.393	T39.394	T39.395	T39.396
Diclofenamide	T50.2X1	T50.2X2	T50.2X3	T50.2X4	T50.2X5	T50.2X6
Diclofensine	T43.291	T43.292	T43.293	T43.294	T43.295	T43.296
Diclonixine	T39.8X1	T39.8X2	T39.8X3	T39.8X4	T39.8X5	T39.8X6
Dicloxacillin	T36.0X1	T36.0X2	T36.0X3	T36.0X4	T36.0X5	T36.0X6
Dicophane	T49.0X1	T49.0X2	T49.0X3	T49.0X4	T49.0X5	T49.0X6
Dicoumarol, dicoumarin, dicumarol	T45.511	T45.512	T45.513	T45.514	T45.515	T45.516
Dicrotophos	T60.0X1	T60.0X2	T60.0X3	T60.0X4	--	--
Dicyanogen (gas)	T65.0X1	T65.0X2	T65.0X3	T65.0X4	--	--
Dicyclomine	T44.3X1	T44.3X2	T44.3X3	T44.3X4	T44.3X5	T44.3X6
Dicycloverine	T44.3X1	T44.3X2	T44.3X3	T44.3X4	T44.3X5	T44.3X6
Dideoxycytidine	T37.5X1	T37.5X2	T37.5X3	T37.5X4	T37.5X5	T37.5X6
Dideoxyinosine	T37.5X1	T37.5X2	T37.5X3	T37.5X4	T37.5X5	T37.5X6
Dieldrin (vapor)	T60.1X1	T60.1X2	T60.1X3	T60.1X4	--	--
Diemal	T42.3X1	T42.3X2	T42.3X3	T42.3X4	T42.3X5	T42.3X6
Dienestrol	T38.5X1	T38.5X2	T38.5X3	T38.5X4	T38.5X5	T38.5X6
Dienoestrol	T38.5X1	T38.5X2	T38.5X3	T38.5X4	T38.5X5	T38.5X6
Dietetic drug NEC	T50.901	T50.902	T50.903	T50.904	T50.905	T50.906
Diethazine	T42.8X1	T42.8X2	T42.8X3	T42.8X4	T42.8X5	T42.8X6
Diethyl						
- barbituric acid	T42.3X1	T42.3X2	T42.3X3	T42.3X4	T42.3X5	T42.3X6
- carbamazine	T37.4X1	T37.4X2	T37.4X3	T37.4X4	T37.4X5	T37.4X6
- carbinol	T51.3X1	T51.3X2	T51.3X3	T51.3X4	--	--

Substance	Poisoning, Accidental (unintentional)	Poisoning, Intentional Self-harm	Poisoning, Assault	Poisoning, Undetermined	Adverse effect	Underdosing
- carbonate	T52.8X1	T52.8X2	T52.8X3	T52.8X4	--	--
- ether (vapor) —see also ether	T41.0X1	T41.0X2	T41.0X3	T41.0X4	T41.0X5	T41.0X6
- oxide	T52.8X1	T52.8X2	T52.8X3	T52.8X4	--	--
- propion	T50.5X1	T50.5X2	T50.5X3	T50.5X4	T50.5X5	T50.5X6
- stilbestrol	T38.5X1	T38.5X2	T38.5X3	T38.5X4	T38.5X5	T38.5X6
- toluamide (nonmedicinal)	T60.8X1	T60.8X2	T60.8X3	T60.8X4	--	--
- - medicinal	T49.3X1	T49.3X2	T49.3X3	T49.3X4	T49.3X5	T49.3X6
Diethylcarbamazine	T37.4X1	T37.4X2	T37.4X3	T37.4X4	T37.4X5	T37.4X6
Diethylene						
- dioxide	T52.8X1	T52.8X2	T52.8X3	T52.8X4	--	--
- glycol (monoacetate) (monobutyl ether) (monoethyl ether)	T52.3X1	T52.3X2	T52.3X3	T52.3X4	--	--
Diethylhexylphthalate	T65.891	T65.892	T65.893	T65.894	--	--
Diethylpropion	T50.5X1	T50.5X2	T50.5X3	T50.5X4	T50.5X5	T50.5X6
Diethylstilbestrol	T38.5X1	T38.5X2	T38.5X3	T38.5X4	T38.5X5	T38.5X6
Diethylstilboestrol	T38.5X1	T38.5X2	T38.5X3	T38.5X4	T38.5X5	T38.5X6
Diethylsulfone-diethylmethane	T42.6X1	T42.6X2	T42.6X3	T42.6X4	T42.6X5	T42.6X6
Diethyltoluamide	T49.0X1	T49.0X2	T49.0X3	T49.0X4	T49.0X5	T49.0X6
Diethyltryptamine (DET)	T40.991	T40.992	T40.993	T40.994	--	--
Difebarbamate	T42.3X1	T42.3X2	T42.3X3	T42.3X4	T42.3X5	T42.3X6
Difencloxazine	T40.2X1	T40.2X2	T40.2X3	T40.2X4	T40.2X5	T40.2X6
Difenidol	T45.0X1	T45.0X2	T45.0X3	T45.0X4	T45.0X5	T45.0X6
Difenoxin	T47.6X1	T47.6X2	T47.6X3	T47.6X4	T47.6X5	T47.6X6
Difetarsone	T37.3X1	T37.3X2	T37.3X3	T37.3X4	T37.3X5	T37.3X6
Diffusin	T45.3X1	T45.3X2	T45.3X3	T45.3X4	T45.3X5	T45.3X6
Diflorasone	T49.0X1	T49.0X2	T49.0X3	T49.0X4	T49.0X5	T49.0X6
Diflos	T44.0X1	T44.0X2	T44.0X3	T44.0X4	T44.0X5	T44.0X6
Diflubenzuron	T60.1X1	T60.1X2	T60.1X3	T60.1X4	--	--
Diflucortolone	T49.0X1	T49.0X2	T49.0X3	T49.0X4	T49.0X5	T49.0X6
Diflunisal	T39.091	T39.092	T39.093	T39.094	T39.095	T39.096
Difluoromethyldopa	T42.8X1	T42.8X2	T42.8X3	T42.8X4	T42.8X5	T42.8X6
Difluorophate	T44.0X1	T44.0X2	T44.0X3	T44.0X4	T44.0X5	T44.0X6
Digestant NEC	T47.5X1	T47.5X2	T47.5X3	T47.5X4	T47.5X5	T47.5X6
Digitalin (e)	T46.0X1	T46.0X2	T46.0X3	T46.0X4	T46.0X5	T46.0X6
Digitalis (leaf) (glycoside)	T46.0X1	T46.0X2	T46.0X3	T46.0X4	T46.0X5	T46.0X6
- lanata	T46.0X1	T46.0X2	T46.0X3	T46.0X4	T46.0X5	T46.0X6
- purpurea	T46.0X1	T46.0X2	T46.0X3	T46.0X4	T46.0X5	T46.0X6
Digitoxin	T46.0X1	T46.0X2	T46.0X3	T46.0X4	T46.0X5	T46.0X6
Digitoxose	T46.0X1	T46.0X2	T46.0X3	T46.0X4	T46.0X5	T46.0X6
Digoxin	T46.0X1	T46.0X2	T46.0X3	T46.0X4	T46.0X5	T46.0X6
Digoxine	T46.0X1	T46.0X2	T46.0X3	T46.0X4	T46.0X5	T46.0X6
Dihydralazine	T46.5X1	T46.5X2	T46.5X3	T46.5X4	T46.5X5	T46.5X6
Dihydrazine	T46.5X1	T46.5X2	T46.5X3	T46.5X4	T46.5X5	T46.5X6
Dihydrocodeine	T40.2X1	T40.2X2	T40.2X3	T40.2X4	T40.2X5	T40.2X6
Dihydrocodeinone	T40.2X1	T40.2X2	T40.2X3	T40.2X4	T40.2X5	T40.2X6
Dihydroergocornine	T46.7X1	T46.7X2	T46.7X3	T46.7X4	T46.7X5	T46.7X6
Dihydroergocristine (mesilate)	T46.7X1	T46.7X2	T46.7X3	T46.7X4	T46.7X5	T46.7X6
Dihydroergokryptine	T46.7X1	T46.7X2	T46.7X3	T46.7X4	T46.7X5	T46.7X6
Dihydroergotamine	T46.5X1	T46.5X2	T46.5X3	T46.5X4	T46.5X5	T46.5X6
Dihydroergotoxine	T46.7X1	T46.7X2	T46.7X3	T46.7X4	T46.7X5	T46.7X6
- mesilate	T46.7X1	T46.7X2	T46.7X3	T46.7X4	T46.7X5	T46.7X6
Dihydrohydroxycodeinone	T40.2X1	T40.2X2	T40.2X3	T40.2X4	T40.2X5	T40.2X6
Dihydrohydroxymorphinone	T40.2X1	T40.2X2	T40.2X3	T40.2X4	T40.2X5	T40.2X6
Dihydroisocodeine	T40.2X1	T40.2X2	T40.2X3	T40.2X4	T40.2X5	T40.2X6
Dihydromorphine	T40.2X1	T40.2X2	T40.2X3	T40.2X4	--	--
Dihydromorphinone	T40.2X1	T40.2X2	T40.2X3	T40.2X4	T40.2X5	T40.2X6
Dihydrostreptomycin	T36.5X1	T36.5X2	T36.5X3	T36.5X4	T36.5X5	T36.5X6
Dihydrotachysterol	T45.2X1	T45.2X2	T45.2X3	T45.2X4	T45.2X5	T45.2X6
Dihydroxyaluminum aminoacetate	T47.1X1	T47.1X2	T47.1X3	T47.1X4	T47.1X5	T47.1X6

Substance	Poisoning, Accidental (unintentional)	Poisoning, Intentional Self-harm	Poisoning, Assault	Poisoning, Undetermined	Adverse effect	Underdosing
Dihydroxyaluminum sodium carbonate	T47.1X1	T47.1X2	T47.1X3	T47.1X4	T47.1X5	T47.1X6
Dihydroxyanthraquinone	T47.2X1	T47.2X2	T47.2X3	T47.2X4	T47.2X5	T47.2X6
Dihydroxycodeinone	T40.2X1	T40.2X2	T40.2X3	T40.2X4	T40.2X5	T40.2X6
Dihydroxypropyl theophylline	T50.2X1	T50.2X2	T50.2X3	T50.2X4	T50.2X5	T50.2X6
Diiodohydroxyquin	T37.8X1	T37.8X2	T37.8X3	T37.8X4	T37.8X5	T37.8X6
- topical	T49.0X1	T49.0X2	T49.0X3	T49.0X4	T49.0X5	T49.0X6
Diiodohydroxyquinoline	T37.8X1	T37.8X2	T37.8X3	T37.8X4	T37.8X5	T37.8X6
Diiodotyrosine	T38.2X1	T38.2X2	T38.2X3	T38.2X4	T38.2X5	T38.2X6
Diisopromine	T44.3X1	T44.3X2	T44.3X3	T44.3X4	T44.3X5	T44.3X6
Diisopropylamine	T46.3X1	T46.3X2	T46.3X3	T46.3X4	T46.3X5	T46.3X6
Diisopropylfluorophos-phonate	T44.0X1	T44.0X2	T44.0X3	T44.0X4	T44.0X5	T44.0X6
Dilantin	T42.0X1	T42.0X2	T42.0X3	T42.0X4	T42.0X5	T42.0X6
Dilaudid	T40.2X1	T40.2X2	T40.2X3	T40.2X4	T40.2X5	T40.2X6
Dilazep	T46.3X1	T46.3X2	T46.3X3	T46.3X4	T46.3X5	T46.3X6
Dill	T47.5X1	T47.5X2	T47.5X3	T47.5X4	T47.5X5	T47.5X6
Diloxanide	T37.3X1	T37.3X2	T37.3X3	T37.3X4	T37.3X5	T37.3X6
Diltiazem	T46.1X1	T46.1X2	T46.1X3	T46.1X4	T46.1X5	T46.1X6
Dimazole	T49.0X1	T49.0X2	T49.0X3	T49.0X4	T49.0X5	T49.0X6
Dimefline	T50.7X1	T50.7X2	T50.7X3	T50.7X4	T50.7X5	T50.7X6
Dimefox	T60.0X1	T60.0X2	T60.0X3	T60.0X4	--	--
Dimemorfan	T48.3X1	T48.3X2	T48.3X3	T48.3X4	T48.3X5	T48.3X6
Dimenhydrinate	T45.0X1	T45.0X2	T45.0X3	T45.0X4	T45.0X5	T45.0X6
Dimercaprol (British anti-lewisite)	T45.8X1	T45.8X2	T45.8X3	T45.8X4	T45.8X5	T45.8X6
Dimercaptopropanol	T45.8X1	T45.8X2	T45.8X3	T45.8X4	T45.8X5	T45.8X6
Dimestrol	T38.5X1	T38.5X2	T38.5X3	T38.5X4	T38.5X5	T38.5X6
Dimetane	T45.0X1	T45.0X2	T45.0X3	T45.0X4	T45.0X5	T45.0X6
Dimethicone	T47.1X1	T47.1X2	T47.1X3	T47.1X4	T47.1X5	T47.1X6
Dimethindene	T45.0X1	T45.0X2	T45.0X3	T45.0X4	T45.0X5	T45.0X6
Dimethisoquin	T49.1X1	T49.1X2	T49.1X3	T49.1X4	T49.1X5	T49.1X6
Dimethisterone	T38.5X1	T38.5X2	T38.5X3	T38.5X4	T38.5X5	T38.5X6
Dimethoate	T60.0X1	T60.0X2	T60.0X3	T60.0X4	--	--
Dimethocaine	T41.3X1	T41.3X2	T41.3X3	T41.3X4	T41.3X5	T41.3X6
Dimethoxanate	T48.3X1	T48.3X2	T48.3X3	T48.3X4	T48.3X5	T48.3X6
Dimethyl						
- arsine, arsinic acid	T57.0X1	T57.0X2	T57.0X3	T57.0X4	--	--
- carbinol	T51.2X1	T51.2X2	T51.2X3	T51.2X4	--	--
- carbonate	T52.8X1	T52.8X2	T52.8X3	T52.8X4	--	--
- diguanide	T38.3X1	T38.3X2	T38.3X3	T38.3X4	T38.3X5	T38.3X6
- ketone	T52.4X1	T52.4X2	T52.4X3	T52.4X4	--	--
- - vapor	T52.4X1	T52.4X2	T52.4X3	T52.4X4	--	--
- meperidine	T40.2X1	T40.2X2	T40.2X3	T40.2X4	T40.2X5	T40.2X6
- parathion	T60.0X1	T60.0X2	T60.0X3	T60.0X4	--	--
- phthlate	T49.3X1	T49.3X2	T49.3X3	T49.3X4	T49.3X5	T49.3X6
- polysiloxane	T47.8X1	T47.8X2	T47.8X3	T47.8X4	T47.8X5	T47.8X6
- sulfate (fumes)	T59.891	T59.892	T59.893	T59.894	--	--
- - liquid	T65.891	T65.892	T65.893	T65.894	--	--
- sulfoxide (nonmedicinal)	T52.8X1	T52.8X2	T52.8X3	T52.8X4	--	--
- - medicinal	T49.4X1	T49.4X2	T49.4X3	T49.4X4	T49.4X5	T49.4X6
- tryptamine	T40.991	T40.992	T40.993	T40.994	--	--
- tubocurarine	T48.1X1	T48.1X2	T48.1X3	T48.1X4	T48.1X5	T48.1X6
Dimethylamine sulfate	T49.4X1	T49.4X2	T49.4X3	T49.4X4	T49.4X5	T49.4X6
Dimethylformamide	T52.8X1	T52.8X2	T52.8X3	T52.8X4	--	--
Dimethyltubocurarinium chloride	T48.1X1	T48.1X2	T48.1X3	T48.1X4	T48.1X5	T48.1X6
Dimeticone	T47.1X1	T47.1X2	T47.1X3	T47.1X4	T47.1X5	T47.1X6
Dimetilan	T60.0X1	T60.0X2	T60.0X3	T60.0X4	--	--
Dimetindene	T45.0X1	T45.0X2	T45.0X3	T45.0X4	T45.0X5	T45.0X6
Dimetotiazine	T43.3X1	T43.3X2	T43.3X3	T43.3X4	T43.3X5	T43.3X6
Dimorpholamine	T50.7X1	T50.7X2	T50.7X3	T50.7X4	T50.7X5	T50.7X6

Substance	Poisoning, Accidental (unintentional)	Poisoning, Intentional Self-harm	Poisoning, Assault	Poisoning, Undetermined	Adverse effect	Underdosing
Dimoxyline	T46.3X1	T46.3X2	T46.3X3	T46.3X4	T46.3X5	T46.3X6
Dinitrobenzene	T65.3X1	T65.3X2	T65.3X3	T65.3X4	--	--
- vapor	T59.891	T59.892	T59.893	T59.894	--	--
Dinitrobenzol	T65.3X1	T65.3X2	T65.3X3	T65.3X4	--	--
- vapor	T59.891	T59.892	T59.893	T59.894	--	--
Dinitrobutylphenol	T65.3X1	T65.3X2	T65.3X3	T65.3X4	--	--
Dinitro (-ortho-) cresol (pesticide) (spray)	T65.3X1	T65.3X2	T65.3X3	T65.3X4	--	--
Dinitrocyclohexylphenol	T65.3X1	T65.3X2	T65.3X3	T65.3X4	--	--
Dinitrophenol	T65.3X1	T65.3X2	T65.3X3	T65.3X4	--	--
Dinoprost	T48.0X1	T48.0X2	T48.0X3	T48.0X4	T48.0X5	T48.0X6
Dinoprostone	T48.0X1	T48.0X2	T48.0X3	T48.0X4	T48.0X5	T48.0X6
Dinoseb	T60.3X1	T60.3X2	T60.3X3	T60.3X4	--	--
Dioctyl sulfosuccinate (calcium) (sodium)	T47.4X1	T47.4X2	T47.4X3	T47.4X4	T47.4X5	T47.4X6
Diodone	T50.8X1	T50.8X2	T50.8X3	T50.8X4	T50.8X5	T50.8X6
Diodoquin	T37.8X1	T37.8X2	T37.8X3	T37.8X4	T37.8X5	T37.8X6
Dionin	T40.2X1	T40.2X2	T40.2X3	T40.2X4	T40.2X5	T40.2X6
Diosmin	T46.991	T46.992	T46.993	T46.994	T46.995	T46.996
Dioxane	T52.8X1	T52.8X2	T52.8X3	T52.8X4	--	--
Dioxathion	T60.0X1	T60.0X2	T60.0X3	T60.0X4	--	--
Dioxin	T53.7X1	T53.7X2	T53.7X3	T53.7X4	--	--
Dioxopromethazine	T43.3X1	T43.3X2	T43.3X3	T43.3X4	T43.3X5	T43.3X6
Dioxyline	T46.3X1	T46.3X2	T46.3X3	T46.3X4	T46.3X5	T46.3X6
Dipentene	T52.8X1	T52.8X2	T52.8X3	T52.8X4	--	--
Diperodon	T41.3X1	T41.3X2	T41.3X3	T41.3X4	T41.3X5	T41.3X6
Diphacinone	T60.4X1	T60.4X2	T60.4X3	T60.4X4	--	--
Diphemanil	T44.3X1	T44.3X2	T44.3X3	T44.3X4	T44.3X5	T44.3X6
- metilsulfate	T44.3X1	T44.3X2	T44.3X3	T44.3X4	T44.3X5	T44.3X6
Diphenadione	T45.511	T45.512	T45.513	T45.514	T45.515	T45.516
- rodenticide	T60.4X1	T60.4X2	T60.4X3	T60.4X4	--	--
Diphenhydramine	T45.0X1	T45.0X2	T45.0X3	T45.0X4	T45.0X5	T45.0X6
Diphenidol	T45.0X1	T45.0X2	T45.0X3	T45.0X4	T45.0X5	T45.0X6
Diphenoxylate	T47.6X1	T47.6X2	T47.6X3	T47.6X4	T47.6X5	T47.6X6
Diphenylamine	T65.3X1	T65.3X2	T65.3X3	T65.3X4	--	--
Diphenylbutazone	T39.2X1	T39.2X2	T39.2X3	T39.2X4	T39.2X5	T39.2X6
Diphenylchloroarsine, not in war	T57.0X1	T57.0X2	T57.0X3	T57.0X4	--	--
Diphenylhydantoin	T42.0X1	T42.0X2	T42.0X3	T42.0X4	T42.0X5	T42.0X6
Diphenylmethane dye	T52.1X1	T52.1X2	T52.1X3	T52.1X4	--	--
Diphenylpyraline	T45.0X1	T45.0X2	T45.0X3	T45.0X4	T45.0X5	T45.0X6
Diphtheria						
- antitoxin	T50.Z11	T50.Z12	T50.Z13	T50.Z14	T50.Z15	T50.Z16
- toxoid	T50.A91	T50.A92	T50.A93	T50.A94	T50.A95	T50.A96
- - with tetanus toxoid	T50.A21	T50.A22	T50.A23	T50.A24	T50.A25	T50.A26
- - - with pertussis component	T50.A11	T50.A12	T50.A13	T50.A14	T50.A15	T50.A16
- vaccine	T50.A91	T50.A92	T50.A93	T50.A94	T50.A95	T50.A96
- - combination						
- - - including pertussis	T50.A11	T50.A12	T50.A13	T50.A14	T50.A15	T50.A16
- - - without pertussis	T50.A21	T50.A22	T50.A23	T50.A24	T50.A25	T50.A26
Diphylline	T50.2X1	T50.2X2	T50.2X3	T50.2X4	T50.2X5	T50.2X6
Dipipanone	T40.491	T40.492	T40.493	T40.494	--	--
Dipivefrine	T49.5X1	T49.5X2	T49.5X3	T49.5X4	T49.5X5	T49.5X6
Diplovax	T50.B91	T50.B92	T50.B93	T50.B94	T50.B95	T50.B96
Diprophylline	T50.2X1	T50.2X2	T50.2X3	T50.2X4	T50.2X5	T50.2X6
Dipropyline	T48.291	T48.292	T48.293	T48.294	T48.295	T48.296
Dipyridamole	T46.3X1	T46.3X2	T46.3X3	T46.3X4	T46.3X5	T46.3X6
Dipyrone	T39.2X1	T39.2X2	T39.2X3	T39.2X4	T39.2X5	T39.2X6
Diquat (dibromide)	T60.3X1	T60.3X2	T60.3X3	T60.3X4	--	--
Disinfectant	T65.891	T65.892	T65.893	T65.894	--	--
- alkaline	T54.3X1	T54.3X2	T54.3X3	T54.3X4	--	--
- aromatic	T54.1X1	T54.1X2	T54.1X3	T54.1X4	--	--

Substance	Poisoning, Accidental (unintentional)	Poisoning, Intentional Self-harm	Poisoning, Assault	Poisoning, Undetermined	Adverse effect	Underdosing
- intestinal	T37.8X1	T37.8X2	T37.8X3	T37.8X4	T37.8X5	T37.8X6
Disipal	T42.8X1	T42.8X2	T42.8X3	T42.8X4	T42.8X5	T42.8X6
Disodium edetate	T50.6X1	T50.6X2	T50.6X3	T50.6X4	T50.6X5	T50.6X6
Disoprofol	T41.291	T41.292	T41.293	T41.294	T41.295	T41.296
Disopyramide	T46.2X1	T46.2X2	T46.2X3	T46.2X4	T46.2X5	T46.2X6
Distigmine (bromide)	T44.0X1	T44.0X2	T44.0X3	T44.0X4	T44.0X5	T44.0X6
Disulfamide	T50.2X1	T50.2X2	T50.2X3	T50.2X4	T50.2X5	T50.2X6
Disulfanilamide	T37.0X1	T37.0X2	T37.0X3	T37.0X4	T37.0X5	T37.0X6
Disulfiram	T50.6X1	T50.6X2	T50.6X3	T50.6X4	T50.6X5	T50.6X6
Disulfoton	T60.0X1	T60.0X2	T60.0X3	T60.0X4	--	--
Dithiazanine iodide	T37.4X1	T37.4X2	T37.4X3	T37.4X4	T37.4X5	T37.4X6
Dithiocarbamate	T60.0X1	T60.0X2	T60.0X3	T60.0X4	--	--
Dithranol	T49.4X1	T49.4X2	T49.4X3	T49.4X4	T49.4X5	T49.4X6
Diucardin	T50.2X1	T50.2X2	T50.2X3	T50.2X4	T50.2X5	T50.2X6
Diupres	T50.2X1	T50.2X2	T50.2X3	T50.2X4	T50.2X5	T50.2X6
Diuretic NEC	T50.2X1	T50.2X2	T50.2X3	T50.2X4	T50.2X5	T50.2X6
- benzothiadiazine	T50.2X1	T50.2X2	T50.2X3	T50.2X4	T50.2X5	T50.2X6
- carbonic acid anhydrase inhibitors	T50.2X1	T50.2X2	T50.2X3	T50.2X4	T50.2X5	T50.2X6
- furfuryl NEC	T50.2X1	T50.2X2	T50.2X3	T50.2X4	T50.2X5	T50.2X6
- loop (high-ceiling)	T50.1X1	T50.1X2	T50.1X3	T50.1X4	T50.1X5	T50.1X6
- mercurial NEC	T50.2X1	T50.2X2	T50.2X3	T50.2X4	T50.2X5	T50.2X6
- osmotic	T50.2X1	T50.2X2	T50.2X3	T50.2X4	T50.2X5	T50.2X6
- purine NEC	T50.2X1	T50.2X2	T50.2X3	T50.2X4	T50.2X5	T50.2X6
- saluretic NEC	T50.2X1	T50.2X2	T50.2X3	T50.2X4	T50.2X5	T50.2X6
- sulfonamide	T50.2X1	T50.2X2	T50.2X3	T50.2X4	T50.2X5	T50.2X6
- thiazide NEC	T50.2X1	T50.2X2	T50.2X3	T50.2X4	T50.2X5	T50.2X6
- xanthine	T50.2X1	T50.2X2	T50.2X3	T50.2X4	T50.2X5	T50.2X6
Diurgin	T50.2X1	T50.2X2	T50.2X3	T50.2X4	T50.2X5	T50.2X6
Diuril	T50.2X1	T50.2X2	T50.2X3	T50.2X4	T50.2X5	T50.2X6
Diuron	T60.3X1	T60.3X2	T60.3X3	T60.3X4	--	--
Divalproex	T42.6X1	T42.6X2	T42.6X3	T42.6X4	T42.6X5	T42.6X6
Divinyl ether	T41.0X1	T41.0X2	T41.0X3	T41.0X4	T41.0X5	T41.0X6
Dixanthogen	T49.0X1	T49.0X2	T49.0X3	T49.0X4	T49.0X5	T49.0X6
Dixyrazine	T43.3X1	T43.3X2	T43.3X3	T43.3X4	T43.3X5	T43.3X6
D-lysergic acid diethylamide	T40.8X1	T40.8X2	T40.8X3	T40.8X4	T40.8X5	--
DMCT	T36.4X1	T36.4X2	T36.4X3	T36.4X4	T36.4X5	T36.4X6
DMSO—see Dimethyl sulfoxide						
DNBP	T60.3X1	T60.3X2	T60.3X3	T60.3X4	--	--
DNOC	T65.3X1	T65.3X2	T65.3X3	T65.3X4	--	--
Dobutamine	T44.5X1	T44.5X2	T44.5X3	T44.5X4	T44.5X5	T44.5X6
DOCA	T38.0X1	T38.0X2	T38.0X3	T38.0X4	T38.0X5	T38.0X6
Docusate sodium	T47.4X1	T47.4X2	T47.4X3	T47.4X4	T47.4X5	T47.4X6
Dodicin	T49.0X1	T49.0X2	T49.0X3	T49.0X4	T49.0X5	T49.0X6
Dofamium chloride	T49.0X1	T49.0X2	T49.0X3	T49.0X4	T49.0X5	T49.0X6
Dolophine	T40.3X1	T40.3X2	T40.3X3	T40.3X4	T40.3X5	T40.3X6
Doloxene	T39.8X1	T39.8X2	T39.8X3	T39.8X4	T39.8X5	T39.8X6
Domestic gas (after combustion) —see Gas, utility						
- prior to combustion	T59.891	T59.892	T59.893	T59.894	--	--
Domiodol	T48.4X1	T48.4X2	T48.4X3	T48.4X4	T48.4X5	T48.4X6
Domiphen (bromide)	T49.0X1	T49.0X2	T49.0X3	T49.0X4	T49.0X5	T49.0X6
Domperidone	T45.0X1	T45.0X2	T45.0X3	T45.0X4	T45.0X5	T45.0X6
Dopa	T42.8X1	T42.8X2	T42.8X3	T42.8X4	T42.8X5	T42.8X6
Dopamine	T44.991	T44.992	T44.993	T44.994	T44.995	T44.996
Doriden	T42.6X1	T42.6X2	T42.6X3	T42.6X4	T42.6X5	T42.6X6
Dormiral	T42.3X1	T42.3X2	T42.3X3	T42.3X4	T42.3X5	T42.3X6
Dormison	T42.6X1	T42.6X2	T42.6X3	T42.6X4	T42.6X5	T42.6X6
Dornase	T48.4X1	T48.4X2	T48.4X3	T48.4X4	T48.4X5	T48.4X6
Dorsacaine	T41.3X1	T41.3X2	T41.3X3	T41.3X4	T41.3X5	T41.3X6

Substance	Poisoning, Accidental (unintentional)	Poisoning, Intentional Self-harm	Poisoning, Assault	Poisoning, Undetermined	Adverse effect	Underdosing
Dosulepin	T43.011	T43.012	T43.013	T43.014	T43.015	T43.016
Dothiepin	T43.011	T43.012	T43.013	T43.014	T43.015	T43.016
Doxantrazole	T48.6X1	T48.6X2	T48.6X3	T48.6X4	T48.6X5	T48.6X6
Doxapram	T50.7X1	T50.7X2	T50.7X3	T50.7X4	T50.7X5	T50.7X6
Doxazosin	T44.6X1	T44.6X2	T44.6X3	T44.6X4	T44.6X5	T44.6X6
Doxepin	T43.011	T43.012	T43.013	T43.014	T43.015	T43.016
Doxifluridine	T45.1X1	T45.1X2	T45.1X3	T45.1X4	T45.1X5	T45.1X6
Doxorubicin	T45.1X1	T45.1X2	T45.1X3	T45.1X4	T45.1X5	T45.1X6
Doxycycline	T36.4X1	T36.4X2	T36.4X3	T36.4X4	T36.4X5	T36.4X6
Doxylamine	T45.0X1	T45.0X2	T45.0X3	T45.0X4	T45.0X5	T45.0X6
Dramamine	T45.0X1	T45.0X2	T45.0X3	T45.0X4	T45.0X5	T45.0X6
Drano (drain cleaner)	T54.3X1	T54.3X2	T54.3X3	T54.3X4	--	--
Dressing, live pulp	T49.7X1	T49.7X2	T49.7X3	T49.7X4	T49.7X5	T49.7X6
Drocode	T40.2X1	T40.2X2	T40.2X3	T40.2X4	T40.2X5	T40.2X6
Dromoran	T40.2X1	T40.2X2	T40.2X3	T40.2X4	T40.2X5	T40.2X6
Dromostanolone	T38.7X1	T38.7X2	T38.7X3	T38.7X4	T38.7X5	T38.7X6
Dronabinol	T40.711	T40.712	T40.713	T40.714	T40.715	T40.716
Droperidol	T43.591	T43.592	T43.593	T43.594	T43.595	T43.596
Dropropizine	T48.3X1	T48.3X2	T48.3X3	T48.3X4	T48.3X5	T48.3X6
Drostanolone	T38.7X1	T38.7X2	T38.7X3	T38.7X4	T38.7X5	T38.7X6
Drotaverine	T44.3X1	T44.3X2	T44.3X3	T44.3X4	T44.3X5	T44.3X6
Drotrecogin alfa	T45.511	T45.512	T45.513	T45.514	T45.515	T45.516
Drug NEC	T50.901	T50.902	T50.903	T50.904	T50.905	T50.906
- specified NEC	T50.991	T50.992	T50.993	T50.994	T50.995	T50.996
DTIC	T45.1X1	T45.1X2	T45.1X3	T45.1X4	T45.1X5	T45.1X6
Duboisine	T44.3X1	T44.3X2	T44.3X3	T44.3X4	T44.3X5	T44.3X6
Dulcolax	T47.2X1	T47.2X2	T47.2X3	T47.2X4	T47.2X5	T47.2X6
Duponol (C) (EP)	T49.2X1	T49.2X2	T49.2X3	T49.2X4	T49.2X5	T49.2X6
Durabolin	T38.7X1	T38.7X2	T38.7X3	T38.7X4	T38.7X5	T38.7X6
Dyclone	T41.3X1	T41.3X2	T41.3X3	T41.3X4	T41.3X5	T41.3X6
Dyclonine	T41.3X1	T41.3X2	T41.3X3	T41.3X4	T41.3X5	T41.3X6
Dydrogesterone	T38.5X1	T38.5X2	T38.5X3	T38.5X4	T38.5X5	T38.5X6
Dye NEC	T65.6X1	T65.6X2	T65.6X3	T65.6X4	--	--
- antiseptic	T49.0X1	T49.0X2	T49.0X3	T49.0X4	T49.0X5	T49.0X6
- diagnostic agents	T50.8X1	T50.8X2	T50.8X3	T50.8X4	T50.8X5	T50.8X6
- pharmaceutical NEC	T50.901	T50.902	T50.903	T50.904	T50.905	T50.906
Dyflos	T44.0X1	T44.0X2	T44.0X3	T44.0X4	T44.0X5	T44.0X6
Dymelor	T38.3X1	T38.3X2	T38.3X3	T38.3X4	T38.3X5	T38.3X6
Dynamite	T65.3X1	T65.3X2	T65.3X3	T65.3X4	--	--
- fumes	T59.891	T59.892	T59.893	T59.894	--	--
Dyphylline	T44.3X1	T44.3X2	T44.3X3	T44.3X4	T44.3X5	T44.3X6
Ear drug NEC	T49.6X1	T49.6X2	T49.6X3	T49.6X4	T49.6X5	T49.6X6
Ear preparations	T49.6X1	T49.6X2	T49.6X3	T49.6X4	T49.6X5	T49.6X6
Echothiophate, echothiopate, ecothiopate	T49.5X1	T49.5X2	T49.5X3	T49.5X4	T49.5X5	T49.5X6
Econazole	T49.0X1	T49.0X2	T49.0X3	T49.0X4	T49.0X5	T49.0X6
Ecothiopate iodide	T49.5X1	T49.5X2	T49.5X3	T49.5X4	T49.5X5	T49.5X6
Ecstasy	T43.641	T43.642	T43.643	T43.644	T43.645	T43.646
Ectylurea	T42.6X1	T42.6X2	T42.6X3	T42.6X4	T42.6X5	T42.6X6
Edathamil disodium	T45.8X1	T45.8X2	T45.8X3	T45.8X4	T45.8X5	T45.8X6
Edecrin	T50.1X1	T50.1X2	T50.1X3	T50.1X4	T50.1X5	T50.1X6
Edetate, disodium (calcium)	T45.8X1	T45.8X2	T45.8X3	T45.8X4	T45.8X5	T45.8X6
Edoxudine	T49.5X1	T49.5X2	T49.5X3	T49.5X4	T49.5X5	T49.5X6
Edrophonium	T44.0X1	T44.0X2	T44.0X3	T44.0X4	T44.0X5	T44.0X6
- chloride	T44.0X1	T44.0X2	T44.0X3	T44.0X4	T44.0X5	T44.0X6
EDTA	T50.6X1	T50.6X2	T50.6X3	T50.6X4	T50.6X5	T50.6X6
Eflornithine	T37.2X1	T37.2X2	T37.2X3	T37.2X4	T37.2X5	T37.2X6
Efloxate	T46.3X1	T46.3X2	T46.3X3	T46.3X4	T46.3X5	T46.3X6
Elase	T49.8X1	T49.8X2	T49.8X3	T49.8X4	T49.8X5	T49.8X6
Elastase	T47.5X1	T47.5X2	T47.5X3	T47.5X4	T47.5X5	T47.5X6

Substance	Poisoning, Accidental (unintentional)	Poisoning, Intentional Self-harm	Poisoning, Assault	Poisoning, Undetermined	Adverse effect	Underdosing
Elaterium	T47.2X1	T47.2X2	T47.2X3	T47.2X4	T47.2X5	T47.2X6
Elcatonin	T50.991	T50.992	T50.993	T50.994	T50.995	T50.996
Elder	T62.2X1	T62.2X2	T62.2X3	T62.2X4	--	--
- berry, (unripe)	T62.1X1	T62.1X2	T62.1X3	T62.1X4	--	--
Electrolyte balance drug	T50.3X1	T50.3X2	T50.3X3	T50.3X4	T50.3X5	T50.3X6
Electrolytes NEC	T50.3X1	T50.3X2	T50.3X3	T50.3X4	T50.3X5	T50.3X6
Electrolytic agent NEC	T50.3X1	T50.3X2	T50.3X3	T50.3X4	T50.3X5	T50.3X6
Elemental diet	T50.901	T50.902	T50.903	T50.904	T50.905	T50.906
Elliptinium acetate	T45.1X1	T45.1X2	T45.1X3	T45.1X4	T45.1X5	T45.1X6
Embramine	T45.0X1	T45.0X2	T45.0X3	T45.0X4	T45.0X5	T45.0X6
Emepronium (salts)	T44.3X1	T44.3X2	T44.3X3	T44.3X4	T44.3X5	T44.3X6
- bromide	T44.3X1	T44.3X2	T44.3X3	T44.3X4	T44.3X5	T44.3X6
Emetic NEC	T47.7X1	T47.7X2	T47.7X3	T47.7X4	T47.7X5	T47.7X6
Emetine	T37.3X1	T37.3X2	T37.3X3	T37.3X4	T37.3X5	T37.3X6
Emollient NEC	T49.3X1	T49.3X2	T49.3X3	T49.3X4	T49.3X5	T49.3X6
Emorfazone	T39.8X1	T39.8X2	T39.8X3	T39.8X4	T39.8X5	T39.8X6
Emylcamate	T43.591	T43.592	T43.593	T43.594	T43.595	T43.596
Enalapril	T46.4X1	T46.4X2	T46.4X3	T46.4X4	T46.4X5	T46.4X6
Enalaprilat	T46.4X1	T46.4X2	T46.4X3	T46.4X4	T46.4X5	T46.4X6
Encainide	T46.2X1	T46.2X2	T46.2X3	T46.2X4	T46.2X5	T46.2X6
Endocaine	T41.3X1	T41.3X2	T41.3X3	T41.3X4	T41.3X5	T41.3X6
Endosulfan	T60.2X1	T60.2X2	T60.2X3	T60.2X4	--	--
Endothall	T60.3X1	T60.3X2	T60.3X3	T60.3X4	--	--
Endralazine	T46.5X1	T46.5X2	T46.5X3	T46.5X4	T46.5X5	T46.5X6
Endrin	T60.1X1	T60.1X2	T60.1X3	T60.1X4	--	--
Enflurane	T41.0X1	T41.0X2	T41.0X3	T41.0X4	T41.0X5	T41.0X6
Enhexymal	T42.3X1	T42.3X2	T42.3X3	T42.3X4	T42.3X5	T42.3X6
Enocitabine	T45.1X1	T45.1X2	T45.1X3	T45.1X4	T45.1X5	T45.1X6
Enovid	T38.4X1	T38.4X2	T38.4X3	T38.4X4	T38.4X5	T38.4X6
Enoxacin	T36.8X1	T36.8X2	T36.8X3	T36.8X4	T36.8X5	T36.8X6
Enoxaparin (sodium)	T45.511	T45.512	T45.513	T45.514	T45.515	T45.516
Enpiprazole	T43.591	T43.592	T43.593	T43.594	T43.595	T43.596
Enprofylline	T48.6X1	T48.6X2	T48.6X3	T48.6X4	T48.6X5	T48.6X6
Enprostil	T47.1X1	T47.1X2	T47.1X3	T47.1X4	T47.1X5	T47.1X6
ENT preparations (anti-infectives)	T49.6X1	T49.6X2	T49.6X3	T49.6X4	T49.6X5	T49.6X6
Enterogastrone	T38.891	T38.892	T38.893	T38.894	T38.895	T38.896
Enviomycin	T36.8X1	T36.8X2	T36.8X3	T36.8X4	T36.8X5	T36.8X6
Enzodase	T45.3X1	T45.3X2	T45.3X3	T45.3X4	T45.3X5	T45.3X6
Enzyme NEC	T45.3X1	T45.3X2	T45.3X3	T45.3X4	T45.3X5	T45.3X6
- depolymerizing	T49.8X1	T49.8X2	T49.8X3	T49.8X4	T49.8X5	T49.8X6
- fibrolytic	T45.3X1	T45.3X2	T45.3X3	T45.3X4	T45.3X5	T45.3X6
- gastric	T47.5X1	T47.5X2	T47.5X3	T47.5X4	T47.5X5	T47.5X6
- intestinal	T47.5X1	T47.5X2	T47.5X3	T47.5X4	T47.5X5	T47.5X6
- local action	T49.4X1	T49.4X2	T49.4X3	T49.4X4	T49.4X5	T49.4X6
- proteolytic	T49.4X1	T49.4X2	T49.4X3	T49.4X4	T49.4X5	T49.4X6
- thrombolytic	T45.3X1	T45.3X2	T45.3X3	T45.3X4	T45.3X5	T45.3X6
EPAB	T41.3X1	T41.3X2	T41.3X3	T41.3X4	T41.3X5	T41.3X6
Epanutin	T42.0X1	T42.0X2	T42.0X3	T42.0X4	T42.0X5	T42.0X6
Ephedra	T44.991	T44.992	T44.993	T44.994	T44.995	T44.996
Ephedrine	T44.991	T44.992	T44.993	T44.994	T44.995	T44.996
Epichlorhydrin, epichlorohydrin	T52.8X1	T52.8X2	T52.8X3	T52.8X4	--	--
Epicillin	T36.0X1	T36.0X2	T36.0X3	T36.0X4	T36.0X5	T36.0X6
Epiestriol	T38.5X1	T38.5X2	T38.5X3	T38.5X4	T38.5X5	T38.5X6
Epilim—see Sodium valproate						
Epimestrol	T38.5X1	T38.5X2	T38.5X3	T38.5X4	T38.5X5	T38.5X6
Epinephrine	T44.5X1	T44.5X2	T44.5X3	T44.5X4	T44.5X5	T44.5X6
Epirubicin	T45.1X1	T45.1X2	T45.1X3	T45.1X4	T45.1X5	T45.1X6
Epitiostanol	T38.7X1	T38.7X2	T38.7X3	T38.7X4	T38.7X5	T38.7X6

Substance	Poisoning, Accidental (unintentional)	Poisoning, Intentional Self-harm	Poisoning, Assault	Poisoning, Undetermined	Adverse effect	Underdosing
Epitizide	T50.2X1	T50.2X2	T50.2X3	T50.2X4	T50.2X5	T50.2X6
EPN	T60.0X1	T60.0X2	T60.0X3	T60.0X4	--	--
EPO	T45.8X1	T45.8X2	T45.8X3	T45.8X4	T45.8X5	T45.8X6
Epoetin alpha	T45.8X1	T45.8X2	T45.8X3	T45.8X4	T45.8X5	T45.8X6
Epomediol	T50.991	T50.992	T50.993	T50.994	T50.995	T50.996
Epoprostenol	T45.521	T45.522	T45.523	T45.524	T45.525	T45.526
Epoxy resin	T65.891	T65.892	T65.893	T65.894	--	--
Eprazinone	T48.4X1	T48.4X2	T48.4X3	T48.4X4	T48.4X5	T48.4X6
Epsilon amino-caproic acid	T45.621	T45.622	T45.623	T45.624	T45.625	T45.626
Epsom salt	T47.3X1	T47.3X2	T47.3X3	T47.3X4	T47.3X5	T47.3X6
Eptazocine	T40.491	T40.492	T40.493	T40.494	T40.495	T40.496
Equanil	T43.591	T43.592	T43.593	T43.594	T43.595	T43.596
Equisetum	T62.2X1	T62.2X2	T62.2X3	T62.2X4	--	--
- diuretic	T50.2X1	T50.2X2	T50.2X3	T50.2X4	T50.2X5	T50.2X6
Ergobasine	T48.0X1	T48.0X2	T48.0X3	T48.0X4	T48.0X5	T48.0X6
Ergocalciferol	T45.2X1	T45.2X2	T45.2X3	T45.2X4	T45.2X5	T45.2X6
Ergoloid mesylates	T46.7X1	T46.7X2	T46.7X3	T46.7X4	T46.7X5	T46.7X6
Ergometrine	T48.0X1	T48.0X2	T48.0X3	T48.0X4	T48.0X5	T48.0X6
Ergonovine	T48.0X1	T48.0X2	T48.0X3	T48.0X4	T48.0X5	T48.0X6
Ergot NEC	T64.81	T64.82	T64.83	T64.84	--	--
- derivative	T48.0X1	T48.0X2	T48.0X3	T48.0X4	T48.0X5	T48.0X6
- medicinal (alkaloids)	T48.0X1	T48.0X2	T48.0X3	T48.0X4	T48.0X5	T48.0X6
- prepared	T48.0X1	T48.0X2	T48.0X3	T48.0X4	T48.0X5	T48.0X6
Ergotamine	T46.5X1	T46.5X2	T46.5X3	T46.5X4	T46.5X5	T46.5X6
Ergotocine	T48.0X1	T48.0X2	T48.0X3	T48.0X4	T48.0X5	T48.0X6
Ergotrate	T48.0X1	T48.0X2	T48.0X3	T48.0X4	T48.0X5	T48.0X6
Eritrityl tetranitrate	T46.3X1	T46.3X2	T46.3X3	T46.3X4	T46.3X5	T46.3X6
Erythrityl tetranitrate	T46.3X1	T46.3X2	T46.3X3	T46.3X4	T46.3X5	T46.3X6
Erythrol tetranitrate	T46.3X1	T46.3X2	T46.3X3	T46.3X4	T46.3X5	T46.3X6
Erythromycin (salts)	T36.3X1	T36.3X2	T36.3X3	T36.3X4	T36.3X5	T36.3X6
- ophthalmic preparation	T49.5X1	T49.5X2	T49.5X3	T49.5X4	T49.5X5	T49.5X6
- topical NEC	T49.0X1	T49.0X2	T49.0X3	T49.0X4	T49.0X5	T49.0X6
Erythropoietin	T45.8X1	T45.8X2	T45.8X3	T45.8X4	T45.8X5	T45.8X6
- human	T45.8X1	T45.8X2	T45.8X3	T45.8X4	T45.8X5	T45.8X6
Escin	T46.991	T46.992	T46.993	T46.994	T46.995	T46.996
Esculin	T45.2X1	T45.2X2	T45.2X3	T45.2X4	T45.2X5	T45.2X6
Esculoside	T45.2X1	T45.2X2	T45.2X3	T45.2X4	T45.2X5	T45.2X6
ESDT (ether-soluble tar distillate)	T49.1X1	T49.1X2	T49.1X3	T49.1X4	T49.1X5	T49.1X6
Eserine	T49.5X1	T49.5X2	T49.5X3	T49.5X4	T49.5X5	T49.5X6
Esflurbiprofen	T39.311	T39.312	T39.313	T39.314	T39.315	T39.316
Eskabarb	T42.3X1	T42.3X2	T42.3X3	T42.3X4	T42.3X5	T42.3X6
Eskalith	T43.8X1	T43.8X2	T43.8X3	T43.8X4	T43.8X5	T43.8X6
Esmolol	T44.7X1	T44.7X2	T44.7X3	T44.7X4	T44.7X5	T44.7X6
Estanozolol	T38.7X1	T38.7X2	T38.7X3	T38.7X4	T38.7X5	T38.7X6
Estazolam	T42.4X1	T42.4X2	T42.4X3	T42.4X4	T42.4X5	T42.4X6
Estradiol	T38.5X1	T38.5X2	T38.5X3	T38.5X4	T38.5X5	T38.5X6
- with testosterone	T38.7X1	T38.7X2	T38.7X3	T38.7X4	T38.7X5	T38.7X6
- benzoate	T38.5X1	T38.5X2	T38.5X3	T38.5X4	T38.5X5	T38.5X6
Estramustine	T45.1X1	T45.1X2	T45.1X3	T45.1X4	T45.1X5	T45.1X6
Estriol	T38.5X1	T38.5X2	T38.5X3	T38.5X4	T38.5X5	T38.5X6
Estrogen	T38.5X1	T38.5X2	T38.5X3	T38.5X4	T38.5X5	T38.5X6
- with progesterone	T38.5X1	T38.5X2	T38.5X3	T38.5X4	T38.5X5	T38.5X6
- conjugated	T38.5X1	T38.5X2	T38.5X3	T38.5X4	T38.5X5	T38.5X6
Estrone	T38.5X1	T38.5X2	T38.5X3	T38.5X4	T38.5X5	T38.5X6
Estropipate	T38.5X1	T38.5X2	T38.5X3	T38.5X4	T38.5X5	T38.5X6
Etacrynate sodium	T50.1X1	T50.1X2	T50.1X3	T50.1X4	T50.1X5	T50.1X6
Etacrynic acid	T50.1X1	T50.1X2	T50.1X3	T50.1X4	T50.1X5	T50.1X6
Etafedrine	T48.6X1	T48.6X2	T48.6X3	T48.6X4	T48.6X5	T48.6X6
Etafenone	T46.3X1	T46.3X2	T46.3X3	T46.3X4	T46.3X5	T46.3X6

Substance	Poisoning, Accidental (unintentional)	Poisoning, Intentional Self-harm	Poisoning, Assault	Poisoning, Undetermined	Adverse effect	Underdosing
Etambutol	T37.1X1	T37.1X2	T37.1X3	T37.1X4	T37.1X5	T37.1X6
Etamiphyllin	T48.6X1	T48.6X2	T48.6X3	T48.6X4	T48.6X5	T48.6X6
Etamivan	T50.7X1	T50.7X2	T50.7X3	T50.7X4	T50.7X5	T50.7X6
Etamsylate	T45.7X1	T45.7X2	T45.7X3	T45.7X4	T45.7X5	T45.7X6
Etebenecid	T50.4X1	T50.4X2	T50.4X3	T50.4X4	T50.4X5	T50.4X6
Ethacridine	T49.0X1	T49.0X2	T49.0X3	T49.0X4	T49.0X5	T49.0X6
Ethacrynic acid	T50.1X1	T50.1X2	T50.1X3	T50.1X4	T50.1X5	T50.1X6
Ethadione	T42.2X1	T42.2X2	T42.2X3	T42.2X4	T42.2X5	T42.2X6
Ethambutol	T37.1X1	T37.1X2	T37.1X3	T37.1X4	T37.1X5	T37.1X6
Ethamide	T50.2X1	T50.2X2	T50.2X3	T50.2X4	T50.2X5	T50.2X6
Ethamivan	T50.7X1	T50.7X2	T50.7X3	T50.7X4	T50.7X5	T50.7X6
Ethamsylate	T45.7X1	T45.7X2	T45.7X3	T45.7X4	T45.7X5	T45.7X6
Ethanol	T51.0X1	T51.0X2	T51.0X3	T51.0X4	--	--
- beverage	T51.0X1	T51.0X2	T51.0X3	T51.0X4	--	--
Ethanolamine oleate	T46.8X1	T46.8X2	T46.8X3	T46.8X4	T46.8X5	T46.8X6
Ethaverine	T44.3X1	T44.3X2	T44.3X3	T44.3X4	T44.3X5	T44.3X6
Ethchlorvynol	T42.6X1	T42.6X2	T42.6X3	T42.6X4	T42.6X5	T42.6X6
Ethebenecid	T50.4X1	T50.4X2	T50.4X3	T50.4X4	T50.4X5	T50.4X6
Ether (vapor)	T41.0X1	T41.0X2	T41.0X3	T41.0X4	T41.0X5	T41.0X6
- anesthetic	T41.0X1	T41.0X2	T41.0X3	T41.0X4	T41.0X5	T41.0X6
- divinyl	T41.0X1	T41.0X2	T41.0X3	T41.0X4	T41.0X5	T41.0X6
- ethyl (medicinal)	T41.0X1	T41.0X2	T41.0X3	T41.0X4	T41.0X5	T41.0X6
- - nonmedicinal	T52.8X1	T52.8X2	T52.8X3	T52.8X4	--	--
- petroleum—see Ligroin						
- solvent	T52.8X1	T52.8X2	T52.8X3	T52.8X4	--	--
Ethiazide	T50.2X1	T50.2X2	T50.2X3	T50.2X4	T50.2X5	T50.2X6
Ethidium chloride (vapor)	T59.891	T59.892	T59.893	T59.894	--	--
Ethinamate	T42.6X1	T42.6X2	T42.6X3	T42.6X4	T42.6X5	T42.6X6
Ethinylestradiol, ethinyloestradiol	T38.5X1	T38.5X2	T38.5X3	T38.5X4	T38.5X5	T38.5X6
- with						
- - levonorgestrel	T38.4X1	T38.4X2	T38.4X3	T38.4X4	T38.4X5	T38.4X6
- - norethisterone	T38.4X1	T38.4X2	T38.4X3	T38.4X4	T38.4X5	T38.4X6
Ethiodized oil (131 I)	T50.8X1	T50.8X2	T50.8X3	T50.8X4	T50.8X5	T50.8X6
Ethion	T60.0X1	T60.0X2	T60.0X3	T60.0X4	--	--
Ethionamide	T37.1X1	T37.1X2	T37.1X3	T37.1X4	T37.1X5	T37.1X6
Ethioniamide	T37.1X1	T37.1X2	T37.1X3	T37.1X4	T37.1X5	T37.1X6
Ethisterone	T38.5X1	T38.5X2	T38.5X3	T38.5X4	T38.5X5	T38.5X6
Ethobral	T42.3X1	T42.3X2	T42.3X3	T42.3X4	T42.3X5	T42.3X6
Ethocaine (infiltration) (topical)	T41.3X1	T41.3X2	T41.3X3	T41.3X4	T41.3X5	T41.3X6
- nerve block (peripheral) (plexus)	T41.3X1	T41.3X2	T41.3X3	T41.3X4	T41.3X5	T41.3X6
- spinal	T41.3X1	T41.3X2	T41.3X3	T41.3X4	T41.3X5	T41.3X6
Ethoheptazine	T40.491	T40.492	T40.493	T40.494	T40.495	T40.496
Ethopropazine	T44.3X1	T44.3X2	T44.3X3	T44.3X4	T44.3X5	T44.3X6
Ethosuximide	T42.2X1	T42.2X2	T42.2X3	T42.2X4	T42.2X5	T42.2X6
Ethotoin	T42.0X1	T42.0X2	T42.0X3	T42.0X4	T42.0X5	T42.0X6
Ethoxazene	T37.91	T37.92	T37.93	T37.94	T37.95	T37.96
Ethoxazorutoside	T46.991	T46.992	T46.993	T46.994	T46.995	T46.996
2-Ethoxyethanol	T52.3X1	T52.3X2	T52.3X3	T52.3X4	--	--
Ethoxzolamide	T50.2X1	T50.2X2	T50.2X3	T50.2X4	T50.2X5	T50.2X6
Ethyl						
- acetate	T52.8X1	T52.8X2	T52.8X3	T52.8X4	--	--
- alcohol	T51.0X1	T51.0X2	T51.0X3	T51.0X4	--	--
- - beverage	T51.0X1	T51.0X2	T51.0X3	T51.0X4	--	--
- aldehyde (vapor)	T59.891	T59.892	T59.893	T59.894	--	--
- - liquid	T52.8X1	T52.8X2	T52.8X3	T52.8X4	--	--
- aminobenzoate	T41.3X1	T41.3X2	T41.3X3	T41.3X4	T41.3X5	T41.3X6
- aminophenothiazine	T43.3X1	T43.3X2	T43.3X3	T43.3X4	T43.3X5	T43.3X6
- benzoate	T52.8X1	T52.8X2	T52.8X3	T52.8X4	--	--

Substance	Poisoning, Accidental (unintentional)	Poisoning, Intentional Self-harm	Poisoning, Assault	Poisoning, Undetermined	Adverse effect	Underdosing
- biscoumacetate	T45.511	T45.512	T45.513	T45.514	T45.515	T45.516
- bromide (anesthetic)	T41.0X1	T41.0X2	T41.0X3	T41.0X4	T41.0X5	T41.0X6
- carbamate	T45.1X1	T45.1X2	T45.1X3	T45.1X4	T45.1X5	T45.1X6
- carbinol	T51.3X1	T51.3X2	T51.3X3	T51.3X4	--	--
- carbonate	T52.8X1	T52.8X2	T52.8X3	T52.8X4	--	--
- chaulmoograte	T37.1X1	T37.1X2	T37.1X3	T37.1X4	T37.1X5	T37.1X6
- chloride (anesthetic)	T41.0X1	T41.0X2	T41.0X3	T41.0X4	T41.0X5	T41.0X6
- - anesthetic (local)	T41.3X1	T41.3X2	T41.3X3	T41.3X4	T41.3X5	T41.3X6
- - - inhaled	T41.0X1	T41.0X2	T41.0X3	T41.0X4	T41.0X5	T41.0X6
- - local	T49.4X1	T49.4X2	T49.4X3	T49.4X4	T49.4X5	T49.4X6
- - solvent	T53.6X1	T53.6X2	T53.6X3	T53.6X4	--	--
- dibunate	T48.3X1	T48.3X2	T48.3X3	T48.3X4	T48.3X5	T48.3X6
- dichloroarsine (vapor)	T57.0X1	T57.0X2	T57.0X3	T57.0X4	--	--
- estranol	T38.7X1	T38.7X2	T38.7X3	T38.7X4	T38.7X5	T38.7X6
- ether—see also ether	T52.8X1	T52.8X2	T52.8X3	T52.8X4	--	--
- formate NEC (solvent)	T52.0X1	T52.0X2	T52.0X3	T52.0X4	--	--
- fumarate	T49.4X1	T49.4X2	T49.4X3	T49.4X4	T49.4X5	T49.4X6
- hydroxyisobutyrate NEC (solvent)	T52.8X1	T52.8X2	T52.8X3	T52.8X4	--	--
- iodoacetate	T59.3X1	T59.3X2	T59.3X3	T59.3X4	--	--
- lactate NEC (solvent)	T52.8X1	T52.8X2	T52.8X3	T52.8X4	--	--
- loflazepate	T42.4X1	T42.4X2	T42.4X3	T42.4X4	T42.4X5	T42.4X6
- mercuric chloride	T56.1X1	T56.1X2	T56.1X3	T56.1X4	--	--
- methylcarbinol	T51.8X1	T51.8X2	T51.8X3	T51.8X4	--	--
- morphine	T40.2X1	T40.2X2	T40.2X3	T40.2X4	T40.2X5	T40.2X6
- noradrenaline	T48.6X1	T48.6X2	T48.6X3	T48.6X4	T48.6X5	T48.6X6
- oxybutyrate NEC (solvent)	T52.8X1	T52.8X2	T52.8X3	T52.8X4	--	--
Ethylene (gas)	T59.891	T59.892	T59.893	T59.894	--	--
- anesthetic (general)	T41.0X1	T41.0X2	T41.0X3	T41.0X4	T41.0X5	T41.0X6
- chlorohydrin	T52.8X1	T52.8X2	T52.8X3	T52.8X4	--	--
- - vapor	T53.6X1	T53.6X2	T53.6X3	T53.6X4	--	--
- dichloride	T52.8X1	T52.8X2	T52.8X3	T52.8X4	--	--
- - vapor	T53.6X1	T53.6X2	T53.6X3	T53.6X4	--	--
- dinitrate	T52.3X1	T52.3X2	T52.3X3	T52.3X4	--	--
- glycol (s)	T52.8X1	T52.8X2	T52.8X3	T52.8X4	--	--
- - dinitrate	T52.3X1	T52.3X2	T52.3X3	T52.3X4	--	--
- - monobutyl ether	T52.3X1	T52.3X2	T52.3X3	T52.3X4	--	--
- imine	T54.1X1	T54.1X2	T54.1X3	T54.1X4	--	--
- oxide (fumigant) (nonmedicinal)	T59.891	T59.892	T59.893	T59.894	--	--
- - medicinal	T49.0X1	T49.0X2	T49.0X3	T49.0X4	T49.0X5	T49.0X6
Ethylenediamine theophylline	T48.6X1	T48.6X2	T48.6X3	T48.6X4	T48.6X5	T48.6X6
Ethylenediaminetetra-acetic acid	T50.6X1	T50.6X2	T50.6X3	T50.6X4	T50.6X5	T50.6X6
Ethylenedinitrilotetra-acetate	T50.6X1	T50.6X2	T50.6X3	T50.6X4	T50.6X5	T50.6X6
Ethylestrenol	T38.7X1	T38.7X2	T38.7X3	T38.7X4	T38.7X5	T38.7X6
Ethylhydroxycellulose	T47.4X1	T47.4X2	T47.4X3	T47.4X4	T47.4X5	T47.4X6
Ethylidene						
- chloride NEC	T53.6X1	T53.6X2	T53.6X3	T53.6X4	--	--
- diacetate	T60.3X1	T60.3X2	T60.3X3	T60.3X4	--	--
- dicoumarin	T45.511	T45.512	T45.513	T45.514	T45.515	T45.516
- dicoumarol	T45.511	T45.512	T45.513	T45.514	T45.515	T45.516
- diethyl ether	T52.0X1	T52.0X2	T52.0X3	T52.0X4	--	--
Ethylmorphine	T40.2X1	T40.2X2	T40.2X3	T40.2X4	T40.2X5	T40.2X6
Ethylnorepinephrine	T48.6X1	T48.6X2	T48.6X3	T48.6X4	T48.6X5	T48.6X6
Ethylparachlorophen-oxyisobutyrate	T46.6X1	T46.6X2	T46.6X3	T46.6X4	T46.6X5	T46.6X6
Ethynodiol	T38.4X1	T38.4X2	T38.4X3	T38.4X4	T38.4X5	T38.4X6
- with mestranol diacetate	T38.4X1	T38.4X2	T38.4X3	T38.4X4	T38.4X5	T38.4X6
Etidocaine	T41.3X1	T41.3X2	T41.3X3	T41.3X4	T41.3X5	T41.3X6
- infiltration (subcutaneous)	T41.3X1	T41.3X2	T41.3X3	T41.3X4	T41.3X5	T41.3X6
- nerve (peripheral) (plexus)	T41.3X1	T41.3X2	T41.3X3	T41.3X4	T41.3X5	T41.3X6
Etidronate	T50.991	T50.992	T50.993	T50.994	T50.995	T50.996

Substance	Poisoning, Accidental (unintentional)	Poisoning, Intentional Self-harm	Poisoning, Assault	Poisoning, Undetermined	Adverse effect	Underdosing
Etidronic acid (disodium salt)	T50.991	T50.992	T50.993	T50.994	T50.995	T50.996
Etifoxine	T42.6X1	T42.6X2	T42.6X3	T42.6X4	T42.6X5	T42.6X6
Etilefrine	T44.4X1	T44.4X2	T44.4X3	T44.4X4	T44.4X5	T44.4X6
Etilfen	T42.3X1	T42.3X2	T42.3X3	T42.3X4	T42.3X5	T42.3X6
Etinodiol	T38.4X1	T38.4X2	T38.4X3	T38.4X4	T38.4X5	T38.4X6
Etiroxate	T46.6X1	T46.6X2	T46.6X3	T46.6X4	T46.6X5	T46.6X6
Etizolam	T42.4X1	T42.4X2	T42.4X3	T42.4X4	T42.4X5	T42.4X6
Etodolac	T39.391	T39.392	T39.393	T39.394	T39.395	T39.396
Etofamide	T37.3X1	T37.3X2	T37.3X3	T37.3X4	T37.3X5	T37.3X6
Etofibrate	T46.6X1	T46.6X2	T46.6X3	T46.6X4	T46.6X5	T46.6X6
Etofylline	T46.7X1	T46.7X2	T46.7X3	T46.7X4	T46.7X5	T46.7X6
- clofibrate	T46.6X1	T46.6X2	T46.6X3	T46.6X4	T46.6X5	T46.6X6
Etoglucid	T45.1X1	T45.1X2	T45.1X3	T45.1X4	T45.1X5	T45.1X6
Etomidate	T41.1X1	T41.1X2	T41.1X3	T41.1X4	T41.1X5	T41.1X6
Etomide	T39.8X1	T39.8X2	T39.8X3	T39.8X4	T39.8X5	T39.8X6
Etomidoline	T44.3X1	T44.3X2	T44.3X3	T44.3X4	T44.3X5	T44.3X6
Etoposide	T45.1X1	T45.1X2	T45.1X3	T45.1X4	T45.1X5	T45.1X6
Etorphine	T40.2X1	T40.2X2	T40.2X3	T40.2X4	T40.2X5	T40.2X6
Etoval	T42.3X1	T42.3X2	T42.3X3	T42.3X4	T42.3X5	T42.3X6
Etozolin	T50.1X1	T50.1X2	T50.1X3	T50.1X4	T50.1X5	T50.1X6
Etretinate	T50.991	T50.992	T50.993	T50.994	T50.995	T50.996
Etryptamine	T43.691	T43.692	T43.693	T43.694	T43.695	T43.696
Etybenzatropine	T44.3X1	T44.3X2	T44.3X3	T44.3X4	T44.3X5	T44.3X6
Etynodiol	T38.4X1	T38.4X2	T38.4X3	T38.4X4	T38.4X5	T38.4X6
Eucaine	T41.3X1	T41.3X2	T41.3X3	T41.3X4	T41.3X5	T41.3X6
Eucalyptus oil	T49.7X1	T49.7X2	T49.7X3	T49.7X4	T49.7X5	T49.7X6
Eucatropine	T49.5X1	T49.5X2	T49.5X3	T49.5X4	T49.5X5	T49.5X6
Eucodal	T40.2X1	T40.2X2	T40.2X3	T40.2X4	T40.2X5	T40.2X6
Euneryl	T42.3X1	T42.3X2	T42.3X3	T42.3X4	T42.3X5	T42.3X6
Euphthalmine	T44.3X1	T44.3X2	T44.3X3	T44.3X4	T44.3X5	T44.3X6
Eurax	T49.0X1	T49.0X2	T49.0X3	T49.0X4	T49.0X5	T49.0X6
Euresol	T49.4X1	T49.4X2	T49.4X3	T49.4X4	T49.4X5	T49.4X6
Euthroid	T38.1X1	T38.1X2	T38.1X3	T38.1X4	T38.1X5	T38.1X6
Evans blue	T50.8X1	T50.8X2	T50.8X3	T50.8X4	T50.8X5	T50.8X6
Evipal	T42.3X1	T42.3X2	T42.3X3	T42.3X4	T42.3X5	T42.3X6
- sodium	T41.1X1	T41.1X2	T41.1X3	T41.1X4	T41.1X5	T41.1X6
Evipan	T42.3X1	T42.3X2	T42.3X3	T42.3X4	T42.3X5	T42.3X6
- sodium	T41.1X1	T41.1X2	T41.1X3	T41.1X4	T41.1X5	T41.1X6
Exalamide	T49.0X1	T49.0X2	T49.0X3	T49.0X4	T49.0X5	T49.0X6
Exalgin	T39.1X1	T39.1X2	T39.1X3	T39.1X4	T39.1X5	T39.1X6
Excipients, pharmaceutical	T50.901	T50.902	T50.903	T50.904	T50.905	T50.906
Exhaust gas (engine) (motor vehicle)	T58.01	T58.02	T58.03	T58.04	--	--
Ex-Lax (phenolphthalein)	T47.2X1	T47.2X2	T47.2X3	T47.2X4	T47.2X5	T47.2X6
Expectorant NEC	T48.4X1	T48.4X2	T48.4X3	T48.4X4	T48.4X5	T48.4X6
Extended insulin zinc suspension	T38.3X1	T38.3X2	T38.3X3	T38.3X4	T38.3X5	T38.3X6
External medications (skin) (mucous membrane)	T49.91	T49.92	T49.93	T49.94	T49.95	T49.96
- dental agent	T49.7X1	T49.7X2	T49.7X3	T49.7X4	T49.7X5	T49.7X6
- ENT agent	T49.6X1	T49.6X2	T49.6X3	T49.6X4	T49.6X5	T49.6X6
- ophthalmic preparation	T49.5X1	T49.5X2	T49.5X3	T49.5X4	T49.5X5	T49.5X6
- specified NEC	T49.8X1	T49.8X2	T49.8X3	T49.8X4	T49.8X5	T49.8X6
Extrapyramidal antagonist NEC	T44.3X1	T44.3X2	T44.3X3	T44.3X4	T44.3X5	T44.3X6
Eye agents (anti-infective)	T49.5X1	T49.5X2	T49.5X3	T49.5X4	T49.5X5	T49.5X6
Eye drug NEC	T49.5X1	T49.5X2	T49.5X3	T49.5X4	T49.5X5	T49.5X6
FAC (fluorouracil + doxorubicin + cyclophosphamide)	T45.1X1	T45.1X2	T45.1X3	T45.1X4	T45.1X5	T45.1X6
Factor						
- I (fibrinogen)	T45.8X1	T45.8X2	T45.8X3	T45.8X4	T45.8X5	T45.8X6
- III (thromboplastin)	T45.8X1	T45.8X2	T45.8X3	T45.8X4	T45.8X5	T45.8X6

Substance	Poisoning, Accidental (unintentional)	Poisoning, Intentional Self-harm	Poisoning, Assault	Poisoning, Undetermined	Adverse effect	Underdosing
- VIII (antihemophilic Factor) (concentrate)	T45.8X1	T45.8X2	T45.8X3	T45.8X4	T45.8X5	T45.8X6
- IX complex	T45.7X1	T45.7X2	T45.7X3	T45.7X4	T45.7X5	T45.7X6
- - human	T45.8X1	T45.8X2	T45.8X3	T45.8X4	T45.8X5	T45.8X6
Famotidine	T47.0X1	T47.0X2	T47.0X3	T47.0X4	T47.0X5	T47.0X6
Fat suspension, intravenous	T50.991	T50.992	T50.993	T50.994	T50.995	T50.996
Fazadinium bromide	T48.1X1	T48.1X2	T48.1X3	T48.1X4	T48.1X5	T48.1X6
Febarbamate	T42.3X1	T42.3X2	T42.3X3	T42.3X4	T42.3X5	T42.3X6
Fecal softener	T47.4X1	T47.4X2	T47.4X3	T47.4X4	T47.4X5	T47.4X6
Fedrilate	T48.3X1	T48.3X2	T48.3X3	T48.3X4	T48.3X5	T48.3X6
Felodipine	T46.1X1	T46.1X2	T46.1X3	T46.1X4	T46.1X5	T46.1X6
Felypressin	T38.891	T38.892	T38.893	T38.894	T38.895	T38.896
Femoxetine	T43.221	T43.222	T43.223	T43.224	T43.225	T43.226
Fenalcomine	T46.3X1	T46.3X2	T46.3X3	T46.3X4	T46.3X5	T46.3X6
Fenamisal	T37.1X1	T37.1X2	T37.1X3	T37.1X4	T37.1X5	T37.1X6
Fenazone	T39.2X1	T39.2X2	T39.2X3	T39.2X4	T39.2X5	T39.2X6
Fenbendazole	T37.4X1	T37.4X2	T37.4X3	T37.4X4	T37.4X5	T37.4X6
Fenbutrazate	T50.5X1	T50.5X2	T50.5X3	T50.5X4	T50.5X5	T50.5X6
Fencamfamine	T43.691	T43.692	T43.693	T43.694	T43.695	T43.696
Fendiline	T46.1X1	T46.1X2	T46.1X3	T46.1X4	T46.1X5	T46.1X6
Fenetylline	T43.691	T43.692	T43.693	T43.694	T43.695	T43.696
Fenflumizole	T39.391	T39.392	T39.393	T39.394	T39.395	T39.396
Fenfluramine	T50.5X1	T50.5X2	T50.5X3	T50.5X4	T50.5X5	T50.5X6
Fenobarbital	T42.3X1	T42.3X2	T42.3X3	T42.3X4	T42.3X5	T42.3X6
Fenofibrate	T46.6X1	T46.6X2	T46.6X3	T46.6X4	T46.6X5	T46.6X6
Fenoprofen	T39.311	T39.312	T39.313	T39.314	T39.315	T39.316
Fenoterol	T48.6X1	T48.6X2	T48.6X3	T48.6X4	T48.6X5	T48.6X6
Fenoverine	T44.3X1	T44.3X2	T44.3X3	T44.3X4	T44.3X5	T44.3X6
Fenoxazoline	T48.5X1	T48.5X2	T48.5X3	T48.5X4	T48.5X5	T48.5X6
Fenproporex	T50.5X1	T50.5X2	T50.5X3	T50.5X4	T50.5X5	T50.5X6
Fenquizone	T50.2X1	T50.2X2	T50.2X3	T50.2X4	T50.2X5	T50.2X6
Fentanyl (analogs)	T40.411	T40.412	T40.413	T40.414	T40.415	T40.416
Fentazin	T43.3X1	T43.3X2	T43.3X3	T43.3X4	T43.3X5	T43.3X6
Fenthion	T60.0X1	T60.0X2	T60.0X3	T60.0X4	--	--
Fenticlor	T49.0X1	T49.0X2	T49.0X3	T49.0X4	T49.0X5	T49.0X6
Fenylbutazone	T39.2X1	T39.2X2	T39.2X3	T39.2X4	T39.2X5	T39.2X6
Feprazone	T39.2X1	T39.2X2	T39.2X3	T39.2X4	T39.2X5	T39.2X6
Fer de lance (bite) (venom)	T63.061	T63.062	T63.063	T63.064	--	--
Ferric—see also Iron						
- chloride	T45.4X1	T45.4X2	T45.4X3	T45.4X4	T45.4X5	T45.4X6
- citrate	T45.4X1	T45.4X2	T45.4X3	T45.4X4	T45.4X5	T45.4X6
- hydroxide						
- - colloidal	T45.4X1	T45.4X2	T45.4X3	T45.4X4	T45.4X5	T45.4X6
- - polymaltose	T45.4X1	T45.4X2	T45.4X3	T45.4X4	T45.4X5	T45.4X6
- pyrophosphate	T45.4X1	T45.4X2	T45.4X3	T45.4X4	T45.4X5	T45.4X6
Ferritin	T45.4X1	T45.4X2	T45.4X3	T45.4X4	T45.4X5	T45.4X6
Ferrocholinate	T45.4X1	T45.4X2	T45.4X3	T45.4X4	T45.4X5	T45.4X6
Ferrodextrane	T45.4X1	T45.4X2	T45.4X3	T45.4X4	T45.4X5	T45.4X6
Ferropolimaler	T45.4X1	T45.4X2	T45.4X3	T45.4X4	T45.4X5	
Ferrous—see also Iron						
- phosphate	T45.4X1	T45.4X2	T45.4X3	T45.4X4	T45.4X5	T45.4X6
- salt	T45.4X1	T45.4X2	T45.4X3	T45.4X4	T45.4X5	T45.4X6
- - with folic acid	T45.4X1	T45.4X2	T45.4X3	T45.4X4	T45.4X5	T45.4X6
Ferrous fumerate, gluconate, lactate, salt NEC, sulfate (medicinal)	T45.4X1	T45.4X2	T45.4X3	T45.4X4	T45.4X5	T45.4X6
Ferrovanadium (fumes)	T59.891	T59.892	T59.893	T59.894	--	--
Ferrum—see Iron						
Fertilizers NEC	T65.891	T65.892	T65.893	T65.894	--	--
- with herbicide mixture	T60.3X1	T60.3X2	T60.3X3	T60.3X4	--	--
Fetoxilate	T47.6X1	T47.6X2	T47.6X3	T47.6X4	T47.6X5	T47.6X6

Substance	Poisoning, Accidental (unintentional)	Poisoning, Intentional Self-harm	Poisoning, Assault	Poisoning, Undetermined	Adverse effect	Underdosing
Fiber, dietary	T47.4X1	T47.4X2	T47.4X3	T47.4X4	T47.4X5	T47.4X6
Fiberglass	T65.831	T65.832	T65.833	T65.834	--	--
Fibrinogen (human)	T45.8X1	T45.8X2	T45.8X3	T45.8X4	T45.8X5	T45.8X6
Fibrinolysin (human)	T45.691	T45.692	T45.693	T45.694	T45.695	T45.696
Fibrinolysis						
- affecting drug	T45.601	T45.602	T45.603	T45.604	T45.605	T45.606
- inhibitor NEC	T45.621	T45.622	T45.623	T45.624	T45.625	T45.626
Fibrinolytic drug	T45.611	T45.612	T45.613	T45.614	T45.615	T45.616
Filix mas	T37.4X1	T37.4X2	T37.4X3	T37.4X4	T37.4X5	T37.4X6
Filtering cream	T49.3X1	T49.3X2	T49.3X3	T49.3X4	T49.3X5	T49.3X6
Fiorinal	T39.011	T39.012	T39.013	T39.014	T39.015	T39.016
Firedamp	T59.891	T59.892	T59.893	T59.894	--	--
Fish, noxious, nonbacterial	T61.91	T61.92	T61.93	T61.94	--	--
- ciguatera	T61.01	T61.02	T61.03	T61.04	--	--
- scombroid	T61.11	T61.12	T61.13	T61.14	--	--
- shell	T61.781	T61.782	T61.783	T61.784	--	--
- specified NEC	T61.771	T61.772	T61.773	T61.774	--	--
Flagyl	T37.3X1	T37.3X2	T37.3X3	T37.3X4	T37.3X5	T37.3X6
Flavine adenine dinucleotide	T45.2X1	T45.2X2	T45.2X3	T45.2X4	T45.2X5	T45.2X6
Flavodic acid	T46.991	T46.992	T46.993	T46.994	T46.995	T46.996
Flavoxate	T44.3X1	T44.3X2	T44.3X3	T44.3X4	T44.3X5	T44.3X6
Flaxedil	T48.1X1	T48.1X2	T48.1X3	T48.1X4	T48.1X5	T48.1X6
Flaxseed (medicinal)	T49.3X1	T49.3X2	T49.3X3	T49.3X4	T49.3X5	T49.3X6
Flecainide	T46.2X1	T46.2X2	T46.2X3	T46.2X4	T46.2X5	T46.2X6
Fleroxacin	T36.8X1	T36.8X2	T36.8X3	T36.8X4	T36.8X5	T36.8X6
Floctafenine	T39.8X1	T39.8X2	T39.8X3	T39.8X4	T39.8X5	T39.8X6
Flomax	T44.6X1	T44.6X2	T44.6X3	T44.6X4	T44.6X5	T44.6X6
Flomoxef	T36.1X1	T36.1X2	T36.1X3	T36.1X4	T36.1X5	T36.1X6
Flopropione	T44.3X1	T44.3X2	T44.3X3	T44.3X4	T44.3X5	T44.3X6
Florantyrone	T47.5X1	T47.5X2	T47.5X3	T47.5X4	T47.5X5	T47.5X6
Floraquin	T37.8X1	T37.8X2	T37.8X3	T37.8X4	T37.8X5	T37.8X6
Florinef	T38.0X1	T38.0X2	T38.0X3	T38.0X4	T38.0X5	T38.0X6
- ENT agent	T49.6X1	T49.6X2	T49.6X3	T49.6X4	T49.6X5	T49.6X6
- ophthalmic preparation	T49.5X1	T49.5X2	T49.5X3	T49.5X4	T49.5X5	T49.5X6
- topical NEC	T49.0X1	T49.0X2	T49.0X3	T49.0X4	T49.0X5	T49.0X6
Flowers of sulfur	T49.4X1	T49.4X2	T49.4X3	T49.4X4	T49.4X5	T49.4X6
Floxuridine	T45.1X1	T45.1X2	T45.1X3	T45.1X4	T45.1X5	T45.1X6
Fluanisone	T43.4X1	T43.4X2	T43.4X3	T43.4X4	T43.4X5	T43.4X6
Flubendazole	T37.4X1	T37.4X2	T37.4X3	T37.4X4	T37.4X5	T37.4X6
Fluclorolone acetonide	T49.0X1	T49.0X2	T49.0X3	T49.0X4	T49.0X5	T49.0X6
Flucloxacillin	T36.0X1	T36.0X2	T36.0X3	T36.0X4	T36.0X5	T36.0X6
Fluconazole	T37.8X1	T37.8X2	T37.8X3	T37.8X4	T37.8X5	T37.8X6
Flucytosine	T37.8X1	T37.8X2	T37.8X3	T37.8X4	T37.8X5	T37.8X6
Fludeoxyglucose (18F)	T50.8X1	T50.8X2	T50.8X3	T50.8X4	T50.8X5	T50.8X6
Fludiazepam	T42.4X1	T42.4X2	T42.4X3	T42.4X4	T42.4X5	T42.4X6
Fludrocortisone	T50.0X1	T50.0X2	T50.0X3	T50.0X4	T50.0X5	T50.0X6
- ENT agent	T49.6X1	T49.6X2	T49.6X3	T49.6X4	T49.6X5	T49.6X6
- ophthalmic preparation	T49.5X1	T49.5X2	T49.5X3	T49.5X4	T49.5X5	T49.5X6
- topical NEC	T49.0X1	T49.0X2	T49.0X3	T49.0X4	T49.0X5	T49.0X6
Fludroxycortide	T49.0X1	T49.0X2	T49.0X3	T49.0X4	T49.0X5	T49.0X6
Flufenamic acid	T39.391	T39.392	T39.393	T39.394	T39.395	T39.396
Fluindione	T45.511	T45.512	T45.513	T45.514	T45.515	T45.516
Flumequine	T37.8X1	T37.8X2	T37.8X3	T37.8X4	T37.8X5	T37.8X6
Flumethasone	T49.0X1	T49.0X2	T49.0X3	T49.0X4	T49.0X5	T49.0X6
Flumethiazide	T50.2X1	T50.2X2	T50.2X3	T50.2X4	T50.2X5	T50.2X6
Flumidin	T37.5X1	T37.5X2	T37.5X3	T37.5X4	T37.5X5	T37.5X6
Flunarizine	T46.7X1	T46.7X2	T46.7X3	T46.7X4	T46.7X5	T46.7X6
Flunidazole	T37.8X1	T37.8X2	T37.8X3	T37.8X4	T37.8X5	T37.8X6

Substance	Poisoning, Accidental (unintentional)	Poisoning, Intentional Self-harm	Poisoning, Assault	Poisoning, Undetermined	Adverse effect	Underdosing
Flunisolide	T48.6X1	T48.6X2	T48.6X3	T48.6X4	T48.6X5	T48.6X6
Flunitrazepam	T42.4X1	T42.4X2	T42.4X3	T42.4X4	T42.4X5	T42.4X6
Fluocinolone (acetonide)	T49.0X1	T49.0X2	T49.0X3	T49.0X4	T49.0X5	T49.0X6
Fluocinonide	T49.0X1	T49.0X2	T49.0X3	T49.0X4	T49.0X5	T49.0X6
Fluocortin (butyl)	T49.0X1	T49.0X2	T49.0X3	T49.0X4	T49.0X5	T49.0X6
Fluocortolone	T49.0X1	T49.0X2	T49.0X3	T49.0X4	T49.0X5	T49.0X6
Fluohydrocortisone	T38.0X1	T38.0X2	T38.0X3	T38.0X4	T38.0X5	T38.0X6
- ENT agent	T49.6X1	T49.6X2	T49.6X3	T49.6X4	T49.6X5	T49.6X6
- ophthalmic preparation	T49.5X1	T49.5X2	T49.5X3	T49.5X4	T49.5X5	T49.5X6
- topical NEC	T49.0X1	T49.0X2	T49.0X3	T49.0X4	T49.0X5	T49.0X6
Fluonid	T49.0X1	T49.0X2	T49.0X3	T49.0X4	T49.0X5	T49.0X6
Fluopromazine	T43.3X1	T43.3X2	T43.3X3	T43.3X4	T43.3X5	T43.3X6
Fluoracetate	T60.8X1	T60.8X2	T60.8X3	T60.8X4	--	--
Fluorescein	T50.8X1	T50.8X2	T50.8X3	T50.8X4	T50.8X5	T50.8X6
Fluorhydrocortisone	T50.0X1	T50.0X2	T50.0X3	T50.0X4	T50.0X5	T50.0X6
Fluoride (nonmedicinal) (pesticide) (sodium) NEC	T60.8X1	T60.8X2	T60.8X3	T60.8X4	--	--
- hydrogen—see Hydrofluoric acid						
- medicinal NEC	T50.991	T50.992	T50.993	T50.994	T50.995	T50.996
- - dental use	T49.7X1	T49.7X2	T49.7X3	T49.7X4	T49.7X5	T49.7X6
- not pesticide NEC	T54.91	T54.92	T54.93	T54.94	--	--
- stannous	T49.7X1	T49.7X2	T49.7X3	T49.7X4	T49.7X5	T49.7X6
Fluorinated corticosteroids	T38.0X1	T38.0X2	T38.0X3	T38.0X4	T38.0X5	T38.0X6
Fluorine (gas)	T59.5X1	T59.5X2	T59.5X3	T59.5X4	--	--
- salt—see Fluoride (s)						
Fluoristan	T49.7X1	T49.7X2	T49.7X3	T49.7X4	T49.7X5	T49.7X6
Fluormetholone	T49.0X1	T49.0X2	T49.0X3	T49.0X4	T49.0X5	T49.0X6
Fluoroacetate	T60.8X1	T60.8X2	T60.8X3	T60.8X4	--	--
Fluorocarbon monomer	T53.6X1	T53.6X2	T53.6X3	T53.6X4	--	--
Fluorocytosine	T37.8X1	T37.8X2	T37.8X3	T37.8X4	T37.8X5	T37.8X6
Fluorodeoxyuridine	T45.1X1	T45.1X2	T45.1X3	T45.1X4	T45.1X5	T45.1X6
Fluorometholone	T49.0X1	T49.0X2	T49.0X3	T49.0X4	T49.0X5	T49.0X6
Fluorophosphate insecticide	T60.0X1	T60.0X2	T60.0X3	T60.0X4	--	--
Fluorosol	T46.3X1	T46.3X2	T46.3X3	T46.3X4	T46.3X5	T46.3X6
Fluorouracil	T45.1X1	T45.1X2	T45.1X3	T45.1X4	T45.1X5	T45.1X6
Fluorphenylalanine	T49.5X1	T49.5X2	T49.5X3	T49.5X4	T49.5X5	T49.5X6
Fluothane	T41.0X1	T41.0X2	T41.0X3	T41.0X4	T41.0X5	T41.0X6
Fluoxetine	T43.221	T43.222	T43.223	T43.224	T43.225	T43.226
Fluoxymesterone	T38.7X1	T38.7X2	T38.7X3	T38.7X4	T38.7X5	T38.7X6
Flupenthixol	T43.4X1	T43.4X2	T43.4X3	T43.4X4	T43.4X5	T43.4X6
Flupentixol	T43.4X1	T43.4X2	T43.4X3	T43.4X4	T43.4X5	T43.4X6
Fluphenazine	T43.3X1	T43.3X2	T43.3X3	T43.3X4	T43.3X5	T43.3X6
Fluprednidene	T49.0X1	T49.0X2	T49.0X3	T49.0X4	T49.0X5	T49.0X6
Fluprednisolone	T38.0X1	T38.0X2	T38.0X3	T38.0X4	T38.0X5	T38.0X6
Fluradoline	T39.8X1	T39.8X2	T39.8X3	T39.8X4	T39.8X5	T39.8X6
Flurandrenolide	T49.0X1	T49.0X2	T49.0X3	T49.0X4	T49.0X5	T49.0X6
Flurandrenolone	T49.0X1	T49.0X2	T49.0X3	T49.0X4	T49.0X5	T49.0X6
Flurazepam	T42.4X1	T42.4X2	T42.4X3	T42.4X4	T42.4X5	T42.4X6
Flurbiprofen	T39.311	T39.312	T39.313	T39.314	T39.315	T39.316
Flurobate	T49.0X1	T49.0X2	T49.0X3	T49.0X4	T49.0X5	T49.0X6
Fluroxene	T41.0X1	T41.0X2	T41.0X3	T41.0X4	T41.0X5	T41.0X6
Fluspirilene	T43.591	T43.592	T43.593	T43.594	T43.595	T43.596
Flutamide	T38.6X1	T38.6X2	T38.6X3	T38.6X4	T38.6X5	T38.6X6
Flutazolam	T42.4X1	T42.4X2	T42.4X3	T42.4X4	T42.4X5	T42.4X6
Fluticasone propionate	T38.0X1	T38.0X2	T38.0X3	T38.0X4	T38.0X5	T38.0X6
Flutoprazepam	T42.4X1	T42.4X2	T42.4X3	T42.4X4	T42.4X5	T42.4X6
Flutropium bromide	T48.6X1	T48.6X2	T48.6X3	T48.6X4	T48.6X5	T48.6X6
Fluvoxamine	T43.221	T43.222	T43.223	T43.224	T43.225	T43.226
Folacin	T45.8X1	T45.8X2	T45.8X3	T45.8X4	T45.8X5	T45.8X6

Substance	Poisoning, Accidental (unintentional)	Poisoning, Intentional Self-harm	Poisoning, Assault	Poisoning, Undetermined	Adverse effect	Underdosing
Folic acid	T45.8X1	T45.8X2	T45.8X3	T45.8X4	T45.8X5	T45.8X6
- with ferrous salt	T45.2X1	T45.2X2	T45.2X3	T45.2X4	T45.2X5	T45.2X6
- antagonist	T45.1X1	T45.1X2	T45.1X3	T45.1X4	T45.1X5	T45.1X6
Folinic acid	T45.8X1	T45.8X2	T45.8X3	T45.8X4	T45.8X5	T45.8X6
Folium stramoniae	T48.6X1	T48.6X2	T48.6X3	T48.6X4	T48.6X5	T48.6X6
Follicle-stimulating hormone, human	T38.811	T38.812	T38.813	T38.814	T38.815	T38.816
Folpet	T60.3X1	T60.3X2	T60.3X3	T60.3X4	--	--
Fominoben	T48.3X1	T48.3X2	T48.3X3	T48.3X4	T48.3X5	T48.3X6
Food, foodstuffs, noxious, nonbacterial, NEC	T62.91	T62.92	T62.93	T62.94	--	--
- berries	T62.1X1	T62.1X2	T62.1X3	T62.1X4	--	--
- fish—see also Fish	T61.91	T61.92	T61.93	T61.94	--	--
- mushrooms	T62.0X1	T62.0X2	T62.0X3	T62.0X4	--	--
- plants	T62.2X1	T62.2X2	T62.2X3	T62.2X4	--	--
- seafood	T61.91	T61.92	T61.93	T61.94	--	--
- - specified NEC	T61.8X1	T61.8X2	T61.8X3	T61.8X4	--	--
- seeds	T62.2X1	T62.2X2	T62.2X3	T62.2X4	--	--
- shellfish	T61.781	T61.782	T61.783	T61.784	--	--
- specified NEC	T62.8X1	T62.8X2	T62.8X3	T62.8X4	--	--
Fool's parsley	T62.2X1	T62.2X2	T62.2X3	T62.2X4	--	--
Formaldehyde (solution), gas or vapor	T59.2X1	T59.2X2	T59.2X3	T59.2X4	--	--
- fungicide	T60.3X1	T60.3X2	T60.3X3	T60.3X4	--	--
Formalin	T59.2X1	T59.2X2	T59.2X3	T59.2X4	--	--
- fungicide	T60.3X1	T60.3X2	T60.3X3	T60.3X4	--	--
- vapor	T59.2X1	T59.2X2	T59.2X3	T59.2X4	--	--
Formic acid	T54.2X1	T54.2X2	T54.2X3	T54.2X4	--	--
- vapor	T59.891	T59.892	T59.893	T59.894	--	--
Foscarnet sodium	T37.5X1	T37.5X2	T37.5X3	T37.5X4	T37.5X5	T37.5X6
Fosfestrol	T38.5X1	T38.5X2	T38.5X3	T38.5X4	T38.5X5	T38.5X6
Fosfomycin	T36.8X1	T36.8X2	T36.8X3	T36.8X4	T36.8X5	T36.8X6
Fosfonet sodium	T37.5X1	T37.5X2	T37.5X3	T37.5X4	T37.5X5	T37.5X6
Fosinopril	T46.4X1	T46.4X2	T46.4X3	T46.4X4	T46.4X5	T46.4X6
- sodium	T46.4X1	T46.4X2	T46.4X3	T46.4X4	T46.4X5	T46.4X6
Fowler's solution	T57.0X1	T57.0X2	T57.0X3	T57.0X4	--	--
Foxglove	T62.2X1	T62.2X2	T62.2X3	T62.2X4	--	--
Framycetin	T36.5X1	T36.5X2	T36.5X3	T36.5X4	T36.5X5	T36.5X6
Frangula	T47.2X1	T47.2X2	T47.2X3	T47.2X4	T47.2X5	T47.2X6
- extract	T47.2X1	T47.2X2	T47.2X3	T47.2X4	T47.2X5	T47.2X6
Frei antigen	T50.8X1	T50.8X2	T50.8X3	T50.8X4	T50.8X5	T50.8X6
Freon	T53.5X1	T53.5X2	T53.5X3	T53.5X4	--	--
Fructose	T50.3X1	T50.3X2	T50.3X3	T50.3X4	T50.3X5	T50.3X6
Frusemide	T50.1X1	T50.1X2	T50.1X3	T50.1X4	T50.1X5	T50.1X6
FSH	T38.811	T38.812	T38.813	T38.814	T38.815	T38.816
Ftorafur	T45.1X1	T45.1X2	T45.1X3	T45.1X4	T45.1X5	T45.1X6
Fuel						
- automobile	T52.0X1	T52.0X2	T52.0X3	T52.0X4	--	--
- - exhaust gas, not in transit	T58.01	T58.02	T58.03	T58.04	--	--
- - vapor NEC	T52.0X1	T52.0X2	T52.0X3	T52.0X4	--	--
- gas (domestic use) —see also Carbon, monoxide, fuel, utility	T59.891	T59.892	T59.893	T59.894	--	--
- - utility	T59.891	T59.892	T59.893	T59.894	--	--
- - - in mobile container	T59.891	T59.892	T59.893	T59.894	--	--
- - - incomplete combustion of—see Carbon, monoxide, fuel, utility						
- - - piped (natural)	T59.891	T59.892	T59.893	T59.894	--	--
- industrial, incomplete combustion	T58.8X1	T58.8X2	T58.8X3	T58.8X4	--	--
Fugillin	T36.8X1	T36.8X2	T36.8X3	T36.8X4	T36.8X5	T36.8X6
Fulminate of mercury	T56.1X1	T56.1X2	T56.1X3	T56.1X4	--	--
Fulvicin	T36.7X1	T36.7X2	T36.7X3	T36.7X4	T36.7X5	T36.7X6
Fumadil	T36.8X1	T36.8X2	T36.8X3	T36.8X4	T36.8X5	T36.8X6

Substance	Poisoning, Accidental (unintentional)	Poisoning, Intentional Self-harm	Poisoning, Assault	Poisoning, Undetermined	Adverse effect	Underdosing
Fumagillin	T36.8X1	T36.8X2	T36.8X3	T36.8X4	T36.8X5	T36.8X6
Fumaric acid	T49.4X1	T49.4X2	T49.4X3	T49.4X4	T49.4X5	T49.4X6
Fumes (from)	T59.91	T59.92	T59.93	T59.94	--	--
- carbon monoxide—see Carbon, monoxide						
- charcoal (domestic use)—see Charcoal, fumes						
- chloroform—see Chloroform						
- coke (in domestic stoves, fireplaces)—see Coke fumes						
- corrosive NEC	T54.91	T54.92	T54.93	T54.94	--	--
- ether—see ether						
- freons	T53.5X1	T53.5X2	T53.5X3	T53.5X4	--	--
- hydrocarbons	T59.891	T59.892	T59.893	T59.894	--	--
- - petroleum (liquefied)	T59.891	T59.892	T59.893	T59.894	--	--
- - - distributed through pipes (pure or mixed with air)	T59.891	T59.892	T59.893	T59.894	--	--
- lead—see lead						
- metal—see Metals, or the specified metal						
- nitrogen dioxide	T59.0X1	T59.0X2	T59.0X3	T59.0X4	--	--
- pesticides—see Pesticides						
- petroleum (liquefied)	T59.891	T59.892	T59.893	T59.894	--	--
- - distributed through pipes (pure or mixed with air)	T59.891	T59.892	T59.893	T59.894	--	--
- polyester	T59.891	T59.892	T59.893	T59.894	--	--
- specified source NEC—see also substance specified	T59.891	T59.892	T59.893	T59.894	--	--
- sulfur dioxide	T59.1X1	T59.1X2	T59.1X3	T59.1X4	--	--
Fumigant NEC	T60.91	T60.92	T60.93	T60.94	--	--
Fungi, noxious, used as food	T62.0X1	T62.0X2	T62.0X3	T62.0X4	--	--
Fungicide NEC (nonmedicinal)	T60.3X1	T60.3X2	T60.3X3	T60.3X4	--	--
Fungizone	T36.7X1	T36.7X2	T36.7X3	T36.7X4	T36.7X5	T36.7X6
- topical	T49.0X1	T49.0X2	T49.0X3	T49.0X4	T49.0X5	T49.0X6
Furacin	T49.0X1	T49.0X2	T49.0X3	T49.0X4	T49.0X5	T49.0X6
Furadantin	T37.91	T37.92	T37.93	T37.94	T37.95	T37.96
Furazolidone	T37.8X1	T37.8X2	T37.8X3	T37.8X4	T37.8X5	T37.8X6
Furazolium chloride	T49.0X1	T49.0X2	T49.0X3	T49.0X4	T49.0X5	T49.0X6
Furfural	T52.8X1	T52.8X2	T52.8X3	T52.8X4	--	--
Furnace (coal burning) (domestic), gas from	T58.2X1	T58.2X2	T58.2X3	T58.2X4	--	--
- industrial	T58.8X1	T58.8X2	T58.8X3	T58.8X4	--	--
Furniture polish	T65.891	T65.892	T65.893	T65.894	--	--
Furosemide	T50.1X1	T50.1X2	T50.1X3	T50.1X4	T50.1X5	T50.1X6
Furoxone	T37.91	T37.92	T37.93	T37.94	T37.95	T37.96
Fursultiamine	T45.2X1	T45.2X2	T45.2X3	T45.2X4	T45.2X5	T45.2X6
Fusafungine	T36.8X1	T36.8X2	T36.8X3	T36.8X4	T36.8X5	T36.8X6
Fusel oil (any) (amyl) (butyl) (propyl), vapor	T51.3X1	T51.3X2	T51.3X3	T51.3X4	--	--
Fusidate (ethanolamine) (sodium)	T36.8X1	T36.8X2	T36.8X3	T36.8X4	T36.8X5	T36.8X6
Fusidic acid	T36.8X1	T36.8X2	T36.8X3	T36.8X4	T36.8X5	T36.8X6
Fytic acid, nonasodium	T50.6X1	T50.6X2	T50.6X3	T50.6X4	T50.6X5	T50.6X6
GABA	T43.8X1	T43.8X2	T43.8X3	T43.8X4	T43.8X5	T43.8X6
Gadopentetic acid	T50.8X1	T50.8X2	T50.8X3	T50.8X4	T50.8X5	T50.8X6
Galactose	T50.3X1	T50.3X2	T50.3X3	T50.3X4	T50.3X5	T50.3X6
b-Galactosidase	T47.5X1	T47.5X2	T47.5X3	T47.5X4	T47.5X5	T47.5X6
Galantamine	T44.0X1	T44.0X2	T44.0X3	T44.0X4	T44.0X5	T44.0X6
Gallamine (triethiodide)	T48.1X1	T48.1X2	T48.1X3	T48.1X4	T48.1X5	T48.1X6
Gallium citrate	T50.991	T50.992	T50.993	T50.994	T50.995	T50.996
Gallopamil	T46.1X1	T46.1X2	T46.1X3	T46.1X4	T46.1X5	T46.1X6
Gamboge	T47.2X1	T47.2X2	T47.2X3	T47.2X4	T47.2X5	T47.2X6
Gamimune	T50.Z11	T50.Z12	T50.Z13	T50.Z14	T50.Z15	T50.Z16
Gamma globulin	T50.Z11	T50.Z12	T50.Z13	T50.Z14	T50.Z15	T50.Z16
Gamma-aminobutyric acid	T43.8X1	T43.8X2	T43.8X3	T43.8X4	T43.8X5	T43.8X6
Gamma-benzene hexachloride (medicinal)	T49.0X1	T49.0X2	T49.0X3	T49.0X4	T49.0X5	T49.0X6

Substance	Poisoning, Accidental (unintentional)	Poisoning, Intentional Self-harm	Poisoning, Assault	Poisoning, Undetermined	Adverse effect	Underdosing
- nonmedicinal, vapor	T53.6X1	T53.6X2	T53.6X3	T53.6X4	--	--
Gamma-BHC (medicinal) —see also **Gamma- benzene hexachloride**	T49.0X1	T49.0X2	T49.0X3	T49.0X4	T49.0X5	T49.0X6
Gamulin	T50.Z11	T50.Z12	T50.Z13	T50.Z14	T50.Z15	T50.Z16
Ganciclovir (sodium)	T37.5X1	T37.5X2	T37.5X3	T37.5X4	T37.5X5	T37.5X6
Ganglionic blocking drug NEC	T44.2X1	T44.2X2	T44.2X3	T44.2X4	T44.2X5	T44.2X6
- specified NEC	T44.2X1	T44.2X2	T44.2X3	T44.2X4	T44.2X5	T44.2X6
Ganja	T40.711	T40.712	T40.713	T40.714	T40.715	T40.716
Garamycin	T36.5X1	T36.5X2	T36.5X3	T36.5X4	T36.5X5	T36.5X6
- ophthalmic preparation	T49.5X1	T49.5X2	T49.5X3	T49.5X4	T49.5X5	T49.5X6
- topical NEC	T49.0X1	T49.0X2	T49.0X3	T49.0X4	T49.0X5	T49.0X6
Gardenal	T42.3X1	T42.3X2	T42.3X3	T42.3X4	T42.3X5	T42.3X6
Gardepanyl	T42.3X1	T42.3X2	T42.3X3	T42.3X4	T42.3X5	T42.3X6
Gas NEC	T59.91	T59.92	T59.93	T59.94	--	--
- acetylene	T59.891	T59.892	T59.893	T59.894	--	--
- - incomplete combustion of	T58.11	T58.12	T58.13	T58.14	--	--
- air contaminants, source or type not specified	T59.91	T59.92	T59.93	T59.94	--	--
- anesthetic	T41.0X1	T41.0X2	T41.0X3	T41.0X4	T41.0X5	T41.0X6
- blast furnace	T58.8X1	T58.8X2	T58.8X3	T58.8X4	--	--
- butane - see butane						
- carbon monoxide - see Carbon, monoxide						
- chlorine	T59.4X1	T59.4X2	T59.4X3	T59.4X4	--	--
- coal	T58.2X1	T58.2X2	T58.2X3	T58.2X4	--	--
- cyanide	T57.3X1	T57.3X2	T57.3X3	T57.3X4	--	--
- dicyanogen	T65.0X1	T65.0X2	T65.0X3	T65.0X4	--	--
- domestic - see Domestic gas						
- exhaust	T58.01	T58.02	T58.03	T58.04	--	--
- from utility (for cooking, heating, or lighting) (after combustion) – see Carbon, monoxide, fuel, utility						
- - prior to combustion	T59.891	T59.892	T59.893	T59.894	--	--
- from wood- or coal-burning stove or fireplace	T58.2X1	T58.2X2	T58.2X3	T58.2X4	--	--
- fuel (domestic use) (after combustion) - see also Carbon, monoxide, fuel						
- - industrial use	T58.8X1	T58.8X2	T58.8X3	T58.8X4	--	--
- - prior to combustion	T59.891	T59.892	T59.893	T59.894	--	--
- - utility	T59.891	T59.892	T59.893	T59.894	--	--
- - - in mobile container	T59.891	T59.892	T59.893	T59.894	--	--
- - - incomplete combustion of – see Carbon, monoxide, fuel, utility						
- - - piped (natural)	T59.891	T59.892	T59.893	T59.894	--	--
- garage	T58.01	T58.02	T58.03	T58.04	--	--
- hydrocarbon NEC	T59.891	T59.892	T59.893	T59.894	--	--
- - incomplete combustion of – see Carbon, monoxide, fuel, utility						
- - liquefied - see butane						
- - - piped	T59.891	T59.892	T59.893	T59.894	--	--
- hydrocyanic acid	T65.0X1	T65.0X2	T65.0X3	T65.0X4	--	--
- illuminating (after combustion)	T58.11	T58.12	T58.13	T58.14	--	--
- - prior to combustion	T59.891	T59.892	T59.893	T59.894	--	--
- incomplete combustion, any – see Carbon, monoxide						
- kiln	T58.8X1	T58.8X2	T58.8X3	T58.8X4	--	--
- lacrimogenic	T59.3X1	T59.3X2	T59.3X3	T59.3X4	--	--
- liquefied petroleum - see butane						
- marsh	T59.891	T59.892	T59.893	T59.894	--	--
- motor exhaust, not in transit	T58.01	T58.02	T58.03	T58.04	--	--
- mustard, not in war	T59.891	T59.892	T59.893	T59.894	--	--
- natural	T59.891	T59.892	T59.893	T59.894	--	--
- nerve, not in war	T59.91	T59.92	T59.93	T59.94	--	--

Substance	Poisoning, Accidental (unintentional)	Poisoning, Intentional Self-harm	Poisoning, Assault	Poisoning, Undetermined	Adverse effect	Underdosing
- oil	T52.0X1	T52.0X2	T52.0X3	T52.0X4	--	--
- petroleum (liquefied) (distributed in mobile containers)	T59.891	T59.892	T59.893	T59.894	--	--
- - piped (pure or mixed with air)	T59.891	T59.892	T59.893	T59.894	--	--
- piped (manufactured) (natural) NEC	T59.891	T59.892	T59.893	T59.894	--	--
- producer	T58.8X1	T58.8X2	T58.8X3	T58.8X4	--	--
- propane - see propane						
- refrigerant (chlorofluoro-carbon)	T53.5X1	T53.5X2	T53.5X3	T53.5X4	--	--
- - not chlorofluoro-carbon	T59.891	T59.892	T59.893	T59.894	--	--
- sewer	T59.91	T59.92	T59.93	T59.94	--	--
- specified source NEC	T59.91	T59.92	T59.93	T59.94	--	--
- stove (after combustion)	T58.11	T58.12	T58.13	T58.14	--	--
- - prior to combustion	T59.891	T59.892	T59.893	T59.894	--	--
- tear	T59.3X1	T59.3X2	T59.3X3	T59.3X4	--	--
- therapeutic	T41.5X1	T41.5X2	T41.5X3	T41.5X4	T41.5X5	T41.5X6
- utility (for cooking, heating, or lighting) (piped) NEC	T59.891	T59.892	T59.893	T59.894	--	--
- - in mobile container	T59.891	T59.892	T59.893	T59.894	--	--
- - incomplete combustion of – see Carbon, monoxide, fuel, utilty						
- - piped (natural)	T59.891	T59.892	T59.893	T59.894	--	--
- water	T58.11	T58.12	T58.13	T58.14	--	--
- - incomplete combustion of – see Carbon, monoxide, fuel, utility						
Gaseous substance—see Gas						
Gasoline	T52.0X1	T52.0X2	T52.0X3	T52.0X4	--	--
- vapor	T52.0X1	T52.0X2	T52.0X3	T52.0X4	--	--
Gastric enzymes	T47.5X1	T47.5X2	T47.5X3	T47.5X4	T47.5X5	T47.5X6
Gastrografin	T50.8X1	T50.8X2	T50.8X3	T50.8X4	T50.8X5	T50.8X6
Gastrointestinal drug	T47.91	T47.92	T47.93	T47.94	T47.95	T47.96
- biological	T47.8X1	T47.8X2	T47.8X3	T47.8X4	T47.8X5	T47.8X6
- specified NEC	T47.8X1	T47.8X2	T47.8X3	T47.8X4	T47.8X5	T47.8X6
Gaultheria procumbens	T62.2X1	T62.2X2	T62.2X3	T62.2X4	--	--
Gefarnate	T44.3X1	T44.3X2	T44.3X3	T44.3X4	T44.3X5	T44.3X6
Gelatin (intravenous)	T45.8X1	T45.8X2	T45.8X3	T45.8X4	T45.8X5	T45.8X6
- absorbable (sponge)	T45.7X1	T45.7X2	T45.7X3	T45.7X4	T45.7X5	T45.7X6
Gelfilm	T49.8X1	T49.8X2	T49.8X3	T49.8X4	T49.8X5	T49.8X6
Gelfoam	T45.7X1	T45.7X2	T45.7X3	T45.7X4	T45.7X5	T45.7X6
Gelsemine	T50.991	T50.992	T50.993	T50.994	T50.995	T50.996
Gelsemium (sempervirens)	T62.2X1	T62.2X2	T62.2X3	T62.2X4	--	--
Gemeprost	T48.0X1	T48.0X2	T48.0X3	T48.0X4	T48.0X5	T48.0X6
Gemfibrozil	T46.6X1	T46.6X2	T46.6X3	T46.6X4	T46.6X5	T46.6X6
Gemonil	T42.3X1	T42.3X2	T42.3X3	T42.3X4	T42.3X5	T42.3X6
Gentamicin	T36.5X1	T36.5X2	T36.5X3	T36.5X4	T36.5X5	T36.5X6
- ophthalmic preparation	T49.5X1	T49.5X2	T49.5X3	T49.5X4	T49.5X5	T49.5X6
- topical NEC	T49.0X1	T49.0X2	T49.0X3	T49.0X4	T49.0X5	T49.0X6
Gentian	T47.5X1	T47.5X2	T47.5X3	T47.5X4	T47.5X5	T47.5X6
- violet	T49.0X1	T49.0X2	T49.0X3	T49.0X4	T49.0X5	T49.0X6
Gepefrine	T44.4X1	T44.4X2	T44.4X3	T44.4X4	T44.4X5	T44.4X6
Gestonorone caproate	T38.5X1	T38.5X2	T38.5X3	T38.5X4	T38.5X5	T38.5X6
Gexane	T49.0X1	T49.0X2	T49.0X3	T49.0X4	T49.0X5	T49.0X6
Gila monster (venom)	T63.111	T63.112	T63.113	T63.114	--	--
Ginger	T47.5X1	T47.5X2	T47.5X3	T47.5X4	T47.5X5	T47.5X6
- Jamaica—see Jamaica, ginger						
Gitalin	T46.0X1	T46.0X2	T46.0X3	T46.0X4	T46.0X5	T46.0X6
- amorphous	T46.0X1	T46.0X2	T46.0X3	T46.0X4	T46.0X5	T46.0X6
Gitaloxin	T46.0X1	T46.0X2	T46.0X3	T46.0X4	T46.0X5	T46.0X6
Gitoxin	T46.0X1	T46.0X2	T46.0X3	T46.0X4	T46.0X5	T46.0X6
Glafenine	T39.8X1	T39.8X2	T39.8X3	T39.8X4	T39.8X5	T39.8X6
Glandular extract (medicinal) NEC	T50.Z91	T50.Z92	T50.Z93	T50.Z94	T50.Z95	T50.Z96

Substance	Poisoning, Accidental (unintentional)	Poisoning, Intentional Self-harm	Poisoning, Assault	Poisoning, Undetermined	Adverse effect	Underdosing
Glaucarubin	T37.3X1	T37.3X2	T37.3X3	T37.3X4	T37.3X5	T37.3X6
Glibenclamide	T38.3X1	T38.3X2	T38.3X3	T38.3X4	T38.3X5	T38.3X6
Glibornuride	T38.3X1	T38.3X2	T38.3X3	T38.3X4	T38.3X5	T38.3X6
Gliclazide	T38.3X1	T38.3X2	T38.3X3	T38.3X4	T38.3X5	T38.3X6
Glimidine	T38.3X1	T38.3X2	T38.3X3	T38.3X4	T38.3X5	T38.3X6
Glipizide	T38.3X1	T38.3X2	T38.3X3	T38.3X4	T38.3X5	T38.3X6
Gliquidone	T38.3X1	T38.3X2	T38.3X3	T38.3X4	T38.3X5	T38.3X6
Glisolamide	T38.3X1	T38.3X2	T38.3X3	T38.3X4	T38.3X5	T38.3X6
Glisoxepide	T38.3X1	T38.3X2	T38.3X3	T38.3X4	T38.3X5	T38.3X6
Globin zinc insulin	T38.3X1	T38.3X2	T38.3X3	T38.3X4	T38.3X5	T38.3X6
Globulin						
- antilymphocytic	T50.Z11	T50.Z12	T50.Z13	T50.Z14	T50.Z15	T50.Z16
- antirhesus	T50.Z11	T50.Z12	T50.Z13	T50.Z14	T50.Z15	T50.Z16
- antivenin	T50.Z11	T50.Z12	T50.Z13	T50.Z14	T50.Z15	T50.Z16
- antiviral	T50.Z11	T50.Z12	T50.Z13	T50.Z14	T50.Z15	T50.Z16
Glucagon	T38.3X1	T38.3X2	T38.3X3	T38.3X4	T38.3X5	T38.3X6
Glucocorticoids	T38.0X1	T38.0X2	T38.0X3	T38.0X4	T38.0X5	T38.0X6
Glucocorticosteroid	T38.0X1	T38.0X2	T38.0X3	T38.0X4	T38.0X5	T38.0X6
Gluconic acid	T50.991	T50.992	T50.993	T50.994	T50.995	T50.996
Glucosamine sulfate	T39.4X1	T39.4X2	T39.4X3	T39.4X4	T39.4X5	T39.4X6
Glucose	T50.3X1	T50.3X2	T50.3X3	T50.3X4	T50.3X5	T50.3X6
- with sodium chloride	T50.3X1	T50.3X2	T50.3X3	T50.3X4	T50.3X5	T50.3X6
Glucosulfone sodium	T37.1X1	T37.1X2	T37.1X3	T37.1X4	T37.1X5	T37.1X6
Glucurolactone	T47.8X1	T47.8X2	T47.8X3	T47.8X4	T47.8X5	T47.8X6
Glue NEC	T52.8X1	T52.8X2	T52.8X3	T52.8X4	--	--
Glutamic acid	T47.5X1	T47.5X2	T47.5X3	T47.5X4	T47.5X5	T47.5X6
Glutaral (medicinal)	T49.0X1	T49.0X2	T49.0X3	T49.0X4	T49.0X5	T49.0X6
- nonmedicinal	T65.891	T65.892	T65.893	T65.894	--	--
Glutaraldehyde (nonmedicinal)	T65.891	T65.892	T65.893	T65.894	--	--
- medicinal	T49.0X1	T49.0X2	T49.0X3	T49.0X4	T49.0X5	T49.0X6
Glutathione	T50.6X1	T50.6X2	T50.6X3	T50.6X4	T50.6X5	T50.6X6
Glutethimide	T42.6X1	T42.6X2	T42.6X3	T42.6X4	T42.6X5	T42.6X6
Glyburide	T38.3X1	T38.3X2	T38.3X3	T38.3X4	T38.3X5	T38.3X6
Glycerin	T47.4X1	T47.4X2	T47.4X3	T47.4X4	T47.4X5	T47.4X6
Glycerol	T47.4X1	T47.4X2	T47.4X3	T47.4X4	T47.4X5	T47.4X6
- borax	T49.6X1	T49.6X2	T49.6X3	T49.6X4	T49.6X5	T49.6X6
- intravenous	T50.3X1	T50.3X2	T50.3X3	T50.3X4	T50.3X5	T50.3X6
- iodinated	T48.4X1	T48.4X2	T48.4X3	T48.4X4	T48.4X5	T48.4X6
Glycerophosphate	T50.991	T50.992	T50.993	T50.994	T50.995	T50.996
Glyceryl						
- gualacolate	T48.4X1	T48.4X2	T48.4X3	T48.4X4	T48.4X5	T48.4X6
- nitrate	T46.3X1	T46.3X2	T46.3X3	T46.3X4	T46.3X5	T46.3X6
- triacetate (topical)	T49.0X1	T49.0X2	T49.0X3	T49.0X4	T49.0X5	T49.0X6
- trinitrate	T46.3X1	T46.3X2	T46.3X3	T46.3X4	T46.3X5	T46.3X6
Glycine	T50.3X1	T50.3X2	T50.3X3	T50.3X4	T50.3X5	T50.3X6
Glyclopyramide	T38.3X1	T38.3X2	T38.3X3	T38.3X4	T38.3X5	T38.3X6
Glycobiarsol	T37.3X1	T37.3X2	T37.3X3	T37.3X4	T37.3X5	T37.3X6
Glycols (ether)	T52.3X1	T52.3X2	T52.3X3	T52.3X4	--	--
Glyconiazide	T37.1X1	T37.1X2	T37.1X3	T37.1X4	T37.1X5	T37.1X6
Glycopyrrolate	T44.3X1	T44.3X2	T44.3X3	T44.3X4	T44.3X5	T44.3X6
Glycopyrronium	T44.3X1	T44.3X2	T44.3X3	T44.3X4	T44.3X5	T44.3X6
- bromide	T44.3X1	T44.3X2	T44.3X3	T44.3X4	T44.3X5	T44.3X6
Glycoside, cardiac (stimulant)	T46.0X1	T46.0X2	T46.0X3	T46.0X4	T46.0X5	T46.0X6
Glycyclamide	T38.3X1	T38.3X2	T38.3X3	T38.3X4	T38.3X5	T38.3X6
Glycyrrhiza extract	T48.4X1	T48.4X2	T48.4X3	T48.4X4	T48.4X5	T48.4X6
Glycyrrhizic acid	T48.4X1	T48.4X2	T48.4X3	T48.4X4	T48.4X5	T48.4X6
Glycyrrhizinate potassium	T48.4X1	T48.4X2	T48.4X3	T48.4X4	T48.4X5	T48.4X6
Glymidine sodium	T38.3X1	T38.3X2	T38.3X3	T38.3X4	T38.3X5	T38.3X6

Substance	Poisoning, Accidental (unintentional)	Poisoning, Intentional Self-harm	Poisoning, Assault	Poisoning, Undetermined	Adverse effect	Underdosing
Glyphosate	T60.3X1	T60.3X2	T60.3X3	T60.3X4	--	--
Glyphylline	T48.6X1	T48.6X2	T48.6X3	T48.6X4	T48.6X5	T48.6X6
Gold						
- colloidal (l98Au)	T45.1X1	T45.1X2	T45.1X3	T45.1X4	T45.1X5	T45.1X6
- salts	T39.4X1	T39.4X2	T39.4X3	T39.4X4	T39.4X5	T39.4X6
Golden sulfide of antimony	T56.891	T56.892	T56.893	T56.894	--	--
Goldylocks	T62.2X1	T62.2X2	T62.2X3	T62.2X4	--	--
Gonadal tissue extract	T38.901	T38.902	T38.903	T38.904	T38.905	T38.906
- female	T38.5X1	T38.5X2	T38.5X3	T38.5X4	T38.5X5	T38.5X6
- male	T38.7X1	T38.7X2	T38.7X3	T38.7X4	T38.7X5	T38.7X6
Gonadorelin	T38.891	T38.892	T38.893	T38.894	T38.895	T38.896
Gonadotropin	T38.891	T38.892	T38.893	T38.894	T38.895	T38.896
- chorionic	T38.891	T38.892	T38.893	T38.894	T38.895	T38.896
- pituitary	T38.811	T38.812	T38.813	T38.814	T38.815	T38.816
Goserelin	T45.1X1	T45.1X2	T45.1X3	T45.1X4	T45.1X5	T45.1X6
Grain alcohol	T51.0X1	T51.0X2	T51.0X3	T51.0X4	--	--
Gramicidin	T49.0X1	T49.0X2	T49.0X3	T49.0X4	T49.0X5	T49.0X6
Granisetron	T45.0X1	T45.0X2	T45.0X3	T45.0X4	T45.0X5	T45.0X6
Gratiola officinalis	T62.2X1	T62.2X2	T62.2X3	T62.2X4	--	--
Grease	T65.891	T65.892	T65.893	T65.894	--	--
Green hellebore	T62.2X1	T62.2X2	T62.2X3	T62.2X4	--	--
Green soap	T49.2X1	T49.2X2	T49.2X3	T49.2X4	T49.2X5	T49.2X6
Grifulvin	T36.7X1	T36.7X2	T36.7X3	T36.7X4	T36.7X5	T36.7X6
Griseofulvin	T36.7X1	T36.7X2	T36.7X3	T36.7X4	T36.7X5	T36.7X6
Growth hormone	T38.811	T38.812	T38.813	T38.814	T38.815	T38.816
Guaiac reagent	T50.991	T50.992	T50.993	T50.994	T50.995	T50.996
Guaiacol derivatives	T48.4X1	T48.4X2	T48.4X3	T48.4X4	T48.4X5	T48.4X6
Guaifenesin	T48.4X1	T48.4X2	T48.4X3	T48.4X4	T48.4X5	T48.4X6
Guaimesal	T48.4X1	T48.4X2	T48.4X3	T48.4X4	T48.4X5	T48.4X6
Guaiphenesin	T48.4X1	T48.4X2	T48.4X3	T48.4X4	T48.4X5	T48.4X6
Guamecycline	T36.4X1	T36.4X2	T36.4X3	T36.4X4	T36.4X5	T36.4X6
Guanabenz	T46.5X1	T46.5X2	T46.5X3	T46.5X4	T46.5X5	T46.5X6
Guanacline	T46.5X1	T46.5X2	T46.5X3	T46.5X4	T46.5X5	T46.5X6
Guanadrel	T46.5X1	T46.5X2	T46.5X3	T46.5X4	T46.5X5	T46.5X6
Guanatol	T37.2X1	T37.2X2	T37.2X3	T37.2X4	T37.2X5	T37.2X6
Guanethidine	T46.5X1	T46.5X2	T46.5X3	T46.5X4	T46.5X5	T46.5X6
Guanfacine	T46.5X1	T46.5X2	T46.5X3	T46.5X4	T46.5X5	T46.5X6
Guano	T65.891	T65.892	T65.893	T65.894	--	--
Guanochlor	T46.5X1	T46.5X2	T46.5X3	T46.5X4	T46.5X5	T46.5X6
Guanoclor	T46.5X1	T46.5X2	T46.5X3	T46.5X4	T46.5X5	T46.5X6
Guanoctine	T46.5X1	T46.5X2	T46.5X3	T46.5X4	T46.5X5	T46.5X6
Guanoxabenz	T46.5X1	T46.5X2	T46.5X3	T46.5X4	T46.5X5	T46.5X6
Guanoxan	T46.5X1	T46.5X2	T46.5X3	T46.5X4	T46.5X5	T46.5X6
Guar gum (medicinal)	T46.6X1	T46.6X2	T46.6X3	T46.6X4	T46.6X5	T46.6X6
Hachimycin	T36.7X1	T36.7X2	T36.7X3	T36.7X4	T36.7X5	T36.7X6
Hair						
- dye	T49.4X1	T49.4X2	T49.4X3	T49.4X4	T49.4X5	T49.4X6
- preparation NEC	T49.4X1	T49.4X2	T49.4X3	T49.4X4	T49.4X5	T49.4X6
Halazepam	T42.4X1	T42.4X2	T42.4X3	T42.4X4	T42.4X5	T42.4X6
Halcinolone	T49.0X1	T49.0X2	T49.0X3	T49.0X4	T49.0X5	T49.0X6
Halcinonide	T49.0X1	T49.0X2	T49.0X3	T49.0X4	T49.0X5	T49.0X6
Halethazole	T49.0X1	T49.0X2	T49.0X3	T49.0X4	T49.0X5	T49.0X6
Hallucinogen NOS	T40.901	T40.902	T40.903	T40.904	T40.905	T40.906
- specified NEC	T40.991	T40.992	T40.993	T40.994	T40.995	T40.996
Halofantrine	T37.2X1	T37.2X2	T37.2X3	T37.2X4	T37.2X5	T37.2X6
Halofenate	T46.6X1	T46.6X2	T46.6X3	T46.6X4	T46.6X5	T46.6X6
Halometasone	T49.0X1	T49.0X2	T49.0X3	T49.0X4	T49.0X5	T49.0X6
Haloperidol	T43.4X1	T43.4X2	T43.4X3	T43.4X4	T43.4X5	T43.4X6
Haloprogin	T49.0X1	T49.0X2	T49.0X3	T49.0X4	T49.0X5	T49.0X6

Substance	Poisoning, Accidental (unintentional)	Poisoning, Intentional Self-harm	Poisoning, Assault	Poisoning, Undetermined	Adverse effect	Underdosing
Halotex	T49.0X1	T49.0X2	T49.0X3	T49.0X4	T49.0X5	T49.0X6
Halothane	T41.0X1	T41.0X2	T41.0X3	T41.0X4	T41.0X5	T41.0X6
Haloxazolam	T42.4X1	T42.4X2	T42.4X3	T42.4X4	T42.4X5	T42.4X6
Halquinols	T49.0X1	T49.0X2	T49.0X3	T49.0X4	T49.0X5	T49.0X6
Hamamelis	T49.2X1	T49.2X2	T49.2X3	T49.2X4	T49.2X5	T49.2X6
Haptendextran	T45.8X1	T45.8X2	T45.8X3	T45.8X4	T45.8X5	T45.8X6
Harmonyl	T46.5X1	T46.5X2	T46.5X3	T46.5X4	T46.5X5	T46.5X6
Hartmann's solution	T50.3X1	T50.3X2	T50.3X3	T50.3X4	T50.3X5	T50.3X6
Hashish	T40.711	T40.712	T40.713	T40.714	T40.715	T40.716
Hawaiian Woodrose seeds	T40.991	T40.992	T40.993	T40.994	--	--
HCB	T60.3X1	T60.3X2	T60.3X3	T60.3X4	--	--
HCH	T53.6X1	T53.6X2	T53.6X3	T53.6X4	--	--
- medicinal	T49.0X1	T49.0X2	T49.0X3	T49.0X4	T49.0X5	T49.0X6
HCN	T57.3X1	T57.3X2	T57.3X3	T57.3X4	--	--
Headache cures, drugs, powders NEC	T50.901	T50.902	T50.903	T50.904	T50.905	T50.906
Heavenly Blue (morning glory)	T40.991	T40.992	T40.993	T40.994	--	--
Heavy metal antidote	T45.8X1	T45.8X2	T45.8X3	T45.8X4	T45.8X5	T45.8X6
Hedaquinium	T49.0X1	T49.0X2	T49.0X3	T49.0X4	T49.0X5	T49.0X6
Hedge hyssop	T62.2X1	T62.2X2	T62.2X3	T62.2X4	--	--
Heet	T49.8X1	T49.8X2	T49.8X3	T49.8X4	T49.8X5	T49.8X6
Helenin	T37.4X1	T37.4X2	T37.4X3	T37.4X4	T37.4X5	T37.4X6
Helium (nonmedicinal) NEC	T59.891	T59.892	T59.893	T59.894	--	--
- medicinal	T48.991	T48.992	T48.993	T48.994	T48.995	T48.996
Hellebore (black) (green) (white)	T62.2X1	T62.2X2	T62.2X3	T62.2X4	--	--
Hematin	T45.8X1	T45.8X2	T45.8X3	T45.8X4	T45.8X5	T45.8X6
Hematinic preparation	T45.8X1	T45.8X2	T45.8X3	T45.8X4	T45.8X5	T45.8X6
Hematological agent	T45.91	T45.92	T45.93	T45.94	T45.95	T45.96
- specified NEC	T45.8X1	T45.8X2	T45.8X3	T45.8X4	T45.8X5	T45.8X6
Hemlock	T62.2X1	T62.2X2	T62.2X3	T62.2X4	--	--
Hemostatic	T45.621	T45.622	T45.623	T45.624	T45.625	T45.626
- drug, systemic	T45.621	T45.622	T45.623	T45.624	T45.625	T45.626
Hemostyptic	T49.4X1	T49.4X2	T49.4X3	T49.4X4	T49.4X5	T49.4X6
Henbane	T62.2X1	T62.2X2	T62.2X3	T62.2X4	--	--
Heparin (sodium)	T45.511	T45.512	T45.513	T45.514	T45.515	T45.516
- action reverser	T45.7X1	T45.7X2	T45.7X3	T45.7X4	T45.7X5	T45.7X6
Heparin-fraction	T45.511	T45.512	T45.513	T45.514	T45.515	T45.516
Heparinoid (systemic)	T45.511	T45.512	T45.513	T45.514	T45.515	T45.516
Hepatic secretion stimulant	T47.8X1	T47.8X2	T47.8X3	T47.8X4	T47.8X5	T47.8X6
Hepatitis B						
- immune globulin	T50.Z11	T50.Z12	T50.Z13	T50.Z14	T50.Z15	T50.Z16
- vaccine	T50.B91	T50.B92	T50.B93	T50.B94	T50.B95	T50.B96
Hepronicate	T46.7X1	T46.7X2	T46.7X3	T46.7X4	T46.7X5	T46.7X6
Heptabarb	T42.3X1	T42.3X2	T42.3X3	T42.3X4	T42.3X5	T42.3X6
Heptabarbital	T42.3X1	T42.3X2	T42.3X3	T42.3X4	T42.3X5	T42.3X6
Heptabarbitone	T42.3X1	T42.3X2	T42.3X3	T42.3X4	T42.3X5	T42.3X6
Heptachlor	T60.1X1	T60.1X2	T60.1X3	T60.1X4	--	--
Heptalgin	T40.2X1	T40.2X2	T40.2X3	T40.2X4	T40.2X5	T40.2X6
Heptaminol	T46.3X1	T46.3X2	T46.3X3	T46.3X4	T46.3X5	T46.3X6
Herbicide NEC	T60.3X1	T60.3X2	T60.3X3	T60.3X4	--	--
Heroin	T40.1X1	T40.1X2	T40.1X3	T40.1X4	T40.1X5	--
Herplex	T49.5X1	T49.5X2	T49.5X3	T49.5X4	T49.5X5	T49.5X6
HES	T45.8X1	T45.8X2	T45.8X3	T45.8X4	T45.8X5	T45.8X6
Hesperidin	T46.991	T46.992	T46.993	T46.994	T46.995	T46.996
Hetacillin	T36.0X1	T36.0X2	T36.0X3	T36.0X4	T36.0X5	T36.0X6
Hetastarch	T45.8X1	T45.8X2	T45.8X3	T45.8X4	T45.8X5	T45.8X6
HETP	T60.0X1	T60.0X2	T60.0X3	T60.0X4	--	--
Hexachlorobenzene (vapor)	T60.3X1	T60.3X2	T60.3X3	T60.3X4	--	--
Hexachlorocyclohexane	T53.6X1	T53.6X2	T53.6X3	T53.6X4	--	--

Substance	Poisoning, Accidental (unintentional)	Poisoning, Intentional Self-harm	Poisoning, Assault	Poisoning, Undetermined	Adverse effect	Underdosing
Hexachlorophene	T49.0X1	T49.0X2	T49.0X3	T49.0X4	T49.0X5	T49.0X6
Hexadiline	T46.3X1	T46.3X2	T46.3X3	T46.3X4	T46.3X5	T46.3X6
Hexadimethrine (bromide)	T45.7X1	T45.7X2	T45.7X3	T45.7X4	T45.7X5	T45.7X6
Hexadylamine	T46.3X1	T46.3X2	T46.3X3	T46.3X4	T46.3X5	T46.3X6
Hexaethyl tetraphos-phate	T60.0X1	T60.0X2	T60.0X3	T60.0X4	--	--
Hexafluorenium bromide	T48.1X1	T48.1X2	T48.1X3	T48.1X4	T48.1X5	T48.1X6
Hexafluronium (bromide)	T48.1X1	T48.1X2	T48.1X3	T48.1X4	T48.1X5	T48.1X6
Hexa-germ	T49.2X1	T49.2X2	T49.2X3	T49.2X4	T49.2X5	T49.2X6
Hexahydrobenzol	T52.8X1	T52.8X2	T52.8X3	T52.8X4	--	--
Hexahydrocresol (s)	T51.8X1	T51.8X2	T51.8X3	T51.8X4	--	--
- arsenide	T57.0X1	T57.0X2	T57.0X3	T57.0X4	--	--
- arseniurated	T57.0X1	T57.0X2	T57.0X3	T57.0X4	--	--
- cyanide	T57.3X1	T57.3X2	T57.3X3	T57.3X4	--	--
- - gas	T59.891	T59.892	T59.893	T59.894	--	--
- Fluoride (liquid)	T57.8X1	T57.8X2	T57.8X3	T57.8X4	--	--
- - vapor	T59.891	T59.892	T59.893	T59.894	--	--
- phophorated	T60.0X1	T60.0X2	T60.0X3	T60.0X4	--	--
- sulfate	T57.8X1	T57.8X2	T57.8X3	T57.8X4	--	--
- sulfide (gas)	T59.6X1	T59.6X2	T59.6X3	T59.6X4	--	--
- - arseniurated	T57.0X1	T57.0X2	T57.0X3	T57.0X4	--	--
- sulfurated	T57.8X1	T57.8X2	T57.8X3	T57.8X4	--	--
Hexahydrophenol	T51.8X1	T51.8X2	T51.8X3	T51.8X4	--	--
Hexalen	T51.8X1	T51.8X2	T51.8X3	T51.8X4	--	--
Hexamethonium bromide	T44.2X1	T44.2X2	T44.2X3	T44.2X4	T44.2X5	T44.2X6
Hexamethylene	T52.8X1	T52.8X2	T52.8X3	T52.8X4	--	--
Hexamethylmelamine	T45.1X1	T45.1X2	T45.1X3	T45.1X4	T45.1X5	T45.1X6
Hexamidine	T49.0X1	T49.0X2	T49.0X3	T49.0X4	T49.0X5	T49.0X6
Hexamine (mandelate)	T37.8X1	T37.8X2	T37.8X3	T37.8X4	T37.8X5	T37.8X6
Hexanone, 2-hexanone	T52.4X1	T52.4X2	T52.4X3	T52.4X4	--	--
Hexanuorenium	T48.1X1	T48.1X2	T48.1X3	T48.1X4	T48.1X5	T48.1X6
Hexapropymate	T42.6X1	T42.6X2	T42.6X3	T42.6X4	T42.6X5	T42.6X6
Hexasonium iodide	T44.3X1	T44.3X2	T44.3X3	T44.3X4	T44.3X5	T44.3X6
Hexcarbacholine bromide	T48.1X1	T48.1X2	T48.1X3	T48.1X4	T48.1X5	T48.1X6
Hexemal	T42.3X1	T42.3X2	T42.3X3	T42.3X4	T42.3X5	T42.3X6
Hexestrol	T38.5X1	T38.5X2	T38.5X3	T38.5X4	T38.5X5	T38.5X6
Hexethal (sodium)	T42.3X1	T42.3X2	T42.3X3	T42.3X4	T42.3X5	T42.3X6
Hexetidine	T37.8X1	T37.8X2	T37.8X3	T37.8X4	T37.8X5	T37.8X6
Hexobarbital	T42.3X1	T42.3X2	T42.3X3	T42.3X4	T42.3X5	T42.3X6
- rectal	T41.291	T41.292	T41.293	T41.294	T41.295	T41.296
- sodium	T41.1X1	T41.1X2	T41.1X3	T41.1X4	T41.1X5	T41.1X6
Hexobendine	T46.3X1	T46.3X2	T46.3X3	T46.3X4	T46.3X5	T46.3X6
Hexocyclium	T44.3X1	T44.3X2	T44.3X3	T44.3X4	T44.3X5	T44.3X6
- metilsulfate	T44.3X1	T44.3X2	T44.3X3	T44.3X4	T44.3X5	T44.3X6
Hexoestrol	T38.5X1	T38.5X2	T38.5X3	T38.5X4	T38.5X5	T38.5X6
Hexone	T52.4X1	T52.4X2	T52.4X3	T52.4X4	--	--
Hexoprenaline	T48.6X1	T48.6X2	T48.6X3	T48.6X4	T48.6X5	T48.6X6
Hexylcaine	T41.3X1	T41.3X2	T41.3X3	T41.3X4	T41.3X5	T41.3X6
Hexylresorcinol	T52.2X1	T52.2X2	T52.2X3	T52.2X4	--	--
HGH (human growth hormone)	T38.811	T38.812	T38.813	T38.814	T38.815	T38.816
Hinkle's pills	T47.2X1	T47.2X2	T47.2X3	T47.2X4	T47.2X5	T47.2X6
Histalog	T50.8X1	T50.8X2	T50.8X3	T50.8X4	T50.8X5	T50.8X6
Histamine (phosphate)	T50.8X1	T50.8X2	T50.8X3	T50.8X4	T50.8X5	T50.8X6
Histoplasmin	T50.8X1	T50.8X2	T50.8X3	T50.8X4	T50.8X5	T50.8X6
Holly berries	T62.2X1	T62.2X2	T62.2X3	T62.2X4	--	--
Homatropine	T44.3X1	T44.3X2	T44.3X3	T44.3X4	T44.3X5	T44.3X6
- methylbromide	T44.3X1	T44.3X2	T44.3X3	T44.3X4	T44.3X5	T44.3X6
Homochlorcyclizine	T45.0X1	T45.0X2	T45.0X3	T45.0X4	T45.0X5	T45.0X6
Homosalate	T49.3X1	T49.3X2	T49.3X3	T49.3X4	T49.3X5	T49.3X6
Homo-tet	T50.Z11	T50.Z12	T50.Z13	T50.Z14	T50.Z15	T50.Z16

Substance	Poisoning, Accidental (unintentional)	Poisoning, Intentional Self-harm	Poisoning, Assault	Poisoning, Undetermined	Adverse effect	Underdosing
Hormone	T38.801	T38.802	T38.803	T38.804	T38.805	T38.806
- adrenal cortical steroids	T38.0X1	T38.0X2	T38.0X3	T38.0X4	T38.0X5	T38.0X6
- androgenic	T38.7X1	T38.7X2	T38.7X3	T38.7X4	T38.7X5	T38.7X6
- anterior pituitary NEC	T38.811	T38.812	T38.813	T38.814	T38.815	T38.816
- antidiabetic agents	T38.3X1	T38.3X2	T38.3X3	T38.3X4	T38.3X5	T38.3X6
- antidiuretic	T38.891	T38.892	T38.893	T38.894	T38.895	T38.896
- cancer therapy	T45.1X1	T45.1X2	T45.1X3	T45.1X4	T45.1X5	T45.1X6
- follicle stimulating	T38.811	T38.812	T38.813	T38.814	T38.815	T38.816
- gonadotropic	T38.891	T38.892	T38.893	T38.894	T38.895	T38.896
- - pituitary	T38.811	T38.812	T38.813	T38.814	T38.815	T38.816
- growth	T38.811	T38.812	T38.813	T38.814	T38.815	T38.816
- luteinizing	T38.811	T38.812	T38.813	T38.814	T38.815	T38.816
- ovarian	T38.5X1	T38.5X2	T38.5X3	T38.5X4	T38.5X5	T38.5X6
- oxytocic	T48.0X1	T48.0X2	T48.0X3	T48.0X4	T48.0X5	T48.0X6
- parathyroid (derivatives)	T50.991	T50.992	T50.993	T50.994	T50.995	T50.996
- pituitary (posterior) NEC	T38.891	T38.892	T38.893	T38.894	T38.895	T38.896
- - anterior	T38.811	T38.812	T38.813	T38.814	T38.815	T38.816
- specified, NEC	T38.891	T38.892	T38.893	T38.894	T38.895	T38.896
- thyroid	T38.1X1	T38.1X2	T38.1X3	T38.1X4	T38.1X5	T38.1X6
Hornet (sting)	T63.451	T63.452	T63.453	T63.454	--	--
Horse anti-human lymphocytic serum	T50.Z11	T50.Z12	T50.Z13	T50.Z14	T50.Z15	T50.Z16
Horticulture agent NEC	T65.91	T65.92	T65.93	T65.94	--	--
- with pesticide	T60.91	T60.92	T60.93	T60.94	--	--
Human						
- albumin	T45.8X1	T45.8X2	T45.8X3	T45.8X4	T45.8X5	T45.8X6
- growth hormone (HGH)	T38.811	T38.812	T38.813	T38.814	T38.815	T38.816
- immune serum	T50.Z11	T50.Z12	T50.Z13	T50.Z14	T50.Z15	T50.Z16
Hyaluronidase	T45.3X1	T45.3X2	T45.3X3	T45.3X4	T45.3X5	T45.3X6
Hyazyme	T45.3X1	T45.3X2	T45.3X3	T45.3X4	T45.3X5	T45.3X6
Hycodan	T40.2X1	T40.2X2	T40.2X3	T40.2X4	T40.2X5	T40.2X6
Hydantoin derivative NEC	T42.0X1	T42.0X2	T42.0X3	T42.0X4	T42.0X5	T42.0X6
Hydeltra	T38.0X1	T38.0X2	T38.0X3	T38.0X4	T38.0X5	T38.0X6
Hydergine	T44.6X1	T44.6X2	T44.6X3	T44.6X4	T44.6X5	T44.6X6
Hydrabamine penicillin	T36.0X1	T36.0X2	T36.0X3	T36.0X4	T36.0X5	T36.0X6
Hydralazine	T46.5X1	T46.5X2	T46.5X3	T46.5X4	T46.5X5	T46.5X6
Hydrargaphen	T49.0X1	T49.0X2	T49.0X3	T49.0X4	T49.0X5	T49.0X6
Hydrargyri amino-chloridum	T49.0X1	T49.0X2	T49.0X3	T49.0X4	T49.0X5	T49.0X6
Hydrastine	T48.291	T48.292	T48.293	T48.294	T48.295	T48.296
Hydrazine	T54.1X1	T54.1X2	T54.1X3	T54.1X4	--	--
- monoamine oxidase inhibitors	T43.1X1	T43.1X2	T43.1X3	T43.1X4	T43.1X5	T43.1X6
Hydrazoic acid, azides	T54.2X1	T54.2X2	T54.2X3	T54.2X4	--	--
Hydriodic acid	T48.4X1	T48.4X2	T48.4X3	T48.4X4	T48.4X5	T48.4X6
Hydrocarbon gas	T59.891	T59.892	T59.893	T59.894	--	--
- incomplete combustion of—see Carbon, monoxide, fuel, utility						
- liquefied (mobile container)	T59.891	T59.892	T59.893	T59.894	--	--
- - piped (natural)	T59.891	T59.892	T59.893	T59.894	--	--
Hydrochloric acid (liquid)	T54.2X1	T54.2X2	T54.2X3	T54.2X4	--	--
- medicinal (digestant)	T47.5X1	T47.5X2	T47.5X3	T47.5X4	T47.5X5	T47.5X6
- vapor	T59.891	T59.892	T59.893	T59.894	--	--
Hydrochlorothiazide	T50.2X1	T50.2X2	T50.2X3	T50.2X4	T50.2X5	T50.2X6
Hydrocodone	T40.2X1	T40.2X2	T40.2X3	T40.2X4	T40.2X5	T40.2X6
Hydrocortisone (derivatives)	T38.0X1	T38.0X2	T38.0X3	T38.0X4	T38.0X5	T38.0X6
- aceponate	T49.0X1	T49.0X2	T49.0X3	T49.0X4	T49.0X5	T49.0X6
- ENT agent	T49.6X1	T49.6X2	T49.6X3	T49.6X4	T49.6X5	T49.6X6
- ophthalmic preparation	T49.5X1	T49.5X2	T49.5X3	T49.5X4	T49.5X5	T49.5X6
- topical NEC	T49.0X1	T49.0X2	T49.0X3	T49.0X4	T49.0X5	T49.0X6
Hydrocortone	T38.0X1	T38.0X2	T38.0X3	T38.0X4	T38.0X5	T38.0X6
- ENT agent	T49.6X1	T49.6X2	T49.6X3	T49.6X4	T49.6X5	T49.6X6

Substance	Poisoning, Accidental (unintentional)	Poisoning, Intentional Self-harm	Poisoning, Assault	Poisoning, Undetermined	Adverse effect	Underdosing
- ophthalmic preparation	T49.5X1	T49.5X2	T49.5X3	T49.5X4	T49.5X5	T49.5X6
- topical NEC	T49.0X1	T49.0X2	T49.0X3	T49.0X4	T49.0X5	T49.0X6
Hydrocyanic acid (liquid)	T57.3X1	T57.3X2	T57.3X3	T57.3X4	--	--
- gas	T65.0X1	T65.0X2	T65.0X3	T65.0X4	--	--
Hydroflumethiazide	T50.2X1	T50.2X2	T50.2X3	T50.2X4	T50.2X5	T50.2X6
Hydrofluoric acid (liquid)	T54.2X1	T54.2X2	T54.2X3	T54.2X4	--	--
- vapor	T59.891	T59.892	T59.893	T59.894	--	--
Hydrogen	T59.891	T59.892	T59.893	T59.894	--	--
- arsenide	T57.0X1	T57.0X2	T57.0X3	T57.0X4	--	--
- arseniureted	T57.0X1	T57.0X2	T57.0X3	T57.0X4	--	--
- chloride	T57.8X1	T57.8X2	T57.8X3	T57.8X4	--	--
- cyanide (salts)	T57.3X1	T57.3X2	T57.3X3	T57.3X4	--	--
- - gas	T57.3X1	T57.3X2	T57.3X3	T57.3X4	--	--
- Fluoride	T59.5X1	T59.5X2	T59.5X3	T59.5X4	--	--
- - vapor	T59.5X1	T59.5X2	T59.5X3	T59.5X4	--	--
- peroxide	T49.0X1	T49.0X2	T49.0X3	T49.0X4	T49.0X5	T49.0X6
- phosphureted	T57.1X1	T57.1X2	T57.1X3	T57.1X4	--	--
- sulfide	T59.6X1	T59.6X2	T59.6X3	T59.6X4	--	--
- - arseniureted	T57.0X1	T57.0X2	T57.0X3	T57.0X4	--	--
- sulfureted	T59.6X1	T59.6X2	T59.6X3	T59.6X4	--	--
Hydromethylpyridine	T46.7X1	T46.7X2	T46.7X3	T46.7X4	T46.7X5	T46.7X6
Hydromorphinol	T40.2X1	T40.2X2	T40.2X3	T40.2X4	--	--
Hydromorphinone	T40.2X1	T40.2X2	T40.2X3	T40.2X4	T40.2X5	T40.2X6
Hydromorphone	T40.2X1	T40.2X2	T40.2X3	T40.2X4	T40.2X5	T40.2X6
Hydromox	T50.2X1	T50.2X2	T50.2X3	T50.2X4	T50.2X5	T50.2X6
Hydrophilic lotion	T49.3X1	T49.3X2	T49.3X3	T49.3X4	T49.3X5	T49.3X6
Hydroquinidine	T46.2X1	T46.2X2	T46.2X3	T46.2X4	T46.2X5	T46.2X6
Hydroquinone	T52.2X1	T52.2X2	T52.2X3	T52.2X4	--	--
- vapor	T59.891	T59.892	T59.893	T59.894	--	--
Hydrosulfuric acid (gas)	T59.6X1	T59.6X2	T59.6X3	T59.6X4	--	--
Hydrotalcite	T47.1X1	T47.1X2	T47.1X3	T47.1X4	T47.1X5	T47.1X6
Hydrous wool fat	T49.3X1	T49.3X2	T49.3X3	T49.3X4	T49.3X5	T49.3X6
Hydroxide, caustic	T54.3X1	T54.3X2	T54.3X3	T54.3X4	--	--
Hydroxocobalamin	T45.8X1	T45.8X2	T45.8X3	T45.8X4	T45.8X5	T45.8X6
Hydroxyamphetamine	T49.5X1	T49.5X2	T49.5X3	T49.5X4	T49.5X5	T49.5X6
Hydroxycarbamide	T45.1X1	T45.1X2	T45.1X3	T45.1X4	T45.1X5	T45.1X6
Hydroxychloroquine	T37.8X1	T37.8X2	T37.8X3	T37.8X4	T37.8X5	T37.8X6
Hydroxydihydrocodeinone	T40.2X1	T40.2X2	T40.2X3	T40.2X4	T40.2X5	T40.2X6
Hydroxyestrone	T38.5X1	T38.5X2	T38.5X3	T38.5X4	T38.5X5	T38.5X6
Hydroxyethyl starch	T45.8X1	T45.8X2	T45.8X3	T45.8X4	T45.8X5	T45.8X6
Hydroxymethylpenta-none	T52.4X1	T52.4X2	T52.4X3	T52.4X4	--	--
Hydroxyphenamate	T43.591	T43.592	T43.593	T43.594	T43.595	T43.596
Hydroxyphenylbutazone	T39.2X1	T39.2X2	T39.2X3	T39.2X4	T39.2X5	T39.2X6
Hydroxyprogesterone	T38.5X1	T38.5X2	T38.5X3	T38.5X4	T38.5X5	T38.5X6
- caproate	T38.5X1	T38.5X2	T38.5X3	T38.5X4	T38.5X5	T38.5X6
Hydroxyquinoline (derivatives) NEC	T37.8X1	T37.8X2	T37.8X3	T37.8X4	T37.8X5	T37.8X6
Hydroxystilbamidine	T37.3X1	T37.3X2	T37.3X3	T37.3X4	T37.3X5	T37.3X6
Hydroxytoluene (nonmedicinal)	T54.0X1	T54.0X2	T54.0X3	T54.0X4	--	--
- medicinal	T49.0X1	T49.0X2	T49.0X3	T49.0X4	T49.0X5	T49.0X6
Hydroxyurea	T45.1X1	T45.1X2	T45.1X3	T45.1X4	T45.1X5	T45.1X6
Hydroxyzine	T43.591	T43.592	T43.593	T43.594	T43.595	T43.596
Hyoscine	T44.3X1	T44.3X2	T44.3X3	T44.3X4	T44.3X5	T44.3X6
Hyoscyamine	T44.3X1	T44.3X2	T44.3X3	T44.3X4	T44.3X5	T44.3X6
Hyoscyamus	T44.3X1	T44.3X2	T44.3X3	T44.3X4	T44.3X5	T44.3X6
- dry extract	T44.3X1	T44.3X2	T44.3X3	T44.3X4	T44.3X5	T44.3X6
Hypaque	T50.8X1	T50.8X2	T50.8X3	T50.8X4	T50.8X5	T50.8X6
Hypertussis	T50.Z11	T50.Z12	T50.Z13	T50.Z14	T50.Z15	T50.Z16
Hypnotic	T42.71	T42.72	T42.73	T42.74	T42.75	T42.76
- anticonvulsant	T42.71	T42.72	T42.73	T42.74	T42.75	T42.76

Substance	Poisoning, Accidental (unintentional)	Poisoning, Intentional Self-harm	Poisoning, Assault	Poisoning, Undetermined	Adverse effect	Underdosing
- specified NEC	T42.6X1	T42.6X2	T42.6X3	T42.6X4	T42.6X5	T42.6X6
Hypochlorite	T49.0X1	T49.0X2	T49.0X3	T49.0X4	T49.0X5	T49.0X6
Hypophysis, posterior	T38.891	T38.892	T38.893	T38.894	T38.895	T38.896
Hypotensive NEC	T46.5X1	T46.5X2	T46.5X3	T46.5X4	T46.5X5	T46.5X6
Hypromellose	T49.5X1	T49.5X2	T49.5X3	T49.5X4	T49.5X5	T49.5X6
Ibacitabine	T37.5X1	T37.5X2	T37.5X3	T37.5X4	T37.5X5	T37.5X6
Ibopamine	T44.991	T44.992	T44.993	T44.994	T44.995	T44.996
Ibufenac	T39.311	T39.312	T39.313	T39.314	T39.315	T39.316
Ibuprofen	T39.311	T39.312	T39.313	T39.314	T39.315	T39.316
Ibuproxam	T39.311	T39.312	T39.313	T39.314	T39.315	T39.316
Ibuterol	T48.6X1	T48.6X2	T48.6X3	T48.6X4	T48.6X5	T48.6X6
Ichthammol	T49.0X1	T49.0X2	T49.0X3	T49.0X4	T49.0X5	T49.0X6
Ichthyol	T49.4X1	T49.4X2	T49.4X3	T49.4X4	T49.4X5	T49.4X6
Idarubicin	T45.1X1	T45.1X2	T45.1X3	T45.1X4	T45.1X5	T45.1X6
Idrocilamide	T42.8X1	T42.8X2	T42.8X3	T42.8X4	T42.8X5	T42.8X6
Ifenprodil	T46.7X1	T46.7X2	T46.7X3	T46.7X4	T46.7X5	T46.7X6
Ifosfamide	T45.1X1	T45.1X2	T45.1X3	T45.1X4	T45.1X5	T45.1X6
Iletin	T38.3X1	T38.3X2	T38.3X3	T38.3X4	T38.3X5	T38.3X6
Ilex	T62.2X1	T62.2X2	T62.2X3	T62.2X4	--	--
Illuminating gas (after combustion)	T58.11	T58.12	T58.13	T58.14	--	--
- prior to combustion	T59.891	T59.892	T59.893	T59.894	--	--
Ilopan	T45.2X1	T45.2X2	T45.2X3	T45.2X4	T45.2X5	T45.2X6
Iloprost	T46.7X1	T46.7X2	T46.7X3	T46.7X4	T46.7X5	T46.7X6
Ilotycin	T36.3X1	T36.3X2	T36.3X3	T36.3X4	T36.3X5	T36.3X6
- ophthalmic preparation	T49.5X1	T49.5X2	T49.5X3	T49.5X4	T49.5X5	T49.5X6
- topical NEC	T49.0X1	T49.0X2	T49.0X3	T49.0X4	T49.0X5	T49.0X6
Imidazole-4-carboxamide	T45.1X1	T45.1X2	T45.1X3	T45.1X4	T45.1X5	T45.1X6
Imipenem	T36.0X1	T36.0X2	T36.0X3	T36.0X4	T36.0X5	T36.0X6
Imipramine	T43.011	T43.012	T43.013	T43.014	T43.015	T43.016
Iminostilbene	T42.1X1	T42.1X2	T42.1X3	T42.1X4	T42.1X5	T42.1X6
Immu-G	T50.Z11	T50.Z12	T50.Z13	T50.Z14	T50.Z15	T50.Z16
Immuglobin	T50.Z11	T50.Z12	T50.Z13	T50.Z14	T50.Z15	T50.Z16
Immune						
- globulin	T50.Z11	T50.Z12	T50.Z13	T50.Z14	T50.Z15	T50.Z16
- serum globulin	T50.Z11	T50.Z12	T50.Z13	T50.Z14	T50.Z15	T50.Z16
Immunoglobin human (intravenous) (normal)	T50.Z11	T50.Z12	T50.Z13	T50.Z14	T50.Z15	T50.Z16
- unmodified	T50.Z11	T50.Z12	T50.Z13	T50.Z14	T50.Z15	T50.Z16
Immunosuppressive drug	T45.1X1	T45.1X2	T45.1X3	T45.1X4	T45.1X5	T45.1X6
Immu-tetanus	T50.Z11	T50.Z12	T50.Z13	T50.Z14	T50.Z15	T50.Z16
Indalpine	T43.221	T43.222	T43.223	T43.224	T43.225	T43.226
Indanazoline	T48.5X1	T48.5X2	T48.5X3	T48.5X4	T48.5X5	T48.5X6
Indandione (derivatives)	T45.511	T45.512	T45.513	T45.514	T45.515	T45.516
Indapamide	T46.5X1	T46.5X2	T46.5X3	T46.5X4	T46.5X5	T46.5X6
Indendione (derivatives)	T45.511	T45.512	T45.513	T45.514	T45.515	T45.516
Indenolol	T44.7X1	T44.7X2	T44.7X3	T44.7X4	T44.7X5	T44.7X6
Inderal	T44.7X1	T44.7X2	T44.7X3	T44.7X4	T44.7X5	T44.7X6
Indian						
- hemp	T40.711	T40.712	T40.713	T40.714	T40.715	T40.716
- tobacco	T62.2X1	T62.2X2	T62.2X3	T62.2X4	--	--
Indigo carmine	T50.8X1	T50.8X2	T50.8X3	T50.8X4	T50.8X5	T50.8X6
Indobufen	T45.521	T45.522	T45.523	T45.524	T45.525	T45.526
Indocin	T39.2X1	T39.2X2	T39.2X3	T39.2X4	T39.2X5	T39.2X6
Indocyanine green	T50.8X1	T50.8X2	T50.8X3	T50.8X4	T50.8X5	T50.8X6
Indometacin	T39.391	T39.392	T39.393	T39.394	T39.395	T39.396
Indomethacin	T39.391	T39.392	T39.393	T39.394	T39.395	T39.396
- farnesil	T39.4X1	T39.4X2	T39.4X3	T39.4X4	T39.4X5	T39.4X6
Indoramin	T44.6X1	T44.6X2	T44.6X3	T44.6X4	T44.6X5	T44.6X6
Industrial						

Substance	Poisoning, Accidental (unintentional)	Poisoning, Intentional Self-harm	Poisoning, Assault	Poisoning, Undetermined	Adverse effect	Underdosing
- alcohol	T51.0X1	T51.0X2	T51.0X3	T51.0X4	--	--
- fumes	T59.891	T59.892	T59.893	T59.894	--	--
- solvents (fumes) (vapors)	T52.91	T52.92	T52.93	T52.94	--	--
Influenza vaccine	T50.B91	T50.B92	T50.B93	T50.B94	T50.B95	T50.B96
Ingested substance NEC	T65.91	T65.92	T65.93	T65.94	--	--
INH	T37.1X1	T37.1X2	T37.1X3	T37.1X4	T37.1X5	T37.1X6
Inhalation, gas (noxious) —see Gas Inhibitor						
- angiotensin-converting enzyme	T46.4X1	T46.4X2	T46.4X3	T46.4X4	T46.4X5	T46.4X6
- carbonic anhydrase	T50.2X1	T50.2X2	T50.2X3	T50.2X4	T50.2X5	T50.2X6
- fibrinolysis	T45.621	T45.622	T45.623	T45.624	T45.625	T45.626
- monoamine oxidase NEC	T43.1X1	T43.1X2	T43.1X3	T43.1X4	T43.1X5	T43.1X6
- - hydrazine	T43.1X1	T43.1X2	T43.1X3	T43.1X4	T43.1X5	T43.1X6
- postsynaptic	T43.8X1	T43.8X2	T43.8X3	T43.8X4	T43.8X5	T43.8X6
- prothrombin synthesis	T45.511	T45.512	T45.513	T45.514	T45.515	T45.516
Ink	T65.891	T65.892	T65.893	T65.894	--	--
Inorganic substance NEC	T57.91	T57.92	T57.93	T57.94	--	--
Inosine pranobex	T37.5X1	T37.5X2	T37.5X3	T37.5X4	T37.5X5	T37.5X6
Inositol	T50.991	T50.992	T50.993	T50.994	T50.995	T50.996
- nicotinate	T46.7X1	T46.7X2	T46.7X3	T46.7X4	T46.7X5	T46.7X6
Inproquone	T45.1X1	T45.1X2	T45.1X3	T45.1X4	T45.1X5	T45.1X6
Insect (sting) , venomous	T63.481	T63.482	T63.483	T63.484	--	--
- ant	T63.421	T63.422	T63.423	T63.424	--	--
- bee	T63.441	T63.442	T63.443	T63.444	--	--
- caterpillar	T63.431	T63.432	T63.433	T63.434	--	--
- hornet	T63.451	T63.452	T63.453	T63.454	--	--
- wasp	T63.461	T63.462	T63.463	T63.464	--	--
Insecticide NEC	T60.91	T60.92	T60.93	T60.94	--	--
- carbamate	T60.0X1	T60.0X2	T60.0X3	T60.0X4	--	--
- chlorinated	T60.1X1	T60.1X2	T60.1X3	T60.1X4	--	--
- mixed	T60.91	T60.92	T60.93	T60.94	--	--
- organochlorine	T60.1X1	T60.1X2	T60.1X3	T60.1X4	--	--
- organophosphorus	T60.0X1	T60.0X2	T60.0X3	T60.0X4	--	--
Insular tissue extract	T38.3X1	T38.3X2	T38.3X3	T38.3X4	T38.3X5	T38.3X6
Insulin (amorphous) (globin) (isophane) (Lente) (NPH) (Semilente) (Ultralente)	T38.3X1	T38.3X2	T38.3X3	T38.3X4	T38.3X5	T38.3X6
- defalan	T38.3X1	T38.3X2	T38.3X3	T38.3X4	T38.3X5	T38.3X6
- human	T38.3X1	T38.3X2	T38.3X3	T38.3X4	T38.3X5	T38.3X6
- injection, soluble	T38.3X1	T38.3X2	T38.3X3	T38.3X4	T38.3X5	T38.3X6
- - biphasic	T38.3X1	T38.3X2	T38.3X3	T38.3X4	T38.3X5	T38.3X6
- intermediate acting	T38.3X1	T38.3X2	T38.3X3	T38.3X4	T38.3X5	T38.3X6
- protamine zinc	T38.3X1	T38.3X2	T38.3X3	T38.3X4	T38.3X5	T38.3X6
- slow acting	T38.3X1	T38.3X2	T38.3X3	T38.3X4	T38.3X5	T38.3X6
- zinc						
- - protamine injection	T38.3X1	T38.3X2	T38.3X3	T38.3X4	T38.3X5	T38.3X6
- - suspension (amorphous) (crystalline)	T38.3X1	T38.3X2	T38.3X3	T38.3X4	T38.3X5	T38.3X6
Interferon (alpha) (beta) (gamma)	T37.5X1	T37.5X2	T37.5X3	T37.5X4	T37.5X5	T37.5X6
Intestinal motility control drug	T47.6X1	T47.6X2	T47.6X3	T47.6X4	T47.6X5	T47.6X6
- biological	T47.8X1	T47.8X2	T47.8X3	T47.8X4	T47.8X5	T47.8X6
Intranarcon	T41.1X1	T41.1X2	T41.1X3	T41.1X4	T41.1X5	T41.1X6
Intravenous						
- amino acids	T50.991	T50.992	T50.993	T50.994	T50.995	T50.996
- fat suspension	T50.991	T50.992	T50.993	T50.994	T50.995	T50.996
Inulin	T50.8X1	T50.8X2	T50.8X3	T50.8X4	T50.8X5	T50.8X6
Invert sugar	T50.3X1	T50.3X2	T50.3X3	T50.3X4	T50.3X5	T50.3X6
Inza—see Naproxen						
Iobenzamic acid	T50.8X1	T50.8X2	T50.8X3	T50.8X4	T50.8X5	T50.8X6
Iocarmic acid	T50.8X1	T50.8X2	T50.8X3	T50.8X4	T50.8X5	T50.8X6
Iocetamic acid	T50.8X1	T50.8X2	T50.8X3	T50.8X4	T50.8X5	T50.8X6
Iodamide	T50.8X1	T50.8X2	T50.8X3	T50.8X4	T50.8X5	T50.8X6

Substance	Poisoning, Accidental (unintentional)	Poisoning, Intentional Self-harm	Poisoning, Assault	Poisoning, Undetermined	Adverse effect	Underdosing
Iodide NEC—see also Iodine	T49.0X1	T49.0X2	T49.0X3	T49.0X4	T49.0X5	T49.0X6
- mercury (ointment)	T49.0X1	T49.0X2	T49.0X3	T49.0X4	T49.0X5	T49.0X6
- methylate	T49.0X1	T49.0X2	T49.0X3	T49.0X4	T49.0X5	T49.0X6
- potassium (expectorant) NEC	T48.4X1	T48.4X2	T48.4X3	T48.4X4	T48.4X5	T48.4X6
Iodinated						
- contrast medium	T50.8X1	T50.8X2	T50.8X3	T50.8X4	T50.8X5	T50.8X6
- glycerol	T48.4X1	T48.4X2	T48.4X3	T48.4X4	T48.4X5	T48.4X6
- human serum albumin (131I)	T50.8X1	T50.8X2	T50.8X3	T50.8X4	T50.8X5	T50.8X6
Iodine (antiseptic, external) (tincture) NEC	T49.0X1	T49.0X2	T49.0X3	T49.0X4	T49.0X5	T49.0X6
- 125—see also Radiation sickness, and Exposure to radioactivce isotopes	T50.8X1	T50.8X2	T50.8X3	T50.8X4	T50.8X5	T50.8X6
- - therapeutic	T50.991	T50.992	T50.993	T50.994	T50.995	T50.996
- 131—see also Radiation sickness, and Exposure to radioactivce isotopes	T50.8X1	T50.8X2	T50.8X3	T50.8X4	T50.8X5	T50.8X6
- - therapeutic	T38.2X1	T38.2X2	T38.2X3	T38.2X4	T38.2X5	T38.2X6
- diagnostic	T50.8X1	T50.8X2	T50.8X3	T50.8X4	T50.8X5	T50.8X6
- for thyroid conditions (antithyroid)	T38.2X1	T38.2X2	T38.2X3	T38.2X4	T38.2X5	T38.2X6
- solution	T49.0X1	T49.0X2	T49.0X3	T49.0X4	T49.0X5	T49.0X6
- vapor	T59.891	T59.892	T59.893	T59.894	--	--
Iodipamide	T50.8X1	T50.8X2	T50.8X3	T50.8X4	T50.8X5	T50.8X6
Iodized (poppy seed) oil	T50.8X1	T50.8X2	T50.8X3	T50.8X4	T50.8X5	T50.8X6
Iodobismitol	T37.8X1	T37.8X2	T37.8X3	T37.8X4	T37.8X5	T37.8X6
Iodochlorhydroxyquin	T37.8X1	T37.8X2	T37.8X3	T37.8X4	T37.8X5	T37.8X6
- topical	T49.0X1	T49.0X2	T49.0X3	T49.0X4	T49.0X5	T49.0X6
Iodochlorhydroxyquinoline	T37.8X1	T37.8X2	T37.8X3	T37.8X4	T37.8X5	T37.8X6
Iodocholesterol (131I)	T50.8X1	T50.8X2	T50.8X3	T50.8X4	T50.8X5	T50.8X6
Iodoform	T49.0X1	T49.0X2	T49.0X3	T49.0X4	T49.0X5	T49.0X6
Iodohippuric acid	T50.8X1	T50.8X2	T50.8X3	T50.8X4	T50.8X5	T50.8X6
Iodopanoic acid	T50.8X1	T50.8X2	T50.8X3	T50.8X4	T50.8X5	T50.8X6
Iodophthalein (sodium)	T50.8X1	T50.8X2	T50.8X3	T50.8X4	T50.8X5	T50.8X6
Iodopyracet	T50.8X1	T50.8X2	T50.8X3	T50.8X4	T50.8X5	T50.8X6
Iodoquinol	T37.8X1	T37.8X2	T37.8X3	T37.8X4	T37.8X5	T37.8X6
Iodoxamic acid	T50.8X1	T50.8X2	T50.8X3	T50.8X4	T50.8X5	T50.8X6
Iofendylate	T50.8X1	T50.8X2	T50.8X3	T50.8X4	T50.8X5	T50.8X6
Ioglycamic acid	T50.8X1	T50.8X2	T50.8X3	T50.8X4	T50.8X5	T50.8X6
Iohexol	T50.8X1	T50.8X2	T50.8X3	T50.8X4	T50.8X5	T50.8X6
Ion exchange resin						
- anion	T47.8X1	T47.8X2	T47.8X3	T47.8X4	T47.8X5	T47.8X6
- cation	T50.3X1	T50.3X2	T50.3X3	T50.3X4	T50.3X5	T50.3X6
- cholestyramine	T46.6X1	T46.6X2	T46.6X3	T46.6X4	T46.6X5	T46.6X6
- intestinal	T47.8X1	T47.8X2	T47.8X3	T47.8X4	T47.8X5	T47.8X6
Iopamidol	T50.8X1	T50.8X2	T50.8X3	T50.8X4	T50.8X5	T50.8X6
Iopanoic acid	T50.8X1	T50.8X2	T50.8X3	T50.8X4	T50.8X5	T50.8X6
Iophenoic acid	T50.8X1	T50.8X2	T50.8X3	T50.8X4	T50.8X5	T50.8X6
Iopodate, sodium	T50.8X1	T50.8X2	T50.8X3	T50.8X4	T50.8X5	T50.8X6
Iopodic acid	T50.8X1	T50.8X2	T50.8X3	T50.8X4	T50.8X5	T50.8X6
Iopromide	T50.8X1	T50.8X2	T50.8X3	T50.8X4	T50.8X5	T50.8X6
Iopydol	T50.8X1	T50.8X2	T50.8X3	T50.8X4	T50.8X5	T50.8X6
Iotalamic acid	T50.8X1	T50.8X2	T50.8X3	T50.8X4	T50.8X5	T50.8X6
Iothalamate	T50.8X1	T50.8X2	T50.8X3	T50.8X4	T50.8X5	T50.8X6
Iothiouracil	T38.2X1	T38.2X2	T38.2X3	T38.2X4	T38.2X5	T38.2X6
Iotrol	T50.8X1	T50.8X2	T50.8X3	T50.8X4	T50.8X5	T50.8X6
Iotrolan	T50.8X1	T50.8X2	T50.8X3	T50.8X4	T50.8X5	T50.8X6
Iotroxate	T50.8X1	T50.8X2	T50.8X3	T50.8X4	T50.8X5	T50.8X6
Iotroxic acid	T50.8X1	T50.8X2	T50.8X3	T50.8X4	T50.8X5	T50.8X6
Ioversol	T50.8X1	T50.8X2	T50.8X3	T50.8X4	T50.8X5	T50.8X6
Ioxaglate	T50.8X1	T50.8X2	T50.8X3	T50.8X4	T50.8X5	T50.8X6
Ioxaglic acid	T50.8X1	T50.8X2	T50.8X3	T50.8X4	T50.8X5	T50.8X6
Ioxitalamic acid	T50.8X1	T50.8X2	T50.8X3	T50.8X4	T50.8X5	T50.8X6

Substance	Poisoning, Accidental (unintentional)	Poisoning, Intentional Self-harm	Poisoning, Assault	Poisoning, Undetermined	Adverse effect	Underdosing
Ipecac	T47.7X1	T47.7X2	T47.7X3	T47.7X4	T47.7X5	T47.7X6
Ipecacuanha	T48.4X1	T48.4X2	T48.4X3	T48.4X4	T48.4X5	T48.4X6
Ipodate, calcium	T50.8X1	T50.8X2	T50.8X3	T50.8X4	T50.8X5	T50.8X6
Ipral	T42.3X1	T42.3X2	T42.3X3	T42.3X4	T42.3X5	T42.3X6
Ipratropium (bromide)	T48.6X1	T48.6X2	T48.6X3	T48.6X4	T48.6X5	T48.6X6
Ipriflavone	T46.3X1	T46.3X2	T46.3X3	T46.3X4	T46.3X5	T46.3X6
Iprindole	T43.011	T43.012	T43.013	T43.014	T43.015	T43.016
Iproclozide	T43.1X1	T43.1X2	T43.1X3	T43.1X4	T43.1X5	T43.1X6
Iprofenin	T50.8X1	T50.8X2	T50.8X3	T50.8X4	T50.8X5	T50.8X6
Iproheptine	T49.2X1	T49.2X2	T49.2X3	T49.2X4	T49.2X5	T49.2X6
Iproniazid	T43.1X1	T43.1X2	T43.1X3	T43.1X4	T43.1X5	T43.1X6
Iproplatin	T45.1X1	T45.1X2	T45.1X3	T45.1X4	T45.1X5	T45.1X6
Iproveratril	T46.1X1	T46.1X2	T46.1X3	T46.1X4	T46.1X5	T46.1X6
Iron (compounds) (medicinal) NEC	T45.4X1	T45.4X2	T45.4X3	T45.4X4	T45.4X5	T45.4X6
- ammonium	T45.4X1	T45.4X2	T45.4X3	T45.4X4	T45.4X5	T45.4X6
- dextran injection	T45.4X1	T45.4X2	T45.4X3	T45.4X4	T45.4X5	T45.4X6
- nonmedicinal	T56.891	T56.892	T56.893	T56.894	--	--
- salts	T45.4X1	T45.4X2	T45.4X3	T45.4X4	T45.4X5	T45.4X6
- sorbitex	T45.4X1	T45.4X2	T45.4X3	T45.4X4	T45.4X5	T45.4X6
- sorbitol citric acid complex	T45.4X1	T45.4X2	T45.4X3	T45.4X4	T45.4X5	T45.4X6
Irrigating fluid (vaginal)	T49.8X1	T49.8X2	T49.8X3	T49.8X4	T49.8X5	T49.8X6
- eye	T49.5X1	T49.5X2	T49.5X3	T49.5X4	T49.5X5	T49.5X6
Isepamicin	T36.5X1	T36.5X2	T36.5X3	T36.5X4	T36.5X5	T36.5X6
Isoaminile (citrate)	T48.3X1	T48.3X2	T48.3X3	T48.3X4	T48.3X5	T48.3X6
Isoamyl nitrite	T46.3X1	T46.3X2	T46.3X3	T46.3X4	T46.3X5	T46.3X6
Isobenzan	T60.1X1	T60.1X2	T60.1X3	T60.1X4	--	--
Isobutyl acetate	T52.8X1	T52.8X2	T52.8X3	T52.8X4	--	--
Isocarboxazid	T43.1X1	T43.1X2	T43.1X3	T43.1X4	T43.1X5	T43.1X6
Isoconazole	T49.0X1	T49.0X2	T49.0X3	T49.0X4	T49.0X5	T49.0X6
Isocyanate	T65.0X1	T65.0X2	T65.0X3	T65.0X4	--	--
Isoephedrine	T44.991	T44.992	T44.993	T44.994	T44.995	T44.996
Isoetarine	T48.6X1	T48.6X2	T48.6X3	T48.6X4	T48.6X5	T48.6X6
Isoethadione	T42.2X1	T42.2X2	T42.2X3	T42.2X4	T42.2X5	T42.2X6
Isoetharine	T44.5X1	T44.5X2	T44.5X3	T44.5X4	T44.5X5	T44.5X6
Isoflurane	T41.0X1	T41.0X2	T41.0X3	T41.0X4	T41.0X5	T41.0X6
Isoflurophate	T44.0X1	T44.0X2	T44.0X3	T44.0X4	T44.0X5	T44.0X6
Isomaltose, ferric complex	T45.4X1	T45.4X2	T45.4X3	T45.4X4	T45.4X5	T45.4X6
Isometheptene	T44.3X1	T44.3X2	T44.3X3	T44.3X4	T44.3X5	T44.3X6
Isoniazid	T37.1X1	T37.1X2	T37.1X3	T37.1X4	T37.1X5	T37.1X6
- with						
- - rifampicin	T36.6X1	T36.6X2	T36.6X3	T36.6X4	T36.6X5	T36.6X6
- - thioacetazone	T37.1X1	T37.1X2	T37.1X3	T37.1X4	T37.1X5	T37.1X6
Isonicotinic acid hydrazide	T37.1X1	T37.1X2	T37.1X3	T37.1X4	T37.1X5	T37.1X6
Isonipecaine	T40.491	T40.492	T40.493	T40.494	T40.495	T40.496
Isopentaquine	T37.2X1	T37.2X2	T37.2X3	T37.2X4	T37.2X5	T37.2X6
Isophane insulin	T38.3X1	T38.3X2	T38.3X3	T38.3X4	T38.3X5	T38.3X6
Isophorone	T65.891	T65.892	T65.893	T65.894	--	--
Isophosphamide	T45.1X1	T45.1X2	T45.1X3	T45.1X4	T45.1X5	T45.1X6
Isopregnenone	T38.5X1	T38.5X2	T38.5X3	T38.5X4	T38.5X5	T38.5X6
Isoprenaline	T48.6X1	T48.6X2	T48.6X3	T48.6X4	T48.6X5	T48.6X6
Isopromethazine	T43.3X1	T43.3X2	T43.3X3	T43.3X4	T43.3X5	T43.3X6
Isopropamide	T44.3X1	T44.3X2	T44.3X3	T44.3X4	T44.3X5	T44.3X6
- iodide	T44.3X1	T44.3X2	T44.3X3	T44.3X4	T44.3X5	T44.3X6
Isopropanol	T51.2X1	T51.2X2	T51.2X3	T51.2X4	--	--
Isopropyl						
- acetate	T52.8X1	T52.8X2	T52.8X3	T52.8X4	--	--
- alcohol	T51.2X1	T51.2X2	T51.2X3	T51.2X4	--	--
- - medicinal	T49.4X1	T49.4X2	T49.4X3	T49.4X4	T49.4X5	T49.4X6
- ether	T52.8X1	T52.8X2	T52.8X3	T52.8X4	--	--

Substance	Poisoning, Accidental (unintentional)	Poisoning, Intentional Self-harm	Poisoning, Assault	Poisoning, Undetermined	Adverse effect	Underdosing
Isopropylaminophenazone	T39.2X1	T39.2X2	T39.2X3	T39.2X4	T39.2X5	T39.2X6
Isoproterenol	T48.6X1	T48.6X2	T48.6X3	T48.6X4	T48.6X5	T48.6X6
Isosorbide dinitrate	T46.3X1	T46.3X2	T46.3X3	T46.3X4	T46.3X5	T46.3X6
Isothipendyl	T45.0X1	T45.0X2	T45.0X3	T45.0X4	T45.0X5	T45.0X6
Isotretinoin	T50.991	T50.992	T50.993	T50.994	T50.995	T50.996
Isoxazolyl penicillin	T36.0X1	T36.0X2	T36.0X3	T36.0X4	T36.0X5	T36.0X6
Isoxicam	T39.391	T39.392	T39.393	T39.394	T39.395	T39.396
Isoxsuprine	T46.7X1	T46.7X2	T46.7X3	T46.7X4	T46.7X5	T46.7X6
Ispagula	T47.4X1	T47.4X2	T47.4X3	T47.4X4	T47.4X5	T47.4X6
- husk	T47.4X1	T47.4X2	T47.4X3	T47.4X4	T47.4X5	T47.4X6
Isradipine	T46.1X1	T46.1X2	T46.1X3	T46.1X4	T46.1X5	T46.1X6
I-thyroxine sodium	T38.1X1	T38.1X2	T38.1X3	T38.1X4	T38.1X5	T38.1X6
Itraconazole	T37.8X1	T37.8X2	T37.8X3	T37.8X4	T37.8X5	T37.8X6
Itramin tosilate	T46.3X1	T46.3X2	T46.3X3	T46.3X4	T46.3X5	T46.3X6
Ivermectin	T37.4X1	T37.4X2	T37.4X3	T37.4X4	T37.4X5	T37.4X6
Izoniazid	T37.1X1	T37.1X2	T37.1X3	T37.1X4	T37.1X5	T37.1X6
- with thioacetazone	T37.1X1	T37.1X2	T37.1X3	T37.1X4	T37.1X5	T37.1X6
Jalap	T47.2X1	T47.2X2	T47.2X3	T47.2X4	T47.2X5	T47.2X6
Jamaica						
- dogwood (bark)	T39.8X1	T39.8X2	T39.8X3	T39.8X4	T39.8X5	T39.8X6
- ginger	T65.891	T65.892	T65.893	T65.894	--	--
- - root	T62.2X1	T62.2X2	T62.2X3	T62.2X4	--	--
Jatropha	T62.2X1	T62.2X2	T62.2X3	T62.2X4	--	--
- curcas	T62.2X1	T62.2X2	T62.2X3	T62.2X4	--	--
Jectofer	T45.4X1	T45.4X2	T45.4X3	T45.4X4	T45.4X5	T45.4X6
Jellyfish (sting)	T63.621	T63.622	T63.623	T63.624	--	--
Jequirity (bean)	T62.2X1	T62.2X2	T62.2X3	T62.2X4	--	--
Jimson weed (stramonium)	T62.2X1	T62.2X2	T62.2X3	T62.2X4	--	--
- seeds	T62.2X1	T62.2X2	T62.2X3	T62.2X4	--	--
Josamycin	T36.3X1	T36.3X2	T36.3X3	T36.3X4	T36.3X5	T36.3X6
Juniper tar	T49.1X1	T49.1X2	T49.1X3	T49.1X4	T49.1X5	T49.1X6
Kallidinogenase	T46.7X1	T46.7X2	T46.7X3	T46.7X4	T46.7X5	T46.7X6
Kallikrein	T46.7X1	T46.7X2	T46.7X3	T46.7X4	T46.7X5	T46.7X6
Kanamycin	T36.5X1	T36.5X2	T36.5X3	T36.5X4	T36.5X5	T36.5X6
Kantrex	T36.5X1	T36.5X2	T36.5X3	T36.5X4	T36.5X5	T36.5X6
Kaolin	T47.6X1	T47.6X2	T47.6X3	T47.6X4	T47.6X5	T47.6X6
- light	T47.6X1	T47.6X2	T47.6X3	T47.6X4	T47.6X5	T47.6X6
Karaya (gum)	T47.4X1	T47.4X2	T47.4X3	T47.4X4	T47.4X5	T47.4X6
Kebuzone	T39.2X1	T39.2X2	T39.2X3	T39.2X4	T39.2X5	T39.2X6
Kelevan	T60.1X1	T60.1X2	T60.1X3	T60.1X4	--	--
Kemithal	T41.1X1	T41.1X2	T41.1X3	T41.1X4	T41.1X5	T41.1X6
Kenacort	T38.0X1	T38.0X2	T38.0X3	T38.0X4	T38.0X5	T38.0X6
Keratolytic drug NEC	T49.4X1	T49.4X2	T49.4X3	T49.4X4	T49.4X5	T49.4X6
- anthracene	T49.4X1	T49.4X2	T49.4X3	T49.4X4	T49.4X5	T49.4X6
Keratoplastic NEC	T49.4X1	T49.4X2	T49.4X3	T49.4X4	T49.4X5	T49.4X6
Kerosene, kerosine (fuel) (solvent) NEC	T52.0X1	T52.0X2	T52.0X3	T52.0X4	--	--
- insecticide	T52.0X1	T52.0X2	T52.0X3	T52.0X4	--	--
- vapor	T52.0X1	T52.0X2	T52.0X3	T52.0X4	--	--
Ketamine	T41.291	T41.292	T41.293	T41.294	T41.295	T41.296
Ketazolam	T42.4X1	T42.4X2	T42.4X3	T42.4X4	T42.4X5	T42.4X6
Ketazon	T39.2X1	T39.2X2	T39.2X3	T39.2X4	T39.2X5	T39.2X6
Ketobemidone	T40.491	T40.492	T40.493	T40.494	--	--
Ketoconazole	T49.0X1	T49.0X2	T49.0X3	T49.0X4	T49.0X5	T49.0X6
Ketols	T52.4X1	T52.4X2	T52.4X3	T52.4X4	--	--
Ketone oils	T52.4X1	T52.4X2	T52.4X3	T52.4X4	--	--
Ketoprofen	T39.311	T39.312	T39.313	T39.314	T39.315	T39.316
Ketorolac	T39.8X1	T39.8X2	T39.8X3	T39.8X4	T39.8X5	T39.8X6
Ketotifen	T45.0X1	T45.0X2	T45.0X3	T45.0X4	T45.0X5	T45.0X6

Substance	Poisoning, Accidental (unintentional)	Poisoning, Intentional Self-harm	Poisoning, Assault	Poisoning, Undetermined	Adverse effect	Underdosing
Khat	T43.691	T43.692	T43.693	T43.694	--	--
Khellin	T46.3X1	T46.3X2	T46.3X3	T46.3X4	T46.3X5	T46.3X6
Khelloside	T46.3X1	T46.3X2	T46.3X3	T46.3X4	T46.3X5	T46.3X6
Kiln gas or vapor (carbon monoxide)	T58.8X1	T58.8X2	T58.8X3	T58.8X4	--	--
Kitasamycin	T36.3X1	T36.3X2	T36.3X3	T36.3X4	T36.3X5	T36.3X6
Konsyl	T47.4X1	T47.4X2	T47.4X3	T47.4X4	T47.4X5	T47.4X6
Kosam seed	T62.2X1	T62.2X2	T62.2X3	T62.2X4	--	--
Krait (venom)	T63.091	T63.092	T63.093	T63.094	--	--
Kwell (insecticide)	T60.1X1	T60.1X2	T60.1X3	T60.1X4	--	--
- anti-infective (topical)	T49.0X1	T49.0X2	T49.0X3	T49.0X4	T49.0X5	T49.0X6
Labetalol	T44.8X1	T44.8X2	T44.8X3	T44.8X4	T44.8X5	T44.8X6
Laburnum (seeds)	T62.2X1	T62.2X2	T62.2X3	T62.2X4	--	--
- leaves	T62.2X1	T62.2X2	T62.2X3	T62.2X4	--	--
Lachesine	T49.5X1	T49.5X2	T49.5X3	T49.5X4	T49.5X5	T49.5X6
Lacidipine	T46.5X1	T46.5X2	T46.5X3	T46.5X4	T46.5X5	T46.5X6
Lacquer	T65.6X1	T65.6X2	T65.6X3	T65.6X4	--	--
Lacrimogenic gas	T59.3X1	T59.3X2	T59.3X3	T59.3X4	--	--
Lactated potassic saline	T50.3X1	T50.3X2	T50.3X3	T50.3X4	T50.3X5	T50.3X6
Lactic acid	T49.8X1	T49.8X2	T49.8X3	T49.8X4	T49.8X5	T49.8X6
Lactobacillus						
- acidophilus	T47.6X1	T47.6X2	T47.6X3	T47.6X4	T47.6X5	T47.6X6
- - compound	T47.6X1	T47.6X2	T47.6X3	T47.6X4	T47.6X5	T47.6X6
- bifidus, lyophilized	T47.6X1	T47.6X2	T47.6X3	T47.6X4	T47.6X5	T47.6X6
- bulgaricus	T47.6X1	T47.6X2	T47.6X3	T47.6X4	T47.6X5	T47.6X6
- sporogenes	T47.6X1	T47.6X2	T47.6X3	T47.6X4	T47.6X5	T47.6X6
Lactoflavin	T45.2X1	T45.2X2	T45.2X3	T45.2X4	T45.2X5	T45.2X6
Lactose (as excipient)	T50.901	T50.902	T50.903	T50.904	T50.905	T50.906
Lactuca (virosa) (extract)	T42.6X1	T42.6X2	T42.6X3	T42.6X4	T42.6X5	T42.6X6
Lactucarium	T42.6X1	T42.6X2	T42.6X3	T42.6X4	T42.6X5	T42.6X6
Lactulose	T47.3X1	T47.3X2	T47.3X3	T47.3X4	T47.3X5	T47.3X6
Laevo—see Levo-						
Lanatosides	T46.0X1	T46.0X2	T46.0X3	T46.0X4	T46.0X5	T46.0X6
Lanolin	T49.3X1	T49.3X2	T49.3X3	T49.3X4	T49.3X5	T49.3X6
Largactil	T43.3X1	T43.3X2	T43.3X3	T43.3X4	T43.3X5	T43.3X6
Larkspur	T62.2X1	T62.2X2	T62.2X3	T62.2X4	--	--
Laroxyl	T43.011	T43.012	T43.013	T43.014	T43.015	T43.016
Lasix	T50.1X1	T50.1X2	T50.1X3	T50.1X4	T50.1X5	T50.1X6
Lassar's paste	T49.4X1	T49.4X2	T49.4X3	T49.4X4	T49.4X5	T49.4X6
Latamoxef	T36.1X1	T36.1X2	T36.1X3	T36.1X4	T36.1X5	T36.1X6
Latex	T65.811	T65.812	T65.813	T65.814	--	--
Lathyrus (seed)	T62.2X1	T62.2X2	T62.2X3	T62.2X4	--	--
Laudanum	T40.0X1	T40.0X2	T40.0X3	T40.0X4	T40.0X5	T40.0X6
Laudexium	T48.1X1	T48.1X2	T48.1X3	T48.1X4	T48.1X5	T48.1X6
Laughing gas	T41.0X1	T41.0X2	T41.0X3	T41.0X4	T41.0X5	T41.0X6
Laurel, black or cherry	T62.2X1	T62.2X2	T62.2X3	T62.2X4	--	--
Laurolinium	T49.0X1	T49.0X2	T49.0X3	T49.0X4	T49.0X5	T49.0X6
Lauryl sulfoacetate	T49.2X1	T49.2X2	T49.2X3	T49.2X4	T49.2X5	T49.2X6
Laxative NEC	T47.4X1	T47.4X2	T47.4X3	T47.4X4	T47.4X5	T47.4X6
- osmotic	T47.3X1	T47.3X2	T47.3X3	T47.3X4	T47.3X5	T47.3X6
- saline	T47.3X1	T47.3X2	T47.3X3	T47.3X4	T47.3X5	T47.3X6
- stimulant	T47.2X1	T47.2X2	T47.2X3	T47.2X4	T47.2X5	T47.2X6
L-dopa	T42.8X1	T42.8X2	T42.8X3	T42.8X4	T42.8X5	T42.8X6
Lead (dust) (fumes) (vapor) NEC	T56.0X1	T56.0X2	T56.0X3	T56.0X4	--	--
- acetate	T49.2X1	T49.2X2	T49.2X3	T49.2X4	T49.2X5	T49.2X6
- alkyl (fuel additive)	T56.0X1	T56.0X2	T56.0X3	T56.0X4	--	--
- anti-infectives	T37.8X1	T37.8X2	T37.8X3	T37.8X4	T37.8X5	T37.8X6
- antiknock compound (tetraethyl)	T56.0X1	T56.0X2	T56.0X3	T56.0X4	--	--
- arsenate, arsenite (dust) (herbicide) (insecticide) (vapor)	T57.0X1	T57.0X2	T57.0X3	T57.0X4	--	--

Substance	Poisoning, Accidental (unintentional)	Poisoning, Intentional Self-harm	Poisoning, Assault	Poisoning, Undetermined	Adverse effect	Underdosing
- carbonate	T56.0X1	T56.0X2	T56.0X3	T56.0X4	--	--
- - paint	T56.0X1	T56.0X2	T56.0X3	T56.0X4	--	--
- chromate	T56.0X1	T56.0X2	T56.0X3	T56.0X4	--	--
- - paint	T56.0X1	T56.0X2	T56.0X3	T56.0X4	--	--
- dioxide	T56.0X1	T56.0X2	T56.0X3	T56.0X4	--	--
- inorganic	T56.0X1	T56.0X2	T56.0X3	T56.0X4	--	--
- iodide	T56.0X1	T56.0X2	T56.0X3	T56.0X4	--	--
- - pigment (paint)	T56.0X1	T56.0X2	T56.0X3	T56.0X4	--	--
- monoxide (dust)	T56.0X1	T56.0X2	T56.0X3	T56.0X4	--	--
- - paint	T56.0X1	T56.0X2	T56.0X3	T56.0X4	--	--
- organic	T56.0X1	T56.0X2	T56.0X3	T56.0X4	--	--
- oxide	T56.0X1	T56.0X2	T56.0X3	T56.0X4	--	--
- - paint	T56.0X1	T56.0X2	T56.0X3	T56.0X4	--	--
- paint	T56.0X1	T56.0X2	T56.0X3	T56.0X4	--	--
- salts	T56.0X1	T56.0X2	T56.0X3	T56.0X4	--	--
- specified compound NEC	T56.0X1	T56.0X2	T56.0X3	T56.0X4	--	--
- tetra-ethyl	T56.0X1	T56.0X2	T56.0X3	T56.0X4	--	--
Lebanese red	T40.711	T40.712	T40.713	T40.714	T40.715	T40.716
Lefetamine	T39.8X1	T39.8X2	T39.8X3	T39.8X4	T39.8X5	T39.8X6
Lenperone	T43.4X1	T43.4X2	T43.4X3	T43.4X4	T43.4X5	T43.4X6
Lente lietin (insulin)	T38.3X1	T38.3X2	T38.3X3	T38.3X4	T38.3X5	T38.3X6
Leptazol	T50.7X1	T50.7X2	T50.7X3	T50.7X4	T50.7X5	T50.7X6
Leptophos	T60.0X1	T60.0X2	T60.0X3	T60.0X4	--	--
Leritine	T40.2X1	T40.2X2	T40.2X3	T40.2X4	T40.2X5	T40.2X6
Letosteine	T48.4X1	T48.4X2	T48.4X3	T48.4X4	T48.4X5	T48.4X6
Letter	T38.1X1	T38.1X2	T38.1X3	T38.1X4	T38.1X5	T38.1X6
Lettuce opium	T42.6X1	T42.6X2	T42.6X3	T42.6X4	T42.6X5	T42.6X6
Leucinocaine	T41.3X1	T41.3X2	T41.3X3	T41.3X4	T41.3X5	T41.3X6
Leucocianidol	T46.991	T46.992	T46.993	T46.994	T46.995	T46.996
Leucovorin (factor)	T45.8X1	T45.8X2	T45.8X3	T45.8X4	T45.8X5	T45.8X6
Leukeran	T45.1X1	T45.1X2	T45.1X3	T45.1X4	T45.1X5	T45.1X6
Leuprolide	T38.891	T38.892	T38.893	T38.894	T38.895	T38.896
Levalbuterol	T48.6X1	T48.6X2	T48.6X3	T48.6X4	T48.6X5	T48.6X6
Levallorphan	T50.7X1	T50.7X2	T50.7X3	T50.7X4	T50.7X5	T50.7X6
Levamisole	T37.4X1	T37.4X2	T37.4X3	T37.4X4	T37.4X5	T37.4X6
Levanil	T42.6X1	T42.6X2	T42.6X3	T42.6X4	T42.6X5	T42.6X6
Levarterenol	T44.4X1	T44.4X2	T44.4X3	T44.4X4	T44.4X5	T44.4X6
Levdropropizine	T48.3X1	T48.3X2	T48.3X3	T48.3X4	T48.3X5	T48.3X6
Levobunolol	T49.5X1	T49.5X2	T49.5X3	T49.5X4	T49.5X5	T49.5X6
Levocabastine (hydrochloride)	T45.0X1	T45.0X2	T45.0X3	T45.0X4	T45.0X5	T45.0X6
Levocarnitine	T50.991	T50.992	T50.993	T50.994	T50.995	T50.996
Levodopa	T42.8X1	T42.8X2	T42.8X3	T42.8X4	T42.8X5	T42.8X6
- with carbidopa	T42.8X1	T42.8X2	T42.8X3	T42.8X4	T42.8X5	T42.8X6
Levo-dromoran	T40.2X1	T40.2X2	T40.2X3	T40.2X4	T40.2X5	T40.2X6
Levoglutamide	T50.991	T50.992	T50.993	T50.994	T50.995	T50.996
Levoid	T38.1X1	T38.1X2	T38.1X3	T38.1X4	T38.1X5	T38.1X6
Levo-iso-methadone	T40.3X1	T40.3X2	T40.3X3	T40.3X4	T40.3X5	T40.3X6
Levomepromazine	T43.3X1	T43.3X2	T43.3X3	T43.3X4	T43.3X5	T43.3X6
Levonordefrin	T49.6X1	T49.6X2	T49.6X3	T49.6X4	T49.6X5	T49.6X6
Levonorgestrel	T38.4X1	T38.4X2	T38.4X3	T38.4X4	T38.4X5	T38.4X6
- with ethinylestradiol	T38.5X1	T38.5X2	T38.5X3	T38.5X4	T38.5X5	T38.5X6
Levopromazine	T43.3X1	T43.3X2	T43.3X3	T43.3X4	T43.3X5	T43.3X6
Levoprome	T42.6X1	T42.6X2	T42.6X3	T42.6X4	T42.6X5	T42.6X6
Levopropoxyphene	T40.491	T40.492	T40.493	T40.494	T40.495	T40.496
Levopropylhexedrine	T50.5X1	T50.5X2	T50.5X3	T50.5X4	T50.5X5	T50.5X6
Levoproxyphylline	T48.6X1	T48.6X2	T48.6X3	T48.6X4	T48.6X5	T48.6X6
Levorphanol	T40.491	T40.492	T40.493	T40.494	T40.495	T40.496
Levothyroxine	T38.1X1	T38.1X2	T38.1X3	T38.1X4	T38.1X5	T38.1X6

Substance	Poisoning, Accidental (unintentional)	Poisoning, Intentional Self-harm	Poisoning, Assault	Poisoning, Undetermined	Adverse effect	Underdosing
- sodium	T38.1X1	T38.1X2	T38.1X3	T38.1X4	T38.1X5	T38.1X6
Levsin	T44.3X1	T44.3X2	T44.3X3	T44.3X4	T44.3X5	T44.3X6
Levulose	T50.3X1	T50.3X2	T50.3X3	T50.3X4	T50.3X5	T50.3X6
Lewisite (gas), not in war	T57.0X1	T57.0X2	T57.0X3	T57.0X4	--	--
Librium	T42.4X1	T42.4X2	T42.4X3	T42.4X4	T42.4X5	T42.4X6
Lidex	T49.0X1	T49.0X2	T49.0X3	T49.0X4	T49.0X5	T49.0X6
Lidocaine	T41.3X1	T41.3X2	T41.3X3	T41.3X4	T41.3X5	T41.3X6
- regional	T41.3X1	T41.3X2	T41.3X3	T41.3X4	T41.3X5	T41.3X6
- spinal	T41.3X1	T41.3X2	T41.3X3	T41.3X4	T41.3X5	T41.3X6
Lidofenin	T50.8X1	T50.8X2	T50.8X3	T50.8X4	T50.8X5	T50.8X6
Lidoflazine	T46.1X1	T46.1X2	T46.1X3	T46.1X4	T46.1X5	T46.1X6
Lighter fluid	T52.0X1	T52.0X2	T52.0X3	T52.0X4	--	--
Lignin hemicellulose	T47.6X1	T47.6X2	T47.6X3	T47.6X4	T47.6X5	T47.6X6
Lignocaine	T41.3X1	T41.3X2	T41.3X3	T41.3X4	T41.3X5	T41.3X6
- regional	T41.3X1	T41.3X2	T41.3X3	T41.3X4	T41.3X5	T41.3X6
- spinal	T41.3X1	T41.3X2	T41.3X3	T41.3X4	T41.3X5	T41.3X6
Ligroin (e) (solvent)	T52.0X1	T52.0X2	T52.0X3	T52.0X4	--	--
- vapor	T59.891	T59.892	T59.893	T59.894	--	--
Ligustrum vulgare	T62.2X1	T62.2X2	T62.2X3	T62.2X4	--	--
Lily of the valley	T62.2X1	T62.2X2	T62.2X3	T62.2X4	--	--
Lime (chloride)	T54.3X1	T54.3X2	T54.3X3	T54.3X4	--	--
Limonene	T52.8X1	T52.8X2	T52.8X3	T52.8X4	--	--
Lincomycin	T36.8X1	T36.8X2	T36.8X3	T36.8X4	T36.8X5	T36.8X6
Lindane (insecticide) (nonmedicinal) (vapor)	T53.6X1	T53.6X2	T53.6X3	T53.6X4	--	--
- medicinal	T49.0X1	T49.0X2	T49.0X3	T49.0X4	T49.0X5	T49.0X6
Liniments NEC	T49.91	T49.92	T49.93	T49.94	T49.95	T49.96
Linoleic acid	T46.6X1	T46.6X2	T46.6X3	T46.6X4	T46.6X5	T46.6X6
Linolenic acid	T46.6X1	T46.6X2	T46.6X3	T46.6X4	T46.6X5	T46.6X6
Linseed	T47.4X1	T47.4X2	T47.4X3	T47.4X4	T47.4X5	T47.4X6
Liothyronine	T38.1X1	T38.1X2	T38.1X3	T38.1X4	T38.1X5	T38.1X6
Liotrix	T38.1X1	T38.1X2	T38.1X3	T38.1X4	T38.1X5	T38.1X6
Lipancreatin	T47.5X1	T47.5X2	T47.5X3	T47.5X4	T47.5X5	T47.5X6
Lipo-alprostadil	T46.7X1	T46.7X2	T46.7X3	T46.7X4	T46.7X5	T46.7X6
Lipo-Lutin	T38.5X1	T38.5X2	T38.5X3	T38.5X4	T38.5X5	T38.5X6
Lipotropic drug NEC	T50.901	T50.902	T50.903	T50.904	T50.905	T50.906
Liquefied petroleum gases	T59.891	T59.892	T59.893	T59.894	--	--
- piped (pure or mixed with air)	T59.891	T59.892	T59.893	T59.894	--	--
Liquid						
- paraffin	T47.4X1	T47.4X2	T47.4X3	T47.4X4	T47.4X5	T47.4X6
- petrolatum	T47.4X1	T47.4X2	T47.4X3	T47.4X4	T47.4X5	T47.4X6
- - topical	T49.3X1	T49.3X2	T49.3X3	T49.3X4	T49.3X5	T49.3X6
- specified NEC	T65.891	T65.892	T65.893	T65.894	--	--
- substance	T65.91	T65.92	T65.93	T65.94	--	--
Liquor creosolis compositus	T65.891	T65.892	T65.893	T65.894	--	--
Liquorice	T48.4X1	T48.4X2	T48.4X3	T48.4X4	T48.4X5	T48.4X6
- extract	T47.8X1	T47.8X2	T47.8X3	T47.8X4	T47.8X5	T47.8X6
Lisinopril	T46.4X1	T46.4X2	T46.4X3	T46.4X4	T46.4X5	T46.4X6
Lisuride	T42.8X1	T42.8X2	T42.8X3	T42.8X4	T42.8X5	T42.8X6
Lithane	T43.8X1	T43.8X2	T43.8X3	T43.8X4	T43.8X5	T43.8X6
Lithium	T56.891	T56.892	T56.893	T56.894	--	--
- gluconate	T43.591	T43.592	T43.593	T43.594	T43.595	T43.596
- salts (carbonate)	T43.591	T43.592	T43.593	T43.594	T43.595	T43.596
Lithonate	T43.8X1	T43.8X2	T43.8X3	T43.8X4	T43.8X5	T43.8X6
Liver						
- extract	T45.8X1	T45.8X2	T45.8X3	T45.8X4	T45.8X5	T45.8X6
- - for parenteral use	T45.8X1	T45.8X2	T45.8X3	T45.8X4	T45.8X5	T45.8X6
- fraction 1	T45.8X1	T45.8X2	T45.8X3	T45.8X4	T45.8X5	T45.8X6
- hydrolysate	T45.8X1	T45.8X2	T45.8X3	T45.8X4	T45.8X5	T45.8X6
Lizard (bite) (venom)	T63.121	T63.122	T63.123	T63.124	--	--

Substance	Poisoning, Accidental (unintentional)	Poisoning, Intentional Self-harm	Poisoning, Assault	Poisoning, Undetermined	Adverse effect	Underdosing
LMD	T45.8X1	T45.8X2	T45.8X3	T45.8X4	T45.8X5	T45.8X6
Lobelia	T62.2X1	T62.2X2	T62.2X3	T62.2X4	--	--
Lobeline	T50.7X1	T50.7X2	T50.7X3	T50.7X4	T50.7X5	T50.7X6
Local action drug NEC	T49.8X1	T49.8X2	T49.8X3	T49.8X4	T49.8X5	T49.8X6
Locorten	T49.0X1	T49.0X2	T49.0X3	T49.0X4	T49.0X5	T49.0X6
Lofepramine	T43.011	T43.012	T43.013	T43.014	T43.015	T43.016
Lolium temulentum	T62.2X1	T62.2X2	T62.2X3	T62.2X4	--	--
Lomotil	T47.6X1	T47.6X2	T47.6X3	T47.6X4	T47.6X5	T47.6X6
Lomustine	T45.1X1	T45.1X2	T45.1X3	T45.1X4	T45.1X5	T45.1X6
Lonidamine	T45.1X1	T45.1X2	T45.1X3	T45.1X4	T45.1X5	T45.1X6
Loperamide	T47.6X1	T47.6X2	T47.6X3	T47.6X4	T47.6X5	T47.6X6
Loprazolam	T42.4X1	T42.4X2	T42.4X3	T42.4X4	T42.4X5	T42.4X6
Lorajmine	T46.2X1	T46.2X2	T46.2X3	T46.2X4	T46.2X5	T46.2X6
Loratidine	T45.0X1	T45.0X2	T45.0X3	T45.0X4	T45.0X5	T45.0X6
Lorazepam	T42.4X1	T42.4X2	T42.4X3	T42.4X4	T42.4X5	T42.4X6
Lorcainide	T46.2X1	T46.2X2	T46.2X3	T46.2X4	T46.2X5	T46.2X6
Lormetazepam	T42.4X1	T42.4X2	T42.4X3	T42.4X4	T42.4X5	T42.4X6
Lotions NEC	T49.91	T49.92	T49.93	T49.94	T49.95	T49.96
Lotusate	T42.3X1	T42.3X2	T42.3X3	T42.3X4	T42.3X5	T42.3X6
Lovastatin	T46.6X1	T46.6X2	T46.6X3	T46.6X4	T46.6X5	T46.6X6
Lowila	T49.2X1	T49.2X2	T49.2X3	T49.2X4	T49.2X5	T49.2X6
Loxapine	T43.591	T43.592	T43.593	T43.594	T43.595	T43.596
Lozenges (throat)	T49.6X1	T49.6X2	T49.6X3	T49.6X4	T49.6X5	T49.6X6
LSD	T40.8X1	T40.8X2	T40.8X3	T40.8X4	T40.8X5	--
L-Tryptophan—see amino acid						
Lubricant, eye	T49.5X1	T49.5X2	T49.5X3	T49.5X4	T49.5X5	T49.5X6
Lubricating oil NEC	T52.0X1	T52.0X2	T52.0X3	T52.0X4	--	--
Lucanthone	T37.4X1	T37.4X2	T37.4X3	T37.4X4	T37.4X5	T37.4X6
Luminal	T42.3X1	T42.3X2	T42.3X3	T42.3X4	T42.3X5	T42.3X6
Lung irritant (gas) NEC	T59.91	T59.92	T59.93	T59.94	--	--
Luteinizing hormone	T38.811	T38.812	T38.813	T38.814	T38.815	T38.816
Lutocylol	T38.5X1	T38.5X2	T38.5X3	T38.5X4	T38.5X5	T38.5X6
Lutromone	T38.5X1	T38.5X2	T38.5X3	T38.5X4	T38.5X5	T38.5X6
Lututrin	T48.291	T48.292	T48.293	T48.294	T48.295	T48.296
Lye (concentrated)	T54.3X1	T54.3X2	T54.3X3	T54.3X4	--	--
Lygranum (skin test)	T50.8X1	T50.8X2	T50.8X3	T50.8X4	T50.8X5	T50.8X6
Lymecycline	T36.4X1	T36.4X2	T36.4X3	T36.4X4	T36.4X5	T36.4X6
Lymphogranuloma venereum antigen	T50.8X1	T50.8X2	T50.8X3	T50.8X4	T50.8X5	T50.8X6
Lynestrenol	T38.4X1	T38.4X2	T38.4X3	T38.4X4	T38.4X5	T38.4X6
Lyovac Sodium Edecrin	T50.1X1	T50.1X2	T50.1X3	T50.1X4	T50.1X5	T50.1X6
Lypressin	T38.891	T38.892	T38.893	T38.894	T38.895	T38.896
Lysergic acid diethylamide	T40.8X1	T40.8X2	T40.8X3	T40.8X4	T40.8X5	--
Lysergide	T40.8X1	T40.8X2	T40.8X3	T40.8X4	T40.8X5	--
Lysine vasopressin	T38.891	T38.892	T38.893	T38.894	T38.895	T38.896
Lysol	T54.1X1	T54.1X2	T54.1X3	T54.1X4	--	--
Lysozyme	T49.0X1	T49.0X2	T49.0X3	T49.0X4	T49.0X5	T49.0X6
Lytta (vitatta)	T49.8X1	T49.8X2	T49.8X3	T49.8X4	T49.8X5	T49.8X6
Mace	T59.3X1	T59.3X2	T59.3X3	T59.3X4	--	--
Macrogol	T50.991	T50.992	T50.993	T50.994	T50.995	T50.996
Macrolide						
- anabolic drug	T38.7X1	T38.7X2	T38.7X3	T38.7X4	T38.7X5	T38.7X6
- antibiotic	T36.3X1	T36.3X2	T36.3X3	T36.3X4	T36.3X5	T36.3X6
Mafenide	T49.0X1	T49.0X2	T49.0X3	T49.0X4	T49.0X5	T49.0X6
Magaldrate	T47.1X1	T47.1X2	T47.1X3	T47.1X4	T47.1X5	T47.1X6
Magic mushroom	T40.991	T40.992	T40.993	T40.994	--	--
Magnamycin	T36.8X1	T36.8X2	T36.8X3	T36.8X4	T36.8X5	T36.8X6
Magnesia magma	T47.1X1	T47.1X2	T47.1X3	T47.1X4	T47.1X5	T47.1X6
Magnesium NEC	T56.891	T56.892	T56.893	T56.894	--	--

Substance	Poisoning, Accidental (unintentional)	Poisoning, Intentional Self-harm	Poisoning, Assault	Poisoning, Undetermined	Adverse effect	Underdosing
- carbonate	T47.1X1	T47.1X2	T47.1X3	T47.1X4	T47.1X5	T47.1X6
- citrate	T47.4X1	T47.4X2	T47.4X3	T47.4X4	T47.4X5	T47.4X6
- hydroxide	T47.1X1	T47.1X2	T47.1X3	T47.1X4	T47.1X5	T47.1X6
- oxide	T47.1X1	T47.1X2	T47.1X3	T47.1X4	T47.1X5	T47.1X6
- peroxide	T49.0X1	T49.0X2	T49.0X3	T49.0X4	T49.0X5	T49.0X6
- salicylate	T39.091	T39.092	T39.093	T39.094	T39.095	T39.096
- silicofluoride	T50.3X1	T50.3X2	T50.3X3	T50.3X4	T50.3X5	T50.3X6
- sulfate	T47.4X1	T47.4X2	T47.4X3	T47.4X4	T47.4X5	T47.4X6
- thiosulfate	T45.0X1	T45.0X2	T45.0X3	T45.0X4	T45.0X5	T45.0X6
- trisilicate	T47.1X1	T47.1X2	T47.1X3	T47.1X4	T47.1X5	T47.1X6
Malathion (medicinal)	T49.0X1	T49.0X2	T49.0X3	T49.0X4	T49.0X5	T49.0X6
- insecticide	T60.0X1	T60.0X2	T60.0X3	T60.0X4	--	--
Male fern extract	T37.4X1	T37.4X2	T37.4X3	T37.4X4	T37.4X5	T37.4X6
M-AMSA	T45.1X1	T45.1X2	T45.1X3	T45.1X4	T45.1X5	T45.1X6
Mandelic acid	T37.8X1	T37.8X2	T37.8X3	T37.8X4	T37.8X5	T37.8X6
Manganese (dioxide) (salts)	T57.2X1	T57.2X2	T57.2X3	T57.2X4	--	--
- medicinal	T50.991	T50.992	T50.993	T50.994	T50.995	T50.996
Mannitol	T47.3X1	T47.3X2	T47.3X3	T47.3X4	T47.3X5	T47.3X6
- hexanitrate	T46.3X1	T46.3X2	T46.3X3	T46.3X4	T46.3X5	T46.3X6
Mannomustine	T45.1X1	T45.1X2	T45.1X3	T45.1X4	T45.1X5	T45.1X6
MAO inhibitors	T43.1X1	T43.1X2	T43.1X3	T43.1X4	T43.1X5	T43.1X6
Mapharsen	T37.8X1	T37.8X2	T37.8X3	T37.8X4	T37.8X5	T37.8X6
Maphenide	T49.0X1	T49.0X2	T49.0X3	T49.0X4	T49.0X5	T49.0X6
Maprotiline	T43.021	T43.022	T43.023	T43.024	T43.025	T43.026
Marcaine	T41.3X1	T41.3X2	T41.3X3	T41.3X4	T41.3X5	T41.3X6
- infiltration (subcutaneous)	T41.3X1	T41.3X2	T41.3X3	T41.3X4	T41.3X5	T41.3X6
- nerve block (peripheral) (plexus)	T41.3X1	T41.3X2	T41.3X3	T41.3X4	T41.3X5	T41.3X6
Marezine	T45.0X1	T45.0X2	T45.0X3	T45.0X4	T45.0X5	T45.0X6
Marihuana	T40.711	T40.712	T40.713	T40.714	T40.715	T40.716
Marijuana	T40.711	T40.712	T40.713	T40.714	T40.715	T40.716
Marine (sting)	T63.691	T63.692	T63.693	T63.694	--	--
- animals (sting)	T63.691	T63.692	T63.693	T63.694	--	--
- plants (sting)	T63.711	T63.712	T63.713	T63.714	--	--
Marplan	T43.1X1	T43.1X2	T43.1X3	T43.1X4	T43.1X5	T43.1X6
Marsh gas	T59.891	T59.892	T59.893	T59.894	--	--
Marsilid	T43.1X1	T43.1X2	T43.1X3	T43.1X4	T43.1X5	T43.1X6
Matulane	T45.1X1	T45.1X2	T45.1X3	T45.1X4	T45.1X5	T45.1X6
Mazindol	T50.5X1	T50.5X2	T50.5X3	T50.5X4	T50.5X5	T50.5X6
MCPA	T60.3X1	T60.3X2	T60.3X3	T60.3X4	--	--
MDMA	T43.641	T43.642	T43.643	T43.644	T43.645	T43.646
Meadow saffron	T62.2X1	T62.2X2	T62.2X3	T62.2X4	--	--
Measles virus vaccine (attenuated)	T50.B91	T50.B92	T50.B93	T50.B94	T50.B95	T50.B96
Meat, noxious	T62.8X1	T62.8X2	T62.8X3	T62.8X4	--	--
Meballymal	T42.3X1	T42.3X2	T42.3X3	T42.3X4	T42.3X5	T42.3X6
Mebanazine	T43.1X1	T43.1X2	T43.1X3	T43.1X4	T43.1X5	T43.1X6
Mebaral	T42.3X1	T42.3X2	T42.3X3	T42.3X4	T42.3X5	T42.3X6
Mebendazole	T37.4X1	T37.4X2	T37.4X3	T37.4X4	T37.4X5	T37.4X6
Mebeverine	T44.3X1	T44.3X2	T44.3X3	T44.3X4	T44.3X5	T44.3X6
Mebhydrolin	T45.0X1	T45.0X2	T45.0X3	T45.0X4	T45.0X5	T45.0X6
Mebumal	T42.3X1	T42.3X2	T42.3X3	T42.3X4	T42.3X5	T42.3X6
Mebutamate	T43.591	T43.592	T43.593	T43.594	T43.595	T43.596
Mecamylamine	T44.2X1	T44.2X2	T44.2X3	T44.2X4	T44.2X5	T44.2X6
Mechlorethamine	T45.1X1	T45.1X2	T45.1X3	T45.1X4	T45.1X5	T45.1X6
Mecillinam	T36.0X1	T36.0X2	T36.0X3	T36.0X4	T36.0X5	T36.0X6
Meclizine (hydrochloride)	T45.0X1	T45.0X2	T45.0X3	T45.0X4	T45.0X5	T45.0X6
Meclocycline	T36.4X1	T36.4X2	T36.4X3	T36.4X4	T36.4X5	T36.4X6
Meclofenamate	T39.391	T39.392	T39.393	T39.394	T39.395	T39.396
Meclofenamic acid	T39.391	T39.392	T39.393	T39.394	T39.395	T39.396
Meclofenoxate	T43.691	T43.692	T43.693	T43.694	T43.695	T43.696

Substance	Poisoning, Accidental (unintentional)	Poisoning, Intentional Self-harm	Poisoning, Assault	Poisoning, Undetermined	Adverse effect	Underdosing
Meclozine	T45.0X1	T45.0X2	T45.0X3	T45.0X4	T45.0X5	T45.0X6
Mecobalamin	T45.8X1	T45.8X2	T45.8X3	T45.8X4	T45.8X5	T45.8X6
Mecoprop	T60.3X1	T60.3X2	T60.3X3	T60.3X4	--	--
Mecrilate	T49.3X1	T49.3X2	T49.3X3	T49.3X4	T49.3X5	T49.3X6
Mecysteine	T48.4X1	T48.4X2	T48.4X3	T48.4X4	T48.4X5	T48.4X6
Medazepam	T42.4X1	T42.4X2	T42.4X3	T42.4X4	T42.4X5	T42.4X6
Medicament NEC	T50.901	T50.902	T50.903	T50.904	T50.905	T50.906
Medinal	T42.3X1	T42.3X2	T42.3X3	T42.3X4	T42.3X5	T42.3X6
Medomin	T42.3X1	T42.3X2	T42.3X3	T42.3X4	T42.3X5	T42.3X6
Medrogestone	T38.5X1	T38.5X2	T38.5X3	T38.5X4	T38.5X5	T38.5X6
Medroxalol	T44.8X1	T44.8X2	T44.8X3	T44.8X4	T44.8X5	T44.8X6
Medroxyprogesterone acetate (depot)	T38.5X1	T38.5X2	T38.5X3	T38.5X4	T38.5X5	T38.5X6
Medrysone	T49.0X1	T49.0X2	T49.0X3	T49.0X4	T49.0X5	T49.0X6
Mefenamic acid	T39.391	T39.392	T39.393	T39.394	T39.395	T39.396
Mefenorex	T50.5X1	T50.5X2	T50.5X3	T50.5X4	T50.5X5	T50.5X6
Mefloquine	T37.2X1	T37.2X2	T37.2X3	T37.2X4	T37.2X5	T37.2X6
Mefruside	T50.2X1	T50.2X2	T50.2X3	T50.2X4	T50.2X5	T50.2X6
Megahallucinogen	T40.901	T40.902	T40.903	T40.904	T40.905	T40.906
Megestrol	T38.5X1	T38.5X2	T38.5X3	T38.5X4	T38.5X5	T38.5X6
Meglumine						
- antimoniate	T37.8X1	T37.8X2	T37.8X3	T37.8X4	T37.8X5	T37.8X6
- diatrizoate	T50.8X1	T50.8X2	T50.8X3	T50.8X4	T50.8X5	T50.8X6
- iodipamide	T50.8X1	T50.8X2	T50.8X3	T50.8X4	T50.8X5	T50.8X6
- iotroxate	T50.8X1	T50.8X2	T50.8X3	T50.8X4	T50.8X5	T50.8X6
MEK (methyl ethyl ketone)	T52.4X1	T52.4X2	T52.4X3	T52.4X4	--	--
Meladinin	T49.3X1	T49.3X2	T49.3X3	T49.3X4	T49.3X5	T49.3X6
Meladrazine	T44.3X1	T44.3X2	T44.3X3	T44.3X4	T44.3X5	T44.3X6
Melaleuca alternifolia oil	T49.0X1	T49.0X2	T49.0X3	T49.0X4	T49.0X5	T49.0X6
Melanizing agents	T49.3X1	T49.3X2	T49.3X3	T49.3X4	T49.3X5	T49.3X6
Melanocyte-stimulating hormone	T38.891	T38.892	T38.893	T38.894	T38.895	T38.896
Melarsonyl potassium	T37.3X1	T37.3X2	T37.3X3	T37.3X4	T37.3X5	T37.3X6
Melarsoprol	T37.3X1	T37.3X2	T37.3X3	T37.3X4	T37.3X5	T37.3X6
Melia azedarach	T62.2X1	T62.2X2	T62.2X3	T62.2X4	--	--
Melitracen	T43.011	T43.012	T43.013	T43.014	T43.015	T43.016
Mellaril	T43.3X1	T43.3X2	T43.3X3	T43.3X4	T43.3X5	T43.3X6
Meloxine	T49.3X1	T49.3X2	T49.3X3	T49.3X4	T49.3X5	T49.3X6
Melperone	T43.4X1	T43.4X2	T43.4X3	T43.4X4	T43.4X5	T43.4X6
Melphalan	T45.1X1	T45.1X2	T45.1X3	T45.1X4	T45.1X5	T45.1X6
Memantine	T43.8X1	T43.8X2	T43.8X3	T43.8X4	T43.8X5	T43.8X6
Menadiol	T45.7X1	T45.7X2	T45.7X3	T45.7X4	T45.7X5	T45.7X6
- sodium sulfate	T45.7X1	T45.7X2	T45.7X3	T45.7X4	T45.7X5	T45.7X6
Menadione	T45.7X1	T45.7X2	T45.7X3	T45.7X4	T45.7X5	T45.7X6
- sodium bisulfite	T45.7X1	T45.7X2	T45.7X3	T45.7X4	T45.7X5	T45.7X6
Menaphthone	T45.7X1	T45.7X2	T45.7X3	T45.7X4	T45.7X5	T45.7X6
Menaquinone	T45.7X1	T45.7X2	T45.7X3	T45.7X4	T45.7X5	T45.7X6
Menatetrenone	T45.7X1	T45.7X2	T45.7X3	T45.7X4	T45.7X5	T45.7X6
Meningococcal vaccine	T50.A91	T50.A92	T50.A93	T50.A94	T50.A95	T50.A96
Menningovax (-AC) (-C)	T50.A91	T50.A92	T50.A93	T50.A94	T50.A95	T50.A96
Menotropins	T38.811	T38.812	T38.813	T38.814	T38.815	T38.816
Menthol	T48.5X1	T48.5X2	T48.5X3	T48.5X4	T48.5X5	T48.5X6
Mepacrine	T37.2X1	T37.2X2	T37.2X3	T37.2X4	T37.2X5	T37.2X6
Meparfynol	T42.6X1	T42.6X2	T42.6X3	T42.6X4	T42.6X5	T42.6X6
Mepartricin	T36.7X1	T36.7X2	T36.7X3	T36.7X4	T36.7X5	T36.7X6
Mepazine	T43.3X1	T43.3X2	T43.3X3	T43.3X4	T43.3X5	T43.3X6
Mepenzolate	T44.3X1	T44.3X2	T44.3X3	T44.3X4	T44.3X5	T44.3X6
- bromide	T44.3X1	T44.3X2	T44.3X3	T44.3X4	T44.3X5	T44.3X6
Meperidine	T40.491	T40.492	T40.493	T40.494	T40.495	T40.496
Mephebarbital	T42.3X1	T42.3X2	T42.3X3	T42.3X4	T42.3X5	T42.3X6

Substance	Poisoning, Accidental (unintentional)	Poisoning, Intentional Self-harm	Poisoning, Assault	Poisoning, Undetermined	Adverse effect	Underdosing
Mephenamin (e)	T42.8X1	T42.8X2	T42.8X3	T42.8X4	T42.8X5	T42.8X6
Mephenesin	T42.8X1	T42.8X2	T42.8X3	T42.8X4	T42.8X5	T42.8X6
Mephenhydramine	T45.0X1	T45.0X2	T45.0X3	T45.0X4	T45.0X5	T45.0X6
Mephenoxalone	T42.8X1	T42.8X2	T42.8X3	T42.8X4	T42.8X5	T42.8X6
Mephentermine	T44.991	T44.992	T44.993	T44.994	T44.995	T44.996
Mephenytoin	T42.0X1	T42.0X2	T42.0X3	T42.0X4	T42.0X5	T42.0X6
- with phenobarbital	T42.3X1	T42.3X2	T42.3X3	T42.3X4	T42.3X5	T42.3X6
Mephobarbital	T42.3X1	T42.3X2	T42.3X3	T42.3X4	T42.3X5	T42.3X6
Mephosfolan	T60.0X1	T60.0X2	T60.0X3	T60.0X4	--	--
Mepindolol	T44.7X1	T44.7X2	T44.7X3	T44.7X4	T44.7X5	T44.7X6
Mepiperphenidol	T44.3X1	T44.3X2	T44.3X3	T44.3X4	T44.3X5	T44.3X6
Mepitiostane	T38.7X1	T38.7X2	T38.7X3	T38.7X4	T38.7X5	T38.7X6
Mepivacaine	T41.3X1	T41.3X2	T41.3X3	T41.3X4	T41.3X5	T41.3X6
- epidural	T41.3X1	T41.3X2	T41.3X3	T41.3X4	T41.3X5	T41.3X6
Meprednisone	T38.0X1	T38.0X2	T38.0X3	T38.0X4	T38.0X5	T38.0X6
Meprobam	T43.591	T43.592	T43.593	T43.594	T43.595	T43.596
Meprobamate	T43.591	T43.592	T43.593	T43.594	T43.595	T43.596
Meproscillarin	T46.0X1	T46.0X2	T46.0X3	T46.0X4	T46.0X5	T46.0X6
Meprylcaine	T41.3X1	T41.3X2	T41.3X3	T41.3X4	T41.3X5	T41.3X6
Meptazinol	T39.8X1	T39.8X2	T39.8X3	T39.8X4	T39.8X5	T39.8X6
Mepyramine	T45.0X1	T45.0X2	T45.0X3	T45.0X4	T45.0X5	T45.0X6
Mequitazine	T43.3X1	T43.3X2	T43.3X3	T43.3X4	T43.3X5	T43.3X6
Meralluride	T50.2X1	T50.2X2	T50.2X3	T50.2X4	T50.2X5	T50.2X6
Merbaphen	T50.2X1	T50.2X2	T50.2X3	T50.2X4	T50.2X5	T50.2X6
Merbromin	T49.0X1	T49.0X2	T49.0X3	T49.0X4	T49.0X5	T49.0X6
Mercaptobenzothiazole salts	T49.0X1	T49.0X2	T49.0X3	T49.0X4	T49.0X5	T49.0X6
Mercaptomerin	T50.2X1	T50.2X2	T50.2X3	T50.2X4	T50.2X5	T50.2X6
Mercaptopurine	T45.1X1	T45.1X2	T45.1X3	T45.1X4	T45.1X5	T45.1X6
Mercumatilin	T50.2X1	T50.2X2	T50.2X3	T50.2X4	T50.2X5	T50.2X6
Mercuramide	T50.2X1	T50.2X2	T50.2X3	T50.2X4	T50.2X5	T50.2X6
Mercurochrome	T49.0X1	T49.0X2	T49.0X3	T49.0X4	T49.0X5	T49.0X6
Mercurophylline	T50.2X1	T50.2X2	T50.2X3	T50.2X4	T50.2X5	T50.2X6
Mercury, mercurial, mercuric, mercurous (compounds) (cyanide) (fumes) (nonmedicinal) (vapor) NEC	T56.1X1	T56.1X2	T56.1X3	T56.1X4	--	--
- ammoniated	T49.0X1	T49.0X2	T49.0X3	T49.0X4	T49.0X5	T49.0X6
- anti-infective						
- - local	T49.0X1	T49.0X2	T49.0X3	T49.0X4	T49.0X5	T49.0X6
- - systemic	T37.8X1	T37.8X2	T37.8X3	T37.8X4	T37.8X5	T37.8X6
- - topical	T49.0X1	T49.0X2	T49.0X3	T49.0X4	T49.0X5	T49.0X6
- chloride (ammoniated)	T49.0X1	T49.0X2	T49.0X3	T49.0X4	T49.0X5	T49.0X6
- - fungicide	T56.1X1	T56.1X2	T56.1X3	T56.1X4	--	--
- diuretic NEC	T50.2X1	T50.2X2	T50.2X3	T50.2X4	T50.2X5	T50.2X6
- fungicide	T56.1X1	T56.1X2	T56.1X3	T56.1X4	--	--
- organic (fungicide)	T56.1X1	T56.1X2	T56.1X3	T56.1X4	--	--
- oxide, yellow	T49.0X1	T49.0X2	T49.0X3	T49.0X4	T49.0X5	T49.0X6
Mersalyl	T50.2X1	T50.2X2	T50.2X3	T50.2X4	T50.2X5	T50.2X6
Merthiolate	T49.0X1	T49.0X2	T49.0X3	T49.0X4	T49.0X5	T49.0X6
- ophthalmic preparation	T49.5X1	T49.5X2	T49.5X3	T49.5X4	T49.5X5	T49.5X6
Meruvax	T50.B91	T50.B92	T50.B93	T50.B94	T50.B95	T50.B96
Mesalazine	T47.8X1	T47.8X2	T47.8X3	T47.8X4	T47.8X5	T47.8X6
Mescal buttons	T40.991	T40.992	T40.993	T40.994	--	--
Mescaline	T40.991	T40.992	T40.993	T40.994	--	--
Mesna	T48.4X1	T48.4X2	T48.4X3	T48.4X4	T48.4X5	T48.4X6
Mesoglycan	T46.6X1	T46.6X2	T46.6X3	T46.6X4	T46.6X5	T46.6X6
Mesoridazine	T43.3X1	T43.3X2	T43.3X3	T43.3X4	T43.3X5	T43.3X6
Mestanolone	T38.7X1	T38.7X2	T38.7X3	T38.7X4	T38.7X5	T38.7X6
Mesterolone	T38.7X1	T38.7X2	T38.7X3	T38.7X4	T38.7X5	T38.7X6
Mestranol	T38.5X1	T38.5X2	T38.5X3	T38.5X4	T38.5X5	T38.5X6

Substance	Poisoning, Accidental (unintentional)	Poisoning, Intentional Self-harm	Poisoning, Assault	Poisoning, Undetermined	Adverse effect	Underdosing
Mesulergine	T42.8X1	T42.8X2	T42.8X3	T42.8X4	T42.8X5	T42.8X6
Mesulfen	T49.0X1	T49.0X2	T49.0X3	T49.0X4	T49.0X5	T49.0X6
Mesuximide	T42.2X1	T42.2X2	T42.2X3	T42.2X4	T42.2X5	T42.2X6
Metabutethamine	T41.3X1	T41.3X2	T41.3X3	T41.3X4	T41.3X5	T41.3X6
Metactesylacetate	T49.0X1	T49.0X2	T49.0X3	T49.0X4	T49.0X5	T49.0X6
Metacycline	T36.4X1	T36.4X2	T36.4X3	T36.4X4	T36.4X5	T36.4X6
Metaldehyde (snail killer) NEC	T60.8X1	T60.8X2	T60.8X3	T60.8X4	--	--
Metals (heavy) (nonmedicinal)	T56.91	T56.92	T56.93	T56.94	--	--
- dust, fumes, or vapor NEC	T56.91	T56.92	T56.93	T56.94	--	--
- light NEC	T56.91	T56.92	T56.93	T56.94	--	--
- - dust, fumes, or vapor NEC	T56.91	T56.92	T56.93	T56.94	--	--
- specified NEC	T56.891	T56.892	T56.893	T56.894	--	--
- thallium	T56.811	T56.812	T56.813	T56.814	--	--
Metamfetamine	T43.621	T43.622	T43.623	T43.624	T43.625	T43.626
Metamizole sodium	T39.2X1	T39.2X2	T39.2X3	T39.2X4	T39.2X5	T39.2X6
Metampicillin	T36.0X1	T36.0X2	T36.0X3	T36.0X4	T36.0X5	T36.0X6
Metamucil	T47.4X1	T47.4X2	T47.4X3	T47.4X4	T47.4X5	T47.4X6
Metandienone	T38.7X1	T38.7X2	T38.7X3	T38.7X4	T38.7X5	T38.7X6
Metandrostenolone	T38.7X1	T38.7X2	T38.7X3	T38.7X4	T38.7X5	T38.7X6
Metaphen	T49.0X1	T49.0X2	T49.0X3	T49.0X4	T49.0X5	T49.0X6
Metaphos	T60.0X1	T60.0X2	T60.0X3	T60.0X4	--	--
Metapramine	T43.011	T43.012	T43.013	T43.014	T43.015	T43.016
Metaproterenol	T48.291	T48.292	T48.293	T48.294	T48.295	T48.296
Metaraminol	T44.4X1	T44.4X2	T44.4X3	T44.4X4	T44.4X5	T44.4X6
Metaxalone	T42.8X1	T42.8X2	T42.8X3	T42.8X4	T42.8X5	T42.8X6
Metenolone	T38.7X1	T38.7X2	T38.7X3	T38.7X4	T38.7X5	T38.7X6
Metergoline	T42.8X1	T42.8X2	T42.8X3	T42.8X4	T42.8X5	T42.8X6
Metescufylline	T46.991	T46.992	T46.993	T46.994	T46.995	T46.996
Metetoin	T42.0X1	T42.0X2	T42.0X3	T42.0X4	T42.0X5	T42.0X6
Metformin	T38.3X1	T38.3X2	T38.3X3	T38.3X4	T38.3X5	T38.3X6
Methacholine	T44.1X1	T44.1X2	T44.1X3	T44.1X4	T44.1X5	T44.1X6
Methacycline	T36.4X1	T36.4X2	T36.4X3	T36.4X4	T36.4X5	T36.4X6
Methadone	T40.3X1	T40.3X2	T40.3X3	T40.3X4	T40.3X5	T40.3X6
Methallenestril	T38.5X1	T38.5X2	T38.5X3	T38.5X4	T38.5X5	T38.5X6
Methallenoestril	T38.5X1	T38.5X2	T38.5X3	T38.5X4	T38.5X5	T38.5X6
Methamphetamine	T43.621	T43.622	T43.623	T43.624	T43.625	T43.626
Methampyrone	T39.2X1	T39.2X2	T39.2X3	T39.2X4	T39.2X5	T39.2X6
Methandienone	T38.7X1	T38.7X2	T38.7X3	T38.7X4	T38.7X5	T38.7X6
Methandriol	T38.7X1	T38.7X2	T38.7X3	T38.7X4	T38.7X5	T38.7X6
Methandrostenolone	T38.7X1	T38.7X2	T38.7X3	T38.7X4	T38.7X5	T38.7X6
Methane	T59.891	T59.892	T59.893	T59.894	--	--
Methanethiol	T59.891	T59.892	T59.893	T59.894	--	--
Methaniazide	T37.1X1	T37.1X2	T37.1X3	T37.1X4	T37.1X5	T37.1X6
Methanol (vapor)	T51.1X1	T51.1X2	T51.1X3	T51.1X4	--	--
Methantheline	T44.3X1	T44.3X2	T44.3X3	T44.3X4	T44.3X5	T44.3X6
Methanthelinium bromide	T44.3X1	T44.3X2	T44.3X3	T44.3X4	T44.3X5	T44.3X6
Methaphenilene	T45.0X1	T45.0X2	T45.0X3	T45.0X4	T45.0X5	T45.0X6
Methapyrilene	T45.0X1	T45.0X2	T45.0X3	T45.0X4	T45.0X5	T45.0X6
Methaqualone (compound)	T42.6X1	T42.6X2	T42.6X3	T42.6X4	T42.6X5	T42.6X6
Metharbital	T42.3X1	T42.3X2	T42.3X3	T42.3X4	T42.3X5	T42.3X6
Methazolamide	T50.2X1	T50.2X2	T50.2X3	T50.2X4	T50.2X5	T50.2X6
Methdilazine	T43.3X1	T43.3X2	T43.3X3	T43.3X4	T43.3X5	T43.3X6
Methedrine	T43.621	T43.622	T43.623	T43.624	T43.625	T43.626
Methenamine (mandelate)	T37.8X1	T37.8X2	T37.8X3	T37.8X4	T37.8X5	T37.8X6
Methenolone	T38.7X1	T38.7X2	T38.7X3	T38.7X4	T38.7X5	T38.7X6
Methergine	T48.0X1	T48.0X2	T48.0X3	T48.0X4	T48.0X5	T48.0X6
Methetoin	T42.0X1	T42.0X2	T42.0X3	T42.0X4	T42.0X5	T42.0X6
Methiacil	T38.2X1	T38.2X2	T38.2X3	T38.2X4	T38.2X5	T38.2X6

Substance	Poisoning, Accidental (unintentional)	Poisoning, Intentional Self-harm	Poisoning, Assault	Poisoning, Undetermined	Adverse effect	Underdosing
Methicillin	T36.0X1	T36.0X2	T36.0X3	T36.0X4	T36.0X5	T36.0X6
Methimazole	T38.2X1	T38.2X2	T38.2X3	T38.2X4	T38.2X5	T38.2X6
Methiodal sodium	T50.8X1	T50.8X2	T50.8X3	T50.8X4	T50.8X5	T50.8X6
Methionine	T50.991	T50.992	T50.993	T50.994	T50.995	T50.996
Methisazone	T37.5X1	T37.5X2	T37.5X3	T37.5X4	T37.5X5	T37.5X6
Methisoprinol	T37.5X1	T37.5X2	T37.5X3	T37.5X4	T37.5X5	T37.5X6
Methitural	T42.3X1	T42.3X2	T42.3X3	T42.3X4	T42.3X5	T42.3X6
Methixene	T44.3X1	T44.3X2	T44.3X3	T44.3X4	T44.3X5	T44.3X6
Methobarbital, methobarbitone	T42.3X1	T42.3X2	T42.3X3	T42.3X4	T42.3X5	T42.3X6
Methocarbamol	T42.8X1	T42.8X2	T42.8X3	T42.8X4	T42.8X5	T42.8X6
- skeletal muscle relaxant	T48.1X1	T48.1X2	T48.1X3	T48.1X4	T48.1X5	T48.1X6
Methohexital	T41.1X1	T41.1X2	T41.1X3	T41.1X4	T41.1X5	T41.1X6
Methohexitone	T41.1X1	T41.1X2	T41.1X3	T41.1X4	T41.1X5	T41.1X6
Methoin	T42.0X1	T42.0X2	T42.0X3	T42.0X4	T42.0X5	T42.0X6
Methopholine	T39.8X1	T39.8X2	T39.8X3	T39.8X4	T39.8X5	T39.8X6
Methopromazine	T43.3X1	T43.3X2	T43.3X3	T43.3X4	T43.3X5	T43.3X6
Methorate	T48.3X1	T48.3X2	T48.3X3	T48.3X4	T48.3X5	T48.3X6
Methoserpidine	T46.5X1	T46.5X2	T46.5X3	T46.5X4	T46.5X5	T46.5X6
Methotrexate	T45.1X1	T45.1X2	T45.1X3	T45.1X4	T45.1X5	T45.1X6
Methotrimeprazine	T43.3X1	T43.3X2	T43.3X3	T43.3X4	T43.3X5	T43.3X6
Methoxa-Dome	T49.3X1	T49.3X2	T49.3X3	T49.3X4	T49.3X5	T49.3X6
Methoxamine	T44.4X1	T44.4X2	T44.4X3	T44.4X4	T44.4X5	T44.4X6
Methoxsalen	T50.991	T50.992	T50.993	T50.994	T50.995	T50.996
Methoxyaniline	T65.3X1	T65.3X2	T65.3X3	T65.3X4	--	--
Methoxybenzyl penicillin	T36.0X1	T36.0X2	T36.0X3	T36.0X4	T36.0X5	T36.0X6
Methoxychlor	T53.7X1	T53.7X2	T53.7X3	T53.7X4	--	--
Methoxy-DDT	T53.7X1	T53.7X2	T53.7X3	T53.7X4	--	--
2-Methoxyethanol	T52.3X1	T52.3X2	T52.3X3	T52.3X4	--	--
Methoxyflurane	T41.0X1	T41.0X2	T41.0X3	T41.0X4	T41.0X5	T41.0X6
Methoxyphenamine	T48.6X1	T48.6X2	T48.6X3	T48.6X4	T48.6X5	T48.6X6
Methoxypromazine	T43.3X1	T43.3X2	T43.3X3	T43.3X4	T43.3X5	T43.3X6
5-Methoxypsoralen (5-MOP)	T50.991	T50.992	T50.993	T50.994	T50.995	T50.996
8-Methoxypsoralen (8-MOP)	T50.991	T50.992	T50.993	T50.994	T50.995	T50.996
Methscopolamine bromide	T44.3X1	T44.3X2	T44.3X3	T44.3X4	T44.3X5	T44.3X6
Methsuximide	T42.2X1	T42.2X2	T42.2X3	T42.2X4	T42.2X5	T42.2X6
Methyclothiazide	T50.2X1	T50.2X2	T50.2X3	T50.2X4	T50.2X5	T50.2X6
Methyl						
- acetate	T52.4X1	T52.4X2	T52.4X3	T52.4X4	--	--
- acetone	T52.4X1	T52.4X2	T52.4X3	T52.4X4	--	--
- acrylate	T65.891	T65.892	T65.893	T65.894	--	--
- alcohol	T51.1X1	T51.1X2	T51.1X3	T51.1X4	--	--
- aminophenol	T65.3X1	T65.3X2	T65.3X3	T65.3X4	--	--
- amphetamine	T43.621	T43.622	T43.623	T43.624	T43.625	T43.626
- androstanolone	T38.7X1	T38.7X2	T38.7X3	T38.7X4	T38.7X5	T38.7X6
- atropine	T44.3X1	T44.3X2	T44.3X3	T44.3X4	T44.3X5	T44.3X6
- benzene	T52.2X1	T52.2X2	T52.2X3	T52.2X4	--	--
- benzoate	T52.8X1	T52.8X2	T52.8X3	T52.8X4	--	--
- benzol	T52.2X1	T52.2X2	T52.2X3	T52.2X4	--	--
- bromide (gas)	T59.891	T59.892	T59.893	T59.894	--	--
- - fumigant	T60.8X1	T60.8X2	T60.8X3	T60.8X4	--	--
- butanol	T51.3X1	T51.3X2	T51.3X3	T51.3X4	--	--
- carbinol	T51.1X1	T51.1X2	T51.1X3	T51.1X4	--	--
- carbonate	T52.8X1	T52.8X2	T52.8X3	T52.8X4	--	--
- CCNU	T45.1X1	T45.1X2	T45.1X3	T45.1X4	T45.1X5	T45.1X6
- cellosolve	T52.91	T52.92	T52.93	T52.94	--	--
- cellulose	T47.4X1	T47.4X2	T47.4X3	T47.4X4	T47.4X5	T47.4X6
- chloride (gas)	T59.891	T59.892	T59.893	T59.894	--	--
- chloroformate	T59.3X1	T59.3X2	T59.3X3	T59.3X4	--	--
- cyclohexane	T52.8X1	T52.8X2	T52.8X3	T52.8X4	--	--

Substance	Poisoning, Accidental (unintentional)	Poisoning, Intentional Self-harm	Poisoning, Assault	Poisoning, Undetermined	Adverse effect	Underdosing
- cyclohexanol	T51.8X1	T51.8X2	T51.8X3	T51.8X4	--	--
- cyclohexanone	T52.8X1	T52.8X2	T52.8X3	T52.8X4	--	--
- cyclohexyl acetate	T52.8X1	T52.8X2	T52.8X3	T52.8X4	--	--
- demeton	T60.0X1	T60.0X2	T60.0X3	T60.0X4	--	--
- dihydromorphinone	T40.2X1	T40.2X2	T40.2X3	T40.2X4	T40.2X5	T40.2X6
- ergometrine	T48.0X1	T48.0X2	T48.0X3	T48.0X4	T48.0X5	T48.0X6
- ergonovine	T48.0X1	T48.0X2	T48.0X3	T48.0X4	T48.0X5	T48.0X6
- ethyl ketone	T52.4X1	T52.4X2	T52.4X3	T52.4X4	--	--
- glucamine antimonate	T37.8X1	T37.8X2	T37.8X3	T37.8X4	T37.8X5	T37.8X6
- hydrazine	T65.891	T65.892	T65.893	T65.894	--	--
- iodide	T65.891	T65.892	T65.893	T65.894	--	--
- isobutyl ketone	T52.4X1	T52.4X2	T52.4X3	T52.4X4	--	--
- isothiocyanate	T60.3X1	T60.3X2	T60.3X3	T60.3X4	--	--
- mercaptan	T59.891	T59.892	T59.893	T59.894	--	--
- morphine NEC	T40.2X1	T40.2X2	T40.2X3	T40.2X4	T40.2X5	T40.2X6
- nicotinate	T49.4X1	T49.4X2	T49.4X3	T49.4X4	T49.4X5	T49.4X6
- paraben	T49.0X1	T49.0X2	T49.0X3	T49.0X4	T49.0X5	T49.0X6
- parafynol	T42.6X1	T42.6X2	T42.6X3	T42.6X4	T42.6X5	T42.6X6
- parathion	T60.0X1	T60.0X2	T60.0X3	T60.0X4	--	--
- peridol	T43.4X1	T43.4X2	T43.4X3	T43.4X4	T43.4X5	T43.4X6
- phenidate	T43.631	T43.632	T43.633	T43.634	T43.635	T43.636
- prednisolone	T38.0X1	T38.0X2	T38.0X3	T38.0X4	T38.0X5	T38.0X6
- - ENT agent	T49.6X1	T49.6X2	T49.6X3	T49.6X4	T49.6X5	T49.6X6
- - ophthalmic preparation	T49.5X1	T49.5X2	T49.5X3	T49.5X4	T49.5X5	T49.5X6
- - topical NEC	T49.0X1	T49.0X2	T49.0X3	T49.0X4	T49.0X5	T49.0X6
- propylcarbinol	T51.3X1	T51.3X2	T51.3X3	T51.3X4	--	--
- rosaniline NEC	T49.0X1	T49.0X2	T49.0X3	T49.0X4	T49.0X5	T49.0X6
- salicylate	T49.2X1	T49.2X2	T49.2X3	T49.2X4	T49.2X5	T49.2X6
- sulfate (fumes)	T59.891	T59.892	T59.893	T59.894	--	--
- - liquid	T52.8X1	T52.8X2	T52.8X3	T52.8X4	--	--
- sulfonal	T42.6X1	T42.6X2	T42.6X3	T42.6X4	T42.6X5	T42.6X6
- testosterone	T38.7X1	T38.7X2	T38.7X3	T38.7X4	T38.7X5	T38.7X6
- thiouracil	T38.2X1	T38.2X2	T38.2X3	T38.2X4	T38.2X5	T38.2X6
Methylamphetamine	T43.621	T43.622	T43.623	T43.624	T43.625	T43.626
Methylated spirit	T51.1X1	T51.1X2	T51.1X3	T51.1X4	--	--
Methylatropine nitrate	T44.3X1	T44.3X2	T44.3X3	T44.3X4	T44.3X5	T44.3X6
Methylbenactyzium bromide	T44.3X1	T44.3X2	T44.3X3	T44.3X4	T44.3X5	T44.3X6
Methylbenzethonium chloride	T49.0X1	T49.0X2	T49.0X3	T49.0X4	T49.0X5	T49.0X6
Methylcellulose	T47.4X1	T47.4X2	T47.4X3	T47.4X4	T47.4X5	T47.4X6
- laxative	T47.4X1	T47.4X2	T47.4X3	T47.4X4	T47.4X5	T47.4X6
Methylchlorophenoxy-acetic acid	T60.3X1	T60.3X2	T60.3X3	T60.3X4	--	--
Methyldopa	T46.5X1	T46.5X2	T46.5X3	T46.5X4	T46.5X5	T46.5X6
Methyldopate	T46.5X1	T46.5X2	T46.5X3	T46.5X4	T46.5X5	T46.5X6
Methylene						
- blue	T50.6X1	T50.6X2	T50.6X3	T50.6X4	T50.6X5	T50.6X6
- chloride or dichloride (solvent) NEC	T53.4X1	T53.4X2	T53.4X3	T53.4X4	--	--
Methylenedioxyamphetamine	T43.621	T43.622	T43.623	T43.624	T43.625	T43.626
Methylenedioxymethamphetamine	T43.641	T43.642	T43.643	T43.644	T43.645	T43.646
Methylergometrine	T48.0X1	T48.0X2	T48.0X3	T48.0X4	T48.0X5	T48.0X6
Methylergonovine	T48.0X1	T48.0X2	T48.0X3	T48.0X4	T48.0X5	T48.0X6
Methylestrenolone	T38.5X1	T38.5X2	T38.5X3	T38.5X4	T38.5X5	T38.5X6
Methylethyl cellulose	T50.991	T50.992	T50.993	T50.994	T50.995	T50.996
Methylhexabital	T42.3X1	T42.3X2	T42.3X3	T42.3X4	T42.3X5	T42.3X6
Methylmorphine	T40.2X1	T40.2X2	T40.2X3	T40.2X4	T40.2X5	T40.2X6
Methylparaben (ophthalmic)	T49.5X1	T49.5X2	T49.5X3	T49.5X4	T49.5X5	T49.5X6
Methylparafynol	T42.6X1	T42.6X2	T42.6X3	T42.6X4	T42.6X5	T42.6X6
Methylpentynol, methylpentynol	T42.6X1	T42.6X2	T42.6X3	T42.6X4	T42.6X5	T42.6X6
Methylphenidate	T43.631	T43.632	T43.633	T43.634	T43.635	T43.636

Substance	Poisoning, Accidental (unintentional)	Poisoning, Intentional Self-harm	Poisoning, Assault	Poisoning, Undetermined	Adverse effect	Underdosing
Methylphenobarbital	T42.3X1	T42.3X2	T42.3X3	T42.3X4	T42.3X5	T42.3X6
Methylpolysiloxane	T47.1X1	T47.1X2	T47.1X3	T47.1X4	T47.1X5	T47.1X6
Methylprednisolone—see Methyl, prednisolone						
Methylrosaniline	T49.0X1	T49.0X2	T49.0X3	T49.0X4	T49.0X5	T49.0X6
Methylrosanilinium chloride	T49.0X1	T49.0X2	T49.0X3	T49.0X4	T49.0X5	T49.0X6
Methyltestosterone	T38.7X1	T38.7X2	T38.7X3	T38.7X4	T38.7X5	T38.7X6
Methylthionine chloride	T50.6X1	T50.6X2	T50.6X3	T50.6X4	T50.6X5	T50.6X6
Methylthioninium chloride	T50.6X1	T50.6X2	T50.6X3	T50.6X4	T50.6X5	T50.6X6
Methylthiouracil	T38.2X1	T38.2X2	T38.2X3	T38.2X4	T38.2X5	T38.2X6
Methyprylon	T42.6X1	T42.6X2	T42.6X3	T42.6X4	T42.6X5	T42.6X6
Methysergide	T46.5X1	T46.5X2	T46.5X3	T46.5X4	T46.5X5	T46.5X6
Metiamide	T47.1X1	T47.1X2	T47.1X3	T47.1X4	T47.1X5	T47.1X6
Meticillin	T36.0X1	T36.0X2	T36.0X3	T36.0X4	T36.0X5	T36.0X6
Meticrane	T50.2X1	T50.2X2	T50.2X3	T50.2X4	T50.2X5	T50.2X6
Metildigoxin	T46.0X1	T46.0X2	T46.0X3	T46.0X4	T46.0X5	T46.0X6
Metipranolol	T49.5X1	T49.5X2	T49.5X3	T49.5X4	T49.5X5	T49.5X6
Metirosine	T46.5X1	T46.5X2	T46.5X3	T46.5X4	T46.5X5	T46.5X6
Metisazone	T37.5X1	T37.5X2	T37.5X3	T37.5X4	T37.5X5	T37.5X6
Metixene	T44.3X1	T44.3X2	T44.3X3	T44.3X4	T44.3X5	T44.3X6
Metizoline	T48.5X1	T48.5X2	T48.5X3	T48.5X4	T48.5X5	T48.5X6
Metoclopramide	T45.0X1	T45.0X2	T45.0X3	T45.0X4	T45.0X5	T45.0X6
Metofenazate	T43.3X1	T43.3X2	T43.3X3	T43.3X4	T43.3X5	T43.3X6
Metofoline	T39.8X1	T39.8X2	T39.8X3	T39.8X4	T39.8X5	T39.8X6
Metolazone	T50.2X1	T50.2X2	T50.2X3	T50.2X4	T50.2X5	T50.2X6
Metopon	T40.2X1	T40.2X2	T40.2X3	T40.2X4	T40.2X5	T40.2X6
Metoprine	T45.1X1	T45.1X2	T45.1X3	T45.1X4	T45.1X5	T45.1X6
Metoprolol	T44.7X1	T44.7X2	T44.7X3	T44.7X4	T44.7X5	T44.7X6
Metrifonate	T60.0X1	T60.0X2	T60.0X3	T60.0X4	--	--
Metrizamide	T50.8X1	T50.8X2	T50.8X3	T50.8X4	T50.8X5	T50.8X6
Metrizoic acid	T50.8X1	T50.8X2	T50.8X3	T50.8X4	T50.8X5	T50.8X6
Metronidazole	T37.8X1	T37.8X2	T37.8X3	T37.8X4	T37.8X5	T37.8X6
Metycaine	T41.3X1	T41.3X2	T41.3X3	T41.3X4	T41.3X5	T41.3X6
- infiltration (subcutaneous)	T41.3X1	T41.3X2	T41.3X3	T41.3X4	T41.3X5	T41.3X6
- nerve block (peripheral) (plexus)	T41.3X1	T41.3X2	T41.3X3	T41.3X4	T41.3X5	T41.3X6
- topical (surface)	T41.3X1	T41.3X2	T41.3X3	T41.3X4	T41.3X5	T41.3X6
Metyrapone	T50.8X1	T50.8X2	T50.8X3	T50.8X4	T50.8X5	T50.8X6
Mevinphos	T60.0X1	T60.0X2	T60.0X3	T60.0X4	--	--
Mexazolam	T42.4X1	T42.4X2	T42.4X3	T42.4X4	T42.4X5	T42.4X6
Mexenone	T49.3X1	T49.3X2	T49.3X3	T49.3X4	T49.3X5	T49.3X6
Mexiletine	T46.2X1	T46.2X2	T46.2X3	T46.2X4	T46.2X5	T46.2X6
Mezereon	T62.2X1	T62.2X2	T62.2X3	T62.2X4	--	--
- berries	T62.1X1	T62.1X2	T62.1X3	T62.1X4	--	--
Mezlocillin	T36.0X1	T36.0X2	T36.0X3	T36.0X4	T36.0X5	T36.0X6
Mianserin	T43.021	T43.022	T43.023	T43.024	T43.025	T43.026
Micatin	T49.0X1	T49.0X2	T49.0X3	T49.0X4	T49.0X5	T49.0X6
Miconazole	T49.0X1	T49.0X2	T49.0X3	T49.0X4	T49.0X5	T49.0X6
Micronomicin	T36.5X1	T36.5X2	T36.5X3	T36.5X4	T36.5X5	T36.5X6
Midazolam	T42.4X1	T42.4X2	T42.4X3	T42.4X4	T42.4X5	T42.4X6
Midecamycin	T36.3X1	T36.3X2	T36.3X3	T36.3X4	T36.3X5	T36.3X6
Mifepristone	T38.6X1	T38.6X2	T38.6X3	T38.6X4	T38.6X5	T38.6X6
Milk of magnesia	T47.1X1	T47.1X2	T47.1X3	T47.1X4	T47.1X5	T47.1X6
Millipede (tropical) (venomous)	T63.411	T63.412	T63.413	T63.414	--	--
Miltown	T43.591	T43.592	T43.593	T43.594	T43.595	T43.596
Milverine	T44.3X1	T44.3X2	T44.3X3	T44.3X4	T44.3X5	T44.3X6
Minaprine	T43.291	T43.292	T43.293	T43.294	T43.295	T43.296
Minaxolone	T41.291	T41.292	T41.293	T41.294	T41.295	T41.296
Mineral						
- acids	T54.2X1	T54.2X2	T54.2X3	T54.2X4	--	--

Substance	Poisoning, Accidental (unintentional)	Poisoning, Intentional Self-harm	Poisoning, Assault	Poisoning, Undetermined	Adverse effect	Underdosing
- oil (laxative) (medicinal)	T47.4X1	T47.4X2	T47.4X3	T47.4X4	T47.4X5	T47.4X6
- - emulsion	T47.2X1	T47.2X2	T47.2X3	T47.2X4	T47.2X5	T47.2X6
- - nonmedicinal	T52.0X1	T52.0X2	T52.0X3	T52.0X4	--	--
- - topical	T49.3X1	T49.3X2	T49.3X3	T49.3X4	T49.3X5	T49.3X6
- salt NEC	T50.3X1	T50.3X2	T50.3X3	T50.3X4	T50.3X5	T50.3X6
- spirits	T52.0X1	T52.0X2	T52.0X3	T52.0X4	--	--
Mineralocorticosteroid	T50.0X1	T50.0X2	T50.0X3	T50.0X4	T50.0X5	T50.0X6
Minocycline	T36.4X1	T36.4X2	T36.4X3	T36.4X4	T36.4X5	T36.4X6
Minoxidil	T46.7X1	T46.7X2	T46.7X3	T46.7X4	T46.7X5	T46.7X6
Miokamycin	T36.3X1	T36.3X2	T36.3X3	T36.3X4	T36.3X5	T36.3X6
Miotic drug	T49.5X1	T49.5X2	T49.5X3	T49.5X4	T49.5X5	T49.5X6
Mipafox	T60.0X1	T60.0X2	T60.0X3	T60.0X4	--	--
Mirex	T60.1X1	T60.1X2	T60.1X3	T60.1X4	--	--
Mirtazapine	T43.021	T43.022	T43.023	T43.024	T43.025	T43.026
Misonidazole	T37.3X1	T37.3X2	T37.3X3	T37.3X4	T37.3X5	T37.3X6
Misoprostol	T47.1X1	T47.1X2	T47.1X3	T47.1X4	T47.1X5	T47.1X6
Mithramycin	T45.1X1	T45.1X2	T45.1X3	T45.1X4	T45.1X5	T45.1X6
Mitobronitol	T45.1X1	T45.1X2	T45.1X3	T45.1X4	T45.1X5	T45.1X6
Mitoguazone	T45.1X1	T45.1X2	T45.1X3	T45.1X4	T45.1X5	T45.1X6
Mitolactol	T45.1X1	T45.1X2	T45.1X3	T45.1X4	T45.1X5	T45.1X6
Mitomycin	T45.1X1	T45.1X2	T45.1X3	T45.1X4	T45.1X5	T45.1X6
Mitopodozide	T45.1X1	T45.1X2	T45.1X3	T45.1X4	T45.1X5	T45.1X6
Mitotane	T45.1X1	T45.1X2	T45.1X3	T45.1X4	T45.1X5	T45.1X6
Mitoxantrone	T45.1X1	T45.1X2	T45.1X3	T45.1X4	T45.1X5	T45.1X6
Mivacurium chloride	T48.1X1	T48.1X2	T48.1X3	T48.1X4	T48.1X5	T48.1X6
Miyari bacteria	T47.6X1	T47.6X2	T47.6X3	T47.6X4	T47.6X5	T47.6X6
Moclobemide	T43.1X1	T43.1X2	T43.1X3	T43.1X4	T43.1X5	T43.1X6
Moderil	T46.5X1	T46.5X2	T46.5X3	T46.5X4	T46.5X5	T46.5X6
Mofebutazone	T39.2X1	T39.2X2	T39.2X3	T39.2X4	T39.2X5	T39.2X6
Mogadon—see Nitrazepam						
Molindone	T43.591	T43.592	T43.593	T43.594	T43.595	T43.596
Molsidomine	T46.3X1	T46.3X2	T46.3X3	T46.3X4	T46.3X5	T46.3X6
Mometasone	T49.0X1	T49.0X2	T49.0X3	T49.0X4	T49.0X5	T49.0X6
Monistat	T49.0X1	T49.0X2	T49.0X3	T49.0X4	T49.0X5	T49.0X6
Monkshood	T62.2X1	T62.2X2	T62.2X3	T62.2X4	--	--
Monoamine oxidase inhibitor NEC	T43.1X1	T43.1X2	T43.1X3	T43.1X4	T43.1X5	T43.1X6
- hydrazine	T43.1X1	T43.1X2	T43.1X3	T43.1X4	T43.1X5	T43.1X6
Monobenzone	T49.4X1	T49.4X2	T49.4X3	T49.4X4	T49.4X5	T49.4X6
Monochloroacetic acid	T60.3X1	T60.3X2	T60.3X3	T60.3X4	--	--
Monochlorobenzene	T53.7X1	T53.7X2	T53.7X3	T53.7X4	--	--
Monoethanolamine	T46.8X1	T46.8X2	T46.8X3	T46.8X4	T46.8X5	T46.8X6
- oleate	T46.8X1	T46.8X2	T46.8X3	T46.8X4	T46.8X5	T46.8X6
Monooctanoin	T50.991	T50.992	T50.993	T50.994	T50.995	T50.996
Monophenylbutazone	T39.2X1	T39.2X2	T39.2X3	T39.2X4	T39.2X5	T39.2X6
Monosodium glutamate	T65.891	T65.892	T65.893	T65.894	--	--
Monosulfiram	T49.0X1	T49.0X2	T49.0X3	T49.0X4	T49.0X5	T49.0X6
Monoxide, carbon—see Carbon, monoxide						
Monoxidine hydrochloride	T46.1X1	T46.1X2	T46.1X3	T46.1X4	T46.1X5	T46.1X6
Monuron	T60.3X1	T60.3X2	T60.3X3	T60.3X4	--	--
Moperone	T43.4X1	T43.4X2	T43.4X3	T43.4X4	T43.4X5	T43.4X6
Mopidamol	T45.1X1	T45.1X2	T45.1X3	T45.1X4	T45.1X5	T45.1X6
MOPP (mechloreth-amine + vincristine + prednisone + procarbazine)	T45.1X1	T45.1X2	T45.1X3	T45.1X4	T45.1X5	T45.1X6
Morfin	T40.2X1	T40.2X2	T40.2X3	T40.2X4	T40.2X5	T40.2X6
Morinamide	T37.1X1	T37.1X2	T37.1X3	T37.1X4	T37.1X5	T37.1X6
Morning glory seeds	T40.991	T40.992	T40.993	T40.994	--	--
Moroxydine	T37.5X1	T37.5X2	T37.5X3	T37.5X4	T37.5X5	T37.5X6
Morphazinamide	T37.1X1	T37.1X2	T37.1X3	T37.1X4	T37.1X5	T37.1X6
Morphine	T40.2X1	T40.2X2	T40.2X3	T40.2X4	T40.2X5	T40.2X6

Substance	Poisoning, Accidental (unintentional)	Poisoning, Intentional Self-harm	Poisoning, Assault	Poisoning, Undetermined	Adverse effect	Underdosing
- antagonist	T50.7X1	T50.7X2	T50.7X3	T50.7X4	T50.7X5	T50.7X6
Morpholinylethylmorphine	T40.2X1	T40.2X2	T40.2X3	T40.2X4	--	--
Morsuximide	T42.2X1	T42.2X2	T42.2X3	T42.2X4	T42.2X5	T42.2X6
Mosapramine	T43.591	T43.592	T43.593	T43.594	T43.595	T43.596
Moth balls—see also Pesticides	T60.2X1	T60.2X2	T60.2X3	T60.2X4	--	--
- naphthalene	T60.2X1	T60.2X2	T60.2X3	T60.2X4	--	--
- paradichlorobenzene	T60.1X1	T60.1X2	T60.1X3	T60.1X4	--	--
Motor exhaust gas	T58.01	T58.02	T58.03	T58.04	--	--
Mouthwash (antiseptic) (zinc chloride)	T49.6X1	T49.6X2	T49.6X3	T49.6X4	T49.6X5	T49.6X6
Moxastine	T45.0X1	T45.0X2	T45.0X3	T45.0X4	T45.0X5	T45.0X6
Moxaverine	T44.3X1	T44.3X2	T44.3X3	T44.3X4	T44.3X5	T44.3X6
Moxisylyte	T46.7X1	T46.7X2	T46.7X3	T46.7X4	T46.7X5	T46.7X6
Mucilage, plant	T47.4X1	T47.4X2	T47.4X3	T47.4X4	T47.4X5	T47.4X6
Mucolytic drug	T48.4X1	T48.4X2	T48.4X3	T48.4X4	T48.4X5	T48.4X6
Mucomyst	T48.4X1	T48.4X2	T48.4X3	T48.4X4	T48.4X5	T48.4X6
Mucous membrane agents (external)	T49.91	T49.92	T49.93	T49.94	T49.95	T49.96
- specified NEC	T49.8X1	T49.8X2	T49.8X3	T49.8X4	T49.8X5	T49.8X6
Multiple unspecified drugs, medicaments and biological substances	T50.911	T50.912	T50.913	T50.914	T50.915	T50.916
Mumps						
- immune globulin (human)	T50.Z11	T50.Z12	T50.Z13	T50.Z14	T50.Z15	T50.Z16
- skin test antigen	T50.8X1	T50.8X2	T50.8X3	T50.8X4	T50.8X5	T50.8X6
- vaccine	T50.B91	T50.B92	T50.B93	T50.B94	T50.B95	T50.B96
Mumpsvax	T50.B91	T50.B92	T50.B93	T50.B94	T50.B95	T50.B96
Mupirocin	T49.0X1	T49.0X2	T49.0X3	T49.0X4	T49.0X5	T49.0X6
Muriatic acid—see Hydrochloric acid						
Muromonab-CD3	T45.1X1	T45.1X2	T45.1X3	T45.1X4	T45.1X5	T45.1X6
Muscle-action drug NEC	T48.201	T48.202	T48.203	T48.204	T48.205	T48.206
Muscle affecting agents NEC	T48.201	T48.202	T48.203	T48.204	T48.205	T48.206
- oxytocic	T48.0X1	T48.0X2	T48.0X3	T48.0X4	T48.0X5	T48.0X6
- relaxants	T48.201	T48.202	T48.203	T48.204	T48.205	T48.206
- - central nervous system	T42.8X1	T42.8X2	T42.8X3	T42.8X4	T42.8X5	T42.8X6
- - skeletal	T48.1X1	T48.1X2	T48.1X3	T48.1X4	T48.1X5	T48.1X6
- - smooth	T44.3X1	T44.3X2	T44.3X3	T44.3X4	T44.3X5	T44.3X6
Muscle relaxant—see Relaxant, muscle						
Muscle-tone depressant, central NEC	T42.8X1	T42.8X2	T42.8X3	T42.8X4	T42.8X5	T42.8X6
- specified NEC	T42.8X1	T42.8X2	T42.8X3	T42.8X4	T42.8X5	T42.8X6
Mushroom, noxious	T62.0X1	T62.0X2	T62.0X3	T62.0X4	--	--
Mussel, noxious	T61.781	T61.782	T61.783	T61.784	--	--
Mustard (emetic)	T47.7X1	T47.7X2	T47.7X3	T47.7X4	T47.7X5	T47.7X6
- black	T47.7X1	T47.7X2	T47.7X3	T47.7X4	T47.7X5	T47.7X6
- gas, not in war	T59.91	T59.92	T59.93	T59.94	--	--
- nitrogen	T45.1X1	T45.1X2	T45.1X3	T45.1X4	T45.1X5	T45.1X6
Mustine	T45.1X1	T45.1X2	T45.1X3	T45.1X4	T45.1X5	T45.1X6
M-vac	T45.1X1	T45.1X2	T45.1X3	T45.1X4	T45.1X5	T45.1X6
Mycifradin	T36.5X1	T36.5X2	T36.5X3	T36.5X4	T36.5X5	T36.5X6
- topical	T49.0X1	T49.0X2	T49.0X3	T49.0X4	T49.0X5	T49.0X6
Mycitracin	T36.8X1	T36.8X2	T36.8X3	T36.8X4	T36.8X5	T36.8X6
- ophthalmic preparation	T49.5X1	T49.5X2	T49.5X3	T49.5X4	T49.5X5	T49.5X6
Mycostatin	T36.7X1	T36.7X2	T36.7X3	T36.7X4	T36.7X5	T36.7X6
- topical	T49.0X1	T49.0X2	T49.0X3	T49.0X4	T49.0X5	T49.0X6
Mycotoxins	T64.81	T64.82	T64.83	T64.84	--	--
- aflatoxin	T64.01	T64.02	T64.03	T64.04	--	--
- specified NEC	T64.81	T64.82	T64.83	T64.84	--	--
Mydriacyl	T44.3X1	T44.3X2	T44.3X3	T44.3X4	T44.3X5	T44.3X6
Mydriatic drug	T49.5X1	T49.5X2	T49.5X3	T49.5X4	T49.5X5	T49.5X6
Myelobromal	T45.1X1	T45.1X2	T45.1X3	T45.1X4	T45.1X5	T45.1X6
Myleran	T45.1X1	T45.1X2	T45.1X3	T45.1X4	T45.1X5	T45.1X6
Myochrysin (e)	T39.2X1	T39.2X2	T39.2X3	T39.2X4	T39.2X5	T39.2X6

Substance	Poisoning, Accidental (unintentional)	Poisoning, Intentional Self-harm	Poisoning, Assault	Poisoning, Undetermined	Adverse effect	Underdosing
Myoneural blocking agents	T48.1X1	T48.1X2	T48.1X3	T48.1X4	T48.1X5	T48.1X6
Myralact	T49.0X1	T49.0X2	T49.0X3	T49.0X4	T49.0X5	T49.0X6
Myristica fragrans	T62.2X1	T62.2X2	T62.2X3	T62.2X4	--	--
Myristicin	T65.891	T65.892	T65.893	T65.894	--	--
Mysoline	T42.3X1	T42.3X2	T42.3X3	T42.3X4	T42.3X5	T42.3X6
Nabilone	T40.711	T40.712	T40.713	T40.714	T40.715	T40.716
Nabumetone	T39.391	T39.392	T39.393	T39.394	T39.395	T39.396
Nadolol	T44.7X1	T44.7X2	T44.7X3	T44.7X4	T44.7X5	T44.7X6
Nafcillin	T36.0X1	T36.0X2	T36.0X3	T36.0X4	T36.0X5	T36.0X6
Nafoxidine	T38.6X1	T38.6X2	T38.6X3	T38.6X4	T38.6X5	T38.6X6
Naftazone	T46.991	T46.992	T46.993	T46.994	T46.995	T46.996
Naftidrofuryl (oxalate)	T46.7X1	T46.7X2	T46.7X3	T46.7X4	T46.7X5	T46.7X6
Naftifine	T49.0X1	T49.0X2	T49.0X3	T49.0X4	T49.0X5	T49.0X6
Nail polish remover	T52.91	T52.92	T52.93	T52.94	--	--
Nalbuphine	T40.491	T40.492	T40.493	T40.494	T40.495	T40.496
Naled	T60.0X1	T60.0X2	T60.0X3	T60.0X4	--	--
Nalidixic acid	T37.8X1	T37.8X2	T37.8X3	T37.8X4	T37.8X5	T37.8X6
Nalorphine	T50.7X1	T50.7X2	T50.7X3	T50.7X4	T50.7X5	T50.7X6
Naloxone	T50.7X1	T50.7X2	T50.7X3	T50.7X4	T50.7X5	T50.7X6
Naltrexone	T50.7X1	T50.7X2	T50.7X3	T50.7X4	T50.7X5	T50.7X6
Namenda	T43.8X1	T43.8X2	T43.8X3	T43.8X4	T43.8X5	T43.8X6
Nandrolone	T38.7X1	T38.7X2	T38.7X3	T38.7X4	T38.7X5	T38.7X6
Naphazoline	T48.5X1	T48.5X2	T48.5X3	T48.5X4	T48.5X5	T48.5X6
Naphtha (painters') (petroleum)	T52.0X1	T52.0X2	T52.0X3	T52.0X4	--	--
- solvent	T52.0X1	T52.0X2	T52.0X3	T52.0X4	--	--
- vapor	T52.0X1	T52.0X2	T52.0X3	T52.0X4	--	--
Naphthalene (non-chlorinated)	T60.2X1	T60.2X2	T60.2X3	T60.2X4	--	--
- chlorinated	T60.1X1	T60.1X2	T60.1X3	T60.1X4	--	--
- - vapor	T60.1X1	T60.1X2	T60.1X3	T60.1X4	--	--
- insecticide or moth repellent	T60.2X1	T60.2X2	T60.2X3	T60.2X4	--	--
- - chlorinated	T60.1X1	T60.1X2	T60.1X3	T60.1X4	--	--
- vapor	T60.2X1	T60.2X2	T60.2X3	T60.2X4	--	--
- - chlorinated	T60.1X1	T60.1X2	T60.1X3	T60.1X4	--	--
Naphthol	T65.891	T65.892	T65.893	T65.894	--	--
Naphthylamine	T65.891	T65.892	T65.893	T65.894	--	--
Naphthylthiourea (ANTU)	T60.4X1	T60.4X2	T60.4X3	T60.4X4	--	--
Naprosyn—see Naproxen						
Naproxen	T39.311	T39.312	T39.313	T39.314	T39.315	T39.316
Narcotic (drug)	T40.601	T40.602	T40.603	T40.604	T40.605	T40.606
- analgesic NEC	T40.601	T40.602	T40.603	T40.604	T40.605	T40.606
- antagonist	T50.7X1	T50.7X2	T50.7X3	T50.7X4	T50.7X5	T50.7X6
- specified NEC	T40.691	T40.692	T40.693	T40.694	T40.695	T40.696
- synthetic	T40.491	T40.492	T40.493	T40.494	T40.495	T40.496
Narcotine	T48.3X1	T48.3X2	T48.3X3	T48.3X4	T48.3X5	T48.3X6
Nardil	T43.1X1	T43.1X2	T43.1X3	T43.1X4	T43.1X5	T43.1X6
Nasal drug NEC	T49.6X1	T49.6X2	T49.6X3	T49.6X4	T49.6X5	T49.6X6
Natamycin	T49.0X1	T49.0X2	T49.0X3	T49.0X4	T49.0X5	T49.0X6
Natrium cyanide—see Cyanide (s)						
Natural						
- blood (product)	T45.8X1	T45.8X2	T45.8X3	T45.8X4	T45.8X5	T45.8X6
- gas (piped)	T59.891	T59.892	T59.893	T59.894	--	--
- - incomplete combustion	T58.11	T58.12	T58.13	T58.14	--	--
Nealbarbital	T42.3X1	T42.3X2	T42.3X3	T42.3X4	T42.3X5	T42.3X6
Nectadon	T48.3X1	T48.3X2	T48.3X3	T48.3X4	T48.3X5	T48.3X6
Nedocromil	T48.6X1	T48.6X2	T48.6X3	T48.6X4	T48.6X5	T48.6X6
Nefopam	T39.8X1	T39.8X2	T39.8X3	T39.8X4	T39.8X5	T39.8X6
Nematocyst (sting)	T63.691	T63.692	T63.693	T63.694	--	--
Nembutal	T42.3X1	T42.3X2	T42.3X3	T42.3X4	T42.3X5	T42.3X6

Substance	Poisoning, Accidental (unintentional)	Poisoning, Intentional Self-harm	Poisoning, Assault	Poisoning, Undetermined	Adverse effect	Underdosing
Nemonapride	T43.591	T43.592	T43.593	T43.594	T43.595	T43.596
Neoarsphenamine	T37.8X1	T37.8X2	T37.8X3	T37.8X4	T37.8X5	T37.8X6
Neocinchophen	T50.4X1	T50.4X2	T50.4X3	T50.4X4	T50.4X5	T50.4X6
Neomycin (derivatives)	T36.5X1	T36.5X2	T36.5X3	T36.5X4	T36.5X5	T36.5X6
- with						
- - bacitracin	T49.0X1	T49.0X2	T49.0X3	T49.0X4	T49.0X5	T49.0X6
- - neostigmine	T44.0X1	T44.0X2	T44.0X3	T44.0X4	T44.0X5	T44.0X6
- ENT agent	T49.6X1	T49.6X2	T49.6X3	T49.6X4	T49.6X5	T49.6X6
- ophthalmic preparation	T49.5X1	T49.5X2	T49.5X3	T49.5X4	T49.5X5	T49.5X6
- topical NEC	T49.0X1	T49.0X2	T49.0X3	T49.0X4	T49.0X5	T49.0X6
Neonal	T42.3X1	T42.3X2	T42.3X3	T42.3X4	T42.3X5	T42.3X6
Neoprontosil	T37.0X1	T37.0X2	T37.0X3	T37.0X4	T37.0X5	T37.0X6
Neosalvarsan	T37.8X1	T37.8X2	T37.8X3	T37.8X4	T37.8X5	T37.8X6
Neosilversalvarsan	T37.8X1	T37.8X2	T37.8X3	T37.8X4	T37.8X5	T37.8X6
Neosporin	T36.8X1	T36.8X2	T36.8X3	T36.8X4	T36.8X5	T36.8X6
- ENT agent	T49.6X1	T49.6X2	T49.6X3	T49.6X4	T49.6X5	T49.6X6
- ophthalmic preparation	T49.5X1	T49.5X2	T49.5X3	T49.5X4	T49.5X5	T49.5X6
- topical NEC	T49.0X1	T49.0X2	T49.0X3	T49.0X4	T49.0X5	T49.0X6
Neostigmine bromide	T44.0X1	T44.0X2	T44.0X3	T44.0X4	T44.0X5	T44.0X6
Neraval	T42.3X1	T42.3X2	T42.3X3	T42.3X4	T42.3X5	T42.3X6
Neravan	T42.3X1	T42.3X2	T42.3X3	T42.3X4	T42.3X5	T42.3X6
Nerium oleander	T62.2X1	T62.2X2	T62.2X3	T62.2X4	--	--
Nerve gas, not in war	T59.91	T59.92	T59.93	T59.94	--	--
Nesacaine	T41.3X1	T41.3X2	T41.3X3	T41.3X4	T41.3X5	T41.3X6
- infiltration (subcutaneous)	T41.3X1	T41.3X2	T41.3X3	T41.3X4	T41.3X5	T41.3X6
- nerve block (peripheral) (plexus)	T41.3X1	T41.3X2	T41.3X3	T41.3X4	T41.3X5	T41.3X6
Netilmicin	T36.5X1	T36.5X2	T36.5X3	T36.5X4	T36.5X5	T36.5X6
Neurobarb	T42.3X1	T42.3X2	T42.3X3	T42.3X4	T42.3X5	T42.3X6
Neuroleptic drug NEC	T43.501	T43.502	T43.503	T43.504	T43.505	T43.506
Neuromuscular blocking drug	T48.1X1	T48.1X2	T48.1X3	T48.1X4	T48.1X5	T48.1X6
Neutral insulin injection	T38.3X1	T38.3X2	T38.3X3	T38.3X4	T38.3X5	T38.3X6
Neutral spirits	T51.0X1	T51.0X2	T51.0X3	T51.0X4	--	--
- beverage	T51.0X1	T51.0X2	T51.0X3	T51.0X4	--	--
Niacin	T46.7X1	T46.7X2	T46.7X3	T46.7X4	T46.7X5	T46.7X6
Niacinamide	T45.2X1	T45.2X2	T45.2X3	T45.2X4	T45.2X5	T45.2X6
Nialamide	T43.1X1	T43.1X2	T43.1X3	T43.1X4	T43.1X5	T43.1X6
Niaprazine	T42.6X1	T42.6X2	T42.6X3	T42.6X4	T42.6X5	T42.6X6
Nicametate	T46.7X1	T46.7X2	T46.7X3	T46.7X4	T46.7X5	T46.7X6
Nicardipine	T46.1X1	T46.1X2	T46.1X3	T46.1X4	T46.1X5	T46.1X6
Nicergoline	T46.7X1	T46.7X2	T46.7X3	T46.7X4	T46.7X5	T46.7X6
Nickel (carbonyl) (tetra-carbonyl) (fumes) (vapor)	T56.891	T56.892	T56.893	T56.894	--	--
Nickelocene	T56.891	T56.892	T56.893	T56.894	--	--
Niclosamide	T37.4X1	T37.4X2	T37.4X3	T37.4X4	T37.4X5	T37.4X6
Nicofuranose	T46.7X1	T46.7X2	T46.7X3	T46.7X4	T46.7X5	T46.7X6
Nicomorphine	T40.2X1	T40.2X2	T40.2X3	T40.2X4	--	--
Nicorandil	T46.3X1	T46.3X2	T46.3X3	T46.3X4	T46.3X5	T46.3X6
Nicotiana (plant)	T62.2X1	T62.2X2	T62.2X3	T62.2X4	--	--
Nicotinamide	T45.2X1	T45.2X2	T45.2X3	T45.2X4	T45.2X5	T45.2X6
Nicotine (insecticide) (spray) (sulfate) NEC	T60.2X1	T60.2X2	T60.2X3	T60.2X4	--	--
- from tobacco	T65.291	T65.292	T65.293	T65.294	--	--
- - cigarettes	T65.221	T65.222	T65.223	T65.224	--	--
- not insecticide	T65.291	T65.292	T65.293	T65.294	--	--
Nicotinic acid	T46.7X1	T46.7X2	T46.7X3	T46.7X4	T46.7X5	T46.7X6
Nicotinyl alcohol	T46.7X1	T46.7X2	T46.7X3	T46.7X4	T46.7X5	T46.7X6
Nicoumalone	T45.511	T45.512	T45.513	T45.514	T45.515	T45.516
Nifedipine	T46.1X1	T46.1X2	T46.1X3	T46.1X4	T46.1X5	T46.1X6
Nifenazone	T39.2X1	T39.2X2	T39.2X3	T39.2X4	T39.2X5	T39.2X6
Nifuraldezone	T37.91	T37.92	T37.93	T37.94	T37.95	T37.96

Substance	Poisoning, Accidental (unintentional)	Poisoning, Intentional Self-harm	Poisoning, Assault	Poisoning, Undetermined	Adverse effect	Underdosing
Nifuratel	T37.8X1	T37.8X2	T37.8X3	T37.8X4	T37.8X5	T37.8X6
Nifurtimox	T37.3X1	T37.3X2	T37.3X3	T37.3X4	T37.3X5	T37.3X6
Nifurtoinol	T37.8X1	T37.8X2	T37.8X3	T37.8X4	T37.8X5	T37.8X6
Nightshade, deadly (solanum) —see also Belladonna	T62.2X1	T62.2X2	T62.2X3	T62.2X4	--	--
- berry	T62.1X1	T62.1X2	T62.1X3	T62.1X4	--	--
Nikethamide	T50.7X1	T50.7X2	T50.7X3	T50.7X4	T50.7X5	T50.7X6
Nilstat	T36.7X1	T36.7X2	T36.7X3	T36.7X4	T36.7X5	T36.7X6
- topical	T49.0X1	T49.0X2	T49.0X3	T49.0X4	T49.0X5	T49.0X6
Nilutamide	T38.6X1	T38.6X2	T38.6X3	T38.6X4	T38.6X5	T38.6X6
Nimesulide	T39.391	T39.392	T39.393	T39.394	T39.395	T39.396
Nimetazepam	T42.4X1	T42.4X2	T42.4X3	T42.4X4	T42.4X5	T42.4X6
Nimodipine	T46.1X1	T46.1X2	T46.1X3	T46.1X4	T46.1X5	T46.1X6
Nimorazole	T37.3X1	T37.3X2	T37.3X3	T37.3X4	T37.3X5	T37.3X6
Nimustine	T45.1X1	T45.1X2	T45.1X3	T45.1X4	T45.1X5	T45.1X6
Niridazole	T37.4X1	T37.4X2	T37.4X3	T37.4X4	T37.4X5	T37.4X6
Nisentil	T40.2X1	T40.2X2	T40.2X3	T40.2X4	T40.2X5	T40.2X6
Nisoldipine	T46.1X1	T46.1X2	T46.1X3	T46.1X4	T46.1X5	T46.1X6
Nitramine	T65.3X1	T65.3X2	T65.3X3	T65.3X4	--	--
Nitrate, organic	T46.3X1	T46.3X2	T46.3X3	T46.3X4	T46.3X5	T46.3X6
Nitrazepam	T42.4X1	T42.4X2	T42.4X3	T42.4X4	T42.4X5	T42.4X6
Nitrefazole	T50.6X1	T50.6X2	T50.6X3	T50.6X4	T50.6X5	T50.6X6
Nitrendipine	T46.1X1	T46.1X2	T46.1X3	T46.1X4	T46.1X5	T46.1X6
Nitric						
- acid (liquid)	T54.2X1	T54.2X2	T54.2X3	T54.2X4	--	--
- - vapor	T59.891	T59.892	T59.893	T59.894	--	--
- oxide (gas)	T59.0X1	T59.0X2	T59.0X3	T59.0X4	--	--
Nitrimidazine	T37.3X1	T37.3X2	T37.3X3	T37.3X4	T37.3X5	T37.3X6
Nitrite, amyl (medicinal) (vapor)	T46.3X1	T46.3X2	T46.3X3	T46.3X4	T46.3X5	T46.3X6
Nitroaniline	T65.3X1	T65.3X2	T65.3X3	T65.3X4	--	--
- vapor	T59.891	T59.892	T59.893	T59.894	--	--
Nitrobenzene, nitrobenzol	T65.3X1	T65.3X2	T65.3X3	T65.3X4	--	--
- vapor	T65.3X1	T65.3X2	T65.3X3	T65.3X4	--	--
Nitrocellulose	T65.891	T65.892	T65.893	T65.894	--	--
- lacquer	T65.891	T65.892	T65.893	T65.894	--	--
Nitrodiphenyl	T65.3X1	T65.3X2	T65.3X3	T65.3X4	--	--
Nitrofural	T49.0X1	T49.0X2	T49.0X3	T49.0X4	T49.0X5	T49.0X6
Nitrofurantoin	T37.8X1	T37.8X2	T37.8X3	T37.8X4	T37.8X5	T37.8X6
Nitrofurazone	T49.0X1	T49.0X2	T49.0X3	T49.0X4	T49.0X5	T49.0X6
Nitrogen	T59.0X1	T59.0X2	T59.0X3	T59.0X4	--	--
- mustard	T45.1X1	T45.1X2	T45.1X3	T45.1X4	T45.1X5	T45.1X6
Nitroglycerin, nitro-glycerol (medicinal)	T46.3X1	T46.3X2	T46.3X3	T46.3X4	T46.3X5	T46.3X6
- nonmedicinal	T65.5X1	T65.5X2	T65.5X3	T65.5X4	--	--
- - fumes	T65.5X1	T65.5X2	T65.5X3	T65.5X4	--	--
Nitroglycol	T52.3X1	T52.3X2	T52.3X3	T52.3X4	--	--
Nitrohydrochloric acid	T54.2X1	T54.2X2	T54.2X3	T54.2X4	--	--
Nitromersol	T49.0X1	T49.0X2	T49.0X3	T49.0X4	T49.0X5	T49.0X6
Nitronaphthalene	T65.891	T65.892	T65.893	T65.894	--	--
Nitrophenol	T54.0X1	T54.0X2	T54.0X3	T54.0X4	--	--
Nitropropane	T52.8X1	T52.8X2	T52.8X3	T52.8X4	--	--
Nitroprusside	T46.5X1	T46.5X2	T46.5X3	T46.5X4	T46.5X5	T46.5X6
Nitrosodimethylamine	T65.3X1	T65.3X2	T65.3X3	T65.3X4	--	--
Nitrothiazol	T37.4X1	T37.4X2	T37.4X3	T37.4X4	T37.4X5	T37.4X6
Nitrotoluene, nitrotoluol	T65.3X1	T65.3X2	T65.3X3	T65.3X4	--	--
- vapor	T65.3X1	T65.3X2	T65.3X3	T65.3X4	--	--
Nitrous						
- acid (liquid)	T54.2X1	T54.2X2	T54.2X3	T54.2X4	--	--
- - fumes	T59.891	T59.892	T59.893	T59.894	--	--
- ether spirit	T46.3X1	T46.3X2	T46.3X3	T46.3X4	T46.3X5	T46.3X6

Substance	Poisoning, Accidental (unintentional)	Poisoning, Intentional Self-harm	Poisoning, Assault	Poisoning, Undetermined	Adverse effect	Underdosing
- oxide	T41.0X1	T41.0X2	T41.0X3	T41.0X4	T41.0X5	T41.0X6
Nitroxoline	T37.8X1	T37.8X2	T37.8X3	T37.8X4	T37.8X5	T37.8X6
Nitrozone	T49.0X1	T49.0X2	T49.0X3	T49.0X4	T49.0X5	T49.0X6
Nizatidine	T47.0X1	T47.0X2	T47.0X3	T47.0X4	T47.0X5	T47.0X6
Nizofenone	T43.8X1	T43.8X2	T43.8X3	T43.8X4	T43.8X5	T43.8X6
Noctec	T42.6X1	T42.6X2	T42.6X3	T42.6X4	T42.6X5	T42.6X6
Noludar	T42.6X1	T42.6X2	T42.6X3	T42.6X4	T42.6X5	T42.6X6
Nomegestrol	T38.5X1	T38.5X2	T38.5X3	T38.5X4	T38.5X5	T38.5X6
Nomifensine	T43.291	T43.292	T43.293	T43.294	T43.295	T43.296
Nonoxinol	T49.8X1	T49.8X2	T49.8X3	T49.8X4	T49.8X5	T49.8X6
Nonylphenoxy (polyethoxy-ethanol)	T49.8X1	T49.8X2	T49.8X3	T49.8X4	T49.8X5	T49.8X6
Noptil	T42.3X1	T42.3X2	T42.3X3	T42.3X4	T42.3X5	T42.3X6
Noradrenaline	T44.4X1	T44.4X2	T44.4X3	T44.4X4	T44.4X5	T44.4X6
Noramidopyrine	T39.2X1	T39.2X2	T39.2X3	T39.2X4	T39.2X5	T39.2X6
- methanesulfonate sodium	T39.2X1	T39.2X2	T39.2X3	T39.2X4	T39.2X5	T39.2X6
Norbormide	T60.4X1	T60.4X2	T60.4X3	T60.4X4	--	--
Nordazepam	T42.4X1	T42.4X2	T42.4X3	T42.4X4	T42.4X5	T42.4X6
Norepinephrine	T44.4X1	T44.4X2	T44.4X3	T44.4X4	T44.4X5	T44.4X6
Norethandrolone	T38.7X1	T38.7X2	T38.7X3	T38.7X4	T38.7X5	T38.7X6
Norethindrone	T38.4X1	T38.4X2	T38.4X3	T38.4X4	T38.4X5	T38.4X6
Norethisterone (acetate) (enantate)	T38.4X1	T38.4X2	T38.4X3	T38.4X4	T38.4X5	T38.4X6
- with ethinylestradiol	T38.5X1	T38.5X2	T38.5X3	T38.5X4	T38.5X5	T38.5X6
Noretynodrel	T38.5X1	T38.5X2	T38.5X3	T38.5X4	T38.5X5	T38.5X6
Norfenefrine	T44.4X1	T44.4X2	T44.4X3	T44.4X4	T44.4X5	T44.4X6
Norfloxacin	T36.8X1	T36.8X2	T36.8X3	T36.8X4	T36.8X5	T36.8X6
Norgestrel	T38.4X1	T38.4X2	T38.4X3	T38.4X4	T38.4X5	T38.4X6
Norgestrienone	T38.4X1	T38.4X2	T38.4X3	T38.4X4	T38.4X5	T38.4X6
Norlestrin	T38.4X1	T38.4X2	T38.4X3	T38.4X4	T38.4X5	T38.4X6
Norlutin	T38.4X1	T38.4X2	T38.4X3	T38.4X4	T38.4X5	T38.4X6
Normal serum albumin (human) , salt-poor	T45.8X1	T45.8X2	T45.8X3	T45.8X4	T45.8X5	T45.8X6
Normethandrone	T38.5X1	T38.5X2	T38.5X3	T38.5X4	T38.5X5	T38.5X6
Normison—see Benzodiazepines						
Normorphine	T40.2X1	T40.2X2	T40.2X3	T40.2X4	--	--
Norpseudoephedrine	T50.5X1	T50.5X2	T50.5X3	T50.5X4	T50.5X5	T50.5X6
Nortestosterone (furanpropionate)	T38.7X1	T38.7X2	T38.7X3	T38.7X4	T38.7X5	T38.7X6
Nortriptyline	T43.011	T43.012	T43.013	T43.014	T43.015	T43.016
Noscapine	T48.3X1	T48.3X2	T48.3X3	T48.3X4	T48.3X5	T48.3X6
Nose preparations	T49.6X1	T49.6X2	T49.6X3	T49.6X4	T49.6X5	T49.6X6
Novobiocin	T36.5X1	T36.5X2	T36.5X3	T36.5X4	T36.5X5	T36.5X6
Novocain (infiltration) (topical)	T41.3X1	T41.3X2	T41.3X3	T41.3X4	T41.3X5	T41.3X6
- nerve block (peripheral) (plexus)	T41.3X1	T41.3X2	T41.3X3	T41.3X4	T41.3X5	T41.3X6
- spinal	T41.3X1	T41.3X2	T41.3X3	T41.3X4	T41.3X5	T41.3X6
Noxious foodstuff	T62.91	T62.92	T62.93	T62.94	--	--
- specified NEC	T62.8X1	T62.8X2	T62.8X3	T62.8X4	--	--
Noxiptiline	T43.011	T43.012	T43.013	T43.014	T43.015	T43.016
Noxytiolin	T49.0X1	T49.0X2	T49.0X3	T49.0X4	T49.0X5	T49.0X6
NPH Iletin (insulin)	T38.3X1	T38.3X2	T38.3X3	T38.3X4	T38.3X5	T38.3X6
Numorphan	T40.2X1	T40.2X2	T40.2X3	T40.2X4	T40.2X5	T40.2X6
Nunol	T42.3X1	T42.3X2	T42.3X3	T42.3X4	T42.3X5	T42.3X6
Nupercaine (spinal anesthetic)	T41.3X1	T41.3X2	T41.3X3	T41.3X4	T41.3X5	T41.3X6
- topical (surface)	T41.3X1	T41.3X2	T41.3X3	T41.3X4	T41.3X5	T41.3X6
Nutmeg oil (liniment)	T49.3X1	T49.3X2	T49.3X3	T49.3X4	T49.3X5	T49.3X6
Nutritional supplement	T50.901	T50.902	T50.903	T50.904	T50.905	T50.906
Nux vomica	T65.1X1	T65.1X2	T65.1X3	T65.1X4	--	--
Nydrazid	T37.1X1	T37.1X2	T37.1X3	T37.1X4	T37.1X5	T37.1X6
Nylidrin	T46.7X1	T46.7X2	T46.7X3	T46.7X4	T46.7X5	T46.7X6
Nystatin	T36.7X1	T36.7X2	T36.7X3	T36.7X4	T36.7X5	T36.7X6
- topical	T49.0X1	T49.0X2	T49.0X3	T49.0X4	T49.0X5	T49.0X6
Nytol	T45.0X1	T45.0X2	T45.0X3	T45.0X4	T45.0X5	T45.0X6

Substance	Poisoning, Accidental (unintentional)	Poisoning, Intentional Self-harm	Poisoning, Assault	Poisoning, Undetermined	Adverse effect	Underdosing
Obidoxime chloride	T50.6X1	T50.6X2	T50.6X3	T50.6X4	T50.6X5	T50.6X6
Octafonium (chloride)	T49.3X1	T49.3X2	T49.3X3	T49.3X4	T49.3X5	T49.3X6
Octamethyl pyrophos-phoramide	T60.0X1	T60.0X2	T60.0X3	T60.0X4	--	--
Octanoin	T50.991	T50.992	T50.993	T50.994	T50.995	T50.996
Octatropine methyl-bromide	T44.3X1	T44.3X2	T44.3X3	T44.3X4	T44.3X5	T44.3X6
Octotiamine	T45.2X1	T45.2X2	T45.2X3	T45.2X4	T45.2X5	T45.2X6
Octoxinol (9)	T49.8X1	T49.8X2	T49.8X3	T49.8X4	T49.8X5	T49.8X6
Octreotide	T38.991	T38.992	T38.993	T38.994	T38.995	T38.996
Octyl nitrite	T46.3X1	T46.3X2	T46.3X3	T46.3X4	T46.3X5	T46.3X6
Oestradiol	T38.5X1	T38.5X2	T38.5X3	T38.5X4	T38.5X5	T38.5X6
Oestriol	T38.5X1	T38.5X2	T38.5X3	T38.5X4	T38.5X5	T38.5X6
Oestrogen	T38.5X1	T38.5X2	T38.5X3	T38.5X4	T38.5X5	T38.5X6
Oestrone	T38.5X1	T38.5X2	T38.5X3	T38.5X4	T38.5X5	T38.5X6
Ofloxacin	T36.8X1	T36.8X2	T36.8X3	T36.8X4	T36.8X5	T36.8X6
Oil (of)	T65.891	T65.892	T65.893	T65.894	--	--
- bitter almond	T62.8X1	T62.8X2	T62.8X3	T62.8X4	--	--
- cloves	T49.7X1	T49.7X2	T49.7X3	T49.7X4	T49.7X5	T49.7X6
- colors	T65.6X1	T65.6X2	T65.6X3	T65.6X4	--	--
- fumes	T59.891	T59.892	T59.893	T59.894	--	--
- lubricating	T52.0X1	T52.0X2	T52.0X3	T52.0X4	--	--
- Niobe	T52.8X1	T52.8X2	T52.8X3	T52.8X4	--	--
- vitriol (liquid)	T54.2X1	T54.2X2	T54.2X3	T54.2X4	--	--
- - fumes	T54.2X1	T54.2X2	T54.2X3	T54.2X4	--	--
- wintergreen (bitter) NEC	T49.3X1	T49.3X2	T49.3X3	T49.3X4	T49.3X5	T49.3X6
Oily preparation (for skin)	T49.3X1	T49.3X2	T49.3X3	T49.3X4	T49.3X5	T49.3X6
Ointment NEC	T49.3X1	T49.3X2	T49.3X3	T49.3X4	T49.3X5	T49.3X6
Olanzapine	T43.591	T43.592	T43.593	T43.594	T43.595	T43.596
Oleander	T62.2X1	T62.2X2	T62.2X3	T62.2X4	--	--
Oleandomycin	T36.3X1	T36.3X2	T36.3X3	T36.3X4	T36.3X5	T36.3X6
Oleandrin	T46.0X1	T46.0X2	T46.0X3	T46.0X4	T46.0X5	T46.0X6
Oleic acid	T46.6X1	T46.6X2	T46.6X3	T46.6X4	T46.6X5	T46.6X6
Oleovitamin A	T45.2X1	T45.2X2	T45.2X3	T45.2X4	T45.2X5	T45.2X6
Oleum ricini	T47.2X1	T47.2X2	T47.2X3	T47.2X4	T47.2X5	T47.2X6
Olive oil (medicinal) NEC	T47.4X1	T47.4X2	T47.4X3	T47.4X4	T47.4X5	T47.4X6
Olivomycin	T45.1X1	T45.1X2	T45.1X3	T45.1X4	T45.1X5	T45.1X6
Olsalazine	T47.8X1	T47.8X2	T47.8X3	T47.8X4	T47.8X5	T47.8X6
Omeprazole	T47.1X1	T47.1X2	T47.1X3	T47.1X4	T47.1X5	T47.1X6
OMPA	T60.0X1	T60.0X2	T60.0X3	T60.0X4	--	--
Oncovin	T45.1X1	T45.1X2	T45.1X3	T45.1X4	T45.1X5	T45.1X6
Ondansetron	T45.0X1	T45.0X2	T45.0X3	T45.0X4	T45.0X5	T45.0X6
Ophthaine	T41.3X1	T41.3X2	T41.3X3	T41.3X4	T41.3X5	T41.3X6
Ophthetic	T41.3X1	T41.3X2	T41.3X3	T41.3X4	T41.3X5	T41.3X6
Opiate NEC	T40.601	T40.602	T40.603	T40.604	T40.605	T40.606
- antagonists	T50.7X1	T50.7X2	T50.7X3	T50.7X4	T50.7X5	T50.7X6
Opioid NEC	T40.2X1	T40.2X2	T40.2X3	T40.2X4	T40.2X5	T40.2X6
Opipramol	T43.011	T43.012	T43.013	T43.014	T43.015	T43.016
Opium alkaloids (total)	T40.0X1	T40.0X2	T40.0X3	T40.0X4	T40.0X5	T40.0X6
- standardized powdered	T40.0X1	T40.0X2	T40.0X3	T40.0X4	T40.0X5	T40.0X6
- tincture (camphorated)	T40.0X1	T40.0X2	T40.0X3	T40.0X4	T40.0X5	T40.0X6
Oracon	T38.4X1	T38.4X2	T38.4X3	T38.4X4	T38.4X5	T38.4X6
Oragrafin	T50.8X1	T50.8X2	T50.8X3	T50.8X4	T50.8X5	T50.8X6
Oral contraceptives	T38.4X1	T38.4X2	T38.4X3	T38.4X4	T38.4X5	T38.4X6
Oral rehydration salts	T50.3X1	T50.3X2	T50.3X3	T50.3X4	T50.3X5	T50.3X6
Orazamide	T50.991	T50.992	T50.993	T50.994	T50.995	T50.996
Orciprenaline	T48.291	T48.292	T48.293	T48.294	T48.295	T48.296
Organidin	T48.4X1	T48.4X2	T48.4X3	T48.4X4	T48.4X5	T48.4X6
Organonitrate NEC	T46.3X1	T46.3X2	T46.3X3	T46.3X4	T46.3X5	T46.3X6
Organophosphates	T60.0X1	T60.0X2	T60.0X3	T60.0X4	--	--

Substance	Poisoning, Accidental (unintentional)	Poisoning, Intentional Self-harm	Poisoning, Assault	Poisoning, Undetermined	Adverse effect	Underdosing
Orimune	T50.B91	T50.B92	T50.B93	T50.B94	T50.B95	T50.B96
Orinase	T38.3X1	T38.3X2	T38.3X3	T38.3X4	T38.3X5	T38.3X6
Ormeloxifene	T38.6X1	T38.6X2	T38.6X3	T38.6X4	T38.6X5	T38.6X6
Ornidazole	T37.3X1	T37.3X2	T37.3X3	T37.3X4	T37.3X5	T37.3X6
Ornithine aspartate	T50.991	T50.992	T50.993	T50.994	T50.995	T50.996
Ornoprostil	T47.1X1	T47.1X2	T47.1X3	T47.1X4	T47.1X5	T47.1X6
Orphenadrine (hydrochloride)	T42.8X1	T42.8X2	T42.8X3	T42.8X4	T42.8X5	T42.8X6
Ortal (sodium)	T42.3X1	T42.3X2	T42.3X3	T42.3X4	T42.3X5	T42.3X6
Orthoboric acid	T49.0X1	T49.0X2	T49.0X3	T49.0X4	T49.0X5	T49.0X6
- ENT agent	T49.6X1	T49.6X2	T49.6X3	T49.6X4	T49.6X5	T49.6X6
- ophthalmic preparation	T49.5X1	T49.5X2	T49.5X3	T49.5X4	T49.5X5	T49.5X6
Orthocaine	T41.3X1	T41.3X2	T41.3X3	T41.3X4	T41.3X5	T41.3X6
Orthodichlorobenzene	T53.7X1	T53.7X2	T53.7X3	T53.7X4	--	--
Ortho-Novum	T38.4X1	T38.4X2	T38.4X3	T38.4X4	T38.4X5	T38.4X6
Orthotolidine (reagent)	T54.2X1	T54.2X2	T54.2X3	T54.2X4	--	--
Osmic acid (liquid)	T54.2X1	T54.2X2	T54.2X3	T54.2X4	--	--
- fumes	T54.2X1	T54.2X2	T54.2X3	T54.2X4	--	--
Osmotic diuretics	T50.2X1	T50.2X2	T50.2X3	T50.2X4	T50.2X5	T50.2X6
Otilonium bromide	T44.3X1	T44.3X2	T44.3X3	T44.3X4	T44.3X5	T44.3X6
Otorhinolaryngological drug NEC	T49.6X1	T49.6X2	T49.6X3	T49.6X4	T49.6X5	T49.6X6
Ouabain (e)	T46.0X1	T46.0X2	T46.0X3	T46.0X4	T46.0X5	T46.0X6
Ovarian						
- hormone	T38.5X1	T38.5X2	T38.5X3	T38.5X4	T38.5X5	T38.5X6
- stimulant	T38.5X1	T38.5X2	T38.5X3	T38.5X4	T38.5X5	T38.5X6
Ovral	T38.4X1	T38.4X2	T38.4X3	T38.4X4	T38.4X5	T38.4X6
Ovulen	T38.4X1	T38.4X2	T38.4X3	T38.4X4	T38.4X5	T38.4X6
Oxacillin	T36.0X1	T36.0X2	T36.0X3	T36.0X4	T36.0X5	T36.0X6
Oxalic acid	T54.2X1	T54.2X2	T54.2X3	T54.2X4	--	--
- ammonium salt	T50.991	T50.992	T50.993	T50.994	T50.995	T50.996
Oxamniquine	T37.4X1	T37.4X2	T37.4X3	T37.4X4	T37.4X5	T37.4X6
Oxanamide	T43.591	T43.592	T43.593	T43.594	T43.595	T43.596
Oxandrolone	T38.7X1	T38.7X2	T38.7X3	T38.7X4	T38.7X5	T38.7X6
Oxantel	T37.4X1	T37.4X2	T37.4X3	T37.4X4	T37.4X5	T37.4X6
Oxapium iodide	T44.3X1	T44.3X2	T44.3X3	T44.3X4	T44.3X5	T44.3X6
Oxaprotiline	T43.021	T43.022	T43.023	T43.024	T43.025	T43.026
Oxaprozin	T39.311	T39.312	T39.313	T39.314	T39.315	T39.316
Oxatomide	T45.0X1	T45.0X2	T45.0X3	T45.0X4	T45.0X5	T45.0X6
Oxazepam	T42.4X1	T42.4X2	T42.4X3	T42.4X4	T42.4X5	T42.4X6
Oxazimedrine	T50.5X1	T50.5X2	T50.5X3	T50.5X4	T50.5X5	T50.5X6
Oxazolam	T42.4X1	T42.4X2	T42.4X3	T42.4X4	T42.4X5	T42.4X6
Oxazolidine derivatives	T42.2X1	T42.2X2	T42.2X3	T42.2X4	T42.2X5	T42.2X6
Oxazolidinedione (derivative)	T42.2X1	T42.2X2	T42.2X3	T42.2X4	T42.2X5	T42.2X6
Ox bile extract	T47.5X1	T47.5X2	T47.5X3	T47.5X4	T47.5X5	T47.5X6
Oxcarbazepine	T42.1X1	T42.1X2	T42.1X3	T42.1X4	T42.1X5	T42.1X6
Oxedrine	T44.4X1	T44.4X2	T44.4X3	T44.4X4	T44.4X5	T44.4X6
Oxeladin (citrate)	T48.3X1	T48.3X2	T48.3X3	T48.3X4	T48.3X5	T48.3X6
Oxendolone	T38.5X1	T38.5X2	T38.5X3	T38.5X4	T38.5X5	T38.5X6
Oxetacaine	T41.3X1	T41.3X2	T41.3X3	T41.3X4	T41.3X5	T41.3X6
Oxethazine	T41.3X1	T41.3X2	T41.3X3	T41.3X4	T41.3X5	T41.3X6
Oxetorone	T39.8X1	T39.8X2	T39.8X3	T39.8X4	T39.8X5	T39.8X6
Oxiconazole	T49.0X1	T49.0X2	T49.0X3	T49.0X4	T49.0X5	T49.0X6
Oxidizing agent NEC	T54.91	T54.92	T54.93	T54.94	--	--
Oxipurinol	T50.4X1	T50.4X2	T50.4X3	T50.4X4	T50.4X5	T50.4X6
Oxitriptan	T43.291	T43.292	T43.293	T43.294	T43.295	T43.296
Oxitropium bromide	T48.6X1	T48.6X2	T48.6X3	T48.6X4	T48.6X5	T48.6X6
Oxodipine	T46.1X1	T46.1X2	T46.1X3	T46.1X4	T46.1X5	T46.1X6
Oxolamine	T48.3X1	T48.3X2	T48.3X3	T48.3X4	T48.3X5	T48.3X6
Oxolinic acid	T37.8X1	T37.8X2	T37.8X3	T37.8X4	T37.8X5	T37.8X6
Oxomemazine	T43.3X1	T43.3X2	T43.3X3	T43.3X4	T43.3X5	T43.3X6

Substance	Poisoning, Accidental (unintentional)	Poisoning, Intentional Self-harm	Poisoning, Assault	Poisoning, Undetermined	Adverse effect	Underdosing
Oxophenarsine	T37.3X1	T37.3X2	T37.3X3	T37.3X4	T37.3X5	T37.3X6
Oxprenolol	T44.7X1	T44.7X2	T44.7X3	T44.7X4	T44.7X5	T44.7X6
Oxsoralen	T49.3X1	T49.3X2	T49.3X3	T49.3X4	T49.3X5	T49.3X6
Oxtriphylline	T48.6X1	T48.6X2	T48.6X3	T48.6X4	T48.6X5	T48.6X6
Oxybate sodium	T41.291	T41.292	T41.293	T41.294	T41.295	T41.296
Oxybuprocaine	T41.3X1	T41.3X2	T41.3X3	T41.3X4	T41.3X5	T41.3X6
Oxybutynin	T44.3X1	T44.3X2	T44.3X3	T44.3X4	T44.3X5	T44.3X6
Oxychlorosene	T49.0X1	T49.0X2	T49.0X3	T49.0X4	T49.0X5	T49.0X6
Oxycodone	T40.2X1	T40.2X2	T40.2X3	T40.2X4	T40.2X5	T40.2X6
Oxyfedrine	T46.3X1	T46.3X2	T46.3X3	T46.3X4	T46.3X5	T46.3X6
Oxygen	T41.5X1	T41.5X2	T41.5X3	T41.5X4	T41.5X5	T41.5X6
Oxylone	T49.0X1	T49.0X2	T49.0X3	T49.0X4	T49.0X5	T49.0X6
- ophthalmic preparation	T49.5X1	T49.5X2	T49.5X3	T49.5X4	T49.5X5	T49.5X6
Oxymesterone	T38.7X1	T38.7X2	T38.7X3	T38.7X4	T38.7X5	T38.7X6
Oxymetazoline	T48.5X1	T48.5X2	T48.5X3	T48.5X4	T48.5X5	T48.5X6
Oxymetholone	T38.7X1	T38.7X2	T38.7X3	T38.7X4	T38.7X5	T38.7X6
Oxymorphone	T40.2X1	T40.2X2	T40.2X3	T40.2X4	T40.2X5	T40.2X6
Oxypertine	T43.591	T43.592	T43.593	T43.594	T43.595	T43.596
Oxyphenbutazone	T39.2X1	T39.2X2	T39.2X3	T39.2X4	T39.2X5	T39.2X6
Oxyphencyclimine	T44.3X1	T44.3X2	T44.3X3	T44.3X4	T44.3X5	T44.3X6
Oxyphenisatine	T47.2X1	T47.2X2	T47.2X3	T47.2X4	T47.2X5	T47.2X6
Oxyphenonium bromide	T44.3X1	T44.3X2	T44.3X3	T44.3X4	T44.3X5	T44.3X6
Oxypolygelatin	T45.8X1	T45.8X2	T45.8X3	T45.8X4	T45.8X5	T45.8X6
Oxyquinoline (derivatives)	T37.8X1	T37.8X2	T37.8X3	T37.8X4	T37.8X5	T37.8X6
Oxytetracycline	T36.4X1	T36.4X2	T36.4X3	T36.4X4	T36.4X5	T36.4X6
Oxytocic drug NEC	T48.0X1	T48.0X2	T48.0X3	T48.0X4	T48.0X5	T48.0X6
Oxytocin (synthetic)	T48.0X1	T48.0X2	T48.0X3	T48.0X4	T48.0X5	T48.0X6
Ozone	T59.891	T59.892	T59.893	T59.894	--	--
PABA	T49.3X1	T49.3X2	T49.3X3	T49.3X4	T49.3X5	T49.3X6
Packed red cells	T45.8X1	T45.8X2	T45.8X3	T45.8X4	T45.8X5	T45.8X6
Padimate	T49.3X1	T49.3X2	T49.3X3	T49.3X4	T49.3X5	T49.3X6
Paint NEC	T65.6X1	T65.6X2	T65.6X3	T65.6X4	--	--
- cleaner	T52.91	T52.92	T52.93	T52.94	--	--
- fumes NEC	T59.891	T59.892	T59.893	T59.894	--	--
- lead (fumes)	T56.0X1	T56.0X2	T56.0X3	T56.0X4	--	--
- solvent NEC	T52.8X1	T52.8X2	T52.8X3	T52.8X4	--	--
- stripper	T52.8X1	T52.8X2	T52.8X3	T52.8X4	--	--
Palfium	T40.2X1	T40.2X2	T40.2X3	T40.2X4	--	--
Palm kernel oil	T50.991	T50.992	T50.993	T50.994	T50.995	T50.996
Paludrine	T37.2X1	T37.2X2	T37.2X3	T37.2X4	T37.2X5	T37.2X6
PAM (pralidoxime)	T50.6X1	T50.6X2	T50.6X3	T50.6X4	T50.6X5	T50.6X6
Pamaquine (naphthoute)	T37.2X1	T37.2X2	T37.2X3	T37.2X4	T37.2X5	T37.2X6
Panadol	T39.1X1	T39.1X2	T39.1X3	T39.1X4	T39.1X5	T39.1X6
Pancreatic						
- digestive secretion stimulant	T47.8X1	T47.8X2	T47.8X3	T47.8X4	T47.8X5	T47.8X6
- dornase	T45.3X1	T45.3X2	T45.3X3	T45.3X4	T45.3X5	T45.3X6
Pancreatin	T47.5X1	T47.5X2	T47.5X3	T47.5X4	T47.5X5	T47.5X6
Pancrelipase	T47.5X1	T47.5X2	T47.5X3	T47.5X4	T47.5X5	T47.5X6
Pancuronium (bromide)	T48.1X1	T48.1X2	T48.1X3	T48.1X4	T48.1X5	T48.1X6
Pangamic acid	T45.2X1	T45.2X2	T45.2X3	T45.2X4	T45.2X5	T45.2X6
Panthenol	T45.2X1	T45.2X2	T45.2X3	T45.2X4	T45.2X5	T45.2X6
- topical	T49.8X1	T49.8X2	T49.8X3	T49.8X4	T49.8X5	T49.8X6
Pantopon	T40.0X1	T40.0X2	T40.0X3	T40.0X4	T40.0X5	T40.0X6
Pantothenic acid	T45.2X1	T45.2X2	T45.2X3	T45.2X4	T45.2X5	T45.2X6
Panwarfin	T45.511	T45.512	T45.513	T45.514	T45.515	T45.516
Papain	T47.5X1	T47.5X2	T47.5X3	T47.5X4	T47.5X5	T47.5X6
- digestant	T47.5X1	T47.5X2	T47.5X3	T47.5X4	T47.5X5	T47.5X6
Papaveretum	T40.0X1	T40.0X2	T40.0X3	T40.0X4	T40.0X5	T40.0X6

Substance	Poisoning, Accidental (unintentional)	Poisoning, Intentional Self-harm	Poisoning, Assault	Poisoning, Undetermined	Adverse effect	Underdosing
Papaverine	T44.3X1	T44.3X2	T44.3X3	T44.3X4	T44.3X5	T44.3X6
Para-acetamidophenol	T39.1X1	T39.1X2	T39.1X3	T39.1X4	T39.1X5	T39.1X6
Para-aminobenzoic acid	T49.3X1	T49.3X2	T49.3X3	T49.3X4	T49.3X5	T49.3X6
Para-aminophenol derivatives	T39.1X1	T39.1X2	T39.1X3	T39.1X4	T39.1X5	T39.1X6
Para-aminosalicylic acid	T37.1X1	T37.1X2	T37.1X3	T37.1X4	T37.1X5	T37.1X6
Paracetaldehyde	T42.6X1	T42.6X2	T42.6X3	T42.6X4	T42.6X5	T42.6X6
Paracetamol	T39.1X1	T39.1X2	T39.1X3	T39.1X4	T39.1X5	T39.1X6
Parachlorophenol (camphorated)	T49.0X1	T49.0X2	T49.0X3	T49.0X4	T49.0X5	T49.0X6
Paracodin	T40.2X1	T40.2X2	T40.2X3	T40.2X4	T40.2X5	T40.2X6
Paradione	T42.2X1	T42.2X2	T42.2X3	T42.2X4	T42.2X5	T42.2X6
Paraffin (s) (wax)	T52.0X1	T52.0X2	T52.0X3	T52.0X4	--	--
- liquid (medicinal)	T47.4X1	T47.4X2	T47.4X3	T47.4X4	T47.4X5	T47.4X6
- - nonmedicinal	T52.0X1	T52.0X2	T52.0X3	T52.0X4	--	--
Paraformaldehyde	T60.3X1	T60.3X2	T60.3X3	T60.3X4	--	--
Paraldehyde	T42.6X1	T42.6X2	T42.6X3	T42.6X4	T42.6X5	T42.6X6
Paramethadione	T42.2X1	T42.2X2	T42.2X3	T42.2X4	T42.2X5	T42.2X6
Paramethasone	T38.0X1	T38.0X2	T38.0X3	T38.0X4	T38.0X5	T38.0X6
- acetate	T49.0X1	T49.0X2	T49.0X3	T49.0X4	T49.0X5	T49.0X6
Paraoxon	T60.0X1	T60.0X2	T60.0X3	T60.0X4	--	--
Paraquat	T60.3X1	T60.3X2	T60.3X3	T60.3X4	--	--
Parasympatholytic NEC	T44.3X1	T44.3X2	T44.3X3	T44.3X4	T44.3X5	T44.3X6
Parasympathomimetic drug NEC	T44.1X1	T44.1X2	T44.1X3	T44.1X4	T44.1X5	T44.1X6
Parathion	T60.0X1	T60.0X2	T60.0X3	T60.0X4	--	--
Parathormone	T50.991	T50.992	T50.993	T50.994	T50.995	T50.996
Parathyroid extract	T50.991	T50.992	T50.993	T50.994	T50.995	T50.996
Paratyphoid vaccine	T50.A91	T50.A92	T50.A93	T50.A94	T50.A95	T50.A96
Paredrine	T44.4X1	T44.4X2	T44.4X3	T44.4X4	T44.4X5	T44.4X6
Paregoric	T40.0X1	T40.0X2	T40.0X3	T40.0X4	T40.0X5	T40.0X6
Pargyline	T46.5X1	T46.5X2	T46.5X3	T46.5X4	T46.5X5	T46.5X6
Paris green	T57.0X1	T57.0X2	T57.0X3	T57.0X4	--	--
- insecticide	T57.0X1	T57.0X2	T57.0X3	T57.0X4	--	--
Parnate	T43.1X1	T43.1X2	T43.1X3	T43.1X4	T43.1X5	T43.1X6
Paromomycin	T36.5X1	T36.5X2	T36.5X3	T36.5X4	T36.5X5	T36.5X6
Paroxypropione	T45.1X1	T45.1X2	T45.1X3	T45.1X4	T45.1X5	T45.1X6
Parzone	T40.2X1	T40.2X2	T40.2X3	T40.2X4	T40.2X5	T40.2X6
PAS	T37.1X1	T37.1X2	T37.1X3	T37.1X4	T37.1X5	T37.1X6
Pasiniazid	T37.1X1	T37.1X2	T37.1X3	T37.1X4	T37.1X5	T37.1X6
PBB (polybrominated biphenyls)	T65.891	T65.892	T65.893	T65.894	--	--
PCB	T65.891	T65.892	T65.893	T65.894	--	--
PCP						
- meaning pentachlorophenol	T60.1X1	T60.1X2	T60.1X3	T60.1X4	--	--
- - fungicide	T60.3X1	T60.3X2	T60.3X3	T60.3X4	--	--
- - herbicide	T60.3X1	T60.3X2	T60.3X3	T60.3X4	--	--
- - insecticide	T60.1X1	T60.1X2	T60.1X3	T60.1X4	--	--
- meaning phencyclidine	T40.991	T40.992	T40.993	T40.994	--	--
Peach kernel oil (emulsion)	T47.4X1	T47.4X2	T47.4X3	T47.4X4	T47.4X5	T47.4X6
Peanut oil (emulsion) NEC	T47.4X1	T47.4X2	T47.4X3	T47.4X4	T47.4X5	T47.4X6
- topical	T49.3X1	T49.3X2	T49.3X3	T49.3X4	T49.3X5	T49.3X6
Pearly Gates (morning glory seeds)	T40.991	T40.992	T40.993	T40.994	--	--
Pecazine	T43.3X1	T43.3X2	T43.3X3	T43.3X4	T43.3X5	T43.3X6
Pectin	T47.6X1	T47.6X2	T47.6X3	T47.6X4	T47.6X5	T47.6X6
Pefloxacin	T37.8X1	T37.8X2	T37.8X3	T37.8X4	T37.8X5	T37.8X6
Pegademase, bovine	T50.Z91	T50.Z92	T50.Z93	T50.Z94	T50.Z95	T50.Z96
Pelletierine tannate	T37.4X1	T37.4X2	T37.4X3	T37.4X4	T37.4X5	T37.4X6
Pemirolast (potassium)	T48.6X1	T48.6X2	T48.6X3	T48.6X4	T48.6X5	T48.6X6
Pemoline	T50.7X1	T50.7X2	T50.7X3	T50.7X4	T50.7X5	T50.7X6
Pempidine	T44.2X1	T44.2X2	T44.2X3	T44.2X4	T44.2X5	T44.2X6
Penamecillin	T36.0X1	T36.0X2	T36.0X3	T36.0X4	T36.0X5	T36.0X6
Penbutolol	T44.7X1	T44.7X2	T44.7X3	T44.7X4	T44.7X5	T44.7X6

Substance	Poisoning, Accidental (unintentional)	Poisoning, Intentional Self-harm	Poisoning, Assault	Poisoning, Undetermined	Adverse effect	Underdosing
Penethamate	T36.0X1	T36.0X2	T36.0X3	T36.0X4	T36.0X5	T36.0X6
Penfluridol	T43.591	T43.592	T43.593	T43.594	T43.595	T43.596
Penflutizide	T50.2X1	T50.2X2	T50.2X3	T50.2X4	T50.2X5	T50.2X6
Pengitoxin	T46.0X1	T46.0X2	T46.0X3	T46.0X4	T46.0X5	T46.0X6
Penicillamine	T50.6X1	T50.6X2	T50.6X3	T50.6X4	T50.6X5	T50.6X6
Penicillin (any)	T36.0X1	T36.0X2	T36.0X3	T36.0X4	T36.0X5	T36.0X6
Penicillinase	T45.3X1	T45.3X2	T45.3X3	T45.3X4	T45.3X5	T45.3X6
Penicilloyl polylysine	T50.8X1	T50.8X2	T50.8X3	T50.8X4	T50.8X5	T50.8X6
Penimepicycline	T36.4X1	T36.4X2	T36.4X3	T36.4X4	T36.4X5	T36.4X6
Pentachloroethane	T53.6X1	T53.6X2	T53.6X3	T53.6X4	--	--
Pentachloronaphthalene	T53.7X1	T53.7X2	T53.7X3	T53.7X4	--	--
Pentachlorophenol (pesticide)	T60.1X1	T60.1X2	T60.1X3	T60.1X4	--	--
- fungicide	T60.3X1	T60.3X2	T60.3X3	T60.3X4	--	--
- herbicide	T60.3X1	T60.3X2	T60.3X3	T60.3X4	--	--
- insecticide	T60.1X1	T60.1X2	T60.1X3	T60.1X4	--	--
Pentaerythritol	T46.3X1	T46.3X2	T46.3X3	T46.3X4	T46.3X5	T46.3X6
- chloral	T42.6X1	T42.6X2	T42.6X3	T42.6X4	T42.6X5	T42.6X6
- tetranitrate NEC	T46.3X1	T46.3X2	T46.3X3	T46.3X4	T46.3X5	T46.3X6
Pentaerythrityl tetranitrate	T46.3X1	T46.3X2	T46.3X3	T46.3X4	T46.3X5	T46.3X6
Pentagastrin	T50.8X1	T50.8X2	T50.8X3	T50.8X4	T50.8X5	T50.8X6
Pentalin	T53.6X1	T53.6X2	T53.6X3	T53.6X4	--	--
Pentamethonium bromide	T44.2X1	T44.2X2	T44.2X3	T44.2X4	T44.2X5	T44.2X6
Pentamidine	T37.3X1	T37.3X2	T37.3X3	T37.3X4	T37.3X5	T37.3X6
Pentanol	T51.3X1	T51.3X2	T51.3X3	T51.3X4	--	--
Pentapyrrolinium (bitartrate)	T44.2X1	T44.2X2	T44.2X3	T44.2X4	T44.2X5	T44.2X6
Pentaquine	T37.2X1	T37.2X2	T37.2X3	T37.2X4	T37.2X5	T37.2X6
Pentazocine	T40.491	T40.492	T40.493	T40.494	T40.495	T40.496
Pentetrazole	T50.7X1	T50.7X2	T50.7X3	T50.7X4	T50.7X5	T50.7X6
Penthienate bromide	T44.3X1	T44.3X2	T44.3X3	T44.3X4	T44.3X5	T44.3X6
Pentifylline	T46.7X1	T46.7X2	T46.7X3	T46.7X4	T46.7X5	T46.7X6
Pentobarbital	T42.3X1	T42.3X2	T42.3X3	T42.3X4	T42.3X5	T42.3X6
- sodium	T42.3X1	T42.3X2	T42.3X3	T42.3X4	T42.3X5	T42.3X6
Pentobarbitone	T42.3X1	T42.3X2	T42.3X3	T42.3X4	T42.3X5	T42.3X6
Pentolonium tartrate	T44.2X1	T44.2X2	T44.2X3	T44.2X4	T44.2X5	T44.2X6
Pentosan polysulfate (sodium)	T39.8X1	T39.8X2	T39.8X3	T39.8X4	T39.8X5	T39.8X6
Pentostatin	T45.1X1	T45.1X2	T45.1X3	T45.1X4	T45.1X5	T45.1X6
Pentothal	T41.1X1	T41.1X2	T41.1X3	T41.1X4	T41.1X5	T41.1X6
Pentoxifylline	T46.7X1	T46.7X2	T46.7X3	T46.7X4	T46.7X5	T46.7X6
Pentoxyverine	T48.3X1	T48.3X2	T48.3X3	T48.3X4	T48.3X5	T48.3X6
Pentrinat	T46.3X1	T46.3X2	T46.3X3	T46.3X4	T46.3X5	T46.3X6
Pentylenetetrazole	T50.7X1	T50.7X2	T50.7X3	T50.7X4	T50.7X5	T50.7X6
Pentylsalicylamide	T37.1X1	T37.1X2	T37.1X3	T37.1X4	T37.1X5	T37.1X6
Pentymal	T42.3X1	T42.3X2	T42.3X3	T42.3X4	T42.3X5	T42.3X6
Peplomycin	T45.1X1	T45.1X2	T45.1X3	T45.1X4	T45.1X5	T45.1X6
Peppermint (oil)	T47.5X1	T47.5X2	T47.5X3	T47.5X4	T47.5X5	T47.5X6
Pepsin	T47.5X1	T47.5X2	T47.5X3	T47.5X4	T47.5X5	T47.5X6
- digestant	T47.5X1	T47.5X2	T47.5X3	T47.5X4	T47.5X5	T47.5X6
Pepstatin	T47.1X1	T47.1X2	T47.1X3	T47.1X4	T47.1X5	T47.1X6
Peptavlon	T50.8X1	T50.8X2	T50.8X3	T50.8X4	T50.8X5	T50.8X6
Perazine	T43.3X1	T43.3X2	T43.3X3	T43.3X4	T43.3X5	T43.3X6
Percaine (spinal)	T41.3X1	T41.3X2	T41.3X3	T41.3X4	T41.3X5	T41.3X6
- topical (surface)	T41.3X1	T41.3X2	T41.3X3	T41.3X4	T41.3X5	T41.3X6
Perchloroethylene	T53.3X1	T53.3X2	T53.3X3	T53.3X4	--	--
- medicinal	T37.4X1	T37.4X2	T37.4X3	T37.4X4	T37.4X5	T37.4X6
- vapor	T53.3X1	T53.3X2	T53.3X3	T53.3X4	--	--
Percodan	T40.2X1	T40.2X2	T40.2X3	T40.2X4	T40.2X5	T40.2X6
Percogesic—see also acetaminophen	T45.0X1	T45.0X2	T45.0X3	T45.0X4	T45.0X5	T45.0X6
Percorten	T38.0X1	T38.0X2	T38.0X3	T38.0X4	T38.0X5	T38.0X6

Substance	Poisoning, Accidental (unintentional)	Poisoning, Intentional Self-harm	Poisoning, Assault	Poisoning, Undetermined	Adverse effect	Underdosing
Pergolide	T42.8X1	T42.8X2	T42.8X3	T42.8X4	T42.8X5	T42.8X6
Pergonal	T38.811	T38.812	T38.813	T38.814	T38.815	T38.816
Perhexiline	T46.3X1	T46.3X2	T46.3X3	T46.3X4	T46.3X5	T46.3X6
Perhexiline (maleate)	T46.3X1	T46.3X2	T46.3X3	T46.3X4	T46.3X5	T46.3X6
Periactin	T45.0X1	T45.0X2	T45.0X3	T45.0X4	T45.0X5	T45.0X6
Pericyazine	T43.3X1	T43.3X2	T43.3X3	T43.3X4	T43.3X5	T43.3X6
Periclor	T42.6X1	T42.6X2	T42.6X3	T42.6X4	T42.6X5	T42.6X6
Perindopril	T46.4X1	T46.4X2	T46.4X3	T46.4X4	T46.4X5	T46.4X6
Perisoxal	T39.8X1	T39.8X2	T39.8X3	T39.8X4	T39.8X5	T39.8X6
Peritoneal dialysis solution	T50.3X1	T50.3X2	T50.3X3	T50.3X4	T50.3X5	T50.3X6
Peritrate	T46.3X1	T46.3X2	T46.3X3	T46.3X4	T46.3X5	T46.3X6
Perlapine	T42.4X1	T42.4X2	T42.4X3	T42.4X4	T42.4X5	T42.4X6
Permanganate	T65.891	T65.892	T65.893	T65.894	--	--
Permethrin	T60.1X1	T60.1X2	T60.1X3	T60.1X4	--	--
Pernocton	T42.3X1	T42.3X2	T42.3X3	T42.3X4	T42.3X5	T42.3X6
Pernoston	T42.3X1	T42.3X2	T42.3X3	T42.3X4	T42.3X5	T42.3X6
Peronine	T40.2X1	T40.2X2	T40.2X3	T40.2X4	--	--
Perphenazine	T43.3X1	T43.3X2	T43.3X3	T43.3X4	T43.3X5	T43.3X6
Pertofrane	T43.011	T43.012	T43.013	T43.014	T43.015	T43.016
Pertussis						
- immune serum (human)	T50.Z11	T50.Z12	T50.Z13	T50.Z14	T50.Z15	T50.Z16
- vaccine (with diphtheria toxoid) (with tetanus toxoid)	T50.A11	T50.A12	T50.A13	T50.A14	T50.A15	T50.A16
Peruvian balsam	T49.0X1	T49.0X2	T49.0X3	T49.0X4	T49.0X5	T49.0X6
Peruvoside	T46.0X1	T46.0X2	T46.0X3	T46.0X4	T46.0X5	T46.0X6
Pesticide (dust) (fumes) (vapor) NEC	T60.91	T60.92	T60.93	T60.94	--	--
- arsenic	T57.0X1	T57.0X2	T57.0X3	T57.0X4	--	--
- chlorinated	T60.1X1	T60.1X2	T60.1X3	T60.1X4	--	--
- cyanide	T65.0X1	T65.0X2	T65.0X3	T65.0X4	--	--
- kerosene	T52.0X1	T52.0X2	T52.0X3	T52.0X4	--	--
- mixture (of compounds)	T60.91	T60.92	T60.93	T60.94	--	--
- naphthalene	T60.2X1	T60.2X2	T60.2X3	T60.2X4	--	--
- organochlorine (compounds)	T60.1X1	T60.1X2	T60.1X3	T60.1X4	--	--
- petroleum (distillate) (products) NEC	T60.8X1	T60.8X2	T60.8X3	T60.8X4	--	--
- specified ingredient NEC	T60.8X1	T60.8X2	T60.8X3	T60.8X4	--	--
- strychnine	T65.1X1	T65.1X2	T65.1X3	T65.1X4	--	--
- thallium	T60.4X1	T60.4X2	T60.4X3	T60.4X4	--	--
Pethidine	T40.491	T40.492	T40.493	T40.494	T40.495	T40.496
Petrichloral	T42.6X1	T42.6X2	T42.6X3	T42.6X4	T42.6X5	T42,6X6
Petrol	T52.0X1	T52.0X2	T52.0X3	T52.0X4	--	--
- vapor	T52.0X1	T52.0X2	T52.0X3	T52.0X4	--	--
Petrolatum	T49.3X1	T49.3X2	T49.3X3	T49.3X4	T49.3X5	T49.3X6
- hydrophilic	T49.3X1	T49.3X2	T49.3X3	T49.3X4	T49.3X5	T49.3X6
- liquid	T47.4X1	T47.4X2	T47.4X3	T47.4X4	T47.4X5	T47.4X6
- - topical	T49.3X1	T49.3X2	T49.3X3	T49.3X4	T49.3X5	T49.3X6
- nonmedicinal	T52.0X1	T52.0X2	T52.0X3	T52.0X4	--	--
- red veterinary	T49.3X1	T49.3X2	T49.3X3	T49.3X4	T49.3X5	T49.3X6
- white	T49.3X1	T49.3X2	T49.3X3	T49.3X4	T49.3X5	T49.3X6
Petroleum (products) NEC	T52.0X1	T52.0X2	T52.0X3	T52.0X4	--	--
- benzine (s) —see Ligroin						
- ether—see Ligroin						
- jelly—see Petrolatum						
- naphtha—see Ligroin						
- pesticide	T60.8X1	T60.8X2	T60.8X3	T60.8X4	--	--
- solids	T52.0X1	T52.0X2	T52.0X3	T52.0X4	--	--
- solvents	T52.0X1	T52.0X2	T52.0X3	T52.0X4	--	--
- vapor	T52.0X1	T52.0X2	T52.0X3	T52.0X4	--	--
Peyote	T40.991	T40.992	T40.993	T40.994	--	--
Phanodorm, phanodorn	T42.3X1	T42.3X2	T42.3X3	T42.3X4	T42.3X5	T42.3X6

Substance	Poisoning, Accidental (unintentional)	Poisoning, Intentional Self-harm	Poisoning, Assault	Poisoning, Undetermined	Adverse effect	Underdosing
Phanquinone	T37.3X1	T37.3X2	T37.3X3	T37.3X4	T37.3X5	T37.3X6
Phanquone	T37.3X1	T37.3X2	T37.3X3	T37.3X4	T37.3X5	T37.3X6
Pharmaceutical						
- adjunct NEC	T50.901	T50.902	T50.903	T50.904	T50.905	T50.906
- excipient NEC	T50.901	T50.902	T50.903	T50.904	T50.905	T50.906
- sweetener	T50.901	T50.902	T50.903	T50.904	T50.905	T50.906
- viscous agent	T50.901	T50.902	T50.903	T50.904	T50.905	T50.906
Phemitone	T42.3X1	T42.3X2	T42.3X3	T42.3X4	T42.3X5	T42.3X6
Phenacaine	T41.3X1	T41.3X2	T41.3X3	T41.3X4	T41.3X5	T41.3X6
Phenacemide	T42.6X1	T42.6X2	T42.6X3	T42.6X4	T42.6X5	T42.6X6
Phenacetin	T39.1X1	T39.1X2	T39.1X3	T39.1X4	T39.1X5	T39.1X6
Phenadoxone	T40.2X1	T40.2X2	T40.2X3	T40.2X4	--	--
Phenaglycodol	T43.591	T43.592	T43.593	T43.594	T43.595	T43.596
Phenantoin	T42.0X1	T42.0X2	T42.0X3	T42.0X4	T42.0X5	T42.0X6
Phenaphthazine reagent	T50.991	T50.992	T50.993	T50.994	T50.995	T50.996
Phenazocine	T40.491	T40.492	T40.493	T40.494	T40.495	T40.496
Phenazone	T39.2X1	T39.2X2	T39.2X3	T39.2X4	T39.2X5	T39.2X6
Phenazopyridine	T39.8X1	T39.8X2	T39.8X3	T39.8X4	T39.8X5	T39.8X6
Phenbenicillin	T36.0X1	T36.0X2	T36.0X3	T36.0X4	T36.0X5	T36.0X6
Phenbutrazate	T50.5X1	T50.5X2	T50.5X3	T50.5X4	T50.5X5	T50.5X6
Phencyclidine	T40.991	T40.992	T40.993	T40.994	T40.995	T40.996
Phendimetrazine	T50.5X1	T50.5X2	T50.5X3	T50.5X4	T50.5X5	T50.5X6
Phenelzine	T43.1X1	T43.1X2	T43.1X3	T43.1X4	T43.1X5	T43.1X6
Phenemal	T42.3X1	T42.3X2	T42.3X3	T42.3X4	T42.3X5	T42.3X6
Phenergan	T42.6X1	T42.6X2	T42.6X3	T42.6X4	T42.6X5	T42.6X6
Pheneticillin	T36.0X1	T36.0X2	T36.0X3	T36.0X4	T36.0X5	T36.0X6
Pheneturide	T42.6X1	T42.6X2	T42.6X3	T42.6X4	T42.6X5	T42.6X6
Phenformin	T38.3X1	T38.3X2	T38.3X3	T38.3X4	T38.3X5	T38.3X6
Phenglutarimide	T44.3X1	T44.3X2	T44.3X3	T44.3X4	T44.3X5	T44.3X6
Phenicarbazide	T39.8X1	T39.8X2	T39.8X3	T39.8X4	T39.8X5	T39.8X6
Phenindamine	T45.0X1	T45.0X2	T45.0X3	T45.0X4	T45.0X5	T45.0X6
Phenindione	T45.511	T45.512	T45.513	T45.514	T45.515	T45.516
Pheniprazine	T43.1X1	T43.1X2	T43.1X3	T43.1X4	T43.1X5	T43.1X6
Pheniramine	T45.0X1	T45.0X2	T45.0X3	T45.0X4	T45.0X5	T45.0X6
Phenisatin	T47.2X1	T47.2X2	T47.2X3	T47.2X4	T47.2X5	T47.2X6
Phenmetrazine	T50.5X1	T50.5X2	T50.5X3	T50.5X4	T50.5X5	T50.5X6
Phenobal	T42.3X1	T42.3X2	T42.3X3	T42.3X4	T42.3X5	T42.3X6
Phenobarbital	T42.3X1	T42.3X2	T42.3X3	T42.3X4	T42.3X5	T42.3X6
- with						
- - mephenytoin	T42.3X1	T42.3X2	T42.3X3	T42.3X4	T42.3X5	T42.3X6
- - phenytoin	T42.3X1	T42.3X2	T42.3X3	T42.3X4	T42.3X5	T42.3X6
- sodium	T42.3X1	T42.3X2	T42.3X3	T42.3X4	T42.3X5	T42.3X6
Phenobarbitone	T42.3X1	T42.3X2	T42.3X3	T42.3X4	T42.3X5	T42.3X6
Phenobutiodil	T50.8X1	T50.8X2	T50.8X3	T50.8X4	T50.8X5	T50.8X6
Phenoctide	T49.0X1	T49.0X2	T49.0X3	T49.0X4	T49.0X5	T49.0X6
Phenol	T49.0X1	T49.0X2	T49.0X3	T49.0X4	T49.0X5	T49.0X6
- disinfectant	T54.0X1	T54.0X2	T54.0X3	T54.0X4	--	--
- in oil injection	T46.8X1	T46.8X2	T46.8X3	T46.8X4	T46.8X5	T46.8X6
- medicinal	T49.1X1	T49.1X2	T49.1X3	T49.1X4	T49.1X5	T49.1X6
- nonmedicinal NEC	T54.0X1	T54.0X2	T54.0X3	T54.0X4	--	--
- pesticide	T60.8X1	T60.8X2	T60.8X3	T60.8X4	--	--
- red	T50.8X1	T50.8X2	T50.8X3	T50.8X4	T50.8X5	T50.8X6
Phenolic preparation	T49.1X1	T49.1X2	T49.1X3	T49.1X4	T49.1X5	T49.1X6
Phenolphthalein	T47.2X1	T47.2X2	T47.2X3	T47.2X4	T47.2X5	T47.2X6
Phenolsulfonphthalein	T50.8X1	T50.8X2	T50.8X3	T50.8X4	T50.8X5	T50.8X6
Phenomorphan	T40.2X1	T40.2X2	T40.2X3	T40.2X4	--	--
Phenonyl	T42.3X1	T42.3X2	T42.3X3	T42.3X4	T42.3X5	T42.3X6
Phenoperidine	T40.491	T40.492	T40.493	T40.494	--	--

Substance	Poisoning, Accidental (unintentional)	Poisoning, Intentional Self-harm	Poisoning, Assault	Poisoning, Undetermined	Adverse effect	Underdosing
Phenopyrazone	T46.991	T46.992	T46.993	T46.994	T46.995	T46.996
Phenoquin	T50.4X1	T50.4X2	T50.4X3	T50.4X4	T50.4X5	T50.4X6
Phenothiazine (psychotropic) NEC	T43.3X1	T43.3X2	T43.3X3	T43.3X4	T43.3X5	T43.3X6
- insecticide	T60.2X1	T60.2X2	T60.2X3	T60.2X4	--	--
Phenothrin	T49.0X1	T49.0X2	T49.0X3	T49.0X4	T49.0X5	T49.0X6
Phenoxybenzamine	T46.7X1	T46.7X2	T46.7X3	T46.7X4	T46.7X5	T46.7X6
Phenoxyethanol	T49.0X1	T49.0X2	T49.0X3	T49.0X4	T49.0X5	T49.0X6
Phenoxymethyl penicillin	T36.0X1	T36.0X2	T36.0X3	T36.0X4	T36.0X5	T36.0X6
Phenprobamate	T42.8X1	T42.8X2	T42.8X3	T42.8X4	T42.8X5	T42.8X6
Phenprocoumon	T45.511	T45.512	T45.513	T45.514	T45.515	T45.516
Phensuximide	T42.2X1	T42.2X2	T42.2X3	T42.2X4	T42.2X5	T42.2X6
Phentermine	T50.5X1	T50.5X2	T50.5X3	T50.5X4	T50.5X5	T50.5X6
Phenthicillin	T36.0X1	T36.0X2	T36.0X3	T36.0X4	T36.0X5	T36.0X6
Phentolamine	T46.7X1	T46.7X2	T46.7X3	T46.7X4	T46.7X5	T46.7X6
Phenyl						
- butazone	T39.2X1	T39.2X2	T39.2X3	T39.2X4	T39.2X5	T39.2X6
- enediamine	T65.3X1	T65.3X2	T65.3X3	T65.3X4	--	--
- hydrazine	T65.3X1	T65.3X2	T65.3X3	T65.3X4	--	--
- - antineoplastic	T45.1X1	T45.1X2	T45.1X3	T45.1X4	T45.1X5	T45.1X6
- mercuric compounds—see Mercury						
- salicylate	T49.3X1	T49.3X2	T49.3X3	T49.3X4	T49.3X5	T49.3X6
Phenylalanine mustard	T45.1X1	T45.1X2	T45.1X3	T45.1X4	T45.1X5	T45.1X6
Phenylbutazone	T39.2X1	T39.2X2	T39.2X3	T39.2X4	T39.2X5	T39.2X6
Phenylenediamine	T65.3X1	T65.3X2	T65.3X3	T65.3X4	--	--
Phenylephrine	T44.4X1	T44.4X2	T44.4X3	T44.4X4	T44.4X5	T44.4X6
Phenylethylbiguanide	T38.3X1	T38.3X2	T38.3X3	T38.3X4	T38.3X5	T38.3X6
Phenylmercuric						
- acetate	T49.0X1	T49.0X2	T49.0X3	T49.0X4	T49.0X5	T49.0X6
- borate	T49.0X1	T49.0X2	T49.0X3	T49.0X4	T49.0X5	T49.0X6
- nitrate	T49.0X1	T49.0X2	T49.0X3	T49.0X4	T49.0X5	T49.0X6
Phenylmethylbarbitone	T42.3X1	T42.3X2	T42.3X3	T42.3X4	T42.3X5	T42.3X6
Phenylpropanol	T47.5X1	T47.5X2	T47.5X3	T47.5X4	T47.5X5	T47.5X6
Phenylpropanolamine	T44.991	T44.992	T44.993	T44.994	T44.995	T44.996
Phenylsulfthion	T60.0X1	T60.0X2	T60.0X3	T60.0X4	--	--
Phenyltoloxamine	T45.0X1	T45.0X2	T45.0X3	T45.0X4	T45.0X5	T45.0X6
Phenyramidol, phenyramidon	T39.8X1	T39.8X2	T39.8X3	T39.8X4	T39.8X5	T39.8X6
Phenytoin	T42.0X1	T42.0X2	T42.0X3	T42.0X4	T42.0X5	T42.0X6
- with Phenobarbital	T42.3X1	T42.3X2	T42.3X3	T42.3X4	T42.3X5	T42.3X6
pHisoHex	T49.2X1	T49.2X2	T49.2X3	T49.2X4	T49.2X5	T49.2X6
Pholcodine	T48.3X1	T48.3X2	T48.3X3	T48.3X4	T48.3X5	T48.3X6
Pholedrine	T46.991	T46.992	T46.993	T46.994	T46.995	T46.996
Phorate	T60.0X1	T60.0X2	T60.0X3	T60.0X4	--	--
Phosdrin	T60.0X1	T60.0X2	T60.0X3	T60.0X4	--	--
Phosfolan	T60.0X1	T60.0X2	T60.0X3	T60.0X4	--	--
Phosgene (gas)	T59.891	T59.892	T59.893	T59.894	--	--
Phosphamidon	T60.0X1	T60.0X2	T60.0X3	T60.0X4	--	--
Phosphate	T65.891	T65.892	T65.893	T65.894	--	--
- laxative	T47.4X1	T47.4X2	T47.4X3	T47.4X4	T47.4X5	T47.4X6
- organic	T60.0X1	T60.0X2	T60.0X3	T60.0X4	--	--
- solvent	T52.91	T52.92	T52.93	T52.94	--	--
- tricresyl	T65.891	T65.892	T65.893	T65.894	--	--
Phosphine	T57.1X1	T57.1X2	T57.1X3	T57.1X4	--	--
- fumigant	T57.1X1	T57.1X2	T57.1X3	T57.1X4	--	--
Phospholine	T49.5X1	T49.5X2	T49.5X3	T49.5X4	T49.5X5	T49.5X6
Phosphoric acid	T54.2X1	T54.2X2	T54.2X3	T54.2X4	--	--
Phosphorus (compound) NEC	T57.1X1	T57.1X2	T57.1X3	T57.1X4	--	--
- pesticide	T60.0X1	T60.0X2	T60.0X3	T60.0X4	--	--
Phthalates	T65.891	T65.892	T65.893	T65.894	--	--
Phthalic anhydride	T65.891	T65.892	T65.893	T65.894	--	--

Substance	Poisoning, Accidental (unintentional)	Poisoning, Intentional Self-harm	Poisoning, Assault	Poisoning, Undetermined	Adverse effect	Underdosing
Phthalimidoglutarimide	T42.6X1	T42.6X2	T42.6X3	T42.6X4	T42.6X5	T42.6X6
Phthalylsulfathiazole	T37.0X1	T37.0X2	T37.0X3	T37.0X4	T37.0X5	T37.0X6
Phylloquinone	T45.7X1	T45.7X2	T45.7X3	T45.7X4	T45.7X5	T45.7X6
Physeptone	T40.3X1	T40.3X2	T40.3X3	T40.3X4	T40.3X5	T40.3X6
Physostigma venenosum	T62.2X1	T62.2X2	T62.2X3	T62.2X4	--	--
Physostigmine	T49.5X1	T49.5X2	T49.5X3	T49.5X4	T49.5X5	T49.5X6
Phytolacca decandra	T62.2X1	T62.2X2	T62.2X3	T62.2X4	--	--
- berries	T62.1X1	T62.1X2	T62.1X3	T62.1X4	--	--
Phytomenadione	T45.7X1	T45.7X2	T45.7X3	T45.7X4	T45.7X5	T45.7X6
Phytonadione	T45.7X1	T45.7X2	T45.7X3	T45.7X4	T45.7X5	T45.7X6
Picoperine	T48.3X1	T48.3X2	T48.3X3	T48.3X4	T48.3X5	T48.3X6
Picosulfate (sodium)	T47.2X1	T47.2X2	T47.2X3	T47.2X4	T47.2X5	T47.2X6
Picric (acid)	T54.2X1	T54.2X2	T54.2X3	T54.2X4	--	--
Picrotoxin	T50.7X1	T50.7X2	T50.7X3	T50.7X4	T50.7X5	T50.7X6
Piketoprofen	T49.0X1	T49.0X2	T49.0X3	T49.0X4	T49.0X5	T49.0X6
Pilocarpine	T44.1X1	T44.1X2	T44.1X3	T44.1X4	T44.1X5	T44.1X6
Pilocarpus (jaborandi) extract	T44.1X1	T44.1X2	T44.1X3	T44.1X4	T44.1X5	T44.1X6
Pilsicainide (hydrochloride)	T46.2X1	T46.2X2	T46.2X3	T46.2X4	T46.2X5	T46.2X6
Pimaricin	T36.7X1	T36.7X2	T36.7X3	T36.7X4	T36.7X5	T36.7X6
Pimeclone	T50.7X1	T50.7X2	T50.7X3	T50.7X4	T50.7X5	T50.7X6
Pimelic ketone	T52.8X1	T52.8X2	T52.8X3	T52.8X4	--	--
Pimethixene	T45.0X1	T45.0X2	T45.0X3	T45.0X4	T45.0X5	T45.0X6
Piminodine	T40.2X1	T40.2X2	T40.2X3	T40.2X4	T40.2X5	T40.2X6
Pimozide	T43.591	T43.592	T43.593	T43.594	T43.595	T43.596
Pinacidil	T46.5X1	T46.5X2	T46.5X3	T46.5X4	T46.5X5	T46.5X6
Pinaverium bromide	T44.3X1	T44.3X2	T44.3X3	T44.3X4	T44.3X5	T44.3X6
Pinazepam	T42.4X1	T42.4X2	T42.4X3	T42.4X4	T42.4X5	T42.4X6
Pindolol	T44.7X1	T44.7X2	T44.7X3	T44.7X4	T44.7X5	T44.7X6
Pindone	T60.4X1	T60.4X2	T60.4X3	T60.4X4	--	--
Pine oil (disinfectant)	T65.891	T65.892	T65.893	T65.894	--	--
Pinkroot	T37.4X1	T37.4X2	T37.4X3	T37.4X4	T37.4X5	T37.4X6
Pipadone	T40.2X1	T40.2X2	T40.2X3	T40.2X4	--	--
Pipamazine	T45.0X1	T45.0X2	T45.0X3	T45.0X4	T45.0X5	T45.0X6
Pipamperone	T43.4X1	T43.4X2	T43.4X3	T43.4X4	T43.4X5	T43.4X6
Pipazetate	T48.3X1	T48.3X2	T48.3X3	T48.3X4	T48.3X5	T48.3X6
Pipemidic acid	T37.8X1	T37.8X2	T37.8X3	T37.8X4	T37.8X5	T37.8X6
Pipenzolate bromide	T44.3X1	T44.3X2	T44.3X3	T44.3X4	T44.3X5	T44.3X6
Piperacetazine	T43.3X1	T43.3X2	T43.3X3	T43.3X4	T43.3X5	T43.3X6
Piperacillin	T36.0X1	T36.0X2	T36.0X3	T36.0X4	T36.0X5	T36.0X6
Piperazine	T37.4X1	T37.4X2	T37.4X3	T37.4X4	T37.4X5	T37.4X6
- estrone sulfate	T38.5X1	T38.5X2	T38.5X3	T38.5X4	T38.5X5	T38.5X6
Piper cubeba	T62.2X1	T62.2X2	T62.2X3	T62.2X4	--	--
Piperidione	T48.3X1	T48.3X2	T48.3X3	T48.3X4	T48.3X5	T48.3X6
Piperidolate	T44.3X1	T44.3X2	T44.3X3	T44.3X4	T44.3X5	T44.3X6
Piperocaine	T41.3X1	T41.3X2	T41.3X3	T41.3X4	T41.3X5	T41.3X6
- infiltration (subcutaneous)	T41.3X1	T41.3X2	T41.3X3	T41.3X4	T41.3X5	T41.3X6
- nerve block (peripheral) (plexus)	T41.3X1	T41.3X2	T41.3X3	T41.3X4	T41.3X5	T41.3X6
- topical (surface)	T41.3X1	T41.3X2	T41.3X3	T41.3X4	T41.3X5	T41.3X6
Piperonyl butoxide	T60.8X1	T60.8X2	T60.8X3	T60.8X4	--	--
Pipethanate	T44.3X1	T44.3X2	T44.3X3	T44.3X4	T44.3X5	T44.3X6
Pipobroman	T45.1X1	T45.1X2	T45.1X3	T45.1X4	T45.1X5	T45.1X6
Pipotiazine	T43.3X1	T43.3X2	T43.3X3	T43.3X4	T43.3X5	T43.3X6
Pipoxizine	T45.0X1	T45.0X2	T45.0X3	T45.0X4	T45.0X5	T45.0X6
Pipradrol	T43.691	T43.692	T43.693	T43.694	T43.695	T43.696
Piprinhydrinate	T45.0X1	T45.0X2	T45.0X3	T45.0X4	T45.0X5	T45.0X6
Pirarubicin	T45.1X1	T45.1X2	T45.1X3	T45.1X4	T45.1X5	T45.1X6
Pirazinamide	T37.1X1	T37.1X2	T37.1X3	T37.1X4	T37.1X5	T37.1X6
Pirbuterol	T48.6X1	T48.6X2	T48.6X3	T48.6X4	T48.6X5	T48.6X6

Substance	Poisoning, Accidental (unintentional)	Poisoning, Intentional Self-harm	Poisoning, Assault	Poisoning, Undetermined	Adverse effect	Underdosing
Pirenzepine	T47.1X1	T47.1X2	T47.1X3	T47.1X4	T47.1X5	T47.1X6
Piretanide	T50.1X1	T50.1X2	T50.1X3	T50.1X4	T50.1X5	T50.1X6
Piribedil	T42.8X1	T42.8X2	T42.8X3	T42.8X4	T42.8X5	T42.8X6
Piridoxilate	T46.3X1	T46.3X2	T46.3X3	T46.3X4	T46.3X5	T46.3X6
Piritramide	T40.491	T40.492	T40.493	T40.494	--	--
Piromidic acid	T37.8X1	T37.8X2	T37.8X3	T37.8X4	T37.8X5	T37.8X6
Piroxicam	T39.391	T39.392	T39.393	T39.394	T39.395	T39.396
- beta-cyclodextrin complex	T39.8X1	T39.8X2	T39.8X3	T39.8X4	T39.8X5	T39.8X6
Pirozadil	T46.6X1	T46.6X2	T46.6X3	T46.6X4	T46.6X5	T46.6X6
Piscidia (bark) (erythrina)	T39.8X1	T39.8X2	T39.8X3	T39.8X4	T39.8X5	T39.8X6
Pitch	T65.891	T65.892	T65.893	T65.894	--	--
Pitkin's solution	T41.3X1	T41.3X2	T41.3X3	T41.3X4	T41.3X5	T41.3X6
Pitocin	T48.0X1	T48.0X2	T48.0X3	T48.0X4	T48.0X5	T48.0X6
Pitressin (tannate)	T38.891	T38.892	T38.893	T38.894	T38.895	T38.896
Pituitary extracts (posterior)	T38.891	T38.892	T38.893	T38.894	T38.895	T38.896
- anterior	T38.811	T38.812	T38.813	T38.814	T38.815	T38.816
Pituitrin	T38.891	T38.892	T38.893	T38.894	T38.895	T38.896
Pivampicillin	T36.0X1	T36.0X2	T36.0X3	T36.0X4	T36.0X5	T36.0X6
Pivmecillinam	T36.0X1	T36.0X2	T36.0X3	T36.0X4	T36.0X5	T36.0X6
Placental hormone	T38.891	T38.892	T38.893	T38.894	T38.895	T38.896
Placidyl	T42.6X1	T42.6X2	T42.6X3	T42.6X4	T42.6X5	T42.6X6
Plague vaccine	T50.A91	T50.A92	T50.A93	T50.A94	T50.A95	T50.A96
Plant						
- food or fertilizer NEC	T65.891	T65.892	T65.893	T65.894	--	--
- - containing herbicide	T60.3X1	T60.3X2	T60.3X3	T60.3X4	--	--
- noxious, used as food	T62.2X1	T62.2X2	T62.2X3	T62.2X4	--	--
- - berries	T62.1X1	T62.1X2	T62.1X3	T62.1X4	--	--
- - seeds	T62.2X1	T62.2X2	T62.2X3	T62.2X4	--	--
- - specified type NEC	T62.2X1	T62.2X2	T62.2X3	T62.2X4	--	--
Plasma	T45.8X1	T45.8X2	T45.8X3	T45.8X4	T45.8X5	T45.8X6
- expander NEC	T45.8X1	T45.8X2	T45.8X3	T45.8X4	T45.8X5	T45.8X6
- protein fraction (human)	T45.8X1	T45.8X2	T45.8X3	T45.8X4	T45.8X5	T45.8X6
Plasmanate	T45.8X1	T45.8X2	T45.8X3	T45.8X4	T45.8X5	T45.8X6
Plasminogen (tissue) activator	T45.611	T45.612	T45.613	T45.614	T45.615	T45.616
Plaster dressing	T49.3X1	T49.3X2	T49.3X3	T49.3X4	T49.3X5	T49.3X6
Plastic dressing	T49.3X1	T49.3X2	T49.3X3	T49.3X4	T49.3X5	T49.3X6
Plegicil	T43.3X1	T43.3X2	T43.3X3	T43.3X4	T43.3X5	T43.3X6
Plicamycin	T45.1X1	T45.1X2	T45.1X3	T45.1X4	T45.1X5	T45.1X6
Podophyllotoxin	T49.8X1	T49.8X2	T49.8X3	T49.8X4	T49.8X5	T49.8X6
Podophyllum (resin)	T49.4X1	T49.4X2	T49.4X3	T49.4X4	T49.4X5	T49.4X6
Poison NEC	T65.91	T65.92	T65.93	T65.94	--	--
Poisonous berries	T62.1X1	T62.1X2	T62.1X3	T62.1X4	--	--
Pokeweed (any part)	T62.2X1	T62.2X2	T62.2X3	T62.2X4	--	--
Poldine metilsulfate	T44.3X1	T44.3X2	T44.3X3	T44.3X4	T44.3X5	T44.3X6
Polidexide (sulfate)	T46.6X1	T46.6X2	T46.6X3	T46.6X4	T46.6X5	T46.6X6
Polidocanol	T46.8X1	T46.8X2	T46.8X3	T46.8X4	T46.8X5	T46.8X6
Poliomyelitis vaccine	T50.B91	T50.B92	T50.B93	T50.B94	T50.B95	T50.B96
Polish (car) (floor) (furni-ture) (metal) (porcelain) (silver)	T65.891	T65.892	T65.893	T65.894	--	--
- abrasive	T65.891	T65.892	T65.893	T65.894	--	--
- porcelain	T65.891	T65.892	T65.893	T65.894	--	--
Poloxalkol	T47.4X1	T47.4X2	T47.4X3	T47.4X4	T47.4X5	T47.4X6
Poloxamer	T47.4X1	T47.4X2	T47.4X3	T47.4X4	T47.4X5	T47.4X6
Polyaminostyrene resins	T50.3X1	T50.3X2	T50.3X3	T50.3X4	T50.3X5	T50.3X6
Polycarbophil	T47.4X1	T47.4X2	T47.4X3	T47.4X4	T47.4X5	T47.4X6
Polychlorinated biphenyl	T65.891	T65.892	T65.893	T65.894	--	--
Polycycline	T36.4X1	T36.4X2	T36.4X3	T36.4X4	T36.4X5	T36.4X6
Polyester fumes	T59.891	T59.892	T59.893	T59.894	--	--
Polyester resin hardener	T52.91	T52.92	T52.93	T52.94	--	--

Substance	Poisoning, Accidental (unintentional)	Poisoning, Intentional Self-harm	Poisoning, Assault	Poisoning, Undetermined	Adverse effect	Underdosing
- fumes	T59.891	T59.892	T59.893	T59.894	--	--
Polyestradiol phosphate	T38.5X1	T38.5X2	T38.5X3	T38.5X4	T38.5X5	T38.5X6
Polyethanolamine alkyl sulfate	T49.2X1	T49.2X2	T49.2X3	T49.2X4	T49.2X5	T49.2X6
Polyethylene adhesive	T49.3X1	T49.3X2	T49.3X3	T49.3X4	T49.3X5	T49.3X6
Polyferose	T45.4X1	T45.4X2	T45.4X3	T45.4X4	T45.4X5	T45.4X6
Polygeline	T45.8X1	T45.8X2	T45.8X3	T45.8X4	T45.8X5	T45.8X6
Polymyxin	T36.8X1	T36.8X2	T36.8X3	T36.8X4	T36.8X5	T36.8X6
- B	T36.8X1	T36.8X2	T36.8X3	T36.8X4	T36.8X5	T36.8X6
- - ENT agent	T49.6X1	T49.6X2	T49.6X3	T49.6X4	T49.6X5	T49.6X6
- - topical NEC	T49.0X1	T49.0X2	T49.0X3	T49.0X4	T49.0X5	T49.0X6
- E sulfate (eye preparation)	T49.5X1	T49.5X2	T49.5X3	T49.5X4	T49.5X5	T49.5X6
Polynoxylin	T49.0X1	T49.0X2	T49.0X3	T49.0X4	T49.0X5	T49.0X6
Polyoestradiol phosphate	T38.5X1	T38.5X2	T38.5X3	T38.5X4	T38.5X5	T38.5X6
Polyoxymethyleneurea	T49.0X1	T49.0X2	T49.0X3	T49.0X4	T49.0X5	T49.0X6
Polysilane	T47.8X1	T47.8X2	T47.8X3	T47.8X4	T47.8X5	T47.8X6
Polytetrafluoroethylene (inhaled)	T59.891	T59.892	T59.893	T59.894	--	--
Polythiazide	T50.2X1	T50.2X2	T50.2X3	T50.2X4	T50.2X5	T50.2X6
Polyvidone	T45.8X1	T45.8X2	T45.8X3	T45.8X4	T45.8X5	T45.8X6
Polyvinylpyrrolidone	T45.8X1	T45.8X2	T45.8X3	T45.8X4	T45.8X5	T45.8X6
Pontocaine (hydrochloride) (infiltration) (topical)	T41.3X1	T41.3X2	T41.3X3	T41.3X4	T41.3X5	T41.3X6
- nerve block (peripheral) (plexus)	T41.3X1	T41.3X2	T41.3X3	T41.3X4	T41.3X5	T41.3X6
- spinal	T41.3X1	T41.3X2	T41.3X3	T41.3X4	T41.3X5	T41.3X6
Porfiromycin	T45.1X1	T45.1X2	T45.1X3	T45.1X4	T45.1X5	T45.1X6
Posterior pituitary hormone NEC	T38.891	T38.892	T38.893	T38.894	T38.895	T38.896
Pot	T40.711	T40.712	T40.713	T40.714	T40.715	T40.716
Potash (caustic)	T54.3X1	T54.3X2	T54.3X3	T54.3X4	--	--
Potassic saline injection (lactated)	T50.3X1	T50.3X2	T50.3X3	T50.3X4	T50.3X5	T50.3X6
Potassium (salts) NEC	T50.3X1	T50.3X2	T50.3X3	T50.3X4	T50.3X5	T50.3X6
- aminobenzoate	T45.8X1	T45.8X2	T45.8X3	T45.8X4	T45.8X5	T45.8X6
- aminosalicylate	T37.1X1	T37.1X2	T37.1X3	T37.1X4	T37.1X5	T37.1X6
- antimony ' tartrate'	T37.8X1	T37.8X2	T37.8X3	T37.8X4	T37.8X5	T37.8X6
- arsenite (solution)	T57.0X1	T57.0X2	T57.0X3	T57.0X4	--	--
- bichromate	T56.2X1	T56.2X2	T56.2X3	T56.2X4	--	--
- bisulfate	T47.3X1	T47.3X2	T47.3X3	T47.3X4	T47.3X5	T47.3X6
- bromide	T42.6X1	T42.6X2	T42.6X3	T42.6X4	T42.6X5	T42.6X6
- canrenoate	T50.0X1	T50.0X2	T50.0X3	T50.0X4	T50.0X5	T50.0X6
- carbonate	T54.3X1	T54.3X2	T54.3X3	T54.3X4	--	--
- chlorate NEC	T65.891	T65.892	T65.893	T65.894	--	--
- chloride	T50.3X1	T50.3X2	T50.3X3	T50.3X4	T50.3X5	T50.3X6
- citrate	T50.991	T50.992	T50.993	T50.994	T50.995	T50.996
- cyanide	T65.0X1	T65.0X2	T65.0X3	T65.0X4	--	--
- ferric hexacyanoferrate (medicinal)	T50.6X1	T50.6X2	T50.6X3	T50.6X4	T50.6X5	T50.6X6
- - nonmedicinal	T65.891	T65.892	T65.893	T65.894	--	--
- Fluoride	T57.8X1	T57.8X2	T57.8X3	T57.8X4	--	--
- glucaldrate	T47.1X1	T47.1X2	T47.1X3	T47.1X4	T47.1X5	T47.1X6
- hydroxide	T54.3X1	T54.3X2	T54.3X3	T54.3X4	--	--
- iodate	T49.0X1	T49.0X2	T49.0X3	T49.0X4	T49.0X5	T49.0X6
- iodide	T48.4X1	T48.4X2	T48.4X3	T48.4X4	T48.4X5	T48.4X6
- nitrate	T57.8X1	T57.8X2	T57.8X3	T57.8X4	--	--
- oxalate	T65.891	T65.892	T65.893	T65.894	--	--
- perchlorate (nonmedicinal) NEC	T65.891	T65.892	T65.893	T65.894	--	--
- - antithyroid	T38.2X1	T38.2X2	T38.2X3	T38.2X4	T38.2X5	T38.2X6
- - medicinal	T38.2X1	T38.2X2	T38.2X3	T38.2X4	T38.2X5	T38.2X6
- Permanganate (nonmedicinal)	T65.891	T65.892	T65.893	T65.894	--	--
- - medicinal	T49.0X1	T49.0X2	T49.0X3	T49.0X4	T49.0X5	T49.0X6
- sulfate	T47.2X1	T47.2X2	T47.2X3	T47.2X4	T47.2X5	T47.2X6
Potassium-removing resin	T50.3X1	T50.3X2	T50.3X3	T50.3X4	T50.3X5	T50.3X6
Potassium-retaining drug	T50.3X1	T50.3X2	T50.3X3	T50.3X4	T50.3X5	T50.3X6

Substance	Poisoning, Accidental (unintentional)	Poisoning, Intentional Self-harm	Poisoning, Assault	Poisoning, Undetermined	Adverse effect	Underdosing
Povidone	T45.8X1	T45.8X2	T45.8X3	T45.8X4	T45.8X5	T45.8X6
- iodine	T49.0X1	T49.0X2	T49.0X3	T49.0X4	T49.0X5	T49.0X6
Practolol	T44.7X1	T44.7X2	T44.7X3	T44.7X4	T44.7X5	T44.7X6
Prajmalium bitartrate	T46.2X1	T46.2X2	T46.2X3	T46.2X4	T46.2X5	T46.2X6
Pralidoxime (iodide)	T50.6X1	T50.6X2	T50.6X3	T50.6X4	T50.6X5	T50.6X6
- chloride	T50.6X1	T50.6X2	T50.6X3	T50.6X4	T50.6X5	T50.6X6
Pramiverine	T44.3X1	T44.3X2	T44.3X3	T44.3X4	T44.3X5	T44.3X6
Pramocaine	T49.1X1	T49.1X2	T49.1X3	T49.1X4	T49.1X5	T49.1X6
Pramoxine	T49.1X1	T49.1X2	T49.1X3	T49.1X4	T49.1X5	T49.1X6
Prasterone	T38.7X1	T38.7X2	T38.7X3	T38.7X4	T38.7X5	T38.7X6
Pravastatin	T46.6X1	T46.6X2	T46.6X3	T46.6X4	T46.6X5	T46.6X6
Prazepam	T42.4X1	T42.4X2	T42.4X3	T42.4X4	T42.4X5	T42.4X6
Praziquantel	T37.4X1	T37.4X2	T37.4X3	T37.4X4	T37.4X5	T37.4X6
Prazitone	T43.291	T43.292	T43.293	T43.294	T43.295	T43.296
Prazosin	T44.6X1	T44.6X2	T44.6X3	T44.6X4	T44.6X5	T44.6X6
Prednicarbate	T49.0X1	T49.0X2	T49.0X3	T49.0X4	T49.0X5	T49.0X6
Prednimustine	T45.1X1	T45.1X2	T45.1X3	T45.1X4	T45.1X5	T45.1X6
Prednisolone	T38.0X1	T38.0X2	T38.0X3	T38.0X4	T38.0X5	T38.0X6
- ENT agent	T49.6X1	T49.6X2	T49.6X3	T49.6X4	T49.6X5	T49.6X6
- ophthalmic preparation	T49.5X1	T49.5X2	T49.5X3	T49.5X4	T49.5X5	T49.5X6
- steaglate	T49.0X1	T49.0X2	T49.0X3	T49.0X4	T49.0X5	T49.0X6
- topical NEC	T49.0X1	T49.0X2	T49.0X3	T49.0X4	T49.0X5	T49.0X6
Prednisone	T38.0X1	T38.0X2	T38.0X3	T38.0X4	T38.0X5	T38.0X6
Prednylidene	T38.0X1	T38.0X2	T38.0X3	T38.0X4	T38.0X5	T38.0X6
Pregnandiol	T38.5X1	T38.5X2	T38.5X3	T38.5X4	T38.5X5	T38.5X6
Pregneninolone	T38.5X1	T38.5X2	T38.5X3	T38.5X4	T38.5X5	T38.5X6
Preludin	T43.691	T43.692	T43.693	T43.694	T43.695	T43.696
Premarin	T38.5X1	T38.5X2	T38.5X3	T38.5X4	T38.5X5	T38.5X6
Premedication anesthetic	T41.201	T41.202	T41.203	T41.204	T41.205	T41.206
Prenalterol	T44.5X1	T44.5X2	T44.5X3	T44.5X4	T44.5X5	T44.5X6
Prenoxdiazine	T48.3X1	T48.3X2	T48.3X3	T48.3X4	T48.3X5	T48.3X6
Prenylamine	T46.3X1	T46.3X2	T46.3X3	T46.3X4	T46.3X5	T46.3X6
Preparation H	T49.8X1	T49.8X2	T49.8X3	T49.8X4	T49.8X5	T49.8X6
Preparation, local	T49.4X1	T49.4X2	T49.4X3	T49.4X4	T49.4X5	T49.4X6
Preservative (nonmedicinal)	T65.891	T65.892	T65.893	T65.894	--	--
- medicinal	T50.901	T50.902	T50.903	T50.904	T50.905	T50.906
- wood	T60.91	T60.92	T60.93	T60.94	--	--
Prethcamide	T50.7X1	T50.7X2	T50.7X3	T50.7X4	T50.7X5	T50.7X6
Pride of China	T62.2X1	T62.2X2	T62.2X3	T62.2X4	--	--
Pridinol	T44.3X1	T44.3X2	T44.3X3	T44.3X4	T44.3X5	T44.3X6
Prifinium bromide	T44.3X1	T44.3X2	T44.3X3	T44.3X4	T44.3X5	T44.3X6
Prilocaine	T41.3X1	T41.3X2	T41.3X3	T41.3X4	T41.3X5	T41.3X6
- infiltration (subcutaneous)	T41.3X1	T41.3X2	T41.3X3	T41.3X4	T41.3X5	T41.3X6
- nerve block peripheral (plexus)	T41.3X1	T41.3X2	T41.3X3	T41.3X4	T41.3X5	T41.3X6
- regional	T41.3X1	T41.3X2	T41.3X3	T41.3X4	T41.3X5	T41.3X6
Primaquine	T37.2X1	T37.2X2	T37.2X3	T37.2X4	T37.2X5	T37.2X6
Primidone	T42.6X1	T42.6X2	T42.6X3	T42.6X4	T42.6X5	T42.6X6
Primula (veris)	T62.2X1	T62.2X2	T62.2X3	T62.2X4	--	--
Prinadol	T40.2X1	T40.2X2	T40.2X3	T40.2X4	T40.2X5	T40.2X6
Priscol, Priscoline	T44.6X1	T44.6X2	T44.6X3	T44.6X4	T44.6X5	T44.6X6
Pristinamycin	T36.3X1	T36.3X2	T36.3X3	T36.3X4	T36.3X5	T36.3X6
Privet	T62.2X1	T62.2X2	T62.2X3	T62.2X4	--	--
- berries	T62.1X1	T62.1X2	T62.1X3	T62.1X4	--	--
Privine	T44.4X1	T44.4X2	T44.4X3	T44.4X4	T44.4X5	T44.4X6
Pro-Banthine	T44.3X1	T44.3X2	T44.3X3	T44.3X4	T44.3X5	T44.3X6
Probarbital	T42.3X1	T42.3X2	T42.3X3	T42.3X4	T42.3X5	T42.3X6
Probenecid	T50.4X1	T50.4X2	T50.4X3	T50.4X4	T50.4X5	T50.4X6
Probucol	T46.6X1	T46.6X2	T46.6X3	T46.6X4	T46.6X5	T46.6X6
Procainamide	T46.2X1	T46.2X2	T46.2X3	T46.2X4	T46.2X5	T46.2X6

Substance	Poisoning, Accidental (unintentional)	Poisoning, Intentional Self-harm	Poisoning, Assault	Poisoning, Undetermined	Adverse effect	Underdosing
Procaine	T41.3X1	T41.3X2	T41.3X3	T41.3X4	T41.3X5	T41.3X6
- benzylpenicillin	T36.0X1	T36.0X2	T36.0X3	T36.0X4	T36.0X5	T36.0X6
- nerve block (periphreal) (plexus)	T41.3X1	T41.3X2	T41.3X3	T41.3X4	T41.3X5	T41.3X6
- penicillin G	T36.0X1	T36.0X2	T36.0X3	T36.0X4	T36.0X5	T36.0X6
- regional	T41.3X1	T41.3X2	T41.3X3	T41.3X4	T41.3X5	T41.3X6
- spinal	T41.3X1	T41.3X2	T41.3X3	T41.3X4	T41.3X5	T41.3X6
Procalmidol	T43.591	T43.592	T43.593	T43.594	T43.595	T43.596
Procarbazine	T45.1X1	T45.1X2	T45.1X3	T45.1X4	T45.1X5	T45.1X6
Procaterol	T44.5X1	T44.5X2	T44.5X3	T44.5X4	T44.5X5	T44.5X6
Prochlorperazine	T43.3X1	T43.3X2	T43.3X3	T43.3X4	T43.3X5	T43.3X6
Procyclidine	T44.3X1	T44.3X2	T44.3X3	T44.3X4	T44.3X5	T44.3X6
Producer gas	T58.8X1	T58.8X2	T58.8X3	T58.8X4	--	--
Profadol	T40.491	T40.492	T40.493	T40.494	T40.495	T40.496
Profenamine	T44.3X1	T44.3X2	T44.3X3	T44.3X4	T44.3X5	T44.3X6
Profenil	T44.3X1	T44.3X2	T44.3X3	T44.3X4	T44.3X5	T44.3X6
Proflavine	T49.0X1	T49.0X2	T49.0X3	T49.0X4	T49.0X5	T49.0X6
Progabide	T42.6X1	T42.6X2	T42.6X3	T42.6X4	T42.6X5	T42.6X6
Progesterone	T38.5X1	T38.5X2	T38.5X3	T38.5X4	T38.5X5	T38.5X6
Progestin	T38.5X1	T38.5X2	T38.5X3	T38.5X4	T38.5X5	T38.5X6
- oral contraceptive	T38.4X1	T38.4X2	T38.4X3	T38.4X4	T38.4X5	T38.4X6
Progestogen NEC	T38.5X1	T38.5X2	T38.5X3	T38.5X4	T38.5X5	T38.5X6
Progestone	T38.5X1	T38.5X2	T38.5X3	T38.5X4	T38.5X5	T38.5X6
Proglumide	T47.1X1	T47.1X2	T47.1X3	T47.1X4	T47.1X5	T47.1X6
Proguanil	T37.2X1	T37.2X2	T37.2X3	T37.2X4	T37.2X5	T37.2X6
Prolactin	T38.811	T38.812	T38.813	T38.814	T38.815	T38.816
Prolintane	T43.691	T43.692	T43.693	T43.694	T43.695	T43.696
Proloid	T38.1X1	T38.1X2	T38.1X3	T38.1X4	T38.1X5	T38.1X6
Proluton	T38.5X1	T38.5X2	T38.5X3	T38.5X4	T38.5X5	T38.5X6
Promacetin	T37.1X1	T37.1X2	T37.1X3	T37.1X4	T37.1X5	T37.1X6
Promazine	T43.3X1	T43.3X2	T43.3X3	T43.3X4	T43.3X5	T43.3X6
Promedol	T40.2X1	T40.2X2	T40.2X3	T40.2X4	--	--
Promegestone	T38.5X1	T38.5X2	T38.5X3	T38.5X4	T38.5X5	T38.5X6
Promethazine (teoclate)	T43.3X1	T43.3X2	T43.3X3	T43.3X4	T43.3X5	T43.3X6
Promin	T37.1X1	T37.1X2	T37.1X3	T37.1X4	T37.1X5	T37.1X6
Pronase	T45.3X1	T45.3X2	T45.3X3	T45.3X4	T45.3X5	T45.3X6
Pronestyl (hydrochloride)	T46.2X1	T46.2X2	T46.2X3	T46.2X4	T46.2X5	T46.2X6
Pronetalol	T44.7X1	T44.7X2	T44.7X3	T44.7X4	T44.7X5	T44.7X6
Prontosil	T37.0X1	T37.0X2	T37.0X3	T37.0X4	T37.0X5	T37.0X6
Propachlor	T60.3X1	T60.3X2	T60.3X3	T60.3X4	--	--
Propafenone	T46.2X1	T46.2X2	T46.2X3	T46.2X4	T46.2X5	T46.2X6
Propallylonal	T42.3X1	T42.3X2	T42.3X3	T42.3X4	T42.3X5	T42.3X6
Propamidine	T49.0X1	T49.0X2	T49.0X3	T49.0X4	T49.0X5	T49.0X6
Propane (distributed in mobile container)	T59.891	T59.892	T59.893	T59.894	--	--
- distributed through pipes	T59.891	T59.892	T59.893	T59.894	--	--
- incomplete combustion	T58.11	T58.12	T58.13	T58.14	--	--
Propanidid	T41.291	T41.292	T41.293	T41.294	T41.295	T41.296
Propanil	T60.3X1	T60.3X2	T60.3X3	T60.3X4	--	--
1-Propanol	T51.3X1	T51.3X2	T51.3X3	T51.3X4	--	--
2-Propanol	T51.2X1	T51.2X2	T51.2X3	T51.2X4	--	--
Propantheline	T44.3X1	T44.3X2	T44.3X3	T44.3X4	T44.3X5	T44.3X6
- bromide	T44.3X1	T44.3X2	T44.3X3	T44.3X4	T44.3X5	T44.3X6
Proparacaine	T41.3X1	T41.3X2	T41.3X3	T41.3X4	T41.3X5	T41.3X6
Propatylnitrate	T46.3X1	T46.3X2	T46.3X3	T46.3X4	T46.3X5	T46.3X6
Propicillin	T36.0X1	T36.0X2	T36.0X3	T36.0X4	T36.0X5	T36.0X6
Propiolactone	T49.0X1	T49.0X2	T49.0X3	T49.0X4	T49.0X5	T49.0X6
Propiomazine	T45.0X1	T45.0X2	T45.0X3	T45.0X4	T45.0X5	T45.0X6
Propionaldehyde (medicinal)	T42.6X1	T42.6X2	T42.6X3	T42.6X4	T42.6X5	T42.6X6
Propionate (calcium) (sodium)	T49.0X1	T49.0X2	T49.0X3	T49.0X4	T49.0X5	T49.0X6

Substance	Poisoning, Accidental (unintentional)	Poisoning, Intentional Self-harm	Poisoning, Assault	Poisoning, Undetermined	Adverse effect	Underdosing
Propion gel	T49.0X1	T49.0X2	T49.0X3	T49.0X4	T49.0X5	T49.0X6
Propitocaine	T41.3X1	T41.3X2	T41.3X3	T41.3X4	T41.3X5	T41.3X6
- infiltration (subcutaneous)	T41.3X1	T41.3X2	T41.3X3	T41.3X4	T41.3X5	T41.3X6
- nerve block (peripheral) (plexus)	T41.3X1	T41.3X2	T41.3X3	T41.3X4	T41.3X5	T41.3X6
Propofol	T41.291	T41.292	T41.293	T41.294	T41.295	T41.296
Propoxur	T60.0X1	T60.0X2	T60.0X3	T60.0X4	--	--
Propoxycaine	T41.3X1	T41.3X2	T41.3X3	T41.3X4	T41.3X5	T41.3X6
- infiltration (subcutaneous)	T41.3X1	T41.3X2	T41.3X3	T41.3X4	T41.3X5	T41.3X6
- nerve block (peripheral) (plexus)	T41.3X1	T41.3X2	T41.3X3	T41.3X4	T41.3X5	T41.3X6
- topical (surface)	T41.3X1	T41.3X2	T41.3X3	T41.3X4	T41.3X5	T41.3X6
Propoxyphene	T40.491	T40.492	T40.493	T40.494	T40.495	T40.496
Propranolol	T44.7X1	T44.7X2	T44.7X3	T44.7X4	T44.7X5	T44.7X6
Propyl						
- alcohol	T51.3X1	T51.3X2	T51.3X3	T51.3X4	--	--
- carbinol	T51.3X1	T51.3X2	T51.3X3	T51.3X4	--	--
- hexadrine	T44.4X1	T44.4X2	T44.4X3	T44.4X4	T44.4X5	T44.4X6
- iodone	T50.8X1	T50.8X2	T50.8X3	T50.8X4	T50.8X5	T50.8X6
- thiouracil	T38.2X1	T38.2X2	T38.2X3	T38.2X4	T38.2X5	T38.2X6
Propylaminopheno-thiazine	T43.3X1	T43.3X2	T43.3X3	T43.3X4	T43.3X5	T43.3X6
Propylene	T59.891	T59.892	T59.893	T59.894	--	--
Propylhexedrine	T48.5X1	T48.5X2	T48.5X3	T48.5X4	T48.5X5	T48.5X6
Propyliodone	T50.8X1	T50.8X2	T50.8X3	T50.8X4	T50.8X5	T50.8X6
Propylparaben (ophthalmic)	T49.5X1	T49.5X2	T49.5X3	T49.5X4	T49.5X5	T49.5X6
Propylthiouracil	T38.2X1	T38.2X2	T38.2X3	T38.2X4	T38.2X5	T38.2X6
Propyphenazone	T39.2X1	T39.2X2	T39.2X3	T39.2X4	T39.2X5	T39.2X6
Proquazone	T39.391	T39.392	T39.393	T39.394	T39.395	T39.396
Proscillaridin	T46.0X1	T46.0X2	T46.0X3	T46.0X4	T46.0X5	T46.0X6
Prostacyclin	T45.521	T45.522	T45.523	T45.524	T45.525	T45.526
Prostaglandin (I2)	T45.521	T45.522	T45.523	T45.524	T45.525	T45.526
- E1	T46.7X1	T46.7X2	T46.7X3	T46.7X4	T46.7X5	T46.7X6
- E2	T48.0X1	T48.0X2	T48.0X3	T48.0X4	T48.0X5	T48.0X6
- F2 alpha	T48.0X1	T48.0X2	T48.0X3	T48.0X4	T48.0X5	T48.0X6
Prostigmin	T44.0X1	T44.0X2	T44.0X3	T44.0X4	T44.0X5	T44.0X6
Prosultiamine	T45.2X1	T45.2X2	T45.2X3	T45.2X4	T45.2X5	T45.2X6
Protamine sulfate	T45.7X1	T45.7X2	T45.7X3	T45.7X4	T45.7X5	T45.7X6
- zinc insulin	T38.3X1	T38.3X2	T38.3X3	T38.3X4	T38.3X5	T38.3X6
Protease	T47.5X1	T47.5X2	T47.5X3	T47.5X4	T47.5X5	T47.5X6
Protectant, skin NEC	T49.3X1	T49.3X2	T49.3X3	T49.3X4	T49.3X5	T49.3X6
Protein hydrolysate	T50.991	T50.992	T50.993	T50.994	T50.995	T50.996
Prothiaden—see Dothiepin hydrochloride						
Prothionamide	T37.1X1	T37.1X2	T37.1X3	T37.1X4	T37.1X5	T37.1X6
Prothipendyl	T43.591	T43.592	T43.593	T43.594	T43.595	T43.596
Prothoate	T60.0X1	T60.0X2	T60.0X3	T60.0X4	--	--
Prothrombin						
- activator	T45.7X1	T45.7X2	T45.7X3	T45.7X4	T45.7X5	T45.7X6
- synthesis inhibitor	T45.511	T45.512	T45.513	T45.514	T45.515	T45.516
Protionamide	T37.1X1	T37.1X2	T37.1X3	T37.1X4	T37.1X5	T37.1X6
Protirelin	T38.891	T38.892	T38.893	T38.894	T38.895	T38.896
Protokylol	T48.6X1	T48.6X2	T48.6X3	T48.6X4	T48.6X5	T48.6X6
Protopam	T50.6X1	T50.6X2	T50.6X3	T50.6X4	T50.6X5	T50.6X6
Protoveratrine (s) (A) (B)	T46.5X1	T46.5X2	T46.5X3	T46.5X4	T46.5X5	T46.5X6
Protriptyline	T43.011	T43.012	T43.013	T43.014	T43.015	T43.016
Provera	T38.5X1	T38.5X2	T38.5X3	T38.5X4	T38.5X5	T38.5X6
Provitamin A	T45.2X1	T45.2X2	T45.2X3	T45.2X4	T45.2X5	T45.2X6
Proxibarbal	T42.3X1	T42.3X2	T42.3X3	T42.3X4	T42.3X5	T42.3X6
Proxymetacaine	T41.3X1	T41.3X2	T41.3X3	T41.3X4	T41.3X5	T41.3X6
Proxyphylline	T48.6X1	T48.6X2	T48.6X3	T48.6X4	T48.6X5	T48.6X6
Prozac—see Fluoxetine hydrochloride						
Prunus						

Substance	Poisoning, Accidental (unintentional)	Poisoning, Intentional Self-harm	Poisoning, Assault	Poisoning, Undetermined	Adverse effect	Underdosing
- laurocerasus	T62.2X1	T62.2X2	T62.2X3	T62.2X4	--	--
- virginiana	T62.2X1	T62.2X2	T62.2X3	T62.2X4	--	--
Prussian blue						
- commercial	T65.891	T65.892	T65.893	T65.894	--	--
- therapeutic	T50.6X1	T50.6X2	T50.6X3	T50.6X4	T50.6X5	T50.6X6
Prussic acid	T65.0X1	T65.0X2	T65.0X3	T65.0X4	--	--
- vapor	T57.3X1	T57.3X2	T57.3X3	T57.3X4	--	--
Pseudoephedrine	T44.991	T44.992	T44.993	T44.994	T44.995	T44.996
Psilocin	T40.991	T40.992	T40.993	T40.994	--	--
Psilocybin	T40.991	T40.992	T40.993	T40.994	--	--
Psilocybine	T40.991	T40.992	T40.993	T40.994	--	--
Psoralene (nonmedicinal)	T65.891	T65.892	T65.893	T65.894	--	--
Psoralens (medicinal)	T50.991	T50.992	T50.993	T50.994	T50.995	T50.996
PSP (phenolsulfonphthalein)	T50.8X1	T50.8X2	T50.8X3	T50.8X4	T50.8X5	T50.8X6
Psychodysleptic drug NOS	T40.901	T40.902	T40.903	T40.904	T40.905	T40.906
- specified NEC	T40.991	T40.992	T40.993	T40.994	T40.995	T40.996
Psychostimulant	T43.601	T43.602	T43.603	T43.604	T43.605	T43.606
- amphetamine	T43.621	T43.622	T43.623	T43.624	T43.625	T43.626
- caffeine	T43.611	T43.612	T43.613	T43.614	T43.615	T43.616
- methylphenidate	T43.631	T43.632	T43.633	T43.634	T43.635	T43.636
- specified NEC	T43.691	T43.692	T43.693	T43.694	T43.695	T43.696
Psychotherapeutic drug NEC	T43.91	T43.92	T43.93	T43.94	T43.95	T43.96
- antidepressants—see also Antidepressant	T43.201	T43.202	T43.203	T43.204	T43.205	T43.206
- specified NEC	T43.8X1	T43.8X2	T43.8X3	T43.8X4	T43.8X5	T43.8X6
- tranquilizers NEC	T43.501	T43.502	T43.503	T43.504	T43.505	T43.506
Psychotomimetic agents	T40.901	T40.902	T40.903	T40.904	T40.905	T40.906
Psychotropic drug NEC	T43.91	T43.92	T43.93	T43.94	T43.95	T43.96
- specified NEC	T43.8X1	T43.8X2	T43.8X3	T43.8X4	T43.8X5	T43.8X6
Psyllium hydrophilic mucilloid	T47.4X1	T47.4X2	T47.4X3	T47.4X4	T47.4X5	T47.4X6
Pteroylglutamic acid	T45.8X1	T45.8X2	T45.8X3	T45.8X4	T45.8X5	T45.8X6
Pteroyltriglutamate	T45.1X1	T45.1X2	T45.1X3	T45.1X4	T45.1X5	T45.1X6
PTFE—see Polytetrafluoroethylene						
Pulp						
- devitalizing paste	T49.7X1	T49.7X2	T49.7X3	T49.7X4	T49.7X5	T49.7X6
- dressing	T49.7X1	T49.7X2	T49.7X3	T49.7X4	T49.7X5	T49.7X6
Pulsatilla	T62.2X1	T62.2X2	T62.2X3	T62.2X4	--	--
Pumpkin seed extract	T37.4X1	T37.4X2	T37.4X3	T37.4X4	T37.4X5	T37.4X6
Purex (bleach)	T54.91	T54.92	T54.93	T54.94	--	--
Purgative NEC—see also Cathartic	T47.4X1	T47.4X2	T47.4X3	T47.4X4	T47.4X5	T47.4X6
Purine analogue (antineoplastic)	T45.1X1	T45.1X2	T45.1X3	T45.1X4	T45.1X5	T45.1X6
Purine diuretics	T50.2X1	T50.2X2	T50.2X3	T50.2X4	T50.2X5	T50.2X6
Purinethol	T45.1X1	T45.1X2	T45.1X3	T45.1X4	T45.1X5	T45.1X6
PVP	T45.8X1	T45.8X2	T45.8X3	T45.8X4	T45.8X5	T45.8X6
Pyrabital	T39.8X1	T39.8X2	T39.8X3	T39.8X4	T39.8X5	T39.8X6
Pyramidon	T39.2X1	T39.2X2	T39.2X3	T39.2X4	T39.2X5	T39.2X6
Pyrantel	T37.4X1	T37.4X2	T37.4X3	T37.4X4	T37.4X5	T37.4X6
Pyrathiazine	T45.0X1	T45.0X2	T45.0X3	T45.0X4	T45.0X5	T45.0X6
Pyrazinamide	T37.1X1	T37.1X2	T37.1X3	T37.1X4	T37.1X5	T37.1X6
Pyrazinoic acid (amide)	T37.1X1	T37.1X2	T37.1X3	T37.1X4	T37.1X5	T37.1X6
Pyrazole (derivatives)	T39.2X1	T39.2X2	T39.2X3	T39.2X4	T39.2X5	T39.2X6
Pyrazolone analgesic NEC	T39.2X1	T39.2X2	T39.2X3	T39.2X4	T39.2X5	T39.2X6
Pyrethrin, pyrethrum (nonmedicinal)	T60.2X1	T60.2X2	T60.2X3	T60.2X4	--	--
Pyrethrum extract	T49.0X1	T49.0X2	T49.0X3	T49.0X4	T49.0X5	T49.0X6
Pyribenzamine	T45.0X1	T45.0X2	T45.0X3	T45.0X4	T45.0X5	T45.0X6
Pyridine	T52.8X1	T52.8X2	T52.8X3	T52.8X4	--	--
- aldoxime methiodide	T50.6X1	T50.6X2	T50.6X3	T50.6X4	T50.6X5	T50.6X6
- aldoxime methyl chloride	T50.6X1	T50.6X2	T50.6X3	T50.6X4	T50.6X5	T50.6X6
- vapor	T59.891	T59.892	T59.893	T59.894	--	--

Substance	Poisoning, Accidental (unintentional)	Poisoning, Intentional Self-harm	Poisoning, Assault	Poisoning, Undetermined	Adverse effect	Underdosing
Pyridium	T39.8X1	T39.8X2	T39.8X3	T39.8X4	T39.8X5	T39.8X6
Pyridostigmine bromide	T44.0X1	T44.0X2	T44.0X3	T44.0X4	T44.0X5	T44.0X6
Pyridoxal phosphate	T45.2X1	T45.2X2	T45.2X3	T45.2X4	T45.2X5	T45.2X6
Pyridoxine	T45.2X1	T45.2X2	T45.2X3	T45.2X4	T45.2X5	T45.2X6
Pyrilamine	T45.0X1	T45.0X2	T45.0X3	T45.0X4	T45.0X5	T45.0X6
Pyrimethamine	T37.2X1	T37.2X2	T37.2X3	T37.2X4	T37.2X5	T37.2X6
- with sulfadoxine	T37.2X1	T37.2X2	T37.2X3	T37.2X4	T37.2X5	T37.2X6
Pyrimidine antagonist	T45.1X1	T45.1X2	T45.1X3	T45.1X4	T45.1X5	T45.1X6
Pyriminil	T60.4X1	T60.4X2	T60.4X3	T60.4X4	--	--
Pyrithione zinc	T49.4X1	T49.4X2	T49.4X3	T49.4X4	T49.4X5	T49.4X6
Pyrithyldione	T42.6X1	T42.6X2	T42.6X3	T42.6X4	T42.6X5	T42.6X6
Pyrogallic acid	T49.0X1	T49.0X2	T49.0X3	T49.0X4	T49.0X5	T49.0X6
Pyrogallol	T49.0X1	T49.0X2	T49.0X3	T49.0X4	T49.0X5	T49.0X6
Pyroxylin	T49.3X1	T49.3X2	T49.3X3	T49.3X4	T49.3X5	T49.3X6
Pyrrobutamine	T45.0X1	T45.0X2	T45.0X3	T45.0X4	T45.0X5	T45.0X6
Pyrrolizidine alkaloids	T62.8X1	T62.8X2	T62.8X3	T62.8X4	--	--
Pyrvinium chloride	T37.4X1	T37.4X2	T37.4X3	T37.4X4	T37.4X5	T37.4X6
PZI	T38.3X1	T38.3X2	T38.3X3	T38.3X4	T38.3X5	T38.3X6
Quaalude	T42.6X1	T42.6X2	T42.6X3	T42.6X4	T42.6X5	T42.6X6
Quarternary ammonium						
- anti-infective	T49.0X1	T49.0X2	T49.0X3	T49.0X4	T49.0X5	T49.0X6
- ganglion blocking	T44.2X1	T44.2X2	T44.2X3	T44.2X4	T44.2X5	T44.2X6
- parasympatholytic	T44.3X1	T44.3X2	T44.3X3	T44.3X4	T44.3X5	T44.3X6
Quazepam	T42.4X1	T42.4X2	T42.4X3	T42.4X4	T42.4X5	T42.4X6
Quicklime	T54.3X1	T54.3X2	T54.3X3	T54.3X4	--	--
Quillaja extract	T48.4X1	T48.4X2	T48.4X3	T48.4X4	T48.4X5	T48.4X6
Quinacrine	T37.2X1	T37.2X2	T37.2X3	T37.2X4	T37.2X5	T37.2X6
Quinaglute	T46.2X1	T46.2X2	T46.2X3	T46.2X4	T46.2X5	T46.2X6
Quinalbarbital	T42.3X1	T42.3X2	T42.3X3	T42.3X4	T42.3X5	T42.3X6
Quinalbarbitone sodium	T42.3X1	T42.3X2	T42.3X3	T42.3X4	T42.3X5	T42.3X6
Quinalphos	T60.0X1	T60.0X2	T60.0X3	T60.0X4	--	--
Quinapril	T46.4X1	T46.4X2	T46.4X3	T46.4X4	T46.4X5	T46.4X6
Quinestradiol	T38.5X1	T38.5X2	T38.5X3	T38.5X4	T38.5X5	T38.5X6
Quinestradol	T38.5X1	T38.5X2	T38.5X3	T38.5X4	T38.5X5	T38.5X6
Quinestrol	T38.5X1	T38.5X2	T38.5X3	T38.5X4	T38.5X5	T38.5X6
Quinethazone	T50.2X1	T50.2X2	T50.2X3	T50.2X4	T50.2X5	T50.2X6
Quingestanol	T38.4X1	T38.4X2	T38.4X3	T38.4X4	T38.4X5	T38.4X6
Quinidine	T46.2X1	T46.2X2	T46.2X3	T46.2X4	T46.2X5	T46.2X6
Quinine	T37.2X1	T37.2X2	T37.2X3	T37.2X4	T37.2X5	T37.2X6
Quiniobine	T37.8X1	T37.8X2	T37.8X3	T37.8X4	T37.8X5	T37.8X6
Quinisocaine	T49.1X1	T49.1X2	T49.1X3	T49.1X4	T49.1X5	T49.1X6
Quinocide	T37.2X1	T37.2X2	T37.2X3	T37.2X4	T37.2X5	T37.2X6
Quinoline (derivatives) NEC	T37.8X1	T37.8X2	T37.8X3	T37.8X4	T37.8X5	T37.8X6
Quinupramine	T43.011	T43.012	T43.013	T43.014	T43.015	T43.016
Quotane	T41.3X1	T41.3X2	T41.3X3	T41.3X4	T41.3X5	T41.3X6
Rabies						
- immune globulin (human)	T50.Z11	T50.Z12	T50.Z13	T50.Z14	T50.Z15	T50.Z16
- vaccine	T50.B91	T50.B92	T50.B93	T50.B94	T50.B95	T50.B96
Racemoramide	T40.2X1	T40.2X2	T40.2X3	T40.2X4	--	--
Racemorphan	T40.2X1	T40.2X2	T40.2X3	T40.2X4	T40.2X5	T40.2X6
Racepinefrin	T44.5X1	T44.5X2	T44.5X3	T44.5X4	T44.5X5	T44.5X6
Raclopride	T43.591	T43.592	T43.593	T43.594	T43.595	T43.596
Radiator alcohol	T51.1X1	T51.1X2	T51.1X3	T51.1X4	--	--
Radioactive drug NEC	T50.8X1	T50.8X2	T50.8X3	T50.8X4	T50.8X5	T50.8X6
Radio-opaque (drugs) (materials)	T50.8X1	T50.8X2	T50.8X3	T50.8X4	T50.8X5	T50.8X6
Ramifenazone	T39.2X1	T39.2X2	T39.2X3	T39.2X4	T39.2X5	T39.2X6
Ramipril	T46.4X1	T46.4X2	T46.4X3	T46.4X4	T46.4X5	T46.4X6
Ranitidine	T47.0X1	T47.0X2	T47.0X3	T47.0X4	T47.0X5	T47.0X6
Ranunculus	T62.2X1	T62.2X2	T62.2X3	T62.2X4	--	--

Substance	Poisoning, Accidental (unintentional)	Poisoning, Intentional Self-harm	Poisoning, Assault	Poisoning, Undetermined	Adverse effect	Underdosing
Rat poison NEC	T60.4X1	T60.4X2	T60.4X3	T60.4X4	--	--
Rattlesnake (venom)	T63.011	T63.012	T63.013	T63.014	--	--
Raubasine	T46.7X1	T46.7X2	T46.7X3	T46.7X4	T46.7X5	T46.7X6
Raudixin	T46.5X1	T46.5X2	T46.5X3	T46.5X4	T46.5X5	T46.5X6
Rautensin	T46.5X1	T46.5X2	T46.5X3	T46.5X4	T46.5X5	T46.5X6
Rautina	T46.5X1	T46.5X2	T46.5X3	T46.5X4	T46.5X5	T46.5X6
Rautotal	T46.5X1	T46.5X2	T46.5X3	T46.5X4	T46.5X5	T46.5X6
Rauwiloid	T46.5X1	T46.5X2	T46.5X3	T46.5X4	T46.5X5	T46.5X6
Rauwoldin	T46.5X1	T46.5X2	T46.5X3	T46.5X4	T46.5X5	T46.5X6
Rauwolfia (alkaloids)	T46.5X1	T46.5X2	T46.5X3	T46.5X4	T46.5X5	T46.5X6
Razoxane	T45.1X1	T45.1X2	T45.1X3	T45.1X4	T45.1X5	T45.1X6
Realgar	T57.0X1	T57.0X2	T57.0X3	T57.0X4	--	--
Recombinant (R) —see specific protein						
Red blood cells, packed	T45.8X1	T45.8X2	T45.8X3	T45.8X4	T45.8X5	T45.8X6
Red squill (scilliroside)	T60.4X1	T60.4X2	T60.4X3	T60.4X4	--	--
Reducing agent, industrial NEC	T65.891	T65.892	T65.893	T65.894	--	--
Refrigerant gas (chlorofluoro-carbon)	T53.5X1	T53.5X2	T53.5X3	T53.5X4	--	--
- not chlorofluoro-carbon	T59.891	T59.892	T59.893	T59.894	--	--
Regroton	T50.2X1	T50.2X2	T50.2X3	T50.2X4	T50.2X5	T50.2X6
Rehydration salts (oral)	T50.3X1	T50.3X2	T50.3X3	T50.3X4	T50.3X5	T50.3X6
Rela	T42.8X1	T42.8X2	T42.8X3	T42.8X4	T42.8X5	T42.8X6
Relaxant, muscle						
- anesthetic	T48.1X1	T48.1X2	T48.1X3	T48.1X4	T48.1X5	T48.1X6
- central nervous system	T42.8X1	T42.8X2	T42.8X3	T42.8X4	T42.8X5	T42.8X6
- skeletal NEC	T48.1X1	T48.1X2	T48.1X3	T48.1X4	T48.1X5	T48.1X6
- smooth NEC	T44.3X1	T44.3X2	T44.3X3	T44.3X4	T44.3X5	T44.3X6
Remoxipride	T43.591	T43.592	T43.593	T43.594	T43.595	T43.596
Renese	T50.2X1	T50.2X2	T50.2X3	T50.2X4	T50.2X5	T50.2X6
Renografin	T50.8X1	T50.8X2	T50.8X3	T50.8X4	T50.8X5	T50.8X6
Replacement solution	T50.3X1	T50.3X2	T50.3X3	T50.3X4	T50.3X5	T50.3X6
Reproterol	T48.6X1	T48.6X2	T48.6X3	T48.6X4	T48.6X5	T48.6X6
Rescinnamine	T46.5X1	T46.5X2	T46.5X3	T46.5X4	T46.5X5	T46.5X6
Reserpin (e)	T46.5X1	T46.5X2	T46.5X3	T46.5X4	T46.5X5	T46.5X6
Resorcin, resorcinol (nonmedicinal)	T65.891	T65.892	T65.893	T65.894	--	--
- medicinal	T49.4X1	T49.4X2	T49.4X3	T49.4X4	T49.4X5	T49.4X6
Respaire	T48.4X1	T48.4X2	T48.4X3	T48.4X4	T48.4X5	T48.4X6
Respiratory drug NEC	T48.901	T48.902	T48.903	T48.904	T48.905	T48.906
- antiasthmatic NEC	T48.6X1	T48.6X2	T48.6X3	T48.6X4	T48.6X5	T48.6X6
- anti-common-cold NEC	T48.5X1	T48.5X2	T48.5X3	T48.5X4	T48.5X5	T48.5X6
- expectorant NEC	T48.4X1	T48.4X2	T48.4X3	T48.4X4	T48.4X5	T48.4X6
- stimulant	T48.901	T48.902	T48.903	T48.904	T48.905	T48.906
Retinoic acid	T49.0X1	T49.0X2	T49.0X3	T49.0X4	T49.0X5	T49.0X6
Retinol	T45.2X1	T45.2X2	T45.2X3	T45.2X4	T45.2X5	T45.2X6
Rh (D) immune globulin (human)	T50.Z11	T50.Z12	T50.Z13	T50.Z14	T50.Z15	T50.Z16
Rhodine	T39.011	T39.012	T39.013	T39.014	T39.015	T39.016
RhoGAM	T50.Z11	T50.Z12	T50.Z13	T50.Z14	T50.Z15	T50.Z16
Rhubarb						
- dry extract	T47.2X1	T47.2X2	T47.2X3	T47.2X4	T47.2X5	T47.2X6
- tincture, compound	T47.2X1	T47.2X2	T47.2X3	T47.2X4	T47.2X5	T47.2X6
Ribavirin	T37.5X1	T37.5X2	T37.5X3	T37.5X4	T37.5X5	T37.5X6
Riboflavin	T45.2X1	T45.2X2	T45.2X3	T45.2X4	T45.2X5	T45.2X6
Ribostamycin	T36.5X1	T36.5X2	T36.5X3	T36.5X4	T36.5X5	T36.5X6
Ricin	T62.2X1	T62.2X2	T62.2X3	T62.2X4	--	--
Ricinus communis	T62.2X1	T62.2X2	T62.2X3	T62.2X4	--	--
Rickettsial vaccine NEC	T50.A91	T50.A92	T50.A93	T50.A94	T50.A95	T50.A96
Rifabutin	T36.6X1	T36.6X2	T36.6X3	T36.6X4	T36.6X5	T36.6X6
Rifamide	T36.6X1	T36.6X2	T36.6X3	T36.6X4	T36.6X5	T36.6X6
Rifampicin	T36.6X1	T36.6X2	T36.6X3	T36.6X4	T36.6X5	T36.6X6

Substance	Poisoning, Accidental (unintentional)	Poisoning, Intentional Self-harm	Poisoning, Assault	Poisoning, Undetermined	Adverse effect	Underdosing
- with isoniazid	T37.1X1	T37.1X2	T37.1X3	T37.1X4	T37.1X5	T37.1X6
Rifampin	T36.6X1	T36.6X2	T36.6X3	T36.6X4	T36.6X5	T36.6X6
Rifamycin	T36.6X1	T36.6X2	T36.6X3	T36.6X4	T36.6X5	T36.6X6
Rifaximin	T36.6X1	T36.6X2	T36.6X3	T36.6X4	T36.6X5	T36.6X6
Rimantadine	T37.5X1	T37.5X2	T37.5X3	T37.5X4	T37.5X5	T37.5X6
Rimazolium metilsulfate	T39.8X1	T39.8X2	T39.8X3	T39.8X4	T39.8X5	T39.8X6
Rimifon	T37.1X1	T37.1X2	T37.1X3	T37.1X4	T37.1X5	T37.1X6
Rimiterol	T48.6X1	T48.6X2	T48.6X3	T48.6X4	T48.6X5	T48.6X6
Ringer (lactate) solution	T50.3X1	T50.3X2	T50.3X3	T50.3X4	T50.3X5	T50.3X6
Ristocetin	T36.8X1	T36.8X2	T36.8X3	T36.8X4	T36.8X5	T36.8X6
Ritalin	T43.631	T43.632	T43.633	T43.634	T43.635	T43.636
Ritodrine	T44.5X1	T44.5X2	T44.5X3	T44.5X4	T44.5X5	T44.5X6
Roach killer—see Insecticide						
Rociverine	T44.3X1	T44.3X2	T44.3X3	T44.3X4	T44.3X5	T44.3X6
Rocky Mountain spotted fever vaccine	T50.A91	T50.A92	T50.A93	T50.A94	T50.A95	T50.A96
Rodenticide NEC	T60.4X1	T60.4X2	T60.4X3	T60.4X4	--	--
Rohypnol	T42.4X1	T42.4X2	T42.4X3	T42.4X4	T42.4X5	T42.4X6
Rokitamycin	T36.3X1	T36.3X2	T36.3X3	T36.3X4	T36.3X5	T36.3X6
Rolaids	T47.1X1	T47.1X2	T47.1X3	T47.1X4	T47.1X5	T47.1X6
Rolitetracycline	T36.4X1	T36.4X2	T36.4X3	T36.4X4	T36.4X5	T36.4X6
Romilar	T48.3X1	T48.3X2	T48.3X3	T48.3X4	T48.3X5	T48.3X6
Ronifibrate	T46.6X1	T46.6X2	T46.6X3	T46.6X4	T46.6X5	T46.6X6
Rosaprostol	T47.1X1	T47.1X2	T47.1X3	T47.1X4	T47.1X5	T47.1X6
Rose bengal sodium (131I)	T50.8X1	T50.8X2	T50.8X3	T50.8X4	T50.8X5	T50.8X6
Rose water ointment	T49.3X1	T49.3X2	T49.3X3	T49.3X4	T49.3X5	T49.3X6
Rosoxacin	T37.8X1	T37.8X2	T37.8X3	T37.8X4	T37.8X5	T37.8X6
Rotenone	T60.2X1	T60.2X2	T60.2X3	T60.2X4	--	--
Rotoxamine	T45.0X1	T45.0X2	T45.0X3	T45.0X4	T45.0X5	T45.0X6
Rough-on-rats	T60.4X1	T60.4X2	T60.4X3	T60.4X4	--	--
Roxatidine	T47.0X1	T47.0X2	T47.0X3	T47.0X4	T47.0X5	T47.0X6
Roxithromycin	T36.3X1	T36.3X2	T36.3X3	T36.3X4	T36.3X5	T36.3X6
Rt-PA	T45.611	T45.612	T45.613	T45.614	T45.615	T45.616
Rubbing alcohol	T51.2X1	T51.2X2	T51.2X3	T51.2X4	--	--
Rubefacient	T49.4X1	T49.4X2	T49.4X3	T49.4X4	T49.4X5	T49.4X6
Rubella vaccine	T50.B91	T50.B92	T50.B93	T50.B94	T50.B95	T50.B96
Rubeola vaccine	T50.B91	T50.B92	T50.B93	T50.B94	T50.B95	T50.B96
Rubidium chloride Rb82	T50.8X1	T50.8X2	T50.8X3	T50.8X4	T50.8X5	T50.8X6
Rubidomycin	T45.1X1	T45.1X2	T45.1X3	T45.1X4	T45.1X5	T45.1X6
Rue	T62.2X1	T62.2X2	T62.2X3	T62.2X4	--	--
Rufocromomycin	T45.1X1	T45.1X2	T45.1X3	T45.1X4	T45.1X5	T45.1X6
Russel's viper venin	T45.7X1	T45.7X2	T45.7X3	T45.7X4	T45.7X5	T45.7X6
Ruta (graveolens)	T62.2X1	T62.2X2	T62.2X3	T62.2X4	--	--
Rutinum	T46.991	T46.992	T46.993	T46.994	T46.995	T46.996
Rutoside	T46.991	T46.992	T46.993	T46.994	T46.995	T46.996
Sabadilla (plant)	T62.2X1	T62.2X2	T62.2X3	T62.2X4	--	--
- pesticide	T60.2X1	T60.2X2	T60.2X3	T60.2X4	--	--
Saccharated iron oxide	T45.8X1	T45.8X2	T45.8X3	T45.8X4	T45.8X5	T45.8X6
Saccharin	T50.901	T50.902	T50.903	T50.904	T50.905	T50.906
Saccharomyces boulardii	T47.6X1	T47.6X2	T47.6X3	T47.6X4	T47.6X5	T47.6X6
Safflower oil	T46.6X1	T46.6X2	T46.6X3	T46.6X4	T46.6X5	T46.6X6
Safrazine	T43.1X1	T43.1X2	T43.1X3	T43.1X4	T43.1X5	T43.1X6
Salazosulfapyridine	T37.0X1	T37.0X2	T37.0X3	T37.0X4	T37.0X5	T37.0X6
Salbutamol	T48.6X1	T48.6X2	T48.6X3	T48.6X4	T48.6X5	T48.6X6
Salicylamide	T39.091	T39.092	T39.093	T39.094	T39.095	T39.096
Salicylate NEC	T39.091	T39.092	T39.093	T39.094	T39.095	T39.096
- methyl	T49.3X1	T49.3X2	T49.3X3	T49.3X4	T49.3X5	T49.3X6
- theobromine calcium	T50.2X1	T50.2X2	T50.2X3	T50.2X4	T50.2X5	T50.2X6
Salicylazosulfapyridine	T37.0X1	T37.0X2	T37.0X3	T37.0X4	T37.0X5	T37.0X6
Salicylhydroxamic acid	T49.0X1	T49.0X2	T49.0X3	T49.0X4	T49.0X5	T49.0X6

Substance	Poisoning, Accidental (unintentional)	Poisoning, Intentional Self-harm	Poisoning, Assault	Poisoning, Undetermined	Adverse effect	Underdosing
Salicylic acid	T49.4X1	T49.4X2	T49.4X3	T49.4X4	T49.4X5	T49.4X6
- with benzoic acid	T49.4X1	T49.4X2	T49.4X3	T49.4X4	T49.4X5	T49.4X6
- congeners	T39.091	T39.092	T39.093	T39.094	T39.095	T39.096
- derivative	T39.091	T39.092	T39.093	T39.094	T39.095	T39.096
- salts	T39.091	T39.092	T39.093	T39.094	T39.095	T39.096
Salinazid	T37.1X1	T37.1X2	T37.1X3	T37.1X4	T37.1X5	T37.1X6
Salmeterol	T48.6X1	T48.6X2	T48.6X3	T48.6X4	T48.6X5	T48.6X6
Salol	T49.3X1	T49.3X2	T49.3X3	T49.3X4	T49.3X5	T49.3X6
Salsalate	T39.091	T39.092	T39.093	T39.094	T39.095	T39.096
Salt substitute	T50.901	T50.902	T50.903	T50.904	T50.905	T50.906
Salt-replacing drug	T50.901	T50.902	T50.903	T50.904	T50.905	T50.906
Salt-retaining mineralocorticoid	T50.0X1	T50.0X2	T50.0X3	T50.0X4	T50.0X5	T50.0X6
Saluretic NEC	T50.2X1	T50.2X2	T50.2X3	T50.2X4	T50.2X5	T50.2X6
Saluron	T50.2X1	T50.2X2	T50.2X3	T50.2X4	T50.2X5	T50.2X6
Salvarsan 606 (neosilver) (silver)	T37.8X1	T37.8X2	T37.8X3	T37.8X4	T37.8X5	T37.8X6
Sambucus canadensis	T62.2X1	T62.2X2	T62.2X3	T62.2X4	--	--
- berry	T62.1X1	T62.1X2	T62.1X3	T62.1X4	--	--
Sandril	T46.5X1	T46.5X2	T46.5X3	T46.5X4	T46.5X5	T46.5X6
Sanguinaria canadensis	T62.2X1	T62.2X2	T62.2X3	T62.2X4	--	--
Saniflush (cleaner)	T54.2X1	T54.2X2	T54.2X3	T54.2X4	--	--
Santonin	T37.4X1	T37.4X2	T37.4X3	T37.4X4	T37.4X5	T37.4X6
Santyl	T49.8X1	T49.8X2	T49.8X3	T49.8X4	T49.8X5	T49.8X6
Saralasin	T46.5X1	T46.5X2	T46.5X3	T46.5X4	T46.5X5	T46.5X6
Sarcolysin	T45.1X1	T45.1X2	T45.1X3	T45.1X4	T45.1X5	T45.1X6
Sarkomycin	T45.1X1	T45.1X2	T45.1X3	T45.1X4	T45.1X5	T45.1X6
Saroten	T43.011	T43.012	T43.013	T43.014	T43.015	T43.016
Saturnine—see Lead						
Savin (oil)	T49.4X1	T49.4X2	T49.4X3	T49.4X4	T49.4X5	T49.4X6
Scammony	T47.2X1	T47.2X2	T47.2X3	T47.2X4	T47.2X5	T47.2X6
Scarlet red	T49.8X1	T49.8X2	T49.8X3	T49.8X4	T49.8X5	T49.8X6
Scheele's green	T57.0X1	T57.0X2	T57.0X3	T57.0X4	--	--
- insecticide	T57.0X1	T57.0X2	T57.0X3	T57.0X4	--	--
Schizontozide (blood) (tissue)	T37.2X1	T37.2X2	T37.2X3	T37.2X4	T37.2X5	T37.2X6
Schradan	T60.0X1	T60.0X2	T60.0X3	T60.0X4	--	--
Schweinfurth green	T57.0X1	T57.0X2	T57.0X3	T57.0X4	--	--
- insecticide	T57.0X1	T57.0X2	T57.0X3	T57.0X4	--	--
Scilla, rat poison	T60.4X1	T60.4X2	T60.4X3	T60.4X4	--	--
Scillaren	T60.4X1	T60.4X2	T60.4X3	T60.4X4	--	--
Sclerosing agent	T46.8X1	T46.8X2	T46.8X3	T46.8X4	T46.8X5	T46.8X6
Scombrotoxin	T61.11	T61.12	T61.13	T61.14	--	--
Scopolamine	T44.3X1	T44.3X2	T44.3X3	T44.3X4	T44.3X5	T44.3X6
Scopolia extract	T44.3X1	T44.3X2	T44.3X3	T44.3X4	T44.3X5	T44.3X6
Scouring powder	T65.891	T65.892	T65.893	T65.894	--	--
Sea						
- anemone (sting)	T63.631	T63.632	T63.633	T63.634	--	--
- cucumber (sting)	T63.691	T63.692	T63.693	T63.694	--	--
- snake (bite) (venom)	T63.091	T63.092	T63.093	T63.094	--	--
- urchin spine (puncture)	T63.691	T63.692	T63.693	T63.694	--	--
Seafood	T61.91	T61.92	T61.93	T61.94	--	--
- specified NEC	T61.8X1	T61.8X2	T61.8X3	T61.8X4	--	--
Secbutabarbital	T42.3X1	T42.3X2	T42.3X3	T42.3X4	T42.3X5	T42.3X6
Secbutabarbitone	T42.3X1	T42.3X2	T42.3X3	T42.3X4	T42.3X5	T42.3X6
Secnidazole	T37.3X1	T37.3X2	T37.3X3	T37.3X4	T37.3X5	T37.3X6
Secobarbital	T42.3X1	T42.3X2	T42.3X3	T42.3X4	T42.3X5	T42.3X6
Seconal	T42.3X1	T42.3X2	T42.3X3	T42.3X4	T42.3X5	T42.3X6
Secretin	T50.8X1	T50.8X2	T50.8X3	T50.8X4	T50.8X5	T50.8X6
Sedative NEC	T42.71	T42.72	T42.73	T42.74	T42.75	T42.76
- mixed NEC	T42.6X1	T42.6X2	T42.6X3	T42.6X4	T42.6X5	T42.6X6

Substance	Poisoning, Accidental (unintentional)	Poisoning, Intentional Self-harm	Poisoning, Assault	Poisoning, Undetermined	Adverse effect	Underdosing
Sedormid	T42.6X1	T42.6X2	T42.6X3	T42.6X4	T42.6X5	T42.6X6
Seed disinfectant or dressing	T60.8X1	T60.8X2	T60.8X3	T60.8X4	--	--
Seeds (poisonous)	T62.2X1	T62.2X2	T62.2X3	T62.2X4	--	--
Selegiline	T42.8X1	T42.8X2	T42.8X3	T42.8X4	T42.8X5	T42.8X6
Selenium NEC	T56.891	T56.892	T56.893	T56.894	--	--
- disulfide or sulfide	T49.4X1	T49.4X2	T49.4X3	T49.4X4	T49.4X5	T49.4X6
- fumes	T59.891	T59.892	T59.893	T59.894	--	--
- sulfide	T49.4X1	T49.4X2	T49.4X3	T49.4X4	T49.4X5	T49.4X6
Selenomethionine (75Se)	T50.8X1	T50.8X2	T50.8X3	T50.8X4	T50.8X5	T50.8X6
Selsun	T49.4X1	T49.4X2	T49.4X3	T49.4X4	T49.4X5	T49.4X6
Semustine	T45.1X1	T45.1X2	T45.1X3	T45.1X4	T45.1X5	T45.1X6
Senega syrup	T48.4X1	T48.4X2	T48.4X3	T48.4X4	T48.4X5	T48.4X6
Senna	T47.2X1	T47.2X2	T47.2X3	T47.2X4	T47.2X5	T47.2X6
Sennoside A+B	T47.2X1	T47.2X2	T47.2X3	T47.2X4	T47.2X5	T47.2X6
Septisol	T49.2X1	T49.2X2	T49.2X3	T49.2X4	T49.2X5	T49.2X6
Seractide	T38.811	T38.812	T38.813	T38.814	T38.815	T38.816
Serax	T42.4X1	T42.4X2	T42.4X3	T42.4X4	T42.4X5	T42.4X6
Serenesil	T42.6X1	T42.6X2	T42.6X3	T42.6X4	T42.6X5	T42.6X6
Serenium (hydrochloride)	T37.91	T37.92	T37.93	T37.94	T37.95	T37.96
Serepax—see Oxazepam						
Sermorelin	T38.891	T38.892	T38.893	T38.894	T38.895	T38.896
Sernyl	T41.1X1	T41.1X2	T41.1X3	T41.1X4	T41.1X5	T41.1X6
Serotonin	T50.991	T50.992	T50.993	T50.994	T50.995	T50.996
Serpasil	T46.5X1	T46.5X2	T46.5X3	T46.5X4	T46.5X5	T46.5X6
Serrapeptase	T45.3X1	T45.3X2	T45.3X3	T45.3X4	T45.3X5	T45.3X6
Serum						
- antibotulinus	T50.Z11	T50.Z12	T50.Z13	T50.Z14	T50.Z15	T50.Z16
- anticytotoxic	T50.Z11	T50.Z12	T50.Z13	T50.Z14	T50.Z15	T50.Z16
- antidiphtheria	T50.Z11	T50.Z12	T50.Z13	T50.Z14	T50.Z15	T50.Z16
- antimeningococcus	T50.Z11	T50.Z12	T50.Z13	T50.Z14	T50.Z15	T50.Z16
- anti-Rh	T50.Z11	T50.Z12	T50.Z13	T50.Z14	T50.Z15	T50.Z16
- anti-snake-bite	T50.Z11	T50.Z12	T50.Z13	T50.Z14	T50.Z15	T50.Z16
- antitetanic	T50.Z11	T50.Z12	T50.Z13	T50.Z14	T50.Z15	T50.Z16
- antitoxic	T50.Z11	T50.Z12	T50.Z13	T50.Z14	T50.Z15	T50.Z16
- complement (inhibitor)	T45.8X1	T45.8X2	T45.8X3	T45.8X4	T45.8X5	T45.8X6
- convalescent	T50.Z11	T50.Z12	T50.Z13	T50.Z14	T50.Z15	T50.Z16
- hemolytic complement	T45.8X1	T45.8X2	T45.8X3	T45.8X4	T45.8X5	T45.8X6
- immune (human)	T50.Z11	T50.Z12	T50.Z13	T50.Z14	T50.Z15	T50.Z16
- protective NEC	T50.Z11	T50.Z12	T50.Z13	T50.Z14	T50.Z15	T50.Z16
Setastine	T45.0X1	T45.0X2	T45.0X3	T45.0X4	T45.0X5	T45.0X6
Setoperone	T43.591	T43.592	T43.593	T43.594	T43.595	T43.596
Sewer gas	T59.91	T59.92	T59.93	T59.94	--	--
Shampoo	T55.0X1	T55.0X2	T55.0X3	T55.0X4	--	--
Shellfish, noxious, nonbacterial	T61.781	T61.782	T61.783	T61.784	--	--
Sildenafil	T46.7X1	T46.7X2	T46.7X3	T46.7X4	T46.7X5	T46.7X6
Silibinin	T50.991	T50.992	T50.993	T50.994	T50.995	T50.996
Silicone NEC	T65.891	T65.892	T65.893	T65.894	--	--
- medicinal	T49.3X1	T49.3X2	T49.3X3	T49.3X4	T49.3X5	T49.3X6
Silvadene	T49.0X1	T49.0X2	T49.0X3	T49.0X4	T49.0X5	T49.0X6
Silver	T49.0X1	T49.0X2	T49.0X3	T49.0X4	T49.0X5	T49.0X6
- anti-infectives	T49.0X1	T49.0X2	T49.0X3	T49.0X4	T49.0X5	T49.0X6
- arsphenamine	T37.8X1	T37.8X2	T37.8X3	T37.8X4	T37.8X5	T37.8X6
- colloidal	T49.0X1	T49.0X2	T49.0X3	T49.0X4	T49.0X5	T49.0X6
- nitrate	T49.0X1	T49.0X2	T49.0X3	T49.0X4	T49.0X5	T49.0X6
- - ophthalmic preparation	T49.5X1	T49.5X2	T49.5X3	T49.5X4	T49.5X5	T49.5X6
- - toughened (keratolytic)	T49.4X1	T49.4X2	T49.4X3	T49.4X4	T49.4X5	T49.4X6
- nonmedicinal (dust)	T56.891	T56.892	T56.893	T56.894	--	--
- protein	T49.5X1	T49.5X2	T49.5X3	T49.5X4	T49.5X5	T49.5X6
- salvarsan	T37.8X1	T37.8X2	T37.8X3	T37.8X4	T37.8X5	T37.8X6

Substance	Poisoning, Accidental (unintentional)	Poisoning, Intentional Self-harm	Poisoning, Assault	Poisoning, Undetermined	Adverse effect	Underdosing
- sulfadiazine	T49.4X1	T49.4X2	T49.4X3	T49.4X4	T49.4X5	T49.4X6
Silymarin	T50.991	T50.992	T50.993	T50.994	T50.995	T50.996
Simaldrate	T47.1X1	T47.1X2	T47.1X3	T47.1X4	T47.1X5	T47.1X6
Simazine	T60.3X1	T60.3X2	T60.3X3	T60.3X4	--	--
Simethicone	T47.1X1	T47.1X2	T47.1X3	T47.1X4	T47.1X5	T47.1X6
Simfibrate	T46.6X1	T46.6X2	T46.6X3	T46.6X4	T46.6X5	T46.6X6
Simvastatin	T46.6X1	T46.6X2	T46.6X3	T46.6X4	T46.6X5	T46.6X6
Sincalide	T50.8X1	T50.8X2	T50.8X3	T50.8X4	T50.8X5	T50.8X6
Sinequan	T43.011	T43.012	T43.013	T43.014	T43.015	T43.016
Singoserp	T46.5X1	T46.5X2	T46.5X3	T46.5X4	T46.5X5	T46.5X6
Sintrom	T45.511	T45.512	T45.513	T45.514	T45.515	T45.516
Sisomicin	T36.5X1	T36.5X2	T36.5X3	T36.5X4	T36.5X5	T36.5X6
Sitosterols	T46.6X1	T46.6X2	T46.6X3	T46.6X4	T46.6X5	T46.6X6
Skeletal muscle relaxants	T48.1X1	T48.1X2	T48.1X3	T48.1X4	T48.1X5	T48.1X6
Skin						
- agents (external)	T49.91	T49.92	T49.93	T49.94	T49.95	T49.96
- - specified NEC	T49.8X1	T49.8X2	T49.8X3	T49.8X4	T49.8X5	T49.8X6
- test antigen	T50.8X1	T50.8X2	T50.8X3	T50.8X4	T50.8X5	T50.8X6
Sleep-eze	T45.0X1	T45.0X2	T45.0X3	T45.0X4	T45.0X5	T45.0X6
Sleeping draught, pill	T42.71	T42.72	T42.73	T42.74	T42.75	T42.76
Smallpox vaccine	T50.B11	T50.B12	T50.B13	T50.B14	T50.B15	T50.B16
Smelter fumes NEC	T56.91	T56.92	T56.93	T56.94	--	--
Smog	T59.1X1	T59.1X2	T59.1X3	T59.1X4	--	--
Smoke NEC	T59.811	T59.812	T59.813	T59.814	--	--
Smooth muscle relaxant	T44.3X1	T44.3X2	T44.3X3	T44.3X4	T44.3X5	T44.3X6
Snail killer NEC	T60.8X1	T60.8X2	T60.8X3	T60.8X4	--	--
Snake venom or bite	T63.001	T63.002	T63.003	T63.004	--	--
- hemocoagulase	T45.7X1	T45.7X2	T45.7X3	T45.7X4	T45.7X5	T45.7X6
Snuff	T65.211	T65.212	T65.213	T65.214	--	--
Soap (powder) (product)	T55.0X1	T55.0X2	T55.0X3	T55.0X4	--	--
- enema	T47.4X1	T47.4X2	T47.4X3	T47.4X4	T47.4X5	T47.4X6
- medicinal, soft	T49.2X1	T49.2X2	T49.2X3	T49.2X4	T49.2X5	T49.2X6
- superfatted	T49.2X1	T49.2X2	T49.2X3	T49.2X4	T49.2X5	T49.2X6
Sobrerol	T48.4X1	T48.4X2	T48.4X3	T48.4X4	T48.4X5	T48.4X6
Soda (caustic)	T54.3X1	T54.3X2	T54.3X3	T54.3X4	--	--
- bicarb	T47.1X1	T47.1X2	T47.1X3	T47.1X4	T47.1X5	T47.1X6
- chlorinated—see Sodium, hypochlorite						
Sodium						
- acetosulfone	T37.1X1	T37.1X2	T37.1X3	T37.1X4	T37.1X5	T37.1X6
- acetrizoate	T50.8X1	T50.8X2	T50.8X3	T50.8X4	T50.8X5	T50.8X6
- acid phosphate	T50.3X1	T50.3X2	T50.3X3	T50.3X4	T50.3X5	T50.3X6
- alginate	T47.8X1	T47.8X2	T47.8X3	T47.8X4	T47.8X5	T47.8X6
- amidotrizoate	T50.8X1	T50.8X2	T50.8X3	T50.8X4	T50.8X5	T50.8X6
- aminopterin	T45.1X1	T45.1X2	T45.1X3	T45.1X4	T45.1X5	T45.1X6
- amylosulfate	T47.8X1	T47.8X2	T47.8X3	T47.8X4	T47.8X5	T47.8X6
- amytal	T42.3X1	T42.3X2	T42.3X3	T42.3X4	T42.3X5	T42.3X6
- antimony gluconate	T37.3X1	T37.3X2	T37.3X3	T37.3X4	T37.3X5	T37.3X6
- arsenate	T57.0X1	T57.0X2	T57.0X3	T57.0X4	--	--
- aurothiomalate	T39.4X1	T39.4X2	T39.4X3	T39.4X4	T39.4X5	T39.4X6
- aurothiosulfate	T39.4X1	T39.4X2	T39.4X3	T39.4X4	T39.4X5	T39.4X6
- barbiturate	T42.3X1	T42.3X2	T42.3X3	T42.3X4	T42.3X5	T42.3X6
- basic phosphate	T47.4X1	T47.4X2	T47.4X3	T47.4X4	T47.4X5	T47.4X6
- bicarbonate	T47.1X1	T47.1X2	T47.1X3	T47.1X4	T47.1X5	T47.1X6
- bichromate	T57.8X1	T57.8X2	T57.8X3	T57.8X4	--	--
- biphosphate	T50.3X1	T50.3X2	T50.3X3	T50.3X4	T50.3X5	T50.3X6
- bisulfate	T65.891	T65.892	T65.893	T65.894	--	--
- borate						
- - cleanser	T57.8X1	T57.8X2	T57.8X3	T57.8X4	--	--

Substance	Poisoning, Accidental (unintentional)	Poisoning, Intentional Self-harm	Poisoning, Assault	Poisoning, Undetermined	Adverse effect	Underdosing
- - - eye	T49.5X1	T49.5X2	T49.5X3	T49.5X4	T49.5X5	T49.5X6
- - therapeutic	T49.8X1	T49.8X2	T49.8X3	T49.8X4	T49.8X5	T49.8X6
- bromide	T42.6X1	T42.6X2	T42.6X3	T42.6X4	T42.6X5	T42.6X6
- cacodylate (nonmedicinal) NEC	T50.8X1	T50.8X2	T50.8X3	T50.8X4	T50.8X5	T50.8X6
- - anti-infective	T37.8X1	T37.8X2	T37.8X3	T37.8X4	T37.8X5	T37.8X6
- - herbicide	T60.3X1	T60.3X2	T60.3X3	T60.3X4	--	--
- calcium edetate	T45.8X1	T45.8X2	T45.8X3	T45.8X4	T45.8X5	T45.8X6
- carbonate NEC	T54.3X1	T54.3X2	T54.3X3	T54.3X4	--	--
- chlorate NEC	T65.891	T65.892	T65.893	T65.894	--	--
- - herbicide	T54.91	T54.92	T54.93	T54.94	--	
- chloride	T50.3X1	T50.3X2	T50.3X3	T50.3X4	T50.3X5	T50.3X6
- - with glucose	T50.3X1	T50.3X2	T50.3X3	T50.3X4	T50.3X5	T50.3X6
- chromate	T65.891	T65.892	T65.893	T65.894	--	
- citrate	T50.991	T50.992	T50.993	T50.994	T50.995	T50.996
- cromoglicate	T48.6X1	T48.6X2	T48.6X3	T48.6X4	T48.6X5	T48.6X6
- cyanide	T65.0X1	T65.0X2	T65.0X3	T65.0X4	--	--
- cyclamate	T50.3X1	T50.3X2	T50.3X3	T50.3X4	T50.3X5	T50.3X6
- dehydrocholate	T45.8X1	T45.8X2	T45.8X3	T45.8X4	T45.8X5	T45.8X6
- diatrizoate	T50.8X1	T50.8X2	T50.8X3	T50.8X4	T50.8X5	T50.8X6
- dibunate	T48.4X1	T48.4X2	T48.4X3	T48.4X4	T48.4X5	T48.4X6
- dioctyl sulfosuccinate	T47.4X1	T47.4X2	T47.4X3	T47.4X4	T47.4X5	T47.4X6
- dipantoyl ferrate	T45.8X1	T45.8X2	T45.8X3	T45.8X4	T45.8X5	T45.8X6
- edetate	T45.8X1	T45.8X2	T45.8X3	T45.8X4	T45.8X5	T45.8X6
- ethacrynate	T50.1X1	T50.1X2	T50.1X3	T50.1X4	T50.1X5	T50.1X6
- feredetate	T45.8X1	T45.8X2	T45.8X3	T45.8X4	T45.8X5	T45.8X6
- Fluoride—see Fluoride						
- fluoroacetate (dust) (pesticide)	T60.4X1	T60.4X2	T60.4X3	T60.4X4	--	--
- free salt	T50.3X1	T50.3X2	T50.3X3	T50.3X4	T50.3X5	T50.3X6
- fusidate	T36.8X1	T36.8X2	T36.8X3	T36.8X4	T36.8X5	T36.8X6
- glucaldrate	T47.1X1	T47.1X2	T47.1X3	T47.1X4	T47.1X5	T47.1X6
- glucosulfone	T37.1X1	T37.1X2	T37.1X3	T37.1X4	T37.1X5	T37.1X6
- glutamate	T45.8X1	T45.8X2	T45.8X3	T45.8X4	T45.8X5	T45.8X6
- hydrogen carbonate	T50.3X1	T50.3X2	T50.3X3	T50.3X4	T50.3X5	T50.3X6
- hydroxide	T54.3X1	T54.3X2	T54.3X3	T54.3X4	--	--
- hypochlorite (bleach) NEC	T54.3X1	T54.3X2	T54.3X3	T54.3X4	--	--
- - disinfectant	T54.3X1	T54.3X2	T54.3X3	T54.3X4	--	--
- - medicinal (anti-infective) (external)	T49.0X1	T49.0X2	T49.0X3	T49.0X4	T49.0X5	T49.0X6
- - vapor	T54.3X1	T54.3X2	T54.3X3	T54.3X4	--	--
- hyposulfite	T49.0X1	T49.0X2	T49.0X3	T49.0X4	T49.0X5	T49.0X6
- indigotin disulfonate	T50.8X1	T50.8X2	T50.8X3	T50.8X4	T50.8X5	T50.8X6
- iodide	T50.991	T50.992	T50.993	T50.994	T50.995	T50.996
- - I-131	T50.8X1	T50.8X2	T50.8X3	T50.8X4	T50.8X5	T50.8X6
- - - therapeutic	T38.2X1	T38.2X2	T38.2X3	T38.2X4	T38.2X5	T38.2X6
- iodohippurate (131I)	T50.8X1	T50.8X2	T50.8X3	T50.8X4	T50.8X5	T50.8X6
- iopodate	T50.8X1	T50.8X2	T50.8X3	T50.8X4	T50.8X5	T50.8X6
- iothalamate	T50.8X1	T50.8X2	T50.8X3	T50.8X4	T50.8X5	T50.8X6
- iron edetate	T45.4X1	T45.4X2	T45.4X3	T45.4X4	T45.4X5	T45.4X6
- lactate (compound solution)	T45.8X1	T45.8X2	T45.8X3	T45.8X4	T45.8X5	T45.8X6
- lauryl (sulfate)	T49.2X1	T49.2X2	T49.2X3	T49.2X4	T49.2X5	T49.2X6
- L-triiodothyronine	T38.1X1	T38.1X2	T38.1X3	T38.1X4	T38.1X5	T38.1X6
- magnesium citrate	T50.991	T50.992	T50.993	T50.994	T50.995	T50.996
- mersalate	T50.2X1	T50.2X2	T50.2X3	T50.2X4	T50.2X5	T50.2X6
- metasilicate	T65.891	T65.892	T65.893	T65.894	--	--
- metrizoate	T50.8X1	T50.8X2	T50.8X3	T50.8X4	T50.8X5	T50.8X6
- monofluoroacetate (pesticide)	T60.1X1	T60.1X2	T60.1X3	T60.1X4	--	--
- morrhuate	T46.8X1	T46.8X2	T46.8X3	T46.8X4	T46.8X5	T46.8X6
- nafcillin	T36.0X1	T36.0X2	T36.0X3	T36.0X4	T36.0X5	T36.0X6
- nitrate (oxidizing agent)	T65.891	T65.892	T65.893	T65.894	--	--
- nitrite	T50.6X1	T50.6X2	T50.6X3	T50.6X4	T50.6X5	T50.6X6

Substance	Poisoning, Accidental (unintentional)	Poisoning, Intentional Self-harm	Poisoning, Assault	Poisoning, Undetermined	Adverse effect	Underdosing
- nitroferricyanide	T46.5X1	T46.5X2	T46.5X3	T46.5X4	T46.5X5	T46.5X6
- nitroprusside	T46.5X1	T46.5X2	T46.5X3	T46.5X4	T46.5X5	T46.5X6
- oxalate	T65.891	T65.892	T65.893	T65.894	--	--
- oxide/peroxide	T65.891	T65.892	T65.893	T65.894	--	--
- oxybate	T41.291	T41.292	T41.293	T41.294	T41.295	T41.296
- para-aminohippurate	T50.8X1	T50.8X2	T50.8X3	T50.8X4	T50.8X5	T50.8X6
- perborate (nonmedicinal) NEC	T65.891	T65.892	T65.893	T65.894	--	--
- - medicinal	T49.0X1	T49.0X2	T49.0X3	T49.0X4	T49.0X5	T49.0X6
- - soap	T55.0X1	T55.0X2	T55.0X3	T55.0X4	--	--
- percarbonate—see Sodium, perborate						
- pertechnetate Tc99m	T50.8X1	T50.8X2	T50.8X3	T50.8X4	T50.8X5	T50.8X6
- phosphate						
- - cellulose	T45.8X1	T45.8X2	T45.8X3	T45.8X4	T45.8X5	T45.8X6
- - dibasic	T47.2X1	T47.2X2	T47.2X3	T47.2X4	T47.2X5	T47.2X6
- - monobasic	T47.2X1	T47.2X2	T47.2X3	T47.2X4	T47.2X5	T47.2X6
- phytate	T50.6X1	T50.6X2	T50.6X3	T50.6X4	T50.6X5	T50.6X6
- picosulfate	T47.2X1	T47.2X2	T47.2X3	T47.2X4	T47.2X5	T47.2X6
- polyhydroxyaluminium monocarbonate	T47.1X1	T47.1X2	T47.1X3	T47.1X4	T47.1X5	T47.1X6
- polystyrene sulfonate	T50.3X1	T50.3X2	T50.3X3	T50.3X4	T50.3X5	T50.3X6
- propionate	T49.0X1	T49.0X2	T49.0X3	T49.0X4	T49.0X5	T49.0X6
- propyl hydroxybenzoate	T50.991	T50.992	T50.993	T50.994	T50.995	T50.996
- psylliate	T46.8X1	T46.8X2	T46.8X3	T46.8X4	T46.8X5	T46.8X6
- removing resins	T50.3X1	T50.3X2	T50.3X3	T50.3X4	T50.3X5	T50.3X6
- salicylate	T39.091	T39.092	T39.093	T39.094	T39.095	T39.096
- salt NEC	T50.3X1	T50.3X2	T50.3X3	T50.3X4	T50.3X5	T50.3X6
- selenate	T60.2X1	T60.2X2	T60.2X3	T60.2X4	--	--
- stibogluconate	T37.3X1	T37.3X2	T37.3X3	T37.3X4	T37.3X5	T37.3X6
- sulfate	T47.4X1	T47.4X2	T47.4X3	T47.4X4	T47.4X5	T47.4X6
- sulfoxone	T37.1X1	T37.1X2	T37.1X3	T37.1X4	T37.1X5	T37.1X6
- tetradecyl sulfate	T46.8X1	T46.8X2	T46.8X3	T46.8X4	T46.8X5	T46.8X6
- thiopental	T41.1X1	T41.1X2	T41.1X3	T41.1X4	T41.1X5	T41.1X6
- thiosalicylate	T39.091	T39.092	T39.093	T39.094	T39.095	T39.096
- thiosulfate	T50.6X1	T50.6X2	T50.6X3	T50.6X4	T50.6X5	T50.6X6
- tolbutamide	T38.3X1	T38.3X2	T38.3X3	T38.3X4	T38.3X5	T38.3X6
- (L) -triiodothyronine	T38.1X1	T38.1X2	T38.1X3	T38.1X4	T38.1X5	T38.1X6
- tyropanoate	T50.8X1	T50.8X2	T50.8X3	T50.8X4	T50.8X5	T50.8X6
- valproate	T42.6X1	T42.6X2	T42.6X3	T42.6X4	T42.6X5	T42.6X6
- versenate	T50.6X1	T50.6X2	T50.6X3	T50.6X4	T50.6X5	T50.6X6
Sodium-free salt	T50.901	T50.902	T50.903	T50.904	T50.905	T50.906
Sodium-removing resin	T50.3X1	T50.3X2	T50.3X3	T50.3X4	T50.3X5	T50.3X6
Soft soap	T55.0X1	T55.0X2	T55.0X3	T55.0X4	--	--
Solanine	T62.2X1	T62.2X2	T62.2X3	T62.2X4	--	--
- berries	T62.1X1	T62.1X2	T62.1X3	T62.1X4	--	--
Solanum dulcamara	T62.2X1	T62.2X2	T62.2X3	T62.2X4	--	--
- berries	T62.1X1	T62.1X2	T62.1X3	T62.1X4	--	--
Solapsone	T37.1X1	T37.1X2	T37.1X3	T37.1X4	T37.1X5	T37.1X6
Solar lotion	T49.3X1	T49.3X2	T49.3X3	T49.3X4	T49.3X5	T49.3X6
Solasulfone	T37.1X1	T37.1X2	T37.1X3	T37.1X4	T37.1X5	T37.1X6
Soldering fluid	T65.891	T65.892	T65.893	T65.894	--	--
Solid substance	T65.91	T65.92	T65.93	T65.94	--	--
- specified NEC	T65.891	T65.892	T65.893	T65.894	--	--
Solvent, industrial NEC	T52.91	T52.92	T52.93	T52.94	--	--
- naphtha	T52.0X1	T52.0X2	T52.0X3	T52.0X4	--	--
- petroleum	T52.0X1	T52.0X2	T52.0X3	T52.0X4	--	--
- specified NEC	T52.8X1	T52.8X2	T52.8X3	T52.8X4	--	--
Soma	T42.8X1	T42.8X2	T42.8X3	T42.8X4	T42.8X5	T42.8X6
Somatorelin	T38.891	T38.892	T38.893	T38.894	T38.895	T38.896
Somatostatin	T38.991	T38.992	T38.993	T38.994	T38.995	T38.996

Substance	Poisoning, Accidental (unintentional)	Poisoning, Intentional Self-harm	Poisoning, Assault	Poisoning, Undetermined	Adverse effect	Underdosing
Somatotropin	T38.811	T38.812	T38.813	T38.814	T38.815	T38.816
Somatrem	T38.811	T38.812	T38.813	T38.814	T38.815	T38.816
Somatropin	T38.811	T38.812	T38.813	T38.814	T38.815	T38.816
Sominex	T45.0X1	T45.0X2	T45.0X3	T45.0X4	T45.0X5	T45.0X6
Somnos	T42.6X1	T42.6X2	T42.6X3	T42.6X4	T42.6X5	T42.6X6
Somonal	T42.3X1	T42.3X2	T42.3X3	T42.3X4	T42.3X5	T42.3X6
Soneryl	T42.3X1	T42.3X2	T42.3X3	T42.3X4	T42.3X5	T42.3X6
Soothing syrup	T50.901	T50.902	T50.903	T50.904	T50.905	T50.906
Sopor	T42.6X1	T42.6X2	T42.6X3	T42.6X4	T42.6X5	T42.6X6
Soporific	T42.71	T42.72	T42.73	T42.74	T42.75	T42.76
Soporific drug	T42.71	T42.72	T42.73	T42.74	T42.75	T42.76
- specified type NEC	T42.6X1	T42.6X2	T42.6X3	T42.6X4	T42.6X5	T42.6X6
Sorbide nitrate	T46.3X1	T46.3X2	T46.3X3	T46.3X4	T46.3X5	T46.3X6
Sorbitol	T47.4X1	T47.4X2	T47.4X3	T47.4X4	T47.4X5	T47.4X6
Sotalol	T44.7X1	T44.7X2	T44.7X3	T44.7X4	T44.7X5	T44.7X6
Sotradecol	T46.8X1	T46.8X2	T46.8X3	T46.8X4	T46.8X5	T46.8X6
Soysterol	T46.6X1	T46.6X2	T46.6X3	T46.6X4	T46.6X5	T46.6X6
Spacoline	T44.3X1	T44.3X2	T44.3X3	T44.3X4	T44.3X5	T44.3X6
Spanish fly	T49.8X1	T49.8X2	T49.8X3	T49.8X4	T49.8X5	T49.8X6
Sparine	T43.3X1	T43.3X2	T43.3X3	T43.3X4	T43.3X5	T43.3X6
Sparteine	T48.0X1	T48.0X2	T48.0X3	T48.0X4	T48.0X5	T48.0X6
Spasmolytic						
- anticholinergics	T44.3X1	T44.3X2	T44.3X3	T44.3X4	T44.3X5	T44.3X6
- autonomic	T44.3X1	T44.3X2	T44.3X3	T44.3X4	T44.3X5	T44.3X6
- bronchial NEC	T48.6X1	T48.6X2	T48.6X3	T48.6X4	T48.6X5	T48.6X6
- quaternary ammonium	T44.3X1	T44.3X2	T44.3X3	T44.3X4	T44.3X5	T44.3X6
- skeletal muscle NEC	T48.1X1	T48.1X2	T48.1X3	T48.1X4	T48.1X5	T48.1X6
Spectinomycin	T36.5X1	T36.5X2	T36.5X3	T36.5X4	T36.5X5	T36.5X6
Speed	T43.621	T43.622	T43.623	T43.624	T43.625	T43.626
Spermicide	T49.8X1	T49.8X2	T49.8X3	T49.8X4	T49.8X5	T49.8X6
Spider (bite) (venom)	T63.391	T63.392	T63.393	T63.394	--	--
- antivenin	T50.Z11	T50.Z12	T50.Z13	T50.Z14	T50.Z15	T50.Z16
Spigelia (root)	T37.4X1	T37.4X2	T37.4X3	T37.4X4	T37.4X5	T37.4X6
Spindle inactivator	T50.4X1	T50.4X2	T50.4X3	T50.4X4	T50.4X5	T50.4X6
Spiperone	T43.4X1	T43.4X2	T43.4X3	T43.4X4	T43.4X5	T43.4X6
Spiramycin	T36.3X1	T36.3X2	T36.3X3	T36.3X4	T36.3X5	T36.3X6
Spirapril	T46.4X1	T46.4X2	T46.4X3	T46.4X4	T46.4X5	T46.4X6
Spirilene	T43.591	T43.592	T43.593	T43.594	T43.595	T43.596
Spirit (s) (neutral) NEC	T51.0X1	T51.0X2	T51.0X3	T51.0X4	--	--
- beverage	T51.0X1	T51.0X2	T51.0X3	T51.0X4	--	--
- industrial	T51.0X1	T51.0X2	T51.0X3	T51.0X4	--	--
- mineral	T52.0X1	T52.0X2	T52.0X3	T52.0X4	--	--
- of salt—see Hydrochloric acid						
- surgical	T51.0X1	T51.0X2	T51.0X3	T51.0X4	--	--
Spironolactone	T50.0X1	T50.0X2	T50.0X3	T50.0X4	T50.0X5	T50.0X6
Spiroperidol	T43.4X1	T43.4X2	T43.4X3	T43.4X4	T43.4X5	T43.4X6
Sponge, absorbable (gelatin)	T45.7X1	T45.7X2	T45.7X3	T45.7X4	T45.7X5	T45.7X6
Sporostacin	T49.0X1	T49.0X2	T49.0X3	T49.0X4	T49.0X5	T49.0X6
Spray (aerosol)	T65.91	T65.92	T65.93	T65.94	--	--
- cosmetic	T65.891	T65.892	T65.893	T65.894	--	--
- medicinal NEC	T50.901	T50.902	T50.903	T50.904	T50.905	T50.906
- pesticides—see Pesticides						
- specified content—see specific substance						
Spurge flax	T62.2X1	T62.2X2	T62.2X3	T62.2X4	--	--
Spurges	T62.2X1	T62.2X2	T62.2X3	T62.2X4	--	--
Sputum viscosity-lowering drug	T48.4X1	T48.4X2	T48.4X3	T48.4X4	T48.4X5	T48.4X6
Squill	T46.0X1	T46.0X2	T46.0X3	T46.0X4	T46.0X5	T46.0X6
- rat poison	T60.4X1	T60.4X2	T60.4X3	T60.4X4	--	--
Squirting cucumber (cathartic)	T47.2X1	T47.2X2	T47.2X3	T47.2X4	T47.2X5	T47.2X6

Substance	Poisoning, Accidental (unintentional)	Poisoning, Intentional Self-harm	Poisoning, Assault	Poisoning, Undetermined	Adverse effect	Underdosing
Stains	T65.6X1	T65.6X2	T65.6X3	T65.6X4	--	--
Stannous fluoride	T49.7X1	T49.7X2	T49.7X3	T49.7X4	T49.7X5	T49.7X6
Stanolone	T38.7X1	T38.7X2	T38.7X3	T38.7X4	T38.7X5	T38.7X6
Stanozolol	T38.7X1	T38.7X2	T38.7X3	T38.7X4	T38.7X5	T38.7X6
Staphisagria or stavesacre (pediculicide)	T49.0X1	T49.0X2	T49.0X3	T49.0X4	T49.0X5	T49.0X6
Starch	T50.901	T50.902	T50.903	T50.904	T50.905	T50.906
Stelazine	T43.3X1	T43.3X2	T43.3X3	T43.3X4	T43.3X5	T43.3X6
Stemetil	T43.3X1	T43.3X2	T43.3X3	T43.3X4	T43.3X5	T43.3X6
Stepronin	T48.4X1	T48.4X2	T48.4X3	T48.4X4	T48.4X5	T48.4X6
Sterculia	T47.4X1	T47.4X2	T47.4X3	T47.4X4	T47.4X5	T47.4X6
Sternutator gas	T59.891	T59.892	T59.893	T59.894	--	--
Steroid	T38.0X1	T38.0X2	T38.0X3	T38.0X4	T38.0X5	T38.0X6
- anabolic	T38.7X1	T38.7X2	T38.7X3	T38.7X4	T38.7X5	T38.7X6
- androgenic	T38.7X1	T38.7X2	T38.7X3	T38.7X4	T38.7X5	T38.7X6
- antineoplastic, hormone	T38.7X1	T38.7X2	T38.7X3	T38.7X4	T38.7X5	T38.7X6
- - estrogen	T38.5X1	T38.5X2	T38.5X3	T38.5X4	T38.5X5	T38.5X6
- ENT agent	T49.6X1	T49.6X2	T49.6X3	T49.6X4	T49.6X5	T49.6X6
- ophthalmic preparation	T49.5X1	T49.5X2	T49.5X3	T49.5X4	T49.5X5	T49.5X6
- topical NEC	T49.0X1	T49.0X2	T49.0X3	T49.0X4	T49.0X5	T49.0X6
Stibine	T56.891	T56.892	T56.893	T56.894	--	--
Stibogluconate	T37.3X1	T37.3X2	T37.3X3	T37.3X4	T37.3X5	T37.3X6
Stibophen	T37.4X1	T37.4X2	T37.4X3	T37.4X4	T37.4X5	T37.4X6
Stilbamidine (isetionate)	T37.3X1	T37.3X2	T37.3X3	T37.3X4	T37.3X5	T37.3X6
Stilbestrol	T38.5X1	T38.5X2	T38.5X3	T38.5X4	T38.5X5	T38.5X6
Stilboestrol	T38.5X1	T38.5X2	T38.5X3	T38.5X4	T38.5X5	T38.5X6
Stimulant						
- central nervous system—see also Psychostimulant	T43.601	T43.602	T43.603	T43.604	T43.605	T43.606
- - analeptics	T50.7X1	T50.7X2	T50.7X3	T50.7X4	T50.7X5	T50.7X6
- - opiate antagonist	T50.7X1	T50.7X2	T50.7X3	T50.7X4	T50.7X5	T50.7X6
- - psychotherapeutic NEC—see also Psychotherapeutic drug	T43.601	T43.602	T43.603	T43.604	T43.605	T43.606
- - specified NEC	T43.691	T43.692	T43.693	T43.694	T43.695	T43.696
- respiratory	T48.901	T48.902	T48.903	T48.904	T48.905	T48.906
Stone-dissolving drug	T50.901	T50.902	T50.903	T50.904	T50.905	T50.906
Storage battery (cells) (acid)	T54.2X1	T54.2X2	T54.2X3	T54.2X4	--	--
Stovaine	T41.3X1	T41.3X2	T41.3X3	T41.3X4	T41.3X5	T41.3X6
- infiltration (subcutaneous)	T41.3X1	T41.3X2	T41.3X3	T41.3X4	T41.3X5	T41.3X6
- nerve block (peripheral) (plexus)	T41.3X1	T41.3X2	T41.3X3	T41.3X4	T41.3X5	T41.3X6
- spinal	T41.3X1	T41.3X2	T41.3X3	T41.3X4	T41.3X5	T41.3X6
- topical (surface)	T41.3X1	T41.3X2	T41.3X3	T41.3X4	T41.3X5	T41.3X6
Stovarsal	T37.8X1	T37.8X2	T37.8X3	T37.8X4	T37.8X5	T37.8X6
Stove gas—see Gas, stove						
Stoxil	T49.5X1	T49.5X2	T49.5X3	T49.5X4	T49.5X5	T49.5X6
Stramonium	T48.6X1	T48.6X2	T48.6X3	T48.6X4	T48.6X5	T48.6X6
- natural state	T62.2X1	T62.2X2	T62.2X3	T62.2X4	--	--
Streptodornase	T45.3X1	T45.3X2	T45.3X3	T45.3X4	T45.3X5	T45.3X6
Streptoduocin	T36.5X1	T36.5X2	T36.5X3	T36.5X4	T36.5X5	T36.5X6
Streptokinase	T45.611	T45.612	T45.613	T45.614	T45.615	T45.616
Streptomycin (derivative)	T36.5X1	T36.5X2	T36.5X3	T36.5X4	T36.5X5	T36.5X6
Streptonivicin	T36.5X1	T36.5X2	T36.5X3	T36.5X4	T36.5X5	T36.5X6
Streptovarycin	T36.5X1	T36.5X2	T36.5X3	T36.5X4	T36.5X5	T36.5X6
Streptozocin	T45.1X1	T45.1X2	T45.1X3	T45.1X4	T45.1X5	T45.1X6
Streptozotocin	T45.1X1	T45.1X2	T45.1X3	T45.1X4	T45.1X5	T45.1X6
Stripper (paint) (solvent)	T52.8X1	T52.8X2	T52.8X3	T52.8X4	--	--
Strobane	T60.1X1	T60.1X2	T60.1X3	T60.1X4	--	--
Strofantina	T46.0X1	T46.0X2	T46.0X3	T46.0X4	T46.0X5	T46.0X6
Strophanthin (g) (k)	T46.0X1	T46.0X2	T46.0X3	T46.0X4	T46.0X5	T46.0X6
Strophanthus	T46.0X1	T46.0X2	T46.0X3	T46.0X4	T46.0X5	T46.0X6

Substance	Poisoning, Accidental (unintentional)	Poisoning, Intentional Self-harm	Poisoning, Assault	Poisoning, Undetermined	Adverse effect	Underdosing
Strophantin	T46.0X1	T46.0X2	T46.0X3	T46.0X4	T46.0X5	T46.0X6
Strophantin-g	T46.0X1	T46.0X2	T46.0X3	T46.0X4	T46.0X5	T46.0X6
Strychnine (nonmedicinal) (pesticide) (salts)	T65.1X1	T65.1X2	T65.1X3	T65.1X4	--	--
- medicinal	T48.291	T48.292	T48.293	T48.294	T48.295	T48.296
Strychnos (ignatii) —see Strychnine						
Styramate	T42.8X1	T42.8X2	T42.8X3	T42.8X4	T42.8X5	T42.8X6
Styrene	T65.891	T65.892	T65.893	T65.894	--	--
Succinimide, antiepileptic or anticonvulsant	T42.2X1	T42.2X2	T42.2X3	T42.2X4	T42.2X5	T42.2X6
- mercuric—see Mercury						
Succinylcholine	T48.1X1	T48.1X2	T48.1X3	T48.1X4	T48.1X5	T48.1X6
Succinylsulfathiazole	T37.0X1	T37.0X2	T37.0X3	T37.0X4	T37.0X5	T37.0X6
Sucralfate	T47.1X1	T47.1X2	T47.1X3	T47.1X4	T47.1X5	T47.1X6
Sucrose	T50.3X1	T50.3X2	T50.3X3	T50.3X4	T50.3X5	T50.3X6
Sufentanil	T40.411	T40.412	T40.413	T40.414	T40.415	T40.416
Sulbactam	T36.0X1	T36.0X2	T36.0X3	T36.0X4	T36.0X5	T36.0X6
Sulbenicillin	T36.0X1	T36.0X2	T36.0X3	T36.0X4	T36.0X5	T36.0X6
Sulbentine	T49.0X1	T49.0X2	T49.0X3	T49.0X4	T49.0X5	T49.0X6
Sulfacetamide	T49.0X1	T49.0X2	T49.0X3	T49.0X4	T49.0X5	T49.0X6
- ophthalmic preparation	T49.5X1	T49.5X2	T49.5X3	T49.5X4	T49.5X5	T49.5X6
Sulfachlorpyridazine	T37.0X1	T37.0X2	T37.0X3	T37.0X4	T37.0X5	T37.0X6
Sulfacitine	T37.0X1	T37.0X2	T37.0X3	T37.0X4	T37.0X5	T37.0X6
Sulfadiasulfone sodium	T37.0X1	T37.0X2	T37.0X3	T37.0X4	T37.0X5	T37.0X6
Sulfadiazine	T37.0X1	T37.0X2	T37.0X3	T37.0X4	T37.0X5	T37.0X6
- silver (topical)	T49.0X1	T49.0X2	T49.0X3	T49.0X4	T49.0X5	T49.0X6
Sulfadimethoxine	T37.0X1	T37.0X2	T37.0X3	T37.0X4	T37.0X5	T37.0X6
Sulfadimidine	T37.0X1	T37.0X2	T37.0X3	T37.0X4	T37.0X5	T37.0X6
Sulfadoxine	T37.0X1	T37.0X2	T37.0X3	T37.0X4	T37.0X5	T37.0X6
- with pyrimethamine	T37.2X1	T37.2X2	T37.2X3	T37.2X4	T37.2X5	T37.2X6
Sulfaethidole	T37.0X1	T37.0X2	T37.0X3	T37.0X4	T37.0X5	T37.0X6
Sulfafurazole	T37.0X1	T37.0X2	T37.0X3	T37.0X4	T37.0X5	T37.0X6
Sulfaguanidine	T37.0X1	T37.0X2	T37.0X3	T37.0X4	T37.0X5	T37.0X6
Sulfalene	T37.0X1	T37.0X2	T37.0X3	T37.0X4	T37.0X5	T37.0X6
Sulfaloxate	T37.0X1	T37.0X2	T37.0X3	T37.0X4	T37.0X5	T37.0X6
Sulfaloxic acid	T37.0X1	T37.0X2	T37.0X3	T37.0X4	T37.0X5	T37.0X6
Sulfamazone	T39.2X1	T39.2X2	T39.2X3	T39.2X4	T39.2X5	T39.2X6
Sulfamerazine	T37.0X1	T37.0X2	T37.0X3	T37.0X4	T37.0X5	T37.0X6
Sulfameter	T37.0X1	T37.0X2	T37.0X3	T37.0X4	T37.0X5	T37.0X6
Sulfamethazine	T37.0X1	T37.0X2	T37.0X3	T37.0X4	T37.0X5	T37.0X6
Sulfamethizole	T37.0X1	T37.0X2	T37.0X3	T37.0X4	T37.0X5	T37.0X6
Sulfamethoxazole	T37.0X1	T37.0X2	T37.0X3	T37.0X4	T37.0X5	T37.0X6
- with trimethoprim	T36.8X1	T36.8X2	T36.8X3	T36.8X4	T36.8X5	T36.8X6
Sulfamethoxydiazine	T37.0X1	T37.0X2	T37.0X3	T37.0X4	T37.0X5	T37.0X6
Sulfamethoxypyridazine	T37.0X1	T37.0X2	T37.0X3	T37.0X4	T37.0X5	T37.0X6
Sulfamethylthiazole	T37.0X1	T37.0X2	T37.0X3	T37.0X4	T37.0X5	T37.0X6
Sulfametoxydiazine	T37.0X1	T37.0X2	T37.0X3	T37.0X4	T37.0X5	T37.0X6
Sulfamidopyrine	T39.2X1	T39.2X2	T39.2X3	T39.2X4	T39.2X5	T39.2X6
Sulfamonomethoxine	T37.0X1	T37.0X2	T37.0X3	T37.0X4	T37.0X5	T37.0X6
Sulfamoxole	T37.0X1	T37.0X2	T37.0X3	T37.0X4	T37.0X5	T37.0X6
Sulfamylon	T49.0X1	T49.0X2	T49.0X3	T49.0X4	T49.0X5	T49.0X6
Sulfan blue (diagnostic dye)	T50.8X1	T50.8X2	T50.8X3	T50.8X4	T50.8X5	T50.8X6
Sulfanilamide	T37.0X1	T37.0X2	T37.0X3	T37.0X4	T37.0X5	T37.0X6
Sulfanilylguanidine	T37.0X1	T37.0X2	T37.0X3	T37.0X4	T37.0X5	T37.0X6
Sulfaperin	T37.0X1	T37.0X2	T37.0X3	T37.0X4	T37.0X5	T37.0X6
Sulfaphenazole	T37.0X1	T37.0X2	T37.0X3	T37.0X4	T37.0X5	T37.0X6
Sulfaphenylthiazole	T37.0X1	T37.0X2	T37.0X3	T37.0X4	T37.0X5	T37.0X6
Sulfaproxyline	T37.0X1	T37.0X2	T37.0X3	T37.0X4	T37.0X5	T37.0X6
Sulfapyridine	T37.0X1	T37.0X2	T37.0X3	T37.0X4	T37.0X5	T37.0X6
Sulfapyrimidine	T37.0X1	T37.0X2	T37.0X3	T37.0X4	T37.0X5	T37.0X6
Sulfarsphenamine	T37.8X1	T37.8X2	T37.8X3	T37.8X4	T37.8X5	T37.8X6

Substance	Poisoning, Accidental (unintentional)	Poisoning, Intentional Self-harm	Poisoning, Assault	Poisoning, Undetermined	Adverse effect	Underdosing
Sulfasalazine	T37.0X1	T37.0X2	T37.0X3	T37.0X4	T37.0X5	T37.0X6
Sulfasuxidine	T37.0X1	T37.0X2	T37.0X3	T37.0X4	T37.0X5	T37.0X6
Sulfasymazine	T37.0X1	T37.0X2	T37.0X3	T37.0X4	T37.0X5	T37.0X6
Sulfated amylopectin	T47.8X1	T47.8X2	T47.8X3	T47.8X4	T47.8X5	T47.8X6
Sulfathiazole	T37.0X1	T37.0X2	T37.0X3	T37.0X4	T37.0X5	T37.0X6
Sulfatostearate	T49.2X1	T49.2X2	T49.2X3	T49.2X4	T49.2X5	T49.2X6
Sulfinpyrazone	T50.4X1	T50.4X2	T50.4X3	T50.4X4	T50.4X5	T50.4X6
Sulfiram	T49.0X1	T49.0X2	T49.0X3	T49.0X4	T49.0X5	T49.0X6
Sulfisomidine	T37.0X1	T37.0X2	T37.0X3	T37.0X4	T37.0X5	T37.0X6
Sulfisoxazole	T37.0X1	T37.0X2	T37.0X3	T37.0X4	T37.0X5	T37.0X6
- ophthalmic preparation	T49.5X1	T49.5X2	T49.5X3	T49.5X4	T49.5X5	T49.5X6
Sulfobromophthalein (sodium)	T50.8X1	T50.8X2	T50.8X3	T50.8X4	T50.8X5	T50.8X6
Sulfobromphthalein	T50.8X1	T50.8X2	T50.8X3	T50.8X4	T50.8X5	T50.8X6
Sulfogaiacol	T48.4X1	T48.4X2	T48.4X3	T48.4X4	T48.4X5	T48.4X6
Sulfomyxin	T36.8X1	T36.8X2	T36.8X3	T36.8X4	T36.8X5	T36.8X6
Sulfonal	T42.6X1	T42.6X2	T42.6X3	T42.6X4	T42.6X5	T42.6X6
Sulfonamide NEC	T37.0X1	T37.0X2	T37.0X3	T37.0X4	T37.0X5	T37.0X6
- eye	T49.5X1	T49.5X2	T49.5X3	T49.5X4	T49.5X5	T49.5X6
Sulfonazide	T37.1X1	T37.1X2	T37.1X3	T37.1X4	T37.1X5	T37.1X6
Sulfones	T37.1X1	T37.1X2	T37.1X3	T37.1X4	T37.1X5	T37.1X6
Sulfonethylmethane	T42.6X1	T42.6X2	T42.6X3	T42.6X4	T42.6X5	T42.6X6
Sulfonmethane	T42.6X1	T42.6X2	T42.6X3	T42.6X4	T42.6X5	T42.6X6
Sulfonphthal, sulfonphthol	T50.8X1	T50.8X2	T50.8X3	T50.8X4	T50.8X5	T50.8X6
Sulfonylurea derivatives, oral	T38.3X1	T38.3X2	T38.3X3	T38.3X4	T38.3X5	T38.3X6
Sulforidazine	T43.3X1	T43.3X2	T43.3X3	T43.3X4	T43.3X5	T43.3X6
Sulfoxone	T37.1X1	T37.1X2	T37.1X3	T37.1X4	T37.1X5	T37.1X6
Sulfur, sulfurated, sulfuric, sulfurous, sulfuryl (compounds NEC) (medicinal)	T49.4X1	T49.4X2	T49.4X3	T49.4X4	T49.4X5	T49.4X6
- acid	T54.2X1	T54.2X2	T54.2X3	T54.2X4	--	--
- dioxide (gas)	T59.1X1	T59.1X2	T59.1X3	T59.1X4	--	--
- ether—see Ether (s)						
- hydrogen	T59.6X1	T59.6X2	T59.6X3	T59.6X4	--	--
- medicinal (keratolytic) (ointment) NEC	T49.4X1	T49.4X2	T49.4X3	T49.4X4	T49.4X5	T49.4X6
- ointment	T49.0X1	T49.0X2	T49.0X3	T49.0X4	T49.0X5	T49.0X6
- pesticide (vapor)	T60.91	T60.92	T60.93	T60.94	--	--
- vapor NEC	T59.891	T59.892	T59.893	T59.894	--	--
Sulfuric acid	T54.2X1	T54.2X2	T54.2X3	T54.2X4	--	--
Sulglicotide	T47.1X1	T47.1X2	T47.1X3	T47.1X4	T47.1X5	T47.1X6
Sulindac	T39.391	T39.392	T39.393	T39.394	T39.395	T39.396
Sulisatin	T47.2X1	T47.2X2	T47.2X3	T47.2X4	T47.2X5	T47.2X6
Sulisobenzone	T49.3X1	T49.3X2	T49.3X3	T49.3X4	T49.3X5	T49.3X6
Sulkowitch's reagent	T50.8X1	T50.8X2	T50.8X3	T50.8X4	T50.8X5	T50.8X6
Sulmetozine	T44.3X1	T44.3X2	T44.3X3	T44.3X4	T44.3X5	T44.3X6
Suloctidil	T46.7X1	T46.7X2	T46.7X3	T46.7X4	T46.7X5	T46.7X6
Sulph——see also Sulf-						
Sulphadiazine	T37.0X1	T37.0X2	T37.0X3	T37.0X4	T37.0X5	T37.0X6
Sulphadimethoxine	T37.0X1	T37.0X2	T37.0X3	T37.0X4	T37.0X5	T37.0X6
Sulphadimidine	T37.0X1	T37.0X2	T37.0X3	T37.0X4	T37.0X5	T37.0X6
Sulphadione	T37.1X1	T37.1X2	T37.1X3	T37.1X4	T37.1X5	T37.1X6
Sulphafurazole	T37.0X1	T37.0X2	T37.0X3	T37.0X4	T37.0X5	T37.0X6
Sulphamethizole	T37.0X1	T37.0X2	T37.0X3	T37.0X4	T37.0X5	T37.0X6
Sulphamethoxazole	T37.0X1	T37.0X2	T37.0X3	T37.0X4	T37.0X5	T37.0X6
Sulphan blue	T50.8X1	T50.8X2	T50.8X3	T50.8X4	T50.8X5	T50.8X6
Sulphaphenazole	T37.0X1	T37.0X2	T37.0X3	T37.0X4	T37.0X5	T37.0X6
Sulphapyridine	T37.0X1	T37.0X2	T37.0X3	T37.0X4	T37.0X5	T37.0X6
Sulphasalazine	T37.0X1	T37.0X2	T37.0X3	T37.0X4	T37.0X5	T37.0X6
Sulphinpyrazone	T50.4X1	T50.4X2	T50.4X3	T50.4X4	T50.4X5	T50.4X6
Sulpiride	T43.591	T43.592	T43.593	T43.594	T43.595	T43.596
Sulprostone	T48.0X1	T48.0X2	T48.0X3	T48.0X4	T48.0X5	T48.0X6

Substance	Poisoning, Accidental (unintentional)	Poisoning, Intentional Self-harm	Poisoning, Assault	Poisoning, Undetermined	Adverse effect	Underdosing
Sulpyrine	T39.2X1	T39.2X2	T39.2X3	T39.2X4	T39.2X5	T39.2X6
Sultamicillin	T36.0X1	T36.0X2	T36.0X3	T36.0X4	T36.0X5	T36.0X6
Sulthiame	T42.6X1	T42.6X2	T42.6X3	T42.6X4	T42.6X5	T42.6X6
Sultiame	T42.6X1	T42.6X2	T42.6X3	T42.6X4	T42.6X5	T42.6X6
Sultopride	T43.591	T43.592	T43.593	T43.594	T43.595	T43.596
Sumatriptan	T39.8X1	T39.8X2	T39.8X3	T39.8X4	T39.8X5	T39.8X6
Sunflower seed oil	T46.6X1	T46.6X2	T46.6X3	T46.6X4	T46.6X5	T46.6X6
Superinone	T48.4X1	T48.4X2	T48.4X3	T48.4X4	T48.4X5	T48.4X6
Suprofen	T39.311	T39.312	T39.313	T39.314	T39.315	T39.316
Suramin (sodium)	T37.4X1	T37.4X2	T37.4X3	T37.4X4	T37.4X5	T37.4X6
Surfacaine	T41.3X1	T41.3X2	T41.3X3	T41.3X4	T41.3X5	T41.3X6
Surital	T41.1X1	T41.1X2	T41.1X3	T41.1X4	T41.1X5	T41.1X6
Sutilains	T45.3X1	T45.3X2	T45.3X3	T45.3X4	T45.3X5	T45.3X6
Suxamethonium (chloride)	T48.1X1	T48.1X2	T48.1X3	T48.1X4	T48.1X5	T48.1X6
Suxethonium (chloride)	T48.1X1	T48.1X2	T48.1X3	T48.1X4	T48.1X5	T48.1X6
Suxibuzone	T39.2X1	T39.2X2	T39.2X3	T39.2X4	T39.2X5	T39.2X6
Sweet niter spirit	T46.3X1	T46.3X2	T46.3X3	T46.3X4	T46.3X5	T46.3X6
Sweet oil (birch)	T49.3X1	T49.3X2	T49.3X3	T49.3X4	T49.3X5	T49.3X6
Sweetener	T50.901	T50.902	T50.903	T50.904	T50.905	T50.906
Sym-dichloroethyl ether	T53.6X1	T53.6X2	T53.6X3	T53.6X4	--	--
Sympatholytic NEC	T44.8X1	T44.8X2	T44.8X3	T44.8X4	T44.8X5	T44.8X6
- haloalkylamine	T44.8X1	T44.8X2	T44.8X3	T44.8X4	T44.8X5	T44.8X6
Sympathomimetic NEC	T44.901	T44.902	T44.903	T44.904	T44.905	T44.906
- anti-common-cold	T48.5X1	T48.5X2	T48.5X3	T48.5X4	T48.5X5	T48.5X6
- bronchodilator	T48.6X1	T48.6X2	T48.6X3	T48.6X4	T48.6X5	T48.6X6
- specified NEC	T44.991	T44.992	T44.993	T44.994	T44.995	T44.996
Synagis	T50.B91	T50.B92	T50.B93	T50.B94	T50.B95	T50.B96
Synalar	T49.0X1	T49.0X2	T49.0X3	T49.0X4	T49.0X5	T49.0X6
Synthroid	T38.1X1	T38.1X2	T38.1X3	T38.1X4	T38.1X5	T38.1X6
Synthetic cannabinoids	T40.721	T40.722	T40.723	T40.724	T40.725	T40.726
Syntocinon	T48.0X1	T48.0X2	T48.0X3	T48.0X4	T48.0X5	T48.0X6
Syrosingopine	T46.5X1	T46.5X2	T46.5X3	T46.5X4	T46.5X5	T46.5X6
Systemic drug	T45.91	T45.92	T45.93	T45.94	T45.95	T45.96
- specified NEC	T45.8X1	T45.8X2	T45.8X3	T45.8X4	T45.8X5	T45.8X6
2,4,5-T	T60.3X1	T60.3X2	T60.3X3	T60.3X4	--	--
Tablets—see also specified substance	T50.901	T50.902	T50.903	T50.904	T50.905	T50.906
Tace	T38.5X1	T38.5X2	T38.5X3	T38.5X4	T38.5X5	T38.5X6
Tacrine	T44.0X1	T44.0X2	T44.0X3	T44.0X4	T44.0X5	T44.0X6
Tadalafil	T46.7X1	T46.7X2	T46.7X3	T46.7X4	T46.7X5	T46.7X6
Talampicillin	T36.0X1	T36.0X2	T36.0X3	T36.0X4	T36.0X5	T36.0X6
Talbutal	T42.3X1	T42.3X2	T42.3X3	T42.3X4	T42.3X5	T42.3X6
Talc powder	T49.3X1	T49.3X2	T49.3X3	T49.3X4	T49.3X5	T49.3X6
Talcum	T49.3X1	T49.3X2	T49.3X3	T49.3X4	T49.3X5	T49.3X6
Taleranol	T38.6X1	T38.6X2	T38.6X3	T38.6X4	T38.6X5	T38.6X6
Tamoxifen	T38.6X1	T38.6X2	T38.6X3	T38.6X4	T38.6X5	T38.6X6
Tamsulosin	T44.6X1	T44.6X2	T44.6X3	T44.6X4	T44.6X5	T44.6X6
Tandearil, tanderil	T39.2X1	T39.2X2	T39.2X3	T39.2X4	T39.2X5	T39.2X6
Tannic acid	T49.2X1	T49.2X2	T49.2X3	T49.2X4	T49.2X5	T49.2X6
- medicinal (astringent)	T49.2X1	T49.2X2	T49.2X3	T49.2X4	T49.2X5	T49.2X6
Tannin—see Tannic acid						
Tansy	T62.2X1	T62.2X2	T62.2X3	T62.2X4	--	--
TAO	T36.3X1	T36.3X2	T36.3X3	T36.3X4	T36.3X5	T36.3X6
Tapazole	T38.2X1	T38.2X2	T38.2X3	T38.2X4	T38.2X5	T38.2X6
Tar NEC	T52.0X1	T52.0X2	T52.0X3	T52.0X4	--	--
- camphor	T60.1X1	T60.1X2	T60.1X3	T60.1X4	--	--
- distillate	T49.1X1	T49.1X2	T49.1X3	T49.1X4	T49.1X5	T49.1X6
- fumes	T59.891	T59.892	T59.893	T59.894	--	--
- medicinal	T49.1X1	T49.1X2	T49.1X3	T49.1X4	T49.1X5	T49.1X6

Substance	Poisoning, Accidental (unintentional)	Poisoning, Intentional Self-harm	Poisoning, Assault	Poisoning, Undetermined	Adverse effect	Underdosing
- ointment	T49.1X1	T49.1X2	T49.1X3	T49.1X4	T49.1X5	T49.1X6
Taractan	T43.591	T43.592	T43.593	T43.594	T43.595	T43.596
Tarantula (venomous)	T63.321	T63.322	T63.323	T63.324	--	--
Tartar emetic	T37.8X1	T37.8X2	T37.8X3	T37.8X4	T37.8X5	T37.8X6
Tartaric acid	T65.891	T65.892	T65.893	T65.894	--	--
Tartrate, laxative	T47.4X1	T47.4X2	T47.4X3	T47.4X4	T47.4X5	T47.4X6
Tartrated antimony (anti-infective)	T37.8X1	T37.8X2	T37.8X3	T37.8X4	T37.8X5	T37.8X6
Tauromustine	T45.1X1	T45.1X2	T45.1X3	T45.1X4	T45.1X5	T45.1X6
TCA—see Trichloroacetic acid						
TCDD	T53.7X1	T53.7X2	T53.7X3	T53.7X4	--	--
TDI (vapor)	T65.0X1	T65.0X2	T65.0X3	T65.0X4	--	--
Tear						
- gas	T59.3X1	T59.3X2	T59.3X3	T59.3X4	--	--
- solution	T49.5X1	T49.5X2	T49.5X3	T49.5X4	T49.5X5	T49.5X6
Teclothiazide	T50.2X1	T50.2X2	T50.2X3	T50.2X4	T50.2X5	T50.2X6
Teclozan	T37.3X1	T37.3X2	T37.3X3	T37.3X4	T37.3X5	T37.3X6
Tegafur	T45.1X1	T45.1X2	T45.1X3	T45.1X4	T45.1X5	T45.1X6
Tegretol	T42.1X1	T42.1X2	T42.1X3	T42.1X4	T42.1X5	T42.1X6
Teicoplanin	T36.8X1	T36.8X2	T36.8X3	T36.8X4	T36.8X5	T36.8X6
Telepaque	T50.8X1	T50.8X2	T50.8X3	T50.8X4	T50.8X5	T50.8X6
Tellurium	T56.891	T56.892	T56.893	T56.894	--	--
- fumes	T56.891	T56.892	T56.893	T56.894	--	--
TEM	T45.1X1	T45.1X2	T45.1X3	T45.1X4	T45.1X5	T45.1X6
Temazepam	T42.4X1	T42.4X2	T42.4X3	T42.4X4	T42.4X5	T42.4X6
Temocillin	T36.0X1	T36.0X2	T36.0X3	T36.0X4	T36.0X5	T36.0X6
Tenamfetamine	T43.621	T43.622	T43.623	T43.624	T43.625	T43.626
Teniposide	T45.1X1	T45.1X2	T45.1X3	T45.1X4	T45.1X5	T45.1X6
Tenitramine	T46.3X1	T46.3X2	T46.3X3	T46.3X4	T46.3X5	T46.3X6
Tenoglicin	T48.4X1	T48.4X2	T48.4X3	T48.4X4	T48.4X5	T48.4X6
Tenonitrozole	T37.3X1	T37.3X2	T37.3X3	T37.3X4	T37.3X5	T37.3X6
Tenoxicam	T39.391	T39.392	T39.393	T39.394	T39.395	T39.396
TEPA	T45.1X1	T45.1X2	T45.1X3	T45.1X4	T45.1X5	T45.1X6
TEPP	T60.0X1	T60.0X2	T60.0X3	T60.0X4	--	--
Teprotide	T46.5X1	T46.5X2	T46.5X3	T46.5X4	T46.5X5	T46.5X6
Terazosin	T44.6X1	T44.6X2	T44.6X3	T44.6X4	T44.6X5	T44.6X6
Terbufos	T60.0X1	T60.0X2	T60.0X3	T60.0X4	--	--
Terbutaline	T48.6X1	T48.6X2	T48.6X3	T48.6X4	T48.6X5	T48.6X6
Terconazole	T49.0X1	T49.0X2	T49.0X3	T49.0X4	T49.0X5	T49.0X6
Terfenadine	T45.0X1	T45.0X2	T45.0X3	T45.0X4	T45.0X5	T45.0X6
Teriparatide (acetate)	T50.991	T50.992	T50.993	T50.994	T50.995	T50.996
Terizidone	T37.1X1	T37.1X2	T37.1X3	T37.1X4	T37.1X5	T37.1X6
Terlipressin	T38.891	T38.892	T38.893	T38.894	T38.895	T38.896
Terodiline	T46.3X1	T46.3X2	T46.3X3	T46.3X4	T46.3X5	T46.3X6
Teroxalene	T37.4X1	T37.4X2	T37.4X3	T37.4X4	T37.4X5	T37.4X6
Terpin (cis) hydrate	T48.4X1	T48.4X2	T48.4X3	T48.4X4	T48.4X5	T48.4X6
Terramycin	T36.4X1	T36.4X2	T36.4X3	T36.4X4	T36.4X5	T36.4X6
Tertatolol	T44.7X1	T44.7X2	T44.7X3	T44.7X4	T44.7X5	T44.7X6
Tessalon	T48.3X1	T48.3X2	T48.3X3	T48.3X4	T48.3X5	T48.3X6
Testolactone	T38.7X1	T38.7X2	T38.7X3	T38.7X4	T38.7X5	T38.7X6
Testosterone	T38.7X1	T38.7X2	T38.7X3	T38.7X4	T38.7X5	T38.7X6
Tetanus toxoid or vaccine	T50.A91	T50.A92	T50.A93	T50.A94	T50.A95	T50.A96
- antitoxin	T50.Z11	T50.Z12	T50.Z13	T50.Z14	T50.Z15	T50.Z16
- immune globulin (human)	T50.Z11	T50.Z12	T50.Z13	T50.Z14	T50.Z15	T50.Z16
- toxoid	T50.A91	T50.A92	T50.A93	T50.A94	T50.A95	T50.A96
- - with diphtheria toxoid	T50.A21	T50.A22	T50.A23	T50.A24	T50.A25	T50.A26
- - - with pertussis	T50.A11	T50.A12	T50.A13	T50.A14	T50.A15	T50.A16
Tetrabenazine	T43.591	T43.592	T43.593	T43.594	T43.595	T43.596
Tetracaine	T41.3X1	T41.3X2	T41.3X3	T41.3X4	T41.3X5	T41.3X6

Substance	Poisoning, Accidental (unintentional)	Poisoning, Intentional Self-harm	Poisoning, Assault	Poisoning, Undetermined	Adverse effect	Underdosing
- nerve block (peripheral) (plexus)	T41.3X1	T41.3X2	T41.3X3	T41.3X4	T41.3X5	T41.3X6
- regional	T41.3X1	T41.3X2	T41.3X3	T41.3X4	T41.3X5	T41.3X6
- spinal	T41.3X1	T41.3X2	T41.3X3	T41.3X4	T41.3X5	T41.3X6
Tetrachlorethylene—see Tetrachloroethylene						
Tetrachlormethiazide	T50.2X1	T50.2X2	T50.2X3	T50.2X4	T50.2X5	T50.2X6
2,3,7,8-Tetrachlorodibenzo-p-dioxin	T53.7X1	T53.7X2	T53.7X3	T53.7X4	--	--
Tetrachloroethane	T53.6X1	T53.6X2	T53.6X3	T53.6X4	--	--
- vapor	T53.6X1	T53.6X2	T53.6X3	T53.6X4	--	--
- - paint or varnish	T53.6X1	T53.6X2	T53.6X3	T53.6X4	--	--
Tetrachloroethylene (liquid)	T53.3X1	T53.3X2	T53.3X3	T53.3X4	--	--
- medicinal	T37.4X1	T37.4X2	T37.4X3	T37.4X4	T37.4X5	T37.4X6
- vapor	T53.3X1	T53.3X2	T53.3X3	T53.3X4	--	--
Tetrachloromethane—see Carbon tetrachloride						
Tetracosactide	T38.811	T38.812	T38.813	T38.814	T38.815	T38.816
Tetracosactrin	T38.811	T38.812	T38.813	T38.814	T38.815	T38.816
Tetracycline	T36.4X1	T36.4X2	T36.4X3	T36.4X4	T36.4X5	T36.4X6
- ophthalmic preparation	T49.5X1	T49.5X2	T49.5X3	T49.5X4	T49.5X5	T49.5X6
- topical NEC	T49.0X1	T49.0X2	T49.0X3	T49.0X4	T49.0X5	T49.0X6
Tetradifon	T60.8X1	T60.8X2	T60.8X3	T60.8X4	--	--
Tetradotoxin	T61.771	T61.772	T61.773	T61.774	--	--
Tetraethyl						
- lead	T56.0X1	T56.0X2	T56.0X3	T56.0X4	--	--
- pyrophosphate	T60.0X1	T60.0X2	T60.0X3	T60.0X4	--	--
Tetraethylammonium chloride	T44.2X1	T44.2X2	T44.2X3	T44.2X4	T44.2X5	T44.2X6
Tetraethylthiuram disulfide	T50.6X1	T50.6X2	T50.6X3	T50.6X4	T50.6X5	T50.6X6
Tetrahydroaminoacridine	T44.0X1	T44.0X2	T44.0X3	T44.0X4	T44.0X5	T44.0X6
Tetrahydrocannabinol	T40.711	T40.712	T40.713	T40.714	T40.715	T40.716
Tetrahydrofuran	T52.8X1	T52.8X2	T52.8X3	T52.8X4	--	--
Tetrahydronaphthalene	T52.8X1	T52.8X2	T52.8X3	T52.8X4	--	--
Tetrahydrozoline	T49.5X1	T49.5X2	T49.5X3	T49.5X4	T49.5X5	T49.5X6
Tetralin	T52.8X1	T52.8X2	T52.8X3	T52.8X4	--	--
Tetramethrin	T60.2X1	T60.2X2	T60.2X3	T60.2X4	--	--
Tetramethylthiuram (disulfide) NEC	T60.3X1	T60.3X2	T60.3X3	T60.3X4	--	--
- medicinal	T49.0X1	T49.0X2	T49.0X3	T49.0X4	T49.0X5	T49.0X6
Tetramisole	T37.4X1	T37.4X2	T37.4X3	T37.4X4	T37.4X5	T37.4X6
Tetranicotinoyl fructose	T46.7X1	T46.7X2	T46.7X3	T46.7X4	T46.7X5	T46.7X6
Tetrazepam	T42.4X1	T42.4X2	T42.4X3	T42.4X4	T42.4X5	T42.4X6
Tetronal	T42.6X1	T42.6X2	T42.6X3	T42.6X4	T42.6X5	T42.6X6
Tetryl	T65.3X1	T65.3X2	T65.3X3	T65.3X4	--	--
Tetrylammonium chloride	T44.2X1	T44.2X2	T44.2X3	T44.2X4	T44.2X5	T44.2X6
Tetryzoline	T49.5X1	T49.5X2	T49.5X3	T49.5X4	T49.5X5	T49.5X6
Thalidomide	T45.1X1	T45.1X2	T45.1X3	T45.1X4	T45.1X5	T45.1X6
Thallium (compounds) (dust) NEC	T56.811	T56.812	T56.813	T56.814	--	--
- pesticide	T60.4X1	T60.4X2	T60.4X3	T60.4X4	--	--
THC	T40.711	T40.712	T40.713	T40.714	T40.715	T40.716
Thebacon	T48.3X1	T48.3X2	T48.3X3	T48.3X4	T48.3X5	T48.3X6
Thebaine	T40.2X1	T40.2X2	T40.2X3	T40.2X4	T40.2X5	T40.2X6
Thenoic acid	T49.6X1	T49.6X2	T49.6X3	T49.6X4	T49.6X5	T49.6X6
Thenyldiamine	T45.0X1	T45.0X2	T45.0X3	T45.0X4	T45.0X5	T45.0X6
Theobromine (calcium salicylate)	T48.6X1	T48.6X2	T48.6X3	T48.6X4	T48.6X5	T48.6X6
- sodium salicylate	T48.6X1	T48.6X2	T48.6X3	T48.6X4	T48.6X5	T48.6X6
Theophyllamine	T48.6X1	T48.6X2	T48.6X3	T48.6X4	T48.6X5	T48.6X6
Theophylline	T48.6X1	T48.6X2	T48.6X3	T48.6X4	T48.6X5	T48.6X6
- aminobenzoic acid	T48.6X1	T48.6X2	T48.6X3	T48.6X4	T48.6X5	T48.6X6
- ethylenediamine	T48.6X1	T48.6X2	T48.6X3	T48.6X4	T48.6X5	T48.6X6
- piperazine p-amino-benzoate	T48.6X1	T48.6X2	T48.6X3	T48.6X4	T48.6X5	T48.6X6
Thiabendazole	T37.4X1	T37.4X2	T37.4X3	T37.4X4	T37.4X5	T37.4X6
Thialbarbital	T41.1X1	T41.1X2	T41.1X3	T41.1X4	T41.1X5	T41.1X6

Substance	Poisoning, Accidental (unintentional)	Poisoning, Intentional Self-harm	Poisoning, Assault	Poisoning, Undetermined	Adverse effect	Underdosing
Thiamazole	T38.2X1	T38.2X2	T38.2X3	T38.2X4	T38.2X5	T38.2X6
Thiambutosine	T37.1X1	T37.1X2	T37.1X3	T37.1X4	T37.1X5	T37.1X6
Thiamine	T45.2X1	T45.2X2	T45.2X3	T45.2X4	T45.2X5	T45.2X6
Thiamphenicol	T36.2X1	T36.2X2	T36.2X3	T36.2X4	T36.2X5	T36.2X6
Thiamylal	T41.1X1	T41.1X2	T41.1X3	T41.1X4	T41.1X5	T41.1X6
- sodium	T41.1X1	T41.1X2	T41.1X3	T41.1X4	T41.1X5	T41.1X6
Thiazesim	T43.291	T43.292	T43.293	T43.294	T43.295	T43.296
Thiazides (diuretics)	T50.2X1	T50.2X2	T50.2X3	T50.2X4	T50.2X5	T50.2X6
Thiazinamium metilsulfate	T43.3X1	T43.3X2	T43.3X3	T43.3X4	T43.3X5	T43.3X6
Thiethylperazine	T43.3X1	T43.3X2	T43.3X3	T43.3X4	T43.3X5	T43.3X6
Thimerosal	T49.0X1	T49.0X2	T49.0X3	T49.0X4	T49.0X5	T49.0X6
- ophthalmic preparation	T49.5X1	T49.5X2	T49.5X3	T49.5X4	T49.5X5	T49.5X6
Thioacetazone	T37.1X1	T37.1X2	T37.1X3	T37.1X4	T37.1X5	T37.1X6
- with isoniazid	T37.1X1	T37.1X2	T37.1X3	T37.1X4	T37.1X5	T37.1X6
Thiobarbital sodium	T41.1X1	T41.1X2	T41.1X3	T41.1X4	T41.1X5	T41.1X6
Thiobarbiturate anesthetic	T41.1X1	T41.1X2	T41.1X3	T41.1X4	T41.1X5	T41.1X6
Thiobismol	T37.8X1	T37.8X2	T37.8X3	T37.8X4	T37.8X5	T37.8X6
Thiobutabarbital sodium	T41.1X1	T41.1X2	T41.1X3	T41.1X4	T41.1X5	T41.1X6
Thiocarbamate (insecticide)	T60.0X1	T60.0X2	T60.0X3	T60.0X4	--	--
Thiocarbamide	T38.2X1	T38.2X2	T38.2X3	T38.2X4	T38.2X5	T38.2X6
Thiocarbarsone	T37.8X1	T37.8X2	T37.8X3	T37.8X4	T37.8X5	T37.8X6
Thiocarlide	T37.1X1	T37.1X2	T37.1X3	T37.1X4	T37.1X5	T37.1X6
Thioctamide	T50.991	T50.992	T50.993	T50.994	T50.995	T50.996
Thioctic acid	T50.991	T50.992	T50.993	T50.994	T50.995	T50.996
Thiofos	T60.0X1	T60.0X2	T60.0X3	T60.0X4	--	--
Thioglycolate	T49.4X1	T49.4X2	T49.4X3	T49.4X4	T49.4X5	T49.4X6
Thioglycolic acid	T65.891	T65.892	T65.893	T65.894	--	--
Thioguanine	T45.1X1	T45.1X2	T45.1X3	T45.1X4	T45.1X5	T45.1X6
Thiomercaptomerin	T50.2X1	T50.2X2	T50.2X3	T50.2X4	T50.2X5	T50.2X6
Thiomerin	T50.2X1	T50.2X2	T50.2X3	T50.2X4	T50.2X5	T50.2X6
Thiomersal	T49.0X1	T49.0X2	T49.0X3	T49.0X4	T49.0X5	T49.0X6
Thionazin	T60.0X1	T60.0X2	T60.0X3	T60.0X4	--	--
Thiopental (sodium)	T41.1X1	T41.1X2	T41.1X3	T41.1X4	T41.1X5	T41.1X6
Thiopentone (sodium)	T41.1X1	T41.1X2	T41.1X3	T41.1X4	T41.1X5	T41.1X6
Thiopropazate	T43.3X1	T43.3X2	T43.3X3	T43.3X4	T43.3X5	T43.3X6
Thioproperazine	T43.3X1	T43.3X2	T43.3X3	T43.3X4	T43.3X5	T43.3X6
Thioridazine	T43.3X1	T43.3X2	T43.3X3	T43.3X4	T43.3X5	T43.3X6
Thiosinamine	T49.3X1	T49.3X2	T49.3X3	T49.3X4	T49.3X5	T49.3X6
Thiotepa	T45.1X1	T45.1X2	T45.1X3	T45.1X4	T45.1X5	T45.1X6
Thiothixene	T43.4X1	T43.4X2	T43.4X3	T43.4X4	T43.4X5	T43.4X6
Thiouracil (benzyl) (methyl) (propyl)	T38.2X1	T38.2X2	T38.2X3	T38.2X4	T38.2X5	T38.2X6
Thiourea	T38.2X1	T38.2X2	T38.2X3	T38.2X4	T38.2X5	T38.2X6
Thiphenamil	T44.3X1	T44.3X2	T44.3X3	T44.3X4	T44.3X5	T44.3X6
Thiram	T60.3X1	T60.3X2	T60.3X3	T60.3X4	--	--
- medicinal	T49.2X1	T49.2X2	T49.2X3	T49.2X4	T49.2X5	T49.2X6
Thonzylamine (systemic)	T45.0X1	T45.0X2	T45.0X3	T45.0X4	T45.0X5	T45.0X6
- mucosal decongestant	T48.5X1	T48.5X2	T48.5X3	T48.5X4	T48.5X5	T48.5X6
Thorazine	T43.3X1	T43.3X2	T43.3X3	T43.3X4	T43.3X5	T43.3X6
Thorium dioxide suspension	T50.8X1	T50.8X2	T50.8X3	T50.8X4	T50.8X5	T50.8X6
Thornapple	T62.2X1	T62.2X2	T62.2X3	T62.2X4	--	--
Throat drug NEC	T49.6X1	T49.6X2	T49.6X3	T49.6X4	T49.6X5	T49.6X6
Thrombin	T45.7X1	T45.7X2	T45.7X3	T45.7X4	T45.7X5	T45.7X6
Thrombolysin	T45.611	T45.612	T45.613	T45.614	T45.615	T45.616
Thromboplastin	T45.7X1	T45.7X2	T45.7X3	T45.7X4	T45.7X5	T45.7X6
Thurfyl nicotinate	T46.7X1	T46.7X2	T46.7X3	T46.7X4	T46.7X5	T46.7X6
Thymol	T49.0X1	T49.0X2	T49.0X3	T49.0X4	T49.0X5	T49.0X6
Thymopentin	T37.5X1	T37.5X2	T37.5X3	T37.5X4	T37.5X5	T37.5X6
Thymoxamine	T46.7X1	T46.7X2	T46.7X3	T46.7X4	T46.7X5	T46.7X6

Substance	Poisoning, Accidental (unintentional)	Poisoning, Intentional Self-harm	Poisoning, Assault	Poisoning, Undetermined	Adverse effect	Underdosing
Thymus extract	T38.891	T38.892	T38.893	T38.894	T38.895	T38.896
Thyreotrophic hormone	T38.811	T38.812	T38.813	T38.814	T38.815	T38.816
Thyroglobulin	T38.1X1	T38.1X2	T38.1X3	T38.1X4	T38.1X5	T38.1X6
Thyroid (hormone)	T38.1X1	T38.1X2	T38.1X3	T38.1X4	T38.1X5	T38.1X6
Thyrolar	T38.1X1	T38.1X2	T38.1X3	T38.1X4	T38.1X5	T38.1X6
Thyrotrophin	T38.811	T38.812	T38.813	T38.814	T38.815	T38.816
Thyrotropic hormone	T38.811	T38.812	T38.813	T38.814	T38.815	T38.816
Thyroxine	T38.1X1	T38.1X2	T38.1X3	T38.1X4	T38.1X5	T38.1X6
Tiabendazole	T37.4X1	T37.4X2	T37.4X3	T37.4X4	T37.4X5	T37.4X6
Tiamizide	T50.2X1	T50.2X2	T50.2X3	T50.2X4	T50.2X5	T50.2X6
Tianeptine	T43.291	T43.292	T43.293	T43.294	T43.295	T43.296
Tiapamil	T46.1X1	T46.1X2	T46.1X3	T46.1X4	T46.1X5	T46.1X6
Tiapride	T43.591	T43.592	T43.593	T43.594	T43.595	T43.596
Tiaprofenic acid	T39.311	T39.312	T39.313	T39.314	T39.315	T39.316
Tiaramide	T39.8X1	T39.8X2	T39.8X3	T39.8X4	T39.8X5	T39.8X6
Ticarcillin	T36.0X1	T36.0X2	T36.0X3	T36.0X4	T36.0X5	T36.0X6
Ticlatone	T49.0X1	T49.0X2	T49.0X3	T49.0X4	T49.0X5	T49.0X6
Ticlopidine	T45.521	T45.522	T45.523	T45.524	T45.525	T45.526
Ticrynafen	T50.1X1	T50.1X2	T50.1X3	T50.1X4	T50.1X5	T50.1X6
Tidiacic	T50.991	T50.992	T50.993	T50.994	T50.995	T50.996
Tiemonium	T44.3X1	T44.3X2	T44.3X3	T44.3X4	T44.3X5	T44.3X6
- iodide	T44.3X1	T44.3X2	T44.3X3	T44.3X4	T44.3X5	T44.3X6
Tienilic acid	T50.1X1	T50.1X2	T50.1X3	T50.1X4	T50.1X5	T50.1X6
Tifenamil	T44.3X1	T44.3X2	T44.3X3	T44.3X4	T44.3X5	T44.3X6
Tigan	T45.0X1	T45.0X2	T45.0X3	T45.0X4	T45.0X5	T45.0X6
Tigloidine	T44.3X1	T44.3X2	T44.3X3	T44.3X4	T44.3X5	T44.3X6
Tilactase	T47.5X1	T47.5X2	T47.5X3	T47.5X4	T47.5X5	T47.5X6
Tiletamine	T41.291	T41.292	T41.293	T41.294	T41.295	T41.296
Tilidine	T40.491	T40.492	T40.493	T40.494	--	--
Timepidium bromide	T44.3X1	T44.3X2	T44.3X3	T44.3X4	T44.3X5	T44.3X6
Timiperone	T43.4X1	T43.4X2	T43.4X3	T43.4X4	T43.4X5	T43.4X6
Timolol	T44.7X1	T44.7X2	T44.7X3	T44.7X4	T44.7X5	T44.7X6
Tin (chloride) (dust) (oxide) NEC	T56.6X1	T56.6X2	T56.6X3	T56.6X4	--	--
- anti-infectives	T37.8X1	T37.8X2	T37.8X3	T37.8X4	T37.8X5	T37.8X6
Tincture, iodine—see Iodine						
Tindal	T43.3X1	T43.3X2	T43.3X3	T43.3X4	T43.3X5	T43.3X6
Tinidazole	T37.3X1	T37.3X2	T37.3X3	T37.3X4	T37.3X5	T37.3X6
Tinoridine	T39.8X1	T39.8X2	T39.8X3	T39.8X4	T39.8X5	T39.8X6
Tiocarlide	T37.1X1	T37.1X2	T37.1X3	T37.1X4	T37.1X5	T37.1X6
Tioclomarol	T45.511	T45.512	T45.513	T45.514	T45.515	T45.516
Tioconazole	T49.0X1	T49.0X2	T49.0X3	T49.0X4	T49.0X5	T49.0X6
Tioguanine	T45.1X1	T45.1X2	T45.1X3	T45.1X4	T45.1X5	T45.1X6
Tiopronin	T50.991	T50.992	T50.993	T50.994	T50.995	T50.996
Tiotixene	T43.4X1	T43.4X2	T43.4X3	T43.4X4	T43.4X5	T43.4X6
Tioxolone	T49.4X1	T49.4X2	T49.4X3	T49.4X4	T49.4X5	T49.4X6
Tipepidine	T48.3X1	T48.3X2	T48.3X3	T48.3X4	T48.3X5	T48.3X6
Tiquizium bromide	T44.3X1	T44.3X2	T44.3X3	T44.3X4	T44.3X5	T44.3X6
Tiratricol	T38.1X1	T38.1X2	T38.1X3	T38.1X4	T38.1X5	T38.1X6
Tisopurine	T50.4X1	T50.4X2	T50.4X3	T50.4X4	T50.4X5	T50.4X6
Titanium (compounds) (vapor)	T56.891	T56.892	T56.893	T56.894	--	--
- dioxide	T49.3X1	T49.3X2	T49.3X3	T49.3X4	T49.3X5	T49.3X6
- ointment	T49.3X1	T49.3X2	T49.3X3	T49.3X4	T49.3X5	T49.3X6
- oxide	T49.3X1	T49.3X2	T49.3X3	T49.3X4	T49.3X5	T49.3X6
- tetrachloride	T56.891	T56.892	T56.893	T56.894	--	--
Titanocene	T56.891	T56.892	T56.893	T56.894	--	--
Titroid	T38.1X1	T38.1X2	T38.1X3	T38.1X4	T38.1X5	T38.1X6
Tizanidine	T42.8X1	T42.8X2	T42.8X3	T42.8X4	T42.8X5	T42.8X6
TMTD	T60.3X1	T60.3X2	T60.3X3	T60.3X4	--	--
TNT (fumes)	T65.3X1	T65.3X2	T65.3X3	T65.3X4	--	--

Substance	Poisoning, Accidental (unintentional)	Poisoning, Intentional Self-harm	Poisoning, Assault	Poisoning, Undetermined	Adverse effect	Underdosing
Toadstool	T62.0X1	T62.0X2	T62.0X3	T62.0X4	--	--
Tobacco NEC	T65.291	T65.292	T65.293	T65.294	--	--
- cigarettes	T65.221	T65.222	T65.223	T65.224	--	--
- Indian	T62.2X1	T62.2X2	T62.2X3	T62.2X4	--	--
- smoke, second-hand	T65.221	T65.222	T65.223	T65.224	--	--
Tobramycin	T36.5X1	T36.5X2	T36.5X3	T36.5X4	T36.5X5	T36.5X6
Tocainide	T46.2X1	T46.2X2	T46.2X3	T46.2X4	T46.2X5	T46.2X6
Tocoferol	T45.2X1	T45.2X2	T45.2X3	T45.2X4	T45.2X5	T45.2X6
Tocopherol	T45.2X1	T45.2X2	T45.2X3	T45.2X4	T45.2X5	T45.2X6
- acetate	T45.2X1	T45.2X2	T45.2X3	T45.2X4	T45.2X5	T45.2X6
Tocosamine	T48.0X1	T48.0X2	T48.0X3	T48.0X4	T48.0X5	T48.0X6
Todralazine	T46.5X1	T46.5X2	T46.5X3	T46.5X4	T46.5X5	T46.5X6
Tofisopam	T42.4X1	T42.4X2	T42.4X3	T42.4X4	T42.4X5	T42.4X6
Tofranil	T43.011	T43.012	T43.013	T43.014	T43.015	T43.016
Toilet deodorizer	T65.891	T65.892	T65.893	T65.894	--	--
Tolamolol	T44.7X1	T44.7X2	T44.7X3	T44.7X4	T44.7X5	T44.7X6
Tolazamide	T38.3X1	T38.3X2	T38.3X3	T38.3X4	T38.3X5	T38.3X6
Tolazoline	T46.7X1	T46.7X2	T46.7X3	T46.7X4	T46.7X5	T46.7X6
Tolbutamide (sodium)	T38.3X1	T38.3X2	T38.3X3	T38.3X4	T38.3X5	T38.3X6
Tolciclate	T49.0X1	T49.0X2	T49.0X3	T49.0X4	T49.0X5	T49.0X6
Tolmetin	T39.391	T39.392	T39.393	T39.394	T39.395	T39.396
Tolnaftate	T49.0X1	T49.0X2	T49.0X3	T49.0X4	T49.0X5	T49.0X6
Tolonidine	T46.5X1	T46.5X2	T46.5X3	T46.5X4	T46.5X5	T46.5X6
Toloxatone	T42.6X1	T42.6X2	T42.6X3	T42.6X4	T42.6X5	T42.6X6
Tolperisone	T44.3X1	T44.3X2	T44.3X3	T44.3X4	T44.3X5	T44.3X6
Tolserol	T42.8X1	T42.8X2	T42.8X3	T42.8X4	T42.8X5	T42.8X6
Toluene (liquid)	T52.2X1	T52.2X2	T52.2X3	T52.2X4	--	--
- diisocyanate	T65.0X1	T65.0X2	T65.0X3	T65.0X4	--	--
Toluidine	T65.891	T65.892	T65.893	T65.894	--	--
- vapor	T59.891	T59.892	T59.893	T59.894	--	--
Toluol (liquid)	T52.2X1	T52.2X2	T52.2X3	T52.2X4	--	--
- vapor	T52.2X1	T52.2X2	T52.2X3	T52.2X4	--	--
Toluylenediamine	T65.3X1	T65.3X2	T65.3X3	T65.3X4	--	--
Tolylene-2,4-diisocyanate	T65.0X1	T65.0X2	T65.0X3	T65.0X4	--	--
Tonic NEC	T50.901	T50.902	T50.903	T50.904	T50.905	T50.906
Topical action drug NEC	T49.91	T49.92	T49.93	T49.94	T49.95	T49.96
- ear, nose or throat	T49.6X1	T49.6X2	T49.6X3	T49.6X4	T49.6X5	T49.6X6
- eye	T49.5X1	T49.5X2	T49.5X3	T49.5X4	T49.5X5	T49.5X6
- skin	T49.91	T49.92	T49.93	T49.94	T49.95	T49.96
- specified NEC	T49.8X1	T49.8X2	T49.8X3	T49.8X4	T49.8X5	T49.8X6
Toquizine	T44.3X1	T44.3X2	T44.3X3	T44.3X4	T44.3X5	T44.3X6
Toremifene	T38.6X1	T38.6X2	T38.6X3	T38.6X4	T38.6X5	T38.6X6
Tosylchloramide sodium	T49.8X1	T49.8X2	T49.8X3	T49.8X4	T49.8X5	T49.8X6
Toxaphene (dust) (spray)	T60.1X1	T60.1X2	T60.1X3	T60.1X4	--	--
Toxin, diphtheria (Schick Test)	T50.8X1	T50.8X2	T50.8X3	T50.8X4	T50.8X5	T50.8X6
Toxoid						
- combined	T50.A21	T50.A22	T50.A23	T50.A24	T50.A25	T50.A26
- diphtheria	T50.A91	T50.A92	T50.A93	T50.A94	T50.A95	T50.A96
- tetanus	T50.A91	T50.A92	T50.A93	T50.A94	T50.A95	T50.A96
Trace element NEC	T45.8X1	T45.8X2	T45.8X3	T45.8X4	T45.8X5	T45.8X6
Tractor fuel NEC	T52.0X1	T52.0X2	T52.0X3	T52.0X4	--	--
Tragacanth	T50.991	T50.992	T50.993	T50.994	T50.995	T50.996
Tramadol	T40.421	T40.422	T40.423	T40.424	T40.425	T40.426
Tramazoline	T48.5X1	T48.5X2	T48.5X3	T48.5X4	T48.5X5	T48.5X6
Tranexamic acid	T45.621	T45.622	T45.623	T45.624	T45.625	T45.626
Tranilast	T45.0X1	T45.0X2	T45.0X3	T45.0X4	T45.0X5	T45.0X6
Tranquilizer NEC	T43.501	T43.502	T43.503	T43.504	T43.505	T43.506
- with hypnotic or sedative	T42.6X1	T42.6X2	T42.6X3	T42.6X4	T42.6X5	T42.6X6

Substance	Poisoning, Accidental (unintentional)	Poisoning, Intentional Self-harm	Poisoning, Assault	Poisoning, Undetermined	Adverse effect	Underdosing
- benzodiazepine NEC	T42.4X1	T42.4X2	T42.4X3	T42.4X4	T42.4X5	T42.4X6
- butyrophenone NEC	T43.4X1	T43.4X2	T43.4X3	T43.4X4	T43.4X5	T43.4X6
- carbamate	T43.591	T43.592	T43.593	T43.594	T43.595	T43.596
- dimethylamine	T43.3X1	T43.3X2	T43.3X3	T43.3X4	T43.3X5	T43.3X6
- ethylamine	T43.3X1	T43.3X2	T43.3X3	T43.3X4	T43.3X5	T43.3X6
- hydroxyzine	T43.591	T43.592	T43.593	T43.594	T43.595	T43.596
- major NEC	T43.501	T43.502	T43.503	T43.504	T43.505	T43.506
- penothiazine NEC	T43.3X1	T43.3X2	T43.3X3	T43.3X4	T43.3X5	T43.3X6
- phenothiazine-based	T43.3X1	T43.3X2	T43.3X3	T43.3X4	T43.3X5	T43.3X6
- piperazine NEC	T43.3X1	T43.3X2	T43.3X3	T43.3X4	T43.3X5	T43.3X6
- piperidine	T43.3X1	T43.3X2	T43.3X3	T43.3X4	T43.3X5	T43.3X6
- propylamine	T43.3X1	T43.3X2	T43.3X3	T43.3X4	T43.3X5	T43.3X6
- specified NEC	T43.591	T43.592	T43.593	T43.594	T43.595	T43.596
- thioxanthene NEC	T43.591	T43.592	T43.593	T43.594	T43.595	T43.596
Tranxene	T42.4X1	T42.4X2	T42.4X3	T42.4X4	T42.4X5	T42.4X6
Tranylcypromine	T43.1X1	T43.1X2	T43.1X3	T43.1X4	T43.1X5	T43.1X6
Trapidil	T46.3X1	T46.3X2	T46.3X3	T46.3X4	T46.3X5	T46.3X6
Trasentine	T44.3X1	T44.3X2	T44.3X3	T44.3X4	T44.3X5	T44.3X6
Travert	T50.3X1	T50.3X2	T50.3X3	T50.3X4	T50.3X5	T50.3X6
Trazodone	T43.211	T43.212	T43.213	T43.214	T43.215	T43.216
Trecator	T37.1X1	T37.1X2	T37.1X3	T37.1X4	T37.1X5	T37.1X6
Treosulfan	T45.1X1	T45.1X2	T45.1X3	T45.1X4	T45.1X5	T45.1X6
Tretamine	T45.1X1	T45.1X2	T45.1X3	T45.1X4	T45.1X5	T45.1X6
Tretinoin	T49.0X1	T49.0X2	T49.0X3	T49.0X4	T49.0X5	T49.0X6
Tretoquinol	T48.6X1	T48.6X2	T48.6X3	T48.6X4	T48.6X5	T48.6X6
Triacetin	T49.0X1	T49.0X2	T49.0X3	T49.0X4	T49.0X5	T49.0X6
Triacetoxyanthracene	T49.4X1	T49.4X2	T49.4X3	T49.4X4	T49.4X5	T49.4X6
Triacetyloleandomycin	T36.3X1	T36.3X2	T36.3X3	T36.3X4	T36.3X5	T36.3X6
Triamcinolone	T38.0X1	T38.0X2	T38.0X3	T38.0X4	T38.0X5	T38.0X6
- ENT agent	T49.6X1	T49.6X2	T49.6X3	T49.6X4	T49.6X5	T49.6X6
- hexacetonide	T49.0X1	T49.0X2	T49.0X3	T49.0X4	T49.0X5	T49.0X6
- ophthalmic preparation	T49.5X1	T49.5X2	T49.5X3	T49.5X4	T49.5X5	T49.5X6
- topical NEC	T49.0X1	T49.0X2	T49.0X3	T49.0X4	T49.0X5	T49.0X6
Triampyzine	T44.3X1	T44.3X2	T44.3X3	T44.3X4	T44.3X5	T44.3X6
Triamterene	T50.2X1	T50.2X2	T50.2X3	T50.2X4	T50.2X5	T50.2X6
Triazine (herbicide)	T60.3X1	T60.3X2	T60.3X3	T60.3X4	--	--
Triaziquone	T45.1X1	T45.1X2	T45.1X3	T45.1X4	T45.1X5	T45.1X6
Triazolam	T42.4X1	T42.4X2	T42.4X3	T42.4X4	T42.4X5	T42.4X6
Triazole (herbicide)	T60.3X1	T60.3X2	T60.3X3	T60.3X4	--	--
Tribenoside	T46.991	T46.992	T46.993	T46.994	T46.995	T46.996
Tribromacetaldehyde	T42.6X1	T42.6X2	T42.6X3	T42.6X4	T42.6X5	T42.6X6
Tribromoethanol, rectal	T41.291	T41.292	T41.293	T41.294	T41.295	T41.296
Tribromomethane	T42.6X1	T42.6X2	T42.6X3	T42.6X4	T42.6X5	T42.6X6
Trichlorethane	T53.2X1	T53.2X2	T53.2X3	T53.2X4	--	--
Trichlorethylene	T53.2X1	T53.2X2	T53.2X3	T53.2X4	--	--
Trichlorfon	T60.0X1	T60.0X2	T60.0X3	T60.0X4	--	--
Trichlormethiazide	T50.2X1	T50.2X2	T50.2X3	T50.2X4	T50.2X5	T50.2X6
Trichlormethine	T45.1X1	T45.1X2	T45.1X3	T45.1X4	T45.1X5	T45.1X6
Trichloroacetic acid, Trichloracetic acid	T54.2X1	T54.2X2	T54.2X3	T54.2X4	--	--
- medicinal	T49.4X1	T49.4X2	T49.4X3	T49.4X4	T49.4X5	T49.4X6
Trichloroethane	T53.2X1	T53.2X2	T53.2X3	T53.2X4	--	--
Trichloroethanol	T42.6X1	T42.6X2	T42.6X3	T42.6X4	T42.6X5	T42.6X6
Trichloroethyl phosphate	T42.6X1	T42.6X2	T42.6X3	T42.6X4	T42.6X5	T42.6X6
Trichloroethylene (liquid) (vapor)	T53.2X1	T53.2X2	T53.2X3	T53.2X4	--	--
- anesthetic (gas)	T41.0X1	T41.0X2	T41.0X3	T41.0X4	T41.0X5	--
- vapor NEC	T53.2X1	T53.2X2	T53.2X3	T53.2X4	--	--
Trichlorofluoromethane NEC	T53.5X1	T53.5X2	T53.5X3	T53.5X4	--	--
Trichloronate	T60.0X1	T60.0X2	T60.0X3	T60.0X4	--	--
2,4,5-Trichlorophen-oxyacetic acid	T60.3X1	T60.3X2	T60.3X3	T60.3X4	--	--

Substance	Poisoning, Accidental (unintentional)	Poisoning, Intentional Self-harm	Poisoning, Assault	Poisoning, Undetermined	Adverse effect	Underdosing
Trichloropropane	T53.6X1	T53.6X2	T53.6X3	T53.6X4	--	--
Trichlorotriethylamine	T45.1X1	T45.1X2	T45.1X3	T45.1X4	T45.1X5	T45.1X6
Trichomonacides NEC	T37.3X1	T37.3X2	T37.3X3	T37.3X4	T37.3X5	T37.3X6
Trichomycin	T36.7X1	T36.7X2	T36.7X3	T36.7X4	T36.7X5	T36.7X6
Triclobisonium chloride	T49.0X1	T49.0X2	T49.0X3	T49.0X4	T49.0X5	T49.0X6
Triclocarban	T49.0X1	T49.0X2	T49.0X3	T49.0X4	T49.0X5	T49.0X6
Triclofos	T42.6X1	T42.6X2	T42.6X3	T42.6X4	T42.6X5	T42.6X6
Triclosan	T49.0X1	T49.0X2	T49.0X3	T49.0X4	T49.0X5	T49.0X6
Tricresyl phosphate	T65.891	T65.892	T65.893	T65.894	--	--
- solvent	T52.91	T52.92	T52.93	T52.94	--	--
Tricyclamol chloride	T44.3X1	T44.3X2	T44.3X3	T44.3X4	T44.3X5	T44.3X6
Tridesilon	T49.0X1	T49.0X2	T49.0X3	T49.0X4	T49.0X5	T49.0X6
Tridihexethyl iodide	T44.3X1	T44.3X2	T44.3X3	T44.3X4	T44.3X5	T44.3X6
Tridione	T42.2X1	T42.2X2	T42.2X3	T42.2X4	T42.2X5	T42.2X6
Trientine	T45.8X1	T45.8X2	T45.8X3	T45.8X4	T45.8X5	T45.8X6
Triethanolamine NEC	T54.3X1	T54.3X2	T54.3X3	T54.3X4	--	--
- detergent	T54.3X1	T54.3X2	T54.3X3	T54.3X4	--	--
- trinitrate (biphosphate)	T46.3X1	T46.3X2	T46.3X3	T46.3X4	T46.3X5	T46.3X6
Triethanomelamine	T45.1X1	T45.1X2	T45.1X3	T45.1X4	T45.1X5	T45.1X6
Triethylenemelamine	T45.1X1	T45.1X2	T45.1X3	T45.1X4	T45.1X5	T45.1X6
Triethylenephosphoramide	T45.1X1	T45.1X2	T45.1X3	T45.1X4	T45.1X5	T45.1X6
Triethylenethiophosphoramide	T45.1X1	T45.1X2	T45.1X3	T45.1X4	T45.1X5	T45.1X6
Trifluoperazine	T43.3X1	T43.3X2	T43.3X3	T43.3X4	T43.3X5	T43.3X6
Trifluoroethyl vinyl ether	T41.0X1	T41.0X2	T41.0X3	T41.0X4	T41.0X5	T41.0X6
Trifluperidol	T43.4X1	T43.4X2	T43.4X3	T43.4X4	T43.4X5	T43.4X6
Triflupromazine	T43.3X1	T43.3X2	T43.3X3	T43.3X4	T43.3X5	T43.3X6
Trifluridine	T37.5X1	T37.5X2	T37.5X3	T37.5X4	T37.5X5	T37.5X6
Triflusal	T45.521	T45.522	T45.523	T45.524	T45.525	T45.526
Trihexyphenidyl	T44.3X1	T44.3X2	T44.3X3	T44.3X4	T44.3X5	T44.3X6
Triiodothyronine	T38.1X1	T38.1X2	T38.1X3	T38.1X4	T38.1X5	T38.1X6
Trilene	T41.0X1	T41.0X2	T41.0X3	T41.0X4	T41.0X5	T41.0X6
Trilostane	T38.991	T38.992	T38.993	T38.994	T38.995	T38.996
Trimebutine	T44.3X1	T44.3X2	T44.3X3	T44.3X4	T44.3X5	T44.3X6
Trimecaine	T41.3X1	T41.3X2	T41.3X3	T41.3X4	T41.3X5	T41.3X6
Trimeprazine (tartrate)	T44.3X1	T44.3X2	T44.3X3	T44.3X4	T44.3X5	T44.3X6
Trimetaphan camsilate	T44.2X1	T44.2X2	T44.2X3	T44.2X4	T44.2X5	T44.2X6
Trimetazidine	T46.7X1	T46.7X2	T46.7X3	T46.7X4	T46.7X5	T46.7X6
Trimethadione	T42.2X1	T42.2X2	T42.2X3	T42.2X4	T42.2X5	T42.2X6
Trimethaphan	T44.2X1	T44.2X2	T44.2X3	T44.2X4	T44.2X5	T44.2X6
Trimethidinium	T44.2X1	T44.2X2	T44.2X3	T44.2X4	T44.2X5	T44.2X6
Trimethobenzamide	T45.0X1	T45.0X2	T45.0X3	T45.0X4	T45.0X5	T45.0X6
Trimethoprim	T37.8X1	T37.8X2	T37.8X3	T37.8X4	T37.8X5	T37.8X6
- with sulfamethoxazole	T36.8X1	T36.8X2	T36.8X3	T36.8X4	T36.8X5	T36.8X6
Trimethylcarbinol	T51.3X1	T51.3X2	T51.3X3	T51.3X4	--	--
Trimethylpsoralen	T49.3X1	T49.3X2	T49.3X3	T49.3X4	T49.3X5	T49.3X6
Trimeton	T45.0X1	T45.0X2	T45.0X3	T45.0X4	T45.0X5	T45.0X6
Trimetrexate	T45.1X1	T45.1X2	T45.1X3	T45.1X4	T45.1X5	T45.1X6
Trimipramine	T43.011	T43.012	T43.013	T43.014	T43.015	T43.016
Trimustine	T45.1X1	T45.1X2	T45.1X3	T45.1X4	T45.1X5	T45.1X6
Trinitrine	T46.3X1	T46.3X2	T46.3X3	T46.3X4	T46.3X5	T46.3X6
Trinitrobenzol	T65.3X1	T65.3X2	T65.3X3	T65.3X4	--	--
Trinitrophenol	T65.3X1	T65.3X2	T65.3X3	T65.3X4	--	--
Trinitrotoluene (fumes)	T65.3X1	T65.3X2	T65.3X3	T65.3X4	--	--
Trional	T42.6X1	T42.6X2	T42.6X3	T42.6X4	T42.6X5	T42.6X6
Triorthocresyl phosphate	T65.891	T65.892	T65.893	T65.894	--	--
Trioxide of arsenic	T57.0X1	T57.0X2	T57.0X3	T57.0X4	--	--
Trioxysalen	T49.4X1	T49.4X2	T49.4X3	T49.4X4	T49.4X5	T49.4X6
Tripamide	T50.2X1	T50.2X2	T50.2X3	T50.2X4	T50.2X5	T50.2X6

Substance	Poisoning, Accidental (unintentional)	Poisoning, Intentional Self-harm	Poisoning, Assault	Poisoning, Undetermined	Adverse effect	Underdosing
Triparanol	T46.6X1	T46.6X2	T46.6X3	T46.6X4	T46.6X5	T46.6X6
Tripelennamine	T45.0X1	T45.0X2	T45.0X3	T45.0X4	T45.0X5	T45.0X6
Triperiden	T44.3X1	T44.3X2	T44.3X3	T44.3X4	T44.3X5	T44.3X6
Triperidol	T43.4X1	T43.4X2	T43.4X3	T43.4X4	T43.4X5	T43.4X6
Triphenylphosphate	T65.891	T65.892	T65.893	T65.894	--	--
Triple						
- bromides	T42.6X1	T42.6X2	T42.6X3	T42.6X4	T42.6X5	T42.6X6
- carbonate	T47.1X1	T47.1X2	T47.1X3	T47.1X4	T47.1X5	T47.1X6
- vaccine						
- - DPT	T50.A11	T50.A12	T50.A13	T50.A14	T50.A15	T50.A16
- - including pertussis	T50.A11	T50.A12	T50.A13	T50.A14	T50.A15	T50.A16
- - MMR	T50.B91	T50.B92	T50.B93	T50.B94	T50.B95	T50.B96
Triprolidine	T45.0X1	T45.0X2	T45.0X3	T45.0X4	T45.0X5	T45.0X6
Trisodium hydrogen edetate	T50.6X1	T50.6X2	T50.6X3	T50.6X4	T50.6X5	T50.6X6
Trisoralen	T49.3X1	T49.3X2	T49.3X3	T49.3X4	T49.3X5	T49.3X6
Trisulfapyrimidines	T37.0X1	T37.0X2	T37.0X3	T37.0X4	T37.0X5	T37.0X6
Trithiozine	T44.3X1	T44.3X2	T44.3X3	T44.3X4	T44.3X5	T44.3X6
Tritiozine	T44.3X1	T44.3X2	T44.3X3	T44.3X4	T44.3X5	T44.3X6
Tritoqualine	T45.0X1	T45.0X2	T45.0X3	T45.0X4	T45.0X5	T45.0X6
Trofosfamide	T45.1X1	T45.1X2	T45.1X3	T45.1X4	T45.1X5	T45.1X6
Troleandomycin	T36.3X1	T36.3X2	T36.3X3	T36.3X4	T36.3X5	T36.3X6
Trolnitrate (phosphate)	T46.3X1	T46.3X2	T46.3X3	T46.3X4	T46.3X5	T46.3X6
Tromantadine	T37.5X1	T37.5X2	T37.5X3	T37.5X4	T37.5X5	T37.5X6
Trometamol	T50.2X1	T50.2X2	T50.2X3	T50.2X4	T50.2X5	T50.2X6
Tromethamine	T50.2X1	T50.2X2	T50.2X3	T50.2X4	T50.2X5	T50.2X6
Tronothane	T41.3X1	T41.3X2	T41.3X3	T41.3X4	T41.3X5	T41.3X6
Tropacine	T44.3X1	T44.3X2	T44.3X3	T44.3X4	T44.3X5	T44.3X6
Tropatepine	T44.3X1	T44.3X2	T44.3X3	T44.3X4	T44.3X5	T44.3X6
Tropicamide	T44.3X1	T44.3X2	T44.3X3	T44.3X4	T44.3X5	T44.3X6
Trospium chloride	T44.3X1	T44.3X2	T44.3X3	T44.3X4	T44.3X5	T44.3X6
Troxerutin	T46.991	T46.992	T46.993	T46.994	T46.995	T46.996
Troxidone	T42.2X1	T42.2X2	T42.2X3	T42.2X4	T42.2X5	T42.2X6
Tryparsamide	T37.3X1	T37.3X2	T37.3X3	T37.3X4	T37.3X5	T37.3X6
Trypsin	T45.3X1	T45.3X2	T45.3X3	T45.3X4	T45.3X5	T45.3X6
Tryptizol	T43.011	T43.012	T43.013	T43.014	T43.015	T43.016
TSH	T38.811	T38.812	T38.813	T38.814	T38.815	T38.816
Tuaminoheptane	T48.5X1	T48.5X2	T48.5X3	T48.5X4	T48.5X5	T48.5X6
Tuberculin, purified protein derivative (PPD)	T50.8X1	T50.8X2	T50.8X3	T50.8X4	T50.8X5	T50.8X6
Tubocurare	T48.1X1	T48.1X2	T48.1X3	T48.1X4	T48.1X5	T48.1X6
Tubocurarine (chloride)	T48.1X1	T48.1X2	T48.1X3	T48.1X4	T48.1X5	T48.1X6
Tulobuterol	T48.6X1	T48.6X2	T48.6X3	T48.6X4	T48.6X5	T48.6X6
Turpentine (spirits of)	T52.8X1	T52.8X2	T52.8X3	T52.8X4	--	--
- vapor	T52.8X1	T52.8X2	T52.8X3	T52.8X4	--	--
Tybamate	T43.591	T43.592	T43.593	T43.594	T43.595	T43.596
Tyloxapol	T48.4X1	T48.4X2	T48.4X3	T48.4X4	T48.4X5	T48.4X6
Tymazoline	T48.5X1	T48.5X2	T48.5X3	T48.5X4	T48.5X5	T48.5X6
Typhoid-paratyphoid vaccine	T50.A91	T50.A92	T50.A93	T50.A94	T50.A95	T50.A96
Typhus vaccine	T50.A91	T50.A92	T50.A93	T50.A94	T50.A95	T50.A96
Tyropanoate	T50.8X1	T50.8X2	T50.8X3	T50.8X4	T50.8X5	T50.8X6
Tyrothricin	T49.6X1	T49.6X2	T49.6X3	T49.6X4	T49.6X5	T49.6X6
- ENT agent	T49.6X1	T49.6X2	T49.6X3	T49.6X4	T49.6X5	T49.6X6
- ophthalmic preparation	T49.5X1	T49.5X2	T49.5X3	T49.5X4	T49.5X5	T49.5X6
Ufenamate	T39.391	T39.392	T39.393	T39.394	T39.395	T39.396
Ultraviolet light protectant	T49.3X1	T49.3X2	T49.3X3	T49.3X4	T49.3X5	T49.3X6
Undecenoic acid	T49.0X1	T49.0X2	T49.0X3	T49.0X4	T49.0X5	T49.0X6
Undecoylium	T49.0X1	T49.0X2	T49.0X3	T49.0X4	T49.0X5	T49.0X6
Undecylenic acid (derivatives)	T49.0X1	T49.0X2	T49.0X3	T49.0X4	T49.0X5	T49.0X6
Unna's boot	T49.3X1	T49.3X2	T49.3X3	T49.3X4	T49.3X5	T49.3X6

Substance	Poisoning, Accidental (unintentional)	Poisoning, Intentional Self-harm	Poisoning, Assault	Poisoning, Undetermined	Adverse effect	Underdosing
Unsaturated fatty acid	T46.6X1	T46.6X2	T46.6X3	T46.6X4	T46.6X5	T46.6X6
Uracil mustard	T45.1X1	T45.1X2	T45.1X3	T45.1X4	T45.1X5	T45.1X6
Uramustine	T45.1X1	T45.1X2	T45.1X3	T45.1X4	T45.1X5	T45.1X6
Urapidil	T46.5X1	T46.5X2	T46.5X3	T46.5X4	T46.5X5	T46.5X6
Urari	T48.1X1	T48.1X2	T48.1X3	T48.1X4	T48.1X5	T48.1X6
Urate oxidase	T50.4X1	T50.4X2	T50.4X3	T50.4X4	T50.4X5	T50.4X6
Urea	T47.3X1	T47.3X2	T47.3X3	T47.3X4	T47.3X5	T47.3X6
- peroxide	T49.0X1	T49.0X2	T49.0X3	T49.0X4	T49.0X5	T49.0X6
- stibamine	T37.4X1	T37.4X2	T37.4X3	T37.4X4	T37.4X5	T37.4X6
- topical	T49.8X1	T49.8X2	T49.8X3	T49.8X4	T49.8X5	T49.8X6
Urethane	T45.1X1	T45.1X2	T45.1X3	T45.1X4	T45.1X5	T45.1X6
Urginea (maritima) (scilla) —see Squill						
Uric acid metabolism drug NEC	T50.4X1	T50.4X2	T50.4X3	T50.4X4	T50.4X5	T50.4X6
Uricosuric agent	T50.4X1	T50.4X2	T50.4X3	T50.4X4	T50.4X5	T50.4X6
Urinary anti-infective	T37.8X1	T37.8X2	T37.8X3	T37.8X4	T37.8X5	T37.8X6
Urofollitropin	T38.811	T38.812	T38.813	T38.814	T38.815	T38.816
Urokinase	T45.611	T45.612	T45.613	T45.614	T45.615	T45.616
Urokon	T50.8X1	T50.8X2	T50.8X3	T50.8X4	T50.8X5	T50.8X6
Ursodeoxycholic acid	T50.991	T50.992	T50.993	T50.994	T50.995	T50.996
Ursodiol	T50.991	T50.992	T50.993	T50.994	T50.995	T50.996
Urtica	T62.2X1	T62.2X2	T62.2X3	T62.2X4	--	--
Utility gas—see Gas, utility						
Vaccine NEC	T50.Z91	T50.Z92	T50.Z93	T50.Z94	T50.Z95	T50.Z96
- antineoplastic	T50.Z91	T50.Z92	T50.Z93	T50.Z94	T50.Z95	T50.Z96
- bacterial NEC	T50.A91	T50.A92	T50.A93	T50.A94	T50.A95	T50.A96
- - with						
- - - other bacterial component	T50.A21	T50.A22	T50.A23	T50.A24	T50.A25	T50.A26
- - - pertussis component	T50.A11	T50.A12	T50.A13	T50.A14	T50.A15	T50.A16
- - - viral-rickettsial component	T50.A21	T50.A22	T50.A23	T50.A24	T50.A25	T50.A26
- - mixed NEC	T50.A21	T50.A22	T50.A23	T50.A24	T50.A25	T50.A26
- BCG	T50.A91	T50.A92	T50.A93	T50.A94	T50.A95	T50.A96
- cholera	T50.A91	T50.A92	T50.A93	T50.A94	T50.A95	T50.A96
- diphtheria	T50.A91	T50.A92	T50.A93	T50.A94	T50.A95	T50.A96
- - with tetanus	T50.A21	T50.A22	T50.A23	T50.A24	T50.A25	T50.A26
- - - and pertussis	T50.A11	T50.A12	T50.A13	T50.A14	T50.A15	T50.A16
- influenza	T50.B91	T50.B92	T50.B93	T50.B94	T50.B95	T50.B96
- measles	T50.B91	T50.B92	T50.B93	T50.B94	T50.B95	T50.B96
- - with mumps and rubella	T50.B91	T50.B92	T50.B93	T50.B94	T50.B95	T50.B96
- meningococcal	T50.A91	T50.A92	T50.A93	T50.A94	T50.A95	T50.A96
- mumps	T50.B91	T50.B92	T50.B93	T50.B94	T50.B95	T50.B96
- paratyphoid	T50.A91	T50.A92	T50.A93	T50.A94	T50.A95	T50.A96
- pertussis	T50.A11	T50.A12	T50.A13	T50.A14	T50.A15	T50.A16
- - with diphtheria	T50.A11	T50.A12	T50.A13	T50.A14	T50.A15	T50.A16
- - - and tetanus	T50.A11	T50.A12	T50.A13	T50.A14	T50.A15	T50.A16
- - with other component	T50.A11	T50.A12	T50.A13	T50.A14	T50.A15	T50.A16
- plague	T50.A91	T50.A92	T50.A93	T50.A94	T50.A95	T50.A96
- poliomyelitis	T50.B91	T50.B92	T50.B93	T50.B94	T50.B95	T50.B96
- poliovirus	T50.B91	T50.B92	T50.B93	T50.B94	T50.B95	T50.B96
- rabies	T50.B91	T50.B92	T50.B93	T50.B94	T50.B95	T50.B96
- respiratory syncytial virus	T50.B91	T50.B92	T50.B93	T50.B94	T50.B95	T50.B96
- rickettsial NEC	T50.A91	T50.A92	T50.A93	T50.A94	T50.A95	T50.A96
- - with						
- - - bacterial component	T50.A21	T50.A22	T50.A23	T50.A24	T50.A25	T50.A26
- Rocky Mountain spotted fever	T50.A91	T50.A92	T50.A93	T50.A94	T50.A95	T50.A96
- rubella	T50.B91	T50.B92	T50.B93	T50.B94	T50.B95	T50.B96
- sabin oral	T50.B91	T50.B92	T50.B93	T50.B94	T50.B95	T50.B96
- smallpox	T50.B11	T50.B12	T50.B13	T50.B14	T50.B15	T50.B16
- TAB	T50.A91	T50.A92	T50.A93	T50.A94	T50.A95	T50.A96

Substance	Poisoning, Accidental (unintentional)	Poisoning, Intentional Self-harm	Poisoning, Assault	Poisoning, Undetermined	Adverse effect	Underdosing
- tetanus	T50.A91	T50.A92	T50.A93	T50.A94	T50.A95	T50.A96
- typhoid	T50.A91	T50.A92	T50.A93	T50.A94	T50.A95	T50.A96
- typhus	T50.A91	T50.A92	T50.A93	T50.A94	T50.A95	T50.A96
- viral NEC	T50.B91	T50.B92	T50.B93	T50.B94	T50.B95	T50.B96
- yellow fever	T50.B91	T50.B92	T50.B93	T50.B94	T50.B95	T50.B96
Vaccinia immune globulin	T50.Z11	T50.Z12	T50.Z13	T50.Z14	T50.Z15	T50.Z16
Vaginal contraceptives	T49.8X1	T49.8X2	T49.8X3	T49.8X4	T49.8X5	T49.8X6
Valerian						
- root	T42.6X1	T42.6X2	T42.6X3	T42.6X4	T42.6X5	T42.6X6
- tincture	T42.6X1	T42.6X2	T42.6X3	T42.6X4	T42.6X5	T42.6X6
Valethamate bromide	T44.3X1	T44.3X2	T44.3X3	T44.3X4	T44.3X5	T44.3X6
Valisone	T49.0X1	T49.0X2	T49.0X3	T49.0X4	T49.0X5	T49.0X6
Valium	T42.4X1	T42.4X2	T42.4X3	T42.4X4	T42.4X5	T42.4X6
Valmid	T42.6X1	T42.6X2	T42.6X3	T42.6X4	T42.6X5	T42.6X6
Valnoctamide	T42.6X1	T42.6X2	T42.6X3	T42.6X4	T42.6X5	T42.6X6
Valproate (sodium)	T42.6X1	T42.6X2	T42.6X3	T42.6X4	T42.6X5	T42.6X6
Valproic acid	T42.6X1	T42.6X2	T42.6X3	T42.6X4	T42.6X5	T42.6X6
Valpromide	T42.6X1	T42.6X2	T42.6X3	T42.6X4	T42.6X5	T42.6X6
Vanadium	T56.891	T56.892	T56.893	T56.894	--	--
Vancomycin	T36.8X1	T36.8X2	T36.8X3	T36.8X4	T36.8X5	T36.8X6
Vapor—see also Gas	T59.91	T59.92	T59.93	T59.94	--	--
- kiln (carbon monoxide)	T58.8X1	T58.8X2	T58.8X3	T58.8X4	--	--
- lead—see lead						
- specified source NEC	T59.891	T59.892	T59.893	T59.894	--	--
Vardenafil	T46.7X1	T46.7X2	T46.7X3	T46.7X4	T46.7X5	T46.7X6
Varicose reduction drug	T46.8X1	T46.8X2	T46.8X3	T46.8X4	T46.8X5	T46.8X6
Varnish	T65.4X1	T65.4X2	T65.4X3	T65.4X4	--	--
- cleaner	T52.91	T52.92	T52.93	T52.94	--	--
Vaseline	T49.3X1	T49.3X2	T49.3X3	T49.3X4	T49.3X5	T49.3X6
Vasodilan	T46.7X1	T46.7X2	T46.7X3	T46.7X4	T46.7X5	T46.7X6
Vasodilator						
- coronary NEC	T46.3X1	T46.3X2	T46.3X3	T46.3X4	T46.3X5	T46.3X6
- peripheral NEC	T46.7X1	T46.7X2	T46.7X3	T46.7X4	T46.7X5	T46.7X6
Vasopressin	T38.891	T38.892	T38.893	T38.894	T38.895	T38.896
Vasopressor drugs	T38.891	T38.892	T38.893	T38.894	T38.895	T38.896
Vecuronium bromide	T48.1X1	T48.1X2	T48.1X3	T48.1X4	T48.1X5	T48.1X6
Vegetable extract, astringent	T49.2X1	T49.2X2	T49.2X3	T49.2X4	T49.2X5	T49.2X6
Venlafaxine	T43.211	T43.212	T43.213	T43.214	T43.215	T43.216
Venom, venomous (bite) (sting)	T63.91	T63.92	T63.93	T63.94	--	--
- amphibian NEC	T63.831	T63.832	T63.833	T63.834	--	--
- animal NEC	T63.891	T63.892	T63.893	T63.894	--	--
- ant	T63.421	T63.422	T63.423	T63.424	--	--
- arthropod NEC	T63.481	T63.482	T63.483	T63.484	--	--
- bee	T63.441	T63.442	T63.443	T63.444	--	--
- centipede	T63.411	T63.412	T63.413	T63.414	--	--
- fish	T63.591	T63.592	T63.593	T63.594	--	--
- frog	T63.811	T63.812	T63.813	T63.814	--	--
- hornet	T63.451	T63.452	T63.453	T63.454	--	--
- insect NEC	T63.481	T63.482	T63.483	T63.484	--	--
- lizard	T63.121	T63.122	T63.123	T63.124	--	--
- marine						
- - animals	T63.691	T63.692	T63.693	T63.694	--	--
- - - bluebottle	T63.611	T63.612	T63.613	T63.614	--	--
- - - jellyfish NEC	T63.621	T63.622	T63.623	T63.624	--	--
- - - Portuguese Man-o-war	T63.611	T63.612	T63.613	T63.614	--	--
- - - sea anemone	T63.631	T63.632	T63.633	T63.634	--	--
- - - specified NEC	T63.691	T63.692	T63.693	T63.694	--	--
- - fish	T63.591	T63.592	T63.593	T63.594	--	--
- - plants	T63.711	T63.712	T63.713	T63.714	--	--

Substance	Poisoning, Accidental (unintentional)	Poisoning, Intentional Self-harm	Poisoning, Assault	Poisoning, Undetermined	Adverse effect	Underdosing
- - sting ray	T63.511	T63.512	T63.513	T63.514	--	--
- millipede (tropical)	T63.411	T63.412	T63.413	T63.414	--	--
- plant NEC	T63.791	T63.792	T63.793	T63.794	--	--
- - marine	T63.711	T63.712	T63.713	T63.714	--	--
- reptile	T63.191	T63.192	T63.193	T63.194	--	--
- - gila monster	T63.111	T63.112	T63.113	T63.114	--	--
- - lizard NEC	T63.121	T63.122	T63.123	T63.124	--	--
- scorpion	T63.2X1	T63.2X2	T63.2X3	T63.2X4	--	--
- snake	T63.001	T63.002	T63.003	T63.004	--	--
- - African NEC	T63.081	T63.082	T63.083	T63.084	--	--
- - American (North) (South) NEC	T63.061	T63.062	T63.063	T63.064	--	--
- - Asian	T63.081	T63.082	T63.083	T63.084	--	--
- - Australian	T63.071	T63.072	T63.073	T63.074	--	--
- - cobra	T63.041	T63.042	T63.043	T63.044	--	--
- - coral snake	T63.021	T63.022	T63.023	T63.024	--	--
- - rattlesnake	T63.011	T63.012	T63.013	T63.014	--	--
- - specified NEC	T63.091	T63.092	T63.093	T63.094	--	--
- - taipan	T63.031	T63.032	T63.033	T63.034	--	--
- specified NEC	T63.891	T63.892	T63.893	T63.894	--	--
- spider	T63.301	T63.302	T63.303	T63.304	--	--
- - black widow	T63.311	T63.312	T63.313	T63.314	--	--
- - brown recluse	T63.331	T63.332	T63.333	T63.334	--	--
- - specified NEC	T63.391	T63.392	T63.393	T63.394	--	--
- - tarantula	T63.321	T63.322	T63.323	T63.324	--	--
- sting ray	T63.511	T63.512	T63.513	T63.514	--	--
- toad	T63.821	T63.822	T63.823	T63.824	--	--
- wasp	T63.461	T63.462	T63.463	T63.464	--	--
Venous sclerosing drug NEC	T46.8X1	T46.8X2	T46.8X3	T46.8X4	T46.8X5	T46.8X6
Ventolin—see Albuterol						
Veramon	T42.3X1	T42.3X2	T42.3X3	T42.3X4	T42.3X5	T42.3X6
Verapamil	T46.1X1	T46.1X2	T46.1X3	T46.1X4	T46.1X5	T46.1X6
Veratrine	T46.5X1	T46.5X2	T46.5X3	T46.5X4	T46.5X5	T46.5X6
Veratrum						
- album	T62.2X1	T62.2X2	T62.2X3	T62.2X4	--	--
- alkaloids	T46.5X1	T46.5X2	T46.5X3	T46.5X4	T46.5X5	T46.5X6
- viride	T62.2X1	T62.2X2	T62.2X3	T62.2X4	--	--
Verdigris	T60.3X1	T60.3X2	T60.3X3	T60.3X4	--	--
Veronal	T42.3X1	T42.3X2	T42.3X3	T42.3X4	T42.3X5	T42.3X6
Veroxil	T37.4X1	T37.4X2	T37.4X3	T37.4X4	T37.4X5	T37.4X6
Versenate	T50.6X1	T50.6X2	T50.6X3	T50.6X4	T50.6X5	T50.6X6
Versidyne	T39.8X1	T39.8X2	T39.8X3	T39.8X4	T39.8X5	T39.8X6
Vetrabutine	T48.0X1	T48.0X2	T48.0X3	T48.0X4	T48.0X5	T48.0X6
Vidarabine	T37.5X1	T37.5X2	T37.5X3	T37.5X4	T37.5X5	T37.5X6
Vienna						
- green	T57.0X1	T57.0X2	T57.0X3	T57.0X4	--	--
- - insecticide	T60.2X1	T60.2X2	T60.2X3	T60.2X4	--	--
- red	T57.0X1	T57.0X2	T57.0X3	T57.0X4	--	--
- - pharmaceutical dye	T50.991	T50.992	T50.993	T50.994	T50.995	T50.996
Vigabatrin	T42.6X1	T42.6X2	T42.6X3	T42.6X4	T42.6X5	T42.6X6
Viloxazine	T43.291	T43.292	T43.293	T43.294	T43.295	T43.296
Viminol	T39.8X1	T39.8X2	T39.8X3	T39.8X4	T39.8X5	T39.8X6
Vinbarbital, vinbarbitone	T42.3X1	T42.3X2	T42.3X3	T42.3X4	T42.3X5	T42.3X6
Vinblastine	T45.1X1	T45.1X2	T45.1X3	T45.1X4	T45.1X5	T45.1X6
Vinburnine	T46.7X1	T46.7X2	T46.7X3	T46.7X4	T46.7X5	T46.7X6
Vincamine	T45.1X1	T45.1X2	T45.1X3	T45.1X4	T45.1X5	T45.1X6
Vincristine	T45.1X1	T45.1X2	T45.1X3	T45.1X4	T45.1X5	T45.1X6
Vindesine	T45.1X1	T45.1X2	T45.1X3	T45.1X4	T45.1X5	T45.1X6
Vinesthene, vinethene	T41.0X1	T41.0X2	T41.0X3	T41.0X4	T41.0X5	T41.0X6

Substance	Poisoning, Accidental (unintentional)	Poisoning, Intentional Self-harm	Poisoning, Assault	Poisoning, Undetermined	Adverse effect	Underdosing
Vinorelbine tartrate	T45.1X1	T45.1X2	T45.1X3	T45.1X4	T45.1X5	T45.1X6
Vinpocetine	T46.7X1	T46.7X2	T46.7X3	T46.7X4	T46.7X5	T46.7X6
Vinyl						
- acetate	T65.891	T65.892	T65.893	T65.894	--	--
- bital	T42.3X1	T42.3X2	T42.3X3	T42.3X4	T42.3X5	T42.3X6
- bromide	T65.891	T65.892	T65.893	T65.894	--	--
- chloride	T59.891	T59.892	T59.893	T59.894	--	--
- ether	T41.0X1	T41.0X2	T41.0X3	T41.0X4	T41.0X5	T41.0X6
Vinylbital	T42.3X1	T42.3X2	T42.3X3	T42.3X4	T42.3X5	T42.3X6
Vinylidene chloride	T65.891	T65.892	T65.893	T65.894	--	--
Vioform	T37.8X1	T37.8X2	T37.8X3	T37.8X4	T37.8X5	T37.8X6
- topical	T49.0X1	T49.0X2	T49.0X3	T49.0X4	T49.0X5	T49.0X6
Viomycin	T36.8X1	T36.8X2	T36.8X3	T36.8X4	T36.8X5	T36.8X6
Viosterol	T45.2X1	T45.2X2	T45.2X3	T45.2X4	T45.2X5	T45.2X6
Viper (venom)	T63.091	T63.092	T63.093	T63.094	--	--
Viprynium	T37.4X1	T37.4X2	T37.4X3	T37.4X4	T37.4X5	T37.4X6
Viquidil	T46.7X1	T46.7X2	T46.7X3	T46.7X4	T46.7X5	T46.7X6
Viral vaccine NEC	T50.B91	T50.B92	T50.B93	T50.B94	T50.B95	T50.B96
Virginiamycin	T36.8X1	T36.8X2	T36.8X3	T36.8X4	T36.8X5	T36.8X6
Virugon	T37.5X1	T37.5X2	T37.5X3	T37.5X4	T37.5X5	T37.5X6
Viscous agent	T50.901	T50.902	T50.903	T50.904	T50.905	T50.906
Visine	T49.5X1	T49.5X2	T49.5X3	T49.5X4	T49.5X5	T49.5X6
Visnadine	T46.3X1	T46.3X2	T46.3X3	T46.3X4	T46.3X5	T46.3X6
Vitamin NEC	T45.2X1	T45.2X2	T45.2X3	T45.2X4	T45.2X5	T45.2X6
- A	T45.2X1	T45.2X2	T45.2X3	T45.2X4	T45.2X5	T45.2X6
- B NEC	T45.2X1	T45.2X2	T45.2X3	T45.2X4	T45.2X5	T45.2X6
- - nicotinic acid	T46.7X1	T46.7X2	T46.7X3	T46.7X4	T46.7X5	T46.7X6
- B1	T45.2X1	T45.2X2	T45.2X3	T45.2X4	T45.2X5	T45.2X6
- B2	T45.2X1	T45.2X2	T45.2X3	T45.2X4	T45.2X5	T45.2X6
- B6	T45.2X1	T45.2X2	T45.2X3	T45.2X4	T45.2X5	T45.2X6
- B12	T45.2X1	T45.2X2	T45.2X3	T45.2X4	T45.2X5	T45.2X6
- B15	T45.2X1	T45.2X2	T45.2X3	T45.2X4	T45.2X5	T45.2X6
- C	T45.2X1	T45.2X2	T45.2X3	T45.2X4	T45.2X5	T45.2X6
- D	T45.2X1	T45.2X2	T45.2X3	T45.2X4	T45.2X5	T45.2X6
- D2	T45.2X1	T45.2X2	T45.2X3	T45.2X4	T45.2X5	T45.2X6
- D3	T45.2X1	T45.2X2	T45.2X3	T45.2X4	T45.2X5	T45.2X6
- E	T45.2X1	T45.2X2	T45.2X3	T45.2X4	T45.2X5	T45.2X6
- E acetate	T45.2X1	T45.2X2	T45.2X3	T45.2X4	T45.2X5	T45.2X6
- hematopoietic	T45.8X1	T45.8X2	T45.8X3	T45.8X4	T45.8X5	T45.8X6
- K NEC	T45.7X1	T45.7X2	T45.7X3	T45.7X4	T45.7X5	T45.7X6
- K1	T45.7X1	T45.7X2	T45.7X3	T45.7X4	T45.7X5	T45.7X6
- K2	T45.7X1	T45.7X2	T45.7X3	T45.7X4	T45.7X5	T45.7X6
- PP	T45.2X1	T45.2X2	T45.2X3	T45.2X4	T45.2X5	T45.2X6
- ulceroprotectant	T47.1X1	T47.1X2	T47.1X3	T47.1X4	T47.1X5	T47.1X6
Vleminckx's solution	T49.4X1	T49.4X2	T49.4X3	T49.4X4	T49.4X5	T49.4X6
Voltaren—see Diclofenac sodium						
Warfarin	T45.511	T45.512	T45.513	T45.514	T45.515	T45.516
- rodenticide	T60.4X1	T60.4X2	T60.4X3	T60.4X4	--	--
- sodium	T45.511	T45.512	T45.513	T45.514	T45.515	T45.516
Wasp (sting)	T63.461	T63.462	T63.463	T63.464	--	--
Water						
- balance drug	T50.3X1	T50.3X2	T50.3X3	T50.3X4	T50.3X5	T50.3X6
- distilled	T50.3X1	T50.3X2	T50.3X3	T50.3X4	T50.3X5	T50.3X6
- gas—see Gas, water						
- - incomplete combustion of—see Carbon, monoxide, fuel, utility						
- hemlock	T62.2X1	T62.2X2	T62.2X3	T62.2X4	--	--
- moccasin (venom)	T63.061	T63.062	T63.063	T63.064	--	--
- purified	T50.3X1	T50.3X2	T50.3X3	T50.3X4	T50.3X5	T50.3X6

Substance	Poisoning, Accidental (unintentional)	Poisoning, Intentional Self-harm	Poisoning, Assault	Poisoning, Undetermined	Adverse effect	Underdosing
Wax (paraffin) (petroleum)	T52.0X1	T52.0X2	T52.0X3	T52.0X4	--	--
- automobile	T65.891	T65.892	T65.893	T65.894	--	--
- floor	T52.0X1	T52.0X2	T52.0X3	T52.0X4	--	--
Weed killers NEC	T60.3X1	T60.3X2	T60.3X3	T60.3X4	--	--
Welldorm	T42.6X1	T42.6X2	T42.6X3	T42.6X4	T42.6X5	T42.6X6
White						
- arsenic	T57.0X1	T57.0X2	T57.0X3	T57.0X4	--	--
- hellebore	T62.2X1	T62.2X2	T62.2X3	T62.2X4	--	--
- lotion (keratolytic)	T49.4X1	T49.4X2	T49.4X3	T49.4X4	T49.4X5	T49.4X6
- spirit	T52.0X1	T52.0X2	T52.0X3	T52.0X4	--	--
Whitewash	T65.891	T65.892	T65.893	T65.894	--	--
Whole blood (human)	T45.8X1	T45.8X2	T45.8X3	T45.8X4	T45.8X5	T45.8X6
Wild						
- black cherry	T62.2X1	T62.2X2	T62.2X3	T62.2X4	--	--
- poisonous plants NEC	T62.2X1	T62.2X2	T62.2X3	T62.2X4	--	--
Window cleaning fluid	T65.891	T65.892	T65.893	T65.894	--	--
Wintergreen (oil)	T49.3X1	T49.3X2	T49.3X3	T49.3X4	T49.3X5	T49.3X6
Wisterine	T62.2X1	T62.2X2	T62.2X3	T62.2X4	--	--
Witch hazel	T49.2X1	T49.2X2	T49.2X3	T49.2X4	T49.2X5	T49.2X6
Wood alcohol or spirit	T51.1X1	T51.1X2	T51.1X3	T51.1X4	--	--
Wool fat (hydrous)	T49.3X1	T49.3X2	T49.3X3	T49.3X4	T49.3X5	T49.3X6
Woorali	T48.1X1	T48.1X2	T48.1X3	T48.1X4	T48.1X5	T48.1X6
Wormseed, American	T37.4X1	T37.4X2	T37.4X3	T37.4X4	T37.4X5	T37.4X6
Xamoterol	T44.5X1	T44.5X2	T44.5X3	T44.5X4	T44.5X5	T44.5X6
Xanthine diuretics	T50.2X1	T50.2X2	T50.2X3	T50.2X4	T50.2X5	T50.2X6
Xanthinol nicotinate	T46.7X1	T46.7X2	T46.7X3	T46.7X4	T46.7X5	T46.7X6
Xanthotoxin	T49.3X1	T49.3X2	T49.3X3	T49.3X4	T49.3X5	T49.3X6
Xanthinol nicotinate	T46.7X1	T46.7X2	T46.7X3	T46.7X4	T46.7X5	T46.7X6
Xantocillin	T36.0X1	T36.0X2	T36.0X3	T36.0X4	T36.0X5	T36.0X6
Xenon (127Xe) (133Xe)	T50.8X1	T50.8X2	T50.8X3	T50.8X4	T50.8X5	T50.8X6
Xenysalate	T49.4X1	T49.4X2	T49.4X3	T49.4X4	T49.4X5	T49.4X6
Xibornol	T37.8X1	T37.8X2	T37.8X3	T37.8X4	T37.8X5	T37.8X6
Xigris	T45.511	T45.512	T45.513	T45.514	T45.515	T45.516
Xipamide	T50.2X1	T50.2X2	T50.2X3	T50.2X4	T50.2X5	T50.2X6
Xylene (vapor)	T52.2X1	T52.2X2	T52.2X3	T52.2X4	--	--
Xylocaine (infiltration) (topical)	T41.3X1	T41.3X2	T41.3X3	T41.3X4	T41.3X5	T41.3X6
- nerve block (peripheral) (plexus)	T41.3X1	T41.3X2	T41.3X3	T41.3X4	T41.3X5	T41.3X6
- spinal	T41.3X1	T41.3X2	T41.3X3	T41.3X4	T41.3X5	T41.3X6
Xylol (vapor)	T52.2X1	T52.2X2	T52.2X3	T52.2X4	--	--
Xylometazoline	T48.5X1	T48.5X2	T48.5X3	T48.5X4	T48.5X5	T48.5X6
Yeast	T45.2X1	T45.2X2	T45.2X3	T45.2X4	T45.2X5	T45.2X6
- dried	T45.2X1	T45.2X2	T45.2X3	T45.2X4	T45.2X5	T45.2X6
Yellow						
- fever vaccine	T50.B91	T50.B92	T50.B93	T50.B94	T50.B95	T50.B96
- jasmine	T62.2X1	T62.2X2	T62.2X3	T62.2X4	--	--
- phenolphthalein	T47.2X1	T47.2X2	T47.2X3	T47.2X4	T47.2X5	T47.2X6
Yew	T62.2X1	T62.2X2	T62.2X3	T62.2X4	--	--
Yohimbic acid	T40.991	T40.992	T40.993	T40.994	T40.995	T40.996
Zactane	T39.8X1	T39.8X2	T39.8X3	T39.8X4	T39.8X5	T39.8X6
Zalcitabine	T37.5X1	T37.5X2	T37.5X3	T37.5X4	T37.5X5	T37.5X6
Zaroxolyn	T50.2X1	T50.2X2	T50.2X3	T50.2X4	T50.2X5	T50.2X6
Zephiran (topical)	T49.0X1	T49.0X2	T49.0X3	T49.0X4	T49.0X5	T49.0X6
- ophthalmic preparation	T49.5X1	T49.5X2	T49.5X3	T49.5X4	T49.5X5	T49.5X6
Zeranol	T38.7X1	T38.7X2	T38.7X3	T38.7X4	T38.7X5	T38.7X6
Zerone	T51.1X1	T51.1X2	T51.1X3	T51.1X4	--	--
Zidovudine	T37.5X1	T37.5X2	T37.5X3	T37.5X4	T37.5X5	T37.5X6
Zimeldine	T43.221	T43.222	T43.223	T43.224	T43.225	T43.226
Zinc (compounds) (fumes) (vapor) NEC	T56.5X1	T56.5X2	T56.5X3	T56.5X4	--	--

Substance	Poisoning, Accidental (unintentional)	Poisoning, Intentional Self-harm	Poisoning, Assault	Poisoning, Undetermined	Adverse effect	Underdosing
- anti-infectives	T49.0X1	T49.0X2	T49.0X3	T49.0X4	T49.0X5	T49.0X6
- antivaricose	T46.8X1	T46.8X2	T46.8X3	T46.8X4	T46.8X5	T46.8X6
- bacitracin	T49.0X1	T49.0X2	T49.0X3	T49.0X4	T49.0X5	T49.0X6
- chloride (mouthwash)	T49.6X1	T49.6X2	T49.6X3	T49.6X4	T49.6X5	T49.6X6
- chromate	T56.5X1	T56.5X2	T56.5X3	T56.5X4	--	--
- gelatin	T49.3X1	T49.3X2	T49.3X3	T49.3X4	T49.3X5	T49.3X6
- oxide	T49.3X1	T49.3X2	T49.3X3	T49.3X4	T49.3X5	T49.3X6
- - plaster	T49.3X1	T49.3X2	T49.3X3	T49.3X4	T49.3X5	T49.3X6
- peroxide	T49.0X1	T49.0X2	T49.0X3	T49.0X4	T49.0X5	T49.0X6
- pesticides	T56.5X1	T56.5X2	T56.5X3	T56.5X4	--	--
- phosphide	T60.4X1	T60.4X2	T60.4X3	T60.4X4	--	--
- pyrithionate	T49.4X1	T49.4X2	T49.4X3	T49.4X4	T49.4X5	T49.4X6
- stearate	T49.3X1	T49.3X2	T49.3X3	T49.3X4	T49.3X5	T49.3X6
- sulfate	T49.5X1	T49.5X2	T49.5X3	T49.5X4	T49.5X5	T49.5X6
- - ENT agent	T49.6X1	T49.6X2	T49.6X3	T49.6X4	T49.6X5	T49.6X6
- - ophthalmic solution	T49.5X1	T49.5X2	T49.5X3	T49.5X4	T49.5X5	T49.5X6
- - topical NEC	T49.0X1	T49.0X2	T49.0X3	T49.0X4	T49.0X5	T49.0X6
- undecylenate	T49.0X1	T49.0X2	T49.0X3	T49.0X4	T49.0X5	T49.0X6
Zineb	T60.0X1	T60.0X2	T60.0X3	T60.0X4	--	--
Zinostatin	T45.1X1	T45.1X2	T45.1X3	T45.1X4	T45.1X5	T45.1X6
Zipeprol	T48.3X1	T48.3X2	T48.3X3	T48.3X4	T48.3X5	T48.3X6
Zofenopril	T46.4X1	T46.4X2	T46.4X3	T46.4X4	T46.4X5	T46.4X6
Zolpidem	T42.6X1	T42.6X2	T42.6X3	T42.6X4	T42.6X5	T42.6X6
Zomepirac	T39.391	T39.392	T39.393	T39.394	T39.395	T39.396
Zopiclone	T42.6X1	T42.6X2	T42.6X3	T42.6X4	T42.6X5	T42.6X6
Zorubicin	T45.1X1	T45.1X2	T45.1X3	T45.1X4	T45.1X5	T45.1X6
Zotepine	T43.591	T43.592	T43.593	T43.594	T43.595	T43.596
Zovant	T45.511	T45.512	T45.513	T45.514	T45.515	T45.516
Zoxazolamine	T42.8X1	T42.8X2	T42.8X3	T42.8X4	T42.8X5	T42.8X6
Zuclopenthixol	T43.4X1	T43.4X2	T43.4X3	T43.4X4	T43.4X5	T43.4X6
Zygadenus (venenosus)	T62.2X1	T62.2X2	T62.2X3	T62.2X4	--	--
Zyprexa	T43.591	T43.592	T43.593	T43.594	T43.595	T43.596

Accident - *continued*

    |nontraffic V74.3
    |while boarding or alighting V74.4
  |two wheeled motor vehicle (traffic)
    V72.9
    |nontraffic V72.3
    |while boarding or alighting V72.4
  |van (traffic) V73.9
    |nontraffic V73.3
    |while boarding or alighting V73.4
|driver
  |collision (with)
    |animal (traffic) V70.5
      |being ridden (traffic) V76.5
        |nontraffic V76.0
      |nontraffic V70.0
    |animal-drawn vehicle (traffic) V76.5
      |nontraffic V76.0
    |bus (traffic) V74.5
      |nontraffic V74.0
    |car (traffic) V73.5
      |nontraffic V73.0
    |motor vehicle NOS (traffic) V79.40
      |nontraffic V79.00
      |specified type NEC (traffic)
        V79.49
        |nontraffic V79.09
    |pedal cycle (traffic) V71.5
      |nontraffic V71.0
    |pickup truck (traffic) V73.5
      |nontraffic V73.0
    |railway vehicle (traffic) V75.5
      |nontraffic V75.0
    |specified vehicle NEC (traffic)
      V76.5
      |nontraffic V76.0
    |stationary object (traffic) V77.5
      |nontraffic V77.0
    |streetcar (traffic) V76.5
      |nontraffic V76.0
    |three wheeled motor vehicle (traffic)
      V72.5
      |nontraffic V72.0
    |truck (traffic) V74.5
      |nontraffic V74.0
    |two wheeled motor vehicle (traffic)
      V72.5
      |nontraffic V72.0
    |van (traffic) V73.5
      |nontraffic V73.0
  |noncollision accident (traffic) V78.5
    |nontraffic V78.0
  |noncollision accident (traffic) V78.9
    |nontraffic V78.3
    |while boarding or alighting V78.4
  |nontraffic V79.3
|hanger-on
  |collision (with)
    |animal (traffic) V70.7
      |being ridden (traffic) V76.7
        |nontraffic V76.2
      |nontraffic V70.2
    |animal-drawn vehicle (traffic) V76.7
      |nontraffic V76.2
    |bus (traffic) V74.7
      |nontraffic V74.2
    |car (traffic) V73.7
      |nontraffic V73.2
    |pedal cycle (traffic) V71.7
      |nontraffic V71.2
    |pickup truck (traffic) V73.7
      |nontraffic V73.2
    |railway vehicle (traffic) V75.7
      |nontraffic V75.2

Accident - *continued*

    |specified vehicle NEC (traffic)
      V76.7
      |nontraffic V76.2
    |stationary object (traffic) V77.7
      |nontraffic V77.2
    |streetcar (traffic) V76.7
      |nontraffic V76.2
    |three wheeled motor vehicle (traffic)
      V72.7
      |nontraffic V72.2
    |truck (traffic) V74.7
      |nontraffic V74.2
    |two wheeled motor vehicle (traffic)
      V72.7
      |nontraffic V72.2
    |van (traffic) V73.7
      |nontraffic V73.2
  |noncollision accident (traffic) V78.7
    |nontraffic V78.2
|passenger
  |collision (with)
    |animal (traffic) V70.6
      |being ridden (traffic) V76.6
        |nontraffic V76.1
      |nontraffic V70.1
    |animal-drawn vehicle (traffic) V76.6
      |nontraffic V76.1
    |bus (traffic) V74.6
      |nontraffic V74.1
    |car (traffic) V73.6
      |nontraffic V73.1
    |motor vehicle NOS (traffic) V79.50
      |nontraffic V79.10
      |specified type NEC (traffic)
        V79.59
        |nontraffic V79.19
    |pedal cycle (traffic) V71.6
      |nontraffic V71.1
    |pickup truck (traffic) V73.6
      |nontraffic V73.1
    |railway vehicle (traffic) V75.6
      |nontraffic V75.1
    |specified vehicle NEC (traffic)
      V76.6
      |nontraffic V76.1
    |stationary object (traffic) V77.6
      |nontraffic V77.1
    |streetcar (traffic) V76.6
      |nontraffic V76.1
    |three wheeled motor vehicle (traffic)
      V72.6
      |nontraffic V72.1
    |truck (traffic) V74.6
      |nontraffic V74.1
    |two wheeled motor vehicle (traffic)
      V72.6
      |nontraffic V72.1
    |van (traffic) V73.6
      |nontraffic V73.1
  |noncollision accident (traffic) V78.6
    |nontraffic V78.1
|specified type NEC V79.88
  |military vehicle V79.81
|cable car, not on rails V98.0
  |on rails *see* Accident, transport,
  streetcar occupant
car occupant V49.9
  |ambulance occupant *see* Accident,
  transport, ambulance occupant
  |collision (with)
    |animal (traffic) V40.9
      |being ridden (traffic) V46.9
      |nontraffic V46.3

Accident - *continued*

      |while boarding or alighting V46.4
      |nontraffic V40.3
      |while boarding or alighting V40.4
    |animal-drawn vehicle (traffic) V46.9
      |nontraffic V46.3
      |while boarding or alighting V46.4
    |bus (traffic) V44.9
      |nontraffic V44.3
      |while boarding or alighting V44.4
    |car (traffic) V43.92
      |nontraffic V43.32
      |while boarding or alighting V43.42
    |motor vehicle NOS (traffic) V49.60
      |nontraffic V49.20
      |specified type NEC (traffic) V49.69
        |nontraffic V49.29
    |pedal cycle (traffic) V41.9
      |nontraffic V41.3
      |while boarding or alighting V41.4
    |pickup truck (traffic) V43.93
      |nontraffic V43.33
      |while boarding or alighting V43.43
    |railway vehicle (traffic) V45.9
      |nontraffic V45.3
      |while boarding or alighting V45.4
    |specified vehicle NEC (traffic) V46.9
      |nontraffic V46.3
      |while boarding or alighting V46.4
    |sport utility vehicle (traffic) V43.91
      |nontraffic V43.31
      |while boarding or alighting V43.41
    |stationary object (traffic) V47.9
      |nontraffic V47.3
      |while boarding or alighting V47.4
    |streetcar (traffic) V46.9
      |nontraffic V46.3
      |while boarding or alighting V46.4
    |three wheeled motor vehicle (traffic)
      V42.9
      |nontraffic V42.3
      |while boarding or alighting V42.4
    |truck (traffic) V44.9
      |nontraffic V44.3
      |while boarding or alighting V44.4
    |two wheeled motor vehicle (traffic)
      V42.9
      |nontraffic V42.3
      |while boarding or alighting V42.4
    |van (traffic) V43.94
      |nontraffic V43.34
      |while boarding or alighting V43.44
  |driver
    |collision (with)
      |animal (traffic) V40.5
        |being ridden (traffic) V46.5
          |nontraffic V46.0
        |nontraffic V40.0
      |animal-drawn vehicle (traffic) V46.5
        |nontraffic V46.0
      |bus (traffic) V44.5
        |nontraffic V44.0
      |car (traffic) V43.52
        |nontraffic V43.02
      |motor vehicle NOS (traffic) V49.40
        |nontraffic V49.00
        |specified type NEC (traffic)
          V49.49
          |nontraffic V49.09
      |pedal cycle (traffic) V41.5
        |nontraffic V41.0
      |pickup truck (traffic) V43.53
        |nontraffic V43.03
      |railway vehicle (traffic) V45.5

Accident - *continued*
- |streetcar (traffic) V26.9
  - |nontraffic V26.2
  - |while boarding or alighting V26.3
- |three wheeled motor vehicle (traffic) V22.9
  - |nontraffic V22.2
  - |while boarding or alighting V22.3
- |truck (traffic) V24.9
  - |nontraffic V24.2
  - |while boarding or alighting V24.3
- |two wheeled motor vehicle (traffic) V22.9
  - |nontraffic V22.2
  - |while boarding or alighting V22.3
- |van (traffic) V23.9
  - |nontraffic V23.2
  - |while boarding or alighting V23.3
- |driver
  - |collision (with)
    - |animal (traffic) V20.4
      - |being ridden (traffic) V26.4
      - |nontraffic V20.0
    - |animal-drawn vehicle (traffic) V26.4
      - |nontraffic V26.0
      - |nontraffic V26.0
    - |bus (traffic) V24.4
      - |nontraffic V24.0
    - |car (traffic) V23.4
      - |nontraffic V23.0
    - |motor vehicle NOS (traffic) V29.40
      - |nontraffic V29.00
      - |specified type NEC (traffic) V29.49
        - |nontraffic V29.09
    - |pedal cycle (traffic) V21.4
      - |nontraffic V21.0
    - |pickup truck (traffic) V23.4
      - |nontraffic V23.0
    - |railway vehicle (traffic) V25.4
      - |nontraffic V25.0
    - |specified vehicle NEC (traffic) V26.4
      - |nontraffic V26.0
    - |stationary object (traffic) V27.4
      - |nontraffic V27.0
    - |streetcar (traffic) V26.4
      - |nontraffic V26.0
    - |three wheeled motor vehicle (traffic) V22.4
      - |nontraffic V22.0
    - |truck (traffic) V24.4
      - |nontraffic V24.0
    - |two wheeled motor vehicle (traffic) V22.4
      - |nontraffic V22.0
    - |van (traffic) V23.4
      - |nontraffic V23.0
  - |noncollision accident (traffic) V28.4
    - |nontraffic V28.0
- |noncollision accident (traffic) V28.9
  - |nontraffic V28.2
  - |while boarding or alighting V28.3
- |nontraffic V29.3
- |passenger
  - |collision (with)
    - |animal (traffic) V20.5
      - |being ridden (traffic) V26.5
        - |nontraffic V26.1
      - |nontraffic V20.1
    - |animal-drawn vehicle (traffic) V26.5
      - |nontraffic V26.1
    - |bus (traffic) V24.5
      - |nontraffic V24.1

Accident - *continued*
- |car (traffic) V23.5
  - |nontraffic V23.1
- |motor vehicle NOS (traffic) V29.50
  - |nontraffic V29.10
  - |specified type NEC (traffic) V29.59
    - |nontraffic V29.19
- |pedal cycle (traffic) V21.5
  - |nontraffic V21.1
- |pickup truck (traffic) V23.5
  - |nontraffic V23.1
- |railway vehicle (traffic) V25.5
  - |nontraffic V25.1
- |specified vehicle NEC (traffic) V26.5
  - |nontraffic V26.1
- |stationary object (traffic) V27.5
  - |nontraffic V27.1
- |streetcar (traffic) V26.5
  - |nontraffic V26.1
- |three wheeled motor vehicle (traffic) V22.5
  - |nontraffic V22.1
- |truck (traffic) V24.5
  - |nontraffic V24.1
- |two wheeled motor vehicle (traffic) V22.5
  - |nontraffic V22.1
- |van (traffic) V23.5
  - |nontraffic V23.1
- |noncollision accident (traffic) V28.5
  - |nontraffic V28.1
- |specified type NEC V29.88
- |military vehicle V29.81
- |motor vehicle NEC occupant (traffic) V89.2
- |occupant (of)
  - |aircraft (powered) V95.9
    - |fixed wing
      - |commercial *see* Accident, transport, aircraft, occupant, powered, fixed wing, commercial
      - |private *see* Accident, transport, aircraft, occupant, powered, fixed wing, private
    - |nonpowered V96.9
    - |specified NEC V95.8
  - |airport battery-powered vehicle *see* Accident, transport, industrial vehicle occupant
  - |all-terrain vehicle (ATV) *see* Accident, transport, all-terrain vehicle occupant
  - |animal-drawn vehicle *see* Accident, transport, animal-drawn vehicle occupant
  - |automobile *see* Accident, transport, car occupant
  - |balloon V96.00
  - |battery-powered vehicle *see* Accident, transport, industrial vehicle occupant
  - |bicycle *see* Accident, transport, pedal cyclist
    - |motorized *see* Accident, transport, motorcycle rider
  - |boat NEC *see* Accident, watercraft
  - |bulldozer *see* Accident, transport, construction vehicle occupant
  - |bus *see* Accident, transport, bus occupant
  - |cable car (on rails) *see also* Accident, transport, streetcar occupant
    - |not on rails V98.0
  - |car *see also* Accident, transport, car

Accident - *continued*
- occupant
  - |cable (on rails) *see also* Accident, transport, streetcar occupant
    - |not on rails V98.0
  - |coach *see* Accident, transport, bus occupant
  - |coal-car *see* Accident, transport, industrial vehicle occupant
  - |digger *see* Accident, transport, construction vehicle occupant
  - |dump truck *see* Accident, transport, construction vehicle occupant
  - |earth-leveler *see* Accident, transport, construction vehicle occupant
  - |farm machinery (self-propelled) *see* Accident, transport, agricultural vehicle occupant
  - |forklift *see* Accident, transport, industrial vehicle occupant
  - |glider (unpowered) V96.20
    - |hang V96.10
    - |powered (microlight) (ultralight) *see* Accident, transport, aircraft, occupant, powered, glider
  - |glider (unpowered) NEC V96.20
  - |hang-glider V96.10
  - |harvester *see* Accident, transport, agricultural vehicle occupant
  - |heavy (transport) vehicle *see* Accident, transport, truck occupant
  - |helicopter *see* Accident, transport, aircraft, occupant, helicopter
  - |ice-yacht V98.2
  - |kite (carrying person) V96.8
  - |land-yacht V98.1
  - |logging car *see* Accident, transport, industrial vehicle occupant
  - |mechanical shovel *see* Accident, transport, construction vehicle occupant
  - |microlight *see* Accident, transport, aircraft, occupant, powered, glider
  - |minibus *see* Accident, transport, pickup truck occupant
  - |minivan *see* Accident, transport, pickup truck occupant
  - |moped *see* Accident, transport, motorcycle
  - |motor scooter *see* Accident, transport, motorcycle
  - |motorcycle (with sidecar) *see* Accident, transport, motorcycle
  - |off-road motor-vehicle (see also Accident, transport, all-terrain vehicle occupant) V86.99
- |off-road motor-vehicle (see also Accident, transport, all-terrain vehicle occupant) V86.99
- |pedal cycle *see also* Accident, transport, pedal cyclist
- |pick-up (truck) *see* Accident, transport, pickup truck occupant
- |railway (train) (vehicle) (subterranean) (elevated) *see* Accident, transport, railway vehicle occupant
- |rickshaw *see* Accident, transport, pedal cycle
  - |motorized *see* Accident, transport, three-wheeled motor vehicle
  - |pedal driven *see* Accident, transport, pedal cyclist
- |road-roller *see* Accident, transport, construction vehicle occupant

Accident - *continued*

    |nontraffic V05.09

    |traffic V05.19

  |streetcar V06.99

    |nontraffic V06.09

    |traffic V06.19

  |stationary object V00.822

  |two |or three-wheeled motor

    vehicle V02.99

    |nontraffic V02.09

    |traffic V02.19

  |vehicle V09.9

    |animal-drawn V06.99

      |nontraffic V06.09

      |traffic V06.19

    |motor

      |nontraffic V09.00

      |traffic V09.20

 |fall V00.821

 |nontraffic V09.1

  |involving motor vehicle NEC

    V09.00

 |traffic V09.3

  |involving motor vehicle NEC

    V09.20

|flat-bottomed NEC V00.388

 |collision (with) V09.9

  |animal being ridden or animal

    drawn vehicle V06.99

    |nontraffic V06.09

    |traffic V06.19

  |bus or heavy transport V04.99

    |nontraffic V04.09

    |traffic V04.19

  |car V03.99

    |nontraffic V03.09

    |traffic V03.19

  |pedal cycle V01.99

    |nontraffic V01.09

  |traffic V01.19

  |pick-up truck or van V03.99

    |nontraffic V03.09

    |traffic V03.19

  |railway (train) (vehicle) V05.99

    |nontraffic V05.09

    |traffic V05.19

  |stationary object V00.382

  |streetcar V06.99

    |nontraffic V06.09

    |traffic V06.19

  |two |or three-wheeled motor

    vehicle V02.99

    |nontraffic V02.09

    |traffic V02.19

  |vehicle V09.9

    |animal-drawn V06.99

      |nontraffic V06.09

      |traffic V06.19

    |motor

      |nontraffic V09.00

      |traffic V09.20

 |fall V00.381

 |nontraffic V09.1

  |involving motor vehicle NEC

    V09.00

 |snow

  |board *see* Accident, transport,

    pedestrian, conveyance, snow

    board

  |ski | *see* Accident, transport,

    pedestrian, conveyance, skis

    (snow)

 |traffic V09.3

  |involving motor vehicle NEC

Accident - *continued*

    V09.20

|gliding type NEC V00.288

 |collision (with) V09.9

  |animal being ridden or animal

    drawn vehicle V06.99

    |nontraffic V06.09

    |traffic V06.19

  |bus or heavy transport V04.99

    |nontraffic V04.09

    |traffic V04.19

  |car V03.99

    |nontraffic V03.09

    |traffic V03.19

  |pedal cycle V01.99

    |nontraffic V01.09

    |traffic V01.19

  |pick-up truck or van V03.99

    |nontraffic V03.09

    |traffic V03.19

  |railway (train) (vehicle) V05.99

    |nontraffic V05.09

    |traffic V05.19

  |stationary object V00.282

  |streetcar V06.99

    |nontraffic V06.09

    |traffic V06.19

  |two |or three-wheeled motor

    vehicle V02.99

    |nontraffic V02.09

    |traffic V02.19

  |vehicle V09.9

    |animal-drawn V06.99

      |nontraffic V06.09

      |traffic V06.19

    |motor

      |nontraffic V09.00

      |traffic V09.20

 |fall V00.281

 |heelies *see* Accident, transport,

    pedestrian, conveyance, heelies

 |ice skate *see* Accident, transport,

    pedestrian, conveyance, ice skate

 |nontraffic V09.1

  |involving motor vehicle NEC

    V09.00

 |sled *see* Accident, transport,

    pedestrian, conveyance, sled

 |traffic V09.3

  |involving motor vehicle NEC

    V09.20

  |wheelies *see* Accident, transport,

    pedestrian, conveyance, heelies

|heelies V00.158

 |colliding with stationary object

    V00.152

 |fall V00.151

|hoverboard

 |collision with

  |animal being ridden or animal

    drawn   vehicle V06.938

    |nontraffic V06.038

    |traffic V06.138

  |bus or heavy transport V04.938

    |nontraffic V04.038

    |traffic V04.138

  |car V03.938

    |nontraffic V03.038

    |traffic V03.138

  |pedal cycle V01.938

    |nontraffic V01.038

    |traffic V01.138

  |pick-up or van V03.938

    |nontraffic V03.038

Accident - *continued*

    |traffic V03.138

  |railway (train) (vehicle) V05.938

    |nontraffic V05.038

    |traffic V05.138

  |streetcar V06.938

    |nontraffic V06.038

    |traffic V06.138

  |three wheeled motor vehicle V02.938

    |nontraffic V02.038

    |traffic V02.138

  |two wheeled motor vehicle V02.938

    |nontraffic V02.038

    |traffic V02.138

  |vehicle, nonmotor, specified NEC

    V06.938

    |nontraffic V06.038

    |traffic V06.138

 |fall V00.848

|Segway

 |collision with

  |animal being ridden or animal drawn

    vehicle V06.938

    |nontraffic V06.038

    |traffic V06.138

  |bus or heavy transport V04.938

    |nontraffic V04.038

    |traffic V04.138

  |car V03.938

    |nontraffic V03.038

    |traffic V03.138

  |pedal cycle V01.938

    |nontraffic V01.038

    |traffic V01.138

  |pick up or van V03.938

    |nontraffic V03.038

    |traffic V03.138

  |railway (train) (vehicle) V05.938

    |nontraffic V05.038

    |traffic V05.138

  |streetcar V06.938

    |nontraffic V06.038

    |traffic V06.138

  |three wheeled motor vehicle V02.938

    |nontraffic V02.038

    |traffic V02.138

  |two wheeled motor vehicle V02.938

    |nontraffic V02.038

    |traffic V02.138

  |vehicle, nonmotor, specified NEC

    V06.938

    |nontraffic V06.038

    |traffic V06.138

 |fall V00.848

 |standing

  |electric scooter

   |collision with

    |animal being ridden or animal drawn

      vehicle V06.931

      |nontraffic V06.031

      |traffic V06.131

    |bus or heavy transport V04.931

      |nontraffic V04.031

      |traffic V04.131

    |car V03.931

      |nontraffic V03.031

      |traffic V03.131

    |pedal cycle V01.931

      |nontraffic V01.031

      |traffic V01.131

    |pick up or van V03.931

      |nontraffic V03.031

      |traffic V03.131

    |railway (train) (vehicle) V05.931

Accident - *continued*

|animal being ridden or animal
 drawn vehicle V06.99
 |nontraffic V06.09
 |traffic V06.19
|bus or heavy transport V04.99
 |nontraffic V04.09
 |traffic V04.19
|car V03.99
 |nontraffic V03.09
 |traffic V03.19
|pedal cycle V01.99
 |nontraffic V01.09
 |traffic V01.19
|pick-up truck or van V03.99
 |nontraffic V03.09
 |traffic V03.19
|railway (train) (vehicle) V05.99
 |nontraffic V05.09
 |traffic V05.19
|streetcar V06.99
 |nontraffic V06.09
 |traffic V06.19
|stationary object V00.142
|two or three-wheeled motor
 vehicle V02.99
 |nontraffic V02.09
 |traffic V02.19
|vehicle V09.9
 |animal-drawn V06.99
  |nontraffic V06.09
  |traffic V06.19
 |motor
  |nontraffic V09.00
  |traffic V09.20
|fall V00.141
|nontraffic V09.1
 |involving motor vehicle NEC
  V09.00
|traffic V09.3
 |involving motor vehicle NEC
  V09.20
|skate board V00.138
 |collision (with) V09.9
 |animal being ridden or animal
  drawn vehicle V06.92
  |nontraffic V06.02
  |traffic V06.12
 |bus or heavy transport V04.92
  |nontraffic V04.02
  |traffic V04.12
 |car V03.92
  |nontraffic V03.02
  |traffic V03.12
 |pedal cycle V01.92
  |nontraffic V01.02
  |traffic V01.12
 |pick-up truck or van V03.92
  |nontraffic V03.02
  |traffic V03.12
 |railway (train) (vehicle) V05.92
  |nontraffic V05.02
  |traffic V05.12
 |streetcar V06.92
  |nontraffic V06.02
  |traffic V06.12
 |stationary object V00.132
 |two or three-wheeled motor
  vehicle V02.92
  |nontraffic V02.02
  |traffic V02.12
 |vehicle V09.9
  |animal-drawn V06.92
   |nontraffic V06.02

Accident - *continued*

  |traffic V06.12
  |motor
   |nontraffic V09.00
   |traffic V09.20
 |nontraffic V09.1
  |involving motor vehicle NEC
   V09.00
 |traffic V09.3
  |involving motor vehicle NEC
   V09.20
|sled V00.228
 |collision (with) V09.9
 |animal being ridden or animal
  drawn vehicle V06.99
  |nontraffic V06.09
  |traffic V06.19
 |bus or heavy transport V04.99
  |nontraffic V04.09
  |traffic V04.19
 |car V03.99
  |nontraffic V03.09
  |traffic V03.19
 |pedal cycle V01.99
  |nontraffic V01.09
  |traffic V01.19
 |pick-up truck or van V03.99
  |nontraffic V03.09
  |traffic V03.19
 |railway (train) (vehicle) V05.99
  |nontraffic V05.09
  |traffic V05.19
 |streetcar V06.99
  |nontraffic V06.09
  |traffic V06.19
 |stationary object V00.222
 |two or three-wheeled motor
  vehicle V02.99
  |nontraffic V02.09
  |traffic V02.19
 |vehicle V09.9
  |animal-drawn V06.99
   |nontraffic V06.09
   |traffic V06.19
  |motor
   |nontraffic V09.00
   |traffic V09.20
 |fall V00.221
 |nontraffic V09.1
  |involving motor vehicle NEC
   V09.00
 |traffic V09.3
  |involving motor vehicle NEC
   V09.20
|skis (snow) V00.328
 |collision (with) V09.9
 |animal being ridden or animal
  drawn vehicle V06.99
  |nontraffic V06.09
  |traffic V06.19
 |bus or heavy transport V04.99
  |nontraffic V04.09
  |traffic V04.19
 |car V03.99
  |nontraffic V03.09
  |traffic V03.19
 |pedal cycle V01.99
  |nontraffic V01.09
  |traffic V01.19
 |pick-up truck or van V03.99
  |nontraffic V03.09
  |traffic V03.19
 |railway (train) (vehicle) V05.99
  |nontraffic V05.09

Accident - *continued*

  |traffic V05.19
 |streetcar V06.99
  |nontraffic V06.09
  |traffic V06.19
 |stationary object V00.322
 |two or three-wheeled motor
  vehicle V02.99
  |nontraffic V02.09
  |traffic V02.19
 |vehicle V09.9
  |animal-drawn V06.99
   |nontraffic V06.09
   |traffic V06.19
  |motor
   |nontraffic V09.00
   |traffic V09.20
 |fall V00.321
 |nontraffic V09.1
  |involving motor vehicle NEC
   V09.00
 |traffic V09.3
  |involving motor vehicle NEC
   V09.20
|snow board V00.318
 |collision (with) V09.9
 |animal being ridden or animal
  drawn vehicle V06.99
  |nontraffic V06.09
  |traffic V06.19
 |bus or heavy transport V04.99
  |nontraffic V04.09
  |traffic V04.19
 |car V03.99
  |nontraffic V03.09
  |traffic V03.19
 |pedal cycle V01.99
  |nontraffic V01.09
  |traffic V01.19
 |pick-up truck or van V03.99
  |nontraffic V03.09
  |traffic V03.19
 |railway (train) (vehicle) V05.99
  |nontraffic V05.09
  |traffic V05.19
 |streetcar V06.99
  |nontraffic V06.09
  |traffic V06.19
 |stationary object V00.312
 |two or three-wheeled motor
  vehicle V02.99
  |nontraffic V02.09
  |traffic V02.19
 |vehicle V09.9
  |animal-drawn V06.99
   |nontraffic V06.09
   |traffic V06.19
  |motor
   |nontraffic V09.00
   |traffic V09.20
 |fall V00.311
 |nontraffic V09.1
  |involving motor vehicle NEC
   V09.00
 |traffic V09.3
  |involving motor vehicle NEC
   V09.20
|specified type NEC V00.898
 |collision (with) V09.9
 |animal being ridden or animal
  drawn vehicle V06.99
  |nontraffic V06.09
  |traffic V06.19
 |bus or heavy transport V04.99

Accident - *continued*

    |nontraffic V04.09
    |traffic V04.19
  |car V03.99
    |nontraffic V03.09
    |traffic V03.19
  |pedal cycle V01.99
    |nontraffic V01.09
    |traffic V01.19
  |pick-up truck or van V03.99
    |nontraffic V03.09
    |traffic V03.19
  |railway (train) (vehicle) V05.99
    |nontraffic V05.09
    |traffic V05.19
  |streetcar V06.99
    |nontraffic V06.09
    |traffic V06.19
  |stationary object V00.892
  |two or three-wheeled motor
    vehicle V02.99
    |nontraffic V02.09
    |traffic V02.19
  |vehicle V09.9
    |animal-drawn V06.99
      |nontraffic V06.09
      |traffic V06.19
    |motor
      |nontraffic V09.00
      |traffic V09.20
  |fall V00.891
  |nontraffic V09.1
    |involving motor vehicle NEC
      V09.00
  |traffic V09.3
    |involving motor vehicle NEC
      V09.20
|traffic V09.3
  |involving motor vehicle V09.20
    |military V09.21
    |specified type NEC V09.29
|wheelchair (powered) V00.818
  |collision (with) V09.9
    |animal being ridden or animal
      drawn vehicle V06.99
      |nontraffic V06.09
      |traffic V06.19
    |bus or heavy transport V04.99
      |nontraffic V04.09
      |traffic V04.19
    |car V03.99
      |nontraffic V03.09
      |traffic V03.19
    |pedal cycle V01.99
      |nontraffic V01.09
      |traffic V01.19
    |pick-up truck or van V03.99
      |nontraffic V03.09
      |traffic V03.19
    |railway (train) (vehicle) V05.99
      |nontraffic V05.09
      |traffic V05.19
    |streetcar V06.99
      |nontraffic V06.09
      |traffic V06.19
    |stationary object V00.812
    |two or three-wheeled motor
      vehicle V02.99
      |nontraffic V02.09
      |traffic V02.19
    |vehicle V09.9
      |animal-drawn V06.99
        |nontraffic V06.09
        |traffic V06.19

Accident - *continued*

    |motor
      |nontraffic V09.00
      |traffic V09.20
  |fall V00.811
  |nontraffic V09.1
    |involving motor vehicle NEC
      V09.00
  |traffic V09.3
    |involving motor vehicle NEC
      V09.20
  |wheeled shoe V00.158
    |colliding with stationary object
      V00.152
    |fall V00.151
|on foot *see also* Accident, pedestrian
  |collision (with)
    |animal being ridden or animal drawn
      vehicle V06.90
      |nontraffic V06.00
      |traffic V06.10
    |bus or heavy transport V04.90
      |nontraffic V04.00
      |traffic V04.10
    |car V03.90
      |nontraffic V03.00
      |traffic V03.10
    |pedal cycle V01.90
      |nontraffic V01.00
      |traffic V01.10
    |pick-up truck or van V03.90
      |nontraffic V03.00
      |traffic V03.10
    |railway (train) (vehicle) V05.90
      |nontraffic V05.00
      |traffic V05.10
    |streetcar V06.90
      |nontraffic V06.00
      |traffic V06.10
    |two or three-wheeled motor vehicle
      V02.90
      |nontraffic V02.00
      |traffic V02.10
    |vehicle V09.9
      |animal-drawn V06.90
        |nontraffic V06.00
        |traffic V06.10
      |motor
        |nontraffic V09.00
        |traffic V09.20
    |nontraffic V09.1
      |involving motor vehicle V09.00
        |military V09.01
        |specified type NEC V09.09
    |traffic V09.3
      |involving motor vehicle V09.20
        |military V09.21
        |specified type NEC V09.29
  |person NEC (unknown way or
    transportation) V99
  |collision (between)
    |bus (with)
      |heavy transport vehicle (traffic)
        V87.5
      |nontraffic V88.5
    |car (with)
      |nontraffic V88.5
      |bus (traffic) V87.3
      |nontraffic V88.3
      |heavy transport vehicle (traffic)
        V87.4
      |nontraffic V88.4
    |pick-up truck or van (traffic) V87.2
      |nontraffic V88.2

Accident - *continued*

    |train or railway vehicle (traffic)
      V87.6
    |nontraffic V88.6
    |two-or three-wheeled motor vehicle
      (traffic) V87.0
    |nontraffic V88.0
  |motor vehicle (traffic) NEC V87.7
    |nontraffic V88.7
  |two-or three-wheeled vehicle (with)
    (traffic)
    |motor vehicle NEC V87.1
    |nontraffic V88.1
  |nonmotor vehicle (collision)
    (noncollision) (traffic) V87.9
    |nontraffic V88.9
|pickup truck occupant V59.9
  |collision (with)
    |animal (traffic) V50.9
      |being ridden (traffic) V56.9
        |nontraffic V56.3
        |while boarding or alighting V56.4
      |nontraffic V50.3
      |while boarding or alighting V50.4
    |animal-drawn vehicle (traffic) V56.9
      |nontraffic V56.3
      |while boarding or alighting V56.4
    |bus (traffic) V54.9
      |nontraffic V54.3
      |while boarding or alighting V54.4
    |car (traffic) V53.9
      |nontraffic V53.3
      |while boarding or alighting V53.4
    |motor vehicle NOS (traffic) V59.60
      |nontraffic V59.20
      |specified type NEC (traffic) V59.69
        |nontraffic V59.29
    |pedal cycle (traffic) V51.9
      |nontraffic V51.3
      |while boarding or alighting V51.4
    |pickup truck (traffic) V53.9
      |nontraffic V53.3
      |while boarding or alighting V53.4
    |railway vehicle (traffic) V55.9
      |nontraffic V55.3
      |while boarding or alighting V55.4
    |specified vehicle NEC (traffic) V56.9
      |nontraffic V56.3
      |while boarding or alighting V56.4
    |stationary object (traffic) V57.9
      |nontraffic V57.3
      |while boarding or alighting V57.4
    |streetcar (traffic) V56.9
      |nontraffic V56.3
      |while boarding or alighting V56.4
    |three wheeled motor vehicle (traffic)
      V52.9
      |nontraffic V52.3
      |while boarding or alighting V52.4
    |truck (traffic) V54.9
      |nontraffic V54.3
      |while boarding or alighting V54.4
    |two wheeled motor vehicle (traffic)
      V52.9
      |nontraffic V52.3
      |while boarding or alighting V52.4
    |van (traffic) V53.9
      |nontraffic V53.3
      |while boarding or alighting V53.4
  |driver
    |collision (with)
      |animal (traffic) V50.5
        |being ridden (traffic) V56.5
          |nontraffic V56.0

Accident - *continued*

 |nontraffic V50.0
 |animal-drawn vehicle (traffic) V56.5
  |nontraffic V56.0
 |bus (traffic) V54.5
  |nontraffic V54.0
 |car (traffic) V53.5
  |nontraffic V53.0
 |motor vehicle NOS (traffic) V59.40
  |nontraffic V59.00
  |specified type NEC (traffic)
   V59.49
   |nontraffic V59.09
 |pedal cycle (traffic) V51.5
  |nontraffic V51.0
 |pickup truck (traffic) V53.5
  |nontraffic V53.0
 |railway vehicle (traffic) V55.5
  |nontraffic V55.0
 |specified vehicle NEC (traffic)
   V56.5
  |nontraffic V56.0
 |stationary object (traffic) V57.5
  |nontraffic V57.0
 |streetcar (traffic) V56.5
  |nontraffic V56.0
 |three wheeled motor vehicle (traffic)
   V52.5
  |nontraffic V52.0
 |truck (traffic) V54.5
  |nontraffic V54.0
 |two wheeled motor vehicle (traffic)
   V52.5
  |nontraffic V52.0
 |van (traffic) V53.5
  |nontraffic V53.0
 |noncollision accident (traffic) V58.5
  |nontraffic V58.0
|noncollision accident (traffic) V58.9
 |nontraffic V58.3
 |while boarding or alighting V58.4
|nontraffic V59.3
|hanger-on
 |collision (with)
  |animal (traffic) V50.7
   |being ridden (traffic) V56.7
    |nontraffic V56.2
   |nontraffic V50.2
  |animal-drawn vehicle (traffic) V56.7
   |nontraffic V56.2
  |bus (traffic) V54.7
   |nontraffic V54.2
  |car (traffic) V53.7
   |nontraffic V53.2
  |pedal cycle (traffic) V51.7
   |nontraffic V51.2
  |pickup truck (traffic) V53.7
   |nontraffic V53.2
  |railway vehicle (traffic) V55.7
   |nontraffic V55.2
  |specified vehicle NEC (traffic)
    V56.7
   |nontraffic V56.2
  |stationary object (traffic) V57.7
   |nontraffic V57.2
  |streetcar (traffic) V56.7
   |nontraffic V56.2
  |three wheeled motor vehicle (traffic)
    V52.7
   |nontraffic V52.2
  |truck (traffic) V54.7
   |nontraffic V54.2
  |two wheeled motor vehicle (traffic)
    V52.7

 |nontraffic V52.2
 |van (traffic) V53.7
  |nontraffic V53.2
 |noncollision accident (traffic) V58.7
  |nontraffic V58.2
|passenger
 |collision (with)
  |animal (traffic) V50.6
   |being ridden (traffic) V56.6
    |nontraffic V56.1
   |nontraffic V50.1
  |animal-drawn vehicle (traffic) V56.6
   |nontraffic V56.1
  |bus (traffic) V54.6
   |nontraffic V54.1
  |car (traffic) V53.6
   |nontraffic V53.1
  |motor vehicle NOS (traffic) V59.50
   |nontraffic V59.10
   |specified type NEC (traffic)
    V59.59
    |nontraffic V59.19
  |pedal cycle (traffic) V51.6
   |nontraffic V51.1
  |pickup truck (traffic) V53.6
   |nontraffic V53.1
  |railway vehicle (traffic) V55.6
   |nontraffic V55.1
  |specified vehicle NEC (traffic)
    V56.6
   |nontraffic V56.1
  |stationary object (traffic) V57.6
   |nontraffic V57.1
  |streetcar (traffic) V56.6
   |nontraffic V56.1
  |three wheeled motor vehicle (traffic)
    V52.6
   |nontraffic V52.1
  |truck (traffic) V54.6
   |nontraffic V54.1
  |two wheeled motor vehicle (traffic)
    V52.6
   |nontraffic V52.1
  |van (traffic) V53.6
   |nontraffic V53.1
  |noncollision accident (traffic) V58.6
   |nontraffic V58.1
 |specified type NEC V59.88
  |military vehicle V59.81
 |quarry truck *see* Accident, transport,
  industrial vehicle occupant
|race car *see* Accident, transport, motor
  vehicle NEC occupant
|railway vehicle occupant V81.9
 |collision (with) V81.3
  |motor vehicle (non-military) (traffic)
   V81.1
   |military V81.83
   |nontraffic V81.0
  |rolling stock V81.2
  |specified object NEC V81.3
 |during derailment V81.7
 |with antecedent collision *see*
   Accident, transport, railway vehicle
   occupant, collision
 |explosion V81.81
 |fall (in railway vehicle) V81.5
  |during derailment V81.7
   |with antecedent collision *see*
     Accident, transport, railway
     vehicle occupant, collision
  |from railway vehicle V81.6
   |during derailment V81.7

 |with antecedent collision *see*
   Accident, transport, railway
   vehicle occupant, collision
 |while boarding or alighting V81.4
 |fire V81.81
 |object falling onto train V81.82
 |specified type NEC V81.89
 |while boarding or alighting V81.4
|ski lift V98.3
|snowmobile occupant (nontraffic) V86.92
 |driver V86.52
 |hanger-on V86.72
 |passenger V86.62
 |traffic V86.32
  |driver V86.02
  |hanger-on V86.22
  |passenger V86.12
 |while boarding or alighting V86.42
|specified NEC V98.8
|sport utility vehicle occupant *see also*
  Accident, transport, pickup truck
  occupant
|streetcar occupant V82.9
 |collision (with) V82.3
  |motor vehicle (traffic) V82.1
   |nontraffic V82.0
  |rolling stock V82.2
 |during derailment V82.7
  |with antecedent collision *see*
    Accident, transport, streetcar
    occupant, collision
 |fall (in streetcar) V82.5
  |during derailment V82.7
   |with antecedent collision *see*
     Accident, transport, streetcar
     occupant, collision
  |from streetcar V82.6
   |during derailment V82.7
    |with antecedent collision *see*
      Accident, transport, streetcar
      occupant, collision
   |while boarding or alighting V82.4
  |while boarding or alighting V82.4
 |specified type NEC V82.8
 |while boarding or alighting V82.4
|three-wheeled motor vehicle occupant
  V39.9
 |collision (with)
  |animal (traffic) V30.9
   |being ridden (traffic) V36.9
    |nontraffic V36.3
    |while boarding or alighting V36.4
   |nontraffic V30.3
   |while boarding or alighting V30.4
  |animal-drawn vehicle (traffic) V36.9
   |nontraffic V36.3
   |while boarding or alighting V36.4
  |bus (traffic) V34.9
   |nontraffic V34.3
   |while boarding or alighting V34.4
  |car (traffic) V33.9
   |nontraffic V33.3
   |while boarding or alighting V33.4
  |motor vehicle NOS (traffic) V39.60
   |nontraffic V39.20
   |specified type NEC (traffic) V39.69
    |nontraffic V39.29
  |pedal cycle (traffic) V31.9
   |nontraffic V31.3
   |while boarding or alighting V31.4
  |pickup truck (traffic) V33.9
   |nontraffic V33.3
   |while boarding or alighting V33.4

Accident - *continued*
　|railway vehicle (traffic) V35.9
　　|nontraffic V35.3
　　|while boarding or alighting V35.4
　|specified vehicle NEC (traffic) V36.9
　　|nontraffic V36.3
　　|while boarding or alighting V36.4
　|stationary object (traffic) V37.9
　　|nontraffic V37.3
　　|while boarding or alighting V37.4
　|streetcar (traffic) V36.9
　　|nontraffic V36.3
　　|while boarding or alighting V36.4
　|three wheeled motor vehicle (traffic)
　　　V32.9
　　|nontraffic V32.3
　　|while boarding or alighting V32.4
　|truck (traffic) V34.9
　　|nontraffic V34.3
　　|while boarding or alighting V34.4
　|two wheeled motor vehicle (traffic)
　　　V32.9
　　|nontraffic V32.3
　　|while boarding or alighting V32.4
　|van (traffic) V33.9
　　|nontraffic V33.3
　　|while boarding or alighting V33.4
　|driver
　　|collision (with)
　　　|animal (traffic) V30.5
　　　　|being ridden (traffic) V36.5
　　　　　|nontraffic V36.0
　　　　|nontraffic V30.0
　　　|animal-drawn vehicle (traffic) V36.5
　　　　|nontraffic V36.0
　　　|bus (traffic) V34.5
　　　　|nontraffic V34.0
　　　|car (traffic) V33.5
　　　　|nontraffic V33.0
　　　|motor vehicle NOS (traffic) V39.40
　　　　|nontraffic V39.00
　　　　|specified type NEC (traffic)
　　　　　　V39.49
　　　　　|nontraffic V39.09
　　　|pedal cycle (traffic) V31.5
　　　　|nontraffic V31.0
　　　|pickup truck (traffic) V33.5
　　　　|nontraffic V33.0
　　　|railway vehicle (traffic) V35.5
　　　　|nontraffic V35.0
　　　|specified vehicle NEC (traffic)
　　　　　V36.5
　　　　|nontraffic V36.0
　　　|stationary object (traffic) V37.5
　　　　|nontraffic V37.0
　　　|streetcar (traffic) V36.5
　　　　|nontraffic V36.0
　　　|three wheeled motor vehicle (traffic)
　　　　　V32.5
　　　　|nontraffic V32.0
　　　|truck (traffic) V34.5
　　　　|nontraffic V34.0
　　　|two wheeled motor vehicle (traffic)
　　　　　V32.5
　　　　|nontraffic V32.0
　　　|van (traffic) V33.5
　　　　|nontraffic V33.0
　　|noncollision accident (traffic) V38.5
　　　|nontraffic V38.0
　|noncollision accident (traffic) V38.9
　　|nontraffic V38.3
　　|while boarding or alighting V38.4
　|nontraffic V39.3
　|hanger-on

Accident - *continued*
　|collision (with)
　　|animal (traffic) V30.7
　　　|being ridden (traffic) V36.7
　　　　|nontraffic V36.2
　　　|nontraffic V30.2
　　|animal-drawn vehicle (traffic) V36.7
　　　|nontraffic V36.2
　　|bus (traffic) V34.7
　　　|nontraffic V34.2
　　|car (traffic) V33.7
　　　|nontraffic V33.2
　　|pedal cycle (traffic) V31.7
　　　|nontraffic V31.2
　　|pickup truck (traffic) V33.7
　　　|nontraffic V33.2
　　|railway vehicle (traffic) V35.7
　　　|nontraffic V35.2
　　|specified vehicle NEC (traffic)
　　　　V36.7
　　　|nontraffic V36.2
　　|stationary object (traffic) V37.7
　　　|nontraffic V37.2
　　|streetcar (traffic) V36.7
　　　|nontraffic V36.2
　　|three wheeled motor vehicle (traffic)
　　　　V32.7
　　　|nontraffic V32.2
　　|truck (traffic) V34.7
　　　|nontraffic V34.2
　　|two wheeled motor vehicle (traffic)
　　　　V32.7
　　　|nontraffic V32.2
　　|van (traffic) V33.7
　　　|nontraffic V33.2
　|noncollision accident (traffic) V38.7
　　|nontraffic V38.2
　|passenger
　　|collision (with)
　　　|animal (traffic) V30.6
　　　　|being ridden (traffic) V36.6
　　　　　|nontraffic V36.1
　　　　|nontraffic V30.1
　　　|animal-drawn vehicle (traffic) V36.6
　　　　|nontraffic V36.1
　　　|bus (traffic) V34.6
　　　　|nontraffic V34.1
　　　|car (traffic) V33.6
　　　　|nontraffic V33.1
　　　|motor vehicle NOS (traffic) V39.50
　　　　|nontraffic V39.10
　　　　|specified type NEC (traffic)
　　　　　　V39.59
　　　　　|nontraffic V39.19
　　　|pedal cycle (traffic) V31.6
　　　　|nontraffic V31.1
　　　|pickup truck (traffic) V33.6
　　　　|nontraffic V33.1
　　　|railway vehicle (traffic) V35.6
　　　　|nontraffic V35.1
　　　|specified vehicle NEC (traffic) V36.6
　　　　|nontraffic V36.1
　　　|stationary object (traffic) V37.6
　　　　|nontraffic V37.1
　　　|streetcar (traffic) V36.6
　　　　|nontraffic V36.1
　　　|three wheeled motor vehicle
　　　　　(traffic) V32.6
　　　　|nontraffic V32.1
　　　|truck (traffic) V34.6
　　　　|nontraffic V34.1
　　　|two wheeled motor vehicle (traffic)
　　　　　V32.6
　　　　|nontraffic V32.1

Accident - *continued*
　　|van (traffic) V33.6
　　　|nontraffic V33.1
　|noncollision accident (traffic) V38.6
　　|nontraffic V38.1
　|specified type NEC V39.89
　　|military vehicle V39.81
　|tractor (farm) (and trailer) *see* Accident,
　　　transport, agricultural vehicle occupant
　|tram *see* Accident, transport, streetcar
　　|in mine or quarry *see* Accident,
　　　transport, industrial vehicle occupant
　|trolley *see* Accident, transport, streetcar
　　|in mine or quarry *see* Accident,
　　　transport, industrial vehicle occupant
　|truck (heavy) occupant V69.9
　　|collision (with)
　　　|animal (traffic) V60.9
　　　　|being ridden (traffic) V66.9
　　　　　|nontraffic V66.3
　　　　　|while boarding or alighting V66.4
　　　　|nontraffic V60.3
　　　　|while boarding or alighting V60.4
　　　|animal-drawn vehicle (traffic) V66.9
　　　　|nontraffic V66.3
　　　　|while boarding or alighting V66.4
　　　|bus (traffic) V64.9
　　　　|nontraffic V64.3
　　　　|while boarding or alighting V64.4
　　　|car (traffic) V63.9
　　　　|nontraffic V63.3
　　　　|while boarding or alighting V63.4
　　　|motor vehicle NOS (traffic) V69.60
　　　　|nontraffic V69.20
　　　　|specified type NEC (traffic) V69.69
　　　　　|nontraffic V69.29
　　　|pedal cycle (traffic) V61.9
　　　　|nontraffic V61.3
　　　　|while boarding or alighting V61.4
　　　|pickup truck (traffic) V63.9
　　　　|nontraffic V63.3
　　　　|while boarding or alighting V63.4
　　　|railway vehicle (traffic) V65.9
　　　　|nontraffic V65.3
　　　　|while boarding or alighting V65.4
　　　|specified vehicle NEC (traffic) V66.9
　　　　|nontraffic V66.3
　　　　|while boarding or alighting V66.4
　　　|stationary object (traffic) V67.9
　　　　|nontraffic V67.3
　　　　|while boarding or alighting V67.4
　　　|streetcar (traffic) V66.9
　　　　|nontraffic V66.3
　　　　|while boarding or alighting V66.4
　　　|three wheeled motor vehicle (traffic)
　　　　　V62.9
　　　　|nontraffic V62.3
　　　　|while boarding or alighting V62.4
　　　|truck (traffic) V64.9
　　　　|nontraffic V64.3
　　　　|while boarding or alighting V64.4
　　　|two wheeled motor vehicle (traffic)
　　　　　V62.9
　　　　|nontraffic V62.3
　　　　|while boarding or alighting V62.4
　　　|van (traffic) V63.9
　　　　|nontraffic V63.3
　　　　|while boarding or alighting V63.4
　　|driver
　　　|collision (with)
　　　　|animal (traffic) V60.5
　　　　　|being ridden (traffic) V66.5
　　　　　　|nontraffic V66.0
　　　　　|nontraffic V60.0

Accident - *continued*
  |nontraffic V58.0
 |noncollision accident (traffic) V58.9
  |nontraffic V58.3
  |while boarding or alighting V58.4
 |nontraffic V59.3
 |hanger-on
  |collision (with)
   |animal (traffic) V50.7
    |being ridden (traffic) V56.7
     |nontraffic V56.2
    |nontraffic V50.2
   |animal-drawn vehicle (traffic) V56.7
    |nontraffic V56.2
   |bus (traffic) V54.7
    |nontraffic V54.2
   |car (traffic) V53.7
    |nontraffic V53.2
   |pedal cycle (traffic) V51.7
    |nontraffic V51.2
   |pickup truck (traffic) V53.7
    |nontraffic V53.2
   |railway vehicle (traffic) V55.7
    |nontraffic V55.2
   |specified vehicle NEC (traffic)
    V56.7
    |nontraffic V56.2
   |stationary object (traffic) V57.7
    |nontraffic V57.2
   |streetcar (traffic) V56.7
    |nontraffic V56.2
   |three wheeled motor vehicle (traffic)
    V52.7
    |nontraffic V52.2
   |truck (traffic) V54.7
    |nontraffic V54.2
   |two wheeled motor vehicle (traffic)
    V52.7
    |nontraffic V52.2
   |van (traffic) V53.7
    |nontraffic V53.2
  |noncollision accident (traffic) V58.7
   |nontraffic V58.2
 |passenger
  |collision (with)
   |animal (traffic) V50.6
    |being ridden (traffic) V56.6
     |nontraffic V56.1
    |nontraffic V50.1
   |animal-drawn vehicle (traffic) V56.6
    |nontraffic V56.1
   |bus (traffic) V54.6
    |nontraffic V54.1
   |car (traffic) V53.6
    |nontraffic V53.1
   |motor vehicle NOS (traffic) V59.50
    |nontraffic V59.10
    |specified type NEC (traffic)
     V59.59
     |nontraffic V59.19
   |pedal cycle (traffic) V51.6
    |nontraffic V51.1
   |pickup truck (traffic) V53.6
    |nontraffic V53.1
   |railway vehicle (traffic) V55.6
    |nontraffic V55.1
   |specified vehicle NEC (traffic)
    V56.6
    |nontraffic V56.1
   |stationary object (traffic) V57.6
    |nontraffic V57.1
   |streetcar (traffic) V56.6
    |nontraffic V56.1
   |three wheeled motor vehicle (traffic)
    V52.6

Accident - *continued*
   |nontraffic V52.1
   |truck (traffic) V54.6
    |nontraffic V54.1
   |two wheeled motor vehicle (traffic)
    V52.6
    |nontraffic V52.1
   |van (traffic) V53.6
    |nontraffic V53.1
  |noncollision accident (traffic) V58.6
   |nontraffic V58.1
 |specified type NEC V59.88
  |military vehicle V59.81
 |watercraft occupant *see* Accident,
  watercraft
|vehicle NEC V89.9
 |animal-drawn NEC *see* Accident,
  transport, animal-drawn vehicle
  occupant
 |special
  |agricultural *see* Accident, transport,
   agricultural vehicle occupant
  |construction *see* Accident, transport,
   construction vehicle occupant
  |industrial *see* Accident, transport,
   industrial vehicle occupant
  |three-wheeled NEC (motorized) *see*
   Accident, transport, three-wheeled
   motor vehicle occupant
|watercraft V94.9
 |causing
  |drowning *see* Drowning, due to,
   accident to, watercraft
  |injury NEC V91.89
   |crushed between craft and object
    V91.19
   |powered craft V91.13
    |ferry boat V91.11
    |fishing boat V91.12
    |jet skis V91.13
    |liner V91.11
    |merchant ship V91.10
    |passenger ship V91.11
   |unpowered craft V91.18
    |canoe V91.15
    |inflatable V91.16
    |kayak V91.15
    |sailboat V91.14
    |surf-board V91.18
    |windsurfer V91.18
  |fall on board V91.29
   |powered craft V91.23
    |ferry boat V91.21
    |fishing boat V91.22
    |jet skis V91.23
    |liner V91.21
    |merchant ship V91.20
    |passenger ship V91.21
   |unpowered craft
    |canoe V91.25
    |inflatable V91.26
    |kayak V91.25
    |sailboat V91.24
  |fire on board causing burn V91.09
   |powered craft V91.03
    |ferry boat V91.01
    |fishing boat V91.02
    |jet skis V91.03
    |liner V91.01
    |merchant ship V91.00
    |passenger ship V91.01
   |unpowered craft V91.08
    |canoe V91.05
    |inflatable V91.06

Accident - *continued*
    |kayak V91.05
    |sailboat V91.04
    |surf-board V91.08
    |water skis V91.07
    |windsurfer V91.08
  |hit by falling object V91.39
   |powered craft V91.33
    |ferry boat V91.31
    |fishing boat V91.32
    |jet skis V91.33
    |liner V91.31
    |merchant ship V91.30
    |passenger ship V91.31
   |unpowered craft V91.38
    |canoe V91.35
    |inflatable V91.36
    |kayak V91.35
    |sailboat V91.34
    |surf-board V91.38
    |water skis V91.37
    |windsurfer V91.38
  |specified type NEC V91.89
   |powered craft V91.83
    |ferry boat V91.81
    |fishing boat V91.82
    |jet skis V91.83
    |liner V91.81
    |merchant ship V91.80
    |passenger ship V91.81
   |unpowered craft V91.88
    |canoe V91.85
    |inflatable V91.86
    |kayak V91.85
    |sailboat V91.84
    |surf-board V91.88
    |water skis V91.87
    |windsurfer V91.88
 |due to, caused by cataclysm *see* Forces of
  nature, by type
 |military NEC V94.818
  |with civilian watercraft V94.810
  |civilian in water injured by V94.811
 |nonpowered, struck by
  |nonpowered vessel V94.22
  |powered vessel V94.21
 |specified type NEC V94.89
 |striking swimmer
  |powered V94.11
  |unpowered V94.12
Acid throwing (assault) Y08.89
Activity (involving) (of victim at time of
 event) Y93.9
 |aerobic and step exercise (class) Y93.A3
 |alpine skiing Y93.23
 |animal care NEC Y93.K9
 |arts and handcrafts NEC Y93.D9
 |athletics NEC Y93.79
 |athletics played as a team or group NEC
  Y93.69
 |athletics played individually NEC Y93.59
 |baking Y93.G3
 |ballet Y93.41
 |barbells Y93.B3
 |BASE (Building, Antenna, Span, Earth)
  jumping Y93.33
 |baseball Y93.64
 |basketball Y93.67
 |bathing (personal) Y93.E1
 |beach volleyball Y93.68
 |bike riding Y93.55
 |blackout game Y93.85
 |boogie boarding Y93.18
 |bowling Y93.54

|boxing Y93.71
|brass instrument playing Y93.J4
|building construction Y93.H3
|bungee jumping Y93.34
|calisthenics Y93.A2
|canoeing (in calm and turbulent water) Y93.16
|capture the flag Y93.6A
|cardiorespiratory exercise NEC Y93.A9
|caregiving (providing) NEC Y93.F9
  |bathing Y93.F1
  |lifting Y93.F2
|cellular
  |communication device Y93.C2
  |telephone Y93.C2
|challenge course Y93.A5
|cheerleading Y93.45
|choking game Y93.85
|circuit training Y93.A4
|cleaning
  |floor Y93.E5
|climbing NEC Y93.39
  |mountain Y93.31
  |rock Y93.31
  |wall Y93.31
|clothing care and maintenance NEC Y93.E9
|combatives Y93.75
|computer
  |keyboarding Y93.C1
  |technology NEC Y93.C9
|confidence course Y93.A5
|construction (building) Y93.H3
|cooking and baking Y93.G3
|cool down exercises Y93.A2
|cricket Y93.69
|crocheting Y93.D1
|cross country skiing Y93.24
|dancing (all types) Y93.41
|digging
  |dirt Y93.H1
|dirt digging Y93.H1
|dishwashing Y93.G1
|diving (platform) (springboard) Y93.12
  |underwater Y93.15
|dodge ball Y93.6A
|downhill skiing Y93.23
|drum playing Y93.J2
|dumbbells Y93.B3
|electronic
  |devices NEC Y93.C9
    |hand held interactive Y93.C2
  |game playing (using) (with)
    |interactive device Y93.C2
    |keyboard or other stationary device Y93.C1
|elliptical machine Y93.A1
|exercise(s)
  |machines ((primarily) for)
    |cardiorespiratory conditioning Y93.A1
    |muscle strengthening Y93.B1
  |muscle strengthening (non-machine) NEC Y93.B9
|external motion NEC Y93.I9
  |rollercoaster Y93.I1
|fainting game Y93.85
|field hockey Y93.65
|figure skating (pairs) (singles) Y93.21
|flag football Y93.62
|floor mopping and cleaning Y93.E5
|food preparation and clean up Y93.G1
|football (American) NOS Y93.61
  |flag Y93.62
  |tackle Y93.61

|touch Y93.62
|four square Y93.6A
|free weights Y93.B3
|frisbee (ultimate) Y93.74
|furniture
  |building Y93.D3
  |finishing Y93.D3
  |repair Y93.D3
|game playing (electronic)
  |using keyboard or other stationary device Y93.C1
  |using interactive device Y93.C2
|gardening Y93.H2
|golf Y93.53
|grass drills Y93.A6
|grilling and smoking food Y93.G2
|grooming and shearing an animal Y93.K3
|guerilla drills Y93.A6
|gymnastics (rhythmic) Y93.43
|handball Y93.73
|handcrafts NEC Y93.D9
|hand held interactive electronic device Y93.C2
|hang gliding Y93.35
|hiking (on level or elevated terrain) Y93.01
|hockey (ice) Y93.22
  |field Y93.65
|horseback riding Y93.52
|household (interior) maintenance NEC Y93.E9
|ice NEC Y93.29
  |dancing Y93.21
  |hockey Y93.22
  |skating Y93.21
|inline roller skating Y93.51
|ironing Y93.E4
|judo Y93.75
|jumping (off) NEC Y93.39
  |BASE (Building, Antenna, Span, Earth) Y93.33
  |bungee Y93.34
  |jacks Y93.A2
  |rope Y93.56
|jumping jacks Y93.A2
|jumping rope Y93.56
|karate Y93.75
|kayaking (in calm and turbulent water) Y93.16
|keyboarding (computer) Y93.C1
|kickball Y93.6A
|knitting Y93.D1
|lacrosse Y93.65
|land maintenance NEC Y93.H9
|landscaping Y93.H2
|laundry Y93.E2
|machines (exercise)
  |primarily for cardiorespiratory conditioning Y93.A1
  |primarily for muscle strengthening Y93.B1
|maintenance
  |exterior building NEC Y93.H9
  |household (interior) NEC Y93.E9
  |land Y93.H9
  |property Y93.H9
|marching (on level or elevated terrain) Y93.01
|martial arts Y93.75
|microwave oven Y93.G3
|milking an animal Y93.K2
|mopping (floor) Y93.E5
|mountain climbing Y93.31
|muscle strengthening

  |exercises (non-machine) NEC Y93.B9
  |machines Y93.B1
|musical keyboard (electronic) playing Y93.J1
|Nordic skiing Y93.24
|obstacle course Y93.A5
|oven (microwave) Y93.G3
|packing up and unpacking in moving to a new residence Y93.E6
|parasailing Y93.19
|pass out game Y93.85
|percussion instrument playing NEC Y93.J2
|personal
  |bathing and showering Y93.E1
  |hygiene NEC Y93.E8
  |showering Y93.E1
|physical games generally associated with school recess, summer camp and children Y93.6A
|physical training NEC Y93.A9
|piano playing Y93.J1
|pilates Y93.B4
|platform diving Y93.12
|playing musical instrument
  |brass instrument Y93.J4
  |drum Y93.J2
  |musical keyboard (electronic) Y93.J1
  |percussion instrument NEC Y93.J2
  |piano Y93.J1
  |string instrument Y93.J3
  |winds instrument Y93.J4
|property maintenance
  |exterior NEC Y93.H9
  |interior NEC Y93.E9
|pruning (garden and lawn) Y93.H2
|pull-ups Y93.B2
|push-ups Y93.B2
|racquetball Y93.73
|rafting (in calm and turbulent water) Y93.16
|raking (leaves) Y93.H1
|rappelling Y93.32
|refereeing a sports activity Y93.81
|residential relocation Y93.E6
|rhythmic gymnastics Y93.43
|rhythmic movement NEC Y93.49
|riding
  |horseback Y93.52
  |rollercoaster Y93.I1
|rock climbing Y93.31
|rollercoaster riding Y93.I1
|roller skating (inline) Y93.51
|rough housing and horseplay Y93.83
|rowing (in calm and turbulent water) Y93.16
|rugby Y93.63
|running Y93.02
|SCUBA diving Y93.15
|sewing Y93.D2
|shoveling Y93.H1
  |dirt Y93.H1
  |snow Y93.H1
|showering (personal) Y93.E1
|sit-ups Y93.B2
|skateboarding Y93.51
|skating (ice) Y93.21
  |roller Y93.51
|skiing (alpine) (downhill) Y93.23
  |cross country Y93.24
  |Nordic Y93.24
  |water Y93.17
|sledding (snow) Y93.23
|sleeping (sleep) Y93.84
|smoking and grilling food Y93.G2

Assault (homicidal) - *continued*
|steam X98.0
Assault (homicidal) - *continued*
|striking against
 |other person Y04.2
 |sports equipment Y08.09
  |baseball bat Y08.02
  |hockey stick Y08.01
|struck by
 |sports equipment Y08.09
  |baseball bat Y08.02
  |hockey stick Y08.01
|submersion *see* Assault, drowning
|violence Y09
|weapon Y09
 |blunt Y00
 |cutting or piercing *see* Assault, cutting or
  piercing instrument
 |firearm *see* Assault, firearm
|wound Y09
 |cutting *see* Assault, cutting or piercing
  instrument
 |gunshot *see* Assault, firearm
 |knife X99.1
Assault (homicidal) - *continued*
|piercing *see* Assault, cutting or piercing
 instrument
|puncture *see* Assault, cutting or piercing
 instrument
|stab *see* Assault, cutting or piercing
 instrument
Attack by mammals NEC W55.89
Avalanche *see* Landslide
Aviator's disease *see* Air, pressure

B

**Barotitis, barodontalgia, barosinusitis,
 barotrauma (otitic) (sinus)** *see* Air,
 pressure
Battered (baby) (child) (person) (syndrome)
 X58
Bayonet wound W26.1
|in
 |legal intervention *see* Legal, intervention,
  sharp object, bayonet
 |war operations *see* War operations,
  combat
|stated as undetermined whether accidental
 or intentional Y28.8
|suicide (attempt) X78.2
Bean in nose *see* categories T17 and T18
Bed set on fire NEC *see* Exposure, fire,
 uncontrolled, building, bed
Beheading (by guillotine)
|homicide X99.9
|legal execution *see* Legal, intervention
Bending, injury in (prolonged) (static)
 X50.1
Bends *see* Air, pressure, change
Bite, bitten by
|alligator W58.01
|arthropod (nonvenomous) NEC W57
|bull W55.21
|cat W55.01
|cow W55.21
|crocodile W58.11
|dog W54.0
|goat W55.31
|hoof stock NEC W55.31
|horse W55.11
|human being (accidentally) W50.3
 |with intent to injure or kill Y04.1

Bite, bitten by - *continued*
 |as, or caused by, a crowd or human
  stampede (with fall) W52
 |assault Y04.1
 |homicide (attempt) Y04.1
 |in
  |fight Y04.1
|insect (nonvenomous) W57
|lizard (nonvenomous) W59.01
|mammal NEC W55.81
 |marine W56.31
|marine animal (nonvenomous) W56.81
|millipede W57
|moray eel W56.51
|mouse W53.01
|person(s) (accidentally) W50.3
 |with intent to injure or kill Y04.1
 |as, or caused by, a crowd or human
  stampede (with fall) W52
 |assault Y04.1
 |homicide (attempt) Y04.1
 |in
  |fight Y04.1
|pig W55.41
|raccoon W55.51
|rat W53.11
|reptile W59.81
 |lizard W59.01
 |snake W59.11
 |turtle W59.21
  |terrestrial W59.81
|rodent W53.81
 |mouse W53.01
 |rat W53.11
 |specified NEC W53.81
 |squirrel W53.21
|shark W56.41
|sheep W55.31
|snake (nonvenomous) W59.11
|spider (nonvenomous) W57
|squirrel W53.21
Blast (air) in war operations *see* War
 operations, blast
Blizzard X37.2
Blood alcohol level Y90.9
|less than 20mg/100ml Y90.0
|presence in blood, level not specified Y90.9
|20-39mg/100ml Y90.1
|40-59mg/100ml Y90.2
|60-79mg/100ml Y90.3
|80-99mg/100ml Y90.4
|100-119mg/100ml Y90.5
|120-199mg/100ml Y90.6
|200-239mg/100ml Y90.7
Blow X58
|by law-enforcing agent, police (on duty)
 see Legal, intervention, manhandling
 |blunt object *see* Legal, intervention, blunt
  object
Blowing up *see* Explosion
Brawl (hand) (fists) (foot) Y04.0
Breakage (accidental) (part of) ladder
 (causing fall) W11
|scaffolding (causing fall) W12
Broken
|glass, contact with *see* Contact, with, glass
|power line (causing electric shock) W85
Bumping against, into (accidentally)
|object NEC W22.8
 |with fall *see* Fall, due to, bumping
  against, object
 |caused by crowd or human stampede (with
  fall) W52
 |sports equipment W21.9

Bumping - *continued*
|person(s) W51
 |with fall W03
  |due to ice or snow W00.0
 |assault Y04.2
 |caused by, a crowd or human stampede
  (with fall) W52
 |homicide (attempt) Y04.2
|sports equipment W21.9
Burn, burned, burning (accidental) (by)
 (from) (on)
|acid NEC *see* Table of Drugs and
 Chemicals
|bed linen *see* Exposure, fire, uncontrolled,
 in building, bed
|blowtorch X08.8
 |with ignition of clothing NEC X06.2
  |nightwear X05
|bonfire, campfire (controlled) *see also*
 Exposure, fire, controlled, not in building
 |uncontrolled *see* Exposure, fire,
  uncontrolled, not in building
|candle X08.8
 |with ignition of clothing NEC X06.2
  |nightwear X05
|caustic liquid, substance (external) (internal)
 NEC *see* Table of Drugs and Chemicals
|chemical (external) (internal) *see also*
 Table of Drugs and Chemicals
 |in war operations *see* War operations. fire
|cigar(s) or cigarette(s) X08.8
 |with ignition of clothing NEC X06.2
  |nightwear X05
|clothes, clothing NEC (from controlled fire)
 X06.2
 |with conflagration *see* Exposure, fire,
  uncontrolled, building
 |not in building or structure *see*
  Exposure, fire, uncontrolled, not in
  building
|cooker (hot) X15.8
 |stated as undetermined whether accidental
  or intentional Y27.3
 |suicide (attempt) X77.3
|electric blanket X16
|engine (hot) X17
|fire, flames *see* Exposure, fire
|flare, Very pistol *see* Discharge, firearm
 NEC
|heat
 |from appliance (electrical) (household)
  X15.8
 |cooker X15.8
 |hotplate X15.2
 |kettle X15.8
 |light bulb X15.8
 |saucepan X15.3
 |skillet X15.3
 |stove X15.0
 |stated as undetermined whether
  accidental or intentional Y27.3
 |suicide (attempt) X77.3
 |toaster X15.1
|in local application or packing during
 medical or surgical procedure Y63.5
|heating
 |appliance, radiator or pipe X16
|homicide (attempt) *see* Assault, burning
|hot
 |air X14.1
 |cooker X15.8
 |drink X10.0
 |engine X17
 |fat X10.2

Burn, burned, burning - *continued*
|fluid NEC X12
|food X10.1
|gases X14.1
|heating appliance X16
|household appliance NEC X15.8
|kettle X15.8
|liquid NEC X12
|machinery X17
|metal (molten) (liquid) NEC X18
|object (not producing fire or flames) NEC
   X19
|oil (cooking) X10.2
|pipe(s) X16
|radiator X16
|saucepan (glass) (metal) X15.3
|stove (kitchen) X15.0
|substance NEC X19
   |caustic or corrosive NEC *see* Table of
  Drugs and Chemicals
|toaster X15.1
|tool X17
|vapor X13.1
|water (tap) *see* Contact, with, hot, tap
   water
|hotplate X15.2
  |suicide (attempt) X77.3
|ignition *see* Ignition
|in war operations *see* War operations, fire
|inflicted by other person X97
  |by hot objects, hot vapor, and steam *see*
     Assault, burning, hot object
|internal, from swallowed caustic, corrosive
   liquid, substance *see* Table of Drugs and
   Chemicals
|iron (hot) X15.8
  |stated as undetermined whether accidental
     or intentional Y27.3
  |suicide (attempt) X77.3
|kettle (hot) X15.8
  |stated as undetermined whether accidental
     or intentional Y27.3
  |suicide (attempt) X77.3
|lamp (flame) X08.8
  |with ignition of clothing NEC X06.2
  |nightwear X05
|lighter (cigar) (cigarette) X08.8
  |with ignition of clothing NEC X06.2
  |nightwear X05
|lightning *see* subcategory T75.0
  |causing fire *see* Exposure, fire
|liquid (boiling) (hot) NEC X12
  |stated as undetermined whether accidental
     or intentional Y27.2
  |suicide (attempt) X77.2
|local application of externally applied
   substance in medical or surgical care
   Y63.5
|on board watercraft
  |due to
  |accident to watercraft V91.09
    |powered craft V91.03
     |ferry boat V91.01
     |fishing boat V91.02
     |jet skis V91.03
     |liner V91.01
     |merchant ship V91.00
     |passenger ship V91.01
    |unpowered craft V91.08
     |canoe V91.05
     |inflatable V91.06
     |kayak V91.05
     |sailboat V91.04
     |surf-board V91.08

Burn, burned, burning - *continued*
    |water skis V91.07
    |windsurfer V91.08
  |fire on board V93.09
   |ferry boat V93.01
   |fishing boat V93.02
   |jet skis V93.03
   |liner V93.01
   |merchant ship V93.00
   |passenger ship V93.01
   |powered craft NEC V93.03
   |sailboat V93.04
    |specified heat source NEC on board
     V93.19
   |ferry boat V93.11
   |fishing boat V93.12
   |jet skis V93.13
   |liner V93.11
   |merchant ship V93.10
   |passenger ship V93.11
   |powered craft NEC V93.13
   |sailboat V93.14
|machinery (hot) X17
|matches X08.8
  |with ignition of clothing NEC X06.2
  |nightwear X05
|mattress *see* Exposure, fire, uncontrolled,
  building, bed
|medicament, externally applied Y63.5
|metal (hot) (liquid) (molten) NEC X18
|nightwear (nightclothes, nightdress, gown,
  pajamas, robe) X05
|object (hot) NEC X19
|pipe (hot) X16
  |smoking X08.8
   |with ignition of clothing NEC X06.2
   |nightwear X05
|powder *see* Powder burn
|radiator (hot) X16
|saucepan (hot) (glass) (metal) X15.3
  |stated as undetermined whether accidental
     or intentional Y27.3
  |suicide (attempt) X77.3
|self-inflicted X76
  |stated as undetermined whether accidental
     or intentional Y26
|steam X13.1
  |pipe X16
  |stated as undetermined whether
     accidental or intentional Y27.8
  |stated as undetermined whether accidental
     or intentional Y27.0
  |suicide (attempt) X77.0
|stove (hot) (kitchen) X15.0
  |stated as undetermined whether accidental
     or intentional Y27.3
  |suicide (attempt) X77.3
|substance (hot) NEC X19
  |boiling X12
  |stated as undetermined whether
     accidental or intentional Y27.2
  |suicide (attempt) X77.2
  |molten (metal) X18
|suicide (attempt) NEC X76
  |hot
  |household appliance X77.3
  |object X77.9
|stated as undetermined whether accidental
   or intentional Y27.0
|therapeutic misadventure
  |heat in local application or packing during
    medical or surgical procedure Y63.5
  |overdose of radiation Y63.2
|toaster (hot) X15.1

Burn, burned, burning - *continued*
  |stated as undetermined whether accidental
     or intentional Y27.3
  |suicide (attempt) X77.3
|tool (hot) X17
|torch, welding X08.8
  |with ignition of clothing NEC X06.2
  |nightwear X05
|trash fire (controlled) *see* Exposure, fire,
   controlled, not in building
  |uncontrolled *see* Exposure, fire,
    uncontrolled, not in building
|vapor (hot) X13.1
  |stated as undetermined whether accidental
     or intentional Y27.0
  |suicide (attempt) X77.0
|Very pistol *see* Discharge, firearm NEC
Butted by animal W55.82
|bull W55.22
|cow W55.22
|goat W55.32
|horse W55.12
|pig W55.42
|sheep W55.32

C

Caisson disease
| *see* Air, pressure, change
Campfire (exposure to) (controlled) *see*
  also Exposure, fire, controlled, not in
  building
|uncontrolled *see* Exposure, fire,
   uncontrolled, not in building
Capital punishment (any means) *see* Legal,
  intervention
Car sickness T75.3
Casualty (not due to war) NEC X58
|war *see* War operations
Cat
|bite W55.01
|scratch W55.03
Cataclysm, cataclysmic (any injury) NEC
  see Forces of nature
Catching fire *see* Exposure, fire
Caught
|between
Caught - *continued*
|folding object W23.0
|objects (moving) (stationary and moving)
  W23.0
  |and machinery *see* Contact, with, by
    type of machine
  |stationary W23.1
|sliding door and door frame W23.0
|by, in
|machinery (moving parts of) *see* Contact,
   with, by type of machine
|washing-machine wringer W23.0
|under packing crate (due to losing grip)
  W23.1
**Cave-in caused by cataclysmic earth surface
  movement or eruption** *see* Landslide
Change(s) in air pressure
| *see* Air, pressure, change
**Choked, choking (on) (any object except
  food or vomitus)** food (bone) (seed) *see*
  categories T17 and T18
|vomitus T17.81-
Civil insurrection *see* War operations
Cloudburst (any injury) X37.8
**Cold, exposure to (accidental) (excessive)
  (extreme) (natural) (place) NEC** *see*
  Exposure, cold

Collapse
|building W20.1
    |burning (uncontrolled fire) X00.2
Collapse - continued0
|dam or man-made structure (causing earth
    movement) X36.0
|machinery see Contact, with, by type of
    machine
|structure W20.1
    |burning (uncontrolled fire) X00.2
Collision (accidental) NEC see also
    Accident, transport V89.9
|pedestrian W51
    |with fall W03
        |due to ice or snow W00.0
    |involving pedestrian conveyance see
        Accident, transport, pedestrian,
        conveyance
    |and
        |crowd or human stampede (with fall)
            W52
        |object W22.8
            |with fall see Fall, due to, bumping
                against, object
|person(s) see Collision, pedestrian
|transport vehicle NEC V89.9
    |and
        |avalanche, fallen or not moving see
            Accident, transport
        |falling or moving see Landslide
        |landslide, fallen or not moving see
            Accident, transport
        |falling or moving see Landslide
    |due to cataclysm see Forces of nature, by
        type
    |intentional, purposeful suicide (attempt)
        see Suicide, collision
Combustion, spontaneous see Ignition
**Complication (delayed) of or following
    (medical or surgical procedure)** Y84.9
|with misadventure see Misadventure
|amputation of limb(s) Y83.5
|anastomosis (arteriovenous) (blood vessel)
    |(gastrojejunal) (tendon) (natural or
    |artificial material) Y83.2
|aspiration (of fluid) Y84.4
    |tissue Y84.8
|biopsy Y84.8
|blood
    |sampling Y84.7
    |transfusion
        |procedure Y84.8
|bypass Y83.2
|catheterization (urinary) Y84.6
    |cardiac Y84.0
|colostomy Y83.3
|cystostomy Y83.3
|dialysis (kidney) Y84.1
|drug see Table of Drugs and Chemicals
|due to misadventure see Misadventure
|duodenostomy Y83.3
|electroshock therapy Y84.3
|external stoma, creation of Y83.3
|formation of external stoma Y83.3
|gastrostomy Y83.3
|graft Y83.2
|hypothermia (medically-induced) Y84.8
|implant, implantation (of)
    |artificial
        |internal device (cardiac pacemaker)
            (electrodes in brain) (heart valve
            prosthesis) (orthopedic) Y83.1
        |material or tissue (for anastomosis or
            bypass) Y83.2

Complication - *continued*
    |with creation of external stoma Y83.3
    |natural tissues (for anastomosis or bypass)
        Y83.2
        |with creation of external stoma Y83.3
|infusion
    |procedure Y84.8
|injection see Table of Drugs and Chemicals
    |procedure Y84.8
|insertion of gastric or duodenal sound Y84.5
|insulin-shock therapy Y84.3
|paracentesis (abdominal) (thoracic)
    (aspirative) Y84.4
|procedures other than surgical operation see
    Complication of or following, by type of
    procedure
|radiological procedure or therapy Y84.2
|removal of organ (partial) (total) NEC
    Y83.6
|sampling
    |blood Y84.7
    |fluid NEC Y84.4
    |tissue Y84.8
|shock therapy Y84.3
|surgical operation NEC see also
    Complication of or following, by type of
    operation Y83.9
    |reconstructive NEC Y83.4
        |with
            |anastomosis, bypass or graft Y83.2
            |formation of external stoma Y83.3
    |specified NEC Y83.8
|transfusion see also Table of Drugs and
    Chemicals
    |procedure Y84.8
|transplant, transplantation (heart) (kidney)
    (liver) (whole organ, any) Y83.0
    |partial organ Y83.4
|ureterostomy Y83.3
|vaccination see also Table of Drugs and
    Chemicals
    |procedure Y84.8
Compression
|divers' squeeze see Air, pressure, change
|trachea by
    |food (lodged in esophagus) see categories
        T17 and T18
    |vomitus (lodged in esophagus) T17.81-
Conflagration see Exposure, fire,
    uncontrolled
Constriction (external)
|hair W49.01
|jewelry W49.04
|ring W49.04
|rubber band W49.03
|specified item NEC W49.09
|string W49.02
|thread W49.02
Contact (accidental) with
|abrasive wheel (metalworking) W31.1
|alligator W58.09
    |bite W58.01
    |crushing W58.03
    |strike W58.02
|amphibian W62.9
    |frog W62.0
    |toad W62.1
|animal (nonvenomous) NEC W64
    |marine W56.89
        |bite W56.81
        |dolphin see Contact, with, dolphin
        |fish NEC see Contact, with, fish
        |mammal see Contact, with, mammal,
            marine

Contact (accidental) - *continued*
    |orca see Contact, with, orca
    |sea lion see Contact, with, sea lion
    |shark see Contact, with, shark
    |strike W56.82
|animate mechanical force NEC W64
|arrow W21.89
    |not thrown, projected or falling W45.8
|arthropods (nonvenomous) W57
|axe W27.0
|band-saw (industrial) W31.2
|bayonet see Bayonet wound
|bee(s) X58
|bench-saw (industrial) W31.2
|bird W61.99
    |bite W61.91
    |chicken see Contact, with, chicken
    |duck see Contact, with, duck
    |goose see Contact, with, goose
    |macaw see Contact, with, macaw
    |parrot see Contact, with, parrot
    |psittacine see Contact, with, psittacine
    |strike W61.92
    |turkey see Contact, with, turkey
|blender W29.0
|boiling water X12
    |stated as undetermined whether
        accidental or intentional Y27.2
    |suicide (attempt) X77.2
|bore, earth-drilling or mining (land)
    (seabed) W31.0
|buffalo see Contact, with, hoof stock
    NEC
|bull W55.29
    |bite W55.21
    |gored W55.22
    |strike W55.22
|bumper cars W31.81
|camel see Contact, with, hoof stock NEC
|can
    |lid W26.8
    |opener W27.4
        |powered W29.0
|cat W55.09
    |bite W55.01
    |scratch W55.03
|caterpillar (venomous) X58
|centipede (venomous) X58
|chain
    |hoist W24.0
        |agricultural operations W30.89
    |saw W29.3
|chicken W61.39
    |peck W61.33
    |strike W61.32
|chisel W27.0
|circular saw W31.2
|cobra X58
|combine (harvester) W30.0
|conveyer belt W24.1
|cooker (hot) X15.8
    |stated as undetermined whether
        accidental or intentional Y27.3
    |suicide (attempt) X77.3
|coral X58
|cotton gin W31.82
|cow W55.29
    |bite W55.21
    |strike W55.22
|crane W24.0
    |agricultural operations W30.89
|crocodile W58.19
    |bite W58.11
    |crushing W58.13

Contact (accidental) - *continued*
　|strike W58.12
　|dagger W26.1
　　|stated as undetermined whether
　　　accidental or intentional Y28.2
　　|suicide (attempt) X78.2
　|dairy equipment W31.82
　|dart W21.89
　　|not thrown, projected or falling W45.8
　|deer *see* Contact, with, hoof stock NEC
　|derrick W24.0
　　|agricultural operations W30.89
　　　|hay W30.2
　|dog W54.8
　　|bite W54.0
　　|strike W54.1
　|dolphin W56.09
　　|bite W56.01
　　|strike W56.02
　|donkey *see* Contact, with, hoof stock
　　　NEC
　|drill (powered) W29.8
　　|earth (land) (seabed) W31.0
　　|nonpowered W27.8
　|drive belt W24.0
　　|agricultural operations W30.89
　|dry ice *see* Exposure, cold, man-made
　|dryer (clothes) (powered) (spin) W29.2
　|duck W61.69
　　|bite W61.61
　　|strike W61.62
　|earth (-)
　　|drilling machine (industrial) W31.0
　　|scraping machine in stationary use
　　　W31.83
　|edge of stiff paper W26.2
　|electric
　　|beater W29.0
　　|blanket X16
　　|fan W29.2
　　　|commercial W31.82
　　|knife W29.1
　　|mixer W29.0
　|elevator (building) W24.0
　　|agricultural operations W30.89
　　　|grain W30.3
　|engine(s), hot NEC X17
　|excavating machine W31.0
　|farm machine W30.9
　|feces *see* Contact, with, by type of animal
　|Fer de lance X58
　|fish W56.59
　　|bite W56.51
　　|shark *see* Contact, with, shark
　　|strike W56.52
　|flying horses W31.81
　|forging (metalworking) machine W31.1
　|fork W27.4
　|forklift (truck) W24.0
　　|agricultural operations W30.89
　|frog W62.0
　|garden
　　|cultivator (powered) W29.3
　　　|riding W30.89
　　|fork W27.1
　|gas turbine W31.3
　|Gila monster X58
　|giraffe *see* Contact, with, hoof stock NEC
　|glass (sharp) (broken) W25
　　|with subsequent fall W18.02
　　|assault X99.0
　　|due to fall *see* Fall, by type

Contact (accidental) - *continued*
　|stated as undetermined whether
　　accidental or intentional Y28.0
　|suicide (attempt) X78.0
　|goat W55.39
　　|bite W55.31
　　|strike W55.32
　|goose W61.59
　　|bite W61.51
　　|strike W61.52
　|hand
　　|saw W27.0
　　|tool (not powered) NEC W27.8
　　　|powered W29.8
　|harvester W30.0
　|hay-derrick W30.2
　|heat NEC X19
　　|from appliance (electrical) (household)
　　　see Contact, with, hot, household
　　　appliance
　　　|heating appliance X16
　|heating
　　|appliance (hot) X16
　　|pad (electric) X16
　|hedge-trimmer (powered) W29.3
　|hoe W27.1
　|hoist (chain) (shaft) NEC W24.0
　　|agricultural W30.89
　|hoof stock NEC W55.39
　　|bite W55.31
　　|strike W55.32
　|hornet(s) X58
　|horse W55.19
　　|bite W55.11
　　|strike W55.12
　|hot
　　|air X14.1
　　　|inhalation X14.0
　　|cooker X15.8
　　|drinks X10.0
　　|engine X17
　　|fats X10.2
　　|fluids NEC X12
　　　|assault X98.2
　　　|suicide (attempt) X77.2
　　　|undetermined whether accidental or
　　　　intentional Y27.2
　　|food X10.1
　　|gases X14.1
　　　|inhalation X14.0
　　|heating appliance X16
　　|household appliance X15.8
　　　|assault X98.3
　　　|cooker X15.8
　　　|hotplate X15.2
　　　|kettle X15.8
　　　|light bulb X15.8
　　　|object NEC X19
　　　　|assault X98.8
　　　　|stated as undetermined whether
　　　　　accidental or intentional Y27.9
　　　　|suicide (attempt) X77.8
　　　|saucepan X15.3
　　　|skillet X15.3
　　　|stove X15.0
　　　|stated as undetermined whether
　　　　accidental or intentional Y27.3
　　　|suicide (attempt) X77.3
　　　|toaster X15.1
　　|kettle X15.8
　　|light bulb X15.8
　　|liquid NEC *see also* Burn X12
　　　|drinks X10.0

Contact (accidental) - *continued*
　|stated as undetermined whether
　　accidental or intentional Y27.2
　|suicide (attempt) X77.2
　|tap water X11.8
　　|stated as undetermined whether
　　　accidental or intentional Y27.1
　　|suicide (attempt) X77.1
　|machinery X17
　|metal (molten) (liquid) NEC X18
　|object (not producing fire or flames)
　　　NEC X19
　|oil (cooking) X10.2
　|pipe X16
　|plate X15.2
　|radiator X16
　|saucepan (glass) (metal) X15.3
　|skillet X15.3
　|stove (kitchen) X15.0
　|substance NEC X19
　|tap-water X11.8
　　|assault X98.1
　　|heated on stove X12
　　　|stated as undetermined whether
　　　　accidental or intentional Y27.2
　　　|suicide (attempt) X77.2
　　|in bathtub X11.0
　　　|running X11.1
　　|stated as undetermined whether
　　　accidental or intentional Y27.1
　　|suicide (attempt) X77.1
　|toaster X15.1
　|tool X17
　|vapors X13.1
　　|inhalation X13.0
　|water (tap) X11.8
　　|boiling X12
　　　|stated as undetermined whether
accidental or intentional Y27.2
　　　　|suicide (attempt) X77.2
　　|heated on stove X12
　　　|stated as undetermined whether
accidental or intentional Y27.2
　　　　|suicide (attempt) X77.2
　　|in bathtub X11.0
　　　|running X11.1
　　|stated as undetermined whether
accidental or intentional Y27.1
　　　|suicide (attempt) X77.1
　|hotplate X15.2
　|ice-pick W27.4
　|insect (nonvenomous) NEC W57
　|kettle (hot) X15.8
　|knife W26.0
　　|assault X99.1
　　|electric W29.1
　　|stated as undetermined whether
accidental or intentional Y28.1
　　　|suicide (attempt) X78.1
　|lathe (metalworking) W31.1
　　|turnings W45.8
　　|woodworking W31.2
　|lawnmower (powered) (ridden) W28
　　|causing electrocution W86.8
　　　|suicide (attempt) X83.1
　　|unpowered W27.1
　|lift, lifting (devices) W24.0
　　|agricultural operations W30.89
　　|shaft W24.0
　|liquefied gas *see* Exposure, cold, man-
made
　|liquid air, hydrogen, nitrogen *see*
　　Exposure, cold, man-made
　|lizard (nonvenomous) W59.09

Contact (accidental) - *continued*
- |bite W59.01
- |strike W59.02
- |llama *see* Contact, with, hoof stock NEC
- |macaw W61.19
  - |bite W61.11
  - |strike W61.12
- |machine, machinery W31.9
  - |abrasive wheel W31.1
  - |agricultural including animal-powered
    W30.9
    - |combine harvester W30.0
    - |grain storage elevator W30.3
    - |hay derrick W30.2
    - |power take-off device W30.1
    - |reaper W30.0
    - |specified NEC W30.89
    - |thresher W30.0
    - |transport vehicle, stationary W30.81
  - |band saw W31.2
  - |bench saw W31.2
  - |circular saw W31.2
  - |commercial NEC W31.82
  - |drilling, metal (industrial) W31.1
  - |earth-drilling W31.0
  - |earthmoving or scraping W31.89
  - |excavating W31.89
  - |forging machine W31.1
  - |gas turbine W31.3
  - |hot X17
  - |internal combustion engine W31.3
  - |land drill W31.0
  - |lathe W31.1
  - |lifting (devices) W24.0
  - |metal drill W31.1
  - |metalworking (industrial) W31.1
  - |milling, metal W31.1
  - |mining W31.0
  - |molding W31.2
  - |overhead plane W31.2
  - |power press, metal W31.1
  - |prime mover W31.3
  - |printing W31.89
  - |radial saw W31.2
  - |recreational W31.81
  - |roller-coaster W31.81
  - |rolling mill, metal W31.1
  - |sander W31.2
  - |seabed drill W31.0
  - |shaft
    - |hoist W31.0
    - |lift W31.0
  - |specified NEC W31.89
  - |spinning W31.89
  - |steam engine W31.3
  - |transmission W24.1
  - |under cutter W31.0
  - |water driven turbine W31.3
  - |weaving W31.89
  - |woodworking or forming (industrial)
    W31.2
- |mammal (feces) (urine) W55.89
  - |bull *see* Contact, with, bull
  - |cat *see* Contact, with, cat
  - |cow *see* Contact, with, cow
  - |goat *see* Contact, with, goat
  - |hoof stock *see* Contact, with, hoof stock
  - |horse *see* Contact, with, horse
  - |marine W56.39
    - |dolphin *see* Contact, with, dolphin
    - |orca *see* Contact, with, orca
    - |sea lion *see* Contact, with, sea lion
    - |specified NEC W56.39
      - |bite W56.31
      - |strike W56.32

Contact (accidental) - *continued*
- |pig *see* Contact, with, pig
- |raccoon *see* Contact, with, raccoon
- |rodent *see* Contact, with, rodent
- |sheep *see* Contact, with, sheep
- |specified NEC W55.89
  - |bite W55.81
  - |strike W55.82
- |marine
  - |animal W56.89
    - |bite W56.81
    - |dolphin *see* Contact, with, dolphin
    - |fish NEC *see* Contact, with, fish
    - |mammal *see* Contact, with, mammal,
  - marine
    - |orca *see* Contact, with, orca
    - |sea lion *see* Contact, with, sea lion
    - |shark *see* Contact, with, shark
    - |strike W56.82
- |meat
  - |grinder (domestic) W29.0
    - |industrial W31.82
    - |nonpowered W27.4
  - |slicer (domestic) W29.0
    - |industrial W31.82
- |merry go round W31.81
- |metal, hot (liquid) (molten) NEC X18
- |millipede W57
- |nail W45.0
  - |gun W29.4
- |needle (sewing) W27.3
  - |hypodermic W46.0
    - |contaminated W46.1
- |object (blunt) NEC
  - |hot NEC X19
  - |legal intervention *see* Legal,
    intervention, blunt object
  - |sharp NEC W45.8
    - |inflicted by other person NEC W45.8
      - |stated as
        - |intentional homicide (attempt) *see*
          Assault, cutting or piercing
          instrument
      - |legal intervention *see* Legal,
        intervention, sharp object
      - |self-inflicted X78.9
- |orca W56.29
  - |bite W56.21
  - |strike W56.22
- |overhead plane W31.2
- |paper (as sharp object) W26.2
- |paper-cutter W27.5
- |parrot W61.09
  - |bite W61.01
  - |strike W61.02
- |pig W55.49
  - |bite W55.41
  - |strike W55.42
- |pipe, hot X16
- |pitchfork W27.1
- |plane (metal) (wood) W27.0
  - |overhead W31.2
- |plant thorns, spines, sharp leaves or other
  mechanisms W60
- |powered
  - |garden cultivator W29.3
  - |household appliance, implement, or
    machine W29.8
  - |saw (industrial) W31.2
    - |hand W29.8
- |printing machine W31.89
- |psittacine bird W61.29
  - |bite W61.21
  - |macaw *see* Contact, with, macaw

Contact (accidental) - *continued*
- |parrot *see* Contact, with, parrot
  - |strike W61.22
- |pulley (block) (transmission) W24.0
  - |agricultural operations W30.89
- |raccoon W55.59
  - |bite W55.51
  - |strike W55.52
- |radial-saw (industrial) W31.2
- |radiator (hot) X16
- |rake W27.1
- |rattlesnake X58
- |reaper W30.0
- |reptile W59.89
  - |lizard *see* Contact, with, lizard
  - |snake *see* Contact, with, snake
  - |specified NEC W59.89
    - |bite W59.81
    - |crushing W59.83
    - |strike W59.82
  - |turtle *see* Contact, with, turtle
- |rivet gun (powered) W29.4
- |road scraper *see* Accident, transport,
  construction vehicle
- |rodent (feces) (urine) W53.89
  - |bite W53.81
  - |mouse W53.09
    - |bite W53.01
  - |rat W53.19
    - |bite W53.11
  - |specified NEC W53.89
    - |bite W53.81
  - |squirrel W53.29
    - |bite W53.21
- |roller coaster W31.81
- |rope NEC W24.0
  - |agricultural operations W30.89
- |saliva *see* Contact, with, by type of
  animal
- |sander W29.8
  - |industrial W31.2
- |saucepan (hot) (glass) (metal) X15.3
- |saw W27.0
  - |band (industrial) W31.2
  - |bench (industrial) W31.2
  - |chain W29.3
  - |hand W27.0
- |sawing machine, metal W31.1
- |scissors W27.2
- |scorpion X58
- |screwdriver W27.0
  - |powered W29.8
- |sea
  - |anemone, cucumber or urchin (spine)
    X58
  - |lion W56.19
    - |bite W56.11
    - |strike W56.12
- |serpent *see* Contact, with, snake, by type
- |sewing-machine (electric) (powered)
  W29.2
  - |not powered W27.8
- |shaft (hoist) (lift) (transmission) NEC
  W24.0
  - |agricultural W30.89
- |shark W56.49
  - |bite W56.41
  - |strike W56.42
- |sharp object(s) W26.9
  - |specified NEC W26.8
- |shears (hand) W27.2
  - |powered (industrial) W31.1
    - |domestic W29.2
- |sheep W55.39

Drowning (accidental) - *continued*

 |passenger ship V90.31
 |fishing boat V90.32
 |jet skis V90.33
 |unpowered V90.38
  |canoe V90.35
  |inflatable V90.36
  |kayak V90.35
  |sailboat V90.34
  |water skis V90.37
 |overturning V90.09
 |powered V90.03
  |merchant ship V90.00
  |passenger ship V90.01
  |fishing boat V90.02
  |jet skis V90.03
 |unpowered V90.08
  |canoe V90.05
  |inflatable V90.06
  |kayak V90.05
  |sailboat V90.04
 |sinking V90.19
 |powered V90.13
  |merchant ship V90.10
  |passenger ship V90.11
  |fishing boat V90.12
  |jet skis V90.13
 |unpowered V90.18
  |canoe V90.15
  |inflatable V90.16
  |kayak V90.15
  |sailboat V90.14
 |specified type NEC V90.89
 |powered V90.83
  |merchant ship V90.80
  |passenger ship V90.81
  |fishing boat V90.82
  |jet skis V90.83
 |unpowered V90.88
  |canoe V90.85
  |inflatable V90.86
  |kayak V90.85
  |sailboat V90.84
  |water skis V90.87
 |avalanche *see* Landslide
 |cataclysmic
 |earth surface movement NEC *see*
  Forces of nature, earth movement
 |storm *see* Forces of nature, cataclysmic
  storm
 |cloudburst X37.8
 |cyclone X37.1
 |fall overboard (from) V92.09
 |powered craft V92.03
 |ferry boat V92.01
 |liner V92.01
 |merchant ship V92.00
 |passenger ship V92.01
 |fishing boat V92.02
 |jet skis V92.03
 |unpowered craft V92.08
 |canoe V92.05
 |inflatable V92.06
 |kayak V92.05
 |sailboat V92.04
 |surf-board V92.08
 |water skis V92.07
 |windsurfer V92.08
 |resulting from
 |accident to watercraft *see* Drowning,
  due to, accident to, watercraft
 |being washed overboard (from)
  V92.29
 |powered craft V92.23

Drowning (accidental) - *continued*

 |ferry boat V92.21
 |liner V92.21
 |merchant ship V92.20
 |passenger ship V92.21
 |fishing boat V92.22
 |jet skis V92.23
 |unpowered craft V92.28
 |canoe V92.25
 |inflatable V92.26
 |kayak V92.25
 |sailboat V92.24
 |surf-board V92.28
 |water skis V92.27
 |windsurfer V92.28
 |motion of watercraft V92.19
 |powered craft V92.13
 |ferry boat V92.11
 |liner V92.11
 |merchant ship V92.10
 |passenger ship V92.11
 |fishing boat V92.12
 |jet skis V92.13
 |unpowered craft
 |canoe V92.15
 |inflatable V92.16
 |kayak V92.15
 |sailboat V92.14
 |hurricane X37.0
 |jumping into water from watercraft
  (involved in accident) *see also*
  Drowning, due to, accident to,
  watercraft
 |without accident to or on watercraft
  W16.711-
tidal wave NEC *see* Forces of nature, tidal
 wave
 |torrential rain X37.8
 |following
 |fall
 |into
 |bathtub W16.211
 |bucket W16.221
 |fountain *see* Drowning, following,
  fall, into, water, specified NEC
 |quarry *see* Drowning, following, fall,
  into, water, specified NEC
 |reservoir *see* Drowning, following,
  fall, into, water, specified NEC
 |swimming-pool W16.011
 |striking
 |bottom W16.021
 |wall W16.031
 |stated as undetermined whether
  accidental or intentional Y21.3
 |suicide (attempt) X71.2
 |water NOS W16.41
 |natural (lake) (open sea) (river)
  (stream) (pond) W16.111
 |striking
 |bottom W16.121
 |side W16.131
 |specified NEC W16.311
 |striking
 |bottom W16.321
 |wall W16.331
 |overboard NEC *see* Drowning, due to,
  fall overboard
 |jump or dive
 |from boat W16.711
 |striking bottom W16.721
 |into
 |fountain *see* Drowning, following,
  jump or dive, into, water, specified NEC

Drowning (accidental) - *continued*

 |quarry *see* Drowning, following, jump
  or dive, into, water, specified NEC
 |reservoir *see* Drowning, following,
  jump or dive, into, water, specified NEC
 |swimming-pool W16.511
 |striking
 |bottom W16.521
 |wall W16.531
 |suicide (attempt) X71.2
 |water NOS W16.91
 |natural (lake) (open sea) (river)
  (stream) (pond) W16.611
 |specified NEC W16.811
 |striking
 |bottom W16.821
 |wall W16.831
 |striking bottom W16.621
 |homicide (attempt) X92.9
 |in
 |bathtub (accidental) W65
 |assault X92.0
 |following fall W16.211
 |stated as undetermined whether
  accidental or intentional Y21.1
 |stated as undetermined whether
  accidental or intentional Y21.0
 |suicide (attempt) X71.0
 |lake *see* Drowning, in, natural water
 |natural water (lake) (open sea) (river)
  (stream) (pond) W69
 |assault X92.3
 |following
 |dive or jump W16.611
 |striking bottom W16.621
 |fall W16.111
 |striking
 |bottom W16.121
 |side W16.131
 |stated as undetermined whether
  accidental or intentional Y21.4
 |suicide (attempt) X71.3
 |quarry *see* Drowning, in, specified place
  NEC
 |quenching tank *see* Drowning, in,
  specified place NEC
 |reservoir *see* Drowning, in, specified
  place NEC
 |river *see* Drowning, in, natural water
 |sea *see* Drowning, in, natural water
 |specified place NEC W73
 |assault X92.8
 |following
 |dive or jump W16.811
 |striking
 |bottom W16.821
 |wall W16.831
 |fall W16.311
 |striking
 |bottom W16.321
 |wall W16.331
 |stated as undetermined whether
  accidental or intentional Y21.8
 |suicide (attempt) X71.8
 |stream *see* Drowning, in, natural water
 |swimming-pool W67
 |assault X92.1
 |following fall X92.2
 |following
 |dive or jump W16.511
 |striking
 |bottom W16.521
 |wall W16.531
 |fall W16.011

Drowning (accidental) - *continued*
|striking
|bottom W16.021
|wall W16.031
|stated as undetermined whether
accidental or intentional Y21.2
|following fall Y21.3
|suicide (attempt) X71.1
|following fall X71.2
|war operations *see* War operations,
restriction of airway
|resulting from accident to watercraft see
Drowning, due to, accident, watercraft
|self-inflicted X71.9
|stated as undetermined whether accidental
or intentional Y21.9
|suicide (attempt) X71.9

E

Earth (surface) movement NEC *see* Forces
of nature, earth movement
Earth falling (on) W20.0
|caused by cataclysmic earth surface
movement or eruption *see* Landslide
Earthquake (any injury) X34
Effect(s) (adverse) of
|air pressure (any) *see* Air, pressure
|cold, excessive (exposure to) *see* Exposure,
cold
|heat (excessive) *see* Heat
|hot place (weather) *see* Heat
|insolation X30
Effect(s) - *continued*
|late *see* Sequelae
|motion *see* Motion
|nuclear explosion or weapon in war
operations *see* War operations, nuclear
weapon
|radiation *see* Radiation
|travel *see* Travel
Electric shock (accidental) (by) (in) *see*
Exposure, electric current
Electrocution (accidental) *see* Exposure,
electric current
**Endotracheal tube wrongly placed during
anesthetic procedure**
Entanglement
|in
|bed linen, causing suffocation *see*
category T71
|wheel of pedal cycle V19.88
Entry of foreign body or material *see*
Foreign body
Environmental pollution related condition
|see Z57
Execution, legal (any method) *see* Legal,
intervention
Exhaustion
|cold *see* Exposure, cold
|due to excessive exertion *see also*
Overexertion X50.9
|heat *see* Heat
**Explosion (accidental) (of) (with secondary
fire)** W40.9
|acetylene W40.1
|aerosol can W36.1
|air tank (compressed) (in machinery) W36.2
|aircraft (in transit) (powered) NEC V95.9
|balloon V96.05
|fixed wing NEC (private) V95.25
|commercial V95.35
|glider V96.25
|hang V96.15

Explosion (accidental) - *continued*
|powered V95.15
|helicopter V95.05
|in war operations *see* War operations,
destruction of aircraft
|microlight V95.15
|nonpowered V96.9
|specified NEC V96.8
|powered NEC V95.8
|stated as
|homicide (attempt) Y03.8
|suicide (attempt) X83.0
|ultralight V95.15
|anesthetic gas in operating room W40.1
|antipersonnel bomb W40.8
|assault X96.0
|homicide (attempt) X96.0
|suicide (attempt) X75
|assault X96.9
|bicycle tire W37.0
|blasting (cap) (materials) W40.0
|boiler (machinery), not on transport vehicle
W35
|on watercraft *see* Explosion, in,
watercraft
|butane W40.1
|caused by other person X96.9
|coal gas W40.1
|detonator W40.0
|dump (munitions) W40.8
|dynamite W40.0
|in
|assault X96.8
|homicide (attempt) X96.8
|legal intervention
|injuring
|bystander Y35.112
|law enforcement personnel Y35.111
|suspect Y35.113
|suicide (attempt) X75
|explosive (material) W40.9
|gas W40.1
|in blasting operation W40.0
|specified NEC W40.8
|in
|assault X96.8
|homicide (attempt) X96.8
|legal intervention
|injuring
|bystander Y35.192
|law enforcement personnel
Y35.191
|suspect Y35.193
|suicide (attempt) X75
|factory (munitions) W40.8
|fertilizer bomb W40.8
|assault X96.3
|homicide (attempt) X96.3
|suicide (attempt) X75
|firearm (parts) NEC W34.19
|airgun W34.110
|BB gun W34.110
|gas, air or spring-operated gun NEC
W34.118
|handgun W32.1
|hunting rifle W33.12
|larger firearm W33.10
|specified NEC W33.19
|machine gun W33.13
|paintball gun W34.111
|pellet gun W34.110
|shotgun W33.11
|Very pistol [flare] W34.19
|fire-damp W40.1

Explosion (accidental) - *continued*
|fireworks W39
|gas (coal) (explosive) W40.1
|cylinder W36.9
|aerosol can W36.1
|air tank W36.2
|pressurized W36.3
|specified NEC W36.8
|gasoline (fumes) (tank) not in moving motor
vehicle W40.1
|bomb W40.8
|assault X96.1
|homicide (attempt) X96.1
|suicide (attempt) X75
|in motor vehicle *see* Accident, transport,
by type of vehicle
|grain store W40.8
|grenade W40.8
|in
|assault X96.8
|homicide (attempt) X96.8
|legal intervention
|injuring
|bystander Y35.192
|law enforcement personnel Y35.191
|suspect Y35.193
|suicide (attempt) X75
|handgun (parts) *see* Explosion, firearm,
handgun (parts) homicide (attempt)
X96.9
|antipersonnel bomb *see* Explosion,
antipersonnel bomb
|fertilizer bomb *see* Explosion, fertilizer
bomb
|gasoline bomb *see* Explosion, gasoline
bomb
|letter bomb *see* Explosion, letter bomb
|pipe bomb *see* Explosion, pipe bomb
|specified NEC X96.8
|hose, pressurized W37.8
|hot water heater, tank (in machinery) W35
|on watercraft *see* Explosion, in,
watercraft
|in, on
|dump W40.8
|factory W40.8
|mine (of explosive gases) NEC W40.1
|watercraft V93.59
|powered craft V93.53
|ferry boat V93.51
|fishing boat V93.52
|jet skis V93.53
|liner V93.51
|merchant ship V93.50
|passenger ship V93.51
|sailboat V93.54
|letter bomb W40.8
|assault X96.2
|homicide (attempt) X96.2
|suicide (attempt) X75
|machinery *see also* Contact, with, by type
of machine
|on board watercraft *see* Explosion, in,
watercraft
|pressure vessel *see* Explosion, by type of
vessel
|methane W40.1
|mine W40.1
|missile NEC W40.8
|mortar bomb W40.8
|in
|assault X96.8
|homicide (attempt) X96.8
|legal intervention

Explosion (accidental) - *continued*
  |injuring
    |bystander Y35.192
    |law enforcement personnel Y35.191
    |suspect Y35.193
  |suicide (attempt) X75
|munitions (dump) (factory) W40.8
|pipe, pressurized W37.8
  |bomb W40.8
    |assault X96.4
    |homicide (attempt) X96.4
    |suicide (attempt) X75
|pressure, pressurized
  |cooker W38
  |gas tank (in machinery) W36.3
  |hose W37.8
  |pipe W37.8
  |specified device NEC W38
  |tire W37.8
    |bicycle W37.0
  |vessel (in machinery) W38
|propane W40.1
|self-inflicted X75
|shell (artillery) NEC W40.8
  |during war operations *see* War
    operations, explosion
  |in
    |legal intervention
      |injuring
        |bystander Y35.122
        |law enforcement personnel Y35.121
        |suspect Y35.123
    |war *see* War operations, explosion
|spacecraft V95.45
|steam or water lines (in machinery) W37.8
|stove W40.9
|stated as undetermined whether accidental
  or intentional Y25
|suicide (attempt) X75
|tire, pressurized W37.8
  |bicycle W37.0
|undetermined whether accidental or
  intentional Y25
|vehicle tire NEC W37.8
  |bicycle W37.0
|war operations *see* War operations,
  explosion
Exposure (to) X58
|air pressure change *see* Air, pressure
|cold (accidental) (excessive) (extreme)
    (natural) (place) X31
  |assault Y08.89
  |due to
    |man-made conditions W93.8
      |dry ice (contact) W93.01
        |inhalation W93.02
      |liquid air (contact) (hydrogen)
        (nitrogen) W93.11
        |inhalation W93.12
      |refrigeration unit (deep freeze) W93.2
      |suicide (attempt) X83.2
    |weather (conditions) X31
  |homicide (attempt) Y08.89
  |self-inflicted X83.2
|due to abandonment or neglect X58
|electric current W86.8
  |appliance (faulty) W86.8
    |domestic W86.0
  |caused by other person Y08.89
  |conductor (faulty) W86.1
  |control apparatus (faulty) W86.1
  |electric power generating plant,
    distribution station W86.1

Exposure (to) - *continued*
  |electroshock gun *see* Exposure, electric
    current, taser
  |high-voltage cable W85
  |homicide (attempt) Y08.89
  |legal execution *see* Legal, intervention,
    specified means NEC
  |lightning *see* subcategory T75.0
  |live rail W86.8
  |misadventure in medical or surgical
    procedure in electroshock therapy
    Y63.4
  |motor (electric) (faulty) W86.8
    |domestic W86.0
  |self-inflicted X83.1
  |specified NEC W86.8
    |domestic W86.0
  |stun gun *see* Exposure, electric current,
    taser
  |suicide (attempt) X83.1
  |taser W86.8
    |assault Y08.89
    |legal intervention *see* category Y35
    |self-harm (intentional) X83.8
    |undetermined intent Y33
  |third rail W86.8
  |transformer (faulty) W86.1
  |transmission lines W85
|environmental tobacco smoke X58
|excessive
  |cold *see* Exposure, cold
  |heat (natural) NEC X30
  |man-made W92
|factor(s) NOS X58
  |environmental NEC X58
    |man-made NEC W99
    |natural NEC *see* Forces of nature
  |specified NEC X58
|fire, flames (accidental) X08.8
  |assault X97
  |campfire *see* Exposure, fire, controlled,
    not in building
  |controlled (in)
    |with ignition (of) clothing *see also*
      Ignition, clothes X06.2
      |nightwear X05
    |bonfire *see* Exposure, fire, controlled,
      not in building
    |brazier (in building or structure) *see*
      also Exposure, fire, controlled,
      building
      |not in building or structure *see*
        Exposure, fire, controlled, not in
        building
    |building or structure X02.0
      |with
        |fall from building X02.3
        |injury due to building collapse
          X02.2
        |from building X02.5
        |smoke inhalation X02.1
      |hit by object from building X02.4
      |specified mode of injury NEC X02.8
    |fireplace, furnace or stove *see*
      Exposure, fire, controlled, building
    |not in building or structure X03.0
      |with
        |fall X03.3
        |smoke inhalation X03.1
      |hit by object X03.4
      |specified mode of injury NEC X03.8
    |trash *see* Exposure, fire, controlled, not
      in building

Exposure (to) - *continued*
  |fireplace *see* Exposure, fire, controlled,
    building
  |fittings or furniture (in building or
    structure) (uncontrolled) *see* Exposure,
    fire, uncontrolled, building
  |forest (uncontrolled) *see* Exposure, fire,
    uncontrolled, not in building
  |grass (uncontrolled) *see* Exposure, fire,
    uncontrolled, not in building
  |hay (uncontrolled) *see* Exposure, fire,
    uncontrolled, not in building
  |homicide (attempt) X97
  |ignition of highly flammable material X04
  |in, of, on, starting in
    |machinery *see* Contact, with, by type of
      machine
    |motor vehicle (in motion) *see also*
      Accident, transport, occupant by type
      of vehicle V87.8
      |with collision *see* Collision
    |railway rolling stock, train, vehicle
      V81.81
      |with collision *see* Accident, transport,
        railway vehicle occupant
    |street car (in motion) V82.8
      |with collision *see* Accident, transport,
        streetcar occupant
    |transport vehicle NEC *see also*
      Accident, transport
      |with collision *see* Collision
    |war operations *see also* War operations,
      fire
      |from nuclear explosion *see* War
        operations, nuclear weapons
    |watercraft (in transit) (not in transit)
      V91.09
      |localized *see* Burn, on board
        watercraft, due to, fire on board
      |powered craft V91.03
        |ferry boat V91.01
        |fishing boat V91.02
        |jet skis V91.03
        |liner V91.01
        |merchant ship V91.00
        |passenger ship V91.01
      |unpowered craft V91.08
        |canoe V91.05
        |inflatable V91.06
        |kayak V91.05
        |sailboat V91.04
        |surf-board V91.08
        |waterskis V91.07
        |windsurfer V91.08
  |lumber (uncontrolled) *see* Exposure, fire,
    uncontrolled, not in building
  |mine (uncontrolled) *see* Exposure, fire,
    uncontrolled, not in building
  |prairie (uncontrolled) *see* Exposure, fire,
    uncontrolled, not in building
  |resulting from
    |explosion *see* Explosion
    |lightning X08.8
  |self-inflicted X76
  |specified NEC X08.8
  |started by other person X97
  |stove *see* Exposure, fire, controlled,
    building
  |stated as undetermined whether accidental
    or intentional Y26
  |suicide (attempt) X76
  |tunnel (uncontrolled) *see* Exposure, fire,
    uncontrolled, not in building
  |uncontrolled

Exposure (to) - *continued*
|in building or structure X00.0
  |with
    |fall from building X00.3
    |injury due to building collapse
      X00.2
    |jump from building X00.5
    |smoke inhalation X00.1
  |bed X08.00
    |due to
      |cigarette X08.01
      |specified material NEC X08.09
  |furniture NEC X08.20
    |due to
      |cigarette X08.21
      |specified material NEC X08.29
  |hit by object from building X00.4
  |sofa X08.10
    |due to
      |cigarette X08.11
      |specified material NEC X08.19
  |specified mode of injury NEC X00.8
|not in building or structure (any) X01.0
  |with
    |fall X01.3
    |smoke inhalation X01.1
  |hit by object X01.4
  |specified mode of injury NEC X01.8
|undetermined whether accidental or
  intentional Y26
|forces of nature NEC *see* Forces of nature
|G-forces (abnormal) W49.9
|gravitational forces (abnormal) W49.9
|heat (natural) NEC *see* Heat
|high-pressure jet (hydraulic) (pneumatic)
  W49.9
|hydraulic jet W49.9
|inanimate mechanical force W49.9
|jet, high-pressure (hydraulic) (pneumatic)
  W49.9
|lightning *see* subcategory T75.0
  |causing fire *see* Exposure, fire
|mechanical forces NEC W49.9
  |animate NEC W64
  |inanimate NEC W49.9
|noise W42.9
  |supersonic W42.0
|noxious substance *see* Table of Drugs and
  Chemicals
|pneumatic jet W49.9
|prolonged in deep-freeze unit or refrigerator
  W93.2
|radiation *see* Radiation
|smoke *see also* Exposure, fire
  |tobacco, second hand Z77.22
|specified factors NEC X58
|sunlight X32
  |man-made (sun lamp) W89.8
    |tanning bed W89.1
|supersonic waves W42.0
|transmission line(s), electric W85
|vibration W49.9
|waves
  |infrasound W49.9
  |sound W42.9
  |supersonic W42.0
|weather NEC *see* Forces of nature Y99.9
|child assisting in compensated work for
  family Y99.8
|civilian activity done for financial or other
  compensation Y99.0
|civilian activity done for income or pay
  Y99.0

Exposure (to) - *continued*
|family member assisting in compensated
  work for other family member Y99.8
|hobby not done for income Y99.8
|leisure activity Y99.8
|military activity Y99.1
|off-duty activity of military personnel Y99.8
|recreation or sport not for income or while a
  student Y99.8
|specified NEC Y99.8
|student activity Y99.8
|volunteer activity Y99.2

F

Factors, supplemental
|alcohol
  |blood level
    |less than 20mg/100ml Y90.0
    |presence in blood, level not specified
      Y90.9
    |20-39mg/100ml Y90.1
    |40-59mg/100ml Y90.2
    |60-79mg/100ml Y90.3
    |80-99mg/100ml Y90.4
    |100-119mg/100ml Y90.5
    |120-199mg/100ml Y90.6
    |200-239mg/100ml Y90.7
    |240mg/100ml or more Y90.8
  |presence in blood, but level not specified
    Y90.9
|environmental-pollution-related condition
  |see Z57
|nosocomial condition Y95
|work-related condition Y99.0
Failure
|in suture or ligature during surgical
  procedure Y65.2
|mechanical, of instrument or apparatus
  (any) (during any medical or surgical
  procedure) Y65.8
|sterile precautions (during medical and
  surgical care) *see* Misadventure, failure,
  sterile precautions, by type of procedure
|to
  |introduce tube or instrument Y65.4
    |endotracheal tube during anesthesia
      Y65.3
  |make curve (transport vehicle) NEC *see*
    Accident, transport
  |remove tube or instrument Y65.4
Fall, falling (accidental) W19
|building W20.1
  |burning (uncontrolled fire) X00.3
|down
  |embankment W17.81
  |escalator W10.0
  |hill W17.81
  |ladder W11
  |ramp W10.2
  |stairs, steps W10.9
|due to
  |bumping against
    |object W18.00
      |sharp glass W18.02
      |specified NEC W18.09
      |sports equipment W18.01
    |person W03
      |due to ice or snow W00.0
      |on pedestrian conveyance *see*
        Accident, transport, pedestrian,
        conveyance
  |collision with another person W03
    |due to ice or snow W00.0

Fall, falling (accidental) - *continued*
  |involving pedestrian conveyance *see*
    Accident, transport, pedestrian,
    conveyance
  |grocery cart tipping over W17.82
  |ice or snow W00.9
    |from one level to another W00.2
    |on stairs or steps W00.1
    |involving pedestrian conveyance *see*
      Accident, transport, pedestrian,
      conveyance
    |on same level W00.0
  |slipping (on moving sidewalk) W01.0
    |with subsequent striking against object
      W01.10
      |furniture W01.190
      |sharp object W01.119
        |glass W01.110
        |power tool or machine W01.111
        |specified NEC W01.118
      |specified NEC W01.198
  |striking against
    |object W18.00
      |sharp glass W18.02
      |specified NEC W18.09
      |sports equipment W18.01
    |person W03
      |due to ice or snow W00.0
      |on pedestrian conveyance *see*
        Accident, transport, pedestrian,
        conveyance
|earth (with asphyxia or suffocation (by
  pressure)) *see* Earth, falling
|from, off, out of
  |aircraft NEC (with accident to aircraft
    NEC) V97.0
    |while boarding or alighting V97.1
  |balcony W13.0
  |bed W06
  |boat, ship, watercraft NEC (with drowning
    or submersion) *see* Drowning, due to,
    fall overboard
    |with hitting bottom or object V94.0
  |bridge W13.1
  |building W13.9
    |burning (uncontrolled fire) X00.3
  |cavity W17.2
  |chair W07
  |cherry picker W17.89
  |cliff W15
  |dock W17.4
  |embankment W17.81
  |escalator W10.0
  |flagpole W13.8
  |furniture NEC W08
  |grocery cart W17.82
  |haystack W17.89
  |high place NEC W17.89
    |stated as undetermined whether
      accidental or intentional Y30
  |hole W17.2
  |incline W10.2
  |ladder W11
  |lifting device W17.89
  |machine, machinery *see also* Contact,
    with, by type of machine
    |not in operation W17.89
  |manhole W17.1
  |mobile elevated work platform [MEWP]
    W17.89
  |motorized mobility scooter W05.2
  |one level to another NEC W17.89
    |intentional, purposeful, suicide (attempt)
      X80

Fall, falling (accidental) - *continued*
  |stated as undetermined whether
    accidental or intentional Y30
|pit W17.2
|playground equipment W09.8
  |jungle gym W09.2
  |slide W09.0
  |swing W09.1
|quarry W17.89
|railing W13.9
|ramp W10.2
|roof W13.2
|scaffolding W12
|scooter (nonmotorized) W05.1
  |motorized mobility W05.2
|sky lift W17.89
|stairs, steps W10.9
  |curb W10.1
  |due to ice or snow W00.1
  |escalator W10.0
  |incline W10.2
  |ramp W10.2
  |sidewalk curb W10.1
  |specified NEC W10.8
  |standing
    |electric scooter V00.841
    |micro-mobility pedestrian conveyance
      V00.848
|stepladder W11
|storm drain W17.1
|streetcar NEC V82.6
  |with antecedent collision *see* Accident,
    transport, streetcar occupant
  |while boarding or alighting V82.4
|structure NEC W13.8
  |burning (uncontrolled fire) X00.3
|table W08
|toilet W18.11
  |with subsequent striking against object
    W18.12
|train NEC V81.6
  |during derailment (without antecedent
    collision) V81.7
    |with antecedent collision *see*
      Accident, transport, railway vehicle
      occupant
  |while boarding or alighting V81.4
|transport vehicle after collision *see*
  Accident, transport, by type of vehicle,
  collision
|tree W14
|vehicle (in motion) NEC *see also*
  Accident, transport V89.9
  |motor NEC *see also* Accident,
    transport, occupant, by type of vehicle
    V87.8
  |stationary W17.89
    |while boarding or alighting *see*
      Accident, transport, by type of
      vehicle, while boarding or alighting
|viaduct W13.8
|wall W13.8
|watercraft *see also* Drowning, due to, fall
  overboard
  |with hitting bottom or object V94.0
|well W17.0
|wheelchair, non-moving W05.0
  |powered *see* Accident, transport,
    pedestrian, conveyance occupant,
    specified type NEC
|window W13.4
|in, on
  |aircraft NEC V97.0
    |with accident to aircraft V97.0

Fall, falling (accidental) - *continued*
  |while boarding or alighting V97.1
|bathtub (empty) W18.2
  |filled W16.212
    |causing drowning W16.211
|escalator W10.0
|incline W10.2
|ladder W11
|machine, machinery *see* Contact, with, by
  type of machine
|object, edged, pointed or sharp (with cut)
  see Fall, by type
|playground equipment W09.8
  |jungle gym W09.2
  |slide W09.0
  |swing W09.1
|ramp W10.2
|scaffolding W12
|shower W18.2
  |causing drowning W16.211
|staircase, stairs, steps W10.9
  |curb W10.1
  |due to ice or snow W00.1
  |escalator W10.0
  |incline W10.2
  |specified NEC W10.8
|streetcar (without antecedent collision)
  V82.5
  |with antecedent collision *see* Accident,
    transport, streetcar occupant
  |while boarding or alighting V82.4
|train (without antecedent collision) V81.5
  |with antecedent collision *see* Accident,
    transport, railway vehicle occupant
  |during derailment (without antecedent
    collision) V81.7
    |with antecedent collision *see*
      Accident, transport, railway vehicle
      occupant
  |while boarding or alighting V81.4
|transport vehicle after collision *see*
  Accident, transport, by type of vehicle,
  collision
|watercraft V93.39
  |due to
    |accident to craft V91.29
      |powered craft V91.23
        |ferry boat V91.21
        |fishing boat V91.22
        |jet skis V91.23
        |liner V91.21
        |merchant ship V91.20
        |passenger ship V91.21
      |unpowered craft
        |canoe V91.25
        |inflatable V91.26
        |kayak V91.25
        |sailboat V91.24
    |powered craft V93.33
      |ferry boat V93.31
      |fishing boat V93.32
      |jet skis V93.33
      |liner V93.31
      |merchant ship V93.30
      |passenger ship V93.31
    |unpowered craft V93.38
      |canoe V93.35
      |inflatable V93.36
      |kayak V93.35
      |sailboat V93.34
      |surf-board V93.38
      |windsurfer V93.38
|into
  |cavity W17.2

Fall, falling (accidental) - *continued*
  |dock W17.4
|fire *see* Exposure, fire, by type
|haystack W17.89
|hole W17.2
|lake *see* Fall, into, water
|manhole W17.1
|moving part of machinery *see* Contact,
  with, by type of machine
|ocean *see* Fall, into, water
|opening in surface NEC W17.89
|pit W17.2
|pond *see* Fall, into, water
|quarry W17.89
|river *see* Fall, into, water
|shaft W17.89
|storm drain W17.1
|stream *see* Fall, into, water
|swimming pool *see also* Fall, into, water,
  in, swimming pool
  |empty W17.3
|tank W17.89
|water W16.42
  |causing drowning W16.41
  |from watercraft *see* Drowning, due to,
    fall overboard
  |hitting diving board W21.4
  |in
    |bathtub W16.212
      |causing drowning W16.211
    |bucket W16.222
      |causing drowning W16.221
    |natural body of water W16.112
      |causing drowning W16.111
      |striking
        |bottom W16.122
          |causing drowning W16.121
        |side W16.132
          |causing drowning W16.131
    |specified water NEC W16.312
      |causing drowning W16.311
      |striking
        |bottom W16.322
          |causing drowning W16.321
        |wall W16.332
          |causing drowning W16.331
    |swimming pool W16.012
      |causing drowning W16.011
      |striking
        |bottom W16.022
          |causing drowning W16.021
        |wall W16.032
          |causing drowning W16.031
    |utility bucket W16.222
      |causing drowning W16.221
  |well W17.0
|involving
  |bed W06
  |chair W07
  |furniture NEC W08
  |glass *see* Fall, by type
  |playground equipment W09.8
    |jungle gym W09.2
    |slide W09.0
    |swing W09.1
  |roller blades *see* Accident, transport,
    pedestrian, conveyance
  |skateboard(s) *see* Accident, transport,
    pedestrian, conveyance
  |skates (ice) (in line) (roller) *see* Accident,
    transport, pedestrian, conveyance
  |skis *see* Accident, transport, pedestrian,
    conveyance
  |table W08

Fall, falling (accidental) - *continued*
|wheelchair, non-moving W05.0
  |powered *see* Accident, transport,
    pedestrian, conveyance, specified type
    NEC
|object *see* Struck by, object, falling
|off
  |toilet W18.11
  |with subsequent striking against object
    W18.12
|on same level W18.30
  |due to
    |specified NEC W18.39
    |stepping on an object W18.31
|out of
  |bed W06
  |building NEC W13.8
  |chair W07
  |furniture NEC W08
  |wheelchair, non-moving W05.0
    |powered *see* Accident, transport,
      pedestrian, conveyance, specified type
      NEC
  |window W13.4
|over
  |animal W01.0
  |cliff W15
  |embankment W17.81
  |small object W01.0
|rock W20.8
|same level W18.30
  |from
    |being crushed, pushed, or stepped on by
      a crowd or human stampede W52
    |collision, pushing, shoving, by or with
      other person W03
    |slipping, stumbling, tripping W01.0
  |involving ice or snow W00.0
    |involving skates (ice) (roller),
      skateboard, skis *see* Accident,
      transport, pedestrian, conveyance
|snowslide (avalanche) *see* Landslide
|stone W20.8
|structure W20.1
  |burning (uncontrolled fire) X00.3
|through
  |bridge W13.1
  |floor W13.3
  |roof W13.2
  |wall W13.8
  |window W13.4
|timber W20.8
|tree (caused by lightning) W20.8
|while being carried or supported by other
  person(s) W04
Fallen on by
|animal (not being ridden) NEC W55.89
Felo-de-se *see* Suicide
Fight (hand) (fists) (foot) *see* Assault, fight
Fire (accidental) *see* Exposure, fire
Firearm discharge *see* Discharge, firearm
Fireball effects from nuclear explosion in
war operations *see* War operations,
  nuclear weapons
Fireworks (explosion) W39
Flash burns from explosion *see* Explosion
Flood (any injury) (caused by) X38
|collapse of man-made structure causing
  earth movement X36.0
|tidal wave *see* Forces of nature, tidal wave

Food (any type) in
|air passages (with asphyxia, obstruction, or
  suffocation) *see* categories T17 and T18
|alimentary tract causing asphyxia (due to
  compression of trachea) *see* categories
  T17 and T18
Forces of nature X39.8
|avalanche X36.1
  |causing transport accident *see* Accident,
    transport, by type of vehicle
|blizzard X37.2
|cataclysmic storm X37.9
  |with flood X38
  |blizzard X37.2
  |cloudburst X37.8
  |cyclone X37.1
  |dust storm X37.3
  |hurricane X37.0
  |specified storm NEC X37.8
  |storm surge X37.0
  |tornado X37.1
  |twister X37.1
  |typhoon X37.0
|cloudburst X37.8
|cold (natural) X31
|cyclone X37.1
|dam collapse causing earth movement
  X36.0
|dust storm X37.3
|earth movement X36.1
  |earthquake X34
  |caused by dam or structure collapse X36.0
|earthquake X34
|flood (caused by) X38
  |dam collapse X36.0
  |tidal wave *see* Forces of nature, tidal
    wave
|heat (natural) X30
|hurricane X37.0
|landslide X36.1
|volcanic eruption X35
Foreign body
|aspiration *see* Index to Diseases and
    Injuries, Foreign body, respiratory tract
|embedded in skin W45
|entering through skin W45.8
  |can lid W26.8
  |nail W45.0
  |paper W26.2
  |specified NEC W45.8
  |splinter W45.8
Forest fire (exposure to) *see* Exposure, fire,
  uncontrolled, not in building
Found injured X58
|from exposure (to) *see* Exposure
|on
  |highway, road (way), street V89.9
  |railway right of way V81.9
Fracture (circumstances unknown or
unspecified) X58
|due to specified cause NEC X58
Freezing *see* Exposure, cold **Frostbite** X31
|due to man-made conditions *see* Exposure,
  cold, man-made **Frozen** *see* Exposure,
  cold

G

Gored by bull W55.22
Gunshot wound W34.00

H

Hailstones, injured by X39.8
Hanged herself or himself *see* Hanging, self-
  inflicted
Hanging (accidental) *see also* category T71
|legal execution *see* Legal, intervention,
  specified means NEC
Heat (effects of) (excessive) X30
|due to
  |man-made conditions W92
    |on board watercraft V93.29
      |fishing boat V93.22
      |merchant ship V93.20
      |passenger ship V93.21
      |sailboat V93.24
      |specified powered craft NEC V93.23
  |weather (conditions) X30
|from
  |electric heating apparatus causing burning
    X16
  |nuclear explosion in war operations *see*
    War operations, nuclear weapons
  |inappropriate in local application or packing
    in medical or surgical procedure Y63.5
Hemorrhage
|delayed following medical or surgical
  treatment without mention of
  misadventure *see* Index to Diseases and
  Injuries, Complication(s)
|during medical or surgical treatment as
  misadventure *see* Index to Diseases and
  Injuries, Complication(s)
High
|altitude (effects) *see* Air, pressure, low
|level of radioactivity, effects *see* Radiation
|pressure (effects) *see* Air, pressure, high
|temperature, effects *see* Heat
Hit, hitting (accidental) by *see* Struck by
Hitting against *see* Striking against
Homicide (attempt) (justifiable) *see* Assault
Hot
|place, effects *see also* Heat
|weather, effects X30
House fire (uncontrolled) *see* Exposure, fire,
  uncontrolled, building
Humidity, causing problem X39.8
Hunger X58
Hurricane (any injury) X37.0
Hypobarism, hypobaropathy *see* Air,
  pressure, low

I

Ictus
|caloris *see also* Heat
|solaris X30
Ignition (accidental) *see also* Exposure, fire
  X08.8
|anesthetic gas in operating room W40.1
|apparel X06.2
  |from highly flammable material X04
  |nightwear X05
|bed linen (sheets) (spreads) (pillows)
  (mattress) *see* Exposure, fire,
  uncontrolled, building, bed
|benzine X04
|clothes, clothing NEC (from controlled fire)
  X06.2
  |from
    |highly flammable material X04
|ether X04
  |in operating room W40.1
|explosive material *see* Explosion
|gasoline X04
|jewelry (plastic) (any) X06.0

Ignition (accidental) - *continued*
|kerosene X04
|material
||explosive *see* Explosion
||highly flammable with secondary
|||explosion X04
|nightwear X05
|paraffin X04
|petrol X04

Immersion (accidental) *see also* Drowning
|hand or foot due to cold (excessive) X31

Implantation of quills of porcupine W55.89

Inanition (from) (hunger) X58
|thirst X58

Inappropriate operation performed
|correct operation on wrong side or body part
||(wrong side) (wrong site) Y65.53
|operation intended for another patient done
||on wrong patient Y65.52
|wrong operation performed on correct
||patient Y65.51

Inattention after, at birth (homicidal intent)
|(infanticidal intent) X58

Incident, adverse
|device
||anesthesiology Y70.8
|||accessory Y70.2
|||diagnostic Y70.0
|||miscellaneous Y70.8
|||monitoring Y70.0
|||prosthetic Y70.2
|||rehabilitative Y70.1
|||surgical Y70.3
|||therapeutic Y70.1
||cardiovascular Y71.8
|||accessory Y71.2
|||diagnostic Y71.0
|||miscellaneous Y71.8
|||monitoring Y71.0
|||prosthetic Y71.2
|||rehabilitative Y71.1
|||surgical Y71.3
|||therapeutic Y71.1
||gastroenterology Y73.8
|||accessory Y73.2
|||diagnostic Y73.0
|||miscellaneous Y73.8
|||monitoring Y73.0
|||prosthetic Y73.2
|||rehabilitative Y73.1
|||surgical Y73.3
|||therapeutic Y73.1
||general
|||hospital Y74.8
||||accessory Y74.2
||||diagnostic Y74.0
||||miscellaneous Y74.8
||||monitoring Y74.0
||||prosthetic Y74.2
||||rehabilitative Y74.1
||||surgical Y74.3
||||therapeutic Y74.1
|||surgical Y81.8
||||accessory Y81.2
||||diagnostic Y81.0
||||miscellaneous Y81.8
||||monitoring Y81.0
||||prosthetic Y81.2
||||rehabilitative Y81.1
||||surgical Y81.3
||||therapeutic Y81.1
||gynecological Y76.8
|||accessory Y76.2
|||diagnostic Y76.0

Incident, adverse - *continued*
|||miscellaneous Y76.8
|||monitoring Y76.0
|||prosthetic Y76.2
|||rehabilitative Y76.1
|||surgical Y76.3
|||therapeutic Y76.1
||medical Y82.9
|||specified type NEC Y82.8
||neurological Y75.8
|||accessory Y75.2
|||diagnostic Y75.0
|||miscellaneous Y75.8
|||monitoring Y75.0
|||prosthetic Y75.2
|||rehabilitative Y75.1
|||surgical Y75.3
|||therapeutic Y75.1
||obstetrical Y76.8
|||accessory Y76.2
|||diagnostic Y76.0
|||miscellaneous Y76.8
|||monitoring Y76.0
|||prosthetic Y76.2
|||rehabilitative Y76.1
|||surgical Y76.3
|||therapeutic Y76.1
||ophthalmic Y77.8
|||accessory Y77.2
|||contact lens (rigid gas permeable) (soft
||(hydrophilic)) Y77.11
|||diagnostic Y77.0
|||miscellaneous Y77.8
|||monitoring Y77.0
|||prosthetic Y77.2
|||rehabilitative Y77.19
|||surgical Y77.3
|||therapeutic Y77.19
||orthopedic Y79.8
|||accessory Y79.2
|||diagnostic Y79.0
|||miscellaneous Y79.8
|||monitoring Y79.0
|||prosthetic Y79.2
|||rehabilitative Y79.1
|||surgical Y79.3
|||therapeutic Y79.1
||otorhinolaryngological Y72.8
|||accessory Y72.2
|||diagnostic Y72.0
|||miscellaneous Y72.8
|||monitoring Y72.0
|||prosthetic Y72.2
|||rehabilitative Y72.1
|||surgical Y72.3
|||therapeutic Y72.1
||personal use Y74.8
|||accessory Y74.2
|||diagnostic Y74.0
|||miscellaneous Y74.8
|||monitoring Y74.0
|||prosthetic Y74.2
|||rehabilitative Y74.1
|||surgical Y74.3
|||therapeutic Y74.1
||physical medicine Y80.8
|||accessory Y80.2
|||diagnostic Y80.0
|||miscellaneous Y80.8
|||monitoring Y80.0
|||prosthetic Y80.2
|||rehabilitative Y80.1
|||surgical Y80.3
|||therapeutic Y80.1

Incident, adverse - *continued*
|||plastic surgical Y81.8
|||accessory Y81.2
|||diagnostic Y81.0
|||miscellaneous Y81.8
|||monitoring Y81.0
|||prosthetic Y81.2
|||rehabilitative Y81.1
|||surgical Y81.3
|||therapeutic Y81.1
||radiological Y78.8
|||accessory Y78.2
|||diagnostic Y78.0
|||miscellaneous Y78.8
|||monitoring Y78.0
|||prosthetic Y78.2
|||rehabilitative Y78.1
|||surgical Y78.3
|||therapeutic Y78.1
||urology Y73.8
|||accessory Y73.2
|||diagnostic Y73.0
|||miscellaneous Y73.8
|||monitoring Y73.0
|||prosthetic Y73.2
|||rehabilitative Y73.1
|||surgical Y73.3
|||therapeutic Y73.1

Incineration (accidental) *see* Exposure, fire

Infanticide *see* Assault

Infrasound waves (causing injury) W49.9

Ingestion
|foreign body (causing injury) (with
||obstruction) *see* Foreign body,
||alimentary canal
|poisonous
||plant(s) X58
||substance NEC *see* Table of Drugs and
||Chemicals

Inhalation
|excessively cold substance, man-made *see*
||Exposure, cold, man-made
|food (any type) (into respiratory tract) (with
||asphyxia, obstruction respiratory tract,
||suffocation) *see* categories T17 and T18
|foreign body *see* Foreign body, aspiration
|gastric contents (with asphyxia, obstruction
||respiratory passage, suffocation) T17.81-
|hot air or gases X14.0
|liquid air, hydrogen, nitrogen W93.12
||suicide (attempt) X83.2
|steam X13.0
||assault X98.0
||stated as undetermined whether accidental
|||or intentional Y27.0
||suicide (attempt) X77.0
|toxic gas *see* Table of Drugs and Chemicals
|vomitus (with asphyxia, obstruction
||respiratory passage, suffocation) T17.81-

Injury, injured (accidental(ly)) NOS X58
|by, caused by, from
||assault *see* Assault
||law-enforcing agent, police, in course of
|||legal intervention *see* Legal intervention
||suicide (attempt) X83.8
|due to, in
||civil insurrection *see* War operations
||fight *see also* Assault, fight Y04.0
||war operations *see* War operations
|homicide *see also* Assault Y09
|inflicted (by)
||in course of arrest (attempted),
|||suppression of disturbance,
|||maintenance of order, by law-enforcing
|||agents *see* Legal intervention

Injury, injured (accidental(ly)) NOS -
continued
  |other person
    |stated as
      |accidental X58
      |intentional, homicide (attempt) *see*
        Assault
      |undetermined whether accidental or
        intentional Y33
  |purposely (inflicted) by other person(s) *see*
    Assault
  |self-inflicted X83.8
  |stated as accidental X58
  |specified cause NEC X58
  |undetermined whether accidental or
    intentional Y33
Insolation, effects X30
Insufficient nourishment X58
Interruption of respiration (by)
  |food (lodged in esophagus) *see* categories
    T17 and T18
  |vomitus (lodged in esophagus) T17.81-
Intervention, legal *see* Legal intervention
Intoxication
  |drug *see* Table of Drugs and Chemicals
  |poison *see* Table of Drugs and Chemicals

J

Jammed (accidentally)
  |between objects (moving) (stationary and
    moving) W23.0
  |stationary W23.1
Jumped, jumping
  |before moving object NEC X81.8
  |motor vehicle X81.0
  |subway train X81.1
  |train X81.1
  |undetermined whether accidental or
    intentional Y31
  |from
  |boat (into water) voluntarily, without
    accident (to or on boat) W16.712
    |with
      |accident to or on boat *see* Accident,
        watercraft
      |drowning or submersion W16.711
        |suicide (attempt) X71.3
      |striking bottom W16.722
        |causing drowning W16.721
  |building *see also* Jumped, from, high
    place W13.9
    |burning (uncontrolled fire) X00.5
  |high place NEC W17.89
    |suicide (attempt) X80
    |undetermined whether accidental or
      intentional Y30
  |structure *see also* Jumped, from, high
    place W13.9
    |burning (uncontrolled fire) X00.5
  |into water W16.92
    |causing drowning W16.91
    |from, off watercraft *see* Jumped, from,
      boat
    |in
      |natural body W16.612
        |causing drowning W16.611
        |striking bottom W16.622
          |causing drowning W16.621
      |specified place NEC W16.812
        |causing drowning W16.811
        |striking
          |bottom W16.822

Jumped, jumping - *continued*
          |causing drowning W16.821
        |wall W16.832
          |causing drowning W16.831
    |swimming pool W16.512
      |causing drowning W16.511
      |striking
        |bottom W16.522
          |causing drowning W16.521
        |wall W16.532
          |causing drowning W16.531
  |suicide (attempt) X71.3

K

Kicked by
  |animal NEC W55.82
  |person(s) (accidentally) W50.1
    |with intent to injure or kill Y04.0
    |as, or caused by, a crowd or human
      stampede (with fall) W52
    |assault Y04.0
    |homicide (attempt) Y04.0
    |in
      |fight Y04.0
      |legal intervention
        |injuring
Kicked by |*(continued)*
        |bystander Y35.812
        |law enforcement personnel Y35.811
        |suspect Y35.813
Kicking
  |against
    |object W22.8
      |sports equipment W21.9
      |stationary W22.09
        |sports equipment W21.89
    |person *see* Striking against, person
    |sports equipment W21.9
  |carpet stretcher with knee X50.3
Killed, killing (accidentally) NOS *see also*
  Injury X58
  |in
    |action *see* War operations
    |brawl, fight (hand) (fists) (foot) Y04.0
      |by weapon *see also* Assault
        |cutting, piercing *see* Assault, cutting
          or piercing instrument
        |firearm *see* Discharge, firearm, by
      type, homicide
  |self
    |stated as
      |accident NOS X58
      |suicide *see* Suicide
      |undetermined whether accidental or
      intentional Y33
Kneeling (prolonged) (static) X50.1
Knocked down (accidentally) (by) NOS X58
  |animal (not being ridden) NEC *see also*
    Struck by, by type of animal
  |crowd or human stampede W52
  |person W51
    |in brawl, fight Y04.0
  |transport vehicle NEC *see also* Accident,
    transport V09.9

L

Laceration NEC *see* Injury
Lack of
  |care (helpless person) (infant) (newborn)
    X58

Lack of - *continued*
  |food except as result of abandonment or
    neglect X58
  |due to abandonment or neglect X58
  |water except as result of transport accident
    X58
  |due to transport accident *see* Accident,
    transport, by type
  |helpless person, infant, newborn X58
Landslide (falling on transport vehicle)
  X36.1
  |caused by collapse of man-made structure
    X36.0
Late effect *see* Sequelae
Legal
  |execution (any method) *see* Legal,
    intervention
  |intervention (by)
    |baton *see* Legal, intervention, blunt
      object, baton
    |bayonet *see* Legal, intervention, sharp
      object, bayonet
    |blow *see* Legal, intervention,
      manhandling
    |blunt object
      |baton
        |injuring
          |bystander Y35.312
          |law enforcement personnel Y35.311
          |suspect Y35.313
      |injuring
        |bystander Y35.302
        |law enforcement personnel Y35.301
        |suspect Y35.303
      |specified NEC
        |injuring
          |bystander Y35.392
          |law enforcement personnel Y35.391
          |suspect Y35.393
      |stave
        |injuring
          |bystander Y35.392
          |law enforcement personnel Y35.391
          |suspect Y35.393
    |bomb *see* Legal, intervention, explosive
    |cutting or piercing instrument *see* Legal,
      intervention, sharp object
    |dynamite *see* Legal, intervention,
      explosive, dynamite
    |explosive(s)
      |dynamite
        |injuring
          |bystander Y35.112
          |law enforcement personnel Y35.111
          |suspect Y35.113
      |grenade
        |injuring
          |bystander Y35.192
          |law enforcement personnel Y35.191
          |suspect Y35.193
      |injuring
        |bystander Y35.102
        |law enforcement personnel Y35.101
        |suspect Y35.103
      |mortar bomb
        |injuring
          |bystander Y35.192
          |law enforcement personnel Y35.191
          |suspect Y35.193
      |shell
        |injuring
          |bystander Y35.122
          |law enforcement personnel Y35.121
          |suspect Y35.123

M

Military operations - *continued*
  |improvised explosive device [IED]
    (person-borne) (roadside) (vehicle-
    borne) Y37.23
  |land mine Y37.29-
  |marine mine (at sea) (in harbor) Y37.02
  |marine weapon Y37.00-
    |specified NEC Y37.09-
  |sea-based artillery shell Y37.03
  |specified NEC Y37.29-
  |torpedo Y37.04-
 |fire Y37.30-
  |specified NEC Y37.39-
 |firearms
  |discharge Y37.43
  |pellets Y37.42-
 |flamethrower Y37.33-
 |fragments (from) (of)
  |improvised explosive device [IED]
    (person-borne) (roadside) (vehicle-
    borne) Y37.26
  |munitions Y37.25-
  |specified NEC Y37.29
  |weapons Y37.27-
 |friendly fire Y37.92-
 |hand to hand (unarmed) combat Y37.44-
 |hot substances *see* Military operations, fire
 |incendiary bullet Y37.32-
 |nuclear weapon (effects of) Y37.50
  |acute radiation exposure Y37.54-
  |blast pressure Y37.51
  |direct blast Y37.51-
  |direct heat Y37.53-
  |fallout exposure Y37.54
  |fireball Y37.53-
  |indirect blast (struck or crushed by blast
    debris) (being thrown by blast) Y37.52
  |ionizing radiation (immediate exposure)
    Y37.54-
  |nuclear radiation Y37.54
  |radiation
    |ionizing (immediate exposure) Y37.54
    |nuclear Y37.54-
    |thermal Y37.53-
  |specified NEC Y37.59-
  |secondary effects Y37.54
  |thermal radiation Y37.53-
 |restriction of air (airway)
  |intentional Y37.46-
  |unintentional Y37.47-
 |rubber bullets Y37.41-
 |shrapnel NOS Y37.29-
 |suffocation *see* Military operations,
  restriction of airways
 |unconventional warfare NEC Y37.7X-
 |underwater blast NOS Y37.00-
 |warfare
  |conventional NEC Y37.49-
  |unconventional NEC Y37.7X-
 |weapons
  |biological weapons Y37.6X
  |chemical Y37.7X-
  |nuclear (effects of) Y37.50-
    |acute radiation exposure Y37.54
    |blast pressure Y37.51-
    |direct blast Y37.51
    |direct heat Y37.53-
    |fallout exposure Y37.54
    |fireball Y37.53-
    |indirect blast (struck or crushed by blast
    debris) (being thrown by blast) Y37.52
    |radiation
      |ionizing (immediate exposure) Y37.54
      |nuclear Y37.54-

Military operations - *continued*
    |thermal Y37.53-
  |secondary effects Y37.54
  |specified NEC Y37.59-
 |of mass destruction [WMD] Y37.91-
 |weapon of mass destruction [WMD]
  Y37.91-
**Misadventure(s) to patient(s) during
surgical or medical care** Y69
 |contaminated medical or biological
  substance (blood, drug, fluid) Y64.9
  |administered (by) NEC Y64.9
    |immunization Y64.1
    |infusion Y64.0
    |injection Y64.1
    |specified means NEC Y64.8
    |transfusion Y64.0
    |vaccination Y64.1
 |excessive amount of blood or other fluid
  during transfusion or infusion Y63.0
 |failure
  |in dosage Y63.9
    |electroshock therapy Y63.4
    |inappropriate temperature (too hot or too
      cold) in local application and packing
      Y63.5
    |infusion
      |excessive amount of fluid Y63.0
      |incorrect dilution of fluid Y63.1
    |insulin-shock therapy Y63.4
    |nonadministration of necessary drug or
      biological substance Y63.6
    |overdose *see* Table of Drugs and
      Chemicals
    |radiation, in therapy Y63.2
  |radiation
    |overdose Y63.2
  |specified procedure NEC Y63.8
  |transfusion
    |excessive amount of blood Y63.0
 |mechanical, of instrument or apparatus
  (any) (during any procedure) Y65.8
 |sterile precautions (during procedure)
  Y62.9
  |aspiration of fluid or tissue (by puncture
    or catheterization, except heart) Y62.6
  |biopsy (except needle aspiration) Y62.8
    |needle (aspirating) Y62.6
  |blood sampling Y62.6
  |catheterization Y62.6
    |heart Y62.5
  |dialysis (kidney) Y62.2
  |endoscopic examination Y62.4
  |enema Y62.8
  |immunization Y62.3
  |infusion Y62.1
  |injection Y62.3
  |needle biopsy Y62.6
  |paracentesis (abdominal) (thoracic)
    Y62.6
  |perfusion Y62.2
  |puncture (lumbar) Y62.6
  |removal of catheter or packing Y62.8
  |specified procedure NEC Y62.8
  |surgical operation Y62.0
  |transfusion Y62.1
  |vaccination Y62.3
 |suture or ligature during surgical
  procedure Y65.2
 |to introduce or to remove tube or
  instrument *see* Failure, to
 |hemorrhage *see* Index to Diseases and
  Injuries, Complication(s)
 |inadvertent exposure of patient to radiation

Misadventure(s) to patient(s) - *continued*
  Y63.3
 |inappropriate
  |operation performed *see* Inappropriate
    operation performed
  |temperature (too hot or too cold) in local
    application or packing Y63.5
 |infusion *see also* Misadventure, by type,
  infusion Y69
  |excessive amount of fluid Y63.0
  |incorrect dilution of fluid Y63.1
  |wrong fluid Y65.1
 |mismatched blood in transfusion Y65.0
 |nonadministration of necessary drug or
  biological substance Y63.6
 |overdose *see* Table of Drugs and Chemicals
  |radiation (in therapy) Y63.2
 |perforation *see* Index to Diseases and
  Injuries, Complication(s)
 |performance of inappropriate operation *see*
  Inappropriate operation performed
 |puncture *see* Index to Diseases and Injuries,
  Complication(s)
 |specified type NEC Y65.8
  |failure
    |suture or ligature during surgical
      operation Y65.2
    |to introduce or to remove tube or
      instrument *see* Failure, to
  |infusion of wrong fluid Y65.1
  |performance of inappropriate operation
    see Inappropriate operation performed
  |transfusion of mismatched blood Y65.0
  |wrong
    |fluid in infusion Y65.1
    |placement of endotracheal tube during
      anesthetic procedure Y65.3
Misadventure(s) to patient(s) - *continued*
 |transfusion *see* Misadventure, by type,
  transfusion
  |excessive amount of blood Y63.0
  |mismatched blood Y65.0
 |wrong
  |drug given in error *see* Table of Drugs
    and Chemicals
  |fluid in infusion Y65.1
  |placement of endotracheal tube during
    anesthetic procedure Y65.3
Mismatched blood in transfusion Y65.0
Motion sickness T75.3
Mountain sickness W94.11
Mudslide (of cataclysmic nature) *see*
  Landslide
Murder (attempt) *see* Assault

N

Nail
 |contact with W45.0
Nail - *continued*
  |gun W29.4
 |embedded in skin W45.0
Neglect (criminal) (homicidal intent) X58
Noise (causing injury) (pollution) W42.9
 |supersonic W42.0
Nonadministration (of)
 |drug or biological substance (necessary)
  Y63.6
 |surgical and medical care Y66
Nosocomial condition Y95

O

Object
|falling
|from, in, on, hitting
||machinery *see* Contact, with, by type of
   machine
|set in motion by
||accidental explosion or rupture of pressure
   vessel W38
||firearm *see* Discharge, firearm, by type
||machine (ry) *see* Contact, with, by type of
   machine
Overdose (drug) *see* Table of Drugs and
   Chemicals
|radiation Y63.2
Overexertion X50.9
|from
||prolonged static or awkward postures
   X50.1
||repetitive movements X50.3
||specified strenuous movements or
   postures NEC X50.9
||strenuous movement or load X50.0
Overexposure (accidental) (to)
|cold *see also* Exposure, cold X31
||due to man-made conditions *see*
   Exposure, cold, man-made
|heat *see also* Heat X30
|radiation *see* Radiation
|radioactivity W88.0
|sun (sunburn) X32
|weather NEC *see* Forces of nature
|wind NEC *see* Forces of nature
Overheated *see* Heat
Overturning (accidental)
|machinery *see* Contact, with, by type of
   machine
Overturning - *continued*
|transport vehicle NEC *see also* Accident,
   transport V89.9
|watercraft (causing drowning, submersion)
   see also Drowning, due to, accident to,
   watercraft, overturning
||causing injury except drowning or
   submersion *see* Accident, watercraft,
   causing, injury NEC

P

Parachute descent (voluntary) (without
   accident to aircraft) V97.29
|due to accident to aircraft *see* Accident,
   transport, aircraft
Pecked by bird W61.99
Perforation during medical or surgical
   treatment as misadventure *see* Index to
   Diseases and Injuries, Complication(s)
Perpetrator, perpetration, of assault,
   maltreatment and neglect (by) Y07.9
|boyfriend Y07.03
|brother Y07.410
||stepbrother Y07.435
|coach Y07.53
|cousin
||female Y07.491
||male Y07.490
|daycare provider Y07.519
||at-home
|||adult care Y07.512
|||childcare Y07.510
||care center
|||adult care Y07.513

Perpetrator, perpetration, of assault,
maltreatment and neglect - *continued*
|||childcare Y07.511
|family member NEC Y07.499
|father Y07.11
||adoptive Y07.13
||foster Y07.420
||stepfather Y07.430
|foster father Y07.420
|foster mother Y07.421
|girl friend Y07.04
|healthcare provider Y07.529
||mental health Y07.521
||specified NEC Y07.528
|husband Y07.01
|instructor Y07.53
|mother Y07.12
||adoptive Y07.14
||foster Y07.421
||stepmother Y07.433
|multiple perpetrators Y07.6
|nonfamily member Y07.50
||specified NEC Y07.59
|nurse Y07.528
|occupational therapist Y07.528
|partner of parent
||female Y07.434
||male Y07.432
|physical therapist Y07.528
|sister Y07.411
|speech therapist Y07.528
|stepbrother Y07.435
|stepfather Y07.430
|stepmother Y07.433
|stepsister Y07.436
|teacher Y07.53
|wife Y07.02
Piercing *see* Contact, with, by type of object
   or machine
Pinched
|between objects (moving) (stationary and
   moving) W23.0
||stationary W23.1
Pinned under machine (ry) *see* Contact,
   with, by type of machine
Place of occurrence Y92.9
|abandoned house Y92.89
|airplane Y92.813
|airport Y92.520
|ambulatory health services establishment
   NEC Y92.538
|ambulatory surgery center Y92.530
|amusement park Y92.831
|apartment (co-op) *see* Place of occurrence,
   residence, apartment
|assembly hall Y92.29
|bank Y92.510
|barn Y92.71
|baseball field Y92.320
|basketball court Y92.310
|beach Y92.832
|boarding house *see* Place of occurrence,
   residence, boarding house
|boat Y92.814
|bowling alley Y92.39
|bridge Y92.89
|building under construction Y92.61
|bus Y92.811
||station Y92.521
|cafe Y92.511
|campsite Y92.833
|campus *see* Place of occurrence, school
|canal Y92.89
|car Y92.810

Place of occurrence - *continued*
|casino Y92.59
|children's home *see* Place of occurrence,
   residence, institutional, orphanage
|church Y92.22
|cinema Y92.26
|clubhouse Y92.29
|coal pit Y92.64
|college (community) Y92.214
|condominium *see* Place of occurrence,
   residence, apartment
|construction area *see* Place of occurrence,
   industrial and construction area
|convalescent home *see* Place of occurrence,
   residence, institutional, nursing home
|court-house Y92.240
|cricket ground Y92.328
|cultural building Y92.258
||art gallery Y92.250
||museum Y92.251
||music hall Y92.252
||opera house Y92.253
||specified NEC Y92.258
||theater Y92.254
|dancehall Y92.252
|day nursery Y92.210
|dentist office Y92.531
|derelict house Y92.89
|desert Y92.820
|dock NOS Y92.89
|dockyard Y92.62
|doctor's office Y92.531
|dormitory *see* Place of occurrence,
   residence, institutional, school dormitory
|dry dock Y92.62
|factory (building) (premises) Y92.63
|farm (land under cultivation) (outbuildings)
   Y92.79
||barn Y92.71
||chicken coop Y92.72
||field Y92.73
||hen house Y92.72
||house *see* Place of occurrence, residence,
   house
||orchard Y92.74
||orchard Y92.74
||specified NEC Y92.79
|football field Y92.321
|forest Y92.821
|freeway Y92.411
|gallery Y92.250
|garage (commercial) Y92.59
||boarding house Y92.044
||military base Y92.135
||mobile home Y92.025
||nursing home Y92.124
||orphanage Y92.114
||private house Y92.015
||reform school Y92.155
|gas station Y92.524
|gasworks Y92.69
|golf course Y92.39
|gravel pit Y92.64
|grocery Y92.512
|gymnasium Y92.39
|handball court Y92.318
|harbor Y92.89
|harness racing course Y92.39
|healthcare provider office Y92.531
|highway (interstate) Y92.411
|hill Y92.828
|hockey rink Y92.330
|home *see* Place of occurrence, residence
|hospice *see* Place of occurrence, residence,
   institutional, nursing home

Prolonged
|sitting in transport vehicle *see* Travel, by
 type of vehicle
|stay in
 |high altitude as cause of anoxia,
  barodontalgia, barotitis or hypoxia
  W94.11
 |weightless environment X52
Pulling, excessive *see also* Overexertion
 X50.9
Puncture, puncturing *see also* Contact, with,
 by type of object or machine
|by
 |plant thorns, spines, sharp leaves or other
  mechanisms NEC W60
|during medical or surgical treatment as
 misadventure *see* Index to Diseases and
 Injuries, Complication(s)
Pushed, pushing (accidental) (injury in)
|by other person(s) (accidental) W51
 |with fall W03
  |due to ice or snow W00.0
 |as, or caused by, a crowd or human
  stampede (with fall) W52
 |before moving object NEC Y02.8
  |motor vehicle Y02.0
  |subway train Y02.1
  |train Y02.1
 |from
  |high place NEC
   |in accidental circumstances W17.89
   |stated as
    |intentional, homicide (attempt) Y01
    |undetermined whether accidental or
     intentional Y30
  |transport vehicle NEC *see also*
   Accident, transport V89.9
   |stated as
    |intentional, homicide (attempt)
     Y08.89
|overexertion X50.9

R

Radiation (exposure to)
|arc lamps W89.0
|atomic power plant (malfunction) NEC
 W88.1
|complication of or abnormal reaction to
 medical radiotherapy Y84.2
|electromagnetic, ionizing W88.0
|gamma rays W88.1
|in
 |war operations (from or following nuclear
  explosion) *see* War operations
|inadvertent exposure of patient (receiving
 test or therapy) Y63.3
|infrared (heaters and lamps) W90.1
 |excessive heat from W92
|ionized, ionizing (particles, artificially
 accelerated) |radioisotopes W88.1
 |specified NEC W88.8
 |x-rays W88.0
|isotopes, radioactive *see* Radiation,
 radioactive isotopes
|laser(s) W90.2
 |in war operations *see* War operations
|misadventure in medical care Y63.2
|light sources (man-made visible and
 ultraviolet) W89.9
 |natural X32
 |specified NEC W89.8
 |tanning bed W89.1
 |welding light W89.0

Radiation (exposure to) - *continued*
|man-made visible light W89.9
 |specified NEC W89.8
 |tanning bed W89.1
 |welding light W89.0
|microwave W90.8
|misadventure in medical or surgical
 procedure Y63.2
|natural NEC X39.08
 |radon X39.01
|overdose (in medical or surgical procedure)
 Y63.2
|radar W90.0
|radioactive isotopes (any) W88.1
 |atomic power plant malfunction W88.1
 |misadventure in medical or surgical
  treatment Y63.2
|radiofrequency W90.0
|radium NEC W88.1
|sun X32
|ultraviolet (light) (man-made) W89.9
 |natural X32
 |specified NEC W89.8
 |tanning bed W89.1
 |welding light W89.0
|welding arc, torch, or light W89.0
 |excessive heat from W92
|x-rays (hard) (soft) W88.0
Range disease W94.11
Rape (attempted) T74.2-
Rat bite W53.11
Reaching (prolonged) (static) X50.1
Reaction, abnormal to medical procedure
 see also Complication of or following, by
 type of procedure Y84.9
|with misadventure *see* Misadventure
|biologicals *see* Table of Drugs and
 Chemicals
|drugs *see* Table of Drugs and Chemicals
|vaccine *see* Table of Drugs and Chemicals
Recoil
|airgun W34.110
|BB gun W34.110
|firearm NEC W34.19
Recoil - *continued*
|gas, air or spring-operated gun NEC
 W34.118
|handgun W32.1
|hunting rifle W33.12
|larger firearm W33.10
 |specified NEC W33.19
|machine gun W33.13
|paintball gun W34.111
|pellet W34.110
|shotgun W33.11
|Very pistol [flare] W34.19
Reduction in
|atmospheric pressure
 | *see* Air, pressure, change
Rock falling on or hitting (accidentally)
 (person) W20.8
|in cave-in W20.0
Run over (accidentally) (by)
|animal (not being ridden) NEC W55.89
|machinery *see* Contact, with, by specified
 type of machine
|transport vehicle NEC *see also* Accident,
 transport V09.9
 |intentional homicide (attempt) Y03.0
 |motor NEC V09.20
  |intentional homicide (attempt) Y03.0
Running
|before moving object X81.8
 |motor vehicle X81.0

Running off, away
|animal (being ridden) *see also* Accident,
 transport V80.918
 |not being ridden W55.89
|animal-drawn vehicle NEC *see also*
 Accident, transport V80.928
|highway, road (way), street
 |transport vehicle NEC *see also* Accident,
  transport V89.9
Rupture pressurized devices *see* Explosion,
 by type of device

S

Saturnism *see* Table of Drugs and
 Chemicals, lead

Scald, scalding (accidental) (by) (from) (in)
 X19
|air (hot) X14.1
|gases (hot) X14.1
|homicide (attempt) *see* Assault, burning,
 hot object
|inflicted by other person
 |stated as intentional, homicide (attempt)
  see Assault, burning, hot object
|liquid (boiling) (hot) NEC X12
 |stated as undetermined whether accidental
  or intentional Y27.2
 |suicide (attempt) X77.2
|local application of externally applied
 substance in medical or surgical care
 Y63.5
|metal (molten) (liquid) (hot) NEC X18
|self-inflicted X77.9
|stated as undetermined whether accidental
 or intentional Y27.8
|steam X13.1
 |assault X98.0
 |stated as undetermined whether accidental
  or intentional Y27.0
 |suicide (attempt) X77.0
|suicide (attempt) X77.9
|vapor (hot) X13.1
Scald, scalding - *continued*
|assault X98.0
|stated as undetermined whether accidental
 or intentional Y27.0
|suicide (attempt) X77.0
Scratched by
|cat W55.03
|person(s) (accidentally) W50.4
 |with intent to injure or kill Y04.0
 |as, or caused by, a crowd or human
  stampede (with fall) W52
 |assault Y04.0
 |homicide (attempt) Y04.0
 |in
  |fight Y04.0
  |legal intervention
   |injuring
    |bystander Y35.892
    |law enforcement personnel Y35.891
    |suspect Y35.893
    |unspecified person Y35.899
Seasickness T75.3
Self-harm NEC *see also* External cause by
 type, undetermined whether accidental or
 intentional
|intentional *see* Suicide
|poisoning NEC *see* Table of drugs and
 biologicals, accident

Self-inflicted (injury) NEC *see also* External
cause by type, undetermined whether
accidental or intentional
|intentional *see* Suicide
|poisoning NEC *see* Table of drugs and
biologicals, accident
Sequelae (of)
|accident NEC *see* W00-X58 with 7th
character S
|assault (homicidal) (any means) *see* X92-
Y08 with 7th character S
|homicide, attempt (any means) *see* X92-
Y08 with 7th character S
|injury undetermined whether accidentally or
purposely inflicted *see* Y21-Y33 with
7th character S
|intentional self-harm (classifiable to X71-
X83) *see* X71-X83 with 7th character S
|legal intervention *see* with 7th character S
Y35
|motor vehicle accident *see* V00-V99 with
7th character S
|suicide, attempt (any means) *see* X71-X83
with 7th character S
|transport accident *see* V00-V99 with 7th
character S
|war operations *see* War operations
Shock
|electric *see* Exposure, electric current
|from electric appliance (any) (faulty) W86.8
|domestic W86.0
|suicide (attempt) X83.1
Shooting, shot (accidental(ly)) *see also*
Discharge, firearm, by type
|herself or himself *see* Discharge, firearm by
type, self-inflicted
|homicide (attempt) *see* Discharge, firearm
by type, homicide
|in war operations *see* War operations
|inflicted by other person *see* Discharge,
firearm by type, homicide
|accidental *see* Discharge, firearm, by type
of firearm
|legal
|execution *see* Legal, intervention, firearm
|intervention *see* Legal, intervention,
firearm
|self-inflicted *see* Discharge, firearm by
type, suicide
|accidental *see* Discharge, firearm, by type
of firearm
|suicide (attempt) *see* Discharge, firearm by
type, suicide
Shoving (accidentally) by other person *see*
Pushed, by other person
Sickness
|alpine W94.11
|motion *see* Motion
|mountain W94.11
Sinking (accidental)
|watercraft (causing drowning, submersion)
see also Drowning, due to, accident to,
watercraft, sinking
|causing injury except drowning or
submersion *see* Accident, watercraft,
causing, injury NEC
Siriasis X32
Sitting (prolonged) (static) X50.1
Slashed wrists *see* Cut, self-inflicted
**Slipping (accidental) (on same level) (with
fall)** W01.0
|on
|ice W00.0
|with skates *see* Accident, transport,
pedestrian, conveyance

Slipping (accidental) - *continued*
|mud W01.0
|oil W01.0
|snow W00.0
|with skis *see* Accident, transport,
pedestrian, conveyance
|surface (slippery) (wet) NEC W01.0
|without fall W18.40
|due to
|specified NEC W18.49
|stepping from one level to another
W18.43
|stepping into hole or opening W18.42
|stepping on object W18.41
Sliver, wood, contact with W45.8
Smoldering (due to fire) *see* Exposure, fire
Sodomy (attempted) by force T74.2-
Sound waves (causing injury) W42.9
|supersonic W42.0
Splinter, contact with W45.8
Stab, stabbing *see* Cut
Standing (prolonged) (static) X50.1
Starvation X58
Status of external cause Y99.9
|child assisting in compensated work for
family Y99.8
|civilian activity done for financial or other
compensation Y99.0
|civilian activity done for income or pay
Y99.0
|family member assisting in compensated
work for other family member Y99.8
|hobby not done for income Y99.8
|leisure activity Y99.8
|military activity Y99.1
|off-duty activity of military personnel Y99.8
|recreation or sport not for income or while a
student Y99.8
|specified NEC Y99.8
|student activity Y99.8
|volunteer activity Y99.2
Stepped on
|by
|animal (not being ridden) NEC W55.89
|crowd or human stampede W52
|person W50.0
Stepping on
|object W22.8
|with fall W18.31
|sports equipment W21.9
|stationary W22.09
|sports equipment W21.89
|person W51
|by crowd or human stampede W52
|sports equipment W21.9
Sting
|arthropod, nonvenomous W57
|insect, nonvenomous W57
Storm (cataclysmic) *see* Forces of nature,
cataclysmic storm
Straining, excessive *see also* Overexertion
X50.9
Strangling *see* Strangulation
Strangulation (accidental) *see* category T71
Strenuous movements *see also* Overexertion
X50.9
Striking against
|airbag (automobile) W22.10
|driver side W22.11
|front passenger side W22.12
|specified NEC W22.19
|bottom when
|diving or jumping into water (in) W16.822
|causing drowning W16.821

Striking against - *continued*
|from boat W16.722
|causing drowning W16.721
|natural body W16.622
|causing drowning W16.821
|swimming pool W16.522
|causing drowning W16.521
|falling into water (in) W16.322
|causing drowning W16.321
|fountain *see* Striking against, bottom
when, falling into water, specified
NEC
|natural body W16.122
|causing drowning W16.121
|reservoir *see* Striking against, bottom
when, falling into water, specified
NEC
|specified NEC W16.322
|causing drowning W16.321
|swimming pool W16.022
|causing drowning W16.021
|diving board (swimming-pool) W21.4
|object W22.8
|with
|drowning or submersion *see* Drowning
|fall *see* Fall, due to, bumping against,
object
|caused by crowd or human stampede (with
fall) W52
|furniture W22.03
|lamppost W22.02
|sports equipment W21.9
|stationary W22.09
|sports equipment W21.89
|wall W22.01
|person(s) W51
|with fall W03
|due to ice or snow W00.0
|as, or caused by, a crowd or human
stampede (with fall) W52
|assault Y04.2
|homicide (attempt) Y04.2
|sports equipment W21.9
|wall (when) W22.01
|diving or jumping into water (in) W16.832
|causing drowning W16.831
|swimming pool W16.532
|causing drowning W16.531
|falling into water (in) W16.332
|causing drowning W16.331
|fountain *see* Striking against, wall
when, falling into water, specified
NEC
|natural body W16.132
|causing drowning W16.131
|reservoir *see* Striking against, wall
when, falling into water, specified
NEC
|specified NEC W16.332
|causing drowning W16.331
|swimming pool W16.032
|causing drowning W16.031
|swimming pool (when) W22.042
|causing drowning W22.041
|diving or jumping into water W16.532
|causing drowning W16.531
|falling into water W16.032
|causing drowning W16.031
Struck (accidentally) by
|airbag (automobile) W22.10
|driver side W22.11
|front passenger side W22.12
|specified NEC W22.19
|alligator W58.02

Struck (accidentally) by - *continued*
| animal (not being ridden) NEC W55.89
| avalanche *see* Landslide
| ball (hit) (thrown) W21.00
  | assault Y08.09
  | baseball W21.03
  | basketball W21.05
  | golf ball W21.04
  | football W21.01
  | soccer W21.02
  | softball W21.07
  | specified NEC W21.09
  | volleyball W21.06
| bat or racquet
  | baseball bat W21.11
    | assault Y08.02
  | golf club W21.13
    | assault Y08.09
  | specified NEC W21.19
    | assault Y08.09
  | tennis racquet W21.12
    | assault Y08.09
| bullet *see also* Discharge, firearm by type
  | in war operations *see* War operations
| crocodile W58.12
| dog W54.1
| flare, Very pistol *see* Discharge, firearm NEC
| hailstones X39.8
| hockey (ice) | field
    | puck W21.221
    | stick W21.211
  | puck W21.220
  | stick W21.210
    | assault Y08.01
| landslide *see* Landslide
| law-enforcement agent (on duty) *see* Legal, intervention, manhandling
  | with blunt object *see* Legal, intervention, blunt object
| lightning *see* subcategory T75.0
  | causing fire *see* Exposure, fire
| machine *see* Contact, with, by type of machine
| mammal NEC W55.89
  | marine W56.32
| marine animal W56.82
| missile
  | firearm *see* Discharge, firearm by type
  | in war operations *see* War operations, missile
| object W22.8
  | blunt W22.8
    | assault Y00
    | suicide (attempt) X79
    | undetermined whether accidental or intentional Y29
  | falling W20.8
    | from, in, on
      | building W20.1
        | burning (uncontrolled fire) X00.4
      | cataclysmic
        | earth surface movement NEC *see* Landslide
        | storm *see* Forces of nature, cataclysmic storm
      | cave-in W20.0
      | earthquake X34
      | machine (in operation) *see* Contact, with, by type of machine
      | structure W20.1
        | burning X00.4
      | transport vehicle (in motion) *see* Accident, transport, by type of vehicle

Struck (accidentally) by - *continued*
| watercraft V93.49
  | due to
    | accident to craft V91.39
      | powered craft V91.33
        | ferry boat V91.31
        | fishing boat V91.32
        | jet skis V91.33
        | liner V91.31
        | merchant ship V91.30
        | passenger ship V91.31
      | unpowered craft V91.38
        | canoe V91.35
        | inflatable V91.36
        | kayak V91.35
        | sailboat V91.34
        | surf-board V91.38
        | windsurfer V91.38
    | powered craft V93.43
      | ferry boat V93.41
      | fishing boat V93.42
      | jet skis V93.43
      | liner V93.41
      | merchant ship V93.40
      | passenger ship V93.41
    | unpowered craft V93.48
      | sailboat V93.44
      | surf-board V93.48
      | windsurfer V93.48
| moving NEC W20.8
| projected W20.8
  | assault Y00
  | in sports W21.9
    | assault Y08.09
  | ball W21.00
    | baseball W21.03
    | basketball W21.05
    | football W21.01
    | golf ball W21.04
    | soccer W21.02
    | softball W21.07
    | specified NEC W21.09
    | volleyball W21.06
  | bat or racquet
    | baseball bat W21.11
      | assault Y08.02
    | golf club W21.13
      | assault Y08.09
    | specified NEC W21.19
      | assault Y08.09
    | tennis racquet W21.12
      | assault Y08.09
  | hockey (ice)
    | field
      | puck W21.221
      | stick W21.211
    | puck W21.220
    | stick W21.210
      | assault Y08.01
  | specified NEC W21.89
| set in motion by explosion *see* Explosion
| thrown W20.8
  | assault Y00
  | in sports W21.9
    | assault Y08.09
  | ball W21.00
    | baseball W21.03
    | basketball W21.05
    | football W21.01
    | golf ball W21.04
    | soccer W21.02
    | soft ball W21.07
    | specified NEC W21.09
    | volleyball W21.06

Struck (accidentally) by - *continued*
| bat or racquet
  | baseball bat W21.11
    | assault Y08.02
  | golf club W21.13
    | assault Y08.09
  | specified NEC W21.19
    | assault Y08.09
  | tennis racquet W21.12
    | assault Y08.09
| hockey (ice)
  | field
    | puck W21.221
    | stick W21.211
  | puck W21.220
  | stick W21.210
    | assault Y08.01
  | specified NEC W21.89
| other person(s) W50.0
  | with
    | blunt object W22.8
      | intentional, homicide (attempt) Y00
      | sports equipment W21.9
      | undetermined whether accidental or intentional Y29
    | fall W03
      | due to ice or snow W00.0
  | as, or caused by, a crowd or human stampede (with fall) W52
  | assault Y04.2
  | homicide (attempt) Y04.2
  | in legal intervention
    | injuring
      | bystander Y35.812
      | law enforcement personnel Y35.811
      | suspect Y35.813
  | sports equipment W21.9
| police (on duty) *see* Legal, intervention, manhandling
  | with blunt object *see* Legal, intervention, blunt object
| sports equipment W21.9
  | assault Y08.09
  | ball W21.00
    | baseball W21.03
    | basketball W21.05
    | football W21.01
    | golf ball W21.04
    | soccer W21.02
    | soft ball W21.07
    | specified NEC W21.09
    | volleyball W21.06
  | bat or racquet
    | baseball bat W21.11
      | assault Y08.02
    | golf club W21.13
      | assault Y08.09
    | specified NEC W21.19
    | tennis racquet W21.12
      | assault Y08.09
  | cleats (shoe) W21.31
  | foot wear NEC W21.39
  | football helmet W21.81
  | hockey (ice)
    | field
      | puck W21.221
      | stick W21.211
    | puck W21.220
    | stick W21.210
      | assault Y08.01
  | skate blades W21.32
  | specified NEC W21.89
    | assault Y08.09
| thunderbolt *see* subcategory T75.0

Struck (accidentally) by - *continued*
|causing fire *see* Exposure, fire
|transport vehicle NEC *see also* Accident,
   transport V09.9
|intentional, homicide (attempt) Y03.0
|motor NEC *see also* Accident, transport
   V09.20
|homicide Y03.0
Struck (accidentally) by - *continued*
|vehicle (transport) NEC *see* Accident,
   transport, by type of vehicle
|stationary (falling from jack, hydraulic
   lift, ramp) W20.8
Stumbling
|over
   |animal NEC W01.0
      |with fall W18.09
   |carpet, rug or (small) object W22.8
      |with fall W18.09
   |person W51
      |with fall W03
         |due to ice or snow W00.0
|without fall W18.40
   |due to
      |specified NEC W18.49
      |stepping from one level to another
         W18.43
      |stepping into hole or opening W18.42
      |stepping on object W18.41
Submersion (accidental) *see* Drowning
Suffocation (accidental) (by external means)
   (by pressure) (mechanical) *see also*
   category T71
|due to, by
   |avalanche *see* Landslide
   |explosion *see* Explosion
   |fire *see* Exposure, fire
   |food, any type (aspiration) (ingestion)
      (inhalation) *see* categories T17 and
      T18
   |ignition *see* Ignition
   |landslide *see* Landslide
   |machine (ry) *see* Contact, with, by type of
      machine
   |vomitus (aspiration) (inhalation) T17.81-
|in
   |burning building X00.8
Suicide, suicidal (attempted) (by) X83.8
|blunt object X79
|burning, burns X76
   |hot object X77.9
      |fluid NEC X77.2
      |household appliance X77.3
      |specified NEC X77.8
      |steam X77.0
      |tap water X77.1
      |vapors X77.0
|caustic substance *see* Table of Drugs and
   Chemicals
|cold, extreme X83.2
|collision of motor vehicle with
   |motor vehicle X82.0
   |specified NEC X82.8
   |train X82.1
   |tree X82.2
|crashing of aircraft X83.0
|cut (any part of body) X78.9
|cutting or piercing instrument X78.9
   |dagger X78.2
   |glass X78.0
   |knife X78.1
   |specified NEC X78.8
   |sword X78.2
|drowning (in) X71.9

Suicide, suicidal - *continued*
   |bathtub X71.0
   |natural water X71.3
   |specified NEC X71.8
   |swimming pool X71.1
      |following fall X71.2
|electrocution X83.1
|explosive(s) (material) X75
|fire, flames X76
|firearm X74.9
   |airgun X74.01
   |handgun X72
   |hunting rifle X73.1
   |larger X73.9
      |specified NEC X73.8
   |machine gun X73.2
   |shotgun X73.0
   |specified NEC X74.8
|hanging X83.8
|hot object *see* Suicide, burning, hot object
|jumping
   |before moving object X81.8
      |motor vehicle X81.0
      |subway train X81.1
      |train X81.1
   |from high place X80
|late effect of attempt *see* X71-X83 with 7th
   character S
|lying before moving object, train, vehicle
   X81.8
|poisoning *see* Table of Drugs and
   Chemicals
|puncture (any part of body) *see* Suicide,
   cutting or piercing instrument
|scald *see* Suicide, burning, hot object
|sequelae of attempt *see* X71-X83 with 7th
   character S
|sharp object (any) *see* Suicide, cutting or
   piercing instrument
|shooting *see* Suicide, firearm
|specified means NEC X83.8
|stab (any part of body) *see* Suicide, cutting
   or piercing instrument
|steam, hot vapors X77.0
|strangulation X83.8
|submersion *see* Suicide, drowning
|suffocation X83.8
|wound NEC X83.8
Sunstroke X32
Supersonic waves (causing injury) W42.0
Surgical procedure, complication of
   (delayed or as an abnormal reaction
   without mention of misadventure)
   see also Complication of or following, by
   type of procedure
Surgical procedure |*(continued)*
|due to or as a result of misadventure *see*
   Misadventure
Swallowed, swallowing
|foreign body *see* Foreign body, alimentary
   canal
|poison *see* Table of Drugs and Chemicals
|substance
   |caustic or corrosive *see* Table of Drugs
      and Chemicals
   |poisonous *see* Table of Drugs and
      Chemicals

T

Tackle in sport W03
Terrorism (involving) Y38.80
   |biological weapons Y38.6X-
   |chemical weapons Y38.7X-

Terrorism - *continued*
   |conflagration Y38.3X-
   |drowning and submersion Y38.89-
   |explosion Y38.2X-
      |destruction of aircraft Y38.1X
      |marine weapons Y38.0X-
   |fire Y38.3X-
   |firearms Y38.4X-
   |hot substances Y38.3X-
   |lasers Y38.89-
   |nuclear weapons Y38.5X-
   |piercing or stabbing instruments Y38.89-
   |secondary effects Y38.9X-
   |specified method NEC Y38.89-
   |suicide bomber Y38.81-
Thirst X58
Threat to breathing
   |aspiration *see* Aspiration
   |due to cave-in, falling earth or substance
      NEC *see* category T71
Thrown (accidentally)
   |against part (any) of or object in transport
      vehicle (in motion) NEC *see also*
      Accident, transport
   |from
      |high place, homicide (attempt) Y01
      |machinery *see* Contact, with, by type of
         machine
      |transport vehicle NEC *see also* Accident,
         transport V89.9
   |off *see* Thrown, from
Thunderbolt *see* subcategory T75.0
   |causing fire *see* Exposure, fire
Tidal wave (any injury) NEC *see* Forces of
   nature, tidal wave
Took
   |overdose (drug) *see* Table of Drugs and
      Chemicals
   |poison *see* Table of Drugs and Chemicals
Tornado (any injury) X37.1
Torrential rain (any injury) X37.8
Torture X58
Trampled by animal NEC W55.89
Trapped (accidentally)
   |between objects (moving) (stationary and
      moving) *see* Caught
   |by part (any) of
      |motorcycle V29.88
      |pedal cycle V19.88
      |transport vehicle NEC *see also* Accident,
         transport V89.9
Travel (effects) (sickness) T75.3
Tree falling on or hitting (accidentally)
   (person) W20.8
Tripping
   |over
      |animal W01.0
         |with fall W01.0
      |carpet, rug or (small) object W22.8
         |with fall W18.09
      |person W51
         |with fall W03
            |due to ice or snow W00.0
   |without fall W18.40
      |due to
         |specified NEC W18.49
         |stepping from one level to another
            W18.43
         |stepping into hole or opening W18.42
         |stepping on object W18.41
Twisted by person(s) (accidentally) W50.2
   |with intent to injure or kill Y04.0
   |as, or caused by, a crowd or human
      stampede (with fall) W52

War operations - *continued*
　|unconventional warfare NEC Y36.7X-
　|underwater blast NOS Y36.00-
　|warfare
　　|conventional NEC Y36.49-
　　|unconventional NEC Y36.7X-
　|weapons
　　|biological weapons Y36.6X-
　　|chemical Y36.7X-
　　|nuclear (effects of) Y36.50-
　　　|acute radiation exposure Y36.54
　　　|blast pressure Y36.51-
　　　|direct blast Y36.51
　　　|direct heat Y36.53-
　　　|fallout exposure Y36.54
　　　|fireball Y36.53-
　　　|indirect blast (struck or crushed by blast
　　　　debris) (being thrown by blast)
　　　　Y36.52
　　　|radiation
　　　　|ionizing (immediate exposure) Y36.54
　　　　|nuclear Y36.54-
　　　　|thermal Y36.53-
　　　|secondary effects Y36.54
　　　|specified NEC Y36.59-
　　|of mass destruction [WMD] Y36.91
　|weapon of mass destruction [WMD] Y36.91
Washed
　|away by flood *see* Flood
　|off road by storm (transport vehicle) *see*
　　Forces of nature, cataclysmic storm
Weather exposure NEC *see* Forces of nature
Weightlessness (causing injury) (effects of)
　(in spacecraft, real or simulated) X52
Work related condition Y99.0
Wound (accidental) NEC *see also* Injury
　X58
　|battle *see also* War operations Y36.90
　|gunshot *see* Discharge, firearm by type
Wreck transport vehicle NEC *see also*
　Accident, transport V89.9
Wrong
　|device implanted into correct surgical site
　　Y65.51
　|fluid in infusion Y65.1
　|procedure (operation) on correct patient
　　Y65.51
　|patient, procedure performed on Y65.52

List of Three Digit Categories

CHAPTER 1: CERTAIN INFECTIOUS AND PARASITIC DISEASES (A00-B99)

A00 Cholera
A01 Typhoid and paratyphoid fevers
A02 Other salmonella infections
A03 Shigellosis
A04 Other bacterial intestinal infections
A05 Other bacterial foodborne intoxications, not elsewhere classified
A06 Amebiasis
A07 Other protozoal intestinal diseases
A08 Viral and other specified intestinal infections
A09 Infectious gastroenteritis and colitis unspecified
A15 Respiratory tuberculosis
A17 Tuberculosis of nervous system
A18 Tuberculosis of other organs
A19 Miliary tuberculosis
A20 Plague
A21 Tularemia
A22 Anthrax
A23 Brucellosis
A24 Glanders and melioidosis
A25 Rat-bite fever
A26 Erysipeloid
A27 Leptospirosis
A28 Other zoonotic bacterial diseases, not elsewhere classified
A30 Leprosy (Hansen's disease)
A31 Infection due to other mycobacteria
A32 Listeriosis
A33 Tetanus neonatorum
A34 Obstetrical tetanus
A35 Other tetanus
A36 Diphtheria
A37 Whooping cough
A38 Scarlet fever
A39 Meningococcal infection
A40 Streptococcal sepsis
A41 Other sepsis
A42 Actinomycosis
A43 Nocardiosis
A44 Bartonellosis
A46 Erysipelas
A48 Other bacterial diseases, not elsewhere classified
A49 Staphylococcal infection of unspecified site
A50 Congenital syphilis
A51 Early syphilis
A52 Late syphilis
A53 Other and unspecified syphilis
A54 Gonococcal infection

A55 Chlamydial lymphogranuloma (venereum)
A56 Other sexually transmitted chlamydial diseases
A57 Chancroid
A58 Granuloma inguinale
A59 Trichomoniasis
A60 Anogenital herpesviral [herpes simplex] infections
A63 Other predominantly sexually transmitted diseases, not elsewhere classified
A64 Unspecified sexually transmitted disease
A65 Nonvenereal syphilis
A66 Yaws
A67 Pinta [carate]
A68 Relapsing fevers
A69 Other spirochetal infections
A70 Chlamydia psittaci infections
A71 Trachoma
A74 Other diseases caused by chlamydiae
A75 Typhus fever
A77 Spotted fever [tick-borne rickettsioses]
A78 Q fever
A79 Other rickettsioses
A80 Acute poliomyelitis
A81 Atypical virus infections of central nervous system
A82 Rabies
A83 Mosquito-borne viral encephalitis
A84 Tick-borne viral encephalitis
A85 Other viral encephalitis, not elsewhere classified
A86 Unspecified viral encephalitis
A87 Viral meningitis
A88 Other viral infections of central nervous system, not elsewhere classified
A89 Unspecified viral infection of central nervous system
A90 Dengue fever [classical dengue]
A91 Dengue hemorrhagic fever
A92 Other mosquito-borne viral fevers
A93 Other arthropod-borne viral fevers, not elsewhere classified
A94 Unspecified arthropod-borne viral fever
A95 Yellow fever
A96 Arenaviral hemorrhagic fever
A98 Other viral hemorrhagic fevers, not elsewhere classified
A99 Unspecified viral hemorrhagic fever
B00 Herpesviral [herpes simplex] infections
B01 Varicella [chickenpox]
B02 Zoster [herpes zoster]
B03 Smallpox
B04 Monkeypox
B05 Measles
B06 Rubella [German measles]

B07 Viral warts
B08 Cowpox
B09 Other human herpesviruses
B10 Other human herpesviruses
B15 Acute hepatitis A
B16 Acute hepatitis B
B17 Other acute viral hepatitis
B18 Chronic viral hepatitis
B19 Unspecified viral hepatitis
B20 Human immunodeficiency virus [HIV] disease
B25 Cytomegaloviral disease
B26 Mumps
B27 Infectious mononucleosis
B30 Viral conjunctivitis
B33 Other viral diseases, not elsewhere classified
B34 Viral infection of unspecified site
B35 Dermatophytosis
B36 Other superficial mycoses
B37 Candidiasis
B38 Coccidioidomycosis
B39 Histoplasmosis
B40 Blastomycosis
B41 Paracoccidioidomycosis
B42 Sporotrichosis
B43 Chromomycosis and pheomycotic abscess
B44 Aspergillosis
B45 Cryptococcosis
B46 Zygomycosis
B47 Mycetoma
B48 Other mycoses, not elsewhere classified
B49 Unspecified mycosis
B50 Plasmodium falciparum malaria
B51 Plasmodium vivax malaria
B52 Plasmodium malariae malaria
B53 Other specified malaria
B54 Unspecified malaria
B55 Leishmaniasis
B56 African trypanosomiasis
B57 Chagas' disease
B58 Toxoplasmosis
B59 Pneumocystosis
B60 Other protozoal diseases, not elsewhere classified
B64 Unspecified protozoal disease
B65 Schistosomiasis [bilharziasis]
B66 Other fluke infections
B67 Echinococcosis
B68 Taeniasis
B69 Cysticercosis
B70 Diphyllobothriasis and sparganosis
B71 Other cestode infections
B72 Dracunculiasis

B73 Onchocerciasis

B74 Filariasis

B75 Trichinellosis

B76 Hookworm diseases

B77 Ascariasis

B78 Strongyloidiasis

B79 Trichuriasis

B80 Enterobiasis

B81 Other intestinal helminthiases, not elsewhere classified

B82 Unspecified intestinal parasitism

B83 Other helminthiases

B85 Pediculosis and phthiriasis

B86 Scabies

B87 Myiasis

B88 Other infestations

B89 Unspecified parasitic disease

B90 Sequelae of tuberculosis

B91 Sequelae of poliomyelitis

B92 Sequelae of leprosy

B94 Sequelae of other and unspecified infectious and parasitic diseases

B95 Streptococcus, Staphylococcus, and Enterococcus as the cause of diseases classified elsewhere

B96 Other bacterial agents as the cause of diseases classified elsewhere

B97 Viral agents as the cause of diseases classified elsewhere

B99 Other and unspecified infectious diseases

CHAPTER 2: NEOPLASMS (C00-D49)

C00 Malignant neoplasm of lip

C01 Malignant neoplasm of base of tongue

C02 Malignant neoplasm of other and unspecified parts of tongue

C03 Malignant neoplasm of gum

C04 Malignant neoplasm of floor of mouth

C05 Malignant neoplasm of palate

C06 Malignant neoplasm of other and unspecified parts of mouth

C07 Malignant neoplasm of parotid gland

C08 Malignant neoplasm of other and unspecified major salivary glands

C09 Malignant neoplasm of tonsil

C10 Malignant neoplasm of oropharynx

C11 Malignant neoplasm of nasopharynx

C12 Malignant neoplasm of pyriform sinus

C13 Malignant neoplasm of hypopharynx

C14 Malignant neoplasm of other and ill-defined sites in the lip, oral cavity and pharynx

C15 Malignant neoplasm of esophagus

C16 Malignant neoplasm of stomach

C17 Malignant neoplasm of small intestine

C18 Malignant neoplasm of colon

C19 Malignant neoplasm of rectosigmoid junction

C20 Malignant neoplasm of rectum

C21 Malignant neoplasm of anus and anal canal

C22 Malignant neoplasm of liver and intrahepatic bile ducts

C23 Malignant neoplasm of gallbladder

C24 Malignant neoplasm of other and unspecified parts of biliary tract

C25 Malignant neoplasm of pancreas

C26 Malignant neoplasm of other and ill-defined digestive organs

C30 Malignant neoplasm of nasal cavity and middle ear

C31 Malignant neoplasm of accessory sinuses

C32 Malignant neoplasm of larynx

C33 Malignant neoplasm of trachea

C34 Malignant neoplasm of bronchus and lung

C37 Malignant neoplasm of thymus

C38 Malignant neoplasm of heart, mediastinum and pleura

C39 Malignant neoplasm of other and ill-defined sites in the respiratory system and intrathoracic organs

C40 Malignant neoplasm of bone and articular cartilage of limbs

C41 Malignant neoplasm of bone and articular cartilage of other and unspecified sites

C43 Malignant melanoma of skin

C44 Other and unspecified malignant neoplasm of skin

C45 Mesothelioma

C46 Kaposi's sarcoma

C47 Malignant neoplasm of peripheral nerves and autonomic nervous system

C48 Malignant neoplasm of retroperitoneum and peritoneum

C49 Malignant neoplasm of other connective and soft tissue

C4A Merkel cell carcinoma

C50 Malignant neoplasm of breast

C52 Malignant neoplasm of vagina

C53 Malignant neoplasm of cervix uteri

C54 Malignant neoplasm of corpus uteri

C55 Malignant neoplasm of uterus, part unspecified

C56 Malignant neoplasm of ovary

C57 Malignant neoplasm of other and unspecified female genital organs

C58 Malignant neoplasm of placenta

C60 Malignant neoplasm of penis

C61 Malignant neoplasm of prostate

C62 Malignant neoplasm of testis

C63 Malignant neoplasm of other and unspecified male genital organs

C64 Malignant neoplasm of kidney, except renal pelvis

C65 Malignant neoplasm of renal pelvis

C66 Malignant neoplasm of ureter

C67 Malignant neoplasm of bladder

C68 Malignant neoplasm of other and unspecified urinary organs

C69 Malignant neoplasm of eye and adnexa

C70 Malignant neoplasm of meninges

C71 Malignant neoplasm of brain

C72 Malignant neoplasm of spinal cord, cranial nerves and other parts of central nervous system

C73 Malignant neoplasm of thyroid gland

C74 Malignant neoplasm of adrenal gland

C75 Malignant neoplasm of other endocrine glands and related structures

C76 Malignant neoplasm of other and ill-defined sites

C77 Secondary and unspecified malignant neoplasm of lymph nodes

C78 Secondary malignant neoplasm of respiratory and digestive organs

C79 Secondary malignant neoplasm of other and unspecified sites

C7A Malignant neuroendocrine tumors

C7B Secondary neuroendocrine tumors

C80 Malignant neoplasm without specification of site

C81 Hodgkin lymphoma

C82 Follicular lymphoma

C83 Non-follicular lymphoma

C84 Mature T/NK-cell lymphomas

C85 Other specified and unspecified types of non-Hodgkin lymphoma

C86 Other specified types of T/NK-cell lymphoma

C88 Malignant immunoproliferative diseases and certain other B-cell lymphomas

C90 Multiple myeloma and malignant plasma cell neoplasms

C91 Lymphoid leukemia

C92 Myeloid leukemia

C93 Monocytic leukemia

C94 Other leukemias of specified cell type

C95 Leukemia of unspecified cell type

C96 Other and unspecified malignant neoplasms of lymphoid, hematopoietic and related tissue

D00 Carcinoma in situ of oral cavity, esophagus and stomach

D01 Carcinoma in situ of other and unspecified digestive organs

D02 Carcinoma in situ of middle ear and respiratory system

D03 Melanoma in situ

D04 Carcinoma in situ of skin

D05 Carcinoma in situ of breast

D06 Carcinoma in situ of cervix uteri

D07 Carcinoma in situ of other and unspecified genital organs

D09 Carcinoma in situ of other and unspecified sites

D10 Benign neoplasm of mouth and pharynx

D11 Benign neoplasm of major salivary glands

D12	Benign neoplasm of colon, rectum, anus and anal canal
D13	Benign neoplasm of other and ill-defined parts of digestive system
D14	Benign neoplasm of middle ear and respiratory system
D15	Benign neoplasm of other and unspecified intrathoracic organs
D16	Benign neoplasm of bone and articular cartilage
D17	Benign lipomatous neoplasm
D18	Hemangioma and lymphangioma, any site
D19	Benign neoplasm of mesothelial tissue
D20	Benign neoplasm of soft tissue of retroperitoneum and peritoneum
D21	Other benign neoplasms of connective and other soft tissue
D22	Melanocytic nevi
D23	Other benign neoplasms of skin
D24	Benign neoplasm of breast
D25	Leiomyoma of uterus
D26	Other benign neoplasms of uterus
D27	Benign neoplasm of ovary
D28	Benign neoplasm of other and unspecified female genital organs
D29	Benign neoplasm of male genital organs
D30	Benign neoplasm of urinary organs
D31	Benign neoplasm of eye and adnexa
D32	Benign neoplasm of meninges
D33	Benign neoplasm of brain and other parts of central nervous system
D34	Benign neoplasm of thyroid gland
D35	Benign neoplasm of other and unspecified endocrine glands
D36	Benign neoplasm of other and unspecified sites
D37	Neoplasm of uncertain behavior of oral cavity and digestive organs
D38	Neoplasm of uncertain behavior of middle ear and respiratory and intrathoracic organs
D39	Neoplasm of uncertain behavior of female genital organs
D3A	Benign carcinoid tumor of unspecified site
D40	Neoplasm of uncertain behavior of male genital organs
D41	Neoplasm of uncertain behavior of urinary organs
D42	Neoplasm of uncertain behavior of meninges
D43	Neoplasm of uncertain behavior of brain and central nervous system
D44	Neoplasm of uncertain behavior of endocrine glands
D45	Polycythemia vera
D46	Myelodysplastic syndromes
D47	Other neoplasms of uncertain behavior of lymphoid, hematopoietic and related tissue
D48	Neoplasm of uncertain behavior of other and unspecified sites
D49	Neoplasms of unspecified behavior

CHAPTER 3: DISEASES OF THE BLOOD AND BLOOD-FORMING ORGANS AND CERTAIN DISORDERS INVOLVING THE IMMUNE MECHANISM (D50-D89)

D50	Iron deficiency anemia
D51	Vitamin B12 deficiency anemia
D52	Folate deficiency anemia
D53	Other nutritional anemias
D55	Anemia due to enzyme disorders
D56	Thalassemia
D57	Sickle-cell disorders
D58	Other hereditary hemolytic anemias
D59	Acquired hemolytic anemia
D60	Acquired pure red cell aplasia [erythroblastopenia]
D61	Other aplastic anemias and other bone marrow failure syndromes
D62	Acute posthemorrhagic anemia
D63	Anemia in chronic diseases classified elsewhere
D64	Other anemias
D65	Disseminated intravascular coagulation [defibrination syndrome]
D66	Hereditary factor VIII deficiency
D67	Hereditary factor IX deficiency
D68	Other coagulation defects
D69	Purpura and other hemorrhagic conditions
D70	Neutropenia
D71	Functional disorders of polymorphonuclear neutrophils
D72	Other disorders of white blood cells
D73	Diseases of spleen
D74	Methemoglobinemia
D75	Other and unspecified diseases of blood and blood-forming organs
D76	Other specified diseases with participation of lymphoreticular and reticulohistiocytic tissue
D77	Other disorders of blood and blood-forming organs in diseases classified elsewhere
D78	Intraoperative and postprocedural complications of the spleen
D80	Immunodeficiency with predominantly antibody defects
D81	Combined immunodeficiencies
D82	Immunodeficiency associated with other major defects
D83	Common variable immunodeficiency
D84	Other immunodeficiencies
D86	Sarcoidosis
D89	Other disorders involving the immune mechanism, not elsewhere classified

CHAPTER 4: ENDOCRINE, NUTRITIONAL AND METABOLIC DISEASES (E00-E89)

E00	Congenital iodine-deficiency syndrome
E01	Iodine-deficiency related thyroid disorders and allied conditions
E02	Subclinical iodine-deficiency hypothyroidism
E03	Other hypothyroidism
E04	Other nontoxic goiter
E05	Thyrotoxicosis [hyperthyroidism]
E06	Thyroiditis
E07	Other disorders of thyroid
E08	Diabetes mellitus due to underlying condition
E09	Drug or chemical induced diabetes mellitus
E10	Type 1 diabetes mellitus
E11	Type 2 diabetes mellitus
E13	Other specified diabetes mellitus
E15	Nondiabetic hypoglycemic coma
E16	Other disorders of pancreatic internal secretion
E20	Hypoparathyroidism
E21	Hyperparathyroidism and other disorders of parathyroid gland
E22	Hyperfunction of pituitary gland
E23	Hypofunction and other disorders of the pituitary gland
E24	Cushing's syndrome
E25	Adrenogenital disorders
E26	Hyperaldosteronism
E27	Other disorders of adrenal gland
E28	Ovarian dysfunction
E29	Testicular dysfunction
E30	Disorders of puberty, not elsewhere classified
E31	Polyglandular dysfunction
E32	Diseases of thymus
E34	Other endocrine disorders
E35	Disorders of endocrine glands in diseases classified elsewhere
E36	Intraoperative complications of endocrine system
E40	Kwashiorkor
E41	Nutritional marasmus
E42	Marasmic kwashiorkor
E43	Unspecified severe protein-calorie malnutrition
E44	Protein-calorie malnutrition of moderate and mild degree
E45	Retarded development following protein-calorie malnutrition
E46	Unspecified protein-calorie malnutrition
E50	Vitamin A deficiency
E51	Thiamine deficiency
E52	Niacin deficiency [pellagra]
E53	Deficiency of other B group vitamins

E54 Ascorbic acid deficiency

E55 Vitamin D deficiency

E56 Other vitamin deficiencies

E58 Dietary calcium deficiency

E59 Dietary selenium deficiency

E60 Dietary zinc deficiency

E61 Deficiency of other nutrient elements

E63 Other nutritional deficiencies

E64 Sequelae of malnutrition and other nutritional deficiencies

E65 Localized adiposity

E66 Overweight and obesity

E67 Other hyperalimentation

E68 Sequelae of hyperalimentation

E70 Disorders of aromatic amino-acid metabolism

E71 Disorders of branched-chain amino-acid metabolism and fatty-acid metabolism

E72 Other disorders of amino-acid metabolism

E73 Lactose intolerance

E74 Other disorders of carbohydrate metabolism

E75 Disorders of sphingolipid metabolism and other lipid storage disorders

E76 Disorders of glycosaminoglycan metabolism

E77 Disorders of glycoprotein metabolism

E78 Disorders of lipoprotein metabolism and other lipidemias

E79 Disorders of purine and pyrimidine metabolism

E80 Disorders of porphyrin and bilirubin metabolism

E83 Disorders of mineral metabolism

E84 Cystic fibrosis

E85 Amyloidosis

E86 Volume depletion

E87 Other disorders of fluid, electrolyte and acid-base balance

E88 Other and unspecified metabolic disorders

E89 Postprocedural endocrine and metabolic complications and disorders, not elsewhere classified

CHAPTER 5: MENTAL, BEHAVIORAL AND NEURODEVELOPMENTAL DISORDERS (F01-F99)

F01 Vascular dementia

F02 Dementia in other diseases classified elsewhere

F03 Unspecified dementia

F04 Amnestic disorder due to known physiological condition

F05 Delirium due to known physiological condition

F06 Unspecified dementia

F07 Other mental disorders due to known physiological condition

F09 Personality and behavioral disorders due to known physiological condition

F10 Alcohol related disorders

F11 Opioid related disorders

F12 Cannabis related disorders

F13 Sedative, hypnotic, or anxiolytic related disorders

F14 Cocaine related disorders

F15 Other stimulant related disorders

F16 Hallucinogen related disorders

F17 Nicotine dependence

F18 Inhalant related disorders

F19 Other psychoactive substance related disorders

F21 Schizotypal disorder

F22 Delusional disorders

F23 Brief psychotic disorder

F24 Shared psychotic disorder

F25 Schizoaffective disorders

F28 Other psychotic disorder not due to a substance or known physiological condition

F29 Unspecified psychosis not due to a substance or known physiological condition

F30 Manic episode

F31 Bipolar disorder

F32 Major depressive disorder, single episode

F33 Major depressive disorder, recurrent

F34 Persistent mood [affective] disorders

F39 Unspecified mood [affective] disorder

F40 Phobic anxiety disorders

F41 Other anxiety disorders

F42 Obsessive-compulsive disorder

F43 Reaction to severe stress, and adjustment disorders

F44 Dissociative and conversion disorders

F45 Somatoform disorders

F48 Other nonpsychotic mental disorders

F50 Eating disorders

F51 Sleep disorders not due to a substance or known physiological condition

F52 Sexual dysfunction not due to a substance or known physiological condition

F53 Mental and behavioral disorders associated with the puerperium, not elsewhere classified

F54 Psychological and behavioral factors associated with disorders or diseases classified elsewhere

F55 Abuse of non-psychoactive substances

F59 Unspecified behavioral syndromes associated with physiological disturbances and physical factors

F60 Specific personality disorders

F63 Impulse disorders

F64 Gender identity disorders

F65 Paraphilias

F66 Other sexual disorders

F68 Other disorders of adult personality and behavior

F69 Unspecified disorder of adult personality and behavior

F70 Mild intellectual disabilities

F71 Moderate mental retardation

F72 Severe intellectual disabilities

F73 Profound intellectual disabilities

F78 Other intellectual disabilities

F79 Unspecified intellectual disabilities

F80 Specific developmental disorders of speech and language

F81 Specific developmental disorders of scholastic skills

F82 Specific developmental disorder of motor function

F84 Pervasive developmental disorders

F88 Other disorders of psychological development

F89 Unspecified disorder of psychological development

F90 Attention-deficit hyperactivity disorders

F91 Conduct disorders

F93 Emotional disorders with onset specific to childhood

F94 Disorders of social functioning with onset specific to childhood and adolescence

F95 Tic disorder

F98 Other behavioral and emotional disorders with onset usually occurring in childhood and adolescence

F99 Mental disorder not otherwise specified

CHAPTER 6: DISEASES OF THE NERVOUS SYSTEM (G00-G99)

G00 Bacterial meningitis, not elsewhere classified

G01 Meningitis in bacterial diseases classified elsewhere

G02 Meningitis in other infectious and parasitic diseases classified elsewhere

G03 Meningitis due to other and unspecified causes

G04 Encephalitis, myelitis and encephalomyelitis

G05 Encephalitis, myelitis and encephalomyelitis in diseases classified elsewhere

G06 Intracranial and intraspinal abscess and granuloma

G07 Intracranial and intraspinal abscess and granuloma in diseases classified elsewhere

G08 Intracranial and intraspinal phlebitis and thrombophlebitis

G09 Sequelae of inflammatory diseases of central nervous system

G10 Huntington's disease

G11 Hereditary ataxia

G12	Spinal muscular atrophy and related syndromes
G13	Systemic atrophies primarily affecting central nervous system in diseases classified elsewhere
G14	Postpolio syndrome
G20	Parkinson's disease
G21	Secondary parkinsonism
G23	Other degenerative diseases of basal ganglia
G24	Dystonia
G25	Other extrapyramidal and movement disorders
G26	Extrapyramidal and movement disorders in diseases classified elsewhere
G30	Alzheimer's disease
G31	Other degenerative diseases of nervous system, not elsewhere classified
G32	Other degenerative disorders of nervous system in diseases classified elsewhere
G35	Multiple sclerosis
G36	Other acute disseminated demyelination
G37	Other demyelinating diseases of central nervous system
G40	Epilepsy and recurrent seizures
G43	Migraine
G44	Other headache syndromes
G45	Transient cerebral ischemic attacks and related syndromes
G46	Vascular syndromes of brain in cerebrovascular diseases
G47	Sleep disorders
G50	Disorders of trigeminal nerve
G51	Facial nerve disorders
G52	Disorders of other cranial nerves
G53	Cranial nerve disorders in diseases classified elsewhere
G54	Nerve root and plexus disorders
G55	Mononeuropathies of upper limb
G56	Mononeuropathies of lower limb
G57	Mononeuropathy in diseases classified elsewhere
G58	Other mononeuropathies
G59	Hereditary and idiopathic neuropathy
G60	Disorders of trigeminal nerve
G61	Inflammatory polyneuropathy
G62	Other and unspecified polyneuropathies
G63	Polyneuropathy in diseases classified elsewhere
G64	Other disorders of peripheral nervous system
G65	Sequelae of inflammatory and toxic polyneuropathies
G70	Myasthenia gravis and other myoneural disorders
G71	Primary disorders of muscles
G72	Other and unspecified myopathies
G73	Malignant neoplasm of thyroid gland
G80	Cerebral palsy
G81	Hemiplegia and hemiparesis

G82	Paraplegia (paraparesis) and quadriplegia (quadriparesis)
G83	Other paralytic syndromes
G89	Pain, not elsewhere classified
G90	Disorders of autonomic nervous system
G91	Hydrocephalus
G92	Toxic encephalopathy
G93	Other disorders of brain
G94	Other disorders of brain in diseases classified elsewhere
G95	Other and unspecified diseases of spinal cord
G96	Other disorders of central nervous system
G97	Intraoperative and postprocedural complications and disorders of nervous system, not elsewhere classified
G98	Other disorders of nervous system not elsewhere classified
G99	Other disorders of nervous system in diseases classified elsewhere

CHAPTER 7: DISEASES OF THE EYE AND ADNEXA (H00-H59)

H00	Hordeolum and chalazion
H01	Other inflammation of eyelid
H02	Other disorders of eyelid
H04	Disorders of lacrimal system
H05	Disorders of orbit
H10	Conjunctivitis
H11	Other disorders of conjunctiva
H15	Disorders of sclera
H16	Keratitis
H17	Corneal scars and opacities
H18	Other disorders of cornea
H20	Iridocyclitis
H21	Other disorders of iris and ciliary body
H22	Disorders of iris and ciliary body in diseases classified elsewhere
H25	Age-related cataract
H26	Other cataract
H27	Other disorders of lens
H28	Cataract in diseases classified elsewhere
H30	Chorioretinal inflammation
H31	Other disorders of choroid
H32	Chorioretinal disorders in diseases classified elsewhere
H33	Retinal detachments and breaks
H34	Retinal vascular occlusions
H35	Other retinal disorders
H36	Retinal disorders in diseases classified elsewhere
H40	Glaucoma
H42	Glaucoma in diseases classified elsewhere
H43	Disorders of vitreous body
H44	Disorders of globe
H46	Optic neuritis

H47	Other disorders of optic [2nd] nerve and visual pathways
H49	Paralytic strabismus
H50	Other strabismus
H51	Other disorders of binocular movement
H52	Disorders of refraction and accommodation
H53	Visual disturbances
H54	Blindness and low vision
H55	Nystagmus and other irregular eye movements
H57	Other disorders of eye and adnexa
H59	Intraoperative and postprocedural complications and disorders of eye and adnexa, not elsewhere classified

CHAPTER 8: DISEASES OF THE EAR AND MASTOID PROCESS (H60-H95)

H60	Otitis externa
H61	Other disorders of external ear
H62	Disorders of external ear in diseases classified elsewhere
H65	Nonsuppurative otitis media
H66	Suppurative and unspecified otitis media
H67	Otitis media in diseases classified elsewhere
H68	Eustachian salpingitis and obstruction
H69	Other and unspecified disorders of Eustachian tube
H70	Mastoiditis and related conditions
H71	Cholesteatoma of middle ear
H72	Perforation of tympanic membrane
H73	Other disorders of tympanic membrane
H74	Other disorders of middle ear mastoid
H75	Other disorders of middle ear and mastoid in diseases classified elsewhere
H80	Otosclerosis
H81	Disorders of vestibular function
H82	Vertiginous syndromes in diseases classified elsewhere
H83	Other diseases of inner ear
H90	Conductive and sensorineural hearing loss
H91	Other and unspecified hearing loss
H92	Otalgia and effusion of ear
H93	Other disorders of ear, not elsewhere classified
H94	Other disorders of ear in diseases classified elsewhere
H95	Intraoperative and postprocedural complications and disorders of ear and mastoid process, not elsewhere classified

CHAPTER 9: DISEASES OF THE CIRCULATORY SYSTEM (I00-I99)

I00	Rheumatic fever without heart involvement
I01	Rheumatic fever with heart involvement

I02 Rheumatic chorea

I05 Rheumatic mitral valve diseases

I06 Rheumatic aortic valve diseases

I07 Rheumatic tricuspid valve diseases

I08 Multiple valve diseases

I09 Other rheumatic heart diseases

I10 Essential (primary) hypertension

I11 Hypertensive heart disease

I12 Hypertensive chronic kidney disease

I13 Hypertensive heart and chronic kidney disease

I15 Secondary hypertension

I16 Hypertensive crisis

I20 Angina pectoris

I21 Acute myocardial infarction

I22 Subsequent ST elevation (STEMI) and non-ST elevation (NSTEMI) myocardial infarction

I23 Certain current complications following ST elevation (STEMI) and non-ST elevation (NSTEMI) myocardial infarction (within the 28 day period)

I24 Other acute ischemic heart diseases

I25 Chronic ischemic heart disease

I26 Pulmonary embolism

I27 Other pulmonary heart diseases

I28 Other diseases of pulmonary vessels

I30 Acute pericarditis

I31 Other diseases of pericardium

I32 Pericarditis in diseases classified elsewhere

I33 Acute and subacute endocarditis

I34 Nonrheumatic mitral valve disorders

I35 Nonrheumatic aortic valve disorders

I36 Nonrheumatic tricuspid valve disorders

I37 Nonrheumatic pulmonary valve disorders

I38 Endocarditis, valve unspecified

I39 Endocarditis and heart valve disorders in diseases classified elsewhere

I40 Acute myocarditis

I41 Myocarditis in diseases classified elsewhere

I42 Cardiomyopathy

I43 Cardiomyopathy in diseases classified elsewhere

I44 Atrioventricular and left bundle-branch block

I45 Other conduction disorders

I46 Cardiac arrest

I47 Paroxysmal tachycardia

I48 Atrial fibrillation and flutter

I49 Other cardiac arrhythmias

I50 Heart failure

I51 Complications and ill-defined descriptions of heart disease

I52 Other heart disorders in diseases classified elsewhere

I60 Nontraumatic subarachnoid hemorrhage

I61 Nontraumatic intracerebral hemorrhage

I62 Other and unspecified nontraumatic intracranial hemorrhage

I63 Cerebral infarction

I65 Occlusion and stenosis of precerebral arteries, not resulting in cerebral infarction

I66 Occlusion and stenosis of cerebral arteries, not resulting in cerebral infarction

I67 Other cerebrovascular diseases

I68 Cerebrovascular disorders in diseases classified elsewhere

I69 Sequelae of cerebrovascular disease

I70 Atherosclerosis

I71 Aortic aneurysm and dissection

I72 Other aneurysm

I73 Other peripheral vascular diseases

I74 Arterial embolism and thrombosis

I75 Atheroembolism

I76 Other disorders of arteries and arterioles

I77 Diseases of capillaries

I78 Disorders of arteries, arterioles and capillaries in diseases classified elsewhere

I79 Disorders of arteries, arterioles and capillaries in diseases classified elsewhere

I80 Phlebitis and thrombophlebitis

I81 Portal vein thrombosis

I82 Other venous embolism and thrombosis

I83 Varicose veins of lower extremities

I84 Unspecified thrombosed hemorrhoids

I85 Esophageal varices

I86 Varicose veins of other sites

I87 Other disorders of veins

I88 Nonspecific lymphadenitis

I89 Other noninfective disorders of lymphatic vessels and lymph nodes

I95 Hypotension

I96 Gangrene, not elsewhere classified

I97 Intraoperative and postprocedural complications and disorders of circulatory system, not elsewhere classified

I99 Other and unspecified disorders of circulatory system

CHAPTER 10: DISEASES OF THE RESPIRATORY SYSTEM (J00-J99)

J00 Acute nasopharyngitis [common cold]

J01 Acute sinusitis

J02 Acute nasopharyngitis [common cold]

J03 Acute tonsillitis

J04 Acute laryngitis and tracheitis

J05 Acute obstructive laryngitis [croup] and epiglottitis

J06 Acute upper respiratory infections of multiple and unspecified sites

J09 Influenza due to certain identified influenza viruses

J10 Influenza due to other identified influenza virus

J12 Viral pneumonia, not elsewhere classified

J13 Pneumonia due to Streptococcus pneumoniae

J14 Pneumonia due to Hemophilus influenzae

J15 Bacterial pneumonia, not elsewhere classified

J16 Pneumonia due to other infectious organisms, not elsewhere classified

J17 Pneumonia in diseases classified elsewhere

J18 Pneumonia, unspecified organism

J20 Acute bronchitis

J21 Acute bronchiolitis

J22 Unspecified acute lower respiratory infection

J30 Vasomotor and allergic rhinitis

J31 Chronic rhinitis, nasopharyngitis and pharyngitis

J32 Chronic sinusitis

J33 Nasal polyp

J34 Other and unspecified disorders of nose and nasal sinuses

J35 Chronic diseases of tonsils and adenoids

J36 Peritonsillar abscess

J37 Chronic laryngitis and laryngotracheitis

J38 Diseases of vocal cords and larynx, not elsewhere classified

J39 Other diseases of upper respiratory tract

J40 Bronchitis, not specified as acute or chronic

J41 Simple and mucopurulent chronic bronchitis

J42 Unspecified chronic bronchitis

J43 Emphysema

J44 Other chronic obstructive pulmonary disease

J45 Asthma

J47 Bronchiectasis

J60 Coalworker's pneumoconiosis

J61 Pneumoconiosis due to asbestos and other mineral fibers

J62 Pneumoconiosis due to dust containing silica

J63 Pneumoconiosis due to other inorganic dusts

J64 Unspecified pneumoconiosis

J65 Pneumoconiosis associated with tuberculosis

J66 Airway disease due to specific organic dust

J67 Hypersensitivity pneumonitis due to organic dust

J68 Respiratory conditions due to inhalation of chemicals, gases, fumes and vapors

J69 Pneumonitis due to solids and liquids

J70 Respiratory conditions due to other external agents

J80	Acute respiratory distress syndrome	**K40**	Inguinal hernia	**L01**	Impetigo
J81	Pulmonary edema	**K41**	Femoral hernia	**L02**	Cutaneous abscess, furuncle and carbuncle
J82	Pulmonary eosinophilia, not elsewhere classified	**K42**	Umbilical hernia	**L03**	Cellulitis and acute lymphangitis
J84	Other interstitial pulmonary diseases	**K43**	Ventral hernia	**L04**	Acute lymphadenitis
J85	Abscess of lung and mediastinum	**K44**	Diaphragmatic hernia	**L05**	Pilonidal cyst and sinus
J86	Pyothorax	**K45**	Other abdominal hernia	**L08**	Other local infections of skin and subcutaneous tissue
J90	Pleural effusion, not elsewhere classified	**K46**	Unspecified abdominal hernia	**L08**	Other specified local infections of the skin and subcutaneous tissue
J91	Pleural effusion in conditions classified elsewhere	**K50**	Crohn's disease [regional enteritis]	**L10**	Pemphigus
J92	Pleural plaque	**K51**	Ulcerative colitis	**L11**	Other acantholytic disorders
J93	Pneumothorax and air leak	**K52**	Other and unspecified noninfective gastroenteritis and colitis	**L12**	Pemphigoid
J94	Other pleural conditions	**K55**	Vascular disorders of intestine	**L13**	Other bullous disorders
J95	Intraoperative and postprocedural complications and disorders of respiratory system, not elsewhere classified	**K56**	Paralytic ileus and intestinal obstruction without hernia	**L14**	Bullous disorders in diseases classified elsewhere
		K57	Diverticular disease of intestine	**L20**	Atopic dermatitis
J96	Respiratory failure, not elsewhere classified	**K58**	Irritable bowel syndrome	**L21**	Seborrheic dermatitis
J98	Other respiratory disorders	**K59**	Fissure and fistula of anal and rectal regions	**L22**	Diaper dermatitis
J99	Respiratory disorders in diseases classified elsewhere	**K60**	Abscess of anal and rectal regions	**L23**	Allergic contact dermatitis
		K61	Other diseases of anus and rectum	**L24**	Irritant contact dermatitis
		K62	Other diseases of intestine	**L25**	Unspecified contact dermatitis
		K63	Hemorrhoids and perianal venous thrombosis	**L26**	Exfoliative dermatitis
		K65	Peritonitis	**L27**	Dermatitis due to substances taken internally

CHAPTER 11: DISEASES OF THE DIGESTIVE SYSTEM (K00-K95)

K00	Disorders of tooth development and eruption	**K66**	Other disorders of peritoneum	**L28**	Lichen simplex chronicus and prurigo
		K67	Disorders of peritoneum in infectious diseases classified elsewhere	**L29**	Pruritus
K01	Embedded and impacted teeth	**K68**	Disorders of retroperitoneum	**L30**	Other and unspecified dermatitis
K02	Dental caries	**K70**	Alcoholic liver disease	**L40**	Psoriasis
K03	Other diseases of hard tissues of teeth	**K71**	Toxic liver disease	**L41**	Parapsoriasis
K04	Diseases of pulp and periapical tissues	**K72**	Hepatic failure, not elsewhere classified	**L42**	Pityriasis rosea
K05	Gingivitis and periodontal diseases	**K73**	Chronic hepatitis, not elsewhere classified	**L43**	Lichen planus
K06	Other disorders of gingiva and edentulous alveolar ridge	**K74**	Fibrosis and cirrhosis of liver	**L44**	Other papulosquamous disorders
		K75	Other inflammatory liver diseases	**L45**	Papulosquamous disorders in diseases classified elsewhere
K08	Other disorders of teeth and supporting structures	**K76**	Other diseases of liver		
K09	Cysts of oral region, not elsewhere classified	**K77**	Liver disorders in diseases classified elsewhere	**L49**	Exfoliation due to erythematous conditions according to extent of body surface involved
K11	Diseases of salivary glands	**K80**	Cholelithiasis	**L50**	Urticaria
K12	Stomatitis and related lesions	**K81**	Cholecystitis	**L51**	Erythema multiforme
K13	Other diseases of lip and oral mucosa	**K82**	Other diseases of gallbladder	**L52**	Erythema nodosum
K14	Diseases of tongue	**K83**	Other diseases of biliary tract	**L53**	Other erythematous conditions
K20	Esophagitis	**K85**	Acute pancreatitis	**L54**	Erythema in diseases classified elsewhere
K21	Gastro-esophageal reflux disease	**K86**	Other diseases of pancreas		
K22	Other diseases of esophagus	**K87**	Disorders of gallbladder biliary tract and pancreas in diseases classified elsewhere	**L55**	Sunburn
K23	Disorders of esophagus in diseases classified elsewhere	**K90**	Intestinal malabsorption	**L56**	Other acute skin changes due to ultraviolet radiation
K25	Gastric ulcer	**K91**	Intraoperative and postprocedural complications and disorders of digestive system, not elsewhere classified	**L57**	Skin changes due to chronic exposure to nonionizing radiation
K26	Duodenal ulcer			**L58**	Radiodermatitis
K27	Peptic ulcer, site unspecified	**K92**	Other diseases of digestive system	**L59**	Other disorders of skin and subcutaneous tissue related to radiation
K28	Gastrojejunal ulcer	**K94**	Complications of artificial openings of the digestive system		
K29	Gastritis and duodenitis	**K95**	Complications of bariatric procedures	**L60**	Nail disorders
K30	Functional dyspepsia			**L62**	Nail disorders in diseases classified elsewhere
K31	Other diseases of stomach and duodenum				
K35	Acute appendicitis			**L63**	Alopecia areata
K36	Other appendicitis	**CHAPTER 12: DISEASES OF THE SKIN AND SUBCUTANEOUS TISSUE (L00-L99)**		**L64**	Androgenic alopecia
K37	Unspecified appendicitis			**L65**	Other nonscarring hair loss
K38	Other diseases of appendix	**L00**	Staphylococcal scalded skin syndrome	**L66**	Cicatricial alopecia [scarring hair loss]

L67 Hair color and hair shaft abnormalities

L68 Hypertrichosis

L70 Acne

L71 Rosacea

L72 Follicular cysts of skin and subcutaneous tissue

L73 Other follicular disorders

L74 Eccrine sweat disorders

L75 Apocrine sweat disorders

L76 Intraoperative and postprocedural complications of skin and subcutaneous tissue

L80 Vitiligo

L81 Other disorders of pigmentation

L82 Seborrheic keratosis

L83 Acanthosis nigricans

L84 Corns and callosities

L85 Other epidermal thickening

L86 Keratoderma in diseases classified elsewhere

L87 Transepidermal elimination disorders

L88 Pyoderma gangrenosum

L89 Pressure ulcer

L90 Atrophic disorders of skin

L91 Hypertrophic disorders of skin

L92 Granulomatous disorders of skin and subcutaneous tissue

L93 Lupus erythematosus

L94 Other localized connective tissue disorders

L95 Vasculitis limited to skin, not elsewhere classified

L97 Non-pressure chronic ulcer of lower limb, not elsewhere classified

L98 Other disorders of skin and subcutaneous tissue, not elsewhere classified

L99 Other disorders of skin and subcutaneous tissue in diseases classified elsewhere

CHAPTER 13: DISEASES OF THE MUSCULOSKELETAL SYSTEM AND CONNECTIVE TISSUE (M00-M99)

M00 Pyogenic arthritis

M01 Direct infections of joint in infectious and parasitic diseases classified elsewhere

M02 Postinfective and reactive arthropathies

M04 Autoinflammatory syndromes

M05 Rheumatoid arthritis with rheumatoid factor

M06 Other rheumatoid arthritis

M07 Enteropathic arthropathies

M08 Juvenile arthritis

M10 Idiopathic gout unspecified site

M11 Other crystal arthropathies

M12 Other and unspecified arthropathy

M13 Other arthritis

M14 Arthropathies in other diseases classified elsewhere

M15 Polyosteoarthritis

M16 Osteoarthritis of hip

M17 Osteoarthritis of knee

M18 Osteoarthritis of first carpometacarpal joint

M19 Other and unspecified osteoarthritis

M1A Idiopathic chronic gout unspecified site without tophus (tophi)

M20 Acquired deformities of fingers and toes

M21 Other acquired deformities of limbs

M22 Disorder of patella

M23 Internal derangement of knee

M24 Other specific joint derangements

M25 Other joint disorder, not elsewhere classified

M26 Dentofacial anomalies [including malocclusion]

M27 Other diseases of jaws

M30 Polyarteritis nodosa and related conditions

M31 Other necrotizing vasculopathies

M32 Systemic lupus erythematosus (SLE)

M33 Dermatopolymyositis

M34 Systemic sclerosis [scleroderma]

M35 Other systemic involvement of connective tissue

M36 Systemic disorders of connective tissue in diseases classified elsewhere

M40 Kyphosis and lordosis

M41 Scoliosis

M42 Spinal osteochondrosis

M43 Other deforming dorsopathies

M45 Ankylosing spondylitis

M46 Other inflammatory spondylopathies

M47 Spondylosis

M48 Other spondylopathies

M49 Spondylopathies in diseases classified elsewhere

M50 Cervical disc disorders

M51 Thoracic, thoracolumbar, and lumbosacral intervertebral disc disorders

M53 Other and unspecified dorsopathies, not elsewhere classified

M54 Dorsalgia

M60 Myositis

M61 Calcification and ossification of muscle

M62 Other disorders of muscle

M63 Disorders of muscle in diseases classified elsewhere

M65 Synovitis and tenosynovitis

M66 Spontaneous rupture of synovium and tendon

M67 Other disorders of synovium and tendon

M70 Soft tissue disorders related to use, overuse and pressure

M71 Other bursopathies

M72 Fibroblastic disorders

M75 Shoulder lesions

M76 Enthesopathies, lower limb, excluding foot

M77 Other enthesopathies

M79 Other and unspecified soft tissue disorders, not elsewhere classified

M80 Osteoporosis with current pathological fracture

M81 Osteoporosis without current pathological fracture

M83 Puerperal osteomalacia

M84 Disorder of continuity of bone

M85 Other disorders of bone density and structure

M86 Osteomyelitis

M87 Osteonecrosis

M88 Osteitis deformans [Paget's disease of bone]

M89 Other disorders of bone

M90 Osteopathies in diseases classified elsewhere

M91 Juvenile osteochondrosis of hip and pelvis

M92 Other juvenile osteochondrosis

M93 Other osteochondropathies

M94 Other disorders of cartilage

M95 Other acquired deformities of musculoskeletal system and connective tissue

M96 Intraoperative and postprocedural complications and disorders of musculoskeletal system, not elsewhere classified

M97 Periprosthetic fracture around internal prosthetic joint

M99 Biomechanical lesions, not elsewhere classified

CHAPTER 14: DISEASES OF THE GENITOURINARY SYSTEM (N00-N99)

N00 Acute nephritic syndrome

N01 Rapidly progressive nephritic syndrome

N02 Recurrent and persistent hematuria

N03 Chronic nephritic syndrome

N04 Nephrotic syndrome

N05 Unspecified nephritic syndrome

N06 Isolated proteinuria with specified morphological lesion

N07 Hereditary nephropathy, not elsewhere classified

N08 Glomerular disorders in diseases classified elsewhere

N10 Acute tubulointerstitial nephritis

N11 Chronic tubulointerstitial nephritis

N12 Tubulo-interstitial nephritis not specified as acute or chronic

N13 Obstructive and reflux uropathy

N14 Drug- and heavy-metal-induced tubulointerstitial and tubular conditions

N15 Other renal tubulointerstitial diseases

N16	Renal tubulointerstitial disorders in diseases classified elsewhere	**N74**	Female pelvic inflammatory disorders in diseases classified elsewhere	**O11**	Pre-existing hypertension with pre-eclampsia
N17	Acute kidney failure	**N75**	Diseases of Bartholin's gland	**O12**	Gestational [pregnancy-induced] edema and proteinuria without hypertension
N18	Chronic kidney disease (CKD)	**N76**	Other inflammation of vagina and vulva		
N19	Unspecified kidney failure	**N77**	Vulvovaginal ulceration and inflammation in diseases classified elsewhere	**O13**	Gestational [pregnancy-induced] hypertension without significant proteinuria
N20	Calculus of kidney and ureter				
N21	Calculus of lower urinary tract	**N80**	Endometriosis	**O14**	Pre-eclampsia
N22	Calculus of urinary tract in diseases classified elsewhere	**N81**	Female genital prolapse	**O15**	Eclampsia
		N82	Fistulae involving female genital tract	**O16**	Unspecified maternal hypertension
N23	Unspecified renal colic	**N83**	Noninflammatory disorders of ovary, fallopian tube and broad ligament	**O20**	Hemorrhage in early pregnancy
N25	Disorders resulting from impaired renal tubular function			**O21**	Excessive vomiting in pregnancy
		N84	Polyp of female genital tract	**O22**	Venous complications and hemorrhoids in pregnancy
N26	Unspecified contracted kidney	**N85**	Other noninflammatory disorders of uterus, except cervix		
N27	Small kidney of unknown cause			**O23**	Infections of genitourinary tract in pregnancy
N28	Other disorders of kidney and ureter, not elsewhere classified	**N86**	Erosion and ectropion of cervix uteri		
		N87	Dysplasia of cervix uteri	**O24**	Diabetes mellitus in pregnancy, childbirth, and the puerperium
N29	Other disorders of kidney and ureter in diseases classified elsewhere	**N88**	Other noninflammatory disorders of cervix uteri		
				O25	Malnutrition in pregnancy, childbirth and the puerperium
N30	Cystitis	**N89**	Other noninflammatory disorders of vagina		
N31	Neuromuscular dysfunction of bladder, not elsewhere classified			**O26**	Maternal care for other conditions predominantly related to pregnancy
		N90	Other noninflammatory disorders of vulva and perineum		
N32	Other disorders of bladder			**O28**	Abnormal findings on antenatal screening of mother
N34	Urethritis and urethral syndrome	**N91**	Absent, scanty and rare menstruation		
N35	Urethral stricture	**N92**	Excessive, frequent and irregular menstruation	**O29**	Complications of anesthesia during pregnancy
N36	Other disorders of urethra				
N37	Urethral disorders in diseases classified elsewhere	**N93**	Other abnormal uterine and vaginal bleeding	**O30**	Multiple gestation
				O31	Complications specific to multiple gestation
N39	Other disorders of urinary system	**N94**	Pain and other conditions associated with female genital organs and menstrual cycle		
N40	Enlarged prostate			**O32**	Maternal care for malpresentation of fetus
N41	Inflammatory diseases of prostate				
N42	Other and unspecified disorders of prostate	**N95**	Menopausal and other perimenopausal disorders	**O33**	Maternal care for disproportion
				O34	Maternal care for abnormality of pelvic organs
N43	Hydrocele and spermatocele	**N96**	Recurrent pregnancy loss		
N44	Noninflammatory disorders of testis	**N97**	Female infertility	**O35**	Maternal care for known or suspected fetal abnormality and damage
N45	Orchitis and epididymitis	**N98**	Complications associated with artificial fertilization		
N46	Male infertility			**O36**	Maternal care for other fetal problems
N47	Disorders of prepuce	**N99**	Intraoperative and postprocedural complications and disorders of genitourinary system, not elsewhere classified	**O40**	Polyhydramnios
N48	Other disorders of penis			**O41**	Other disorders of amniotic fluid and membranes
N49	Inflammatory disorders of male genital organs, not elsewhere classified				
				O42	Premature rupture of membranes
N50	Other and unspecified disorders of male genital organs	**CHAPTER 15: PREGNANCY, CHILDBIRTH AND THE PUERPERIUM (O00-O9A)**		**O43**	Placental disorders
				O44	Placenta previa
N51	Disorders of male genital organs in diseases classified elsewhere			**O45**	Premature separation of placenta [abruptio placentae]
		O00	Ectopic pregnancy		
N52	Male erectile dysfunction	**O00**	Anencephaly and similar malformations	**O46**	Antepartum hemorrhage, not elsewhere classified
N53	Other male sexual dysfunction	**O01**	Hydatidiform mole		
N60	Benign mammary dysplasia	**O02**	Other abnormal products of conception	**O47**	False labor
N61	Inflammatory disorders of breast	**O03**	Spontaneous abortion	**O48**	Late pregnancy
N62	Hypertrophy of breast	**O04**	Complications following (induced) termination of pregnancy	**O60**	Preterm labor
N63	Unspecified lump in breast			**O61**	Failed induction of labor
N64	Other disorders of breast	**O07**	Failed attempted termination of pregnancy	**O62**	Abnormalities of forces of labor
N65	Deformity and disproportion of reconstructed breast			**O63**	Long labor
		O07	Other congenital malformations of nervous system	**O64**	Obstructed labor due to malposition and malpresentation of fetus
N70	Salpingitis and oophoritis				
N71	Acute inflammatory disease of uterus	**O08**	Complications following ectopic and molar pregnancy	**O65**	Obstructed labor due to maternal pelvic abnormality
N72	Inflammatory disease of cervix uteri				
N73	Other female pelvic inflammatory diseases	**O09**	Supervision of high risk pregnancy	**O66**	Other obstructed labor
		O10	Pre-existing hypertension complicating pregnancy, childbirth and the puerperium	**O67**	Labor and delivery complicated by intrapartum hemorrhage, not elsewhere classified

O68 Labor and delivery complicated by abnormality of fetal acid-base balance

O69 Labor and delivery complicated by umbilical cord complications

O70 Perineal laceration during delivery

O71 Other obstetric trauma

O72 Postpartum hemorrhage

O73 Retained placenta and membranes, without hemorrhage

O74 Complications of anesthesia during labor and delivery

O75 Other complications of labor and delivery, not elsewhere classified

O76 Abnormality in fetal heart rate and rhythm complicating labor and delivery

O77 Other fetal stress complicating labor and delivery

O80 Encounter for full-term uncomplicated delivery

O82 Encounter for cesarean delivery without indication

O85 Puerperal sepsis

O86 Other puerperal infections

O87 Venous complications and hemorrhoids in the puerperium

O88 Obstetric embolism

O89 Complications of anesthesia during the puerperium

O90 Complications of the puerperium, not elsewhere classified

O91 Infections of breast associated with pregnancy, the puerperium and lactation

O92 Other disorders of breast and disorders of lactation associated with pregnancy and the puerperium

O94 Sequelae of complication of pregnancy, childbirth, and the puerperium

O98 Maternal infectious and parasitic diseases classifiable elsewhere but complicating pregnancy, childbirth and the puerperium

O99 Other maternal diseases classifiable elsewhere but complicating pregnancy, childbirth and the puerperium

O9A Maternal malignant neoplasms, traumatic injuries and abuse classifiable elsewhere but complicating pregnancy, childbirth and the puerperium

CHAPTER 16: CERTAIN CONDITIONS ORIGINATING IN THE PERINATAL PERIOD (P00-P96)

P00 Newborn (suspected to be) affected by maternal conditions that may be unrelated to present pregnancy

P01 Newborn (suspected to be) affected by maternal complications of pregnancy

P02 Newborn (suspected to be) affected by complications of placenta, cord and membranes

P03 Newborn (suspected to be) affected by other complications of labor and delivery

P04 Newborn (suspected to be) affected by noxious substances transmitted via placenta or breast milk

P05 Disorders of newborn related to slow fetal growth and fetal malnutrition

P07 Disorders of newborn related to short gestation and low birth weight, not elsewhere classified

P08 Disorders of newborn related to long gestation and high birth weight

P09 Abnormal findings on neonatal screening

P10 Intracranial laceration and hemorrhage due to birth injury

P11 Other birth injuries to central nervous system

P12 Birth injury to scalp

P13 Birth injury to skeleton

P14 Birth injury to peripheral nervous system

P15 Other birth injuries

P19 Metabolic acidemia in newborn

P22 Respiratory distress of newborn

P23 Congenital pneumonia

P24 Neonatal aspiration

P25 Interstitial emphysema and related conditions originating in the perinatal period

P26 Pulmonary hemorrhage originating in the perinatal period

P27 Chronic respiratory disease originating in the perinatal period

P28 Other respiratory conditions originating in the perinatal period

P29 Cardiovascular disorders originating in the perinatal period

P35 Congenital viral diseases

P36 Bacterial sepsis of newborn

P37 Other congenital infectious and parasitic diseases

P38 Omphalitis of newborn

P39 Other infections specific to the perinatal period

P50 Newborn affected by intrauterine (fetal) blood loss

P51 Umbilical hemorrhage of newborn

P52 Intracranial nontraumatic hemorrhage of newborn

P53 Hemorrhagic disease of newborn

P54 Other neonatal hemorrhages

P55 Hemolytic disease of newborn

P56 Hydrops fetalis due to hemolytic disease

P57 Kernicterus

P58 Neonatal jaundice due to other excessive hemolysis

P59 Neonatal jaundice from other and unspecified causes

P60 Disseminated intravascular coagulation of newborn

P61 Other perinatal hematological disorders

P70 Transitory disorders of carbohydrate metabolism specific to newborn

P71 Transitory neonatal disorders of calcium and magnesium metabolism

P72 Other transitory neonatal endocrine disorders

P74 Other transitory neonatal electrolyte and metabolic disturbances

P76 Other intestinal obstruction of newborn

P77 Necrotizing enterocolitis of newborn

P78 Other perinatal digestive system disorders

P80 Hypothermia of newborn

P81 Other disturbances of temperature regulation of newborn

P83 Other conditions of integument specific to newborn

P84 Other problems with newborn

P90 Convulsions of newborn

P91 Other disturbances of cerebral status of newborn

P92 Feeding problems of newborn

P93 Reactions and intoxications due to drugs administered to newborn

P94 Disorders of muscle tone of newborn

P95 Stillbirth

P96 Other conditions originating in the perinatal period

CHAPTER 17: CONGENITAL MALFORMATIONS, DEFORMATIONS AND CHROMOSOMAL ABNORMALITIES (Q00-Q99)

Q01 Encephalocele

Q02 Microcephaly

Q03 Congenital hydrocephalus

Q04 Other congenital malformations of brain

Q05 Spina bifida

Q06 Other congenital malformations of spinal cord

Q10 Congenital malformations of eyelid, lacrimal apparatus and orbit

Q11 Anophthalmos, microphthalmos and macrophthalmos

Q12 Congenital lens malformations

Q13 Congenital malformations of anterior segment of eye

Q14 Congenital malformations of posterior segment of eye

Q15 Other congenital malformations of eye

Q16 Congenital malformations of ear causing impairment of hearing

Q17 Other congenital malformations of ear

Q18 Other congenital malformations of face and neck

Q20 Congenital malformations of cardiac chambers and connections

Q21 Congenital malformations of cardiac septa

Q22 Congenital malformations of pulmonary and tricuspid valves

Q23 Congenital malformations of aortic and mitral valves

Q24 Other congenital malformations of heart

Q25	Congenital malformations of great arteries	Q71	Reduction defects of upper limb	R10	Abdominal and pelvic pain
Q26	Congenital malformations of great veins	Q72	Reduction defects of lower limb	R11	Nausea and vomiting
Q27	Other congenital malformations of peripheral vascular system	Q73	Reduction defects of unspecified limb	R12	Heartburn
		Q74	Other congenital malformations of limb(s)	R13	Aphagia and dysphagia
Q28	Other congenital malformations of circulatory system			R14	Flatulence and related conditions
		Q75	Other congenital malformations of skull and face bones	R15	Fecal incontinence
Q30	Congenital malformations of nose			R16	Hepatomegaly and splenomegaly, not elsewhere classified
Q31	Congenital malformations of larynx	Q76	Congenital malformations of spine and bony thorax		
Q32	Congenital malformations of trachea and bronchus	Q77	Osteochondrodysplasia with defects of growth of tubular bones and spine	R17	Unspecified jaundice
				R18	Ascites
Q33	Congenital malformations of lung	Q78	Other osteochondrodysplasias	R19	Other symptoms and signs involving the digestive system and abdomen
Q34	Other congenital malformations of respiratory system	Q79	Congenital malformations of musculoskeletal system, not elsewhere classified		
Q35	Cleft palate			R20	Disturbances of skin sensation
Q36	Cleft lip	Q80	Congenital ichthyosis	R21	Rash and other nonspecific skin eruption
Q37	Cleft palate with cleft lip	Q81	Epidermolysis bullosa	R22	Localized swelling, mass and lump of skin and subcutaneous tissue
Q38	Other congenital malformations of tongue, mouth and pharynx	Q82	Other congenital malformations of skin		
		Q83	Congenital malformations of breast	R23	Other skin changes
Q39	Congenital malformations of esophagus	Q84	Other congenital malformations of integument	R25	Abnormal involuntary movements
Q40	Other congenital malformations of upper alimentary tract			R26	Abnormalities of gait and mobility
		Q85	Phakomatoses, not elsewhere classified	R27	Other lack of coordination
Q41	Congenital absence, atresia and stenosis of small intestine	Q86	Congenital malformation syndromes due to known exogenous causes, not elsewhere classified	R29	Other symptoms and signs involving the nervous and musculoskeletal systems
Q42	Congenital absence, atresia and stenosis of large intestine			R30	Pain associated with micturition
		Q87	Other specified congenital malformation syndromes affecting multiple systems	R31	Hematuria
Q43	Other congenital malformations of intestine			R32	Unspecified urinary incontinence
Q44	Congenital malformations of gallbladder, bile ducts and liver	Q89	Other congenital malformations, not elsewhere classified	R33	Retention of urine
		Q90	Down syndrome	R34	Polyuria
Q45	Other congenital malformations of digestive system	Q91	Trisomy 18 and Trisomy 13	R35	Polyuria
		Q92	Other trisomies and partial trisomies of the autosomes, not elsewhere classified	R36	Urethral discharge
Q50	Congenital malformations of ovaries, fallopian tubes and broad ligaments			R37	Sexual dysfunction, unspecified
Q51	Congenital malformations of uterus and cervix	Q93	Monosomies and deletions from the autosomes, not elsewhere classified	R39	Other and unspecified symptoms and signs involving the genitourinary system
Q52	Other congenital malformations of female genitalia	Q95	Balanced rearrangements and structural markers, not elsewhere classified		
				R40	Somnolence, stupor and coma
Q53	Undescended and ectopic testicle	Q96	Turner's syndrome	R41	Other symptoms and signs involving cognitive functions and awareness
Q54	Hypospadias	Q97	Other sex chromosome abnormalities, female phenotype, not elsewhere classified		
Q55	Other congenital malformations of male genital organs			R42	Dizziness and giddiness
		Q98	Other sex chromosome abnormalities, male phenotype, not elsewhere classified	R43	Disturbances of smell and taste
Q56	Indeterminate sex and pseudohermaphroditism			R44	Other symptoms and signs involving general sensations and perceptions
		Q99	Other chromosome abnormalities, not elsewhere classified		
Q60	Renal agenesis and other reduction defects of kidney			R45	Symptoms and signs involving emotional state
Q61	Cystic kidney disease			R46	Symptoms and signs involving appearance and behavior
Q62	Congenital obstructive defects of renal pelvis and congenital malformations of ureter	**CHAPTER 18: SYMPTOMS, SIGNS AND ABNORMAL CLINICAL AND LABORATORY FINDINGS, NOT ELSEWHERE CLASSIFIED (R00-R99)**		R47	Speech disturbances, not elsewhere classified
				R48	Dyslexia and other symbolic dysfunctions, not elsewhere classified
Q63	Other congenital malformations of kidney	R00	Abnormalities of heart beat		
Q64	Other congenital malformations of urinary system	R01	Cardiac murmurs and other cardiac sounds	R49	Voice and resonance disorders
Q65	Congenital deformities of hip			R50	Fever of other and unknown origin
Q66	Congenital deformities of feet	R03	Abnormal blood-pressure reading, without diagnosis	R51	Headache
Q67	Congenital musculoskeletal deformities of head, face, spine and chest			R52	Pain, unspecified
		R04	Hemorrhage from respiratory passages	R53	Malaise and fatigue
Q68	Other congenital musculoskeletal deformities	R05	Cough	R54	Age-related physical debility
		R06	Abnormalities of breathing	R55	Syncope and collapse
Q69	Polydactyly	R07	Pain in throat and chest	R56	Convulsions, not elsewhere classified
Q70	Syndactyly	R09	Other symptoms and signs involving the circulatory and respiratory system	R57	Shock, not elsewhere classified
				R58	Hemorrhage not elsewhere classified
				R59	Enlarged lymph nodes

R60 Edema, not elsewhere classified

R61 Generalized hyperhidrosis

R62 Lack of expected normal physiological development in childhood and adults

R63 Symptoms and signs concerning food and fluid intake

R64 Cachexia

R65 Symptoms and signs specifically associated with systemic inflammation and infection

R68 Other general symptoms and signs

R70 Elevated erythrocyte sedimentation rate and abnormality of plasma viscosity

R71 Abnormality of red blood cells

R73 Elevated blood glucose level

R74 Abnormal serum enzyme levels

R75 Inconclusive laboratory evidence of human immunodeficiency virus [HIV]

R76 Other abnormal immunological findings in serum

R77 Other abnormalities of plasma proteins

R78 Findings of drugs and other substances, not normally found in blood

R79 Other abnormal findings of blood chemistry

R80 Proteinuria

R81 Glycosuria

R82 Other and unspecified abnormal findings in urine

R83 Abnormal findings in cerebrospinal fluid

R84 Abnormal findings in specimens from respiratory organs and thorax

R85 Abnormal findings in specimens from digestive organs and abdominal cavity

R86 Abnormal findings in specimens from male genital organs

R87 Abnormal findings in specimens from female genital organs

R88 Abnormal findings in other body fluids and substances

R89 Abnormal findings in specimens from other organs, systems and tissues

R90 Abnormal findings on diagnostic imaging of central nervous system

R91 Abnormal findings on diagnostic imaging of lung

R92 Abnormal and inconclusive findings on diagnostic imaging of breast

R93 Abnormal findings on diagnostic imaging of other body structures

R94 Abnormal results of function studies

R97 Abnormal tumor markers

R99 Ill-defined and unknown cause of mortality

CHAPTER 19: INJURY, POISONING AND CERTAIN OTHER CONSEQUENCES OF EXTERNAL CAUSES (S00-T88)

S00 Superficial injury of head

S00 Insect bite (nonvenomous) of scalp, initial encounter

S01 Open wound of head

S02 Fracture of skull and facial bones

S03 Dislocation and sprain of joints and ligaments of head

S04 Injury of cranial nerve

S05 Injury of eye and orbit

S06 Intracranial injury

S07 Crushing injury of head

S08 Avulsion and traumatic amputation of part of head

S09 Other and unspecified injuries of head

S10 Superficial injury of neck

S10 Abrasion of unspecified part of neck, initial encounter

S11 Open wound of neck

S12 Fracture of cervical vertebra and other parts of neck

S13 Dislocation and sprain of joints and ligaments at neck level

S14 Injury of nerves and spinal cord at neck level

S15 Injury of blood vessels at neck level

S16 Injury of muscle, fascia and tendon at neck level

S17 Crushing injury of neck

S19 Other specified and unspecified injuries of neck

S20 Superficial injury of thorax

S20 Abrasion of unspecified parts of thorax, initial encounter

S21 Open wound of thorax

S22 Fracture of rib(s), sternum and thoracic spine

S23 Dislocation and sprain of joints and ligaments of thorax

S24 Injury of nerves and spinal cord at thorax level

S25 Injury of blood vessels of thorax

S26 Injury of heart

S27 Injury of other and unspecified intrathoracic organs

S28 Crushing injury of thorax, and traumatic amputation of part of thorax

S29 Other and unspecified injuries of thorax

S30 Superficial injury of abdomen, lower back, pelvis and external genitals

S30 Blister (nonthermal) of lower back and pelvis, initial encounter

S31 Open wound of abdomen, lower back, pelvis and external genitals

S32 Fracture of lumbar spine and pelvis

S33 Dislocation and sprain of joints and ligaments of lumbar spine and pelvis

S34 Injury of lumbar and sacral spinal cord and nerves at abdomen, lower back and pelvis level

S35 Injury of blood vessels at abdomen, lower back and pelvis level

S36 Injury of intra-abdominal organs

S36 Injury of intra-abdominal organs

S37 Injury of urinary and pelvic organs

S38 Crushing injury and traumatic amputation of abdomen, lower back, pelvis and external genitals

S39 Other and unspecified injuries of abdomen, lower back, pelvis and external genitals

S40 Superficial injury of shoulder and upper arm

S41 Open wound of shoulder and upper arm

S42 Fracture of shoulder and upper arm

S43 Dislocation and sprain of joints and ligaments of shoulder girdle

S44 Injury of nerves at shoulder and upper arm level

S45 Injury of blood vessels at shoulder and upper arm level

S46 Injury of muscle, fascia and tendon at shoulder and upper arm level

S47 Crushing injury of shoulder and upper arm

S48 Traumatic amputation of shoulder and upper arm

S49 Other and unspecified injuries of shoulder and upper arm

S50 Superficial injury of elbow and forearm

S51 Open wound of elbow and forearm

S52 Fracture of forearm

S53 Dislocation and sprain of joints and ligaments of elbow

S54 Injury of nerves at forearm level

S55 Injury of blood vessels at forearm level

S56 Injury of muscle, fascia and tendon at forearm level

S57 Crushing injury of elbow and forearm

S58 Traumatic amputation of elbow and forearm

S59 Other and unspecified injuries of elbow and forearm

S60 Superficial injury of wrist, hand and fingers

S61 Open wound of wrist, hand and fingers

S62 Fracture at wrist and hand level

S63 Dislocation and sprain of joints and ligaments at wrist and hand level

S64 Injury of nerves at wrist and hand level

S65 Injury of blood vessels at wrist and hand level

S66 Injury of muscle, fascia and tendon at wrist and hand level

S67 Crushing injury of wrist, hand and fingers

S68 Traumatic amputation of wrist, hand and fingers

S69 Other and unspecified injuries of wrist, hand and finger(s)

S70 Superficial injury of hip and thigh

S71 Open wound of hip and thigh

S72 Fracture of femur

S73 Dislocation and sprain of joint and ligaments of hip

S74 Injury of nerves at hip and thigh level

S75 Injury of blood vessels at hip and thigh level

S76 Injury of muscle, fascia and tendon at hip and thigh level

S77 Crushing injury of hip and thigh

S78 Traumatic amputation of hip and thigh

S79 Other and unspecified injuries of hip and thigh

S80 Superficial injury of knee and lower leg

S81 Open wound of knee and lower leg

S82 Fracture of lower leg, including ankle

S83 Dislocation and sprain of joints and ligaments of knee

S84 Injury of nerves at lower leg level

S85 Injury of blood vessels at lower leg level

S86 Injury of muscle, fascia and tendon at lower leg level

S87 Crushing injury of lower leg

S88 Traumatic amputation of lower leg

S89 Other and unspecified injuries of lower leg

S90 Superficial injury of ankle, foot and toes

S91 Open wound of ankle, foot and toes

S92 Fracture of foot and toe, except ankle

S93 Dislocation and sprain of joints and ligaments at ankle, foot and toe level

S93 Dislocation and sprain of joints and ligaments at ankle, foot and toe

S94 Injury of nerves at ankle and foot level

S95 Injury of blood vessels at ankle and foot level

S96 Injury of muscle and tendon at ankle and foot level

S97 Crushing injury of ankle and foot

S98 Traumatic amputation of ankle and foot

S99 Other and unspecified injuries of ankle and foot

T07 Unspecified multiple injuries

T14 Injury of unspecified body region

T15 Foreign body on external eye

T16 Foreign body in ear

T17 Foreign body in respiratory tract

T18 Foreign body in alimentary tract

T19 Foreign body in genitourinary tract

T20 Burn and corrosion of head, face, and neck

T21 Burn and corrosion of trunk

T22 Burn and corrosion of shoulder and upper limb, except wrist and hand

T23 Burn and corrosion of wrist and hand

T24 Burn and corrosion of lower limb, except ankle and foot

T25 Burn and corrosion of ankle and foot

T26 Burn and corrosion confined to eye and adnexa

T27 Burn and corrosion of respiratory tract

T28 Burn and corrosion of other internal organs

T30 Burn and corrosion, body region unspecified

T31 Burns classified according to extent of body surface involved

T32 Corrosions classified according to extent of body surface involved

T33 Superficial frostbite

T34 Frostbite with tissue necrosis

T36 Poisoning by, adverse effect of and underdosing of systemic antibiotics

T37 Poisoning by, adverse effect of and underdosing of other systemic anti-infectives and antiparasitics

T38 Poisoning by, adverse effect of and underdosing of hormones and their synthetic substitutes and antagonists, not elsewhere classified

T39 Poisoning by, adverse effect of and underdosing of nonopioid analgesics, antipyretics and antirheumatics

T40 Poisoning by, adverse effect of and underdosing of narcotics and psychodysleptics [hallucinogens]

T41 Poisoning by, adverse effect of and underdosing of anesthetics and therapeutic gases

T42 Poisoning by, adverse effect of and underdosing of antiepileptic, sedative-hypnotic and antiparkinsonism drugs

T43 Poisoning by, adverse effect of and underdosing of psychotropic drugs, not elsewhere classified

T44 Poisoning by, adverse effect of and underdosing of drugs primarily affecting the autonomic nervous system

T45 Poisoning by, adverse effect of and underdosing of primarily systemic and hematological agents, not elsewhere classified

T46 Poisoning by, adverse effect of and underdosing of agents primarily affecting the cardiovascular system

T47 Poisoning by, adverse effect of and underdosing of agents primarily affecting the gastrointestinal system

T48 Poisoning by, adverse effect of and underdosing of agents primarily acting on smooth and skeletal muscles and the respiratory system

T49 Poisoning by, adverse effect of and underdosing of topical agents primarily affecting skin and mucous membrane and by ophthalmological, otorhinolaryngological and dental drugs

T50 Poisoning by, adverse effect of and underdosing of diuretics and other and unspecified drugs, medicaments and biological substances

T51 Toxic effect of alcohol

T52 Toxic effect of organic solvents

T53 Toxic effect of halogen derivatives of aliphatic and aromatic hydrocarbons

T54 Toxic effect of corrosive substances

T55 Toxic effect of soaps and detergents

T56 Toxic effect of metals

T57 Toxic effect of other inorganic substances

T58 Toxic effect of carbon monoxide

T59 Toxic effect of other gases, fumes and vapors

T60 Toxic effect of pesticides

T61 Toxic effect of noxious substances eaten as seafood

T62 Toxic effect of other noxious substances eaten as food

T63 Toxic effect of contact with venomous animals and plants

T64 Toxic effect of aflatoxin and other mycotoxin food contaminants

T65 Toxic effect of other and unspecified substances

T66 Radiation sickness, unspecified

T67 Effects of heat and light

T68 Hypothermia

T69 *Other effects of reduced temperature*

T70 Effects of air pressure and water pressure

T71 Asphyxiation

T73 Effects of other deprivation

T74 Adult and child abuse, neglect and other maltreatment, confirmed

T75 Other and unspecified effects of other external causes

T76 Adult and child abuse, neglect and other maltreatment, suspected

T78 Adverse effects, not elsewhere classified

T79 Certain early complications of trauma, not elsewhere classified

T80 Complications following infusion, transfusion and therapeutic injection

T81 Complications of procedures, not elsewhere classified

T82 Complications of cardiac and vascular prosthetic devices, implants and grafts

T83 Complications of genitourinary prosthetic devices, implants and grafts

T84 Complications of internal orthopedic prosthetic devices, implants and grafts

T85 Complications of other internal prosthetic devices, implants and grafts

T86 Complications of transplanted organs and tissue

T87 Complications peculiar to reattachment and amputation

T88 Other complications of surgical and medical care, not elsewhere classified

CHAPTER 20: EXTERNAL CAUSES OF MORBIDITY (V00-Y99)

V00 Pedestrian conveyance accident

V01 Pedestrian injured in collision with pedal cycle

V03 Pedestrian injured in collision with car, pick-up truck or van

V05 Pedestrian injured in collision with railway train or railway vehicle

V06 Pedestrian injured in collision with other nonmotor vehicle

V09	Pedestrian injured in other and unspecified transport accidents	V83	Occupant of special vehicle mainly used on industrial premises injured in transport accident	W26	Contact with knife, sword or dagger
V10	Pedal cycle rider injured in collision with pedestrian or animal	V86	Occupant of special all-terrain or other off-road motor vehicle, injured in transport accident	W27	Contact with nonpowered hand tool
V13	Pedal cycle rider injured in collision with car, pick-up truck or van	V87	Traffic accident of specified type but victim's mode of transport unknown	W28	Contact with powered lawn mower
V15	Pedal cycle rider injured in collision with railway train or railway vehicle	V88	Nontraffic accident of specified type but victim's mode of transport unknown	W29	Contact with other powered hand tools and household machinery
V17	Pedal cycle rider injured in collision with fixed or stationary object	V89	Motor- or nonmotor-vehicle accident, type of vehicle unspecified	W30	Contact with agricultural machinery
V18	Pedal cycle rider injured in noncollision transport accident	V90	Drowning and submersion due to accident to watercraft	W31	Contact with other and unspecified machinery
V19	Pedal cycle rider injured in other and unspecified transport accidents	V91	Other injury due to accident to watercraft	W32	Accidental handgun discharge and malfunction
V20	Motorcycle rider injured in collision with pedestrian or animal	V92	Drowning and submersion due to accident on board watercraft, without accident to watercraft	W33	Accidental rifle, shotgun and larger firearm discharge and malfunction
V21	Motorcycle rider injured in collision with pedal cycle	V93	Other injury due to accident on board watercraft, without accident to watercraft	W34	Accidental discharge and malfunction from other and unspecified firearms and guns
V23	Motorcycle rider injured in collision with car, pick-up truck or van	V94	Other and unspecified water transport accidents	W35	Explosion and rupture of boiler
V25	Motorcycle rider injured in collision with railway train or railway vehicle	V95	Accident to powered aircraft causing injury to occupant	W36	Explosion and rupture of gas cylinder
V26	Motorcycle rider injured in collision with other nonmotor vehicle	V96	Accident to nonpowered aircraft causing injury to occupant	W38	Explosion and rupture of other specified pressurized devices
V27	Motorcycle rider injured in collision with fixed or stationary object	V97	Other specified air transport accidents	W39	Discharge of firework
V28	Motorcycle rider injured in noncollision transport accident	V98	Other specified transport accidents	W40	Explosion of other materials
V29	Motorcycle rider injured in other and unspecified transport accidents	V99	Unspecified transport accident	W42	Exposure to noise
V40	Car occupant injured in collision with pedestrian or animal	W01	Fall on same level from slipping, tripping and stumbling	W45	Foreign body or object entering through skin
V43	Car occupant injured in collision with car, pick-up truck or van	W03	Other fall on same level due to collision with another person	W46	Contact with hypodermic needle
V45	Car occupant injured in collision with railway train or railway vehicle	W05	Fall from non-moving wheelchair, nonmotorized scooter and motorized mobility scooter	W49	Exposure to other inanimate mechanical forces
V46	Car occupant injured in collision with other nonmotor vehicle	W06	Fall from bed	W50	Accidental hit, strike, kick, twist, bite or scratch by another person
V47	Car occupant injured in collision with fixed or stationary object	W07	Fall from chair	W51	Accidental striking against or bumped into by another person
V48	Car occupant injured in noncollision transport accident	W08	Fall from other furniture	W52	Crushed, pushed or stepped on by crowd or human stampede
V49	Car occupant injured in other and unspecified transport accidents	W09	Fall on and from playground equipment	W53	Contact with rodent
V57	Occupant of pick-up truck or van injured in collision with fixed or stationary object	W10	Fall on and from stairs and steps	W54	Contact with dog
V58	Occupant of pick-up truck or van injured in noncollision transport accident	W11	Fall on and from ladder	W55	Contact with other mammals
V59	Occupant of pick-up truck or van injured in other and unspecified transport accidents	W12	Fall on and from scaffolding	W57	Bitten or stung by nonvenomous insect and other nonvenomous arthropods
V69	Occupant of heavy transport vehicle injured in other and unspecified transport accidents	W13	Fall from, out of or through building or structure	W59	Contact with other nonvenomous reptiles
V78	Bus occupant injured in noncollision transport accident	W14	Fall from tree	W64	Exposure to other animate mechanical forces
V80	Animal-rider or occupant of animal-drawn vehicle injured in transport accident	W15	Fall from cliff	W65	Accidental drowning and submersion while in bath-tub
		W16	Fall, jump or diving into water	W67	Accidental drowning and submersion while in swimming-pool
V81	Occupant of railway train or railway vehicle injured in transport accident	W17	Other fall from one level to another	W69	Accidental drowning and submersion while in natural water
		W18	Other slipping, tripping and stumbling and falls	W74	Unspecified cause of accidental drowning and submersion
V82	Occupant of powered streetcar injured in transport accident	W19	Unspecified fall	W85	Exposure to electric transmission lines
		W20	Struck by thrown, projected or falling object	W86	Exposure to other specified electric current
		W21	Striking against or struck by sports equipment	W88	Exposure to ionizing radiation
		W22	Striking against or struck by other objects	W89	Exposure to man-made visible and ultraviolet light
		W23	Caught, crushed, jammed or pinched in or between objects	W90	Exposure to other nonionizing radiation
				W92	Exposure to excessive heat of man-made origin
		W24	Contact with lifting and transmission devices, not elsewhere classified	W93	Exposure to excessive cold of man-made origin
				W94	Exposure to high and low air pressure and changes in air pressure

W99 Exposure to other man-made environmental factors

X00 Exposure to uncontrolled fire in building or structure

X01 Exposure to uncontrolled fire, not in building or structure

X02 Exposure to controlled fire in building or structure

X03 Exposure to controlled fire, not in building or structure

X04 Exposure to ignition of highly flammable material

X05 Exposure to ignition or melting of nightwear

X06 Exposure to ignition or melting of other clothing and apparel

X08 Exposure to other specified smoke, fire and flames

X11 Contact with hot tap-water

X12 Contact with other hot fluids

X19 Contact with other heat and hot substances

X30 Exposure to excessive natural heat

X31 Exposure to excessive natural cold

X34 Earthquake

X35 Volcanic eruption

X36 Avalanche, landslide and other earth movements

X37 Cataclysmic storm

X38 Flood

X39 Exposure to other forces of nature

X50 Overexertion and strenuous or repetitive movements

X52 Prolonged stay in weightless environment

X58 Exposure to other specified factors

X71 Intentional self-harm by drowning and submersion

X72 Intentional self-harm by handgun discharge

X73 Intentional self-harm by rifle, shotgun and larger firearm discharge

X74 Intentional self-harm by other and unspecified firearm and gun discharge

X75 Intentional self-harm by explosive material

X76 Intentional self-harm by smoke, fire and flames

X77 Intentional self-harm by steam, hot vapors and hot objects

X78 Intentional self-harm by sharp object

X80 Intentional self-harm by jumping from a high place

X81 Intentional self-harm by jumping or lying in front of moving object

X82 Intentional self-harm by crashing of motor vehicle

X83 Intentional self-harm by other specified means

X92 Assault by drowning and submersion

X93 Assault by handgun discharge

X94 Assault by rifle, shotgun and larger firearm discharge

X95 Assault by other and unspecified firearm and gun discharge

X96 Assault by explosive material

X97 Assault by smoke, fire and flames

X98 Assault by steam, hot vapors and hot objects

X99 Assault by sharp object

Y00 Assault by blunt object

Y01 Assault by pushing from high place

Y02 Assault by pushing or placing victim in front of moving object

Y03 Assault by crashing of motor vehicle

Y04 Assault by bodily force

Y07 Perpetrator of assault, maltreatment and neglect

Y08 Assault by other specified means

Y09 Assault by unspecified means

Y22 Handgun discharge, undetermined intent

Y23 Rifle, shotgun and larger firearm discharge, undetermined intent

Y24 Other and unspecified firearm discharge, undetermined intent

Y25 Contact with explosive material, undetermined intent

Y26 Exposure to smoke, fire and flames, undetermined intent

Y27 Contact with steam, hot vapors and hot objects, undetermined intent

Y28 Contact with sharp object, undetermined intent

Y30 Falling, jumping or pushed from a high place, undetermined intent

Y31 Falling, lying or running before or into moving object, undetermined intent

Y32 Crashing of motor vehicle, undetermined intent

Y33 Other specified events, undetermined intent

Y35 Legal intervention

Y36 Operations of war

Y38 Terrorism

Y62 Failure of sterile precautions during surgical and medical care

Y63 Failure in dosage during surgical and medical care

Y64 Contaminated medical or biological substances

Y65 Other misadventures during surgical and medical care

Y69 Unspecified misadventure during surgical and medical care

Y83 Surgical operation and other surgical procedures as the cause of abnormal reaction of the patient, or of later

Y84 Other medical procedures as the cause of abnormal reaction of the patient, or of later complication, without

Y92 Place of occurrence of the external cause

Y93 Activity codes

Y99 External cause status

CHAPTER 21: FACTORS INFLUENCING HEALTH STATUS AND CONTACT WITH HEALTH SERVICES (Z00-Z99)

Z00 Encounter for general examination without complaint, suspected or reported diagnosis

Z01 Encounter for other special examination without complaint, suspected or reported diagnosis

Z02 Encounter for administrative examination

Z03 Encounter for medical observation for suspected diseases and conditions ruled out

Z04 Encounter for examination and observation for other reasons

Z05 Encounter for observation and evaluation of newborn for suspected diseases and conditions ruled out

Z08 Encounter for follow-up examination after completed treatment for malignant neoplasm

Z09 Encounter for follow-up examination after completed treatment for conditions other than malignant neoplasm

Z11 Encounter for screening for infectious and parasitic diseases

Z12 Encounter for screening for malignant neoplasms

Z13 Encounter for screening for other diseases and disorders

Z14 Genetic carrier

Z15 Genetic susceptibility to disease

Z16 Resistance to antimicrobial drugs

Z17 Estrogen receptor status

Z18 Retained foreign body fragments

Z19 Hormone sensitivity malignancy status

Z20 Contact with and (suspected) exposure to communicable diseases

Z21 Asymptomatic human immunodeficiency virus [HIV] infection status

Z22 Carrier of infectious disease

Z23 Encounter for immunization

Z28 Immunization not carried out and underimmunization status

Z29 Encounter for other prophylactic measures

Z30 Encounter for contraceptive management

Z31 Encounter for procreative management

Z32 Encounter for pregnancy test and childbirth and childcare instruction

Z33 Pregnant state

Z34 Encounter for supervision of normal pregnancy

Z36 Encounter for antenatal screening of mother

Z37 Outcome of delivery

Z38 Liveborn infants according to place of birth and type of delivery

Z39 Encounter for maternal postpartum care and examination

Z3A   Weeks of gestation

Z40   Encounter for prophylactic surgery

Z41   Encounter for procedures for purposes other than remedying health state

Z42   Encounter for plastic and reconstructive surgery following medical procedure

Z43   Encounter for attention to artificial openings

Z44   Encounter for fitting and adjustment of external prosthetic device

Z45   Encounter for adjustment and management of implanted device

Z46   Encounter for fitting and adjustment of other devices

Z47   Orthopedic aftercare

Z48   Encounter for other postprocedural aftercare

Z49   Encounter for attention to artificial openings

Z51   Encounter for other aftercare and medical care

Z52   Donors of organs and tissues

Z53   Persons encountering health services for specific procedures and treatment, not carried out

Z55   Problems related to education and literacy

Z56   Problems related to employment and unemployment

Z57   Occupational exposure to risk factors

Z59   Problems related to housing and economic circumstances

Z60   Problems related to social environment

Z62   Problems related to upbringing

Z63   Other problems related to primary support group, including family circumstances

Z64   Problems related to certain psychosocial circumstances

Z65   Problems related to other psychosocial services

Z65   Problems related to other psychosocial circumstances

Z68   Body mass index [BMI]

Z69   Encounter for mental health services for victim and perpetrator of abuse

Z70   Counseling related to sexual attitude, behavior and orientation

Z71   Persons encountering health services for other counseling and medical advice, not elsewhere classified

Z72   Problems related to lifestyle

Z73   Problems related to life management difficulty

Z74   Problems related to care provider dependency

Z75   Problems related to medical facilities and other health care

Z76   Persons encountering health services in other circumstances

Z77   Other contact with and (suspected) exposures hazardous to health

Z78   Other specified health status

Z79   Long term (current) drug therapy

Z80   Family history of primary malignant neoplasm

Z81   Family history of mental and behavioral disorders

Z82   Family history of certain disabilities and chronic diseases (leading to disablement)

Z83   Family history of other specific disorders

Z84   Family history of other conditions

Z85   Personal history of malignant neoplasm

Z86   Personal history of certain other diseases

Z87   Personal history of other diseases and conditions

Z88   Allergy status to drugs, medicaments and biological substances

Z89   Acquired absence of limb

Z90   Acquired absence of organs, not elsewhere classified

Z91   Personal risk factors, not elsewhere classified

Z92   Personal history of medical treatment

Z93   Artificial opening status

Z94   Transplanted organ and tissue status

Z95   Presence of cardiac and vascular implants and grafts

Z96   Presence of other functional implants

Z97   Presence of other devices

Z98   Other postprocedural states

Z99   Dependence on enabling machines and devices, not elsewhere classified

CHAPTER 22: CODES FOR SPECIAL PURPOSES (U00-U85)

U07   Emergency use of U07

U09   Post COVID-19 condition